Canadian Contributors (by Chapter)

CHAPTER 1
Jayne Elliott
Cynthia Toman
Lynnette Leeseberg Stamler

CHAPTER 2
Lynnette Leeseberg Stamler
Lise Talbot

CHAPTER 3
Joanne Profetto-McGrath
Judy Worrell

CHAPTER 4
Marjorie McIntyre
Carol McDonald

CHAPTER 5
Donna Goodridge

CHAPTER 6
D. Shelley Raffin Bouchal
Christina Preto

CHAPTER 7
Jamie Crawley
Lucia Yiu

CHAPTER 8
Lucia Yiu

CHAPTER 9
Donna M. Wilson
Corrine Truman

CHAPTER 10
Ellen Rukholm
Denise Newton Mathur

CHAPTER 11
Lynnette Leeseberg Stamler

CHAPTER 12
Jean Hughes

CHAPTER 13
Kristen Knibbs

CHAPTER 14
Ellen Rukholm

CHAPTER 15
Diane Groll
Lucia Yiu

CHAPTER 16
Sharon McMahon

CHAPTER 17
Sharon McMahon
Lucia Yiu

CHAPTER 18
Sharon McMahon

CHAPTER 19
Sandra P. Hirst

CHAPTER 20
Mary-Anne Andrusyszyn
Yolanda Babenko-Mould
Kristen Lethbridge

CHAPTER 21
Mitzi G. Mitchell

CHAPTER 22
Geraldine (Jody) Macdonald
Sheila O'Keefe-McCarthy

CHAPTER 23
Diane Clare

CHAPTER 24
Beth Swart

CHAPTER 25
Linda Ferguson

CHAPTER 26
Linda West
Katherine A. Hungerford
Lucia Yiu

CHAPTER 27
Carol Ann Sherman

CHAPTER 28
Carol Ann Sherman
Madeleine Buck

CHAPTER 29
Ann Fisk

CHAPTER 30
Madeleine Buck

CHAPTER 31
Beth Swart

CHAPTER 32
Donna Moralejo

CHAPTER 33
Donna Goodridge

CHAPTER 34
Michael McGillion
Judy Watt-Watson
Tricia Kavanagh

CHAPTER 35
Sherry Espin

CHAPTER 36
Kimberly A. McAlpine
Lucia Yiu

CHAPTER 37
Diana McMillan

CHAPTER 38
Madeleine Buck
Linda West

CHAPTER 39
Caroline Marchionni

CHAPTER 40
Laura MacIsaac

CHAPTER 41
Laura MacIsaac

CHAPTER 42
Athea McBean

CHAPTER 43
Debbie Fraser Askin

CHAPTER 44
Joanne E. Toornstra

CHAPTER 45
Carol McDonald

CHAPTER 46
Joanne Olson
Margaret B. Clark

CHAPTER 47
Madeleine Buck

CHAPTER 48
D. Shelley Raffin Bouchal
Nancy J. Moules

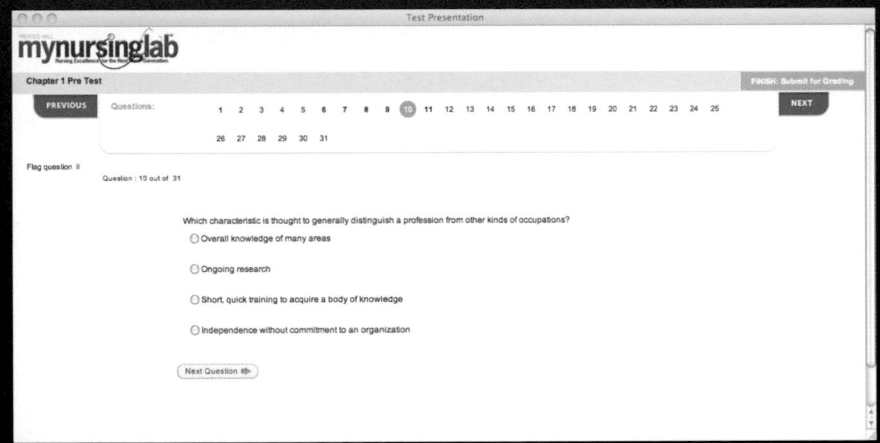

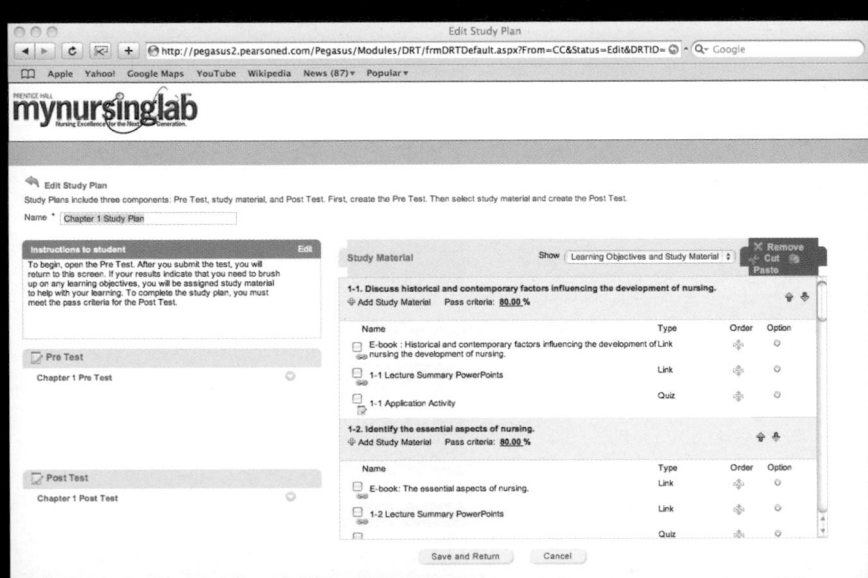

Improve Results!

The Study Plan lets you practise with a variety of tools to help you master nursing principles.

Animated and video tutorials and activities bring topics to life.

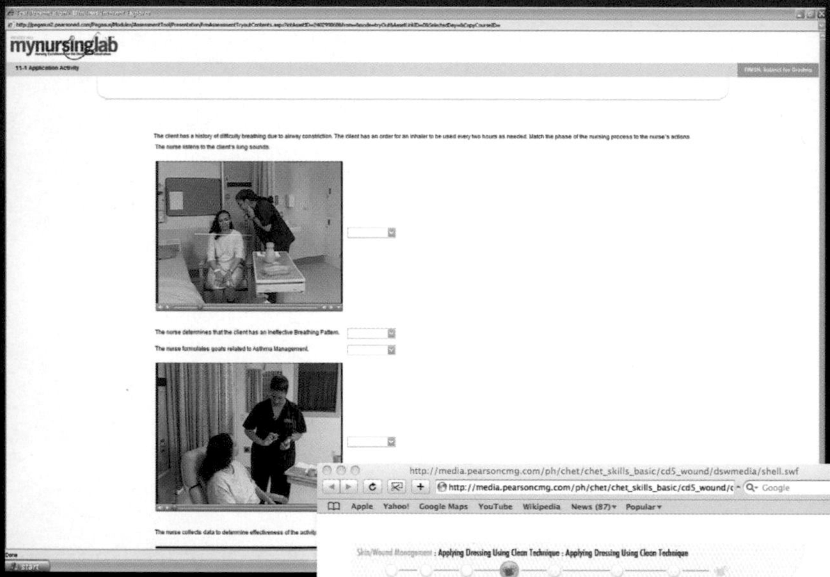

Nursing Skills Videos

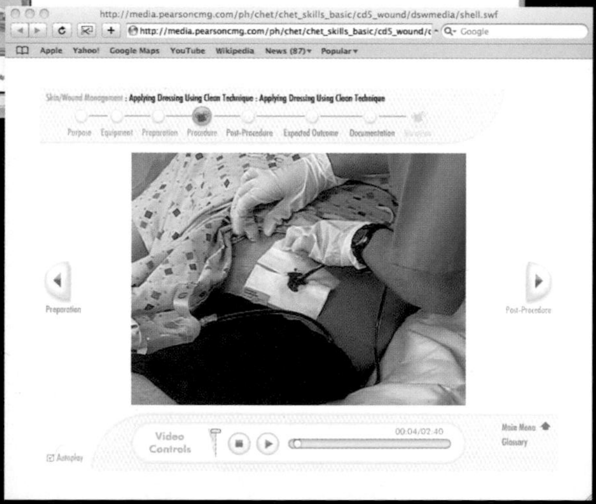

Interactive Exercises, such as Care Plans and Case Studies

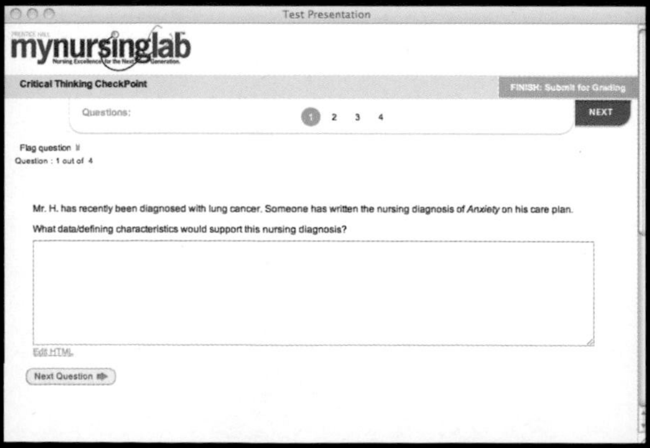

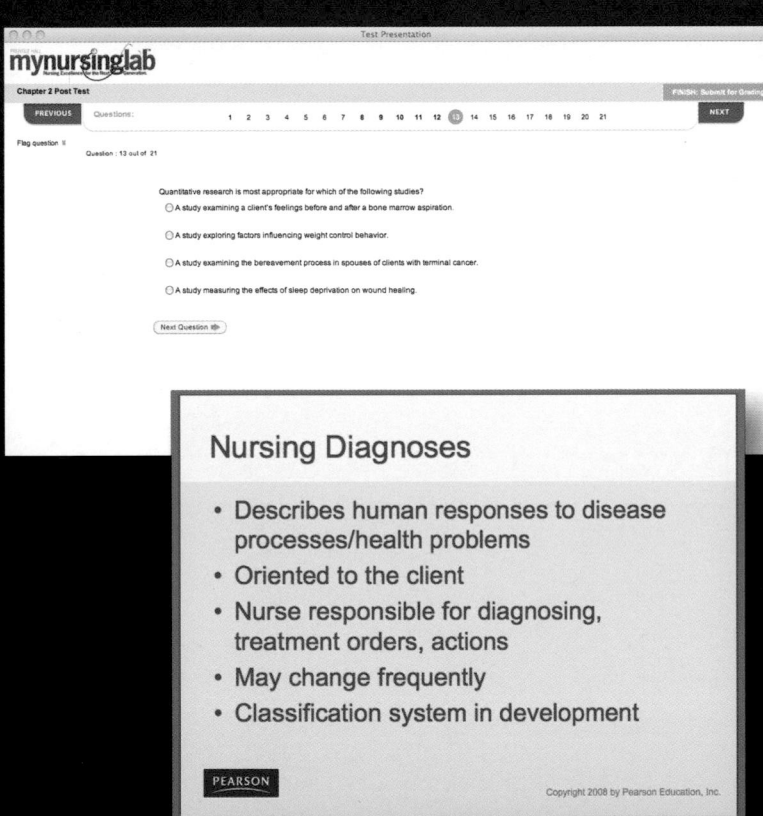

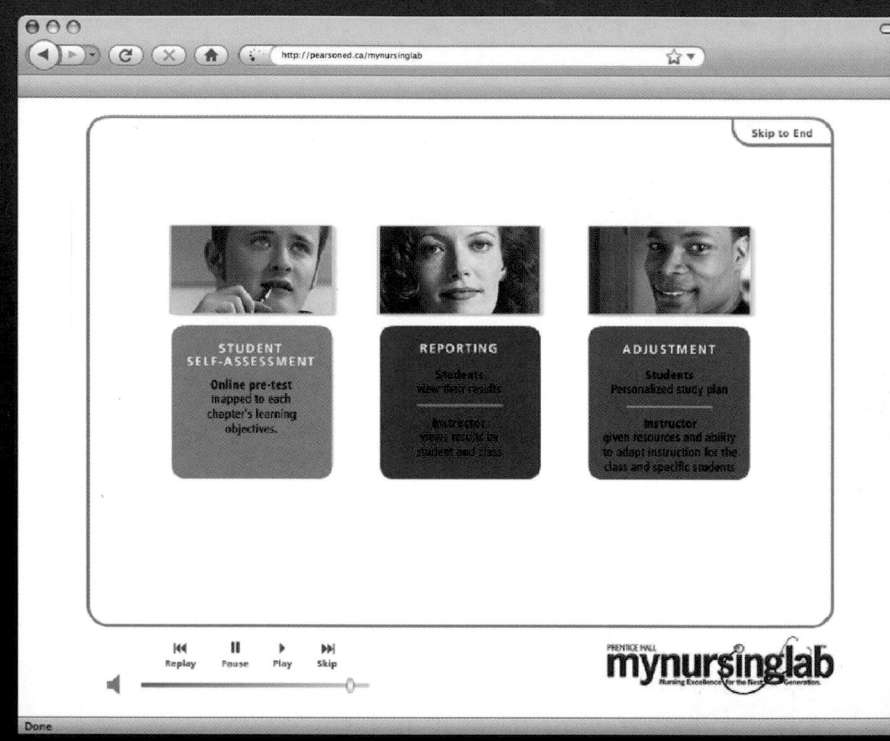

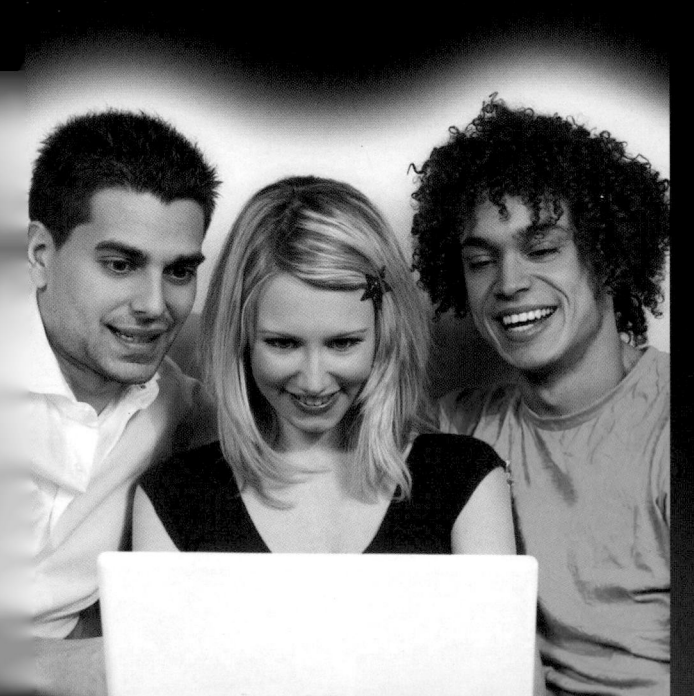

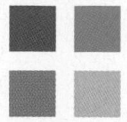

SECOND CANADIAN EDITION

Fundamentals of Canadian Nursing

Concepts, Process, and Practice

SECOND CANADIAN EDITION

Fundamentals of Canadian Nursing

Concepts, Process, and Practice

Barbara Kozier, MN, RN

Glenora Erb, BScN, RN

Audrey Berman, PhD, RN, AOCN

Shirlee J. Snyder, EdD, RN

D. Shelley Raffin Bouchal, RN, BScN, MN, PhD

Sandra Hirst, RN, BScN, MSc, PhD, GNC(C)

Lucia Yiu, RN, BSc, BA, MScN
Associate Professor
Faculty of Nursing
University of Windsor

Lynnette Leeseberg Stamler, RN, PhD
Professor and Assistant Dean
College of Nursing
University of Saskatchewan

Madeleine Buck, RN, BScN, MScN
Assistant Director
School of Nursing
McGill University
Clinical Associate, McGill University Health Centre

Pearson Canada
Toronto

Lucia Yiu dedicates this edition to her daughters (Tamara, Camillia, and Tiffany Matuk), parents, siblings, friends, colleagues, and students. They value education as an investment for the future. They believe that through diligence, commitment, and high standards, each person can make a difference.

Lynnette Stamler dedicates this edition to her biological sisters, Karen and Marilyn, her many nonbiological sisters through marriage and friendship, and students and colleagues. Each has contributed to my learning and joy in nursing and teaching. All have supported me in many ways along the journey.

Madeleine Buck dedicates this edition to the Highlands Hope Nurse Counsellor Network of Tanzania. The knowledge, skill, creativity, and dedication of these nurses in dealing with the HIV/AIDS pandemic and other heath-related issues is truly commendable.

Audrey Berman dedicates this edition to the real heroes in nursing education: the faculty. These men and women elect to spend their professional energies transmitting their knowledge, skills, and caring not just to clients, but to the extensions of their arms and minds—the generations of nurses to come. They are my colleagues, my friends, and my family.

Shirlee Snyder dedicates this edition to her husband, Terry J. Schnitter, for his unconditional love and support, and to her stepdaughter, Kelly, an awesome young woman, and caring mother, wife, and daughter who is diligently working on achieving her goal of becoming a nurse.

Library and Archives Canada Cataloguing in Publication

Fundamentals of Canadian nursing : concepts, process and practice / Barbara Kozier ... [et al.]. — 2nd Canadian ed.

Includes index.
Originally publ. under title: Fundamentals of nursing, the nature of nursing practice in Canada.
ISBN 978-0-13-613537-1

1. Nursing—Canada—Textbooks. 2. Nursing—Textbooks.
I. Kozier, Barbara

RT41.F86 2010 610.7 C2008-901788-9

Care has been taken to confirm the accuracy of information presented in this book. The authors, editors, and the publisher, however, cannot accept any responsibility for errors or omissions or for consequences from the application of the information in this book and make no warranty, expressed or implied, with respect to its contents.

The authors and publisher have exerted every effort to ensure that drug selections and dosages set forth in this text are in accord with current recommendations and practice at the time of publication. However, in view of ongoing research, changes in government regulations, and the constant flow of information relating to drug therapy and drug reactions, the reader is urged to check the package inserts of all drugs for any change in indications of dosage and for added warnings and precautions. This is particularly important when the recommended agent is a new or infrequently employed drug.

ISBN-13: 978-0-13-613537-1

ISBN-10: 0-13-613537-4

Vice President, Editorial Director: Gary Bennett

Acquisitions Editor: Michelle Sartor

Marketing Manager: Colleen Gauthier

Developmental Editor: Maurice Esses

Production Editor: Leanne Rancourt

Copy Editor: Dawn Hunter

Proofreaders: Valerie Adams, Marg Butka

Production Coordinators: Trish Ciardullo, Lynn O'Rourke

Composition: Joan Wilson, Hermia Chung, Nelson Gonzalez

Photo/Permissions Research: Lisa Brant

Art Director: Julia Hall

Cover/Interior Design: Miguel Acevedo

Cover Image: Veer

2 3 4 5 13 12 11 10

Printed and bound in United States.

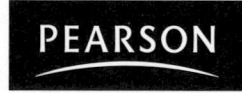

PEARSON

Canadian Contributors

Mary-Anne Andrusyszyn, BScN, RN, MScN, edD
Professor and A/Director
School of Nursing
University of Western Ontario

Debbie Fraser Askin, MN, RNC
Associate Professor
Faculty of Nursing
University of Manitoba

Yolanda Babenko-Mould, RN, BScN, MScN, PhD(c)
Doctoral Candidate
School of Nursing
University of Western Ontario

D. Shelley Raffin Bouchal, RN, BScN, MN, PhD
Assistant Professor
Faculty of Nursing
University of Calgary

Diane Clare, RN, BN, MEd, EdD
Rural Nursing Coordinator—Streaming Video Program
Nursing Department
Red River College

Margaret B. Clark
Teaching Chaplain and Clinical Pastoral Education [CPE] Supervisor
Spiritual Care and Cultural Services
University of Alberta and Stollery Children's Hospitals

Jamie Crawley, RN, BScN, BA, MBA/HCM, PhD(c)
Lecturer
Faculty of Nursing
University of Windsor

Jayne Elliott, PhD (History)
Research Facilitator/Administrator
AMS Nursing History Research Unit
School of Nursing
University of Ottawa

Sherry Espin, RN, PhD
Associate Professor
School of Nursing
Ryerson University

Linda Ferguson, RN, PhD
Director, Centre for the Advancement of the Study of Nursing Education & Interprofessional Education
Professor, College of Nursing
University of Saskatchewan

Ann Fisk, RN, MEd
Instructor, Nursing Department
Red Deer College (University of Alberta Collaborative Baccalaureate Nursing Program)

Donna Goodridge, RN, BA, BN, MN, PhD, CHPCN(c)
Assistant Professor
College of Nursing
University of Saskatchewan

Diane Groll, BA, BSc, MScN, PhD
Assistant Professor
Faculty of Nursing
Queen's University

Sandra Hirst, RN, BScN, MSc, PhD, GNC(C)
Associate Professor
Faculty of Nursing
University of Calgary

Jean Hughes, RN, PhD
Associate Professor
School of Nursing
Dalhousie University

Katherine A. Hungerford, RN, BScN, MEd
Sessional Instructor
Faculty of Nursing
University of Windsor

Tricia Kavanagh, RN, PhD(c)
Pain Research Centre
Lawrence S. Bloomberg Faculty of Nursing
University of Toronto

Kristin Knibbs, BScN, MN
College of Nursing
University of Saskatchewan

Kristen Lethbridge, BScN, RN, MScN, PhD(c)
Doctoral Candidate
School of Nursing
University of Western Ontario

Geraldine (Jody) Macdonald, RN, BScN, Med, EdD
Senior Lecturer, Lead Teacher, UG Program and Coordinator, Clinical Nursing Field, MN Program
Lawrence S. Bloomberg Faculty of Nursing
University of Toronto

Laura MacIsaac, RN, BScN, CNN(C)
Stroke Specialist Case Manager
Kingston General Hospital
Kingston, Ontario

Caroline Marchionni, RN, BSc, MSc(A) Administration, MSc(A) Nursing
Nurse Clinician
Montreal Neurological Hospital

Denise Newton Mathur, RN, BA (Anthropology), MA (Humanities)
Lecturer
School of Nursing
Laurentian University

Kimberly A. McAlpine, RN(EC), MSc(N)
Primary Health Care Nurse Practitioner
Sandwich Community Health Centre Inc.
Windsor, Ontario

Athea McBean, RN, MSc(A)
Clinical Nurse Specialist, Cardiology
Sir Mortimer B. Davis Jewish General Hospital
Faculty Lecturer, School of Nursing
McGill University

Carol McDonald, RN, PhD
Assistant Professor
Coordinator, Nurse Educator
MN Program Stream
School of Nursing
University of Victoria

Michael McGillion, RN, PhD
Assistant Professor
Lawrence S. Bloomberg Faculty of Nursing
University of Toronto

Marjorie McIntyre, BScN, MScN, PhD
Associate Professor
School of Nursing
University of Victoria

Sharon McMahon, RN, BScN, BA, Med, EdD
Associate Professor
Faculty of Nursing
University of Windsor

Diana McMillan, PhD
Assistant Professor
Faculty of Nursing
University of Manitoba

Mitzi G. Mitchell, RN, GNC(C), BScN, BA (Soc), MHSc, MN, DNS(c), PhD(c),
Lecturer
School of Nursing
York University

Donna Moralejo, RN, PhD
Associate Professor
School of Nursing
Memorial University of Newfoundland

Nancy J. Moules, RN, BN, MN, PhD
Associate Professor
Faculty of Nursing
University of Calgary

Sheila O'Keefe-McCarthy, RN, BScN, MN, CNCC(C), PhD(c)
Lawrence S. Bloomberg Faculty of Nursing
University of Toronto

Joanne Olson, PhD
Professor and Associate Dean
Undergraduate Programs
Faculty of Nursing
University of Alberta

Christina Preto, BA, LLB, MSc (Bioethics)
The W. Maurice Young Centre for Applied Ethics
University of British Columbia

Joanne Profetto-McGrath, RN, Med, PhD
Associate Professor and Interim Dean
PI-Building Provider Capacity Research Program
Senior Research Fellow—KUSP
Faculty of Nursing
University of Alberta

Ellen Rukholm, RN, BScn, MScn, PhD, FCAHS
Professor Emerita
School of Nursing
Laurentian University
Executive Director/Directrice générale, CASN/ACESI

Carol Ann Sherman, RN, MSc(N)
Faculty Lecturer
School of Nursing
McGill University

Beth Swart, BScN, MES
Professor
School of Nursing
Ryerson University

Lise Talbot, RN, PhD
Vice-doyenne aux sciences de la santé
Faculté de médecine et des sciences de la santé
Université de Sherbrooke

Cynthia Toman, RN, PhD (History)
Assistant Professor, School of Nursing
Assistant Director, AMS Nursing History Research Unit
University of Ottawa

Joanne E. Toornstra, RN, BScN, MEd
Faculty Lecturer
Faculty of Nursing
University of Alberta

Corrine Truman, RN, PhD
Performance Measurement and Evaluation Consultant
Health Services Planning & Information
Capital Health
Edmonton, Alberta

Judy Watt-Watson, RN, PhD
Professor
Lawrence S. Bloomberg Faculty of Nursing
University of Toronto

Linda West, RN, BA, MBA, PhD
Interim Vice-President Human Resources
Regina Qu'Appelle Health Region

Donna M. Wilson, RN, PhD
Professor and Caritas Nurse Scientist
Faculty of Nursing
University of Alberta

Judy Worrell, RN MN(c)
Faculty of Nursing
University of Alberta

U.S. Contributors

Paul Arnstein, RN, PhD, APRN-BC
Associate Professor
Boston College

Jean Benzel-Lindley, PhD, RN
Course Coordinator
School of Nursing
Nevada State College

Sherrilyn Coffman, DNS, RN, CPN
Associate Professor
School of Nursing
Nevada State College

Barbara D'Anna, DSL, RN, MSN, CNOR
Assistant Professor
Anne Arundel Community College

Karen DeAngelis, RN, BSN, MSN, EdD
Acting Director of Nursing 2004
Lanier Village Estates

Ardys Dunn, PhD, PNP
Professor
Samuel Merritt College

Karen Fontaine, RN, MSN
Professor
Purdue University Calumet

Cory Hartley, MSN, BSN
3M Company

Judith Herrmann, PhD, MS, BSN
Assistant Director and Assistant Professor of Nursing
University of Delaware

Chris Jackson, PhD, MSN, BSN
Associate Professor
Eastern University

Jackie Jones, RN, MSN, EdD
Assistant Professor
North Georgia College and State University

Lindsay McCrea, MS, CS, CWOCN, FNP
Assistant Professor
Samuel Merritt College

Helda Pinzon-Perez, PhD, CHES, RMT
Associate Professor
California State University

Ann Rogers, PhD, RN, FAAN
Associate Professor
School of Nursing
University of Pennsylvania

Barbara Steuble, PhD, MSN, BSN
Assistant Professor
Samuel Merritt College

Elizabeth Taylor, PhD
Associate Professor
Loma Linda College

Tamara Zurakoski, PhD, CRNP
Lecturer/Clinical Specialist
School of Nursing
University of Pennsylvania

Canadian Reviewers

Kay Barrington, RN, BVocEd, MEd
Nurse Educator and Program Coordinator
Centre for Nursing Studies
St. John's, Newfoundland

Virginia Birnie, RN, BSc(N), MScN
Nursing Faculty
Camosun College

Ann Brokenshire, RN, BScN, MEd
Instructor
School of Nursing
Ryerson University

Carol Butler, RN, BScN, MScN, MEd
Professor
School of Nursing
Fanshawe College

Beryl Cable-Williams, RN, MN, PhD(pc)
Trent/Fleming School of Nursing

Sandra Carter, RN, BN, MN
Nursing Faculty
Centre for Nursing Studies
St. John's, Newfoundland

Linda Cooper, PhD, RN
Professor
School of Nursing
Ryerson University

Paula Crawford-Dickinson, RN, BScN, BA, BHA, MN-ACNP, CNN(C)
Professor
School of Nursing
George Brown College

Margaret Mui Cunningham, RN, MScN
Clinical Associate
School of Nursing
University of British Columbia

Kim English, RN, BScN, MN
Faculty
Trent/Fleming School of Nursing

Lori Haller, BScN, MScN, EdD(in progress)
Associate Professor
Faculty of Nursing
University of New Brunswick

Carmen Hust, RN, MScN
School of Nursing
Algonquin College

P. Dianne Iverson, Dip. Ed., RN, BA, MN
Professor of Nursing
Department of Health Sciences
St. Lawrence College

Tanya Johnson, RN, BScN, MScN
School of Nursing
York University

Sandra Kostashuk, RN, BScN, MAdEd
Faculty and Coordinator Year 1 BScN Program
School of Nursing
Grant MacEwan College

Catherine Little, RN, BScN, MEd
Department of Practical Nursing
Mohawk College

Lisa Little, RN, BScN, MHS
Senior Nurse Consultant
Canadian Nurses Association

Sandra Madorin, RN, BScN, MScN
Department of Health Sciences
Georgian College

Marlene Mercer, RN, MN
Assistant Professor
School of Nursing
Dalhousie University

Beverley O'Malley. MAM(Health), BScN, RN
Faculty, working with internationally educated nurses seeking to re-enter the nursing workforce in Canada. Approved by the College of LPN's BC as a curriculum evaluator for LPN education programs
Kwantlen University College

Linda Patrick, RN, PhD
Associate Professor
Faculty of Nursing
University of Windsor

Eva Peisachovich, RN, BScN, MScN
School of Nursing
York University

Denyse Pharand, RN, PhD
Assistant Professor
School of Nursing
University of Ottawa

Wanda Pierson, RN, MScN, MA, PhD
Chair
Nursing Department
Langara College

Jason Powell, RN, BScN, MScN
ENC—PhD Nursing student (UWO—Nursing Education)
Department of Nursing
Humber College

Carol Sime, RN, MEd
Coordinator
Practical Nursing Program
Centennial College

Rick Vanderlee, RN, EdD
Director
School of Nursing
Nipissing University

Dawn Witherspoon, BScN, MDDE
Department of Practical Nursing—Distance
NorQuest College

Contents

Preface xix

Special Features xxix

UNIT 1 THE FOUNDATION OF NURSING IN CANADA 1

Chapter 1
Historical and Contemporary Nursing Practice 2

Historical Nursing Practice *3*
Contemporary Nursing Practice *8*
Roles and Functions of the Nurse *14*
Nursing Profession *15*
Factors Influencing Contemporary Nursing Practice *17*
Nursing Organizations *18*

Chapter 2
Nursing Education in Canada 26

Nursing Education *27*
Types of Educational Programs *27*
Nursing Associations and Their Influence on Education *30*
Issues Facing Nursing Education *31*

Chapter 3
Nursing Research in Canada 38

Nursing Research *39*

Chapter 4
Nursing Philosophies, Theories, Concepts, Frameworks, and Models 55

What Is Philosophy? *56*
Philosophy's Three Primary Areas of Inquiry *56*
Paradigms or World Views *56*
Philosophy in Nursing *57*
Overview of Selected Nursing Philosophies *58*
Concepts and Theories *59*
Overview of Selected Nursing Theories *60*

Chapter 5
Values, Ethics, and Advocacy 72

Values *73*
Ethics *78*
Moral Theories *78*
Nursing Codes of Ethics *81*
Ethical Decision Making *81*
Selected Ethical Issues in Nursing *82*
Nursing and Advocacy *84*
Enhancing Ethical Practice *85*

Chapter 6
Accountability and Legal Aspects of Nursing 90

Relationship of Nurses and the Law *91*
Contractual Arrangements in Nursing *95*
Areas of Potential Tort Liability in Nursing *99*
Selected Legal Aspects of Nursing Practice *104*
Legal Protections in Nursing Practice *106*
Reporting Crimes, Torts, and Unsafe Practices *108*
Legal Responsibilities of Students *108*

UNIT 2 CONTEMPORARY HEALTH CARE IN CANADA 115

Chapter 7
Health, Wellness, and Illness 116

Concepts of Health, Wellness, and Well-Being *117*
Models of Health and Wellness *119*
Health-Promotion Models *121*
Illness and Disease *123*
What Makes Canadians Healthy? *125*
Summary *125*

Chapter 8
Health Promotion 131

Development of Health-Promotion Initiatives in Canada *132*
Defining Health Promotion *137*
Types of Health-Promotion Programs *138*
Sites for Health-Promotion Activities *139*
Pender's Health-Promotion Model *139*
The Transtheoretical Model: Stages of Health Behaviour Change *141*
The Nursing Process and the Role of the Nurse in Health Promotion *143*
Promoting Canadians' Health *147*

Chapter 9
The Canadian Health-Care System 152

Rights and Health Care *154*
Categories of Health Care *156*
Types of Health-Care Organizations and Care Settings *158*
Providers of Health Care *163*
Factors Affecting the Health-Care System *164*
Contemporary Frameworks for Care *168*
Models for the Delivery of Nursing *169*

Chapter 10
Culture Care 173

Canada's Cultural Mosaic *174*
Definitions and Concepts Related to Culture *178*
Culturally Sensitive and Safe Care *181*
Selected Cultural Parameters for Nursing *184*
Providing Culturally Competent Care *190*

Chapter 11
Individual Care 198

Individual Health *199*
Applying Theoretical Frameworks to Individuals *204*

Chapter 12
Nursing Care of Families 211

What Is Family? *212*
Family Nursing *212*
Development of Family Nursing *213*
Shifting Focus to Family Involvement in Health Care *215*
Canadian Families: A Demographic Snapshot *215*
Understanding Families *218*
Nursing Care of Families *222*
Evaluating Nursing Care of Families *228*

Chapter 13
Community-Based Nursing 235

Health-Care Reform *236*
Community-Based Health Care *238*
Continuity of Care *246*

Chapter 14
Rural and Remote Health Care 252

Definition of *Rural* *253*
Rural Health: Place, Space, and Time *253*
Elements of a Rural Health Framework *254*
Health of Rural Residents *256*
Health-Care Delivery *262*

Chapter 15
Complementary and Alternative Health Modalities 271

Basic Concepts *272*
Complementary Health Modalities *272*
Nursing Role in Complementary and Alternative Health Modalities *283*

UNIT 3 LIFESPAN AND DEVELOPMENTAL STAGES 289

Chapter 16
Concepts of Growth and Development 290

Factors Influencing Growth and Development *291*
Stages of Growth and Development *292*
Growth and Development Theories *292*
Applying Growth and Development Concepts to Nursing Practice *302*

Chapter 17
Development from Conception through Adolescence 307

Conception and Prenatal Development *308*
Neonates and Infants (Birth to 1 Year) *309*
Toddlers (1 to 3 Years) *315*
Preschoolers (4 to 5 Years) *319*
School-Age Children (6 to 12 Years) *322*
Adolescence (12 to 18 Years) *324*

Chapter 18
Young and Middle-Aged Adulthood 333

Young Adults (20 to 40 Years) *334*
Middle-Aged Adults (40 to 65 Years) *338*

Chapter 19
Older Adults 347

Characteristics of Older Adults in Canada *348*
Attitudes toward Aging *349*
Gerontological Nursing in Canada *350*
Care Settings for Older Adults *350*
Theories of Aging *350*
Physiological Aging *351*
Psychosocial Aging *355*
Cognitive Abilities and Aging *357*
Moral Development *357*
Spiritual Development *358*
Health Assessment and Promotion *358*

UNIT 4 INTEGRAL ASPECTS OF NURSING 367

Chapter 20
Critical Thinking 368

Critical Thinking *369*
Critical-Thinking Abilities *370*
Attitudes That Foster Critical Thinking *371*
Standards of Critical Thinking *374*
Developing Critical-Thinking Attitudes and Skills *377*

Chapter 21
Caring, Comforting, and Communicating 383

Caring *384*
Comforting *384*
Communicating *386*
The Helping Relationship *397*
Group Communication *400*
Communication and the Nursing Process *402*
Communication among Health Professionals *407*

Chapter 22
The Nursing Process 412

Overview of the Nursing Process *415*
Assessing *417*
Diagnosing *429*
Planning *439*
Implementing *456*
Evaluating *458*
Nursing Process Summarized *464*

Chapter 23
Documenting and Reporting 470

Ethical and Legal Considerations *471*
Purposes of Client Records *472*
Documentation Systems *473*
Documenting Nursing Activities *480*
Guidelines for Recording *486*
Reporting *490*
Conferring *491*

Chapter 24
Nursing Informatics 496

Computers in Nursing Practice *498*
Informatics in Nursing Education *505*
Informatics in Nursing Administration *507*
Computers in Nursing Research *508*
Conclusion *509*

Chapter 25
Teaching and Learning 514

Teaching *515*
Learning *516*
Nurse as Educator *520*

Chapter 26
Leading, Managing, and Delegating 536

The Nurse as Leader 537
The Nurse as Manager 540
The Nurse as Delegator 543
Change 544

UNIT 5 NURSING ASSESSMENT AND CLINICAL STUDIES 551

Chapter 27
Health Assessment 552

Physical Health Assessment 553
General Survey 561
The Integument 564
Head 572
The Neck 594
Thorax and Lungs 599
Cardiovascular and Peripheral Vascular Systems 609
The Breasts and Axillae 618
Abdomen 622
Musculoskeletal System 630
Neurological System 633
The Female Genitals and Inguinal Lymph Nodes 646
The Male Genitals and Inguinal Area 650
The Anus and Rectum 654

Chapter 28
Vital Signs 661

Body Temperature 662
Pulse 672
Respirations 682
Blood Pressure 686
Oxygen Saturation 696

Chapter 29
Hygiene 704

Skin 705
Feet 720
Nails 726
Mouth 727
Hair Care 737
Eyes 743
Ears 746
Nose 749
Supporting a Hygienic Environment 749

Chapter 30
Safety 762

Factors Affecting Safety 764
Assessing 766
Diagnosing 768
Planning 768
Implementing 768
Evaluating 790

Chapter 31
Medication Administration 795

Key Concepts in Pharmacology 796
Drug Legislation 796
Effects of Drugs 799
Actions of Drugs in the Body 801
Factors Affecting Medication Action 802
Routes of Administration 804
Medication Prescription 806
Systems of Measurement 809
Administering Medications Safely 812
Administering Enteral Medications 818
Parenteral Medications 825
Topical Medications 856

Chapter 32
Infection Prevention and Control 877

Health-Care-Associated Infections 878
Types of Organisms Causing Infections 880
Body Defences against Infection 880
Pathophysiology of Infection 883
The Clinical Spectrum of Infection 883
Infection: An Imbalance between Microorganisms and Defences 884
The Chain of Infection 885
Breaking the Chain: Prevention and Control of Health-Care-Associated Infections 888
Routine Practices and Additional Precautions 911
Practical Issues for Implementation of Precautions 914
Nursing Responsibility for Infection Prevention and Control 916
Occupational Health Issues Related to Infection 919
Roles of the Infection-Control Practitioner 920
Infection Prevention and Control Is a Shared Responsibility 921

Chapter 33
Skin Integrity and Wound Care 927

Skin Function and Integrity 928
Types of Wounds 928
Pressure Ulcers 928
Lower Extremity Ulcers 934
Wound Healing 934
Assessing 940
Diagnosing 945
Planning 946
Implementing 947

Evaluating 967
Heat and Cold Applications 968

Chapter 34
Pain Management 978

The Nature of Pain 979
Pain Mechanisms 982
Assessing 988
Diagnosing 993
Planning 994
Implementing 996
Evaluating 1010

Chapter 35
Caring for Perioperative Clients 1017

Types of Surgery 1018
Preoperative Phase 1021
Intraoperative Phase 1032
Postoperative Phase 1034

UNIT 6 PROMOTING PHYSIOLOGICAL HEALTH 1059

Chapter 36
Sensory Perception 1060

Components of the Sensory-Perceptual Process 1061
Sensory Alterations 1061
Factors Affecting Sensory Function 1063
Assessing 1064
Diagnosing 1066
Planning 1067
Implementing 1067
Evaluating 1074

Chapter 37
Rest and Sleep 1080

Physiology of Sleep 1081
Normal Sleep Patterns and Requirements 1083
Factors Affecting Sleep 1085
Common Sleep Disorders 1087
Sleep Deprivation 1089
Assessing 1089
Diagnosing 1091
Planning 1091
Implementing 1094
Evaluating 1097

Chapter 38
Activity and Exercise 1103

Normal Movement 1104
Exercise 1110
Factors Affecting Body Alignment and Activity 1114
Effects of Immobility 1115
Assessing 1121
Diagnosing 1124
Planning 1125
Implementing 1125
Evaluating 1159

Chapter 39
Nutrition 1166

Essential Nutrients: Macronutrients 1167
Essential Nutrients: Micronutrients 1170
Energy Balance 1171
Factors Affecting Nutrition 1172
Nutritional Variations throughout the Lifespan 1176
Standards for a
Healthy Diet 1180
Vegetarian Diets 1184
Altered Nutrition 1185
Assessing 1186
Diagnosing 1196
Planning 1196
Implementing 1198
Evaluating 1218

Chapter 40
Fecal Elimination 1225

Physiology of Defecation 1226
Factors That Affect Defecation 1228
Common Fecal Elimination Problems 1231
Bowel Diversion Ostomies 1234
Assessing 1236
Diagnosing 1238
Planning 1240
Implementing 1242
Evaluating 1259

Chapter 41
Urinary Elimination 1263

Physiology of Urinary Elimination 1264
Factors Affecting Voiding 1266
Altered Urine Production 1269
Altered Urinary Elimination 1269

Chapter 42
Oxygenation and Circulation 1308

Physiology of the Respiratory System 1309
Physiology of the Cardiovascular System 1312
Factors Affecting Respiratory and Cardiovascular Function 1317
Alterations in Function 1320

Chapter 43
Fluid, Electrolyte, and Acid-Base Balance 1367

Body Fluids and Electrolytes *1368*
Acid-Base Balance and pH *1377*
Factors Affecting Body Fluid, Electrolytes, and the Acid-Base Balance *1378*
Disturbances in Fluid, Electrolyte, and Acid-Base Balance *1380*

UNIT 7 PROMOTING PSYCHOSOCIAL HEALTH 1429

Chapter 44
Self-Concept 1430

Self-Concept *1431*
Formation of Self-Concept *1431*
Components of Self-Concept *1433*
Factors That Affect Self-Concept *1435*
Nursing Management *1436*

Chapter 45
Sexuality and Sexual Health Practices 1446

Sexual Orientation *1447*
Gender Identity *1448*
Sexual Health *1448*
Sexuality throughout Life *1449*
Factors Influencing Sexuality *1451*
Sexual Desire and Pleasure *1453*
Sexual Arousal Disorders *1456*
Nursing Management *1456*

Chapter 46
Spirituality 1471

Spirituality, Religion, and Faith *1472*
Spiritual, Religious, and Faith Development *1473*
Spiritual and Religious Care *1475*
Spiritual Health and the Nursing Process *1478*

Chapter 47
Stress and Coping 1489

Concept of Stress *1490*
Models of Stress *1490*
Indicators of Stress *1494*
Coping *1496*
Assessing *1499*
Diagnosing *1500*
Planning *1501*
Implementing *1503*
Evaluating *1507*

Chapter 48
Loss, Grieving, and Death 1512

Loss and Grief *1513*
Dying and Death *1518*

Appendix A
Laboratory Values 1540

Appendix B
Formulae 1547

Appendix C
Vital Signs 1548

Appendix D
2007–2008 NANDA International Approved Nursing Diagnoses 1550

Index 1552

Photo Credits 1593

Preface

In *Toward 2020: Visions of Nursing,* Villeneuve and MacDonald (2006) foresee a dramatic change in the future for nurses, their roles, and the care they will provide.

Scarce funding and the longer life expectancy of Canadians will increase the current shift of financial and human resources for health-care from hospital to community settings. The primary health-care system will broaden: self-care and patient-led care will be the norm. Nurses will be part of an expanding interprofessional health team. Together with physicians, allied health workers, and human-service workers, nurses will provide holistic care within a shared-care model. The demands on the nursing profession will be greater than ever before. Therefore, nurse educators should do their best to equip students to meet the challenges of the evolving practice of nursing.

Within the context of the current and future health-care system, the second Canadian edition of *Fundamentals of Canadian Nursing: Concept, Process, and Practice* is intended to prepare undergraduate nursing students as they embark on their nursing careers. This textbook provides students with a fundamental understanding of what is required for contemporary professional nursing practice in Canada. Building on the first edition, we have placed more emphasis on needed *skills,* such as communication, critical thinking, decision making, use of the nursing process, development of interpersonal relationships, teaching, leading and managing change, use of technology, application of primary health-care principles, and engaging in collaborative practice. We have also devoted more attention to important *concepts,* such as caring, wellness, health promotion, disease prevention, complementary and alternative health modalities, rural health, multiculturalism, growth and development, nursing theories, nursing informatics, nursing research and education, ethics, accountability, and advocacy. Furthermore, throughout the text, we have highlighted basic nursing care for clients across the lifespan from hospital to community settings in the culturally diverse Canadian health-care system. In all areas, we have integrated the most recent literature and best-practice guidelines .

Nurses provide care in all settings. In this text, the term *client* is used in a broad and general context. More specifically, those living in the community are described as *clients*; those in the hospital are *patients*, and those living in long-term-care facilities are *residents.*

Contributors from across Canada were invited to help make this edition relevant to all Canadian nurses. This book has become a vehicle for us to share our knowledge, experiences, and expertise, and to help prepare the future generation of nurses. Every effort has been made to preserve the spirit of the original text prepared by the U.S. authors. Based on feedback from reviewers, faculty, and students using the text, extensive changes have been made in this edition to reflect the latest research and best nursing practice for Canadian nurses. This edition also has a significant increase in new photos to illustrate key concepts, and the presentation of clinical skills has been reorganized for increased clarity. We have made every effort to ensure that the level of specificity and readability is appropriate for beginning nursing students. We believe this text will provide a strong foundation for advanced nursing studies.

Pedagogical Approach

Primary Health Care, Critical Thinking, Nursing Process, and *Lifespan* are themes that frame our pedagogical approach to student learning, and we have threaded these throughout the book. These themes, defined below, guide the provision of client-centred care:

Primary Health Care is a philosophy and an approach to providing the best care possible through health promotion, intersectoral cooperation, public participation, appropriate technology, and accessibility. According to Health Canada (2006), primary health care (PHC) is "essential (promotive, preventive, curative, rehabilitative, and supportive) care that focuses on preventing illness and promoting health. ... It includes all services that play a part in health, such as income, housing, education, and environment" (p. 10).

Health Canada. (2006). *About PHC,* p. 10. Retrieved January 10, 2008, from http://www.hc-sc.gc.ca/hcs-sss/prim/about-apropos/index_e.html#1

Villeneuve, M., & MacDonald, J. (2006). *Toward 2020: Visions for Nursing.* Ottawa, ON: Canadian Nurses Association.

The five principles of PHC are:

- *Accessibility*—essential health care universally available to all clients in an acceptable and affordable way, regardless of geographical location.
- *Public participation*—clients participate in making decisions about their own health.
- *Health promotion*—activities that aim to empower clients to understand what determines their health and develop skills to improve and maintain their health and well-being.
- *Appropriate technology*—technology and modes of care appropriately adapted to the community's social, economic, and cultural development.
- *Intersectoral cooperation*—multidisciplinary health activities that aim at improving economic and social development.

Critical Thinking is essential for safe and competent nursing practice. It is a cognitive process that includes creativity, problem solving, and decision making. Nurses use critical thinking to make reasoned and informed decisions as they implement interventions in the practice setting. They make reliable observations, reason inductively and deductively, draw sound conclusions, make valid inferences, differentiate fact from opinion, evaluate the information sources, clarify concepts, and select appropriate actions.

Nursing Process is a systematic approach to clinical reasoning where the nurse will assess, analyze, plan, implement, and evaluate client care. Its purposes are to identify a client's health status (actual or potential health problems or needs or strengths), to establish plans to meet the identified needs, and to deliver specific nursing interventions to meet those needs. The nursing process is cyclical: it follows a logical sequence, but more than one component may be involved at any one time.

Lifespan refers to the period from conception to death. The developmental stages are continuous, predictable, and orderly, and are influenced by maturational, environmental, and genetic factors. Erikson described the following eight stages of development throughout lifespan:

Infancy	0–1.5 years	trust and mistrust
Early childhood	1.5–3 years	autonomy vs. shame and doubt
Late childhood	3–5 years	initiative vs. guilt
School age	6–12 years	industry vs. inferiority
Adolescence	12–20 years	identity vs. role confusion
Young adulthood	18–25 years	intimacy vs. isolation
Adulthood	25–65 years	generativity vs. stagnation
Maturity	65–death	integrity vs. despair

Chapter Organization and Content

For this second Canadian edition, we have reordered some of the chapters, added a new chapter (*Chapter 19: Older Adults*), and rewrote *Chapter 13: Community Health Nursing*. We also thoroughly revised the others, with major revisions in *Chapter 30: Safety*, *Chapter 32: Infection Prevention Control*, and *Chapter 33: Skin Integrity and Wound Care*.

This textbook is divided into 7 units. The following description highlights the key concepts presented and summarizes some of the significant changes that were made for this edition.

Unit 1—The Foundation of Nursing in Canada (Chapters 1–6) introduces the nature of the nursing profession, from the history of nursing to its current practice, education, and research. We expanded on the licensed (registered) practical nurses, and registered psychiatric nurses in *Chapter 1: Historical and Contemporary Nursing Practice*. The educational preparation and programs for various nursing programs have been broadened and updated in *Chapter 2: Nursing Education in Canada*. *Chapter 3: Nursing Research in Canada* has a new section on critiquing research. A new table for comparison of nursing theories has been added in *Chapter 4: Nursing Philosophies, Theories, Concepts, Frameworks, and Models*. *Chapter 5: Values, Ethics, and Advocacy* includes the top ten ethical concerns of Canadians and a discussion of the new Code of Ethics from the Canadian Nurses Association. There is more emphasis in *Chapter 6: Accountability and Legal Aspects of Nursing* on advocacy, accountability, and privacy legislation as required by the nursing discipline. Here we also stress evidence-informed practice and nursing outcomes.

Unit 2—Contemporary Health Care in Canada (Chapters 7–15) describes health-care practice in today's multicultural environments. Basic concepts of health, illness, and wellness have been expanded in *Chapter 7*. *Chapter 8: Health Promotion* has an updated section on the historical development of health promotion in Canada. Political leadership and issues such as wait times are discussed in *Chapter 9: The Canadian Health-Care System*. There is also more attention given to diverse and vulnerable clients (such as aboriginal and immigrant populations) with an emphasis on best practices for culturally safe care in *Chapter 10: Culture Care*. This new edition thoroughly updates the discussion of nursing care for individuals in *Chapter 11* and families in *Chapter 12*. The previously separate chapter on Home Care Nursing is now included as part of *Chapter 13: Community-Based Nursing*, which now also includes the 2008 Standards for Canadian Community Health Nursing Practice. More emphasis has been placed on Northern nursing in *Chapter 14: Rural and Remote Health Care*. *Chapter 15: Complementary and Alternative Health Modalities* now has more contemporary holistic care practices, with an emphasis on the role of the nurse.

Unit 3—Lifespan and Developmental Stages (Chapters 16–19) describes clients' various developmental stages and their specific health needs throughout the lifespan. In updating chapters in this unit, we added new concept maps to illustrate the major developmental theories. And as mentioned above, we created a new chapter, *Chapter 19: Older Adults*, to reflect the growing health needs of the aging population.

Unit 4—Integral Aspects of Nursing (Chapters 20–26) describes the fundamental nursing tools required for practice, including critical thinking and decision making, caring and communication, the nursing process, documenting and reporting, teaching and learning, and leading and managing change. These tools provide a foundation for the fundamental skills chapters presented in the remaining units of the text. *Chapter 22* presents the nursing process, which forms the main framework for the basic management of client care. NANDA taxonomy is used throughout this book with a new appendix listing the 2007–2008 NANDA-approved nursing diagnoses. *Chapter 24: Nursing Informatics* updates the use of computers in nursing and distinguishes among the various types of electronic patient records. This chapter also highlights the use of the NurseONE portal for nursing information. Contemporary change theories, managing the millennium generation, and the leadership roles in nursing are new to *Chapter 26: Leading, Managing, and Delegating.*

Unit 5—Nursing Assessment and Clinical Skills (Chapters 27–35) provides fundamental knowledge to guide the provision of care described in the remainder of the book. *Chapter 27: Health Assessment* and *Chapter 28: Vital Signs* prepare students with an understanding of assessment techniques, procedures, and normal findings throughout the lifespan. These chapters include the most recent Canadian screening guidelines for a range of prevalent and significant illnesses affecting our nation. The latest Canadian Hypertension Education Program guidelines for blood pressure measurement and monitoring are also included. The remaining chapters in this Unit focus on integral components of care in relation to hygiene, safety, medication administration, infection prevention and control, skin integrity and wound care, pain management, and caring for perioperative clients. As mentioned above, *Chapter 30: Safety, Chapter 32: Infection Prevention Control,* and *Chapter 33: Skin Integrity and Wound Care* have been completely rewritten. And the other chapters have been thoroughly revised. Significant changes and important updates have been made with regard to Health Canada infection prevention and control guidelines, immunization guidelines, general safety issues throughout the lifespan, patient safety within the health-care sector, Safer Healthcare Now! initiatives, the classification of pressure ulcers using the latest 2007 National Pressure Ulcer Advisory Panel revisions that include 6 (rather than 4) stages of pressure ulcers, Canadian Association of Wound Care guidelines, medication administration procedures that incorporate the Institute for Safe Medication Practices guidelines, the latest "10 Rights" of medication administration (increased from 5), and current pain assessment tools and pain management approaches.

Unit 6—Promoting Physiological Health (Chapters 36–43) discusses such physiologic concepts as sensory perception; rest and sleep; activity and exercise; nutrition; fecal elimination; urinary elimination; fluid, electrolytes, and acid-base balance; and oxygenation and circulation. *Chapter 36: Sensory Perception* highlights the links between medications and sensory perceptions, and the implications for patient safety. Rest and sleep as part of normal development and health (as well as illness) are discussed in *Chapter 37: Rest and Sleep.* The latest Canadian guidelines for activity and exercise and a significant discussion on the safety of nurses in caring for immobile patients augment *Chapter 38: Activity and Exercise.* Eating Well with Canada's Food Guide, and a discussion on obesity trends in Canadians, trans-fat updates, and the latest recommendations in monitoring nutritional health are highlighted in *Chapter 39: Nutrition. Chapter 40: Fecal Elimination* and *Chapter 41: Urinary Elimination* provide the most recent guidelines to ensure healthy fecal and urinary elimination patterns, including the care of clients with altered function. More scientific and biological detail is provided in *Chapter 42: Oxygenation and Circulation* and *Chapter 43: Fluid, Electrolyte, and Acid-Base Balance* to ensure that nurses can better understand the complexities that can arise in these areas when caring for clients. Safer Healthcare Now! recommendations for preventing ventilator-associated pneumonia, closed airway suction, and continuous positive airway pressure (CPAP) augment this chapter.

Unit 7—Promoting Psychosocial Health (Chapters 44–48) covers a wide range of areas that affect one's health. Self-concept, sexuality, spirituality, stress and coping, and loss, grieving, and death are all areas that a nurse should consider to care effectively for a client. *Chapter 45: Self-Concept* has new discussions of locus of control content and the importance of congruence of self-appraisal. *Chapter 45: Sexuality and Sexual Health Practices* strengthens and updates the material on breast health, prostate examination, HIV, Hepatitis B, and other STIs. *Chapter 46: Spirituality* examines spiritual care in both health and illness and considers the meanings of spiritual health in the 21st century. Lifespan considerations of stress and coping are emphasized in *Chapter 47: Stress and Coping.* Issues around nutrition and hydration of the dying patient as well as pain management and home care at the time of death are highlighted in *Chapter 48: Loss, Grieving, and Death.*

Four new **Appendices** are provided near the end of the book. They summarize important information about vital signs, normal laboratory values, formulae, and NANDA International nursing diagnoses to help students access important facts and terms in a user-friendly manner. The book ends with a robust **Index** in which key terms and the pages on which they are defined are boldfaced for easy reference.

Special Features in the Chapters

We have carefully prepared special features to facilitate learning and to highlight the 4 themes that form the framework for this edition—namely, *Primary Health Care*, *Critical Thinking*, *Nursing Process*, and *Lifespan*. Complete lists of many of these individual types of special features are provided following this preface.

Objectives are listed at the beginning of each chapter to outline skills and knowledge to be learned.

Key Terms are boldfaced where they are defined in the body of the text. They are also listed near the end of each chapter and are boldfaced for easy reference in the index.

An **Evidence-Informed Practice** box in each chapter highlights current evidence that informs nursing practice and relates relevant Canadian research to the nursing profession and its clinical practice. Systematic reviews are included where appropriate.

Evidence-Informed Practice

How Can Employers Promote Empowerment for New Graduate Nurses?

The nursing shortage and projected retirement of nurses in the next few years have resulted in the need for enhanced recruitment and retention of nurses. A high priority among health-care organizations is the development of strategies to improve working conditions and to provide a supportive environment for new graduate nurses.

A predictive, nonexperimental survey design investigated factors that promote empowerment among new graduate nurses (Cho, Laschinger, & Wong, 2006). This study tested the relationships among structural empowerment, six areas of work life, emotional exhaustion, and organizational commitment. Structural empowerment measured employees' perceptions of access to opportunity, information, support, and resources. The six areas of work life included workload, control, rewards, community, fairness, and values. Emotional exhaustion measured how often an individual experienced feelings of disengagement and burnout in his or her work. Organizational commitment measured the psychological link between the employee and the organization.

The researchers found that structural empowerment had a positive effect on the areas of work life and a negative effect on emotional exhaustion. They concluded that increasing access to job flexibility, strong interpersonal relationships, information, support, and learning opportunities are potential strategies to retain new graduate nurses.

NURSING IMPLICATIONS: This study suggests the importance of a positive work environment to ensuring commitment of new graduates and resulting retention of staff. The following strategies would contribute:

- Use multiple communication techniques: regular staff meetings, forums, electronic messages, brown bag lunches, and written updates.
- Use support staff to reduce nursing time spent on non-nursing tasks.
- Provide orientation, emotional support, assistance, and collaborative learning opportunities.
- Give new graduates opportunities for leadership roles and involvement in decision making.
- Offer choices and alternatives for flexibility in jobs (job sharing, innovative scheduling).
- Build strong interpersonal relationships through team building and mentoring programs.

Source: Based on "Workplace Empowerment, Work Engagement and Organizational Commitment of New Graduate Nurses," by J. Cho, H. K. S. Laschinger, and C. Wong, 2006, *Canadian Journal of Nursing Leadership, 19*(3), pp. 43–60.

A **Case Study** in each chapter presents an actual or hypothetical scenario that is applicable to Canadian nursing. The *critical thinking questions* in each Case Study guide students to reflect on one or more of the following themes: primary health care, nursing process, lifespan, and critical thinking. Suggested answers are available on the MyNursingLab (www.mynursinglab.com)

Nursing and Canadian Society boxes found in selected chapters, present facts about Canadian society and their implications for nursing.

NURSING AND CANADIAN SOCIETY

Fact	Implications for Nursing Practice
1960: The Canadian Bill of Rights barred discrimination by federal agencies on the grounds of race, national origin, colour, religion or gender. 1961: Changes to Canada's Immigration Act meant that fewer immigrants were European and the mix of source countries shifted to nations in southern Europe, Asia, and the West Indies.	These rights are legally protected. Nurses must have knowledge of the ethnic and cultural makeup of the Canadian population and use that knowledge to provide culturally competent and safe care.
1969: The Official Languages Act was enacted to protect minority language rights.	Clients have the right to have health care services provided in either official language in any part of Canada.
1971: The federal government announced its policy of multiculturalism.	People are encouraged to retain their cultural beliefs and practices, rather than being assimilated into the mainstream culture. This means that nurses need to be culturally sensitive and incorporate appropriate measures into health-care assessment and delivery.
1982: The Canadian Charter of Rights and Freedoms considered multiculturalism to be constitutional and protected equality rights without discrimination (in particular based on race, national or ethnic origin, colour, religion, gender, age, or mental or physical disability). Section 27 explicitly stated that the Charter will be interpreted in a manner consistent with the preservation and enhancement of the multicultural heritage of Canadians; by virtue of this section of the Charter, Canada became a constitutional multicultural stage.	The Charter entrenches equality rights without discrimination, again obligating nurses to provide culturally competent and safe care grounded in respect for the self and client.
1982: The Canada Act replaced the British North America Act as Canada's constitution and also recognized the three main groups of Aboriginal peoples in Canada: First Nations, Metis, and Inuit.	This policy acknowledged the rights of the Aboriginal peoples in Canada. Nurses must have knowledge of and respect for the customs and beliefs of Metis, First Nations, and Inuit, and integrate that knowledge into the provision of culturally safe care.
1986: The Employment Equity Act was established to achieve equality in the workplace so that no persons would be denied employment opportunities or benefits for reasons unrelated to ability; it established the principle that employment equity means more than treating persons in the same way but also requires special measures and the accommodation of differences; it identified four groups thought to experience disadvantage in employment: women, Aboriginal peoples, persons with disability, and persons in a visible minority (Canadian Human Rights Commission, n.d.).	This policy recognizes the challenges faced by Aboriginal peoples and other groups in seeking and maintaining employment, and hence the impact of unemployment on poverty and self-esteem. In assessing, planning, and providing care, it is the nurse's responsibility to consider the impact of poverty and self-esteem on the health and well-being of all peoples, especially those identified in the Act.
Previous censuses have shown that the Aboriginal population is growing much faster than the total population. Given the younger age of the Aboriginal population, this trend is expected to continue (Statistics Canada, 2008d).	This rapid increase in the Aboriginal populations will have an impact on health-care services for both the young and older adults.
Approximately two-fifths of the Canadian population have one origin other than British, French, or Aboriginal.	The fact that the Canadian population is increasing in diversity has implications for how nurses incorporate the changes in practice needed to address this diversity. The importance of culture is highlighted in the fact that this topic is listed in the 2006 Canadian Nurses Association (CNA) *Blueprint for the Registered Nurse Examination*, which parallels nursing competencies and standards of practice.

Reflect on Primary Health Care boxes engage students to reflect on the clinical application of one or more of the five principles of primary health care in relation to chapter-specific topics.

REFLECT ON PRIMARY HEALTH CARE

Health promotion is a principle of primary health care. Nurses adopt the primary health care approach to provide promotive, preventive, curative, rehabilitative, and supportive or palliative care to their clients. The focus of their care is on preventing illness and promoting health. In promoting the health of individuals, families, group, and communities, nurses must help their clients understand factors that determine their health and develop effective skills to improve and maintain their own health and well-being. Consider how you can work with your clients and interdisciplinary health-care providers to provide health-promotion services that are culturally sensitive and accessible to your clients. Also, examine whether the educational material is written in a language and at a level that can be understood by clients from another culture.

Case Study 21

You are the nursing student assigned to care for Mr. Manasovitz, a 45-year-old man, who will be returning from the recovery room after undergoing the removal of a mass from his abdomen. While you are preparing his room for his return, the nurse and physician arrive to talk with Mrs. Manasovitz about her husband's surgery. The physician explains that the mass was malignant and invasive. Mr. Manasovitz is a candidate for chemotherapy, but his prognosis is guarded because of the extent of the tumour growth. Mrs. Manasovitz looks away, closes her eyes, and only nods her head "yes." As the physician leaves, the nurse approaches Mrs. Manasovitz, sits next to her, and puts her arm around Mrs. Manasovitz, who begins to cry. The nurse uses a soothing voice to tell Mrs. Manasovitz that it is okay to cry and provides assurance by remaining with her. The two of them sit in silence until Mrs. Manasovitz is able to express her feelings. The nurse listens attentively. Later, the nurse offers to get a cup of coffee for Mrs. Manasovitz and offers to assist her at this difficult time.

Critical Thinking Questions

1. Interpret Mrs. Manasovitz's nonverbal behaviour in response to the news about her husband's surgery.
2. Evaluate the nurse's response to Mrs. Manasovitz on the basis of the concepts of caring and comforting.
3. Why is it important for the nurse to effectively communicate with Mrs. Manasovitz at this time?
4. The nurse was described as listening attentively to Mrs. Manasovitz. Cite actions that portray attentive listening.
5. Think about your past experiences when you or a family member has been ill. What relationship characteristics did you most value on the part of the nurse caring for you?

After working through these questions, go to the MyNursingLab at **http://www.mynursinglab.com** to check your answers.

Numerous **Skill** boxes throughout the book provide step-by-step directions, along with rationales, for a wide range of clinical topics. Each skill includes a purpose statement, an assessment focus, a list of equipment, and an evaluation focus. Reference to infection prevention and control issues for each skill has been integrated. For this edition, we have highlighted the rationales by the use of colour. We have also included more photos and figures, and we label them with circled red numbers to make the presentation easier to follow.

SKILL 27.7

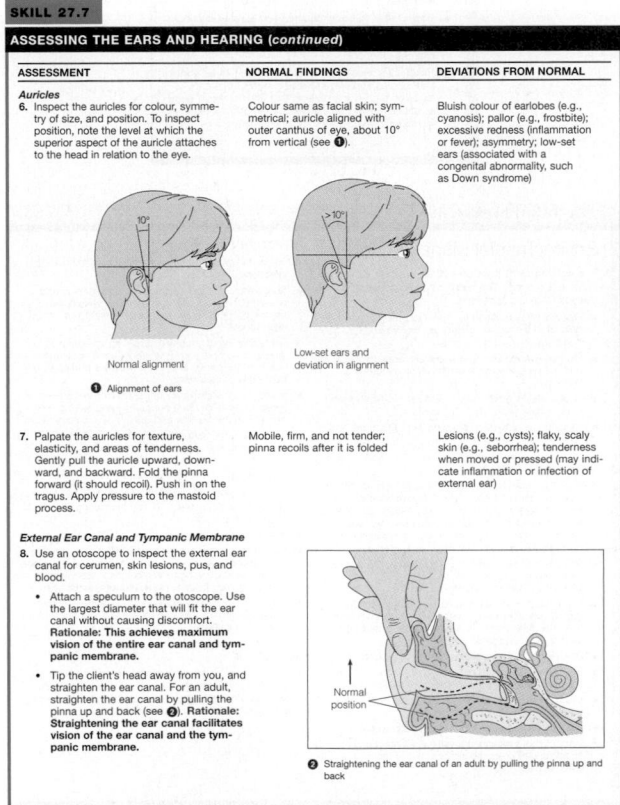

ASSESSING THE EARS AND HEARING (*continued*)

ASSESSMENT	NORMAL FINDINGS	DEVIATIONS FROM NORMAL
Auricles		
6. Inspect the auricles for colour, symmetry of size, and position. To inspect position, note the level at which the superior aspect of the auricle attaches to the head in relation to the eye.	Colour same as facial skin; symmetrical; auricle aligned with outer canthus of eye, about 10° from vertical (see ❶).	Bluish colour of earlobes (e.g., cyanosis); pallor (e.g., frostbite); excessive redness (inflammation or fever); asymmetry; low-set ears (associated with a congenital abnormality, such as Down syndrome)

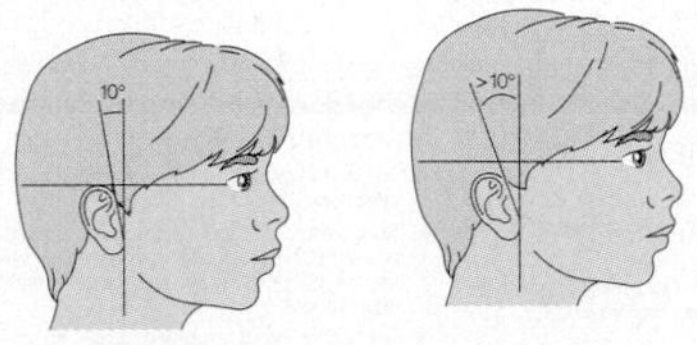

Normal alignment

Low-set ears and deviation in alignment

❶ Alignment of ears

ASSESSMENT	NORMAL FINDINGS	DEVIATIONS FROM NORMAL
7. Palpate the auricles for texture, elasticity, and areas of tenderness. Gently pull the auricle upward, downward, and backward. Fold the pinna forward (it should recoil). Push in on the tragus. Apply pressure to the mastoid process.	Mobile, firm, and not tender; pinna recoils after it is folded	Lesions (e.g., cysts); flaky, scaly skin (e.g., seborrhea); tenderness when moved or pressed (may indicate inflammation or infection of external ear)

External Ear Canal and Tympanic Membrane

8. Use an otoscope to inspect the external ear canal for cerumen, skin lesions, pus, and blood.

- Attach a speculum to the otoscope. Use the largest diameter that will fit the ear canal without causing discomfort. **Rationale: This achieves maximum vision of the entire ear canal and tympanic membrane.**
- Tip the client's head away from you, and straighten the ear canal. For an adult, straighten the ear canal by pulling the pinna up and back (see ❷). **Rationale: Straightening the ear canal facilitates vision of the ear canal and the tympanic membrane.**

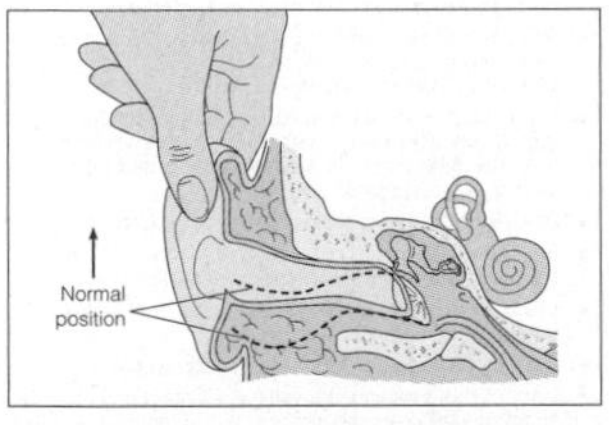

❷ Straightening the ear canal of an adult by pulling the pinna up and back

Lifespan Considerations boxes indicate how nursing care should be adapted for infants, children, adolescents, and older adults.

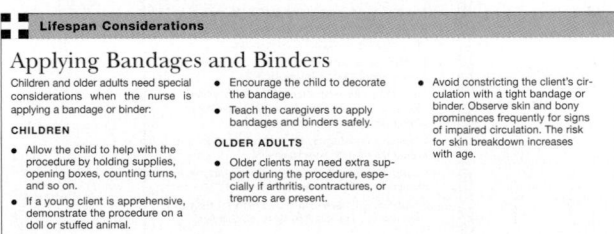

Lifespan Considerations

Applying Bandages and Binders

Children and older adults need special considerations when the nurse is applying a bandage or binder:

CHILDREN

- Allow the child to help with the procedure by holding supplies, opening boxes, counting turns, and so on.
- If a young client is apprehensive, demonstrate the procedure on a doll or stuffed animal.
- Encourage the child to decorate the bandage.
- Teach the caregivers to apply bandages and binders safely.

OLDER ADULTS

- Older clients may need extra support during the procedure, especially if arthritis, contractures, or tremors are present.
- Avoid constricting the client's circulation with a tight bandage or binder. Observe skin and bony prominences frequently for signs of impaired circulation. The risk for skin breakdown increases with age.

Clinical Alerts provide students with tips on nursing responsibilities and precautions, along with the underlying rationales, when caring for clients in various clinical situations.

CLINICAL ALERT

Whenever mercury-in-glass thermometers are encountered, the nurse should recommend their immediate replacement with less hazardous thermometers and their safe disposal.

Home Care Considerations boxes guide students to consider client issues for successful home recovery and living.

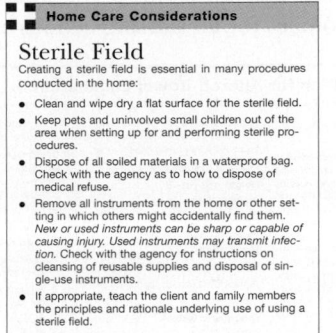

Home Care Considerations

Sterile Field

Creating a sterile field is essential in many procedures conducted in the home:

- Clean and wipe dry a flat surface for the sterile field.
- Keep pets and uninvolved small children out of the area when setting up for and performing sterile procedures.
- Dispose of all soiled materials in a waterproof bag. Check with the agency as to how to dispose of medical refuse.
- Remove all instruments from the home or other setting in which others might accidentally find them. *New or used instruments can be sharp or capable of causing injury. Used instruments may transmit infection.* Check with the agency for instructions on cleansing of reusable supplies and disposal of single-use instruments.
- If appropriate, teach the client and family members the principles and rationale underlying use of using a sterile field.

Clinical Manifestations list the signs and symptoms in bullet format to give students a quick and easy reference to key manifestations of illness.

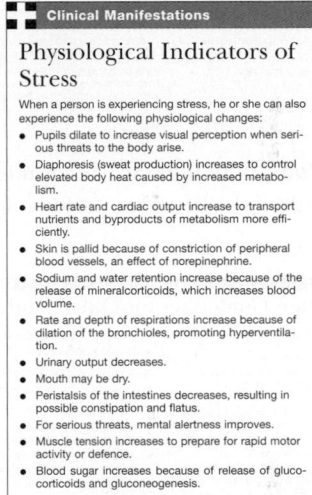

Clinical Manifestations

Physiological Indicators of Stress

When a person is experiencing stress, he or she can also experience the following physiological changes:

- Pupils dilate to increase visual perception when serious threats to the body arise.
- Diaphoresis (sweat production) increases to control elevated body heat caused by increased metabolism.
- Heart rate and cardiac output increase to transport nutrients and byproducts of metabolism more efficiently.
- Skin is pallid because of constriction of peripheral blood vessels, an effect of norepinephrine.
- Sodium and water retention increase because of the release of mineralcorticoids, which increases blood volume.
- Rate and depth of respirations increase because of dilation of the bronchioles, promoting hyperventilation.
- Urinary output decreases.
- Mouth may be dry.
- Peristalsis of the intestines decreases, resulting in possible constipation and flatus.
- For serious threats, mental alertness improves.
- Muscle tension increases to prepare for rapid motor activity or defence.
- Blood sugar increases because of release of glucocorticoids and gluconeogenesis.

Practice Guidelines provide clear, succinct summaries of correct and incorrect clinical actions.

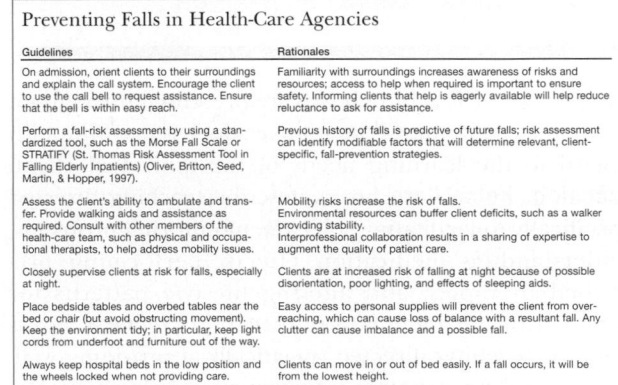

PRACTICE GUIDELINES 30.1

Preventing Falls in Health-Care Agencies

Guidelines	Rationales
On admission, orient clients to their surroundings and explain the call system. Encourage the client to use the call bell to request assistance. Ensure that the bell is within easy reach.	Familiarity with surroundings increases awareness of risks and resources; access to help when required is important to ensure safety. Informing clients that help is eagerly available will help reduce reluctance to ask for assistance.
Perform a fall-risk assessment by using a standardized tool, such as the Morse Fall Scale or STRATIFY (St. Thomas Risk Assessment Tool in Falling Elderly Inpatients) (Oliver, Britton, Seed, Martin, & Hopper, 1997).	Previous history of falls is predictive of future falls; risk assessment can identify modifiable factors that will determine relevant, client-specific, fall-prevention strategies.
Assess the client's ability to ambulate and transfer. Provide walking aids and assistance as required. Consult with other members of the health-care team, such as physical and occupational therapists, to help address mobility issues.	Mobility risks increase the risk of falls. Environmental resources can buffer client deficits, such as a walker providing stability. Interprofessional collaboration results in a sharing of expertise to augment the quality of patient care.
Closely supervise clients at risk for falls, especially at night.	Clients are at increased risk of falling at night because of possible disorientation, poor lighting, and effects of sleeping aids.
Place bedside tables and overbed tables near the bed or chair (but avoid obstructing movement). Keep the environment tidy; in particular, keep light cords from underfoot and furniture out of the way.	Easy access to personal supplies will prevent the client from overreaching, which can cause loss of balance with a resultant fall. Any clutter can cause imbalance and a possible fall.
Always keep hospital beds in the low position and the wheels locked when not providing care.	Clients can move in or out of bed easily. If a fall occurs, it will be from the lowest height.

continued

A **Sample Care Plan** in selected chapters provides assessment data, nursing diagnoses, client goals, desired outcomes, and *nursing interventions* (known as *therapeutic plans* in Quebec) relevant to the scenario presented in the chapter. Rationales for all nursing actions are included.

Sample Care Plan for Altered Bowel Elimination

ASSESSMENT DATA

Nursing Assessment

Mrs. Emma Brown is 78 years old. She has been a widow for 9 months. She lives alone in a low-income housing complex for older people. Her two children live with their families in a city approximately 240 km away. She always enjoyed cooking for her family; however, now that she is alone, she does not cook for herself. As a result, she has developed irregular eating patterns and tends to prepare soup-and-toast meals. She gets little exercise and has bouts of insomnia since her husband's death. For the past month, Mrs. Brown has been having a problem with constipation. She states she has a bowel movement about every 3 to 4 days and her stools are hard and painful to excrete. Mrs. Brown decides to attend the health fair sponsored by the housing complex and seeks assistance from the public health nurse.

Physical Examination

Height: 162 cm

Weight: 65 kg

Temperature: 36.2°C

Pulse: 82 bpm

Respirations: 20/min

Blood pressure: 128/74 mm Hg

Active bowel sounds, abdomen slightly distended

Diagnostic Data

CBC: Hgb 108 g/L

Urinalysis negative

Nursing Diagnosis

Constipation related to low-fibre diet and inactivity (as evidenced by infrequent, hard stools; painful defecation; abdominal distension)

Client Goals

Mrs. Brown will (1) establish a regular pattern of bowel elimination, (2) develop and maintain an exercise program, and (3) initiate nutritional alterations that will enhance regular bowel elimination.

Desired Health Outcomes

1. Increases daily fluid intake to 2000 mL unless contraindicated
2. Includes fibre in at least one meal per day
3. Walks for 20 minutes at least three times per week
4. Verbalizes relief of constipation by the second week

NURSING INTERVENTIONS AND SELECTED ACTIVITIES WITH RATIONALE* *[IN ITALICS]*

Constipation and Impaction Management

• Identify factors (e.g., medications, activity level, diet) that can cause or contribute to constipation.	*Assessing causative factors is an essential first step in teaching and planning for improved bowel elimination.*
• Encourage increased fluid intake, unless contraindicated.	*Sufficient fluid intake is necessary for the bowel to absorb sufficient amounts of liquid and promote proper stool consistency.*
• Evaluate her medication profile for gastrointestinal side effects.	*Constipation is a common side effect of many drugs, including opioid analgesics and antacids.*
• Teach Mrs. Brown how to keep a food diary.	*An appraisal of food intake will help identify whether Mrs. Brown is eating a well-balanced diet and consuming adequate amounts of fluid and fibre. Excessive meat or refined food intake will produce small, hard stools.*

(continue)

Health-Promotion Guidelines provide guidelines for promoting the health of clients at various stages of their development.

Health-Promotion Guidelines for Older Adults

The following are important to the health of older adults:

HEALTH TESTS AND SCREENING

- Routine physical examination (annually for females; every 2 to 3 years or as directed by health-care provider for males)
- Immunizations as recommended, such as a tetanus booster every 10 years, pneumococcal vaccinations, and annual influenza vaccine
- Regular dental assessments (e.g., yearly)
- Tonometry for signs of glaucoma and examination for other eye disease every 2 to 3 years or annually, if indicated
- Testicular and breast self-examination monthly
- Screenings for cardiovascular disease (e.g., blood pressure measurement; electrocardiogram and cholesterol test, as directed by the health-care provider)
- Screenings for colorectal, breast, cervical, uterine, ovarian, and prostate cancers
- Screening for tuberculosis every 2 years

SAFETY

- Home safety measures to prevent falls, fire, burns, scalds, and electrocution
- Motor vehicle safety reinforcement, especially when driving at night
- Precautions to prevent pedestrian accidents
- Education about medications

NUTRITION AND EXERCISE

- Importance of a well-balanced diet with fewer calories to accommodate lower metabolic rate and decreased physical activity
- Importance of sufficient amounts of vitamin D and calcium to prevent osteoporosis
- Regular program of moderate exercise to maintain joint mobility, muscle tone, and bone calcification

ELIMINATION

- Importance of adequate roughage in the diet, adequate exercise, and at least 1500 mL of fluid daily to prevent constipation

SOCIAL INTERACTIONS

- Intellectual and recreational pursuits
- Personal relationships that promote discussion of feelings, concerns, and fears
- Assessment of risk factors for abuse and neglect
- Availability of social community centres, programs, and support groups for older adults

Three types of Teaching boxes are presented throughout the book. **Teaching: Clinical** boxes discuss teaching with regard to the learning needs of the individual client. **Teaching: Home Care** boxes describe teaching directed specifically to facilitating self-care, monitoring problems, understanding medication effects, performing prescribed therapies, and altering lifestyle patterns for clients living in their home. **Teaching: Wellness** boxes describe teaching directed specifically at providing wellness or health-promotion information to help clients live healthier lives.

TEACHING: CLINICAL

Teaching Tools for Children

The use of the following teaching aids can help focus children's attention:

- *Visits.* Visiting the hospital and treatment rooms; seeing people dressed in uniforms, scrub suits, protective gear.
- *Dress-up.* Touching and dressing up in the clothing they will see and wear.
- *Colouring books.* Using colouring books to prepare for treatments, surgery, or hospitalization; shows what rooms, people, and equipment will look like.
- *Storybooks.* Storybooks describe how the child will feel, what will be done, and what the place will look like. Parents can read these stories to children several times before the experience. Younger children like this repetition.
- *Dolls.* Practising procedures on dolls or teddy bears that they will later experience gives a sense of mastery of the situation. Custom dolls are often available for inserting tubes and giving injections, for example.
- *Puppet play.* Puppets can be used in role-play situations to provide information and show the child what the experience will be like; they help the child express emotions.
- *Health fairs.* Health fairs can educate children about their bodies and ways to stay healthy. Fairs can focus on high-risk problems that children face, such as accidents and poisoning, and on other topics identified in the community as a concern.

TEACHING: HOME CARE

Environmental Management

The way the client takes care of an infection after going home is important. The nurse can help by teaching the client how to do it correctly:

- Discuss injury proofing the home to prevent the possibility of further tissue injury (e.g., use of padding, handrails, removal of hazards).
- Explore ways to control the environmental temperature and airflow (especially if client has an airborne pathogen).
- Determine the advisability of visitors and family members in close proximity to the client.
- Describe ways to manipulate the bed, the room, and other household facilities.

INFECTION CONTROL

- Based on assessment of client and family knowledge, teach proper hand hygiene (e.g. before handling foods, before eating, after toileting, before and after any required home care treatment, and after touching any body substances, such as wound drainage) and related hygiene measures to all family members.
- Promote nail care: keep fingernails short, clean, and well manicured to eliminate rough edges or hangnails, which can harbour microorganisms.
- Instruct not to share personal care items, such as toothbrush, washcloths, and towels, and describe the rationale of how infections can be transmitted from shared personal items.
- Discuss antimicrobial soaps and effective disinfectants.
- Ensure access to and proper use of gloves and other barriers as indicated by the type of infection or risk.
- Discuss the relationship among hygiene, rest, activity, and nutrition in the chain of infection.
- Instruct about proper administration of medication.
- Instruct about cleaning reusable equipment and supplies. Use soap and water, and disinfect with a chlorine bleach solution.

INFECTION PREVENTION

- Teach the client and family members how to avoid infections.
- Suggest techniques for safe food preservation and preparation (e.g., wash raw fruits and vegetables before eating them, refrigerate all opened and unpackaged foods).
- Remind to avoid coughing, sneezing, or breathing directly on others. Cover the mouth and nose with a tissue or the sleeve to prevent the transmission of airborne microorganisms.
- Inform of the importance of maintaining sufficient fluid intake to promote urine production and output. This helps flush the bladder and urethra of microorganisms.
- Emphasize the need for proper immunizations of all family members.

WOUND CARE

- Teach the client and family the signs of wound healing and of wound infection and why monitoring of the wound is important.
- Delineate the factors that promote wound healing.
- Explain the proper technique for changing the dressing and disposing of the soiled one. Reinforce need to place contaminated dressings and other disposable items containing body fluids in moisture-proof plastic bags.
- Advise to put used needles in a puncture-resistant container with a screw-top lid. Label so as not to discard in the garbage.

REFERRALS

- Provide appropriate information regarding how to access community resources, home care agencies, sources of supplies, and community or public health departments for immunizations.

TEACHING: WELLNESS

Preventing Transmission of STIs

Clients need to know how to prevent STIs:

- Talk openly with partners about how to have safe sex and honestly discuss any history of an STI.
- Use condoms in all sexual relationships.
- Abstain from sexual activity with a partner *known* to have or *suspected* of having an STI.
- Report to a health-care facility for examination whenever in doubt about possible exposure or when signs of an STI are evident.
- When an STI is diagnosed, notify all partners and encourage them to seek treatment.
- Consider the use of vaccinations now available for hepatitis B and human papillomavirus (HPV).
- Women should have regular Pap tests for the early detection of STI-related cervical cell changes.

Three types of Assessment boxes are provided throughout the book. **Assessment: Home Care** boxes give guidelines to assess the needs of clients or families or caregivers and to consider the available community resources for discharge and home care planning. **Assessment: Interview** boxes provide examples of interviewing questions to help elicit relevant assessment data from the client. **Assessment: Developmental Guidelines** boxes provide critical assessment questions relevant to the growth and developmental needs of the client.

ASSESSMENT: HOME CARE

Nutrition

Before discharging clients, nurses need to assess their nutrition needs and any problems:

CLIENT AND ENVIRONMENT

- *Self-care abilities:* Assess the ability to feed self, to purchase food, and to prepare meals.
- *Adaptive feeding aids required:* Determine the need for special drinking cups, plates, or feeding utensils (see feeding aids later in chapter).
- *Instructional needs:* Consider nutritional requirements (e.g., *Eating Well with Canada's Food Guide*, dietary guidelines, special diet); adaptive aids available; recommended lifestyle variations; and management of enteral or parenteral nutrition.
- *Physical environment:* Assess for the adequacy of water, electricity, refrigeration, and telephone facilities; and for the presence of a clean, secure area to store and set up enteral or parenteral equipment, as needed.
- *Abilities to manage enteral or parenteral nutrition* (discussed later in chapter): Assess for the cognitive abilities to manage procedures and follow a prescribed schedule; the adequacy of manual dexterity to open sterile packages and handle equipment; the adequacy of visual acuity to read numbers on syringes and pumps; the ability to prepare formulas; and the ability to evaluate the status of the enteral or parenteral access device and report problems.

FAMILY

- *Caregiver availability, skills, and willingness:* Assess for primary and secondary persons able to assist with food purchase, meal preparation, and feeding and who are able to comprehend and administer special diets or the enteral or parenteral nutrition required.
- *Family role changes and coping:* Consider the effect on parenting and spousal roles, financial resources, and social roles.
- *Alternative potential primary or respite caregivers:* Assess, for example, other family members, volunteers, church members, paid caregivers, or housekeeping services, available community respite care (adult daycare, senior centres), and so on.

COMMUNITY

- *Current knowledge, use, and experience with community resources:* Determine the familiarity with nutritional counselling services; home health agencies for enteral or parenteral nutrition support; dietitian or nutritionist for planning appropriate meals for prescribed diet, planning ways to include ethnic food preferences into the diet, and providing written meal plans; medical equipment and supply sources; financial assistance services; support and educational services, such as the following:
  - Weight-management programs (e.g., Weight Watchers, Curves)
  - Dietitians of Canada for information on all nutrition topics
  - Health Canada
  - Meals on Wheels

ASSESSMENT: INTERVIEW

Preoperative Assessment Data

The following information must be gathered in the nursing history before surgery:

- *Current health status.* Essential information includes general health status and the presence of any chronic diseases, such as diabetes or asthma, that may affect the client's response to surgery or anaesthesia. Note any physical limitations that may affect the client's mobility or ability to communicate after surgery, as well as any prostheses, such as hearing aids or contact lenses.
- *Allergies.* Include allergies to prescription and nonprescription drugs, food allergies, and allergies to tape, latex, soaps, or antiseptic agents. Some food allergies indicate a potential reaction to drugs or substances used during surgery or diagnostic procedures; for example, an allergy to seafood alerts the nurse to a potential allergy to iodine-based dyes or soaps commonly used in hospitals; people who are allergic to foods, such as kiwi, banana, avocados, and chestnuts, may also have an allergy to latex in what is called latex-food syndrome.
- *Medications.* List all current medications (prescribed and OTC). It may be vital to maintain a blood level of some medications (e.g., anticonvulsants) throughout the surgical experience; others, such as anticoagulants or Aspirin, increase the risks of surgery and anaesthesia and need to be discontinued several days before surgery. It is important to include in the list any herbal remedies the client currently takes.
- *Previous surgeries and anaesthetic history.* Previous surgical and anaesthetic (general and local) experiences can influence the client's physical and psychological responses to surgery or may reveal unexpected responses to anaesthesia, such as cardiac arrest or malignant hyperthermia crisis.
- *Mental status.* The client's mental status and ability to understand and respond appropriately can affect the entire perioperative experience. Note any developmental disabilities, mental health problems, history of dementia, or excessive anxiety related to the procedure.
- *Understanding of the surgical procedure and anaesthesia.* The client should have a good understanding of the planned procedure and what to expect during and after surgery, as well as the expected outcome of the procedure.
- *Smoking.* Smokers may have more difficulty clearing respiratory secretions after surgery, increasing the risk of postoperative complications, such as pneumonia and atelectasis. Smoking also results in reduced oxygen-carrying capacity, increasing the risk of hypoxemia and delayed wound healing. Nicotine stimulates the surgical stress response, leading to increased workload for the heart.
- *Alcohol and other mind-altering substances.* Use of substances that affect the central nervous system, liver, or other body systems can affect the client's response to anaesthesia, surgery, and postoperative recovery.
- *Coping.* Clients with a healthy self-concept who have successfully employed appropriate coping mechanisms in the past are better able to deal with the stressors associated with surgery.
- *Social resources.* Determine the availability of family or other caregivers as well as the client's social support network. These resources are important to the client's recovery, particularly for the client undergoing same-day or short-stay surgery.
- *Cultural and spiritual considerations.* Culture and spirituality influence the client's response to surgery; respecting cultural and spiritual beliefs and practices can reduce preoperative anxiety and improve recovery.

ASSESSMENT: DEVELOPMENTAL GUIDELINES

The Infant

In these five developmental areas, does the infant do the following?

1. **PHYSICAL DEVELOPMENT**
   - Demonstrate physical growth (weight, length, head and chest circumference) within the normal range
   - Manifest appropriately sized fontanelles for age
   - Exhibit vital signs within normal range for age
2. **MOTOR DEVELOPMENT**
   - Perform gross and fine motor milestones within the normal range for age
   - Exhibit reflexes appropriate for age
3. **SENSORY DEVELOPMENT**
   - Follow a moving object within normal range for age
   - Respond to sounds, such as talking or clapping hands
4. **PSYCHOSOCIAL DEVELOPMENT**
   - Interact appropriately with parent through body movements and vocalizations
5. **DEVELOPMENT IN ACTIVITIES OF DAILY LIVING**
   - Eat and drink appropriate amounts of breast milk, formula, or solid foods
   - Exhibit an elimination pattern within normal range for age
   - Exhibit rest and sleep patterns appropriate for age

Sample **Concept Maps** show the schematic relationships of various concepts and elements of the nursing process and nursing care plans.

CONCEPT MAP

Chest Pain

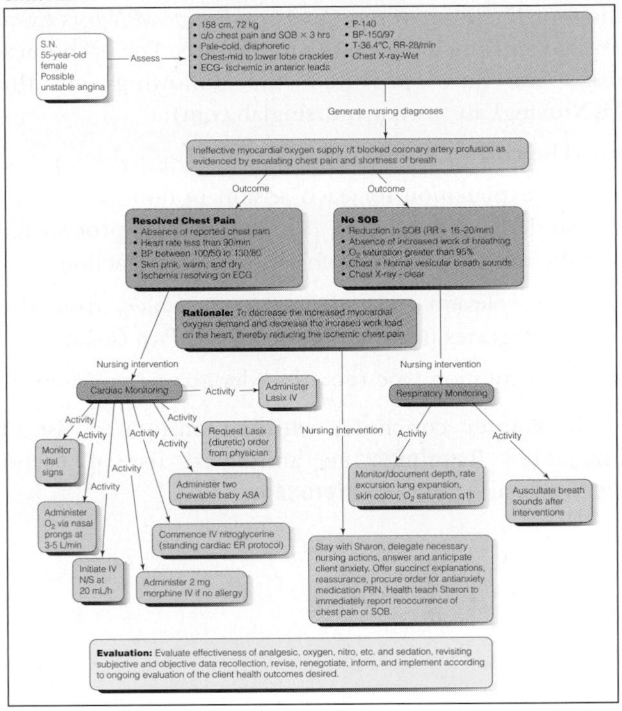

Chapter Highlights near the end of each chapter summarize the key points presented.

CHAPTER HIGHLIGHTS

- Definitions of *family* should include shifting social norms in family structure and each family's mode of describing themselves.
- Nursing care of families is based on relational practices that involve family members in care, respond to their concerns, provide them with information, and/or offer emotional support.
- Family expectations of health-care providers can include a desire for access to information about diagnosis and treatment, a trust that their ill family member will receive good care and be treated compassionately, the recognition of their own involvement in care, and preparation for their roles at home.
- The genogram inquiry helps the nurse demonstrate a concern for all family members, to document relevant information about those involved in the health situation, to appreciate developmental transitions in the family, and to begin to understand family relationships.
- The ecomap inquiry helps the nurse understand sources of family support or stress by tracing external connections to employment, health-care services, and recreational and religious communities.
- Reflective questions invite family members to think differently about themselves, health and illness concerns, and options for addressing concerns.
- Illness narratives help nurses more fully understand the reciprocal influences between health and the family and can assist families to make sense of the illness experience.
- Commendations acknowledge and convey respect for family capability and strengths.
- Families vary in their desire to be directly involved in caregiving activities, and some may need encouragement to take a respite from prolonged caregiving.
- Nurses can evaluate nursing care of families by reflecting on their efforts to invite family questions and concerns, by involving family members in decision making, and by asking the family directly about their experience of the family–nurse relationship.

Near the end of each chapter, **Assess Your Learning** presents 10 multiple-choice questions to help reinforce concepts and clinical application. These questions are modelled on those in the Canadian Registered Nurses Examination (CRNE). An actual CRNE question from the fourth edition of the *Canadian Registered Nurses Exam Prep Guide* is included in many chapters. For each question, we have provided the following on the MyNursingLab (www.mynursinglab.com):

- The correct answer
- An explanation for each answer option that guides students through the decision-making process for the most appropriate answer or nursing action.
- The relevant *nursing competency category* from the 4 categories provided in the CRNE *Prep Guide.*
- The question type (i.e., Knowledge or Application)

Each chapter concludes with an annotated list of **Suggested Readings**, an annotated list of useful **Weblinks**, and a list of **References**.

ASSESS YOUR LEARNING

1. The individual who has strong feelings of independence is meeting which of the following levels within Maslow's hierarchy of needs?

- **a.** Self-actualization
- **b.** Self-esteem
- **c.** Love and belonging
- **d.** Closeness

2. The way an individual interprets the environment can be considered part of which of the following dimensions of individuality?

- **a.** Self-identity
- **b.** Total character
- **c.** Perceptions
- **d.** Values

3. Mr. Greer, who has metastatic cancer of the liver and is severely jaundiced, asks you to assist him in planning a cruise 9 months in the future. You assess that he is using a coping mechanism. You remember that one purpose of coping mechanisms is to do which of the following?

- **a.** Protect the person
- **b.** Provide feedback
- **c.** Stimulate the endocrine system
- **d.** Change society

4. Developmental theories are useful because they do which of the following?

- **a.** Provide a basis for comparison with the individual characteristics
- **b.** Provide a set of rules for structuring individual care
- **c.** Focus on year-by-year changes in the individual
- **d.** Are not affected by the situation the individual is experiencing

5. When a father prepares to leave for work in the morning, his 3-year-old son starts to cry and scream. The father picks him up and delays leaving for a while. The child's behaviour most reflects which part of the family system?

- **a.** Input
- **b.** Throughput
- **c.** Output
- **d.** Feedback

6. Maslow would identify which of the following as belonging on the first (lowest, bottom) level of his hierarchy of needs?

- **a.** Ability to move around
- **b.** Recognition as a member of a peer group
- **c.** Feelings of independence
- **d.** Safety from physical harm

7. Baljit, a student nurse, has recently learned about the use of holistic thinking in nursing. When interviewing a client, which of the following rationales will he use in planning his questions?

- **a.** Individual processes are detached from each other.
- **b.** The reason for consulting the health professional is of primary importance.
- **c.** Each individual is more than the sum of his or her parts.
- **d.** The individual and the immediate environment are the focus of care.

8. Mr. Hannah, 28 years old, has been HIV positive for 5 years. Recently, he has been admitted to the hospital with a confirmed diagnosis of *Pneumocystis carinii* [now known as *Pneumocystis jirovecii*]. Mr. Hannah tells the nurse that he notices people seem to avoid coming into his room and that he is lonely. What strategy should the nurse use to provide support to the client?

- **a.** Explain to him the reason he is isolated is due to his susceptibility to infections.
- **b.** Explain to him that people do not come in to his room because they are afraid of getting HIV.
- **c.** Ask him if any of his family can come to the hospital to keep him company.
- **d.** Spend time talking with him during and between care activities.

9. Sarah, your friend, is trying to make some changes to her lifestyle. You support her by giving positive feedback because positive feedback does what?

- **a.** Inhibits change
- **b.** Stimulates change
- **c.** Maintains homeostasis
- **d.** Regulates change

10. Which of the following best describes psychological homeostasis or emotional well-being?

- **a.** It is inherited from parents.
- **b.** It is dependent on a person's role in family life.
- **c.** It is acquired or learned from living and interacting with others.
- **d.** It is totally independent from a person's culture.

After working through these questions, go to the MyNursingLab at ***http://www.mynursinglab.com*** *to check your answers and see explanations.*

ADDITIONAL RESOURCES AND SUPPLEMENTS

Aside from the robust MyNursingLab (www.mynursinglab.com) described at the front this book, we have provided the following additional resources and supplements to support the new edition.

Clinical Reference Card

Each copy of the book is accompanied by a 6-page laminated Clinical Reference Card, which is intended to serve as a handy reference when engaged in clinical work. The contents include brief summaries of such topics as the normal ranges of vital signs for various age groups, common laboratory values, the pain scale, the Glasgow Coma Scale, and the framework for head-to-toe assessment. The last section consists of an erasable notes section where students can customize the card for their own use by jotting down key points or data that they want to remember.

Instructor's Resource CD-ROM

An Instructor's Resource CD-ROM provides instructors with the following supplements to aid in presenting classes, fostering class discussion, creating tests, and encouraging learning: An **Instructor's Manual** prepared by Thomas Gantert (Fanshawe College), which includes answers to all the questions in the book, along with other material to help design classes

PowerPoint Slides prepared by Thomas Gantert (Fanshawe College), which illuminate and build upon key concepts in the text.

An **Image Library**, which provides electronic files of all the figures, photos, and tables in the book.

A new computerized **Testbank** prepared by Sandy Stewart (Camoson College), Sandra Carter (Centre for Nursing Studies), Ruth Stewart (Grant MacEwan College), and Virginia Birnie (Camosun College). It is available in 2 formats: **Pearson TestGen** and **Pearson MyTest**. Both formats are powerful programs that enable instructors to view and edit existing questions, create new questions, and generate quizzes, tests, exams, or homework. TestGen and MyTest also allow instructors to administer tests on a local area network, have the tests graded electronically, and have the results prepared in electronic or printed reports.

Acknowledgements

We wish to extend our sincere thanks to the many talented and committed people involved in the development of this second Canadian edition. We are especially grateful to

- The students and colleagues who provided valuable suggestions for developing this edition.
- The Canadian contributors, who worked diligently to provide content in their areas of expertise (listed on pages vii–viii).
- The Canadian reviewers, who provided critical appraisal to strengthen this text (listed on pages xi–xii).
- The editors and contributors of the U.S. eighth edition for setting high standards for the book.
- The expert guidance and ongoing support from the editorial and production teams at Pearson Education Canada: Maurice Esses, Lori Will, Michelle Sartor, Marisa D'Andrea, Dawn Hunter, Leanne Rancourt, Lorna Weisbrod and Lisa Little and many others who worked scrupulously behind the scenes to help realize this project.

We would like to thank the following instructors for their invaluable work on the supplements for this edition:

- Thomas Gantert (Fanshawe College) for preparing the *Instructor's Manual* and the *PowerPoint Slides*.
- Virginia Birnie (Camosun College), Sandra Carter (Centre for Nursing Studies), Ruth Stewart (Grant MacEwan College), and Sandy Stewart (Camosun College) for preparing the *Pearson TestGen* (i.e., the computerized Testbank).
- Michelle Acorn, Ute Beffert, Judy Bornais, Claudette Cartier, Linda Chipp, Diane Clare, Helene Deutsch, Jayne Elliott, Ann Fisk, Donna Goodridge, Elaine Howarth, Caroline Marchionni, Donna Moralejo, Harry Peery, Joanne Profetto-McGrath, and Judy Sabiston for helping to create the robust MyNursingLab for this edition.

We also wish to acknowledge the work of the Canadian editors and contributors of the first Canadian edition who provided a foundation upon which we have created this edition:

- Sandra Hirst, RN, BscN, MSc, PhD, GNC(C) (Associate Professor, Faculty of Nursing, University of Calgary)
- D. Shelley Raffin Bouchal, RN, BScN, MN, PhD (Assistant Professor, Faculty of Nursing, University of Calgary)
- Barbara J. Astle, RN, MN
- Cydnee Blake, RN, MN
- Christine Ceci, RN, PhD
- Roberta deJong, RN, MN
- Margaret Edwards, RN, PhD
- Bonnie Friesen, RN, MN
- Dorothy Hughes, RN, PhD
- Carol McDonald, RN, PhD
- Meg McDonagh, RN, MN, ENC (c)
- Marjorie McIntyre, BScN, MScN, PhD
- Nancy J. Moules, RN, BN, MN, PhD
- Florence Myrick, RN, PhD
- Kathleen Oberle, RN, BScN, MN, PhD
- Heather L. Orstead, RN, BN, ET
- Harry Plummer, RN, PhD
- James A Rankin, RN, BSc,MSc PhD
- Sandra M. Reilly, RN, BSN, MEd, EdD
- Marlene Reimer, RN, PhD, NNC(C)
- Dianne M. Tapp, RN, BScN, MN, PhD
- Sandra C. Tenov, RN, BScN, MEd, PhD
- Karen L. Then, RN, BN, MN, PhD
- Elizabeth Thomlinson , RN, PhD
- Ardene Robinson Vollman, RN, PhD
- Lorraine Watson, RN, BN, MEd, PhD
- Leanne Wyrostok , RN, BN, MN

Lucia Yiu

Lynnette Leeseberg Stamler

Madeleine Buck

Special Features

Assessment: Developmental Guidelines

The Infant 314
The Toddler 318
The Preschooler 321
The School-Age Child 323
The Adolescent 327
The Young Adult 337
The Middle-Aged Adult 342
The Older Adult 358

Assessment: Home Care

Hygiene 708
Wound Care and Prevention of Pressure Ulcers 946
Pain 997
Surgical Clients 1039
Sensory-Perception Disturbances 1067
Ability and Activity Problems 1126
Nutrition 1199
Fecal Elimination 1241
Urinary Elimination 1282
Oxygenation 1331
Fluid, Electrolyte, and Acid-Base Balance 1397
Stress and Coping 1504

Assessment: Interview

Complementary and Alternative Health Modalities 283
Learning Needs and Characteristics 521
Data Collection for Hygiene Practices 707
Foot Hygiene 721
Nail Hygiene 726
Oral Hygiene 728
Hair Care 737
Eyes 743
Clients at Risk for Infections 917
History of the Current Pain Experience 990
Preoperative Assessment Data 1022
Sensory-Perceptual Functioning 1065
Sleep Disturbances 1090
Activity and Exercise 1121
Fecal Elimination 1237
Urinary Elimination 1272
Oxygenation and Circulation 1323
Fluid, Electrolyte, and Acid-Base Balance 1390
Personal Identity 1438
Role Performance 1438
Body Image 1438
Sexual Health History 1458
Spirituality 1479
Stress and Coping Patterns 1500
Loss and Grieving 1517
The Dying Individual 1526

Case Study

Case Study 1 21
Case Study 2 34
Case Study 3 51
Case Study 4 67
Case Study 5 86
Case Study 6 109
Case Study 7 127
Case Study 8 148
Case Study 9 169
Case Study 10 192
Case Study 11 208
Case Study 12 228
Case Study 13 248
Case Study 14 264
Case Study 15 284
Case Study 16 303
Case Study 17 328
Case Study 18 343
Case Study 19 362
Case Study 20 379
Case Study 21 408
Case Study 22 464
Case Study 23 492
Case Study 24 510
Case Study 25 532
Case Study 26 547
Case Study 27 656
Case Study 28 699
Case Study 29 758
Case Study 30 790
Case Study 31 872
Case Study 32 922
Case Study 33 972
Case Study 34 1011
Case Study 35 1054
Case Study 36 1076
Case Study 37 1098
Case Study 38 1160
Case Study 39 1219
Case Study 40 1259

Case Study 41 1303
Case Study 42 1362
Case Study 43 1425
Case Study 44 1442
Case Study 45 1467
Case Study 46 1484
Case Study 47 1508
Case Study 48 1534

Clinical Alert

5 Values, Ethics, and Advocacy 81
23 Documenting and Reporting 471
23 Documenting and Reporting 490
26 Leading, Managing, and Delegating 545
27 Health Assessment 624
27 Health Assessment 634
27 Health Assessment 635
28 Vital Signs 667
28 Vital Signs 671
28 Vital Signs 673
28 Vital Signs 685
28 Vital Signs 688
28 Vital Signs 695
30 Safety 776
30 Safety 779
30 Safety 783
30 Safety 785
31 Medication Administration 815
31 Medication Administration 835
31 Medication Administration 857
31 Medication Administration 857
32 Infection Prevention and Control 909
33 Skin Integrity and Wound Care 932
33 Skin Integrity and Wound Care 937
33 Skin Integrity and Wound Care 945
34 Pain Management 982
34 Pain Management 999
35 Caring for Perioperative Clients 1029
35 Caring for Perioperative Clients 1034
35 Caring for Perioperative Clients 1046
36 Sensory Perception 1065
36 Sensory Perception 1066
37 Rest and Sleep 1082
37 Rest and Sleep 1083
37 Rest and Sleep 1083
37 Rest and Sleep 1084
38 Activity and Exercise 1129
38 Activity and Exercise 1147
39 Nutrition 1180
39 Nutrition 1184
39 Nutrition 1201
39 Nutrition 1214
40 Fecal Elimination 1231
40 Fecal Elimination 1234
41 Urinary Elimination 1271
41 Urinary Elimination 1284
43 Fluid, Electrolyte, and Acid-Base Balance 1384
43 Fluid, Electrolyte, and Acid-Base Balance 1412
43 Fluid, Electrolyte, and Acid-Base Balance 1413
43 Fluid, Electrolyte, and Acid-Base Balance 1421
44 Self-Concept 1435
44 Self-Concept 1437
45 Sexuality and Sexual Health Practices 1460
47 Stress and Coping 1495
47 Stress and Coping 1505

Clinical Manifestations

Fever 664
Hypothermia 665
Pain Management 981
Sensory Deprivation 1062
Sensory Overload 1062
Hypoxia 1320
Physiological Indicators of Stress 1494

Concept Map

Overview of Growth and Development Psychosocial Theories and Theorists 298
Chest Pain 444
Ineffective Airway Clearance (Gas Exchange) 447
Sensory-Perceptual Disturbances 1076

Evidence-Informed Practice

Do Fourth-Year Baccalaureate Students Have a More Realistic Picture of Nursing Practice Than First-Year Students? 16
How Can Nurses in Rural and Remote Areas Access Continuing Education? 33
How Can Employers Promote Empowerment for New Graduate Nurses? 42
What Are Caregiver Perceptions of Unsupportive Interactions with Others? 43
Is It Important That Residents Feel They Are Listened to by Staff? 65
What Is Ethical Practice in Nursing? 78
What Are the Issues of Informed Consent? 98
How Can Nurses Help Prevent Falls at Home? 124
Do Parents Use Child Safety Restraint Systems Correctly? 138
Do Persons with Chronic Diseases Identify Barriers and Facilitators to Health Care? 166
What Are the Stories about Cancer among the Woodland Cree of Northern Saskatchewan? 180
Does the Use of Humour Have a Place in a Palliative Care Unit? 203
How Does Family Nursing Relate to Care Involving Mental Illness? 214
Can Immunization Programs Be Successful in Nontraditional Settings? 243
How Do Nurses Define Rural Nursing Practice? 263

How Commonly Known Are Natural Health Product–Drug Interactions? 276
What Impact Does Financial Stress Have on the Health of Canadians? 297
How Does Hearing Impairment Influence Growth and Development? 311
What Are the Experiences of Canadians Living with Mental Health Problems? 341
How Does Ethnicity Influence Perceptions of Health? 349
Do Concept Maps Improve Critical Thinking? 370
What Is an Effective Strategy to Elicit Patient Treatment Preferences? 405
How Reliable Is the Breastfeeding Self-Efficacy Scale in Nursing Assessment? 464
Can Electronic Patient Records Help Capture Client Information? 479
How Can Parents Be Supported at Home Following Surgery on Their Children? 502
Dietary Strategies for Coping with Inflammatory Bowel Disease 527
Organizational Trust and Empowerment: What Are the Effects on Staff Nurse Commitment? 542
Do Routine Screening Programs Have a Positive or Negative Psychological Impact? 634
How Do Beverages and Respiratory Rates Affect Oral Temperature Readings? 667
Does Bath Grab Bar Placement Matter for Older Adults? 718
What Safety Hazards Do Older Adults Deal with When Attempting to Maintain Their Health by Regular Walking? 774
Do Look-Alike Vials Lead to Significant Errors in Heparin Administration? 817
How Well Do Health-Care Workers Wash Their Hands? 879
How Are Skin Tears Best Prevented and Treated? 959
Can a Self-Management Program Help Clients Cope with Chronic Cardiac Pain? 1001
When Should Feeding Be Resumed Following Surgery? 1020
Which Stroke Impairments Predict Discharge Function, Length of Stay, and Discharge Destination in Stroke Rehabilitation? 1072
How Does Violence against Women Affect Their Sleep? 1086
Does Stretching before Exercise Reduce Muscle Soreness? 1110
How Can Nurses Use Nutrition to Prevent Constipation in Older Adults? 1168
Can Chronic Diarrhea in HIV Clients Be Controlled through a Behavioural and Dietary Intervention That Uses Normal Foods? 1251
What Self-Care Strategies Do Individuals with Urinary Incontinence Employ and What Factors Influence the Choice and Maintenance of Strategies? 1285
Do Nurses Implement Smoking Cessation Best Practice Guidelines? 1318
What Are Best Practice Guidelines for Maintaining Vascular Access Devices? 1403
What Influences Adolescents' Self-Esteem? 1435
Lesbian Disclosure: Disrupting the Taken for Granted 1447
What Does Spiritual Nursing Care Mean? 1482
What Are the Links between Maternal Stress during Pregnancy and Behavioural Disturbances in Children? 1500
What Guides Clinicians in Their Grief Work with Families? 1519

Health-Promotion Guidelines

Health-Promotion Guidelines for Neonates and Infants 315
Health-Promotion Guidelines for Toddlers 318
Health-Promotion Guidelines for Preschoolers 321
Health-Promotion Guidelines for School-Age Children 324
Health-Promotion Guidelines for Adolescents 328
Health-Promotion Guidelines for Young Adults 338
Health-Promotion Guidelines for Middle-Aged Adults 342
Health-Promotion Guidelines for Older Adults 359

Home Care Considerations

Pulse 681
Respirations 686
Blood Pressure 696
Pulse Oximetry 699
Hearing Aids 747
Using a Bed or Chair Exit Safety Monitoring Device 779
Implementing Seizure Precautions 781
Applying Restraints 790
Administering Medication 823
Administering an Intradermal Injection 838
Subcutaneous Injections 841
Administering IV Antibiotics 855
Metered-Dose Inhalers 870
Sterile Field 900
Wound Care 961
Applying Bandages and Binders 967
Antiembolism Stockings 1032
Removing Sutures or Staples 1053
Positioning, Moving, and Turning Clients 1141
Administering an Enema 1250
Drainable Bowel Diversion Ostomy Appliances 1257
Collecting Urine 1276
Catheterization 1295
Oxygen Equipment 1342
Suctioning a Tracheostomy or Endotracheal Tube 1356

Lifespan Considerations

Physical Activity and Health 122
Factors Affecting Health Promotion and Illness Prevention 148
Complementary and Alternative Health Modalities 279
Health-Care Decisions for Children and Older Adults 376
Communication with Older Adults 403
Computer Use 505
Special Teaching Considerations 522
General Survey 562
Assessing the Skin 568
Assessing the Hair 570
Assessing the Nails 572
Assessing the Skull and Face 574
Assessing the Eyes and Vision 582
Assessing the Ears and Hearing 587
Assessing the Nose and Sinuses 589
Assessing the Mouth and Oropharynx 594
Assessing the Neck 599
Assessing the Thorax and Lungs 608
Assessing the Heart and Central Vessels 615
Assessing the Peripheral Vascular System 617
Assessing the Breasts and Axillae 621
Assessing the Abdomen 630
Assessing the Musculoskeletal System 633
Assessing the Neurological System 645
Assessing the Female Genitals and Inguinal Lymph Nodes 647
Assessing the Male Genitals and Inguinal Area 653
Assessing the Rectum and Anus 656
Assessing Body Temperature 671
Assessing the Pulse 681
Assessing Respirations 685
Blood Pressure 695
Pulse Oximetry 699
Bathing 706
Implementing Seizure Precautions 780
Restraints 789
Administering Oral Medications 823
Administering an Intradermal Injection 838
Intramuscular Injections 848
Administering Ophthalmic Medications 861
Administering Otic Medications 864
Administering Rectal Medications 868
Administering Metered-Dose Inhalers and Nebulizers 871
Infections 887
Pressure Ulcer and Wound Care 961
Applying Bandages and Binders 967
PCA Pump 1006
Pain Management 1011
Preoperative Teaching 1027
Antiembolism Stockings 1032
Postoperative Care 1035
Positioning, Moving, and Turning Clients 1141
Assisting the Client to Ambulate 1152
Inserting a Nasogastric Tube 1208
Administering a Tube Feeding 1216
Administering an Enema 1250
Factors Affecting Voiding 1267
Catheterization 1295
Sputum and Throat Specimens 1325
Oxygen Delivery Equipment 1341
Suctioning a Tracheostomy or Endotracheal Tube 1356
Fluid and Electrolyte Balance 1379
Enhancing Self-Esteem 1441
Sexuality 1451
Stress and Coping 1491

Nursing and Canadian Society

1 Principles of Primary Health Care 19
2 Nursing Education in Canada 32
3 Nursing Research in Canada 41
4 Nursing Philosophies, Theories, Concepts, Frameworks, and Models 58
5 Top 10 Health-Care Ethics Challenges Facing the Canadian Public 73
6 Accountability and Legal Aspects of Nursing 92
7 Health, Wellness, and Illness 118
8 Health Promotion 136
9 The Canadian Health-Care System 168
10 Culture Care 177
11 Individual Care 199
12 Nursing Care of Families 216
13 Community-Based Nursing 239
14 Rural and Remote Health Care 255
15 Complementary and Alternative Health Modalities 273
17 Development from Conception through Adolescence 327
19 Older Adults 348
23 Documenting and Reporting 471
30 Safety 763
45 Sexuality and Sexual Health Practices 1458
46 Spirituality 1471
47 Stress and Coping 1498
48 Loss, Grieving, and Death 1529

Practice Guidelines

Preventing Falls in Health-Care Agencies 776
Applying Restraints 785
Administering Medications by Nasogastric or Gastrostomy Tube 824
Applying Skin Preparations 858
Assessing Common Pressure Sites 941
Cleansing Wounds 959
Bandaging 963

Providing Passive ROM Exercises 1148
Giving and Removing a Bedpan 1244
Using Antidiarrheal Medications 1247
Maintaining Normal Voiding Habits 1284
Bladder Training 1286
Preventing Catheter-Associated Urinary Infections 1296
Facilitating Fluid Intake 1399
Restricting Fluid Intake 1400
Vein Selection 1402
Caring for Clients with a Venous Access Device 1404

Reflect on Primary Health Care

1 Principles of Primary Health Care 12
2 Nursing Education in Canada 30
5 Values, Ethics, and Advocacy 84
7 Health, Wellness, and Illness 117
8 Health Promotion 137
11 Individual Care 199
15 Complementary and Alternative Health Modalities 284
16 Concepts of Growth and Development 303
17 Development from Conception through Adolescence 309
18 Young and Middle-Aged Adulthood 336
19 Older Adults 362
20 Critical Thinking 379
21 Caring, Comforting, and Communicating 405
22 The Nursing Process 445
23 Documenting and Reporting 472
24 Nursing Informatics 501
25 Teaching and Learning 530
26 Leading, Managing, and Delegating 537
29 Hygiene 709
30 Safety 765
31 Medication Administration 856
32 Infection Prevention and Control 916
33 Skin Integrity and Wound Care 956
34 Pain Management 980
35 Caring for Perioperative Clients 1018
36 Sensory Perception 1069
38 Activity and Exercise 1104
40 Fecal Elimination 1238
42 Oxygenation and Circulation 1336
44 Self-Concept 1434
45 Sexuality and Sexual Health Practices 1460
46 Spirituality 1479
47 Stress and Coping 1499

Sample Care Plans

Sample Care Plan for Amanda Aquilini 452
Sample Care Plan for Acute Pain 994
Sample Care Plan for Sensory-Perceptual Alteration 1074
Sample Care Plan for Rest and Sleep 1092
Sample Care Plan for Nutrition 1197
Sample Care Plan for Altered Bowel Elimination 1240
Sample Care Plan for Urinary Elimination 1280
Sample Care Plan for Ineffective Airway Clearance 1329
Sample Care Plan for Chronic Low Self-Esteem 1439
Sample Care Plan for Spiritual Distress 1483
Sample Care Plan for Ineffective Coping 1502

Skill

SKILL 27.1 Assessing General Appearance and Mental Status 561
SKILL 27.2 Assessing the Skin 566
SKILL 27.3 Assessing the Hair 569
SKILL 27.4 Assessing the Nails 571
SKILL 27.5 Assessing the Skull and Face 573
SKILL 27.6 Assessing the Eye Structures and Visual Acuity 576
SKILL 27.7 Assessing the Ears and Hearing 583
SKILL 27.8 Assessing the Nose and Sinuses 588
SKILL 27.9 Assessing the Mouth and Oropharynx 590
SKILL 27.10 Assessing the Neck 596
SKILL 27.11 Assessing the Thorax and Lungs 603
SKILL 27.12 Assessing the Heart and Central Vessels 612
SKILL 27.13 Assessing the Peripheral Vascular System 615
SKILL 27.14 Assessing the Breasts and Axillae 618
SKILL 27.15 Assessing the Abdomen 624
SKILL 27.16 Assessing the Musculoskeletal System 631
SKILL 27.17 Assessing the Neurological System 637
SKILL 27.18 Assessing the Female Genitals and Inguinal Lymph Nodes 646
SKILL 27.19 Assessing the Male Genitals and Inguinal Area 651
SKILL 27.20 Assessing the Anus and Rectum 654
SKILL 28.1 Assessing Body Temperature 669
SKILL 28.2 Assessing a Peripheral Pulse 675
SKILL 28.3 Assessing an Apical Pulse 678
SKILL 28.4 Assessing an Apical-Radial Pulse 680
SKILL 28.5 Assessing Respirations 684
SKILL 28.6 Assessing Blood Pressure 692
SKILL 28.7 Measuring Oxygen Saturation 697
SKILL 29.1 Bathing an Adult or a Pediatric Client 713
SKILL 29.2 Providing Perineal-Genital Care 718
SKILL 29.3 Providing Foot Care 724
SKILL 29.4 Brushing and Flossing the Teeth 731
SKILL 29.5 Providing Oral Care for an Unconscious Client 735
SKILL 29.6 Providing Hair Care for Clients 739
SKILL 29.7 Shampooing the Hair of a Client Confined to Bed 741

SKILL 29.8 Removing, Cleaning, and Inserting a Hearing Aid 747
SKILL 29.9 Changing an Unoccupied Bed 751
SKILL 29.10 Changing an Occupied Bed 755
SKILL 30.1 Using a Bed or Chair Exit Safety Monitoring Device 777
SKILL 30.2 Implementing Seizure Precautions 779
SKILL 30.3 Applying Restraints 787
SKILL 31.1 Administering Oral Medications 819
SKILL 31.2 Preparing Medications from Ampules 831
SKILL 31.3 Preparing Medications from Vials 832
SKILL 31.4 Mixing Medications by Using One Syringe 834
SKILL 31.5 Administering an Intradermal Injection for Skin Tests 836
SKILL 31.6 Administering a Subcutaneous Injection 839
SKILL 31.7 Administering an Intramuscular Injection 846
SKILL 31.8 Adding Medications to Intravenous Fluid Containers 849
SKILL 31.9 Administering Intravenous Medications Using IV Push 853
SKILL 31.10 Administering Ophthalmic Instillations 858
SKILL 31.11 Administering Otic Instillations 861
SKILL 31.12 Administering Vaginal Instillations 865
SKILL 32.1 Handwashing 892
SKILL 32.2 Donning and Removing Personal Protective Equipment (Gloves, Gown, Mask, Eyewear) 896
SKILL 32.3 Establishing and Maintaining a Sterile Field 901
SKILL 32.4 Donning and Removing Sterile Gloves (Open Method) 905
SKILL 32.5 Donning a Sterile Gown and Sterile Gloves (Closed Method) 907
SKILL 33.1 Obtaining a Wound Drainage Specimen for Culture 944
SKILL 33.2 Applying and Removing a Moist Transparent Wound Barrier Dressing 955
SKILL 33.3 Applying a Hydrocolloid Dressing 956
SKILL 33.4 Irrigating a Wound 960
SKILL 35.1 Teaching Moving, Leg Exercises, Deep Breathing, and Coughing 1024
SKILL 35.2 Applying Antiembolism Stockings 1030
SKILL 35.3 Managing Gastrointestinal Suction 1043
SKILL 35.4 Cleaning a Closed Wound and Applying a Sterile Dressing 1047
SKILL 37.1 Providing a Back Massage 1095
SKILL 38.1 Moving a Client up in Bed 1135
SKILL 38.2 Turning a Client to a Lateral or Prone Position in Bed 1136
SKILL 38.3 Logrolling a Client 1138
SKILL 38.4 Assisting the Client to Sit on the Side of the Bed 1139
SKILL 38.5 Transferring between Bed and Chair 1142
SKILL 38.6 Transferring between Bed and Stretcher 1145
SKILL 38.7 Assisting the Client to Ambulate 1149
SKILL 39.1 Obtaining a Capillary Blood Specimen to Measure Blood Glucose 1194
SKILL 39.2 Inserting a Nasogastric Tube 1205
SKILL 39.3 Removing a Nasogastric Tube 1209
SKILL 39.4 Administering a Tube Feeding 1211
SKILL 39.5 Administering a Gastrostomy or Jejunostomy Feeding 1214
SKILL 40.1 Administering an Enema 1248
SKILL 40.2 Changing a One-Piece, Drainable Bowel Diversion Ostomy Appliance 1255
SKILL 41.1 Collecting a Urine Specimen for Culture and Sensitivity by Clean Catch 1275
SKILL 41.2 Applying an External (Condom) Catheter 1287
SKILL 41.3 Performing Urethral Urinary Catheterization 1291
SKILL 41.4 Performing Bladder Irrigation 1298
SKILL 42.1 Administering Oxygen by Cannula, Facemask, or Face Tent 1338
SKILL 42.2 Administering Air by Continuous Positive Airway Pressure (CPAP) 1343
SKILL 42.3 Providing Tracheostomy Care 1346
SKILL 42.4 Oropharyngeal, Nasopharyngeal, and Nasotracheal Suctioning 1351
SKILL 42.5 Suctioning a Tracheostomy or Endotracheal Tube 1353
SKILL 42.6 Applying a Sequential Compression Device 1359
SKILL 43.1 Starting an Intravenous Infusion 1407
SKILL 43.2 Monitoring an Intravenous Infusion 1414
SKILL 43.3 Changing an Intravenous Container, Tubing, and Dressing 1416
SKILL 43.4 Discontinuing a Peripheral Intravenous Infusion 1418
SKILL 43.5 Changing a Peripheral Intravenous Catheter to an Intermittent Infusion Lock 1419
SKILL 43.6 Initiating, Maintaining, and Terminating a Blood Transfusion by Using a Y-Set 1422

Teaching: Clinical

Teaching Clients with Low Literacy Levels 523
Developing Written Teaching Aids 523
Sample Teaching Plan: Wound Care 526
Teaching Tools for Children 529

Why Do People Have Fevers? 665
Foot Care 725
Using a Metered-Dose Inhaler 869
Skin Integrity 946
Client Self-Management of Pain by Using a PCA Pump 1007
Preoperative Instructions 1024
Preventing Back Injuries 1130
Active ROM Exercises 1147
Controlling Orthostatic Hypotension 1152
Using Canes 1153
Using Walkers 1154
Using Crutches 1155
Assessing Stool for Occult Blood 1239
Managing Diarrhea 1243
Pelvic Floor Muscle Exercises (Kegels) 1287
Clean Intermittent Self-Catheterization 1297
Abdominal (Diaphragmatic) and Pursed-Lip Breathing 1333
Controlled and Huff Coughing 1333
Using Cough Medications 1334
Using an Incentive Spirometer 1335

Teaching: Home Care

Temperature 669
Hygiene 717
Environmental Management 919
Monitoring Pain 997
PCA Pump 1007
Postoperative Instructions 1028
Gastrointestinal Suction 1045
Cleaning a Closed Wound 1049
Activity and Exercise 1126
Tube Feedings 1217
Fecal Elimination 1242
Urinary Elimination 1282
Fluid, Electrolyte, and Acid-Base Balance 1398

Teaching: Wellness

Maintaining a Healthy Blood Pressure 687
Measures to Prevent Tooth Decay 730
Safety Measures throughout the Lifespan 769
Preventing Poisoning 781
Reducing Electrical Hazards 783
Preventing Sensory Impairments 1068
Promoting Rest and Sleep 1095
Nutrition for Older Adults 1181
Nutrition Recommendations for Canadians 1184
Healthy Nutrition 1199
Healthy Defecation 1242
Promoting Healthy Breathing 1331
Promoting a Healthy Heart 1331
Promoting Healthy Fluid and Electrolyte Balance 1399
Preventing Transmission of STIs 1463
Breast Awareness and Mammography 1464
Testicular Self-Examination 1464
Supporting Religious Practices 1481

UNIT 1

The Foundation of Nursing in Canada

CHAPTER 1
Historical and Contemporary Nursing Practice

CHAPTER 2
Nursing Education in Canada

CHAPTER 3
Nursing Research in Canada

CHAPTER 4
Nursing Philosophies, Theories, Concepts, Frameworks, and Models

CHAPTER 5
Values, Ethics, and Advocacy

CHAPTER 6
Accountability and Legal Aspects of Nursing

Chapter 1

Historical and Contemporary Nursing Practice

Nurses have traditionally composed the largest portion of health-care workers in Canada. As such, they have enabled and participated in shaping the Canadian health-care system and have exerted a significant impact on the health of individuals, families, and communities. Although public surveys identify nurses as the most trusted of health-care providers, gloomy forecasts of massive nursing shortfalls persist. Nurses perceive their work as undervalued while others deem it as too expensive in the face of persistent cost-cutting measures and concerns over the viability of state-supported health and medical care. At the same time, nurses struggle to articulate what nurses actually do (Nelson & Gordon, 2006). Nursing policymakers, educators, and union leaders are challenged with defining and defending a unique role for nurses among other health-care professionals and within a rapidly changing health-care system (Villeneuve & MacDonald, 2006).

OBJECTIVES

After studying this chapter, you should be able to

1. Explain major trends in the writing of nursing history
2. Discuss the range of people who provided nursing care in different periods in Canadian history
3. Compare different settings in which nursing has been provided by Canadian nurses
4. Explain the usefulness of nursing history for understanding current practice issues
5. Analyze the influence of changing social, political, and economic conditions over time
6. Describe the scope and standards of nursing practice
7. Evaluate the expanded career goals and their functions
8. Examine the criteria of a profession and the professionalization of nursing

Historical Nursing Practice

In the past, Canadian nurses were on the front lines during cholera, influenza, and polio epidemics, as they were for more recent outbreaks of contagious diseases, such as the SARS (severe acute respiratory syndrome) outbreak in 2003 (MacDougall, 2007). They served in military medical units during the South African War, World War I and II, and the Korean War, leaving a rich heritage for Canadian nurses who continue to play important roles in international conflicts. Nurses and their work were critical to the rapid expansion in the number and size of hospitals, and they continue to facilitate the spread and acceptance of medical technology both within and outside hospitals. Since the late nineteenth century, public health nurses have provided essential health and medical care to isolated populations in both rural and urban centres, a legacy taken up by street nurses caring for people on new frontiers.

As these situations suggest, nursing takes place within broad cultural, sociopolitical, and economic contexts that also influence both its practitioners and its practice. Nursing evolved similarly in most Western nations, partially shaped by societal events and such changes as industrialization, urbanization, wars, cycles of economic depression and expansion, and the women's movement. Developments in scientific and technological knowledge and the consolidation of Western medicine have changed conceptualizations of health and illness, as well as the meanings associated with them. Historical research contributes to nursing knowledge in two main ways: (1) it develops in-depth analyses of these complex relationships, and (2) it creates enhanced understandings of the past that inform both present and future situations.

Early historians of nursing focused primarily on questions about professionalization, education, and leadership, tending to see their history as a steady march of progress through time. Although indebted to these writers, who have preserved vast amounts of source material, historians since the 1980s have examined the profession more critically—paying closer attention to issues that complicate and add greater complexity to their analyses. It is important, for example, to understand who was considered a "nurse" and what nursing work encompassed in a particular historical period. Answers to these questions are contingent on who was available to work as a nurse, what status or value society attributed to nurses' (and women's) work, and how nurses were compensated for that work during a specific timeframe. Including gender, race, ethnicity, and class in historical analyses raises important questions about the social arrangements and relations of power that shaped who was included or excluded as a nurse. Although for the most part nurses have worked as subordinates within health-care systems, they often held positions of privilege, increased social status, and respect in comparison with other female workers. Analyzing nurses as agents of the state allows us to ask in what ways they did (and do) enable and influence larger social, political, and economic agendas through their participation in systems of health care. Knowledge of how nursing developed in specific contexts or sets of circumstances permits nurses to better understand their present situation and, particularly, to see how contemporary concerns might relate to larger social-structural conditions.

Before the establishment of training schools in Canada, women provided most of the nursing care, either for family members and acquaintances or for strangers in their communities. Some took on these roles as charitable acts of kindness; others, self-identifying as nurses in the pre-training era, developed midwifery practices or hired themselves out as "monthly" nurses to care for women in their homes for a month after giving birth (Young, 2004). First Nations women provided much needed help to new, white settler societies as they spread across the frontier—a history too long ignored because the skilled medical care of these women, particularly in midwifery and childhood diseases, was critical to the very survival of these new communities. Women who were members of religious groups were also early skilled caregivers, dating to the first group of European nuns who arrived in what is now Quebec (in 1639) with a mission to provide care for the bodies and souls of both settlers and native inhabitants. These women cared for the sick and destitute where they landed, but many soon followed the new immigrants west and founded hospitals, some of which have survived into the present (see Figure 1.1).

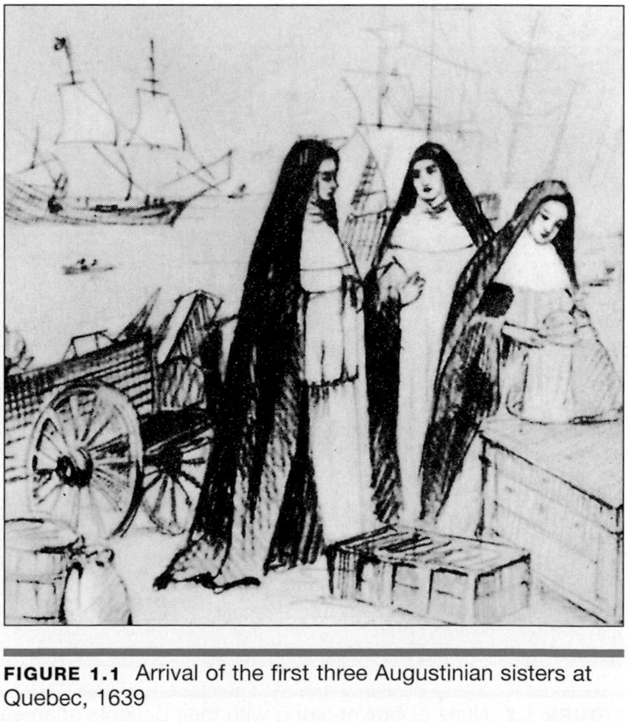

FIGURE 1.1 Arrival of the first three Augustinian sisters at Quebec, 1639

Immigration, growing urbanization, and changing concepts around the transmission and treatment of diseases contributed to the push for formally trained nurses by the late nineteenth century. Early Canadian towns and cities were plagued by inadequate sanitation and sewage systems. Waves of infectious diseases, such as typhus, influenza, and smallpox, regularly devastated both immigrant and native populations (Cassel, 1994). Wealthy patrons initially established hospitals during the late nineteenth century as philanthropic institutions that served the increasingly visible sick poor. Measures to improve and protect the delivery of food and water supplies, a gradual acceptance of germ theory in disease transmission, and the availability of anaesthesia all helped to increase confidence in the idea of scientific medicine. Although cures for many illnesses often lagged far behind identification of causes, perceptions of increased therapeutic efficacy inclined the better-off classes to choose care in medical institutions over treatments (including surgeries) in their homes. Hospital administrators increasingly relied on these paying patients to offset the costs of caring for the poor (Gagan & Gagan, 2002). Significantly, the advent of trained nurses lent both efficiency and respectability to this shift toward hospital care.

Two main influences have shaped formally prepared nursing in Canada. The British system, associated primarily with Florence Nightingale during the mid-nineteenth century, has attracted the most historical attention, even if her vision for an independent nursing force complementary to, and not dependent on, hospital administration was never fully realized. French-Canadian religious communities, which also contributed significantly to the development of trained nurses, blended religious and work life to own and manage hospitals and training schools across the country. The Quiet Revolution in Quebec during the 1960s, in reaction to the hegemony of the church over French-Canadian society, brought in a period of rapid secularization with closer government control over institutions, eroding the nuns' authority within their institutions and shifting nursing education into the public sphere (Charles, 2003; Violette, 2005; Paul, 2005); see Figure 1.2. Both systems built on religious and cultural ideals of respectable femininity that integrated contemporary ideas about scientific thinking with womanly, selfless devotion to duty and service.

The first official training school was established at St. Catharines, Ontario, in 1874 by Dr. Theophilus Mack. Over the next decades, the number of nurses rose dramatically from only 300 at the turn of the twentieth century to 20 000 by the end of World War I (McPherson, 1996). Student nurses formed the major part of the hospital workforce until the 1940s, with the expectation that they would become self-employed as private duty nurses outside the hospital on graduation. The apprenticeship training system was the predominant model of nursing education in both large and small hospitals across the country until the 1970s. Several universities did offer combined programs whereby it was possible to earn a degree in nursing, such as the first degree program established at the University of British Columbia in 1919; the focus of these programs was often on preparing nurses to be supervisors, educators, and public health nurses.

Nursing became one of the few respectable opportunities for paid work available to women in the first half of the twentieth century. The vast majority of student placements in nursing schools were reserved for young, white women whose families could afford to do without their financial

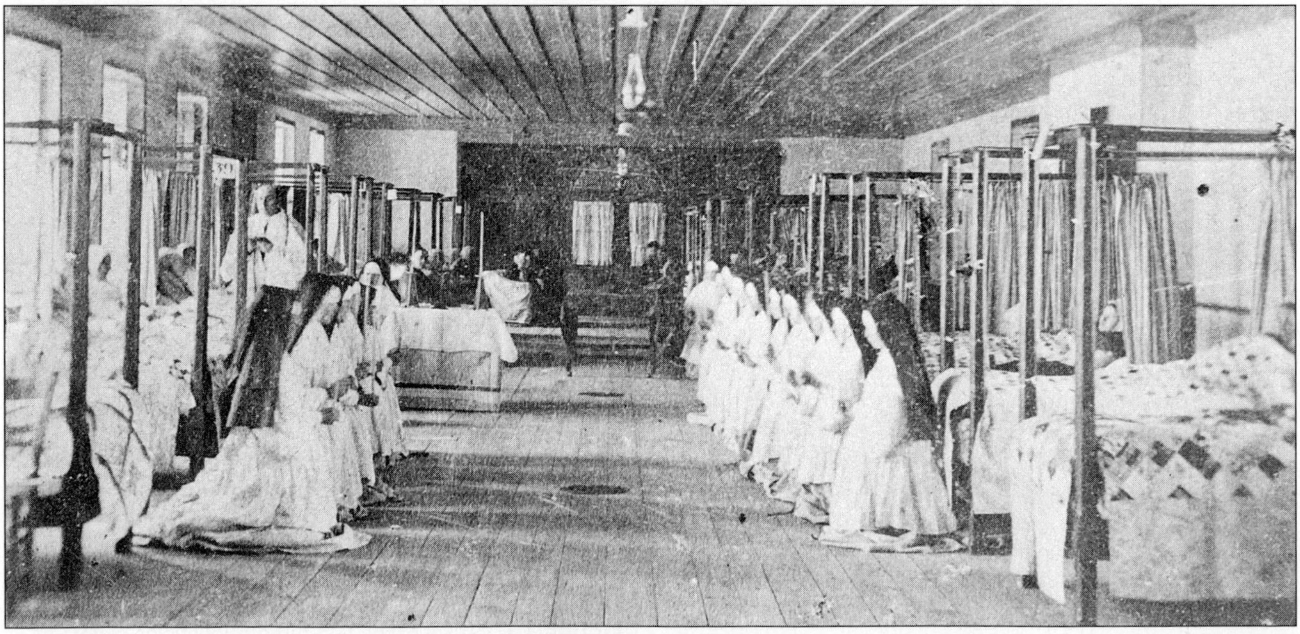

FIGURE 1.2 Nuns at prayer along with their patients at an early Hotel Dieu hospital

contribution, at least for the duration of their training. Two men appear in the 1899 graduating class of Victoria General Hospital in Halifax (Nursing Education in Nova Scotia, n.d.), but men in general have remained vastly underrepresented in the ranks of an occupation strongly tied to the concept, promoted sometimes by nurses themselves, that nursing is women's work (McPherson, 1996). Despite the Canadian Nurses Association's official policy of nondiscrimination in place since the 1940s, few black nurses gained entrance to training programs until the 1970s (McPherson, 1996). In British Columbia, a few nursing students of Asian background were admitted during the late 1930s for the explicit purpose of nursing among their own ethnic communities. And in 1954, Jean Cuthand Goodwill became the first Aboriginal woman to graduate from nursing school in Saskatchewan, but again, not until the 1970s was a concerted effort made to recruit First Nations and Inuit students into nursing (McBain, 2005); see Figures 1.3 and 1.4.

Various professionalization movements throughout the twentieth century also intensified debates over who was, or could become, a nurse. In the early decades, nursing leaders attempted to distance skilled nursing work from domestic caregiving and midwifery. Following a successful campaign by physicians to gain control over medical practice, nurses sought to establish control over nursing through the standardization of educational curricula and the legal authority to credential graduates of recognized hospital-based training programs. Most provinces brought in nurse registration between 1910 and 1922, thus separating trained nurses from others who used the term *nurse* (Mansell, 2003). Newfoundland and Labrador nurses obtained registration in 1954, Northwest Territories nurses in 1975, and Yukon nurses in 1992.

Most nurses worked in private duty after graduation during the first half of the twentieth century, but changing concepts in public health provided other opportunities. Women's groups were instrumental in pushing for reform, particularly in maternal and child health, and initiated many services that provincial health authorities later took over. Poor health status (and subsequent rejection) of wartime recruits because of preventable and treatable illnesses they had contracted in childhood, the devastating impact of the influenza epidemic (1917–1918), and a high rate of tuberculosis and venereal diseases among returning World War I soldiers in 1918 fuelled demands for increased state responsibility in matters of health. Specially trained nurses were dispersed into schools and homes across Canada, in both urban and rural districts. Nurses, as women, met gendered expectations that they were the ideal people to bring the new "gospel of good health" to mothers and their families. By helping to spread new scientific theories of health, including those on social and mental hygiene, nurses were responsible for Canadianizing new immigrants through the promotion of white, middle-class, urban-based ideals on health, which they found that their clients sometimes could not, or would not, meet.

The Victorian Order of Nurses was founded in 1897, but other organizations, such as the Margaret Scott Nursing Mission in Winnipeg, the Alberta District Nursing Service, the Newfoundland Outport Nursing and Industrial Association (NONIA), and the Medical Service to Settlers in Quebec, emerged to meet these public health needs. Several provincial divisions of the

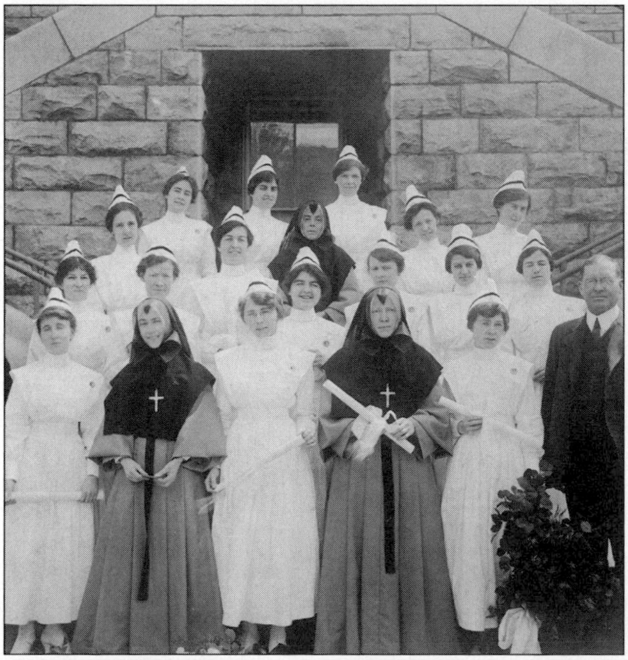

FIGURE 1.3 Ottawa General Hospital graduation 1912

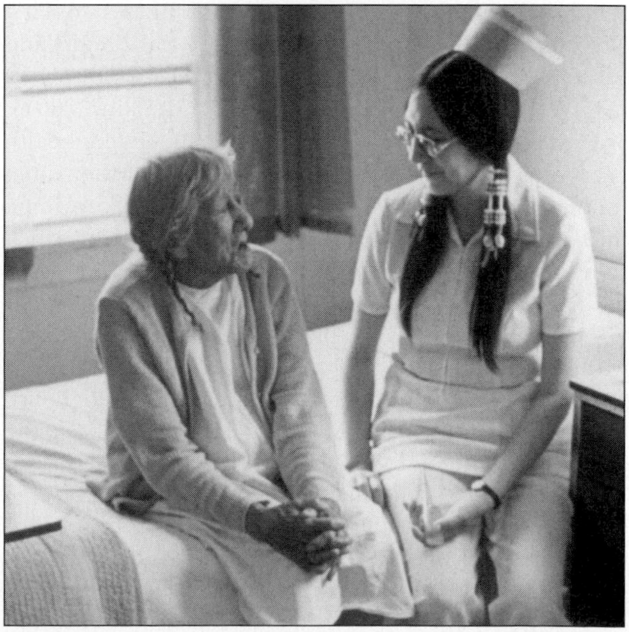

FIGURE 1.4 Aboriginal nurse with a patient at Blood Hospital, Cardston, Alberta

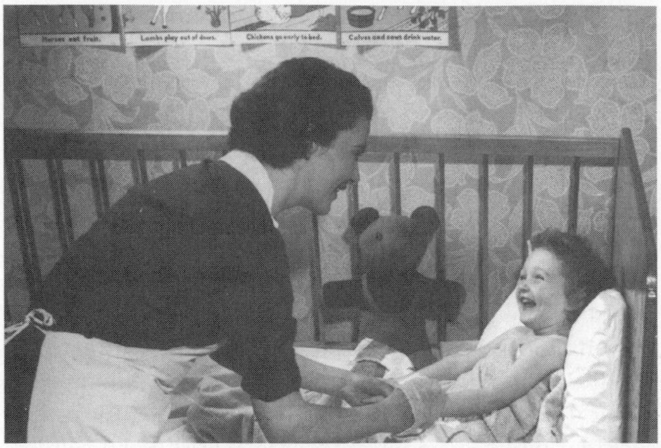

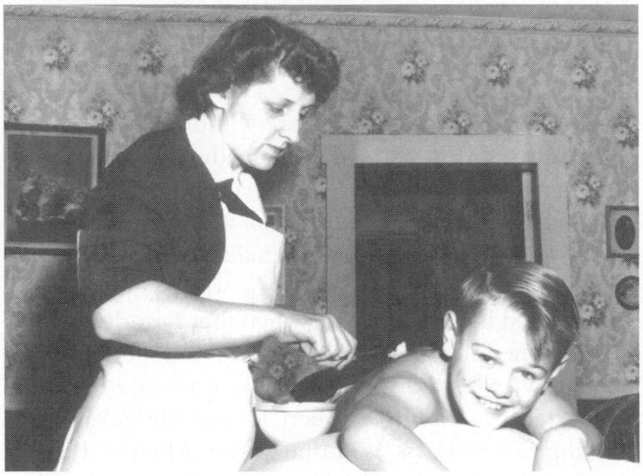

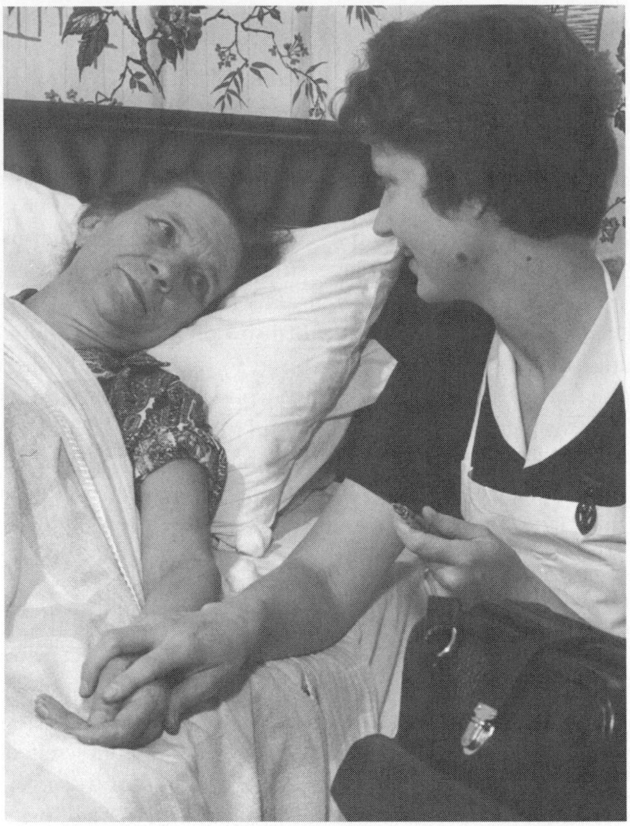

FIGURE 1.5 Three patients of Victorian Order of Nurses (VON) cared for in their own homes. The VON still provides community and home care services across Canada.

Canadian Red Cross Society began outpost programs in isolated parts of their territories (Elliott, 2004; McKay, 2007; Penney, 1996; Richardson, 1998; Rousseau & Daigle, 2000). The federal health department did not regularly supply nursing stations and nurses to First Nations and Inuit populations in the sub-Arctic and Arctic regions of the country until after World War II (McPherson, 2003; Meijer-Drees & McBain, 2001). Together, these nurses brought much-needed health care to areas underserved by physicians, and they often found they needed to undertake such tasks as providing midwifery, stitching wounds, or pulling teeth, for which they had received little training (see Figures 1.5, 1.6, 1.7, and 1.8).

Several small groups of civilian nurses volunteered with the Canadian militia during the Northwest Rebellion (1885), with the Northwest Mounted Police during the Klondike Gold Rush (1898), and with the British Expeditionary Force during the South African War (1899–1902), but they were not officially part of the Canadian military. With the formation of the first permanent nursing service as part of the Canadian Army Medical Corps (CAMC) in 1904, civilian nurses became fully integrated into the Canadian armed forces as soldiers, enlisting as lieutenants with the specially created officer's rank and title of *nursing sister*, serving under the supervision of higher-ranked matrons. During 1944, Matron-in-Chief Elizabeth Smellie became the first woman in the world to rise to the rank of a full colonel. Initially, nursing sisters were the only women to serve in the military and they readily filled every available position in the Canadian armed forces throughout both world wars—even creating long waiting lists to get into

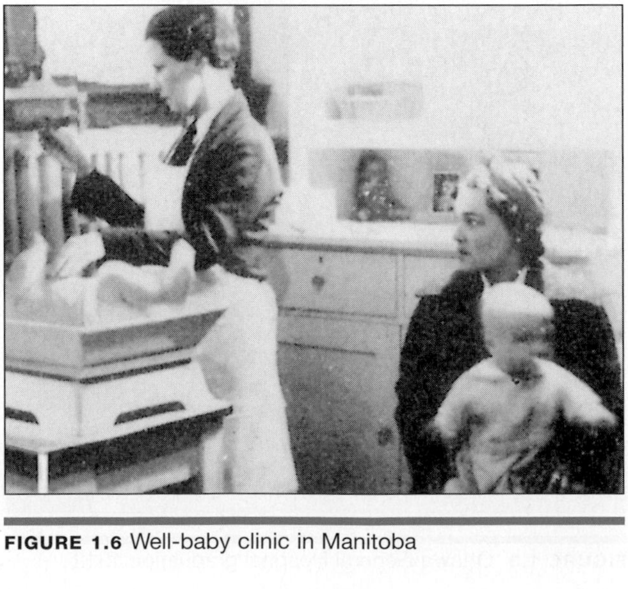

FIGURE 1.6 Well-baby clinic in Manitoba

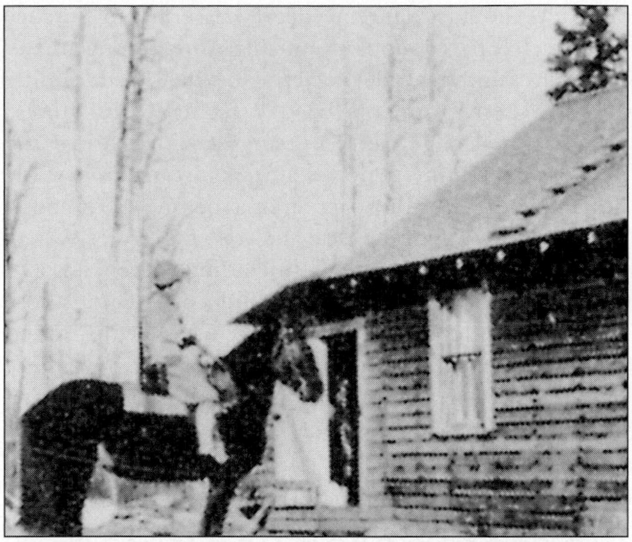

FIGURE 1.7 District nurse at Old Pendryl Cottage, Alberta

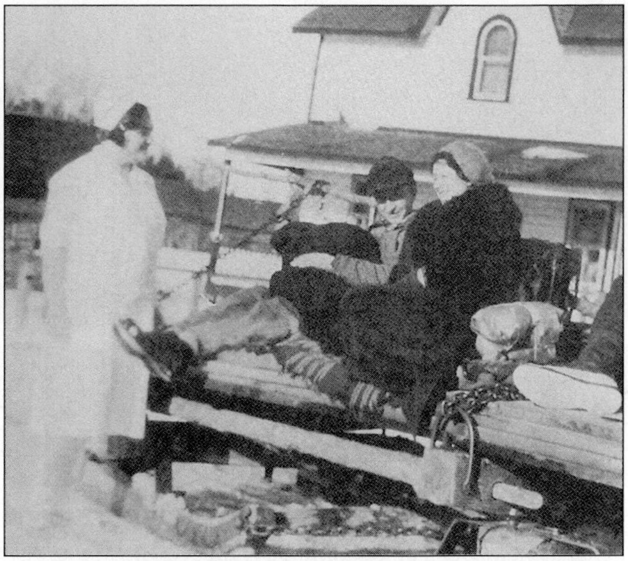

FIGURE 1.8 Red Cross Nurse Gertrude Leroy Miller discharging a patient from the nursing outpost at Wilberforce, Ontario, in the 1930s

the military. Canadian military nurses served with NATO forces in Europe during the 1950s and with the Allied Forces during the Korean War (1950–1953), as well as with peacekeeping forces during the 1990s and beyond.

At least 3141 nursing sisters served during World War I and 4079 during World War II. They called themselves soldiers and understood their work as winning the war through the salvage of damaged men. They actively sought opportunities to move closer to the front lines, readily accepting increased risk and danger as part of the job. Some died in both wars because of enemy action and military-related illnesses and accidents; two were prisoners of war under the Japanese army in Hong Kong for almost two years during World War II; others were torpedoed, bombed, and strafed—and survived to tell about the experiences. Some of them left personal accounts of these experiences; some questioned the contradictory values of caring and saving lives in the midst of organizations designed for the destruction of lives. The armed forces valued their knowledge and skills highly, reluctantly moving them forward as they demonstrated improved outcomes for the soldiers under their care than less-trained personnel could achieve. The military was adamant, however, that nurses were temporary—only for the duration of the war, regardless of what nurses preferred regarding military careers (Toman, 2007); see Figures 1.9, 1.10, and 1.11.

During the 1930s, the private duty market for nurses shrunk because of both an oversupply of graduate nurses and the widespread economic depression that left at least 30% of the Canadian population unemployed. But a boom in hospital construction and the growing use of medical technologies, among other factors, increased the need for nurses again, precipitating a nursing shortage that continued into the 1970s. The nursing leadership campaigned to move nurses' training into educational institutions and gradually weaned hospital administrators from depending on student labour, opening up further employment opportunities for graduate nurses within hospitals. Although hospitals soon became the preferred employer for nurses, the shortage was so great that hospitals had to make substantial changes in the workplace to attract new students for training and married nurses back into the workforce.

Changes in medical and surgical therapeutics were central forces in defining the nature and scope of nursing practices. By accepting delegated medical tasks, nurses have been instrumental in facilitating the spread and acceptance of many technologies that range from thermometers in the early twentieth century, through routine blood tests in the 1940s and 1950s, to the complex systems of medical monitoring in place today (Sandelowski, 2000; Toman, 2001). An increasingly specialized nursing workforce has resulted in a hierarchical relationship among nurses, and between nurses and lesser-skilled auxiliary workers, whose positions emerged initially to help address the shortage of trained nurses.

Each of these issues lies within a body of historical research that offers alternative perspectives through which we can question who and what is determining today's nursing practice. On the one hand, the wider socioeconomic and political milieu has shaped nurses and their work; on the other hand, nurses have participated in shaping the health-care system and the role of nursing within it. Curiosity about the roots of the nursing profession has merit in itself, but many would argue that the value of nursing history lies in its relevance to current issues in professional practice. Much more research is needed, for example, about the transfer of nursing education from hospital training to community colleges

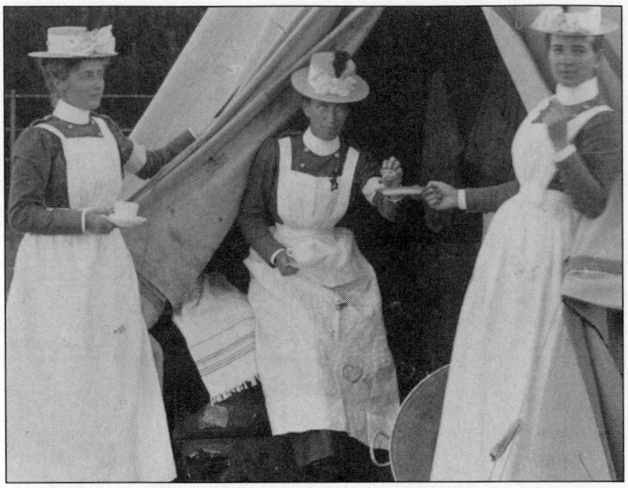

FIGURE 1.9 Canadian civilian nurses with the British Expeditionary Force in South Africa (1899–1902)

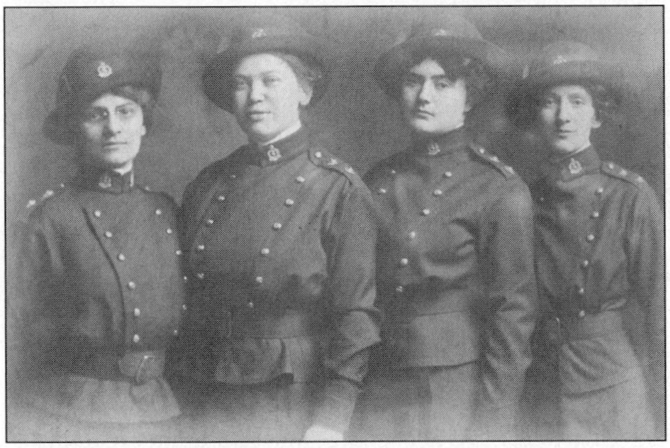

FIGURE 1.10 World War I Nursing Sister Mabel Lucas Rutherford (left) and three colleagues in their dress uniforms

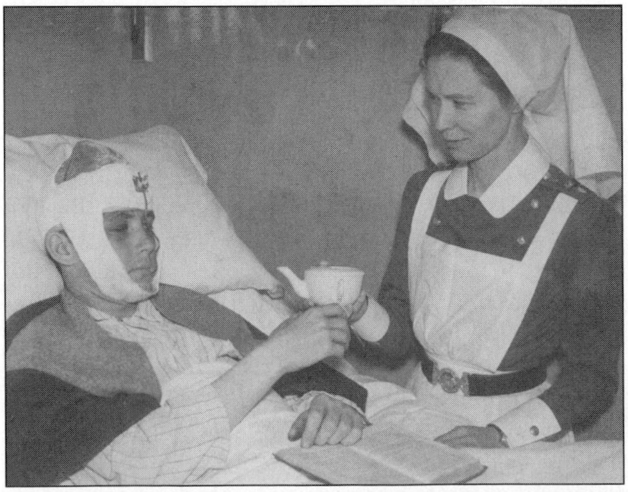

FIGURE 1.11 World War II Nursing Sister Dorothy Macham attending to wounded soldier

and how the baccalaureate degree as entry to practice has affected perceptions of nursing work among nurses themselves and the wider society. Hospital-based training and work environments tried to standardize nurses, nurses' knowledge, and nursing care, creating the illusion of a homogeneous nursing workforce while devaluing the vast diversity among people performing nursing work. A more critical analysis of the roles of gender, class, race, and ethnicity (including whiteness), and the way they have worked to include or exclude those wanting to enter the profession, is necessary to understand who became nurses in Canada and how these influences still shape who become nurses in today's multicultural health-care context.

Contemporary Nursing Practice

An in-depth study of contemporary nursing practice includes a look at selected definitions of nursing, a framework for the Canadian health system, the goals of the nurse within this system, the acts that legislate health care and nursing practice, and the scope and standards of practice. This chapter will concentrate on definitions and the goals and roles of nursing. For the Canadian health system, see Chapter 9, and for legal issues see Chapter 6.

Definitions of Nursing

To understand what nursing is, we must first define the word. Many definitions exist, some of which misrepresent the complex knowledge and skill of professional nursing. Common dictionary definitions, for example, still refer to the nurse as "a person, usually a woman, trained to care for the sick" (Cayne, 1988). Today, however, many men are choosing to become nurses, and nurses also provide preventive and health-promoting care to well clients. This section gives several definitions of nursing, and Chapter 4 provides other definitions created by nursing theorists.

Florence Nightingale described nursing in 1860 as the "use of fresh air, light, warmth, cleanliness, quiet and the proper selection and administration of diet" (Nightingale, 1938, p. 8). She considered a clean, well-ventilated, and quiet environment essential for recovery. Often considered the first nurse theorist, Nightingale raised the status of nursing through education. Nurses were no longer untrained housekeepers but people educated in the care of the sick.

Virginia Henderson was one of the first modern nurses to define nursing. In 1960, she wrote, "the unique function of the nurse is to assist the individual, sick or well, in the performance of those activities contributing to health or its recovery (or to peaceful death) that he would perform unaided if he had the necessary strength, will, or knowledge, and to do this in such a way as to help him gain independence as rapidly as possible" (Henderson, 1966, p. 3). Like Nightingale, Henderson described nursing in relation to the client and the client's environment. Unlike Nightingale, Henderson saw the nurse as concerned with both well and ill individuals, acknowledged that nurses interact with clients even when recovery may not be feasible, and mentioned the teaching and advocacy roles of the nurse.

Professional nursing associations have also examined nursing and developed their definitions of it. In 1987, the Canadian Nurses Association (CNA) described nursing practice as a dynamic, caring, helping relationship in which the nurse helps the client to achieve and maintain optimal health (CNA, 1987). Currently, the CNA refers to the International Council of Nurses (2001) definition:

> *Nursing encompasses autonomous and collaborative care of individuals of all ages, families, groups and communities, sick or well and in all settings. Nursing includes the promotion of health, prevention of illness, and the care of ill, disabled and dying people. Advocacy, promotion of a safe environment, research, participation in shaping health policy and in patient and health systems management, and education are also key nursing roles.*

In the latter half of the twentieth century, a number of nurse theorists developed their own theoretical definitions of nursing. Theoretical definitions are important because they go beyond simplistic common definitions. They describe what nursing is and the interrelationship among nurses, nursing, the client, and the intended client outcome—health. See Chapters 4 and 21. Several themes are common to all the various definitions of nursing: see Box 1.1.

Caring is described as the "essence of nursing" (Leininger, 1984). It is a complex concept that has multiple aspects: affective, cognitive, and ethical. Research to explore the meaning of caring in nursing has been increasing because nursing, more than any other profession, has "the distinction of being responsible for the caring that clients receive in the health-care system" (Miller, 1995, p. 29). Details about caring are discussed in Chapter 21. See also Watson's assumptions of caring in Chapter 4, Box 4.2 (page 63).

BOX 1.1 THEMES COMMON TO DEFINITIONS

Although several different definitions of nursing have been made over the years, they do share some common themes.

- Nursing is caring.
- Nursing is an art.
- Nursing is a science.
- Nursing is client centred.
- Nursing is holistic.
- Nursing is adaptive.
- Nursing is concerned with health promotion, health maintenance, and health restoration.
- Nursing is a helping profession.

Recipients of Nursing

Nurses work with many and varied recipients of care. The recipients can be individuals, families, groups, communities, and populations. Even when planning and implementing care to various recipients, it is important for the nurse to recognize that these recipients live within a larger society—for instance, individuals are connected to families, groups live in the community, and multiple communities exist within a given population. Groups are collections of individuals with a shared goal or purpose, and communities may be defined by geography, culture, or other characteristics.

In this book, we have generally identified the recipient of care as the individual (see Chapter 11). We have, however, also provided some beginning information on families and working with families in providing nursing care (see Chapter 12). When referring to individuals who are receiving nursing care, the literature refers to them as consumers, patients, residents, clients, and other terminology. A **consumer** is an individual, a group of people, or a community that uses a service or commodity. People who use health-care products or services are consumers of health care.

A **patient** is a person who is waiting for or undergoing medical treatment and care. The word *patient* comes from a Latin word meaning "to suffer" or "to bear." Traditionally, the person receiving health care has been called a patient. Usually, people become patients when they seek assistance because of illness or for surgery. Some nurses believe that the word *patient* implies passive acceptance of the decisions and care of health professionals. Additionally, with the emphasis on health promotion and prevention of illness, many recipients of nursing care are not ill. Moreover, nurses interact with family members and significant others to provide support, information, and comfort in addition to caring for the patient.

For these reasons, nurses also refer to recipients of health care as clients. A **client** is a person who engages the advice or services of another who is qualified to provide this service. The term *client* presents the receivers of health care as collaborators in the care, that is, as people who are also responsible for their own health. Thus, the health status of a client is the responsibility of the individual in collaboration with health professionals. In this book, we have generally used the term *patient* to describe the individual admitted to an acute-care facility or otherwise seeking care, the term *resident* for an individual cared for in a long-term-care facility, and the term *client* to describe another recipient of nursing care. Many times the topics discussed in this book are equally applicable to clients, patients, and residents. When this is the case, readers may see references to more than one recipient of care in the same paragraph.

Scope of Nursing

Nursing practice involves four areas: promoting health and wellness, preventing illness, restoring health, and caring for the dying. Within each of these areas, nurses seek to articulate and follow best practices in terms of their care. The Registered Nurses' Association of Ontario has led the way in developing a series of best practices documents (see the Weblinks section in this chapter). Reference to appropriate best practices documents can be found in chapters throughout the book.

PROMOTING HEALTH AND WELLNESS "Wellness is a process that engages people in activities and behaviours that enhance quality of life and maximize personal potential" (Anspaugh, Hamrick, & Rosata, 2003, p. 490). Nurses promote wellness in clients who are both healthy and ill. This promotion may involve individual and community activities to enhance healthy lifestyles, such as improving nutrition and physical fitness, preventing problematic drug and alcohol use, restricting smoking, and preventing accidents and injury in the home and workplace. See Chapters 8 and 13 for further discussion.

PREVENTING ILLNESS The goal of illness-prevention programs is to maintain optimal health by preventing disease. Examples of nursing activities that prevent illness include immunizations, prenatal and infant care, and prevention of sexually transmitted infections.

RESTORING HEALTH Restoring health focuses on the ill client, and it extends from early detection of disease through helping the client during the recovery period. Examples of nursing activities focused on restoring health include the following:

- Providing direct care to the ill person, such as administering medications, baths, and specific procedures and treatments
- Performing diagnostic and assessment procedures, such as measuring blood pressure and examining feces for occult blood
- Consulting with other health-care professionals about client problems
- Teaching clients about recovery activities, such as exercises that will accelerate recovery after a stroke
- Rehabilitating clients to their optimal functional level following physical or mental illness, injury, or chemical addiction

CARING FOR THE DYING This area of nursing practice involves comforting and caring for people of all ages who are dying. It includes helping clients live as comfortably as possible until death and helping the support people cope with death. Nurses carrying out these activities work in homes, hospitals, and extended-care facilities. Some agencies, called *hospices,* are specifically designed for this purpose.

Nursing Settings

Canada has three categories of regulated nurses: registered nurses (RNs), licensed (registered) practical nurses, and registered psychiatric nurses (see Box 1.2 for definitions of each category of regulated nurses). The Canadian Institute for Health Information reported that Canada had 351 048 regulated nurses in 2006. Of these, 325 299 were employed within nursing, of which RNs represented 77.8%, practical nurses were 20.7%, and psychiatric nurses 1.6% (Canadian Institute for Health Information [CIHI], 2007). In the past, the acute-care hospital was the primary practice setting open to most nurses. In 2006, approximately 59% of regulated nurses worked in hospitals, but the rest worked in clients' homes, community agencies, ambulatory clinics, and nursing practice centres (CIHI, 2007). Figure 1.12 shows nurses in a variety of settings.

Nurses have different degrees of nursing autonomy and nursing responsibility in the various settings. They may provide direct care, teach clients and support people, serve as nursing advocates and agents of change, and help determine health policies affecting consumers in the community and in hospitals.

BOX 1.2 DEFINITIONS AND ROLES OF CATEGORIES OF NURSES

Registered nurses (RN) are regulated health care professionals. They work in different domains of nursing practice including direct care (clinical), education, administration and research.

Registered psychiatric nurses (RPN) are members of a distinct profession that provides services to individuals whose primary care needs relate to mental and developmental health. RPNs are regulated as a distinct profession in only four provinces in Canada: British Columbia, Alberta, Saskatchewan and Manitoba.

Licensed practical nurses (LPN) are regulated health professionals who work in partnership with other members of the health care team to provide nursing services to individuals, families and groups of all ages. In Ontario, this category of nursing is called registered practical nurse (RPN).

Source: From *Health Personnel Trends in Canada 1995 to 2004* (pp. 79, 201, 213), by the Canadian Institute for Health Information, 2006, Ottawa: Author. Reprinted with permission.

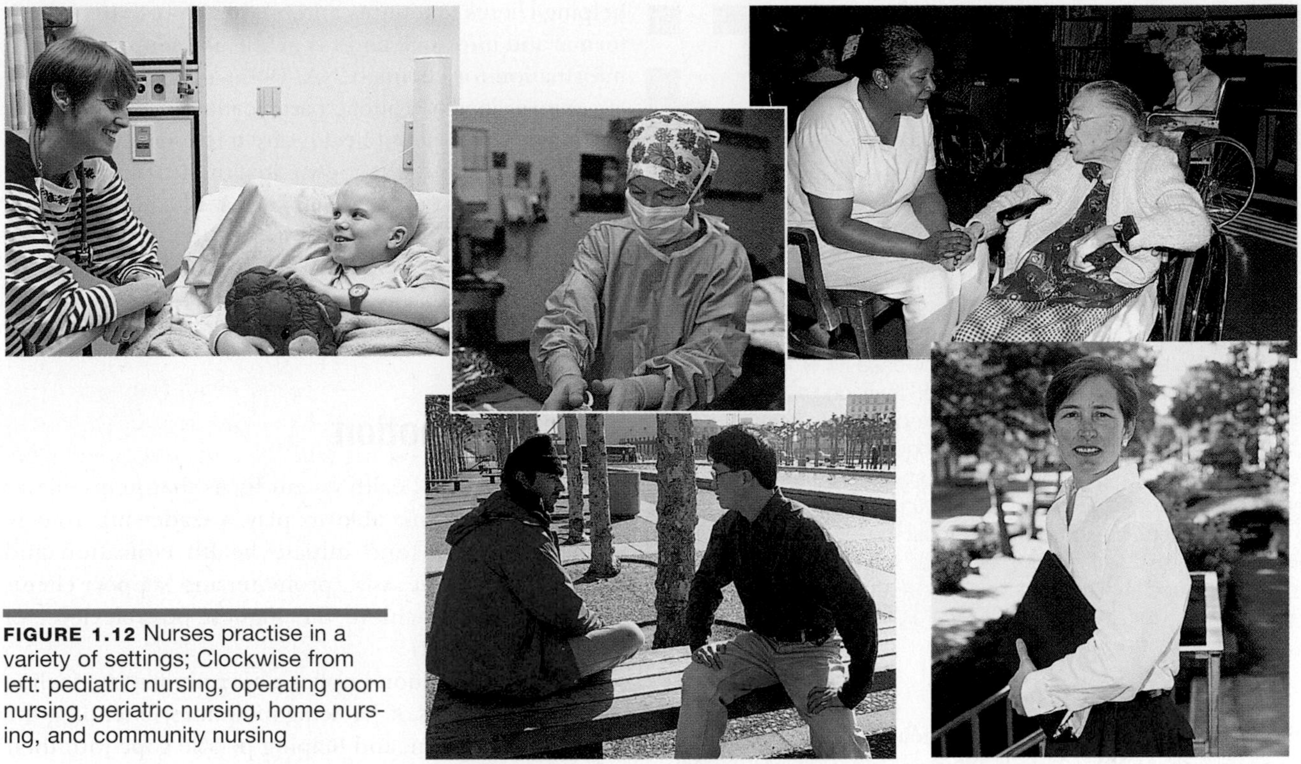

FIGURE 1.12 Nurses practise in a variety of settings; Clockwise from left: pediatric nursing, operating room nursing, geriatric nursing, home nursing, and community nursing

The CNA maintains that an individual's health affects the quality of that person's life. Health is influenced not only by the health-care system but also by human biology, lifestyle choices, and the environment. With this in mind, the CNA advocates a framework to provide direction for the Canadian health-care system that includes (1) the *conditions* of the Canada Health Act; and (2) the *principles* of primary health care.

The Canada Health Act (1984) lists the conditions or national standards that provincial and territorial health insurance plans must respect in order to receive federal cash contributions: public administration, accessibility, comprehensiveness, universality, and portability. The CNA believes that these conditions are essential to Canada's health-care system.

1. *Public administration* means that federal, provincial, and territorial health insurance programs should be nonprofit programs operated by public authorities who are appointed by government (Canada, House of Commons, 1984). (See Chapter 9 for more information on Canada's health-care system.)
2. *Accessibility* means that Canadians have reasonable access to essential health services, with no financial barriers, such as user fees, to impede this access.
3. *Comprehensiveness* means that federal and provincial or territorial health insurance together should cover the full continuum of health services for all Canadians, including health promotion, the prevention of disease and disability, the treatment of disease and disability, restoration, rehabilitation, and support.
4. *Universal coverage* means that all Canadians are entitled to essential health services, regardless of gender, culture, income, language, education, marital status, or age.
5. *Portability* means that Canadians should be covered equally for health services wherever they are in Canada.

Primary Health Care

Primary health care is essential (promotive, preventive, curative, rehabilitative, and supportive) care that focuses on preventing illness and promoting health. It is both a philosophy of health care and an approach to providing health services. Primary health care has been adopted by the World Health Organization and by Canada as the key to a healthy society. Clients of primary health care can be individuals, families, groups, communities, and populations (CNA, 2005; World Health Organization [WHO], 1982).

The principles of primary health care are accessibility, public participation, health promotion, appropriate technology, and intersectoral cooperation. They are outlined in the Reflect on Primary Health Care box.

Taken together, the conditions of the Canada Health Act and the principles of primary health care serve as a solid framework for health-care delivery and the future development of Canada's health-care system. The conditions outlined in the Canada Health Act and the

REFLECT ON PRIMARY HEALTH CARE

Principles of Primary Health Care

Accessibility means that essential health care is universally available to all clients in an acceptable and affordable way, "with no unreasonable geographic or financial barrier" (p. 1). *Public participation* means clients should be encouraged to participate in making decisions about their own health. *Health promotion* means that the health-care system should increase its emphasis on helping clients stay well rather than on treating clients when they are ill. *Appropriate technology* means that technology and modes of care should be appropriately adapted to the community's social, economic, and cultural development. *Intersectoral cooperation* recognizes that health activities must be undertaken concurrently with measures aimed at improving economic and social development (CNA, 2005).

principles required for primary health care are congruent with the CNA's beliefs about nursing practice. All nurses, therefore, play a vital role in the implementation of the conditions of the Canada Health Act and the principles of primary health care (CNA, 1995; WHO, 1982).

PRIMARY CARE AND PRIMARY NURSING Primary health care should not be confused with *primary care* or *primary nursing*. Primary care is provider driven and is the entry point to the health-care system. Primary nursing is a system of delivering nursing services whereby a nurse is responsible for planning the 24-hour care of a specific patient. Both these concepts are illness-oriented concepts. For more information on primary health care and primary care, see Chapter 13.

The Role of the Nurse

The goal of nursing is to improve the health of clients through partnerships with clients, other health-care providers, related community agencies, and government. Nursing practice involves a variety of roles, including direct-care provider, educator, administrator, consultant, policy adviser, and researcher. The principles of primary health care apply to nurses in all these roles (CNA, 1995). Nurses are encouraged to examine their own practice and places of work in light of the pillars of the Canada Health Act and the principles of primary health care (CNA, 2003).

To ensure that Canadians have *reasonable access* to essential health services, nurses provide more options for accessing health services by (1) acting as an entry point for clients into the health-care system; (2) providing nursing care and treatment for health problems; (3) helping clients to identify and use health resources, both formal and informal; and (4) acting as a source of health information for clients (CNA, 1995).

Nurses increase public participation in planning and making decisions about health care by (1) involving clients in decisions about their own health; (2) encouraging clients to take action for their own health; (3) involving clients in identifying their own health-care needs; (4) involving clients in planning, using, and evaluating their own health-care services; and (5) encouraging and using community-development approaches (CNA, 1995).

Health Promotion

In keeping with a health-system focus that helps clients stay well, nurses are able to play a leadership role in health promotion and initiate health education and other activities that assist, promote, and support clients as they strive to achieve the highest possible level of health (CNA, 1992).

Health promotion implies a commitment to dealing with the challenges of reducing inequities, extending the scope of prevention, and helping people cope with their circumstances. It means fostering public participation, strengthening community health services, and coordinating public health policy. Moreover, it means creating environments conducive to health in which people are better able to take care of themselves and to offer one another support in solving and managing collective health problems (CNA, 1995).

Health status is influenced by social norms, cultural values, economic and environmental conditions and policies, and life practices, such as food and exercise choices, the following of safety precautions, and the problematic use of tobacco, alcohol, and other drugs. The CNA believes that consideration of these influences is essential in the development of effective health-promotion initiatives. Health-promotion initiatives must be widely targeted, begin with the very young, and extend throughout the lifespan. The CNA supports the concept that health-promotion strategies should be initiated collaboratively by a variety of appropriate bodies, including health, social, and educational agencies, to meet the identified needs of individuals, families, and communities. It is the belief of the CNA that emphasis on health promotion strengthens and complements the health-care system (CNA, 1992).

Nurses must provide leadership for health promotion. This guiding should be done through positive role modelling and personal demonstration of healthy life practices, as well as by assisting, promoting, and supporting clients, individuals, groups, and communities in self-help activities to understand and achieve their highest possible level of health. Educational curricula for nurses should emphasize the importance of this leadership role and provide the opportunity for related skill development (CNA, 1995).

As part of the goal to ensure that *technology* and *modes of care* are based on health needs and are appropriate to the community's social, economic, and cultural development, nurses (1) strive to provide cost-effective care that is based on client needs, research evidence, and measurable health outcomes; and (2) participate with other health-care professionals in developing, implementing, and evaluating technology and modes of care to ensure their appropriateness and cost-effectiveness (CNA, 1995).

In cooperation with clients, with each other, with professionals from other sectors, and with governments, nurses coordinate client care and strive to integrate health services. Nurses participate with clients in designing public health policies and will continue to do so to achieve health for all. Nurses will continue to work with clients and other health providers to implement the principles of primary health care. The CNA will support them in this endeavour and will monitor the progress of primary health care in Canada (CNA, 1995).

Nurse Practice Acts

Nurse practice acts, or legal acts for professional nursing practice, regulate the practice of nursing in the United States and Canada. Each province and territory in Canada has its own act for each of the regulated nursing groups. Although nurse practice acts differ in various jurisdictions, they all have a common purpose—to protect the public. See Chapter 6 for additional information on scopes of practice and nurse practice acts.

One of the ways that the public is protected is through regulation. The primary purpose of regulation is to protect the public from professionals who are "unqualified, incompetent, or unethical" (Registered Nurses Association of British Columbia [RNABC], 1999). Professions can be regulated in one of two ways: by the government or by the profession itself. In Canada, in all provinces and territories except Ontario, professional organizations function as the self-regulators for registered nurses. In Ontario, the regulatory body and the professional association are separate nursing organizations. Self-regulation means provincial and territorial governments delegate to professional bodies, through legislative acts, the power to determine who may enter and remain in the profession and under what circumstances. Self-regulation is a privilege granted by governments to professional organizations, but "to maintain this privilege, a profession must maintain the trust of the public" (RNABC, p. 6).

One way in which nurses in Canada are regulated is through title control. "The use of such titles as 'registered nurse,' 'RN,' and 'nurse' is protected by legislation. Only individuals who are currently registered with a nursing regulatory body may use these titles" (CNA, 2001, p. 6). Similarly, practical nurses and psychiatric nurses in Canada have title protection. Nurse practitioners are also regulated by the provincial and territorial regulatory bodies.

Nursing regulatory bodies, including the International Council of Nurses (ICN), the CNA, and the provincial and territorial professional organizations, work together to develop frameworks for regulatory matters, such as standards of practice, scope of practice, and continuing competence. *Standards of practice* "reflect the values of the nursing profession, clarify what the profession expects of its members, define the expectations of the public/employers, and provide a benchmark below which performance is unacceptable" (CNA, 2001, p. 6). The *scope of practice* refers to the activities that RNs are educated and authorized to perform as set out in legislation and complemented by standards, guidelines, and policy positions of provincial and territorial nursing regulatory bodies (CNA, 2007, p. 13). *Continuing competence,* as defined by the CNA and the Canadian Association of Schools of Nursing, is "the ongoing ability of a nurse to integrate and apply the knowledge, skills, judgement and personal attributes required to practice safely and ethically in a designated role and setting" (CNA, 2004, p. 1).

Differences in the regulation of professionals in Canada can often be traced to the differences in provincial and territorial legislation. Other health-care workers, such as licensed practical nurses (LPNs), which are called registered practical nurses (RPNs) in Ontario, and registered psychiatric nurses (RPNs in the four Western provinces), are regulated under separate legislation. Nonregulated workers also work in the health-care system. See Chapter 6 for more information on legislation.

Nursing Practice Standards

Nursing practice standards are mandatory for a self-regulating profession. The overall purpose of practice standards is to provide a guideline for determining the quality of nursing care a patient/client receives.

The **nursing practice standards** "represent acceptable requirements for determining the quality of nursing care a patient/client receives" (College and Association of Registered Nurses of Alberta [CARNA], 2003, p. 1). Each jurisdiction compiles its own nursing standards in conjunction with the legislation governing nursing practice in that jurisdiction (see Chapter 6). The CARNA *Nursing Practice Standards* note that the standards

- "apply at all times to all nurses regardless of role
- provide guidelines to assist nurses in decision-making
- support nurses by outlining practice expectations of the profession
- inform the public and others about what they can expect from practising nurses
- are used as a legal reference for reasonable and prudent practice" (CARNA, 2003, p. 2)

Roles and Functions of the Nurse

Nurses assume a number of roles when they provide care for clients. Often, nurses carry out these roles concurrently. For example, the nurse may act as a counsellor while providing physical care and teaching aspects of that care. The roles required at a specific time depend on the needs of the client and aspects of the particular environment. Some of the roles of nurses are described below.

Caregiver

The caregiver role has traditionally included those activities that assist the client physically and psychologically while preserving the client's dignity. The required nursing actions may involve full care for the completely dependent client, partial care for the partially dependent client, and supportive-educative care to assist clients in attaining their highest possible level of health and wellness. Caregiving encompasses the physical, psychosocial, developmental, and spiritual levels. A nurse may provide care directly or delegate it to other caregivers.

Communicator

Communication is integral to all nursing roles. Nurses communicate with the client, support people, other health professionals, and people in the community.

Nurses identify client problems and then communicate these verbally or in writing to other members of the health team. The quality of a nurse's communication is an important factor in nursing care. The nurse must be able to communicate clearly and accurately in order for a client's health-care needs to be met. See Chapter 21.

Educator

As a teacher, the nurse helps clients learn about health and the health-care procedures they need to perform to restore or maintain health. In collaboration with the client, the nurse determines the client's learning needs and readiness to learn, sets specific learning goals and teaching strategies, enacts teaching strategies, and measures learning. Nurses also teach other health-care providers to whom they delegate care, and they share their expertise with other nurses and health-care professionals. See Chapter 25 for additional details about the teaching and learning process.

Client Advocate

A client advocate acts to protect the client. In this role, the nurse may represent the client's needs and wishes to other health-care professionals, such as relaying the client's request for information to the physician. They also assist clients in exercising their rights and help them speak up for themselves. See Chapter 5.

Counsellor

Counselling is the process of helping a client recognize and cope with stressful psychological or social problems, develop improved interpersonal relationships, and promote personal growth. It involves providing emotional, intellectual, and psychological support. In contrast to the psychotherapist, who counsels individuals with identified problems, the nurse counsels primarily healthy individuals with normal adjustment difficulties. The nurse focuses on helping the person develop new attitudes, feelings, and behaviours, rather than on promoting intellectual growth. The nurse encourages the client to look at alternative behaviours, recognize the choices, and develop a sense of control.

Change Agent

The nurse acts as a change agent when assisting clients to make modifications in their own behaviour. Nurses also often act to make changes in a system, such as clinical care, if it is not helping a client return to health. Nurses are continually dealing with change in the health-care system. Technological change, change in the age of the client population, and changes in medications are just a few of the changes nurses deal with daily. See Chapter 26 for additional information about change.

Leader

The leadership role can be employed at different levels: individual client, family, groups of clients, colleagues, or the community. Effective leadership is a learned process requiring an understanding of the needs and goals that motivate people, the knowledge to apply the leadership skills, and the interpersonal skills to influence others. The leadership role of the nurse is discussed in Chapter 26.

Manager

The nurse manages the nursing care of individuals, families, and communities. The nurse-manager also delegates nursing activities to ancillary workers and other nurses, and supervises and evaluates their performance. Managing requires knowledge about organizational structure and dynamics, authority and accountability, leadership, change theory, advocacy, delegation, supervision, and evaluation. See Chapter 26 for additional details.

BOX 1.3 Selected Expanded Career Roles for Nurses

NURSE PRACTITIONER

A nurse practitioner is a registered nurse who has an advanced education and is a graduate of a nurse practitioner program. Nurses can be primary health-care nurse practitioners who work with clients of all ages or can specialize in a single area in acute or community care.

Core Competencies

- Have a direct patient-care focus, conduct advanced assessments, make appropriate diagnoses, and use intervention skills
- Be able to work in a collaborative health-care delivery environment
- Make appropriate consultations and referrals; health promotion
- Have the ability to deal with multiple system levels simultaneously
- Conduct critical analysis of research literature and other forms of evidence
- Work to enhance the visibility and understanding of the nurse practitioner role

CLINICAL NURSE SPECIALIST

The clinical nurse specialist is a registered nurse or registered psychiatric nurse who has an advanced degree or expertise in a specialized area of practice (e.g., gerontology, oncology, mental health, primary health care) and provides direct client care, educates others, consults, conducts research, and manages care.

NURSE MIDWIFE

The nurse midwife is a registered nurse who has completed a program in midwifery and is certified. The nurse gives prenatal and postnatal care and manages deliveries in normal pregnancies. The midwife practises in association with a health-care agency and can obtain medical services if complications occur.

NURSE ADMINISTRATOR

The nurse administrator manages client care, including the delivery of nursing services. The administrator may have a middle-management position, such as nurse manager or supervisor, or a more senior management position, such as director of nursing services. The functions of nurse administrators include budgeting, staffing, and planning programs. The educational preparation for nurse administrator positions is at least a baccalaureate degree in nursing and frequently a master's or doctoral degree.

NURSE RESEARCHER

Nurse researchers investigate nursing problems to improve nursing care and to refine and expand nursing knowledge. They are employed in academic institutions, teaching hospitals, and research centres. Nurse researchers usually have advanced education at the doctoral level.

NURSE EDUCATOR

Nurse educators are employed in nursing programs, at educational institutions, and in hospital or institutional (e.g., long-term care) staff education. Many have advanced degrees in nursing or education.

Researcher/Research Consumer

Nurses use research to improve client care. In a clinical area, nurses need to (1) have awareness of the process and language of research, (2) be sensitive to issues related to protecting the rights of human subjects, (3) participate in the identification of significant researchable problems, and (4) be discriminating consumers of research findings. (See Chapter 3 for more information on nursing research.)

Expanded Career Roles

Nurses are fulfilling expanded career roles, such as those of nurse practitioner, clinical nurse specialist, nurse midwife, nurse administrator, nurse educator, and nurse researcher, that allow greater independence and autonomy. See Box 1.3.

Nursing Profession

Nursing is gaining recognition as a profession. A **profession** has been defined as an occupation that requires extensive education or a calling that requires special knowledge, skill, and preparation. A profession is generally distinguished from other kinds of occupations by (1) its requirement of prolonged, specialized training to acquire a body of knowledge pertinent to the role to be performed, and (2) an orientation of the individual toward service, either to a community or to an organization. The standards of education and practice for the profession are determined by the members of the profession, rather than by outsiders. The education of the professional involves a complete socialization process, more far-reaching in its social and attitudinal aspects and its technical features than is usually required in other kinds of occupations.

Self-regulation is based on the belief that the profession of nursing has the special knowledge required to set standards of practice and to assess the conduct of its members through peer review. As members of the nursing profession, nurses are bound by the ethical values of the profession to base their practice on relevant and current knowledge. Although not all professional organizations use the same criteria for identifying a profession, most include that a profession has a formal base of knowledge, requires significant educational preparation to be admitted to the profession, maintains control over the standards by which new applicants are evaluated, uses the knowledge for the direct benefit of the public, is self-regulating, and maintains a code of ethics (Ross-Kerr, 2003). See Chapter 5 for more information on codes of ethics for nursing.

Criteria of a Profession

SPECIALIZED BODY OF KNOWLEDGE As a profession, nursing is establishing a well-defined body of knowledge and expertise. A number of nursing conceptual frameworks (discussed in Chapter 4) contribute to the knowledge base of nursing and give direction to nursing practice, education, and ongoing research.

Increasing research in nursing is contributing to nursing practice and nursing knowledge. In the 1980s, increased federal funding and professional support helped establish centres for nursing research. Most early research was directed to the study of nursing education. In the 1960s, studies were often related to the nature of the knowledge base underlying nursing practice. Since the 1970s, nursing research has focused on practice-related issues. Nursing research as a dimension of the nurse's role is discussed further in Chapter 3.

SPECIALIZED EDUCATION Specialized education is an important aspect of professional status. In modern times, the trend in education for professions has shifted toward programs in colleges and universities. Many nursing educators believe that the undergraduate nursing curriculum should include liberal arts education, in addition to the biological and social sciences and the nursing discipline.

The CNA recommends the baccalaureate degree as the level of education required for entry to practice as a registered nurse. (See Chapter 2 for more information on nursing education at all levels.)

SERVICE ORIENTATION A service orientation differentiates nursing from an occupation pursued primarily for profit. Many consider altruism (selfless concern for others) the hallmark of a profession. Nursing has a tradition of service to others. This service, however, must be guided by certain rules, policies, or codes of ethics. Nursing is an important component of the health-care delivery system.

PROFESSIONAL ORGANIZATION Operation under the umbrella of a professional organization differentiates a profession from an occupation. For registered nurses, the CNA, in addition to the provincial and territorial nursing organizations, performs the self-regulatory functions.

AUTONOMY AND SELF-REGULATION A profession is autonomous if it regulates itself and sets standards for its members. Providing autonomy is one of the purposes of a professional association. If nursing is to have professional status, it must function autonomously in the formation of policy and in the control of its activities. To be autonomous, a professional group must be granted legal authority to define the scope of its practice, describe its particular functions and roles, and determine its goals and responsibilities in delivery of its services. (See Chapter 6 for additional information on scopes of practice and legislated authority.)

CODE OF ETHICS Nurses have traditionally placed a high value on the worth and dignity of others. The nursing profession requires integrity of its members; that is, a member is expected to do what is considered right.

Ethical codes change as the needs and values of society change. Nursing has developed its own codes of ethics. It is within the nursing educational program that the nurse develops, clarifies, and internalizes professional values. Specific professional nursing values are stated in nursing codes of ethics (see Chapter 5), in standards of nursing practice (discussed earlier in this chapter), and in the legal system itself (see Chapter 6).

> **Evidence-Informed Practice**
>
> ### Do Fourth-Year Baccalaureate Students Have a More Realistic Picture of Nursing Practice Than First-Year Students?
>
> In light of the nursing shortage, it was recognized that not only does Canada need to attract students into nursing programs but it also needs retain them in the profession after they graduate. Grainger and Bolan (2006) wondered if attitudes and understanding of nursing would change as students moved through a baccalaureate program in nursing. Questionnaires were completed by 213 first-year students and 150 fourth-year students. Not surprisingly, the researchers found that fourth-year students had a more realistic picture of the roles of nurses, but some were also more disillusioned about the profession.
>
> **NURSING IMPLICATIONS:** **This research suggests that nurse educators need to examine the curricula to ensure that students gain a realistic picture of nursing but remain enthusiastic about their chosen profession.**
>
> Source: Based on "Perceptions of Nursing as a Career Choice of Students in the Baccalaureate Program," by P. Grainger and C. Bolan, 2006, *Nurse Education Today, 26*, pp. 38–44.

Socialization to Nursing

Socialization can be defined simply as the process by which people (1) learn to become members of groups and society, and (2) learn the social rules defining relationships into which they will enter. Socialization involves learning to behave, feel, and see the world in a manner similar to other persons occupying the same role (Hardy & Conway, 1988). The goal of professional socialization is to instill in individ-

BOX 1.4 BENNER'S STAGES OF NURSING EXPERTISE

STAGE I, NOVICE
No experience (e.g., nursing student). Performance is limited, inflexible, and governed by context-free rules and regulations, rather than experience.

STAGE II, ADVANCED BEGINNER
Demonstrates marginally acceptable performance. Recognizes the meaningful "aspects" of a real situation. Has experienced enough real situations to make judgements about them.

STAGE III, COMPETENT PRACTITIONER
Has two or three years of experience. Demonstrates organizational and planning abilities. Differentiates important factors from less important aspects of care. Coordinates multiple complex care demands.

STAGE IV, PROFICIENT PRACTITIONER
Has three to five years of experience. Perceives a situation as a whole, rather than in terms of parts, as in Stage II. Uses maxims as guides for what to consider in a situation. Has holistic understanding of the client, which improves decision making. Focuses on long-term goals.

STAGE V, EXPERT PRACTITIONER
Performance is fluid, flexible, and highly proficient; no longer requires rules, guidelines, or maxims to connect an understanding of the situation to appropriate action. Demonstrates highly skilled intuitive and analytical abilities in new situations. Is inclined to take a certain action because "it feels right."

Source: From *Novice to Expert: Excellence and Power in Clinical Nursing Practice,* by P. Benner, 1984, Menlo Park, CA: Addison-Wesley Nursing, pp. 21–34. Reprinted with permission.

uals the norms, values, attitudes, and behaviours deemed essential for the survival of the profession.

Various models of the socialization process have been developed. Benner's model (1984) describes five levels of proficiency in nursing based on the Dreyfus general model of skill acquisition (Dreyfus & Dreyfus, 1980). The five stages, which have implications for teaching and learning, are novice, advanced beginner, competent practitioner, proficient practitioner, and expert practitioner. Benner writes that experience is essential for the development of professional expertise. See Box 1.4.

One of the most powerful mechanisms of professional socialization is interaction with fellow students (Hardy & Conway, 1988). Within this student culture, students collectively set the level and direction of their scholastic efforts. They develop perspectives about the situation in which they are involved, the goals they are trying to achieve, and the kinds of activities that are expedient and proper, and they establish a set of practices congruent with all of these. Students become bound together by feelings of mutual cooperation, support, and solidarity.

Factors Influencing Contemporary Nursing Practice

To understand nursing as it is practised today and as it will be practised tomorrow requires an understanding of some of the social forces influencing this profession. These forces usually affect the entire health-care system, and as a major component of that system, nursing cannot avoid the effects.

Economics

Greater financial support provided through public and private health insurance programs has increased the demand for nursing care. Health-care services, such as emergency room care, mental health counselling, and preventive physical examinations, are increasingly being used by people who could not afford them in the past.

These changes present challenges to nurses. Currently, the health-care industry is shifting its emphasis from inpatient care to outpatient care with preadmission testing, increased outpatient same-day surgery, post-hospitalization rehabilitation, home health care, health maintenance, physical fitness programs, and community health education programs. As a result, more nurses are being employed in community-based health settings, such as home health agencies, hospices, and community clinics. These changes in employment for nurses have implications for nursing education, nursing research, and nursing practice.

Consumer Demands

Consumers of nursing services (the public) have become an increasingly effective force in changing nursing practice. On the whole, people are better educated and have more knowledge about health and illness than in the past. Consumers also have become more aware of others' needs for care. The ethical and moral issues raised by poverty and neglect have made people more vocal about the needs of minority groups and the poor.

The public's concepts of health and nursing have also changed. Most now believe that health is a right of all people, not just a privilege of the rich. The media emphasize the message that individuals must assume responsibility for their own health by obtaining a physical examination regularly, checking for signs of cancer and cardiovascular disease, and maintaining their mental well-being by balancing work and recreation. Interest in health and nursing services is therefore greater than ever. Furthermore, many people now want more than freedom from disease—they want energy, vitality, and a feeling of wellness.

Increasingly, the consumer has become an active participant in making decisions about health and nursing care. Planning committees concerned with providing nursing services to a community usually have an active consumer membership. Recognizing the legitimacy of public input, many federal, provincial, and territorial nursing associations and regulatory agencies have consumer representatives on their governing boards.

Family Structure

Family structures influence the need for and provision of nursing services. More people are living away from the extended family and the nuclear family, and the family breadwinner is no longer necessarily the husband. Many single men and women rear children, and in many two-parent families, both parents work. It is also common for young parents to live at great distances from their own parents. These young families need support services, such as daycare centres. For additional information about the family, see Chapter 12.

Science and Technology

Advances in science and technology affect nursing practice. For example, people with *acquired immune deficiency syndrome (AIDS)* are receiving new drug therapies to prolong life and delay the onset of AIDS-associated diseases. Nurses must be knowledgeable about the action of such drugs and the needs of clients receiving them. Nurses acquire knowledge and skills as they adapt to meet the new needs of clients.

In some settings, technological advances have required that nurses become highly specialized. Nurses frequently have to use sophisticated computerized equipment to provide care for clients. In addition, information technology advances have given the nurse and the client access to much more information. Nurses and clients must view this information with a critical eye. As technologies change, nursing education changes, and nurses require more advanced education to provide effective, safe nursing practice.

The need for long-distance monitoring of astronauts and spacecraft, lighter materials, and miniaturization of equipment in the space program has created advanced technologies. Health care has benefited as these new technologies have been adapted to such health-care aids as Viewstar (an aid for those with visual impairments), the insulin infusion pump, the voice-controlled wheelchair, magnetic resonance imaging (MRI), laser surgery, filters for intravenous fluid control devices, and monitoring systems for intensive care.

Demography

Demography is the study of population, including statistics about distribution by age and place of residence, mortality (death), and morbidity (incidence of disease). From demographic data, the needs of the population for nursing services can be assessed:

- The total population in Canada is increasing. The proportion of older adults has also increased, creating a growing need for nursing services for this group. This change in demographics has also highlighted differences in generations. For instance, as the baby boomer generation ages, a variety of social processes, including health care, have been influenced.
- The population is shifting from rural to urban settings. This shift signals increased needs for nursing related to problems caused by pollution and other effects on the environment by concentrations of people. Yet the rural population still needs access to care.
- Mortality and morbidity studies reveal the presence of risk factors. Many of these risk factors (e.g., smoking) are major causes of death and disease that can be prevented through changes in lifestyle. The nurse's role in assessing risk factors and helping clients make healthy lifestyle changes is discussed in Chapter 8.

The Women's Movement

The women's movement brought public attention to both women's and human rights. People are seeking equality in all areas, particularly educational, political, economic, and social equality. Because the majority of nurses are women, this movement has altered nursing's perspectives on economic and educational needs. As a result, nurses are increasingly asserting themselves as professional people who have a right to equality with men in health professions and are demanding more autonomy in client care.

Nursing Organizations

As nursing has developed, an increasing number of nursing organizations have been formed at the local, provincial and territorial, national, and international levels. The organizations that involve most Canadian registered nurses are the CNA and the ICN. Increasingly, nursing specialty organizations are being formed, for example, the Canadian Association of Nurses in Oncology. In addition, many nurses are part of unions. Participation in the activities of nursing associations enhances the growth of involved individuals and helps nurses collectively influence policies that affect nursing practice. Psychiatric and practical nurses are also part of nursing organizations, as described shortly.

Canadian Nurses Association

The CNA is a federation of 11 provincial and territorial nursing associations representing more than 133 500 registered nurses. The CNA's mission states that it is "the national professional voice of registered nurses, supporting them in their practice and advocating for healthy public policy and a quality, publicly funded not-for-profit health system" (CNA, 2008). Toward this end, it promotes high standards of practice, education, research, and administration. In most provinces and territories, the regulatory body and the professional association are within the same organization. In Ontario, the College of Nurses of Ontario (regulatory body) and the Registered Nurses' Association of Ontario (RNAO) are separate organizations (see Table 1.1).

The CNA is the national nursing association of Canada. Nurses do not join the CNA independently but obtain membership by paying a fee to the provincial or territorial organizations. In November 1985, the Ordre des infirmières et infirmiers du Québec (the Quebec Nurses Association, or OIIQ) withdrew from the CNA. This parallels the history that is noted in the Nursing and Canadian Society box. The CNA has developed national standards and a code of ethics, and it offers support to all provincial and territorial organizations. Through the national testing services, the CNA prepares licensure examinations. These examinations are available to all provinces and territories and provide a national standard for licensure of registered nurses. Certification in specific clinical specialties can also be obtained through the CNA (see Chapter 2). Through the Canadian Nurses Foundation, research grants, fellowships, and scholarships are offered to Canadian nurses. The official journal of the CNA, *Canadian Nurse,* is published monthly and sent to each nurse member.

International Council of Nurses

The ICN was established in 1899. Nurses from Great Britain, the United States, and Canada were among the founding members. The council is a federation of national registered nurses' associations, such as the CNA and the American Nurses Association.

Through the ICN, member national associations can work together for the mission of representing nursing worldwide, advancing the profession, and influencing health policy. The five core values of the ICN are visionary leadership, inclusiveness, flexibility, partnership, and achievement (ICN, n.d.). The official journal of the ICN is *International Nursing Review.*

Sigma Theta Tau International Honor Society of Nursing

The Sigma Theta Tau International Honor Society of Nursing (STTI) was founded in 1922 and is headquartered in Indianapolis, Indiana. The Greek letters stand for the Greek words *storga, tharos,* and *tima,* meaning

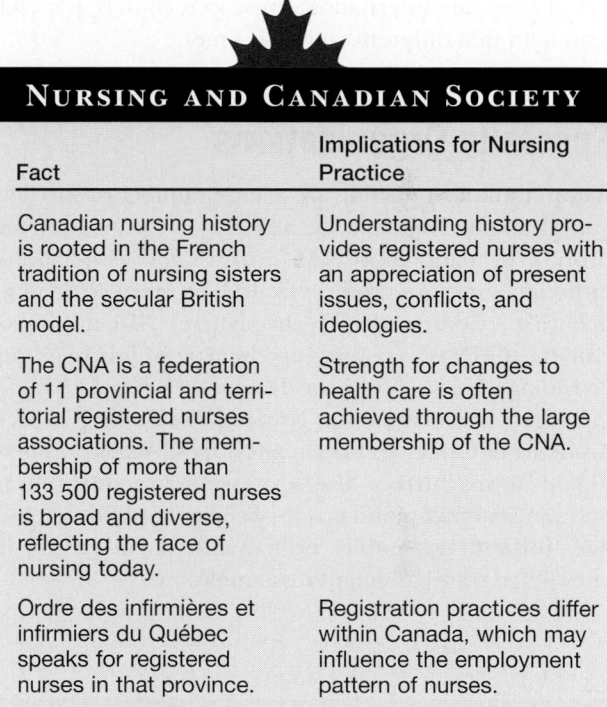

Nursing and Canadian Society

Fact	Implications for Nursing Practice
Canadian nursing history is rooted in the French tradition of nursing sisters and the secular British model.	Understanding history provides registered nurses with an appreciation of present issues, conflicts, and ideologies.
The CNA is a federation of 11 provincial and territorial registered nurses associations. The membership of more than 133 500 registered nurses is broad and diverse, reflecting the face of nursing today.	Strength for changes to health care is often achieved through the large membership of the CNA.
Ordre des infirmières et infirmiers du Québec speaks for registered nurses in that province.	Registration practices differ within Canada, which may influence the employment pattern of nurses.

TABLE 1.1 Provincial and Territorial Registered Nursing Associations

Geographic Area	Nursing Association	Website
British Columbia	College of Registered Nurses of British Columbia	http://www.crnbc.ca
Alberta	College and Association of Registered Nurses of Alberta	http://www.nurses.ab.ca
Saskatchewan	Saskatchewan Registered Nurses' Association	http://www.srna.org
Manitoba	College of Registered Nurses of Manitoba	http://www.crnm.mb.ca
Ontario	Registered Nurses' Association of Ontario	http://www.rnao.org
	College of Nurses of Ontario	http://www.cno.org
Quebec	Ordre des infirmières et infirmiers du Québec	http://www.oiiq.org
New Brunswick	Nurses Association of New Brunswick	http://www.nanb.nb.ca
Nova Scotia	College of Registered Nurses of Nova Scotia	http://www.crnns.ca
Newfoundland and Labrador	Association of Registered Nurses of Newfoundland and Labrador	http://www.arnnl.nf.ca
Prince Edward Island	Association of Registered Nurses of Prince Edward Island	http://www.arnpei.ca
Northwest Territories	Registered Nurses Association of Northwest Territories and Nunavut	http://www.rnantnu.ca
Yukon	Yukon Registered Nurses Association	http://www.yrna.ca

"love," "courage," and "honour." The society is a member of the Association of College Honor Societies. The society's purpose is professional, rather than social. Membership is attained through academic achievement. Nursing students in baccalaureate programs and in master's, doctoral, and postdoctoral programs are eligible to be selected for membership. In addition, community nurses with a "minimum of a baccalaureate degree or equivalent, and demonstrated achievement in nursing" can apply to become members (Sigma Theta Tau International, 2007). STTI became an international organization with the creation of a chapter at the University of Western Ontario. Now chapters span the globe and there are seven STTI chapters in Canada.

The official journal of STTI, *Journal of Nursing Scholarship,* is published quarterly. The journal publishes scholarly articles of interest to nurses. STTI also organizes at least one international research conference each year, held in a different city each time.

Specialty Organizations

Within Canadian nursing are a large number of specialty organizations. These may be linked to the provincial, territorial, or national (CNA) professional associations. Although some are groups of nurses in specialized practice (e.g., Community Health Nurses Association of Canada [CHNAC]), others are by type of job (e.g., the Provincial Nurse Educator Interest Group [PNEIG], Canadian Association for Nursing Research [CANR], Academy of Canadian Executive Nurses [ACEN]). These organizations further the profession by contributing position statements and group-specific standards of practice, influencing public policy, and participating in knowledge translation and dissemination.

Licensed (Registered) Practical Nurses

Practical nurses are licensed in all provinces and territories except Ontario, where they are registered. The national organization—Practical Nurses Canada—states it is the national voice of practical nurses in Canada. Its membership list includes three provincial associations and the student nursing organization. Individual practical nurses from nonmember organizations can join PN Canada. Its website (see the Weblinks section of this chapter) lists a mission, values, and a code of ethics. The associations belonging to PN Canada are asterisked in Table 1.2. Of the territories, only Yukon has a professional association for LPNs and it is in the beginning stages. In addition, the practical nurse regulatory bodies have a national organization: the Canadian Council for Practical Nurse Regulators. It notes that there are national commonalities, but the organizations are different in all jurisdictions.

Registered Psychiatric Nurses

In the four Western provinces, another category of nurses is the registered psychiatric nurse. The Canadian Institute for Health Information's definition of a registered psychiatric nurse is found in Box 1.2 (page 10). The Registered Psychiatric Nurses of Canada organization comprises the regulatory bodies or associations from all four provinces. It also liaises with other psychiatric nursing organizations globally. The provincial and national organizations are listed in Table 1.3.

TABLE 1.2 Provincial and Territorial Practical Nurse Professional Organizations

Geographic Area	Organization	Website
British Columbia*	College of Licensed Practical Nurses of British Columbia	http://www.clpnbc.org
Alberta	College of Licensed Practical Nurses of Alberta	http://www.clpna.com/dnn/
Saskatchewan	Saskatchewan Association of Licensed Practical Nurses	http://www.salpn.com
Manitoba	College of Licensed Practical Nurses of Manitoba	http://www.clpnm.ca
Ontario*	Registered Practical Nurses Association of Ontario	http://www.rpnao.org
Quebec	Ordre des infirmières et infirmiers auxiliaires du Québec	http://www.oiiaq.org
New Brunswick	Association of New Brunswick Licensed Practical Nurses	http://www.anblpn.ca
Nova Scotia	College of Licensed Practical Nurses of Nova Scotia	http://www.clpnns.ca
Newfoundland and Labrador	College of Licensed Practical Nurses of Newfoundland and Labrador	http://www.clpnnl.ca
Prince Edward Island*	Licensed Practical Nursing Association of Prince Edward Island	http://www.lpna.ca
Yukon	Yukon Practical Nurses Association	Early stages of development; no website yet

TABLE 1.3 Canadian Psychiatric Nursing Professional Organizations

Jurisdiction	Organization	Website
National	Registered Psychiatric Nurses of Canada	http://www.rpnc.ca
British Columbia	College of Registered Psychiatric Nurses of British Columbia	http://www.crpnbc.ca
Alberta	College of Registered Psychiatric Nurses of Alberta	http://www.crpna.ab.ca
Saskatchewan	Registered Psychiatric Nurses Association of Saskatchewan	http://www.rpnas.com
Manitoba	College of Registered Psychiatric Nurses of Manitoba	http://www.crpnm.mb.ca

Unions

The majority of today's nurses are union members by virtue of their employment. The Canadian Federation of Nurses Unions (CFNU) is a group representing nine provincial unions and one students' association and speaking for 158 000 members. Created in 1981 as the National Federation of Nurses Unions, its goal is "protecting the health of patients and our national health system, and promoting nurses and the nursing profession at the national level—and doing it effectively" (Canadian Federation of Nurses Unions [CFNU], 2007). Depending on the worksite and collective agreements, the union may include registered nurses, licensed (registered) practical nurses, and registered psychiatric nurses within the membership.

Case Study 1

The supply of nurses in Canada has historically been partially shaped by constraints over who could train as a nurse and who could practise in certain areas, such as pediatrics, obstetrics, psychiatric hospitals, and the military. The following cases illustrate some criteria that have been used in the past to include or exclude people as nurses.

Edith Anderson Monture was a member of the Upper Mohawk band of the Six Nations of the Grand River Reserve near Brantford, Ontario. She was denied entrance to nursing schools in Canada, but she graduated first in her class from the New Rochelle Hospital School of Nursing in New York in 1914. Following volunteer service with the American Expeditionary Force in World War I, she returned to the hospital on the Six Nations Reserve, where she worked as a nurse and midwife until her retirement in 1955 (Moses, 2005).

Estelle Tritt applied for training at the Montreal General Hospital School of Nursing and was told that they didn't take Jewish nurses because "they get married too soon" (Toman, 2007, p. 47). She subsequently applied successfully to the Women's General Hospital at Westmount, Quebec, and graduated from training in 1941. After working at the Jewish General Hospital in Montreal to gain the required years of graduate experience, Tritt was accepted as a military nurse (nursing sister) with the Royal Canadian Army Medical Corps and served overseas during World War II.

This memo was sent to Helen Mussallem, CEO of Canadian Nurses Association, January 18, 1966: "The Surgeon General stated today that he has not changed his mind: 'male nurses will not get commissions in the medical services (nursing). . . . ' His main objection is that 'the men would stay in nursing and would possibly become Matron in the Armed Services. This would not be good in a male oriented service'" (Library and Archives Canada, MG 28, I248, Vol. 78, File 30–3-8).

Critical Thinking Questions

1. The preferred candidates for nursing students until the mid-twentieth century were young, white, Canadian-born women. What are the different factors in these examples that have historically determined who could be a nurse?
2. In what ways are these criteria still influencing the composition of the nursing workforce? What has changed regarding the manifestations of such criteria? What additional characteristics are shaping the nursing profession? To what extent is the profession more inclusive now, and how might some people still face barriers?

After working through these questions, go to the MyNursingLab at **http://www.mynursinglab.com** to check your answers.

KEY TERMS

consumer
patient
client
nursing practice standards
profession
socialization
demography

CHAPTER HIGHLIGHTS

- Knowledge of how larger and changing sociocultural and political contexts have influenced the development of nurses and their practice in the past is key to understanding the relevance of history to present-day concerns in nursing.
- *Nursing* has many definitions and descriptions, but the essence of nursing is caring for and caring about people.
- The scope of nursing practice is outlined by the professional associations (or organizations) of each province and territory. It describes what it is that nurses in a particular province or territory have the legislated authority to do.
- Although traditionally the majority of nurses were employed in hospital settings, today the numbers of nurses working in home health care, ambulatory care, and community health settings are increasing.
- Standards of clinical nursing practice reflect the values of the profession and clarify what professional organizations expect of their members.
- Every nurse can function in a variety of roles that are not exclusive; in reality, the functions often occur together and serve to clarify the nurse's activities. These roles include caregiver, communicator, teacher, client advocate, counsellor, change agent, leader, and research consumer.
- A desired goal of nursing is professionalism, which requires specialized education; a unique body of knowledge, including specific skills and abilities; ongoing research; a code of ethics; autonomy; a service orientation; and a professional organization.
- Socialization is a lifelong process by which people become functioning participants of a society or a group. Although several models of the socialization process have been developed, Benner's five stages of novice, advanced beginner, competent practitioner, proficient practitioner, and expert practitioner can serve as guidelines to establish the phase and extent of an individual's socialization in nursing.
- Participation in the activities of nursing associations and other professional and nonprofessional groups enhances the growth of involved individuals and helps nurses collectively influence policies affecting nursing practice.

ASSESS YOUR LEARNING

1. What is the primary purpose of historical research on the nursing profession?
   a. It showcases the wonderful achievements of nurses in the past.
   b. It provides alternative perspectives for understanding nursing issues.
   c. It proves that nursing has been a true profession for a long time.
   d. It justifies nurses' demand for greater respect and improved salaries.

2. Which of the following statements is true about Canadian nursing?
   a. Before the establishment of the first training school, there were no nurses to care for the needs of the public.
   b. Nursing has always been an equal opportunity profession, genderblind, open to all ethnic groups.
   c. Nurses have traditionally relied on hospitals as their main place of work.
   d. The nursing workforce has experienced recurring periods of oversupply and shortages.

3. What factors exerted a major influence on the shift of medical and nursing care from private homes into hospitals around the beginning of the twentieth century?
   a. The discovery of the germ theory and anaesthesia
   b. The availability of universal health-care insurance to pay for hospital care
   c. Campaigns by the Canadian Red Cross
   d. A lack of nurses because of the high numbers that enlisted for the war

4. How has the rise in use of medical technology shaped nurses and their practice?
   a. Medical technology has reduced the number of nurses needed by making their work less intensive and time-consuming.
   b. Medical technology has led to increased specialization among nurses that differentiates them from personnel with less training.
   c. Increased medical technology caused hospital programs to close and nurses' training to move into educational institutions.

d. Medical technology has had very little effect on nurses or their practice.

5. Which of the following activities would be considered in the category of restoring health?
a. Running a newborn clinic at the local public health facility
b. Administering medications in an orthopedic unit
c. Facilitating a parenting class at the hospital
d. Starting a seniors' walking program at the mall

6. Which of the following describes the principle of comprehensiveness in the Canada Health Act?
a. All levels of health care are available to the residents of a particular jurisdiction.
b. Individuals who move within Canada are covered at all times.
c. There are no user fees for basic services within the jurisdiction.
d. The administration of the plan is devolved to the local authorities.

7. What is the primary purpose of nursing practice standards for a profession?
a. To provide a guideline to determine the boundaries of practice
b. To provide a guideline for delivering safe, ethical, and competent patient care
c. To help nursing students determine what they are allowed to do
d. To serve as a handout for all new patients or clients so that they understand the nursing profession

8. Benner's stages of nursing expertise were primarily developed to do which of the following?
a. Assist nursing students to plot their progress to graduation
b. Ensure performance appraisal forms measure performance against nursing expertise
c. Describe the characteristics of nurses as they move from novice to expert
d. Assist nurse managers to ensure they hire only nurses who are experts

9. Which of the following is a definition of primary health care?
a. Essential care that focuses on preventing illness and promoting health
b. A system in which physicians provide diagnosis and treatment for specific health challenges
c. A system of delivering nursing care to patients and clients
d. A way to ensure that all patients have access to the latest medical advances

10. Many theorists have defined nursing. What is the commonality in all the definitions?
a. Delivery of holistic, adaptive, and client-centred care
b. Delivery of care to a passive recipient
c. Assistant to the physician while delivering care
d. A profession of entrepreneurs delivering independent care

After working through these questions, go to the MyNursingLab at ***http://www.mynursinglab.com*** *to check your answers and see explanations.*

SUGGESTED READINGS

Canadian Nurses Association. (1988). *Health for all Canadians: A call for health-care reform.* Ottawa: Author.

The authors appeal to the Canadian government for the reform of the Canadian health-care system to support the tenets of the Canada Health Act.

Epp, J. (1986). *Achieving health for all: A framework for health promotion.* Ottawa: Health and Welfare Canada.

The authors offer a framework for health promotion that could provide health care for all Canadians through a change in focus from illness care to health promotion.

Bates, C., Dodd, D., & Rousseau, N. (Eds.). (2005). *On all frontiers: Four centuries of Canadian nursing.* Ottawa: University of Ottawa Press & Canadian Museum of Civilization.

This book provides the most recent comprehensive survey of Canadian nursing history, including early lay nursing, midwifery, and a strong section on the contribution of religious sisterhoods.

McKay, M. (2008). Community health nursing in Canada. In L. L. Stamler & L. Yiu (Eds.), *Community health nursing: A Canadian perspective* (2nd ed.) (pp. 1–19). Toronto: Pearson Education.

The author provides a historical overview of the development of community health nursing in Canada.

McPherson, K. (1996). *Bedside matters: The transformation of Canadian nursing, 1900–1990.* Toronto: Oxford University Press.

This author offers an analysis of the position of different generational cohorts of primarily Canadian hospital nurses in the health-care system, and their strategies to improve that position, from a gendered, racialized, and class perspective.

World Health Organization. (1987). *Primary health care: Report of the international conference on primary health care. Alma-Ata, USSR.* Geneva, Switzerland: Author.

This report of the meeting in Alma-Ata, September 12, 1978, expresses the need for urgent action by all governments, all health and development workers, and the world community to protect and promote the health of all the world's people. The conference strongly reaffirmed two things: (1) health, which is a state of complete physical, mental, and social well-being, and not merely the absence of disease or infirmity, is a fundamental human right, and (2) the attainment of the highest possible level of health is a most important worldwide social goal, the realization of which requires the action of many other social and economic sectors in addition to the health sector.

WEBLINKS

Canadian Association for the History of Nursing (CAHN)

http://www.cahn-achn.ca

The Canadian Association for the History of Nursing provides a forum for those interested in the history of nursing through annual conferences, bi-annual newsletters, and financial support of nursing history scholarship. It also promotes the preservation of historical nursing materials through its Guide to Canadian Nursing Archival Resources.

Associated Medical Services Nursing History Research Unit

http://www.health.uottawa.ca/nursinghistory/

The Associated Medical Services Nursing History Unit is the only funded academic centre in Canada dedicated to the production and dissemination of new knowledge in nursing history. It educates graduate students through academic programs and summer research practicums, publishes new research, hosts conferences and seminars, establishes links with international nursing history units, and maintains a comprehensive bibliography on Canadian nursing history.

Registered Nurses' Association of Ontario

http://www.rnao.org/bestpractices

This group has led the way in developing a series of best practices documents. Thirty-five different publications are available, offering guidelines on such subjects as clinical practice and healthy work environments.

Practical Nurses Canada

http://www.pncanada.ca

This organization presents itself as the national association representing provincial licensed practical nurse organizations and affiliated individuals.

REFERENCES

Anspaugh, D. L., Hamrick, M. H., & Rosata, F. D. (2003). *Wellness: Concepts and applications.* New York: McGraw-Hill.

Benner, P. (1984). *From novice to expert: Excellence and power in clinical nursing practice.* Menlo Park, CA: Addison-Wesley Nursing.

Canada Health Act of 1984, R.S., 1985, c. C-6. Ottawa: Government of Canada.

Canada, House of Commons (1984). *An Act Relating to Cash Contributions by Canada in Respect of Insured Health Services Provided Under Provincial Health Care Insurance Plans and Amounts Payable by Canada in Respect of Extended Health Care Services and to Amend and Repeal Certain Acts in Consequence Thereof (The Canada Health Act).* Ottawa: Government of Canada.

Canadian Federation of Nurses Unions. (2007). *About us.* Retrieved May 14, 2007, from http://www.nursesunions.ca/content.php?sec=1

Canadian Institute for Health Information. (2007). *Highlights from the regulated nursing workforce in Canada, 2006.* Ottawa: Author.

Canadian Nurses Association. (1987). *A definition of nursing practice: Standards for nursing practice.* Ottawa: Author.

Canadian Nurses Association. (1992). *Policy statement on health promotion.* Ottawa: Author.

Canadian Nurses Association. (1995). *The Role of the nurse in primary health care.* Ottawa: Author.

Canadian Nurses Association. (2001). Issues and trends in Canadian nursing. Self-regulation: Safeguarding the privilege. *Nursing Now, 10,* 5–8.

Canadian Nurses Association. (2003). Primary health care—The time has come. *NursingNow: Issues and Trends in Canadian Nursing, 16*(September), 1–4.

Canadian Nurses Association. (2004). *CNA and CASN Joint Position Statement: Promoting continuing competency for registered nurses.* Ottawa: Author.

Canadian Nurses Association. (2005). *Primary health care: A summary of the issues.* Ottawa: Author.

Canadian Nurses Association. (2007). *Framework for the practice of registered nurses in Canada.* Ottawa: Author. Retrieved August 9, 2008, from http://www.cna-aiic.ca/CNA/documents/pdf/publications/RN_Framework_Practice_2007_e.pdf

Canadian Nurses Association. (2008). *Vision and mission.* Retrieved September 6, 2008, from http://cna-aiic.ca/CNA/about/mission/default_e.aspx

Canadian Nurses Association. (1984). Canada Health Act: CNA appears before Commons committee. *Canadian Nurse, 80,* 8–9.

Cassel, J. (1994). Public health in Canada. In Dorothy Porter (Ed.), *The History of Public Health and the Modern State* (pp. 276–312). London, UK: Wellcome Institute Series in the History of Medicine.

Cayne, B. S. (Ed.). (1988). *New Lexicon Webster's Dictionary of the English Language* (Rev. ed.). New York: Lexicon Publications.

Charles, A. (2003). Women's work in eclipse: Nuns in Quebec hospitals, 1940–1980. In G. Feldberg, M. Ladd-Taylor, A. Li, & K. McPherson, (Eds.), *Women, health and nation: Canada and the United States since 1945* (pp. 264–291). Montreal: McGill-Queen's University Press.

College and Association of Registered Nurses of Alberta. (2003). *Nursing practice standards.* Retrieved January 26, 2008, from http://www.nurses.ab.ca/Carna-Admin/Uploads/Nursing%20Practice%20Standards_1.pdf

Dreyfus, S. E., & Dreyfus, H. L. (1980, February). *A five-stage model of the mental activities involved in directed skill acquisition.* Unpublished report supported by the Air Force Office of Scientific Research (AFSC), USAF (Contract F49620-79-C-0063), University of California at Berkeley.

Elliott, J. (2004). Blurring the boundaries of space: Shaping nursing lives at the Red Cross outposts in Ontario, 1922–1945. *Canadian Bulletin of Medical History, 21*(2), 303–325.

Gagan, D., & Gagan, R. (2002). *For patients of moderate means: A social history of the voluntary public hospital in Canada, 1890–1950.* Montreal: McGill-Queen's University Press.

Hardy, M. E., & Conway, M. E. (1988). *Role theory: Perspectives for healthy professionals* (2nd ed.). Norwalk, CT: Appleton & Lange.

Henderson, V. (1966). *The nature of nursing: A definition and its implications for practice, research, and education.* New York: Macmillan.

International Council of Nurses (n.d.). *About the International Council of Nurses.*

Retrieved April 14, 2008, from http://www.icn.ch/abouticn.htm

International Council of Nurses. (2001). The ICN definition of nursing. Retrieved September 6, 2008, from http://www.icn.ch/definition.htm

Leininger, M. (1984). *Care: The essence of nursing and health.* Thorofare, NJ: Slack.

Library and Archives Canada. (1966). MG 28, I248, Vol. 78, File 30–3-8. Memo to file from Helen Mussallem, January 18, 1966.

MacDougall, H. (2007). Toronto's health department in action: Influenza in 1919 and SARS in 2003. *Journal of the History of Medicine and Allied Sciences, 62,* 56–89.

Mansell, D. (2003). *Forging the future in Canada: A history of nursing in Canada.* Ann Arbor, MI: Thomas Press.

McBain, L. (2005). Jean Cuthand Goodwill. In C. Bates, D. Dodd, & N. Rousseau (Eds.), *On all frontiers: Four centuries of Canadian nursing* (p. 116). Ottawa: University of Ottawa Press & Canadian Museum of Civilization.

McKay, M. (2007). "The tubercular cow must go": Business, politics, and Winnipeg's milk supply, 1894–1922. *Canadian Bulletin of Medical History, 23*(2), 255–380.

McPherson, K. (1996). *Bedside matters: The transformation of Canadian nursing, 1900–1990.* Toronto: Oxford University Press.

McPherson, K. (2003). Nursing and colonization: The work of Indian health service nurses in Manitoba, 1945–1970. In G. Feldberg, M. Ladd-Taylor, A. Li, & K. McPherson (Eds.), *Women, health and nation: Canada and the United States since 1945* (pp. 223–246). Montreal: McGill-Queen's University Press.

Meijer-Drees, L., & McBain, L. (2001). Nursing and native peoples in northern Saskatchewan: 1930s–1950s. *Canadian Bulletin of Medical History, 18*(1), 43–65.

Miller, K. L. (1995). Keeping the care in nursing care: Our biggest challenge. *Journal of Nursing Administration, 25*(11), 29–32.

Moses, J. (2005). Charlotte Edith Anderson Monture (1890–1996). In C. Bates, D. Dodd, & N. Rousseau (Eds.), *On all frontiers: Four centuries of Canadian nursing* (p. 86). Ottawa: University of Ottawa Press & Canadian Museum of Civilization.

Nelson, S., & Gordon, S. (Eds.). (2006). *The complexities of care: Nursing reconsidered.* Ithaca, NY: Cornell University Press.

Nightingale, F. (1938). *Notes on nursing: What it is, and what it is not.* New York, NY: D Appleton-Century Company.

Nursing Education in Nova Scotia (n.d.). *1899 Graduating class photo.* Retrieved March 30, 2008, from http://www.msvu.ca/library/archives/nhdp/schools/VGH.htm

Paul, P. (2005). Religious nursing orders of Canada: A presence on all western frontiers. In C. Bates, D. Dodd, & N. Rousseau (Eds.), *On all frontiers: Four centuries of Canadian nursing* (pp. 125–138). Ottawa: University of Ottawa Press & Canadian Museum of Civilization.

Penney, S. M. (1996). *A century of caring: 1897–1997, the history of the Victorian Order of Nurses for Canada.* Ottawa: VON Canada.

Registered Nurses Association of British Columbia. (1999). *Nursing self-regulation: Nurses governing nurses in the public interest.* Vancouver: Author.

Richardson, S. (1998). Frontier health care: Alberta's district and municipal nursing services, 1919 to 1976. *Alberta History, 46,* 2–9.

Ross-Kerr, J. C. (2003). Professionalization in Canadian nursing. In J. C. Ross-Kerr & M. Wood (Eds.), *Canadian nursing: Issues and perspectives* (4th ed.) (pp. 29–38). Toronto: Mosby.

Rousseau, N., & Daigle, J. (2000). Medical service to settlers: The gestation and establishment of a nursing service in Quebec, 1932–1943. *Nursing History Review, 8,* 95–116.

Sandelowski, M. (2000). *Devices and desires: Gender, technology and American nursing.* Chapel Hill, NC: University of North Carolina Press.

Sigma Theta Tau International. (2007). *Membership: Apply now.* Retrieved September 22, 2007, from http://www.nursingsociety.org/Membership/ApplyNow/Pages/applynow.aspx

Toman, C. (2001). Blood work: Canadian nursing and blood transfusion, 1942–1990. *Nursing History Review, 9,* 51–78.

Toman, C. (2007). *An officer and a lady: Canadian military nurses and the Second World War.* Vancouver: UBC Press.

Villeneuve, M., & MacDonald, J. (2006). *Towards 2020: Visions for nursing.* Ottawa: Canadian Nurses Association.

Violette, B. (2005). Healing the body and saving the soul: Nursing sisters and the first Catholic hospitals in Quebec (1639–1880). In C. Bates, D. Dodd, & N. Rousseau (Eds.), *On all frontiers: Four centuries of Canadian nursing* (pp. 57–71). Ottawa: University of Ottawa Press & Canadian Museum of Civilization.

World Health Organization (Division of Health Manpower Development). (1982). *Report of a meeting on nursing in support of the goal health for all by the year 2000.* November 16–20, 1981. Geneva, Switzerland: WHO.

Young, J. (2004). "Monthly" nurses, "sick" nurses, and midwives in 19th-century Toronto, 1830–1891. *Canadian Bulletin of Medical History, 21,* 281–302.

Chapter 2

Nursing Education in Canada

In the early twentieth century in Canada, nursing was conceptualized in various ways according to the religion, geographical location, class, status, race, ethinicity, and sexual orientation of the people who practised the profession. Nursing was/is also largely conceptualized by society based on the same factors (broader perspective). While religious groups contributed significantly to nursing education development, Cohen (2000) proposed that the Catholic church, among other agents, was one force that slowed the introduction of science into nursing and the attribution of satisfactory wages. Whatever the influences, nursing education has moved from the traditional focus of teaching knowledge and skills for work in hospital settings to the knowledge education of today. Nursing education is controlled from within the profession through provincial and territorial organizations of nursing and national accrediting bodies.

In Canada, the first training program for nurses was offered at the General and Marine Hospital in St. Catharines, Ontario, in 1874. It became the norm for hospitals to have their own schools of nursing. The training programs of the 1920s, 1930s, and 1940s were characterized by limited coordination of classroom and clinical teaching, long hours, night duty without supervision, and numerous housekeeping chores (Baumgart & Larsen, 1992). The medical staff and nursing supervisors provided the instruction and they were identified as clinical teachers.

Today, as nursing responds to new scientific knowledge and technological, cultural, political, and socioeconomic changes in society, nursing education curricula are continually being revised to meet the needs of very complex clinical situations for patients and a changing environment for nurses. Programs of nursing study are increasingly based on a broad knowledge of biological, social, and physical sciences, as well as the liberal arts and humanities. Nursing curricula now have a greater focus on critical thinking and the application of nursing and supporting knowledge to health prevention and promotion, health maintenance, and health restoration, as provided in college and university settings.

This chapter was written in honour and memory of Dr. Patricia L. Griffin, Executive Director, Canadian Association of Schools of Nursing, 2005–2007.

OBJECTIVES

After studying this chapter, you should be able to

1. Describe the different types of nursing education programs
2. Identify aspects of the baccalaureate level for entry to professional nursing practice
3. Explain the importance of continuing nursing education
4. Describe the role of national nursing associations in shaping nursing education in Canada
5. Analyze issues influencing nursing education in Canada

Nursing Education

Today, provincial and territorial laws and union regulations in Canada recognize five distinct groups within the profession of nursing. Not every province or territory recognizes all groups: All provinces and territories recognize the *registered nurse* (*RN*) and the *licensed practical nurse* (*LPN;* called a *registered practical nurse* in Ontario only [*RPN*]). All jurisdictions except Yukon recognize the *nurse practitioner* (*NP*). In addition, the four Western provinces recognize the *registered psychiatric nurse* (*RPN*). Further, Quebec distinguishes RNs by type of education: diploma or baccalaureate. Responsibilities differ for the five groups. Definitions and roles for the RN, LPN or RPN, and RPN can be found in Chapter 1, Box 1.2 (page 10).

Currently, two *major* educational routes lead to RN licensure: diploma and baccalaureate programs. University **baccalaureate nursing degrees** are currently offered by universities, university colleges, and polytechnical institutes. Many community colleges partner with universities to offer baccalaureate programs. Generic programs involve admitting students directly into the nursing program and having them graduate with a degree or diploma. Programs also exist for students with a previous degree (not in nursing), or part thereof, in which the nursing content has been reconfigured so that students can graduate with a nursing degree in approximately two calendar years. These are variously called generic master's, second entry, compressed, or accelerated programs. A listing of the programs offered by members of the Canadian Association of Schools of Nursing (CASN) can be found in the Weblinks section of this chapter. In addition, many colleges provide diploma education, the majority of which are in Quebec. In some provinces and territories, such as Ontario, polytechnical institutes provide undergraduate degrees. Basic educational programs for practical nurses are generally offered in colleges. No national list exists for practical nursing programs, however, provincial or territorial lists can often be found on the provincial or territorial regulatory websites (see Chapter 1, Table 1.1, page 19). Psychiatric nurses can complete their basic education at the diploma or degree levels, depending on the province. A national listing of psychiatric nursing education programs can be found in the Weblinks section of this chapter.

Graduates of all programs take a **licensing examination** for their group (e.g., RN, LPN or RPN, RPN) provided by the appropriate regulatory authority and, if successful, are licensed within their group. The Canadian Registered Nurse Examination (CRNE) is a multiple-choice test that measures the applicant's ability to work with content that matches the competencies expected of a new graduate nurse. The CRNE question format is the basis for the Assess Your Learning questions at the end of each chapter in this book. CRNE results are reported to candidates as pass or fail. National examinations for all the groups of nurses are administered by the provincial or territorial regulatory authority. The successful candidate becomes licensed in that province or territory, even though the examinations are of national origin. To practise nursing in another province or territory, the nurse must receive reciprocal licensure by applying to that province's or territory's professional association. Both licensure and registration must be renewed each year to remain valid.

Nurses who have been educated in other countries (**internationally educated nurses**, or IENs) apply to have their credentials assessed and are usually granted registration after successfully completing these examinations. Increasingly, the trend has been to provide IENs with entry programs tailored to them to assist them in learning about nursing in Canada's health-care system, cultural (health-care) expectations, and English language used in health-care situations. These programs are completed before writing the Canadian examinations and include both classroom and clinical practice experience.

The legal right to practise nursing within all the groups requires not only a passing grade in licensing examinations but also verification that the graduate has completed a prescribed course of study from an approved program in nursing.

Minimum standards for basic nursing education are established in each province and territory and monitored by the provincial or territorial nursing regulatory bodies. Schools that meet these minimum standards are granted provincial or territorial approval. In addition to provincial or territorial approval in Canada for baccalaureate nursing education, the Canadian Association of Schools of Nursing (CASN) grants accreditation that is focused on standards of excellence for nursing education.

Types of Educational Programs

Hospital Diploma Programs

Florence Nightingale developed a nursing program based on religious, military, and, what is called today, public health and insisted on the moral superiority of her recruits (Cohen, 2000). After Florence Nightingale established the first school of nursing—the Nightingale Training School for Nurses—at St. Thomas's Hospital in England in 1860, the concept travelled quickly to North America. Hospital administrators welcomed the idea of training schools as a source of free or inexpensive staffing for the hospital. Nursing education in the early years largely took the form of apprenticeships. Along with minimal formal classroom instruction, students learned by doing, that is, by providing care to patients in hospitals. The curricula were not standardized and no accreditation was available at that time. Programs were designed to meet the service needs of the hospital, not the educational needs of the students.

Mack Training School at the General and Marine Hospital in St. Catharines, Ontario, opened in 1874 as the first Canadian school of nursing patterned after the Nightingale school. The number of diploma programs rose quickly after these initial programs.

Over the years, as the health-care system, medical care, and knowledge have changed, so have the groups of regulated nurses and the curricula of their educational programs. This evolution contributes to changes in the nurses and their practice in a synergistic manner. For example, as new knowledge and procedures emerge, decisions are made as to the best worker to practise those procedures and use the knowledge. In turn, curricula are revised and implemented, ensuring that the graduates are ready for the health-care world of tomorrow. The overall goal is the health of Canadians and the world.

In Chapter 1, we discussed the number of regulated nurses in Canada and their distribution by category. In this chapter, we examine the educational background of those nurses. The highest level of education in nursing reported by all regulated nurses in 2006 is seen in Table 2.1. These statistics exclude education in disciplines other than nursing. For example, the Canadian Institute for Health Information (CIHI, 2007) lists 382 nurses with a doctoral degree in nursing in Canada in 2006. If doctoral degrees in other disciplines were included, the number would be higher, although still a very small percentage of the total nursing population.

Educational Programs Leading to or Continuing from Basic Registered Nursing Education

COLLEGE DIPLOMA PROGRAMS Mussalem (1960) identified the problems in hospital-based **diploma programs** in nursing caused by the hospital's control over education. Students were used as the primary service providers, and their education was controlled by the hospital. Community college nursing education programs began to appear in the 1960s, also offering diploma preparation. It was not until the 1970s that most diploma nursing programs had moved into community colleges (Baumgart & Larsen, 1992). Today, the majority of colleges are in partnership with universities to provide a common curriculum leading to a baccalaureate degree in nursing. In Quebec, the DEC-BACC program (3 years in a collège d'enseignement général et professionnel, plus 2 years in a university) was first implemented in 2004, with the first cohort of new graduates in 2006. A DEC-BACC is a diplôme d'études collégiales-baccalaurate integrated program. Although the idea behind the collaboration is interesting, the integration of programs and resources between colleges and universities is not attained in all provinces or territories.

BACCALAUREATE DEGREE PROGRAMS In 1919, the first baccalaureate degree program in nursing in English was established at the University of British Columbia in Vancouver, followed by McGill School (Montreal) of Graduate Nurses in 1920 (Street, 1973). The first baccalaureate in French was developed by Institut Marguerite d'Youville in 1938. With the establishment of these programs, nursing moved into the university sector.

In 1932, the Canadian Nurses Association (CNA) and the Canadian Medical Association (CMA) commissioned Dr. George Weir to conduct a study of nursing education in Canada. He found that education was secondary to hospital service as a priority in the schools. Dr. Weir recommended, in the *Survey of Nursing Education in Canada* (1932), that nurses be given a liberal education in addition to a technical one and that university training programs award degrees.

The 1950s saw the greatest expansion of university schools of nursing. Students enrolled in the university for 1 year for non-nursing courses and then moved to a hospital-based model for the practical experience. A fifth year at the university completed what was labelled a "sandwich" program. The university had control over the academic courses and awarded the degree, while the hospital monitored the clinical practice of the nursing student.

It was not until the 1960s that the number of students enrolled in these baccalaureate programs increased markedly. Currently, baccalaureate programs are offered by universities or university-colleges alone or in collabora-

TABLE 2.1 Educational Preparation of the Regulated Nursing Workforce (in percentages)

Education	Registered Nurse	Licensed (Registered) Practical Nurses	Registered Psychiatric Nurses
Diploma	64.2	100.0	94.2
Baccalaureate	33.1		5.5
Master's/doctorate	2.7		0.3

Source: From *Highlights from the Regulated Nursing Workforce in Canada, 2006,* by the Canadian Institute for Health Information, 2007, Ottawa: Author. Reprinted with permission.

tion with other postsecondary institutions, depending on the province or territory. In some provinces, specific colleges have degree-granting status and they independently offer baccalaureate programs. The curricula offer courses in the liberal arts, sciences, humanities, and nursing. The usual degree awarded is a bachelor of science in nursing (BScN, BSN) or a bachelor of nursing (BN).

Most baccalaureate programs also admit registered nurses who have diplomas. Some programs have specifically designed curricula to meet the needs of these students. Some universities also offer nursing students the opportunity to pursue a self-paced or independent study program. Many programs offer distance and online courses that can be accessed by nursing students. Many accept transfer credits from other accredited colleges and universities and offer students the opportunity for prior learning assessment and recognition (PLAR) when the students believe they have acquired the required competency. These programs are referred to as BScN completion, BN transition, or postdiploma programs.

The newest type of program is one in which the students come with all or part of a university degree in another discipline. These are variously called second entry, second degree, accelerated, or compressed programs. Usually 2 to 3 years long, they build on the courses already completed and compress the structure of the nursing curriculum.

Because of changes in the practice environment, the nurse who holds a baccalaureate degree is beginning to reap the rewards of greater autonomy and responsibility, participation in institutional decision making, and career advancement. These changes provide an incentive for nurses with diplomas to continue their formal preparation in baccalaureate completion (transition) programs.

Today, universities and colleges have control over all components of education, and nursing students receive a liberal education combined with a professional one. The majority of these programs are 4 academic years long, an academic year being approximately 8 calendar months. Many educational institutions offer students the opportunity for accelerated completion of the program. Requirements for university admission include a Grade 12 or a high-school diploma with specific prerequisites, such as chemistry and biology.

GRADUATE NURSING EDUCATION Most graduate programs are conducted by departments within the graduate school or faculty of a university, and the applicant must first meet requirements established by the graduate school. Although graduate schools differ, for Canadian students, common requirements for admission to graduate programs in nursing include the following:

- The applicant must be a registered nurse and licensed or eligible for licensure within the program's province or territory.
- The applicant generally must hold a baccalaureate degree in nursing from a recognized university.
- The applicant must give evidence of scholastic ability.
- Letters of recommendation from supervisors, nursing faculty, or nursing colleagues indicating the applicant's ability to do graduate study are required.

MASTER'S PROGRAMS The growth of university nursing programs encouraged the development of graduate study in nursing. In Canada, the first master's program in nursing was established at the University of Western Ontario in London in 1959. This was followed by a program at McGill University in Montreal in 1961 and a French program at Université de Montréal in 1962.

Master's programs may be course based or a combination of course work and thesis research. Programs generally take from 1 to 2 years to complete. Degrees most frequently granted are the master in nursing (MN), master of science in nursing (MScN), and master of science (MS or MSc).

Master's degree programs provide specialized knowledge and skills that enable nurses to assume advanced roles in practice, education, administration, and research.

NURSE PRACTITIONER PROGRAMS "A nurse practitioner (NP) is a registered nurse (RN) with additional education and experience in health assessment, diagnosis and management of illnesses and injuries, including ordering tests and prescribing drugs"(Canadian Nurses Association & Canadian Institute for Health Information [CNA & CIHI], 2005, p. 2). Originally meant to prepare nurses to work in northern nursing stations, nurse practitioner programs were available as early as 1967 at Dalhousie University. However, these programs did not survive largely because of societal factors, such as a perceived oversupply of physicians, lack of corresponding legislation, and lack of support from policymakers in medicine and in nursing (CNA & CIHI, 2006). Currently, all provinces and territories with the exception of Yukon have legislation and regulations regarding NP status in place or in progress. Although NP programs in some provinces are offered at the postdiploma (RN) level, there is a growing trend to have NP programs offered at the master's level. In 2005, 61% of licensed NPs had a baccalaureate degree, and 22.9% reported a master's degree or higher level of education (CNA & CIHI, 2006).

DOCTORAL PROGRAMS Doctorally and postdoctorally prepared nurses are needed in both academic and practice settings to educate nurses at the baccalaureate and master's levels. The number of these programs is increasing in Canada. One of the primary benefits of doctorally prepared nurses is that they can undertake research, which advances nursing knowledge and evidence-informed practice. As of 2004, approximately 0.1% of registered nurses reported being educated at the doctoral level in the discipline (CIHI, 2005) and even fewer at the postdoctoral level. Until recently, nurses were limited in their choice of doctoral programs in nursing and many completed a doctor of philosophy (PhD) degree in other disciplines, such as sociology, psychology, or education. Doctoral programs in nursing, which award PhDs, began in the 1960s in the United States. These programs further prepare the nurse for advanced clinical practice, administration, education, and research. Today, doctoral and postdoctoral education for nurses within their own discipline is available in Canadian universities and research centres.

Content and approach vary among doctoral and postdoctoral programs. Some focus on the usual clinical areas, such as acute care or gerontology nursing, and others emphasize such nontraditional areas as transcultural nursing. Some programs emphasize theory development, but all emphasize research.

LICENSED PRACTICAL NURSING PROGRAMS Practical nurses are educated and licensed or registered in all provinces and territories. Although LPNs/RPNs have programs of varying lengths, the trend is moving to a 2-year program leading to a diploma in practical nursing. Entrance requirements vary across the provinces and territories but usually include a high-school diploma. Practical nursing educational programs have a tradition of being very innovative in providing education at multiple sites within each jurisdiction. Bridging programs for practical nurses who want to obtain their baccalaureate in nursing are becoming more formalized. One of the leaders in this effort is Ontario, where several programs have recently been initiated.

REGISTERED PSYCHIATRIC NURSING PROGRAMS RPNs are educated and licensed in the four Western provinces. Educational programs specific to psychiatric nursing began in Canada in the 1920s. Application requirements generally include a high school diploma. RPNs are educated at the diploma or baccalaureate level. A significant number of RPNs go on to complete graduate-level education, although no graduate programs specific to psychiatric nursing are currently available.

Nursing Associations and Their Influence on Education

Several national nursing associations have influenced nursing education in Canada through their funding of research, pilot education projects, and policy development. These include the CNA, Practical Nurses Canada, Registered Psychiatric Nurses of Canada, and the Canadian Association of Schools of Nursing (CASN). Although the organizations for practical and psychiatric nurses tend to more strongly influence the education of their own constituents, the CNA and CASN have influenced registered nursing education at all levels. See the Reflect on Primary Health Care box.

> **REFLECT ON PRIMARY HEALTH CARE**
>
> Schools of nursing in Canada generally use a conceptual framework as a guide for their curriculum. Some schools of nursing have chosen to use primary health care as one of the foundations for their conceptual framework or their curricula.

Canadian Nurses Association

As early as 1895, a desire was expressed to create a group that would facilitate the integration of francophones and nurses from all provinces and that would represent the nurses of Canada. In 1908, the Canadian National Association of Trained Nurses (Cohen, 2000) became that organization. From this beginning, the CNA is now a federation of 11 provincial and territorial registered nurses' associations, representing more than 133 500 Canadian RNs (CNA, 2007) (see Chapter 1). Quebec nurses do not belong to the CNA.

The CNA has influenced nursing education in Canada in several key areas. Its co-sponsorship of the Weir Report (1932) is one example. In addition, in 1948, the CNA, with financing from the Red Cross, established the Metropolitan School of Nursing in Windsor, Ontario (Jensen, 2007). This demonstration school was Canada's first independent school of nursing, separated financially and physically from the hospital. This pioneer project led to the establishment of the first nursing program in an educational setting in Canada at the Ryerson Institute of Technology in 1963. The growth of similar independent schools of nursing in Canada was delayed until the community college was developed in the 1970s and 1980s. As education is under provincial and territorial jurisdiction, it is through the provincial and territorial registered nurses associations that approval of basic nursing education programs occurs. Approval by the provincial or territorial body ensures that programs meet minimal standards and allows graduates from a specific program, on graduation, to write the CRNE or the Ordre des infirmières et infirmiers du Québec exams in Quebec. This approval must be renewed on a regular basis. Recently, the CNA, in conjunction with the provincial and territorial bodies, completed a project on entry-level competencies. From this project, each jurisdiction completed and endorsed a set of competencies for new RN graduates. Schools of nursing use these competencies as a basis for their curricula, and the CRNE is based on the national competencies.

Another influence of the CNA on nursing education is *certification*, which is a voluntary and periodic process (recertification) by which an organized specialty group verifies that a registered nurse has demonstrated competence in a nursing specialty by having met identified standards of that specialty. Certification was initiated by a CNA membership request in June 1980 through a biennial resolution that directed the board of directors to study the feasibility of developing examinations for certification in major nursing specialties. In 1982, the board of directors adopted a policy of accreditation in nursing as well as a recommendation that the CNA promote the development of certification in nursing specialties (CNA, 1982). The first certification was offered in occupational health nursing. Currently, certification is offered in 17 specialty areas: cardiovascular, community health, critical care, critical care pediatrics, emergency, gastroenterology, gerontology, hospice palliative care, nephrology, neuroscience, occupational health, oncology, orthopedics, perinatal, perioperative, psychiatric or mental health, and rehabilitation. In Quebec, the two first specialty certifications will be available in mental health and in the prevention and control of infections.

The Canadian Association of Schools of Nursing

In 1942, the Provisional Council of University Schools and Departments was formed. The name of the organization was changed in 1971 to the Canadian Association of University Schools of Nursing, with a mandate in 1973 to provide accreditation to university nursing programs in Canada. In 2002, in recognition of the collaborative partnerships that had evolved as part of the entry to practice legislation in several provinces, the name was revised to the Canadian Association of Schools of Nursing (CASN) (Canadian Association of Schools of Nursing [CASN], 2006a). Today, the 91 member schools deliver all or part of a baccalaureate degree in nursing. The purpose of the CASN is *to lead nursing education and nursing scholarship in the interest of healthier Canadians.* To that end, the CASN (1) speaks for Canadian nursing education and scholarship; (2) establishes and promotes national standards of excellence for nursing education; (3) promotes the advancement of nursing knowledge; (4) facilitates the integration of theory, research, and practice; (5) contributes to public policy; and (6) provides a national forum for issues in nursing education and research (CASN, 2006b).

Through its baccalaureate accreditation program, revised in 2005, the CASN provides national standards of excellence for programs of baccalaureate nursing education to use in self and peer evaluation. Although accreditation is voluntary in most jurisdictions, some have mandated that CASN accreditation function as approval in that province or territory. Ontario was the first province to do so. The CASN has also published several position papers on nursing education topics, which schools use to plan curricula and shape new programs. The CASN is a founding member of the Global Alliance for Nursing Education and Scholarship (GANES), an organization that provides a global forum to discuss issues of concern for nursing education programs worldwide.

Canadian Nursing Students' Association

The Canadian Nursing Students' Association (CNSA) is a national organization. With more than 20 000 members, the CNSA is an affiliate member of the CNA and Practical Nurses Canada. The CNSA has a close working relationship with the CASN and is a co-chair of the New Health Professionals Network (CNSA, 2004). The CNSA maintains an influence on nursing education through its partnership with other national and international organizations.

Issues Facing Nursing Education

Nursing education is facing a number of formidable and complex issues, partly because the changes that are generally occurring within Canadian society and education have implications for professional nursing practice. Nurses must be knowledgeable about both the changes in and the issues facing education. They must be able to use critical thinking skills to talk about these issues so that they can actively engage in addressing them, for their resolution will help to shape the nursing profession.

Changes in Health-Care Needs

Shifts are occurring within health care in Canada today. Whether or not a person agrees with the futuristic pictures painted in such documents as *Toward 2020* (Villeneuve & MacDonald, 2006), it is clear that nursing in the future will be different from what we see today. One anticipated change is the shift away from acute-care services toward primary health care. The second is the shift toward community-based care, including home care services, for clients. Clients are being discharged from hospital with higher acuity levels and more complex care needs. Nurses need to work collaboratively and interprofessionally. A third shift is the aging of the Canadian population. Partly because of these shifts, nurses are involved in new roles, such as acting as case manager, program manager, or community developer. These new roles are in addition to the administrative functions that many nurses are currently performing, such as participating on boards, chairing committees, and preparing budgets. These shifts influence the content of nursing education programs, for students require skills to support these roles.

Entry to Practice

In 1982, the CNA approved the following policy statement regarding the future educational requirements for RNs: "The Canadian Nurses Association believes that by the year 2000 the minimum educational requirement for entry into the practice of nursing should be the successful completion of a baccalaureate degree in nursing" (CNA, 1982).

The CNA's position was based on an examination of the future health needs of the country and the type of nursing services that would be required to meet them. Nurses' associations in every province and territory supported this policy (see the Nursing and Canadian Society box). In 2004, CASN and the CNA issued a joint statement supporting the baccalaureate degree as the **entry-to-practice** credential in Canada (CASN & CNA, 2004).

In 1991, Premier McKenna of New Brunswick became the first premier to commit his government to support the baccalaureate degree as entry point into nursing by the year 2000. The following year, 1992, Prince Edward Island became the first province to achieve the goal of a baccalaureate degree as the minimal level of entry into nursing. However, in March 2000, Manitoba's government announced a 23-month diploma program as part of their five-point plan to address the nursing shortage. This move was in direct opposition to the CNA entry-to-practice position. A month earlier, Saskatchewan nurses saw a compromise reached among the provincial government, the Saskatchewan Registered Nurses' Association (SRNA), and the Nursing Education Program of Saskatchewan (NEPS) that protected the nursing degree but offered options regarding accelerated completion of the nursing program. RNs and nursing students had made strong protests over the provincial government's plan to restore diploma education as the entry-level requirement. In 2007, only Quebec and Manitoba did not endorse the baccalaureate as entry to practice. Legislation is in place to change entry to practice to baccalaureate in Alberta by 2010.

A Shortage Crisis

The number of places for nursing students in educational facilities across Canada has risen slightly in recent years, yet the number of graduates remains inadequate to replace those nurses who are leaving the profession and to meet the health needs of clients. The number of nursing graduates peaked in the early 1970s and has substantively decreased since then. By the end of 2006, the CNA estimated that around 5800 Canadian-educated graduates wrote the CRNE (CNA, 2007), and more than 3700 wrote the Quebec registration exam in 2007 (Ordre des infirmières et infirmiers du Québec, 2007, 2008). The number of graduates remains lower than required.

A number of initiatives are addressing this trend. The CNA assumed a lead role with other nursing and non-nursing groups as the secretariat of the study entitled *The Nursing Labour Market in Canada: An Occupational Sector Study* (CNA, 1999). The goal of the study was to produce an integrated labour market strategy for the three regulated nursing groups in Canada (LPNs/RPNs, RPNs, and RNs). The second-entry programs described earlier were implemented partially because of the nursing shortage.

The nursing shortage is a global concern. The issue includes such questions as, What is the best educational preparation for a nurse? Should we re-examine the scopes of practice? What are the ethical implications of recruitment of nurses from other countries?

Changing Demographics in Nursing Programs

Student populations in nursing programs are changing. Aboriginal students, older students, male students, and students with disabilities are enrolling in increasing numbers. In addition, more students are working throughout their programs to obtain the funds required for tuition and living expenses. These changes mean that nurse educators have to address the needs of diverse groups of learners, and nursing programs will have to continue to change. More options are being explored that permit

NURSING AND CANADIAN SOCIETY

Fact	Implications for Nursing Practice
The baccalaureate requirement as entry to practice for registered nurses has been adopted throughout Canada by the majority of provincial and territorial nurses' associations.	Students and RNs need to be aware that opportunities and graduate study will be open to those with a baccalaureate degree in nursing.
Nurses in Canada can obtain a PhD or a post-doctoral within their discipline at a number of Canadian universities.	PhD preparation supports nurses becoming educators and researchers by providing the theoretical knowledge and the practical experience for the roles.
Nursing specialty certification is offered through the CNA certification program.	Employment and personal satisfaction at work may be supported by certification.

part-time study and allow students to work while attending school. Many programs are now offering distributed learning courses as an alternative to traditional modes of learning.

Until recently, few Aboriginal people from Northern Canada entered the nursing profession. To provide for Inuit nurses, Nunavut Arctic College in Iqaluit and the School of Nursing at Dalhousie University collaborated on a 4-year baccalaureate program. The program admitted its first class of Inuit students in October 1999. Another solution has been to work within established programs, offering support to Aboriginal students. One such program is Native Access Program to Nursing/Medicine (NAPN/M) at the University of Saskatchewan, begun in 1985. Congruent with the province having the highest population percentage of Aboriginal persons, this nursing program offered support to more than 116 Aboriginal baccalaureate nursing students and 9 medical students (College of Nursing, University of Saskatchewan, n.d.).

The average age of nurse educators in Canada is moving toward retirement, and active efforts to recruit more are underway. Current initiatives include additional PhD programs in nursing. Serious questions are being asked of nursing programs about where they will recruit future faculty members and how they will be prepared to teach.

Technological Advancements

The growth of technology is influencing nursing education. Advances in web-based technology and computer-assisted instruction offer the potential for flexible, self-directed, interactive learning activities for students in on-site nursing programs. Computer-mediated distance education also makes it possible for nursing programs to offer courses over a large geographic area through the use of a computer network or the internet. This method is a relative newcomer to nursing education. However, by 2004, 41 programs were offered in full or part by distance technology. Twenty of these were baccalaureate, 16 were master's programs, and 5 were PhD programs. Some programs may also include videoconferencing and other means of distance learning. For nurses who already hold a degree, computer-mediated instruction supports continuing education opportunities.

Another technological advancement important to nursing is the use of high-fidelity simulation within nursing education programs. Considered an adjunct learning opportunity for students, these highly technical mannequins allow nursing students and graduates to practise specific skills in a safe environment. The use of additional virtual technology offers further opportunities to engage learners in realistic situations where critical thinking and problem-solving skills can be practised.

Evidence-Informed Practice

How Can Nurses in Rural and Remote Areas Access Continuing Education?

Penz et al. (2007) undertook a national survey to examine the practice of registered nurses in rural and remote areas of Canada. As part of the survey, nurses were asked about participation in continuing education. Sixty-seven percent of respondents perceived barriers to participation. An open-ended question was used to ask the respondents to identify the barriers. After content analysis, three main themes were identified: (1) rural community and work life—which included isolation, low numbers of staff, and availability of education; (2) time constraints; and (3) financial constraints. The researchers further examined the demographic characteristics of those who perceived barriers and found that they "included those who were between 30 and 59 years of age, were single, divorced, widowed, had obtained a higher degree of nursing education, at the baccalaureate, master's, or doctoral level, had dependent children or relatives, worked in full-time or permanent positions, and did not feel they had enough opportunities or employer encouragement to attend CE activities" (p. 63).

NURSING IMPLICATIONS: Participation in continuing education could be increased with attention to the identified barriers. However, employer support is necessary to address most of the identified barriers.

Source: Based on "Barriers to Participating in Continuing Education Activities among Rural and Remote Nurses," by K. Penz, C. D'Arcy, N. Stewart, J. Kosteniuk, D. Morgan, and B. Smith, 2007, *Journal of Continuing Education in Nursing, 38*(2), pp. 58–66.

Interprofessional Education

Nurses have long recognized that they need to work with other health professionals to deliver quality care to their patients. More recently, however, health professionals and other stakeholders, such as government, have advanced the notion that if health professionals are educated together, they will have a greater understanding of the roles each plays and be able to work together more effectively in the health-care workplace. Several health educational programs have already pioneered work in this area, and Health Canada has initiated the Interprofessional Education for Collaborative Patient-Centred Practice (IECPCP) program. The IECPCP program, among other activities, has funded 20 research programs at various sites in Canada to pilot, implement, and evaluate strategies to increase **interprofessional education** and evaluate its effectiveness (Health Canada, 2007). Results from these studies will surely influence how nursing and other health professional education is planned, implemented, and delivered.

Continuing Education to Maintain Competency

To provide competent nursing care (see Box 2.1), an RN must continually enhance the knowledge, skills, and critical thinking required to meet client needs in a changing health-care system. Each jurisdiction and group of nurses has put in place continuing competency requirements for licence or registration renewal. Continuing education or lifelong learning is a strategy to achieve this goal. The CNA interprets **continuing nursing education** as consisting of planned learning experiences undertaken following a basic nursing education. Acknowledging the need to ensure safe practice, the CNA published *A National Framework for Continuing Competency Programs for Registered Nurses* in September 2000. The framework represents a consensus of nursing regulatory bodies in all provinces and territories, including Quebec.

Continuing education is the responsibility of each practising nurse and the employer. The CNA advocates the voluntary participation of nurses in continuing education in which they select learning activities based on their own experiences, learning styles, and practice requirements. Constant updating and growth are essential to keep on top of scientific and technological changes, as well as changes within the nursing profession. A variety of educational and health-care institutions conduct continuing education programs. They are usually designed to meet one or more of the following needs: (1) to keep nurses abreast of new techniques and competence; (2) to help nurses attain expertise in a specialized area of practice, such as intensive care nursing or community nursing; and (3) to provide nurses with information essential to nursing practice, for example, knowledge about the legal aspects of nursing.

Mandatory versus voluntary continuing education has been a topic of interest to practising nurses, educators, administrators, professional and regulatory associations, unions, and governments. Most registered, psychiatric, and licensed practical nursing jurisdictions in Canada view continuing education itself as voluntary and a strong link in a mandatory continuing competency or professional development program.

BOX 2.1 EDUCATIONAL SUPPORT FOR COMPETENT NURSING PRACTICE

The competence of RNs is an essential element of safe and quality nursing practice. Competence is defined as a way to act with the necessary knowledge and skills in a certain context (Le Boterf, 2006; Tardif, 1997).

Competence is one of the main aspects to consider when evaluating quality of care. To practise safely and competently, RNs comply with professional standards, base their practice on relevant knowledge, and, in adherence with the *Code of Ethics for Registered Nurses*, acquire new skills and knowledge in their area of practice on a continuing basis.

BOX 2.2 IN-SERVICE PROGRAMS

In-service programs are run by employers to provide information to employees and have the following characteristics:

- They may address client needs and emerging trends.
- They are usually conducted within a facility.
- Attendance may be mandatory.

In-Service Education

An **in-service education** program is administered by an employer and is designed to upgrade the knowledge or skills of employees (see Box 2.2). For example, an employer might offer an in-service program to inform nurses about a new piece of equipment, about specific isolation practices, or about methods of implementing a nurse theorist's conceptual framework for nursing. Some in-service programs are mandatory, such as cardiopulmonary resuscitation and fire safety programs.

Case Study 2

A friend, knowing that you are a nursing student, tells you that he or she is considering nursing school and wants your advice.

Critical Thinking Questions

1. What questions would you ask before responding?
2. What did you consider when choosing your nursing educational program?

After working through these questions, go to the MyNursingLab at **http://www.mynursinglab.com** to check your answers.

KEY TERMS

baccalaureate nursing degrees
licensing examination
internationally educated nurses
diploma programs
master's programs
entry to practice
interprofessional education
continuing nursing education
in-service education

CHAPTER HIGHLIGHTS

- Nursing education has changed dramatically since the mid-nineteenth century. Early apprenticeship programs established in the nineteenth century were designed to meet the service needs of the hospital, not the educational needs of the students. Today, nursing education is provided primarily in college and university settings independent of hospitals' needs.
- Although baccalaureate programs began in the early twentieth century, baccalaureate education began to take hold only after the release of the Weir Report in 1932. Master's and doctoral programs in nursing grew significantly in the latter part of the twentieth century. Admission requirements, lengths of programs, curricula, and costs for these programs vary considerably.
- Nursing education curricula are continually being revised in response to new scientific knowledge and technological, cultural, political, and socioeconomic changes in society.
- Continuing education is the responsibility of each practising nurse to keep abreast of scientific and technological changes, as well as changes within the nursing profession.

ASSESS YOUR LEARNING

1. The first English university nursing educational program was opened in 1919 at which of the following?
a. The University of Western Ontario
b. McGill University
c. University of British Columbia
d. University of Toronto

2. What was one of the greatest influences on the evolution of registered nursing education programs in Canadian history?
a. The requirements of the regulatory bodies
b. The introduction of the nursing unions
c. The recommendations of the Weir Report
d. The creation of the Mack Training School

3. Which of the following would be the best example of continuing education?
a. A course on leadership offered at a college or university
b. A course given by the employer on the new electronic charting
c. CPR recertification offered by a community agency
d. A course in fitness offered through community services

4. Can a student from another discipline and another university become a registered nurse, and how is this possible?
a. Yes, with an accelerated or compressed degree in nursing
b. No, there are no specific programs available for this student
c. Yes, but the student will need to return to university for a refresher course
d. Yes, if they succeed in passing the national examination

5. The term *entry to practice* refers to which of the following?
a. The amount of time spent in training for the profession
b. The courses required by the educational institution
c. The level of education required to achieve licensure
d. The curriculum required by the accreditation process

6. Which of the following is the purpose of achieving certification?
a. Advanced standing in a graduate nursing program
b. As a requirement for becoming a head or charge nurse
c. To acquire new skills in assessment and evaluation
d. To gain specialized knowledge in a specific area of nursing

7. Accreditation of baccalaureate nursing programs is the mandate of which of the following?
a. CASN

b. CNA
c. Each school of nursing
d. The provincial or territorial governments

8. A nurse who has a nurse practitioner designation has completed additional education to do which of the following?
   a. Prescribe common drugs and order common diagnostic tests
   b. Serve as principal investigator on a funded research project
   c. Teach in graduate nursing programs
   d. Provide high-level leadership in a practice setting

9. Which of the following has responsibility for continuing education?
   a. The college or university
   b. The employing agency
   c. The practising nurse
   d. The professional organization

10. The major impetus for moving nursing education programs away from the hospital setting was which of the following?
   a. To demonstrate the value of apprenticeship models of education to postsecondary institutions
   b. To force physicians to come to the university to teach
   c. To enable the profession to gain control over the educational process
   d. To remove the influence of religious groups over nursing

After working through these questions, go to the MyNursingLab at ***http://www.mynursinglab.com*** *to check your answers and see explanations.*

SUGGESTED READINGS

Canadian Nurses Association press release. (1932). Some features of the report on the survey of nursing education in Canada. *Canadian Nurse, XXVII,* 127–131.

This summary of the *Survey of Nursing Education in Canada,* commonly called the Weir Report, was released to the press in February 1932. It provides a brief historical overview of the status of nursing education in Çanada and the focus on hospital training. It is considered a key stimulus for the movement of nursing education into academic facilities.

WEBLINKS

Canadian Association of Schools of Nursing

http://www.casn.ca/media.php?mid=200

The Canadian Association of Schools of Nursing is a voluntary association representing all universities and colleges that offer undergraduate and graduate programs in nursing. This site lists the programs offered by its members.

Canadian Nurses Association

http://www.cna-nurses.ca

This is the website for the national nursing association in Canada.

Canadian Nursing Students' Association

http://www.cnsa.ca

The site is host to the national association for nursing students in Canada.

Practical Nurses Canada

http://www.pncanada.ca

This site is the national organization of practical nurse organizations across Canada.

Registered Psychiatric Nurses of Canada

http://www.rpnc.ca/pages/education/education.php

This site of the Registered Psychiatric Nurses of Canada has a national listing of psychiatric nursing education programs.

REFERENCES

Baumgart, A. J., & Larsen, J. (Eds.). (1992). *Canadian nursing faces the future* (2nd ed.). Toronto: C. V. Mosby.

Canadian Association of Schools of Nursing. (2006a). *CASN/ACESI historical milestones.* Retrieved May 22, 2007, from http://www.casn.ca/content.php?doc=98

Canadian Association of Schools of Nursing. (2006b). *CASN/ACESI mission.* Retrieved May 22, 2007, from http://www.casn.ca/content.php?sec=1

Canadian Association of Schools of Nursing & Canadian Nurses Association. (2004). *Educational preparation for entry to practice.* Retrieved May 22, 2007, from http://www.casn.ca/media.php?mid=202

Canadian Institute for Health Information. (2005). *Workforce trends of registered nurses in Canada, 2005.* Ottawa: Author.

Canadian Institute for Health Information. (2007). *Highlights from the regulated nursing workforce in Canada, 2006.* Ottawa: Author

Canadian Nurses Association. (1982). *The definition and purposes of the CNA certification program.* Ottawa: Author.

Canadian Nurses Association. (1999). *The nursing labour market in Canada: An occupational sector study.* Ottawa: Author.

Canadian Nurses Association. (2000). *A national framework for continuing competency programs for registered nurses.* Ottawa: Author.

Canadian Nurses Association. (2007). *CRNE bulletin (#10).* Retrieved April 14, 2008, from http://www.cna-nurses.ca/CNA/documents/pdf/publications/CRNE-Bulletin-September-2007-e.pdf

Canadian Nurses Association & Canadian Institute for Health Information. (2005). *The supply and regulation of nurse practitioners in Canada.* Ottawa: Author.

Canadian Nurses Association & Canadian Institute for Health Information. (2006). *The regulation and supply of nurse practitioners in Canada: 2006 Update.* Ottawa: Author.

Canadian Nursing Students' Association. (2004). *The Canadian Nursing Students' Association.* Retrieved May 22, 2007, from http://www.cnsa.ca

Cohen, Y. (2000). *Profession infirmière: Une histoire des soins dans les hôpitaux du Québec.* Montréal: Les presses de l'Université de Montréal.

College of Nursing, University of Saskatchewan. (n.d.). *Native access program to nursing/medicine.* Retrieved April 14, 2008, from http://www.usask.ca/nursing/napn/index.htm

Health Canada. (2007). *Interprofessional education for collaborative patient-centred practice.* Retrieved May 22, 2007, from http://www.hc-sc.gc.ca/hcs-sss/hhr-rhs/strateg/interprof/index_e.htmlHealth

Jensen, P. M. (2007). *Nursing.* Canadian Encyclopedia Historica. Retrieved May 22, 2007, from http://www.thecanadianencyclopedia.com/index.cfm?PgNm=TCE&Params=A1SEC825469

Le Boterf, G. (2006). *Contruire les compétences individuelles et collectives* (4e éd.). Paris, France: Éditions d'Organisation.

Mussalem, H. (1960). *Spotlight on nursing education.* Ottawa: Canadian Nurses Association.

Ordre des infirmières et infirmiers du Québec. (2007). Dossiers de l'OIIQ. *Le Scribe,* 9(3), 2, retrieved April 20, 2008, from http://www.oiiq.org/uploads/periodiques/Scribe/scribev9no3.pdf

Ordre des infirmières et infirmiers du Québec. (2008). Dossiers de l'OIIQ. *Le Scribe,* 10(1), 2, retrieved April 20, 2008, from http://www.oiiq.org/uploads/periodiques/Scribe/scribev10no1.pdf

Street, M. M. (1973). *Watch-fires on the mountains: The life and writings of Ethel Johns.* Toronto: University of Toronto Press.

Tardif, J. (1997). *Pour un enseignement stratégique: l'apport de la psychologie cognitive.* Montréal: Éditions Logiques Inc.

Villeneuve, M., & MacDonald, J. (2006). *Toward 2020: Visions for nursing.* Ottawa: Canadian Nurses Association.

Weir, G. M. (1932). *Survey of nursing education in Canada.* Toronto: University of Toronto Press.

Chapter 3

Nursing Research in Canada

Nurses are actively generating, publishing, and applying research in practice to improve client care and enhance nursing's scientific knowledge base. The use of research has three main benefits for clients: it helps nurses understand the client's situation more thoroughly, assess more accurately, and intervene more effectively. *Nursing research* findings not only improve client care but also affect the health-care system itself. For example, research studies have demonstrated the cost-effectiveness of registered nurses as health-care providers.

OBJECTIVES

After studying this chapter, you should be able to

1. Summarize the concepts and language of research
2. Identify common research methods used in clinical inquiries
3. Describe the way that theory, research, and practice interrelate
4. State the significance of research to the practice of nursing
5. List seven ways the nurse can participate in research activities in practice
6. Differentiate the quantitative approach and the qualitative approach in nursing research
7. Analyze the nurse's role in protecting the rights of human subjects in research
8. Outline the 11 steps of the research process

Nursing Research

The Canadian Nurses Association (CNA) is committed to promoting research as the foundation for clinical practice. Reading research, evaluating the results of research studies, and, where appropriate, integrating new findings into practice are necessary competencies of professional nursing practice (see Box 3.1). Nurses who base their clinical decisions on current, scientifically obtained evidence are being professionally accountable. **Research-based nursing practice** simply means nursing practice that is informed by valid and reliable research findings obtained from scientific investigations. The term *evidence-based practice,* or evidence-based decision making, is gaining popularity in nursing and, in some cases, is preferred to research-based practice. **Evidence-based practice** or **evidence-informed practice** is "broadly defined as the use of the best clinical evidence in making patient care decisions" (Loiselle, Profetto-McGrath, Polit, & Beck, 2007, p. 4). In recent years, the emphasis has increased on integrating appropriate evidence into practice to inform decisions and policymaking, advance the quality of care, and achieve the best possible outcomes for patients, regardless of setting. Although evidence generated by findings from research studies is of primary importance, it is not the only source of knowledge used by nurses. Carper (1978) identified four patterns of nursing knowledge that are essential to nurses: empirical, aesthetic, personal, and moral.

BOX 3.1 COMPETENCIES RELATED TO USE OF EVIDENCE IN PRACTICE

The Canadian Nurses Association's Canadian Registered Nurse Examination (2007) includes the following competencies:

PROFESSIONAL PRACTICE COMPETENCIES:

PP-38 provides rationale for nursing care actions and decisions based on theoretical and evidence-based knowledge from nursing, health sciences, and related disciplines.

PP-40 reads and participates in critiquing evidence-based literature in nursing, health sciences, and related disciplines (i.e., research articles and reports).

NURSING PRACTICE HEALTH AND WELLNESS COMPETENCIES:

HW-13 incorporates research findings about health risks and risk reduction into plan of care.

HW-18 provides evidence-based health-related information to the person.

NURSING PRACTICE ALTERATIONS IN HEALTH COMPETENCIES:

AH-22 uses evidence-based information to assist the person to understand interventions and their relationship to expected outcomes (e.g., possible risks and benefits, discomforts, inconveniences, costs).

Source: From *Canadian Registered Nurse Examination Competences,* by the Canadian Nurses Association, 2007, Ottawa: Author. Copyright 2007 by the Canadian Nurses Association.

When nurses have a question they want to answer to provide better care to their clients, they can do nursing research. **Nursing research** is the systematic, objective investigation of phenomena (experiences, events, or circumstances) of importance to nursing, with the goal of improving practice. Research can be classified, according to the purpose of the study, as *basic* or *applied.* **Basic research** is concerned with generating knowledge and is sometimes called pure research. **Applied research** is concerned with using knowledge to solve immediate problems. Nurse researchers employ a variety of research approaches to substantiate existing knowledge and to discover new knowledge. The two primary approaches are termed *qualitative* and *quantitative.*

Research is different from problem solving. **Problem solving** is specific to a given situation in which alternatives are explored and chosen, and immediate action is taken. Knowledge gained from research is transferable to other situations. The body of knowledge called nursing science and the growth and development of professional nursing depend on research undertaken by nurses.

Although the focus for *all* nurses is the use of research findings in practice, the level of participation in research depends on the nurse's educational level, position, experience, and practical environment. Refer to "Developing Research-Based Practice" in this chapter for specific examples of ways in which nurses participate in research.

The History

As early as 1854, Florence Nightingale demonstrated the importance of research in the delivery of nursing care. When Nightingale arrived in the Crimea in November 1854, she found the military hospital barracks overcrowded, filthy, rat- and flea-infested, and lacking in food, drugs, and essential medical supplies. As a result of these conditions, men died from starvation and such diseases as dysentery, cholera, and typhus (Woodham-Smith, 1950). By systematically collecting, organizing, and reporting data, Nightingale was able to institute sanitary reforms and significantly reduce mortality rates from contagious diseases. Although the Nightingale tradition influenced the establishment of Canadian nursing schools, the research approach did not take hold until the beginning of the twentieth century.

Nursing research has become a significant activity in Canada. The First National Nursing Research Conference was held in 1971 in Ottawa. It was organized by the University of British Columbia School of Nursing and supported by the federal Department of Health and Welfare. Only one of the invited speakers, Dr. Faye Abdellah, was a nurse. This international nursing leader offered a historical perspective of nursing research in the United States. As a result of the conference, the first Centre for Nursing Research in Canada was established at McGill University in Montreal with monies from the federal government.

Historically, research activity in nursing developed slowly as the result of a gradual increase in the number of nurses with research expertise. Because nurses were not prepared to conduct research, many early studies in nursing were conducted by members of other disciplines. Today, nursing research is developing at a more rapid pace, and most nursing research is initiated in university settings because of faculty members' preparation as researchers.

In 2000, Donaldson reviewed breakthroughs in research over four decades and noted that many nurse scientists have played a key role in shaping nursing practice. The breakthroughs have occurred in diverse areas, including personal and family health, child development, dementia care, and pain management.

Linking Theory, Practice, and Research

An interrelationship exists among nursing research, theory, and practice. Research can be used to demonstrate that one nursing practice intervention is more effective than another. Examples of changes in nursing practice motivated by research include the following:

- Changes to the use of indwelling catheters and the management of incontinence among older adults to promote quality of life (Fultz & Herzog, 2001; Newman, 2006)
- Inclusion of patients in the decision-making process to facilitate full participation in the treatment plan (Florin, Ehrenberg, & Ehnfors, 2006)
- Implementation of multiple strategies, including the use of technology to enhance patient learning (Lewis, 2003)
- Development of least-restraint policies to reduce falls (Rask et al., 2007)
- Development of patient-education material to promote successful postoperative pain management (Richards & Hubbert, 2007)

Research ideas, while often born in practice, also come from the nursing literature and nursing theory. Published articles about nursing research may stimulate questions, which lead to interest in further studies. Nursing theorists also generate research questions, since they piece together ideas that explain why something happens. Their explanations are tested, through research, to see if they are credible enough to be useful in clinical practice.

Hospitals and health-care agencies have begun to formally define the link between nursing research and practice. The strategies include the cross-appointment of faculty among hospitals, health-care agencies, and universities; the implementation of programs to develop staff nurses as users of research in their practice; the establishment of ethics committees to review research proposals; the appointment of unit research coordinators; the establishment of nursing research committees; the development of strategic plans for nursing research; and the use of evidence-based decision-making models in practice settings. These strategies create an environment to support evidence-informed practice.

Support for Nursing Research

Nursing research costs money. Computer and library services, data collection, statistical consultation, employment of research assistants, and release time for researchers from their regular work responsibilities can be expensive. While funding sources have developed, financial support is still difficult to obtain, especially for new researchers. Collaborative, interdisciplinary studies have a greater chance of receiving financial support than research conducted only by registered nurses. Insufficient funds to support research are an obstacle for nursing research.

One of the earliest funding sources for nurse researchers was the Alberta Foundation for Nursing Research (AFNR), established by the Alberta government in the 1980s. It existed for a decade and was the only Canadian foundation specifically designed to fund nursing research. It served as the model for subsequent research funding for nurses and was instrumental in the development of graduate programs, especially doctoral programs, in this country.

Today, funds for nursing research come from several nursing sources. At the provincial and territorial level, research funding varies a great deal across the country. A few provincial nursing associations have developed some capacity for the funding of nursing research. Nationally, the Canadian Nurses Foundation funds research. Specialty groups, such as the Canadian Gerontological Nursing Association, also provide financial assistance for their members to conduct research.

Several non-nursing provincial, territorial, and federal agencies accept proposals that meet their funding guidelines when submitted by qualified nurse researchers. These include the Social Sciences and Humanities Research Council (SSHRC), Canadian Health Services Research Foundation (CHSRF), and the Canadian Institutes of Health Research (CIHR). The SSHRC is a federal agency that promotes and supports university-based research in social sciences and humanities, including health. The CHSRF was founded by Industry Canada under the Canada Corporation Act. Its mandate is to sponsor applied health systems research and to facilitate its use in evidence-based decision making. Although not composed solely of nurses, it has strong relevance to the profession because it administers the Nursing Research Fund. The fund's objectives are to develop nursing's research capacity, to sponsor research on nursing issues, and to disseminate nursing research knowledge.

The CIHR was established by an Act of Parliament in 2000 and is Canada's foremost federal agency for health research. Its predecessor was the Medical Research Council. Its goal is to excel in the creation of new knowledge and its translation into improved health for Canadians. The CIHR's goal is based on a broad definition of health and includes biomedical and clinical research, health systems and services research, and population health research. These areas are of interest to nurse researchers. Other recent funding endeavours include the Canadian Foundation for Innovation (CFI), a nonprofit corporation funded by the federal government beginning in 1997 to enable Canada's research community to conduct research and develop technology.

The CHSRF and CNA have allocated significant funds for the development of the Canadian Nursing Knowledge Network (CNKN). This initiative will enhance the CNA's capacity to disseminate relevant research to nurses. Foundations and voluntary associations, such as the Canadian Cancer Society and the Kidney Foundation of Canada, are other sources of funds for nurse researchers. (See the Nursing and Canadian Society box.)

NURSING AND CANADIAN SOCIETY

Fact	Implications for Nursing Practice
The Canadian Association of Nurse Researchers (CANR) is a national organization with representation from every province and territory.	Nurses need to participate in associations that promote the use of research in practice.
The CHSRF (1) funds management and policy research in health services and nursing; (2) supports the synthesis and dissemination of research results; and (3) supports the use of research results by managers and decision makers.	Nurses interested in research need to be aware of funding opportunities.
In 1969, Moyra Allen of McGill University founded the first Canadian scholarly nursing journal. Initially known as *Nursing Papers*, the journal is now known as the *Canadian Journal of Nursing Research*.	The reading of research studies promotes knowledge of Canadian nursing and how to meet the health-care needs of clients.

Approaches to Nursing Research

The two predominant research approaches are quantitative and qualitative. *Quantitative research* is generally considered objective and uses data-gathering techniques that can be verified by others. *Qualitative research* is more subjective, which means that qualitative researchers study things in their natural settings, attempting to make sense of phenomena in terms of the meanings people bring to them. Although today both approaches are valued within the nursing research community, in the past, nurse researchers primarily conducted quantitative research.

These approaches originate from different philosophical perspectives and use different methods for the collection and analysis of data.

QUANTITATIVE RESEARCH **Quantitative research** is a systematic, logical approach to studying phenomena that lend themselves to precise measurement by using quantification and statistical analysis (Berman, Snyder, Kozier, & Erb, 2008). The quantitative approach is most frequently associated with **logical positivism**, a philosophical doctrine that asserts that scientific knowledge is the only kind of factual knowledge. Quantitative research is often viewed as hard science and tends to emphasize deductive reasoning and the *measurable* attributes of human experience. Data are usually collected by using structured methods and procedures and are analyzed by using a number of statistical procedures.

The following are examples of research questions that lend themselves to a quantitative approach:

- What is the effect of nurse home visits on the parenting ability of teen mothers?
- Does rocking in older adults elicit the physiological changes of the relaxation response?
- What is the effect of social support intervention on coping in nurses working in intensive care units?

QUALITATIVE RESEARCH **Qualitative research** is "associated with naturalistic inquiry, which explores the subjective and complex experiences of human beings" (Berman et al., 2008, p. 32). The collection of rich narrative material and analysis take place simultaneously by using an inductive approach to analysis. In the qualitative approach, no formal instruments are used; instead, loosely structured narrative data are collected. Using the inductive method, data are analyzed by identifying themes and patterns that emerge. This approach is most often associated with the **naturalistic paradigm**, which began as a countermovement to positivism. This perspective assumes that multiple perspectives of reality exist, each within a context.

The qualitative approach explores complex human experiences and focuses on the holistic aspects of these experiences from the perspectives of those who are living them (Loiselle et al., 2007). The qualitative approach

Evidence-Informed Practice

How Can Employers Promote Empowerment for New Graduate Nurses?

The nursing shortage and projected retirement of nurses in the next few years have resulted in the need for enhanced recruitment and retention of nurses. A high priority among health-care organizations is the development of strategies to improve working conditions and to provide a supportive environment for new graduate nurses.

A predictive, nonexperimental survey design investigated factors that promote empowerment among new graduate nurses (Cho, Laschinger, & Wong, 2006). This study tested the relationships among structural empowerment, six areas of work life, emotional exhaustion, and organizational commitment. Structural empowerment measured employees' perceptions of access to opportunity, information, support, and resources. The six areas of work life included workload, control, rewards, community, fairness, and values. Emotional exhaustion measured how often an individual experienced feelings of disengagement and burnout in his or her work. Organizational commitment measured the psychological link between the employee and the organization.

The researchers found that structural empowerment had a positive effect on the areas of work life and a negative effect on emotional exhaustion. They concluded that increasing access to job flexibility, strong interpersonal relationships, information, support, and learning opportunities are potential strategies to retain new graduate nurses.

NURSING IMPLICATIONS: This study suggests the importance of a positive work environment to ensuring commitment of new graduates and resulting retention of staff. The following strategies would contribute:

- Use multiple communication techniques: regular staff meetings, forums, electronic messages, brown bag lunches, and written updates.
- Use support staff to reduce nursing time spent on non-nursing tasks.
- Provide orientation, emotional support, assistance, and collaborative learning opportunities.
- Give new graduates opportunities for leadership roles and involvement in decision making.
- Offer choices and alternatives for flexibility in jobs (job sharing, innovative scheduling).
- Build strong interpersonal relationships through team building and mentoring programs.

Source: Based on "Workplace Empowerment, Work Engagement and Organizational Commitment of New Graduate Nurses," by J. Cho, H. K. S. Laschinger, and C. Wong, 2006, *Canadian Journal of Nursing Leadership, 19*(3), pp. 43–60.

would be appropriate for the following types of research questions:

- What is the nature of the bereavement process in spouses of clients with terminal cancer?
- What is the nature of adjustment after a mastectomy?
- What is the impact of eating disorders on family life?

The Research Process

Loiselle et al. (2007) defined **research** as "systematic inquiry that uses disciplined methods to answer questions or solve problems" (p. 4). Whether a quantitative or qualitative approach is used, all research must be meticulously planned, systematically implemented, and carefully analyzed. To achieve this goal, researchers adhere to a formal course of action known as the research process. This process has 11 steps, beginning with the formulation of the research problem and ending with the communication of the research. However, sometimes variation exists in the terms given to these steps, depending on the nature of the study.

1. STATE A RESEARCH PROBLEM The investigator's initial task is to narrow a broad area of interest to a circumscribed **research problem** that specifies exactly the situation that needs to be described, explained, or predicted. The ideas for research may arise from recurrent problems encountered in practice, questions that are difficult to resolve because of contradictions in the literature, or areas in which minimal or no research has been done.

In formulating a research problem, Loiselle et al. (2007) suggest five important considerations: significance, usefulness, researchability, feasibility, and ethical soundness. A research problem has *significance* if it has the potential to contribute to nursing science by enhancing client care, testing or generating a theory, or resolving a day-to-day clinical problem. The question "So what?" must be answered adequately to determine whether a research problem is significant.

The *usefulness* of a study relates to the potential usefulness in clinical practice of the findings. Not only should the problem be significant, but it must also be relevant and applicable to nursing practice.

Researchability means that the problem can be subjected to scientific investigation by using appropriate and sound methodology. Many significant problems that produce ambiguity and uncertainty in clinical situations are not amenable to research. For instance, "Should nurses support voluntary euthanasia?" is a relevant, timely, and difficult question, but it cannot be answered through research.

Feasibility pertains to practical issues, such as availability of time and the material and human resources needed to investigate a research problem or question.

Evidence-Informed Practice

What Are Caregiver Perceptions of Unsupportive Interactions with Others?

The role of caregiver to family members with a chronic illness or disability is assumed predominantly by women. Female caregivers find it beneficial to have the support of other family members, friends, and the wider community, which then increases the demand on these resources. Research reveals that female caregivers often experience unsupportive interactions or "unhelpful interactions and behaviours that occur in relationships which are also sources of support." Such interaction can have a negative influence on both their support satisfaction and their psychological health.

The purpose of this ethnographic study by Neufeld, Harrison, Hughes, and Stewart (2007) was to identify unsupportive interactions as perceived by female caregivers in their social networks of family and friends and with professionals, across varied contexts: two situations involving caregiving as mothers, and two involving caregiving of adult family members. Data collection comprised an initial individual interview, a second interview employing a card sort technique, and final interview to provide feedback on a topology of unsupportive interactions. The results revealed three types of unsupportive interactions common across varying contexts and networks: (1) *negative interactions,* such as minimizing, blaming, and showing disrespect; (2) *ineffective* interactions in terms of inadequate information or professional support; and (3) interactions in which *expected support was absent*. The topology derived from this study provides a solid foundation for tailoring individual support interventions for female (and potentially male) caregivers by helping to identify potentially unhelpful actions. Future research includes the application of an ecological perspective to examine the multiple levels of influence on caregivers in their social environment, as well as further exploration of the reflective process female caregivers use to support change when faced with unsupportive interactions.

NURSING IMPLICATIONS: Consideration of the similarities of unsupportive interactions for caregivers will help nurses and allied health professionals plan appropriate, non-disease-specific support interventions.

Source: Based on "Non-supportive Interactions in the Experience of Women Family Caregivers," by A. Neufeld, M. J. Harrison, K. D. Hughes, and M. J. Stewart, 2007, *Health and Social Care in the Community, 15*(6), pp. 530–541.

Conducting a study involves the use of space, money, equipment, supplies, computers, subjects, research assistants, and consultants.

A study is *ethically sound* if ethical issues are addressed by adhering to rigorous procedures and appropriate ethical reviews, where needed. See "Protecting the Rights of Human Subjects" later in this chapter for details concerning the ethical principles guiding research in Canada.

In quantitative approaches, research problems contain *dependent* and *independent variables,* except for descriptive research, which has no dependent variables. The **dependent variable** is the behaviour, characteristic, or outcome that the researcher wants to explain or predict. The **independent variable** is the presumed cause of, or influence on, the dependent variable. Qualitative studies do not contain variables.

2. DEFINE THE STUDY'S PURPOSE OR RATIONALE The statement of the **study's purpose** indicates what the researcher intends to do with the research problem identified. The study purpose includes *what* the researcher will do, *who* the subjects will be, and *where* the data will be collected.

3. REVIEW THE LITERATURE Before progressing with the development of the research design, the investigator determines what is known and what is not known about the problem. A thorough **review of the literature** provides the foundation on which to build new knowledge. Through a literature review, a researcher may also acquire information about available techniques, instruments, and methods of data analysis that have been used in prior research, as well as potential flaws or problems and how to avoid them. The literature review helps to determine the best approach for studying the problem (Gillis & Jackson, 2002).

4. FORMULATE THE RESEARCH QUESTION OR HYPOTHESIS Once nurse researchers have identified a research problem and are knowledgeable of the literature, they formulate a **research question**. The question may be stated in one of three ways: a statement, a question, or a hypothesis. If researchers are going to describe something, they may make a statement, such as, "The purpose of this study is to identify gender differences in the nursing care of patients admitted to rehabilitation units." They could also ask a question, such as, "What are the communication styles of nurses that produce client satisfaction with nursing care?"

If conducting an experiment, researchers must have a **hypothesis** as to what the outcome will be so that hypothesis-testing statistics can be applied. For example, "Family members of palliative care patients attending support groups will demonstrate more positive coping strategies than those who do not attend" is a testable hypothesis. In whichever way a research question is stated, it must be clearly expressed.

Wood and Ross-Kerr (2006) identify three levels of questions: level one questions relate to topics with little or no prior knowledge, which leads to an exploration; level two questions are useful when a topic has already been well described and any variables arising from the descriptions prompt the researcher to consider relationships between these variables; level three questions build on previous research and look for causal relationships.

5. SELECT A RESEARCH DESIGN A **research design** is the "overall plan for obtaining answers to the research questions" (Loiselle et al., 2007, p. 57). The choice of design depends on the nature of the problem. Level one questions lend themselves to various qualitative designs, while levels two and three are more appropriate for quantitative designs. Sometimes a combination of approaches is used. The research design includes the study setting, the sample, and the type of data to be collected, as well as strategies to reduce bias.

Quantitative research design has three categories:

1. **Experimental design**. The investigator manipulates the independent variable by administering an experimental treatment to some subjects while withholding it from others. The conditions are tightly controlled to objectively test the hypothesis in order to predict cause-and-effect relationships (Potter, Perry, Ross-Kerr, & Wood, 2006).
2. **Quasi-experimental design**. The investigator manipulates the independent variable but without either the randomization or the control that characterizes true experiments. This design is common in health-care studies because random assignment to treatment and control groups is not always feasible in a clinical setting (Potter et al., 2006).
3. **Nonexperimental design**. The investigator does not manipulate the independent variable. Researchers use nonexperimental designs to measure characteristics and determine relationships or correlations among these variables (Loiselle et al., 2007).

As noted earlier, **qualitative designs** seek to derive meaning and understanding from human experience. In such disciplines as nursing, where it is necessary to know what the participant is experiencing, a qualitative design may be the preferred method of identifying data. A qualitative design differs from a quantitative design in the phenomenon studied, the data collection and analysis procedures, and the interpretation of the data. Often, data collection and analysis are done simultaneously. Qualitative designs do not have identifiable measurable variables, and data are not processed through statistical analysis.

Ethnography, grounded theory, and phenomenology are some of the commonly used qualitative methods. **Ethnographic research** is used to describe social behaviours within a particular group or setting. The goal is to understand the culture and norms from the participant's viewpoint (Potter et al., 2006). Studies related to the nursing care or health practices of a particular culture would be examples of ethnographic nursing research. **Grounded theory** research is used to develop nursing theory from collected data. Theory may be generated for relatively new areas, where very little is known, or for more familiar areas, where a fresh viewpoint is sought. **Phenomenology** is a philosophical research method that regards each human as having a unique experience. The researcher uses in-depth conversations to attempt to derive meaning from individuals' descriptions of their experiences (Potter et al., 2006).

In selecting the approach, the researcher should try to identify factors that may affect the study's results. Sometimes, these factors are called limitations. The researcher should acknowledge the limitations of the study, as much as possible, before the data are collected.

6. SELECT THE POPULATION, SAMPLE, AND SETTING At this stage, the researcher chooses the study population, selects a sample, and decides on the setting where the sample can be found. The **population** includes all members of the group who meet the criteria for the study. The **sample** is the segment of the population from whom the data will actually be collected.

7. CONDUCT A PILOT STUDY In quantitative studies, a **pilot study** is a small-scale trial done before the actual study begins. The research procedure is conducted on a few subjects to determine the feasibility of the data collection plan, identify flaws, and refine the proposed plan to strengthen the research methodology (Berman et al., 2008).

8. COLLECT THE DATA When designing a study, researchers must consider how the data will be collected. The most commonly used methods of collecting data in nursing are questionnaires, rating scales, interviews, observation, and biophysical measures.

In quantitative designs, the validity and reliability of measurement tools need to be established before the start of data collection. **Validity** is the degree to which an instrument measures what it is supposed to measure. If a nurse measures anxiety, how can the nurse be sure that what is being measured is not fear or stress, which are related concepts? **Reliability** is the degree of consistency with which an instrument measures a concept or variable. If an instrument is reliable, repeated measurements of the same variable should yield similar or nearly similar results.

9. ANALYZE THE DATA In this step, the collected data are organized, coded, and analyzed for the purpose of answering the research question or testing the hypothesis. Even before data collection is initiated, there must be a systematic plan for analyzing the results. Measurement is a critical part of the research process. Measurement is not a feature of qualitative designs; the discussion here is relevant to quantitative designs. Variables are important components of measurement. The identified research question helps the researcher identify the variables and possible relationships among them. The variables must be clearly defined, observable, and measurable to permit the results of a study to be interpretable. Regardless of the method of measurement used, it must have evidence of objectivity. This means that the system of measurement must be so clear that anyone following the prescribed rules will assign the same or similar score to what was observed.

Data analysis can involve descriptive or inferential statistics. **Descriptive statistics**, procedures that summarize large volumes of data, are used to describe and synthesize data, showing patterns and trends. Descriptive statistics include measures of central tendency and measures of variability.

Measures of central tendency describe the centre of a distribution of data, denoting where most of the subjects lie. These include the mean, median, and mode. **Measures of variability** indicate the degree of dispersion or spread of the data. These include the range, variance, and standard deviation. See Box 3.2 for definitions of these measures. Typically, in a research report, the mean and standard deviation are reported together to give the reader an idea of the nature of the data distribution.

The following is an example: Systolic blood pressure = 130 ± 30. The two statistics reported are the mean and the standard deviation. The number 130 indicates the mean systolic blood pressure, whereas 30 represents 1 standard deviation (SD) from the mean. Hence, 1 SD from the mean would include blood pressure from 100 mm Hg to 160 mm Hg (1 SD less than to 1 SD more than the mean).

Nurse researchers attempt to determine (after data have been analyzed) whether the results are *statistically significant*. Underlying this statement is the notion of *probability*. By convention, p (probability) less than .05 is considered the acceptable level of significance; a p value greater than .05 is considered statistically insignificant. In research, the desire is to generalize beyond the sample; there is a need to determine the probability that the results were due to chance or a fluke, rather than a true occurrence in the population. Hence, a p value of .05 means that the probability of the findings being caused by chance alone is 5 in 100 (Berman et al., 2008).

In qualitative studies, data analysis is often done simultaneously with data collection, which enables the researcher to focus and shape the study as it proceeds. The researcher consistently thinks about the data, works to organize it, and tries to discover meaning in it.

BOX 3.2 DEFINITIONS OF MEASURES OF CENTRAL TENDENCY AND VARIABILITY

CENTRAL TENDENCY

Mean: The sum of all scores divided by the number of subjects; commonly symbolized as *X* or *M*

Median: The middle score or value in a distribution of scores; the value above and below which 50% of the scores lie

Mode: The score or value that occurs most frequently in a distribution of scores

VARIABILITY

Range: The difference between the highest and the lowest values in a distribution of scores

Variance: The square of the standard deviation

Standard deviation: The average to which scores deviate from the mean; commonly symbolized as *SD* or *S;* the most frequently used measure of variability

10. INTERPRET THE FINDINGS In either quantitative or qualitative research, when interpreting the results of the data analysis, the researcher first reports the findings that are directly related to the research question. Sometimes, the researcher uncovers unexpected findings, and these are also reported. Hirst (2000) articulated a definition of resident abuse as perceived by those living and working within long-term care institutions and unexpectedly found that older adults were devalued in these same facilities.

Conclusions are then drawn: what do these findings mean? At this point, researchers can be subjective and insert some of their own thinking into the research report. The results of the current research are compared with previous studies that investigated the same or similar phenomena. The researcher should discuss any problems encountered in the course of the study or any limitations that may have influenced the findings.

After the findings are interpreted, the researcher should indicate the implications for nursing. **Implications** are suggestions for ways of thinking about the phenomenon in the future. Nursing research may unearth indications for changes to nursing practice, administration, or education. For example, in a review of research literature on the impact of international placements on nursing students, the findings suggested that students become more sensitive to cultural issues and cross–cultural care as a result of these experiences (Button, Green, Tengnah, Johansson, & Baker, 2005). An implication is that nurse educators need to provide culturally diverse opportunities for students. In a study examining what percentage of clients had postoperative pain at home and what impact pain had on their activity, the findings identified that clients had received no information on how to cope with pain and were not knowledgeable about analgesic use (Collins & MacDonald, 2000). These findings indicate a need for educational resources on the management of postoperative pain following discharge from hospital to be given to clients.

11. COMMUNICATE THE RESEARCH Implicit in conducting research is the requirement to share with others the knowledge generated, primarily through publication in professional journals or by reporting the results orally or in poster format at professional conferences. Interpreting the results, communicating the findings, and suggesting directions for further study conclude the research process.

In Canada, nursing research findings can be communicated in numerous ways. At the local, provincial or territorial, and national levels, nursing associations and special interest groups use their newsletters, publications, annual meetings, and conferences to promote nursing research and to disseminate findings. The best method of reaching a large number of nurses is through publication in nursing journals (see Box 3.3 for examples). *Canadian Nurse* (*L'infirmière Canadienne*) publishes news items on research activities, abstracts of Canadian research articles, and articles that report research findings.

Developing Research-Based Practice

The nurse needs to be research minded, that is, aware of and open to nursing research. Nurses should critically read, interpret, and evaluate research evidence for applicability to their nursing practice. When reviewing research articles or reports, consider the philosophical view taken in the study; for example, where does knowledge exist? Does it exist in patients' experiences (qualitative) or in logical reasoning of the researcher (quantitative)? Nursing has possibilities for both.

Research-based practice enables nurses to provide high-quality, cost-effective care. Through clinical practice, nurses can identify nursing problems that need to be investigated. Nurses can participate in the implementation of research studies by helping principal researchers collect data in clinical settings. They can also help disseminate research-based knowledge by sharing useful findings with colleagues. Nurses with graduate education also assume the role of clinical experts on clinical practice teams, integrate research findings into practice, design studies, and collaborate with other researchers (Potter et al., 2006).

Research utilization involves a number of activities by nurses to link research findings to practice. To do so, nurses need to access current research findings and critique this literature to determine its appropriateness for a particular clinical setting.

BOX 3.3 EXAMPLES OF RESEARCH JOURNALS IN NURSING

These are just a few of the nursing journals available:

- *Western Journal of Nursing Research*
- *Canadian Journal of Nursing Leadership*
- *Canadian Journal of Public Health*
- *Canadian Nurse/L'infirmière Canadienne*
- *Clinical Nursing Research*
- *Nursing Research*
- *International Journal of Nursing Studies*
- *Nursing Science Quarterly*
- *Qualitative Health Research*
- *Biological Research for Nursing*

Locating Nursing Research Findings

The journal *Nursing Research* was established in 1952 in the United States to serve as a vehicle to communicate nurses' research and scholarly productivity (Donahue, 1985). The publication of many other nursing research journals followed, some devoted to research and others combining clinical, theory, and research publications. Journals are available in the libraries of academic institutions and large hospitals and many journals are now published online on the World Wide Web.

The most efficient way to access research articles is to conduct a search on an index of journal articles (Potter et al., 2006). Examples of these indexes include the Cumulative Index to Nursing and Allied Health Literature (CINAHL), International Nursing Index, MEDLINE, and PubMed. Computerized search assistance is available in health-care libraries; the trick to finding relevant articles is to identify the key words to be used for the search. It may take several computer searches using different key terms and databases to locate the articles. Increasingly, these searches can be done through the World Wide Web. The Canadian Research Information Database (CRID) is a resource for researchers and others interested in accessing the results of research in Canada on the web. In searching the web, be aware of the credibility of the source and when the site was last updated.

The Cochrane Library is a collection of databases with high-quality evidence obtained through systematic reviews. Results from several similar randomized trials are brought together and combined to produce an overall statistic by using exact methodology. This process facilitates evidence-informed decision making for clinical treatment.

The Virginia Henderson International Nursing Library is sponsored by Sigma Theta Tau International and provides online access to reliable nursing information. It also includes the Registry of Nursing Research Database, with up-to-date study and conference abstracts.

The Canadian Nurses Association (CNA), Health Canada, and the First Nations and Inuit Health Branch of Health Canada have created NurseONE, a secure web-based resource to provide nurses "with access to current and reliable information to support their nursing practice, manage their careers, and connect with colleagues and health-care experts." (CNA, n.d., p. 1). It supports an evidence-based approach to care by providing easily accessed digital libraries, online journals, electronic material, and databases that are all approved by the CNA.

Critiquing Research

Critiquing involves intensive scrutiny of a study, including its strengths and weaknesses, its statistical and clinical significance, and the generalizability of the results.

Loiselle et al. (2007) suggest different approaches to critiquing quantitative and qualitative research. For quantitative research, using the IMRAD format (i.e., introduction, method, results, and discussion) will address the study components found in most research reports. See Table 3.1 for relevant questions about each of these components.

TABLE 3.1 Critique of a Quantitative Research Report

Aspect of the Report	Questions to Consider
Title	Does the title inform you of the research problem and study population?
Abstract	Does the abstract summarize the main features of the article?
Introduction	
Problem Statement	Is the problem clear, easy to identify? Does the problem statement identify key concepts and population? Is the problem significant for nursing? Is a quantitative approach suitable? Does the research problem fit the methods?
Literature Review	Is the literature review current and complete? Is it based mostly on primary sources? Does the literature review summarize what is known about the dependent and independent variables and how they are related? Does it provide a solid framework for the new study?
Conceptual Framework	Are key concepts fully defined from a theoretical perspective? Is a theoretical framework described? Is it appropriate? If no theoretical framework is present, does the report justify the absence?
Hypothesis or Research Questions	Are research questions or hypotheses clear and explicit? If not, is there a rationale for their absence? Is there consistency among the questions and hypotheses, the literature review, and the conceptual framework?
Method	
Research Design	Was a rigorous design used given the study purpose? Were appropriate comparisons made for ease of interpretation of the findings? Was there evidence of efforts to minimize threats to internal and external validity?
Population and Sample	Were the population and sample identified and described? Was the sampling design devised to promote a representative sample? Was sample size sufficient? Was a sample size estimate done by using power analysis?
Data Collection and Measurement	Was there congruence between the operational and conceptual definitions? Were key variables defined in an operational manner? Were the instruments well described? Did the report provide evidence of high reliability and validity of data?
Procedures	Was the intervention (if used) described and correctly implemented? Were data collected to minimize bias? Was staff that collected the data trained? Were procedures used to safeguard rights of study participants? Was there an ethics review?
Results	
Data Analysis	Did the analyses deal with each research question or hypotheses? Were statistical methods matched to measurement level of the variables and number of groups being compared?
Findings	Were findings summarized by using tables and figures? Do findings demonstrate sound evidence about the research questions?
Discussion	
Interpretation of Findings	Are major findings interpreted, discussed, and related to prior research and the conceptual framework used? Was there consistency between interpretations and results or limitations of the study?
Implications	Does the article provide details about generalizability of the findings?
Overall	
Presentation	Was the report well organized and did it provide adequate detail for critical analysis? Was the study understandable? Was it written in a way so as to make the findings accessible to practising nurses?
Summary Assessment	Despite identified limitations, do the findings appear valid? Does the study contribute to evidence that can be meaningfully used in nursing practice or the discipline of nursing?

Source: Adapted from *Canadian Essentials of Nursing Research,* 2nd ed., (pp. 438–439), by C. G. Loiselle, J. Profetto-McGrath, D. F. Polit, and C. T. Beck, 2007, Philadelphia, PA: Lippincott Williams & Wilkins.

Qualitative research reports are generally less structured and organized according to the themes. However, a similar approach can be used to critique qualitative research (see Table 3.2).

TABLE 3.2 Critique of a Qualitative Research Report

Aspect of the Report	Questions to Consider
Title	Does the title suggest main phenomenon and the group or community under study?
Abstract	Does the abstract summarize the main features of the article?
Introduction	
Statement of the Problem	Is there a clear identification of the phenomenon of interest? Is the problem clearly stated and easy to identify? Is the problem significant for nursing? Does the research problem fit the methods? Is the qualitative approach suitable?
Literature Review	Does the literature review summarize knowledge related to the problem? Is the literature review current and complete? Does the literature review set down a basis for the new study?
Conceptual Underpinnings	Are key concepts fully defined from a theoretical perspective? Does the report identify the philosophical or ideological basis, conceptual framework, and research tradition? Is the approach congruent with the research questions?
Research Questions	Are research questions clear and explicit? If not, is there a rationale for their absence?
Method	
Research Design and Tradition	Does the research tradition fit with data collection and analysis methods? Was sufficient time spent in the field or with study participants? Did the researcher build on early understanding by adapting the design in the field? Was there evidence of reflective thought by the researcher? Was the number of contacts with participants sufficient?
Sample and Setting	Were the population, sample, and setting identified and described? Was an appropriate approach used to access participants? Was an optimum sampling method used? Was the sample sufficient? Was there saturation of data?
Data Collection Procedures	Was the data gathered in an appropriate manner? Were two or more methods of data gathering used to achieve triangulation? Were the right questions or observations used? Were these recorded appropriately? Was sufficient data collected for depth and richness? Was there a clear description of data collection and recording procedures? Were steps taken to minimize bias or altered behaviour? Were procedures used to safeguard rights of study participants? Was there an ethics review?
Enhancement of Rigour	Was there a description of methods used to promote trustworthiness of the analysis? Were sufficient methods used to enhance credibility? Were research procedures and decision processes documented to be auditable and confirmable?
Results	
Data Analysis	Were methods of data management and analysis clearly described? Did the analysis approach fit with the research tradition, nature, and type of data gathered? Did the analysis produce a tangible output (theory, taxonomy, thematic pattern, etc.)?
Findings	Were the findings summarized with use of quotes? Do the themes capture the meaning of the data? Did the researcher seem to conceptualize the themes or patterns in the data? Did the analysis come up with a thought-provoking and meaningful picture of the phenomenon?
Theoretical Integration	Are there logical connections among the themes or patterns and do these connect to form a meaningful whole? Were figures, maps, or models effectively used to summarize conceptualization? Are the themes or patterns logically linked to a conceptual framework or ideology (if one was use to guide the study)?

(continued)

TABLE 3.2 Critique of a Qualitative Research Report (*continued*)

Discussion	
Interpretation of Findings	Is the interpretation of the findings situated in an appropriate context (e.g., group, cultural, or social)? Are major findings interpreted, discussed, and related to prior research? Is there consistency of the interpretations and the study's limitations? Does the report discuss transferability of findings?
Implications	Are the implications of the study for clinical practice or future study discussed? Are the implications reasonable?
Overall	
Presentation	Was the report well organized and did it provide adequate detail for critical analysis? Were the methods, findings, and interpretations richly described?
Summary Assessment	Do the findings seem trustworthy? Does the study contribute to meaningful evidence that can be used in nursing practice or the discipline of nursing?

Source: Adapted from *Canadian Essentials of Nursing Research*, 2nd ed. (pp. 442–444), by C. G. Loiselle, J. Profetto-McGrath, D. F. Polit, and C. T. Beck, 2007, Philadelphia, PA: Lippincott Williams & Wilkins.

In general, the critique should include consideration of the following:

- Amount of detail about the method, ethical considerations, and interpretation of findings
- Clarity of language
- Objectivity and lack of bias in presentation
- Organization and logical presentation of ideas
- Correct use of grammar and rules of good writing
- Sensitivity to gender, race, and ethnicity
- Appropriateness of title to capture key concepts and target population
- Adequacy of summary of research problem, study methods, and key findings (Loiselle et al., 2007)

Protecting the Rights of Human Subjects

When research is conducted on human participants, the researcher and the nurse have a responsibility to protect the research participant from harm that may result from participation in the study. The nurse, as client advocate, must ensure that clients' rights are protected.

All institutions in which research is conducted should have, or have access to, a committee of qualified individuals called a research ethics board (REB) to approve the research activity and to ensure that the rights of participants are protected. The principle of protecting rights is enforced to some extent by major granting agencies, such as the CIHR and the SSHRC, who make their funding contingent on REB review. REBs have the authority to require modifications to proposed research and can terminate research that is not conducted according to specific requirements. Also offering guidance to nurse researchers in Canada are the CNA's *Code of Ethics for Registered Nurses* (2008) and the Canadian Institutes of Health Research, Natural Sciences and Engineering Research Council of Canada, and Social Science and Humanities Research Council of Canada's *Tri-Council Policy Statement on Ethical Conduct for Research Involving Humans* (1998 with 2000, 2002, and 2005 amendments).

All nurses who practise in settings in which research is being conducted with human subjects, or who participate in such research as data collectors or collaborators, play an important role in safeguarding the rights of human subjects. The *Tri-Council Policy* is based on the following guiding ethical principles.

RESPECT FOR HUMAN DIGNITY Respect for human **dignity** means protecting the interests of the person in all spheres: physical, psychological, and cultural. This cardinal principle forms the basis of ethical obligations in modern research.

RESPECT FOR FREE AND INFORMED CONSENT It is presumed that individuals have the capacity and right to make free and informed decisions. Obtaining **informed consent** is the responsibility of the principal investigator. It is a contract between the investigator and the participant. All clients must be informed about the consequences of consenting to serve as research participants. The client needs to be able to judge whether a reasonable balance exists between the risks of participating in the study and the potential benefits.

Informed consent may appear to be straightforward and easy to implement, but this is not always true. Sometimes, researchers avoid informed consent, believing that the client's knowledge of being observed could alter behaviour and distort the findings. It is the nurse's responsibility to safeguard participants' human rights and ensure that informed consent takes place before their involvement in any research study.

Informed consent includes written and oral explanations. It should be in the participant's preferred language and at an appropriate educational level. Documenting informed consent by obtaining a participant's consent in writing is important. Participants who can only give oral permission must have their consent witnessed by a third person. If the participant is a minor, or is not capable of consenting because of mental or physical disability, a legally authorized representative, such as a parent or guardian, may sign the consent. Consent must be voluntary and informed, and no additional risk, discomfort, or invasion of privacy to that stated in the consent document can take place. In addition, the participant must be guaranteed that refusal to take part in or withdraw from the study will not jeopardize the quality of nursing care.

RESPECT FOR VULNERABLE PERSONS Greater ethical obligations toward vulnerable people and those who have diminished competence or decision-making capacity must be met. Children, people in institutions, and others are entitled to special protection against abuse and exploitation. In research, this often means that special procedures are needed to protect the interests of vulnerable people.

RESPECT FOR PRIVACY AND CONFIDENTIALITY The principle of respect for privacy and confidentiality is considered fundamental to human dignity in many cultures. Standards of privacy and confidentiality protect personal information and enable a client to participate without worrying about later embarrassment. The anonymity of a study participant is ensured if the investigator cannot link a specific subject to the information reported. **Confidentiality** means that any information a subject provides will not be made public or available to others without the subject's consent. Investigators must inform research subjects about the measures that provide for these rights. Such measures may include the use of pseudonyms or code numbers or the reporting of only aggregate or group data in published research.

RESPECT FOR JUSTICE AND INCLUSIVENESS The ethics review process is required to have fair methods and standards for reviewing research protocols so that no segment of the population is unfairly burdened with the harms of research and those who are vulnerable are not exploited for the advancement of knowledge. Conversely, justice also implies a duty to ensure that some individuals and groups are not neglected or discriminated against with respect to inclusion in research studies.

BALANCING HARMS AND BENEFITS Minimizing harm, or **nonmaleficence**, is the duty to avoid, prevent, or minimize harms to others. A research subject should not be exposed to the possibility of injury beyond everyday situations. The risk can be physical, emotional, legal, financial, or social. For instance, withholding standard care from a client in labour for the purpose of studying the course of natural childbirth clearly poses a potential physical danger. Risks can be less overt and involve psychological factors, such as exposure to stress or anxiety, or social factors, such as loss of confidentiality or loss of privacy. This means that research should involve the smallest number of human subjects and smallest number of tests on subjects that will ensure scientifically valid data.

Maximizing benefit, or **beneficence**, is the duty to benefit others and maximize the net benefits. This is particularly relevant in social science disciplines, like social work and nursing, in which the advancement of knowledge can produce benefits for society.

RIGHT TO FULL DISCLOSURE Even though it may be possible to collect data about a client as part of everyday care without the client's particular knowledge or consent, to do so is considered unethical. **Full disclosure** is a basic right. It means that deception, either by withholding information about a client's participation in a study or by giving the client false or misleading information about what participating in the study will involve, will not occur.

RIGHT OF SELF-DETERMINATION Many clients in dependent positions, such as people in nursing homes, feel pressured to participate in studies. They feel that they must please the doctors and nurses who are responsible for their treatment and care. The **right of self-determination** means that subjects should feel free from constraints, coercion, or any undue influence to participate in a study. Masked inducements, for instance, suggesting to potential participants that by taking part in the study they might become famous, make an important contribution to science, or receive special attention, must be strictly avoided. Nurses must be assertive in advocating for this essential right.

Case Study 3

A research study is being implemented on the unit as Jamie, a third-year baccalaureate nursing student in a large university in Western Canada, starts his adult health course rotation. He participates in the orientation session held by the researchers to inform the staff about their study. The purpose of the study is to understand the presurgical experiences of the patients. Jamie is interested in working with the researchers.

Critical Thinking Questions

1. Identify the responsibilities of beginning nurses in relation to nursing research.
2. What questions might Jamie ask of the researchers as he explores his possible interest in the study?
3. How might Jamie ensure that he protects the rights of his patients, if they decide to participate in the study?

After working through these questions, go to the MyNursingLab at **http://www.mynursinglab.com** to check your answers.

KEY TERMS

research-based nursing practice
evidence-based practice
evidence-informed practice
nursing research
basic research
applied research
problem solving
quantitative research
logical positivism
qualitative research
naturalistic paradigm
research
research problem
dependent variable
independent variable
study purpose
review of the literature
research question
hypothesis
research design
experimental design
quasi-experimental design
nonexperimental design
qualitative designs
ethnographic research
grounded theory
phenomenology
population
sample
pilot study
validity
reliability
descriptive statistics
measures of central tendency
measures of variability
mean
median
mode
range
variance
standard deviation
implications
critiquing
dignity
informed consent
confidentiality
nonmaleficence
beneficence
full disclosure
right of self-determination

CHAPTER HIGHLIGHTS

- Nurses are now generating new knowledge and applying research in practice to improve client care.
- Nurses at all levels are participating in nursing research activities. All nurses practising in settings in which research is conducted have a role in safeguarding the clients' rights.
- The use of research will help nurses understand the client's situation more thoroughly, assess more accurately, and intervene more effectively.
- The Canadian Nurses Association is a leader in the promotion of evidence-based nursing practice.
- Most nursing research is initiated in university settings because of the preparation of faculty members as researchers.
- In Canada today, nursing research faces both capabilities and constraints for its ongoing development.
- The nurse has a duty to protect the rights of the research participants.
- A need exists for nursing research on a wide range of nursing questions.
- Qualitative and quantitative methods are employed in nursing research.

- Seven ways that nurses can participate in research are by (1) identifying nursing problems that need to be investigated, (2) helping principal researchers collect data in clinical settings, (3) disseminating research-based knowledge by sharing useful findings with colleagues, (4) assuming the role of clinical expert on clinical practice teams, (5) integrating research findings into practice, (6) designing studies, and (7) collaborating with other researchers.
- Research utilization involves a number of activities by nurses to link research findings to practice. To do so, nurses need to access current research findings and critique this literature to determine its appropriateness for a particular clinical setting.

ASSESS YOUR LEARNING

1. Which of the following is an example of a strategy employed to link theory, practice, and research in nursing?
  a. Ensuring that nursing research is exclusively conducted by qualified, university-based scientists
  b. Implementing cross-appointments of faculty among hospitals, health-care agencies, and universities
  c. Promoting studies that focus on nursing as a distinct discipline rather than interdisciplinary studies
  d. Establishing concise health information systems containing only essential medical data for ease of use

2. Which of the following research roles is expected of a baccalaureate nurse working as a staff nurse in an acute-care hospital?
  a. Designing studies and collaborating with other researchers
  b. Assuming the role of clinical expert on clinical practice teams
  c. Identifying nursing problems that need to be investigated
  d. Submitting research proposals to the hospital ethics board for approval

3. As a student or staff nurse seeking guidance from published research, you would do which of the following?
  a. Accept the findings without question, since the study has been published
  b. Compare the study subjects with your patients to determine if the findings are applicable
  c. Look for another study since you need at least two sources to ensure the findings are consistent
  d. Write to the researchers for the raw data so you can analyze the data yourself

4. Which of the following studies would best lend itself to a quantitative research approach?
  a. A study measuring the effects of preoperative teaching on postoperative wound healing
  b. A study examining perceptions of adolescents with type 1 diabetes mellitus
  c. A study exploring factors influencing social isolation among seniors living alone in the community
  d. A study describing the experience of adjustment following sudden infant death

5. Which of the following studies would best lend itself to a qualitative research approach?
  a. A study measuring nutrition and weight changes in clients with cancer
  b. A study examining the relationships between urinary infections and indwelling catheters
  c. A study examining the relationships among infant, mother, and contextual factors and mother–low-birth-weight-infant interaction
  d. A study exploring the caregiving role adult daughters play when a parent is hospitalized for a cardiac condition

6. The nurse is conducting a research project on differences in long-term psychological functioning in young women following alternative pregnancy resolution decisions (abortion, adoption, keeping the baby). After identifying the problem, what is the next step in the research process?
  a. Select the population and sample
  b. Review the literature
  c. Identify data collection methods
  d. Conduct a pilot study

7. The choice of a research design is determined by which of the following?
  a. The preferences of the researcher conducting the research
  b. The availability of tested measurement instruments for the variables of interest
  c. The availability of potential subjects to participate in the study
  d. The nature of the problem being investigated

8. In ensuring the principle of self-determination related to participation in research studies for residents in a long-term-care facility, the nurse should do which of the following?
  a. Contribute to the research process by offering staff assistance to gather all the data from the residents
  b. Insist on personally gathering the informed consent from the residents
  c. Recognize that the residents are in a dependent position and should not be coerced into participating
  d. Refuse to allow researchers into the facility, since the residents are in no condition to consent

9. You work as a nurse on a special assessment unit in a rehabilitation hospital with children who have developmental disorders. You have been asked to help identify potential participants for an institutionally approved research study on independent community living options for adolescents with Down syndrome. One of your clients is an 18-year-old who has told you previously that he wants to move out of his parents' home and live independently, but his parents are against such a move. How would you protect the rights of the client in this case?

a. Discuss your dilemma with the client and his family together

b. Refer the client's name to the researcher and leave the decision up to her

c. Talk to your nursing manager and seek her advice in this matter

d. Talk to the client alone and ask him what he would like to do about participation in the study

10. The nurse is developing a workshop on teenage pregnancy for school children from 12 to 14 years of age. What is the best way to gather information for the presentation?

a. Ask parents what they think teenagers should know about pregnancy.

b. Do an internet search of websites for pregnant teenagers.

c. Conduct a literature review of research on teenage pregnancy.

d. Consult other nurses who work with pregnant teenagers.

After working through these questions, go to the MyNursingLab at ***http://www.mynursinglab.com*** *to check your answers and see explanations.*

SUGGESTED READINGS

Canadian Nurses Association. (2004). *Everyday ethics: Putting the code into practice* (2nd ed.). Ottawa: Author.

This publication gives historical and situational information related to the CNA Code of Ethics. It is also a helpful guide in using the Code of Ethics.

Forbes, D., & Phillipchuk, D. (2001). The dissemination and use of nursing research. *Canadian Nurse, 97*(7), 18–22.

The authors describe a project of the College and Association of Registered Nurses of Alberta to identify how research findings could be more effectively disseminated and used in clinical practice. From a series of five workshops, participants identified that they often had insufficient time to read research articles and implement new ideas. They also identified that sharing of ideas and successful approaches to using research in practice contributed to their own evidence-based practice.

Stajduhar, K. I., Bidgood, D., Meagher, C., Morris, V., Shaw, A. L., Showler, C., & Short, S. J. (2002). Bringing nursing research alive in the practice setting. *Canadian Nurse, 98*(10), 14–18.

The authors present the benefits and challenges that front-line nurses recognized in implementing a study on injection drug use. They identify that research informs their practice and see the value of doing research to learn about research. They describe their greatest challenge as overcoming their own bias toward research.

WEBLINKS

Canadian Nurses Association

http://www.cna-nurses.ca

Through its search mechanism, the CNA provides access to research initiatives specific to the practice of nursing.

Canadian Institutes of Health Research

http://www.cihr-irsc.gc.ca

The CIHR is a primary funding source for Canadian nurse researchers.

Canadian Consortium for Health Promotion Research

http://iuhpeconference.org/consortium/

The focus of the consortium is to improve health-promotion research, policy, and practice in Canada by linking research, capacity development, and information dissemination.

Canadian Cochrane Centre

http://www.ccnc.cochrane.org

The centre's mandate is to promote health-care decisions based on accurate knowledge (evidence-based health care), through the dissemination and application of systematic reviews of health-care interventions. This site provides evidence-based resources.

Social Sciences and Humanities Research Council of Canada

http://www.sshrc.ca

This council is an arm's-length federal agency that promotes and supports university-based research and training in the social sciences and humanities.

NurseONE Portal

http://www.nurseone-inf-fusion.ca

This web-based resource was developed by the CNA, Health Canada, and the First Nations and Inuit Health Branch of Health Canada. It provides a variety of resources to support evidence-based clinical practice for Canadian nurses.

REFERENCES

Berman, A., Snyder, S. J., Kozier, B., & Erb, G. (2008). *Kozier and Erb's fundamentals of nursing* (8th ed.). Upper Saddle River, NJ: Pearson/Prentice Hall.

Button, L., Green, B., Tengnah, C., Johansson, I., & Baker, C. (2005). The impact of international placements on nurses' personal and professional lives: Literature review. *Journal of Advanced Nursing, 50*(3), 315–324.

Canadian Institutes of Health Research, Natural Sciences and Engineering Research Council of Canada, & Social Science and Humanities Research Council of Canada. (1998 with 2000, 2002, and 2005 amendments). *Tri-council policy statement: Ethical conduct for research involving humans.* Ottawa: Author.

Canadian Nurses Association (n.d.). NurseONE: The Canadian nurses portal. Ottawa: Author. Retrieved August 13, 2008, from http://www.cna-aiic.ca/CNA/documents/pdf/publications/Portal_Overview_2_e.pdf

Canadian Nurses Association. (2007). *Canadian registered nurse examination competences.* Ottawa: Author.

Canadian Nurses Association. (2008). *Code of ethics for registered nurses.* Ottawa: Author

Carper, B. (1978). Fundamental patterns of knowing in nursing. *Advances in Nursing Science 1*(1), 13–23.

Collins, M., & MacDonald, V. (2000). Managing postoperative pain at home. *Canadian Nurse, 96*(7), 26–29.

Donahue, M. P. (1985). *Nursing: The finest art.* St. Louis, MO: Mosby.

Donaldson, S. K. (2000). Breakthroughs in scientific research: The discipline of nursing, 1960–1999. *Annual Review of Nursing Research, 18,* 247–311.

Florin, J., Ehrenberg, A., & Ehnfors, M. (2006). Patient participation in clinical decision-making in nursing: A comparative study of nurses' and patients' perceptions. *Journal of Clinical Nursing, 15*(12), 1498–1508.

Fultz, N. H., & Herzog, A. R. (2001). Self-reported social and emotional impact of urinary incontinence. *Journal of the American Geriatrics Society, 49,* 892–899.

Gillis, A., & Jackson, W. (2002). *Research for nurses: Methods and interpretation.* Philadelphia, PA: Davis.

Hirst, S. (2000). Resident abuse: An insider's perspective. *Geriatric Nursing, 21,* 38–42.

Lewis, C. (2003). Computers in patient education. *CIN: Computers, Informatics, Nursing, 21*(2), 88–96.

Loiselle, C. G., Profetto-McGrath, J., Polit, D. F., & Beck, C. T. (2007). *Canadian essentials of nursing research* (2nd ed.). Philadelphia, PA: Lippincott Williams & Wilkins.

Newman, D. K. (2006). Urinary incontinence, catheters, and urinary tract infections: An overview of CMS Tag F 315. *Ostomy Wound Management, 52*(12), 34–36, 38, 40–44.

Potter, P., Perry, A., Ross-Kerr, J., & Wood, M. (2006). *Canadian fundamentals of nursing* (3rd ed.). Toronto: Harcourt Canada.

Rask, K., Parmelee, P. A., Taylor, J. A., Green, D., Brown, H., Hawley, J., et al. (2007). Implementation and evaluation of a nursing home fall management program. *Journal of the American Geriatric Society, 55*(3), 342–349.

Richards, J., & Hubbert, A. O. (2007). Experiences of expert nurses in caring for patients with postoperative pain. *Pain Management Nursing, 8*(1), 17–24.

Wood, M. J., & Ross-Kerr, J. C. (2006). *Basic steps in planning nursing research: From question to proposal* (6th ed.). Sudbury, MA: Jones and Bartlett Publishers.

Woodham-Smith, C. (1950). *Florence Nightingale.* London, UK: Constable & Co.

Chapter 4

Nursing Philosophies, Theories, Concepts, Frameworks, and Models

Philosophical thinking is an indispensable feature of our everyday lives. When people reflect on the meaning of their experiences, consider how they might evaluate the *truth* of an observation, or try to determine the *best* course of action in a particular situation, they are engaging in philosophical thought. The word *philosophy*, translated from its original Greek, means simply "love of wisdom." Philosophical thinking is also what people draw on to make their way, as wisely as they can, through their lives. To be wise means, in part, to use knowledge well. Therefore, nurses should be committed to using philosophical thinking to improve their understanding of the particular values, beliefs, and assumptions that inform their thinking and influence what they say and do.

Philosophical thinking provides the foundation for the development and analysis of the concepts (including conceptual models and conceptual frameworks) and theories used to articulate knowledge of the discipline. **Concept** is another word for idea. Nurses make use of concepts to highlight the ideas that are important to the discipline. A **conceptual framework**, viewed simply, is a cluster of related concepts around a particular topic. A **conceptual model** is a diagram or illustration showing graphically how concepts within a particular cluster are positioned in relationship to each other. A

OBJECTIVES

After studying this chapter, you should be able to

1. Identify the purposes and essential elements of theories in nursing
2. Examine the purposes and benefits of philosophies in nursing
3. Describe three main areas of philosophical inquiry and two research traditions
4. Compare selected philosophical approaches in relation to the questions they pose for nursing
5. Identify selected theoretical works in terms of how nursing is conceptualized and the assumptions underpinning these conceptualizations
6. Define the terms *philosophy*, *paradigm*, *assumption*, *concept*, *conceptual framework*, *conceptual model*, and *theory*

theory goes beyond conceptual models and frameworks to show the nature and significance of relationships among concepts. Theories offer ways of looking at (conceptualizing) a discipline—such as nursing—in clear explicit terms that can be communicated to others.

Philosophical and theoretical thinking support the discipline's professionalism and collegial status with other health professionals. Nurses must communicate clearly what makes their place in the interdisciplinary team important. To achieve this clarity, concepts and theories are used to organize and analyze nursing knowledge. To use this knowledge wisely, the philosophical beliefs and assumptions that are the foundation for its creation and use must be made clear.

What Is Philosophy?

Although the word *philosophy* has an ordinary, everyday meaning, in the sense that people say they each have their own philosophy, or set of beliefs and assumptions, about the world and their place in it, philosophy is also a scientific discipline. *Science* here means the systematic formulation of a body of knowledge. In a formal sense, philosophy is a scientific discipline that raises, explores, and attempts to answer questions bearing on "our ideas about our experience, the universe, and human affairs" (Fry, 1992, p. 87). In philosophy, people use critical analysis in pursuit of goals.

Philosophical thinking can assist with the following:

- Identifying and questioning assumptions
- Clarifying how concepts are used and how they have meaning
- Assessing arguments made to defend or critique particular ways of thinking

Philosophy's Three Primary Areas of Inquiry

Philosophy's three primary areas of inquiry are ontology, epistemology, and ethics. These terms refer to areas of inquiry somewhat familiar to most of people. **Ontology** investigates the nature of being. It asks such questions as, What is the nature of reality? What is the meaning and purpose of our existence? What does it mean to be a person? **Epistemology** investigates the nature of knowledge. How do we know something? What are the limits of knowledge? On what grounds can we say something is true? What is the difference between what is believed to constitute knowledge and what is described as opinion? **Ethics** explores the nature of moral conduct and judgment. What is good? How should people behave or react in particular circumstances? How should people judge the actions of others? The ways in which we answer these kinds of ontological, epistemological, and ethical questions reflect our basic assumptions and beliefs about the world.

Paradigms or World Views

A **paradigm** (or world view) is a particular way of thinking based on a specific set of beliefs, values, and assumptions. Each person's world view influences how he or she perceives, comprehends, and interprets the world. It shapes people's understanding of events and the means used to seek knowledge. Nevertheless, people are often unaware of their underlying beliefs, values, and assumptions. In particular, **assumptions** often operate unconsciously and are beliefs that are taken for granted, without evidence that has been systematically generated.

Many social arrangements rest solely on assumptions. For example, the idea that nursing is "women's work" relies on an assumption that particular kinds of work are best suited for women and other kinds of work are more appropriate for men. This assumption is often based on other unexamined beliefs about what is sometimes described as women's natural capacity for caring and nurturing. To critique this assumption requires examining particular beliefs and values: such notions as caring, men's and women's "proper" positions in society, the difference between men and women, and the social value attributed to various kinds of work. This kind of inquiry might suggest that women's historical association with activities of care is a reflection not so much of women's essential nature but rather of the ways in which social roles and responsibilities have been allocated throughout history. Philosophical inquiry helps to make explicit what underlies the assumption that nursing is women's work.

Empiricist and Interpretive Traditions

Though many world views or paradigms exist, two ways of understanding the world have been particularly influential in nursing: the empiricist and the interpretive traditions. According to the **empiricist tradition**, a single reality exists independently of our knowledge of it. The world exists separate from human knowers. Knowledge can be obtained by observation and experiment—in other words, by means of the **scientific method**. Truth can be determined by comparing knowledge claims against this independently existing reality. In making discoveries about this world as it really is, scientists can and should prevent subjective biases and beliefs from influencing their perceptions. According to this tradition, it is possible to produce objective knowledge of the world.

By contrast, according to the **interpretive tradition**, no single fixed reality exists against which knowledge can be measured. Knowledge of the world independent of theorizing about it is not possible. Knowledge of the world is always mediated through assumptions. In fact, some scholars in the interpretive tradition argue that the nature of human understanding is itself interpretive and that it is our nature as human beings to create meaning from our experiences.

Each of these two philosophical traditions includes many variations. People who work in one of these traditions often express their beliefs and assumptions somewhat differently. Therefore, simply labelling a work as empiricist or interpretive is of limited use. It is much more fruitful to consider the specific beliefs and assumptions that underlie a particular work.

Both the empiricist and the interpretive traditions have strong adherents, but the point here is not to suggest the rightness or wrongness of either tradition. Rather, it is to recognize that world views provide a general orientation to the world, a way to organize perceptions and experience. In knowledge-generating activities, paradigmatic views influence directions for research and study, problem identification, and guidelines for inquiry and action. Because writers often do not make their world views explicit, readers of nursing research and theory should carefully consider exactly what assumptions are in play.

Philosophy in Nursing

Philosophy is an essential feature of all scientific disciplines, and nursing is no exception. The study of philosophy in nursing enables nurses to further their understanding of the values, beliefs, assumptions, and knowledge that constitute the discipline. Generally speaking, the study of philosophy in nursing can be understood as the "philosophical inquiry about nursing's social and humanitarian roles, its form of thought, nature, scope, purpose, methods, language, moral presuppositions, and knowledge claims" (Fry, 1999, p. 6). Philosophy in nursing involves consideration of the same sorts of ontological, epistemological, and ethical questions mentioned earlier in the chapter. Here, we formulate how these questions are studied in relation to the art, science, and practice of nursing. Thus, an ontological inquiry will consider the nature of nursing; an epistemological inquiry will consider nursing knowledge; an ethical inquiry will consider the moral questions that arise in nursing. Nurses use philosophy to think, to examine assumptions, to analyze concepts, and to carefully consider arguments. In this sense, philosophical inquiry in nursing is an invaluable practical activity in which all nurses should participate.

Developing a particular philosophy of nursing involves careful clarification and reflection on what nurses are trying to do, why they do it, and what knowledge they use. A useful philosophy of nursing will help accomplish these goals. First, it will identify the central phenomena of the discipline. Second, it will relate nursing to a particular world view or philosophical tradition. Third, it will offer some criteria concerning knowledge development in the discipline (Salsberry, 1994). Formulating a philosophy of nursing is about making nurses' frame of reference for being in the world explicit (Smith, 1994).

Scientific inquiry is still the predominant mode of inquiry in nursing. However, science cannot answer some nursing questions (Kikuchi, 1992). Scientific inquiry is directed toward the material world, to what can be measured or is observable through the senses. Thus, techniques of science cannot answer some questions concerning the nature of nursing, the moral ground of nursing practice, or the particular meanings of nurse–patient relationships. Interpretive approaches as well as empiricist approaches are important in nursing philosophy.

Philosophical thinking in nursing has developed on many fronts, and nurses have used philosophy in many different ways (see the Nursing and Canadian Society box). Since the 1980s, nurses have published many articles and books about nursing philosophy, and they have organized many conferences around philosophical themes. In 1988, the Institute for Philosophical Nursing Research was founded at the University of Alberta. If the philosophy of nursing is understood as simply an activity that uses philosophical methods and raises certain kinds of questions about the discipline of nursing, it is possible to appreciate the necessity to support within nursing a number of different approaches to philosophy.

NURSING AND CANADIAN SOCIETY

Fact	Implications for Nursing Practice
In 1988, the Institute for Philosophical Nursing Research was founded at the University of Alberta.	The aim of the institute is to provide leadership in the pursuit of philosophical nursing knowledge that underlies the advancement of the nursing practice.
Philosophical methods raise certain kinds of questions about the discipline of nursing.	Nurses can appreciate the necessity to support within nursing a number of different approaches to philosophy.
Techniques of science cannot answer some questions concerning the nature of nursing, the moral ground of nursing practice, or the particular meanings of nurse–patient relationships.	The CNA's (2002) position statement *Evidence-Based Decision-Making and Nursing Practice* provides directive to nurses concerning the need for scientific evidence to underlie practice.

Overview of Selected Nursing Philosophies

The work of selected nurse philosophers demonstrates the ways in which philosophy can be used in nursing and the kinds of questions a philosophical perspective can address. In the survey that follows, selected nurse philosophers are organized into four groups, according to the types of topics they might address (see Table 4.1). This survey is, of necessity, a partial one, but a range of philosophical positions are included.

Some nurse philosophers directly address nursing philosophy itself as a topic for discussion. For example, Kikuchi (1992) argued for a place for philosophical inquiry in nursing by reasoning that science cannot answer all of nursing's questions. In a later paper, Kikuchi and Simmons (1994) presented a philosophical argument against the appropriateness of particular philosophies for nursing. Salsberry (1994) claimed that a philosophy of nursing will identify the central phenomena of the discipline and relate nursing to a particular world view or philosophical tradition. Smith (1994) asserted that arriving at a philosophy of nursing makes explicit our frame of reference for being in the world. Edwards (1997) explored what constitutes a philosophy of nursing, considering not only what should be included under this heading but also how it should be included. For Edwards, a philosophy of nursing should include an analysis of the concepts deemed to be central to the discipline. Such analysis would include ontological and epistemological values and logic. Johnson (1994) took up the question of what is meant by the art of nursing by using a philosophical method of argument to arrive at a definition of nursing as an art associated with expressive, creative, and intuitive abilities.

Beginning from a different philosophical perspective, Bishop and Scudder (1999) used an interpretive approach to articulate a meaning of nursing from the point of view of practising nurses. Their interpretation focused on nursing as the practice of caring, as a way of being for others, and as a relationship. In all these papers, the authors did not insist that they were offering correct knowledge as found in a scientific paper. Rather, they presented arguments, defended positions, and invited readers to consider the persuasiveness of their analyses and conclusions.

A second group of nurse philosophers used philosophy to address nursing research questions. Often, these inquiries took a phenomenological approach, which means that the researcher investigated and described particular phenomena as they are consciously experienced in nursing practice. Topics of this kind of research range from experiences of illness or grief to experiences of homelessness. For example, Cameron (1992) considered the meanings that the question, "How are you?" can

TABLE 4.1 Selected Nurse Philosophers

Topics They Might Address	Nurse Philosophers	Approach to Inquiry
Argument	Kikuchi, J., & Simmons, H. Johnson, J.	Philosophical Analysis Philosophical Analysis
Epistemology	Edwards, S. Purkis, M. E. Neslon, S.	Philosophical Analysis Philosophical Analysis Philosophical Analysis
Research	Cameron, B.	Interpretive Phenomenology
Ethics	Gadow, S. Bergum, V. Storch, J.	Relational Ethics Relational Ethics Bioethics

have in the context of a nurse–patient relationship, showing that nurses should not take their understanding of these words for granted. Bergum (1989) philosophically explored women's experiences of becoming mothers. These kinds of philosophical writings stimulate nurses to reflect on the meanings of experiences and phenomena that they sometimes assume they already understand. In other words, these types of philosophical inquiries expand thinking by giving us more to think about.

A third group of nurse philosophers asked epistemological questions about the practice of nursing. Some of these writers explicitly drew on other philosophers or philosophical traditions to explicate nursing practice. Purkis (1997) used ideas from the writings of the French philosopher Michel Foucault (1926–1984), such as the disciplined and disciplining gaze (how nurses communicate what counts as health and its promotion) of the nurse, to reflect on the implications of health-promotion discourses and practice. Lawler (1997) also drew on Foucault's writings to suggest that the disciplines of science and economics have influenced how people speak and think about nursing. In particular, the world views that prevail in science and economics do not recognize the importance of relationship and contexts, concepts that nurses consider central to the practice of nursing.

In the area of ethics, a fourth group of nurse philosophers addressed ethical questions about the practice of nursing. Gadow (1994) suggested that the inability of patients to determine the meaning of their own experiences is a moral issue for nursing. Liaschenko (1997) suggested that serious ethical dilemmas can arise for nurses because of the systems and structures that contribute to the powerlessness that some nurses experience in practice.

Even this abbreviated discussion of nurse philosophers reveals that nursing philosophy can be approached in many ways. Note, however, that although they are often not stated, philosophical ideas are an integral component of nursing practice, research, and theory development. Foregrounding, or making explicit philosophical thinking, furthers our understanding of current nursing practices and develops the profession more effectively for the future.

Concepts and Theories

Philosophical thinking provides the foundation for the development and critical analysis of nursing knowledge. Nursing knowledge is organized and communicated by using concepts, models, frameworks, and theories. A theory of nursing will address the subject matter of the discipline of nursing in accordance with a particular philosophical world view. For example, a theory of nursing will include some conceptualization of the nature of nursing, its scope, and purpose. It will identify and describe the central nursing concepts, such as person, health, nursing, and environment, and also propose how these phenomena can be known. It may also address ethical concerns by specifying how to understand moral phenomena encountered in nursing practice. The building blocks of theories are concepts.

Concepts are abstract ideas or mental images of phenomena. They are words that bring forth mental pictures of the properties and meanings of objects, events, or things. Concepts can be (1) readily observable, or *concrete,* ideas, such as thermometer, rash, and lesion; (2) indirectly observable, or *inferential,* ideas, such as pain and temperature; or (3) non-observable, or *abstract,* ideas, such as equilibrium, adaptation, stress, and powerlessness. Many concepts apply to nursing: concepts about human beings, health, helping relationships, and communication. Nursing theories address and specify relationships among four major abstract concepts referred to as the **metaparadigm** of nursing—the most global philosophical or conceptual framework of a profession. A metaparadigm is a higher level of abstraction than a paradigm. It identifies the concepts central to the discipline without relating them to the assumptions of a particular world view. Although consensus exists that the following four concepts make up nursing's metaparadigm (Fawcett, 2005), others have proposed an alternative metaparadigm (Newman, Sime, & Corcoran-Perry, 1981; Parse, 1987):

1. *Person* or *client,* the recipient of nursing care (includes individuals, families, groups, and communities)
2. *Environment,* the internal and external surroundings that affect the client, which includes people in the physical environment, such as families, friends, and significant others
3. *Health,* the degree of wellness or well-being that the client experiences
4. *Nursing,* the attributes, characteristics, and actions of the nurse providing care on behalf of, or in conjunction with, the client

Each nurse theorist's definitions of nursing's major concepts vary in accordance with their world view, their philosophy, and their experience in nursing. Nursing theories serve several purposes (see Box 4.1).

The terms *theory* and *conceptual framework* are often used interchangeably in nursing literature. Strictly speaking, they differ in their levels of abstraction; a conceptual framework is more abstract than a theory. As noted earlier, a conceptual framework is a group of related concepts. It provides an overall view or orientation to focus thoughts. A conceptual framework can be visualized as an umbrella under which many concepts can exist. A theory is a supposition or system of ideas that is proposed to explain a given phenomenon. For example, Newton proposed his theory of gravity to explain why objects always fall from a tree to the ground. A theory

BOX 4.1 PURPOSES OF NURSING THEORIES AND CONCEPTUAL FRAMEWORKS

Nursing theories and conceptual frameworks provide direction and guidance for (1) structuring professional nursing practice, education, and research; and (2) differentiating the focus of nursing from other professions.

IN PRACTICE

- Help nurses to describe, explain, and predict everyday experiences
- Guide assessment, intervention, and evaluation of nursing care
- Provide a rationale for collecting reliable and valid data about the health status of clients, which are essential for effective decision making and implementation
- Help establish criteria to measure the quality of nursing care
- Help build a common nursing terminology to use in communicating with other health professionals: ideas are developed and words defined
- Enhance the autonomy (independence and self-governance) of nursing by defining its own independent functions

IN EDUCATION

- Provide a general focus for curriculum design
- Guide curricular decision making

IN RESEARCH

- Offer a framework for generating knowledge and new ideas
- Assist in discovering knowledge gaps in the specific field of study
- Offer a systematic approach to identify questions for study, select variables, interpret findings, and validate nursing interventions

goes one step beyond a conceptual framework by relating concepts through definitions that state significant relationships between concepts.

The major purpose of a conceptual framework is to give clear and explicit direction to the three areas of nursing: practice, education, and research. A theory, in contrast, is more limited in scope. Its primary purpose is to generate knowledge in a field. A theory explores phenomena, expresses relationships among facts, generates a hypothesis, and predicts future events and relationships.

Because the primary purpose of nursing theory is to generate scientific knowledge, nursing theory and nursing research are closely related. Nursing knowledge is generated within empiricist and interpretive research traditions. Empiricist approaches can be theory generating or theory testing, whereas interpretive approaches expose understandings of an experience. Scientific knowledge is derived from testing hypotheses (assumptions) generated by theories for nursing. Research determines the utility of those hypotheses, and research findings may be developed into theories for nursing. In the research process, comparisons are made between the observed outcomes of research and the relationship predicted by the hypotheses.

Overview of Selected Nursing Theories

Theory development gained momentum in the 1960s and has progressed markedly since then. Because opinions on the nature and structure of nursing vary, theories continue to be developed. Each theory bears the name of the person or group who developed it and reflects the beliefs of the developer.

The following nursing theories vary considerably in their (1) level of abstraction; (2) conceptualization of the client, health or illness, and nursing; and (3) ability to describe, explain, or predict. Some theories are broad in scope; others are limited. See Table 4.2 for a summary.

Only brief summaries of the theorists' central theme and basic assumptions are included here. For more detailed information on how specific theories are used in current nursing practice, please see Alligood and Tomey (2006) and Tomey and Alligood (2006) in the Suggested Readings section of this chapter.

Nightingale's Environmental Theory

Florence Nightingale, often considered the first nurse theorist, defined nursing more 100 years ago as "the act of utilizing the environment of the patient to assist him in his recovery" (Nightingale, 1860/1957). She linked health with five environmental factors: (1) pure or fresh air, (2) pure water, (3) efficient drainage, (4) cleanliness, and (5) light, especially direct sunlight. Deficiencies in these five factors produced lack of health, or illness.

These environmental factors attain significance when we consider that sanitation conditions in the hospitals of the mid-nineteenth century were extremely poor and that women working in the hospitals were often unreliable, uneducated, and incompetent.

In addition to those factors, Nightingale also stressed the importance of keeping the client warm, maintaining a noise-free environment, and attending to the client's diet in terms of assessing intake, timeliness of the meal, and its effect on the person.

Nightingale set the stage for further work in the development of nursing theories. Her general concepts about ventilation, cleanliness, quiet, warmth, and diet

TABLE 4.2 Selected Nurse Theorists' Conceptualization of Nursing, Health, Environment, and Human Beings

Nightingale	• *Nursing* is the act of using the environment of the patient to assist in recovery. • *Health* is linked to five *environmental* factors: fresh air, pure water, efficient drainage, cleanliness, and light. A deficiency in any of these factors is linked to illness. • *Human beings* are described as recipients of compassionate care.
Peplau	• *Nursing* is a therapeutic relationship between the nurse and the client. • *Health* includes interpersonal and intrapersonal experiences. • *Environment* includes the client's internal experiences and the relational environment in which he or she lives. • *Human beings* are conceptualized as subjects of their own experience rather than as objects of professional care.
Henderson	• *Nursing* is assisting sick or well individuals to gain independence in meeting their fundamental needs, or accompanying the client to a peaceful death. • *Health* is linked to the 14 fundamental needs identified by Henderson. • *Environment* is understood as the physicality of the client and his or her immediate physical surroundings. *Nurses* manage the environment as a way of moving the client toward performing activities unaided. • *Human* beings are physical beings who experience a variety of needs and are in relation with others for the purpose of meeting those needs.
Roy	• *Nursing* is the promotion of client adaptation in experiences of health, quality of life, and death with dignity. • *Health* is the way in which human beings interact with and adapt to environmental stimuli. • *Environment* is understood as the variable and constantly changing stimuli to which a person must adapt. • *Human beings* are seen as interacting with their physical and social environments and in relationship with the world and with God: "Persons are seen as adapting to those stimuli present as a result of his/her position on the health-illness continuum" (Roy & Andrews in Fawcett, 2005, p. 367).
Watson	• *Nursing* is an intentional consciousness of caring enacted between a nurse and another, transcending the boundaries of time, space, and physicality. • *Health* "refers to unity and harmony within the mind, body and soul. Health is also associated with the degree of congruence between the self as perceived and the self as experienced" (Watson, 1988, p. 48). • Environment, both internal and external, are interdependent and strongly influence health and illness. Healing environments comprise physical and nonphysical energies and consciousness, whereby wholeness, comfort, beauty, dignity, and peace are potentiated. • *Human beings* physically are confined in space and time, whereas the mind and soul are not.
Parse	• *Nursing* is co-creating a situation in which clients choose and bear responsibility for patterns of health. • *Health* is a continuously changing process, the quality of life co-created by human beings in relation with the universe. • *Environment* is understood as the world in which lived experiences unfold. • *Human beings* are open, indivisible, freely choosing beings who co-create patterns of relating.
Leininger	• *Nursing* is "a learned humanistic and scientific profession and discipline which is focused on human care phenomenon and activities to help people maintain or regain their wellbeing or health in culturally meaningful ways" (Leininger & McFarland, 2006, p. 7). • *Health* is a culturally defined, valued, and practised state of well-being that reflects people's abilities to perform their daily activities. • *Environment* is the physical, ecological, sociopolitical, and cultural context of events or experiences. • *Human beings,* families, clans, and collective groups are constituted within cultural contexts, including values, beliefs, and life ways.
Newman	• *Nursing* is the study of caring in the human health experience. • *Health* is conceptualized as expanding consciousness that occurs when a person gains insight from a disturbance in the flow of daily living. The process of evolution of consciousness is also the process of health. • *Environment* is unbroken wholeness in which health and illness are viewed as a single process. • *Human beings* are continuous with the undivided wholeness of the universe and can be identified by their patterns of consciousness: "The person does not *possess* consciousness, the person *is* consciousness" (Newman in Fawcett, 2005, p. 452).
Campbell (UBC Model)	• *Nursing* is the activities that help patients to learn and maximize their coping abilities to manage critical situations within their life cycle. • *Health* is stability—preferably at the most optimum level possible within the situation. • *Environment* is anything that is outside the individual's system. • *Person* refers to individuals, each of whom shares nine basic needs. The individual meets those needs through coping mechanisms.
Allen (McGill Model)	• *Nursing* is the response of the profession to individuals' search for healthy living. • *Health* is a social process. Health can be described, measured, and modified. • *Environment* is the social context in which learning takes place. • *Person* in this model refers to the family or other social group.

remain integral parts of nursing and health care today. Dunphy (2006) reminds us that in addition to manifesting these core ideals of health, Nightingale, as an original nurse-activist, demonstrated the ways in which the values of caring can be transformed into an activism capable of transforming an "unjust health care system . . . into a more humanistic and just one" (p. 54). In this way, Nightingale was a role model for showing through practice that actions driven by caring and compassion bring about justice.

Peplau's Interpersonal Relations Model

Hildegard Peplau, a psychiatric nurse, introduced her interpersonal concepts in 1952. Central to Peplau's theory is the use of a therapeutic relationship between the nurse and the client. Though now a taken-for-granted practice in nursing, in the early 1950s the idea of engaging with clients as subjects, rather than treating them as objects, was revolutionary, Despite the early resistance to her approach, Peplau's work is responsible for the integration of the therapeutic relationship, the nurse–client relationship into nursing theory. Traces of Peplau's emphasis on the nurse–client relationship can be found in all the major theoretical works today.

Nurses enter into a personal relationship with an individual when the need is present. The nurse–client relationship evolves in four phases:

1. *Orientation.* During this phase, the client seeks help, and the nurse helps the client to understand the problem and the extent of the need for help.
2. *Working phase: identification.* During this phase, the client may assume a posture of dependence, interdependence, or independence in relation to the nurse (relatedness); the nurse uses her or his professional knowledge "to aid the patience [*sic*] to make full use of the relationship, in order to solve the health problem" (Fawcett, 2005, p. 535). The nurse's focus is on helping the client understand the interpersonal meaning of their situation or behaviour (Peplau, 1952).
3. *Working phase: exploitation.* In this phase, the client derives full value from what the nurse offers through the relationship. The client uses available services on the basis of self-interest and needs. Power shifts from the nurse to the client.
4. *Termination.* In this final phase, the nurse–client relationship has closure (Peplau, 1952). Termination is seen as the endpoint of a time-limited relationship and calls for a marking of the end of the relationship.

To help clients fulfill their needs, nurses assume many roles: stranger, teacher, resource person, surrogate, leader, and counsellor. Peplau's model continues to be used by clinicians and has contributed significantly to the use of therapeutic relationships and the nurse as a therapeutic tool in many areas of nursing practice.

Henderson's Definition of Nursing

In 1966, Virginia Henderson formulated a definition of the unique function of nursing. This definition was a major stepping stone in the emergence of nursing as a discipline separate from medicine. Like Nightingale, Henderson described nursing in relation to the client and the client's environment. Unlike Nightingale, Henderson saw the nurse as concerned with both well and ill individuals, acknowledged that nurses interact with clients even when recovery may not be feasible, and mentioned the teaching and advocacy roles of the nurse.

Henderson conceptualized the nurse's role as helping sick or well individuals to gain independence in meeting these 14 fundamental needs (1966, 1991, p. 22–23):

1. *Breathe normally*
2. *Eat and drink adequately*
3. *Eliminate body wastes*
4. *Move and maintain desirable positions*
5. *Sleep and rest*
6. *Select suitable clothes, dress and undress*
7. *Maintain body temperature within a normal range by adjusting clothing and modifying the environment*
8. *Keep the body clean and well groomed and protect the integument*
9. *Avoid dangers in the environment and avoid injuring others*
10. *Communicate with others in expressing emotions, needs, fears, or opinions*
11. *Worship according to one's faith*
12. *Work in such a way that there is a sense of accomplishment*
13. *Play or participate in various forms of recreation*
14. *Learn, discover, or satisfy the curiosity that leads to normal development and health, and use the available health facilities*

Henderson published many works and continues to be cited in current nursing literature. Her emphasis on the importance of nursing's independence from, and interdependence with, other health-care disciplines is well recognized. In Henderson's later work (1991), she questioned whether nurses continue to value engagement with clients in the palliative experience or if the profession has shifted toward a medical approach in which the focus is prolonging life, even when death is inevitable.

Roy's Adaptation Model

Sister Callista Roy's adaptation model was first published in book form in 1976. She defined *adaptation* as "the process and outcome whereby the thinking and feeling person uses conscious awareness and choice to create human and environmental integration" (Roy, 1997, p. 44).

Roy later restated her scientific and philosophical assumptions for the twenty-first century. These assumptions focused on the increasing complexity of person and environment, self-organization, and the relationship among human beings, the universe, and what can be considered a supreme being or God. Her philosophical assumptions were refined by using major characteristics of "creation spirituality"—a view that "persons and the earth are one, and that they are in God and of God" (Roy, 1997, p. 46). "Roy's vision for the future emphasizes the principle that people and the earth have common patterns and integral relationships" (Roy & Zhan, 2006, p. 270). In this way Roy moved past her earlier supposition that the system acts to maintain itself, shifting the emphasis to the "purposefulness of human existence in a universe that is creative" (p. 270).

Roy focused on the individual as a biopsychosocial adaptive system that employs a feedback cycle of input (stimuli), throughput (control processes), and output (behaviours or adaptive responses). Both the individual and the environment are sources of stimuli that require modification to promote adaptation, an ongoing purposive response. "Central to Roy's theoretical model is the belief that adaptive responses support health, which is defined as a state and a process of being and becoming integrated and whole" (Roy & Zahn, 2006, p. 270). Although Roy originally conceptualized her model in regard to the health of the individual, more recently the modes of the model have been expanded to speak to groups as well as individuals. Each person's or group's adaptation level is unique and constantly changing.

Individuals and groups respond to needs (stimuli) in one of four modes:

1. The *physiological mode* involves the body's basic physiological needs and ways of adapting to fluid and electrolytes, activity and rest, circulation and oxygen, nutrition and elimination, protection, the senses, and neurological and endocrine functions.
2. The *self-concept mode* includes two components: the *physical* self, which involves sensation and body image, and the *personal* self, which involves self-ideal, self-consistency, and the moral-ethical self.
3. The *role function mode* is determined by the need for social integrity and refers to the performance of duties based on given positions within society.
4. The *interdependence mode* involves a person's relations with significant others and support systems that provide help, affection, and attention.

The goal of Sister Callista Roy's model is to enhance life processes through adaptation in these four adaptive modes.

Watson's Human Caring Theory

Jean Watson (1979) believed the practice of caring is central to nursing; it is the unifying focus for practice. Her major assumptions about caring are shown in Box 4.2. Watson originally referred to the nursing interventions related to human care as *carative factors,* a guide Watson refers to as the "core of nursing." Watson later expanded each of the carative factors to become *clinical caritas processes.* Watson explains: "What differs in the *clinical caritas* framework is that a decidedly spiritual dimension and an overt evocation of love and caring are merged for a new paradigm for this millennium" (Watson, 2006, p. 298). *Caritas* originates with a Greek word meaning "to cherish or appreciate."

Watson (1979) outlined the original carative factors with the addition of the clinical caritas processes in 2001 (Watson, 2001):

1. Forming a humanistic-altruistic system of values becomes a practice of loving kindness and equanimity within the context of caring consciousness.
2. Instilling faith and hope becomes being authentically present and enabling and sustaining the deep belief system and subjective world of self and the one being cared for.
3. Cultivating sensitivity to ourselves and others becomes cultivation of our own spiritual practices

BOX 4.2 WATSON'S ASSUMPTIONS OF CARING

- Human caring in nursing is not just an emotion, concern, attitude, or benevolent desire. Caring connotes a personal response.
- Caring is an intersubjective (between human subjects) human process and is the moral ideal of nursing.
- Caring can be effectively demonstrated only interpersonally.
- Effective caring promotes health and individual or family growth.
- Caring promotes health more than does curing.
- Caring responses accept people not only as they are now but also for what they may become.
- A caring environment offers the development of potential while allowing the person to choose the best action at a given time.
- Caring occasions involve action and choice by nurse and client. If the caring occasion is transpersonal, the limits of openness expand, as do human capacities.
- The most abstract characteristic of a caring person is that the person is somehow responsive to another person as a unique individual, perceives the other's feelings, and sets one person apart from another.
- Human caring involves values, a will and a commitment to care, knowledge, caring actions, and consequences.
- The ideal and value of caring is a starting point, a stance, and an attitude that has to become a will, an intention, a commitment, and a conscious judgment that manifests itself in concrete acts.

and transpersonal self, going beyond the ego self, opening to others with sensitivity and compassion.

4. Developing a helping-trust (human care) relationship becomes developing and sustaining a helping-trusting authentic caring relationship.
5. Promoting and accepting the expression of positive and negative feelings becomes being present to and supportive of the expression of positive and negative feelings as a connection with deeper spirit of self and the one being cared for.
6. Systematic use of a creative problem-solving caring process becomes creative use of self and all ways of knowing as part of the caring process, to engage in artistry of caring-healing practices.
7. Promotion of transpersonal teaching-learning becomes engaging in a genuine teaching-learning experience that attends to unity of being and meaning, attempting to stay within others' frames of reference.
8. Providing a supportive, protective, or corrective mental, physical, sociocultural, and spiritual environment becomes creating a healing environment at all levels (a physical and nonphysical, subtle environment of energy and consciousness whereby wholeness, beauty, comfort, dignity, and peace are potentiated).
9. Assisting with the gratification of human needs becomes assisting with basic needs with an intentional caring consciousness administering human care essentials, which potentiate alignment of mind-body-spirit, wholeness and unity of being in all aspects of care, and tending to both embodied spirit and spiritual emergence.
10. Allowing for existential-phenomenological-spiritual forces becomes opening and attending to spiritual-mysterious and existential dimensions of our own life-death, and soul care for self and the one being cared for.

In addition to the carative factors or caritas processes, three major ideas underpin all of Watson's work: (1) the transpersonal caring relationship, (2) the caring moment or caring occasion, and (3) the caring (healing) consciousness.

Although numerous theorists include the idea of caring in their work, Watson's work spoke particularly of *transpersonal caring*, in which the nurse seeks to "connect with and embrace the spirit or soul of the other" through genuine and authentic engagement (2006, p. 299). The *caring moment* is understood to be "the moment of coming together" of the nurse and the client in which each person brings all of his or her experiential history with an intention of care and a possibility of connection. "If the caring moment is transpersonal, each feels a connection with the other at the spirit level; thus, the moment transcends time and space, opening up new possibilities for healing and human connection at a deeper level than physical interaction" (p. 300). The relationship between the nurse and client is affected by the nurse's consciousness in the moment and thus transpersonal caring within a caring moment is manifest in an intentional *consciousness of caring or healing* by the nurse. For Watson, the process of an intentional (consciousness) transpersonal caring occasion transcended time, space, and physicality: the effect of a caring interaction can go beyond the time and space boundaries of a given caring moment.

Watson's theory of human caring has received worldwide recognition and is a major force in redefining nursing as a *caring-healing health* model. Watson (2006) described her theory as building on nursing's disciplinary heritage, while simultaneously challenging nursing to mature in its own discipline and to affect health-care providers beyond disciplinary boundaries in a caring model of health.

Parse's Theory of Human Becoming

Parse first published her theory in 1981 in *Man-Living-Health: A Theory for Nursing* and later retitled her work as a theory of human becoming, substituting the term *human* for *man*. Parse proposed three assumptions about human becoming (1995):

1. Human becoming is freely choosing personal *meaning* in situations in the intersubjective process of relating value priorities.
2. Human becoming is co-creating *rhythmic patterns* or relating in mutual process with the universe.
3. Human becoming is *co-transcending* multidimensionally with the emerging possibilities.

These three assumptions focus on the concepts of meaning, rhythmicity, and co-transcendence:

- Meaning arises from a person's interrelationship with the world and refers to happenings to which the person attaches varying degrees of significance.
- Rhythmicity is the movement toward greater diversity.
- Co-transcendence is the process of reaching out beyond the self.

Parse's theory of human becoming emphasizes how individuals choose and bear responsibility for patterns of personal health. Parse contends that the client, not the nurse, is the authority figure and decision maker. The nurse's role involves helping individuals and families in choosing the possibilities for changing the health process. Specifically, the nurse's role consists of illuminating meaning (uncovering what was and what will be), synchronizing rhythms (leading through discussion to recognize harmony), and mobilizing transcendence (dreaming of possibilities and planning to reach them).

The Parse nurse uses "true presence" in the nurse–client process. "In true presence, the nurse's whole being is immersed with the client as the other illuminates the meanings of his or her situation and moves beyond the moment" (Parse, 1994, p. 18).

Leininger's Cultural Care Diversity and Universality Theory

Madeleine Leininger, a well-known nurse anthropologist, first published her cultural care diversity and universality theory in 1985 in the journal *Nursing and Health Care* and explained it further in 1988 and then in 1991, in her book *Culture Care Diversity and Universality: A Theory of Nursing*.

Leininger stated that *care* is the essence of nursing and the dominant, distinctive, and unifying feature of nursing. She emphasized that human caring, although a universal phenomenon, varies among cultures in its expressions, processes, and patterns; it is largely culturally derived. Leininger's work draws on the premise that people of different cultures are capable of informing caregivers of the kind of care they need. McFarland points out that Leininger's theory is the "only nursing theory explicitly focused on culture and care of diverse cultures" (2006, p. 477). Leininger defined culture, culture care, culture care diversity, culture care universality, generic care, and professional care. Her sunrise model, which depicts her theory, is presented in Chapter 10. For nurses to assist people of diverse cultures, Leininger also presented three intervention modes:

- Culture care preservation and maintenance
- Culture care accommodation, negotiation, or both
- Culture care restructuring and repatterning

Margaret Newman and Expansion of Consciousness

Margaret Newman's theory was influenced by her early life experiences in caring for her mother, when she began to think of health as other than the absence of disease. Following her undergraduate and graduate nursing education, informed by Martha Rogers, Newman proposed that illness reflects the life pattern of the person and that illness and health are part of a unitary life process, one no more important than the other. As she continued to develop her theory in the 1970s, Newman articulated the central thesis of her work that health is the expansion of consciousness (Newman, 1986).

When challenged about the scientific basis for her theory, Newman interestingly sidestepped the controversy of the scientification of nursing theory and instead claimed that her work "is not necessarily about science but rather about *meaning:* the meaning of life and health . . . found in the evolving process of expanding consciousness" (Newman, 1986, p. 4). Newman suggested that the use of the theory of health as expanded consciousness requires education in a curriculum that disrupts a view of health and illness as dichotomous or even as disparate ends of a continuum and instead has a "view of disease as a meaningful aspect of health. Furthermore the nurse has to let go of wanting to control the situation. The client's choices have to be respected and supported, even when those choices conflict with the nurse's personal values" (Fawcett, 2005, p. 462).

Evidence-Informed Practice

Is It Important That Residents Feel They Are Listened to by Staff?

Canadian researchers Jonas-Simpson, Mitchell, Fisher, Jones, and Linscott (2006) interviewed 20 residents in long-term-care settings to ask about the experience of being listened to. The residents were male and female and were in institutional settings because of either social support or physical support needs. The research questions, interview questions, and method of analysis were all guided by Parse's theory of human becoming. The results of the study revealed that these participants found that being listened to was critical to quality of life. They described the feelings in themselves when they perceived that others listened to them, as well as the relationships sustained through listening, and, finally, how being listened to gave them a sense of being a "bit important" in a large setting.

NURSING IMPLICATIONS: Developing strong listening skills and conveying that what an individual has to say is important to the nurse strengthens the nurse–resident relationship, contributes to the resident feeling nurtured, and enhances the quality of the resident's life. This research supports the use of true presence while delivering nursing care.

Source: Based on "The Experience of Being Listened to: A Qualitative Study of Older Adults in Long-Term-Care Settings," by C. M. Jonas-Simpson, G. J. Mitchell, A. Fisher, G. Jones, and J. Linscott, 2006, *Journal of Gerontological Nursing, 32*(1), pp. 46–53.

Campbell's UBC (University of British Columbia) Model of Nursing

Margaret Campbell (1987) developed the UBC model of nursing. Campbell guided nurse practitioners, researchers, and educators to look to the following elements of a model to guide their practice: "the view of the client" or "the recipient of care" and "the role and function of nursing in relation to the recipient of care and as a distinct and separate member of the team of health care professionals" (p. 5). In the UBC model, the major theme is a behavioural system with interacting and interdependent subsystems, each representing a basic human need. Campbell viewed human beings as having nine basic human needs, constantly striving to satisfy these needs by using a range of coping behaviours, both innate and acquired. According to this model, environment is that which lies outside the boundary of the system. The nurse is seen as nurturing "individuals experiencing critical periods so that they may develop and use a range of coping behaviours that will permit them to satisfy their basic human needs, to achieve stability and to reach optimum health" (Campbell, 1987, p. 10).

Margaret Campbell developed this model on the basis of several assumptions about Canadian society. She assumed that society views optimal health as a desirable goal for all of its members and that members of society would assume responsibility for utilizing behaviours that promote and maintain positive health. She further assumed that society expects its members will behave in ways that will not be harmful to themselves or others in the satisfaction of their needs. She assumed that society expects health-care professionals to function competently and ethically. Lastly, Campbell assumed that society expects the UBC model for nursing, or any model for nursing, to be congruent with the values of that society. These assumptions about the values that Canadians hold and the beliefs about nursing that Campbell identified then guided her to conceptualize the UBC model in a particular way.

The UBC model in Figure 4.1 shows the nine subsystems that make up the behavioural system, with each subsystem representing one basic need. This illustration also shows how each of these subsystems relates to the others and how they interrelate to the system as whole, a feature of significance to nursing. For example, whatever happens to one subsystem (including nursing interventions) can influence the system as a whole. Figure 4.2 shows the structure of each of the subsystems. Each subsystem is responsible for the satisfaction of one of the basic needs. Each subsystem consists of (1) an inner region that includes the need and the abilities to meet that need, and (2) an outer region that includes the need-related goal and the forces influencing attainment of that goal. Figure 4.3 shows how the parts of a subsystem relate to one another. The determinants of coping behaviours are both cognitive (knowing what to do) and executive (carry the needed action out). Forces influence movement toward or away from desired goals. It is the understanding of the detailed structure and function of a particular subsystem, and its interrelation with other subsystems and with the behavioural system as a whole, that guides the nurse in making decisions relative to providing care.

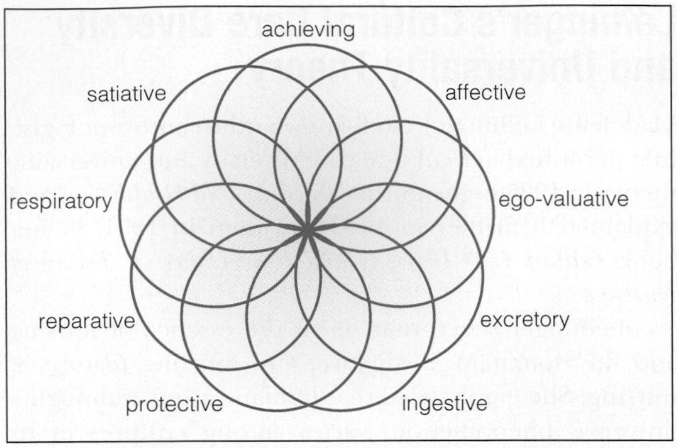

FIGURE 4.1 The Nine Basic Needs of the Individual
(From **The UBC Model for Nursing: Directions for Practice** *(p. 32), by M. Campbell, 1987, Vancouver: University of British Columbia School of Nursing.)*

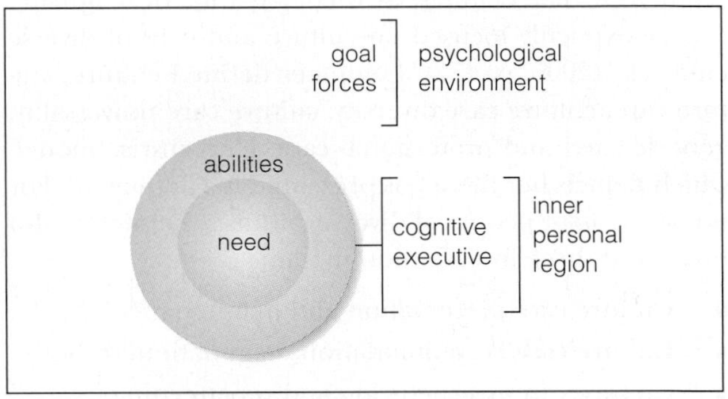

FIGURE 4.2 Structure of a Subsystem: The Parts
(From **The UBC Model for Nursing: Directions for Practice** *(p. 33), by M. Campbell, 1987, Vancouver: University of British Columbia School of Nursing.)*

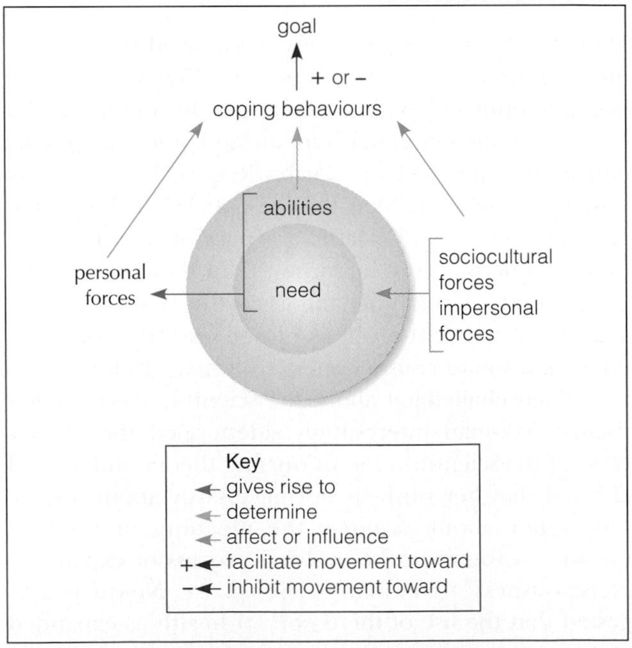

FIGURE 4.3 Structure of a Subsystem: Interrelationship of the Parts
(From **The UBC Model for Nursing: Directions for Practice** *(p. 34), by M. Campbell, 1987, Vancouver: University of British Columbia School of Nursing.)*

Allen's McGill Model of Nursing (1986)

Another example of a nursing model is the McGill model developed by Moyra Allen (1986). In this model, the theme for nursing is the nature of healthy living. This model serves as the curriculum model for the McGill School of Nursing. Allen saw the search for healthy living as a quest. The focus of this model is the family or other social group in which learning is initiated, nurtured, and directed. The environment is the context in which this learning takes place. This context could be the home, workplace, community group, hospital, or clinic. Health, according to Allen, is something that can be measured and can be modified. In Allen's model, nursing is a professional response to the person's natural response to healthy living. The goal of nursing is to assist people to enhance their problem-solving skills in dealing with health matters.

The McGill model of nursing has been credited with developing a unique role for nurses on an interdisciplinary team by providing a framework for the conceptualizing of the nurse's role, the assessment of families' needs, and the development of a nursing knowledge base (Feeley & Gerez-Lirette, 1992). The McGill model of nursing has been identified as appropriate for community health nursing in that it concentrates on health promotion and brings together elements underlying a family-development view of care. In more recent years, the focus of clinical practice with families has been shifting from a deficit-based to a strength-based perspective, a perspective that is central to the McGill model of nursing (Feeley & Gottlieb, 2000).

Sister Simone Roach's Attributes of Professional Caring

In her 1992 book *The Human Act of Caring*, Dr. Simone Roach puts forth the notion that "caring is an essential ingredient in human development and survival" (p. 2). Roach claims that nurses' professional caring has five important attributes: compassion, competence, confidence, conscience, and commitment. In her 2002 book she added the sixth attribute of comportment (see Box 4.3 for a description of each).

BOX 4.3 ROACH'S ATTRIBUTES OF PROFESSIONAL CARING

Roach claims that nurses' professional caring has six important attributes:

- *Compassion:* a sensitivity to the pain and brokenness of the other; a quality of presence that allows one to share with and make room for the other
- *Competence:* having the knowledge, judgment, skills, energy, experience, and motivation required to respond adequately to the demands of the professional responsibilities
- *Confidence:* the self-belief that fosters trusting relationships
- *Conscience:* a state of moral awareness that grows with experience
- *Commitment:* a complex, affective response characterized by convergence between desires and obligations and by the deliberate choice to act in accordance with them
- *Comportment:* use of dress, language, and personal bearing to communicate caring and respect for the dignity of both the patient and the nurse

Source: From *The Human Art of Caring: A Blueprint for the Health Professions* (2nd revised edition), by S. Roach, 2002, Ottawa: Canadian Hospital Association Press.

Case Study 4

Kaili is a 32-year-old man with HIV. His first AIDS-defining illness caused his weight to drop from 80 kg to 54 kg because of intractable diarrhea. The physician thought caloric intake was of primary importance and urged Kaili to eat whatever he desired. Medications for the diarrhea were also prescribed, but Kaili was not happy with the side effects of the medication. Since Kaili was getting worse, the nurse argued that he needed intravenous feedings and his oral intake should be restricted to bland foods until the diarrhea stopped. Then, the nurse noted, additional foods could be added one at a time according to Kaili's tolerance of them. Kaili has many family and friends, who offered to manage his intake.

The physician's stance was that AIDS was similar to advanced cancer in terms of quality of life; he would not order intravenous feedings, just as he would not for someone with advanced cancer. The nurse argued that this was Kaili's first AIDS infection, and his prognosis was better than an individual with advanced cancer. The nurse wanted to stop the diarrhea and supplement nutrition in the meantime. Kaili's friends and family were pleased with the nurse's approach, but Kaili was not as easily convinced.

Critical Thinking Questions

1. What concepts are present in this case?
2. How are the nurse and physician defining the paradigm? What are their main perspectives?
3. How might Florence Nightingale analyze this situation?
4. Which of the nursing models in this chapter best supports the nurse's plan of care?

After working through these questions, go to the MyNursingLab at **http://www.mynursinglab.com** to check your answers.

KEY WORDS

concept
conceptual framework
conceptual model
theory
ontology
epistemology
ethics
paradigm
assumptions
empiricist tradition
scientific method
interpretive tradition
metaparadigm

CHAPTER HIGHLIGHTS

- As an increasingly emerging profession, nursing is now deeply involved in identifying its own unique knowledge base—that is, the body of knowledge essential to nursing practice, or a nursing science.
- Nurses must communicate exactly what makes their place in the interdisciplinary team unique and important.
- Theories offer ways of conceptualizing a discipline in clear, explicit terms that can be communicated to others.
- Because opinions about the nature and structure of nursing vary, theories continue to be developed. Each nursing theory bears the name of the person or group who developed it and reflects the beliefs of the developer.
- The theories vary considerably in (1) their level of abstraction; (2) their conceptualization of the client, health and illness, and nursing; and (3) their ability to describe, explain, or predict. Some theories are broad in scope; others are limited.
- Nursing theories serve several essential purposes, some of which are to differentiate the focus of nursing from other professions; to structure professional nursing practice, education, and research; to help build a common nursing terminology to use in communicating with other health professionals; and to enhance autonomy of nursing through defining its own independent functions.
- Because the primary purpose of nursing theory is to generate scientific knowledge, nursing theory and nursing research are closely related. Scientific knowledge is derived from testing hypotheses generated by theories for nursing. Research determines the utility of those hypotheses, and research findings may be developed into theories for nursing.
- The major distinction between a theory and a conceptual framework or model is the level of abstraction, with the conceptual framework being more abstract than the theory. A conceptual model is a system of related concepts or a conceptual diagram. Its major purpose is to give clear and explicit direction to the three areas of nursing: practice, education, and research. A theory generates knowledge in a field.
- Nursing theories address and specify relationships among four major concepts, the building blocks of theory: nursing, health and illness, environment, and the person or client.
- Each nurse theorist's definitions of these four major concepts vary in accordance with personal philosophy, scientific orientation, experience in nursing, and how that experience has affected the theorist's view of nursing.
- Conceptual models for nursing relate to the nursing process in that they are operationalized or made real by the use of the nursing process. How nurses view human beings influences how they assess and intervene.
- Today, models for nursing are being refined in accordance with societal needs and with their tested usefulness.

ASSESS YOUR LEARNING

1. Nursing theory is important to the development of the nursing discipline for what reason?
   - **a.** It specifies the direction of the research efforts in the profession.
   - **b.** It tells us exactly how to act in various situations.
   - **c.** It articulates the role of nurses and differentiates nursing from other professions.
   - **d.** It helps us to question our assumptions.
2. Which of the following types of concepts might *caring* be conceptualized as?
   - **a.** Concrete
   - **b.** Inferential
   - **c.** Metaparadigm
   - **d.** Abstract
3. While Jane and Marcy are studying for a nursing exam, Marcy asks what the difference is between a theory and a conceptual framework. Which of these statements made by Jane would reflect an accurate understanding of the two terms?
   - **a.** "A theory explicitly states the relationship between concepts, while a conceptual framework is a group of related concepts."

b. "Theory is also used interchangeably with the term *conceptual model.*"

c. "There is absolutely no difference between the terms *theory* and *conceptual framework;* the terms are used interchangeably."

d. "A theory is broader in scope and its purpose is to generate knowledge, while a conceptual framework is more limited in scope and its purpose is to give direction to nursing research, practice, and education."

4. A nurse is taking care of a pediatric patient who has undergone surgery for a ruptured appendix. Postoperatively, the nurse is reluctant to administer any analgesics to her patient because she believes children experience less pain than adults. Her belief exemplifies which of the following?

a. A philosophical inquiry

b. An ethical opinion

c. An assumption

d. A physiological fact

5. In 1978 the nursing scholar Carper identified four patterns of nursing knowledge, including empirics, esthetics, personal knowledge, and ethics. What area of philosophical inquiry does this represent?

a. Ontology

b. Epistemology

c. Paradigm

d. Scientific method

6. Nurse John has been working with Lana, an inpatient with a history of depression and suicide ideation, for the past two weeks. In conversation, Lana has demonstrated readiness for discharge and has asked John to help her access services in the community to help her cope when she goes home. According to Peplau's interpersonal relations model, John and Lana are demonstrating which phase of the nurse–patient relationship?

a. Orientation

b. Identification

c. Exploitation

d. Termination

7. The metaparadigm of nursing is the global framework of the profession. The abstract concepts generally agreed on as the metaparadigm include which of the following?

a. Caring, health, environment, patient

b. Person, nursing, health, environment

c. Health, caring, patient, nursing

d. Research, practice, education

8. While in discussion regarding the care of a patient, your nursing colleague states, "I just really think we need to identify the stressors affecting Mr. Megron's health, and then we can help him adapt to his new health situation." What theorist might you suspect your colleague follows in her nursing practice?

a. Roy

b. Henderson

c. Parse

d. Nightingale

9. Many of the nursing theorists use the concept of caring as a strong element within their theory. Which of the following theorists is best known for her theory on caring?

a. Florence Nightingale

b. Jean Watson

c. Virginia Henderson

d. Madeleine Leininger

10. The UBC (University of British Columbia) model of nursing could be considered which type of theory?

a. Systems

b. Interpersonal

c. Caring

d. Developmental

After working through these questions, go to the MyNursingLab at ***http://www.mynursinglab.com*** *to check your answers and see explanations.*

SUGGESTED READINGS

Alligood, M. & Tomey, A. (2006). *Nursing theory: Utilization and application* (3rd ed.). St. Louis, MO: Mosby.

This is an excellent source for examining how selected nursing theories contribute to and drive nursing practice.

Arndt, M. J. (1995). Parse's theory of human becoming in practice with hospitalized adolescents. *Nursing Science Quarterly, 8*(2), 86–90.

This author applies Parse's theory of human becoming to the care of hospitalized adolescents and their families. Four scenarios are included to illustrate the practice methodology of this theory: an 18-year-old boy with Hirschsprung's disease; a 17-year-old boy with acute myelogenous leukemia; an 18-year-old girl with acute myeloblastic leukemia; and a 15-year-old girl admitted for surgery for an abdominal mass.

Gless, P. A. (1995). Applying the Roy adaptation model to the care of clients with quadriplegia. *Rehabilitation Nursing, 20*(1), 11–16.

Gless states that clients with quadriplegia can benefit from a holistic approach to care that focuses on promoting positive coping and adaptation, an approach that the Roy adaptation model delineates. This article discusses major assumptions of Roy's adaptation model and offers a case study to show the effectiveness of using the nursing process within the model's guidelines to help a client with quadriplegia adapt to living in a long-term-care facility. Roy's five steps of the nursing process (assessment of stimuli, nursing diagnosis, goal setting, nursing interventions, and evaluation) are applied to the physiologic, self-concept, role-function, and interdependent adaptive modes.

Marckx, B. B. (1995). Watson's theory of caring: A model for implementation in practice. *Journal of Nursing Care Quality, 9*(4), 43–54.

Marckx introduces Jean Watson's theory of human caring in nursing as an innovative approach to improving care for residents in a special dementia unit. Specific examples of ways that Watson's model can be applied in typical nurse–client situations are presented. Implementation strategies with creative visual aids are included, and research tools for the evaluation of outcomes are described.

Tomey, A., & Alligood, M. (2006). *Nurse theorists and their work* (6th ed.). St. Louis, MO: Mosby.

This beginning text presents many of the nurse theorists in terms of background, their theory, critique, and acceptance by the nursing community.

Wright, P. S., Piazza, D., Holcombe, J., & Foote, A. (1994). A comparison of three theories of nursing used as a guide for the nursing care of an 8-year-old child with leukemia. *Journal of Pediatric Oncology Nursing, 11,* 14–19.

These authors evaluate three nursing theories that can be used to provide a framework for holistic pediatric oncology nursing practice: the Roy adaptation model, the Neuman systems model, and the Orem general theory of nursing. The authors compare the theories in terms of the metaparadigm of nursing and present a critique. Four comparative tables are included. The decision of which theory to use is left to the individual nurse.

WEBLINKS

The Nursing Theory Page

http://www.sandiego.edu/academics/nursing/theory/

This site was developed by the Faculty of Nursing, University of Alberta, and provides an overview of a number of different nursing theorists. It is now hosted by the Hahn School of Nursing and Health Sciences at the University of San Diego, California.

Clayton State University Department of Nursing: Nursing Theory Links Page

http://healthsci.clayton.edu/eichelberger/nursing.htm

This site provides access to the writings of a number of different nursing theorists.

Information and Resources for Nurses Worldwide

http://www.nurses.info/nursing_theory_accepted_theories.htm

This webpage has links to numerous sites for nursing theory and nurse theorists.

International Consortium of the Parse Scholars' Home Page

http://www.humanbecoming.org

This is a webpage for Dr. Rosemarie Parse, author of Illumination: The human becoming theory in practice and research.

Health as Expanding Consciousness

http://www.healthasexpandingconsciousness.org

This website features Dr. Margaret Newman's theory of nursing health as expanding consciousness.

REFERENCES

Allen, M. (1986). A developmental health model: Nursing as continuous inquiry (audio tape). In series *Nursing Theory Congress. Theoretical pluralism: Direction for a practice discipline.* Markham, ON: Audio Archives of Canada.

Alligood, M. & Tomey, A. (2006). *Nursing theory: Utilization and application* (3rd ed.). St. Louis, M): Mosby.

Bishop, A., & Scudder, J. (1999). A philosophical interpretation of nursing. *Scholarly Inquiry for Nursing Practice, 13*(1), 17–27.

Bergum, V. (1989). *Woman to mother: A Transformation.* Granby, MA: Bergin & Garvey.

Campbell, M. (1987). *The UBC model for nursing: Directions for practice.* Vancouver: University of British Columbia School of Nursing.

Cameron, B. (1992). The nursing "how are you?" *Phenomenology & Pedagogy, 10,* 173–185.

Canadian Nurses Association. (2002). *Evidence-based decision-making and nursing practice.* Ottawa: Author.

Dunphy, L. (2006). Florence Nightingale's legacy of caring and its applications. In M. E. Parker (Ed.), *Nursing theories and nursing practice* (pp. 39–57). Philadelphia, PA: Davis.

Edwards, S. (1997). What is philosophy of nursing? *Journal of Advanced Nursing, 25,* 1089–1093.

Fawcett, J. (2005). *Contemporary nursing knowledge: Analysis and evaluation of nursing models and theories.* Philadelphia, PA: Davis.

Feeley N., & Gerez-Lirette T. (1992). Development of professional practice based on the McGill model of nursing in an ambulatory care setting. *Journal of Advanced Nursing, 17*(7), 801–808.

Feeley, N., & Gottlieb, L. N. (2000). Nursing approaches for working with family strengths and resources. *Journal of Family Nursing, 6*(1), 9–24.

Fry, S. (1992). Neglect of philosophical inquiry in nursing: Cause and effect. In J. Kikuchi & H. Simmons (Eds.), *Philosophic inquiry in nursing* (pp. 85–96). Newbury Park, CA: Sage.

Fry, S. (1999). The philosophy of nursing. *Scholarly Inquiry for Nursing Practice, 13*(1), 5–15.

Gadow, S. (1994). Whose body? Whose story? The question about narrative in women's health care. *Soundings, 77*(3/4), 295–307.

Henderson, V. (1966). *The nature of nursing: A definition and its implications for practice, research, and education.*

Riverside, NJ: Macmillan.

Henderson, V. A. (1991). *The nature of nursing: Reflections after 25 years.* New York: National League for Nursing Press. Pub. No. 15–2346.

Johnson, J. A. (1994). Dialectical examination of nursing art. *Advances in Nursing Science, 17*(1), 1–14.

Kikuchi, J. (1992). Nursing questions that science cannot answer. In J. Kikuchi & H. Simmons (Eds.), *Philosophic inquiry in nursing* (pp. 26–37). Newbury Park, CA: Sage.

Kikuchi, J. & Simmons, H. (1994). A pragmatic philosophy of nursing: Threat or promise? In J. Kikuchi & H. Simmons (Eds.), *Developing a philosophy of nursing* (pp. 79–94). Thousand Oaks, CA: Sage.

Lawler, J. (1997). *The body in nursing.* Melbourne, AU: Churchill Livingstone.

Leininger, M. M. (1985). Transcultural care diversity and universality: A theory of nursing. *Nursing and Health Care, 6,* 208–212.

Leininger, M. M. (1988). Leininger's theory of nursing: Cultural care, diversity and universality. *Nursing Science Quarterly, 1*(4), 152–160.

Leininger, M. M. (Ed.). (1991). *Culture care diversity and universality: A theory of nursing.* New York: National League for Nursing Press. Pub. No. 15–2402.

Leininger, M., & McFarland, M. (2006) *Cultural care, diversity and universality: A worldwide nursing theory.* Sudbury, ON: Jones and Bartlett.

Liaschenko, J. (1997). Ethics and the geography of nurse–patient relationship: Spatial vulnerabilities and gendered space. *Scholarly Inquiry for Nursing Practice, 11*(1), 45–59.

McFarland, M. (2006). Part two: Application of Leininger's theory of culture care diversity and universality. In M. E. Parker (Ed.), *Nursing theories and nursing practice* (pp. 321–333). Philadelphia, PA: Davis.

Newman, M. (1986). *Health as expanding consciousness.* St. Louis, MO: Mosby.

Newman, M., Sime, A., & Corcoran-Perry, S. (1991). The focus of the discipline of nursing. *Advances in Nursing Science, 14*(1), 1–6.

Nightingale, F. (1957). *Notes on nursing.* Philadelphia, PA: Lippincott. (Original work published 1860).

Parse, R. R. (1981). *Man-living-health: A theory of nursing.* New York: Wiley.

Parse, R. R. (1987). *Nursing science: Major paradigms, theories, and critiques.* Philadelphia, PA: Saunders.

Parse, R. R. (1994). Quality of life: Sciencing and living the art of human becoming. *Nursing Science Quarterly, 7*(1), 16–21.

Parse, R. R. (Ed.). (1995). *Illumination: The human becoming theory in practice and research.* New York: National League for Nursing Press. Pub. No. 15–2670.

Peplau, H. E. (1952). *Interpersonal relations in nursing.* New York: Putnam.

Purkis, M. E. (1997). The "social determinants" of practice: A critical analysis of the discourse of health promotion. *Canadian Journal of Nursing Research, 29*(1), 47–62.

Roach, Sr. S. (2002). *The human act of caring: A blueprint for the health professions* (2nd Rev. Ed.). Ottawa: Canadian Hospital Association Press.

Roy, C. (1976). *Introduction to nursing: An adaptation model.* Englewood Cliffs, NJ: Prentice-Hall.

Roy, C. (1997). Future of the Roy model: Challenge to redefine adaptation. *Nursing Science Quarterly, 10*(1), 42–48.

Roy, C., & Zahn, L. (2006). Sister Callista Roy's adaptation model and its applications. In M. E. Parker (Ed.), *Nursing theories and nursing practice* (pp. 268–280). Philadelphia, PA: Davis.

Salsberry, P. (1994). A philosophy of nursing: What it is? What it is not? In J. Kikuchi & H. Simmons (Eds.), *Developing a philosophy of nursing* (pp. 11–19). Thousand Oaks, CA: Sage.

Smith, M. (1994). Arriving at a philosophy of nursing: Discovering? Constructing? Evolving? In J. Kikuchi & H. Simmons (Eds.), *Developing a philosophy of nursing* (pp. 43–59). Thousand Oaks, CA: Sage.

Tomey, A., & Alligood, M. (2006). *Nursing theorists and their work* (6th ed.). St. Louis, MO: Mosby.

Watson, J. (1979). *Nursing: The philosophy and science of caring.* Boston: Little, Brown.

Watson, J. (1988). *Nursing: Human science and human care: A theory of nursing.* New York: National League for Nursing Press. Pub. No. 15–2236.

Watson, J. (2001) Jean Watson: Theory of human caring. In M. E. Parker (Ed.), *Nursing theories and nursing practice* (pp. 343–354). Philadelphia, PA: Davis

Watson, J. (2006). Part one: Jean Watson's theory of human caring. In M. E. Parker (Ed.), *Nursing theories and nursing practice* (pp. 295–302). Philadelphia, PA: Davis.

Chapter 5

Values, Ethics, and Advocacy

In their daily work, nurses deal with intimate and fundamental human events, such as birth, death, and suffering. They must evaluate the morality of their own actions when they face the many ethical issues that surround such sensitive areas. Because of the special nature of the nurse–client relationship, nurses are the ones who support and advocate for clients and families who are facing difficult choices and for those who are living with the results of choices that others make for and about them. The nurse is frequently confronted with decisions about the rightness or wrongness of particular actions within a given context. It is essential, therefore, that nurses have a strong grounding in ethics and a sound approach to ethical decision making.

Ethical issues in nursing evolve to reflect the challenges facing society. Although numerous ethical challenges affect patients and families in health-care settings, a panel of Canadian clinical bioethicists identified 10 that they felt were the most pressing (Breslin, MacRae, Bell, & Singer, 2005). The Nursing and Canadian Society box lists these by rank. Nurses face many of these challenges on a daily basis.

OBJECTIVES

After studying this chapter, you should be able to

1. Explain how values, moral frameworks, and codes of ethics affect moral decisions
2. Explain how nurses can use their knowledge of values and values clarification to facilitate ethical decision making by clients
3. Identify the moral issues and principles involved when presented with an ethical situation
4. Explain the uses and limitations of professional codes of ethics
5. Analyze some common ethical issues facing health-care professionals
6. Describe ways in which nurses can enhance their ethical decision making and practice
7. Discuss the advocacy role of the nurse

NURSING AND CANADIAN SOCIETY

Top 10 Health-Care Ethics Challenges Facing the Canadian Public

Rank	Scenario	Implications for Nursing Practice
1	"Disagreement between patients/families and health care professionals about treatment decisions" (Breslin et al., 2005)	Ongoing dialogue about treatment between patients or families and providers is a key component of nursing care.
2	"Waiting lists" (Breslin et al., 2005)	Demand for nurses specializing in perioperative, rehabilitation, and surgical nursing will continue to increase.
3	"Access to needed health care resources for the aged, chronically ill and mentally ill" (Breslin et al., 2005)	Nurses with the skills and abilities to provide care to these vulnerable populations across diverse settings is essential.
4	"Shortage of family physicians or primary care teams in both rural and urban settings" (Breslin et al., 2005)	Expanded nursing practice and roles, such as the nurse practitioner, will form a cornerstone of our health-care system.
5	"Medical error" (Breslin et al., 2005)	Accountability for individual nursing practice and the recognition of systemic causes of medical error will gain importance.
6	"Withholding/withdrawing life-sustaining treatment in the context of terminal or serious illness" (Breslin et al., 2005)	Earlier and improved communication between health-care providers and patients or families can prevent the use of unwanted and inappropriate therapies. Nurses are key players in discussions with families and other providers about withholding or withdrawing therapies.
7	"Achieving informed consent" (Breslin et al., 2005)	Nurses are in a position to assess whether the patient and family have fully understood the procedure for which they gave consent, and nurses can advocate for additional discussion.
8	"Ethical issues related to subject participation in research" (Breslin et al., 2005)	Nursing research often deals with vulnerable populations, such as children, those with dementia, or those who are incarcerated. Nursing researchers abide by guidelines for ethical conduct of research.
9	"Substitute decision making" (Breslin et al., 2005)	When patients are physically or cognitively compromised and unable to consent to medical interventions, nurses work with substitute decision makers, such as family members, to promote sound ethical decisions.
10	"The ethics of surgical innovation and incorporating new technologies for patient care" (Breslin et al., 2005)	Nurses should engage in dialogue with other health-care providers to consider the implications of new technologies from an ethical perspective.

Source: Based on "Top 10 Health Care Ethics Challenges Facing the Public: Views of Toronto Bioethicists," by J. M. Breslin, S. K. MacRae, J. Bell, and P. A. Singer, 2005, *BMC Medical Ethics, 6*, p. 5, table 1.

According to the Canadian Nurses Association (2004), nurses have increasingly expressed concern about their ability to deliver safe care in today's health-care system. The potential for compromised safety creates new moral problems and intensifies old ones, making it critical for nurses to make sound moral decisions. Therefore, nurses need to (1) develop sensitivity to the ethical dimensions of nursing practice, (2) examine their own and their clients' values, (3) understand how values influence their decisions, and (4) think ahead to the kinds of moral problems they are likely to face. This chapter explores the influences of values and moral frameworks on the ethical dimensions of nursing practice and on the nurse's role as a client advocate.

Values

Values are enduring beliefs or attitudes about the worth of a person, an object, an idea, or an action. Values are important because they influence decisions and actions, including nurses' ethical decision making. Even though they may be unspoken and perhaps even unconsciously held, values underlie all moral dilemmas. Of course, not all values are moral values. For example, people hold values about work, family, religion, politics, money, and relationships, to name just a few. Values are often taken for granted. In the same way that people are not aware of their breathing, they usually do not think about their values; they simply accept them and act on them.

A **value set** is the small group of values held by an individual. People organize their sets of values internally along a continuum from most important to least important, forming a **value system**. Value systems are basic to a way of life, give direction to life, and form the basis of behaviour—especially behaviour that is based on decisions or choices.

Values consist of beliefs and attitudes, which are related, but not identical, to values. People have many different beliefs and attitudes but only a small number of values. **Beliefs** (or opinions) are interpretations or conclusions that people accept as true. They are based more on faith than on fact and may or may not be true. Beliefs do not necessarily involve values. For example, the statement "If I study hard I will get a good grade" expresses a belief that does not involve a value. By contrast, the statement "Good grades are really important to me, and I must study hard to obtain good grades" involves both a value and a belief.

Attitudes are mental positions or feelings toward a person, an object, or an idea (e.g., acceptance, compassion, openness). Typically, an attitude lasts over time, whereas a belief may last only briefly. Attitudes are often judged as bad or good, positive or negative, whereas beliefs are judged as correct or incorrect. Attitudes have thinking and behavioural aspects. Attitudes vary greatly among individuals. For example, some clients may feel strongly about their need for privacy, whereas others may dismiss it as unimportant.

Values Transmission

Values are learned through observation and experience. As a result, they are heavily influenced by a person's sociocultural environment—that is, by societal traditions; by cultural, ethnic, and religious groups; and by family and peer groups. For example, if a parent consistently demonstrates honesty in dealing with others, his or her child will probably begin to value honesty. Nurses should keep in mind the influence of values on health. For example, some cultures value treatment by a folk healer over that by a health-care provider. For additional information about cultural values related to health and illness, see Chapter 10.

PERSONAL VALUES Although people derive values from society and their individual subgroups, they internalize some or all of these values and perceive them as **personal values**. People need societal values in order to feel accepted, and they need personal values to have a sense of individuality.

PROFESSIONAL VALUES Nurses' **professional values** are acquired during socialization into nursing from codes of ethics, nursing experiences, teachers, and peers. The College of Nurses of Ontario (2005) identifies the following values as being most important to nursing care: client well-being, client choice, privacy and confidentiality, respect for life, the maintaining of commitments, truthfulness, and fairness. The Registered Nurses' Association of Ontario (2006) has framed its Client-Centred Care Best Practice Guidelines Program around a widely accepted set of professional values (see Box 5.1). In client-centred care, the client is viewed as a whole person and the approach involves advocacy, empowerment, and respect for the client's autonomy, voice, self-determination, and participation in decision making. Table 5.1 lists the values and professional behaviours associated with these values.

Values Clarification

Values clarification is a process by which people identify, examine, and develop their own individual values. A principle of values clarification is that no one set of values is right for everyone. When people can identify their values, they can retain or change them and thus act based on freely chosen, rather than unconscious, values. Values clarification promotes personal growth by fostering awareness, empathy, and insight. Therefore, it is an important step for nurses to take in dealing with ethical problems.

Often, values clarification is an internal process not apparent to the person. In some cases, a values clarification exercise can be useful in helping individuals or groups to become more aware of their values and how they may influence their actions. For example, asking a client to agree or disagree with a list of statements or to rank in order of importance a list of beliefs can assist the nurse and client to make the client's values more open so they can be considered in planning the client's care. See Table 5.2 on page 76 for an example of a general values clarification exercise.

BOX 5.1 CLIENT-CENTRED BEST PRACTICE RECOMMENDATION

Nurses embrace as foundational to client-centred care the following values and beliefs:

- Respect
- Human dignity
- Clients are experts for their own lives
- Clients as leaders
- Clients' goals coordinate care of the health-care team
- Continuity and consistency of care and caregiver
- Timeliness
- Responsiveness
- Universal access to care

These values and beliefs must be incorporated into, and demonstrated throughout, every aspect of client care and service.

Source: *Client Centred Care Best Practice Guidelines*, by the Registered Nurses' of Ontario, 2006, Toronto: Author.

TABLE 5.1 Essential Nursing Values and Behaviours

Values	Professional Behaviors
Altruism is a concern for the welfare and well-being of others. In professional practice, altruism is reflected by the nurse's concern for the welfare of patients, other nurses, and other health care providers. *Autonomy* is the right to self-determination. Professional practice reflects autonomy when the nurse respects patients' rights to make decisions about their health care. *Human dignity* is respect for the inherent worth and uniqueness of individuals and populations. In professional practice, human dignity is reflected when the nurse values and respects all patients and colleagues. *Integrity* is acting in accordance with an appropriate code of ethics and accepted standards of practice. Integrity is reflected in professional practice when the nurse is honest and provides care based on an ethical framework that is accepted within the profession. *Social justice* is upholding moral, legal, and humanistic principles. This value is reflected in professional practice when the nurse works to ensure equal treatment under the law and equal access to quality health care.	• Demonstrates understanding of cultures, beliefs, and perspectives of others. • Advocates for patients, particularly the most vulnerable. • Takes risks on behalf of patients and colleagues. • Mentors other professionals. • Plans care in partnership with patients. • Honors the right of patients and families to make decisions about health care. • Provides information so patients can make informed choices. • Provides culturally competent and sensitive care. • Protects the patient's privacy. • Preserves the confidentiality of patients and health care providers. • Designs care with sensitivity to individual patient needs. • Provides honest information to patients and the public. • Documents care accurately and honestly. • Seeks to remedy errors made by self or others. • Demonstrates accountability for own actions. • Supports fairness and nondiscrimination in the delivery of care. • Promotes universal access to health care. • Encourages legislation and policy consistent with the advancement of nursing care and health care.

Source: From *The Essentials of Baccalaureate Education for Professional Nursing Practice* (pp. 8–9), American Association of Colleges of Nursing, 1998, Washington, DC: Author. Reprinted with permission.

CLARIFYING THE NURSE'S VALUES Nurses and nursing students need to examine the values they hold about life, death, health, and illness (College of Nurses of Ontario, 2005). One strategy for gaining awareness of personal values is to consider your own attitudes about specific issues, such as abortion or euthanasia, asking, Can I accept this, or live with this? Why does this bother me? What would I do or want done in this situation? Nurses use critical thinking (see Chapter 20) to reflect on various viewpoints and previous experiences that may have influenced their own values.

CLARIFYING CLIENT VALUES To plan effective care, nurses need to identify clients' values as they influence and relate to a particular health problem. For example, a client with failing eyesight will probably place a high value on the ability to see, and a client with chronic pain will value comfort. Normally, people take such things for granted. The nurse needs to ask such questions as, "What really matters to you in this situation?" "What would have to happen to make this seem like a good experience for you?" "What do you think you want to have happen here?" "Who do you want to make decisions for you?" "What do you want from me as a nurse?" The reflective nurse will soon recognize that without an understanding of a client's values, it is impossible to answer the questions. Therefore, this understanding is foundational for ethical practice. For information about health beliefs and values, see Chapter 7.

When clients hold unclear or conflicting values that are detrimental to their health, the nurse should use values clarification as an intervention. Examples of behaviours that may indicate the need for clarification of health values are listed in Table 5.3 on page 77.

The following process may help clients clarify their values:

1. *List alternatives.* Make sure that the client is aware of all alternative actions. Ask, "Are you considering other courses of action?" "Tell me about them."
2. *Examine possible consequences of choices.* Make sure the client has thought about the possible results of each action. Ask, "What do you think you will gain from doing that?" "What benefits do you foresee?"
3. *Choose freely.* To determine whether the client chose freely, ask, "Did you have any say in that decision?" "Do you have a choice?"
4. *Feel good about the choice.* To determine how the client feels, ask, "How do you feel about that decision (or action)?" Because some clients may not feel satisfied with their decision, a more sensitive question may be "Some people feel good after a decision is made; others feel bad. How do you feel?"

TABLE 5.2 Questionnaire for Personal Values Clarification

1 = Things I value very much 2 = Things I value 3 = Things I don't value very much

	Help Society	Do something which contributes to improving the world we live in
	Help Others	Be directly included in helping other people, either individually or in small groups
	Work Ethics	Feeling satisfied from a job well done
	Enjoyment of Life	Enjoying life, having fun in life
	Honesty	Being able to tell people what I really think and believe; having them be honest with me
	Approval	Having other people like me
	Competition	Engage in activities which pit my abilities against others
	Make Decisions	Have the power to decide courses of action
	Respect	Having other people think highly of me and hold me in good esteem
	Leadership	Be in a position to influence the attitudes or opinions of other people
	Knowledge	Understanding gained through study and/or experience
	Work Mastery	Become an expert in whatever work I do
	Peace	Living in a peaceful, harmonious society and environment
	Creativity	Have the opportunity to create new things, ideas, products, works of art
	Freedom	Being able to do or say what I want.
	Good Character	Knowing inside that I do the right, moral, just thing
	Loyalty	Sticking with people who are close to me and/or believe in what I do
	Justice	Being fair and just and having others treat me fairly and justly
	Stability	Have a routine and duties that are largely predictable
	Safety	Be assured of being safe and free from harm
	Recognition	Be publicly recognized
	Children	Having happy, healthy children
	Excitement	Experience a high degree of (or frequent) excitement
	Adventure	Have duties which require frequent risk-taking
	Power	Having authority over others
	Economic Security	Having enough money to buy whatever I want
	Leisure	Having time for hobbies, sports, other activities
	Inner Harmony	Being at peace with one's self
	Wealth	Profit, gain, making a lot of money
	Trustworthiness	Having people trust me and being able to trust them
	Challenge	Do activities that use my physical and/or mental capabilities
	Independence	Be able to determine the nature of my day without significant direction from others
	Change and Variety	Varied, frequently changing responsibilities and settings
	Moral Fulfillment	Feel that whatever I do contributes to a set of moral standards that I feel are very important
	Community	Being a part of a close and supportive community
	Caring	Experiencing love and affection daily
	Health	Being free from disease or sickness, feeling good physically
	Religion/Spirituality	Doing what's right according to my religious and/or spiritual beliefs
	Family	Making sure my family members are healthy and safe
	Friendship	Having good, reliable friends I can count on

Now, list your top five essential values (from those rated 1 above).

MY 5 MOST ESSENTIAL VALUES

1.
2.
3.
4.
5.

Source: From *Questionnaire for Values Clarification,* Johns Hopkins Bloomberg School of Public Health Center for Communication Programs, copyright 2002.

5. *Affirm the choice.* Ask, "How will you discuss this with others (family, friends)?"

6. *Act on the choice.* To determine whether the client is prepared to act on the decision, ask, for example, "Will it be difficult to tell your partner about this?"

TABLE 5.3 Client Behaviours That May Indicate Unclear Values

Behaviour	Example
Ignoring a health professional's advice	A client with heart disease who values hard work ignores advice to exercise regularly.
Inconsistent communication or behaviour	A pregnant woman says she wants a healthy baby, but continues to drink alcohol and smoke tobacco.
Numerous admissions to a health agency for the same problem	A middle-aged, obese woman repeatedly seeks help for back pain but does not lose weight.
Confusion or uncertainty about which course of action to take	A woman wants to obtain a job to meet financial obligations, but also wants to stay at home to care for her ailing husband.

7. *Act with a pattern.* To determine whether the client consistently behaves in a certain way, ask, "How many times have you done that before?" or "Would you act that way again?"

When implementing these seven steps to clarify values, the nurse helps the client to think through each question but does not impose personal values. The nurse rarely, if ever, offers an opinion when the client asks for it—and then only with great care or when the nurse is an expert in the content area. Because each situation is different, what the nurse would choose in his or her own life may not be relevant to the client's circumstances.

Thus, if the client asks the nurse, "What would you have done in my situation?" it is best to redirect the question back to the client rather than answering from a personal view.

CLARIFYING VALUES AND OBLIGATIONS IN CARE SITUATIONS Nurses need to understand their own values in the broader sense, but they also need to identify values that are relevant in individual care situations. They need to ask, What factors in this situation might affect how I think about "right" action? Are there particular contextual features that might change my views? For example, the nurse might value autonomy as a general rule but might question this value if it means supporting a client's decision to commit suicide.

Because of their unique position in the health-care hierarchy, nurses often experience conflicts among their loyalties and obligations to clients, families, other health-care providers, employing institutions, and licensing bodies. Client needs may conflict with institutional policies, physician preferences, needs of the client's family, or even laws. According to the CNA's code of ethics, the nurse's first loyalty is to the client. However, it is not always easy to determine which action best serves the client's needs. For instance, a nurse may think that a client needs to be provided with the most current evidence-based information, but that information may conflict with the physician's advice; if the client goes against that advice, it may damage the physician–client relationship. The nurse will then have to decide what the greater good is in the situation.

Ethical Obligations

Making a commitment to treat others with respect and to uphold the values of well-being, choice, and dignity are fundamental to nursing. Nurses have an obligation to maintain commitments that they assume as regulated health professionals, such as keeping promises, being honest, and meeting implicit or explicit obligations toward their clients, themselves, one another, the nursing profession, other members of the health-care team, and quality practice settings (College of Nurses of Ontario, 2005). However, despite such clear moral commitments, nurses may still face situations in which the right action is not easily identified (Oberle & Hughes, 2001; Redman & Fry, 2000). A good decision is one that is in the client's best interests and at the same time preserves the integrity of all involved. Nurses have **ethical obligations**, or responsibilities imposed as a result of ethical imperatives, to their clients, to the agency that employs them, and to other health-care professionals. Unfortunately, there will be times when some of these obligations appear to be in conflict, as when the nurse feels a strong duty to follow institutional policy but at the same time feels that the policy does not serve the best interests of the client. For example, in a study of ethical issues in Canadian public health nursing, one participant described a situation with a pregnant teenage client who already had another small child. She was booked for a prenatal visit with her doctor but had no means of transportation and had no money for taxi fare. The nurse was expecting to drive past the clinic and would have been pleased to take the client to her appointment but was aware of the rule prohibiting nurses from using their own cars to transport patients. She felt conflicted by the obligation to be a "good employee" and the obligation to meet the client's needs (Oberle & Tenove, 2000). Making choices between conflicting values and obligations can be a significant source of stress for nurses (Oberle & Tenove, 2000).

Ethics

The term **ethics** has several meanings in common use. It refers to (1) a method of inquiry that helps people understand the morality of human behaviour (i.e., it is the study of morality), (2) the practices or beliefs of a certain group (e.g., medical ethics, nursing ethics), and (3) formal statements about expected standards of moral behaviour of a particular group. Thus, it is generally used to refer to a broader understanding of moral life through the application of theories and sets of principles that give structure to morality (Yeo & Moorehouse, 1996).

Nurses are often faced with moral quandaries in practice, that is, with decisions about *ought, should, good,* and *bad*. For example, the nurse might have to decide about whether or not to use physical restraints on clients who are confused and in danger of hurting themselves. The question is whether taking away a person's free choice is truly in that person's best interests and, therefore, whether the nurse *ought* or *ought not* to do it. The nurse's action will be guided by his or her individual belief system (morality) and by the broadly accepted standards of the society and the profession (as articulated in ethics theory and codes of ethics). A **code of ethics** is a formalized statement of a group's beliefs.

When faced with difficult decisions, it is important that the nurse be able to distinguish between *ethics* and *law*. Laws do reflect the moral values of a society, and they offer guidance in determining what is moral. However, an action can be legal but not moral. For example, an order for full resuscitation of a dying client is legal, but the nurse could question whether the act is moral. Conversely, an action can be moral but illegal. If a child at home stops breathing, it is moral but not legal to exceed the speed limit when driving to the hospital. The legal aspects of nursing practice are covered in Chapter 6.

Moral Theories

Moral theories, which are a set of abstract principles, provide different lenses through which nurses can view and clarify disturbing client-care situations. Nurses can use moral theories in developing explanations for their ethical decisions and actions and in discussing problem situations with others. Three types of moral theories are widely used, and they can be differentiated by their emphasis on (1) consequences, (2) principles and duties, or (3) relationships.

Evidence-Informed Practice

What Is Ethical Practice in Nursing?

The purpose of this qualitative descriptive study by Varcoe et al. (2004) was to explore, from the perspective of nurses, the meaning of ethics and the enactment of ethical practice in nursing. Eighty-seven Canadian nurses were interviewed in 19 focus groups of three to nine nurses each.

The nurses described ethics in their practice as both relational and highly contextual. Nurses worked between and in relation to family members, patients, and other health-care providers, and within a context laden with values that often contradicted their own. Conflict and tension were frequent. Nurses enacted their roles as moral agents with caution and compromise, suggesting limited support and leadership for ethical practice. Although most nurses did not have the opportunity to discuss ethical concerns, those who did reported these activities to be personally and professionally sustaining. The authors note that nurses need to understand ethical theory through connection with their everyday practice. Ethical theory for nursing practice needs to help nurses understand the organizational and societal forces affecting their practice, and provide guidance for negotiating power relationships, negotiating competing interests, and affecting the larger social and political context of practice.

NURSING IMPLICATIONS: Everyday nursing practice is highly charged with ethical issues. Nurses must be aware of their roles as moral agents within the larger health-care environment and develop opportunities to reflect on the ethical nature of their practice.

Source: Based on "Ethical Practice in Nursing: Working the In-Betweens," by C. Varcoe, G. Doane, P. Rodney, J. L. Storch, K. Mahoney, G. McPherson, et al., 2004, *Journal of Advanced Nursing, 45*(3), pp. 316–325.

Consequence-based (teleological) theories look to an action's outcomes (consequences) in judging whether that action is right or wrong. **Utilitarianism**, one form of consequentialist theory, views a good act as one that brings the most good and the least harm for the greatest number of people. This is called the principle of **utility**. This approach is often used in making decisions about the funding and delivery of health care. Teleological theories focus on issues of fairness.

Principles-based (deontological) theories involve logical and formal processes and emphasize individual rights, duties, and obligations. The morality of an action is determined not by its consequences but by whether it is done according to an impartial, objective principle. For example, following the rule "Do not lie," a nurse might believe he or she should tell the truth to a dying client, even though the physician has given instruction not to do so. There are many deontological theories; each justifies the rules of acceptable behaviour differently.

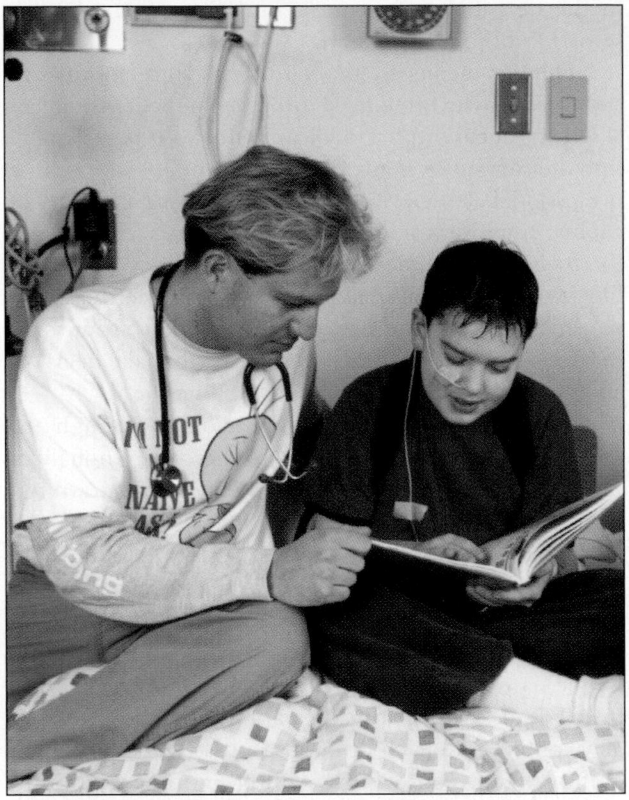

FIGURE 5.1 Relational caring is a professional relationship

Relationships-based (caring) theories stress courage, generosity, commitment, and the need to nurture and maintain relationships (see Figure 5.1). Unlike the two preceding theories, which frame problems in terms of justice (fairness) and formal reasoning, caring theories (see Chapter 4) judge actions according to a perspective of caring and responsibility. Principles-based theories stress individual rights, but caring theories promote the common good or the welfare of the group.

A moral theory guides moral decisions, but it does not determine the outcome. Imagine a situation in which a frail, elderly client has made it clear that he does not want further surgery, but the family and surgeon insist. Three nurses have each decided that they will not help with preparations for surgery and that they will work through proper channels to try to prevent it. Using consequence-based reasoning, Nurse A thinks, "Surgery will cause him more suffering; he probably will not survive it anyway, and the family may even feel guilty later." Using principles-based reasoning, Nurse B thinks, "This violates the principle of autonomy. This man has a right to decide what happens to his body." Using caring-based reasoning, Nurse C thinks, "My relationship to this client commits me to protecting him and meeting his needs, and I feel such compassion for him. I must try to help the family understand that he needs their support." Each perspective is based on the nurse's moral framework.

Principle-Based Ethics

Principle-based ethics is the most widely known approach to health-care ethics. This approach was first described in Beauchamp and Childress's 1979 book *Principles of Biomedical Ethics.* Their idea was that when health-care providers encountered an ethical problem, they would examine the situation, decide which ethical principles applied, and use them to make a decision. Their belief was that principles would be useful because even if people disagreed about which action was right in a situation, they might be able to agree on the principles that applied. Such an agreement could serve as the basis for a solution that was acceptable to all parties. For example, most people would agree with the principle that nurses are obligated to respect their clients, even if they disagree as to whether the nurse should deceive a particular client about the prognosis. The original principles of bioethics were *autonomy,* beneficence, nonmaleficence, and *justice* (Beauchamp & Childress, 2001). Later, principles of *fidelity* and *veracity* were added, and autonomy was expanded to *respect for persons.* These principles are very useful in discussions about ethical dimensions of particular care situations in nursing, although it is increasingly being realized that the biomedical ethics paradigm falls short of recognizing concepts important to nursing, such as nurturance, compassion, and communication (Ferrell, 2006).

The principle of **autonomy (respect for persons)** states that individuals have the right to make choices about their own lives. It also means showing respect for others and accepting them as unique individuals with personal histories that influence their decision making. In health care, this means that health-care providers must honour the person's right to choose methods or approaches to diagnosis and treatment. Choices must be free and informed, that is, made without coercion and with the benefit of all necessary information. Some patients are unable to make their own decisions (for example, cognitively impaired elderly persons, young children, or comatose patients); health-care professionals are obligated to try to make decisions that, to the best of their knowledge, the persons would make for themselves. Usually, the nurse gains information about the person's preferences from that person's family.

Nonmaleficence is the duty to do no harm. Although this would seem to be a simple principle to follow, in reality, it is complex. Harm can mean intentional harm, risk of harm, and unintentional harm. In nursing, intentional harm is never acceptable; nurses must not deliberately harm patients. However, nurses sometimes inflict harm during a nursing intervention that is intended to be helpful. Causing such harm would not be unethical as such. For example, a nurse may be required to carry out treatments that cause pain or discomfort, such as administering chemotherapy that has the side effects of severe nausea and vomiting. If the principle of nonmaleficence were taken on the surface, it would appear to dictate that the nurse should not carry out such actions. On reflection, however, the nurse would realize that failure to administer the drugs would cause the patient greater harm by allowing the cancer to progress unchecked. Similarly, nurses are often in the position of trying to mobilize patients after surgery, even when they are in pain and resist movement. Again, the nurse must realize that the effects of immobility are potentially more harmful than the increased discomfort. The nurse must consider the risk of harm from various sources and consider which action would be the most beneficial to the patient. Thus, the nurse must examine potential harms *and* benefits in considering whether the acts of harm were unethical. Unintentional harm is often unpredictable and could result from a lack of specific knowledge about a patient or from unexpected consequences of certain actions. Harm of that nature would be an error but would not necessarily have ethical implications, as the intent was positive.

Beneficence is the obligation to "do good." Nurses have a duty to implement actions that benefit their clients, that is, to act in the client's best interests. However, what is considered "good" in any situation is not always clear. Is it better, for instance, to tell a patient the truth about the diagnosis of a terminal disease or withhold the information? Which would be of greater benefit? An important question that arises in discussions of benefit is, who defines "good"? Should it be the health professional or the patient and family? For example, a nurse might believe that it is in a patient's best interests to get up and walk, whereas the patient might believe otherwise. The nurse must then consider whose beliefs should prevail in this instance. When health-care providers make decisions for clients without seeking their input, it is called **paternalism**. In the past, a paternalistic attitude was accepted; people expected doctors and nurses to make decisions for them. Today, clients are respected as having the ability to make decisions for themselves, and paternalism is not considered ethical. Nurses who want to make decisions for patients "in their best interests" must question whether they are being paternalistic.

Justice is often referred to as fairness. In health care, justice issues arise most often in deciding how scarce resources should be used. Such questions as who should get a heart for transplantation, whether a patient should be discharged to make room for another patient who seems more ill, or whether funding should be directed to heart-health programs or home care for the seniors require justice-based decisions. Nurses make justice decisions all the time in prioritizing care. For example, a nurse making home visits finds one client tearful and depressed and knows that staying for 30 minutes more to talk would help. However, that would take time from another client, who is diabetic and needs a great deal of teaching and observation. Many factors must be weighed in the decision, and a nurse must be prepared to do some hard thinking.

Fidelity means to be faithful to agreements and promises. Nurses often make promises to patients, such as "I'll be right back with a medication for your pain," or "I'll find out for you." Clients take such promises seriously. As professional caregivers, nurses have responsibilities to clients, employers, government, and society, as well as to themselves. Sometimes, these responsibilities are in conflict, as when institutional policy suggests one thing, and the nurse believes the patient would benefit from something else. Nurses need to be prepared to make decisions about where their primary responsibilities lie.

Veracity refers to telling the truth. Although this seems straightforward, in practice, choices are not always clear. Should a nurse tell the truth when it is known that it will cause harm? Does a nurse tell a lie if the lie will relieve anxiety and fear? These kinds of decisions form the basis for many moral dilemmas in nursing.

Although bioethics principles are meant to help the health-care provider make decisions, it is never quite as simple as deciding which principle applies in any one case. Often, several principles apply, and the principles may conflict with each other. If a nurse working in community health observes a young mother exhibiting inappropriate parenting practices, does the nurse respect the mother's autonomy and right to care for her child as she sees fit (respecting autonomy), or does the nurse intervene and insist that changes be made (beneficence)? Does a nurse restrain confused senior patients to keep them from hurting themselves (nonmaleficence) or let them wander and risk a serious fall (respecting autonomy)? Such questions are very difficult and require active reflection. The nurse who is insensitive to or unaware of the ethical dimensions of such practice decisions is less likely to choose the most ethically sound course of action.

Nursing Ethics and Relational Ethics

Some authors believe that nursing's ethical foundation must be based on caring and, therefore, nursing is better served by an approach that takes into account the relationship between nurse and patient (Gastmans, 2006). Some also suggest that caring is a **virtue**, that is, an "excellence of character" (Begley, 2005) or a highly valued personality characteristic that predisposes a person to act in a certain way, and that nurses must possess the virtue of caring if they are to make ethical decisions in practice (Benner, 1997; Salsberry, 1992; van Hooft, 1999).

Ethical theories coming from these perspectives are called **relational ethics theories** or **ethics of care**. These theories suggest that we all have a moral obligation to others simply because we are human and that we ought to act in others' best interests. Actions are judged according to whether they demonstrate caring and responsibility. Bioethics theory tends to consider situations more in the abstract, whereas relational theories take into account the individual's personal story or *narrative*. Thus, they are more concrete and rooted in the client's own reality.

Relational ethics theory seems to fit well with the caring concepts that are central to nursing, as it demands that clients be affirmed as persons, not objects (Marck, 2000a, 2000b). However, it is important to remember that caring is not unique to nursing and that some have criticized the caring perspective for (1) reinforcing the stereotype of women as caretakers and (2) overlooking other important moral principles, such as fairness and autonomy (Bowden, 1995). Nonetheless, nursing scholars seem to be in agreement that the commitment to others that is reflected in an attitude of caring is the basis, if not the whole, of nursing ethics (Marck, 2000b).

Nursing Codes of Ethics

No single theory of ethical decision making is universally applicable to nursing. However, within the profession, norms of practice can be used to help the nurse make moral decisions. These norms are reflected in a professional code of ethics, which is a set of ethical principles that (1) is shared by members of the group, (2) reflects their moral judgments over time, and (3) serves as a standard for their professional actions. Codes of ethics usually have higher requirements than do legal standards. Nursing codes of ethics have the following purposes:

- To inform the public about the minimum standards of the profession and help them understand professional nursing conduct
- To provide a sign of the profession's commitment to the public it serves
- To outline the major ethical considerations of the profession
- To provide general guidelines for professional behaviour
- To guide the profession in self-regulation
- To remind nurses of the special responsibility they assume when caring for clients

Codes of ethics for nursing have been developed at the international level by the International Council of Nurses (ICN), and at the national level by different countries. The ICN (2006) Code of Ethics for Nurses notes that nurses have four fundamental responsibilities: to promote health, to prevent illness, to restore health, and to alleviate suffering. The Canadian Nurses Association (CNA) *Code of Ethics for Registered Nurses* (2008) articulates the value system held by the nursing profession in Canada and, as such, serves as a blueprint for ethical practice by Canadian nurses. However, the Code cannot provide answers to particular care decisions. Instead, the Code reflects the mandate of professional nursing and the elements that must be considered in making ethical practice decisions. Nurses are responsible for being familiar with the code that governs their practice. Box 5.2 describes the nursing values that are the foundation for the Canadian Nurses Association's Code of Ethics. See the Weblinks section of this chapter for a link to the complete Code of Ethics.

BOX 5.2 CANADIAN NURSES ASSOCIATION'S CODE OF ETHICS FOR REGISTERED NURSES

The CNA *Code of Ethics for Registered Nurses* (2008) outlines the values that should guide Canadian nursing practice. Each value is accompanied by an itemized list of ethical responsibilities:

1. *Providing safe, compassionate, competent and ethical care:* Nurses provide safe, compassionate, competent and ethical care.
2. *Promoting health and well-being:* Nurses work with people to enable them to attain their highest possible level of health and well-being.
3. *Promoting and respecting informed decision-making:* Nurses recognize, respect and promote a person's right to be informed and make decisions.
4. *Preserving dignity:* Nurses recognize and respect the intrinsic worth of each person.
5. *Maintaining privacy and confidentiality:* Nurses recognize the importance of privacy and confidentiality and safeguard personal, family and community information obtained in the context of a professional relationship.
6. *Promoting justice:* Nurses uphold principles of justice by safeguarding human rights, equity and fairness and by promoting the public good.
7. *Being accountable:* Nurses are accountable for their actions and answerable for their practice.

Source: *Code of Ethics for Registered Nurses,* by the Canadian Nurses Association, 2008, Ottawa: Author. Reprinted with permission.

CLINICAL ALERT

Ethical behaviour is contextual; what is an ethical action or decision in one situation may not be ethical in a different situation.

Ethical Decision Making

In this chapter, we have discussed several types of ethics theory (teleological, deontological, and relational ethics). In addition, we have discussed codes of ethics and the impact of personal and professional values on decision making. How can these various parts be brought together to help a nurse develop a plan to enhance ethical practice? Providing ethical care requires considerable thought and reflection, and ethical decision making can be enhanced if nurses have an understanding of the values that drive their practice.

Making Ethical Decisions

Responsible ethical reasoning is rational and systematic. It should be based on ethical principles and codes rather than solely on emotions, intuition, fixed policies, or precedent (that is, an earlier similar occurrence). Two decision-making models are shown in Box 5.3.

A good decision is one that is in the client's best interest and also preserves the integrity of all involved. Nurses have ethical obligations to their clients, to the agency that employs them, and to health-care providers. Therefore, nurses must weigh competing factors when making ethical decisions. See Box 5.4 for examples. Although ethical reasoning is principle based and has the client's well-being at its centre, being involved in ethical problems and dilemmas is stressful for a client who has not responded to mainstream therapies. Although legal issues are involved, the nurse must determine if, ethically, the client should be made aware of a potentially effective alternative. Another example is individual nurses' decisions regarding honouring picket lines during employee strikes. The nurse may experience conflict, feeling the need to support co-workers in their efforts to improve working conditions, feeling the need to ensure clients receive care and are not abandoned, and feeling loyalty to the hospital employer.

BOX 5.3 ETHICAL DECISION-MAKING MODELS

These two decision-making models can be used in clinical practice to facilitate ethical choices:

THOMPSON AND THOMPSON (1985)

- Review the situation to determine health problems, decision needs, ethical components, and key individuals.
- Gather additional information to clarify the situation.
- Identify the ethical issues in the situation.
- Define personal and professional moral positions.
- Identify moral positions of key individuals involved.
- Identify value conflicts, if any.
- Determine who should make the decision.
- Identify the range of actions with anticipated outcomes.
- Decide on a course of action and carry it out.
- Evaluate/review the results of the decision/action.

CASSELLS AND REDMAN (1989)

- Identify the moral aspects of nursing care.
- Gather relevant facts related to a moral issue.
- Clarify and apply personal values.
- Understand ethical theories and principles.
- Utilize competent interdisciplinary resources.
- Propose alternative actions.
- Apply nursing codes of ethics to help guide actions.
- Choose and implement resolutive action.
- Participate actively in resolving the issue.
- Apply . . . laws governing nursing practice.
- Evaluate the resolutive action taken.

Sources: From *Bioethical Decision-Making for Nurses* (p. 99), by J. B. Thompson and H. O. Thompson, 1985, Norwalk, CT: Appleton-Century-Croft; and "Preparing Students to be Moral Agents in Clinical Nursing Practice," by J. Cassells and B. Redman, 1989, *Nursing Clinics of North America, 24*(2), pp. 463–473. Reprinted with permission.

BOX 5.4 EXAMPLES OF NURSES' OBLIGATIONS IN ETHICAL DECISIONS

Nurses must meet a variety of obligations in making ethical decisions:

- Maximize the client's well-being.
- Balance the client's need for autonomy with family members' responsibilities for the client's well-being.
- Support each family member and enhance the family support system.
- Carry out agency policies.
- Protect other clients' well-being.
- Protect the nurse's own standards of care.

Decision Making in Practice

A decision-making framework can help the nurse in making ethical decisions. Frameworks must take into account the facts, beliefs, and values inherent in the situation. Knowing the kinds of questions to ask in a situation is essential if the nurse is to get the necessary information.

Selected Ethical Issues in Nursing

In the past, nurses did not consider themselves to be **moral agents**. Moral agents have the capacity for making moral judgments and for taking actions that are consistent with morality. With changes in the profession, nurses' awareness of ethical issues in practice is growing. Nurses are beginning to realize that many problems at the institutional level are really ethical issues. For example, workload becomes an ethical issue for nurses when a unit is insufficiently staffed to enable them to uphold the values of well-being and respect. When nurses are too busy to listen to patients or to employ comfort strategies, then professional values are being violated. The current and projected shortage of registered nurses in Canada has serious implications for the safe and ethical care of patients (Canadian Federation of Nurses Unions, 2008). The health human resource crisis is of such importance that the ICN has launched a new international centre aimed at informing policymaking and building capacity in the areas of nursing human resources planning, management, and development. Rodney and Varcoe (2001) argue that such problems *must* be examined from an ethics perspective and that nurses must begin to understand that striving for better working conditions is part of nursing's moral imperative. If the quality of work life is unsatisfactory, and the standard of care is compromised, nurses' moral base is eroded.

Developing and maintaining a trusting, caring, and supportive relationship with a client is the foundation of nursing ethics (Gastmans, Dierckx de Casterle, & Schotsmans, 1998). The CNA's Code of Ethics for Registered Nurses (2008) indicates the values held by the profession. However, the Code acknowledges that "given the complexity of ethical situations, the code can only outline nurses' ethical responsibilities and guide nurses in their reflection and decision-making. It cannot ensure ethical practice" (p. 4). Thus, it points again to the need for nurses to have a clear understanding of their own values.

Nurses must consider how their values might affect the care they give to clients. Certainly, every caregiving situation has moral components and will be affected by the values, beliefs, and attitudes of all those involved. However, some kinds of care situations cause nurses to pay particular attention to their own values. Abortion, end-of-life issues, and the withdrawing and withholding of food and fluids are examples of issues in which values are central.

The unprecedented advances in medical technology over the past four decades have engendered significant changes in professional, social, and legal expectations about care outcomes (Ferrell, 2006). Ethical issues related to **medical futility**, defined as life-sustaining care that is unlikely to result in meaningful survival, continue to present challenges in nursing practice. Euthanasia and the withholding or withdrawal of life-sustaining treatment are frequently cited by Canadian nurses as ethical issues (Oberle & Hughes, 2001). Often, the problem is that the family or the physician wants aggressive care to continue, whereas nurses believe that the client's dignity is being eroded by continued treatment. Sometimes, the opposite applies; nurses believe that treatment should continue, and others want it to be terminated. Either way, the situation can cause the nurse moral distress, particularly if he or she feels powerless to affect the decision making.

Redman and Fry (2000) analyzed numerous published reports of studies of ethical conflict in nursing and determined that the most common disagreements centre on decisions about the medical treatment of patients. When such disagreement exists, communication and problem-solving skills are particularly important. The nurse can use a framework to analyze the problem on the basis of understanding the patient's and family's wishes and can use values cited in the CNA Code of Ethics (2008) to develop an argument for approaching the problem from a nursing ethics perspective. Nurses need to be prepared to explore, with the physician, patient, and family, why they each believe that a particular pathway should be followed and work with them to come to a common understanding that is acceptable to all. Sometimes, agreement is not possible, and nurses must look carefully at their own frame of reference and why they believe the treatment decisions are incorrect. Please see Box 5.5 for additional discussion. The question that must be asked in every instance is, whose needs are being met? If the nurses place priority on their own values above those of the patients (which may be contrary to the CNA Code of Ethics for Nurses), they may be unable

BOX 5.5 VARIATIONS IN APPLYING MORAL PRINCIPLES

Although a moral principle may exist and be valued in different cultures, the degree to which it is valued and the manner in which it is used in health care may be quite variable. Nurses must become familiar with how moral principles are viewed within the cultural groups with which they practice.

Principle	Examples of Ethnic and Cultural Variations
Autonomy	Family members, rather than the patient, receive information on the patient's condition and take primary responsibility for decision making. The family and community are viewed as affected by the patient's condition and decisions as much as the individual is affected: Chinese, Koreans, Mexican Americans, Bosnian Americans. (In Canada, data on ethnicity is not collected in the same way it is in the United States, so comparable Canadian data are not available for all principles.)
Veracity	Prefer patient not to be told directly of a life-threatening condition: Hispanics, Asians, Pakistanis, Bosnian Americans, Italian Americans, Canadian Aboriginals.
Nonmaleficence	Discussion of advance directives and such issues as cardiopulmonary resuscitation may be viewed as physically and emotionally harmful to the patient: Filipino, Canadian Aboriginals, Chinese.
Beneficence	Health-care providers should promote patient well-being and hope: Asian cultures, Canadian Aboriginals, Russians.

Sources: From "Bioethics for Clinicians: 18. Aboriginal Cultures," by J. H. Ellerby, J. McKenzie, S. McKay, G. J. Gariepy, and J. M. Kaufert, 2000, *Canadian Medical Association Journal, 163,* pp. 845–850; "Cultural Diversity at the End of Life: Issues and Guidelines for Family Physicians," by H. R. Searight and J. Gafford, 2005, *American Family Physician, 71,* 515–522; "It's Like Playing with Your Destiny: Bosnian Immigrants' Views of Advance Directives and End-of-Life Decision-Making," by H. R. Searight and J. Gafford, 2005, *Journal of Immigrant Health, 7*(3), pp. 195–203.

to resolve the dilemma and may continue to experience moral distress. Thus, the importance of values clarification again becomes evident. Discussion with clients and other health-care providers about differences in values can help ease the tension that such situations produce (CNA, 2008).

The increasing cultural diversity evident in both patient and family and nursing populations in Canada can create ethically charged situations. Differences in values, lifestyle, and background demand ongoing dialogue to achieve common understandings about issues with ethical implications. For the internationally educated nurse (IEN), the process of integration and transition into practice in a new culture can be overwhelming, given unfamiliar technology and significant differences in health care (McGuire & Murphy, 2005).

Most of the issues just considered are centred on acute-care settings. It is important to recognize that nurses in other areas of practice also experience ethical issues, although the problems may not be as obviously dramatic as the life-and-death concerns of acute-care nurses (Oberle & Tenove, 2000). MacPhail (1996) examined ethics in community nursing and found relationship, trust, and advocacy to be central to community health nursing practice. For example, nurses in the study talked about difficulties in working with individuals who had chosen to adopt at-risk lifestyles, such as problematic drug use and prostitution. How could they provide support for the person without appearing to condone or support the lifestyle? How could they honour autonomy and at the same time try to change the individuals' behaviours? How could they maintain trust while adhering to legal requirements to report certain practices, such as child abuse? This study demonstrated that community health nursing is rooted in relationships and that the nurses who fail to attend to the ethical dimensions of relationships will be unable to provide effective care. These issues must be considered within the context of the broader society (see the Reflect on Primary Health Care box).

REFLECT ON PRIMARY HEALTH CARE

Practising in an ethical manner includes looking at ethical issues in a broader context. For example, examining the principles of primary health care (accessibility, public participation, health promotion, appropriate technology, and intersectoral collaboration) with an ethical lens will encourage the nurse to explore at a societal level such issues as those mentioned in this section and the Nursing and Canadian Society box (p. 73).

Nursing and Advocacy

Within the powerful institutional machinery of the health-care system is the significant potential for the client to be a relatively powerless player in his or her own care (Hewitt, 2002). The notion of **advocacy** in nursing is closely tied to empowering clients through the provision of information, support, and intervention. One definition of advocacy is "acting to the limit of professional ability to provide for the client's interests and needs as the patient defines them" (Dubler, 1992). Curtin (1979) defined advocacy as the moral art in nursing that evolves from shared vulnerability, past experiences, and humanity in the nurse–patient relationship. The overall goal of a client advocate is to protect clients' rights.

An advocate is one who expresses and defends the cause of another. Three primary elements constitute advocacy by the nurse, according to Tschudin and Hunt (1994). The first is that the nurse's position is proactive, rather than passive and subordinate. Second, the nurse speaks up and acts on behalf of the patient. Finally, some kind of difficulty or conflict exists that necessitates the need for advocacy.

Nurses are frequently placed in an advocacy role when clients and families are unable, or unwilling, to speak up for themselves. Nurses must ensure that clients and families have the necessary information to enable them to consider options and must provide them with support when they make decisions. Sometimes, the nurse must defend the client's or family's views when others are trying to coerce them into making a different decision. This is often a difficult role for the nurse because it may pit the nurse against other members of the health-care team. However, the nurse must be guided by the professional code, which places choice, dignity, and well-being as the highest values. To be an effective advocate involves the following:

- Recognizing that the rights and values of clients and families must take precedence when they conflict with those of health-care providers
- Being aware that conflicts may arise over issues that require consultation, confrontation, or negotiation
- Being assertive and using excellent communication techniques

Advocacy may be required at the broader, systems level as well. For example, the CNA Code of Ethics (2008) articulates a value of **quality practice environments**, that is, environments conducive to safe, competent, and ethical care. Nurses may have to be involved in political action when underfunding threatens the integrity of the health-care system. It is a nurse's moral obligation to work to ensure that the best possible conditions exist for the clients' health-care needs to be met. This is another demanding role for nurses, one with which many nurses are unfamiliar. Nurses may choose not to act because it is too much trouble or they are reluctant to engage with unfamiliar administrative personnel or agencies. However, providing ethical care for clients is not an easy task, and nurses must be prepared to take action to ensure quality care.

Advocacy is an important role for nurses. Nonetheless, nurses must be careful not to suggest (or believe) that they are the only advocates for the client. The term *advocacy* is potentially divisive; that is, it could cause conflict in itself because it suggests that the client needs to be protected. Not all clients feel the need for protection, and the nurse must honour their right to self-determination. As well, other health-care providers, such as physicians, may resent the implication that clients need to be protected from them. Physicians, too, consider themselves to be client advocates, as do many other concerned professionals, such as social workers and physiotherapists. The nurse has a moral obligation to the client but also an obligation to keep the health-care team functioning cohesively. Therefore, the nurse must be sensitive to the implications of such terms as *advocacy* and use them carefully. The basic values in client advocacy are shown in Box 5.6.

Enhancing Ethical Practice

It should be noted that decisions about a client's care are not made by nurses alone. Although the nurse's input is important, in reality, several people are usually involved in making an ethical decision. Therefore, collaboration, communication, and compromise are important skills for health professionals. When nurses do not have the autonomy to act on their moral or ethical choices, compromise becomes essential. Integrity-preserving compromises are most likely to be produced by collaborative decision making. The mnemonic device LEARN can remind nurses to work toward collaboration in ethical decisions (Berlin & Fowkes, 1983):

L isten to others.

E xplain your perceptions.

A cknowledge and discuss differences.

R ecommend alternatives.

N egotiate agreement.

As should be evident from the preceding discussion, excellent ethical decision-making skills require considerable reflection and practice. Rodney and Starzomski (1993), Davis and Aroskar (1991), and Wilkinson (1996) described a number of strategies to help nurses overcome possible organizational and social constraints that may hinder the ethical practice of nursing:

- Become aware of your own values and the ethical aspects of nursing.
- Be familiar with the code of ethics that is to guide your practice.
- Learn about and respect the values, opinions, and responsibilities of other health-care professionals.
- Participate in or establish ethics rounds. Ethics rounds, using hypothetical or real cases, incorporate the traditional teaching approach for clinical rounds but focus on the ethical dimensions of client care, rather than clinical diagnosis and treatment.
- Serve on institutional ethics committees.

In addition, the researchers stressed the importance of striving for collaborative practice in which nurses function effectively in cooperation with clients and other health-care professionals. Ethical practice does not just happen—it takes a great deal of work. Every nurse has an obligation to understand the ethical foundations of practice and to make a conscious effort to examine and reflect on the ethical dimensions of each caregiving encounter. It is only with an understanding of the ethical components of a situation that nurses can meet their obligation to act in the best interests of the client.

BOX 5.6 BASIC VALUES IN CLIENT ADVOCACY

The basic values in client advocacy are the following:

- The client is a holistic, autonomous being who has the right to make choices and decisions.
- Clients have the right to expect a nurse–client relationship that is based on shared respect, trust, collaboration in solving problems related to health and health-care needs, and consideration of their thoughts and feelings.
- It is the nurse's responsibility to ensure the client has access to health-care services that meet health needs.

Case Study 5

At a Canadian acute-care hospital, nurses expressed concern with the care of a 98-year-old Asian woman. She had been in a nursing home for several years and had been bedridden because of severe arthritis. As a result, she had numerous contractures that made it difficult to position her, and her skin had broken down in several areas. She was responding only to painful stimuli, and the nurses observed indications of considerable pain whenever she was moved. She had a pulmonary infection and was receiving triple antibiotic therapy. The antibiotics gave her severe diarrhea, which necessitated more frequent moving and bathing. The antibiotics had not been effective, and the order was due for renewal. The nurses expressed the view that the antibiotics ought to be discontinued and that further aggressive care should be terminated. In their view, continuing treatment was robbing the patient of the possibility of a dignified death. Nurses wanted a DNR (do not resuscitate) order instituted. The patient's daughter adamantly disagreed, saying that it was her obligation to see that her mother got every possible treatment. In their culture, she argued, it was a demonstration of respect to try to preserve life at all costs.

What could the nurses do? They wanted to respect the daughter's wishes, but they believed that treatment was causing harm to the patient and that it was wrong to continue to use scarce resources trying to preserve life in this futile situation. They felt constrained by the desire to respect cultural differences but also felt strongly that the patient was being harmed, even tortured, by nursing actions. Because of their distress, they put pressure on the physician to have the DNR order instituted and discontinue therapy. The physician was reluctant. A consultation with the clinical ethics committee was called by the unit manager.

Critical Thinking Questions

1. How can this situation be explored by applying ethical principles?
2. What are the goals of care? Are these goals shared by the patient? the nurses? other health-care professionals?
3. How does a focus on relationships improve your ethical understanding of the situation?
4. How would everyone (client, family, caregivers, institutions, organization, society) be affected by the decision?
5. What external conditions must be considered?
6. What (and whose) values must be considered?

After working through these questions, go to the MyNursingLab at **http://www.mynursinglab.com** to check your answers.

KEY TERMS

values
value set
value system
beliefs
attitudes
personal values
professional values
values clarification
ethical obligations
ethics
code of ethics
moral theories
consequence-based (teleological) theories
utilitarianism
utility
principles-based (deontological) theories
relationships-based (caring) theories
autonomy (respect for persons)
nonmaleficence
beneficence
paternalism
justice
fidelity
veracity
virtue
relational ethics theories or ethics of care
moral agents
medical futility
advocacy
quality practice environments

CHAPTER HIGHLIGHTS

- Values are enduring beliefs that give direction and meaning to life and guide a person's behaviour.
- Values clarification is a process in which people identify, examine, and develop their own values.
- Nursing ethics refers to the moral problems that arise in nursing practice and to ethical decisions that nurses make.
- Morality refers to what is right and wrong in conduct, character, or attitude.
- Moral issues are those that arouse conscience, are concerned with important values and norms, and evoke such words as *good, bad, right, wrong, should,* and *ought.*

- Three common moral frameworks (approaches) are consequence-based (teleological), principles-based (deontological), and relationships-based (caring) theories.
- Moral principles (e.g., autonomy, beneficence, nonmaleficence, justice, fidelity, and veracity) are broad, general philosophical concepts that can be used to make and explain moral choices.
- A professional code of ethics is a formal statement of a group's ideals and values that serves as a standard and guideline for the group's professional actions and informs the public of its commitment.
- Ethical problems are created as a result of changes in society, advances in technology, conflicts within nursing itself, and nurses' conflicting loyalties and obligations (e.g., to clients, families, employers, primary-care providers, and other nurses).
- Nurses' ethical decisions are influenced by their moral theories and principles, personal and professional values, and nursing codes of ethics.
- The goal of ethical reasoning, in the context of nursing, is to reach a mutual, peaceful agreement that is in the best interests of the client; reaching the agreement may require compromise.
- Nurses are responsible for determining their own actions and for supporting clients who are making moral decisions or for whom decisions are being made by others.
- Nurses can enhance their ethical practice and client advocacy by clarifying their own values, understanding the values of other health-care professionals, becoming familiar with nursing codes of ethics, and participating in ethics committees and rounds.
- Client advocacy involves concern for and actions on behalf of another person or organization in order to bring about change.
- The functions of the advocacy role are to inform, support, and mediate.

ASSESS YOUR LEARNING

1. When an ethical issue arises, one of the most important nursing responsibilities in managing client-care situations is which of the following?
   - **a.** Being able to defend the morality of your own actions
   - **b.** Remaining neutral and detached when making ethical decisions
   - **c.** Ensuring that a team is responsible for deciding ethical questions
   - **d.** Following the client's and family's wishes exactly

2. Which of the following situations is most clearly a violation of the underlying principles associated with professional nursing ethics?
   - **a.** The hospital policy permits use of internal fetal monitoring during labour. However, literature both supports and refutes the value of this practice.
   - **b.** When asked about the purpose of a medication, a nurse colleague responds, "Oh, I never look them up. I just give what is prescribed."
   - **c.** The nurses on the unit agree to sponsor a fundraising event to support a labour strike proposed by fellow nurses at another facility.
   - **d.** A client reports that he didn't quite tell the doctor the truth when asked if he was following his therapeutic diet at home.

3. Following a motor vehicle collision, the parents refuse to permit withdrawal of life support from their child, who has no apparent brain function. Although the nurse believes the child should be allowed to die and organ donation considered, the nurse supports the parents' decision. Which moral principle provides the basis for the nurse's actions?
   - **a.** Respect for autonomy
   - **b.** Nonmaleficence
   - **c.** Beneficence
   - **d.** Justice

4. Which of the following statements would be *most* helpful when a nurse is assisting clients in clarifying their values?
   - **a.** "That was not a good decision. Why did you think it would work?"
   - **b.** "The most important thing is to follow the plan of care. Did you follow all your doctor's orders?"
   - **c.** "Some people might have made a different decision. What led you to make your decision?"
   - **d.** "If you had asked me, I would have given you my opinion about what to do. Now, how do you feel about your choice?"

5. After recovering from her hip replacement, an older client wants to go home. The family wants the client to go to a nursing home. If the nurse were acting as a client advocate, the nurse would perform which of the following?
   - **a.** Inform the family that the client has a right to decide on her own.
   - **b.** Ask the primary-care provider to discharge the client to her home.
   - **c.** Suggest the client hire a lawyer to protect her rights.
   - **d.** Help the client and family communicate their views to each other.

6. Mr. Goldman, 78 years old, was admitted with congestive heart failure. His wife tells the nurse that

she is afraid her husband's condition is deteriorating, and despite several requests, the physician has not been in to see him. Which of the following is the most appropriate nursing action?
a. Assess Mr. Goldman and inform the couple that the physician will be contacted to convey their concerns.
b. Explain to Mrs. Goldman that she may speak with the physician later during rounds.
c. Reassure Mrs. Goldman that her husband is receiving appropriate care.
d. Inform Mrs. Goldman that the nurse-in-charge will be notified of her concerns.

7. You are assigned to care for Martin Seymour, a 77-year-old man with advanced cancer of the pancreas. His physician is concerned that Martin will become delirious if he is given an analgesic and has not left any orders for pain control. As a patient advocate, which of the following is your best course of action in this situation?
a. Administer opioids until pain relief is achieved
b. Help Martin to relax through guided imagery
c. Describe the patient's complaints of pain to the physician and request the patient be reassessed as soon as possible
d. Confront the physician about the inappropriateness of care she is providing

8. A daughter does not want her mother to learn of the mother's diagnosis of advanced cancer. She asks you to tell her mother that you don't know why she is in the hospital if her mother asks you. In this situation, you are being asked to compromise which ethical principle?
a. Principle of beneficence
b. Principle of nonmaleficence
c. Principle of veracity
d. Principle of fidelity

9. Which of the following is defined as the professional obligation of a nurse to assume responsibility for his or her own actions?
a. Individuality
b. Accountability
c. Bioethics
d. Utilitarianism

10. Which activity reflects the nurse's role as advocate?
a. Conducting a research study into the benefits of exercise
b. Notifying the supervisor about a client's adverse drug reaction
c. Facilitating client decision making
d. Assessing changes in blood pressure

After working through these questions, go to the MyNursingLab at ***http://www.mynursinglab.com*** *to check your answers and see explanations.*

SUGGESTED READINGS

Canadian Nurses Association. (series). *Ethics in practice.* Ottawa: Author.

This series of articles is available on the Canadian Nurses Association's website. Various issues are addressed in a clear, readable, and practical format. Topics include whistle-blowing, advance directives, and the use of restraints.

Canadian Nurses Association. (2002). *Ethical research guidelines for registered nurses.* Ottawa: Author.

This publication was prepared by the CNA in response to a need identified by nurses in practice for guidance around ethics in research. It details a nurse's obligations with respect to supporting and conducting research with patients or clients, and includes a series of case studies to demonstrate practical applications.

Canadian Nurses Association. (2003). *Position statement: Patient safety.* Retrieved January 29, 2007, from http://www.cna-nurses.ca/CNA/documents/pdf/publications/PS70_Patient-Safety_en.pdf

The Canadian Nurses Association has published position statements on a variety of topics. This one talks about issues related to patient safety and the nurse's role.

Canadian Nurses Association. (2004). *Everyday ethics: Putting the code into practice* (2nd ed.). Ottawa: Author.

This document was developed as a study guide to be used as an adjunct to the 2002 CNA Code of Ethics. It provides the nurse with clear explanations and examples of how the Code might be used in practice.

WEBLINKS

Nursing Ethics.ca

http://www.nursingethics.ca

This site lists Canadian resources related to ethical practice.

Canadian Nurses Association's Code of Ethics

http://www.cna-aiic.ca/CNA/practice/ethics/code/default_e-aspx

This site provides access to the Code of Ethics for the CNA and links to provincial and territorial websites for related documentation.

Centre for Applied Ethics

http://www.ethics.ubc.ca/newsletter/index.html

Established in 1993 by the University of British Columbia, the Centre for Applied Ethics is an interdisciplinary research centre that studies a variety of topics, including health-care practices. Its newsletter is available on the site.

Canadian Bioethics Society

http://www.bioethics.ca

The Canadian Bioethics Society was established in 1988 by the union of the Canadian Society of Bioethics and the Canadian Society for Medical Bioethics. Its members include health-care administrators, lawyers, nurses, philosophers, physicians, theologians, and others interested in the ethical dimensions of health care.

REFERENCES

Beauchamp, T. L., & Childress, J. F. (1979). *Principles of biomedical ethics.* New York: Oxford University Press.

Beauchamp, T. L., & Childress, J. F. (2001). *Principles of biomedical ethics* (5th ed.). New York: Oxford University Press.

Begley, A. M. (2005). Practising virtue: A challenge to the view that a virtue centred approach to ethics lacks practical content. *Nursing Ethics, 12*(6), 622–637.

Benner, P. (1997). A dialogue between virtue ethics and care ethics. *Theoretical Medicine, 18,* 47–61.

Berlin, E. A., & Fowkes, W. C. (1983). Teaching framework for cross-cultural care: Application in family practice. *Western Journal Medicine, 139*(6), 934–938.

Bowden, P. L. (1995). The ethics of nursing care and "the ethic of care." *Nursing Inquiry, 2*(1), 10–21.

Breslin, J. M., MacRae, S. K., Bell, J., & Singer, P. A. (2005). Top 10 health care ethics challenges facing the public: Views of Toronto bioethicists. *BMC Medical Ethics, 6,* 5.

Canadian Federation of Nurses Unions. (2008). *Nursing health human resources in Canada: The time for action was yesterday!* Retrieved March 14, 2008, from http://www.nursesunions.ca/content.php?doc=90

Canadian Nurses Association. (2004). *Everyday ethics: Putting the code into practice* (2nd ed.). Ottawa: Author.

Canadian Nurses Association. (2008). *Code of ethics for registered nurses.* Ottawa: Author.

College of Nurses of Ontario. (2005). *Practice standard: Ethics.* Retrieved November 30, 2008, from http://www.cno.org/docs/prac/41034_Ethics.pdf

Curtin, L. L. (1979). The nurse as advocate: A philosophical foundation for nursing. *Advances in Nursing Science, 1*(3), 1–10.

Davis, A. J., & Aroskar, M. A. (1991). *Ethical dilemmas and nursing practice* (3rd ed.). East Norwalk, CT: Appleton & Lange.

Dubler N. (1992). Individual advocacy as a governing principle. *Journal of Case Management, 1*(3), 82–86.

Ferrell, B. R. (2006). Understanding the moral distress of nurses witnessing medically futile care. *Oncology Nursing Forum, 33*(5), 922–930.

Gastmans, C., Dierckx de Casterle, B., & Schotsmans, P. (1998). Nursing considered as moral practice: A philosophical-ethical interpretation on nursing. *Kennedy Institute of Ethics, 8,* 43–69.

Gastmans, C. (2006). The care perspective in healthcare ethics. In Anne J. Davis, Verena Tschudin, & Louise de Raeve (Eds.), *Essentials of teaching and learning in nursing ethics: Perspectives and methods* (pp. 76–89). Toronto: Churchill Livingstone Elsevier.

Hewitt, J. (2002). A critical review of the arguments debating the role of the nurse advocate. *Journal of Advanced Nursing, 37*(5), 439–455.

International Council of Nurses. (2006). *The ICN code for nurses.* Geneva, Switzerland: Imprimerie Fornara.

MacPhail, S. (1996). *Ethical issues in community nursing.* Unpublished doctoral dissertation, University of Alberta.

Marck, P. (2000a). Recovering ethics after "technics": Developing critical text on technology. *Nursing Ethics, 7*(1), 5–14.

Marck, P. (2000b). Nursing in a technological world: Searching for healing communities. *Advances in Nursing Science, 23,* 63–81.

McGuire, M., & Murphy, S. (2005). The internationally educated nurse. *Canadian Nurse, 101,* 25–29.

Oberle, K., & Tenove, S. (2000). Ethical issues in public health nursing. *Nursing Ethics, 7,* 425–438.

Oberle, K., & Hughes, D. (2001). Doctors' and nurses' perceptions of ethical problems in end-of-life decisions. *Journal of Advanced Nursing, 33,* 707–715.

Redman, B. K., & Fry, S. (2000). Nurses' ethical conflicts: What is really known about them? *Nursing Ethics, 7,* 360–366.

Registered Nurses' of Ontario. (2006). *Client Centred Care Best Practice Guidelines.* Toronto: Author.

Rodney, P., & Starzomski, R. (1993, October). Constraints on the moral agency of nurses. *Canadian Nurse, 89,* 23–26.

Rodney, P., & Varcoe, C. (2001). Towards ethical inquiry in the economic evaluation of nursing practice. *Canadian Journal of Nursing Research, 33*(1), 35–57.

Salsberry, P. (1992). Caring, virtue theory, and a foundation for nursing ethics. *Scholarly Inquiry for Nursing Practice: An International Journal, 6,* 155–167.

Tschudin, V., & Hunt, G. (1994). Dissatisfaction: With professional relationships, with the status quo and with health care in general. *Nursing Ethics: An International Journal for Health Care Professionals, 1*(2), 69–70.

van Hooft, S. (1999). Acting for the virtue of caring in nursing. *Nursing Ethics, 6,* 189–201.

Wilkinson, J. M. (1996). *Toward a context-sensitive theory of nursing ethics: Classification and comparison of nurses' narratives from four time periods (1934, 1979, 1989 and 1995).* Doctoral dissertation, University of Kansas.

Yeo, M., & Moorhouse, A. (Eds.). (1996). *Concepts and cases in nursing ethics* (2nd ed.). Peterborough, ON: Broadview Press.

Chapter 6

Accountability and Legal Aspects of Nursing

Nursing practice is governed by many legal concepts. It is important for nurses to know the basics of the Canadian legal system and its relationship to the profession of nursing. Accountability is an essential concept of professional nursing practice and the law. Knowledge of laws that regulate and affect nursing practice is needed for two reasons:

1. To ensure that the nurse's decisions and actions are consistent with current legal principles
2. To protect the nurse from liability

OBJECTIVES

After studying this chapter, you should be able to

1. Describe the history and sources of Canadian law
2. Identify regulatory considerations in nursing and their impact on the practice of nursing in Canada
3. Identify selected aspects of professional regulation and their role in governing the practice of nursing, including expanding the scope of nursing practice
4. Discuss measures of accountability and discipline in nursing practice
5. Identify the two interdependent legal roles of provider of service and employer or contractor for service in nursing
6. Discuss areas of potential tort liability in nursing
7. Discuss informed consent, confidentiality, problematic substance use, and chemical dependency
8. Discuss legal issues and safe practices in documentation, telephone advice, incident reports, and reports of unsafe practices
9. Identify ways nurses and nursing students can minimize their chances of liability
10. Discuss legal protections of nurses in practice

Relationship of Nurses and the Law

Laws can be defined as "those rules made by humans which regulate social conduct in a formally prescribed and legally binding manner" (Bernzweig, 1996, p. 3).

Functions of the Law in Nursing

The law serves a number of functions in nursing:

- It provides a framework for establishing which nursing actions in the care of clients are legal.
- It outlines the responsibilities that govern nursing practice and nurses' relationships with physicians, other health-care practitioners, and the care system.
- It helps establish the boundaries of independent nursing action.
- It assists nurses in ensuring that they are consistent, competent, and safe in providing quality care that serves society while preserving individual rights and human dignity.

History and Source of Canada's Laws

Historically, Canadian law is derived from two distinct European systems, namely English common law and French civil law. Quebec follows the civil law system, while the other Canadian provinces and territories follow the common law legal tradition.

THE COMMON LAW TRADITION In the English **common law** tradition, legal principles and rules evolve through the courts. Judges interpret and apply principles from similar decisions in previous cases (*precedents*) to the particular case before them to reach a decision. For this reason, common law is sometimes called *case law* or *judge-made law*. In reality, no two cases are identical and the common law develops through judges making distinctions between cases and determining when an earlier case is not applicable to the case being considered. In this way, the common law at once provides some consistency and predictability regarding what legal solution will be appropriate in a given instance, and is flexible enough to allow for the particulars of a specific situation to be considered (Keatings & Smith, 2000).

The hierarchy within the courts has important implications for how the common law develops. Each province and territory has a lower-level trial court and a higher-level appeal court. The decisions of higher courts are binding on the lower courts in the same jurisdiction. Decisions in one jurisdiction, province, or territory are not binding in another jurisdiction, province, or territory, but such decisions are often treated as a persuasive source of law. This is particularly true when lower courts in one jurisdiction are considering a judgment from a higher-level court in a different jurisdiction. In contrast, a decision from the Supreme Court of Canada is binding on all other courts in the country (Keatings & Smith, 2000).

THE CIVIL LAW TRADITION The tradition of **civil law**, with its Roman roots, is quite different. A key distinguishing feature is that instead of emerging through the courts, laws are written down in what is referred to as a code. This code provides all citizens with an accessible and written collection of the laws that apply to them and that judges must follow. Quebec's Civil Code, first enacted in 1866 just before Confederation, is amended periodically and underwent a major revision in 1994. Like other civil codes, it contains a comprehensive statement of rules and general principles. Unlike common law courts, courts in a civil law system first look to the Code, and then refer to previous decisions for consistency.

STATUTORY LAW The distinction between the common and civil law traditions reveals two different sources of legal authority: (1) case law or judge-made law and (2) the Civil Code. Parliament and the provincial or territorial legislatures are another key source of Canadian law. Parliament has the power to pass laws for all of Canada, while the legislatures of each province and territory pass laws of a more local nature. Laws enacted by either of these legislative bodies are called *statutes, legislation,* or *acts*. When Parliament or one of the legislatures enacts legislation, that legislation then supersedes any case law dealing with the same subject. In Quebec, much legislation exists to cover areas not dealt with in the Civil Code.

Responsibility for the Canadian health-care system is shared between the federal and provincial or territorial governments, according to the division of powers set out in the *Constitution Act, 1867*. As a leading constitutional scholar notes, "health is an 'amorphous topic' which is distributed to the federal parliament or provincial legislatures depending on the purpose and effect of the particular health matter at issue" (Hogg, 1997, p. 445). However, despite the federal government having some jurisdiction in this area, health care and its delivery is interpreted as largely within provincial and territorial authority. For example, regulation of health-care professionals is a responsibility of the provinces and territories, and is one that, as will be discussed here, has in many instances been delegated by the provinces and territories to the provincial and territorial professional organizations.

Tort law refers to that body of the law through which a person who suffers injury caused by another person is able to claim compensation for that injury. Tort law is divided into two main categories: intentional torts and negligence. When a person proves that he or she has suffered harm caused by another, either through intentional action or through negligence, that person will have a claim for damages (compensation) against the person who caused the harm (called the *tortfeasor*). The goal of compensation in tort law is to put the person who suffered the harm back in the position he or she would have been in had the tortfeasor not acted. This is a guiding principle and is clearly more feasible in some cases than in others. Negligence and those intentional torts most applicable to the nursing context are discussed in greater detail later in this chapter. Please see Table 6.1 for examples of laws that affect nurses and nursing practice.

Regulatory Considerations in Nursing

Like most professions, nursing is a vocation requiring advanced education and training (*Black's Law Dictionary*, 2004). Professionals have "an exclusive right to practise a particular profession. This in theory protects the public from those not qualified to practise. . . . In Canada, the law prevents unqualified individuals from claiming to be members of a professional body, or in some cases, from practising the skills which are specifically identified with the particular professional body" (Morris, Ferguson, & Dykeman, 1999, p. 37). Although it gets its authority from the provincial and territorial governments, the profession itself is self-governing (see the Nursing and Canadian Society box). Each province and territory has a professional regulatory body that, depending on the jurisdiction, is called a college or an association (see Table 1.1 on page 19 for a list of the provincial and territorial nursing regulatory bodies). The following section reviews the roles and responsibilities of these provincial and territorial professional bodies and their impact on the practice of nursing in Canada.

TABLE 6.1 Selected Categories of Laws Affecting Nurses

Category	Examples
Constitutional	Due process Equal protection
Statutory (legislative)	Nurse practice acts Good Samaritan/ Emergency medical aid acts Child and adult abuse laws Living wills Sexual harassment laws
Criminal (public)	Murder, manslaughter Theft Arson Active euthanasia Sexual assault Illegal possession of controlled drugs
Contracts (private or civil)	Nurse and client Nurse and employer Nurse and insurance Client and agency
Torts (private or civil)	Negligence Libel and slander Invasion of privacy Assault and battery False imprisonment Abandonment

NURSING AND CANADIAN SOCIETY

Fact	Implications for Nursing Practice
The focus of nurse regulation is public protection. This regulation assures the public that they are receiving safe and ethical care from competent, qualified registered nurses.	Regulation defines the practice and boundaries of the nursing profession, including the requirements and qualifications to practise.
The regulatory system for nursing in Canada reflects the country's federal and provincial or territorial government structure.	One way that nurses are regulated is through *title control*. Registered nurse (RN) and nurse practitioner (NP), registered (licensed) practical nurse (RPN/LPN), and registered psychiatric nurse (RPN) are protected by legislation. Only nurses currently registered with a nursing regulatory body can use these titles.
Canadian public interest is best served when regulatory bodies adopt a framework that strengthens clinical nursing practice and leadership and promotes public safety.	A regulatory framework used by many of the provincial or territorial nursing regulatory bodies that embodies such principles as promoting good practice, preventing poor practice, and intervening in unacceptable practice.

Source: Based on "Understanding Self-Regulation," by the Canadian Nurses Association, 2007, February, *Nursing Now: Issues and Trends in Canadian Nursing, 21*, pp. 1–5.

PROVINCIAL AND TERRITORIAL REGULATORY BODIES

In Canada, the regulation of nursing is a function of provincial and territorial law. Nurses have been granted an exclusivity of practice (a right of self-government or self-regulation) and an obligation to monitor and discipline their own membership (Canadian Nurses Association [CNA], 2007). The provincial and territorial nursing **regulatory bodies**, such as the College of Registered Nurses of British Columbia (CRNBC), the College and Association of Registered Nurses of Alberta (CARNA), the Saskatchewan Registered Nurses' Association (SRNA), or the College of Nurses of Ontario (CNO), are given their authority by the provincial and territorial governments through legislation. Through such legislation and the associated regulations, these bodies are charged with regulating entry into the profession, setting standards of competent practice, establishing continuing competence or education and quality assurance improvement programs, and drafting bylaws for the general and day-to-day governance of the profession. (See the Nursing and Canadian Society box for additional information.)

The laws regulating nursing in the provinces and territories (other than Ontario and Quebec) are fairly uniform. Several provinces have umbrella legislation containing general provisions regarding all recognized health professionals within the province, as well as companion legislation relating specifically to nursing (see examples of the legislation for each province and territory listed in Table 6.2). In Ontario, the Regulated Health Professions Act and the Nursing Act govern the nursing profession (Keatings & Smith, 2000). This legislation makes the CNO the governing body responsible for the regulation of nursing in the province. Section 11 of the Nursing Act prohibits anyone from declaring himself or herself as competent to practise as a registered nurse unless the CNO has certified that person.

As further examples, Alberta and British Columbia both have legislation called the Health Professions Act. These acts provide a common regulatory structure for the governance of health professions within the provinces. Regulations (or subordinate legislation) are enacted under the Health Professions Act that designate nursing as a regulated profession under the act with its own self-governing body. In British Columbia, for example, the Nurses (Registered) and Nurse Practitioner Regulation was approved by Cabinet in 2005. This regulation not only governs registered nurses but also establishes nurse practitioners as a recognized category of registered nurse under the new CRNBC. The Nurses (Registered) and Nurse Practitioner Regulation sets out reserved titles and the scope of practice for CRNBC registrants, including reserved actions for general and certified registered nurse practice as well as nurse practitioner practice. As explained on the CRNBC website, under the province's Health Professions Act, the CRNBC is responsible for serving and protecting the public, and for exercising its powers in the public interest. To fulfill that role, the act

TABLE 6.2 Nursing Legislation in Canadian Provinces and Territories

Province or Territory	Health Care and Nursing Legislation for *Registered Nurses (RN)*
British Columbia	Health Professions Act
Alberta	Health Professions Act and Nursing Professions Act
Northwest Territories and Nunavut	Nursing Profession Act and Nunavut Nursing Professions Act
Saskatchewan	The Registered Nurses Act
Manitoba	The Registered Nurses Act
New Brunswick	Nurses Act
Nova Scotia	Registered Nurses Act
Prince Edward Island	Registered Nurses Act
Newfoundland and Labrador	Registered Nurses Act
Ontario	Regulated Health Professions Act, Nursing Act, and Health Professions Procedural Code
Quebec	Professional Code of Quebec and Nurses Act
Yukon	Registered Nurses Profession Act
Province or Territory	**Health Care and Nursing Legislation for *Licensed Practical Nurses (LPN)***
British Columbia	Health Professions Act and CLPNBC bylaws
Alberta	Health Professions Act and Health Disciplines Act
Northwest Territories and Nunavut	Licensed Practical Nurses Act
Saskatchewan	Licensed Practical Nurses Act
Manitoba	Licensed Practical Nurses Act
New Brunswick	Licensed Practical Nurses Act
Nova Scotia	Licensed Practical Nurses Act
Prince Edward Island	Licensed Practical Nurses Act
Newfoundland and Labrador	Licensed Practical Nurses Act
Ontario (Registered Practical Nurse)	Regulated Health Professions Act, Nursing Act, and Health Professions Procedural Code
Quebec	Professional Code of Quebec, Nurses Act, and Licensed Practical Nurses Act
Province or Territory	**Health Care and Nursing Legislation for *Registered Psychiatric Nurses***
British Columbia	Health Professions Act and Registered Psychiatric Nurses Act
Alberta	Health Professions Act and Health Disciplines Act
Saskatchewan	Registered Psychiatric Nurses Act
Manitoba	Registered Psychiatric Nurses Act

Source: Updated and adapted from "The Canadian Legal System," by M. Keatings and O. Smith, 2000. In M. Keatings and O. Smith (Eds.), *Ethical and Legal Issues in Canadian Nursing* (pp. 51–94). Toronto: W.B. Saunders.

empowers the CRNBC to make bylaws to govern registrants, though most of the bylaws still do require government approval.

SELECTED ASPECTS OF PROFESSIONAL REGULATION
Credentialing is the process of determining and maintaining competence in nursing practice. The law prohibits individuals from declaring themselves to be *nurses* or *registered nurses* unless they are registered with a provincial or territorial nursing body. Writing the registered nurse licensing examination in all provinces and territories, except Quebec, is the first step to becoming a registered nurse and starts lifelong continuing education and professional standards portfolios. The credentialing process is one way in which the nursing profession sets and maintains standards of practice and accountability for the educational preparation of its members. Credentialing includes licensure, registration, certification, and accreditation.

Licensure and registration together are a way to protect the public from unsafe practitioners and to assure employers that the nurse has met minimum requirements for entry to practice. The term **registration** means the listing of an individual's name on an official roster. In Canada, practising nurses in all provinces and territories are required by law to be registered or to hold a valid permit or licence with their provincial or territorial nursing association. Registration usually occurs every year. Only those who are registered are entitled to call themselves registered nurses, licensed (registered) practical nurses, or registered psychiatric nurses, or to use the initials RN, LPN, or RPN. To be registered, the nurse must have completed a basic course of nursing studies in an approved program of the registering body and have passed the national qualifying exams.

Certification is a voluntary practice that proves that a nurse has met minimum standards of nursing competence in specialty areas, such as perinatal nursing, pediatrics, mental health, gerontology, or critical care nursing. Certification enhances a nurse's confidence and proficiency in a specialty area. Certification is a commitment to the leading edge in national health-care standards. It gives national scope to the principle of continued competence encouraged by provincial and territorial quality assurance programs. The Canadian Nurses Association (CNA) offers certification in 17 areas.

Programs in nursing education must receive approval from their regulatory body in order for their graduates to write the registration examination and apply for registration. Approval is based on standards that the school and program must meet. Accreditation for baccalaureate programs is completed by the Canadian Association of Schools of Nursing (CASN). Please see Chapter 2 for additional information.

EXPANDING THE ROLE OF REGISTERED NURSES
The various acts and regulations that govern the practice of nursing in Canada are also responsible for setting the scope and nature of nursing in Canada. Recently, the development of policy and legislation to expand the scope of RNs' practice has become a prominent issue across the country. Diverse models have been used to provide authority to RNs performing extended or expanded roles. Diagnostic and treatment functions have been delegated by government to the medical profession through legislation (CNA, 2002a). The CNA formed a committee of provincial and territorial representatives to establish a framework to guide the development and implementation of legislation dealing with nursing roles that require additional regulation (i.e., primary care functions). In 2002, the CNA (2002c) published a second edition of its *Advanced Nursing Practice: A National Framework,* which includes information about various aspects of advanced nursing practice (ANP), such as competencies, educational preparation, and regulation. The CNA is also playing a leading role in ensuring that the national dialogue in this area continues, an illustration of which is the *Report of 2005 Dialogue on Advanced Nursing Practice* (2006). This report "provides an understanding of [the] history, the factors that must shape ANP and strategies for effectively moving forward" (p. 2), and emphasizes the important role of RNs in advanced practice roles in improving access to and outcomes of care in Canada's health-care system.

Accountability and Discipline in Nursing

In addition to the elements just outlined, the nursing regulatory bodies are also responsible for ensuring that standards are established and maintained. This task includes investigating complaints regarding the level of practice or other competency issues of individual registrants and, where appropriate, addressing them through disciplinary action.

STANDARDS AND BEST PRACTICES The establishment of nursing practice standards is essential for a self-regulating profession. In assessing the quality of care provided by nurses, it is crucial to have objective criteria by which to judge whether the care given is good, adequate, or unsafe. Nursing practice standards are generally broad in nature to capture the varied roles and practice settings in which nurses practise. For example, the Registered Nurses' Association of Ontario (RNAO) has produced a variety of documents that explain practice standards and expectations, such as *Therapeutic Nurse-Client Relationship, Culturally Sensitive Care,* and *Documentation.*

Standards are also used as a template for nurses to assess their own nursing practice annually in order to determine their professional development goals and meet continuing competence requirements set out by the provincial or territorial body. It is the responsibility of all regulated members to understand their associations practice standards and apply them to their nursing practices, specific to their areas of practice and roles. Standards are based on the values of the profession, articulated in the *Code of Ethics for Registered Nurses* and codes of ethics for other categories of nurses. Together, ethics and standards provide the basis for nursing practice in Canada.

COMPLAINT PROCESS Each provincial and territorial nursing body has a mechanism in place to review the conduct of its members to ensure safe and ethical nursing practice. They are required to investigate complaints against RNs and discipline those members who fail to meet the standards of the profession. The regulatory body may receive complaints about nurses from a variety of sources, including the public, hospitals or other employers, and other nurses or health-care providers. Occasionally, nurses may decide to self-report if they are concerned that they are not able to practise safely. The complaint process comprises a number of steps, including the complaint intake or receipt and initial assessment, the investigation process, the review process, and possibly a hearing and an appeal. Although variations exist across jurisdictions, so too do many similarities. Nurses are encouraged to check with their provincial or territorial association to determine the process to follow. The disciplinary role is central to the regulatory body's duty to protect the public, is taken very seriously, and can have significant consequences for the registrant. When a case involves either civil or criminal wrongs, further legal consequences can follow, separate and apart from the provincial and territorial regulatory body discipline process.

Contractual Arrangements in Nursing

Legal Roles of Nurses

Nurses have two separate but interdependent legal roles, each with rights and associated responsibilities: (1) provider of service and (2) employee or contractor for service.

PROVIDER OF SERVICE The nurse is expected to provide safe and competent care so that no harm (physical, psychological, or material) comes to the recipient of the service. A nurse, for example, has an obligation to practise and direct the practice of others under the nurse's supervision so that harm or injury to the client is prevented and standards of care are maintained. When **delegating care** to others, the nurse is responsible for ensuring that this delegation is appropriate and that those delegated to (e.g., family, other health-care members, students) have the skills to fulfill the functions (CNA, 2002a). Nurses are obligated to follow physicians' orders, unless they believe that these orders have the potential to harm or injure the patient. The nurse must then carefully assess the situation and obtain clarification from the physician, if necessary. If the physician confirms the order and the nurse still believes the order to be unsafe, informing the supervisor is the next responsibility. The nurse also needs to carefully document, in chronological order, the steps taken. At this point, resolving the problem of the questionable order should be the supervisor's responsibility. It is imperative that a nurse speak out and investigate orders that are believed to be unsafe, as the nurse who carries out the order could be held legally responsible for any harm suffered by the patient.

The **standards of care** by which a nurse acts or fails to act are legally defined by nurse practice acts and by the rule of reasonable and prudent action—what a sensible and careful professional with similar preparation and experience would do in similar circumstances. The **contractual obligations** of a nurse toward the patient may be either implied, such as to render safe and competent care, or be more specifically stated, such as they might be within a contract for private employment, specifying what types of services will be provided, when, and for what payment. Employment contracts are discussed further in the following section.

EMPLOYEE OR CONTRACTOR FOR SERVICE Nurses, whether in independent practice or as employees, have employment contracts. A **contract** is an agreement between two or more persons that creates an obligation to do or not do a particular thing (*Black's Law Dictionary*, 2004). For a contract to exist (Parisi, 1999), the following conditions must be met:

- Each contract must have a lawful purpose.
- Each party entering the contract must be competent and understand the subject matter.
- Each party must understand the obligations of the contract.
- Each party must have obligations and benefits derived from the contract.
- At minimum, all employment contracts must meet the standards set forth in provincial, territorial, and federal labour standards and codes.

Employment contracts can be oral, written, or implied. If a union is not involved, the nurse and the employer can negotiate an individual employment contract that sets forth the rights and obligations of each party. A nurse who is employed directly by a client (a nurse in private practice) usually has a written contract with that client in which the nurse agrees to provide professional services for a certain fee. In a unionized organization, the terms and conditions of employment are those of the union contract with the employer. Verbal employment contracts can be problematic because they lack proof of the terms negotiated.

Contractual relationships vary among practice settings. An independent nurse practitioner is a contractor for service, whose contractual relationship with the client is an independent one. The nurse employed by a hospital functions within an employer–employee relationship, in which the nurse represents and acts for the hospital and, therefore, must function within the employer's policies. If an employee commits a wrongful action, employers are normally held legally responsible because of a doctrine called **vicarious liability**. This principle does not usually apply to independent practitioners (Canadian Nurses Protective Society [CNPS], 1998).

Nurses need to be familiar with their terms of employment and the laws that dictate responsibility if a lawsuit is initiated. A nurse found liable in a civil lawsuit would usually be covered by the employer's liability insurer, who would cover the legal fees, court costs, and damages (CNPS, 1998). For example, in the case of *Joseph Brant Memorial Hospital v. Koziol* (1978), a patient died from aspiration following back surgery. In this case, the nurse did not rouse him to cough or deep breathe, and the record did not document care. The nursing care was found to be below the standard and the hospital was held vicariously liable. In another Ontario case, a hospital was held vicariously liable for the negligence of two obstetrical nurses—one an inexperienced junior nurse, and the other her supervisor. In this case, the fact that severe decelerations in the fetal heart monitor were not reported to the staff obstetrician resulted in a delayed caesarean section and ultimately in a severely compromised infant. In its decision, the court noted that

> *nurses are professionals who also possess special skills and knowledge and the same principles apply as in the case of doctors, residents and interns. They have a duty to use those skills in making appropriate assessments of patients and to communicate accurately those assessments to physicians. In this case the nurses were employees of the . . . Hospital and if they breached their duty to exercise appropriate skill and care in making interpretations and communicating information to physicians and damage results, the hospital will be liable. (Granger (Litigation guardian of) v. Ottawa General Hospital, 1996; cited in Sneiderman, Irvine, & Osborne, 2003)*

Ultimately, the court held that the nurses had breached their duty of care and the hospital was held vicariously liable for their negligence. Moreover, in dismissing the case against the defendant physicians, the court emphasized that it was inappropriate to expect the physicians to double check the work of other members of the health-care team; instead, it was held that

> *the staff obstetrician should be entitled to rely upon the information being given to him or her by the staff nurse on the understanding that the nurse, assigned by the hospital to these duties, has been properly trained, is sufficiently experienced and knows what he or she is doing at all times within the scope of his or her professional responsibilities (Granger (Litigation guardian of) v. Ottawa General Hospital, 1996; cited in Sneiderman et al., 2003)*

The doctrine of vicarious liability does not imply that the nurse cannot be held liable as an individual. And it does not imply that the doctrine will prevail if the employee's actions are extraordinarily inappropriate, that is, beyond those expected or foreseen by the employer. For example, if the nurse hits a client in the face, the employer could avoid liability because such conduct is beyond the bounds of expected behaviour. Criminal acts, such as taking tranquilizers for personal use from a client's supply, would also be considered extraordinarily inappropriate behaviour. Nurses can be held liable for failure to act as well. For example, a nurse who sees another nurse hitting a patient and fails to do anything to protect the patient may also be considered negligent. See Box 6.1 for information on legal protection for nurses.

The nurse in the role of employee or contractor for service has obligations to the employer, the patient, and other personnel. The nursing care provided must be within the limitations and terms specified. The nurse has an obligation to contract only for those responsibilities that he or she is competent to discharge.

The nurse is expected to respect the rights and responsibilities of other health-care participants. For example, although the nurse has a responsibility to explain nursing activities to a patient, the nurse does not have the right to comment on medical practice in a way that disturbs the client or denounces the physician. At the same time, the nurse has the right to expect reasonable and prudent conduct from other health professionals. Please see Table 6.3 for examples of roles, responsibilities, and rights of nurses.

BOX 6.1 LEGAL PROTECTION IN AN EMPLOYEE–EMPLOYER RELATIONSHIP

Nurses should be aware of the liability protection they have:

- Nurses should seek written confirmation of their employment status and professional liability coverage.
- Nurses should ensure that the employer is notified immediately if they are sued or involved in a potential liability situation.
- Nurses should be aware of the process and cooperate with the employer's insurer and lawyer representing (defending) them in a legal suit.
- Nurses who practice as independent practitioners should contact their insurer, if they have one, and CNPS to discuss their existing liability protection.

Source: From "Vicarious Liability," by the Canadian Nurses Protective Society, 1998, *infoLAW*, 7(1). Reprinted with permission of Canadian Nurses Protective Society.

TABLE 6.3 Legal Roles, Responsibilities, and Rights

Role	Responsibilities (Obligations)	Rights
Provider of service	To provide safe and competent care commensurate with the nurse's preparation, experience, and circumstances To inform clients of the consequences of various alternatives and outcomes of care To provide adequate supervision and evaluation of others for whom the nurse is responsible To remain competent	The right to adequate and qualified assistance as necessary The right to reasonable and prudent conduct from clients, e.g., provision of accurate information as required
Employee or contractor for service	To fulfill the obligations of contracted service with the employer To respect the employer To respect the rights and responsibilities of other health-care providers	The right to adequate working conditions (e.g., safe equipment and facilities) The right to compensation for services rendered The right to reasonable and prudent conduct by other health-care providers
Citizen	To protect the rights of the recipients of care	The right to respect of the nurse's own rights and responsibilities by others Right to physical safety

Consent Issues

Patients are entitled to make decisions about their health care and have the right to be given all available information relevant to such decisions. Obtaining consent is not a discrete event; rather, it is a process that should occur throughout the relationship between the patient and all health-care providers.

Consent has three components: (1) disclosure, (2) capacity, and (3) voluntariness. **Disclosure** refers to the provision of information, including the risks of treatment, alternative treatment and its associated facts and risks, and the effects and risks of no treatment. **Capacity** refers to the patient's ability to understand the relevant information and appreciate the consequences of the decision. **Voluntariness** refers to the patient's right to come to a decision without force, coercion, or manipulation from others (Etchells, Sharpe, Walsh, Williams, & Singer, 1999). When these three requirements are met, that is, when a patient has received all the information, when the patient has the capacity to make the decision, and when the patient is free from coercion, the patient is in a position to provide what is called **informed consent** to the medical treatment.

Consent is of two types: express and implied. **Express consent** is a clear statement by the patient and can be either oral or written. "It is important to remember that the patient has the right to withdraw consent or revoke a previously given consent at any time, even orally, provided he/she is mentally competent to do so" (Keatings & Smith, 2000, p. 186). **Implied consent** exists when the individual's nonverbal behaviour indicates willingness. Examples of implied consent include the following:

- In emergency situations, when the individual cannot provide express consent
- During surgery, when additional procedures are needed that are consistent with the procedure already consented to
- In therapy, when the person continues to participate without withdrawing previously provided consent

In such situations, the CNPS (1994) suggests that provincial and territorial legislation, including hospital or institutional policies and procedures, be followed. For treatments that entail risk or more than mild discomfort, express rather than implied consent should be obtained (Etchells, Sharpe, Walsh, et al., 1999).

OBTAINING CONSENT AND DISCLOSING INFORMATION Obtaining consent to medical or nursing care is a legal requirement. Under common law, treating a competent patient without obtaining any consent, or treating a patient who is refusing treatment, constitutes **battery**, whereas treating a patient without obtaining fully informed consent constitutes **negligence** (Parisi, 1999).

Obtaining informed consent for specific *medical* and *surgical* treatments is the responsibility of a physician. Although this responsibility is delegated to nurses in some agencies and no laws prohibit the nurse from being part of the information-giving process, the practice, nevertheless, is highly undesirable. The nurse does not perform direct medical procedures and may not have the detailed medical knowledge of the physician performing the procedure. Also, it is not the nurse's responsibility to "supply the gaps or deficiencies in the physician's dialogue with the patient"; however, it is the responsibility of the nurse to "respond appropriately and ensure that when information gaps occur the physician is

Evidence-Informed Practice

What Are the Issues of Informed Consent?

As part of a larger qualitative study examining cancer care communication with patients, Oliffe, Thorne, Hislop, and Armstrong (2007) examined data to determine how patients of various ethnicities perceived the communication. Two important themes emerged: (1) the content and volume of the information, and (2) the role of family members in receiving and sharing information. The first theme reflects the widely held Western view that information is always a good thing, but respondents suggested that too much information could contribute to a loss of hope. The second theme contrasted the Western value of patient autonomy with that of respecting the patient's familial web. Respondents suggested that listening to the family for more knowledge about the patient before giving potentially distressing news was important.

NURSING IMPLICATIONS: While informed consent is both a value and a legal expectation, we need to understand that the meaning of the term informed consent can be "mediated by culture and context" (p. 13). The authors suggest that nurses consider that "consent becomes a process that requires repeated attempts to ascertain what the patient (and family) wants to know and how involved they want to be in the process" (p. 13) in order to prevent harm based on ignorance while respecting potential harm from unwanted information.

Source: Based on "'Truth-Telling' and Cultural Assumptions in an Era of Informed Consent," by J. Oliffe, S. Thorne, T. G. Hislop, and E. Armstrong, 2007, *Family and Community Health, 30*(1), pp. 5–15.

alerted in time to put things right" (Sneiderman et al., 2003, p. 164). Often, the nurse's responsibility is to witness the giving of informed consent for medical procedures, which involves the following:

- Witnessing the exchange between the client and the physician
- Establishing that the client really did understand, that is, was truly informed

Obtaining informed consent for *nursing* procedures is the responsibility of the nurse. This applies, in particular, to nurse-midwives and nurse practitioners in performing procedures in their advanced practices. However, it also applies to other nurses performing direct care, such as inserting nasogastric tubes or starting an intravenous infusion. It can be a challenge to determine the amount and type of information required for the client to make an informed decision. The client should have the following general information:

- The purposes of the treatment
- What he or she can expect to feel or experience
- The intended benefits of the treatment
- The possible risks or negative outcomes of the treatment
- The advantages and disadvantages of possible alternatives to the treatment (including no treatment)

THE THREE ELEMENTS OF INFORMED CONSENT: A CLOSER LOOK As discussed, for a patient's consent to treatment to be valid, it must be given voluntarily. To give informed consent voluntarily, the patient must not feel coerced. Sometimes, fear of disapproval from a health professional can be the motivation for giving consent; such consent is not voluntarily given.

It is also important that the patient be **informed**, that is, that he or she is provided with all the necessary information and understands it all. Technical words and language barriers can inhibit understanding. If a patient cannot read, the consent form must be read to the patient before it is signed. If the patient does not speak the same language as the health professional who is providing the information, the help of an interpreter must be acquired.

If given sufficient information, a **competent** adult is assumed to be able to make decisions regarding health. A competent adult is a person over 18 years of age (ages vary across jurisdictions) who is conscious and oriented. A patient who is confused, disoriented, or sedated is not considered functionally competent.

Informed consent regulations were originally written with acute-care settings in mind. Nonetheless, ensuring informed consent is equally important in providing nursing care in the home and community. Because the provision of home care often occurs over an extended period of time, the nurse has multiple opportunities to ensure that the client agrees to the plan of treatment. A challenge to informed consent in the home, however, is that the plan may affect other members of the family, and, if so, they need to be consulted.

In many areas of health-care law and capacity, consent becomes a confusing issue. The first is related to minors. Canadian common law does not specify an age below which a person is not presumed capable (Etchells, Sharpe, Elliot, & Singer, 1999). Some provinces have legislation that lowers the age of consent below 18 years. A minor can give consent if it is determined that the person has adequate knowledge and judgment (is able to reasonably foresee consequences of a decision or lack of a decision) (Sharpe, 1993). Some provinces have legislation that establishes the age of consent to treatment; health-care providers should be aware of the legislative requirements of their own province or territory.

It is also important to remember that capacity can change over time. A patient who is confused, disoriented, or sedated is not considered functionally competent; however, this state may be temporary and requires careful skilled assessment. Individuals who are unconscious or injured in such a way that they are unable to give consent require substitute consent from another individual.

Statutes tend to provide a hierarchy of **substitute decision makers**. Priority is given to a court-appointed substitute decision maker or person with power of attorney for personal care or proxy. If these do not exist, authority falls to a spouse, and then to various family members in accordance with the statutory list (CNPS, 2004, p. 2). The substitute decision maker should be the person with the best knowledge of the patient's specific wishes or of the patient's values and beliefs. In general, close relatives are preferred as substitute decision makers as they "know the patient best" and are able to make a decision that would be as close to the patient's as possible. Most jurisdictions have enacted legislation to deal with substitute consent and to allow people to create a legally valid personal or advance directive or to appoint a health-care agent (Downie & Caulfield, 1999). Although not all provinces and territories have enacted comprehensive legislation, the courts are likely to apply many of the principles embodied in existing legislation (Morris et al., 1999).

In the case of a patient with a mental illness, capacity to consent may or may not be valid, depending on whether the mental illness makes that patient unable to appreciate the nature, quality, and consequences of the proposed treatment. In this case, patients who refuse treatment can have their capacity questioned by the clinician. These patients require careful assessment to screen for incapacity (a full discussion of which is beyond the scope of this text). If the clinician remains unsure, expert assessments can go to hospital ethics committees or legal review boards (Etchells, Sharpe, Elliot, et al., 1999). Provincial and territorial mental health acts or similar statutes generally provide direction and specify the rights of people with mental illness under the law, as well as the rights of the professionals caring for such patients.

Areas of Potential Tort Liability in Nursing

Tort Law

A **tort** is a civil wrong committed against a person or a person's property. Battery and the failure to obtain informed consent, discussed earlier, are examples of torts. Torts are usually litigated in court by civil action between individuals. In other words, the person claimed to be responsible for the tort is sued for damages. Tort liability is based on fault, that is, something that was done incorrectly (an unreasonable act of commission) or something that should have been done but was not (omission). Torts can be broadly categorized as either negligence or intentional.

NEGLIGENCE In the nursing context, negligence consists of conduct and behaviour that falls below the standard expected of an ordinary, reasonable, and prudent nurse. Such conduct places another person at risk for harm. Failing to obtain informed consent, failing to follow proper procedure in moving a patient, or administering the wrong dosage of medication all constitute examples of negligence in nursing. Four elements must be present in a negligence lawsuit against a nurse:

1. *Duty.* The nurse must have a relationship with the client that involves providing care. Such duty is evident when the nurse has been assigned to care for a client in the home, hospital, or community by virtue of employment. In contrast, a nurse in private practice may have the option of deciding whether to accept a patient for care; as such, the duty is established when the nurse takes on an individual as a patient.
2. *Breach.* A standard of care must be expected in the specific situation that the nurse did not observe. This is the failure to act as a reasonable, prudent nurse under the circumstances. The practice is measured against that of similar nurses, unless the nurse undertakes a practice outside the usual nursing role. In such an instance, the nurse may be held to a higher standard based on advanced training. The standard can come from documents published by national or professional organizations, provincial or territorial nursing practice standards, institutional policies and procedures, or textbooks or journals, or it may be stated by expert witnesses.
3. *Harm.* The client must have sustained injury, damage, or harm. The plaintiff will be asked to document physical injury, medical costs, loss of wages, pain and suffering, and any other damages.
4. *Causation.* It must be proved that the harm occurred as a *direct result* of the nurse's failure to follow the standard and the nurse could have (or should have) known that failure to follow the standard could result in such harm.

A claim of negligence will usually centre on factors 2 and 4, that is, issues of what constituted the appropriate standard of care, and whether such standard was breached and whether the breach directly caused the harm to the plaintiff will be the issues most in question. To avoid charges of negligence, nurses need to recognize those nursing situations in which negligent actions are most likely to occur and to take measures to prevent them (see Box 6.2). A common situation is *medication error.* Because of the large number of medications taken by patients, and the numerous commercial names commonly used for the various drugs, safety precautions assume greater importance to ensure that the patient receives the right drug, in the proper dose, at the right time, and in the proper manner. Medication errors include failing to read the medication label, misreading or incorrectly calculating the dosage, failing to identify the client correctly, preparing the wrong concentration,

BOX 6.2 BASIC NURSING CARE ERRORS RESULTING IN NEGLIGENCE

Three kinds of nursing errors can result in negligence. Examples of each kind of error are listed below.

ASSESSMENT ERRORS

- Failing to gather and chart client information adequately
- Failing to recognize the significance of certain information (e.g., laboratory values, vital signs)

PLANNING ERRORS

- Failing to chart each identified problem
- Failing to use language in the care plan that other caregivers understand
- Failing to ensure continuity of care by ignoring the care plan
- Failing to give discharge instructions that the client understands

INTERVENTION ERRORS

- Failing to interpret and carry out a doctor's orders
- Failing to perform nursing tasks correctly
- Failing to pursue the physician if the physician doesn't respond to calls or failing to notify the nurse-manager if the physician is unavailable

or administering a medication by the wrong route (e.g., intravenously instead of intramuscularly). Nurses always need to check medications very carefully (see Chapter 31). Even after checking, the nurse should recheck the medication order and the medication before administering it if, for example, the client states, "I did not have a green pill before."

A nurse's responsibility for adverse effects and critical incidents (National Steering Committee on Patient Safety, 2002) will be weighed in accordance with the provincial or territorial body's governing professional nursing standard. Health-care employers often have policies and procedures for medication administration and standards for documentation that include the steps to follow once an error has been discovered. Such standards also include the requirement to keep up to date with the latest professional and technological developments, such as new intravenous tubing or intravenous pumps. Additional education should be taken as required to maintain expertise to the appropriate standard.

A nurse must administer medications according to the ten *rights* of medication administration (see Chapter 31). Nurses must take action to ensure that they do not misread, mishear, or misunderstand the drug that they are giving. For example, such a drug as hydromorphone can easily be mistaken for morphine. This error is known as confirmation bias: seeing what you expect to see (Borg, 2008).

Despite this diligence, medication errors still occur. Such was the case in which a 67-year-old man in the emergency department was given 10 mg of hydromorphone IM instead of 10 mg of morphine. He was given this drug just before discharge as the patient declined to stay for observation. Hydromporphone that was packaged in a similar way to morphine was mistakenly selected from the opioid cupboard. The dose given to the patient (who was opioid naive) was equivalent to about 60 mg to 70 mg of morphine. Within 1 hour of the patient's discharge, the opioid count revealed the error. The hospital took immediate action to find the patient; unfortunately, he arrested and died in another rural hospital. Possible legal investigations in such a case may or may not lead to legal proceedings and penalties. In 2004, the Institute for Safe Medication Practices Canada generated a detailed report with recommendations for practitioners and institutions; "unfortunately in the years since the report morphine/hydromorphone substitution errors continue to be made" (Borg, 2008, p. 35).

Patients often fall accidentally, sometimes with resultant injury. Some falls can be prevented by elevating the side rails on the cribs, beds, and stretchers for babies, small children, and, when necessary, adults. If a nurse leaves the rails down, or leaves a baby unattended on a bath table, that nurse may be found liable in negligence if the patient falls and is injured as a direct result. Most hospitals and nursing homes have policies regarding the use of safety devices, such as side rails and restraints. The nurse needs to be familiar with these policies and to take precautions to prevent accidents. Information about providing a safe environment for patients can be found in Chapter 30.

In some instances, ignoring a patient's complaints can constitute negligence. The nurse who does not report a client's complaint of acute abdominal pain is negligent and may be found liable for the ensuing appendix rupture and death. By failing to take vital signs and to check the dressing of a patient who has just had abdominal surgery, a nurse omits important assessments. If the patient hemorrhages and dies, the nurse may be found liable for negligence.

The case of *Downey v. Rothwell* (1974) is a good and often cited example of negligence in the nursing context. In this case, a 35-year-old plaintiff who had a history of grand mal epileptic seizures and recently had discontinued her anticonvulsant prescription for phenobarbital, suffered a severe arm injury after falling off an examining room table. Mrs. Downey was under the care of an RN (of 40 years experience) who had worked in this doctor's clinic for the past 22 years. The client informed the nurse that she was experiencing the sensation (called an aura) of having an epileptic seizure. The nurse remained in the room with the client for about a half an hour. When nothing happened, however, the nurse left the room to locate Mrs. Downey's file, leaving her unattended. During this time, the client experienced a severe seizure, fell onto the floor, and broke her arm. The nurse, having the knowledge about epileptic seizures, should have recognized an aura and remained with the client, ensuring her safety on the examination table.

In this case, the judge concluded that leaving the client unattended constituted a breach of the standard of care expected of an RN. A nursing instructor who testified as an expert witness and textbook materials were both presented to establish the appropriate standard of care. These sources were unanimous in stating that the nurse in this situation should have remained with the client. The nurse was found to be negligent, and for that negligence, her employers were made vicariously liable.

INTENTIONAL TORTS Negligence is different from **intentional torts**. The main difference is that negligent acts are unintentional, and intentional torts are committed on purpose by the tortfeasor. Another difference is that harm is a required element in negligence, while no harm need be suffered by the plaintiff for a defendant to be found liable of an intentional tort. Also, because no standard of care is involved, no expert witnesses are needed. Assault, battery, false imprisonment, and invasion of privacy are some of the intentional torts most likely to be relevant in the nursing context.

Assault can be described as an attempt or threat to touch another person unjustifiably. Assault precedes battery; it is the act that causes the person to believe a battery is about to occur. For example, the person who threatens someone by making a menacing gesture with a club or a closed fist is guilty of assault. A nurse who threatens a client with an injection after the client refuses to take the medication orally would be committing assault.

Battery is intentional harmful or offensive contact with another person (or the person's clothes or even something the person is carrying), without that person's consent. It is not necessary that a battery actually result in harm to the plaintiff, instead, "offensive contact is enough, however trivial it may seem, for it may trigger retaliatory measures by persons whose dignity and self respect are threatened" by the contact (Linden & Feldthusen, 2006, p. 44). "[B]attery is . . . a tort or legal wrong which protects people's 'dignitary interests,' their rights to personal autonomy and to freedom from wanton, humiliating or otherwise unwelcome interference" (Sneiderman et al., 2003, p. 160). In the previous example, if the nurse followed through on the threat and gave the injection without the client's consent, the nurse would be committing battery. Liability applies even though the physician ordered the medication or the activity and even if the client benefits from the nurse's action. Case law also indicates that it is battery "where a nurse in good faith administers a vaccination believing wrongly that there has been consent" (*Toews v. Weisner,* [2001, BCSC] as cited by Linden & Feldthusen, 2006).

A good example of a case involving battery is *Malette v. Shulman* (1990), from the Ontario Court of Appeal. In this case, an unconscious patient arrived in the emergency department following a car accident. The physician determined that the patient required a blood transfusion to survive and proceeded to transfuse her even after being advised that she carried a card in her wallet that identified her as a Jehovah's Witness. The card indicated that, on the basis of her religious convictions, she did not want to be given blood under any circumstances. The card was neither dated nor witnessed. The patient survived and successfully sued the physician for battery. Although this case did not involve nurses, it serves to highlight the fact that even though consent is often deemed to be implied in emergency situations, such consent may in some circumstances be set aside when a strong indication exists that the patient would not have consented to the treatment.

Battery clearly exists when consent is not obtained for treatment. However, the courts will also consider as battery treatments given that either go beyond or are different from that for which consent was obtained (such as when the wrong disc is operated on), or when consent is obtained through fraud or misrepresentation (Linden & Feldthusen, 2006). In contrast, when a patient has consented to treatment but then complains that he or she was not given adequate information, for example, as to the risks associated with the procedure, the plaintiff would properly bring the claim of negligence. As noted earlier, for consent to be valid, the patient must be competent to give consent. It can be very difficult to determine whether clients who are very old, who have specific mental disorders, or who take particular medications are competent to agree to treatments. If the nurse is uncertain whether a client refusing a treatment is competent, the supervisor and physician should be consulted to ensure that the treatment is ethically and legally permissible.

False imprisonment is the intentional confining of a person within fixed boundaries, without that person's consent. As others have explained, the name is somewhat misleading. Linden and Feldthusen (2006) explain as follows:

> *Firstly, there is no need for any prison to be involved. Although one can certainly imprison someone by incarceration behind prison walls, it can also be accomplished in other ways [for example, one can imprison someone in a psychiatric hospital, room, car, or boat]. Secondly, the confinement cannot be "false" in the sense of being unreal. The word "false" is intended to impart the notion of unauthorized or wrongful detention. (p. 50)*

The plaintiff does not need to prove damages to successfully bring a false imprisonment action, but must show that he or she "was intentionally restrained and that no reasonable avenue of escape was available. [Moreover], the plaintiff need not be conscious of the confinement" at the time it occurred (Picard & Robertson, 1996, p. 338).

The 1994 case *Lebel v. Roe* in Yukon provides a good example of false imprisonment in the nursing context. In that case, a patient agreed to be admitted to a psychiatric facility after being advised (incorrectly) by a mental health nurse that she would be apprehended by the RCMP if she refused to come voluntarily. The court awarded the patient $5000, holding that the nurse ought to have known her statement was incorrect, that her statement resulted in the patient believing that her freedom was restricted, and that her admission to the facility constituted false imprisonment (as discussed by Picard & Robertson, 1996, p. 339). Although nurses may suggest under certain circumstances that a patient remain in the hospital room or in bed, the patient must not be detained against his or her will. The patient has a right to leave, even though it may be detrimental to health.

If the patient insists on leaving, most institutions require that the patient sign a release stating that the agency will not be held responsible for any resulting harm. As with all situations, the nurse should try to inform the patient of potential risks and alternative courses of actions. The use of force to detain someone against his or her will can constitute battery, and even the threat of restraint made to detain the patient can be considered assault. The nurse must be cautious with the use of restraints (see Chapter 30).

Invasion of privacy is a developing area of Canadian law: "although the right to privacy is well-entrenched in American tort law, the Canadian and English courts have been reluctant to recognize a separate common law right to privacy . . . [however,] we seem to be drifting closer to the American model" (Linden & Feldthusen, 2006, p. 59). The American model outlines four distinct privacy torts: (1) intrusion on the plaintiff's seclusion or private affairs, (2) public disclosure of embarrassing private facts about the plaintiff, (3) publicity that places the plaintiff in a false light in the public eye, and (4) appropriation of the plaintiff's name or likeness for the defendant's advantage (Linden & Feldthusen, 2006, p. 59).

Canadian courts have generally recognized invasions of privacy that fall under the fourth category only; however, a very recent Ontario case, *Somwar v. McDonald's Restaurants of Canada* (2006), suggests that in light of technological advancements that allow for easy (proper and improper) collection, access, and dissemination of personal information, the courts may well be more willing to recognize invasion of privacy as a distinct tort. This case was not in the medical context, but it does demonstrate that the longstanding position of the courts in this area might be changing. The case involved an action for invasion of privacy as a result of an unauthorized credit check by the plaintiff's employer. The defendant employer sought to have the claim dismissed on the ground that Ontario law did not recognize such a cause of action. However, the judge found that "it is not settled law in Ontario that there is no tort of invasion of privacy" (*Somwar v. McDonald's Restaurants of Canada,* 2006) and refused to strike the claim.

In his decision, he commented as follows:

> *With advancements in technology, personal data of an individual can now be collected, accessed (properly and improperly), and disseminated more easily than ever before. There is a resulting increased concern in our society about the risk of unauthorized access to an individual's personal information. The traditional torts such as nuisance, trespass, and harassment may not provide adequate protection against infringement of an individual's privacy interests. Protection of those privacy interests by providing a common law remedy for their violation would be consistent with Charter values and an "incremental revision" and logical extension of the existing jurisprudence. Even if the plaintiff's claim for invasion of privacy were classified as "novel" (which, in any event, is not a proper basis for dismissing it) the foregoing analysis leads me to conclude that the time has come to recognize invasion of privacy as a tort in its own right. (Somwar v. McDonald's Restaurants of Canada, 2006)*

This case is discussed by Linden & Feldthusen (2006, p. 60).

A number of Canadian provinces have also implemented privacy legislation that make it a "tort, actionable without proof of damage, for a person, willfully and without a claim of right, to violate the privacy of another" (Privacy Act, RSBC, 1996, as cited by Linden & Feldthusen, 2006). Despite these legislative advances, in most cases, although the possibility of pursuing a civil claim for breach of privacy exists, it seems that "professional disciplinary proceedings remain by far the more realistic deterrent to this variety of nursing malpractice" (Sneiderman et al., 2003, p. 179).

One important exception exists to the courts' hesitation in awarding liability for invasions of privacy: breach of confidentiality will give rise to legal remedy against, for example, a nurse or other health-care provider who divulges confidential patient information (Sneiderman et al., 2003). In nursing, liability can result if the nurse breaches confidentiality by passing along confidential patient information to others who are not directly involved in care of that patient or by intruding into the patient's private domain. In this context, a delicate balance must be maintained between the need for a number of people to contribute to the diagnosis and treatment of a client and the client's right to confidentiality. In most situations, necessary discussion about a client's medical condition is considered appropriate, but unnecessary discussions and gossip are considered a breach of confidentiality. Necessary discussion involves only those engaged in the client's care. In some instances, however, a statutorily imposed duty exists to report what would normally constitute confidential information. Most provinces and territories have a variety of statutes that impose a duty to report some confidential patient information. Four major categories are (1) vital statistics, such as births and deaths, (2) infections and communicable diseases, such as diphtheria, syphilis, and typhoid fever, (3) child or elder abuse, and (4) violent incidents, such as gunshot wounds and knife wounds.

THE PROCESS OF ACTION (LAWSUIT) In Canada, a court action, or a *lawsuit,* is not usually the first step in attempting to resolve contractual, tort, or other legal disputes (Keatings & Smith, 2000). Resolving the problem often begins with informal discussions between the parties; complaint mechanisms, such as mediation or arbitration, may occur later. Engaging in discussion early may prevent the need to go to court. The following is a brief and general description of the litigation process:

1. Court actions are controlled by what are termed the *rules of civil procedures* (Keatings & Smith, 2000) or the rules of court, which regulate how court actions occur. A legal action is generally initiated by filing a *Writ of Summons* and a *Statement of Claim* by a lawyer on behalf of the plaintiff. This document claims that the plaintiff's legal rights have been infringed on by one or more people, referred to as *defendants.*
2. In turn, the defendant has the right to file a *Statement of Defence* in response to the plaintiff's claim, within a specified time. This statement is necessary for the defendant to participate in the action. The statement of defence is filed with the court and served on the plaintiff. Collectively, the Statements of Claim and Defence are known as *pleadings* (Keatings & Smith, 2000).
3. Both parties engage in pretrial activities, such as examinations for *discovery* (in which one party asks the other party questions under oath) and discovery of documents, in an effort to gain all the facts of the situation.
4. A civil action may be tried by judge alone, or by judge and jury, according to the wishes of either party to the action. However, depending on its nature or complexity, a case may be limited to being heard by judge alone (Keatings & Smith, 2000). During the trial, a plaintiff must offer evidence of the defendant's wrongdoing. This duty of proving an assertion is the *burden of proof.* The defendant has opportunities to make counterclaims or provide justification for his or her actions.
5. The judge renders a decision, or the jury renders a verdict. If the outcome is not acceptable to one of the parties, it may be possible to appeal the decision to a higher court.

Patient Safety: A Recent Report

Significant attention has recently been focused on issues related to patient safety in Canada's health-care system, because "the costs of unsafe health care—both personal and fiscal—to individuals, their families and their communities and to the state are massive" (Downie, Lahey, Ford, Gibson, Thomson, Ward, et al., 2006). In 2006, a report entitled *Patient Safety Law: From Silos to Systems,* funded by Health Canada, "explored the use of legal instruments by governments to improve patient safety" (Downie et al., 2006, p. 1). The report provides an overview of the various legal tools in Canada that, in patchwork fashion, address issues of patient safety. It also identifies strengths and weaknesses for each area, as well as for the system as a whole. Some of the elements reviewed include approaches to institutional, professional, and products regulation in Canada, as well as adverse event reporting frameworks and relevant aspects of the complaint and inquiry processes and available compensation systems. The authors' comments provide some helpful insights into some of the problems and suggest some possible solutions:

> *Having taken a system governance perspective, we identified a body of law that can be described as patient safety law, in that it functions to protect the patient by reducing unsafe acts within the health care system. The different areas of law that affect patient safety (e.g., tort law, professional regulation, institutional regulation) are not usually conceived of as an integrated system of law. However, conceiving of patient safety law as an integrated entity has value since it allows the discussion to move away from thinking in terms of narrow siloed categories of law to thinking of the larger systemic objectives the legal framework should enable regarding the governance of patient safety. (Downie et al., 2006, p. 2)*

How the various recommendations made in this report are implemented, and whether the additional research it calls for is executed, remains to be seen; however, the report clearly highlights that a more holistic, system-wide approach to patient safety is in line with international trends and would address some of the gaps identified in our current approach.

Adverse Event Reporting

One of the key areas addressed in the report on patient safety was **adverse event reporting**. Although "adverse events reporting systems are a structural facet of safety regulation in other sectors . . . they are a relatively recent innovation in the health care system" (Downie et al., 2006, p. 56). In some provinces (including Saskatchewan and Quebec), adverse event reporting frameworks have been established through legislative initiatives. The first example of this was Saskatchewan's Regional Health Services Act, passed in 2002, which gave rise to mandatory reporting of adverse events to the provincial health department. In 2004, with the addition of the Critical Incident Regulation under the act, the requirements and details of the reporting structure were made clearer and more complete. Under this framework, for example, health-care organizations and the regional health authorities to which they report "are required to give notice of critical incidents arising from their operations within three business days, or as soon as possible thereafter" to the Department of Health (Downie et al., 2006, p. 56). Notification must be followed up by a detailed written report. The *Saskatchewan Critical Incident Reporting Guideline* (Government of Saskatchewan, 2004) offers some additional insight into what is required under the framework. The guideline defines a **critical incident** as "a serious adverse health event including, but not limited to, the actual or potential loss of life, limb or function related to a health service provided by, or a program operated by, a regional health authority (RHA) or health care organization (HCO)" (p. 1). Some of the categories under which a reportable incident can arise include "surgical events, product or device events, patient protection events, care management events, environmental events and criminal events" (Downie et al., p. 56).

Although developments and initiatives, such as those in Saskatchewan, Quebec, and pending legislation in Manitoba, suggest that improvements are underway, the concern expressed in the report of the National Steering Committee on Patient Safety (2002) that Canada is behind several other countries in the development of such mechanisms has not yet been fully addressed. Some of the recommendations made in the committee's report specifically address the issue of how to improve the reporting of adverse events:

- The adoption of nonpunitive reporting policies within a quality improvement framework across the system that encourage and reward reporting, with limited exceptions.
- The review and revision of legislation across all Canadian jurisdictions in order to protect patient safety data and reports from disclosure in legal proceedings. Facts relating to the event should be recorded on the patient's health record and should not be privileged. De-identified information could be entered into a provincial or territorial or national database to facilitate the sharing of lessons learned across jurisdictions (Downie et al., 2006, p. 59).

The recommendations indicate a tension between litigation and quality assurance or improvement systems. The former does not encourage openness or transparency in the wake of an adverse event, as this has the potential to expose those health-care providers and institutions involved to liability; in contrast, to fully identify, understand, learn from, and thereby reduce future likelihood of adverse events, mechanisms are needed that will encourage reporting and open discussion of such events. Ultimately, such a system will help increase patient safety, as well as the accountability of both individuals and organizations within the health-care system.

Selected Legal Aspects of Nursing Practice

Confidentiality and Privacy

As discussed earlier, fundamental to the nurse–patient relationship is the professional obligation to respect patient confidentiality. Confidentiality brings with it both moral and legal obligations for nurses. Whenever possible, nurses uphold confidentiality, except when harm might result to the patient or others or when statute law or legislation requires disclosure (i.e., suspected child abuse, infectious disease, information for workers' compensation boards, or a court order). The CNA Code of Ethics (2008) states: "When nurses are required to disclose information for a particular purpose, they disclose only the amount of information necessary for that purpose and inform only those necessary. The attempt is to do so in ways that minimize any potential harm to the individual, family or community" (p. 15). Legally, the betrayal of a patient's confidence is covered under the area of professional misconduct and may result in discipline by the provincial or territorial conduct committee of the professional nursing association.

Confidential information is "intimate or private knowledge" protected under a duty of confidentiality. **Confidentiality** can be summarized as the duty of someone (a professional) who has received confidential information in trust to protect that information and disclose it to others only with permission, or when rules or laws authorize its disclosure. Confidential information can come directly from the patient, received through written documents, electronic data, or come from a third party. A common rule frequently noted in policy is that all knowledge is considered confidential unless otherwise stated by the patient.

Often, the notion of confidential information is discussed within the framework of the legal right to *privacy*. In simple terms, **privacy** is about people, while confidentiality is about duty to protect information. Privacy is about a person's right to control the intrusion of others into his or her life. In other words it concerns what information a health-care provider can have. A patient's right to privacy means that he or she has the right to disclose details of his or her life, illness, feelings, finances, and family interactions, or *not* to disclose them. Confidentiality is about what a nurse does with the information. When patients give their personal information to a nurse, they trust that the nurse will disclose it only to appropriate members of the health-care team. Maintaining patient confidentiality is an important element of trust and as such is a moral obligation of nurses.

Many key documents have been written in the development and evolution of public policy concerning informational privacy. In 1996 the Canadian Standards Association developed the *Model Code for the Protection of Personal Information.* This document stemmed from principles of fair information practices that significantly influenced policy development in Canada and elsewhere. Privacy legislation was then introduced at both the federal and the provincial or territorial levels to protect Canadians' personal information. The Personal Information and Protection of Electronic Documents Act (PIPEDA) was ratified in January 2001. It applies in all provinces and territories unless they have introduced substantially similar privacy legislation (Office of the Privacy Commissioner of Canada, 2004).

The primary legal consideration with respect to any information that the nurse obtains from a patient during the course of the professional relationship is that such information is confidential and cannot be disclosed to anyone who has no valid purpose for requesting it. The rule has some exceptions, both in the common law and as provided by statute. But in many provinces, if an unauthorized person accesses a patient's health record, or if health information is inappropriately released, a breach of patient's privacy rights can result in legal liability for the custodian of the records and the individuals involved in the incident. Because of that risk, it is important for all nurses, health-care professionals, and employees to be aware of current developments in and comply with the legislated requirements of Canadian privacy law.

Problematic Substance Use and Chemical Dependency

Problematic substance use and chemical dependency are serious problems, endangering the safety of the public and the health of nurses. Many factors in the workplace are linked to nurses' problematic substance use: shift work, stress, long working hours, and access to a large variety of pharmacological substances all contribute to the risk (Adlersberg & Mackinnon, 2004). Prevention, early recognition, and effective treatment programs are essential to promote the health of nurses and ensure public safety.

RNs have a professional responsibility to protect patients from harm. Education and prevention of problematic substance use must begin in schools of nursing and nurses' workplaces to heighten awareness and promote early detection. Denying that a problem exists is a common first sign of problematic substance use. Admitting there is a problem may be the hardest step. It is not uncommon for co-workers to explain or excuse unacceptable behaviour, rather than consider the possibility of problematic drug or alcohol use (CNA, 2002b). Nurses need to be aware of signs of a potential problem (see Box 6.3). Consultation with licensing bodies is available to help deal with suspected problems. Guidance for RNs is also provided by the CNA Code of Ethics and CNA Position Statement on Substance Misuse and Chemical Dependency by Nurses (2002b). Nurses must adhere to the reporting requirements of the licensing bodies.

Employers must have sound policies and procedures for identifying and intervening in situations involving a possibly impaired nurse. The primary concern is for the protection of clients, but it is also critically important that the nurse's problem be identified quickly so that appropriate treatment may be instituted. Box 6.3 lists behaviours that may be seen in the impaired nurse. The guidelines presented in the box can be used to report the nurse suspected of chemical impairment.

A variety of programs have been developed to help nurses recover from a problematic substance use. Nurses need the same caring attitude from peers as that shown to patients. The goal is to have nurses enter rehabilitative treatment. Employee and family assistance programs can provide support and direction for nurses who require assistance to deal with their substance involvement. Rehabilitation is a complex process. A work re-entry plan can assist nurses to return to their job and provide safe and competent care.

BOX 6.3 BEHAVIOURAL INDICATORS OF CHEMICAL MISUSE

Nurses need to be aware of the signs of problematic drug or alcohol use.

- Increased isolation from colleagues, friends, and family
- Frequent reports of illness, minor accidents, and emergencies
- Complaints about poor work performance
- Inability to meet schedules and deadlines
- Tendency to avoid new and challenging assignments
- Mood swings, irritability, and depression
- Request for night shifts
- Social avoidance of staff
- Illogical and sloppy charting
- Excessive errors
- Increasing carelessness about personal appearance
- Medication errors that require many changes in charting
- Arriving early or staying late for no reason
- Volunteering to administer client medications, especially pain medications

Source: Adapted from *Nurse's Legal Handbook,* 5th ed., by Springhouse Corporation, 2004, Springhouse, PA: Springhouse.

Legal Protections in Nursing Practice

Professional Liability Insurance

All nurses are advised to have professional liability insurance. Despite the high level of competence promoted and maintained, excellent communication with clients, and increasing awareness of the risks involved in giving care, a lawsuit can still be initiated by a client. "Nurses who are employees are covered by their employer's insurance through the operation of vicarious liability" (CNPS, 1995, p. 2). An employment relationship must have existed at the time of the incident and the defendant employee must have been sued for work done within the scope of his or her employment. The determination regarding whether an employer–employee relationship existed will be identified by the courts (CNPS, 2006). Nurses in independent practice do not have this protection; they are held directly accountable for their practice and thus require their own insurance.

In Canada, legal support and liability protection insurance can be obtained through the CNPS, a nonprofit society established in 1988. As a member in good standing in most provincial and territorial associations, nurses are able to obtain the services of the CNPS free of charge. Nurses in British Columbia and Quebec are not included in the CNPS and are covered by other insurance agents. CNPS Plus offers additional insurance to all registered nurses at an annual premium. This added insurance, originally designed for independent practitioners, nurse practitioners, and independent contractors, offers insurance for malpractice coverage, business protection, professional discipline costs, and directors' and officers' liability coverage (CNPS, 2008).

Nurses often provide nursing services outside of employment-related activities, such as being available for first aid at children's sport or social activities or providing health screening and education at health fairs. Neighbours or friends may seek advice about illnesses or treatment for themselves or family members. In the latter situation, the nurse may be tempted to give advice; however, it is always advisable for the nurse to refer the friend or neighbour to the family physician.

Nurses may also act as **good Samaritans** by providing emergency assistance at an accident scene. This type of professional activity is not covered by an employer's insurance policy because the care given was not the responsibility of the employer. The good Samaritan/emergency medical aid acts are designed to protect those acting reasonably, without gross negligence. While the *Code of Ethics for Registered Nurses* (CNA, 2008) no longer specifically mentions emergency care, it does note that "during a natural or human-made disaster, including a communicable disease outbreak, nurses have a duty to provide care, using appropriate safety measures" (p. 9).

To encourage citizens to be good Samaritans, most provinces and territories have now enacted legislation releasing a good Samaritan from legal liability for injuries caused in such circumstances, even if the injuries resulted from negligence of the person offering emergency aid. The Alberta Emergency Medical Act established in 1980 protects physicians and other registered health-discipline members, including RNs, unless gross negligence is involved. The act covers people who give help in an emergency, at a level that would be provided by a reasonably careful person under similar circumstances (Phillips, 2006). Manitoba, Ontario, New Brunswick, and Nunavut do not have good Samaritan legislation, although New Brunswick does protect physicians who voluntary give first aid or emergency treatment outside of a hospital or doctor's office from liability, under the Medical Act of 1981 (Phillips, 2006).

It is vital for the good Samaritan to consider that once he or she has begun to help the victim, he or she has entered into a nurse–client relationship with that person and is bound by a duty of care to that person. "You now have a duty, in law, to the injured person to continue to treat that person until you are relieved by another competent professional, the preference being one with medical training, or until the person is out of immediate danger" (Phillips, 2006, p. 2).

Carrying Out a Physician's Orders

Nurses are expected to analyze the procedures and medications ordered by physicians. It is the nurse's responsibility to seek clarification of ambiguous or seemingly erroneous orders from the prescribing physician or covering on-call physician.

Nurses are not absolved of responsibility for their actions simply because they are following a physician's order. The law states that nurses must understand the cause and effect of the treatment. If nurses carry out treatment they know is wrong, they are guilty of negligence.

If the order is neither ambiguous nor erroneous, the nurse is responsible for carrying it out. For example, if the physician orders oxygen to be administered at 4 L per minute, the nurse must administer oxygen at that rate, and not at 2 L or 6 L per minute. If the orders state that the client is not to have solid food after a bowel resection, the nurse must ensure that no solid food is given to the client.

To protect themselves legally, nurses must question several categories of orders:

1. *Question any order a client questions.* For example, if a client who has been receiving intramuscular injections tells the nurse that the doctor changed the order from an injectable to an oral medication, the nurse should recheck the order before giving the medication.
2. *Question any order if the patient's condition has changed.* The nurse is considered responsible for notifying the physician of any significant changes in the

patient's condition, whether the physician requests notification or not. For example, if a client who is receiving an intravenous infusion suddenly develops a rapid pulse, chest pain, and a cough, the nurse must notify the physician immediately and question continuance of the ordered rate of infusion. If a patient who is receiving morphine for pain develops severely depressed respirations, the nurse must withhold the medication and notify the physician.

3. *Question and record verbal orders to avoid miscommunications.* In addition to recording the time, the date, the physician's name, and the orders, the nurse documents the circumstances that occasioned the call to the physician, reads the orders back to the physician, and documents that the physician confirmed the orders as the nurse read them back.
4. *Question any order that is illegible, unclear, or incomplete.* Misinterpretations in the name of a drug or in dose, for example, can easily occur with handwritten orders. The nurse is responsible for ensuring that the order is interpreted the way it was intended and that it is a safe and appropriate order.

Providing Safe, Competent Nursing Care

Competent practice is a major legal safeguard for nurses. Nurses need to provide care that is within the legal boundaries of their practice and within the boundaries of agency policies and procedures. Nurses, therefore, must be familiar with their various job descriptions, which may be different across agencies. All nurses are responsible for ensuring that their various educational qualifications and experiences are adequate to meet the responsibilities delineated in their job description.

Competency also involves care that protects clients from harm. Nurses need to anticipate sources of client injury, educate clients about hazards, and implement measures to prevent injury. Nursing competency is one measure of accountability that allows the nurse to uphold the special knowledge, training, and skills associated with nursing. Because of this knowledge, patients rely on the nurse to provide the standard of care a reasonable, prudent nurse with similar training would in similar circumstances. If the nurse breaches this knowledge, he or she could injure the client and incur liability.

Application of the nursing process is another essential aspect of providing safe and effective client care. All assessments and care must be documented accurately. Effective communication can also protect the nurse from negligence claims. Nurses need to approach every client with sincere concern and include the client in conversations. In addition, nurses should always acknowledge when they do not know the answer to a client's questions, telling the client they will find out the answer and then following through.

Ways to take legal precautions are summarized in Box 6.4.

BOX 6.4 LEGAL PRECAUTIONS FOR NURSES

Nurses can do several things to protect themselves legally:

- Function within the scope of your education, job description, and jurisdiction's nurse practice act.
- Follow the procedures and policies of the employing agency.
- Build and maintain good rapport with clients. Keeping clients informed about diagnostic and treatment plans, giving feedback on their progress, and showing concern for the outcome of their care can prevent a sense of powerlessness and a buildup of hostility in the client.
- Always identify clients, particularly before initiating major interventions (e.g., surgical or other invasive procedures, or when administering medications or blood transfusions).
- Observe and monitor the client accurately. Record and communicate to the physician any significant changes in the client's condition.
- Promptly and accurately document all assessments and care given. Records must show that the nurse provided and supervised the client's care at regular intervals (the frequency of required reporting varies with the agency).
- Be alert when implementing nursing interventions and give each task your full attention and skill.
- Perform procedures appropriately. Negligent incidents during procedures generally relate to equipment failure, improper technique, and improper performance of the procedure. For instance, the nurse must know how to safeguard the client in the event that a respirator or other equipment fails.
- Make sure the correct medications are given in the correct dose, by the right route, at the scheduled time, and to the right client. See Chapter 31 for more detailed information about the administration of medications.
- When delegating nursing responsibilities, make sure that the person who is delegated a task understands what to do and that the person has the required knowledge and skill. As the delegating nurse, you can be held liable for harm caused by the person to whom the care was delegated.
- Protect clients from injury. Inform clients of hazards and use appropriate safety devices and measures to prevent falls, burns, or other injuries.
- Report all incidents involving clients. Prompt reports enable those responsible to attend to the client's well-being, to analyze why the incident occurred, and to prevent recurrences.
- Always check any order that a client questions and ensure that verbal orders are accurate and documented appropriately. Question and confirm standing orders if you are inexperienced in a particular area.
- Know your own strengths and weaknesses. Ask for assistance and supervision in situations for which you feel inadequately prepared.
- Maintain your clinical competence. For students, this demands study and practice before caring for clients. For graduate nurses, it means continued study, including maintaining and updating clinical knowledge and skills.

Quality Documentation

The client's medical record is a legal document and can be produced in court as evidence. Licensing bodies have documentation standards in place to which nurses are held accountable. Failure to meet these standards can result in disciplinary action against the nurse (CNPS, 2007). The courts look to the chart as a chronological record of all aspects of care from admission until discharge. Nursing documentation is often used as a means of reconstructing events surrounding the care given and dates and times, as a way of refreshing the memories of a witness, because often several months or years elapse before the lawsuit goes to trial. The effectiveness of a witness's testimony can depend on the accuracy of such records. Nurses, therefore, need to keep accurate and complete records of nursing care provided to clients.

Nurses have obligations to perform certain nursing acts, such as taking vital signs. In the eyes of the court, failure to document these acts may suggest that the act was not performed. Omissions can constitute negligence and be the basis for tort liability. Insufficient or inaccurate assessments and documentation can hinder proper diagnosis and treatment and result in injury to the client.

Electronic documentation carries a higher risk of breach of confidentiality. Policies and procedures, as well as specific technologies, are required to protect the confidentiality of the client's health record and system security. This is especially true of the transfer of information. See Chapter 23 for types of records and facts about recording.

Reporting Crimes, Torts, and Unsafe Practices

Nurses may need to report nursing colleagues or other health professionals for practices that endanger the health and safety of clients. For instance, problematic alcohol and drug use, theft from a client or agency, and unsafe nursing practice should be reported. Reporting a colleague is not easy. The person reporting may feel disloyal, incur the disapproval of others, or feel that chances for promotion are endangered. When reporting an incident or series of incidents, the nurse must be careful to describe observed behaviour only and not make inferences as to what might be happening. Box 6.5 outlines guidelines for reporting a crime, tort, or unsafe practice. Reporting these events is referred to as *whistle-blowing.*

"**Whistle-blowers** are people who expose negligence, abuses, [and] dangers, such as professional misconduct or incompetence in the organization in which they work" (Hardingham, 1999, p. 1). The decision to be a whistle-blower is never an easy one, unless there is a legal obligation (such as in the cases of child abuse or the abuse of vulnerable adults). Reporting it should be considered as the step to take when all else has failed. Nurses may be the first to come upon unsafe practice or to identify actual or potential hazards. It can be a difficult situation, where the nurse is caught between the values and standards of the profession and the values and norms of the employing organization. The CNA's Code of Ethics (CNA, 2008) can be used as a guideline. Four values in the Code are especially relevant to nurses deciding whether to blow the whistle:

- Promoting health and well-being
- Preserving dignity
- Maintaining privacy and confidentiality
- Being accountable

BOX 6.5 GUIDELINES FOR REPORTING A CRIME, TORT, OR UNSAFE PRACTICE

Nurses should follow these guidelines when reporting a crime, tort, or unsafe practice:

- Write a clear description of the situation you believe you should report.
- Make sure that your statements are accurate.
- Make sure you are credible. Obtain support from at least one trustworthy person before filing the report.
- Report the matter by starting at the lowest possible level in the agency hierarchy.
- Assume responsibility for reporting the individual by being open about it. Sign your name to the letter.
- See the problem through once you have reported it.

Legal Responsibilities of Students

Nursing students are responsible for their own actions and liable for their own acts of negligence committed during the course of clinical experiences. When they perform duties that are within the scope of professional nursing, such as administering an injection, they generally share the responsibility with the instructor, health-care facility, and educational institution. Communication among all individuals must be clear and unambiguous in relation to goals and objectives to be achieved in order to meet the students' needs during the clinical experience. "Student nurses are not held to a standard of perfection; rather, they are held to the standard of their peers" (Phillips, 2007, p. 2).

In cases arising from negligent acts by nursing students, the student was traditionally treated as an employee of the hospital, which was held liable under the doctrine of *respondent superior.* Today, nursing students are not usually considered employees of the agencies in which they receive clinical experience because nursing programs usually contract with agencies to provide clinical experiences for students.

Managing legal risks means considering first the competence of the student. Ensuring that the clinical experience is safe is shared by the student, the educational institution, the health-care agency, and the instructor or preceptor accompanying the student. Before the student enters clinical practice, the educator must be aware of the student's capabilities and whether the curriculum is current and relevant.

Students in clinical situations must be assigned activity within their capabilities and be given reasonable guidance and supervision. Nursing instructors are responsible for assigning students to the care of clients and for providing reasonable supervision. Failure to provide reasonable supervision or the assignment of a client to a student who is not prepared and competent can be a basis for liability.

To fulfill responsibilities to clients and to minimize chances for liability, nursing students need to do the following:

- Make sure they are prepared to carry out the necessary care for assigned clients.
- Ask for additional help or supervision in situations for which they feel inadequately prepared.
- Comply with the policies of the agency in which they obtain their clinical experience.
- Comply with the policies and definitions of responsibility supplied by the school of nursing.

Students who work as part-time or temporary nursing assistants or aides must also remember that legally they can perform only those tasks that appear in the job description of a nurse's aide or assistant. Even though a student may have received instruction and acquired competence in administering injections or suctioning a tracheostomy tube, the student cannot legally perform these tasks while employed as an aide or assistant. While acting as a paid worker, the student is covered for negligent acts by the employer, not by the school of nursing.

Case Study 6

Mrs. Jiminez in the Royal Victoria Hospital in Montreal is not progressing well following extensive surgery for gastrointestinal cancer. She has experienced severe weight loss and has little desire to eat. Dr. Jones, the physician, has elected to place a subclavian catheter in order to administer total parenteral nutrition. Dr. Jones telephones the nursing unit and requests that the nurse obtain the patient's informed consent for this invasive procedure. The nurse completes the procedural consent form according to the physician's orders and goes to Mrs. Jiminez's room.

The nurse informs Mrs. Jiminez that the physician plans to place a catheter into her subclavian vein so that additional nutrients can be administered to her. The nurse further explains that these nutrients will help Mrs. Jiminez heal and regain her strength. In making decisions, Mrs. Jiminez often relies on her eldest son because "he knows best." Mrs. Jiminez asks, "Will it hurt? I'm so tired of all this pain, I'm not sure I want anything else done." The nurse replies, "Oh, don't worry, we'll make sure you don't feel a thing. Your doctor will be here shortly and he is expecting this permit to be signed, so will you please sign it now?"

Critical Thinking Questions

1. When the nurse takes the consent form into Mrs. Jiminez's room for her to sign, is the patient actually signing a valid consent?
2. What is the difference between informed consent and signing a consent form?
3. Evaluate the nurse's approach to Mrs. Jiminez regarding this invasive procedure.
4. Who is responsible for obtaining the consent?

After working through these questions, go to the MyNursingLab at **http://www.mynursinglab.com** to check your answers.

KEY TERMS

laws
common law
civil law
tort law
regulatory bodies
credentialing
licensure
registration
certification
delegating care
standards of care
contractual obligations
contract
contractual relationships
vicarious liability
disclosure
capacity
voluntariness
informed consent
express consent
implied consent
battery
negligence
informed
competent
substitute decision makers
tort
intentional torts
assault
false imprisonment
invasion of privacy
adverse event reporting
critical incident

confidential information
confidentiality
privacy
good Samaritan
whistle-blowers

CHAPTER HIGHLIGHTS

- Accountability is an essential concept of professional nursing practice.
- Nurses need to understand laws that regulate and affect nursing practice to ensure that their actions are consistent with current legal principles and to protect themselves from liability.
- In Canada the regulation of nursing is a function of the provinces and territories.
- Nursing has been granted an exclusivity of practice (a right of self-government or self-regulation).
- Professional regulation in nursing practice is determined and maintained by credentialing, licensure and registration, and certification, which protect the public's welfare and safety.
- Standards of practice published by provincial and territorial nursing associations and agency policies, procedures, and job descriptions further delineate the scope of a nurse's practice.
- The nurse has specific legal obligations and responsibilities to clients, employers, and the profession. As a citizen, the nurse has the rights and responsibilities shared by all individuals in the society.
- Nursing regulatory bodies are also responsible for accountability and discipline in nursing.
- Legal roles in nursing vary according to nurses' roles as provider of service and employee or contractor for service.
- Nurses can be held liable for unintentional torts, such as negligence, and for intentional torts, such as invasion of privacy, assault, and battery.
- Negligence of nurses can be established when (1) the nurse (defendant) owed a duty to the client, (2) the nurse failed to carry out that duty according to standards, (3) the client (plaintiff) was injured, and (4) the client's injury was caused by the nurse's failure to follow the standard.
- The nurse is responsible for ensuring that the informed consent of a client is complete before nursing treatment regimens and procedures begin.
- Informed consent implies that (1) the consent was given voluntarily, (2) the client had the capacity and competency to understand, and (3) the client was given enough information with which to make an informed decision.
- Good Samaritan and emergency medical aid acts protect health professionals from claims of malpractice when they offer assistance at the scene of an emergency, provided that no willful wrongdoing or gross departure from normal standards of care take place.
- Nurses can obtain professional liability insurance through the Canadian Nurses Protective Society.
- Selected legal aspects of nursing practice include issues of confidentiality and privacy, informed consent, the carrying out of physicians' orders, quality documentation, and problematic substance use.
- Problematic substance use and chemical dependency in health-care workers can occur because of the high levels of stress involved in many health-care settings and the easy access to addictive drugs. Chemical impairment includes the problematic use of alcohol and addictive drugs. The nurse needs to know the proper methods for reporting nursing colleagues whose practice is chemically impaired.
- Nursing students need to make certain that they are prepared to provide the necessary care to assigned clients and to ask for help or supervision in situations for which they feel inadequately prepared.

ASSESS YOUR LEARNING

1. Which of the following is most accurate regarding an unintentional tort?
   a. Unintentional torts are commonly regarded as acts of battery.
   b. Unintentional torts are the least common of the torts committed by nurses.
   c. Unintentional torts are commonly regarded as acts of negligence.
   d. Unintentional torts are wrongful acts but could not lead a client to use these in a lawsuit.
2. How is common law established?
   a. By legislators, but enforced by an administrative agency
   b. By judicial decisions to resolve legal disputes
   c. By federal legislators in response to provincial or territorial needs for social regulation
   d. By provincial or territorial nursing bodies and medical boards who develop practice standards
3. Which of the following is true for licensure in Canadian nursing?
   a. It is a legal method to control the quality of the nursing profession by establishing a minimum standard.
   b. It is established and governed by the federal government.

c. It applies only to those nurses returning to the profession who have completed a refresher course.
d. It is not a qualification for membership in each provincial or territorial nursing association.

4. Which of the following is most accurate regarding nursing liability?
a. Nursing liability refers to not accepting responsibility for your own actions.
b. Nursing liability refers to a nurse's legal responsibility for harm caused to a patient by an inappropriate nursing action or by a failure to perform a required nursing action.
c. Nurses can deny responsibility for a harmful act or inaction on the grounds that someone else was also involved.
d. Nurses can be held legally liable even though they were not a part of the care.

5. Mrs. Jack, who is alert and oriented, refuses to take an antipsychotic medication that you, the nurse, bring to her. She states, "I don't like the way it makes me feel." What would be the most legally prudent action that you could take?
a. Tell Mrs. Jack that the medication is prescribed for her and she should take it.
b. Crush her medication and administer it in her food.
c. Ask her son to convince her to take the medication.
d. Withhold the medication, talk to Mrs. Jack about the importance of taking the medication, document the incident, and notify the physician.

6. Which of the following is an accurate reflection of provincial or territorial documentation standards?
a. Failure to meet these standards would not destroy the nurse's defence in a lawsuit as he or she would be protected by the professional association.
b. The courts look only at the medical charting done by the physician, not the nurse's charting.
c. Failure to meet these standards could result in disciplinary action against individual nurses.
d. Documentation is used strictly as a means of communication between health-care professionals and is not used by the courts in a lawsuit.

7. Which characteristic related to the frequency and detail of charting are irrelevant?
a. The complexity of the client's health
b. Facility or agency policies and procedures
c. The degree to which the client's condition puts him or her at risk
d. The time of the shift and availability of staff to chart

8. *Capacity* in informed consent is most accurately defined as which of the following?
a. A one-time event that is decided by the courts
b. Only the ability to understand the procedure that the physician will be doing
c. An understanding of the nature of the decision to be made and the consequences of the decision, including the decision to decline the treatment
d. After each decision, the nurse must reassess the client's capacity

9. You are the nurse working with a student who informs you that she does not fully understand when a nurse might be liable in her day-to-day practice. Which of the following would suggest a situation of potential liability for a nurse?
a. A child admitted to your unit is too weak to be weighed. The nurse obtains a verbal estimate from the mother, documents the situation and the child's estimated weight, and ensures that the procedure is done when safe to do so.
b. Your patient Mr. Jones, who is very obese, has come to your unit postoperatively after abdominal surgery. As you care for him the next day, he continues to refuse to move out of bed and walk. You document the situation, inform the charge nurse, and continue to encourage Mr. Jones by exploring other related range of motion exercises and teaching related to the importance of walking after surgery.
c. While admitting Mrs. White, 78 years old, to your unit, the daughter informs you that her mother sometimes coughs and even chokes when she is eating. At dinner you inform the care aide that Mrs. White can feed herself and can be left alone as long as she sits up to eat.
d. You question the physician about an order for an antihypertensive medication dose that seems rather high to you. After checking with the pharmacist, who feels the dose is high but safe, you give the medication, document the patient's response to the medication (low blood pressure), and ensure that the risk for falls is noted on the patient's care plan.

10. A personal care attendant introduces herself to Rita, 18 years old, by saying that she is the nurse who will give her a bath today. The nurse provides feedback to the attendant based on which of the following principles?
a. Clients should be able to address by name those caring for them.
b. Young people do not understand the various levels of nursing staff.
c. All health-care workers giving basic care to clients may introduce themselves as a member of the care team.
d. Clients should know the title and responsibilities of those providing their care.

After working thourgh these questions, go to the MyNursingLab at ***http://www.mynursinglab.com*** *to check your answers and see explanations.*

SUGGESTED READINGS

Keatings, M., & Smith, O. (2000). *Ethical and legal issues in Canadian nursing* (2nd ed.). Toronto: W.B. Saunders.

This is a classic textbook that covers ethical and legal issues in Canada specifically for nurses. The book uses Canadian cases and identifies the relationship between ethical and legal issues that are common in nursing practice.

Kerr, L., & Ross-Kerr, J. (2003). The practicing nurse and the law. In J. Ross-Kerr & M. Wood (Eds.), *Canadian nursing: Issues and perspectives* (4th ed.) (pp. 195–208). Toronto: Mosby.

This chapter provides an overview of the law and the principal areas of nurses' involvement in the legal system. It emphasizes areas of concern related to legal issues in Canada.

McIntyre, M., Thomlinson, B., & McDonald, C. (2006). *Realities of Canadian nursing: Professional practice and power issues* (2nd ed.). Philadelphia, PA: Lippincott.

Throughout the book, the authors reveal a critical analysis of the tensions and contradictions that exist between nurses' legislated mandate to self-regulate and the changing nature of the realities of nurses' work.

WEBLINKS

Canadian Nurses Protective Society

http://www.cnps.ca

The Canadian Nurses Protective Society website offers information about several legal issues and liability protection for nurses who are members in a provincial or territorial nursing association in Canada.

Canadian Nurses Association: Certification

http://www.cna-nurses.ca/CNA/nursing/certification/default_e.aspx

This portion of the Canadian Nurses Association website offers a historical perspective of certification in Canada.

CASN Accreditation Program

http://www.casn.ca/content.php?sec=5

This website offers information about the accreditation standards and policies of the Canadian Association of Schools of Nursing.

University of Toronto Joint Centre for Bioethics

http://www.utoronto.ca/jcb/outreach/living_wills.htm

This website allows you to download a blank living will (which includes legal information specific to each province and territory, as well as further information on personal care decisions).

REFERENCES

Adlersberg, M. & MacKinnon, J. (2004). Registered nurses and substance misuse or abuse: RNABC's role. *Nursing BC, 36*(2), 13–15.

Bernzweig, F. (1996). *The nurse's liability for malpractice: A programmed course* (6th ed.). St. Louis, MO: Mosby.

Black's law dictionary (8th ed.). (2004). St. Paul, MN: Thomson West Publishing.

Borg, E. (2008). Hydromorphone: Handle with care. *Canadian Nurse, 104*(1), 35.

Canadian Nurses Association. (2002a). *Position statement on advanced nursing practice.* Ottawa: Author.

Canadian Nurses Association. (2002b). *Substance misuse and chemical dependency by nurses.* Ottawa: Author.

Canadian Nurses Association. (2002c). *Advanced nursing practice: A national framework.* Ottawa: Author.

Canadian Nurses Association. (2006). *Dialogue on advanced nursing practice.* Retrieved December 5, 2007, from http://www.cna-nurses.ca/CNA/practice/advanced/dialogue/default_e.aspx

Canadian Nurses Association. (2007). Understanding self regulation. *Nursing Now: Issues and Trends in Canadian Nursing, 21,* 1–5.

Canadian Nurses Association. (2008). *Code of ethics for registered nurses.* Centennial Edition. Ottawa: Author.

Canadian Nurses Protective Society. (1994). Consent to treatment: The role of the nurse. *InfoLaw, 3*(2). Ottawa: Author.

Canadian Nurses Protective Society. (1995). *Independent practice: Legal considerations. 4*(1). Ottawa: Author.

Canadian Nurses Protective Society. (1998). Vicarious liability. *InfoLaw,* 7(1). Ottawa: Author.

Canadian Nurses Protective Society. (2004). *Consent for the incapable adult.* Ottawa: Author.

Canadian Nurses Protective Society. (2006). *Collaborative practice: Are nurses employees or self-employed?* Ottawa: Author.

Canadian Nurses Protective Society. (2007). *Quality documentation: Your best defence.* Ottawa: Author.

Canadian Nurses Protective Society. (2008). *CNPS Plus: An optional extended protection plan for Canadian nurses.* Retrieved March 14, 2008, from http://www.cnps.ca/cnps_plus/index_e.html

Canadian Standards Association. (1996). *Model code for the protection of personal information.* Rexdale, ON: Author. CAN/CSA-Q830-96.

Downey v. Rothwell (1974). 5W.W.R. 311, 49 D.L.R. (3d) 82 (Alta, S.C.)

Downie, J., & Caulfield, T. (1999). *Canadian health law and policy.* Toronto: Butterworths.

Downie, J., Lahey, W., Ford, D., Gibson, E., Thomson, M., Ward, T., et al. (2006). *Patient safety law: From silos to systems (final report), country report: Canada.* Ottawa: Health Canada (Project number: HPRP 6795-15-5760009).

Etchells, E., Sharpe, G., Elliott, C., & Singer, P. (1999). Capacity. In P. Singer (Ed.), *Bioethics at the bedside: A clinician's guide* (pp. 17–24). Ottawa: Canadian Medical Association.

Etchells, E., Sharpe, G., Walsh, P., Williams, J., & Singer, P. (1999). Consent. In P. Singer (Ed.), *Bioethics at the bedside: A clinician's guide* (pp. 1–7). Ottawa: Canadian Medical Association.

Government of Saskatchewan. (2004). *Saskatchewan critical incident reporting guideline.* Regina, SK: Author.

Hardingham, L. (1999). I see and am silent/I see and speak out: The ethical dilemma of whistle-blowing. In *Ethics in Practice* (pp. 1–4). Ottawa: Canadian Nurses Association.

Hogg, P. W. (1997). *Constitutional law of Canada* (4th ed.). Scarborough, ON: Carswell.

Institute for Safe Medication Practices Canada. (2004). *Event analysis report: hydromorphone/morphine event Red Deer Regional Hospital.* Red Deer, AB: Author.

Joseph Brant Memorial Hospital v. Koziol, [1978] 1 SCR 491.

Keatings, M., & Smith, O. (2000). The Canadian legal system. In M. Keatings & O. Smith (Eds.), *Ethical and legal issues in Canadian nursing* (pp. 51–94). Toronto: W.B. Saunders.

Lebel v. Roe, [1994] Y.J. No. 62.

Linden, A. M., & Feldthusen, B. (2006). *Canadian tort law* (8th ed.). Toronto: LexisNexis Canada.

Malette v. Shulman (1990), 67 D.L.R. (4th) 321 (Ont. C.A.).

Morris, J., Ferguson, M., & Dykeman, M. (1999). *Canadian nurses and the law.* Toronto: Butterworths.

National Steering Committee on Patient Safety. (2002). *Building a safer system: A national integrated strategy for improving patient safety in Canadian health care.* Ottawa: Author.

Office of the Privacy Commissioner of Canada. (2004). *Fact sheet: Questions and answers regarding the application of PIPEDA, Alberta and British Columbia's Personal Information Protection Act (PIPAs).* Retrieved July 5, 2006, from http://www.privcom.gc.ca/

Parisi, L. (1999). Legal framework for health-care services. In J. Hibbard & D. Smith (Eds.), *Nursing management in Canada* (2nd ed.) (pp. 43–64). Toronto: W.B. Saunders.

Phillips, E. (2006). *Is there a risk in being a good Samaritan?* Retrieved March 3, 2007, from http://www.cnps.ca/members/publications/articles/good_sam/good_sam_e.html

Phillips, E. (2007). *Managing legal risks in preceptorships.* Retrieved March 3, 2007, from http://www.cnps.ca/members/publications/articles/preceptor/preceptor_e.html

Picard, E., & Robertson, G. (1996). *Legal liability of doctors and hospitals in Canada* (3rd ed.). Toronto: Carswell.

Sharpe, G. (1993). Consent and minors. *Health Law Canada, 13,* 197–207.

Sneiderman, B., Irvine, J. C., & Osborne, P. (2003). *Canadian medical law: An introduction for physicians, nurses and other health care professionals* (3rd ed.). Scarborough, ON: Thomson Canada.

Somwar v. McDonald's Restaurants of Canada Ltd., [2006] O.J. No. 64 (Ont. S.C.J.).

UNIT 2

Contemporary Health Care in Canada

CHAPTER 7
Health, Wellness, and Illness

CHAPTER 8
Health Promotion

CHAPTER 9
The Canadian Health-Care System

CHAPTER 10
Culture Care

CHAPTER 11
Individual Care

CHAPTER 12
Nursing Care of Families

CHAPTER 13
Community-Based Nursing

CHAPTER 14
Rural and Remote Health Care

CHAPTER 15
Complementary and Alternative Health Modalities

Chapter 7

Health, Wellness, and Illness

For many years, the focus for health was on treatments and cures for diseases. Today, the emphasis is on promoting health and wellness in individuals, families, and communities. People's health beliefs influence their health practices. Similarly, nurses' understanding of health and wellness will determine the scope and nature of their nursing practice. Throughout this chapter, the word *clients* will refer to patients in the hospital setting and clients in the community setting.

OBJECTIVES

After studying this chapter, you should be able to

1. Differentiate among health, wellness, and well-being
2. Explain the health and wellness models
3. Discuss primary prevention, secondary prevention, and tertiary prevention
4. Differentiate illness from disease and acute illness from chronic illness
5. Describe the effects of illness on the roles and functions of individuals and families
6. Discuss factors that determine health

Concepts of Health, Wellness, and Well-Being

Health, wellness, and well-being have many definitions and interpretations. A nurse must be familiar with their conceptual commonalities and consider how each term is individualized with specific clients.

Health

Health is a state of being well and using every power possessed to the fullest extent (Nightingale, 1969). The World Health Organization ([WHO], 1948) defines health as "a state of complete physical, mental, and social well-being, and not merely the absence of disease or infirmity." This definition reflects concern for the individual as a total person functioning physically, psychologically, and socially within his or her environment. People's lives and health are affected by all interaction, including interaction with the environment and such elements of it as climate, food, shelter, clean air, and water; and interaction with family, employers and co-workers, friends, and associates (see the Reflect on Primary Health Care box).

Health has also been defined in terms of roles and performance. Talcott Parsons (1951) conceptualized health as the ability to maintain normal roles. Marc Lalonde (1974), in his report *A New Perspective on the Health of Canadians,* presented the *health field concept,* which included human biology, environment, lifestyle, and health-care organizations. This landmark document shifted the focus of care from treatment to the importance of lifestyle and environmental factors on health (see Figure 8.1 on page 132, Lalonde's health field concept).

REFLECT ON PRIMARY HEALTH CARE

Many Canadians and people in other developed countries view having clean air and water, taking time off to manage stress, being physically active to prevent disease, and so on, as ways to achieve good health, wellness, and quality of life. Those who live in poverty and those who live in developing countries see that being healthy comes from having adequate food and proper nutrition, safe water and basic sanitation, education, basic health care for mothers and children, immunization, and from controlling and treating illnesses, including injuries and communicable diseases. The WHO (1978) articulated these as essential *elements of primary health care* for program planning and policy development. Consider how these elements are related to the determinants of health outlined in Table 7.2 on page 126.

Source: Based on *The Declaration of Alma-Ata,* by the World Health Organization, 1978, Geneva, Switzerland: Author.

BOX 7.1 DEVELOPING A PERSONAL DEFINITION OF HEALTH

The following questions can help nurses develop a personal definition of health:

- Is health more than the absence of disease symptoms?
- Are health and wellness the same?
- Are disease and illness different?
- Is health static or changing?
- Are wellness, health, and illness separate entities or points along a continuum?
- Is health the ability of an individual to adapt to the environment?
- Is health a condition of a person's actualization?
- Is health the effective functioning of self-care activities?
- Is health socially determined?
- How do you rate your health and why?

PERSONAL DEFINITION OF HEALTH Health is a highly individualized perception. People may say they feel healthy even though they have physical challenges that some would consider illnesses. A person can view health as having fewer symptoms of disease and pain, being active, or remaining in good spirits. It is a way of life through which the body, mind, and emotions interrelate harmoniously.

Many factors affect individual definitions of health, including an individual's previous experiences, expectations of self, age, and sociocultural influences. Nurses should be aware of their own personal definitions of health and appreciate that other people will have their unique definitions. People's definitions of health influence their behaviour related to health and illness. By understanding clients' perceptions of health and illness, nurses can provide more meaningful assistance to help them regain or attain a state of health. See Box 7.1 on developing a personal definition of health.

Wellness and Well-Being

Wellness is a state of well-being, which is also a component of health. The basic concept of wellness includes developing self-awareness or self-responsibility to reach an ultimate goal of optimal health and happiness. Wellness is a dynamic and growing process that involves daily decision making in the areas of nutrition, stress management, physical fitness, preventive health care, and emotional health (see the Nursing and Canadian Society box).

Well-being is a "subjective perception of vitality and feeling well. . . . [It] can be described objectively, experienced, and measured . . . and can be plotted on a continuum" (Hood & Leddy, 2003, p. 264). Anspaugh, Hamrick, and Rosato (2006) described seven overlapping components of wellness, as shown in Figure 7.1:

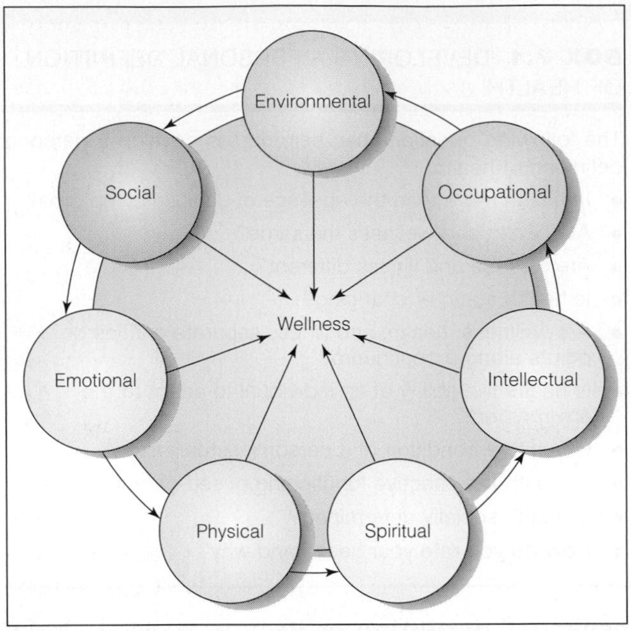

FIGURE 7.1 The seven components of wellness
(From **Wellness: Concepts and Applications,** *6th ed. (p. 4), by D. J. Anspaugh, M. H. Hamrick, and F. D. Rosato, 2006, New York: McGraw-Hill. Reprinted by permission.)*

1. *Social.* The ability to interact successfully with people and within the environment of which each person is a part, to develop and maintain intimacy with significant others, and to develop respect and tolerance for those with different opinions and beliefs.
2. *Emotional.* The ability to manage stress and to express emotions appropriately. Emotional wellness involves the ability to recognize, accept, and express feelings and to accept limitations.
3. *Intellectual.* The ability to learn and use information effectively for personal, family, and career development. Intellectual wellness involves striving for continued growth and learning to deal with new challenges effectively.
4. *Spiritual.* The belief in some force (nature, science, religion, or a higher power) that provides meaning and purpose to life. It includes a person's own morals, values, and ethics.
5. *Occupational.* The ability to achieve a balance between work and leisure. A person's beliefs about education, employment, and home influence personal satisfaction and relationships with others.
6. *Environmental.* The ability to promote health measures that improve the standard of living and quality of life in the community in such areas as food, water, and air quality.
7. *Physical.* The ability to carry out daily tasks, achieve fitness (e.g., pulmonary, cardiovascular, gastrointestinal), maintain adequate nutrition and proper body fat, avoid problematic drug and alcohol use, avoid using tobacco products, and generally practise positive lifestyle habits.

NURSING AND CANADIAN SOCIETY

Facts	Implications for Nursing Practice
The popularity of tattoos and body piercings is on the rise. It is possible to transmit herpes, hepatitis B, hepatitis C, human immunodeficiency virus (HIV), acquired immune deficiency syndrome (AIDS), staphylococcus, and streptococcus via breaks in the skin and equipment that is not cleaned and sterilized appropriately (Health Canada, 2006a).	Nurses play a preventive role by educating individuals before and after the tattoo or piercing about, for instance, the need to examine the facility, equipment, and person performing the tattoo or piercing for cleanliness; the importance of the use of gloves and infection control; and how to care for their tattoo or piercing and reduce their risk for infection.
Statistics Canada reports that two out of every three adults in Canada are overweight or obese. The number of obese children has tripled in the past 25 years. Obesity increases a person's risk for developing hypertension, type 2 diabetes, coronary heart disease, breast or colon cancer, sleep apnea, low self-esteem, and depression (Health Canada, 2006b).	Nurses should assess their clients' perceptions of their susceptibility to obesity and determine ways to incorporate physical activity into everyday life. For example, nurses can stress the importance of clients' reading labels on food products to determine which products are healthier; teach them appropriate food portions; and help them avoid fad diets that promise extreme weight loss.
The use of headphones to listen to portable music players at volume levels greater than 70 dBA (A-weighted decibel) can cause permanent hearing loss, depending on the duration of listening time. Early signs of hearing loss include a buzzing or ringing in the ears and thinking that those around you are always mumbling when they speak (Health Canada, 2006c).	Nurses should be aware of the popular use of portable music players among members of the younger population, inform them of their risk for potential hearing loss, and suggest ways to reduce this risk, such as by lowering the volume of music, reducing exposure time to loud music or noise, being aware of the early signs of hearing loss, and getting appropriate follow-up testing.
Poor oral health can lead to cavities and gum disease, affecting a person's ability to chew and digest food properly and reducing self-esteem. Gum disease left untreated can lead to infections that can cause heart disease and, in pregnant women, pre-term delivery (Health Canada, 2006d).	Nurses should educate clients regarding the benefits of preventive action, such as appropriate oral hygiene and proper dental care. Proper care includes attending dental appointments, eating a healthy diet, and helping younger children with their dental health.

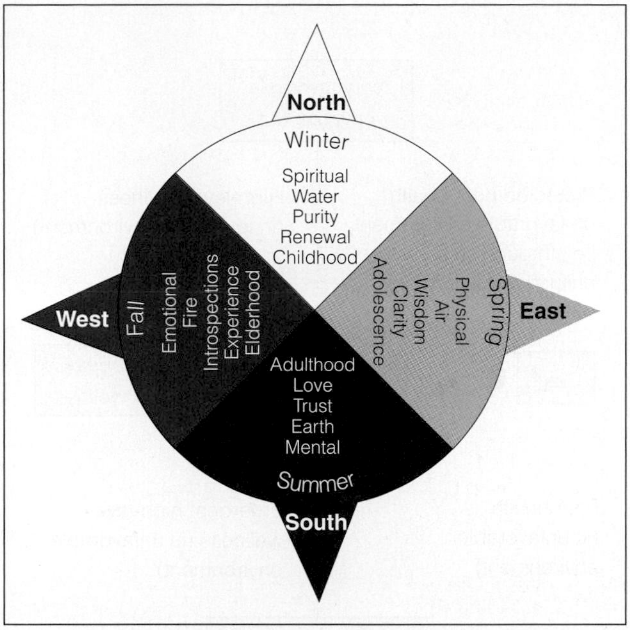

FIGURE 7.2 Aboriginal medicine wheel

ABORIGINAL VIEWS OF WELLNESS Hales and Lauzon (2007) described the holistic world view of health and wellness of Aboriginal people by using the medicine wheel. The **medicine wheel** has many variations, but they all emphasize "the way of good life" or "everyday good living" in the context of human behaviour and interaction. The term *medicine* refers to spiritual energy and healing or enlightened experience. Aboriginal people see the "interconnectedness between the physical and spiritual world, between the mind, body, and spirit" (p. 4) and create healing by guiding decisions and actions toward balance and harmony. The medicine wheel has four colours representing north, south, east, and west (see Figure 7.2). "The teachings are about walking the earth in a peaceful and good way; they assist in helping to seek healthy minds (East), strong inner spirits (South), inner peace (West), strong, healthy bodies (North). A Medicine Wheel [is viewed] as a mirror within which everything about the human condition is reflected back. It requires courage to look into the mirror and really see what is being reflected back about an individual's life" (p. 4).

Models of Health and Wellness

Smith's Models of Health

Smith (1981) organized the different approaches around four models that describe broad theories of health: the eudaimonistic, adaptive, role-performance, and clinical models. Each model has its own outcomes and provides a unique dimension of health. Nurses can move between and among the models as the clients' needs change. As such, circumstances determine which model will work best. For example, the clinical model emphasizes physiological needs, whereas role-performance structures nursing interventions around social relations. Both largely work to restore equilibrium for patients. Conversely, the other two models, adaptive and eudaimonistic, focus on the growth that occurs during changes in people's lives.

EUDAIMONISTIC MODEL Smith (1981) viewed health as "the condition of actualization or realization of . . . [intrinsic] potential. Illness is a condition that impedes or prevents self-actualization" (p. 45). Exemplified by Maslow's work (1954, 1962a, 1962b, 1970), this approach measures health as the "fulfillment" and "complete development" of individuals. This model takes a holistic view in which the task of the health professional is "to attempt to assist the individual toward self-fulfillment" (Smith, p. 45).

ADAPTIVE MODEL The adaptive model views health as "the condition of the organism in which it can engage in effective interaction with its physical and social environments. . . . Disease is a breakdown in the ability of the organism to cope with certain changes in its environment" (Smith, p. 45). Health, therefore, is a creative process, and disease is a failure in adaptation. The aim of treatment is to restore the person's ability to adapt or cope. Extreme good health is the result of flexible adaptation to and interaction with the environment to maximum advantage. The model focuses on restoration of the body by adapting to dangers in the environment and on adaptation, that is, survival, growth, or mastery.

ROLE-PERFORMANCE MODEL In the role-performance model, health is defined as an individual's ability to fulfill societal roles, that is, to perform his or her work. People usually fulfill several roles (e.g., mother, daughter, and friend). In this model, people who fulfill their roles are healthy even if they have clinical illness. For example, a man who works all day at his job may be considered healthy, even though an X-ray of his lung indicates a tumour. Sickness is the inability to perform a work role. This model assumes that individuals in optimal health function at optimal capacity. When multirole performance is expected, however, the model fails to address role conflict and the relative importance of different roles.

CLINICAL MODEL In the clinical model, people are viewed as physiologic systems with related functions; health is identified by the absence of signs and symptoms of disease or injury. In this model, the opposite of health is disease or injury. When the signs and symptoms are no longer present, health-care providers consider the individual's health restored. This model has the narrowest interpretation of health and has minimal interest in improving the body's ultimate performance.

Agent-Host-Environment Model

The agent-host-environment model (see Figure 7.3) is used to identify risk factors that result from the interaction of agent, host, and environment. Health is an ever-changing state, and the goal is to promote and maintain health. When the variables are in balance, health is maintained; when variables are not in balance, disease occurs. The model has three dynamic, interactive elements:

1. *Agent.* Any environmental factor or stressor (biological, chemical, mechanical, physical, or psychosocial) that by its presence or absence (e.g., lack of essential nutrients) can lead to illness or disease.
2. *Host.* A person or people who may or may not be at risk of acquiring a disease. Family history, age, and lifestyle habits influence the host's reaction to an agent.
3. *Environment.* Includes all factors external to the host that may or may not predispose the person to the development of the disease. The physical environment includes climate, living conditions, sound (noise) levels, and economic level. The social environment can include interactions with others and life events, such as the death of a spouse.

Dunn's High-Level Wellness Grid

Dunn (1959) described a health grid in which a health axis and an environmental axis intersect. The grid shows the interaction of the environment with the illness-wellness continuum (see Figure 7.4). The health axis extends from peak wellness to death, and the environmental axis extends from very favourable to very unfavourable. The intersection of the two axes forms the four quadrants of health and wellness:

1. *High-level wellness in a favourable environment.* An example in this quadrant is a person who implements healthy lifestyle behaviours and has the biopsychosocial, spiritual, and economic resources to support this lifestyle.

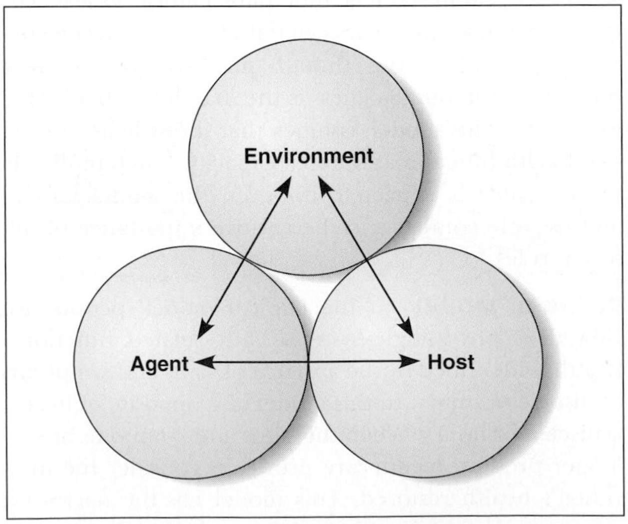

FIGURE 7.3 The agent-host-environment triangle

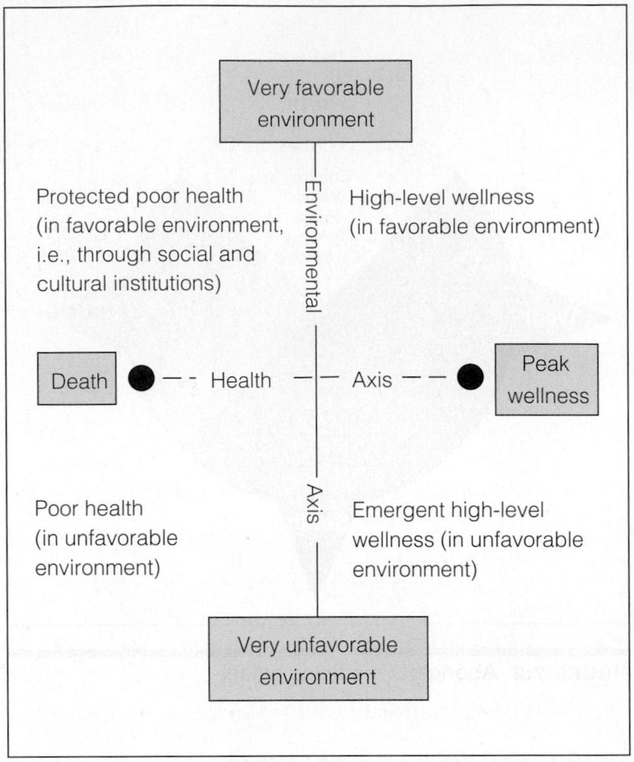

FIGURE 7.4 Dunn's health grid: Its axes and quadrants
(From "High-Level Wellness for Man and Society," by H. L. Dunn, 1959, American Journal of Public Health, 49, p. 788. Reprinted with permission.)

2. *Emergent high-level wellness in an unfavourable environment.* In this quadrant, an example is a woman who has the knowledge to implement healthy lifestyle practices but does not implement adequate self-care practices because of family responsibilities, job demands, or other factors.
3. *Protected poor health in a favourable environment.* An example in this quadrant is an ill person (e.g., one with multiple fractures or severe hypertension) whose needs are met by the health-care system and who has access to appropriate medications, diet, and health-care instruction.
4. *Poor health in an unfavourable environment.* In this quadrant, an example is a young child who has asthma and is living in an abandoned warehouse.

Travis's Illness-Wellness Continuum

Travis's illness-wellness continuum (see Figure 7.5) ranges from high-level wellness to premature death (Travis & Ryan, 2001), shown by two arrows pointing in opposite directions and joined at a neutral point. People move back and forth within the continuum. Movement to the right of the neutral point indicates increasing levels of health and well-being. This improvement is achieved in three steps: (1) awareness, (2) education, and (3) growth. In contrast, movement to the left of the neutral point indicates decreasing levels of health.

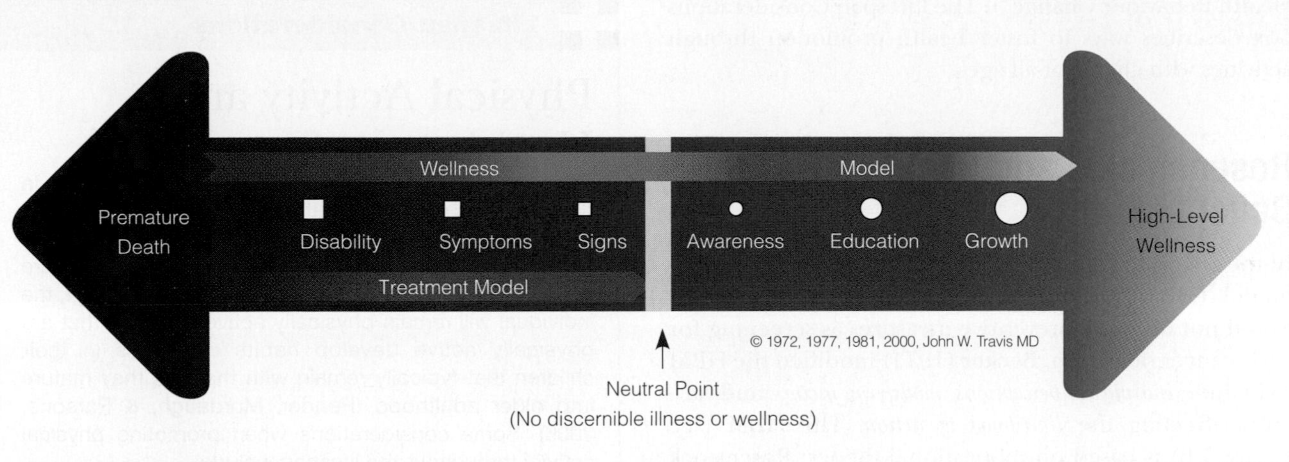

FIGURE 7.5 Illness-wellness continuum
(From **Wellness Workbook,** *by J. W. Travis and R. S. Ryan, 1988, Berkeley, CA: Ten Speed Press Copyright 1981, 1988 by John W. Travis, MD. http://www.thewellspring.com. Reprinted with permission.)*

Travis and Ryan believed it is possible to be physically ill and at the same time oriented toward wellness, or to be physically healthy and at the same time function from an illness perspective.

Levels of Prevention

Prevention refers to avoiding the development of disease and occurs in three levels: primary, secondary, and tertiary (Leavell & Clark, 1965). Table 7.1 summarizes the levels and their foci, and provides examples of prevention activities. The level can occur at various points during the course of a disease and can overlap in practice. For example, a client may have experienced a heart attack, and a goal of secondary prevention is to give cardiac medications immediately to limit disability. The teaching (e.g., lifestyle changes) given to the client to prevent new complications will be similar to the health-education activities in primary prevention, and the goal of the client to return home with follow-up appointments, such as for cardiac rehabilitation, is tertiary prevention.

Health-Promotion Models

Several theories and models of health beliefs and behaviours have been developed to help determine whether an individual is likely to participate in disease-prevention activities. They are useful tools in developing programs for helping people change to healthier lifestyles and develop positive attitudes toward preventive health measures (See Chapter 8, in the sections "Pender's Health-Promotion Model" and "The Transtheoretical Model: Stages of

TABLE 7.1 Levels of Prevention, Foci, and Activities

Level	Focus	Examples of Activities
Primary prevention	Focuses on health promotion and protection against specific health problems or disease. Precedes disease or dysfunction and is applied to generally healthy individuals or groups.	• the teaching of accident and poisoning prevention, immunizations, family planning, nutrition, exercise, stress management, home and occupational safety • lifestyle and nutrition teaching to prevent cancer or heart disease
Secondary prevention	Focuses on early identification or detection of health problems and prompts intervention to alleviate health problems and limit future disability.	• screening for developmental delays, screening for blood pressure; tuberculosis skin test; clinical breast examination and testicular examination; annual physical and dental examination
Tertiary prevention	Focuses on restoration and rehabilitation to an optimal level of functioning. Begins after an illness, when a defect or disability is stabilized or determined to be irreversible.	• the teaching of foot care to diabetic clients • the teaching of range of motion exercises for post-stroke patients

Health Behaviour Change"). The Lifespan Considerations box describes ways to foster health promotion through activities with clients of all ages.

Rosenstock's and Becker's Health Belief Model

In the 1950s, Rosenstock (1974) proposed a health belief model (HBM) to predict which individuals would or would not use such preventive measures as screening for early cancer detection. Becker (1974) modified the HBM to include *individual perceptions, modifying factors,* and variables affecting the *likelihood of action.* The HBM (see Figure 7.6) is based on motivational theory: Rosenstock assumed that good health is an objective common to all people; Becker added "positive health motivation" as a consideration.

INDIVIDUAL PERCEPTIONS Individual perceptions include the following:

- *Perceived susceptibility.* A family history of a certain disorder, such as diabetes or heart disease, may make the individual feel at high risk for having a heart attack.
- *Perceived seriousness.* The perception of the individual that the illness may cause death or have serious consequences, such as concern about having a heart attack and the subsequent financial and lifestyle challenges.
- *Perceived threat.* Perceived susceptibility and perceived seriousness combine to determine the total perceived threat of an illness to a specific individual. For example, a person who has high cholesterol, does not exercise, and is the sole financial provider for the family may have an increased perceived threat of having a heart attack.

MODIFYING FACTORS Factors that modify a person's perceptions include the following:

- *Demographic variables.* Demographic variables include age, gender, race, and ethnicity. An infant, for example, does not perceive the importance of a healthy diet. An adolescent may perceive peer approval as more important than family approval and, subsequently, participate in risk-taking activities or adopt unhealthy eating and sleeping patterns.
- *Sociopsychological variables.* Social pressure or influence from peers or other reference groups (e.g., self-help or vocational groups) may encourage preventive health behaviours even when individual motivation is low. The expectations of others may motivate people, for example, not to drive after drinking alcohol.
- *Structural variables.* Knowledge about the target disease and prior contact with it are structural variables that are presumed to influence preventive behaviours. For example, people with prior skin

Lifespan Considerations

Physical Activity and Health

Cardiovascular complications can begin early in childhood if children are eating a diet high in salt and fat and are not participating in physical activity. Staying fit and active early in life can positively influence future health behaviours and the likelihood that, as an adult, the individual will remain physically active. Families that are physically active develop habits of fitness in their children that typically remain with them as they mature into older adulthood (Pender, Murdaugh, & Parsons, 2006). Some considerations when promoting physical activity throughout the lifespan include:

CHILDREN

- Females are most influenced by female role models, such as family or adult friends who exercise, demonstrate enjoyment of the activity, and preference for that activity.
- Males are influenced by male role models engaging in physical fitness, such as adult family members or friends showing enjoyment of the activity, and self-efficacy to participate.
- Socioeconomic status can affect a child's ability to participate in organized recreational activities.
- Lack of transportation to and from events can be a barrier to participation.
- Older siblings who are physically active can have a positive influence on activity and health.

ADOLESCENTS

- Females who perceive themselves as being less athletic are less likely to participate in physical activity.
- For males, personal interest in sports and sports media and competence are powerful influencers of exercise.
- Access to recreational facilities and less television viewing can affect physical fitness for both sexes.

ADULTS

- Previous levels of exercise predict continued and future participation in physical activity.
- Family obligations and work stressors influence their ability to remain fit.
- Feelings of self-efficacy and spousal or peer support highly influence the initiation of or long-term commitment to physical activity.
- Cost, time, and access to facilities are potential barriers to participation.

OLDER ADULTS

- Fear of hurting themselves, limited access and transportation to facilities, and restricted financial resources are potential barriers to physical activity.
- Most feel that remaining active will improve mental alertness and reduce feelings of social isolation.
- Activities that build on existing skills and competencies of older adults are most beneficial.

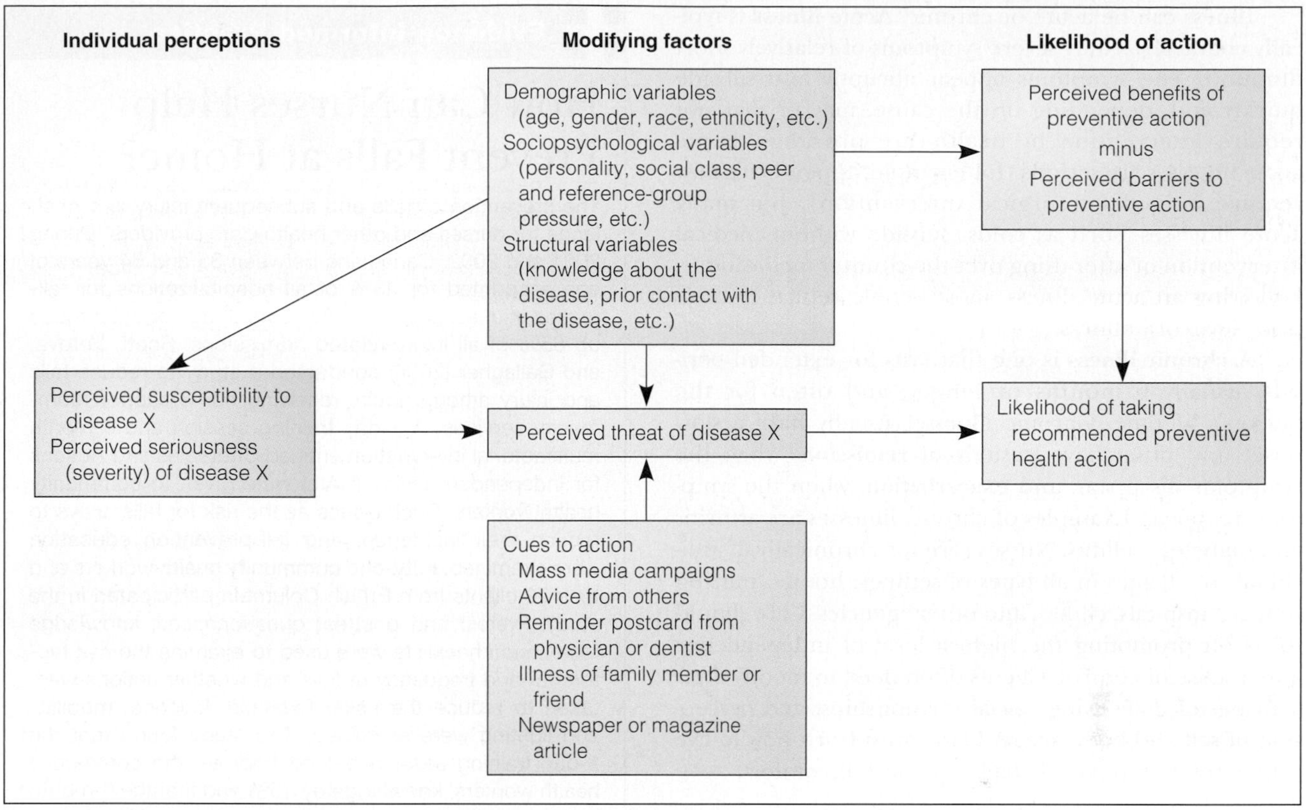

FIGURE 7.6 The health belief model

(From "Selected Psychosocial Models and Correlates Of Individual Health-Related Behaviours," by Marshall H. Becker, Don P. Haefner, Stanislav V. Kasl, John P. Kirscht, Lois A. Maiman, and Irwin M. Rosenstock, 1977, **Medical Care**, *15(5 Suppl), pp. 27–46. Reprinted with permission.)*

cancer may use sunscreen with a high sun protection factor (SPF) before going outside.

- *Cues to action.* Cues can be either internal or external. Internal cues include thoughts about an ill family member. External cues include internet and television advertisements.

LIKELIHOOD OF ACTION The likelihood of a person taking recommended preventive health action depends on the perceived benefits of the action minus the perceived barriers to the action.

- *Perceived benefits of the action.* Examples include refraining from smoking to prevent lung cancer, and eating nutritious foods and avoiding snacks to maintain weight control.
- *Perceived barriers to action.* Examples include cost, inconvenience, unpleasantness, and lifestyle changes.

Pender, Murdaugh, and Parsons (2006) modified the HBM to develop a health-promotion model. According to Pender, the HBM explains health-protecting or preventive behaviours but does not emphasize health-promoting behaviours (see Chapter 8, the section "Pender's Health-Promotion Model").

Illness and Disease

Illness is a highly personal state in which the person's physical, emotional, intellectual, social, developmental, or spiritual functioning is thought to be diminished. It is not synonymous with disease and may or may not be related to disease. An individual can have a disease, such as diabetes, and not feel ill. Similarly, a person with a headache can feel ill or uncomfortable, yet have no discernible disease. Illness is highly subjective; only the person experiencing it can say that he or she is ill.

Disease can be described as an alteration in bodily functions resulting in a reduction of capacities or a shortening of the normal lifespan. People once thought disease was caused by "forces" or spirits. This belief was replaced by causation theory, in which multiple factors interact to cause disease and determine an individual's response to treatment.

The causation of a disease is called its **etiology**. For example, a virus is the biologic agent of severe acute respiratory syndrome (SARS). However, other etiological factors, such as age, nutritional status, and occupation, are involved in the development of SARS and the course of infection.

Illness can be acute or chronic. **Acute illness** is typically characterized by severe symptoms of relatively short duration. The symptoms appear abruptly and subside quickly and, depending on the cause, may or may not require intervention by health-care providers. Some acute illnesses are serious (for example, appendicitis may require immediate surgical intervention), but many acute illnesses, such as colds, subside without medical intervention or after using over-the-counter medications. Following an acute illness, most people return to their prior level of wellness.

A **chronic illness** is one that lasts for extended periods, usually 6 months or longer, and often for the person's lifetime. Chronic illnesses usually have a slow onset and often have periods of **remission**, when the symptoms disappear, and **exacerbation**, when the symptoms reappear. Examples of chronic illnesses are arthritis and diabetes mellitus. Nurses care for chronically ill individuals of all ages in all types of settings: homes, nursing homes, hospitals, clinics, and other agencies. Care should focus on promoting the highest level of independence and a sense of control. Clients often need to modify their activities of daily living, social relationships, and perception of self and body image. Many must learn how to live with increasing physical challenges and discomfort.

Evidence-Informed Practice

How Can Nurses Help Prevent Falls at Home?

The prevention of falls and subsequent injury is a challenge for nurses and other health-care providers. During 2001 and 2002, Canadians between 35 and 64 years of age accounted for 45% of all hospitalizations for fall-related injuries, and those 65 years of age or older made up 85% of all injury-related admissions. Scott, Votova, and Gallagher (2006) conducted a study to reduce falls and injury among adults receiving home support community services. A 1-day training session and 6-month multifactorial intervention entitled Strategies and Actions for Independent Living (SAIL) were given to community health workers. Such issues as the risk for falls, ways to reduce their incidence, and fall-prevention education were examined. Fifty-one community health workers and their 70 clients from British Columbia participated in the study. Pretest and posttest questionnaires, knowledge tests, and checklists were used to examine the risk factors for and frequency of falls and whether actions were taken to reduce the risks. Exercise, balance, mobility, and lighting were examined. The study found that the 1-day training session helped improve the community health workers' knowledge by 25% and that the 6-month multifactorial interventions contributed to a 43% reduction in total falls and a 39% decrease in the number of falls within the 6-month intervention period.

NURSING IMPLICATIONS: Reduction in falls can enhance older adults' self-confidence, mobility, exercise, and socialization, as they become less fearful of falling again. Home health nurses play a key role in fall prevention by working collaboratively with other health-care providers to reduce falls and related injuries at home. They can act as facilitators and trainers by educating older adults and conducting home assessments to identify risks for falls. Home health nurses can also act as researchers to determine the best evidence for effective interventions.

Source: Based on "Falls Prevention Training for Community Health Workers: Strategies and Actions for Independent Living (SAIL)," by V. J. Scott, K. Votova, and E. Gallagher, 2006, *Journal of Gerontological Nursing, 32*(10), pp. 48–56.

Effects of Illness

Illness changes the diagnosed individual and his or his family. The changes vary depending on the nature, severity, and duration of the illness; the attitudes associated with the illness; financial demands; adjustments to usual roles; and so on.

IMPACT ON THE CLIENT Ill clients may experience behavioural and emotional changes, and changes in lifestyle, self-concept, and body image. Behavioural and emotional changes associated with short-term illness are generally mild and short-lived. The individual, for example, may become irritable and lack the energy or desire to interact in the usual fashion with family members or friends. Heightened responses are likely with severe, life-threatening, chronic, or disabling illnesses. Anxiety, fear, anger, withdrawal, denial, a sense of hopelessness, and powerlessness are all common responses to severe or disabling illnesses. For example, a client who receives a diagnosis of cancer, AIDS, or a disabling neurologic disease may, over time, experience episodes of denial, fear, and hopelessness.

Certain illnesses can also change the client's body image or physical appearance, especially if it entails severe scarring or the loss of a limb. The client's self-esteem and self-concept may also be affected (e.g., loss of bodily function, increased dependence on others, unemployment, and strained relationships with others). In addition to participating in treatments and taking medications, the ill person may need to change his or her diet and activity, exercise, rest, and sleep patterns.

Ill individuals are vulnerable to loss of **autonomy**, which is the state of being independent and self-directed without outside control. Nurses need to support the clients' right to self-determination and autonomy by providing them with sufficient information to participate in decision making and maintain feelings of control. Nurses can help their clients express their thoughts and provide care to help them effectively cope with change by

- Providing explanations about any necessary adjustments to the client and their significant others
- Making arrangements, wherever possible, to accommodate the client's lifestyle
- Actively listening to clients as they share their feelings about various changes

- Reinforcing and incorporating desirable changes as a permanent part of the client's lifestyle

IMPACT ON THE FAMILY A person's illness affects not only the person who is ill but also the family or significant others. The kind of effect and its extent depend chiefly on three factors: (1) the member of the family who is ill, (2) the seriousness and length of the illness, and (3) the cultural and social customs the family follows.

The changes that can occur in the family include the following:

- Role changes
- Task reassignments and increased demands on time
- Increased stress because of anxiety about the outcome of the illness for the client and conflict about new responsibilities
- Financial problems
- Loneliness as a result of separation and pending loss
- Change in social customs

> **BOX 7.2** WHAT MAKES CANADIANS HEALTHY?
>
> This story from the Public Health Agency of Canada speaks to the complex set of factors that determine health conditions.
>
> *Why is Jason in the hospital?* Because he has a bad infection in his leg.
>
> *But why does he have an infection?* Because he has a cut on his leg, and it got infected.
>
> *But why does he have a cut on his leg?* Because he was playing in the junk yard next to his apartment building, and there was some sharp, jagged steel there that he fell on.
>
> *But why was he playing in a junk yard?* Because his neighbourhood is kind of rundown. A lot of kids play there, and there is no one to supervise them.
>
> *But why does he live in that neighbourhood?* Because his parents can't afford a nicer place to live.
>
> *But why can't his parents afford a nicer place to live?* Because his Dad is unemployed and his Mom is sick.
>
> *But why is his Dad unemployed?* Because he doesn't have much education and he can't find a job.
>
> *But why . . . ?*
>
> Source: *What Makes Canadians Healthy or Unhealthy?* by Public Health Agency of Canada, 2004, retrieved October 11, 2007, from http://www.phac-aspc.gc.ca/ph-sp/determinants/determinants-eng.php. Adapted and reproduced with permission.

What Makes Canadians Healthy?

Everything in the ecosystem and society affects the health of individuals, families, and communities (Mahler, 1977). Nurses must maintain a spirit of inquiry and inquisitiveness about the world and the root causes of what determines good health. Box 7.2 describes a simple story that speaks to the complex set of factors that determines the health conditions surrounding individuals, families, communities, and nations.

Upstream and Downstream Views

Imagine standing on the edge of a swift-running river. You hear a child's cry for help coming from the river. You jump in and save the drowning child. Shortly afterward, you hear another cry for help, jump in again, and save yet another child. This is repeated several more times but not always with the same success. Although busy with your efforts to rescue these children, there are intervals when you have no one to rescue. Rather than going upstream to find out why these children fall into the stream, you occupy yourself doing other things. Consequently, because of your inaction, you never find out that the children who fell in the river slipped on the riverbank while playing dangerously close to the water.

This metaphor speaks about the importance of looking beyond the immediate event when studying health. In the analogy of drowning children, nurses make a difference every day in the lives of "drowning" patients with medical problems. The emphasis, however, is usually on episodic nursing care. They are downstream thinkers and act on the immediate problem at hand. Instead, nurses must examine problems as upstream thinkers and be advocates for health. They should invest not only in the biological but also in the psychological, cultural, spiritual, and sociological factors associated with health.

Determinants of Health

Many variables influence a person's health status, beliefs, and behaviours. These factors may or may not be under conscious control. People usually control their health behaviours and lifestyle choices. In contrast, people have little or no choice over their genetic makeup, age, sex, culture, and, sometimes, geographic environments. Table 7.2 presents factors that determine the health of Canadians and their underlying premises.

Summary

Nurses play an important role in providing anticipatory guidance to help clients attain optimal health. It has been suggested that health-care systems in the year 2020 will provide "seamless movement" within self-care strategies, health promotion, and community-based primary health-care teams (Villeneuve & Macdonald, 2006, p. 94). It will be the norm for health-care providers and

TABLE 7.2 Determinants That Influence Health and Their Premises

Key Determinant	Underlying Premises
Income and social status	Health status improves with higher income and greater social status. High income determines living conditions, such as safe housing and the ability to buy sufficient amounts of good food. The healthiest populations are those in societies that are prosperous and have an equitable distribution of wealth. Research indicates that higher income and status generally result in more control over life circumstances.
Social support networks	Support from families, friends, and communities is associated with better health. Caring social support networks are important for helping people solve problems and deal with adversity, as well as for maintaining a sense of mastery and control over life circumstances.
Education and literacy	Health status improves with higher levels of education. Education is closely tied to socioeconomic status, and effective education for children and lifelong learning for adults are key contributors to health. Education equips people with the knowledge and skills necessary for problem solving and helps provide a sense of control, better job opportunities, and higher income levels. It improves people's ability to access and understand information to help keep them healthy.
Employment and working conditions	Unemployment, underemployment, and stressful or unsafe working conditions are associated with poor health. People who have more control over their work circumstances and fewer stress-related job demands are healthier and often live longer.
Social environments	The importance of social support also extends to the broader community. Civic vitality refers to the strength of social networks within a community, region, province or territory, or country. It is reflected in the institutions, organizations, and informal giving practices that people create to share resources and build attachments with others. A society's array of values and norms influence the health and well-being of individuals and populations through social stability, recognition of diversity, safety, good working relationships, and cohesive communities.
Physical environments	Contaminants in our air, water, food, and soil can cause a variety of adverse health effects, including cancer, birth defects, respiratory illness, and gastrointestinal ailments. Factors related to housing, indoor air quality, and the design of communities and transportation systems can significantly influence our physical and psychological well-being.
Personal health practices and coping skills	Personal health practices and coping skills refer to actions through which individuals can prevent diseases and promote self-care, cope with challenges, develop self-reliance, and make choices that enhance health. Personal life choices are greatly influenced by the socioeconomic environments in which people live, learn, work, and play. Through research in such areas as heart disease and disadvantaged childhood, we have more evidence that powerful biochemical and physiological pathways link the individual socioeconomic experience to vascular conditions and other adverse health events.
Healthy child development	Evidence on the effects of early experiences on brain development, school readiness, and health in later life has sparked growing interest in early child development as a powerful determinant of health. A young person's development is greatly affected by his or her attachment to significant others, housing and neighbourhood, family income and parents' level of education, access to nutritious foods and physical recreation, genetic makeup, and access to dental and medical care.
Biology and genetic endowment	The basic biology and organic makeup of the human body are a fundamental determinant of health. Genetic endowment provides an inherited predisposition to a wide range of individual responses that affect health status.
Health services	Health services, particularly those designed to maintain and promote health, to prevent disease, and to restore health and function contribute to population health.
Gender	Gender refers to the array of society-determined roles, personality traits, attitudes, behaviours, values, relative power, and influence that society ascribes to the two sexes on a differential basis.
Culture	Some people or groups may face additional health risks because of a socioeconomic environment that is largely determined by dominant cultural values that contribute to the perpetuation of such conditions as marginalization, stigmatization, loss or devaluation of language and culture, and lack of access to culturally appropriate health care and services.

Source: Adapted from *Population Health Approach: What Determines Health?* by the Public Agency of Canada, 2004, retrieved March 14, 2008, from http://www.phac-aspc.gc.ca/ph-sp/phdd/determinants/determinants.html#evidence. Reproduced with permission of the Minister of Public Works and Government Services Canada, 2007.

clients to share the responsibility for health and wellness. An understanding of various approaches to health will enhance health-care providers' ability to impart knowledge on health, identify the root causes of the problem, reduce barriers, and support positive actions toward good health (see Case Study 7).

Case Study 7

Russel and Rayne have both suffered heart attacks; they live near downtown Toronto and are members of the Anishnawbe First Nation people. Russel, on advice from his traditional healer and physician, requested a healing ceremony, started exercising, reduced his salt and fat intake, entered stress-reduction classes, and returned to work 6 weeks after his heart attack. He has a positive outlook, is doing well, and talks about being "well." Rayne also changed his dietary habits and started exercising; however, he has been unable to quit smoking even though he wants to and has been advised to do so. Rayne is frequently despondent, very fearful of having another heart attack, has not yet returned to work, and frequently talks about being "ill."

Critical Thinking Questions

1. How does Russel's psychological dimension of health status differ from Rayne's?
2. Both Russel and Rayne have heart disease. Russel considers himself well whereas Rayne considers himself ill. Explain this phenomenon based on Dunn's high-level wellness grid.
3. What external factors may have influenced Russel's decision to implement positive health behaviours?
4. What factors may have prevented Rayne from developing the same positive outlook and taking the same actions as Russel did regarding his illness?
5. What nursing interventions would be most beneficial to Rayne regarding his smoking problem?
6. What would be some cultural considerations when teaching Russel and Rayne?

After working through these questions, go to the MyNursingLab at **http://www.mynursinglab.com** to check your answers.

KEY TERMS

health
wellness
well-being
medicine wheel
illness
disease
etiology
acute illness
chronic illness
remission
exacerbation
autonomy

CHAPTER HIGHLIGHTS

- Nurses need to clarify their understanding of health because their personal definitions of health largely determine the scope and nature of their nursing practice.
- Perspectives on health have changed; instead of being the absence of disease, health has come to mean the fulfillment of a person's maximum potential for physical, psychosocial, and spiritual functioning.
- Notions of health are highly individual; the nurse works with the client and the client's perception of health to provide meaningful assistance.
- Wellness can be described as an active, seven-dimensional process of becoming aware of and making choices to move toward a higher level of well-being. The seven dimensions of wellness are physical, social, emotional, intellectual, spiritual, occupational, and environmental.
- Well-being can be described as a subjective perception of balance, harmony, and vitality. It is a state, rather than a process.
- Most people describe health as freedom from the symptoms of disease, the ability to be active, and a state of being in good spirits.
- Various models explain health. Smith organized the approaches around four models: clinical, role-performance, adaptive, and eudaimonistic.
- Health belief and behaviour models, such as Rosenstock's and Becker's health belief model (HBM), have been developed to help determine whether an individual is likely to participate in disease-prevention and health-promotion activities.

- Illness is usually associated with disease but may occur independently. Illness is a personal experience in which the person feels unhealthy or ill. Disease alters bodily functions and results in a reduction of capacities or a shortened lifespan.
- An individual's usual pattern of behaviour changes with illness, which may disrupt a person's autonomy, lifestyle, roles, and finances.
- The illness of one member of a family affects all other members.
- Various determinants significantly affect the health of individuals, families, and communities.

ASSESS YOUR LEARNING

1. Mr. Smith is a 72-year-old man who lives alone in an apartment. He describes himself as healthy, self-sufficient, and financially secure. Mr. Smith has no living relatives and states that he often feels sad and lonely. He does his shopping at a grocery store across the street and eats a well-balanced diet. Which health determinant may have the most influence on Mr. Smith's ability to maintain his health over the next few years?
a. Income and social status
b. Social support networks
c. Physical environment
d. Gender

2. Modified social relationships, change in body image, and feelings of hopelessness best describe which of the following?
a. Disability
b. Disease
c. Chronic illness
d. Acute illness

3. A person who is worried about her own health, because her mom and grandmother both developed breast cancer, has individual perceptions about which of the following, which may subsequently influence her future prevention activities?
a. Perceived susceptibility
b. Perceived seriousness
c. Sociopsychological variables
d. Demographic variables

4. Which of the following is defined as a "subjective perception of vitality and feeling well; it can be described objectively, experienced, and measured, and can be plotted on a continuum"?
a. Health
b. Perception
c. Wellness
d. Well-being

5. Mr. Street is a middle-aged homeless man who has come into the clinic with a generalized body rash. Mr. Street has strong body odour and appears very dirty. Which of the following concepts is most important for the nurse to understand?
a. Mr. Street needs education on proper bathing and hygiene practices.
b. Education regarding self-care hygiene practices is not going to be enough to change Mr. Street's behaviours.
c. Homeless people are always very dirty and there is nothing that can be done to change that.
d. Homeless people often don't care as much about their hygiene as the rest of the population.

6. Ms. Run, age 52 years, has an annual mammography for breast cancer. She does not have a diagnosis of breast cancer or a family history of this type of cancer. This screening is an example of what type of prevention?
a. Primary prevention
b. Secondary prevention
c. Tertiary prevention
d. Health promotion

7. A new mom brings her newborn daughter to your wellness clinic for a checkup. In the course of the assessment, you notice that mom holds the baby only when necessary and does not communicate with or look at her new baby. Believing this new family to be at risk, you offer support services of home care visits and counselling. Which of the following determinants of health is most at risk in this situation?
a. Physical environment
b. Healthy child development
c. Gender
d. Income and social status

8. Mrs. Jog has been exercising and calorie counting ever since her diagnosis of hypertension last fall. She has set a goal of reducing her blood pressure over the next 6 months. Her strategy is an example of which of the following?
a. Primary prevention
b. Secondary prevention
c. Tertiary prevention
d. Health promotion

9. Mr. Chan was recently diagnosed with diabetes mellitus. He is confident that he can control his blood sugar with diet and exercise alone. He recently checked out a video on the management of diabetes at a community diabetic health education

centre. Mr. Chan's actions are most representative of which one of the following models?
a. Health belief model
b. Clinical model
c. Role-performance model
d. Agent-host-environment model

10. Mrs. Jones sees a nurse at the local diabetes centre. She states, "I feel healthy, even though I have diabetes." Which of the following responses by the nurse is consistent with the generally recognized definition of health?
a. "Health is influenced mainly by biology."
b. "The definition of health is a personal belief."
c. "Health is a state of complete physical, mental, and social well-being."
d. "Health is defined as the absence of disease."

After working through these questions, go to the MyNursingLab at ***http://www.mynursinglab.com*** *to check your answers and see explanations.*

SUGGESTED READINGS

Public Health Agency of Canada & Canadian Institute for Health Information. (2006, September). *How healthy are rural Canadians? An assessment of their health status and health determinants: Summary report.* Ottawa: Authors.

This report presented the results of a research program on the health status and determinants of health in rural populations and discussed programs and policies that will address the health needs of this population.

Wardle, J., Haase, A., Steptoe, A., Nillapun, M., Jonwutiwes, K., & Bellisle, F. (2004). Gender difference in food choice: The contribution of health beliefs and dieting. *Annals of Behavioral Medicine, 27*(2), 107–116.

This study examined food-choice behaviours in a large sample of young adults from 23 countries and tested two possible explanatory mechanisms for women's greater likelihood of dieting and women's greater beliefs in the importance of healthy diets. Health beliefs were found to explain 40% of the variation in dietary selections.

WEBLINKS

Canadian Health Network

http://www.canadian-health-network.ca

Funded by and in partnership with Health Canada, this website links to a wide range of complementary and alternative health information, including the Natural Health Products Directorate.

Canadian Holistic Nurses Association

http://www.chna.ca

This site presents the philosophy and objectives of the Canadian Holistic Nurses Association (CHNA) and information on the levels of training for a Holistic Nursing Specialty.

Health Canada

http://www.hc-sc.gc.ca

This government client-centred website provides a collection of health-related resources and services.

Registered Nurses' Association of Ontario

http://www.rnao.org

This organization is the professional association advocating for registered nurses in Ontario. Part of its support for nurses is the creation of evidence-based Best Practice Guidelines to promote the health and safety of clients and improve client care.

REFERENCES

Anspaugh, D. J., Hamrick, M. H., & Rosato, F. D. (2006). *Wellness: Concepts and applications* (6th ed.). New York: McGraw-Hill.

Becker, M. (Ed.). (1974). *The health belief model and personal health behavior.* Thorofare, NJ: Charles B. Slack.

Dunn, H. L. (1959). High-level wellness for man and society. *American Journal of Public Health, 49,* 786–788.

Hales, D., & Lauzon, L. (2007). *An invitation to health.* Toronto, ON: Thomas and Nelson.

Health Canada. (2006a). *It's your health: Tattooing and piercing.* Retrieved October 11, 2007, from http://www.hc-sc.gc.ca/iyh-vsv/life-vie/tat_e.html

Health Canada. (2006b). *It's your health: Obesity.* Retrieved October 11, 2007, from http://www.hc-sc.gc.ca/iyh-vsv/life-vie/obes_e.html

Health Canada. (2006c). *It's your health: Personal stereo systems and the risk of hearing loss.* Retrieved October 11, 2007, from http://www.hc-sc.gc.ca/iyh-vsv/life-vie/stereo-baladeur_e.html

Health Canada. (2006d). *It's your health: The effects of oral health on overall health.* Retrieved October 11, 2007, from http://www.hc-sc.gc.ca/iyh-vsv/life-vie/dent_e.html

Hood, L., & Leddy, S. K. (2003). *Leddy & Pepper's conceptual bases of professional nursing* (5th ed.). Philadelphia: Lippincott Williams & Wilkins.

Lalonde, M. (1974). *A new perspective on the health of Canadians.* Ottawa: Government of Canada.

Leavell, H. R., & Clark, E. G. (1965). *Preventive medicine for the doctor in his community* (3rd ed.). New York: McGraw-Hill.

Mahler, H. (1977, November). *What is health for all?* Geneva, Switzerland: World Health Organization.

Maslow, A. (1954). Normality, health and values. *Main Currents, 10,* 75–81.

Maslow, A. (1962a). Health as transcendence of the environment. *Journal of Humanistic Psychology, 2,* 1–7.

Maslow, A. (1962b). *Toward a psychology of being.* Princeton, NJ: Van Nostrand.

Maslow, A. (1970). *Motivation and personality* (2nd ed.). New York: Harper & Row.

Nightingale, F. (1969). *Notes on nursing: What it is, and what it is not.* New York: Dover Books. (Original work published 1860).

Parsons, T. (1951). *The social system.* Glencoe, IL: Free Press.

Pender, N. J., Murdaugh, C. L., & Parsons, M. J. (2006). *Health promotion in nursing practice* (5th ed.). Upper Saddle River, NJ: Prentice Hall.

Rosenstock, I. M. (1974). Historical origins of the health belief model. In M. H. Becker (Ed.), *The health belief model and personal health behavior* (pp. 27–59). Thorofare, NJ: Charles B. Slack.

Smith, J. A. (1981). The idea of health: A philosophical inquiry. *Advances in Nursing Science, 3*(3), 43–50.

Travis, J. W., & Ryan, R. S. (2001). *Simply well.* Berkeley, CA: Ten Speed Press.

Villeneuve, M., & Macdonald, J. (2006). *Toward 2020: Visions for Nursing.* Ottawa: Canadian Nurses Association.

World Health Organization. (1948). *Preamble to the constitution of the World Health Organization as adopted by the International Health Conference.* New York, June 19–22, 1946; signed on July 22, 1946 by the representatives of 61 States (Official Records of the World Health Organization, no. 2, p. 100) and entered into force on April 7, 1948.

Chapter 8

Health Promotion

Health promotion is a cornerstone of professional nursing practice (Community Health Nurses Association of Canada, 2003). In the past two decades, the public has become increasingly aware of the relationship between lifestyle and illness. As people begin to adopt health-promoting habits, such as getting more physically active, balancing stress and relaxation, maintaining good nutrition, and controlling the use of tobacco, alcohol, and other drugs, nurses must understand what health promotion is in order to effectively promote health and prevent illness.

OBJECTIVES

After studying this chapter, you should be able to

1. Examine the development of health-promotion initiatives in Canada
2. Discuss the essential components of the following health-promotion models and documents: Lalonde Report, *Ottawa Charter for Health Promotion*, Epp's health-promotion framework, population health-promotion model, the *Jakarta Declaration*, and Pender's health-promotion model
3. Differentiate health promotion from health protection and health education
4. Identify various sites and types of health-promotion programs
5. Explain the six stages of change in Prochaska's transtheoretical model
6. Discuss the role of the nurse when using nursing process to assess a client's health and develop, implement, and evaluate plans for health promotion

Development of Health-Promotion Initiatives in Canada

Health promotion has a long tradition, dating back to 4000 B.C.E. and the Egyptians' sewage disposal system, feeding of the poor, and warnings about excessive alcohol consumption. Florence Nightingale was the very first nurse to promote clean air and hygiene during the Crimean War in the 1800s. In the early 1900s, public health movements in Canada focused on the control of communicable diseases. At the turn of the twentieth century, this work was exemplified by the Victorian Order of Nurses and public health nurses promoting nutrition and maternal and child health among the poor (Stamler & Yiu, 2008). See Chapter 1.

Changing Focus in Public Health (Post–World War II)

Since World War II, Canadians and people in other industrialized countries have benefited from marked improvement in health as a result of advances in scientific medicine and technology. Mandatory public health measures, such as immunization, sanitation, water purification, and the pasteurization of milk, to control communicable diseases have prevented many illnesses and deaths. Union movements helped improve working conditions and income; economic improvement in turn led to better housing and living conditions and improved nutrition. As Canadians enjoyed longer life expectancy, chronic diseases (e.g., cancer and heart disease) and accidents gradually replaced tuberculosis, diarrhea, and influenza as the leading causes of death. Public health practice has now begun shifting its emphasis from infection control to health-promotion activities by addressing risk factors that contribute to various diseases, such as tobacco use, lack of physical activity, and poor eating habits (Stamler & Yiu, 2008).

Lalonde Report (1974)

With the passing of the Canada Health Act in 1968, governments became responsible for financing a universal health-care system with services that are accessible to all Canadians. By the late 1970s, they were troubled by the increasing gaps between escalating health-care costs and limited health outcomes. In an effort to control the escalating health-care costs, they began exploring factors that influenced the health of Canadians. This led to the first landmark health-promotion document in Canada, *A New Perspective on the Health of Canadians* (Lalonde, 1974), known as the Lalonde Report.

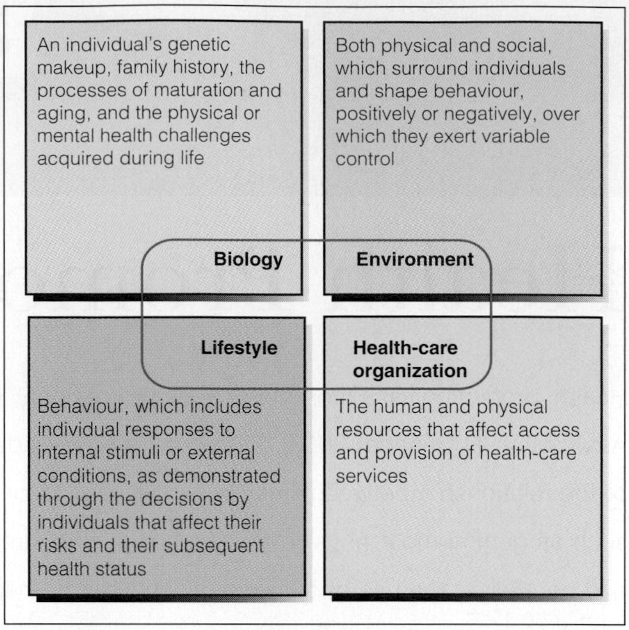

An individual's genetic makeup, family history, the processes of maturation and aging, and the physical or mental health challenges acquired during life
Both physical and social, which surround individuals and shape behaviour, positively or negatively, over which they exert variable control
Biology
Environment
Lifestyle
Health-care organization
Behaviour, which includes individual responses to internal stimuli or external conditions, as demonstrated through the decisions by individuals that affect their risks and their subsequent health status
The human and physical resources that affect access and provision of health-care services

FIGURE 8.1 Lalonde's health field concept

Lalonde conceptualized the **health field concept**, which listed biology, lifestyles, environment, and health-care organizations as the four elements that determine health (see Figure 8.1). The concept marked a shift from a medical to a behavioural approach to health and put the emphasis on individuals' responsibility for their own health. Nevertheless, this approach was heavily criticized for blaming the victims for their poor health and failing to recognize the socioeconomic barriers to people making healthy lifestyle choices.

The Epp Report (1986)

By the mid-1980s, health promotion had become a global discussion following the declaration of "Health for All by the Year 2000" by the World Health Organization (1978) at the Alma-Ata conference in Russia. In 1986, Canada hosted the first international conference on health promotion in Ottawa and released Jake Epp's (1986) *Achieving Health for All: A Framework for Health Promotion* (Figure 8.2). Epp identified three *health-promotion challenges*:

1. *Reducing inequities.* Members of disadvantaged groups have significantly shorter life expectancies, poorer health, and a higher prevalence of disability than the average Canadian.
2. *Increasing prevention.* Various forms of preventable diseases and injuries continue to undermine the health and quality of life of many Canadians.
3. *Enhancing coping.* Many Canadians suffer from various forms of chronic disease, disability, or

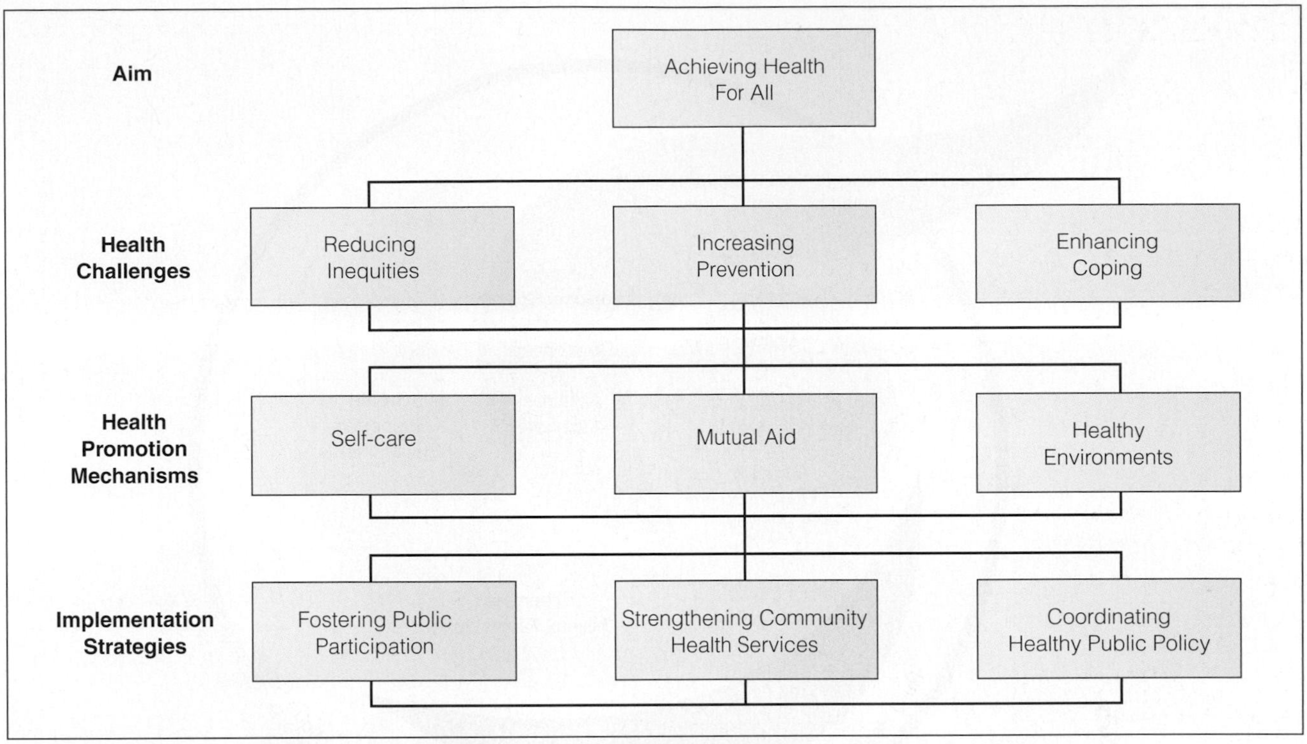

FIGURE 8.2 A framework for health promotion
(From **Achieving Health for All: A Framework for Health Promotion** *(p. 8), 1986, by J. Epp, Ottawa: Health Canada. Copyright 1986 by Minister of Public Works and Government Services. Reprinted with permission.)*

emotional stress, and they lack adequate community support to cope and live meaningful, productive, and dignified lives.

Epp (1986) proposed three *health-promotion mechanisms* to overcome these challenges:

1. Self-care, or the decisions and actions individuals take in the interest of their own health
2. Mutual aid, or the actions people take to help one another cope
3. Healthy environments, or the creation of conditions and surroundings conducive to health

Epp (1986) also suggested three key *health-promotion implementation strategies*:

1. Fostering public participation
2. Strengthening community health services
3. Coordinating healthy public policy

Epp (1986) stressed the importance of *public participation* in implementing health-promotion programs. He believed that decisions about health should not belong exclusively to either the experts or the governments, and what people needed were *partnerships in health* with all stakeholders. Communities began to see health as their prerogative and took collective action on what they saw as priorities for their well-being. This led to the *healthy communities* movement to improve social and working environments; it was initiated in Toronto in 1984 and later spread worldwide (Raeburn & Rootman, 1998).

Ottawa Charter for Health Promotion (1986)

The *Ottawa Charter for Health Promotion* (World Health Organization, Health and Welfare Canada, & Canadian Public Health Association, 1986), shown in Figure 8.3, was conceived and signed by delegates from 38 countries at the end of the 1986 First International Conference on Health Promotion in Ottawa. This charter addresses the importance of a socioenvironmental approach to achieving equity in health. It viewed health as a "resource for everyday living" and identified the fundamental conditions or prerequisites for health as peace, shelter, education, food, income, social justice, equity, sustainable resources, and a stable ecosystem. The charter also stressed that individuals, government, and nongovernment sectors must work in partnership for health. It outlined five health-promotion strategies:

1. Build healthy public policy.
2. Create supportive environments.
3. Strengthen community action.
4. Develop personal skills.
5. Reorient health services.

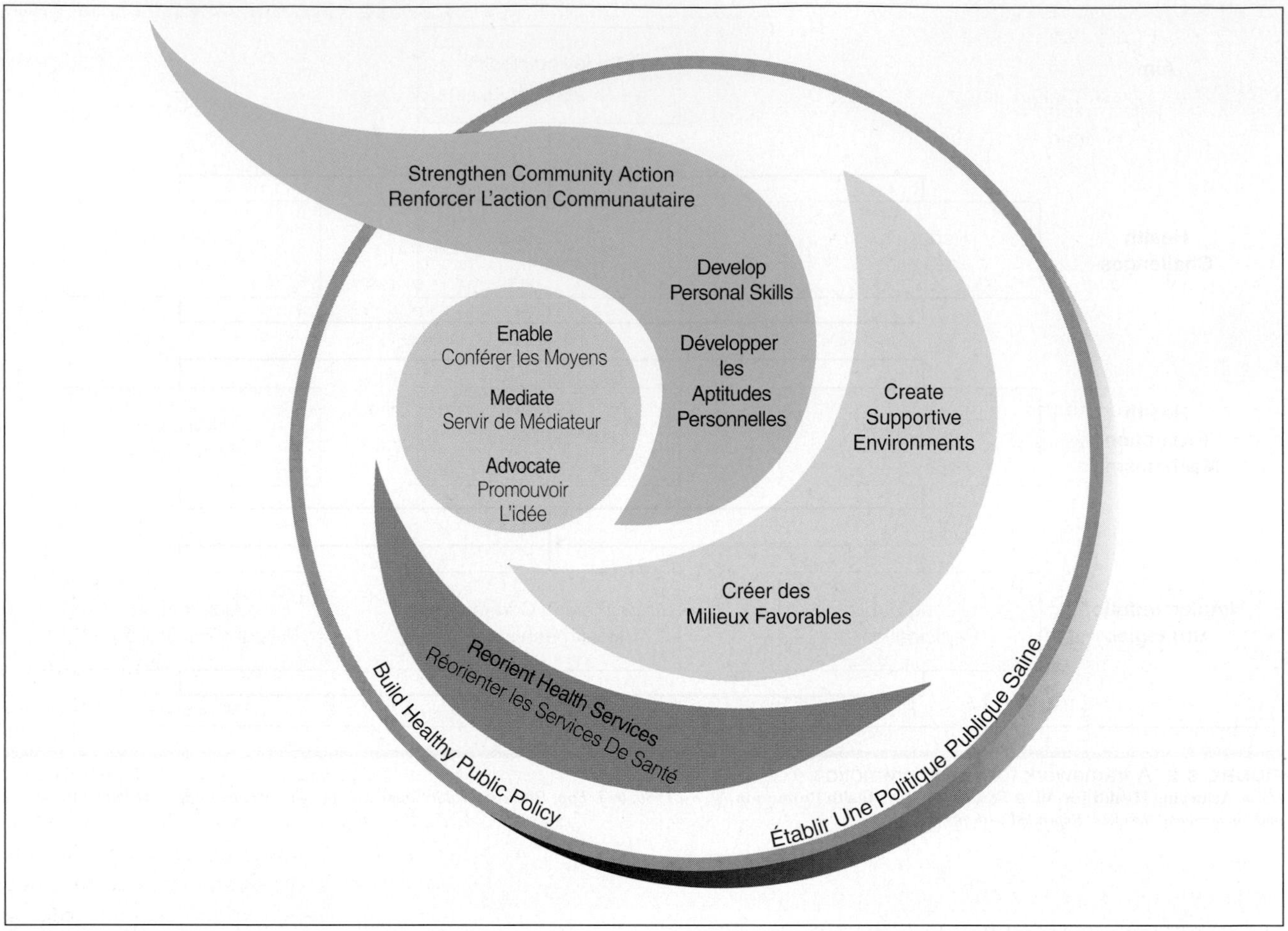

FIGURE 8.3 The *Ottawa Charter for Health Promotion*
(From **The Ottawa Charter for Health Promotion,** *by the World Health Organization, Health and Welfare Canada, and Canadian Public Health Association, 1986, Geneva, Switzerland: World Health Organization. Retrieved July 28, 2006, from http://www.who.int/healthpromotion/conferences/previous/ottawa/en/index4.html)*

Strategies for Population Health (1994)

Between 1991 and 1996, the progress of health promotion was set back by the severe global economic recession. The need for all health services to demonstrate evidence of health outcomes, accountability, cost-effectiveness, and efficiency was more important than ever. The Canadian Institute of Advanced Research released a report, *Strategies for Population Health: Investing in Health of Canadians* (Federal, Provincial, and Territorial Advisory Committee on Population Health, 1994), which set the *determinants of health* at the centre of the *framework for population health* (Figure 8.4). In this framework, the 12 determinants of health were divided into five groups that lent direction to population health initiatives (see Table 8.1). All known individual and collective factors, including their conditions and the interactions that determine people's health, must be considered in planning action to improve health. Information and research are part of community action research. Tracking results and outcomes through research and information augments the broad, long-term effects of health initiatives and enables the formulation of public policy.

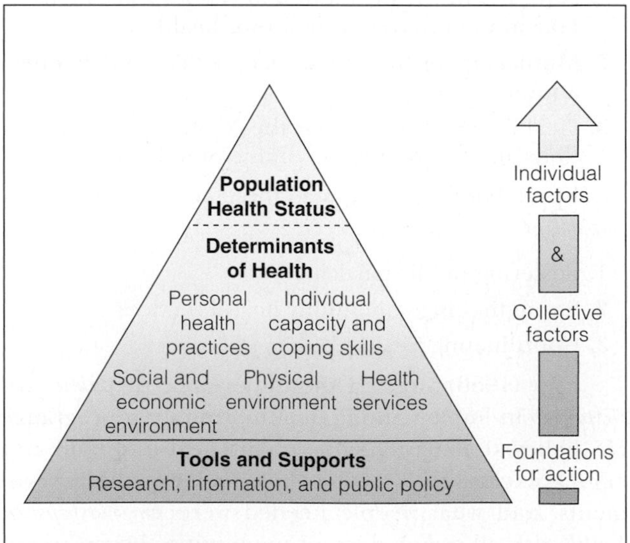

FIGURE 8.4 Framework for population health
(From **Population Health Approach: Underlying Premises and Evidence Table,** *by Health Canada, 2002, Ottawa: Author. Copyright 2002 by the Minister of Public Works and Government Services Canada. Adapted and reproduced with permission.)*

TABLE 8.1 Population Health Initiatives and Determinants of Health

Population Health Initiatives	Determinants of Health
Social and economic environments	Education Employment and working conditions Income and social status Social support networks Social environments
Individual capacity and coping skills	Healthy child development Biology and genetic endowment Gender
Health services	Health services
Physical environments	Physical environments
Personal health practices	Personal health practices and coping skills Culture

Population Health-Promotion Model (1996)

Hamilton and Bhatti (1996) developed a population health-promotion model, shown in Figure 8.5, to improve population health. The model integrated the concepts of health-promotion strategies from the *Ottawa Charter for Health Promotion,* the determinants of health from the *Strategies for Population Health,* and the levels of potential clients for intervention. These clients may be individuals, families, communities, groups, or societies. This model presented four key questions for examination when implementing health-promotion actions: (1) *what* action are we taking, (2) *how* can we take action, (3) *with whom* can we act, and (4) *why* take such an action. It also emphasized the importance of research and evidence-based decision making.

Jakarta Declaration and *Toronto Charter for a Healthy Canada* (since 1997)

In the late 1990s, poverty, social and economic inequities, globalization, and environmental degradation gained increasing recognition as threats to health. Social determinants of health became the key themes in health-promotion discussions and resulted in the adoption of the 1997 *Jakarta Declaration on Health Promotion* (World Health Organization [WHO], 1997). Canada, together with other nations, affirmed social justice, equity, and sustainability as new commitments for health promotion at local, national, and international levels. The *Jakarta Declaration* endorsed the *Ottawa Charter for Health Promotion,* as its principles were grounded in primary health care, social justice, and community empowerment; and it presented five priorities for health promotion in the twenty-first century:

1. Promote social responsibility for health.
2. Increase investment for health development.
3. Consolidate and expand partnerships for health.
4. Increase community capacity and empower the individual.
5. Secure an infrastructure for health promotion.

Building on the *Jakarta Declaration,* the 2002 *Toronto Charter for a Healthy Canada* (Raphael & Curry-Stevens, 2003) addressed social determinants of health, their implications, and policy development in such areas as early childhood development, education, employment and working conditions, food security, health-care services, housing shortages, income and its equitable distribution, social safety nets, social exclusion, unemployment, and job security. Today, the challenges facing health-promotion initiatives involve helping communities to take responsibility for their own health, using new technologies (e.g., the internet and telehealth) to reach the population being served, and attaining evidence or measurable outcomes within the fiscal constraints. The emergence of new communicable diseases, such as the West Nile virus, bovine spongiform encephalitis (mad cow disease), and severe acute respiratory syndrome (SARS), and threats of bioterrorism and natural disasters also have put more demands on the public health system in Canada (Kirby, 2003). The Public Health Agency of Canada was launched in September 2004 with the mandate to protect and promote the health of the public.

Canada has established itself as the world leader in health promotion. The current health-promotion focus is on building an infrastructure for collaborative research in health among various disciplines and on developing knowledge and translating it to practice. Policies are being created to address major health issues, such as tobacco and drug use, obesity, mental health, poverty, early childhood development, diabetes, heart disease, and Aboriginal peoples' health. To improve the

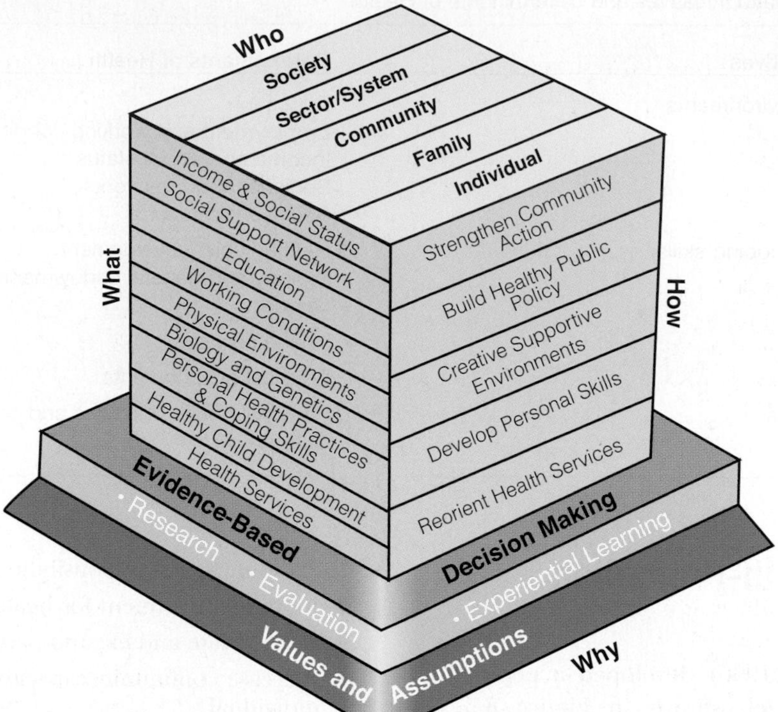

FIGURE 8.5 An integrated model of population health and health promotion
(Adapted from **Population Health Promotion: An Integrated Model of Population Health and Health Promotion,** *by N. Hamilton and T. Bhatti, 1996, Ottawa: Health Canada, Health Promotion and Development Division. Copyright 1996 by the Minister of Public Works and Government Services Canada. Adapted and reproduced with permission.)*

health of Canadians, nurses must understand the implications of various health-promotion initiatives for their practice (O'Neill & Dupéré, 2005), as shown in the Nursing and Canadian Society box.

Nursing and Canadian Society

Fact	Implications for Nursing Practice
The 1974 *New Perspective on the Health of Canadians,* also known as the Lalonde Report, is often cited as the beginning of health promotion.	Nurses must appreciate and understand the historical development and achievements of health promotion in order to promote its vision and future directions, and continue to explore what determines Canadians' health.
Jake Epp's *Achieving Health for All: A Framework for Health Promotion* (1986) reinforced the WHO's goal of health for all by 2000.	Nurses must continue to investigate ongoing health-promotion challenges and mechanisms to plan and implement participatory actions to achieve equity in health.
The 1986 *Ottawa Charter for Health Promotion* marked the shift from traditional treatment and prevention health care to health-promotion strategies that feature empowerment.	Nurses must focus on the broader definitions of health, go beyond health education, and work with intersectoral partners to empower clients to take control of their lives through policy changes and supportive environments.
Hamilton and Bhatti's 1996 population health-promotion model outlined who, what, where, and how to promote population health and stressed the importance of evidence-based practice.	Nurses must acquire the knowledge and skills needed to promote health for individuals, families, groups, and communities in various settings. Accountable actions and ongoing monitoring and evaluation while striving for evidence-based outcomes must be emphasized.
The 2002 *Toronto Charter for a Healthy Canada* expanded on the 1997 *Jakarta Declaration on Health Promotion* to address the importance of social determinants of health, their implications, and policy development.	Nurses must advocate and be politically active from local to international levels to address the broader determinants of health and work and move toward sustainability, social justice, and equity in health.

Defining Health Promotion

What, then, is health promotion? **Health promotion** is "a *strategy* that aims at informing, influencing, and assisting both individuals and organizations so that they will accept more responsibility and be more active in matters affecting mental and physical health" (Lalonde, 1974, p. 66). It involves any *activity* or *program* designed to improve the social and environmental living conditions that enhance people's well-being (Labonte, 1992). Health promotion is also a *process* of enabling or empowering people to increase control over and to improve their health by maximizing positive changes to their physical, economic, social, and political environments (Epp 1986; Health Canada, 2005; WHO, 1984). **Empowerment** is "a social action process in which individuals and groups act to gain mastery over their lives in the context of changing their social and political environment" (Wallerstein & Bernstein, 1994, p. 142). Health promotion, therefore, is a philosophy, a process, and a multisectoral and sociocultural approach that aims to enhance the health and well-being of individuals and communities through policy formulation, supportive environments, and health education (see the Reflect on Primary Health Care box).

Health promotion is not synonymous with health education. WHO (1998) defined **health education** as "consciously constructed opportunities for learning designed to facilitate changes in behavior towards a predetermined goal, and involving some form of communication designed to improve health literacy, knowledge, and life skills conducive to individual and community health" (p. 14). Health education, therefore, is a strategy of health promotion; it is concerned with the communication of information and the fostering of motivation, skills, and confidence to take action to improve health.

REFLECT ON PRIMARY HEALTH CARE

Health promotion is a principle of primary health care. Nurses adopt the primary health care approach to provide promotive, preventive, curative, rehabilitative, and supportive or palliative care to their clients. The focus of their care is on preventing illness and promoting health. In promoting the health of individuals, families, group, and communities, nurses must help their clients understand factors that determine their health and develop effective skills to improve and maintain their own health and well-being. Consider how you can work with your clients and interdisciplinary health-care providers to provide health-promotion services that are culturally sensitive and accessible to your clients. Also, examine whether the educational material is written in a language and at a level that can be understood by clients from another culture.

Central to health promotion is prevention. Leavell and Clark (1965) described *three levels of prevention* during a course of disease progression (see Chapter 7 for primary, secondary, and tertiary levels of prevention). The notions of *health promotion, health protection,* and *disease prevention* are significantly different. Pender, Murdaugh, and Parsons (2006) define health promotion as "behaviour motivated by the desire to increase well-being and actualize human health potential." **Health protection** involves activities focused on preventing, avoiding, or minimizing injuries that individuals have little or no control over and preventable illnesses. **Disease prevention** is concerned with taking measures to prevent and control common risk factors for diseases. Behaviours in both *health protection* and *disease prevention* are "motivated by a desire to actively avoid illness, detect it early, or maintain functioning within the constraints of illness" (p. 7). The major difference in these terms lies with the underlying *motivation* for the individual behaviour (see Table 8.2).

TABLE 8.2 Differences between Health Promotion and Health Protection and Disease Prevention

	Health Promotion	Health Protection and Disease Prevention
Aim	To attain a higher level of wellness by modifying own behaviours and improving social, environmental, and economic conditions	To increase resistance to harm by modifying the environment to minimize preventable illness or injury
Motivation	Motivated by personal, positive desire for wellness	Motivated by avoidance of harm or illness
Examples of activity focus	• Stress management • Physical activity • Nutrition • Parenting on child health • Sexual health (e.g., HIV, sexually transmitted infections [STIs]) • Problematic substance use, tobacco and alcohol use • Chronic disease management • Injury prevention	• Emergency responses • Vehicle, water, food, and drug safety • Infectious disease control • Occupational health safety • Early detection of cancer (e.g., breast health) • Health hazard investigation (e.g., chemical, radiation, and water)

Activities for health promotion, health protection, and disease prevention are complementary processes and are carried out for numerous reasons. For example, suppose a 40-year-old male begins a program of walking five kilometres each day. If the goal of his program is to decrease his risk of cardiovascular disease, then the activity is considered disease prevention. By contrast, if the motivation for walking is to increase his overall health and feeling of well-being, then it is considered health-promotion behaviour.

Health promotion can be offered to all clients regardless of their age or state of health. Age-specific health-promotion activities are discussed in Chapters 16 to 19. See Box 8.1 for some sample activities.

Types of Health-Promotion Programs

Information dissemination uses a variety of media to educate the public and raise their awareness about the risks of particular lifestyle choices and personal behaviours, as well as the benefits of changing those behaviours and improving the quality of life. Billboards, posters, brochures, newspaper features, books, and health fairs all offer opportunities for the dissemination of health-promotion information. See Box 8.1 for health-promotion teaching topics and the Evidence-Informed Practice box for an example.

Health risk appraisal and **wellness assessment programs** are used to apprise individuals of the risk factors that are inherent in their lives in order to motivate them to reduce specific risks and develop positive health habits. Wellness assessment programs focus on more positive methods of enhancement, in contrast to the risk-factor approach used in health appraisal.

Lifestyle and behaviour change programs require the active participation of the individuals and are geared

Evidence-Informed Practice

Do Parents Use Child Safety Restraint Systems Correctly?

Motor vehicle accidents are the leading cause of death and injury in children under 14 years of age in Canada. Snowdon, Polgar, Patrick, and Stamler (2006) surveyed 1263 parents of children aged birth to 9 years in two Ontario communities on their use of child safety restraint systems; only 68% of 2199 children had the correct seats for their weight, and the rate of premature transitioning into safety seats inappropriate for the child's height and weight increased with the age of the child. Data showed that parents had limited knowledge concerning the correct use of safety seats and tended to use nonprofessionals for vehicle safety information.

NURSING IMPLICATIONS: Nurses play a critical role in health promotion through safety promotion and injury prevention in childrearing families. They can prevent premature deaths by reinforcing the mandatory child safety restraint systems, providing the needed information to enhance parents' awareness of the importance of securing children safely in vehicles and using the correct safety seat for the child's height, weight, and age.

Source: Based on "Parents' Knowledge about and Use of Child Safety Systems," by A. Snowdon, J. Polgar, L. Patrick, and L. Stamler, 2006, *Canadian Journal of Nursing Research, 38*(2), pp. 98–114.

BOX 8.1 EXAMPLES OF HEALTH-PROMOTION TEACHING TOPICS FOR VARIOUS AGE GROUPS

Nurses can use the following age-specific topics to teach clients about health-promotion strategies:

Infants
- Infant–parent attachment and bonding
- Breastfeeding
- Activities to stimulate development
- Activity and sleep patterns
- Immunizations
- Safety promotion and injury prevention

Children
- Nutrition
- Dental health
- Vision, hearing, speech
- Discipline
- Activity and sleep patterns
- Immunizations
- Safety promotion and injury prevention

Adolescents
- Communicating with teens
- Hormonal changes
- Nutrition
- Exercise and rest
- Peer group influences
- Self-concept and body image
- Sexuality and sexual health
- Accident prevention

Adults
- Smoking cessation
- Alcohol and drug use
- Family relationships
- Lifestyles
- Weight control
- Stress and coping
- Regular health screening and examination
- Workplace safety

Older Adults
- Adequate sleep
- Dental and oral health
- Foot health
- Hearing aid use
- Immunizations
- Medication management
- Mental health
- Nutrition
- Exercise
- Safety promotion and injury prevention

toward enhancing their quality of life and extending their lifespan. Individuals generally consider lifestyle changes after they have been informed of the need to change their health behaviours and have become aware of the potential benefits of the process. These programs are available, both on group and on individual bases, and they address such issues as stress management, nutrition awareness, weight control, smoking cessation, and exercise.

Environmental control programs address contaminants in the air, food, and water that will affect the health of future generations. The most common concerns of community groups are toxic and nuclear wastes, nuclear power plants, air and water pollution, and herbicide and pesticide spraying.

Sites for Health-Promotion Activities

Health-promotion programs and activities can be offered to individuals and families in the home or in the community setting, such as in schools, hospitals, or worksites. Individual teaching or home visits can be costly, while group teaching is more cost-effective and can offer a setting for socialization and peer support.

Community health-promotion programs are frequently offered by health units, community health centres, and nonprofit health agencies. They may include immunization programs or blood pressure screenings, fire prevention information, bicycle safety programs for children, or a safe-driving campaign for young adults.

School health-promotion programs form a foundation of good health practices for children of all ages. They are cost-effective and offer a convenient setting for health-promotion programs. The school nurse works with teachers to plan and deliver information on various health topics, such as basic nutrition, dental care, activity and play, problematic drug and alcohol use, domestic violence, child abuse, and issues related to sexuality and pregnancy.

Worksite programs may include programs that address air quality, accident prevention, back-saving programs, blood pressure screening, fitness information, and relaxation techniques. Benefits to the employees can include an increased feeling of well-being, fitness, weight control, and decreased stress. Benefits to the employers can include an increase in productivity and morale, a decrease in absenteeism, and a lower rate of employee turnover, all of which can help to decrease business and health-care costs.

Effective health-promotion activities must be guided by models or conceptual frameworks for practice. The rest of this chapter presents two common practice models in health promotion, as well as the use of the nursing process in health promotion.

Pender's Health-Promotion Model

Nola Pender's revised health-promotion model (HPM), shown in Figure 8.6, considers the motivational source for behaviour change to be based on how the client perceives the benefits of changing the given health behaviour. Unlike the health belief model (see Chapter 7 for Rosenstock's and Becker's health belief model), the HPM does not include "fear" or "threat" as a motivating source for changing health behaviour (Pender et al., 2006, p. 48). Variables in the revised HPM are described here.

Individual Characteristics and Experiences

The importance of an individual's unique personal factors or characteristics and experiences depends on the target behaviour for health promotion. Personal factors are categorized as biological (e.g., age, strength, balance), psychological (e.g., self-esteem, self-motivation), and sociocultural (e.g., race, ethnicity, education, socioeconomic status). Some personal factors can influence health behaviours, while others, such as age, cannot be changed. Prior related behaviour includes previous experience, knowledge, and skill in health-promoting actions. Individuals who received benefits from previous health-promoting behaviours will engage in future health-promoting behaviours. In contrast, a person with a history of barriers to achieving the behaviour remembers the "hurdles" and will avoid making changes. Nurses can assist by focusing on the positive benefits of the behaviour, teaching how to overcome the barriers, and providing positive feedback for the client's successes.

Nursing interventions usually focus on factors that can be modified. It is just as important, however, to focus on factors that cannot be changed, such as family history. For instance, nurses could direct more support and information to women with a strong family history of breast cancer by emphasizing the importance of early detection and treatment and offering more hope for a cure. Helping to transform that fear into hope for early detection can make a difference in health attitudes and behaviours.

Behaviour-Specific Cognitions and Affect

Behaviour-specific cognitions and affect have major motivational significance for acquiring and maintaining health-promoting behaviours. Behaviour-specific cognitions and affect constitute a critical core for participation because they can be modified through nursing interventions. They include the following:

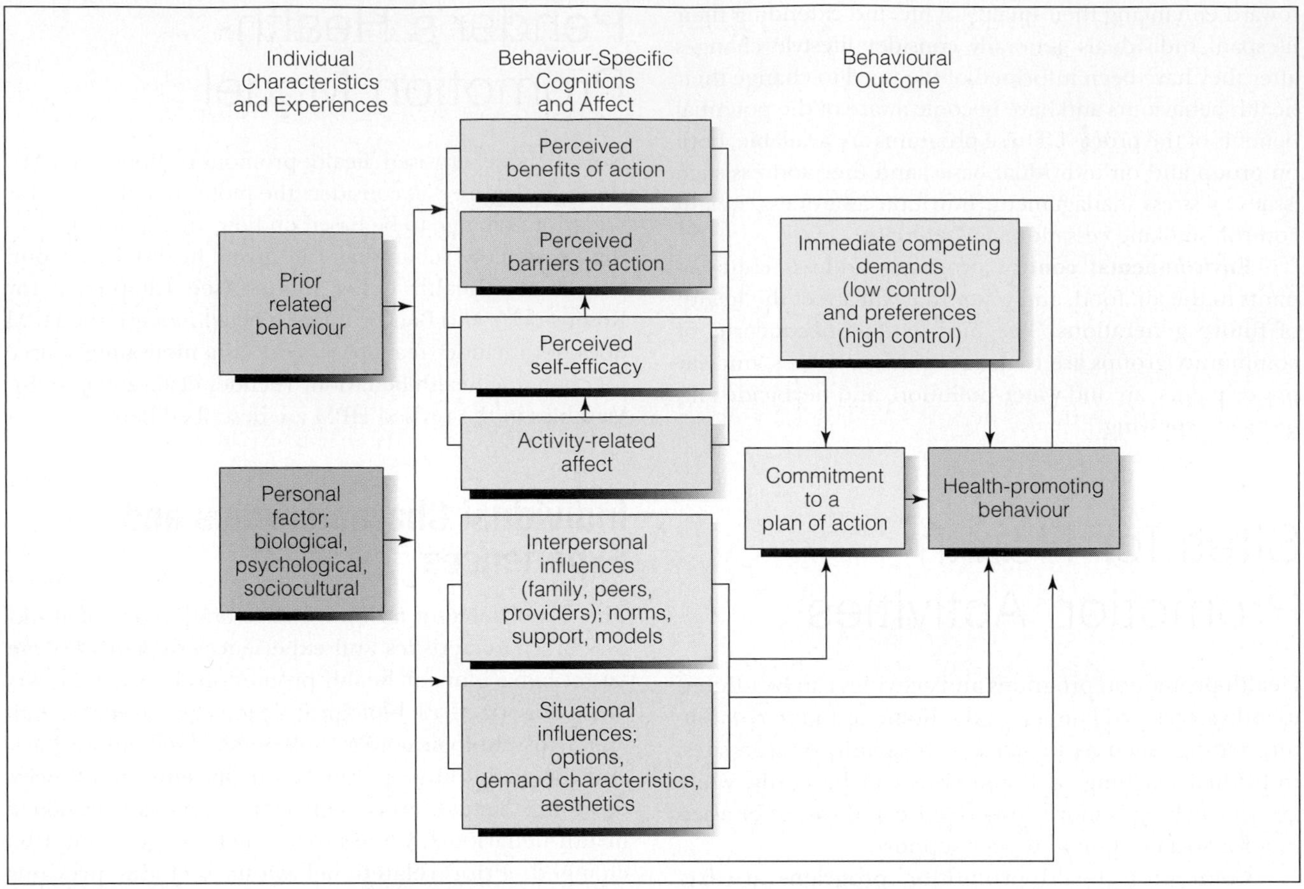

FIGURE 8.6 The health-promotion model (revised)
(From ***Health Promotion in Nursing Practice,*** *5th ed. (p. 50), by N. J. Pender, C. L. Murdaugh, and M. A. Parsons, 2006, Upper Saddle River, NJ: Prentice Hall. Copyright 2006 by Prentice Hall. Reprinted with permission.)*

- *Perceived benefits of action:* Anticipated benefits or outcomes (e.g., physical fitness, stress reduction) affect the person's plan to participate in health-promoting behaviours and may facilitate continued practice. Prior positive experience with the behaviour or observations of others engaged in the behaviour is a motivational factor.
- *Perceived barriers to action:* A person's perceptions about available time, inconvenience, expense, and difficulty performing the activity can act as barriers (imagined or real) to the individual's commitment to a plan of action.
- *Perceived self-efficacy:* This concept refers to the person's conviction in successfully carrying out the behaviour needed to achieve a desired outcome, such as maintaining an exercise program to lose weight. Often people who have serious doubts about their capabilities decrease their efforts and give up, whereas those with a strong sense of efficacy exert greater effort to master problems or challenges.
- *Activity-related affect:* The subjective feelings, such as reaction to the thought of the behaviour, perceived enjoyment, or unpleasant activities, that occur before, during, and following an activity can influence whether a person will repeat the behaviour or maintain the behaviour. A positive affect or emotional response to a behaviour is likely to be repeated, and behaviours associated with a negative affect are usually avoided.
- *Interpersonal influences:* Interpersonal influences are a person's perceptions concerning the behaviours, beliefs, or attitudes of others. Family, peers, and health professionals are sources of interpersonal influences that can shape a person's health-promoting behaviours. Interpersonal influences include the expectations of significant others, social support (e.g., emotional encouragement), and learning done through observing others or modelling.
- *Situational influences:* Situational influences have direct and indirect effects on health-promoting behaviours. They include perceptions of available options, demand characteristics, and the aesthetic features of the environment. An example of an individual's perception of available options is easy access to healthful alternatives, such as vending machines and restaurants that provide healthful menu options. Demand characteristics can directly affect healthy behaviours through policies, such as a company regulation that demands safety equipment to be worn or that establishes a nonsmoking environment. Individuals are more apt to perform health-promotion behaviours if they are comfortable in the environment versus feeling alienated. Environments that are considered safe as well as

those that are interesting are also desirable aesthetic features that facilitate health-promotion behaviours.

Commitment to a Plan of Action

Commitment to a plan of action involves dedication and the identification of specific strategies for carrying out and reinforcing the behaviour. Strategies are important because commitment alone often results in good intentions but not actual performance of the behaviour.

Immediate Competing Demands and Preferences

Competing demands are those behaviours over which an individual has a low level of control. For example, an unexpected work or family responsibility may compete with a planned visit to the health club and not responding to this responsibility may cause a more negative outcome than missing the exercise routine. *Competing preferences* are behaviours over which an individual has a high level of control; however, this control depends on the individual's ability to be self-regulating or to not give in. For example, a person who chooses a high-fat food over a low-fat food because it tastes better has given in to an urge based on a competing preference.

Behavioural Outcome

Health-promoting behaviour, the outcome of the health-promotion model, is directed toward the client attaining positive health outcomes, such as improved health, enhanced functional ability, and better quality of life at all stages of development (Pender et al., 2006).

The Transtheoretical Model: Stages of Health Behaviour Change

Health behaviour change is a cyclic phenomenon in which people progress through several stages. In the first stage, the person does not think seriously about changing a behaviour; by the time the person reaches the final stage, he or she is successfully maintaining the change in behaviour. If the person does not succeed in changing behaviour, relapse occurs. The Prochaska's transtheoretical model (TTM) (Prochaska, Redding, & Evers, 2002), shown in Figure 8.7 and commonly known as *change theory*, describes six stages of change.

Precontemplation Stage

In the precontemplation stage, the person does not think about changing his or her behaviour in the future 6 months. They may be uninformed or underinformed about the consequences of the risk behaviours. Or the person may have tried changing and been unsuccessful and now sees the behaviour as their fate or feels that change is hopeless. Individuals in this stage tend to avoid reading, talking, or thinking about their high-risk behaviours.

Contemplation Stage

During the contemplation stage, the person acknowledges having a problem, seriously considers changing a specific behaviour, actively gathers information, and verbalizes plans to change the behaviour in the near future (e.g., next 6 months). The person, however, may not be ready to commit to action. Some people may stay in the contemplative stage for months or years before taking action. When contemplators begin the transition to the preparation stage, their thinking is clearly marked by two changes: focusing on the solution rather than the problem and thinking more about the future than the past.

Preparation Stage

The preparation stage occurs when the person intends to take action in the immediate future (e.g., within the next month). Some people in this stage may have already started making small behavioural changes, such as buying a self-help book. At this stage, the person makes the final specific plans to accomplish the change.

Action Stage

The action stage occurs when the person actively implements the behavioural and cognitive strategies of their action plan to interrupt previous health-risk behaviours and adopt new ones. This stage requires the greatest commitment of time and energy.

Maintenance Stage

During the maintenance stage, the person strives to prevent relapse by integrating newly adopted behaviours into his or her lifestyle. This stage lasts until the person no longer experiences temptation to return to previous unhealthy behaviours. Without a strong commitment to maintenance, the person will relapse, usually to the precontemplation or contemplation stage.

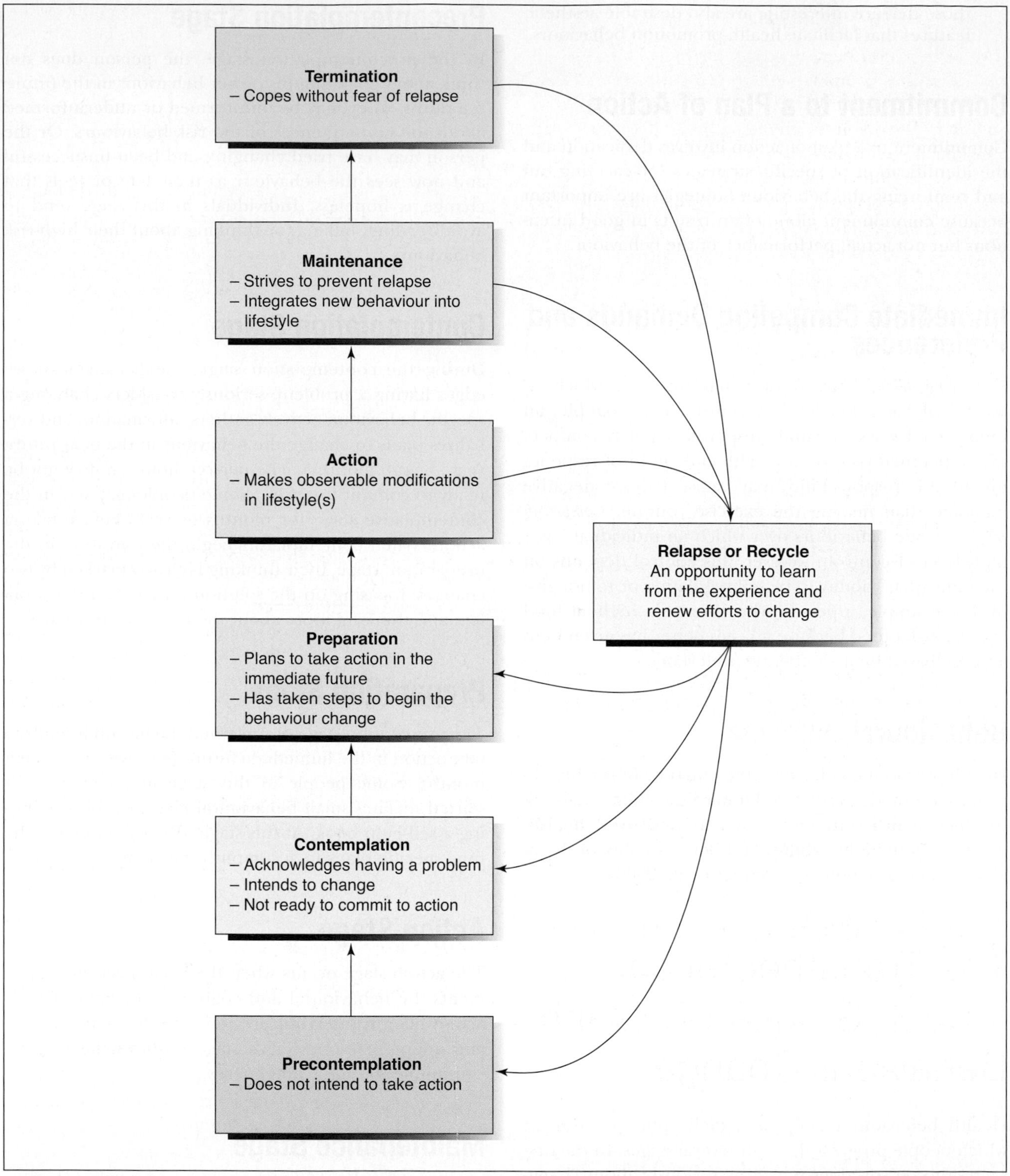

FIGURE 8.7 The transtheoretical model: Stages of change. The stages of change are rarely linear. It is more common for people to recycle several times through the stages. The person who takes action and has a relapse (recycles through some or all of the stages) is more apt to be successful the next time than the individual who never takes action.

(Based on content from **Changing for Good** *by James O. Prochaska, John C. Norcross, and Carlo C. DiClimente, 1994, New York: HarperCollins Publishers. Copyright 1994 by James O. Prochaska, John C. Norcross, and Carlo C. DiClimente; "The Transtheoretical Model and Stages of Change," by James O. Prochaska, Colleen A. Redding, and Kerry E. Evers in* **Health Behaviors and Health Education: Theory, Research, and Practice,** *3rd ed., by Karen Glanz, Barbara K. Rimer, and Frances Marcus Lewis (Eds.), 2002, San Francisco, CA: Jossey-Bass.)*

Termination Stage

The termination stage is the ultimate goal, at which the individual has complete confidence that the problem is no longer a temptation or threat. It is as if they had never acquired the habit in the first place. Experts debate whether some behaviours can be terminated versus requiring continual maintenance.

These six stages are cyclical; people generally move through one stage before progressing to the next. However, at any point a person can relapse or recycle to any previous stage. In fact, the average successful self-changer recycles through the stages several times before they exit the cycle. Most individuals who relapse return to the contemplation stage. During this time they can think about what they have learned and plan for the next action.

The Nursing Process and the Role of the Nurse in Health Promotion

The increasing emphasis on health promotion has created opportunities for nurses to work with individuals, families, groups, and communities in diverse settings. The **role of the nurse in health promotion** may involve advocacy, consultation, teaching, facilitation, or coordination of health services. The nurse applies the nursing process to assess clients' health and assist them in setting goals and plans and to take responsibility for positive health changes. Refer to Chapter 22, the section "Overview of the Nursing Process."

Assessing the Health of Individuals

A thorough assessment of the individual's health status is basic to health promotion. Components of this assessment are the health history and physical examination, lifestyle assessment, spiritual health assessment, social support systems review, health-risk appraisal, health beliefs review, and life stress review.

HEALTH HISTORY AND PHYSICAL EXAMINATION The health history and physical examination discussed in Chapter 27 provide guidelines for detecting any existing problems. The medical history, age, gender, race, ethnicity, and culture of the individual must be considered when collecting data. For example, an environmental safety assessment and immunization history must be appropriate to the person's age and gender. Also, when doing a nutritional assessment, the nurse must consider how age, lifestyle, and cultural practices influence the dietary patterns of the client (see Chapter 10, the section "Selected Cultural Parameters for Nursing").

LIFESTYLE ASSESSMENT **Lifestyle assessment** focuses on the personal lifestyle and habits of the client as they affect health, such as physical activity, nutritional practices, stress management, and such habits as smoking, alcohol consumption, and drug use. Lifestyle assessment provides a basis for decisions related to desired behaviour and lifestyle change.

SPIRITUAL HEALTH ASSESSMENT **Spiritual health** is the ability to develop our inner nature to its fullest potential, including the ability to discover and articulate a basic purpose in life, to learn how to experience love, joy, peace, and fulfillment, and how to help ourselves and others achieve their fullest potential (Pender et al., 2006). Individuals' spiritual beliefs can affect their interpretation of events in their life and, therefore, an assessment of spiritual well-being is a part of evaluating their overall health (see Chapter 46).

SOCIAL SUPPORT SYSTEMS REVIEW Through interpersonal relationships, individuals and groups can provide comfort, assistance, encouragement, and information. **Social support** fosters successful coping and promotes satisfying and effective living. **Social support systems** create an environment that encourages healthy behaviours, promotes self-esteem and wellness, and provides feedback that the person's actions will lead to desirable outcomes. Examples of social support systems include family, peer support groups, computer-based support groups, community organized religious support systems (e.g., churches), and self-help groups (e.g., Alcoholics Anonymous, Weight Watchers). The nurse and client discuss and evaluate the adequacy of the client's support system and, if necessary, mutually plan options for enhancing the support system.

HEALTH-RISK APPRAISAL The principle behind health-risk appraisal (HRA) is that each person faces certain health hazards and that average risks are applicable to a client if the health professional knows the client's characteristics and the mortality of a large group of cohorts with similar characteristics (Pender et al., 2006). The objectives of most HRAs are twofold:

1. To assess risk factors that may lead to health problems
2. To change health behaviours that place the client at risk of developing an illness

Risk factors are features that can cause a client to be vulnerable to developing a specific health problem, such as cancer. An **at-risk aggregate** refers to a subgroup within the community or population that is at greater risk of illness or poor recovery.

HRAs focus on the assessment of lifestyle factors and health behaviours. Risk factors can be categorized according to (1) age, (2) genetic factors, (3) biological characteristics, (4) personal health habits, (5) lifestyle, and (6) environment. Clients cannot control some of the risk factors, such as age, gender, and family history;

others, such as blood pressure, stress, and cigarette smoking, can be partially or totally controlled.

HEALTH BELIEFS REVIEW Assessment of clients' health-care beliefs reveals how much the clients believe or perceive they can influence or control health through personal behaviours. Some cultures have a strong belief in fate: "Whatever will be, will be." An example is diabetic teaching, which often requires many lifestyle changes in diet and exercise, and close control of blood glucose levels to prevent complications. If the person believes he or she has no control over the outcome, it is difficult to motivate the client to make the necessary changes. Awareness of these differences in beliefs can provide a better indication of readiness and motivation on the part of the client to engage in healthy behaviours.

LIFE STRESS REVIEW Abundant literature and a variety of stress-related tools can measure the impact of stress on mental and physical well-being. High levels of stress are associated with an increased possibility of illness (see Chapter 47, the section "Concept of Stress").

VALIDATING ASSESSMENT DATA Following the collection of assessment data, the nurse and client jointly review the client's current health practices and attitudes. This allows for validation of the information by the client and may increase awareness of the need to change behaviour. The nurse and client should consider the following:

- Any existing health problems
- The client's perceived degree of control over his or her health status
- The client's level of physical fitness and nutritional status
- Illnesses for which the client is at risk
- Any health beliefs related to cultural and spiritual practices
- The client's current health practices
- Any sources of stress and the client's ability to handle stress
- The client's social support systems
- The information the client needs to enhance his or her health-care practices

Diagnosing

Wellness nursing diagnoses, or *strength-oriented diagnoses,* provide a clear focus for planning interventions and can be applied at all levels of prevention. When the nurse and client conclude that the client has positive function in a certain pattern area, such as adequate nutrition or effective coping, the nurse can use this information to help the client reach a higher level of functioning. Examples of wellness diagnoses are the following:

- Health-seeking behaviours, such as physical fitness
- Effective breastfeeding
- Anticipatory grieving

Planning

Health-promotion plans need to be mutually developed according to the needs, desires, and priorities of the client. The client chooses the health-promotion goals; the frequency, duration, and course of actions; and the method of evaluation. The nurse acts as a resource person, an adviser, and a counsellor. The nurse provides information, emphasizes the importance of small steps in making behavioural changes, and helps the client to set realistic and measurable goals.

Pender et al. (2006) outline several steps in the process of planning health promotion, which are carried out jointly by the nurse and the client (see Box 8.2 for an example of an individual prevention and health-promotion plan):

1. *Review and summarize the data from the assessment.* The nurse shares with the client a summary of the data collected from the various assessments (e.g., physical health and fitness, nutrition, sources of stress, spirituality, health practices).
2. *Reinforce strengths and competencies.* The nurse and the client come to consensus about areas in which the client is doing well and areas that need work.
3. *Identify health-care goals.* The client selects two or three priority goals and reviews the behaviour change options. These goals are formulated during the planning phase and a date is determined for attaining them.
4. *Identify behavioural or health outcomes.* For each of the selected goals or areas in step 3, the nurse and client determine what specific behavioural changes are needed to bring about the desired outcome. For example, to reduce the risk of cardiovascular disease, the client may need to change behaviours, such as stopping smoking, losing weight, and increasing his or her activity level.
5. *Develop a behaviour change plan.* A constructive program of change is based on client ownership of the behaviour changed (Pender et al., 2006). Clients may need help in examining value-behaviour inconsistencies and in selecting behavioural options that are most appealing and that they are most willing to try. The client's priorities will reflect personal values, activity preferences, and expectations of success.
6. *Reiterate the benefits of change.* The benefits will probably need to be reiterated even though the client is committed to the change. The health-related and non-health-related benefits should be kept before the client as central motivating factors.
7. *Address environmental and interpersonal facilitators and barriers to change.* Environmental and interpersonal factors and available resources that support positive change should be explored and used to reinforce the client's efforts to change his or her lifestyle. All people experience barriers, some of which can be anticipated and planned for, thereby making the change more likely to occur.

BOX 8.2 EXAMPLE OF AN INDIVIDUAL PREVENTION AND HEALTH-PROMOTION PLAN

Designed for: James Moore
Home Address: 714 George
Home Telephone Number: 222-3333
Occupation (if employed): Building services supervisor
Work Telephone Number: 445-6666
Cultural Identification: African Canadian
Birth Date: 3/14/59 Date of Initial Plan: 1/15/2010

Client strengths	Satisfactory peer relationships, spiritual strength, adequate sleep pattern
Major risk factors	Elevated cholesterol, mild obesity, sedentary lifestyle, moderate life change, multiple daily hassles
Nursing diagnoses (derived from assessment of functional health patterns)	Deficient Diversional Activity Imbalanced Nutrition: More than Body Requirements Caregiver Role Strain (elderly mother)
Medical diagnoses (if any)	Mild hypertension
Age-specific screening recommendations	Blood pressure, cholesterol, fecal occult blood, malignant skin lesions, depression
Desired behavioural and health outcomes	Become a regular exerciser (3×/week), lower my blood pressure, weigh 75 kg

Personal Health Goals (1 = highest priority)	Selected Behaviours to Accomplish Goals	Stage of Change	Strategies/Interventions for Change
1. Achieve desired body weight	Begin a progressive walking program	Planning	Counterconditioning Reinforcement management Client contracting
	Decrease caloric intake while maintaining good nutrition	Action (eating 4 fruits and 4 vegetables daily; using low-fat dairy products for last 2 months)	Stimulus control Cognitive restructuring
2. Decrease risk for hypertension-related disorders	Change from high- to low-sodium snacks	Contemplation	Consciousness raising Learning facilitation
3. Learn to manage stress effectively	Attend relaxation classes and use home relaxation tapes	Contemplation	Consciousness raising Self-re-evaluation Simple relaxation therapy
4. Increase leisure-time activities	Join a local bowling league	Contemplation	Support system enhancement

Source: From *Health Promotion in Nursing Practice*, 5th ed. (pp. 129–130), by N. J. Pender, C. L. Murdaugh, and M. A. Parsons, 2006, Upper Saddle River, NJ: Prentice Hall. Reprinted with permission.

8. *Determine a time frame for implementation.* Setting a time frame helps the client target when to develop the needed knowledge and skills for implementation of a new behaviour. The time frame may be several weeks or months. Scheduling short-term goals and rewards can offer encouragement to achieve long-term objectives. Clients may need help to be realistic and to deal with one behaviour at a time.
9. *Commit to behaviour change.* Commitments to changing behaviours are usually verbal, but increasingly a formal, written behavioural contract is being used to motivate the client to follow through with selected actions. Motivation to follow through is provided by a positive reinforcement or reward stated in the contract. *Contracting* is based on the belief that all people have the potential for growth and the right of self-determination, even though their choices may be different from the norm.

Implementing

Implementing is the "doing" part of behaviour change. Self-responsibility is emphasized in implementing the plan. Depending on the client's needs, the nursing strategies may include supporting, teaching, consulting, coordinating, facilitating, counselling, and modelling to enhance behaviour change.

PROVIDING AND FACILITATING SUPPORT The focus of providing support is on the desired behaviour change. The nurse must be nonjudgmental when offering support, whether on an individual basis or in a group setting. The nurse can also facilitate the development of support networks for the client, such as family members and friends.

Individual Counselling Sessions Counselling sessions may be routinely scheduled as part of the plan or may be provided if the client encounters difficulty in carrying out interventions or meets insurmountable barriers to change. The nurse acts as a facilitator, supporting the client's decision making in regard to the health-promotion plan.

Telephone or Computer Counselling Telephone or computer counselling may be provided to the client to help in answering questions, reviewing goals and strategies, and reinforcing progress. This form of support can be useful and convenient for the busy client who may not have the time for regular in-person sessions.

Group Support Group sessions provide an opportunity for participants to learn the experiences of others in changing behaviour. Regular group contacts give individuals a renewed commitment to their goals.

Facilitating Social Support Social networks, such as family and friends, can facilitate or impede the efforts directed toward prevention and health promotion. The nurse's role is to communicate the client's needs and goals, and assist the client to assess, modify, and develop the social support necessary to achieve the desired change.

PROVIDING HEALTH EDUCATION Health education programs on a variety of health-promotion topics can be provided to groups, individuals, or communities. The health-promotion topics must be based on the health needs of the people. Specific health-promotion goals must be set and outcomes evaluated after the program implementation.

ENHANCING BEHAVIOUR CHANGE Whether people will make and maintain changes to improve health or prevent disease depends on many interrelated factors. To help clients succeed in implementing behaviour changes, the nurse needs to understand the stages of change and effective interventions that focus on moving the individual through the stages of change. Figure 8.8 provides suggested strategies for helping clients, depending on their stage of change. Guidelines for assisting the client toward behaviour change are in Box 8.3. The nursing goal is not necessarily to change behaviour but to advance the client to the next stage of change.

HARM REDUCTION **Harm reduction** is a health-promotion approach that aims to minimize harm or reduce the negative consequences of risk behaviour by keeping people as safe and healthy as possible in their current lifestyle realities (Canadian Nurses Association [CNA], 2002). The nurse provides the needed knowledge, skills, resources, and support to those who are at risk, to reduce

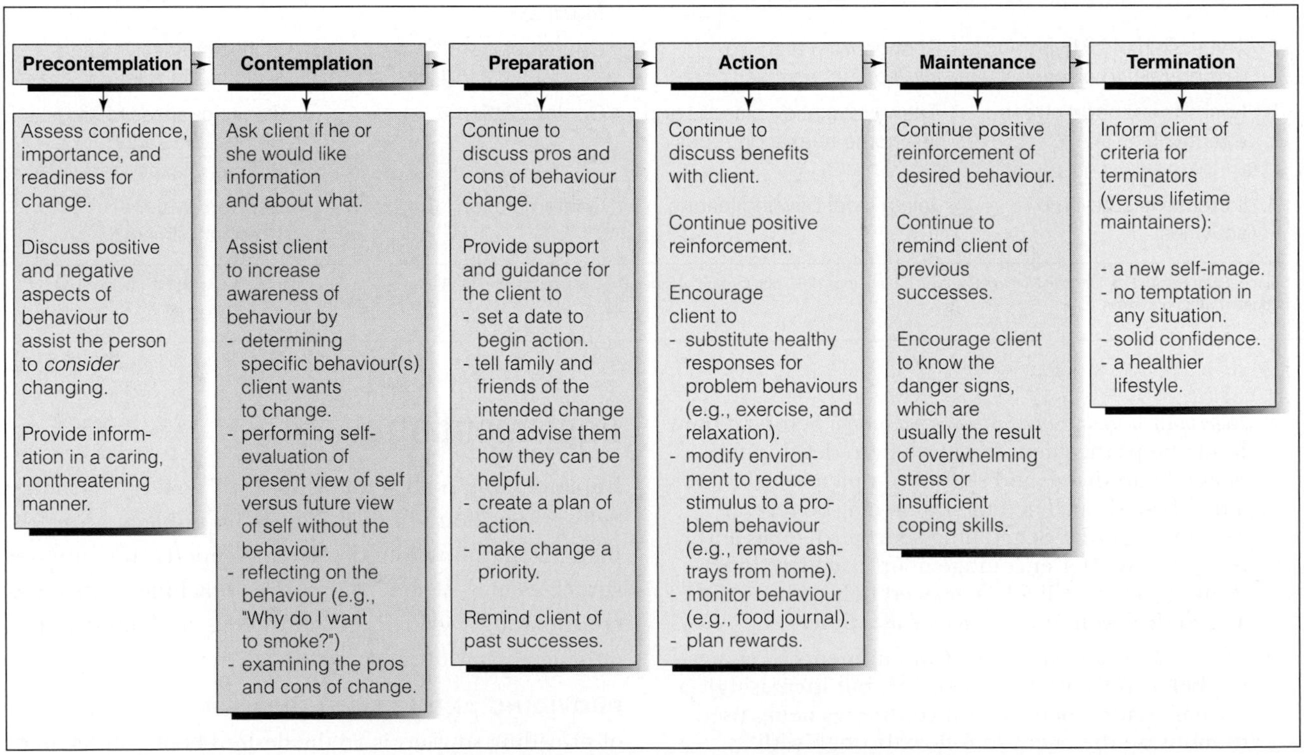

FIGURE 8.8 Strategies to promote behavioural change for each stage of change
(Data are from "The Transtheorectical Model and Stages of Change," by James O. Prochaska, Colleen A. Redding, and Kerry E. Evers in **Health Behaviors and Health Education: Theory, Research, and Practice,** *3rd ed., by Karen Glanz, Barbara K. Rimer, and Frances Marcus Lewis (Eds.), 2002, San Francisco, CA: Jossey-Bass;* **Changing for Good** *by James O. Prochaska, John C. Norcross, and Carlo C. DiClimente, 1994, New York: HarperCollins Publishers. Copyright 1994 by James O. Prochaska, John C. Norcross, and Carlo C. DiClimente;* **Health Behavior Change: A Guide for Practitioners** *by S. Rollnick, P. Mason, and C. Butler, 1999, Edinburgh, UK: Churchill Livingstone; "Patient Teaching to Promote Behavioral Change," by L. Saarmann, J. Daugherty, and B. Riegel, 2000,* **Nursing Outlook,** *48(6), 281–287.)*

BOX 8.3 GUIDELINES FOR ENHANCING BEHAVIOUR CHANGE

Nurses can use the following guidelines to help clients move to the next stage of change to achieve the desired outcome:

ESTABLISH A RAPPORT AND SET THE AGENDA

- Establish a trusting relationship with the client.
- Identify the client's presenting problem or current situation and concerns.
- Ask which behaviour he or she feels most ready to *think* about changing and focus on one specific behaviour at a time.

ASSESS IMPORTANCE, CONFIDENCE, AND READINESS

- Assess the importance the client gives to the behaviour change and his or her confidence level and readiness for change.
- *Importance* refers to the personal value of change. Ask, "How do you feel at the moment about [state the change]?" "How important is it to you to [state the change]?" "On a scale of 1 to 10, with 1 being 'not important' and 10 'very important,' what number would you give yourself?"
- *Confidence* relates to the mastering of the skills needed to achieve the behaviour and the situations in which behaviour change will be challenging to the client. Ask, "If you decided right now to change, how confident would you feel about succeeding?"

EXCHANGE INFORMATION AND REDUCE RESISTANCE

- Present information in a nonjudgmental manner and avoid using the word *you* too much. Referring to other people (versus *you*) and what happens to them makes the information less threatening to the client. Ask for the client's interpretation of the information presented.
- Reduce resistance to change by
  - Emphasizing personal choice and control
  - Re-examining the client's feelings about importance and confidence regarding making the specific change
  - Reflecting, understanding, and respecting how the client feels

Source: Adapted from *Health Behavior Change: A Guide for Practitioners,* by S. Rollnick, P. Mason, and C. Butler, 1999, Edinburgh, UK: Churchill Livingstone. Adapted with permission from Elsevier.

the harm done to those engaging in these behaviours and the overall community. Examples of harm reduction are the PARTY programs to promote responsible drinking and the needle exchange program to prevent the spread of AIDS or hepatitis C.

Some nurses may experience value conflicts and be concerned that they are not providing health-promoting behaviours with this approach. Regardless, they need to recognize that clients have rights to accessible, nonjudgmental, and noncoercive treatments (see Chapter 5, the section "Ethical Decision Making"), and that prevention activities are best aimed at people engaging in high-risk behaviours (CNA, 2002).

ROLE MODELLING Through observing a role model during the early stages of learning and change, the client acquires ideas for behaviour and coping strategies for specific problems. The nurse and client should mutually select role models with whom the client can identify and whom he or she respects. Nurses can be models of wellness by demonstrating good health habits.

Evaluating

Evaluation of the plan is an ongoing, collaborative effort between the nurse and the client, both during the attainment of short-term goals and after the completion of long-term goals. During evaluation, the client may decide to continue with the plan, reorder priorities, change strategies, or revise the health-promotion contract.

Promoting Canadians' Health

Canada has been at the forefront of influencing health promotion. Canadian nurses must understand the historical development of health promotion and its significant contributions nationally and internationally. The goal of nursing is to promote clients' health and to reduce inequities in health. Canadian nurses must, therefore, possess the necessary knowledge and skills in health promotion to address the social determinants of health, to promote positive behaviour change in their clients, and to develop healthy public policies at the community level. Through the use of the nursing process (see Chapter 22, the section "Overview of the Nursing Process"), nurses work with individual clients of all ages, families, groups, and communities and help them attain the highest level of functioning (see Chapter 7, the section "Health"; Chapter 22, the section "Overview of the Nursing Process"; and the Lifespan Considerations box in this chapter).

Lifespan Considerations

Factors Affecting Health Promotion and Illness Prevention

CHILDREN

Childhood obesity is becoming a serious health problem. In 2004, Statistics Canada reported that 26% of children and youth aged 2 to 17 years were overweight, and 8% were obese. Between 1979 and 2004, rates of overweight and obesity among 2- to 5-year-olds increased by 21%; they doubled among 6- to 17-year-olds and tripled among adolescents aged 12 to 17 years (Shields, 2005).

Obesity and overweight in children contribute to long-term health problems, such as heart disease and diabetes mellitus. Healthy eating habits and adequate exercise patterns form the basis for healthy growth and prevention of too much weight gain in children. It is the responsibility of parents and caregivers to provide children with healthy food choices and an environment that makes eating a pleasure. Adults must be role models for their children, eating well and exercising regularly themselves.

OLDER ADULTS

In older adults, health promotion and illness prevention are important, but often the focus is on learning to adapt to and live with increasing changes and limitations. Maximizing strengths continues to be of prime importance in maintaining optimal function and quality of life. Factors to be aware of that might indicate a need for additional information or resources include these:

- An increase in physical limitations
- The presence of one or more chronic illnesses
- A change in cognitive status
- Difficulty in accessing health-care services because of transportation problems
- A poor support system
- The need for environmental modifications for safety and to maintain independence
- An attitude of hopelessness and depression, which decreases the motivation to use resources or learn new information

Case Study 8

The Canadian Medical Association conducted a telephone survey with 293 parents of children under the age of 18, between June 20 and July 9, 2006. Parents were asked to rate the overall health of their children. Although only 6% of parents gave the overall health of Canadian children an A grade, at least 40% gave their own children's level of physical activity and diet an A grade. Only 9% of parents considered their children overweight or obese, as compared with the 26% of children reported by Statistics Canada. Although these parents, regardless of their cultural backgrounds and socioeconomic status, tended to see their own children as healthier than other Canadian children, they endorsed implementing measures that would improve the health, diet, and physical activity of Canadian children.

Critical Thinking Questions

1. Why do parents see their own children as healthier than is reported by the government?
2. Discuss your roles in the prevention of childhood obesity.
3. Review key elements in the health-promotion documents in this chapter. Discuss possible health-promotion approaches to preventing obesity in children.

After working through these questions, go to the MyNursingLab at **http://www.mynursinglab.com** to check your answers.

Sources: Based on *2006 National Report Card: General Population. Final Summary Report* by Canadian Medical Association, 2006, Ottawa: Ipsos-Reid Corporation; "Overweight and Obesity among Children and Youth," by M. Shields, 2005, *Health Reports, 17*(2), Catalogue No. 82–003-XIE, Ottawa: Statistics Canada.

KEY TERMS

health field concept
health promotion
empowerment
health education
health protection
disease prevention
information dissemination
health risk appraisal
wellness assessment programs
lifestyle and behaviour change programs
environmental control programs

role of the nurse in health promotion
lifestyle assessment
spiritual health
social support
social support systems
risk factors
at-risk aggregate
wellness nursing diagnoses
harm reduction

CHAPTER HIGHLIGHTS

- Canada is a world leader in health promotion and has taken a sociocultural approach to examining what determines health.
- Five key documents have influenced health promotion in Canada: the Lalonde Report, the *Ottawa Charter for Health Promotion, Achieving Health for All,* the *Jakarta Declaration on Health Promotion,* and the *Toronto Charter for a Healthy Canada.*
- Health promotion is defined as client behaviour directed toward developing well-being and actualizing human health potential. Health protection is client behaviour geared toward preventing illness, detecting it early, or maintaining function.
- Health-promotion activities are directed toward developing client resources that maintain or enhance well-being. Health-protection activities are geared toward preventing specific diseases, such as immunization to prevent poliomyelitis.
- Health promotion includes (1) information dissemination, (2) health appraisal and wellness assessment, (3) lifestyle and behaviour change, and (4) environmental control programs. These programs can be carried out in the home, schools, community centres, hospitals, and worksites.
- Pender's health-promotion model depicts the multidimensional nature of persons interacting with their interpersonal and physical environments as they pursue health. The major motivational variables that are modifiable through nursing interventions include perceived benefits of action, perceived barriers to action, perceived self-efficacy, activity-related affect, interpersonal influences, and situational influences.
- Prochaska et al. proposed a six-stage model for health behaviour change: (1) precontemplation, (2) contemplation, (3) preparation, (4) action, (5) maintenance, and (6) termination. If a person is not successful in changing behaviour, relapse occurs. At any point in these stages, people can move to any previous stage. An understanding of these stages enables the nurse to provide appropriate nursing interventions.
- The nurse's role in health promotion is to act as a facilitator of the process of assessing, planning, implementing, evaluating, and understanding health. Nurses seek opportunities to strengthen the profession's influence on health promotion, disseminate information that promotes an educated public, and help individuals and communities to change long-standing adverse health behaviours.
- A complete and accurate assessment of the individual's health status is basic to health promotion. Assessments or reviews of a client's spiritual health, social support, health beliefs, and life stress are also important because they affect a person's health.
- Health-promotion activities are mutually planned and directed according to the client's needs, desires, and priorities.
- The nurse provides ongoing support and supplies additional information and education in order to help individuals change their lifestyles or health behaviours.
- During the evaluation phase of the health-promotion process, the nurse assists clients in determining whether they will continue with the plan, reorder priorities, or revise the plan.
- As role models for their clients, nurses should develop attitudes and behaviours that reflect healthy lifestyles.

ASSESS YOUR LEARNING

1. Which of the following is the aim of health promotion?
   - **a.** Reduce premature death
   - **b.** Empower and expand positive potential for health
   - **c.** Minimize the occurrence of harms to health and well-being
   - **d.** Avoid illness and maintain health functioning
2. Which of the following is a health-promotion priority today?
   - **a.** Securing an infrastructure for health promotion and consolidating and expanding partnerships for health
   - **b.** Developing personal skills and orienting health services
   - **c.** Developing population health models
   - **d.** Creating new determinants of health
3. Using a condom during sexual activity is an example of which if the following?
   - **a.** Health promotion
   - **b.** Health protection
   - **c.** Disease prevention
   - **d.** Empowerment

4. What is the best way for the nurse to promote safe sexual practices in a group of adolescents?
   a. Provide condoms.
   b. Encourage abstinence.
   c. Teach ways to prevent pregnancy.
   d. Teach safe sex practices.

5. Which of the following statements reflects the contemplation stage of behaviour change?
   a. "I currently do not exercise 30 minutes three times a week and do not intend to start in the next 6 months."
   b. "I have tried several times to exercise 30 minutes three times a week but am seriously thinking of trying again in the next month."
   c. "I currently do not exercise 30 minutes three times a week, but I am thinking about starting to do so in the next 6 months."
   d. "I have exercised 30 minutes three times a week regularly for more than 6 months."

6. A female client is 20 kg overweight. She previously attended two programs that guaranteed weight loss. Although she lost the weight, she gained it back and more after each program. She tells you, "I was just born to be fat. I don't have the willpower." According to Pender's health-promotion model, the nurse should focus on which of the following behaviour-specific cognition and affect variables for this client?
   a. Perceived barriers to action
   b. Perceived self-efficacy
   c. Interpersonal influences
   d. Situational influences

7. If a client fails to follow the information or teaching provided, how should the nurse respond?
   a. Give up, since the client does not want to change his behaviour.
   b. Tell the client that he must follow your instructions.
   c. Act as the role model for the client so that he can imitate the expected behaviour.
   d. Assess what the barriers are and allow the client to determine what he can or will do.

8. Which of the following individuals would have an increased possibility of illness in the near future?
   a. A 25-year-old man who recently married his high school sweetheart
   b. A 35-year-old man who was fired from his job
   c. A 40-year-old woman who started a nursing program
   d. A 50-year-old woman whose husband died a month ago

9. A client is very worried about how his business is doing while he is hospitalized. He spends much time on the phone and with colleagues instead of resting. To promote the client's health, what should the nurse do first?
   a. Assess the client's physiological needs.
   b. Assess the client's perception of his health status.
   c. Discuss with the client the plans for the needed behavioural change.
   d. Eliminate stress and distraction by offering the client a private room.

10. Which of the following provides data that indicate whether the person has an increased chance of acquiring a specific disease?
   a. Lifestyle assessment
   b. Health risk appraisal
   c. Health beliefs review
   d. Health education

After working through these questions, go to the MyNursingLab at ***http://www.mynursinglab.com*** *to check your answers and see explanations.*

SUGGESTED READINGS

Maville, J. A., & Huerta, C. G. (2008). *Health promotion in nursing* (2nd ed.). Clifton Park, NY: Thomson Delmar Learning.

This book provides a comprehensive view of health promotion. It includes conceptual frameworks, theoretical approaches to health promotion, relevant nursing concepts, and health-promotion interventions and strategies throughout the life cycle.

O'Neill, M., Pederson, A., Dupéré, S., & Rootman, I. (2007). *Health promotion in Canada: Critical perspectives* (2nd ed.). Toronto: Canadian Scholars' Press.

This book provides a detailed account of health promotion, both globally and nationally. It challenges the readers to analyze various issues and perspectives related to the current state of health promotion and for the future of humanity.

WEBLINKS

Centre for Health Promotion: University of Toronto

http://www.utoronto.ca/chp/

This health-promotion site is internationally recognized for leading and linking community and academia into partnership in education, evaluation, and research. It develops and evaluates innovative health-promotion approaches and best practice guidelines and conducts various health promotion educational programs.

Public Health Agency of Canada

http://www.phac-aspc.gc.ca/new_e.html

The role of this federal website is to promote and protect the health of Canadians through leadership, partnership, innovation, and action in public health through dissemination of latest comprehensive information, resources, and government releases.

Health Canada

http://www.hc-sc.gc.ca

A federal government site that provides health information, related issues, and resources to help Canadians to maintain and improve their health.

Ontario Ministry of Health Promotion

http://www.mhp.gov.on.ca/english/about.asp

Established in 2005, this site provides information that targets specific sectors of society. It aims to help Ontarians live healthier by making healthy choices and choosing healthy lifestyles.

REFERENCES

Canadian Nurses Association. (2002). *Hepatitis C—A nursing guide.* Ottawa: Author.

Community Health Nurses Association of Canada. (2003). *Community health nursing standards of practice.* Retrieved March 21, 2008, from http://www.chnac.ca/index.php?option=com_content&task=view&id=19&Itemid=36

Epp, J. (1986). *Achieving health for all: A framework for health promotion.* Ottawa: Health and Welfare Canada.

Federal, Provincial, and Territorial Advisory Committee on Population Health. (1994). *Toward a healthy future: Second report on the health of Canadians.* Ottawa: Minister of Public Works and Government Services Canada.

Hamilton, N., & Bhatti, T. (1996). *Population health promotion: An integrated model of population health and health promotion.* Ottawa: Health Canada, Health Promotion and Development Division.

Health Canada. (2005). *Health protection and promotion.* Retrieved November 20, 2007, from http://www.hc-sc.gc.ca/sr-sr/activ/protection/index_e.html

Kirby, M. (2003, November). *Reforming health protection and promotion in Canada: Time to act. The standing Senate committee on social affairs, science and technology.* Retrieved November 20, 2006, from http://www.parl.gc.ca/37/2/parlbus/commbus/senate/com-e/soci-e/rep-e/repfinnov03-e.htm

Labonte, R. (1992). *Determinants of health: Empowering strategies for nursing practice.* Vancouver, BC: Registered Nurses Association of British Columbia.

Lalonde, M. (1974). *A new perspective on the health of Canadians.* Ottawa: Government of Canada.

Leavell, H. R., & Clark, E. G. (1965). *Preventive medicine for the doctor in the community* (3rd ed.). New York: McGraw-Hill.

O'Neill, M., & Dupéré, S. (2005, April). Health promotion: The next generations. *Reviews of Health Promotion and Education Online,* Article 10. Retrieved July 6, 2006, from http://www.rhpeo.org/reviews/2005/10/index.htm

Pender, N. J., Murdaugh, C. L., & Parsons, M. A. (2006). *Health promotion in nursing practice* (5th ed.). Upper Saddle River, NJ: Prentice Hall.

Prochaska, J. O., Redding, C. A., & Evers, K. E. (2002). The transtheoretical model and stages of change (pp. 99–120). In K. Glanz, B. K. Rimer, & F. M. Lewis (Eds.), *Health behavior and health education: Theory, research, and practice* (3rd ed.). San Francisco, CA: Jossey-Bass.

Raeburn J., & Rootman, I. (1998). *People-centered health promotion.* Chichester, UK: John Wiley & Sons.

Raphael, D., & Curry-Stevens, A. (2003). *The Toronto charter for a healthy Canada.* Toronto: York University School of Health Policy and Management and the Centre for Social Justice. Retrieved November 20, 2006, from http://quartz.atkinson.yorku.ca/QuickPlace/draphael/Main.nsf/h_Index/DD7BEC96FA3D0DAF85256CD9005F5534/?OpenDocument

Shields, M. (2005). *Measured obesity: Overweight Canadian children and adolescents. Nutrition: Findings from the Canadian community health survey: Issue no. 1.* Ottawa: Statistics Canada. Retrieved September 5, 2008, from http://www.calgaryhealthregion.ca/programs/childobesity/pdf/cobesity%5B1%5D.pdf.

Stamler, L., & Yiu, L. (2008). *Community health nursing: A Canadian perspective* (2nd ed.). Toronto: Pearson Education Canada.

Wallerstein, N., & Bernstein, E. (1994). Introduction to community empowerment, participatory education, and health. *Health Education Quarterly, 21*(2), 141–148.

World Health Organization. (1978). *The declaration of Alma-Ata.* Geneva, Switzerland: Author.

World Health Organization. (1984). *Health promotion: A discussion document on the concepts and principles.* Copenhagen, Denmark: WHO Regional Office for Europe.

World Health Organization. (1997). *The Jakarta declaration.* Geneva, Switzerland: Author.

World Health Organization. (1998). *Health Promotion Glossary.* Geneva, Switzerland: Author. Retrieved November 19, 2006, from http://www.who.int/hpr/NPH/docs/hp_glossary_en.pdf

World Health Organization, Health and Welfare Canada, & Canadian Public Health Association. (1986). *Ottawa charter for health promotion.* Ottawa: Canadian Public Health Association.

Chapter 9

The Canadian Health-Care System

A **health-care system** is the sum of health-care services provided by all disciplines. In Canada, the health-care system is considered a major contributor to the well-being of its populace. Although other comparisons can be made, the health-care system is often used to define Canada against other countries, countries in which health care is neither as advanced nor as accessible to their citizens. Health care is big business. It is a major source of employment, both directly and indirectly, as many companies supply goods and services to the health-care system. It is also a major source of government spending. Traditionally, the primary purpose of a health-care system has been to provide care to the ill and injured. However, health promotion, illness prevention, wellness initiatives, technological advancements that permit earlier detection of and intervention for health problems, and many other developments are changing the health-care system. The roles of nurses are also changing, both in response to health-care system changes and because of the need for ongoing beneficial health-care and system reforms.

OBJECTIVES

After studying this chapter, you should be able to

1. Relate the history of the Canadian health-care system
2. Outline the five criteria or principles of the Canada Health Act (1984)
3. Highlight the four essential elements of the patient's bill of rights and the social values underpinning it and a publicly funded health system
4. List the three original elements that composed Canada's social safety network
5. Define the impact of urgency-of-need determinations on gaining access to publicly funded health-care services
6. Describe the functions and purposes of the health-care sectors outlined in this chapter
7. Differentiate primary, secondary, tertiary, and quaternary health-care services
8. Report on the social, political, technological, and other factors that affect health-care delivery and influence health system reform
9. Identify the distinct roles and functions of 10 other health-care professionals and paraprofessionals
10. Describe four contemporary models of nursing care

This large and complex system of health care did not emerge suddenly or without precedent. The British North America Act (1867) established Canada as a country and laid out the respective jurisdictions of the federal and provincial governments. Responsibility for health, education, and social services was delegated to the provinces. As Canada grew through immigration, high birthrates, and industrialization, the population became more urbanized. Poor housing and sanitation, crowded living conditions, poverty, and a volatile economy contributed to already high rates of morbidity and mortality. In response, public health legislation was enacted to deal with infectious diseases, maternal and child health, workplace safety, and environmental sanitation. Churches and charities continued to provide hospital care (as they did before Confederation), and voluntary organizations began to emerge. Some of these organizations continue to serve the health of the public today (e.g., Victorian Order of Nurses, Children's Aid Societies, Canadian Mental Health Association). Municipal governments also became involved, often to assist those who were poverty stricken. The union movement and fraternal brotherhoods established benevolent funds, which members contributed to and could access in the event they were unable to work. These funds were the precursors to today's employment insurance program and workers' compensation.

The two World Wars (1914–1918 and 1939–1945) were instrumental in highlighting the importance of a social safety network. Many injured soldiers with permanent disabilities returned, needing health care and other forms of assistance. The wars also created a demand for services by the soldiers' widows, children, and senior parents, who had lost their sources of support. In 1927, the federal government implemented a cost-sharing pension program for senior persons in need. Rural municipalities were the first given the power by the Government of Canada to levy taxes to pay for physicians (through the Municipality Act, 1916) and then hospital services (through the Municipal Medical and Hospital Services Act, 1939). The Family Allowance Act (1945), however, was the first universal social program in Canada. It provided every Canadian family with a stipend for each child regardless of family income. Other universal programs that formed the Canadian social safety network included Old Age Security (through the Old Age Security Act, 1952, 1975) and the Canada Pension Plan (which came into force in 1966). Today, a comprehensive range of programs are in place, although many are no longer universal. The Canadian health-care system is one exception. It was designed as a universal program through the Hospital Insurance and Diagnostic Services Act (1957), which brought uniform coverage for these services across Canada, with the 1966 Medical Care Act extending this coverage to include physicians' services. In 1984, the Canada Health Act was passed, in large part to ensure universal health-care accessibility by outlawing extra-billing and other co-payments or user charges for insured health-care services. Each province and territory today has a health-care insurance plan that continues to be governed by the Canada Health Act (1984). This act provides for federal cost sharing, whereby the Government of Canada pays a proportion of the provincial or territorial costs of provided health care, on the condition that five criteria are met: **public administration**, **comprehensiveness**, **universality**, **portability**, and **accessibility** (see Table 9.1).

Although this social safety network was developed to meet the needs of individuals requiring assistance and to address the social values of compassion and equity, many social, economic, and other developments, including rising costs and demands for services, have challenged each program. In response to these developments, the provinces and territories have been restructuring their programs, including their health-care systems, although much of this redevelopment has been done to accommodate evidence-based practice and technological developments, allowing health care to be delivered in new ways with better outcomes. For instance, surgical and other developments have resulted in more people having day surgery, when only a few short years ago, they would have been admitted to hospital for a few days or even weeks. Complication rates and recovery times are much better with laparoscopic and other modern forms of surgery. Another major development factor has been changing views of how health is determined and how disease and injury are prevented. Intersectoral collaboration and public participation are strategies being used to create more equitable distribution of increasingly scarce resources and services. Efforts are being made to curb costs and make more effective use of health personnel and infrastructure through such initiatives as regionalization, integration, and devolution or shifting of hospital care to community agencies and families.

Increasingly, Canadians are paying out of pocket or contributing to supplementary insurance plans that cover enhanced (i.e., nonessential or additional and uninsured) health-care services; prescription drugs and home care supplies; vision, hearing, and dental care; care in long-term-care and other continuing-care facilities; and complementary therapies. These costs can be considerable, with low-income Canadians disproportionately disadvantaged by this shift, not only in health-care venues but also in health-care costs. Concern is growing over the right of all Canadians to access health care under uniform terms and conditions.

TABLE 9.1 Canada Health Act

1. Public administration	The public administration criterion, set out in section 8 of the Canada Health Act, applies to provincial and territorial health-care insurance plans. The act specifically states that to satisfy the criterion respecting public administration, the health-care insurance plan of each province or territory "must be administered and operated on a non-profit basis by a public authority appointed or designated by the government of the province; the public authority must be responsible to the provincial government for that administration and operation; and the public authority must be subject to audit of its accounts and financial transactions by such authority as is charged by law with the audit of the accounts of the province."
2. Comprehensiveness	The comprehensiveness criterion of the Canada Health Act requires that, in order to be eligible for federal cash transfer payments, the health-care insurance plan of each province or territory "must insure all insured health services provided by hospitals, medical practitioners or dentists [i.e., such as in the case of surgical-dental services that require a hospital setting] and, where the law of the province so permits, similar or additional services rendered by other health care practitioners."
3. Universality	Under the universality criterion, "the health care insurance plan of a province must entitle one hundred per cent of the insured persons of the province to the insured health services provided for by the plan on uniform terms and conditions."
4. Portability	To satisfy the criterion of portability, "the health care insurance plan of a province must not impose any minimum period of residence in the province, or waiting period, in excess of three months before residents of the province are eligible for or entitled to insured health services; must provide for and be administered and operated so as to provide for the payment of amounts for the cost of insured health services provided to insured persons while temporarily absent from the province on the basis that (i) where the insured services are provided in Canada, payment of health services is at the rate that is approved by the health care insurance plan of the province in which the services are provided, unless the provinces concerned agree to apportion the cost between them in a different manner, or (ii) where the insured health services are provided out of Canada, payment is made on the basis of the amount that would have been paid by the province for similar services rendered in the province, with due regard, in the case of hospital services, to the size of the hospital, standards of service and other relevant factors; and must provide for and be administered and operated so as to provide for the payment, during any minimum period of residence, or any waiting period, imposed by the health care insurance plan of another province, of the cost of insured health services provided to persons who have ceased to be insured persons by reason of having become residents of that other province, on the same basis as though they had not ceased to be residents of the province."
5. Accessibility	The intent of the accessibility criterion is to ensure that residents of a province or territory have reasonable access to insured hospital, medical, and surgical-dental services on uniform terms and conditions, unprecluded or unimpeded, either directly or indirectly, by charges (user charges or extra-billing) or other means (e.g., discrimination on the basis of age, health status, or financial circumstances). In addition, the health-care insurance plans of the province or territory must provide reasonable compensation to physicians and dentists for all the insured health-care services they provide; and payment to hospitals to cover the cost of insured health-care services.

Note: Since 1984, slight changes through re-interpretation of the act have occurred. These changes are outlined in Health Canada's annual reports on the Canada Health Act. One such change outlined in the Canada Health Act Annual Report 2001–2002 *was that reasonable access in terms of physical availability of medically necessary services has been interpreted under the Canada Health Act by using the "where and as available" rule. Thus, residents of a province or territory are entitled to have access on uniform terms and conditions to insured health-care services at the setting "where" the services are provided and "as" the services are available in that setting.*

Source: © Adapted and Reproduced with the permission of the Minister of Public Works and Government Services Canada, 2003. Health Canada assumes no responsibility for any errors or omissions which may have occurred in the adaptation of its material.

Rights and Health Care

The movement for **clients' rights** in health care arose in the late 1960s. Its broad goal was to improve the quality of health care, largely by making the health-care system and health-care professionals more aware of and responsive to client needs. Ultimately, clients wanted assurance of self-determination and control over their own bodies when they were ill. Informed consent, confidentiality, and the right of the client to accept or refuse treatment are all aspects of this self-determination. The need for clients' rights continues because of (1) their vulnerability when ill, (2) the complexity of relationships in health-care settings, and (3) the considerable uncertainty, coupled with differing value judgments, over the expected and probable outcomes of health care. Today, the goals of health normally include maximized autonomy and independence for the client, with good health considered a joint responsibility of the client, the health-care providers, and society. These goals cannot be met, however, unless clients accept active responsibility for their health and health care, and unless clients and care providers have respect for each other.

When people are ill, they are frequently unable to assert their rights as they would if they were healthy. Asserting rights requires energy, mental competency, some knowledge about the health problem and their care options, and an underlying awareness of a person's rights in the situation. In 1972 (revised in 1989), the Consumers' Association of Canada published the *Consumer Rights to Health Care* (see Table 9.2). Additional bills of rights have been developed since, which indicates continuing concern over the rights of clients to considerate and respectful care; the consideration of privacy for clients, including confidentiality of all records and communications regarding their care; and the right to make decisions about their care, including the right to refuse a treatment or plan of care. These concerns are occurring despite clients in all parts of Canada having the legislated right to make a statement about their care preferences, such as through a living will or advance directive, preferences that should be adhered to by all health-care organizations and health-care professionals, if permitted by law. Client preferences for assisted suicide and other illegal or criminal actions cannot be carried out.

It is widely understood now that clients have the right to refuse treatment, even when it is life saving; the right to review their health-care records and have them explained; the right to receive publicly funded health care, provided it is reasonable and appropriate; and the right to be informed of any business or other arrangements among institutions or people involved in their care. In addition, clients have the right to be informed of resources that can be used to resolve a dispute or grievance and of health-care agency policies and practices that relate to their care, treatment, and responsibilities, and to be informed of any charges or costs associated with their care options. Furthermore, clients have the right to have options explained when hospital care is no longer appropriate and to expect a reasonable continuity of care both within and across health-care settings when they are moved. Clients can also refuse to participate in any research study.

TABLE 9.2 Consumer Rights to Health Care

1. Right to be informed	(a) about preventative health care, including education on nutrition, drug use, birth control, appropriate education (b) about the health-care system, including the extent of government insurance coverage for services, supplemental insurance plans, the referral system to auxiliary health and social facilities and services in the community (c) about the individual's own diagnosis and specific treatment program, including prescribed surgery and medication, options, effects, and side effects (d) about the specific costs of procedures, services, and professional fees undertaken on behalf of the individual consumer
2. Right to be respected as the individual with the major responsibility for their own health care	(a) right that confidentiality of health records be maintained (b) right to refuse experimentation, undue painful prolongation of life, or participation in teaching programs (c) right of adult to refuse treatment, right to die with dignity
3. Right to participate in decision making affecting their health	(a) through consumer representation at each level of government in planning and evaluating the system of health services, the types and qualities of service and the conditions under which health services are delivered (b) with the health professionals and the personnel involved in their direct health care
4. Right to equal access to health care (health education, prevention, treatment and rehabilitation) regardless of the individual's economic status, gender, age, creed, ethnic origin, and location	(a) right to access to adequately qualified health personnel (b) right to a second opinion (c) right to prompt response in emergencies

Source: *Consumer Rights to Health Care,* by the Consumers' Association of Canada, 1989, Ottawa: Author.

Health-care professionals are obliged to advise clients of their rights to make informed choices about their treatment and care. The client should be asked about any advance directive (e.g., not to be resuscitated in the event of a cardiac arrest), and this information must be placed on the health-care record. If the law, the health-care organization's policies and programs or services, or the health-care professional's moral stance limits the implementation of any advance directive, the client has a right to be informed of this before any problem arises. See details about advance directives in Chapter 48.

If a client lacks decision-making capacity, is legally incompetent, or is a minor, these rights can be exercised on the client's behalf by a designated surrogate or proxy decision maker. Nurses are often advocates for clients in these and other situations. Nursing organizations, such as the Canadian Nurses Association (CNA), have also been advocates for clients and society through lobbying and through the development of position statements, such as the 2000 *Framework for Canada's Health System* (Canadian Nurses Association [CNA], 2000a)

Categories of Health Care

Health-care services are commonly categorized according to type and level. In Canada, health-care services are also categorized on the basis of urgency of need.

Types of Health Care

Four types of health-care services are often described: (1) health promotion and illness prevention, (2) diagnosis and treatment, (3) rehabilitation and health restoration, and (4) hospice palliative or end-of-life care. These can be linked to the levels of prevention discussed in Chapter 7.

HEALTH PROMOTION AND ILLNESS PREVENTION

In 1981, one of the most influential organizations globally, the World Health Organization (WHO), developed an aim that by the year 2000, all persons would be able to lead socially and economically productive lives. The overall goal was to ensure health for all individuals by increasing access to and distribution of health-care services; however, universal health care was not guaranteed. This lofty goal was developed in keeping with a series of Canadian documents that emphasized health and wellness, as opposed to illness care, and thus illustrated rising interest in and awareness of the importance of health promotion; the documents included Marc Lalonde's (1974) *A New Perspective on the Health Of Canadians*, the *Ottawa Charter for Health Promotion* (World Health Organization, Health and Welfare Canada, & Canadian Public Health Association, 1986), and Jake Epp's (1986) *Achieving Health for All: A Framework for Health Promotion.* (See Chapter 8 for a more detailed discussion on health promotion.)

Since the 1980s, more and more people have been recognizing the advantages of staying healthy and avoiding illness. Health-promotion programs address determinants of health, such as lifestyle, as well as physical, psychological, and social environments. **Health promotion** activities emphasize the important role that clients have in maintaining their own health, while encouraging them to maintain the highest level of wellness they can achieve. Recent transitions in health care also reflect a growing support for community-based nursing and health care that capitalizes on health promotion.

The health-care system also offers **illness prevention** and injury prevention programs. These may be directed at the client or the community and involve such practices as providing immunizations, identifying risk factors for illnesses (e.g., dietary habits or blood lipid levels for cardiovascular disease), and helping people take measures to prevent both acute and chronic illnesses from occurring. Illness prevention also includes environmental programs to reduce the incidence of illness or disability. Environmental protective measures are often legislated by governments and lobbied for by citizens' groups. (See further issues of safety in Chapter 30.)

DIAGNOSIS AND TREATMENT

Traditionally, the greatest emphasis of the health-care system has been on the **diagnosis** and **treatment** of illnesses. Physicians' offices and hospitals, on an inpatient and an outpatient or ambulatory care basis, are the major settings for these services. Community-based organizations are also increasingly providing these services. For example, community health centres and primary health clinics may provide maternal and childcare, mental health services, and care of clients with chronic health conditions (e.g., diabetes mellitus). Limited diagnostic technology may be available in these centres and clinics, but referrals for laboratory or diagnostic imaging services are offered. Some shopping malls and high-density commercial or residential areas have walk-in clinics that provide a wide range of services without appointment. Voluntary human immunodeficiency virus (HIV) testing and counselling is another example of a service that has shifted from traditional health-care settings to community-based organizations.

REHABILITATION AND HEALTH RESTORATION

Rehabilitation and **health restoration** is a process of restoring ill or injured people to more optimal levels of health and functioning. Rehabilitative care emphasizes the importance of assisting clients to function adequately in the physical, mental, social, economic, and vocational areas of their lives. The goal of rehabilitation is to help people move to their previous level of health (i.e., to their previous capabilities) or the highest level they are capable of given their current health status. Often, the aim is for the person to become independent, although this aim is impossible for some. If the person is hospitalized, rehabilitation will begin in the hospital and may continue in a subacute-care unit or rehabilitative hospital. Increasingly, with hospital stays that typically last fewer than 7 days and the majority of surgeries and other treatments done on an ambulatory care or outpatient basis, rehabilitation is taking place in the home. Rehabilitation can occur through such simple means as having the client resume self-care, but some clients will need extensive rehabilitative treatment and follow-up once their health has been restored or stabilized.

HOSPICE PALLIATIVE OR END-OF-LIFE CARE The term **hospice palliative care** refers to the provision of humane, compassionate care to the dying (see Chapter 48). Some nurses and other professionals specialize in hospice palliative care, with that care limited often to persons experiencing difficult dying processes, such as those with incurable cancer. Nurses who specialize in hospice palliative care may become credentialed through the CNA; these specialists are recognized as having advanced competencies in hospice palliative care nursing through the additional designation of CHPCN(C): Certified in Hospice and Palliative Care Nursing (Canada).

Approximately 5% to 10% of decedents in Canada received specialized hospice palliative care services, with the remaining 90% to 95% of decedents typically having received some assistance while terminally ill from nurses and others who are not hospice palliative care specialists. Increasingly, family members are providing **end-of-life care** in the home assisted by home care nurses. Some dying processes, however, such as those associated with a long decline in health through advanced aging or serious progressive chronic illnesses, require much more support, which is more often provided in a hospice or extended-care facility, such as a long-term-care facility. Nurses who provide hospice palliative or end-of-life care may do so within private residences, in local hospitals and other care facilities, or in specialized care settings, such as a freestanding hospice in the community or a palliative care unit in a hospital or nursing home.

Levels of Health Care

Health-care services can also be categorized according to the complexity or level of the services provided: primary, secondary, tertiary, or quaternary. See Table 9.3 for the levels of care and the kinds of services that may be provided by nurses at these levels. Services provided within one level of care can often be coordinated and implemented in many different health-care settings besides hospitals. Nurses play a key role in health-promotion activities and in providing primary health care, whether in the hospital or the community. Planning for nursing services in an institution or community must be approached with levels of care required in mind.

Categories of Need for Health Care

Although all Canadians can access the health-care system if they require any of the many insured services available, an assessment of their urgency of need for health care is the major defining criterion in Canada affecting the speed at which health care is provided and thus obtained. Physicians and nurse practitioners, as well as triage nurses in emergency departments, are charged with the responsibility of determining how urgent each presenting person's need for health care is. Different systems of classifying the nature of illnesses exist, but most are oriented to identifying whether the person has one of three categories of need:

TABLE 9.3 Levels of Health Care Classified According to Increasing Complexity

Primary care (first point of contact)	Health promotion Preventive care (e.g., immunizations, prenatal or well-baby clinics) Health education Environmental protection and risk assessment Early detection and treatment (e.g., physician office nursing and telehealth nursing) Long-term care Emergency room care
Secondary care (care from specialist following referral)	Diagnosis and treatment (complex)
Tertiary (settings of highly specialized skills, technology, supports)	Acute care Care of the dying in hospital palliative care units or hospices Rehabilitation
Quaternary (centres of highly specialized care)	Transplant perioperative and postsurgical nursing

1. *Urgent:* An urgent health problem is one that requires immediate treatment to save a life or prevent serious complications, such as in cases of myocardial infarction (acute heart attack) or a cardiovascular accident (stroke).
2. *Emergent:* An emergent health problem is one where diagnostic and often treatment services are required in the next few days or weeks, such as when there is a possibility of cancer, multiple sclerosis, or any other condition that could become serious in the near future.
3. *Elective:* An elective or nonurgent health problem is one that will progress slowly, if at all, or one that could resolve without health-care intervention. Knee and hip replacements for arthritic joints are common elective procedures. It normally takes many years for arthritis to progress to a state where a joint replacement requiring major surgery is indicated. Waiting for this surgery for a few weeks is not normally a health hazard, as the disease continues to progress slowly or not at all. In addition, waiting for this surgery allows time for the person to make living or other arrangements, as their postoperative recovery will be many weeks or months in length. A high proportion, as many as half, of all persons who are booked for elective surgeries and elective diagnostic tests do not choose to have these procedures performed. Unfortunately, many of these people do not call to cancel their booked appointments, leaving gaps in operating room and diagnostic imaging schedules, unless someone else can quickly fill in.

This determination of need, a resource-allocation and planning process, although difficult to understand for ill clients who want to have their health problem immediately diagnosed and addressed, is important for ensuring health-system efficiency and for containing health-care costs. People who have emergent and elective health-care needs have their names added to a waiting list, with their urgency of need clearly listed. People who have an urgent health problem are often sent directly to the emergency department or operating room, with arrangements made for care while they are in transit.

One example of a system for classifying the nature of illnesses is the Canadian Triage and Acuity Scale used by the Canadian Institute for Health Information (2005) to assess the appropriate and inappropriate use of emergency departments. For example, the Canadian Institute for Health Information (CIHI) reports that in 2004, more than one half of the visits to Canadian emergency rooms were for health problems of a less urgent nature. As well, almost 20% of adults who visited emergency rooms in 2004, when surveyed, indicated they could have received treatment for their condition at a physician's office (CIHI, 2005).

Waiting lists have been a long-standing method in Canada of ensuring both appropriate access to health care and effective use of expensive and sometimes scarce health resources, which typically is the newest diagnostic machinery. Although quality of life may be affected while waiting for emergent or elective diagnostic tests, surgery, or other treatments, the health of the individual is not normally affected. However, considerable concern over waiting too long for health care has arisen in recent years. This concern is valid when the health of an individual is affected by the wait. For instance, if the delay is too long in obtaining a joint replacement and the affected person develops a secondary health problem because of that delay, such as a bed sore or severe depression, then the wait clearly was too long. A considerable number of research investigations and other attempts at tracking waiting times and identifying appropriate waits for select health-care services have been conducted. This work is ongoing, as are approaches to reduce wait times for health care.

Despite waiting lists, the vast majority of Canadians needing health care get same-day service, as they can call a telehealth line for health care advice and information or can see a health-care provider in a physician's office, medi-clinic, community or health-care centre, or hospital emergency department. Blood work and X-rays or other common diagnostic tests will also be taken that same day if these are indicated. Furthermore, same-day service is provided if the health problem is urgent and also, in many cases, when it is emergent.

Types of Health-Care Organizations and Care Settings

In Canada, health-care organizations are numerous and care settings varied. Some organizations provide many services; for example, a hospital provides a wide range of inpatient and outpatient or ambulatory care services, including emergency room services. Some of these services can be obtained through community-based agencies. For example, specialized hospice palliative care can be provided in a hospital, the home, or another community setting, such as a hospice or long-term-care facility. The **continuum of care** refers to care given in a variety of settings from the onset of the health challenge to the point where the recipient of care no longer requires it.

A client can be categorized as either an inpatient or an outpatient. An *inpatient* is admitted to hospital and is expected to remain for 1 or more days of care. With technological and other advances, most hospital stays now are shorter than 7 days. A client who is an *outpatient* similarly requires health care but does not stay more than a few hours in hospital. The majority of diagnostic tests and treatments, including most surgical procedures, are done on an outpatient basis now. Although this shift to ambulatory care has greatly increased the efficiency of the health-care system, this shift has major implications for clients and their families; for instance, a person can become ill, undergo a number of diagnostic tests that diagnose a type and stage of cancer, have regular blood work and other cancer clinic examinations, receive monthly chemotherapy treatments, and then have 2 weeks of daily radiation for palliative pain-reduction and never once be a hospital inpatient. Traditional nursing roles and responsibilities have changed and are continuing to change in response to the considerable and ongoing shift of client care from the hospital to the home or community.

Clients, particularly those with severe or chronic and incurable health conditions requiring various forms of care over an extended time, often receive their care through a number of health-care organizations. This care and the location of this care will depend on their care needs, the availability of family or friends to assist them, the number and type of services or care agencies within their immediate community, supplementary insurance coverage, and many other potential factors. To address the health and health-care needs of an entire population, a wide range of health-care organizations have developed in Canada.

Public Health

Public health, a subset of community health, includes services that are numerous and varied, as they typically focus on promoting health and preventing illness. Depending on the needs of the people in the immediate community, public health offices may offer immunization programs for travellers, children, and adults; well-baby clinics and prenatal health programs; cancer screening and screening for other conditions, such as communicable diseases; education and support for persons living with a chronic mental or physical illness; a wide range of school programs, such as health education to prevent teenage pregnancy and other common age-based health issues, such as sports injuries; alcohol, drug, and gambling addiction detection and abuse services; water and air testing services; and so on. In some areas, the local public health office is also the site where people can request home care services for a person who needs assistance in the home and where home care employees report to work.

Public health services are provided through government (official) departments established at the local, regional (in some provinces with regionalization), provincial or territorial, and federal levels. Although their aims have considerable similarity, the health programs and services at the federal, provincial or territorial, regional, and local rural or urban levels vary according to the public health needs of the people over whom they have jurisdiction.

At the federal level, Health Canada (2008) is charged with the responsibility of "helping Canadians maintain and improve their health, while respecting individual choices and circumstances," and its goal is "for Canada to be among the countries with the healthiest people in the world." Public health is of concern to most Health Canada branches and agencies, which conduct and disseminate research findings. They are further engaged in policy and program development (or refinement) with regard to meeting the long-term needs of Canadians for health care, as well as protecting Canadians from avoidable risks through disease prevention and wellness initiatives. Health Canada is also charged with providing health-care services directly in some areas to First Nations and Inuit peoples. The federal government also administers a number of veterans' health services in Canada and has other departments that directly or indirectly support the health and well-being of Canadians. In 2004, the Public Health Agency of Canada (2008) was created by the federal government to "promote and protect the health of Canadians through leadership, partnership, innovation and action in public health." This agency focuses on health promotion, chronic disease prevention and control, infectious disease prevention and control, emergency preparedness and response, and public health practices to renew the public health system of Canada and enhance the sustainability of the health-care system. Among other services, the Public Health Agency of Canada is responsible for the National Microbiology Laboratory, the Laboratory for Foodborne Zoonoses, and the Pandemic Preparedness Secretariat.

In addition to the Office of the Chief Dental Officer, a Healthy Environments and Consumer Safety Branch, a Health Policy Branch, and a Health Products and Food Branch, the federal minister of health is also responsible for the Canadian Institutes of Health Research (2007), Canada's major agency for funding and directing health research. Thirteen institutes are charged with fostering needed research in defined areas and the use of that research in practice or policy initiatives; one of these is the Institute of Population and Public Health. The research that is conducted through this institute and the others is commonly oriented to health promotion and illness prevention or management. Nurses are often research team members or principal investigators, as well as institute board members and members of the scientific teams that judge the quality and importance of the many research proposals that are submitted in competition for potential funding.

Much intergovernment communication and program coordination occurs between Health Canada, the Public Health Agency, and provincial or territorial health departments. Contact is both at the political or top level through the elected and appointed federal and provincial or territorial ministers of health and chief public health officer, and at the front lines with the ongoing work of the many nurses and other personnel hired to support their department's mandate.

Provincial and territorial health departments are as broadly oriented as the federal health department is to public health and thus to supporting both health and wellness through health promotion and effective health care, although their mandates are confined to policies and programs or services on a provincial or territorial basis. Although all provinces and territories have similar public health and other health-care services, some differences exist. Some provinces, for instance, have established agencies specifically for drug, alcohol, or gambling abuse.

Regional health departments and local agencies traditionally have responsibility for developing programs and providing the services that meet the health needs of people living in or travelling through a defined geographic area, by providing the necessary staff and facilities to carry out these programs, continually evaluating the need for and effectiveness of their programs, and monitoring changing health needs. Client and service utilization information collected at this level is crucial for provincial or territorial and federal monitoring of public health and the efficacy of health care.

Nurses work at all levels of public health service, as direct-care providers, care coordinators, department or office managers, and policymakers. Nurses who are certified in community health nursing have met specific eligibility requirements, passed a written examination, and met a national standard of competency in public health and home care nursing. In Canada, expertise in this speciality is recognized with the initials CCHN(C)—Certified in Community Health Nursing (Canada)—granted by the CNA. (See Chapters 1 and 2 for more information on certification and competency, and Chapter 13 for more information on public health nursing.)

Home Care

Home care services are provided to people living outside hospitals and long-term-care facilities who need temporary or permanent assistance with health-care needs, such as complex dressing changes, or with activities of daily living, such as bathing. Home care was traditionally provided to seniors and younger persons with disabilities. Earlier discharge of clients from hospital has made home care an increasingly important aspect of the health-care delivery system. The home is now a common care-delivery site, with expectations that care at this site will increase. In addition, the scope of services offered in the home has broadened. Home care organizations provide education and comprehensive care to acute, chronic, and terminally ill clients. Nurses and nursing aides or assistants are the most common home care employees. See Chapter 13.

Community Health Centres

Community health centres are found in many Canadian communities. Most of these ambulatory care centres have a wide range of health-promotive, diagnostic, and treatment services. These facilities normally provide medical, nursing, nutrition, social work, laboratory, and radiological services. Some provide services to people who require minor surgical procedures that can be performed outside hospitals. After surgery, the client returns home that day. These centres offer three main advantages: (1) they are more accessible to clients and thus help in obtaining necessary and timely health care, (2) they are more holistic in their approach to health and illness, as they typically focus on more than just the presenting symptoms or health problem, and (3) they free costly and scarce hospital services for more seriously ill clients. Nurses in community care centres may have basic or advanced education. Nurse practitioners and clinical nurse specialists are often needed for their specialized knowledge and skills. The term *community health centre* has replaced the term *clinic* in many places.

Physician Offices

In Canada, the physician's office is the traditional primary-care setting in which first contact between clients and the health-care system has occurred. Although the majority of physicians have their own office or work with several other physicians in a group practice, the trend now is toward community health centres and primary care clinics in which physicians work with an interdisciplinary team comprising nurse practitioners and other health or social service professionals. Community health centres and primary care clinics are expected to provide a holistic range of health services, as compared with the more limited set of medical services that are often provided by physicians in their offices, in keeping with the fee-for-service schedule of payments that is negotiated by medical groups with their provincial or territorial health departments.

Clients most often go to physician offices for illness diagnosis and treatment, and also for routine health monitoring and ongoing chronic illness management. Medication prescriptions, either new or refills, are a common outcome of visits to physician offices, along with referrals for laboratory and other diagnostic tests, and referrals to medical specialists or other specialists. Increasingly, the aim of health care is to prevent illnesses through improving health and through better management of health problems to prevent acute episodes of illness and disease progression.

Nurses employed in physician offices have a variety of roles and responsibilities. Some nurses carry out traditional functions, including client registration, preparing clients for examination, obtaining information, and providing information to clients and other persons or organizations. Other functions can include obtaining specimens, assisting with procedures, and providing some treatments. In contrast, nurse practitioners and clinical nurse specialists may be employed to provide primary care to clients in stable or unstable health. Nurse practitioners diagnose health conditions that require intervention and plan and provide this intervention or make referrals to other professionals (CNA, 2002). They typically prescribe medications. Nurse practitioners and clinical nurse specialists (although their scope of practice is more limited) are expected to have a holistic and wellness orientation.

General or Specialist Clinics

The term *clinic* refers to health-care organizations that are managed by a group of physicians or nurses, with these normally situated either in a hospital or in a community setting. Many provide a distinct and specialized type of health service, such as breastfeeding support, midwifery, diabetes mellitus education and ongoing care, and burn and wound care. If based in a hospital, these clinics may still be called an outpatient or ambulatory care clinic, as they usually serve only persons not currently admitted to hospital as inpatients. Nurses in these clinics have a wide range of functions, in keeping with their education and their level of skills and knowledge.

Occupational Health Clinics

The occupational health clinic or office is gaining importance as a common setting for employee health care. Employee health has long been recognized as significant to workplace productivity. Today, more companies encourage workplace wellness by providing exercise facilities and having on-site offices for the coordination or provision of a wide range of health-promotion activities.

Community nurses in the occupational health setting have a variety of roles. Worker safety has been a traditional concern of occupational health nurses. Today, nursing functions in occupational health care may include work safety and health education; pre-employment and annual employee health screening for tuberculosis, hearing loss, vision or eye problems; and immunization information. Other functions may include screening for such health problems as hypertension and obesity, assessing disability and readiness to return to work, providing workplace discord counselling and crisis intervention, and planning pre-retirement or retirement programs. Businesses are realizing that occupational health clinics can be a significant factor in staff attraction and staff retention.

In Canada, occupational health nurses are typically registered nurses holding a diploma or degree in nursing. They may also have a certificate, diploma, or degree in occupational health and safety from a college or university. Nurses who are certified in occupational health nursing have met specific eligibility requirements, passed a written examination, and met a national standard of competency in occupational health. In Canada, expertise unique to this specialty is recognized with the initials COHN(C)—Certified in Occupational Health Nursing (Canada)—granted by the CNA. (See Chapters 1 and 2 for more information on certification and competency.)

Hospitals

Hospitals traditionally have provided a broad range of services for ill, injured, and dying persons. Most hospitals are open to any person needing the type of care that is provided there. However, military hospitals provide care only to military personnel and their dependants. Although hospitals are chiefly viewed as institutions that provide health care, they have other functions, such as being a resource for health-related research and for nursing education.

Hospitals can be classified by the services they provide. General hospitals admit clients requiring a variety of services; most often these are medical, surgical, obstetric, pediatric, and psychiatric or mental health services. Hospitals are becoming more specialized, however, such as when one hospital in a region becomes a maternal and child centre, with no other hospitals in that region offering these services. Some hospitals only offer a specialty service, such as psychiatric or pediatric care.

Hospitals are usually described as acute-care or chronic-care (i.e., long-term-care) facilities. An acute-care hospital provides assistance to clients who are acutely ill and whose need for hospitalization is relatively short term, for example, a few hours or days. Increasingly, with health-care advances, acute-care clients are requiring only a few hours of observation following surgery, other treatments, diagnostic procedures, or examinations. Long-term-care hospitals, such as auxiliary care hospitals, provide care for extended periods, sometimes for years or the remainder of the client's life.

The variety of health-care services that hospitals provide usually depends on their size and their location. Hospitals vary considerably in size, from small rural hospitals with only a few inpatient beds to large urban hospitals that may have as many as 1000 beds. Large urban hospitals typically have a wide range of inpatient services, one or more large capacity emergency departments, advanced diagnostic facilities and laboratories, day surgery units, pharmacy services, intensive- and coronary-care services, and outpatient or ambulatory care clinics. Some large hospitals also have ultra-specialized or quaternary services, such as spinal cord injury or burn units, organ transplantation programs, oncology services, and kidney dialysis units. In addition, some hospitals have problematic substance use treatment units or health-promotion units. Small rural hospitals are often limited to some inpatient beds, basic radiology and laboratory services, and first-response emergency services. The number of services that a rural hospital provides is directly related to its size, the educational and practice qualifications of the hospital's staff and physicians, the number of people who rely on it for health care, and its distance from an urban centre.

Hospitals in Canada have undergone massive changes over time, but particularly since the mid-1990s. One the most common changes has been a reduction in the number of inpatient beds, offset by an increase in outpatient and day surgery services. Some hospitals began providing innovative services, such as fitness classes, daycare for older people or terminally ill persons, and nutrition classes. Some hospitals even established alternative birth centres to make birthing more of a normal and natural life event. Within some provinces, regional health authorities have been given the responsibility for such changes and for the overall planning and provision of health-care services in their region. In others, the provincial or territorial government and local hospital or health-care boards are responsible for operating, planning, and policymaking for hospitals.

Another change relates to the client population. Most clients admitted to hospitals today are seriously ill and require complex nursing care for some time on an inpatient basis; others are less ill and may be treated on an outpatient or ambulatory care basis. With the increasing acuity (or severity) of illness among clients, general hospitals have virtually become complex-care centres.

Nurses in hospitals have multiple responsibilities, including coordinating client care, assessing and monitoring client health, providing a wide range of direct-care services, conducting research studies, orienting new staff, and educating staff for continuing competency. Management roles are often fulfilled by nurses, with nurses having responsibility for a hospital unit or department, increasingly as top-level executives.

Extended-Care (Continuing-Care) Facilities

Extended-care or continuing-care facilities (complex-care facilities in British Columbia) have more traditionally been called nursing homes or long-term-care facilities. Extended-care facilities include skilled nursing homes (for intermediate-level care) and extended-care facilities (for long-term care); typically these provide personal care for those who are chronically ill and unable to care for themselves without assistance. A new type of extended-care facility is one offering subacute care. Subacute care was developed for acute-care hospital clients who no longer need acute care but require additional rehabilitation for a few weeks before they return home. These facilities can become the client's home and, consequently, the people who live there are frequently referred to as residents, rather than as patients or clients.

Because long-term disability occurs most often among the seniors, extended-care facilities have programs that are largely oriented to the needs of this age group. These facilities are intended for people who require not only basic personal services (bathing, hygiene, assistance with daily activities, and so on) but also some regular nursing care and occasional medical attention.

Like those working in hospitals, nurses working in extended-care facilities have a wide range of possible responsibilities. Some assist clients with their daily activities and provide care when necessary, while others coordinate care and rehabilitation activities, and still others manage part or all of the facility.

Retirement Homes, Lodges, and Assisted-Living Centres

Retirement homes, lodges, assisted-living centres, and other forms of housing for seniors who require little, if any, assistance consist of separate houses, condominiums, or apartments for residents. Residents live relatively independently; however, many of these facilities offer meals, laundry services, the assurance of nursing care if needed, transportation, and social activities. Some centres have additional capacity to care for residents experiencing short-term or long-term illnesses. However, some facilities, such as lodges, admit and retain only residents who are able to dress themselves and are ambulatory.

Nurses in retirement and assisted-living centres provide limited care to residents; usually their work is related to the administration of medications, minor treatments, staff or client supervision, or the administration and management of the facility.

Rehabilitation Centres

Rehabilitation centres may be independent-living community centres, entire hospitals, or special units in hospitals or other health-care facilities. However, because rehabilitation ideally starts the moment the client enters the hospital, hospital nurses who are employed on pediatric, psychiatric, medical or surgical, and all other units help to rehabilitate clients.

Rehabilitation centres play an important role in helping clients to restore their health and recuperate.

Drug and alcohol rehabilitation centres, for example, help clients free themselves from drug or alcohol dependence and assist them to re-enter the community and function to the best of their abilities. Today, the concept of rehabilitation is applied to all illnesses (physical and mental), to injuries, and to chemical addictions. Nurses in the rehabilitation setting coordinate client activities and ensure that clients are complying with their treatments. This type of nursing often requires specialized skills and knowledge.

Daycare Centres

Daycare centres serve many functions and many age groups. Some daycare centres provide care for children with disabilities while their parents work. Other centres provide care for adults who cannot be left at home alone but do not need to be in an institution. Eldercare centres generally provide care involving socializing, exercise programs, and stimulation. Some centres provide counselling and physical therapy. Others provide hospice palliative care. Nurses who are employed in daycare centres may provide medications, treatments, and counselling, or perform other functions, such as management and education.

Rural Primary Care

Rural primary care hospitals were created in some provinces during the process of health-system reform in the 1990s. They provide emergency care to clients in rural areas who require stabilization before transfer to a larger hospital. Usually, basic laboratory and radiological services are also available.

Hospice Palliative Care Services

Traditionally, a hospice was a place for travellers to rest. Recently, the term has come to mean a homelike health-care facility for the dying (see Chapter 48 for more information on hospice care). Hospice palliative care, more broadly, is a type of care that may be offered in any setting, such as a home, nursing home, or hospital. Its central concept, as distinct from the acute-care model, is not saving life but improving or maintaining the quality of life until death. Cicely Saunders, founder of St. Christopher's Hospice in London, England, believed that the physical and social environments of dying people are as important as medical interventions on their behalf. Nurses who work in hospice palliative care may or may not have advanced education and preparation for this important work. Some nurses obtain CHPCN(C) designation.

Crisis Centres

Crisis centres provide emergency services to clients experiencing life crises. These centres may operate out of a hospital or a community organization, and most provide 24-hour telephone service. Some also provide direct counselling to people at the centre or in their homes. The primary purpose of a crisis centre is to help people cope with an immediate crisis and provide guidance and support for their long-term therapy.

Nurses working in crisis centres need well-developed communication and counselling skills. The nurse must immediately identify the person's problem, offer assistance to help the person cope or obtain needed help, and perhaps later direct the person to resources for long-term support.

Telehealth

Telephone advice services are now common across Canada. Nurses who are hired to provide telephone advice are often seasoned nurses, ones who can ask key questions to elicit needed information and can supply appropriate answers to the wide range of persons calling in with health concerns. These nurses also advise callers how to manage nonurgent situations at home and, in some instances, how and when to seek appropriate medical or hospital care. These services are typically available 24 hours a day, 7 days a week. Telehealth services greatly assist people at home who have a health concern and little or no knowledge about it. The number of visits to hospital emergency departments is greatly reduced in areas with telehealth, a benefit for both those who do not need to go to the emergency department and those who do need care in emergency departments.

Mutual Support and Self-Help Groups

Canada has hundreds of mutual support or self-help groups that focus on nearly every major health problem or life crisis that people can experience. Such groups arose largely because people felt their needs were not being met by the existing health-care system. Alcoholics Anonymous, which was formed in 1935, served as the model for many of these groups.

Providers of Health Care

The providers of health care, collectively referred to as the health-care team or health professionals, are health

TABLE 9.4 Roles of Selected Health-Care Team Members

Physician	Physicians prevent, diagnose, and treat human illness and assist in rehabilitation after the onset of disease or injury.
Dentist	Dentists diagnose, prevent, and treat diseases, conditions, and disorders of the teeth, mouth, and surrounding tissues and structures.
Pharmacist	Pharmacists help people to make the best use of their medications and to safely achieve desired health outcomes. Their professional practice emphasizes drug therapy management of diseases and symptoms and the promotion of wellness and disease prevention.
Dietitian or nutritionist	Dietitians plan, implement, and manage nutrition and food service programs in a variety of settings.
Physiotherapist	Physiotherapists or physical therapists are primary care health professionals who analyze the impact of injury, disease and/or disorders on movement and function.
Respiratory therapist	Respiratory therapists are health-care professionals who assist physicians with the diagnosis and treatment of lung disorders.
Occupational therapist	The primary goal of an occupational therapist is to enable people to participate in the activities of everyday life.
Paramedical technologist	These are workers who assist or complete diagnostic tests—such as radiology, laboratory, or nuclear medicine.
Social worker	Social workers promote social change aimed at improving conditions that affect the health and well-being of individuals, families, groups, and communities.
Alternative care providers	Chiropractors, herbalists, acupuncture, for example.

Source: *Health Personnel Trends in Canada 1995 to 2004*, by the Canadian Institute for Health Information, 2006, Ottawa: Author.

personnel from a variety of disciplines who coordinate their knowledge and skills to assist clients, families, groups, and communities. Their mutual goal is to restore a client's health and promote wellness. The choice of personnel for a particular client depends on the needs of the client. The roles of the categories of nurses are found in Chapter 1; Table 9.4 defines the role of selected other health professionals: **physicians**, **dentists**, **pharmacists**, **dietitians**, **nutritionists**, **physiotherapists**, **respiratory therapists**, **occupational therapists**, **paramedical technologists**, **social workers**, and **alternative care providers.**

Factors Affecting the Health-Care System

Today, people have greater knowledge about their health and health care than in previous years. They also have higher expectations about the health services they receive. Canadians expect up-to-date, effective, appropriate, and mistake-free health care. In the past, physicians made necessary health-care decisions; today, people usually want to be involved in these decisions, if not be solely responsible for them. Most citizens have also become aware that their lifestyle and their home or work environment have profound effects on their health. As a result, they desire more information and services related to health promotion and illness prevention. A considerable number of other factors are also affecting the health-care system.

Advancements in Technology and Evidence-Based Care

Scientific knowledge and technology related to health care are rapidly increasing. Improved diagnostic and treatment procedures, highly sophisticated equipment, and more knowledgeable health-care professionals create better outcomes for those who are seriously ill and allow for earlier diagnosis of health conditions that might otherwise have remained undetected until late in the illness, when death was inevitable or major surgery and long hospitalizations were needed. New medications are continually being developed to treat and prevent both chronic and acute health problems. The higher prevention, cure, and remission rates with cancer are but one example of the life-saving impact of these advancements.

Surgical procedures involving the heart, lungs, brain, and liver that were nonexistent as little as 10 years ago are common today. Recovery following major surgery has also improved in terms of both health outcomes and speed of recovery. Laser, laparoscopic, and microscopic procedures have streamlined the treatment of illnesses that required major surgery not long ago. Some surgeries no longer need to be done, as minimally invasive or nonsurgical techniques and medications have made them unnecessary. A prime example is gallbladder removal, which used to be a major surgical procedure involving a 10-day hospital stay and a high probability of wound infections and pneumonia. Although gallbladder disease is still one of the most common diseases in

Canada, it can now be treated either with medications to dissolve the stones causing gallbladder disease or through laparoscopic gallbladder removal, a day surgery procedure. Computers that improve client care and can store and retrieve large volumes of information in databases are common place in health-care organizations now. Health-care research is also greatly advanced, with the knowledge gained important for evidence-based practice improvements by current health-care professionals and in the education of new health-care professionals.

Clients are now more likely to be treated in the community or to recover at home after receiving acute care in hospital. For example, 30 years ago a person having cataract surgery had to remain in bed in the hospital for 10 days; today, most cataract removals are performed on an outpatient basis, with the person returning home with instructions for postsurgical care and medical follow-up. As a result of this shift out of hospital, some direct and indirect costs have been passed to the client or his or her family. These include the cost of medications and supplies that would be provided at no charge if hospitalized. Lost time from work and interrupted careers are indirect costs, as family members normally are needed for transportation purposes and for providing both pre- and post-treatment care in the home. Family caregiving may be long term, with the informal caregiver burden also linked to health issues for family members providing 24-hour 7-day-a-week care for chronically ill or dying loved ones.

Technological advances and specialized treatments or procedures also come with a high price tag for the health-care system, a prime economic concern. This cost is offset, however, by the cost savings that normally result from health-care advancements. However, it is much easier to cost out the price of a new diagnostic machine than it is to calculate the savings that arise from preventing some illnesses and treating others earlier.

Economics

Paying for health care has been an issue since 1966, when the Medical Care Act (the precursor of the 1984 Canada Health Act) was passed, containing a promise of 50/50 cost sharing between the federal and provincial governments. The health-care system is very much affected by the country's total economic status. Inflation and the economic recessions of the 1970s and 1990s brought increasing concern about escalating health-care costs. Canada's health-care costs have increased considerably since 1966, and they continue to increase above inflation. Many factors contribute to this increase, including the cost of not doing more to prevent illnesses and injuries, and the high cost of delivering health care in Canada. Although 80% of citizens live in urban centres, 20% live in rural and remote areas across 95% of Canada's land surface.

Other reasons for this sizeable increase in costs include the following:

- The cost of drugs and health-care supplies have been increasing substantially.
- Existing equipment and facilities are continually becoming obsolete as research uncovers better health-care methods.
- Additional space, sophisticated equipment, and other technologies are required to provide modern evidence-based care.
- Inflation increases all costs, including health-care provider wages and benefits.
- The number of people working within the health-care system has increased.
- The total population has grown and so the demand for health-care services has increased.
- Health-system inefficiency, notably minimal home care and extended-care services that would permit more care out of hospitals, have become common.
- Changes in illnesses have occurred; more clients have multiple illnesses and more are acquiring infections that delay hospital discharge.

Growth and Demographic Changes

In 1966 and 1984, when the two acts that sequentially formed the current health-care system were passed, the population of Canada was 20 million and 26 million, respectively. Today, there are 31 million Canadians, each of whom can be expected to see a physician at least once a year. Approximately 10% of Canadian citizens of all ages will require some additional health care, either in a hospital or in another care setting.

The characteristics of the Canadian family have also changed considerably in the last few decades. The numbers of single-parent families and alternative family structures have increased markedly. Most single-parent families are headed by women, many of whom work in low-paying jobs; they typically require assistance with childcare or when a child is sick at home. Divorce continues to be common, with more divorced or never-married persons entering old age without the assistance of children or spouses. Considerable geographic mobility also means family members may not be available to help. The birthrate is low, with immigration needed to maintain youth and working-age population levels.

Recognition of the cultural and ethnic diversity of Canada is also increasing. In 2000, the CNA (2000b) published *Cultural Diversity: Changes and Challenges* and, in 2004, a position statement entitled *Promoting Culturally Competent Care,* which acknowledge the increasingly diverse clients that nurses work with. Health-care professionals and organizations are aware of this diversity and are meeting the challenges presented by persons who have different languages, diets, social customs, illnesses, and health-care practices and beliefs. For example, more organizations are employing translators or ensuring they are available, and more are hosting workshops and other educational opportunities to increase cultural knowledge and respect.

Uneven Distribution of Services

Some problems in the distribution of health services across Canada exist. Two main considerations are (1) uneven distribution and (2) increased specialization. In some areas, particularly remote and rural locations, the numbers of health-care professionals and services available locally are insufficient to meet the health-care needs of individuals, families, and communities. Rural clients, such as Inuit and other northern residents, may need to travel long distances to obtain the services they require. For instance, small rural hospitals may no longer offer surgical or childbirthing services; this may be because of personnel and equipment shortages or health-care specialization.

Health-care organizations are becoming more specialized, with cancer care and many other services only provided in a select few larger organizations where economies of scale can reduce costs and where frequency of care delivery helps to ensure competent health-care practice. Because of the highly specialized techniques and new knowledge that have emerged over the past 30 years of research, an increasing number of health-care personnel provide only specialized services. They may be highly specialized technicians or technologists who have relatively narrow, exacting jobs, such as orthotic technologists, biomedical electronic technologists, and nuclear medicine technologists. Increased specialization is evident also among physicians, nurses, and other health-care professionals. This specialization, although beneficial in some regards, leads to fragmentation of care and to other concerns. To clients, it may mean receiving care from 5 to 30 different people during a hospitalization. This seemingly endless stream of personnel can be confusing and frightening. It can also lead to errors.

Providing safe care is very important. The Canadian Patient Safety Institute was established in 2003 as an independent nonprofit corporation, operating collaboratively with health professionals and organizations, regulatory bodies, and governments to build and advance a safer health-care system for Canadians (Canadian Patient Safety Institute, 2005). Nursing has contributed to these efforts through such initiatives as the CNA's *Position Statement on Patient Safety* (2003), and the *Patient Safety Resource Guide* (CNA, 2007). The Canadian Council on Health Services Accreditation is a national nongovernment body that assesses health-care organizations' ability to meet or exceed expected standards. This organization has health-care excellence as its aim. Health-care consumers are also more aware of patient safety issues because of media attention and are looking at health-care institutions to implement safety policies.

Access to Health Care

Rural or remote residency has been associated with higher rates of risk factors, illnesses, and death (CIHI, 2006). Reduced access to health care as compared with urban Canadians may be responsible for these higher rates. Low income is another common factor associated with greater health care needs (CIHI, 2004). Access to and thus use of health-care services is adversely affected by low-paying jobs, unemployment, and poverty. Although Canadians do not have to pay to see a physician or to be hospitalized, taking a day off for a medical appointment could be a day without pay for someone in a low-paying job without sick days. The transportation costs to access health care and the costs of out-of-hospital care are also disproportionately higher for persons with low incomes. Government assistance may be available, but the eligibility for programs and benefits varies con-

Evidence-Informed Practice

Do Persons with Chronic Diseases Identify Barriers and Facilitators to Health Care?

Spenceley (2005) conducted a systemic review of research examining barriers and facilitators to formal health services for Canadians with chronic disease. Thirty-one studies conducted between 1990 and 2002 were reviewed. The theme of the results was symmetry or balance. For instance, an identified barrier was lack of symmetry between client and provider, including fear of privacy violations; gender mismatches; and cultural, generational, or belief differences. In contrast, examples of facilitators included a trusting provider relationship, personal follow-up contact by provider, the sensitivity of the provider to client culture, or informal advocates who "knew the system." The research expressed surprise at the paucity of Canadian research examining geographic barriers to access, even in our least populous areas.

NURSING IMPLICATIONS: Nurses and other health providers need to examine their practice to ensure that the services available are sufficient and available to meet the client needs.

Source: Based on "Access to Health Services by Canadians Who Are Chronically Ill," by S. M. Spenceley, 2005, *Western Journal of Nursing Research, 27*(4), pp. 465–486.

siderably across provinces and territories. (See Chapter 14 for more information on rural health care.)

Climate Change

Awareness of climate change or global warming has grown. Examples of weather emergencies include Hurricane Katrina and the tsunami in Indonesia. These events cause considerable health impacts, and we can expect to see pandemics, heat waves, and more violent weather (Office of the Auditor General of Canada, 2006).

Population Aging and an Increasing Number of Older Adults

An increase in the number of older people is anticipated: from 3.9 million in 2000 to 6.9 million by 2021 (Statistics Canada, 2002). Seniors aged 85 and older are the fastest-growing population group; seniors in this age group are more likely to need assistance to remain in their own homes or to accomplish activities of daily living. Most seniors live independently; only 7% live in extended-care or other seniors' facilities. Chronic illnesses are more prevalent among seniors, although 3 of every 4 seniors aged 65 to 74 and 2 of every 3 seniors aged 75 and older rate their health as good, very good, or excellent (Public Health Agency of Canada, 2005). Considerable concern exists over the use of health services by seniors, despite 86% of the Canadian population being younger and potentially as likely to need health care. Some differences in health-care needs are becoming evident, as most persons living in extended-care facilities and 80% of all persons who require end-of-life care are seniors. Some differences in health-services use are also becoming more evident, such as seniors having higher rates of home care and longer hospital stays when admitted to hospital.

Older people are increasingly productive and active into advanced old age. They fulfill many important responsibilities, through volunteering, holding political office, heading boards or corporations, caring for grandchildren and ill family members or friends, and, increasingly, through maintaining paid employment (Health Canada, 2002). The feeling of being a useful citizen is essential to health. Special programs are being designed in communities so that the talents and skills of this group will not be lost to society. Other programs, such as seniors' daycare, are being designed for health-promotion purposes and for earlier detection and proactive management of health problems. These programs are often used by women, as they are more likely to live longer and to live alone.

Women's Health

The women's movement has been instrumental in changing health-care practices. Examples are the provision of childbirth services in more relaxed settings, such as birthing centres, and the provision of overnight facilities for parents in children's hospitals. Traditionally, many health-care concerns that are unique to women, both young and old, have been overlooked, as the focus of attention has been on reproductive aspects of health. One of Health Canada's responses in this area is the Gender-Based Analysis initiative, which recognizes the variety of factors that contribute to gender differences in terms of health and health care, as well as providing evidence of the effects of gender on the determinants of health (Health Canada, 2006).

Homeless Populations

The growing number of homeless individuals and families is a health problem, too. The homeless differ from those who are poor. The homeless are socially isolated, lack any type of permanent residence, and are often disaffiliated from family or friends. Because of the conditions in which homeless people live (e.g., in shelters, in parks, in tents, in cars, or on the streets), existing health challenges are often exacerbated and new health challenges, such as frost bite, malnutrition, and injuries, often emerge. For more information on poverty and homelessness, see Crowe (2008) in the Suggested Readings section.

Factors contributing to homelessness include the high cost of housing and the change from inpatient to outpatient care services provided by mental health organizations. Some homeless people have physical, mental, social, or emotional health challenges. Limited access to health-care services significantly contributes to their generally poor health. Tuberculosis, for instance, is more common among homeless people.

Political and Other Leadership

Other important forces of change with regard to the health-care system are political, nursing, and other leaders. A change in political party at the provincial, territorial, and federal levels is certain to bring about reforms, through task forces or commission reports (see the Nursing and Canadian Society box). Increasingly, leaders are using visions for health promotion and sustainable health care, coupled with evidence from research to plan policy and programs that incrementally change the Canadian health-care system.

NURSING AND CANADIAN SOCIETY

Fact	Implications for Nursing Practice
The five criteria of the Canada Health Act (CHA) are the cornerstone of the Canadian health-care system.	Nurses need to understand the criteria of the Canada Health Act and the health-care system to deliver effective quality care within it.
The Canadian health-care system has evolved into its present form over 6 decades. Saskatchewan, in 1947, was the first province to establish public, universal hospital insurance. Ten years later, the Canadian government passed legislation to permit the federal government to share in the cost of provincial hospital insurance plans. By 1961, all provinces and territories had public insurance plans that provided comprehensive coverage for in-hospital care.	Nurses' roles as client advocates are important in today's health-care system to ensure that the health-care needs of all people are served.
Canada's health expenditures stand fifth of all industrialized nations and Canada's system is the highest of all publicly funded universal health-care systems worldwide.	Nurses have a responsibility to be fiscally accountable.
Recent federal initiatives have included the Commission on the Future of Health Care, chaired by Roy Romanow, and the Standing Senate Committee on Social Affairs, Science and Technology (the Health of Canadians-the Federal Role), chaired by the Honourable Michael Kirby.	Nurses need to understand government initiatives that will affect health care.

Contemporary Frameworks for Care

A number of newer approaches to client care support continuity of care and cost-effectiveness. They include case management and patient-focused care. Continuity of care across organizations and care providers is increasingly important, as is cost-effectiveness.

Case Management

Case management describes a range of models for integrated health-care services for individuals or groups. Case management may involve nurse-physician teams that assume collaborative responsibility for planning, assessing needs, coordinating, implementing, and evaluating care for groups of clients, from preadmission to discharge or transfer and recuperation.

Nurse **case managers** may be hired by a hospital or another health-care organization to perform similar functions. They generally coordinate care for a specific client population, such as clients with chronic obstructive lung disease or chronic mental health problems. A critical component of their role is collaboration with other health-care professionals and the client to achieve established outcomes.

Case management can be used as a cost-containment strategy, as earlier discharge from hospital and avoidance of hospitalization can save costs. Case management often uses **critical pathways** to track the client's progress. A critical pathway is a plan or tool for the managed care of a client that specifies interdisciplinary assessments, interventions, treatments, and outcomes for specific health-related conditions across time. Critical pathways are also called critical paths, interdisciplinary plans, anticipated recovery plans, interdisciplinary care plans, and action plans. These plans can be developed for surgical procedures, emergency care, trauma care, and many other health-related interventions. They are usually used for high-volume-case types or situations that have relatively predictable outcomes. The pathways are designed in collaboration with members of the health-care team who are involved in managing the case type, and the pathways are considered best practices based on a body of evidence in that field. It is important to exercise clinical judgment when applying standard protocols and to refrain from using them as a checklist for all clients. Critical pathways are presented in later chapters.

Patient-Focused Care

Patient-focused care is a delivery model that emphasizes the client and his or her needs. The supposition is that if activities normally provided by auxiliary personnel (e.g., physical therapy, respiratory therapy, ECG testing, phlebotomy or blood draws) are moved closer to the client, the number of personnel and the number of steps involved to get the work done are decreased. Patient-focused care units often have their own admitting, pharmacy, laboratory, and radiology areas, although variations exist. For instance, breast screening vans go out to rural areas, and some regional rehabilitation teams or programs make regular rounds to satellite centres.

Cross-training, development of multiskilled workers who can perform tasks or functions in more than one discipline, is an essential element of patient-focused care. For example, a health-care worker may be taught to obtain a 12-lead ECG and perform phlebotomy, or individuals who are already certified in one profession can take on a second certification, such as medical laboratory and X-ray technology, nursing and respiratory therapy, and physical and occupational therapy. Because patient-focused care can result in the blurring of role boundaries, collaboration is vital during the design and implementation process.

A recent initiative is **interprofessional collaboration**, which has long been a topic in the practice arena and is now gaining momentum in the education arena. In light of this, Health Canada developed the Interprofessional Education for Collaborative Patient-Centred Practice (IECPCP) initiative in 2005. "Collaborative patient-centred practice is designed to promote the active participation of several health care disciplines and professions. It enhances patient-, family-, and community-centred goals and values, provides mechanisms for continuous communication among health care providers, optimizes staff participation in clinical decision making (within and across disciplines), and fosters respect for the contributions of all providers" (Health Canada, 2007, p. 1).

Models for the Delivery of Nursing

Contemporary configurations for the delivery of nursing include collaborative arrangements, such as managed care, case management, and patient-focused care discussed earlier. Frequently, delivery methods comprise components of more than one configuration. Box 9.1 describes the most common delivery methods used in acute-care settings: the **case method**, the **functional method**, **team nursing**, and **primary nursing**.

BOX 9.1 NURSING DELIVERY METHODS USED IN HEALTH-CARE SETTINGS

Case method	• One nurse is assigned to and is responsible for the comprehensive care of a group of clients over the course of a shift.
Functional method	• The method focuses on the jobs to be completed (e.g., vital signs, medication administration). • Personnel with less preparation than the professional nurse perform less complex care. • It gives authority and responsibility to the person assigning the work, for example, the nurse manager or team leader.
Team nursing	• The delivery of individualized nursing care to clients is done by a nursing team, led by a professional nurse. • The team consists of registered nurses, licensed (or registered) practical nurses, psychiatric nurses and assistive personnel.
Primary nursing	• One nurse is responsible for the total care of clients, 24 hours a day, 7 days a week. • Associates provide care when the primary nurse is not available.

Case Study 9

Rebecca Konapinksi is leaving the hospital after having major surgery. She is leaving the hospital with a drain that will stay in place for about 10 days. It is obvious in talking to her that she is apprehensive and worried about who will change her dressing when she gets home. Her two children are young and her husband travels a great deal.

Critical Thinking Questions

1. What is meant by continuum of health-care service delivery?
2. How might Rebecca's family and friends provide health-care services to her?
3. How would a nurse provide health care to her?

After working through these questions, go to the MyNursingLab at **http://www.mynursinglab.com** to check your answers.

KEY TERMS

health-care system
public administration
comprehensiveness
universality
portability
accessibility
clients' rights
health promotion
illness prevention
diagnosis
treatment
rehabilitation
health restoration
hospice palliative care
end-of-life care
continuum of care
physician
dentist
pharmacist
dietitian
nutritionist
physiotherapist
respiratory therapist
occupational therapist
paramedical technologist
social worker
alternative care providers
case management
case manager
critical pathways
patient-focused care
interprofessional collaboration
case method
functional method
team nursing
primary nursing

CHAPTER HIGHLIGHTS

- The health-care system has developed into a large, complex organization comprising a wide variety of organizations, services, and health-care providers. At the heart of this system is the client.
- Health care must be considered a right of all people living in Canada.
- Health-care services can be categorized as primary, secondary, tertiary, or quaternary, and grouped by type of service: (1) health promotion and illness prevention, (2) diagnosis and treatment, (3) rehabilitation, and (4) hospice palliative and end-of-life care.
- Hospitals provide a wide variety of services on an inpatient and outpatient basis. Hospitals can be categorized as acute care or extended care. Many other settings, such as clinics, offices, and daycare centres, also provide health care.
- Various providers of health care coordinate their skills to assist clients. Their mutual goal is to restore a client's health and promote wellness. This coordination can occur even when hospice palliative care is provided.
- The many factors affecting health-care delivery include health-care consumers, women's health, an increasingly larger population, advances in knowledge and technology, economic factors, fragmentation of care, increased costs, health care of the homeless, uneven distribution of health services, demographic changes, and access barriers to health care.
- A number of different nursing models are used, including the case method, the functional method, team nursing, and primary nursing.

ASSESS YOUR LEARNING

1. Alicia, a 24-year-old from Ontario was vacationing in British Columbia when she injured herself. She was given immediate medical treatment at the nearest hospital and was not charged any additional cost for her treatment though she lives out of province. This example best demonstrates which of the five principles of the Canada Health Act?
   a. Comprehensiveness
   b. Universality
   c. Portability
   d. Accessibility

2. John is diagnosed with a condition requiring a blood transfusion. John declines the transfusion because of his religious beliefs. This exemplifies which right of health-care consumers?
   a. Right to be informed
   b. Right to be respected as the individuals with the major responsibility for their own health care
   c. Right to participate in decision making that affects their health care
   d. Right to equal access to health care

3. Which types of health-care services have traditionally been emphasized within the Canadian health-care system?
   a. Diagnosis and treatment
   b. Rehabilitation and health restoration
   c. Health promotion and illness prevention
   d. Hospice palliative and end-of-life care

4. Which of these examples is considered part of primary health care services?
   a. A visit to an orthopedic specialist
   b. Screening for scoliosis
   c. Emergency room care
   d. Diagnostic imaging

5. Part of the responsibility of a registered nurse is to understand the role of health-care personnel involved in the different dimensions of client care. Wendy, an experienced RN, is working on a busy cardiology ward. One of her patients is being discharged home with a prescription for eight new cardiac drugs to add to his health-care regime. Which health-care provider might best be suited for the role of complex medication education?
   a. The registered nurse
   b. The pharmacist
   c. The social worker
   d. The physician

6. The Canadian health-care system is being affected by a number of societal and demographic factors. Which of the following statements is *true*?
   a. Most of the older people in Canada are no longer independent, with the majority living in extended-care facilities.
   b. Reduced access to health care by the rural populations in Canada may be a factor associated with higher rates of illness and death.
   c. Canadians are realizing the health-care system may not meet all their needs and therefore have lower expectations regarding the care and delivery of health services.
   d. Advancements in technology have decreased the amount of time spent in hospital and concurrently decreased care requirements from community health agencies and individual clients.

7. Team nursing is just one of many models used for the delivery of nursing care. Which of the following statements best describes team nursing?
   a. It allows for delegation of tasks to other members of the health-care team.
   b. It plans and delivers care for a group of patients on a 24/7 basis.
   c. It has the potential to result in the fragmentation of nursing care.
   d. It is the first point of contact for most patients within the health-care system.

8. Brian, a registered nurse, is asked to explain urgency-of-need categories in the Canadian health system. Which of these statements made by Brian suggests he does not fully understand how this system functions?
   a. "The urgency of need for health care is the key standard in the determination of the speed at which health care is delivered."
   b. "The urgency-of-need system is both a planning and a resource-allocation process."
   c. "Patients whose conditions are classified as emergent are often sent directly to the emergency room or operation room for care."
   d. "Waiting lists are the accepted standard of ensuring suitable access to health care and effective use of resources."

9. Over the past decade, there has been a greater shift from inpatient hospital care to care in the outpatient or community arena. This change has also resulted in which of the following?
   a. An increase in out-of-pocket expenses for individual consumers and families
   b. A decrease in the availability of treatments requiring sophisticated equipment
   c. A decreased requirement for nurses to work in the hospital setting
   d. A decrease in the number of extended-care facilities required for the population

10. Which of the following is an example of an illness- and injury-prevention program?
   a. Analysis of motor vehicle collisions
   b. Use of occupational protective equipment
   c. Teaching crutch walking in an ambulatory care clinic
   d. Support group for women with breast cancer

After working through these questions, go to the MyNursingLab at ***http://www.mynursinglab.com*** *to check your answers and see explanations.*

SUGGESTED READINGS

Crowe, C. (2008). Poverty, hunger and homelessness. In L. L. Stamler & L. Yiu (Eds.), *Community health nursing: A Canadian perspective* (2nd ed.) (pp. 377–384). Toronto: Pearson Education Canada.

This chapter is written by a nurse advocate for the homeless.

Paluck, E., Williamson, D., Milligan, C. D., & Frankish, C. J. (2001). The use of population health and health promotion research by health regions in Canada. *Canadian Journal of Public Health, 92*(1), 19–23.

This study looks at the use of evidence-based decision making by using population health data by region in Canada.

Shamian, J., & Griffin, P. (2003). Translating research into health policy. *Canadian Journal of Nursing Research, 35*(3), 45–52.

These authors talk about the Office of Nursing Policy in Health Canada and the increase in funding for nursing research. They propose that the most important aspect of nursing research is its influence on changing and developing health policy based on that evidence.

WEBLINKS

Canadian Council on Health Services Accreditation

http://www.cchsa.ca

The Canadian Council on Health Services Accreditation is a national nongovernment body that assesses health-care organizations' ability to meet or exceed expected standards.

Canadian Healthcare Association

http://www.cha.ca

The Canadian Healthcare Association is a federation of provincial and territorial hospital and health-care organizations.

Canadian Nurses Association

http://www.cna-aiic.ca

This site provides access to the position statements and other publications of this national nursing organization.

Canadian Occupational Health Nurses Association

http://www.cohna-aciist.ca

The site is sponsored by and speaks for Occupational Health Nurses in Canada.

Canadian Public Health Association

http://www.cpha.ca

The Canadian Public Health Association advocates for improvements to health care according to the principles of disease prevention, health promotion and protection, and healthy public policy.

Commission on the Future of Health Care in Canada

http://www.hc-sc.gc.ca/english/care/romanow/index1.html

Chaired by Roy Romanow, the mandate of the Commission on the Future of Health Care in Canada was "to ensure that our health system meets the challenges of the 21st century." The site provides access to the work of the Commission.

Health Canada

http://www.hc-sc.gc.ca

This is a site of the federal government and provides access to national legislation, policy statements, and related health-care information.

REFERENCES

Canada Health Act (R.S., 1985, c. C-6).

Canadian Institute for Health Information. (2004). *Improving the health of Canadians.* Ottawa: Author.

Canadian Institute for Health Information. (2005). *Understanding emergency department wait time.* Ottawa: Author.

Canadian Institute for Health Information. (2006). *How healthy are rural Canadians? An assessment of their health status and health determinants.* Ottawa: Author.

Canadian Institutes of Health Research. (2007). *CIHR institutes.* Retrieved December 10, 2007, from http://www.cihr-irsc.gc.ca/e/9466.html

Canadian Nurses Association. (2000a) *Position statement. Framework for Canada's health system.* Retrieved December 10, 2007, from http://cna-aiic.ca/CNA/documents/pdf/publications/PS41_Framework_Canadas_Health_System_June_2000_e.pdf

Canadian Nurses Association. (2000b). *Cultural diversity: Challenges and changes. NursingNow, 7.* Retrieved April 15, 2008, from http://www.cna-aiic.ca/CNA/documents/pdf/publications/CulturalDiversity_February2000_e.pdf

Canadian Nurses Association. (2002). *Fact sheet: Role of the nurse practitioner around the world.* Ottawa: Author.

Canadian Nurses Association. (2003). *Position statement: Patient safety.* Ottawa: Author.

Canadian Nurses Association. (2004). *Position statement: Promoting culturally competent care.* Ottawa: Author.

Canadian Nurses Association. (2007). *Patient safety resource guide.* Retrieved December 10, 2007, at http://www.cna-nurses.ca/cna/practice/environment/safety/guide/default_e.aspx

Canadian Patient Safety Institute. (2005). *About us.* Retrieved December 10, 2007, from http://www.patientsafetyinstitute.ca/about.html

Consumers' Association of Canada. (1989). *Consumer rights to health care.* Ottawa: Author.

Epp, J. (1986). *Achieving health for all: a framework for health promotion.* Ottawa: Health and Welfare Canada.

Health Canada. (2002). *Canada's aging population.* Ottawa: Author.

Health Canada. (2006). *Gender-based analysis.* Retrieved December 10, 2007, from http://www.hc-sc.gc.ca/hl-vs/pubs/women-femmes/gender-sexes_e.html

Health Canada. (2007). *Interprofessional education for collaborative patient-centred practice.* Retrieved September 6, 2008, from http://www.hc-sc.gc.ca/hcs-sss/hhr-rhs/strateg/interprof/index-eng.php

Health Canada. (2008). *About Health Canada.* Retrieved December 10, 2007, from http://www.hc-sc.gc.ca/ahc-asc/index_e.html

Lalonde, M. (1974). *A new perspective on the health of Canadians.* Ottawa: Government of Canada.

Office of the Auditor General of Canada. (2006). *2006 report on climate change.* Ottawa: Author.

Public Health Agency of Canada. (2005). *Canada's seniors at a glance.* Retrieved December 10, 2007, from http://www.phac-aspc.gc.ca/seniors-aines/pubs/seniors_at_glance/poster2_e.html

Public Health Agency of Canada. (2008). *About the agency: Mission, vision and values.* Retrieved December 10, 2007, from http://www.phac-aspc.gc.ca/about_apropos/index.html

Statistics Canada. (2002). *Profile of the Canadian population by age and sex: Canada ages.* Retrieved December 10, 2007, from http://www12.statcan.ca/english/census01/products/analytic/companion/age/contents.cfm

World Health Organization. (1981). *Global strategy for health for all by the year 2000.* Geneva: Author.

World Health Organization, Health and Welfare Canada, & Canadian Public Health Association. (1986). *Ottawa charter for health promotion.* Ottawa: Canadian Public Health Association.

Chapter 10

Culture Care

In this chapter, we explore all the diverse elements of Canadian culture. We examine culture as a concept and the cultural perspectives that can be used to guide nursing practice. Cultural knowledge, sensitivity, and resources are then applied to primary care and health promotion. A transcultural care perspective is an essential component of care not only for nurses but also for all health-care professionals who need to deliver quality health care to their clients. Madeleine Leininger (2006), a well-known nurse and cultural anthropologist, noted that "culture was the broadest, most comprehensive, holistic, and universal feature of human beings and care was predicted to be embedded in culture" (p. 3). Therefore, it is imperative that Canadian nurses be informed and become culturally sensitive and competent in order to safely care for the diverse ethnic and Aboriginal populations in Canada.

OBJECTIVES

After studying this chapter, you should be able to

1. Describe the concept of culture
2. Describe cultural diversity and vulnerability in relation to the client, the nurse, and health
3. Differentiate cultural awareness, cultural sensitivity, cultural competence, and cultural safety
4. Identify seven characteristics of culture and describe how they pertain to nursing
5. Identify components of Leininger's sunrise model, Purnell and Paulanka's model for cultural competence, Giger and Davidhizar's transcultural assessment model, and the medicine wheel
6. Describe and apply guidelines for culturally sensitive, safe, and competent health care
7. Describe four cultural barriers to health care and identify ways to overcome them
8. Analyze the different health views of culturally diverse clients: traditional healing, biomedical, and holistic
9. Identify factors related to communication with culturally diverse clients and colleagues
10. Assess clients from a cultural perspective and plan culturally competent, sensitive, and safe client care

Canada's Cultural Mosaic

It is important to understand the history of the peoples in Canada in order to truly comprehend and appreciate their diverse ethnic and cultural origins. Examining the historical context and national policies of Canada that affect immigrants, refugees, and Aboriginal peoples provides nurses with insight into the evolution of Canada's cultural mosaic, and ultimately lays the foundation to think critically about providing culturally safe, culturally competent care.

Canada has a long history of migrations and immigration; individuals from diverse backgrounds and cultures have come to Canada and called it home. The original inhabitants here were the indigenous or Aboriginal peoples. Theories conflict about when and how Aboriginal peoples arrived in this part of North America. One theory is the Bering land bridge theory, which speculates that the First Nations peoples crossed a land bridge between what is now Alaska and Asia. However, the Aboriginal peoples and their traditional teachings maintain that they are the first peoples of Canada and have existed here from the very beginning. Despite attempts to totally assimilate Aboriginal groups, they remain as distinct in language, culture, and ethnicity as are the more recent immigrants to Canada.

Early in the seventeenth century, Europeans established settlements primarily in Quebec, New Brunswick, and Nova Scotia. They also moved westward into Ontario, the Prairie provinces, and British Columbia. With the defeat of the French General Montcalm by the British General Wolfe in 1769, Canada became a British colony. By 1891, Canada's population growth was small compared with that in the United States. Canada's population of 4.8 million persons was distributed unevenly across its vast territory, with the majority concentrated in Ontario, Quebec, and the Atlantic region. With the completion of the transcontinental railway in 1885, all of Canada became accessible, from the east coast to the west coast. This allowed settlers to travel more easily and provided a means for farmers to export their grain. In addition, the dispossession of Aboriginal land rights through the signing of the seven numbered treaties in the 1870s enabled the federal government to open up the West to agricultural settlement. The closing of the American frontier meant that Canada could attract immigrants from the United States, Britain, and Europe.

During the twentieth century, three major migrations helped shape the present composition of the Canadian population. The first occurred between 1901 and 1912, when almost 3 million people arrived, mainly from Britain and northern European countries. By 1911, immigrants accounted for 22% of the population, compared with 13% in 1901. Between 1919 and 1931, only 1.2 million immigrants arrived in Canada. This decline occurred for several reasons: Canadians were involved in social policies that influenced the character of the country, including its immigration policy; the years between World War I and II was a period of immigration restriction and reduction; the Canadian government increased sanctions regarding certain immigrant groups; and the war-torn conditions of Europe left many individuals without the means to immigrate to other countries.

The second group of immigrants came after World War II, when hundreds of thousands of people in Europe were displaced from their homelands or were refugees. More than 1 million immigrants arrived in Canada between 1946 and 1955, with most of them still coming from Britain and other European countries. The third major migration began in 1977 and continues today. Between 2001 and 2006, more than 1 million immigrants were accepted into Canada.

In proportion to its population, Canada permits about twice as many people as does the United States. Consequently, the proportion of foreign-born individuals in Canada is more than 20%, while the proportion in the United States is 12.5%. Only Australia rivals Canada in its proportion of first-generation immigrants: 22.2% (Chui, Tran, & Maheux, 2007). The Atlantic provinces are the only areas in which people of British origin are the majority ethnic group, while Quebec retains French as the most common ethnic origin of its population. Statistics Canada projects that by 2030, immigration may be the only source of population growth in Canada (Chui, Tran, & Maheux, 2007).

New immigrants tend to settle in geographical areas that have individuals from their homeland; in a new country, the presence of others from a familiar linguistic, religious, and cultural background makes the transition to a new way of life easier. The vast majority, 97.2%, of immigrants entering Canada between 2001 and 2006 (Chui, Tran, & Maheux, 2007) settled in urban areas, with more than half in the large cities of Toronto, Montreal, and Vancouver.

Historical events and immigration patterns and policies have shaped the ethnocultural composition of Canada. In the beginning, Canada was dominated by French and British cultures, as a consequence of colonization. These two groups remain unassimilated by each other. Aboriginal peoples were also not completely assimilated, even though numerous government policies attempted to do that. Today, Canada is a multicultural nation in which a plethora of languages, religions, belief systems, values, and life patterns prevail.

Demographic Profile

A demographic profile of Canada includes statistical descriptions and analyses of its population; for example, the number of people in the country or in a region, or the number of people who speak both official languages. See Table 10.1 for information about the Aboriginal population.

In terms of the whole population, the results of the 2006 census (Chui, Tran, & Maheux, 2007; Martel &

TABLE 10.1 Population by Aboriginal Group, 2006 Census

Region	Total Population	Aboriginal Identity Population[1]	Aboriginal Population: North American Indian	Aboriginal Population: Métis	Aboriginal Population: Inuit	Non-Aboriginal Identity Population
Canada	31 241 030	1 172 785	698 025	389 780	50 480	30 068 240
Newfoundland and Labrador	500 610	23 455	7 765	6 470	4 715	477 160
Prince Edward Island	134 205	1 730	1 225	385	30	132 475
Nova Scotia	903 090	24 175	15 240	7 680	325	878 920
New Brunswick	719 650	17 650	12 385	4 270	185	701 995
Quebec	7 435 905	108 425	65 085	27 980	10 950	7 327 475
Ontario	12 028 895	242 495	158 395	73 605	2 035	11 786 405
Manitoba	1 133 515	175 395	100 640	71 805	565	958 115
Saskatchewan	953 850	141 890	91 400	48 120	215	811 960
Alberta	3 256 355	188 365	97 275	85 495	1 610	3 067 990
British Columbia	4 074 385	196 075	129 580	59 445	795	3 878 310
Yukon	30 190	7 580	6 280	800	255	22 615
Northwest Territories	41 060	20 635	12 640	3 580	4 160	20 420
Nunavut	29 325	24 915	100	130	24 635	4 405

1. Includes the Aboriginal groups (North American Indian, Métis and Inuit), multiple Aboriginal responses and Aboriginal responses not included elsewhere.

Source: Adapted from *Aboriginal Identity Population by Age Groups, Median Age and Sex, 2006 Counts, for Canada, Provinces and Territories and Census Metropolitan Areas and Census Agglomerations—20% Sample Data*, by Statistics Canada (2008). Retrieved May 16, 2008, from http://www12.statcan.ca/english/census06/data/highlights/Aboriginal/pages/Page.cfm?Lang=E&Geo=CMA&Code=10&Table=1&Data=Count&Sex=1&Age=1&StartRec=1&Sort=2&Display=Page&CSDFilter=250

Caron-Malenfant, 2007a, 2007b; Statistics Canada, 2008a, 2008c, 2008d) identify the following points:

- Canada's population has more than doubled in the past 50 years, from just more than 14 million in 1951 to just more than 31 million in 2006.
- The People's Republic of China was the main source country of immigrants to Canada in 2001 and again in 2006. In 2006, 14% of recent immigrants came from China, while India counted for 11.6%, followed by the Philippines (7%) and Pakistan (5.2%). Six of the top 10 countries of birth of all newcomers in the 2006 census were in Asia and the Middle East.
- Canada's national median age reached an all-time high of 39.5 years in 2006, rising steadily since 1966. Statistics Canada's demographic projection is that by 2031 the median age of the population will be 44 years.
- In 2006, the median age of Canada's workforce increased to 41.2 from 39.5 in 2001. This rise is especially strong in the percentage of workers that are more than 55 years of age, which increased to 15.3% from 11.7% in 2001.
- Chinese is the most common language spoken at home, after English and French.
- Aboriginal people are a young and urban population. The median age of the Aboriginal population is 24.7 years, 14 years younger than the non-Aboriginal population.
- Older Canadians are shaping national demographics: between 2001 and 2006, the population older than 80 years increased by 25%. Statistics Canada projects that the number of seniors (65 years of age and older) could outpace the number of children younger than 15 years of age within the next 10 years.
- The increase in visible minority populations has outpaced the natural population increase, increasing by 27.2% compared with the total population increase of 5.4%. In 2006, visible minorities accounted for 16.2% of the population, compared with 11.2% in 1996.
- Since the end of World War II, a substantial proportion of immigrants, in excess of 500 000 in total, have been refugees, coming from Hungary in 1956; Czechoslovakia in 1968; Southeast Asia, the Middle East, South and Central America, Africa, and, more recently, from Bosnia and Somalia.
- Discerning whether an individual is an immigrant or a refugee, that is, whether or not the move to Canada was a choice or forced is a consideration in providing culturally safe care.

Language

During each of the census periods, Canadians were asked to identify their mother tongue, which was defined as "the first language that a person learned at home in childhood and still understands" (Corbeil & Blaser, 2007). In 2006, more than 200 languages were reported, including Aboriginal languages. English was most commonly spoken at home, by 67%, whereas 21% of the population reported that French was most commonly spoken at home. One in five of the population in 2006

population reported that French was most commonly spoken at home. One in five of the population in 2006 was an allophone (i.e., mother tongue other than English or French). For allophones, one of the seven grouped Chinese languages was the most common mother tongue (18.6%), followed by Italian (6.6%), Punjabi (5.9%), Spanish (5.8%), German (5.4%), Tagalog (4.8%), and Arabic (4.7%) (Corbeil & Blaser, 2007).

According to the 2006 census, 81% of the new immigrants who had arrived in the previous five years were unable to speak either one of the two official languages (Corbeil & Blaser, 2007). This number was larger than at any other time in the twentieth century, a situation that put a strain on certain services, such as English or French language training and translation services, and posed challenges in the delivery of health care. Most of these individuals were women who lived in large households in urban centres, in large ethnic communities. Statistics Canada (Schellenberg & Maheux, 2007) conducted a longitudinal survey of immigrants to Canada and 32% of immigrants who sought employment in Canada identified language as a major barrier to employment.

Religion

The 2001 census identified 33 religions in Canada where at least 0.1% of the population reported an affiliation. Historically, the major religious denominations in Canada have been Christians, either Catholic or Protestant. In 2001, Statistics Canada determined that 43.6% of the population identified themselves as Roman Catholic and 29% as Protestant. The other religions most commonly cited were Muslim, Judaism, Buddhism, Hinduism, and Sikhism, with all but Judaism increasing significantly since 1991. About 16% reported that they had no religious affiliation, a significant rise from 1971 (12%) (Statistics Canada, 2003).

Visible Minorities

In Canada, non-British and non-French immigrants remained on the fringes of mainstream society until the middle of the twentieth century. The 2006 census collected information on members of visible minority groups in Canada, defined by the Employment Equity Act as "persons, other than aboriginal people, who are non-Caucasian in race, or non-white in colour" (Statistics Canada, 2008b). In 2006, over 5 million persons identified themselves as members of visible minority groups, representing 16.2% of the Canadian population. The numbers of visible minorities have steadily increased over the past 25 years. Indeed, visible minorities represented 4.7% of Canadians in 1981, 9.4% in 1991, 11.2% in 1996, 13.4% in 2001, and 16.2% in 2006. Ontario is home to more than half of the visible minority population (Statistics Canada, 2008c).

The rise of the visible minority population was five times the increase in the general population since 2001 (Statistics Canada, 2008c). The largest visible minority population is the South Asian group (4% of total population), followed by the Chinese (3.9%) and Blacks (2.5%). Other visible minority groups included Filipinos, who represented 8.1% of the visible minority population, Latin Americans (6.0%), Arabs (5.2%), Southeast Asians (4.7%), West Asians (3.1%), Koreans (2.8%), and Japanese (1.6%) (see Table 10.2).

The Toronto, Montreal, and Vancouver census metropolitan areas (CMAs) were home to 68.9% of the recent immigrants in 2006. Between 2001 and 2006, higher proportions of recent immigrants chose to settle in smaller CMAs. Fully 16.6% of newcomers in 2006 settled in the CMAs of Calgary, Ottawa-Gatineau, Edmonton, Winnipeg, Hamilton, and London. In 2001, by comparison, 14.3% of newcomers lived in these CMAs (Statistics Canada, 2008c).

Canada's Multicultural Policy

The multicultural policy in Canada was initiated in 1971 as a guideline for federal government policy and reflects the evolving nature of Canadian society. In 1988, the Multiculturalism Act was passed, guaranteeing multiculturalism as a legal entity and affirming its importance to Canada. As a policy promoting tolerance and diversity, multiculturalism was to be the opposite of assimilation, for to assimilate is to lose those characteristics that distinguish a group from the culture that surrounds it. Canada has been called a mosaic or an ethnically plural

TABLE 10.2 Visible minority population, by place of origin, 1996 Census and 2006 Census

	1996 Census	2006 Census
Total population	28 528 125	31 241 030
Visible minority population	3 197 480	5 068 095
South Asian	670 590	1 262 865
Chinese	860 150	1 216 565
Black	573 860	783 795
Filipino	234 195	410 700
Latin American	176 970	304 245
Arab/West Asian	244 665	422 245
Southeast Asian	172 765	239 935
Korean	64 835	141 890
Japanese	68 135	81 300
Multiple visible minority	61 575	133 120
Visible minority (not included elsewhere)	69 745	71 420

Source: Adapted from Statistics Canada (2001). Total population by Visible Minority Population for Canada, 1996, from http://www.statcan.ca/english/census96/feb17/vmcan.htm, and Statistics Canada (2009). 2006 Census of Population from http://www40.statcan.gc.ca/l01/cst01/demo50a-eng.htm

society because of the way it has absorbed immigrants. It has supported people in retaining a distinct sense of cultural identity. This is in contrast to the melting pot of the United States, where immigrants are assimilated into the mainstream of that culture. (See the Nursing and Canadian Society box for a summary of Canadian legislation and important facts on multiculturalism in Canada.)

An ethnocultural profile of Canada today shows a nation that has become increasingly multi-ethnic and multicultural. This portrait is diverse and varies from province to territory, city to city, and community to com-

NURSING AND CANADIAN SOCIETY

Fact	Implications for Nursing Practice
1960: The Canadian Bill of Rights barred discrimination by federal agencies on the grounds of race, national origin, colour, religion or gender. 1961: Changes to Canada's Immigration Act meant that fewer immigrants were European and the mix of source countries shifted to nations in southern Europe, Asia, and the West Indies.	These rights are legally protected. Nurses must have knowledge of the ethnic and cultural makeup of the Canadian population and use that knowledge to provide culturally competent and safe care.
1969: The Official Languages Act was enacted to protect minority language rights.	Clients have the right to have health-care services provided in either official language in any part of Canada.
1971: The federal government announced its policy of multiculturalism.	People are encouraged to retain their cultural beliefs and practices, rather than being assimilated into the mainstream culture. This means that nurses need to be culturally sensitive and incorporate appropriate measures into health-care assessment and delivery.
1982: The Canadian Charter of Rights and Freedoms considered multiculturalism to be constitutional and protected equality rights without discrimination (in particular based on race, national or ethnic origin, colour, religion, gender, age, or mental or physical disability). Section 27 explicitly stated that the Charter will be interpreted in a manner consistent with the preservation and enhancement of the multicultural heritage of Canadians; by virtue of this section of the Charter, Canada became a constitutional multicultural stage.	The Charter entrenches equality rights without discrimination, again obligating nurses to provide culturally competent and safe care grounded in respect for the self and client.
1982: The Canada Act replaced the British North America Act as Canada's constitution and also recognized the three main groups of Aboriginal peoples in Canada: First Nations, Metis, and Inuit.	This policy acknowledged the rights of the Aboriginal peoples in Canada. Nurses must have knowledge of and respect for the customs and beliefs of Metis, First Nations, and Inuit and integrate that knowledge into the provision of culturally safe care.
1986: The Employment Equity Act was established to achieve equality in the workplace so that no persons would be denied employment opportunities or benefits for reasons unrelated to ability; it established the principle that employment equity means more than treating persons in the same way but also requires special measures and the accommodation of differences; it identified four groups thought to experience disadvantage in employment: women, Aboriginal peoples, persons with disability, and persons in a visible minority (Canadian Human Rights Commission, n.d.).	This policy recognizes the challenges faced by Aboriginal peoples and other groups in seeking and maintaining employment, and hence the impact of unemployment on poverty and self-esteem. In assessing, planning, and providing care, it is the nurse's responsibility to consider the impact of poverty and self-esteem on the health and well-being of all peoples, especially those identified in the act.
Previous censuses have shown that the Aboriginal population is growing much faster than the total population. Given the younger age of the Aboriginal population, this trend is expected to continue (Statistics Canada, 2008d).	This rapid increase in the Aboriginal populations will have an impact on health-care services for both young and older adults.
Approximately two-fifths of the Canadian population have one origin other than British, French, or Aboriginal.	The fact that the Canadian population is increasing in diversity has implications for how nurses incorporate the changes in practice needed to address this diversity. The importance of culture is highlighted in the fact that this topic is listed in the 2006 Canadian Nurses Association (CNA) *Blueprint for the Registered Nurse Examination*, which parallels nursing competencies and standards of practice.

munity. Immigration over the past 100 years has shaped Canada, with each new wave of immigrants adding to the nation's ethnic and cultural composition. Half a century ago, most immigrants came from Europe; now most are from several parts of Asia. The number of visible minority groups in Canada is growing. Canadians listed more than 200 ethnic groups in answering the 2006 census question on ethnic ancestry, thus reflecting a varied and rich cultural mosaic (Statistics Canada, 2008c).

Culture as a Concept

COMPONENTS OF CULTURE Cultures are complex. Their facets relate to all aspects of life: language, art, music, values systems (beliefs, morals, rules), religion, philosophy, family interaction, patterns of behaviour, childrearing practices, rituals or ceremonies, recreation and leisure activities, festivals and holidays, nutrition, food preferences, and health practices. Many parts of culture (e.g., health and illness practices; attitudes about touch, territory, and privacy; childbirth; and death and dying practices) affect nursing practice.

Religious values are part of cultural values, and they can influence dietary restrictions, family planning, the use of blood transfusions, and death-related practices, such as autopsy, organ donation, cremation, and prolonging life. Understanding the unique values and belief systems of particular religious groups is important in providing culturally safe care. For example, many Orthodox Jews believe in prolonging life as much as possible and don't believe in cremation; some Aboriginal peoples practise traditional healing methods, such as use of the sweat lodge; many Jehovah's Witnesses will not accept blood transfusions; and many Jewish and Muslim dietary practices prohibit eating pork or pork products. These are just a few examples; however, in providing culturally safe care, the important nursing action is to conduct a cultural assessment and ask the client about his or her preferences.

CHARACTERISTICS OF CULTURE Culture exhibits the following characteristics:

- *Culture is learned.* It is neither instinctive nor innate. It is learned through life experiences from birth.
- *Culture is taught.* It is transmitted from parents, extended family, and peers to children over successive generations. Verbal and nonverbal communication patterns transmit culture.
- *Culture is social.* It originates and develops through people's interactions: families, groups, and communities.
- *Culture is adaptive.* Customs, beliefs, and practices change as people adapt to the social environment and as people's biological and psychological needs change. For example, the idea of the extended family still exits; however, the means by which families interact and communicate has been transformed, despite large geographical distances, by the World Wide Web, which facilitates instant visual and verbal communication. Messages can now be transmitted instantaneously around the world to children, grandchildren, brothers, sisters, mothers, fathers, grandmothers, grandfathers, aunts, and uncles.
- *Culture is shared.* This is true to varying degrees. Even though values, beliefs, and traditions may be shared, unique differences still exist for each individual within a cultural group.
- *Culture is difficult to articulate.* Members of a specific cultural group often find it difficult to explain their own culture. Many of the values and behaviours are habitual and are carried out subconsciously.
- *Culture exists at many levels.* Culture is most easily identified at a visible level. Rituals (e.g., funerals), dress, and celebrations are visual cues to culture that are easily revealed. Often, it is more difficult to find out about the more abstract concepts, such as values, beliefs, and traditions.

Definitions and Concepts Related to Culture

All groups of people face similar issues in adapting to their environment: providing nutrition and shelter, caring for and educating children, dividing labour, organizing socially, controlling disease, and maintaining health. Humans adapt to varying environments by developing cultural solutions to meet these needs. Understanding the cultural dimension of people is the focus of the field of anthropology. Cultural anthropologists attempt to understand culture by studying both similarities and differences among human groups. Nurses can use the cultural information gained by cultural anthropologists to understand and help clients (individuals, their families, groups, or communities) to achieve optimum health.

Culture is a universal experience, but no two cultures are exactly alike. Two important terms identify the differences and similarities among peoples of different cultures. **Culture-universals** are the commonalities of values, norms of behaviour, and life patterns among different cultures. **Culture-specifics** are those values, beliefs, and patterns of behaviour that tend to be unique to a designated culture, rather than shared with members of other cultures. For example, Aboriginal peoples' powwows, the date on and the way in which Chinese New Year is celebrated, East Indian Diwali celebrations, Robbie Burns Day for the Scottish, and Saint-Jean-Baptiste Day for the Québécois are all culture-specifics.

The terms *culture, diversity, ethnicity,* and *race* are often used interchangeably, but they are not synonymous. **Culture** is defined as "the learned, shared, and transmitted values, beliefs, norms, and lifeway practices of a particular group that guide thinking, decisions, and actions in patterned ways" (Leininger, 1988, p. 158). Because cultural patterns are learned, it is important for nurses to note that all members of a particular group may not share identical cultural experiences. Thus, individual members of a cultural group will be somewhat different from their own cultural counterparts (Waxler-Morrison, Anderson, & Richardson, 1990). For example, generations have different appreciations of music according to exposure within their peer group—swing from the 1940s, jive from the 1950s, rock and roll from the 1960s, and so on. Large cultural groups often have cultural subgroups or subsystems. A **subculture** usually comprises people who have a distinct identity and yet are also related to a larger cultural group.

Bicultural "is used to describe a person who crosses two cultures, lifestyles, and sets of values" (Giger & Davidhizar, 2004, p. 67). For example, a young man whose father is Cree and whose mother is European Canadian may maintain his traditional Cree heritage while also being influenced by his mother's cultural values.

Diversity refers to the "fact or state of being different" (Steinmetz & Braham, 1993, p. 141). Many factors account for differences: race, gender, sexual orientation, culture, ethnicity, socioeconomic status, educational attainment, religious affiliation, ability, and so on. Diversity, therefore, occurs not only between cultural groups but also within a cultural group.

The term **ethnic** refers to a group of people who share a common and distinctive culture and who are members of a specific group. Although ethnicity has sometimes been used to identify race, Giger and Davidhizar (2004) suggest that it is "a common social and cultural heritage that is passed on to successive generations" (p. 67). The characteristics of the group give an individual a sense of **cultural identity**. Other factors that help define ethnicity may include religion and the geographic background of the family.

Race is a controversial term. For some people the definition of race includes having common characteristics, such as skin colour, bone structure, facial features, hair texture, and blood type. The term *race* becomes problematic when it leads to negative stereotyping. Different ethnic groups can belong to the same race, and different cultures can be found within the same ethnic group. For example, the terms *Caucasian* and *European Canadian* describe the race of people whose origins are in Europe. Whereas British Canadians are a subgroup of European Canadians, Scottish Canadians (an ethnic subgroup of British Canadians) may have cultural practices different from other British Canadians. It is important to understand that not all people of the same race have the same culture. Culture should not be confused with either race or ethnic group. Race, culture, and ethnic origin are three different terms that are often used interchangeably; however, it is inappropriate to do so.

It is helpful to differentiate the terms *acculturation* and *ethnic identity*. **Acculturation**, **assimilation**, and **colonization** are processes and policies that focus on the absorption of people into a dominant culture. In Canada, an example of assimilation would be the forced integration of Aboriginal peoples into the European-Canadian culture. Assimilation was an explicit policy of the Canadian government that led to the removal of Aboriginal children from their homes and families and their subsequent institutionalization in residential schools. Doane and Varcoe (2005), citing Potthast-Jutkeit (1997) in describing colonization, talk about attending to the ways in which colonization has shaped and continues to influence families around the globe. Through colonial rule, "many cultures have had to cope with the imposition of Christian-European family norms and with the values of their colonizers" (p. 128). The purpose of acculturation, assimilation, or colonization is to impose the values, attitudes, beliefs, or practices of a dominant group in society on a minority group. It is often defined in terms of such observable factors as dress, food, and language. Individuals who are acculturated may no longer eat foods associated with their culture or always wear traditional dress (Lynam, 1992). **Ethnic identity**, in contrast, refers to a subjective perspective of the person's heritage and to a sense of belonging to a group that is distinguishable from other groups. Thus, people may be visibly acculturated to the mainstream culture but retain an identity that differs from the mainstream.

The cultural beliefs and practices regarding health and illness of North America's many different ethnic and cultural groups are important considerations for nurses in planning nursing care. The study of anthropology by nurses, which looks at the origin, behaviour, and physical, social, and cultural development of human beings, is an important contribution to nursing (Leininger, 1970). Leininger defines **transcultural nursing** as a "field of nursing [that] focus[es] on the comparative study and analysis of different cultures and subcultures in the world with respect to their caring behaviors, nursing care, and health-illness values, beliefs, and patterns of behaviors with the goal of developing a scientific and humanistic body of knowledge in order to provide culture-specific and culture-universal nursing care practice" (p. 8).

Cultural awareness, cultural sensitivity, and cultural safety are prerequisites for the provision of culturally competent nursing care. **Cultural awareness** is the conscious and informed recognition of the differences and similarities between different cultural or ethnic groups. Cultural awareness is not knowledge derived solely from myths and stereotypes. **Cultural sensitivity** is the respect and appreciation for cultural behaviours based on an understanding of the other person's experience and perspective. According to Papps and Ramsden (1996), "it is consumers or patients who decide whether they feel safe with the care that has been given. Cultural safety within nursing addresses power relationships between the service provider and the people who use the service. . . . Someone who feels unsafe will not be able to take full

Evidence-Informed Practice

What Are the Stories about Cancer among the Woodland Cree of Northern Saskatchewan?

When doing research with indigenous communities, Smith (1999, p. 128) stated that "in many projects the process is far more important than the outcome. Processes are expected to be respectful, to enable people, to heal and to educate." Roberts's (2006) research focus was on how the Woodland Cree of Northern Saskatchewan perceive cancer as a whole: their internalization, their diagnosis, and treatment experiences, as well as their world view of health and illness. Community participants included Elders, cancer survivors, and family members. The interviews were either in Cree or in English and the methodology was narrative inquiry, the collection of stories. Each step of the research process was intended to benefit the participants, the same way the nursing process is expected to benefit clients.

NURSING IMPLICATIONS: Through research such as this, nurses can begin to understand how cultural perspectives influence clients' views of health and health challenges.

Source: Based on "Caught Between Two Worlds: An Aboriginal Researchers' Experience Researching in Her Home Community," by R. Roberts, 2006, *Pimatisiwin, 3*(2), pp. 101–108.

advantage of the primary health care service offered and may, therefore, avoid the service until dramatic and expensive secondary or tertiary intervention is required" (p. 494). **Cultural safety** is focused on self-knowledge or self-reflection. A nurse who understands his or her own culture and the theory of power relations can be culturally safe in any human context (Nursing Council of New Zealand, 2005). Culturally safe care emphasizes the provision of nursing care that takes into account all that makes human beings unique and avoids stereotyping.

Cultural competence is "knowing, utilizing, and appreciating the culture of another in assisting with the resolution of a problem" (DeSantis & Lowe, 1992, p. 1). The culturally competent nurse, therefore, works within the cultural belief system of the client to respond effectively in cross-cultural situations (Campbell & Campbell, 1996). To provide culturally competent care, nurses need data about the client's personal and cultural views regarding health and illness. To make valid assessments, nurses need to try to see and hear the world as their clients do. When developing care plans, nurses need to consider the client's world and daily experiences. Although a client's needs and behaviours can be better understood when participants' cultural health norms are identified, nurses must take care to avoid stereotyping clients by culture norms. Care must be individualized.

Culture shock can occur when members of one culture are abruptly moved to another culture or setting. **Culture shock** is the state of being disoriented or unable to respond to a different cultural environment because of its sudden strangeness, unfamiliarity, and incompatibility with the person's perceptions and expectations (Leininger, 1978). For example, when immigrants first enter Canada or the United States, language and behaviour differences may initially cause them difficulty in carrying out normal activities. People can also experience culture shock when they are abruptly thrust into the health-care subculture. Nursing students, for example, may experience culture shock when they enter nursing school and must learn medical terminology (a new language) and provide care for clients in clinical environments with which they are unfamiliar. Expressions of culture shock can range from silence and immobility to agitation. The CNA has developed a position statement on delivering culturally competent care (Canadian Nurses Association [CNA], 2004) to assist nurses in ensuring their care is appropriate.

Health-Care Concerns

Nurses must consider cultural and ethnic factors in providing quality nursing care. A group's world view shapes its health culture—the values, beliefs, and practices it holds about health promotion, disease prevention, illness treatment, and the expectations that guide the nurse–client encounter.

People who belong to the same ethnic group may have little in common in their lifestyles, beliefs, and values. For example, a Canadian of East Indian ancestry could be a third-generation Canadian who cannot speak a word of Hindi, a recently arrived lawyer from New Delhi, or an ethnic refugee from a small mountain village in northern India. Socioeconomic status, length of time in Canada, educational level, age, sex, and country of origin will influence the perspectives of health and health behaviours. However, some genetically acquired biological traits, such as differences in skin pigmentation, body build, and metabolism, can have a bearing on a person's health. For example, individuals who trace their ancestry to Black racial groups of Africa, among others, are predisposed to a genetic blood condition known as sickle-cell anemia.

It is important for nurses to explore the cultural and ethnic beliefs and the health-care practices of all Canadians. The Canadian health-care system is rooted in Western biomedical principles, in which outcome is oriented toward the effective diagnosis and treatment of disease. Clients from a non-dominant culture may view nurses of the predominant culture as a threat to their traditional ways of dealing with health-care concerns. For example, a young woman may be perceived by an older Asian male as an inappropriate person to provide personal nursing care because of status difference.

Language differences can present another barrier to effective nursing care. Ethnic minority immigrants may not be able to read and write in either official language of Canada. Written instructions from a nurse may be misunderstood or not fully understood.

Health-care professionals are not expected to know and understand *all* cultures of the world; it is possible, however, for them to develop an in-depth understanding of three or four cultures and to learn about other cultures over time (Leininger, 1993). It is also important for nurses to understand their own cultural beliefs and biases.

Nurses need to be aware that although people from a given ethnic group share certain beliefs, values, and experiences, often there is also widespread intra-ethnic diversity. Major differences within ethnic groups may be due to such factors as age, sex, level of education, socioeconomic status, religious affiliation, and area of origin in the home country (rural or urban). Such factors influence the client's beliefs about health and illness, health and illness practices, help-seeking behaviours, and expectations of health professionals (Anderson, Waxler-Morrison, Richardson, Herbert, & Murphy, 1990). For these reasons, nurses should make special effort to avoid ethnic stereotyping (Papps & Ramsden, 1996)

Two transcultural health-care systems generally exist side by side, with limited awareness of the other by practitioners in either system: an indigenous health-care system and a professional health-care system (Leininger, 1993). The *indigenous health-care system* refers to traditional folk methods of health care, such as folk medicines and other home treatments. The more recent *professional health-care system* refers to a structured system maintained by individuals who have engaged in a formal program of study. The indigenous system is the older system and often provided health care long before a professional system entered the culture. According to Leininger, few professional health-care workers are knowledgeable about the indigenous health-care system or its practitioners. Some professionals regard the indigenous system as unscientific or "primitive," or even as "quackery." Leininger emphasizes that the goal of health care should be to use the best of both systems and that health professionals need to consider ways to interface with the two systems for the benefit of the people served. "Every culture has health, caring, and caring processes, techniques, and practices viewed as important to the people" (Leininger, 1993, p. 38).

Leininger produced the sunrise model to depict her theory of cultural care diversity and universality (Figure 10.1). This model emphasizes that health and care are influenced by elements of the social structure, such as technology, religious and philosophical factors, kinship and social systems, cultural values, political and legal factors, economic factors, and educational factors. These social factors are addressed within environmental contexts, language expressions, and ethnohistory. Each of these systems is part of the social structure of any society; health-care expressions, patterns, and practices are also integral parts of these aspects of social structure (Leininger, 1993).

Since the development of Leininger's sunrise model, several other models have been developed. All of these models address similar elements of culture pertinent to nursing care. Some focus on broad concepts, such as an emphasis on understanding of personal biases, prejudices, values, and beliefs, combined with an understanding of power, trust, and equity; the possession of cultural resources and cultural knowledge (Srivastava, 2007); and emphasis on learning the practices and beliefs that are attributed to particular cultures (Purnell & Paulanka, 2005). Others introduce notions of time, space (Giger & Davidhizar, 2004; Spector, 2004), and communication (Andrews & Boyle, 2003). Although these models have elements in common, each model emphasizes slightly different attributes that can guide the nurse to assess patient, family, or community culture. However, health-care providers should use these models in conjunction with a cultural safety lens to avoid a checklist approach. The assumption that checklists and learning about rituals and practices in general will provide insight into the complexity of social human behaviour is risky. Cultural safety takes into consideration power relations and the uniqueness of human beings and avoids stereotyping.

Culturally Sensitive and Safe Care

Several national and provincial nursing groups have developed position statements and best practices for delivery of appropriate cultural care. Examples are the Canadian Nurses Association (2004) *Position Statement: Promoting Culturally Competent Care* and the Registered Nurses' Association of Ontario (2007) *Embracing Cultural Diversity in Health Care: Developing Cultural Competence.* The College of Nurses of Ontario's *Practice Guideline for Culturally Sensitive Care* (2008) emphasizes the following elements for providing culturally sensitive care:

1. *Being culturally knowledgeable:* It is impossible to possess in-depth knowledge about all cultures; however, it is possible to have a general understanding of how cultures can affect health practices and beliefs
2. *Being client-centred:* Client-centred care requires that nurses recognize the client's culture, the nurse's own culture, and how both affect the nurse–client relationship—the focus of care is always the client's needs. Each client and each situation is unique and requires individual assessment and planning.
3. *Being self-reflective:* Self-reflection is a fundamental element of providing culturally sensitive, competent, and safe care. Nurses may fall into the trap of

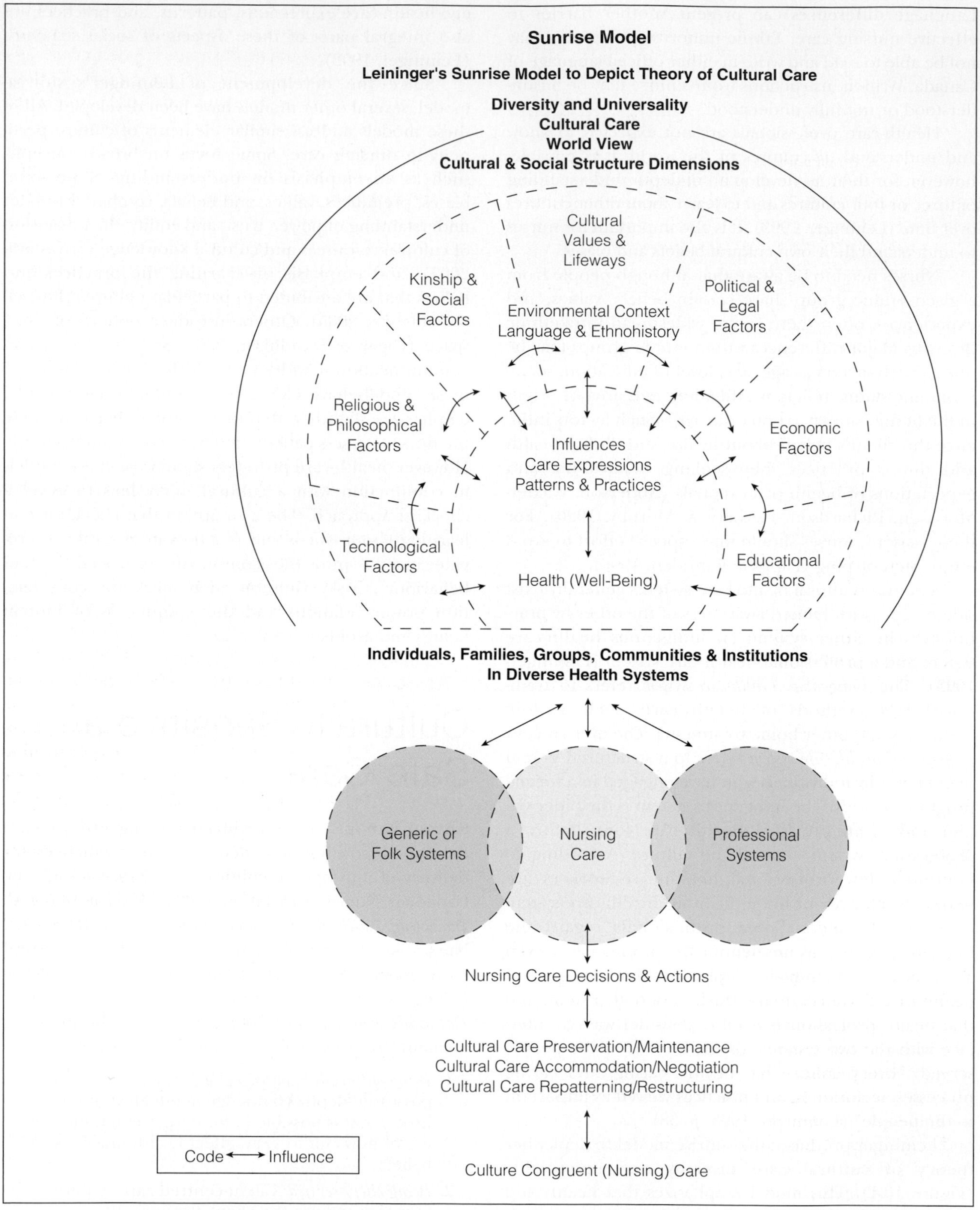

FIGURE 10.1 Leininger's Sunrise Model
(Source:* Culture care diversity and universality: A theory of nursing, *by M. Leininger, 1991, New York: National League for Nursing, p. 43. Pub. No. 15–2402. Reprinted with permission.)

thinking they know a culture and therefore know what is best for the client, or nurses might impose their beliefs and values on the client or presuppose that their own values are the same as the clients'. Understanding the self as distinct from others in the broadest sense is critical in the provision of culturally safe care.

4. *Recognizing potential conflict between the culture of the nursing profession's values and beliefs and client cultural values and beliefs:* The nursing profession itself has a culture that can come into conflict with the cultural values and beliefs of clients. When beliefs and values come into conflict, it is the nurse's role to reflect on her professional beliefs and values and to explore and reframe the treatment or therapy in a culturally appropriate way that meets the client's goal of care.
5. *Facilitating client choice:* This is part of the nurse's role in providing quality care. A client's choice could place other clients at risk or be threatening to their care. In such situations, it is the nurse's responsibility to balance these demands. The nurse attempts to meet some of the client's wishes while at the same time protecting other clients.
6. *Incorporating client's cultural preferences:* Adding these into the client's nursing care plan can facilitate the client's physical, emotional, or spiritual health, taking into consideration whether or not the practices are harmful to the client or other clients. Endorsement of one client's cultural beliefs, practices, or values does not mean the nurse adopts these views or requires other clients to do so.
7. *Accommodating client cultural beliefs and practices:* This can be done by finding ways to minimize risks or remove obstacles.

Barriers to Cultural Sensitivity and Safety

Many factors can be barriers to providing culturally sensitive or culturally congruent care to clients and their support people. These issues can also affect communication and working relationships with other health-care personnel. Ethnocentrism, stereotyping, prejudice, and discrimination are some of these elements.

Ethnocentrism refers to the view that the beliefs and values of one person's own culture are superior to those of other cultures. In health care, ethnocentrism can include the view that the only valid health-care beliefs and practices are those held by the professionals in the health-care system. Nurses who take a transcultural view, however, value their own beliefs and practices while respecting the beliefs and practices of others. It is important for nurses to realize that although many people of diverse racial and religious backgrounds have combined their traditional health practices with Western health practices, other people may be unable or unwilling to do so.

Most people are gradually exposed to their culture's beliefs, values, and practices over a period of years, starting at birth. Ethnocentrism is thought to result from lack of exposure or knowledge of other cultures. **Ethnorelativity** is the ability to appreciate and respect the viewpoints of other cultures.

Stereotyping occurs when the assumption is made that all members of a culture or ethnic group are alike. For example, a nurse may assume that all Italians express pain volubly or that all Chinese people like rice. Stereotyping may be based on generalizations founded in research, or it may be unrelated to reality. For example, research indicates that Italians are likely to express pain verbally; however, an Italian client may not verbalize pain. Stereotyping that is unrelated to reality can be either positive or negative and is frequently an outcome of racism or discrimination. Nurses need to realize that not all people of a specific group have the same health beliefs, practices, and values. It is, therefore, essential to identify a specific client's beliefs, needs, and values, rather than assuming they are the same as those attributable to the larger group.

Prejudice is a strongly held opinion about some topic or group of people. A prejudice may be positive or negative. A positive prejudice often stems from a strong sense of ethnocentrism (Eliason, 1993). Prejudice may also derive from ignorance, misinformation, past experience, or fear. Types of negative prejudice include ageism, which is negative attitudes toward older adults; sexism, meaning negative attitudes toward women; and homophobia, which is negativism toward lesbians and gay men.

Banks and Banks (1989, p. 37) define **discrimination** as "the differential treatment of individuals or groups based on categories such as race, ethnicity, gender, social class, or exceptionality." For example, a nurse takes a child who is waiting in an emergency department ahead of another child. The child taken ahead appears clean, is neatly dressed, and is smiling; the other child appears dirty, is wearing worn clothes, and is angry. **Racism** is a form of discrimination related to ethnocentrism in which a person believes that race is the primary determinant of human traits and capacities and that racial differences result in an inherent superiority of a particular race.

Conveying Cultural Sensitivity

It is important for nurses to be culturally sensitive and to convey this sensitivity to clients, support people, and other health-care personnel. Some ways to do so include the following:

- Always address clients by their last names (e.g., Mrs. Aylia, Dr. Rush) until they give you permission to use other names. In some cultures, the more formal style of address is a sign of respect, whereas the use of first names may be considered disrespectful. It is important to ask clients how they want to be addressed.

- When meeting a person for the first time, introduce yourself by your full name and explain your role in the person's health care. This helps establish a relationship and provides an opportunity for clients and nurses to learn the pronunciation of one another's names.
- Be genuine with people, and be honest about the knowledge you lack about their culture.
- Use language that is culturally sensitive; for example, use terms such as *gay, lesbian, bisexual, transgendered,* or *two-spirited* rather than *homosexual*; do not use *man* or *mankind* when referring to a woman; *African Canadian* is preferred by some over *Black,* and *Latin American* is preferred over *Hispanic. Asian* is more acceptable than *Oriental* (Eliason, 1993). In Canada, use the term *Aboriginal* to refer to First Nations, Inuit, and Metis. Even better, ask the person what term they prefer. Members of some ethnic groups may prefer the appellation of *Hispanic* or *Oriental,* for example.
- Find out what the clients know about their health problems, illnesses, and treatments. Assess whether this information is congruent with the predominant health-care culture. If the beliefs and practices are incongruent, establish whether this will have a negative effect on the client's health.
- Do not make any assumptions about the client, and always ask about anything you do not understand.
- Respect the client's values, beliefs, and practices, even if they differ from your own or from those of the predominant culture. If you don't agree with them, it is important to respect the client's rights to hold these beliefs. It is important for the client to feel safe in the nurse–client relationship.
- Show respect for the client's support people. In some cultures, men in the family make decisions affecting the client, while in other cultures, women make the decisions.
- Make a concerted effort to earn the client's trust, but do not be surprised if it develops slowly or not at all.

Selected Cultural Parameters for Nursing

This section outlines selected cultural and ethnic phenomena of significance to nursing.

Health Beliefs and Practices

The **scientific** or **biomedical health belief** is based on the belief that life and life processes are controlled by physical and biochemical processes that can be manipulated (Andrews & Boyle, 2003). The client with this view will believe that illness is caused by germs, viruses, bacteria, or a breakdown of the human machine, the body. This client will expect a pill, treatment, or surgery to cure health problems.

The **holistic health belief** holds that the forces of nature must be maintained in balance or harmony. Human life is one aspect of nature that must be in harmony with the rest of nature. When the natural balance or harmony is disturbed, illness results. The medicine wheel is an ancient symbol used by First Nations members of North and South America to express many concepts. For health and wellness, the medicine wheel teaches that the four aspects of the individual's nature—the physical, the mental, the emotional, and the spiritual—must be in balance. The medicine wheel can also be used to express the individual's relationship with the environment as a dimension of wellness.

The concept of yin and yang in the Chinese culture and the hot-cold theory of illness in many Spanish cultures are examples of holistic health beliefs. When a Chinese client has a yin illness or a cold illness, the treatment may include a yang or hot food (e.g., hot tea). For example, a Chinese client who has been diagnosed with cancer, a yin disease, will want to eat cultural foods that have yang properties.

What is considered hot or cold varies considerably across cultures. In many cultures, the mother who has just delivered a baby should be offered warm or hot foods and kept warm with blankets because childbirth is seen as a cold condition. Conventional scientific thought recommends cooling the body to reduce a fever. The physician may order liquids for the client and cool compresses to be applied to the forehead, the axillae, or the groin. Galanti (2004) states that many cultures believe that the best way to treat a fever is to "sweat it out." Clients from these cultures may want to cover up with several blankets, take hot baths, and drink hot beverages. Giger and Davidhizar (2004) state that the nurse must keep in mind that a treatment strategy that is consistent with the client's beliefs may have a better chance of being successful. For example, the Latin American client who avoids spicy foods when experiencing a stomach disturbance may be eating foods consistent with the bland diet that is normally prescribed by physicians.

Sociocultural forces, such as politics, economics, geography, religion, and the predominant health-care system, can influence the client's health status and health-care behaviour. For example, people who have limited access to scientific health care may turn to traditional medicine or healing. **Traditional medicine** is defined as those beliefs and practices relating to illness prevention and healing that derive from cultural traditions, rather than from modern medicine's scientific base. Many students might recall special teas or cures used by older family members to prevent or treat colds, fevers, indigestion, and other common health problems. People continue to use chicken soup as a treatment for the flu.

Why do individuals use these traditional healing methods? Traditional medicine, in contrast to biomedical health care, is thought to be more humanistic. The consultation and treatment takes place in the community of the recipient, frequently in the home of the healer. It is less expensive than scientific or biomedical care because the health problem is identified primarily through conversation with the client and the family. The healer often prepares the treatments, for example, teas to be ingested, poultices to be applied, or charms or amulets to be worn. A frequent component of treatment is some ritual practice on the part of the healer or the client to cause healing to occur. Because traditional healing practices are culturally based, they are often more comfortable and less frightening for the client.

It is important for the nurse to obtain information about traditional healing practices that may have been used before the client sought Western medical treatment. Often, clients are reluctant to share home remedies with health-care professionals for fear of being laughed at or rebuked. The nurse should remember that treatments once considered to be traditional treatments, including acupuncture, therapeutic touch, and massage, are now being investigated for their therapeutic effect. On the other hand, herbal remedies sometimes interact with cardiac medications with deleterious effects on a person's health, ranging from discomfort to death.

Family Patterns

The family is the basic unit of society. Cultural values can determine communication within the family group, the norm for family size, and the roles of specific family members. In some families, the man is considered the provider and decision maker. The woman may need to consult her family before making decisions about her medical treatment or the treatment of her children (Galanti, 2004). Some families are matriarchal; that is, the mother or grandmother is viewed as the leader of the family and is usually the decision maker. The nurse needs to identify who has the authority to make decisions in a client's family. If the decision maker is someone other than the client, the nurse needs to include that person in health-care discussions.

The value placed on children and older people within a society is culturally derived. In some cultures, older people are considered the holders of the culture's wisdom and are, therefore, highly respected. Responsibility for caring for elder relatives is determined by cultural practices. In many cultures, older relatives who cannot live independently often live with a married son or daughter and his or her family.

Cultural gender-role behaviour may also affect nurse–client interaction. In some countries, men dominate and women have little status. Men from these countries may not accept instruction from a female nurse or physician but are receptive to the same instruction given by a male physician or nurse (Galanti, 2004). Some cultures have a prevailing concept of machismo, or male superiority. Machismo requires that the adult man provide for and protect his family, including extended family members. The woman is expected to maintain the home and raise the children.

Cultural family values may also dictate the extent of the family's involvement in the hospitalized client's care. In some cultures, the nuclear and the extended family will want to visit for long periods and participate in care. In other cultures, the entire clan may want to visit and participate in the client's care (Galanti, 2004). This can cause concern on nursing units with strict visiting policies. The nurse should evaluate the positive benefits of family participation in the client's care and modify visiting policies as appropriate.

Cultures that value the needs of the extended family as much as those of the individual may hold the belief that personal and family information must stay within the family. Some cultural groups are very reluctant to disclose family information to outsiders, including health-care professionals. This attitude can present difficulties for health-care professionals who require knowledge of family interaction patterns to help clients with emotional problems.

Naming systems in many cultures differ from those in North America. In some cultures (e.g., Japanese and Vietnamese), the family name comes first and the given name second. One or two names may or may not be added between the family and given names. Other nomenclature may be used to delineate sex and child or adult status. For example, in traditional Japanese culture, adults address other adults by their surname followed by *san,* meaning *Mr., Mrs.,* or *Miss.* An example is "Maurakami san." The children are referred to by their first names followed by *kun* for boys and *chan* for girls. Sikhs and Hindus traditionally have three names. Hindus have a personal name, a complementary name, and then a family name. Sikhs have a personal name, the title *Singh* for men and *Kaur* for women, and then the family name. Names by marriage also vary. In Central America, a woman who marries retains her father's name and takes her husband's. For example, if Louisa Viccario marries Carlos Gonzales, she becomes Louisa Viccario de Gonzales. The connecting *de* means "belonging to." Nurses need to become familiar with appropriate ways to address clients.

Communication Style

Communication and culture are closely interconnected. Through communication, culture is transmitted from one generation to the next, and knowledge about the culture is transmitted within the group and to those outside the group. Communicating with clients of various ethnic and cultural backgrounds is critical to providing culturally competent, safe nursing care. A therapeutic nurse–client relationship is grounded in meaningful communication between the nurse and the client. Cultural variations in both verbal and nonverbal communication can require the development of a communication plan that incorporates the client as an informed partner in care.

VERBAL COMMUNICATION The most obvious cultural difference is in verbal communication: vocabulary, grammatical structure, voice qualities, intonation, rhythm, speed, pronunciation, and silence (Giger & Davidhizar, 2004). In North America, the predominant language is English; however, immigrant groups who speak English still encounter language differences because English words can have different meanings in different English-speaking cultures. For example, in Canada a *boot* is a type of footwear that comes to the ankle or higher; in England, a *boot* can also be the trunk of a car. Similarly, great differences exist between the French spoken in Canada and that spoken in France. In Canada, the French language has evolved, assimilating First Nations and English terms. In Quebec, nurses must meet the French-language requirements and need to be aware of the language diversity that exists within the province.

Initiating verbal communication may be influenced by cultural values. The busy nurse may want to complete nursing admission assessments quickly. The client, however, may be offended when the nurse immediately asks personal questions. In some cultures, it is believed that social courtesies should be established before business or personal topics are discussed. Discussing general topics can convey that the nurse is interested in the client and has time for the client. This enables the nurse to develop a rapport with the client before progressing to more personal discussion.

Verbal communication becomes even more difficult when an interaction involves people who speak different languages. Both clients and health professionals experience frustration when they are unable to communicate verbally with each other. For clients who have limited knowledge of English, the nurse should avoid slang words, medical terminology, and abbreviations. Augmenting spoken conversation with gestures or pictures can increase the client's understanding. The nurse should speak slowly, in a respectful manner, and at a normal volume. Speaking loudly does not help the client understand and may be offensive. The nurse must also frequently validate the client's understanding of what is being communicated. The nurse must be wary of interpreting a client's smiling and nodding to mean that the client understands; the client may only be trying to please the nurse while not understanding what is being said.

For the client who speaks a different language, an interpreter may be necessary. Galanti (2004) notes that cultural rules often dictate who can discuss what with whom. Guidelines for using an interpreter are shown in Box 10.1. Whenever possible, professional health-care interpreters should be used.

Interpreters should be objective individuals who can provide accurate interpretation of the client's information and of the health professional's questions, information, and instruction. Many institutions that are located in culturally diverse communities have interpreters available on staff or maintain a list of employees who are fluent in other languages. Embassies, consulates, ethnic churches, ethnic clubs, or telephone companies may also be able to provide interpretation services. Nurses and other health personnel can use pictures and gestures to augment verbal communication.

Nurses who speak a second language may be asked to interpret for others. Some nursing schools and health-

BOX 10.1 USING AN INTERPRETER

When using an interpreter, nurses should use the following guidelines:

- Avoid asking a member of the client's family, especially a child or spouse, to act as interpreter. Some clients, not wanting family members to know about their problems, may not provide complete or accurate information.
- Be sure to obtain client consent to use an interpreter or for any other arrangement for communication.
- Avoid complicated language as the client may have limited understanding of or vocabulary in English related to health problems.
- Be aware of sex, age, dialect, and religious differences; it is preferable to use an interpreter of the same sex as the client to avoid embarrassment and faulty translation of sexual matters.
- Avoid an interpreter who is politically or socially incompatible with the client. For example, a Bosnian Serb may not be the best interpreter for a Muslim, even if he speaks the language.
- Address the questions to the client, *not* to the interpreter.
- Ask the interpreter to interpret as closely as possible the words used—the interpreter's role is to be the voice of the client.
- Speak slowly and distinctly. Do *not* use metaphors, for example, "Does it swell like a grapefruit?" or "Is the pain stabbing like a knife stab?"
- Observe the facial expressions and body language that the client assumes when listening and talking to the interpreter.
- Ask the interpreter to share any insights about the client; however, be sure these are perceived to be insights and not facts or the client's actual beliefs.
- Explain to the client and the interpreter that all communication is confidential—no client information will be disclosed to anyone.
- Write down key points, directions, and/or appointment times so they are not confused or forgotten.
- Ask the client to repeat in his or her own words all instructions and information.
- Determine from the interpreter whether or not any aspects of the interaction were difficult.

care institutions do not permit nursing students to interpret for a procedure consent because a lack of knowledge about the procedure may lead the student to give inaccurate information. The student should check the institution's policy before agreeing to interpret for institutional staff and physicians.

Nurses and other health-care providers must remember that clients for whom English is a second language may lose command of their English when they are in stressful situations. Clients who have used English comfortably for years in social and business communication may forget and revert back to their primary language when they are ill or distressed. It is important for the nurse to assure the client that this is normal and to promote behaviours to facilitate verbal communication.

NONVERBAL COMMUNICATION To communicate effectively with culturally diverse clients, the nurse needs to be aware of two aspects of nonverbal communication behaviours: (1) what nonverbal behaviours mean to the client, and (2) what specific nonverbal behaviours mean in the client's culture. It is not required that the nurse be knowledgeable about the nonverbal behaviour patterns of all cultures; however, before assigning meaning to nonverbal behaviour, the nurse must consider the possibility that the behaviour may have a different meaning for the client and the family. Furthermore, to provide safe and effective care, nurses who work with specific cultural groups should learn more about cultural behaviour and communication patterns within these cultures.

Nonverbal communication can include the use of silence, touch, eye movement, facial expressions, and body posture. Some cultures are quite comfortable with long periods of silence, whereas others consider it appropriate to speak before the other person has finished talking. Many people value silence and view it as essential to understanding a person's needs or use silence to preserve privacy. Some cultures view silence as a sign of respect, whereas to other people, silence may indicate agreement (Giger & Davidhizar, 2004).

Touching involves learned behaviours that can have both positive and negative meanings. In the North American culture, a firm handshake is a recognized form of greeting that reflects cordiality (Giger & Davidhizar, 2004). In some European cultures, greetings may include a kiss on one or both cheeks along with the handshake. In some societies, touch is considered magical, and because of the belief that the soul can leave the body on physical contact, casual touching is forbidden. Vietnamese Canadians may find touching of the head or shoulders to be anxiety producing because of such a belief (Giger & Davidhizar, 2004). Nurses should, therefore, touch a client's head only with permission. The sex of the person touching and being touched often has cultural significance.

Cultures also dictate what forms of touch are appropriate for individuals of the same sex and opposite sex. In many cultures, for example, a kiss is not appropriate for a public greeting between persons of the opposite sex, even those who are family members; however, a kiss on the cheek is acceptable as a greeting among individuals of the same sex. The nurse should watch interaction among clients and families for cues to the appropriate degree of touch in that culture. The nurse can also assess the client's response to touch when providing nursing care, for example, by noting the client's reaction to the physical examination or a bath.

Facial expression can also vary between cultures. Giger and Davidhizar (2004) state that Italian, Jewish, Black, and Spanish-speaking persons are more likely to smile readily and use facial expression to communicate feelings, whereas Irish, English, and northern European people tend to have less facial expression and are less open in their response, especially to strangers. Facial expressions can also convey a meaning opposite to what is felt or understood.

Eye movement during communication has cultural foundations. In Western cultures, direct eye contact is regarded as important and generally shows that the other is attentive and listening. It conveys self-confidence, openness, interest, and honesty. Lack of eye contact may be interpreted as secretiveness, shyness, guilt, lack of interest, or even a sign of a mental health problem. However, other cultures view eye contact as impolite or an invasion of privacy. For Cree Nation members, continuous direct eye contact is considered impolite and an invasion of privacy (Yonge & Bernard, 1998). The nurse should not misinterpret the character of the client who avoids eye contact.

Body posture and gesture are also culturally learned. Finger pointing, the V sign with the index and middle fingers, and the thumbs-up sign have different meanings. For example, the V sign means victory in some cultures, but it is an offensive gesture in other cultures (Galanti, 2004). In the Hmong culture, bowing the head slightly when entering the room where an elder is present and using both hands to give something to someone are considered signs of respect (Rairdan & Higgs, 1992).

Communication is an essential part of establishing a relationship with clients and their families. It is also important for developing effective working relationships with health-care colleagues. However, it is important to remember that although nonverbal communication may vary considerably between cultures, "it is impossible to become an authority on your own culture(s), let alone someone else's and it is counter to the concept of cultural safety, where differences within cultures, not just between them is acknowledged and respected. What cultural safety asks us to do when we face a nursing situation outside of our sphere of cultural experience is to 'ask'" (Hughes & Farrow, 2006, p. 13). To enhance their practice, nurses can observe the communication patterns of clients and colleagues and be aware of their own communication behaviours.

Space Orientation

Space is a relative concept that includes the individual, the body, the surrounding environment, and objects within that environment. The relationship between the individual's own body and objects and persons within a space is learned and is influenced by culture. For example, in nomadic societies space is not owned; it is occupied temporarily until the tribe moves on. In Western societies, people tend to be more territorial, as reflected in such phrases as "This is my space" or "Get out of my space." In Western cultures, spatial distances are defined as the intimate zone, the personal zone, and the social and public zones. The size of these areas may vary with the specific culture. Nurses move through all three zones as they provide care for clients. The nurse needs to be aware of the client's response to movement toward him or her. The client may physically withdraw or back away if the nurse is perceived as being too close. The nurse will need to explain to the client why there is a need to be close. To assess the lungs with a stethoscope, for example, the nurse needs to move into the client's intimate space. The nurse should first explain the procedure and await permission to continue.

Residents in long-term-care facilities or patients who are hospitalized for an extended time may want to personalize their space. They may want to arrange their room differently or control the placement of objects on their bedside cabinet or overbed table. The nurse should be responsive to clients' needs to have some control over their space. When there are no medical contraindications, clients should be permitted and encouraged to wear their own clothing and have objects of personal significance. Wearing cultural dress or having personal and cultural items in the environment can increase self-esteem by promoting not only the client's individuality but also his or her cultural identity. Of course, the nurse should caution the client about responsibility for loss of personal items.

Time Orientation

Time orientation refers to an individual's focus on the past, the present, or the future. Most cultures combine all three time orientations, but one orientation is more likely to dominate. The North American focus on time tends to be directed to the future, emphasizing time and schedules (Galanti, 2004). Nursing students know what times they must be in class or clinical. They know what courses they will take in future semesters. European Canadians often plan for next week, their vacation, or their retirement. Other cultures may have a different concept of time. Members of First Nations communities may be perceived as being present oriented and to not be concerned with the future. However, other values, such as family and community, may override or come into conflict with European views or orientations regarding time. For example, going to class or to a doctor's appointment may take a backseat if a family member becomes ill. The first obligation is always to family and community. Often no explanations are given, perhaps because none are expected within the Aboriginal culture. The First Nations peoples' cultural belief in the seven generations means that whatever is done today must be considered in light of its impact in the next seven generations. This belief is particularly important with regard to the environment. Another belief is to share what you have. Beliefs about time are grounded in values about courage, respect, honesty, humility, love, truth, and wisdom, beliefs that could come into conflict with health-care provider health-promotion efforts if they are not understood (Laurentian University, 2007).

The culture of nursing and health care values time. Appointments are scheduled, and treatments are prescribed with time parameters (e.g., changing a dressing once a day). Medication orders include how often the medicine is to be taken and when (e.g., digoxin 0.25 mg, once a day, in the morning). Nurses need to be aware of the meaning of time for clients. Giger and Davidhizar (2004) state that when caring for clients who are "present-oriented," it is important to avoid fixed schedules. The nurse can offer a time range for activities and treatments. For example, instead of telling the client to take digoxin every day at 10 a.m., the nurse might tell the client to take it every day in the morning, or every day after getting out of bed.

Nutritional Patterns

Most cultures have staple foods, that is, foods that are plentiful or readily accessible in the environment. For example, the staple food of most Asians is rice; of Italians, pasta; and of Eastern Europeans, wheat. Even clients who have been in Canada for several generations often continue to eat the foods of their cultural homelands.

The way food is prepared and served is also related to cultural practices. For example, in Canada, a traditional food served for the Thanksgiving holiday is stuffed turkey; however, in different regions of the country, the contents of the stuffing may vary. The variation may be influenced by ethnic preference or by regional tradition, such as including oysters, fruit, or nuts, or using rice instead of bread.

The ways in which staple foods are prepared also vary. For example, some Asian cultures prefer steamed rice; others prefer boiled rice. Southern Asians from India prepare unleavened bread from wheat flour, rather than the leavened bread of European Canadians.

Food-related cultural behaviours can include whether to breastfeed or bottle-feed infants and when to introduce solid foods to them. Food can also be considered part of the remedy for illness. Foods classified as hot foods or foods that are hot in temperature may be used to treat illnesses that are classified as cold illnesses, as noted earlier. For example, corn meal (a hot food) may be used to treat arthritis (a cold illness). Each culture group defines what it considers to be hot and cold entities.

Religious practice associated with specific cultures also affects diet. Some Roman Catholics avoid meat on certain days, such as Ash Wednesday and Good Friday, and some Protestant faiths prohibit meat, tea, coffee, or alcohol. Both Orthodox Judaism and Islam prohibit the ingestion of pork or pork products. Orthodox Jews observe kosher customs, eating certain foods only if they are inspected by a rabbi and prepared according to dietary laws. For example, the eating of milk products and meat products at the same meal is prohibited. Some Buddhists, Hindus, and Sikhs are strict vegetarians. The nurse must be sensitive to such religious dietary practices.

Pain Responses

It has been demonstrated that beliefs about and responses to pain vary among ethnic and racial groups. Cultural response to pain must be viewed in relation to both the actual perception of pain and the meaning or significance of pain to the client and family. In some cultures, pain is considered a punishment for bad deeds; the individual is, therefore, to tolerate pain without complaint in order to atone for sins. In other cultures, self-infliction of pain is a sign of mourning or grief. In other groups, pain is anticipated as a part of the ritualistic practices of passage ceremonies and, therefore, tolerance of pain signifies strength and endurance. In some cultures, boys especially are taught "to take pain like a man" and that "big boys don't cry," but in other cultures, the expression of pain elicits attention and sympathy.

Galanti (2004) notes that nurses and clients may assess pain differently. Nurses and physicians may underestimate or overestimate (and treat accordingly) their client's pain in relation to the client's expression of pain and their own cultural context. Client responses to pain should be assessed within the context of their culture. If the client does not complain of pain, it should not be assumed that the client is not experiencing pain. The nurse must be aware of what conditions are likely to cause pain and offer clients pain relief, as appropriate.

Treatment for pain may also vary with culture. In European Canadian cultures, medication is typically used for pain relief. In other cultures, heat, cold, relaxation, or other techniques and treatments may be used.

Death and Dying Practices

Death is a universal experience, and people want to die with dignity. Various cultural and religious traditions and practices associated with death, dying, and the grieving process help people cope with these experiences. Nurses are often present through the dying process and at the moment of death, especially when it occurs in a healthcare facility. Knowledge of the client's religious and cultural heritage helps nurses provide individualized care to clients and their families, even though they may not participate in the rituals associated with death. It is important for the nurse to ask the family if any special customs or practices are required prior to and after the death of the client.

Dying in solitude is unacceptable in most cultures. In many cultures, people prefer a peaceful death at home rather than in the hospital. Some ethnic groups may request that health professionals not reveal the prognosis to dying clients. They believe the person's last days should be free of worry and pain. People in other cultures prefer that a family member (preferably a male in some cultures) be told the diagnosis so that the client can be tactfully informed by a family member in gradual stages or not told at all. Nurses also need to determine whom to call and when, as the client's death draws near.

Beliefs and attitudes about death, its cause, and the soul also vary among cultures. Unnatural deaths, or bad deaths, are sometimes distinguished from good deaths. In some cultures, the death of a person who has behaved well in life is considered less threatening because that person will be reincarnated into a good life next time.

Beliefs about preparation of the body, autopsy, organ donation, cremation, and prolonging life can be closely allied to the person's religion. *Autopsy*, for example, may be prohibited, opposed, or discouraged by Eastern Orthodox religions, Muslims, Jehovah's Witnesses, and Orthodox Jews. Some religions prohibit the removal of body parts and dictate that all body parts be given appropriate burial. *Organ donation* is prohibited by Jehovah's Witnesses and Muslims, whereas Buddhists in North America consider it an act of mercy and encourage it. *Cremation* is discouraged, opposed, or prohibited by the Mormon, Eastern Orthodox, Islamic, and Jewish faiths. Hindus, in contrast, prefer cremation and cast the ashes in a holy river. *Prolongation of life* is generally encouraged; however, some religions, such as Christian Science, are unlikely to use medical means to prolong life, and the Jewish faith generally opposes prolonging life after irreversible brain damage. In terminal illness, Buddhists may permit euthanasia.

Nurses also need to be knowledgeable about the client's death-related rituals, such as last rites and administration of Holy Communion, chanting at the bedside, and other rituals, such as special procedures for washing, dressing, positioning, and shrouding the dead. For example, certain people may want to retain their native customs, in which family members of the same sex wash and prepare the body for burial and cremation. Muslims customarily turn the body to face Mecca. Nurses need to ask family members about their preference and verify who will carry out these activities. Burial clothes and other cultural or religious items are often important symbols for the funeral. For example, faithful Mormons are often dressed in their temple clothes. Some First Nations people may be dressed in elaborate apparel and jewellery and wrapped in new blankets along with money. The nurse must ensure that any ritual items present in the health-care agency are given to the family or to the funeral home.

Providing Culturally Competent Care

Students in Canadian nursing programs are expected to learn about cultural diversity, and all nurses are expected to provide care, regardless of the culture of the client. The CNA notes that "cultural effectiveness is essential to the accurate assessment of client health status, needs and goals" (CNA, 2000, p. 2). Competencies expected of Canadian nurses include "demonstrating consideration for client diversity, providing culturally sensitive care (e.g., openness, sensitivity, recognizing culturally based practices and values); and incorporating cultural practices into health promotion activities" (CNA, 2000, p. 1).

All phases of the nursing process are affected by the client's and the nurse's cultural values, beliefs, and behaviours. As the client's culture and the nurse's culture come together in the nurse–client relationship, a unique cultural environment is created that can improve or impair the client's outcome. Self-awareness of personal biases can enable nurses to develop modifying behaviours or (if they are unable to do so) to remove themselves from situations where care may be compromised. Nurses can become more aware of their own culture through a values clarification (see Chapter 5). The nurse must also consider the cultural values of the health-care setting because those too can influence the client's outcome. As an example, see Box 10.2 for recommendations for working with Aboriginal clients

To obtain cultural assessment data, the nurse uses broad statements and open-ended questions that encourage clients to express themselves fully (see Box 10.3 for examples). The important principle to remember when conducting an assessment is that "the client is the teacher and expert regarding his or her culture, and the nurse is the learner" (Rosenbaum, 1995, p. 188). At this stage, the nurse draws no conclusions but obtains information from the client.

Many cultural assessment tools are available. The nurse needs to use a tool appropriate to the situation and adapt it as required. For example, a nurse in an emergency department of an urban hospital may need a different format from a nurse working in a home care setting. Nurses need to ensure they collect enough basic cultural data to identify patterns of behaviour that may either facilitate or interfere with a nursing strategy or treatment plan.

BOX 10.2 GUIDE FOR HEALTH PROFESSIONALS WORKING WITH ABORIGINAL PEOPLES

According to the Society of Obstetricians and Gynaecologists of Canada (2000), health professionals should do the following:

1. Have a basic understanding of the appropriate names with which to refer to the various groups of Aboriginal peoples in Canada
2. Have a basic understanding of the current sociodemographics of Aboriginal peoples in Canada
3. Familiarize themselves with the traditional geographic territories and language groups of Aboriginal peoples
4. Have a basic understanding of the disruptive impact of colonization on the health and well-being of Aboriginal peoples
5. Recognize that the current sociodemographic challenges facing many Aboriginal individuals and communities have a significant impact on health status
6. Recognize the need to provide health services for Aboriginal peoples as close to home as possible
7. Have a basic understanding of governmental obligations and policies regarding the health of Aboriginal peoples in Canada
8. Recognize the need to support Aboriginal individuals and communities in the process of self-determination

Source: Adapted from *Policy Statement: A Guide for Health Professionals Working with Aboriginal Peoples* (p. 5), by the Society of Obstetricians and Gynaecologists of Canada, 2000. Retrieved May 16, 2008, from http://www.sogc.org/guidelines/public/100E-PS1-December2000.pdf

Anderson and colleagues (1990) and the College of Nurses of Ontario (2008) emphasize the following points relevant to cultural assessment:

- A cultural assessment takes time and usually needs to extend over several sessions.
- The nurse's recognition of his or her own ethnicity and social background is essential. Even when the nurse and client share the same ethnic background, the nurse should expect differences in beliefs and values.
- Self-reflection assists nurses in determining values and biases that could influence interventions and their effect on the client. Self-reflection causes nurses to look at their responses to different situations and think about why they reacted in the manner they did. Nurses continually reflect on their reaction to their own culture and to clients' cultures to give culturally appropriate, safe care.
- The *process* of assessment is important. How and when questions are asked requires sensitivity and clinical judgment.
- The timing and phrasing of questions need to be adapted to the individual. Timing is important in introducing questions. Sensitivity is needed in phrasing questions.
- Trust must be established before clients can be expected to volunteer and share sensitive information. The nurse, therefore, needs to spend time with clients, introduce some social conversation,

BOX 10.3 EXAMPLES OF OPEN-ENDED QUESTIONS FOR A CULTURAL ASSESSMENT

CULTURAL AFFILIATION
I am interested in learning about your cultural heritage. Can you tell me about your cultural group, where you were born, and how long you have lived in this country?

BELIEFS ABOUT CURRENT ILLNESS
What do you call your problem? What name do you give it? What do you think has caused it? Why did it start when it did? What does your sickness do to your body? How severe is it? What do you fear most about your sickness? What are the chief problems your sickness has caused for you personally, for your family, and at work?

COMMUNICATION
What languages do you speak at home? What languages are you most comfortable speaking? In what language(s) can you read and write? How would you like us to address you? by your first name? by your last name? Would you like an interpreter?

HEALTH-CARE PRACTICES
What kinds of things do you do to maintain health? For example, what types of food do you eat to maintain health? What foods do you eat during illness, and how is food prepared? What other activities do you or your family do to keep people healthy (e.g., wearing amulets, religious or spiritual practices)? How do you know when you are healthy?

ILLNESS BELIEFS AND CARE PRACTICES
What kinds of things do you do to treat illness? Do you use traditional healers (shaman, curandero, priest, spiritualist, minister, monk)? Who determines when a person is sick? How would you describe your past experiences with cultural healers and Western health professionals? What special remedies are generally used for the illness you have? What remedies are you currently using (e.g., herbal remedies, potions, massage, wearing of talismans, copper bracelets, or charms)? What remedies have you used in the past, and which did you find helpful? What remedies or treatments are you considering now, and how can we help? Is the care we are giving you what you think it should be? How would you like us to care for you?

FAMILY LIFE AND SUPPORT SYSTEM
I would like to learn about your family. Who are the members of your family? What family duties do women and men usually perform in your culture? Whom do you consult when making health-care decisions (e.g., another family member, cultural or religious leader)? Who will be able to help you during and after treatment? Do you need help to contact these people?

Sources: Based on *Transcultural Concepts in Nursing Care* (4th ed.), M. M. Andrews and J. S. Boyle, 2003, Philadelphia, PA: Lippincott; "Culture, Illness and Care," by A. Kleinman, L. Eisenberg, and B. Good, 1978, *Annals of Internal Medicine, 88*, pp. 251–258; "A Cultural Assessment Guide: Learning Cultural Sensitivity," by J. N. Rosenbaum, 1991, *Canadian Nurse, 88*, pp. 32–33; and *Cross-Cultural Caring: A Handbook for Health Professionals in Western Canada*, by N. Waxler-Morrison, J. Anderson, and E. Richardson (Eds.), 1990, Vancouver: UBC Press.

and convey a genuine desire to understand their values and beliefs.

Before a cultural assessment begins, the nurse determines what language the client speaks and the client's degree of fluency in English. The nurse can also learn about the client's communication patterns and space orientation by observing both verbal and nonverbal communication. For example, does the client do the speaking or defer to another? What nonverbal communication behaviours does the client exhibit (e.g., touching, eye contact)? What significance do these behaviours have for the nurse–client interaction? What is the client's proximity to other people and objects within the environment? How does the client react to the nurse's movement toward him or her? What cultural objects within the environment have importance for health promotion or health maintenance?

To provide *culturally congruent care* that benefits, satisfies, and is meaningful to the people nurses serve, Leininger (1991) conceptualizes three major modes to guide nursing judgments, decisions, and actions:

1. *Cultural care preservation and maintenance.* The nurse accepts and complies with the client's cultural beliefs. For example, the nurse provides herbal tea to ease a "nervous stomach," a practice the client says has worked well in the past.
2. *Cultural care accommodation and negotiation.* The nurse plans, negotiates, and accommodates the client's culturally specific food preferences, religious practices, kinship needs, childcare practices, and treatment practices.
3. *Cultural care repatterning or restructuring.* The nurse is knowledgeable about culture care and develops ways to repattern or restructure nursing care without violating either the client's beliefs or the nurse's standards of practice.

Cultural care preservation may involve the use of cultural health-care practices, such as giving herbal tea, chicken soup, or hot foods to the ill client. Accommodating the client's viewpoint and negotiating appropriate care require expert communication skills, such as responding empathetically, validating information, and effectively summarizing content.

Negotiation is a collaborative process. It acknowledges that the nurse–client relationship is reciprocal and that differences exist between the nurse and client about notions of health, illness, and treatment. The nurse attempts to bridge the gap between his or her (scientific and cultural) perspectives and the client's (cultural) perspectives. During the negotiation process, the nurse first elicits the client's views and acknowledges these views; then, if appropriate, the nurse provides relevant scientific information. If the client's views reveal that certain behaviours would not affect the client's condition adversely, then the nurse incorporates these views in planning care. If the client's views can lead to harmful behaviours, then the nurse attempts to shift the client's perspectives to the scientific view.

Negotiation, therefore, occurs when cultural treatment practices conflict with those of the health-care system and when the cultural practices are considered harmful to the client's well-being. The nurse must determine precisely how the client is managing the illness, what practices could be harmful, and which practices can be safely combined with Western medicine. For example, reducing dosages of an antihypertensive medication or replacing insulin therapy with herbal measures can be detrimental. In situations where harm may occur, the nurse needs to inform the client about possible outcomes.

When a client chooses to follow only cultural practices and refuses all prescribed medical or nursing interventions, nursing goals for the client need to be adjusted. Anderson and colleagues (1990) point out that monitoring the client's condition to identify changes in health state and to recognize impending crises before they become irreversible may be all that is realistically achievable. At a time of crisis, the nurse may then have the opportunity to renegotiate the original care approach.

Transcultural nursing care is challenging. It requires discovery of the meaning of the client's behaviour, flexibility, creativity, and knowledge to adapt nursing interventions. For example, a culturally sensitive nurse knows that a Chinese woman who has just given birth and refuses to eat fruits and vegetables, refuses to drink the cold water at her bedside, stays in bed, and refuses to take sitz baths, baths, or showers needs to increase her yang forces. The nurse will make plans to adapt nursing interventions accordingly.

Nurses also need to identify community resources that are available to assist clients of diverse cultures. Nurses should try to learn from each transcultural nursing situation that they encounter to improve the delivery of culture-specific care to future clients. Box 10.4 offers suggestions for providing culturally competent nursing care.

BOX 10.4 PROVIDING CULTURALLY COMPETENT CARE TO FAMILIES

To offer culturally competent nursing care, nurses can use the following suggestions:

- Learn the rituals, customs, and practices of the major cultural groups with whom you come into contact. Learn to appreciate the richness of diversity as an asset, rather than a hindrance, in your practice.
- Identify personal biases, attitudes, prejudices, and stereotypes.
- Include cultural assessment of the client and family as part of overall assessment.
- Recognize that it is the client's (or family's) right to make his or her own health-care choices.
- Convey respect and cooperate with traditional helpers and caregivers.

Case Study 10

Rose Maniwaki is a 65-year-old Aboriginal person with a history of diabetes. She was diagnosed with gestational diabetes during her first pregnancy in her early twenties. She has had six pregnancies and, during each, her diabetes was significantly aggravated. She is now fully insulin dependent with type II diabetes and is clinically obese (175 cm tall, 110 kg). Her diabetes is extremely difficult to control. She has had her right foot amputated below the knee and has had a prosthesis since age 60. She has osteoarthritis, osteoporosis, and high blood pressure.

Rose is a widow. Her husband died in his forties of uncontrolled diabetes combined with alcoholism. She lives in a small, poorly insulated, mouldy, overcrowded, two-bedroom house in a First Nations community in northern Ontario. After her husband's death, she raised her children alone on social assistance and is now raising five grandchildren so her daughter can attend nursing school in a community 400 km away. Two of Rose's other children are dead—one from suicide, the other from a drunk driving car accident. Her other surviving children have left northern Ontario, and she has had little or no contact with them. Rose is also struggling with alcoholism.

Rose experiences depression and takes Prozac to help with her health problems and sense of loss. The Prozac does not help very much. Rose uses sleeping pills to assist with sleep. Rose attended residential school from age 6 to 13 and, therefore, is not as connected to her family and community as she might otherwise be. She has had trouble connecting with her culture and its values. However, there is a new community health centre with a traditional circular healing room where traditional healers are available alongside a nurse practitioner, nurses, community health representatives, a nutritionist, and a social worker. Rose has been coming to the health centre on a more or less regular basis and has found herself drawn to the traditional healers.

Rose has come to the health centre because she is experiencing breakdown of her stump, which is cracked and painful, as well as draining pus. The nurse practitioner advises her that she may need to travel south to the hospital if the infection persists. Rose has no other family members in the community and worries about who would care for her grandchildren if she has to fly out for hospital care. Rose has brought one of her granddaughters with her to the clinic. Rose's granddaughter is extremely overweight—and, given her family history, at high risk for diabetes.

Through her involvement at the community health centre and interactions with the traditional healers, Rose has begun to become more active in the community and has joined a women's drumming group. She has found the regular gatherings of her drumming group, comprising women of varying ages, to be very helpful in her struggle with alcoholism and depression. Her drumming group gave the opening welcome to an evening heart health talk held in her community for First Nations women and Rose discovered that diabetes is a major risk factor.

As a result of her experiences at the community health centre and in her drumming group, Rose has become involved in self-governance and has joined a group in the local band office, particularly focusing on health issues, such as diabetes, alcoholism, and depression.

Critical Thinking Questions

1. Using the nursing process, develop a plan of care for Rose and her family (assessment, nursing diagnosis, planning, intervention, and evaluation; see Chapter 22).
   a. How would you integrate knowledge of colonization and residential schools into Rose and her family's care?
   b. How would you integrate Rose's newly discovered appreciation of traditional healing to her plan of care?
   c. As a health-care provider, what questions would you ask Rose about her family, her community, her diabetes?

After working through these questions, go to the MyNursingLab at **http://www.mynursinglab.com** to check your answers.

KEY TERMS

culture-universals
culture-specifics
culture
subculture
bicultural
diversity
ethnic
cultural identity
race
acculturation
assimilation
colonization
ethnic identity
transcultural nursing
cultural awareness
cultural sensitivity
cultural safety
cultural competence
culture shock
ethnocentrism
ethnorelativity
stereotyping
prejudice
discrimination
racism
scientific or biomedical health belief
holistic health belief
traditional medicine

CHAPTER HIGHLIGHTS

- Canadians come from a variety of ethnic and cultural backgrounds, and many Canadians retain at least some of their traditional values, beliefs, and practices.
- Many groups in Canada are bicultural; that is, they embrace two cultures: their original ethnic culture and a Canadian culture.
- An individual's ethnic and cultural background can influence beliefs, values, and practices.
- Through acculturation, most ethnic and cultural groups in Canada modify some of their traditional cultural characteristics.
- Personal characteristics also modify an individual's cultural values, beliefs, and practices.
- Health beliefs and practices, family patterns, communication style, space and time orientation, nutritional patterns, pain response, and death and dying practices influence the relationship between the nurse and the client who have individual cultural backgrounds.
- When assessing a client, the nurse considers the client's cultural values, beliefs, and practices related to health and health care.
- Self-reflection is a critical component of providing culturally safe health care.

ASSESS YOUR LEARNING

1. Canada's population has more than doubled in the past 50 years, because of which of the following?
   a. Immigration
   b. Longer life expectancy
   c. Higher birthrates
   d. Immunization

2. The Canada Act, which replaced the British North America Act in 1982, recognized what specific groups in Canada?
   a. Immigrants from Europe
   b. Aboriginal groups: First Nations, Métis, and Inuit
   c. British and French descendants of the first European immigrants
   d. New immigrants to Canada from Asia

3. Cultural safety focuses on which of the following?
   a. Transcultural nursing theories
   b. Cultural awareness
   c. Cultural competence
   d. Self-reflection and power

4. An example of stereotyping is which of the following?
   a. Holding a strong opinion against an individual or group of individuals
   b. Giving preferential treatment to individuals or groups of individuals based on gender, social class, or ethnicity
   c. Assuming that all members of a group are alike
   d. Seeing your one own group as superior to another

5. You are about to begin assisting a young woman from a Middle Eastern country with her morning care; she suddenly appears to be very uncomfortable and asks if she can do it later. In keeping with the College of Nurses of Ontario's *Guidelines for Culturally Sensitive Care,* which of the following would you do?
   a. Immediately pack up your equipment and tell her you will be back later.
   b. Explain that you are very busy and that this is the only time that her morning care can be done.
   c. Discuss with the client when she would like to do her morning care and incorporate it in your nursing care plan.
   d. Tell the client that if she does not do it now, she will have to wait until tomorrow.

6. You are assigned to care for an older Aboriginal man. In keeping with his traditions, he would like to do a "smudge," that is, ignite a very small quantity of tobacco that he keeps in a pouch with him at all times. What should you do?
   a. Explain that there is a no smoking bylaw and that he cannot smoke at any time.
   b. Inform him that lighting fires in the hospital is against the law.
   c. Insist that he give you his tobacco since smoking is bad for him.
   d. Ask him what a smudge is and why he wants to do it.

7. In the scenarios in questions 5 and 6, what is the most important aspect of providing culturally competent nursing care?
   a. The client feels safe in the nurse–client relationship.
   b. You feel that you have done everything to make the client like you.
   c. You learn something new every day.
   d. Your clients' preferences are as important as your own.

8. You are assigned to care for a client who does not speak or understand English, the only language that you speak and understand. The client is accompanied by his young grandson, who appears to be about 8 years of age. In this instance you would require which of the following?
   a. An older member of the family to act as an interpreter
   b. A professional health-care interpreter
   c. No additional help—the grandson will be the best person to interpret
   d. The use of nonverbal methods of communication, such as drawing pictures or gesturing

9. You are working in a community agency and one of your clients is consistently late for appointments. This is very distressing to you, since you are very busy and cannot always accommodate the client when she does eventually appear. You are aware that not all cultures have the same time orientation as Western cultures, that is, to be on time and to keep their scheduled appointments. However, you are not sure whether that is the only reason for the lateness. What should you do?
   a. Tell the client that you are very busy and that she should let you know in advance if she is going to be late for the appointment.
   b. In a calm and nonthreatening manner you ask the client why she is always late for appointments and ask if you can assist her in any way to keep the scheduled appointments.
   c. Explain to the client that time is very important in Western or Canadian culture.

d. Offer to get her a watch so she can keep track of the time.

10. You are assigned two patients who have had abdominal surgery; one patient is constantly complaining about pain, while the other patient does not tell you he is experiencing pain, but you can tell by his facial expressions that he is. Which of the following is true?

a. You know that varying beliefs and responses pertaining to pain exist in different cultures and that pain should always be assessed within the context of the patient's culture.

b. You believe that every patient should be cared for equally and according to Western beliefs and values.

c. You insist that the patient who is more vocal about their pain keep quiet since he is disturbing the other patients.

d. You ask their physicians to increase their analgesic.

After working through these questions, go to the MyNursingLab at ***http://www.mynursinglab.com*** *to check your answers and see explanations.*

SUGGESTED READINGS

Abdullah, S. N. (1995). Towards an individualized client's care: Implications for education. The transcultural approach. *Journal of Advanced Nursing, 22,* 715–720.

Individualized care cannot be achieved without considering the factors associated with the personal being, such as culture, beliefs, and traditions. This article has nurses look at their own values as a step to providing unbiased nursing care.

Browne, A., & Fiske, J. (2001). First Nations women's encounters with mainstream health care services. *Western Journal of Nursing Research, 23*(2), 126–147.

This research examines mainstream health-care encounters from the viewpoint of First Nations women from a reserve community in northwestern Canada. The women's narratives identified their encounters as being shaped by racism, discrimination, and structural inequities that contribute to their marginalization from mainstream society.

Spector, R. E. (2004). *Cultural diversity in health and illness* (6th ed.). Upper Saddle River, NJ: Pearson Prentice Hall.

This useful text begins with sections on creating self-awareness in providers of their own and their familial beliefs and practices regarding health and illness. The author discusses general information on health traditions and health care. Specific views of specific cultural groups are outlined. A guide to heritage assessment and health traditions is included.

WEBLINKS

Canadian Heritage Multiculturalism

http://www.canadianheritage.gc.ca/progs/multi/index_e.cfm

This site has multiple links to governmental, nongovernmental, Canadian, and international organizations.

Virtual Museum Canada

http://www.virtualmuseum.ca/English/index_flash.html

This site is the result of a partnership between Canada's museum community and the Department of Canadian Heritage. Through the internet, the user can celebrate the stories and treasures that have helped to define Canada.

Indian and Northern Affairs Canada

http://www.ainc-inac.gc.ca

This site describes the First Nations peoples and their cultures. The Indian Act, the Oka Crisis, and the Royal Commission on Aboriginal Peoples are among some of the topics addressed through the publications available on the site.

Aboriginal Nurses Association of Canada

http://www.anac.on.ca

This is the website of the only professional Aboriginal nursing organization in Canada. It contains information on history, statistics, and current events and initiatives.

First Nations and Inuit Branch

http://www.hc-sc.gc.ca/fnih-spni/index_e.html

This government site gives information on history, health challenges, funding, and programming focused on Canada's Aboriginal groups.

Health Canada's Food Guide

http://www.hc-sc.gc.ca/fn-an/pubs/fnim-pnim/index_e.html
http://www.hc-sc.gc.ca/fn-an/food-guide-aliment/index_e.html

At the first site, you will find culturally appropriate information for using Canada's Food Guide *with Aboriginal groups, in a publication called* Eating Well with Canada's Food Guide: First Nations, Inuit and Métis. *The second link is to the original* Canada's Food Guide.

REFERENCES

Anderson, J. M., Waxler-Morrison, N., Richardson, E., Herbert, C., & Murphy, M. (1990). Delivering culturally sensitive health care. In N. Waxler-Morrison, J. Anderson, & E. Richardson (Eds.), *Cross-cultural caring: A handbook for health professionals in Western Canada* (pp. 245–267). Vancouver, BC: UBC Press.

Andrews, M. M., & Boyle, J. S. (2003). *Transcultural concepts in nursing care* (4th ed.). Philadelphia, PA: Lippincott.

Banks, J., & Banks, C. (1989). *Multicultural education and perspectives.* Boston, MA: Allyn & Bacon.

Campbell, J., & Campbell, D. (1996). Cultural competence in the care of abused women. *Journal of Nurse-Midwifery, 41*(6), 457–461.

Canadian Human Rights Commission. (n.d.). *Human rights in Canada: A historical perspective.* Retrieved May 18, 2008, from http://www.chrc-ccdp.ca/en/timePortals/milestones/118mile.asp

Canadian Multiculturalism Act. RS 1985, c.24 (4th Supp). *Statutes of Canada.* Ottawa: Queen's Printer. pp. 835–841.

Canadian Nurses Association. (2000). Cultural diversity—Changes and challenges. *Nursing Now: Issues and Trends in Canadian Nursing.* Ottawa: Author. Retrieved December 14, 2007, from: http://www.cna-aiic.ca/CNA/documents/pdf/publications/CulturalDiversity_February2000_e.pdf

Canadian Nurses Association. (2004). *Position Statement: Promoting Culturally Competent Care.* Retrieved December 14, 2007, from: http://www.cna-nurses.ca/CNA/issues/position/practice/default_e.aspx

Canadian Nurses Association. (2006). *Blueprint for the Canadian Registered Nurse Examination.* Ottawa: Author.

Chui, T., Tran, K., & Maheux, H. (2007). *Immigration in Canada: A portrait of the foreign-born population, 2006 census: Findings.* Retrieved May 18, 2008, from http://www12.statcan.ca/english/census06/analysis/immcit/index.cfm

College of Nurses of Ontario. (2008). *Practice Guideline for Culturally Sensitive Care.* Retrieved December 14, 2007, from http://www.cno.org/docs/prac/41040_CulturallySens.pdf

Corbeil, J.-P., & Blaser, C. (2007). *The evolving linguistic portrait, 2006 census: Findings.* Retrieved May 18, 2008, from http://www12.statcan.ca/english/census06/analysis/language/index.cfm

DeSantis, L., & Lowe, J. (1992). Moving from cultural sensitivity to cultural competence in nursing practice: Pitfalls and progress. Paper presented at the 18th Annual Transcultural Nursing Society Conference, Miami, FL, October 22–24, 1992.

Doane, G. & Varcoe, C. (2005). *Family nursing as relational inquiry.* Philadelphia, PA: Lippincott, Williams, Wilkins

Eliason, M. J. (1993). Ethics and transcultural nursing care. *Nursing Outlook, 4,* 225–228.

Galanti, G. (2004). *Caring for patients from different cultures* (3rd ed.). Philadelphia, PA: University of Pennsylvania Press.

Giger, J. N., & Davidhizar, R. (2004). *Transcultural nursing: Assessment and interventions* (4th ed.). St. Louis, MO: Mosby.

Hughes, M., & Farrow, T. (2006). Preparing for cultural safety assessment. *Kai Tiaki Nursing New Zealand,* Feb. 2006, pp. 12–14.

Laurentian University. (2007). *Interprofessional collaboration: Culturally informed Aboriginal health care.* Sudbury, ON: Author.

Leininger, M. M. (1970). *Nursing and anthropology: Two worlds to blend.* New York: Wiley.

Leininger, M. M. (1978). *Transcultural nursing: Concepts, theories, and practices.* New York: Wiley.

Leininger, M. M. (1988). Leininger's theory of nursing: Cultural care diversity and universality. *Nursing Science Quarterly, 14,* 152–160.

Leininger, M. M. (Ed.). (1991). *Culture care diversity and universality: A theory of nursing.* New York: National League for Nursing Press. Pub. No. 15–2402.

Leininger, M. M. (1993). Towards conceptualization of transcultural health care systems: Concepts and a model. *Journal of Transcultural Nursing, 4,* 32–40.

Leininger, M. M. (2006). *Culture care diversity and universality: A worldwide nursing theory.* (2nd ed.). Toronto: Jones and Barlett Publishers.

Lynam, M. J. (1992). Towards the goal of providing culturally sensitive care: Principles upon which to build nursing curricula. *Journal of Advanced Nursing, 17,* 149–157.

Martel, L., & Caron-Malenfant. (2007a). *Portrait of the Canadian population in 2006, Findings.* Retrieved May 18, 2008, from http://www12.statcan.ca/english/census06/analysis/popdwell/index.cfm

Martel, L., & Caron-Malenfant. (2007b). *Portrait of the Canadian population in 2006, age and sex: Findings.* Retrieved May 18, 2008, from http://www12.statcan.ca/english/census06/analysis/agesex/index.cfm

Nursing Council of New Zealand. (2005). *Guidelines for cultural safety, the Treaty of Waitangi and Maori health in nursing education and practice.* Wellington, NZ: Author. Retrieved May 16, 2008, from http://www.nursingcouncil.org.nz/Cultural%20Safety.pdf

Purnell, L., & Paulanka, B. (2005). *Transcultural health care: A culturally competent approach.* Philadelphia, PA: Davis.

Papps, E., & Ramsden, I. (1996). Cultural safety in nursing: The New Zealand experience. *International Journal for Quality in Health Care, 8*(5), 491–497.

Potthast-Jukeit, B. (1997). The history of the family and colonialism. *The History of the Family, 2*(2), 115–121.

Rairdan, B., & Higgs, Z. R. (1992). When your patient is a Hmong refugee. *American Journal of Nursing, 92,* 52–55.

Registered Nurses' Association of Ontario. (2007). *Best practice guideline: Embracing cultural diversity in health care: Developing Cultural Competence.* Toronto: Author

Rosenbaum, J. N. (1995). Teaching cultural sensitivity. *Journal of Nursing Education, 34,* 188–189.

Schellenberg, G., & Maheux, H. (2007). *Immigrants' perspectives on their first four years in Canada: Highlights from three waves of the longitudinal survey of immigrants to Canada.* Retrieved May 18, 2008, from http://www.statcan.ca/english/freepub/11-008-XIE/2007000/11-008-XIE20070009627.htm

Smith, L. T. (1999). *Decolonizing methodologies: Research and indigenous peoples.* London, UK: Zed.

Spector, R. E. (2004). *Cultural diversity in health and illness* (6th ed.). Upper Saddle River, NJ: Pearson Prentice Hall.

Srivastava, R. H. (2007). *The healthcare professional's guide to clinical cultural competence.* Toronto: Mosby Elsevier Canada.

Statistics Canada. (2003). *Religions in Canada.* Retrieved May 18, 2008, from http://www12.statcan.ca/english/census01/Products/Analytic/companion/rel/contents.cfm

Statistics Canada. (2008a). *Canada's changing labour force, 2006 census: Findings.* Retrieved May 18, 2008, from http://www12.statcan.ca/english/census06/analysis/labour/index.cfm

Statistics Canada. (2008b). *Visible minority population and population group reference guide, 2006 census.* Retrieved May 17, 2008, from http://www12.statcan.ca/english/census06/reference/reportsandguides/visible-minorities.cfm

Statistics Canada. (2008c). *Canada's ethnocultural mosaic, 2006 census: Findings.* Retrieved May 17, 2008, from http://www12.statcan.ca/english/census06/analysis/ethnicorigin/index.cfm

Statistics Canada. (2008d). Aboriginal peoples in Canada in 2006: Inuit, Métis and First Nations, 2006 census. *The Daily,* January 15. Retrieved May 18, 2008, from http://www.statcan.ca/Daily/English/080115/d080115a.htm

Steinmetz, S., & Braham, C. G. (Eds.). (1993). *Random House Webster's dictionary.* New York: Ballantine Reference Library.

Waxler-Morrison, N., Anderson, J., & Richardson, E. (Eds.). (1990). *Cross-cultural caring: A handbook for health professionals in Western Canada.* Vancouver, BC: UBC Press.

Yonge, O., & Bernard, M. (1998). The Cree living in urban settings. In R. E. Davidhizar & J. N. Giger (Eds.), *Canadian transcultural nursing: Assessment and intervention* (pp. 179–196). St. Louis, MO: Mosby.

Chapter 11

Individual Care

Nurses assess and plan health care for individuals. Care of the individual is enhanced when the nurse understands the concepts of individuality, holism, homeostasis, human needs, and systems theory. The beliefs and values of each person and the support they receive come in large part from the family and are reinforced by the community. Thus, an understanding of family dynamics and the context of the community assists the nurse in planning care. For additional information on the family and community, see Chapters 12 and 13. To assist clients toward health, nurses must understand them as individuals. The nurse uses knowledge of individuality, holism, homeostasis, human needs, and systems theory in the context of the client's situation, whomever the client may be (individual, family, group, community, population). This text is primarily concerned with individual clients.

This application of knowledge is known as client-centred care and is the centrepiece of the profession and of this text. As outlined in Chapter 1, the individual recipient of care may be called a patient, resident, or client. This terminology has been a topic of some controversy, with several organizations using both patient and client in their published documents. For example, the Saskatchewan Registered Nurses' Association (2005) refers to *patients* in their *Nurse Practitioner Scope of Practice,* and the College of Nurses of Ontario (2004) refers to *patient safety movement*. Conversely, the *Best Practice Guidelines* of the Registered Nurses' Association of Ontario kept the title *Client Centred Care* when they revised the guideline in 2006. Wing (1997) actually asked individuals attending a back-pain clinic and contends that the majority of individuals seeking care prefer to be called *patients*. He makes the point that the health professional should follow the person's lead and use the terminology preferred by the individual. In this text, we have chosen to refer to the individual seeking care, especially within an acute-care setting as a *patient*, and the person living in a long-term-care setting as a *resident*. We have referred to *clients* as those individuals receiving care in community settings. Sometimes concepts that are developed for individuals can be applied to communities and vice versa (see the Reflect on Primary Health Care box).

OBJECTIVES

After studying this chapter, you should be able to

1. Explain the relationship of individuality and holism to nursing practice
2. Compare and contrast the elements of physiologic and psychological homeostasis
3. Identify six common factors that can make an individual more vulnerable to some health problems and describe a nursing implication for each
4. Identity Maslow's five categories in the hierarchy of human needs
5. Discuss how a nurse might use the three selected types of theories to begin to assess an individual's health needs

REFLECT ON PRIMARY HEALTH CARE

Often the principles of primary health are considered in light of the health of communities and populations. However, each of the principles can be applied to the individual seeking care. For instance, accessibility may be difficult even when the service is present if it has limited hours or affordable public transport to get to the service is lacking. Public participation may refer to the individual's contributions to decisions about his or her health care.

It is important to remember, as you read this chapter, that you are an individual and are influenced by the same factors as your clients. For example, when reading the Nursing and Canadian Society box, do you identify in your home community with the nursing implications presented?

NURSING AND CANADIAN SOCIETY

Fact	Implications for Nursing Practice
In a list of European and North American countries, only Iceland has a smaller population density per square kilometre than Canada (Statistics Canada, 2005).	Access to health care may be difficult for some people in Canada.
The trend was to higher levels of education in the population from 1986 to 2006. For example, persons with a high school diploma rose from 20% to 24%. In the same population, persons with a college certificate or degree went from 10.4% to 32%, and those with a completed bachelor's degree went from 6% to 23% (Statistics Canada, 2004a, 2008).	Nurses may expect that patients come with higher levels of health-care knowledge and also expect to be provided with more information about health and health care.
By 2006, the total population had increased by 5.4% since 2001. One-person households, however, increased by 13.5% between 1996–2001 and by 11.8% from 2001–2006 (Statistics Canada, 2004b, 2007a, b).	More people are living alone in Canada and may not have readily available assistance from family members.

Individual Health

Concept of Individuality

To help clients attain, maintain, or regain an optimal level of health, nurses need to understand clients as individuals. Each individual is a unique being who is different from every other human being, with a different genetic makeup, life experiences, and environmental interactions.

Dimensions of individuality include the person's total character, self-identity, and perceptions. The person's *total character* encompasses behaviours, emotional states, attitudes, values, motives, abilities, habits, and appearances. The person's *self-identity* encompasses perception of self as a separate and distinct entity, alone and in interactions with others. Identity is often threatened by actual or perceived alterations in wellness. Some changes are minor and may be considered merely inconveniences; others can compromise existence in profound ways. The person's *perceptions* encompass the way the person interprets the environment or situation, directly affecting how the person thinks, feels, and acts in any given situation.

Nurses' and clients' perceptions determine their subjective realities at the time of their interaction. Differences can exist in the two views of reality that will influence communication, acceptance of each other, and whether the client's health-care needs are being met. Sometimes, the views of nurses and clients differ because of their own unique experiences.

When providing care, nurses need to focus on the client within both a total care and an individualized care context. In the total care context, the nurse considers all the principles and areas that apply when taking care of any client of that age and condition. In the individualized care context, the nurse becomes acquainted with the client as an individual, referring to the total care principles and using the principles that apply to this person at this time. For example, a nurse who is advising the mother of a preschooler understands that the child's desire to explore the world is a developmental stage that all preschoolers experience. However, the preschooler diagnosed with attention deficit disorder with hyperactivity may have an increased risk of accidents and injuries when interacting with the environment, because of impulsivity and poor self-control.

Concept of Holism

Nurses are concerned with the individual as a whole, complete, or holistic person, not as an assembly of parts and processes. The terms **holistic** and **holism** are derived from the Greek word meaning "whole." The term *holism* itself

BOX 11.1 FACTORS INFLUENCING THE IMPACT OF ILLNESS ON THE INDIVIDUAL

Holism can help nurses understand how different factors and relationships can change the way illness affects an individual. Some of these factors follow:

- The meaning of the illness to the individual
- The nature of the illness, which can range from minor to life threatening
- The duration of the illness, which ranges from short to long term
- The residual effects of the illness, including none to permanent disability
- The financial and social impact of the illness on the individual's ability to work
- The impact of the illness on the individual's family

was coined by Jan Smuts, a South African scholar and political leader, in his book *Holism and Evolution* (1926). In holistic theory, a living organism is seen as an interacting, unified whole that is more than the mere sum of its parts. Viewed in this light, any disturbance in one part is a disturbance of the whole system or being (see Box 11.1).

When applied in nursing, the concept of holism emphasizes that nurses must keep the whole person in mind and strive to understand how one area of concern relates to the whole person. The nurse must also consider the relationship of the individual to the external environment and to others. For example, in helping a man who is grieving over the death of his spouse, the nurse explores the impact of the loss on the whole person (i.e., on the man's appetite, rest and sleep patterns, energy level, sense of well-being, mood, usual activities, family relationships, and relationships with others). Nursing interventions are directed toward restoring overall harmony, so they depend on the man's sense of purpose and meaning of his life. Nursing theorists, such as Parse and Newman (see Chapter 4 for additional information), based their theories on looking at the whole person.

Concept of Homeostasis

The concept of homeostasis was first introduced by Cannon (1939) to describe the relative constancy of the internal processes of the body, such as blood oxygen and carbon dioxide levels, blood pressure, body temperature, blood glucose, and fluid and electrolyte balance. To Cannon, the word *homeostasis* did not imply something stagnant, set, or immobile; it meant a condition that might vary but remained relatively constant. Cannon viewed the human being as separate from the external environment and constantly endeavouring to maintain physiologic **equilibrium**, or balance, through adaptation to that environment. **Homeostasis**, then, is the tendency of the body to maintain a state of balance or equilibrium while continually changing.

PHYSIOLOGIC HOMEOSTASIS Physiologic homeostasis means that the internal environment of the body is relatively stable and constant. All cells of the body require a relatively constant environment to function; thus, the body's internal environment must be maintained within narrow limits. Homeostatic mechanisms have four main characteristics:

1. They are self-regulating.
2. They are compensatory.
3. They tend to be regulated by negative feedback systems.
4. They can require several feedback mechanisms to correct only one physiologic imbalance.

Self-regulation means that homeostatic mechanisms come into play automatically in the healthy person. However, if a person is ill or if an organ, such as a lung, is injured, the homeostatic mechanisms may not be able to respond to the stimulus as they would normally. Homeostatic mechanisms are **compensatory** (counterbalancing) because they tend to counteract conditions that are abnormal for the person. An example is a sudden drop in temperature. The compensatory mechanisms are that the peripheral blood vessels constrict, thereby diverting most of the blood internally, and muscular activity increases and shivering occurs to create heat. Through these mechanisms the body temperature remains stable, despite the cold.

Feedback is the mechanism by which some of the output of a system is fed back into the system as input. This input influences the behaviour of the system and its future output. **Negative feedback** inhibits change; **positive feedback** stimulates change. Most biological systems are controlled by negative feedback to bring the system back to stability. This type of feedback system senses and counteracts any deviations from normal. Negative feedback is a common control mechanism for hormone levels. For example, an increase in the production of parathyroid hormone is stimulated by a drop in blood calcium, but when additional parathyroid hormone raises the level of blood calcium, the hormone's production is then inhibited. As noted, several negative feedback systems can be required to correct one physiologic imbalance. For example, with hypoxia (shortage of oxygen), the concentration of red blood cells increases and the heart rate becomes faster to transport the blood and available oxygen around the body adequately.

The two major homeostatic regulators are the autonomic nervous system and the endocrine system. In addition, the cardiovascular system, the renal system, the respiratory system, and the gastrointestinal system are important in maintaining homeostasis. See Figure 11.1.

PSYCHOLOGICAL HOMEOSTASIS The term *psychological homeostasis* refers to emotional or psychological balance or a state of mental well-being. Each person has certain psychological needs, such as the need for love, security, and self-esteem, that must be met to maintain

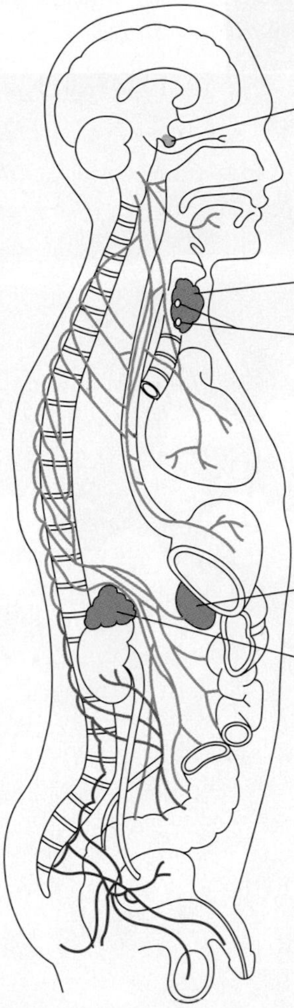

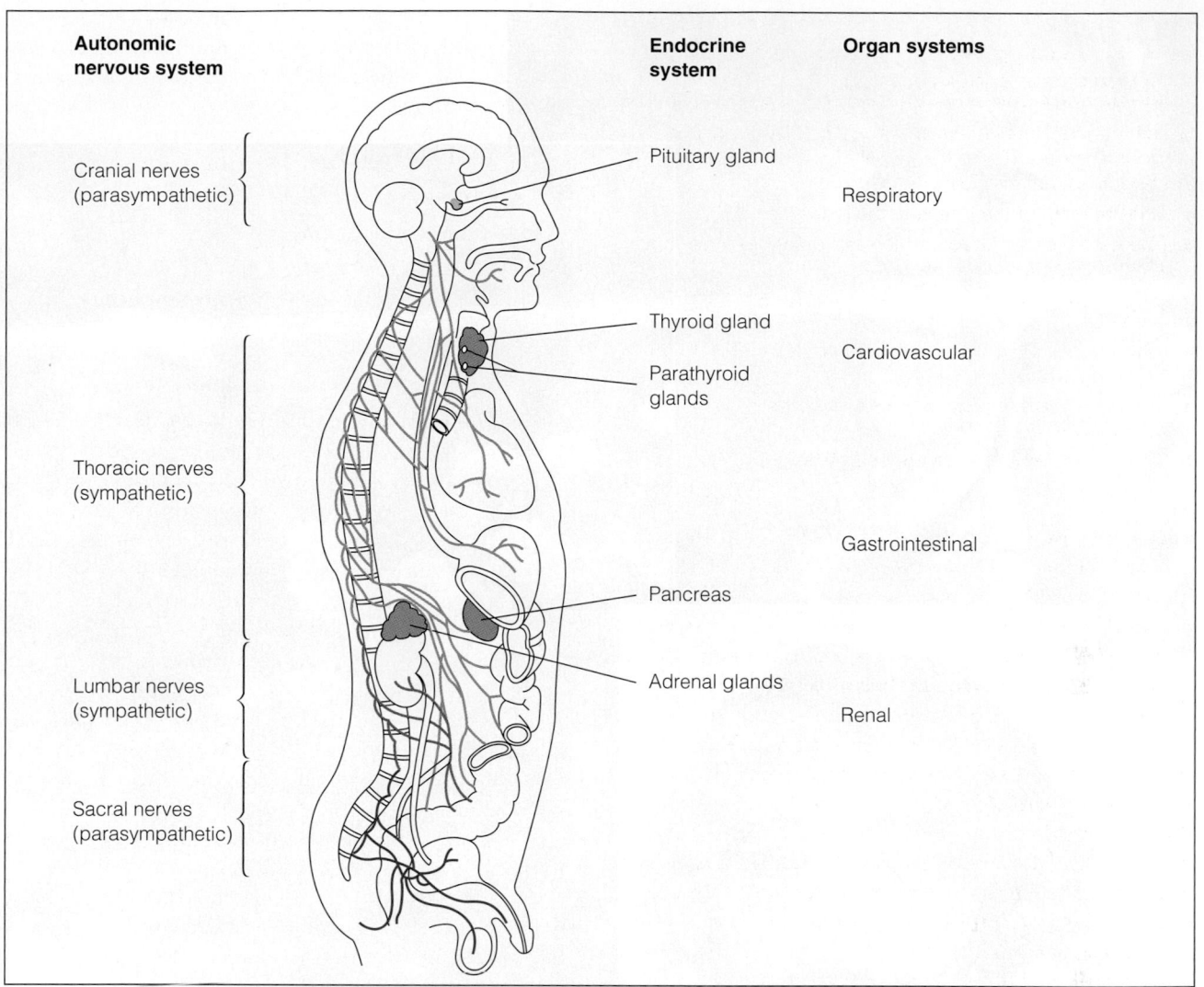

FIGURE 11.1 The homeostatic regulators of the body: autonomic nervous system, endocrine system, and specific organ systems

psychological homeostasis. When one or more of these needs is not met or is threatened, certain coping mechanisms are activated to protect the person and return him or her to psychological homeostasis (see Chapter 47 for additional information on stress and coping).

Psychological homeostasis is acquired or learned through the experience of living and interacting with others. In addition, societal norms and culture influence behaviour. Some prerequisites for a person to develop psychological homeostasis can be summarized as follows:

- *A stable physical environment in which the person feels safe and secure.* For example, the basic needs for food, shelter, and clothing must be met consistently from birth onward.
- *A stable psychological environment from infancy onward, so that feelings of trust and love develop.* Growing children and adolescents also need kind but firm and consistent discipline, encouragement, and support to be their own unique selves.
- *A social environment that includes adults who are healthy role models.* Children learn the customs and values of society from these individuals.
- *A life experience that provides satisfaction.* Throughout life, people encounter many frustrations. They deal with these better if enough satisfying experiences have occurred to counterbalance the frustrating ones.

An example of the importance of psychological homeostasis is the training of athletes. A winning attitude and feeling supported by coaches, family, and friends may be as important as strength and speed training.

Assessing the Health of Individuals

A thorough assessment of the individual's health status is basic to health promotion (see Figure 11.2). Components of this system may include the health history and physical examination, physical fitness assessment, lifestyle assess-

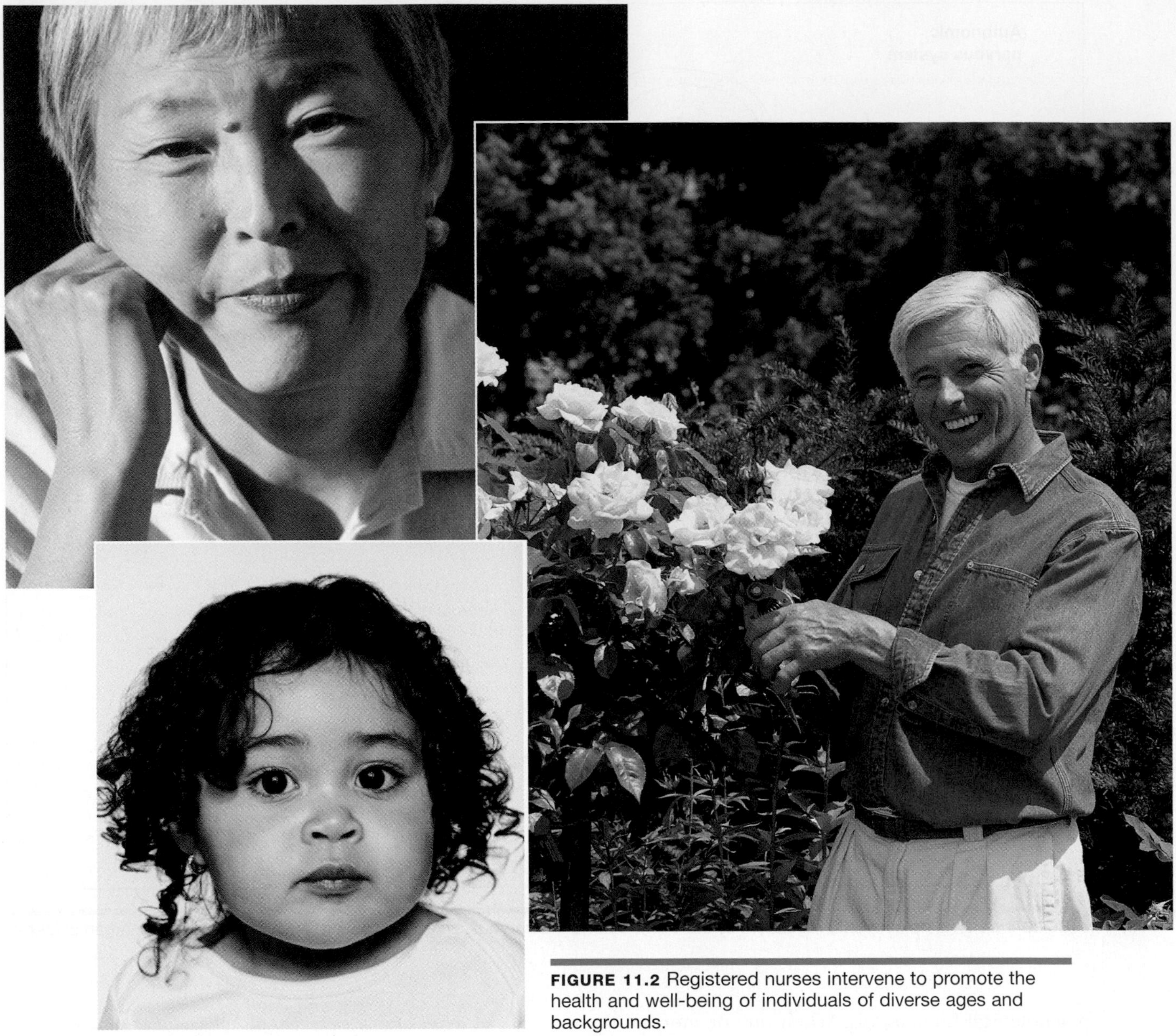

FIGURE 11.2 Registered nurses intervene to promote the health and well-being of individuals of diverse ages and backgrounds.

ment, health-risk appraisal, health beliefs review, spiritual health assessment, social support systems review, and life-stress review. Details about selected assessments are discussed in Chapters 7, 8, 27, 46, and 47.

HEALTH APPRAISAL The *health appraisal* begins with a complete health history. The health history is one of the most effective ways of identifying existing or potential health problems (see Chapter 27). If further evaluation is indicated, a referral is made to the appropriate health-care professional. When the focus is on health, the appraisal includes information on lifestyle behaviours and health beliefs. The nurse uses data from the health appraisal to formulate a health profile. The health profile provides the data necessary to determine wellness or to establish a nursing diagnosis and to plan appropriate nursing interventions to promote optimal health through lifestyle modification.

HEALTH BELIEFS To promote health, the nurse must understand the health beliefs of individuals. Health beliefs may reflect a lack of information or misinformation about health or disease. They may also include folklore and practices from different cultures. Many clients may have outdated information about health, illness, treatment, and prevention. The nurse is frequently in a position to give the latest information or to correct misconceptions. For additional information on health beliefs, see Chapters 7, 8, and 10.

COPING MECHANISMS Individual coping mechanisms are the behaviours individuals use to deal with stress or changes. Coping mechanisms can be viewed as an active method of problem solving developed to meet life's challenges. See Box 11.2 for some health-promoting coping mechanisms. The coping mechanisms individuals develop reflect their own resourcefulness. Individuals

BOX 11.2 HEALTH-PROMOTING COPING MECHANISMS

The following coping mechanisms can be beneficial when they promote health:

- Problem solving
- Positive thinking
- A sense of personal control over own life
- Delayed gratification
- Good health behaviours (e.g., exercise, good nutrition)
- Social support relationships

may use the same coping patterns rather consistently over time or may change their coping strategies when new demands are made on them.

Nurses working with individuals realize the importance of assessing coping mechanisms as a way of determining how individuals relate to stress. Also important are the resources available to the individual. Internal resources, such as knowledge, skills, effective communication patterns, and a sense of purpose, assist in the problem-solving process. Age and the individual's developmental stage often bring with them experiences that may or may not support positive coping strategies. In addition, external support systems promote coping and adaptation. For additional information on coping, please see Chapter 47.

Evidence-Informed Practice

Does the Use of Humour Have a Place in a Palliative Care Unit?

Nurse researchers Dean and Gregory (2005) examined the use of humour in an inpatient palliative care setting. One author followed six nurses during their day-to-day activities 2 times weekly for 12 weeks and described their activities. Other data included conversations with clients, family members, nurses, physicians, a social worker, and a physiotherapist. Analysis of the data revealed that humour is an important part of all aspects within the palliative care unit. Humour helped clients and staff to build relationships and contend with circumstances. The authors noted that use and receptivity of humour was affected by differences in the current state of affairs (e.g., a new diagnosis or immediately following a dose of chemotherapy), ethnicity, gender, amount of stress, and general personality.

NURSING IMPLICATIONS: It is important to assess the individual and the current situation and decide whether or not to use humour. Humour should be combined with caring and sensitivity to produce a "powerful therapeutic asset."

Source: Based on "More Than Trivial: Strategies for Using Humor in Palliative Care," by R. A. K. Dean and D. M. Gregory, 2005, *Cancer Nursing, 28*(4), 292–300.

RISK FOR HEALTH PROBLEMS Risk assessment helps the nurse identify individuals at higher risk than the general population of developing specific health problems, such as stroke, diabetes, and lung cancer. The vulnerability of individuals to health problems may be based on age, hereditary or genetic factors, gender or race, cultural factors, sociological factors, and lifestyle practices.

DEVELOPMENTAL FACTORS Individuals at both ends of the age continuum are at risk of developing health problems. Young children lack the knowledge, skills, and experience to establish a repertoire of coping strategies. Many older adults feel a lack of purpose and decreased self-esteem. These feelings, in turn, reduce their motivation to engage in health-promoting behaviours, such as exercise or community and family involvement.

HEREDITARY FACTORS Individuals born into families with a history of certain diseases, such as diabetes or cardiovascular disease, are at greater risk of developing these conditions. A detailed individual and family history, including genetically transmitted disorders, is essential to the identification of individuals at risk. These data are used not only to monitor the health of individuals but also to recommend modifications in health practices that potentially reduce the risk, minimize the consequences, or postpone the development of genetically related conditions.

GENDER OR RACE Some individuals may be at risk of developing a disease by reason of gender or race. Males, for example, are at greater risk of having cardiovascular disease at an earlier age than are females, and females are at greater risk of developing osteoporosis, particularly after menopause. Although it is sometimes difficult to separate genetic factors from cultural ones, certain risk factors seem to be related to race. Sickle-cell anemia, for example, is a hereditary disease predominantly affecting people of African descent. Indigenous people seem more susceptible to certain diseases, such as diabetes, than the general population.

CULTURAL FACTORS Culture creates an atmosphere that influences the health beliefs and practices of an individual. To provide culturally sensitive care, nurses need to recognize and understand a broad spectrum of cultural values, beliefs, and practices (see Chapter 10).

SOCIOLOGICAL FACTORS The individual's health is influenced by a variety of sociological factors. One of the most noteworthy is poverty. Poverty is a major problem that affects the health of the individual. If an individual is born into or grows up in a single-parent family headed by a female, then the risk of poverty increases. Other factors include the person's roles within society, at work, and in the community, and personal interests and activities.

Lifestyle Factors It has become clear that many diseases are preventable, that the effects of some diseases can be minimized, and that the onset of disease can be delayed through lifestyle modifications. Cancer, cardiovascular disease, adult-onset diabetes, and tooth decay are among lifestyle diseases. The incidence of lung cancer, for example, would be greatly reduced if people stopped smoking. Good nutrition, dental hygiene, and use of fluoride—in the water supply, in toothpaste, as topical supplements—have been shown to reduce caries (dental decay).

One of the most important lifestyle issues today is obesity. Obesity has become pandemic in Canada and the negative health effects of obesity are many and varied. Other important lifestyle considerations are exercise, stress management, and rest. Today, nurses have the knowledge to prevent or minimize the effects of some of the main causes of disease, disability, and death. The challenge is to disseminate information about prevention and to motivate individuals to make lifestyle changes before the onset of illness.

Nursing Process

Nurses committed to individualized care involve the client in the nursing process. The process is discussed in Chapter 22. Data gathered during an individual assessment can lead to different nursing diagnoses. Planned nursing interventions that are needed to assist the individual to health and that enhance personal well-being are identified on the basis of a diagnosis. Evaluation determines whether the planned interventions have led to the achievement of the established goals and outcomes.

Applying Theoretical Frameworks to Individuals

A variety of theoretical frameworks provide the nurse with a holistic overview of health promotion for the individual across the lifespan. Major theoretical frameworks that nurses use in promoting the health of the *individual* are needs theories, developmental stage theories, and systems theories.

Needs Theories

In needs theories, human needs are ranked on an ascending scale according to how essential the needs are for survival. Abraham Maslow, perhaps the most renowned needs theorist, ranks human needs on five levels in ascending order (1970):

1. *Physiological needs.* Such needs as air, food, water, shelter, rest, sleep, activity, and temperature maintenance are crucial for survival.
2. *Safety and security needs.* The need for safety has both physical and psychological aspects. The person needs to feel safe, both in the physical environment and in relationships.
3. *Love and belonging needs.* The third level of needs includes giving and receiving affection, attaining a place in a group, and maintaining the feeling of belonging.
4. *Self-esteem needs.* The individual needs both self-esteem (i.e., feelings of independence, competence, and self-respect) and esteem from others (i.e., recognition, respect, and appreciation).
5. *Self-actualization.* When the need for self-esteem is satisfied, the individual strives for self-actualization, the innate need for a person to develop his or her maximum potential and realize abilities and qualities. (See Box 11.3.)

KALISH'S HIERARCHY OF NEEDS Richard Kalish (1977) adapted Maslow's hierarchy of needs into six levels, rather than five. He suggests an additional category of needs

BOX 11.3 MASLOW'S CHARACTERISTICS OF A SELF-ACTUALIZED PERSON

According to Maslow, a self-actualized person has the following characteristics:

- Is realistic, sees life clearly, and is objective about observations
- Judges people correctly
- Has superior perception, is more decisive
- Has a clear notion of right and wrong
- Is usually accurate in predicting future events
- Understands art, music, politics, and philosophy
- Possesses humility, listens to others carefully
- Is dedicated to some work, task, duty, or vocation
- Is highly creative, flexible, spontaneous, courageous, and willing to make mistakes
- Is open to new ideas
- Is self-confident and has self-respect
- Has low degree of self-conflict; personality is integrated
- Respects self, does not need fame, possesses a feeling of self-control
- Is highly independent, desires privacy
- Can appear remote and detached
- Is friendly, loving, and governed more by inner directives than by society
- Can make decisions contrary to popular opinion
- Is problem centred rather than self-centred
- Accepts the world for what it is

Source: Based on Chapter 3, "The Study of Self-Actualization," from *The Third Force: The Psychology of Abraham Maslow*, by Frank Goble. Copyright © 1970 by Thomas Jefferson Research Center. Reprinted by permission of Viking Penguin, a division of Penguin Books U.S.A., Inc.

between the physiological needs and the safety and security needs. This category, referred to as *stimulation needs*, includes sex, activity, exploration, manipulation, and novelty. See Figure 11.3. Kalish emphasizes that children need to explore and manipulate their environments to achieve optimal growth and development. He notes that adults, too, often seek novel adventures or stimulating experiences before considering their safety or security needs. Maslow, by contrast, includes the pursuit of knowledge and aesthetic needs in the category of self-actualization needs.

CHARACTERISTICS OF BASIC NEEDS All people have the same basic needs; however, a person's perception of a need varies according to learning and the standards of his or her culture. For example, professional achievement may be important in one culture or subculture and unimportant in another. People's needs have the following characteristics:

- People meet their own needs relative to their own priorities. For example, during a drought, a mother might give up her share of water or food and risk starvation or die so that her child can live.
- Although basic needs generally must be met, some needs can be deferred. An example is the need for independence. During an acute illness, the individual may prefer to be somewhat dependent on health professionals and other caregivers, and then resume the desire for independence after recovery.
- Failure to meet needs results in one or more homeostatic imbalances, which can eventually result in illness.
- A need can make itself felt by either external or internal stimuli. An example is the need for food. A person may experience hunger as a result of thinking about food (internal stimulation) or as a result of seeing a beautiful cake (external stimulation).
- A person who perceives a need can respond in several ways to meet it. The choice of response is largely a result of learned experiences, lifestyle, and the values of the culture. For example, the professional woman who comes home from work feeling tired may meet the need for relaxation by walking around the park. Many people's food choices at mealtimes and snack times are based on past experiences, lifestyle, and culture.
- Needs are interrelated. Some needs cannot be met unless related needs are also met. The need for hydration can be seriously altered if the need for elimination of urine is not also met. Likewise, the need for security can be markedly altered if the need for oxygen is threatened by a respiratory obstruction.

Needs can be satisfied in healthy and unhealthy ways. Ways of meeting basic needs are considered healthy when they are not harmful to others or to the self, conform to the individual's sociocultural values, and are within the law. Conversely, unhealthy behaviour may be harmful to others or to the self, does not conform to the individual's sociocultural values, or is not within the law. Maslow found that people who satisfy their basic needs appropriately are healthier, happier, and more effective than those whose needs are frustrated (Goble, 1970).

Throughout their lifetime, individuals strive to meet needs. A person's perception of a need and his or her response to satisfy a need can be influenced by ethnocultural standards, by external and internal stimuli (e.g., hunger), and by self-determined priorities (e.g., stopping smoking). Positive factors that affect the satisfying of needs are an individual's healthy position on the wellness–illness continuum, the presence of supportive relationships, a good self-concept, and the satisfactory achievement of developmental stages. For example, if an infant achieves the developmental task of learning to trust, then the basic needs of feeling loved and secure are readily resolved.

Knowledge of the theoretical bases of human needs assists nurses in responding therapeutically to a client's behaviours and in understanding themselves and their

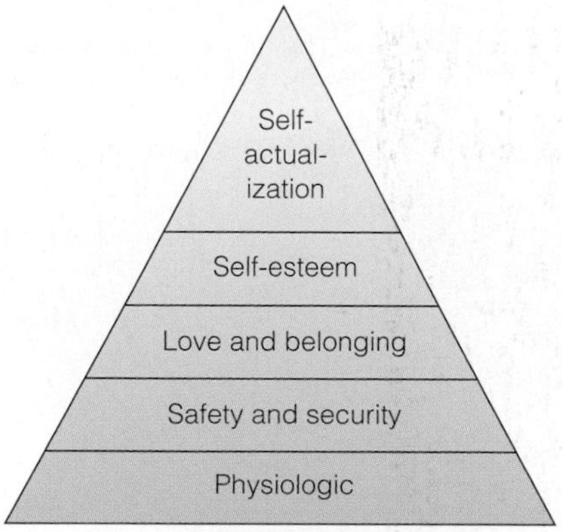

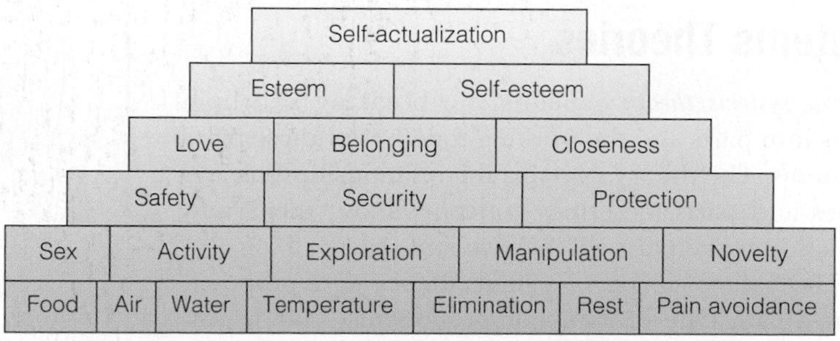

FIGURE 11.3 Maslow's needs and Kalish's adaptation

Source: **The Psychology of Human Behavior,** *5th ed., by R. A. Kalish, 1983. Copyright © 1983 by Wadsworth, Inc. Reprinted with permission of Brooks/Cole Publishing Company, Monterey, CA 93940.*

own responses to needs. Human needs serve as a framework for assessing behaviours, assigning priorities to desired outcomes, and planning nursing interventions. For example, an adult with poor self-esteem would have difficulty becoming self-actualized. Therefore, nursing interventions would focus on increasing the client's self-esteem.

Developmental Stage Theories

Developmental stage theories related to individuals categorize a person's behaviours or tasks into approximate age ranges or in terms that describe the features of an age group. The age ranges of the stages do not take into account individual differences; however, the categories do describe characteristics associated with the majority of individuals at periods when distinctive developmental changes occur and with the specific tasks that must be accomplished. Because human development is highly complex and multifaceted, developmental stage theories describe only one aspect of development, such as cognitive, psychosexual, psychosocial, moral, or faith development. Stage theories emphasize a definite, predictable sequence of development that is orderly and continuous. Each stage is affected by those stages preceding it and affects those stages that follow. For example, an adolescent who is unable to establish a stable sense of personal identity may have difficulty in later developmental stages with adult roles and career aspirations. See Chapter 16 for further information about developmental stages.

Developmental stage theories allow nurses to describe the typical behaviours of an individual within a certain age group, explain the significance of those behaviours, predict behaviours that might occur in a given situation, and provide a rationale to control behavioural manifestations. Individuals can be compared with a representative group of people at the same time or be compared at different times. During care, the nurse's knowledge of stage theories can be used in parental and client education, counselling, and anticipatory guidance.

Systems Theories

General systems theory explains the breaking of whole things into parts and the working together of those parts in systems. The theory explains the relationship between wholes and parts, describes concepts about them, and predicts how the parts will behave and react.

The basic concepts of systems theory were proposed in the 1950s. One of its major proponents, Ludwig von Bertalanffy (1968) introduced systems theory as a universal theory that could be applied to many fields of study. Systems theory is applied in health professions when curricula are focused on body systems, such as respiratory, cardiac, or gastrointestinal. Nurses are increasingly using systems theory to understand not only biological systems but also systems in families, communities, and nursing and health care. General systems theory provides a way of examining interrelationships and deriving principles. Systems theory can also be used in nursing theories and curricula, such as Campbell's UBC model (see Chapter 4).

A **system** is a set of interacting identifiable parts or components. A system can be an individual, a family, or a community. The fundamental components of a system are matter, energy, and communication. Without any one of these, a system does not exist. The individual is a human system with matter (the body), energy (chemical or thermal), and communication (e.g., the nervous system). The **boundary** of a system, such as the skin in the human system, is a real or imaginary line that differentiates one system from another system or a system from its environment.

Systems can be complex and, therefore, are often studied as *subsystems.* Each subsystem belongs to a higher system. In the individual or human system, the subsystems (or lower-level systems) are the organ systems, such as the respiratory system and the digestive system; the *suprasystems* are the family systems. See Figure 11.4 for a hierarchy of the human system.

Because all the parts of a system are interrelated, the whole system responds to changes in one of its parts. This interrelatedness is the basis for nursing's holistic view of the client. For example, a tumour of the liver affects the whole individual, that is, the person may be nauseated, tired, anxious, and so on. A psychological problem, such as stress or anxiety, can also manifest itself in physiological symptoms, such as sleeplessness, nausea, or changes in cardiac function.

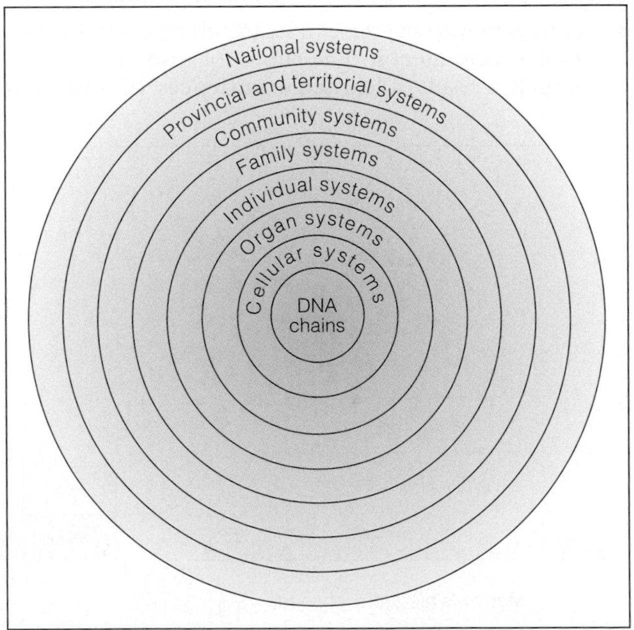

FIGURE 11.4 A common system hierarchy

Systems come in two general types: closed and open. A **closed system** does not exchange energy, matter, or information with its environment. An example of a closed system is a chemical reaction that takes place in a test tube. In reality, outside the laboratory, no closed systems exist. In an **open system**, energy, matter, and information move into and out of the system through the system boundary. All living systems, such as plants, animals, people, families, and communities, are open systems, since their survival depends on a continuous exchange of energy. They are, therefore, in a constant state of change.

Because humans are biopsychosocial beings, their biological, psychological, social, and spiritual components can be regarded as systems with hierarchic, interrelated subsystems.

The *biological system* can be subdivided into the neurological, musculoskeletal, respiratory, circulatory, gastrointestinal, and urinary subsystems, among others. Each subsystem can, in turn, be subdivided. For example, the urinary system consists of the kidneys, the ureters, and the bladder; the circulatory system consists of the heart and the blood vessels. The biological system can also be subdivided into categories of needs or functional health patterns or activities of daily living, such as nutrition and hydration, sleep or rest, activity or exercise, elimination, and so on.

The *psychological, social,* and *spiritual systems* are a focus of research in several disciplines. Although the interrelatedness of the systems is clearly evident, the explicit delineation of specific susbsystems, the exact relationships among them, and their influence on health are still not well understood (Belar, 2003). Topics within these systems include thinking, feeling, faith, empathy, coping, hardiness, quality of life, self-efficacy, power, and social support. Nurse researchers and theorists have used research results on these topics as a basis for theory development and improving practice.

For its functioning, an open system depends on the quality and quantity of its input, output, and feedback. **Input** consists of information, material, or energy that enters the system. After the input is absorbed by the system, it is processed in a way useful to the system. This transformation is called **throughput**. For example, food is input to the digestive system; it is digested (throughput) so that it can be used by the body. **Output** from a system is energy, matter, or information given out by the system as a result of its processes. Output from the digestive system is feces, nutrients, and caloric energy.

Feedback, as discussed for homeostasis in an individual, is a process that enables a system to regulate itself by redirecting the output of a system to affect the input of the same system, thus forming a feedback loop (Figure 11.5). Numerous examples of this feedback mechanism are found within individual, family, and community systems. In the individual, for example, the autonomic nervous system relies on a feedback system to balance the effects of the sympathetic and parasympathetic centres, which modify heart and respiratory rates. In the family system, parents provide feedback to children to modify behaviour. In the community, laws, rules, and regulations guide the behaviour of citizens.

Human systems theories assert that the individual is an open system in constant interaction with a changing environment. People interact with the environment by adjusting themselves to it or adjusting it to themselves. For instance, increasing environmental (societal) emphasis on physical activity has caused many Canadians to increase their own activity levels and to encourage family members to do so as well. Constant input into the system and feedback to it maintain the system in a state of dynamic equilibrium (homeostasis). This premise directs the nurse to look at environmental factors influencing the system and to plan nursing interventions to help the client maintain homeostasis. For example, the individual who is experiencing severe anxiety may be taught a variety of stress-management techniques.

The family unit can also be viewed as a system. Its members are interdependent, working toward specific purposes and goals. Many families are described as *open systems,* for they are continually interacting with and influenced by other systems in the community. Boundaries regulate the input from other systems that interact with the family system; they also regulate output from the family system to the community or to society. Boundaries protect the family from the demands and influences of other systems. Open families are likely to welcome input from without, encouraging individual members to adapt beliefs and practices to meet the changing demands of society. Such families are more likely to seek out health-care information and use community resources. These families are adaptable and, therefore, better prepared to cope with changes in lifestyle needed to restore, maintain, or promote health.

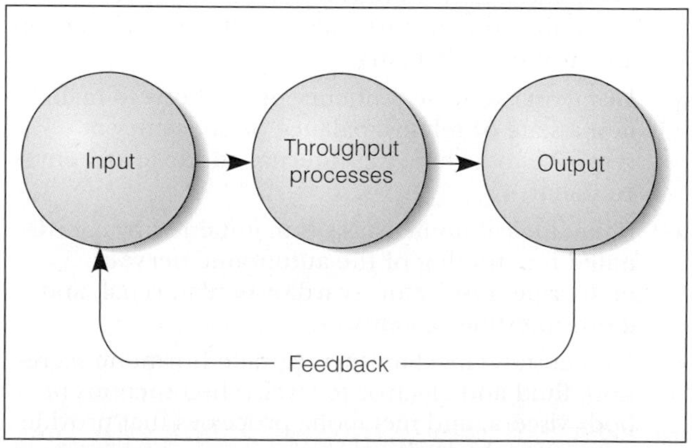

FIGURE 11.5 An open system with a feedback mechanism

Case Study 11

Aliyah is a young mother of three children who lives in Windsor, Ontario. She has developed a severe arthritic condition that has affected her ability to work and adequately care for her family. Her illness has created a financial hardship for the family and has strained their roles. She has given up her position as a secretary at an automotive plant. Aliyah and her husband have custody of their children from previous marriages, as well as a daughter together. She is reluctant to seek assistance from outside sources because she fears interference from her ex-spouse concerning her children.

Critical Thinking Skills

1. What type of assessment data might you collect?
2. When dealing with Aliyah's physical problem, why must the nurse be concerned about the other issues occurring in Aliyah's life?
3. Explore Aliyah's situation from the perspective of Maslow.
4. What suggestions might you give Aliyah to help her cope with her condition?

After working through these questions, go to the MyNursingLab at **http://www.mynursinglab.com** to check your answers.

KEY TERMS

holistic
holism
equilibrium
homeostasis
self-regulation
compensatory
feedback
negative feedback
positive feedback
system
boundary
closed system
open system
input
throughput
output

CHAPTER HIGHLIGHTS

- Nursing involves viewing the client as an individual and in a holistic way.
- To ensure holistic health care, the nurse considers all the components of health (health promotion, health maintenance, health education and illness prevention, and restorative-rehabilitative care) and recognizes that disturbance in one part of a person affects the whole being.
- Homeostasis is the tendency of the body to maintain a state of relative balance or constancy in response to a changing internal and external environment.
- Physiological homeostasis is maintained by coordinated functioning of the autonomic nervous, endocrine, respiratory, cardiovascular, renal, and gastrointestinal systems.
- Homeostatic mechanisms regulate hormone secretion, fluid and electrolyte levels, the functions of body viscera, and metabolic processes that provide energy for the body.
- Psychological homeostasis, or emotional well-being, is acquired or learned through the experience of living and interacting with others.
- Although each individual has unique characteristics, certain needs are common to all people.
- A variety of social, psychological, and nursing theoretical frameworks provide the nurse with a holistic overview of the health promotion of individuals and families across the lifespan.
- Maslow's hierarchy of human needs consists of five categories: physiological (survival) needs, safety needs, love and belonging needs, self-esteem needs, and self-actualization needs.
- People vary in how they rank their needs at any given moment.
- Needs satisfaction can be altered by illness, significant relationships, self-concept, and developmental levels.

ASSESS YOUR LEARNING

1. The individual who has strong feelings of independence is meeting which of the following levels within Maslow's hierarchy of needs?
   a. Self-actualization
   b. Self-esteem
   c. Love and belonging
   d. Closeness

2. The way an individual interprets the environment can be considered part of which of the following dimensions of individuality?
   a. Self-identity
   b. Total character
   c. Perceptions
   d. Values

3. Mr. Greer, who has metastatic cancer of the liver and is severely jaundiced, asks you to assist him in planning a cruise 9 months in the future. You assess that he is using a coping mechanism. You remember that one purpose of coping mechanisms is to do which of the following?
   a. Protect the person
   b. Provide feedback
   c. Stimulate the endocrine system
   d. Change society

4. Developmental theories are useful because they do which of the following?
   a. Provide a basis for comparison with the individual characteristics
   b. Provide a set of rules for structuring individual care
   c. Focus on year-by-year changes in the individual
   d. Are not affected by the situation the individual is experiencing

5. When a father prepares to leave for work in the morning, his 3-year-old son starts to cry and scream. The father picks him up and delays leaving for a while. The child's behaviour most reflects which part of the family system?
   a. Input
   b. Throughput
   c. Output
   d. Feedback

6. Maslow would identify which of the following as belonging on the first (lowest, bottom) level of his hierarchy of needs?
   a. Ability to move around
   b. Recognition as a member of a peer group
   c. Feelings of independence
   d. Safety from physical harm

7. Baljit, a student nurse, has recently learned about the use of holistic thinking in nursing. When interviewing a client, which of the following rationales will he use in planning his questions?
   a. Individual processes are detached from each other.
   b. The reason for consulting the health professional is of primary importance.
   c. Each individual is more than the sum of his or her parts.
   d. The individual and the immediate environment are the focus of care.

8. Mr. Hannah, 28 years old, has been HIV-positive for 5 years. Recently, he has been admitted to the hospital with a confirmed diagnosis of *Pneumocystis carinii* [now known as *Pneumocystis jiroveci*]. Mr. Hannah tells the nurse that he notices people seem to avoid coming into his room and that he is lonely. What strategy should the nurse use to provide support to the client?
   a. Explain to him the reason he is isolated is due to his susceptibility to infections.
   b. Explain to him that people do not come in to his room because they are afraid of getting HIV.
   c. Ask him if any of his family can come to the hospital to keep him company.
   d. Spend time talking with him during and between care activities.

9. Sarah, your friend, is trying to make some changes to her lifestyle. You support her by giving positive feedback because positive feedback does what?
   a. Inhibits change
   b. Stimulates change
   c. Maintains homeostasis
   d. Regulates change

10. Which of the following best describes psychological homeostasis or emotional well-being?
   a. It is inherited from parents.
   b. It is dependent on a person's role in family life.
   c. It is acquired or learned from living and interacting with others.
   d. It is totally independent from a person's culture.

*After working through these questions, go to the MyNursingLab at **http://www.mynursinglab.com** to check your answers and see explanations.*

SUGGESTED READINGS

Bergh, I., Jakobsson, E., Sjöström, B., & Steen, B. (2005). Ways of talking about experiences of pain among older patients following orthopaedic surgery. *Journal of Advanced Nursing, 52*(4), 351–361.

In this article the authors examined how 60 Swedish older adult patients with hip fracture or replacement surgery described their pain. They based the study on the understanding that the verbal description of pain is the best indicator of the pain experience. They conclude that "exploring the ways older patients talk about pain is expected to result in a better understanding of the older patient's need of empathic individualized care and in the optimization of pain management" (p. 351).

Suhonen, R., Välimäki, M., & Leino-Kilpi, H. (2005). Individualized care, quality of life and satisfaction with nursing care. *Journal of Advanced Nursing, 50*(3), 283–292.

These authors studied patients having surgery, their perceptions of individualized care, and its effect on patient satisfaction and quality of life. They found that the greater the individualization perceived by the patients, the greater their satisfaction with care. There was less indication that individualized care affected quality of life from the patients' perspective.

Swenson, S. L., Zettler, P., & Lo, B. (2005). "She gave it her best shot right away": Patient experiences of biomedical and patient-centered communication. *Patient Education and Counseling, 61*, 200–211.

In this study, patients were shown two videos of physicians interviewing patients and using either a patient-centred or biomedical approach. The patients were then interviewed about their perceptions. Results indicated that different patients liked different styles, according to their personal values and expectations. Understanding the diversity of patients is important to giving individualized care.

WEBLINKS

Public Health Agency of Canada

http://www.phac-aspc.gc.ca

This site provides current Canadian-specific information about many health topics.

Statistics Canada

http://www.statcan.ca

This site provides a variety of federal government statistics related to Canadian life and health.

REFERENCES

Belar, C. (2003). Concepts and models. In S. Llewelyn & P. Kennedy, *Handbook of clinical health psychology* (pp. 7–19). Chichester, UK: John Wiley & Sons.

Cannon, W. B. (1939). *The wisdom of the body* (2nd ed.). New York: Norton

College of Nurses of Ontario. (2004). The patient safety movement—The basics. Retrieved January 8, 2008, from http://www.cno.org/pubs/mag/2004/09Sept/features/patientsafety/index.htm

Goble, R. G. (1970). *The third force: the psychology of Abraham Maslow.* Richmond Hill, ON: Simon & Schuster.

Kalish, R. (1977). *The later years: Social applications of gerontology.* Montery, CA: Brooks/Cole.

Maslow, A. H. (1970). *Motivation and personality* (2nd ed.). New York: Harper & Row.

Registered Nurses' Association of Ontario. (2006). *Best practice guideline: Client centred care.* Toronto: Author.

Saskatchewan Registered Nurses' Association. (2005). *Registered nurse (nurse practitioner) RN (NP) scope of practice and the law.* Retrieved January 8, 2008, from INK "http://www.srna.org/nurse_practitioner/documents/2005_RNNP_scope_of_practice.pdf"

Smuts, J. (1926). *Holism and evolution.* New York: Macmillan.

Statistics Canada. (2004a). *Population 15 years and over by highest degree, certificate or diploma (1986–2001).* Retrieved September 12, 2006, from http://www40.statcan.ca/101/cst01.educ42.htm

Statistics Canada. (2004b). *Household type, in private households, 2001 counts, for Canada, provinces and territories—20% sample data.* Retrieved September 18, 2006, from http://www12.statcan.ca/english/census01/products/highlight/PrivateHouseholds/Page.cfm?Lang=E&Geo=PR&View=1a&Table=3&StartRec=1&Sort=11&B1=Change

Statistics Canada. (2005). *Population density, births and deaths for selected countries.* Retrieved September 12, 2006, from http://www40.statcan,ca/101/dem001a.htm

Statistics Canada. (2007a). 2006 census: Families, marital status, households and dwelling characteristics. *The Daily,* September 12. Retrieved February 4, 2008, from http://www.statcan.ca/Daily/English/070912/d070912a.htm

Statistics Canada. (2007b). *Portrait of the Canadian population in 2006: National portrait.* Retrieved September 7, 2008, from http://www12.statcan.ca/english/census06/analysis/popdwell/index.cfm

Statistics Canada. (2008). *Number and proportion of persons aged 25 to 64 by level of educational attainment and age groups, Canada, 2006.* Retrieved September 7, 2008, from http://www12.statcan.ca/english/census06/analysis/education/tables/table2.htm

von Bertalanffy, L. (1968). *General systems theory: Foundation, development, applications.* New York: Braziller.

Wing, P. (1997). Patient or client? If in doubt, ask. *Canadian Medical Association Journal, 157*(3), 287–289.

Chapter 12

Nursing Care of Families

Whenever concerns related to health and illness arise, both individuals and those who are involved in their lives are affected. Usually these are family members. Nurses encounter family members in every practice setting, including home care, community clinics, and hospitals. As health-care services have shifted away from institutional care with shorter hospital stays, family members are increasingly called on to provide care at home. Care can involve emotional support, symptom monitoring, and such technical procedures as dressing changes or dialysis and intravenous therapies. Family members can be a tremendous resource to nurses through their knowledge of patient preferences and usual patterns of response to difficulties. However, family members do not always hold similar views about caregiving roles. Nurses are challenged to invite and respect all views of family members and provide them with information and emotional support. Nurses are also challenged to involve family members in decision making, in ways that respect the rights and wishes of patients, and to prepare family members with appropriate knowledge, skills, and supports for caregiving roles.

OBJECTIVES

After studying this chapter, you should be able to

1. Define *family* in a way that accounts for diverse forms of structure and relationship
2. Describe three factors influencing the shift in nursing perspective from the individual to the person in the context of the family
3. Outline historical developments in family nursing
4. Discuss the impact of trends in health-care services on family involvement
5. Propose possible family member expectations for their involvement in care
6. Analyze demographic trends in Canadian families that influence health and family structure
7. Identify three questions to be posed during a genogram and ecomap inquiry
8. Formulate questions aimed at exploring reciprocal influences between health and illness and the family
9. Describe relational practices that foster a collaborative stance with family members
10. Explain five relational practices that can be integrated when providing nursing care with families

What Is Family?

Standards of family structure have shifted dramatically over the past three decades. Couples now often postpone childbearing until after completing their postsecondary education and establishing careers. Rising rates of divorce and remarriage have resulted in more blended and lone-parent families. Increased family mobility has also shifted the roles of extended family members. These changes challenge definitions of **family** that were based on long held assumptions (see Box 12.1). Persons choosing to define themselves as family may or may not be bound by blood or legal status. The Vanier Institute of the Family (n.d.) uses a definition that attempts to be open to and respectful of the many different ways families organize themselves:

> *The Vanier Institute of the Family defines family as any combination of two or more persons who are bound together over time by ties of mutual consent, birth and/or adoption, or placement and who, together, assume responsibilities for variant combinations of some of the following:*
>
> - *Physical maintenance and care of group members*
> - *Addition of new members through procreation or adoption*
> - *Socialization of children*
> - *Social control of members*
> - *Production, consumption, distribution of goods and services, and*
> - *Affective nurturance—love*

In clinical practice, it is helpful to the nurse to understand how members of a particular family identify themselves in relation to each other. Who is in *this* family? How do *these* family members view their relationships, priorities, concerns, responsibilities, and preferences? To establish a therapeutic relationship with a family, nurses need to be respectful of the ways that families describe themselves and to appreciate that "the family is who they say they are" (Wright & Leahey, 2005a, p. 60).

BOX 12.1 TYPES OF FAMILIES IN TODAY'S SOCIETY

Family can be described in different ways according to the characteristics of its members (e.g., age, ethnicity, number, sexual orientation, employment), their relationship (e.g., marital, cohabitation, biological, blended, adoptive), or their generation (*nuclear*: parent and child; *extended*: aunts, uncles, cousins; *intergenerational*: grandparents, great-grandparents).

- Traditional: both parents reside in the home with children; mother assumes nurturing role and father provides economic necessities
- Two career: both husband and wife are employed
- Lone parent: one parent with a child or children
- Adolescent: an infant is born to adolescent parents
- Blended: families who join together to form a new one
- Cohabiting: unrelated individuals or families who live under one roof
- Adoptive: children are adopted by parent(s)
- Mixed race: parents or children of different ethnicities
- Nuclear: parent(s) and child(ren) from same generation
- Mixed generation: parent(s) and child(ren) from several generations
- Gay or lesbian: a same-sex couple

Family Nursing

Family nursing refers to relational practices that involve family members in care, respond to their concerns, or provide information and emotional support. Care of family members calls for nursing practices that occur within conversation and relationship, across every health-care setting.

When nurses encounter families in their day-to-day practice, each encounter affords a possibility for the nursing of families. Family members may be present when the home care nurse visits. They may be maintaining a rotating vigil at the bedside of an ill family member, and the nurse may have several brief conversations during a shift. The nurse may conduct a more formal family assessment interview on the patient's admission to an outpatient or inpatient facility. The nurse may be involved in a family conference with family and other health-care team members to facilitate decision making, treatment planning, or discharge. In some situations, the nurse has little or no direct contact with family members of the individual client, yet the needs and concerns of family members can still be addressed in their absence.

Frequently in nursing, the individual is the focus of care and the extent to which family members are encouraged to be involved in health-care encounters varies. Many agencies now provide structural supports to include family members and value their presence and contribution to care. These supports include open or flexible visiting policies; comfortable waiting rooms and access to overnight facilities, refreshments, and telephones; and increased access to information from health-care professionals.

Nursing of families challenges nurses to shift their perspective from thinking of the client as an individual to "thinking family" or "thinking interactionally" (Wright & Leahey, 2005a, p. 11). This means that the nurse must forge a collaborative relationship not only with the patient but also with the people who are involved with the patient during the health-care encounter. Involvement of family members helps the nurse better understand the meaning of illness to the patient and family, and the possibilities for support during recovery, health maintenance, or health promotion. Unfortunately, despite the growing recognition of the importance of family in health care, limited transfer of family theory to nursing practice has taken place (e.g.,

Segaric & Hall, 2005). This gap may, in part, be due to conceptual confusion. Few practice areas view the family as the context for the patient or view the family as the unit of care. However, nurses need family theory to provide truly relevant care, given that the family is the fundamental unit of society with norms, values, and roles distinct from that of the individual (Dwairy, 2002).

Four theoretical frameworks have contributed to family nursing practice. Systems theories help nurses understand the family as a group of interconnected individuals (e.g., Wright & Leahey, 2005a). Symbolic interaction theoretical frameworks help nurses to focus on both the individual and the family and on how they relate (e.g., Forchuk & Dorsay, 1995). Developmental theories assist in understanding how families manage with developmental tasks, and social exchange theories assist nurses in considering what resources they can offer that families will view as beneficial (e.g., Byrd, 2006).

In some practice settings, the client is conceptualized as the **person in the context of the family**. Here the individual is viewed as the primary focus of nursing concern and the family as a significant contextual influence in health, illness, and recovery. Nursing care is focused on *both* individuals (foreground) and families (background). Family members are viewed as being connected to the person and relevant to the health concerns of the individual and his or her environment. For example, participation of family members in decisions related to discharge planning can provide emotional support and instrumental assistance to the individuals when they return home. Likewise, family members can be a valuable resource to both the patient and the health-care team for decision making around serious illness (Heyland, Tranmer, O'Callaghan, & Gafni, 2003).

Though the individual is the focus of care, evidence shows that there should also be varying degrees of intent to nurse family members by attending to the impact of the health situation on the family. For example, nurses can *reduce family stress* by providing education to parents of neonatal or pediatric patients around their children's painful procedures or changes in appearance, behaviour, or emotions (Board & Ryan-Wegner, 2003; Davidson et al., 2007). Similarly, nurses can lessen the anxiety of children whose parent is in ICU by helping them to prepare for visiting their parent in hospital (Davidson et al., 2007).

Nurses can also *improve the health* of family members caring for loved ones with dementia by teaching them personal coping strategies (Selwood, Johnston, Katona, Lyketsos, & Livingston, 2007). Likewise, nurses can *acknowledge families* by including them in discharge planning discussions and showing concern for its impact on the demands of family caregivers (their time, energy, and health) when the patient returns home (Davidson et al., 2007). As Friedemann (1995) argued, "All nursing is family nursing and is practised in all clinical settings" (p. 34). She proposed that nurses cannot contribute to the healing of persons without attention to the contexts and relationships in which they live.

Nursing practice may also focus on the **family unit as the client of care**. Attention is simultaneously directed toward the individual *and* family—with the family in the foreground. The family unit is assisted to make changes in family relationships and processes around the difficulties they encounter (Wright, Watson, & Bell, 1996). Heightened attention is given to reciprocity within relationships between family members, between the family and the nurse, and between illness and the family. This work typically requires advanced practice skills. Family systems nursing (Wright & Leahey, 1990) is an example of family nursing specialization that addresses the complex functions of the family unit and shifts nursing attention between various family subsystems (such as the parent–child relationship or the marital relationship) and other higher systems levels (such as health-care agencies, schools, community clinics) as needed (Friedemann, 1995) (see Chapter 11 for a review of general systems theory).

Development of Family Nursing

Historically, nurses have encountered family members by virtue of their shared presence in homes, communities, and hospitals. However, although the interest in the family as a focus of nursing care extends back to the earliest traditions of modern nursing (Whall & Fawcett, 1991), it is important to note that the family unit and its activities (including childrearing) were considered private matters, rather than a public societal concern, until very recently (Hart, 1991).

During the early decades of the twentieth century, there was interest, both within the clinical practice and within the nursing curricula domains, in having nurses (public health and private duty nurses) provide care to families at home *or* assist families to care for loved ones and also provide them with respite from caregiving activities. Public health nurses have a longstanding tradition of educating families to address the health needs of all family members. In Canada by the 1920s, reliance on hospital services was growing and demand for home health care by private duty nurses was diminishing (McPherson, 1996). By the 1940s and 1950s, private duty nursing had declined dramatically and was coupled with federal and provincial or territorial legislation that increased construction of public hospitals across the country. This was followed by the advent of the Canadian system of medicare, which provided public health-care insurance for medical and hospital services. Illness care became increasingly entrenched within hospitals.

Focus on Individuals in Hospital Care

The rise of scientific biomedicine and the organizational efficiencies of hospital care contributed to a focus on the individual. The client was viewed as the individual patient with a particular pathology, who required diagnosis and treatment. As medicine focused on curing disease, nurses contributed greatly to the organizational efficiencies that supported these activities (McPherson, 1996). Families were considered less relevant and rarely involved in hospital care. However, in recent years, attention has increasingly focused on the psychosocial aspects of health and illness and recognized the importance of the influence of family (Firth, 2006). In addition, many changes in practice and policy within the health-care system have been guided by nurses' responsiveness to the needs, requests, and expectations of families.

Family Care Traditions in Public Health, Maternal and Child, Pediatric, and Mental Health Nursing

Throughout these developments, public health nurses, maternal and child nurses, and pediatric nurses maintained an enduring interest in family care. Hospitals were challenged to provide structural support for family involvement. In maternity settings, couples demanded the presence of fathers in the delivery room. Mothers objected to postpartum separation from their newborns, leading to rooming-in practices, with infants cared for at the mother's bedside. In pediatric settings, parents desired round the clock access to their children through flexible visiting policies. Nursing research in the 1970s and 1980s addressed such topics as parent–infant attachment, maternal role attainment, childbearing or childrearing transitions in the family life cycle with little emphasis on parenting (Gage, Everett, & Bullock, 2006), and the impact of pediatric illness on family members. Although much of this early work focused on maternal–child relationships, emphasis on the roles of fathers and husbands has increased. Family nursing research has broadened its focus to include more theory development (e.g., a typology of family health nursing practice: Macduff, 2006), best practices and standards (e.g., meeting needs of families of patients with parenteral nutrition: Sexton, Coad, & Holden, 2005; diabetes: Cole & Chesla, 2006; cancer care: Given & Sherwood, 2006), and an examination of best ways to work *with* families, for example, through negotiation (Corlett & Twycross, 2006) or family-centred care (Shields, Pratt, & Hunter, 2006).

The importance of family in mental health nursing is a relatively recent acknowledgement. Families often feel rejection or stigma when their loved one is diagnosed with a *mental illness*, and many try to conceal the diagnosis and avoid involvement in care (Phelan, Bromet, & Link, 1998). Even when families try to contact care providers for information and emotional support (Doornbos, 2001, 2002), they are often unsuccessful as staff often place their loyalty with the patient (Sjöbloom, Pejlert, & Asplund, 2005). Only recently has nursing research begun to understand the experience (Wade, 2006) and needs (Clarke, 2006) of families whose loved ones have a mental health problem and begun to explore the effects of different models of family nursing care delivery (Goudreau, Duhamel, & Ricard, 2006).

Evidenced-Informed Practice

How Does Family Nursing Relate to Care Involving Mental Illness?

The purpose of the qualitative, descriptive study by Ward-Griffin, Schofield, Vos, and Coatsworth-Puspoky (2005) was to explore the perspectives of individuals who were caring for a family member with a mental illness, with particular attention to housing, quality of supports, and formal care services. Eleven focus groups with family caregivers (N = 75) were conducted. Both individual and team thematic analyses were undertaken until interpretations of the experiences of the participants were inductively developed and conceptualized into a holistic interpretation. Findings revealed that family caregivers formed a "circle of care" around the individual with the mental illness, trying to provide both support for independence and protection for safety. However, findings also suggested that this "circle of care" eventually led to a "vicious cycle" of caregiving. Three major themes were identified: witnessing inadequacies, working behind the scenes, and creating a better world.

NURSING IMPLICATIONS: This research highlights the need for health providers to acknowledge their own beliefs and attitudes about family caregiving and mental illness. It also underscores the need for nurses to assist families in both providing care and gaining respite from their caregiving duties. Finally, this research highlights the need for changes to the health-care system (both policies and services) if primary health care is to become a reality for families of people with mental illness.

Source: Based on "Canadian Families Caring for Members with Mental Illness: A Vicious Cycle," by C. Ward-Griffin, R. Schofield, S. Vos, and R. Coatsworth-Puspoky, 2005, *Journal of Family Nursing, 11*(2), pp. 140–161.

Family Nursing in Critical Care Settings

During the last four decades of the twentieth century, acute-care hospitals introduced specialized critical care units. Nurses recognized the impact on family members of carrying out highly invasive and technological procedures under tenuous life-and-death circumstances. Nursing research reflected a desire to understand and assist with the emotional distress, uncertainty, and informational needs of family members under these extraordinary circumstances (Myers, Eichhorn, & Guzzetta, 2000). Again, nurses were challenged to humanize these environments by finding ways to enable family access to patients and information and to facilitate family involvement in decision making (Davidson et al., 2007).

Shifting Focus to Family Involvement in Health Care

During the 1990s, Canadian hospitals changed dramatically because of increasing political pressure for fiscal restraint within the public health-care system. The length of hospital stays was considerably reduced, reserved for management of acute episodic events, urgent diagnostic assessment, and treatment requiring intensive physiological monitoring. Outpatient services, home care, and community service increased as alternatives. These changes were coupled with the shifting demographics of the Canadian population. Average life expectancy is increasing, and key causes of death and disability have shifted to chronic illnesses (heart disease, cancer, and respiratory diseases), prompting a change in the direction of care from one that focuses on hospital and professionals to one that focuses on home and family.

More than at any time in the past, family members are now implicitly expected to be involved in the complex ongoing medical management of an ill family member at home (Mayer, 2001). Health-care providers rely on family members to assist with the administration of medication regimes, symptom management, dressing changes, and even such technical procedures as intravenous therapies, feeding systems, respiratory ventilators, and home dialysis. To be effective, the relationship between health-care providers and family members must be collaborative and reciprocal—each needs the support of the other (Ting, 2007).

Family Expectations for Involvement in Care

Recent clinical practice guidelines (e.g., Davidson et al., 2007) offer examples of family's hopes and expectations for involvement in care. Family members want to be able to *communicate* with health-care professionals about the ill person's condition. They want *access to information* about test results, diagnosis, treatment plans, and prognosis. Family members want to be able to *trust* that the ill person will be given good care and treated compassionately. They may feel compelled to be vigilant and protect the ill family member at a time of vulnerability. Family members want *recognition* that they are included and valued. Emotional attachment to the ill person can be a powerful motive for their involvement in providing care, but they also seek recognition of their own emotional distress. Finally, family members want *information and preparation* for their roles so they can confidently provide ongoing physical and emotional care. Unfortunately, evidence shows that, regardless of culture, most caregivers provide ongoing care without support from any professional caregivers (Navaie-Waliser, Feldman, Gould, Levine, Kuerbis, & Donelan, 2001, 2002).

Canadian Contributions to the Field of Family Nursing

Canadian nurses have made significant contributions to the field of family nursing (Bell, 1996). The Calgary family assessment model (Wright & Leahey, 2005a) was first published in 1984, updated, and then enhanced with the Calgary family intervention model in subsequent editions of the landmark text *Nurses and families: A guide to family assessment and intervention*. The International Family Nursing Conference, first held in Calgary, Alberta, in 1989, continues to meet regularly. The *Journal of Family Nursing* was first published in 1995 under the editorship of Dr. Janice Bell, University of Calgary. Nursing education programs increasingly offer family nursing in both undergraduate and specialized graduate programs in Canadian universities.

Canadian Families: A Demographic Snapshot

Canada has a growing population of about 33 million people (Statistics Canada, 2008a). However, its growth is not sustained from within. Indeed, Canada has a declining fertility rate (1.5 children per woman compared with a replacement rate of 2.1 children) and a population of seniors whose numbers will surpass those of the child population (under 15 years) by 2027. Canada's growth is largely due to immigration, with the rate being roughly twice that of United States and the second-largest among the G8 countries (Martel & Caron-Malenfant, 2007). More than one in five Canadians was born in another country and about 43% of Canada's population has origins other than Aboriginal, French, or English (Chui, Tran, & Maheux, 2007). The following depiction of Canadian demographics is based on an analysis of data from Statistics Canada and the Vanier Institute of the Family (*Family facts*, n.d.; Sauvé, 2004, 2006).

Cultural Diversity

Canada is heavily influenced by diverse ethnic, religious, and cultural traditions. In 2006 more than 1.1 million Canadians (3.8% of the Canadian population) reported some Aboriginal ancestry (including First Nations, Inuit, and Metis) (Statistics Canada, 2008b). The Aboriginal community is generally younger than their non-Aboriginal counterparts with one-third of its population under the age of 24 years. Although some Aboriginal people live on designated reserves, 54% live in urban areas with the highest concentrations located in the Northern and Prairie communities west of Ontario (10% of Winnipeg's population is Aboriginal). Immigrants represent a significant proportion of the Canadian population. In 2006, the total number of immigrants in Canada was estimated at 6.1 million, representing 19.8% of Canada's total population. Each year, Canada welcomes between 200 000 and 300 000 immigrants and refugees into the country. Before 1970, Canadian culture was powerfully shaped by European immigration. However, post-1970 statistics reveal that the majority of immigrants now come from Asia (Chui, Tran, & Maheux, 2007).

Mobility

Canadian families are characterized by high mobility (see the Nursing and Canadian Society box). According to the 2006 census, approximately 41% of Canadian residents over 5 years of age had moved within the past 5 years (Statistics Canada, 2006). About 15% moved to another location within their municipality, while almost 3% moved to another province or territory (Statistics Canada, 2008c). This fact is noteworthy since mobility occurred most often for those 15 to 44 years, during a time when families tend to be young and vulnerable. Mobility can be very stressful, as families join new communities; establish friendships, school relationships, and employment; or handle long-distance relationships (e.g., with an older parent or a spouse who works away from home). Many young families also experience difficulty with employment when they move, as their usual supports (e.g., parents, grandparents, friends) are no longer available to assist (e.g., for childcare).

Trends in Marriage, Divorce, Common Law Relationships, and Parenting

As with other social structures, the family (nearly 9 million in Canada) is experiencing a number of significant changes (Statistics Canada, 2007a, 2007b). Although married-couple families accounted for nearly 69% of families in 2006, their numbers are falling (down from 71% in 2001 and 80% in 1986). Conversely, the number of common law families (15.5%) is on the rise (up from 13.8% in 2001). The number of lone-parent families (15.9%), although on the rise over the past 20 years (15.7% in 2001), seems to have stabilized. Although women head 8 out of 10 of these families, the percentage of families headed by men has increased significantly (20% in 2006). Same-sex couples accounted for 0.6% of all families in 2006—54% of these couples were male, nearly 17% were married, and 9% had children under the age of 25 years. For the first time, Canada had more unmarried than married people older than 15 years of age and more families without children. (See Box 12.2 for the top 10 trends for Canadian families.)

NURSING AND CANADIAN SOCIETY

Fact	Implications for Nursing Practice
The average age of first marriages had been rising but seems to have stabilized (28.5 years for women, 30.6 years for men in 2003). (Sauvé, 2004). There are increasing numbers of young children with older mothers (nearly 8% of children aged 4 years had mothers in their 40s) (Sauvé, 2006).	Assessments should address the impact of family developmental tasks on health maintenance routines and practices.
Changes to the Divorce Act in 1985 resulted in a peak in divorce rates in the decade that followed (38% in 2003) (*Family Facts*, n.d.). However, divorce rates are currently declining (Statistics Canada, 2007a).	Genogram inquiries should routinely include consideration of stepparenting and blended family arrangements.
More than 9 out of 10 individuals with special needs or disabilities live with their families (Statistics Canada, 2007a). Seventeen percent of families are headed by a member aged at least 65 years. The numbers are expected to climb to 30% in 2026 (Sauvé, 2006).	Assessments should address the need for respite care and home care support for family members who are willing and able to fulfill ongoing caregiving responsibilities.
Canadian families are highly mobile—between 2001 and 2006, about 41% of all Canadian residents moved to a different location (Statistics Canada 2008c).	Assessments should explore the availability of family members to provide emotional and instrumental assistance during health difficulties.

BOX 12.2 THE TOP 10 TRENDS FOR CANADIAN FAMILIES

1. Fewer couples are getting legally married.
2. More couples are breaking up.
3. Families are getting smaller.
4. Children experience more transitions as parents change their marital status.
5. Canadians are generally satisfied with life.
6. Family violence is under-reported.
7. Multiple-earner families are now the norm.
8. Women still do most of the juggling involved in balancing work and home.
9. Inequality is worsening.
10. The future will have more aging families.

Source: From *Profiling Canada's Families III,* by Roger Sauvé, 2004, Ottawa: Vanier Institute of the Family. Printed from The Vanier Institute of the Family's website at http://www.vifamily.ca. © 2007. Reproduced with permission from The Vanier Institute of the Family.

The average age of marriage has increased and although about 38% of marriages ended in divorce in 2003, divorce rates are declining. The drop is mostly because of lower rates of marriage, increasing numbers of common law relationships, and the drop that followed the peak caused by the 1985 changes to the Divorce Act (Statistics Canada, 2007a). In 2001, 63% of all Canadian families (married or common law) had children (any age) living at home (*Family facts,* n.d.), and in 2006 nearly 26% of all young adults aged 25 to 29 years lived at home with their parents (Statistics Canada, 2007a). In 2001, more than 500 000 Canadian families were stepfamilies or blended families, in which at least one child was being raised by a biological or adoptive parent and a stepparent, up from approximately 430 000 in 1995 (*Family facts,* n.d.). In addition, approximately 3000 domestic adoptions (some of which were within blended families) and 2000 international adoptions occurred, while nearly 66 000 children were in foster care or available for adoption.

Income

Seven out of 10 couples with children in Canada are dual-income families. Between 1989 and 2003 the average disposable income per Canadian household (after transfers and income taxes) increased by only 3% in real terms (Sauvé, 2004). However, total spending jumped by 17% over the same period. In 1989, the typical household was able to put aside 13% of its disposable income but by 2003 this was down to only 1%, the lowest level in more than 40 years (Sauvé, 2004). Although more than 76% of female lone parents with school-age children were employed, employment does not guarantee prosperity. Indeed, more than half (56%) of the female lone-parent families lived below the poverty line (officially known as low-income cutoffs; Canadian Council on Social Development, 2005). The number of lone-parent women living below the poverty line was more than double the number of families living in poverty for all other groups: male lone parents (24%), two-parent families (12%), couples without children (11%), and older adults (7%). Nearly 1 in 10 Canadians receives social assistance or welfare and has an income well below the poverty line. Reduced access to employment insurance and the lack of affordable housing and dependable childcare force many families to rely on social assistance at some time (Morisette & Ostrovsky, 2007). However, reduced social assistance rates in recent years have meant that the average family on welfare now earns income that is far below the poverty line and that 41% of low-income children live in families where at least one parent works full time all year while the family still lives in poverty (Campaign 2000, 2008; Morisette & Ostrovsky, 2007).

It is not known how many homeless people live in Canada, but estimates range from 150 000 to 250 000, including many families (Housing & Homelessness Branch, Human Resources & Social Development Canada, 2006). However, as most homeless families do not go to shelters or facilities, their numbers are not included in homeless counts and they remain almost invisible (Federation of Canadian Municipalities, 2004). Instead, they live in unsafe, overcrowded housing, with friends and family, or in cheap motels. These families are often headed by lone-parent mothers who are struggling with mental health issues, addiction problems, or violence. Families who do access shelters are often forced to split up, with fathers going to a different location.

Families Providing Care

More than 8 out of 10 Canadians over the age of 85 years have some form of disability and more than 9 out of 10 individuals with special needs or disabilities live with their families in their own, their parents, or their children's home. Although many persons with disabilities are capable of caring for themselves, when they do require assistance, they most often turn to their families (McCloskey, 2005). Families continue to provide much of the care required for aging or disabled family members. Although many do not identify themselves as such, this is a very large population. Almost 700 000 Canadians spend more than 10 hours every week caring for seniors, and close to 3 million Canadians provide support to family members with disabilities (Canadian Association for Community Care, 2001). Caregivers make a significant contribution to the health and well-being of the country; indeed, they are the very foundation of the nation's long-term-care system (Gibson & Houser, 2007). It is estimated that Canadian caregivers contribute more than $5 billion worth of free services annually (Fast, Eales, & Keating, 2001).

Although older adults often serve as caregivers for their partners, women between the ages of 35 and 54 years are most likely to provide unpaid care to seniors, and they do so while maintaining other career and family responsibilities. Little is known about young children who serve as caregivers, for example, to a lone parent with a debilitating mental illness, out of fear of having the family separated if authorities are informed.

Caregiving affords many personal rewards; however, it also comes with numerous physical, psychological, social, and financial risks that are absorbed by the family and friends providing care (Gibson & Houser, 2007; Neufeld & Harrison, 2000). Unfortunately, limited health-care resources or government financial supports and the lack of employment flexibility or respite alternatives tends to isolate caregivers, which, in turn, increases their distress and burnout (Canadian Caregiver Coalition, 2003). Yet, without their help, the current health-care system would not function. Nurses are in a position to afford them much-needed support.

Understanding Families

Nursing care of families begins with understanding the family at a particular point in time, that is, *who* is involved and *how*. It is not realistic to expect that the nurse will fix the past, present, or future problems confronting the family. However, it is reasonable to expect that the nurse will help the family to navigate their way through a particular difficulty with a health problem or life transition. The focus of these encounters is the family's hopes and expectations for the present situation and ways the nurse can assist with reciprocal influences between the family and their health or illness concern (see Figure 12.1).

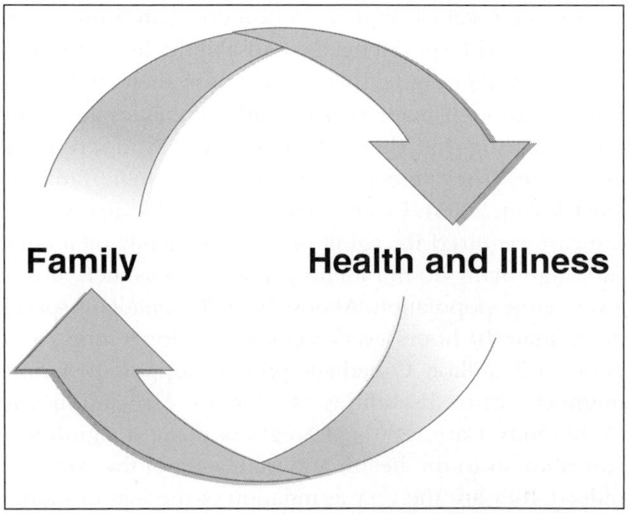

FIGURE 12.1 Reciprocal influence between family and health or illness

Illness affects the family, and the family affects the illness. By exploring both segments of this reciprocal loop in clinical conversation, the nurse can uncover many areas of inquiry that inform the nurse and create openings for addressing concerns of family members.

Who Is Involved in the Situation?

Family supports can assist the patient at the clinic, at the bedside, or in the home. However, a variety of reasons (work commitments, transportation difficulties, child-care responsibilities, economic constraints, or their own poor health) can prevent the nurse from actually meeting with the family members. In addition, family members may not want to be involved or the patient may not want to have them involved. However, if the nurse does not engage family members in conversation when encountering them, or does not ask about them in their absence, it becomes impossible to understand the possibilities for family support or the constraints and limits for family involvement.

At a minimum, the nurse can acknowledge the presence of family members and engage them by inviting their questions and concerns, explaining the value of family to patient health, and welcoming their participation. More specifically, the nurse can ask what family members understand of the health situation; provide clear, honest information; answer questions; and strive for consensus (Davidson et al., 2007).

Unfortunately, much of this information is often lost because it is not recorded or communicated. More structured documentation about the family can be facilitated by a genogram inquiry (Hanson & Boyd, 1996; Wright & Leahey, 2005a). The **genogram** is a concise visual depiction of the family structure and relevant situational information that can be sketched on nursing admission forms, progress notes, or Kardex cards and used with numerous areas of nursing, such as postpartum families (Holtslander, 2005) or in pediatrics (Martinez, D'Artois, & Rennick, 2007).

Mapping out a genogram can be brief (minutes) or the focus of an entire family assessment interview (see Box 12.3). The nurse can introduce the genogram by explaining that it helps the health team understand the family situation and provide more effective care, for example, by identifying others who might be involved in the care, have access to information, or assist with discharge planning.

Figure 12.2 illustrates an example of a detailed genogram and common conventions for constructing these diagrams. The situation involves a family in which the father, Ron, is hospitalized following a heart attack. He is a long-haul truck driver and divorced from Susan, with whom he had two children (Scott and Evan). Ron is now married to Elaine, a licensed practical nurse. Together they have a daughter, Katie. Elaine is the main caregiver for her mother, the only living grandparent in the family, who lives a 45-minute drive away. The family resides in a small city in which one of the main industries is closing. Ron does most of his driving for this company.

BOX 12.3 FAMILY ASSESSMENT GUIDE

For each of the areas assessed, the nurse should consider strengths, limitations, and opportunities.

FAMILY STRUCTURE

- Size and type: nuclear, extended, or alternative family
- Age and sex of family members

FAMILY ROLES AND FUNCTIONS

- Family members working outside the home; type of work and satisfaction with it
- Household roles and responsibilities and how tasks are distributed
- Ways childrearing responsibilities are shared
- Major decision maker and methods of decision making
- Family members' satisfaction with roles, the way tasks are divided, and the way decisions are made

PHYSICAL HEALTH STATUS

- Current physical health status of each member
- Perceptions of own health and other family members' health
- Preventive health practices (e.g., status of immunizations, oral hygiene practices, regularity and frequency of visits to the dentist, regularity of visual examinations)
- Routine health care, when and why physician last seen

INTERACTION PATTERNS

- Ways of expressing affection, love, sorrow, anger, and so on
- Most significant family member in person's life
- Openness of communication with all family members

FAMILY VALUES

- Cultural and religious orientations; degree to which cultural practices are followed
- Use of leisure time and whether leisure time is shared with total family unit
- Family's view of education, teachers, and the school system
- Health values: how much emphasis is put on exercise, diet, preventive health care

COPING RESOURCES

- Degree of emotional support offered to one another
- Availability of support persons and affiliations outside the family (e.g., friends, religious memberships)
- Methods of handling stressful situations and conflicting goals of family members
- Financial ability to meet current and future needs

The nurse can introduce the genogram with basic questions about individuals' ages, interests, and occupations. Age-appropriate questions can also be directed to young children about school, friends, and favourite games or toys. Beginning questions usually focus on the family members currently residing together or who are involved in some way in the health-care situation. However, inquiry should also explore other family relationships that seem to be relevant to the current situation. For example, in Figure 12.2, the genogram inquiry uncovered the 8-year-old daughter's worries about her father's health, Ron's significant family history with heart disease, and Elaine's caregiving responsibilities for her aging mother. The genogram inquiry may reveal recent losses in the family or significant family events that may contribute to concurrent stress or difficulties confronted by the family. Asking questions about relationships with previous marital partners who are involved in ongoing co-parenting responsibilities can also be important. For example, the nurse could ask Ron how his ex-wife, Susan, believes that Scott and Evan have been reacting to the news of their father's heart attack. This discussion builds an understanding not only of Ron's relationship with his two sons, but also of the nature of his relationship with his ex-wife. It is important that the genogram questions explore and focus on family concerns and the impact of

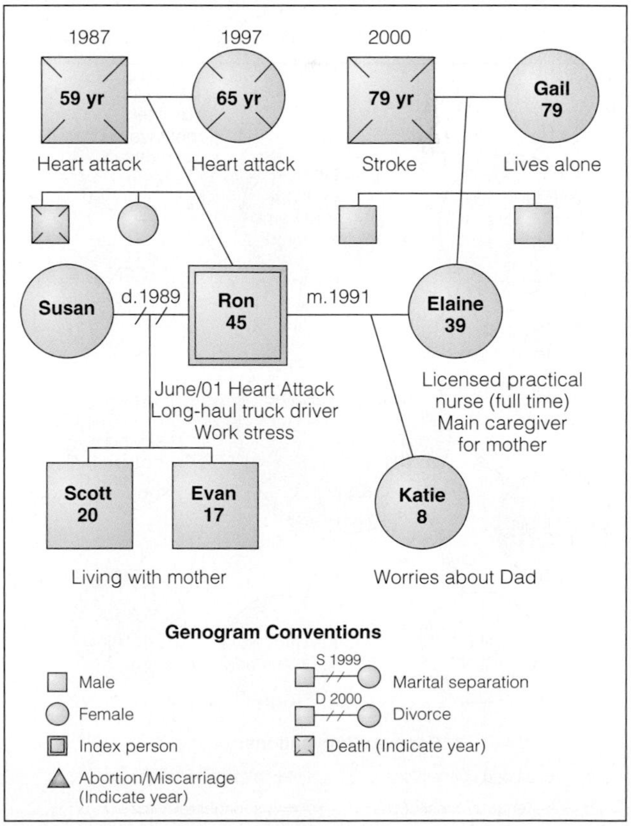

FIGURE 12.2 Family genogram

the health problem on family members and their relationships. As they explore the genogram information together, the nurse and family members can become more engaged and committed to working together. Initiating a genogram inquiry can be an intervention that encourages the nurse *and* family to "think family" and to consider the impact of the situation on all family members.

The context and external environment of the family can similarly be explored by sketching an **ecomap** (Figure 12.3). This diagram uses symbols to depict the family's connections to larger systems, including community agencies, health-care providers, work, religion, friends, and other meaningful parts of their lives (Bomar, 1996; Wright & Leahey, 2005a). The symbols are able to express relationships in ways that may be inadequately portrayed in words (Ray & Street, 2005). The genogram of family members sharing a household is sketched at the centre of the diagram. Ecomap questions could include the following examples:

- *To understand how connected the family is with other resources*: Are there any other clinics, health-care professionals, or community agencies that are involved with your family regarding this health concern?
- *To understand the family's level of satisfaction*: Which of these contacts have been most or least helpful to you?
- *To understand the family's support network*: Are there any other self-help groups, religious groups, or personal relationships outside your family that either have been supportive to you or have contributed to your stress?

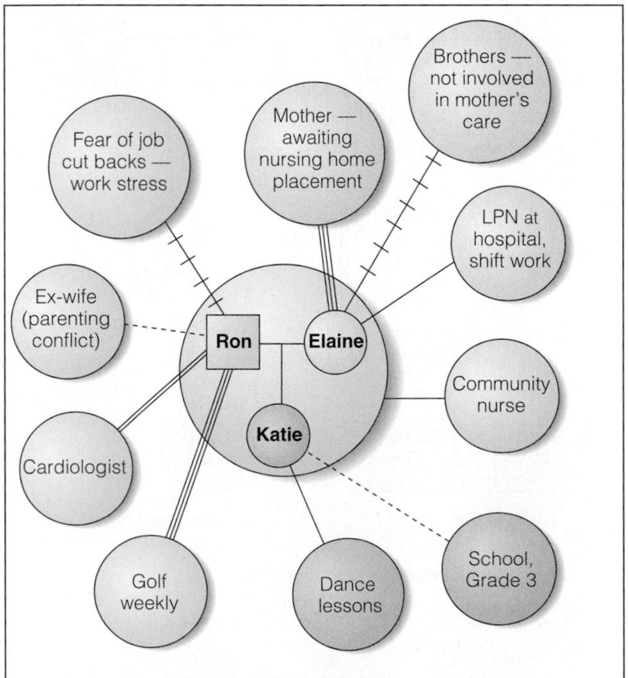

FIGURE 12.3 Family ecomap

The ecomap can also depict the dynamic nature of the relationships and stressors with extended family members, work colleagues, or friends. For example, Figure 12.3 helps highlight many external demands on Elaine. In addition to coping with her husband's heart attack, she does shift work and is a caregiver for her mother. She is also dealing with the often difficult transition of placing her mother in a nursing home, with little apparent support from her brothers.

Each circle on the ecomap represents an outside contact with either an individual or the entire family. However, the number of identified contacts in the social network should not be assumed to indicate that support is provided or received or that such contacts are easily accessible (Bomar, 1996). Straight lines are drawn to indicate the intensity of helpful relationships (for either party); dotted lines indicate ambivalent relationships; and slashed (or jagged) lines indicate difficult or stressful relationships. The ecomap can heighten the nurse's awareness of the possibility of social isolation or of family overload with multiple overlapping connections with health-care professionals or agencies. It also provides an opportunity to explore the nature and quality of these networks.

How Does Illness Affect the Family?

Exploring the impact of illness on the family increases the nurse's appreciation of the distress and suffering of all family members, including the person who is experiencing the health problem (Wright & Leahey, 2005a). The long-term impact of illness demands differs when the family is confronted with recovery from an acute illness episode and when the family faces these responsibilities on an ongoing basis, as in the case of a chronic or debilitating illness (Hopkins & Brett, 2005). Instrumental functioning of the family (i.e., activities of daily living) can be affected. Indeed, family members caring for an ill or a recovering loved one at home may need to assist with hygiene, mobilization, medication administration, changes in meal preparation, or follow-up visits to doctors and clinics.

Illness can also affect expressive functioning and communications within the family. Anxiety, depression, and uncertainty can cause distress for the ill person and, in some cases, can be an even greater burden for others in the family. For example, if one partner struggles with physical limitations and is unable to carry on a usual routine, the other partner may be pressed to take on new responsibilities for childcare, household maintenance, or employment. Family members often feel compelled to be strong and portray an optimistic outlook for others. In reality, they may be concerned about the implications of the loss of physical functioning in their loved one, the implications of a poor prognosis, or the possibility of premature death.

It can be painful for family members to discuss their distress and worries. As a result, communication patterns and family roles can shift dramatically, depending on whether members address their concerns openly together or conceal their worries and suffer in silence. Every new diagnosis, change in treatment plan, or contact with a new health-care setting potentially has an impact on other family members, including a heightened vulnerability to illness (Goodwin, Wickramaratne, Nomura, & Weissman, 2007).

Nurses need to encourage productive conversations that explore family understandings of the impact of illness. Such conversations can help reveal family values (e.g., family beliefs about appropriate roles and responsibilities for different members, family beliefs about why people get ill and strategies for healing), which, in turn, can assist in understanding their decisions. The nurse who initiates these conversations in the presence of other family members creates an opportunity for each to listen to the others' concerns. Such discussions can help family members become mutually supportive.

The nurse can help family members who are hesitant to raise sensitive matters by asking them to *meet together,* and then introducing topics and helping them explore the issues. Alternatively, the nurse can *meet privately* with individual members, with the understanding that some highly stigmatized behaviour and health conditions are disclosed at considerable risk to those affected. For example, the nurse who observes that a mother, who has brought her child to the pediatric emergency room, is very anxious and hesitant to discuss her child's bruising, may realize that the mother's behaviour is consistent with domestic violence. In such a case, the nurse would realize that to build trust with the mother, he or she would need to engage her in private discussion. Therefore, the nurse would reassure the mother by first attending to the child's health problem, and then opening a discussion about family stress and its effects, including the possibility of mistreatment and abuse. The nurse would also provide time for the mother to reflect on and acknowledge the implications of such a discussion, and then reassure her that immediate and ongoing assistance is available (Dowd, Kennedy, Knapp, & Stallbaumer-Rouyer, 2002).

Not all situations require the same approach. For example, when working within circumstances involving a sexually transmitted disease, such as HIV/AIDS, nurses need to be sensitive to the fact that making a disclosure to family is not only challenging but may also require different approaches, according to gender, sexual orientation, and cultural background (Korner, 2007). For example, a discussion of positive HIV test results with an undeclared bisexual married man attending an infertility clinic will address very different issues (e.g., coming to terms with the diagnosis, coming to terms with bisexuality, figuring out how to tell his wife, facing the possibility of his marriage breaking up, forming a health treatment plan) than will a discussion of the same results with an openly gay couple who requested HIV testing (e.g., coming to terms with the diagnosis, facing the implications for the relationship, forming a health treatment plan). Examples of questions that may be helpful for exploring the impact of illness on the family are provided in Box 12.4.

How Does the Family Affect the Illness?

Just as the illness has an influence on each family member, each family member also has an influence on the illness (Firth, 2006). This statement does not mean that the person can control the illness or determine health outcomes. Family members cope with and respond to the illness in many different ways—each journey is unique and different from that of the patient. However, the need for support, information, valuing, and respect is the same. Therapeutic conversation in this domain helps uncover ways family members have found to manage the demands of the illness in their daily lives. They may view a health concern as a challenge and embrace changes necessitated by health maintenance or illness management. They may be overwhelmed by illness demands that compound other concurrent life stressors. A new diagnosis may challenge family members to seek new information and to figure out what this means for their lives. Family members may develop expertise in their vigilance for the return of troublesome symptoms or potential complications.

Family members typically attempt to offer help and encouragement to the ill or recovering person while also attempting to manage their own distress. On occasion, the ill person sees family offers of support as intrusive,

BOX 12.4 EXAMPLES OF QUESTIONS THAT EXPLORE IMPACT OF ILLNESS ON THE FAMILY

The nurse can use these questions to help a family work through the illness of a family member:

- What do you think has been the most difficult change that each of you has had to deal with since the heart attack? How do your views compare with those of the other members of your family?
- Of all your family members, who do you think is worrying the most about what this new diagnosis means?
- Of all the things that you or your family are confronting as you prepare for discharge, which ones do you think we could try to address today?
- What do you anticipate will cause the most difficulty for each member of your family when you return home?
- Which member of your family is most likely to initiate discussions of difficulties or concerns as they arise at home?

paternalistic, or as a limitation to their independence. Conversations about these attempts to influence their loved one's illness can help family members to understand their sense of helplessness, to explore how they would most prefer to be involved, to limit the caregiving burden, and to enable family members to show their caring in a manner that is experienced as supportive. Illness often compounds other life stressors. For example, marital discord, difficulties with parenting of teenagers, unemployment, and conflict within the extended family can interfere with family coping and increase the complexity of family involvement during health-care encounters. In such circumstances, the nurse might have a discussion with the family to explore their responses to the illness in question. The nurse might also explore the family's capacities, resources, and so on, and ways in which they might be used to overcome their sense of helplessness. Learning about the family's resourcefulness provides the nurse with opportunities to help members recognize their own strengths to build new ways of coping. These conversations help the nurse understand the family's usual ways of managing difficulties and introduce ideas that may be different from those that the family has already attempted. Exploration of family strengths in illness management is an often-neglected domain of inquiry. Examples of questions that explore family influence on the illness are posed in Box 12.5.

Nursing Care of Families

As stated earlier, nursing care of families is exercised almost exclusively through relational practices. Even if only one or two family members are directly involved in the health-care encounter, the nurse–family relationship is more complex than is the relationship with individual clients. The nurse needs to engage and understand each family member to elicit concerns and invite questions. Family members and patients may hold similar or different perspectives and may require different supports. The nurse needs to not only appreciate these multiple perspectives but also attempt to respond in ways that account for them. Nurses can enhance their family nursing practice by using the guidelines in Box 12.6.

BOX 12.5 EXAMPLES OF QUESTIONS THAT EXPLORE THE IMPACT OF THE FAMILY ON ILLNESS

These questions can help debrief families when someone experiences an illness:

- What has been the most helpful thing that your family has done for you that has made a difference to this hospitalization?
- What have each of you learned about limiting stress that will be most useful to you when you return home?
- How have each of your family members been most helpful to you as you have been preparing for discharge?
- Of all of the lifestyle changes that have been recommended to you, which ones do you believe each of your family members will be able to implement most successfully?
- How would you like each of your family members to be involved in your recovery at home?

BOX 12.6 FAMILY NURSING PRACTICES

Good family nursing practices include the following:

- Engaging in a collaborative relational stance
- Asking reflective questions
- Enabling access to the patient
- Eliciting illness narratives
- Commending family and individual strengths
- Offering information
- Creating and encouraging family support
- Suggesting respite from caregiving

Engaging in a Collaborative Relational Stance

Relational practices are influenced by nurses' beliefs about the kinds of obligations people have toward family members, about expectations of family members, and about the skills and knowledge that nurses bring to family encounters. Many of these ideas are presupposed in nursing practice, for example, the idea that recovery from an acute episode of illness will affect family members. However, ideas about whether nurses are responsible for caring for family members and what ought to be done may be less clear. The nurse's stance toward the family is influenced by the habits, practices, concerns, and skills the nurse brings to the situation (Browning & Warren, 2006). In family nursing, **relational stance** refers to the thoughtful and purposeful choices that nurses make in clinical practice about the ways that they will engage and involve families and respond to their concerns (Walker & Dewar, 2001; Tapp, 2000). Families feel engaged when information is shared and they are included in decision making, when they have someone to contact when needed, and when services are responsive to their needs (Walker & Dewar, 2001).

It is often assumed that a good nursing relationship with the patient and family will increase the effectiveness of nurses' work with them. Robinson's (1996) research challenged nurses to reconsider relational practices as creating a context or climate which, in itself, is an "intervention." This research described examples of relational practices that were noticed by family members in a study of women and families experiencing chronic illnesses. The family participants described the nurse as a *curious listener,* who found a balance between listening and asking good questions that focused conversation and brought into the open significant differences in family perspectives. They viewed the nurse as a *compassionate stranger,* someone who was deeply interested in the family's situation, yet who had some objectivity and could offer a new point of view that was impartial to various family members. Families valued the nurse as a *nonjudgmental collaborator* whose avoidance of blaming and criticism helped family members speak with less reservation. This collaborative stance helped families to realize what they needed to do and then to do it together. Families appreciated the nurse as a *mirror for family strengths,* whose positive orientation toward strengths, resources, and possibilities fostered family confidence and capability.

Collaboration entails working with the family to create shared understandings of the difficulties they are encountering. Together, the family and the nurse generate other possibilities for dealing with health concerns or illness. A **collaborative relational stance** is one that values the multiple ideas and perspectives that are inevitably encountered within the family and demonstrates respect for family strengths and capabilities in addressing health concerns and living with illness (see Box 12.7). It is through the process of "shaping mutuality" that a nurse and family caregiver learn to collaborate and achieve their individual goals and desired outcomes, both for the patient and for themselves (Jeon, 2004).

Asking Reflective Questions

Studies have consistently shown that families find nurses particularly helpful when nurses ask good questions (Tapp, 1997; Wright et al., 1996). The best questions enable families to think differently about themselves, about other family members, and about health and illness—both in the present and in the future (Firth, 2006). Wright et al. (1996) described this practice as "asking questions that invite reflection" (p. 116) to promote understanding of events and relationships of everyday life. Wright and Leahey (2005a) described **reflective questions** as interventive because they not only *provide information* to the nurse but also *facilitate changes in the family* as new information emerges in conversations. Family members come to understand one another, their difficulties, and possible solutions differently as they listen to one another's responses to reflective questions. Table 12.1 summarizes examples of types of reflective questions: **difference questions**, **behavioural effect questions**, **hypothetical or future-oriented questions**, and **triadic questions** (Wright & Leahey, 2005a). In addition, the three most common errors in family nursing are included, along with strategies for avoiding such mistakes (Wright & Leahey, 2005b).

BOX 12.7 QUESTIONS INVITING NURSING REFLECTION ON RELATIONAL STANCE

A collaborative relational stance is important in the nurse–family relationship. Use the questions that follow to evaluate your own relational stance:

- To what extent am I imposing my beliefs on the family?
- To what extent did I elicit the patient's and family members' expectations, hopes, questions, and ideas?
- How frequently are decisions about the patient's health care made mutually by the patient, family, and myself?
- Do my actions and comments acknowledge the strengths and abilities of this family?
- What can I learn from this family about their experiences in living with this health problem?

Source: From "Family-Nurse Relationships: Core Assumptions and Clinical Implications," by M. Leahey and S. Harper-Jaques, 1996, *Journal of Family Nursing, 2*(2), pp. 133–151.

Enabling Access to the Hospitalized Patient

Within inpatient practice settings, an issue commonly encountered by families is that of limited visiting hours (Farrell, Joseph, & Schwartz-Barcott, 2005). Hospital policies regarding visiting hours may impose constraints for family members who want to be present at the patient's bedside. The reasons for limiting family access can include concerns for patient rest and privacy, infection control, limited space at the bedside, patient instability, and the possible impact of viewing procedures on family members. Nurses may not be comfortable when family members observe their performance of bedside care or technical procedures. Nurses may believe that the impact of an emotionally distraught family member at the bedside can upset the patient. Sometimes, the patient may request limitations to family visiting.

Family members may want to be present to provide emotional support to the ill person, to protect the ill person from harm through possible mistakes or careless treatment by health-care providers, or to quell their own emotional distress (Mitchell, Courtney, & Coyer, 2003). Access to the patient often means access to information. Family members who are present at the bedside may have more opportunities to consult directly with the health team. When family members are able to access the patient, they also have more opportunity to understand their loved one's condition, which, in turn, can help them gain confidence as they see the patient progress in strength and recovery or assist them to prepare for difficulties and loss. Nurses have a responsibility to facilitate that understanding. Families want different kinds of information in different situations. For example, when removing life supports from a patient, families want (1) assurances that the patient will not be abandoned before death, (2) assurances that the patient will be comfortable

TABLE 12.1 Types of Reflective Questions

Types of Questions	Examples
Difference Question Explores differences among people, relationships, time, ideas, or beliefs	Who do you think will be most affected by this new diagnosis of heart disease when you return home? What impact has this experience with the heart attack had on your relationship as a couple?
Behavioural Effect Question Explores the effect of one family member's behaviour on another	When your daughter Katie is worried about her Dad's health, what do you tell her? How does Ron show his stress when his work is demanding? What impact does this have on you, Elaine? What impact does it have on Katie?
Hypothetical or Future-Oriented Question Explores family options and alternative actions or implications in the future	What do you predict will be the most difficult change for you as you try to implement lifestyle changes? How do you anticipate your family's daily routine to be different when you are discharged home?
Triadic Question Posed to a third person about the relationship between the other two people	Ron, what impact has this hospitalization had on Elaine's relationship with Katie? Elaine, how are you hoping Ron's relationship with Katie might be different since the heart attack?
Most Common Errors	**How to Avoid**
Failing to create a context for change (being curious about the problem), the foundation of the therapeutic relationship	• Show interest • Obtain a clear understanding of the most pressing concern • Validate each family member's experience • Acknowledge suffering and the sufferer
Taking sides	• Maintain curiosity • Identify all the perspectives (identifying does not equate with condoning) • Remember that all members experience some suffering during a family illness or problem • Give equal time to each concern and each member • Treat all information as a new discovery • Avoid having private conversations in which one family member reports on another
Giving too much advice	• Give advice, opinions, and recommendations only after a thorough assessment • Offer advice without believing the ideas are best or better • Ask more questions instead of giving statements during initial conversations

Source: Adapted from *Nurses and Families: A Guide to Family Assessment and Intervention,* by L. M. Wright and M. Leahey, 2005, Philadelphia, PA: F.A. Davis. Reprinted with permission from F. A. Davis Company, Philadelphia, PA. Additional information is taken from "The Three Most Common Errors in Family Nursing: How to Avoid or Sidestep," by L. M. Wright and M. Leahey, 2005, *Journal of Family Nursing*, 11, p. 90.

and will not suffer, and (3) support for family's decisions about end-of-life care, including support for family's decision to withdraw or not to withdraw life support (Stapleton, Engelberg, Wenrich, Goss, & Curtis, 2006).

Nurses interpret hospital policy and unit guidelines and often have discretion to flex visiting rules when warranted in particular situations or to collectively generate a unit culture that is more family friendly. Many nurses argue that visiting hours require balancing the visitors' needs for information and access to a loved one with the nurses' need to safely manage the care of a critically ill individual (Farrell et al., 2005). Studies of the effects of visiting on mental status and various physiological systems have shown no physiological rationale for restricting visitors and some reasons for making visiting hours more flexible, even in ICU (e.g., Griffin, 2003; Lee et al., 2007). Many pediatric settings and, increasingly, adult ICU and emergency settings show positive effects on the family when they have open, unrestricted visiting policies, even during resuscitation (e.g., Myers et al., 2000). However, these situations require adequate preparation of the family, availability of support personnel to help the family through a crisis situation, and family debriefing and support following a crisis (Benner, Hooper-Kyriakidis, & Stannard, 1999). In addition, patients, families, and staff do not always share the same views around visiting hours (Tanner, 2005), so it is important to check with the patient, where possible, when discussing visitation.

Eliciting Illness Narratives

Nurses access the beliefs and meanings that people hold about their day-to-day experience of illness through illness narratives, rather than medical narratives (Morris, 1998). **Medical narratives** provide clinicians with information relevant to the nature and course of physical symptoms, diagnosis, and treatment of a disease process and concurrent or past illness problems for the person or other family members. In contrast, **illness narratives** seek understanding of the person's and family's experience of illness in the ordinary acts of everyday living; the influence of illness on relationships with family, friends, and workmates; the person's ability to gain influence over the impact of illness in their lives; and the stories told of encounters with the health-care system. Both medical and illness narratives are important and useful, and nurses must be able to conduct both forms of inquiry. Table 12.2 offers examples of questions that illustrate differences between medical and illness narratives.

Eliciting illness narratives with families is an important relational practice. These stories help the nurse understand family strengths and difficulties and also help patients and their families come to terms with their own experiences. In the telling of these stories, people reach a new understanding of their experiences with illness. Family members are better able to appreciate what is happening and to realize that their experiences are both similar and different. Family members may describe the telling of illness stories as therapeutic in itself (e.g., Berg, 2006). However, illness conversations face many constraints. Family members may want to maintain privacy or may not want to burden friends or other family members. Although people expect to tell health-care professionals their medical story, they are often surprised that health-care professionals are interested in illness stories. However, when asked, they often relate encounters with health-care systems that contributed to difficult illness experiences.

When nurses elicit illness stories, they are drawn into the richly contextualized lives of the people they encounter. It becomes much more difficult to objectify or depersonalize people and, in turn, much easier to recognize the strengths, resourcefulness, and capabilities of the family members. Illness stories enable nurses to offer family commendations that acknowledge their efforts to maintain health or manage illness.

Commending Family and Individual Strengths

Nurses may adopt the stance that patients and families have strengths and capabilities, that they have solved problems before and are resourceful and only temporarily in need of assistance from health-care professionals (McElheran & Harper-Jaques, 1994). This stance heightens the nurse's ability to recognize and elicit examples of the family's resourcefulness throughout their work together. Examples of strength and capability appear in the illness narratives as people and families tell of the ways in which they have been able to manage or live with a health problem or illness. Other examples are evident in the day-to-day situations and conversations that occur as nurses and families work together. When nurses acknowledge strengths directly to the family, the practice of offering commendations emerges. This practice can help families recognize their own strengths and realize that these can be transferred to other situations and are valued by other health-care professionals. Commendations are not always experienced as warm and gentle. Indeed, although considered constructive, they can also

TABLE 12.2 Examples of Questions to Elicit Medical and Illness Narratives

Medical Narrative	Illness Narrative
Could you describe the onset of the chest pain?	What does it mean to you when the chest pains come and are so unpredictable?
Have you had any acute health problems or chronic illnesses in the past?	Of all of the health problems that you have encountered in the past, what has been the most difficult thing you have had to deal with?
Does your extended family have any previous history of heart disease?	What have you learned from your parents' experiences with heart disease that might be helpful during your own recovery?
Have you had any cardiac diagnostic tests done in the past?	Based on the diagnostic tests that you have had done, what are your predictions about your health in the future?
Which of the following cardiac risk factors would apply to you: smoker, sedentary lifestyle, high-fat diet?	Tell me how it has been for you and your family as you have tried to incorporate the lifestyle changes that have been recommended.

be experienced as provocative, potent, and powerful (Limacher & Wright, 2006).

Commendations are statements of praise that "highlight strengths, support movement of the nurse-patient-family system in ways that meet the family's needs and assist the nurse in engaging the patient and family at levels of interaction that are not problem saturated, but are resource focused" (McElheran & Harper-Jaques, 1994, p. 7). When health problems occur, families may be overwhelmed by difficulties and feel unable to cope with the uncertainty or transitions they are facing. Commendations can help change the view that families have of themselves or their situations and support their confidence in one another. Commendations support the idea that the patient and the family are active participants who are in charge of their health or life situation and can offer hope for the future (McElheran & Harper-Jaques, 1994). This practice can encourage families to continue seeking further options to discover their own solutions to problems (Wright & Leahey, 2005a). Commendations can also enhance connection in the family–nurse relationship as the nurse conveys respect for and appreciation of the family's contributions and efforts in difficult situations.

Commendations should echo the family's own language and fit with their values and perceptions of their experiences. When the nurse does not know the family well, commendations can be offered as "beginning impressions" of what they have been doing well. Commendations can be introduced by such comments as "What I've noticed about your family (or about what you've told me) is that . . . ," "I'm really impressed by the way that . . . ," "I appreciate how you have been able to . . . ," "I'm wondering if your talent in this situation is the way that you . . . " It may be helpful to offer a commendation before offering an opinion or idea that might be difficult for family members to accept, with such comments such as "You have all really pulled together in wonderful ways to understand your son's illness. Unfortunately, as there is no cure for his illness, he will need increasing amounts of care . . . care that is often painful." Commendations offered at the end of a conversation can highlight change or support family choices that have emerged within the discussion through such comments as "It is quite remarkable how many decisions you have made today, given that, when we started our discussion, you each said that you were in no position to make any decisions."

Offering Information

Families indicate that obtaining information about the health situation greatly assists them to make decisions, to cope more effectively, and to be able to support their ill family member appropriately (Davidson et al., 2007). Nurses play an important role in providing information for health promotion, recovery, and health maintenance, or during acute episodes of illness. Health-promotion messages within the media and public domain are often confusing or contradictory. Illness care operates within an increasingly technical biomedical domain with a specialized jargon. Nurses are positioned in the middle of these public and biotechnical discourses and can help families interpret this information. Also, nurses typically know the health-care system well and can offer information to help people access appropriate services effectively. They can, for example, provide handouts of resource lists, teach steps for navigating bureaucratic systems, make advance contact with services when referring, and make follow-up phone calls to families. These actions foster a sense of partnership with families and facilitate service access.

Family members other than the ill individual can play an important role in garnering information about diagnosis, treatment, and health maintenance. The ill person may be less able to seek out or comprehend new information because of illness, effects of medications, or invasive diagnostics and treatment. By informing and educating family members, the nurse helps them understand illness events, anticipate likely events on a trajectory of illness, and prepare for their caregiving roles (Levine, 1998).

Nurses often make assumptions about the kind of information that would be most helpful to particular people or families. Frequently, these assumed essentials concern the details of the disease process, medication management, and activity guidelines. However, it is important to discuss with the family the kind of information they believe would be most helpful. Other concerns may be far more pressing, such as how to provide emotional support at home or how to arrange for transportation to a follow-up appointment and how to pay for it—concerns that families can be hesitant to raise on their own. Many nurses believe that more information will result in decreased anxiety but it is not always so. Nurses can be very helpful to families by assisting them to identify the amount of information they want now and to locate other sources of information (such as self-help or support groups, public service groups, websites, or community resource centres) that they can access at other times. The challenge is to offer resources (information and support) that address family questions and needs in a timely fashion (as needed) and in suitable ways (e.g., plain language).

Creating and Encouraging Family Support

When nurses are "thinking family" (Wright & Leahey, 2005a), they are more likely to be aware that all family members may be in need of support. The health-care literature often conceptualizes **family support** as a form of social support—the provision of emotional, instrumental, informational, and appraisal assistance that helps to buffer stress. It is not unidirectional, but rather **reciprocal** (mutual) as individuals attempt to be supportive of one another. Therefore, in health care, the focus does not remain solely on the patient but, instead, on identified caregivers and other family members as well.

Social support is not simply nice to have; it plays a critical role in psychological health (Deci, La Guardia, Moller, Scheiner, & Ryan, 2006). *Giving* support has been found to be a stronger predictor of psychological health than the act of *receiving* support (Deci et al., 2006). Further, the number of contacts within a social network is less important than the *perceived quality* of social relationships and the extent to which they are experienced as supportive (Bomar, 1996).

Nurses provide family support as they involve family members in care and respond to their concerns and questions. Nurses can help family members to listen to one another's concerns, feelings, and stories and make meaning of illness and health-care encounters, thus increasing the possibility for them to be supportive of one another (Wright & Leahey, 2005a).

Family members may seek guidance about how they can be supportive of the ill person. These needs typically arise at times when family members are also experiencing distress, concern, and need for emotional support. Nurses can help family members discuss their preferences about the kind of assistance or support they desire from one another (Tapp, 1997). For example, following an acute episode of illness, the patient may want to regain a sense of independence. Family members may have difficulty gauging how much assistance is desired or appropriate. If the ill person views needing help as a sign of weakness, offers of assistance from family members may be unwelcome.

As another example, following diagnosis of diabetes, family members frequently attempt to be helpful through watchful monitoring of medications, activity, or diet, while the ill person may find these reminders unhelpful or intrusive. At the same time, it can be hurtful to family members when their well-intended efforts are rebuffed, especially if they view the ill person as not attending responsibly to health-maintenance activities.

The ill person may be self-absorbed with the experience of illness and recovery and less aware of the impacts on other family members. Illness conversations can be constrained by a desire to maintain a positive attitude. Family members may be reluctant to discuss their own needs or frustrations, especially if their distress is motivated by worries about the future or prognosis. These difficulties can contribute to significant family conflict. By using reflective questions, the nurse can assist family members to explore their perceptions and concerns, come to appreciate the perspective of other members, and discuss how each person would prefer to both receive and offer assistance.

Suggesting Respite from Caregiving

Families differ in their desire to be directly involved in caregiving. For example, Benner and colleagues (1999) suggested that family members of chronically ill patients who are hospitalized may want to participate in familiar caregiving rituals (such as grooming, assisting with meals, comfort measures) to maintain a connection. Others may be exhausted from caregiving at home and welcome respite from these demands. It is important to encourage family participation in caregiving to the extent that they desire, but this should be facilitated following careful exploration of both patient and family preferences. Such discussions are not always easy. Indeed, evidence suggests that nurses and families have difficulty discussing family participation in caretaking activities (e.g., Roden, 2005).

A study by Ward-Griffin (1999) explored transitions in caregiving between community nurses and family members caring for an older person at home. Initially, family members were encouraged to be involved and were grateful to be of assistance. They became knowledgeable and skillful in these activities as the nurse shifted care to the family caregiver at a comfortable pace. However, family members gradually reported feeling overwhelmed as nurses reduced their time and involvement. Eventually, many family caregivers reported that the amount of care they were expected to provide led to physical and emotional exhaustion, social isolation, and strained family relationships. This report highlights the potential for caregiver burden. Another study, by Leenerts and Teel (2006), explored communication skills used by nurses to create partnerships with older spouse caregivers of persons with dementia. Conversations that resulted in partnerships depended on one theme only: relational conversation, that is, conversation that included listening with intent, affirming emotions, creating relational images, and planning enactment.

Financial constraints can make it difficult for families to secure respite from caregiving. Research shows that caregivers who are poor, married, have a poor health status, provide care for a long time, care for patients with poor performance status, and who pay high medical expenses are more likely to lose their family savings (Yun et al., 2005). Household income may be reduced because of the ill person's inability to work, or family members may be forfeiting income in order to be available to an ill family member. Finances can limit options to compensate a replacement caregiver or to allow for a vacation. Additionally, it can be difficult for family members to allow themselves to take respite from caregiving without guilt (Wright & Leahey, 2005a). The ill person may be reluctant to accept an alternative caregiver. A primary caregiver may be reluctant to request assistance from, or disagree with, extended family members. Possible constraints should be explored with the family, perhaps by discussing the implications should the caregiver become rundown or get ill or measures that would give the caregiver comfort if respite care were provided.

Many possible options are available for **respite care**. Regularly obtaining a few hours away from home may be sufficient in some instances. Others may prefer an extended vacation for several weeks. Some may desire respite for brief one- or two-day periods. Respite programs may be available either to provide care in home or for temporary inpatient placement. Unfortunately, respite care is not available in all provinces and territories or in many rural areas. Hence, for many families, respite care must be provided by other family members or friends.

Evaluating Nursing Care of Families

Relational practices are inherent in nurses' efforts to evaluate their clinical practice with families. Every encounter with patients and families provides opportunities for the nurse to invite their viewpoint. The nurse can reflect on the extent to which information was communicated to families, how families were involved in decision making, and the ways that patient and family expectations, hopes, questions, and ideas were discussed (Leahey & Harper-Jaques, 1996) and met, or not, and barriers that might have surfaced. The nurse can also solicit feedback from the patient and family about their experience of the family–nurse relationship (see Box 12.8). Their comments and suggestions can provide useful opportunities for fostering ongoing development in clinical skills that enable nursing care of families to be provided in a respectful and healing manner.

BOX 12.8 EVALUATING THE NURSING CARE OF FAMILIES

Gaining feedback from the patient and family about their experience of the family–nurse relationship is important for professional development. These questions can assist in getting started:

- Of all the issues that we have talked about today, which of these ideas, if any, seemed most useful to you? In what way is it useful?
- What else could we have talked about that would be more helpful?
- Which family member do you think has benefited most from our conversation? How?
- If I were to encounter another family in a similar situation tomorrow, what do you think I should be sure to talk with them about?
- What advice would you give to me about working with other families who might run into this situation?
- Is there anything in our work together that supported your confidence in dealing with this difficulty?

Case Study 12

At the morning change of shift report on the medical unit of a large city hospital where you work, you are warned about John's "demanding family." The family has recently immigrated to Canada looking for a safer country to call home. They speak English as a second language. The father, although a teacher in his home country, has been working as a dishwasher or cleaner on nightshift when he can find a job. John, his Canadian name, is a 1-year-old boy who has been hospitalized for the past week for diagnostic tests that have attempted to locate the cause for his progressive neurological deficits. Test results have been inconclusive. The mother has not left John's side since his admission. Each morning, when the father arrives, with limited English, he interrogates the nurse about John's progress overnight and the plan of action for the day. The nurses are concerned by what they describe as "overly strict" parenting practices with John, and the wife's subservient attitude toward her husband. The father approaches you as you begin your shift.

Critical Thinking Questions

1. How might the family's cultural background be affecting their response to this health situation?
2. How would you engage this family to foster a more productive and collaborative relationship?
3. How would you attempt to address their concerns?
4. What is the relationship between the health problem and the family members?
5. How might the family's cultural background be affecting the parenting practices? How would you engage the family in a discussion about this matter?

After working through these questions, go to the MyNursingLab at **http://www.mynursinglab.com** to check your answers.

KEY TERMS

family
family nursing
person in the context of the family
family unit as the client of care
genogram
ecomap
relational stance
collaborative relational stance
reflective questions
difference questions
behavioural effect questions
hypothetical or future-oriented questions
triadic questions
medical narratives
illness narratives
commendations
family support
reciprocity
respite care

CHAPTER HIGHLIGHTS

- Definitions of *family* should include shifting social norms in family structure and each family's mode of describing themselves.
- Nursing care of families is based on relational practices that involve family members in care, respond to their concerns, provide them with information, and/or offer emotional support.
- Family expectations of health-care providers can include a desire for access to information about diagnosis and treatment, a trust that their ill family member will receive good care and be treated compassionately, the recognition of their own involvement in care, and preparation for their roles at home.
- The genogram inquiry helps the nurse demonstrate a concern for all family members, to document relevant information about those involved in the health situation, to appreciate developmental transitions in the family, and to begin to understand family relationships.
- The ecomap inquiry helps the nurse understand sources of family support or stress by tracing external connections to employment, health-care services, and recreational and religious communities.
- Reflective questions invite family members to think differently about themselves, health and illness concerns, and options for addressing concerns.
- Illness narratives help nurses more fully understand the reciprocal influences between health and the family and can assist families to make sense of the illness experience.
- Commendations acknowledge and convey respect for family capability and strengths.
- Families vary in their desire to be directly involved in caregiving activities, and some may need encouragement to take a respite from prolonged caregiving.
- Nurses can evaluate nursing care of families by reflecting on their efforts to invite family questions and concerns, by involving family members in decision making, and by asking the family directly about their experience of the family–nurse relationship.

ASSESS YOUR LEARNING

1. Chris is a 42-year-old father who is terminally ill. He continues to want to drive his children to school but his wife, Sula, fears that his illness makes him unsafe. Sula asks the nurse to reinforce her view. Which of the following responses by the nurse best reflects a family nursing approach?
   a. "You have raised an important issue. However, this is a private family matter and if nursing became involved it would be interfering."
   b. "You both have very legitimate concerns. Can we talk about some ways for you, Chris, to maintain independence despite your illness and for you, Sula, to ensure that everyone is safe?"
   c. "Chris, your wife is only looking out for your best interests. I know it is a painful reality, but you are too ill to be driving."
   d. "Sula, I think driving is only one of many issues that you and Chris are going to have to address around your husband's illness. I'd like to refer you for counselling."

2. Skyla is a 35-year-old Aboriginal woman with rapidly advancing cancer. She has the choice of following the usual course of treatment, known to have mixed outcomes, or trying an experimental treatment with little or no clear outcome data. The patient asks the nurse to help her plan for a discussion of the dilemma with her family. Which of the following responses by the nurse best indicates the use of a difference question?
   a. "Who do you think will be most affected by these treatment choices?"
   b. "Are you nervous about your family's reaction?"
   c. "Your decision is very personal—no one but you can decide."
   d. "What effect do you think your cultural beliefs will have on your decision?"

3. Eight-year-old Darren was diagnosed with kidney disease 2 years ago. He lives with his parents and 5-year-old sister in a small rural community 4 hours away from the closest tertiary health centre. Since his diagnosis, Darren has been seen at the health centre eight times—three times for admission. At first, the entire family came to the hospital but now Darren and his mother travel to the city, while Dad and sister stay home for work and school. Darren has been hospitalized this admission for 3 weeks. The nurse notices that Darren's mother is becoming exhausted; however, when invited to take breaks, she politely, but firmly, refuses. Which of the following statements best explains the mother's reaction as a family caregiver?
   - **a.** The mother fears that Darren will not receive good care or be treated compassionately.
   - **b.** The mother has become overly possessive of Darren since his hospitalization.
   - **c.** The mother would actually be relieved if the nurse ordered her to take a break.
   - **d.** The mother wants to ensure that hospital staff regard her as a good mother.

4. Tracy, an 8-year-old girl with chronic lower respiratory tract disease, is hospitalized with a respiratory infection. Even though she is very ill, the nurse notices that Tracy tries to help her mother, who has been at her bedside night and day, by doing simple tasks. Which of the following statements best explains Tracy's demonstration of social support?
   - **a.** The nurse knows that Tracy's psychological development will be compromised if she continues to take on caregiving responsibilities at such a young age.
   - **b.** The nurse knows that she will have to explain to Tracy that, while her gestures are very thoughtful, when she thinks her mother needs help she should call the nurse as Tracy is too ill.
   - **c.** The nurse appreciates that relationships are reciprocal and even though Tracy is young and ill, both she and her mother gain strength when they each give and receive support.
   - **d.** The nurse knows that Tracy is a born helper and she should be encouraged to help out on the unit whenever possible.

5. During rounds, the nurse discusses her concerns about a patient's wife, who has been at her husband's bedside round the clock over the past 2 months. Misha has a terminal illness and is not expected to live more than a few weeks. He is a 36-year-old father of three young children, and he immigrated to Canada 4 years ago with his family and parents. He had high hopes of setting up his own engineering business but found himself driving a taxi. Misha has been the sole breadwinner for the family. The nurse notes that the family is in need of additional supports. Which of the following approaches best reflects family-centred nursing?
   - **a.** The nurse is sympathetic to Misha's situation and makes the hospital environment as comfortable as possible for his wife.
   - **b.** The nurse works with Misha's wife to connect her with support services for the family situation.
   - **c.** The nurse calls regular family meetings and together they plan and carry out a family plan of care.
   - **d.** The nurse introduces Misha's wife to another wife on the unit whose husband has a similar terminal illness.

6. Ashley Jackson recently lost her job as a line worker when the candy factory where she had worked for the past 6 years closed. Her oldest son, Tremaine, aged 4 years, has asthma and needs weekly visits to the community health clinic to get established on a new treatment regime. The family has missed the last three appointments, due to the cost of transportation, but Ashley denies any financial difficulty when asked directly. Which of the following statements best explains the nurse's decision to conduct an ecomap inquiry with the mother rather than pointing out to Ashley the cost to the health system of missed appointments?
   - **a.** It assists the nurse to understand sources of family stress and supports by tracing external connections in the community.
   - **b.** It assists the nurse to understand developmental transitions in the family.
   - **c.** It assists the nurse to understand family relationships.
   - **d.** It assists the nurse to gather a family health history.

7. Grandparents Hester and Randy Bishop have had custody of their grandchildren (ages 10, 12, and 14 years) for 13 months. The mother, who has been receiving treatment for a drug addiction, comes to visit her 12-year-old daughter, Sarah, who has been hospitalized for minor surgery. Which of the following initial actions best reflects a family nursing response to the mother?
   - **a.** "I can see that you care about your daughter but as you do not have custody, I'll have to ask you to leave."
   - **b.** "I can see that you have made good progress with your addiction and so I think it is important that you visit your daughter. If your parents do not want to meet with you, then I will stay with you and your daughter during the visit."
   - **c.** "I can see that it is very important to you that your daughter and family see that you care about Sarah and are making a real effort to address your addiction. However, this may not be an easy visit for your family. What challenges do you think your daughter and parents might have around accepting your visit?"
   - **d.** "I'll have to ask your daughter and, if she agrees to see you, then you are welcome to visit."

8. The community health nurse is doing a hospital discharge follow-up visit with 74-year-old Mrs. Pineau. She recently suffered a stroke that has left her with some cognitive impairment and short-term memory loss. She can still carry out many activities of daily living (e.g., shopping, cooking, and going to the bank) with minimal assistance. In discussion with Mrs. Pineau, the nurse learns that she has one son, who rarely visits and does not appear to be very supportive. Mrs. Pineau mentions that she is going to give her life savings to her son so he can buy the house that he has been talking about. Which of the following immediate actions best reflects a family nursing approach?
   - **a.** The nurse calls for a thorough assessment of Mrs. Pineau's mental competence.
   - **b.** The nurse tells Mrs. Pineau that her intentions may not be a good idea and that she should call her lawyer to discuss the matter.
   - **c.** The nurse invites Mrs. Pineau to discuss her intentions more fully and how she thinks all family members, including her son, might view the decision.
   - **d.** The nurse calls individual family members to tell them of Mrs. Pineau's intentions.

9. Mabel, 70 years old, was diagnosed with Alzheimer dementia 2 years ago. She and her husband, Harold, were adamant that they would stay in their home despite the fact that their two children lived a 5-hour drive away and could only visit once per month. Mabel has been cared for by her husband with the help of home care services (personal care workers under the direction of community health nurses). Mabel's memory loss has now progressed to the point that her husband is exhausted with the caregiving responsibilities. Yet, he fiercely denies that the care is a burden. Which of the following statements by the community health nurse best demonstrates a reflective response?
   - **a.** "I know that you love your wife very much but her care is wearing you out."
   - **b.** "I can see by the loving care you give to your wife that she means the world to you. If she could talk, what do you think she would be telling your children?"
   - **c.** "I think your wife would be best cared for in a nursing home."
   - **d.** "Maybe it is time for your children to move closer so that they can help you care for your wife."

10. Eric is a 14-year-old boy who was diagnosed with cystic fibrosis during infancy. His parents appear to be coping well, but they state that there are times when they feel very alone when dealing with the chronic aspects of Eric's condition. Which of the following responses by the nurse best reflects a family nursing approach?
   - **a.** "You seem lonely and depressed; talking to a counsellor may relieve some of your concerns."
   - **b.** "You appear to be coping well. Although things may seem difficult now, they will improve."
   - **c.** "Many families who have children with cystic fibrosis experience similar feelings of loneliness. Would you like me to arrange for you to talk with one of those families?"
   - **d.** "You should join the Cystic Fibrosis Association. It always needs volunteers and it can help you meet people."

After working through these questions, go to the MyNursingLab at ***http://www.mynursinglab.com*** *to check your answers and see explanations.*

SUGGESTED READINGS

Shields, L., Pratt, J., & Hunter, J. (2006). Family centred care: a review of qualitative studies. *Journal of Clinical Nursing, 15*(10), 1317–1323.

This article systematically reviewed qualitative studies involving the use of family-centred care in children's hospitals. Although family-centred care has become a cornerstone of pediatric practice, its effectiveness is not known. Findings revealed a common thread of negotiation between staff and families and that the perceptions held by both parents and staff influenced the delivery of family-centred care. A subtheme was discovered regarding the cost of family-centred care: the cost affected both families and staff and it included both financial and emotional factors.

Willis, L., Demiris, G., & Oliver, D. P. (2007). Internet use by hospice families and providers: A review. *Journal of Medical Systems, 31*(2), 97–101.

This literature review explores the current evidence related to use of the internet by hospice patients or families and palliative care or hospice professionals. Participants in the studies included patients, caregivers and family members, and health-care professionals. Findings overall indicate that internet-based interventions are effective.

WEBLINKS

The Vanier Institute of the Family

http://www.vifamily.ca

The Vanier Institute is a national charitable organization dedicated to promoting the well-being of Canadian families through research, consultation, and policy development. The website links to online publications related to contemporary family trends and such issues as aging, divorce, employment, and family income.

Department of Justice Canada

http://www.canada.justice.gc.ca/en/ps/sup/stat.htm

This Government of Canada website provides information about legal issues, programs and services of interest to families (such as child custody, access, and support), fact sheets on family violence and child abuse, and links to research publications on these topics.

Canadian Council on Social Development

http://www.ccsd.ca

The website of this national nonprofit organization provides information and publications relevant to the social and economic security of Canadian families.

Family Nursing Resources

http://www.eFamilyNursing.com

This website markets educational products (books and videotapes) to family nursing educators and students.

REFERENCES

Bell, J. M. (1996). Signal events in family nursing. *Journal of Family Nursing, 2*(4), 347–349.

Benner, P., Hooper-Kyriakidis, P., & Stannard, D. (1999). *Clinical wisdom and interventions in critical care: A thinking-in-action approach.* Philadelphia, PA: W.B. Saunders.

Berg, S. (2006). In their own voices: families discuss end-of-life decision making—part 2. *Pediatric Nursing, 32*(3), 237, 238–242.

Board, R., & Ryan-Wenger, N. (2003). Stressors and stress symptoms of mothers with children in the PICU. *Journal of Pediatric Nursing, 18*(3), 195–202.

Bomar, P. J. (Ed.). (1996). *Nurses and family health promotion.* Philadelphia, PA: Saunders.

Browning, G., & Warren, N. A. (2006). Unmet needs of family members in the medical intensive care waiting room. *Critical Care Nursing Quarterly, 29*(1), 86–95.

Byrd, M. E. (2006). Social exchange as a framework for client-nurse interaction during public health nursing maternal-child home visits. *Public Health Nursing, 23*(3), 271–276.

Campaign 2000. (2008). Work isn't working for Ontario families: New report. Retrieved May 16, 2008, from http://action.web.ca/home/c2000/alerts.shtml?preview=1&sh_itm=1edb14b8d114c92ddf2f8bc3092b0de5&AA_EX_Session=47c840b7eedfcc97eec7a30d8586a8c9

Canadian Association for Community Care. (2001). *Give me a break! Helping family caregivers of seniors overcome barriers to respite.* Ottawa: Author.

Canadian Caregiver Coalition. (2003). *Caring together: Caregiver recognition is sound social policy.* Policy Paper Series Number 2. Ottawa: Author.

Canadian Council on Social Development. (2005). *Poverty lines 2004.* Retrieved May 2, 2008, from http://www.ccsd.ca/factsheets/fs_lico04_bt.htm

Chui, T., Tran, K., & Maheux, H. (2007). *Immigration in Canada: A portrait of the foreign-born population, 2006 census: Findings.* Retrieved May 18, 2008, from http://www12.statcan.ca/english/census06/analysis/immcit/index.cfm

Clarke, C. (2006). Relating with professionals. *Journal of Psychiatric Mental Health Nursing, 13*(5), 522–526.

Cole, I., & Chesla, C. A. (2006). Interventions for the family with diabetes. *Nursing Clinics of North America, 41*(4), 625–639, vii.

Corlett, J., & Twycross, A. (2006). Negotiation of care by children's nurses: lessons from research. *Paediatric Nursing, 18*(8), 34–37.

Davidson, J. E., Powers, K., Hedayat, K. M., Tieszenm M., Kon, A. A., Shepard, E., et al. (2007). Clinical practice guidelines for support of the family in the patient-centered intensive care unit: American College of Critical Care Medicine Task Force 2004–2005. *Critical Care Medicine, 35*(2), 605–622.

Deci, E. L., La Guardia, J. G., Moller, A. C., Scheiner, M. J., & Ryan, R. M. (2006). On the benefits of giving as well as receiving autonomy support: Mutuality in close friendships. *Personality and Social Psychology Bulletin, 32*(3), 313–327.

Doornbos, M. M. (2001). Professional support for family caregivers of people with serious and persistent mental illnesses. *Journal of Psychosocial Nursing and Mental Health Services, 39*(12), 38–45.

Doornbos, M. M. (2002). Family caregivers and the mental health care system: Reality and dreams. *Archives of Psychiatric Nursing, 16*(1), 39–46.

Dowd, M. D., Kennedy, C., Knapp, J. F., & Stallbaumer-Rouyer, J. (2002). Mothers' and health care providers' perspectives on screening for intimate partner violence in a pediatric emergency department. *Archives of Pediatric Adolescent Medicine, 156*(8), 794–799.

Dwairy, M. (2002). Foundations of psychosocial dynamic personality theory of collective people. *Clinical Psychology Review, 22*(3), 345–362.

Family facts. (n.d.). Vanier Institute of the Family. Retrieved May 20, 2007, from http://www.vifamily.ca/library/facts/facts.html

Farrell, M. E., Joseph, D. H., & Schwartz-Barcott, D. (2005). Visiting hours in the ICU: Finding the balance among patient, visitor and staff needs. *Nursing Forum, 40*(1), 18–28.

Fast, J., Eales, J. & Keating, N. (2001). *Economic impact of health, income security, and labour policies on informal caregivers of frail seniors.* Ottawa: Status of Women. Retrieved April 4, 2008, from http://www.swccfc.gc.ca/pubs/pubspr/0662654765/200103_0662654765_e.pdf

Federation of Canadian Municipalities. (2004). *Quality of life in Canadian communities: theme report 1: Incomes, shelter and necessities.* Retrieved April 6, 2006, from http://www.fcm.ca/english/qol/nov172004.pdf

Firth, P. (2006). Patients and their families. *Recent Results Cancer Research,* 168, 61–71.

Forchuk, C., & Dorsay, J. P. (1995). Hildegard Peplau meets family systems nursing: Innovation in theory-based practice. *Journal of Advanced Nursing, 21*(1), 110–115.

Friedemann, M. (1995). *The framework of systemic organization: A conceptual approach to families and nursing.* Thousand Oaks, CA: Sage.

Gage, J. D., Everett, K. D., & Bullock, L. (2006). Integrative review of parenting in nursing research. *Journal of Nursing Scholarship, 38*(1), 56–62.

Gibson, M. J., & Houser, A. (2007). *Valuing the invaluable: A new look at the economic value of family caregiving.* Washington, DC: AARP Public Policy Institute. Retrieved June 14, 2006, from http://www.aarp.org/research/housing-mobility/caregiving/ib82_caregiving.html

Given, B., & Sherwood, P. R. (2006). Family care for the older person with cancer. *Seminars in Oncology Nursing, 22*(1), 43–50.

Goodwin, R. D., Wickramaratne, P., Nomura, Y., & Weissman, M. M. (2007). Familial depression and respiratory illness in children. *Archives of Pediatric Adolescent Medicine, 161*(5), 487–494.

Goudreau, J., Duhamel, F., & Ricard, N. (2006). The impact of a family systems nursing educational program on the practice of psychiatric nurses: A pilot study. *Journal of Family Nursing, 12*(3), 292–306.

Griffin, T. (2003). Facing challenges to family-centered care. I: Conflicts over visitation. *Pediatric Nursing, 29*(2), 135–137.

Hanson, S. M. H., & Boyd, S. T. (1996). *Family health care nursing: Theory, practice, research.* Philadelphia, PA: Davis.

Hart, S. N. (1991). From property to person status. *American Psychologist, 46,* 53–59.

Heyland, D. K., Tranmer, J., O'Callaghan, C. J., & Gafni, A. (2003). The seriously ill hospitalized patient: Preferred role in end-of-life decision making? *Journal of Critical Care, 18*(1), 3–10.

Holtslander, L. (2005). Clinical application of the 15-minute family interview: Addressing the needs of postpartum families. *Journal of Family Nursing, 11*(1), 5–18.

Hopkins, R. O., & Brett, S. (2005). Chronic neurocognitive effects of critical illness. *Current Opinion in Critical Care, 11*(4), 369–375.

Housing & Homelessness Branch, Human Resources & Social Development Canada. (2006). *Homelessness by cities.* Retrieved May 20, 2007, from http://intraspec.ca/homelessCanada_news-and-reports.php#homeless-counts

Jeon, Y. H. (2004). Shaping mutuality: Nurse-family caregiver interactions in caring for older people with depression. *International Journal of Mental Health Nursing, 13*(2), 126–134.

Korner, H. (2007). Negotiating cultures: disclosure of HIV-positive status among people from minority ethnic communities in Sydney. *Culture, Health and Sexuality, 9*(2), 137–152.

Leahey, M., & Harper-Jaques, S. (1996). Family-nurse relationships: Core assumptions and clinical implications. *Journal of Family Nursing, 2*(2), 133–151.

Lee, M. D., Friedenberg, A. S., Mukpo, D. H., Conray, K., Palmisciano, A., & Levy, M. M. (2007). Visiting hours policies in New England intensive care units: Strategies for improvement. *Critical Care Medicine, 35*(2), 497–501.

Leenerts, M. H., & Teel, C. S. (2006). Relational conversation as method for creating partnerships: Pilot study. *Journal of Advanced Nursing, 54*(4), 467–476.

Levine, C. (1998). *Rough crossings: Family caregivers' odysseys through the health care system.* New York: United Hospital Fund of New York.

Limacher, L. H., & Wright, L. M. (2006). Exploring the therapeutic family intervention of commendations: Insights from research. *Journal of Family Nursing, 12*(3), 307–331.

Macduff, C. (2006). An analysis of a typology of family health nursing practice. *Nurse Research, 14*(1), 34–47.

Martel, L., & Caron-Malenfant. (2007). *Portrait of the Canadian population in 2006, Findings.* Retrieved May 18, 2008 from http://www12.statcan.ca/english/census06/analysis/popdwell/index.cfm

Martinez, A. M, D'Artois, D., & Rennick, J. E. (2007). Does the 15-minute (or less) family interview influence family nursing practice? *Journal of Family Nursing, 13*(2), 157–178.

Mayer, G. G. (2001). Families as hospital care givers: A self-service approach to the nursing shortage. *Journal of Nursing Administration, 31*(10), 457–458.

McCloskey, D. (2005). Caregiving and Canadian families. *Transition, 35*(2). Retrieved May 20, 2007, from http://www.vifamily.ca/library/transition/352/352.html

McElheran, N., & Harper-Jaques, S. (1994). Commendations: A resource intervention for clinical practice. *Clinical Nurse Specialist, 8*(1), 7–10.

McPherson, K. (1996). *Bedside matters: The transformation of Canadian nursing, 1900–1990.* Toronto: Oxford University Press.

Mitchell, M. L, Courtney, M., & Coyer, F. (2003). Understanding uncertainty and minimizing families' anxiety at the time of transfer from intensive care. *Nursing Health Sciences, 5*(3), 207–217.

Morisette, R., & Ostrovsky, Y. (2007). *Income instability of lone parents, singles and two-parent families in Canada, 1984 to 2004.* Statistics Canada Analytical Studies Branch Research Paper Series No. 297. Retrieved April 4, 2008, from http://www.statcan.ca/english/research/11F0019MIE/11F0019MIE2007297.pdf

Morris, D. B. (1998). *Illness and culture in the postmodern age.* Berkeley, CA: University of California Press.

Myers, T. A., Eichhorn, D. J., & Guzzetta, C. E. (2000). Family presence during invasive procedures and resuscitation. *American Journal of Nursing, 100,* 32–43.

Navaie-Waliser, M., Feldman, P. H., Gould, D. A., Levine, C., Kuerbis, A. N., & Donelan, K. (2001). The experiences and challenges of informal caregivers: Common themes and differences among whites, Blacks, and Hispanics. *Gerontologist, 41*(6), 733–741.

Navaie-Waliser, M., Feldman, P. H., Gould, D. A., Levine, C., Kuerbis, A. N., & Donelan, K. (2002). When the caregiver needs care: The plight of vulnerable caregivers. *American Journal of Public Health, 92*(3), 409–413.

Neufeld, N., & Harrison, J. (2000). Family caregiving: Issues in gaining access to support. In M. J. Stewart (Ed.), *Chronic conditions and caregiving in Canada: Social support strategies* (pp. 249–273). Toronto: University of Toronto Press.

Phelan J. C., Bromet, E. J., & Link, B. G. (1998). Psychiatric illness and family stigma. *Schizophrenia Bulletin, 24*(1), 115–126.

Ray, R. A., & Street, A. F. (2005). Ecomapping: An innovative research tool for nurses. *Journal of Advanced Nursing, 50*(5), 545–552.

Robinson, C. A. (1996). Health care relationships revisited. *Journal of Family Nursing, 2*(2), 152–173.

Roden, J. (2005). The involvement of parents and nurses in the care of acutely-ill children in a non-specialist paediatric setting. *Journal of Child Health Care, 9*(3), 222–240.

Sauvé, R. (2004). *Profiling Canada's families III.* Ottawa: Vanier Institute of the Family.

Sauvé, R. (2006). *Contemporary family trends: The effects of the changing age structure on households and families to 2026.* Ottawa: Vanier Institute of the Family.

Segaric, C. A., & Hall, W. A. (2005). The family theory-practice gap: A matter of clarity? *Nursing Inquiry, 12*(3), 210–218.

Selwood, A., Johnston, K., Katona, C., Lyketsos, C., & Livingston, G. (2007). Systematic review of the effect of psychological interventions on family caregivers of people with dementia. *Journal of Affective Disorders, 101*(1–3), 75–89.

Sexton, E., Coad, J., & Holden, C. (2005). Review of homecare packages for paediatric HPN patients. *British Journal of Nursing, 14*(20), 1080–1085.

Shields, L., Pratt, J., & Hunter, J. (2006). Family centred care: a review of qualitative studies. *Journal of Clinical Nursing, 15*(10), 1317–1323.

Sjöblom, L. M., Pejlert, A., & Asplund, K. (2005). Nurses' view of the family in psychiatric care. *Journal of Clinical Nursing, 14*(5), 562–569.

Stapleton, R. D., Engelberg, R.A., Wenrich, M. D., Goss, C. H., & Curtis, J. R. (2006). Clinician statements and family satisfaction with family conferences in the intensive care unit. *Critical Care Medicine, 34*(6), 1679–1685.

Statistics Canada. (2006). *Report on the demographic situation in Canada 2003 and 2004.* Retrieved September 13, 2007, from http://www.statcan.ca/english/freepub/91-209-XIE/91-209-XIE2003000.pdf

Statistics Canada. (2007a). *Family portrait: Continuity and change in Canadian families and households in 2006, 2006 census.* Catalogue no. 97-553-XIE. Ottawa: Ministry of Industry. Retrieved September 13, 2007, from http://www12.statcan.ca/english/census06/analysis/famhouse/index.cfm

Statistics Canada. (2007b). *Canada* (table). *2006 community profiles.* 2006 Census. Catalogue no. 92-591-XWE. Retrieved May 14, 2008, from http://www12.statcan.ca/english/census06/data/profiles/community/Index.cfm?Lang=E

Statistics Canada. (2008a). Canada's population estimates. *The Daily,* June 25, 2008. Retrieved September 17, 2008, from http://www.statcan.ca/Daily/English/080625/d080625b.htm

Statistics Canada. (2008b). Aboriginal peoples in Canada in 2006: Inuit, Métis and First Nations, 2006 census. *The Daily,* January 15. Retrieved May 18, 2008, from http://www.statcan.ca/Daily/English/080115/d080115a.htm

Statistics Canada. (2008c). *Report on the demographic situation in Canada, 2005 and 2006.* Retrieved September 17, 2008 from http://www.statcan.ca/english/freepub/91-209-XIE/91-209-XIE2004000.pdf

Tanner, J. (2005). Visiting time preferences of patients, visitors and staff. *Nursing Times, 101*(27), 38–42.

Tapp, D. M. (1997). *Exploring therapeutic conversations between nurses and families experiencing ischemic heart disease.* Unpublished doctoral dissertation, University of Calgary, Alberta.

Tapp, D. M. (2000). The ethics of relational stance in family nursing: Resisting the view of "nurse as expert." *Journal of Family Nursing, 6*(1), 69–91.

Vanier Institute of the Family. (n.d.). *Definition of family.* Retrieved June 20, 2007, from http://www.vifamily.ca/about/definition.html

Ting, J. (2007). Family orientated delivery of routine nursing care in hospital. *Australia Nursing Journal, 14*(10), 27.

Wade, J. (2006). "Crying alone with my child": Parenting a school age child diagnosed with bipolar disorder. *Issues in Mental Health Nursing, 27*(8), 885–903.

Walker, E., & Dewar, B. J. (2001). How do we facilitate carers' involvement in decision making? *Journal of Advanced Nursing, 34*(3), 329–337.

Ward-Griffin, C. (1999). Nurse-family caregiver relationships: Moving beyond the rhetoric of shared care. *Registered Nurse,* November/December, 8–10.

Whall, A. L., & Fawcett, J. (1991). The family as a focal phenomenon in nursing. In A. L. Whall & J. Fawcett (Eds.), *Family theory development in nursing: State of the science and art* (pp. 7–29). Philadelphia, PA: Davis.

Wright, L. M., & Leahey, M. (1990). Trends in nursing of families. *Journal of Advanced Nursing, 15,* 148–154.

Wright, L. M., & Leahey, M. (2005a) *Nurses and families: A guide to family assessment and intervention.* Philadelphia, PA: Davis.

Wright, L. M, & Leahey, M. (2005b). The three most common errors in family nursing: How to avoid or sidestep. *Journal of Family Nursing, 11*(2), 90–101.

Wright, L. M., Watson, W. L., & Bell, J. M. (1996). *Beliefs: The heart of healing in families and illness.* New York: Basic Books.

Yun, Y. H., Rhee, Y. S., Kang, I. O., Lee, J. S., Bang, S. M., Lee, W. S., et al. (2005). Economic burdens and quality of life of family caregivers of cancer patients. *Oncology, 68*(2–3), 107–114.

Chapter 13

Community-Based Nursing

The Canadian health-care system is changing. Escalating health-care costs, expanding technology, changing demographics, shorter hospital stays, and diminishing access to health care are some of the factors motivating this change. One of the greatest changes has been the shift of health-care delivery from institutions to the community and home environments (Coyte & McKeever, 2001). Health care, once delivered predominantly in hospital settings, is now routinely provided in the home and other community-based environments. Though acute-care institutions will undoubtedly remain a vital component of the health-care system, their prominence may be lessened in the future. The trend toward community-based care will play a significant role in the future of Canada's health-care system.

Hunt (2005) suggested that over the past decade, every employment setting has seen an increase in the number of registered nurses; however, the greatest increase has occurred in community-based settings. Despite this significant shift in care delivery, governments still struggle to provide comprehensive, cost-effective health services to Canadians.

The trend continues toward an integrated health-care system, one that is community-based, multidisciplinary, and collaborative. With the shift from institutional to community-based care come changes in the roles and responsibilities of health-care professionals.

OBJECTIVES

After studying this chapter, you should be able to

1. Discuss factors influencing health-care reform
2. Identify the five essential aspects of the Alma-Ata Declaration, particularly primary health care and its impact on community health nursing
3. Describe community-based health care
4. List and describe the Community Health Nurses Association of Canada's community health nursing standards of practice
5. Describe the role of a community health nurse, a home health nurse, and a public health nurse, and describe the environments in which they practise
6. Explain essential aspects of cooperative partnerships in health care: definitions, objectives, benefits, and the nurse's role
7. Delineate the role of the nurse in providing continuity of care
8. Compare and contrast community-based nursing and traditional institutional-based nursing

Health-Care Reform

Health-care consumers are playing a more prominent role than ever in health-care delivery. In the report *An Ounce of Prevention: Strengthening the Balance in Health Care Reform,* the Canadian Public Health Association (CPHA) suggested that though developments in health over the past century have been remarkable, if medicare is to remain sustainable, we must "build on the opportunities afforded by past successes, improved information, knowledge and research capacities, and technological advances" (Canadian Public Health Association Board of Directors, 2000, p. vii). This reform of the health-care system could be addressed through legislative initiatives and restructuring responses suited to provincial and territorial systems. Whatever the approach, agreement exists that care must shift from a strict illness focus to one that includes determinants of health (see Chapter 7) and features service in a community-based environment. The CPHA also asserted that the creation of sustainable health care that provides the Canadian population with lasting health gains can be achieved only through a system that concentrates on doing the following:

- Focusing on the broader determinants of health (such as socioeconomic status and education)
- Maintaining the vision and values that form the basis of our current medicare system
- Recognizing that increased privatization will only shift rather than contain future health-care costs
- Investing in and developing a range of health-care services, from public health and community care to hospitals and long-term-care facilities

The Canadian Nurses Association (CNA) (2003) endorsed a restructured health-care system based on the principles of primary health care as the most effective way to achieve optimal health care for the population. Specifically, the CNA recommended that governments commit to a strong publicly funded health-care system that permits accessibility to essential health services, allows for public participation in health decisions, and emphasizes health promotion and the adoption of a community health approach.

Storch (2006) stressed the importance of "thinking outside the box" when it comes to health-care reform. She asserted that nurses are, and should be, at the forefront of health-care change. As highly educated, caring professionals, nurses have a responsibility to influence change by attending to the history, current status, and future projections of health care. By taking action individually and collectively, the nursing profession has the power to bring greater attention to the social determinants of health and to ensure more effective delivery of care under the primary health-care philosophy.

The precursor to much of Canada's health-care reform was the 1978 International Conference on Primary Health Care. This meeting in the World Health Assembly resulted in a report known as the Declaration of Alma-Ata (so named for the geographic location in which the conference was held). In this report, the term *primary heath care* was coined by the World Health Organization (WHO) and the United Nations International Children's Emergency Fund (UNICEF). Subsequently, five principles central to the care delivery philosophy were outlined (see Box 13.1). These principles are still commonly referred to today.

Primary health care is defined as

> *essential health care based on practical, scientifically sound, and socially acceptable methods and technology made universally accessible to individuals and families in the community through their full participation and at a cost that the community and country can afford to maintain at every stage of their development in the spirit of self-reliance and self-determinations. (World Health Organization [WHO] & United Nations International Children's Emergency Fund [UNICEF], 1978, ¶ 7)*

Deep concern for the health of the world's population, specifically short life expectancies and high mortality rates among children, led to the formation of the global health strategy of *primary health care* (PHC). All members of the WHO were encouraged to take actions toward the attainment of "health for all by the year 2000" through an adequate food supply, safe water, adequate sanitation, maternal and child health care, immunization, the prevention and control of endemic diseases, the provision of essential drugs, health education, and the treatment of common diseases and injuries.

BOX 13.1 FIVE PRINCIPLES OF PRIMARY HEALTH CARE

The following five principles of primary health care are used by the Canadian Nurses Association:

1. *Accessibility:* A continuing and organized supply of essential health services is available to all people with no unreasonable geographic or financial barriers.
2. *Public participation:* Individuals and communities have the right and responsibility to be active partners in making decisions about their health care and the health of their communities.
3. *Health promotion:* The process of enabling people to increase control over and to improve their health.
4. *Appropriate technology:* This includes methods of care, service delivery, procedures and equipment that are socially acceptable and affordable.
5. *Intersectoral cooperation:* Commitment from all sectors (government, community and health) is essential for meaningful action on health determinants.

Source: From *Primary Health Care: A Summary of the Issues,* by the Canadian Nurses Association, 2005, Ottawa: Author.

The Declaration of Alma-Ata (WHO & UNICEF, 1978) emphasized health or well-being as a fundamental right and a worldwide social goal. It was an attempt to address inequality in the health status of persons in all countries and to target governments that needed to be responsible for policies that would promote economic, social, and health development, which were considered basic to the achievement of "health for all." PHC extends beyond traditional health-care services. It involves issues of the environment, agriculture, housing, and other social, economic, and political issues, such as poverty, transportation, unemployment, and economic development. A major feature of PHC is that consumers, governments at all levels, and public institutions are involved in the planning and delivery of health care. Similarly, the roles of physicians and nurses change. For PHC to be realized, and health-care reform to be successful, health care needs to be organized in such a way that it spans geographical boundaries, bridges service sectors, and creates seamless linkages within and across disciplines serving the public. Additionally, it requires health-care providers, nurses included, to develop specialized skills in working with individuals, families, and communities that enable them to collaborate with, rather than merely provide care to, clients.

In *Building on Values: The Future of Health Care in Canada*, Roy Romanow stressed "the need to change the scopes and patterns of practice of health care providers to reflect changes in how health care services are delivered, particularly through new approaches to primary health care" (2002, p. xxvii). This notion was echoed by Storch (2006), who suggested that nurses are natural leaders in the move to what was expected to be less costly, community-based, and client-driven care. Box 13.2 outlines three strategic areas for health reform.

The distinction between primary health care (PHC) and primary care (PC) is an important one. PHC differs from PC in that although PC includes the need to practise in the context of family and community, the emphasis is on the delivery of personal health services by clinicians. PC addresses personal health services and not population-focused public health services.

BOX 13.2 THREE STRATEGIC AREAS FOR HEALTH-CARE REFORM

The Canadian Nurses Association views the following three strategic areas as required for health-care reform:

1. A publicly funded system best serves the health of Canadians. It offers clear advantages in terms of access to health services and cost containment for the system as a whole.
2. The success of the health-care system is critically dependent on a vibrant nursing workforce. Targeted investments for recruitment and retention are useful for achieving this.
3. A primary health-care approach provides an excellent framework for health-care reform in Canada. The five principles of primary health care, accessibility, public participation, prevention and health promotion, appropriate technology, and intersectoral cooperation, offer a framework for rebuilding the health-care system in Canada.

Barnes et al. (1995) stated that PHC is community driven and involves a "bottom-up" approach that requires active community involvement in decision making to improve health. PC, conversely, is expert driven and involves a "top-down" approach by health professionals who advise individuals and communities about what is best for their health. Other differences are shown in Table 13.1.

PHC and PC also have similarities. Both systems acknowledge the prevention and promotion components of health and well-being. Both systems strive for universal access to and affordability of health care, support empowerment of the client, and target those at risk for preventable health problems.

TABLE 13.1 Differences between Primary Care and Primary Health Care

Primary Care	Primary Health Care
• Community participation is provider directed.	• Community participation is client directed.
• The professional's role is as expert, provider, authority, team leader.	• The professional's role is as facilitator, consultant, resource.
• Collaboration occurs among members of the health-care team.	• Collaboration goes beyond the health-care sector.
• The individual or family is the focus.	• The community or some aggregate is the focus.
• Access is limited.	• Access is universal.
• Health care is available within given health-care institutions.	• Health care is available where people live and work.
• Empowerment is a provider-assisted process.	• Empowerment is a collaborative, enabling process.

Source: Adapted from "Primary Health Care and Primary Care: A Confusion of Philosophies," by Barnes et al., 1995, *Nursing Outlook, 43*(1), pp. 7–16.

Over the past 30 years, Canadians have embraced the notions of PHC and the resulting strategies for health promotion that have arisen from them (Epp, 1986). See Chapter 8 for more details. Canadian consumers also effect major changes in the delivery of health care as they increase their knowledge of health promotion, illness prevention, and treatment options. The resulting expectation of collaboration in decision making about their own, their families, and, to some extent, their communities' health has changed the role of the health-care consumer and, as a result, that of the health-care professional.

Community-Based Health Care

Community-based health care (CBHC) is a system that provides health-related services within the context of people's daily lives—that is, in places where people spend their time in the community. Care can be delivered in a variety of settings, including, but not limited to, homes, shelters, workplaces, schools, and seniors' centres. In contrast to the traditional health-care system that focused primarily on the ill and the injured, community-based care is holistic. It involves a broad range of services designed not only to restore health but also to promote health and prevent illness in the public.

In the past two decades, the delivery of nursing services in the community has increased observably. A number of factors have contributed to this trend, among them rising health-care costs, an aging population, and a growing emphasis on preventing illness and enhancing quality of life. CBHC is not simply an adjunct to acute care; in fact, many individuals use community health-care services in an effort to avoid hospitalization altogether.

In the context of CBHC, the term *client* is often defined more broadly than in acute care. Community-based care can be delivered to an individual, a family, a group, or an entire population. In each case, the individual or group of people with which the nurse is working is considered the client.

In Canada, health-care delivery is a provincial and territorial concern, and the manner in which health regions finance and deliver CBHC differs widely across the provinces and territories (Coyte & McKeever, 2001).

However, the following features are common to all regions:

- A focus on health promotion and maintenance, education and management, and coordination and continuity of care within the community environment
- A focus on the health needs of individuals, families, and communities
- Integration of community-based care into larger health-system offerings

Nursing practice is seen as autonomous, with decisions for care made by collaboration between the nurse and client, and made congruent with personal and societal values and beliefs of both. Several components make up community-based care:

- Self-care, with the client and family assuming primary decision making for their health care
- A focus on preventive care, whether at the primary, secondary, or tertiary level
- A realization that care must be provided within the context of the community; that health and the social environment are interactive and must take into account the culture, values, and resources of the individual, family, and community
- The need for continuity of care to counteract the fragmentation of care currently existing in the health-care system
- Collaboration among health-care providers and across sectors resulting in shared responsibility for communication in order to optimize the client's health

Approaches in Community-Based Health Care

As greater emphasis is placed on the general health of the community, in contrast to the traditional system that focused on care of ill and injured individuals, new approaches to health-care delivery emerge (see the Nursing and Canadian Society box). Some of these are an integrated health-care system, community initiatives, community coalitions, and outreach programs:

- An *integrated health-care system* is one that makes all levels of prevention—primary, secondary, and tertiary—available in an integrated form. (See Chapter 7 for descriptions of these levels.) The goals are to facilitate continuity of care, recovery, positive health outcomes, and the long-term benefits of modifying harmful lifestyles through health promotion and disease prevention. In many parts of the country, hospitals are reflecting this concept by redefining themselves as "health-care organizations" or "integrated health-care systems." Movement of clients between settings is coordinated to minimize any disruption in service, also referred to as seamless care.
- *Community initiatives* are being sponsored by some hospitals or local community agencies. These initiatives, called "healthy cities" or "healthier communities," rely on members of the community to establish health priorities, set measurable goals, and determine actions required to attain these goals. Although health-care professionals and organizations may be involved in these activities, the goal is for the community to assume responsibility for the direction, coordination, and implementation of health-care services in consultation with its resident members.

- *Community coalitions* bring together individuals and groups for the shared purpose of improving the community's health. Nurses are major participants and contributors in these coalitions and often assume leadership roles. Community coalitions may focus on a single or multifaceted problem and can be health promotive, illness and injury preventive, or restorative in nature. Examples include the establishment of an abuse prevention program, a gang prevention program, an older adult assessment program, and an immunization program for a high-risk group.
- *Outreach programs* that use lay health workers are a method of linking underserved or high-risk populations (such as immigrant populations, homeless people, or single parents) with the formal health-care system. They can minimize or reduce barriers to health care, increase access to services, and thus improve the health status of the community. They involve partnerships among nurses, community members, and lay health workers who assist their neighbours through outreach networks. Nurses often provide training, consultation, and support to these individuals, who then assume responsibility for contact with marginalized individuals and groups in their community.

Community Health Nursing

As CBHC becomes more widespread, the requirement for nursing care delivered in the community also increases. As a result, it is important that the practice of community health nurses be distinguished and their practice competencies defined.

The Community Health Nurses Association of Canada (CHNAC) is a national federation of community health nurses that promotes community health nursing and the health of communities. As such, they have defined the scope of and established standards of practice for community health nurses.

According to the CHNAC, **community health nurses (CHNs)** "are registered nurses whose practice specialty promotes the health of individuals, families, communities, and populations, and an environment that supports health. . . . The practice of community health nurses combines nursing theory and knowledge, social sciences and public health science with primary health care" (2008, p. 6).

It is under this broad umbrella of CHNs that home health nurses and public health nurses practice. A **home health nurse (HHN)** "is a community health nurse who combines knowledge from primary health care (including determinants of health), nursing science, and theory and knowledge of the social sciences" to focus on "prevention, health restoration, maintenance, or palliation." (CHNAC, 2008, p. 8). Home health nurses provide care in the client's home, school or workplace.

In contrast, a **public health nurse (PHN)** "is a community health nurse who combines knowledge from public health science, primary health care (including determinants of health), nursing science, and theory and knowledge from the social sciences" and "focuses on promoting, protecting, and preserving the health of populations" (CHNAC, 2008, p. 8). PHNs practise in a variety of settings, including but not limited to, "community health centres, schools, street clinics, youth centres, and nursing outposts" (p. 8). However, it is their focus on the health promotion of populations that distinguishes their practice. In contrast to HHNs, who work mainly with individuals and families, the focus of PHNs' practice is at the larger population level. PHNs do recognize that the health of a population is inextricably linked to that of its constituent members and, as a result, PHNs may work with individuals and families to realize the ultimate goal of population health.

Nursing and Canadian Society

Facts	Implications for Nursing Practice
The Victorian Order of Nurses Canada delivers more than 50 different home nursing, health-promotion, support, and other services to 1 million Canadians and their families every year in 1300 communities, coast to coast.	Nurses need to be aware of resources that are available to clients under their care so that supplied services meet identified needs.
The Canadian government is strengthening the population health concept, recognizing that it is a major component of the new health-for-all policy for the twenty-first century.	Nurses need to be aware that nursing the community is different from nursing *in* the community. The former focuses on population health and the latter on individuals.
A World Health Organization meeting in Canada in 1986 produced the *Ottawa Charter for Health Promotion*. The Charter highlighted the importance of strengthening community action, reorienting health services to place greater emphasis on health promotion, and the necessity for intersectoral action for health.	The nurse will need to involve individual and community-focused strategies in order to ensure health for all. An individual action may be referring a client to a weight-loss program; while a community-focused strategy may be providing support to new mothers who want to establish a cooperative babysitting service.

Regardless of their place of work, CHNs are drawn to the specialty for similar reasons. Nurses enter into and continue in community practice because of their increased initiative and the high levels of autonomy and professional status inherent in community health nursing (Best & Thurston, 2006; Thurtle, 2005). The CNA has also acknowledged the specialized knowledge and skill inherent in working with communities. They now offer a certification exam in community health nursing.

Based on the CNA's *Code of Ethics for Registered Nurses* (2008), CHNAC (2008) developed a list of values and beliefs common to CHNs. These values and beliefs include caring, the principles of PHC, multiple ways of knowing, individual and community partnership, and empowerment. Based on these values and beliefs, as well as nursing knowledge and community partnerships, five interrelated standards of practice were defined: promoting health, building individual and community capacity, building relationships, facilitating access and equity, and demonstrating professional responsibility and accountability. The Canadian community health nursing practice model (seen in Figure 13.1) illustrates the dynamic nature of community health nursing practice. The model includes the practice standards, client groups, values and beliefs, and CHN process demonstrating their interrelatedness as vital components of CHN practice (CHNAC, 2008).

Community-Based Settings

Traditionally, community nursing services have been provided by regional and provincial or territorial health departments. Primary settings included schools (school health nursing), workplaces (occupational health nursing), and homes (home care nursing). Over the years, numerous other settings have been established: daycare centres, seniors' centres, storefront clinics, homeless shelters, mental health centres, crisis centres, drug rehabilitation programs, ambulatory care centres, nurse-managed care centres, churches, and others.

Regardless of the practice setting, several overreaching roles are shared by all CHNs:

- *Advocate:* Advocacy involves supporting the client's choices in health care and includes discussion about client rights and the provision of assistance in accessing community resources. The role of advocate can be particularly challenging when family members' or other caregivers' views differ from those of the client. In the event of conflict, it is the nurse's responsibility to ensure the client's rights and desires are upheld.
- *Caregiver:* The role of caregiver is one common to every nursing specialty. In community health, this role may or may not include the provision of direct client care. The CHN may provide direct care, such as ostomy care, intravenous therapy, or complex dressing changes. However, much of the CHNs time can also be spent teaching the client or family and friends to provide required care. In home care, additional nursing care, such as bathing, feeding, and maintaining a clean and safe environment, may be provided by care aides or practical nurses.
- *Educator:* In the role of educator, a CHN focuses on illness care, prevention of health problems, and the promotion of optimal wellness. The context of health education will vary, depending largely on the practice setting and client population with which the CHN works. Teaching can take the form of group presentations (as seen in school health or occupational health) or individual client teaching (as seen in home care). The role of educator is critical to community health nursing; informing clients enables them to become active participants in their

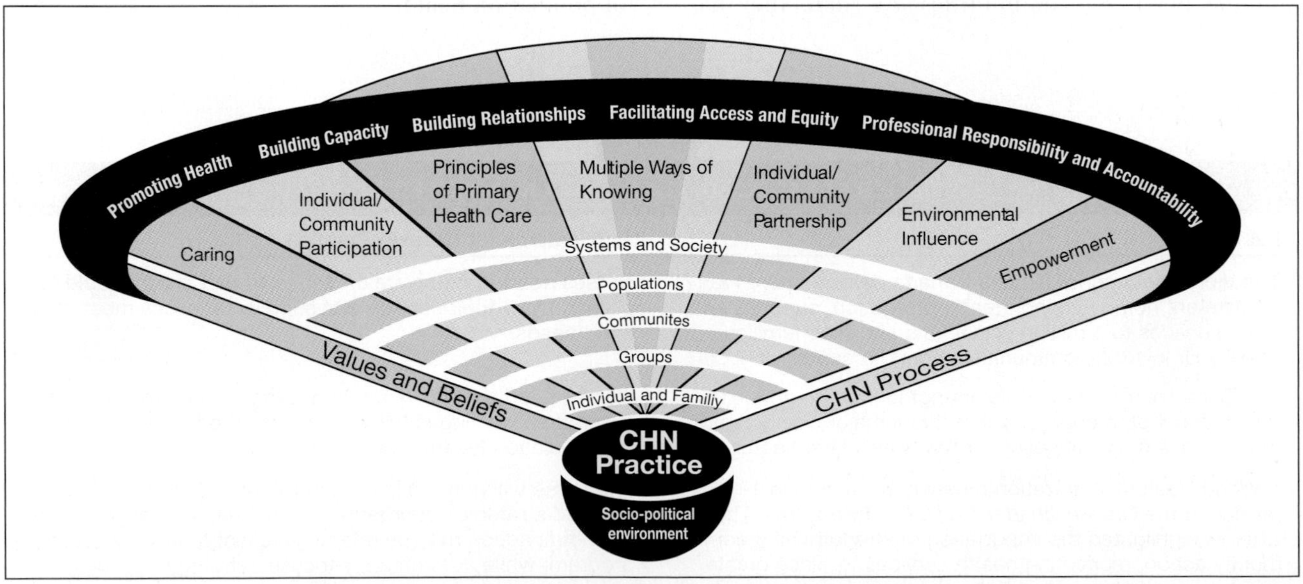

FIGURE 13.1 The Canadian community health nursing practice model
(From **Canadian Community Health Nursing Standards of Practice,** *by the Community Health Nurses Association of Canada, 2008, Toronto: Author.)*

own health care. As such, it is imperative that every CHN have knowledge of teaching and learning principles and be skilled in the use of strategies that facilitate learning (see Chapter 25 for additional information).

- *Case manager or coordinator:* Ultimately, it is often the CHN who is responsible for the assessment of actual and potential health problems, the coordination of care plans, and the evaluation of client outcomes. When multiple professions are involved in the delivery of care, the role of case manager can shift among the professions, depending on the needs of the client. Some of the professions with which CHNs routinely collaborate include occupational therapy, physical therapy, medicine, pharmacy, nutrition, education, and social work.
- *Health promoter:* Health promotion is certainly within the role of every nurse. However, for many CHNs, health promotion constitutes the majority of their practice. For some, health promotion occurs at the population level through such activities as policy development or social marketing campaign; for others, it occurs at the individual or small group level through such activities as prenatal classes and cooking cooperatives.

COMMUNITY HEALTH CENTRE NURSING Community health nursing centres provide PC to specific populations and are managed by advance practice nurses, such as nurse practitioners and CHNs. These nurses provide services from health promotion, to screening, to PC. Although the nurses are the primary providers of care to clients visiting the centre, consultation with other health professionals, including physicians, is available as needed. Nursing centres can be located at any community site, including both urban and rural areas.

There are various categories of community nursing centres (Riesch, 1992):

- *Community outreach centres:* freestanding clinics similar to the traditional community public health clinics
- *Institution-based centres:* centres associated with a large parent organization, such as a hospital, a corporation, or an academic institution
- *Wellness centres:* centres that provide such services as health promotion, health maintenance, education, counselling, and screening

Telehealth projects use communication and information technology to provide health information and health-care services to people in rural, remote, or underserved areas. Video conferences or video clinics enable health-care workers to provide distant consultation and to assess and treat ambulatory clients who have a variety of health-care needs. These video conferences are similar to any outpatient clinic visit, except that the client and health-care specialist are kilometres apart. A related development to telehealth is *telenursing,* in which nurses provide client teaching and health promotion to distant clients. Hader (2005) suggests that nurses must learn to use technology in a manner that can enhance the quality of care, while making every attempt to ensure that the essence of nursing, the relationship between nurse and client, is not disrupted.

PARISH NURSING Parish nursing was first established in Canada in 1992. Since then, the specialty has become more common as faith communities seek to sustain and improve the health of their members. "A parish nurse is a registered nurse with specialized knowledge, who is called to ministry and affirmed by a faith community to promote health, healing and wholeness" (Canadian Association for Parish Nursing Ministry, 2004, ¶ 1). Though by definition a parish nurse is a holistic practitioner, the focus is on the spiritual component of health promotion, not necessarily hands-on care. Initially, parish nurses were volunteers, but now, some are employees paid by the congregation or an affiliated institution, such as a health system or community agency.

The International Parish Nurse Resource Centre (n.d.) describes the roles of the parish nurse as follows:

- *Personal health counsellor,* who discusses health issues and problems with individuals and makes home, hospital, and nursing home visits as needed
- *Health educator,* who educates and supports individuals through health education activities that promote an understanding of the relationship among values, attitudes, lifestyle, faith, and well-being
- *Referral source,* who acts as a liaison to other congregational and community resources
- *Facilitator,* who recruits and coordinates volunteers within the congregation, and develops support groups
- *Integrator* of faith and health
- *Community assessor and evaluator,* who uses health promotion, illness prevention, treatment, and rehabilitative services to improve the health of parish members

Buijs and Olson (2001) stated that "with specialized knowledge in health promotion, parish nurses build on the capacities of individuals, families, faith communities, and the broader community when connecting people to resources that address physical, social, economic, mental, and spiritual determinants of health" (p. 17). With their focus on health promotion and spirituality, parish nurses exemplify holistic practice.

SCHOOL HEALTH NURSING School health services are provided at the individual, family, and community levels in an effort to ensure an optimal level of health within the school community. A school health nurse will work within the school and surrounding community by using primarily health-promotion and illness prevention strategies. As a part of an interprofessional team, he or she is responsible for the assessment, planning, implementation, and evaluation of school health programs. Within this context, a school health nurse provides direct care to

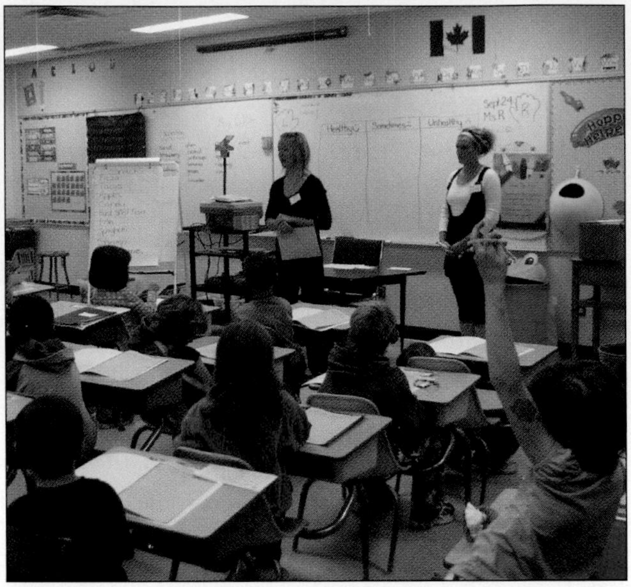

FIGURE 13.2 A school health nurse provides health-promotion teaching in the classroom.

students, provides leadership in the development and implementation of health policy and services, promotes a healthy school environment, and acts as a liaison among the school, family, community, and health-care system (see Figure 13.2).

OCCUPATIONAL HEALTH NURSING Employers of all sizes are increasingly concerned with the health and safety of their employees. As a result, the need for health services in the workplace is greater than ever before. According to the Canadian Occupational Health Nurses Association, "the primary role of the occupational health nurse is to coordinate the delivery of comprehensive, equitable, quality occupational health services for workers and worker groups" (2003, p. 2). Within this role, nurses may be charged with the development of programs aimed at safety and accident prevention, at the prevention and control of contagious diseases, and at lifestyle modification, and offer acute emergency care. Typically, the work of an occupational health nurse also includes multidisciplinary teamwork; workplace health services often involve the collaboration of occupational health nurses, physicians, human resource members, and specialized physical and occupational therapists.

FORENSIC NURSING For as long as victims of violence have presented at emergency rooms and clinics, nurses have treated and documented these patients' injuries. However, forensic nursing is a relatively new specialty in community health nursing, and it constitutes an important link for medico-legal investigation. Forensic nurses may deliver comprehensive equitable treatment to victims of crime (when working as sexual assault nurse examiners) or to perpetrators of crime (when working as forensic outreach nurses). In either case, it is their focus on the health of those affected by crime that distinguishes their practice (Pyrek, 2006).

HOME CARE NURSING Home care nursing is the delivery of health-care services in the client's home environment, often with the effect of delaying or alleviating the need for long-term-care or acute-care alternatives.

Traditionally, home care services were provided primarily by the Victoria Order of Nurses (VON), a nonprofit home-visiting organization. However, the delivery of home care has begun to change, and services are now delivered by a variety of agencies (see Box 13.3).

The types of clients who receive home care services are highly varied. A home care nurse can provide health promotion, such as postnatal visits; acute health care, such as wound infection management; chronic health care, such as diabetes medication management; or palliative care at the end of life.

Home care nurses function highly independently in the community, visiting clients in their home. Because the home is the family's territory, power and control issues in delivering nursing care differ from those in institutional settings. For example, entry into a home is granted, not assumed; therefore, the development of trust and rapport are crucial. As well, unlike in hospital settings, the family and client set their own priorities and schedules in their home. Health care is often provided with other family members present, and they may participate to varying degrees in care delivery.

Home care nurses have identified significant advantages in caring for individuals and families in the home. The intimacy of the environment fosters familiarity, sharing, connections, and caring between clients and families and the nurse. Behaviours are more natural, cultural beliefs and practices are more visible, and multigenerational interactions are more readily displayed. Home care nurses are more able to complete assessments that extend beyond the client themselves. As a guest in the client's home, nurses are able to assess the living environment, support systems, and daily activities in a way institution-based care providers cannot (see Figure 13.3).

BOX 13.3 HOME CARE AGENCIES

A variety of agencies can provide home care services:

- *Public or government agencies* are operated by provincial and territorial or local governments and financed primarily by public funds.
- *Voluntary or private nonprofit agencies,* such as the Victorian Order of Nurses, are supported by donations, endowments, charities, and third-party reimbursement.
- *Private, proprietary agencies,* such as ParaMed, are for-profit organizations that are governed by either individual owners or national corporations. Some of these agencies participate in third-party reimbursement; others rely on private payment for service.

As a result, home care nurses often uncover health-related issues other than those for which they were referred. These issues can include situations of abuse, neglect, or extreme poverty. It may be necessary for the home care nurse to provide additional services or to refer the client to another professional who can best meet these needs.

More than any other care providers, home care nurses have firsthand knowledge of the burden of caregiving. In the interest of cutting health-care costs, policymakers, third-party payers, and medical providers are placing increasingly complex responsibilities on clients' families and friends (Coyte & McKeever, 2001). Caregiving demands can extend for months or years, placing the caregivers themselves, many of whom are older adults, at risk for physiological and psychosocial health problems.

Home care is not included in the Canada Health Act. Subsequently, its services are not insured in the same way as are physician's services, for example. Home care is delivered by public, private nonprofit, and private for-profit agencies in Canada, with the proportion of private versus public services varying by province and territory. Home health-care services are reimbursed by three mechanisms: (1) provincial or territorial and municipal government funds, (2) private insurance, and (3) private payment by home care recipients. Within public home care agencies, professional services (e.g., nursing, therapies) are generally provided free up to an identified figure per month, while user fees may apply to support services (personal care, house cleaning, transportation). User fees are generally allocated on a sliding scale based on income, as determined by income tax returns. Clients may or may not be responsible for the cost of supplies, equipment, and medications.

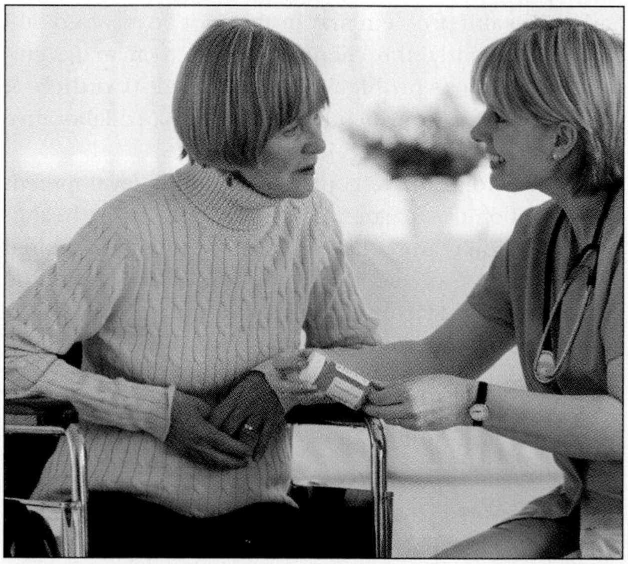

FIGURE 13.3 A home care nurse provides direct client care in the home.

Evidence-Informed Practice

Can Immunization Programs Be Successful in Nontraditional Settings?

Low vaccination coverage in areas with a high burden of vaccine-preventable diseases can pose a significant health risk to the community. Poverty, homelessness, poor nutrition and hygiene, shelter overcrowding, and problematic substance use are but a few of the factors that place residents of the downtown eastside (DTES) of Vancouver at risk. In these 10 square blocks, the infection rates resulting from four vaccine-preventable pathogens (hepatitis A, hepatitis B, influenza, and *streptococcal pneumoniae*) were particularly high—in some cases, 14 times that of the rest of British Columbia, and the highest in Canada. It was necessary to examine new immunization strategies. High-risk populations often have barriers to accessing health services, such as a lack of telephones and a lack of access to transportation. For these reasons, initiatives that work well in other populations can fail. On this basis, teams of two nurses and one community volunteer began an immunization blitz in the DTES (Weatherill, Buxton, & Daly, 2004). They immunized individuals in nontraditional settings, including hotels, food banks, drop-in centres, pubs, and parks. Results were encouraging. During the 5-week immunization blitz, 8723 persons were immunized (with only a 12% refusal rate). Nurses found the experience rewarding and felt they were making a real difference in the health of the DTES community. The immunization initiative was intended to reduce morbidity and mortality associated with vaccine-preventable diseases in a high-risk population. The reduction of hepatitis A and pneumonia diagnoses are preliminary indicators of the program's success.

NURSING IMPLICATIONS: Vaccination coverage can be increased in high-risk, inner-city populations by using alternative delivery programs. Public health nursing outreach in nontraditional settings has the potential to decrease the risk associated with vaccine-preventable diseases, by facilitating immunization in a population that often faces significant barriers to accessing health-care services.

Source: Based on "Immunization Programs in Non-traditional Settings," by S. Weatherill, J. Buxton, and P. Daly, 2004, *Canadian Journal of Public Health, 95*(2), pp. 133–136.

Safety Concerns in Community Health Nursing

Any time a nurse visits the home of a client, whether the client is known to the nurse or not, precautions should be taken to ensure nurse safety. Many clients live in neighbourhoods that may present safety concerns for a visiting nurse. It is important that CHNs are vigilant with their use of safety precautions, regardless of their familiarity with the neighbourhood or the client. For example, it is important that mechanisms be in place to inform colleagues of the visit destination and expected time of return. Safety-related policy and procedures vary across health regions. It is the responsibility of the CHN to become familiar with regulations in his or her place of work.

Community and Public Health Workforce Competencies

The CNA (1998) in its document *Nursing with Communities—Making the Transition* suggested that the knowledge and skills required of CHNs has steadily grown since public health certificates were first offered in Canadian universities in 1920. Today, nurses practising in community-based integrated health-care systems require highly specialized knowledge and skills.

In 1998, the Pew Health Professions Commission in the United States developed 21 competencies for the twenty-first century. These recommendations cross professional boundaries and offer strategic direction for all health professions. They include a focus in the following areas: ethics, evidence-informed practice, critical thinking, determinants of health, PHC, population health promotion, client-centred collaboration, interdisciplinary practice, and public policy advocacy.

In Canada, similar efforts are underway to develop public health workforce core competencies. A draft set of these competencies was released in early 2006. Since then, they have undergone a review process, including input from the public health workforce, resulting in a full release in 2007. The competencies transcend the boundaries of specific disciplines within public health; they reflect the common knowledge, skills, and abilities of public health workers; and they reflect the public health approach to health issues (Public Health Agency of Canada, 2007). In all, 44 competencies divided among seven domains are included (see Box 13.4).

BOX 13.4 PUBLIC HEALTH WORKFORCE CORE COMPETENCY DOMAINS

The 44 competencies of public health-care workers are divided among the following seven domains:

1. Core Public Health Sciences
2. Assessment and Analysis
3. Policy and Program Planning, Implementation and Evaluation
4. Partnerships, Collaboration and Advocacy
5. Diversity and Inclusiveness
6. Communication
7. Leadership

Source: *Core Competencies for Public Health in Canada, Release 1.0*, by the Public Health Agency of Canada, 2007, Ottawa: Author.

The Community Health Nurse as a Collaborator

CHNs routinely collaborate with clients, peers, and other health-care professionals. They frequently collaborate about client care but can also be involved in collaboration on bioethical issues, legislation, and health-related research with other professional organizations. Box 13.5 outlines selected aspects of the nurse's role as a collaborator.

COLLABORATIVE PARTNERSHIP IN HEALTH CARE

The traditional hierarchical relationship that has dominated health-care delivery emerged from an illness focus in which the health professional assumed the role of expert. This model of care delivery is no longer functional in our changing health-care system. As the boundaries of each health-care profession change, and as consumers play an increasingly active role in care delivery, a collaborative approach is required. **Collaborative partnership** is defined as "the pursuit of person-centered goals through a dynamic process that requires the active participation and agreement of all partners. The relationship is one of partnership and the way of working together is collaborative, hence the term *collaborative partnership*" (Gottlieb & Feeley, 2006, p. 8).

In the collaborative partnership model of health care, the client shares responsibility for his or her health, and the nurse acknowledges that clients have knowledge and capabilities that can be used to understand and manage their illness in a meaningful way. The relationship between the nurse and client is reciprocal and mutual; goals and plans of care are jointly determined. Within this context, the role of the nurse is one of facilitator. He or she encourages clients to share their perceptions and expertise. Joint decisions are made in an effort to develop the client's autonomy and self-efficacy. In the end, the health problem may or may not be resolved but, more importantly, the client's capacity to manage current and future problems is enhanced (Gottlieb & Feeley, 2006). The principles integral to a collaborative partnership are described in Box 13.6.

Six key forces have contributed to the development of a collaborative partnership approach within health-care systems in many countries including, but not limited to, Australia, Canada, the United Kingdom, and the United States: (1) consumerism and patient rights, (2) PHC and health promotion, (3) accessibility of health information, (4) changes in thinking about nursing and ethical care, (5) the shift from hospital-based to home-based care, and (6) knowledge about how people change (Gottlieb & Feeley, 2006).

INTERPROFESSIONAL COOPERATION IN HEALTH CARE It is the position of the CNA (2005) that every Canadian is entitled to health care within a system that has the capacity to help them meet their needs. The

BOX 13.5 THE COMMUNITY HEALTH NURSE AS A COLLABORATOR

The community health nurse's role as a collaborator covers many different aspects:

WITH CLIENTS

- Acknowledges, supports, and encourages clients' active involvement in health-care decisions
- Encourages a sense of client autonomy and an equal position with other members of the health-care team
- Helps clients set goals and objectives for health care that are mutually agreed on
- Provides client consultation in a collaborative fashion

WITH PEERS

- Shares personal expertise with other nurses and elicits the expertise of others to ensure quality client care
- Develops a sense of trust and mutual respect with peers that recognizes their unique contributions

WITH OTHER HEALTH-CARE PROFESSIONALS

- Recognizes the contribution that individual members of the interdisciplinary team can make by virtue of their expertise and view of the situation
- Listens to each individual's views
- Shares health-care responsibilities in exploring options, setting goals, and making decisions with clients and families
- Participates in collaborative interdisciplinary research to increase knowledge of a practice problem or situation

WITH PROFESSIONAL NURSING ORGANIZATIONS

- Seeks out opportunities to collaborate with and within professional organizations
- Serves on committees in local, provincial or territorial, and national nursing organizations or specialty groups
- Supports professional organizations in political action to create solutions for professional and health-care concerns

WITH LEGISLATORS

- Offers expert opinions on legislative initiatives related to health care
- Collaborates with other health-care providers and consumers on health-care legislation to best serve the needs of the public

BOX 13.6 PRINCIPLES OF THE COLLABORATIVE PARTNERSHIP

The following 10 principles are essential in a collaborative partnership:

1. Both person and nurse want to and agree to enter into a collaborative relationship.
2. The collaborative partnership can assume many forms depending on the person's preferences, abilities, and circumstances.
3. The nurse continually assesses the conditions that influence collaboration and adjusts the form that the collaborative partnership takes to best fit the person's needs and abilities and the situation.
4. The collaborative partnership is purposeful and goal directed.
5. To achieve mutually agreed-on goals, both the nurse and the person need to have as thorough an understanding of the situation as is possible at that point in time. This involves sharing with one another the other's unique perspective.
6. In a collaborative partnership, the person is the essential and primary sources of information.
7. Both person and nurse contribute resources that are used collaboratively.
8. Collaboration, in some situations, involves sharing a very different perspective with a person, challenging his view, or inviting him to see something different.
9. The collaborative partnership may change within an encounter and across encounters as the situation changes or as the person's needs or abilities evolve.
10. A collaborative partnership approach requires a varied repertoire of communication and interpersonal skills.

Source: From *The Collaborative Partnership Approach to Care: A Delicate Balance*, by L. Gottlieb and N. Feeley, 2006, Toronto: Mosby Elsevier Canada.

responsiveness of the health-care system is directly related to the effectiveness of cooperation among health professionals. This **interprofessional cooperation** is a hallmark of PHC and involves the development of a common purpose or care outcome, the acceptance and recognition of complementary skills and expertise among different providers, and the effective coordination and ongoing communication among providers (Enhancing Interdisciplinary Collaboration in Primary Health Care Initiative [EICP Initiative], 2006).

As the scope of health professionals, including CHNs, changes, it is increasingly important that the foundations of interprofessional cooperation be defined. The principles that form the basis of interprofessional cooperation in PHC in Canada reflect shared values among various professions and create a system-wide approach to the delivery of policies, programs, and services (EICP Initiative, 2006):

- Patient or client engagement
- Population health approach

- Best possible care and services
- Access
- Trust and respect
- Effective communication

COMPETENCIES BASIC TO COLLABORATION Key elements necessary for collaboration include effective communication skills, mutual respect and trust, and a decision-making process.

COMMUNICATION Collaborating to solve complex problems requires effective communication skills. Effective *communication* can occur only if the involved parties are committed to understanding one another's professional roles and appreciating one another as individuals. Instead of focusing on distinctions, health professionals must concentrate on their common ground—the client's needs.

MUTUAL RESPECT AND TRUST *Mutual respect* occurs when two or more people show or feel honour or esteem toward one another. *Trust* occurs when a person is confident in the actions of another person. Both mutual respect and trust imply a mutual process and outcome. They must be expressed both verbally and nonverbally.

DECISION MAKING The *decision-making* process at the team level involves shared responsibility for the outcome. Obviously, to create a solution, the team must follow each step of the decision-making process, beginning with a clear definition of the problem. Team decision making must be directed at the objectives of the specific effort. It requires full consideration and respect of diverse viewpoints. Members must be able to verbalize their perspectives in a nonthreatening environment. An important aspect of decision making is the interdisciplinary team focus on the client's priority needs and the organization of interventions accordingly. The discipline best able to address the client's needs is given priority in planning. Nurses, by the nature of their holistic practice, are well suited for interprofessional cooperation.

Continuity of Care

A major responsibility of the CHN is to ensure continuity of care. **Continuity of care** is the coordination of health-care services by health-care providers for clients moving from one health-care setting to another and among health-care professionals. Continuity ensures uninterrupted health services as the client moves from one level of care to another, for example, from an acute-care hospital to home, or from home to a long-term-care facility. This link is of increasing importance as changes in the health-care system, nursing roles, interprofessional relationships, and client populations continue. In an integrated review of continuity of care, Sparbel and Anderson found that although the concept was not consistently or well defined, it was "strongly affected by a variety of communication and systems factors" (2000, p. 22). To provide continuity of care, nurses need to do the following:

- Involve the client and family or significant other in all phases (assessing, planning, implementing, and evaluating care) of entry and exit from one setting to another.
- Collaborate and communicate with other health-care professionals as needed.
- Ensure that required services for positive outcomes are both available and coordinated to provide seamless care (Sparbel & Anderson, 2000).

Case management is an integrative health-care model that tracks a client through a variety of care settings to ensure care continuity. Weil and Karls (as cited in McWilliam, 2000) addressed potential duplication and care fragmentation while ensuring clients receive "services in a supportive, effective, and cost-efficient manner" (p. 146). The following are the three models of case management used in Canada:

1. *The brokerage or service management model,* wherein health professionals are designated to assess client needs, implement service, and evaluate client progress while ensuring cost-effectiveness and, ideally, cost reduction
2. *Integrated team or provider-driven model,* wherein one professional provider is designated as primary caregiver to provide the leadership for care, while a team delivers services with the goal of achieving care continuity
3. *Self-managed care or client-centred model,* wherein clients assume, with caregiver support, personal control over care decisions

Discharge Planning

Discharge planning is frequently viewed as synonymous with continuity of care. Traditional discharge planning has referred to discharge from the hospital to home. However, discharges occur from many other settings. Discharge planning can be viewed as the process of preparing a client to transition between care environments in the same facility. For example, a client with a cerebral vascular accident may move from a medical unit to a rehabilitation unit, or a client with multiple traumas may move from an emergency to an intensive care unit. The term *discharge planning* can also refer to the movement of a client from one care environment to another entirely. For example, an older adult client may transition to long-term care when he or she is no longer able to live at home. The focus of discharge planning is always at the individual client and family level, but each agency generally has its own policies and procedures to guide the process. Many agencies have *discharge planners,* a health or social services professional who coordinates the transition and acts as a link between the discharging and the receiving facilities. Often, a nurse assumes the responsibility of providing continuity of care.

Discharge planning needs to begin when a client is admitted to an agency, especially in hospitals where the lengths of stays are considerably shortened. Effective discharge planning involves (1) ongoing assessment to obtain comprehensive information about the client's ongoing needs, (2) statements of nursing care, and (3) plans to ensure the client's and caregivers' needs are met. In some situations, discharge planning necessitates health team and family conferences. At a health team conference, health professionals focus on ways to individualize care for the client. At a family conference, both health professionals and the family discuss family issues related to the client. Both types of conferences give the client, family, and health-care professionals the opportunity to mutually plan care and set goals.

Nurses preparing to discharge clients need to assess the following parameters:

- The client's personal and health data
- The client's knowledge of the disease processes, including signs and symptoms, treatment, and services
- The client's ability to perform the activities of daily living
- Any physical, cognitive, or other functional limitations the client may have
- The caregiver's responses and abilities
- The adequacy of the client's financial resources

BOX 13.7 DISCHARGE PLANNING: HOME ASSESSMENT PARAMETERS

When planning the discharge of a client, the nurse needs to assess the client's strengths and deficits.

PERSONAL AND HEALTH DATABASE

Age; gender; height and weight; cultural data; medical history; current health status; surgery

ABILITIES TO PERFORM ACTIVITIES OF DAILY LIVING (ADLs)

Abilities for dressing; eating; toileting; hygienic care (tub, shower, or sponge bathing, oral care); ambulating (with or without aids, such as a cane, crutches, walker, wheelchair); transferring (from bed to chair, in and out of a bath, in and out of a car); preparing meals; using transportation; and shopping

DISABILITIES AND LIMITATIONS

Sensory losses (auditory, visual); motor losses (paralysis, amputation); communication disorders; mental confusion or depression; incontinence; and so on

CAREGIVERS' RESPONSES AND ABILITIES

Principal caregiver's relationship to client; thoughts and feelings about client's discharge; expectations for recovery; health and coping abilities; comfort with performing needed care

FINANCIAL RESOURCES

Financial resources and needs (note equipment, supplies, medications, special foods required)

COMMUNITY SUPPORTS

Family members, friends, neighbours, volunteers; resources, such as the Victorian Order of Nurses and Meals on Wheels; nutrition services; health centres; CHNs; day programs; legal assistance; home care; respite care

HOME HAZARD APPRAISAL

Safety precautions, self-care barriers, and home hazards. Assess the following:

- *Walkways and stairways (inside and outside).* Note uneven sidewalks or paths, broken or loose steps, absence of handrails or placement on only one side of stairways, insecure handrails, congested hallways or other traffic areas, and adequacy of lighting at night.
- *Floors.* Note uneven and highly polished or slippery floors and any unanchored rugs or mats.
- *Furniture.* Note hazardous placement of furniture with sharp corners. Note chairs or stools that are too low to get into and out of or that provide inadequate support.
- *Bathrooms.* Note presence of grab bars around tubs and toilets, nonslip surfaces in tubs and shower stalls, hand-held showerhead, adequacy of night lighting, need for raised toilet seat or bath chair in tub or shower, ease of access to shelves, and water temperature regulated at a maximum of 48°C.
- *Kitchen.* Note pilot lights (gas stove) in need of repair, inaccessible storage areas, and hazardous furniture.
- *Bedrooms.* Note adequacy of lighting, in particular the availability of night-lights and accessibility of light switches; ease of access to commode, urinal, or bedpan; and need for hospital bed or bed rails.
- *Electrical.* Note unanchored or frayed electrical cords and outlets that are overloaded and/or near water.
- *Fire protection.* Note the presence or absence of smoke detectors, fire extinguisher, and fire escape plan, improper storage of combustibles (e.g., gasoline) or corrosives (e.g., rust remover [phosphoric acid]), and accessibility of emergency telephone numbers (fire, police).
- *Toxic substances.* Note improperly labelled cleaning solutions.
- *Communication devices.* Note presence of methods to call for help, such as a telephone or internal intercom in the bedroom and elsewhere (e.g., kitchen), and access to emergency telephone numbers.
- *Medications.* Note medications kept beyond date of expiry, adequacy of lighting for medication cabinet or storage, and method of disposal of sharp objects, such as needles used for injections.
- *Pets.* Note the presence of any pets, whether the pet supports the client (such as a dog that barks when someone knocks on door) or is often in the way, the safety for home care workers entering home, and food supplies for pet and owner.

NEED FOR HEALTH-CARE ASSISTANCE

Home-delivered meals; special dietary needs; volunteers for telephone reassurance, friendly visiting, transportation, shopping; assistance with bathing; assistance with housekeeping; assistance with wound care, ostomies, tubes, intravenous medications, and so on

- Community supports
- Hazards or barriers that the home environment presents
- The need for health-care assistance in the home

It is important that assessment focus equally on the client's strengths and deficits, as well as his or her home, family, and community environments. Since all these factors play a part in the optimal care of the client, the nurse must build on strengths while attending to the deficits that currently impede optimal health. The diagnoses and plan of care establish nursing activities necessary before the client is discharged. These activities most often include (1) teaching the client to cope with continuing self-care at home, and (2) a home care referral (see Box 13.7).

Clients need help to understand their situation, to make health-care decisions, and to learn new health behaviours. As a result of shortened hospital stays, it is often unrealistic to try to teach clients everything they need to know. Referral to a home health agency for follow-up teaching may be necessary (see Chapter 25 for details about effective teaching strategies).

Referrals

Regardless of the setting from and to which clients are moving, the referral process is a systematic problem-solving approach that ensures appropriate and timely information is communicated in order to assist the client in accessing resources that meet his or her health-care needs. During the referral, pertinent information about the client's health, care needs, and social environment is communicated between discharging and care-providing agencies. An effective referral involves all of the following: information is reliable and up to date, the referral is practical and timely, the referral is individualized, and the referral is coordinated and mutually agreed on (Hunt, 2005). McWilliam noted that "accessing, coordinating and monitoring the multiple services and providers involved in care, especially when the client moves to the community, is both complex and costly" (2000, p. 146).

Referrals need to present as much information as possible about the client and the hospitalization. Most agencies have well-established protocols and detailed referral forms for this purpose. The assessment guide in Box 13.7 can also be used, but increasingly, nurses must learn to both assess and clearly articulate those assessments to multiple audiences, including families and health-care providers. Beyond this, nurses are often called on to examine client and family needs at a larger systems level to assist in the deliberations around the provision of health-care services in a community to ensure that the full spectrum of client needs can be addressed and met in the spirit of PHC. Education in public health policy and strategies to influence and effect change is essential.

Case Study 13

Mr. Yao is a 67-year-old male with a 20-year history of hypertension and diabetes mellitus. He has recently undergone amputation of three toes because of poor circulation. Since he is progressing well and his blood glucose is within normal limits, he is being discharged home from hospital. He has been referred to home care, which will assign a nurse to change his foot dressings, administer intravenous antibiotics, and monitor his blood glucose levels.

Critical Thinking Questions

1. How will the nurse's role differ when delivering care in the client's home instead of the hospital?
2. What factors within the home environment might affect Mr. Yao's care?
3. What financial savings might be derived from caring for a client at home rather than in a hospital or other institution?

After working through these questions, go to the MyNursingLab at **http://www.mynursinglab.com** to check your answers.

KEY TERMS

primary health care (PHC)
community-based health care (CBHC)
community health nurse (CHN)
home health nurse (HHN)
public health nurse (PHN)
collaborative partnership
interprofessional cooperation
continuity of care

CHAPTER HIGHLIGHTS

- Health-care costs, access to health care, and the quality of health care are major areas of concern in the current health-care system.
- The Canadian Nurses Association's position and the Alma-Ata Declaration have set forth recommendations for health-care reform that focus on accessibility

of health-care services, health promotion and disease prevention, public participation, the use of appropriate technology, and intersectoral cooperation.

- Clients support an increased emphasis on health-care measures that promote wellness and do so at individual, family, group, and community levels.
- Community-based health care, similar to primary health care, provides health-related services in places where people spend their time—in homes, in shelters, in long-term-care residences, at work, in schools, in seniors' centres, and so on.
- Community-based health care is client driven and involves a broad range of services designed to promote health, prevent illness, restore health, and protect the public.
- Public health nursing and home health nursing, subsets of community health nursing, are becoming increasingly prominent specialties in health-care delivery.
- CHNs practise in a variety of settings and provide a variety of services: community health centre nursing, parish nursing, school health nursing, occupational health nursing, home care nursing, and forensic nursing.
- Various approaches are emerging to address community-based care: an integrated health-care system, community initiatives, community coalitions, and outreach programs using lay health workers.
- Community-based nursing directs nursing care toward a specific population or group. It is not confined to one practice setting; it extends beyond institutional boundaries to involve a network of nursing services: nursing wellness centres, ambulatory care, long-term care, home health, and hospice care.
- To practise in community-based health-care systems, nurses will need to learn new knowledge and competencies, such as determinants of a healthy community, primary and secondary preventive strategies, health-promotion strategies, collaborative and interdisciplinary teamwork, information management, and so on. Education in public health policy and strategies to influence and effect change is also essential.
- Intrasectoral and intersectoral cooperation are essential components of community-based care. Key elements of cooperation include effective communication skills, mutual respect and trust, and a good decision-making process.
- It is predicted that nurses will emerge as community health-care leaders. Because primary health care is directed toward the community and client, nurses' roles will change to those of facilitator, consultant, and resource, rather than those of expert provider and team leader.
- A major responsibility of the nurse is to ensure continuity of care as clients move from one level of care to another.
- Continuity of care extends beyond the individual and includes a series of actions both within and outside an individual agency, which involve (1) discharge planning that begins when clients are admitted to an agency, (2) collaboration with the client and support persons, and (3) interdisciplinary cooperation.

ASSESS YOUR LEARNING

1. Based on a community needs assessment, a public health nurse develops a program to prevent childhood obesity. Which of the following strategies is most appropriate for successful implementation?
   - **a.** Provide information to the teacher for classroom use
   - **b.** Involve parents, teachers, and children in program development
   - **c.** Ask the school administration to remove all vending machines
   - **d.** Initiate an exercise program for obese children during recess

2. In contrast to a home health nurse, the practice of public health nurses is characterized by which of the following?
   - **a.** Their focus on prevention
   - **b.** Their focus on the health of populations
   - **c.** Their work in school health, occupational health, and home care
   - **d.** Their work with marginalized groups

3. Which statement best describes the concept of primary health care?
   - **a.** It is medical care provided at the initial point of contact within the health-care system.
   - **b.** It is synonymous with community-based nursing.
   - **c.** It is more relevant for developing countries than for industrialized nations.
   - **d.** It is a philosophy of care delivery that can be applied in any sector.

4. A community health nurse involved in political action to reduce homelessness through increased availability of affordable housing would most likely employ which of the following primary health care principles?
   - **a.** Accessibility, health promotion, and public participation
   - **b.** Illness and injury prevention, and political action
   - **c.** Social justice and equity

   d. Appropriate use of technology, and community organization

5. Discharge planning can include a referral to a home care nurse. Which of the following best describes the expectations of the referral?
   a. The home care nurse will deliver all care himself or herself.
   b. The discharge assessment of service needs will be followed exactly.
   c. The home care nurse will coordinate the health-care service needs of the client.
   d. The discharge plan is developed solely by the discharge planner and the client.

6. The Victorian Order of Nurses exemplifies which of the following types of home care agencies?
   a. Public or government agency
   b. Voluntary or private nonprofit agency
   c. Private proprietary agency
   d. Private cooperative agency

7. An older adult client is being discharged from the home care services program. Which of the following strategies is most appropriate to ensure a successful transition?
   a. Make one last home visit to review client teaching
   b. Call the client's family physician to advise him or her of the change
   c. Schedule a case conference with the client, his or her family, and relevant health professionals
   d. Provide the client with a list of applicable community resources

8. At the end of the postpartum home visiting period with a first-time mom, which of the following is the most important for the nurse to assess?
   a. Mom has been given the answers to all of her breastfeeding questions.
   b. Mom and baby are no long experiencing difficulty with breastfeeding.
   c. Mom feels confident that she can access the necessary resources to deal with current and future difficulties with breastfeeding.
   d. Baby is gaining weight appropriately.

9. Which of the following best exemplifies the three competencies basic to collaboration in the care of a home care client?
   a. The CHN questioning the appropriateness of a prescription from the client's attending physician
   b. The CHN involving physical therapy and occupational therapy in the client's plan of care
   c. The CHN informing the client's family of changes made to the client's plan of care
   d. The CHN calling a case planning meeting for the client, his or her family, and all of the health professionals involved in the client's plan of care when issues arise

10. A young woman receiving services from an occupational health nurse for an injury sustained at work has assumed personal control over her plan of care in consultation with the occupational health nurse and other health-care providers. Which of the following best describes the model of case management being employed?
   a. Brokerage or service management model
   b. Integrated team or provider-driven model
   c. Self-managed care or client-centred model
   d. Collaborative care model

After working through these questions, go to the MyNursingLab at ***http://www.mynursinglab.com*** *to check your answers and see explanations.*

SUGGESTED READINGS

Community Health Nurses Association of Canada. (2008). *Canadian community health nursing standards of practice.* Toronto: Author. Retrieved September 9, 2008, from http://www.chnac.ca/images/downloads/standards/chn_standards_of_practice_mar08_english.pdf

The community health nursing standards document outlines the practice expectations of community health nurses within Canada.

Schoenfeld, B., & MacDonald, M. (2002). Saskatchewan public health nursing survey [Electronic version]. *Canadian Journal of Public Health, 93*(6), 452–456.

This Canadian study replicates a study completed 10 years earlier and examines issues related to the practice of public health nurses.

Underwood, J. (2003). *The value of nurses in the community.* Ottawa: Canadian Nurses Association.

In this article, the author examines issues related to community health nursing practice and makes recommendations for community health service delivery in Canada.

WEBLINKS

Victorian Order of Nurses Canada

http://www.von.ca

The Victorian Order of Nurses Canada (VON Canada) is a registered charity and national health-care organization that has been caring for Canadians in their homes and communities since 1897. The site provides information about the VON, the services offered, and how to access them.

Health Canada

http://www.hc-sc.gc.ca/

Health Canada is a national government agency. Its website provides links to current health-related programs and documents.

Department of Justice Canada: Canada Health Act

http://laws.justice.gc.ca/en/C-6/index.html

This Department of Justice site provides access to federal legislation, including the Canada Health Act and regulations concerning billing.

Canadian Public Health Association

http://www.cpha.ca

The Canadian Public Health Association (CPHA) is a national, independent, nonprofit association representing public health interests in Canada.

Canadian Home Care Association

http://www.cdnhomecare.ca

The Canadian Home Care Association represents more than 600 Canadian organizations that are involved in home care and community care.

REFERENCES

Barnes, D., Eribes, C., Juarbe, T., Nelson, M., Proctor, S., Sawyer, L., et al. (1995). Primary health care and primary care: A confusion of philosophies. *Nursing Outlook, 43*(1), 7–16.

Best, M., & Thurston, N. (2006). Canadian public health nurses' job satisfaction. *Public Health Nursing, 23*(3), 250–255.

Buijs, R., & Olson, J. (2001). Parish nurses influencing determinants of health. *Journal of Community Health Nursing, 18*(1), 13–23.

Canadian Association for Parish Nursing Ministry. (2004). *Parish nursing.* Ingersoll, ON: Author. Retrieved January 10, 2007, from http://www.capnm.ca/core_competencies.htm

Canadian Nurses Association. (1998). *Nursing with communities: Making the transition.* Ottawa: Author.

Canadian Nurses Association. (2003). *Primary health care: The time has come.* Ottawa: Author.

Canadian Nurses Association. (2005). *Interprofessional collaboration.* Ottawa: Author.

Canadian Nurses Association. (2008). *Code of ethics for registered nurses.* Ottawa: Author.

Canadian Occupational Health Nurses Association. (2003). *Occupational health nursing practice standards.* Ottawa: Author. Retrieved December 14, 2006, from http://www.cohna-aciist.ca/english/

Canadian Public Health Association Board of Directors. (2000). *An ounce of prevention: Strengthening the balance in health care reform.* Ottawa: Author.

Community Health Nurses Association of Canada. (2008). *Canadian community health nursing standards of practice.* Toronto: Author. Retrieved September 9, 2008, from http://www.chnac.ca/images/downloads/standards/chn_standards_of_practice_mar08_english.pdf

Coyte, P., & McKeever. (2001). Home care in Canada: Passing the buck. *Canadian Journal of Nursing Research, 33*(2), 11–25.

Enhancing Interdisciplinary Collaboration in Primary Health Care Initiative. (2006). *The principles and framework for interdisciplinary collaboration in primary health care.* Ottawa: Author.

Epp, J. (1986). *Achieving health for all: A framework for health promotion.* Ottawa: Health and Welfare Canada.

Gottlieb, L., & Feeley, N. (2006). *The collaborative partnership approach to care: A delicate balance.* Toronto: Mosby Elsevier.

Hader, R. (2005). Forge the connection between technology and compassion. *Nursing Management, 36*(12), 4.

Hunt, R. (2005). *Introduction to community-based nursing* (3rd ed.). Philadelphia, PA: Lippincott Williams & Wilkins.

International Parish Nurse Resource Centre. (n.d.). *History of parish nursing.* Retrieved December 11, 2006, from http://ipnrc.parishnurses.org/

McWilliam, C. L. (2000). Homecare: National perspectives and policies. In M. J. Stewart (Ed.), *Community nursing: Promoting Canadians' health* (2nd ed.) (pp. 143–155). Toronto: WB Saunders.

Pew Health Professions Commission. (1998). *Recreating health professional practice for a new century.* San Francisco, CA: Author.

Public Health Agency of Canada. (2007). *Core competencies for public health in Canada, Release 1.0.* Ottawa: Author.

Pyrek, K. (2006). *Forensic nursing.* Boca Raton, FL: Taylor & Francis Group.

Riesch, S. K. (1992). Nursing centers: An analysis of the anecdotal literature. *Journal of Professional Nursing, 8*(1), 16–25.

Romanow, R. (2002). *Building on values: The future of health care in Canada.* Ottawa: Commission on the Future of Health Care in Canada.

Sparbel, K., & Anderson, M. (2000). Integrated literature review of continuity of care: Part 1, conceptual issues. *Journal of Nursing Scholarship, 32*(1), 17–24.

Storch, J. (2006). Canadian health care system. In M. McIntyre, E. Thomlinson, & C. McDonald (Eds.), *Realities of Canadian nursing: Professional, practice, and power issues* (pp. 29–53). Philadelphia, PA: Lippincott Williams & Wilkins.

Thurtle, V. (2005). Why do nurses enter community and public health practice? [Electronic version]. *Community Practitioner, 78*(4), 140–145.

World Health Organization & United Nations International Children's Emergency Fund. (1978). *Declaration of Alma-Ata: Health for all by the year 2000.* Geneva, Switzerland: Author.

Chapter 14

Rural and Remote Health Care

Canada was originally a predominantly **rural** (a word to describe places like the countryside, towns, and small cities outside urban centres), agrarian-based nation, and it remained so until societal changes following World Wars I and II resulted in the growth of industry in urban centres. This growth led to the migration of rural residents to find employment in these industrial centres. In 1901, 37% of the population lived in urban centres, as compared with 80% in 2006 (Statistics Canada, 2007a). Urban populations surpassed rural ones in the 1921 to 1931 period; before that time, agriculture and natural resources were dominant industries. In **agriculture** assets come from cultivating soil, producing crops, and raising livestock. **Natural resources** are assets supplied by nature, such as oil, coal, water, and timber, that can be used to create wealth. Since that time, the number of census farms has steadily declined, most recently with a 7.1% drop from 2001 to 2006 (Statistics Canada, 2007a).

Although approximately 20% of Canadians continue to live in rural and **remote** regions, those areas located far from urban and even rural centres, the realities of rural life belie the myth of a tranquil, healthy existence. Many rural communities in Canada are confronted by demographic,

OBJECTIVES

After studying this chapter, you should be able to

1. Describe the issues related to establishing universal definitions of *rural, remote*, and *isolated* communities
2. Describe the geographical characteristics of rural, remote, and isolated communities and associated health-care issues
3. Describe the cultural groups that populate rural, remote, and isolated communities and their associated health-care issues
4. Describe the predominant occupational trends in rural, remote, and isolated communities and the associated health-care issues
5. Summarize the health concerns of individuals, families, and communities within rural, remote, and isolated contexts
6. Identify existing and emerging health-care delivery issues within rural, remote, and isolated contexts
7. Analyze the broad scope of rural, remote, and isolated nursing practice
8. Examine topics of concern to nurses in rural, remote, and isolated practice

ecological, economic, and social challenges related to geographical **isolation** (a state of complete physical separation from other regions), boom-bust cycles, a reliance on nonrenewable natural resources, chronic high unemployment, the vulnerability of single-industry communities, aging populations, and so on (Pong, 2007). Correspondingly, nursing practice is affected by the diversity found within this huge geographical region of Canada. Health-care delivery is further complicated by incomplete and sometimes conflicting data on the health status of residents in these regions.

Definition of *Rural*

One obstacle identified by researchers is the lack of consensus regarding the definition of the term *rural* (MacLeod et al., 2004). A common definition could facilitate comparison of study findings and experiences by researchers, clinicians, health policymakers, and health-care delivery agencies (Thomlinson, McDonagh, Crooks, & Lees, 2004).

Statistics Canada and the Rural Secretariat used six definitions to outline how *rural* could be defined (du Plessis, Beshiri, Bollman, & Clemenson, 2001) and suggested that the appropriate definition be chosen based on the particular question being asked. The first five of the six definitions are based on census geography that includes enumeration areas, census subdivisions, census consolidated subdivisions, and census divisions. The sixth uses postal codes. The six definitions follow (du Plessis et al., p.7):

1. *Census rural area:* individuals living outside places of 1000 people or more or outside places with densities of 400 or more people per square kilometre.
2. *Rural and small town:* people living in towns outside the commuting zone of larger urban centres of 10 000 or greater in population. People can then be placed into four subgroups according to the size of commuting flow and the amount of influence of a larger urban centre (metropolitan influence zone).
3. *Organisation for Economic Co-operation and Development (OECD) rural communities:* people in communities of fewer than 150 individuals per square kilometre. People living in the countryside, towns, and small cities.
4. *OECD predominantly rural regions:* people living in census divisions with more than 50% of the population living in OECD rural communities. It includes all census divisions without a major city.
5. *Nonmetropolitan regions (Beale Code Approach):* people living outside metropolitan regions with urban centres of 50 000 or more population.
6. *Rural postal codes:* people who have a 0 (zero) as the second character in their postal code.

Each definition is built around different criteria, such as population size, density, labour market, or settlement context. Choosing a definition is important because how *rural* is defined can profoundly affect research results, policy development and use, program administration, and even how funding is distributed by governments at all levels (a **policy** is a plan or a course of action that the government follows). So, understanding the limitations and benefits of definitions based on geographical scale (local, community, or regional), a geographical dimension (population size, density, labour market), a rural small town, or degrees of rurality, and whether more than one definition is used is important. Du Plessis and her colleagues (2001) identified some limitations of geographical definitions: the use of only one definition cannot capture the complexity of rurality, a common definition is lacking, qualitative data is disregarded, and definitions are preset.

MacLeod et al. (2004), in their study of rural and remote nursing practice, chose to define remote as "the territories" and "nursing stations or outposts." **Northern**, for Canada, can be defined as the region north of the north–south line developed in the working papers by the Geography Division of Statistics Canada (McNiven, 1999). Kulig et al. (2008) identified four themes that define rurality from a nursing perspective: community characteristics, geographical location, human and technical resources, and nursing practice characteristics. Geographical isolation, economic and labour force characteristics, access to goods and services, and availability of health care are elements that factor into whether an area is considered rural, remote, or isolated.

Rural Health: Place, Space, and Time

Theoretical justifications for the study of place and nursing are slowly emerging from the nursing literature (Andrews, 2006). In health geography, **place** can be viewed as having social or physical attributes, and notions of space and time can be either conceptualized as internal or external to place (Angus, Kontos, Dyck, McKeever, & Poland, 2005; Davies, Day, & Williamson, 2004).

Carolan, Andrews, and Hodnett (2006) described some of the elements of place from a health geography perspective and debate the fit with nursing. These authors described *place* in several ways in relation to nursing, including as "situatedness" or being in, and feeling, place; creating a healing place; place in terms of disembodiment or displacement and the nurse's "place" involving issues of workplace, power, and gender (p. 203).

Health care includes space and time in terms of the uniqueness and peculiarities of place. Rural health often involves the dynamics of journey—place is joined by space and time to other places when issues of distance, transportation, and access to health-care professionals and services arise. Places are not isolated points or spots on a map but are interconnected in multiple ways. Other views of place address place as "not opposite to space, but connected to and produced by spatial practices and logics" (Kelly, 2003, p. 2280). The spatialization of place can come from theoretical conceptualization or from consideration of spatial-structure practices that are economic and political. Malone (2003), in discussing distal nursing, depicted place and nursing as physical, narrative, and moral closeness.

The characteristics or attributes of *rural place* can contribute to the uniqueness and peculiarities of being rural, and a framework to guide the assessment, planning, implementation, and evaluation of rural health care for individuals, families, and communities is critical. In particular, such a framework helps us to understand and provide the optimum care possible to rural residents in relation to research, policy, and practice. The Canadian Nurses Association (CNA) and the Canadian Medical Association developed a rural health framework that can be found at the CNA website, listed in the Weblinks section of this chapter.

Elements of a Rural Health Framework

The Canada Health Act provides for the "right to health care for all." The five federally defined principles that comprise the core of this act are universality, accessibility, portability, comprehensiveness, and public administration. Rural, remote, and isolated communities are confronted by challenges in gaining access to **equitable health care**, that is, the same or comparable health care as is provided elsewhere (Racher & Vollman, 2002; Strasser, 2003). Canadians may believe the principles to be sound; however, at the same time, they have a desire to eliminate deficits, reduce the debt load, and lower taxes (Kelly, 2003). It is a balancing act to maintain high-quality health-care systems and manage the conflicting demands of the public. Acury et al. (2005) put forth a framework that incorporated geography and spatial behaviour as enabling factors in rural health-care utilization, controlling for demographic, social, cultural, and health status factors. These authors, in a survey of 1059 adults in 12 rural communities, found that several geographical and spatial behaviour factors, including having a driver's licence, using provided rides, and being within a reasonable distance for regular care, were significantly related to health-care utilization for regular health appointments and chronic care. Geographical and spatial behaviour are important to consider as factors in rural health-care utilization.

Geography

Even though Canada is the second-largest country in the world in size of landmass, it has a relatively small population, the majority of which is concentrated close to the Canada–United States border. According to Statistics Canada (2007a), Canada's population is now more than 31 million, an increase of 5.4% since the 2001 census. This increase represents a higher rate of population growth than in any other G8 country, and two-thirds of that growth has been attributed to international immigration. In 2006, 68% of the Canadian population lived in census metropolitan areas, and almost 80% lived in urban centres of 10 000 persons or more. Since 2001, the rural population also increased slightly (1%) to just fewer than 6 million people, a change from the previous census period, which saw rural population decline. From 2001 to 2006, the largest growth in rural populations (4%) occurred in the rural–urban fringe zones—the areas close to urban centres (Statistics Canada, 2007a).

Although rural populations have shown a slight increase across Canada, regional variations exist. For example, rural areas in the Atlantic provinces and Saskatchewan declined in population, while the Northwest Territories, Nunavut, and Alberta had the fastest-growing rural populations (Statistics Canada, 2007a). For the first time, the population of the territories surpassed 100 000 people, nearly half of whom live in the three capital cities. Small rural towns and hamlets increased in some cases by as much as 20% over the previous census. The population increase in Nunavut was due to natural increase from 2001 to 2006, when the fertility rate was twice the national average (3.1 versus 1.5 children per woman). Indeed, the Aboriginal population has the fastest-growing natural increase (Statistics Canada, 2007a). In Canada, the **Aboriginal population** includes those who can trace their origins to First Nations, Inuit, or Metis.

These regional variations, combined with the concentration of population in the four major urban regions of the Golden Horseshoe in southern Ontario, Montreal and its surroundings, British Columbia's lower mainland and southern Vancouver Island, and the Calgary–Edmonton area, contribute to issues for the delivery of health care to rural residents (see the Nursing and Canadian Society box).

Nursing and Canadian Society

Fact	Implications for Nursing Practice
Almost 6 million Canadians live in rural and remote areas of the country.	Particular geographical factors influence access to health-care services. For example, distance and lack of resources affect emergency care for persons involved in farming and resource industry accidents.
In the 2001 Speech from the Throne, the government declared it was committed to rural Canada and rural Canadians and would work with communities to develop successful solutions to the challenges they face.	Nurses working in rural areas need to participate in policy and program development initiatives of various governmental departments, recognizing how these actions affect health and health-care delivery within their communities.
The Aboriginal population is the fastest-growing population in Canada, with most being youth and children living in underserviced Northern, rural, and remote communities.	Nurses working in Northern, rural, and remote communities need to participate in policy and program initiatives to address health-care inequities.

It is difficult to specifically locate where the North begins. General agreement exists that great distances and difficult terrain often separate the communities in Northern Canada. With relatively few roads through a large geographical area, travel is still often dependent on weather. For example, winter roads built on the ice and snow can only be built when the weather is cold enough to permit travel across the frozen expanses of northern lakes and rivers. This, in turn, affects the type of goods transported into Northern communities. These factors are not as important in areas of Canada with an integrated highway system.

Enormous diversity exists within Canada in rural and Northern communities. This becomes particularly evident when examining the vastly different geographical regions of the country: the coastal towns and fishing villages in the Atlantic provinces; the rural farming and lumbering communities in Quebec; the mining and forestry industries in Northern Ontario; the rolling prairie lands; the Northern isolated communities set on the tundra; and the orchards and semi-arid farmlands and ranches of the interior of British Columbia. This lack of geographical homogeneity adds to the complexity of health-care issues and delivery systems across the country.

Demography

The ethnic composition of rural areas differs from urban areas. Rural Canada has the lowest proportion of immigrants, including new immigrants and visible minorities; 95.9% live in urban regions (Statistics Canada, 2008a). Many (46%) (Statistics Canada, 2008b) Canadians who identify themselves as First Nations, Inuit, and Metis live in remote, Northern, and rural areas of the country. The majority of Aboriginal communities (64%) are non-isolated; 14% are semi-isolated; and 22% are isolated or remote isolated. As well, many of the people living in the rural communities of several provinces, such as Ontario, Quebec, and New Brunswick, are francophone. The particular health issues related to these populations have important implications.

Most rural communities have large populations of children and youth (0 to 19 years) and seniors (older than 60 years), in comparison with a somewhat smaller population of working-age people (20 to 59 years). However, overall they are, for the most part, older than urban populations. Factors that contribute to the bimodal population age pattern include the aging of the rural population, out migration of rural youth for education and employment, and in migration of retirees (Pong, 2007). In the main, rural unemployment rates are higher and education and income levels are lower. Lower income and a lack of education, combined with large numbers of young and old people, may well contribute to the lower health status of rural and Northern communities.

Economic conditions vary by region and the degree of reliance on single industries, such as agriculture and natural resources. Declining economic conditions have also precipitated a decrease in population in some rural regions, such as in Saskatchewan and Newfoundland and Labrador. Huge disparities within a region can be related to migration caused by changes in the primary industry or industries of a region. Currently, mining is booming in Northern rural communities across the country, whereas the forestry industry is in serious decline, resulting in migration from small towns into larger urban centres.

Over time, a significant reduction in the number of family farms has been associated with a decrease in population. However, the decline in farms in 2006 was slower than it was in 2001; although fewer farms remain, an increased number of farms are reporting larger areas or higher gross farm receipts (Statistics Canada, 2007c). The majority of these larger farms are family corporations. Despite overall recent improvements in the farming economy, the countrywide trend has been for older farm operators to retire but for fewer of their children to continue with the family farm. The consequent decrease in population has a significant economic and sociocultural impact on the residents and communities in rural areas.

Occupations

Although the term *rural* is often equated with agriculture, other major industries in rural regions include mining, fishing, logging and forestry, and resource extraction, such as for oil and potash. In addition, rural communities have a variety of merchants, service dealers, and support services (see Box 14.1). In 2001, managerial and professional occupations were more concentrated in urban regions than in rural regions, while the concentration of unskilled occupations was sizeably higher in predominantly rural regions (Magnusson & Alasia, 2004).

According to a study by Rupnik, Thompson-James, and Bollman (2001), from 1970 to 2000, rural families had the lowest average incomes. In 1997, the average income for rural families was $48 850, whereas the average family income in the most populated areas was $59 920. By using 2000 data, Singh (2004) demonstrated that within each province and territory, incomes in rural regions were lower than those in urban regions. Furthermore, he showed that the income gap widened somewhat between 1980 and 2000. An additional study looking at areas within the provinces only (Alasia & Rothwell, 2004) also demonstrated that the between-province income disparity decreased over the 1990s, while the within-province disparities increased substantially. In other words, income disparity is shifting from a provincial to a rural-urban divide.

The economy of many rural and Northern communities is based on a single resource, which has implications in times of economic downturns and in times of growth and expansion. Rural employment has matched urban areas since 2001, after lagging throughout the previous decade. Employment in small towns and rural areas rose 1.3% in 2005, compared with the 1.4% gain in urban Canada. The biggest employment increases occurred in northern Manitoba, followed by Athabasca, Alberta, driven by the development of the oil sands. Mining has had a recovery, which has helped Northern Ontario and interior British Columbia, and it has offset somewhat the forestry sector downturn. Cape Breton led the Atlantic region in job growth. Despite a declining rural population, rural Saskatchewan experienced revitalization in farming. However, improvements in employment are not uniform across rural areas in Canada, as shown by the downturn in the forestry sector, with lumber and paper mills closing in Northern Ontario, Quebec, and New Brunswick (Statistics Canada, 2007b).

BOX 14.1 MAJOR OCCUPATIONS IN RURAL REGIONS

Rural communities support many different occupations. These are a few of the major ones:

Agriculture	Mining
Logging	Fishing
Oil and potash extraction	Tourism
Merchants	Service sector

Health of Rural Residents

Health Issues

Although there is a perception that rural residents are healthier than their urban counterparts, statistics demonstrate that, for the majority, this is not the case (Pong, 2007). Pong et al. (2006) recently completed the first report produced at the pan-Canadian level that provides a broad picture of the health of rural populations. They did so by analyzing data from three different sources: the Canadian annual mortality database, the Canadian Community Health Survey, and the Cancer Registry (see Box 14.2). Some of the findings affirmed previously identified health-related factors, such as the prevalence of smoking and obesity, as compared with urbanites (Mitura & Bollman, 2003, 2004). Other health influences, such as eating habits and physical activity, showed lower practice levels in rural communities. These statistics are supported by research examining the perceptions of rural women, who identified that they felt more vulnerable because of living in the rural North (Leipert & Reutter, 2005).

Higher overall rural mortality risks were attributed to such causes as **circulatory diseases** (those that affect the heart, arteries, capillaries, or veins), **respiratory diseases** (those that affect the nose, throat, larynx, trachea, bronchi, or lungs), **injuries** (harm, hurt, trauma, or a wound that is caused accidentally or deliberately), and **suicide** (the act of a person deliberately causing his or her own death). Indeed, people living in rural areas farthest from urban centres were at the greatest risk for all causes. Respiratory disease risks were, for the most part, significantly higher in rural areas, except for women living in more rural areas, who reported a prevalence of asthma significantly lower than their urban counterparts. Interestingly, the incidence rates of most cause-specific cancers were lower in rural areas than in urban areas.

Women living in the most rural areas reported a higher prevalence of diabetes and also had higher risks of dying from diabetes or from the complications of the disease compared with those living in urban areas. Canadians living in rural areas experienced higher prevalence of **arthritis** (inflammation of a joint) and rheumatism than those living in urban areas for both sexes. Pong et al.'s (2006) full report can be found at the Centre for Rural and Northern Health Research (CRaNHR) and the Canadian Institute for Health Information (CIHI) websites.

BOX 14.2 HEALTH CONCERNS FOR RURAL RESIDENTS

Rural residents face a number of health concerns:

- Respiratory problems
- Circulatory diseases
- Stress related to farm production and declining income
- Pesticide use
- Chemical contaminants
- Skin diseases
- Zoonoses
- Mental health issues
- Water safety around dugouts and ponds
- Machinery injuries
- Injuries from livestock
- Safe play spaces for children
- Water supply safety
- Hearing protection
- Eyesight protection
- Suicide
- Injuries
- Motor vehicle collisions
- Problematic substance use

Pampalon, Martinez, and Hamel (2006) conducted a study that looked at the health status of rural populations and the major determinants of health in Quebec. Similar to Pong et al. (2006), these researchers found that health varied within rural areas and, generally speaking, the closer residents lived to urban centres, the better their health. They further stated that what really discriminates urban from rural and areas within rural regions are health determinants (socioeconomic) and the presence of specific health conditions, such as respiratory disease, trauma (motor vehicle accidents and suicide), breast cancer, heart disease, infant mortality, smoking, and obesity.

RESPIRATORY PROBLEMS Respiratory disease is a common health problem among agrarian rural dwellers, and rates of respiratory diseases are significantly higher across the board in rural communities, compared with urban centres, according to Pong et al. (2006). Exposure to grain dust, wood smoke, agricultural chemicals for crop production, and noxious gases emitted from silos or oil and gas wells have all been implicated as having immediate or long-term adverse effects on the health of this population. Depending on the specific chemical and length of exposure, ill effects resulting from inhalation of toxic substances can result in systemic problems, such as headaches, blurred vision, or possibly convulsions. Asthma is particularly prevalent in southern Alberta, an area noted for its wind and cattle feedlots; however, in the pan-Canadian health report, this regional rural difference does not show up in the overall health of rural residents, highlighting the need for both pan-Canadian and regional health and illness data.

CHEMICALS Chemical contaminants can cause a variety of clinical manifestations, depending on the agent, source, amount, and route of absorption. Skin disorders, such as dermatitis, are a common problem for those working with chemicals without the use of personal protective equipment, such as gloves and coveralls. Canadian studies of pesticide use among farmers have found an increased risk of cancers among those exposed (Bushy, 2000). Gastrointestinal problems from acute or insidious poisoning through ingestion of contaminated food or water supplies are also concerns encountered particularly after crop spraying. Arbuckle, Bruce, Ritter, and Hall (2006) recommend that people who apply pesticides and their families should be counselled on hygienic practices (e.g., removing footwear and washing soiled hands before entering the home) to reduce indirect sources of exposure to herbicides.

CANCER Some epidemiological evidence supports regional variation in the prevalence of some cancers among rural populations. For example, rates of skin cancer, especially of the lip, are higher for men living in rural areas (Pong et al., 2006). Lip cancer is linked to increased exposure to the sun and its ultraviolet (UV) radiation among farmers and others who work in the sun without adequate UVB protection. Cervical cancer rates were significantly higher for women in the two most rural categories, compared with urban areas, in the 20- to 44-year age group, and the rate of having a Pap test was lower (Pong, 2007). As well, cancer was more prevalent in the Aboriginal population. However, according to Pong et al. (2006) in the pan-Canadian study of rural health, in general, no significant differences exist between rural and urban residents in terms of cause-specific cancers.

WATER SAFETY Water safety is a twofold concern: first, irrigation ditches, dugouts, and northern lakes and rivers are common sites of drowning; second, contaminated wells and creeks that supply drinking water for rural residents pose health risks. For example, preschoolers may fall into the water, whereas adults may drown when the vehicles they are riding in break through the ice.

The events in Walkerton, Ontario; North Battleford, Saskatchewan (Charrois, Graham, Hrudey, & Froese, 2004); and Kashechewan in Northern Ontario serve as examples of the enormous challenges Canadian rural society faces in terms of potable drinking water. Infrastructure to support potable water is either deteriorating or has never met rigorous health standards. In Walkerton, *E. coli* bacterial contamination of the water transportation system caused seven deaths and made 2300 other residents ill. Vincente and Christoffersen (2006) examined the sequence of events in Walkerton and revealed an interaction among all levels in a complex community system, including "physical factors, unsafe practices of individual workers, inadequate oversight and enforcement by local government and a provincial regulatory agency and budget reductions imposed by the provincial government" (p. 93). Many remote and Northern residents continue to obtain their drinking water from sources that are not treated to remove bacteria and parasites. This fact, coupled with inadequate sewage disposal, has resulted in outbreaks of infection that are most harmful to infants, children, older adults, and persons who are immunocompromised.

ZOONOSES Other risks for rural and remote residents are zoonoses. These are diseases that are communicated from animals to humans. One of the more common zoonoses is brucellosis, which is contracted from cattle, swine, and goats. Humans acquire this disease, known as undulant fever, from ingestion of unpasteurized dairy products. Another zoonosis seen in rural and northern areas is rabies, which is often transmitted from foxes, raccoons, and skunks. Although tularemia is spread by insects in some locales in Canada, it can be transmitted from seals and, therefore, can be contracted by hunters in the northern and eastern coastal regions (Lochhaas, 1987).

Bovine spongiform encephalopathy (BSE) is a progressive, fatal disease of the nervous system of cattle. It is one member of a family of diseases known as transmissible spongiform encephalopathies (TSEs). Other TSEs include scrapie in sheep, chronic wasting disease (CWD) in deer and elk, and Creutzfeldt-Jakob disease (CJD) in humans. Although the exact cause of BSE is unknown, it is associated with the accumulation of abnormal proteins, or BSE prions, in the brain. No treatment or vaccine is currently available for the disease (Agriculture and Food, Alberta, 2007; Barnett & McLean, 2005; Canadian Food Inspection Agency, 2005).

In Northern and Arctic regions, trichinosis is a parasitic infection that is commonly found in wild game, such as bears, cougars, and walruses. From 1970 to 1997, Labrador, Quebec, the Northwest Territories (including present-day Nunavut), and Yukon had the highest number of reported cases of trichinosis, numbering more than 100 (Appleyard & Gajadhar, 2000). Hantavirus is a recent health concern that is prevalent in arid rural areas. This pathogen is spread through droppings from deer mice.

AGRICULTURAL INJURIES In the 2006 census, 13 801 farms reported farm-related injuries in the previous 12 months. This represents 6.0% of all Canadian farms. Comparisons by farm type of all farms reporting injuries show that livestock operations have a higher proportion of injuries than crop operations. Other than poultry and egg operations, all livestock operations had a higher incidence of injury than their overall share of operations by farm type. For farms reporting operator injuries, field crop farms report the highest incidence of injury, with 34.0% of farms. Beef farms rank ahead of all other farm types in injuries to other family members, with 32.0% of the farms reporting them. The picture changes in the case of farms reporting injuries to other persons. After field crop farms—which report 20.1% of the injuries to other persons—are greenhouse, nursery, and floriculture operations (15.0%), likely because this farm type uses more hired labour (Statistics Canada, 2007d).

Maltais (2007) determined that nearly two agriculture injuries in five are fractures (20.70%) or open wounds (19.79%), as reported by farm operators in Canada in 2001. The majority of farm injuries (51.95%) are musculoskeletal (fractures, dislocations, sprains or strains, and back injuries). Reported injury cases are more frequent for men (4.04%) than for women (1.89%). Operators aged 66 and older have a slightly lower percentage of injuries (2.95%) than other age classes, which have fairly similar injury frequencies (varying between 3.23% and 3.76%).

When injuries occur, farm income is jeopardized because operators of small family farms are not usually covered by workers' compensation. Farm injury-prevention programs should stress gender sensitivity (e.g., women completing tasks by using machinery designed for men's generally larger bodies) by using education, regulation, or engineering approaches (Dimich-Ward et al., 2007). As well, Maltais (2007) suggested that prevention programs should focus on men under 55 years of age who work part time on their farm; primary operators of farms specializing in horse or sheep production or those who have a large cattle herd; farm operators who have more than 160 hectares under cultivation; and those who have gross farm receipts less than $500 000.

PRIMARY INDUSTRY INJURIES The most dangerous industry to work in from 1996 to 2005 was mining, quarrying, and oil wells (49.9 fatalities per 100 000 workers); followed by logging and forestry (42.9 per 100 000 workers); fishing and trapping (35.6 per 100 000 workers); agriculture (28.1 fatalities per 100 000 workers); and construction (20.6 fatalities per 100 000 workers) (Sharpe & Hardt, 2006). From 1996 to 2005, primary industry occupations had the highest fatality rate at 19.5 per 100 000 workers. Occupational health and safety programs should ensure that appropriate safety equipment is available, properly maintained, and used correctly. Such programs have done much to reduce the incidence of occupational injuries and fatalities in these primary industries.

SAFE PLAY AREAS FOR CHILDREN Agricultural injuries and fatalities are an important health issue for preschool children. Brison et al. (2006) analyzed pan-Canadian data related to fatal injuries in children aged 1 to 6 years and found that death caused by fatal farm injuries was almost double all-cause unintentional fatal injury. Three major causes were identified: being run over as a bystander, being run over as an extra rider, and drowning. The implications for providing health care include restricting preschool-age children's access to agriculture work sites and developing and delivering communication strategies to educate families as to the lethal danger exposure the work site engenders. Designated safe play areas for small children living on farms are rare but needed. Once children reach school age, statistics show a decrease in agriculture-related injuries and fatalities, until children are 10 years of age or older. At that age, many farm children begin to help with work. Schools not only provide farm children with an education but also serve to protect them from farm hazards for several hours a day.

MOTOR VEHICLE COLLISIONS When discussing motor vehicles, the ones most commonly considered are cars, trucks, and motorcycles. However, farm vehicles, such as tractors, all-terrain vehicles (ATVs), dirt bikes, and snowmobiles are also included in this category, even though they are primarily used for off-road activities. Close to 40% of all motor vehicle collisions (MVCs) occur in rural areas and small towns, and they are the most important cause of injury mortality (Pong et al., 2006). Conditions thought to affect the mortality rate of rural and northern regions include the following:

- Road conditions: narrow gravel roads, rock cuts, winter ice and snow
- High traffic speeds
- Wildlife or livestock on the roads
- Lower rates of seat belt and child restraint use
- The practice of riding in the back of open pick-up trucks
- Limited emergency medical personnel
- Greater distances to emergency medical services

In addition to the majority of collisions involving more than one vehicle, single-vehicle rollovers are common. These may be the result of high speed and loose gravel on country roads. ATV rollovers occur in the process of carrying out farm or ranch work. Numerous injuries are incurred when ATV, dirt bike, and snowmobile riders encounter barbed-wire fences, especially while travelling at high speeds. In northern areas, snowmobile mishaps are the leading cause of injury and death.

Another factor related to the increased mortality in MVCs in rural areas is the distance that must be travelled to get either the necessary resources to the person in need or the injured individual to the appropriate level of care. In trauma care, the first hour following a traumatic event is commonly referred to as the "golden hour," since the care delivered to the victim during this initial phase strongly influences patient outcome.

MVCs caused 2578 deaths in Canada in 2005, and 1606 of these were in rural areas (Transport Canada, 2005). Of those drivers who were fatally injured, most had been drinking and driving and had an average blood alcohol level of twice the legal limit. Compared with the 2578 deaths in 2005, some 4063 fatalities occurred in 1986. This decrease can be attributed to a combination of factors: better engineering of vehicles and roads, advances in medical care, increased public awareness campaigns, and education regarding traffic safety through such initiatives as Mission Possible, supported by the Canadian Automobile Association; the Heroes program from the Canadian Injury Prevention Foundation; and the Prevent Alcohol and Risk-Related Trauma in Youth (PARTY) program in Alberta and Ontario.

HEARING LOSS Many rural residents are at increased risk for noise-induced hearing loss. Working with heavy equipment, such as grain dryers, tractors, combines, and augers, can lead to intense exposure to loud noises for long periods. Pig farmers are especially at risk during feeding time when they are exposed to high-pitched squeals (Winters et al., 2005).

In addition to these occupational risks for hearing loss, rural dwellers may also suffer from presbycusis, hearing loss that accompanies aging, and sociocusis, hearing loss that results from recreational activities, such as listening to loud music or the gunshots during skeet shooting. Prevention of hearing loss and preservation of residual hearing may be accomplished through occupational health and safety education regarding these issues:

- Reducing the length of exposure to harmful noise
- Surrounding the sound with a sound-dampening enclosure
- Isolating the sound by placing a barrier around the driver, such as a tightly enclosed tractor or heavy machinery cab
- Wearing proper hearing-protection equipment (Winters et al., 2005)

Otitis media (middle-ear infection) and resultant hearing loss are endemic in Aboriginal children in Northern Canada, with the prevalence in some communities as much as 40 times greater than in urban southern communities (Bowd, 2005). Causes include increased susceptibility to infection because of immunity deficits, a decline in breastfeeding, cigarette smoke exposure, and poor diet. Hearing impairment can affect learning and literacy and have profound economic and social costs. Public health-care providers need to be informed and provide care that includes traditional knowledge and practices.

LOSS OF EYESIGHT Loss of sight and eye injuries are health concerns for both rural and urban populations. However, because of the very nature of the work performed by rural residents, more eye injuries are treated in rural acute-care facilities. Farmers, ranchers, loggers, and sawmill workers often have foreign bodies, such as gravel and wood chips, lodged in their eyes. Farmers are at increased risk of getting chemical spray in their eyes when applying a variety of fertilizers, herbicides, and pesticides. Those who work in the oil industry on the rigs or as heavy-duty mechanics require medical attention regularly for a variety of chemicals splashed into their eyes. For example, one particularly caustic substance known as "big orange" is a powerful engine degreaser that quickly causes sloughing of delicate ophthalmic tissues if it is not vigorously and immediately flushed.

Rural dwellers suffer a significant number of eye injuries from blunt trauma. These injuries occur as a result of a direct blow to the eye, such as when an animal pushes a person into a fence or throws a rider to the ground, or when a stone from a slingshot or a softball directly strikes the eye. Penetrating eye injuries are more likely to cause permanent loss of vision. When a projectile enters the eye, it may go right through or remain embedded within the globe. Examples of penetrating eye trauma include a pellet from a BB gun or a projectile, such as a solder pin, thrown off a running piece of machinery on the farm or in the oil and gas industry.

Flash burns are one of the more common injuries seen among welders. A similar type of burn also occurs when persons are in the sun for long periods without proper eye protection from UV rays. This injury can manifest as snow blindness in trappers or outfitters, especially in springtime, or in any other rural or remote-area resident who is not wearing protective eye lenses.

MENTAL HEALTH ISSUES Mental health issues are those that affect an individual's mood, behaviour, thinking, and perceptions. The problem may be the result of an organic process, such as Alzheimer's disease, or be of a functional nature, such as depression. The number of Canadians who seek care related to mental health issues is unknown (Canadian Institute for Health Information, 2001). However, the Canadian Mental Health Association (2008) notes that "20% of Canadians will personally experience a mental illness in their lifetime."

Mental health problems affect more people than does breast cancer, Alzheimer's disease, or diabetes (Alberta Health and Wellness, 1999). Even though Pong et al. (2006) reported that across Canada, suicide continues to be a major risk for rural and remote residents, their study did not find a high prevalence of depression, compared with their urban counterparts. Pong et al. suggested that this finding can be explained methodologically as the data for suicide and depression were obtained from two different sources at two different times. As well, factors such as personal stigma, visibility, and confidentiality may have affected self-reported responses to questions regarding depression. Despite stressors related to the diverse workplaces of rural residents, regional studies by Elgar, Arlett, and Groves (2003) and Patten, Stuart, Russell, Maxwell, & Arboleda-Florez (2003) confirmed that rural residents do not experience depression at a greater level than urbanites. Several factors differentiate rural mental health issues and care from urban ones and may affect whether or not residents seek care:

- The lack of infrastructure to support and mobilize resources
- Different situational variables precipitating a mental health event or crisis, such as drought conditions during which farmers are unable to produce crops
- The lack of anonymity in rural communities
- The stigma still associated with mental health problems
- Concern regarding confidentiality

PROBLEMATIC SUBSTANCE USE The onset of problematic substance use can be inadvertent and insidious. Commonly misused substances include tobacco, alcohol, opioids, and a wide range of illicit drugs, such as cannabis and hallucinogens. In addition, the inhalation of various aerosol products, glues, and gasoline is a growing problem among Canadian youth, especially in the more remote regions. One example that recently received much attention from the media was the problem of children in Davis Inlet in Labrador sniffing gasoline, while many parents were misusing alcohol.

Substance use may begin in response to curiosity, in an attempt to achieve peer approval, as is often the case with tobacco and alcohol use among youth, or as a means of achieving an altered mental state in an attempt to escape situations or events. Problematic substance use refers to the inappropriate use of prescription drugs and nonprescription drugs (including alcohol) and the use of illicit drugs.

Alcohol continues to be the primary drug leading to health-related problems (Centre for Addiction and Mental Health, 2002). Problematic alcohol use causes chronic disease, permanent disabilities, and fatalities that result from sensory and motor impairment. This, in turn, leads to a variety of traumatic injuries and deaths as a result of falls, drowning, and MVCs. Multiple social and economic factors contribute to the fact that the Canadian Aboriginal population is at increased risk of death through alcohol and suicide (Health Canada, 2001).

SUICIDE In the past decade the incidence of suicide among rural youth has increased, with the highest rate occurring among the Canadian Aboriginal population. This rate is estimated to be two to four times that of the non-Aboriginal population (Langlois & Morrison, 2002). The national suicide rates for 2000–2004 ranged from 11.3 to 11.9 per 100 000 (Statistics Canada, 2008c). In 1998, the latest year for comparative statistics, Quebec and Alberta led the country with the highest age-standardized suicide rates at 21 and 16 per 100 000 population aged 10 or older, respectively (Langlois & Morrison). Pong et al. (2006) reported that low-income single men and women in the 15 to 24 age group living in the most rural and remote communities are at greatest risk of dying from suicide, with rates four times as high for men as for women.

Factors that are believed to contribute to a high incidence of suicide are depression; problematic substance use; changing family, community, and economic dynamics; cultural changes that emphasize the valuing of increased personal freedom and heterogeneity; declining religious affiliations; and Western society's tendency to view suicide as a terminal means of problem solving. Although these factors are also influential in urban settings, rural communities tend to be more isolated from formalized health and social services. The lack of anonymity within small communities and the fear of being stigmatized with a mental health problem pressure some rural and Northern residents to keep their problems to themselves.

Special Concerns in Aboriginal Communities

The problems that exist for rural residents are magnified for those who live in First Nations communities (Health Canada, 2000). High infant morbidity and mortality and significantly higher accident and injury rates among all ages contribute to lowered life expectancies. Lack of clean water and sewage systems, inadequate housing, and high unemployment are contributing factors. Diabetes is a major health issue—the prevalence being three to five times as high as in other communities; and the death rate is six times the Canadian average (Barton, Anderson, & Thommasen, 2004). **Diabetes** is a metabolic disease in which high blood glucose levels are caused by defects in insulin secretion, action, or both. Type 2 diabetes has been found in children younger than 10 years at diagnosis (Young et al., 2002).

The most common causes of death for First Nations people aged 1 to 44 years were poisoning and injury. Children under 10 years died predominantly from unintentional injuries. Suicide and self-injury were the leading cause of death for youth and adults up to 44 years. Suicide accounted for 22% of deaths in youth and 16% in early adulthood. Potential years of life lost from injury were considerably higher than for all other causes of death and close to 3.5 times that for the general Canadian population. MVCs were a leading cause of death for all First Nations age groups. Circulatory disease was the main cause of death for the First Nations aged 45 years and older (Health Canada, 2000). Social disruption, lack of hope for the future, problematic substance use, and family violence have all been suggested as underlying or related factors for suicide. Efforts to combat these problems include community mobilization and awareness campaigns.

Kirmayer, Simpson, and Cargo (2003) suggested that even though direct causal links are a challenge to show quantitatively, obvious and convincing evidence shows that a long history of cultural oppression and marginalization has played a role in the high levels of mental health problems found in many Aboriginal communities. On the positive side, evidence also shows that fortifying an ethnocultural sense of identity, community unity, and political empowerment can assist in improving mental health in Aboriginal communities. Mental health promotion that emphasizes youth and community empowerment through individual and community-based initiatives, as well as larger political and cultural processes, is likely to have broad effects on mental health and general well-being in Aboriginal communities.

Tradition and healing are central to current efforts by Aboriginal peoples to confront historical injustices and suffering brought on by **colonialism**, when European settlers arrived in Canada and assumed control of the land and its resources. Aboriginal peoples in Canada are involved in healing their own traditions, repairing the ruptures and discontinuity in the sharing of traditional knowledge and values, and asserting their collective identity and power (Kirmayer et al., 2003).

According to Llewellyn (2002), residential schools were established by the Canadian government in the late nineteenth century and were in operation until the 1980s to provide education to First Nations children. They were administered by Christian churches: Methodist (United Church of Canada), Presbyterian, Anglican, and several Roman Catholic orders. The policies by which the schools were run came from the Canadian government; however, day-to-day management lay with the religious organizations. The government used these schools to implement its policy of assimilation. "Settlers demanded that the colonial government respond to the so called Indian problem," which arose with the arrival and spread of British settlers into First Nations lands (p. 256). The idea behind the assimilation policy was to integrate First Nations into the settlers' culture, and the most expedient way to do this was through the establishment of schools and the enforcement of the English language as the only mode of communication. These schools created and enforced situations that led to detachment, humiliation, and feelings of helplessness and powerlessness (Dyck, 1997; Knockwood, 1992). The removal of children from their families; the destruction of First Nations languages, culture, and spirituality; and the physical and emotional abuse the children endured are at the core of many of the health and social challenges that face First Nations and their communities today.

Llewellyn (2002) presents arguments in support of and against the use of litigation to resolve the more than 100 years of abuse perpetrated by the policies and practices of residential schools. Llewellyn introduces and makes a case for **restorative justice**, an approach to justice that involves righting the wrong, as much as possible, through reconciliation, healing, and building peace within communities, which builds on and learns from the successes and failures of the South African Truth and Reconciliation Commission. "The idea of such a process has been supported by a variety of groups, including the

Royal Commission on Aboriginal Peoples, the Assembly of First Nations, the Law Commission of Canada and several of the church organizations implicated in residential school cases" (p. 289). Health-care providers working in rural, remote, and isolated communities must be knowledgeable about this issue and the impact it has had on the culture, spirituality, health, and well-being of Aboriginal people. Health-care workers must also be able to provide culturally safe care.

Health-Care Delivery

Health-Care Delivery Issues

Many factors contribute to making the delivery of appropriate and cost-effective health services to rural, remote, and Northern populations a challenge (see Box 14.3). Accessibility to equitable health-care services is at the heart of health-care delivery issues. A major factor is the need to deliver a variety of health services to a population that is sparsely distributed over a large geographical area, with a limited number of health-care professionals. Current and impending shortages of health-care professionals will only exacerbate an already challenging health human resources problem (MacLeod et al., 2004; Pong & Russell, 2003; Rukholm, 2006). The inclusion of health issues of rural, remote, and Northern residents within general statistics contributes to difficulties in being able to focus on specific concerns affecting these populations. The recent work of Pong et al. (2006) was a beginning step in addressing the challenge of adequate and useful statistical data to affect health-care policy and practice in rural, remote, and isolated communities across Canada. Hanlon and Halseth (2005) provided a regional analysis highlighting the challenges of service delivery and raising policy questions for an aging population in rural and remote locations in British Columbia.

BOX 14.3 NURSING AND HEALTH-CARE DELIVERY ISSUES

Nursing in rural and remote areas can be affected by a number of delivery issues:

- Data gaps and inadequate information about the health status of rural residents
- Distance
- Sparse population
- Limited infrastructure, including transportation and communication
- Limited health-care resources and access to technology
- Educational preparation for generalist-specialist practice
- Recruitment and retention of professionals
- Ethical issues (lack of anonymity, confidentiality, resources)
- Changing demographics and care requirements of the community

Health-care providers in rural, remote, and Northern areas must possess a broad generalized knowledge base to meet the diverse health-care needs of the residents. **Interdisciplinary or interprofessional approaches**, in which nurses interact with many other health-care professionals from all areas, have been suggested as one way to increase the effectiveness of health-care delivery (MacLeod et al. 2004). MacLeod et al. suggested that nurses working in rural, remote, and Northern communities often interact with other health-care professionals at a distance. These researchers further stated that "new models of interprofessional practice can be developed that are supportive of the varied strengths of and resources available to rural and remote communities" (p. 4). Hayward (2005) described the facilitation of interdisciplinary practice through the provision of a mobile service to older adults in rural seniors' centres and in the home by students and faculty in nursing, physical therapy, occupational therapy, pharmacy, and dietetics, as well as other disciplines.

Halseth and Williams (1999) described one rural community's approach to community participation and empowerment in decision making and health-care delivery through the establishment of a community-based resource centre for health and wellness. Community participation involved local residents in defining the health and social services for their community—a different approach from the usual traditional delivery of health care.

RURAL, REMOTE, AND NORTHERN NURSING PRACTICE Nurses practise in multiple settings in rural, remote, and Northern sites; they provide acute and extended care, community health services, home care, occupational health services, and mental health services, and, in some provinces and territories, they are taking on **expanded practice** roles, in which nursing goes beyond the traditional nursing roles. Often, these nurses, especially in remote communities, work alone (MacLeod et al., 2004).

Nursing Practice Issues

In the past the majority of research regarding rural and remote nursing has come from Australia and the United States. During the last few years, there has been an explosion of Canadian research focusing on rural nursing practice (Kulig, Nahachewsky, Thomlinson, MacLeod, & Curran, 2004; Leipert & Reutter, 2003; Paluck, Allerdings, Kealy, & Dorgan, 2006; Thomlinson et al., 2004), nurses (Kulig, et al., 2003; MacLeod et al., 2004; Stewart et al., 2005), nurse practitioners (Way, Jones, Baskerville, & Busing, 2001), and nursing education and professional development (Kosteniuk, D'Arcy, Stewart, & Smith, 2006; Rukholm, 2004). Issues that arose in the

Evidence-Informed Practice

How Do Nurses Define Rural Nursing Practice?

Kulig et al. (2008) surveyed 3933 registered nurses (RNs) to identify how they defined *rurality*. These RNs were sampled randomly from the Canadian population of nurses by using a Statistics Canada definition of rurality. In addition, the sample included RNs working in outpost settings and in the territories. Four themes emerged from content analysis of the data: community characteristics, geographical location, human and technical resources, and nursing practice characteristics. Community characteristics had both positive (lifestyle) and challenging (access to facilities and services) aspects. The researchers suggested that their findings challenge the idea of "developing a national numerical index of rurality based on distance to services" (p. 31). Accessibility of human and technological resources was evident across definitions of rurality, no matter the location. Nursing practice characteristics in rural settings had both positive and negative attributes, such as "independence" versus "lack of supports" (p. 31).

NURSING IMPLICATIONS: The implications of rurality for nurses included being very cognizant of the "content areas that describe rural communities, geographical location, health human and technological resources and the characteristics of nursing practice." Study findings highlighted the importance of calling attention to the positive elements of both rural communities and rural nursing practice for the recruitment of RNs (p. 31).

Source: Based on "How Do Registered Nurses Define Rurality?" by J. Kulig et al., 2008, *Australian Journal of Rural Health, 16*(1), pp. 28–32.

MacLeod et al. (2004) pan-Canadian study of rural nursing practice and rural nurses included the following:

- Managers and policymakers need to better understand the realities of rural and remote practice to develop a "rural lens" that could be used as part of a pan-Canadian rural and remote nursing strategy.
- Nurses' personal and professional roles are inseparable in small communities.
- Many rural nurses work alone, indicating a need for at-a-distance, face-to-face, and technological supports.
- Understanding of nurses and their partnerships with their communities could aid recruitment and retention.
- Support for new ways of interprofessional practice is essential.
- Particular attention must be paid to and support given to nurses in Aboriginal communities to provide culturally competent, appropriate care.
- Retirement and migration need to be addressed by providing relevant continuing education.
- The distinctiveness of rural and remote nursing practice cannot be captured until unique personal identifiers are created along with relevant urban rural indicators (MacLeod et al., 2004, p. v).

Rural nursing in Canada has lacked a consistent definition and has not yet been formally recognized as a distinct specialized area of nursing practice (Rennie, Baird-Crooks, Remus, & Engels, 2000). Although some claim that the only difference between rural and urban nursing is the environment in which nursing is practised, others disagree. Scharff (1998) claims that rural nursing is distinctive in terms of "its boundaries, intersections, dimensions, and even its very core" (p. 20). Describing the core of nursing as care and the unique relationship between the nurse and the patient, Scharff is adamant that "what happens at the core of rural nursing is something apart from what happens at the core of nursing anywhere else" (p. 20). This caring is based on interpersonal knowledge of the patients and clients, their families, and their communities, as well as the relationship that exists between the nurses and their co-workers.

In 2001, nursing researchers from across Canada, in collaboration with a geographer, began a major study on the nature of rural and remote nursing. Stewart et al. (2005) and MacLeod et al. (2004) made admirable progress in this regard and also provided direction for education, research, and practice pertaining to rural and remote nursing. With regard to research utilization or knowledge transfer, work by Olade (2003) found that less than one quarter of the 106 rural nurses she surveyed had favourable attitudes toward the use of nursing research in practice. These findings point to the need to establish and sustain linkages between researchers and rural nurses, in particular, for distance research, research relevance to practice issues, and practitioner knowledge about research. Even though some caution regarding the findings is advised, since the instrument used by Olade to measure research utilization has been critiqued for lack of construct validity and inadequate reliability by Frasure (2008), the findings are important and should be studied further.

Rural nurses in Canada, the United States, and Australia share many common characteristics. Nurses are often described as highly visible members of the community, resourceful, flexible, autonomous, self-reliant, and effective team members (MacLeod et al., 2004). Above all else, rural nurses are described as *generalists* and *specialist-generalists*. The need to maintain general practice skills covering all ages and all the conditions that clients or patients can present with is a major challenge for rural nurses.

The high visibility of the nurse in the community (a key factor that affects nursing practice) and the resultant lack of anonymity mean that nurses may never be off duty and may be consulted by friends and neighbours wherever they go (MacLeod et al., 2004; Nickel, 2004). This lack of anonymity presents particular problems when these same friends and neighbours present with injuries and life-threatening illnesses. Other characteristics of rural practice are the following:

- Greater autonomy because there are fewer nurses and other health professionals
- Greater knowledge of the client's or patient's home and family conditions
- Closer interface with other health-care professionals
- Greater opportunity to affect health-care planning and policy at the local level because of the recognized role as a resource on health care and the prominence in the community

EDUCATION FOR RURAL AND REMOTE PRACTICE

As early as 1975, a course in rural hospital nursing was offered at the Foothills Hospital School of Nursing in Calgary (Reimer & Mills, 1988). Across the country, some undergraduate nursing programs are beginning to include theory and clinical practice specific to rural nursing in their curricula. Other programs continue to use rural placements as practicum sites, with a lesser emphasis placed on the setting itself. The recruitment and retention of nurses for practise in rural, remote, and Northern regions of Canada have been persistent problems, and these continue to grow in importance (MacLeod et al., 2004; O'Brien-Pallas, Alksnis, & Wang, 2003; Rukholm et al., 2006). It is anticipated that with the projected national nursing shortage, an even greater emphasis on preparing and attracting nurses to practise in these areas will be needed. Nursing leaders and educators have a role in the education and psychological preparation of nurses to work in these diverse settings. It is essential that more nursing students be educated to practise in rural and remote acute-care and community settings.

Postdiploma education for Northern, remote, and expanded practice nursing has a somewhat longer history. The Dalhousie Outpost Nursing (OPN) program began in 1967 with a mandate to educate nurses for the roles and responsibilities inherent in nursing practice in Northern and remote Canadian communities. The OPN program closed in 1997 when federal funding was withdrawn and reallocated to regional initiatives (Martin-Misener, Vuckic, & May, 1999). Although the number of programs being offered across the country for nurses working in rural, remote, and Aboriginal communities has increased, not enough nurses are graduating from nursing programs to fill the gaps left by retirements and migration (O'Brien-Pallas et al., 2003; Pong & Russell, 2003; Rukholm et al., 2006). New programs have recently emerged from many universities. One example is the University of Northern British Columbia, which is offering a one-year certificate program in rural and Northern nursing for experienced registered nurses, with an option to complete an undergraduate degree in nursing. As well, a graduate program with a focus on rural and Northern nursing is offered through a blended-mode (face to face and internet) delivery at Laurentian University in Northern Ontario. Laurentian also offers a unique interdisciplinary program at the doctoral level in rural and Northern health, focusing on health services and health policy. Aboriginal nursing–specific programs are reported by 8 of the 91 Canadian Association of Schools of Nursing members (Gregory, 2007).

TELEHEALTH AND RURAL AND REMOTE PRACTICE

Telehealth (the sharing of nursing information by using electronic means, such as a telephone or the internet, to answer consumers' questions), **telemedicine** (the use of technology to transmit electronic medical data about clients to persons at distant locations), and blended-mode learning (a combination of face to face, videoconferencing, internet, paper-based, and web casting) have mushroomed with technological advances and increased access to high-speed internet connections and videoconferencing capacity (Atack, 2003; Atack & Rankin, 2002; Carter & Rukholm, 2002; Carter et al., 2006; Pong & Russell, 2003; Rukholm et al., 2006).

Jennett and Andruchuk (2001) identified practical issues specific to the successful integration of telehealth into the Canadian system at national, regional, provincial, and territorial levels. Five critical issues for the best possible implementation of telehealth programs are environment readiness; needs-based planning with an array of different partnerships; technological equipment; phased application; and evaluation. Application of change theory and the transformation of the culture of teaching and learning are also important. Consideration of sustainability, technological supports, and attention to best practices, lessons learned, buy-in, and so on, are all important to the success and sustainability of telehealth programs (Hogenbirk, Montgomery, Boydell, Pong, & Cudney, 2006; Ohinmaa, Hailey, & Roine, 2001).

Russell and Perris (2003) reported on a 6-month telementoring initiative in a Canadian community nursing agency. The online discussions focused on collaborative learning and professional development that showed improved asynchronous communication and problem-solving skills as a result of online discussions and fostered "communal opportunistic learning and professional development" (p. 227).

Case Study 14

Mr. Donaldson is a 45-year-old farmer who presented to the emergency department with cellulitis in his right leg, secondary to a puncture wound from the tine of a pitchfork. He runs a family grain-and-cattle operation about 50 kilometres from town and the nearest hospital. He is given the choice of being admitted to hospital or returning to hospital every eight hours for a one-hour antibiotic treatment and for a daily dressing change. He is told he must limit his activity and keep his leg elevated as much as possible.

Critical Thinking Questions

1. What issues should the nurse discuss with Mr. Donaldson to assist him in choosing his treatment options?
2. How might the patient's regime vary from that in an urban setting?
3. How might Mr. Donaldson's occupation influence his recovery?
4. What health-care delivery issues common to rural and remote residents affect Mr. Donaldson's treatment?

After working through these questions, go to the MyNursingLab at **http://www.mynursinglab.com** to check your answers.

KEY TERMS

rural
agriculture
natural resources
remote
isolation
policy
Northern
place
equitable health care
Aboriginal population
circulatory diseases
respiratory diseases
injuries
suicide
arthritis
diabetes
colonialism
restorative justice
interdisciplinary or interprofessional approaches
expanded practice
telehealth
telemedicine

CHAPTER HIGHLIGHTS

- Consensus on clear, comprehensive definitions for *rural*, *remote*, and *Northern* areas is required to allow for data collection on health-care information of residents in these regions of the country.
- Great diversity in the geography of Canada contributes to particular regional issues.
- Rural and remote residents have higher infant mortality, lower life expectancy, and higher rates of injuries and death than urban residents.
- Common health concerns include respiratory illnesses, chemical exposures, circulatory diseases, hearing and sight problems, and zoonoses.
- Water safety concerns include the contamination of drinking water supplies and drowning in ditches, dugouts, rivers, and lakes.
- Injuries and deaths within rural and remote primary industries are a significant factor in the health care of rural populations.
- Children are at particular risk for injury or death because of the lack of designated safe play areas for young children.
- Numerous factors contribute to high mortality rates from motor vehicle collisions.
- Social and economic factors contribute to increased mortality and morbidity within the Aboriginal population in Canada.
- Challenges to health-service delivery are sparse population, distance, and difficulties in recruiting and retaining health-care professionals.
- Knowledge about the impact of residential schools on the culture, spirituality, health, and well-being of Aboriginal people must be considered in the delivery of culturally safe health care.
- A major challenge for rural nurses is to attain and maintain practice skills for providing care for all ages and health conditions.
- Key characteristics of rural and remote practice are lack of anonymity, greater autonomy, and broad generalist practice.

ASSESS YOUR LEARNING

1. Rural communities are characterized by which of the following?
   a. Lower incomes and generally higher rates of cancer as compared with urban centres
   b. A range of incomes and generally lower rates of cancer as compared with urban centres
   c. Higher incomes and cancer rates generally similar to urban communities
   d. Lower incomes and cancer rates similar to urban communities in general

2. Originally, the Canadian economy was mainly which of the following?
   a. Agrarian, natural-resource based, and rural
   b. An even blend of rural agrarian and urban industry
   c. Urban with some agriculture and industry
   d. Urban based on a skilled knowledge industry
3. For which of the following reasons have rural populations declined in the past century?
   a. Few new immigrants choose to live in rural areas.
   b. Rural Aboriginal populations are not increasing.
   c. Urban residents have a higher birth rate than rural residents.
   d. An increase in farming technology means there is less rural opportunity.
4. Which of the following are the main causes of mortality in rural and Northern communities?
   a. Motor vehicle collisions, respiratory diseases, suicide, and circulatory diseases
   b. Injuries, poisonings, arthritis, and cancer
   c. Cardiovascular disease, cancer, arthritis, and accidents
   d. Injuries, suicide, circulatory and respiratory diseases
5. You are the nurse in a rural First Nations community in Northern Ontario. Lately, there have been a number of serious motor vehicle collisions, including one that killed four local teenagers. Problematic substance use was part of the causes of the accidents. What should be your next step?
   a. Approach the local high school to lecture on the dangers of smoking and substance use
   b. Approach the local high school and invite students to participate in a quit smoking contest you have designed
   c. Meet with a group of local teenagers and community elders and work with them to develop a video game they created on stopping drinking and driving
   d. Meet with the high school principal to tell him or her about the dangers of substance use, drinking, and fatal accidents
6. As a nurse working in a rural and remote community in Saskatchewan, you know that farm injuries are a major health issue. Preschool children are particularly at high risk of fatal injuries. You have been approached by the wife of a local farmer who wants you to help her organize a safe play area for preschool children. What should be your next step?
   a. Arrange to meet with the farmers at a local fall fair to talk with them about the hazards of farming
   b. Post signs in the community about farm hazards and invite parents to come to a meeting
   c. Talk to the town mayor, the school principal, and other civic leaders, along with parents, and tell them they must recognize farm hazards for children
   d. Invite parents, teachers, the school principal, the mayor, and other civic leaders to a meeting to talk about safe play areas for preschool children
7. Following a detached retina, Mr. Boucher, 78 years old and a retired farmer, must adapt to his blindness while continuing to live in the country with his wife. What factor should the nurse consider to help them rearrange the inside of their house?
   a. The distance separating the couple from their neighbours
   b. The family's beliefs
   c. The availability of resources
   d. Mrs. Boucher's level of literacy
8. You are the new nurse working alone in an Aboriginal community that is experiencing a high incidence of suicide. You have read about the effects of colonization and the resultant marginalization experienced by everyone in the community. You would decide to do which of the following?
   a. Post signs warning Aboriginal youth in the community about the dangers of alcohol
   b. Meet with the elders in the community to ask for their advice on how to proceed with a community plan to work with the seniors who experienced colonization
   c. Meet with the elders in the community to ask their advice on how to work with 15- to 19-year-olds for a community suicide-prevention plan
   d. Call your supervisor, and if she can't help, call the local family physician for advice
9. Providing health care to inhabitants of rural and remote communities experiencing motor vehicle collisions is challenging because of which of the following?
   a. So many new immigrants live in rural communities.
   b. The primary industries are fishing, farming, mining, and forestry.
   c. The population is sparsely distributed over a wide geographical area.
   d. The nurse must be flexible and friendly with local inhabitants.
10. Children in Northern Aboriginal communities are at increased risk for type 2 diabetes. As the nurse in the community, you want to raise awareness about this health risk. What should be your next step?
   a. Talk with the teenagers in the community because they may have younger siblings
   b. Meet with the school principal and launch a poster contest featuring student-drawn pictures of healthy foods
   c. Ask the children to draw pictures of their healthy community and post these on the walls
   d. Ask the children to draw and post pictures of healthy foods that come from their community

After working through these questions, go to the MyNursingLab at ***http://www.mynursinglab.com*** *to check your answers and see explanations.*

SUGGESTED READINGS

Winters, C., & Lee, H. (Eds.). (2006). *Rural nursing: Concepts, theory, and practice.* New York: Springer Publishing.

This text represents 30 years of work by nurse academics at Montana State University. A conceptual framework for rural nursing practices that draws together research, theory, and stories from rural nursing practice is presented. The authors formulate a basis for comprehending the special elements of rural nursing and health.

WEBLINKS

Canadian Association for Rural and Remote Nursing

http://www.carrn.com

The site provides access to the Canadian Association for Rural and Remote Nursing. The association is meant to be a voice for rural and remote nursing and to promote the speciality.

Centre for Rural and Northern Health Research

http://www.cranhr.ca

This research centre has two sites: one at Lakehead University in Thunder Bay, Ontario, and the other at Laurentian University in Sudbury, Ontario.

Canadian Rural Health Research Society

http://crhrs-scrsr.usask.ca

The Canadian Rural Health Research Society offers the opportunity for researchers engaged in rural, remote, and Northern health research to network with researchers of many disciplines.

Government of Canada: Canadian Rural Partnership

http://www.rural.gc.ca/home_e.phtml

This site provides access to knowledge, information, programs, and services for and about rural and remote Canada.

International Council of Nurses Rural and Remote Nurses Network

http://www.icn.ch/rrn_network.htm

This site provides a global forum for discussing issues related to rural and remote nursing.

NurseONE

http://www.nurseone.ca

Developed by the Canadian Nurses Association with support from the First Nations and Inuit Health Branch of Health Canada, NurseONE is a source of reliable information systematically organized for nurses. It includes important nursing links to nursing in First Nations and Inuit communities, health news, other news sources, and much more.

Health Canada: Office of Nursing Services

http://www.hc-sc.gc.ca/ahc-asc/branch-dirgen/fnihb-dgspni/ons-bsi/index_e.html

This office provides support to the First Nations and Inuit Health Branch of Health Canada.

Society of Rural Physicians of Canada

http://www.srpc.ca

The Society of Rural Physicians of Canada (SRPC) is the national voice of Canadian rural physicians. Founded in 1992, the SRPC's mission is to provide leadership for rural physicians and to promote sustainable conditions and equitable health care for rural communities. The site provides information about the society and its resources.

The Development of a Multistakeholder Framework/Index of Rurality

http://cna-aiic.ca/CNA/documents/pdf/publications/Final_Report_e.pdf

This report describes the rural health framework developed by the Canadian Nurses Association (CNA) and the Canadian Medical Association.

REFERENCES

Acury, T., Gesler, W., Preisser, J. L., Sherman, J., Spencer, J., & Perrin, J. (2005). The effects of geography and spatial behavior on health care utilization among the residents of a rural region. *Health Services Research, 40*(1), 135–155.

Agriculture and Food, Alberta. (2007). *Bovine spongiform encephalopathy (BSE) fact sheet.* Retrieved May, 2007, from http://www1.agric.gov.ab.ca/$department/deptdocs.nsf/all/cpv8104?opendocument

Alasia, A., & Rothwell, N. (2004). The rural/urban divide is not changing: Income disparities persist. *Rural and Small Town Canada Analysis Bulletin, 4*(4).

Alberta Health and Wellness. (1999). *Report on the health of Albertans: Looking through a wider lens.* Edmonton, AB: Government of Alberta, Alberta Health and Wellness.

Andrews, G. (2006). Geographies of health in nursing. *Health & Place, 12,* 110–118.

Angus, J., Kontos, P., Dyck, I., McKeever, P., & Poland, B. (2005). The personal significance of home: Habitus and the experience of receiving long-term home care. *Sociology of Health & Illness, 27*(2), 161–187.

Appleyard, G. D., & Gajadhar, A. A. (2000). A review of trichinellosis in people and wildlife in Canada. *Canadian Journal of Public Health, 91,* 293–297.

Arbuckle, T. E., Bruce, D., Ritter, L., & Hall, J. C. (2006). Indirect sources of herbicide exposure for families on Ontario farms. *Journal of Exposure Science and Environmental Epidemiology, 16,* 98–104.

Atack, L. (2003). Becoming a web-based learner: Registered nurses experiences. *Journal of Advanced Nursing, 44*(3), 289–297.

Atack, L., & Rankin, J. (2002). A descriptive study of registered nurses' experiences with web-based learning. *Journal of Advanced Nursing, 40*(2), 457–465.

Barnett, F., & McLean, G. (2005). Care management of Creutzfeldt-Jakob disease within the United Kingdom. *Journal of Nursing Management, 13,* 111–118.

Barton, S., Anderson, N., & Thommasen, H. (2004). The diabetes experiences of Aboriginal people living in a rural Canadian community. *Australian Journal of Rural Health, 13,* 242–246.

Bowd, A. D. (2005). Otitis media: Health and social consequences for Aboriginal youth in Canada's North. *International Journal of Circumpolar Health, 64*(1), 5–15.

Brison, R., Pickett, W., Berg, W., Linneman, J., Zentner, J., & Marlenga, B. (2006). Fatal agricultural injuries in preschool children: Risks, injury patterns and strategies for prevention. *Canadian Medical Association Journal, 174*(12), 1723–1726.

Bushy, A. (2000). Behavioral health care: Rural issues and strategies. In A. Bushy (Ed.), *Orientation to nursing in the rural community* (pp. 107–123). Thousand Oaks, CA: Sage Publications.

Canadian Food Inspection Agency. (2005). *Technical overview of BSE in Canada—March 2005.* Retrieved May 16, 2007, http://www.inspection.gc.ca/english/anima/heasan/disemala/bseesb/200503canadae.shtml

Canadian Institute for Health Information. (2001). *Health care in Canada.* Ottawa: Canadian Institute for Health Information and Statistics Canada.

Canadian Mental Health Association. (2008). *Fast facts: Mental health/mental illness.* Retrieved May 16, 2008, from http://www.cmha.ca/bins/content_page.asp?cid=6-20-23-43

Carolan, M., Andrews, G., & Hodnett, E. (2006). Writing place: A comparison of nursing research and health geography. *Nursing Inquiry, 13*(3), 203–219.

Carter, L., & Rukholm, E. (2002). Online scholarly discourse: Lessons learned for continuing and nurse educators. *Canadian Journal of University Continuing Education, 28*(2), 33–50.

Carter, L., Rukholm, E., Mossey, S., Viverais-Dresler, G., Bakker, D., & Sheehan, C. (2006). Critical thinking in the online nursing educational setting: Raising the bar. *Canadian Journal of University Continuing Education, 32*(1), 27–46.

Centre for Addiction and Mental Health. (2002). *Alcohol, tobacco and other drug use among Ontario students.* Sheet #2. Toronto: Author.

Charrois, J., Graham, D., Hrudey, S., & Froese, K. (2004). Disinfection by-products in small Alberta community drinking water supplies. *Journal of Toxicology and Environmental Health, 67,* 1797–1803.

Davies, G., Day, R., & Williamson, S. (2004). The geography of health knowledge/s (Editorial). *Health & Place, 10,* 293–297.

Dimich-Ward, H., Guernsey, J. R., Pickett, W., Rennie, D., Hartling, L., & Brison, R. J. (2007). Gender differences in the occurrence of farm related injuries. *Occupational and Environmental Medicine, 61,* 52–56.

du Plessis, V., Beshiri, R., Bollman, R. D., & Clemenson, H. (2001). Definitions of rural. *Rural and Small Town Canada Analysis Bulletin, 3*(3).

Dyck, N. (1997). *Differing visions: Administering Indian residential schooling in Prince Albert 1867–1995.* Halifax, NS: Fernwood Publishing.

Elgar, F., Arlet, C., & Groves, R. (2003). Stress, coping and behavioral problems among rural and urban adolescents. *Journal of Adolescence, 26,* 574–585.

Frasure, J. (2008). Analysis of instruments measuring nurses' attitudes towards research utilization: A systematic review. *Journal of Advanced Nursing, 61*(1), 5–15.

Gregory, D. (2007). *Against the odds: An update on Aboriginal nursing in Canada.* Report funded by Canadian Association of Schools of Nursing under the auspices of Health Canada (First Nations and Inuit Health Branch). Lethbridge, AB: University of Lethbridge.

Halseth, G., & Williams, A. (1999). Guthrie House: A rural community organizing for wellness. *Health & Place, 5,* 27–44.

Hanlon, N., & Halseth, G. (2005). The greying of resource communities in northern British Columbia: Implications for health care delivery in already-underserviced communities. *Canadian Geographer, 49*(1), 1–24.

Hayward, K. (2005). Facilitating interdisciplinary practice through mobile service provision to the rural older adult. *Geriatric Nursing, 26*(1), 29–33.

Health Canada. (2000). *Highlights of First Nations health statistics: Statistical profile on the health of First Nations in Canada for the year 2000.* Retrieved September 14, 2008, from http://www.hc-sc.gc.ca/fniah-spnia/pubs/abor-autoch/stats_profil_eng.php

Health Canada. (2001). *Preventing substance use problems among young people—A compendium of best practices.* Retrieved June 2, 2007, http://www.hc-sc.gc.ca/hl-vs/pubs/adp-apd/prevent/pattern-tendance_e.html

Hogenbirk, J., Montgomery, P., Boydell, K., Pong, R., & Cudney, D. (2006). *Using telehealth to augment delivery of mental health services by family health teams: Potential barriers and possible solutions: Final report.* Sudbury, ON: Centre for Rural and Northern Health Research. Retrieved May 16, 2007, from http://www.cranhr.ca/onlrpts.html#TMH

Jennett, P., & Andruchuk, K. (2001). Telehealth: "Real life" implementation issues. *Computer Methods and Programs in Biomedicine, 64,* 169–174.

Kelly, S. (2003). Bioethics and rural health: Theorizing place, space, and subjects. *Social Science and Medicine, 56,* 2277–2288.

Kirmayer, L., Simpson, C., & Cargo, M. (2003). Healing traditions: Culture, community and mental health promotion with Canadian Aboriginal peoples. *Australasian Psychiatry, 11*(S1), 15–23.

Knockwood, I. (1992). *Out of the depths: The experience of Mi'kmaw children at the Indian residential school at Shubenacadie, Nova Scotia.* Lockeport, NS: Roseway Publishing.

Kosteniuk, J., D'Arcy, C., Stewart, N., & Smith, B. (2006). Central and peripheral information source use among rural and remote registered nurses. *Journal of Advanced Nursing, 55*(1), 100–114.

Kulig, J., Thomlinson, E., Curran, F., Nahachewsky, D., MacLeod, M., Stewart, N., et al. (2003). *Rural and remote nursing practice: An analysis of policy documents.* Retrieved May 16, 2007, from http://www.ruralnursing.unbc.ca/reports/jkulig/jkulig_report.php

Kulig, J., Nahachewsky, D., Thomlinson, E., MacLeod, M., & Curran, F. (2004). Maximizing the involvement of rural nurses in policy. *Canadian Journal of Nursing Leadership, 17*(1), 88–96.

Kulig, J., Andrews, M., Stewart, N., Pitblado, R., MacLeod, M., Bentham, D., et al. (2008). How do rural nurses define rurality? *Australian Journal of Rural Health, 16*(1), 28–32.

Langlois, S., & Morrison, P. (2002). Suicide deaths and suicide attempts. *Health Reports, 13*(2), 9–22.

Leipert, B., & Reutter, L. (2003). Women's health in northern British Columbia: The role of geography and gender. *Canadian Journal of Rural Medicine, 10*(4), 241–253.

Leipert, B., & Reutter, L. (2005). Developing resilience: How women maintain their health in northern geographically isolated settings. *Qualitative Health Research, 15*(1), 49–65.

Llewlleyn, J. (2002). Dealing with the legacy of native residential school abuse in Canada: Litigation, ADR, and restorative justice. *University of Toronto Law Journal, 52*, 253–300.

Lochhaas, T. (Ed.). (1987). *Mosby's medical dictionary* (2nd ed.). Toronto: Mosby.

MacLeod, M., Kulig, J., Stewart, N., Pitblado, R., Banks, K., D'Arcy, C., et al. (2004). *The nature of nursing practice in rural and remote Canada.* Ottawa: Canadian Health Services Research Foundation.

Magnusson, E., & Alasia, A. (2004). Occupational patterns with industry groups: A rural-urban comparison. *Rural and Small Town Canada Analysis Bulletin, 5*(6).

Malone, R. E. (2003). Distal nursing. *Social Science and Medicine, 56*(11), 2317–2326.

Maltais, V. (2007). Risk factors associated with farm injuries in Canada 1991 to 2001. *Agriculture and Rural Working Paper Series.* Ottawa: Agriculture Division, Statistics Canada.

Martin-Misener, R., Vuckic, A., & May, R. (1999). Lessons learned from the Dalhousie Outpost Nursing program. In W. Ramp, J. Kulig, I. Townsend, & V. McGowan (Eds.), *Health in rural settings: Contexts for action* (pp. 203–210). Lethbridge, AB: University of Lethbridge Press.

McNiven, C. (1999). North is that direction. *Canadian Social Trends* (Autumn), 8–11. Ottawa: Statistics Canada.

Mitura, V., & Bollman, R. (2003). The health of rural Canadians: A rural-urban comparison of health indicators. *Rural and Small Town Canada Analysis Bulletin, 4*(6), 1–23.

Mitura, V., & Bollman, R. (2004). Health status and behaviours of Canada's youth: A rural-urban comparison. *Rural and Small Town Canada Analysis Bulletin, 5*(3), 1–22.

Nickel, M-B. (2004). Professional boundaries: The dilemma of dual and multiple relationships in rural clinical practice. *Counseling and Clinical Psychology Journal, 1*(1), 17–22.

O'Brien-Pallas, L., Alksnis, C., & Wang, S. (2003). *Bringing the future into focus: Projecting RN retirement in Canada.* Ottawa: Canadian Institute for Health Information.

Ohinmaa, A., Hailey, D., & Roine, R. (2001). Elements for assessment of telemedicine applications. *International Journal of Technology Assessment in Health Care, 17*(2), 190–202.

Olade, R. A. (2003). Attitudes and factors affecting research utilization. *Nursing Forum, 38*(4), 5–15.

Paluck, E., Allerdings, M., Kealy, K., & Dorgan, H. (2006). Health promotion needs of women living in rural areas: An exploratory study. *Canadian Journal of Rural Medicine, 11*(92), 111–116.

Pampalon, R., Martinez, J., & Hamel, D. (2006). Does living in rural areas make a difference for health in Quebec? *Health & Place, 12,* 421–435.

Patten, S., Stuart, H., Russell, M., Maxwell, C., & Arboleda-Florez, J. (2003). Epidemiology of major depression in a predominantly rural health region. *Social Psychiatry Psychiatric Epidemiology, 38,* 360–365.

Pong, R., & Russell, N. (2003). *A review and synthesis of strategies and policy recommendations on the rural health workforce.* Retrieved May, 16, 2007, from http://www.laurentian.ca/Laurentian/Home/Departments/CRaNHR/reports.htm

Pong, R., DesMeules, M., Legace, C., Heng, D., Manuel, D., Pitblado, R., et al. (2006). *How healthy are rural Canadians? An assessment of their health status and health determinants.* Ottawa: Canadian Institutes for Health Information.

Pong, R. (2007). *Rural poverty and health: What do we know?* Paper presented to the Standing Senate Committee on Agriculture and Forestry. Ottawa, ON.

Racher, F., & Vollman, A. (2002). Exploring dimensions of access to health services: Implications for nursing research and practice. *Research and Theory for Nursing Practice: An International Journal, 16*(2), 77–90.

Reimer, M., & Mills, C. (1988). Rural hospital nursing as an elective. *Journal of Rural Health, 4*(2), 5–8.

Rennie, D., Baird-Crooks, K., Remus, G., & Engel, J. (2000). Rural nursing in Canada. In A. Bushy (Ed.), *Orientation to nursing in the rural community* (pp. 217–231). Thousand Oaks, CA: Sage.

Rukholm, E. (2004). Professional development opportunities. In L. McGillis Hall (Ed.), *Quality work environments for nurse and patient safety* (pp. 163–180). Sudbury, MA: Jones & Bartlett.

Rukholm, E. (2006). *Recruitment and retention of RNs and RPNs in Northeastern Ontario.* A report for the Nursing Secretariat, Ontario Ministry of Health and Long-Term Care. Toronto: Ministry of Health and Long-Term Care. Available at the CRaNHR website at http://www.cranhr.ca/

Rukholm, E., Carter, L., Librion-Grenier, L., Schroeder, C., Wheelwright, M., Hladin, N., et al. (2006). *Converting stroke best practices nursing education into a province wide tele-educational module: An evaluation report.* Toronto: Ontario Ministry of Health and Long-Term Care.

Rupnik, C., Thompson-James, M., & Bollman, R. (2001). Measuring economic well-being of rural Canadians using income indicators. *Rural and Small Town Canada Analysis Bulletin, 2*(5).

Russell, A., & Perris, K. (2003). Telementoring in community nursing: A shift from dyadic to communal models of learning and professional development. *Mentoring and Tutoring, 11*(2), 227–237.

Scharff, J. E. (1998). The distinctive nature and scope of rural nursing practice: Philosophical bases. In H. J. Lee (Ed.), *Conceptual basis of rural nursing* (pp. 19–38). New York: Springer Publishing.

Sharpe, A., & Hardt, J. (2006). *Five deaths a day: Workplace fatalities in Canada, 1993–2005.* Ottawa: Center for the Study of Living Standards.

Singh, V. (2004). The rural-urban income gap within provinces: An update to 2000. *Rural and Small Town Analysis Bulletin, 5*(7).

Statistics Canada. (2007a). Portrait of the Canadian population in 2006. *Population and dwelling counts, 2006 census.* Ottawa: Author.

Statistics Canada. (2007b). Study: Recent trends in Canadian lumber industry. *The Daily,* June 7. Retrieved May 16, 2008, from http://www.statcan.ca/Daily/English/070607/d070607a.htm

Statistics Canada. (2007c). 2006 census of agriculture: Farm operations and operators. *The Daily,* May 16. Retrieved September 10, 2008, from http://www.statcan.ca/Daily/English/070516/d070516a.htm

Statistics Canada. (2007d). *2006 census of agriculture.* Retreived September 10, 2008, from http://www.statcan.ca/english/agcensus2006/index.htm

Statistics Canada. (2008a). *Canada's ethnocultural mosaic, 2006 census: Findings.* Retrieved September 10, 2008, from http://www12.statcan.ca/english/census06/analysis/ethnicorigin/index.cfm

Statistics Canada. (2008b). *Aboriginal peoples in Canada in 2008, Inuit, Métis and First Nations, 2006 census: Findings.* Retrieved September 10, 2008, from http://www12.statcan.ca/english/

census06/analysis/aboriginal/index.cfm

Statistics Canada. (2008c). *Suicide and suicide rate, by sex and age group.* Retrieved May 19, 2008, from http://www40.statcan.ca/l01/cst01/perhlth66a.htm

Stewart, N., D'Arcy, C., Pitblado, R., Forbes, D., Morgan, D., Remus, G., et al. (2005). *Report of the national survey of nursing practice in rural and remote Canada.* Saskatoon, SK: University of Saskatchewan, Applied Research/Psychiatry and College of Nursing. Retrieved May 16, 2007, from http://www.ruralnursing.unbc.ca/pubandpresent.php?download=SurveyReportEnglish.pdf

Strasser, R. (2003). Rural health around the world: Challenges and solutions. *Family Practice, 20*(4), 457–463.

Thomlinson, E., McDonagh, M., Crooks, K., & Lees, M. (2004). Health beliefs of rural Canadians: Implications for practice. *Australian Journal of Rural Health, 12,* 258–263.

Transport Canada. (2005). *Canadian motor vehicle traffic collision statistics.* Ottawa: Author. Retrieved June 2, 2001, from http://www.tc.gc.ca/pol/en/t-facts_e/Highways_ Data_ Menu.htm

Vicente, K., & Christoffersen, K. (2006). The Walkerton *E. coli* outbreak: A test of Rasmussen's framework for risk management in a dynamic society. *Theoretical Issues in Ergonomics Science,* 7(2), 93–112.

Way, D., Jones, L., Baskerville, B., & Busing, N. (2001). Primary health care services provided by nurse practitioners and family physicians in shared practice. *Canadian Medical Association Journal, 165*(9), 1210–1214.

Winters, M., MacIntyre, E., Peters, C., Thom, J., Teschke, K., & Davies, H. (2005). *Noise and hearing loss in farming.* Retrieved February 10, 2008, from http://www.cher.ubc.ca/PDFs/FARSHAFinalRevised.pdf

Young, T. K., Marens, P. J., Taback, S. P., Sellers, E. A. C., Dean, H. J., Cheang, M., et al. (2002). Type 2 diabetes mellitus in children prenatal and early infancy risk factors among Native Canadians. *Archive of Pediatric and Adolescent Medicine, 156,* 651–655.

Chapter 15

Complementary and Alternative Health Modalities

Today, more and more Canadians are using complementary and alternative health modalities (CAHM); however, many nurses are unprepared to help clients obtain alternative medical therapies and, as a result, may lack information or even harbour misinformation (Keimig & Braun, 2004). In response to this trend, Health Canada (2005) is gauging the awareness, attitudes, knowledge, and behaviours among Canadians pertaining to natural health products (NHPs). Most provincial and territorial nursing associations also have developed position statements on the provision of holistic therapies. Thus, nurses must understand the different interventions that complement Western medicine and their potential risks and benefits. They must also practise within their professional guidelines to provide safe and effective nursing care.

In this chapter, the terms *complementary medicine* and *alternative medicine* are used to describe as many as 1800 therapies that have been practised around the world for centuries. Many of these modalities originated from ancient medical systems of Egyptians, Chinese, Asian Indians, Greeks, and Aboriginal peoples. **Complementary medicine** is used *together with* conventional or Western medicine. For example, the scent of essential oils from flowers or herbs used in aromatherapy can help promote relaxation and well-being. **Alternative medicine** is used *in place of* conventional medicine. An example of an alternative therapy is the use of acupuncture for back pain relief instead of surgery, as recommended by the health-care provider. **Integrative medicine** combines treatments from Western medicine and complementary and alternative medicine (CAM) to achieve maximum safety and effectiveness of care (National Institutes of Health, 2008).

OBJECTIVES

After studying this chapter, you should be able to

1. Describe the terms *complementary medicine, alternative medicine,* and *integrative medicine*
2. Explain the basic concepts used in complementary and alternative health modalities: holism, humanism, balance, spirituality, energy, and healing environments
3. Describe the five main categories of complementary and alternative health modalities
4. Describe the principles and clinical application of the complementary and alternative health modalities
5. Describe the role of Health Canada in complementary and alternative medicine
6. Explain why natural health products should be used with care
7. Discuss the role of the nurse in assisting clients with the use of various health modalities

Basic Concepts

Several concepts are common to most alternative health practices. These are holism, humanism, balance, spirituality, energy, and healing environments.

Holism

Holism refers to combined mental, emotional, spiritual, relationship, and environmental components. **Holistic health** involves the total person: the whole of the person's being and the overall quality of life. **Holistic health care** considers all the components of health, health promotion, health maintenance, health education, illness prevention, and restorative care. Interventions are individualized within the entire context of the person's life. The focus of the Canadian Holistic Nurses Association (CHNA) is to enhance the healing of the whole person from birth to death.

Humanism

The **humanist** views the mind and body as indivisible and believes that people have the power to solve their own problems, that people are responsible for the patterns of their lives, and that well-being is a combination of personal satisfaction and contributions to the larger community. Nurses can help consumers assert their right to choose their own healing journey and the quality of their life and death experiences (Fontaine, 2005).

Balance

The concept of **balance** consists of mental, physical, emotional, spiritual, and environmental components. Balance is attained when each component reaches a state of equilibrium. *Physical* aspects include optimal functioning of all body systems. *Emotional* aspects include the ability to feel and express the entire range of human emotions. *Mental* aspects include feelings of self-worth, a positive identity, a sense of accomplishment, and the ability to appreciate and create. *Spiritual* aspects involve moral values, a meaningful purpose in life, and a feeling of connectedness to others and a divine source. *Environmental* aspects include physical, biological, economic, social, and political conditions. Being in balance is a learned skill and must be practised regularly to engage in the process of healthful living.

Spirituality

Spiritual healing techniques and spiritually based health-care systems are among the most ancient healing practices. Spirit is the liveliness and richness of one's life. **Spirituality** (see Chapter 46) includes the drive to become all that we can be, and it is bound to intuition, creativity, and motivation. It is the dimension that involves relationship with the self, with others, and with a higher power. Spirituality gives people meaning and purpose in their lives. It involves finding significant meaning in the entirety of life, including illness and death.

Energy

The concept of energy has been recognized for centuries in most cultures. **Energy** is viewed as the force that integrates and connects the body, mind, and spirit. Chinese Taoist scholars believed that energy was the basic building material of the universe. Albert Einstein and other physicists proved that matter and energy are the same and that energy is not only the raw material of the cosmos but also the glue that holds it together. Scientists look at the universe in terms of the forces of tiny particles of matter. People are beings of energy, living in a universe composed of energy.

Grounding and centring are common terms used in various healing practices. *Grounding* relates to a person's connection with the ground and, in a broader sense, to that person's whole contact with reality. Being grounded suggests stability, security, independence, the presence of a solid foundation, and the ability to live in the present rather than escape into dreams. *Centring* refers to the process of focusing the mind on the centre of energy, allowing the person to operate intuitively, with awareness, and to channel energy throughout the body. When people are centred, they are fully connected to the part of their bodies where all their energies meet.

Healing Environments

Nursing has always focused on creating healing environments for their clients. Nurses create these environments by providing compassionate and holistic care through the use of their hands, heart, and mind. Nurses must also create healing environments for themselves. Working with people can be draining work. Nurses need to learn how to restore their energy and replenish themselves.

Complementary Health Modalities

Ethnocentrism, the assumption that your own cultural or ethnic group is superior to others, has often prevented Western health-care practitioners from learning new ways to promote health and prevent chronic illness.

Health-care providers must therefore learn about various complementary health modalities being practised in other cultures and countries for disease prevention and treatment. The World Health Organization (WHO) (2003) reported that traditional healing practices have been part of the cultures in many developing countries for years and are now spreading rapidly in the industrialized world (see Box 15.1). The *Baseline Natural Health Products Survey Among Consumers* conducted by Health Canada (2005) confirms an increasing use of NHPs among Canadians (see the Nursing and Canadian Society box).

Complementary health modalities have been grouped into five major categories by National Institutes of Health (NIH) National Center for Complementary and Alternative Medicine (NCCAM) in the United States: alternative medical systems, biologically based treatments, manipulative and body-based therapies, energy therapies, and mind-body interventions.

Alternative Medical Systems

A number of health-care practices have been systematized throughout the centuries and throughout the world. These typically include an entire set of values, attitudes, and beliefs that generate a philosophy of life, not simply a group of remedies.

AYURVEDA The Indian system of medicine, Ayurveda, is at least 2500 years old. **Ayurveda** views illness as a state of imbalance among the body's systems. The individual aims to minimize stress by achieving an optimal balance of emotional health, physical health, spiritual health, mental health, and environmental health. Specific lifestyle interventions are a major preventive and therapeutic approach in Ayurveda. Each person is prescribed an individualized diet and exercise program depending on dosha (body) type and the nature of the underlying dosha imbalance. Herbal preparations are added to the

BOX 15.1 USE AND POPULARITY OF TRADITIONAL MEDICINE

The WHO has provided some statistics on the use and popularity of different modalities around the world.

- In China, traditional herbal preparations account for 30%–50% of the total medicinal consumption.
- In Ghana, Mali, Nigeria, and Zambia, the first line of treatment for 60% of children with high fever resulting from malaria is the use of herbal medicines at home.
- WHO estimates that in several African countries traditional birth attendants assist in the majority of births.
- In Europe, North America, and other industrialized regions, over 50% of the population have used complementary or alternative medicine at least once.
- In San Francisco, London, and South Africa, 75% of people living with HIV/AIDS use TM/CAM.
- 70% of the population in Canada have used complementary medicine at least once.
- In Germany, 90% of the population have used a natural remedy at some point in their life. Between 1995 and 2000, the number of doctors who had undergone special training in natural remedy medicine had almost doubled to 10 800.
- In the United States, 158 million of the adult population use complementary medicines and according to the USA Commission for Alternative and Complementary medicines, US$17 billion was spent on traditional remedies in 2000.
- In the United Kingdom, annual expenditure on alternative medicine is US$230 million.
- The global market for herbal medicines currently stands at over US$60 billion annually and is growing steadily.

Source: From "Traditional Medicine," by the World Health Organization, 2003, *Fact sheet No. 134.* Copyright by the World Health Organization. Retrieved on January 25, 2008, from http://www.who.int/mediacentre/factsheets/fs134/en/

NURSING AND CANADIAN SOCIETY

Fact	Implications for Nursing Practice
More than 70% of Canadians consume NHPs, such as vitamins and minerals, herbal remedies, and other complementary or alternative therapies. Many Canadians (77%) use complementary or alternative therapies for disease prevention and health maintenance, and 38% stated they used NHPs on a daily basis.	By understanding the interaction between natural and pharmaceutical products, nurses can offer informed advice to clients about self-care decisions.
Eight in 10 Canadians believe that it is important to respect the role that NHPs play in some cultures.	As the Canadian population becomes increasingly diverse, nurses must be culturally sensitive to the unique health-care practices among various cultural groups.
A majority of Canadians (81%) think the use of NHPs will increase over the next 10 years, and 7 in 10 (72%) believe Canadians have the right to use any NHP they choose.	Nurses need to be aware of their provincial or territorial nursing guidelines regarding alternative and complementary therapies to ensure their advice is ethically sound and their services fall within the scope of practice.
The costs of complementary and alternative therapies are rarely covered by provincial, territorial, or private health insurance plans.	Nurses need to know how to access information on the credentials of therapists and the costs of these therapies.

diet for preventive or regenerative purposes as well as for the treatment of specific disorders. Yoga, breathing exercises, and meditative techniques are also prescribed by the practitioner.

TRADITIONAL CHINESE MEDICINE **Traditional Chinese medicine (TCM)** has been practised in China for more than 3000 years. TCM sees that the body is a delicate balance of yin and yang: two opposing and inseparable forces. Yin represents the cold, slow, or passive principle, while yang represents the hot, excited, or active principle. Health is achieved by maintaining the body in a balanced state and disease is due to an internal imbalance of yin and yang. This imbalance leads to blockage in the flow of qi (pronounced *chee*), or vital energy, and of blood along pathways known as meridians.

TCM views the mind, body, spirit, and emotions as inseparable. The heart is not just a blood pump; it also influences a person's capacity for joy, a sense of purpose in life, and connectedness with others. The kidneys filter fluids, but they also manage the capacity for fear, will and motivation, and faith in life. The lungs breathe in air and breathe out waste products, but they also regulate the capacity to grieve, as well as a person's acknowledgment of the self and of others. The liver cleanses the body, and it also influences feelings of anger, vision, and creativity. The stomach has a part in digestion of food and influences the ability to be thoughtful, kind, and nurturing as well. These are just a few of the mind–body connections that TCM practitioners recognize.

TCM practitioners use a variety of ancient and modern therapeutic methods, including acupuncture, acupressure, herbal medicine, massage, heat therapy, qigong, Tai Chi, and nutritional lifestyle counselling. Multiple herbs in combinations may be used to treat individual clients.

TRADITIONAL ABORIGINAL MEDICINE Spirituality and medicine are inseparable in Aboriginal healing. Medicine women and men see themselves as channels through which the Great Power helps others achieve well-being in mind, body, and spirit. The only healer is the One, who created all things. Medicine people consider that they have certain knowledge to put things together to help the sick person heal and that knowledge has to be dispensed in a certain way, often through ritual or ceremony. Healers use medicine objects to assist them and ceremony treatments, such as the sweat lodge, singing, pipe ceremony, sun dance, and vision quest. Other treatments include smudging, drumming and chanting, healing touch, acupressure, and herbs.

Health is viewed as a balance or harmony of mind and body. The goal is to be in harmony with all things, which means first being in harmony with yourself. If the mind is negative, the body will be drained, making it more vulnerable. When people open up to the universe, learn what is good for them, and find ways to be happier, they can begin to work toward a longer and healthier life (see Chapter 7, the section "Aboriginal Views of Wellness").

HOMEOPATHY **Homeopathy** is a self-healing system, assisted by small doses of remedies or medicines, which is useful in a variety of acute and chronic disorders. It is based on the premises of the *law of similar,* which claims that a natural substance that produces a given symptom in a healthy person cures it in a sick person. If taken in large amounts, these natural compounds will produce symptoms of disease.

Natural healing compounds are prepared through a process of serial dilution. The compound is first dissolved in a water–alcohol mixture called the *mother tincture.* One drop of the tincture is then mixed with 10 drops of water-alcohol, and this process is repeated hundreds or thousands of times depending on the potency being prepared. The homeopathic belief is that the more the substance is diluted, the more potent it becomes as a remedy. It is not presently understood how homeopathic remedies work.

NATUROPATHY **Naturopathic medicine** involves botanical medicine, homeopathy, clinical nutrition, hydrotherapy, naturopathic manipulation, TCM and acupuncture, and prevention and lifestyle counselling. In Canada, practitioners of naturopathic medicine are primary care physicians trained at accredited medical colleges in a four-year, full-time program. British Columbia, Manitoba, New Brunswick, Nova Scotia, Ontario, Quebec, and Saskatchewan require that naturopathic doctors pass licensing board exams in order to practise. A licensing board is in development for Alberta.

The goal is to promote health through diet and exercise rather than through the application of a particular therapy. Faith, hope, and belief feature prominently in the treatment. People are given the responsibility for their own health and well-being, and traditional pharmaceuticals and surgical interventions are rarely used.

Biologically Based Treatments

Botanical (plant) healings are used by 80% of the world's population. These include herbs, aromatherapy, homeopathy, and naturopathy. **Herbal medicine** refers to the use of herbs to treat disease and supplement other treatments. **Herbal therapy** is used to prevent disease or promote health through the routine use of herbs.

HERBAL MEDICINE Herbs have been used by humans since antiquity for the prevention and treatment of illness. Herbs or botanicals are plants that are valued for their medicinal properties, flavour, scent, and so on. Herbs contain dozens of bioactive compounds. Geographic location, harvest season, post-harvest processing, and storage are some of the factors that contribute to the concentration of these bioactive compounds. It is often not clear which of these compounds underlie an herb's medical use. More than 10 000 herbs have been identified as useful for medicinal purposes. See Table 15.1 for some of the more commonly used herbs.

Health Canada (2007) plays a key role in ensuring that Canadians have access to high-quality, safe, and effective NHPs while respecting culturally oriented health-care practices. Under the 2004 Natural Health Products Regulations, **natural health products (NHPs)** include vitamins and minerals, herbal remedies, homeopathic medicines, traditional medicines, probiotics, and other products like amino acids and essential fatty acids.

The determination of the safety and efficacy of herbal products presents a challenge, as herbal experts often disagree on how to interpret the varying evidence available for many types of herbal remedies (WHO, 2003). Most herbs are consumed without untoward reactions when they are taken in small amounts. It is when the product is consumed in excess amounts that problems arise.

A healthy lifestyle is the primary promoter of good health, and conventional medicine may offer the best solutions for many problems. However, with the current proliferation of lay literature on herbal remedies and the wide availability of such products in health food stores, more people are relying on herbal and other less conventional therapies for a wide variety of problems. Health-care professionals must become aware of the use of herbs by their clients and be knowledgeable, using evidence-based practice. The nurse should be using resources such as Health Canada (2008), the Canadian Adverse Reaction Newsletter, and MedEffect Canada.

AROMATHERAPY **Aromatherapy** is the therapeutic use of plant essential oils in which the odour or fragrance plays an important part. The chemicals found in the essential oils are absorbed into the body, resulting in physiological or psychological benefit. The essential oils that are used in aromatherapy are plant oils distilled from flowers, roots, bark, leaves, wood resins, and lemon or orange rinds. The oils are massaged into the skin, inhaled, placed in baths, used as compresses, or mixed into ointments. Different oils calm, stimulate, improve sleep, change eating habits, or boost the immune system. Examples are shown in Table 15.2.

TABLE 15.1 Selected Common Herbal Preparations, Uses, and Precautions

Herb	Uses	Precautions
Echinacea	To boost the immune system and as a natural antibiotic	Long-term use (beyond 8 weeks) can cause hepatotoxicity; it should not be used by individuals with compromised immune systems, autoimmune diseases, or progressive neurological conditions.
Evening primrose	To relieve symptoms of menopause	It should not be taken without consultation by individuals on estrogen replacement therapy, anticoagulants, or blood pressure or blood cholesterol medicine.
Garlic	To lower cholesterol; also believed to have anticancer properties	It can cause a need for an increased dose of antihypertensives.
Ginger	To reduce nausea, motion sickness, and other gastrointestinal disorders	It can enhance the anticoagulant effect of warfarin, leading to an increased risk of bleeding. The use of ginger to prevent morning sickness has not been proven completely safe.
Ginkgo biloba	To enhance memory and enhance peripheral circulation	It may alter the metabolism and effectiveness of some prescription and nonprescription medications, including anticonvulsants, antidepressants, anticoagulants, antihypertensives, insulin, and others. Safety during pregnancy has not been established.
Ginseng	To increase stamina and to boost the immune system	It may affect blood glucose levels and should not be used while pregnant or nursing. It can be toxic in very large quantities.
Melatonin	To use as sleep aid—popular with shift workers or to combat jet lag	It has only minimal effectiveness in helping with sleep problems. People may have allergic reactions and experience mild side effects, such as headache and stomach ache.
Milk thistle	To improve liver functions, reduce gall bladder inflammation, treat psoriasis, lower cholesterol levels, and reduce cancer growth in breast, cervical, and prostate cancers	It reduces the effectiveness of oral contraceptives. It also has a laxative effect and may cause upset stomach, diarrhea, and bloating.
St. John's wort	To use as an antidepressant	It has shown to be effective in some cases of mild to moderate depression but not major depression. It should not be combined with other antidepressant medications.

Evidence-Informed Practice

How Commonly Known Are Natural Health Product–Drug Interactions?

Charrois et al. (2007) identified community pharmacists' familiarity with NHPs and related adverse side effects and their ability to counsel known NHP–drug interactions. A convenience sample of 321 community pharmacists in Alberta and British Columbia participated in the survey. The response rate was 41% (n = 132). Of these, 47% of pharmacists stated that they had identified a potential interaction with NHPs, but only 2% of these respondents reported it to Health Canada. Pharmacists (76%) were most familiar with the interaction between sertraline and St. John's wort, and were least familiar with interactions between NHPs and antiretrovirals.

NURSING IMPLICATIONS: Because more and more Canadians are using NHPs, nurses, as part of the health-care team, must work with physicians and pharmacist and be alert to possible drug interactions and side effects of NHPs experienced by their clients. Nurses are in ideal position to make assessments and help their clients to choose the most appropriate complementary or alternative therapies. Further education regarding NHPs, the related drug interactions, and their role in alternative and complementary health modalities must be encouraged and incorporated in the nursing educational curriculum.

Source: Based on "Community Identification of Natural Health Product-Drug Interactions," by T. L. Charrois, R. L. Hill, D. Vu, B. C. Foster, H. S. Boon, K. Cramer, and S. Vohra, 2007, *Annals of Pharmacotherapy, 41*(7), pp. 1124–1129.

TABLE 15.2 Selected Essential Oils and Their Uses

Oil	Use
Birch	Acts as an anti-inflammatory agent and decongestant, relieves arthritis pain
Chamomile	Soothes muscle pains, acts as a GI antispasmodic, relieves stress, decreases insomnia
Eucalyptus	Decreases fever, relieves pain, acts as an anti-inflammatory and antiviral, boosts immune system
Geranium	Modifies mood, acts as an antidiarrheal agent
Ginger	Helps ward off colds, calm upset stomach, decrease nausea, soothes sprains and muscle spasms.
Jasmine	Uplifts and stimulates, acts as an antidepressant
Lavender	Relieves headache, stress, and insomnia
Peppermint	Relieves nausea, acts as an antipyretic and respiratory aid

Nurses should be aware of the potential complications from using certain oils and caution clients of their usage and storage. Essential oils, other than lavender and tea tree oil, are quite potent and can irritate the skin. They should be diluted with a carrier oil before being used on the skin. Carrier oils, such as sunflower oil, grapeseed oil, and soy oil, contain vitamins, proteins, and minerals that provide added nutrients to the body. Essential oils should not be ingested, because even modest amounts can be fatal. Pregnant women and people with epilepsy should consult a knowledgeable health-care practitioner or qualified aromatherapist before using essential oils. Some oils can trigger bronchial spasms, so people with asthma should consult their primary health-care provider before using oils.

DIETARY THERAPY **Dietary therapy** consists of the consumption of specific types of diets or supplements, including vitamins, minerals, amino acids, herbs and other botanicals, and miscellaneous substances, such as enzymes and fish oils, to prevent or treat illness. Similar to herbal therapy, nutritional therapy aims to help clients obtain or maintain good health. The therapy focuses on eating more fresh vegetables, fruits, and whole grains. A variety of diets are offered for treating cancer, cardiovascular disease, and food allergies. In many cases, diet therapy mirrors traditional dietary and medical advice: reducing excess use of sugar and salt, reducing excess fat, increasing the intake of fruit and vegetables, and stressing the need for a well-balanced diet.

Not all supplements are harmless. Three major concerns exist for clients' use of nutritional supplements: efficacy, consistency, and safety (Health Canada, 2007; WHO, 2003). Insufficient evidence is available to determine the effectiveness of supplements, so nurses should assist clients in gathering reliable information about supplements by using guidelines from the Health Canada's Natural Health Products Directorate. Supplements are manufactured by different companies and often contain a variety of substances in varying amounts. No legal definitions exist for the words *standardized, certified,* or *verified* for supplements. Some supplements cause adverse effects, such as diarrhea or high blood pressure, while others become dangerous when taken in combination with certain medications. Another safety concern with supplements is that they may be contaminated with dangerous substances, such as mould, bacteria, pesticides, and metals (Rolfes, Pinna, & Whitney, 2006). Nurses must assess clients for use of dietary supplements and include teaching about the known benefits and risks of supplements in the care planning.

ORTHOMOLECULAR THERAPY **Orthomolecular medicine** aims to prevent and treat disease by providing the body with optimal amounts of substances that are natural to the body. It is based on the premise that many diseases are caused by molecular imbalances that are correctable by administration of the right nutrient molecules at the right time. Orthomolecular therapy originated in the early 1950s when a few psychiatrists began adding massive doses of vitamin B3 (nicotinic acid or nicotinamide) to their treatment of severe mental health problems, and the therapy was termed *megavitamin therapy*. Later this treatment regimen was expanded to include other vitamins, minerals, hormones, and diets.

The human body has a limited capacity to use vitamins in its metabolic activities. When vitamins are consumed in excess of the body's physiological needs, they function as drugs rather than as vitamins. Nurses need to be aware of the potential complications of ingesting megadoses of vitamins and minerals and be able to advise patients on potential fraudulent or unproven claims. Research is not conclusive on the role of multivitamins and mineral supplements to prevent cancer and chronic illness in adults (Huang et al., 2006).

Manipulative and Body-Based Therapies

Some manual healing methods come from ancient times, and some were developed in the latter half of the twentieth century. These healing practices include chiropractic; massage; acupuncture, acupressure, and reflexology; and hand-mediated biofield therapies.

CHIROPRACTIC THERAPY **Chiropractic therapy** is the third-largest independent health profession in the Western world, after conventional medicine and dentistry. Chiropractic doctors focus on the spine and its relation to the component bone structures, muscles, and nerves. Chiropractors believe that displacements of the spine can result in a variety of symptoms that can be treated by spinal manipulation or adjustment. Three primary goals guide chiropractic intervention. The first goal is to reduce or eliminate pain. The second goal is to correct the spinal dysfunction, thereby restoring biomechanical balance to re-establish shock absorption, leverage, and range of motion. In addition, muscles and ligaments are strengthened by spinal rehabilitative exercises to increase resistance to further injury. The third goal is preventive maintenance to ensure the problem does not recur.

As with any treatment, clients need to be aware of the benefits and limitations of chiropractic care. As holistic practitioners, chiropractors work with many facets of clients' lifestyles. Exercise programs are designed, rehabilitation measures are planned, correct posture and lifting techniques are explained, and activities of daily living are assessed and improved.

MASSAGE Healing through touch, or **massage**, goes back to early civilization. Touch is an important part of healing. One possible explanation is that touch stimulates the production of certain chemicals in the immune system that promote healing.

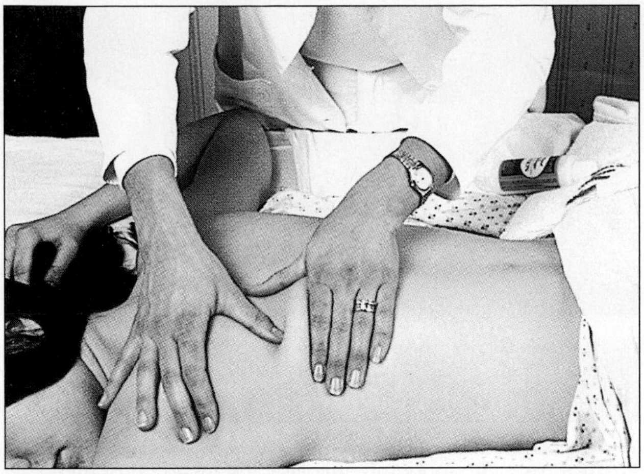

FIGURE 15.1 Massage over the shoulder and back

THERAPEUTIC MASSAGE Physically, massage relaxes muscles and releases the buildup of lactic acid that accumulates during exercise (see Figure 15.1). It can also improve the blood and lymph circulation, stretch joints, and relieve pain and congestion. In the mental-emotional aspect, massage can relieve anxiety and provide a sense of relaxation and well-being. Spiritually, it provides a sense of harmony and balance. The individuals receiving a massage may enter a meditative state, thus relaxing their minds and expanding their awareness. A variety of massage strokes or movements can be used singly or in combination, depending on the outcome desired. These include effleurage (stroking), friction, pressure, and petrissage (kneading, or large, quick pinches of the skin, subcutaneous tissue, and muscle).

ORIENTAL MASSAGE **Tui Na** is a massage treatment that uses acupressure, a modality of Chinese medicine, the purpose of which is to bring the body into balance. The words *Tui Na* translate into "push-grasp" or "poke-pinch" in Chinese. It is a series of pressing, tapping, and kneading with palms, fingertips, knuckles, or implements that help remove blockages along the meridians of the body and stimulate the flow of qi and blood to promote healing. Tui Na ranges from light stroking to deep-tissue work that would be considered too vigorous or too painful for a recreational or relaxing massage.

ACUPUNCTURE, ACUPRESSURE, AND REFLEXOLOGY **Acupuncture** and **acupressure** are techniques of applying pressure or stimulation to specific points on the body, known as acupuncture points, to relieve pain, cure certain illnesses, and promote wellness. Acupuncture uses needles (see Figure 15.2), whereas acupressure uses finger pressure. **Reflexology** is a form of acupressure most commonly performed on the feet, but the hands or ears may also be manipulated. See Figure 15.3 for the foot reflex areas.

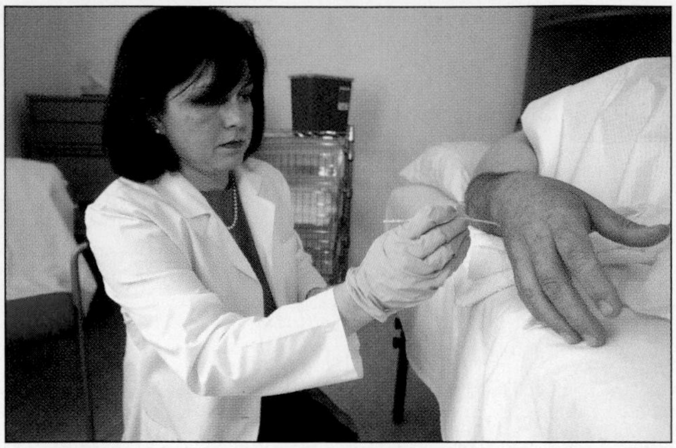

FIGURE 15.2 Acupuncture involves the insertion of thin, sterile needles.

Acupuncture, acupressure, and reflexology are treatments rooted in the traditional Eastern philosophy that qi, or life energy, flows through the body along pathways known as meridians. As vital energy flows through the meridians, it forms tiny whirlpools close to the skin's surface at places called acupuncture points. These points function somewhat like gates to moderate the flow of qi.

When the flow of energy becomes blocked or congested, people experience discomfort or pain on a physical level, may feel frustrated or irritable on an emotional level, and may experience a sense of vulnerability or lack of purpose in life on a spiritual level. The goal of care in wellness acupuncture is to recognize and manage the disruption before illness or disease occurs. Practitioners bring balance to the body's energies, which promotes optimal health and well-being, and facilitates people's own healing capacity (Stibich & Wissow, 2006). A number of clinical trials have reported that acupuncture improves symptoms of osteoarthritis (Novey, 2002), decreases pain (Brinkhaus et al., 2006; Singh et al., 2006), and improves memory, orientation, and the ability to perform the activities of daily living (Yu, Zhang, Liu, Meng, & Han, 2006).

QIGONG AND TAI CHI A number of therapies focus on movement, body awareness, and breathing, and their purpose is to maintain health as well as to correct specific problems. **Qigong** (pronounced *chee goong*) is a Chinese discipline consisting of breathing and mental exercises combined with body movements. **Tai Chi** (pronounced *teye chee*) arose out of qigong and is a discipline that combines physical fitness, meditation, and self-defence. Both disciplines consist of soft, slow, continuous movements that are circular in nature. The slowness of movements requires attentive control that quiets the mind and develops the person's powers of awareness and concentration. The continuous circular nature of the movements develops strength and endurance.

Almost anyone can participate in movement-oriented therapies (see the Lifespan Considerations box). They can be learned by the young and by seniors, by people with physical challenges or who are physically

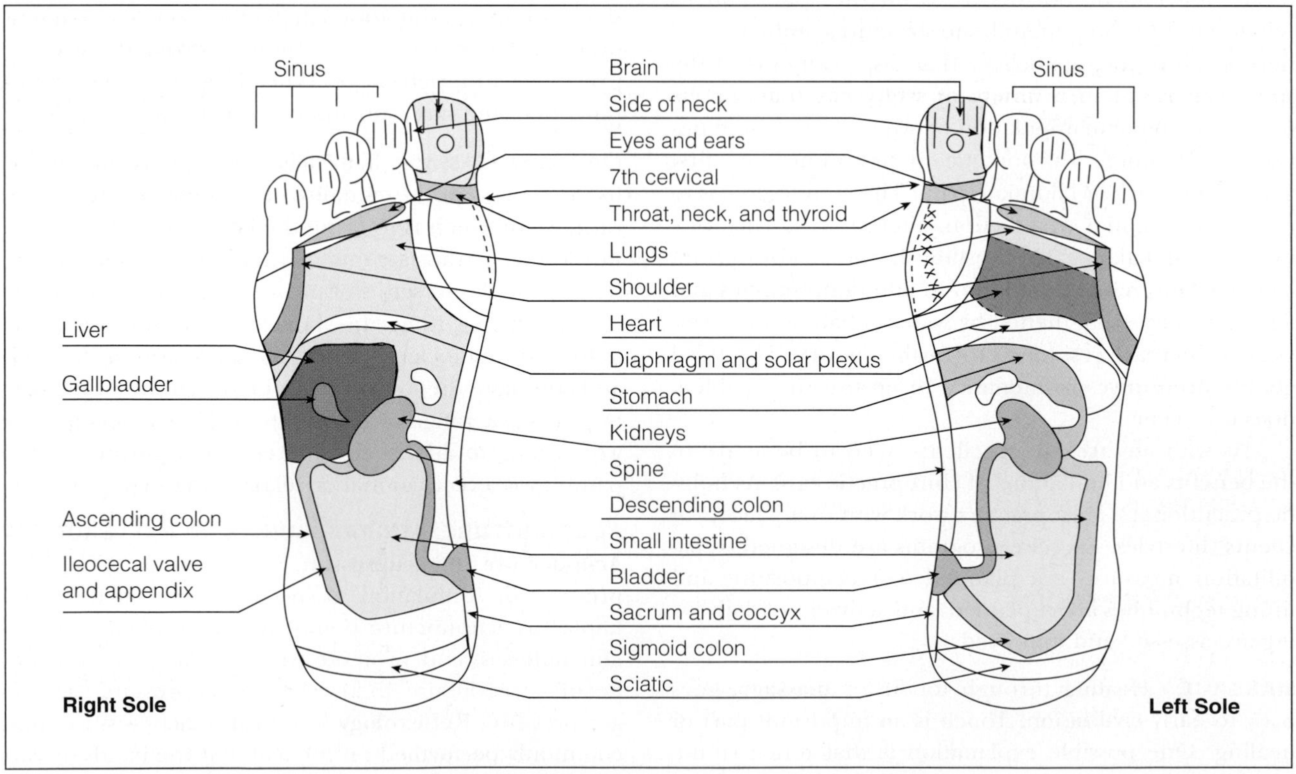

FIGURE 15.3 Foot reflex areas

Lifespan Considerations

CAHM can have various psychological and physiological benefits for clients, regardless of their age. Here are two examples.

BENEFITS OF MASK MAKING FOR CHILDREN WHO ARE CHRONICALLY OR TERMINALLY ILL: Mask making can be used as a therapeutic tool when working with children who are chronically or terminally ill. As a form of art therapy, mask making helps children cope with their illness by "making special," or moving their understanding of the illness and its effects beyond the ordinary, often into the spiritual realm. The process of making the mask can help the child confront the illness, express his or her emotions, develop meaning, and, ultimately, gain a sense of control in an overwhelming situation.

Masks can be made from materials found in the health-care setting—gauze, plastic cups for dispensing medication, plastic covers from IV ports, gloves, and tubing. They can be hung from doors, put on walls, or made into mobiles. Children can be very creative in making masks. After a child's death, the mask can be a way parents and others remember the child (Driessnack, 2004).

BENEFITS OF TAI CHI FOR OLDER ADULTS

The practice of Tai Chi has been found to have the following benefits:

- Tai Chi improves the balance of older adults and reduces the risk of falls (Hakim, Newton, Segal, & DuCette, 2004). This is especially important for people with osteoporosis. Those who have better postural control and increased flexibility reduce their risk of falls and risk of hip fractures, which are a major contributor to dysfunction and death in older women.
- Older adults with moderate sleep complaints improved self-rated sleep quality through a 6-month, low- to moderate-intensity Tai Chi program. Tai Chi appears to be effective as a nonpharmacological approach to sleep enhancement for sleep-disturbed older individuals (Li et al., 2004).
- Older adults who performed Tai Chi had an increase in varicella zoster virus-specific cell-mediated immunity and thus decreased risk for herpes zoster (Irwin, Pike, Cole, & Oxman, 2003).
- Tai Chi exercise intervention is beneficial for retarding bone loss in weight-bearing bones in early postmenopausal women (Chan et al., 2004).

fit, and by those in good health and those recovering from long-term injury or illness. These Eastern practices can be done alone, in pairs, or in large groups.

Energy Therapies

The three most prominent therapies that use the hands to alter the biofield, or energy field, are therapeutic touch (TT), healing touch, and reiki. The goals are to accelerate the person's own healing process and to facilitate healing at all levels of body, mind, emotions, and spirit. These treatments are designed neither to diagnose physical conditions nor to replace conventional surgery, medicine, or drugs in treating organic disease.

THERAPEUTIC TOUCH Noncontact **therapeutic touch (TT)** is a process by which practitioners believe they can transmit energy to a person who is ill or injured to potentiate the healing process. TT involves four steps:

1. *Centring* to achieve a sense of detachment, sensitivity, and balance
2. *Assessing* the client's energy field from head to toe by moving the palms of both hands 5 to 15 centimetres above the client's skin surface
3. *Mobilizing* or unruffling the client's congestive energy field by moving the hands in sweeping motion from the pressure field down along the long bones of the body
4. *Transferring energy* from the practitioner to the client over the identified area of congestion to help the client regain balance in energy field and to promote healing

HEALING TOUCH **Healing touch** is a group of noninvasive energy-based techniques that incorporate TT. Healing touch can be helpful in promoting relaxation, reducing pain, and managing stress.

REIKI **Reiki** (*ray-key*), a Japanese word for "universal life force," is a healing technique that channels life energy to someone through the hands. It is a stress-reduction and relaxation technique that taps into the client's own life-force energy to improve health and enhance quality of life.

BIOELECTROMAGNETIC THERAPIES **Bioelectromagnetic therapies** involve the use of electromagnetic fields, such as pulsed fields, magnetic fields, or alternating current or direct current fields, in people with diseases ranging from asthma and arthritis, through poisoning and tubal pregnancy, to wrinkles. It is thought that some types of illness and pain are associated with imbalances in biological electric and magnetic fields. Bioelectromagnetic therapy realigns the fields to correct imbalances through the application of magnets, the use of lasers or direct electrical stimulation, and even the ingestion of magnetized liquids.

Magnetic therapy is one of the most common of the bioelectromagnetic therapies, and it involves the application of magnets to the body to stimulate the nerves to create a better blood flow to various parts of the body. Common magnetic therapies involve the use of bracelets, mattress pads, necklaces, bands, and so on, with magnets placed in them, which are then worn on the body or, in the case of mattress pads, slept on.

Mind-Body Interventions

YOGA The word **yoga** refers to the uniting of all the powers of the body, mind, and spirit. Yoga is an approach to living a balanced life based on ancient teachings found in Hindu spiritual treatises (the *Upanishads*) written in 800–400 B.C.E. Yoga has many different schools, including Hatha yoga and Kundalini yoga, but the system of Ashtanga yoga is the core from which all other schools have evolved. Each school stresses a different technique, but all have as their goal the mastery of the self. Hatha yoga is a series of gentle stretching exercises using specific *asanas* (postures) and *pranayama* (breathing techniques). Kundalini yoga is a more forceful, highly energizing form that focuses on pushing to the limits. The breathing technique most commonly used in this type of yoga is the "breath of fire," a deep, hard, and fast nostril breath.

The Western approach to yoga tends to be more fitness oriented, with the goal of managing stress, learning to relax, and increasing vitality and well-being. Individuals interested in beginning yoga are advised to explore the specific program offered to ensure that it includes the techniques most suited to their needs.

HYPNOSIS **Hypnosis** is a trance state or an altered state of consciousness in which an individual's concentration is focused and distraction is minimized. People in trances are aware of what is going on around them but choose not to focus on it. They can return to normal awareness whenever they choose. Hypnosis is not a surrender of control; it is only an advanced form of relaxation. It can be used to help people gain self-control, improve self-esteem, and become more autonomous. In some medical facilities, hypnosis is routinely used with a variety of conditions, usually in conjunction with other forms of medical, surgical, psychiatric, or psychological treatment. It can be used with nonmedical clients as well, in working through problems of living or situations of performance anxiety, and in changing bad habits. Depending on the complexity and seriousness of the complaint, treatment typically runs from 2 to 10 sessions.

MEDITATION **Meditation** is a technique used to relax the body and calm the mind. It produces a state of deep peace and rest combined with mental alertness, and it involves both relaxation and focused attention. Anyone can meditate to feel calm, cope with stress, and, for those with spiritual inclinations, feel as one with a higher power or the universe. Meditation can be practised individually or in groups and is easy to learn. It requires no change in belief system and is compatible with most religious practices.

If practised regularly, such as 20 minutes twice a day, meditation produces widespread positive effects on physical and psychological functioning. The autonomic nervous system responds with a decrease in heart rate, lower blood pressure, decreased respiratory rate and oxygen consumption, and a lower arousal threshold. People who meditate say that they have clearer minds and sharper thoughts. Meditation's residual effects—improved stress-coping abilities—are a protection against daily stress and anxiety. All other self-healing methods are improved with the practice of meditation. Skill in meditation is enhanced when the person first masters the skills of breathing, progressive relaxation, and imagery. See Box 15.2 for some of the guidelines for meditation.

PROGRESSIVE RELAXATION Relaxation techniques have been used extensively to reduce high levels of stress and chronic pain. **Progressive relaxation** requires that the client (1) tense and then relax successive muscle groups, and (2) focus attention on discriminating between the feelings experienced when the muscle group is relaxed and when it was tense. Such techniques enable the client to exert control over the body's responses to tension and anxiety by creating a second centre of concentration.

Three requisites to relaxation are correct posture, a mind at rest, and a quiet environment. Procedures for teaching progressive relaxation vary. The method for relaxing muscle groups, the specific muscle groups to be relaxed, the number of sessions involved, and the role of the instructor (taped versus live instructions) can differ. Tensing of muscle groups is often maintained for five to seven seconds and is followed by relaxation of the muscle group at a predetermined cue. To achieve maximum relaxation, various positive and affirmative phrases are used, such as "Let all the tension go" and "Enjoy the feelings as your muscles become relaxed and loose." Guidelines for progressive relaxation are outlined in Box 15.3.

GUIDED IMAGERY Imagery is a two-way communication between the conscious and unconscious mind and

BOX 15.2 GUIDELINES FOR MEDITATION

Practise this process daily for 10- to 20-minute periods:

1. Create a special time and place for meditation. Ideally, choose the early morning or evening, and wait at least two hours after eating so that complete energy is devoted to meditation, rather than to digestive demands. A quiet, comfortable place, devoid of distractions, is essential.
2. Sit either cross-legged on the floor or upright in a straight-backed chair, keeping the spine straight and the body relaxed. Avoid a lying position; this increases the tendency to fall asleep.
3. Support your palms on the thighs, and close your eyes.
4. Follow deep-breathing or progressive relaxation exercises.
5. Focus attention completely on either breathing or a chosen mental image. If using a mantra, repeat the word or phrase either aloud or silently while exhaling. When distracting thoughts appear, allow them to drift into and out of your mind without giving them undue attention; then refocus on your breathing or your mantra.

BOX 15.3 GUIDELINES FOR PROGRESSIVE RELAXATION

Relaxation techniques have been used extensively to reduce high levels of stress and chronic pain. The steps in progressive relaxation are as follows:

- Sit comfortably in a chair, with your feet flat on the ground.
- Tense and tighten your right fist. Focus on the feeling of tension as you do so.
- Allow the muscles in your right fist to relax. Contrast the difference in feeling from tension to relaxation.
- Repeat the preceding two steps for the left fist.
- Now tense and relax both your left and right fists.
- Focus on and relish the feeling of relaxation.
- Now tighten the muscles in both fists and both arms. Feel the tension, fully relax the muscles, and again focus on the sensation of relaxation.
- Progressively tighten and relax each muscle group in the body: toes, ankles, knees, buttocks and groin, stomach and lower back muscles, chest and upper back muscles, shoulders, forehead, and jaw muscles.
- Couple deep breathing with progressive relaxation. While relaxing your muscles, inhale deeply, send the breath to the fist (or other muscle group), and exhale.

The entire exercise should last a minimum of 10 minutes.

involves the whole body and all of its senses. Imagery enables people to open their minds to mental ideas of positive creative images that can foster self-healing and bring about desired achievements. Worry is the most common form of imagery that affects our health. In our imagination we react to current stressors and anticipated dangers. Our bodies become aroused and tense and we activate the fight-or-flight mechanism. **Guided imagery** is a state of focused attention, much like hypnosis, that encourages changes in attitudes, behaviour, and physiological reactions. Guided imagery can help people learn how to stop troublesome thoughts and focus on images that help them relax and decrease the negative impact of stressors.

In guided imagery, the images may be created by the therapist based on the needs and desires of the client. Clients can also create the images as a way to understand the meaning of symptoms or to access inner resources. Imagery stimulates changes in many body functions, such as heart rate, blood pressure, respiratory patterns, brain-wave rhythms and patterns, electrical characteristics of the skin, local blood flow and temperature, gastrointestinal motility and secretions, sexual arousal, and levels of various hormones and neurotransmitters. Table 15.3 describes several types of imagery.

BIOFEEDBACK **Biofeedback** is a technique that brings under conscious control the bodily processes normally thought to be beyond voluntary command. In the past, physiological processes, such as muscle tension, heartbeat, blood flow, peristalsis, and skin temperature, were considered involuntary. However, studies show that these processes are partially subject to voluntary control. The feedback is usually provided through temperature meters that indicate skin temperature changes or an electromyogram (EMG) that shows the electric potential created by the contraction of muscles. Reduced EMG activity reflects muscle relaxation. Biofeedback teaches clients to achieve a generalized state of relaxation, which is characterized by parasympathetic dominance, in opposition to the pattern of physiological arousal manifested in stress-related disorders.

PILATES **Pilates** (pronounced *pih-lah-tes*) is a method of physical movement and exercise designed to stretch, strengthen, and balance the body, in particular the core or centre, including the abdominal region. It is based in principles of yoga, Zen meditation, and ancient Greek and Roman physical regimens. Exercises, coupled with focused breathing patterns, are done on the floor or with simple types of equipment. Benefits include increased

TABLE 15.3 Types of Imagery

Type	Description	Example
Feeling state	Move from a feeling state of tension to one of peace	Imagine self at a beach or floating gently on the water
End-state	Imagine self in the situation wanted	See self as strong and healthy
Energetic	Imagine free-flowing energy	Feel self pulling up energy from the earth through the soles of the feet
Cellular	Imagine events at cellular level	Imagine natural killer cells surrounding and attacking cancer cells
Physiological	Imagine events at the bodily level	Imagine all blood vessels relaxed and wider in order to lower blood pressure
Psychological	Change perception of self	Imagine a dialogue with a person with whom you are in conflict in an effort to find a new solution to the problem
Spiritual	Make contact with God or the Divine	Imagine being held in the hands of God where you are perfectly safe

lung capacity, improved flexibility and joint health, muscular coordination, increased bone density, and better posture and balance. Pilates can help rehabilitate back, knee, hip, shoulder, and stress injuries, and relieve muscle aches.

PRAYER **Prayer** is an active process of communication with God, a saint, or any kind of higher power that answers the prayer. Prayer can be conducted individually or in groups and may even be conducted at a distance by individuals unknown to the person for whom the prayers of healing are made. The universality of prayer is evidenced in all cultures having some form of prayer. Prayer has been and continues to be used in times of difficulty and illness, even in the most secular societies.

Prayer can also be described according to form. *Colloquial prayer* is an informal talk with God, as if talking to a good friend. *Intercessory prayer* is asking God for things for yourself or others. The focus is on what God can provide. Intercessory prayer for others may be called *distant prayer,* if the person being prayed for is remote from the person who is praying. This form of prayer is of interest to researchers, but at the present time scientific evidence is not conclusive. *Ritual prayer* is the use of formal prayers or rituals, such as prayers from a prayer book or the Jewish siddur, or the Catholic practice of saying the rosary. *Meditative prayer,* also known as contemplative prayer, is similar to meditation and is a process of focusing the mind on an aspect of God for a period. Prayer is a self-care strategy that provides comfort, increases hope, and promotes healing and psychological well-being (Dijoseph & Cavendish, 2005; Hampton & Weinert, 2006).

MUSIC THERAPY **Music therapy** consists of listening, rhythm, body movement, and singing. It is used for a variety of reasons in practice settings. Music can alter ordinary levels of consciousness to achieve the mind's fullest potential. Quiet, soothing music without words is often used to induce relaxation and promote self-expression. Musical selections without words are preferred because clients may concentrate on the messages and meaning of words, rather than allowing themselves to flow with the music. Music recordings are often used to relax and distract clients in perioperative holding areas, cardiac care units, birthing rooms, counselling rooms, rehabilitation and physical therapy units, and sleep-induction units.

For individualized therapy, the nurse needs knowledge of the effects that particular types of music produce. Therapeutic music can include mood, choral, classical, romantic, impressionist, country, soft rock, opera, or new age music. To select the appropriate music, the nurse needs to consider the client's preferences as well as the goals of therapy. Additionally, the nurse must consider appropriate times for use and the length of therapy sessions. For example, some people may want to have a music session after a morning shower to balance the body-mind for the day's events. The usual duration of a session is about 20 minutes. Clients are encouraged to let the body respond to the music as it wants, that is, to relax the muscles, lie down, hum, clap, or dance. Some clients may want to make their own recording of musical selections they find appealing.

HUMOUR AND LAUGHTER **Humour** involves the ability to discover, express, or appreciate the comical or absurdly incongruous, to be amused by our own imperfections or the whimsical aspects of life, and to see the funny side of an otherwise serious situation. The use of humour in nursing is defined as helping the client "to perceive, appreciate, and express what is funny, amusing, or ludicrous in order to establish relationships, relieve tension, release anger, facilitate learning, or cope with painful feeling" (Dochterman & Bulechek, 2004, p. 422). Elaboration of these functions of humour in nursing situations follows:

- *Establishing relationships.* Humour decreases the social distance between persons and helps to put people at ease. When tension is decreased, people can focus on the message and on other people rather than on their own feelings. The use of humour helps the nurse establish rapport with clients, an important factor in achieving success in nursing interventions.
- *Relieving tension and anxiety.* The effective use of humour relieves the tension of emotionally charged events. The personal nature of humour, for example, helps clients deal with the impersonal nature of wearing a hospital gown and a numbered ID band and with answering embarrassing questions and undergoing uncomfortable tests. People can also use humour prophylactically to decrease stress.
- *Releasing anger and aggression.* Humour helps individuals act out impulses or feelings in a safe and nonthreatening manner. It dissipates feelings of anger and aggression by focusing on the comic elements of a situation.
- *Facilitating learning.* Many lectures and presentations begin with a joke or cartoon. Humour not only reduces the presenter's anxiety but also gains the audience's attention. People learn more when humour is used and anxiety levels are reduced. People also recall more information when they associate information with a joke. Use of humour in instruction, however, needs to be carefully planned so that it will contribute to learning.
- *Coping with painful feelings.* People may use humour to blunt the immediate effect of situations that are too painful, such as the effect of a threatening diagnosis or treatment. Humour diminishes anxiety and fear and reduces tension, thus enabling the person to confront and deal with the situation.

Humour also has physiological benefits that involve alternating states of stimulation and relaxation. Laughter stimulates increases in respiratory rate, heart rate, muscular tension, and oxygen exchange. A state of relaxation follows laughter, during which heart rate, blood pressure, respiration, and muscle tension decrease. Humour stimulates the production of catecholamines and hormones. It also releases endorphins, thereby increasing pain tolerance.

Many health-care settings are now interested in providing humour as a caring skill and have recognized that "laughter is the best medicine." The nurse needs to use humour effectively and cautiously by considering the feelings of others and cultural variations in what people consider humorous. Humour rooms that are supplied with games, funny audiotapes and videotapes, humorous books, collections of cartoons, and so on, are being created for clients and staff.

ANIMAL-ASSISTED THERAPY **Animal-assisted therapy** is the use of specifically selected animals as a treatment modality in health and human service settings. It has been shown to be a successful intervention for people with a variety of physical or psychological conditions. Throwing an object for a dog to retrieve or brushing the animal increases upper extremity range of motion. Reaching for the object the dog has retrieved improves coordination. Ambulating with a dog improves mobility. Recalling the animal's name helps with memory. Giving simple commands to the animal increases language production. Attending to the animal and the situation increases attention and concentration. Therapeutic horseback riding, or hippotherapy, uses the rhythmic movement of the horse to increase sensory processing and improve posture, balance, and mobility in people with movement dysfunctions.

Resident animals live at long-term health-care facilities. Species include fish, birds, hamsters, gerbils, guinea pigs, rabbits, cats, and dogs. Some staff members report that full-time pets become so perceptive that they actually gravitate to the rooms of people who are the most isolated or depressed. Those residents who have regular visits are more receptive to treatment, have a greater incentive to recover, and have an increased will to live (*Animals in Residential Facilities*, 2003). The contributions companion animals (personal pets) make to the emotional well-being of people include unconditional love and opportunities for affection; achievement of trust, responsibility, and empathy toward others; hope and motivation; and a source of reassurance.

HORTICULTURAL THERAPY **Horticultural therapy**, also called gardening or a healing garden, is an adjunct therapy to occupational and physical therapy. People may view nature, visit a healing garden or a wander garden, or actually participate in gardening. When it is a communal activity, gardening decreases social isolation by fostering interactions with others. Horticultural therapy stimulates the five senses, provides leisure activities, improves motor function, provides a sense of achievement, and improves self-esteem (Detweiler & Warf, 2005; Milligan, Gatrell, & Bingley, 2004).

Nursing Role in Complementary and Alternative Health Modalities

Every year billions of dollars are spent on unproven, fraudulently marketed, and potentially dangerous health products. These are usually promoted to cure or prevent a multitude of diseases or symptoms that are often physiologically unrelated, such as arthritis and indigestion. The nurse must ask the obvious questions: If it is not possible to measure the effect of these treatments, how would the manufacturer and promoter know it is working? Does it sound too good to be true? Do the claims for the product seem exaggerated or unrealistic? Are there simplistic conclusions being drawn from a complex study to sell a product? See the Assessment: Interview box for more questions.

Although the internet can be a valuable source of accurate, reliable information, it also has a wealth of misinformation that may not be obvious. Learn to distinguish hype from evidence-based science. Be skeptical about anecdotal information from persons who have no formal training in nutrition or botanicals, or from personal testimonials (e.g., from store employees, friends, or online chat rooms and message boards) about incredible benefits or results obtained from using a product. Remember that the only way to know if a drug is working or is harmful is through large, preferably placebo-controlled, blind studies.

In Canada, our culturally diverse health-care consumers are demanding a broader range of health options that are familiar to them. Nurses must inquire about

ASSESSMENT: INTERVIEW

Complementary and Alternative Health Modalities

Nurses can use these questions to ask their clients about their use of CAHM:

- Tell me about your use of teas, herbs, vitamins, or other natural products to improve your health.
- What traditional or folk remedies are used in your family?
- Do you meditate, pray, or use relaxation techniques, music, or yoga for healing purposes?
- What alternative therapies have you used (acupuncture, touch therapies, magnets, hypnosis, etc.)?
- Tell me what you know about the benefits and risks of the CAHM you are using.
- Have you discussed your use of CAHM with your health-care provider?

healing practices the client may have used previously (see the Assessment: Interview box). If nurses see themselves as healers, it becomes even more important for them to develop specific healing attitudes and behaviours. The Canadian Nurses Association (1999, 2008) expects nurses to demonstrate safe, competent, and ethical care (see the Reflect on Primary Health Care box). In relation to CAHM, nurses must do the following:

1. Have a strong fundamental, evidence-based knowledge of the human body and various CAHM
2. Demonstrate practice competencies in teaching clients related to the safe and appropriate use of complementary medicine
3. Be nonjudgmental and respectful regarding clients' choices to use any of the CAHM within his or her own cultural context
4. Act as an advocate and facilitator by providing accurate information on CAHM modalities, NHPs, and the risks and benefits as opposed to conventional health-care practices in order to help clients make informed decisions
5. Encourage clients to discuss their use of CAHM with their health-care provider

REFLECT ON PRIMARY HEALTH CARE

To improve the health of clients, nurses act by working in partnerships with clients, other health-care providers, and related community partners. They are the entry point for clients to access the health-care system. They assess the client's health problems, provide accurate information, from conventional Western medicine to available CAHM, and assist the client in making the choice of treatment as desired. Consider how these nursing roles reflect the primary health-care principles of accessibility, intersectoral collaboration, and health promotion.

Case Study 15

Mr. Chou, 67 years old, has been in the hospital for two weeks because of congestive heart failure. His family believes strongly in traditional Chinese medicine, and you notice that they are bringing in herbal teas for Mr. Chou. They would like to bring in an acupuncturist next week.

Critical Thinking Questions

1. What are your attitudes toward methods of healing that are different from Western contemporary medicine?
2. How would you find out whether the herbal teas were effective or detrimental to Mr. Chou's present condition?
3. What do you know about the benefits of acupuncture?
4. How would you deal with this situation with Mr. Chou? with the family? with the agency?

After working through these questions, go to the MyNursingLab at **http://www.mynursinglab.com** to check your answers.

KEY TERMS

complementary medicine
alternative medicine
integrative medicine
holism
holistic health
holistic health care
humanist
balance
spirituality
energy
Ayurveda
traditional Chinese medicine (TCM)
homeopathy
naturopathic medicine
herbal medicine
herbal therapy
natural health products (NHPs)
aromatherapy
dietary therapy
orthomolecular medicine
chiropractic therapy
massage
Tui Na
acupuncture
acupressure
reflexology
qigong
Tai Chi
therapeutic touch (TT)
healing touch
reiki
bioelectromagnetic therapy
yoga
hypnosis
meditation
progressive relaxation
guided imagery
biofeedback
Pilates
prayer
music therapy
humour
animal-assisted therapy
horticultural therapy

CHAPTER HIGHLIGHTS

- Complementary health modalities are practised by a majority of Canadians. Therefore, nurses need to be aware of the different types of therapies and their potential benefits and harms.
- The concepts common to most alternative practices include holism, humanism, balance, spirituality, energy, and healing environments.
- Ancient health-care practices typically include an entire set of values, attitudes, and beliefs that generate a philosophy of life, not simply a group of remedies. Harmony or balance in energy is the emphasis.
- Complementary and alternative health modalities are generally classified into five categories: alternative medical system, biologically based therapies, manipulative and body-based methods, energy therapy, and mind-body interventions.
- Alternative medical systems include Ayurveda, traditional Chinese medicine, traditional Aboriginal medicine, homeopathy, and naturopathy.
- Biologically based treatments include herbal medicine, aromatherapy, dietary therapy, and orthomolecular therapy.
- Manipulative and body-based treatments include chiropractic therapy; massage therapy; Tui Na; acupuncture, acupressure, and reflexology; qigong and Tai Chi.
- Energy therapies include therapeutic touch, healing touch, reiki, and bioelectromagnetic therapies.
- Mind-body interventions include yoga, hypnosis, meditation, progressive relaxation, guided imagery, biofeedback, Pilates, prayer, music therapy, humour, animal-assisted therapy, and horticultural therapy. They all focus on realigning or creating balance in mental and physical processes to bring about healing.
- Although many botanical and nutritional supplements can be helpful in certain conditions, their effectiveness and safety are not all well studied.
- Nurses act as the entry point for clients to access various health services. Nurses can advocate and facilitate their clients' use of natural health products and complementary and alternative modalities within their cultural context as an integral part of care.

ASSESS YOUR LEARNING

1. A nurse is teaching a prenatal class to a group of women about pain relief measures during labour. A young woman states, "I prefer not to use any medication during labour; aromatherapy oils have a calming effect on me." What is the nurse's most appropriate response?
   a. "Aromatherapy oils may work for mild pain but will not reduce labour pain."
   b. "Keep your options open at this point, since aromatherapy may not be sufficient to manage labour pain."
   c. "Aromatherapy oils are a good choice to use with medication for labour pain."
   d. "You need to determine that aromatherapy oils are safe to use during pregnancy."

2. A client asks the nurse the differences between traditional therapies and alternative therapies. Which of the following is the best response?
   a. "Alternative therapies cost less than traditional therapies."
   b. "Alternative therapies are used if traditional therapies are ineffective."
   c. "Alternative therapies can be as effective as traditional therapies for some conditions."
   d. "Alternative therapies use products from nature but traditional therapies do not."

3. Before meeting with a client who has a terminal illness, a new graduate nurse reviews information on spirituality. Which of the following is the best explanation of spirituality?
   a. Something that gives people purpose and meaning in their lives
   b. A formalized religious dogma
   c. A nondenominational community service
   d. People being responsible for their life patterns

4. In which of the following ways do nurses create healing environments?
   a. Using technology to prevent hospital-acquired infections
   b. Empowering clients to make healthy decisions for themselves
   c. Placing aquariums in day rooms of nursing homes
   d. Ensuring that physicians' orders are carried out

5. A client asks the nurse to state one of the primary principles associated with naturopathy. Which of the following is the best response?
   a. "A higher being guides the learning needed to treat disease."
   b. "It focuses on environmental causes when treating illnesses."

c. "It focuses on early detection and treatment of disease."

d. "It is a way of life to maintain health and prevent disease."

6. From the perspective of traditional Chinese medicine (TCM), which is the best definition of disease?
   a. Imbalance or disruption in food digestion
   b. Imbalance or interruption in the flow of qi
   c. Imbalance or disruption in key social relationships
   d. Imbalance or disruption in thoughts or emotions

7. A hospitalized patient is due for surgery tomorrow. You learn that he had not told his physician that he was taking natural health products (NHPs) in addition to his other prescribed medication. What should you do?
   a. You would not be concerned as NHPs are harmless.
   b. You would be concerned as the patient is at risk of uncontrolled bleeding during surgery.
   c. You would report all medications and NHPs the patient is on to the attending physician.
   d. You would offer herbal medicine to the patient to cleanse his digestive system before the surgery.

8. You are caring for James, who has colon cancer and has undergone chemotherapy. His prognosis is unknown. James has experienced much pain. He is depressed and anxious. He asks you for advice regarding the use of therapeutic touch to ease his pain. Which of the following is the most appropriate nursing action?
   a. You cannot endorse the use of any complementary and alternative health modalities.
   b. You ensure that James understands what therapeutic touch is first.
   c. You encourage James to consider music therapy to relieve his pain.
   d. You pray with James so that he will be protected from harm.

9. A 2-month pregnant woman told you that she wants to take ginseng to avoid stretch marks. Which of the following is the most appropriate nursing action?
   a. Advise the mother not to take ginseng as it may be toxic if taken in very large quantities.
   b. Advise against using ginseng as it is not recommended for pregnant and nursing mothers.
   c. Endorse the use of ginseng as it is a well-known and popular Chinese medicine.
   d. Advise the mother on other ways to reduce stretch marks, such as aiming for gradual weight gain during pregnancy.

10. Which of the following would be the most appropriate form of mind and body interventions for older clients who are at risk for falls?
   a. Music therapy
   b. Tai Chi
   c. Diet therapy
   d. Guided imagery

After working through these questions, go to the MyNursingLab at ***http://www.mynursinglab.com*** *to check your answers and see explanations.*

SUGGESTED READINGS

Adams, J., & Tovey, P. (Eds.). (2008). *Complementary and alternative medicine in nursing and midwifery: Towards a critical social science.* New York: Routledge.

This book views CAM within the context of critical social science. It examines the meanings of care of CAM in nursing and midwifery and its role in holistic wellness nursing and public health. A chapter is devoted to CAM in nursing, midwifery, and medicine in Canada.

Snyder, M., & Linquist, R. (Eds.). (2006). *Complementary/alternative therapies in nursing* (5th ed.). New York: Springer.

This practical guide covers the principles, techniques, research, cultural diversity, and health-promotion methods of CAM, and the healing practices for specific illnesses and symptoms. It describes a wide range of alternative therapies, including perspectives on future research and practice.

Yang, K. (2007). Review of yoga programs for four leading risk factors of chronic diseases. *Evidence-Based Complementary and Alternative Medicine, 4*(4), 487–491.

This systematic review of 32 articles published between 1980 and April 2007 found that yoga is generally effective in reducing body weight, blood pressure, glucose levels, and cholesterol levels. However, more studies are needed to determine the effects of long-term adherence to yoga programs and to include the diverse populations at high risk for diabetes.

WEBLINKS

Health Canada

http://www.hc-sc.gc.ca/dhp-mps/prodnatur/index_e.html

As part of the Health Products and Food Branch of Health Canada, the Natural Health Products Directorate (NHPD) is the regulating authority for natural health products for sale in Canada.

Canadian Chiropractic Association

http://www.ccachiro.org

This site provides the general public with information on the role of chiropractic in the health-care system, including its history, training, and scientific research.

Canadian Holistic Nurses Association

http://www.chna.ca

This site presents the philosophy and objectives of the Canadian Holistic Nurses Association (CHNA) and information on the levels of training for a holistic nursing specialty.

The Integrative Health Institute

http://www.mtroyal.ca/integrativehealth/

The Integrative Health Institute, Calgary, provides evidence-based integrative health education, training, and resources to the public and health professionals. It supports the development of complementary and alternative therapies locally, provincially, and nationally.

Canadian Association of Naturopathic Doctors

http://www.naturopathicassoc.ca

This site provides information on ethics and standards, and a roster of naturopathic doctors who are members of the Canadian Naturopathic Association.

REFERENCES

Animals in residential facilities: Guidelines and resources for success. (2003). Renton, WA: Delta Society.

Brinkhaus, B., Witt, C. M., Jena, S., Linde, K., Streng, A., Wagenpfeil, S., et al. (2006). Acupuncture in patients with chronic low back pain. *Archives of Internal Medicine, 166,* 450–457.

Canadian Nurses Association. (1999). Complementary therapies—Finding the right balance. *Nursing Now: Issues and Trends in Canadian Nursing, 6.*

Canadian Nurses Association. (2008). *Nursing in Canada: Canadian registered nurse examination—Competencies.* Retrieved January 22, 2008, from http://www.cna-nurses.ca/CNA/nursing/rnexam/competencies/default_e.aspx

Chan, K., Qin, L., Lau, M., Woo, J., Au, S., Choy, W., et al. (2004). A randomized, prospective study of the effects of Tai Chi Chun exercise on bone mineral density in postmenopausal women. *Archives of Physical Medicine and Rehabilitation, 85,* 717–722.

Detweiler, M. B., & Warf, C. (2005). Dementia wander garden aids post cerebrovascular stroke restorative therapy. *Alternative Therapies in Health and Medicine, 11*(4), 54–58.

Dijoseph, J., & Cavendish, R. (2005). Expanding the dialogue on prayer relevant to holistic care. *Holistic Nursing Practice, 19,* 147–154.

Dochterman, J., & Bulechek, G. B. (Eds.). (2004). *Nursing interventions classification (NIC)* (4th ed.). St. Louis, MO: Mosby.

Driessnack, M. (2004). Remember me: Mask making with chronically and terminally ill children. *Holistic Nursing Practice, 18,* 211–214.

Fontaine, K. L. (2005). *Complementary & alternative therapies for nursing practice* (2nd ed.). Upper Saddle River, NJ: Prentice Hall.

Hakim, R. M., Newton, R. A., Segal, J., & DuCette, J. P. (2004). A group intervention to reduce fall risk factors in community dwelling older adults. *Physical and Occupational Therapy in Geriatrics, 22*(1), 1–20.

Hampton, J. S., & Weinert, C. (2006). An exploration of spirituality in rural women with chronic illness. *Holistic Nursing Practice, 20*(1), 27–33.

Health Canada. (2005). *Baseline natural health products survey among consumers: Final report.* Retrieved January 20, 2008, from http://www.hc-sc.gc.ca/dhp-mps/alt_formats/hpfb-dgpsa/pdf/pubs/eng_cons_survey_e.pdf

Health Canada. (2007). *Natural health products, drug and health products.* Retrieved January 20, 2008, from http://www.hc-sc.gc.ca/dhp-mps/prodnatur/index_e.html

Health Canada. (2008). *Advisories, Warnings and Recalls for Health Professionals.* Retrieved October 15, 2008, from http://www.hc-sc.gc.ca/dhp-mps/medeff/advisories-avis/prof/_2008/index-eng.php

Huang, H. Y., Caballero, B., Chang, S., Alberg, A. J., Semba, R. D., Schneyer, R. F., et al. (2006). The efficacy and safety of multivitamin and mineral supplement use to prevent cancer and chronic disease in adults: A systematic review for a National Institutes of Health state-of-the-science conference. *Annals of Internal Medicine, 145*(5), 372–385.

Irwin, M. R., Pike, J. L., Cole, J. C., & Oxman, M. N. (2003). Effects of a behavioral intervention, tai chi chih, on varicella-zoster virus specific immunity and health functioning in older adults. *Psychosomatic Medicine, 65,* 824–830.

Keimig, T. J., & Braun, C.A. (2004). Student nurses' knowledge and perceptions of alternative and complementary therapies [Online]. *Journal of Undergraduate Nursing Scholarship.* Retrieved January 20, 2008, from http://juns.nursing.arizona.edu/articles/Fall%202004/keimig.htm

Li, F., Fisher, K. J., Harmer, P., Irbe, D., Tearse, R. G., & Weimer, C. (2004). Tai chi and self rated quality of sleep and daytime sleepiness in older adults: A randomized controlled trial. *Journal of the American Geriatrics Society, 52,* 892–900.

Milligan, C., Gatrell, A., & Bingley, A. (2004). Cultivating health. *Social Science & Medicine, 58,* 1781–1793.

National Institutes of Health. (2008). *CMA basics: National Centre for Complementary and Alternative Medicine.* Retrieved January 20, 2008, from http://nccam.nih.gov/health/whatiscam/

Novey, D. W. (2002). Osteoarthritis. *Primary Care, 29,* 263–277.

Rolfes, S. R., Pinna, K., & Whitney, E. (2006). *Understanding normal and clinical nutrition* (7th ed.). Belmont, CA: Thomson.

Singh, B. B., Wu, W. S., Hwang, S. H., Khorsan, R., Der-Martirosian, C., Vinjamury, S. P., et al. (2006). Effectiveness of acupuncture in the treatment of fibromyalgia. *Alternative Therapies in Health and Medicine, 12*(2), 34–41.

Stibich, M., & Wissow, L. (2006). Meaning shift: Findings from wellness acupuncture. *Alternative Therapies in Health and Medicine, 12*(2), 42–48.

World Health Organization. (2003). *Traditional medicine.* Retrieved January 25, 2008, from http://www.who.int/mediacentre/factsheets/fs134/en/

Yu, J., Zhang, X., Liu, C., Meng, Y., & Han, J. (2006). Effect of acupuncture treatment on vascular dementia. *Neurological Research, 28*, 97–103.

UNIT **3**

Lifespan and Developmental Stages

CHAPTER 16
Concepts of Growth and Development

CHAPTER 17
Development from Conception through Adolescence

CHAPTER 18
Young and Middle-Aged Adulthood

CHAPTER 19
Older Adults

Chapter 16

Concepts of Growth and Development

From the moment of conception through to old age, we continue to *grow and develop* until we die. The terms *growth* and *development* are often used interchangeably, but they have different meanings. **Growth** is physical change and increase in size. Indicators of growth include height, weight, bone size, and dentition. Growth rates vary during different stages; for example, the growth rate is rapid during the prenatal, neonatal, infancy, and adolescent stages. **Development** is an increase in the complexity of function and skill progression. It is the capacity and skill of a person to adapt to the environment. Development is the behavioural aspect of growth; for example, a person develops the ability to walk, to talk, and to run. **Developmental milestones** refer to the developmental sequences and patterns that are predictable in a child's growth. These milestones may vary from one culture to another; they are benchmarks for when to expect development tasks to take place (Invest in Kids, 2007).

Growth and development are independent but interrelated processes. For example, an infant's muscles, bones, and nervous system must grow to a certain point before the infant can sit up or walk. Growth generally takes place during the first 20 years of life; development continues after that. Principles of growth and development are shown in Box 16.1.

OBJECTIVES

After studying this chapter, you should be able to

1. Describe the factors that influence human growth and development
2. Discuss the principles and stages of human growth and task development
3. Describe Havighurst's developmental tasks theory
4. Describe the characteristics and implications of Freud's theory of psychosexual development
5. Describe Erikson's eight stages of psychosocial development
6. Compare Peck's and Gould's stages of adult development
7. Explain Piaget's theory of cognitive development
8. Compare Kohlberg's and Gilligan's theories of moral development
9. Compare Fowler's and Westerhoff's stages of spiritual development

BOX 16.1 PRINCIPLES OF GROWTH AND DEVELOPMENT

All humans follow the same pattern of growth and development. The process is independent, interactive, and governed by the following general principles:

- The sequence of each stage is predictable, although the time of onset, the length of the stage, and the effects of each stage vary with the person.
- Each developmental stage has its own characteristics. For example, Piaget suggests that in the sensorimotor stage (birth to 2 years), children learn to coordinate simple motor tasks.
- Growth and development occur
  - in a *cephalocaudal* direction, that is, starting at the head and moving to the trunk, the legs, and the feet. This pattern is particularly obvious at birth, when the head of the infant is disproportionately large.
  - in a proximal to distal direction, that is, from the centre of the body outward (see Figure 16.1). For example, infants can roll over before they can grasp an object with the thumb and second finger.
  - in continuous, orderly, sequential processes influenced by maturational, environmental, and genetic factors.
- Development proceeds from simple to complex or from single acts to integrated acts. To accomplish the integrated act of drinking and swallowing a liquid from a cup, for example, the child must first learn a series of single acts: eye-hand coordination, grasping, hand-mouth coordination, controlled tipping of the cup, and then mouth, lip, and tongue movements to drink and swallow.
- Development becomes increasingly differentiated. *Differentiated development* begins with a generalized response and progresses to a skilled specific response. For example, an infant's initial response to a stimulus involves the total body; a 5-year-old child can respond more specifically with laughter or fear.

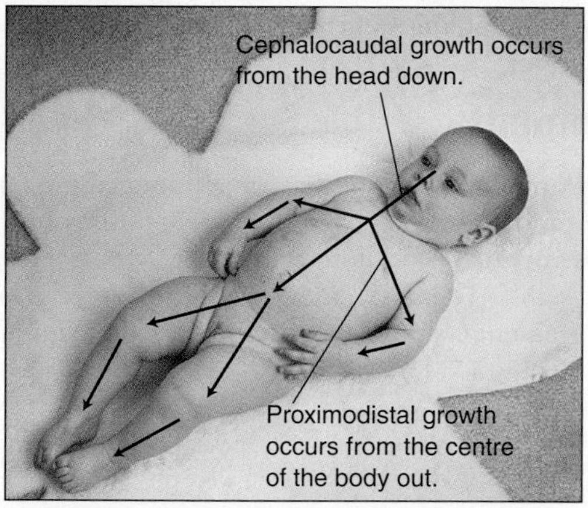
Cephalocaudal growth occurs from the head down.
Proximodistal growth occurs from the centre of the body out.

FIGURE 16.1 Cephalocaudal and proximodistal growth

- Certain stages of growth and development are more critical than others. For example, the first 10 to 12 weeks after conception are critical. The incidence of congenital anomalies as a result of exposure to certain viruses, chemicals, or drugs is greater during this stage than in others.
- The pace of growth and development is uneven. It is known that growth is greater during infancy than during childhood. Asynchronous development is demonstrated by rapid growth of the head during infancy and of the extremities at puberty.

Factors Influencing Growth and Development

Many factors can influence growth and development. Knowledge of these factors helps the nurse to provide anticipatory guidance to promote optimal growth and development of the individual.

Genetic

The genetic inheritance of an individual is established at conception. It remains unchanged throughout life and determines such characteristics as gender, physical characteristics (e.g., eye colour, potential height), and, to some extent, temperament.

Temperament

Temperament (i.e., the way individuals respond to their external and internal environment) sets the stage for the interactive dynamics of growth and development. Temperament may persist throughout the lifespan, though caution must be taken not to irrevocably label or categorize infants and children.

Family

Family provides support and safety for the child. Families are involved in their children's physical and psychological well-being and development (Ball & Bindler, 2006). Children are socialized through family dynamics. The parents set expected behaviours and model appropriate behaviour.

Nutrition

Adequate nutrition is an essential component of growth and development. For example, poorly nourished children are more likely to have infections than are well-nourished children. In addition, poorly nourished children may not attain their full height potential.

Environment

A few environmental factors that can influence growth and development are the child's living conditions (e.g., homelessness), socioeconomic status (e.g., poor versus financially stable), climate, and community (e.g., provides developmental support versus exposes the child to hazards).

Health

Illness or injury can affect growth and development. Being hospitalized is stressful for a child and can affect his or her coping mechanisms. Prolonged or chronic illness may affect normal developmental processes.

Culture

Cultural customs can influence a child's growth and development. Nutritional practices may influence the rate of growth for infants. Childrearing practices may influence development. For example, the Inuit practice of carrying infants on boards often delays walking (Ball & Bindler, 2006).

Stages of Growth and Development

The rate of a person's growth and development is highly individual. However, the sequence of growth and development is predictable. Stages of growth usually correspond to certain developmental changes. See Table 16.1.

Growth and development are commonly thought of as having eight major components: biophysical, psychosocial, cognitive, behavioural, social, ecological, moral, and spiritual. A discussion of some of the major theories relating to these components follows.

Growth and Development Theories

Biophysical Theory

ARNOLD GESELL (1880–1961) Biophysical development theories describe the development and physical changes of the body. These changes are compared against established norms. Arnold Gesell's theory states that development is directed by genetics. He asserts that child development is a maturational process based on an in-born timetable. Although children benefit from experience, they will achieve maturational milestones, such as rolling over, sitting, and walking, at specific times.

Psychosocial Theories

Psychosocial development refers to the development of personality. **Personality** is a complex concept that is difficult to define. It can be considered as the outward (interpersonal) expression of the inner (intrapersonal) self. It encompasses a person's temperament, feelings, character traits, independence, self-esteem, self-concept, behaviour, ability to interact with others, and ability to adapt to life changes.

ROBERT HAVIGHURST (1900–1991) Robert Havighurst believed that learning is basic to life and that people continue to learn throughout life. He described growth and development as occurring during six stages, with tasks to be learned in each (see Table 16.2 on page 294). A **developmental task** is "a task which arises at or about a certain period in the life of an individual, successful achievement of which leads to his happiness and to success with later tasks, while failure leads to unhappiness in the individual, disapproval by society, and difficulty with later tasks" (Havighurst, 1972, p. 2).

Havighurst's developmental tasks provide a framework to evaluate a person's general accomplishments. However, the broad categories limit its usefulness as a tool in assessing specific accomplishments, particularly those of infancy and childhood.

SIGMUND FREUD (1856–1939) Sigmund Freud (1923) introduced a number of concepts about development that are still used today: the unconscious mind, defence mechanisms, and the id, ego, and superego. The **unconscious mind** is the part of a person's mental life that the person is unaware of. This concept of the unconscious is one of Freud's major contributions to the field of psychiatry. **Defence mechanisms**, or **adaptive mechanisms** as they are more commonly called today, are the result of conflicts because of environmental and social restrictions. The **id** is the source of instinctive and unconscious urges, which Freud considered chiefly sexual in nature. The id is also the source of all pleasure and gratification. The **ego** is formed by the person to make effective contact with social and physical needs. Through the ego, the id impulses are satisfied. The **superego** contains the conscience and the ego ideal. The conscience consists of society's "do not's," usually as a result of parental and cultural expectations. The ego ideal comprises the standards of perfection toward which the individual strives. Freud proposed that the underlying motivation to human development is an energy form or life instinct, which he called **libido.**

TABLE 16.1 Stages of Growth and Development

Stage	Age	Significant Characteristics	Nursing Implications
Neonatal	Birth to 28 days	Behaviour is largely reflexive and develops to more purposeful behaviour.	Help parents to identify and meet unmet needs.
Infancy	1 month to 1 year	Physical growth is rapid.	Control the infant's environment so that physical and psychological needs are met.
Toddlerhood	1 to 3 years	Motor development permits increased physical autonomy. Psychosocial skills increase.	Safety and risk-taking strategies must be balanced to permit growth.
Preschool	3 to 6 years	The preschooler's world is expanding. New experiences and the preschooler's social role are tried during play. Physical growth is slower.	Provide opportunities for play and social activity.
School age	6 to 11 years	This stage includes the preadolescent period (10 to 12 years). The peer group increasingly influences behaviour. Physical, cognitive, and social development increase, and communication skills improve.	Allow time and energy for the school-age child to pursue hobbies and school activities. Recognize and support the child's achievements.
Adolescence	12 to 19 years	The self-concept changes with biological development. Values are tested. Physical growth accelerates. Stress increases, especially in the face of conflicts.	Help adolescents to develop coping behaviours. Help adolescents develop strategies for resolving conflicts.
Young adulthood	20 to 39 years	A personal lifestyle develops. The person usually establishes a relationship with a significant other and a commitment to something.	Accept the adult's chosen lifestyle and assist with necessary adjustments relating to health. Recognize the person's commitments. Support change as necessary for health.
Middle adulthood	40 to 64 years	Lifestyle changes because of other changes; for example, children leave home, occupational goals change.	Help clients to plan for anticipated changes in life, to recognize the risk factors related to health, and to focus on strengths rather than weaknesses.
Older adulthood			
Young-old	65 to 74 years	Adaptation to retirement and changing physical abilities is often necessary. Chronic illness may develop.	Help clients to keep physically and socially active and to maintain peer group interactions.
Middle-old	75 to 84 years	Adaptation to decline in speed of movement, reaction time, and sensory abilities, and increasing dependence on others may be necessary.	Help clients to cope with loss (e.g., hearing, sensory abilities, eyesight, death of loved one). Provide necessary safety measures.
Old-old	85 and over	Physical problems may increase.	Assist clients with self-care, as required, and with maintaining as much independence as possible.

According to Freud's theory of psychosexual development, the personality develops in five overlapping stages from birth to adulthood. The libido changes its location of emphasis within the body from one stage to another. Therefore, a particular body area has special significance to a client at a particular stage. The first three stages (oral, anal, and phallic) are called *pregenital stages.* The next stage is the *latency stage.* The culminating stage is the *genital stage.* Table 16.3 on page 295 indicates characteristics for each stage.

If the individual does not achieve a satisfactory resolution at each stage, the personality becomes fixated at that stage. **Fixation** is immobilization or the inability of the personality to proceed to the next stage because of anxiety. For example, nurses can assist an infant's development by making feeding a pleasurable experience and by making toilet training a positive experience, thereby enhancing the child's feeling of self-control. If, however, the toilet training was a negative experience, the resulting conflict or stress can delay or prolong progression

TABLE 16.2 Havighurst's Age Periods and Developmental Tasks

Infancy and Early Childhood

1. Learning to walk
2. Learning to take solid foods
3. Learning to talk
4. Learning to control the elimination of body wastes
5. Learning sex differences and sexual modesty
6. Achieving psychological stability
7. Forming simple concepts of social and physical reality
8. Learning to relate emotionally to parents, siblings, and other people
9. Learning to distinguish right from wrong and developing a conscience

Middle Childhood

1. Learning physical skills necessary for ordinary games
2. Building wholesome attitudes toward oneself as a growing organism
3. Learning to get along with age-mates
4. Learning an appropriate masculine or feminine social role
5. Developing fundamental skills in reading, writing, and arithmetic
6. Developing concepts necessary for everyday living
7. Developing conscience, morality, and a scale of values
8. Achieving personal independence
9. Developing attitudes toward social groups and institutions

Adolescence

1. Achieving new and more mature relations with age-mates of both genders
2. Achieving a masculine or feminine social role
3. Accepting one's physique and using the body effectively
4. Achieving emotional independence from parents and other adults
5. Achieving assurance of economic independence
6. Selecting and preparing for an occupation
7. Preparing for marriage and family life
8. Developing intellectual skills and concepts necessary for civic competence
9. Desiring and achieving socially responsible behaviour
10. Acquiring a set of values and an ethical system as a guide to behaviour

Early Adulthood

1. Selecting a mate
2. Learning to live with a partner
3. Starting a family
4. Rearing children
5. Managing a home
6. Getting started in an occupation
7. Taking on civic responsibility
8. Finding a congenial social group

Middle Age

1. Achieving adult civic and social responsibility
2. Establishing and maintaining an economic standard of living
3. Assisting teenage children to become responsible and happy adults
4. Developing adult leisure-time activities
5. Relating oneself to one's spouse as a person
6. Accepting and adjusting to the physiological changes of middle age
7. Adjusting to aging parents

Later Maturity

1. Adjusting to decreasing physical strength and health
2. Adjusting to retirement and reduced income
3. Adjusting to death of spouse
4. Establishing an explicit affiliation with one's age group
5. Meeting social and civic obligations
6. Establishing satisfactory physical living arrangements

Source: From *Developmental Tasks and Education,* 3rd ed., by Robert J. Havighurst, 1972, New York: Longman. Copyright © 1972 by Longman Publishers, USA. Reprinted with permission.

through a stage or cause a person to regress to a previous stage. Ideally, an individual progresses through each stage with balance among the id, ego, and superego.

ERIK ERIKSON (1902–1996) Erik H. Erikson (1963, 1964) adapted and expanded Freud's theory of development to include the entire lifespan, believing that people continue to develop throughout life. He described eight stages of development. In contrast to Freud, Erikson believed the ego to be the conscious core of the personality. See Table 16.4 on page 296.

Erikson envisioned life as a sequence of developmental stages or levels of achievement. Each stage signals a task that must be achieved. The resolution of the task can be complete, partial, or unsuccessful. Erikson believed that the greater the task achievement, the healthier is the personality of the person; failure to achieve a task influences the person's ability to achieve the next task. These developmental tasks can be viewed as a series of crises, and successful resolution of these crises is supportive to the person's ego. Failure to resolve the crises is damaging to the ego. After attaining one developmental stage, the person may fall back and need to approach it again.

Erikson's eight stages reflect both positive and negative aspects of the critical life periods. The resolution of the conflicts at each stage enables the person to function

TABLE 16.3 Freud's Five Stages of Development

Stage	Age	Characteristics	Implications
Oral	Birth to 1.5 years	Mouth is the centre of pleasure (major source of gratification and exploration). Security is primary need. Major conflict: weaning	Feeding produces pleasure and sense of comfort and safety. Feeding should be pleasurable and provided when required.
Anal	1.5 to 3 years	Anus and bladder are the sources of pleasure (sensual satisfaction, self-control). Major conflict: toilet training	Controlling and expelling feces provide pleasure and sense of control. Toilet training should be a pleasurable experience.
Phallic	4 to 6 years	The child's genitals are the centre of pleasure. Masturbation offers pleasure. Other activities can include fantasy, experimentation with peers, and questioning of adults about sexual topics. Major conflict: the Oedipus or Electra complex, which resolves when the child identifies with parent of same sex. (The Oedipus complex refers to the male child's attraction for his mother and hostile attitudes toward his father. The Electra complex refers to the female's attraction for her father and hostile attitudes toward her mother.)	The child identifies with the parent of the opposite sex and later takes on a love relationship outside the family. Encourage identity.
Latency	6 years to puberty	Energy is directed to physical and intellectual activities. Sexual impulses tend to be repressed. Develop relationships between peers of the same sex.	Encourage child with physical and intellectual pursuits. Encourage sports and other activities with same-sex peers.
Genital	Puberty and after	Energy is directed toward full sexual maturity and function and development of skills needed to cope with the environment.	Encourage separation from parents, achievement of independence, and decision making.

Source: From *Health Promotion Strategies Through the Life Span*, 7th ed. (p. 238), by R. B. Murray and J. P. Zentner, 2001, Upper Saddle River, NJ: Merrill/Prentice Hall. Adapted with permission.

effectively in society. Each stage has its developmental task, and the individual must find a balance between, for example, trust versus mistrust (stage 1) or integrity versus despair (stage 8) (see Figures 16.2 and 16.3).

When using Erikson's developmental framework, nurses should be aware of indicators of positive and negative resolution of each stage and note that the environment is highly influential in development. Nurses can enhance a client's development by being aware of the person's developmental stage and by helping the person develop coping skills relative to stressors experienced at that level and by providing the individual with appropriate opportunities and encouragement. For example, a 10-year-old child can be encouraged to be creative, to finish schoolwork, and to learn how to accomplish these tasks within the limitations imposed by illness.

Erikson emphasized that people must change and adapt their behaviour to maintain control over their lives. In his view, no stage in personality development can be bypassed, but people can become fixated at one stage or regress to a previous stage. For example, a middle-aged woman who has never satisfactorily accomplished the task of resolving identity versus role confusion might regress to an earlier stage when stressed by an illness she cannot cope with.

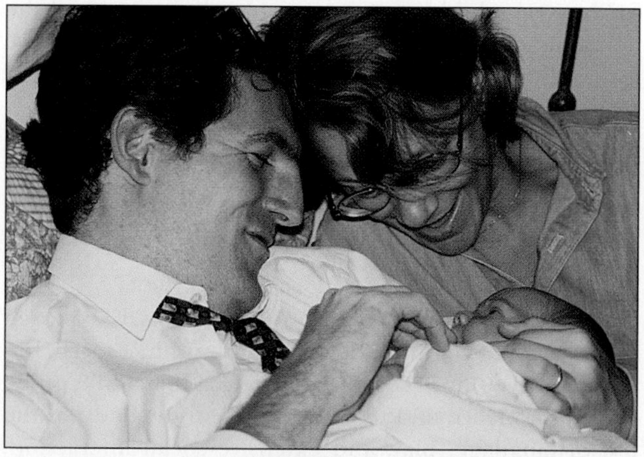

FIGURE 16.2 Trust is established when the infant's basic needs are met.

TABLE 16.4 Erikson's Eight Stages of Development

Stage	Age	Central Task	Indicators of Positive Resolution	Indicators of Negative Resolution
Infancy	Birth to 18 months	Trust versus mistrust	Learning to trust others	Mistrust, withdrawal, estrangement
Early childhood	18 months to 3 years	Autonomy versus shame and doubt	Self-control without loss of self-esteem Ability to cooperate and to express oneself	Compulsive self-restraint or compliance Willfulness and defiance
Late childhood	3 to 6 years	Initiative versus guilt	Learning the degree to which assertiveness and purpose influence the environment Beginning ability to evaluate one's own behaviour	Lack of self-confidence Pessimism, fear of wrongdoing Overcontrol and overrestriction of own activity
School age	6 to 12 years	Industry versus inferiority	Beginning to create, develop, and manipulate Developing sense of competence and perseverance	Loss of hope, sense of being mediocre Withdrawal from school and peers
Adolescence	12 to 18 years	Identity versus role confusion	Coherent sense of self Plans to actualize own abilities	Feelings of confusion, indecisiveness, and possible antisocial behaviour
Young adulthood	18 to 25 years	Intimacy versus isolation	Intimate relationship with another person Commitment to work and relationships	Impersonal relationships Avoidance of relationship, career, or lifestyle commitments
Adulthood	25 to 65 years	Generativity versus stagnation	Creativity, productivity, concern for others	Self-indulgence, self-concern, lack of interests and commitments
Maturity	65 years to death	Integrity versus despair	Acceptance of worth and uniqueness of own life Acceptance of death	Sense of loss, contempt for others

Source: Adapted from *Childhood and Society,* by Erik H. Erikson, 1991, New York: W. W. Norton. Copyright 1950, © 1963 by W. W. Norton & Company, Inc., renewed © 1978, 1991 by Erik H. Erikson. Reprinted by permission of W. W. Norton & Company, Inc.

STELLA CHESS (1914–2007) AND ALEXANDER THOMAS (1914–2003) Stella Chess and Alexander Thomas identified nine temperamental qualities seen in children's behaviour (see Table 16.5). The "goodness of fit" between children's temperamental qualities and the demands of their environment contributes to positive interaction and positive growth and development (Rothbart, 2004). **Goodness of fit** refers to whether parents' expectations of their child's behaviour are consistent with the child's temperament type. When parents understand a child's temperament characteristics, they are better able to shape the environment to meet the child's needs (Ball & Bindler, 2006).

LEV VYGOTSKY (1896–1934) Lev Vygotsky explored the concept of cognitive development within a social, historical, and cultural context. He viewed that adults guide children to learn and that development depends on the use of language, play, and extensive social interaction. His ideas have been used in the treatment of children with learning disorders, autism, mental challenges, and other disabilities (Edwards, 2002). His work also supports the benefit of adult social learning opportunities via group interaction and observation.

ROBERT PECK (1919–2002) Robert Peck believed that physical capabilities and functions decrease with old age, and mental and social capacities tend to increase in the latter part of life (Peck, 1968). He proposed three developmental tasks during old age, in contrast to Erikson's stage of maturity (integrity versus despair):

1. *Ego differentiation versus work-role preoccupation.* An adult's identity and feelings of worth are highly dependent on that person's work role. On retirement, people may experience feelings of worthlessness unless they derive their sense of identity from a number of roles so that one such role can replace the work role or occupation as a source of self-esteem. For example, a man who likes to garden or golf can obtain ego rewards from those activities, replacing rewards formerly obtained from his occupation.
2. *Body transcendence versus body preoccupation.* This task calls for the individual to adjust to decreasing physical capacities and, at the same time, maintain

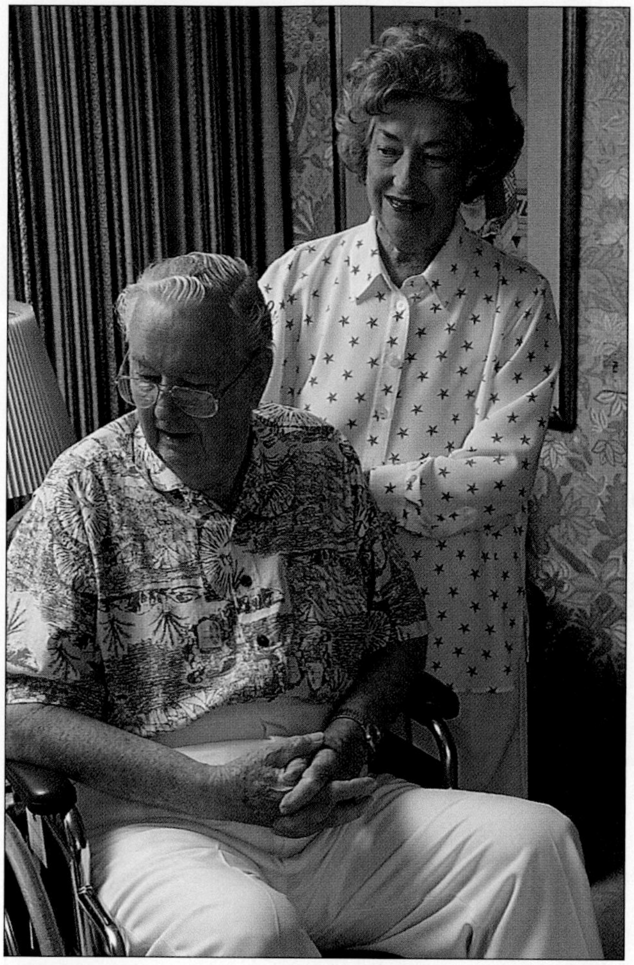

FIGURE 16.3 Assistive devices help maintain independence and self-esteem, which also helps the older adult's ego integrity to adapt and cope with the reality of aging.

TABLE 16.5 Chess ad Thomas's Characteristics of Temperament

Characteristic	Examples of Behaviour Style
Activity level	Active, restless, always on the move versus quiet, inactive
Sensitivity	Apparently oblivious to stimuli versus reacts to minimal stimuli
Intensity	Minimal reaction to stimuli versus strong and intense reaction
Adaptability	Responds smoothly to unexpected events versus resists change
Distractibility	Focuses on tasks versus easily distracted by minimal stimuli
Approach and withdrawal	Jumps right into activities versus hesitant to engage, slow to warm up
Mood	Cheerful, happy versus serious, sombre
Persistence	Sticks to tasks versus easily gives up
Regularity	Demonstrates patterns of behaviour versus random activity

feelings of well-being. Preoccupation with declining body functions reduces happiness and satisfaction with life.

3. *Ego transcendence versus ego preoccupation.* Ego transcendence is the acceptance, without fear, of death as inevitable. This acceptance includes being actively involved in our own future beyond death. Ego preoccupation, by contrast, results in holding onto life and a preoccupation with self-gratification.

ROGER GOULD (B. 1935) Roger Gould (1972) believed that transformation is a central theme during adulthood. He described seven stages of adult development:

- *Stage 1 (ages 16–18).* Individuals consider themselves part of the family, rather than individuals, and want to separate from their parents.
- *Stage 2 (ages 18–22).* Although the individuals have established autonomy, they feel it is in jeopardy; they feel they could be pulled back into their families.
- *Stage 3 (ages 22–28).* Individuals feel established as adults and autonomous from their families. They see themselves as well defined but still feel the need to prove themselves to their parents. They see this as the time for growing and building for the future.
- *Stage 4 (ages 29–34).* Marriage and careers are well established. Individuals question what life is all

Evidence-Informed Practice

What Impact Does Financial Stress Have on the Health of Canadians?

When added to increasing mortgage burdens, escalating personal debt from unrestrained consumer purchasing and spending is creating devastating financial stress across Canada. The increasing frequency of personal bankruptcy, relationship problems, depression, and suicide are direct results of financial debts. Suggestions for health interventions include looking at individual personal spending, deciding on necessities, seeking a mutual plan for saving to eliminating needless purchases, seeking assistance from nonprofit charitable agencies mandated to provide credit counselling and debt-resolution services, learning more about hidden debt-proliferating lifestyle choices and ways to avoid these traps, and teaching children and youth the essential skills of budgeting, how debt begins, and how to manage money responsibly.

NURSING IMPLICATIONS: The nurse must be aware of "debt stress" and help clients to manage their budget to fulfill their life responsibility, according to their adult development and task levels. This may help their clients avoid financial and health crises.

Source: Based on *The High Health Cost of Debt,* by K. Jenkins, 2007, Ottawa: Canadian Health Network, Public Health Agency of Canada. Retrieved April 19, 2007, from http://www.canadian-health-network.ca/servlet/ContentServer?cid=1164718734763&pagena

about and want to be accepted as they are, no longer finding it necessary to prove themselves.

- *Stage 5 (ages 35–43)*. Through self-reflection, individuals question values and life itself. They see time as finite, with little time left to shape the lives of adolescent children.
- *Stage 6 (ages 43–50)*. Personalities are seen as set. Time is accepted as finite. Individuals are interested in social activities with friends and spouse and desire both sympathy and affection from spouse.
- *Stage 7 (ages 50–60)*. This is a period of transformation, with a realization of mortality and a concern for health. There is an increase in warmth and a decrease in negativism. The spouse is seen as a valuable companion (Gould, 1972, pp. 525–527).

The concept map provides an overview of growth and development psychosocial theories and theorists.

CONCEPT MAP

Overview of Growth and Development Psychosocial Theories and Theorists

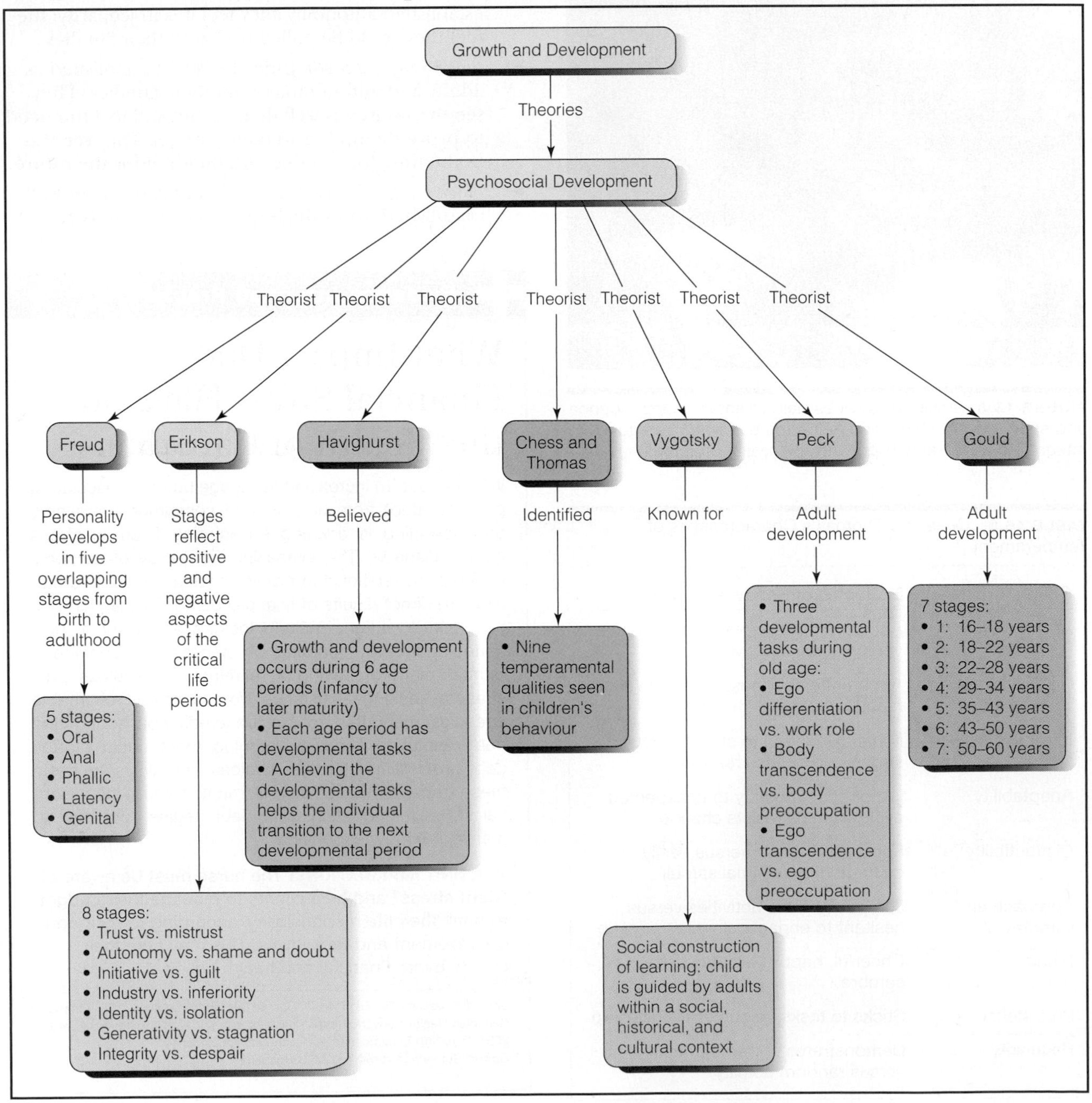

Cognitive Theory

JEAN PIAGET (1896–1980) **Cognitive development** refers to the manner in which people learn to think, reason, and use language. It involves a person's intelligence, perceptual ability, and ability to process information. Cognitive development represents a progression of mental abilities from illogical to logical thinking, from simple to complex problem solving, and from understanding concrete ideas to understanding abstract concepts.

The most widely known cognitive theorist is Jean Piaget. According to Piaget (1966), cognitive development is an orderly, sequential process in which a variety of new experiences (stimuli) must exist before intellectual abilities can develop. Piaget's cognitive developmental process is divided into five major phases: the sensorimotor phase, the preconceptual phase, the intuitive thought phase, the concrete operations phase, and the formal operations phase. A person develops through each of these phases; each phase has its own unique characteristics. See Table 16.6.

In each phase, the person uses three primary abilities: *assimilation, accommodation,* and *adaptation.* **Assimilation** is the process through which humans encounter and react to new situations by using the mechanisms they already possess. In this way, people acquire knowledge and skills as well as insights into the world around them. **Accommodation** is a process of change whereby cognitive processes mature sufficiently to allow the person to solve problems that were unsolvable before. This adjustment is possible chiefly because new knowledge has been assimilated. **Adaptation**, or coping behaviour, is the ability to handle the demands made by the environment.

TABLE 16.6 Piaget's Phases of Cognitive Development

Phases and Stages	Age	Significant Behaviour
Sensorimotor phase	Birth to 2 years	
Stage 1: Use of reflexes	Birth to 1 month	Most action is reflexive
Stage 2: Primary circular reaction	1 to 4 months	Perception of events is centred on the body Objects are extension of self
Stage 3: Secondary circular reaction	4 to 8 months	Acknowledges the external environment Actively makes changes in the environment
Stage 4: Coordination of secondary schemata	8 to 12 months	Can distinguish a goal from a means of attaining it
Stage 5: Tertiary circular reaction	12 to 18 months	Tries and discovers new goals and ways to attain goals Rituals are important
Stage 6: Inventions of new means	18 to 24 months	Interprets the environment by mental image Uses make-believe and pretend play
Preconceptual phase	2 to 4 years	Uses an egocentric approach to accommodate the demands of an environment Everything is significant and relates to "me" Explores the environment Language development is rapid Associates words with objects
Intuitive thought phase	4 to 7 years	Egocentric thinking diminishes Thinks of one idea at a time Includes others in the environment Words express thoughts
Concrete operations phase	7 to 11 years	Solves concrete problems Begins to understand relationships, such as size Understands right and left Cognizant of viewpoints
Formal operations phase	11 to 15 years	Uses rational thinking Reasoning is deductive and futuristic

Source: Adapted from *The Origins of Intelligence in Children*, by J. Piaget, 1966, Madison, CT: International Universities Press, Inc. Copyright © 1966. Used by permission.

Nurses can employ Piaget's theory of cognitive development when developing teaching strategies. For example, a nurse can expect a toddler to be egocentric and literal; therefore, explanations to the toddler should focus on the needs of the toddler, rather than on the needs of others. When teaching adults, nurses may become aware that some adults are more comfortable with concrete thought and are slower to acquire and apply new information than are other adults.

Behaviourist Theory

B. F. SKINNER (1904–1990) Behaviourist theory, or behaviourism, states that learning takes place when an individual's reaction to a stimulus is either positively or negatively reinforced. The more rapid, consistent, and positive the reinforcement is, the more likely a behaviour is to be learned and retained. B. F. Skinner believed that organisms learn as they respond to or operate in their environment. He maintained that rewarded or reinforced behaviour will be repeated; behaviour that is punished will be suppressed. Most of his work was with laboratory animals.

Social Learning Theory

ALBERT BANDURA (B. 1925) Social learning theorists contend that this process of learning by observing and thinking about the behaviour of others may not always lead to change in the individual's behaviour; in contrast, behaviourist theory says that learning will result in a permanent change in behaviour. Albert Bandura believes that learning occurs through imitation and practice and requires more awareness, self-motivation, and self-regulation of the individual, and that the individual actively interacts with the environment to learn new skills and behaviours.

Ecologic Theory

URIE BRONFENBRENNER (1917–2005) Urie Bronfenbrenner viewed the child as interacting with the environment at different levels, or systems. He believed each child brings a unique set of genes—and specific attributes, such as age, gender, health, and other characteristics—to his or her interactions with the environment (Ball & Bindler, 2006).

Ecologic theory has five levels or systems. The *microsystem* includes close relationships the child has on a daily basis (e.g., home, school, friends). The *mesosystem* level includes relationships of microsystems with one another. For example, two common microsystems for children are home and school. The *exosystem* includes those settings that may influence the child but with which the child does not have daily contact (e.g., parent's job, local school board). The *macrosystem* level includes attitudes and beliefs of the child's culture, and the *chronosystem* involves the time period in which the child is growing up as it influences views of health and illness.

Moral Theories

Moral development, a complex process not fully understood, involves learning what ought to be and what ought not to be done. It is more than imprinting parents' rules and virtues or values on children. The term **moral** means "relating to right and wrong." The terms *morality, moral behaviour,* and *moral development* need to be distinguished. **Morality** refers to the requirements necessary for people to live together in society; **moral behaviour** is the way a person perceives those requirements and responds to them; **moral development** is the pattern of change in moral behaviour with age.

LAWRENCE KOHLBERG (1927–1987) Lawrence Kohlberg's theory specifically addressed moral development in children and adults (Berkowitz & Oser, 1985). Kohlberg focused on the reasons an individual makes a decision. He viewed moral development as progressing through three levels and six stages. Levels and stages are not always linked to a certain developmental stage because some people progress to a higher level of moral development than others do.

At Kohlberg's first level, called the *premoral* or *preconventional level,* children are responsive to cultural rules and labels of good and bad, right and wrong. However, children interpret these in terms of the physical consequences of their actions, that is, punishment or reward. At the second level, the *conventional level,* the individual is concerned about maintaining the expectations of the family, group, or nation and sees this as right. The emphasis at this level is on conformity and loyalty to his or her own expectations as well as society's. Level three is called the *postconventional, autonomous,* or *principled level.* At this level, people make an effort to define valid values and principles without regard to outside authority or to the expectations of others. For additional information about Kohlberg's levels, see Table 16.7.

CAROL GILLIGAN (B. 1936) Carol Gilligan (1982) believes that moral development needs to include the concepts of caring and responsibility. She views moral development as proceeding through three levels and two transitions, with each level representing a more complex understanding of the relationship of the self and others and each transition resulting in a crucial re-evaluation of the conflict between selfishness and responsibility (Murray & Zentner, 2001, p. 251).

- *Stage 1, caring for the self.* In this stage, the person is concerned only with caring for the self. The individual feels isolated, alone, and unconnected to others, and has no concern or conflict with the needs of others because the self is the most impor-

TABLE 16.7 Kohlberg's Stages of Moral Development

Level	Stage	Average Age
I. **Preconventional** Person is responsive to cultural rules of labels of good and bad, right or wrong. Externally established rules determine right or wrong actions. Person reasons in terms of punishment, reward, or exchange of favours.	1. **Punishment and Obedient Orientation** Fear of punishment, not respect for authority, is the reason for decisions, behaviour, and conformity.	Toddler to 7 years
Egocentric focus	2. **Instrumental Relativist Orientation** Conformity is based on egocentricity and narcissistic needs. There is no feeling of justice, loyalty, or gratitude. "I'll do something if I get something for it or because it pleases you."	Preschooler through school age
II. **Conventional** Person is concerned with maintaining expectations and rules of the family, group, nation, or society. A sense of guilt has developed and affects behaviour. The person values conformity, loyalty, and active maintenance of social order and control. Conformity means good behaviour or what pleases or helps another and is approved.	3. **Interpersonal Concordance Orientation** Decisions and behaviour are based on concerns about others' reactions; the person wants others' approval or a reward. An empathic response, based on understanding of how another person feels, is a determinant for decisions and behaviour. ("I can put myself in your shoes.")	School age through adulthood (most [Canadian] women are in this stage)
Societal focus	4. **Law-and-Order Orientation** The person wants established rules from authorities, and the reason for decisions and behaviour is that social and sexual rules and traditions demand the response. ("I'll do something because it's the law and my duty.")	Adolescence and adulthood (most men are in this stage)
III. **Postconventional** The person lives autonomously and defines moral values and principles that are distinct from personal identification with group values. He or she lives according to principles that are universally agreed on and that the person considers appropriate for life.	5. **Social Contract Legalistic Orientation** The social rules are not the sole basis for decisions and behaviour because the person believes a higher moral principle applies, such as equality, justice, or due process.	Middle-age or older adult. Only 20% or less of [Canadians] achieve this stage.
Universal focus	6. **Universal Ethical Principle Orientation** Decisions and behaviours are based on internalized rules, on conscience rather than social laws, and on self-chosen ethical and abstract principles that are universal, comprehensive, and consistent.	Middle-age or older adult. Few people attain or maintain this stage. Examples of this stage are seen in times of crisis or extreme situations.

Source: From Health Promotion Strategies Through the Life Span, *7th ed. (pp. 252–253), by R. B. Murray and J. P. Zentner, 2001, Upper Saddle River, NJ: Merrill/Prentice Hall. Adapted with permission.*

tant. The focus of this stage is survival. The end of this stage occurs when the individual begins to view this approach as selfish. At this time, the person also begins to see a need for relationships and connections with other people.

- *Stage 2, caring for others.* The individual recognizes the selfishness of earlier behaviour and begins to understand the need for caring relationships with others. Caring relationships bring with them responsibility. The definition of *responsibility* includes self-sacrifice, where "good" is considered to be "caring for others." The individual now approaches relationships with a focus of not hurting others. This approach causes the individual to be more responsive and submissive to others' needs, excluding any thoughts of meeting his or her own. A transition occurs when the individual recognizes that this approach can cause difficulties with relationships because of the lack of balance between caring for the self and caring for others.
- *Stage 3, caring for the self and others.* A person sees the need for a balance between caring for others and caring for the self. The concept of responsibility now includes responsibility for the self and for other people. Care remains the focus by which decisions are made. However, the person recognizes the interconnections between the self and others and realizes that if his or her own needs are not met, other people may also suffer.

Gilligan believes women often see morality in the integrity of relationships and caring so that the moral problems they encounter are different from those of men. Men tend to consider what is right to be what is just, whereas for women, what is right is taking responsibility for others as a self-chosen decision (Gilligan, 1982). The ethic of justice, or fairness, is based on the idea of equality and equal treatment.

Spiritual Theories

The spiritual component of growth and development refers to individuals' understanding of their relationship with the universe and their perceptions about the direction and meaning of life.

JAMES FOWLER (B. 1940) James Fowler (1981) describes **faith** as a force that gives meaning to a person's life. *Faith* is a form of knowing, a way of being in relation to "an ultimate environment"; it is a relational phenomenon and is "an active 'mode-of-being-in-relation' to another or others in which we invest commitment, belief, love, risk and hope" (Fowler & Keen, 1985). See Table 16.8.

Fowler believes that the development of faith is an interactive process between the person and the environment. In each of Fowler's stages, new patterns of thought, values, and beliefs are added to those already held by the individual; therefore, the stages must follow in sequence.

JOHN WESTERHOFF (B. 1933) Westerhoff (1976) describes faith as a way of being and behaving that evolves from an experienced faith guided by parents and others during a person's infancy and childhood to an owned faith that is internalized in adulthood and serves as a directive for personal action (see Table 16.9). For the client who is ill, faith—whether in a higher authority (e.g., God, Allah, Jehovah), in the client's own self, in the health-care team, or in a combination of all—provides strength and trust.

Applying Growth and Development Concepts to Nursing Practice

Different theories explain one or more aspects of an individual's growth and development. The nurse may find it necessary to apply several theories for an adequate understanding of the growth and development of a client (see the Reflect on Primary Health Care box). Developmental theories can be useful in guiding assessment, explaining behaviour, and providing a direction for nursing interventions. An understanding of a child's intellectual ability helps a nurse to anticipate and explain certain reactions, responses, and needs. Nurses can then encourage client behaviour that is appropriate for that particular developmental stage. In adult care, knowledge about the physical, cognitive, and psychological aspects of the aging process is a fundamental aspect of administering sensitive nursing care.

TABLE 16.8 Fowler's Stages of Spiritual Development

Stage	Age	Description
0. Undifferentiated	0 to 3 years	Infant is unable to formulate concepts about self or the environment
1. Intuitive-projective	4 to 6 years	A combination of images and beliefs given by trusted others, mixed with the child's own experience and imagination
2. Mythic-literal	7 to 12 years	Private world of fantasy and wonder; symbols refer to something specific; dramatic stories and myths used to communicate spiritual meanings
3. Synthetic-conventional	Adolescent or adult	World and ultimate environment is structured by the expectations and judgments of others; interpersonal focus
4. Individuating-reflective	After 18 years	Constructing one's own explicit system; high degree of self-consciousness
5. Paradoxical-consolidative	After 30 years	Awareness of truth from a variety of viewpoints
6. Universalizing	Maybe never	Becoming an incarnation of the principles of love and justice

Sources: Adapted from *Life Maps: Conversations in the Journey of Faith*, by J. Fowler and S. Keen, 1985, Waco, TX: Word Books; and *How to Help Your Child Have a Spiritual Life: A Parents' Guide to Inner Development*, by A. Hollander, 1980, New York: A and W Publishers. Used with permission.

TABLE 16.9 Westerhoff's Four Stages of Faith

Stage	Age	Behaviour
Experience faith	Infancy/early adolescence	Experiences faith through interaction with others who are living a particular faith tradition
Affiliative faith	Late adolescence	Actively participates in activities that characterize a particular faith tradition; experiences awe and wonderment; feels a sense of belonging
Searching faith	Young adulthood	Through a process of questioning and doubting own faith, acquires a cognitive as well as an affective faith
Owned faith	Middle adulthood/old age	Puts faith into personal and social action and is willing to stand up for what the individual believes, even against the nurturing community

Source: Adapted from *Will Our Children Have Faith?* (pp. 79–103), by J. Westerhoff, 1976, New York: Seabury Press.

REFLECT ON PRIMARY HEALTH CARE

By understanding human growth and development, nurses can provide anticipatory *health-promotion* teaching to help clients reach their optimal health. Consider this example: pregnant adolescents tend to make egocentric and lifestyle choices without regard for the future health consequences of the unborn child; nurses can teach pregnant teens that maternal alcohol consumption during pregnancy can negatively alter the growth and developmental potential of the fetus. Find out if pregnant teens have *access* to early prenatal care in your community.

Case Study 16

The client is a 4-month-old child whose parents have recently emigrated from Ghana, Africa. They have been in Canada for about a year. Carol, the mother, attended prenatal classes and followed routine protocols to prepare for a vaginal delivery, which was uneventful. John weighed 2.5 kg at birth and now weighs about 7.3 kg. He is being seen at the well-baby clinic for a routine appointment. His mother comments that John recognizes her voice and is able to roll over, but he still needs two naps a day. She expresses concern that his movements appear clumsy.

Critical Thinking Questions

1. What conclusions can you draw about the child's growth and development on the basis of the data provided?
2. What contextual factors might influence the client's future development?
3. What suggestions would you make to his mother to support John's growth and development?
4. What attitude and cognitive critical thinking skills did you use to answer the questions pertaining to this case?

After working through these questions, go to the MyNursingLab at **http://www.mynursinglab.com** to check your answers.

KEY TERMS

growth
development
developmental milestones
temperament
personality
developmental tasks
unconscious mind
defence mechanisms or adaptive mechanisms
id
ego
superego
libido
fixation
goodness of fit
cognitive development
assimilation
accommodation
adaptation
moral
morality
moral behaviour
moral development
faith

CHAPTER HIGHLIGHTS

- Growth is physical change and an increase in size. The pattern of physiological growth is similar for all people.
- Development is an increase in the complexity of function and skill progression. It is the capacity and skill of the individual to adapt to the environment.
- The rate of a person's growth and development is highly individual, but the sequence of growth and development is predictable.
- Heredity and environment are the primary factors influencing growth and development.
- Components of growth and development are generally categorized as biophysical, psychosocial, cognitive, behavioural, social, ecologic, moral, and spiritual.
- Gesell's biophysical development theory stated that development is directed by genetics.
- Psychosocial development refers to the development of personality. Psychosocial theorists include Havighurst, Freud, Erickson, Chess and Thomas, Vygotsky, Peck, and Gould.
- Havighurst believed that learning is basic to life and that people continue to learn throughout life. His theory describes six age periods, with developmental tasks for each period.
- Cognitive development refers to the manner in which people learn to think, reason, and use language. The most widely known cognitive theorist is Piaget.
- Behaviourist learning theory emphasizes stimulus response and either positive or negative reinforcement as the basis for learning and behaviour change. The most widely known behaviourist theorist is Skinner.
- Social learning theory states that learning can occur by observation. Role modelling and learning from watching role models are a part of social learning theory. Attention and cognitive function, in which the individual thinks about the behaviour of the self and others, as well as the expected rewards and punishments for certain behaviours, are important to social learning. The most widely known social learning theorist is Bandura.
- Ecologic theory sees the child as interacting with the environment at different levels, or systems. Bronfenbrenner described five levels or systems of interaction.
- Moral development, a complex process not fully understood, involves learning what ought to be and what ought not to be done. Kohlberg's theory focuses on the reasons an individual makes a decision. Gilligan's theory included the concepts of caring and responsibility in the stages of moral development, which move through three levels and two transitions.
- The spiritual component of growth and development refers to individuals' understanding of their relationship with the universe and their perceptions about the direction and meaning of life. Fowler and Westerhoff are two theorists who describe stages of spiritual development or faith.
- The nurse's major role is in assessing the client's growth and development to maintain or promote the client's health.

ASSESS YOUR LEARNING

1. Research has shown that the vast majority of young Canadians below the age of 18 who skateboard wear no protective equipment. What would be the most effective strategy a community health nurse could use to decrease the incidence of accidental injuries in this population?

   a. Involve a group of adolescents in creating a video that promotes the use of protective gear for skateboarders.

   b. Lobby government to create a law that makes wearing protecting gear mandatory for skateboarders.

c. Lecture to groups of school-age children and adolescents on the importance of wearing protective gear when skateboarding.

d. Develop an information pamphlet for parents describing the risks of skateboarding and the importance of protective gear.

2. Piaget's cognitive theory has application to pediatric practice. Which of the following is one example of how to integrate Piaget's theory to nursing practice?

a. Making sure 3-year-olds have a clock to see when their pills are due

b. Providing two methods of medicine administration by glass or spoon to preschool children so they have a choice

c. Assimilating family members into the care plan to promote positive outcomes

d. Teaching parents that their child can understand and do simple math

3. Constance, age 12 years, is crying by her locker at school. Her friends are gathered around, trying to "give her some protection." You are the school nurse who is called by the physical education teacher to come and help out. On the way, you reflect on the most likely scenario you will find. Based on the norms of growth and development, you would most likely find which of the following?

a. Constance has begun her menstrual cycle, was unprepared, and is embarrassed and frightened.

b. Students want to focus on Constance's need for peer pressure.

c. Constance has fallen or been injured and collapsed by her locker in pain.

d. Her friends have been trying to protect her from bullies in the school.

4. The parents of a 5-month-old infant and a 3-year-old child ask the nurse about the sequence and timing of developmental milestones. Which of the following is the most appropriate response?

a. "This infant should reach the milestones at the same time as your older child did."

b. "The infant may reach the milestones in a different order from your older child."

c. "The sequence of reaching each milestone should follow the same pattern but may be at a different rate."

d. "There are no predictable patterns. Try to enjoy the uniqueness of each child."

5. The nurse examines a 2-year-old child recently hospitalized with pneumonia. Which patterns of behaviour are most likely to be exhibited by the child?

a. Lies quietly while the nurse listens to the lungs

b. Asks many questions about what the nurse is doing and hearing

c. Fusses, cries, and pushes the nurse away during assessment of the breath sounds

d. Enjoys playing "nurse" with the stethoscope, and listens to self and others' breath sounds

6. A 14-year-old is scheduled to have surgical repair of a spinal curvature (scoliosis). The adolescent will be hospitalized for about 2 weeks. What nursing intervention will be most helpful during the hospital stay?

a. Have peers visit frequently during the day.

b. Instruct parents to room-in with her.

c. Encourage her to go to the recreation room.

d. Encourage her to arrange for her teachers to provide her with homework.

7. A 65-year-old man who recently retired after 40 years of work as an independent contractor is scheduled for a physical examination. The nurse should be concerned about which of the following comments?

a. "My wife and I are planning to drive to Halifax in June to visit our grandkids."

b. "Every day, when I wake up, it's hard to find a reason to get out of bed."

c. "I often take ibuprofen for the pain in my knees."

d. "People still call me for advice on building projects. I may never get to retire!"

8. An 11-year-old child is scheduled for a yearly physical examination. The accompanying parent expresses concern because the child "seems all wrapped up in the soccer teammates and other peers, leaving very little time for the family." Using Havighurst's developmental tasks, what would be the nurse's *best* response?

a. "This is somewhat unusual. Are there problems that we need to discuss?"

b. "Although this is normal for 11-year-olds, this transition can be difficult for families."

c. "Become involved in her life and insist that she set aside time for the family."

d. "This is normal development. You need to let her grow up."

9. A 5-year-old boy arrives for the preadmission workup for a surgical procedure. When the nurse brings in the intravenous (IV) control pump the child states, "I am afraid that it will bite me because I have been bad." Using knowledge of Piaget, Erikson, and Fowler, which of the following is the best nursing action?

a. Reassure the child by providing opportunities for touching and exploring the machine, as well as explaining how it works.

b. Understand that his imagination is out of control. Tell him that his fears are unfounded and that he needs to be a "big boy."

c. Recognize that he is too young to understand and that he needs to be quickly distracted.

d. Acknowledge his need for fantasy by reassuring him that if he is a "good boy" the bad machine will not bite him.

10. Nursing implications associated with the care of people in middle adulthood must consider which of the following?

a. Clients' stage of development encourages them to be self-centred and actively changing.

b. Individuals will be focused on their increasing age and physical limits.

c. Personal lifestyle changes result from physical changes in the self and others.

d. The peer group is vitally important to the accomplishment of the tasks of middle age.

*After working through these questions, go to the MyNursingLab at **http://www.mynursinglab.com** to check your answers and see explanations.*

SUGGESTED READINGS

Berk, L. E. (2004). *Development through the lifespan* (3rd ed.). Boston: Allyn & Bacon.

This text examines physical, cognitive, emotional, and social development from the prenatal period to the end of life, including theory and research in human development and biological and environmental foundations of development.

Thomson, H., & Meggitt, C. (2007). *Human growth and development for health and social care.* London, UK: Hodder Arnold.

This book covers the subject of human growth and development from the physical, psychological, and social perspectives.

WEBLINKS

Canadian Health Network

http://www.canadian-health-network.ca

This site provides accurate Canadian content that focuses on health and wellness. Use the topics list on the left side to find information on children.

Canadian Institute of Child Health

http://www.cich.ca

The site provides information on children's policies, research, and programs pertaining to nurturing, protecting, educating, and empowering children.

Public Health Agency of Canada—Division of Childhood and Adolescence

http://www.phac-aspc.gc.ca/dca-dea/main_e.html

The Division of Childhood and Adolescence serves as a centre of expertise, leadership, and coordination within the federal government and Health Canada for issues, activities, and programs concerning children and youth.

REFERENCES

Ball, J. W., & Bindler, R. C. (2006). *Child health nursing.* Upper Saddle River, NJ: Pearson Education.

Berkowitz, M. W., & Oser, F. (Eds.). (1985). *Moral education: Theory and application.* Hillsdale, NJ: Lawrence Erlbaunt.

Edwards, M. E. (2002). Attachment, mastery, and interdependence: A model of parenting processes. *Family Process, 41*(3), 389–404.

Erikson, E. H. (1963). *Childhood and society* (2nd ed.). New York: Norton.

Erikson, E. H. (1964). *Insight and responsibility: Lectures on the ethical implications of psychoanalytic insight.* New York: Norton.

Fowler, J. W. (1981). *Stages of faith: The psychology of human development and the quest for meaning.* New York: Harper & Row.

Fowler, J., & Keen, S. (1985). *Life maps: Conversations in the journey of faith.* Waco, TX: Word Books.

Freud, S. (1923). *The ego and the id.* London, UK: Hogarth Press.

Gilligan, C. (1982). *In a different voice: Psychological theory and women's development.* Cambridge, MA: Harvard University Press.

Gould, R. L. (1972). The phases of adult life: A study in developmental psychology. *American Journal of Psychiatry, 129,* 33–43.

Havighurst, R. J. (1972). *Developmental tasks and education* (3rd ed.). New York: Longman Publishers.

Invest in Kids. (2007). *Definition of development.* Retrieved March 15, 2007, from http://www.investinkids.ca

Murray, R. B., & Zentner, J. P. (2001). *Health promotion strategies through the life span* (7th ed.). Upper Saddle River, NJ: Prentice Hall.

Peck, R. (1968). Psychological developments in the second half of life. In B. L. Neugarten (Ed.), *Middle age and aging* (pp. 88–92). Chicago: University of Chicago Press.

Piaget, J. (1966). *Origins of intelligence in children.* New York: Norton.

Rothbart, M. K. (2004). Commentary: Differentiated measures of temperament and multiple pathways to childhood disorders. *Journal of Clinical Child and Adolescent Psychology, 33*(1), 82–87.

Westerhoff, J. (1976). *Will our children have faith?* New York: Seabury Press.

Chapter 17

Development from Conception through Adolescence

Knowledge of growth and development is essential for nurses to provide clients with anticipated guidance for optimal developmental milestones. Based on the concepts of growth and development introduced in Chapter 16, this chapter will emphasize health assessment, including health-promotion and protection activities to meet the physical, psychosocial, cognitive, moral, and spiritual developmental needs from infancy through adolescence. Conception and prenatal or intrauterine development lasts approximately nine calendar months (10 lunar months) or 38 to 40 weeks, depending on the method of calculation. A lunar month is 28 days. If the time is calculated from the first day of the last menstrual period, its average length is 10 lunar months, or 40 weeks.

OBJECTIVES

After studying this chapter, you should be able to

1. Identify the characteristic tasks at different stages of development, from infancy through adolescence.
2. Describe expected physical development from infancy through adolescence
3. Trace psychosocial development according to Erikson, from infancy through adolescence
4. Explain cognitive development according to Piaget, from infancy through adolescence
5. Describe spiritual development according to Fowler throughout childhood and adolescence
6. Discuss assessment activities and expected characteristics from birth through late childhood
7. List essential nursing activities to promote and protect the health of infants, toddlers, preschoolers, school-age children, and adolescents

Conception and Prenatal Development

Pregnancy is divided into three periods called **trimesters**, each of which lasts about 3 months. Each trimester includes certain landmarks for changes in the mother and the fetus. The two phases of intrauterine life are the *embryonic phase* in the first trimester and the *fetal phase* in the second and third trimesters.

The fertilized ovum develops into an organism with most of the human features in the *embryonic phase*. The embryo is implanted in the endometrium of the uterus. The *placenta* is a flat, disc-shaped organ that is highly vascular. It normally forms in the upper segment of the endometrium of the uterus. Its functions are to exchange nutrients and gases between the embryo or fetus and the mother to sustain growth in utero.

Within the first three weeks of life, tissues differentiate into three layers—the *ectoderm* (outer layer), *mesoderm* (middle layer), and *endoderm* or *entoderm* (inner layer). The ectoderm and endoderm are formed in the second week; the mesoderm forms in the third week. These layers form all of the body's complex organs and systems as a series of outpouchings, inpouchings, foldings, and tubular formations. Organs are developed between 8 to 12 weeks during this *embryonic phase*. The *fetal phase* is characterized by a period of rapid growth in the size of the fetus. Both genetic and environmental factors affect its growth.

At the end of the second trimester, the fetus resembles a small baby. Because very little fat is present beneath the skin, the skin appears wrinkled, red, and transparent. The underlying blood vessels are visible. A protective covering, called **vernix caseosa**, begins to develop over the skin. This is a white, cheese-like substance that adheres to the skin and can become 3 mm thick by birth. **Lanugo**, a fine downy hair, covers the body. At about 5 months, the mother begins to feel fetal movement and the fetal heartbeat is audible.

At the end of the third trimester, the fetus is approximately 50 cm long and weights 2.7 to 3.8 kg. The lanugo has disappeared, and the skin has a normal colour and appears less wrinkled. More subcutaneous fat makes the baby look more rotund. The baby gains most of its weight during the last 2 months in utero. Box 17.1 lists maternal factors that can lead to a higher risk of a low-birth-weight baby.

BOX 17.1 MATERNAL FACTORS THAT CONTRIBUTE TO A HIGHER RISK OF LOW-BIRTH-WEIGHT BABIES

The following factors can contribute to mothers having low-birth-weight babies:

- Being underweight before pregnancy
- Gaining less than 9 kg during pregnancy
- Not getting adequate prenatal care
- Being age 16 years or younger, or 35 years or older
- Having a low socioeconomic level
- Having poor nutrition during pregnancy
- Using tobacco, drugs, or alcohol during pregnancy
- Having a history of abortion
- Experiencing complications during pregnancy, poor health status, exposure to infections
- Having high stress levels

Source: Adapted from *Health Promotion Strategies Through the Life Span*, 7th ed. (p. 309), by R. B. Murray and J. P. Zentner, 2001, Upper Saddle River, NJ: Prentice Hall. Adapted with permission.

Intrauterine Development

During the intrauterine stage of development, the embryo or fetus relies on the maternal blood flow through the placenta to meet its basic survival needs. The health of the mother is essential for optimal fetal growth and development.

OXYGEN To meet the fetal demands for oxygen, the pregnant mother gradually increases her normal blood flow by about one-third, peaking at about 8 months; increases tidal volume by about 40% with associated increased respiration; and increases her cardiac output significantly. Fetal circulation travels from the placenta through two umbilical arteries, which carry deoxygenated blood away from the fetus. By 20 weeks, the fetal heartbeat is audible through a fetoscope, or as early as the tenth week if a Doppler stethoscope with ultrasound is used.

NUTRITION AND FLUIDS The fetus obtains nourishment from the placental circulation and by swallowing amniotic fluid. Nutritional needs are met when the mother eats a well-balanced diet containing sufficient calories to meet both her needs and those of the fetus.

REST AND ACTIVITY The fetus sleeps most of the time but develops a pattern of sleep and wakefulness that can persist after birth. Fetal activity begins about the fourth lunar month of pregnancy.

ELIMINATION Throughout pregnancy, fetal feces are formed from swallowed amniotic fluid, but normally no stool is passed until after birth. Inadequate oxygenation of the fetus during the third trimester can result in relaxation of the anal sphincter and passage of feces into the amniotic fluid. Urine normally is excreted into the amniotic fluid when the kidneys mature (16 to 20 weeks).

TEMPERATURE MAINTENANCE Although amniotic fluid provides a constant temperature for the fetus, significant changes in maternal temperature (e.g., fever, very high-temperature baths or saunas) can alter the temperature of the amniotic fluid and that of the fetus.

SAFETY Because the body systems form during the embryonic period, the embryo is particularly vulnerable to damage or harm from a **teratogen**—anything that adversely affects normal cellular development in the embryo or fetus (Venes, 2005). Expectant mothers must avoid radiography (X-ray) and medications that are known teratogens.

Maternal, neonatal, and infant mortality are significantly increased with maternal use of drugs or alcohol (Wolfe, Davis, Guydish, & Delucchi, 2005). **Fetal alcohol syndrome** (FAS), a result of alcohol use by the pregnant woman, is impaired mitochondrial development in the fetus that leads to microcephaly, mental retardation, learning disorders, and other central nervous system defects (Kvigne et al., 2004). Smoking has been associated with preterm labour, spontaneous abortion, low-birth-weight infants, sudden infant death syndrome, and learning disorders (Albrecht et al., 2004; Anderson, Johnson, & Batal, 2005). All women of childbearing age should abstain from alcohol and drug use. Those who engage in unprotected sex are at significant risk for sexually transmitted infections (STIs).

REFLECT ON PRIMARY HEALTH CARE

Growth monitoring is an integral part of physical assessment of children. First Nations and Inuit children, Quebec Cree children, and those from the western regions of the Northwest Territories tend to have growth patterns different from children from other Canadian regions; they also are heavier at birth and in early life. Epidemiological data suggest that the variations in growth patterns in these ethnic groups are caused by environmental factors rather than genetic factors. The Canadian Paediatric Society (CPS) saw little purpose in devising a special growth curve for each ethnic group. It recommended the use of the growth charts published by the Centers for Disease Control and Prevention in the United States (see the Weblinks section of this chapter) for *all* Canadian children, regardless of their race and ethnicity. The CPS further emphasized the importance of assessing growth patterns over time to detect deviations, addressing the nature of the problem early, and not focusing on race and ethnicity (First Nations and Inuit Health Committee & Canadian Paediatric Society, 2007). Growth charts are useful health assessment tools for children. Consider how using growth charts is a reflection of the primary health-care principles of *appropriate technology* and *health promotion*.

Neonates and Infants (Birth to 1 Year)

Physical Development

The neonate's basic task is survival, which requires breathing, sleeping, sucking, eating, swallowing, digesting, and eliminating. Newborns and infants undergo significant physiological change in weight, length, head growth, vision, and motor development. Because many of the infant's activities and pleasures are mouth centred, this stage in development is often referred to as the *oral* stage (see Chapter 16, the section on Freud).

WEIGHT At birth, most babies weigh about 2.7 to 3.8 kg. Just after birth, it is normal for most newborns to lose 5% to 10% of their birth weight because of fluid loss. Newborns usually regain that weight in about 1 week. After several days, they gain weight at the rate of 150 g to 210 g weekly for 6 months. By 6 months of age, infants usually reach twice their birth weight, and by 12 months, three times their birth weight. Aboriginal children tend to be heavier at birth and in early life (see the Reflect on Primary Health Care box).

LENGTH The average length of a Canadian newborn is about 50–52 cm. At birth, Black infants tend to be shorter. Female babies, on average, are smaller than male babies. Two lengths are the crown-to-rump length (the sitting length) and the recumbent head-to-heel length (from the top of the head to the base of the heels). See Figure 17.1. Normally, the crown-to-rump length is approximately the same as the head circumference. By 6 months, infants gain another 13.75 cm of length. By 12 months, they add another 7.5 cm. The rate of increase in length is largely influenced by the baby's size at birth and by nutrition.

HEAD AND CHEST CIRCUMFERENCE Assessment of head circumference is of particular importance in infants and children to determine the growth rate of the skull and the brain. An infant's head should be measured at every checkup until the child is 2 years old (Figure 17.2). Normal head circumference (**normocephaly**) is often related to chest circumference. At birth, the

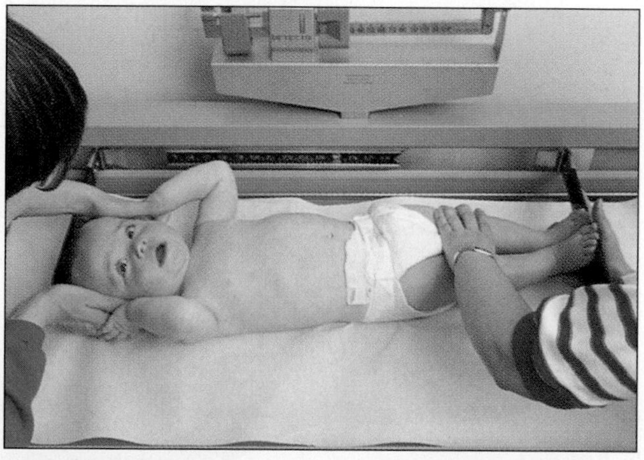

FIGURE 17.1 Measuring an infant head to heel, from the top of the head to the base of the heels

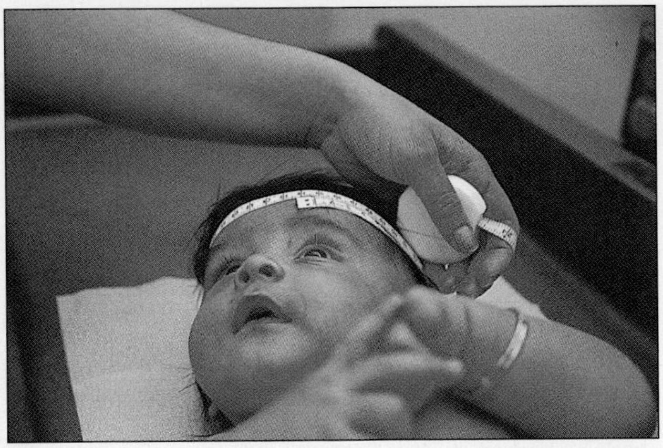

FIGURE 17.2 An infant's head circumference is measured around the skull, above the eyebrows.

average head circumference is 33–35 cm and generally varies only 1 cm or 2 cm. The chest circumference is usually less than the head circumference by about 2.5 cm. As the infant grows, the chest circumference becomes larger than the head circumference. At about 9 or 10 months, both circumferences are about the same, and after 1 year of age, the chest circumference is larger.

HEAD MOULDING The heads of most newborn babies are misshapen because of the moulding of the head that occurs during vaginal deliveries. Moulding of the head is made possible by *fontanelles* (unossified membranous gaps) in the bone structure of the skull and by overriding of the *sutures* (junction lines of the skull bones). Within a week, a newborn's head usually regains its symmetry. The larger anterior fontanelle (4 cm to 6 cm in diameter and diamond-shaped) can increase in size for several months after birth. After 6 months, the size gradually decreases until closure occurs between 9 and 18 months. The posterior fontanelle, between the parietal bones and the occipital bone, closes from 4 to 8 weeks after birth (Figure 17.3).

VISION The newborn can follow large moving objects and blink in response to bright light and sound. A newborn's pupils respond slowly, and the eyes cannot focus on close objects. By 1 month, the infant can focus his or her gaze on objects and follow moving ones. At 4 months, the infant recognizes a parent's smile, although social smiles may appear as early as 2 months. The 4-month-old has almost complete colour vision and follows objects through a 180-degree arc. A 5-month-old infant reaches for objects. Between 6 and 10 months, the infant can fix on an object and follow it in all directions. By 12 months, the infant will have depth perception and recognize drop-offs, such as steps or the edge of the bed.

HEARING Newborns with normal hearing will react with a startle to a loud noise, a reaction called the *Moro reflex*. Within a few days, they are able to distinguish different sounds and may distinguish the difference between the mother's voice and that of another woman. Between 3 and 6 months, the infant will look for sounds, stop an activity to listen, and respond with distress or pleasure to angry or happy voices.

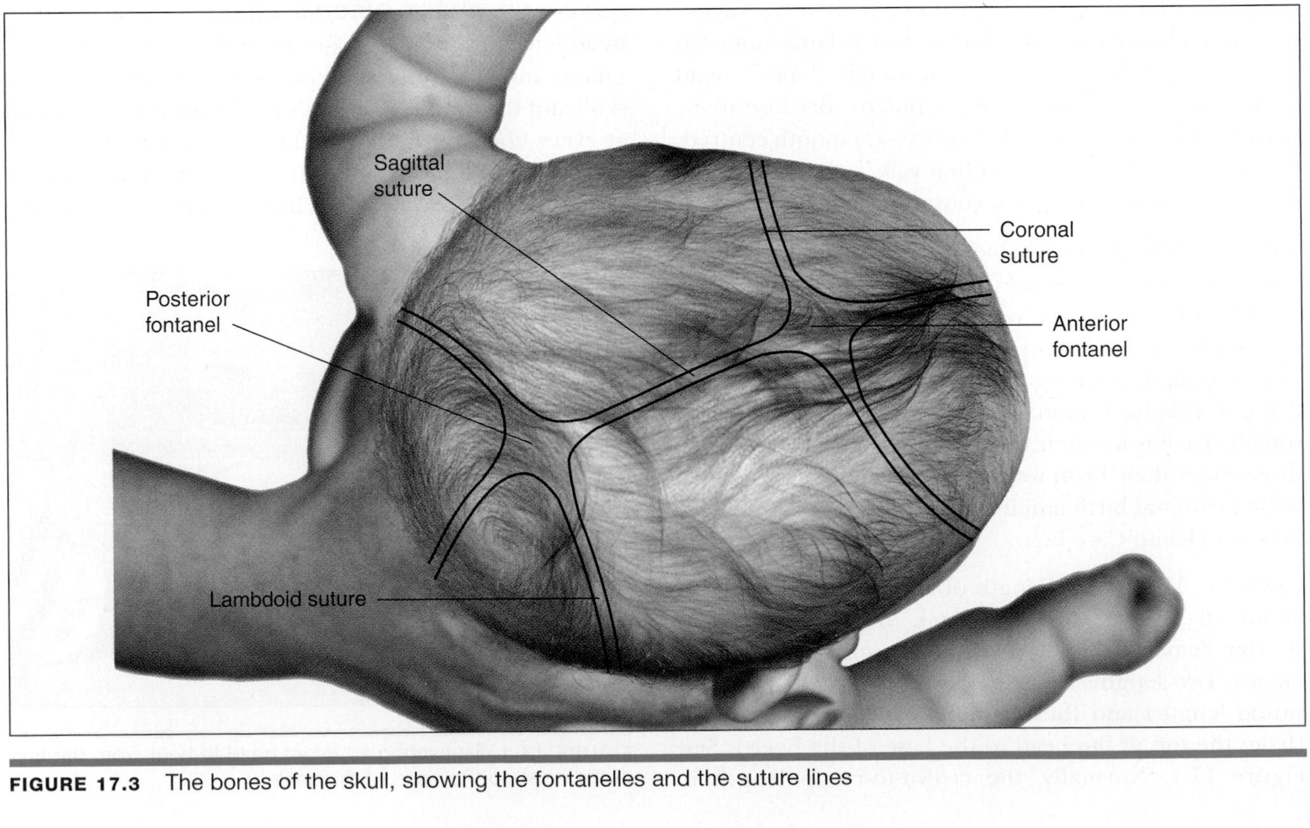

FIGURE 17.3 The bones of the skull, showing the fontanelles and the suture lines

Evidence-Informed Practice

How Does Hearing Impairment Influence Growth and Development?

The incidence of childhood hearing impairment is about 1 per 1000 live births (Canadian Working Group on Childhood Hearing, 2005). It increases to 10 per 1000 with extreme prematurity, severe neonatal jaundice, and congenital facial defects. Between 70% and 90% of children have transient conductive hearing impairment from middle ear infections. Comprehensive hearing screening before 6 months of age is essential. Early identification of hearing impairment leads to improved hearing and facilitates communication development.

NURSING IMPLICATIONS: Nurses must be aware of problems associated with congenital rubella, genetic anomalies, birth asphyxia, severe neonatal jaundice and kernicterus, meningitis or encephalitis, and antibiotics therapy. They must integrate hearing appraisals for all neonates and at-risk children. Timely referral to trained specialists in audiology and speech may prevent cognitive and communication delays.

Source: Based on *Early Hearing and Communication Development*, by the Canadian Working Group on Childhood Hearing, 2005, Ottawa: Minister of Public Works and Government Services Canada. Retrieved June 18, 2007, from www.phac-aspc.gc.ca/publicat/eh-dp/exe_sum-eng.php

SPEECH Between 6 and 9 months, individual words begin to take on meaning and the infant may look at named objects or people. The 9- to 12-month-old infant understands many words (e.g., "no," "hot," "dog"), uses gestures (e.g., waves "bye-bye"), may articulate one or two words with a specific reference (e.g., "mama," "dada"), and may respond to simple commands.

SMELL AND TASTE The senses of smell and taste are functional shortly after birth. Newborns can recognize the smell of their mother's milk and respond to this smell by turning toward their mother.

TOUCH The sense of touch is well developed at birth. Skin-to-skin touching is important for an infant's development. The newborn responds positively to warmth, love, and comfort when touched, held, and cuddled and is also sensitive to temperature extremes and pain.

REFLEXES The reflexes of the newborn are involuntary nervous system responses to stimuli. They are neither learned nor consciously carried out. Reflexes normally present at birth are the rooting, sucking, Moro, palmar grasp, plantar, tonic neck, stepping, and Babinski reflexes. See Box 17.2 for a description of these reflexes. Infant reflexes disappear during the first year of life. In addition, the abilities to yawn, stretch, sneeze, burp, and hiccup are all present at birth.

BOX 17.2 INFANT REFLEXES

From the moment of birth, newborns display the following reflexes of the involuntary nervous system:

- *Sucking reflex:* A feeding reflex occurs when the infant's lips are touched; it persists throughout infancy.
- *Rooting reflex:* A feeding reflex is elicited by touching the baby's cheek, causing the baby's head to turn to the side that was touched; it usually disappears after 4 months.
- *Moro reflex:* This reflex is often assessed to estimate the maturity of the central nervous system. A loud noise, a sudden change in position, or an abrupt jarring of the crib elicits this reflex. The infant reacts by extending both arms and legs outward with the fingers spread, then suddenly retracting the limbs. Often, the infant cries at the same time. This reflex disappears after 4 months.
- *Palmar grasp reflex:* This reflex occurs when a small object is placed against the palm of the hand, causing the fingers to curl around it. This reflex disappears after 3 months.
- *Plantar reflex:* When an object is placed just beneath the toes, they curl around it. This reflex disappears after 8 months.
- *Tonic neck reflex (TNR) or fencing reflex:* When a baby lying on its back turns its head to the right side, for example, the left side of the body shows a flexing of the left arm and the left leg. This postural reflex disappears after 4 months.
- *Stepping reflex (walking or dancing reflex):* This reflex can be elicited by holding the baby upright so that the feet touch a flat surface. The legs then move up and down as if the baby were walking. This reflex usually disappears at about 2 months.
- *Babinski reflex:* A newborn baby has a positive Babinski if when the sole of the foot is stroked, the big toe rises and the other toes fan out. After age 1 year, the infant exhibits a negative Babinski; that is, the toes curl downward. A positive Babinski after age 1 year indicates brain damage.

MOTOR DEVELOPMENT Motor development increases with the infants' abilities to move and to control the body. Initially, body movement is uncoordinated. At 1 month, they lift their head momentarily when prone, turn their head, and have a head lag when pulled to a sitting position. After 6 months, they can sit without support (Figure 17.4). At 9 months, they can sit, reach, grasp a rattle, and transfer it from hand to hand. At 12 months, they can turn the pages of a book, put objects into a container, and walk and dress themselves with some assistance.

Psychosocial Development

According to Erikson (1963), the central crisis at this stage is *trust versus mistrust* (see Table 16.4 on page 296). Resolution of this stage determines how the person approaches subsequent developmental stages. Fulfillment of needs is required for the infant to develop a basic sense of trust. Parents can enhance this sense of trust by (1) responding consistently to an infant's needs,

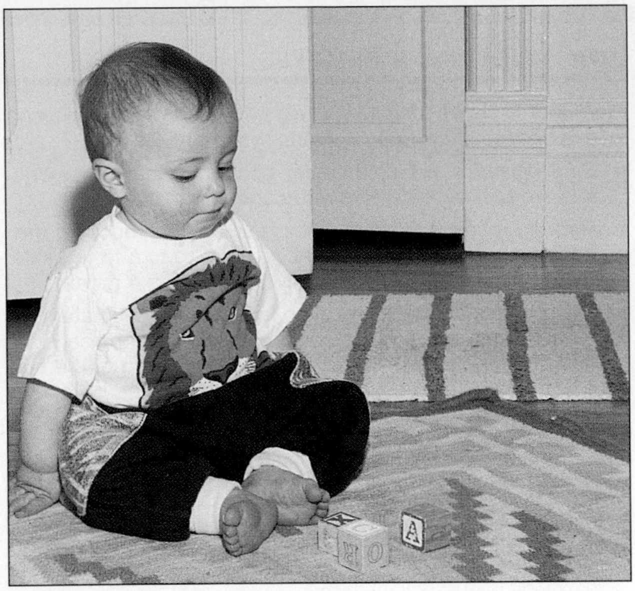

FIGURE 17.4 An infant sits without support at 6 months of age.

(2) providing a predictable environment in which routines are established, and (3) being sensitive to the infant's needs and meeting these needs skillfully and promptly.

Newborns react socially to caregivers by paying attention to the face or voice and by cuddling when held. See Table 17.1 for examples of motor and social development. Mothering behaviour, such as consistent care, handling, stroking, and cuddling, is essential for healthy psychosocial development. By 8 months, most infants tend to attach to their parents and may show displeasure when left with strangers.

Cognitive Development

Piaget (1966) viewed cognitive development as a result of interaction between an individual and the environment. The initial period of cognitive development is the *sensorimotor phase* (see Table 16.6 on page 299). This phase has six stages, three of which take place during the first year. From 4 to 8 months, infants begin to have perceptual recognition. By 6 months, they attend to new stimuli, while familiar objects are looked at for a short time. By 12 months, infants have a concept of both space and time. They experiment to reach a goal, such as a toy on a chair.

Moral Development

Infants associate right and wrong with pleasure and pain. What gives them pleasure is right, since they are too young to reason otherwise. Positive responses from the parents, such as smiles, caresses, and voice tones of approval, in these early months teach that certain behaviours are "good." Pain or harsh voices are associated with "bad" behaviour. In later months and years, children can tell easily and quickly by changes in parental facial expressions and voice tones whether their behaviour is approved or disapproved.

Health Problems

A number of health problems of neonates and infants require interventions from health-care personnel. Safety concerns are of particular importance.

FAILURE-TO-THRIVE SYNDROME **Failure to thrive** is a condition in which an infant falls below the fifth percentile for weight and height on a standard growth chart (Emond, Drewett, Blair, & Emmett, 2007). The two categories for this syndrome are *organic* causes (e.g., cardiac disease) and *inorganic* causes, which usually involve the parent–child relationship. Infants deprived of mothering, especially from months 3 to 15, will not learn to form significant relationships or to trust others. Touch, cuddling, and visual and auditory stimulation are all critical

TABLE 17.1 Examples of Motor and Social Development in Infancy

Age	Motor Development	Social Development
Newborn	Turns head from side to side when in a prone position Grasps by reflex when object is placed in palm of hand	Displays displeasure by crying, and satisfaction by soft vocalizations Attends to adult face and voice by eye contact and quieting
6 months	Lifts chest and shoulders off table when prone, bearing weight on hands Manipulates small objects	Starts to imitate sounds Vocalizes one-syllable sounds: "ma-ma," "da-da"
9 months	Creeps and crawls Beginner pincer grasp with thumb and forefinger	Complies with simple verbal commands Displays fear of being left alone (e.g., going to bed) Waves "bye-bye"
12 months	Walks alone with help Uses spoon to feed self	Clings to mother in unfamiliar situations Demonstrates emotions, such as anger and affection

for infants as they come to know their selves and the environment. Infants who lack a loving, responsive relationship from a caregiver often fail to develop normally. Infants with inorganic failure to thrive show delayed development without any physical cause. They are often malnourished; they fail to gain weight or grow normally.

INFANT COLIC **Colic** is acute abdominal pain caused by periodic contractions of the intestines during the first 3 months of life. Although the direct cause is not known, swallowing air, feeding too rapidly, having allergies, taking in excessive amounts of carbohydrates, experiencing infant emotional distress, and feeling the anxiety of the caregiver may be associated with colic.

The nurse can help relieve colic by assessing the infant during feeding and suggesting possible changes, such as a quiet space and time during and after feeding, changing the formula or nipple, increasing the burping frequency, increasing the infant's water intake, cuddling the infant, and finding the position that provides the infant with the most comfort. Providing parental respite care or support is essential.

CRYING Infants who cry up to 10 to 12 hours a day are described as being *colicky*. A crying or fussy period lasting 1 to 2 hours a day is not uncommon but is a concern and is stressful for the parents or caregivers.

CHILD ABUSE Abuse can take various forms, including physical abuse and neglect, sexual abuse, and emotional abuse and neglect. Deliberate whiplash shaking can lead to **shaken baby syndrome (SBS)**, a constellation of severe injuries, such as cerebral damage, neurological defects, blindness, and mental retardation, in infants. These injuries often occur without external evidence of head injury. Nurses should suspect SBS in infants less than 1 year old who have apnea (a pause in or stoppage of breathing), seizures, lethargy or drowsiness, bradycardia (a slow heart rate), or respiratory difficulty, who are in coma, or who die. Subdural and retinal hemorrhages with the absence of external signs of trauma are hallmarks of the syndrome (Geddes, 2004). Parents need to be aware of the dangers in shaking infants and ask for assistance if they feel they could harm their baby (Health Canada, 2002).

SUDDEN INFANT DEATH SYNDROME The sudden and unexpected death of an infant may be a case of **sudden infant death syndrome (SIDS)**. A postmortem examination usually fails to reveal a cause. The highest incidence of SIDS occurs in the second and fourth months of life, and boys are more susceptible than girls. Research has shown that having the infant sleep on its back greatly decreases the risk of SIDS. Sleeping on the back is preferred as infants may roll onto their stomach from a side-lying position, blocking their breathing (Anderson, Johnson, & Batal, 2005) (see Figure 17.5).

The Canadian Paediatric Society (2004) stated that the risk of SIDS increases when infants sleep in the same bed with adults who smoke cigarettes. These infants are

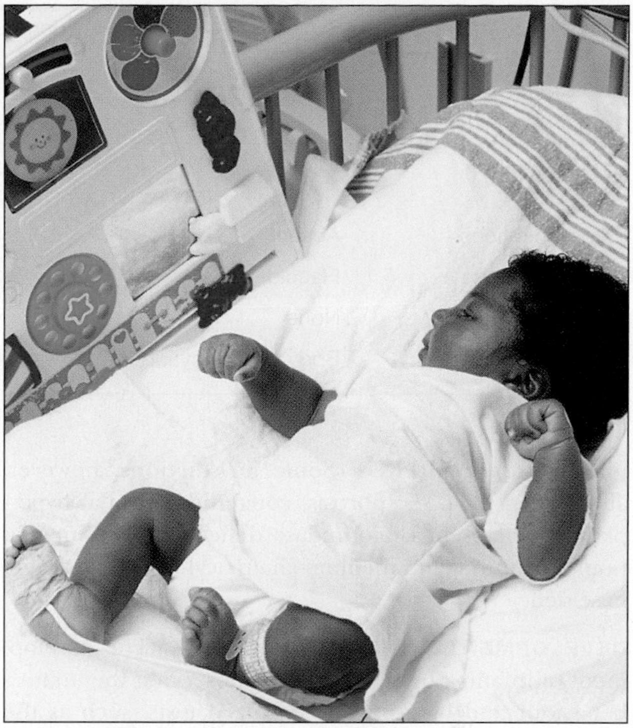

FIGURE 17.5 Place an infant on his or her back for sleeping. Note the infant's tonic neck reflex.

also at risk for asphyxia when bed-sharing with adults who smoke cigarettes, who cannot be easily aroused because of extreme fatigue, or who are impaired by alcohol or drug use. Nurses must assess the cultural practice for sleeping arrangements in the home, discuss the dangers of bed-sharing practices with the parents, and suggest alternatives for a safe sleeping environment for infants.

Health Assessment and Promotion

APGAR SCORING **Apgar** scores are assessed in neonates immediately following birth. These scores provide a numeric indicator of the baby's physiological capacities to adapt to extrauterine life. Each of five signs is assigned a maximum score of 2, so that the total score achievable is 10. A score less than 7 suggests that the baby is having difficulty, and a score less than 4 indicates that the baby's condition is critical. Apgar scoring is usually carried out 60 seconds after birth and is repeated in 5 minutes. Those with very low scores require special resuscitative measures and care. See Table 17.2.

NEWBORN SCREENING According to the Save Babies Through Screening Foundation of Canada (2007), about 132 babies in Canada die unnecessarily each year because of undetected genetic and metabolic disorders. At least 99% of these deaths are preventable with comprehensive newborn screening. Canada lacks federal guidelines for newborn screening. Currently, *all* provinces and territories screen for congenital hypothyroidism and

TABLE 17.2 Apgar Scoring System to Assess the Newborn

	Score		
Sign	0	1	2
1. Heart rate	Absent	Slow (fewer than 100 beats per minute)	More than 100 beats per minute
2. Respirations	Absent	Slow, irregular	Regular rate, crying
3. Muscle tone	Flaccid	Some flexion of extremities	Active movements
4. Reflex irritability	None	Grimace	Cries
5. Colour	Body pale or cyanotic	Body pink, extremities blue	Body completely pink

phenylketonuria (PKU). Some jurisdictions, however, also screen for cystic fibrosis, congenital adrenal hyperplasia, galactosemia, biotinidase deficiency, tyrosinemia, homocystinuria, and medium-chain acyl-CoA dehydrogenase deficiency.

DEVELOPMENTAL SCREENING TESTS The development of infants can be assessed by observing the infant's behaviour and by using standardized tests, such as the **Denver Developmental Screening Test (DDST)**. The DDST is used to screen children from birth to 6 years of age. The test is intended to estimate the abilities of a child compared with those of an average group of children of the same age and ethnic group. Four main areas are screened: (1) *personal-social,* (2) *fine motor adaptive,* (3) *language,* and (4) *gross motor.*

ONGOING NURSING ASSESSMENTS The nurse examines and observes the infant, taking into account variations that occur with developmental age and activity. For example, the pulse/minute of the baby at birth is affected by the child's activity, rising up to 170 when crying and falling to as low as 70 during sleep. The nurse actively listens to the parents for possible problems or areas of concern, and reviews with the parents the expected behaviours or characteristics for the particular age group, reinforcing certain behaviours, responses, and activities of the infant as normal and expected, given individual differences that occur. The nurse assesses maternal bonding and infant attachment and provides anticipatory parental support and guidance as needed. See the Assessment: Developmental Guidelines box.

The first month of life is thought to be critical for physical adjustments to extrauterine life and for the psychosocial adjustment of the parents. From 1 to 12 months, infants experience rapid change, with advances in growth and psychosocial development. For a summary of health and wellness promotion, see the Health-Promotion Guidelines box for neonates and infants. (See Chapter 30, the section called "Promoting Safety across the Lifespan.")

ASSESSMENT: DEVELOPMENTAL GUIDELINES

The Infant

In these five developmental areas, does the infant do the following?

1. **PHYSICAL DEVELOPMENT**
   - Demonstrate physical growth (weight, length, head and chest circumference) within the normal range
   - Manifest appropriately sized fontanelles for age
   - Exhibit vital signs within normal range for age
2. **MOTOR DEVELOPMENT**
   - Perform gross and fine motor milestones within the normal range for age
   - Exhibit reflexes appropriate for age
3. **SENSORY DEVELOPMENT**
   - Follow a moving object within normal range for age
   - Respond to sounds, such as talking or clapping hands
4. **PSYCHOSOCIAL DEVELOPMENT**
   - Interact appropriately with parent through body movements and vocalizations
5. **DEVELOPMENT IN ACTIVITIES OF DAILY LIVING**
   - Eat and drink appropriate amounts of breast milk, formula, or solid foods
   - Exhibit an elimination pattern within normal range for age
   - Exhibit rest and sleep patterns appropriate for age

Health-Promotion Guidelines for Neonates and Infants

The following are important to the health of neonates and infants:

HEALTH EXAMINATIONS

- At birth, 2 weeks, and at 2, 4, 6, and 12 months

PROTECTIVE MEASURES

- Routine immunizations: 5-in-1 (DPTP-Hib) or DTaP-IPV and Hib vaccines protect against diphtheria, tetanus, pertussis, polio, and *Haemophilus influenzae,* type B (Hib) vaccine, hepatitis B vaccine (HepB), varicella vaccine, pneumococcal conjugate vaccine, and meningococcal C conjugate vaccine; influenza vaccine and other vaccines as recommended. Schedules may vary across provinces and territories. See Table 32.9: Routine Immunization Schedules for Infants and Children (page 910).
- Fluoride supplements, if inadequate water fluoridation (less than 0.7 parts per million)
- Screening for congenital hypothyroidism, phenylketonuria (PKU), and other metabolic and congenital disorders, according to jurisdictions
- Prompt attention for illnesses or fever
- Appropriate skin hygiene and clothing

INFANT SAFETY

- Supervision at all times
- Car seat, crib, playpen, bath, sleeping arrangement, and home environment safety measures
- Feeding measures (e.g., avoid propping bottle)
- Toys with no small parts or sharp edges

NUTRITION

- Breastfeeding and bottle-feeding techniques
- Formula preparation
- Feeding schedule
- Introduction of solid foods
- Need for iron supplements at 4 to 6 months. Give iron-fortified formulas to infants who are not breastfed or for infants receiving formula as well as breast milk. By age 6 months, offer iron-rich foods.

ELIMINATION

- Characteristics and frequency of stool and urine elimination
- Diarrhea and dehydration signs

REST AND SLEEP

- Usual sleep and rest patterns

SENSORY STIMULATION

- Touch: holding, cuddling, rocking
- Vision: colourful, moving toys
- Hearing: soothing voice tones, music, singing
- Play: toys appropriate for development

Toddlers (1 to 3 Years)

Toddlers develop from having no voluntary control to learning to walk, speak, and control their bladder and bowels, and acquiring all kinds of information about their environment.

Physical Development

Two-year-old toddlers are usually chubby, with relatively short legs and large heads. Their face appears small when compared with the skull. As the toddler grows, the face seems to grow from under the skull and appears better proportioned. Toddlers have a pronounced lumbar lordosis and a protruding abdomen. The abdominal muscles grow and strengthen gradually and the abdomen flattens.

WEIGHT Two-year-olds can be expected to weigh approximately four times their birth weight, gaining about 2 kg between 1 year and 2 years and about 1 to 2 kg between 2 and 3 years. The 3-year-old weighs about 13.6 kg.

HEIGHT A toddler's height can be measured as height or length. *Height* is measured while the toddler stands. *Length* is measured while the toddler is in a recumbent position. The measurements differ slightly, so nurses must specify which measurement is used. Between 1 and 2 years, the average growth in height is 10 cm to 12 cm, and between 2 and 3 years, it slows to 6 cm to 8 cm.

HEAD CIRCUMFERENCE The head circumference of the toddler increases about 2.5 cm on average during this period. By 24 months, the head is 80% of the average adult size and the brain is 70% of its adult size.

SENSORY ABILITIES Visual acuity is fairly well established at 1 year. Estimates of visual acuity for toddlers are 20/70 at 18 months and 20/40 at 2 years of age. Accommodation to near and far objects is fairly well developed by 18 months and continues to mature with age. At 3 years, the toddler can look away from a toy before reaching out and picking it up. This ability requires the integration of visual and neuromuscular mechanisms.

The senses of hearing, taste, smell, and touch become increasingly developed and associated with one another. Hearing in the 3-year-old is at adult levels. The taste buds of the toddler are sensitive to the natural flavours of food, and the 3-year-old prefers familiar odours and tastes. Touch is a very important sense, and a distressed toddler is often soothed by tactile sensations.

MOTOR ABILITIES *Fine muscle coordination* and *gross motor skills* improve during toddlerhood. At the age of 18 months, toddlers can pick up small beads and place them in a receptacle. They can also hold a spoon and a cup and can walk upstairs with assistance. They will probably crawl down the stairs.

At 2 years, toddlers can hold a spoon and put it into their mouths correctly. They are able to run; their gait is steady; and they can balance on one foot and ride a tricycle. By 3 years, most children are toilet trained, although they still may have the occasional accident when playing or during the night.

Psychosocial Development

According to Freud (1923), the ages of 2 and 3 years represent the *anal phase* when the rectum and anus are particularly significant areas of the body (see Table 16.3 on page 295). Erikson sees the period from 18 months to 3 years as the time when the central developmental task is autonomy versus shame and doubt (see Table 16.4 on page 296).

Toddlers begin to develop their *sense of autonomy* by asserting themselves with the frequent use of the word "no." They are often frustrated by restraints on their behaviour and may have temper tantrums. They learn to gain control over their emotions with guidance from their caregivers. Parents need to have a great deal of patience coupled with an understanding of the importance of this developmental milestone. They need to give the child some measure of control and, at the same time, be consistent in setting limits so that the child learns the results of misbehaviour. The nurse can also assist the parents and caregivers in promoting the toddler's development by suggesting the activities summarized in Box 17.3.

BOX 17.3 FOSTERING THE TODDLER'S PSYCHOSOCIAL DEVELOPMENT

Parents and caregivers can do many things to stimulate a toddler's psychosocial development:

- Provide toys suitable for the toddler, including some toys challenging enough to motivate but not so difficult that the toddler will fail. (Failure will intensify feelings of self-doubt and shame.)
- Make positive suggestions rather than giving commands. Avoid an emotional climate of negativism, blame, and punishment.
- Give the toddler two or three choices, all of which are safe.
- When the toddler has a temper tantrum, make sure he or she is safe, and then turn away.
- Help the toddler develop inner control by setting and enforcing consistent, reasonable limits.
- Praise the toddler's accomplishments; give spontaneous feedback for positive behaviour.

Self-concept is made up of body image, feelings about the self, adaptive and defensive mechanisms, reactions from others, and our own perceptions of these reactions, attitudes, values, and many of life's experiences (Starr, 2004). Children learn to develop a sense of self through their immediate social environment, in which their parents play a significant role. If the children's social interactions with their parents are negative (e.g., constant disapproval regarding eating, toilet training, or other behaviour), the children may begin to see themselves as bad. This perception forms a negative self-concept. Parents need to give toddlers positive input so that they can develop a positive and healthy self-concept. Children with a strong self-concept and security are able to deal with periodic failures later in life without damage to their self-esteem.

Although toddlers like to explore the environment, they always need to have a significant person nearby. Parents need to know that young children experience acute **separation anxiety**—the fear and frustration that come with parental absences. Abandonment is their greatest fear. At this age, the child may also have difficulty accepting a babysitter or strongly resist being left by the parents at a daycare centre or when separated from their parents or admitted to hospital.

Toddlers need room for exploration and interaction with other children and adults. At the same time, they need to know that the parental bond of a loving and close relationship remains secure. They assert their independence by saying "no" or by dawdling. During the toddler stage, receptive and expressive language skills are developing quickly. They can understand words and follow directions long before they can actually speak them.

Regression, or reverting to an earlier development stage, can take the form of bedwetting or using baby talk. Nurses can help parents to understand that this behaviour is normal and indicates that the toddler is trying to establish his or her position in the family.

Cognitive Development

According to Piaget, the toddler completes the fifth and sixth stages of the *sensorimotor phase* and starts the *preconceptual phase* at about 2 years of age. In the fifth stage, the toddler solves problems by a trial-and-error process. By stage 6, toddlers can solve problems mentally. During Piaget's preconceptual phase, toddlers have some symbolic thought; for example, a chair may represent a place of safety, and a blanket may symbolize comfort. Concepts develop in late toddlerhood when the child learns words to represent classes of objects or thoughts. An example of a concrete concept is *table*, representing a number of articles of furniture that may look different but match the characteristics of a table.

Moral Development

According to Kohlberg (1977), the first level of moral development is *preconventional,* when children respond to punishment and reward. During the second year, children begin to know that some activities elicit affection and approval and recognize that certain rituals create feelings of security. Children also sense what attitudes their parents hold about moral matters.

Spiritual Development

Fowler (1981) viewed the toddler's stage of spiritual development as undifferentiated. Toddlers may be aware of some religious practices, but they are primarily involved in acquiring knowledge and learning emotional reactions. A toddler may repeat short prayers at bedtime, conforming to a ritual for praise and affection.

Health Problems

ACCIDENTS Accidents are the leading cause of death for toddlers (Health Council of Canada, 2006), as they are curious and like to feel and taste everything. The most common causes of fatal injuries are automobile accidents, drowning, burns, poisoning, and falls. Parents or other caregivers need to take preventive measures to guard against these threats (see Figure 17.6).

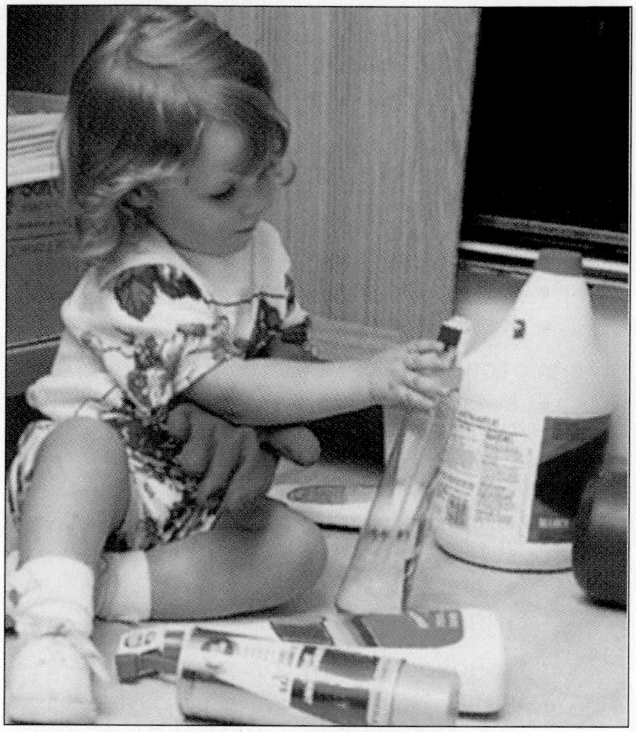

FIGURE 17.6 Keep medicines and other poisonous material locked away.

VISION PROBLEMS Early screening to detect amblyopia and strabismus can correct common problems in toddlers. **Amblyopia** (lazy-eye) is reduced visual acuity in one eye without obvious defect or change in the eye; the brain favours the images from the stronger eye over those from the affected eye. **Strabismus** (cross-eye) is unequally aligned eyes, which distorts vision so that the child's brain suppresses vision in one eye.

DENTAL CARIES Dental caries are common and often a result of the excessive intake of sweets or a prolonged exposure of teeth to carbohydrates, such as through the use of the bottle during naps and at bedtime. Good dental hygiene can prevent dental caries and hence promote proper speech development and nutrition.

RESPIRATORY TRACT AND EAR INFECTIONS Respiratory and middle-ear infections are common during toddlerhood. The incidence increases with exposure to other children and the use of a bottle during naps or at bedtime or if bottles are propped for feedings. Respiratory and ear infections contribute significantly to visits to health-care providers.

Health Assessment and Promotion

Growth and development in the toddler and preschool years provide the basis for a child's future health and well-being. It is essential that nurses provide anticipatory guidance and accurate assessments to promote health and detect problems for early interventions.

Assessment activities for the toddler are similar to those for the infant. Guidelines for growth and development of the toddler are shown in the Assessment: Developmental Guidelines box.

Promoting health and wellness includes such areas as accident prevention, toilet training, and good dental hygiene. See the Health-Promotion Guidelines box for toddlers.

ASSESSMENT: DEVELOPMENTAL GUIDELINES

The Toddler

In these four developmental areas, does the toddler do the following?

1. **PHYSICAL DEVELOPMENT**
   - Demonstrate physical growth (weight, height, and head circumference) within normal range
   - Manifest vital signs within normal range for age
   - Exhibit vision and hearing abilities within normal range
2. **MOTOR DEVELOPMENT**
   - Perform gross and fine motor milestones within the normal range for age. For example, by 3 years of age is the toddler able to do the following?
     - Walk up steps without assistance
     - Balance on one foot, jump, and walk on toes
     - Copy a circle
     - Build a bridge from blocks
     - Ride a tricycle
3. **PSYCHOSOCIAL DEVELOPMENT**
   - Perform psychosocial developmental milestones for age. For example, by 3 years of age is the toddler able to do the following?
     - Express likes and dislikes
     - Display curiosity and ask questions
     - Accept separation from mother for short periods
     - Begin to play and communicate with children and others outside the immediate family
     - Understand such words as *up, down, cold,* and *hungry*
     - Speak in sentences of three to four words
     - Imitate religious rituals of the family
4. **DEVELOPMENT IN ACTIVITIES OF DAILY LIVING**
   - Feed self
   - Eat and drink a variety of foods
   - Begin to develop bowel and bladder control
   - Exhibit a sleep pattern appropriate for age
   - Dress self

Health-Promotion Guidelines for Toddlers

The following are important to the health of toddlers:

HEALTH EXAMINATIONS

- At 15 and 18 months and then as recommended by the health-care provider
- Dental visits starting at age 3 years
- Hearing tests by 18 months or earlier

PROTECTIVE MEASURES

- Routine immunizations: continuing 5-in-1 (DPTP-Hib) or DTaP-IPV and Hib series, measles-mumps-rubella vaccine (MMR), pneumococcal conjugate vaccine, influenza vaccine, varicella vaccine, flu vaccine, and other vaccines as recommended by jurisdiction
- Screenings for tuberculosis (TB) and lead poisoning as recommended
- Fluoride supplements, if inadequate water fluoridation (less than 0.7 parts per million)

TODDLER SAFETY

- Importance of supervision and teaching child to obey instructions
- Home environment safety measures (e.g., lock medicine cabinet)
- Outdoor safety measures (e.g., close supervision near water, use of car seat)
- Appropriate toys with lift locks on toy boxes
- Elimination of toxins in environment (e.g., pesticides, herbicides, mercury, lead, arsenic in playground materials)
- Use of smoke and carbon monoxide detectors in home

NUTRITION

- Importance of nutritious meals and snacks
- Teaching of simple mealtime manners
- Dental care

ELIMINATION

- Toilet training techniques

REST AND SLEEP

- Dealing with sleep disturbances

PLAY

- Provision of adequate space and a variety of activities
- Toys that allow “acting out” behaviours and provide motor and sensory stimulation safety

Preschoolers (4 to 5 Years)

During the preschool period, physical growth slows, but control of the body and coordination increase greatly. Preschoolers' worlds expand as they meet relatives, friends, and neighbours.

Physical Development

By 4 or 5 years, preschool children appear taller and thinner than toddlers because they tend to grow more in height than in weight. The preschooler's brain reaches almost adult size by 5 years. The extremities grow more quickly than the body trunk, making the child's body appear somewhat out of proportion. The posture of preschoolers gradually changes as the pelvis is straightened and the abdominal muscles become stronger: the preschooler appears slender with erect posture.

WEIGHT Weight gain in preschool children is generally slow. By 5 years, they gain about 3 kg to 5 kg and reach between 18 kg and 20 kg.

HEIGHT Preschool children grow about 5 cm to 6.25 cm each year. By age 5, they double their birth length and measure 100 cm.

VISION Preschool children are generally **hyperopic** (farsighted), that is, unable to focus on near objects. As the eye grows in length, it becomes **emmetropic** (it refracts light normally). If the eyes become too long, the child becomes **myopic** (nearsighted), that is, unable to focus on objects that are far away. In severe cases of hyperopia or myopia, glasses may be prescribed. Visual acuity generally improves by the end of the preschool years. Normal vision for the 5-year-old is approximately 20/30. The Snellen E chart can be used to assess the preschooler's vision (see Chapter 27, the section called "Eyes and Vision").

HEARING AND TASTE The hearing of the preschool child has reached optimal levels, and the ability to listen (attending to and comprehending what is said) has matured since the toddler age. As for the sense of taste, preschoolers show their preferences by asking for something "yummy," and they may refuse something they consider "yucky."

MOTOR ABILITIES By age 5, children can wash their hands and face and brush their teeth by themselves. They are self-conscious about exposing their bodies and go to the bathroom without telling others. Typically, preschool children run with increasing skill each year. They can jump three steps and can balance on their toes and dress themselves without assistance.

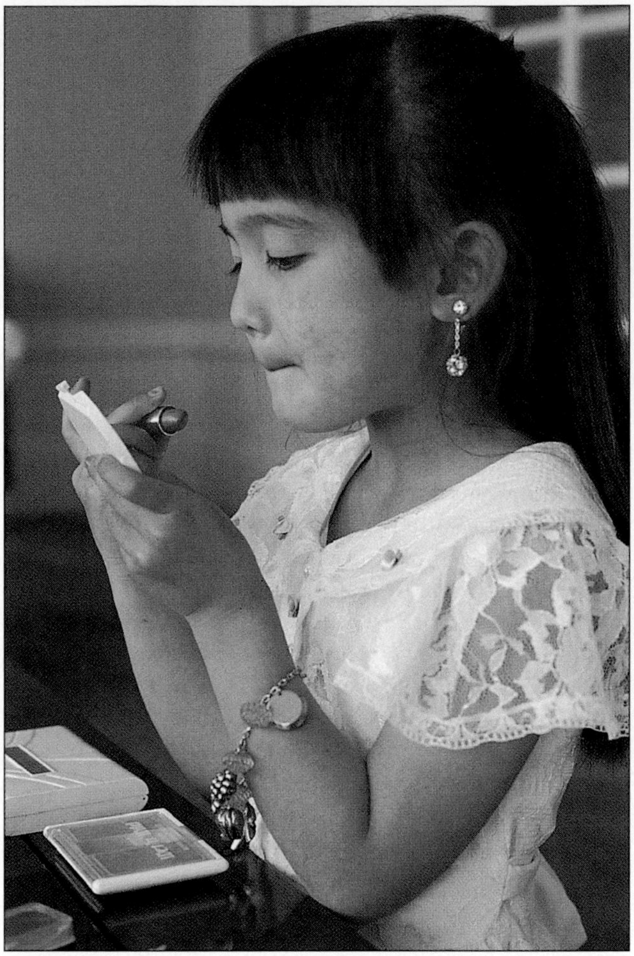

FIGURE 17.7 Preschoolers often identify with the parent of the same sex and like to mimic behaviour.

Psychosocial Development

Erikson (1963) writes that the major developmental crisis of the preschooler is *initiative versus guilt* (see Table 16.4 on page 296). Preschoolers begin to solve problems in accordance with their consciences as their personalities and self-concepts develop.

Parents can enhance the self-concept of the preschooler by providing opportunities for new achievements where the child can learn, repeat, and master. For example, a child obtains a two-wheel bike with safety wheels and quickly learns coordination, balance, use of the brakes, and bicycle safety. Mastery of these tasks provides the child with a sense of accomplishment.

The self-concept of the preschooler is also based on gender identification. Preschoolers are aware of the two sexes. They often imitate sexual stereotypes and usually begin by identifying with the parent of the same sex. They may mimic the parent's behaviour, attitudes, and appearance (Figure 17.7). Parents need to expect that preschoolers will be curious about their own bodies and sexual functions as well as those of others, and they will often ask questions.

Freud (1923) theorizes that the preschooler is in the *phallic stage* of development (see Table 16.3 on page 295). The focus during this stage is the genital area. In the Electra or Oedipus complex (Engel, 1962), the child focuses feelings of love chiefly on the parent of the opposite sex, and the parent of the same sex may receive some hostile feelings. The child begins to develop sexual interests and becomes interested in clothes and hair styles.

Four *adaptive mechanisms* are learned: *identification, introjection, imagination, and repression.* **Identification** occurs when the child perceives the self as similar to another person and behaves like that person. For example, a boy may internalize the attitudes and gender behaviour of his father. **Introjection** is the assimilation of the attributes of others. When preschoolers observe their parents, they assimilate many of their values and attitudes. **Imagination**, or make-believe, is an important part of preschoolers' lives and is culturally and socially dependent. For example, boys can fantasize a stool becomes a robot warrior and girls imagine it a beautiful swan. **Repression** is removing experiences, thoughts, and impulses from awareness. Preschoolers learn to play with a small number of their peers. They gradually learn to play with more people, socialize, and participate more in the family. Associations with neighbours, family guests, and babysitters reinforce social relationships.

In their *speech,* 4-year-old children are often dogmatic; they tend to believe that what they know is right. They can speak and understand 1500 or more words. They love making up their own words and mixing fact and fiction. Exaggeration is common. Their language skills are well developed by age 5. They use words purposefully, ask questions to acquire information, speak as a means of social interaction, and are capable of long conversations.

Preschoolers become increasingly aware of themselves, and they play with their bodies largely out of curiosity. By 5 years of age, they know the correct names for the different body parts and can draw various features of a person. Preschoolers can also describe their feelings, such as sad, happy, or angry. The preschooler begins to learn how to control his or her feelings and behaviour, and uses the same types of *coping mechanisms* in response to stress as the toddler does, although protest behaviour (kicking, screaming) is less likely to occur.

Preschoolers need to feel that they are loved and are an important part of the family. The child who has to compete with siblings for parental attention will often display jealousy or sibling rivalry. Parents and caregivers should be aware that preschoolers need time to adjust to a new baby and may need additional attention or special activities to go through this adjustment period.

Guidance and discipline are important parts of the parental role. As children seek independence from adults, they often test limits by refusing to cooperate and by ignoring parental requests. Such power struggles can be controlled by encouraging children to be responsible for their own behaviour and setting reasonable expectations and consistent limits.

Cognitive Development

According to Piaget (1966), preschoolers gain *intuitive thought* and form concepts by learning through trial and error (see Table 16.6 on page 299). Children are still egocentric, but egocentrism gradually subsides as they encounter wider experiences. Preschoolers become concerned about death as something inevitable and they also associate death with others rather than themselves. Death may still be confused with sleep and "going away" for prolonged periods.

Moral Development

Moral behaviour to a preschooler may mean taking turns at play or sharing. Preschoolers enjoy sharing, helping, protecting, befriending, showing affection, and giving encouragement to others. Children who perceive their parents as strict may become resentful or overly obedient. Preschoolers usually control their behaviour because they want love and approval from their parents. Nurses can encourage parents to give preschoolers recognition for their behaviours. It is also important for parents to answer preschoolers' "why" questions and discuss values with them.

Spiritual Development

According to Fowler (1981), children from the ages of 4 to 6 years are at the *intuitive-projective stage* of spiritual development (see Table 16.8 on page 302). At this stage, faith is primarily taught by parents and teachers through picture books or simple explanations of spiritual matters. Preschoolers' imaginations can envision such ideas as angels or the devil. Children imitate religious behaviour, for example, by bowing their heads in prayer, although they don't understand the meaning of the behaviour.

Health Problems

Health problems in preschoolers are similar to those of toddlers. Respiratory tract problems and communicable diseases, such as fifth disease (a viral disease that causes a distinctive rash on the face, arms, and body), meningitis, and head lice, are common as the preschooler interacts with other children. Accidents and dental caries continue to be problems. Congenital abnormalities, such as cardiac disorders and hernias, are often corrected by this age.

Health Assessment and Promotion

During assessment, the preschooler can often participate in answering questions with assistance from parents or caregivers. They are fairly independent but still need supervision and guidance (see the Assessment: Developmental Guidelines box). Promoting health and wellness includes such areas as preventing accidents, and ensuring dental health, good nutrition, cognitive stimulation, and sufficient sleep. See the Health-Promotion Guidelines box for preschoolers.

ASSESSMENT: DEVELOPMENTAL GUIDELINES

The Preschooler

In these four developmental areas, does the preschooler do the following by age 5?

1. **PHYSICAL DEVELOPMENT**
   - Demonstrate physical growth (weight, height) within normal range
   - Manifest vital signs within normal range for age
   - Exhibit vision and hearing abilities within normal range
2. **MOTOR DEVELOPMENT**
   - Perform gross and fine motor milestones within the normal range for age:
     - Jump rope and skip
     - Climb playground equipment
     - Ride a bicycle with training wheels
     - Print letters and numbers
3. **PSYCHOSOCIAL DEVELOPMENT**
   - Perform psychosocial developmental milestones for age:
     - Separate easily from parents
     - Display imagination and creativity
     - Enjoy playing with peers in cooperative activities
     - Understand right from wrong and respond to others' expectations of behaviour
     - Identify four colours
     - Exhibit increasing vocabulary using complete sentences and all parts of speech
     - Cooperate in doing simple chores (e.g., putting away toys)
     - Demonstrate awareness of sexual differences
4. **DEVELOPMENT IN ACTIVITIES OF DAILY LIVING**
   - Demonstrate development of toilet training
   - Perform simple hygiene measures
   - Dress and undress self
   - Engage in bedtime rituals and demonstrate ability to put self to sleep

Health-Promotion Guidelines for Preschoolers

The following are important to the health of preschoolers:

HEALTH EXAMINATIONS
- Every 1 to 2 years

PROTECTIVE MEASURES
- Routine immunizations: DTaP-IPV, IPV series, MMR, and other immunizations as recommended
- Tuberculin skin test as recommended
- Vision and hearing screening
- Regular dental screenings and fluoride treatment

PRESCHOOLER SAFETY
- Education about simple safety rules (e.g., crossing the street, use of car seat)
- Teaching of ways to play safely (e.g., bicycle and playground safety, use of helmets)
- Education to prevent poisoning

NUTRITION
- Importance of nutritious meals and snacks

ELIMINATION
- Teaching of proper hygiene (e.g., washing hands after using bathroom)

REST AND SLEEP
- Ways to deal with sleep disturbances (e.g., nightmares)

PLAY
- Provision of times for group play activities
- Teaching of simple games that require cooperation and interaction
- Provision of toys and dress-ups for role-playing

School-Age Children (6 to 12 Years)

The school-age period starts about 6 years of age, when the deciduous teeth are shed and ends with the preadolescent (prepuberty) period at about 12 years with the onset of puberty. **Puberty** is the age at which the reproductive organs become functional and secondary sex characteristics develop. The average age of onset of puberty is 10 for girls and 12 for boys. Skills learned and willingness to try new tasks during this stage are particularly important for later life. The period from 6 to 12 years is one of rapid and dramatic change.

Physical Development

The school-age child gains weight rapidly and thus appears less thin than previously. Individual differences because of both genetic and environmental factors are obvious at this time.

WEIGHT At 6 years, boys tend to weigh about 21 kg, about 1 kg more than girls. The weight gain from 6 to 12 years of age averages about 3.2 kg per year, but the major weight gains occur from age 10 to 12 for boys and from 9 to 12 for girls. By 12 years of age, boys and girls weigh 40 kg to 42 kg on average; girls are usually heavier.

HEIGHT At 6 years, both boys and girls are about the same height, 115 cm. They are about 150 cm by 12 years. Before puberty, children of both sexes have a growth spurt—girls between 10 and 12 years and boys between 12 and 14 years. Thus, girls may well be taller than boys at 12 years, but boys are usually stronger.

The extremities tend to grow more quickly than the trunk; thus, school-age children's bodies appear somewhat ill-proportioned. By age 6, the thoracic curvature starts to develop, and the lordosis disappears. Full adult posture is not assumed until after the complete development of the skeletal musculature during the adolescent period.

VISION The depth and distance perception of 6- to 8-year-olds is accurate. By age 6 years, the eye muscles are well developed and coordinated. Because the shape of the eye changes during growth, the farsightedness of the preschool years gradually changes to 20/20 vision during the school-age years; 20/20 vision is usually well established between 9 and 11 years of age.

HEARING AND TOUCH Auditory perception is fully developed in school-age children. They are able to identify fine differences in voices, both in sound and in pitch. They have a well-developed sense of touch for heat and cold on all body surfaces; they are also able to identify an unseen object, such as a pencil or a book, simply by touch. This ability is called **stereognosis.**

PREPUBERTAL CHANGES Little change takes place in the reproductive and endocrine systems until the prepuberty period. At about ages 9 to 13 years, endocrine functions slowly increase, which can result in increased perspiration and more active sebaceous glands. Girls may have sticky vaginal discharge prior to puberty. Menstrual cycles or menses commencing before 10 years are due to improved nourishment and undetected estrogen intake from nonfood sources. Early-onset menses should be followed up with a health practitioner.

MOTOR ABILITIES Between ages 6 and 10, children perfect their muscular skills and coordination. By 9 years, most are becoming skilled in games of interest or school sports, such as football or baseball. Most have sufficient fine motor control for such activities as building models, sewing, or playing musical instruments.

Psychosocial Development

The central task of school-age children is *industry versus inferiority* (Erikson, 1963). At this time, children begin to create and develop a sense of competence and perseverance. They are motivated by activities that provide a sense of worth. They concentrate on mastering skills that will help them function in the adult world. Children who are successful and receive recognition for their efforts feel competent and in control of themselves and of the environment. Children who feel unaccepted by their peers, or who receive negative feedback and little recognition, may feel inferior and worthless (see Table 16.4 on page 296).

Freud (1923) describes a *latency stage* in school-age children. Their focus is on physical and intellectual activities, while sexual tendencies seem to be repressed (see Table 16.3 on page 295). Although the focus of interest for this age group has moved to school, peers, and other activities, the home remains the crucial place for the child's development of high self-esteem.

Cognitive Development

The ages 7 to 11 years mark Piaget's (1966) *concrete operations phase* (see Table 16.6 on page 299). These children change from egocentric interactions to cooperative interactions. They also develop an increased understanding of concepts that are associated with specific objects, for example, associating "conservation" with "wildlife." Logical reasoning develops from intuitive reasoning (e.g., adding and subtracting to obtain an answer to a problem). Children also learn about cause-and-effect relationships (e.g., knowing that a stone will not float because it is heavier than water).

By age 6, children learn the concept of time and can read both digital and numerical clocks. The schedule in school helps them learn the time periods. By age 7 or 8, children usually know the value of money.

Reading skills are usually well developed. What a child reads is largely influenced by the family. By 9 years, most children are self-motivated. They may compete with themselves; they like discussion and debate and like to plan ahead. By 12 years, they are motivated by inner drive rather than by competition with peers.

Moral Development

In Kohlberg's (1977) stage 1 of the *preconventional* level (punishment and obedience), school-age children act to avoid being punished. Some, however, are at stage 2 (*instrumental-relativist orientation*): they do things to benefit themselves but getting a fair share or chance for everyone is important. Between ages of 10 and 13, most children progress to the *conventional* level. This level has two stages: stage 3 is the *interpersonal concordance* (good boy or nice girl) stage, and stage 4 is the *law and order orientation*. The child shifts from the concrete interests of individuals to the interests of groups. The motivation for moral action at this stage is in living up to what significant others think of the child (see Table 16.7 on page 301).

Spiritual Development

According to Fowler (1981), the school-age child is at stage 2 in spiritual development, the *mythic-literal* stage. Children learn to distinguish fantasy from fact. *Spiritual facts* are those beliefs that are accepted by a religious group, whereas *fantasy* is thoughts and images formed in the child's mind. Parents and religious leaders still influence the child more than peers do in spiritual matters (see Table 16.8 on page 302).

Health Problems

Communicable diseases, dental caries, accidents, and the achievement of a healthy weight are health problems for school-agers. The most common nutritional problem among children is obesity, which contributes to the increased incidence of hypertension and type 2 diabetes in childhood (Strock, Cottrell, Abang, Buschbacher, & Hannon, 2005), and increases the risk for diabetes, hypertension, and cardiovascular disease in adulthood.

Health Assessment and Promotion

Comprehensive assessment relies on the nurse's ability to respond to questions from the child, parent, or other caregiver. The nurse provides feedback, encouragement, and support, and builds on the child's strengths. See the Assessment: Developmental Guidelines box for the school-age child.

Promoting health and wellness includes dental examinations and hygiene, immunization, safety measures to prevent accidents, physical fitness, supporting autonomy, self-esteem, and infection control. See the Health-Promotion Guidelines box for school-age children.

ASSESSMENT: DEVELOPMENTAL GUIDELINES

The School-Age Child

In these four developmental areas, does the school-age child do the following?

1. PHYSICAL DEVELOPMENT

- Demonstrate physical growth (weight, height) within normal range
- Manifest vital signs within normal range for age
- Exhibit vision and hearing abilities within normal range
- Demonstrate male or female prepubertal changes within normal range

2. MOTOR DEVELOPMENT

- Possess coordinated motor skills for age
- Do tricks on a bike or climb a tree
- Throw and catch a small ball
- Play a musical instrument

3. PSYCHOSOCIAL DEVELOPMENT

- Meet psychosocial developmental milestones for age
- Make friends of the same sex and establish a peer group
- Become less dependent on family and venture away from them
- Interact well with parents
- Control strong and impulsive feelings
- Participate in organized competitions
- Read, print, and manipulate numbers and letters easily
- Exhibit a concept of money and make change for small amounts of money
- Express self in a logical manner and talk through problems
- Enjoy riddles and read and understand comics
- Invest in a hobby or collection
- Like to help others
- Think of self as likable and healthy

4. DEVELOPMENT IN ACTIVITIES OF DAILY LIVING

- Demonstrate concern for personal cleanliness and appearance
- Express need for privacy

Health-Promotion Guidelines for School-Age Children

The following are important to the health of school-age children:

HEALTH EXAMINATIONS

- Annual physical examination or as recommended

PROTECTIVE MEASURES

- Immunizations as recommended. Human papillomavirus (HPV) vaccination is given only to females aged 9–26 at a three-dose schedule (0, 2, and 6 months)
- Tuberculin skin test as recommended
- Periodic vision, speech, and hearing screenings
- Regular dental screenings and fluoride treatment
- Provision of accurate information about sexual health (e.g., reproduction, AIDS)
- The right gear for the sport: helmets, pads, face and mouth guards

SCHOOL-AGE CHILD SAFETY

- Use of proper sport equipment (e.g., helmets, pads) and booster seat in car, as applicable
- The child takes responsibility for own safety (e.g., participating in bicycle and water safety courses)

NUTRITION

- Importance of eating a balanced diet and not skipping meals
- Minimization of food related to obesity

ELIMINATION

- Utilizing positive approaches for elimination problems (e.g., enuresis)

PLAY AND SOCIAL INTERACTIONS

- Provision of opportunities for a variety of organized group activities
- Acceptance of realistic expectations of child's abilities
- Role model for acceptance of other persons who may be different
- Provision of a home environment that limits television viewing and video games and encourages completion of homework

Adolescence (12 to 18 Years)

Adolescence is the period during which the person becomes physically and psychologically mature and acquires a personal identity. At the end of this critical period, the teen is ready to enter adulthood and assume responsibilities. The length of adolescence is culturally determined to some extent and may extend to 18 or 20 years of age in North America.

Puberty is the first stage of adolescence, in which the sexual organs begin to grow and mature. **Menarche** (onset of menstruation) occurs in girls, **ejaculation** (expulsion of semen) in boys. For girls, puberty normally starts between 10 and 14 years; for boys, between 12 and 16 years. The adolescent period is often subdivided into three stages: early adolescence (ages 12 to 13), middle adolescence (14 to 16 years), and late adolescence (from 17 to 18 or 20 years). Late adolescence is a more stable stage, when adolescents are involved with planning their future and economic independence.

Physical Development

During puberty, growth is accelerated through an *adolescent growth spurt.* Males begin between ages 12 and 16 years; females begin between ages 10 and 14 years. Because the growth spurt begins earlier in girls, many girls surpass boys in height at this time. Boys will catch up and often surpass the girls by the end of this period.

PHYSICAL GROWTH Physical growth continues throughout adolescence. Growth is fastest for boys at about 14 years, and the maximum height is often reached at about 18 or 19 years. Some males add another 1 cm or 2 cm to their height during their 20s as the vertebral column continues to grow gradually. From 10 to 18 years of age, the average Canadian male doubles his weight, gaining about 32 kg, and grows about 41 cm. The fastest rate of growth in girls occurs at about age 12 years; they reach their maximum height at about 15 to 16 years. From ages 10 to 18 years, the average Canadian female gains about 25 kg and grows about 24 cm.

Physical growth is greatly influenced by heredity, nutrition, medical care, illness, physical and emotional environment, family size, race, and culture. Growth is noted first in the musculoskeletal system, which follows a sequential pattern: the head, hands, and feet are the first to grow to adult status, followed by extremities. Because the extremities grow before the trunk, the adolescent looks leggy. After the trunk grows to full size, the shoulders, chest, and hips grow. Skull and facial bones also change proportions—the forehead becomes more prominent, and the jawbones develop.

GLANDULAR CHANGES The eccrine and apocrine glands increase their secretions and become fully functional during puberty. The **eccrine glands**, found over most of the body, produce sweat. The **apocrine glands** develop in the axillae, anal, and genital areas; external auditory canals; and around the umbilicus and areolae of the breasts. Apocrine sweat is released onto the skin in response to emotional stimuli only. **Sebaceous glands** also become active under the influence of androgens in both males and females. The sebaceous glands, which secrete **sebum**, become most active on the face, neck, shoulder, upper back, chest, and genitals.

SEXUAL CHARACTERISTICS **Primary sexual characteristics** relate to the organs necessary for reproduction, such as the testes, penis, vagina, and uterus. **Secondary sexual characteristics** differentiate the male from the female but do not relate directly to reproduction. Examples are pubic hair growth, breast development, and voice changes.

Both primary and secondary sex characteristics develop during puberty. The first noticeable sign that puberty has begun in males is the appearance of pubic hair. The milestone of male puberty is considered to be the first ejaculation, which commonly occurs at about 14 years of age. Fertility follows several months later. Sexual maturity is achieved by age 18 years. Often, the first noticeable sign of puberty in females is the appearance of the *breast bud*, although the appearance of hair along the labia may precede this. The milestone of female puberty is the menarche, which occurs about 2 years after the breast bud appears. At first, menstrual periods are scanty and irregular and may occur without ovulation. Ovulation is usually established 1 to 2 years after menarche. Female internal reproductive organs reach adult size about age 18 to 20 years.

Psychosocial Development

According to Erikson (1963), the psychosocial task of the adolescent is the *establishment of identity*. The danger of this stage is *role confusion* (see Table 16.4 on page 296). The inability to settle on a career path commonly disturbs the adolescent. Less commonly, doubts about sexual identity arise. Adolescents help one another through this identity crisis by forming cliques and a separate youth culture, often excluding all those who are "different" in cultural background, aspects of dress, gestures, and tastes. Hair styling, skin care, and clothes become very important. In-groupers of an adolescent clique can be excessively clannish and cruel in excluding out-groupers; this intolerance is a temporary defence against identity confusion.

The adolescent has unlimited imagination and ambition and aspires to great accomplishments. The sense of industry is re-enacted when the adolescent chooses a career. The extent to which these tasks were achieved earlier influences the adolescent's ability to achieve a healthy self-concept and self-identity.

The adolescent needs to establish a self-concept that accepts both personal strengths and personal weaknesses. Faced with dramatic changes in body structure and function, and greater expectations to assume responsibilities, many adolescents experience temporary difficulty in developing a positive self-image (e.g., preoccupation with acne problem). Adolescents with physical challenges or illnesses are particularly vulnerable to peer rejection or bullying. Those who are accepted, loved, and valued by family and peers generally tend to gain confidence and feel good about themselves. Those who have difficulty forming relationships, or who are perceived by peers as too different and who are not included in adolescent cliques, may develop less favourable self-images and have low self-esteem.

Because sex roles are becoming less defined in Canadian society, adopting masculine and feminine roles is increasingly confusing for today's adolescent. In forming a sexual identity, adolescents first fantasize the male or female role and then enact various aspects of that imagined role. Later, adolescents begin to establish intimacy with a partner or partners. This intimacy lays the groundwork for the commitments of adulthood. Sexual experimentation is not part of true intimacy, but once intimacy is realized, sexual activity follows. Gay and lesbian youth can experience a great deal of confusion during this period as their questions about self and identity may go unanswered.

Many adolescents are sexually active and may engage in masturbation as well as sexual activity, with the same or opposite sex. Garriguet (2005) reported that teen girls with low self-esteem were more likely to have sexual intercourse by age 15 than those with strong self-esteem. The opposite was found in boys. The 2003 Canadian Community Health Survey (Statistics Canada, 2003) reported that the average age at which Canadians have sex for the first time is 16.5 years; 28% of 15- to 17-year-olds indicated sexual intercourse had occurred at least once; one-third of those sexually active between 15 and 24 years of age reported more than one sexual partner in the previous year. About 30% of those with multiple sexual partners had not used a condom. Older teens had sex more often without a condom than younger teens. Those who began sexual intercourse by age 13 had twice the incidence of reporting an STI than those who waited until they were older.

At about the age of 15 years, the *need for independence*, combined with the need for family support, sometimes creates conflict within the adolescent and between the adolescent and the family. The young person may appear hostile or depressed at times during this crisis. Adolescents prefer to be with their peers and may seek advice from adults other than parents. Parents sometimes are bewildered by this stage and instead of reducing controls, they increase them, causing the adolescent to rebel.

Adolescents may develop brief crushes on adults outside the family. They sometimes adopt some of the attributes of the adults with whom they are infatuated. This modelling can be helpful in the maturing process.

Some of the discord in the family at this time is due to the generation gap. Adolescents' values may differ from those of their parents and be difficult for the parents to understand and to accept. Restrictions and guidance need to be presented in a manner that makes adolescents feel loved. They need consistency in guidance, fewer restrictions, and as much independence as they can handle, but they need to know that their parents will assist them when necessary.

Peer groups are defined by like-minded, loosely bonded, and self-identified cohorts who influence one another's ideas, values, behaviours, and lifestyle choices and provide one another with a sense of belonging, pride, social learning, and gender roles (Figure 17.8.). Most peer groups have well-defined, gender-specific modes of acceptable behaviour. Peer groups change with age, starting as single-sex groups, evolving into mixed groups, and finally narrowing to couples who share activities.

For gay and lesbian youth, adolescence is a difficult time. Because peer acceptance is crucial to self-acceptance, lesbian and gay adolescents usually conform to the heterosexual codes and behaviours even though these do not feel natural or correct. Adolescents who are openly gay or lesbian may face not only the ostracism of their peers but also the misunderstanding and hostility of parents, teachers, and other important adults.

Cognitive Development

Adolescents begin Piaget's *formal operations phase* of cognitive development (see Table 16.6 on page 299) with cognitive abilities maturing between the ages of 11 and 15 years. At this stage, adolescents can think beyond the present and are highly idealistic. They become more informed about the world and environment. They use new information to solve everyday problems and communicate with adults on most subjects, such as interest areas and career plans.

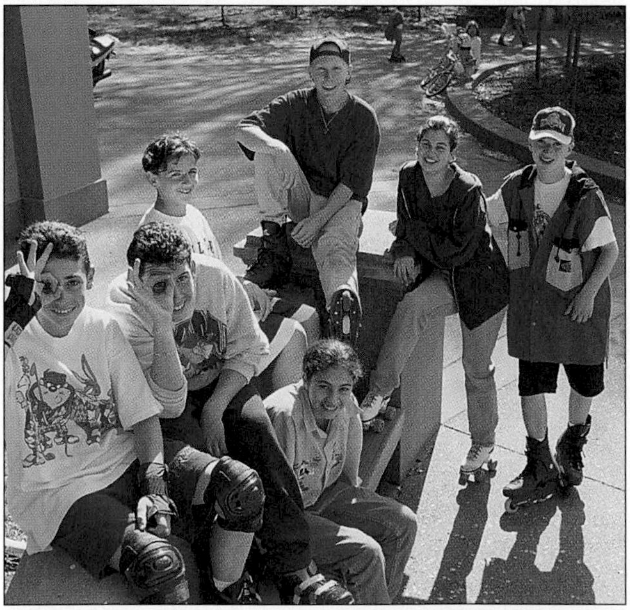

FIGURE 17.8 Adolescent peer group relationships enhance a sense of belonging, self-esteem, and self-identity.

Moral Development

According to Kohlberg (1977), the young adolescent is usually at the *conventional level* of moral development. Although most still want to abide by social order and existing laws, many discard the values they have adopted from parents in favour of those they consider more suitable. In the *postconventional* or *principled level,* they start to question the rules and laws of society, especially if their personal views are in conflict with societal laws and what they perceive as individual rights. Not all adolescents, or even adults, proceed to this postconventional level. See Kohlberg's stages of moral development in Table 16.7 on page 301.

Spiritual Development

According to Fowler (1981), the adolescent reaches the *synthetic-conventional* stage of spiritual development. As they encounter different groups in society, they are exposed to a wide variety of opinions, beliefs, and behaviours regarding religious matters; some may seek advice from a significant other, such as a parent or a minister.

Often, the adolescent believes that various religious beliefs and practices have more similarities than differences. At this stage, the adolescent's focus is on interpersonal, rather than conceptual, matters.

Health Problems

Adolescents can be at risk for unintentional injuries, STIs, inactivity, unhealthy eating, mental health problems, teen pregnancy, and problematic tobacco, alcohol, and other drug use (Canadian Institute for Health Information, 2005). Common problems related to nutrition and self-esteem among adolescents include obesity, anorexia nervosa, and bulimia (see the Nursing and Canadian Society box). Psychological and emotional challenges may lead to mental health problems and the first manifestation of schizophrenia can appear in late adolescence (Toga, Thompson, & Sowell, 2006). Adolescents in communal living, such as in college or university dormitories, may have increased risk for infectious diseases, such as measles, mumps, mononucleosis, and meningitis. Other health problems include acne, cardiovascular disease, tooth decay, gingivitis, misalignment of teeth, neglect, and abuse.

In 2004, three leading causes of death in the 10-to-24 age group are unintentional injuries (e.g., falls, drowning, poisoning, motor vehicle collisions), suicide, and cancer (Public Health Agency of Canada, 2008). The Health Council of Canada (2006) estimated about "1.1 million—or 14 per cent—of Canada's children under age 20 have mental health conditions that affect their lives at home, at school and in the community. . . .

Nursing and Canadian Society

Fact	Implications for Nursing Practice
Six percent of Canadian babies are born underweight (< 2500 g) because of poor maternal diet, lifestyle, poverty, smoking, and dieting (Statistics Canada, 2006).	Preconceptual health and prenatal care are important for healthy pregnancy outcomes.
Cancer is the second-leading cause of death in Canada, though the overall childhood cancer rates have remained unchanged over the last 12 to 16 years (Ritter, 2001).	Nursing health assessment needs to include screening for early detection of cancer among children. The importance of regular physical examination and harm reduction to provide a safe environment must be emphasized.
Rates of overweight and obesity among Canadian youth have more than doubled in the last 25 years. One million young Canadians are overweight, and half a million are obese (Health Council of Canada, 2006; Shields, 2006).	Obesity is a result of the lack of physical activity and poor food choices. The highest nutrient and energy demands occur during the growth spurt in adolescence. Nurses need to consider these when creating a diet and exercise plan to foster adolescents' weight control.
Rates of adolescent pregnancy continue to be high, though pregnancy rates in Canada among 15- to 19-year-olds declined from 68.9 per 1000 in 1997 to 33.9 in 2002 (Dryburgh, 2002).	Nurses can help prevent unintended pregnancy by promoting the use of birth control methods and teaching or counselling teens about themselves (roles, self-concepts, etc.).

In 2002, more than six per cent of youth and young adults experienced a major depressive episode in the previous year, six per cent reported suicidal thoughts, and five per cent had social anxiety disorder" (p. 20). Suicide accounts for 24% of all deaths among 15- to 24-year-olds and is the second-leading cause of death for Canadians between 10 and 24 years (Canadian Mental Health Association [CMHA], 2006).

Teen suicide rates in Canada are similar to those in the United States, with females experiencing more depression and suicidal ideas than males (Cheung & Renaud, 2007). Males act on their thoughts four times more often than females do. Suicide rates increase with age, poverty, Aboriginal and Inuit heritage, seasonal darkness, untreated mental disorders, a history of sexual abuse, and location (CMHA, 2006). Motor vehicle collisions, drug and alcohol overdoses, firearm accidents, and even homicides can be disguised suicides.

Assessment: Developmental Guidelines

The Adolescent

In these three developmental areas, does the adolescent do the following?

1. **PHYSICAL DEVELOPMENT**
   - Exhibit physical growth (weight, height) within normal range for age and gender
   - Demonstrate male or female sexual development consistent with standards
   - Manifest vital signs within normal range for age and gender
   - Exhibit vision and hearing abilities within normal range
2. **PSYCHOSOCIAL DEVELOPMENT**
   - Interact well with parents, teachers, peers, siblings, and persons in authority
   - Like self
   - Think and plan for the future, such as university, a relationship, or a career
   - Choose a lifestyle and interests that fit own identity
   - Determine own beliefs and values
   - Begin to establish a sense of identity in the family
   - Seek help from appropriate persons about problems
3. **DEVELOPMENT IN ACTIVITIES OF DAILY LIVING**
   - Demonstrate knowledge of physical development, menstruation, reproduction, birth control, and methods for the prevention of STIs
   - Exhibit healthy lifestyle practices in nutrition, exercise, recreation, sleep patterns, and personal habits
   - Demonstrate concern for personal cleanliness and appearance
   - Reach out to members of their religious faith, peer group for support
   - Have a comfortable environment to practise the rituals of their faith

Health Assessment and Promotion

Guidelines for growth and development of the adolescent are shown in the Assessment: Developmental Guidelines box on page 327.

Adolescents are usually self-directed in meeting their health needs. Because of maturational changes, however, they need teaching and guidance, such as screening for hearing and vision; information on avoiding tobacco, alcohol, and drug use; and facts about healthy sexual practices, blood pressure maintenance, healthy weights, and immunizations. See the Health-Promotion Guidelines box for adolescents.

Health-Promotion Guidelines for Adolescents

The following are important to the health of adolescents:

HEALTH EXAMINATIONS

- Yearly or as recommended by the health-care provider

PROTECTIVE MEASURES

- Immunizations as recommended, such as adult diphtheria-tetanus and pertussis (DTaP) vaccine; and HepB vaccine, meningococcal vaccine, and human papillomavirus vaccine (HPV) if not yet immunized.
- Screening for TB as recommended
- Vision and hearing screenings
- Regular dental assessments
- Provision of accurate information about sexual issues

ADOLESCENT SAFETY

- Motor vehicle safety (e.g., driver's education course, seat belts, motorcycle helmets)
- Implementation of proper precautions during all athletic activities (e.g., medical supervision, proper equipment, hydration, and nutrients)
- Open lines of communication and being alert to signs of bullying or harassment, problematic substance use, emotional disturbances, and depression

NUTRITION AND EXERCISE

- Importance of healthy snacks and appropriate patterns of food intake and exercise
- Control of factors that may lead to nutritional problems (e.g., obesity, anorexia nervosa, bulimia)
- Balance of sedentary activities with regular exercise

SOCIAL INTERACTIONS

- Encouragement of relationships that respect feelings, concerns, and fears
- Parental encouragement of peer group activities promoting moral and spiritual values
- Parents acting as role models for appropriate social interactions
- Parents provision of a comfortable home environment for appropriate adolescent peer group activities

Case Study 17

Billy is a 6-year-old boy entering Grade 1. He is scared and hesitant to let go of his mother's hand. As the nursing student working in this setting, you have the opportunity to work with Billy and other young children as they start school.

Critical Thinking Questions

1. How would you help Billy's mother reassure him?
2. On the basis of his age, what strategies might you use to teach Billy and his classmates about health promotion?

After working through these questions, go to the MyNursingLab at **http://www.mynursinglab.com** to check your answers.

KEY TERMS

trimesters
vernix caseosa
lanugo
teratogen
fetal alcohol syndrome
normocephaly
failure to thrive
colic
shaken baby syndrome (SBS)
sudden infant death syndrome (SIDS)
Apgar
Denver Developmental Screening Test (DDST)
self-concept
separation anxiety
regression
amblyopia
strabismus
hyperopic
emmetropic
myopic
identification
introjection
imagination
repression
puberty
stereognosis
adolescence
menarche
ejaculation
eccrine glands
apocrine glands
sebaceous glands
sebum
primary sexual characteristics
secondary sexual characteristics
peer groups

CHAPTER HIGHLIGHTS

- Intrauterine development lasts about 9 months.
- Genetic and environmental factors affect the development of the fetus.
- A sense of trust and security in the newborn is essential for subsequent development; the infant derives this sense from parental love, warmth, and prompt attention to physical needs.
- Measurements of length, weight, head and chest circumferences, fontanelle size and status, reflex abilities, and motor development are important indicators of the newborn's growth and health.
- Infants from 1 month to 1 year reveal marked growth in size and stature with appropriate nutrition and care: birth weight doubles by 6 months and triples by 12 months.
- During infancy, motor development is notable: at 3 months, infants can raise their heads from the prone position; at 6 months, they can sit unsupported; and at 12 months, they can stand momentarily and walk with help.
- To develop cognitively, the infant needs a variety of sensory and motor stimuli.
- Early childhood spans the period from 1 to 6 years and is subdivided into the toddler group, age 1 to 3 years, and the preschool group, ages 4 and 5 years.
- During childhood, dramatic changes occur as the child moves from being a dependent person to becoming an independent person entering school.
- As the nervous system develops, body systems mature to the point at which the child can control his or her body, achieve finer muscle control, and perform all the activities of daily living, such as washing and dressing.
- Critical to psychosocial development during childhood is the development of a sense of autonomy and initiative.
- By the end of early childhood, the child has reached the phase of intuitive thought, has developed some internal moral controls, and is at the undifferentiated level of spiritual development.
- School-age children perfect their muscular skills and coordination and develop a sense of competence, perseverance, and self-worth.
- During emotional development, school-age children face Erikson's conflict of industry versus inferiority.
- School-age children begin to understand relationships and change from being egocentric to having cooperative interactions; according to Piaget, they are in the concrete operations phase of cognitive development.
- Most school-age children progress to the conventional level of moral development and to the mythic-literal stage of spiritual development.
- Rapid growth in height, secondary sexual characteristics, sexual maturity, and increasing independence from the family are major landmarks of adolescence.
- Peer groups assume great importance during adolescence; they provide a sense of belonging and self-esteem and facilitate the development of a positive self-concept.
- Adolescents are at Fowler's synthetic-conventional stage of spiritual development.
- Adolescents between the ages of 11 and 15 years begin the formal operations stage of cognitive development; they are able to think logically, rationally, and futuristically and can conceptualize things as they could be, rather than as they are.
- The adolescent is at Kohlberg's conventional level of moral development, and some proceed to the postconventional or principled level.
- The three leading causes of adolescent death are unintentional injuries, suicide, and cancer.
- Adolescents can be at risk for unintentional injuries, STIs, inactivity, unhealthy eating, mental health problems, teen pregnancy, and problematic tobacco, alcohol, and other drug use.

ASSESS YOUR LEARNING

1. What is the most appropriate strategy for teaching kindergarten children effective hand hygiene techniques?
   - **a.** Explaining and demonstrating the proper procedure for hand hygiene.
   - **b.** Involving the children in initiative and imaginative techniques on hand hygiene.
   - **c.** Developing a poster showing colourful bacteria growing on hands.
   - **d.** Providing a video for the children to watch at home.

2. You are involved as a nurse with a new Family Health Network in a community that has many young families and many new babies. Your responsibility is to complete the neonatal assessments of the new babies of the families in your clinic. Newborn health can be appraised through measuring which of the following?
   - **a.** Muscular skills, vocalization, and feeding
   - **b.** Weight, height, fontanelle size, and head circumference
   - **c.** Tolerance for separation, sleep, and number of wet diapers
   - **d.** Assessment of the levels of formal operations and responses to parental smiles

3. You care for the teens in the local high school as the school health nurse, and you are struck by the aspects of development that are common signals pointing to the healthy progress of teens through developmental tasks of adolescence. Looking for the healthy indicators of developmental maturation, you must know that the landmarks of adolescent development into adulthood consist of which of the following?
   - **a.** Increased self-care activities, sexually mature behaviours, close interpersonal relationships outside the family
   - **b.** Peer pressure, a successful part-time job, graduation from secondary school
   - **c.** Synthetic-conventional family dynamics, peer cohesion, and increased size
   - **d.** Cooperative interactions, peer-focused language, and concern about personal health

4. Nurses can meet the health-care needs of adolescents through which of the following?
   - **a.** Encouraging teens to take responsibility for their behaviours and actions based on correct knowledge of health-care measures
   - **b.** Promoting parental accountability for yearly physicals, dental exams, and dietary requirements
   - **c.** Providing many free clinics and lots of pamphlets to teach families about proper health activities
   - **d.** Creating injury-proof strategies and requiring helmets and pads during all sports

5. A parent is worried about his year-old child's vision as he seems to be unable to put his toys into the correct shapes into the holder right on his lap. The parent indicates that the child wants to sit close to the TV screen to watch his favourite cartoon characters and does not seem to respond to smiles on other people's faces. Which of the following is the correct age and characteristic match regarding vision?
   - **a.** At 4 months, infants still have problems focusing on close objects.
   - **b.** At 9 months, infants begin to recognize and stare at colours.
   - **c.** By 12 months, depth perception is developed.
   - **d.** Rooting and Babinski reflexes mature as infants gain visual coordination.

6. Newborn care can create anxiety for new parents. Knowing what you do about new parents and their transition to baby care at home, which is the best choice from the titles below for a presentation you would give just before they are discharged?
   - **a.** *Apgar Scoring: The Way to Help Baby Learn*
   - **b.** *Safety Proofing Baby: Tips from A to Z*
   - **c.** *For Crying Out Loud! Keep That Baby Quiet!*
   - **d.** *Better Not Spoil That Baby: Cleaning Up after Baby*

7. You are in the emergency room and an 18-month-old is rushed in by ambulance with a pulse but absent respirations. You are performing your triage assessment. When should you suspect shaken baby syndrome (SBS)?
   - **a.** The child is 3 months old.
   - **b.** The parents claim the child is a good baby most of the time.
   - **c.** Assessment and diagnostics reveal injury, apnea, lethargy, and retinal hemorrhage.
   - **d.** An Apgar score of 10 is achieved.

8. Toddlers are prone to fatal injuries for which of the following reasons?
   - **a.** Parents and other caregivers provide preventive measures in the home, playground, and daycare settings.
   - **b.** Recurrent respiratory and ear infections create increased risk for health problems.
   - **c.** They are able to walk up and down stairs easily without assistance.
   - **d.** Most are curious about the tastes of everything and often copy others' actions.

9. Immunization for all children up to age 6 should include which of the following?

a. One-time injections to combat measles, tetanus, and polio
b. Sequential injections at specific ages for DPT-Polio, MMR, Hib, Hep B
c. Yearly TB immunizations in any province or territory
d. Examination of the child for allergies after administering the vaccines

10. School-age children enjoy group activities. These may lead to which of the following health problems?
a. MVAs, broken legs, and concussions
b. Head injuries, bullying, and poisoning
c. Lost teeth, eye injuries and abrasions
d. Communicable diseases, such as scabies, head lice, chickenpox

After working through these questions, go to the MyNursingLab at **http://www.mynursinglab.com** *to check your answers and see explanations.*

SUGGESTED READINGS

Bradley, B. (2006). *The baby and childcare encyclopedia.* Toronto: Family Communications Inc.
This collection of parenting tips presents the collected work of many specialists and health-care authorities in Canada.

Saunders, N., & Friedman, J. (2006). *Caring for kids: The complete Canadian guide to children's health.* Toronto: Key Porter.
This is a comprehensive medical guide to health and wellness in children (ages 0–10). The information is based on scientific evidence and is published in cooperation with Toronto's Hospital for Sick Children.

WEBLINKS

Canadian Paediatric Society

http://www.caringforkids.cps.ca

This site provides information about children from Canadian pediatric experts.

Health Canada

http://www.hc-sc.gc.ca/english/index.html

This site provides a search engine to enable the user to access a range of Canadian child health resources.

Centers for Disease Control and Prevention, National Center for Health Statistics

http://www.cdc.gov/growthcharts

This website has downloadable growth charts and information on their use.

Canadian Public Health Association

http://www.drinkingfacts.ca

This site has resources, such as videotape scenarios and true stories of teens with problematic alcohol use, that will be useful for facilitators for discussion purposes.

Ontario Ministry of Health and Long-Term Care

http://www.health.gov.on.ca/english/media/mediafiles/archives/media_06/media_0307_ar.html

The 3-minute 2006 video clip gives an excellent introduction on newborn screening.

Registered Nurses' Association of Ontario

http://www.rnao.org/Page.asp?PageID=924&ContentID=800

This site provides best practice guidelines related to multiple strategies to enhance healthy adolescent development in various life situations and settings.

Public Health Agency of Canada: Healthy Settings for Young People in Canada

http://www.phac-aspc.gc.ca/dca-dea/yjc/summ-eng.php

This cross-national research study is Canada's only national database for health behaviour in school-age children. It aims to explore the health, well-being, and health behaviours of young people (aged 11 to 15 years) and their social settings, specifically, their school environment.

REFERENCES

Albrecht, S. A., Maloni, J. A., Thomas, K. K., Jones, R., Halleran, J., & Osborne, J. (2004). Smoking cessation counseling for pregnant women who smoke: Scientific basis for practice for AWHONN's SUCCESS project. *Journal of Obstetric, Gynecologic & Neonatal Nursing, 33*(3), 298–305.

Anderson, M. E., Johnson, D.C., & Batal, H. A. (2005). Sudden infant death syndrome and prenatal maternal smoking: Rising attributed risk in the back to sleep era. *BMC Medicine, 3*(1), 4.

Canadian Institute for Health Information. (2005). *Improving the health of young Canadians.* Ottawa: Author.

Canadian Mental Health Association. (2006). *Suicide.* Retrieved March 31, 2008, from http://www.ontario.cmha.ca/about_mental_health.asp?cID=7608

Canadian Paediatric Society. (2004). Recommendations for safe sleeping environments for infants and children. *Paediatrics & Child Health, 9*(9), 659–663.

Cheung, A., & Renaud, C. (2007). *Teen suicide rates in Canada similar to US despite universal health care. Insight Wellness News Article.* Retrieved June 19, 2007, from http://www.anxiety-and-depression-solutions.com/articles/news/Teen_suicide_rates_in_Canada_similar_to_US_despite_universal_health_care.php

Dryburgh, H. (2002). Teen pregnancy. *Health Reports, 12*(1), 9–18.

Emond, A., Drewett, R., Blair, P., & Emmett, P. (2007). Postnatal factors associated with failure to thrive in term infants in the Avon Longitudinal Study of Parents and Children. *Child: Care, Health and Development, 33*(3), 351–351.

Engel, G. I. (1962). *Psychological development in health and disease.* Philadelphia, PA: Saunders.

Erikson, E. H. (1963). *Childhood and society* (2nd ed.). New York: Norton.

First Nations and Inuit Health Committee & Canadian Paediatric Society. (2007). Growth assessment in Aboriginal children: Is there need for change? *Paediatric & Child Health, 9*(7), 477–479. Retrieved September 8, 2007, from http://www.cps.ca/english/statements/II/FNIH04-01.htm

Fowler, J. W. (1981). *Stages of faith: The psychology of human development and the quest for meaning.* New York: Harper & Row.

Freud, S. (1923). *The ego and the id.* London, UK: Hogarth Press.

Garriguet, D. (2005). *Early sexual intercourse.* Statistics Canada. Retrieved June 18, 2007, from http://www.statcan.ca/bsolc/english/bsolc?catno=82–003-X20040037837

Geddes, J. F. (2004). The evidence base for shaken baby syndrome. *British Medical Journal, 328,* 719–720.

Health Canada. (2002). *Shaken baby syndrome.* Retrieved September 10, 2007, from http://www.phac-aspc.gc.ca/dca-dea/prenatal/shaken_e.html

Health Council of Canada. (2006). *Their future is now: Healthy choices for Canada's children & youth.* Retrieved April 20, 2007, from http://www.healthcouncilcanada.ca/docs/rpts/2006/HCC_ChildHealth_EN.pdf

Kohlberg, L. (1977). *Recent research in moral development.* New York: Holt, Rinehart, Winston.

Kvigne, V. L., Leonardson, G. R., Neff-Smith, M., Brock, E., Borzelleca, J., & Welty, T. K. (2004). Characteristics of children who have full or incomplete fetal alcohol syndrome. *Journal of Pediatrics, 145*(5), 635–640.

Piaget, J. (1966). *Origins of intelligence in children.* New York: Norton.

Public Health Agency of Canada. (2008). *Leading causes of death and hospitalization in Canada.* Retrieved August 25, 2008, from http://www.phac-aspc.gc.ca/publicat/lcd-pcd97/index-eng.php

Ritter, L. (2001, June 15). No basis for pesticide bans. *National Post.* Retrieved May 15, 2007, from http://www.uoguelph.ca/cntc/announce/june2001.shtml

Save Babies Through Screening Foundation of Canada. (2007). *News.* Retrieved September 10, 2007, from http://www.savebabiescanada.org/News.htm

Shields, M. (2006). Overweight and obesity among children and youth. *Health Reports, 17*(3), 27–42. Statistics Canada, Catalogue no. 82-003-XIE.

Starr, N. B. (2004). Self-perception. In C. E. Burns, A. M. Dunn, M. A. Brady, N. B. Starr, & C. G. Blosser (Eds.), *Pediatric primary care: A handbook for nurse practitioners* (3rd ed.) (pp. 375–339). Philadelphia, PA: W. B. Saunders.

Statistics Canada. (2003). *Canadian community health survey.* Ottawa: Author.

Statistics Canada. (2006). *Pregnancy outcomes by age group, 2004.* Retrieved January 27, 2007, from http://www40.statcan.ca/l01/cst01/hlth65a.htm

Strock, G. A., Cottrell, E. R., Abang, A. E., Buschbacher, R. M., & Hannon, T. S. (2005). Childhood obesity: A simple equation with complex variables. *Journal of Long Term Effects of Medical Implants, 15*(1), 15–32.

Toga, A. W., Thompson, P. M., & Sowell, E. R. (2006). Mapping brain maturation. *Trends in Neurosciences, 29*(3), 148–159.

Venes, D. (Ed.). (2005). *Taber's cyclopedic medical dictionary* (20th ed.). Philadelphia, PA: F. A. Davis.

Wolfe, E. L., Davis, T., Guydish, J., & Delucchi, K. L. (2005). Mortality risk associated with perinatal drug and alcohol use in California. *Journal of Perinatology, 25*(2), 93–100.

Chapter 18

Young and Middle-Aged Adulthood

The adult phase of development encompasses the years from the end of adolescence to death. Because the developmental tasks of young adults differ from those of older adults, adulthood is often divided into three phases: young adulthood, middle adulthood, and late adulthood. Here, young adults are defined as people 20 to 40 years old, middle-aged adults as 40 to 65 years old, and late adulthood refers to life beyond 65 years.

Adult age span includes three very different generations: the **baby boomers** (born in years 1945–1964), **Generation X** (birth years 1965–1978), and **Generation Y** or the *Millennials* (born 1979–2000). A new term, **zoomer**, has been coined by M. Znaimer to describe active adults over 50 (Ross Cravit, 2008). Each cohort has shared specific life events and has its own world view. Baby boomers are characterized by an individualistic outlook, a tendency toward a "workaholic" orientation, a desire to be respected at work, and a feeling of role overload (Hill, 2004; Hu, Herrick, & Hodgin, 2004). Many Generation Xers were raised in two-worker households in which long hours at work were common. They may be less impressed with corporate values, more skeptical, and resistant to authority, but they enjoy challenges and opportunities to creatively solve problems. Generation Y (or Millennials) have come of age in an increasingly multicultural context. They are technologically sophisticated (and dependent) and enjoy public affirmation of their efforts.

Human development is a complex synthesis of physiological, cognitive, psychological, moral, and spiritual development. Nurses should expect individual variations and take these into consideration when applying theories to caregiving.

OBJECTIVES

After studying this chapter, you should be able to

1. Compare and contrast the following generational groups: baby boomers, Generation X, and Generation Y
2. Describe the usual physical developmental changes throughout adulthood
3. Identify tasks characteristic of different stages of development from young to middle adulthood
4. Discuss changes in cognitive development according to Piaget throughout adulthood
5. Differentiate moral development according to Gilligan and Kohlberg throughout adulthood
6. Examine spiritual development according to Fowler throughout adulthood
7. Identify developmental assessment guidelines for young and middle-aged adults
8. Identify selected health problems for adults
9. Analyze selected health problems associated with young and middle-aged adults

Young Adults (20 to 40 Years)

The age at which a person is considered an adult depends on how adulthood is described. Legally, a person in Canada can vote at 18 years. The legal age for alcohol consumption outside the home varies among the provinces and territories from 18 to 21 years. Another criterion of adulthood is financial independence, which is also highly variable. Some adolescents support themselves as early as 16 years of age, usually because of family circumstances. By contrast, some adults are financially dependent on their families for many years.

Adulthood may also be indicated by the person moving away from home and establishing his or her own living arrangements. Some adolescents may leave home because of family problems. In recent years, however, more young adults have been choosing to remain at home. **Boomerang kids** have evolved: young adults who move back into their parents' homes after an initial period of independent living. Contributing to this trend are high housing costs, high divorce rates, high unemployment rates, and many problems resulting from problematic substance use. Some who work full time receive only minimum wages and are unable to earn enough money to be totally independent.

Young adults are typically busy people who juggle many challenges. They are expected to assume new roles at work, at home, and in the community, and to develop interests, values, and attitudes related to these roles.

BOX 18.1 PSYCHOSOCIAL DEVELOPMENT: YOUNG ADULT

Young adults experience a great deal of psychosocial development:

- According to Freud's theory (1923), the young adult is in the genital stage, in which energy is directed toward attaining a mature sexual relationship.
- The young adult is in the intimacy versus isolation phase of Erikson's stages (1963) of development.
- According to Havighurst (1972), the young adult has the following developmental tasks:
  - Selecting a mate
  - Learning to live with a partner
  - Starting a family
  - Rearing children
  - Managing a home
  - Establishing a career
  - Taking on civic responsibility
  - Finding a congenial social group
- The young adult has the following developmental tasks, according to Nelson and Barry (2005):
  - Separation from parents
  - Exploration of new identities for self
  - Personal discovery and self-discovery
  - High-risk behaviour

Physical Development

People in their early 20s are in their prime physically. The musculoskeletal system is well developed and coordinated. This is the period when athletic endeavours reach their peak. All other systems of the body are also functioning efficiently. Emerging adults, however, tend to be high-risk takers (Nelson & Barry, 2005), placing their high-functioning bodies at substantial risk of serious injury. Occupational strain and injuries can threaten their physical functioning.

Although physical changes are minimal during this stage, weight and muscle mass may change as a result of diet and exercise. Gradual physical and psychosocial changes occur naturally in pregnant and lactating women.

Psychosocial Development

In contrast to the minimal growth changes, psychosocial development of the young adult is great. Box 18.1 highlights theorists Freud, Erikson, and Havighurst.

Young adults face new experiences and changes in lifestyle as they mature. They must make choices about education and employment, whether to marry or remain single, about owning a home, and about rearing children. Social activities include forming new friendships and assuming some community responsibilities.

Many young adults have experienced the stress of their parents' divorce. Many have been raised in blended families or stepfamilies. Feelings of being caught between two divorced parents can create heavy burdens. Common stresses experienced in blended families include concerns about adequate financial resources, difficulty deciding how much personal information to share with others, and worries about loyalty and disloyalty to others (Afifi, 2003). These childhood experiences have obvious implications for the development of intimate relationships in young adults. **Intimacy**, according to Erikson (1963), concerns developing affectionate relationships and lengthy attachments and making personal commitments to another that may include marriage or sexual relations (Orshan, 2008).

Occupational choice and education are largely inseparable. Education influences occupational opportunities; conversely, an occupation, once chosen, can determine the education needed and sought. Education enhances employment opportunities and usually ensures economic survival. As the role of women has changed, many have chosen to assume active careers and civic roles in society, in addition to their roles as mother or spouse or both (Figure 18.1).

Remaining single is becoming a chosen lifestyle of young adults, perhaps to pursue an education and then to have the freedom to pursue their chosen vocation.

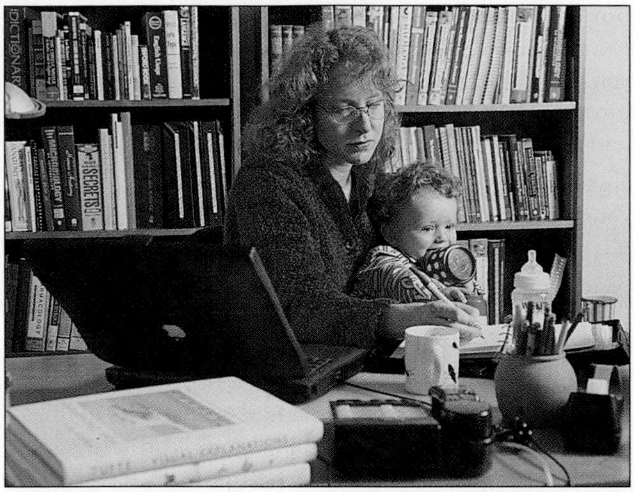

FIGURE 18.1 Many young women combine active careers with motherhood.

Some unmarried individuals choose to live with another person of the opposite or same sex and share living arrangements and expenses. They do not consider themselves to be single.

Although nontraditional lifestyles are becoming more acceptable in society, traditional attitudes can contribute social pressures that lead to stress responses. The multiple roles of adulthood (citizen, worker, taxpayer, homeowner, spouse, daughter or son, brother or sister, parent, friend) can create stress as a result of role conflict, role ambiguity, and role confusion.

Cognitive Development

Young adults in the *formal operations stage* think abstractly and employ logic (Piaget, 1966). Most adults identify strongly with the values and norms of their social group and will act in ways that are consistent with those norms (Pfaffenberger, 2005).

Recently, some researchers in the field of psychology have proposed a concept of postformal thought following Piaget's formal operational stage. **Postformal thought** includes creativity, intuition, and the ability to consider information related to other ideas. Postformal thinkers can comprehend and balance arguments created by both logic and emotion. Only about 10% of adults reach this stage and are able to resolve complex problems. Meditation and other insight-oriented practices facilitate becoming a postformal thinker (Pfaffenberger, 2005).

Moral Development

Young adults who have mastered the previous stages of Kohlberg's theory of moral development may now enter the *postconventional level*. The person is able to separate the self from the expectations and rules of others and to define morality in terms of personal principles. When individuals perceive a conflict with society's rules or laws, they judge according to their own principles. For example, a person may intentionally break the law and join a protest group to stop hunters from killing wild animals, believing that the principle of conservation of wildlife justifies the protest action. This type of reasoning is called *principled reasoning*. Gilligan (1982) argues that as individuals approach young adulthood, each gender tends to define moral problems somewhat differently (see Chapter 16, the section on Gilligan). Men often use an ethic of justice and define moral problems in terms of rules and rights. Women, by contrast, often define moral problems in terms of obligations to care and to avoid hurt.

Spiritual Development

According to Fowler (1981), the *individuating-reflective* period commences around 18 years of age. The religious teaching that the young adult had as a child may now be accepted or redefined as the individual focuses on reality. For example, a 27-year-old adult may ask philosophical questions regarding spirituality and may be self-conscious about spiritual matters.

Health Problems

Young adults are generally healthy. Health problems common in this age group include accidents, suicide, problematic substance use, hypertension, sexually transmitted infections (STIs), interpersonal violence, and certain malignancies. Some of the problems (accidents, problematic substance use, and STIs) are related to lifestyle patterns and most can be prevented through such strategies as education, counselling, and early detection by using problem identification and screening.

INJURIES Among young adults, accidents are responsible for more deaths than all other causes combined. Unintentional injuries, such as motor vehicle accidents, are the leading cause of mortality; other causes of accidental death include drowning, fires, burns, and firearms. Education about safety precautions and accident prevention is a major role of the nurse who is promoting the health of young adults (see Chapter 30, the section "Promoting Safety across the Lifespan").

SUICIDE Suicide is another leading cause of death in young adults. Many suicides are often mistaken for accidental death. Suicide may result from depression, which can have organic or physiological causes and be triggered by problems in relationships; perceived occupational, academic, or financial failure; or trouble coping with the pressures, responsibilities, and heightened expectations of adulthood.

The nurse's role in the prevention of suicide includes providing information about the early signs of suicide and identifying factors indicative of potential problems, such as depression, a variety of physical complaints, including weight changes, sleep disturbances, digestive disorders, decreased interest in social and work roles, dropping grades, and increased social isolation. A young adult identified as at risk for suicide should be referred or escorted immediately to a mental health professional or a crisis centre. (See the Reflect on Primary Health Care box.)

PROBLEMATIC SUBSTANCE USE Problematic substance use is a major threat to health. Alcohol, marijuana, amphetamines, and cocaine, for example, can bring about temporary feelings of well-being that may be appealing to people with adjustment problems. Prolonged use can lead to physical and psychological dependency and subsequent health problems. Alcohol and drug use during pregnancy can lead to fetal damage. Prolonged use of alcohol can lead to cirrhosis of the liver and cancer of the esophagus.

Nursing strategies related to problematic substance use include teaching about the complications of their use, changing individual attitudes toward problematic substance use, and counselling clients to learn effective coping strategies.

Smoking can lead to lung cancer and cardiovascular disease. The nurse's role regarding smoking is to (1) serve as a role model by not smoking; (2) provide educational information regarding the dangers of smoking; (3) help make smoking socially unacceptable; and (4) suggest resources, such as hypnosis, lifestyle training, and behaviour modification, to clients who want to stop smoking. The nurse must understand the process of change as it applies to these health issues.

SEXUALLY TRANSMITTED INFECTIONS Sexually transmitted infections (STIs), such as genital herpes, acquired immune deficiency syndrome (AIDS), syphilis, and gonorrhea, are common infections in young adults. Chlamydia is the most prevalent STI and the most prevalent infectious disease in Canada (Health Canada, 2004). Other STIs, such as gonorrhea, are becoming resistant to antibiotics. Nursing functions are largely educational regarding the use of condoms to reduce the transfer of infections. Transmission of genital warts or other contagious conditions can still be shared as the condom does not cover all the contact area during sexual activity. Correct knowledge about the symptoms of these diseases can help the client obtain early treatment. The nurse must be nonjudgmental, understand the client's lifestyle, and treat any information obtained as confidential.

REFLECT ON PRIMARY HEALTH CARE

Because of the stigma and inadequate support services, almost half of depressed young adults in Canada do not seek or have access to mental health services (Canadian Mental Health Association, 2007). Nurses educate the public, service providers, and politicians about mental health, and lobby for accessible and timely services to meet the needs of the clients and their families. Through these activities, consider how nurses use the primary health-care principles of *health promotion, accessibility, intersectoral cooperation,* and *public participation* to make this happen.

OBESITY IN CHILDBEARING WOMEN Statistics Canada (2006) reported that obesity is a growing health concern in Canada and that 20% of Canadians 18 years or older residing in large census metropolitan areas (CMAs) were obese, compared with 29% who lived outside a CMA in 2004. Approximately 5.5 million or 23% of Canadian adults were obese. Obesity rates are rising among 25- to 34-year-olds, and 23% of Canadian women of childbearing age are obese (Kirkey, 2007). Nutrition assessment, diet teaching, and exercise are important elements in developing an individualized wellness plan for the clients. Women of childbearing age and pregnant women are at risk for various nutritional deficiencies. The nurse must assess and stress the importance of increased calcium, iron, biotin, and folic acid requirements during pregnancy and if the woman is breastfeeding.

ABUSE OF WOMEN The problem of battering, or abuse, affects families at all socioeconomic levels. Stresses that predispose families to abuse may include financial problems, lack of family and community supports, and physical as well as social isolation. A nurse who works with women should explicitly ask if they are frightened or being hurt by someone they know. The nurse should become familiar with community resources, such as women's shelters, social services, and protective services. Besides helping women to regain their self-esteem, the nurse can educate the public that violent behaviour is not acceptable and can provide anger management programs for both genders.

MALIGNANCIES The Canadian Cancer Statistics (Canadian Cancer Society, National Cancer Institute of Canada, Statistics Canada, Provincial/Territorial Cancer Registries, & Public Health Agency of Canada, 2008) showed that the leading cause of cancer morbidity and mortality for both men and women is lung cancer, followed by colorectal cancer. Thirty percent of the newly diagnosed cancers and 18% of deaths occurred in the young and middle-aged adult. Testicular cancer is the most common neoplasm in men aged 20 to 34 years; hence, monthly *testicular self-examination,* a means of early detection of testicular cancer, is recommended (see Chapter 45, the Teaching: Wellness box on testicular self-examination, page 1464). New cancer cases are rising in young women ages 20–39, with breast cancer as the most common cancer in women worldwide, including Canada. Women between 40 and 69 should have a clinical breast examination (CBE) every 2 years, and those between 50 and 69 should also have a mammogram every 2 years (Canadian Cancer Society [CCS], 2008a). After age 69, the woman's health-care provider will determine the need for any further mammograms. All women should be familiar with their breasts and aware of what is normal for them (see Chapter 45).

Young adult females should also be screened for cervical cancer by having a routine **Pap (Papanicolaou) test or smear** during a pelvic examination. A Pap test or smear is done by obtaining and examining cells from the uterine cervical os. Immunization against the human papillomavirus (HPV) shows great promise in preventing cervical cancer for young adults (who have not been sexually active and are between the ages of 9–26). The nurse should also screen for high-risk factors for cervical cancer: sexual activity at an early age, multiple sexual partners, or a history of syphilis, herpes genitalis, or *Trichomonas* vaginitis.

Many young adults are reluctant to have or do screening examinations. Nurses must explain the purposes and procedures to encourage preventive measures. Provinces and territories have varying recommendations for male and female screening examinations across adulthood. Generally, within 3 years of commencing sexual activity, or by age 18, all women should commence Pap tests every 1 to 3 years, depending on the screening guidelines in each province or territory (CCS, 2008b).

ENVIRONMENTAL EXPOSURE Health Canada facilitates biomonitoring of dust, food, water, soil, air, and life forms in various workplaces and communities. Of concern for young adults are such things as heavy metals, dioxins and furans, pesticides, fungicides, herbicides, bleaches, and other carcinogenic agents found in some cleaning solutions, such as polychlorinated biphenyls (PCBs) and aromatic hydrocarbons. Second-hand smoke byproducts contain cotinine, a metabolite of nicotine that is a proven carcinogen.

Moulds release spores and toxins into the air in damp and dark environments. Respiratory responses, like asthma, allergies, and ongoing respiratory infections, get worse inside the home, school, and other buildings with roof leaks, wet basements, water-sodden plaster, and carbon-based building materials.

IMMUNIZATIONS Adult maintenance of immunizations is often overlooked till prompted by travel plans and requirements for access to certain jobs or after a traumatic injury in which tetanus is a worry. Young adults should be encouraged to participate in flu immunization clinics and to adhere to their adult immunization schedule. Adults should retain their immunization documents and follow the recommendations wherever they live. Nurses must ask about allergies before administering immunization agents. HPV vaccines will not prevent genital warts, HIV, other STIs, or pregnancies.

CAFFEINE Health Canada recommends a daily intake of caffeine for women of childbearing years be no more than 300 mg per day from all sources, including teas, coffee, cola, chocolate, herbs, such as guarana and yerba mate, energy drinks, and some over-the-counter medications. Adverse effects of caffeine overload appear after 450 mg per day. Overdose is noted by hyper-alertness, anxiety, rapid heart beat variations, palpitations, tremors, and loss of bone calcium. Everyone should be taught to read labels for caffeine. Caffeine-free products should be encouraged, especially for pregnant or breastfeeding women.

Health Assessment and Promotion

Assessment guidelines for the growth and development of the young adult are shown in the Assessment: Developmental Guidelines box.

Young adults are usually interested in meeting their health needs. However, because of the many stresses and

ASSESSMENT: DEVELOPMENTAL GUIDELINES

The Young Adult

In these three areas, does the young adult do the following?

1. PHYSICAL DEVELOPMENT

- Exhibit weight, BMI, within normal range for age and gender
- Manifest vital signs (e.g., blood pressure) within normal range for age and gender
- Demonstrate visual and hearing abilities within normal range
- Exhibit appropriate knowledge (e.g., about sexually transmitted infections) and attitudes about sexuality

2. PSYCHOSOCIAL DEVELOPMENT

- Feel independent from parents
- Have a realistic self-concept
- Like self and direction of life
- Interact well with family
- Cope with the stresses of change and growth
- Have well-established bonds with significant others and intimacy with a partner or close friends
- Have a meaningful social life
- Demonstrate emotional, social, and economic responsibility for own life
- Have a set of values that guide behaviour

3. ACTIVITIES OF DAILY LIVING

- Have a healthy lifestyle

Health-Promotion Guidelines for Young Adults

HEALTH TESTS AND SCREENINGS

The following are important to the health of young adults:

- Routine physical examination (every 1 to 3 years for females; every 2 to 3 years for males)
- Immunizations as recommended, such as tetanus-diphtheria boosters every 10 years, meningococcal vaccine, hepatitis B vaccine, and human papillomavirus vaccine if not yet given
- Dental assessments yearly (every 6 to 9 months preferred)
- Regular vision and hearing screenings
- Clinical breast examination every 2 years for women over age 40; males as needed
- Once sexually active, pelvic exam and Papanicolaou smear every 1–3 years, depending on provincial/territorial guidelines
- Testicular self-examination monthly; clinical exam yearly
- Screening for cardiovascular disease (e.g., cholesterol, blood sugar, thyroid hormone every 3 years if results are normal; yearly blood pressure to detect hypertension; baseline electrocardiogram at age 30)
- Tuberculosis skin test (as required by employer)
- Yearly rectal exam for hemorrhoids, prostate size, skin changes, STIs; fecal occult blood test using a stool sample if a family history of early onset intestinal cancer
- Smoking: history and counselling as needed to quit; avoidance of tobacco use in any form
- Self-inspection of all skin surfaces for warts, changing moles, freckles, and lesions

SAFETY

- Motor vehicle safety (always buckle up, use designated drivers, maintain brakes and tires, prevent road rage, drive alert and distraction-free, no cell phone use while driving, no speeding or stunt driving)
- Sun and insect bite protection
- Workplace safety measures and equipment (helmet, boots, ladder guards)
- Water safety (e.g., no diving in shallow water)
- Wearing of the right gear for each sport
- Safe sex practices: screen for STIs and HIV if needed, ask about sex-related health conditions *before* having sex, and know correct methods of protection
- Responsible drinking, avoidance of becoming intoxicated, mixing substances, or leaving drinks unattended

NUTRITION AND EXERCISE

- Adequate antioxidants, vitamins and minerals, iron, and calcium intake in diet
- Avoidance of nutritional and exercise factors that may lead to cardiovascular disease (e.g., obesity, cholesterol, fat intake, lack of exercise)

SOCIAL INTERACTIONS

- Relationships that promote discussion of feelings, concerns, and fears
- Short- and long-term goals for interpersonal, work, personal, and career choices

changes that occur throughout this 20-year period, the nurse needs to offer teaching and guidance in several health-care areas. The nurse may want to discuss some or all of the health-promotion topics outlined in the Health-Promotion Guidelines box on young adults.

Middle-Aged Adults (40 to 65 Years)

The middle years, from 40 to 65 years, have been called the years of stability and consolidation. For most people, it is a time when children have grown up and moved away or are moving away from home. Thus, partners generally have more time for and with each other and time to pursue interests they may have deferred for years (Figure 18.2).

Maturity is the state of maximal function and integration, or the state of being fully developed. Mature individuals take many perspectives into account and consider the views of others. Mature adults are open to new experiences and continued growth; they can tolerate ambiguity, are flexible, and can adapt to change. Additionally, they have the quality of self-acceptance, and they are able to be reflective and insightful about life and to see themselves as others see them. Mature adults assume responsibility for themselves and expect others to do the same. They confront the tasks of life in a realistic and mature manner, make decisions, and accept responsibility for those decisions.

Physical Development

A number of changes take place during the middle years. At 40 years, most adults can function as effectively as they did in their 20s. However, between 40 to 65 years, many physical changes take place. See Table 18.1 for a summary of these changes.

Both men and women experience decreasing hormonal production during the middle years. **Menopause** refers to the change of life in women (i.e., when

TABLE 18.1 Physical Changes of the Middle-Aged Adult

Category	Description
Appearance	Hair begins to thin, and grey hair appears. Skin turgor (fullness or elasticity) and moisture decrease, subcutaneous fat decreases, and wrinkling occurs. Fatty tissue is redistributed, resulting in fat deposits in the abdominal area.
Musculoskeletal system	Skeletal muscle bulk decreases at about age 60 years. Thinning of the intervertebral discs causes a decrease in height of about 2 cm or 3 cm. Calcium loss from bone tissue is more common among postmenopausal women. Muscle growth continues in proportion to use.
Cardiovascular system	Blood vessels lose elasticity and become thicker.
Sensory perception	Visual acuity declines, often by the late 40s, especially for near vision (presbyopia). Auditory acuity for high-frequency sounds also decreases (presbycusis), particularly in men. Taste sensations also diminish.
Metabolism	Metabolism slows, resulting in weight gain.
Gastrointestinal system	Gradual decrease in tone of the large intestine may predispose the individual to constipation.
Urinary system	Nephron units of the kidneys are lost during this time, and glomerular filtration rate decreases.
Sexuality	Hormonal changes take place in both men and women.

menstruation ceases). It is said to have occurred when a woman has not had a menstrual period in 1 year. Menopause usually occurs anywhere between ages 40 and 55 years. The average is about 47 years. At this time, ovarian activity declines until ovulation ceases. Common symptoms are hot flashes and chilliness, the breasts may become smaller and flabby, and women tend to gain weight. Insomnia and headaches also occur with relative frequency. Psychologically, menopause can be an anxiety-producing time, especially if the ability to bear children is an integral part of the woman's self-concept.

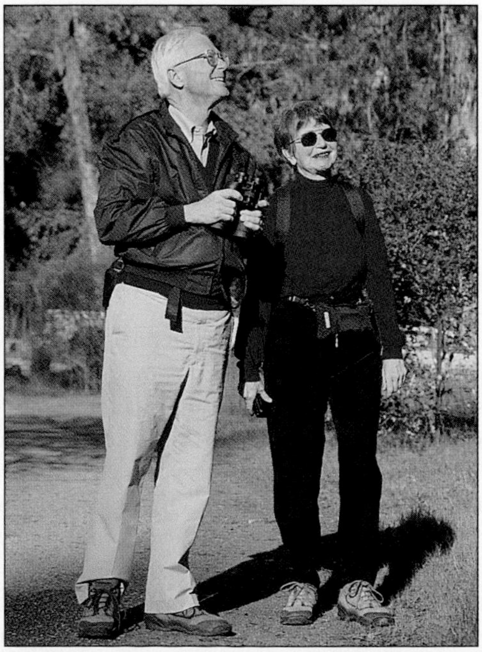

FIGURE 18.2 Middle-aged adults have time to pursue interests that may have been put aside for childcare.

Climacteric (andropause) refers to the change of life in men, when sexual activity decreases. Men do not experience a change comparable with menopause in women. Androgen levels decrease very slowly; however, men can father children even in late life. The psychological problems that men experience are generally related to health status, finances, the fear of getting old, retirement, and boredom. (See Chapter 45, the section on Sexuality Throughout Life: Adulthood.)

Psychosocial Development

Before the mid-twentieth century, middle-aged adults received little attention (Lachman, 2004). Havighurst (1972) outlines seven tasks for this age group (see Box 18.2). Erikson (1963) views the developmental

BOX 18.2 PSYCHOSOCIAL DEVELOPMENT: MIDDLE-AGED ADULT

The middle-aged adult is in the *generativity versus stagnation* phase of Erikson (1963). According to Havighurst (1972), the middle-aged adult has the following developmental tasks:

- Achieving adult civic and social responsibilities
- Establishing and maintaining an economic standard of living
- Assisting teenage children to become responsible and happy adults
- Developing adult leisure-time activities
- Relating to his or her spouse as a person
- Accepting and adjusting to the physiological changes of middle age
- Adjusting to aging parents
- Balancing the needs of children, parents, work, and so on

choice of the middle-aged adult as *generativity versus stagnation.* **Generativity** is defined as the concern for establishing and guiding the next generation. In other words, the concern about providing for the welfare of humankind is as important as the concern of providing for the self. Marriage partners have more time for companionship and recreation, and, thus, marriage can be more satisfying. In middle age, the self seems more altruistic, and concepts of service to others and love and compassion gain prominence. These concepts motivate charitable and altruistic actions, such as church work and fundraising drives. Generative middle-aged persons are able to feel a sense of comfort in their lifestyle and receive gratification from charitable activities.

Erikson (1963) believed that people who are unable to expand their interests at this time and who do not assume the responsibilities of middle age suffer a sense of boredom and impoverishment, that is, stagnation. These people have difficulty accepting their aging bodies and become withdrawn and isolated. They are preoccupied with the self and unable to give to others. Some may regress to younger patterns of behaviour.

The "midlife crisis" occurs when individuals recognize that they have reached the halfway mark of life. They perceive that life is finite and that youthfulness and physical strength can no longer be taken for granted. The universality of the midlife crisis is disputed by some who suggest that some midlifers experience a crisis that promotes further development, while some have consistently functioned in a crisis mode from early life (Lachman, 2004). People usually accept the fact that they are aging; however, a few try to defy the years by the way they dress and even by their actions. Some men and women have extramarital affairs with or marry younger persons; new freedoms to be independent and follow individual interests emerge. Before this period, the marriage partner or lover and other persons were crucial to a definition of the self. Now, the middle-aged person does not make comparisons with others, no longer fears aging or death, relaxes the sense of competitiveness, and enjoys independence and freedom. The person establishes ethical and moral standards that are independent of the standards of others. The focus shifts from inner self and being to others and doing. Religious and philosophical concerns become important.

Cognitive Development

Cognitive processes change little, including reaction time, memory, perception, learning, problem solving, and creativity. Reaction time during the middle years stays much the same or diminishes during the later part of the middle years. Memory and problem solving are maintained through middle adulthood. Learning continues and can be enhanced by increased motivation and thinking activities, puzzles, and problem solving. Genetic, environmental, and personality factors account for the large differences in mental abilities in early and middle adulthood (Edelman & Mandle, 2006). The experiences of the professional, social, and personal life of middle-aged persons will be reflected in their cognitive performance. Thus, approaches to problem solving and task completion will vary considerably in a middle-aged group.

Moral Development

According to Kohlberg (1971, 1981), most adults move beyond the *conventional level* to the *postconventional level.* Kohlberg believed that extensive experience of personal moral choice and responsibility is required before people can reach the postconventional level. Kohlberg found that few of his subjects achieved the third level of moral development. To move from stage 4, a *law and order orientation,* to stage 5, a *social contract orientation,* requires that the individual move to a stage in which rights of others take precedence. Recent research demonstrates that moral development continues through adulthood and that few individuals attain stage 5 before age 40 (Dawson, 2002).

Spiritual Development

Not all adults progress through Fowler's stages (1981) to the fifth, called the *paradoxical-consolidative stage.* At this stage, the individual can view *truth* from a number of viewpoints. Fowler's fifth stage corresponds to Kohlberg's fifth stage. Fowler believes that only some individuals after the age of 30 years reach these levels.

In middle age, people tend to be less dogmatic about religious beliefs, and religion often offers more comfort to the middle-aged person than it did previously. People in this age group often rely on spiritual beliefs to help them deal with illness, death, and tragedy.

Health Problems

Many middle-aged adults remain healthy; however, the risk of developing a health problem increases. Leading causes of death in this age group include motor vehicle and occupational accidents, chronic diseases, such as cancer, and cardiovascular disease. Lifestyle patterns, in combination with aging, family history, developmental stressors (e.g., menopause, climacteric), and situational stressors (e.g., divorce), are often related to the health problems that do arise. Smoking and excessive alcohol consumption place an individual at greater risk of developing chronic respiratory problems, lung cancer, and liver disease. Overeating can result in obesity, diabetes mellitus, atherosclerosis, and associated risks for hypertension and coronary artery disease. The nurse can play an important role in teaching about preventive health care to avoid or minimize the risk of such health problems.

INJURIES Changing physiological factors, such as visual acuity and decreased reaction times, as well as concern over personal and work-related responsibilities, may contribute to the accident rate of middle-aged people. Motor vehicle collisions are the most common cause of accidental death in this age group. Other accidental causes of death for middle-aged adults include falls, fires, burns, poisonings, and drowning. Occupational accidents continue to be a significant safety hazard during the middle years.

CANCER Cancer accounts for considerable mortality and morbidity in both men and women. It is the second leading cause of death among people between the ages of 25 and 64 years in Canada. The patterns of cancer types and incidences for men and women have changed over the past several decades. Men have a high incidence of cancer of the lung and prostate. In women, breast cancer is highest in incidence, followed by cancer of the lung and colon. About 40% of Canadian females and 45% of men will develop cancer in their lifetime, and 1 in 4 Canadians will die from cancer.

As mentioned earlier, females may need to be reminded to perform monthly breast self-examinations and men to perform monthly testicular self-examinations to detect changes. Postmenopausal women should report any vaginal bleeding.

CARDIOVASCULAR DISEASE Coronary artery disease (CAD) is a leading cause of death in Canada. Several factors contribute to the risk of CAD: smoking, obesity, hypertension, hyperlipidemia, diabetes mellitus, sedentary lifestyle, a family history of myocardial infarction or sudden death in a father younger than 55 years old or in a mother younger than 65 years old, and the individual's age. Men over 45 years of age and women over 55 years of age are at greater risk of developing CAD than are younger adults. Physical inactivity places individuals at greater risk of developing CAD than does any other factor (Edelman & Mandle, 2006).

OBESITY Middle-aged adults who gain weight may not be aware of some common facts about this age period. Decreased metabolic activity and decreased physical activity mean a decrease in caloric need. The nurse's role is to counsel clients to prevent obesity by reducing caloric intake and engaging in regular exercise. Clients should also be warned that being overweight is a risk factor for many chronic diseases, such as diabetes and hypertension, and for problems of mobility, such as arthritis. Clients should seek medical advice before considering any major changes in their diets or exercise.

ALCOHOLISM The excessive use of alcohol can result in unemployment, disrupted homes, accidents, and diseases. Nearly 1 in 10 Canadians report problems with their drinking of alcohol. Nurses can help clients by providing information about the dangers of excessive alcohol use, by helping the individual clarify values about health, and by referring the client to a group, such as Alcoholics Anonymous.

MENTAL HEALTH Interpersonal relationship tensions and family violence can place partners at risk of physical harm, stress, and psychological strain. Post-traumatic stress disorder (PTSD) can contribute to mental health problems and physical symptoms. Cultural variations must also be attended to when considering clients' mental health. Developmental stressors, such as menopause, climacteric, aging, impending retirement, and situational stressors, such as divorce, unemployment, and death of a spouse, can precipitate increased anxiety and depression in middle-aged adults. Recent research points to a growing positive correlation between depression and type 2 diabetes (Antai-Otong, 2007; Nichols & Brown, 2003). Clients may benefit from support groups or individual therapy to help them cope with specific crises.

Health Assessment and Promotion

Assessment guidelines for the growth and development of the middle-aged adult are shown in the Assessment: Developmental Guidelines box. The nurse can choose to discuss some or all of the health-promotion topics outlined in Health-Promotion Guidelines box for

Evidence-Informed Practice

What Are the Experiences of Canadians Living with Mental Health Problems?

Kirby and Keon (2006) described the experiences of Canadians living with mental illness from a series of focus group discussions. The devalued feelings of service providers and stories from affected family members across the country were described. Insight into the frustration and confusion of individuals living with mental health disorders is given. Evidence outlines gaps in the determinants of health, such as housing, meaningful work, future educational opportunities, and peer support programs. Stigma and discrimination within the health professions are outlined.

NURSING IMPLICATIONS: Many adults may experience various life crises. When providing care to clients, nurses must be sensitive to clients' mental health needs and the effects of mental illness on their families and communities.

Source: Based on *Out of the Shadows at Last: Transforming Mental Health, Mental Illness and Addiction Services in Canada. Final report of the Standing Senate Committee on Social Affairs, Science and Technology,* by M. J. L. Kirby and W. J. Keon, 2006, Ottawa: Government of Canada.

middle-aged adults and throughout the book. Nurses must consider the variation in health-services utilization and the health-promotion needs for these clients. For example, the 2001 Canadian Community Health Survey showed that members of visible minorities tend to seek medical services less often than other Canadians; their utilization of hospital services and cancer screening services is also significantly less (Quan et al., 2006).

ASSESSMENT: DEVELOPMENTAL GUIDELINES

The Middle-Aged Adult

In these three developmental areas, does the middle-aged adult do the following?

1. **PHYSICAL DEVELOPMENT**

- Exhibit weight within normal range for age and gender
- Manifest vital signs (e.g., blood pressure) within normal range for age and gender
- Manifest visual and hearing abilities within normal range
- Exhibit appropriate knowledge and attitudes about sexuality (e.g., about menopause)
- Verbalize any changes in eating, elimination, sleep, or exercise

2. **PSYCHOSOCIAL DEVELOPMENT**

- Accept the aging body
- Feel comfortable and respect self
- Enjoy new freedom to be independent
- Accept changes in family roles (e.g., having teenage children and aging parents)
- Interact well and share companionable activities with life partner
- Expand and renew previous interests
- Pursue charitable and altruistic activities
- Have a meaningful philosophy of life

3. **DEVELOPMENT IN ACTIVITIES OF DAILY LIVING**

- Follow preventive health practices

Health-Promotion Guidelines for Middle-Aged Adults

The following are important to the health of middle-aged adults:

HEALTH TESTS AND SCREENING

- Routine physical examination (annually for females; every 2 to 3 years or as directed by health-care provider for males)
- Immunizations as recommended, such as a tetanus booster every 10 years and influenza and pneumococcal vaccinations
- Regular dental assessments (e.g., yearly), daily brushing, flossing, gum massage
- Tonometry (to test pressure in the eye) for signs of glaucoma and eye exams for other eye diseases (e.g., macular degeneration) every 2 to 3 years or annually, if indicated
- Screening for breast cancer: clinical breast self-examination at least every 2 years for women over 40, and mammography every 2 years between 50 and 69
- Testicular self-examination monthly
- Screenings for cardiovascular disease (e.g., blood pressure measurement; electrocardiogram and cholesterol test as directed by the health-care provider)
- Screenings for colorectal, cervical, uterine, and prostate cancers
- Screening for tuberculosis every 2 years

SAFETY

- Motor vehicle safety reinforcement, especially when driving at night
- Workplace safety measures (e.g., avoid repetitive strain)
- Home safety measures: keeping hallways and stairways lighted and uncluttered, using smoke and carbon monoxide detectors, using nonskid mats and hand rails in the bathrooms
- The practice of safe sex

NUTRITION AND EXERCISE

- Importance of adequate fibre, protein, calcium, and vitamin D in diet
- Avoidance of overuse of caffeine
- Avoidance of nutritional and exercise factors that may lead to cardiovascular disease (e.g., obesity, sedentary lifestyle); monitoring of cholesterol and lipid levels; avoidance of saturated and trans fat intake
- Vigorous exercise program that emphasizes skill and coordination; daily exercise for a minimum of 30 minutes

SOCIAL INTERACTIONS

- Discussion of feelings, concerns, depression, and fears
- Time to expand and review previous interests
- Retirement planning (financial and possible diversional activities), with partner, if appropriate
- Limited alcohol consumption

Case Study 18

Kintu M., 34, is an Inuit man living in an urban Arctic community with healthy children aged 4, 3, and 1. His partner, Alana, 24, provides home daycare. Kintu works for the territorial government in the logging industry. Both take turns driving transports during the freeze-up to make "a bit more money" for fresh vegetables and milk, which are very expensive. Kintu and Alana consider English to be their mother tongue, they do not speak their native language well, and their children speak only English. Their elders live on the land and are renowned for their knowledge of the environment, culture, hunting and domestic skills, healing, and storytelling. Kintu drives several hours to reach their parents' settlement, where Alana and the children spend their summers. The weeks of continuous summer daylight are the busiest for Kintu, so he stays with his crew, isolated from his family. During these periods, he becomes sleep-deprived, eats poorly, and is lonely. His workplace errors increase, his anger becomes explosive, and his alcohol consumption increases. Today, he has driven off the highway. His load has spilled and the cab of the vehicle is crushed. Kintu is trapped but has radioed in, sounding confused. With GPS tracking, he is rescued and evacuated to the medical centre. He sustained a head injury and many broken bones, and has some vision and memory loss. Police found extensive skid marks showing that Kintu tried to stop suddenly. He says he was not speeding but tried to avoid a herd of deer that ran across the road unexpectedly. Evidence confirms he is not at fault. No one can reach his wife or parents.

He will be off work for at least 16 weeks with benefits, and he must attend the rehabilitation and health centre 1500 km away. His supervisor recommends that Kintu use his time to create a new career track. Kintu is feeling overwhelmed and depressed. The dark season is coming and his family will be coming home soon.

Critical Thinking Questions

1. As the community nurse, describe how you would help Kintu and his family prioritize the stress that is accumulating because of the crash.
2. Apply your knowledge of normal development and state three high-priority goals and resources that you may need to suggest to the M. family as they adapt to this situation in their northern community.
3. State how and why Kintu's and Alana's Inuit heritage may affect the health and well-being of the M. family and how you as a nurse would promote culturally appropriate care.
4. Kintu states he is feeling depressed. State some of the possible causes for his self-reported assessment and how they may make this feeling a health threat for him.

After working through these questions, go to the MyNursingLab at **http://www.mynursinglab.com** to check your answers.

KEY TERMS

baby boomers
Generation X
Generation Y
zoomers
boomerang kids
intimacy
postformal thought
Pap (Papanicolaou) test or smear
maturity
menopause
climacteric
generativity

CHAPTER HIGHLIGHTS

- Three distinct generations are included in adulthood: baby boomers, Generation Xers, and Generation Ys. Each has its own world view.
- Physical growth and development peaks in the middle 20s and then becomes decremental.
- Emerging and young adults develop a self-identity and prepare for intimate relationships with others.
- Moral development continues throughout adulthood.
- Spirituality may be important to young adults but is considered a private matter.
- Health problems for young adults are primarily related to lifestyle and behaviour.
- Midlife adults begin to notice physical changes associated with aging.
- The developmental choice for midlife adults is generativity versus stagnation.
- Adults in midlife must balance the needs of many, including their own parents and children.
- Health decisions made by midlife adults may affect their health in later life.
- A variety of health threats, including cancer and heart disease, begin to affect persons in middle age.
- Physical activity, healthy nutrition choices, and routine care by a health provider are important throughout the adult years.

ASSESS YOUR LEARNING

1. Mrs. Kelly, 52 years old, is experiencing symptoms of menopause, including occasional hot flashes and insomnia. She states that she exercises daily, meditates, and has consulted a naturopath. She asks the nurse what else she could do to handle these life changes. How should the nurse respond?
   - **a.** Refer Mrs. Kelly for a medical check-up.
   - **b.** Advise Mrs. Kelly to take estrogen.
   - **c.** Ask Mrs. Kelly to keep an exercise diary.
   - **d.** Encourage Mrs. Kelly to continue what she has been doing.

2. The adult children of a couple have just helped them celebrate retirement after 35 years of employment. The parents are not concerned and seem ready to make the changes necessary, but their offspring are worried. To help this family adapt to the parents' retirement, you must understand which of the following?
   - **a.** Young adults are concerned about the caregiver burden for themselves very soon.
   - **b.** Old people become worried about their health status, ability to travel, and mental rigidity.
   - **c.** Middle-aged adults can adjust to altered schedules, roles, physical strength, and economic changes.
   - **d.** Retired persons focus on themselves, avoiding relationships with peers of bygone days.

3. You are the occupational health nurse (OHN) in a large manufacturing company and see many employees through the year. Given your mandate, you would be most concerned about which of the following issues for the middle-aged cohort in your workplace?
   - **a.** The promotion of workplace safety
   - **b.** Timetables and output deadlines
   - **c.** Union-related benefits and vacations
   - **d.** Boredom, abuse, and contract performance

4. As a parish nurse, you have the opportunity to provide nursing outreach to many individuals from a variety of cultures and from across all age groups. You are struck by the common traits you are seeing in the healthy and contented adults. With your understanding of the healthy development of the adult, what would you choose as the stage of development that describes this group?
   - **a.** Trust versus mistrust
   - **b.** Industry versus guilt
   - **c.** Autonomy versus dependence
   - **d.** Generativity versus stagnation

5. Mrs. T. has come to the clinic with her husband for a check-up. She has shared with the nurse practitioner that she is afraid her husband may not be able to drive anymore. She became worried the previous week when he did not come home from curling at the usual time. Since then, he has become lost twice more while out on his own. As a nurse in the clinic, taking the history of Mr. and Mrs. T, what would you want to do?
   - **a.** Ask Mr. T. if he and Mrs. T. have had a fight recently.
   - **b.** Ask Mr. T. about any headaches, visual problems, or unusual symptoms.
   - **c.** While separated from the other, ask each about the past 10 days.
   - **d.** Listen to each story, take both people's blood pressures, and ask about time, date, persons, and places.

6. The community health nurse at the nearby Family Wellness Centre has been asked to create a weekly Wellness Program for Working Mothers. Based on the needs of working mothers, which of the following would be the best program?
   - **a.** One that teaches members about health problems of aging, such as cancer
   - **b.** One that focuses on immunizations and smoking cessation
   - **c.** One that encourages personal changes and home safety
   - **d.** One that limits decision making and input to planning

7. The home care nurse is visiting Mr. P. in his home for a wound dressing to a chronic leg ulcer associated with varicose veins because of many hours of standing in his job for more than 30 years. Mr. P. is 56 years of age. He lives alone with his two cats. He complains of having to get up to go to the bathroom several times a night to urinate, which upsets him. He is 26 kg overweight and eats packaged frozen foods. His blood pressure is 190/90. In addition to updating his history and examining the wound while doing a sterile dressing change, which of the following should the nurse consider assessing for?
   - **a.** Personal neglect
   - **b.** Chronic disability criterion
   - **c.** Measures to prevent constipation
   - **d.** Health needs, strengths, and safety

8. Integration of developmental transitions experienced by middle-aged adults is necessary for meaningful health teaching. Most relevant topics would include which of the following?
   - **a.** Accepting an aging body, handling dependent parents, and handling departing children
   - **b.** Wear and tear, interpersonal stress, and sleep deprivation as new parents
   - **c.** Education and career preparation, childbearing roles, and increasing free time

d. Formal operations and the law and order orientation of Havighurst's theory

9. You are a school nurse helping parents to create learning resources for their teen children. Which of the following subjects would be the best choice of mutual interest for both parents and teens?
a. Sexually transmitted infections
b. Abuse and internet crime
c. Anorexia and obesity
d. Rules of the road and drivers' training

10. Motor vehicle safety is an ongoing safety concern. When promoting motor vehicle safety, nurses should suggest which of the following to young adults?
a. "Use designated drivers, day or night, as needed."
b. "Text a cell message while driving to prevent road rage."
c. "Just read and do the computer-simulated games in drivers' ed."
d. "Keep the car clean, waxed, filled up, and environmentally friendly."

After working through these questions, go to the MyNursingLab at ***http://www.mynursinglab.com*** *to check your answers and see explanations.*

SUGGESTED READINGS

Brown, C. G. (2004). Testicular cancer: An overview. *Urologic Nursing, 24*(2), 83–93.

This article provides a review of the epidemiology, risk factors, early detection, signs and symptoms, diagnosis, and treatment of malignant testicular cancer and the nurse's role in educating adult men.

Rederstorff, J. C., Buchanan, N. T., & Settlers, I. H. (2007). The moderating roles of race and gender-role attitudes in the relationship between sexual harassment and psychological well-being. *Psychology of Women Quarterly, 31*(1), 50–61.

This article discusses race, roles, gender expectations, interaction with power, survival of sexual harassment, and strong psychological aspects of self.

WEBLINKS

Canadian Public Health Agency

http://www.phac-aspc.gc.ca/ah-sa-eng.php?rd=adult_eng

This site provides various topics related to adult health, from chronic diseases and infectious diseases, to health promotion, travel health, and adult health projects.

Statistics Canada

http://www.statcan.ca/english/freepub/11-008-XIE/2007004/11-008-XIE200700410311.htm

This link summarizes Warren Clark's Canadian Social Trends study on delayed transitions of young adults.

REFERENCES

Afifi, T. D. (2003). "Feeling caught" in stepfamilies: Managing boundary turbulence through appropriate communication privacy rules. *Journal of Social and Personal Relationships, 20,* 729–755.

Antai-Otong, D.(2007). The art of prescribing—Diabetes and depression: Pharmacologic considerations. *Perspectives in Psychiatric Care, 43*(2), 93–96.

Canadian Cancer Society, National Cancer Institute of Canada, Statistics Canada, Provincial/Territorial Cancer Registries, & Public Health Agency of Canada. (2008). *Canadian cancer statistics, 2008.* Retrieved September 11, 2008, from http://www.cancer.ca/Canada-wide/About%20cancer/Cancer%20statistics/~/media/CCS/Canada%20wide/Files%20List/English%20files%20heading/pdf%20not%20in%20publications%20section/Canadian%20Cancer%20Society%20Statistics%20PDF%202008_614137951.ashx

Canadian Cancer Society. (2008a). Early detection and screening for breast cancer. Retrieved September 11, 2008, from http://www.cancer.ca/Canada-wide/About%20cancer/Types%20of%20cancer/Early%20detection%20and%20screening%20for%20breast%20cancer.aspx?sc_lang=en

Canadian Cancer Society. (2008b). Screening for cervical cancer. Retrieved September 11, 2008, from http://www.cancer.ca/Canada-wide/About%20cancer/Types%20of%20cancer/Screening%20for%20cervical%20cancer.aspx?sc_lang=en%20).%20This%20statement%20seems%20to%20imply%20that%20cervical%20cancer%20screening%20is%20specific%20to%20provincial/%20territorial%20guidelines.

Canadian Mental Health Association. (2007). *Ontario mental health notes (MHN).* Retrieved May 18, 2007, from http://www.ontario.cmha.ca/content/reading_room/mhnotes.asp?

Dawson, T. L. (2002). New tools, new insights: Kohlberg's moral judgement stages revisited. *International Journal of Behavioral Development, 26*(2), 154–166.

Edelman, C. L., & Mandle, C. L. (2006). *Health promotion throughout the life span* (6th ed.). St. Louis, MO: Mosby.

Erikson, E. H. (1963). *Childhood and society* (2nd ed.). New York: Norton.

Fowler, J. W. (1981). *Stages of faith: The psychology of human development and the quest for meaning.* New York: Harper & Row.

Freud, S. (1923). *The ego and the id.* London, UK: Hogarth Press.

Gilligan, C. (1982). *In a different voice: Psychological theory and women's development.* Cambridge, MA: Harvard University Press.

Havighurst, R. J. (1972). *Developmental tasks and education* (3rd ed.). New York: Longman.

Health Canada. (2004). *It's your health: Chlamydia.* Retrieved March 27, 2007, from www.hc-sc.gc.ca/iyh-vsv/alt_formats/cmcd-dcmc/pdf/chlamydia_e.pdf

Hill, K. S. (2004). Defy the decades with multigenerational teams. *Nursing Management, 35*(1), 32–35.

Hu, J., Herrick, C., & Hodgin, K. A. (2004). Managing the multigenerational nursing team. *Health Care Manager, 22*, 334–341.

Kirkey, S. (2007, October 3). Pregnant women shouldn't pack on the pounds. *The Windsor Star,* p. A1.

Kohlberg, L. (1971). *Recent research in moral development.* New York: Holt, Rinehart & Winston.

Kohlberg, L. (1981). *The psychology of moral development: Moral stages and the idea of justice.* San Francisco, CA: Harper & Row.

Lachman, M. E. (2004). Development in midlife. *Annual Review of Psychology, 55*, 305–331.

Nelson, L. J., & Barry, C. M. (2005). Distinguishing features of emerging adulthood: The role of self-classification as an adult. *Journal of Adolescent Research, 20*, 242–262.

Nichols, G. A., & Brown, J. B. (2003). Unadjusted and adjusted prevalence of diagnosed depression in type 2 diabetes. *Diabetes Care, 26*, 744–749.

Orshan, S.A. (2008). *Maternity, newborn, and women's health nursing: Comprehensive care across the lifespan.* Philadelphia, PA: Wolters Kluwer/Lippincott, Williams & Wilkins.

Pfaffenberger, A. H. (2005). Optimal adult development: An inquiry into the dynamics of growth. *Journal of Humanistic Psychology, 45*(3), 279–301.

Piaget, J. (1966). *Origins of intelligence in children.* New York: Norton.

Quan, H., Fong, A., De Coster, C., Wang, J., Musto, R., Noseworthy, T., et al. (2006). Variation in health services utilization among ethnic populations [Electronic version]. *Canadian Medical Association Journal, 174*(6).

Ross Cravit, C. (2008). *Zoomers create a new vision of aging.* Retrieved August 28, 2008, from http://www.carp.ca/article_display.cfm?documentID=3011&CabinetID=263&LibraryID=70&cityID=7

Statistics Canada. (2006, August 22). Health reports: Regional differences in obesity. *The Daily.* Retrieved May 30, 2007, from http://www.statcan.ca/Daily/English/060822/d060822b.htm

Chapter 19

Older Adults

Older adults constitute one of the fastest-growing groups in Canada and their numbers are expected to double by 2025 (Health Canada, 2007). The number of older Canadians increased from 2.4 million to 4.2 million between 1981 and 2005, with their corresponding share of the total population increasing from 9.6% to 13.1%.

OBJECTIVES

After studying this chapter, you should be able to

1. Describe the demographics of the aging population in Canada
2. Discuss the development of the Canadian Gerontological Nursing Association (CGNA)
3. Describe the expected physiological changes throughout older adulthood
4. Describe psychosocial development according to Erikson during older adulthood
5. Discuss changes in cognitive development according to Piaget throughout older adulthood
6. Describe moral development according to Kohlberg throughout older adulthood
7. Examine spiritual development according to Fowler throughout older adulthood
8. Analyze selected health problems associated with older adults
9. Discuss the role of the nurse in promoting the health and well-being of older adults

Characteristics of Older Adults in Canada

Most older adults are women, especially in older age groups. In 2005, women accounted for almost 75% of those aged 90 or older, while they accounted for 52% of persons aged 65 to 69. Many of these older adults are married. The tendency for women to live longer and to marry men older than themselves means that about a third of Canada's older adults are widowed, with more of these likely to be women. Conversely, older men are more likely to have a spouse than are older women (Statistics Canada, 2006).

Most Canadians have a long life expectancy. To provide programs and services that respond to older adults' needs, Health Canada (2007) and the Public Health Agency of Canada (2007) actively engage in research to better understand those needs. Their websites provide a wide range of related health information and research for this population (see also the Nursing and Canadian Society box). Although health problems and disabilities do typically accompany advancing years, most older adults view aging as a positive experience (Clarke, Marshall, Ryff, & Rosenthal, 2000).

NURSING AND CANADIAN SOCIETY

Fact	Implications for Nursing Practice
Health Canada (2007) and the Public Health Agency of Canada (2007) conduct studies to examine health patterns, health and wellness issues, and ways to reduce disability.	Nurses need to be aware of the current literature and be able to identify evidence that supports their work with older adults.
Some associations advocate for older adults, such as the National Seniors Council, the Alzheimer Society of Canada, the Canadian Association on Gerontology, the Canadian Gerontological Nursing Association, and the Canadian Geriatric Society.	Nurses need to network and be aware of the services and resources available not only for themselves but also for their clients.
Older adults welcome new technology into their homes when it meets their needs and is explained clearly to them.	Nurses may work with telehealth and older adults, especially in rural or remote areas of Canada. Some older adults may need education regarding how to obtain reliable health information from the web.

Society uses different terms to describe those over the age of 65 years (e.g., seniors, geriatrics, elderly, older adults, the aged). The term *older adult* will be used in this chapter. The term **frail elderly** describes the older individual who has significant physiological and functional impairment.

The passing of calendar time from one birthday to the next illustrates chronological aging. **Chronological age** has limited significance in terms of health, but because chronological age helps predict many health problems, it has some legal, economic, and social policy uses. It is used to determine eligibility for some programs, such as pensions.

Functional age is more useful than chronological age in that it is based on the fact that aging is a multifaceted, diverse process in which individuals at a specific chronological age are either older or younger than their peers in terms of some relevant skill or experience.

Special Groups of Older Canadians

ABORIGINAL OLDER ADULTS Aboriginal older adults are divided into three groups: First Nations, Inuit, and Metis. More than 39 900 Canadians over the age of 65 identified themselves as Aboriginal in the latest census data (Statistics Canada, 2006). The older adult Aboriginal population tends to be younger on average than the non-Aboriginal older adult population. Language, education, mobility, and cultural identity are factors to consider in working with this group of older adults. For example, many Aboriginal older adults have not finished high school (Statistics Canada, 2006).

FRAIL OLDER ADULTS **Frailty** is a general decline in an older adult's physical functioning that can result in increased vulnerability to illness. Defining characteristics include unintentional loss of more than 10% of body weight in the preceding year, feelings of exhaustion, grip strength in the lowest 20% for age, walking speed in the lowest 20% for age, and low caloric expenditure (< 270 kcal) (Fried et al., 2001). Frailty is not a natural consequence of aging, but rather it is a disease state that responds to intervention by the nurse.

ETHNIC OLDER ADULTS With the shift in immigration patterns from Europe to Asia, Africa, and the Middle East, the Canadian population is becoming increasingly diverse. Chinese people compose the largest ethnic group in Canada (Statistics Canada, 2006). Some ethnic older adults experience barriers to accessing health-care services because of language barriers, lack of knowledge of the services available, and lack of sensitivity on the part of health-care providers to ethnically appropriate care.

Evidence-Informed Practice

How Does Ethnicity Influence Perceptions of Health?

Based on the *Aging in Manitoba* study, Menec, Shooshtari, and Lambert (2007) examined whether self-rated health differed among older Canadians of different ethnic backgrounds and identified possible factors contributing to these differences. The participants consisted of four ethnic groups: British Canadian, Northern or Central European Canadian, Eastern European Canadians, and other. In both 1983 and 1996, older Eastern European Canadian adults rated their health much lower than the British Canadian adults. Analyses showed that the perception of health in these older adults was influenced by their cultural backgrounds and not by their demographic variables, social status, income level, language spoken, or health status.

NURSING IMPLICATIONS: Because the perception of health can be influenced by cultural factors, nurses must consider the ethnic backgrounds of older adult clients and avoid overgeneralizing their health practices across the ethnic groups.

Source: Based on "Ethnic Differences in Self-Rated Health among Older Adults: A Cross-Sectional and Longitudinal Analysis," by V. H. Menec, S. Shooshtari, and P. Lambert, 2007, *Journal of Aging and Health, 19*(1), pp. 62–86.

OLDER ADULTS WITH INTELLECTUAL DISABILITIES Canadians born before 1945 represent the first significantly large group of aging adults who have intellectual disabilities. Little research regarding this subgroup of older adults has been published. The variance in age criterion reported on aging and intellectual disability makes it difficult to accurately estimate the number of older adults living with a lifelong disability. In Canada, Statistics Canada (2001) indicated that approximately 44 770 adults aged 45 to 64 and 11 080 between the ages of 65 and 74 have an intellectual disability. Despite identification difficulties, consensus exists in the literature that the cohort of older adults with such disabilities is increasing (Haveman, 2004).

Attitudes toward Aging

Nurses may have preconceived ideas about older adults. These ideas are influenced by family, colleagues, work experiences, and society, and, unfortunately, they are often negative. The term **ageism** was coined by Robert Butler (1963) to describe the stereotypes that promote negative views of older adults. Images of older adults as frail, dependent, and in need of long-term care have pervaded nursing practice for many years. They are far from the truth (see Table 19.1 for more myths and realities).

Nurses need gerontological knowledge for several reasons:

- To ensure older adults receive appropriate health-care interventions
- To have sufficient knowledge to advocate for care and respect for older adults and refute the myths and stereotypes that can be damaging to them
- To assess the strengths and uniqueness in each older adult

TABLE 19.1 Myths and Realities of Aging

Myth	Reality
People consider themselves to be old at 65.	People feel old based on their health and functional ability, rather than their chronological age.
In today's society, families no longer care for older people.	In North America, 80% of the care of older adults is provided by their families.
As people grow older, it is natural for them to want to withdraw from society.	Because older people are unique individuals, each of them responds differently to society.
By age 70, an individual's psychologic growth is complete.	People never lose their capacity for psychologic growth.
In old age, there is an inevitable decline in all intellectual abilities.	A few areas of cognitive ability decline in older adulthood, but other areas show improvement.
Older adults cannot learn complex new skills.	Older adults are capable of learning new things, but the speed with which they process information slows with age.
Older people decrease the level of their sexual activity because they are less able to perform sexually.	If sexual activity in older people declines, it is because of social reasons (e.g., loss of partner) or risk factors, such as diseases and adverse medication effects.
Most old people are depressed and should be allowed to withdraw from society.	About one-third of older people exhibit depressive symptoms; however, depression is a very treatable condition at any age.

Source: From *Nursing for Wellness in Older Adults,* 4th ed. (p. 10), by C. A. Miller, 2004, Philadelphia, PA: Lippincott Williams & Wilkins. Reprinted with permission.

Gerontological Nursing in Canada

Gerontological nursing has emerged as a separate branch of professional nursing practice. The first North American textbook on gerontological nursing was published in the United States in 1950, but it was more than a decade before gerontological nursing was recognized officially as a specialty within nursing in that country.

In Canada, provincial associations of gerontological nursing emerged in the mid-1970s, the first being established in Ontario, in 1974, as the Gerontological Nursing Association. Although the seeds for a national association were laid in 1983, with the first National Conference on Gerontological Nursing held in Victoria, British Columbia, it was not until 1985 that the Canadian Gerontological Nursing Association was formed. The first Canadian textbook, called *Promoting Healthy Aging: A Nursing and Community Perspective,* was written by Beckingham and Witter DuGas in 1993. Today, national certification in *gerontological nursing* is available through the Canadian Nurses Association.

Care Settings for Older Adults

Any nurse who works with older adults and those important to them might be called a gerontological nurse. **Gerontology** is a term used to describe the study of aging and older adults. Gerontological nurses practice in a variety of settings, including acute-care hospitals, long-term facilities (e.g., nursing homes, auxiliary hospitals), rehabilitation units, community, home, assisted or designated living, adult daycare, and hospice.

Theories of Aging

Biological theories of aging are either intrinsic or extrinsic. *Intrinsic* theory addresses factors within the body; *extrinsic* theory encompasses factors in the environment. Table 19.2 describes some of the common "biological theories" of aging.

TABLE 19.2 Common Biological Theories of Aging

Theory Type	Hypotheses
Wear-and-tear theories	• Proposes that humans, like automobiles, have vital parts that run down with time, leading to aging and death • Proposes that the faster an organism lives, the quicker it dies • Proposes that cells wear out through exposure to internal and external stressors, including trauma, chemicals, and buildup of natural wastes
Endocrine theory	• Proposes that events occurring in the hypothalamus and pituitary are responsible for changes in hormone production and response that result in the organism's decline
Free-radical theory	• Proposes that unstable free radicals (groups of atoms) result from the oxidation of organic materials, such as carbohydrates and proteins; these radicals cause biochemical changes in the cells, and the cells cannot regenerate themselves
Genetic theories	• Proposes that the organism is genetically programmed for a predetermined number of cell divisions, after which the cells/organism dies. • Proposes that when damage to the protein synthesis occurs, faulty proteins will be synthesized and will gradually accumulate, causing a progressive decline in the organism
Cross-linking theories	• Proposes that the irreversible aging of proteins such as collagen is responsible for the ultimate failure of tissues and organs • Proposes that as cells age, chemical reactions create strong bonds, or cross-linkages, between proteins; these bonds cause loss of elasticity, stiffness, and eventual loss of function
Immune theories	• Proposes that the immune system becomes less effective with age, resulting in reduced resistance to infectious disease and viruses • Proposes that a decrease in immune function may result in an increase in autoimmune responses, causing the body to produce antibodies that attack itself

Physiological Aging

Although people age somewhat differently, many changes occur in almost everyone and are considered normal. A more accurate description of these changes is *usual.* Usual aging refers to what happens to most people, including disorders that are common in the aging process. Usual aging does not mean that the changes are unavoidable or desirable.

As the person ages, a number of physical changes occur; some are visible, some are not. See Table 19.3 for a summary of the normal physical changes associated with aging.

Integument

The skin becomes drier and more fragile, the hair loses colour, the fingernails and toenails become thickened and brittle, and in women over 60 years, facial hair increases.

Responses to these changes vary among individuals and cultures. For example, one person may feel distinguished with grey hair, whereas another may feel depressed, interpreting grey hair as a sign of losing youth.

These integumentary changes accompany progressive losses of subcutaneous fat and muscle tissue; muscle atrophy and loss of elastic fibre, resulting in a double

TABLE 19.3 Normal Physical Changes Associated with Aging

PHYSICAL CHANGES	RATIONALE
Integumentary	
Increased skin dryness	Decrease in sebaceous gland activity and tissue fluid
Increased skin pallor	Decreased vascularity
Increased skin fragility	Reduced thickness and vascularity of the dermis; loss of subcutaneous fat
Progressive wrinkling and sagging of the skin	Loss of skin elasticity, increased dryness, and decreased subcutaneous fat
Lentigo senilis (brown age spots) on exposed body parts (e.g., face, hands, arms)	Clustering of melanocytes (pigment-producing cells)
Decreased perspiration	Reduced number and function of sweat glands
Thinning and greying of scalp, pubic, and axillary hair	Progressive loss of pigment cells from the hair bulbs
Slower nail growth and increased thickening with ridges	Increased calcium deposition
Neuromuscular	
Decreased speed and power of skeletal muscle contractions	Decrease in muscle fibres
Slowed reaction time	Diminished conduction speed of nerve fibres and decreased muscle tone
Loss of height (stature)	Atrophy of intervertebral discs, increased flexion at hips and knees
Loss of bone mass	Bone reabsorption outpaces bone reformation
Joint stiffness	Drying and loss of elasticity in joint cartilage
Impaired balance	Decreased muscle strength, reaction time, and coordination, change in centre of gravity
Greater difficulty in complex learning and abstraction	Fewer cells in cerebral cortex
Sensory and Perceptual	
Loss of visual acuity	Degeneration leading to lens opacity (cataracts), thickening, and inelasticity (presbyopia)
Increased sensitivity to glare and decreased ability to adjust to darkness	Changes in the ciliary muscles; rigid pupil sphincter; decrease in pupil size
Arcus senilis (partial or complete glossy white circle around the periphery of the cornea)	Fatty deposits
Presbycusis (progressive loss of hearing)	Changes in the structures and nerve tissues in the inner ear; thickening of the eardrum
Decreased sense of taste, especially the sweet sensations at the tip of the tongue	Decreased number of taste buds in the tongue because of tongue atrophy
Decreased sense of smell	Atrophy of the olfactory bulb at the base of the brain (responsible for smell perception)
Increased threshold for sensations of pain, touch, and temperature	Possible nerve conduction and neuron changes

(continued)

TABLE 19.3 Normal Physical Changes Associated with Aging (continued)

PHYSICAL CHANGES	RATIONALE
Pulmonary	
Decreased ability to expel foreign or accumulated matter	Decreased elasticity and ciliary activity
Decreased lung expansion, less effective exhalation, reduced vital capacity, and increased residual volume	Weakened thoracic muscles; calcification of costal cartilage, making the rib cage more rigid with increased anterior-posterior diameter; dilation from inelasticity of alveoli
Dyspnea (difficult breathing) following intense exercise	Diminished delivery and diffusion of oxygen to the tissues to repay the normal oxygen debt because of exertion or changes in both respiratory and vascular tissues
Cardiovascular	
Reduced cardiac output and stroke volume, particularly during increased activity or unusual demands; may result in shortness of breath on exertion and pooling of blood in the extremities	Increased rigidity and thickness of heart valves (hence decreased filling and emptying abilities); decreased contractile strength
Reduced elasticity and increased rigidity of arteries	Increased calcium deposits in the muscular layer
Increase in diastolic and systolic blood pressure	Inelasticity of systemic arteries and increased peripheral resistance
Orthostatic hypotension	Reduced sensitivity of the blood pressure–regulating baroreceptors
Gastrointestinal	
Delayed swallowing time	Alterations in the swallowing mechanism
Increased tendency for indigestion	Gradual decrease in digestive enzymes, reduction in gastric pH, and slower absorption rate
Increased tendency for constipation	Decreased muscle tone of the intestines; decreased peristalsis; decreased free body fluid
Urinary	
Reduced filtering ability of the kidney and impaired renal function	Decreased number of functioning nephrons (basic functional units of the kidney) and arteriosclerotic changes in blood flow
Less effective concentration of urine	Decreased tubular function
Urinary urgency and urinary frequency	Enlarged prostate gland in men; weakened muscles supporting the bladder or weakness of the urinary sphincter in women
Tendency for nocturnal frequency and retention of residual urine	Decreased bladder capacity and tone
Genitals	
Prostate enlargement (benign) in men	Exact mechanism is unclear; possible endocrine changes
Multiple changes in women (shrinkage and atrophy of the vulva, cervix, uterus, fallopian tubes, and ovaries; reduction in secretions; and changes in vaginal flora)	Diminished secretion of female hormones and more alkaline vaginal pH
Increased time to sexual arousal	Changes in blood supply to penis, clitoris
Decreased firmness of erection, increased refractory period (men)	Changes in blood supply
Decreased vaginal lubrication and elasticity (women)	Loss of estrogen effects
Immunological	
Decreased immune response; lowered resistance to infections	T cells less responsive to antigens; B cells produce fewer antibodies
Poor response to immunization	Immune system changes may precipitate insulin resistance
Decreased stress response	
Endocrine	
Increased insulin resistance	Unclear mechanism
Decreased thyroid function	

chin; sagging of eyelids and earlobes; and wrinkling of skin, especially in areas exposed to the sun. Bony prominences become visible. In older women, the breasts become smaller and may sag; if large and pendulous, they may cause chafing where the skin surfaces touch. Loss of subcutaneous fat decreases the older adult's tolerance of the cold.

Neuromusculoskeletal

With aging comes gradual reduction in the speed and power of skeletal or voluntary muscle contractions and sustained muscular effort. Exercise can strengthen weakened muscles, and up to about age 50 years, the skeletal muscles can increase in bulk and density. After that time, a steady decrease in muscle fibres occurs, ultimately leading to the typical wasted appearance of the very old person. Thus, older adults often complain about their lack of strength and how quickly they tire. Activities can still be carried out but at a slower pace. Often, balance is impaired with age. Prolonged muscle efforts may be sustained by older people, provided they take rest pauses and avoid peak performance.

Reaction time slows with age. It can be delayed further by decreased muscle tone as a result of diminished physical activity. Older people compensate for this reaction difference by being cautious—for instance, in their driving habits.

A slight loss in overall stature occurs with age. This can be exaggerated by muscular weakness, resulting in a stooping posture called **kyphosis**. **Osteoporosis**, a decrease in bone density, along with increased brittleness of bone, makes the older adult prone to serious fractures, some of which may be spontaneous (**pathological fractures**). Osteoporosis occurs more frequently in people with insufficient intake of dietary calcium, in women after menopause, and in individuals who are immobilized or physically inactive.

Some degenerative joint changes occur, making movement stiffer and more restricted. Stiffness is aggravated by inactivity; for example, if a person sits too long. Physical activity and proper nutrition will slow bone density loss and decrease muscle atrophy and stiffness (see Figure 19.1).

Sensory and Perceptual

Each of the senses becomes less efficient in older adulthood. Changes in vision associated with aging include the obvious changes around the eye, such as the shrunken appearance of the eyes because of loss of orbital fat, the slowed blink reflex, and the looseness of the eyelids, particularly the lower lid, due to poorer muscle tone. Other changes result in loss of visual acuity, less power of adaptation to darkness and dim light, decrease

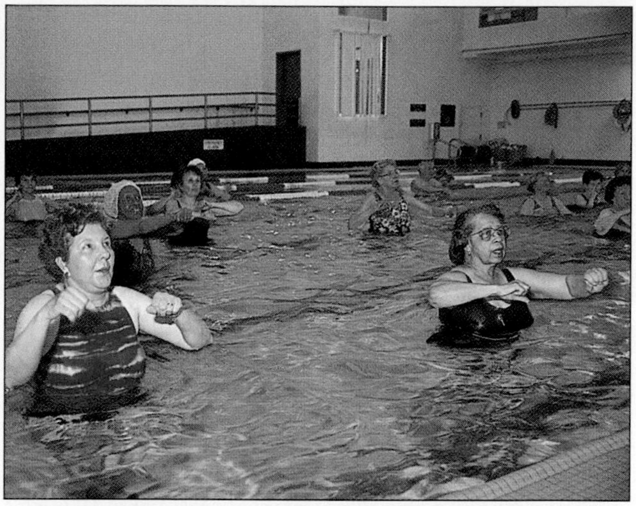

FIGURE 19.1 A regular program of exercise is important for maintenance of joint mobility and muscle tone. It can also promote socialization.

in accommodation to near and far objects, loss of peripheral vision, and difficulty in discriminating similar colours, especially blues, greens, and purples.

Presbyopia, the inability of the eye to focus or accommodate because of a loss of flexibility of the lens, causes a decrease in near vision. This generally starts around age 40. Visual acuity lessens gradually after age 50 and more rapidly after age 70 (Tabloski, 2006).

By 80 years, adults have some lens opacity (**cataracts**) that reduces visual acuity and causes glare to be a problem. Surgical removal of cataracts is common. Changes in the ciliary muscles, which control the shape of the lens, reduce the power of the lens to adjust to near and far vision. The pupil's diameter is reduced, and the amount of light entering the eye is thereby restricted. This slows the reaction time to decreases in light, a problem compounded with night driving. Diminished retinal function and reduced peripheral vision also occur.

The loss of hearing ability, called **presbycusis**, affects people over age 65 years. Gradual loss of hearing is more common among men, perhaps because men are more frequently in noisy work environments. Hearing loss is greater in the higher frequencies than the lower. Thus, older adults with hearing loss usually hear speakers with low, distinct voices best. Older adults may have more difficulty compensating for hearing loss than the young, who pay closer attention to the lip movements of the speaker.

Older people have a poorer sense of taste and smell and are less stimulated by food than the young. This change significantly affects their appetite, contributing to poor nutrition.

Loss of skin receptors takes place gradually, producing an increased threshold for sensations of pain, touch, and temperature. The older person may not be able to distinguish hot from cold or sense the intensity of heat.

Stimuli causing severe pain in a younger person may cause only minor sensation or pressure in the older individual. This places the older adult at higher risk for burns and other injuries.

Pulmonary

Respiratory efficiency is reduced with age. At about age 55, respiratory muscles begin to weaken and the chest wall gradually becomes stiffer (decreasing compliance). These changes result from age-associated kyphoscoliosis (curvature of the spine), calcification of intercostal cartilage, and arthritis of the costovertebral joints. With age, the muscles used in breathing, such as the diaphragm, tend to weaken. People experience increased rigidity of the trachea and connecting airways because of a loss of muscle tone. As a consequence of the age-related changes in the lung tissues and the chest wall, the pulmonary system of older adults is less able to provide adequate gas exchange. The person inhales a smaller volume of air because of the musculoskeletal changes in the chest wall that reduce the size of the chest. Total lung volume is not significantly reduced but rather it is redistributed. A greater volume of residual air is left in the lungs after expiration, and the capacity to cough efficiently decreases because of weaker expiratory muscles. In individuals who do not smoke or have a lung disorder, the muscles of breathing and the lungs continue to function well enough to meet the needs of the body during ordinary daily activities.

Dyspnea (difficult breathing) occurs frequently with increased activity, such as running for a bus or carrying heavy parcels upstairs. Older adults may also have more difficulty breathing at high altitudes.

Cilia, which line the trachea, are less effective with age. Mucus secretions tend to collect more readily in the respiratory tree. Thus, susceptibility to respiratory infections increases in older adults. From about the fifth decade on, a consistent increase occurs in the incidence of respiratory diseases, such as chronic obstructive lung disease and pneumonia.

Cardiovascular

The working capacity of the heart diminishes with age. This is particularly evident when increased demands are made on the heart muscles, such as during periods of exercise or emotional stress. The heart rate at normal rest does not change with age. However, the heart rate is slow to respond to stress and slow to return to normal after periods of physical activity.

Changes in the arteries occur concurrently. Reduced arterial elasticity may result in diminished blood supply to, for instance, the legs and the brain, resulting in pain in the calf muscles on exertion and dizziness, respectively.

Blood pressure measurements often indicate a significant increase in systolic and a slight increase in diastolic pressures. There may be a delay in the circulatory adjustments required when a person quickly stands up from a lying position. The delay results in an abrupt drop in systolic blood pressure known as **orthostatic hypotension.**

Gastrointestinal

The digestive system is impaired by aging. Gradual decreases in digestive enzymes occur; examples are ptyalin in salivary secretions, which converts starch; pepsin and trypsin, which digest protein; and lipase, a fat-splitting enzyme.

The number of absorbing cells in the intestinal tract decreases, as does the gastric pH. These factors lower the absorption rate, slowing the absorption of nutrients and drugs. The muscle tone of the intestines also decreases, causing a decrease in peristalsis and elimination. These changes in muscle tone, digestive juices, and intestinal activity may lead to indigestion and constipation in the older adult.

Urinary

The excretory function of the kidney diminishes with age, but usually not significantly below normal levels unless a disease process intervenes. The kidney's filtering abilities may also be impaired; thus, waste products may be filtered and excreted more slowly.

More noticeable changes are those related to the bladder. Complaints of urinary urgency and urinary frequency are common. The capacity of the bladder and its ability to completely empty diminish with age. Many older adults need to get up during the night to void (**nocturnal frequency**) and may experience retention of residual urine, predisposing them to bladder infections.

Genitals

Degenerative changes in the gonads are gradual in men. Production of testosterone continues, and the testes can produce sperm well into old age, although the number of sperm produced gradually decreases. In women, the degenerative changes in the ovaries are noticed by the abrupt cessation of menses in middle age during menopause.

Changes in the gonads of older women result from diminished secretion of the ovarian hormones. Some changes, such as the shrinking of the uterus and ovaries, go unnoticed. Other changes are obvious. The breasts atrophy, and lubricating vaginal secretions are reduced. Reduced natural lubrication is the cause of painful intercourse, which often necessitates the use of lubricating gels.

Immune

With age, the immune system becomes less effective. The consequence is an increase in the incidence and severity of urinary tract infections, cancers, and infectious diseases, like pneumonia. The effect of immune system changes is so all-encompassing that it has led some to hypothesize that the aging process is due to immune senescence.

Psychosocial Aging

A number of theories explain psychosocial aging. According to **disengagement theory**, aging involves mutual withdrawal (disengagement) between the older person and others in that person's environment. This withdrawal relieves the older person of some of society's pressures and gradually reduces the number of people with whom the older person interacts. According to **activity theory**, the best way to age is to stay active physically and mentally, and according to **continuity theory**, people maintain their values, habits, and behaviours in old age. A person who is accustomed to having people around will continue to do so, and the person who prefers not to be involved with others will more likely disengage. This theory accounts for the great variety of behaviour seen in older people. The most recent theories regard older adults as capable of maintaining control over their own lives and playing an active role in politics and the economy.

According to Erikson, the developmental task at this time is *integrity versus despair.* People who attain ego integrity view life with a sense of wholeness and derive satisfaction from past accomplishments. They view death as an acceptable completion of life. According to Erikson, people who develop integrity accept events in one's life cycle (Erikson, 1982). By contrast, people who despair often believe they have made poor choices during life and wish they could live life over. Robert Butler sees integrity as bringing serenity and wisdom, and despair as resulting in the inability to accept fate. Despair gives rise to feelings of frustration, discouragement, and a sense that life has been worthless (Butler, 1963).

Peck (1968) proposes the following developmental tasks of the older adult in contrast to Erikson's task of ego integrity versus despair:

1. Ego differentiation versus work-role preoccupation
2. Body transcendence versus body preoccupation
3. Ego transcendence versus ego preoccupation

For details about these tasks see Chapter 16, in the section "Growth and Development Theories." Havighurst (1972) and Duvall (1977) have further defined the developmental tasks of the older adult (see Box 19.1).

BOX 19.1 DEVELOPMENTAL TASKS OF THE OLDER ADULT

According to Havighurst (1972) and Duvall (1977), the older adult has the following developmental tasks:

65 TO 75 YEARS

- Adjusting to decreasing physical strength and health
- Adjusting to retirement and lower and fixed income
- Adjusting to the death of parents, spouses, and friends
- Adjusting to new relationships with adult children
- Adjusting to leisure time
- Adjusting to slower physical and cognitive responses
- Keeping active and involved
- Making satisfying living arrangements as aging progresses

75 YEARS AND OLDER

- Adapting to living alone
- Safeguarding physical and mental health
- Adjusting to the possibility of moving into a nursing home
- Remaining in touch with other family members
- Finding meaning in life
- Adjusting to one's own death

Source: From *Health Promotion Strategies Through the Life Span,* 7th ed., by R. B. Murray and J. P. Zentner, 2001, Upper Saddle River, NJ: Prentice Hall.

Retirement

Today, a majority of the people over 65 years are not working. Many provinces have already eliminated the mandatory retirement age, and many people who are healthy continue to work on a full- or part-time basis. Work offers a better income, a sense of self-worth, and the chance to continue established routines. Some need to work for economic reasons.

Retirement can be a time when deferred projects or recreational activities can be pursued. Older adults find outlets in travelling, volunteer services, intellectual pursuits, or hobbies (Figure 19.2).

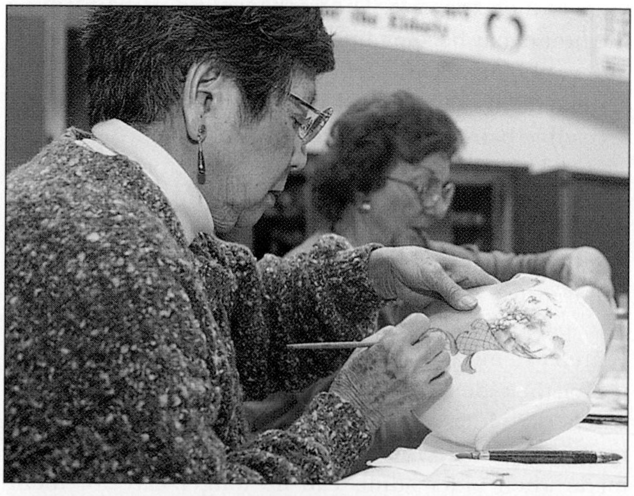

FIGURE 19.2 Many older adults find creative outlets during retirement.

The lifestyle of later years is, to a large degree, formulated in youth. People who attempt suddenly to refocus and enrich their lives at retirement usually have difficulty. Those who learned early in life to live well-balanced and fulfilling lives are generally more successful in retirement. The person who has been concerned only with the accomplishments of the children or who has been concerned only with the paycheque can be left with a feeling of emptiness when children leave and the job no longer exists. The later years can foster a sense of integrity and continuity, or they can be years of despair.

Economic Change

The financial needs of older adults vary considerably. Though most need less money for living expenses, and although some own their homes, costs continue to rise, making it difficult for some to manage. Adequate financial resources enable the older person to remain independent.

Problems with income are often related to low retirement benefits, lack of pension plans, and the increased length of the retirement years. Older members of minority groups often have greater financial problems. Older women usually have lower incomes than men, primarily because of their time out of the workforce and gender discrimination in pay scales.

Nurses should be aware of the costs of health care. For example, while assisting an older adult to plan a diet, consider which foods the client can afford to buy. The physician can order lower-priced medications. Supplies used in an older adult's care should be as economical as possible.

Relocation

During late adulthood, many people relocate. A variety of factors can lead to this decision. The house may be too large or too expensive. The work involved in maintaining the house may become burdensome or impossible. Some older persons with decreased mobility want living arrangements that are all on one floor or need more accessible bathroom facilities.

Making the decision to move is often stressful. The older adult may be moving to an apartment, which may mean leaving the comfort of the family home and the neighbours of several decades. Some move nearer to their children for support. For some, relocation is voluntary. The person may be seeking a more moderate climate geared to a more leisurely lifestyle. Adjustment will be easier for the older person making a voluntary move.

Some older people must relocate to long-term-care facilities. The decision to enter a facility is frequently made when older adults can no longer care for themselves, often because of mobility problems and memory impairment. All provide meals but vary in other services, such as assistance with hygiene and dressing, physical therapy, recreational activities, and medical and nursing supervision.

Independence and Self-Esteem

Aging in place describes a process that enables older adults to age within the comfort and familiarity of their own homes. It is important to them to be able to look after themselves even if they have to struggle to do so. To maintain the older adult's sense of self-respect, nurses and family members need to encourage them to do as much as possible for themselves, provided that safety is maintained.

Some older adults experience discomfort when doing activities they enjoyed in their younger years. Assistive devices are items that ease the strains of daily activities at home, at work, or at play. They include medical equipment and mobility aids. These devices can help older adults improve their quality of life and maintain their independence.

Social Relationships

Grandparenting offers many older adults an enjoyable role in later life. More women than men experience grandparenting (Kemp, 2003). However, the role is changing; increasingly they are assuming responsibility for raising their grandchildren because the parents are unable to provide care because of problematic substance use, poverty, or other problems.

Older adults with increased social contacts tend to receive more support and usually demonstrate health-promotive behaviours. The death of family and friends, retirement, and relocation can reduce social contacts. Diminished social contact leads to social isolation, diminished social support, and decreased well-being. Living alone is a common experience for older adults and can present challenges. Older people who live alone may describe feelings of loneliness and isolation. Eating for most persons is a social activity; some older adults who live alone do not prepare balanced meals, and undernutrition becomes a concern.

Relatively little is known about the nature of relationships as they evolve over time in older lesbians and gay men. Although older lesbian and gay adults experience the same bodily changes with aging and many of the same emotions as do older heterosexual adults, they may, in addition, face unique challenges, such as the loss of a partner through HIV infection and a higher risk of social isolation. Nurses can offer informational and emotional support that may be beneficial to older adults.

Death and Grieving

Well-adjusted aging couples usually thrive on each other's companionship. When a mate dies, the partner experiences loss, emptiness, and loneliness. Many are capable and manage to live alone; however, reliance on younger family members increases with advancing age and when ill health occurs.

More women than men face bereavement and solitude because women usually live longer. Older people are often reminded of their own mortality by the death of friends. It is a time when life is reviewed with happiness or regret. Independence established before the loss of a mate makes this adjustment period easier. A person who has successful relationships with children and grandchildren, meaningful friendships, economic security, ongoing interests, and a peaceful philosophy of life copes more easily with bereavement. See Chapter 48.

Cognitive Abilities and Aging

Intellectual capacity includes perception, cognitive agility, memory, and learning. **Perception,** or the ability to interpret the environment, depends on the acuteness of the senses. If the aging person's senses are impaired, the ability to perceive the environment and react appropriately is diminished. Changes in the nervous system can also affect perceptual capacity.

Changes in the cognitive structures occur with age: neurons are progressively lost. Blood flow to the brain decreases, the meninges appear to thicken, and brain metabolism slows. Overall, the older adult maintains problem-solving, judgment, creativity, and other well-practised cognitive skills. Intellectual loss generally reflects a disease process, such as atherosclerosis, which causes the blood vessels to narrow and diminishes perfusion of nutrients to the brain. Most older adults do not experience cognitive impairments.

Memory is also a component of intellectual capacity that involves the following steps:

1. Momentary perception of stimuli from the environment, referred to as **sensory memory**, occurs.
2. Storage in **short-term memory** (information held in the brain for immediate use or what a person has in mind at a given moment) takes place. An example of this type of memory is calling information for a telephone number and remembering the number for only the brief time needed to dial it. Short-term memory that deals with activities or the recent past (minutes to a few hours) is often referred to as **recent memory.**
3. Encoding, by which information leaves short-term memory and enters **long-term memory**, the repository for information stored for periods longer than 72 hours and usually weeks and years, is the final stage. Memories of childhood friends, teachers, and events are stored in long-term memory. Older people who remember the flowers in their wedding bouquet or the names of the boys on their dance card are drawing from long-term memory.

In older adults, retrieval of information from long-term memory can be slower, especially if the information is not frequently used. Most age-related differences occur in short-term memory. Older adults tend to forget the recent past. This forgetfulness can be improved by the use of memory aids, making lists, and placing objects in consistent locations.

Older people need additional time for learning, largely because of the problem of retrieving information. Motivation is also important. Older adults have more difficulty than younger ones in learning information they do not consider meaningful. It is suggested that the older person remain mentally active to maintain cognitive ability at the highest possible level. Lifelong mental activity, particularly verbal activity, helps the older person retain a high level of cognitive function and may help maintain long-term memory. Cognitive impairment that interferes with normal life is not part of normal aging. A decline in intellectual abilities that interferes with social or occupational functions should be regarded as abnormal. In such instances, family members should be advised to seek prompt medical evaluation.

Moral Development

According to Kohlberg (1981), moral development is completed in the early adult years. Most older people stay at Kohlberg's conventional level of moral development (see Table 16.7 on page 301), and some are at the preconventional level. An older person at the preconventional level obeys rules to avoid pain and the displeasure of others. At stage 1, a person defines good and bad in relation to the self, whereas older people at stage 2 may act to meet another's needs as well as their own. Older adults at the conventional level follow society's rules of conduct in response to the expectations of others.

The value and belief patterns that are important to older adults may have little or no significance to younger people because they developed during a time that was very different from today. In addition, a large number of today's older adults are either foreign-born or first-generation citizens. Cultural background, life experiences, gender, religion, and socioeconomic status influence people's values. The nurse must identify and consider the specific values of the older client when nursing care is planned.

Spiritual Development

Older adults can contemplate new religious and philosophical views and try to understand ideas missed previously or interpreted differently. The older person also derives a sense of worth by sharing experiences or views. In contrast, the older adult who has not matured spiritually may feel despair as the drive for economic and professional success wanes.

Many older people have strong religious convictions and continue to attend religious services. Involvement in religion often helps the older adult to resolve issues related to the meaning of life, to adversity, or to good fortune.

According to Fowler and Keen (1985), some people enter the sixth stage of spiritual development, *universalizing* (see Table 16.8 on page 302). People whose spiritual development reaches this level think and act in a way that exemplifies love and justice.

Health Assessment and Promotion

A primary role of nurses is to promote healthy aging, the goals of which are to maintain physical and emotional health, to avoid ailments, and to remain active and independent. For most people, maintaining general good health requires more effort as they age. Health-promotive behaviours have been shown to reduce the risk of developing several disorders that commonly occur with age. These behaviours include following a nutritious diet, exercising regularly, ceasing to smoke, reducing alcohol consumption, and remaining mentally active. Through acquiring the needed knowledge, either from health-care providers, support groups, or credible internet sources, older adults can exert some control over what happens to them as they age.

The initial step in promoting health is a detailed assessment of the older adult. This may be more comprehensive than one conducted on a younger adult, because of the increased medical and health complexity of an older client. Often a team approach is helpful. Assessment by the nurse requires an ability to listen to the older client, to ask questions, to obtain data from multiple sources, and to recognize normal aging changes and be able to differentiate them from abnormal ones (see the Assessment: Developmental Guidelines box and the Health-Promotion Guidelines box for older adults).

A number of assessment tools or guidelines have been developed to help nurses. Exactly what tools are used depends on the purpose of the evaluation and the setting. Assessment activities may include measurement of weight, height, and vital signs; observation of the skin for hydration status or the presence of lesions; examination of visual acuity using the Snellen chart; examination of hearing acuity using the whisper, Weber, and Rinne tests (see Chapter 27); and questions about the following:

- Usual dietary pattern
- Any problems with bowel or urinary elimination
- Activity or exercise and sleep and rest patterns
- Family and social activities and interests
- Any problems with reading, writing, or problem solving
- Adjustment to retirement or loss of partner
- Economic situation
- Mental and emotional status

ASSESSMENT: DEVELOPMENT GUIDELINES

The Older Adult

In these developmental areas, does the older adult do the following?

1. **PHYSICAL DEVELOPMENT**
   - Adjust to physiological changes (e.g., appearance, sensory and perceptual, musculoskeletal, neurological, cardiovascular)
   - Adapt lifestyle to diminishing energy and ability
   - Maintain vital signs (especially blood pressure) within normal range for age and gender
2. **PSYCHOSOCIAL DEVELOPMENT**
   - Manage retirement years in a satisfying manner
   - Participate in social and leisure activities
   - Have a social network of friends and support persons
   - View life as worthwhile
   - Have high self-esteem
   - Gain support from value system or spiritual philosophy
   - Accept and adjust to the death of significant others
3. **DEVELOPMENT IN ACTIVITIES OF DAILY LIVING**
   - Exhibit healthy practices in nutrition, exercise, recreation, sleep patterns, and personal habits
   - Have the ability to care for self or to secure appropriate help with activities of daily living
   - Have satisfactory living arrangements and income to meet changing needs

Health-Promotion Guidelines for Older Adults

The following are important to the health of older adults:

HEALTH TESTS AND SCREENING

- Routine physical examination (annually as directed by health-care provider)
- Immunizations as recommended, such as a tetanus booster every 10 years, pneumococcal vaccinations, and annual influenza vaccine
- Regular dental assessments (e.g., yearly)
- Tonometry for signs of glaucoma and examination for other eye disease every 2 to 3 years or annually, if indicated
- Testicular self-examination and breast awareness regularly
- Screenings for cardiovascular disease (e.g., blood pressure measurement; electrocardiogram and cholesterol test, as directed by the health-care provider)
- Screenings for colorectal, cervical, uterine, ovarian, and prostate cancers
- Mammogram every 2 years until age 69 and as directed later

SAFETY

- Home safety measures to prevent falls, fire, burns, scalds, and electrocution
- Motor vehicle safety reinforcement, especially when driving at night
- Precautions to prevent pedestrian accidents
- Education about medications

NUTRITION AND EXERCISE

- Importance of a well-balanced diet with fewer calories to accommodate lower metabolic rate and decreased physical activity
- Importance of sufficient amounts of vitamin D and calcium to prevent osteoporosis
- Regular program of moderate exercise to maintain joint mobility, muscle tone, and bone calcification

ELIMINATION

- Importance of adequate roughage in the diet, adequate exercise, and at least 1500 mL of fluid daily to prevent constipation

SOCIAL INTERACTIONS

- Intellectual and recreational pursuits
- Personal relationships that promote discussion of feelings, concerns, and fears
- Assessment of risk factors for abuse and neglect
- Availability of community centres, programs, and support groups for older adults

Several areas of assessment may require special attention. A mental status assessment is a structured approach to collecting data about an older adult's cognitive functioning. Nurses frequently work with such standardized screening tools as the mini-mental status exam.

Another area is medication use:

- Review all prescription, over-the-counter, and nontraditional medications.
- Identify whether the older adult is able to take medications correctly.
- Identify the older adult's understandings of the reasons for the medications.

A third area of assessment may be pain management. Chapter 34 provides a description of pain management. However, older adults with cognitive impairment may require special attention as to the presence of pain.

Health Problems

Health problems that older adults may experience include accidents, chronic disabling diseases, mental health problems, problematic drug use, dementia, abuse, cancer, and emergencies. Leading causes of death in people ages 65 years and over are cancer, heart disease, cerebrovascular disease (stroke), chronic lower respiratory lung disease, diabetes, influenza, accidents, and so on (Wilkins, 2002).

ACCIDENTS Older adults have a disproportionate share of accidents that cause injury and even death. Many of these accidents are directly related to the physiological changes that accompany normal aging. Because vision is limited, reflexes are slowed, and bones are brittle, caution is required in climbing stairs, driving a car, and even walking. Driving, particularly night driving, requires caution because accommodation of the eye to light is impaired and peripheral vision is diminished. Older persons need to remember to turn their head before changing lanes, and they should not rely on side vision, for example, when crossing a street.

Fires are a hazard for the older adult with a failing memory. The older person may forget that the stove is on or may not extinguish a cigarette or candle completely. Because of reduced sensitivity to pain and heat, care must be taken to prevent burns when the person has hot baths or uses heating devices.

Many older adults suffer and die each year from hypothermia. **Hypothermia** is a body temperature below normal. A lowered metabolism and loss of normal insulation from thinning subcutaneous tissue decrease the older client's ability to retain heat.

Because older clients who take analgesics or sedatives may become lethargic or confused, they should be monitored regularly. Other nonpharmaceutical measures to induce sleep should be used whenever possible. Nurses can help older clients make the home environment safe. Specific hazards can be identified and corrected; for example, hand rails can be installed on staircases. Guidelines for accident prevention for the older adult are detailed in Chapter 30, Table 30.1: Risk Factors and Preventive Measures for Falls (page 775), and the section "Preventing Specific Hazards."

CHRONIC DISABLING ILLNESSES Many older adults function well without impairments within the community; others are afflicted with one or more chronic illnesses that may seriously impair their functioning. Chronic conditions are more prevalent among older adults than among those in middle age. Examples of these are arthritis, rheumatism, osteoporosis, heart disease, stroke, chronic obstructive lung disease, diabetes, hypertension, hearing and visual alterations, and cognitive dysfunctions. In addition, acute illnesses, such as pneumonia; fractures; and trauma from falls, motor vehicle collisions, or other incidents, can create chronic health problems. The presence of chronic conditions varies regionally; for example, the prevalence of high blood pressure is higher in the Atlantic region than in the rest of Canada, as is the prevalence of arthritis in Ontario. Chronic illness brings about many changes to the client and to family members: the client, for example, may need increasing help with the activities of daily living, such as ambulation, feeding, and hygiene; health-care expenses often escalate; family roles may need to be altered; and family members may need to change their lifestyle to meet caregiving needs.

STROKES Most strokes are blood clots that get stuck in the small blood vessels in the brain that supply neurons with oxygen and other necessities. When this happens, neurons die from lack of oxygen. If this occurs often, the older adult may develop multi-infarct dementia. They become disoriented and wander off, perhaps getting lost. Others may have difficulty forming new memories.

Sometimes, a long interruption of blood flow to the brain is caused by a large clot in a major blood vessel (ischemic stroke) or the bursting of a blood vessel in the brain. The older adult may feel dizziness, numbness, and weak, often on one side of the body only. Some will have obvious problems with their vision or producing or understanding speech. Treatment for strokes involves controlling high blood pressure, which, along with age, is the major risk factor. Other contributing factors include smoking, drinking, and diabetes.

CARDIAC DISEASE The most common types of heart disease are coronary artery disease (CAD) and heart failure. In CAD, the lumens of the coronary arteries are narrowed by fatty fibrous or calcium plaques, which reduce the blood volume that can flow through. Heart failure occurs when the heart muscle fails to pump enough blood to meet the body's metabolic demands.

OSTEOARTHRITIS Osteoarthritis (OA) is the most common joint disorder. Although it primarily affects women, men can be diagnosed with it. Accumulated wear and tear causes deterioration of the articular cartilage. In OA, stiffness that comes with inactivity can be relieved by activity; however, this same activity causes pain, which is relieved by rest.

MENTAL HEALTH PROBLEMS Although, in general, older Canadians report a high level of life satisfaction, depression is found in about 10% to 20% of the older adult population. Approximately 50% of those aged over 80 are depressed and about 80% to 90% of the long-term-care residents have a mental disorder. It is difficult to diagnose mental health problems in older adults: many are not willing to disclose their illness, and their mental condition may also be masked or confused by their physiological changes. Older adults are burdened by the stigma of both mental illness and old age (Government of Canada, 2006).

Older adults with mental health problems will show signs and symptoms that include a lack of interest in people and things, trouble sleeping, significant changes in appetite, visible sadness, withdrawal from social activities, and feelings of worthlessness. Often, the depression they experience is triggered by personal losses, such as the loss of a spouse or a home. The challenges of living with a chronic disease condition can also initiate depression.

Some older adults may use alcohol to help them cope with the changes and problems of their older years. Mental health problems may be a cause of suicide. Although the mortality rate of suicide is relatively small in older adults, the rate for men 65 years and older is consistently higher than men in all age groups (Government of Canada, 2006).

Nurses may need to monitor those older adults who live alone, have recently experienced multiple losses, have a history of alcohol abuse, have a history of suicide attempts, or have a debilitating or life-threatening disease. Possible sources of help include self-help groups, peer support programs, home care services, and primary health-care services.

PROBLEMATIC DRUG USE Older adults who suffer from acute or chronic diseases may require medication. They may also purchase over-the-counter (OTC) drugs to cope with common discomforts related to aging, such as constipation and joint pain. Self-administration of medication can lead to misuse situations, including taking too much or too little medication, combining alcohol and medication, combining prescribed medications with OTC drugs, taking medications at the wrong time, taking someone else's medication, or noncompliance. Other potential misuse situations occur when more than one physician prescribes medications and the client fails to tell each doctor what has been previously prescribed.

Additionally, the pharmacodynamics of drugs are altered in older adults. The variations in absorption, distribution, metabolism, and excretion of drugs are related to physiological changes associated with aging. These variations are discussed in Chapter 31.

DEMENTIA **Dementia** is a general term for a permanent or progressive organic mental disorder that is characterized by personality changes, confusion, disorientation, deterioration of intellectual functioning, and impaired control of memory, judgment, and impulses. The most common type of dementia is Alzheimer's disease, or as it is more commonly known as nowadays, SDAT (Senile Dementia of the Alzheimer's Type). Its cause is unknown. SDAT affects about 750 000 people in Canada (Canadian Study of Health and Aging Working Group, 1994). By 2011, it is estimated that 111 430 Canadians (60% males and 40% females) will develop SDAT or a related disease, and by 2031, that number is expected to rise to 750 000 Canadians (Alzheimer's Society, 2007).

The symptoms of SDAT have been grouped into three or four stages and vary somewhat from client to client. The most prominent symptoms are cognitive dysfunctions, including decline in memory, learning, attention, judgment, orientation, and language skills. Loss of memory capacity alone does not constitute a diagnosis of SDAT. Dr. Alois Alzheimer first identified the disease in 1906. He described the two hallmarks of the disease: plaques—numerous tiny dense deposits scattered throughout the brain—which become toxic to brain cells at excessive levels, and tangles, which interfere with vital processes, eventually choking off the living cells. As well, when brain cells degenerate and die, the brain markedly shrinks in some regions. The symptoms are progressive, and all victims experience a steady decline in cognitive and physical abilities, lasting between 7 and 15 years and ending in death. In the last stage, the resident needs total assistance, is unable to communicate, is incontinent, and may be unable to walk.

Nurses may use the term *dementia* when an older patient is actually experiencing **delirium**. This common, but reversible, disorder involves fluctuations in consciousness. It may be manifested as confusion, disorientation to place, person, and time, and sometimes by bizarre behaviour. Delirium can be triggered by lack of sleep, sensory overload, sensory deprivation, relocation, and adverse drug interactions. Nurses need to be able to identify when delirium is superimposed on dementia—failure to do so has significant consequences (see Chapter 36, the section "Helping the Confused Client").

SDAT has no cure or specific treatment. Many older adults with SDAT are cared for in the home. The burden of care is frequently on women who are themselves aging. The caregivers often drive themselves to physical and emotional exhaustion while they render continuous care and experience the anguish of seeing a loved one turned into a person who no longer remembers who he or she is. The nurse's responsibility is to provide supportive nursing care, accurate information, and referral assistance.

OLDER ADULT ABUSE In 2005, older adults constituted 2% of all victims of violent crime. As with other victims of crime, older adults were more likely to be victimized by their adult children, current or ex-spouses, siblings, or friends. Half of the family violence experienced by older adults resulted in minor physical injuries that were sustained from the aggressor's use of physical force. "Four in ten homicides against seniors were committed by a family member (44%). Another one-third of seniors were killed by an acquaintance (31%), 17% by a stranger, and the remaining homicides were unsolved" (Ogrodnik, 2007, p. 7).

Older adult abuse or neglect can occur in private homes, older adults' apartments, and health-care facilities. Older adults living at home may be ashamed to admit that their children have abused them. They frequently lack financial resources or the mental capacity to report the situation.

Three elements compose the assessment process: the older client, the health-care provider, and the context in which abuse or neglect may occur. The nurse may ask the client to describe a typical day. In describing such a typical day, the older adult may reveal that he or she is left alone for long periods without access to food. Other questions may include, Who makes the decisions about your life? Has anyone forced you to do something that you do not want to do?

The nurse needs to ask about family structure and relationships, caregiving, and lifestyle practices. To determine whether the abuse or the neglect is unintentional or not, the nurse must decide if the caregiver understands the care requirements of the older adult. Genograms and ecomaps are helpful assessment tools. The nurse assesses situational factors, since they have the potential of contributing to abuse or neglect. Such factors include the caregiver's workload and the resources available. The interview with the care provider may include the following questions:

- What kind of care does your mother (father) require?
- What do you expect her to do for herself?
- What services do you have available to help you provide care?
- What other responsibilities do you have, inside and outside the home?

The care provider's dependence on the older adult may be addressed by asking these questions:

- Who owns the home where you and your mother live?
- Do you have power of attorney or enduring power of attorney?
- How is your mother's pension cheque deposited?

REFLECT ON PRIMARY HEALTH CARE

As older Canadians enjoy longer lives, they are faced with the burden of chronic illness associated with the aging process, the risk of suffering from mental health problems, and possible abuse because of their physical and mental vulnerabilities. Nurses apply the *health-promotion* principle to educate the older adults, the caregivers, and the health-care providers so that they will have a better understanding of the aging process and realistic expectations of care for older adults. Furthermore, as nurses invite their input as well as that of others in the interdisciplinary team, they can develop a seamless approach to promoting quality-of-life care and respite service for the older adults and their caregivers. Reflect on how these *public participation* and *intersectoral cooperation* approaches can lead to one-stop shopping or multiservice agencies in many communities (e.g., Community Care Access Centres in Ontario).

Nurses can educate responsible relatives about the needs of older adults and the resources available to provide increased support (see the Reflect on Primary Health Care box). They should report abuse to the appropriate agency. Nurses should be familiar with the laws of their jurisdiction regarding the reporting of suspected or known abuse. The legally competent adult cannot be forced to leave the abusive situation and may decide to stay. If the client is not legally competent, court proceedings to attain guardianship can be initiated.

CANCER Cancer is a significant health concern for older Canadians. Lung cancer is the second leading cause of death among older men, and the sixth leading cause among older women. Breast, prostate, and colorectal cancers are also leading causes of mortality. When assessing an older adult, the nurse should review the warning signs of cancer: change in bowel or bladder habits, a sore that does not heal, unusual vaginal bleeding or discharge, abdominal discomfort, thickening or lump in the breast or elsewhere, obvious changes in a wart or mole, and a nagging cough or hoarseness. Diagnosis is often complicated by the presence of co-existing chronic conditions and by common misperceptions about aging held by health-care professionals.

EMERGENCIES In 2003, such disasters as the forest fires in British Columbia and the SARS outbreak put some older adults at risk of injury and even death. Health Canada, in association with the World Health Organization and the Government of Manitoba, hosted an international workshop in Winnipeg in 2007 that identified older adults as one of the vulnerable priority groups in emergency situations.

Older people have experiences that can provide useful coping strategies for the community. Researchers found that after the 1997 Red River flood in Manitoba, older adults coped with the stressors around them more effectively than did younger survivors.

Nursing Interventions

Communicating with older adults can be challenging for nurses (see Chapter 21 for Lifespan Considerations: Communication with Older Adults, page 403). To support nurses in their work with older adults, the Registered Nurses' Association of Ontario (RNAO) developed a number of guidelines related to the care of older clients. These guidelines are intended to help nurses make evidence-based decisions specific to their practice circumstances. The following selected guidelines are available on the RNAO website to all nurses:

- Nursing management of hypertension
- Prevention of falls and injuries in the older adult
- Screening for delirium, dementia, and depression in older adults
- Stroke assessment across the continuum of care

Case Study 19

Alice Green, a 68-year-old female, has had a bone density scan as part of a regular physical exam and has been told that she has severe osteoporosis. Her physician has ordered a medication that is supposed to maintain bone mass in clients with osteoporosis. Alice lives alone in her own home and is able to perform activities of daily living independently.

Critical Thinking Questions

1. How would you define osteoporosis to Mrs. Green?
2. What risk factors related to osteoporosis should be included in an assessment of Mrs. Green?
3. Which of the risk factors are modifiable or can be altered by a change in lifestyle?
4. What medication teaching is essential when a client is taking medications to increase or maintain bone mass in osteoporosis?
5. What preventive measures should be taught to decrease risks of fractures and to maintain bone mass?

After working through these questions, go to the MyNursingLab at **http://www.mynursinglab.com** to check your answers.

KEY TERMS

frail elderly
chronological age
functional age
frailty
ageism
gerontology
kyphosis
osteoporosis
pathological fractures
presbyopia
cataracts
presbycusis
dyspnea
orthostatic hypotension
nocturnal frequency
disengagement theory
activity theory
continuity theory
perception
sensory memory
short-term memory
recent memory
long-term memory
hypothermia
dementia
delirium

CHAPTER HIGHLIGHTS

- Older adults experience many physical changes associated with aging. All body systems undergo change: integumentary, neuromusculoskeletal, sensory and perceptual, pulmonary, cardiovascular, gastrointestinal, immune, urinary, and genital.
- Several types of theories have been proposed to account for the biological aging process: wear-and-tear, endocrine, free-radical, genetics cross-linking, and immune theories.
- The older adult has to adjust to possible psychosocial changes, including retirement (which necessitates financial and social adjustments), relocation, increasing dependence on others, and coping with losses and death.
- Psychosocial theories about aging include the disengagement, activity, and continuity theories. Such theories reflect the controversial nature of our understanding of older adults.
- Nurses need to advocate for older adults and to help dispel the myths and stereotypes associated with aging and older adults.
- Health-promotion information for all adults needs to include positive health practices that can promote health and wellness. These include (1) recommended physical, visual, hearing, and dental assessments; (2) screenings for cardiovascular disease and cancer; (3) clinical breast examinations and testicular self-examinations; (4) immunizations; (5) Papanicolaou smears for women; (6) safety precautions to prevent accidents; (7) appropriate nutrition and exercise; (8) measures to prevent constipation; and (9) strong social interactions.
- Health problems of older adults include accidents, chronic disabling diseases, problematic drug use, mental health problems, older adult abuse, and cancer.
- The Canadian Gerontological Nursing Association speaks for many registered nurses committed to promoting the health and well-being of older adults and those who work with them.

ASSESS YOUR LEARNING

1. In view of the increased incidence of prostate cancer among older Canadian men, which of the following topics would be important to include in a health promotion presentation to a group of men?
- **a.** Signs and symptoms of prostate cancer.
- **b.** Screening practices for prostate cancer.
- **c.** Treatment for prostate cancer.
- **d.** Rising mortality rates of prostate cancer.

2. Mrs. Weathers, an 83-year-old long-term-care resident has Alzheimer's (SDAT). She has recently been diagnosed with pneumonia. When the nurse offers Mrs. Weathers, her 1200h antibiotic, she yells, "Get out, get out." Which of the following would be the most appropriate action for the nurse?
- **a.** Break open the capsule and place the powder in her lunch.
- **b.** Leave the medication on the bedside table and let her take it when she is ready.
- **c.** Quietly leave the room and return in 15 minutes to offer the medication.
- **d.** Emphasize to Mrs. Weathers that she must take the medication.

3. Mrs. Chino has recently been admitted to a long-term-care facility. She refuses to interact with other residents, appears sad, and has not been eating. How should the nurse intervene?
- **a.** Ask other residents to visit Mrs. Chino.
- **b.** Speak with Mrs. Chino about her feelings.
- **c.** Suggest that the physician prescribe an antidepressant.
- **d.** Take Mrs. Chino to social events in the facility.

4. Activity theory suggests that activity is which of the following?

a. Constrained by economic circumstances
b. Used by the individual to stay healthy
c. Maintained throughout the lifespan
d. Reduced according to age

5. Which of the following statements about abuse of older adults is true?

a. Trusteeship reduces the occurrence of older adult abuse.
b. Most abuse is committed by daughters and daughters-in-law.
c. Nurses must be familiar with national laws regarding the reporting of abuse of older adults.
d. Older clients should be assessed for the presence of abuse.

6. Six months ago, Mr. Harry experienced a right-sided cerebrovascular accident. When the home care nurse visits, she observes that Mr. Harry is reluctant to perform the exercises suggested by the physiotherapist when Mr. Harry was in hospital. How should the nurse intervene?

a. Encourage the client to perform the exercises on a regular basis.
b. Help the client to verbalize his feelings.
c. Refer the client to mental health services.
d. Talk to his wife about the reason why her husband is reluctant.

7. Usual physical changes associated with aging include which of the following?

a. Decreased muscle mass and tone
b. Orthostatic hypertension
c. Increased cardiac output
d. Urinary incontinence and frequency

8. Mrs. Wu has been a widow for about 7 months. She recently sold her house and moved into a seniors' complex, following the advice of her daughter, who lives about 600 km away. Influencing her decision was the fact that she has never driven a car. The nurse should be aware of what?

a. Mrs. Wu may be vulnerable to social isolation.
b. Mrs. Wu may be subject to abuse by her daughter.
c. Mrs. Wu may be experiencing dementia.
d. Retirement may be stressful to Mrs. Wu.

9. Mr. Ken, an 82-year-old retired engineer, likes to ride his bicycle to the library twice a week. What might this indicate to the nurse?

a. Chronological age is a more accurate indicator of abilities than is functional age.
b. Functional age is the same as chronological age.
c. Functional age is a more accurate indicator of abilities than is chronological age.
d. This is an example of continuity theory.

10. Mrs. Treathing, who is on a number of medications, was admitted to a long-term-care facility with Alzheimer's disease (SDAT) about 6 months ago. Over the past several days, she has demonstrated bizarre behaviour, hallucinations, and increased verbal rambling. How should the nurse intervene?

a. Ask other residents to visit Mrs. Treathing as she is experiencing sensory deprivation because of lack of social interaction.
b. Assess Mrs. Treathing for signs of adverse effects from the medications she is taking.
c. Inform the other staff of the changes in Mrs. Treathing's behaviour.
d. Request that a sedative be given to reduce Mrs. Treathing's aggressive behaviour.

After working through these questions, go to the MyNursingLab at ***http://www.mynursinglab.com*** *to check your answers and see explanations.*

SUGGESTED READINGS

Markle-Reid, M., Weir, R., Browne, G., Roberts, J., Gafni, A., & Henderson, S. (2006). Health promotion for frail older home care clients. *Nursing and Healthcare Management and Policy, 54*(3), 381–395.

This paper reports that older adults functioned better when proactive nursing health-promotion intervention was offered in addition to home care for older adults than when home care services alone were offered.

Wallace, M. (2008). *Essentials of gerontological nursing/Meredith Wallace.* New York: Springer.

This book describes the normal changes of aging, health assessment, and health promotion of older adults. Also included are medication usage, cognitive and psychological issues in aging, ethical issues of aging and independence, quality-of-life care, environments of care, end-of-life care, and future trends in geriatric nursing.

WEBLINKS

Canadian Association on Gerontology

http://www.cagacg.ca

The Canadian Association on Gerontology is a national, multidisciplinary, scientific, and educational association established to provide leadership in matters related to the aging population. Its website identifies its mandate, publications, annual conference, and educational support to students.

Canadian Gerontological Nursing Association

http://www.cgna.net

This site provides an introduction to the Canadian Gerontological Nursing Association, including its mission, role, and standards.

Public Health Agency of Canada, Division of Aging and Seniors

http://www.hc-sc.gc.ca/seniors-aines/index.htm

The Division of Aging and Seniors, Health Canada, provides federal leadership in areas pertaining to aging and older adults. The division serves as a portal for information and a centre for expertise.

Registered Nurses' Association of Ontario: Best Practice Guidelines

http://www.rnao.org/bestpractices/index.asp

This site provides access to the best practice guidelines developed by the Registered Nurses' Association of Ontario, including its best practice guidelines for "Screening for Delirium, Dementia, and Depression in Older Adults" (November 2003).

REFERENCES

Alzheimer's Society. (2007). Alzheimer's disease statistics. Retrieved August 26, 2008, from http://www.alzheimer.ca/english/disease/stats-people.htm

Beckingham, A. C., & Witter DuGas, B. (1993). *Promoting healthy aging: A nursing and community perspective.* St. Louis, MO: Mosby-Year Book.

Butler, R. (1963). The life review: An interpretation of reminiscence in the aged. *Psychiatry, 26,* 65–76.

Canadian Study of Health & Aging Working Group. (1994). Canadian study of health and aging: Study methods and prevalence of dementia. *Canadian Medical Association Journal, 150,* 899–912.

Clarke, P. J., Marshall, V., W., Ryff, C., & Rosenthal, C. J. (2000). Well-being in Canadian seniors: Findings from the Canadian study of health and aging. *Canadian Journal on Aging, 19,* 139–159.

Duvall, E. M. (1977). *Family development* (5th ed.). Philadelphia, PA: Lippincott.

Erikson, E. H. (1982). *The life cycle completed: A review.* New York, NY: Norton.

Fowler, J., & Keen, S. (1985). *Life maps: Conversations in the journey of faith.* Waco, TX: Word Books.

Fried L. P., Tangen, C., Walston, J., Newman, A., Hirsch, C. Gottdiener, J., et al. (2001). Frailty in older adults: Evidence for a phenotype. *The Journals of Gerontology Series A: Biological Sciences and Medical Sciences, 56,* M146–M157.

Government of Canada. (2006). *The human face of mental health and mental illness in Canada, 2006.* Retrieved October 15, 2007, from http://www.phac-aspc.gc.ca/publicat/human-humain06/pdf/human_face_e.pdf

Haveman, M. J. (2004). Disease epidemiology and aging people with intellectual disabilities. *Journal of Policy and Practice in Intellectual Disabilities, 1*(1), 16–23.

Havighurst, R. J. (1972). *Developmental tasks and education* (3rd ed.). New York, NY: Longman.

Health Canada. (2007). *Healthy living: Seniors.* Retrieved October 16, 2007, from http://www.hc-sc.gc.ca/hl-vs/seniors-aines/index_e.html

Kemp, C. L. (2003). The social demographic contours of contemporary grandparenthood: Mapping patterns in Canada and the United States. *Journal of Comparative Family Studies, 34,* 187–212.

Kohlberg, L. (1981). *The psychology of moral development: Moral stages and the idea of justice.* San Francisco, CA: Harper & Row.

Ogrodnik, L. (2007). *Family violence in Canada: A statistical profile, 2007.* Ottawa: Statistics Canada: Canadian Centre for Justice Statistics. Cat. No. 85-224-XIE.

Peck, R. (1968). Psychological development in the second half of life. In B. L. Neugarten (Ed.), *Middle age and aging* (pp. 137–147). Chicago, IL: University of Chicago Press.

Public Health Agency of Canada. (2007). *Seniors health.* Retrieved October 16, 2007, from http://www.phac-aspc.gc.ca/sh-sa_e.html

Statistics Canada. (2001). *Participation and activity limitation survey.* Ottawa: Minister of Supply and Services. Cat. No. 89-578-X.

Statistics Canada. (2006). *Portrait of the Canadian population in 2006, 2006 Census.* Ottawa: Minister of Supply and Services. Cat. No. 9705550-XIE.

Tabloski, P. A. (2006). *Gerontological nursing.* Upper Saddle River, NJ: Pearson Prentice Hall.

Wilkins, K. (2002). *Health reports—Supplement: Predictors of death in seniors.* Retrieved September 7, 2008, from http://www.statcan.ca/english/freepub/82-003-SIE/2005000/pdf/82-003-SIE20050007447.pdf

UNIT 4

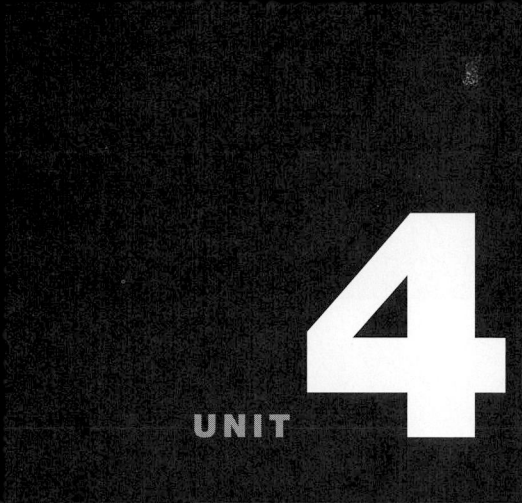

Integral Aspects of Nursing

CHAPTER 20
Critical Thinking

CHAPTER 21
Caring, Comforting, and Communicating

CHAPTER 22
Nursing Process

CHAPTER 23
Documenting and Reporting

CHAPTER 24
Nursing Informatics

CHAPTER 25
Teaching and Learning

CHAPTER 26
Leading, Managing, and Delegating

Chapter 20

Critical Thinking

The nature of the nursing discipline and the complexity of nurses' work mandate that nurses be *critical thinkers.* Nurses help clients solve problems or issues by critically analyzing contributing factors. *Critical thinking* allows the nurse and client to make better decisions. Critical thinking, problem solving, and decision making are interrelated processes. Creativity in problem solving and decision making can enhance the effectiveness of proposed solutions or decisions.

Nurses use critical thinking to make meaningful observations, draw sound conclusions, create new information and ideas, evaluate lines of reasoning, question prevailing assumptions, and improve self-knowledge. The Canadian Association of Schools of Nursing (1998) promotes and supports the use of critical thinking. It acknowledges the importance and relevance of critical thinking to the discipline and practice of nursing.

OBJECTIVES

After studying this chapter, you should be able to

1. Describe the characteristics, skills, and attitudes of critical thinking
2. Describe the significance of developing critical-thinking abilities to practise safe and competent nursing care
3. Discuss the relationship among critical thinking, the nursing process, and the problem-solving and decision-making processes
4. Discuss ways of demonstrating critical thinking in nursing practice

Critical Thinking

The thinking process that guides nursing practice must be organized, purposeful, and disciplined, rather than random or undirected. Simpson and Courtney (2002) explain **critical thinking** as "a process, an orientation of the mind, . . . including both the cognitive and affective domains of reasoning" (p. 91). Parse (1996) describes critical thinking as "carefully choosing a direction in light of personal tacit and explicit knowing" (p. 139). Critical thinking involves calling into question the assumptions that underlie usual ways of thinking about people and acting in situations, and then being prepared to think and act differently on the basis of this critical questioning (Brookfield, 1987). Assumptions are those unquestioned givens that are taken for granted as being self-evident truths. Critical thinking is "the art of thinking about thinking" (Paul, 1988, pp. 2–3). It is purposeful thinking wherein the thinker systematically and habitually imposes criteria and intellectual standards on thinking. The thinker is aware of and takes charge of the thinking process, guiding it according to these standards (Paul, 1993).

Critical thinking is a complex process, and within health sciences literature are different conceptualizations of critical thinking. In nursing, critical thinking moves beyond thinking to include purposeful action. An international panel of nursing experts from nine countries who participated in examining conceptualizations of critical thinking developed the following consensus statement:

> *Critical thinking is an essential component of professional accountability and quality nursing care. Critical thinkers in nursing exhibit these habits of the mind: confidence, contextual perspective, creativity, flexibility, inquisitiveness, intellectual integrity, intuition, open-mindedness, perseverance, and reflection. Critical thinkers in nursing practice the cognitive skill of analyzing, applying standards, discriminating, information seeking, logical reasoning, predicting and transforming knowledge. (Scheffer & Rubenfeld, 2000, p. 357)*

Critical thinking is essential for safe and competent nursing practice. Oermann and Gaberson (2006) stated that "critical thinking is needed to make reasoned and informed judgments in the practice setting; by using critical thinking, the nurse decides what to do or believe in a given situation" (p. 114). As they plan and deliver care, nurses are expected to help clients solve problems by critically analyzing contributing factors. This critical analysis, or critical thinking, allows the nurse and client to make better decisions, particularly when neither clear answers nor standardized procedures are available and when conflicting forces make decisions complex. Nurses, therefore, need to embrace the attitudes that promote critical thinking and master critical-thinking skills to process and evaluate information from a variety of sources:

- *Nurses use knowledge from other disciplines.* Nurses deal holistically with human responses. They must draw meaningful information from other disciplines (i.e., make multidisciplinary and interdisciplinary connections) to understand the meaning of client data and plan effective interventions. Using insights from different disciplines to shed light on issues requires critical thought. For example, registered nurses might use information from nutrition, physiology, and physics to promote wound healing and prevent further injury to a client with a pressure ulcer. In preparation for practice, nursing students take courses in the biological and social sciences and humanities so they can acquire a strong foundation on which to build their nursing science knowledge and skill.
- *Nurses deal with change in stressful environments.* Nurses work in rapidly changing situations. Treatments, medications, and technology change constantly, and client conditions can change from minute to minute. Routine actions, therefore, may not be adequate to address all issues. For example, familiarity with the mechanics of drawing up medication in a syringe will not help the nurse deal with a client who is afraid of needles or with one who refuses a medication. When unexpected situations such as these arise, critical thinking enables the nurse to recognize important cues, such as cultural values and beliefs; draw on relevant knowledge; and adapt interventions to meet specific client needs.
- *Nurses make important decisions.* During the course of a workday, nurses make many vital decisions. These decisions often determine the well-being of clients and even their very survival, so it is important that the decisions be sound. Nurses use critical-thinking skills to collect, compile, and interpret the information needed to make decisions. For example, nurses must use prudent judgment to decide which observations to report to the appropriate member of the health-care team immediately and which can be noted in the patient record for the appropriate member of the health-care team to address later, during the routine client visit.

Creativity—original thinking—is a major component of critical thinking. When nurses incorporate creativity into their thinking, they are able to find unique solutions to unique problems. Creative thinking is thinking that results in the development of new ideas and products (Reilly & Oermann, 1992). Creativity in problem solving and decision making is the ability to develop and implement new and better solutions or ideas (Sullivan & Decker, 2005).

A creative thinker uses a combination of knowledge and imagination in practice (Simpson & Courtney, 2002). Students who engage in the creative-thinking process of reflection can develop links between theoretical classroom and clinical practice concepts by analyzing problems and synthesizing information (Kalischuk &

Thorpe, 2002). This process can support students' creation of new meanings about nursing practice with client and families (see the Evidence-Informed Practice box).

Creative thinking may be further enhanced through students' creation of concept maps. **Concept maps** essentially consist of pieces of information or ideas presented in a visual scheme with links or relationships among them. Development of concept maps or concept mapping helps move students from thinking about health issues in a linear manner to being able to visualize the interactions and overlapping of structures, resources, strengths, and issues that influence client, family, or community health (Hsu & Hsieh, 2005). Visual mapping of relationships enables students to develop and clarify links among key pieces of information. As more information is gathered about a client, family, or community, or as the student gains knowledge and experience, the concept maps become more detailed and integrated.

Critical thinking is an essential component of nursing practice. Nurses' work environments are always changing; thus, critical thinking is a vital part of providing competent client care (Brunt, 2005; Ignatavicius, 2001; Martin, 2002). Critical-thinking skills are developed over time through practice and with constructive feedback. Nurses must assess clients and be knowledgeable about their health histories. Additionally, nurses must seek out relevant resources and research-based evidence to guide their practice.

Ignatavicius (2001, p. 38) identifies several characteristics of an *expert critical thinker.* As you read this list, consider its fit with your personality and how you act in clinical situations:

- *Outcomes directed*
- *Open to new ideas*
- *Flexible*
- *Willing to change, risk taker*
- *Innovative*
- *Creative*
- *Analytical*
- *Communicator*
- *Assertive*
- *Persistent*
- *Caring*
- *Energetic*
- *Knowledgeable*
- *Resourceful*
- *Observant*
- *Intuitive*
- *Out of box thinker*

Evidence-Informed Practice

Do Concept Maps Improve Critical Thinking?

Using a descriptive exploratory design, Hicks-Moore and Pasterik (2006) incorporated both quantitative and qualitative methods to assess second-year baccalaureate students' level of critical thinking in their concept maps (CM) during a clinical practicum course. The holistic critical-thinking scoring rubric (HCTSR) was used to examine students' CM within the following six competencies: interpretation, analysis, evaluation, inference, explanation, and self-regulation. Eighteen students submitted a CM, and 8 of those students participated in a focus group. In addition, 3 clinical teachers were involved in a separate focus group. Content analysis of focus group discussions revealed that students felt that using CM enhanced their abilities to work with clients and prioritize care. One student commented, "It was a great way to frame everything holistically, so you didn't look at individual things or look at the client in silos" (p. 7). Clinical teachers noted that students' use of CM supported their abilities to interconnect key aspects of the client's health situation. CM allowed instructors to understand how students approached client problems, data analysis, and rationale for client care.

NURSING IMPLICATIONS: Concept mapping is a useful tool to enhance students' abilities to organize and prioritize client care and to increase confidence to carry out competencies that support effective and quality client care.

Source: Based on "Evaluating Critical Thinking in Clinical Concept Maps: A Pilot Study," by S. L. Hicks-Moore and P. Pasterik, 2006, *International Journal of Nursing Education Scholarship, 3*(1), Article 27. Retrieved April 10, 2008, from http://www.bepress.com/ijnes/vol3/iss1/art27/

Critical-Thinking Abilities

Complex thinking processes, such as critical analysis, problem solving, and decision making, require critical thinking. These cognitive abilities include critical analysis, inductive and deductive reasoning, making valid inferences, differentiating facts from opinions, evaluating the credibility of information sources, clarifying concepts, and recognizing assumptions.

Critical analysis involves the use of questions that can be applied to a particular situation or idea to determine essential, and discard superfluous information and ideas. The questions are *not* sequential steps; rather, they form a set of criteria for judging an idea. Not all questions will need to be applied to every situation, but being aware of all the questions and choosing those appropriate to a given situation is important.

Socrates (born about 470 B.C.E.) was a Greek philosopher who developed the Socratic method of question and answer. Box 20.1 lists the Socratic questions to use in critical analysis. **Socratic questions** can be used to look beneath the surface, recognize and examine assumptions, search for inconsistencies, examine multiple points of view, and differentiate what is known from what is believed. Nurses can employ Socratic questioning when listening to an end-of-shift report, reviewing

BOX 20.1 SOCRATIC QUESTIONS

Nurses can use Socratic questions to help them think critically:

QUESTIONS ABOUT THE QUESTION (OR PROBLEM)

- Is this question clear, understandable, and correctly identified?
- Is this question important?
- Could this question be broken down into smaller parts?
- How might ________ state this question?

QUESTIONS ABOUT ASSUMPTIONS

- You seem to be assuming ________; is that so?
- What could you assume instead? Why?
- Does this assumption always hold true?

QUESTIONS ABOUT POINT OF VIEW

- You seem to be using the perspective of ________. Why?
- What would someone who disagrees with your perspective say?
- Can you see this any other way?

QUESTIONS ABOUT EVIDENCE AND REASONS

- What evidence do you have for that?
- Is there any reason to doubt that evidence?
- How do you know?
- What would change your mind?

QUESTIONS ABOUT IMPLICATIONS AND CONSEQUENCES

- What effect would that have?
- What is the probability that will actually happen?
- What are the alternatives?
- What are the implications of that?

Source: "The Thinker's Guide to the Art of Socratic Questioning," by R. Paul and L. Elder, 2006. Retrieved October 21, 2008, from http://www.criticalthinking.org/files/SocraticQuestioning2006.pdf

TABLE 20.1 Differentiating Types of Statements

Statement	Description	Example
Facts	Can be corroborated through investigation	Blood pressure is affected by blood volume.
Inferences	Conclusions drawn from the facts, going beyond facts to make a statement about something not currently known	If blood volume is decreased (e.g., in hemorrhagic shock), blood pressure will drop.
Judgments	Evaluation of facts or information that reflect values or other criteria; a type of opinion	It is harmful to the client's health if his or her blood pressure drops too low.
Opinions	Beliefs formed over time include judgments that may fit facts or be in error	Nursing intervention can assist in maintaining the client's blood pressure within normal limits.

a client health history or progress notes, planning care, or discussing a client's care with the client, colleagues, and other health professionals (Paul, 1993).

Two other skills used in complex thinking are inductive and deductive reasoning. In **inductive reasoning**, generalizations are formed from a set of facts or observations. When viewed together, certain bits of information suggest a particular interpretation proceeding from the specific to the general. For example, the nurse who observes that a patient has dry skin, poor tissue turgor, sunken eyes, and dark amber urine may make the generalization that the patient is dehydrated.

Deductive reasoning, by contrast, is reasoning from a general to a specific conclusion. If you begin with the premise that the sum of the angles in any triangle is always 180 degrees, you can then conclude that the sum of the angles in the triangle you happen to have is also 180 degrees. A nurse might start with a premise that all children love apple juice. If the client is a child, then the child will love apple juice. This is an example in which the premise is not always valid and, thus, the conclusion also may not be valid.

Nurses use critical thinking to help analyze situations and establish which premises are valid. By using critical thinking, the nurse also differentiates facts, inferences, judgments, and opinions (see Table 20.1).

Attitudes That Foster Critical Thinking

Certain attitudes are crucial to critical thinking. These *affective* dimensions are based on the assumption that a rational person is motivated to develop, learn, and grow. A critical thinker, according to Paul (1993), works to develop the following attitudes or traits: independence of thought, fair-mindedness, insight, intellectual humility, intellectual courage, integrity, perseverance, confidence, curiosity, and contextual awareness.

Independence of Thought

Critical thinking requires that individuals think for themselves. People acquire many beliefs in their childhood that are not necessarily based on reason. These provide an explanation they can comprehend or offer rational reasons for believing. Rewards may have been associated with believing. Alternatively, these beliefs may be an outcome of not questioning the authorities promoting them. As critical thinkers mature and acquire knowledge and experience, they examine their beliefs and assumptions in light of new evidence. Critical thinkers consider a wide range of ideas, learn from them, and then make their own judgments about them.

Fair-Mindedness

Critical thinkers are fair-minded, assessing all viewpoints against the same standards and not basing judgments on personal or group bias or prejudice (Catalano, 2003). Fair-mindedness helps people consider opposing points of view and try to understand new ideas fully before rejecting or accepting them. Critical thinkers strive to be open to the possibility that new evidence or information could change their minds.

Insight

Critical thinkers are open to the possibility that their personal biases or social pressures and customs could unduly affect their thinking. They actively try to examine their own biases and bring them to awareness each time they think or make a decision. For example, consider a nurse who spent extensive time trying to teach a client how to prevent a recurrence of some problem but was mystified when the client appeared uninterested and did not follow the nurse's advice. The nurse's egocentric tendency to assume that all clients would be motivated and interested in preventive care (just because the nurse was) resulted in an inaccurate assessment of the client's desire and readiness to learn; both the nurse's and the client's time was wasted. Had the nurse assessed the client's understandings about what caused the disease, and considered the client's cultural background, beliefs, and perhaps even the client's support systems (that is, had the nurse collected sufficient evidence), the nurse might have developed more meaningful insights about the issues of immediate concern to the client, identified a more relevant problem, and developed an appropriate care plan.

Intellectual Humility

Intellectual humility means having an awareness of the limits of your own knowledge. Critical thinkers are willing to admit what they do not know; they are willing to seek new information and rethink their conclusions in light of new knowledge. They never assume that what everybody knows to be right will always be right, because new evidence may emerge. A hospital nurse might be unable to imagine how the 80-year-old wife will care for her husband, who has recently had a stroke. However, the nurse also recognizes that it is not really possible to know what the couple can achieve without further assessment.

Intellectual Courage

With an attitude of courage, people are willing to consider and examine their own ideas or views, especially those to which they have a strong negative reaction. This type of courage comes from recognizing that beliefs or assumptions are sometimes false or misleading. Values, assumptions, and beliefs are not always acquired rationally (see Chapter 5).

Rational beliefs are those that have been examined and found to be supported by solid reasons and data. After such examination, it is inevitable that some ideas, previously held to be true, are found to contain questionable elements and that some truth may emerge from ideas considered dangerous or false. Courage is needed to be true to new thinking in such cases, especially if social penalties for nonconformity are severe. As an example, some nurses may believe that allowing family members to observe an emergency (such as cardiopulmonary resuscitation) would be psychologically harmful to the family and that members would get in the healthcare team's way. Others may feel that blanket exclusion of family members was unnecessary and extremely stressful for some of them. As a result, nurses can initiate research to demonstrate that the family can be present without detrimental effects to the nurse, the client, or the family.

Integrity

Intellectual integrity requires that individuals apply the same rigorous standards of proof to their own knowledge and beliefs as they apply to the knowledge and beliefs of others. Critical thinkers question their own knowledge and beliefs or assumptions as quickly and thoroughly as they challenge those of another. They are readily able to admit and evaluate inconsistencies within their own beliefs and between their own beliefs and those of another. For example, a nurse might believe that wound care always requires sterile technique. Reading an evidence-based article on the use and outcomes of clean technique for some wounds leads the critically thinking nurse to reconsider.

Perseverance

Nurses who are critical thinkers show perseverance in seeking effective solutions to client and nursing problems. This determination enables them to clarify concepts and sort out related issues, in spite of difficulties and frustrations. Confusion and frustration are uncomfortable, but critical thinkers resist the temptation to find a quick and easy answer. Important questions tend to be complex and confusing and, therefore, often require a great deal of thought and research to arrive at an answer. The nurse needs to continue to address the issue until it is resolved and to resist the temptation to come to a hasty conclusion on a complex issue.

Confidence

Critical thinkers believe that well-reasoned thinking will lead to trustworthy conclusions. Therefore, they cultivate an attitude of confidence in the reasoning process and examine emotion-laden arguments by using the standards for evaluating thought, by asking questions, such as, Is that argument fair? Is it based on sufficient evidence?

The critical thinker develops skill in both inductive reasoning and deductive reasoning. As a critical thinker gains greater awareness of the thinking process and more experience in improving such thinking, confidence in the thinking process will grow. This confident thinker will not be afraid of disagreement and, indeed, will be concerned when all agree too quickly. Such an individual can serve as a role model to colleagues, inspiring and encouraging them to think critically as well.

REASONING PROCESS Clear reasoning is particularly important when problems are complex, lack clarity, and have multiple potential solutions (Oermann & Gaberson, 2006). Oermann and Gaberson (2006) refer to the works of Paul (1993) and Paul and Elder (2005) when summarizing the eight elements of reasoning composing the critical-thinking process:

1. Purpose of the critical thinking
2. Question, issue, or problem that requires resolution
3. Assumptions about the problem
4. Analysis of own and others' points of view
5. Data and evidence to support
6. Concepts and theories used in thinking
7. Inferences and conclusions based on given data
8. Implications and consequences of reasoning

Comer (2005) likens the clinical reasoning process to investigative detective work in which students use the nursing process as an investigative tool to support critical-thinking skills. Students identify a clinical issue to investigate and approach the client's health situation as a mystery to be solved. Comer suggests that students develop a table with investigative headings and columns of assessment data (see Table 20.2).

Clinical detective conclusions: Ineffective airway clearance is related to inadequate hydration, secondary to failure to drink fluids and the presence of postoperative pain, as evidenced by lab results, poor skin turgor, and complaints of thirst and discomfort at the incision site. Goal: patient will drink 250 mL of water every 4 hours for 24 hours. Analgesics will reduce incisional pain and increase mobility.

Curiosity

The internal conversation going on within the mind of a critical thinker is filled with questions: Why do we believe this? What causes that? Does it have to be this way? Could something else work? What would happen if we did it another way? Who says that is so? The curious individual

TABLE 20.2 Clinical Detective Tool

Clinical Mystery	Nursing Diagnosis	Suspects	Investigative Criteria	Findings of Investigation	Hypothesis	Culprit
Why is my patient not coughing up secretions even though his breathing is noisy?	Ineffective airway clearance	Inadequate hydration Ineffective cough	CVP Hgb Bun Creat	CVP = 4 cm H_2O Hgb = 161 g/L Bun = 12 mmol/L Creat = 135 μmol/L	The ineffective airway clearance is likely related to: Inadequate hydration Decreased mobility	Inadequate hydration: patient not drinking adequate amount of fluid Postoperative incisional pain
		Lack of adequate mobility post-operatively	Turgor Intake Output	Poor skin turgor I-500 mL O-750 mL States: I'm just not thirsty		
		Possible postoperative pain	O_2 Sat	O_2 Sat = 96% on 2L nasal prongs		

Source: Adapted from "Clinical Reasoning: Turning Your Students into Clinical Detectives," by S. Comer, 2005, *Nurse Educator, 30*(6), pp. 235–237.

may value tradition but is not afraid to examine traditions to be sure they are still valid. Ruggiero (2006) suggests the following strategies to develop a sense of curiosity and creativity: force uncommon responses, use free association, use analogy, look for unusual combinations, visualize the solution, construct pro and con arguments, and construct relevant scenarios. These strategies can be practised by students as a means to stimulate imagination and discover solutions. The nurse can, for example, apply these questions and strategies to the issue of moving responsibility for a procedure, such as drawing arterial blood samples, among the nursing, respiratory therapy, or laboratory department staff.

Contextual Awareness

Although critical thinking is a rational process, it also entails a contextual dimension in which personal assumptions and actions are questioned within particular contexts. Forneris and Peden-McAlpine (2006) said that *context* is "the nature of the world in a given moment and includes culture, knowledge, underlying assumptions, facts, rules and principles shaping how knowledge is constructed" (p. 2). They suggested that contextual learning contributes to the development of critical-thinking attributes that support students' awareness and consideration of context, dialogue, reflection, and time in the caring interaction with clients and families. We will define **context** as the unique experiences that individuals or clients bring with them to their specific situations or circumstances. Being conscious of context can be called **contextual awareness**. **Assumptions** are those unquestioned givens taken for granted as being self-evident truths about others or situations that we encounter.

Standards of Critical Thinking

How can people know whether their thinking is critical thinking? Paul and Elder (2005) proposed that thinkers can use universal standards, as shown in Table 20.3. Explicitly stating the standards for critical thinking promotes the reliability and validity of the thinking and, thus, makes appropriate action more likely.

TABLE 20.3 Universal Intellectual Standards

Standard	Sample Question
Clarity	What is an example of this?
Accuracy	How can I find out if that is true?
Relevance	How does that help me with the issue?
Logicalness	Does that follow from the evidence?
Breadth	Do I need to consider another point of view?
Precision	Can I be more specific?
Significance	Which of these facts is most important?
Completeness	Have I missed any important aspects?
Fairness	Am I considering the thinking of others?
Depth	What makes this a difficult problem?

Source: From *A Guide for Educators to Critical Thinking Competency Standards* (p. 57), by R. Paul and L. Elder, 2005, Dillon Beach, CA: Foundation for Critical Thinking. Adapted with permission.

Applying Critical Thinking to Nursing Practice

Nurses function effectively some part of every day without thinking critically. Many small decisions are based primarily on habit, with minimal thinking involved; examples include selecting what clothes to wear, choosing which route to take to work, and deciding what to eat for lunch. Psychomotor skills in nursing often involve minimal thinking, such as operating a familiar piece of equipment. But the higher-order skills of critical thinking are needed as soon as a new idea or situation is encountered or a less-than-routine decision must be made.

The **nursing process** is a systematic, rational method of planning and providing individualized nursing care. The phases of the nursing process—assessing, diagnosing, planning, implementing, and evaluating—are discussed in detail in Chapter 22. The phases of the nursing process and their application to a clinical example of critical thinking are shown in Table 20.4, which demonstrates the use of critical thinking with individual clients. In addition, a nurse employs critical thinking when setting priorities for the day. When analyzing a situation and planning strategies for conflict resolution or change, the nurse manager also uses critical thinking. Nurses use critical thinking in nursing practice primarily when solving problems and making decisions. Problem solving and decision making are described in more detail in the sections that follow.

Problem Solving

Critical thinking, problem solving, and decision making are interrelated processes. In comparison, critical thinking is a broader process that relies on examination of knowledge and assumptions, and exploration of alternatives that can include both problem solving and decision making. Problem solving and decision making are often used interchangeably; however, they are different. **Problem solving** involves working through a process of recognizing, defining, and then solving a problem. Many alternative solutions may be considered and implemented in resolving the problem. In *decision making*, alternatives are examined and the one most appropriate to the situation is selected. Decision making may or may

TABLE 20.4 Phases of the Nursing Process and Clinical Examples of Critical Thinking

Nursing Process	Clinical Application
Assessing	*Data:* A 45-year-old Aboriginal male states he has a severe headache; 10 kg overweight; blood pressure 180/95 mmHg. States he has been taking high blood pressure pills only when he has a headache. Is self-employed as a gardener; lives with wife, mother-in-law, and four children. Given these data, a critical thinker is aware that more data must be obtained about the client's cultural health values and reasons for stated behaviour. Failure to think critically and to obtain additional data leads to inaccurate goals, diagnosis, and interventions.
Goal setting	*Goal:* To increase compliance with medication regimen in order to relieve headaches and prevent a cerebrovascular accident (CVA). Thinking critically, a nurse will try to determine the client's goals and to agree to mutual goals.
Diagnosing	A critical thinker will defer identifying the client's diagnosis until more data are obtained and the client's priorities are known. This delay prevents a premature diagnosis based on insufficient data.
Diagnosing	As a critical thinker, the nurse is aware that the client's point of view may differ from the nurse's. Although the nurse may support the Western medical belief system that puts high priority on preventing disease, the critical thinker is also aware that the client may hold diverse views of health and illness, therapy, and preventive measures.
Diagnosing	The critical thinker recognizes that the client's erratic use of the prescribed medication may have multiple causes (e.g., troublesome side effects, or belief that illness is due to God's will and is not preventable) and will not infer a diagnosis with etiology until more data are obtained. Failure to think critically can lead to interpretations that are irrelevant, inadequate, and superficial (e.g., an erroneous interpretation that the client's problem is lack of sufficient knowledge).
Diagnosing	The critical thinker makes assumptions in accordance with a broad, unbiased database and mutually sets client goals. The critical thinker avoids making unverified assumptions, such as that an increase in knowledge will increase this client's compliance or that this client is motivated to prevent a CVA.
Planning	The critical thinker uses concepts about motivation, change theory, and multicultural nursing to understand the client's behaviour and motivation to change. Failure to think critically can lead to exclusive reliance on a simplistic concept, such as "knowledge creates change."
Implementing	The critical thinker considers the implications and consequences of selected nursing strategies before implementing plans of care. Plans of care, including goals and outcomes, are based on ongoing assessment of the client's cultural values, beliefs, and needs. Failure to think critically may lead to ineffective interventions, such as client teaching that focuses only on resolving a knowledge deficit about the prescribed medication. The critical thinker recognizes that a knowledge deficit may or may not be one of several problems.
Evaluating	The critical thinker bases evaluation of client outcomes and the effectiveness of nursing interventions on well-developed, measurable criteria and considers rationally whether outcomes have been validated. Failure to think critically may lead to client noncompliance and an inference that the client did not learn effectively and needs further instruction.

not involve a problem (Ignatavicius, 2001; Sullivan & Decker, 2005).

In problem solving, the nurse obtains information that clarifies the nature of the problem and suggests possible solutions. The nurse then carefully evaluates the possible solutions, chooses the best one to implement, and continues to monitor outcomes and the effectiveness of the solution. The nurse does not discard the other possible solutions but holds them in reserve in the event that the first solution is ineffective. In the same way, depending on the client context, an alternative solution may be more appropriate. Therefore, problem solving for one situation contributes to the nurse's body of knowledge for problem solving in other similar situations (Sullivan & Decker, 2005). Some approaches to problem solving are described next.

TRIAL AND ERROR One way to solve problems is through **trial and error**; that is, a number of approaches are tried until a solution is found. However, knowing why a solution was effective may be difficult to determine if alternatives are not considered systematically. Trial-and-error methods in nursing care can be dangerous because the client might suffer harm if a particular solution or approach is inappropriate (Sullivan & Decker, 2005).

INTUITION **Intuition** is the understanding or learning of things without the conscious use of reasoning. It is also known as sixth sense, hunch, instinct, feeling, or suspicion. As a problem-solving approach, some people view intuition as a form of guessing, and, as such, an inappropriate basis for nursing decisions. However, others view intuition as an essential and legitimate aspect of clinical judgment acquired through knowledge and experience. The nurse must first have the knowledge base necessary to practise in the clinical area and then use that knowledge in clinical practice. Clinical experience allows the nurse to recognize cues and patterns and begin to reach correct conclusions.

Experience is important in improving intuition because the rapidity of the judgment depends on the nurse having seen similar client situations many times before. Sometimes, nurses use the words "I had a feeling" to describe a leap (or a condensing) in the critical-thinking element of considering evidence. These nurses are able to judge quickly and decisively which evidence is most important and to act on that limited evidence. The reliability of intuitive decision making increases as the nurse gains experience in the clinical application of theory. Ruth-Sahd and Hendy (2005) examined the use of intuition by novice nurses in relation to their personal, interpersonal, and professional experiences. Nurses who were older, had experienced more personal/family hospitalizations, and perceived greater social support from colleagues, family, and friends, relied more often on the use of intuition to inform client care decision making than did other nurses.

Decision Making

Decision making is a critical-thinking process for weighing and choosing the best actions to meet a desired goal (Sullivan & Decker, 2005). Decisions must be made whenever several mutually exclusive choices exist. For example, the individual who wants to become a nurse in Canada can choose from many different university programs throughout the country. To make an appropriate decision, a prospective student must evaluate the programs and consider personal circumstances, as well as any other relevant data that may influence the choice.

Nurses make decisions in their personal and professional lives. For example, when faced with meeting several clients' needs at the same time, the nurse must decide which client to assist first. When a client is trying to make a decision about what course of treatment to follow, the nurse may need to provide the client with information or resources (see the Lifespan Considerations box). From a more personal perspective, the nurse must decide whether to work in a hospital or a community and in an urban or a rural setting. Decision making is an important process and takes place at many levels.

Lifespan Considerations

Health-Care Decisions for Children and Older Adults

CHILDREN

Parents most often make decisions about the health care of children. Growing children can participate in those decisions in age-appropriate ways. As described by Piaget (1966), children's ability to reason and critically think about themselves and their situation develops gradually (see Chapter 16).

At each stage, nurses should be aware of the ways children think and sensitive to how children can be involved in health-care decisions:

- Infants progress from reflexive behaviour to simple, repetitive behaviour and then to imitative behaviours, learning the concepts of cause and effect and object permanence. Though not involved in making decisions, they need to be comforted and secure as care is given.
- Toddlers and preschoolers are very egocentric and engage in magical thinking. They cannot reason out the implications of care but need explanations in language they can understand. Play therapy and the use of dolls and toys can help them adjust to care, and they can sometimes be given options (e.g., do you want your dressing changed before breakfast or after?).
- School-age children tend to be concrete thinkers. They benefit from simple, direct explanations; hands-on exploration of equipment and materials; and the chance to help the care provider as appropriate during procedures. Involving these children in care can increase cooperation and decrease anxiety.
- Adolescents are increasingly able to think abstractly and may make many of their own health-care decisions. They should be actively consulted as a part of the family system.

OLDER ADULTS

It is important to include all adult clients in decision making and planning nursing care, but it is especially difficult to do this when working with elders who have impaired cognitive abilities, such as Alzheimer's disease. The nurse should allow them as much control and input as possible, keeping things simple and direct so they understand. Older adults with impairments are usually unable to perform multiple tasks or to think of more than one step at a time. The nurse must have patience and be willing to calmly repeat instructions if necessary. Presenting and discussing issues in basic terms helps to maintain respect and dignity and allows older adults to participate in their own care for as long as possible. If the older adult is unable to perform self-care activities, such as bathing, or health-related activities, such as a dressing change, the nurse seeks appropriate alternative methods for assisting the older adult with these.

The Canadian Nurses Association (2008) emphasized the importance of critical thinking when problem solving and making decisions in nursing practice. This value is also underscored by the College of Nurses of Ontario (CNO) and a decision-making framework was developed for practice. This decision-making framework consists of the following key questions that students and entry-level registered nurses can consider after a client assessment has been completed (College of Nurses of Ontario [CNO], 2005):

1. Do I need assistance to analyze the assessment data?
2. Based on the assessment data, what are the possible options of care and the indications and contraindications for each?
3. Am I satisfied that the proposed care is appropriate for the client, given the particular circumstances and the range of alternative options available?
4. Do I have the authority to provide the proposed care?
5. Am I competent to provide the proposed care?
6. Has the nursing care provided achieved the desired outcomes?

Sullivan and Decker (2005, p. 108) identify a seven-step decision-making process:

1. *Identify the purpose:* The nurse identifies why a decision is needed and what needs to be determined.
2. *Set the criteria:* To set the criteria for decision making, three questions must be answered: what needs to be achieved? What needs to be preserved? What needs to be avoided? For example, for a client with pain, the criteria would be as follows:
   a. What needs to be achieved? Relief of pain
   b. What needs to be preserved? Physical functioning, cognitive functioning, psychological functioning, client comfort
   c. What needs to be avoided? Central nervous system depression, respiratory depression, nausea
3. *Weight the criteria:* The decision maker sets priorities or ranks activities or services in order of importance from least important to most important as they relate to the specific situation. Because the weighting is specific to the situation, an activity can be ranked as most important in one situation and of less importance in another situation.
4. *Seek alternatives:* After establishing and weighting the criteria, the decision maker identifies all possible ways to meet the criteria. In clinical situations, the alternatives may be selected from a range of nursing interventions or client care strategies.
5. *Test alternatives:* The nurse analyzes the alternatives to ensure that he or she has an objective rationale in relation to the established criteria for choosing one strategy over another.
6. *Troubleshoot:* The nurse tries to determine what might go wrong as a result of a decision and develops plans to prevent, minimize, or overcome any problems.
7. *Evaluate the action:* The nurse determines how effective the strategies were and whether they achieved the initial purpose.

The decision-making process and the nursing process share similarities. The nurse uses decision making in all steps of the nursing process. The steps of these two processes are compared in Table 20.5.

TABLE 20.5 Comparison between the Nursing Process and the Decision-Making Process

Nursing Process	Decision-Making Process*
Assess	Identify the purpose
Diagnose	
Plan	Set the criteria Weight the criteria Seek and examine alternatives
Implement	Test alternatives Troubleshoot
Evaluate	Evaluate the action

Note: The decision-making process parallels the nursing process but is also used during each phase of the process.

Developing Critical-Thinking Attitudes and Skills

After gaining an appreciation of what it means to think critically, solve problems, and make decisions, nurses need to become aware of their own thinking style and abilities. Acquiring critical-thinking skills and a critical attitude becomes a matter of practice. Critical thinking is a process that should not be reduced to a singular definition but described according to its "components and central features, phases, and characteristics by which it might be recognized . . . all of which result in a change in belief or course of action" (Riddell, 2007, p. 122). These key components encompass the process of reflection, appraisal of assumptions, inquiry, interpretation, analysis, reasoning, judgment, and contextual considerations (Riddell, 2007).

Critical thinking is not an either/or phenomenon; people develop and use it more or less effectively along a continuum. Some people make better evaluations than others do; some people believe information from nearly any source; still others seldom believe anything without carefully evaluating the credibility of the information. Critical thinking is not easy. Solving problems and making decisions is risky. Sometimes, the outcome is not what was desired. With effort and practice, however, almost everyone can achieve some level of critical thinking and become an effective problem solver and decision maker.

Making Self-Assessments

The nurse should reflect on some of the attitudes discussed earlier that facilitate critical thinking, such as attitudes of curiosity, fair-mindedness, humility, courage, perseverance, and contextual awareness. A nurse might benefit from a rigorous personal assessment to determine which attitudes he or she already possesses and which need to be cultivated. This could also be done with a partner or as a group. The nurse first determines which attitudes are held strongly and form a base for thinking and which are held minimally or not at all. The nurse also needs to reflect on situations in which he or she made decisions that were later regretted and to analyze thinking processes and attitudes or ask a trusted colleague to assess them. Identifying weak or vulnerable skills and attitudes is also important.

Reflection, at every step of critical thinking and nursing care, helps examine the ways in which the nurse gathers and analyzes data, makes decisions, and determines the effectiveness of interventions. Reflection requires the nurse to pause in order to consider his or her beliefs, knowledge, values, and abilities in the situation at hand. The purpose of this reflection is to determine whether the current course of action is the best one and to improve future actions. Figure 20.1 is a visual depiction of the interactive loops of concepts used in critical thinking. Note that the action of reflection appears as part of three of the steps shown: the starting points, processes, and outcomes.

Tolerating Dissonance and Ambiguity

How recent nursing graduates cope with ambiguity in practice and uncertainty becomes the precursor to initiating their critical-thinking process (Boychuk Duchscher, 2003). Nurses, therefore, need to take deliberate efforts to cultivate critical-thinking attitudes. For example, to develop fair-mindedness, a nurse could deliberately seek out information that is opposed to his or her own views; this provides practice in understanding and learning to be open to other viewpoints. It is a human tendency to seek out information that corresponds to previously held

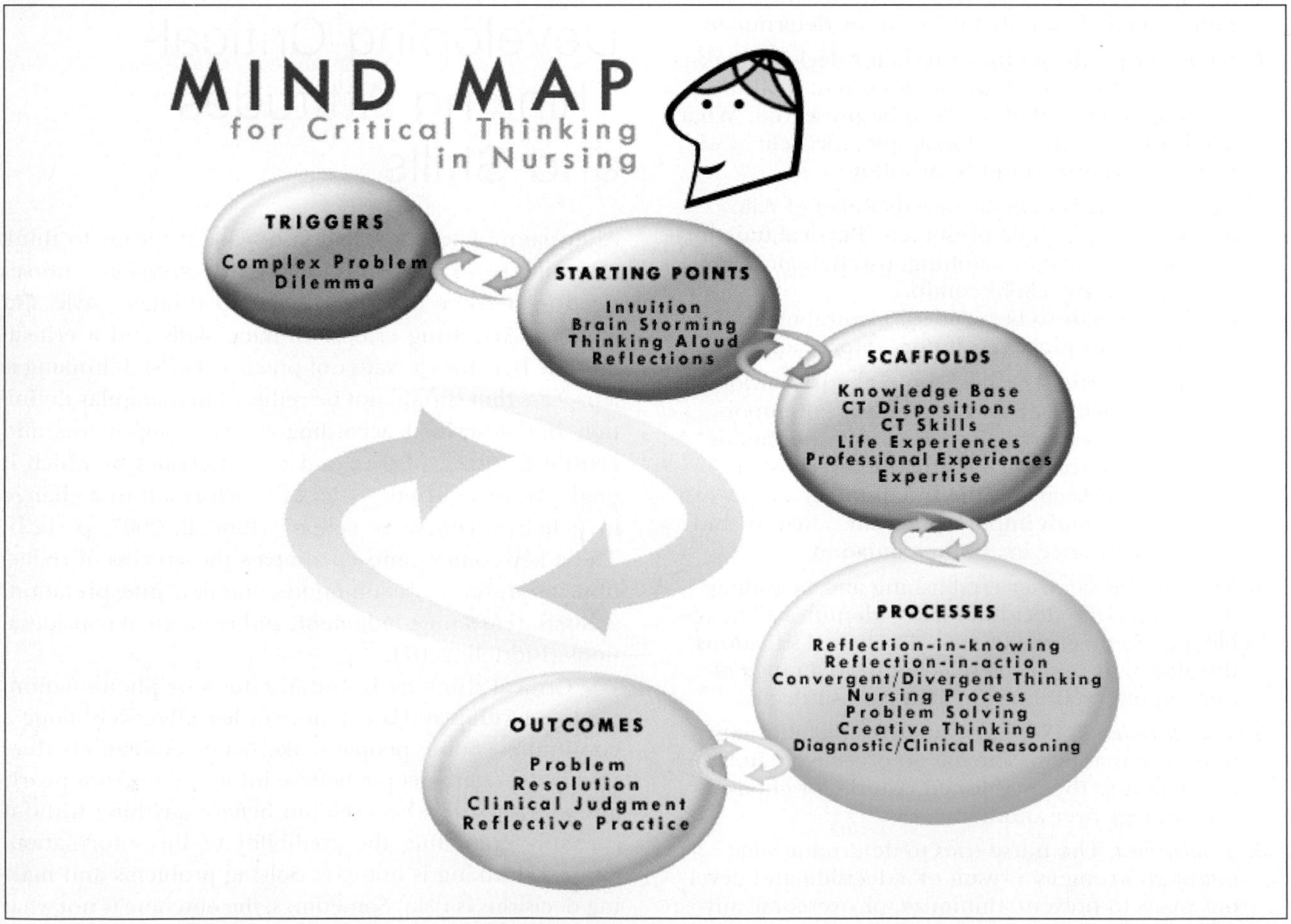

FIGURE 20.1 Mind map for critical thinking in nursing

Source: Duphome, P. & Giddens, J. (2004). **Critical thinking in nursing resource.** *Funded by an intramural grant of the College of Nursing, University of New Mexico.*

beliefs and to ignore evidence that may contradict cherished ideas. Nurses should increase their tolerance for ideas that contradict previously held beliefs, and they should practise suspending judgment.

Suspending judgment means tolerating ambiguity for a time. If an issue is complex, it may not be resolved quickly or neatly, and judgment should be postponed. For a while, the nurse will need to say, "I don't know" and be comfortable with that answer until more is known. Although postponing judgment may not be feasible in emergency situations, where fast action is required, it is often feasible in other situations.

Seeking Situations in Which Good Thinking Is Practised

Nurses will find it valuable to attend conferences in clinical or educational settings that support open examination of all sides of issues and respect opposing viewpoints. Cultivating a questioning attitude, by using either Socratic questioning or another technique, is vital (see the Reflect on Primary Health Care box). Nurses need to review the standards for evaluating thinking and apply them to their own thinking. If nurses are aware of their own thinking and assumptions—while they are doing the thinking—they can detect thinking errors.

Creating Environments That Support Critical Thinking

A nurse cannot develop or maintain critical-thinking attitudes in a vacuum. Nurses in leadership positions must be particularly aware of the climate for thinking that they establish, and they must actively create a stimulating environment that encourages differences of opinion and fair examination of ideas and options. As leaders, nurses should encourage colleagues to examine evidence carefully before they come to conclusions and to avoid *group think,* the tendency to defer unthinkingly to the will of the group.

REFLECT ON PRIMARY HEALTH CARE

Nurses apply critical-thinking skills as they use *primary health-care approach* to care for their clients. This activity involves knowing *what* are the health-promotion needs of their clients; *how, where,* and *when* to engage their clients and the members of the multidisciplinary team for input regarding their clients' needs, strengths, and barriers; and *what* and *how* to adapt the resources or appropriate technology in order to design services and care that will meet the clients' socioeconomic and cultural needs.

Case Study 20

You are taking the bus to downtown Windsor, an area that is unfamiliar to you. As a nursing student involved in a community health practice experience, you assess the neighbourhood along the bus route. There is graffiti on both residential and commercial buildings, trash is blowing along the road outside a number of premises, and some shops are closed, with boarded-up windows. You see a home with the front porch falling away, another home with a few broken windows, and a home with a roof that is missing many shingles. In your assessment, you notice that children reside in each of these residences, as older bikes and a few toys are scattered around each property. As the bus passes a gas station and convenience store, you notice a group of youth painting a mural depicting community development on the side of the gas station wall. When you pass by a city park in this neighbourhood, you see a child under 10 years old playing on a rusty swing set, while his young mother is close by, rocking her newborn. In the distance, a woman is pushing a grocery cart that is filled with items in garbage bags. The woman looks to be in her 50s and has a slow gait as she struggles with the cart. On your return to your nursing program, you meet with the community health faculty adviser to discuss the neighbourhood assessment experience.

Critical Thinking Questions*

1. What conclusions do you draw about this neighbourhood based on your assessment?
2. What further information would be relevant to support your conclusions?
3. How can a nursing student begin to address some of the actual and potential issues assessed within the neighbourhood?
4. What assumptions do you hold about this neighbourhood and the people you saw who reside in the area?
5. Do any of your assumptions reflect biases or prejudices?
6. What critical-thinking skills were used to respond to this case study?

* Questions adapted from *Critical Thinking in Nursing: Case Studies across the Curriculum*, by C. Green, 2000, Upper Saddle River, NJ: Prentice Hall Health.

After working through these questions, go to the MyNursingLab at **http://www.mynursinglab.com** to check your answers.

KEY TERMS

critical thinking
creativity
concept maps
critical analysis
Socratic questions
inductive reasoning
deductive reasoning
context
contextual awareness
assumptions
nursing process
problem solving
trial and error
intuition
decision making

CHAPTER HIGHLIGHTS

- Nurses need critical-thinking skills and attitudes to be safe, competent, skillful practitioners. Critical thinking is a purposeful mental activity in which ideas are produced and evaluated and judgments are made.
- Critical thinking is reasonable, rational, reflective, autonomous, creative, and fair and inspires an attitude of inquiry that focuses on deciding what to believe or do.
- Critical thinkers have certain attitudes and traits: independence of thought, fair-mindedness, insight, intellectual humility, intellectual courage, integrity, perseverance, confidence, curiosity, and contextual awareness.
- Nurses use critical thinking as they apply knowledge from other subjects and fields to nursing practice, deal with change in stressful environments, and make important decisions related to client care. When nurses incorporate creativity into their thinking, they are able to find unique solutions to unique problems.
- Critical thinking consists of high-level cognitive processes that include problem solving and decision making. Three problem-solving methods are trial and error, intuition, and the nursing process.
- The elements of reasoning include (1) the purpose of critical thinking, (2) the question, issue, or problem, (3) assumptions, (4) analysis of points of view, (5) information, data, and evidence, (6) concepts and theories, (7) inferences and conclusions, and (8) implications and consequences. Critical thinkers consider these elements when solving problems and making decisions.
- The nursing process and critical thinking are interrelated and interdependent, but they are not identical. Both involve problem solving, decision making, and creativity.
- Decisions must be made whenever several mutually exclusive choices exist. Nurses must make decisions in both their personal and professional lives. The steps of the decision-making process are identifying the purpose of the decision, setting the criteria, weighting the criteria, seeking alternatives, testing alternatives, troubleshooting, and evaluating the action.
- Almost everyone has at least some level of critical-thinking skill, and that skill can be developed with practice. Some guidelines to enhance critical-thinking skills and attitudes include making a self-assessment, tolerating dissonance and ambiguity, seeking situations in which good thinking is practised, and creating environments that support critical thinking.

ASSESS YOUR LEARNING

1. Mr. Richard runs into the emergency department. He screams, "My wife is bleeding! She is going to die! Quick, do something! She is losing our baby in the car!" What should the nurse do as a priority?
   - **a.** Ask Mr. Richard to say where the car is and then conduct a summary assessment of the situation.
   - **b.** Tell a colleague to perform a vaginal examination as quickly as possible.
   - **c.** Inform the physician of the urgency of the situation and suggest that the operating room be prepared.
   - **d.** Tell Mr. Richard that he must calm down because his screaming is only making the situation worse and his cooperation is required.
2. A patient with diarrhea has a physician's order for a bulk laxative daily. The nurse, not realizing that bulk laxatives can help solidify certain types of diarrhea, concludes that the physician does not know the patient has diarrhea. This statement is an example of which of the following?
   - **a.** A fact
   - **b.** An inference
   - **c.** A judgment
   - **d.** An opinion
3. A patient reports feeling hungry but does not eat when food is served. Using critical-thinking skills, the nurse should do which of the following?
   - **a.** Assess why the patient is not eating the food provided.
   - **b.** Continue to leave the food at the bedside until the patient is hungry enough to eat.
   - **c.** Notify the health-care provider that tube feeding may be needed soon.
   - **d.** Believe the patient is not really hungry.

4. The patient who is short of breath benefits from the head of the bed being elevated. Because this position can result in skin breakdown in the sacral area, the nurse decides to study the amount of sacral pressure occurring in other positions. This decision is an example of which of the following?
   a. The scientific method
   b. The trial-and-error method
   c. Intuition
   d. The nursing process
5. In the decision-making process, the nurse sets and weights the criteria, examines alternatives, and performs which of the following before implementing the plan?
   a. Re-examines the purpose for making the decision
   b. Consults the client and family members to determine their view of the criteria
   c. Identifies and considers various means for reaching the outcomes
   d. Determines the logical course of action should intervening problems arise
6. Mrs. Tanner is an 87-year-old woman who had hip replacement surgery 2 weeks ago. Today is Mrs. Tanner's fourth day at the rehabilitation centre. Her long-term plan is to return home after 6 weeks of therapy. Today is your first day caring for this patient. You have returned Mrs. Tanner to her room and helped her into bed for the night. Mrs. Tanner had a difficult time at physiotherapy this afternoon, and you have just spent an hour with her, listening to her concerns about getting up and around on her own in the future. Before leaving the room, what should you do?
   a. Inform Mrs. Tanner you will also be caring for her tomorrow and wish her goodnight.
   b. Tell Mrs. Tanner you will turn out the lights and leave the door ajar as you leave.
   c. Ensure Mrs. Tanner's call bell is within reach and the bedside rails are in the upright position.
   d. Knowing Mrs. Tanner has an as-needed order for a sleeping pill, ask if she feels she will need a pill tonight.
7. Mr. Avery is a 72-year-old man who had a heart attack 3 weeks ago. He has been started on one Aspirin a day, a new anticoagulant, and a different blood pressure (BP) medication. He continues to receive oxygen via nasal prongs. Next week he will be going home. You enter his room to do his morning assessment, including his vital signs (BP, pulse, temperature, respirations, oxygen saturation). Mr. Avery tells you he is having trouble catching his breath. You take his pulse and note it is above the normal range. His respirations seem laboured. What should your next steps be?
   a. Find your clinical instructor or the nurse assigned to this patient and report these findings.
   b. Leave Mr. Avery, find a peer, and discuss what you should do.
   c. Stay with Mr. Avery, continue with your assessment, and document and report the complete set of vitals.
   d. Push the call bell to get help as Mr. Avery is having another heart attack.
8. You are asked to interview Mrs. Crocker, a 92-year-old woman who has just today come to the long-term-care facility to live. You need to take a complete history from her. Which of the following should you do?
   a. Ensure you have the proper health history forms, enter the room, pull up a chair and sit down, introduce yourself, and begin the history.
   b. Ensure you have the proper health history forms, knock, enter the room, introduce yourself, and explain what you would like to do.
   c. Enter the room, find Mrs. Crocker sleeping, and decide to wait until tomorrow or the next day to complete the history.
   d. Ensure you have the proper health history forms, enter the room, introduce yourself, stand at Mrs. Crocker's bedside, and complete the forms.
9. Nancy Crane is the manager of the transplant unit. She is concerned about having adequate staffing on the unit for the summer as several nurses have requested the same weekends off. How might the problem best be resolved?
   a. Call a unit meeting to consider what solutions the nursing staff might propose.
   b. Propose that no holidays be permitted during the peak summer months.
   c. Ask each nurse for his or her preferences and have a lottery.
   d. Let everyone take the holidays they want and see what happens.
10. Your classmate, Lydia, shares with you that she recently found a small lump in her breast and that she doesn't want to get a mammogram or see her nurse practitioner. She tells you her grandmother had breast cancer. She asks for your advice on what she should do. What is your best course of action?
    a. Ask if she would like to go for a walk and talk about her discovery.
    b. Tell her not to worry about it, that it's probably nothing, but to keep an eye on it.
    c. Offer to find some reading materials for her about mammograms and breast cancer.
    d. Ask how you can support her in making a decision to deal with the issue.

After working through these questions, go to the MyNursingLab at ***http://www.mynursinglab.com*** *to check your answers and see explanations.*

SUGGESTED READINGS

Riddell, T. (2007). Critical assumptions: Thinking critically about critical thinking. *Journal of Nursing Education, 46,* 121–126.

This author provides an overview of critical thinking and challenges readers to examine their assumptions about critical thinking. The underlying assumptions that critical thinking can be learned and that the ability improves clinical competence are questioned.

Vaughn L., & MacDonald, C. (2007). *The power of critical thinking* (Canadian ed.). Toronto, ON: Oxford University Press.

This easy-to-read Canadian textbook introduces the deductive and inductive reasoning process with illustrative examples and exercises to help students apply concepts in various situations.

WEBLINKS

The Critical Thinking Community

http://www.criticalthinking.org

This is the Critical Thinking Community website, based on Dr. Richard Paul and Dr. Linda Elder's work on their critical concepts and tools.

The Critical Thinking Consortium

http://www.tc2.ca

This is a Canadian consortium of educational associations that promote critical thinking through research, professional development and publications.

"A Practical Guide to Critical Thinking"

http://www.skepdic.com/essays/haskins.pdf

This paper is written as a guide to critical thinking and how to develop reasoning skills and arguments.

Registered Nurses' Association of Ontario: Nursing Best Practice Guidelines

http://www.rnao.org

This site has a number of published guidelines, as well as a Toolkit and Educator's Resource to support implementation of best practices.

REFERENCES

Boychuk Duchscher, J. E. (2003). Critical thinking: Perceptions of newly graduated female baccalaureate nurses. *Journal of Nursing Education, 42*(1), 14–27.

Brookfield, S. D. (1987). *Developing critical thinking. Challenging adults to explore alternative ways of thinking and acting.* San Francisco, CA: Jossey-Bass.

Brunt, B. A. (2005). Models, measurement, and strategies in developing critical-thinking skills. *The Journal of Continuing Education in Nursing, 36,* 255–262.

Canadian Association of Schools of Nursing. (1998). *Position paper on baccalaureate education.* Ottawa: Author.

Canadian Nurses Association. (2008). *Canadian Registered Nurse Examination.* Retrieved October 22, 2008, from http://www.cna-nurses.ca/CNA/nursing/rnexam/default_e.aspx

Catalano, J. T. (2003). *Nursing now! Today's issues, tomorrow's trends* (3rd ed.). Philadelphia, PA: Davis.

College of Nurses of Ontario. (2005). *Entry to practice competencies.* Toronto, ON: Author.

Comer, S. (2005). Clinical reasoning. Turning your students into clinical detectives. *Nurse Educator, 30*(6), 235–237.

Forneris, S. G., & Peden-McAlpine, C. J. (2006). Contextual learning: A reflective learning intervention for nursing education. *International Journal of Nursing Education Scholarship, 3*(1), Article 17. Retrieved June 20, 2007, from http://www.bepress.com/ijnes/v013/iss1/art17/

Hsu, L., & Hsieh, S. (2005). Concept maps as an assessment tool in a nursing course. *Journal of Professional Nursing, 21*(3), 141–149.

Ignatavicius, D. D. (2001). Critical thinking skills for at-the-bedside success. *Nursing Management, 32*(1), 37–39.

Kalischuk, G. R., & Thorpe, K. (2002). Thinking creatively: From nursing education to practice. *Journal of Continuing Education in Nursing, 33*(4), 155–163.

Martin, C. (2002). The theory of critical thinking of nursing. *Nursing Education Perspectives, 23*(5), 243–247.

Oermann, M. H., & Gaberson, K. B. (2006). *Evaluation and testing in nursing education* (2nd ed.). New York, NY: Springer Publishing Company.

Parse, R. R. (1996). Critical thinking: What is it? *Nursing Science Quarterly, 9*(4), 139.

Paul, R. W. (1988). *What, then, is critical thinking?* From the Eighth Annual and Sixth International Conference on Critical Thinking and Educational Reform. Rohnert Park, CA: Center for Critical Thinking and Moral Critique, Sonoma State University.

Paul, R. W. (1993). *Critical thinking: How to prepare students for a rapidly changing world.* Santa Rosa, CA: Foundation for Critical Thinking.

Paul, R., & Elder, L. (2005). *A guide for educators to critical thinking competency standards.* Dillon Beach, CA: Foundation for Critical Thinking.

Piaget, J. (1966). *Origins of intelligence in children.* New York, NY: Norton.

Reilly, D. E., & Oermann, M. H. (1992). Cognitive learning in the clinical setting. In *Clinical teaching in nursing education* (2nd ed.) (pp. 207–246). New York: National League for Nursing.

Riddell, T. (2007). Critical assumptions: Thinking critically about critical thinking. *Journal of Nursing Education, 46,* 121–126.

Ruggiero, V. R. (2006). *The art of thinking: A guide to critical and creative thought* (8th ed.). New York, NY: Pearson Education.

Ruth-Sahd, L. A., & Hendy, H. M. (2005). Predictors of novice nurses' use of intuition to guide patient care decisions. *Journal of Nursing Education, 44,* 450–458.

Simpson, E., & Courtney, M. (2002). Critical thinking in nursing education: Literature review. *International Journal of Nursing Practice, 8*(2), 89–98.

Scheffer, B. K., & Rubenfeld, M. G. (2000). A consensus statement on critical thinking in nursing. *Journal of Nursing Education, 39,* 352–362.

Sullivan, E. J., & Decker, P. J. (Eds.) (2005). Thinking critically, making decisions, problem solving. In *Effective leadership and management in nursing* (6th ed.) (pp. 100–120). Upper Saddle River, NJ: Pearson Prentice Hall.

Chapter 21

Caring, Comforting, and Communicating

Many students enter the nursing profession because they want to care for people. In this caring profession, communication is a critical skill; it is the process by which people meet their survival needs, build relationships, and experience joy. In nursing, communication is used to gather information, to teach and persuade, and to express caring and comfort. Comforting is the process by which nurses help clients and their significant others face the distresses and discomforts they may encounter. Communication is an integral part of the nurse–client relationship. In caring for clients, nurses need strong communication skills to effectively convey client needs and wants to the interdisciplinary team.

OBJECTIVES

After studying this chapter, you should be able to

1. Discuss various descriptions, actions, and outcomes associated with caring
2. Describe the concept of comforting
3. List four essential aspects of the communication process
4. Analyze nine factors that influence the communication process
5. Differentiate verbal and nonverbal communication
6. Describe four phases of the helping relationship
7. Identify 10 features of effective groups

Caring

Caring is considered by many nurses to be an essential aspect of nursing. Madeleine Leininger (2001) stated that "*caring* is the essence of nursing and the dominant, distinctive, and unifying feature of nursing" (p. 35). She said that there can be no cure without caring but that there can be caring without curing. She emphasized that human caring, although a universal phenomenon, varies among cultures in its expressions, processes, and patterns; it is largely culturally divided.

The outcomes of caring are varied. Caring can promote self-actualization, promote individual growth, preserve human dignity and worth, augment self-healing, and relieve distress. Conversely, caring may not evoke a tangible outcome. It may not be a means to an end and may be regarded as an end in itself. The goodness of caring is often found in the process itself—that of engagement and connection between the nurse and the client (Cronin & Rawlings-Anderson, 2004). Caring includes assistive, supportive, and facilitative acts for individuals or groups.

Culture Care Diversity and Universality (Leininger)

Leininger (2001) stated that caring, as nurturing behaviour, has been present throughout history and is one of the most critical factors in helping people maintain or regain health. Her theory of culture care diversity and universality is based on the assumption that nurses must understand various cultures in order to function effectively.

To provide care that is congruent with cultural values, beliefs, and practices, the nurse must understand these differences and similarities. To understand the care desired by clients and "enter their broader worldview," the nurse requires knowledge of the culture and local language (Leininger, 2001, p. 58). Culturally congruent care is provided in three major ways: (1) by preserving the client's familiar lifeways, (2) by making accommodations in care that are satisfying to clients, and (3) by repatterning nursing care to help the client move toward wellness (Leininger).

Theory of Human Care (Watson)

Jean Watson (1985, 1999a, 1999b) believed the practice of caring is central to nursing. She described caring as being grounded in a set of universal human values: kindness, concern, and love of the self and others. It is the moral ideal of nursing and it involves the will to care, the intent to care, and the caring actions. Caring actions include communication, positive regard, support, or physical interventions by the nurse. Caring goes beyond the notions of curing at all costs. Within the caring situation, the nurse enters into the experience of the client, and the client can enter into the nurse's experience. The nurse maintains professional objectivity; both the nurse and the client seek a sense of harmony within the mind, body, and soul, thereby actualizing the real self.

The Primacy of Caring (Benner and Wrubel)

Benner and Wrubel (1989) viewed caring as the essence of excellence in nursing. Nursing is described as a relationship in which caring is primary because it sets up the possibility of giving and receiving help. Caring practice requires attending to the particular client over time, determining what matters to the person, and using this knowledge in clinical judgments.

A caring relationship requires a certain amount of openness and capacity to respond to care on the part of the client. In caring practice, being with someone can be just as important as doing something for that person, if not more so. As the nurse gains expertise, he or she learns how to be with people, to respect who they are and where they are at, and to stop doing for them. Thus, caring practice involves client advocacy and provides the necessary conditions to help the client grow and develop (Gordon, Benner, & Noddings, 1996).

Caring: The Human Mode of Being (Roach)

Simone Roach (2002) viewed caring as the human mode of being, or the "most common, authentic criterion of humanness" (p. 28). Most persons are caring and develop their caring abilities by being true to self, being real, and being who they truly are. Roach defined the following attributes as the six Cs of caring: compassion, competence, confidence, conscience, commitment, and comportment (see Box 21.1). Each of the six Cs reflects specific values and includes virtuous actions by which a nurse can demonstrate caring behaviours.

Comforting

Comforting is a characteristic unique to nursing and an essential aspect of caring. Making the client as comfortable as possible has been a frequent nursing action since the days of Nightingale. Although nurses have always provided comfort measures that give strength, solace, support, encouragement, hope, and assistance, the concepts of comfort and comforting have not been developed or structured for nursing science (Donahue, 1989).

BOX 21.1 THE SIX Cs OF CARING IN NURSING

COMPASSION
Awareness of one's relationship to others, sharing their joys, sorrows, pain, and accomplishments. Participation in the experience of another.

COMPETENCE
Having the knowledge, judgment, skills, energy, experience, and motivation to respond adequately to others within the demands of professional responsibilities.

CONFIDENCE
The quality that fosters trusting relationships. Comfort with self, client, and family.

CONSCIENCE
Morals, ethics, and an informed sense of right and wrong. Awareness of personal responsibility.

COMMITMENT
Convergence between one's desires and obligations and the deliberate choice to act in accordance with them.

COMPORTMENT
Appropriate bearing, demeanour, dress, and language that are in harmony with a caring presence. Presenting oneself as someone who respects others and demands respect.

Source: Adapted from *Caring: The Human Mode of Being,* 2nd ed., by M. S. Roach, 2002, Ottawa: CHA Press.

The Comforting Process

Comforting is a process that "includes discrete, transitory actions, such as touching, or broad, longer lasting interventions, such as listening" (Morse, 1996, p. 6). The comforting role of a nurse is in working with the client to assist them in becoming comfortable. The comforting process is *client led* because it occurs in response to cues presented by the client; however, it is generally *nurse controlled* because nurses select the appropriate comfort measures and adjust them according to the needs of the client. Thus, comforting is an active process and, whenever possible, involves the cooperative actions of both clients and nurses.

Comfort

The desired outcome of comforting is **comfort**. The origin of the word *comfort* is the Latin word *confortare,* meaning "to strengthen greatly." Comfort implies a renewal, an amplification of power or sense of control, an invigorating influence, a positive mindset, and a readiness for action. It enables the client to perform the usual activities of daily life.

COMFORT NEEDS Kolcaba (1991, 1995) identified comfort needs within four contexts:

- *Physical comfort needs* relate to bodily sensations and the physiological problems associated with the medical diagnosis.
- *Psychospiritual comfort needs* relate to the internal awareness of self, including esteem, concept, sexuality, and meaning in life. They can also include the person's relationship to a higher order or being.
- *Social comfort needs* relate to interpersonal, family, and social relationships.
- *Environmental comfort needs* relate to the external background of human experience and can include light, noise, ambience, colour, temperature, and natural versus synthetic elements.

INTENSITY (TYPE) OF COMFORT Three types of comfort described by Kolcaba (1991) are relief, ease, and transcendence. **Relief** from discomfort is the experience of having a specific need met. Relief may be incomplete, partial, or temporary, lasting only a short time until discomfort arises again. It enables the client to return to former functions or to have a peaceful death. **Ease** refers to a state of calm or peaceful contentment in which the client can perform activities efficiently. This state of comfort can exist without a prior state of discomfort or can indicate complete relief from discomforts that are lasting, rather than temporary relief from severe discomforts. **Transcendence** refers to the state in which the client is invigorated or inspired to reach for extraordinary performance as an end state, rather than ordinary performance, which is the end state for relief and ease. Extraordinary performance requires unusual effort by the client to shed preoccupation with pain, disability, or other difficulties. For example, transcendence may be necessary when illness and injury cause a permanent change in the body, such as with clients who have debilitating arthritis and pain or a spinal cord injury.

COMFORT MEASURES Comfort measures may be provided both directly to the client and indirectly through other personnel, family, or environment. Examples of indirect actions include maintaining a quiet environment, coordinating the activities of other health-care personnel, and supporting the client's family members or significant others. Comfort measures are initiated when the nurse perceives client distress or discomfort or the client indicates a specific need for comforting. Because discomfort comes in such diverse states, nurses need to be creative and innovative in providing specific, individualized care.

Comfort care may require simple physical actions, such as providing a warm blanket, offering a cup of tea, or applying lotion to dry skin. However, it also requires nursing knowledge and skills specific to the client's medical and nursing problems. Examples include interventions for skin breakdown, pain, infection, airway clearance, confusion, and so on.

Comfort measures also encompass the client's psychospiritual, social, and environmental realms. Examples of psychospiritual comfort measures are talking in soothing tones, acknowledging and accepting feelings, offering a presence, and encouraging decision making. Social measures can include supporting family and friends and encouraging their visits. Environmental comfort measures can involve merely opening a window or removing clutter. Because the goal of any comforting measure is enhanced comfort, success in comfort care is evaluated by comparing comfort levels before and after intervention. Absolute or total comfort in a hospital setting is often not possible. Nurses are, therefore, challenged to encourage and inspire clients to rise above adversities.

Communicating

The term *communication* has various meanings depending on the context in which it is used. To some, communication is the interchange of information between two or more people; in other words, it is the exchange of ideas or thoughts. This kind of communication uses such methods as talking and listening or writing and reading; however, painting, dancing, storytelling, and body gestures are also means of communication.

Communication involves the interchange of ideas or thoughts, a transmission of feelings, or a more personal and social interaction between two or more people. Communication is often synonymous with relating. Frequently, one member of a couple comments that the other is not communicating (e.g., some teenagers complain about a generation gap—being unable to communicate with understanding or feeling to a parent or authority figure). Communication is a basic component of human relationships, including nursing.

The *intent* of any communication is to elicit a response. When individuals communicate, they have a purpose. Thus, communication is a process. It has two main purposes: (1) to influence others and (2) to obtain information. Helpful communication encourages a sharing of information, thoughts, or feelings between two or more people. Unhelpful communication hinders or blocks the transfer of information and feelings.

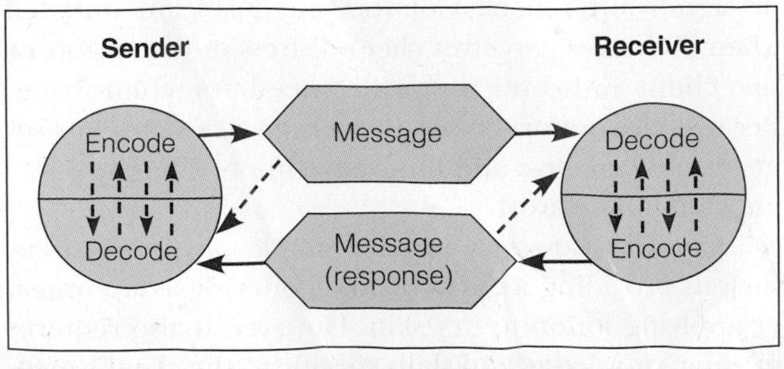

FIGURE 21.1 The communication process. The dashed arrows indicate intrapersonal communication (self-talk). The solid lines indicate interpersonal communication.

Effective communication is essential for the establishment of a nurse–client relationship. Nurses who communicate effectively are better able to initiate change that promotes health, establish a trusting therapeutic relationship with a client and support persons, and prevent legal problems associated with nursing practice.

Communication can occur on an intrapersonal level within a single individual, as well as on interpersonal and group levels. Intrapersonal communication is the communication that you have with yourself; another name is *self-talk*. Both the sender and the receiver of a message usually engage in this type of communication. It involves thinking about the message before it is sent, while it is being sent, and after it is sent, and it occurs constantly. Consequently, intrapersonal communication can interfere with a person's ability to hear a message as the sender intended.

The Communication Process

Communication involves a sender, a message, a receiver, and a response or feedback. Communication is a reciprocal process that involves the sending and receiving of messages between more than at least two individuals (Verderber & Verderber, 2001).

Communication is a two-way process involving the sending and the receiving of a message (see Figure 21.1). Because the intent of communication is to elicit a response, the process is ongoing; the receiver of the message then becomes the sender of a response, and the original sender then becomes the receiver.

SENDER The **sender**, a person or group who wants to convey a message to another, can be considered the *source-encoder.* This term suggests that the person or group sending the message must have an idea or reason for communicating (source) and must put the idea or feeling into a form that can be transmitted. **Encoding** involves the selection of specific signs or symbols (codes) to transmit the message, such as which language and words to use, how to arrange the words, and what tone of voice and gestures to use. For example, if the receiver speaks English, the sender usually selects English words. If the message is "Mr. Johnson, smoking is not permitted in patient rooms in this hospital," the tone of voice selected will be one of firmness, and a shake of the head or a pointing index finger can reinforce it. The nurse must not only deal with dialects and foreign languages but also must cope with two language approaches—the lay-person's and the health professional's.

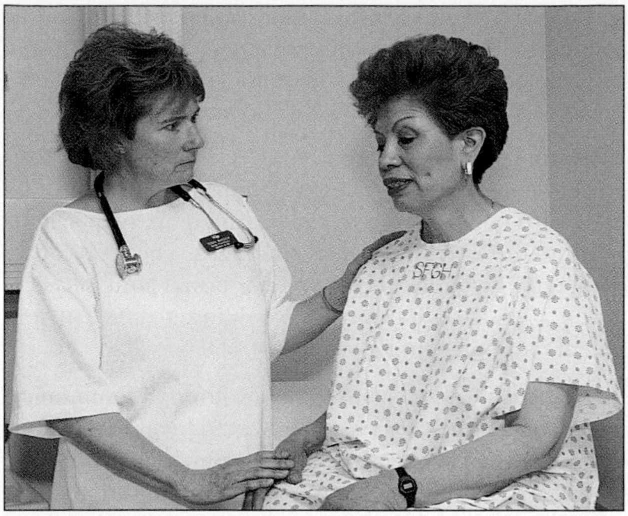

FIGURE 21.2 Appropriate forms of touch can communicate caring.

MESSAGE The **message** refers to what is actually said or written, the body language that accompanies the words, and how the message is transmitted. The medium used to convey the message is the channel. It is important for the channel to be appropriate for the message, and it should help make the intent of the message clearer.

Talking face to face with a person can be more effective in some instances than telephoning or writing a message. Recording messages on tape or communicating by radio or television may be more appropriate for larger audiences. Written communication is often appropriate for long explanations or for a communication that needs to be preserved. The nonverbal channel of touch is often highly effective (see Figure 21.2).

RECEIVER The **receiver** is the listener, who must listen, observe, and attend. This person is the *decoder,* who must perceive what the sender intended (interpretation). Perception uses all the senses to receive verbal and nonverbal messages. To **decode** means to relate the message perceived to the receiver's storehouse of knowledge and experience and to sort out the meaning of the message. Whether the message is decoded accurately by the receiver, according to the sender's intent, depends largely on their similarities in knowledge and experience and sociocultural background. If the meaning of the decoded message matches the intent of the sender, then the communication has been effective. Ineffective communication occurs when the message sent is misinterpreted by the receiver. For example, Mr. Johnson may perceive the message accurately—"No smoking is allowed in my room." However, if experience has taught him that he can smoke in his room if a certain nurse is on duty, he will interpret the intent of the message differently.

RESPONSE *Response* is the message that the receiver returns to the sender. It is also called **feedback**. Feedback can be verbal, nonverbal, or both. Nonverbal examples are a nod of the head or a yawn. Either way, feedback allows the sender to correct or reword a message. In the case of Mr. Johnson, the receiver may appear irritated or say, "Well, the nurse on evening shift lets me smoke." The sender then knows the message was interpreted accurately. However, now the original sender becomes the receiver, who is required to decode and respond.

Modes of Communication

Communication is generally carried out in two different modes: verbal and nonverbal. **Verbal communication** uses the spoken or written word; **nonverbal communication** uses other forms, such as gestures or facial expressions and touch. Although both kinds of communication occur concurrently, the majority of communication is nonverbal. Learning about nonverbal communication is thus important for nurses in developing effective communication patterns and relationships with clients.

Another form of communication has evolved with technology—**electronic communication**. The most common form of electronic communication is email, in which an individual can send a message, by computer, to another person or group of people. Nurses must decide when it is appropriate and not appropriate to use email when communicating with clients.

VERBAL COMMUNICATION Verbal communication is largely conscious because people choose the words they use. The words used vary among individuals according to culture, socioeconomic background, age, and education. As a result, countless possibilities exist for the ways ideas are exchanged. An abundance of words can be used to form messages. In addition, a wide variety of feelings can be conveyed when people talk.

When choosing words to say or write, nurses need to consider (1) pace and intonation, (2) simplicity, (3) clarity and brevity, (4) timing and relevance, (5) adaptability, (6) credibility, and (7) humour.

PACE AND INTONATION The manner of speech, as in the pace or rhythm and intonation, will modify the feeling and impact of the message. The intonation can express enthusiasm, sadness, anger, or amusement. The pace of speech can indicate interest, anxiety, boredom, or fear.

SIMPLICITY Many complex technical terms become natural to nurses; however, laypersons often misunderstand these terms. Words such as *vasoconstriction* or *cholecystectomy* are meaningful to the nurse and easy to use but are ill advised when communicating with clients. Nurses need to select simple, appropriate, and understandable terms based on the age, knowledge, culture, and education of the client. For example, instead of saying to a client, "The nurses will be catheterizing you tomorrow for a urinalysis," it may be more appropriate and understandable to say, "Tomorrow we need to get a sample of your urine, so we will collect it by putting a small tube into your bladder." The latter statement is more likely to elicit a response from the client as to why it is needed and whether it will be uncomfortable because the client understands the message being conveyed by the nurse.

Clarity and Brevity Clarity is saying precisely what is meant and brevity is using the fewest words necessary. The result is a message that is simple and clear. An aspect of this is congruence, or consistency, in which the nurse's behaviour or nonverbal communication matches the words spoken. When the nurse tells the client, "I am interested in hearing what you have to say," the nonverbal behaviour would include the nurse facing the client, making eye contact, and leaning forward. The goal is to communicate clearly so that all aspects of a situation or circumstance are understood. To ensure clarity in communication, nurses also need to speak slowly and enunciate carefully.

Timing and Relevance No matter how clearly or simply words are stated or written, the timing needs to be appropriate to ensure that words are heard, and the messages are related to the person or to the person's interests and concerns. This involves sensitivity to the client's needs and concerns. For example, a client who is enmeshed in fear of cancer may not hear the nurse's explanations about the expected procedures before and after gallbladder surgery. In this situation, it is better for the nurse first to encourage the client to express concerns, and then to deal with those concerns. The necessary explanations can be provided at another time when the client is able to listen.

Another problem in timing is asking several questions at once. For example, a nurse enters a client's room and says in one breath, "Good morning, Mrs. Brody. How are you this morning? Did you sleep well last night? Is your partner coming to see you before your surgery?" The client no doubt wonders which question to answer first, if any. A related pattern of poor timing is to ask a question and then not wait for an answer before making another comment.

Adaptability Spoken messages need to be altered in accordance with behavioural cues from the client. This adjustment is referred to as *adaptability*. What the nurse says and how it is said must be individualized and carefully considered. This requires astute assessment and sensitivity on the part of the nurse. For example, a nurse who usually smiles, appears cheerful, and greets the client every afternoon with an enthusiastic "Hi, Mrs. Brown!" notices that she is not smiling and appears distressed. It is important for the nurse to modify tone of speech and express concern in facial expression while moving toward the client.

Credibility *Credibility* means "worthiness of belief, trustworthiness, and reliability." Nurses foster credibility by being consistent, dependable, and honest. The nurse needs to be knowledgeable about what is being discussed and to have accurate information. Nurses should convey confidence and certainty in what they are saying while being able to acknowledge their limitations. "I don't know the answer to that, but I will find someone who does."

Humour The use of humour can be a positive and powerful tool in the nurse–client relationship, but it must be used with care. Humour can be used to help clients adjust to difficult and painful situations. The physical act of laughter can be both an emotional and physical release, reducing tension by providing a different perspective and promoting a sense of well-being.

NONVERBAL COMMUNICATION Nonverbal communication is sometimes called *body language*. It includes gestures, body movements, use of touch, and physical appearance, including adornment. Nonverbal communication often tells others more about what a person is *feeling* than what is actually said (Figure 21.3). Nonverbal communication either reinforces or contradicts what is said verbally. For example, if a nurse says to a client, "I'd be happy to sit here and talk to you for a while" and yet glances nervously at a watch every few seconds, the actions contradict the verbal message. The client is more likely to believe the nonverbal behaviour, which conveys "I am very busy and need to leave."

Observing and interpreting the client's nonverbal behaviour is an essential skill for nurses to develop. To observe nonverbal behaviour efficiently requires a systematic assessment of the person's overall physical appearance, posture, gait, facial expressions, and gestures. Whatever is observed, the nurse needs to exercise caution in interpretation, always clarifying any observation with the client.

Transculturally, nonverbal communication varies widely. Even in such behaviours as smiling and handshaking, cultures differ. For example, to many Hispanics, smiling and handshaking are an integral part of an interaction and essential to establishing trust. The same behaviour might be perceived by a Russian as insolent and frivolous.

The nurse cannot always be sure of the correct interpretation of the feelings expressed nonverbally. The same feeling can be expressed nonverbally in more than one way, even within the same cultural group. For example, anger may be communicated by aggressive or excessive body motion, or it may be communicated by frozen stillness. In some cultures, a smile may be used to conceal anger. Therefore, the interpretation of such observations requires validation with the client. For example, the nurse might say, "You look as if you have been crying. Can you tell me more about that?"

Personal Appearance Clothing and adornments can be rich sources of information about a client. Although choice of apparel is highly personal, it can convey social and financial status, culture, religion, group association, and self-concept. Charms and amulets may be worn for decorative or for health protection purposes. When the

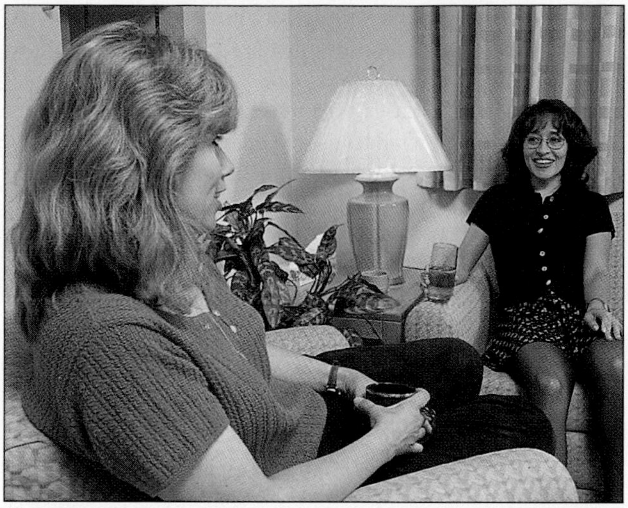
A

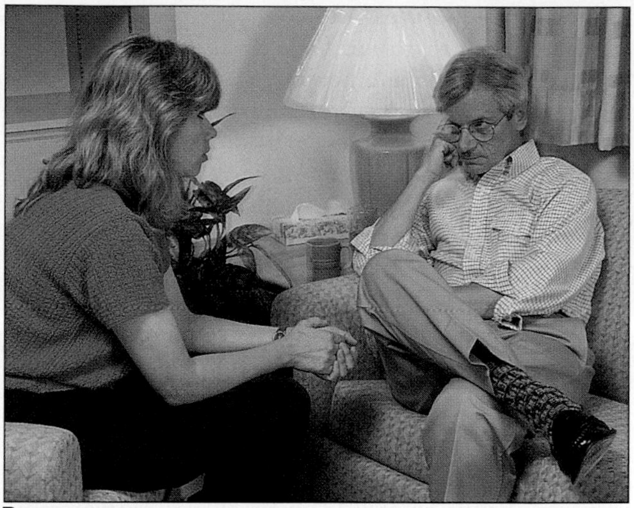
B

FIGURE 21.3 Nonverbal communication sometimes conveys meaning more effectively than words. **A.** The postures of these women indicate openness to communication. **B.** The listener's posture suggests resistance to communication.

symbolic meaning of an object is unfamiliar, the nurse can inquire about its significance, which may foster rapport with the client.

How a person dresses is often an indicator of how the person feels. Someone who is tired or ill may not have the energy or the desire to maintain normal grooming. When a person known for immaculate grooming becomes lax about appearance, the nurse may suspect a loss of self-esteem or a physical illness. The nurse must validate these observed nonverbal data by asking the client. For acutely ill clients in hospital or home care settings, a change in grooming habits may signal that the client is feeling better. A man may request a shave or a woman may request a shampoo and some makeup.

Posture and Gait The ways people walk and carry themselves are often reliable indicators of self-concept, current mood, and health. Erect posture and an active, purposeful stride suggest a feeling of well-being. Slouched posture and a slow, shuffling gait suggest depression or physical discomfort. Tense posture and a rapid, determined gait suggest anxiety or anger. The posture of people when they are sitting or lying can also indicate feelings or mood. Again, the nurse clarifies the meaning of the observed behaviour by describing to the client what the nurse sees and then asking what it means or whether the nurse's interpretation is correct. For example, "You look as if it really hurts to move. Are you in pain? What would help make you feel more comfortable?"

Facial Expression No part of the body is as expressive as the face (see Figure 21.4). Feelings of surprise, fear, anger, disgust, happiness, and sadness can be conveyed by facial expressions. Although the face can express the person's genuine emotions, it is also possible to control these muscles so the emotion expressed does not reflect what the person is feeling. Many facial expressions convey a universal meaning. The smile expresses happiness. Contempt is conveyed by the mouth turned down, the head tilted back, and the eyes directed down the nose. No single expression can be interpreted accurately, however, without considering other reinforcing physical cues, the setting in which it occurs, the expression of others in the same setting, and the cultural background of the client.

Nurses need to be aware of their own expressions and what they are communicating to clients. Clients are quick to notice the nurse's facial expression, particularly when a client feels unsure or uncomfortable. The client who questions the nurse about a feared diagnostic result will watch whether the nurse maintains eye contact or looks away when answering. The client who has had disfiguring surgery will examine the nurse's face for signs of disgust. It is impossible to control all facial expression,

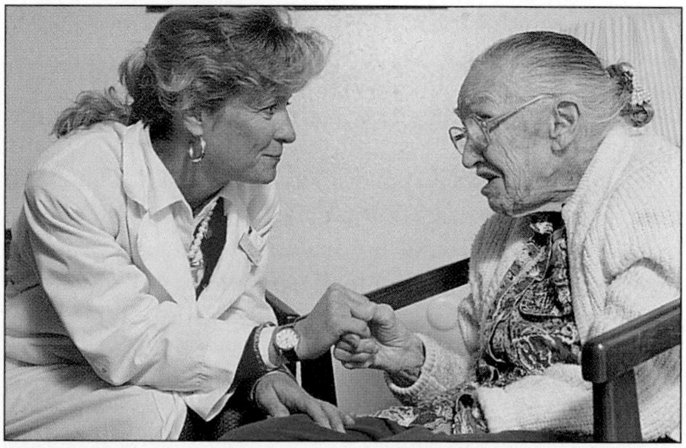

FIGURE 21.4 The nurse's facial expression communicates warmth and caring.

but the nurse must learn to control expressions of feelings like fear or disgust in some circumstances.

Eye contact is another essential element of facial communication. In many cultures, mutual eye contact acknowledges recognition of the other person and a willingness to maintain communication. Often, a person initiates contact with another person with a glance, capturing the person's attention before communicating. A person who feels weak or defenceless often averts the eyes or avoids eye contact; the communication received may be too embarrassing or too dominating.

Gestures Hand and body gestures can emphasize and clarify the spoken word, or they can occur without words to indicate a particular feeling or to give a sign. A parent awaiting information about his child in surgery may wring his hands or pick his nails. A gesture may more clearly indicate the size or shape of an object. A wave goodbye and the motioning of a visitor toward a chair are gestures that have relatively universal meanings. Some gestures, however, are culture specific. The North American gesture meaning "shoo" or "go away" means "come here" or "come back" in some Asian cultures. In the Hmong culture, it is considered rude to point at something with your toe.

For people with special communication problems, such as the deaf, the hands are invaluable in communication. Many deaf people learn sign language. Ill persons who are unable to reply verbally can similarly devise a communication system by using the hands. The client may be able to raise an index finger once for "yes" and twice for "no." Other signals can often be devised by the client and the nurse to denote other meanings.

ELECTRONIC COMMUNICATION Computers are increasingly playing a big role in nursing practice. Many health-care agencies are moving toward electronic medical records in which nurses document their assessments and nursing care. Electronic mail (email) can be used in health-care facilities for many purposes: to schedule and confirm appointments, to report lab results, to conduct client education, and to follow up with discharged clients (Austin, 2006). Email is the most common form of electronic communication. It is important for the nurse to know the advantages and disadvantages of email and also other guidelines to ensure client confidentiality.

Advantages Email is a fast, efficient way to communicate, and it is legible. It provides a record of the date and time of the message that was sent or received. Some health facilities provide information to their clients on how they can reach, via email, specified staff members. This improves communication and continuity of client care.

Disadvantages The disadvantage or negative aspect of email is the risk to client confidentiality. Organizations must apply reasonable and appropriate safeguards when emailing protected health information. The health-care agency needs to have an email encryption system to ensure security. An agency may have its own system or outsource an encryption service.

Not everyone has a computer. Although access to a computer may be available, not everyone has the necessary computer skills. Email can enhance communication with some clients but not all clients. Other forms of communication will be needed for clients who have limited abilities with speaking English or French, reading, writing, or using a computer.

When Not to Use Email Austin (2006) lists the following situations in which it is best to avoid using email:

- When the information is urgent and the client's health could be in jeopardy if he or she doesn't read it immediately
- Highly confidential information (e.g., HIV status, mental health, chemical dependency)
- Abnormal lab data: if the information is confusing and could prompt many questions by the client, it is better to either see or telephone the person

Other Guidelines Agencies usually develop standards and guidelines for the use of email in health care. It is important to know, per the agency's guidelines, what can be emailed to clients. Usually, clients need to sign an email consent form first. This form provides information about the risks of email and authorizes the health agency to communicate with the client at a specified email address.

Instead of identifying the email as "confidential" in the subject line, Austin (2006) advises including a disclaimer that the message is to be read only by the person to whom it is addressed and that no one else is authorized to read the message. Additionally, the disclaimer should state that if the email is sent to anyone else by mistake, he or she should contact the sender.

Information sent to a client via email is considered part of the client's medical record. Therefore, a copy of the email needs to be put in the client's chart. Emails, like other documentation in the client's record, can be used as evidence during litigation.

Email is another form of communication that can enhance effective relationships with clients. It is not, however, a substitute for effective verbal and nonverbal communication. Nurses need to use their professional judgment about what forms of communication will best meet their client's health needs.

Factors Influencing the Communication Process

Many factors influence the communication process. Some of these are development, gender, values and perceptions, personal space, territoriality, roles and relationships, environment, congruence, and attitudes.

DEVELOPMENT Language, psychosocial, and intellectual development move through stages across the lifespan. Knowledge of a client's developmental stage will allow the nurse to modify the message accordingly. The use of dolls and games with simple language can help explain a procedure to an 8-year-old. With adolescents who have developed more abstract thinking skills, a more detailed explanation can be given, whereas a well-educated, middle-aged business executive may want to have detailed technical information provided. Older clients are apt to have had a wider range of experiences with the health-care system, which can influence their response or understanding. With aging also come changes in vision and hearing acuity that can affect nurse–client interactions.

GENDER From an early age, females and males communicate differently. Girls tend to use language to seek confirmation, minimize differences, and establish intimacy. Boys use language to establish independence and negotiate status within a group. These differences can continue into adulthood so that the same communication may be interpreted differently by a man and a woman.

VALUES AND PERCEPTIONS Values are the standards that influence behaviour, and perceptions are the personal view of an event. Because each person has unique personality traits, values, and life experiences, each will perceive and interpret messages and experiences differently. For example, if the nurse draws the curtains around a crying woman and leaves her alone, the woman may interpret this as "The nurse thinks that I will upset others and that I shouldn't cry" or "The nurse respects my need to be alone." It is important for the nurse to be aware of a client's values and to validate or correct perceptions to avoid creating barriers in the nurse–client relationship.

PERSONAL SPACE **Personal space** is the distance people prefer in interactions with others. Middle-class North Americans use definite distances in various interpersonal relationships, along with specific voice tones and body language. Communication, thus, alters in accordance with four distances, each with a close and a far phase. Tamparo and Lindh (2008) listed the following example:

1. Intimate: Touching to 0.5 m
2. Personal: 0.5 m to 1.3 m
3. Social: 1.3 m to 4 m
4. Public: 4 m and beyond

Intimate distance communication is characterized by body contact, heightened sensations of body heat and smell, and vocalizations that are low. Intimate distance is frequently used by nurses. Examples include cuddling a baby, touching the sightless client, positioning clients, observing an incision, and restraining a toddler for an injection. It is a natural protective instinct for people to maintain a certain amount of space immediately around them, and the amount varies with individuals and cultures. When someone who wants to communicate steps too close, the receiver automatically steps back a pace or two. In their therapeutic roles, nurses often are required to violate this personal space. However, it is important for them to be aware when this will occur and to forewarn the client. In many instances, the nurse can respect (not come as close as) a person's intimate distance. In other instances, the nurse can come within intimate distance to communicate warmth and caring.

Personal distance is less overwhelming than intimate distance. Physical contact, such as a handshake or touching a shoulder, is possible. More of the person is perceived at a personal distance so that nonverbal behaviours, such as body stance or full facial expressions, are seen with less distortion. Much communication between nurses and clients happens at this distance. Examples occur when nurses are sitting with clients, giving medications, or establishing an intravenous infusion. Communication at a close personal distance can convey involvement by facilitating the sharing of thoughts and feelings. At the outer extreme of 1.3 m, however, less involvement is conveyed. Bantering and some social conversations are usually at this distance.

Social distance is characterized by a clear visual perception of the whole person. This communication is formal and is limited to seeing and hearing. It is expedient in communicating with several people at the same time or within a short time. Examples occur when nurses make rounds or wave a greeting to someone. Social distance is important in accomplishing the business of the day. However, it is frequently misused. For example, the nurse who stands in the doorway and asks a client, "How are you today?" will receive a more noncommittal reply than the nurse who moves to a personal distance to inquire.

Public distance requires loud, clear vocalizations with careful enunciation. Although the faces and forms of people are seen at public distance, individuality is lost. Instead, the perception is of the group of people or the community.

TERRITORIALITY **Territoriality** is a concept of the space and things that an individual considers as belonging to the self. Territories marked off by people can be visible to others. For example, patients in a hospital often consider their territory as bounded by the curtains around the bed unit or by the walls of a private room. This human tendency to claim territory must be recognized by all health-care workers. Patients often feel the need to defend their territory when it is invaded by others; for example, when a visitor or nurse removes a chair to use at another bed, the visitor has inadvertently violated the territoriality of the client whose chair was removed. Nurses need to obtain permission from patients to remove, rearrange, or borrow objects in their hospital area.

ROLES AND RELATIONSHIPS The roles and the relationship between sender and receiver affect the communication process. Such roles as nursing student and instructor, client and physician, or parent and child affect the content and responses in the communication process. Choice of words, sentence structure, and tone of voice vary considerably from role to role. In addition, the specific relationship between the communicators is significant. The nurse who meets with a client for the first time communicates differently from the nurse who has previously developed a longer relationship with the client.

Effective communication skills are the foundation for positive relationships (Hartrick, 2002). Nurse–client relationships involve negotiation and engagement in order to determine the plans and boundaries needed for therapeutic relationships (Chitty, 2005). They must be discovered, defined, and negotiated. Each relationship is unique and, therefore, is an open forum for discovery and change. By embracing negotiation as a necessary condition of therapeutic relationships, both novices and advanced nurses will enhance their nursing practice.

ENVIRONMENT People usually communicate most effectively in a comfortable environment. Temperature extremes, excessive noise, and a poorly ventilated environment can all interfere with communication. Also, lack of privacy can interfere with a client's communication about matters the client considers private. For example, a client who is worried about the ability of his partner to care for him after discharge from hospital may not want to discuss this concern with a nurse within hearing of other clients in the room. Environmental distraction can impair and distort communication.

CONGRUENCE In **congruent communication**, the verbal and nonverbal aspects of the message match. Clients more readily trust the nurse when they perceive the nurse's communication as congruent. This will also help to prevent miscommunication. When teaching a client how to care for a colostomy, the nurse might say, "You won't have any problem with this." If the nurse looks worried or disgusted while saying this, the client is less likely to trust the words.

INTERPERSONAL ATTITUDES Attitudes convey beliefs, thoughts, and feelings about people and events. Attitudes are communicated convincingly and rapidly to others. Such attitudes as caring, warmth, respect, and acceptance facilitate communication, whereas condescension, lack of interest, and coldness inhibit communication.

Caring and *warmth* convey a feeling of emotional closeness, in contrast to an impersonal approach. Caring is more enduring and intense than warmth. It conveys deep and genuine concern for the person, whereas warmth conveys friendliness and consideration, shown by acts of smiling and attention to physical comforts (Brammer & MacDonald, 2002). Caring involves encouraging expression of and accepting clients' feelings and thoughts. It requires psychological energy and poses the risk of gaining little in return.

Respect is an attitude that emphasizes the other person's worth and individuality. It conveys that the person's hopes and feelings are special and unique, even though similar to others in many ways. A nurse conveys respect by listening open-mindedly to what the other person is saying, even if the nurse disagrees.

Acceptance emphasizes neither approval nor disapproval. The nurse willingly receives the client's honest feelings and actions without judgment. An accepting attitude encourages clients to express personal feelings freely and to be themselves. The nurse may need to restrict acceptance in situations in which clients' actions are harmful to themselves or to others.

Therapeutic Communication

Unlike the social relationship, which may not have a specific purpose or direction, **therapeutic communication** between the nurse and the client is goal-directed and can promote understanding between them.

Nurses need to respond not only to the content of a client's verbal message but also to the feelings and thoughts expressed. It is important to understand how the client views the situation and feels about it before responding. Sometimes, people can convey a thought in words while their emotions contradict the words. For example, a client says, "I am glad my spouse has left me; my spouse was very cruel." However, the nurse observes that the client is in tears as this is said. To respond to the client's *words,* the nurse might simply rephrase, saying "You are pleased that your spouse has left you." To respond to the client's *feelings,* the nurse would need to acknowledge the tears in the client's eyes, saying, for example, "You seem saddened by all this." Such a response helps the client to focus on feelings. In some instances, the nurse may need to know more about the client and resources for coping with these feelings.

Strong emotions are often draining. People usually need time to deal with feelings before they can cope with other matters, such as learning new skills or planning for the future. This is most evident in hospitals when patients learn that they have a terminal illness. Some require hours, days, or even weeks before they are ready to start other tasks. Some need time to themselves, and others need someone to listen; some need assistance identifying and verbalizing feelings, and others need assistance making decisions about future action.

ATTENTIVE LISTENING **Attentive listening** is listening actively by using all the senses, as opposed to listening passively with just the ears. Attentive listening is an active process that requires energy and concentration. It involves paying attention to the total message, both verbal and nonverbal, and noting whether these communica-

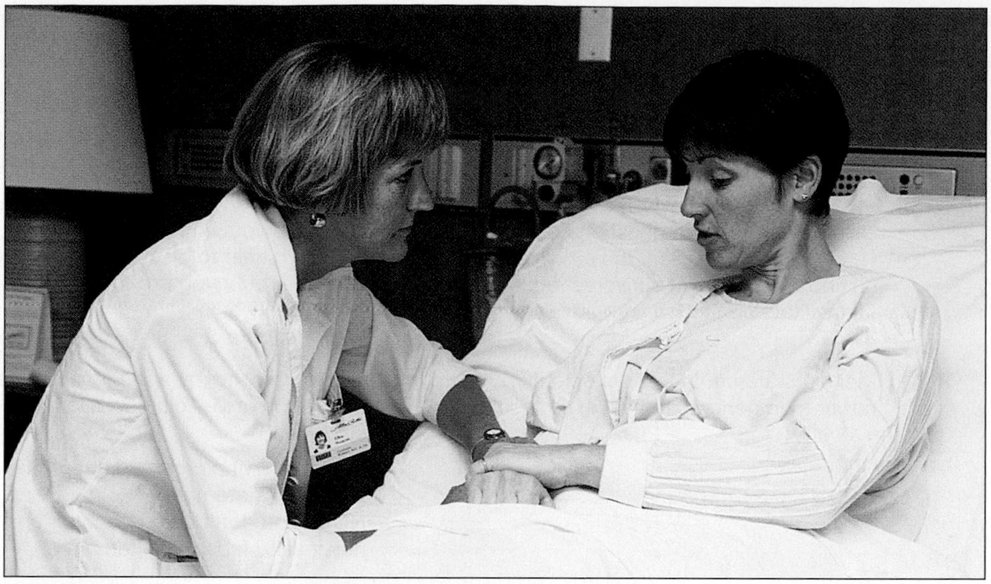

FIGURE 21.5 The nurse conveys attentive listening and actions of physical presence.

tions are congruent. The listener does not select or listen solely to what the listener wants to hear; the nurse focuses not on the nurse's own needs but, rather, on the client's needs. Attentive listening conveys an attitude of caring and interest, thereby encouraging the client to talk.

Attentive listening also involves listening for key themes in the communication. Nurses must be aware of their own biases and careful not to react quickly to the message. The speaker should not be interrupted and the nurse (the responder) should take time to think about the message before responding. As a listener, the nurse also should ask questions either to obtain additional information or to clarify.

Attentive listening is a highly developed skill, and it can be learned with practice. A nurse can convey attentiveness in listening to clients in various ways. Common responses are nodding the head, uttering "uh huh" or "mmm," repeating the words that the client has used, or saying, "I see what you mean" (see Figure 21.5).

PHYSICAL ATTENDING Egan (2006) has outlined five specific ways to convey physical attending, which he defines as the manner of being present to another or being with another. Listening is what a person does while attending. The five actions of physical attending, which convey a "posture of involvement" and specifically focus on comforting a client are shown in Box 21.2. Therapeutic communication techniques facilitate communication and focus on the client's concerns (as described in Table 21.1).

BOX 21.2 ACTIONS OF PHYSICAL ATTENDING

Use of the following actions of physical attending can help nurses to comfort a client:

- *Face the other person squarely.* This position says, "I am available to you." Moving to the side lessens the degree of involvement.
- *Adopt an open posture.* The nondefensive position is one in which neither arms nor legs are crossed. It conveys that the person wants to encourage the passage of communication, as the open door of a home or an office does.
- *Lean toward the person.* People move naturally toward each other when they want to say or hear something—by moving to the front of a class, by moving a chair nearer a friend, or by leaning across a table with arms propped in front. The nurse conveys involvement by leaning forward, closer to the client.
- *Maintain good eye contact.* Mutual eye contact, preferably at the same level, recognizes the other person and denotes willingness to maintain communication. Eye contact neither glares at nor stares down another person but is natural.
- *Try to be relatively relaxed.* Total relaxation is not feasible when the nurse is listening with intensity, but the nurse can show relaxation by taking time in responding, allowing pauses as needed, balancing periods of tension with relaxation, and using gestures that are natural.

These five attending postures need to be adapted to the specific needs (and culture) of clients in a given situation. For example, leaning forward may not be appropriate at the beginning of an interview. It may be reserved until a closer relationship develops between the nurse and the client. The same applies to eye contact, which is generally uninterrupted when the communicators are very involved in the interaction.

TABLE 21.1 Therapeutic Communication Techniques

Technique	Description	Examples
Using silence	Accepting pauses or silences that extend for several seconds or minutes without interjecting any verbal response.	Sitting quietly (or walking with the client) and waiting attentively until the client is able to put thoughts and feelings into words.
Providing general leads	Using statements or questions that (1) encourage the client to verbalize; (2) choose a topic of conversation; and (3) facilitate continued verbalization.	"Perhaps you would like to talk about…" "Would it help to discuss your feelings?" "Where would you like to begin?" "And then what?" "Tell me more . . . ."
Being specific and tentative	Making statements that are specific, rather than general, tentative, or absolute.	"You scratched my arm." (specific statement) NOT: "You are as clumsy as an ox." (general statement) "You seem unconcerned about Mary." (tentative statement) NOT: "You don't care about her and you never will." (absolute statement)
Using open-ended questions	Asking broad questions that lead or invite the client to explore (elaborate, clarify, describe, compare, or illustrate) thoughts or feelings. Open-ended questions specify only the topic to be discussed and invite answers that are longer than one or two words.	"I'd like to hear more about that." "Tell me about . . . ." "How have you been feeling lately?" "What brought you to the hospital?" "What is your opinion?" "You said you were frightened yesterday. How do you feel now?"
Using touch	Providing appropriate forms of touch to reinforce caring feelings. Because tactile contacts vary considerably among individuals, families, and cultures, the nurse must be sensitive to the differences in attitudes and practices of clients and self.	Putting an arm over the client's shoulder, with permission. Placing your hand over the client's hand, with permission.
Restating or paraphrasing	Actively listening for the client's basic message and then repeating those thoughts and/or feelings in similar words. This conveys that the nurse has listened and understood the client's basic message and also offers clients a clearer idea of what they have said.	*Client*: "I couldn't manage to eat any dinner last night—not even the dessert." *Nurse*: "You had difficulty eating yesterday." *Client*: "Yes, I was very upset after my family left." *Client*: "I have trouble talking to strangers." *Nurse*: "You find it difficult talking to people you do not know?"
Seeking clarification	A method of making the client's broad overall meaning of the message more understandable. It is used when paraphrasing is difficult or when the communication is rambling or garbled. To clarify the message, the nurse can restate the basic message or confess confusion and ask the client to repeat or restate the message.	"I'm puzzled." "I'm not sure I understand that." "Would you please say that again?" "Would you tell me more?"
	Nurses can also clarify their own message with statements.	"I meant this rather than that." "I guess I didn't make that clear—I'll go over it again."
Checking perception or seeking consensual validation	A method similar to clarifying that verifies the meaning of specific words, rather than the overall meaning of a message.	*Client*: "My husband never gives me any presents." *Nurse*: "You mean he has never given you a present for your birthday or Christmas?" *Client*: "Well—not never. He does get me something for my birthday and Christmas, but he never thinks of giving me anything at any other time."

(continued)

TABLE 21.1 Therapeutic Communication Techniques *(continued)*

Technique	Description	Examples
Offering the self	Suggesting a presence, interest, or wish to understand the client without making any demands or attaching conditions that the client must comply with to receive the nurse's attention.	"I'll stay with you until your daughter arrives." "We can sit here quietly for a while; we don't need to talk unless you would like to." "I'll help you dress to go home."
Giving information	Providing, in a simple and direct manner, specific factual information the client may or may not request. When information is not known, the nurse states this and indicates who has it or when the nurse will obtain it.	"Your surgery is scheduled for 11 a.m. tomorrow." "You will feel a pulling sensation when the tube is removed from your abdomen." "I do not know the answer to that, but I will find out from Mrs. King, the nurse in charge."
Acknowledging	Giving recognition, in a nonjudgmental way, of a change in behaviour, an effort the client has made, or a contribution to a communication. Acknowledgment may be with or without understanding and verbal or nonverbal.	"You trimmed your beard and moustache and washed your hair." "I notice you keep squinting your eyes. Are you having difficulty seeing?" "You walked twice as far today with your walker."
Clarifying time or sequence	Helping the client clarify an event, situation, or happening in relationship to time.	*Client*: "I vomited this morning." *Nurse*: "Was that after breakfast?" *Client*: "I feel that I have been asleep for weeks." *Nurse*: "You had your operation Monday, and today is Tuesday."
Presenting reality	Helping the client to differentiate the real from the unreal.	"That telephone ring came from the program on television." "That's not a dead mouse in the corner; it is a discarded washcloth." "Your magazine is here in the drawer. It has not been stolen."
Focusing	Helping the client expand on and develop a topic of importance. It is important for the nurse to wait until the client finishes stating the main concerns before attempting to focus. The focus may be an idea or a feeling; however, the nurse often emphasizes a feeling to help the client recognize an emotion disguised behind words.	*Client*: "My wife says she will look after me, but I don't think she can, what with the children to take care of, and they're always after her about something—clothes, homework, what's for dinner that night." *Nurse*: "You are worried about how well she can manage."
Reflecting	Directing ideas, feelings, questions, or content back to clients to enable them to explore their own ideas and feelings about a situation.	*Client*: "What can I do?" *Nurse*: "What do you think would be helpful?" *Client*: "Do you think I should tell my husband?" *Nurse*: "You seem unsure about telling your husband."
Summarizing and planning	Stating the main points of a discussion to clarify the relevant points discussed. This technique is useful at the end of an interview or to review a health teaching session. It often acts as an introduction to future care planning.	"During the past half hour we have talked about . . ." "Tomorrow afternoon we may explore this further." "In a few days I'll review what you have learned about the actions and effects of your insulin."

Barriers to Communication

Nurses need to recognize barriers or nontherapeutic responses to effective communication. See Table 21.2.

Failure to listen, improperly decoding the client's intended message, and placing the nurse's needs above the client's needs are major barriers to communication.

TABLE 21.2 Barriers to Communication

Barrier	Description	Examples
Stereotyping	Offering generalized and oversimplified beliefs about groups of people that are based on experiences too limited to be valid. These responses categorize clients and negate their uniqueness as individuals.	"Two-year-olds are brats." "Women are complainers." "Men don't cry." "Most people don't have any pain after this type of surgery."
Agreeing and disagreeing	Akin to judgmental responses, agreeing and disagreeing imply that the client is either right or wrong and that the nurse is in a position to judge this. These responses deter clients from thinking through their position and may cause a client to become defensive.	*Client*: "I don't think Dr. Broad is a very good doctor. He doesn't seem interested in his patients." *Nurse*: "Dr. Broad is head of the Department of Surgery and is an excellent surgeon."
Being defensive	Attempting to protect a person or health-care services from negative comments. These responses prevent the client from expressing true concerns. The nurse is saying, "You have no right to complain." Defensive responses protect the nurse from admitting weaknesses in the health-care services, including personal weaknesses.	*Client*: "Those night nurses must just sit around and talk all night. They didn't answer my light for over an hour." *Nurse*: "I'll have you know we literally run around on nights. You're not the only client, you know."
Challenging	Giving a response that makes clients prove their statement or point of view. These responses indicate that the nurse is failing to consider the client's feelings, making the client feel it necessary to defend a position.	*Client*: "I felt nauseated after that red pill." *Nurse*: "Surely you don't think I gave you the wrong pill?" *Client*: "I feel as if I am dying." *Nurse*: "How can you feel that way when your pulse is 60?" *Client*: "I believe my husband doesn't love me." *Nurse*: "You can't say that; why, he visits you every day."
Probing	Asking for information chiefly out of curiosity, rather than with the intent to assist the client. These responses are considered prying and violate the client's privacy. Asking "why" is often probing and places the client in a defensive position.	*Client*: "I was speeding along the street and didn't see the stop sign." *Nurse*: "Why were you speeding?" *Client*: "I didn't ask the doctor when he was here." *Nurse*: "Why didn't you?"
Testing	Asking questions that make the client admit to something. These responses permit the client only limited answers and often meet the nurse's need, rather than the client's.	"Who do you think you are?" (forces people to admit their status is only that of client) "Do you think I am not busy?" (forces the client to admit that the nurse really is busy)
Rejecting	Refusing to discuss certain topics with the client. These responses often make clients feel that the nurse is rejecting not only their communication but also the clients themselves.	"I don't want to discuss that. Let's talk about . . ." "Let's discuss other areas of interest to you rather than the two problems you keep mentioning." "I can't talk now. I'm on my way for coffee break."
Changing topics and subjects	Directing the communication into areas of self-interest, rather than considering the client's concerns, is often a self-protective response to a topic that causes anxiety. These responses imply that what the nurse considers important will be discussed and that clients should not discuss certain topics.	*Client*: "I'm separated from my wife. Do you think I should have sexual relations with another woman?" *Nurse*: "You like gardening. This sunshine is good for my roses. I have a beautiful rose garden."

(continued)

TABLE 21.2 Barriers to Communication *(continued)*

Barrier	Description	Examples
Unwarranted reassurance	Using clichés or comforting statements of advice as a means to reassure the client. These responses block the fears, feelings, and other thoughts of the client.	"You'll feel better soon." "I'm sure everything will turn out all right." "Don't worry."
Passing judgment	Giving opinions and approving or disapproving responses, moralizing, or implying one's own values. These responses imply that the client must think as the nurse thinks, fostering client dependence.	"That's good (bad)." "You shouldn't do that." "That's not good enough." "What you did was wrong (right)."
Giving common advice	Telling the client what to do. These responses deny the client's right to be an equal partner. Note that giving expert, rather than common, advice is therapeutic.	*Client*: "Should I move from my home to a nursing home?" *Nurse*: "If I were you, I'd go to a nursing home where you'll get your meals cooked for you."

The Helping Relationship

Nurse–client relationships are referred to by some as *interpersonal relationships,* by others as *therapeutic relationships,* and by still others as *helping relationships.* Helping is a growth-facilitating process that strives to achieve two basic goals (Egan, 2006):

1. Helping clients manage their problems in living more effectively and develop unused or underused opportunities more fully
2. Helping clients become better at helping themselves in their everyday lives

A helping relationship can develop over weeks of working with a client, or over minutes. The keys to the helping relationship are (1) the development of trust and acceptance between the nurse and the client, and (2) an underlying belief that the nurse cares about and wants to help the client.

The helping relationship is influenced by the personal and professional characteristics of the nurse and the client. Age, gender, appearance, diagnosis, education, values, ethnic and cultural background, personality, expectations, and setting can all affect the development of the nurse–client relationship. Consideration of all these factors, combined with good communication skills and sincere interest in the client's welfare, will enable the nurse to create a helping relationship. Characteristics of helping relationships are described in Box 21.3.

BOX 21.3 CHARACTERISTICS OF A HELPING RELATIONSHIP

A helping relationship has the following characteristics:

- It is an intellectual and emotional bond between the nurse and the client and is focused on the client.
- It respects the client as an individual, including
  a. Maximizing the client's abilities to participate in decision making and treatments
  b. Considering ethnic and cultural aspects
  c. Considering family relationships and values
- It respects client confidentiality.
- It focuses on the client's well-being.
- It is based on mutual trust, respect, and acceptance.

Phases of the Helping Relationship

The helping relationship process can be described in terms of four sequential phases, each characterized by identifiable tasks and skills. The relationship must progress through the stages in succession because each builds on the one before. Nurses can identify the progress of a relationship by understanding these phases: preinteraction phase, introductory phase, working (maintaining) phase, and termination phase. Table 21.3 summarizes the tasks and skills required.

PREINTERACTION PHASE Before an interview and in most situations, the nurse has information about the client before the first face-to-face meeting. Such information can include the client's name, address, age, medical history, and social history. Planning for the initial visit may generate some anxious feelings in the nurse. If the nurse recognizes these feelings and identifies specific information to be discussed, positive outcomes can evolve.

INTRODUCTORY PHASE The introductory phase, also referred to as the *orientation phase* or the *prehelping phase,* is important because it sets the tone for the rest of the relationship. During this initial encounter, the client and the nurse closely observe each other and form judg-

TABLE 21.3 Tasks and Skills for Each Phase of the Helping Relationship

Phase	Tasks	Skills
Preinteraction phase	The nurse reviews pertinent knowledge, considers potential areas of concern, and develops plans for interaction.	Recognizing limitations and seeking assistance, as required.
Introductory phase		
1. Opening the relationship	Both client and nurse identify each other by name. When the nurse initiates the relationship, it is important to explain the nurse's role to give the client an idea of what to expect. When the client initiates the relationship, the nurse needs to help the client express concerns and reasons for seeking help. Vague, open-ended questions, such as "What's on your mind today?" are helpful at this stage.	A relaxed, attending attitude to put the client at ease. It is not easy for all clients to receive help.
2. Clarifying the problem	Because the client initially may not see the problem clearly, the nurse's major task is to help clarify the problem.	Attentive listening, paraphrasing, clarifying, and other effective communication techniques discussed in this chapter. A common error at this stage is to ask too many questions of the client.
3. Structuring and formulating the contract (obligations to be met by both the nurse and client)	Nurse and client develop a degree of trust and verbally agree about (1) location, frequency, and length of meetings, (2) overall purpose of the relationship, (3) how confidential material will be handled, (4) tasks to be accomplished, and (5) duration and indications for termination of the relationship.	Communication skills listed above and ability to overcome resistive behaviours if they occur.
Working phase	Nurse and client accomplish the tasks outlined in the introductory phase, enhance trust and rapport, and develop caring.	
1. Exploring and understanding thoughts and feelings	The nurse assists the client to explore thoughts and feelings and acquires an understanding of the client. The client explores thoughts and feelings associated with problems, develops the skill of listening, and gains insight into personal behaviour.	Listening and attending skills, empathy, respect, genuineness, concreteness, self-disclosure, and confrontation. Skills acquired by the client are nondefensive listening and self-understanding.
2. Facilitating and taking action	The nurse plans programs within the client's capabilities and considers long- and short-term goals. The client needs to learn to take risks (i.e., accept that either failure or success may be the outcome). The nurse needs to reinforce successes and help the client recognize failures realistically.	Decision-making and goal-setting skills. Also, for the nurse, reinforcement skills; for the client, risk taking.
Termination phase	Nurse and client accept feelings of loss. The client accepts the end of the relationship without feelings of anxiety or dependence.	For the nurse, summarizing skills. For the client, abilities to handle problems independently.

ments about the other's behaviour. The three stages of this introductory phase are opening the relationship, clarifying the problem, and structuring and formulating the contract (Brammer & MacDonald, 2002). Other important tasks of the introductory phase include getting to know each other and developing a degree of trust.

After introductions, the nurse may initially engage in some social interaction to put the client at ease. For example, the nurse and client may talk about what a nice day it is and what they would like to do if at home.

During the initial parts of the introductory phase, the client may display some resistive behaviours. *Resistive behaviours* are those that inhibit involvement, cooperation, or change. They may be due to difficulty in acknowledging the need for help and, thus, a dependent role, fear of exposing and facing feelings, anxiety about the discomfort involved in changing problem-causing behaviour patterns, and fear or anxiety in response to the nurse's approach, which may, in the client's opinion, be inappropriate.

Resistive behaviours can be overcome by conveying a caring attitude, genuine interest in the client, and competence. These behaviours of the nurse also foster the development of trust in the relationship. *Trust* can be described as a reliance on someone without doubt or question, or the belief that the other person is capable of assisting in times of distress and, in all likelihood, will do so. To trust another person involves risk; clients become vulnerable when they share thoughts, feelings, and attitudes with the nurse. Trust, however, enables the client to express thoughts and feelings openly.

By the end of the introductory phase, clients should begin to

- Develop trust in the nurse
- View the nurse as a competent professional capable of helping
- View the nurse as honest, open, and concerned about their welfare
- Believe the nurse will try to understand and respect their cultural values and beliefs
- Believe the nurse will respect client confidentiality
- Feel comfortable talking with the nurse about feelings and other sensitive issues
- Understand the purpose of the relationship and the roles
- Feel that they are active participants in developing a mutually agreeable plan of care

WORKING PHASE During the working phase of a helping relationship, the nurse and the client begin to view each other as unique individuals. They begin to appreciate this uniqueness and care about each other. Caring is sharing deep and genuine concern about the welfare of another person. Once caring develops, the potential for empathy increases.

The working phase has two major stages: *exploring and understanding thoughts and feelings*, and *facilitating and taking action*. The nurse helps the client to explore thoughts, feelings, and actions and helps the client plan a program of action to meet established goals.

EXPLORING AND UNDERSTANDING THOUGHTS AND FEELINGS The nurse requires the following skills for this phase of the helping relationship:

- *Empathetic listening and responding.* Nurses must listen attentively and communicate (respond) in ways that indicate they have listened to what was said and understand how the client feels. The nurse responds to content or feelings, or both, as appropriate. The nurse's nonverbal behaviours are also important. Nonverbal behaviours indicating empathy include moderate head nodding, a steady gaze, moderate gesturing, and little activity or body movement. **Empathy** is an emotional response experienced by the helper and an *intellectual* process through which the helper tries to have a correct understanding of another person's emotional state and point of view (Egan, 2006). Empathetic listening focuses on a kind of way of being with clients to develop an understanding of them and their world. This understanding, however, must also be communicated effectively to the client—an empathetic response. The end result of empathy is comforting and caring for the client and a helping, healing relationship.
- *Respect.* The nurse must show respect for the client's willingness to be available, as well as a desire to work with the client, and a manner that conveys the idea of taking the client's point of view seriously.
- *Genuineness.* The genuine person is spontaneous, is nondefensive, displays few discrepancies, and uses self-disclosure appropriately (Egan, 2006). Personal statements can be helpful in solidifying the rapport between the nurse and the client. Nurses need to exercise caution when making references about themselves. These statements must be used with discretion.
- *Concreteness.* The nurse must assist the client to be concrete and specific, rather than to speak in generalities. When the client says, "I'm stupid and clumsy," the nurse narrows the topic to the specific by pointing out, "You tripped on the scatter rug."
- *Confrontation.* The nurse points out discrepancies among thoughts, feelings, and actions that inhibit the client's self-understanding or exploration of specific areas. This is done empathetically, not judgmentally.

During this first stage of the working phase, the intensity of interaction increases, and such feelings as anger, shame, or self-consciousness may be expressed. If the nurse is skilled in this stage, and if the client is willing to pursue self-exploration, the outcome is a beginning of understanding on the part of the client about behaviour and feelings.

FACILITATING AND TAKING ACTION Ultimately, the client must make decisions and take action to become more effective. The responsibility for action belongs to the client. The nurse, however, collaborates in these decisions, provides support, and may offer options or information.

TERMINATION PHASE The termination phase of the relationship is often expected to be difficult and filled with ambivalence. On the one hand, if the previous phases have evolved effectively, the client generally has a positive outlook and feels able to handle problems independently. On the other hand, because caring attitudes have developed, it is natural to expect some feelings of loss, and each person needs to develop a way of saying goodbye.

Many methods can be used to terminate relationships. Summarizing or reviewing the process can produce a sense of accomplishment. This can include sharing reminiscences of how things were at the beginning of the relationship and comparing them with how they are now. It is also helpful for both the nurse and the client to express their feelings about termination openly and honestly. Thus, termination discussions need to start in advance of the termination interview. This allows time for the client to adjust to independence. In some situations, referrals are necessary, or it may be appropriate to offer an occasional standby meeting to give support as needed. Follow-up phone calls are another intervention that eases the client's transition to independence.

Developing Helping Relationships

Whatever the practice setting, the nurse establishes some type of helping relationship in which mutual goals (outcomes) are set with the client or, if the client is unable to participate, with support persons. The following are key elements for developing a helping relationship:

- Listen actively and identify what the person is feeling.
- Put yourself in the other person's shoes (i.e., empathize).
- Be honest and genuine.
- Be aware of cultural differences.
- Maintain client confidentiality.
- Know your role and limitations and refer client to the appropriate health-care professional as needed.

Group Communication

People are born into a group (i.e., a family) and interact with others at all stages of life in various groups: peer groups, work groups, recreational groups, religious groups, and so on. A **group** is two or more people who have shared needs and goals, who take each other into account in their actions and who, thus, are held together and set apart from others by virtue of their interactions. Groups exist to help people achieve goals (outcomes) that would be unattainable by individual effort alone. For example, groups can often solve problems more effectively than one person by pooling the ideas and expertise of several individuals; in addition, information can be disseminated to groups more quickly than to individuals.

Group Dynamics

The communication that takes place between members of any group is known as **group dynamics**. The manner of this communication will be determined by a number of interrelated factors and variables. Members of the group will have an effect on the group dynamics on the basis of their motivation for participating and their similarity to other group members and the goal of that group.

The unique dynamics of each group will influence its maturation or group process, as well as the effectiveness of the group. Three main functions are required for any group to be effective: (1) it must maintain a degree of group unity or cohesion, (2) it needs to develop and modify its structure to improve its effectiveness, and (3) it must accomplish its goals. The characteristics of an effectively functioning group are shown in Table 21.4.

Types of Health-Care Groups

Much of a nurse's professional life is spent in a wide variety of groups, ranging from *dyads* (two-person groups) to large professional organizations. As a participant in a group, the nurse may be required to fulfill different roles: member or leader, teacher or learner, adviser or advisee, and so on.

Common types of health-care groups include task groups, teaching and learning groups, self-help groups, self-awareness or growth groups, therapy groups, and work-related social support groups. Among the characteristics of these various types of groups and the nurse's role are similarities and differences.

TASK GROUPS The task group is one of the most common types of work-related groups to which nurses belong. Examples are health-care planning committees, nursing service committees, nursing team meetings, nursing care conference groups, and hospital staff meetings. The focus of such groups is the completion of a specific task, and the format is defined at the outset by the leader or members. The methods vary according to the task to be performed.

The leader of a task group, usually called the *chairperson,* must be accepted by the members as an appropriate leader and, therefore, should be an expert in the area of task emphasis. The chairperson's role is to identify the specific task, clarify communication, and assist in expressing opinions and offering solutions. *Committee members* are generally selected in terms of their individual functional role and employment status rather than in terms of their personal characteristics. Member participation is determined by the task. A target date for termination of the group is usually set in advance.

TEACHING AND LEARNING GROUPS The major purpose of teaching and learning groups is to impart information to the participants. Examples of teaching groups include continuing education and client health-care groups. Numerous subjects are often handled via the group teaching format: childbirth techniques; birth control methods; effective parenting; nutrition; management of chronic illness, such as diabetes; exercise for middle-aged and older adults; and instructions to family members about follow-up care for discharged clients. A nurse who leads a group in which the primary purpose is to teach or learn must be skilled in the teaching-learning process discussed in Chapter 25 (see Figure 21.6).

TABLE 21.4 Comparative Features of Effective and Ineffective Groups

Factor	Effective Groups	Ineffective Groups
Atmosphere	Comfortable and relaxed: it is a working atmosphere in which people demonstrate their interest and involvement.	Tense: lacks privacy or voluntary commitment to the group.
Purpose	Goals, tasks, and outcomes are clarified, understood, and modified so that members of the group can commit themselves to purposes through cooperation.	The purposes are unclear, misunderstood, or imposed.
Leadership and member participation	Leadership is democratic with a shift in leadership from time to time depending on knowledge or experience.	Authoritarian: the leader may dominate the group, or the members may defer unduly. Member participation is unequal, with some members dominating.
Communication	Open: ideas and feelings are encouraged.	Closed: only idea production is encouraged. Feelings are ignored. Members may have "hidden agendas" (personal goals at cross-purposes with group goals).
Decision making	Done by the group, although various decision-making procedures appropriate to the situation may be instituted.	Done by the highest authority in the group, or one or two strong members of the group, with minimal involvement by members. Disagreements are ignored.
Cohesion	Facilitated through valuing other group members, open expression of feelings, trust, and support.	The leader claims full credit for achievements. Comments are critical and focus on personal characteristics.
Conflict tolerance	The reasons for disagreements or conflicts are carefully examined, and the group seeks to resolve them.	Fear of conflict prevents decisions and growth.
Power	Determined by the members' abilities and the information they possess. Power is shared.	Determined by position in the group. Obedience to authority is strong. The issue is who is in control based on individual emotional needs of members.
Problem solving	High: constructive criticism is frequent, frank, relatively comfortable, and oriented toward problem solving.	Low: criticism may be destructive, taking the form of either overt or covert personal attacks.
Creativity	Encouraged.	Discouraged.

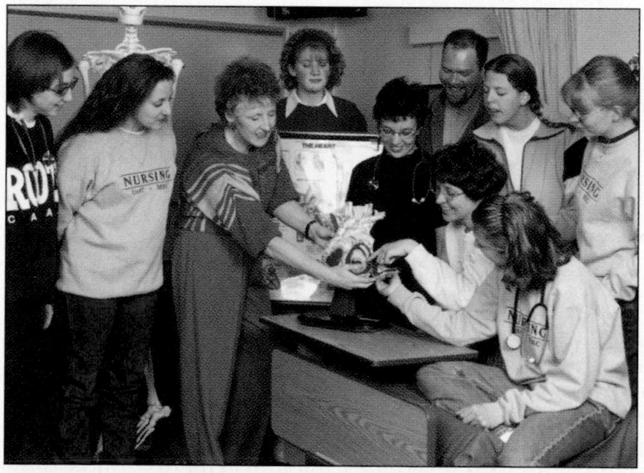

FIGURE 21.6 Teaching can occur within groups.

SELF-HELP GROUPS A self-help group is a small, voluntary organization composed of individuals who share a similar health, social, or daily living concern. These groups are based on the helper-therapy principle: Those who help are helped most. One of the central beliefs of the self-help movement is that people who experience a particular social or health concern have an understanding of the condition that those without it do not.

Self-help groups are available for a range of concerns (e.g., stillbirth, parenting, adolescent pregnancy, divorce, problematic drug use, cancer, menopause, mental illness, diabetes, acquired immune deficiency syndrome [AIDS], women's health, caring for the elderly, and grief). Alcoholics' Anonymous was the first self-help group. The positive aspects of self-help groups are outlined in Box 21.4.

BOX 21.4 POSITIVE ASPECTS OF SELF-HELP GROUPS

Self-help groups have many positive aspects:

- Members can experience almost instant kinship because the essence of the group is the idea that "you are not alone."
- Members can talk about their feelings and listen to the concerns of others, knowing they all share this experience.
- The group atmosphere is generally one of acceptance, support, encouragement, and caring.
- Many members act as role models for newer members and can inspire them to attempt tasks they might consider impossible.
- The group provides the opportunity for people to help as well as to *be* helped—a critical component in restoring self-esteem.

The major functions of the nurse's role in self-help groups include the following:

- Helping clients form such groups by identifying key people who can act as facilitators
- Sharing expertise with clients and helping them gain appropriate knowledge and skills
- Informing clients and support persons about existing self-help groups available to them
- Participating as a member of a self-help group when this is appropriate; the nurse's role is that of a resource person, that is, being "on tap but not on top"
- Helping out in times of crisis

SELF-AWARENESS OR GROWTH GROUPS The purpose of self-awareness or growth groups is to develop or use interpersonal strengths. The overall aim is to improve the person's functioning in the group to which they return, whether job, family, or community. From the beginning, broad goals are usually apparent, for example, to study communication patterns, group process, or problem solving. Because the focus of these groups is interpersonal concerns around current situations, the work of the group is oriented to reality testing with a here-and-now emphasis. Members are responsible for correcting inefficient patterns of relating and communicating with each other. They learn group process through participation and involvement and guided exercises.

THERAPY GROUPS Therapy groups work toward self-understanding, more satisfactory ways of relating or handling stress, and changing patterns of behaviour toward health. Members of the therapy group are referred to as clients or, in some settings, as patients. They are selected by health-care professionals after extensive selection interviews that consider the pattern of personalities, behaviours, needs, and identification of group therapy as the treatment of choice. Duration of therapy groups is not usually set. A termination date is usually mutually determined by the therapist and members.

WORK-RELATED SOCIAL SUPPORT GROUPS Many nurses, for example, hospice, emergency, and acute-care nurses, experience high levels of vocational stress. Various types of group support can buffer such stress. Group members who know about the work of others can encourage and challenge members to be more creative and enthusiastic about their work and to achieve more. For example, a nurse may help another team member consider alternative strategies for intervention. Members also can share the joys of success and the frustration of failure through active listening without giving advice or making judgments.

Communication and the Nursing Process

Communication is an integral part of the nursing process. Nurses use communication skills in each phase of the nursing process. Communication is also important when caring for clients who have communication problems.

Assessing

To assess the client's communication, the nurse determines communication impairments or barriers and communication style. Remember that culture can influence when and how a client speaks. Obviously, language varies according to age and development. With children, the nurse observes sounds, gestures, and vocabulary.

IMPAIRMENTS TO COMMUNICATION Various barriers can alter a client's ability to send, receive, or comprehend messages. These include language deficits, sensory deficits, cognitive impairments, structural deficits, and paralysis. The nurse must assess each client to determine their presence.

LANGUAGE DEFICITS Determine the client's primary language for communicating and whether a fluent interpreter is required. Some clients who use English as a second language may have language skills that are inadequate to meet their needs.

SENSORY DEFICITS The ability to hear, see, feel, and smell are important adjuncts to communication. Deafness can significantly alter the message the client receives; impaired vision alters the ability to observe nonverbal behaviour, such as a smile or a gesture; the inability to feel and smell can impair the client's capabilities to report injuries or detect the smoke from a fire. For clients with severe hearing impairments, follow these steps:

- Look for a MedicAlert bracelet (or necklace or tag) indicating hearing loss.
- Determine whether the client wears a hearing aid and whether it is functioning.
- Observe whether the client is attempting to see your face to read your lips.
- Observe whether the client is using his or her hands to communicate with sign language.

Cognitive Impairments Any disorder that impairs cognitive functioning (e.g., cerebrovascular disease, Alzheimer's disease, and brain tumours or injuries) can affect a client's ability to use and understand language (see the Lifespan Considerations box). These clients lose the ability to speak, have impaired articulation, or may not be able to find the correct words. Certain medications, such as sedatives, antidepressants, and neuroleptics, can also impair speech, causing the client to use incomplete sentences or to slur words.

The nurse assesses whether the client responds when asked a question and, if so, the nurse then assesses the following: Is the client's speech fluent or hesitant? Does the client use words correctly? Can the client comprehend instructions as evidenced by following directions? Can the client repeat words or phrases? In addition, the nurse assesses the client's ability to understand written words: Can the client follow written directions? Can the client respond correctly by pointing to a written word? Can the client read aloud? Can the client recognize words or letters if unable to read whole sentences? The nurse uses large, clearly written words when trying to establish abilities in this area.

When the client is unconscious, the nurse looks for any indication that suggests comprehension of what is communicated (e.g., tries to arouse the client verbally and through touch). The nurse can ask a closed question, such as "Can you hear me?" and watch for a nonverbal response, such as a nod of the head for yes or a shake for no, or the nurse can ask for a hand squeeze or blink of the eyes once for yes or twice for no.

Structural Deficits Structural deficits of the oral and nasal cavities and respiratory system can alter a person's ability to speak clearly and spontaneously. Examples include cleft palate, artificial airways, such as an endotracheal tube or tracheostomy, and laryngectomy (removal of the larynx). Extreme dyspnea (shortness of breath) can also impair speech patterns.

Paralysis If verbal impairment is combined with paralysis of the upper extremities that impairs the client's ability to write, the nurse should determine whether the client can point, nod, shrug, blink, or squeeze a hand. Any of these could be used to devise a communication system.

STYLE OF COMMUNICATION In assessing communication style, the nurse considers both verbal and nonverbal communication. In addition to physical barriers, some psychological illnesses (e.g., depression or psychosis) influence the ability to communicate. The client may demonstrate constant verbalization of the same words or phrases, a loose association of ideas, or flight of ideas.

Verbal Communication When assessing verbal communication, the nurse focuses on three areas: the content

Lifespan Considerations

Communication with Older Adults

Older adults may have physical or cognitive problems that necessitate nursing interventions for improvement of communication skills. Some of the common problems are as follows:

- Sensory deficits, such as vision and hearing
- Cognitive impairment, as in dementia
- Neurological deficits from strokes or other neurological conditions, such as aphasia (expressive or receptive) and lack of movement
- Psychosocial problems, such as depression

Recognizing specific needs and obtaining appropriate resources for clients can greatly increase their socialization and quality of life. Interventions directed toward improving communication in clients with these special needs are as follows:

- Make sure that assistive devices, glasses, and hearing aids are being used and are in good working order.
- Make referrals to appropriate resources, such as speech therapy.
- Make use of communications aids, such as communication boards, computers, or pictures, when possible.
- Keep environmental distractions to a minimum.
- Speak in short, simple sentences, one subject at a time. Reinforce or repeat what is said when necessary.
- Always face the person when speaking. Coming up behind someone can startle him or her.
- Include family and friends in conversation.
- Use reminiscing, either in individual conversations or in groups, to maintain memory connections and to enhance self-identity and self-esteem in the older adult.
- When verbal expression and nonverbal expression are incongruent, believe the nonverbal. Clarification of this and attentiveness to their feelings will help promote a feeling of caring and acceptance.
- Find out what has been important and has meaning to the person and try to maintain these things as much as possible. Even simple things, such as bedtime rituals, become important if they are lost in a hospital or extended-care setting.

of the message, the themes, and verbalized emotions. In addition, the nurse considers the following:

- Whether the communication pattern is slow, rapid, quiet, spontaneous, hesitant, evasive, and so on
- The vocabulary of the individual, particularly any changes from the vocabulary normally used; for example, a person who normally never swears may indicate increased stress or illness by an uncharacteristic use of profanity
- The presence of hostility, aggression, assertiveness, reticence, hesitance, anxiety, or loquaciousness (incessant verbalization) in communication
- Difficulties with verbal communication, such as slurring, stuttering, an inability to pronounce a particular sound, a lack of clarity in enunciation, an inability to speak in sentences, loose association of ideas, flight of ideas, or an inability to find or name words or identify objects
- Refusal or inability to speak

Nonverbal Communication Consider nonverbal communication in relation to the client's culture. Pay particular attention to facial expression, gestures, body movements, affect, tone of voice, posture, and eye contact.

Diagnosing

Impaired communication can be used as a nursing diagnosis when "an individual experiences, or could experience, a decreased ability to receive, process, transmit, and use a system of symbols—anything that has meaning (i.e., transmits meaning)" (Wilkinson, 2005, p. 80). Communication problems can be *receptive* (e.g., difficulty hearing) or *expressive* (e.g., difficulty speaking).

Wilkinson (2005) points out that the *impaired verbal communication* diagnosis may not be useful when an individual's communication problems are caused by a psychiatric illness or a coping problem. In those instances, the diagnosis of *fear* or *anxiety* may be more appropriate. Other nursing diagnoses (Carpenito-Moyet, 2008) used for clients experiencing communication problems that involve impaired verbal communication as the etiology could include the following:

- *Anxiety* related to impaired verbal communication
- *Powerlessness* related to impaired verbal communication
- *Self-esteem, chronic low* related to impaired verbal communication
- *Social isolation* related to impaired verbal communication

Planning

When a nursing diagnosis related to impaired communication has been made, the nurse and client determine goals or outcomes and begin planning ways to promote effective communication. The overall client goal for persons with *impaired verbal communication* is to reduce or resolve the factors impairing the communication. Specific nursing interventions will be planned from the stated etiology. Examples of outcome criteria to evaluate the effectiveness of nursing interventions and achievement of client goals follow:

- The client communicates that needs are being met.
- He or she begins to establish a method of communication:
  a. Signals yes or no to direct questions by using vocalization or an agreed-on physical cue (e.g., eye blink, hand squeeze)
  b. Uses verbal or nonverbal techniques to indicate needs
- The client perceives the message accurately, as evidenced by appropriate verbal or nonverbal responses.
- He or she communicates effectively in any of the following ways:
  a. Using the predominant language
  b. Using a translator or an interpreter
  c. Using sign language
  d. Using a word board or a picture board
  e. Using a computer
- The client regains maximum communication abilities.
- He or she expresses minimum fear, anxiety, frustration, and depression.
- The client uses resources appropriately.

Implementing

Nursing interventions to facilitate communication with clients who have problems with speech or language include manipulating the environment, providing support, employing measures to enhance communication, and educating the client and support person.

MANIPULATE THE ENVIRONMENT A quiet environment with limited distractions will make the most of the communication efforts of both the client and the nurse and increase the possibility of effective communication. Sufficient light will help in conveying nonverbal messages, which is especially important if visual or auditory acuity is impaired. Initially, the nurse needs to provide a calm, relaxed environment that will help reduce any anxiety the client may have. Any factor that affects communication can create feelings of frustration, anxiety, depression, or hostility in the client. Effective communication normally contributes to clients' sense of security and feelings that they are not alone, so communication problems can cause some clients to feel isolated and confused.

PROVIDE SUPPORT The nurse should convey encouragement to the client and provide nonverbal reassurance, perhaps by touch, if appropriate. If the nurse does not understand, it is critical to let the client know so that the nurse can provide clarification with other words or through some other means of communication. When speaking with a client who has difficulty understanding, the nurse should check frequently to determine what the client has heard and understood. The use of open-ended questions will help the nurse obtain accurate information about the effectiveness of communication. For example, Maria Perez, who has limited English skills, is being taught about a diet related to her Crohn's disease. If the nurse asks, "Do you understand what to eat?" Maria may nod her head yes. However, this does not give her nurse confirmation that the message given has been received. Rather, the nurse needs to say, "What do you think will be good for you to eat when you go home?" The nurse's body language (e.g., gestures, posture, facial expression, and eye contact) should convey acceptance and approval.

EMPLOY MEASURES TO ENHANCE COMMUNICATION Determine how the client can best receive messages: by listening, by looking, through touch, or through an interpreter. Ways to enhance communication include keeping words simple and concrete and discussing topics of interest to the client. It is often helpful to use alternative communication strategies, such as word boards, pictures, or paper and pencil (see the Reflect on Primary Health Care box).

Often, interpreters can help a client and nurse to communicate when the client lacks fluency in the predominant language. Some hospitals have a list of interpreters for various languages who can assist at the bedside. If the client's support person offers to interpret, it is important to ask the client's permission, for the sake of confidentiality. Then, instruct the person to translate as precisely as possible, without interpretation.

EDUCATE THE CLIENT AND SUPPORT PERSONS Sometimes, clients and support people can be prepared in advance for communication problems, for example, before an intubation or throat surgery. By explaining anticipated problems, the client is often less anxious when problems do arise.

REFLECT ON PRIMARY HEALTH CARE

In providing a holistic and caring approach in nursing practice, nurses work with clients, their significant others, and members of the multidisciplinary team to gather the needed information for nursing care planning (*intersectoral cooperation*). Effective communication skills are used to elicit input so that a plan of care can be mutually developed (*public participation*). In caring for acutely ill clients, nurses must consider how best to use *technology* to help them provide the needed quality of life, care, and comfort.

Evidence-Informed Practice

What Is an Effective Strategy to Elicit Patient Treatment Preferences?

Sidani, Epstein, and Miranda (2006) described a strategy that operationalizes an integrated patient-centred approach in nursing by addressing a clinical problem with patient's choice. A key step is to elicit patient preferences. Patients stated that they feel cared for when they feel respected and heard. The strategy consists of three stages: synthesis of evidence, generation of intervention description, and eliciting preferences.

NURSING IMPLICATIONS: It is important to use evidence-based approaches with patient-centred care in order to enhance the quality of care patients receive. Nurses are encouraged to use this strategy when caring for patients and their families in practice settings to augment the nurse–person relationship.

Source: Based on "Eliciting Patient Treatment Preferences: A Strategy to Integrate Evidence-Based and Patient-Centred Care, by S. Sidani, D. Epstein, and J. Miranda, 2006, *Worldviews on Evidence-Based Nursing, 3*(3), pp. 116–123.

Evaluating

Evaluation is useful for both client and nurse communication.

CLIENT COMMUNICATION To establish whether client goals have been met in relation to communication, the nurse must listen actively, observe nonverbal cues, and use therapeutic communication skills to determine that communication was effective. Examples of evaluative statements indicating goal achievement could be "Using picture board effectively to indicate needs" or "The client stated, 'I listened more closely to my daughter yesterday and found out how she feels about our divorce.'"

NURSE COMMUNICATION For nurses to evaluate the effectiveness of their own communication with clients, process recordings are frequently used. A **process recording** is a verbatim (word-for-word) account of a conversation. It can be taped or written and includes all verbal and nonverbal interactions of both the client and the nurse. One method of writing a process recording is to make two columns on a page. The first column lists what the nurse and the client said along with the associated nonverbal behaviour. The second column contains interpretive comments about the nurse's responses. An example of a process recording is shown in Table 21.5.

Once a process recording has been completed, it should be analyzed in terms of the content and meaning of the interaction based on communication theory. Each of the nurse's statements is interpreted in terms of the communication skill used, with the rationale for and effectiveness of its use. Any barriers to effective

TABLE 21.5 Simple Process Recording

Mary Jane Adams, a nursing aide, reports to Irene Olsen, the staff nurse, that Sandra Barrett, the client in room 815, had finished only her orange juice when Ms. Adams collected the breakfast trays. Mrs. Barrett had been admitted 2 days earlier for diagnostic studies. Concerned about her client, Ms. Olsen walks down the corridor to room 815, knocks, and enters. Mrs. Barrett turns away from the window, tears in her eyes, as Ms. Olsen enters.

Nurse/Client Dialogue	Analysis
Nurse: Good morning, Mrs. Barrett.	Acknowledging.
Client: Hello.	
Nurse: I understand you didn't eat your breakfast.	Making a specific statement but ignoring the nonverbal.
Client: I wasn't hungry.	
Nurse: Is something wrong?	Asking a closed question that fails to facilitate exploration.
Client: No. (Eyes fill with tears.)	
Nurse: You look sad, as if you're about to cry.	Giving feedback.
Client: (Cries)	
Nurse: I'll sit here awhile with you. (Sits down.)	Offering self.
Client: (Continues to cry.)	
Nurse: (After a 30-second pause) Sometimes it's hard to share the things you're concerned about with someone you don't know well. I'd like to be able to help.	Empathizing. Supporting. Offering self.
Client: (Angrily) You can help me by telling me the truth.	
Nurse: (Leans forward and maintains eye contact.)	Actively listening and demonstrating interest.
Client: Everyone beats around the bush when I ask them what's wrong with me. The nurse manager said, "What do you think is wrong?" That kind of put-off drives me up the wall!	
Nurse: You're angry because you're not getting any answers. It seems as if the staff knows something about your condition and they're keeping it from you.	Paraphrasing.
Client: They all seem to be in cahoots. Nobody tells me anything. (Pause.) (Softly) If the news was good, they wouldn't beat around the bush.	
Nurse: I'm wondering if you're worried that because people haven't answered your question it means that you have a serious illness?	Paraphrasing.
Client: Good news is always easy to give.	
Nurse: Yes, people do seem to be able to deliver good news easier and faster. I also know that we don't have any news—good or bad—to give you because none of the laboratory or x-ray results are back yet. I know that doesn't help answer your questions, but I hope it relieves you a bit from worrying that there is some bad news that's being withheld.	Giving information. Supporting.
Client: Well, when my father-in-law had surgery for a bleeding ulcer, the x-ray and laboratory results were available immediately.	
Nurse: When there's a question of emergency surgery being needed, then test results are asked for immediately. Usually, though, it's preferable to wait for an accurate reading and a thorough written report.	Giving information.
Client: Are you absolutely sure?	
Nurse: You don't sound convinced.	Acknowledging the implied.
Client: Listen, I don't mean to give you a hard time. It's just that . . . it may not seem like an emergency to my doctor or the lab people, but it sure is to me. I can't stand not knowing. I don't know the results of the tests I had yesterday. I don't know how many more tests I have to have. Will I have to have surgery? When can I go home?	

(continued)

communication can be identified, with a possible alternative response noted. The outcome for nurses should be increased awareness and insight regarding their communication strengths, as well as identification of areas for future skills development.

TABLE 21.5 Simple Process Recording (*continued*)

Nurse/Client Dialogue	Analysis
Nurse: The problem you need help with now is finding out the answers to four questions: What are the results of yesterday's tests? Is your doctor considering any other tests for you and, if so, what are they? Is surgery being planned? And when can you go home? Let's try to figure out how you can get the answers to these questions.	Summarizing. Encouraging problem solving. Encouraging collaboration.
Client: Well, I can't call my doctor on the phone. All his receptionist will do is take the message. And, anyway, I'm afraid that he'll be offended if he thinks I'm complaining about him. You won't tell him, will you?	
Nurse: No, not unless you and I decide together that it would be the best solution.	Encouraging further exploration.
Client: I suppose I could try to forget about it and be patient, just like everyone tells me to.	
Nurse: You've tried that, but you're still worried, fearful, and angry. Let's think of some other possibilities.	Focusing on solutions.
Client: Maybe you could call his office for me! Since you're a nurse, they'll probably put your call right through.	
Nurse: So far there are three possible solutions—calling his office yourself, waiting until he comes to visit you later this afternoon, or having me call his office. Are there any other possible solutions that we haven't considered?	
Client: I can't think of any other.	
Nurse: Okay, then, which do you think would be best?	Demonstrating respect for the client.
Client: I guess I'd feel better if you called his office. I just don't want him to think that I'm criticizing him.	
Nurse: You're concerned about what he might think of you because of this phone call. Let's discuss how I should handle the call and what I should say.	Paraphrasing. Encouraging collaboration and problem solving.

Source: Adapted from material by Carol Ren Kneisl, president and educational director, nursing transitions, Williamsville, New York.

Communication among Health Professionals

Effective communication among health professionals is as important as the promotion of therapeutic communication between the nurse and the client. More than 60% of medication errors are caused by mistakes in interpersonal communication (Maxfield, Grenny, McMillan, Patterson, & Switzler, 2005). Nurses tend to communicate differently from physicians. For example, nurses usually strive for consensus whereas physicians focus on ruling out alternatives (Lindeke & Sieckert, 2005). Beyea (2004) describes nurses' communication style as narrative and descriptive versus the physicians' style being focused on a need or problem. These differences can make collaboration more difficult.

Assertive communication promotes client safety. People who use assertive communication are honest, direct, and appropriate while being open to ideas and respecting the rights of others. An important characteristic of assertive communication includes the use of "I" statements versus "you" statements. The "you" statement places blame and puts the listener in a defensive position; the "I" statement encourages discussion. For example, a nurse who states, "I am concerned about . . ." to a physician will be gaining the attention of the doctor while also giving the message of the importance of working together for the benefit of the client. It is then essential for the nurse to be clear, concise, organized, and fully informed when verbally presenting the client concern. Nurses must note the fine line between assertive and aggressive communication. Assertive communication is an open expression of ideas and opinions while respecting the rights, opinions, and ideas of others. Aggressive communication strongly asserts the person's legitimate rights and opinions with little regard or respect for the rights and opinions of others (Catalano, 2006).

Case Study 21

You are the nursing student assigned to care for Mr. Manasovitz, a 45-year-old man, who will be returning from the recovery room after undergoing the removal of a mass from his abdomen. While you are preparing his room for his return, the nurse and physician arrive to talk with Mrs. Manasovitz about her husband's surgery. The physician explains that the mass was malignant and invasive. Mr. Manasovitz is a candidate for chemotherapy, but his prognosis is guarded because of the extent of the tumour growth. Mrs. Manasovitz looks away, closes her eyes, and only nods her head "yes." As the physician leaves, the nurse approaches Mrs. Manasovitz, sits next to her, and puts her arm around Mrs. Manasovitz, who begins to cry. The nurse uses a soothing voice to tell Mrs. Manasovitz that it is okay to cry and provides assurance by remaining with her. The two of them sit in silence until Mrs. Manasovitz is able to express her feelings. The nurse listens attentively. Later, the nurse offers to get a cup of coffee for Mrs. Manasovitz and offers to assist her at this difficult time.

Critical Thinking Questions

1. Interpret Mrs. Manasovitz's nonverbal behaviour in response to the news about her husband's surgery.
2. Evaluate the nurse's response to Mrs. Manasovitz on the basis of the concepts of caring and comforting.
3. Why is it important for the nurse to effectively communicate with Mrs. Manasovitz at this time?
4. The nurse was described as listening attentively to Mrs. Manasovitz. Cite actions that portray attentive listening.
5. Think about your past experiences when you or a family member has been ill. What relationship characteristics did you most value on the part of the nurse caring for you?

After working through these questions, go to the MyNursingLab at **http://www.mynursinglab.com** to check your answers.

KEY TERMS

caring
comforting
comfort
relief
ease
transcendence
communication
sender
encoding
message
receiver
decode
feedback
verbal communication
nonverbal communication
electronic communication
personal space
territoriality
congruent communication
therapeutic communication
attentive listening
empathy
group
group dynamics
process recording

CHAPTER HIGHLIGHTS

- Communication is a critical nursing skill used to gather information, to teach and persuade, and to express caring and comfort.
- Caring is said to be the essence of nursing. It includes assistive, supportive, and facilitative acts for individuals or groups.
- Caring acts promote individual growth, preserve human dignity and worth, augment self-healing, and relieve distress.
- Comforting is a complex process. Enhanced comfort is the desired outcome or product of comforting in which the client experiences relief of discomfort, ease, or transcendence.
- Comfort needs can be viewed in a framework of physical, psychospiritual, social, and environmental needs. Nurses need to be knowledgeable, skilled, and innovative to individualize comforting strategies.
- Caring and comforting are key concepts in the nurse–client process. When patients feel cared for, they report higher levels of health satisfaction and quality of life. Client-centred care is focused on effective nurse–client interaction.
- Communication is a two-way interpersonal process involving the sender of the message and the receiver of the message. It also involves intrapersonal messages, or self-talk, which can affect the message, the interpretation of the message, and the response.
- Because the sender must encode the message and determine the appropriate channels for conveying

it, and because the receiver must perceive the message, decode it, and then respond, the communication process includes four elements: sender, message, receiver, and feedback.

- Verbal communication is effective when the criteria of pace and intonation, simplicity, clarity and brevity, timing, relevance, adaptability, and credibility are met.
- Nonverbal communication often reveals more about a person's thoughts and feelings than verbal communication; it includes personal appearance, posture and gait, facial expressions, and gestures.
- When assessing verbal and nonverbal behaviours, the nurse needs to consider cultural influences and be aware that a single nonverbal expression can indicate any of a variety of feelings and that words can have various meanings.
- When communication is effective, verbal and nonverbal expressions are congruent.
- Electronic communication, particularly email, is evolving in nursing practice. Email has advantages and disadvantages and nurses must be aware of the risk to client confidentiality.
- Many factors influence the communication process: development, gender, values and perceptions, personal space (intimate, personal, social, and public distance), territoriality, roles and relationships, environment, congruence, and attitudes.
- Many techniques facilitate therapeutic communication: attentive listening; paraphrasing; clarifying; using open questions and statements; focusing; being specific; using touch and silence; clarifying reality, time, or sequence; providing general leads; and summarizing.
- Techniques that inhibit communication include offering invalidated reassurance, stating approval or disapproval, giving common (not expert) advice, stereotyping, and being defensive.
- The effective nurse–client relationship is a helping relationship that facilitates growth and provides support, comfort, and hope.
- Four phases of the helping relationship are the preinteraction phase, the introductory phase, the working phase, and the termination phase; each has a specific purpose or goal and requires specific skills of the nurse.
- To help clients with communication problems, the nurse manipulates the environment, provides support, employs measures to enhance communication, and educates the client and support persons.
- Nurses interact with groups of clients and colleagues in a wide variety of settings. To use groups rationally and effectively, nurses must understand the features of effective groups.
- Effective groups produce outstanding results, succeed in spite of difficulties, and have members who feel responsible for the output of the group. They accomplish their goals (outcomes), maintain cohesion, and develop and modify their structure in ways that improve effectiveness.
- Process recordings are frequently made by nurses to evaluate their own communication. With them, nurses can analyze both the process and the content of the communication.
- Effective communication among health professionals is vital and communication styles can differ between nurses and physicians.
- Assertive communication can promote client safety.

ASSESS YOUR LEARNING

1. The interpersonal communication process is situated in the context that includes which of the following components?

a. Social, historical, physical, psychological, and cultural
b. Physical and psychological
c. Cultural and historical
d. Environmental

2. A young woman is crying on a chair beside her bed. As her nurse, which of the following is your most caring response?

a. "You look sad. Why are you crying?"
b. "Are you in pain?"
c. "Tell me more about how you are feeling."
d. "Do you want to go home?"

3. You are a nurse in a fast-paced medical unit. A patient approaches you and asks where his nurse is. Knowing that she is on break, which of the following is your most caring response?

a. "I am not sure, but she will be back soon to assist you."
b. "She is having coffee. She has had a very busy morning."
c. "She is having coffee. Is there anything that I may assist you with?"
d. "She is having coffee and I am very busy. Can you wait until she comes back"?

4. Which of the following describes the comforting process?

a. A simple process of giving and receiving
b. Unique to nursing
c. A complex process
d. Does not last longer than the intervention

5. A health-care team on an acute geriatric unit meets on a weekly basis to review clients' progress. The nurse observes that one team member consistently dominates the discussion. Which of the following actions is most appropriate for the nurse to take?

a. Continue observing and note any changes in behaviour.

b. Discuss these observations with the group.

c. Speak to group members individually to validate these observations.

d. Speak with the individual privately regarding these observations.

6. A colleague says, "You do not know what you are doing!" How would you respond in order to build effective communication?

a. "Of course I do! You don't know what you are saying."

b. "Let's talk about this later."

c. "You have hurt my feelings. I am going to speak with the manager."

d. "Let's go to a quieter area and you can tell me what you mean."

7. What method of communicating is a barrier to communication?

a. Judging

b. Caring

c. Summarizing

d. Clarifying

8. A supervisor states to you that you are spending too much time talking with patients and not enough time training the new staff on the unit. Which of the following is your response?

a. "I will work overtime tonight to make sure they are all trained."

b. "I understand your concerns; however, my priority is to the patients."

c. "I understand. It is important in my role to be with patients and discuss their issues and concerns with them. I will speak with the new staff and schedule training times."

d. "It is my role as a nurse to speak with my patients as much as possible. You know that."

9. After breakfast, a client states that he wants to rest in bed for the morning and not go to physiotherapy. Which of the following is your best response?

a. "It is best if you go. The physiotherapist will help you walk better."

b. "Please tell me more about this."

c. "Are you in pain?"

d. "What would you like me to tell her?"

10. Which of the following best describes each nurse–client relationship?

a. Nurse-centred

b. Power based

c. Open to discovery and change, unique, and client-focused

d. Not based on boundaries

After working through these questions, go to the MyNursingLab at ***http://www.mynursinglab.com*** *to check your answers and see explanations.*

SUGGESTED READINGS

Arnold, E., & Underman Boggs, K. (2007). *Interpersonal relationships: Professional communication skills for nurses* (5th ed.). St. Louis, MO: Saunders-Elsevier.

This easy-to-read book provides an overview of communication principles and strategies, with practical tips on how to interact effectively with clients, families, and other health-care providers.

Preston, P. (2005). Nonverbal communication: Do you really say what you mean? *Journal of Healthcare Management, 50*(2), 83–86.

This article reinforces the role of nonverbal communication in professional image and communication. It includes helpful strategies to improve your ability to read nonverbal cues and to guide your own body language.

WEBLINKS

College and Association of Registered Nurses of Alberta

https://www.nurses.ab.ca/Carna-Admin/Uploads/Professional%20Boundaries%20Guidelines.pdf

This website (similar to various provincial and territorial associations of registered nurses) includes documents that provide interpretations of the expectations of registered nurses in establishing therapeutic relationships and maintaining appropriate boundaries with clients and their significant others.

College of Nurses of Ontario

http://www.cno.org/pubs/publist.html

This website includes documents concerning the nurse–client relationship, such as Therapeutic Nurse–Client Relationship, and Ethics.

Registered Nurses' Association of Ontario

http://www.rnao.org

The following documents are related to the nurse–client relationship: Client Centred Care, Establishing Therapeutic Relationships, and Supporting and Strengthening Families Through Expected and Unexpected Life Events. They are available on this site by clicking Nursing Best Practice Guidelines, then Clinical Practice Guidelines Program, and Guidelines and Fact Sheets.

REFERENCES

Austin, S. (2006). E-mail: So fast, so convenient, so . . . risky? *Nursing, 36*(2), 76–77.

Benner, P., & Wrubel, J. (1989). *The primacy of caring: Stress and coping in health and illness.* Menlo Park, CA: Addison-Wesley.

Beyea, S. C. (2004). Improving verbal communication in clinical care. *AORN Journal, 79*(5), 1053–1057.

Brammer, L. M., & MacDonald, G. (2002). *The helping relationship: Process and skills* (8th ed.). Englewood Cliffs, NJ: Prentice Hall.

Carpenito-Moyet, L. J. (2008). *Nursing diagnosis: Application to clinical practice* (12th ed.). Philadelphia, PA: Lippincott, Wilkins and Wilson.

Catalano, J. T. (2006). *Nursing now! Today's issues, tomorrow's trends* (4th ed.). Philadelphia, PA: Davis.

Chitty, K. K. (2005). *Professional nursing: Concepts & challenges* (4th ed.). St. Louis, MO: Elsevier.

Cronin, P., & Rawlings-Anderson, K. (2004). *Knowledge for contemporary nursing practice.* New York, NY: Mosby.

Donahue, P. (1989). *Nursing: The finest art.* St. Louis, MO: Mosby.

Egan, G. (2006). *The skilled helper: A problem-management approach to helping* (8th ed.). Pacific Grove, CA: Brooks/Cole.

Gordon, S., Benner, P., & Noddings, N. (1996). *Caregiving.* Philadelphia, PA: University of Pennsylvania Press.

Hartrick, G. (2002). Beyond interpersonal communication: The significance of relationship in health promoting practice. In L. Young & C. Hayes (Eds.), *Transforming health promotion practice: Concepts, Issues, and Applications* (pp. 91–105). Philadelphia, PA: Davis.

Kolcaba, K. Y. (1991). A taxonomic structure for the concept of comfort. *Image: Journal of Nursing Scholarship, 23*(4), 237–240.

Kolcaba, K. Y. (1995). Comfort as process and product merged in holistic nursing art. *Journal of Holistic Nursing, 13*(2), 117–131.

Leininger, M. (Ed.). (2001). *Cultural care diversity and universality: A theory of nursing.* Sudbury, MA: Jones & Bartlett.

Lindeke, L. L., & Sieckert, A. M. (2005). Nurse-physician workplace collaboration. *Online Journal of Issues in Nursing, 10*(1), Manuscript 4. Retrieved February 2, 2005, from http://www.nursingworld.org/ojin/topic26/tpc26_4.htm

Maxfield, D., Grenny, J., McMillan, R., Patterson, K., & Switzler, A. (2005). *Silence kills: The seven crucial conversations for healthcare.* Provo, UT: VitalSmarts.

Morse, J. (1996). The science of comforting. *Reflections, 22*(4), 6–7.

Roach, M. S. (2002). *Caring, the human mode of being* (2nd ed.). Ottawa, ON: CHA Press.

Tamparo, C. T., & Lindh, W. Q. (2008). *Therapeutic communications for health professionals* (3rd ed.). Albany, NY: Delmar: Thomson Learning.

Verderber, K. S., & Verderber, R. F. (2001). *Inter-act: Interpersonal communication concepts, skills, and contexts* (9th ed.). Toronto, ON: Wadsworth.

Watson, J. (1985). *Nursing: Human science and human care.* Norwalk, CT: Appleton-Century-Crofts.

Watson, J. (1999a). Postmodern nursing and beyond. In N. Chaska (Ed.), *The nursing profession: Nursing theories and nursing practice* (pp. 343–354). Philadelphia, PA: Davis.

Watson, J. (1999b). *Nursing: Human science and human care: A theory of nursing.* Boston, MA: National League for Nursing.

Wilkinson, J. M. (2005). *Nursing diagnosis handbook with NIC interventions and NOC outcomes* (8th ed.). Upper Saddle River, NJ: Prentice Hall Health.

Chapter 22

The Nursing Process

The **nursing process** is a systematic, client-centred method for planning and providing nursing care. The nursing process entails gathering and analyzing data in order to identify client strengths and potential or actual health problems, and developing and continually reviewing a plan of nursing interventions to achieve mutually agreed-upon outcomes. At every stage of the process, the nurse works closely with the client to tailor care and build a relationship of mutual regard and trust. See Figure 22.1 for the five phases of the nursing process.

OBJECTIVES

After studying this chapter, you should be able to

1. Describe the five phases of the nursing process: assessment, diagnosis, planning, implementation, and evaluation
2. Identify the relevance of each phase of the nursing process in guiding nursing practice
3. Identify guidelines for data collection, and differentiate objective and subjective data and primary and secondary data
4. Describe the characteristics of and formats for writing nursing diagnoses
5. Identify factors that the nurse must consider when setting priorities for client health outcomes, including establishing effective partnership relationships with clients
6. Outline how critical pathways and concept maps are used to create a comprehensive nursing care plan, including documentation
7. Formulate client health outcome evaluation criteria while planning nursing care
8. Analyze the effectiveness of nursing interventions throughout the nursing process
9. Identify the importance of quality improvement processes to guide ongoing improvement in client care
10. Confirm the centrality of critical or constructive thinking in guiding all phases of the nursing process

THE NURSING PROCESS IN ACTION

The nursing process is a systematic, rational method of planning and providing nursing care. Its purpose is to identify a client's health-care status and actual or potential health problems, to establish plans to meet the identified needs, and to deliver specific nursing interventions to address those needs. The nursing process is cyclical; that is, its components follow a logical sequence, but more than one component can be involved at one time. At the end of the first cycle, care may be terminated if goals are achieved, or the cycle may continue with reassessment, or the plan of care may be modified.

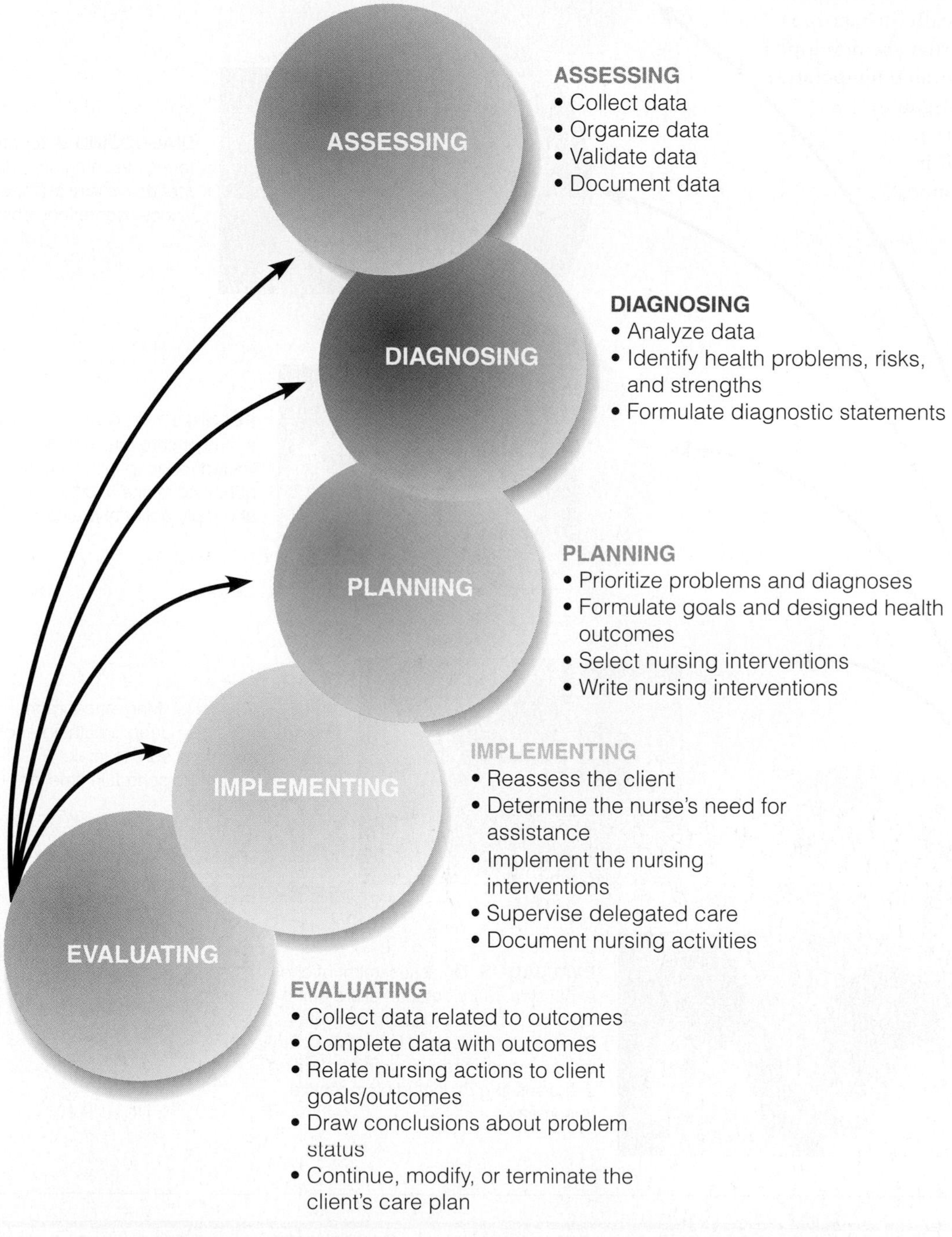
ASSESSING
ASSESSING
• Collect data
• Organize data
• Validate data
• Document data
DIAGNOSING
DIAGNOSING
• Analyze data
• Identify health problems, risks, and strengths
• Formulate diagnostic statements
PLANNING
PLANNING
• Prioritize problems and diagnoses
• Formulate goals and designed health outcomes
• Select nursing interventions
• Write nursing interventions
IMPLEMENTING
IMPLEMENTING
• Reassess the client
• Determine the nurse's need for assistance
• Implement the nursing interventions
• Supervise delegated care
• Document nursing activities
EVALUATING
EVALUATING
• Collect data related to outcomes
• Complete data with outcomes
• Relate nursing actions to client goals/outcomes
• Draw conclusions about problem status
• Continue, modify, or terminate the client's care plan

FIGURE 22.1 The nursing process in action

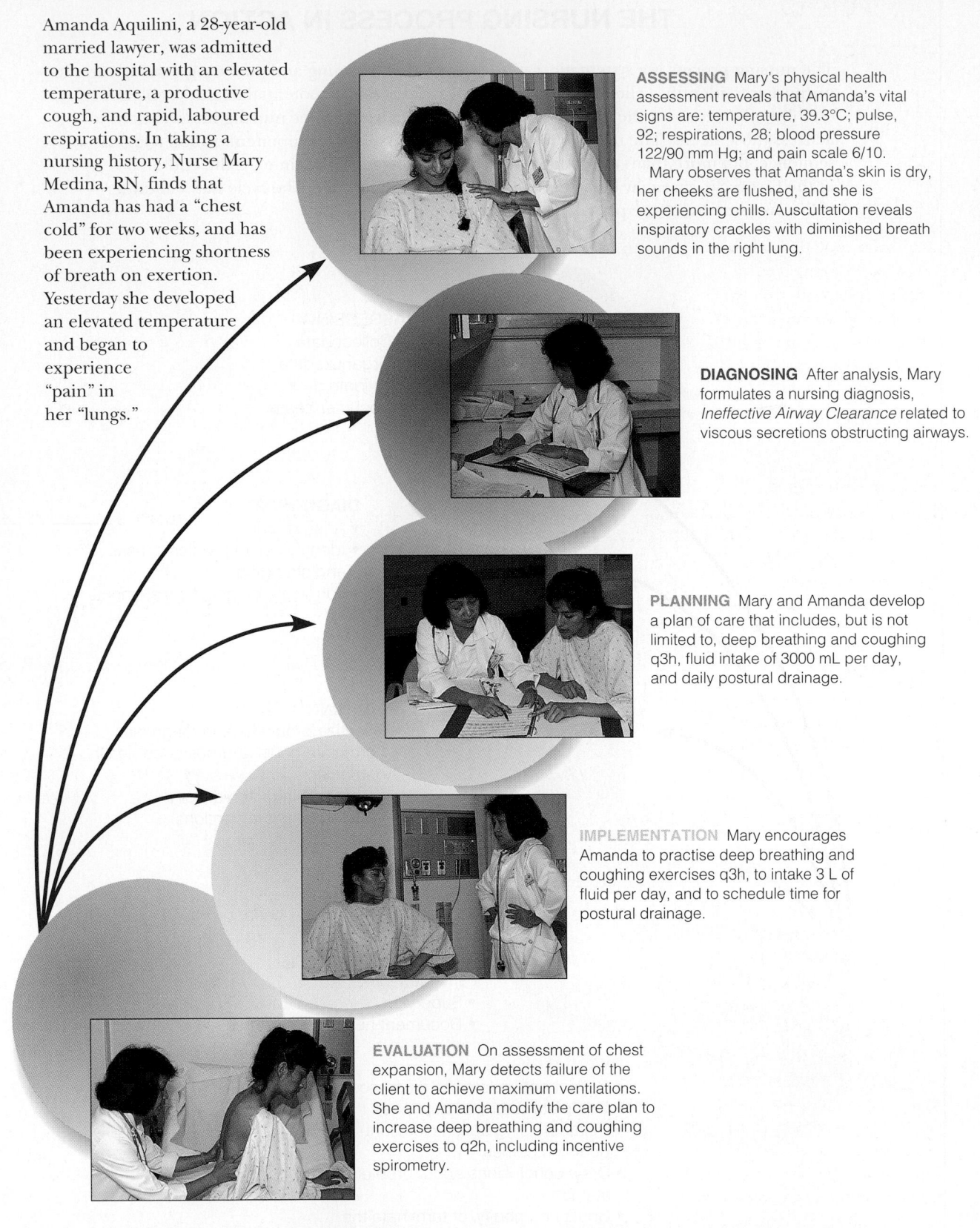

Amanda Aquilini, a 28-year-old married lawyer, was admitted to the hospital with an elevated temperature, a productive cough, and rapid, laboured respirations. In taking a nursing history, Nurse Mary Medina, RN, finds that Amanda has had a "chest cold" for two weeks, and has been experiencing shortness of breath on exertion. Yesterday she developed an elevated temperature and began to experience "pain" in her "lungs."

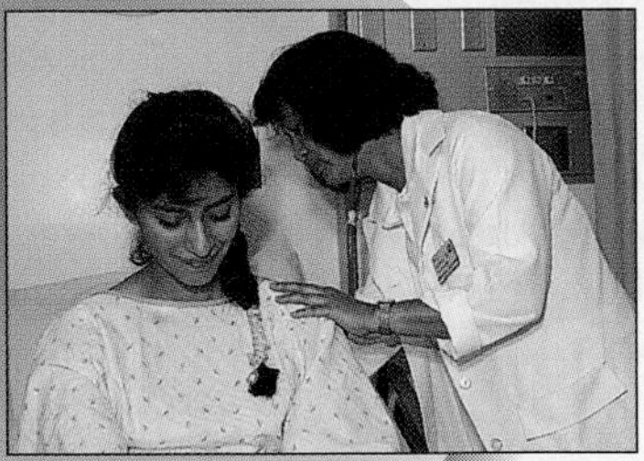

ASSESSING Mary's physical health assessment reveals that Amanda's vital signs are: temperature, 39.3°C; pulse, 92; respirations, 28; blood pressure 122/90 mm Hg; and pain scale 6/10.

Mary observes that Amanda's skin is dry, her cheeks are flushed, and she is experiencing chills. Auscultation reveals inspiratory crackles with diminished breath sounds in the right lung.

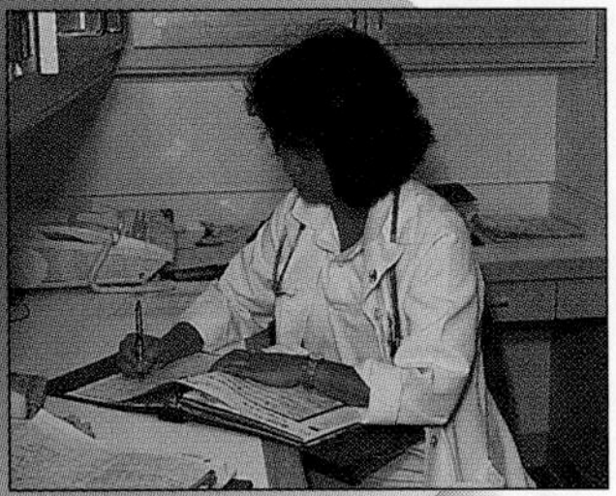

DIAGNOSING After analysis, Mary formulates a nursing diagnosis, *Ineffective Airway Clearance* related to viscous secretions obstructing airways.

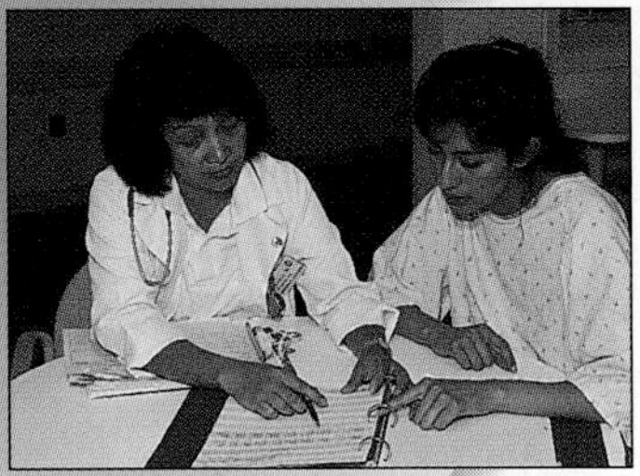

PLANNING Mary and Amanda develop a plan of care that includes, but is not limited to, deep breathing and coughing q3h, fluid intake of 3000 mL per day, and daily postural drainage.

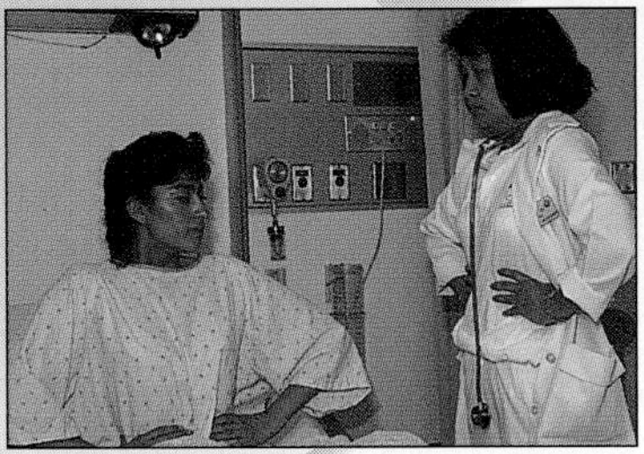

IMPLEMENTATION Mary encourages Amanda to practise deep breathing and coughing exercises q3h, to intake 3 L of fluid per day, and to schedule time for postural drainage.

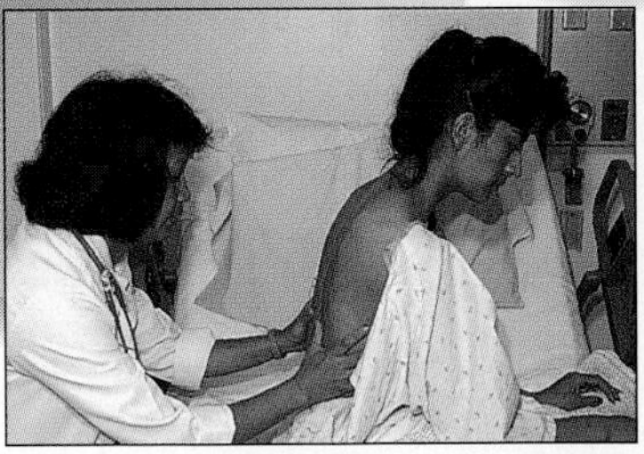

EVALUATION On assessment of chest expansion, Mary detects failure of the client to achieve maximum ventilations. She and Amanda modify the care plan to increase deep breathing and coughing exercises to q2h, including incentive spirometry.

FIGURE 22.1 The nursing process in action (*continued*)

Overview of the Nursing Process

Hall (1955) originated the term *nursing process* in 1955, and Johnson (1959), Orlando (1961), and Wiedenbach (1963) were among the first to use it to refer to a series of phases describing the practice of nursing. Since then, various nurses have described the process of nursing and organized the phases in different ways.

The use of the nursing process in clinical practice gained additional legitimacy in 1973 when the phases were included in the American Nurses Association's *Standards of Nursing Practice.* The standards of practice within the most current *Scope and Standards of Nursing Practice* include the five phases of the nursing process: assessment, diagnosis, planning, implementation, and evaluation (American Nurses Association, 2004).

In Canada, the Canadian Nurses Association (CNA) confirmed the fundamental role of the nursing process in guiding nursing practice in 1986 (Canadian Nurses Association [CNA], 1986). The nursing process remains a fundamental process that facilitates a thoughtful, informed, evidence-based, and ethical nursing practice. This process guides practice with individual, family, group, and community clients in simple to complex practice environments. It is a process that fosters thinking practitioners who make sound judgments (Macdonald, 2002). The College of Nurses of Ontario's (2007) standards of nursing practice support the centrality of the nursing process phases in guiding nursing practice to meet client health outcomes.

Phases of the Nursing Process

Although nurse theorists use different terms to describe the phases of the nursing process, the activities of the nurse using the process are similar. For example, *diagnosis* may also be called *analysis,* and *implementation* may be called *intervention.*

An overview of the five-phase nursing process is shown in Table 22.1.

The phases of the nursing process are not separate entities but overlapping, continuing subprocesses. For example, assessing, which may be considered the first phase of the nursing process, is also carried out during the implementing and evaluating phases (see Figure 22.2). For instance, while actually administering medications (implementing), the nurse continuously notes the client's skin colour, level of consciousness, and so on.

Each phase of the nursing process affects the others; they are closely interrelated. For example, if inadequate data are obtained during assessing, the nursing diagnoses will be incomplete or incorrect; inaccuracy will also be reflected in the planning, implementing, and evaluating phases.

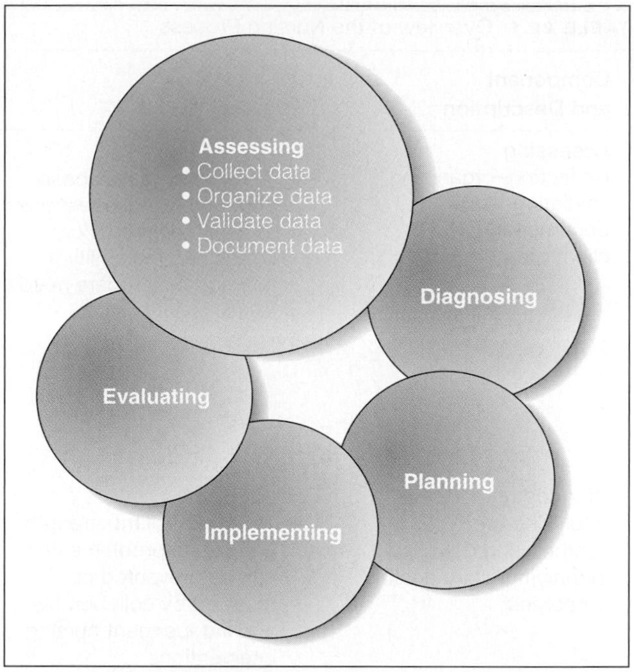

FIGURE 22.2 Assessing: The assessment process involves four closely related activities.

Characteristics of the Nursing Process

The nursing process has distinctive characteristics that enable the nurse to respond to the changing health status of the client. These characteristics include its cyclic and dynamic nature, client centredness, focus on problem solving and decision making, interpersonal and collaborative style, universal applicability, and use of critical thinking:

- Data from each phase provide input into the next phase. Findings from evaluation feed back into assessment. Hence, the nursing process is a regularly repeated event or sequence of events (cyclical) that is continuously changing (dynamic) rather than staying the same (static).
- The nursing process is client centred. The nurse organizes the plan of care according to client problems rather than nursing goals. In the assessment phase, the nurse collects data to determine the client's habits, routines, and needs, enabling the nurse to incorporate client routines into the care plan as much as possible.
- The nursing process is an adaptation of problem-solving technique (see Chapter 20) and systems theory (see Chapter 11). It can be viewed as parallel to but separate from the process used in medicine (the medical model). Both processes (1) begin with data gathering and analysis, (2) base action (intervention or treatment) on a problem statement (nursing diagnosis or medical diagnosis), and (3) include an evaluative component. However, the medical model focuses on physiological systems and the disease process, whereas the nursing process is directed toward a client's responses to disease and illness.

TABLE 22.1 Overview of the Nursing Process

Component and Description	Purpose	Activities
Assessing Collecting, organizing, validating, and documenting client data	• To establish a database about the client's response to health concerns or illness and the ability to manage health-care needs	• Establish a database: – Consult with client to obtain a nursing health history. – Conduct a physical assessment. – Review client records. – Review relevant literature. – Consult support persons. – Consult health-care professionals. • Update data as needed. • Organize data. • Validate data. • Communicate/document data.
Diagnosing Analyzing and synthesizing data and identifying client health outcomes	• To identify client strengths and health problems that can be prevented or resolved by collaborative and independent nursing interventions • To develop a list of nursing diagnoses and collaborative problems that will focus care	• Interpret and analyze data: – Cluster or group data. – Identify gaps and inconsistencies. • Determine client's strengths, risks, and problems. • Formulate nursing diagnoses and collaborative problem statements. • Document nursing diagnoses on the care plan
Planning Determining how to prevent, reduce, or resolve the identified priority client problems; how to support client strengths; and how to implement nursing interventions in an organized, individualized, and goal-directed manner to achieve client health outcomes	• To develop an individualized care plan that specifies client goals and desired health outcomes and related nursing interventions	• Set priorities and goals or health outcomes in collaboration with client. • Write goals/desired outcomes. • Select nursing strategies/interventions. • Consult other health-care professionals. • Write nursing orders and nursing care plan. • Communicate care plan to relevant health-care providers.
Implementing Carrying out (or delegating) and documenting the planned nursing interventions	• To assist the client to meet desired goals and desired health outcomes; promote wellness; prevent illness and disease; restore health; and facilitate coping with altered functioning	• Reassess the client to update the database. • Determine the nurse's need for nursing assistance. • Perform (or delegate) planned nursing interventions. • Communicate what nursing actions were implemented: – Document care and client responses to care. – Give verbal reports, as necessary.
Evaluating Measuring the degree to which goals/outcomes have been achieved and identifying factors that positively or negatively influence this achievement	• To determine whether to continue, modify, or terminate the plan of care	• Collaborate with client and collect data related to desired health outcomes. • Document achievement of health outcomes and modifications of the care plan. • Judge whether goals/outcomes have been achieved. • Relate nursing actions to client health outcomes. • Make decisions about problem status. • Review and modify the care plan as indicated or terminate nursing care.

- Decision making is involved in every phase of the nursing process. Nurses can be highly creative in determining when and how to use data to make decisions. They are not bound by standard responses and can apply their repertoire of skills and knowledge to assist clients. This facilitates tailoring of the nurse's plan of care.
- The nursing process is interpersonal and collaborative. It requires the nurse to communicate directly and consistently with clients to meet their needs. It also requires that nurses collaborate, as members of the health-care team, in a joint effort to provide quality client care.

Assessing

Assessing is the systematic and continuous collection, organization, validation, and documentation of data (information). In effect, assessing is a continuous process carried out during all phases of the nursing process. For example, in the evaluation phase, assessment is done to determine the outcomes of the nursing strategies and to evaluate goal achievement. All phases of the nursing process depend on the accurate and complete collection of data.

The nurse completes a holistic assessment of the client, which may be an individual, a family, a group, or a community. The broad spectrum of determinants of health and how these determinants are affecting human responses are considered during assessment. Assessment comes in four different types: initial assessment, problem-focused assessment, emergency assessment, and time-lapsed reassessment (see Table 22.2). Assessments vary according to their purpose, timing, time available, and client status.

Nursing assessments focus on a client's responses to a health problem. A nursing assessment should include the client's strengths, perceived needs, health problems, related experience, health practices, values, culture, and lifestyle preferences. The nursing assessment includes collaborating with the client to prioritize the client's concerns.

Collecting Data

Data collection is the process of gathering information about a client's health status. It must be both systematic and continuous to prevent the omission of significant data and reflect a client's changing health status.

A **database** is all the information about a client; it includes the nursing health history (see Box 22.1), physical assessment, health-care provider's history and physical examination, results of laboratory and diagnostic tests, and material contributed by other health personnel.

Client data should include past history as well as current problems. For example, a history of an allergic reaction to penicillin is a vital piece of historical data. Past surgical procedures, folk healing practices, and chronic

TABLE 22.2 Types of Assessment

Type	Time Performed	Purpose	Example
Initial assessment	Performed within specified time after admission to a health-care agency	To establish a complete database for problem identification, reference, and future comparison	Nursing admission assessment
Problem-focused assessment	Ongoing process integrated with nursing care	To determine the status of a specific problem identified in earlier assessment of a new problem	Hourly assessment of client's fluid intake and urinary output in an ICU
	Initial assessment when client presents for brief, episodic care	To identify new or evolving problems	Assessment of client's ability to perform self-care while assisting a client to bathe
Emergency assessment	During any physiological or psychological crisis	To identify life-threatening, new, or overlooked problems	Rapid assessment of a person's airway, breathing status, and circulation during a cardiac arrest
			Assessment of suicidal tendencies or potential for violence
Time-lapsed reassessment	Follow-up several months after initial assessment	To compare the client's current status to baseline data previously obtained	Reassessment of a client's functional health patterns in a home care or outpatient setting or in a home or hospital shift change

BOX 22.1 COMPONENTS OF A NURSING HEALTH HISTORY

BIOGRAPHICAL DATA

Client's name, address, age, gender, marital status, occupation, religious preference, next of kin, and usual sources of health care

CHIEF CONCERN OR REASON FOR VISIT

The answer given to the question, "What is troubling you?" or, "What brought you to the hospital or clinic?" The chief concern should be recorded in the client's own words.

HISTORY OF PRESENT ILLNESS OR HEALTH CONCERN

- Symptoms: description of each; steady, episodic, or worsening pattern
- Onset of symptoms: sudden or gradual, how long ago, circumstances at time of onset
- How often the problem occurs
- Exact location of the distress
- Character of the complaint (e.g., intensity of pain or quality of sputum, emesis, or discharge)
- Other phenomena or symptoms associated with the chief concern
- Factors that aggravate or alleviate the problem

PAST HISTORY

- *Medications:* all currently used prescription and over-the-counter medications, such as Aspirin, nasal spray, vitamins, laxatives, birth control pills, or herbal remedies
- *Hospitalization for serious illnesses:* reasons for the hospitalization, dates, surgery performed, course of recovery, and any complications
- *Immunizations:* date of the last tetanus shot, influenza immunization
- *Accidents and injuries:* how, when, and where the incident occurred, type of injury, treatment received, and complications
- *Childhood illnesses,* such as chickenpox, mumps, measles, rubella (German measles), rubeola (red measles), streptococcal infections, scarlet fever, rheumatic fever, and other significant illnesses
- *Allergies:* drugs, animals, insects, or other environmental agents and the type of reaction that occurs
- *Infectious disease exposure*

FAMILY HISTORY OF ILLNESS

To ascertain risk factors for certain diseases, the ages of siblings, parents, and grandparents and their current state of health or (if they are deceased) the cause of death are obtained. Particular attention should be given to such disorders as heart disease, cancer, diabetes, hypertension, obesity, allergies, arthritis, tuberculosis, bleeding, alcoholism, and mental health illnesses.

LIFESTYLE

- *Personal habits:* the amount, frequency, and duration of substance use (tobacco, alcohol, coffee, cola, tea, and illicit or recreational drugs)
- *Diet:* description of a typical diet on a normal day or any special diet, number of meals and snacks per day, who cooks and shops for food, ethnically distinct food patterns, and allergies
- *Sleep and rest patterns:* usual daily sleep and wake times, difficulties sleeping, remedies used for difficulties, napping
- *Activities of daily living (ADL):* any difficulties experienced in the basic activities of eating, grooming, dressing, elimination, and mobility
- *Recreation and hobbies:* exercise activity and tolerance, hobbies and other interests

SOCIAL DATA

- *Family relationships and friendships:* the client's support system in times of stress (who helps in time of need?); what effect the client's illness has on the family; and whether any family problems are affecting the client. See also the discussion of family assessment in Chapter 12
- *Ethnic affiliation:* health customs and beliefs; cultural practices that may affect health care and recovery. See also detailed ethnic and cultural assessment guide in Chapter 10
- *Educational history:* data about the client's highest level of education attained and any past difficulties with learning
- *Occupational history:* current employment status, the number of days missed from work because of illness, history of accidents on the job, occupational hazards with a potential for future disease or accident, the client's need to change jobs because of past illness, the employment status of both spouses or partners and the way childcare is handled, and the client's overall satisfaction with the work
- *Economic status:* financial concerns
- *Home and neighbourhood conditions:* home safety measures and adjustments in physical facilities that may be required to help the client manage a physical disability, activity intolerance, and activities of daily living; the availability of neighbourhood and community services to meet the client's needs

PSYCHOLOGICAL DATA

- *Major stressors* experienced in the past year and the client's perception of them
- *Usual coping pattern* for a serious problem or a high level of stress
- *Communication style:* ability to verbalize appropriate emotion; nonverbal communication, such as eye movements, gestures, use of touch, and posture; interactions with support persons; and the congruence of nonverbal behaviour and verbal expression

PATTERNS OF HEALTH CARE

These are all the health-care resources the client is currently using and has used in the past. These include the family health-care provider, specialists (e.g., ophthalmologist or gynecologist), dentist, alternative practitioners (e.g., herbalist or faith healers), health clinic, or health centre; whether the client considers the care being provided adequate; and whether access to health care is a problem.

diseases are also examples of historical data. Current data relate to present circumstances, such as pain, nausea, sleep patterns, and religious practices. To collect data accurately, both the client and the nurse must actively participate. Data can be subjective or objective and constant or variable, and from a primary or secondary source.

Data can be subjective or objective. **Subjective data** are also referred to as *symptoms.* Subjective data are based on client's perceptions, sensations, feelings, values, beliefs, attitudes, and understanding of personal health status and life situations. They can also include the perceptions of families, significant others, and health-care professionals. **Symptom management** involves preventing and treating the symptoms of a disease, the side effects of treatment, and any other problems related to the treatment or to the disease. Symptom management is a key nursing intervention that directly affects client health outcomes. Examples of subjective symptoms that nurses can influence include pain, fatigue, and nausea (Orchard, Reid-Haughian, & Vanderlee, 2006).

A complete database of both subjective and objective data provides a baseline for determining client's responses to nursing and medical interventions. To identify the key symptoms that should be the primary focus of care, clients are asked to indicate what symptoms are of the most concern. Priority symptom management is then based on the subjective and objective data. See Box 22.2.

Objective data, also referred to as *signs*, are detectable by an observer or can be tested against an accepted standard. They can be seen, heard, felt, or smelled, and they are obtained by observation or physical examination. For example, a discolouration of the skin and a blood pressure reading are objective data. During the physical examination, the nurse obtains the objective data needed to validate subjective data and to complete the assessment phase of the nursing process.

SOURCES OF DATA Sources of data are *primary* or *secondary*. The client is the primary source of data. Family members or other support persons, other health professionals, records and reports, laboratory and diagnostic analyses, and relevant literature are secondary or indirect sources. All sources other than the client are considered secondary sources.

CLIENT The best source of data is usually the client, unless the client is too ill, young, or confused to communicate clearly. The client can usually provide subjective data that no one else can offer.

SUPPORT PEOPLE Family members, friends, and caregivers who know the client well often can supplement or verify information provided by the client. They might convey information about the client's response to illness, the stresses the client was experiencing before the illness, important information about the client's home and/or work environment, family attitudes toward health, wellness, illness, or any prior health directive.

The nurse should also indicate on the nursing history what data was obtained from a support person. Refer to Chapter 34 for an assessment interview for a pain history.

CLIENT RECORDS Client records include information documented by various health-care professionals and data regarding the client's occupation, religion, and marital status. By reviewing such records before interviewing the client, the nurse can avoid asking questions for which answers have already been supplied. Repeated questioning can be stressful and annoying to clients and cause concern about the lack of communication among health-care professionals.

Medical records (e.g., medical history, physical examination, progress notes, and consultations) can provide nurses with information about the client's coping behaviours, health practices, previous illnesses, and allergies.

Records of therapies by other health professionals, such as social workers, dietitians, or physiotherapists, help the nurse obtain relevant data not expressed by the client.

Laboratory records also provide pertinent health information. For example, the determination of blood glucose level allows health professionals to monitor the effects of oral hypoglycemic medications. Any laboratory data about a client must be compared with established norms for that particular test and for the client's age, sex, and so on. Laboratory tests vary among agencies, and norms can, therefore, be different. Some laboratory tests, such as blood gases and pulmonary function tests, vary according to altitude above sea level. Therefore, a nurse relocating from Halifax to Calgary would need to consider these differences when examining the data.

The nurse must always consider the information in client records in light of the present situation. For example, if the most recent health record is 5 years old, it is likely that the client's health practices and coping behaviours have changed.

HEALTH-CARE PROFESSIONALS Nurses, social workers, physicians, and physiotherapists, for example, may have information from either previous or current contact with the client. Sharing of information among professionals is especially important to ensure continuity of care when clients are transferred to and from home and health-care agencies.

LITERATURE The review of nursing and related literature, such as professional journals and reference texts, can provide additional information for the database. A literature review includes but is not limited to the following information:

- Standards or norms against which to compare findings (e.g., height and weight tables, normal developmental tasks for an age group)

BOX 22.2 EXAMPLES OF SUBJECTIVE AND OBJECTIVE DATA

SUBJECTIVE

"I feel exhausted. I can't sleep. It's too noisy in here."

Client states he has a cramping pain in his abdomen. States, "I feel sick to my stomach."

OBJECTIVE

1000h: Client is observed dozing in chair.

Client is reported to be walking in halls at 0200h.

Vomited 100 mL green-tinged fluid.

Abdomen firm and slightly distended.

Active bowel sounds auscultated in all four quadrants.

- Cultural and social health practices
- Clinical practice guidelines
- Research evidence for nursing interventions and evaluation criteria relevant to a client's health problems
- Information about medical diagnoses, treatments, and prognoses

DATA COLLECTION METHODS The primary methods used to collect data are observing, interviewing, and examining. Observation occurs whenever the nurse is in contact with the client or support persons. Interviewing is used mainly while taking the nursing health history. Examining is the major method used in the physical health assessment.

In practice, the nurse uses all three methods simultaneously when assessing clients. For example, during the client interview, the nurse observes, listens, asks questions, and mentally retains information to explore in the physical examination.

OBSERVING To observe is to gather data by using the five senses. Observation is a conscious, deliberate skill that is developed through effort and with an organized approach. Although nurses observe mainly through sight, most of the senses are engaged during careful observations. Examples of client data observed through four of the five senses are shown in Table 22.3.

TABLE 22.3 Observational Skills

Sense	Example of Client Data
Sight	Overall appearance (body size, general weight, posture, grooming); signs of distress or discomfort; facial and body gestures; skin colour and lesions; abnormalities of movement; nonverbal demeanour (e.g., signs of anger or anxiety); religious or cultural artifacts (e.g., books, icons, beads)
Smell	Body or breath odours; factory emissions
Hearing	Lung and heart sounds; bowel sounds; ability to communicate; language spoken; ability to initiate conversation; ability to respond when spoken to; orientation to time, person, and place; thoughts and feelings about self, others, and health status; noise level
Touch	Skin temperature and moisture; muscle strength (e.g., hand grip); pulse rate, rhythm, and volume; palpatory lesions (e.g., lumps, masses, nodules)

Observation has two aspects: (1) noticing the stimuli and (2) selecting, organizing, and interpreting the data. A nurse who observes that a client's face is flushed must relate that observation to, for example, body temperature, activity, environmental temperature, and blood pressure. Errors can occur in selecting, organizing, and interpreting data. For example, a nurse might not notice certain signs, either because they are unexpected or because they do not conform to preconceptions about a client's illness. Nurses often need to focus on specific stimuli to avoid being overwhelmed by a multitude of stimuli. Observing, therefore, involves discriminating among stimuli, that is, distinguishing stimuli in a meaningful manner. For example, nurses caring for newborns learn to ignore the usual sounds of machines in the nursery but respond quickly to an infant's cry or movement.

The experienced nurse is often able to attend to an intervention (e.g., giving a bed bath or monitoring an intravenous infusion) and, at the same time, make important observations (e.g., noting a change in respiratory status or skin colour). The beginning student must learn to make observations and complete tasks simultaneously.

Nursing observations must be organized so that nothing significant is missed. Most nurses develop a particular sequence for observing events, usually focusing on the client first. For example, a nurse walks into a client's room and observes, in the following order:

- The client (e.g., response to greeting, verbalizations)
- Clinical signs of client distress (e.g., pallor or flushing, laboured breathing, and behaviour indicating pain or emotional distress)
- Threats to the client's safety, real or potential (e.g., a lowered side rail, a fire threat)
- The presence and functioning of associated equipment (e.g., intravenous equipment and oxygen)
- The immediate environment (e.g., appropriateness of lighting level, accessibility to personal items), including the people in it and assistive equipment

INTERVIEWING An **interview** is a planned communication or a conversation with a purpose, for example, to get or give information, identify problems of mutual concern, evaluate change, teach, provide support, or provide counselling or therapy. Interviewing is a process that the nurse applies in most phases of the nursing process. During the assessment phase, the primary purpose of the interview is to gather data. One example of the interview is the nursing health history, which is a part of the nursing admission assessment.

Two approaches to interviewing are used: directive and nondirective. The **directive interview** is highly structured and elicits specific information. The nurse establishes the purpose of the interview and guides the interview, at least at the outset, by asking closed questions (see the next section) that call for specific data. The client responds to questions but may have limited opportunity to ask questions or discuss concerns. Nurses frequently use directive interviews to gather and to give information when time is limited (e.g., in an emergency situation).

During a **nondirective interview**, or rapport-building interview, by contrast, the nurse facilitates the client's control of purpose, subject matter, and pacing. *Rapport* is an understanding between two or more people. The nurse encourages communication by asking open-ended questions (see the next section) and providing empathetic responses.

A combination of directive and nondirective approaches is usually appropriate during the information-gathering interview, the goals of which are to collect data and to begin to establish rapport. The nurse begins by asking open-ended questions to determine areas of concern for the client. If, for example, a client expresses worry about surgery, the nurse pauses to explore the client's worry and to provide support. Simply to note the worry, without dealing with it, can leave the impression that the nurse does not care about the client's concerns or dismisses them as unimportant. As the interview evolves, the nurse may use closed questions to obtain more specific data and to complete the nursing health history.

KINDS OF INTERVIEW QUESTIONS Questions are often classified as closed or open-ended and as neutral or leading.

Closed questions, used in the directive interview, are restrictive and generally require only "yes" or "no" or short factual answers giving specific information. Examples of closed questions are: "Did you take this medication?" "Are you having pain now? Show me where it is." "How old are you?" "When did you fall?"

Open-ended questions, associated with the nondirective interview, lead or invite clients to discover and explore (elaborate, clarify, or illustrate) their thoughts or feelings. An open-ended question specifies only the broad topic to be discussed and invites answers longer than one or two words. Such questions give clients the freedom to divulge only the information that they are ready to disclose. Responses may also convey clients' attitudes and beliefs. The open-ended question is useful at the beginning of an interview or to change topics and to elicit attitudes.

Examples of open-ended questions are, "How have you been feeling lately?" "What brought you to the hospital?" "How did you feel in that situation?" Open-ended questions usually begin with *what* or *how*.

Open-ended and closed questions each have advantages and disadvantages. See Box 22.3 for a summary.

The type of question a nurse chooses depends on the needs of the client at the time. For example, the nurse asks closed questions in an emergency or other acute situation when information must be obtained quickly. Nurses often find it necessary to use a combination of closed and open-ended questions throughout an

BOX 22.3 SELECTED ADVANTAGES AND DISADVANTAGES OF OPEN-ENDED AND CLOSED QUESTIONS

OPEN-ENDED QUESTIONS

Advantages

1. They let the interviewee do the talking.
2. The interviewer is able to listen and observe.
3. They are easy to answer and nonthreatening.
4. They reveal what the interviewee thinks is important.
5. They may reveal the interviewee's lack of information, misunderstanding of words, frame of reference, prejudices, or stereotypes.
6. They can provide information the interviewer may not ask for.
7. They can reveal the interviewee's degree of feeling about an issue.
8. They can convey interest and trust because of the freedom they provide.

Disadvantages

1. They take more time.
2. Only brief answers may be given.
3. Valuable information may be withheld.
4. They often elicit more information than necessary.
5. Responses are difficult to document and require skill in recording.
6. The interviewer requires skill in controlling an open-ended interview.
7. Responses require psychological insight and sensitivity from the interviewer.

CLOSED QUESTIONS

Advantages

1. Questions and answers can be controlled more effectively.
2. They require less effort from the interviewee.
3. They may be less threatening, since they do not require explanations or justifications.
4. They take less time.
5. Information can be asked for sooner than it would be volunteered.
6. Responses are easily documented.
7. Questions are easy to use and can be handled by unskilled interviewers.

Disadvantages

1. They may provide too little information and require follow-up questions.
2. They may not reveal how the interviewee feels.
3. They do not allow the interviewee to volunteer possibly valuable information.
4. They may inhibit communication and convey lack of interest by the interviewer.
5. The interviewer may dominate the interview with questions.

Source: From *Interviewing: Principles and Practices* (11th ed.), by C. J. Stewart and W. B. Cash, Jr., 2006, McGraw-Hill. Reprinted with permission from The McGraw-Hill Companies.

interview to accomplish the goals of the interview and obtain needed information.

A **neutral question** is a question the client can answer without direction or pressure from the nurse. Examples are "How do you feel about that?" and "Why do you think you had the operation?" A **leading question**, by contrast, directs the client's answer. The phrasing of the question suggests what answer is expected. Examples are "You're stressed about surgery tomorrow, aren't you?" or "You will take your medicine, won't you?" The leading question gives the client less opportunity to decide whether the answer is true or not. Leading questions create problems if the client, in an effort to please the nurse, gives inaccurate responses. This can result in inaccurate data.

PLANNING THE INTERVIEW AND SETTING Before beginning an interview, the nurse reviews available information, such as the postoperative record, information about the current illness, or literature about the client's health problem. The nurse also reviews the data collection form to make sure that the data to be collected are really needed and will serve some purpose related to the client's care. If a form is not available, most nurses prepare an interview guide to remember areas of information and determine what questions to ask.

Each interview is influenced by time, place, seating arrangement, and distance:

- *Time:* Nurses should try to schedule interviews with hospitalized clients for a time when the client is physically comfortable and free of pain and when interruptions by friends, family, and other health professionals are minimal. Nurses should schedule interviews with clients in their homes at a time mutually selected with the client.
- *Place:* A well-lit, well-ventilated, moderate-sized room that is relatively free of noise, movements, and interruptions encourages communication. In addition, a place where others cannot overhear or see the client is desirable. Most people are inhibited when answering personal questions or expressing strong feelings in the sight or hearing of others.
- *Seating arrangement:* A seating arrangement with the nurse behind a desk and the client seated across creates a formal setting that suggests a business meeting between a superior and a subordinate. In contrast, a seating arrangement in which the parties sit on two chairs placed at right angles to a desk or table or a few feet apart, with no table between, creates a less formal atmosphere, and the nurse and client tend to feel on equal terms. In groups, a horseshoe or circular chair arrangement can avoid a superior or head-of-the-table position. When a client is in bed, the nurse can sit at a 45-degree angle to the bed. This position is less formal and intimidating than standing at the foot of the bed.
- *Distance:* People feel uncomfortable when talking to someone who is too close or too far away. Most people feel comfortable maintaining a distance of about 1 metre during an interview. Communication at a distance greater than this tends to be more impersonal and may suggest a lack of involvement on the part of the nurse. Some clients require more or less personal space depending on their cultural and personal needs.

STAGES OF AN INTERVIEW An interview has three major stages: the opening or introduction, the body or development, and the closing.

The Opening The opening can be the most important part of the interview because what is said and done at that time sets the tone for the remainder of the interview. The purposes of the opening are to establish rapport and orient the interviewee. Either step can come first, depending on the situation, the relationship between the two parties, and the interviewer's choice. The rapport and orientation stages may occur at the same time and are often indistinguishable.

Establishing rapport is a process of creating goodwill and trust. It can begin with a greeting ("Good morning, Mr. Johnson") or a self-introduction ("Good morning. I'm Jennifer Thomas, a nursing student") accompanied by nonverbal gestures, such as a smile, a handshake, and a friendly manner. The nurse continues to develop rapport by asking questions about the person and may proceed with some small talk about the weather, sports, families, and the like. The nurse must be careful not to overdo this stage; too much superficial talk can arouse anxiety about what is to follow and may appear insincere.

In the orientation stage, the nurse explains the purpose and nature of the interview, for example, what information is needed, how long it will take, and what is expected of the client. The nurse usually states that the client has the right not to provide data and tells the client how the information will be used.

The following is an example of an interview introduction:

Step 1—Establish Rapport

Nurse: Hello, Ms. Goodwin, I'm Jim Fellows. I'm a nursing student, and I'll be assisting with your care here.

Client: Hi. Are you a student from the university?

Nurse: Yes, I'm in my final year. Are you familiar with the campus?

Client: Oh, yes! I'm an avid hockey fan. My nephew graduated in 2007, and I often attend hockey games with him.

Nurse: That's great! Sounds like fun.

Client: Yes, I enjoy it very much.

Step 2—Orientation

Nurse: May I sit with you here for about 10 minutes to talk about how I can help you while you're here?

Client: All right. What do you want to know?

Nurse: Well, to plan your care after your operation, I'd like to get some information about your normal daily activities and what you expect here in the hospital. I'd like to make notes while we talk to get the important points and have them available to the other staff who will also look after you.

Client: OK. That's all right with me.

Nurse: If there is anything you don't want to talk about, please feel free to say so, and if there is anything you would rather I didn't write down, just tell me. Is this a good time for you?

Client: Sure, that will be fine.

The Body In the body of the interview, the client communicates what he or she thinks, feels, knows, and perceives in response to questions from the nurse. The nurse can make the transition from the opening stage to this stage by asking an open-ended question that is related to the stated purpose, is easy to answer, and does not embarrass or place stress on the person. For example, "What brought you to the hospital today?"

Effective development of the interview demands that the nurse use communication skills that make both parties feel comfortable and serve the purpose of the interview. See the discussion of communication skills in Chapter 21.

The Closing The nurse usually terminates the interview when the needed information has been obtained. In some cases, however, a client terminates it, for example, when deciding not to give any more information or when unable to offer more information for some other reason—fatigue, for example. The closing is important in maintaining the rapport and trust and in facilitating future interactions. The following techniques are commonly used to close an interview.

1. Offering to answer questions: "Do you have any questions?" Be sure to allow time for the person to answer, or the offer will be regarded as insincere.
2. Conclude by saying, "Well, that's about all I need to know for now" or "Well, those are all the questions I have for now." Preceding a remark with the word "well" generally signals that the end of the interaction is near.
3. Thank the client. "Thank you for your time." "The questions you have answered will be helpful in planning your nursing care."
4. Express concern for the person's welfare and future: "I'll see you on Thursday." "I hope all goes well for you. If you run into additional problems, be sure to get in touch with me."
5. Plan for the next meeting, if there is to be one. Include the day, time, place, topic, and purpose: "Let's get together again tomorrow, here, at 9 a.m. to see how you are managing then."
6. Reveal what will happen next. For example: "Ms. Goodwin, I will be responsible for giving you care three mornings per week while you are here. I will be in to see you Monday, Tuesday, and Wednesday between 8 o'clock and noon. At those times, we can adjust your care, if we need to, and prepare for discharge."
7. Signal that the time is up if a time limit was agreed on or explain why the interview must close at that time: "Well, I see our time is up; it went so quickly today," or "I'm sorry, but we're going to have to end our discussion; I have another appointment in 10 minutes."
8. Provide a summary to verify accuracy and agreement. Summarizing serves several purposes: it helps to terminate the interview, it reassures the client that the nurse has listened, it checks the accuracy of the nurse's perceptions, it clears the way for new ideas, and it helps the client to note progress and forward direction. "Let's review what we have covered in this interview." Summaries are particularly helpful for clients who are anxious or who have difficulty staying with the topic: "Well, it seems to me that you are especially worried about your hospitalization and chest pain because your father died of a heart attack five years ago. Is that correct? I'll discuss this with you again tomorrow, and we'll decide what plans need to be made to help you."

EXAMINING The *physical examination* or physical health assessment is a systematic data collection method that uses observational skills (i.e., the senses of sight, hearing, smell, and touch) to detect health problems. To conduct the examination, the nurse uses techniques of inspection, auscultation, palpation, and percussion. These techniques are discussed in Chapter 27.

The physical assessment is carried out systematically. It can be organized according to the examiner's preference, in a head-to-toe approach, or a body systems approach. Usually, the nurse first records a general impression about the client's overall appearance and health status, for example, age, body size, mental and nutritional status, speech, and behaviour. Then, the nurse takes such measurements as vital signs, height, and weight. The **cephalocaudal** (head-to-toe) approach begins the assessment at the head, progresses to the neck, thorax, abdomen, and extremities, and ends at the toes. The nurse using a body systems approach investigates each system individually, that is, the respiratory system, the circulatory system, the nervous system, and so on. During the physical assessment, the nurse assesses all body parts and compares findings on each side of the body (e.g., lungs). These techniques are discussed in detail in Chapter 27.

Instead of giving a complete examination, the nurse may focus on a specific problem area noted from the nursing assessment, such as the client's inability to urinate. On occasion, the nurse may find it necessary to resolve a client complaint or problem (e.g., shortness of breath) before completing the examination. Alternatively, the nurse may perform a screening examination. A **screening examination**, also called a *review of systems,* is a brief review of essential functioning of various body parts or systems. An example of a screening examination is the nursing admission assessment form shown in Figure 22.3.

ADMISSION DATA

Date 07-12-24 Time 1515h Primary Language English

Arrived Via: ☐ Wheelchair ☐ Stretcher ☑ Ambulatory

From: ☐ Admitting ☐ ER ☑ Home ☐ Nursing Home ☐ Other

Admitting M.D. R. Katz Time Notified 1700h

ORIENTATION TO UNIT

	YES	NO		YES	NO
Arm Band Correct	☒	☐	Visiting Hours	☒	☐
Allergy Band	☒	☐	Smoking Policy	☒	☐
Telephone	☒	☐	TV, Lights, Bed Controls,		
Electrical Policy	☒	☐	Call Lights, Side Rails	☒	☐
Educational Mat©l	☒	☐	Nurses Station	☒	☐
(TV Brochure)	☒	☐			

Family M.D. R. Katz

Weight 57 kg Height 158 cm BP:R — L 122/80

Temp. 39.4°C Pulse 92, weak Resp. 28, shallow

Source Providing Information ☑ Patient ☐ Other

Unable to Obtain History ☐

Reason for Admission (Onset, Duration, Pt.©s Perception)' "Chest cold" X2 weeks S.O.B on exertion. "Lung pain, fever," "Dr. says I have pneumonia."

ALLERGIES & REACTIONS

Drugs Penicillin

Food/Other

Signs & Symptoms rash, nausea

Blood Reaction ☐ Yes ☑ No Dyes/Shellfish ☐ Yes ☑ No

MEDICATIONS

Current Meds	Dose/Freq.	Last Dose
Synthroid	0.1 mg. daily	12-24, 0800h

Disposition of Meds: ☒ Home ☐ Pharmacy ☐ Safe *At Bedside

MEDICAL HISTORY

☑ No Major Problems ☐ Gastro
☐ Cardiac ☐ Arthritis
☐ Hyper/Hypotension ☐ Stroke
☐ Diabetes ☐ Seizures
☐ Cancer ☐ Glaucoma
☐ Respiratory ☑ Other Childbirth-2000

Surgery/Procedures	Date
Appendectomy	1995
Partial thyroidectomy	2000

SPECIAL ASSISTIVE DEVICES

☐ Wheelchair ☐ Contacts ☐ Venous Access Device ☐ Dentures ☐ Partial ☐ Upper ☐ Lower
☐ Braces ☐ Hearing Aid ☐ Epidural Catheter
☐ Cane/Crutches ☐ Prosthesis
☐ Walker ☐ Glasses
☐ Other None

VALUABLES

Patient informed Hospital not responsible for personal belongings.

Valuables Disposition: ☐ Patient ☐ Safe ☐ Given to

Patient/SO Signature None

PSYCHOSOCIAL HISTORY

Recent Stress None

Coping Mechanism Not assessed because of fatigue

Support System Husband, coworkers, friends

Calm: ☑ Yes ☐ No

Anxious: ☐ Yes ☐ No Facial muscles tense; trembling

Religion Catholic, Would want Last Rites

Tobacco Use: ☐ Yes ☑ No

Alcohol Use: ☐ Yes ☑ No

Drug Use: ☐ Yes ☑ No

NEUROLOGICAL

Oriented: ☑ Person ☑ Place ☑ Time ☐ Confused ☐ Sedated ☐ Alert ☐ Restless ☑ Lethargic ☐ Comatose

Pupils: ☑ Equal ☐ Unequal ☑ Reactive ☐ Sluggish ☐ Other 3mm.

Extremity Strength: ☑ Equal ☐ Unequal

Speech: ☑ Clear ☐ Slurred ☐ Other

MUSCULO-SKELETAL

Normal ROM of Extremities ☑ Yes ☐ No

☑ Weakness ☐ Paralysis ☐ Contractures ☐ Joint Swelling ☑ Pain

☐ Other ↓ related to fatigue when coughing

RESPIRATORY

Pattern: ☐ Even ☐ Uneven ☑ Shallow ☑ Dyspnea ☑ Other diminished breath sounds

Breathing Sounds: ☐ Clear ☑ Other inspiratory crackles

Secretions: ☐ None ☑ Other pink, thick sputum

Cough: ☐ None ☑ Productive ☐ Nonproductive

CARDIOVASCULAR

Pulses: Apical Rate 92-W ☑ Reg. ☐ Irregular ☐ Pacemaker

S = Strong W = Weak A = Absent D = Doppler

Radial R 92 L — Pedal R — L —

Edema: ☑ Absent ☐ Present Site

Perfusion: ☐ Warm ☐ Dry ☑ Diaphoretic ☐ Cool (Hot)

GASTROINTESTINAL

Oral Mucosa ☐ Normal ☑ Other pale and dry

Bowel Sounds: ☑ Normal ☐ Other Abd. soft

Wt. Change: ☐ ☑ N/V Stool Frequency/Character 1/day; soft

Last B/M 07-12-23 ☐ Ostomy (type)

Equip.

GENITOURINARY

Urine: Last Voided This morning

☐ Normal ☐ Anuria ☐ Hematuria ☐ Dysuri ☐ Incontinent

☒ Other ↓ amount & frequency since ill

☐ Catheter (type) Other

LMP 07-12-23 ☐ Vaginal/Penile Discharge

Other

SELF CARE

Need Assist with: ☐ Ambulating ☐ Elimination ☐ Meals ☒ Hygiene ☐ Dressing
While fatigued

Amanda Aquilini [F. age 28]
#4637651

NORTH BROWARD HOSPITAL DISTRICT
NURSING ADMINISTRATION ASSESSMENT

FIGURE 22.3 Assessment for Amanda Aquilini. Nursing assessment tool.

NUTRITION

General Appearance: ☑ Well Nourished ☐ Emaciated ☐ Other ______

Appetite: ☐ Good ☐ Fair ☑ Poor -x2 days

Diet Liquid Meal Pattern 3/day

☐ Feeds Self ☐ Assist ☐ Total Feed

SKIN ASSESSMENT

Color: ☐ Normal ☐ Flushed ☑ Pale ☐ Dusky ☐ Cyanotic ☐ Jaundiced ☑ Other Cheeks flushed, hot

General Description Surgical scars: RLQ abdomen; anterior neck

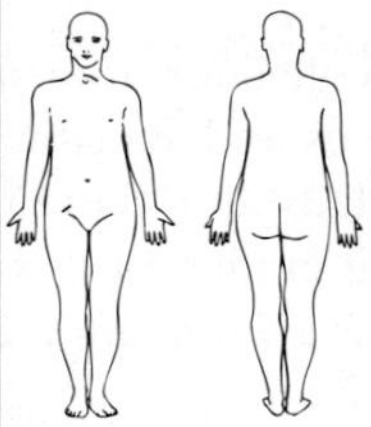

Note Cultures Obtained ______

PRESSURE SORE ™ AT RISK SCREENING CRITERIA

OVERALL SKIN CONDITION

Grade		
	0	Turgor (elasticity adequate, skin warm and moist)
✓	1	Poor turgor, skin cold & dry
	2	Areas mottled, red or denuded
	3	Existing skin ulcer/lesions

BOWEL AND BLADDER CONTROL

Grade		
✓	0	Always able to ask for bedpan
	1	Incontinence of urine
	2	Incontinence of feces
	3	Totally incontinent Confined to bed

REHABILITATIVE STATE

Grade		
	0	Fully ambulatory
✓	1	Ambulated with assistance
	2	Chair to bed ambulation only
	3	Confined to bed
	4	Immobile in bed

NUTRITIONAL STATE

Grade		
	0	Eats all
✓	1	Eats very little
	2	Refuses food often
	3	Tube feeding
	4	Intravenous feeding

MENTAL STATE

Grade		
✓	0	Alert and clear
	1	Confused
	2	Disoriented/senile
	3	Stuporous
	4	Unconscious

CHRONIC DISEASE STATUS (i.e. COPD, ASCVD, Peripheral Vascular Disease, Diabetes, or Renal Disease, Cancer, Motor or Sensory Deficits, Elderly, Other)

Grade		
✓	0	Absent
	1	One Present
	2	Two Present
	3	Three or more Present

TOTAL 3 Refer to Skin Care Protocol

FALLS SCREENING

If one or more of the following are checked institute fall precautions/plan of care

☐ History of Falls ☐ Unsteady Gait ☐ Confusion/Disorientation ☐ Dizziness

If two or more of the following are checked institute fall precautions/plan of care

☐ Age over 80 ☐ Utilizes cane, walker, w/c ☐ Sleeplessness

☐ Impaired vision ☐ Urgency/frequency in elimination

☐ Multiple Diagnoses ☐ Impaired hearing ☐ Medication/Sedative /Diuretic etc.

☐ Inability to understand or follow directions

NURSE SIGNATURE/TITLE	DATE	TIME
Mary Medina, RN	07-12-24	1530h
NURSE SIGNATURE/TITLE	DATE	TIME

EDUCATION/DISCHARGE PLANNING

1. What do you know about your present illness? "Dr. says I have pneumonia." "I will have an I.V."
2. What information do you want or need about your illness? ______
3. Would you like family/SO involved in your care? Husband, Michael
4. How long do you expect to be in the hospital? "1-2 days"
5. What concerns do you have about leaving the hospital? ______

CHECK APPROPRIATE BOX

Will patient need post discharge assistance with ADLs/physical functioning? ☐ Yes ☑ No ☐ Unknown

Does patient have family capable of and willing to provide assistance post discharge?

☑ Yes ☐ No ☐ Unknown ☐ No family

Is assistance needed beyond that which family can provide?

☐ Yes ☑ No ☐ Unknown

Previous admission in the last six months?

☐ Yes ☑ No ☐ Unknown

Patient lives with Husband and 1 child

Planned discharge to Home

Comments: Fatigue and anxiety may have interfered with learning. Re-teach anything covered at admission, later.

Social Services Notified ☐ Yes ☑ No

NARRATIVE NOTES

S--c/O sharp chest pain when coughing and dyspnea on exertion. States unable to carry out regular daily exercise for past week. Coughing relieved "if I sit up and sit still." Nausea associated with coughing. Having occasional "chills." Occasionally becomes frightened, stating, "I can't breathe." Well groomed but "too tired to put on make-up."

O--Chest expansion < 3 cm, no nasal flaring or use of accessory muscles. Breath sounds and insp. crackles in Ⓡ upper and lower chest.

Assesses own supports as "good" (eg, relationship c̄ husband). Is "worried" about daughter. States husband will be out of town until tomorrow. Left 5-year-old daughter with neighbour. Concerned too about her work (is lawyer). "I'll never get caught up." Had water at noon—no food today. Informed of need to save urine for 24 h specimen. IV D_5W LR 1000 mL started in Ⓡarm, 100 mL/h Slow capillary refill. Keeping head of bed↑ to facilitate breathing.

NORTH BROWARD HOSPITAL DISTRICT
NURSING ADMINISTRATION ASSESSMENT

FIGURE 22.3 Assessment for Amanda Aquilini. Nursing assessment tool (*continued*).

Courtesy of North Broward Hospital District, Broward County. Reprinted with permission.

Organizing Data

The nurse uses a written or computerized format that organizes the assessment data systematically. This format is often referred to as a *nursing health history*, *nursing assessment*, or *nursing data base form*. The format can be modified according to the client's physical status, such as one focused on musculoskeletal data for orthopedic clients.

NURSING CONCEPTUAL MODELS Most schools of nursing and health-care agencies have developed their own structured assessment tools. Many of these are based on selected nursing theories (see Chapter 4). Two examples are Gordon's functional health pattern framework and Roy's adaptation model.

Gordon (2006) provides a framework of 11 functional health patterns (see Box 22.4). Gordon uses the word *pattern* to signify a sequence of recurring behaviour. The nurse collects data about dysfunctional as well as functional behaviour. Thus, by using Gordon's framework to organize data, nurses are able to discern emerging patterns.

Roy and Andrews (1999) outline the data to be collected according to the Roy adaptation model and classify observable behaviour into four categories: physiological, self-concept, role function, and interdependence (see Box 22.5).

Figure 22.3 is a concise data collection tool that is organized according to body systems and specific nursing concerns (e.g., screening for falls and allergies); it does not use one particular nursing model. In Box 22.6, the data from Amanda Aquilini is shown after being

BOX 22.4 GORDON'S TYPOLOGY OF 11 FUNCTIONAL HEALTH PATTERNS

The following 11 functional health patterns can be used to organize data:

1. *Health-perception/health-management pattern*. Describes the client's perceived pattern of health and well-being and how health is managed.
2. *Nutritional-metabolic pattern*. Describes the client's pattern of food and fluid consumption relative to metabolic need and pattern indicators of local nutrient supply.
3. *Elimination pattern*. Describes the patterns of excretory function (bowel, bladder, and skin).
4. *Activity-exercise pattern*. Describes the pattern of exercise, activity, leisure, and recreation.
5. *Sleep-rest pattern*. Describes patterns of sleep, rest, and relaxation.
6. *Cognitive-perceptual pattern*. Describes sensory-perceptual and cognitive patterns.
7. *Self-perception/self-concept pattern*. Describes the client's self-concept pattern and perceptions of self (e.g., self-conception/worth, comfort, body image, feeling state).
8. *Role-relationship pattern*. Describes the client's pattern of role participation and relationships.
9. *Sexuality-reproductive pattern*. Describes the client's patterns of satisfaction and dissatisfaction with sexuality pattern; describes reproductive patterns.
10. *Coping/stress-tolerance pattern*. Describes the client's general coping pattern and the effectiveness of the pattern in terms of stress tolerance.
11. *Value-belief pattern.* Describes the patterns of values, beliefs (including spiritual), and goals that guide the client's choices or decisions.

Source: From *Manual of Nursing Diagnosis* (11th ed.) (pp. 1–5), by M. Gordon, 2006, Boston: Jones & Bartlett. Reprinted with permission.

BOX 22.5 ROY'S ADAPTATION MODEL

The Roy adaptation model classifies observable behaviour into the following categories:

ADAPTIVE MODES

1. **Physiological/Physical**
   - Oxygenation
   - Nutrition
   - Elimination
   - Activity and rest
   - Protection
   - Senses
   - Fluid, electrolytes, and acid-base balance
   - Neurological function
   - Endocrine function
2. **Self-Concept/Group Identity**
   - Physical self
   - Personal self
3. **Role Function**
4. **Interdependence**

Source: From *The Roy Adaptation Model* (pp. 102–114), by C. Roy and H. A. Andrews, 1999, Stamford, CT: Appleton & Lange.

BOX 22.6 DATA FOR AMANDA AQUILINI, ORGANIZED ACCORDING TO FUNCTIONAL HEALTH PATTERNS

HEALTH PERCEPTION AND HEALTH MANAGEMENT

- Aware and understands medical diagnosis
- Gives thorough history of illnesses and surgeries
- Complies with Synthroid regimen
- Relates progression of illness in detail
- Expects to have antibiotic therapy and "go home in a day or two"

NUTRITIONAL AND METABOLIC

- 158 cm tall; weighs 57 kg
- Usual eating pattern "3 meals a day"
- "No appetite" since having "cold"
- Has not eaten today; last fluids at noon
- Nauseated
- Oral temp 39.4°C
- Decreased skin turgor

ELIMINATION

- Usually no problem
- Decreased urinary frequency and amount 2–3 days
- Last bowel movement yesterday, formed, "normal"

ACTIVITY AND EXERCISE

- No musculoskeletal impairment
- Difficulty sleeping because of cough
- "Can't breathe lying down"
- States, "I feel weak"
- Short of breath on exertion
- Exercises daily

COGNITIVE AND PERCEPTUAL

- No sensory deficits
- Pupils 3 mm, equal, brisk reaction
- Oriented to time, place, and person
- Responsive but fatigued
- Responds appropriately to verbal and physical stimuli
- Recent and remote memory intact
- States "short of breath" on exertion
- Reports "pain in lungs," especially when coughing
- Experiencing chills
- Reports nausea

SELF-PERCEPTION AND SELF-CONCEPT

- Expresses "concern" and "worry" over leaving daughter with neighbours until husband returns
- Well-groomed, says, "Too tired to put on makeup"

ROLES AND RELATIONSHIPS

- Lives with husband and 7-year-old daughter
- Husband out of town; will be back tomorrow afternoon
- Child with neighbour until husband returns
- States "good" relationships with friends and co-workers
- Working mother, lawyer

COPING AND STRESS

- Anxious: "I can't breathe"
- Facial muscles tense; trembling
- Expresses concerns about work: "I'll never get caught up"

VALUES AND BELIEFS

- Catholic
- Anointing of the sick requested
- Middle-class, professional orientation
- No wish to see chaplain or priest at present

MEDICATION AND HISTORY

- Synthroid 0.1 mg per day
- Client has history of appendectomy, partial thyroidectomy

NURSING PHYSICAL ASSESSMENT

- 28 years old
- Height 158 cm; weight 57 kg
- TPR 39.4°C, 92, 28
- Radial pulses weak, regular
- Blood pressure 122/80 sitting
- Skin hot and pale, cheeks flushed
- Mucous membranes dry and pale
- Respirations shallow; chest expansion < 3 cm
- Cough productive of small amounts of pale pink sputum
- Inspiratory crackles auscultated throughout right upper and lower chest
- Diminished breath sounds on right side
- Abdomen soft, not distended
- Old surgical scars: anterior neck, RLQ abdomen
- Diaphoretic

organized according to Gordon's 11 functional health patterns. Note how the categories in Box 22.6 differ from those in Figure 22.3. As a rule, the nurse organizes the data by using the same model on which the data collection tool is based.

Body Systems Model The body systems model focuses on abnormalities of the following systems:

- Integumentary
- Respiratory
- Cardiovascular
- Nervous
- Musculoskeletal
- Gastrointestinal
- Genitourinary
- Reproductive

Maslow's Hierarchy of Needs Maslow's hierarchy of needs clusters data pertaining to the following:

- Physiological needs (survival needs)
- Safety and security needs
- Love and belonging needs
- Self-esteem needs
- Self-actualization needs

See Chapter 11 for detailed information.

Developmental Theories Several physical, psychosocial, cognitive, and moral developmental theories can be used by the nurse in specific situations. Examples include the following:

- Havighurst's age periods and developmental tasks
- Freud's five stages of development
- Erikson's eight stages of development
- Piaget's phases of cognitive development
- Kohlberg's stages of moral development

See Chapters 16, 17, 18, and 19 for further information.

Validating Data

If the nursing process is to be an effective framework for nursing care, the information gathered during the assessment phase must be complete and accurate. **Validation** is the act of double-checking or verifying data (cues) to confirm that they are accurate and factual. Validating data helps the nurse do the following:

- Ensure that assessment information is complete.
- Ensure that objective and related subjective data agree.
- Obtain additional information that may have been missed initially.
- Differentiate between cues and inferences. **Cues** are subjective or objective data that can be directly heard or observed by the nurse, that is, what the client says or what the nurse can see, hear, feel, smell, or measure. **Inferences** are the nurse's conclusions or interpretation of the cues (e.g., a nurse observes the cues that an incision is red, hot, and swollen; the nurse makes the inference that the incision is infected).
- Avoid jumping to conclusions and focusing too quickly on what seem like obvious problems.

As a rule, the nurse validates data when discrepancies exist between data obtained in the nursing interview (subjective data) and the physical examination (objective data), or when the client's statements differ at different times in the assessment. Guidelines for validating data are shown in Table 22.4.

To collect data accurately, nurses need to be aware of their own biases, values, and beliefs and to separate fact from inference, interpretation, and assumption. For example, a nurse seeing a man holding his arm to his chest might assume that he is experiencing chest pain, when, in fact, he has a painful hand.

To build an accurate database and avoid premature closure, nurses must validate assumptions regarding the client's physical or emotional behaviour. In the previous example, the nurse should ask the client why he is holding his arm to his chest. The client's response may

TABLE 22.4 Validating Assessment Data

Guideline	Example
Compare subjective and objective data to verify the client's statements with your observations.	Client's perceptions of "feeling hot" need to be compared with measurement of the body temperature.
Clarify any ambiguous or vague statements.	*Client:* "I've felt sick on and off for 6 weeks." *Nurse:* "Describe what your sickness is like. Tell me what you mean by 'on and off'."
Be sure your data consist of cues and not inferences.	*Observation:* Dry skin and reduced tissue turgor *Inference:* Dehydration *Action:* Collect additional data that are needed to make the inference in the diagnosing phase. For example, determine the client's fluid intake, amount and appearance of urine, and blood pressure.
Double-check data that are extremely abnormal.	*Observation:* A resting pulse of 50 beats per minute or a blood pressure of 180/96 *Action:* Use another piece of equipment as needed to confirm abnormalities, or ask someone else to collect the same data.
Determine the presence of factors that may interfere with accurate measurement.	A crying infant will have an abnormal respiratory rate and will need quieting before accurate assessment can be made.
Use references (textbooks, journals, research reports) to explain phenomena.	A nurse considers tiny purple or bluish-black swollen areas under the tongue of an older client to be abnormal until reading about physical changes of aging. Such varicosities are not uncommon.

validate the nurse's assumptions or prompt further questioning. Figure 22.3 (pages 424 and 425) shows that the nurse auscultated Amanda Aquilini's heart and lungs to validate her statement that she had "pain" in her "lungs" and "shortness of breath" on exertion. Failure to validate assumptions can lead to an inaccurate or incomplete nursing assessment and could compromise client safety.

Documenting Data

To complete the assessment phase, the nurse records client data. Accurate documentation is essential and should include all data collected about the client's health status. Data are recorded in a factual manner and not interpreted by the nurse. For example, the nurse records the client's breakfast intake (objective data) as "coffee 240 mL, juice 120 mL, 1 egg, and 1 slice of toast," rather than as "appetite good" (a judgment). A judgment or conclusion, such as "appetite good" or "normal appetite," may have different meanings for different people. To increase accuracy, the nurse records subjective data in the client's own words. Restating in other words what someone says increases the chance of changing the original meaning. Details of recording are discussed in Chapter 23.

Diagnosing

Diagnosing is the second phase of the nursing process. In this phase, nurses use critical-thinking skills to interpret assessment data and identify client strengths, problems and health outcomes. Diagnosing is a pivotal step in the nursing process. All activities preceding this phase are directed toward formulating the nursing diagnoses or hypotheses; all the care-planning activities following this phase are based on the nursing diagnoses (see Figure 22.4).

In this phase of the nursing process, the nurse and client identify priority concerns and develop client goals or desired health outcomes and nursing interventions to prevent, reduce, or alleviate the client's health problems and promote health. When evaluating care, the nurse will compare client health outcomes to these predetermined client goals or desired health outcomes.

The First National Conference to identify nursing diagnoses was sponsored by the Saint Louis University School of Nursing and Allied Health Professions in 1973. International recognition came with the First Canadian Conference in Toronto in 1977 and the International Nursing Conference in May 1987 in Calgary, Alberta (Hannah, Reimer, Mills, & Letourneau, 1987). In 1982, the conference group accepted the name North American Nursing Diagnosis Association (NANDA), recognizing the participation and contributions of nurses in

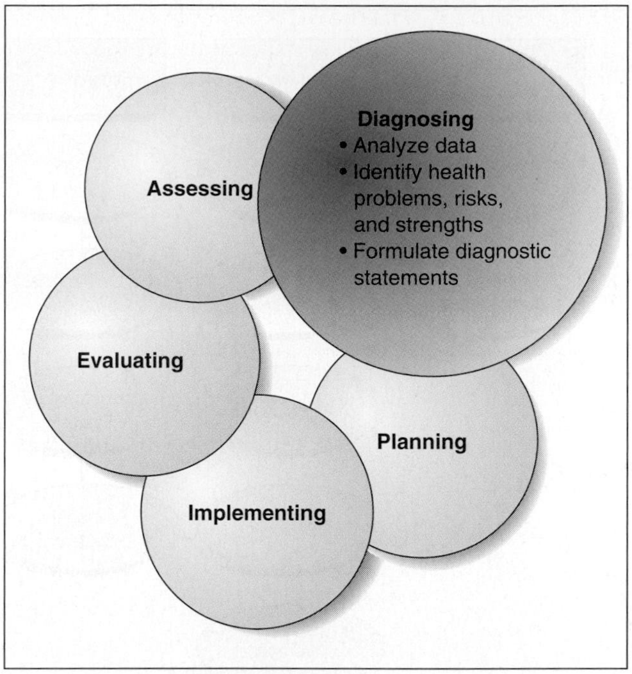
Diagnosing
• Analyze data
• Identify health problems, risks, and strengths
• Formulate diagnostic statements
Assessing
Evaluating
Planning
Implementing

FIGURE 22.4 Diagnosing: The pivotal second phase of the nursing process

the United States and Canada. NANDA, transformed to NANDA International, is the premier international nursing diagnosis association (NANDA International, 2007).

The purpose of NANDA International is to define, refine, and promote a *taxonomy* (a classification system) of nursing diagnostic terminology of general use to professional nurses (see Figure 22.5). The members of NANDA International include staff nurses, clinical specialists, faculty, directors of nursing, deans, theorists, and researchers. The group has currently approved more than 170 nursing diagnosis labels for clinical use and testing (NANDA International, 2007).

Nursing Diagnoses

The nursing diagnosis phase of the nursing process includes identifying one or more nursing diagnoses and collaborating with the client to establish priority health outcomes. **Client health outcomes** are the anticipated, predetermined outcomes that the client selects in collaboration with the nurse to guide and inform nursing practice.

NANDA International Nursing Diagnosis

To use the concept of nursing diagnoses effectively in generating and completing a nursing care plan, the nurse must be familiar with the definitions of terms used, the types, and the components of nursing diagnoses.

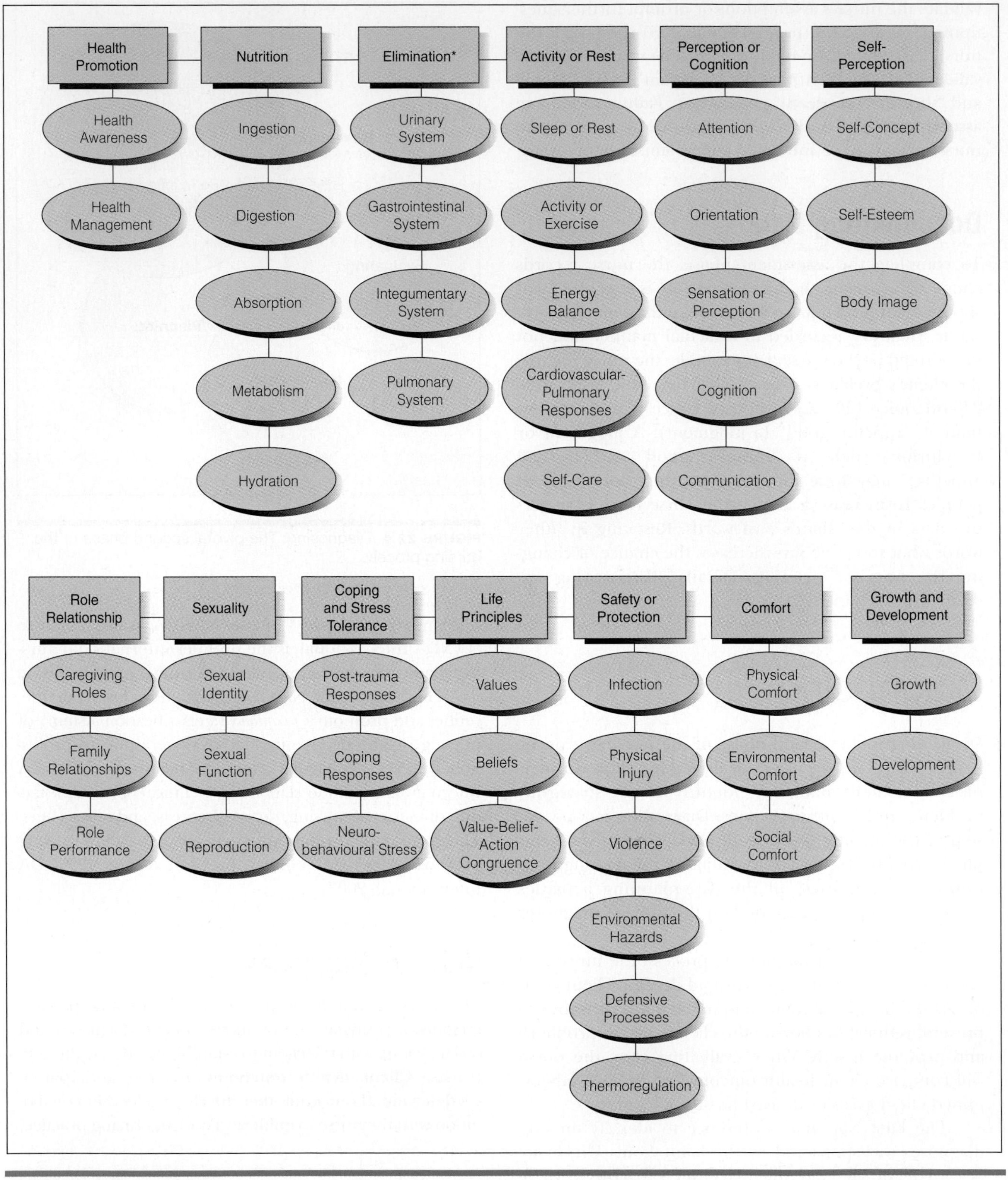

FIGURE 22.5 Taxonomy II

* The 2007–2008 edition of the NANDA International taxonomy diagram is identical to the one shown here except for "Elimination," which now reads "Elimination/Exchange."

Source: From **Definitions and Classifications, 2003–2004,** *by NANDA International, 2003, Philadelphia, PA: Author. Adapted with permission.*

DEFINITIONS The term *diagnosing* refers to the reasoning process, whereas the term *diagnosis* is a statement or conclusion regarding the nature of a phenomenon. The standardized NANDA International names for the diagnoses are called **diagnostic labels**; and the client's problem statement, consisting of the diagnostic label plus **etiology** (causal relationship between a problem and its related risk factors), is called a **nursing diagnosis**.

In 1990, NANDA International adopted an official working definition of nursing diagnosis: "a clinical judgment about individual, family, or community responses to actual and potential health problems/life processes. A nursing diagnosis provides the basis for selection of nursing interventions to achieve outcomes for which the nurse is accountable" (as cited in NANDA International, 2007, p. 332). This definition implies the following:

- The domain of nursing diagnosis includes only those health states that nurses are educated and licensed to treat. For example, generalist nurses are not educated to diagnose or treat such diseases as diabetes mellitus; this task is defined legally as within the practice of medicine. Yet nurses can diagnose and treat *Deficient Knowledge, Ineffective Coping,* or *Imbalanced Nutrition,* all of which are the human responses to the medical diagnosis of diabetes mellitus.
- A nursing diagnosis is a judgment made only after thorough, systematic data collection.
- Nursing diagnoses describe a continuum of health states: deviations from health, presence of risk factors, and areas of enhanced personal growth.

TYPES OF NURSING DIAGNOSES The five types of nursing diagnoses are actual, risk, wellness, possible, and syndrome.

1. An **actual diagnosis** is a client problem that is present at the time of the nursing assessment. Examples are *Ineffective Breathing Pattern* and *Anxiety.* An actual nursing diagnosis is based on the presence of associated signs and symptoms.
2. A **risk nursing diagnosis** is a clinical judgment that a problem does not yet exist, but the presence of **risk factors** indicates that a problem is likely to develop unless the nurse intervenes. For example, all people admitted to a hospital have some possibility of acquiring an infection; however, a client with diabetes or a compromised immune system is at higher risk than others. Therefore, the nurse would appropriately use the label *Risk for Infection* to describe the client's health status.
3. A **wellness nursing diagnosis** "describes human responses to levels of wellness in an individual, family or community that have a readiness for enhancement" (NANDA International, 2007, p. 322). Examples of wellness diagnoses would be *Readiness for Enhanced Spiritual Well-Being* or *Readiness for Enhanced Family Coping.*
4. A **possible nursing diagnosis** is one in which evidence about a health problem is incomplete or unclear. A possible diagnosis requires more data either to support or to refute it. For example, an older widow who lives alone is admitted to the hospital. The nurse notices that she has no visitors and is pleased with attention and conversation from the nursing staff. Until more data are collected, the nurse may write a nursing diagnosis of *Possible Social Isolation* related to unknown etiology.
5. A **syndrome diagnosis** is a diagnosis that is associated with a cluster of other diagnoses (Carpenito-Moyet, 2008). Currently six syndrome diagnoses are on the NANDA International list. *Risk for Disuse Syndrome,* for example, can be experienced by long-term bedridden clients. Clusters of diagnoses associated with this syndrome include *Impaired Physical Mobility, Risk for Impaired Tissue Integrity, Risk for Activity Intolerance, Risk for Constipation, Risk for Infection, Risk for Injury, Risk for Powerlessness, Impaired Gas Exchange,* and so on.

COMPONENTS OF A NANDA INTERNATIONAL NURSING DIAGNOSIS A nursing diagnosis usually has three components: (1) the diagnostic label, (2) the defining characteristics, and (3) related factors. Risk diagnoses have (1) a diagnostic label and (2) risk factors (NANDA International, 2007).

DIAGNOSTIC LABEL (PROBLEM) The problem statement, or diagnostic label, describes the client's health problem or response for which nursing therapy is given. It describes the client's health status clearly and concisely in a few words.

The purpose of the diagnostic label is to direct the formation of client goals and desired health outcomes. It may also suggest some nursing interventions.

To be clinically useful, diagnostic labels need to be specific; when the word *Specify* follows a NANDA International label, the nurse states the area in which the problem occurs, for example, *Deficient Knowledge* (*Medications*) or *Deficient Knowledge* (*Dietary Adjustments*).

Qualifiers are words that have been added to some NANDA International labels to give additional meaning to the diagnostic statement:

- *Deficient* (inadequate in amount, quality, or degree; not sufficient; incomplete)
- *Impaired* (made worse, weakened, damaged, reduced, deteriorated)
- *Decreased* (lesser in size, amount, or degree)
- *Ineffective* (not producing the desired effect)
- *Compromised* (to make vulnerable to threat)

Each diagnostic label approved by NANDA International carries a definition that clarifies its meaning.

DEFINING CHARACTERISTICS **Defining characteristics** are the cluster of signs and symptoms that indicate the presence of a particular diagnostic label. For actual nursing diagnoses, the defining characteristics are in the client's signs and symptoms. For risk nursing diagnoses, no subjective and objective signs are present. Thus, risk factors that cause the client to be more than "normally" vulnerable to the problem are identified instead.

Related Factors and Risk Factors The **related factors** component of a nursing diagnosis identifies one or more probable causes of the health problem, gives direction to the required nursing therapy, and enables the nurse to individualize the client's care. As shown in Table 22.5, the probable causes of *Activity Intolerance* include sedentary lifestyle, generalized weakness, and so on. Differentiating among possible causes in the nursing diagnosis is essential because each may require different nursing interventions.

DIFFERENTIATING NURSING DIAGNOSES FROM MEDICAL DIAGNOSES A nursing diagnosis is a statement of nursing judgment and refers to a condition that nurses are licensed to treat. A medical diagnosis is made by a physician and refers to a condition that only a physician or nurse practitioner can treat. Medical diagnoses refer to disease processes—specific pathophysiological responses that are fairly uniform from one client to another. In contrast, nursing diagnoses describe a client's physical, sociocultural, psychological, and spiritual responses to an illness or a health problem. These responses vary among individuals. A client's medical diagnosis remains the same for as long as the disease process is present, but nursing diagnoses change as the client's responses change, as in the following example:

> *Seventy-year-old Mary Cain and 20-year-old Kristi Vidan both have rheumatoid arthritis. Their disease processes are much the same. X-ray studies show that in both clients, the extent of inflammation and the number of joints involved are similar, and both clients experience almost constant pain. Ms. Cain views her condition as part of the aging process and is responding with acceptance. Ms. Vidan, however, is responding with anger and hostility because she views her disease as a threat to her personal identity, role performance, and self-esteem.*

Nurses have responsibilities related to both medical and nursing diagnoses. Nursing diagnoses relate to the nurse's **independent functions**, that is, the areas of health care that are unique to nursing and separate and distinct from medical management. With regard to medical diagnoses, nurses work collaboratively in carrying out physician-prescribed therapies and treatments.

Nurses may not prescribe *all* the care for a nursing diagnosis, but if the problem is a nursing diagnosis, the nurse can prescribe *most* of the interventions needed for prevention or resolution. For example, most clients with a nursing diagnosis of *Pain* have medical orders for analgesics, but many independent nursing interventions can also alleviate pain (e.g., guided imagery or teaching a client to splint an incision).

DIFFERENTIATING NURSING DIAGNOSES FROM COLLABORATIVE PROBLEMS A collaborative problem is a type of potential problem that nurses manage by using both independent and physician-prescribed interventions. Independent nursing interventions for a collaborative problem focus mainly on monitoring the client's condition and preventing development of a potential complication. Definitive treatment of the condition requires both medical and nursing interventions.

Collaborative problems (see Box 22.7) tend to be present any time a particular disease or treatment is present; that is, each disease or treatment has specific complications that are always associated with it. For example, a statement of collaborative problems is "Potential complications of pneumonia: atelectasis [collapse of all or part of a lung], respiratory failure, pleural effusion [fluid between the two layers that cover and protect the lungs], pericarditis [inflammation of the sac around the heart], and meningitis [inflammation of the membranes that cover the brain and spinal cord]."

Nursing diagnoses, by contrast, involve human responses, which vary greatly from one person to the next. Therefore, the same set of nursing diagnoses cannot be expected to occur with a particular disease or condition; moreover, a single nursing diagnosis may occur as a response to any number of diseases. For example, all postpartum clients have similar collaborative problems (potential complications), such as "Potential complication of childbearing: postpartum hemorrhage,"

TABLE 22.5 Components of a Nursing Diagnosis

Diagnosis and Definition	Related Factors	Defining Characteristics
Activity Intolerance: Insufficient physiological or psychological energy to endure or complete required or desired daily activities	Bed rest or immobility Generalized weakness Imbalance between oxygen supply/demand Sedentary lifestyle	Verbal report of fatigue or weakness Abnormal heart rate or blood pressure response to activity Electrocardiographic changes reflecting arrhythmias or ischemia Exertional discomfort or dyspnea

Source: From *NANDA Nursing Diagnoses: Definitions and Classification, 2007–2008*, by NANDA International, 2007, p. 3, Philadelphia, PA.

BOX 22.7 COLLABORATIVE PROBLEMS

Disease/Situation	Complication		Etiology
Potential complication of childbirth:	hemorrhage	related to	uterine atony retained placental fragments bladder distension
Potential complication of diuretic therapy:	arrhythmia	related to	low serum potassium

but not all new mothers have the same nursing diagnoses. Some might experience *Altered Parenting* (delayed bonding), but most will not; some might have a *Deficient Knowledge* problem, whereas others will not. See Table 22.6 for a comparison of nursing diagnoses, collaborative problems, and medical diagnoses.

The Diagnostic Process

The diagnostic process uses the critical-thinking skills of analysis and synthesis. *Critical thinking* is a cognitive process during which a person reviews data and considers explanations before forming an opinion. *Analysis* is

TABLE 22.6 Comparison of Nursing Diagnoses, Collaborative Problems, and Medical Diagnoses

Category	Nursing Diagnoses	Collaborative Problems	Medical Diagnoses
Example	*Activity Intolerance* related to decreased cardiac output	Potential complication of myocardial infarction: congestive heart failure	Myocardial infarction
Description	Describe human responses to disease process or health problem; consist of a one-, two-, or three-part statement, usually including problem and related factors	Involve human responses—mainly physiological complications of disease, tests, or treatments; consist of a two-part statement of situation/pathophysiology and the potential complication	Describe disease and pathology; do not consider other human responses; usually consist of not more than three words
Orientation and responsibility for diagnosing	Oriented to the individual; nurses responsible for diagnosing	Oriented to pathophysiology; shared responsiblity for diagnosing	Oriented to pathology; physician responsible for diagnosing; diagnosis not within the scope of nursing practice
Treatment orders	Nurse orders most interventions to prevent and treat	Nurse collaborates with physician and other health-care professionals to prevent and treat; require medical orders for definitive treatment	Physician orders primary interventions to prevent and treat
Nursing focus	Treat and prevent	Prevent and monitor for onset or status of condition	Implement medical orders for treatment and monitor status of condition
Nursing actions	Independent	Some independent actions, but primarily for monitoring and preventing	Dependent (primarily)
Duration	Can change frequently	Present when disease or situation is present	Remains the same while disease is present
Classification system	Classification system is developed and being used but is not universally accepted	No universally accepted classification system	Well-developed classification system accepted by the medical profession

paration into components, that is, breaking down whole into its parts (deductive reasoning). *Synthesis* is the opposite, that is, putting together the parts into the whole (inductive reasoning) (see Chapter 20).

The diagnostic process is used continuously by most nurses. An experienced nurse may enter a client's room and immediately observe significant data and draw conclusions about the client. As a result of attaining knowledge, skill, and expertise in the practice setting, the expert nurse may seem to perform these mental processes automatically. Novice nurses, however, need guidelines to understand and formulate nursing diagnoses. The diagnostic process has three steps:

1. Analyzing data
2. Identifying health problems, risks, and strengths
3. Formulating diagnostic statements

ANALYZING DATA In the diagnostic process, analyzing involves the following steps:

1. Compare data against standards (identify significant cues).
2. Cluster cues (generate tentative hypotheses).
3. Identify gaps and inconsistencies.

For experienced nurses, these activities occur continuously rather than sequentially.

COMPARING DATA WITH STANDARDS Nurses draw on knowledge and experience to compare client data with standards and norms and identify significant and relevant cues. A **standard** or **norm** is a generally accepted measure, rule, model, or pattern. The nurse uses a wide range of standards, such as growth and development patterns, normal vital signs, and laboratory values. A cue is any piece of information or data that influences decisions. A cue is considered significant if it does any of the following:

- *The cue points to change in a client's health status or pattern.* These may be positive or negative. For example, the client states: "I have recently experienced shortness of breath while climbing stairs," or "I have not smoked for three months."
- *The cue varies from norms of the client population.* The client's pattern may fit within cultural norms but vary from norms of the general society. The client may consider a pattern—for example, eating very small meals and having little appetite—to be normal. This pattern, however, may not be productive and may require further exploration.
- *The cue indicates a developmental delay.* To identify significant cues, the nurse must be aware of the normal patterns and changes that occur as the person grows and develops. For example, by age 9 months, an infant is usually able to sit without support. The infant who has not accomplished this task needs further assessment for possible developmental delays.

Refer to Table 22.7 for specific examples of client cues and norms to which they may be compared. Significant cues and data clusters for Amanda Aquilini that were extracted from Figure 22.3 (page 424) and the Box 22.4 (page 426) are shown in Table 22.8.

TABLE 22.7 Comparing Cues to Standards and Norms

Type of Cue	Client Cues	Standard/Norm
Deviation from population norms	Height is 158 cm. Woman with small frame Weight 109 kg	The body mass index indicates that the BMI for a woman 158 cm tall who weighs 109 kg is 43.7. Normal BMI ranges from 18.5 to 24.9.
Developmental delay	Child is 18 months old. Parents state child has not yet attempted to speak. Child laughs aloud and makes cooing sounds.	Children usually speak their first word by 10 to 12 months of age.
Changes in client's usual health status	Client states, "I'm just not hungry these days." Ate only 15% of food on breakfast tray Has lost 13 kg in past 3 months	Client usually eats three balanced meals per day. Adults typically maintain stable weight.
Dysfunctional behaviour	Tanya's mother reports that Tanya has not left her room for 2 days. Tanya is age 16. Tanya has stopped attending school and has withdrawn from social contact.	Adolescents usually like to be with their peers; social groups are very important. Functional behaviour includes school attendance.
Changes in client's usual behaviour	Mrs. Stuart reports that lately her husband gets angry easily. "Yesterday he even yelled at the dog." "He just seems so tense."	Mr. Stuart is usually relaxed and easygoing. He is friendly and kind to animals.

TABLE 22.8 Formulating Nursing Diagnoses for Amanda Aquilini

Functional Health Pattern	Client Cue Clusters	Inferences (Tentative Identification of Problems)	Formulating Diagnostic Statements
Health perception/ health management			No problem *Strength:* Shows healthy lifestyle, understanding of and compliance with treatment regimens
Nutritional/metabolic (includes hydration)	"No appetite" since having "cold" Has not eaten today; last fluids at noon today Nauseated ×2 days	*Altered Nutrition: Less than Body Requirements*	***Altered Nutrition: Less than Body Requirements*** related to decreased appetite and nausea and increased metabolism (secondary to disease process) *Strength:* Normal weight for height
	Last fluids at noon today Oral temp 39.4°C Skin hot and pale, cheeks flushed Mucous membranes dry Poor skin turgor *Cues from elimination pattern:* Decreased urinary frequency and amount ×2 days	*Deficient Fluid Volume*	***Deficient Fluid Volume*** related to intake insufficient to replace fluid loss secondary to fever and diaphoresis
Elimination	Decreased urinary frequency and amount × 2 days	Cues consist of elimination data but are actually symptoms of a fluid volume problem in the nutritional/metabolic functional health pattern	No elimination problem
Activity/exercise	States, "I feel weak standing at the sink and in the shower" Short of breath on exertion *Cues from cognitive/ perceptual pattern:* Responsive but fatigued "I can think OK, just weak" *Cues from cardiovascular pattern:* Radial pulses weak, regular Pulse rate 92	*Activity Intolerance*	Activity intolerance related to general weakness, imbalance between oxygen supply/demand *Strength:* No musculo-skeletal impairment, normal energy level is satisfactory, exercises regularly
Sleep/rest	Difficulty sleeping because of cough "Can't breathe lying down"	*Disturbed Sleep Pattern*	***Disturbed Sleep Pattern*** related to cough, pain, orthopnea, fever, and diaphoresis
Cognitive/perceptual	Reports pain in lungs, especially when coughing Responsive but fatigued "I can think OK, just weak"	*Pain* These are cognitive/perceptual data, but they reflect symptoms of problems in the activity/ exercise pattern	***Pain (Chest), Acute*** related to cough secondary to pneumonia *Strength:* No cognitive or sensory deficits

(continued)

TABLE 22.8 Formulating Nursing Diagnoses for Amanda Aquilini (*continued*)

Functional Health Pattern	Client Cue Clusters	Inferences (Tentative Identification of Problems)	Formulating Diagnostic Statements
Self-perception/ self-concept	Expresses "concern" and "worry" over leaving daughter with neighbours until husband returns	Cue is a symptom of a problem in the coping/ stress pattern	No self-perception/self-concept problem
Roles/relationships	Husband out of town; will be back tomorrow afternoon Child with neighbour until husband returns	*Altered Family Processes* related to mother's illness and temporary unavailability of father to provide childcare Cues also related to a problem in the coping/stress pattern	*Risk for Altered Family Processes* related to mother's illness and temporary unavailability of father to provide childcare *Strength:* Neighbours available and willing to help
Coping/stress	Anxious: "I can't breathe" Facial muscles tense; trembling Expresses concerns about work: "I'll never get caught up" *Cues from role/relationship pattern:* Husband out of town; will be back tomorrow afternoon Child with neighbour until husband returns *Cues from self-perception/ self-concept patterns:* Expresses "concern" and "worry" over leaving daughter with neighbours	***Anxiety*** related to difficulty breathing, inability to work, and childcare	***Anxiety*** related to difficulty breathing and concerns over work and parenting roles
Medication/history	No significant cues	No problem	No problem
Physical assessment			
Cardiovascular	Radial pulses weak, regular Pulse rate 92	Cues are symptoms only; symptoms of exercise/rest and oxygenation problems	No cardiovascular problem
Oxygenation	Skin hot, pale, and moist Respirations shallow; chest expansion, 3 cm Cough productive of small amounts of pale pink sputum Inspiratory crackles auscultated throughout right upper and lower chest Diminished breath sounds on right side Mucous membranes pale	***Ineffective Airway Clearance*** related to disease process	***Ineffective Airway Clearance*** related to viscous secretions and shallow chest expansion secondary to pain, deficient fluid volume, and fatigue
Skin	Old surgical scars, anterior neck, RLQ abdomen	No problem now	Old problems; resolved

CLUSTERING CUES Clustering or grouping cues is a process of determining the relatedness of facts and determining whether any patterns are present, whether the data represent isolated incidents, and whether the data are significant. This is the beginning of synthesis.

The nurse may cluster data *inductively* (as in Table 22.8) by combining data from different assessment areas to form a pattern, or the nurse may begin with a framework, such as Gordon's functional health patterns, and cluster the subjective and objective data into the appro-

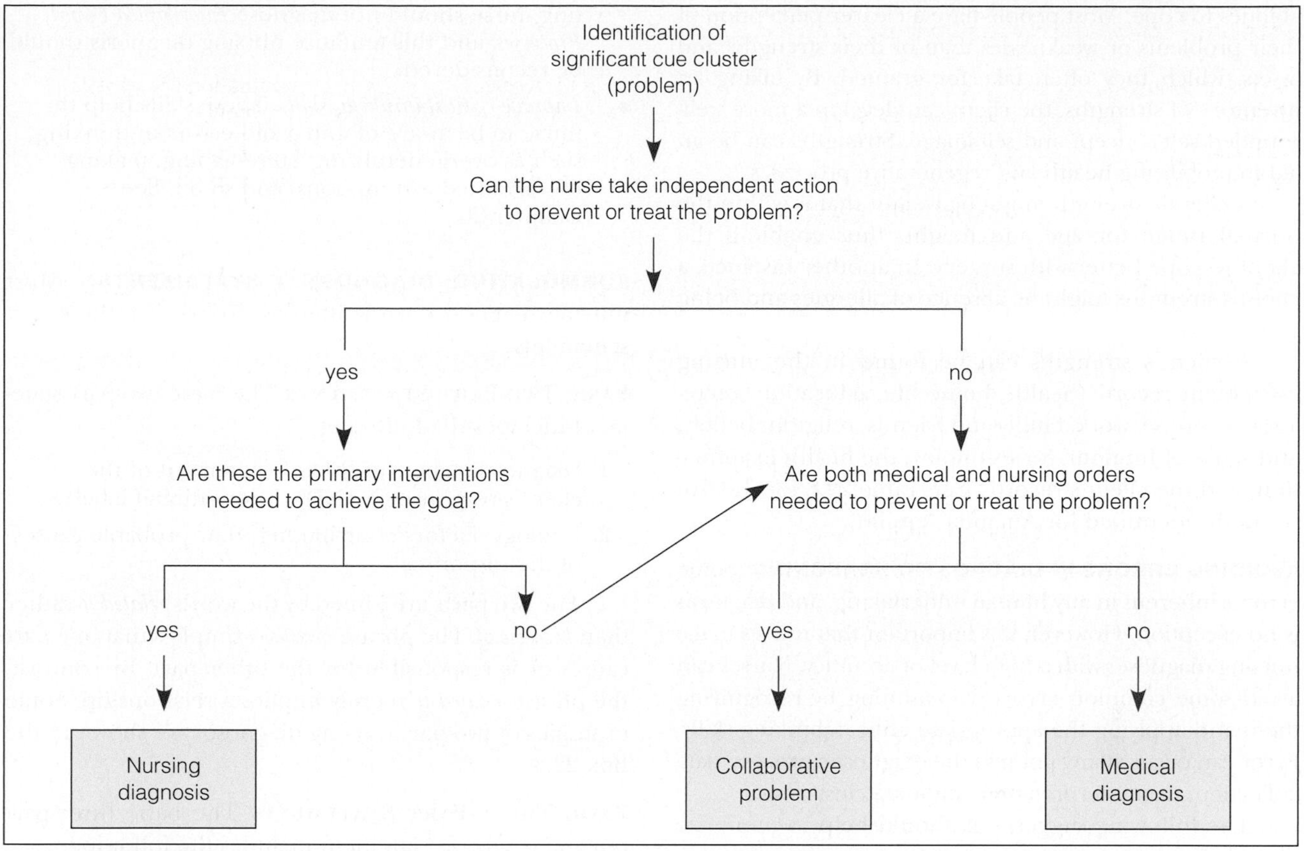

FIGURE 22.6 Decision tree for differentiating among nursing diagnoses, collaborative problems, and medical diagnoses

priate categories (see Box 22.4 on page 426). The latter is a *deductive* approach to data clustering, or pattern formation.

Experienced nurses may cluster data as they collect and interpret it, as evidenced in such remarks or thoughts as, "I'm getting a picture of . . . ," or "This cue doesn't fit the picture." The novice nurse does not have the knowledge base or the clinical experience that aids in recognizing cues. Thus, the novice must take careful assessment notes, search data for abnormal cues, and use textbook resources for comparing the client's cues with the defining characteristics and etiological factors of the accepted nursing diagnoses.

Data clustering involves making inferences about the data. An inference is the nurse's judgment or interpretation of cues. The nurse interprets the possible meaning of the cues and labels the cue clusters with tentative diagnostic hypotheses. Data clustering or grouping for Amanda Aquilini is illustrated in Table 22.8, in which data are clustered according to standardized diagnosis labels.

Identifying Gaps and Inconsistencies in Data Skillful assessment minimizes gaps and inconsistencies in data. However, data analysis should include a final check to ensure that data are complete and correct.

Inconsistencies are conflicting data. Possible sources of conflicting data include measurement error, expectations, and conflicting or unreliable reports. For example, a nurse may learn from the nursing history that the client reports not having seen a doctor in 15 years, yet during the physical health examination, he states, "My doctor takes my blood pressure every week." All inconsistencies must be clarified before a valid pattern can be established.

IDENTIFYING HEALTH PROBLEMS, RISKS, AND STRENGTHS After data are analyzed, the nurse and client can together identify strengths and problems. This is primarily a decision-making process. See Chapter 20.

Determining Problems After grouping and clustering data, the nurse and client together identify tentative diagnoses. In addition, the nurse must determine whether the client's problem is a nursing diagnosis, medical diagnosis, or collaborative problem. See Figure 22.6 for a decision tree to aid in this decision. Also refer to Table 22.6 on page 433.

For examples, refer to the cue clusters and tentative identification of problems for Amanda Aquilini in Table 22.8. In this example, the nurse and client identified nine tentative problems: *Imbalanced Nutrition: Less than Body Requirements; Deficient Fluid Volume; Disturbed Sleep Pattern; Self-Care Deficit; Acute Pain (Chest); Interrupted Family Processes; Anxiety; Activity Intolerance;* and *Ineffective Airway Clearance.*

Determining Strengths At this stage, the nurse and client also establish the client's strengths, resources, and abilities to cope. Most people have a clearer perception of their problems or weaknesses than of their strengths and assets, which they often take for granted. By taking an inventory of strengths, the client can develop a more well-rounded self-concept and self-image. Strengths can be an aid to mobilizing health and regenerative processes.

A client's strength might be weight that is within the normal range for age and height, thus enabling the client to cope better with surgery. In another instance, a client's strengths might be absence of allergies and being a nonsmoker.

A client's strengths can be found in the nursing assessment record (health, home life, education, recreation, exercise, work, family and friends, religious beliefs, and sense of humour, for example), the health examination, and the client's records. See Table 22.8 for the five strengths identified for Amanda Aquilini.

AVOIDING ERRORS IN DIAGNOSTIC REASONING Some error is inherent in any human undertaking, and diagnosis is no exception. However, it is important that nurses make nursing diagnoses with a high level of accuracy. Nurses can avoid some common errors of reasoning by recognizing them and applying the appropriate critical-thinking skills. Error can occur at any point in the diagnostic process: data collection, data interpretation, and data clustering.

The following suggestions should help to minimize diagnostic error:

- *Verify.* Hypothesize possible explanations of the data, but realize that all diagnoses are only tentative until they are verified. Begin and end the diagnostic process by talking with the client and family.
- *Build a good knowledge base, and acquire clinical experience.* Nurses must apply knowledge from many different areas to recognize significant cues and patterns and generate hypotheses about the data.
- *Have a working knowledge of what is normal.* Nurses need to know the population norms for vital signs, laboratory tests, speech development, breath sounds, and so on. In addition, nurses must determine what is normal for a particular person, taking into account age, physical makeup, lifestyle, culture, and the person's own perception of what is normal. For example, high normal blood pressure for adults is in the range of 130–139/85–89 mm Hg (Canadian Hypertension Education Program, 2008). However, a nurse might obtain a reading of 90/50 that is normal for a particular client. The nurse should compare findings with the client's baseline when possible.
- *Consult resources.* Both novices and experienced nurses should consult appropriate resources whenever in doubt about a diagnosis. Professional literature, nursing colleagues, and other professionals are all appropriate resources.
- *Base diagnoses on patterns—that is, on behaviour over time—rather than on an isolated incident.* For example, even though Amanda Aquilini is concerned today about needing to leave her child with a neighbour, it is likely that this concern will be resolved without intervention by the next day. Therefore, the admitting nurse should not diagnose *Interrupted Family Processes,* and this tentative nursing diagnosis should be reconsidered.
- *Improve critical-thinking skills.* These skills help the nurse to be aware of and avoid errors in thinking, such as overgeneralizing, stereotyping, making unwarranted assumptions, and so on. See Chapter 20.

FORMULATING DIAGNOSTIC STATEMENTS Most nursing diagnoses are written as two-part or three-part statements.

BASIC TWO-PART STATEMENTS The basic two-part statement includes the following:

1. Diagnostic label (problem): statement of the client's response (NANDA International label)
2. Etiology: factors contributing to or probable causes of the responses

The two parts are joined by the words *related to* rather than *because of.* The phrase *because of* implies that one part causes or is responsible for the other part. By contrast, the phrase *related to* merely implies a relationship. Some examples of two-part nursing diagnoses are shown in the Box 22.8.

BASIC THREE-PART STATEMENTS The basic three-part nursing diagnosis statement includes the following:

1. Diagnostic label (problem): statement of the client's response (NANDA International label)
2. Etiology: factors contributing to or probable causes of the response
3. Signs and symptoms: defining characteristics manifested by the client

Actual nursing diagnoses can be documented by using the three-part statement (see the Box 22.9) because the signs and symptoms have been identified. This format cannot be used for risk diagnosis because the client does not have signs and symptoms of the diagnosis.

USING DIAGNOSTIC STATEMENTS EFFECTIVELY Beginning nurses often prepare long lists, but checking initial statements (hypotheses) with the client helps both nurse and client narrow down the list to those that are most important in the current clinical context. Next, through negotiating and portioning with the client, the nurse identifies priority client health outcomes to guide nursing care.

BOX 22.8 BASIC TWO-PART DIAGNOSTIC STATEMENT

Diagnostic label		Etiology
Constipation	related to	prolonged laxative use
Ineffective breastfeeding	related to	breast engorgement

BOX 22.9 BASIC THREE-PART DIAGNOSTIC STATEMENT

Diagnostic label		Etiology		Signs and Symptoms
Chronic low self-esteem	related to (r/t)	rejection by husband	as evidenced by (a.e.b.)	hypersensitivity to criticism; states, "I don't know if I can manage by myself" and rejects positive feedback

Planning

Planning is a deliberative, systematic phase of the nursing process that involves decision making and problem solving. In planning, the nurse refers to the client's assessment data, diagnostic statements, and client priorities when designing the nursing interventions required to achieve the client's health outcomes. (See Figure 22.7.) The product of the planning phase is a client care plan.

Although planning is basically the nurse's responsibility, input from the client and support persons is essential if a plan is to be effective. Nurses do not plan *for* the client but encourage the client to participate actively to the extent possible. In a home setting, the client's support people or caregivers are the ones who assist in implementing the plan of care; thus, its effectiveness depends largely on them.

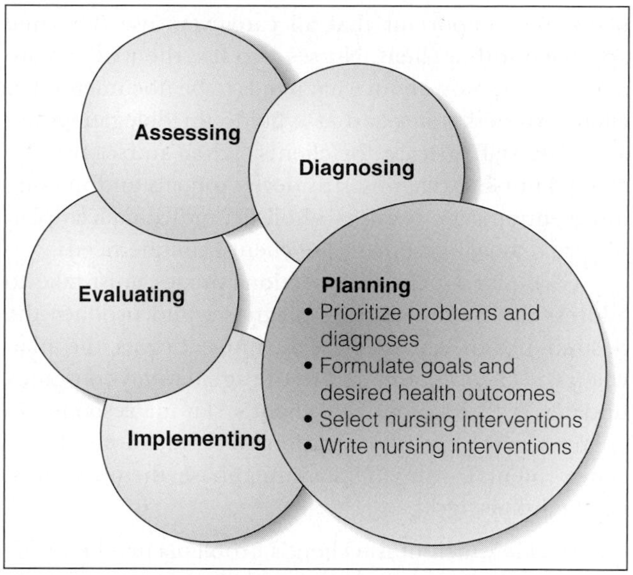
Assessing
Diagnosing
Evaluating
Planning
• Prioritize problems and diagnoses
• Formulate goals and desired health outcomes
• Select nursing interventions
• Write nursing interventions
Implementing

FIGURE 22.7 Planning: The third phase of the nursing process, in which the nurse and client develop a mutually agreed-on plan of care.

Types of Planning

Planning begins with the first client contact and continues until the nurse–client relationship ends, usually when the client is discharged from the health-care agency.

INITIAL PLANNING The nurse who performs the admission assessment usually develops the initial comprehensive plan of care. This nurse has the benefit of the client's body language as well as some intuitive kinds of information that are not available from the written database. Planning should be initiated as soon as possible after the initial assessment, especially because of the trend toward shorter hospital stays.

ONGOING PLANNING As nurses obtain new information and evaluate the client's responses to care, they can individualize the initial care plan further. Ongoing planning also occurs at the beginning of a shift, home visit, or clinic appointment. By using ongoing assessment data, the nurse carries out ongoing planning for the following purposes (Wilkinson, 2007):

1. To determine whether the client's health status has changed
2. To set the priorities for the client's care during the contact period (e.g., shift, home visit)
3. To decide which problems to focus on during the contact period
4. To coordinate the nurse's activities so that more than one problem can be addressed at each client contact

DISCHARGE PLANNING **Discharge planning**, the process of anticipating and planning for needs after discharge, is a crucial part of comprehensive health care and should be addressed in each client's care plan. Because the average stay of clients in acute-care hospitals has become shorter, people are often discharged still needing care. Although many clients are discharged to other agencies (e.g., nursing homes), such care is increasingly being delivered in the home. Effective discharge planning begins at first client contact and involves comprehensive and ongoing assessment to obtain information about the client's ongoing needs.

Developing Nursing Care Plans

The end product of the planning phase of the nursing process is a formal or informal plan of care. An **informal care plan** is a plan of action that exists in the nurse's mind. For example, the nurse may think, "Mrs. Phan is very tired. I will need to reinforce her teaching after she is rested." A **formal care plan** is a written guide that organizes information about the client's care. The most obvious benefit of a formal written care plan is that it provides continuity of care.

Standardized care plans specify the nursing care for groups of clients with common needs (e.g., all clients with myocardial infarction). **Individualized care plans** are tailored to meet the unique needs of a specific client—needs that are not addressed by the standardized plans. It is important that all caregivers use the same approach with a client. Nurses also use the written care plan for direction about what needs to be documented in client progress notes and as a guide for delegating and assigning staff to care for clients. When nurses use the client's nursing diagnoses to develop goals and nursing interventions, the result is a holistic, individualized plan of care that will best meet the client's unique needs.

Care plans include the actions nurses must take to address the client's nursing diagnoses and produce the desired health outcomes. The nurse begins the plan when the client is admitted to the agency and constantly updates it throughout the client's stay in response to changes in the client's condition and evaluations of goal achievement. During the planning phase, the nurse must do the following:

1. Decide which of the client's problems need individualized plans and which problems can be addressed by standardized plans and routine care.
2. Choose and adapt standardized, preprinted interventions and care plans, where appropriate.
3. Write individualized desired health outcomes and nursing interventions for client problems that require nursing attention beyond preplanned, routine care.

The complete plan of care for a client is made up of several different documents that (1) describe the routine care needed to meet basic needs (e.g., bathing, nutrition), (2) address the client's nursing diagnoses and identified health outcomes, and (3) specify nursing responsibilities in carrying out the client's medical plan of care (e.g., keeping the client from eating or drinking before surgery; scheduling a laboratory test). A complete plan of care integrates dependent and independent nursing functions into a meaningful whole and provides a central source of client information. Figure 22.8 illustrates the various documents that may be included in a nursing care plan.

STANDARDIZED APPROACHES TO CARE PLANNING

Most health-care agencies have devised a variety of preprinted, standardized guides for providing essential nursing care to specified groups of clients who have certain needs in common (e.g., all clients with pneumonia). Standards of care, standardized care plans, protocols, policies, and procedures are developed and accepted by the nursing staff to (1) ensure that minimally acceptable standards of care are provided and (2) promote efficient use of nurses' time by removing the need to handwrite common activities that are done over and over for many of the clients with common needs.

Standards of care describe nursing care for groups of clients rather than for individuals, and they describe achievable, rather than ideal, nursing care. They define the interventions for which nurses are held accountable; they do not contain medical orders. Standards of care are usually agency records and not part of the client's care plan, but they may be referred to in the plan (e.g., a nurse might write, "See standards of care for cardiac catheterization"). Standards of care may or may not be organized according to problems or nursing diagnoses.

Standardized care plans are also preplanned, preprinted guides for the nursing care of groups of clients with common needs (e.g., a specific nursing diagnosis, or all the nursing diagnoses associated with a particular medical condition). However, they should not be confused with *standards of care*.

Like standards of care and standardized care plans, **protocols** are preprinted and preplanned to indicate the actions commonly required for a particular group of clients. For example, an agency may have a protocol for admitting a client to the intensive care unit. Protocols may include both medical orders and nursing interventions.

Policies and **procedures** are developed to govern the handling of frequently occurring situations. For example, a hospital may have a policy specifying the number of visitors a client may have. Some policies and procedures are similar to protocols and specify what is to be done, for example, in the case of cardiac arrest. If a policy covers a situation pertinent to client care, it is usually noted on the care plan (e.g., "Make social work referral according to Unit Policy Manual").

A **standing order** is a written document about policies, rules, regulations, or orders regarding client care. Standing orders give nurses the authority to carry out specific actions under certain circumstances, often when a physician is not immediately available. In a hospital critical care unit, a common example is the administration of emergency anti-arrhythmic medications when a client's cardiac monitoring pattern changes. In a home care setting, a physician may write a standing order for the administration of epinephrine for a client who becomes excessively dyspneic.

Nursing care must be individualized to fit the unique needs of each client. In practice, a care plan usually consists of both preprinted and handwritten sections. The nurse uses standardized care plans for predictable, commonly occurring problems and handwrites an individual plan for unusual problems or problems needing special attention. For example, a standardized care plan for all "clients with a medical diagnosis of pneumonia" would probably include a nursing diagnosis of *Deficient Fluid Volume* and direct the nurse to assess the client's hydration status. On a respiratory or medical unit, this would be a common nursing diagnosis; therefore, Amanda Aquilini's nurse was able to obtain a standardized plan directing

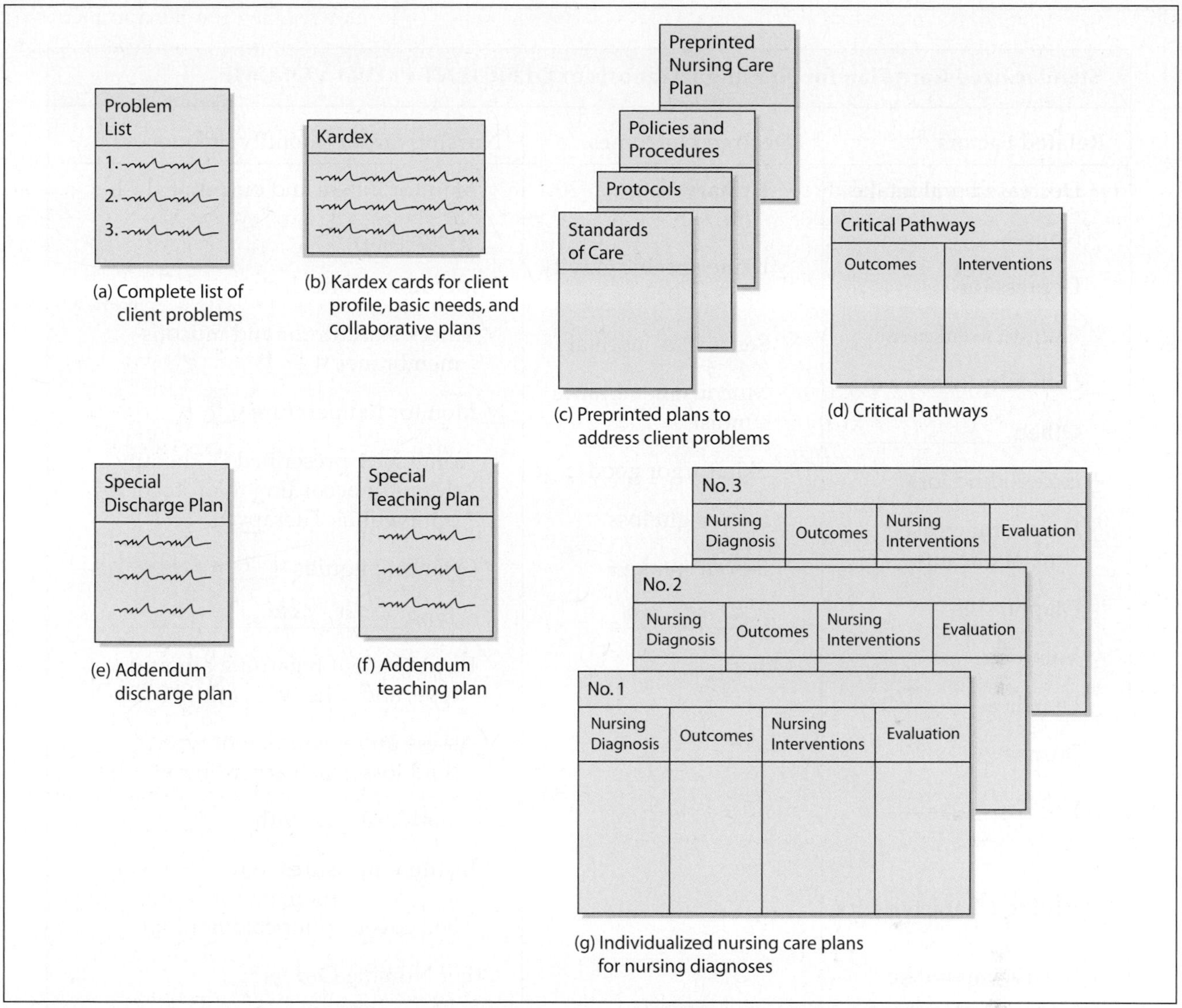

FIGURE 22.8 Documents that may be included in a complete client care plan

Source: From **Nursing Process & Critical Thinking**, *4th ed. (p. 452), by J. M. Wilkinson, 2007, Upper Saddle River, NJ: Prentice Hall. Adapted with permission.*

care commonly needed by clients with *Deficient Fluid Volume.* (See Figure 22.3 on pages 424–425 and Figure 22.9.) However, the nursing diagnosis *Risk for Interrupted Family Processes* would not be common to all clients with pneumonia; it is specific to Amanda. Therefore, the goals and nursing interventions for that diagnosis would need to be handwritten by the nurse.

STUDENT CARE PLANS Because student care plans are a learning activity as well as a plan of care, they may be more lengthy and detailed than care plans used by nurses. To help students learn to write care plans, educators may suggest a five-column format: (1) nursing diagnosis or hypotheses, (2) goals or desired health outcomes, (3) interventions, (4) rationale, and (5) evaluation. A **rationale** is the scientific principle given as the reason for selecting a particular nursing intervention. Students may also be required to cite supporting literature for their stated rationale.

COMPUTERIZED CARE PLANS Computers are increasingly being used to create and store nursing care plans. The computer can generate both standardized and individualized care plans. For an individualized plan, the nurse chooses the appropriate diagnoses from a menu suggested by the computer. The computer then lists possible goals and nursing interventions for those diagnoses; the nurse chooses those appropriate for the client and types in any additional goals and interventions or nursing actions not listed on the menu. The nurse can read the plan on the computer screen or print out an updated working copy each day.

COLLABORATIVE CARE PLANS: CRITICAL PATHWAYS AND CONCEPT MAPS Collaborative care planning is becoming increasingly important given short hospital stays, subspecialization, and escalating health-care costs. Two types of multidisciplinary care plans are commonly used. Both types are standardized plans that outline the

Standardized Care Plan for Nursing Diagnosis of DEFICIENT FLUID VOLUME

Related Factors	Desired Outcomes	Nursing Order (Identify Frequency)
✓ Decreased oral intake	✓ Urinary output > 30 mL/hr	✓ Monitor intake and output q 1 h
✓ Nausea	✓ Urine specific gravity 1.005 ±1.025	✓ Weigh daily
__ Depression	✓ Serum Na^+ normal	✓ Monitor serum electrolyte levels X 1 or until normal
✓ Fatigue, weakness	✓ Mucous membranes moist	✓ Check skin turgor and mucous membranes q 8 h
__ Difficulty swallowing	✓ Skin turgor good	✓ Monitor temperature q 4 h
__ Other:________	✓ No weight loss	✓ Administer prescribed IV therapy (Monitor according to protocol for Intravenous Therapy) 1000 mL D_5 LR at 100 mL/hr
✓ Excess fluid loss	✓ 8-hour intake = 400 mL oral	✓ Offer oral liquids q 1 h
✓ Fever or increased metabolic rate	Other:	Type clear, cold
✓ Diaphoresis		✓ Instruct client regarding amount, type, and schedule of fluid intake
✓ Vomiting		✓ Assess understanding of type of fluid loss; teach accordingly
__ Diarrhea		✓ Mouth care prn with water
__ Burns		✓ Institute measures to reduce fever (e.g., lower room temperature, remove bed covers, offer cold liquids)
__ Other________		Other Nursing Orders: Monitor urine specific gravity q shift
Defining Characteristics		
✓ Insufficient intake		
✓ Negative balance of intake and output		
✓ Dry mucous membranes		
✓ Poor skin turgor		
__ Concentrated urine		
__ Hypernatremia		
✓ Rapid, weak pulse		
__ Falling B/P		
__ Weight loss		

Plan Initiated by: M. Medina RN **Date** 07-12-24

Plan/outcomes evaluated__________ **Date**________

Plan/outcomes evaluated__________ **Date**________

Client: Amanda Aquilini

FIGURE 22.9 A standardized care plan for nursing diagnosis of *Deficient Fluid Volume*

care required for clients with common, predictable—usually medical—conditions (e.g., pneumonia, hip replacement surgery).

Critical Pathways **Critical pathways** are used to plan and direct client care. This multidisciplinary client-centred tool helps the health-care team to deliver care according to the client health outcomes. The document includes the expected outcomes predicted by the client and health-care team (nursing, physiotherapy, medicine, pharmacy, and social work, for instance) to develop and integrate a plan of care as the client progresses through an illness. For example, a pathway for a client suffering from a myocardial infarction, as is the case with Sharon Noble, will recommend daily activities, consults, procedures, management considerations, educational needs, and so on, so that Sharon can progress along the pathway to effective discharge and recovery. Refer to the care pathway created for Sharon in Table 22.9.

Concept Maps **Concept maps** are a diagrammatic representation of the relationships that exist among the client's health outcomes and the interventions. When used in the clinical setting, they act as a tool to help organize complex client data and to help the nurse to critically think through the client presentation while applying the nursing process. Please see the Concept Map box for Ms. Noble.

TABLE 22.9 Acute Coronary Syndrome Care Path for Sharon Noble

Day/Date	Day 1	Day 2	Day 3
Consults	Cardiology	Discharge planner Social work, pastoral	Transfer from ICU Dietary, cardiac educator
Diagnostic tests	ECG, routine blood tests, and chest X-ray	ECG	ECG with chest pain prn
Hygiene	Complete care, bed bath	Bedside basin	Bedside basin, assist client with ADL
Elimination	Bedpan/commode	Bedpan /commode	If no chest pain, use bathroom
Nutrition	Full fluid	Diet as tolerated	Diet as tolerated
Mobility	Complete bed rest	Dangle at bed side	Dangle, sit at side of bed, chair, ambulate in room
Observe/measures	Cardiac monitor and document Vital signs q1h, heart sounds Chest auscultate, neurological assessment	Cardiac monitor and document Vital signs q1h, heart sounds Chest auscultate, IV site	Cardiac monitor and document Vital signs q1h, heart sounds Chest auscultate, IV site
Medication	IV-Nitro/Heparin/Lovenox, ASA, Intergrilin, Beta blockers, ACE inhibitors	CASA, Beta B, ACE inhibitors, Nitrates, Heparin	Reassess-IV Nitro, Heparin, review all meds tolerance
Treatment	O_2 3-5 L	Discontinue when pain free	Reassess O_2 requirements
Psychosocial	Assess anxiety and pain	Assess anxiety and pain	Assess anxiety and pain
Teaching	Instruct, inform, teach care plan Rationale for nursing interventions medications, desired client outcomes	Education, risk factors, provide web resources for patient	Reassess learning needs, involve significant other, ongoing health teaching
Discharge plan	Assess family and supports in anticipation of discharge	Ongoing planning	Initiate discussions re discharge, discuss needed referrals
Client outcomes	Client is chest pain free Systolic BP: 100–140 Heart rate = 55–100 no arrhythmias No SOB, anxiety free	Pain free—tolerates increased activity, stable vital signs Resting respiration rate = 16–20	No reoccurrence of chest pain or SOB with increased ADLs, tolerated ambulation
Other	Thrombolytic ________ Triage ________		

CONCEPT MAP

Chest Pain

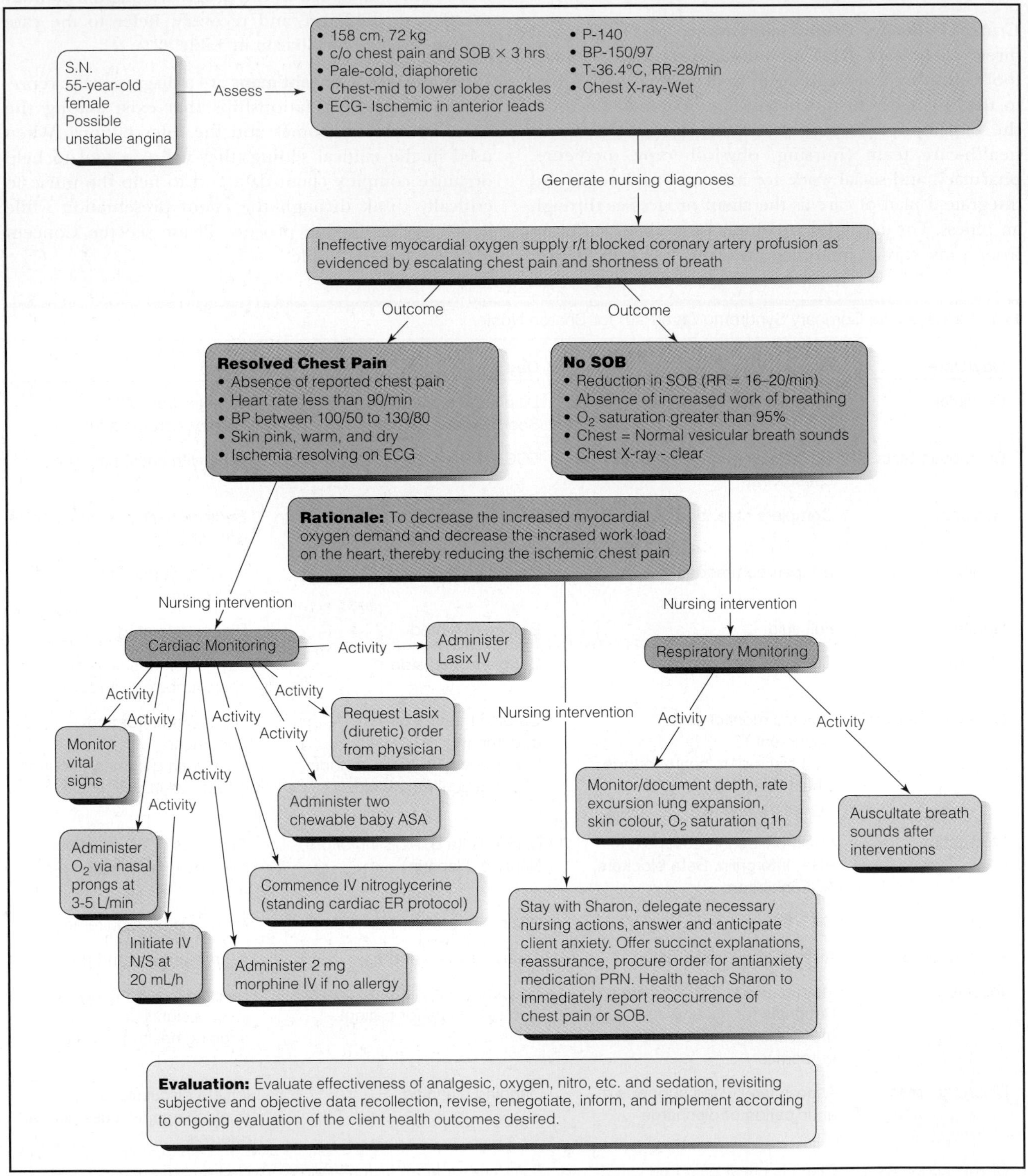

The Planning Process

In the process of developing client care plans, the nurse engages in the following activities:

- Setting priorities
- Establishing client goals or desired health outcomes
- Selecting nursing interventions and activities
- Writing a plan of care

SETTING PRIORITIES Priority setting is the process of establishing a preferential order for nursing diagnoses, client health outcomes, and interventions. The nurse and client begin planning by deciding which nursing diagnosis requires attention first, which second, and so on. Instead of rank-ordering diagnoses, nurses can group them as having high, medium, or low priority. Life-threatening problems, such as loss of respiratory or cardiac function, are designated as *high priority*. Health-threatening problems, such as acute illness and decreased coping ability, are assigned *medium priority* because they may result in delayed development or cause destructive physical or emotional changes. A *low-priority* problem is one that arises from normal developmental needs or that requires only minimal nursing support.

Although not a nursing framework, nurses frequently use Maslow's hierarchy of needs when setting priorities. In Maslow's hierarchy, physiological needs, such as air, food, and water, are basic to life and receive higher priority than the need for security or activity. Growth needs, such as self-esteem, are not perceived as "basic" in this framework. Thus, such nursing diagnoses as *Ineffective Airway Clearance* and *Impaired Gas Exchange* would take priority over such nursing diagnoses as *Anxiety* or *Ineffective Coping*.

It is not necessary to resolve all high-priority diagnoses before addressing others. The nurse may partially address a high-priority diagnosis and then deal with a diagnosis of lesser priority. Furthermore, because clients usually have several problems, the nurse often deals with more than one diagnosis at a time. See Table 22.10 for priorities assigned to Amanda Aquilini's nursing diagnoses.

Priorities change as the client's responses, problems, and therapies change. The nurse must consider a variety of factors when assigning priorities:

1. *The client's health values and beliefs:* Values concerning health may be more important to the nurse than to the client. For example, a client may believe being home for the children to be more urgent than a health problem. When such a difference of opinion exists, the client and nurse should discuss it openly to resolve any conflict. However, in a life-threatening situation, the nurse usually must take the initiative.
2. *The client's priorities:* Involving the client in prioritizing and care planning enhances collaboration. Sometimes, however, the client's perception of what is important conflicts with the nurse's knowledge of potential problems or complications. For example, the client may not regard turning and repositioning in bed as important, preferring to be undisturbed. The nurse, however, aware of the potential complications of prolonged bed rest (e.g., muscle weakness and decubitus ulcers), needs to inform the client and gain the client's agreement to carry out the necessary interventions.
3. *The resources available to the nurse and client:* If money, equipment, or personnel are scarce in a health-care agency, then a problem may be given a lower priority than usual. Nurses in a home setting, for example, do not have the resources of a hospital. If the necessary resources are not available, the solution of that problem might need to be postponed, or the client may need referral. Client resources, such as finances or coping ability, can also influence the setting of priorities.
4. *The urgency of the health problem:* Regardless of the framework used, life-threatening situations require that the nurse assign them high priority. For example, in Table 22.10, although Amanda Aquilini is anxious about childcare, her *Ineffective Airway Clearance* has higher priority (see the Concept Map box Ineffective Airway Clearance on page 447). Situations that affect the integrity of the client, that is, those that could have a negative or destructive effect on the client, also have high priority.
5. *The medical treatment plan:* The priorities for treating health problems must be congruent with treatment by other health-care professionals. For example, a high priority for the client might be to become ambulatory; however, if the physician's therapeutic regimen calls for extended bed rest, then ambulation must assume a lower priority in the nursing care plan. The nurse can provide or teach exercises to facilitate ambulation later, provided the client's health permits. The nursing diagnosis related to ambulation is not ignored; it is merely deferred.

ESTABLISHING CLIENT GOALS OR DESIRED HEALTH OUTCOMES After establishing priorities, the nurse and client set goals for each nursing diagnosis (see the Reflect on Primary Health Care box). On a care plan the **goals** or **desired health outcomes** describe, in terms of observable client responses, what the nurse, through implementation of nursing interventions, hopes the client will achieve. The terms *goal* and *desired health outcome* are used interchangeably in this text, except when discussing and using standardized language. Some references also use the terms *expected outcome, predicted outcome, outcome criterion,* and *objective.*

Some nursing literature differentiates the terms by defining *goals* as broad statements about the client's

REFLECT ON PRIMARY HEALTH CARE

While engaging in the processes of assessing, diagnosing, planning, implementing, and evaluating, the nurse includes the client or patient as a full partner in decision making. During assessment, the nurse talks with the client, observes the client and family or significant others, and analyzes the client's environment, particularly when caring for clients in their homes, workplaces, and education and leisure settings. Next, the nurse engages the client in setting health goals and identifying priority health outcomes. During the planning process, the nurse collaborates with the client in determining mutually agreeable interventions and then continues to work with the client to implement the plan of care collaboratively. Evaluation involves both the expertise of the nurse in assessing how well the client has achieved desired health outcomes and the client's self-assessment. The process will not be effective without the full *participation* of the client. Consider how you involve your clients in planning for their nursing care.

TABLE 22.10 Assigning Priorities to Nursing Diagnoses for Amanda Aquilini

Nursing Diagnosis	Priority	Rationale
Ineffective Airway Clearance related to (1) viscous secretions secondary to deficient fluid volume, and (2) shallow chest expansion secondary to pain and fatigue	High priority	Loss of respiratory functioning is a life-threatening problem. The nurse's primary concern must be to promote Amanda's oxygenation by addressing the related factors.
Deficient Fluid Volume related to intake insufficient to replace fluid loss secondary to fever and diaphoresis	High priority	*Severe Deficient Fluid Volume* is life threatening. Although not that severe for Amanda, it is a high-priority problem because it is also a contributing factor for *Ineffective Airway Clearance.* Collaborative efforts to improve her hydration have already begun (intravenous fluids). The nurse must immediately and continuously assess and promote Amanda's hydration.
Anxiety related to (1) difficulty breathing, and (2) concerns over work and parenting roles	Medium priority	Although Amanda is concerned about work and parenting roles, these are not a threat to life. Also, treatment of her high-priority problem, ***Ineffective Airway Clearance,*** will relieve one of the related factors (dyspnea). Meanwhile, the nurse should provide symptomatic relief of Amanda's anxiety during periods of dyspnea because extreme anxiety could further compromise her oxygenation by causing her to breathe ineffectively and increasing the rate at which she uses oxygen.
Risk for Interrupted Family Processes related to illness and temporary unavailability of father to provide childcare	Low priority	Amanda's child is currently being cared for. If Amanda's husband returns as planned, this risk diagnosis will not develop into an actual diagnosis. No interventions are needed at present except for continued assessment and support.
Imbalanced Nutrition: Less than Body Requirements related to decreased appetite, nausea, and increased metabolism secondary to disease process	Low priority	This problem is not currently health threatening, but it could be if it were to persist. It will almost certainly resolve in a day or two as the medical problem is treated. If the medical problem does not resolve quickly, this will change to a medium priority.
Self-Care Deficit, Bathing/Hygiene related to activity intolerance secondary to ineffective airway clearance and sleep pattern disturbance	Low priority	This problem is caused by other, higher-priority problems; therefore, it will resolve as they resolve. Meanwhile, the nurse needs to assist Amanda with bathing and so on, to support and conserve her energy until she is strong enough to resume her own care.
Disturbed Sleep Pattern related to cough, pain, orthopnea, fever, and diaphoresis	Low priority	Lack of sleep is health threatening. But for the moment, the nurse does not need to address this problem. ***Disturbed Sleep Pattern*** does contribute to Amanda's ***Ineffective Airway Clearance,*** but it is not the main cause. Therefore, measures to promote sleep will be low priority at least until evening. After the nurse has attended to Amanda's oxygenation and hydration needs, this problem priority will change.
Pain (Chest), Acute related to cough secondary to pneumonia	Not on care plan	The nurse did not write ***Pain*** as a problem on the care plan because ***Pain*** is to be addressed as the etiology of ***Disturbed Sleep Pattern*** and ***Ineffective Airway Clearance.*** The related factors to pain (cough and pneumonia) will be treated by medications (collaborative interventions). Independent nursing actions would address the problem rather than the related factors and would be the same as the nursing actions for ***Ineffective Airway Clearance.***

status and *desired health outcomes* as the more specific, observable criteria used to evaluate whether the goals have been met. For example,

Goal (broad): Improve nutritional status

Desired health outcome (specific): Gain 2.5 kg by Jan. 7

When goals are stated broadly, as in this example, the care plan must include *both* goals and desired health outcomes. They are sometimes combined into one statement linked by the words "as evidenced by," as follows: Improve nutritional status as evidenced by weight gain of 2.5 kg by Jan. 7.

CONCEPT MAP

Ineffective Airway Clearance (Gas Exchange)

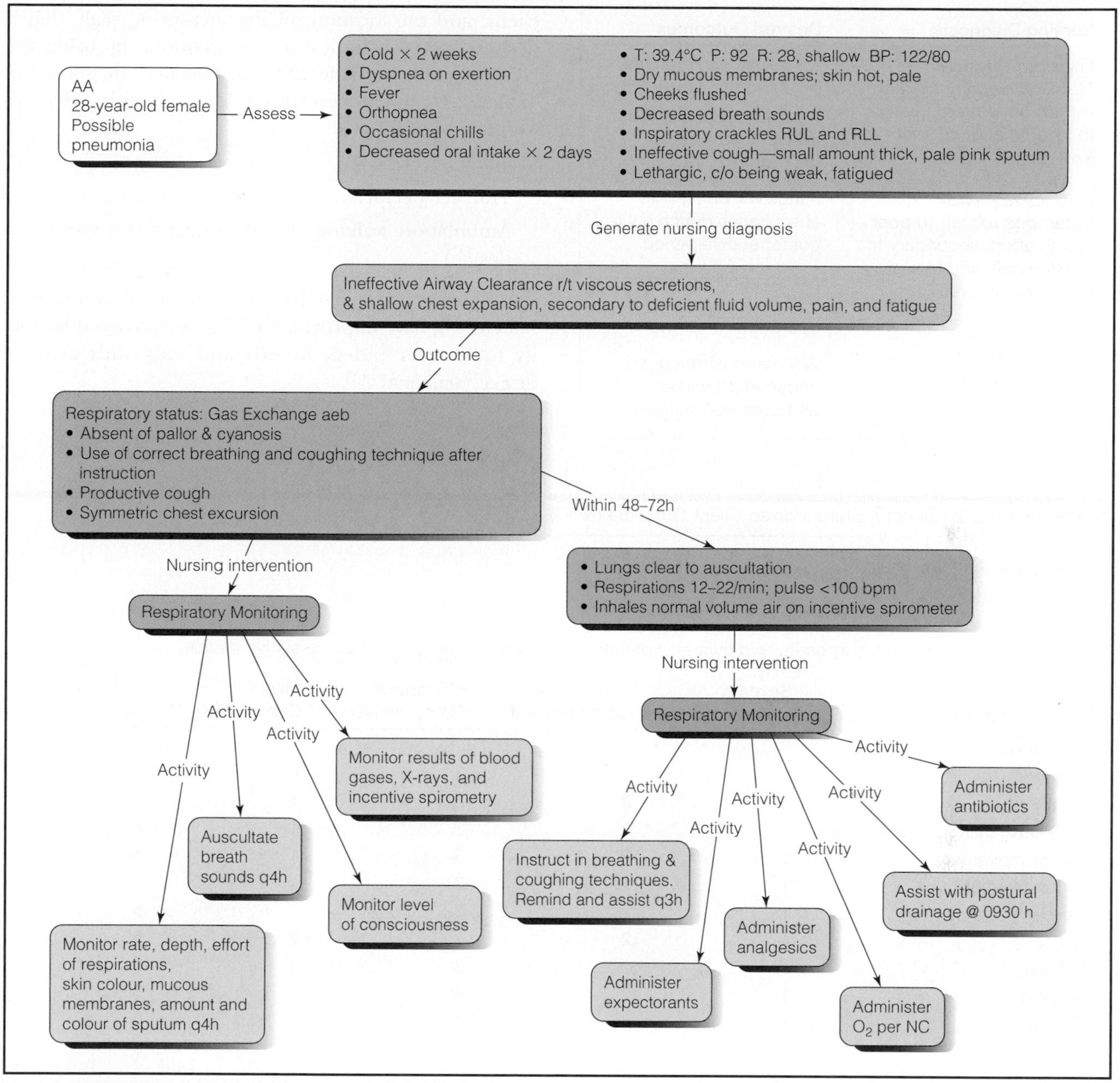

Writing the broad, general goal first can help students think of the specific outcomes that are needed, but the broad goal is just a starting point for planning. It is the specific, observable outcomes that *must* be written on the care plan and used to evaluate client progress. Table 22.11 shows both broad goals and desired health outcomes.

THE NURSING OUTCOMES CLASSIFICATION Standardized nursing language is required if nursing data are to be included in computerized databases that are analyzed and used in nursing decisions. Working toward this end, researchers have developed a taxonomy, the **Nursing Outcomes Classification (NOC)**, for describing client outcomes that respond to nursing interventions. Each NOC outcome includes a definition, a measuring scale, and indicators.

A NOC is similar to a *goal* in traditional language. It is "a measurable patient or family caregiver state, behaviour, or perception that is conceptualized as a variable and is largely influenced by and sensitive to nursing interventions" (Moorhead, Johnson, & Maas, 2004, p. xix). The NOC is broadly stated. In order to be measured, an outcome must be made more specific by identifying the specific indicators that apply to a client. Indicators are similar to desired health outcomes in traditional language. Indicators are also stated in neutral terms, but each outcome includes a five-point scale (a *measure*) that is used to rate the client's status on each

TABLE 22.11 Deriving Desired Client Health Outcomes from Nursing Diagnoses

Nursing Diagnosis	Desired Outcomes
Impaired Physical Mobility: inability to bear weight on left leg, related to inflammation of knee joint	Ambulate with crutches by end of the week Be able to stand without assistance by end of the month
Ineffective Airway Clearance related to poor cough effort, secondary to incision pain and fear of damaging sutures	Lungs will be clear to auscultation during entire postoperative period No skin pallor or cyanosis by 12 hours post-operation Will demonstrate good cough effort within 24 hours after surgery

indicator. When using the NOC taxonomy to write a desired health outcome on a care plan, the nurse writes the label, the indicators that apply to the particular client, and the location on the measuring scale that is desired for each indicator. For example, by using the NOC outcome in Table 22.12 for the client diagnosed in Table 22.13, the individualized desired health outcomes would read as follows:

Mobility Level:

Transfer performance (5, completely independent)

Ambulation: walking (4, independent with assistive device)

Stated in *traditional* language, that goal would read: "Client will have improved mobility as evidenced by ability to transfer independently and walk with assistive device (walker)."

TABLE 22.12 Example of a Standardized Client Outcome (NOC)

Domain I: Functional Health
Class C: Mobility
Outcome: Mobility [0208]
Definition: Ability to move purposefully in own environment independently with or without assistive device

Mobility overall rating	Severely Compromised	Substantially Compromised	Moderately Compromised	Mildly Compromised	Not Compromised
Indicators					
Balance	1	2	3	4	5
Coordination	1	2	3	4	5
Body positioning performance	1	2	3	4	5
Muscle movement	1	2	3	4	5
Joint movement	1	2	3	4	5
Transfer performance	1	2	3	4	5
Gait	1	2	3	4	5
Walking	1	2	3	4	5
Running	1	2	3	4	5
Jumping	1	2	3	4	5
Moves with ease	1	2	3	4	5

Source: From Nursing Outcomes Classification (NOC), *3rd ed. (p. 203), by M. Johnson, M. Maas, and S. Moorhead, Eds., 2004, St. Louis, MO: Mosby. Reprinted with permission.*

TABLE 22.13 Deriving Desired Health Outcomes from Nursing Diagnoses

Nursing Diagnosis	Opposite Healthy Responses (Goals)	Desired Outcomes The client will:
Impaired Physical Mobility: inability to bear weight on left leg, related to inflammation of knee joint	Improved mobility Ability to bear weight on left leg	Ambulate with crutches by end of the week. Stand without assistance by end of the month.
Ineffective Airway Clearance related to poor cough effort, secondary to incision pain and fear of damaging sutures	Effective airway clearance	Have lungs clear to auscultation during entire postoperative period. Have no skin pallor or cyanosis by 12 hours postoperation. Within 24 hours after surgery, demonstrate good cough effort.

PURPOSE OF GOALS OR DESIRED HEALTH OUTCOMES Goals or desired health outcomes serve the following purposes:

1. They provide direction for planning nursing interventions. Ideas for interventions come more easily if the desired health outcomes state clearly and specifically what the nurse hopes the client will achieve.
2. They serve as criteria for evaluating client progress. Although developed in the planning step of the nursing process, desired health outcomes serve as the criteria for judging nursing interventions and client progress in the evaluation step.
3. They enable the client and nurse to determine when the problem has been resolved.
4. They help motivate the client and nurse by providing a sense of achievement. As goals are met, both client and nurse can see that their efforts have been worthwhile. This provides motivation to continue following the plan.

LONG-TERM AND SHORT-TERM GOALS Goals may be short term or long term. A short-term goal might be "Client will raise right arm to shoulder height by Friday." In the same context, a long-term goal might be "Client will regain full use of right arm in six weeks." Short-term goals are useful (1) for clients who require health care for a short time and (2) for those who are frustrated by long-term goals that seem difficult to attain and who need the satisfaction of achieving a short-term goal.

In an acute-care setting, much of the nurse's time is spent on the client's immediate needs, so most goals are short term. However, clients in acute-care settings also need long-term goals to guide planning for their discharge to long-term agencies or home care, especially in a managed care environment. Long-term goals are often used for clients who live at home and have chronic health problems and for clients in nursing homes, extended-care facilities, and rehabilitation centres.

RELATIONSHIP OF GOALS OR DESIRED HEALTH OUTCOMES TO NURSING DIAGNOSES Goals are derived from and relate to the client's nursing diagnoses—primarily from the first clause (diagnostic label). The diagnostic label clause contains the unhealthy response; it states what should change. Therefore, the *essential* client goals are derived from the diagnostic label clause. For example, if the nursing diagnosis is *Risk for Deficient Fluid Volume* related to diarrhea and inadequate intake secondary to nausea, the *essential* goal statement might be "Maintain fluid balance as evidenced by urinary and stool output in balance with fluid intake, normal skin turgor, and moist mucous membranes."

For every nursing diagnosis, the nurse must write at least one desired health outcome that, when achieved, directly demonstrates resolution of the diagnostic label clause.

COMPONENTS OF GOAL OR DESIRED HEALTH OUTCOME STATEMENTS Goal or desired health outcome statements usually have the following four components:

1. *Subject.* The subject, a noun, is the client, any part of the client, or some attribute of the client, such as the client's pulse or urinary output. The subject is often omitted in goals; it is assumed that the subject is the client unless indicated otherwise.
2. *Verb.* The verb specifies an action the client is to perform, for example, what the client is to do, learn, or experience. Verbs that denote directly observable behaviours, such as *administer, demonstrate, show, walk,* must be used. See Box 22.10 for some examples.
3. *Conditions* or *modifiers.* Conditions or modifiers may be added to the verb to explain the circumstances under which the behaviour is to be performed. They explain what, where, when, or how. For example,
   - *Walks with the help of a walker* (how)
   - Lists signs and symptoms of diabetes *after attending two group diabetes classes* (when)
   - *Weight will remain at existing level when at home* (where)
   - Discusses *Canada's Food Guide and recommended daily servings* (what)

   Conditions need not be included if the criterion of performance clearly indicates what is expected.
4. *Criterion of desired performance.* The criterion indicates the standard by which a performance is evaluated or the level at which the client will perform the specified behaviour. These criteria may specify time or speed, accuracy, distance, and quality. To establish a time-achievement criterion, the nurse needs to ask, "How long?" To establish an accuracy criterion, the nurse asks, "How well?" Similarly, the nurse asks, "How far?" and "What is the expected standard?" to establish distance and quality criteria, respectively. Examples follow:
   - Weighs 75 kg *by April* (time)
   - Lists *five out of six* signs of diabetes (accuracy)
   - Walks *one block per day* (time and distance)
   - Administers insulin *using aseptic technique* (quality)

GUIDELINES FOR WRITING GOALS OR DESIRED HEALTH OUTCOMES The following guidelines can help nurses write useful goals and desired health outcomes:

BOX 22.10 EXAMPLES OF ACTION VERBS

Apply	Explain	Share
Assemble	Help	Sit
Breathe	Identify	Sleep
Choose	Inject	State
Compare	List	Talk
Define	Move	Transfer
Demonstrate	Name	Turn
Describe	Prepare	Verbalize
Differentiate	Report	
Discuss	Select	

1. *Write goals and outcomes in terms of client responses, not nurse activities.* Beginning each goal statement with "the client will" can help focus it on client behaviours and responses. Avoid statements that start with *enable, facilitate, allow, let, permit,* or similar verbs followed by the word *client.* These verbs indicate what the nurse hopes to accomplish, not what the client will do.

   Correct: Client will drink 100 mL of water per hour (client behaviour).

   Incorrect: Maintain client hydration (nursing action).

2. *Be sure that desired health outcomes are realistic for the client's capabilities, limitations, and designated time span,* if it is indicated. *Limitations* refer to finances, equipment, family support, social services, physical and mental condition, and time. For example, the outcome "Measures insulin accurately" may be unrealistic for a client who has poor vision because of cataracts.
3. *Ensure that the goals and desired health outcomes are compatible with the therapies of other professionals.* For example, the outcome "Will increase the time spent out of bed by 15 minutes each day" is not compatible with a physician's prescribed therapy of bed rest.
4. *Make sure that each goal is derived from only one nursing diagnosis.* For example, the goal "The client will increase the amount of nutrients ingested and show progress in the ability to feed self" is derived from two nursing diagnoses: *Self-Care Deficit: Feeding* and *Imbalanced Nutrition: Less than Body Requirements.* Keeping the goal statement related to only one diagnosis facilitates evaluation of care by ensuring that planned nursing interventions are clearly related to the diagnosis.
5. *Use observable, measurable terms for outcomes.* Avoid words that are vague and require interpretation or judgment by the observer. For example, such phrases as "increase daily exercise" and "improve knowledge of nutrition" can mean different things to different people. If used in outcomes, these phrases can lead to disagreements about whether the outcome was met. These phrases may be suitable for a broad client goal but are not sufficiently clear and specific to guide the nurse when evaluating client responses.
6. *Make sure the client considers the goals or desired health outcomes important and values them.* Some outcomes, such as those for problems related to self-esteem, parenting, and communication, involve choices that are best made by the client or in collaboration with the client.

Some clients may know what they want to accomplish with regard to their health problems; others may not know all the outcome possibilities. The nurse must actively listen to the client to determine personal values, goals, and desired health outcomes in relation to current health concerns. Clients are usually motivated and expend the necessary energy to reach goals they consider important.

SELECTING NURSING INTERVENTIONS AND ACTIVITIES Nursing interventions and activities are the actions that a nurse performs to achieve client goals. The specific strategies chosen should focus on eliminating or reducing the related factors' contributions to the nursing diagnosis, which is the second clause of the diagnostic statement.

When it is not possible to change the related factors, the nurse chooses interventions to treat the signs and symptoms. Examples of this situation would be *Pain* related to surgical incision and *Anxiety* related to unknown etiology.

Interventions for risk nursing diagnoses should focus on measures to reduce the client's risk factors.

Correct identification of the main related factors during the diagnosing phase provides the framework for choosing successful nursing interventions. For example, the diagnostic label *Activity Intolerance* may have several related factors: pain, weakness, sedentary lifestyle, anxiety, or cardiac arrhythmias. Interventions will vary according to the cause of the problem.

TYPES OF NURSING INTERVENTIONS Nursing interventions are identified and written during the planning step of the nursing process; however, they are actually performed during the implementing step. Nursing interventions include both direct and indirect care, as well as nurse-initiated, physician-initiated, and other provider-initiated treatments. *Direct care* is an intervention performed through interaction with the client. *Indirect care* is an intervention performed away from, but on behalf of, the client, such as interdisciplinary collaboration or management of the care environment.

Independent interventions are those activities that nurses are licensed to initiate on the basis of their knowledge and skills. They include physical care, ongoing assessment, emotional support and comfort, teaching, counselling, environmental management, and making referrals to other health-care professionals.

Dependent interventions are activities carried out under the physician's orders or supervision, or according to specified routines. Physicians' orders commonly include orders for medications, intravenous therapy, diagnostic tests, treatments, diet, and activity. The nurse is responsible for explaining, assessing the need for, and administering the medical orders. Nursing interventions may be written to individualize the medical order based on the client's status. For example, for a medical order of "Progressive ambulation, as tolerated," a nurse might write the following nursing interventions:

1. Dangle for 5 min, 12 h postop.
2. Stand at bedside 24 h postop; observe for pallor, dizziness, and weakness.
3. Check pulse before and after ambulating. Do not progress if pulse > 110.

Collaborative interventions are actions the nurse carries out in collaboration with other health-care team members, such as physical therapists, social workers, dietitians, and physicians. Collaborative nursing activities reflect the overlapping responsibilities of, and collegial relationships among, health personnel. For example, the physician might order physical therapy to teach the client crutch walking. The nurse would be responsible for informing the physical therapy department and for coordinating the client's care to include the physical therapy sessions. When the client returns to the nursing unit, the nurse would assist with crutch walking and collaborate with the physical therapist to evaluate the client's progress.

The amount of time the nurse spends in an independent versus collaborative role or on physician-initiated treatments varies according to the clinical area, type of institution, and specific position of the nurse.

CONSIDERING THE CONSEQUENCES OF EACH STRATEGY Usually, several possible interventions can be identified for each nursing diagnosis. The nurse's task is to choose those that are most likely to achieve the desired client outcomes. The nurse begins by considering the risks and benefits of each activity. An intervention may have more than one consequence. For example, the strategy "Provide accurate information" could result in the following client behaviours:

- Increased anxiety
- Decreased anxiety
- Desire to talk with the physician
- Desire to leave the hospital
- Relaxation

Determining the consequences of each strategy requires nursing knowledge and experience. For example, the nurse's experience may suggest that providing information the night before the client's surgery may increase the client's worry and tension, whereas maintaining the usual rituals before sleep is more effective. The nurse might then consider providing information several days before surgery.

CRITERIA FOR CHOOSING NURSING STRATEGIES After considering the consequences of the alternative nursing strategies, the nurse chooses one or more that are likely to be most effective. Although the nurse bases this decision on knowledge and experience, the client's input is important.

The following criteria can help the nurse choose the best nursing strategy:

- The planned action must be safe and appropriate for the individual's age, health, and condition.
- The planned action must be achievable with the resources available. For example, a home care nurse might want to include a nursing intervention for an older adult client to "Check blood glucose daily"; but, in order for that to occur, either the client must have intact sight, cognition, and memory to carry this out independently, or daily visits from a home care nurse must be available and affordable.
- The planned action must be congruent with the client's values, beliefs, and culture.
- The planned action must be congruent with other therapies (e.g., if the client is not permitted food, the strategy of an evening snack must be deferred until health permits).
- It must be based on evidence from research, expert opinion, and experience.
- It must be within established standards of care as determined by government regulations and professional associations (CNA, provincial or territorial professional associations, specialty organizations, such as the Canadian Association of Neuroscience Nurses) and the policies of the agency.

WRITING A PLAN OF CARE The nurse should use the following guidelines when writing a nursing plan of care:

1. *Date and sign the plan.* The date the plan is written is essential for evaluation, review, and future planning. The nurse's signature demonstrates accountability to the client and to the nursing profession since the effectiveness of nursing actions can be evaluated.
2. *Use category headings,* such as Assessment Data, Nursing Assessment, Nursing Diagnoses, Clients Goals, Desired Health Outcomes, Nursing Interventions, Selected Activities, and Evaluation. *Include a date for the evaluation of each goal.*
3. *Use accepted medical abbreviations and symbols and key words,* rather than complete sentences, to communicate your ideas. For example, write "Turn and reposition q2h," rather than "Turn and reposition the client every two hours." See Table 23.4 on page 488 for a list of commonly used medical abbreviations and Table 23.5 on page 489 for commonly used symbols.
4. *Refer to procedure books or other sources of information* rather than including all the steps on a written plan. For example, write: "See unit procedure book for tracheostomy care," or attach a standard nursing plan about such procedures as radiation-implantation care and preoperative or postoperative care.
5. *Tailor the plan to the unique characteristics of the client* by ensuring that the client's choices, such as preferences about the times of care and the methods used, are included. This reinforces the client's individuality and sense of control. For example, the written nursing intervention "Provide prune juice at breakfast, rather than orange juice" indicates that the client was given a choice of beverages.
6. *Ensure that the nursing plan incorporates preventive and health maintenance aspects as well as restorative ones.* For example, carrying out the order "Provide active-assistance ROM [range-of-motion] exercises to affected limbs q2h" prevents joint contractures and maintains muscle strength and joint mobility.
7. *Ensure that the plan contains orders for ongoing assessment* of the client (e.g., "Inspect incision q8h").
8. *Include collaborative and coordination activities in the plan.* For example, the nurse may write orders to ask a nutritionist or physical therapist about specific aspects of the client's care.

9. *Include plans for the client's discharge and home care needs.* It is often necessary to consult and make arrangements with the community health nurse, social worker, and specific agencies that supply client information and needed equipment. Add teaching and discharge plans as addenda if they are lengthy and complex.

See the Sample Care Plan for Amanda Aquilini.

The Nursing Interventions Classification

Nurse researchers recognized the need for a standardized language to describe the interventions that nurses perform. A taxonomy of nursing interventions referred to as the **Nursing Interventions Classification (NIC)** taxonomy has been developed by the Iowa Intervention Project. This taxonomy consists of three levels: (1) level

Sample Care Plan for Amanda Aquilini

Nursing Diagnosis: Ineffective Airway Clearance related to viscous secretions and shallow chest expansion secondary to deficient fluid volume, pain, and fatigue

Goals/Desired Outcomes	Nursing Interventions	Rationale
Demonstrate adequate air exchange (goal), as evidenced by • Absence of pallor and cyanosis (skin and mucous membranes) • Using correct breathing/coughing technique after instruction • Productive cough • Symmetric chest expansion of at least 4 cm • Reports of chest pain <4 on a 1–10 scale within 30 min after receiving oral analgesics	Monitor respiratory status q4h: rate, depth, effort, skin colour, mucous membranes, amount and colour of sputum. Monitor results of blood gases, chest X-ray studies, and incentive spirometer volume, as available. Monitor level of consciousness. Auscultate lungs q4h. Take vital signs q4h (TPR, BP).	To identify progress toward or deviations from goal. ***Ineffective Airway Clearance*** leads to poor oxygenation, evidenced by pallor, cyanosis, lethargy, and drowsiness. Inadequate oxygenation causes increased pulse rate. Respiratory rate may be decreased by narcotic analgesics. Shallow breathing further compromises oxygenation.
Within 48–72 hours • Lungs clear to auscultation • Respirations 12–22/min, pulse <100 beats/min • Inhaling normal volume of air on incentive spirometer	Instruct in breathing and coughing techniques. Remind to perform, and assist q3h.	To enable client to cough up secretions. May need encouragement and support because of fatigue and pain.
	Administer prescribed expectorant; schedule for maximum effectiveness.	Helps loosen secretions so they can be coughed up and expelled.
	Maintain Fowler's or semi-Fowler's position.	Gravity allows for fuller lung expansion by decreasing pressure of abdomen on diaphragm.
	Administer prescribed analgesics. Notify physician if pain not relieved.	Controls pleuritic pain by blocking pain pathways and altering perception of pain, enabling client to increase thoracic expansion. Unrelieved pain may signal impending complication.
	Administer oxygen by nasal cannula as prescribed. Provide portable oxygen if client goes off unit (e.g., for X-ray examination).	Supplemental oxygen makes more oxygen available to the cells even though less air is being moved by the client, thereby reducing the work of breathing.
	Assist with postural drainage daily at 0930.	Gravity facilitates movement of secretions upward through the respiratory passage.
	Administer prescribed antibiotic to maintain constant blood level. Observe for rash and GI or other side effects.	Resolves infection by bacteriostatic or bactericidal effect, depending on type of antibiotic used. Constant level required to prevent pathogens from multiplying. Allergies to antibiotics are common.

(continued)

Sample Care Plan for Amanda Aquilini (continued)

Nursing Diagnosis: ***Deficient Fluid Volume related to intake insufficient to replace fluid loss***

(See standardized care plan for Deficient Fluid Volume, Figure 22.9, p. 442).

Nursing Diagnosis: Anxiety related to difficulty breathing and concerns over work and parenting roles

Goals/Desired Outcomes	Nursing Interventions	Rationale
Demonstrate decreased anxiety (goal), as evidenced by • Listening to and following instructions for correct breathing and coughing technique, even during periods of dyspnea	When client is dyspneic, stay with her; reassure her you will stay.	Presence of a competent caregiver reduces fear of being unable to breathe. Control of anxiety will help client to maintain effective breathing pattern.
• Verbalizing understanding of condition, diagnostic tests, and treatments (by end of day)	Remain calm; appear confident. Encourage slow, deep breathing.	Reassures client the nurse can help her. Focusing on breathing may help client feel in control and decrease anxiety.
• Decrease in reports of fear and anxiety; none within 12 hours • Voice steady, not shaky • Respiratory rate of 12–22/min • Freely expressing concerns about work and parenting roles, but placing them in perspective in view of her illness	When client is dyspneic, give brief explanations of treatments and procedures. When acute episode is over, give detailed information about nature of condition, treatments, and tests. Reassess whether client needs any information on condition, treatments, or tests.	Anxiety and pain interfere with learning. Knowing what to expect reduces anxiety.
	As client can tolerate, encourage her to express and expand on her concerns about her child and her work. Explore alternatives as needed.	Awareness of source of anxiety enables client to gain control over it.
	Note whether husband returns as scheduled. If not, institute care plan for actual ***Interrupted Family Processes***.	Husband's continued absence would constitute a defining characteristic for this nursing diagnosis.

1: *domains,* (2) level 2: *classes,* and (3) level 3: *interventions.* To view the six domains and 30 classes of interventions within the taxonomy, refer to Table 22.14.

More than 514 interventions (level 3) have been developed. Similar to the NANDA International diagnoses, each broadly stated intervention includes a label (name), a definition, and a list of activities that outline the key actions of nurses in carrying out the intervention. An example appears in Box 22.11.

BOX 22.11 EXAMPLE OF AN NIC NURSING INTERVENTION LABEL

INTERVENTION: TOUCH

DEFINITION: Providing comfort and communication through purposeful tactile contact

ACTIVITIES:

- Observe cultural taboos about touch.
- Put arm around patient's shoulders, as appropriate.
- Hold patient's hand to provide emotional support.
- Apply gentle pressure at wrist, hand, or shoulder of seriously ill patient.
- Rub back in synchrony with patient's breathing, as appropriate.
- Massage around painful area, as appropriate.
- Elicit from parents common actions used to soothe and calm their child.
- Hold infant or child firmly and snugly.
- Encourage parents to touch newborn or ill child.
- Surround premature infant with blanket rolls (nesting).
- Swaddle infant snugly in a blanket to keep arms and legs close to the body.
- Place infant on mother's body immediately after birth.
- Encourage mother to hold, touch, and examine the infant while umbilical cord is being severed.
- Encourage parents to massage infant.
- Demonstrate quieting techniques for infants.
- Provide appropriate pacifier for nonnutritional sucking in newborns.
- Provide oral stimulation exercises before tube feedings in premature infants.

Source: From *Nursing Interventions Classification (NIC),* 4th ed. (p. 738), by J. C. Dochterman and G. M. Bulechek (Eds.), 2004, St. Louis, MO: Mosby. Used with permission.

TABLE 22.14 NIC Taxonomy

Level 1: Domains	Level 2: Classes (lettered for cross-referencing)
Domain 1 *Physiological: Basic* Care that supports physical functioning	A. Activity and Exercise Management: Interventions to organize or assist with physical activity and energy conservation and expenditure B. Elimination Management: Interventions to establish and maintain regular bowel and urinary elimination patterns and manage complications due to altered patterns C. Immobility Management: Interventions to manage restricted body movement and the sequelae D. Nutrition Support: Interventions to modify or maintain nutritional status E. Physical Comfort Promotion: Interventions to promote comfort using physical techniques F. Self-Care Facilitation: Interventions to provide or assist with routine activities of daily living
Domain 2 *Physiological: Complex* Care that supports homeostatic regulation	G. Electrolyte and Acid-Base Management: Interventions to regulate electrolyte/acid-base balance and prevent complications H. Drug Management: Interventions to facilitate desired effects of pharmacological agents I. Neurologic Management: Interventions to optimize neurological functions J. Perioperative Care: Interventions to provide care before, during, and immediately after surgery K. Respiratory Management: Interventions to promote airway patency and gas exchange L. Skin/Wound Management: Interventions to maintain or restore tissue integrity M. Thermoregulation: Interventions to maintain body temperature within a normal range N. Tissue Perfusion Management: Interventions to optimize circulation of blood and fluids to the tissue
Domain 3 *Behavioural* Care that supports psychosocial functioning and facilitates lifestyle changes	O. Behaviour Therapy: Interventions to reinforce or promote desirable behaviours or alter undesirable behaviours P. Cognitive Therapy: Interventions to reinforce or promote desirable cognitive functioning or alter undesirable cognitive functioning Q. Communication Enhancement: Interventions to facilitate delivering and receiving verbal and nonverbal messages R. Coping Assistance: Interventions to assist another to build on own strengths, to adapt to a change in function, or to achieve a higher level of function S. Patient Education: Interventions to facilitate learning T. Psychological Comfort: Interventions to promote comforts using psychological techniques
Domain 4 *Safety* Care that supports protection against harm	U. Crisis Management: Interventions to provide immediate short-term help in both psychological and physiological crises V. Risk Management: Interventions to initiate risk-reduction activities and continue monitoring risks over time
Domain 5 *Family* Care that supports the family unit	W. Childbearing Care: Interventions to assist in understanding and coping with the psychological and physiological changes during the childbearing period X. Lifespan Care: Interventions to facilitate family unit functioning and promote the health and welfare of family members throughout the lifespan
Domain 6 *Health System* Care that supports effective use of the health-care delivery system	Y. Health System Mediation: Interventions to facilitate the interface between patient/family and the health-care system Ya. Health System Management: Interventions to provide and enhance support services for the delivery of care Yb. Information Management: Interventions to facilitate communication among health-care providers
Domain 7 *Community* Care that supports the health of the community	Yc. Community Health Promotion: Interventions that promote the health of the whole community Yd. Community Risk Management: Interventions that assist in detecting or preventing health risks to the whole community Z. Childrearing Care: Interventions to assist in raising children

Source: From *Nursing Interventions Classification (NIC)*, 4th ed. (pp. 112–113), by J. C. Dochterman and G. M. Bulechek (Eds.), 2004, St. Louis, MO: Mosby. Used with permission.

BOX 22.12 EXAMPLES OF NIC INTERVENTIONS LINKED TO THE NANDA INTERNATIONAL NURSING DIAGNOSIS OF DISTURBED SLEEP PATTERN

SLEEP PATTERN, DISTURBED
DEFINITION: "Time limited disruption of sleep (natural, periodic suspension of consciousness) amount and quality" (NANDA International, 2007, p. 170).

Suggested Nursing Interventions for Problem Resolution:	Additional Optional Interventions:
Dementia Management	Anxiety Reduction
Environmental Management	Autogenic Training
Environmental Management: Comfort	Bathing
Hormone Replacement Therapy	Calming Technique
Medication Administration	Coping Enhancement
Medication Management	Energy Management
Medication Prescribing	Exercise Promotion
Phototherapy: Mood/Sleep Regulation	Exercise Therapy: Ambulation
Security Enhancement	Kangaroo Care
Simple Relaxation Therapy	Meditation Facilitation
Sleep Enhancement	Music Therapy
Touch	Nutrition Management
	Pain Management
	Positioning
	Progressive Muscle Relaxation
	Self-Care Assistance: Toileting
	Simple Massage
	Urinary Incontinence Care: Enuresis

Source: From *Nursing Interventions Classification (NIC),* 4th ed. (p. 877), by J. C. Dochterman and G. M. Bulechek (Eds.), 2004, St. Louis, MO: Mosby. Used with permission.

All NIC interventions have been linked to NANDA International nursing diagnostic labels. The nurse can look up a client's nursing diagnosis to see which nursing interventions are suggested. However, each nursing diagnosis contains suggestions for several interventions, so nurses need to select the appropriate interventions based on their judgment and knowledge of the client. For example, the nursing diagnostic label *Sleep Pattern Disturbed* has 12 NIC interventions listed for problem resolution and 18 additional optional interventions. See Box 22.12.

When planning and documenting care in an agency that uses the NIC taxonomy, the nurse chooses from the computer (or writes, if using a manual system) the broad intervention label (e.g., Touch). Not all the activities suggested for the intervention would be needed for every client. The nurse chooses the activities appropriate for the client and individualizes them to fit the resources available in the agency.

When writing individualized nursing interventions on a care plan, the nurse records the activities. The NIC taxonomy provides many benefits to nurse practitioners, nurse educators, nurse administrators, and the nursing profession as a whole (see Box 22.13).

BOX 22.13 BENEFITS OF THE NURSING INTERVENTIONS CLASSIFICATION (NIC)

The NIC taxonomy provides nursing staff with the following benefits:

- Helps demonstrate the impact that nurses have on the health-care delivery system
- Standardizes and defines the knowledge base for nursing curricula and practice
- Facilitates the appropriate selection of a nursing intervention
- Facilitates communication of nursing treatments to other nurses and other providers
- Enables researchers to examine the effectiveness and cost of nursing care
- Assists educators to develop curricula that better articulate with clinical practice
- Facilitates the teaching of clinical decision making to novice nurses
- Assists administrators in planning more effectively for staff and equipment needs
- Facilitates the development and use of nursing information systems
- Communicates the nature of nursing to the public

Source: From *Nursing Interventions Classification (NIC),* 4th ed. (p. vi), by J. C. Dochterman and G. M. Bulechek (Eds.), 2004, St. Louis, MO: Mosby. Used with permission.

Implementing

The nursing process is action oriented, client centred, and goal directed. After developing a plan of care based on the assessing and diagnosing phases, the nurse puts the plan into effect and evaluates the results. On the basis of this evaluation, the plan of care is either continued, modified, or terminated. As in all phases of the nursing process, clients and support persons are encouraged to participate as much as possible.

In the nursing process, implementing is the phase in which the nurse puts the nursing care plan into action. Broadly defined, implementing consists of doing, delegating, and recording. The nurse performs or delegates the nursing interventions that were developed in the planning step and then concludes the implementing step by recording nursing activities and the resulting client responses (Figure 22.10).

Although the nurse may act on the client's behalf (e.g., referring the client to a community health nurse for home care), professional standards support client and family participation as in all phases of the nursing process. The degree of participation depends on the client's health status. For example, an unconscious man is unable to participate in his care and, therefore, needs to have care given to him. By contrast, an ambulatory client may require very little care from the nurse and carry out health-care activities independently.

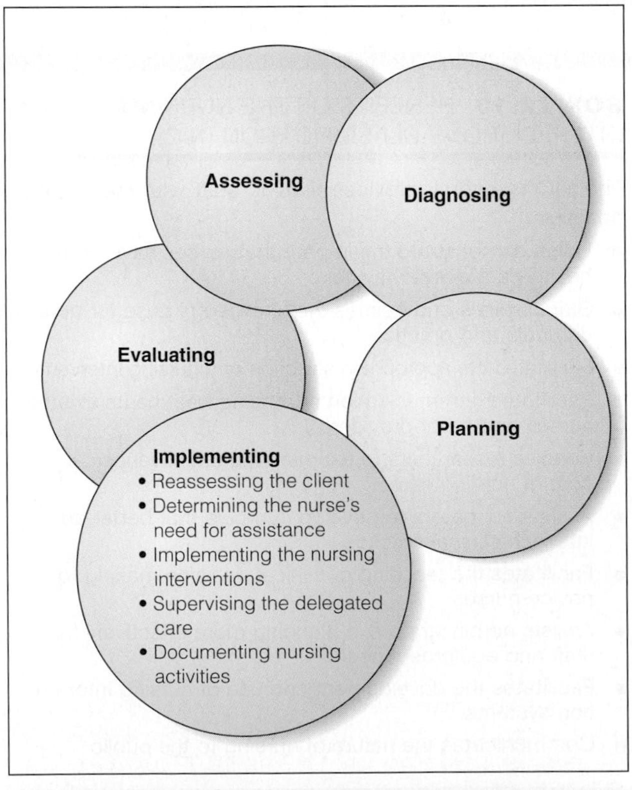
Assessing
Diagnosing
Evaluating
Planning
Implementing
• Reassessing the client
• Determining the nurse's need for assistance
• Implementing the nursing interventions
• Supervising the delegated care
• Documenting nursing activities

FIGURE 22.10 Implementing: The fourth phase of the nursing process, in which the nurse implements the nursing interventions and documents the care provided.

Relationship of Implementing to Other Nursing Process Phases

The first three nursing process phases—assessing, diagnosing, and planning—provide the basis for the nursing actions performed during the implementing step. In turn, the implementing step provides the actual nursing activities and client responses that are evaluated in the final step (evaluating). By using data acquired during assessment, the nurse can individualize the care given in the implementing phase, tailoring the interventions to fit a specific client (e.g., Amanda Aquilini) rather than applying them routinely to categories of clients (e.g., all pneumonia clients).

Ongoing assessment occurs simultaneously with implementation. While implementing the nursing interventions, the nurse continues to reassess the client at every contact, gathering data about the client's responses to the nursing actions and about any new problems that may develop. For example, while bathing an older adult client, the nurse observes a reddened area on the client's sacrum. Or when emptying a catheter bag, the nurse measures 200 mL of strong-smelling, brown urine.

Implementing Skills

To implement the care plan successfully, nurses need good cognitive, interpersonal, and technical skills. The skills are distinct from one another; in practice, however, nurses use them in various combinations and with different emphasis depending on the activity. For instance, when inserting a urinary catheter, the nurse needs cognitive knowledge of the principles and steps of the procedure, technical skill in draping the client and manipulating the equipment, and interpersonal skills to inform and reassure the client.

The **cognitive skills** (intellectual skills) include problem solving, decision making, critical thinking, and creative thinking (see Chapter 20). They are crucial to safe, intelligent nursing care.

Interpersonal skills are necessary for all nursing activities: caring, comforting, referring, counselling, and supporting are just a few. The skills include conveying knowledge, attitudes, feelings, interest, and appreciation of the client's cultural values and lifestyle. Before nurses can be highly skilled in interpersonal relations, they must have self-awareness and sensitivity to others. (See Chapters 21 and 44.)

Technical skills are hands-on skills, such as manipulating equipment, giving injections, and bandaging, moving, lifting, and repositioning clients. These activities are also called procedures or psychomotor skills. The term *psychomotor* includes the interpersonal component, for example, the need to communicate with the client.

Technical skills require knowledge and, frequently, manual dexterity. The number of technical skills expected of a nurse has greatly increased in recent years because of the increased use of technology, especially in acute-care hospitals.

Process of Implementing

The process of implementing normally includes the following:

- Reassessing the client
- Determining the nurse's need for assistance
- Implementing the nursing interventions
- Delegating and supervising
- Communicating the nursing actions

REASSESSING THE CLIENT Just before implementing an order, the nurse must reassess the client to make sure the intervention is still needed. Even though an order is written on the care plan, the client's condition may have changed. For example, Amanda Aquilini had a nursing diagnosis of *Disturbed Sleep Pattern* related to cough, pain, orthopnea (trouble breathing when lying down), fever, and diaphoresis (sweating). During rounds, the nurse discovers that Amanda is sleeping and, therefore, defers the cooling back rub that had been planned as an intervention.

New data may indicate a need to change the priorities of care or the nursing strategies. For example, a nurse begins to teach Ms. Eves, who has diabetes, how to give herself insulin injections. Shortly after beginning the teaching, the nurse realizes that Ms. Eves is not concentrating on the lesson. Subsequent discussion reveals that she is worried about her eyesight and fears she is going blind. Realizing that the client's level of stress is interfering with her learning, the nurse ends the lesson and makes arrangements for the nurse practitioner from the diabetic clinic to meet with her. The nurse also provides supportive communication to help alleviate the client's stress.

DETERMINING THE NURSE'S NEED FOR ASSISTANCE When implementing some nursing strategies, the nurse may require assistance for one of the following reasons:

- The nurse is unable to safely implement the nursing strategies alone (e.g., turning an obese client in bed).
- Assistance would reduce stress on the client (e.g., turning a person who experiences acute pain when moved).
- The nurse lacks the knowledge or skills to implement a particular nursing activity (e.g., a nurse who is not familiar with a particular model of oxygen mask needs assistance the first time it is applied).

IMPLEMENTING NURSING INTERVENTIONS It is important to explain to the client what will be done, what sensations to expect, and what the client is expected to do. For many nursing actions, it is also important to ensure the client's privacy, for example, by closing doors, pulling curtains, or draping the client. The number and kind of nursing activities is almost unlimited. Some examples are caring, communicating, helping, teaching, counselling, acting as a client advocate, leading, and managing. Nurses also coordinate client care. This activity involves scheduling client contacts with other health-care professionals (e.g., laboratory and X-ray technicians, physical and respiratory therapists), departments, or agencies and serving as a liaison among the members of the health-care team.

When implementing interventions, nurses should follow these guidelines:

- Base nursing interventions on scientific knowledge, nursing research, and professional standards of care (evidence-based practice) when these exist. The nurse must be aware of the scientific rationale, as well as possible side effects or complications, of all interventions. For example, a client prefers to take an oral medication after meals; however, this medication is not absorbed well in the presence of food. Therefore, the nurse will need to explain why this preference cannot be honoured.
- Clearly understand the interventions to be implemented and question any that are not understood. The nurse is responsible for intelligent implementation of medical and nursing plans of care. This requires knowledge of each intervention, its purpose in the client's plan of care, any contraindications (e.g., allergies), and changes in the client's condition that may affect the order.
- Adapt activities to the individual client. A client's beliefs, values, age, health status, and environment are factors that can affect the success of a nursing action. For example, the nurse determines that a client chokes when swallowing pills and so consults with the physician to change the order to a liquid form of the medication. Or the nurse recognizes that many Asian persons prefer to drink hot water rather than ice water and, after confirming it with a specific client, supplies this at the bedside.
- Implement safe care. For example, when changing a sterile dressing, the nurse practises sterile technique to prevent infection; when giving a medication, the nurse administers the correct dosage by the ordered route.
- Provide teaching, support, and comfort. See Chapter 25. The nurse should always explain the purpose of interventions, what the client will experience, and how the client can participate. The client must have sufficient knowledge to agree to the plan of care and to be able to assume responsibility for as much self-care as possible. These independent nursing activities enhance the effectiveness of nursing care plans (see Figure 22.11).
- Assume a holistic stance. The nurse must always view the client as a whole and consider the client's responses in that context. For example, whenever possible, the nurse honours the client's expressed preference that interventions be planned for times that fit with the client's usual schedule of visitors, work, sleep, or eating.

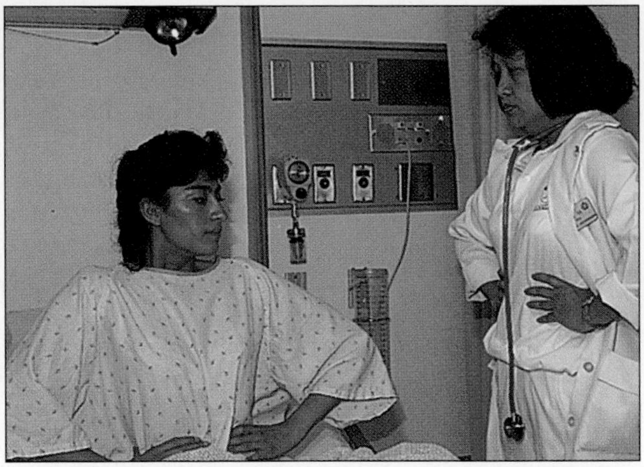

FIGURE 22.11 Amanda agrees to practise deep-breathing exercises q3h during the day. In addition, she verbalizes awareness of the need to increase her fluid intake.

- Respect the dignity of the client and enhance the client's self-esteem. Providing privacy and encouraging clients to make their own decisions are ways of respecting dignity and enhancing self-esteem.
- Encourage clients to participate actively in implementing the nursing interventions. Active participation enhances the client's sense of independence and control. However, clients vary in the degree of participation they desire. Some want total involvement in their care, whereas others prefer little involvement. The amount of desired involvement may be related to the severity of the illness; the client's culture; or the client's fear, understanding of the illness, and understanding of the intervention.

DELEGATING AND SUPERVISING Delegating is another activity that occurs during the planning phase of the nursing process. While choosing and writing nursing interventions on the client's care plan, the nurse must also determine who should actually perform the activity. The ability to delegate client care and assign tasks is a vital skill for registered nurses (RNs) because many health-care agencies have assistive personnel to perform tasks previously done only by RNs. To delegate appropriately, the RN must match the needs of the client and family with the skills, knowledge, and scope of practice of the available caregivers. This requires knowing the background, experience, knowledge, skills, and strengths of each person and understanding which tasks are and are not within their legal scope of practice.

Canadian RNs provide leadership while caring for clients requiring complex care, they collaborate with other professionals to set standards of client care, and they determine the staffing mix that will ensure quality client care (CNA, 2003). Research confirms that a higher RN skill mix decreases mortality rates, lowers rates of hospital readmission 30 days following discharge, and results in lower incidents of pressure ulcers (CNA).

RNs work collaboratively with diverse regulated nursing care providers to achieve the priority goal of attaining optimal client health outcomes (CNA, 2008) and additional goals of preventing errors and ensuring a quality workplace environment. Regulated nursing care providers each have specific educational preparation, scope of practice, and competencies, and are accountable to their own regulatory bodies. RNs, licensed or registered practical nurses, registered psychiatric nurses, and nurses with advanced preparation are all regulated nursing care providers (CNA, 2003).

Unregulated health-care providers are increasingly evident in Canadian health-care settings. RNs are involved in making key decisions that determine the initial and ongoing use of unregulated health-care providers. Unregulated health-care provider standards are varied as they are identified by individual health-care agencies across the provinces and territories (CNA, 2003).

COMMUNICATING THE NURSING ACTIONS After carrying out the nursing interventions, the nurse completes the implementing phase by recording the interventions and client responses in the client record. For information on documenting and reporting, see Chapter 23.

Evaluating

To evaluate is to judge or to appraise. Evaluating is the fifth and last phase of the nursing process. In this context, **evaluation** is a planned, ongoing, purposeful activity in which clients and health-care professionals determine (1) the client's progress toward goal achievement and (2) the effectiveness of the nursing care plan. Evaluation is an important aspect of the nursing process because conclusions drawn from the evaluation determine whether the nursing interventions should be terminated, continued, or changed.

Evaluation may be ongoing, intermittent, or terminal. Evaluation completed immediately after implementing a nursing action enables the nurse to make on-the-spot modifications in an intervention. Evaluation performed at specified intervals (e.g., once a week for the home care client) shows the extent of progress toward goal achievement and enables the nurse to correct any deficiencies and modify the care plan as needed. Evaluation performed at discharge allows the nurse to measure the degree of goal achievement and the client's self-care abilities with regard to follow-up care. Most agencies have a special discharge record for the terminal evaluation.

Through evaluating, nurses accept responsibility for their actions, indicate interest in the results of the nursing actions, and demonstrate a desire not to perpetuate ineffective actions but to adopt more effective ones.

Relationship of Evaluating to Other Nursing Process Phases

Evaluation depends on the effectiveness of the steps that precede it. Assessment data must be accurate and complete so that the nurse can formulate appropriate nursing diagnoses and desired health outcomes. The desired health outcomes must be stated concretely in behavioural terms if they are to be useful for evaluating client responses. Without the implementing phase in which the plan is put into action, there would be nothing to evaluate.

The evaluating and assessing phases overlap. As previously stated, assessment (data collection) is ongoing and continuous at every client contact. However, data are collected for different purposes at different points in the nursing process. During the assessing phase, the nurse collects data for the purpose of making diagnoses. During the evaluating step, the nurse collects data for the purpose of comparing them with preselected goals and judging the effectiveness of the nursing care. The *act* of assessing (data collection) is the same; the differences lie in (1) when the data are collected and (2) how the data are used.

Process of Evaluating Client Responses

The evaluation process has six components (see Figure 22.12). The first component, identify the desired health outcomes (NOC indicators) the nurse will use to measure client goal achievements, is done in the planning stage. The other five are as follows:

1. Collect data related to the desired client health outcomes (NOC indicators).
2. Compare the data with the desired health outcomes (NOC indicators) and judge whether the desired client health outcomes have been achieved.
3. Relate nursing actions to client goals and desired health outcomes.

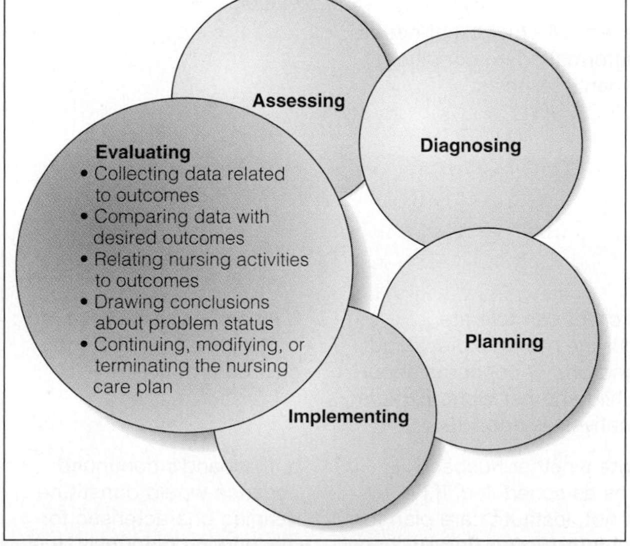

FIGURE 22.12 Evaluating: The final phase of the nursing process, in which the nurse and the client determine the client's progress toward goal achievement and the effectiveness of the plan of care. The plan may be continued, modified, or terminated.

4. Draw conclusions about problem status.
5. Continue, modify, or terminate the client's care plan.

IDENTIFYING DESIRED HEALTH OUTCOMES The desired health outcomes formulated in the diagnosing and planning steps are the criteria used to evaluate the client's response to nursing care. Desired health outcomes serve two purposes: (1) they establish the kind of evaluative data that need to be collected, and (2) they provide a standard against which the data are judged. For example, given the following expected outcomes, any nurse caring for the client would know what data to collect:

- Daily fluid intake will not be less than 2500 mL.
- Urinary output will balance with fluid intake.
- Residual urine will be less than 100 mL.

COLLECTING DATA By using the clearly stated, precise, and measurable desired health outcomes as a guide, the nurse collects data so that conclusions can be drawn about whether goals have been met. It is usually necessary to collect both objective and subjective data.

Some data may require interpretation. Examples of objective data requiring interpretation are the degree of tissue turgor of a dehydrated client or the degree of restlessness of a client with pain. When objective data need interpretation, the nurse may obtain the views of other nurses to substantiate whether change has occurred. Examples of subjective data needing interpretation include complaints of nausea or pain by the client. When interpreting subjective data, the nurse must rely on either (1) the client's statements (e.g., "My pain is worse now than it was after breakfast") or (2) objective indicators of the subjective data even though these indicators may require further interpretation (e.g., decreased restlessness, decreased pulse and respiratory rates, and relaxed facial muscles as indicators of pain relief). Data must be recorded concisely and accurately to facilitate the next part of the evaluating process.

COMPARING DATA WITH OUTCOMES If the first two parts of the evaluation process have been carried out effectively, it is relatively simple to determine whether a desired health outcome has been met. Both the nurse and the client play an active role in comparing the client's actual responses with the desired health outcomes. Did the client drink 3000 mL of fluid in 24 hours? Did the client walk unassisted the specified distance per day? When determining whether a goal has been achieved, the nurse can draw one of three possible conclusions:

1. The goal was met; that is, the client response is the same as the desired health outcome.
2. The goal was partially met; that is, either a short-term goal was achieved but the long-term goal was not, or the desired health outcome was only partially attained.
3. The goal was not met.

After determining whether a goal has been met, the nurse writes an evaluative statement (either on the care plan or in the nurse's notes). An **evaluative statement** consists of two parts: a conclusion and supporting data. The conclusion is a statement that the goal or desired health outcome was met, partially met, or not met. The supporting data are the list of client responses that support the conclusion, for example: Goal met: Oral intake 300 mL more than output; skin turgor good; mucous membranes moist.

See Table 22.15 for evaluative statements for Amanda Aquilini. Data in this table represent Ms. Aquilini's responses to care as observed by the night nurse on the morning after her admission to the unit. In practice, care plans usually do not have a column for evaluative statements; rather, evaluative statements are recorded in the nurses' notes.

RELATING NURSING ACTIONS TO CLIENT GOALS OR OUTCOMES The fourth aspect of the evaluating process is determining whether the nursing actions had any rela-

TABLE 22.15 Modified Care Plan for Amanda Aquilini (One problem only)*

Nursing Diagnosis: *Anxiety* related to difficulty breathing and concern about work and parenting roles.

Desired Outcomes	Evaluative Statements	Nursing Interventions	Rationale
Demonstrates decreased anxiety, as evidenced by		a. When client is dyspneic, stay with her; reassure her you will stay.	a. Reassures client the nurse can help her.
1. Listening to and following instructions for correct breathing and coughing technique, even during periods of dyspnea	1. Goal met. Performed coughing techniques as instructed during periods of dyspnea.	b. Remain calm, appear confident.	b. Presence of a competent caregiver reduces fear of being unable to breathe. Control of anxiety will help client to maintain effective breathing pattern.
		c. Encourage slow, deep breathing.	c. Focusing on breathing may help client feel in control and decrease anxiety.
2. Verbalizing understanding of condition, diagnostic tests, and treatments (by end of day 1)	2. Goal met. See nurse's notes for 3–11 shift. Stated, "I know I need to try to breathe deeply even when it hurts." Demonstrated correct use of incentive spirometer and stated understanding of the need to use it. Understands IV is for hydration and antibiotics. *(Evaluated 07-12-25, JW)*	d. When client is dyspneic, give brief explanations of treatments and procedures.	d. Anxiety and pain interfere with learning. Knowing what to expect reduces anxiety.
		~~e. When acute episode is over, give detailed information about nature of condition, treatments, and tests.~~ Reassess whether client needs any information on condition, treatments, or tests. *(07-12-25, JW).*	e. *Detailed information has been given. Because client shows understanding, there is no need to repeat information.*
3. Decrease in reports of fear and anxiety; none within 12 h	3. Goal met. States, "I know I can get enough air, but it still hurts to breathe."		
4. Voice steady, not shaky	4. Goal met. Speaks in steady voice.		
5. Respiratory rate of 12–22/min	5. Goal not met. Rate 26–36/min.		
6. Freely expressing concerns about work and parenting roles, but placing them in perspective in view of her illness	6. Goal partially met. Discussed only briefly on shift. Not done on night shift because of client's need to rest. *(Evaluated 07-12-25, JW)*	f. As client can tolerate, encourage her to express and expand on her concerns about her child and her work. Explore alternatives as needed.	f. Awareness of source of anxiety enables client to gain control over it.
		g. Note whether husband returns as scheduled. If he does not, institute care plan for actual ***Interrupted Family Process.*** *(Do on 12/25, day shift) (07-12-25, JW)*	g. Husband's continued absence would constitute defining characteristic for this nursing diagnosis. *It is important that this assessment be made right away, so childcare can be arranged if needed*

tion to the outcomes. It should never be assumed that a nursing action was the cause of or the only factor in meeting, partially meeting, or not meeting a goal.

For example, Mrs. Sophi Ringdale was obese and needed to lose 14 kg. When the nurse and client drew up a care plan, one goal was "Lose 1.4 kg in 4 weeks." A nursing strategy in the care plan was "Explain how to plan and prepare a 1000-calorie diet." Four weeks later, the client weighed herself and had lost 1.8 kg. The goal had been met—in fact, exceeded. It is easy to assume that the nursing strategy was highly effective. However, it is important to collect more data before drawing that conclusion. On questioning the client, the nurse might find any of the following: (1) the client planned a 1000-calorie diet and prepared and ate the food; (2) the client planned a 1000-calorie diet but did not prepare the correct food; (3) the client did not understand how to plan a 1000-calorie diet, so she did not bother with it.

If the first possibility is found to be true, the nurse can safely judge that the nursing strategy "Explain how to plan and prepare a 1000-calorie diet" was effective in helping the client lose weight. However, if the nurse learns that either the second or third possibility actually happened, then it must be assumed that the nursing strategy did not affect the outcome. The next step for the nurse is to collect data about what the client actually did to lose weight. It is important to establish the relationship (or lack thereof) of the nursing actions to the client responses.

DRAWING CONCLUSIONS ABOUT THE PROBLEM'S STATUS The nurse uses the judgments about goal achievement to determine whether the care plan was effective in resolving, reducing, or preventing client problems. When goals have been met, the nurse can draw one of the following conclusions about the status of the client's problem:

- The risk problem stated in the nursing diagnosis has been resolved; or the risk nursing diagnosis is being prevented and the risk factors no longer exist. In these instances, the nurse documents that the goals have been met and discontinues the care for the problem.
- The potential problem stated in the nursing diagnosis is being prevented, but the risk factors are still present. In this case, the nurse keeps the problem on the care plan.
- The actual problem still exists even though some goals are being met. For example, a desired health outcome on a client's care plan is "Will ingest 3000 mL of fluid daily." Even though the data may show this outcome has been achieved, other data (dry oral mucous membranes) may indicate that the client still has a *Deficient Fluid Volume.* Therefore, the nursing interventions must be continued even though this one goal was met.

When goals have been partially met, or when goals have not been met, one of two conclusions can be drawn:

1. The care plan may need to be revised since the problem is only partially resolved. The revisions may need to occur during assessing, diagnosing, or planning phases, as well as implementing.
2. The care plan does not need revision because the client merely needs more time to achieve the previously established goals. To make this decision, the nurse must assess why the goals are being only partially achieved, including whether the evaluation was conducted too soon. (See Figure 22.13.)

CONTINUING, MODIFYING, OR TERMINATING THE NURSING CARE PLAN After drawing conclusions about the status of the client's problems, the nurse modifies the care plan as indicated. Depending on the agency, modifications may be made by drawing a single line through portions of the care plan, or marking portions by using a highlighting pen, or writing "Discontinued," "goal met," or "problem resolved" and the date.

Whether or not goals were met, a number of decisions must be made about continuing, modifying, or terminating nursing care for each problem. Before making individual modifications, the nurse must first determine why the plan as a whole was not completely effective. This requires a review of the entire care plan and a critique of the nursing process steps involved in its development. See Table 22.16 for a checklist to use when reviewing a care plan.

Assessing An incomplete or incorrect database influences all subsequent steps of the nursing process and care plan. If data are incomplete, the nurse needs to reassess the client and record the new data. In some instances, new data may indicate the need for new nursing diagnoses, new goals, and new nursing interventions.

Diagnosing If the database is incomplete, new diagnostic statements may be required. If the database is complete, the nurse needs to analyze whether the problems were identified correctly and whether the nursing diagnoses are relevant to that database. After making judgments about the problem's status, the nurse revises or adds new diagnoses as needed to reflect the most recent client data.

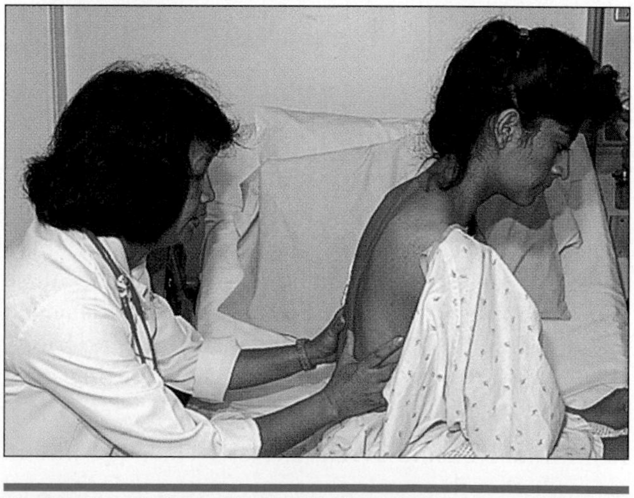

FIGURE 22.13 On assessment of respiratory excursion, Mary detects failure of the client to achieve maximum ventilation. Mary and Amanda re-evaluate the care plan and modify it to increase coughing and deep-breathing exercises to q2h.

TABLE 22.16 Evaluation Checklist

Assessing	Diagnosing	Planning	Implementing
____ Are data complete, accurate, and validated? ____ Do new data require changes in the care plan?	____ Are nursing diagnoses relevant and accurate? ____ Are nursing diagnoses supported by the data? ____ Has problem status changed (i.e., potential, actual, risk)? ____ Are the diagnoses stated clearly and in correct format? ____ Have any nursing diagnoses been resolved?	*Desired health outcomes* ____ Do new nursing diagnoses require new goals? ____ Are goals realistic? ____ Was enough time allowed for goal achievement? ____ Do the goals address all aspects of the problem? ____ Does the client still concur with the goals? ____ Have client priorities changed? *Nursing interventions* ____ Do nursing interventions need to be written for new nursing diagnoses or new goals? ____ Are the nursing interventions related to the stated goals? ____ Is there a rationale to justify each nursing intervention? ____ Are the nursing interventions clear, specific, and detailed? ____ Are new resources available? ____ Do the nursing interventions address all aspects of the client's goals? ____ Were all nursing interventions clearly effective?	____ Was client input obtained at each step of the nursing process? ____ Were goals and nursing interventions acceptable to the client? ____ Did the caregivers have the knowledge and skill to perform the interventions correctly? ____ Were explanations given to the client prior to implementing?

Planning: Desired Health Outcomes If a nursing diagnosis is inaccurate, obviously the goal statement will need revision. If the nursing diagnosis is appropriate, the nurse then checks that the goals are realistic and attainable. Unrealistic goals require correction. The nurse should also determine whether priorities have changed and whether the client still agrees with the priorities. Goals must also be written for any new nursing diagnoses.

Planning: Nursing Interventions The nurse investigates whether the nursing strategies were related to goal achievement and whether the best nursing strategies were selected. Even when diagnoses and goals are appropriate, the nursing strategies selected may not have been the best ones to achieve the goal. New nursing interventions may reflect changes in the amount of nursing care the client needs, scheduling changes, or rearrangement of nursing activities to group similar activities or to permit longer rest or activity periods for the client. If new nursing diagnoses have been written, then new nursing interventions will also be necessary.

Implementing Even if all sections of the care plan appear to be satisfactory, the manner in which the plan was implemented may have interfered with goal achievement. Before selecting new interventions, the nurse should check whether they were carried out. Other personnel may not have carried them out, either because the orders were unclear or because they were unreasonable in terms of external constraints, such as money, staff, time, and equipment.

After making the necessary modifications to the care plan, the nurse implements the modified plan and begins the nursing process cycle again. Refer to Table 22.15 on page 460 to see how the plan for Amanda Aquilini was modified after evaluation of goal achievement and review of the nursing process. A line has been drawn through portions the nurse wanted to delete; additions to the care plan are shown in italics.

EVALUATING THE QUALITY OF NURSING CARE In addition to evaluating goal achievement for individual clients, nurses are also involved in evaluating and modifying the overall quality of care given to groups of clients. This is an essential part of professional accountability.

Quality Assurance A quality assurance program is an ongoing, systematic process designed to evaluate and promote excellence in the health care provided to clients. **Quality assurance** frequently refers to evaluation of the level of care provided in a health-care agency, but it may be limited to the evaluation of the performance of one nurse or more broadly involve the evaluation of the quality of the care in an agency, or even in a province or territory.

Quality assurance requires evaluation of three components of care: structure, process, and outcome. Each type of evaluation requires different criteria and methods, and each has a different focus.

Structure evaluation focuses on the setting in which care is given. It answers the question, What effect does the setting have on the quality of care? Structural standards describe desirable environmental and organizational characteristics that influence care, such as equipment and staffing.

Process evaluation focuses on how the care was given. It answers such questions as these: Is the care relevant to the client's needs? Is the care appropriate, complete, and timely? Process standards focus on the manner in which the nurse uses the nursing process. Some examples of process criteria are "Checks client's identification band before giving medication" and "Performs and records chest assessment, including auscultation, once per shift."

Outcome evaluation focuses on demonstrable changes in the client's health status as a result of nursing care. Outcome criteria are written in terms of client responses or health states, just as they are for evaluation within the nursing process. For example, "How many clients develop pneumonia after undergoing hip repairs?" or "How many clients who have a colostomy experience an infection that delays discharge?"

Quality Improvement A strong national effort is being made in the United States to evaluate and improve the quality of health care based on internal assessment by health-care providers and to increase awareness by the public that medical errors are not uncommon and can be lethal. The Quality of Health Care in America Committee of the Institute of Medicine issued a landmark report: *To Err Is Human: Building a Safer Health System* in 2000 (Institute of Medicine, 2000). The emphases of the report are increasing knowledge related to medical errors and establishing systems for enhancing safe care. Since the report was issued, improved attention to these issues has come from a variety of sources. However, the complexity of the health-care system (including methods of reimbursement), difficulties with leadership, and fear of threats to autonomy have limited progress (Leape & Berwick, 2005).

In Canada, the Canadian Council on Health Services Accreditation (CCHSA), Canadian Patient Safety Institute, and nurse researchers are identifying methods for improving the quality of health care, identifying and measuring nursing-sensitive desired health outcomes, and exploring staff mix and other factors that affect client safety (Affonso & Doran, 2002; Doran et al., 2002; Doran, 2003; McGillis Hall, Doran, & Pink, 2004; McGillis Hall et al., 2005). Additionally, nurse researchers are studying evidence-based nursing interventions that affect client health outcomes (Hodnett, Gates, Hofmeyr, & Sakala, 2006; Hodnett, 2006; Stevens, Croxford et al., 2006; Stevens, McKeever, Guerriere, & Miller, 2006; Stevens, McGrath et al., 2006; Watt-Watson, Chung, Chan, & McGillion, 2004; Watt-Watson, Stevens et al., 2004).

Unlike quality assurance, **quality improvement (QI)** follows client care rather than organizational structure, focuses on process rather than individuals, and uses a systematic approach with the intention of improving the quality of care rather than *ensuring* the quality of care. QI studies often focus on identifying and correcting a system's problems, such as duplication of services in a hospital. QI is also known as continuous quality improvement (CQI), total quality management (TQM), performance improvement (PI), or persistent quality improvement (PQI).

Nursing Audit An **audit** means the examination or review of records. A **retrospective audit** is the evaluation of a client's record after discharge from an agency. *Retrospective* means "relating to past events." A **concurrent audit** is the evaluation of a client's health care while the client is still receiving care from the agency. These evaluations use interviewing, direct observation of nursing care, and review of clinical records to determine whether specific evaluative criteria have been met.

Another type of evaluation of care is the *peer review*. In nurse peer review, nurses functioning in the same capacity (that is, peers) appraise the quality of care or practice performed by other equally qualified nurses. The peer review is based on established standards or criteria and come in two types: individual and nursing audits. The individual peer review focuses on the performance of an individual nurse. The nursing audit focuses on evaluating nursing care through the review of records. The success of these audits depends on accurate documentation.

Evidence-Informed Practice

How Reliable Is the Breastfeeding Self-Efficacy Scale in Nursing Assessment?

The majority of women in developed countries discontinue breastfeeding before the recommended 6 months postpartum. Many known predictors of premature breastfeeding discontinuation are *nonmodifiable* demographic variables, such as maternal age, marital status, educational level, and socioeconomic status. If health professionals are to effectively improve low breastfeeding duration rates, they need to reliably assess high-risk women and identify predisposing factors that are amenable to intervention. One possible *modifiable* variable is breastfeeding confidence. To measure breastfeeding confidence the Breastfeeding Self-Efficacy Scale (BSES) was developed and psychometrically tested on Canadian women. Replicating this original research, further methodological studies have been conducted in several countries, including Australia, China, Italy, Poland, Puerto Rico, Turkey, and the United States. In these studies, BSES scores antenatally and in the early postpartum period have predicted breastfeeding duration at 4, 6, 8, and 16 weeks postpartum. In addition, a significant relationship has been demonstrated between BSES scores and exclusive breastfeeding.

NURSING IMPLICATIONS: These studies provide evidence that the BSES is a fast, accurate, and systematic assessment tool to identify breastfeeding mothers who are high risk to discontinue breastfeeding prematurely. This scale can improve client health outcomes when used by health professionals to (1) assess breastfeeding behaviours and cognitions to individualize confidence-building strategies, and (2) evaluate the effectiveness of various interventions.

Source: Prepared by Dr. Cindy-Lee Dennis. Please refer to selected articles on the breastfeeding self-efficacy scale: Dennis, C.-L. (2006). Identifying predictors of breastfeeding self-efficacy in the immediate postpartum period. *Research in Nursing and Health, 29*(4), 256–268; Kingston, D., Dennis, C.-L., & Sword, W. (2007). Exploring breast-feeding self-efficacy. *Journal of Perinatal and Neonatal Nursing, 21*(2), 207–215; Wutke, K., & Dennis, C.-L. (2007). The reliability and validity of the Polish version of the breastfeeding self-efficacy scale-short form: Translation and psychometric assessment. *International Journal of Nursing Studies, 44*(8), 1439–1446.

Nursing Process Summarized

The nursing process is foundational to nursing practice. Its basic structure can be modified for the split-second decision making sometimes necessary in critical care environments or the complex, long-range planning and evaluation necessary for community health-promotion programs. It is characterized as being the following:

- Open and flexible to meet the unique needs of clients, families, communities, and whole populations
- Cyclic and dynamic, with a built-in plan for evaluation, reassessment, and modification
- Client centred and individualized
- Interpersonal and collaborative as a process and as a means of communication
- Planned and goal directed
- Creative
- Universally applicable

Case Study 22

Ms. Sharon Noble is a 55-year-old woman who lives with her partner, Marielle, in a condominium they own in Barrie, Ontario. They have no children but they do have a close network of friends. Sharon has a business degree and is a self-employed proprietor of Novel-Novels Book Shoppe. She is an agnostic. Her medical care in hospital is covered by the Ontario Health Insurance Plan (OHIP), Liberty Health Insurance, and London Life Insurance.

1. Presenting symptoms: Chest pain and shortness of breath × 3 hours.
2. Vital signs: T-36.4°C, P-140/min, R-28/min at rest. BP-150/97, cloxacillin allergy.
3. Assessment: Visibly short of breath (SOB) at rest, skin cold and clammy, capillary oxygen level is low in blood (saturation 90%) on room air. Chest auscultation: Air entry throughout with medium coarse wet crackles mid- to lower lobes. Apical heart rate very rapid. Baseline cardiac blood work and ECG initiated by RN, chest X-ray requisitioned by RN. O_2 via 5 L nasal prongs commenced. IV of normal saline at 20 mL/h initiated by RN.
4. States, "I have a heaviness that won't let up in the middle of my chest. I feel as if I could be sick to my stomach."
5. Chest pain started after Sharon unloaded 5 heavy boxes of books sent from a publisher. She thought once she stopped it would go away but the intensity of the pressure kept mounting and has lasted 3 hours. She rates her pain (heaviness) as 8/10 using the numeric rating scale.
6. Acute coronary syndrome care path initiated by RN.
7. Client concerns: Sharon is worried about Marielle. Marielle just had cataract surgery and Sharon has been looking after her, instilling the eye drops, shopping, and preparing foods.

Sharon is complaining of increasing chest pain and SOB. She rates her chest pain at 8 out of 10. As nurses we want to give her optimal pain control; what we need to do is make a nursing judgment based on the client presentation (her escalating chest pain and increasing SOB) and our nursing physical assessment. We use objective data to complete the whole picture. Sharon is pale, her skin is cold and clammy, and she is having a lot of chest pain. In assessing why she is experiencing shortness of breath, you can see that her blood pressure is high at 150/97 and her heart rate is rapid at 140/min. The chest assessment reveals air entry throughout the lungs with medium wet crackles mid- to lower lobes.

Sharon's lab reports have been placed on her chart and indicate that her cardiac markers are elevated and the electrocardiogram (ECG) indicates injury to her heart. The chest X-ray indicates that her lungs are wet with fluid. Nurses base their nursing judgments on all the presenting data. As a nurse you correlate how Sharon looks and the way she feels with her physical presentation and compare her lab results with the results of the chest X-ray and the ECG. You understand that Sharon's lung congestion is attributed to her chest pain, the rapid heart rate, and her high blood pressure. Looking at all the data you would assess that Sharon could be experiencing a heart attack (myocardial infarction). We know that Sharon is experiencing chest pain for a few reasons: A blood clot (thrombus) is blocking one or more of her coronary arteries causing lack of oxygen to her heart. The heart muscle is starving for oxygen causing chest pain. The oxygen supply to her heart is less than the demands needed by the body to carry out cellular functioning. This is a medical emergency.

Critical Thinking Questions

1. What questions run through your mind when analyzing Sharon's subjective data?
2. What questions run through your mind when analyzing Sharon's objective data?
3. Considering the above symptoms, explain why Sharon's current condition is a medical emergency.
4. What are your nursing priorities when assessing and caring for Sharon?

After working through these questions, go to the MyNursingLab at **http://www.mynursinglab.com** to check your answers.

KEY TERMS

nursing process
assessing
data collection
database
subjective data
symptom management
objective data
interview
directive interview
nondirective interview
closed questions
open-ended questions
neutral question
leading question
cephalocaudal
screening examination
validation
cues
inferences
client health outcomes
diagnostic label
etiology
nursing diagnosis
actual diagnosis
risk nursing diagnosis
risk factors
wellness nursing diagnosis
possible nursing diagnosis
syndrome diagnosis
qualifiers
defining characteristics
related factors
independent functions
standard
norm
discharge planning
informal care plan
formal care plan
standardized care plans
individualized care plans
protocols
policies
procedures
standing orders
rationale
critical pathway
concept maps
goals
desired health outcomes
Nursing Outcomes Classification (NOC)
Nursing Interventions Classification (NIC)
cognitive skills
interpersonal skills
technical skills
evaluation
evaluative statement
quality assurance
structure evaluation
process evaluation
outcome evaluation
quality improvement (QI)
audit
retrospective audit
concurrent audit

CHAPTER HIGHLIGHTS

- The nursing process is a systematic, client-centred method for structuring the delivery of nursing care. At every stage of the process the nurse works closely with the client to tailor care and build a relationship of mutual regard and trust.
- The goals of the nursing process are to identify a client's actual or potential health-care needs and strengths, to establish plans to meet the identified needs, and to deliver and evaluate specific nursing interventions to meet those needs.
- The nursing process is organized into five interrelated, interdependent phases: assessment, diagnosing, planning, implementing, and evaluating.
- Assessing involves collecting, organizing, validating, and documenting data.
- Assessment involves active participation by client and nurse in obtaining subjective and objective data about the client's health status and assessing the socioenvironmental determinants of health affecting individual, family, group, and community clients.
- The client is the primary source of data. Secondary sources are family, friends, significant other, health-care team members, the health record, and pertinent literature.
- Subjective data are the client's personal perceptions, often gathered during the nursing health history.
- Objective data (e.g., data observed and collected during the physical examination) are detectable by the observer.
- Some data must be validated. Subjective data can be used to validate objective data, and vice versa. Primary and secondary data can also be used to validate each other.
- Nursing models provide frameworks for collecting and organizing client data.
- Diagnosing, or making a nursing diagnosis, is the process of making a clinical judgment (nursing diagnosis or hypothesis) about a client's potential or actual health problems and strengths, and identifying desired health outcomes.
- The critical-thinking skills used in diagnosing include analysis, synthesis, inductive reasoning, and decision making.
- Three phases of the diagnostic process are data analysis; identification of client's health problems, health risks, and strengths; and formulation of diagnostic statements including desired health outcomes.
- It is important to identify client strengths as well as problems.
- Planning involves the nurse, the client, support persons, and other caregivers.
- Planning involves setting priorities, establishing client goals or desired health outcomes, selecting nursing interventions, and writing a plan of care.
- Desired health outcomes describe specific and measureable client responses and help the nurse evaluate the effectiveness of the nursing interventions.
- Nurses initiate and tailor nursing care plans that operationalize critical pathways and concept maps.
- Standardized care plans should be tailored to meet individual, family, group, and community needs.
- Implementation is carrying out or delegating the nursing interventions in collaboration with clients. It incorporates all the activities performed to promote health, prevent complications, treat symptom problems, and facilitate the client's coping with chronic alterations in health status.
- Evaluating is the process of comparing client responses to preselected outcomes to determine whether goals have been met. It includes renegotiating and modifying of unmet goals and re-identifying client health outcomes of the plan of care.
- Nursing interventions and actions promote desired health outcomes.

ASSESS YOUR LEARNING

1. Mrs. Chekov, 25 years old, has undergone a caesarean section. She and her baby have just entered the recovery room. What is the nurse's initial action?
   a. Perform a newborn assessment.
   b. Inspect Mrs. Chekov's dressing and lochia.
   c. Assess Mrs. Chekov's level of pain.
   d. Ask Mrs. Chekov if she would like to feed her baby.

2. An 82-year-old man has been told by his health-care provider that it is no longer safe for him to drive a car. Which statement by the client would indicate the start of positive adaptation to this loss?
   a. "I told the doctor I would stop driving, but I am not going to yet."
   b. "I always knew this day would come, but I hoped it wouldn't be now."
   c. "What does he know? I'm a better driver than he will ever be."
   d. "Well, at least I have friends and family who can take me places."

3. A nursing care plan includes the desired health outcome of "quality of life" for a client with a chronic degenerative illness who is likely to live for many more years. Which of the following is one example that would indicate the outcome has been met?

a. The client demonstrates financial resources to pay for health care for many years.
b. The client spends the majority of his or her time in spiritual reflection.
c. The client has no signs or symptoms of preventative complications of the illness.
d. The client verbalizes satisfaction with current relationships with other persons.

4. Which of the following behaviours is most representative of the *nursing diagnosis* phase of the nursing process?
a. Identifying major problems or needs
b. Organizing data in the client's family history
c. Establishing short-term and long-term goals
d. Administering an antibiotic

5. Which of the following behaviours would indicate that the nurse was using the assessment phase of the nursing process to provide nursing care?
a. Proposing hypotheses
b. Generating desired health outcomes
c. Reviewing results of laboratory tests
d. Documenting care

6. The use of a conceptual or theoretical framework for collecting and organizing assessment data ensures which of the following?
a. Correlation of the data with other members of the health-care team
b. Demonstration of cost-effective care
c. Use of creativity and intuition in creating a plan of care
d. Collection of all necessary information for a thorough appraisal

7. The client with a fractured pelvis requests that family members be allowed to stay overnight in the hospital room. Before determining whether or not this request can be honoured, the nurse should consult which of the following?
a. Hospital policies
b. Standardized care plans
c. Orthopedic protocols
d. Standards of care

8. The nurse selects the nursing diagnosis of *Risk for Impaired Skin Integrity* related to immobility, dry skin, and surgical incision. Which of the following represents a properly stated outcome or goal?
a. The client will turn in bed q2h.
b. The client will report the importance of applying lotion to skin daily.
c. The client will have intact skin during hospitalization.
d. The client will use a pressure-reducing mattress.

9. When initiating the implementation phase of the nursing process, the nurse performs which of the following steps first?
a. Carrying out nursing interventions
b. Determining the need for assistance
c. Reassessing the client
d. Documenting interventions

10. If the nurse planned to evaluate the length of time clients must wait for a nurse to respond to the client need reported over the intercom system on each shift, which of the following processes does this reflect?
a. Structure evaluation
b. Process evaluation
c. Outcome evaluation
d. Audit

After working through these questions, go to the MyNursingLab at ***http://www.mynursinglab.com*** *to check your answers and see explanations.*

SUGGESTED READINGS

Dochterman, J., Titler, M., Wang, J., Reed, D., Pettit, D., Mathew-Wilson, M., et al. (2005). Describing use of nursing interventions for three groups of patients. *Journal of Nursing Scholarship, 37,* 57–66.

This article describes the nursing interventions implemented most frequently during an acute hospital stay for clients with heart failure, hip fractures, or fall risk by use of the Nursing Interventions Classification (NIC).

Kelly, J. H., Weber, J., & Sprengel, A. (2005). Taxonomy of nursing practice: Adding an administrative domain. *International Journal of Nursing Terminologies and Classifications, 16*(3/4), 74–80.

In this article, the authors propose the addition of a fifth domain, administrative, to the taxonomy of nursing practice and introduce the related concept of an organizational nursing diagnosis. The current taxonomy does not include diagnoses that relate to the management or leadership roles of nurses.

Orchard, C., Reid-Haughian, C., & Vanderlee, R. (2006). Health outcomes for better information and care (HOBIC): Integrating patient outcome information into nursing undergraduate curricula. *Canadian Journal of Nursing Leadership 19*(3), 28–33.

In this article, nurse-sensitive outcomes are grouped as activities of daily living, bladder continence, pain symptom, fatigue, dyspnea, nausea, falls, pressure ulcers, and therapeutic self-care. The article identifies the importance of orienting nursing students to focus on client health outcomes in their care of clients.

Wilkinson, J. (2006). *Nursing process and critical thinking* (4th ed.). London, UK: Pearson Education.

This text provides practical examples and critical-thinking exercises to help students apply the five steps of the nursing process to clinical situations.

Wright, L. M., & Leahey, M. (2005). *Nurses and families: A guide to family assessment and intervention* (4th ed.). Philadelphia, PA: Davis.

These well-known Canadian authors use a modified version of the nursing process with emphasis on the assessment and intervention stages in working with families experiencing health problems. This text includes the Calgary family assessment model and the Calgary family intervention model, as well as useful chapters on preparing for, conducting, and recording family interviews. Of practical interest to even the beginning nurse is a chapter on a 15-minute family interview. Case examples reflect the diversities in culture, race, sexual orientation, and family form that practitioners encounter in practice. The effect of terrorism on families is a new feature.

WEBLINKS

Canadian Nurses Association

http://www.cna-nurses.ca/CNA/documents/pdf/publications/PS52_Role_Nurse_Telepractice_Nov_2001_e.pdf

This document presents the Canadian Nurses Association's position statement on the role of the nurse in telepractice.

Canadian Nurses Association and Canadian Federation of Nurses Unions

http://www.cna-nurses.ca/CNA/documents/pdf/publications/PS88-Practice-Environments-e.pdf

This document presents the Canadian Nurses Association's and the Canadian Federation of Nurses Unions' joint position statement on practice environments and their role in maximizing client, nurse, and systems outcomes.

College of Nurses of Ontario

http://www.cno.org/docs/reg/41037_EntryToPracitic_final.pdf

The College of Nurses of Ontario offers this comprehensive guide to its entry-to-practice competencies.

College of Registered Nurses of British Columbia

http://www.crnbc.ca/downloads/375.pdf

The College of Registered Nurses of British Columbia also has online its competencies in the context of entry-level registered nurse practice in British Columbia.

The NIC/NOC Letter

http://www.nursing.uiowa.edu/excellence/nursing_knowledge/clinical_effectiveness/nicnocnews.htm

The NIC/NOC Letter is published by the University of Iowa College for Nursing Center for Classification and Clinical Effectiveness. It is published twice a year, and current and back issues are available at this website.

NANDA International

http://www.nanda.org

Formerly the North American Nursing Diagnosis Association International and now known as NANDA International, this is the premier international nursing diagnosis association. Its website states that it "is committed to increasing the visibility of nursing's contribution to patient care by continuing to develop, refine and classify phenomena of concern to nurses."

REFERENCES

Affonso, D., & Doran, D. M. (2002). Cultivating discoveries in patient safety research: A framework. *Journal International Nursing Perspectives, 2*(1), 33–47.

American Nurses Association. (2004). *Nursing scope and standards of practice.* Kansas City, MO: Author.

Canadian Hypertension Education Program. (2008). Criteria for diagnosis and recommendations for follow-up. Retrieved November 18, 2008, from http://hypertension.ca/chep/recommendations/diagnosis-assessment/follow-up-criteria-for-diagnosis-recommendations/

Canadian Nurses Association. (1986). *Definition of nursing practice, standards of nursing practice.* Ottawa: Author.

Canadian Nurses Association. (2003). *Position statement: Staffing decisions for the delivery of safe nursing care.* Retrieved June 18, 2007, from http://www.cna-aiic.ca http://cna-aiic.ca/CNA/documents/pdf/publications/PS67_Staffing_Decisions_Delivery_Safe_Nursing_Care_June_2003_e.pdf

Carpenito-Moyet, L. J. (2008). *Nursing diagnosis: Application to clinical practice* (12th ed.). Philadelphia, PA: Lippincott, Williams & Wilkins.

College of Nurses of Ontario. (2007). *Standards of nursing practice.* Toronto, ON: Author.

Doran, D. M. (Ed.). (2003). *Nursing sensitive outcomes: State of the science.* Sudbury, MA: Jones & Bartlett.

Doran, D. M., McGillis Hall, L., Sidani, S., O'Brien-Pallas, L., Donner, G., Baker, G. R., et al. (2002). Nursing staff mix and patient outcome achievement: The mediating role of nurse communication. *Journal International Nursing Perspectives, 1*(2–3), 74–83.

Gordon, M. (2006). *Manual of nursing diagnosis* (11th ed.). Boston, MA: Jones & Bartlett.

Hall, L. (1955, June). Quality of nursing care. *Public Health News.* Newark, NJ: State Department of Health.

Hannah, K. J., Reimer, M., Mills, W. C., & Letourneau, S. (1987). *Clinical judgement and decision making: The future with nursing diagnosis.* Toronto: John Wiley & Sons.

Hodnett, E., Gates, S., Hofmeyr, G. J., & Sakala, C. (2006). Continuous support for women during childbirth. *Cochrane Database of Systematic Reviews 2007,* Issue 3. Art. No.: CD003766. DOI: 10.1002/14651858.CD003766.pub2

Hodnett, E. (2006). Support during pregnancy for women at risk of low birthweight babies. *Cochrane Database of Systematic Reviews 2003,* Issue 3. Art. No.: CD000198. DOI: 10.1002/14651858.CD000198.

Institute of Medicine. (2000). *To err is human: Building a safer health system in 2000.* Retrieved April 30, 2008, from http://www.nap.edu/openbook.php?isbn=0309068371

Johnson, D. E. (1959). A philosophy of nursing. *Nursing Outlook, 7,* 198–200.

Leape, L., & Berwick, D. M. (2005). 5 years after to err is human: What have we learned? *Journal of the American Medical Association, 293*(19), 2384–2390.

Macdonald, G. (2002). Transformative unlearning: Safety, discernment and communities of learning. *Nursing Inquiry, 9*(3), 170–178.

McGillis Hall, L., Doran, D., & Pink, G. (2004). Nurse staffing models, nursing hours and patient safety outcomes. *Journal of Nursing Administration.*

McGillis Hall, L., McGilton, K., Krejci, J., Pringle, D., Johnston, E., Fairley, L., & Brown, M. (2005). Determinants of supportive supervisory behaviour in long-term care facilities. *Journal of Nursing Administration, 35*(4), 180–186.

Moorhead, S., Johnson, M., & Maas, M. (Eds.). (2004). *Nursing outcomes classification (NOC)* (3rd ed.). St. Louis, MO: Mosby.

NANDA International. (2007). *NANDA-I nursing diagnoses: Definitions and classification. 2007–2008.* Philadelphia, PA: Author.

Orchard, C., Reid-Haughian, C., & Vanderlee, R. (2006). Health outcomes for better information and care (HOBIC): Integrating patient outcome information into nursing undergraduate curricula. *Canadian Journal of Nursing Leadership, 19*(3), 28–33.

Orlando, I. (1961). The dynamic nurse–patient relationship. New York, NY: Putnam.

Roy, C., & Andrews, H. A. (1999). *The Roy adaptation model* (2nd ed.). Stamford, CT: Appleton & Lange.

Stevens B., Croxford, R., McKeever, P., Yamada, J, Booth, M., Daub, S., et al. (2006). Hospital and home chemotherapy for children with leukemia: A randomized cross-over study. *Pediatric Blood and Cancer, 47,* 285–292.

Stevens, B., McGrath, P., Yamada, J., Gibbins, S., Beyene, J., Breau, L., et al. (2006). Identification of pain indicators for infants at risk for neurological impairment: A Delphi consensus. *BMC Pediatrics, 6,* 1.

Stevens, B., McKeever, P., Guerriere, D., & Miller, K. (2006). The economics and efficacy of home versus hospital breastfeeding support for newborns: A randomized controlled trial. *Journal of Advanced Nursing, 53,* 233–243.

Watt-Watson, J., Chung, F., Chan, V., & McGillion, M. (2004). Pain management following discharge after ambulatory day surgery. *Journal of Nursing Management, 12,* 153–161.

Watt-Watson, J., Stevens, B., Katz, J., Costello, J., Reid, D., & David, T. (2004). Impact of a pain education intervention on postoperative pain management. *Pain, 9,* 73–85.

Wiedenbach, E. (1963). The helping art of nursing. *American Journal of Nursing, 63*(11), 54–57.

Wilkinson, J. M. (2007). *Nursing process and critical thinking.* Upper Saddle River, NJ: Prentice Hall.

Chapter 23

Documenting and Reporting

Effective communication among health-care professionals is vital to the quality of client care. Generally, health-care personnel communicate through discussion, reports, and records. A **discussion** is an informal oral consideration of a subject by two or more health-care personnel to identify a problem or establish strategies to resolve a problem. A **report** is oral, written, or computer-based communication intended to convey information to others. For instance, nurses always report on clients' progress at the end of a hospital work shift. A **record** is written or computer based. The process of making an entry on a client record is called **recording**, **charting**, or **documenting.**

A clinical record, also called a **chart** or **client record**, is a formal, legal document that provides evidence of a client's care. Although health-care organizations use different systems and forms for documentation, all client records have similar information.

OBJECTIVES

After studying this chapter, you should be able to

1. Discuss the purpose of client records
2. List the five common forms included in the client record
3. Explain how common forms in the client record are used to document steps of the nursing process
4. Recognize the seven documentation formats or methods
5. Identify and discuss ethical guidelines and legal requirements for effective documenting and reporting client data
6. List the terminology and abbreviations commonly used for documenting and reporting
7. Describe the nurse's role in documenting, reporting, conferring, and making referrals
8. List four ways to maintain the confidentiality of client records

Ethical and Legal Considerations

The Canadian Nurses Association's (CNA) (2008) *Code of Ethics* outlines values for practice, including safe, competent, ethical, accountable, and confidential care. Documenting and reporting are critical nursing activities guided by the *Code of Ethics*. The client's record is the cornerstone of communication among several disciplines involved in the care of clients. The coordination of this information is vital so that all individuals involved understand and use the information to benefit the client. Nurses must be responsible and accountable for recording and reporting, with full knowledge of professional nursing standards of practice (Canadian Nurses Protective Society, 2007).

The client's record is a legal document. Nurses need to be aware of and follow the legal and ethical standards of documentation, and that documentation needs to be clear, concise, and accurate. Opinions must be avoided unless they are related to nursing or medical diagnoses. Statements made by clients or family members must be quoted with accuracy. Detailed descriptions of what was observed need to be recorded and changes from previous assessments highlighted.

Nurses can be called to court to testify several years after a case has started (see the Nursing and Canadian Society box). Because the nurse's memory may have faded, accurate recording will allow recollection of what occurred and give credible evidence of the care provided. A well-constructed record will allow nurses and other care providers who made the notes to impart their testimony as recorded in their charts. All aspects of the record, including flowsheets, graphic records, and progress and nurses' notes, will provide a complete picture of events for the court. It is illegal for nurses to maintain their own personal journal about clients or client care as it is a breech of confidentiality (Miller & Glusko, 2003).

Each health-care organization has policies about recording and reporting client data, and each nurse is accountable for following these standards, as set out by the regulatory body in each province or territory (Canadian Council of Health Services Accreditation, 2007). As a legal record, a chart or client record is retained by the health agency or held for 10 years by a health professional responsible for the client's care (College of Nurses of Ontario, 2005). Legally, the public can request access to their client records. In Canada, federal privacy legislation, the Personal Information Protection and Electronic Documents Act (2004), applies to provincial and territorial organizations collecting and holding personal information. In addition, provinces and territories apply an additional act to protect the public's privacy. For example, Manitobans are protected by the Freedom of Information and Protection of Privacy Act (1998), and Ontarians are protected by the Personal Health Information Protection Act (2004).

NURSING AND CANADIAN SOCIETY

Fact	Implications for Nursing Practice
A client heath record can be entered into evidence in a court of law.	Nurses have a responsibility to know the legislation, standards, and principles that govern documenting and reporting.
The Canada Health Infoway (2005) aims to put in place some elements of the basic EHR for all Canadians, and by 2010, 50% of Canadians will benefit from better health-care access, quality, and productivity.	Regardless of the documenting and recording system present in any health facility, nurses must apply the same legal principles and regulations to all client health records.
Juries in the Canadian court system are influenced by the overall quality of a client's health record.	Nurses should avoid spelling and grammar mistakes, along with unofficial and confusing abbreviations. A careless entry, poor spelling, and poor grammar tend to prejudice the entire client record, leaving everything suspect of being of poor quality and, therefore, possibly inaccurate.

CLINICAL ALERT

Take safety measures before faxing confidential information. Consent is needed from the client to fax information. Make sure that personally identifiable information (e.g., client name, social insurance number) has been removed. If needed, confirm that the material is being sent to a confidential fax number or call ahead to ensure the person is present to receive the fax. Check that the fax number is correct before pressing the send button.

Ensuring Confidentiality of Electronic Health Records

Because of the increased use of electronic client information, health-care agencies have policies and procedures to ensure the privacy and confidentiality of client information stored in computers. The Canada Health Infoway (2005) is a nonprofit organization supporting the development of technologies, with a mandate to provide electronic health records for 50% of Canadians by 2010. Health facilities in many provinces have begun the transition to electronic health records. Electronic health records are fast becoming a reality for Canadian nurses

(CNA, 2002). The same documenting and recording principles apply regardless of the system of record-keeping used. Health-care agencies are ultimately responsible for the computer information system selected and the overall security of the network.

Nurses are accountable for the integrity and security of client records during use and must adhere to set policies and procedures. The following are some suggestions for ensuring the confidentiality of computerized records:

1. Use a personal password to enter and sign out from computer files. Do not share this password with anyone, including other health-care team members.
2. After logging on, never leave a computer terminal unattended.
3. Do not leave client information displayed on the monitor screen where others can see it. Direct the monitor screen away from the sight of others.
4. Follow agency procedures for documenting sensitive material, such as a diagnosis of acquired immune deficiency syndrome (AIDS).
5. Exit the client record and log off the system when work is completed
6. Use a firewall to protect the server from unauthorized access.
7. Inform the appropriate health-facility managers when a security breach has occurred.

REFLECT ON PRIMARY HEALTH CARE

As nurses work with the interdisciplinary team, their documentation is an important vehicle to communicate and facilitate the type of care needed by their clients. Collaborative effort should be used to develop a documentation of client care with common assessment criteria (e.g., pain assessment scale in palliative clients). The use of electronic health records could also bring experts from a distance, if needed, to engage in multidisciplinary team care planning. Reflect on how both *collaboration* and *appropriate technology* can enhance the nurse's ability to assist clients to *access* the needed care for *optimal health.*

Purposes of Client Records

As legal documents of client care, client records are used by a multidisciplinary health-care team for a number of purposes.

Communication

The client record is the primary communication vehicle for members of the health-care team (see the Reflect on Primary Health Care box). Each health-care professional contributes to the care of the client in various ways and uses the client record to access and document information. Clear, concise, and accurate documentation provides continuity of care and increases the probability of quality health care.

Planning and Continuity of Client Care

Each health-care professional uses data from the client's record to plan care for that client. A physician, for example, may order a specific antibiotic after establishing that the client's temperature is steadily rising and that laboratory tests reveal the presence of a certain microorganism. Nurses apply the nursing process by using baseline and ongoing assessment data to plan care, evaluate the effectiveness, and revise nursing care.

Auditing for Quality Assurance

An audit is a review of records. Client records are regularly audited for quality assurance to evaluate the health-care facility and the care provided by all health-care professionals. Accrediting agencies, such as the Canadian Council of Health Standards Association (CCHSA), may audit client records to determine if a particular health agency is meeting its stated standards (see Chapter 22, the section "Evaluating the Quality of Nursing Care").

Education and Research

Most agencies allow nursing students and health-care providers access to client records. The nursing students or health-care providers are bound by a strict ethical code and legal responsibility to hold all information in confidence and to protect clients' privacy and anonymity by not using identifiable data.

Client records contain valuable information for research and education. They provide a comprehensive view of clients, including medical and nursing diagnoses, signs and symptoms of the condition, diagnostic findings, behaviours, effective treatment strategies, and factors that affect outcomes. These records can assist student learning and understanding of health and illness patterns in various client situations. The treatment plans for a number of clients with the same health problems can yield information helpful in treating other clients. And information from records can assist health-care planners to identify agency needs, such as overutilized and underutilized hospital services.

Documentation Systems

A number of documentation systems are in current use: the source-oriented record; the problem-oriented medical record; the problems, interventions, evaluation (PIE) model; Focus Charting; charting by exception (CBE); computerized documentation; and case management.

Source-Oriented Record

The traditional client record is a **source-oriented record**. Each person or department makes notations in a separate section or sections of the client's chart. For example, the admission department has an admission sheet; the physician has a physician's order sheet and a physician's history sheet; all disciplines record on interdisciplinary notes; and other departments or personnel have their own records. In this type of record, information about a particular problem is distributed throughout the record. For example, if a client had right hemiplegia (paralysis of the left side of the body), data about this problem might be found in the physician's history sheet, on the physician's order sheet, and in the interdisciplinary notes. See Table 23.1 for the components of a source-oriented record.

Narrative charting is a traditional part of the source-oriented record. It consists of written notes that include routine care, normal findings, and client problems. The information has no right or wrong order, although a chronological order is recommended and frequently used. Currently, narrative recording is being replaced by other systems, such as PIE and Focus Charting. Narrative charting is expedient in emergency situations (Figure 23.1). For instance, during emergency situations, a delegated note taker records events in the order they occur.

Many agencies combine narrative charting with another system. For example, an agency using a charting-by-exception system (discussed later) may use narrative charting when describing abnormal findings. When using narrative charting, it is important to organize the information in a clear, coherent manner.

Source-oriented records are convenient because care providers from each discipline can easily locate the forms

TABLE 23.1 Components of the Source-Oriented Record

Form	Information
Admission (face) sheet	Legal name, birth date, age Address Marital status; closest relatives or person to notify in case of emergency Date, time, and admitting diagnosis Food or drug allergies Name of admitting (attending) physician
Initial nursing assessment	Findings from the initial nursing history and physical health assessment
Graphic record	Body temperature, pulse rate, respiratory rate, blood pressure, oxygen saturation, daily weight, and bowel movements
Daily care record	Activity, diet, bathing, and elimination records; may also include restraints, isolation precautions, treatments
Special flowsheets	Examples: 24-hour fluid balance record
Medication record	Name, dosage, route, time, date, site of administered medications Name or initials of person administering the medication
Interdisciplinary notes	Pertinent assessment of client from various disciplines (physicians, physical/respiratory therapists, etc.) Specific nursing care including teaching and client's responses Client's complaints and how client is coping
Medical history and physical examination	Past and family medical history, present medical problems, differential or current diagnoses, findings of physical examination by the physician
Physician's order sheet	Medical orders for medications, treatments, and so on
Consultation records	Reports by medical and clinical specialists
Diagnostic reports	Examples: laboratory reports, X-ray reports, CT scan reports
Client discharge plan and referral summary	Started on admission and completed on discharge; includes nursing problems, general information, and referral data

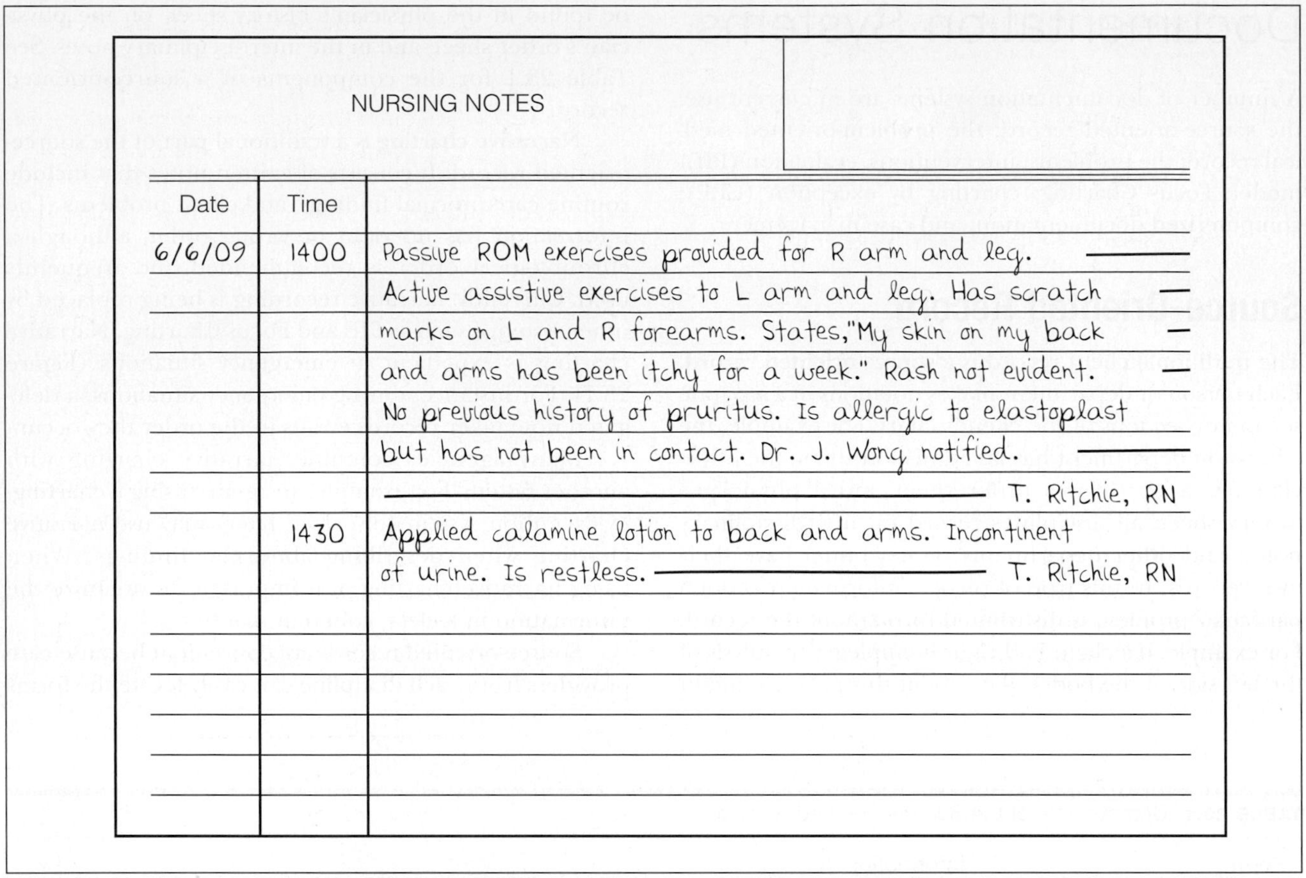
NURSING NOTES

Date	Time	
6/6/09	1400	Passive ROM exercises provided for R arm and leg. Active assistive exercises to L arm and leg. Has scratch marks on L and R forearms. States, "My skin on my back and arms has been itchy for a week." Rash not evident. No previous history of pruritus. Is allergic to elastoplast but has not been in contact. Dr. J. Wong notified. T. Ritchie, RN
	1430	Applied calamine lotion to back and arms. Incontinent of urine. Is restless. T. Ritchie, RN

FIGURE 23.1 An example of narrative notes

on which to record data, and it is easy to trace the information specific to a discipline. The disadvantage is that information about a particular client problem is scattered throughout the chart, so it is difficult to find chronological information on a client's problems and progress.

Problem-Oriented Medical Record

In the **problem-oriented medical record (POMR)**, or **problem-oriented record (POR)**, the data are arranged according to the problems the client has rather than according to the source of the information. Members of the health-care team contribute to the problem list, plan of care, and progress notes. Plans for each active or potential problem are drawn up, and progress notes are recorded for each problem.

The advantages of POR are that (1) it encourages collaboration and (2) the problem list in the front of the chart alerts caregivers to the client's needs and makes it easier to track the status of each problem. Its disadvantages are that (1) caregivers differ in their ability to use the required charting format, (2) it takes constant vigilance to maintain an up-to-date problem list, and (3) it is somewhat inefficient because assessments and interventions that apply to more than one problem must be repeated.

The POR has four basic components:

1. Database
2. Problem list
3. Plan of care
4. Progress notes

In addition, flowsheets and discharge notes are added to the record as needed.

DATABASE The database consists of all information known about the client when the client first enters the health-care agency. It includes the nursing assessment, the physician's history, social and family data, and the results of the physical examination and baseline diagnostic tests. Data are constantly updated as the client's health status changes.

PROBLEM LIST The problem list (Figure 23.2) is derived from the database. It is usually kept at the front of the chart and serves as an index to the numbered entries in the progress notes. Problems are listed in the order in which they are identified, and the list is continually updated as new problems are identified and others resolved. All caregivers can contribute to the problem list, which includes the client's physiological, psychological, social, cultural, spiritual, developmental, and environmental needs. Physicians write problems as medical diagnoses, surgical procedures, or symptoms; nurses write problems as nursing diagnoses.

As the client's condition changes or more data are obtained, it may be necessary to redefine problems. Figure 23.2 illustrates how this has been done for problems 1B, 1C, and 2.

PLAN OF CARE The initial list of orders or plan of care is made with reference to the active problems. Care plans are generated by the person who lists the problems. Physicians write physician's orders or medical care plans; nurses write nursing care plans. The written plan in the record is listed under each problem in the progress notes and is not isolated as a separate list of orders.

PROGRESS NOTES **Progress notes** in the POR are made by all health-care professionals involved in a client's care; they all use the same type of sheet for notes. Progress notes are numbered to correspond to the problems on the problem list and may be lettered for the type of data. For example, **SOAPIER** is an acronym for subjective data, objective data, assessment, planning, interventions, evaluation, and revision.

S: *Subjective data* are obtained from what the client says. They describe the client's perceptions and experience of the problem. When possible, the nurse quotes the client's words; otherwise, they are summarized. Subjective data is included only when it is important and relevant to the problem.

O: *Objective data* consist of information that is measured or observed by use of the senses (e.g., vital signs, labora-

No.	Date Entered	Date Inactive	Client Problem
#1	3/9/09		CVA resulting in Rt hemiplegia and left-sided weakness
#1A	3/9/09		Self-care deficit (hygiene, toileting, grooming, feeding)
#1B	3/9/09		Impaired physical mobility (unable to turn and position self) Redefined 2/7/10
#1C	3/9/09		Total urinary incontinence Redefined 1/17/10
#1D	3/9/09		Progressive dysphasia
#2	3/9/09		Constipation r/t immobility Redefined 6/10/10
#3	3/9/09		History of depression
#4	3/9/09		Essential hypertension
~~#5~~	~~6/6/09~~	~~7/11/09~~	~~Pruritus~~
#2	6/10/09		Risk for constipation r/t insufficient fibre intake
#1C	1/17/10		Urge urinary incontinence at night
#1B	2/7/10		Impaired physical mobility (needs 2-person assistance to transfer and walk)

FIGURE 23.2 A client's problem list in the POR system. Note that problems 1B, 1C, and 2 were redefined on the dates indicated and listed subsequently.

tory and X-ray results). Examples of subjective and objective data are provided in Chapter 22.

A: Assessment is the interpretation or conclusions drawn about the subjective and objective data. The problem list is created from the database; so, the "A" entry should be a statement of the problem. In all subsequent SOAP notes for that problem, the "A" should describe the client's condition and level of progress rather than merely restating the diagnosis or problem.

P: Planning is the plan of care designed to resolve the stated problem. The initial plan is written by the person who enters the problem into the record. All subsequent plans, including revisions, are entered into the progress notes.

Originally, the SOAP format was used, but it was later modified. The acronyms SOAPIE and SOAPIER refer to formats that add interventions, evaluation, and revision.

I: Interventions refer to the specific interventions that have actually been performed by the caregiver.

E: Evaluation includes client responses to nursing interventions and medical treatments. These are primarily reassessment data.

R: Revision reflects care plan modifications suggested by the evaluation. Changes may be made in desired outcomes, interventions, or target dates.

See Figure 23.3 for an example of progress notes that use the SOAP, SOAPIER, and PIE formats.

PIE

The **PIE** charting model is similar to SOAP charting. PIE is an acronym for problems, interventions, and evaluation of nursing care. This system consists of a client care assessment flowsheet and progress notes. The flowsheet

SOAP Format

6/6/09 #5 Generalized pruritus
1400 S— "My skin is itchy on my back and arms, and it's been like this for a week."
O— Skin appears clear—no rash or irritation noted. Marks where client has scratched noted on left and right forearms. Allergic to elastoplast but has not been in contact. No previous history of pruritus.
A— Altered comfort (pruritus): cause unknown.
P— Instructed not to scratch skin.
— Applied calamine lotion to back and arms at 1430 h.
— Cut fingernails.
— Assess further to determine whether recurrence associated with specific drugs or foods.
— Refer to physician and pharmacist for assessment.
T. Ritchie, RN

SOAPIER Format

6/6/09 #5 Generalized pruritus
1400 S— "My skin is itchy on my back and arms, and it's been like this for a week."
O— Skin appears clear—no rash or irritation noted. Marks where client has scratched noted on left and right forearms. Allergic to elastoplast but has not been in contact. No previous history of pruritus.
A— Altered comfort (pruritus): cause unknown.
P— Instruct to not scratch skin.
— Apply calamine lotion as necessary.
— Cut nails to avoid scratches.
— Assess further to determine whether recurrence associated with specific drugs or foods.
— Refer to physician and pharmacist for assessment.
I — Instructed not to scratch skin. Applied calamine lotion to back and arms at 1430 h. Assisted to cut fingernails. Notified physician and pharmacist of problem.
1600 E— States, "I'm still itchy. That lotion didn't help."
R— Remove calamine lotion and apply hydrocortisone cream as ordered.
T. Ritchie, RN

APIE Format

6/6/09 A— Generalized pruritus r/t unknown cause
1400 States, "My skin is itchy on my back and arms, and it's been like this for a week." Skin appears clear. No rash or irritations noted. Marks where client has scratched noted on left and right forearms. Allergic to elastoplast but has not been in contact. No previous history of pruritus.
P— Instruct to not scratch skin.
— Apply calamine lotion as necessary.
— Cut nails to avoid scratches.
— Assess further to determine whether recurrence associated with specific drugs or foods.
— Refer to physician and pharmacist for assessment.
I — Instructed not to scratch skin. Applied calamine lotion to back and arms at 1430 h. Assisted to cut fingernails. Notified physician and pharmacist of problem.
E— States, "I'm still itchy. That lotion didn't help."
T. Ritchie, RN

FIGURE 23.3 Examples of nursing progress notes that use the SOAP, SOAPIER, and PIE formats

covers a 24-hour period and uses specific assessment criteria in a particular format, such as human needs or functional health patterns. After the assessment, the nurse establishes and records specific problems on the progress notes. The *problem statement* is labelled "P" and referred to by number (e.g., P #5). The *interventions* employed to manage the problem are labelled "I" and numbered according to the problem (e.g., I #5). The *evaluation* of the effectiveness of the interventions is also labelled and numbered according to the problem (e.g., E #5).

The PIE system eliminates the traditional care plan and incorporates an ongoing care plan into the progress notes. Therefore, the nurse does not have to create and update a separate plan. A disadvantage is that the nurse must review all the nursing notes before giving care to determine which problems are current and which interventions were effective.

Focus Charting

Focus Charting is intended to make the client and client concerns and strengths the focus of care. Three columns for recording are usually used: date and time, focus, and progress notes (see the example at the end of this section). The *focus* can be a condition, a nursing diagnosis, a behaviour, a sign or symptom, an acute change in the client's condition, or a client's strength. The progress notes are organized into data (D), action (A), and response (R), referred to as DAR or DARP, where (P) stands for future actions or future interventions. The *data category* consists of observations of client status and behaviours, including data from flowsheets (e.g., vital signs, pupil reactivity). The nurse records both subjective and objective data in this section.

The *action category* includes immediate and future nursing actions. It can also include any changes to the plan of care. The *response category* describes the client's response to any nursing and medical care.

The Focus Charting system provides a holistic perspective of the client and the client's needs. It also provides a framework for the progress notes (DAR). The three components do not need to be recorded in order, and each note does not need to have all three categories. Flowsheets and checklists are frequently used in the client's chart to record routine nursing tasks and assessment data.

Date/Hour	Focus	Progress Notes
2/11/10	Pain	**D:** Guarding abdominal incision. Facial grimacing. Rates pain at "8" on scale of 0–10.
0900		**A:** Administered morphine sulphate 4 mg IV.
0930		**R:** Rates pain at "1." States willing to ambulate.

Charting by Exception

Charting by exception (CBE) is a documentation system in which only significant findings or exceptions to norms are recorded by using flowsheets as much as possible. CBE incorporates three key components: clinical observations, nursing interventions, and client response to nursing care (Williams, 2007). For example, CBE uses flowsheets for routine care, and under the principles a nurse would not chart that a wound has not changed (Austin, 2006). CBE has three main aspects:

1. *Unique flowsheets that highlight significant findings and define assessment parameters and findings.* The flowsheets include a sheet for nursing and physician orders to perform assessments or interventions, the graphic record (see Figure 23.4), the fluid balance record, the daily nursing assessments record (Figure 23.5), the client teaching record, the client discharge record, and the skin assessment record.
2. *Documentation by reference to the agency's printed standards of nursing practice,* which eliminates much of the repetitive charting of routine care. An agency using

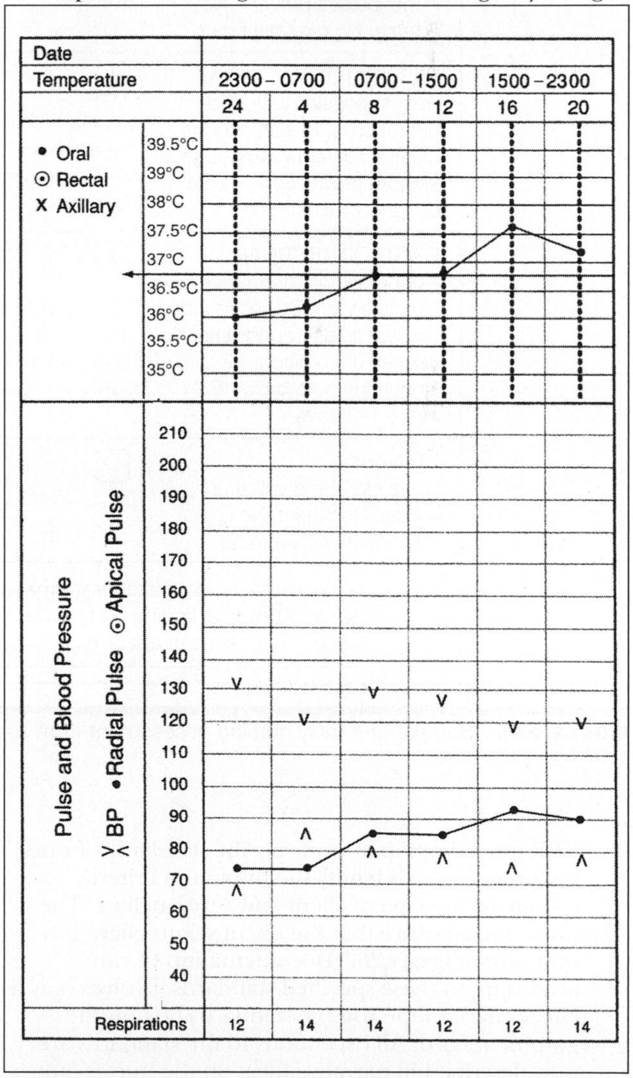

FIGURE 23.4 Sample vital signs graphics record

Medical-Surgical
NURSING ASSESSMENT RECORD

Date: 9/12/2009 0700–1900	Initials: NS	Signature: Nancy Smith RN	
Assessment Parameters	Time: 0800 Notes	Time: 1000 Notes	Time: Notes
NEUROMUSCULAR: Alert and oriented to person, place, and time. Behaviour appropriate to situation. PERL. MAE with symmetry of strength and no muscle weakness. Ambulates independently and performs self-care. Speech clear. Hears normal conversation. Swallows without difficulty. No c/o numbness or tingling, blurred vision, dizziness, or headache.	☑	☑	☐
CARDIOVASCULAR: Regular apical pulse with no extra sounds. Nail beds pink. Pedal pulses present. No edema. No c/o chest pain.	☑	☑	☐
RESPIRATORY: Respirations regular and unlaboured. Breath sounds clear in all fields. No cough or sputum production. No c/o dyspnea.	[*] Coarse crackles aT bases—clears wiTh coughing. Encouraged C + DB	[→]	☐
GASTROINTESTINAL: Abdomen soft, non-tender. No distention. Bowel sounds present in all 4 quadrants. No nausea or vomiting. Continent. Soft, brown BMs every 1–2 days.	[*] Bowel sounds absenT. N/G Tube draining mod. amT lt. brownish fluid	[→]	☐
URINARY: Urine clear and yellow to amber. Continent. No c/o discomfort with voiding.	☑	☑	☐

KEY:
✓ = Assessment matches normal assessment parameters
* = Abnormal finding
→ = No change in abnormal finding since last assessment

FIGURE 23.5 Sample of a daily nursing assessment form used in CBE

CBE must develop its own specific standards of nursing practice that identify the minimum criteria unique to the type of client and care, such as "The nurse must ensure that the unconscious client has oral care at least q2h." Documentation of care according to these specified standards involves only a check mark in the routine standards box on the graphic record. All exceptions to the standards are fully described in narrative form on the nurses' notes.

3. *Bedside accessibility of documentation forms.* In the CBE system, all flowsheets are kept at the client's bedside to allow immediate recording and to eliminate the need to transcribe data from the nurse's worksheet to the permanent record.

Computerized Documentation

Computerized clinical record systems can manage the huge volume of information required in contemporary health care. Nurses use computers to store the client's

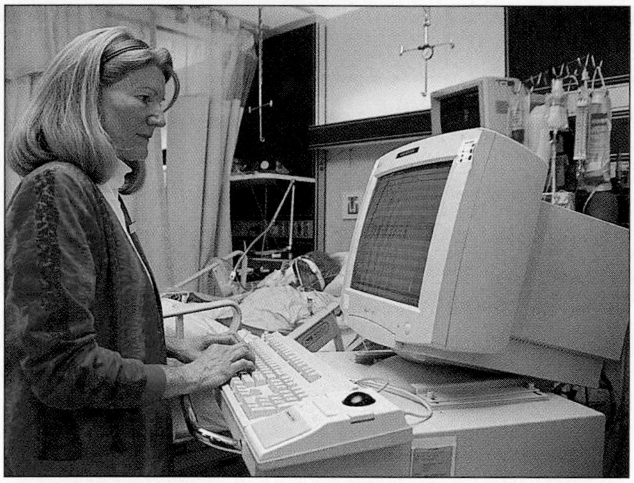

FIGURE 23.6 A bedside computer

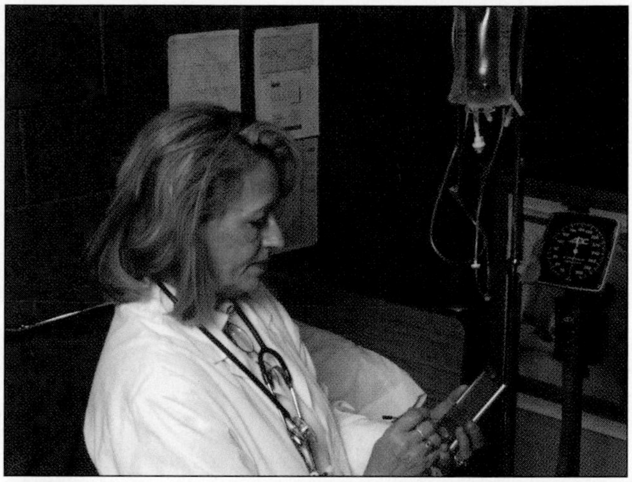

FIGURE 23.7 Electronic client record: A bedside PDA

database, add new data, create and revise care plans, and document client progress. Some institutions have a computer terminal at each client's bedside (see Figure 23.6), or nurses carry a small handheld terminal or personal digital assistant (PDA), enabling the nurse to document care immediately after it is given (see Figure 23.7).

Computerized record systems can generate a work list for the shift with a list of all the treatments, procedures, and medications needed by the client. For example, the nurse can obtain results of a client's blood test, a schedule of all clients on the unit who are to have surgery during the day, a suggested list of interventions for a nursing diagnosis, a graphic chart of a client's vital signs, or a printout of all the progress notes for a client.

Computers make care planning and documentation relatively easy. To record nursing actions and client responses, the nurse either chooses from standardized lists of terms or types narrative information into the computer. Automated speech-recognition technology now allows nurses to enter data by voice for conversion to written documentation.

The computerization of clinical records has made it possible to transmit information from one care setting to another (see Chapter 24, the section "Computers in Nursing Practice," for additional information). Selected pros and cons of computer documentation are shown in Box 23.1.

Evidence-Informed Practice

Can Electronic Patient Records Help Capture Client Information?

Many people with psychiatric illnesses are released from hospital treatment onto the streets or into homeless shelters. It is critical to maintain contact with clients in the month following discharge to continue to develop a trusting therapeutic relationship and the needed follow-up care and treatment. The use of electronic patient records (EPR) can provide a database to enable health-care workers to better track mental health clients and thereby explore ways to improve mental health services at a collective system level (Booth, 2006).

NURSING IMPLICATIONS: Nurses should be involved in the development of electronic records from the program evaluation perspective. They can help provide input on what critical health data to collect for the needed evidence or measurable outcomes for continued improvement of mental health services.

Source: Based on "Using Electronic Patient Records in Mental Health Care to Capture Housing and Homelessness Information of Psychiatric Consumers," by R. G. Booth, 2006, *Issues in Mental Health Nursing, 27*(10), pp. 1067–1077.

Case Management

The case management model emphasizes quality, cost-effective care delivered within an established length of stay. This model uses a multidisciplinary approach to planning and documenting client care by using *critical pathways.* These forms identify the outcomes that certain groups of clients are expected to achieve on each day of care, along with the interventions necessary for each day.

The case management model also incorporates graphics and flowsheets. Progress notes typically use some type of CBE. For example, if goals are met, no further charting is required. Goals that are not met are called **variances**. They are deviations from what is planned on the critical pathway—unexpected occurrences that affect the planned care or the client's responses to care. When a variance occurs, the nurse writes a note documenting the unexpected event, the cause, and the actions taken to correct the situation or justify the actions taken.

BOX 23.1 SELECTED PROS AND CONS OF COMPUTER DOCUMENTATION

The use of computer documentation has advantages and disadvantages:

PROS

- Nurses can use their time efficiently.
- The system links various sources of client information.
- Client information, requests, and results are sent and received quickly.
- Bedside terminals can synthesize information from monitoring equipment.
- Computer records can facilitate a focus on client outcomes.
- Information is legible.
- The system incorporates and reinforces standards of care.
- Standard terminology improves communication.
- Bedside terminals eliminate the need to take notes on a worksheet before recording.
- Bedside terminals permit the nurse to check an order immediately before administering a treatment or medication.
- Links to monitors improve the accuracy of documentation.

CONS

- Client's privacy may be infringed upon if security measures are not used.
- Breakdowns make information temporarily unavailable.
- The system is expensive.
- Extended training periods may be required when a new or updated system is installed.

Critical pathways work best for clients with one or two diagnoses and few individualized needs. Data from clients with multiple diagnoses (e.g., a client with a hip fracture, pneumonia, diabetes, and a pressure sore) or those with an unpredictable course of symptoms (e.g., a neurological client with seizures) are difficult to document on a critical path. See Table 23.2 for an example of how a variance might be documented.

Documenting Nursing Activities

The client record should describe the client's ongoing status and reflect the full range of the nursing process. Regardless of the records system used in an agency, nurses document evidence of the nursing process on a variety of forms throughout the clinical record (see Table 23.3).

Nursing Care Plans

Nursing care plans come in two types: traditional and standardized. The *traditional care plan* is written for each client. The form varies from agency to agency according to the needs of the client and the department. Most forms have three columns: one for nursing diagnoses, a second for expected outcomes, and a third for nursing interventions. (See Chapter 22, the section "Developing Nursing Care Plans" for additional information.)

Standardized care plans have been developed to save documentation time. These plans can be based on an

TABLE 23.2 Example of Variance Documentation (Critical Pathway)

An elderly client has had a below-the-knee amputation. On the third postoperative day, he has a temperature of 38.8°C. Lung sounds are clear, and he is not coughing. The nurse notices redness and skin breakdown over the client's sacrum. The critical pathway outcomes specified for day 3 are "Oral temperature 37.7°C" and "Skin intact over bony prominences." The nurse should chart the following variances:

Date/Time	Variation	Cause	Action Taken/Plans
10/13/09 0900	Elevated temperature	Possible sepsis	4/16-Blood cultures per order. Monitor temp. q1h. Monitor I&O, hydration, and mental status.
10/13/09 1130	Impaired skin integrity: pressure sore on sacrum	Client does not move about in bed unless reminded	4/16-Positioned on L side. Turn side-to-side q2h while awake. On every client contact, remind client to move about in bed. Apply Duoderm daily after bath.

TABLE 23.3 Documentation for the Nursing Process

Step	Documentation Forms
Assessment	Initial assessment form, various flowsheets
Nursing diagnosis	Nursing care plan, Kardex, critical path, interdisciplinary notes, problem list
Planning	Nursing care plan, critical path
Intervention	Interdisciplinary notes, flowsheets
Evaluation	Interdisciplinary notes

institution's standards of practice, thereby helping provide a high quality of nursing care. Standardized plans must be individualized by the nurse in order to adequately address individual client needs.

Kardexes

The **Kardex** is a concise method of organizing and recording data about a client, making information quickly accessible to all health-care professionals. It consists of a series of cards kept in a portable index file or on computer-generated forms. The card for a particular client can be quickly turned up to reveal specific data. The Kardex may or may not become a part of the client's permanent record. In some organizations, it is a temporary worksheet written in pencil for ease in recording frequent changes in details of a client's care. The information on Kardexes may be organized into sections, for example:

- Pertinent information about the client, such as name, room number, age, religion, marital status, admission date, physician's name, diagnosis, type of surgery and date, occupation, and next of kin
- List of medications, with the date of order and the times of administration for each
- List of intravenous fluids, with dates of infusions
- List of daily treatments and procedures, such as irrigations, dressing changes, postural drainage, or measurement of vital signs
- List of diagnostic procedures ordered, such as roentgenography (X-ray photography) or laboratory tests
- Allergies
- Specific data on how the client's physical needs are to be met, such as type of diet, assistance needed with feeding, elimination devices, activity, hygienic needs, and safety precautions (e.g., use of side rails)
- A problem list, stated goals, and a list of nursing approaches to meet the goals and relieve the problems

Flowsheets

Flowsheets enable nurses to record nursing data quickly and concisely and provide an easy-to-read record of the client's condition over time. The time parameters for flowsheets can vary from minutes to months. In a hospital intensive care unit, a client's blood pressure may be monitored by the minute, whereas in an ambulatory clinic, a client's blood glucose level may be recorded once a month.

Flowsheets commonly used are the graphic (clinical) record, the daily nursing care records, the fluid intake and output record, and the medication record.

DAILY NURSING CARE RECORD The daily nursing care is often recorded on a flowsheet or graphic record for diet intake, hygiene, activity, elimination, treatments, protective precautions, diagnostic studies, and so on.

24-HOUR FLUID BALANCE RECORD All routes of fluid intake and all routes of fluid loss or output are measured and recorded on this form. Information about ways to measure and record specific amounts of fluid intake and output are described in Chapter 43.

MEDICATION RECORD Medication flowsheets usually include designated areas for the date of the medication order, the expiration date, the medication name and dose, the frequency of administration and route, time of administration, and the nurse's signature. Some records also include a place to document the client's allergies. (A sample medication record is shown in Figure 31.6: Medication administration record on page 810.)

Progress Notes

Progress notes made by nurses provide information about the progress a client is making toward achieving desired outcomes. Therefore, in addition to assessment and reassessment data, progress notes include information about client problems and nursing interventions. The format used depends on the documentation system in place in the institution, as discussed earlier in this chapter.

Nursing Discharge and Referral Summaries

A discharge note and referral summary are completed when the client is being discharged and transferred to another institution or to a home setting in which a visit by a community health nurse is required (see Figure 23.8 and Chapter 13, the section "Discharge Planning"). Many institutions provide forms for these summaries.

Hôpital général St-Boniface General Hospital

Postpartum Vaginal Delivery Care Map

48 Hour Length of Stay

Approved initiative of the Winnipeg Regional Health Authority

Discharge Teaching Summary
(Fax to Public Health on Discharge)

DISCHARGE TEACHING

	Understanding Indicated By Verbal Response	Task Performed Safely	Repeat Re-demonstrate Remind	Needs Confidence Building
0 - 4 Hours Post Partum				
Mom Self Care: Peri-care				
Normal lochia				
Infant Care: Infant security issues				
Choking baby				
Breastfeeding Initiation				
5 - 12 Hours Post Partum				
Mom Self Care: Involution				
13 - 24 Hours Post Partum				
Mom Self Care: Diet				
Activity / rest				
Elimination				
Medications				
Breast Feeding: Breast care				
Positioning				
Latching				
Duration				
Frequency				
Burping				
Formula Feeding: Amount				
Frequency				
Burping				
Preparation				
Infant Care: Bathing				
Cord care				
Diapering				
Normal stools / voids				
Sleep position				
25 - 48 Hours Post Partum				
Mom Self Care: Sitz bath				
Emotional adjustments: PP depression / blues				
Family planning (method) ______				
Return appointment for self and baby				
Public Health Nurse visit				
Infant Care:				
• **Response to early infant cues and initiates infant care**				
• Jaundice				
• Temperature / sick baby				
• **Describes preparation for infant and safe home environment**				
• **Mom / family aware of conditions that warrant a call to a health care provider**				
• **Aware of need to use car seat**				
• **Vitamin D administration (breast fed infants only)**				
Videos watched (list)				

FORM #0102-3126-8 05/02

FIGURE 23.8 Postpartum Vaginal Delivery Care Map from St. Boniface General Hospital

Source: Courtesy of St. Boniface General Hospital. Wpg, MB. From #0102-3126-8, 05/02.

	Delivery Date/Time: ______________________	**Date:**						
		Time:						
ASSESSMENTS/CONSULTS	**NURSE/MIDWIFE:**							
	• Assess the following q8h: vital signs, breasts, fundus, lochia, perineum, bladder, bowel, lower extremities, discomfort	___	___	___				
	• Assess the following BID: vital signs, breasts, fundus, lochia, perineum, bladder, bowel, lower extremities, discomfort				___	___	___	___
	Consult:							
	• Social work as necessary	___	___	___	___	___	___	___
	☐ Other	___	___	___	___	___	___	___

VITAL SIGNS

D / M / Y							
Time							
Temp Graph 40							
39							
38							
37							
36							
Pulse							
Respirations							
Blood Pressure							
Initial							

ASSESSMENTS/CONSULTS	**NURSE/MIDWIFE:**							
	• Vital signs stable	___	___	___	___	___	___	___
	• Breasts: 3 - 24 hours: soft, nipples comfortable to slightly tender	___	___	___				
	25 - 48 hours: soft to filling, nipples comfortable to slightly tender				___	___	___	___
	• Fundus: 3 - 24 hours: firm, midline at level of umbilicus or slightly below	___	___	___				
	25 - 48 hours: firm, midline at U1 - U2 or lower				___	___	___	___
	• Lochia: 3 - 24 hours: small to moderate rubra with or without small clots	___	___	___				
	25 - 48 hours: small to moderate rubra or serosa, with or without small clots				___	___	___	___
	• Perineum: slight to moderate swelling/bruising, no discharge, if sutured edges well approximated	___	___	___	___	___	___	___
	• Bladder: voids within 6 hours of delivery, first void ≥ 250 cc	___						
	6 - 48 hours; bladder not palpable, voiding QS		___	___	___	___	___	___
	• Bowels: 3 - 24 hours: No BM expected	___	___	___				
	25 - 48 hours: No BM expected or may have 1st BM				___	___	___	___
	• Lower Extremities: nil — scant amount (<+2) pretibial or pedal edema, negative Homans' sign, no calf tenderness on ambulation	___	___	___	___	___	___	___
	• States comfortable, pain at < 2 on pain scale (scale 0 - 10)	___	___	___	___	___	___	___
TESTS	**NURSE/MIDWIFE:**							
	☐ ______________________	___	___	___	___	___	___	___
TREATMENT	**NURSE/MIDWIFE:**							
	■ Straight catheterization prn	___	___	___	___	___	___	___
	■ Foley catheter prn	___	___	___	___	___	___	___
	• Perineal care, ice packs, sitz baths prn	___	___	___	___	___	___	___
	■ Discontinue IV when patient drinking well, voiding QS and afebrile	___	___	___	___	___	___	___
NUTRI-TION	**NURSE/MIDWIFE:**							
	■ Standard diet	___	___	___	___	___	___	___
	☐ Other	___	___	___	___	___	___	___
ACTIVITY/ SAFETY	**NURSE/MIDWIFE:**							
	• Encourage walking in hallway	___	___	___	___	___	___	___
	• Shower	___	___	___	___	___	___	___
	• Tolerates mobilization	___	___	___	___	___	___	___
PSYCHO-SOCIAL	**NURSE/MIDWIFE:**							
	• Assess emotional status, energy level	___	___	___	___	___	___	___
	• Assess parental-infant interaction	___	___	___	___	___	___	___
	• Positive affect	___	___	___	___	___	___	___
	• Cares for own physical needs or requires minimal assistance	___	___	___	___	___	___	___
	• Demonstrates positive parent-infant interaction	___	___	___	___	___	___	___
	Plan Reviewed	___	___	___	___	___	___	___

* Indicates a variance, refer to Variance Record.

FIGURE 23.8 Postpartum Vaginal Delivery Care Map from St. Boniface General Hospital (*continued*)

DELIVERY	DATE	TIME
☐ DELIVERY SPONTANEOUS ☐ FORCEPS TYPE ________ ☐ VACUUM EXTRACTOR		
PERINEUM: ☐ INTACT	☐ EPISIOTOMY ☐ LACERATION	TYPE DEGREE ________

ALLERGIES		
ANAESTHESIA ☐ NONE ☐ EPIDURAL	☐ SPINAL ☐ OTHER	☐ LOCAL

Vital Signs and Assessment (q15 minutes x 4, q30 minutes x 2)

D / M / Y						
Time						
Temperature						
Pulse						
Respirations						
Blood Pressure	/	/	/	/	/	/
Fundus: Height, Position, Tone						
Lochia: Amount, Color						
Bladder						
Perineum						
Motor Function (q1h)	R | L	R | L	R | L	R | L	R | L	R | L
Comments						
Initial						

Fundus Height & Position
- U/U - Umbilicus
- Rt - Right
- Lt - Left
- M - Midline

Fundus Tone
- F - Firm
- B - Boggy
- FM - Firm with Massage

Lochia Amount
- Sc - Scant
- Sm - Small
- Mod - Moderate
- L - Large

Lochia Color
- R - Rubra
- S - Serosa

Bladder
- P - Palpable
- NP - Non Palpable

Perineum
- SW - Swollen
- BR - Bruised
- N - Normal

Motor Function
- 0 - No block or patient has full flexion of foot and knee
- 1 - Partial or just able to move knee
- 2 - Almost complete or able to move foot only
- 3 - Complete or unable to move foot or knee

Note: Use Postpartum Frequent Monitoring Record if required.

Intravenous established @ ____________ by ____________________ (use Fluid Balance Record)

Intravenous discontinued @ ____________ intact / not intact by ____________________

Epidural catheter removed @ ____________ intact / not intact by ____________________

Tests

	D / M / Y / Time	Result	Initial
1. Hemoglobin________	______	______	______
________	______	______	______
________	______	______	______

FIGURE 23.8 Postpartum Vaginal Delivery Care Map from St. Boniface General Hospital (*continued*)

Some records combine the discharge plan, including instructions for care, follow-up appointments, and the final progress note.

If the client is being transferred or going home with visits by a home health nurse, the discharge note takes the form of a referral summary. Regardless of format, discharge and referral summaries usually include some or all of the following:

- Description of the client's physical, mental, and emotional status at discharge or transfer
- Resolved health problems
- Unresolved continuing health problems and continuing care needs, which may include a review-of-systems checklist that considers integumentary, respiratory, cardiovascular, neurological,

Physician/Midwife Assessments

D / M / Y/ Time ______ Signature ______ ☐ Normal ☐ Refer to Variance Record

______ ______ ☐ Normal ☐ Refer to Variance Record

Preparation for Transfer of Care to the Community — Initial

■ Discharge when all outcomes are met

1. Collect live birth registration form .... ______
2. Verify address and phone # for immediate postpartum period .... ______
3. Verify permanent address and phone #
4. Remind re: follow-up appointment with ______
   in 6 or ______ weeks for Mom .... ______
   and with ______ in 7 or ______ days for baby .... ______
5. Discharge prescription given ☐ N/A .... ______
6. Winrho administered ☐ N/A .... ______
7. MMR administered ☐ N/A .... ______
8. Depo-Provera administered ☐ N/A .... ______
9. Give the following discharge instructions:
   ◊ • Caring for Yourself After Having Your Baby .... ______
   ◊ • Caring for Your Newborn Baby at Home.......... ______
10. Mother given phone number for Public Health Nurse or Nursing Station Breast Feeding Hotline (breast fed only).......... ______
11. Complete top section of the Variance Record .... ______
12. Complete the Post Partum Referral form and Discharge Teaching Summary and fax them to the Public Health Office.......... ______
13. Discharge home @ ______ hours of ______ D/M/Y
    ☐ With Newborn ☐ Without Newborn .... ______
    If discharged home without newborn, explain ______

FIGURE 23.8 Postpartum Vaginal Delivery Care Map from St. Boniface General Hospital (*continued*)

musculoskeletal, gastrointestinal, elimination, and reproductive problems

- Treatments that are to be continued (e.g., wound care, oxygen therapy)
- Current medications
- Restrictions that relate to (1) activity, such as lifting, stair climbing, walking, driving, work, (2) diet, and (3) bathing, such as sponge bath, tub, or shower
- Functional and self-care abilities in terms of vision, hearing, speech, mobility with or without aids, meal preparation and eating, preparation and administration of medications, and so on
- Comfort level
- Support networks, including family, significant others, religious adviser, community self-help groups, home care and other community agencies available, and so on
- Client education provided in relation to the disease process, activities and exercise, special diet, medications, specialized care or treatments, follow-up appointments, and so on
- Discharge destination (e.g., home, nursing home) and mode of discharge (e.g., walking, wheelchair, ambulance)
- Referral services (e.g., social worker, home health nurse)

Long-Term-Care Documentation

Nurses need to familiarize themselves with regulations influencing the kind and frequency of documentation required in long-term-care facilities. Usually, the nurse completes a nursing care summary at least once a week for clients requiring skilled care and every 2 to 4 weeks for those requiring intermediate care. Summaries should address the following:

- Specific problems noted in the care plan
- Mental status
- Activities of daily living (ADLs)
- Hydration and nutrition status
- Elimination status
- Safety measures needed (e.g., bed rails)
- Medications
- Treatments
- Preventive measures

Guidelines for documentation in long-term-care facilities are shown in Box 23.2.

Home Care Documentation

Home care is one of the fastest-growing areas in health care in Canada because of an increasing older population and shorter hospitalizations. In home care settings, health-care personnel often document in client-held records that remain at the residence (see Box 23.3). Health-care personnel may access critical information through the use of voicemail, wireless devices, and laptops, which enhances their ability to care for their clients and maintain accurate and current records. In addition, telehealth technologies allow the sharing of professional expertise in urban areas with health-care providers practising in homes and communities in rural and remote locations.

BOX 23.2 LONG-TERM-CARE DOCUMENTATION

Long-term-care facilities require nurses to follow specific guidelines:

- Complete the assessment and screening forms and plan of care within the time period specified by agency policy.
- Document and report any change in the client's condition to the physician and the client's family within 24 hours.
- Document all measures implemented in response to a change in the client's condition.
- Keep a record of any visits and of phone calls from family, friends, and others regarding the client.
- Write nursing summaries and progress notes that comply with the frequency and standards required by agency policy.
- Make sure that progress notes address the client's progress in relation to the goals or outcomes defined in the plan of care.
- Review and revise the plan of care according to agency policies or whenever the client's health status changes.

BOX 23.3 HOME CARE DOCUMENTATION

Home care nurses must follow these documentation guidelines:

- Complete a comprehensive nursing assessment and develop a plan of care.
- Write a progress note at each client visit, noting any changes in the client's condition, nursing interventions performed (including education and instructional brochures and materials provided to the client and home caregiver), client responses to nursing care, and vital signs as indicated.
- Keep a copy of the care plan in the client's home and update it as the client's condition changes.
- Report changes in the plan of care to the appropriate member of the health-care team and document that these were reported.
- Encourage the client or home caregiver to record data when appropriate.
- Write a discharge summary, including the client's health status at discharge, outcomes achieved, and recommendations for further care.

Guidelines for Recording

A client's record is a legal document and can be used to provide evidence in court. Health-care personnel must not only maintain the confidentiality of the client's record but also meet legal standards in the process of recording.

Date and Time

The date and time of each recording is essential not only for legal reasons but also for client safety. Record the time according to the 24-hour clock avoids confusion about whether a time was a.m. or p.m. (Figure 23.9).

Timing

Follow the agency's policy about the frequency of documenting and adjust the frequency as a client's condition indicates; for example, a client whose blood pressure is changing requires more frequent documentation than a client whose blood pressure is constant. As a rule, documenting should be done as soon as possible after an assessment or intervention. No recording should be done *before* providing nursing care. Blanket charting (i.e., charting all events occurring within an extended period of time) is not acceptable.

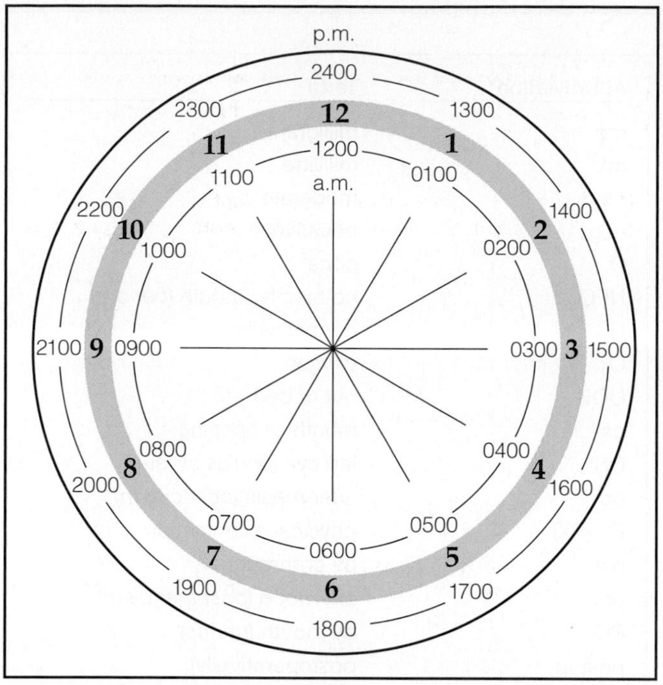

FIGURE 23.9 The 24-hour clock

Legibility

All entries must be legible and easy to read to prevent interpretation errors. Printing or easily understood handwriting is usually permissible.

Permanence

All entries on the client's record are made in dark ink, according to agency policies, so that the record is permanent and changes can be identified. Dark ink reproduces well on microfilm and in duplication processes.

Accepted Terminology and Abbreviations

Use only commonly accepted *abbreviations, symbols,* and *terms* that are specified by the agency. Many abbreviations are standard and used universally. When in doubt about whether to use an abbreviation, write the term out in full until certain about the abbreviation. Abbreviations that are not official can lead to misunderstandings. For example, *D/C* may mean "discharge" or "discontinue"; *od* could mean "once a day" or "right eye." Refer to Table 23.4 and Table 23.5 for the common abbreviations and accepted symbols. Use the metric system to document measurements (e.g., height, weight, volume).

Correct Spelling

Correct spelling is essential for accuracy in recording. Two decidedly different medications may have similar spellings, for example, digitoxin and digoxin.

Signature

Each recording on the nursing notes is signed by the nurse making it. The signature includes the *name* and *title,* for example, "Susan J. Green, RN." The following title abbreviations are often used, but nurses need to follow agency policy about how to sign their names:

RN registered nurse
RNA registered nurse assistant
LPN licensed practical nurse (outside Ontario)
RPN registered practical nurse (Ontario only)
RPN registered psychiatric nurse (Western provinces)
NA nursing assistant
NS nursing student
RA resident attendant
SN student nurse

Accuracy

Check that the correct client's name and identifying information are stamped or written on each page of the clinical record before making any entry. Special care is needed when caring for clients with the same last name. Health facilities may use a brightly coloured warning sticker on the health-care record and information shared by clients with similar names.

Notations on records must be accurate and correct. Accurate notations consist of facts or observations rather than opinions or interpretations. It is more accurate, for example, to write that the client "refused medication" (fact) than to write that the client "was uncooperative" (opinion); or to write that a client "was crying" (observation) is preferable to noting that the client "was depressed" (interpretation). Similarly, when a client expresses worry about the diagnosis or problem, this should be quoted directly on the record: "Stated: 'I'm worried about my leg.'" When describing something, avoid general words, such as *large, good,* or *normal,* which can be interpreted differently. For example, chart specific data, such as "2 cm × 3 cm bruise," rather than "large bruise."

When a *recording mistake* is made, draw one line through it (leave the mistake readable) and write the words *entry mistake* above it with your initials or name (depending on agency policy) and the date and time of correction. Do not erase, blot out, or use correction fluid. The original entry must remain visible.

TABLE 23.4 Commonly Used Abbreviations

Abbreviation	Term
abd	abdomen
ABO	the main blood group system
ac	before meals (*ante cibum*)
ADL	activities of daily living
ad lib	as desired (*ad libitum*)
adm	admitted or admission
am	morning (*ante meridiem*)
amb	ambulatory
amt	amount
approx	approximately (about)
bid	twice daily (*bis in die*)
BM (bm)	bowel movement
BP	blood pressure
BR	bed rest
BRP	bathroom privileges
c̄	with
C	Celsius (centigrade)
CBC	complete blood count
CBR	complete bed rest
CDA	Canadian Diabetic Association
Cl	client
cm	centimetre
c/o	complains of
DAT	diet as tolerated
drsg	dressing
Dx	diagnosis
ECG (EKG)	electrocardiogram
fld	fluid
g	gram
GI	gastrointestinal
GP	general practitioner
gtt	drops (*guttae*)
h	hour (*hora*)
H_2O	water
I&O	intake and output
j	joule
IV	intravenous
kg	kilogram
kJ	kilojoule
L	litre
Lab	laboratory
liq	liquid
LMP	last menstrual period
lt (L)	left
m	metre
meds	medications
mg	milligram
mL	millilitre
mod	moderate
neg	negative
Ø	none
NPO	nothing by mouth (*per ora*)
NS	normal saline
O_2	oxygen
OOB	out of bed
os	mouth or opening
OS	left eye (*oculus sinister*)
pc	after meals (*post cibum*)
PE (PX)	physical examination
per	by or through
pm	afternoon (*post meridiem*)
PO	by mouth (*per os*)
postop	postoperative(ly)
preop	preoperative(ly)
prep	preparation
prn	when necessary (*pro re nata*)
pt	patient
q	every (*quaque*)
qh (q1h)	every hour (*quaque hora*)
q2h, q3h, and so on	every 2 hours, 3 hours, and so on
qid	four times a day (*quater in die*)
req	requisition
Rt (rt, R)	right
S (s̄)	without (*sine*)
SI	Systeme Internationale d'unites (metric system)
spec	specimen
STAT	at once, immediately (*statim*)
tid	three times a day (*ter in die*)
TL	team leader
TLC	tender loving care
TO	telephone order
TPR	temperature, pulse, respirations
VO	verbal order
VS	vital signs
WNL	within normal limits
wt	weight

Note: The Institute for Safe Medication Practice Canada (ISMP) recommends the elimination of specific abbreviations, symbols, and dose designations because they are prone to errors that may cause harm. These symbols include **>, <, @, ss, D/C, hs, OD, OS, os, qd, per os, qhs, Ø, Δ,** and **no.** See Table 31.6 (page 807) for selected examples and visit the ISMP website for a complete listing: http://www.ismp.org/Tools/errorproneabbreviations.pdf

TABLE 23.5 Commonly Used Symbols

Symbol	Term	Symbol	Number
=	equal to	i	1
↑	increased	ii	2
↓	decreased	iii	3
♀	female	iv	4
♂	male	v	5
°	degree	vi	6
#	number; fracture	vii	7
×	times	viii	8
		ix	9
		x	10

Sample Recording

Date: Dec 10/09 Time: 0100

entry mistake AJR

Pulse ~~180 beats per min~~ 108 beats per min

______________ Abby J. Roberts, NS

Write on every line but never between lines. If a *blank* appears in a notation, draw a line through the blank space so that no additional information can be recorded at any other time or by any other person, and sign the notation.

Sample Recording

Date: Nov 7/10 Time: 0730

Urine cloudy, light brown with dark flecks.

No odour. ______________ Lin I. Ma, NS

States "burning pain in pubic region prior to

voiding." ______________ Lin I. Ma, NS

Sequence

Document events in the chronological order in which they occur; for example, record assessments, then the nursing interventions, and then the client's responses. Update problems as needed. Events documented out of sequence must be clearly identified as a late entry, according to agency policy. If alterations are made to the sequence of events, explain that you are making a *late note entry* and include the actual time you are making the note in the client record (Hutchinson & Sharples, 2006).

Appropriateness

Record only information that is significant to the client's health problems and care. Any other personal information that the client conveys is inappropriate for the record. Recording irrelevant information can be considered an invasion of the client's privacy or subject to legal action from the client. A client's disclosure that she was addicted to heroin 20 years ago, for example, *would not* be recorded on the client's medical record unless it had a direct bearing on the client's health.

Completeness

Record only information that is helpful to the client and health-care professionals. Nurses' notes need to reflect the nursing process. Record all assessments, nursing interventions, client problems, client comments and responses to interventions and tests, progress toward goals, and communication with other disciplines.

Care that is *omitted* because of the client's condition or refusal of treatment must also be recorded. It is vitally important to clearly document the events of what happened and why a component of care was omitted. Ensure that the details are specific and state who was notified and outcomes of these actions.

Conciseness

Recordings need to be brief, as well as complete, to save time in communication. For example, write "Perspiring profusely. Respirations shallow, wet, 28 per min." End each thought or sentence with a period.

Legal Prudence

Accurate, complete documentation should give legal protection to the nurse. Admissible in court as a legal document, the nurse's charting should present an accurate, complete representation of the quality of care given. In most instances, failure to completely document the course of a patient's treatment regime can mean that the court will assume the act was not done (Sullivan, 2004). Incompleteness seriously undermines the strength of the evidence, or how convincing it is that the act was actually done.

For the best legal protection, the nurse should not only adhere to professional standards of nursing care but also follow agency policy and procedures for intervention and documentation in all situations—especially in high-risk situations. For example:

December 9, 2010, 1100 hours—Stated "feeling dizzy." Raised side rails, instructed to stay in bed and ring call bell if requiring assistance. ______________ RS Chartrand, RN

December 9, 2010, 1130 hours—Found beside bed on floor. Said, "I climbed over these rails all by myself." When asked about pain, replied, "I feel fine but a little dizzy." Helped into bed. BP 100/60, P90, R24, Dr. RJ Naden notified. ______________ RS Chartrand, RN

Reporting

Reports can be either oral or written. The purpose of reporting is to communicate specific information to a person or group of people. A report should be concise, including only pertinent information and no extraneous detail.

Change-of-Shift Reports

A **change-of-shift report** is a report usually given to nurses starting the next shift. Its purpose is to provide continuity of care for clients by providing the new caregivers with a quick summary of client needs and details of care to be given.

Change-of-shift reports can be written or given orally, either in a face-to-face exchange or by audiotape recording. The face-to-face report permits the listener to ask questions during the report; written and tape-recorded reports are often briefer and less time consuming. Reports are sometimes given at the bedside, and clients as well as nurses can participate in the exchange of information. See the Box 23.4 for key elements of a change-of-shift report and Box 23.5 for a sample change-of-shift report.

CLINICAL ALERT

Be aware of where the shift report takes place in order to maintain client confidentiality. An area that is private and free from interruption is best.

BOX 23.5 SAMPLE CHANGE-OF-SHIFT REPORT

The following sample of a shift-change report uses the key elements listed in Box 23.4:

ROOM 201—C.W.

Admitted last night for pneumonia

Allergic to penicillin

DNR

IV of D5/0.45 NS infusing at 100 mL/h in (L) forearm

Need sputum specimen for C&S

Temp 39.1. Tylenol 325 mg, 2 tablets given at 0600

Lung sounds diminished in lower lobes

ROOM 202—G. H.

Admitted for left total knee arthroplasty on September 14, 2010. POD # 3

Has discharge orders to go to rehab today

Dressing clean, dry, and intact

Regular diet. Taking fluids well.

Had BM yesterday

Pain rating of 4/10—last medicated with oxycodone 2.5 mg with acetaminophen 325 mg, 1 tablet, given at 0400

BOX 23.4 KEY ELEMENTS OF A CHANGE-OF-SHIFT REPORT

The following guidelines are important to follow in all shift-change reports:

- Follow a particular order (e.g., follow room numbers in a hospital).
- Provide basic identifying information for each client (e.g., name, room number, bed designation).
- For new clients, provide the reason for admission or medical diagnosis (or diagnoses), surgery (date), diagnostic tests, plan of therapy, and significant information about the client's support people.
- Include significant changes in the client's condition and present information in order (i.e., assessment, nursing diagnoses, interventions, outcomes, and evaluation). For example, "Mr. Ronald Oakes said he had an aching pain in his left calf at 1400 hours. Inspection revealed no other signs. Calf pain is related to altered blood circulation. Rest and elevation of his legs on a footstool for 30 minutes provided relief."
- Provide exact information, such as "Ms. Jessie Jones received Demerol 100 mg intramuscularly at 2000 hours," *not* "Ms. Jessie Jones received some Demerol during the evening."
- Report the client's need for special emotional support. For example, a client who has just learned that his biopsy results revealed malignancy and who is now scheduled for a laryngectomy needs time to discuss his feelings before preoperative teaching starts.
- Include current nurse-prescribed and physician-prescribed orders.
- Provide a summary of newly admitted clients, including diagnosis, age, general condition, plan of therapy, and significant information about the client's support people.
- Report clients that have been transferred or discharged from the unit.
- Clearly state priorities of care and care that is due after the shift begins. For example, in a 7 a.m. report, the nurse might say, "Mr. Li's vital signs are due at 0730, and his IV bag will need to be replaced by 0800." Give this information at the end of that client's report, as people remember best the first and last information given.
- Be concise. Don't elaborate on background data or routine care (e.g., do not report "Vital signs at 0800 and 1200" when that is the unit standard). Do not report coming and going of visitors unless there is a problem or concern or if the visitors are involved in teaching and care. Social support and visits are the norm.

Telephone Reports

Health-care professionals frequently report about a client by telephone. Nurses inform physicians about a change in a client's condition; a radiologist reports the results of an X-ray study; a nurse may confer with a nurse on another unit about a transferred client.

The nurse receiving a telephone report should document the date and time, the name of the person giving the information, and the information received and should sign the notation. For example:

June 6/09 10:35 a.m. GL Messina, laboratory technician, reported by telephone that Mrs. Sara Ames's hematocrit was 39%. __________
Barbara Ireland, RN

If any doubt exists about the information given over the telephone, the person receiving the information should repeat it back to the sender to ensure accuracy.

When giving a telephone report to a physician, it is important that the nurse be concise and accurate. Begin with your name and relationship to the client (e.g., "This is Jana Gomez; I'm calling from xxx Hospital, Unit xxx, about your patient, Dorothy Mendes. I'm her registered nurse on the 7 p.m. to 7 a.m. shift").

Telephone reports usually include the client's name and medical diagnosis, changes in nursing assessment, vital signs related to baseline vital signs, significant laboratory data, and related nursing interventions. The nurse should have the client's chart ready to give the physician any further information.

After reporting, the nurse should document the date, time, and content of the call. For example:

September 14, 2010, 1200h; Dorothy Mendex admitted to Unit 3000. States has "burning abdominal pain in upper right side of abdomen." BP 120/80, P100, R20 on admission. Demerol 100 mg IM given at 1200h
__________RS Chartrand, RN

September 14, 2010, 1400h; BP 100/40, P120, R30. Pain unchanged. Colour pale and perspiring
__________RS Chartrand, RN

September 14, 2010, 1535h; Dr. Burns called regarding patient's pain, pallor, diaphoresis, and vital signs. Dr. Burns stated will be in to assess in one-half hour
__________RS Chartrand, RN

Telephone Orders

Physicians often order a therapy or medication for a client by telephone. Most agencies have specific policies about telephone orders.

While the physician gives the order, *write* the complete order down and read it back to the physician to ensure accuracy. Question the physician about any order that is ambiguous, unusual (e.g., an abnormally high dosage of a medication), or contraindicated by the client's condition. Then, transcribe the order onto the physician's order sheet, indicating it as a verbal order (VO) or telephone order (TO). See Box 23.6 for selected guidelines.

BOX 23.6 GUIDELINES FOR TELEPHONE ORDERS

With telephone orders, it is especially important to carefully follow these guidelines:

1. Do not accept an order from a prescriber you do not know.
2. Ask the prescriber to speak slowly and clearly.
3. Ask the prescriber to spell out the medication if you are not familiar with it.
4. Question the drug, dosage, or changes if they seem inappropriate for this client.
5. Write down the order or enter it into a computer.
6. Read the order back to the prescriber at the end. Use words for abbreviations (e.g., three times a day for tid).
7. When writing a dosage, always put a number before a decimal (e.g., 0.3 mL) but never put a zero after a decimal (e.g., 6 mg).
8. Write out units (e.g., 20 units of insulin, *not* 20 u of insulin).
9. Follow agency policy about the prescriber protocol for signing telephone orders (e.g., within 24 hours).
10. Never follow a voicemail order. Call the prescriber for a client order. Write it down and read it back for confirmation.

Once the order is transcribed on the physician's order sheet, the order must be countersigned by the physician within a time period described by agency policy. Many acute-care facilities require that this be done within 24 hours.

Conferring

Nurses often confer with colleagues and other health-care providers for advice, information, ideas, or instructions about their client situation in a mentoring relationship, or to elicit or validate data needed to plan nursing care. Two ways nurses share information are through a nursing care conference and nursing rounds.

Nursing Care Conference

A **nursing care conference** is a meeting of a group of nurses to discuss possible solutions to certain problems of a client. The nursing care conference allows each nurse an opportunity to offer an opinion about possible solutions to the problem (e.g., lack of progress toward goal attainment). Other health-care providers may be invited to attend the conference to offer their expertise; for example, a social worker may discuss the family problems of a severely burned child, or a dietitian may discuss the dietary problems of a client who has diabetes. Nursing care conferences are most effective when members on the team will accept and respect each person's contributions and listen with an open mind to what others are saying.

Nursing Rounds

Nursing rounds are procedures in which a group of nurses visits selected clients' bedsides to

- Obtain information that will help plan nursing care
- Provide clients the opportunity to discuss their care
- Evaluate the nursing care the client has received
- Identify alternative nursing possibilities from research and experienced nurses

During rounds, the nurse assigned to the client provides a brief summary of the client's nursing needs and the interventions being implemented. Nursing rounds offer advantages to both clients and nurses: clients can participate in the discussions, and nurses can see the client and the equipment being used. To facilitate client participation in nursing rounds, nurses need to use terms that the client can understand. Medical terminology excludes the client from discussion.

Case Study 23

Mr. Anderson, an 80-year-old male, was admitted for back pain. He has a past medical history of hypertension. He told the admitting nurse that he has lost interest in many of his normal activities because of the constant pain. You read the following documentation entry by a previous nurse:

8—Client is a complainer. I listened to him for 15 minutes with no success.
BP 210/90 and 180/70. P 72, R 18.

12—Refused lunch

2—Client fell out of bed

Critical Thinking Questions

1. What guidelines were *not* used in this documentation?
2. The nursing diagnosis for Mr. Anderson is *acute pain.* What would you expect to document?
3. Using the following pieces of data for Mr. Anderson, sort them into a SOAPIER note:
   a. "I didn't sleep last night."
   b. Positioned on side with pillows behind back
   c. Continues to need analgesic medication to progress toward goal of pain relief
   d. States pain is 8 out of 10
   e. "I feel better." (after interventions)
   f. Last medicated 5 hours previously
   g. Heating pad applied to lower back
   h. BP 210/90, P 72, R 18
   i. Add to plan of care to offer analgesic around the clock q4h versus prn
   j. 6/6/03 #1 Pain
   k. "Sharp, stabbing pain in lower back that radiates to left leg."
   l. Medicated with ordered analgesic
4. Use the same pieces of data and sort them into a DAR note.

After working through these questions, go to the MyNursingLab at **http://www.mynursinglab.com** to check your answers.

KEY TERMS

discussion
report
record
recording
charting
documenting
chart
client record
source-oriented record
narrative charting
problem-oriented medical record (POMR)
problem-oriented record (POR)
progress notes
SOAPIER
PIE
Focus Charting
charting by exception (CBE)
variances
Kardex
flowsheets
change-of-shift report
nursing care conference
nursing rounds

CHAPTER HIGHLIGHTS

- Nurses must accurately document each step of the nursing process on a client record.
- Client records are legal documents and are admissible as evidence in a court of law.
- In source-oriented records, recording is organized around the source of the information.
- In problem-oriented records, recording is organized around client problems.
- Other examples of documentation systems include PIE, Focus Charting, charting by exception, computer documentation, and case management.
- Computer records have simplified nursing documentation. The use of computer terminals at the bedside allows for immediate documentation of nursing actions.
- The case management model focuses on standardized interventions given within a defined time frame.
- The case management record for a client incorporates graphics and flowsheets along with critical pathways that serve as both an abbreviated care plan and a documentation form.
- The Kardex record is used for quick access to current data about clients.
- The content of progress notes should be accurate, sequential, appropriate, complete, concise, legally prudent, and ethical.
- Principles of documentation for long-term care are the same as for acute care; however, documentation in long-term care is (1) less frequent and (2) focuses more on daily functioning, preventive measures, and restorative care.
- In home health care, documentation needs to follow professional, regulatory, and accreditation standards.
- Correctly formatted charting should be legible, use correct terminology and spelling, and include date, time, and appropriate signature.
- Record entries as soon as possible *after* nursing assessments, interventions, and evaluations.
- The nurse has a legal and ethical duty to protect the confidentiality of the client's record; this includes taking special measures to protect information stored in computers.
- The purpose of reporting is to communicate specific information for the goal of improving or maintaining quality of care.

ASSESS YOUR LEARNING

1. The Cameron family is caring for their father at home in the final stage of his life. The family has decided that they will all participate in providing care in order to minimize the caregiver burden for Mrs. Cameron. How should the home care nurse document this?

a. "The agency's standardized palliative care plan will be implemented."

b. "Each family member has agreed to spend one day per week caring for Mr. Cameron."

c. "Mrs. Cameron is unable to cope with the care of her husband without assistance."

d. "A care plan has been developed and presented to the Cameron family."

2. A client frequently refuses his daily medication. The nurse is finishing the narrative charting in the client record and writes the subjective client statement, "Don't come near me with that pill. I hate it. . . . Go away and stop bothering me." Which of the following is the best comment that the nurse could include in the narrative recording?

a. "Client uncooperative again."

b. "Client remains negative about treatment."

c. "Client still very angry with nurse."

d. "Client refuses scheduled medication."

3. Nursing documentation and reporting are guided by which of the following organizations?

a. Canadian Nurses Association, International Council of Nurses, health facility policies

b. Canadian Council of Health Services Accreditation, health facility policies, International Council of Nursing

c. Canadian Nurses Association, health-care policies, provincial or territorial nurses' unions

d. Canadian Nurses Association, Canadian Council of Health Services Accreditation, health-care policies

4. The charting by exception (CBE) method of documenting and reporting is most appropriate and useful for which of the following health-care settings?

a. Acute-care facility

b. Outpost nursing station

c. Primary health-care clinic

d. Long-term-care facility

5. Which of the following is the primary purpose of the client health record?

a. Communication document

b. Nursing process tool

c. Research database

d. Accreditation process

6. When documenting in a client chart (health record), nurses must be sure to include a nursing note related to which of the following?
   a. Routine care
   b. Usual events
   c. Doctor's orders
   d. Treatment refusal

7. Gisele Beulieu, RN, is working evenings on a psychiatric unit in a large urban facility when she receives a telephone call. The caller identifies himself as the husband of one of her patients and wants to know how his wife is doing. Nurse Beulieu is unable to verify the caller's identification. What is the nurse's best response?
   a. "Policy prevents me from providing confidential client information."
   b. "Confidential information can't be provided without patient permission."
   c. "If you want patient information, call back in the morning."
   d. "I don't know who you are, so I can't give you any information."

8. The requirements of documenting and reporting suggest nurses resolve a problem with a chart entry by using which of the following guidelines?
   a. Erase all errors as thoroughly as possible.
   b. Draw a pencil line through the wrong entry and write *entry mistake* above it.
   c. Write *mistaken entry* above the entry.
   d. Write *error* above the entry.

9. Which of the following is a legal comment frequently used to describe nursing care?
   a. Nurses are too busy to chart effectively.
   b. Nurses are often sued for malpractice.
   c. Nurses' routine care that is not documented is assumed to be done.
   d. Nurses' routine care that is not documented is assumed to not be done.

10. Maria Dubois, RN, works on a surgical unit and recently she has been visiting her son (age 18 years) who is receiving treatment on a medical unit in the same facility. While you are caring for her son, you return from lunch and find Nurse Dubois reading her son's chart. Select the best response in this situation?
   a. "Maria, what you are doing is illegal."
   b. "Maria, please read the chart in a private place."
   c. "Maria, as a nurse you know the chart is confidential."
   d. "Maria put that chart back; it's not your business."

After working through these questions, go to the MyNursingLab at ***http://www.mynursinglab.com*** *to check your answers and see explanations.*

SUGGESTED READINGS

Austin, S. (2006). "Ladies & gentlemen of the jury, I present . . . the nursing documentation." *Nursing, 36*(1), 56–62.

The author, a nurse attorney, reviews documentation guidelines to help prevent liability. They are based on actual cases and reflect common allegations of professional negligence.

Monson, M. (2006). Legal checkpoints. Disclosing adverse events: You said it, now write it. *Nursing Management, 37*(8), 16–17, 24.

This article presents practical legal tips on nursing documentation.

Nagle, L. M. (2007). Clinical documentation standards—promise or peril? *Nursing Leadership, 20*(4), 33–36.

The author examines the pros and cons of clinical documentation and concludes that although the electronic health record is the future trend, nurses must take the right steps to ensure that how they document will support management of clinical information.

WEBLINKS

Canadian Council of Health Services Accreditation

http://www.cchsa.ca

This organization helps health service organizations achieve greater degrees of excellence for the benefit of all Canadians. It offers organizations ideas about improving documentation systems and ways to become more consistent in standardizing charting across regions.

Canadian Health Infoway

http://www.infoway-inforoute.ca
http://www.infoway-inforoute.ca/Admin/Upload/Dev/Document/Annual%20Report%2005-06%20EN.pdf

This website presents what is happening in Canada and what the future may hold for electronic health development, telehealth, and teleinformatics.

REFERENCES

Austin, S. (2006). Ladies and gentlemen of the jury, I present . . . the nursing documentation. *Nursing 2006, 36*(1), 56–62.

Canadian Council of Health Services Accreditation. (2007). *Canadian health accreditation report.* Retrieved October 26, 2008, from http://www.accreditation-canada.ca/upload/files/pdf/Media/CHAR/2008_Health_Accreditation_Report_EN.pdf

Canada Health Infoway. (2005). *Executive summary. About Infoway: Vision and mission.* Retrieved November 25, 2005, from http://www.canadahealthinfoway.ca

Canadian Nurses Association. (2002). Demystifying the electronic health record. *Nursing Now, 13.* Ottawa: Author.

Canadian Nurses Association. (2008). *Code of ethics for registered nurses.* Centennial edition. Ottawa: Author.

Canadian Nurses Protective Society. (2007). Quality documentation: Your best defence. *Infolaw, 1*(1).

College of Nurses of Ontario. (2005). *Practice standard: Documentation.* Retrieved June 1, 2007, from http://www.cno.org/docs/prac/41001_documentation.pdf

Freedom of Information and Protection of Privacy Act. (1998). Winnipeg: Government of Manitoba.

Hutchinson, C., & Sharples, C. (2006). Information governance: Practical implications for record-keeping. *Nursing Standard, 20*(36), 59–64.

Miller, J., & Glusko, J. (2003). Legal checkpoints: Standing up to the scrutiny of medical malpractice. *Nursing Management, 34*(10), 20–22.

Personal Health Information Protection Act. (2004). Toronto: Government of Ontario.

Personal Information Protection and Electronic Documents Act. (2004). Ottawa: Government of Canada.

Sullivan, G. (2004). Legally speaking: Does your charting measure up? *RN, 67*(3), 61–65.

Williams, L. (2007). Liability landscape: Are your residents safe and sound when in bed? *Nursing Homes e-newsletter.* Retrieved October 13, 2007, from http://www.nursinghomesmagazine.com/Past_Issues.htm?ID=3244

Chapter 24

Nursing Informatics

Computers have become functional tools for many people, including nurses. Nurses use data and information for decision making and to deliver quality care to their clients. They gather assessment data, integrate information to develop care plans, communicate information to clients and health-care team members, and manage budget and staffing data.

OBJECTIVES

After studying this chapter, you should be able to

1. Define nursing informatics
2. Differentiate among data, information, and knowledge
3. Identify nursing computer applications used in direct client care
4. Discuss advantages of and concerns about electronic health records
5. Describe the issues of privacy, confidentiality, data integrity, and security related to the electronic health record
6. List uses of nursing computer applications
7. Identify ways nursing computer applications can be used by nurse administrators for personnel, facilities management, finance, and quality assurance
8. Examine uses of computers in nursing education
9. Examine the role of nursing informatics in research

Electronic health (ehealth) technologies, including telehealth, virtual education, decision-support systems, and workload measurement through electronic charting are becoming more prevalent in nursing practice (Hannah, 2007). Convergence of information and communications technology allows for rapid and secure transmission of information among health-care professionals through such venues as the internet. It is imperative that nurses understand the opportunities these new technologies provide to enhance their practice.

Informatics refers to the science of computer information systems. **Nursing informatics** is the science of using computer information systems in the practice of nursing. Staggers and Thompson (2002) developed a comprehensive definition of nursing informatics:

> *Nursing informatics is a specialty that integrates nursing science, computer science, and information science to manage and communicate data, information, and knowledge in nursing practice. Nursing informatics facilitates the integration of data, information, and knowledge to support patients, nurses, and other providers in their decision-making in all roles and settings. This support is accomplished through the use of information structures, information processes, and information technology. (2002, p. 262)*

Beyond the definition, the goal of nursing informatics is to improve the health of populations, communities, families, and individuals by optimizing information management and communication. This includes the use of information and technology in providing direct care, in establishing effective administrative systems, in managing and delivering educational experiences, in supporting lifelong learning, and in supporting nursing research (Staggers & Thompson, 2002, p. 260).

Advanced practice in nursing informatics is a growing specialty, as nurses have moved forward to design and adapt computer processes for patient care, education, administration, management, and research. The Canadian Nurses Association (CNA) believes that a "comprehensive, forward-looking, coordinated and collaborative" (2006, p. 3) e-nursing strategy is needed. A specific Canadian e-nursing strategy would facilitate information and technology development initiatives to improve nursing practice and client outcomes. Such a strategy would consider nurses in all domains of practice: clinical practice, education, research, administration, and policy.

Personal digital assistants (PDAs) are handheld computers that can interface with PCs, networks, or phone systems (see Figure 24.1). Smart phones are a combination of a phone and a PDA, as well as other features. PDAs were originally developed as calendar or date books and address books, but nurses increasingly use them as drug and disease database storage devices. Nurses can also record client data as they work; document assessments and treatments quickly and efficiently; and organize, track, and share client data.

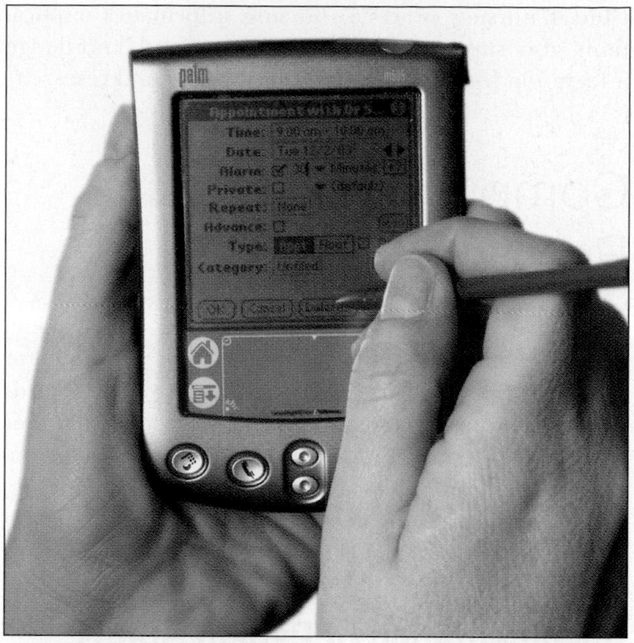

FIGURE 24.1 Nursing informatics applications, such as PDAs, are well suited to assist the nurse in collecting, recording, and using data.

To better understand nursing informatics, an explanation of the interrelationships among data, information, and knowledge is needed. **Data** are raw observations that have not been interpreted, such as age, weight, blood pressure, number of admissions, and number of workload units. **Information** results when data are interpreted, organized, or structured in a meaningful way. For example, data regarding age, disease, blood pressure, or mental status exam score can be integrated to provide information about fall risk. **Knowledge** requires synthesis of information to identify relationships that provide fuller understanding of an issue or subject. For example, once raw data are integrated to provide information about fall risk, the nurse's knowledge about care maps or fall-reduction programs, derived from both practice and the nursing literature, allows for evidence-based decisions that advance effective patient care.

These concepts—data, information, and knowledge—are influenced by nursing informatics applications. Raw data can be collected and stored by using computer systems. Electronic monitoring of vital signs and ECG in intensive care units can be recorded directly to the electronic patient record (EPR). Integration of data to provide useful information is demonstrated when statistics are available on the prevalence of immunizations for a specific disease across communities. Knowledge is enhanced through integration of care maps or decision-support systems, which analyze raw data and nursing assessments to suggest nursing diagnoses and recommended interventions. Beyond clinical nursing practice, nursing informatics applications also support data, information, and knowledge integration for education, administration, and research.

Computers in Nursing Practice

The activities of the registered nurse involve collecting, recording, and using data. Computers are well suited to assist in these functions. Specifically, the nurse records patient information in computer records, accesses other departments' patient information from centralized computers, uses computers to manage patient scheduling, and uses programs for such applications as home health nursing and case management.

Documentation of Patient Status and Medical Record Keeping

A significant part of a nurse's day can be spent recording in patient records or accessing client data from the medical record or elsewhere in the health-care agency. Nurses require access to standardized forms, policies, or procedures and need the capacity to gather broader client information for specific diagnoses. Computers can assist with each of these.

MANAGEMENT INFORMATION SYSTEMS A **management information system (MIS)** is designed to facilitate the organization and application of data used to manage an organization or department. It provides analyses used for strategic planning, decision making, and evaluation of management activities.

HOSPITAL INFORMATION SYSTEMS A **hospital information system (HIS)** is an MIS that focuses on data needed to manage client care activities and health-care organizations. The goal is to provide data needed to determine appropriate actions and control. An HIS will contain subsystems in admissions, medical records (see Figure 24.2), clinical laboratory, pharmacy, order entry, and finance. These record data needed for billing management, quality assurance, scheduling, or inventory. Increasingly, accrediting organizations mandate the use of an HIS and require that reports be submitted by using computerized formats. Eventually, integrated HISs will form the centre of all record keeping and analysis for interdisciplinary health care.

BEDSIDE DATA ENTRY Computerized data entry systems expedite recording of client assessments, medication administration, progress notes, care-plan updates, patient acuity, and (possibly) accrued charges.

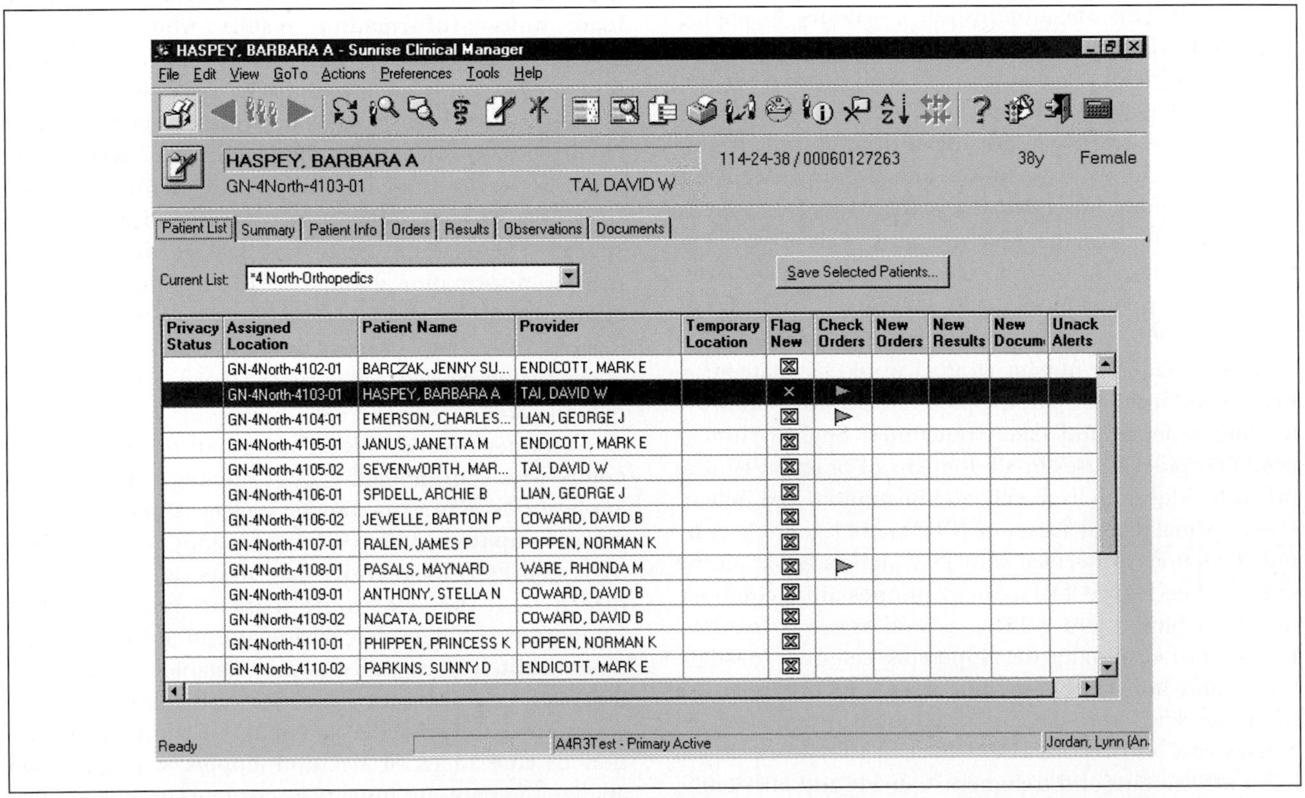

FIGURE 24.2 Client list screen

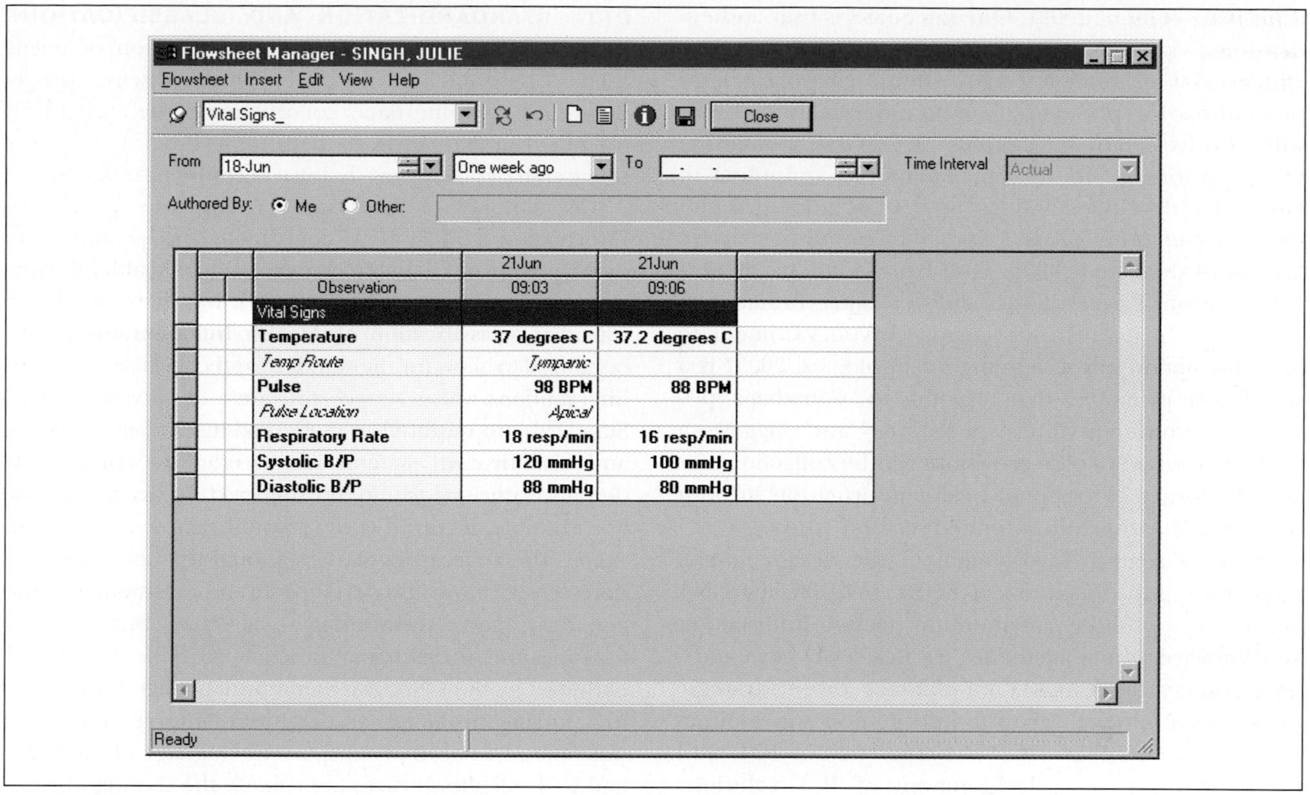

FIGURE 24.3 This screen displays the client's vital signs.

Fixed or handheld terminals, hardwired to the central system or cordless, can transmit data, such as vital signs (see Figure 24.3) to distant sites, linking the client to the agency office. Another type of bedside terminal is the point-of-care or point-of-service computer located near but not necessarily with the patient.

ELECTRONIC HEALTH RECORDS **Electronic health records (EHRs)** permit electronic data retrieval by caregivers, administrators, accreditors, and other persons who require the data and have authorized access. In November 2002, the Romanow Commission issued *Building on Values: The Future of Health Care in Canada,* which emphasized the importance of EHRs as "one of the keys to modernizing Canada's health care system and improving access and outcomes for Canadians" (p. 77). Health Canada (2004) defined the EHR as an individual's health record that is accessible online from many separate, interoperable, automated systems within an electronic network. It is considered to be a comprehensive record garnered from information available from **electronic medical records (EMRs)** and **electronic patient records (EPRs)** for a specific individual.

EMRs are records kept in a clinic, by a family health team, or in a health practitioner's office. The EHR incorporates relevant information from health-care visits and other point-of-service systems, such as pharmacies and diagnostic testing centres. The EHR links institutions. Accurate health information available at the point of care enhances quality of care. Currently, no national standards for EHRs exist—for either the data that should be included or the way the record should be organized.

EPRs are generally understood to be a record of a patient's demographic data, such as name and date of birth, the patient's diagnosis, and details about assessments and interventions provided by health professionals during an episode of care from one health organization. A consumer's copy of the health data, whether paper or electronic, is a personal health record.

Canada remains in a developmental phase, as shifting to the use of EHRs requires considerable investment for the Canadian health-care system. However, benefits far outweigh costs. The Health Council of Canada (2006), established in 2003, identified ways the EHR could improve health care. Reducing errors caused by multiple files and data entry points, avoiding duplication, and improving flow of information will enhance patient safety and increase efficiency. Client health information would be available across the lifespan and clients could participate in their own health care. Supported with federal funding, the nonprofit corporation **Canada Health Infoway** (2005) was mandated to implement development of electronic health systems. The goal is that by 2009, 50% of Canadians will have an EHR.

Concern has been raised in several areas regarding EHRs. Maintaining privacy and security of data is a significant issue (Olsen, 2003). One safeguard is user authentication via passwords or biometric identifiers (fingerprint or retinal scans). Additional policies and procedures for protecting the confidentiality of EHRs will evolve. For example, COACH: Canadian Organization for the Advancement of Computers in Health has developed a widely used set of guidelines outlined in *Guidelines for the Protection of Health Information* last published in 2007. The Pan-Canadian Health Information Privacy and Confidentiality Framework developed through Health Canada (Advisory Committee on Information and Emerging Technologies, 2005) is a set of core principles that responds to "Canadians' privacy and confidentiality expectations" and suggests a "harmonized set of core provisions for the collection, use and disclosure of personal health information in both the publicly and privately funded sectors" (p. 1).

Nurses require involvement in the design, implementation, and evaluation of EHRs. In 2006, the CNA developed a position statement on nursing information and knowledge management (see Box 24.1). Its e-nursing strategy for Canada emphasizes three strategic directions: improved access to information and communications technology (ICT), competency in ICT, and participation in the development of ICT solutions (Canadian Nurses Association [CNA], 2006). One role of the **nurse informaticist**, an expert who combines computer, information, and nursing science, is to develop policies and procedures that advance effective and secure use of computerized health-care records.

DATA STANDARDIZATION AND CLASSIFICATIONS

Nursing benefits from standard classification of terms used to describe and measure clinical, disease, procedure, and outcome data. For nursing to be recognized for the value it adds to patient well-being requires research-based findings that use accepted standards.

A mandate of the Canadian Institute for Health Information (CIHI) is to coordinate and promote the development and maintenance of national health information standards. The CIHI (2004) has developed the **Canadian Classification of Health Interventions (CCI)**, organized to allow for the standardized collection of health interventions across service providers or service settings. Standards are required to guide coding of data elements, and classification systems are needed to consistently describe concepts within nursing and across disciplines. For example, identical coding would denote *exercise* from nurse, physiotherapist, or recreational therapist interventions. The CCI was also developed to be consistent with the concepts and terminology of the International Classification for Nursing Practice (ICNP). The ICNP, endorsed by the CNA, is a common language for describing nursing problems or diagnoses, interventions, and outcomes. Use of the concepts and language of the ICNP and CCI will allow nurses to facilitate the sharing of nursing information. It may take years to determine optimal standards and to choose the determining body. The CNA believes registered nurses should be at the forefront in the collection, storage, and retrieval of data at the national level (see the Reflect on Primary Health Care box).

BOX 24.1 THE CANADIAN NURSES ASSOCIATION IDENTIFIES SEVEN BENEFITS OF THE ELECTRONIC HEALTH RECORD

1. Availability of comprehensive information on the care of clients/patients covering the continuum of health service delivery, across health professionals and over time
2. Convenience and ease of access, transfer and retrieval of information; for example, workload and intervention data can be easily retrieved and aggregated for administrative purposes
3. Ability to dynamically view or display data from different views to support clinical, administrative, and research functions; for example, nurses can easily request data on all of the patient's current medications or all of the patient's test results over a period of time across health organizations; nurses can request necessary data to support the clinical audit and measurement of patient outcomes
4. Provision of a dynamic approach to nursing research and to the development of new nursing knowledge, e.g., the outcome of nursing interventions: what works and what doesn't work under what circumstances
5. Improved data quality and standardization of clinical documentation; data are automatically verified as they are entered to ensure accuracy; data from feeder systems (e.g., admission, discharge and transfer, pharmacy, clinical laboratory, and physician offices) can be entered directly eliminating data entry errors; information is structured and standardized facilitating more effective analysis and communications between health service providers and organizations
6. Improved continuity of client/patient care through the sharing of information between health organizations and health professionals
7. Direct access to knowledge bases and decision-support software tools to support improved decision-making and better client/patient outcomes

Source: From "Demystifying the Electronic Health Record" by the Canadian Nurses Association, 2002, *Nursing Now: Issues and Trends in Canadian Nursing, 13,* p. 3.

REFLECT ON PRIMARY HEALTH CARE

Primary health care is a fundamental component of the Canadian health-care system. With goals of improved accessibility, efficiency, and quality of care, primary health care is critical to the quality and sustainability of health care in Canada. Informatics and communication technologies offer exciting possibilities and are a way to reduce costs and enhance patient safety.

National electronic health records are one such resource essential to information-sharing among health-care providers. These help to improve coordination and avoid repetition (repetition of health histories or similar diagnostic tests). Reflect on how rapid access, using *appropriate technology*, to clinical practice guidelines and electronic references support and strengthen decision making.

In Ontario, the **Health Outcomes for Better Information and Care (HOBIC)** is an initiative for collection and analysis of information on staffing indicators and health outcome measures within different nursing practice settings. HOBIC is part of the Ontario Ministry of Health and Long-Term Care's (2007) information management strategy. Originally known as the Nursing and Health Outcomes Project, it included a feasibility study that was conducted in 16 acute-care, long-term-care, and home care settings across Ontario. Consequently, implementation of the collection of health outcomes data in acute-care, long-term-care, complex continuing care, and home care has begun. Future applications will apply to other health-care sectors and include contributions of interdisciplinary teams. Eventually, the information will be used to direct decisions about appropriate health-care settings and nursing allocation (RNs, RPNs, RPN/LPNs) for improved patient outcomes.

ELECTRONIC ACCESS TO PATIENT DATA Computers are used extensively to assess and monitor patients' conditions. Data accumulated from electronic devices can be stored in the EHR for research purposes. Electronic records require minimum space and can be stored securely or transferred onto different electronic media (e.g., magnetic tape, microfiche). Data can also be transmitted to a consulting specialist in another location over a secure network.

The Computer-Based Patient Record Institute, established in 1992, identified four ways the EMR could improve health care: (1) constant availability of patient health information across the lifespan, (2) ability to monitor quality, (3) access to warehoused (stored) data, and (4) ability for individuals to share in knowledge and activities influencing their own health.

As computers provide access to the EHR, providers can retrieve such data as trends in vital signs or immunization records. The system can be designed to warn providers about conflicting medications or patient parameters indicating dangerous conditions (see Figure 24.4). Sophisticated systems allow replay of audio, graphic, or video data for comparison with current status. Text is legible and can be searched for keywords.

Patient Monitoring and Computerized Diagnostics

Nursing has benefited from the myriad patient monitors available and used across care settings: digital or tympanic thermometers; digital scales; pulse oximetry; electrocardiography (ECG), telemetry, hemodynamic monitoring; apnea monitors; fetal heart monitors; blood glucose analyzers; ventilators; and intravenous (IV) pumps. Some can transmit data to more sophisticated computers or interact with the user via digital displays. Most include error detection, warnings that the instrument is malfunctioning or that the assessed value is outside predetermined parameters. These devices can extend the nurse's observations and supply reliable data.

In specialty areas of health care, patients undergo diagnostic procedures in which computers play a major role. Computerized axial tomography (CAT) scans, magnetic resonance imaging (MRI), and positron emission tomography (PET) scans use computers to perform tests and analyze findings. Blood gas analyzers, pulmonary function test machines, and intracranial pressure monitors all use computer processing and can be linked to store data in the EHR.

Consumer Informatics

Increasingly, patients seek information on the internet about their condition and care or find assistance from lay

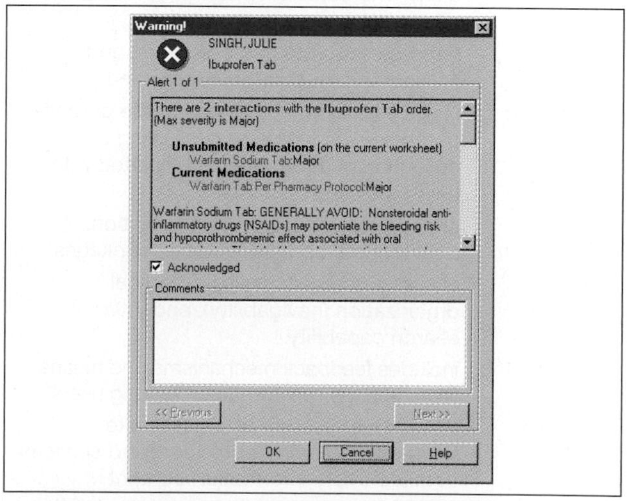

FIGURE 24.4 One of the strengths of an electronic record is its ability to alert the clinician to potential drug interactions by using warnings, such as the one displayed here.

or professionally led online support groups. Nurses can use these sources of information to promote health and guide their clients to reliable health information on the internet. The Health Summit Working Group (Mitretek Systems' Health Information Technology Institute), teamed health-care providers, medical librarians, information resource experts, and consumers to develop a comprehensive set of evaluation criteria (see Table 24.1).

Not all consumers have access to computers and the internet. In 2007, an estimated 19.2 million Canadian households (73%) used the internet for personal reasons (Statistics Canada, 2008). Individuals living in cities are more likely to have internet access than do those in rural areas and small towns. Such factors as income, education, age, and the presence of children in the household all influence internet use. Households with higher annual incomes, individuals with postsecondary education, persons between age 16 and 24, and households with children under 18 were more likely to use the internet regularly (Statistics Canada, 2008).

The Health on the Net (HON) Foundation has developed a code of conduct to standardize the reliability of health information available on the internet. The HON code defines a set of principles to maintain basic ethical standards when presenting health information. Consumers can be confident that the information on sites displaying the HON seal conforms to this standard. Nurses informed about evaluation criteria and the HON seal can more effectively guide clients' acquisition of reliable knowledge, information, and support from the internet.

TABLE 24.1 Criteria for Evaluating Health Information on the Internet

Credibility	includes the source, currency, relevance/utility, and editorial review process for the information.
Content	must be accurate and complete, and an appropriate disclaimer provided.
Disclosure	includes informing the user of the purpose of the site, as well as any profiling or collection of information associated with using the site.
Links	are evaluated according to selection, architecture, content, and back linkages.
Design	encompasses accessibility, logical organization (navigability), and internal search capability.
Interactivity	includes feedback mechanisms and means for exchange of information among users.
Caveats	include clarification of whether site function is to market products and services or is a primary information content provider.

Source: From *Criteria for Assessing the Quality of Health Information on the Internet: Policy Paper*, by Health Summit Working Group, Mitretek Systems, 1999.

Another emerging area is internet-based **patient portals**. Central to patient-centred care are the free flow of information and the patient as the source of control. Patient portals can play a vital role in meeting these goals. The internet provides patients with secure access to relevant health-care information, including individual records, education, and patient support communities and forums. Visiting a patient portal is similar to banking online. The HIS makes such sharing of information possible.

A portal initiative of the Canada Health Infoway (2007) is for family and friends involved in the delivery of health care. The portal will contain information on providing care, respite supports, financial advice, discussion boards, and a **caregiver electronic record (CER)**. The CER can connect caregivers to home and community care supports. Caregivers can track care issues or details about the care they are providing.

Telehealth

One of the most exciting developments in computer-assisted health care is **telehealth**. Canada has provided funding initiatives to encourage and coordinate telehealth development within the country. Telehealth involves using ICTs to deliver health information, services, and expertise over any distance. For example, using

Evidence-Informed Practice

How Can Parents Be Supported at Home Following Surgery on Their Children?

In Young, Siden, and Tredwell's (2007) study, families of children who had been discharged from hospital after scoliosis surgery were assigned to receive videophone or telephone support. Twenty-one families were provided with videophones, and 22 families used traditional telephone. Data times included a day 3 post-discharge contact, any additional calls to the clinic nurse, and a research-generated contact and week 6 interview. Although both forms of contact ensured continuity of professional contact for the families, the value of the technology depended on the characteristics of the family using it.

NURSING IMPLICATIONS: Although new technology may provide increased access for families caring for postsurgical patients at home, it is important to ensure there is a fit between the acceptance of the technology and the family for optimal effect.

Source: Based on "Post-surgical Telehelath Support for Children and Family Care-Givers," by L. Young, H. Siden, and S. Tredwell, 2007, *Journal of Telemedicine and Telecare, 13*(1), pp.15–19

two-way audiovisual connections, an international expert can examine and consult from kilometres away, especially in rural or remote areas where resources and expertise are scarce. Telehealth can be used in (1) teleconsultation, teleimaging, and telepsychiatry, (2) education and training in health disciplines, such as telelearning and telementoring, (3) health information transfer for health-care providers, and (4) health-care information for clients. X-rays, scans, or stored computer data, can all be sent using computers. (See Box 24.2 for more benefits.)

Telehealth is changing the role of the nurse. Nurses are using telehealth technology to provide client-centred care during consultations with clients or health professionals or to teletriage and telecommunicate health-related data. For example, Telehealth Ontario is a telephone service clients can use to receive health advice or information. Software assists the nurse with a series of questions to determine problems or make recommendations to the client.

Innovative programs have been developed to increase the use of telehealth in the health-care sector. In 2006, the Canadian Council on Health Services Accreditation introduced telehealth supplementary criteria as part of the hospital accreditation program, providing a comprehensive assessment of organizations using telehealth to deliver services, maintain communication, or provide consultation and education (Canadian Council on Health Services Accreditation, 2007).

Legal and ethical issues are concerns for nursing telepractice. Who has responsibility for the client? Where should the care provider be licensed? The CNA has developed a position statement on the role of the nurse in telepractice (see Box 24.3). Although telepractice is within the scope of practice, it has yet to be determined which jurisdiction's standards will apply when nurse and client are in different jurisdictions and the interaction occurs on the internet. Each jurisdiction that uses nursing telepractice must also develop policies and procedures to protect client privacy. As these issues are explored, telehealth applications will continue to extend the ability of nursing to provide better access to health-care services.

BOX 24.2 BENEFITS OF TELEHEALTH

Telehealth offers new and exciting ways to improve health care:

- It helps ensure continuity of client care.
- It removes geographical barriers to care.
- It creates centralized health records.
- It allows for collaboration among health-care team members.
- It increases client involvement in care.
- It acts as an education tool.

Evidence-Based Practice

The CNA's position statement *Evidenced-Based Decision Making and Nursing Practice* (2002) states, "Evidence-based decision-making is an important element of quality care in all domains of nursing practice. Evidence-based decision-making is essential to optimize outcomes for patients, improve clinical practice, achieve cost-effective nursing care and ensure accountability and transparency in decision-making" (p. 1). Emerging in the nursing literature are best practice options grounded in viable research. Electronic syntheses of current evidence are accessible from such sources as the Cochrane Library and online databases (CINAHL or OVID).

Nurses must be familiar with online professional resources and search strategies to access such evidence. One such resource is the Registered Nurses' Association of Ontario (RNAO) Best Practice Guidelines. In 1999, the RNAO received provincial government funding to provide Best Practice Guidelines for patient care to Ontario nurses. The RNAO (2008) has more than 30 published guidelines, a toolkit for the implementation of clinical practice guidelines, and an educator's resource for their integration available for download. (See also Box 24.4.)

Practice Management

Computers assist nurses in diverse management functions. In hospitals, data terminals are used to order supplies, tests, meals, and services. Computer tracking can determine the most frequent or costly items used by a particular nursing unit. This information can guide decisions to modify a budget, adjust staffing, relocate supplies, or make other changes.

Computers and handheld devices, such as PDAs, are used extensively for scheduling. Client appointments can be entered or changed. Notes or tags can be attached to appointments, reminding the provider to perform particular services. Schedules can be printed and staffing patterns coordinated. Special requests can be entered and schedules viewed by day, week, month, or year.

Every practice tracks procedures performed by health-care workers, client diagnoses, and time spent with clients to ensure accurate accounting. With managed care, information tracking also determines trends in health problems and the need for providers with specific skills. The use of computerized databases with unique codes for each medication, medical and nursing diagnosis, treatment, and supply allows for optimal management of these data.

BOX 24.3 ROLE OF THE NURSE IN TELEPRACTICE

NURSE–CLIENT RELATIONSHIPS

- As in all areas of nursing practice, the nurse engaged in nursing telepractice establishes a therapeutic nurse–client relationship, using the nursing process, which encompasses client assessment, planning, implementation—through the provision of information, referral, education and support—evaluation and documentation.

COMPETENCIES

- Nurses engaged in telepractice require specialized nursing knowledge and skill. Strong clinical knowledge and assessment skills are critical for a nurse providing services to a client without benefit of face-to-face contact. It is equally important for the nurse to possess competencies relevant to the technologies being used; the ability to determine if nursing telepractice is the appropriate means for meeting the client's needs; and refined communication and documentation skills. As with all nursing practice, nurses engaged in telepractice should consider clients' cultural, spiritual and psychosocial needs and preferences.

LOCUS OF ACCOUNTABILITY

- Nurses engaged in telepractice are considered to be practising in the province/territory where they are located and currently registered, regardless of where the client is located. As such, they must provide nursing telepractice services consistent with the *Code of Ethics for Registered Nurses*, professional practice standards, relevant legislation and practice guidelines of the province/territory in which they are registered and practising. In such a model, the nurse should inform the client with his/her name, professional designation, provincial/territorial regulatory body and place of work. This is to ensure that the client has the option of seeking further information about the nurse should the client wish to file a complaint. In the event complaints are filed, provincial/territorial regulatory bodies have mechanisms in place so that out-of-jurisdiction matters can be handled in the public interest.

SECURITY, CONFIDENTIALITY, AND PRIVACY

- Nurses and employers have a responsibility to develop and/or implement policies ensuring the privacy, security and confidentiality of nurse–client interactions. Of particular importance to nursing telepractice is ensuring that the technologies themselves and client records are secure. The amount and type of security must be appropriate to the technology being used.

INFORMED CONSENT AND CLIENT CHOICE

- Nurses engaged in telepractice, like all nurses, practise within relevant legal authority governing consent to treatment. Whether consent is obtained by implicit or explicit means, it should be based on informed choice. In the case of nursing telepractice, informed choice may require nurses and employers to explain to clients such things as how information will be recorded and stored; who will have access to the information; and who will be present during an interaction. As well, the client has the right to be fully informed about choices regarding nursing telepractice, including the right to seek other methods for care.

PROFESSIONAL PRACTICE ENVIRONMENTS

- Environments fostering professional practice provide for better client outcomes. Ensuring quality professional practice environments that promote safe, competent and ethical nursing telepractice services is a shared responsibility involving practitioners, employers, governments, regulatory bodies, professional associations, educational institutions, unions and the public. Provision of clinical guidelines, standardized protocols and appropriate agency policies and procedures to guide and support nurses' practice and to help reduce liability risk for nurses are important elements of a quality environment for nursing telepractice.

Source: From *The Role of the Nurse in Telepractice*, by the Canadian Nurses Association, 2001. Retrieved from http://www.cna-nurses.ca/CNA/documents/pdf/publications/PS52_Role_Nurse_Telepractice_Nov_2001_e.pdf. Reprinted with permission.

BOX 24.4 HEALTH INFORMATION SERVICES

One major initiative developed by the Canadian Nurses Association is the NurseONE nursing portal. NurseONE is a national, bilingual, web-based health information service for the Canadian nursing community. The goal of NurseONE is to provide quick access to quality, up-to-date health-care information to support nurses in Canada in delivering effective, evidence-based care and to help them manage their careers.

Specific Applications of Computers in Nursing Practice

Computer systems are becoming essential tools for collecting and classifying data used in nursing practice. Specific systems are particularly useful in designated settings.

COMMUNITY AND HOME HEALTH Computer networks are used in innovative ways in home settings. A computer placed in a high-risk client's or family's home allows the client to access information, search the internet, or email a health-care provider with questions or concerns. Clients can also record data about their health status that can be transmitted to the health-care provider at the central network computer. Examples in which using this approach has been successful include monitoring women at risk for preterm labour, persons with AIDS, and clients with Alzheimer's. Home alert systems that allow the client to signal the base station in an emergency are becoming more widely used. Nurses attending clients in their homes often use notebook computer systems to record assessments and transmit data to the main office.

CASE MANAGEMENT Case management refers to the management of health-service delivery. The scope of case management can be broad, encompassing community-based programs, such as home care, child health services, and mental health clinics. Case management involves client-centred services that link clients with health-care and psychosocial services that provide timely, coordinated access to appropriate levels of care. Case managers track a group of clients (the caseload). Software programs allow the case manager to enter and integrate client data with predesigned care-tracking templates with the goal of providing quality and cost-effective interventions and outcomes. Client information is centrally recorded and the following information can be included: (1) intake information and screening, (2) continuous assessment of client needs, (3) planning, (4) coordination and referrals, (5) monitoring and follow-up, (6) discharge planning, and (7) housing assistance. Organizations can use software programs to track and measure outcomes, review trends, and build capacity.

Another supportive service available to community health professionals is CHNET-Works! (Community Health Networks, 2008). This pilot project has as its goal "a network of networks linking community health professionals—practitioners, researchers and decision-makers—from jurisdictions across Canada for the purposes of developing evidence-informed service delivery, planning and policy models in community health. It will involve the creation and transfer of knowledge by facilitating interactions among research, policy and practice experiences" (Community Health Networks, 2008). It includes Fireside Chats, a discussion forum for current and developing issues in community health. Using simultaneous toll-free telephone and internet conference, participants listen to and see the same presentation. Those with high-speed internet connections can link directly to an internet conference, while those without high-speed access can download the presentation.

Informatics in Nursing Education

Computers are used extensively in all aspects of nursing education. Nursing programs require computerized libraries; faculty members use technological teaching strategies in the classroom and when demonstrating and using applications in nursing practice rotations; and academic record keeping is facilitated by database programs.

Lifespan Considerations

Computer Use

CHILDREN AND ADULTS

Computer programs, both CD and internet-based, are available to all ages and for every interest. Issues of concern relate to extended use of computers. Repetitive motion injuries can occur with extensive typing, as can eye strain from computer monitor viewing. Musculoskeletal damage is related to inadequate ergonomic arrangement of desk chairs, surface height, and monitor placement. Those who use computers daily should be evaluated and cautioned regarding these conditions.

Parents should be reminded of potential risks to children from internet contact with strangers and adult-only websites. They also need to monitor children's use of computers to avoid detours from homework into computer games and messaging. All persons must be wary and protect financial and personal information when conducting business via computer.

OLDER ADULTS

Computers are increasingly available to older adults, providing them with communication and exposure to a vast amount of health-care information. Learning how to evaluate information from sites can guard against misinformation. The following factors increase the validity of a site:

- The site lists an author, the author's credentials, or the original source.
- Changes to the information are dated.
- If health-care information is presented, a disclaimer presents limitations and states it is not medical advice.

Computer-assisted programs can be effective teaching aids for older adults. Programs can provide audio or visual instruction and may be interactive. Programs can assist people in understanding medical conditions, medications, or information about procedures and surgeries.

Teaching and Learning

Computers enhance academics for both students and faculty in six major ways: (1) access to and retrieval of literature, (2) evaluation, (3) student and course record management, (4) computer-assisted learning, (5) classroom technologies, and (6) strategies for distance learning. Computers can also be used for teaching clients, as discussed in the Lifespan Considerations box on the previous page.

LITERATURE ACCESS AND RETRIEVAL It is a continuing challenge to stay current in any subject. Computers have significantly improved capacity in this area by presenting catalogues and materials in forms that can be searched systematically. Cumulative indexes of related materials can be electronically searched by currency, language, document type, or other characteristics. Once a list of search matches is displayed, users can select desired citations to print or store. Box 24.5 lists commonly used bibliographic systems and databases.

Complete publications and materials are often available in computerized formats. These include medical textbooks, full text of journals, drug references, digitized X-rays, scans, and graphics. Through the World Wide Web, both classic and current information can be found. Users can access statistics from the Laboratory Centre for Disease Control, census data, and the National Library of Medicine in the United States via computer or PDA.

EVALUATION Computers provide opportunities to direct a variety of learning evaluations. Surveys can be completed online, including anonymous questionnaires for course evaluations. Pools of potential test items can be developed and the computer can generate individual student exams reflecting selection criteria designated by faculty. Answers can be scored electronically and posted immediately by using a program called Gradebook, and question statistics and student results can be analyzed. Although the CNA has yet to move from traditional paper-and-pencil national registration exams to computerized exams, in April 2004, the LeaRN Canadian Registered Nurse Examination (CRNE) Readiness Test was launched. Multiple-choice questions similar to the CRNE provide CRNE candidates the opportunity to take a simulated version of the CRNE exam.

BOX 24.5 COMMON SEARCHABLE HEALTH-RELATED BIBLIOGRAPHIC SYSTEMS AND DATABASES

The following are just a few of the searchable health-related bibliographic systems and databases:

- Acquired Immune Deficiency Syndrome information onLINE (AIDSLINE)
- Centre for Addiction and Mental Health Library Catalogue
- Child and Family Canada
- Statistics Canada
- Cochrane Database of Systematic Reviews
- CANCER LITerature (CANCER LIT)
- Canadian Health Network
- Cumulative Index to Nursing and Allied Health Literature (CINAHL)
- Educational Resources Information Center (ERIC)
- Medical Literature Analysis and Retrieval System (MEDLARS)
- MEDLINE (EBSCOhost)
- Psychological Abstracts (PsychINFO)
- Turning Evidence into Practice (TRIP)

STUDENT AND COURSE RECORD MANAGEMENT Computer spreadsheets assist in maintaining student grades or attendance. Faculty can input student test results into the Gradebook program to calculate percentages, sort student scores, and print results. Scores from multiple exams and marks on essays or other projects are calculated into final grades.

Students are frequently asked to evaluate faculty and courses by using machine-readable forms. These data are scanned into the computer and cumulative results calculated and stored through **data warehousing**, the accumulation of large amounts of data stored over time and available to be examined for output in reports (charts and tables).

Most schools now keep student records on computer. From application through graduation, the registrar's office tracks names, addresses, courses taken, grades, and other pertinent student data. Students may be able to register for classes, check tuition bills, and see their transcripts on campus computer terminals or from any available computer with internet access. In addition, practice education management systems are used for tracking nursing students' clinical education, for example, the Health Sciences Placement Network (HSPnet).

COMPUTER-ASSISTED LEARNING **Computer-assisted learning (CAL)** is individualized self-study using computers to deliver an educational activity. Software programs created by individuals, educational institutions, technology companies, or print publishers help nurses and students learn and demonstrate learning. Learners proceed at their own pace with immediate feedback on their progress. Programs cover topics from drug dosage calculations to ethical decision making and are classified according to format: tutorial, drill and practice, simulation, computer games or edutainment, testing, or problem solving. CAL can contain diagrams, graphics, animation, video, and audio and can be accessed on CD-ROMs or on the internet. All forms of CAL allow rapid access to any section of the program and can be designed to branch to different sections depending on the user's responses.

Tutorials on health assessment, electrocardiogram interpretation, drug interactions, and legal aspects of nursing are examples of these programs. Clinical simulations are valuable, allowing learners to use background knowledge and experiences to test their critical-thinking and problem-solving skills in artificial but realistic situations without risk. **Edutainment** is educational software concealed in a game format. Content or competitive games require the user to strategize and make decisions to reach a goal.

Course syllabi with worksheets or activities to be completed on the computer can be distributed on disk, through a university or college network, or via the internet. Completion of CAL programs may also be appropriate for demonstrating continuing education activities.

CLASSROOM TECHNOLOGY Most new educational buildings are wired to accommodate technology and older buildings are being modified. Many universities are partially or complete laptop institutions. In 1996, Acadia University introduced notebook computers into classrooms, while the University of Ontario Institute of Technology has profiled itself as a laptop-based university since 2003. For faculty, digital projectors and liquid crystal display (LCD) panels are becoming standard. These enhancements allow faculty to employ the full text, video, and audio capabilities of computers in the classroom. Personal response systems or clickers are also used to promote discussion, engage students in active learning activities, and monitor understanding of key concepts.

DISTANCE EDUCATION The integration of information technology and communications technology allows people to communicate effectively across distance and time zones. This ability creates opportunities for **distance education**, which allows instructors and students to be in several different places. Several different distance education delivery systems exist. In one model, students receive course materials, communicate with faculty and other students, and submit assignments through mail, phone or fax, email, a website, and an electronic drop box (a server folder accessible from the internet). This method can be referred to as an asynchronous mode because the persons involved are not interacting in real time.

Interactive videoconferencing, enabled by information technology and telecommunications applications, is also used to allow students at various sites to participate face to face in class discussions. Completely online programs exist for post-RN baccalaureate degrees and master's degrees.

Synchronous distance learning can be accomplished through use of chat and instant messaging. Another computerized delivery of knowledge is ebooks, in which entire textbooks are available on a computer or PDA and can be annotated and searched. PDAs can also contain reference materials, such as drug handbooks, for instant, up-to-date information. As computer technology becomes cost-effective and increases its transmission quality, it is anticipated that more schools will use distance learning strategies to reach students around the globe (see Box 24.6).

Informatics in Nursing Administration

As noted, the volume of data that nurses need to have available and the quantity of data generated by nurses can and must be managed electronically. Nursing administrators require this data to develop strategic plans for the organization.

Human Resources

All employers need to maintain a database for employee records. In addition to demographic and salary data, the database for licensed or certified health-care personnel contains unique fields for such areas as life support certification, health requirements (e.g., tuberculosis testing, hepatitis immunization, rubella titres), and performance appraisals. Administrators can use this human resources database to communicate with employees, examine staffing patterns, and create budget projections.

Medical Records Management

Costs are inherent in and reflected by medical records. It is expensive to keep records, but it is even more expensive if the information cannot be readily accessed. Therefore, nurses require computer programs that allow client records to be searched for such trends as the most common presenting diagnoses, number of cases by diagnosis-related groups, most expensive cases, length of stay, and client outcomes. Nurse informaticists can assist

BOX 24.6 COMPUTERS IN EDUCATION

Computers have contributed to accessible nursing education, and the internet has quickly become the primary medium for delivery of distance education. Online courses are entirely internet-based; the combination of internet-based and classroom-based courses is called web-enhanced or hybrid. Course management software (Blackboard, Web CT, ATutor, Moodle, and Angel) provides an organizing framework for delivery of the internet content of distance courses. Interactive videoconferencing, teleconferencing, and podcasting continue to revolutionize approaches to education.

administrators in the design and implementation of systems that allow for such searches to be generated, analyzed, printed, and distributed.

Facilities Management

Many aspects of managing buildings and non-nursing services can be facilitated by computers. Heating, air conditioning, ventilation, and alarm systems are computer controlled. Security devices, such as identification card readers, bar codes, and magnetic strip readers, permit only authorized personnel to enter client or private areas. Computers also manage and report inventory, tracking everything from pillowcases to syringes.

Budget and Finance

Computerized billing allows claims to be transmitted faster, with a greater likelihood of being complete and accurate compared with handwritten documents. Claims can be paid promptly and the agency will have better control over its financial status. Computers also affect cost savings by reducing the clerical time needed for accounts payable and receivable. In cases in which nursing can directly bill and be reimbursed by payers, the same benefits of computerized accounting apply.

The budget itself is generally a spreadsheet program. This software incorporates tracking as well as forecasting and planning. In uncertain times, the ability to perform what-if calculations is especially valuable.

Quality Assurance and Utilization Reviews

Both internal and external stakeholders in health-care organizations need assurance that the services and activities of the organization generate positive results. Once standards, pathways, key indicators, and other vital data have been identified and described, computers can facilitate accumulation and analysis of data for individuals and groups of clients. Quality is considered a process, not an end point. Applying this perspective, computerized systems are ideal for taking a snapshot of the institution's quality indices.

A utilization review consists of examining trends and looking for the best ways to use resources. For example, would clients who have had a fractured hip repaired have equivalent outcomes at a reduced cost if transferred from the hospital to a skilled nursing facility sooner? Studies can be conducted with computer analyses to answer such questions.

Computers in Nursing Research

Computers are invaluable assistants for both quantitative and qualitative nursing research. In each step of the research process, computers facilitate generation, refinement, analysis, and output. Computer resources are important components of the planning phase for any research project. The computer size and storage capacity must be adequate for the amount of data collected, and proper software programs must be in place to manage and analyze the data. Computerized word processing is also an integral component in the publication and dissemination of research.

Problem Identification

The first step of the research process is to identify and describe the problem of interest. Computers can be useful in locating relevant current literature and related concepts. Perhaps, unknown to the researcher, a solution to the problem has already been found and reported. A search of existing documents and emails to colleagues may help define the problem.

Literature Review

An exhaustive review of the literature can be time-consuming. Without computer access to online or CD-ROM bibliographic databases, the researcher must wade through huge volumes of publications. Most software programs that facilitate searches contain a thesaurus so the most appropriate terms can be selected. If the researcher determines that little has been published on the topic of interest, closely related terms and topics must also be searched. It is not unusual for a researcher to collect more than 100 pertinent articles or books during the literature review. The increase in availability of full-text journal articles online has made the electronic literature search process even more productive.

Electronic citation management software is available to assist in cataloguing references in a personal library database that can be searched and sorted by key words to produce reference lists related to a particular topic. Selected references can then be automatically formatted according to the requirements of the institution or journal.

Research Design

The design of a research study, including the choice of research method, is always driven by the research question. At the design stage, the investigator determines whether to use a qualitative or quantitative approach, what instruments will be used, and the types of analyses that will be carried out on the data to answer the research questions (see Chapter 3 for more information on research design). Computers can be used during this step to search the literature for established instruments or to design and test instruments that need to be developed for the particular study. The investigator would not likely select an instrument or design requiring extensive computer or mathematical analysis if such resources are not available.

Data Collection and Analysis

Once the types of data to be collected have been determined, the investigator will create computerized forms for collecting the data. These can include the informed consent document, a tool to collect demographic data, and recording forms for research variables. If possible, computer-readable forms are created so data can be scanned into the computer or the participant can key in responses directly (e.g., an online survey). This eliminates the errors that can occur if the researcher manually enters data into the computer.

It is particularly important that all variables for analysis are identified in a way the computer can recognize and manipulate. This identification can mean determining how to code the data for optimal manipulation. For example, will age be recorded in specific years or by categories, such as 1–10, 11–15, 16–20? Software programs can assist with the analysis and coding of qualitative data. Such programs as N6 (formerly Nud*ist, an acronym for Non-numerical Unstructured Data with powerful processes of Indexing, Searching, and Theorizing) and Ethnograph assist the researcher in finding and coding sections of text and organizing coded material.

When the variables have been coded, other programs can be used to calculate descriptive and analytic statistics. Calculations that formerly were time-consuming and complex can now be done quickly and accurately by computer programs. Commonly used software programs for quantitative data analysis include SPSS (Statistical Package for the Social Sciences), SAS (Statistical Analysis System), SysSTAT, and MYSTAT. These programs perform analyses and display output in tables, charts, lists, and other easily readable formats.

Research Dissemination

Research is of limited value if the findings are not widely dispersed to practitioners who can use them to improve their practice. Computer word-processing programs are used to author the final reports of research and to send them to various readerships. Many journals now require that manuscripts submitted for publication include both hard copy and electronic versions and the number of electronic journals is increasing. With the rapid growth of email, authors can also send an article or data to interested persons instantly. Computers speed completion of research projects and the availability of the findings to the public.

Computers are frequently used to present research at meetings. Using computer projectors to display screens of data and findings allows the researcher to highlight, modify, and manipulate content in an instant. In computer conferencing, researchers collaborate on a study from distant locations and can examine and analyze the data simultaneously on screen.

Research Grants

Funds are available from a variety of resources in support of nursing research. The budget in a grant application may include a request to purchase computers or software needed to carry out the proposed study. Funds may also be requested for data entry and to run statistical analyses.

Information about available grant funding is easily found online. Government federal grants for nursing projects can be downloaded from internet sites. Forms to be completed are computer generated and often must be submitted to the funding agency in electronic format.

Conclusion

The field of nursing informatics will continue to evolve as advances are made in the underlying disciplines of nursing science, computer science, information science, and telecommunications. Nurses are encouraged to keep abreast of these developments through involvement in such professional organizations as the Canadian Nursing Informatics Association. Nurses must understand the underpinnings of nursing informatics and be ready to take advantage of the opportunities provided by nursing informatics applications to advance the practice of nursing and to provide quality service to the public.

Case Study 24

As a nurse working for a home care agency in a rural town, you want your clients to receive current and accurate health information and care. High-speed computer access is available in your office and many of the residents have computers in their homes.

Critical Thinking Questions

1. You have a difficult clinical case and want to investigate possible interventions. How can computers assist in this endeavour?
2. You decide that sending photos of the client would be useful to your colleagues in providing input. Since time is an issue, you determine it would be expeditious to send them electronically. The client agrees to the photos but is worried about privacy in sending them through the computer. How would you handle this situation?
3. A client shares with you a website promising a cure for the client's illness. How would you respond?
4. You are considering enrolling in an advanced degree program offered online. What would be some of the advantages and disadvantages of such a program?

After working through these questions, go to the MyNursingLab at **http://www.mynursinglab.com** to check your answers.

KEY TERMS

nursing informatics
data
information
knowledge
management information system (MIS)
hospital information system (HIS)
electronic health record (EHR)
electronic medical record (EMR)
electronic patient record (EPR)
Canada Health Infoway
nurse informaticist
Canadian Classification of Health Interventions (CCI)
Health Outcomes for Better Information and Care (HOBIC)
patient portals
caregiver electronic record
telehealth
data warehousing
computer-assisted learning (CAL)
edutainment
distance education

CHAPTER HIGHLIGHTS

- Concerns regarding privacy and confidentiality of health records arise with the use of electronic databases and communications.
- Computers are used extensively to access data through online databases and internet searching. Many nursing journals are electronic.
- Computer-assisted instruction programs include tutorial, drill and practice, and simulations. Programs are also available that simulate the national licensure examination in Canada.
- In distance learning, faculty and students may be located far apart and communicate via computer, phone, fax, and video technologies.
- Bedside entry of nursing data is becoming more prevalent.
- Electronic health records (EHRs) enable longitudinal client data to be collected and made available to health-care providers who require it. Such data warehousing also enables research to be conducted on quality of care, client outcomes, and other parameters. However, no national standards exist for the structure or contents of these records.
- Nurses need to participate in the creation of taxonomies and classifications of electronic data.
- Hospital information systems (HISs) organize data from various areas in the hospital, such as admissions, medical records, clinical laboratory, pharmacy, and finance.
- Computer monitoring and diagnosing of client conditions is widespread. Examples include digital or tympanic thermometers; digital scales; pulse oximetry; ECG, telemetry, and hemodynamic monitoring; apnea monitors; fetal heart monitors; blood glucose analyzers; ventilators; IV pumps; CT scans; and MRI.
- Telehealth, the consultation of the health-care profession by using electronic means of communication, is a growing area generating both excitement and concerns.
- Data terminals in health-care settings allow for the placing of order requests and retrieval of client data. Appointments can be scheduled electronically.
- Computers are used by home health nurses to record client data and to communicate with the

central office. Clients can also have devices in their homes to monitor their own health status and send information about their condition to the nurse.

- Specialized computer software programs enable case managers to track clients' needs, resources, and health-care outcomes.
- Computers are used in nursing administration to manage personnel, human resources, facilities, budgets, quality assurance, utilization reviews, and staffing and scheduling.
- Each step of the nursing research process makes use of informatics technology. In particular, computer systems and applications are used to access literature, analyze data, and report findings.

ASSESS YOUR LEARNING

1. Which of the following best defines *nursing informatics*?
   - **a.** The compilation of information about nursing
   - **b.** The use of computer information systems in the practice of nursing
   - **c.** The results of research in nursing
   - **d.** The ability to take courses in an online format

2. Which of the following is the challenge most associated with the use of an electronic client record system?
   - **a.** Cost
   - **b.** Accuracy
   - **c.** Privacy
   - **d.** Curability

3. Which of the following is associated with electronic (e.g., internet-based) courses?
   - **a.** They take longer.
   - **b.** Everyone has to log on at the same time.
   - **c.** Interpersonal communication is not possible.
   - **d.** It is more difficult to establish a sense of community.

4. Which of the following is the primary advantage of using computers while conducting nursing research?
   - **a.** Locating potential participants
   - **b.** Analyzing the quantitative data
   - **c.** Disseminating the research findings
   - **d.** Designing the steps of the research plan

5. Which of the following is the most appropriate nursing response when a client insists that the practitioner use a treatment method discovered on an internet website?
   - **a.** "The treatment must be examined to see if it is appropriate."
   - **b.** "Most website treatments have not been studied or researched."
   - **c.** "Websites are like advertising; they are biased and may not be legitimate."
   - **d.** "The person who established the website is the only one who can use it on clients."

6. Which of the following is a primary role of the nurse in telehealth practice?
   - **a.** To inform the client's health-care provider of the call
   - **b.** To offer advice about the care being received by a client
   - **c.** To evaluate a previous response received by a client via telehealth
   - **d.** To deliver health information, services, and expertise over any distance

7. The electronic health record can improve patient care for which of the following reasons?
   - **a.** It can be easily transported by the patient and others.
   - **b.** It provides constant availability of patient health information.
   - **c.** It is understood and accepted by everyone.
   - **d.** It is easily accessed by any health professional anywhere in the world.

8. Which of the following classification systems did the Canadian Institute for Health Information develop?
   - **a.** Health on the Net
   - **b.** Canadian Registered Nurse Examination
   - **c.** Canadian Classification of Health Interventions
   - **d.** International Classification for Nursing Practice

9. Synthesis of information is known as which of the following?
   - **a.** Data
   - **b.** Instructions
   - **c.** Statistics
   - **d.** Knowledge

10. Including the source, currency, relevance or utility, and editorial review process for the information on a given website would contribute to which of the following criteria?
   - **a.** Interactivity
   - **b.** Content
   - **c.** Longevity
   - **d.** Validity

*After working through these questions, go to the MyNursingLab at **http://www.mynursinglab.com** to check your answers and see explanations.*

SUGGESTED READINGS

Bartholomew, K., & Curtis, K. (2004). High tech, high touch, why wait? *Nursing Management, 35*, 48, 50–54.

This article describes a variety of technological advances intended to assist the nurse in accurate and timely provision of care. It discusses concerns about why nurses have not moved more quickly to adopt them.

Langowski, C. (2005). The times they are a-changing: Effects of online nursing documentation systems. *Quality Management in Health Care, 14*, 121–125.

The author reports on five research studies aimed at determining whether bedside electronic charting made a difference in quality of documentation and nurses' satisfaction.

WEBLINKS

Canadian Nurses Association (CNA)

http://www.aiic.ca/cna/

The Canadian Nurses Association's (CNA) mission is to advance the quality of nursing in the interest of the public. The CNA is a federation of 11 provincial and territorial nursing associations representing more than 133 700 working registered nurses. The Canadian Nursing Informatics Association is an affiliate member of the CNA.

Canadian Nursing Informatics Association

http://www.cnia.ca/about.htm

This organization provides nursing leadership for the development of nursing and health informatics in Canada.

CHNET-Works

http://www.chnet-works.ca

This is an open electronic space in which community health researchers, decision makers, and practitioners can discuss current issues in community health. Participants can retrieve information, listen to debates among opinion leaders, and participate in online discussions.

Canadian Institute for Health Information (CIHI)

http://cihi.ca

The Canadian Institute for Health Information (CIHI) is an independent, pan-Canadian nonprofit organization that works to improve the health of Canadians and the health-care system through the provision of quality health information. The CIHI is mandated by Canada's health ministers to provide accurate and timely information to inform health policies, to support the Canadian health system, and to increase public awareness of factors affecting good health.

Canadian Society of Telehealth

http://www.cst-sct.org

Canada's first telehealth organization promotes and advocates for the development and implementation of telehealth practices locally and internationally.

COACH: Canada's Health Informatics Association

http://www.coachorg.com

COACH was founded in 1975 and currently has more than 1500 members. This organization aims to promote health informatics within the Canadian health system through education, information, networking, and communication.

Health Canada eHealth Resource Centre

http://www.hc-sc.gc.ca/hcs-sss/ehealth-esante/index_e.html

The eHealth Resource Centre is operated by Health Canada's Health and the Information Highway Division (HIHD). This site provides access to information available from the HIHD and other organizations.

NurseONE Portal

http://www.nurseone-inf-fusion.ca

Developed by the Canadian Nurses Association, this site provides access to reliable, credible, and useful clinical data to enhance evidence-based practice. More recently, e-Therapeutics, the website of the Canadian Pharmacists Association, has linked to the portal, bringing the most current evidence-based drug and therapeutic information to Canadian nurses.

Office of Nursing Policy (ONP)

http://www.hc-sc.gc.ca/hcs-sss/nurs-infirm/index_e.html

Initiated in 1999 by the Minister of Health, the Office of Nursing Policy (ONP) provides evidence-based nursing perspectives on a wide range of policy issues. "The creation of ONP signalled that nursing and nurses' perspectives would be influential in shaping the future of health care in Canada—because optimal nursing care means improved health care and healthier Canadians."

Special Interest Group on Nursing Informatics of the International Medical Informatics Association

http://www.imiani.org

The Special Interest Group on Nursing Informatics of the International Medical Informatics Association is an international nursing organization established in 1983 and dedicated to serving the specific needs of nurses in the field on nursing informatics.

Provincial Nursing Informatics Group

These provincial organizations provide a forum for nursing professionals to communicate and disseminate current developments in health-care information systems.

Nova Scotia Nursing Informatics Group (NSNIG)

http://www.nsnig.ca/aboutNSNIG.html

Ontario Nursing Informatics Group (ONIG)

http://www.onig.on.ca

Saskatchewan Nursing Informatics Association

http://members.fortunecity.com/nurse02/about.html

REFERENCES

Advisory Committee on Information and Emerging Technologies. (2005). *Pan-Canadian health information privacy and confidentiality framework.* Retrieved November 29, 2007, from http://www.hc-sc.gc.ca/hcs-sss/pubs/ehealth-esante/2005-pancanad-priv/index_e.html

Canadian Council on Health Services Accreditation. (2007). New developments to the accreditation program. Retrieved Feb. 3, 2007, from http://www.cchsa.ca/default.aspx?page=46&cat=34

Canada Health Infoway. (2005). *Who we are.* Retrieved February 17, 2007, from http://www.infoway-inforoute.ca/en/WhoWeAre/Overview.aspx

Canada Health Infoway. (2007). *New web portal to help millions of Canadians care for loved ones.* Retrieved January 7, 2008, from http://www.infoway-inforoute.ca/en/News-Events/InTheNews_long.aspx?uid=281

Canadian Institute for Health Information. (2004). *Canadian classification of interventions.* Retrieved January 7, 2008, from http://secure.cihi.ca/cihiweb/dispPage.jsp?cw_page=codingclass_cci_e

Canadian Nurses Association. (2002). *Position statement. Evidenced-based decision making and nursing practice.* Ottawa: Canadian Nurses Association. Retrieved October 3, 2007 from http://www.cna-nurses.ca/CNA/documents/pdf/publications/PS63_Evidence_based_Decision_making_Nursing_Practice_e.pdf

Canadian Nurses Association. (2006). *E-nursing strategy for Canada.* Retrieved February 17, 2007, from http://cna-aiic.ca

COACH: Canada's Health Informatics Association. (2007). *Coach guidelines for the protection of health information.* Toronto: Author.

Community Health Networks. (2008). *CHNET-Works!* Retrieved May 5, 2008, from http://www.chnet-works.ca/

Computer-Based Patient Record Institute. (1992). *Newsletters and membership brochures.* Chicago, IL: Author

Hannah, K. J. (2007). The state of nursing informatics in Canada. *Canadian Nurse, 103*(5), 18–22.

Health Canada. (2004). *Ehealth: Electronic health record.* Retrieved February 17, 2007, from http://www.hc-sc.gc.ca/hcs-sss/ehealth-esante/ehr-dse/index_e.html

Health Council of Canada. (2006). *Healthcare renewal in Canada: Clearing the road to quality.* Retrieved February 17, 2007, from http://www.healthcouncilcanada.ca/en/index.php?option=com_content&task=view&id=70&Itemid=72

Olsen, L. (2003). Privacy and confidentiality in an electronic age. *Chart, 100,* 9

Ontario Ministry of Health and Long-Term Care. (2007). *Health outcomes for better information and care.* Retrieved October 4, 2007, from http://www.health.gov.on.ca/english/providers/project/nursing/nursing_mn.html

Registered Nurses' Association of Ontario. (2008). *Nursing best practice guidelines.* Retrieved October 28, 2008, from http://www.rnao.org

Romanow, R. (2002). *Building on values: The future of health care in Canada.* Retrieved January 7, 2008, from http://www.hc-sc-gc.ca/english/pdf/romonow/pdfs/HCC_Final_Report.pdf

Staggers, N. T., & Thompson, C. B. (2002). The evolution of definitions for nursing informatics: A critical analysis and revised definition. *Journal of the American Medical Informatics Association, 9*(3), 255–261.

Statistics Canada. (2008). "Canadian internet use survey." *The Daily,* June 12. Retrieved October 28, 2008, from http://www.statcan.ca/Daily/English/080612/d080612b.htm

Chapter 25

Teaching and Learning

Client education is a major aspect of nursing practice and an important independent nursing function. Each provincial and territorial nursing association/college in Canada specifies in its standards that teaching is a required competent skill for nursing practice. Best practice guidelines on client-centred care also stress the importance of including teaching in client care; teaching needs to focus on providing information and teaching on issues for which clients have expressed needs and in a manner that is meaningful and relevant to them (Registered Nurses Association of Ontario, 2006). Legislation related to nursing also includes client teaching as a function of nursing, thereby making teaching a legal and professional responsibility.

Client education is multifaceted, involving promoting, protecting, maintaining, and restoring health, and helping clients cope with illness or altered health status. It involves teaching about reducing health risk factors, increasing a person's level of wellness, taking specific protective health measures, coping with diagnostic procedures and treatments, managing symptoms of illness, and optimizing health status. See Box 8.1 on page 138 for examples of health-promotion teaching topics for various age groups.

OBJECTIVES

After studying this chapter, you should be able to

1. Discuss the importance of the nurse's teaching role
2. Compare and contrast andragogy, pedagogy, and geragogy
3. Describe the three main constructs of learning theory
4. Discuss 10 factors that facilitate learning and 4 that interfere with learning throughout the lifespan
5. Use the nursing process to assess, diagnose, develop a plan, implement, and evaluate whether the client has met his or her goals
6. Describe the essential aspects of effective teaching
7. Discuss advantages and disadvantages of selected teaching strategies
8. Identify three methods to evaluate learning

Teaching

Teaching is a system of activities intended to produce learning. The teaching process is intentionally designed to produce specific learning. The teaching-learning process involves dynamic interaction between teacher and learner. Each participant in the process communicates information, emotions, perceptions, and attitudes to the other. The teaching process and the nursing process are much alike. See Table 25.1.

Nurses teach a variety of learners in a range of settings. They teach clients and their families or significant others in the hospital, in the home, or in assisted-living and long-term-care facilities. Nurses teach professional colleagues and subordinate health-care personnel in academic institutions, such as vocational schools, colleges, and universities, and in health-care facilities, such as hospitals or nursing homes.

Teaching Patients and Their Families

Nurses may teach individual clients in one-to-one teaching sessions or in groups. For example, the nurse may teach about wound care while changing a patient's dressing, or teach about diet, exercise, and other lifestyle behaviours that minimize the risk of a heart attack for a patient who has a cardiac problem. Patients are often taught in small groups in preparation for elective surgery in preadmission clinics. The nurse may also be involved in teaching family members or other support people who are caring for the patient. Nurses working in obstetric and pediatric areas teach parents and sometimes grandparents how to care for children.

Because of the decreased length of hospital stays, time constraints on patient education can occur. Nurses need to provide education that will ensure the patient's safe transition from one level of care to another and make appropriate plans for follow-up education in the home. Discharge plans must include both information about what the patient has been taught before transfer or discharge and information about what remains for the patient to learn to perform self-care in the home or other residence (see Chapter 13, the "Discharge Planning" section).

Teaching in the Community

Nurses are often involved in community health education programs. Such teaching activities may be part of the nurse's involvement in an organization, such as the Red Cross or Planned Parenthood, or with other sectors in the community concerned with the well-being of citizens. Community teaching activities may be aimed at large groups of people who have an interest in some aspect of health, such as nutrition classes, cardiopulmonary resuscitation (CPR), cardiac risk factor reduction, or bicycle or swimming safety programs. Community education programs, such as childbirth preparation classes or family planning classes, can also be for small groups or individual learners.

Teaching Health Personnel

Nurses are also involved in the instruction of professional colleagues through continuing education, inservice programs, and staff development. For example, experienced nurses can act as preceptors for students, new graduate nurses, or newly employed nurses. Nurses with specialized knowledge and experience can share that knowledge with nurses who are new to that practice setting. Experienced nurses in practice settings are often involved in the clinical teaching of nursing students. They also teach specialized courses, such as critical care nursing, perioperative nursing, and quality improvement or quality assurance processes.

Nurses can also be involved in teaching other health-care professionals. They may participate in the education of medical students or allied health students. In this capacity, the nurse educator clarifies the role of the nurse for other health professionals or how nurses can assist them in caring for their clients.

TABLE 25.1 Comparison of the Teaching Process and the Nursing Process

Step	Teaching Process	Nursing Process
1	Collect data; analyze client's learning strengths and deficits.	Collect data; analyze client's strengths and deficits.
2	Make educational diagnoses.	Make nursing diagnoses.
3	Prepare teaching plan: • Write learning objectives. • Select content and time frame. • Select teaching strategies.	Plan nursing goals or desired outcomes, and select interventions.
4	Implement teaching plan.	Implement nursing strategies.
5	Evaluate client learning based on achievement of learning objectives.	Evaluate client outcomes based on achievement of goal criteria.

Learning

Like all people, clients have a variety of learning needs. A **learning need** is a desire or a requirement to know something that is presently unknown by the learner. Learning needs include new knowledge but can also include a new or different skill or physical ability, a new understanding about an issue, new beliefs, or a way to change an old behaviour. **Learning** is a change in human disposition or capability that persists and that cannot be accounted for solely by growth.

Learning is a cognitive activity that is represented by a change in behaviour. **Cognitive** refers to the act of knowing or the development of knowledge. See Box 25.1 for attributes of learning.

An important aspect of learning is the individual's desire to learn and to act on the learning, referred to as **compliance**. In the health-care context, compliance is the extent to which a person's behaviour coincides with medical or health advice. Because the term *compliance* may imply that learners are not decision makers about their own health, the term **adherence** is often used to reflect the client's willingness to follow a treatment regimen. Bastable (2008) described both compliance and adherence as the ability to maintain "health-promoting regimens, which are determined largely by a health care provider" (p. 201). Nurses should be cautious about labelling clients as noncompliant. Clients may intend to follow the treatment regimen but may be unable to do so for a number of reasons. Adherence is best illustrated when the person recognizes and accepts the need to learn and then follows through with the appropriate behaviours that reflect the learning. For example, a person diagnosed as having diabetes willingly learns about the special diet needed and then plans and follows the learned diet.

Andragogy is the art and science of teaching adults, in contrast to **pedagogy**, the discipline concerned with helping children learn. **Geragogy** refers to the process involved in stimulating and helping older adults to learn (Hayes, 2005; John, 1988). Nurses can use the following principles of adult learning as a guide for client teaching (Hayes, 2005; Knowles, 1984):

- As people mature, they move from dependence to independence.
- An adult's previous experiences can be used as a resource for learning.
- An adult's readiness to learn is often related to a developmental task or social role.
- An adult is more oriented to learning when the material is useful immediately, not sometime in the future.

BOX 25.1 ATTRIBUTES OF LEARNING

Learning can take many forms, but they all share the same attributes:

- It is an experience that occurs inside the learner.
- It is the discovery of the personal meaning and relevance of ideas.
- It is a consequence of experience.
- It is a collaborative and cooperative process.
- It is an evolutionary process.
- It is a process that is both intellectual and emotional.

Learning Theories

Three main theoretical constructs of learning theory are behaviourism, cognitivism, and humanism. Nurses use behaviourist theory to identify what is to be taught and the reward for correct responses. Cognitive theory will enable nurses to recognize the developmental level of the learner and acknowledge the learner's motivation and environment. When using humanism, nurses focus on the feelings and attitudes of learners and help motivate them to take responsibilities for their own health.

BEHAVIOURISM Edward Thorndike originally advanced behaviourism. His major contribution was that learning should be based on the learner's behaviour. In addition to Thorndike, major behaviourist theorists include Pavlov, Skinner, and Bandura.

In the behaviourist school of thought, an act is called a *response* when it can be traced to the effects of a stimulus. Behaviourists closely observe responses and then manipulate the environment to bring about the intended change. Thus, to modify a person's attitude and response, a behaviourist "would either alter the stimulus condition in the environment or change what happens after a response occurs" (Bastable, 2008, p. 54).

Skinner's (1953) and Pavlov's (1927) work focused on conditioning behavioural responses to a stimulus that caused the response or behaviour. Skinner also introduced the importance of **positive reinforcement** in fostering repetition of an action. Bandura (1971) claimed that most learning comes from observational learning and instruction rather than from overt trial-and-error behaviour. Bandura's research focused on **imitation**, the process by which individuals copy or reproduce what they have observed, and **modelling**, the process by which a person learns by observing the behaviour of others.

Nurses applying behaviouristic theory will do the following:

- Provide sufficient practice time and both immediate and repeat testing and re-demonstration.
- Select teaching strategies that focus attention on desired behaviours.
- Praise the learner for correct behaviour, and provide positive feedback.
- Provide role models of the desired behaviour.

COGNITIVISM Cognitivism or **cognitive theory** depicts learning as a complex cognitive activity, that is, learning is largely a mental, an intellectual, or a thinking process. Based on their personal characteristics and experience, learners perceive their environments selectively. Cognitivists also emphasize the importance of the social, emotional, and physical contexts in which learning occurs, such as the teacher–learner relationship and environment. Developmental readiness and individual readiness (expressed as motivation) are other key factors.

Major cognitive theorists include Piaget, Lewin, and Bloom. Piaget's (1966) five major phases of cognitive development include the sensorimotor phase, the preconceptual phase, the intuitive phase, the concrete operations phase, and the formal intuitive phase. Each phase is discussed in Chapter 16. Lewin (1951) viewed learning as involving four different types of change: change in cognitive structure, change in motivation, change in the sense of belonging to the group, and gain in voluntary muscle control. His widely known theory of change has three basic stages: unfreezing, moving, and refreezing (see Chapter 26, the "Models of Change Management" section).

Bloom (1956) identified three domains or areas of learning: cognitive, affective, and psychomotor. The **cognitive domain** includes six intellectual skills, from the simple to the complex, beginning with knowing, comprehending, and applying. The **affective domain** includes feelings, emotions, interests, attitudes, and appreciations. It involves five major learning categories. The **psychomotor domain** includes motor skills, such as giving an injection.

Nurses should include cognitive and affective domains in every teaching plan, and when teaching a skill, they should include all three domains. For example, teaching a client how to irrigate a colostomy is in the psychomotor domain. But an important part of a teaching plan for a client with a colostomy is to teach why a specific amount of fluid is used and when the irrigation should be carried out; this part is in the cognitive domain. Helping the client accept the colostomy and maintain self-esteem is in the affective domain.

When applying cognitive theory, the nurse will do the following:

- Provide a social, an emotional, and a physical environment conducive to learning.
- Encourage a positive teacher–learner relationship.
- Select multisensory teaching strategies.
- Develop appropriate teaching approaches to target different learning styles.
- Assess a person's developmental and individual readiness to learn, and adapt teaching strategies to the learner's developmental level.
- Select learning outcomes and teaching strategies that encompass the cognitive, affective, and psychomotor domains of learning.

HUMANISM **Humanism** or humanistic learning theory focuses on both the cognitive and the affective qualities of the learner. Prominent members of this school of thought include Abraham Maslow and Carl Rogers. According to humanistic theory, learning is self-motivated, self-initiated, and self-evaluated. Each individual is viewed as a unique composite of biological, psychological, social, cultural, and spiritual factors. Learning focuses on self-development and achieving full potential; it is best when it is relevant to the learner. Autonomy and self-determination are important; the learner identifies the learning needs and takes the initiative to meet these needs. The learner is thus an active participant and takes responsibility for meeting his or her learning needs.

Nurses applying humanistic theory will do the following:

- Encourage the learners to establish goals, and promote self-directed learning.
- Encourage active learning by serving as a facilitator, mentor, or resource for the learner.
- Expose learners to new, relevant information and ask appropriate questions to encourage learners to seek answers.

Factors Affecting Learning

Many factors can facilitate or hinder learning by a client. The nurse should be aware of these factors, particularly when available teaching time is limited.

MOTIVATION **Motivation** to learn is the desire to learn. Motivation is generally greatest when a person experiences a need and believes the need will be met through learning. Often, the nurse's task is to help the client personally work through the problem and identify the need. Sometimes, clients or support people need help identifying relevant situational elements before they can see a need. For instance, clients with heart disease may need to know the effects of smoking before they recognize the need to stop smoking; or adolescents may need to know the consequences of an untreated sexually transmitted disease before they see the need for treatment.

READINESS **Readiness to learn** is the demonstrated behaviours that reflect not only the client's desire or willingness to learn but also his or her ability to learn at a specific time. For example, a client may want to learn self-care during a dressing change, but, when experiencing pain, he may not be able to learn. The nurse can provide pain medication to make the client more comfortable so that he is more able to learn. The nurse's role is often to encourage the development of readiness.

ACTIVE INVOLVEMENT When the learner is actively involved in the process of learning, learning becomes more meaningful, the learning is faster, and retention is better (Figure 25.1). Active learning promotes critical

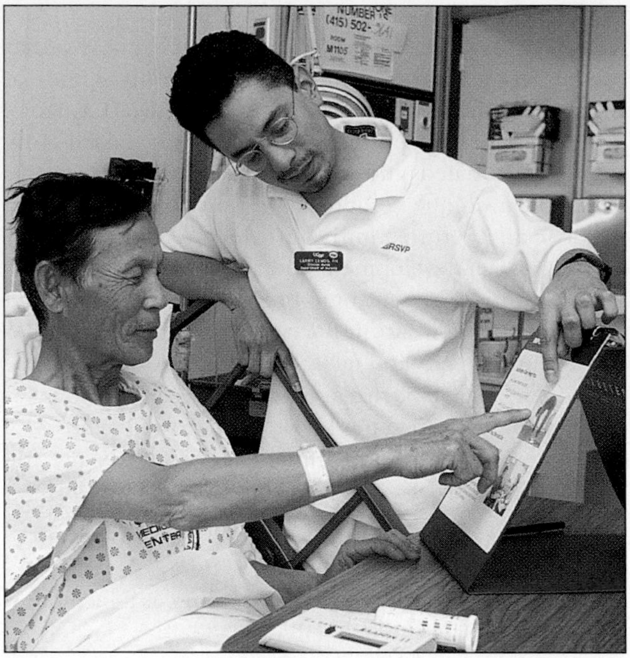

FIGURE 25.1 Learning is facilitated when the client is interested and actively involved.

thinking, enabling learners to problem solve more effectively and to apply the learning to their own situation. For example, clients who are actively involved in learning about their therapeutic diets may be more able to apply the principles being taught to their cultural food preferences and their usual eating habits. Passive learning, such as listening to a lecture or watching a film, does not foster optimal learning.

RELEVANCE The client can learn more easily if he or she can connect or relate the new knowledge or skills to what he or she already knows or has experienced. For example, if a client is diagnosed with hypertension and is overweight and has symptoms of headaches and fatigue, she is more likely to understand the need to lose weight if she remembers having more energy when she weighed less. The nurse needs to validate the relevance of learning with the client throughout the learning process.

FEEDBACK Feedback is information regarding a person's performance in meeting a desired goal, and it needs to be meaningful and given in a timely manner. Feedback that accompanies the practice of psychomotor skills helps the person learn those skills. Support of desired behaviour through praise, positively worded corrections, and suggestions of alternative methods are ways of providing positive feedback. Negative feedback, such as ridicule, anger, or sarcasm, can lead people to withdraw from learning.

NONJUDGMENTAL SUPPORT People learn best when they believe they are accepted and will not be judged. The person who expects to be judged as a "poor" or "good" client will not learn as well as the person who feels no such threat. Once learners have succeeded in accomplishing a task or understanding a concept, they gain self-confidence in their ability to learn. This reduces their anxiety about failure and can motivate greater learning. Nonjudgmental support contributes to a positive and safe climate for learning.

SIMPLE TO COMPLEX Learning is facilitated by material that is logically organized and proceeds from the *simple to the complex*. Such organization enables the learner to comprehend new information, assimilate it with previous learning, and form new understandings. Simple and complex are relative terms depending on the level at which the person is learning. What is simple for one person may be complex for another.

REPETITION Repetition of key concepts and facts facilitates retention of newly learned material. Providing information in several formats, including visual and verbal, and in examples, provides repetition and can reinforce learning. Practice of psychomotor skills, particularly with feedback from the nurse, improves performance of those skills and facilitates their transfer to another setting.

TIMING People retain information and psychomotor skills best when the time between learning and active use of the learning is short; the longer the time interval, the more learning is forgotten. Immediate application facilitates learning. For example, a person who is only shown literature and videotapes about administering insulin and is not permitted to administer the insulin until discharge from the hospital is unlikely to remember what was learned. Learning will be enhanced, however, if the person is encouraged to give injections while in hospital.

ENVIRONMENT An optimal learning environment facilitates learning by reducing distraction and providing physical and psychological comfort. It has a comfortable room temperature, good ventilation, and adequate lighting that is free from glare. Noise can distract the learner and interfere with listening and thinking. To facilitate optimal learning, nurses choose a time or location in which distractions in the environment are limited and interruptions are unlikely.

Privacy is essential for some learning. For example, when a client is learning to irrigate a colostomy, the presence of others can be embarrassing and, thus, interfere with learning. However, when a client is particularly anxious, having a support person present can give the client confidence. Some of the most common barriers to learning are described in Table 25.2.

EMOTIONS Emotions, such as fear, anger, and depression, can impede learning. A high level of anxiety resulting in agitation and the inability to focus or concentrate can also inhibit learning. Clients or families who are experiencing extreme emotional states may not hear spoken words or

TABLE 25.2 Common Barriers to Learning

Barrier	Explanation	Nursing Implications
Acute illness	The client requires all resources and energy to cope with illness.	Defer teaching until the client is less ill. Focus teaching on coping with symptoms.
Pain	Pain decreases a client's ability to concentrate.	Assess and control pain before teaching.
Prognosis	The client can be preoccupied with illness and unable to concentrate on new information.	Defer teaching to a better time. Focus the teaching on coping strategies.
Biorhythms	Mental and physical performances have a circadian rhythm.	Adapt time of teaching to suit the client.
Emotion (e.g., anxiety, denial, depression, grief)	Emotions require energy and distract from learning.	Deal with emotions and possible misinformation first. Provide repetition of content.
Language	The client may not be fluent in the nurse's language.	Obtain the services of an interpreter or a nurse with appropriate language skills. Increase teaching time.
Age		
Older adults	Vision, hearing, and motor control can be impaired in older adults.	Consider sensory and motor deficits in teaching plan.
Children	Children have a shorter attention span.	Plan shorter and more active learning episodes.
Culture or religion	There may be cultural or religious restrictions on certain types of knowledge, for example, birth control information.	Assess the client's cultural or religious needs when planning learning activities.
Physical disability	Visual, hearing, sensory, or motor impairments may interfere with a client's ability to learn.	Plan teaching activities appropriate to learner's physical abilities. For example, provide audio learning tools for the client who is blind, or large-print materials for the client whose vision is impaired.
Mental disability	Impaired cognitive ability may affect the client's capacity for learning.	Assess client's capacity for learning and plan teaching activities to complement the client's ability. Plan more complex learning for the client's caregivers.
Medications, treatment	Drugs and treatments can interfere with the client's ability to concentrate.	Assess the client for the best teaching time. Provide repetition if the client is drowsy or distracted.

may retain only part of the communication. Emotional responses, such as fear and anxiety, may be relieved by information that relieves uncertainty. Medications can be prescribed for extremely distraught clients or families to reduce their anxiety and put them in an emotional state in which understanding or learning can occur.

PHYSIOLOGICAL EVENTS Physiological events, such as a critical illness, pain, or sensory deficits, inhibit learning. Because the client cannot concentrate and apply energy to learning, the learning itself is impaired. The nurse should try to reduce the physiological barriers to learning as much as possible before teaching. Providing analgesics and rest before teaching is often helpful.

CULTURAL BARRIERS Language or values can be cultural barriers to learning. The client who does not understand the nurse's language will learn little. Western medicine may conflict with cultural healing beliefs and practices. Nurses need to be competent in providing culturally safe and sensitive care; otherwise, the client may be partially or totally noncompliant with recommended treatments; for example, clients who come from a culture that does not value slimness may have difficulty learning about a reducing diet.

PSYCHOMOTOR ABILITY Nurses must be aware of a client's psychomotor skills when planning teaching. Psychomotor skills can be affected by health. For example, an older adult who has severe osteoarthritis of the hands may not be able to tie a bandage. The following physical abilities are important for learning psychomotor skills:

1. *Muscle strength.* For example, an older client who cannot rise from a chair because of insufficient leg and muscle strength cannot be expected to learn to lift herself out of a bathtub without assistance.

2. *Motor coordination.* Gross motor coordination is required for such movements as walking, and fine motor coordination is needed when using utensils, such as a fork for eating. For example, a client who has advanced amyotrophic lateral sclerosis (ALS) involving lack of coordination and strength of the lower limbs will probably find it difficult to learn to use a walker.
3. *Energy.* Energy is required for most psychomotor skills, and learning these skills uses more energy. People who are ill or old often have limited energy resources; learning and carrying out these skills must be timed for when the client's energy sources are not depleted.
4. *Sensory acuity.* Sight is used for most learning (e.g., walking with crutches, changing a dressing, drawing a medication into a syringe). Clients who are visually impaired often need the assistance of a support person to carry out such tasks.

Nurse as Educator

Being an educator or teacher is an important and primary role for the nurse. Clients and families have the right to health information in order to make informed decisions about their health. The nurse is in a position to promote healthy lifestyles through the application of health knowledge, the change process, learning theories, and the nursing and teaching processes when teaching clients and their families.

Assessing

A comprehensive assessment of learning needs incorporates data from the nursing history and physical assessment and addresses the client's support system. It also considers client characteristics that can influence the learning process: readiness to learn, motivation to learn, and reading and comprehension level, for example. Assessing a person's stage of change and any barriers to change is also important and often overlooked (see Chapter 8, the section "The Transtheoretical Model: Stages of Health Behaviour Change").

NURSING HISTORY Several elements in the nursing history provide clues to learning needs. These elements include the client's (1) age, (2) understanding and perceptions of the health problem, (3) health beliefs and practices, (4) cultural factors, (5) economic factors, (6) learning style, and (7) support systems. Examples of open-ended interview questions to elicit this information are shown in the Assessment: Interview box.

AGE Age provides information on the person's developmental status that may indicate the need for distinctive health teaching content and teaching approaches. Simple questions to school-age children and adolescents will elicit information on what they know. Observing children at play provides information about their motor and intellectual development as well as their relationships with other children. For older people, conversation and questioning may reveal slow recall or limited psychomotor skills, sensory deficits, and learning difficulties (see the Lifespan Considerations box on page 522).

CLIENT'S UNDERSTANDING OF HEALTH PROBLEM Clients' perceptions of their current health problems and concerns can indicate knowledge deficits or misinformation. In addition, the effects of the problem on the client's usual activities can alert the nurse to other areas requiring instruction. For example, people who cannot manage self-care at home often need information about community resources and services.

HEALTH BELIEFS AND CULTURAL PRACTICES The client's health beliefs and practices must be considered in any teaching plan. The health belief model described in Chapter 7 provides a predictor of preventive health behaviour.

Many cultural groups have their own beliefs and practices, a number of them related to diet, health, illness, and lifestyle. Nurses need to know how the practices and values held by clients affect their learning needs.

Folk beliefs of certain groups can also affect learning. Although the client may readily understand the health-care information being taught, this learning may not be implemented in the home where folk health practices prevail (see Chapter 10, the "Health Beliefs and Practices" section and the section "Transcultural teaching" later in this chapter).

ECONOMIC FACTORS Economic factors can also affect a client's learning. For example, a client who cannot afford to obtain a new sterile syringe for each injection of insulin may find it difficult to learn to administer the insulin when the nurse teaches that a new syringe should be used each time.

LEARNING STYLE Individuals have their own best ways of learning. Some people are visual learners and learn best by watching; others learn by manipulating equipment and discovering how it works. Some people can learn well from reading things presented in an orderly fashion, and others learn best in groups. For some, stressing the thinking part of a skill and its logic will promote learning. For other people, stressing the feeling part or interpersonal aspect motivates and promotes learning.

A client's learning style may be based in his or her cultural background. For example, clients from cultures that have a strong oral tradition may prefer educational videos presented in their language (Munoz & Luckmann, 2005).

The nurse may not have the time to assess each learner's particular learning style and then adapt teaching accordingly; what the nurse can do, however, is to ask clients how they like to learn. Many people know what

ASSESSMENT: INTERVIEW

Learning Needs and Characteristics

The use of opened-ended questions can help nurses find clues to clients' learning needs.

PRIMARY HEALTH PROBLEM

- Tell me what you know about your current health problem. What do you think caused it?
- What concerns do you have about it?
- How has the problem affected what you can or cannot do during your usual activities (e.g., work, recreation, shopping, housework)?
- What do you or did you do at home to relieve the problem? How helpful was it?
- How have the treatments you have started helped your problem?
- What, if any, difficulties have the treatments caused you (e.g., inconvenience, cost, discomfort)?
- Tell me about the tests (surgery, treatments) you are going to have.

HEALTH BELIEFS

- How would you describe your health generally?
- What things do you usually do to keep healthy?
- What health problems do you think you may be at risk for because of family history, age, diet, occupation, inadequate exercise, or habits, such as smoking?
- What changes would you be willing to make to decrease your risk for these problems or to improve your health?

CULTURAL FACTORS

- What language do you use most often when speaking and writing?
- Do you seek the advice of another health practitioner?
- Do you use herbs or other medications or treatments commonly used in your cultural group?
- Does your current doctor know about these?
- What advice or treatments given previously by your doctor conflicted with values or beliefs you consider important?
- When a conflict arose, what did you do?

LEARNING STYLE

- Note the client's age and developmental level.
- What is your highest level of formal education?
- Do you like to read?
- Where do you obtain health information (e.g., physician, nurse, magazines, books, pharmacist, and so on)?
- How do you best learn new things?
  a. By reading about them
  b. By asking questions and discussing them
  c. By watching a demonstration
  d. By using web-based or computer resources
  e. By listening to the teacher
  f. By first being shown how something works and then doing it
  g. By working on your own or in a group
  h. By reflecting on what was learned

CLIENT SUPPORT SYSTEM

- Would you like a family member or friend to help you learn about things that you need to do to take care of yourself?
- Who do you think would be interested in learning with you?

helps them learn, and the nurse can use this information in planning the teaching. In teaching a group, the nurse can use a variety of teaching techniques and vary activities to meet clients' preferred ways of learning. One technique will be effective for some clients, whereas other techniques may be better suited to clients with different learning styles.

Client Support System The nurse explores the client's support system to determine the extent to which others can enhance learning and offer support. Family members or a close friend may help the client perform required skills at home and maintain required lifestyle changes.

PHYSICAL EXAMINATION The visual inspection part of the physical examination provides useful clues to clients' learning needs, such as mental status, energy level, and nutritional status, as well as their physical capacity to learn and to perform self-care activities. For example, visual ability, hearing ability, and muscle coordination affect the selection of content and approaches to teaching.

READINESS TO LEARN A client who is ready may search out information, for instance, by asking questions, reading books or articles, talking to others, and generally showing interest. The person who is not ready to learn is more likely to avoid the subject or situation. In addition, the unready client may change the subject when it is brought up by the nurse. For example, the nurse might say, "I was wondering about a good time to show you how to change your dressing," and the client responds, "Oh, my wife will take care of everything."

The nurse assesses for the following:

- *Physical readiness.* Is the client able to focus on things other than physical status? Is pain, fatigue, or immobility using up all of the client's energy?
- *Emotional readiness.* Is the client emotionally ready to learn self-care activities? Clients who are extremely anxious, depressed, or grieving over their health status are not ready.
- *Cognitive readiness.* Can the client think clearly at this point? Are the effects of anaesthesia and analgesics altering the client's level of consciousness?

Lifespan Considerations

Special Teaching Considerations

OLDER ADULTS

Older adults often have chronic illnesses that require multiple treatments or medications. Health teaching will focus on the same areas as with other ages—health and wellness promotion and prevention of illness and accidents—but often the needs are greatest in learning to manage their lives in order to live with their chronic health conditions and to maintain optimal health and functioning. For older adults to be motivated to learn, the material must be practical and have meaning for them individually, especially if the information is new to them. Special considerations in teaching older adults include the following:

- Health promotion is a priority need and should include these areas:
  - Exercise
  - Nutrition
  - Safety habits
  - Regular health checkups
  - Understanding of medications
- Set achievable goals—involve the client and family in doing this.
- If developing written materials:
  - Use large print (e.g., at least 14-point font) in bulleted format.
  - Use buff-coloured paper (which avoids the glare from white paper).
  - Present the information at a Grade 5 to Grade 6 reading level.
- Increase time for teaching and allow for rest periods as processing of information is slower.
- Ensure that verbal presentation of material is well organized and that there is minimal distraction.
- Repeat information if necessary.
- Use return demonstrations with psychomotor skills, such as teaching someone to learn to do insulin injections.
- Determine where clients obtain most of their health information (e.g., newspapers, magazines, television).
- Use examples that they can relate to in their daily lives.
- Be aware of sensory deficits, such as hearing and vision.
- Use the setting with which the individual is most comfortable—either a group or one-on-one setting.
- If noncompliance is a problem, investigate the cause. It could be due to lack of finances, transportation problems, poor access to medical care, and so on.

Older adults come with a lifetime of experiences and learned knowledge of their own. Respect this and always have them use their strengths to work with any problems. Positive reinforcement and ongoing evaluation of what has been taught are important factors in effective health teaching with older adults.

CHILDREN

It has often been said that the parent is a child's first and most important teacher. Every interaction between a child and a parent (or other adults and children) is a moment in which teaching and learning occurs, often unconsciously. Sometimes the results are ones parents desire and strive for; sometimes they are not what the parent wanted.

To make parents more aware of the teaching they are doing, nurses can point out how the parent is using the concept of a *teaching loop* and how formal teaching strategy can be applied more consciously to many parent–child interactions.

The teaching loop consists of four specific teaching behaviours that give children verbal instruction, role modelling, and positive feedback:

- *Alerting:* Get children's attention by calling their name, touching them, or making a noise.
- *Instructing:* Give the child a short, specific instruction about what is to be done; modelling or demonstrating behaviour can also be done (e.g., "Try it like this...").
- *Performing:* Give the child opportunity to practise the task, play with the toy, and explore the materials being used. Provide enough time but with some structure or direction.
- *Reinforcing:* Give the child feedback; a positive or negative comment (e.g., "You poured the milk very well" or "No, that's not quite right; try turning it this way") that is specific to the task lets children know how they have done and encourages them to continue to learn.

Sources: From *Gerontological Nursing: Promoting Successful Aging with Older Adults,* 3rd ed. (pp. 67–75), by M. Stanley, K. Blair, and P. G. Beare, 2005, Philadelphia, PA: Davis; "Designing Written Medication Instructions: Effective Ways to Help Older Adults Self-Medicate," by K. Hayes, 2005, *Journal of Gerontological Nursing, 31*(5), pp. 5–10, adapted with permission; and "The Observation of Anglo-Mexican and Chinese-American Mothers Teaching Their Young Sons," by D. Steward and M. Steward, 1973, *Child Development*, *44*, pp. 329–337.

Nurses can promote readiness to learn by providing physical and emotional support during the critical stage of recovery. As the client stabilizes physically and emotionally, the nurse can provide opportunities to learn.

MOTIVATION As discussed earlier, motivation relates to whether the client wants to learn and is usually greatest when the client is ready, the learning need is recognized, and the information being offered is meaningful to the client. Nurses can increase a client's motivation in several ways:

- By relating the learning to something the client values and helping the client see the benefits of changing behaviour
- By helping the client make the learning situation pleasant and nonthreatening
- By encouraging self-direction and independence
- By demonstrating a positive attitude about the client's ability to learn
- By offering continuing support and encouragement as the client attempts to learn (i.e., positive reinforcement)

- By creating a learning situation in which the client is likely to succeed (succeeding in small tasks motivates the client to continue learning)

HEALTH LITERACY **Health literacy** is the ability to read, understand, and act on health information, including such tasks as comprehending prescription labels, interpreting appointment slips, completing health insurance forms, and following instructions for diagnostic tests (Redman, 2004). Limited health literacy skills are often greater among certain groups: older adults, people of limited education, poor people, minority populations, and people with limited English proficiency.

Low health literacy skills are associated with poor health outcomes and higher health-care costs. Health Canada (2003) recognized that low literacy has direct and indirect effects on almost all aspects of health. Clients with low literacy skills have less information about health promotion and management of a disease process for themselves and their families. They may be unable to read the educational materials or miss the opportunity for employment where literacy is involved.

It is a challenge for the nurse to teach clients with low or no reading and writing skills. However, such teaching is vitally important because clients with low literacy skills need learning opportunities to improve their health practices (see the Teaching: Clinical box on teaching clients with low literacy levels).

READING LEVEL The nurse should not assume that a client's reading level is equal to the highest grade or level of formal education the client has completed. Most word-processing programs have a feature (called "show readability statistics") under Tools, then Options, and the Spelling and Grammar tab that will calculate the readability of the written material for you. Written health education materials should be written for lower reading levels, such as a Grade 5 or Grade 6 level (Aldridge, 2004). People with good reading skills are not offended by simple reading material and prefer easy-to-read information (see the Teaching: Clinical box on developing written teaching aids).

Box 25.2 describes data clusters on Mr. Steinberg and Mr. Evans. The way these clusters would be used is shown in Box 25.3.

BOX 25.2 DATA CLUSTERS

CLIENT A: MR. STEINBERG
Data cluster: The nurse brings Mr. Steinberg the first dose of a medication ordered by his physician. The nurse asks whether anyone has explained what this medication is and why he is taking it. He says no.

CLIENT B: GEORGE EVANS
Data cluster: George Evans is a 45-year-old man who has come to the clinic for his annual physical examination. He expresses concern about his family history of heart disease and requests information about activities to decrease his risk of heart disease.

TEACHING: CLINICAL

Teaching Clients with Low Literacy Levels

Nurses can use several methods to improve their success in teaching clients with low or no reading and writing skills:

- Use multiple teaching methods: Show pictures. Read important information. Lead a small group discussion. Role-play. Demonstrate a skill. Provide hands-on practice.
- Emphasize key points in simple terms and provide examples.
- Limit the amount of information in a single teaching session by providing short and frequent sessions.
- Associate new information with something the client already knows or associates with his or her job or lifestyle.
- Reinforce information through repetition.
- Involve the client in the teaching.
- Obtain feedback: Ask the client specific questions about the information presented or ask the client to repeat it in his or her own words.
- Avoid handouts with many pages or a classroom lecture format with a large group.

TEACHING: CLINICAL

Developing Written Teaching Aids

When developing any written teaching aids, nurses should consider the following guidelines:

- Keep reading level at or below a Grade 5 level.
- Write abbreviations out in full, and define technical terms.
- Use active, not passive, voice.
- Use easy, common words of one or two syllables (e.g., *use* instead of *utilize,* or *give* instead of *administer*).
- Use the second person (*you*) rather than the third person (*the client*).
- Use a large type size (14 to 16 point), especially for older adults.
- Write short sentences.
- Avoid using all capital letters.
- Place priority information first and repeat more than once.
- Use bold for emphasis.
- Use simple pictures, drawings, or cartoons, if appropriate.
- Leave plenty of white space to create an uncluttered appearance.
- Summarize key points.
- Obtain feedback from nurses and clients.

BOX 25.3 IDENTIFYING NURSING DIAGNOSES, OUTCOMES, AND INTERVENTIONS: CLIENTS REQUIRING TEACHING

CLIENT A: MR. STEINBERG

Nursing Diagnosis or Definition	Sample Desired Outcome (NOC)*/ Definition	Indicator	Selected Interventions (NIC)**/ Definition	Sample NIC Activities
Deficient knowledge (medication information): Related to lack of exposure to newly prescribed medication and absence or deficiency of cognitive information related to specific topic	*Knowledge: medication:* Extent of understanding conveyed about the safe use of medication	*Substantial:* • Identification of correct medication name • Description of medication • Description of side effects of medication • Description of medication precautions	*Teaching prescribed medication:* Preparing a client to safely take prescribed medications and monitor for their effects	• Inform the client of both the generic and brand names of the medication. • Instruct the client on the purpose and action of the medication. • Instruct the client on the dosage, route, and duration of the medication. • Instruct the client on specific precautions to observe when taking the medication (e.g., no driving), as appropriate.

* Bulechek, G. M., Butcher, H. K., & Dochterman, J. C. (Eds.). (2008). *Nursing interventions classification (NIC)*. St. Louis, MO: Mosby Elsevier.
** Moorhead, S., Johnson, M., & Maas, M. (Eds.). (2004). *Nursing outcomes classification (NOC)/Iowa Outcomes Project*. St. Louis, MO: Mosby.

CLIENT B: MR. EVANS

Nursing Diagnosis or Definition	Sample Desired Outcome (NOC)*/ Definition	Indicator	Selected Interventions (NIC)**/ Definition	Sample NIC Activities
Health-seeking behaviour (nutrition, activity, and exercise information): To reduce risk of heart disease; active seeking (by person in stable health) of ways to alter personal health habits or the environment in order to move toward a higher level of health	*Adherence behaviour:* Self-initiated action taken to promote wellness, recovery, and rehabilitation	*Often demonstrated:* • Asks health-related questions when indicated • Seeks health-related information from a variety of sources • Uses strategies to eliminate unhealthy behaviours	*Self-modification assistance:* Reinforcement of self-directed change initiated by the client to achieve personally important goals	• Assist the client in identifying target behaviours that need to change to achieve the desired goal. • Assist the client in identifying a specific goal for change. • Appraise the client's present knowledge and skill level in relationship to the desired change. • Explore with the client potential barriers to changing behaviour.

* Bulechek, G. M., Butcher, H. K., & Dochterman, J. C. (Eds.). (2008). *Nursing interventions classification (NIC)*. St. Louis, MO: Mosby Elsevier.
** Moorhead, S., Johnson, M., & Maas, M. (Eds.). (2004). *Nursing outcomes classification (NOC)/Iowa Outcomes Project*. St. Louis, MO: Mosby.

Diagnosing

Nursing diagnoses for clients with learning needs can be designated in two ways: as the client's primary concern or problem, or as the etiology of a nursing diagnosis associated with the client's response to health alterations or dysfunction.

LEARNING NEED AS THE DIAGNOSTIC LABEL NANDA International (formerly the North American Nursing Diagnosis Association) includes the following diagnostic labels appropriate to a client's learning needs when the learning need is the primary concern:

- *Deficient knowledge:* "absence or deficiency of cognitive information related to a specific topic" (NANDA International, 2007, p. 109). Whenever the diagnostic label *deficient knowledge* is used, either the client is seeking health information or the nurse has identified a learning need. The area of deficiency should always be included in the diagnosis.

The following are examples that use the NANDA International label deficient knowledge as the primary concern:

- *Deficient knowledge: low-cholesterol diet* related to inexperience with newly ordered therapy
- *Deficient knowledge: home safety hazards* related to declining physical mobility

Wilkinson (2005) stresses that if *deficient knowledge* is used as the primary concern, one client goal must be "client will acquire knowledge about." The nurse needs to provide information that has the potential to change the client's behaviour rather than focus on the behaviours caused by the client's lack of knowledge.

A second nursing diagnostic label in which a learning need may be the primary concern or problem is as follows:

- *Health-seeking behaviours:* "active seeking (by a person in stable health) of ways to alter personal health habits and/or the environment in order to move toward a higher level of health" (NANDA International, 2007, p. 88).

When this diagnostic label is used, the client is seeking health information; the client does not have an altered response or dysfunction at the time but is seeking information to improve health or prevent illness. This diagnosis is especially appropriate for clients attending community health education programs. The following are examples that use the NANDA International label *health-seeking behaviour* as the primary concern:

- *Health-seeking behaviour: exercise and activity* related to desire to improve health behaviours and decrease the risk of osteoporosis. This diagnosis is appropriate for the client who has identified a personal health risk for osteoporosis and wants to minimize that risk through exercise.
- *Health-seeking behaviour: home safety hazards* related to desire to minimize risk of injury. This diagnosis is appropriate for parents of a toddler who are seeking information to ensure that their home is safe for their child.

Clinical applications of these kinds of diagnoses are shown in Box 25.3, using the assessment data from Box 25.2.

Planning

Developing a teaching plan is accomplished in a series of steps. Involving the client at this time promotes the formation of a meaningful plan and stimulates client motivation. The client who helps formulate the teaching plan is more likely to achieve the desired outcomes. See the Teaching: Clinical box on page 526 for a sample teaching plan for wound care.

DETERMINING TEACHING PRIORITIES The client's learning needs must be ranked according to priority. The client and the nurse should do this together, with the client's priorities always being considered. Once a client's priorities have been addressed, the client is generally more motivated to concentrate on other identified learning needs. For example, a man who wants to know all about coronary artery disease may not be ready to learn how to change his lifestyle until he meets his own need to learn more about the disease. Nurses can also use theoretical frameworks, such as Maslow's (1970) hierarchy of needs, to establish priorities (see Chapter 11, the section "Needs Theories").

SETTING LEARNING OUTCOMES Learning outcomes can be considered the same as desired outcomes for other nursing diagnoses. They are written in the same way. Like client outcomes, learning outcomes should do the following:

- State the client (learner) behaviour or performance, not nurse behaviour. For example, "Identify personal risk factors for heart disease" (client behaviour), not "Teach the client about cardiac risk factors" (nurse behaviour).
- Reflect an observable, measurable activity. The performance may be visible (e.g., walking) or invisible (e.g., adding a column of figures). However, it is necessary to be able to deduce whether an unobservable activity has been mastered from some performance that represents the activity. Therefore, the performance of an outcome might be written as "selects low-fat foods from a menu" (observable), not "understands low-fat diet" (unobservable). Selected measurable verbs used for learning outcomes are shown in Box 25.4 on page 527. Avoid using such words as *knows, understands, believes,* and *appreciates;* they are neither observable nor measurable.
- Use conditions or modifiers as required to clarify what, where, when, or how the behaviour will be performed. Examples are "demonstrates four-point crutch gait *correctly*" (condition), "irrigates his colostomy *independently* (condition) as taught," or "states *three* (condition) factors that affect blood glucose level."
- Include criteria specifying the time by which learning should have occurred. For example, "the client will state three things that affect blood glucose level *by end of second class on diabetes.*"

Learning outcomes can reflect mastery of concepts, moving from the simple to the complex. For example, the learning outcome "the client will list cardiac risk factors" is a low-level knowledge outcome that simply requires the learner to identify cardiac risk factors; it does not suggest application of the knowledge to the learner's own behaviours. The learning outcome "the client will describe *personal* cardiac risk factors" requires that the learner not

TEACHING: CLINICAL

Sample Teaching Plan: Wound Care

Assessment of learner: A 24-year-old male college student suffered a 7 cm laceration on the lower anterior part of the left leg during a hockey game. The laceration was cleaned, sutured, and bandaged. The client was given an appointment to return to the health clinic in 10 days for suture removal. Client states that he lives in the college dormitory and is able to care for wound if given instructions. Client is able to understand and read English. Assessed to be in the *preparation* and *action* stages of change.

- *Nursing diagnosis:* Deficient knowledge (care of sutured wound) related to no prior experience.
- *Long-term goals:* Client's wound will heal completely without infection or other complications.
- *Intermediate goal:* At clinic appointment, client's wound will be healing without signs of infection, loss of function, or other complication.
- *Short-term goals:* Client will (a) correctly list three signs and symptoms of wound infection and (b) correctly perform a return demonstration of wound cleansing and bandaging.

Behavioural Outcomes	Content Outline	Teaching Methods
On completion of the instructional session, the client will		
1. Describe normal wound healing	I. Normal wound healing	Describe normal wound healing with the use of audiovisuals
2. Describe signs and symptoms of wound infection	II. Infection Signs and symptoms include the wound being warm to the touch, malalignment of the wound edges, and purulent wound drainage. Signs of systemic infection include fever and malaise.	Discuss the mechanism of wound infection. Use audiovisuals to demonstrate infected wound appearance. Provide a handout describing signs and symptoms of wound infection.
3. Identify equipment needed for wound care	III. Wound care equipment a. Cleansing solution as prescribed by physician (e.g., clear water, mild soap and water, or antimicrobial solution) b. Bandaging material: Telfa, gauze wrap, adhesive tape	Demonstrate the equipment needed for cleansing and bandaging wound. Provide a handout listing equipment needed.
4. Demonstrate wound cleansing and bandaging	IV. Demonstration of wound cleansing and bandaging on the client's wound or a mannequin	Demonstrate wound cleansing and bandaging on the client's wound or a mannequin. Provide a handout describing the procedure for cleansing and bandaging the wound.
5. Describe appropriate action if questions or complications arise	V. Resources available for client's questions include health clinic and emergency department	Discuss available resources. Provide a handout listing available resources and a follow-up treatment plan.
6. Identify date, time, and location of follow-up appointment for suture removal	VI. Follow-up treatment plan; where and when	Provide written instructions.

Evaluation: The client will do the following:

1. Correctly describe normal wound healing and signs and symptons of wound infection.
2. Return demonstration of wound cleansing and bandaging.
3. State contact person and telephone number to obtain assistance.
4. State date, time, and location of follow-up appointment.

only know cardiac risk factors but also know personal behaviours that increase risk for cardiac disease.

In writing learning outcomes, the nurse must be specific about what behaviours and knowledge (cognitive, psychomotor, and affective) the learner must have to be able to positively influence his or her health state. In most cases, the learning needs are more complex than simple acquisition of knowledge and include the application of that knowledge to the learner (refer back to Box 25.3 on page 524).

CHOOSING CONTENT What is to be taught is determined by learning outcomes. For instance, "identify

BOX 25.4 EXAMPLES OF VERBS FOR WRITING LEARNING OUTCOMES

Cognitive Domain	Affective Domain	Psychomotor Domain
Compares	Accepts	Assembles
Describes	Attends	Calculates
Evaluates	Chooses	Changes
Explains	Discusses	Demonstrates
Identifies	Displays	Measures
Labels	Initiates	Moves
Lists	Joins	Organizes
Names	Participates	Shows
Plans	Shares	
Selects	Uses	
States		
Writes		

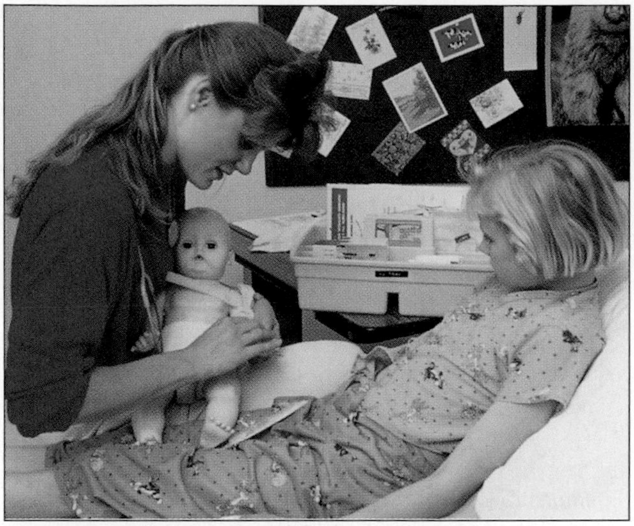

FIGURE 25.2 Teaching materials and strategies should be suited to the client's age and learning abilities.

appropriate sites for insulin injection" means the nurse must include content about the body sites suitable for insulin injections. Nurses can select among many sources of information, including books, nursing journals, and other nurses and health-care professionals. Whatever sources the nurse chooses, content should be

- Accurate and current
- Based on learning outcomes
- Adjusted for the learner's age, developmental stage, culture, and ability

Evidence-Informed Practice

Dietary Strategies for Coping with Inflammatory Bowel Disease

In this qualitative study in southern Ontario, Fletcher and Schneider (2006) addressed the learning needs of women with inflammatory bowel disease. Clients who live with this chronic debilitating gastrointestinal disorder must learn to manage the symptoms of the disease. Besides controlling food consumption, women in this study also had to learn about managing their stress, making lifestyle choices, identifying individual trigger foods, and making healthy eating choices.

NURSING IMPLICATIONS: Nurses must provide clients with evidence-informed information on specific dietary strategies and teach their clients ways to develop lifelong strategies for living with their chronic illness.

Source: Based on "Is There Any Food I Can Eat? Living with Inflammatory Bowel Disease and/or Irritable Bowel Syndrome," by P. C. Fletcher and M. A. Schneider, 2006, *Clinical Nurse Specialist, 20*(5), pp. 241–247.

- Selected with consideration of how much time and what resources are available for teaching

SELECTING TEACHING STRATEGIES The method of teaching that the nurse chooses should be suited to the individual and to the material to be learned (Figure 25.2). For example, the person who cannot read needs material presented in other ways; a one-to-one presentation session with question and answer is usually the best strategy for teaching a client how to give an injection; and group discussion is a useful way of discussing effective coping strategies. See Table 25.3 for selected teaching strategies.

TEACHING TOOLS Having the right tools facilitates teaching. Tools can include handouts, equipment and supplies, photo albums, overhead transparencies, flip charts, bulletin boards, models of the human body, audio and videotapes, closed-circuit television, and computer programs. Tools need to be carefully selected for the individual client on the basis of the nurse's assessment.

ORGANIZING LEARNING EXPERIENCES To save nurses time in constructing their own teaching guides, some health agencies have developed teaching guides for teaching sessions that nurses commonly give. These guides standardize content and teaching methods and make it easier for the nurse to plan and implement client teaching. Standardized teaching plans also ensure consistency of content for the learner, thereby decreasing the risk of confusion if different practices are taught. For example, when teaching infant bathing, the nurses on the unit should be consistent about which soaps are appropriate for the infant's bath and which are not. Whether the nurse is implementing a plan devised by another or developing an individualized teaching plan, some guidelines can help the nurse organize the learning experience:

TABLE 25.3 Selected Teaching Strategies

Strategy	Major Type of Learning	Characteristics
Explanation or description (e.g., lecture)	Cognitive	• Teacher controls content and pace. • Learner is passive and, therefore, retains less information than when actively participating. • Feedback is determined by teacher. • Can be given to individual or group.
One-to-one discussion	Affective, cognitive	• Encourages participation by learner. • Permits reinforcement and repetition at learner's level. • Permits introduction of sensitive subjects.
Answering questions	Cognitive	• Learner guides content taught. • Learner may need to overcome cultural perception that asking questions is impolite. • Can be used with individuals and groups.
Demonstration	Psychomotor	• Can be used with individuals, small or large groups. • Does not permit use of equipment by learners; learner is passive.
Discovery	Cognitive, affective	• Teacher guides problem-solving situation. • Learner is active participant. • Retention of information is high.
Group discussions	Affective, cognitive	• Learner can obtain assistance from supportive group. • Group members learn from one another. • Teacher needs to keep the discussion focused.
Practice	Psychomotor	• Allows repetition and immediate feedback. • Permits hands-on experience.
Printed and audiovisual materials	Cognitive	• Forms include books, pamphlets, films, programmed instruction, and computer learning. • Learners can proceed at their own speed. • Nurse can act as resource person. • Learner can learn independently.
Role-playing	Affective, cognitive	• Permits expression of attitudes, values, and emotions. • Can assist in development of communication skills. • Teacher must create supportive, safe environment for learners.
Modelling	Affective, psychomotor	• Nurse sets example by attitude, psychomotor skill.
Computer-assisted learning programs	All types of learning	• Learner is active. • Learner controls pace. • Provides immediate reinforcement and review. • Use with individuals or groups.

- Start with something the learner is concerned about; for example, before learning how to self-administer insulin, an adolescent wants to know how to adjust his or her lifestyle and still play sports.
- Review what the learner knows, and then proceed to the unknown. This approach gives the learner confidence. Sometimes, you will not know the client's knowledge or skill base and will need to elicit this information, either by asking questions or by having the client fill out a form, such as a pretest.
- Address early in the teaching session any area that is causing the client anxiety. A high level of anxiety can impair concentration in other areas. For example, a woman highly anxious about turning her husband in bed might not be able to learn about bathing him until she has successfully learned to turn him.
- Teach the basics before proceeding to the variations or adjustments. It is confusing to learners to have to consider possible adjustments and variations before they master the basic concepts. For example, when teaching a female client how to insert a retention catheter, it is best to teach the basic procedure before teaching any adjustments that might be needed if the catheter stops draining after insertion.
- Schedule time for review of content and to answer questions learners may have.

Implementing

The nurse must be flexible in implementing any teaching plan and revise the plan as needed. The client's needs may change, or external factors may intervene. For instance, the nurse and the client, Mr. Brown, have planned to irrigate his colostomy at 10 a.m., but when the time comes, Mr. Brown wants additional information before actually doing it himself. In this case, the nurse alters the teaching plan and discusses the desired information, provides written information, and defers teaching the psychomotor skill until the next day. It is also important for nurses to use teaching techniques that enhance learning and reduce or eliminate any barrier to learning, such as pain or fatigue. Refer back to Table 25.2 on page 519 for barriers to learning.

GUIDELINES FOR TEACHING Knowledge alone is not enough to motivate a person to change a behaviour. Do not assume that providing information will automatically result in clients changing their behaviour. Learning what needs to be done to change behaviour and acting on that knowledge are two different processes (Saarmann, Daugherty, & Riegel, 2000, p. 281). The stages of change, the person's willingness and perceived need to change, and barriers to change are important elements to reflect on when implementing a teaching plan (see Chapter 8, the section "The Transtheoretical Model: Stages of Health Behaviour Change").

When implementing a teaching plan, the nurse may find the following guidelines helpful:

1. Assess the characteristics of the learners and, before the teaching session, identify factors that will affect their learning.
2. Determine the outcomes jointly with the client (learner). Reassess learning activities and replace them if they are ineffective. Active learner involvement can enhance learning.
3. The optimal time for each session depends largely on the learner. Whenever possible, ask the client for help to choose the best time, for example, when he or she feels most rested.
4. Establish a rapport between teacher and learner. A relationship that is both accepting and constructive will best assist learning. The nurse should take time to establish a rapport before teaching.
5. Be sensitive to any signs that the pace is too fast or too slow. A client who appears confused or does not comprehend material when questioned may be finding the pace too fast. When the client appears bored and loses interest, the pace may be too slow, the learning period may be too long, or the client may be tired.
6. Build on the client's previous learning and encourage the client to learn and develop new skills. For example, a person whose spouse is diabetic may already have some knowledge of diabetes on which the nurse can build.
7. Communicate clearly and concisely. The words used need to have the same meaning to the learner as to the teacher. Using a layperson's vocabulary enhances communication. Even such words as *urine* or *feces* may be unfamiliar to clients, and abbreviations, such as RR (recovery room) or PAR (postanaesthesia room), are often misunderstood.
8. Use teaching aids that can help focus a learner's attention. To ensure the transfer of learning, the nurse should use the type of supplies or equipment the client will eventually use. Before the teaching session, the nurse needs to assemble all equipment and visual aids and ensure that all audiovisual equipment is functioning effectively (see the Teaching: Clinical box on teaching tools for children).
9. Create an environment conducive to learning. If in the hospital, and if possible, the patient should be out of bed for learning activities. Most people associate their bed with rest and sleep, not with learning.
10. Use multiple senses in teaching to enhance learning. For example, when teaching about changing a surgical dressing, the nurse can tell the client about the procedure (hearing), show how to change the dressing (sight), and let the client manipulate the equipment (touch).
11. Provide a context for learning. For example, learning to select low-sodium foods can be done very effectively in a tour of a grocery store.

TEACHING: CLINICAL

Teaching Tools for Children

The use of the following teaching aids can help focus children's attention:

- *Visits.* Visiting the hospital and treatment rooms; seeing people dressed in uniforms, scrub suits, protective gear.
- *Dress-up.* Touching and dressing up in the clothing they will see and wear.
- *Colouring books.* Using colouring books to prepare for treatments, surgery, or hospitalization; shows what rooms, people, and equipment will look like.
- *Storybooks.* Storybooks describe how the child will feel, what will be done, and what the place will look like. Parents can read these stories to children several times before the experience. Younger children like this repetition.
- *Dolls.* Practising procedures on dolls or teddy bears that they will later experience gives a sense of mastery of the situation. Custom dolls are often available for inserting tubes and giving injections, for example.
- *Puppet play.* Puppets can be used in role-play situations to provide information and show the child what the experience will be like; they help the child express emotions.
- *Health fairs.* Health fairs can educate children about their bodies and ways to stay healthy. Fairs can focus on high-risk problems that children face, such as accidents and poisoning, and on other topics identified in the community as a concern.

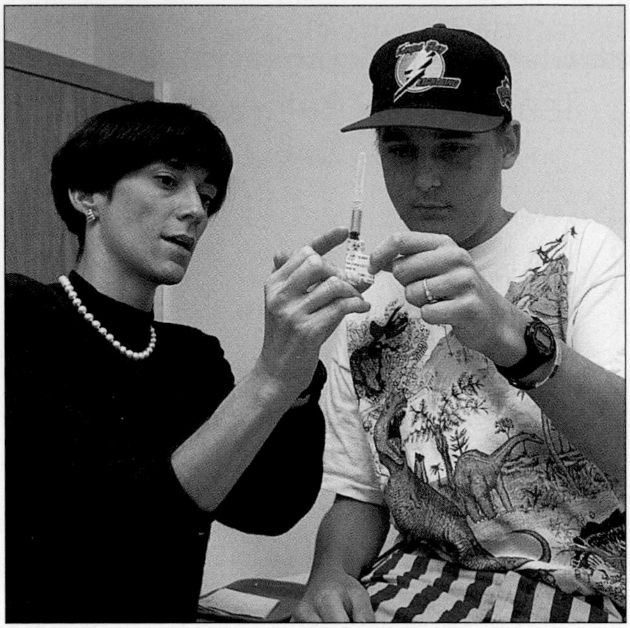

FIGURE 25.3 Teaching activities may need to include hands-on client participation.

12. Provide opportunities for clients to explore the content themselves. Ways to increase learning include stimulating motivation and self-direction, for example, (1) by providing specific, realistic, achievable outcomes; (2) by giving feedback; and (3) by helping the learner derive satisfaction from learning. The nurse can also encourage self-directed independent learning by encouraging the client to explore different sources for the information required. Teaching activities may need to be replaced or supplemented to attain learning outcomes. Figure 25.3 illustrates that actual handling of the syringe may be more effective than explanation alone.
13. Use repetition to reinforce learning. Summarizing content, rephrasing (using other words), and teaching the material in another way are means of repeating and clarifying content. For instance, after discussing the kinds of foods that can be included in a diet, the nurse describes the foods again but in the context of the three meals eaten during one day.

SPECIAL TEACHING STRATEGIES Nurses can choose from a number of special teaching strategies that are appropriate for the learner and the learning outcomes.

CLIENT CONTRACTING Client contracting involves establishing a learning contract with a client that specifies certain outcomes and when they are to be met. Here is an example of a self-contract:

> *I, Amy Martin, will exercise strenuously for 20 minutes three times per week for a period of two weeks and will then buy myself six yellow roses.*
> *Amy Martin*
> *July 30, 2009*

The contract, drawn up and signed by the client and the nurse, can specify the learning outcomes, the responsibilities of the client and the nurse, and the methods of follow-up and evaluation. The contract can be changed in two ways: (1) if the client meets the contract outcomes and wants to negotiate new learning outcomes, and (2) if the client decides that it is not possible to meet the existing learning outcomes and wants to revise them (Rankin, Stallings, & London, 2005). A learning contract allows for freedom, mutual respect, and mutual responsibility and encourages clients to accept responsibility for learning.

GROUP TEACHING Group instruction is economical and provides members with an opportunity to share with and learn from others. A small group allows for discussion in which everyone can participate. A large group often necessitates a lecture technique or use of films, videos, slides, or role-playing by teachers. It is important that all members involved in group instruction have a need in common (e.g., prenatal health or preoperative instruction).

COMPUTER-ASSISTED INSTRUCTION The internet has become a part of the lives of many Canadians, allowing them to communicate and obtain information quickly. The internet has also become an important source of health information, screening tools, health services, and support groups; and many individuals are now accessing the internet before consulting health-care professionals about their health issues. Nurses therefore need to be aware of such technology and be competent in integrating it into their teaching (but see the Reflect on Primary Health Care box).

Computer-assisted instruction (CAI) can be used to teach the application of information, new information, or complex problem-solving skills. CAI is often used for continuing education of health-care professionals. It works most effectively for individuals when using a computer. The learners are able to set the pace that meets

REFLECT ON PRIMARY HEALTH CARE

Client education is a central activity of nursing. Nurses use various teaching strategies to equip their clients with the needed knowledge and thus develop skills to improve and maintain their health. *Health promotion* therefore involves health education. Health education, in turn, calls for nurses to be innovative and to adapt delivery of care to meet client's social, economic, and cultural needs. Consider this example: in developing countries, where high-tech teaching supplies and visual models are often not affordable, nurses incorporate the principle of *appropriate technology* by teaching school children to draw in the sand in the schoolyard in the absence of papers or pencils. Nurses can also use available materials, such as twigs, stones, and vegetables, to create homemade teaching models if commercial models or charts are unavailable.

their learning needs. Others create simulation situations, such as a virtual nursing unit with client charts and assessment data, that require critical thinking as a basis for developing professional skills.

Computer simulations are becoming a common teaching strategy in student learning situations, such as nursing labs. Simulations provide not only a safe environment but also a realistic scenario for student learning, without jeopardizing the safety of a real client. Simulations can also standardize teaching and evaluation.

DISCOVERY OR PROBLEM SOLVING In using the discovery or problem-solving technique, the nurse presents some initial information and then a situation related to the information. The learner applies the new information to the situation and decides what to do. Learners can work alone or in groups. The nurse guides the learners through the thinking process necessary to reach the best action to take in the situation. This method may also be referred to as anticipatory problem solving. For example, the nurse might ask parents with a newborn and a 2-year-old at home to identify ways of addressing issues of sibling rivalry with the toddler.

BEHAVIOUR MODIFICATION The behaviour modification system for changing behaviour has as its basic assumptions (1) that human behaviours are learned and can be selectively strengthened, weakened, eliminated, or replaced, and (2) that a person's behaviour is under conscious control. Under this system, desirable behaviour is regarded, and undesirable behaviour is ignored. The client's response is the key to behaviour change. For example, clients trying to quit smoking are not criticized when they smoke, but they are praised or rewarded when they go without a cigarette for a certain time.

TRANSCULTURAL TEACHING The nurse and clients of different cultural and ethnic backgrounds have additional barriers to overcome in the teaching-learning process. These barriers can include language and communication problems, differing concepts of time, conflicting cultural healing practices, beliefs that may positively or negatively affect learning, or unique high-risk or high-frequency health problems that can be addressed with health-promotion instruction. Nurses should consider the following guidelines when teaching clients from various ethnic backgrounds:

- *Obtain teaching materials, pamphlets, and instructions in languages used by clients.* Nurses who are unable to read the foreign language material for themselves can have the interpreter read the material to clients.
- *Use visual aids, such as pictures, charts, or diagrams, to communicate meaning.* Audiovisual material can be helpful if English is spoken clearly and slowly. Even if understanding the verbal message is a problem for the client, seeing a skill or procedure may be helpful. In some instances, an interpreter can be asked to clarify the visual aid.
- *Use concrete rather than abstract words.* Use simple language (short sentences, short words), and present only one idea at a time.
- *Avoid the use of medical terminology or health-care language,* such as "taking your vital signs" or "apical pulse." Rather, nurses should say they are going to take a blood pressure reading or listen to the client's heart.
- If understanding another's pronunciation is a problem, validate brief information in writing.
- *Use humour very cautiously.* Meaning can change in the translation process.
- *Do not use slang words or colloquialisms.* These may be interpreted literally.
- *Do not assume that a client who nods, uses eye contact, or smiles is indicating an understanding of what is being taught.* These responses may simply be the client's way of indicating respect.
- *Invite and encourage questions during teaching.* Urge clients to ask questions to clarify information.
- When explaining procedures or functioning related to personal areas of the body, it may be appropriate to have the teaching done by a nurse (and interpreter if needed) of the same sex.
- *Include the family in planning and teaching.* This promotes trust and mutual respect. Ask the client to identify the appropriate family member and incorporate that person into the planning and teaching to promote adherence and support of health teaching.
- *Consider the client's time orientation.* The client may be more oriented to the present than the future, so teaching preventative health behaviours may be difficult.
- *Identify cultural health practices and beliefs.* Noncompliance with health teaching may be related to conflict with folk medicine beliefs, lack of understanding, or conflict with cultural beliefs.

Evaluating

Evaluating is both an ongoing and a final process in which the client, the nurse, and often the support people determine what has been learned.

EVALUATING LEARNING The process of evaluation is the same as evaluating client achievement of desired outcomes for other nursing diagnoses. Learning is measured against the predetermined learning outcomes selected in the planning phase of the teaching process. Thus, the outcomes serve not only to direct the teaching plan but also to provide outcome criteria for evaluation. For example, the outcome "selects foods that are low in carbohydrates" can be evaluated by asking the client to name such foods or to select low-carbohydrate foods from a list.

The best method of evaluation depends on the type of learning. In *cognitive learning,* the client demonstrates acquisition of knowledge. Examples of the evaluation tools for cognitive learning include the following:

- Direct observation of behaviour (e.g., observing the client selecting the solution to a problem by using the new knowledge)
- Oral questioning (e.g., asking the client to restate information or provide correct verbal responses to questions)
- Self-reports and self-monitoring, which can be useful during follow-up phone calls and home visits

The acquisition of *psychomotor skills* is best evaluated by observing how well the client carries out a procedure, such as changing a dressing or carrying out a urinary self-catheterization.

Affective learning is more difficult to evaluate. Whether attitudes or values have been learned can be inferred by listening to the client's responses to questions, noting how the client speaks about relevant subjects, and by observing the client's behaviour that expresses feelings and values. For example, do clients who state that they value health actually report use of condoms every time they have sex with a new partner?

Following evaluation, the nurse may find it necessary to modify or repeat the teaching plan if the outcomes have not been met or have been met only partially. For the hospitalized client, follow-up teaching in the home or by phone may be needed.

Behaviour change does not always take place immediately after learning. Often, individuals accept change intellectually first and then change their behaviour only periodically (for example, Mrs. Green, who knows that she must lose weight, diets and exercises off and on). The nurse can assist clients with behaviour change by allowing for client vacillation and by providing encouragement.

EVALUATING TEACHING It is important for nurses to evaluate their own teaching and the content of the teaching program. Evaluation should include a consideration of all factors: the timing, the teaching strategies, the amount of information, whether the teaching was helpful, and so on. The nurse may find, for example, that the client was overwhelmed with too much information, was bored, or was motivated to learn more. Both the client and the nurse should evaluate the learning experience. The client can tell the nurse what was helpful, interesting, and so on. Feedback questionnaires and videotapes of the learning sessions can also be useful.

The nurse should not feel ineffective as a teacher if the client forgets some of what is taught. Forgetting is normal and should be anticipated. Having the client write down information, repeating it during teaching, giving handouts on the information, and having the client be active in the learning process all promote retention.

Documenting

Documentation of the teaching process is essential because it provides a legal record that the teaching took place and communicates the teaching to other health-care professionals. If teaching is not documented, then, legally, it did not occur.

It is also important to document the responses of the client and support people to teaching activities. What did the client or support person say or do to indicate that learning had occurred? Has the client demonstrated mastery of a skill or the acquisition of knowledge? The nurse records this evidence of learning in the client's chart.

Many agencies have multiple-copy client teaching forms that include the medical and nursing diagnoses, the treatment plan, and the client education. After the teaching session is completed, the client and the nurse sign the form and a copy of the form is given to the client as a record of teaching and as reinforcement of the content taught. A second copy of the completed and signed form is placed in the client's chart. The parts of the teaching process that should be documented in the client's chart include the following:

- Diagnosed learning needs
- Learning outcomes
- Topics taught
- Client outcomes
- Need for additional teaching
- Resources provided

The written teaching plan that the nurse uses as a resource to guide future teaching sessions might also include these elements:

- Actual information and skills taught
- Teaching strategies used
- Time framework and content for each class
- Teaching outcomes and methods of evaluation

Case Study 25

Mrs. Marcos is a 59-year-old bank vice-president who is heavily relied on by her boss and co-workers. She moved to Canada from the Philippines 5 years ago. Three days ago, she was admitted to the hospital with complaints of shortness of breath and mild chest pain. A diagnostic evaluation indicates that she has significant coronary artery disease but has not yet suffered a heart attack. Her physician has indicated that Mrs. Marcos will need to make significant lifestyle changes to reduce her heart attack risk. As her nurse, you recognize Mrs. Marcos's need to learn about her disease process, diet, exercise, and stress reduction. As you begin teaching Mrs. Marcos, you note that she is very pleasant and frequently nods her head, but she also seems preoccupied and is readily distracted.

Critical Thinking Questions

1. How would you evaluate Mrs. Marcos's readiness to learn?
2. Mrs. Marcos is obviously a well-educated client. Of what benefit would a learning needs assessment be?
3. You recognize that you have a great deal of information to teach Mrs. Marcos and you are concerned that you will not be able to teach it all. What can you do to help Mrs. Marcos and still feel that you have accomplished your teaching goals?
4. How will you know if your teaching is effective?
5. How might your teaching differ if you were teaching Mrs. Marcos at home, rather than in a hospital or acute-care setting?

After working through these questions, go to the MyNursingLab at **http://www.mynursinglab.com** to check your answers.

KEY TERMS

client education
teaching
learning need
learning
cognitive
compliance
adherence
andragogy
pedagogy
geragogy
positive reinforcement
imitation
modelling
cognitive theory
cognitive domain
affective domain
psychomotor domain
humanism
motivation
readiness to learn
health literacy

CHAPTER HIGHLIGHTS

- Teaching clients and families about their health needs is a major role of the nurse. Nurses also teach colleagues, other health-care professionals, subordinates, nursing and other health-care students, and groups in community education programs.
- Learning is represented by a change in behaviour.
- Three main theories of learning are behaviourism, cognitivism, and humanism.
- Bloom has identified three learning domains: cognitive, affective, and psychomotor.
- A number of factors facilitate learning: motivation, readiness, active involvement, relevance, feedback, nonjudgmental support, the progression from simple to complex concepts, repetition, timing, and environment.
- Such factors as emotions, certain physiological events, cultural barriers, and psychomotor deficits can impede learning.
- The teaching process, like the nursing process, consists of six activities: assessing the learner, diagnosing learning needs, developing a teaching plan, implementing the plan, evaluating learning outcomes and teaching effectiveness, and documenting instructional activities.
- Learning outcomes guide the content of the teaching plan and are written in terms of client or learner behaviour.
- Teaching strategies should be suited to the client, the material to be learned, and the teacher. They should be adjusted to the client's developmental level and health status.
- A teaching plan is a written plan consisting of learning outcomes, content to teach, a time frame for teaching, and strategies to use in teaching the content. The plan must be revised when the client's needs change or the teaching strategies prove ineffective.
- Adaptations in teaching will facilitate learning for clients who have low or no reading skills, or are older or from different cultural backgrounds.
- Evaluation of the teaching-learning process is both an ongoing and a final process.
- Documentation of client teaching is essential to communicate the teaching to other health-care professionals and to provide a record for legal and accreditation purposes.

ASSESS YOUR LEARNING

1. A community health nurse is giving a presentation to a parenting group. Which of the following actions would provide the nurse with the best initial feedback on the nurse's teaching skills?
   - **a.** Elicit the group's feelings about the presentation.
   - **b.** Observe the group's nonverbal behaviour.
   - **c.** Ask the group to complete a feedback questionnaire.
   - **d.** Administer a quiz on the content of the presentation.

2. Which of the following activities would be classified as learning in the affective domain of Bloom's taxonomy?
   - **a.** Learning how to calculate an appropriate drug dosage
   - **b.** Learning to accept the loss of a limb
   - **c.** Learning how to insert a catheter
   - **d.** Reading handout material on the symptoms of congestive heart failure

3. Which of the following is the best way to help a newly diagnosed diabetic client to learn the dietary requirements associated with the disease?
   - **a.** Provide a videotape that addresses the dietary requirements associated with the disease.
   - **b.** Ask a nutritionist to visit the client to present information and handouts about the diabetic diet.
   - **c.** Ask the client to make a list of favourite foods and how to work them into the diet.
   - **d.** Have the client attend a group meeting for diabetic clients to discuss adapting to this chronic health condition.

4. A nurse is scheduling a teaching situation. Which of the following clients is most ready to learn?
   - **a.** A 45-year-old man whose doctor just informed him that he has cancer
   - **b.** A 3-year-old child whose parents have read her a storybook about going to the hospital
   - **c.** A 60-year-old female who received medication 5 minutes ago for relief of abdominal pain
   - **d.** A 70-year-old man, recovering from a stroke, who has returned from physical therapy

5. How can the nurse best assess a client's style of learning?
   - **a.** Ask the client how he or she learns best.
   - **b.** Use a variety of teaching strategies.
   - **c.** Observe the client's interactions with others.
   - **d.** Ask family members.

6. A 74-year-old client who takes multiple medications tells the nurse, "I have no idea what that little yellow pill is for." What is the best nursing diagnosis for this client?
   - **a.** *Deficient knowledge: medication information*
   - **b.** *Health-seeking behaviour: disease information*
   - **c.** *Deficient knowledge: medication information*
   - **d.** *Noncompliance: medication self-administration*

7. A nurse is talking with a client who is scheduled to have a diagnostic procedure. Which comment by the client indicates a teachable moment?
   - **a.** "I've had this procedure done before."
   - **b.** "Will this procedure hurt?"
   - **c.** "I'm trying not to think about it."
   - **d.** "I have an appointment with another person right now."

8. A client needs to learn to self-administer insulin injections. Which statement may reflect low literacy skills?
   - **a.** "I will read the information later—I'm too tired right now."
   - **b.** "I've watched my brother give his own shots. I know how to do it."
   - **c.** "I'm afraid of injections. Do I have to give my own shots?"
   - **d.** "Do you have a video showing how I should give myself the shot?"

9. A client has a learning outcome of "select foods that are low in fat." Which of the following statements reflects that the client has met this learning outcome?
   - **a.** "I understand the importance of maintaining a low-fat diet."
   - **b.** "I feel better about myself now."
   - **c.** "I was able to choose a low-fat lunch off the restaurant menu."
   - **d.** "Since I changed my diet, my husband is also losing weight."

10. A client's learning outcome is "client will state medication name, purpose, and appropriate precautions." Which of the following documented statements reflects evidence of learning?
    - **a.** Taught name, purpose, and precautions for the new cardiac medication; client seemed to understand.
    - **b.** Written information about the medication provided and reviewed; correct responses were given to follow-up questions.
    - **c.** Written information read to client; stated he would read it when he got home.
    - **d.** Information about the medication taught to client; client stated he understood it.

After working through these questions, go to the MyNursingLab at ***http://www.mynursinglab.com*** *to check your answers and see explanations.*

SUGGESTED READINGS

Bastable, S. B. (2008). Nurse as educator: Principles of teaching and learning for nursing practice (3rd ed.). Boston: Jones and Barlett Publishers.

This book focuses on patient education and has extensive information on assessment of clients with a variety of conditions in a variety of settings. It also contains excellent information on instructional methods, instructional materials, and evaluation of learning outcomes.

DeYoung, D. (2009). *Teaching strategies for nurse educators.* Upper Saddle River, NJ: Prentice Hall.

This book presents an overview of teaching and learning theory, motivation, and behaviour change in a multicultural context. It also examines clinical teaching, traditional and activity-based teaching strategies, distance learning, and computer teaching strategies.

McDonald, M. E. (2007). *The nurse educator's guide to assessing learning outcomes* (2nd ed.). Sudbury, MA: Jones and Bartlett Publishers.

This guide provides systematic assessment of learning outcomes, from setting instructional objectives, to assessing critical thinking, and developing evaluative questions and interpreting test results.

Oermann, M. H., & Heinrich, K. T. (Eds.). (2007). *Annual review of nursing education: Challenges and new directions in nursing: Volume 5.* New York: Springer Publishing.

This book describes trends and innovative strategies related to curriculum designs and development. It provides strategies for effective teaching in all settings, including how to solve various difficult teaching situations.

Rankin, S. H., Stallings, K. D., & London, F. (2005). Patient education in health and illness (5th ed.). Philadelphia, PA: Lippincott Williams & Wilkins.

This book contains excellent information on educational theories for teaching and motivating clients. It also focuses on teaching clients who have different cultural backgrounds and beliefs. It specifically addresses issues of health promotion in communities.

WEBLINKS

ABC Canada Literacy Foundation

http://www.abc-canada.org

This foundation is a Canada-wide educational organization that focuses on literacy skills. This site identifies literacy statistics, an overview of related workplace issues, and publications.

Canadian Nurses Association

http://www.cna-aiic.ca/cna/

Through this site, the user has access to resources of the Canadian Nurses Association in which the role of the nurse as client teacher is identified.

Diabetes Nursing Interest Group of the Registered Nurses' Association of Ontario

http://www.dnig.org

This site provides networking opportunities for nurses who are involved in diabetes education and care.

Canadian Public Health Association (CPHA)

http://www.cpha.ca/en/pls.aspx

As part of its National Literacy and Health Program, the CPHA established the Plain Language Service (PLS) to support health-care professionals in the preparation of clear and easily understood written print and internet materials.

REFERENCES

Aldridge, M. D. (2004). Writing and designing readable patient education materials. *Nephrology Nursing Journal, 31*(4), 373–377.

Bandura, A. (1971). Analysis of modeling processes. In A. Bandura (Ed.). *Psychological modeling: Conflicting theories* (pp. 1–62). New York: Aldine-Atherton.

Bastable, S. (2008). *Nurse as educator: Principles of teaching and learning for nursing practice* (3rd ed.). Boston, MA: Jones & Bartlett.

Bloom, B. S. (Ed.). (1956). *Taxonomy of educational objectives. Book 1, Cognitive domain.* New York: Longman.

Hayes, K. (2005). Designing written medication instructions: Effective ways to help older adults self-medicate. *Journal of Gerontological Nursing, 31*(5), 5–10.

Health Canada. (2003). *How does literacy affect the health of Canadians?* Ottawa: Author.

John, M. T. (1988). *Geragogy: A theory for teaching the elderly.* New York: Haworth Press.

Knowles, M. S. (1984). *Andragogy in action.* San Francisco, CA: Jossey-Bass.

Lewin, K. (1951). *Field theory in social science.* New York: Harper and Row.

Maslow, A. H. (1970). *Motivation and personality.* New York: Harper and Row.

Munoz, C., & Luckmann, J. (2005). *Transcultural communication in nursing* (2nd ed.). Clifton Park, NY: Delmar Learning.

NANDA International. (2007). *Nursing diagnoses: Definitions and classification, 2007–2008.* Philadelphia, PA: Author.

Pavlov, I. P. (1927). *Conditioned reflexes* (G. V. Anrep, Trans.). London, UK: Oxford University Press.

Piaget, J. (1966). *Origins of intelligence in children.* New York: Norton.

Rankin, S. H., Stallings, K. D., & London, F. (2005). *Patient education in health and illness* (5th ed.). Philadelphia, PA: Lippincott Williams & Wilkins.

Redman, B. K. (2004). *Advances in patient education.* New York: Springer.

Registered Nurses' Association of Ontario. (2006). *Client centred care. Nursing best practice guidelines: Shaping the future of nursing.* Toronto: Author.

Saarmann, L., Daugherty, J., & Riegel, B. (2000). Patient teaching to promote behavioral change. *Nursing Outlook, 48*, 281–287.

Skinner, B. F. (1953). *Science and human behavior.* New York: Macmillan.

Wilkinson, J. M. (2005). *Nursing diagnosis handbook with NIC interventions and NOC outcomes* (8th ed.). Upper Saddle River, NJ: Prentice Hall Health.

Chapter 26

Leading, Managing, and Delegating

In the rapidly changing and increasingly complex Canadian health-care delivery system, with its worsening nursing shortage, nursing leadership to ensure provision of safe and competent quality care is more important than ever (Canadian Nurses Association [CNA], 2003). In the document *Toward 2020: Visions for Nursing,* the Canadian Nurses Association (CNA) envisions nurses as working with an ever-increasing multidisciplinary team of health-care providers. The CNA stressed that nurse leaders "must focus on health and the health system, not [just] on nurses and nursing. . . . Nurses will be expected to be strong advocates for patients, facilities, communities, and social issues" (Villeneuve & MacDonald, 2006, p. 84). The next generation of nurses must work efficiently and effectively to meet the public expectations and, most importantly, to become effective leaders and direct positive change.

OBJECTIVES

After studying this chapter, you should be able to

1. Compare and contrast leadership and management
2. Differentiate formal from informal leaders
3. Compare and contrast four different leadership styles
4. Identify the characteristics of an effective leader
5. Differentiate the three levels of management
6. Describe the seven skills and competencies needed by a nurse manager
7. Describe the four functions of management
8. Describe four models or processes used in change management
9. Discuss the roles and functions of nurse leaders and managers in planning for and implementing change

The Nurse as Leader

The nurse is often in a leadership position and frequently delegates aspects of care to others. Nursing offers opportunities for nurses to become leaders at many levels. In numerous situations, the nurse also functions as a manager and as a change agent. The professional nurse frequently assumes the roles of leader and manager. These two roles are linked; that is, managers must have leadership abilities, and leaders often manage, but the two roles differ.

A **leader** influences others to work together to accomplish a specific goal. Leaders are often visionary; they are informed, articulate, confident, and self-aware. Leaders also have excellent interpersonal skills and are astute listeners and communicators. They have initiative and the ability and confidence to innovate, change, motivate, facilitate, and mentor others (see the Reflect on Primary Health Care box).

A **manager** is an employee of an organization who is given authority, power, and responsibility for planning, organizing, coordinating, and directing the work of others, and for establishing and evaluating standards. Managers understand organizational structure and culture. They control human, financial, and material resources. Managers set goals, make decisions, and solve problems. They initiate and implement change.

The purposes of nursing leadership vary according to the level of application and include (1) improving the health status of individuals or families, (2) increasing the effectiveness and level of satisfaction among professional colleagues, and (3) improving the attitudes of citizens and legislators toward the nursing profession and their expectations of it.

As managers, nurses are responsible for planning, organizing, and coordinating client care. Nurses, as managers, ensure that the right things are done at the right time in the right way by the right people. They focus on the task and concentrate on activities to increase productivity, while leaders focus on relationships and address the needs of people with whom they are working.

As a manager, the nurse is responsible for (1) efficiently accomplishing the goals of the organization, (2) efficiently using the organization's resources, (3) ensuring effective client care, and (4) ensuring compliance with institutional, professional, regulatory, and governmental standards of care. Table 26.1 compares the leader and manager roles, and Figure 26.1 illustrates some of the leading and managing roles.

REFLECT ON PRIMARY HEALTH CARE

Nurses work in multiple roles with various health-care providers in the multidisciplinary teams to provide care for well and ill clients (*intersectoral collaboration*). Within their organizations, nurse leaders play a formal role to guide their teams in assessing the effectiveness of care, implementing evidence-based practice, and constructing process improvement strategies. These nurse leaders may be team leaders or institutional leaders. As well, they may also be informal (volunteer) leaders associated with professional health and social service organizations or community boards. They assist in strategic planning to create positive change. Find out who the nurse leaders are in your community and the role they play in creating change in their practice locations.

Leadership

Leadership can be formal or informal. The **formal leader**, or appointed leader, is selected by an organization and given official authority to make decisions and act. An **informal leader** is not officially appointed to

TABLE 26.1 Comparison of Leader and Manager Roles

Leaders	Managers
May or may not be officially appointed to the position	Are appointed officially to the position
Have power and authority to enforce decisions only as long as followers are willing to be led	Have power and authority to enforce decisions
Influence others toward goal setting, either formally or informally	Carry out predetermined policies, rules, and regulations
Are interested in risk taking and exploring new ideas	Maintain an orderly, controlled, rational, and equitable structure
Relate to people personally in an intuitive and empathetic manner	Relate to people according to their roles
Feel rewarded by personal achievements	Feel rewarded when fulfilling organizational mission or goals
May or may not be successful as managers	Are managers as long as the appointment holds
Manage relationships	Manage resources
Focus on people	Focus on systems

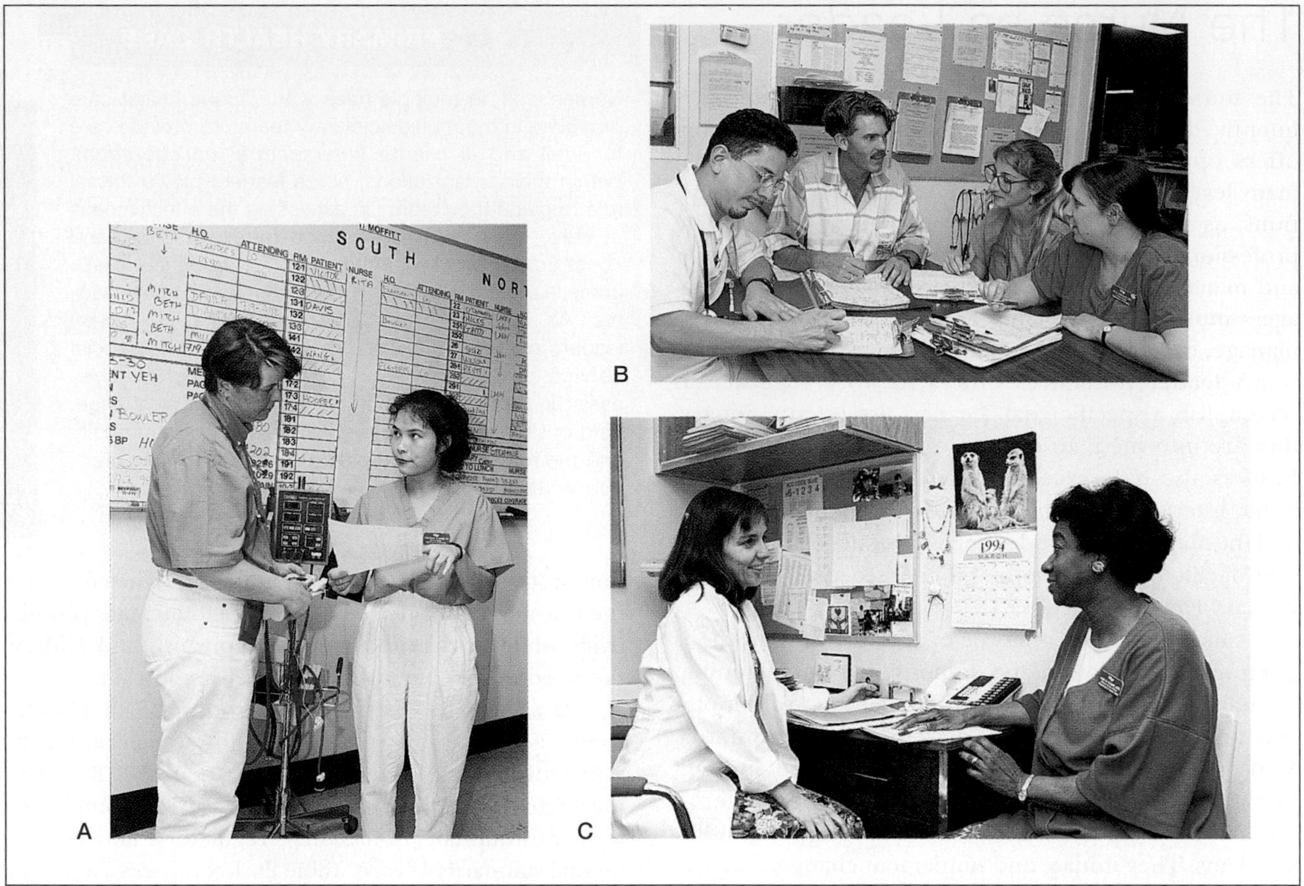

FIGURE 26.1 Nurses as leaders and managers. **A:** The nurse manager discusses work assignments during the change-of-shift report. **B:** The nurse delegates basic client care activities to other care providers. **C:** The nurse consults the social worker during discharge planning.

direct activities of others but is selected by the group as its leader because of seniority, age, special abilities, or a charismatic personality and plays an important role in influencing colleagues, co-workers, or other group members to achieve the group's goals.

Leadership Theory

Early leadership theories focused on what leaders are (trait theories), what leaders do (behavioural theories), and how leaders adapt their leadership style according to the situation (contingency theories). Theories about **leadership style** describe traits, behaviours, motivations, and choices used by individuals to effectively influence others.

CLASSICAL LEADERSHIP THEORIES The *trait theorists* found that leaders often possess specific traits and abilities, including good judgment, decisiveness, knowledge, adaptability, integrity, tact, popularity, nonconformity, and cooperativeness. The *behaviourists* believed that through education, training, and life experiences, effective leaders develop a particular style of leadership. These styles have been characterized as autocratic, democratic, laissez-faire, and bureaucratic.

Autocratic (authoritarian, directive) leaders make decisions for the group. The leader believes individuals are externally motivated and incapable of independent decision making. Similar to a dictator, the autocratic leader determines policies and gives orders and directions to the group. Under this type of leadership, the group may feel secure because procedures are well defined and activities are predictable. Productivity may also be high. However, the group's needs for creativity, autonomy, and self-motivation are not met, and the degree of openness and trust between the leader and the group members is minimal or absent. Members are often dissatisfied with this type of leadership; however, at times an autocratic style is the most effective. When urgent decisions are necessary (e.g., a cardiac arrest, a unit fire, or a mass casualty event), one person must assume the responsibility to make decisions without being challenged by other team members. When group members are unable or do not want to participate in making a decision, the authoritarian style solves the problem and enables the individual or group to move on. This style can also be effective when a project must be completed quickly and efficiently.

Democratic (participative, consultative) leaders encourage group discussion and decision making. This type of leader assumes individuals are internally motivated, capable of making decisions, and value independence. Group productivity and satisfaction are high as group members contribute to the work effort. The democratic leader acts as a catalyst or facilitator, actively guiding the group toward achieving the group's goals. Providing constructive criticism, offering information, making suggestions, and asking questions become the focus of the participative leader. This type of leadership demands that the leader have faith in the group members to accomplish the goals. Although democratic leadership has been shown to be less efficient and more cumbersome than authoritarian leadership, it allows more self-motivation and more creativity among group members. It also calls for a great deal of cooperation and coordination among group members. This style of leadership can be extremely effective in the health-care setting.

The **laissez-faire (nondirective, permissive, ultraliberal) leader** presupposes the group is internally motivated and recognizes the group's need for autonomy and self-regulation. The leader assumes a hands-off approach. However, group members can act independently and at cross-purposes because of a lack of cooperation and coordination. A laissez-faire style is most effective for groups whose members have both personal and professional maturity so that once the group has made a decision, the members become committed to it and have the required expertise to implement it. Individual group members then perform tasks in their area of expertise, while the leader acts as a resource person. Table 26.2 compares the authoritarian, democratic, and laissez-faire leadership styles.

The **bureaucratic leader** presumes the group is externally motivated. However, the bureaucrat does not trust himself or herself or others to make decisions. Instead, the bureaucrat relies on the organization's rules, policies, and procedures to direct the group's work efforts. Group members are usually dissatisfied with the leader's inflexibility and impersonal relations with them.

According to *contingency theorists,* effective leaders adapt their style of leadership to the situation. A popular contingency theory is **situational leadership**. Important aspects of situational leadership are (1) the task behaviours and relationship behaviours of the leader, (2) consideration of the staff members' abilities, (3) the nature of the task to be done, and (4) the context or environment in which the task takes place. The *task orientation* focuses on activities that encourage group productivity. The *relationship orientation* is concerned with interpersonal relationships and focuses on activities that meet group members' needs.

Situational leaders adapt their leadership style to the readiness and willingness of the individual or group to perform the assigned task. When employees are insecure, unable, or unwilling to perform the task, the leader uses a highly directive style, providing specific instructions and close supervision. If the group is motivated and willing but unable to perform the task, the leader again uses a highly directive style but in this case, explains decisions and provides the opportunity for clarification. When the group is able but unwilling or lacking in confidence, the leader shares ideas and facilitates decision making. For a group that is willing, able, and confident to perform the task, the leader delegates, turning responsibility for decision making and implementation over to the group.

CONTEMPORARY LEADERSHIP THEORIES Contemporary theorists have described charismatic leaders, transactional leaders, transformational leaders, connective leaders, and shared leadership.

Charismatic leadership is rare and is characterized by an emotional relationship between the leader and the group members. The charming personality of the leader evokes strong feelings of commitment to both the leader and the leader's cause and beliefs. The followers of a charismatic leader often overcome extreme hardship to achieve the group's goals because of their faith in the leader.

Transactional leadership has a relationship with followers based on an exchange for some resource valued by the follower. These incentives are used to promote loyalty and performance. For example, to ensure adequate staffing on the night shift, the nurse manager entices a staff nurse to work the night shift in exchange for a weekend shift off. The transactional leader represents the traditional manager, focused on the day-to-day tasks of achieving organizational goals and understanding and meeting the needs of the group.

In contrast, **transformational leadership** fosters creativity, risk taking, commitment, and collaboration by empowering the group to share in the organization's vision. The leader inspires others with a clear, attractive,

TABLE 26.2 Comparison of Authoritarian, Democratic, and Laissez-Faire Leadership Styles

	Authoritarian (autocratic)	Democratic (participative)	Laissez-Faire (permissive)
Degree of control	Makes decisions alone	Collaborative	No control
Leader activity level	High	High	Minimal
Assumption of responsibility	Primarily the leader	Shared	Relinquished
Output of the group	High quantity, good quality	Creative, high quality	Variable, may be of poor quality
Efficiency	Very efficient	Less efficient than authoritarian	Inefficient

and attainable goal and enlists them to participate in attaining the goal. Through shared values, honesty, trust, and continual learning, the leader empowers the group. Independence, individual growth, and change are facilitated.

Shared leadership recognizes that a professional workforce is made up of many leaders. No one person is considered to have knowledge or ability beyond that of other members of the work group. Appropriate leadership is thought to emerge in relation to the challenges that confront the work group. Examples of shared leadership in nursing are self-directed work teams, shared governance, and co-leadership. **Shared governance** is a method that aims to distribute decision making among a group of people.

Effective Leadership

Much has been written about effective leadership and style; some descriptive statements about effective leaders are listed in Box 26.1. Leadership is a learned process. To be an effective leader requires an understanding of such factors as the needs, goals, and rewards that motivate people; knowledge of leadership skills and of the group's activities; and possession of interpersonal skills to influence others. Principles of effective leadership include vision, influence, and power.

BOX 26.1 CHARACTERISTICS OF EFFECTIVE LEADERS

Effective leaders have the following characteristics:

- They use a leadership style that is natural to them.
- They use a leadership style appropriate to the task and the members.
- They assess the effects of their behaviour on others and the effects of others' behaviour on themselves.
- They are sensitive to forces acting for and against change.
- They express an optimistic view about human nature.
- They are energetic.
- They are open and encourage openness so that real issues are confronted.
- They facilitate personal relationships.
- They plan and organize activities of the group.
- They are consistent in behaviour toward group members.
- They delegate tasks and responsibilities to develop members' abilities, not merely to get tasks done.
- They involve members in all decisions.
- They value and use group members' contributions.
- They encourage creativity.
- They encourage feedback about their leadership style.
- They assess for and promote the use of current technology.

Vision is a mental image of a possible and desirable future state. Leaders transform visions into realistic goals and communicate their visions to others, who accept them as their own.

Influence is an informal strategy used to gain the cooperation of others without exercising formal authority. Influence is exercised through persuasion and excellent communication skills; it is based on a trusting relationship with the followers.

Power is the capacity to act or to influence others to act to achieve something. There are five sources of power: position power, personal power, task power, relationship power, and knowledge power. **Positional power** is related to the authority associated with a role or title and includes the power to manage people or command resources. **Personal power** is associated with admiration by others, which comes from having such attributes as strength of character, passion, inspiration, or wisdom. **Task power** is the ability to influence who is able to help with a process or task. **Relationship power** pertains to the respect others have for a person's personal abilities, knowledge, or skills (Blanchard, 2003; Sullivan & Decker, 2005).

The Nurse as Manager

The manager's job is to accomplish the work of the organization. To this end, managers perform a number of roles and functions that vary with the type of organization and the level of management.

Levels of Management

Traditional management is divided into three levels of responsibility. **First-level managers** are responsible for managing the work of nonmanagerial personnel and the day-to-day activities of a specific work group or groups. Their primary responsibility is for motivating staff to achieve the organization's goals. This level of manager represents staff and reports to upper administration and vice versa.

Middle-level managers supervise a number of first-level managers and are responsible for the activities in the departments they supervise. Middle-level managers serve as liaisons between first-level managers and upper-level managers.

Upper-level managers are organizational executives who are primarily responsible for establishing goals and developing strategic plans. Nurse executives are responsible for the managing of nursing within an organization, the practice of nursing, and the management of client services. This may include ensuring that nursing standards are met and promoting collaborative practices to provide effective client care.

Management Functions

Four management functions have been described: planning, organizing, directing, and coordinating. These four functions help to achieve the broad goal of quality client care.

PLANNING **Planning** is an ongoing process that involves (1) assessing a situation, (2) establishing goals and objectives based on assessment of a situation or future trends, and (3) developing a plan of action that identifies priorities, delineates who is responsible, determines deadlines, and describes how the intended outcome is to be achieved and evaluated. In short, it involves deciding what to do; when, where, and how to do it; who will do it; and with what resources. Distribution of money, personnel, equipment, and physical space are included in resource allocation. An upper-level manager, such as a nurse executive, spends considerable time planning the department's goals and services and determining numbers and types of nurses and other personnel needed to provide these services. A first-level manager, such as a staff nurse, spends less time planning but manages each client by use of the nursing process.

An example of the planning function is **risk management**: having in place a system to reduce danger to clients and staff. The steps of risk management include anticipating and seeking sources of risk; analyzing, classifying, and prioritizing risks; developing a plan to avoid and manage risk; gathering data that indicate success at avoiding or minimizing risk; and evaluating and modifying risk-reduction programs. Central to the process of risk management is communication among all involved persons.

ORGANIZING After identifying the work and evaluating human and material resources, the manager arranges the work into smaller units. **Organizing** is an ongoing process that involves determining responsibilities, communicating expectations, and establishing the chain of command for authority and communication. Although upper-level managers delegate much of the work, responsibility, and accountability for the work to others, they need to ensure that department objectives, priorities, job descriptions, lines of communication, nursing standards, procedures, and policies clearly describe the expectations.

DIRECTING **Directing** is the process of getting the organization's work accomplished. Directing involves assigning and communicating expectations about the task to be completed; providing instruction and guidance; and ongoing decision making. Upper-level managers devote less time to directing than to planning, organizing, and controlling. Directing at this level of management generally involves supervision of the next level of managers, such as those in middle management (e.g., supervisors, assistant or associate directors, or assistant administrators). Unit managers (charge nurses) and staff nurses devote more time to the directing function. For example, charge nurses direct shift work by assigning clients and scheduling meal and break times. Staff nurses direct the care of clients by ordering nursing care, communicating care in written care plans and shift reports, and supervising care that is given by others.

COORDINATING **Coordinating** is the process of ensuring that plans are carried out and evaluating outcomes. The manager measures results or actions against standards or desired outcomes and then reinforces effective actions or changes ineffective ones. For example, an upper-level manager evaluates the effectiveness of recruitment, staff turnover, and budget performance. The charge nurse appraises staff performance. The staff nurse determines whether nursing interventions have helped the client achieve desired outcomes.

Principles of Management

A manager has authority, accountability, and responsibility.

Authority is the official power to act; it is the legitimate right to direct the work of others (Marquis & Huston, 2005). It is an integral component of managing. Authority is conveyed through leadership actions; it is determined largely by the situation, and it is always associated with responsibility and accountability. The manager must accept the authority granted.

Accountability is a person's ability and willingness to assume responsibility for his or her own actions and to accept the consequences of his or her behaviour. Accountability can be viewed as hierarchic, starting at the individual level, moving to the institutional or professional level, and ending at the societal level. At the individual or client level, accountability is reflected in the nurse's ethical integrity. At the institutional level, it is reflected in the statement of philosophy and objectives of the nursing department and nursing policies. At the professional level, it is reflected in standards of practice developed by national or provincial or territorial nursing associations. At the societal level, it is reflected in legislated nurse practice acts.

Responsibility is an obligation to complete a task. Managers are responsible for the utilization of resources, communication to subordinates, and implementation of organizational goals and objectives.

Skills and Competencies of Nurse Managers

To be effective managers, nurses need to be able to think critically, communicate well, manage resources effectively and efficiently, enhance employee performance, build and manage teams, manage conflict, manage time effectively, delegate effectively, and initiate and manage change. (Refer to Chapter 8, the section "The Transtheoretical Model: Stages of Health Behaviour Change.")

THINKING CRITICALLY **Critical thinking** is a creative cognitive process that includes creativity, problem solving, and decision making (Sullivan & Decker, 2005). The nurse manager reasons with logic, exploring the assumptions, the alternatives, and the consequences of actions. See Chapter 20 for further discussion of critical thinking and decision making.

COMMUNICATING Managers report that they spend their day communicating. Good communication is essential to other critical interpersonal skills and often determines the manager's success as a leader. Managers use both verbal and written communication. Effective managers communicate assertively, expressing their ideas clearly, accurately, and honestly. Managers use **networking**, a process whereby professional links are established, through which people can share ideas, knowledge, and information; offer support and direction to one another; and facilitate accomplishment of professional goals.

MANAGING RESOURCES One of the greatest responsibilities of managers is their accountability for human, fiscal, and material resources. Budgeting and determining variances between the actual and the budgeted expenses are crucial skills for any manager.

In managing human resources, managers need to consider generational reactions to change. For the first time in nursing history, four generations of nurses are working in the health-care system (Martin, 2004). Judith Berg (2006) broadly categorized today's nurses into the "Silent Generation," "Baby Boomers," "Generation X," and the "Millennial Generation." The following describes the characteristics of each generation:

Silent generation (1933–1944): These nurses have a traditional work ethic and good critical-thinking skills. They are disciplined and loyal team players. They share their knowledge and expertise readily with their colleagues.

Baby boomers (1945–1964): These nurses make up most of the nursing community. They are extremely hard-working and have been the driving force of much of the progress in nursing in the past 20 years.

Generation X (1965–1978): These nurses are independent, resilient, confident, and committed to colleagues and clients before an employer. They like to share their expertise with their colleagues and clients. Their care tends to be guided more by their clients' desire than by rules and policies in the organization.

Millennial generation or Generation Y (1979–2000): These nurses grew up with technologies and are at ease with computers, video games, and cell phones. They can multitask, and they can establish rapport easily with team members, patients, and families.

ENHANCING EMPLOYEE PERFORMANCE Employee performance can be enhanced in several ways. The manager can provide day-to-day coaching or serve as a mentor or preceptor. A **mentor** is an experienced and knowledgeable person who provides a supportive environment to facilitate the novice's entry into the system to attain professional outcomes (CNA, 2004). The mentor explains the expectations of the role and the intricacies of the culture. The mentor is a role model and a counsellor.

In the clinical area, the term **preceptor** is used to describe mentoring relationships in which the experienced nurse assists the new nurse or student in acquiring practical nursing skill and judgment, in gaining an understanding of the routines, policies, and procedures of the institution and the unit, and in being socialized into the profession (CNA, 2004).

BUILDING AND MANAGING TEAMS In addition to personnel development, the manager is responsible for building and managing the work team. Familiarity with group processes and the roles that group members play facilitates the manager's ability to lead the group and enhances development of the group into a work team. Groups develop in stages, during which roles and relationships are established. (Detailed information about group stages and roles is discussed in Chapter 21, in the section "Group Communication.")

Evidence-Informed Practice

Organizational Trust and Empowerment: What Are the Effects on Staff Nurse Commitment?

Laschinger and Finegan (2005) explored whether nurses would feel empowered when they had access to information, received support, had the resources required for their work, and had opportunities for education. Two hundred and seventy-three staff nurses were randomly selected from urban teaching hospitals in Ontario to participate in this study. Results revealed that managers who increase access to information, support, resources, flexible job activities, strong alliances, and opportunities to learn and grow can create healthy nursing work environments.

NURSING IMPLICATIONS: Affective commitment to an organization has been related to a sense of empowerment. Nurse managers can create high-trust and high-respect work environments by empowering nurses through providing information, support and guidance, educational opportunities, and resources.

Source: Based on "Using Empowerment to Build Trust and Respect in the Workplace: A Strategy for Addressing the Nursing Shortage," by H. K. S. Laschinger and J. Finegan, 2005, *Nursing Economics, 23*(1), pp. 6–13.

Evaluating the group's work is another responsibility of the manager. Effectiveness, efficiency, and productivity are three outcome measures that are frequently used. In health care, **effectiveness** is a measure of the quality or quantity of services provided. **Efficiency** is a measure of the resources used in the provision of nursing services. In nursing, **productivity** is a performance measure of both the effectiveness and the efficiency of nursing care. Productivity is frequently measured in the amount of nursing resources used per client or in terms of required versus actual hours of care provided.

MANAGING CONFLICT Nurse managers are frequently in a position to manage conflict among people, groups, or teams. Conflict can arise from differing values, philosophies, or personalities. In health care, it can also arise through competition for resources. When conflict among nurses is left unresolved, it can have serious consequences. Collegial relationships based on trust and respect are important to ensuring safe client care. Unresolved conflict—and the lack of communication, support, and trust that often ensues—can leave clients and nurses vulnerable to unnecessary risk (College of Nurses of Ontario [CNO], 2006a). It is an expectation that nurses will demonstrate effective conflict-resolution skills. Communication strategies, such as actively listening, attending to nonverbal behaviours, and addressing behaviours in a nonjudgmental manner, all contribute to promoting respect and collegiality among team members. However, these strategies are only the first step in resolving the conflict. Nurses need to explore and understand the root cause of conflict and abusive behaviour. The CNO's (2006b) *Conflict Prevention and Management Practice Guideline* is a helpful tool for nurses to investigate.

Nurses can use many methods to manage conflict, and each has its advantages and disadvantages. Among the most common are compromise, negotiation, and collaboration. The new nurse manager may require training to become proficient in the use of these methods. Basic principles for all types of conflict management include demonstrating respect for all parties, avoiding blaming others, allowing full discussion, using ground rules during meetings to promote fairness, encouraging active listening, identifying the themes in the discussion, and exploring alternative solutions (Carroll, 2006).

MANAGING TIME The effective nurse manager uses time effectively and helps others to do the same. Many factors inhibit good use of time, such as preference for doing things the nurse likes to do before things the nurse prefers not to have to do, emergencies or crises that divert the nurse's attention, and unrealistic demands from others. Strategies that the manager, and all nurses, can employ to use time well involve setting goals and priorities, delegating appropriately, examining how time is used, minimizing paperwork (automating whenever possible), and using regular schedules that avoid interruptions and set time limits on activities (Sullivan & Decker, 2005).

The Nurse as Delegator

Delegation is the transference of responsibility and authority for the performance of an activity to a competent individual. The delegator retains accountability for the outcome. Delegation is a tool that allows the manager to devote more time to tasks that cannot be delegated. It also enhances the skills and abilities of the delegatee, which builds self-esteem, promotes morale, and enhances teamwork and attainment of the organization's goals. In nursing, delegation refers to indirect care—the intended outcome is achieved through the work of someone supervised by the nurse—and involves defining the task, determining who can perform the task, describing the expectation, seeking agreement, meeting timelines, monitoring performance, and providing feedback to the delegatee regarding performance (Sullivan & Decker, 2005).

Registered nurses (RNs) increasingly delegate components of nursing care to other health-care workers, especially with the increased use of unregulated care providers (UCP), including personal support workers (PSW). An RN who delegates a task to another health-care worker is accountable for selecting an appropriately skilled caregiver and for continued evaluation of the client's care. The delegatee assumes responsibility for the actual performance of the task or procedure. Guidelines for delegating nursing tasks and procedures appear in Box 26.2.

Tasks that can be delegated to UCPs can vary by province or territory and organization. Each provincial and territorial nursing association/college has specific guidelines for RNs to follow. Principles guiding the nurse's decision to delegate that ensure the safety and quality of outcomes are listed in Box 26.3. The UCP cannot delegate tasks to another person.

Once the decision has been made to delegate, the nurse must communicate clearly to the UCP and verify that the UCP understands the following:

- The specific tasks to be done for each client
- When each task is to be done
- The expected outcomes for each task, including parameters outside of which the UCP must immediately report to the nurse (and any action that must urgently be taken)
- Who is available to serve as a resource if needed
- When and in what format (written or verbal) a report on the tasks is expected

BOX 26.2 EXAMPLES OF TASKS THAT CAN AND CANNOT BE DELEGATED TO UNREGULATED CARE PROVIDERS

As the following lists show, not all tasks can be delegated.

TASKS THAT CAN BE DELEGATED TO UNREGULATED CARE PROVIDERS

- Taking vital signs
- Measuring and recording intake and output
- Client transfers and ambulation
- Conducting postmortem care
- Bathing
- Feeding
- Giving gastrostomy feedings in established systems
- Attending to safety
- Weighing
- Performing simple dressing changes
- Suctioning chronic tracheostomies
- Performing basic life support (CPR)

TASKS THAT CANNOT BE DELEGATED TO UNREGULATED CARE PROVIDERS

- Assessment
- Interpretation of data
- Making of a nursing diagnosis
- Creation of a nursing care plan
- Evaluation of care effectiveness
- Care of invasive lines
- Administration of parenteral medications
- Insertion of nasogastric tubes
- Client education
- Performance of triage
- Giving of telephone advice

BOX 26.3 PRINCIPLES USED BY THE NURSE TO DETERMINE DELEGATION TO UNREGULATED CARE PROVIDERS

The following principles should inform every decision to delegate:

1. The nurse must assess the individual client before delegating tasks.
2. The client must be medically stable or in a chronic condition and not fragile.
3. The task must be considered routine for this client.
4. The task must not require a substantial amount of scientific knowledge or technical skill.
5. The task must be considered safe for this client.
6. The task must have a predictable outcome.
7. The nurse must know the agency's procedures and policies about delegation.
8. The nurse must know the scope of practice and the customary knowledge, skills, and job description for each health-care discipline represented on his or her team.
9. The nurse must be aware of individual variations in work abilities. Along with different categories of caregivers are individual variations. Each individual has different experiences and may not be capable of performing every task cited in the job description.
10. When unsure about a UCP's abilities to perform a task, the nurse should observe while the person performs it, or demonstrate it to the person and get a return demonstration before allowing the person to perform it independently.
11. The nurse must clarify reporting expectations to ensure the task is accomplished.
12. The nurse should create an atmosphere that fosters communication, teaching, and learning. For example, staff should be encouraged to ask questions and be listened to carefully regarding their concerns, and the nurse should make use of every opportunity to teach.

Change

Change is the process of making something different from what it was (Sullivan & Decker, 2005). Change can involve gaining new knowledge or skills, or adapting what is currently known in light of new information. Change can involve individual clients, families, communities, organizations, nursing as a profession, and the entire health-care delivery system. Change is an integral aspect of nursing, and nurses are often **change agents**, that is, individuals who initiate, motivate, and implement change. Change agents have the following characteristics:

- They have excellent communication and interpersonal skills with individuals, groups, administration, and all levels of the organization involved in change.
- They have knowledge of available resources and how to use them: people, time, money, facilities, and information.
- They are skilled in problem solving.
- They are skilled in teaching.
- They are respected by those involved in the change.
- They have the ability to encourage and nurture those going through change.
- They are self-confident, are able to take risks, and can inspire trust in themselves and others.

- They are able to make decisions.
- They have a broad base of knowledge.
- They have a good sense of timing.

Types of Change

Three types of change often take place in organizations: developmental, planned, and unplanned.

Developmental change refers to anticipated and predictable changes that occur as the organization grows and as its operation becomes more complex (Hibberd & Smith, 2006). For example, the nurse leader must be acutely aware of and respond to the needs of the organization that has been growing from a staff of 20 to 100 over a short time. The needs can include providing the human, financial, and technological resources to support the day-to-day operation of the organization, and space for the staff, equipment, and clients being served. Also, the organization needs an adequate computer system to support organizational communication and a documentation system.

Unplanned change (or spontaneous change) is an alteration imposed by external events or persons. It occurs when unexpected events force a reaction. *Drift* is a type of unplanned change in which change occurs without effort on anyone's part. *Situational,* or *natural, change* can also be considered unplanned and occurs without any control by the person or group affected. An example is the change that occurs because of a war or a natural disaster. Not all situational changes are negative. For example, when severe acute respiratory syndrome (SARS) hit Canada in 2003, many health agencies reacted by changing their policies and practices (screening visitors and using masks) to protect the public (Hibberd & Smith, 2006).

Planned change is an intended, purposive attempt by an individual, group, organization, or larger social system to achieve the desired change. These changes may be specific to the organization (e.g., visiting schedules), cross-institutional (e.g., merging of linen services), or system-wide (e.g., restructuring of health services). Problem-solving skills, decision-making skills, and interpersonal skills are important factors for effective planned change.

Change can also be considered covert or overt. A *covert change* is hidden or occurs without the individual's awareness. For example, a person can become increasingly deaf without being aware of this fact. *Overt change* is change a person is aware of. Examples are the development of abdominal pain and of shortness of breath while walking up stairs. People who experience overt change may also experience anxiety. Overt change often necessitates behavioural changes that are at variance with the person's needs or goals. An example is a diagnosis of cancer and the subsequent need for therapy even though it interferes with the person's work and family life.

CLINICAL ALERT

In using any change models, managers need to consider that change does not occur in a linear fashion. The change can move back and forth through the stages several times. The manager cannot assume how ready staff members might be for change; they need to weigh the benefits or cost of a particular stage before deciding to practice the behaviour. Change involves emotion, cognition, and behaviour (Prochaska, Redding, & Evers, 2002).

Models of Change Management

LEWIN'S THEORY OF CHANGE According to Lewin (1951), change involves three stages—unfreezing, moving, and refreezing—and it requires a change agent to implement planned change. During the *unfreezing stage,* the change agent will identify the desired change and the related driving and restraining forces, generate alternative solutions, and motivate the participants to change. In the second stage, the *moving stage,* the change agent helps the participants to see that the status quo is undesirable, and together they carry out actions to resolve the identified problem. In the final stage, *refreezing,* the change agent will integrate and stabilize the change and withdraw when change is completed.

QUINN'S THEORY OF CHANGE Quinn (2000a, 2000b) reported that when organizations experience changes, the staff will often experience burnout and a lack of energy, and feel trapped, hopeless, or frustrated. Although most people will cope with these changes by resigning themselves to it or by trying to find a way out around the problem, Quinn aimed to engage people to understand and accept the need for change. This process of change can be a slow and painful one, but the participants are engaged for a "deep change"; that is, they are mobilized to surrender their present selves and to adapt and emerge to a new culture at the collective and individual level.

PROCHASKA'S TRANSTHEORETICAL MODEL Prochaska's transtheoretical model is useful for explaining the readiness for change. The six stages of change are cyclical: precontemplation, contemplation, preparation, action, maintenance, and termination. (Please refer to description in Chapter 8, the section "The Transtheoretical Model: Stages of Health Behaviour Change.")

KOTTER'S EIGHT-STEP CHANGE PROCESS To combat common organization behaviours and resistance to change, Kotter and Rathgeber (2006) provide the following eight steps to guide leaders and managers in leading change successfully:

Set the Stage

1. *Create a sense of urgency:* Help others see the need for change and the importance of acting immediately.
2. *Pull together the guiding team:* Form a powerful group to guide the change. Members of this group need

to possess leadership skills, credibility, communications ability, authority, and analytical skills.

Decide What to Do

3. *Develop the change vision and strategy*: Allow everyone to share his or her vision regarding how to transform the past into a reality for the future.

Make It Happen

4. *Communicate for understanding and buy-in:* Ensure as many people as possible will understand and accept the proposed vision and the strategy.
5. *Empower others to act*: Facilitate the process to achieve the vision by removing barriers and providing the needed resources and support.
6. *Produce short-term wins*: Create some visible successes as quickly as possible.
7. *Don't let up*: Institute the change tirelessly until the vision is achieved.

Make It Stick

8. *Create a new culture*: Foster the new ways of behaving and help the group to develop it into a part of their culture.

The key to effective change management is the ability to balance the amount of threat produced with enough psychological safety to allow the change to be accepted. The art of change management lies in the strategies managers develop to create enough safety for their staff to embrace the change (Schein, 1996). An important aspect of planning change is establishing the likelihood of the acceptance of the change and then determining the criteria by which that acceptance can be identified. Accepting change often takes time, particularly when it does not fit into a person's attitudinal framework. The course of acceptance is easier for people if they are involved in the process. If possible, change should be instituted on a small scale before full implementation. To facilitate acceptance of the change, the change agent also needs to identify common driving and restraining forces (see Box 26.4). Guidelines for dealing with resistance are found in Box 26.5.

BOX 26.4 COMMON DRIVING AND RESTRAINING FORCES

Identifying driving and restraining forces can help the change agent make acceptance of the change possible.

DRIVING FORCES

- Perception that the change is challenging
- Economic gain
- Perception that the change will improve the situation
- Visualization of the future impact of change
- Potential for self-growth, recognition, achievement, and improved relationships

RESTRAINING FORCES

- Fear that something of personal value will be lost (e.g., threat to job security or self-esteem)
- Misunderstanding of the change and its implications
- Low tolerance for change related to intellectual or emotional insecurity
- Perception that the change will not achieve goals; failure to see the big picture
- Lack of time or energy
- Perceived loss of freedom to engage in particular behaviours

BOX 26.5 GUIDELINES FOR DEALING WITH RESISTANCE

The following guidelines are useful for dealing with resistance to change:

1. Communicate with those who oppose the change. Get to the root of their reasons for opposition.
2. Clarify information and provide accurate information.
3. Be open to revisions but clear about what must remain.
4. Present the negative consequences of resistance (threats to organizational survival, compromised client care, and so on).
5. Emphasize the positive consequences of the change and how the individual or group will benefit. However, do not spend too much energy on rational analysis of why the change is good and why the arguments against it do not hold up. People's resistance frequently flows from feelings that are not rational.
6. Keep resisters involved in face-to-face contact with supporters. Encourage proponents to empathize with opponents, recognize valid objections, and relieve unnecessary fears.
7. Maintain a climate of trust, support, and confidence.
8. Follow the *politics of change:* (a) Analyze the organizational chart; know the formal lines of authority. Identify informal lines as well. (b) Identify key persons who will be affected by the change. Pay attention to those immediately above and below the point of change. (c) Find out as much as possible about these key people. What interests them, gets them excited, turns them off? What is on their personal and organizational agendas? Who typically aligns with whom on important decisions? (d) Begin to build a coalition of support before you start the change process. Identify the key people who will most likely support your idea and those who are most likely to be persuaded easily. Talk informally with them to flush out possible objections to your idea and potential opponents. What will the costs and benefits be to them—especially in political terms? Can your idea be modified in ways that retain your objectives but appeal to more key people?

Source: From *Effective Leadership and Management in Nursing,* 6th ed., by E. J. Sullivan and P. J. Decker, 2005. Copyright © 2005 by Upper Saddle River, NJ: Prentice Hall. Adapted with permission.

Considerable research has looked at change and change management during the past decade. Before implementing a change, nurse leaders and managers need to understand why reactions to change vary so much. When planning for change, consider that it is neither good nor bad, but it is different for each person affected by it. Some staff will be energized when considering a change, and other staff will feel threatened or anxious, or have a sense of loss of the familiar. Some may even experience a grief reaction (White, 2004).

A Vision for Change

As nurses work at the forefront of the health-care system, they are affected by change; nobody can avoid it. Knowledgeable nurses make rational plans to deal with opportunities both to initiate and guide needed change and to respond to change that affects them in the workplace, in government, in organizations, and in the community. To recognize these opportunities for change and respond to the factors that influence nursing from without, it is helpful to consider the history of nursing, current trends in nursing, and present political, social, technological, and economic issues.

Grossman and Valiga (2005) stated that "professional nurses can no longer think of themselves as 'just nurses'" (p. 66). The CNA stated that it is time for a shift of focus to have a new generation of nurse leaders and managers (Villeneuve & MacDonald, 2006). One of the visions for the year 2020 is to have at least 20% of nursing leaders from the Aboriginal and visible minority populations, and at least 10% of nursing leaders be male. The nursing curriculum must foster opportunity to develop skills required for nursing leadership (Villeneuve & MacDonald). Nurses can learn and grow to be leaders by doing the following:

- Seize opportunities created by change
- Enable others to influence change
- Support each other, especially younger nurses
- Practice personal accountability
- Put the *Code of Ethics for Registered Nurses* to work every day
- Apply research; participate in research
- Embrace lifelong learning
- Build strategic relationships
- Cultivate flexibility and innovation
- Advocate for improved client care (CNA, 2005, p. 4)

Case Study 26

You have just interviewed for two nursing positions and are trying to decide which job to pursue. During your first interview for a team member position, the nurse manager, Mr. Caruso, was cheerful, spoke highly of his current staff, complimented them on their ability to set goals and participate in decision making, listened to your ideas, and explored ways that you could contribute to this team's effectiveness. The second nurse manager, Mrs. Turner, was also cheerful and talkative. She provided you with a job description as a primary nurse caregiver, explained her expectations of you as a new employee, and spoke of new programs she was attempting to implement. Both nurse managers talked about changes taking place in their facilities and the need for employees to remain flexible.

Critical Thinking Questions

1. On the basis of the brief data provided, speculate about the leadership style of each of these nurse managers.
2. Think about managers (or leaders) you have known and admired. What characteristics did they have that you would like to integrate into your own management style?
3. Both nurse managers spoke of changes that were taking place in their facility. As a nurse, how can you assist your peers who are unhappy and seem to resist change even when it is positive?
4. What factors should you consider before making a decision about accepting a position in a team nursing environment as opposed to a primary nursing environment?

After working through these questions, go to the MyNursingLab at http://www.mynursinglab.com to check your answers.

KEY TERMS

leader
manager
formal leader
informal leader
leadership style
autocratic (authoritarian, directive) leaders
democratic (participative, consultative) leaders
laissez-faire (nondirective, permissive, ultraliberal) leader
bureaucratic leader
situational leadership
charismatic leadership

transactional leadership
transformational leadership
shared leadership
shared governance
vision
influence
power
positional power
personal power
task power
relationship power
first-level managers
middle-level managers
upper-level managers
planning
risk management
organizing
directing
coordinating
authority
accountability
responsibility
critical thinking
networking
Silent generation
baby boomers
Generation X
Millennial generation
mentor
preceptor
effectiveness
efficiency
productivity
delegation
change
change agent
developmental change
unplanned change
planned change

CHAPTER HIGHLIGHTS

- The professional nurse frequently assumes the roles of leader and manager. Leaders influence others to accomplish a specific goal, whereas managers are employees of an organization with responsibility and accountability for accomplishing the tasks of the organization.
- Several leadership styles have been described: autocratic, democratic, laissez-faire, and bureaucratic. These styles are often blended to fit the situation. Nurses need to know which style is most consistent with their behaviour and learn to incorporate aspects of other styles into their practice.
- Descriptions of leadership, including charismatic, transactional, transformational, connective, and shared, address the traits, behaviours, and relationships between leaders and followers.
- Four major management functions are planning, organizing, directing, and coordinating.
- Nurse managers work in the organizational framework of the employing agency. Principles of management include authority, accountability, and responsibility.
- The skills and competencies required by nurse managers are thinking critically, communicating, managing resources, enhancing employee performance, building and managing teams, managing conflict, and managing time.
- Networking is the establishment of professional linkages to obtain information, share ideas, and facilitate the accomplishment of professional goals. Nurses can develop professional networks throughout their careers in a variety of settings, including school, work, professional organizations, and social groups.
- Delegation is a management tool that a manager can use to improve productivity. The manager transfers responsibility and authority to another but retains accountability for the task.
- Nurses frequently act as change agents in relation to clients, families, work settings, and communities. Change is stressful and may be resisted.
- The three types of organizational changes are developmental change, unplanned change, and planned change.
- Planned change requires problem-solving skills, decision-making skills, and interpersonal competence. Nurse leaders and managers must be able to understand the driving and restraining forces and engage their staff to a balance in the change process.
- Lewin's change theory addressed the unfreezing, moving, and freezing stages. Quinn's change theory stressed the need to transform the old self to a new self at the organizational and individual level. Prochaska addressed the importance of readiness for change. Kotter described 8 steps of change from setting the stage to making it happen and making it stick.

ASSESS YOUR LEARNING

1. As *leaders,* nurses influence which of the following?
   a. Clients and their family members
   b. Physicians and other health-care professionals
   c. Politicians
   d. A wide range of people seeking health care or with concerns about health and/or health care

2. Which of the following are three characteristics of successful leaders?
   a. Knowing when to talk, knowing when to listen, and having excellent interpersonal skills
   b. Having a goal, having power over people, and having the resources to succeed
   c. Having a leadership position, creating a vision, and supporting the people

d. Having the ability to motivate, trusting in destiny, and enjoying the process

3. Which of the following is a leadership style that has been described as autocratic?

a. Deprived
b. Exploitive
c. Directive
d. Enlightened

4. A nurse is assigned a new role as a manager of an outpatient department where many issues have been identified. Which of the following would be important as the first goal to achieve?

a. Work all of the unit shifts
b. Set up a meeting with staff
c. Request feedback from team
d. Review the unit budget

5. Both responsibility and which of the following come with the leadership position?

a. Power
b. Dependence
c. Wealth
d. Anxiety

6. A client hospitalized with a stroke is being admitted to home care. Who will be the most likely person to coordinate home care services for the client?

a. Registered nurse
b. Physician
c. Physiotherapist
d. Dietitian

7. What should a staff nurse know before delegating tasks to an ancillary health care worker?

a. The worker should have practised each procedure beforehand.
b. The worker's level of knowledge must be verified before delegation.
c. Workers must be directly supervised in all aspects of nursing care.
d. Workers can perform procedures if they are guided by a registered nurse.

8. Which of the following approaches best illustrates transformational leadership?

a. The leader stimulates group interest in establishing unit goals that contribute to the agency's mission.
b. The leader forms subgroups or task forces that make decisions about unit problems.
c. The leader provides funding for continuing education conferences to staff who have not used any sick leave.
d. The leader adjusts his or her strategies to fit the current situation.

9. After taking the client's history, the nurse recognizes that the client is at risk of developing an infection. Which of the following should the nurse know about the problem?

a. It is the responsibility of the client's physician.
b. It is always a nursing diagnosis.
c. It is a collaborative problem.
d. It is a concern that should be left for the next day shift.

10. The RN stroke coordinator at a Community Care Access Centre explains there will be a move toward best practice guidelines in the management of stroke care and takes the time to facilitate information sessions regarding this change. Several physicians are resistant to the changes. Which strategy would help the nurse encourage change?

a. Request feedback from stakeholders, hold the information sessions to share the feedback, and determine which change theory to apply.
b. Use the information sessions to inform the audience, gather input, and record questions from the attendees.
c. Introduce the changes, complete research, and use the information sessions to inform the audience about the change.
d. Apply a change theory to the process, complete a current literature search, and use the information sessions as a beginning step.

After working through these questions, go to the MyNursingLab at ***http://www.mynursinglab.com*** *to check your answers and see explanations.*

SUGGESTED READINGS

Canadian Nurses Association. (2005). Nursing leadership in a changing world. *Nursing Now: Issues and Trends in Canadian Nursing, 18.* Retrieved October 25, 2007, from http://cna-aiic.ca/CNA/documents/pdf/publications/NN_Nursing_Leadership_05_e.pdf

This article examines what leadership is and should be in today's changing health-care environment.

Registered Nurses' Association of Ontario. (2006). *Healthy work environments best practice guidelines: Developing and sustaining nursing leadership.* Toronto: Author.

This document outlines evidence-based guidelines to promote a healthy working environment.

Villeneuve, M., & MacDonald, J. (2006). *Toward 2020: Visions for nursing.* Ottawa: Canadian Nurses Association. Retrieved October 25, 2007, from http://www.cna-nurses.ca/CNA/documents/pdf/publications/Toward-2020-e.pdf

This document provides a snapshot of where nursing is today and sets a vision for the future of nursing.

WEBLINKS

Canadian Nurses Association

http://www.cna-aiic.ca

This website provides information regarding the Canadian Nurses Association, its policies and guidelines, current news, and links to provincial and territorial sites.

International Council of Nurses

http://www.icn.ch

The website of the International Council of Nurses includes guidelines for improving health-care practices related to multiple issues, links to national and international organizations, and current news and updates.

College of Nurses of Ontario

http://www.cno.org

This website provides nurses with information on the standards of practice for nursing in Ontario, the roles of the CNO, the policies and guidelines, current activities, and educational material.

Registered Nurses' Association of Ontario

http://www.rnao.org

The Registered Nurses' Association of Ontario provides on its website information on health and nursing policy, nursing best practice guidelines, educational material, and information on the Centre for Nursing Excellency.

Better Management.com

http://www.bettermanagement.com/Seminars/VideoInterview/launchInterview.aspx?LibraryID=14177

Arthur, J., & Rathgeber, H. (2006). The risk of uncertainty: managing communication and change for positive action. *Better Management Series.*

This video webcast presents ways to identify risks and needs in the organization and strategies to change the organization culture and attitude as leaders manage and communicate change effectively.

Kotter Associates

http://www.ouricebergismelting.com/html/seminars.html

This site links to various web seminars on leadership and organizational change.

REFERENCES

Blanchard, K. (2003). Taking the lead when you're not in charge. *The Blanchard Management Report.* Issue #164. Retrieved April 25, 2008, from http://www.kenblanchard.com/ignite/ignite_volume3_2003.html

Berg, J. (2006). Strengths of the ages [Electronic version]. *The Spectrum: Career management, 4.* Retrieved October 25, 2007, from http://community.nursingspectrum.com/MagazineArticles/article.cfm?AID=20490

Canadian Nurses Association. (2003). *Succession planning for nursing leadership.* Retrieved October 25, 2007, from http://cna-aiic.ca/CNA/documents/pdf/publications/succession_planning_e.pdf

Canadian Nurses Association. (2004). *Achieving excellence in nursing practice: A guide to preceptorship and mentorship.* Retrieved October 25, 2007, from http://www.cna-nurses.ca/CNA/nursing/education/mentorship/default_e.aspx

Canadian Nurses Association. (2005). Nursing leadership in a changing world. *Nursing Now: Issues and Trends in Canadian Nursing, 18.* Retrieved October 25, 2007, from http://cna-aiic.ca/CNA/documents/pdf/publications/NN_Nursing_Leadership_05_e.pdf

Carroll, P. (2006). *Nursing leadership and management: A practical guide.* Clifton Park, NY: Thomson Delmar Learning.

College of Nurses of Ontario. (2006a). *Therapeutic nurse-client relationship.* Toronto: Author.

College of Nurses of Ontario. (2006b). *Practice guideline: Conflict prevention and management guideline.* Toronto: Author.

Grossman, S., & Valiga, T. (2005). *The new leadership challenge: Creating a preferred future for nursing* (2nd ed.). Philadelphia, PA: Davis.

Hibberd, J. M., & Smith, D. L. (2006). *Nursing leadership and management in Canada.* Toronto: Elsevier Mosby.

Kotter, J., & Rathgeber, H. (2006). *Our icebergs are melting.* New York: St. Martin's Press.

Lewin, K. (1951). *Field theory in social science.* New York: Harper & Row.

Marquis B., & Huston, C. J. (2005). *Leadership roles and management functions in nursing* (4th ed.). Philadelphia: Lippincott.

Martin, C. (2004). Bridging the generation gap(s). *Nursing 2007, 34*(12), 62–63.

Prochaska, J. O., Redding, C. A., & Evers, K. E. (2002). The transtheorectical model and stages of change. In K. Glanz, B. K. Rimer, & F. M. Lewis (Eds.), *Health behavior and health education: Theory, research, and practice* (3rd ed.) (pp. 99–120). San Francisco, CA: Jossey-Bass.

Quinn, R. E. (2000a). *Change the world: How ordinary people can accomplish extraordinary results.* San Francisco, CA: Jossey-Bass.

Quinn, R. E. (2000b). Changing others through changing ourselves. *Journal of Management Inquiry, 9*(2), 147–165.

Schein, E. H. (1996). Kurt Lewin's change theory in the field and in the classroom: Notes toward a model of managed learning. *Systems Practice, 9,* 27–47.

Sullivan, E. J., & Decker, P. J. (2005). *Effective leadership and management in nursing* (6th ed.). Upper Saddle River, NJ: Prentice-Hall.

Villeneuve, M., & MacDonald, J. (2006). *Toward 2020: Visions for nursing.* Ottawa: Canadian Nurses Association. Retrieved October 25, 2007, from http://www.cna-nurses.ca/CNA/documents/pdf/publications/Toward-2020-e.pdf

White, A. (2004). Anticipate responses to change. *Nursing Management, 35,* 11–13.

UNIT 5

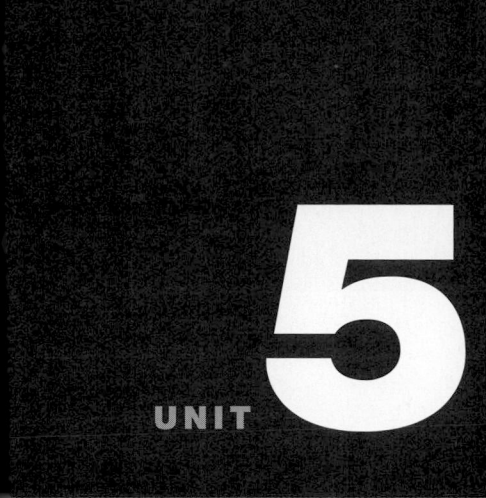

Nursing Assessment and Clinical Studies

CHAPTER 27
Health Assessment

CHAPTER 28
Vital Signs

CHAPTER 29
Hygiene

CHAPTER 30
Safety

CHAPTER 31
Medication Administration

CHAPTER 32
Infection Prevention and Control

CHAPTER 33
Skin Integrity and Wound Care

CHAPTER 34
Pain Management

CHAPTER 35
Caring for Perioperative Clients

Chapter 27

Health Assessment

Assessing a client's health status is a major component of nursing care and has two aspects: (1) the nursing health history discussed in Chapter 22, and (2) the physical assessment discussed in this chapter. A physical examination can be any of three types: (1) a complete assessment (e.g., when a client is admitted to a health-care agency); (2) examination of a body system (e.g., the cardiovascular system); (3) examination of a body area (e.g., the lungs, when difficulty with breathing is observed). *Note:* Some nurses consider *assessment* to be the broad term used in applying the nursing process to health data and *examination* to be the physical process used to gather the data. In this text, the terms *assessment* and *examination* are sometimes used interchangeably, referring to both a critical investigation and an evaluation of client status.

OBJECTIVES

After studying this chapter, you should be able to

1. Identify the purposes of the physical health examination
2. Identify expected outcomes of the health assessment
3. Identify the steps in selected assessment procedures
4. Describe the suggested sequencing to conduct a physical health assessment in an orderly manner
5. Discuss variations in examination techniques appropriate for clients of different ages
6. Explain the four methods of examination
7. Explain the significance of selected physical findings

Physical Health Assessment

A complete health assessment can be conducted starting at the head and proceeding in a systematic manner downward to the toes (head-to-toe assessment). However, the procedure can vary according to the age of the individual, the severity of the illness, the preferences of the nurse, and the location of the examination. Whatever order a nurse chooses to perform an assessment, it is important to be consistent each time it is done. A consistent approach that is routinely practised reduces the likelihood of forgetting or omitting certain parts of the assessment. In addition, consistency in examination facilitates systematic documentation of the findings. The order of head-to-toe assessment is given in Box 27.1. Regardless of what procedure is used, the client's energy and time need to be considered. The health assessment is, therefore, conducted in a systematic and efficient manner that requires the fewest position changes for the client.

The sequence of the assessment differs with children and adults. With children, always proceed from the least invasive or uncomfortable to the more invasive. Examination of the head and neck, heart, lungs, and range of motion can be done early in the process, while the ears, mouth, abdomen, and genitals should be left for the end of the exam.

Frequently, nurses assess a specific body area instead of the entire body. These specific assessments are made in relation to client concerns, the nurse's own observation of problems, the client's presenting problem, nursing interventions provided, and medical therapies. Examples of these situations and assessments are provided in Table 27.1.

A physical health examination can be done for many different reasons:

- To obtain baseline data about the client's functional abilities
- To supplement, confirm, or refute data obtained in the nursing history
- To obtain data that will help the nurse establish nursing diagnoses and a plan of care
- To evaluate the physiological outcomes of health care and, thus, the progress of a client's health problem
- To make clinical judgments about a client's health status
- To identify areas for health promotion and disease prevention

Nurses use national guidelines and evidence-based practice to focus health assessment on specific conditions. For example, when screening for cancer, nurses should keep in mind the Canadian Cancer Society screening guidelines (Box 27.2).

Preparing the Client

Before the assessment, the nurse should explain when and where it will take place, why it is important, and what will happen during the assessment. Often clients are anxious about what the nurse will find. They can be reassured during the examination by explanations at

BOX 27.1 HEAD-TO-TOE FRAMEWORK

- General survey
- Vital signs
- Head
  - Hair, scalp, cranium, face
  - Eyes and vision
  - Ears and hearing
  - Nose and sinuses
  - Mouth and oropharynx
  - Cranial nerves
- Neck
  - Muscles
  - Lymph nodes
  - Trachea
  - Thyroid gland
  - Carotid arteries
  - Neck veins
- Upper extremities
  - Skin and nails
  - Muscle strength and tone
  - Joint range of motion
  - Brachial and radial pulses
  - Biceps tendon reflexes
  - Tendon reflexes
  - Sensation
- Chest and back
  - Skin
  - Breasts and axillae
  - Chest shape and size
  - Lungs
  - Heart
  - Spinal column
- Abdomen
  - Skin
  - Abdominal sounds
  - Specific organs (e.g., liver, bladder)
- Genitals
  - Testicles
  - Vagina
  - Urethra
- Anus and rectum
- Lower extremities
  - Skin and toenails
  - Gait and balance
  - Joint range of motion
  - Femoral, popliteal, posterior tibial, and pedal pulses
  - Tendon and plantar reflexes
  - Sensation

TABLE 27.1 Nursing Assessments Addressing Specific Client Situations

Situation	Physical Assessment
The client complains of abdominal pain.	Inspect, auscultate, percuss, and palpate the abdomen; assess vital signs.
The client is admitted with a head injury.	Assess level of consciousness by using Glasgow Coma Scale (see Table 27.12, p. 635); assess pupils for reaction to light and accommodation; assess vital signs.
The nurse prepares to administer a cardiotonic drug to a client.	Assess apical pulse and compare with baseline data.
The nurse administers postural drainage.	Auscultate lungs before and after the procedure.
The client has just had a cast applied to the lower leg.	Assess peripheral perfusion of toes, capillary blanch test, pedal pulse, if able, and vital signs.
The client's fluid intake is minimal.	Assess tissue turgor, fluid intake and output, and vital signs.

BOX 27.2 CANADIAN CANCER SOCIETY SELECTED EARLY DETECTION AND SCREENING GUIDELINES

Type of Cancer	Screening	Signs and Symptoms	At-Risk Populations and Risk Factors
Prostate cancer The most common cancer in Canadian men	Men over the age of 50 should discuss the risks and benefits of prostate specific antigen (PSA) blood test with their doctor. PSA can be false positive because of prostate problems other than cancer. Men with prostate cancer can have normal PSA levels. Digital rectal examinations can also help to detect prostate cancer.	None in early stages; need to urinate often, especially at night; intense need to urinate (urgency); difficulty in starting or stopping the urine flow; inability to urinate; weak, decreased, or interrupted urine stream; a sense of incompletely emptying the bladder; burning or pain during urination; blood in the urine or semen; painful ejaculation	Being older than 65 years, family history, African ancestry; obesity, physical inactivity, a high-fat diet, and working with cadmium (a metal) are under investigation as possible risk factors
Breast cancer The most common cancer in Canadian women; less than 1% of breast cancers occur in men	Women 40–49: clinical breast exam at least every two years; discussion of benefits and risks of mammography in relation to risks of breast cancer Women 50–69: clinical breast exam at least every 2 years; mammogram every 2 years Women > 70: tailored depending on risk	Lump or swelling in the axilla; changes in breast size or shape; dimpling or puckering of the skin (sometimes called orange peel); redness, swelling, and increased warmth in the affected breast; inverted nipple; crusting or scaling on the nipple	Family history of breast cancer (especially in a mother, sister, or daughter diagnosed before menopause or if mutations on BRCA1 or BRCA2 genes are present); family history of ovarian cancer; previous breast disorders with biopsies showing abnormal cells; no pregnancies or having a first pregnancy after age 30; beginning to menstruate at an early age; having a later than average menopause; dense breast tissue; taking hormone replacement therapy (estrogen plus progestin) for more than 5 years; radiation treatment to the chest area; obesity (especially after menopause), alcohol, and the use of oral contraceptives are associated with a slight increase in breast cancer risk; the effects of smoking, diet, and physical activity are under study

(continued)

(continued)

BOX 27.2 CANADIAN CANCER SOCIETY SELECTED EARLY DETECTION AND SCREENING GUIDELINES

Type of Cancer	Screening	Signs and Symptoms	At-Risk Populations and Risk Factors
Lung cancer The leading cause of cancer death in Canadians	Screening tests are still being tested in clinical trials	Cough or change in cough; hemoptysis (the coughing up of blood from the respiratory tract); shortness of breath; hoarseness; weight loss	Smoking; second-hand smoke; exposure to asbestos, arsenic, chromium, nickel (especially if a smoker); exposure to radon; air pollution; family history of lung cancer
Colorectal Cancer The second leading cause of death from cancer in Canadians	Fecal occult blood test (FOBT) at least every 2 years in men and women age 50 and older of average risk; individualized plan for high-risk clients; follow-up for a positive FOBT could include a colonoscopy, a double-contrast barium enema and a sigmoidoscopy	General discomfort in the abdomen (gas pains, bloating, fullness, or cramps); change in bowel habits, such as diarrhea or constipation, for no apparent reason; bright red or very dark blood in the stool; stools that are narrower than usual; vomiting; feeling very tired; weight loss	Age: particularly after 50; polyps; high-fat diet; obesity; physical inactivity; alcohol consumption; inflammatory bowel disease (ulcerative colitis or Crohn's disease); smoking; family history of colorectal cancer in close relatives (parents, siblings, or children) increases risk, especially if the relatives developed cancer before the age of 45; having familial adenomatous polyposis or hereditary nonpolyposis colon cancer; people of Ashkenazi (Eastern European Jewish) descent
Cervical cancer Rates are declining, owing to early screening; introduction of human papilloma-virus vaccine may reduce incidence even further	Sexually active women: Papanicolaou (Pap) every 1 to 3 years depending on provincial or territorial guidelines; women who are not sexually active continue to require Pap testing; colposcopy and biopsy follow a positive Pap	Abnormal bleeding or bloodstained discharge from the vagina between periods; unusually long or heavy periods; bleeding after sexual intercourse; pain during sexual intercourse; watery discharge from the vagina; increased amount of discharge from the vagina; bleeding from the vagina after menopause	Infection of the cervix with human papillomavirus (HPV); becoming sexually active at a young age; multiple sex partners or a partner who has had multiple partners; smoking; suppression of the immune system by drugs after an organ transplant or a condition, such as AIDS

Source: Summarized from the Canadian Cancer Society's website at http://www.cancer.ca. See the Canadian Cancer Society's website for other cancer type screening, risk factors, and epidemiology.

each step. Instruct the client that all information gathered and documented during the assessment is kept confidential.

Health assessments are usually painless; however, it is important to determine in advance any positions that are contraindicated for a particular client. The nurse helps the client, as needed, to undress and put on a gown. Clients should empty their bladders before the examination. Doing so helps them feel more relaxed and makes palpation of the abdomen and the pubic area more comfortable. If a urinalysis is required, the urine should be collected at the time the client empties his or her bladder. Since an empty rectum facilitates rectal examination, the client should be encouraged to defecate before a complete examination.

When assessing adults, it is important to recognize that people of the same age can differ markedly. Box 27.3 provides special considerations for assessing older adults.

Preparing the Environment

It is important to prepare the environment before starting the assessment. The time for the physical assessment should be convenient to both the client and the nurse. The environment should be well lit and the equipment should be systematically arranged for the examination. A disorganized environment does not convey professional competence to the client.

BOX 27.3 HEALTH ASSESSMENT OF THE OLDER ADULT

Health assessments are often carried out on older adults. Keep these guidelines in mind when examining these clients:

- Be aware of normal physiological changes that occur with age.
- Expose only areas of the body to be examined in order to avoid chilling the client.
- Permit ample time for the client to answer your questions and assume the required positions.
- Be aware of cultural differences. The client may want a family member present during disrobing.
- Arrange for an interpreter if the client's language differs from yours.
- Adapt assessment techniques to any sensory impairment; for example, make sure clients have their eyeglasses or hearing aids.
- If a client is frail, it is wise to plan several assessment times to avoid overtiring him or her.

It is important to provide the client with privacy. Most people are embarrassed if their bodies are exposed or if others can overhear or view them during the assessment. Family and friends should not be present unless the client specifically asks for someone to be present in the room. A client who is physically relaxed will usually experience little discomfort. The room should be warm and comfortable for the client.

Positioning

Several positions are frequently required during the physical assessment. It is important to consider the client's ability to assume a position. The client's physical condition, energy level, and age should also be taken into consideration. Some positions are embarrassing and uncomfortable and, therefore, should not be maintained for long. The assessment is organized so that several body areas can be assessed in one position, thus minimizing the number of position changes needed (see Table 27.2).

Draping

Drapes should be arranged so that the area to be assessed is exposed and other body areas are covered. Exposure of the body is frequently embarrassing to clients. Drapes provide not only a degree of privacy but also warmth. Drapes are made of paper, cloth, or bed linen.

Instrumentation

All equipment required for the health assessment should be clean, in good working order, and readily accessible. Equipment is frequently set up on trays, ready for use. Photographs of various instruments are shown in Table 27.3.

Methods of Examination

Four primary techniques are used in the physical examination: inspection, palpation, percussion, and auscultation. These techniques are discussed throughout this chapter as they apply to each body system.

INSPECTION **Inspection** is a visual examination, that is, an assessment by observing with the eyes. It should be deliberate, purposeful, and systematic. The nurse inspects with the naked eye and with a lighted instrument, such as an otoscope (used to view the ear). In addition to visual observations, olfactory (smell) and auditory (hearing) cues are noted. Nurses frequently use visual inspection to assess moisture, colour, and texture of body surfaces, as well as shape, position, size, colour, and symmetry of the body. Lighting must be sufficient for the nurse to see clearly; either natural or artificial light can be used. When using the auditory senses, it is important to have a quiet environment for accurate hearing. Observation can be combined with the other assessment techniques.

PALPATION **Palpation** is the examination of the body by using the sense of touch. The pads of the fingers are used because their concentration of nerve endings makes them highly sensitive to tactile discrimination. Palpation is used to determine (1) texture (e.g., of the hair); (2) temperature (e.g., of a skin area); (3) vibration (e.g., of a joint); (4) position, size, consistency, and mobility of organs or masses; (5) distension (e.g., of the urinary bladder); (6) pulsation; and (7) the presence of pain on pressure.

There are two types of palpation: light and deep. *Light* (superficial) *palpation* should always precede *deep*

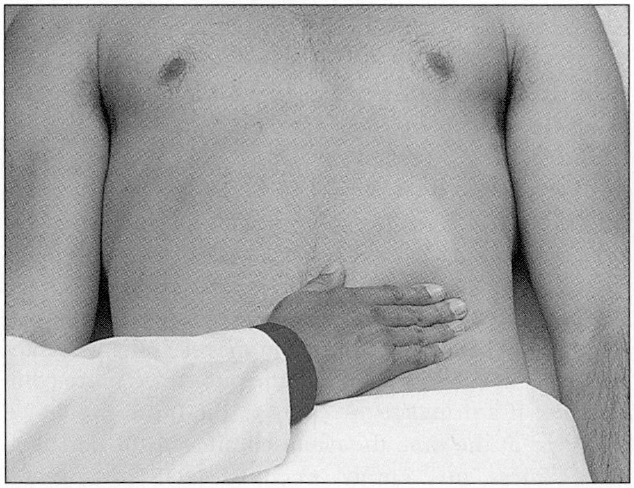

FIGURE 27.1 The position of the hand for light palpation

TABLE 27.2 Client Positions and Body Areas Assessed

Position	Description	Areas Assessed	Cautions
Dorsal recumbent 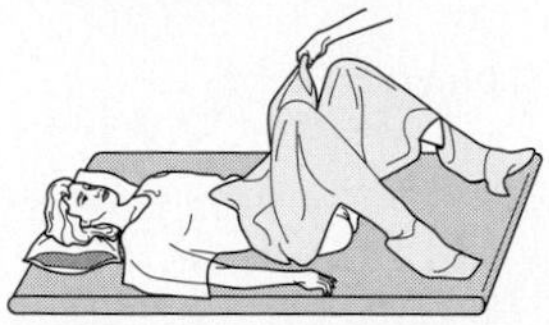	Back-lying position with knees flexed and hips externally rotated; small pillow under the head; soles of feet on the surface	Female genitals, rectum, and female reproductive tract	May be contraindicated for clients who have cardiopulmonary problems.
Supine (horizontal recumbent) 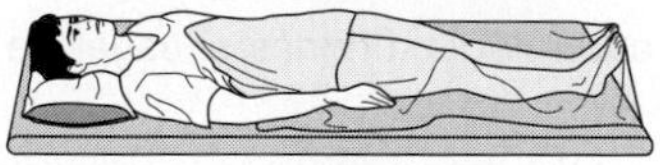	Back-lying position with legs extended; with or without pillow under the head	Head, neck, axillae, anterior thorax, lungs, breasts, heart, vital signs, abdomen, extremities, peripheral pulses	Tolerated poorly by clients with cardio-vascular or respiratory problems.
Sitting 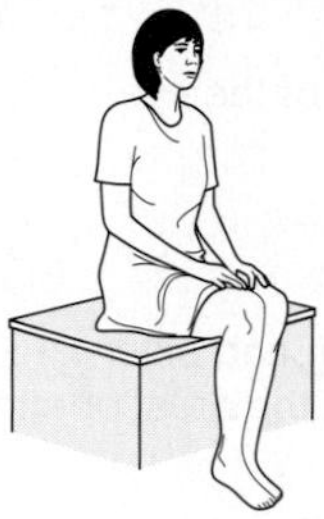	A seated position, back unsupported and legs hanging freely	Head, neck, posterior and anterior thorax, lungs, breasts, axillae, heart, vital signs, upper and lower extremities, reflexes	Older adults and weak clients may require support.
Lithotomy 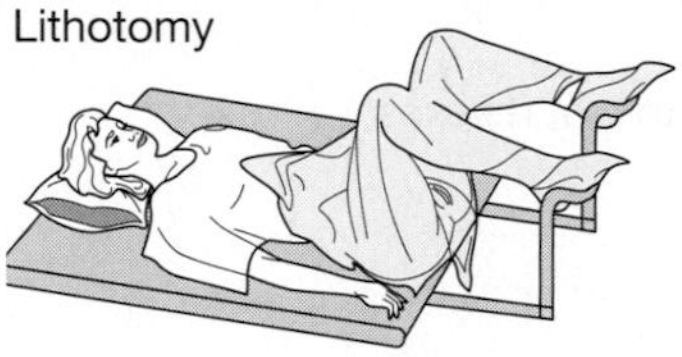	Back-lying position with feet supported in stirrups; the hips should be in line with the edge of the table	Female genitals, rectum, and female reproductive tract	May be uncomfortable and tiring for older adults and often embarrassing.
Sims' 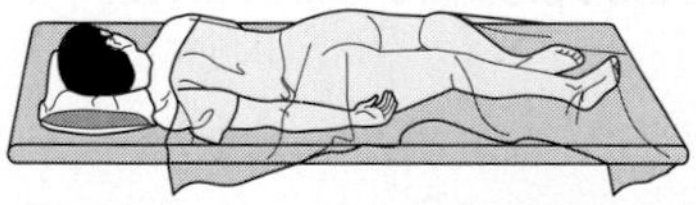	Side-lying position with lowermost arm behind the body, uppermost leg flexed at hip and knee, upper arm flexed at shoulder and elbow	Rectum, vagina	Difficult for older adults and people with limited joint movement.
Prone 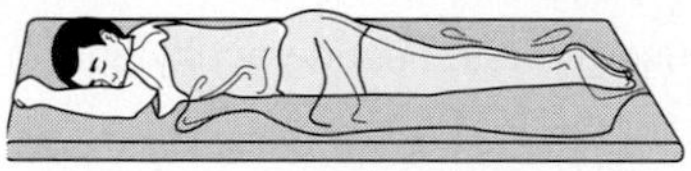	Lies on abdomen with head turned to the side, with or without a small pillow	Posterior thorax, hip joint movement	Often not tolerated by older adults and people with cardiovascular or respiratory problems.

palpation because heavy pressure on the fingertips can dull the sense of touch. For light palpation, the nurse extends the fingers of the dominant hand parallel to the skin surface and presses gently while moving the hand in a circle (Figure 27.1). The skin is slightly depressed in light palpation. If it is necessary to determine the details of a mass, the nurse presses lightly several times, rather than holding the pressure constant. See Box 27.4 for the characteristics of masses.

Deep palpation is done with two hands (bimanually) or one hand. In deep bimanual palpation, the nurse extends the dominant hand as for light palpation, and then places the fingerpads of the nondominant hand on the dorsal surface of the distal interphalangeal joint of

BOX 27.4 CHARACTERISTICS OF MASSES

Nurses should note the following characteristics of any masses:

- Location: Site on the body, dorsal or ventral surface
- Size: Measure in centimetres
- Shape: Oval, round, elongated, irregular
- Consistency: Soft, firm, hard
- Surface: Smooth, nodular
- Mobility: Fixed, mobile
- Pulsatility: Present, absent
- Tenderness: Degree of tenderness to palpation

TABLE 27.3 Equipment and Supplies Used for a Health Examination

Instruments and Supplies		Purpose
Flashlight or penlight	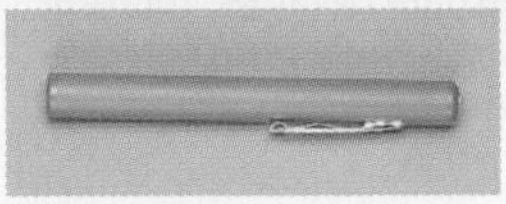	To assist viewing of the pharynx and cervix or to determine the reactions of the pupils of the eye
Laryngeal or dental mirror	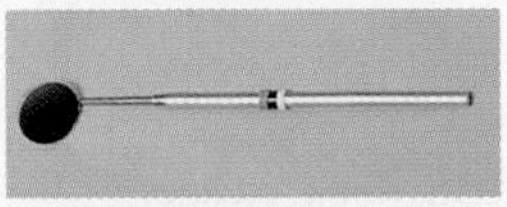	To observe the pharynx and oral cavity
Nasal speculum	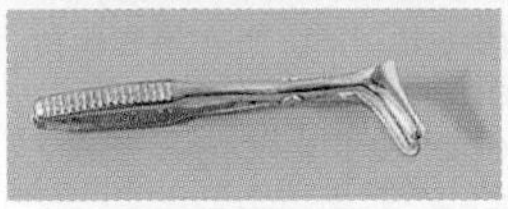	To permit visualization of the lower and middle turbinates; usually a penlight is used for illumination
Ophthalmoscope	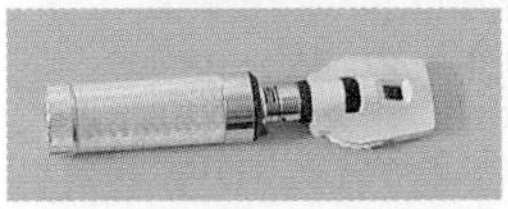	A lighted instrument to visualize the interior of the eye
Otoscope	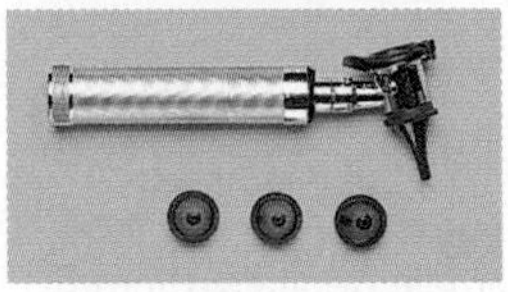	A lighted instrument to visualize the eardrum and external auditory canal (a nasal speculum can be attached to the otoscope to inspect the nasal cavities)
Percussion (reflex) hammer	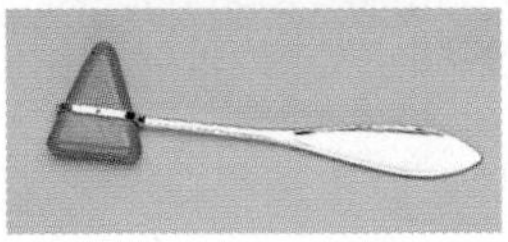	An instrument with a rubber head to test reflexes
Sphygmomanometer and cuff (see Figure 28.19, p. 690)		To measure the blood pressure
Stethoscope (see Figure 4 in Skill 28.3, p. 679)		To auscultate body sounds (e.g., blood pressure, chest, bowel sounds)
Thermometer (see Figures 28.5 through 28.9, p. 668–669)		To measure body temperature
Tuning fork	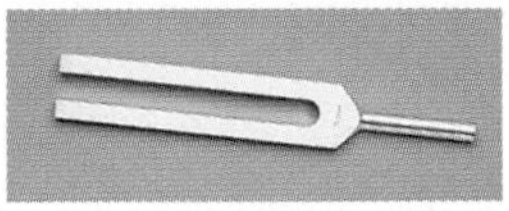	A two-pronged metal instrument used to test hearing acuity and vibratory sense
Vaginal speculum (various sizes) (see Figure 27.38, p. 649)		To assess the cervix and the vagina
Assorted containers and slides		For specimens
Cotton applicators	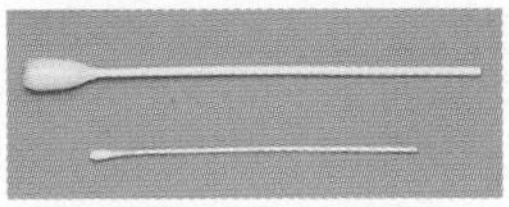	To obtain specimens; to test sensory function
Disposable pads	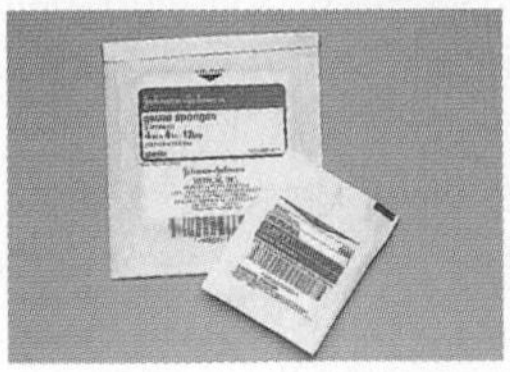	To absorb liquid

(continued)

TABLE 27.3 Equipment and Supplies Used for a Health Examination (*continued*)

Instruments and Supplies	Purpose
Drapes	To cover the client
Gloves (sterile and unsterile) 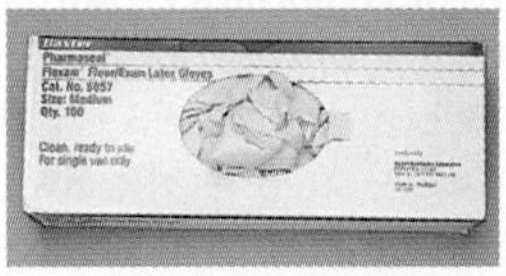	To protect the nurse and client
Lubricant 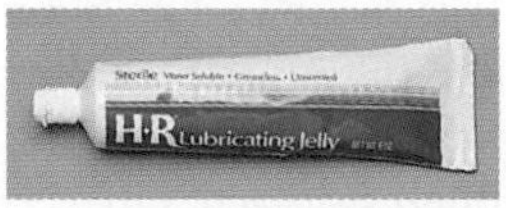	To ease insertion of instruments (e.g., vaginal speculum)
Tongue blades (depressors) 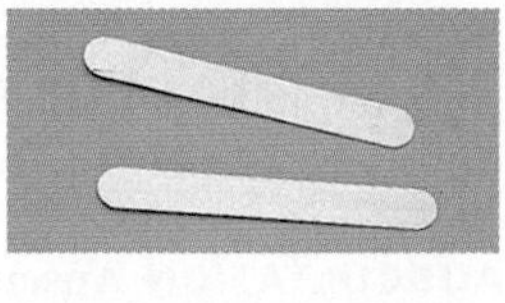	To depress the tongue during assessment of the mouth and pharynx

the middle three fingers of the dominant hand (Figure 27.2). The top hand applies pressure while the lower hand remains relaxed to perceive the tactile sensations. For deep palpation by using one hand, the fingerpads of the dominant hand press over the area to be palpated. Often, the other hand is used to support a mass or organ from below (Figure 27.3). Deep palpation is done only with extreme caution and with a qualified instructor because pressure can damage internal organs. It is not indicated in clients who have acute abdominal pain or pain that is not yet diagnosed.

To test skin temperature, it is best to use the dorsum or back of the hand and fingers where the skin is thinnest. To test for vibration, the nurse should use the palmar surface of the hand. General guidelines for palpation include the following:

- The nurse's hands should be clean and warm and the fingernails short.
- Areas of tenderness should be palpated last.
- Deep palpation, if indicated, should be done after superficial palpation.

The effectiveness of palpation depends largely on the client's level of relaxation. Nurses can assist a client to relax by (1) gowning and draping the client appropriately, (2) positioning the client comfortably, (3) ensuring that their own hands are warm before beginning, and (4) communicating with the client during the exam. During palpation, the nurse should be sensitive to the client's verbal and facial expressions indicating discomfort.

PERCUSSION **Percussion** is the act of striking the body surface to elicit sounds that can be heard or vibrations

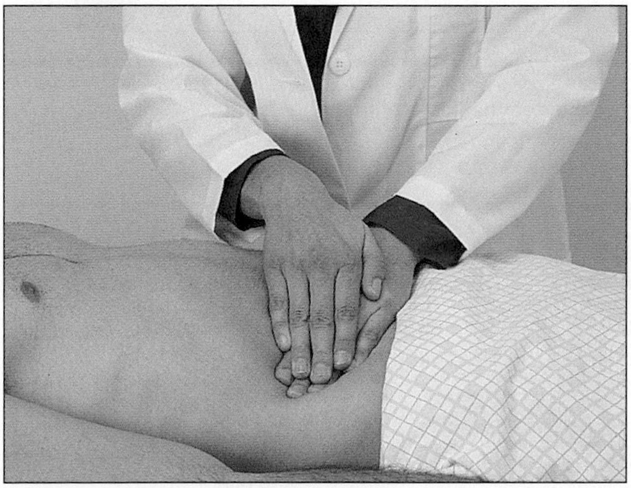

FIGURE 27.2 The position of the hands for deep bimanual palpation

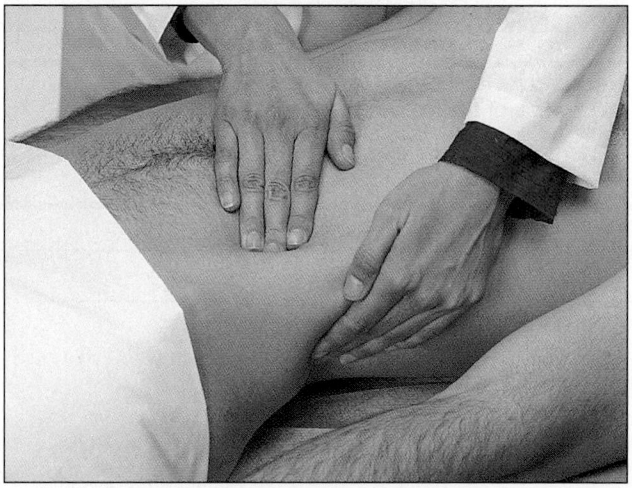

FIGURE 27.3 Deep palpation by using the lower hand to support the body while the upper hand palpates the organ

that can be felt. Percussion has two types: direct and indirect. In *direct percussion,* the nurse strikes the area to be percussed directly with the pads of two, three, or four fingers or with the pad of the middle finger. The strikes are rapid, and the movement is from the wrist. See Figure 27.4. This technique is not generally used to percuss the thorax but is useful in percussing an adult's sinuses.

The second type, *indirect percussion,* is the striking of an object (e.g., a finger) held against the body area to be examined. In this technique, the middle finger of the nondominant hand, referred to as the **pleximeter**, is placed firmly on the client's skin. Only the distal phalanx and joint of this finger should be in contact with the skin. The nurse strikes the pleximeter at the distal interphalangeal joint with the tip of the flexed middle finger of the other hand. The tip of the middle finger that strikes the pleximeter is known as the **plexor** (Figure 27.5). Some nurses may find a point between the distal and proximal joints to be a more comfortable pleximeter point. The motion comes from the wrist; the forearm remains stationary. The angle between the plexor and the pleximeter should be 90 degrees, and the taps must be firm, rapid, and short to obtain a clear sound.

Percussion is used to determine the size and shape of internal organs by establishing their borders. It indicates whether tissue is fluid filled, air filled, or solid. Percussion elicits five types of sound: flatness, dullness, resonance, hyperresonance, and tympany. **Flatness** is an extremely dull sound produced by very dense tissue, such as muscle or bone. **Dullness** is a thud-like sound produced by dense tissue, such as the liver, spleen, or heart. **Resonance** is a hollow sound, such as that produced by lungs filled with air. **Hyperresonance** is not present in a healthy individual. It is described as booming and can be heard over a diseased lung (e.g., in the client with emphysema). **Tympany** is a musical or drum-like sound produced from an air-filled stomach. On a continuum, flatness reflects the most dense tissue (the least amount of air) and tympany the least dense tissue (the greatest amount of air). A percussion sound is described according to its intensity, pitch, duration, and quality. See Table 27.4.

AUSCULTATION **Auscultation** is the process of listening to sounds produced within the body. Auscultation may be direct or indirect. *Direct auscultation* is the use of the unaided ear, for example, to listen to a respiration

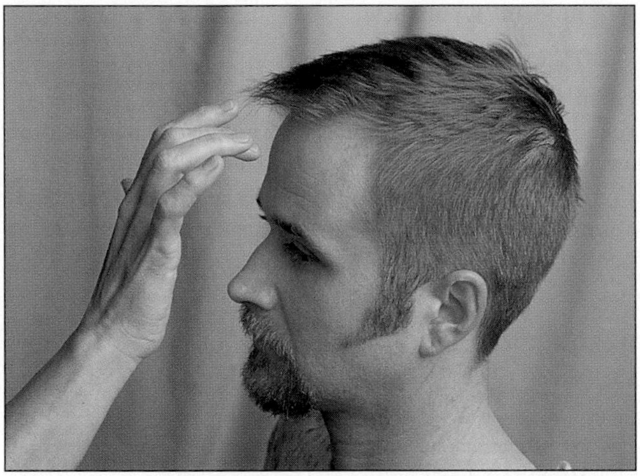

FIGURE 27.4 Direct percussion: Using one hand to strike the surface of the body

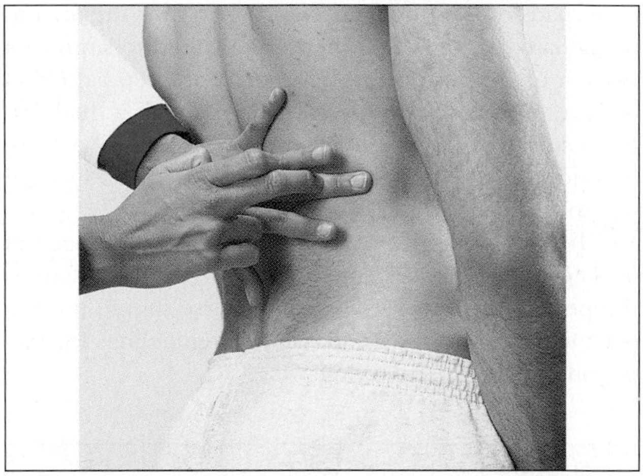

FIGURE 27.5 Indirect percussion: Using the finger of one hand to tap the finger of the other hand

TABLE 27.4 Percussion Sounds and Tones

Sound	Intensity	Pitch	Duration	Quality	Example of Location
Flatness	Soft	High	Short	Extremely dull	Muscle, bone
Dullness	Medium	Medium	Moderate	Thud-like	Liver, heart
Resonance	Loud	Low	Long	Hollow	Normal lung
Hyperresonance	Very loud	Very low	Very long	Booming	Emphysematous lung
Tympany	Loud	High (distinguished mainly by musical timbre)	Moderate	Musical	Stomach filled with gas (air)

wheeze or the grating of a moving joint. *Indirect auscultation* is the use of a stethoscope to listen to sounds from within the body, such as bowel sounds or valve sounds of the heart. A stethoscope amplifies the sounds and conveys them to the nurse's ears.

The stethoscope should be 30 cm to 35 cm long with an internal diameter of about 0.3 cm. It should have both a flat-disc and a bell-shaped diaphragm. (See Figure 4 in Skill 28.3, page 679) The flat-disc diaphragm is best for transmitting high-pitched sounds (e.g., bronchial sounds), and the bell-shaped diaphragm is best for transmitting low-pitched sounds, such as heart sounds. The earpieces of the stethoscope should fit comfortably into the ears, with the earpieces facing forward. The diaphragm of the stethoscope is placed firmly but lightly against the client's skin. If a client is very hairy, it may be necessary to dampen the hairs with a moist cloth so that they will lie flat against the skin and not cause scratching sounds.

Auscultated sounds are described according to their pitch, intensity, duration, and quality. The **pitch** is the frequency of the vibrations (the number of vibrations per second). Low-pitched sounds, such as some heart sounds, have fewer vibrations per second than high-pitched sounds, such as bronchial sounds. The **intensity** (amplitude) refers to the loudness or softness of a sound. Some body sounds are loud, for example, bronchial sounds heard from the trachea; others are soft, for example, normal breath sounds heard in the lungs. The **duration** of a sound is its length (long or short). The **quality** of a sound is a subjective description, for example, whistling, gurgling, or snapping.

General Survey

A physical assessment begins with a general survey, which involves observation of the client's general appearance and behaviour and measurement of vital signs, height, and weight. Many components of the general survey are assessed while taking the client's health history, such as the client's body build, posture, hygiene, and mental status.

Appearance and Behaviour

The general appearance and behaviour of an individual must be assessed in relationship to current circumstances. For example, an individual who has recently experienced a personal loss may appropriately appear depressed. The client's age, gender, and ethnicity or race are useful factors in interpreting findings that suggest increased risk for known conditions. Skill 27.1 describes how to assess general appearance and mental status.

SKILL 27.1

ASSESSING GENERAL APPEARANCE AND MENTAL STATUS

Equipment: None

IMPLEMENTATION

Performance

1. Before performing the procedure, introduce yourself and verify the client's identity by using agency protocol. Explain to the client what you are going to do, why it is necessary, and how he or she can cooperate. Discuss how the results will be used in planning further care or treatments.
2. Perform hand hygiene and observe other appropriate infection prevention and control procedures.
3. Provide for client privacy.

ASSESSMENT	NORMAL FINDINGS	DEVIATIONS FROM NORMAL
General Appearance		
4. Observe body build, height, and weight in relation to the client's age, lifestyle, and health.	Varies with lifestyle	Excessively thin or obese
5. Observe the client's posture and gait, standing, sitting, and walking.	Relaxed, erect posture; coordinated movement	Tense, slouched, bent posture; uncoordinated movement; tremors
6. Observe the client's overall hygiene and grooming. Relate these to the person's activities before the assessment.	Clean, neat	Dirty, unkempt
7. Note body and breath odour in relation to activity level.	No body odour or minor body odour relative to work or exercise; no breath odour	Foul body odour; ammonia odour; acetone breath odour; foul breath

(continued)

SKILL 27.1

ASSESSING GENERAL APPEARANCE AND MENTAL STATUS (*continued*)

ASSESSMENT	NORMAL FINDINGS	DEVIATIONS FROM NORMAL
8. Observe for signs of distress in posture.	No distress noted	Bending over because of abdominal pain; wincing, frowning, or laboured breathing
9. Note obvious signs of health or illness (e.g., in skin colour or breathing).	Healthy appearance	Pallor, weakness, lesions, obvious illness
10. Assess the client's attitude.	Cooperative, able to follow directions	Negative, hostile, withdrawn
11. Note the client's affect or mood; assess the appropriateness of the client's response and level of orientation to time, place, persons, and situation.	Appropriate to situation, orientated	Inappropriate to situation, not orientated
12. Listen for quantity of speech (amount and pace), quality (loudness, clarity, inflection), and organization (coherence of thought, overgeneralization, vagueness).	Understandable, moderate pace; exhibits thought association	Rapid or slow pace; overly loud or soft; uses generalizations; lacks association
13. Listen for relevance and organization of thoughts.	Logical sequence; makes sense; has sense of reality	Illogical sequence; flight of ideas; confusion; vague

EVALUATION

- Perform a detailed follow-up examination of other individual systems based on findings that deviated from expected or normal for the client.
- Report significant deviations from normal to the appropriate members of the health-care team.

Lifespan Considerations

General Survey

INFANTS

- Observation of children's behaviour can provide important data for the general survey, including physical development, neuromuscular function, and social and interactional skills.
- It may be helpful to have parents hold older infants and very young children for part of the assessment.
- Measure the height of children under age 2 in the supine position with knees fully extended.
- Weigh without clothing.
- Include a measurement of head circumference until age 2. Standardized growth charts include head circumference up to age 3.

CHILDREN

- Anxiety in preschool-age children can be decreased by letting them handle and become familiar with the examination equipment.
- School-age children may be very modest and shy about exposing parts of their body.
- Adolescents should be examined without parents present.
- Weigh children without shoes and with as little clothing as possible.

OLDER ADULTS

- Allow extra time for clients to answer questions.
- Adapt questioning techniques as appropriate for clients with hearing or visual limitations.
- Older adults with osteoporosis can lose several centimetres in height. Be sure to document height and ask if they are aware of becoming shorter.
- When asking about weight loss, be specific about amount and time frame (e.g., "Have you lost more than 10 kilograms in the last 2 months?").

Vital Signs

Vital signs are measured (1) to establish baseline data against which to compare future measurements and (2) to detect actual and potential health problems. Refer to Chapter 28 for measurements of temperature, pulse, respirations, blood pressure, and oxygen saturation. See Chapter 34 for pain assessment.

Height, Weight, Body Mass Index, and Waist Circumference

In adults, the ratio of weight to height provides a general measure of health. By asking clients about their height and weight before actually measuring them, the nurse obtains some idea of the person's self-image. Excessive discrepancies between the client's responses and the measurements may provide clues to actual or potential problems in self-concept. It is also important that the nurse and client be aware of any significant unintentional weight gain or loss.

The nurse measures height with a measuring stick attached to weight scales or to a wall. The client removes his or her shoes and stands erect, with heels together, buttocks and the back of the head against the measuring stick, and eyes looking straight ahead. The nurse raises the L-shaped sliding arm on the measuring stick until it rests on top of the client's head, or the nurse places a small flat object, such as a ruler or book, on the client's head. The edge of the flat object should abut the measuring guide.

Weight is usually measured when a client is admitted to a health agency and often regularly, for example, each morning before breakfast. The nurse should use the same scale each time (because there may be some variation among scales), take the measurements at the same time each day, and make sure the client wears the same kind of clothing and no shoes. The client stands on a platform, and the weight is read from a digital display panel or a balancing arm. Clients who cannot stand are weighed on chair (Figure 27.6) or bed scales. The bed scales (Figure 27.7) have canvas straps or a stretcher-like apparatus. A machine lifts the client above the bed, and the weight is reflected either on a digital display panel or on a balance arm like that of a standing scale. Some agencies have beds with built-in scales.

Standardized charts have the average heights and weights of children and adults. It is important to remember that these averages provide only general guidelines for assessing growth, development, and nutritional status.

Body mass index (BMI) is a useful indicator of the overall health status of adults aged 20 to 65 years. BMI does not apply to infants, children, adolescents, pregnant and breastfeeding women, and adults over the age of 65. BMI is calculated by taking the weight of the individual in kilograms and dividing it by the height in metres squared. The formula is BMI = weight (kg)/height (m^2).

For example, an individual weighing 75 kg and measuring 150 cm tall would have a BMI of 33.3, which, as may be seen in Table 39.6 (page 1192), would put him

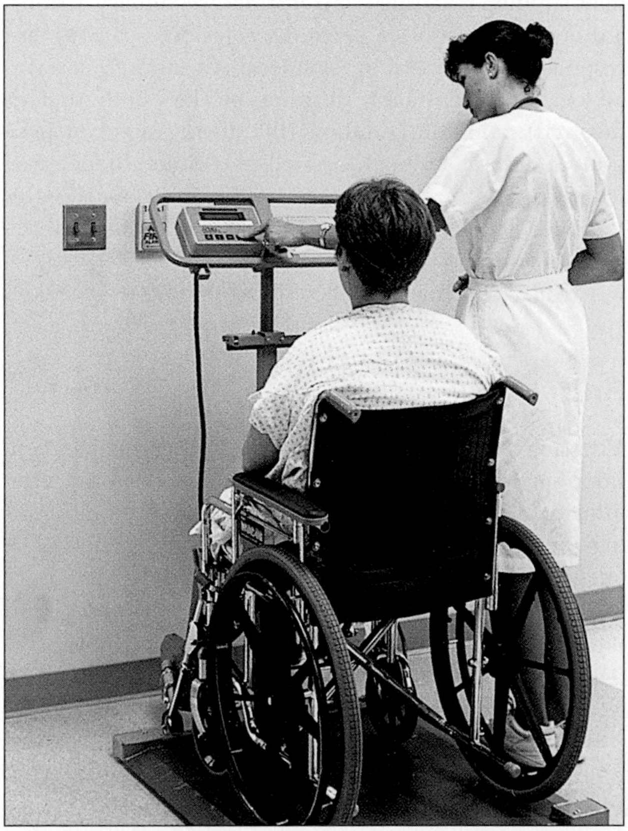

FIGURE 27.6 A chair scale

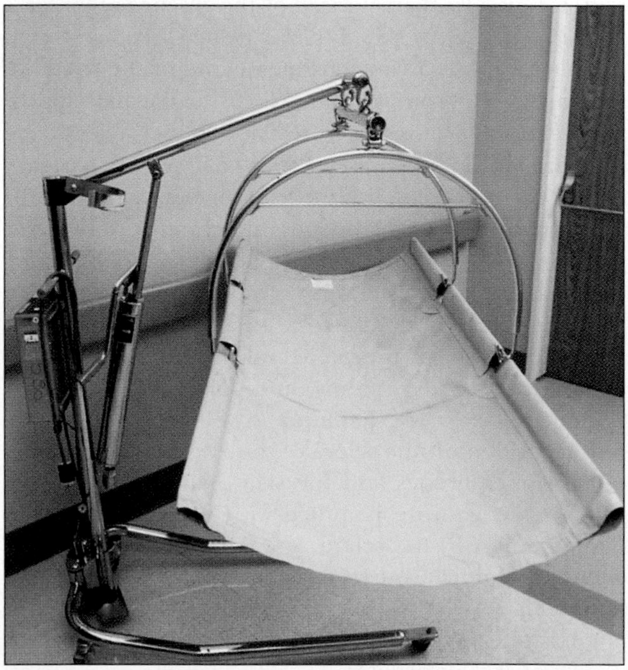

FIGURE 27.7 A bed scale

or her at high risk for health problems. See Table 39.5 (page 1191) for the BMI nomogram and more discussion of BMI.

Because adipose tissue located in the visceral area of the abdomen places the individual at risk, measurement of waist circumference is now becoming a part of the general health assessment. Chapter 39 discusses waist circumference and its influences on health in greater detail. See Figure 39.7 (page 1192) for the waist circumference measurement technique.

The Integument

The integument includes the skin, hair, and nails. The examination begins with a generalized inspection by using a good source of lighting, preferably indirect natural sunlight.

Skin

Assessment of the skin involves inspection and palpation. In some instances, the nurse may also need to use the olfactory sense to detect unusual skin odours; these are usually most evident in the skin folds or in the axillae. Pungent body odour is frequently related to poor hygiene, **hyperhidrosis** (excessive perspiration), or **bromhidrosis** (foul-smelling perspiration). The entire skin surface can be assessed at one time or as each aspect of the body is assessed.

Pallor is the result of inadequate circulating blood or hemoglobin and subsequent reduction in tissue oxygenation. It may be difficult to determine in clients with dark skin. It is usually characterized by the absence of underlying red tones in the skin and may be most readily seen in the buccal mucosa (mucous membrane of the inside of the cheek). In brown-skinned clients, pallor may appear as a yellowish-brown tinge; in black-skinned clients, the skin may appear ashen grey. Pallor in all people is usually most evident in areas with the least pigmentation, such as the conjunctiva, oral mucous membranes, nail beds, palms of the hand, and soles of the feet.

Cyanosis (a bluish tinge) is most evident in the nail beds, lips, and buccal mucosa. In dark-skinned clients, close inspection of the palpebral conjunctiva (the lining of the eyelids), palms, and soles may also show evidence of cyanosis. **Jaundice** (a yellowish tinge) may first be evident in the sclera of the eyes and then in the mucous membranes and the skin. Nurses should take care not to confuse jaundice with the normal yellow pigmentation in the sclera of a dark-skinned or Black client. If jaundice is suspected, the posterior part of the hard palate should also be inspected for a yellowish colour tone. **Erythema** is a redness associated with a variety of skin disorders.

Dark-skinned clients have areas of lighter pigmentation, such as the palms, lips, and nail beds. Localized areas of hyperpigmentation (increased pigmentation) and hypopigmentation (decreased pigmentation) may also occur as a result of changes in the distribution of **melanin** (the dark pigment) or in the function of the melanocytes in the epidermis. An example of hyperpigmentation in a defined area is a birthmark; an example of hypopigmentation is vitiligo. **Vitiligo**, seen as patches of hypopigmented skin, is caused by the destruction of melanocytes in the area. **Albinism** is the complete or partial lack of melanin in the skin, hair, and eyes. Other localized colour changes can indicate a problem, such as edema or a localized infection. **Edema** is the presence of excess interstitial fluid. When edema is present, the tissues appear swollen and the skin is shiny, taut, and blanched. If the edema is accompanied by inflammation, the skin will appear reddened (erythematous). Generalized edema is most often an indication of impaired venous circulation and, in some cases, reflects cardiac dysfunction or vein abnormalities.

A skin lesion is an alteration in a client's normal skin appearance. **Primary skin lesions** are those that appear initially in response to some change in the external or internal environment of the skin (Figure 27.8 ❶–❽). **Secondary skin lesions** are those that do not appear initially but result from changes to the primary lesion, such as those caused by trauma or infection of the primary lesion. For example, a vesicle or blister (primary lesion) may rupture and cause an erosion (secondary lesion). Table 27.5 describes secondary lesions. Nurses are responsible for describing skin lesions accurately in terms of location (e.g., face), distribution (i.e., body regions involved), and configuration (the arrangement or position of several lesions), as well as colour, shape, size, firmness, texture, and characteristics of individual lesions.

See Chapter 33 for discussion of skin assessment relative to wounds and pressure ulcers.

Skill 27.2 on page 566 describes how to assess the skin.

Hair

Assessing a client's hair includes inspecting the hair, considering developmental changes, and determining the individual's hair-care practices and the factors influencing them. Much of the information about hair can be obtained by questioning the client.

Normal hair is resilient and evenly distributed. In people with kwashiorkor (severe protein deficiency), the hair colour is faded and appears reddish or bleached, and the texture is coarse and dry. Some therapies cause **alopecia** (hair loss), and some disease conditions affect the coarseness of hair. For example, hypothyroidism can cause very thin and brittle hair.

Macule, Patch Flat, unelevated change in colour. Macules are 1 mm to 1 cm in size and circumscribed. Examples: freckles, measles, petechiae, flat moles. Patches are larger than 1 cm and may have an irregular shape. Examples: port wine birthmark, vitiligo (white patches), rubella. ❶

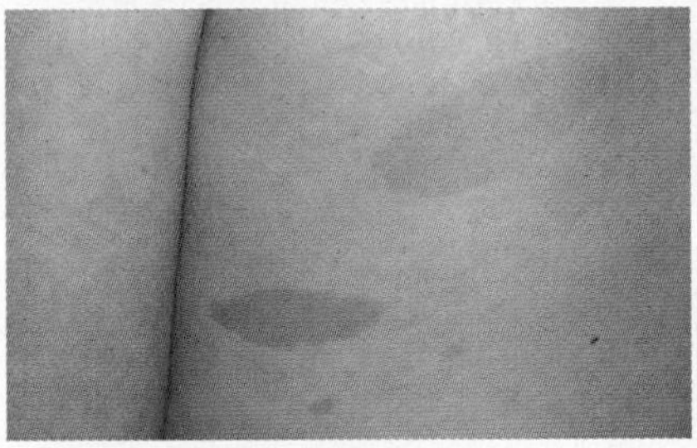

❶ Multiple café-au-lait macules

Papule Circumscribed, solid elevation of skin. Papules are less than 1 cm. Examples: warts, acne, pimples, elevated moles. ❷

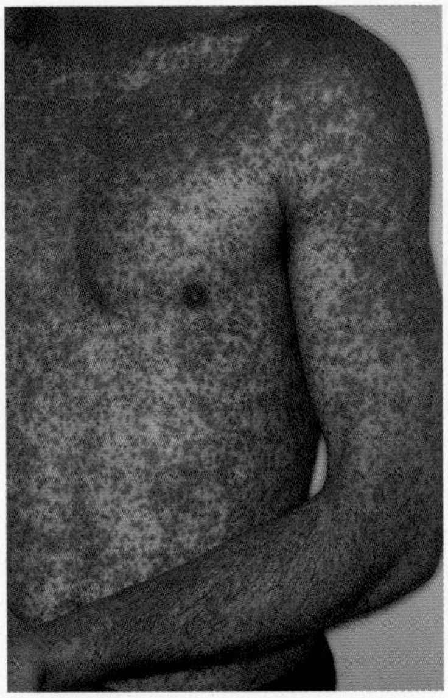

❷ Papular drug eruption

Plaque Plaques are larger than 1 cm. Examples: psoriasis, rubeola. ❸

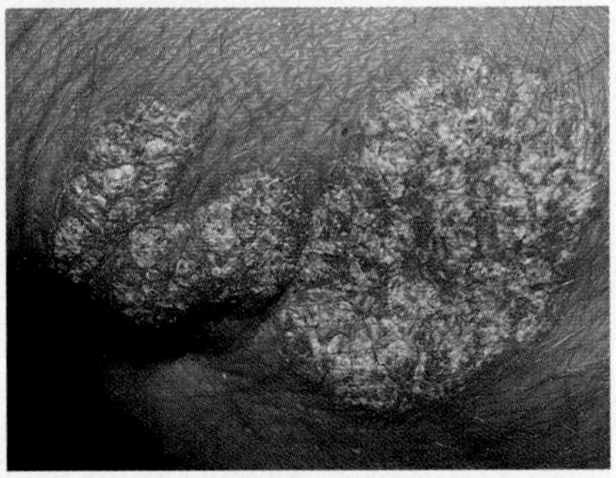

❸ Psoriasis vulgaris

Nodule, Tumour Elevated, solid, hard mass that extends deeper into the dermis than a papule. Nodules have a circumscribed border and are 0.5 cm to 2 cm. Examples: squamous cell carcinoma, fibroma. Tumours are larger than 2 cm and may have an irregular border. Examples: malignant melanoma, hemangioma. ❹

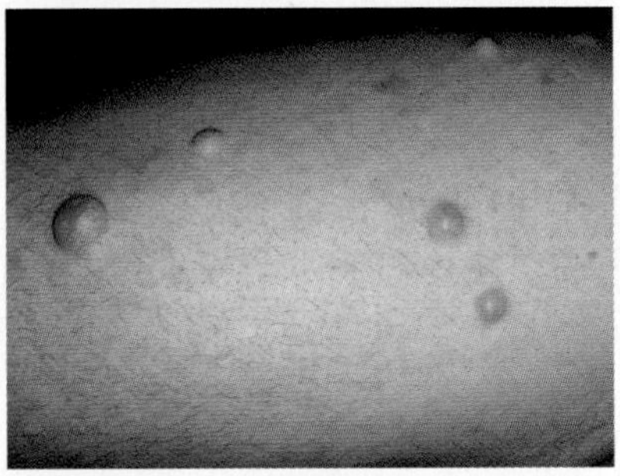

❹ Peripheral neurofibromas

Pustule Vesicle or bulla filled with pus. Examples: acne vulgaris, impetigo. ❺

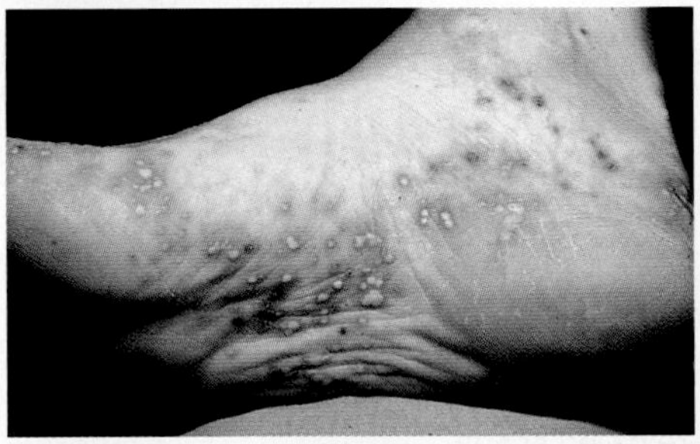

❺ Chronic pustular psoriasis

Vesicle, Bulla A circumscribed, round or oval, thin, translucent mass filled with serous fluid or blood. Vesicles are less than 0.5 cm. Examples: herpes simplex, early chicken pox, small burn blister. Bullae are larger than 0.5 cm. Examples: large blister, second-degree burn, herpes simplex. ❻

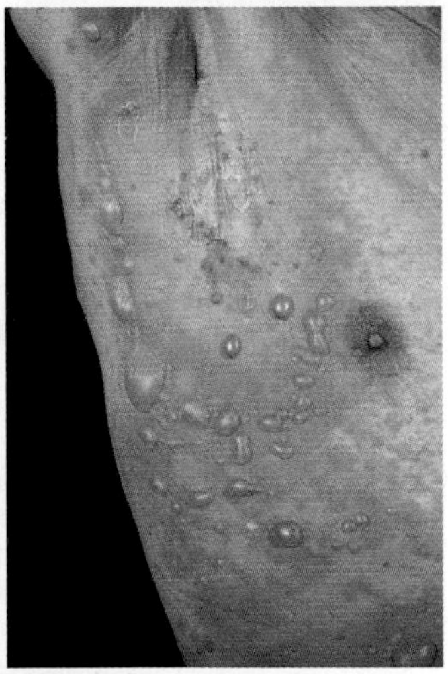

❻ Bullous pemphigoid

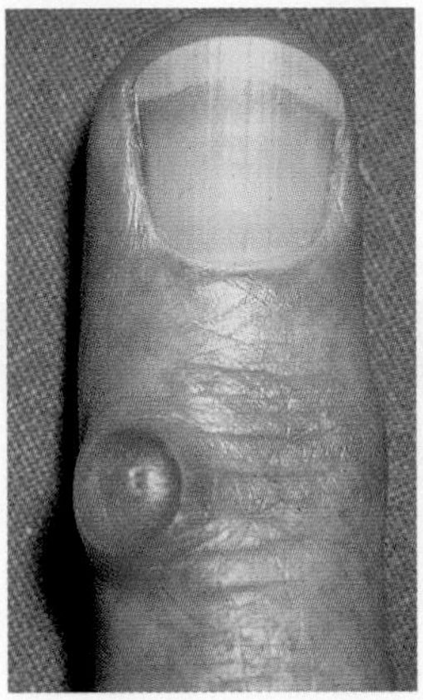

❼ Digital mucous cyst

Cyst A 1 cm or larger, elevated, encapsulated, fluid-filled or semisolid mass arising from the subcutaneous tissue or dermis. Examples: sebaceous and epidermoid cysts, chalazion of the eyelid. ❼

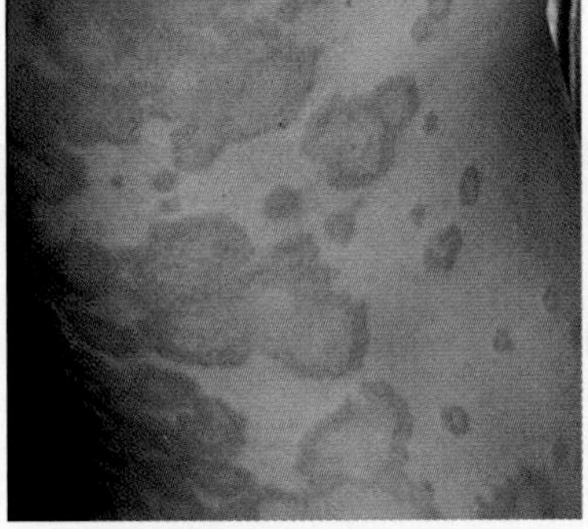

❽ Allergic wheals, urticaria

Wheal A reddened, localized collection of edema fluid; irregular in shape. Size varies. Examples: hives, mosquito bites. ❽

FIGURE 27.8 Primary skin lesions

TABLE 27.5 Secondary Skin Lesions

Atrophy 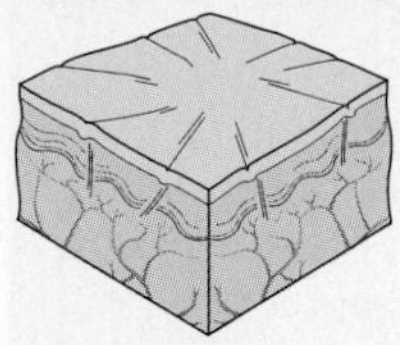	A translucent, dry, paperlike, sometimes wrinkled skin surface resulting from thinning or wasting of the skin caused by loss of collagen and elastin. **Examples** Striae, aged skin	**Ulcer** 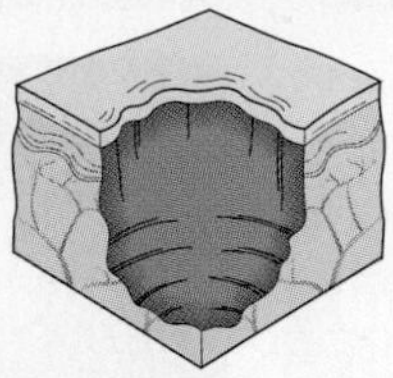	Deep, irregularly shaped area of skin loss extending into the dermis or subcutaneous tissue. May bleed. May leave scar. **Examples** Decubitus ulcers (pressure ulcers), stasis ulcers, chancres
Erosion 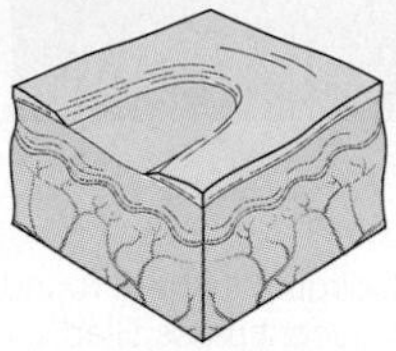	Wearing away of the superficial epidermis causing a moist, shallow depression. Because erosions do not extend into the dermis, they heal without scarring. **Examples** Scratch marks, ruptured vesicles	**Fissure** 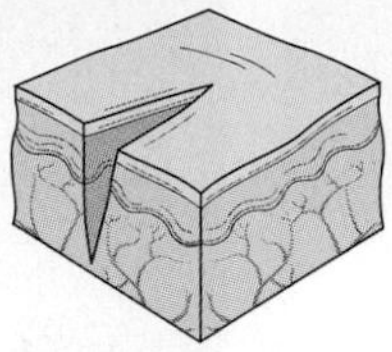	Linear crack with sharp edges extending into the dermis **Examples** Cracks at the corners of the mouth or in the hands, athlete's foot
Lichenification 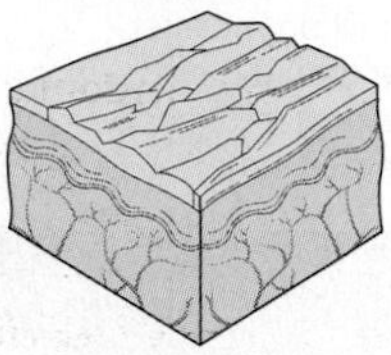	Rough, thickened, hardened area of epidermis resulting from chronic irritation, such as scratching or rubbing. **Example** Chronic dermatitis	**Scar** 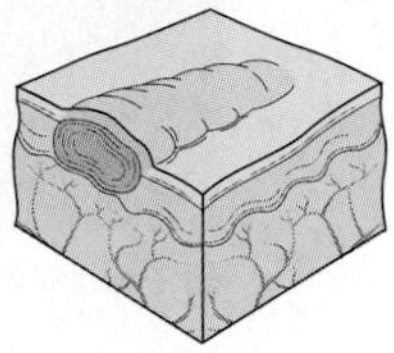	Flat, irregular area of connective tissue left after a lesion or wound has healed. New scars may be red or purple; older scars may be silvery or white. **Examples** Healed surgical wound or injury, healed acne
Scales 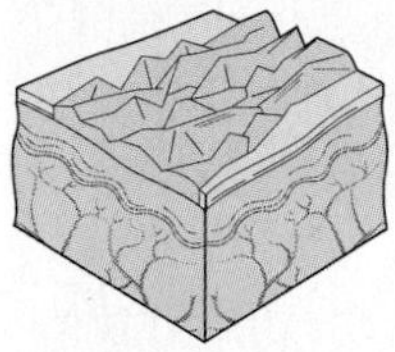	Shedding flakes of greasy, keratinized skin tissue. Colour may be white, grey, or silver. Texture may vary from fine to thick. **Examples** Dry skin, dandruff, psoriasis, and eczema	**Keloid** 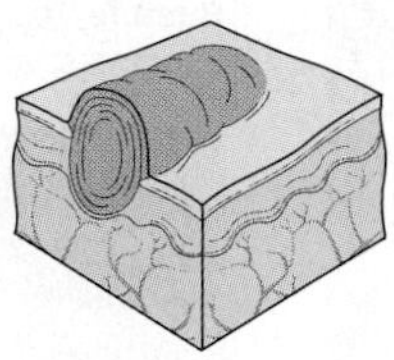	Elevated, irregular, darkened area of excess scar tissue caused by excessive collagen formation during healing. Extends beyond the site of the original injury. Higher incidence in Black people. **Examples** Keloid from ear piercing or surgery
Crust 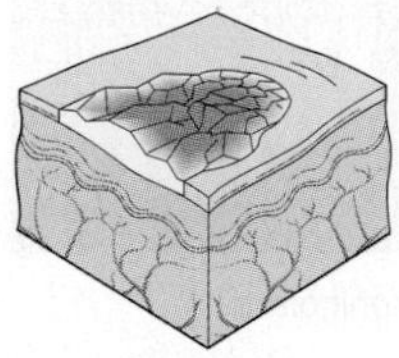	Dry blood, serum, or pus left on the skin surface when vesicles or pustules burst. Can be red-brown, orange, or yellow. Large crusts that adhere to the skin surface are called scabs. **Examples** Eczema, impetigo, herpes, or scabs following abrasion	**Excoriation** 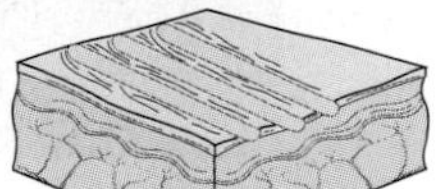	Linear erosion. **Examples** Scratches, some chemical burns

SKILL 27.2

ASSESSING THE SKIN

PLANNING

- Review the characteristics of primary and secondary lesions if necessary (see Figure 27.8 and Table 27.5).
- Ensure that adequate lighting is available.

Equipment

- Millimetre ruler
- Clean gloves
- Magnifying glass

IMPLEMENTATION

Performance

1. Before performing the procedure, introduce yourself and verify the client's identity by using agency protocol. Explain to the client what you are going to do, why it is necessary, and how he or she can cooperate. Discuss how the results will be used in planning further care or treatments.
2. Perform hand hygiene and observe other appropriate infection prevention and control procedures.

(continued)

SKILL 27.2

ASSESSING THE SKIN (*continued*)

3. Provide for client privacy.
4. Inquire whether the client has any history of the following: pain or itching; presence and spread of lesions, bruises, abrasions, pigmented spots; previous experience with skin problems; associated clinical signs; family history; presence of skin problems in other family members; related systemic conditions; use of medications, lotions, home remedies; excessively dry or moist feel to the skin; tendency to bruise easily; association of the problem to season of year, stress, occupation, medications, recent travel, housing, and so on; recent contact with allergens (e.g., metal paint).

ASSESSMENT	NORMAL FINDINGS	DEVIATIONS FROM NORMAL
5. Inspect skin colour (best assessed under natural light and on areas not exposed to the sun).	Varies from light to deep brown; from ruddy pink to light pink; from yellow overtones to olive	Pallor, cyanosis, jaundice, erythema
6. Inspect uniformity of skin colour.	Generally uniform except in areas exposed to the sun; areas of lighter pigmentation (palms, lips, nail beds) in dark-skinned people	Areas of either hyperpigmentation or hypopigmentation
7. Assess edema, if present (i.e., location, colour, temperature, shape, and the degree to which the skin remains indented or pitted when pressed by a finger). Measuring the circumference of the extremity with a millimetre tape may be useful for future comparison.	No edema	See the scale for grading edema in ❶.
8. Inspect, palpate, and describe skin lesions. Apply gloves if lesions are open or draining. Palpate lesions to determine shape and texture. Describe lesions according to location, distribution, colour, configuration, size, shape, type, or structure (see Box 27.5, p. 569).	Freckles, some birthmarks, some flat and raised nevi; no abrasions or other lesions	Various interruptions in skin integrity; irregular, multicoloured, or raised nevi
9. Observe and palpate skin moisture.	Moisture in skin folds and the axillae (varies with environmental temperature and humidity, body temperature, and activity)	Excessive moisture (e.g., in hyperthermia); excessive dryness (e.g., in dehydration)
10. Palpate skin temperature. Compare the two feet and the two hands, using the backs of your fingers.	Uniform; within normal range	Generalized hyperthermia (e.g., in fever); generalized hypothermia (e.g., in shock); localized hyperthermia (e.g., in infection); localized hypothermia (e.g., in arteriosclerosis)
11. Note skin turgor (fullness or elasticity) by lifting and pinching the skin on an extremity.	When pinched, skin springs back to previous state; may be slower in older adults	Skin stays pinched or tented or moves back slowly (e.g., in dehydration)

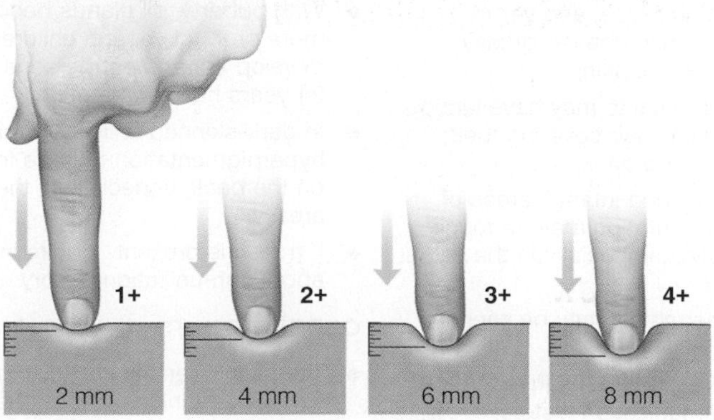

❶ Scale for grading edema

(continued)

SKILL 27.2

ASSESSING THE SKIN (*continued*)

12. Document findings in the client record by using forms or checklists supplemented by narrative notes when appropriate. Draw location of skin lesions on body surface diagrams, shown in ❷.

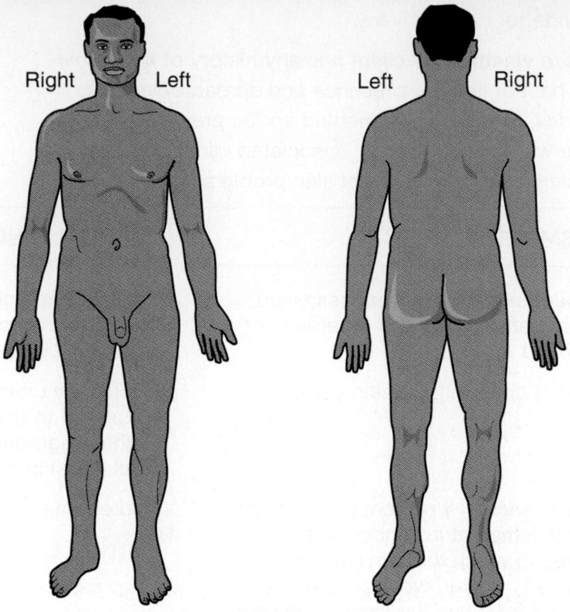

❷ Diagram for charting skin lesions

EVALUATION

- Perform a detailed follow-up examination of other individual systems based on findings that deviated from expected on normal for the client. Relate findings to previous assessment data if available.
- Report significant deviations from normal to the appropriate members of the health-care team.

Lifespan Considerations

Assessing the Skin

INFANTS

- Physiological jaundice may appear in newborns 2 to 3 days after birth and usually lasts about 1 week. Pathological jaundice, or that which indicates a disease, appears within 24 hours of birth and may last more than 8 days.
- Newborns may have milia (whiteheads), small white nodules over the nose and face, and vernix caseosa (white cheesy, greasy material on the skin).
- Premature infants may have lanugo, a fine downy hair covering their shoulders and back.
- In dark-skinned infants, areas of hyperpigmentation may be found on the back, especially in the sacral area.
- Diaper dermatitis may be seen in infants.
- If a rash is present, inquire in detail about immunization history.
- Assess skin turgor by pinching the skin on the abdomen.

CHILDREN

- Children normally have minor skin lesions (e.g., bruising or abrasions) on arms and legs because of their high activity level. Lesions on other parts of the body may be signs of disease or abuse, and a thorough history should be taken.
- Secondary skin lesions may occur frequently as children scratch or expose a primary lesion to microbes.
- With puberty, oil glands become more productive, and children may develop acne. Most persons 12 to 24 years have some acne.
- In dark-skinned children, areas of hyperpigmentation may be found on the back, especially in the sacral area.
- If a rash is present, inquire in detail about immunization history.

OLDER ADULTS

- The skin loses its elasticity and wrinkles. Wrinkles first appear on the skin of the face and neck.
- The skin appears thin and translucent because of loss of dermis and subcutaneous fat.
- The skin is dry and flaky because sebaceous and sweat glands are less active.
- The skin takes longer to return to its natural shape after being tented between the thumb and finger.
- Because of the normal loss of peripheral skin turgor in older adults, assess for hydration by checking skin turgor over the sternum or clavicle.
- Flat, tan- to brown-coloured macules, referred to as *senile lentigines* or *melanotic freckles,* are normally apparent on the back of the hands and other skin areas that are exposed to the sun. These macules may be as large as 1 cm to 2 cm.
- *Seborrheic keratosis* (warty lesions) with irregularly shaped borders and a scaly surface often occur on the face, shoulders, and trunk. These benign lesions begin as yellowish to tan and progress to a dark brown or black.

(continued)

Lifespan Considerations (*continued*)

- Vitiligo tends to increase with age and is thought to result from an autoimmune response.
- *Acrochordons* (cutaneous tags) are most commonly seen in the neck and axillary regions. These skin lesions vary in size and are soft, often flesh coloured, and pedicled (on a stem or stalk of tissue).
- *Telangiectasias* (visible, bright red, fine, dilated blood vessels) commonly occur as a result of the thinning of the dermis and the loss of support for the blood vessel walls.
- *Actinic keratoses* (pink to slightly red lesions with indistinct borders) may appear at about age 50 years, often on the face, ears, backs of the hands, and arms. They can become malignant if untreated.

BOX 27.5 DESCRIBING SKIN LESIONS

Describe lesions according to the following characteristics:

- *Type or structure.* Skin lesions are classified as *primary* (those that appear initially in response to some change in the external or internal environment of the skin) and *secondary* (those that result from modifications, such as chronicity, trauma, or infection, of the primary lesion). For example, a pustule (primary lesion) can burst and cause a secondary crust lesion.
- *Size, shape, and texture.* Note size in millimetres and whether the lesion is circumscribed or irregular; round or oval shaped; flat, elevated, or depressed; solid, soft, or hard; rough or thickened; fluid filled; or has flakes.
- *Colour.* Lesions can have no discolouration; one discrete colour (e.g., red, brown, or black); several colours, as with *ecchymosis* (a bruise), in which an initial dark red or blue fades to yellow. When colour changes are limited to the edges of a lesion, they are described as *circumscribed;* when spread over a large area, they are described as *diffuse.*
- *Distribution.* Distribution is described according to the location of the lesions on the body and symmetry or asymmetry of findings in comparable body areas.
- *Configuration.* Configuration refers to the arrangement of lesions in relation to one another. Configurations of lesions can be annular (arranged in a circle), be clustered together or grouped, be linear (arranged in a line), be arc or bow shaped, merge together or be indiscrete, follow the course of cutaneous nerves, or be meshed in the form of a network.

Skill 27.3 describes how to assess the hair.

SKILL 27.3

ASSESSING THE HAIR

Equipment: Clean gloves

IMPLEMENTATION

Performance

1. Before performing the procedure, introduce yourself and verify the client's identity by using agency protocol. Explain to the client what you are going to do, why it is necessary, and how he or she can cooperate. Discuss how the results will be used in planning further care or treatments.
2. Perform hand hygiene, apply gloves, and observe other appropriate infection prevention and control procedures.
3. Provide for client privacy.

ASSESSMENT	NORMAL FINDINGS	DEVIATIONS FROM NORMAL
4. Inspect the evenness of growth over the scalp.	Evenly distributed hair	Patches of hair loss (i.e., alopecia)
5. Inspect hair thickness or thinness.	Thick hair	Very thin hair (as in hypothyroidism)
6. Inspect hair texture and oiliness.	Silky, resilient hair	Brittle hair (as in hypothyroidism); excessively oily or dry hair
7. Note presence of infections or infestations by parting the hair in several areas, checking behind the ears and along the hairline at the neck.	No infection or infestation	Flaking, sores, lice, nits (louse eggs), and ringworm

(continued)

SKILL 27.3

ASSESSING THE HAIR (*continued*)

ASSESSMENT	NORMAL FINDINGS	DEVIATIONS FROM NORMAL
8. Inspect amount of body hair.	Variable	**Hirsutism** (abnormal hairiness) in women and children; naturally absent or sparse leg hair (poor circulation)

9. Document findings in the client record by using handwritten or electronic forms and checklists supplemented by narrative notes when appropriate.

EVALUATION

Report significant deviations from normal to the appropriate members of the health-care team.

Lifespan Considerations

Assessing the Hair

INFANTS

- It is normal for infants to have either very little or a great deal of body and scalp hair.

CHILDREN

- As puberty approaches, axillary and pubic hair will appear.

OLDER ADULTS

- The age at which the scalp hair greys is influenced largely by genetic factors.
- There may be loss of scalp, pubic, and axillary hair.
- In older women, some facial hair becomes coarse.
- Hairs of the eyebrows, ears, and nostrils become bristle-like and coarse in older adults.

Nails

Nails are inspected for nail plate shape, angle between the nail and the nail bed, nail texture, nail bed colour, and the intactness of the tissues around the nails. The parts of the nail are shown in Figure 27.9.

The nail plate is normally colourless and a convex curve. The angle between the nail and the nail bed is normally 160 degrees (Figure 27.10A). One nail abnormality is the spoon shape, in which the nail curves upward from the nail bed (Figure 27.10B). This condition, called **koilonychia,** may be seen in clients with iron deficiency anemia. **Clubbing** is a condition in which the angle between the nail and the nail bed is 180 degrees or greater (Figure 27.10C and 27.10D). Clubbing can be caused by a long-term lack of oxygen and may be seen in clients with cardiac conditions.

Nail texture is normally smooth. Excessively thick nails can appear in the elderly, in the presence of poor circulation, or in relation to a chronic fungal infection. Excessively thin nails or the presence of grooves or furrows can reflect prolonged iron deficiency anemia. *Beau's lines* are horizontal depressions in the nail that can result from injury or severe illness (Figure 27.10E).

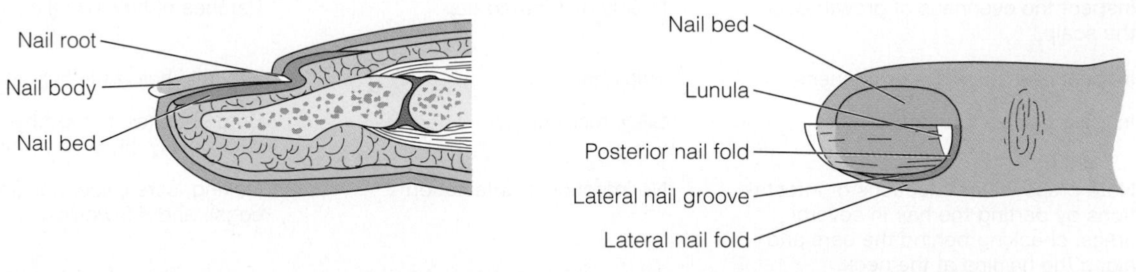

FIGURE 27.9 The parts of a nail

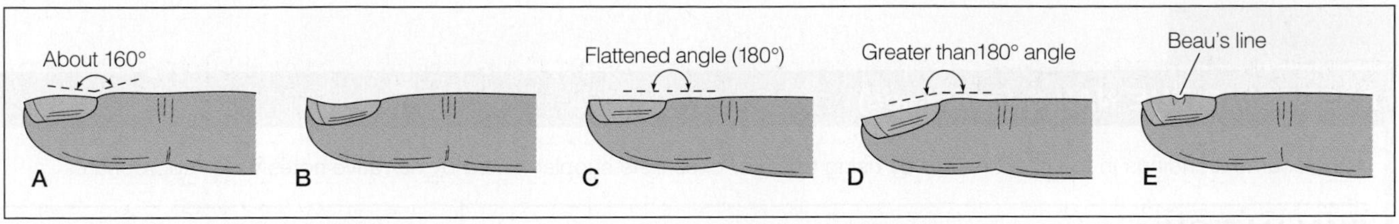

FIGURE 27.10 **A:** A normal nail, showing the convex shape and the nail plate angle of about 160 degrees; **B:** a spoon-shaped nail, which may be seen in clients with iron deficiency anemia; **C:** early clubbing; **D:** late clubbing (may be caused by long-term lack of oxygen); **E:** Beau's line on nail (may result from severe injury or illness)

The nail bed is highly vascular, a characteristic that accounts for its pink colour in Caucasian people. A bluish or purplish tint to the nail bed may reflect cyanosis, and pallor may reflect poor arterial circulation. Should the client report a history of onychomycosis (nail fungus), a referral to a podiatrist or dermatologist for treatment of nail fungus may be appropriate. Symptoms of nail fungus include brittleness, discolouration, thickening, distortion of nail shape, crumbling of the nail, and loosening (detaching) of the nail.

The tissue surrounding the nails is normally intact epidermis. **Paronychia** is an inflammation of the tissues surrounding a nail (often referred to as an "ingrown nail"). The tissues appear inflamed and swollen and tenderness is usually present. A **blanch test** can be carried out to test the capillary refill of peripheral circulation. Normal nail bed capillaries blanch when pressed but quickly turn pink or their usual colour when pressure is released. A slow rate of capillary refill may indicate circulatory problems.

Skill 27.4 describes how to assess the nails.

SKILL 27.4

ASSESSING THE NAILS

Equipment: None

IMPLEMENTATION

Performance

1. Before performing the procedure, introduce yourself and verify the client's identity by using agency protocol. Explain to the client what you are going to do, why it is necessary, and how he or she can cooperate. Discuss how the results will be used in planning further care or treatments. In most situations, clients with artificial nails or polish on fingernails or toenails are not required to remove these for assessment. If the assessment cannot be conducted because of the presence of polish or artificial nails, document this in the record.
2. Perform hand hygiene and observe other appropriate infection prevention and control procedures.
3. Provide for client privacy.
4. Inquire whether the client has any history of the following: diabetes mellitus, peripheral circulatory disease, previous injury, or severe illness.

ASSESSMENT	NORMAL FINDINGS	DEVIATIONS FROM NORMAL
5. Inspect fingernail plate shape to determine its curvature and angle.	Convex curvature; angle between nail and nail bed of about 160° (Figure 27.10A)	Spoon nail (Figure 27.10B); clubbing (180 degrees or greater) (Figure 27.10C and 27.10D)
6. Inspect fingernail and toenail texture.	Smooth texture	Excessive thickness or thinness or presence of grooves or furrows; Beau's lines (Figure 27.10E); discoloured or detached nail, often caused by fungus
7. Inspect fingernail and toenail bed colour.	Highly vascular and pink; dark-skinned clients may have brown or black pigmentation in longitudinal streaks	Bluish or purplish tint (may reflect cyanosis); pallor (may reflect poor arterial circulation)
8. Inspect tissues surrounding nails.	Intact epidermis	Hangnails; paronychia (inflammation)
9. Perform a blanch test to test capillary refill. Press two or more nails between your thumb and index finger; look for blanching and return of usual colour to nail bed.	Prompt return of pink or usual colour, generally less than 2 to 3 seconds.	Delayed return of pink or usual colour (may indicate circulatory impairment)

(continued)

SKILL 27.4

ASSESSING THE NAILS (*continued*)

10. Document findings in the client record by using forms or checklists supplemented by narrative notes when appropriate.

EVALUATION

- Perform a detailed follow-up examination of other individual systems based on findings that deviated from expected or normal for the client. Relate findings to previous assessment data if available.
- Report significant deviations from normal to the appropriate members of the health-care team.

Lifespan Considerations

Assessing the Nails

INFANTS

- Newborns nails grow very quickly, are extremely thin, and tear easily.

CHILDREN

- Bent, bruised, or ingrown toenails can indicate shoes that are too tight.
- Nail biting should be discussed with a family member.

OLDER ADULTS

- The nails grow more slowly and thicken.
- Longitudinal bands commonly develop in older adults, and the nails tend to split.
- Bands across the nails may indicate protein deficiency; white spots, zinc deficiency; and spoon-shaped nails, iron deficiency.
- Toenail fungus is more common and difficult to eliminate (although not dangerous to health).

Head

Assessment of the head includes inspection, palpation, and percussion. The nurse examines the skull, face, eyes, ears, nose, sinuses, mouth, and pharynx.

Skull and Face

Normal skulls come in a range of shapes. A normal head size is referred to as **normocephalic**. Names of areas of the head are derived from names of the underlying bones: frontal, parietal, occipital, mastoid process, mandible, maxilla, and zygomatic (Figure 27.11).

Skill 27.5 describes how to assess the skull and face.

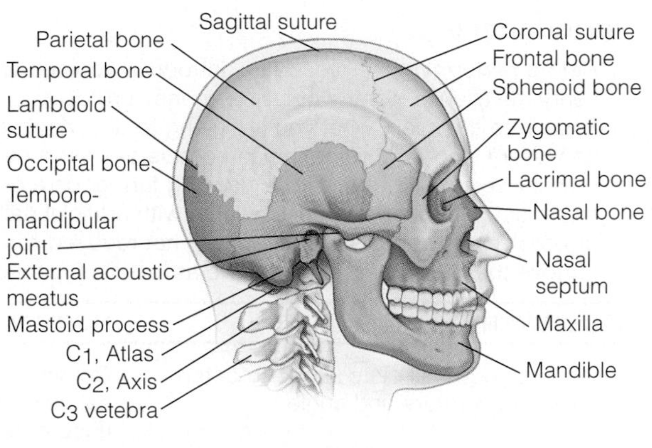

FIGURE 27.11 The bones of the head

Eyes and Vision

To maintain optimum vision, people need to have their eyes examined regularly throughout life. It is recommended that people under age 40 have their eyes tested every 3 to 5 years, or more frequently if there is a family history of diabetes, hypertension, blood dyscrasia, or eye disease (e.g., glaucoma). After age 40, an eye examination is recommended every 2 years to rule out the possibility of glaucoma.

An eye assessment should be carried out as part of the client's initial physical examination; periodic reassessments need to be made for clients in long-term care. Examination of the eyes includes assessment of **visual acuity** (the degree of detail the eye can discern in an image), ocular movement, **visual fields** (the area an individual can see when looking straight ahead), and external structures. If the client wears contact lenses or has an artificial eye, consideration should be given to individual hygiene practices. For the anatomic structures of the eye, see Figure 27.12 and Figure 27.13.

Many people wear eyeglasses or contact lenses to correct common refractive errors of the lens of the eye. These errors include **myopia** (nearsightedness), **hyperopia** (farsightedness), and **presbyopia** (loss of elasticity of the lens and, thus, loss of ability to see close objects). Presbyopia begins at about 45 years of age. People with presbyopia have difficulty reading newsprint. Often, two corrective lenses (bifocals) are required—one for near vision or reading, the other for far vision. **Astigmatism**, an uneven curvature of the cornea that prevents horizontal and verti-

SKILL 27.5

ASSESSING THE SKULL AND FACE

Equipment: None

IMPLEMENTATION

Performance

1. Before performing the procedure, introduce yourself and verify the client's identity by using agency protocol. Explain to the client what you are going to do, why it is necessary, and how he or she can cooperate. Discuss how the results will be used in planning further care or treatments.
2. Perform hand hygiene and observe other appropriate infection prevention and control procedures.
3. Provide for client privacy.
4. Inquire whether the client has any past problems with lumps or bumps, itching, scaling, or dandruff; any history of loss of consciousness, dizziness, seizures, headache, facial pain, or injury; when and how any lumps occurred; the length of time any other problem existed; any known cause of the problem; and associated symptoms, treatment, and recurrences.

ASSESSMENT	NORMAL FINDINGS	DEVIATIONS FROM NORMAL
5. Inspect the skull for size, shape, and symmetry. If the skull is of abnormal size, measure its circumference just above the eyebrows.	Rounded (normocephalic and symmetric, with frontal, parietal, and occipital prominences); smooth skull contour	Lack of symmetry; increased skull size with more prominent nose and forehead; longer mandible (may indicate excessive growth hormone or increased bone thickness)
6. Palpate the skull for nodules or masses and depressions. Use a gentle rotating motion with the fingertips. Begin at the front and palpate down the midline, then palpate each side of the head.	Smooth, uniform consistency; absence of nodules or masses	Sebaceous cysts; local deformities from trauma; masses, nodules
7. Inspect the facial features (e.g., symmetry of structures and of the distribution of hair).	Symmetric or slightly asymmetric facial features; palpebral fissures equal in size; symmetric nasolabial folds; even distribution of hair	Increased or uneven distribution of facial hair; thinning of eyebrows; asymmetric features; exophthalmos (bulging eyes); myxedema facies; moon face
8. Inspect the eyes for edema and hollowness.	No edema or hollowness	Periorbital edema; sunken eyes
9. Note symmetry of facial movements. Ask the client to elevate the eyebrows, frown, lower the eyebrows, close the eyes tightly, puff the cheeks, and smile and show the teeth. See Skill 27.17 (p. 637), Assessing the Neurological System.	Symmetric facial movements	Asymmetric facial movements (e.g., eye on affected side cannot close completely); drooping of lower eyelid and mouth; involuntary facial movements (i.e., tics or tremors)

10. Document findings in the client record by using forms or checklists supplemented by narrative notes when appropriate.

EVALUATION

- Perform a detailed follow-up examination of other systems based on findings that deviated from expected or normal for the client. Relate findings to previous assessment data if available.
- Report significant deviations from normal to the appropriate members of the health-care team.

Lifespan Considerations

Assessing the Skull and Face

INFANTS

- Newborns delivered vaginally can have elongated, moulded heads, which take on more rounded shapes after a week or two. Infants born by caesarean section tend to have smooth, rounded heads.
- The posterior fontanel (soft spot) is about 1 cm in size and usually closes by 8 weeks. The anterior fontanel is larger, about 2 cm to 3 cm in size. It closes by 18 months.
- Newborns can lift their heads slightly and turn them from side to side. Voluntary head control is well established by 4 to 6 months.
- Occipital flattening of positional origin results when an infant spends prolonged periods with the head in the same position against a flat surface. Flattening can occur before birth from wedging against a maternal pelvic bone, or it can occur postnatally.

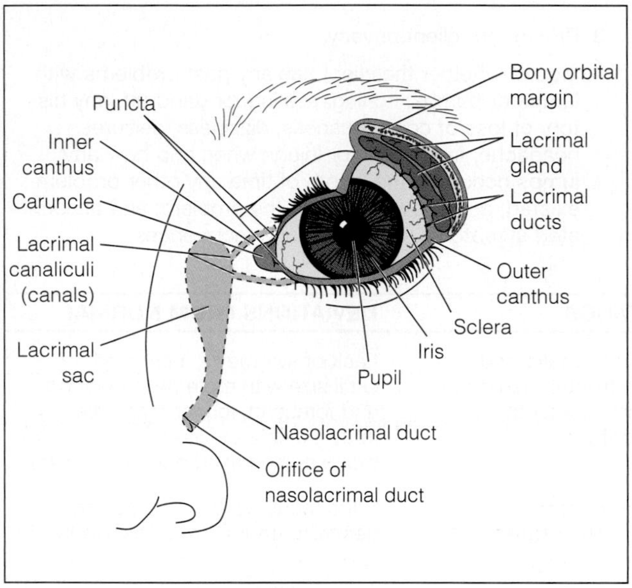

FIGURE 27.12 The external structures and lacrimal apparatus of the left eye

cal rays from focusing on the retina, is a common problem that can occur in conjunction with myopia and hyperopia.

Three types of eye charts are available to test visual acuity (Figure 27.14). A child acquires normal 20/20 vision by 6 years of age. Visual acuity can be tested on a standard Snellen chart. Visual acuity is documented as two numbers (e.g., 20/20). The first number indicates the distance of the client from the chart (i.e., 20 feet, which is about 6 metres), and the second number indicates the distance at which a normal eye can read the chart. For example, a test result of 20/200 means that at 20 feet, the client can read the chart that a person with normal vision could read at 200 feet. In other words, the larger the second number, or denominator, the worse the visual acuity. People with denominators of 40 or more on the Snellen chart, with or without corrective lenses, need to be referred to an ophthalmologist.

Common inflammatory visual problems that nurses encounter in clients include conjunctivitis, dacryocystitis, hordeolum, iritis, and contusions or hematomas of the eyelids and surrounding structures. **Conjunctivitis**

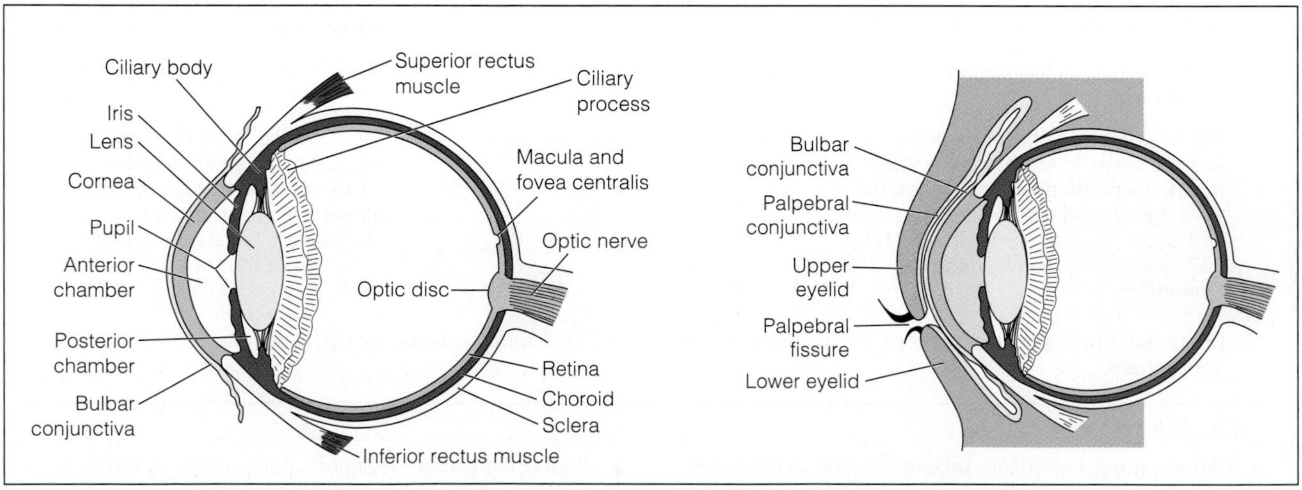

FIGURE 27.13 Anatomic structures of the right eye, lateral view

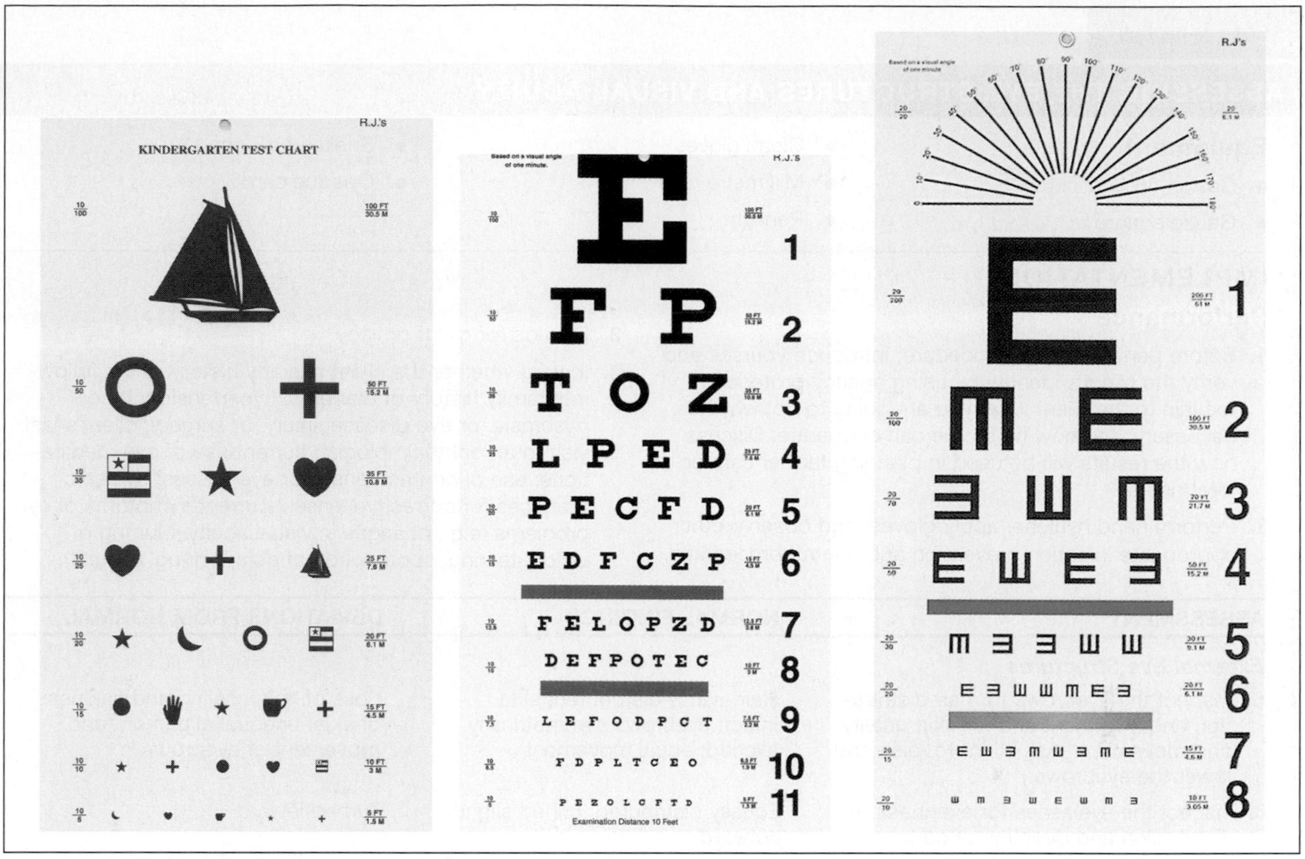

FIGURE 27.14 Three types of eye charts; the preschool children's chart (left), Snellen standard chart (centre), and the Snellen E chart for clients unable to read (right).

(inflammation of the bulbar and palpebral conjunctiva) can result from foreign bodies, chemicals, allergenic agents, bacteria, or viruses. Redness, itching, tearing, and discharge occur. During sleep, the eyelids may become encrusted and matted together. **Dacryocystitis** (inflammation of the lacrimal sac) is manifested by tearing and a discharge from the nasolacrimal duct. **Hordeolum (sty)** is a redness, swelling, and tenderness of the hair follicle and glands that empty at the edge of the eyelids. *Iritis* (inflammation of the iris) can be caused by local or systemic infections and results in pain, tearing, and photophobia (sensitivity to light). Contusions or hematomas are "black eyes" resulting from injury.

Cataracts are an opacity of the lens of the eye. Most cataracts occur in individuals over the age of 65 years. However, cataracts also occur in infants because of a malformation of the lens, for example, if a mother contracts rubella in the first trimester of pregnancy. A common treatment is removal of the lens and replacement of the lens with an implant. **Glaucoma** is a disruption in the circulation of the aqueous fluid, which causes an increase in intraocular pressure and a reduced blood supply to the optic disc. Glaucoma is the most common cause of blindness in people over 40 years. It can be managed if diagnosed early. Danger signs of glaucoma include blurred or foggy vision, loss of peripheral vision, difficulty focusing on close objects, difficulty adjusting to dark rooms, and seeing rainbow-coloured rings around lights.

Eyelids that lie at or below the pupil margin are referred to as *ptosis* and are usually associated with aging, edema from drug allergy or systemic disease (e.g., kidney disease), congenital lid muscle dysfunction, neuromuscular disease (e.g., myasthenia gravis), and third cranial nerve impairment. Eversion, an outturning of the eyelid, is called ectropion; inversion, an inturning of the lid, is called entropion. These abnormalities are often associated with scarring injuries or the aging process.

The pupils are black, are equal in size (about 3 mm to 7 mm in diameter), and have round, smooth borders. **Mydriasis** (enlarged pupils) can indicate injury or glaucoma or result from certain drugs (e.g., atropine). **Miosis** (constricted pupils) can indicate an inflammation of the iris or result from such drugs as morphine or pilocarpine. The pupils can become slightly irregular and smaller in older adults, making it more difficult to examine the eyes. **Anisocoria** (unequal pupils) can result from a central nervous system disorder; however, slight variations may be normal. The iris is normally flat and round. A bulging toward the cornea can indicate increased intraocular pressure.

Skill 27.6 describes how to assess a client's eye structures and visual acuity.

SKILL 27.6

ASSESSING THE EYE STRUCTURES AND VISUAL ACUITY

Equipment

- Cotton tip applicator
- Gauze square
- Clean gloves
- Millimetre ruler
- Penlight
- Snellen or E chart
- Opaque card

IMPLEMENTATION

Performance

1. Before performing the procedure, introduce yourself and verify the client's identity by using agency protocol. Explain to the client what you are going to do, why it is necessary, and how he or she can cooperate. Discuss how the results will be used in planning further care or treatments.
2. Perform hand hygiene, apply gloves, and observe other appropriate infection prevention and control procedures.
3. Provide for client privacy.
4. Inquire whether the client has any history of the following: family history of diabetes, hypertension, blood dyscrasia, or eye disease, injury, or surgery; client's last visit to an ophthalmologist; current use of eye medications; use of contact lenses or eyeglasses; hygienic practices for corrective lenses; current symptoms of eye problems (e.g., changes in visual acuity, blurring of vision, tearing, spots, photophobia, itching, or pain).

ASSESSMENT	NORMAL FINDINGS	DEVIATIONS FROM NORMAL
External Eye Structures		
5. Inspect the eyebrows for hair distribution and alignment and for skin quality and movement. (Ask client to raise and lower the eyebrows.)	Hair evenly distributed; skin intact; eyebrows symmetrically aligned; equal movement	Loss of hair; scaling and flakiness of skin; unequal alignment and movement of eyebrows
6. Inspect the eyelashes for evenness of distribution and direction of curl.	Equally distributed; curled slightly outward	Turned inward
7. Inspect the eyelids for surface characteristics (e.g., skin quality and texture), position in relation to the cornea, ability to blink, and frequency of blinking. For proper visual examination of the upper eyelids, elevate the eyebrows with your thumb and index fingers, and have the client close the eyes (see ❶). Inspect the lower eyelids while the client's eyes are closed.	Skin intact; no discharge; no discolouration; lids close symmetrically; approximately 15 to 20 involuntary blinks per minute; bilateral blinking; when lids open, no visible sclera above corneas, and upper and lower borders of cornea are slightly covered	Redness, swelling, flaking, crusting, plaques, discharge, nodules, lesions; lids close asymmetrically, incompletely, or painfully; rapid, monocular, absent, or infrequent blinking; ptosis, ectropion, or entropion; rim of sclera visible between lid and iris (possible hyperthyroidism)

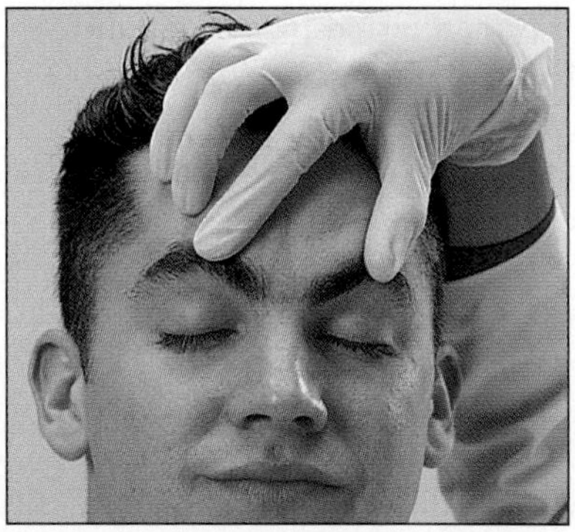

❶ Inspecting the upper eyelids

ASSESSMENT	NORMAL FINDINGS	DEVIATIONS FROM NORMAL
8. Inspect the bulbar conjunctiva (lying over the sclera) for colour, texture, and the presence of lesions. Retract the eyelids with your thumb and index finger, exerting pressure over the upper and lower bony orbits and ask the client to look up, down, and from side to side.	Transparent; capillaries sometimes evident; sclera appears white (yellowish in dark-skinned clients)	Jaundiced sclera (e.g., in liver disease); excessively pale sclera (e.g., in anemia); reddened sclera; lesions or nodules (may indicate damage by mechanical, chemical, allergenic, or bacterial agents)

(continued)

SKILL 27.6

ASSESSING THE EYE STRUCTURES AND VISUAL ACUITY (*continued*)

ASSESSMENT	NORMAL FINDINGS	DEVIATIONS FROM NORMAL
9. Inspect the palpebral conjunctiva (lining of the eyelids) by everting the lids. Note colour, texture, and the presence of lesions. Evert both lower lids and ask the client to look up. Then gently retract the lower lids with the index fingers.	Shiny, smooth, and pink or red	Extremely pale (possible anemia); extremely red (inflammation); nodules or other lesions
10. Evert the upper lids if a problem (e.g., a foreign body) is suspected. • Ask the client to look down while keeping the eyes slightly open. **Rationale: Closing the eyelids contracts the orbicular muscle, which prevents lid eversion.** • Gently grasp the client's eyelashes with the thumb and index finger. Pull the lashes gently downward. **Rationale: Upward or outward pulling on the eyelashes causes muscle contraction.** • Place a cotton-tipped applicator stick about 1 cm above the lid margin, and push it gently downward while holding the eyelashes (see ❷). **Rationale: These actions evert the lid, that is, flip the lower part of the lid over on top of itself.** • Hold the margin of the everted lid or the eyelashes against the ridge of the upper bony orbit with the applicator stick or the thumb (see ❸). • Inspect the conjunctiva for colour, texture, lesions, and foreign bodies. • To return the lid to its normal position, gently pull the lashes forward and ask the client to look up and blink.	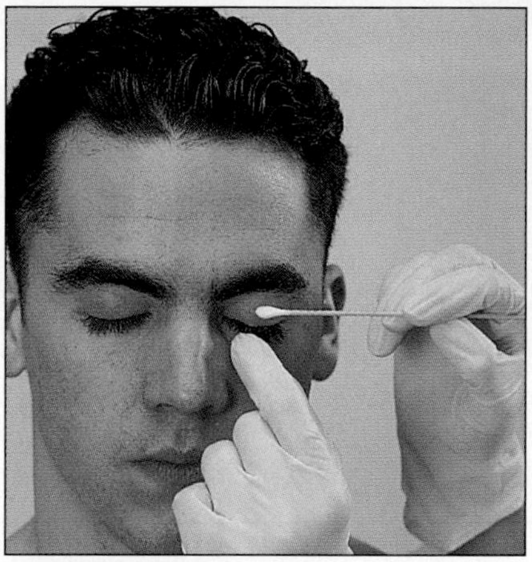 ❷ Everting the upper eyelid 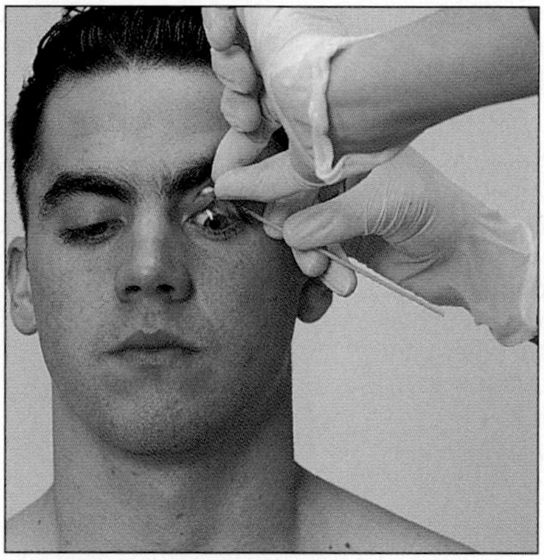 ❸ Holding the margin of the everted upper eyelid	
11. Inspect and palpate the lacrimal gland. • Use the tip of your index finger to palpate the lacrimal gland (see ❹). • Observe for edema between the lower lid and the nose.	No edema or tenderness over lacrimal gland	Swelling or tenderness over lacrimal gland
12. Inspect and palpate the lacrimal sac and nasolacrimal duct. • Observe for evidence of increased tearing. • Use the tip of your index finger to palpate inside the lower orbital rim near the inner canthus (see ❺).	No edema or tearing	Evidence of increased tearing; regurgitation of fluid on palpation of lacrimal sac

(*continued*)

SKILL 27.6

ASSESSING THE EYE STRUCTURES AND VISUAL ACUITY (*continued*)

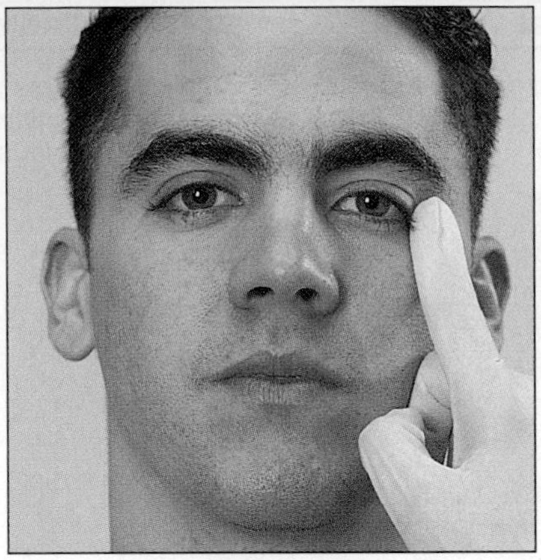

❹ Palpating the lacrimal gland

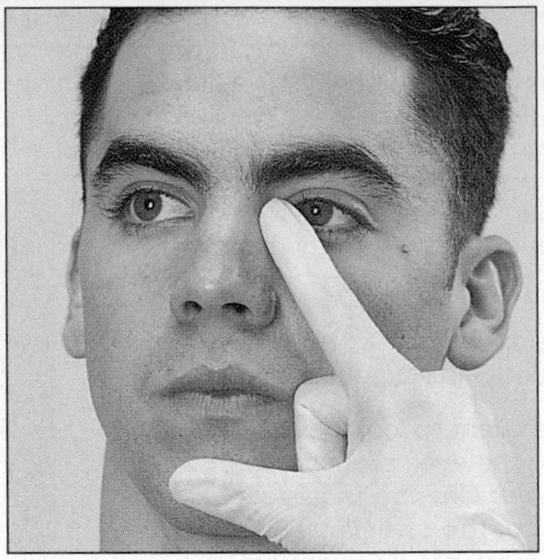

❺ Palpating the lacrimal sac and the nasolacrimal duct

ASSESSMENT	NORMAL FINDINGS	DEVIATIONS FROM NORMAL
13. Inspect the cornea for clarity and texture. Ask the client to look straight ahead. Hold a penlight at an oblique angle to the eye, and move the light slowly across the corneal surface. Tangential lighting best shows corneal regularity.	Transparent, shiny, and smooth; details of the iris are visible; in older people, a thin, greyish-white ring around the margin, called arcus senilis, may be evident	Opaque; surface not smooth (may be the result of trauma or abrasion); arcus senilis in clients under age 40
14. Perform the corneal sensitivity (reflex) test to determine the function of the trigeminal (fifth cranial) nerve. Ask the client to keep both eyes open and look straight ahead. Extend your hand behind the client's field of vision, then bring the gauze toward the outer canthus. Lightly touch the cornea with a corner of the gauze (see ❻). This test is not done on clients wearing contact lenses.	Client blinks when the cornea is touched, indicating that the trigeminal nerve is intact	One or both eyelids fail to respond

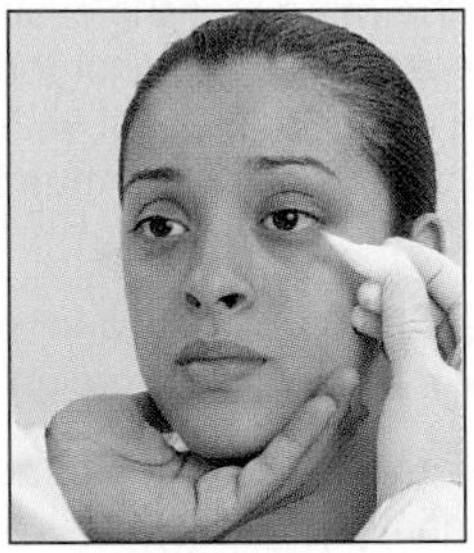

❻ Testing the corneal reflex

ASSESSMENT	NORMAL FINDINGS	DEVIATIONS FROM NORMAL
15. Inspect the anterior chamber for transparency and depth. Use the same oblique lighting as used to test the cornea.	Transparent; no shadows of light on iris; depth of about 3 mm	Cloudy; crescent-shaped shadows on far side of iris; shallow chamber (possible glaucoma)
16. Inspect the pupils for colour, shape, and symmetry of size. Pupil charts are available in some agencies. See ❼ for variations in pupil diameters.	Black in colour; equal in size; normally 3 to 7 mm in diameter; round, smooth border; iris flat and round	Cloudiness, mydriasis, miosis, anisocoria; bulging of iris toward cornea

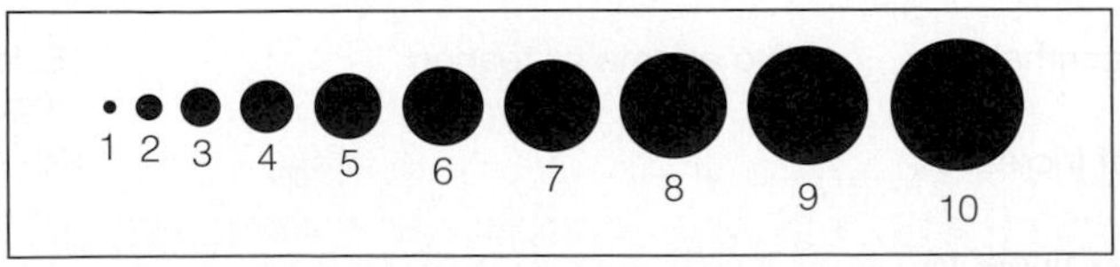

❼ Variations in pupil diameters in millimetres

(continued)

SKILL 27.6

ASSESSING THE EYE STRUCTURES AND VISUAL ACUITY (*continued*)

ASSESSMENT	NORMAL FINDINGS	DEVIATIONS FROM NORMAL
17. Assess each pupil's direct and consensual reaction to light to determine the function of the oculomotor (third) and trochlear (fourth cranial) nerves. • Partially darken the room. • Ask the client to look straight ahead. • By using a penlight and approaching from the side, shine a light on the pupil. • Observe the response of the illuminated pupil. It should constrict (direct response). • Shine the light on the pupil again, and observe the response of the other pupil. It should also constrict (consensual response).	Illuminated pupil constricts (direct response); nonilluminated pupil constricts (consensual response)	Neither pupil constricts; unequal responses; absent responses
18. Assess each pupil's reaction to accommodation. • Hold an object (a penlight or pencil) about 10 cm from the bridge of the client's nose. • Ask the client to look first at the top of the object and then at a distant object (e.g., the far wall) behind the penlight. Alternate the gaze from the near to the far object. • Observe the pupil response. The pupils should constrict when looking at the near object and dilate when looking at the far object. • Next, move the penlight or pencil toward the client's nose. The pupils should converge. To record normal assessment of the pupils, use the abbreviation PERRLA (pupils equally round and react to light and accommodation).	Pupils constrict when looking at near object; pupils dilate when looking at far object; pupils converge when near object is moved toward nose	One or both pupils fail to constrict, dilate, or converge
19. Assess peripheral visual fields to determine function of the retina and neuronal visual pathways to the brain and optic (second cranial) nerve. • Have the client sit directly facing you at a distance of 60 cm to 90 cm. • Ask the client to cover the right eye with a card and look directly at your nose. • Cover or close your eye directly opposite the client's covered eye (i.e., your left eye), and look directly at the client's nose. • Hold an object (e.g., a penlight or pencil) in your fingers, extend your arm, and move the object into the visual field from various points in the periphery (see ❽). The object should be at an equal distance from the client and you. Ask the client to tell you when the moving object is first spotted. a. To test the temporal field of the left eye, extend and move your right arm in from the client's right periphery. Temporally, peripheral objects can be seen at right angles (90 degrees) to the central point of vision. b. To test the superior (upward) field of the left eye, extend and move the right arm down from the upward periphery. The upward field of vision is normally 50 degrees because the orbital ridge is in the way. c. To test the inferior (downward) field of the left eye, extend and move the right arm up from the lower periphery. The downward field of vision is normally 70 degrees because the cheekbone is in the way. d. To test the nasal field of the left eye, extend and move your left arm in from the periphery. The nasal field of vision is normally 50 degrees away from the central point of vision because the nose is in the way. • Repeat the above steps for the right eye, reversing the process.	When looking straight ahead, client can see objects in the periphery	Visual field smaller than normal (possible glaucoma); one-half vision in one or both eyes (indicates nerve damage)

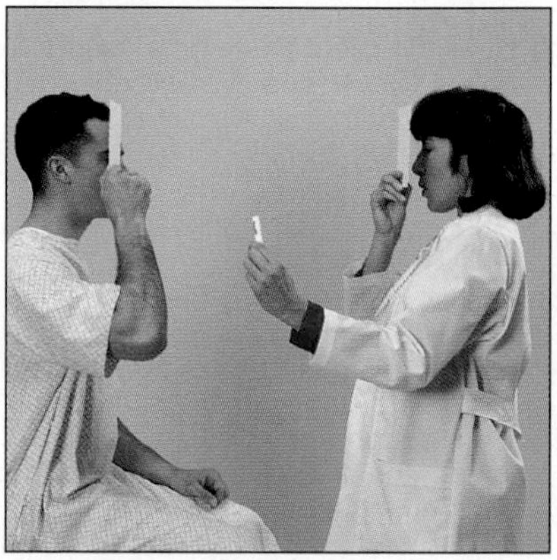

❽ Assessing the client's left peripheral visual field

(continued)

SKILL 27.6

ASSESSING THE EYE STRUCTURES AND VISUAL ACUITY (*continued*)

ASSESSMENT	NORMAL FINDINGS	DEVIATIONS FROM NORMAL
Extraocular Muscle Tests		
20. Assess six ocular movements to determine eye alignment and coordination. These can be performed on clients over 6 months of age.	Both eyes coordinated, move in unison, with parallel alignment	Eye movements not coordinated or parallel; one or both eyes fail to follow a penlight in specific directions (e.g., strabismus or cross-eye); **nystagmus** (rapid involuntary rhythmic eye movement) other than at end point may indicate neurological impairment

- Stand directly in front of the client and hold the penlight at a comfortable distance, such as 30 cm in front of the client's eyes.
- Ask the client to hold the head in a fixed position facing you and to follow the movements of the penlight with the eyes only.
- Move the penlight in a slow, orderly manner through the six cardinal fields of gaze, that is, from the centre of the eye along the lines of the arrows in ❾ and back to the centre.
- Stop the movement of the penlight periodically so that nystagmus can be detected.

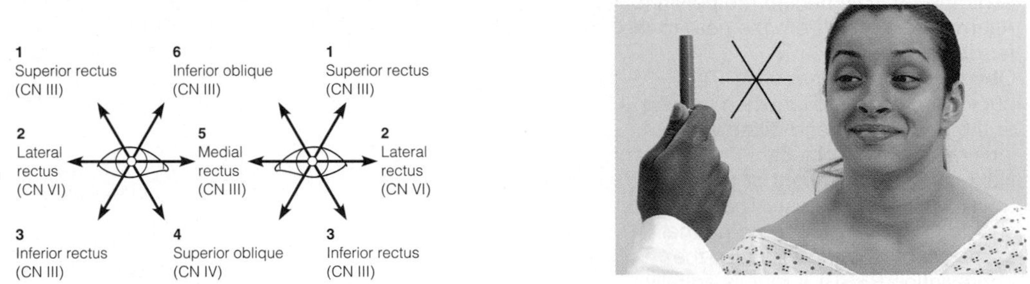

❾ The six muscles that govern eye movement

ASSESSMENT	NORMAL FINDINGS	DEVIATIONS FROM NORMAL
21. Assess for location of light reflex by shining penlight on pupil in corneal surface (Hirschberg test).	Light falls symmetrically on both pupils (e.g., at 6 o'clock on both pupils)	Light falls off centre on one eye (indicates misalignment)
22. Have the client fixate on a near or far object. Cover one eye and observe for movement in the uncovered eye (cover test).	Uncovered eye does not move	If misalignment is present, when dominant eye is covered, the uncovered eye will move to focus on object
Visual Acuity		
23. Assess near vision by providing adequate lighting and asking the client to read from a magazine or newspaper held at a distance of 36 cm (14 in.). If the client normally wears corrective lenses, the glasses or lenses should be worn during the test.	Able to read newsprint	Difficulty reading newsprint unless because of aging process
24. Assess distance vision by asking the client to wear corrective lenses, unless they are used for reading only (i.e., for distances of only 36 cm).	20/20 vision on Snellen-type chart	Denominator of 40 or more on Snellen-type chart with corrective lenses

(continued)

SKILL 27.6

ASSESSING THE EYE STRUCTURES AND VISUAL ACUITY (*continued*)

ASSESSMENT	NORMAL FINDINGS	DEVIATIONS FROM NORMAL
• Ask the client to stand or sit 6 m (20 ft) from a Snellen or character chart (see ⑩), cover the eye not being tested, and identify the letters or characters on the chart. • Take three readings: right eye, left eye, both eyes. • Record the readings of each eye and both eyes (i.e., the smallest line from which the person is able to read one half or more of the letters). At the end of each line of the chart are standardized numbers (fractions). The top line is 20/200. The numerator (top number) is always 20, the distance the person stands from the chart. The denominator (bottom number) is the distance from which the normal eye can read the chart. Therefore, a person who has 20/40 vision, can see at 20 feet from the chart what a normal-sighted person can see at 40 feet from the chart. Visual acuity is recorded as "s̄-c" (without correction), or "c̄-c" (with correction). You can also indicate how many letters were misread in the line (e.g., "visual acuity 20/40, 2 c̄-c" indicates that two letters were misread in the 20/40 line by a client wearing corrective lenses).		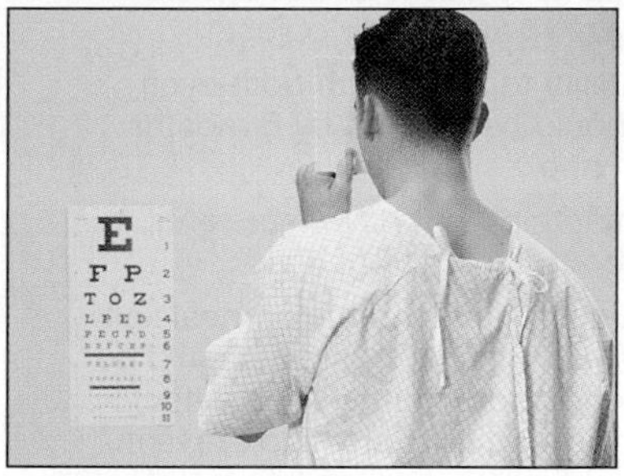 ⑩ Testing distance vision
25. If the client is unable to see even the top line (20/200) of the Snellen-type chart, perform functional vision tests (see Box 27.6).		Functional vision only (e.g., light perception, hand movements, counting fingers at 30 cm)

26. Document findings in the client record by using forms or checklists supplemented by narrative notes when appropriate.

EVALUATION

- Perform a detailed follow-up examination of neurological and other systems based on findings that deviated from expected or normal for the client. Relate findings to previous assessment data if available.
- Report significant deviations from normal to the appropriate members of the health-care team. Persons with denominators of 40 or more on the Snellen or character chart, with or without corrective lenses, may need to be referred to an optometrist or ophthalmologist.

BOX 27.6 PERFORMING FUNCTIONAL VISION TESTS

LIGHT PERCEPTION
Shine a penlight into the client's eye from a lateral position, and then turn the light off. Ask the client to tell you when the light is on or off. If the client knows when the light is on or off, the client has light perception, and the vision is recorded as "LP."

HAND MOVEMENTS (H/M)
Hold your hand 30 cm from the client's face and move it slowly back and forth, stopping it periodically. Ask the client to tell you when your hand stops moving. If the client knows when your hand stops moving, record the vision as "H/M 30 cm."

COUNTING FINGERS (C/F)
Hold up some of your fingers 30 cm from the client's face, and ask the client to count your fingers. If the client can do so, note on the vision record "C/F 30 cm."

Lifespan Considerations

Assessing the Eyes and Vision

INFANTS

- Infants 4 weeks of age should gaze at and follow objects.
- Ability to focus with both eyes should be present by 6 months of age.
- Infants do not have tears until about 3 months of age.
- A cover test and the corneal light reflex (Hirschberg) test should be conducted on infants to detect misalignment early and prevent amblyopia.
- Visual acuity is about 20/300 at 4 months and progressively improves.

CHILDREN

- Epicanthal folds, common in persons of Asian cultures, may cover the medial canthus and cause eyes to appear misaligned. Epicanthal folds may also be seen in young children of any race before the bridge of the nose begins to elevate.
- Preschool children's acuity can be checked with picture cards or the E chart. Acuity should approach 20/20 by 6 years of age.
- A cover test and the corneal light reflex (Hirschberg) test should be conducted on young children to detect misalignment early and prevent amblyopia.
- Always perform the acuity test with glasses on if a child has a prescription to wear lenses.
- Children should be tested for colour vision deficit. From 8% to 10% of Caucasian males and from 0.5% to 1% of Caucasian females have this deficit; it is much less common in non-Caucasian children. The Ishihara or Hardy-Rand-Rittler test can be used.

OLDER ADULTS

Visual Acuity

- Visual acuity decreases as the lens ages, becomes more opaque, and loses elasticity (presbyopia).
- The ability of the iris to accommodate to darkness and dim light diminishes.
- Peripheral vision diminishes.
- The adaptation to light (glare) and dark decreases.
- Accommodation to far objects often improves, but accommodation to near objects decreases.
- Colour vision declines; older people are less able to perceive purple colours and to discriminate pastel colours.
- Many older people wear corrective lenses; they are most likely to have hyperopia. Visual changes are due to loss of elasticity (presbyopia) and transparency of the lens.
- The number of vitreous floaters increases with age.

External Eye Structures

- The skin around the orbit of the eye may darken.
- The eyes may appear dry and lustreless because of the decrease in tear production from the lacrimal glands.
- The eyeball may appear sunken because of the decrease in orbital fat.
- Skin folds of the upper lids may seem more prominent, and the lower lids may sag.
- **Arcus senilis** (a thin, greyish-white arc or ring) appears around part or all of the cornea. It results from an accumulation of a lipid substance on the cornea. The cornea tends to cloud with age.
- The iris may appear pale with brown discolourations as a result of pigment degeneration.
- The conjunctiva of the eye may appear paler than in younger adults and may take on a slightly yellow appearance because of the deposition of fat.
- Pupil reaction to light and accommodation is normally symmetrically equal but may be less brisk.
- The pupils can appear smaller in size, unequal, and irregular in shape because of sclerotic changes in the iris.

Ears and Hearing

Assessment of the ear includes direct inspection and palpation of the external ear, inspection of the remaining parts of the ear by an **otoscope**, and determination of auditory acuity. The ear is usually assessed during an initial physical examination; periodic reassessments may be necessary for long-term clients or those with hearing problems.

The ear is divided into three parts: external ear, middle ear, and inner ear. Most of the structures mentioned next are illustrated in Figure 27.15. The external ear includes the **auricle** or **pinna**, the external auditory canal, and the **tympanic membrane**, or eardrum. Landmarks of the auricle include the **lobule** (earlobe), **helix** (the posterior curve of the auricle's upper aspect), **antihelix** (the anterior curve of the auricle's upper aspect), **tragus** (the cartilaginous protrusion at the entrance to the ear canal), **triangular fossa** (a depression of the antihelix), and **external auditory meatus** (the entrance to the ear canal). Although not part of the ear, the **mastoid**, a bony prominence behind the ear, is another important landmark. The external ear canal is curved, is about 2.5 cm long in the adult, and ends at the tympanic membrane. The tympanic membrane separates the external ear from the middle ear. It is covered with skin that has many fine hairs, glands, and nerve endings. The glands secrete **cerumen** (earwax), which lubricates and protects the canal.

The curvature of the external ear canal differs with age. In the infant and toddler, the canal has an upward curvature. By the age of 3, the ear canal assumes the more downward curvature of adulthood.

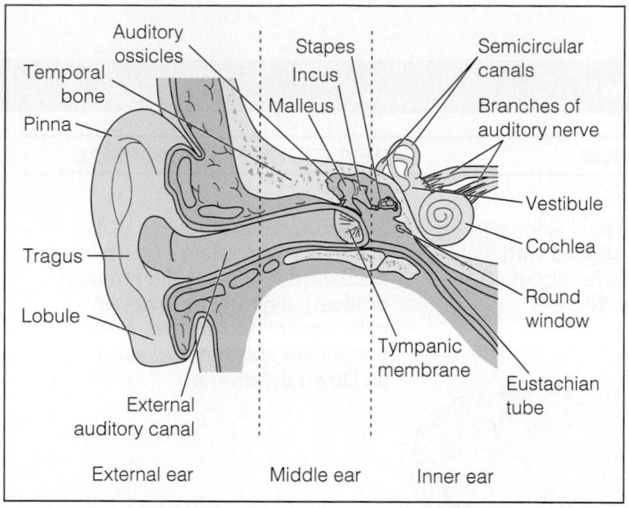

FIGURE 27.15 Anatomic structures of the external, middle, and inner ear

The middle ear is an air-filled cavity that starts at the tympanic membrane and contains three **ossicles** (bones of sound transmission): the **malleus** (hammer), which is the most easily seen, the **incus** (anvil), and the **stapes** (stirrup). The **eustachian tube**, another part of the middle ear, connects the middle ear to the nasopharynx. The tube stabilizes the air pressure between the external atmosphere and the middle ear, thus preventing rupture of the tympanic membrane and discomfort produced by marked pressure differences.

The inner ear contains the **cochlea**, a seashell-shaped structure essential for sound transmission and hearing, and the **vestibule** and **semicircular canals**, which contain the organs of equilibrium.

Sound transmission and hearing are complex processes. In brief, sound can be transmitted by air conduction or bone conduction. Air-conducted transmission occurs by this process:

1. A sound stimulus enters the external canal and reaches the tympanic membrane.
2. The sound waves vibrate the tympanic membrane and reach the ossicles.
3. The sound waves travel from the vibrating ossicles to the opening in the inner ear (oval window).
4. The cochlea receives the sound vibrations.
5. The stimulus travels to the auditory nerve (the eighth cranial nerve) and the cerebral cortex.

Bone-conducted sound transmission occurs when skull bones transport the sound directly to the auditory nerve.

Audiometric evaluations, which measure hearing at various decibels, are recommended for older adults. A common hearing deficit with age is loss of ability to hear high-frequency sounds, such as *f, s, sh,* and *ph.* This neurosensory hearing deficit does not respond well to the use of a hearing aid.

Conduction hearing loss is the result of interrupted transmission of sound waves through the outer and middle ear structures. Possible causes are a tear in the tympanic membrane or an obstruction, because of swelling or other causes, in the auditory canal. **Sensorineural hearing loss** is the result of damage to the inner ear, the auditory nerve, or the hearing centre in the brain. **Mixed hearing loss** is a combination of conduction and sensorineural loss.

Skill 27.7 describes how to assess the ears and hearing.

SKILL 27.7

ASSESSING THE EARS AND HEARING

PLANNING

It is important to conduct the ear and hearing examination in a quiet area. In addition, the location should allow the client to be positioned sitting or standing at the same level as the nurse.

Equipment

- Otoscope with several sizes of ear specula

IMPLEMENTATION

Performance

1. Before performing the procedure, introduce yourself and verify the client's identity by using agency protocol. Explain to the client what you are going to do, why it is necessary, and how he or she can cooperate. Discuss how the results will be used in planning further care or treatments.
2. Perform hand hygiene and observe other appropriate infection prevention and control procedures.
3. Provide for client privacy.
4. Inquire whether the client has a family history of hearing problems or loss; presence of any ear problems; medication history, especially if there are complaints of ringing in ears; any hearing difficulty: its onset, factors contributing to it, and how it interferes with activities of daily living; use of a corrective hearing device: when and from whom it was obtained.
5. Position the client comfortably, seated if possible.

(continued)

SKILL 27.7

ASSESSING THE EARS AND HEARING (*continued*)

ASSESSMENT	NORMAL FINDINGS	DEVIATIONS FROM NORMAL
Auricles		
6. Inspect the auricles for colour, symmetry of size, and position. To inspect position, note the level at which the superior aspect of the auricle attaches to the head in relation to the eye.	Colour same as facial skin; symmetrical; auricle aligned with outer canthus of eye, about 10° from vertical (see ❶).	Bluish colour of earlobes (e.g., cyanosis); pallor (e.g., frostbite); excessive redness (inflammation or fever); asymmetry; low-set ears (associated with a congenital abnormality, such as Down syndrome)

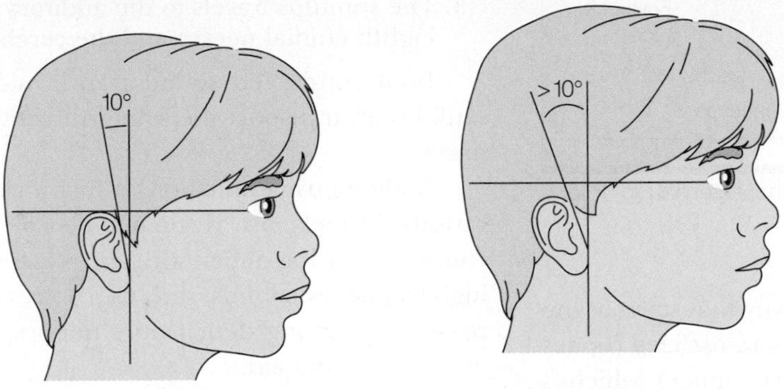

Normal alignment

Low-set ears and deviation in alignment

❶ Alignment of ears

ASSESSMENT	NORMAL FINDINGS	DEVIATIONS FROM NORMAL
7. Palpate the auricles for texture, elasticity, and areas of tenderness. Gently pull the auricle upward, downward, and backward. Fold the pinna forward (it should recoil). Push in on the tragus. Apply pressure to the mastoid process.	Mobile, firm, and not tender; pinna recoils after it is folded	Lesions (e.g., cysts); flaky, scaly skin (e.g., seborrhea); tenderness when moved or pressed (may indicate inflammation or infection of external ear)

External Ear Canal and Tympanic Membrane

8. Use an otoscope to inspect the external ear canal for cerumen, skin lesions, pus, and blood.

- Attach a speculum to the otoscope. Use the largest diameter that will fit the ear canal without causing discomfort. **Rationale: This achieves maximum vision of the entire ear canal and tympanic membrane.**
- Tip the client's head away from you, and straighten the ear canal. For an adult, straighten the ear canal by pulling the pinna up and back (see ❷). **Rationale: Straightening the ear canal facilitates vision of the ear canal and the tympanic membrane.**

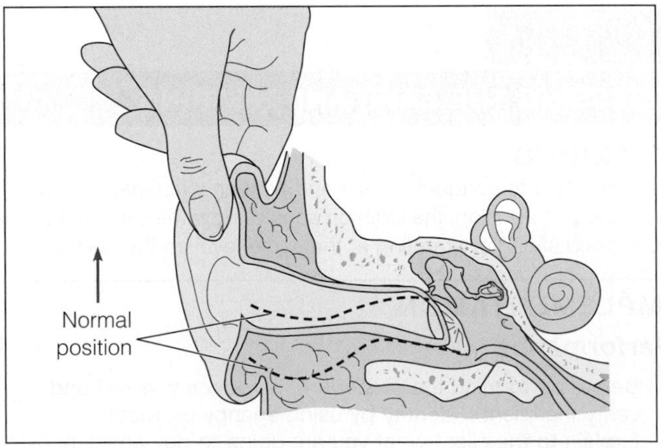

❷ Straightening the ear canal of an adult by pulling the pinna up and back

(continued)

SKILL 27.7

ASSESSING THE EARS AND HEARING (*continued*)

ASSESSMENT	NORMAL FINDINGS	DEVIATIONS FROM NORMAL
• Hold the otoscope either (a) right side up, with your fingers between the otoscope handle and the client's head or (b) upside down, with your fingers and the ulnar surface of your hand against the client's head (see ❸). **Rationale: This stabilizes the head and protects the eardrum and canal from injury if a quick head movement occurs.** • Gently insert the tip of the otoscope into the ear canal, avoiding pressure by the speculum against either side of the ear canal. **Rationale: The inner two-thirds of the ear canal is bony; if the speculum is pressed against either side, the client will experience discomfort.**	Distal third contains hair follicles and glands; dry cerumen, greyish-tan colour; or sticky, wet cerumen in various shades of brown	Redness and discharge; scaling; excessive cerumen obstructing canal 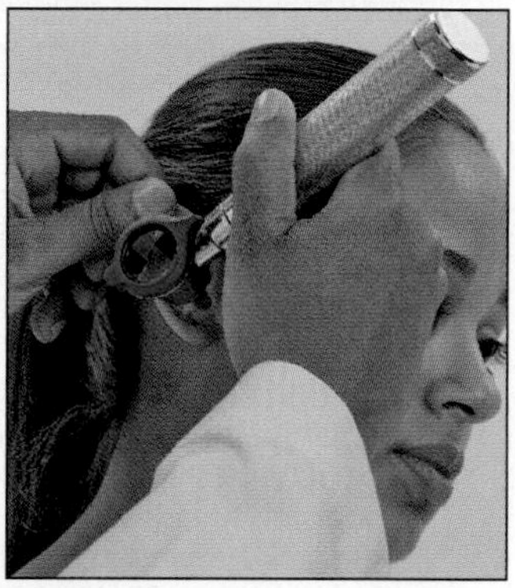 ❸ Inserting an otoscope
9. Inspect the tympanic membrane for colour and gloss.	Pearly grey colour, semi-transparent, light reflex at 5 o'clock in right ear and 7 o'clock in left eart (see ❹) 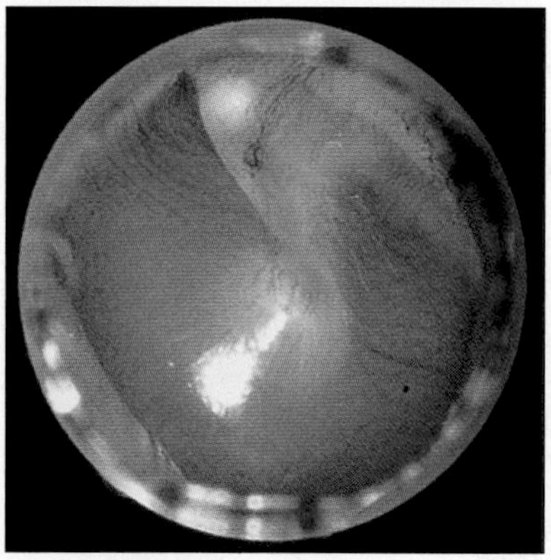 ❹ Normal tympanic membrane with light reflex at 7 o'clock (left ear)	Pink to red, some opacity; yellow-amber, white, blue, or deep red; dull surface

Gross Hearing Acuity Tests

ASSESSMENT	NORMAL FINDINGS	DEVIATIONS FROM NORMAL
10. Assess client's response to normal voice tones. If client has difficulty hearing the normal voice, proceed with the following tests.	Normal voice tones audible	Normal voice tones not audible (e.g., requests nurse to repeat words or statements, leans toward the speaker, turns the head, cups the ears, or speaks in loud voice)

(continued)

SKILL 27.7

ASSESSING THE EARS AND HEARING (*continued*)

ASSESSMENT	NORMAL FINDINGS	DEVIATIONS FROM NORMAL
10A. Perform the watch tick test. The ticking of a watch has a higher pitch than the human voice. Have the client occlude one ear. Out of the client's sight, place a ticking watch 2 cm to 3 cm from the unoccluded ear. Ask what the client can hear. Repeat with the other ear.	Able to hear ticking in both ears	Unable to hear ticking in one or both ears
10B. *Tuning Fork Tests* Perform Weber's test to assess bone conduction by examining the lateralization (sideward transmission) of sounds. • Hold the tuning fork at its base. Activate it by tapping the fork gently against the back of your hand near the knuckles or by stroking the fork between your thumb and index fingers. It should be made to ring softly. • Place the base of the vibrating fork on top of the client's head (see ❺) and ask where the client hears the noise.	Sound is heard in both ears or is localized at the centre of the head (Weber negative)	Sound is heard better in impaired ear, indicating a bone-conductive hearing loss, or sound is heard better in ear without a problem, indicating a sensorineural disturbance (Weber positive)
Conduct the Rinne test to compare air conduction to bone conduction. • Ask the client to block the hearing in one ear intermittently by moving a fingertip in and out of the ear canal. • Hold the handle of the activated tuning fork on the mastoid process of one ear (see ❻) until the client states that the vibration can no longer be heard. • Immediately hold the vibrating fork prongs in front of the client's ear canal (see ❼). • Push aside the client's hair if necessary. Ask whether the client now hears the sound. Sound conducted by air is heard more readily than sound conducted by bone. The tuning fork vibrations conducted by air are normally heard longer.	Air-conducted (AC) hearing is greater than bone-conducted (BC) hearing, that is, AC > BC (positive Rinne)	Bone conduction time is equal to or longer than the air conduction time, that is, BC > AC or BC = AC (negative Rinne; indicates a conductive hearing loss)

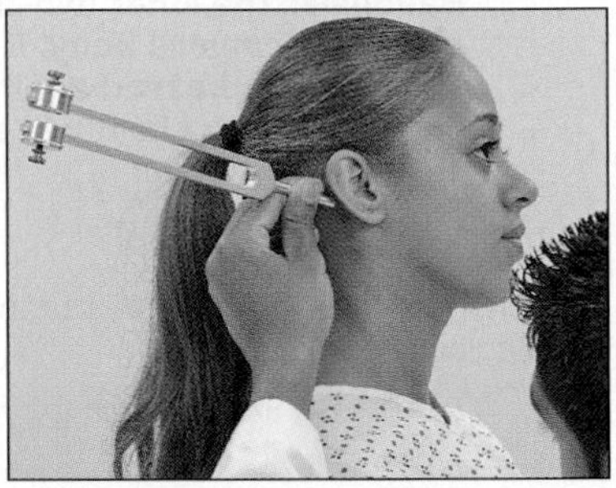

❻ Base of the tuning fork on the mastoid process (Rinne test)

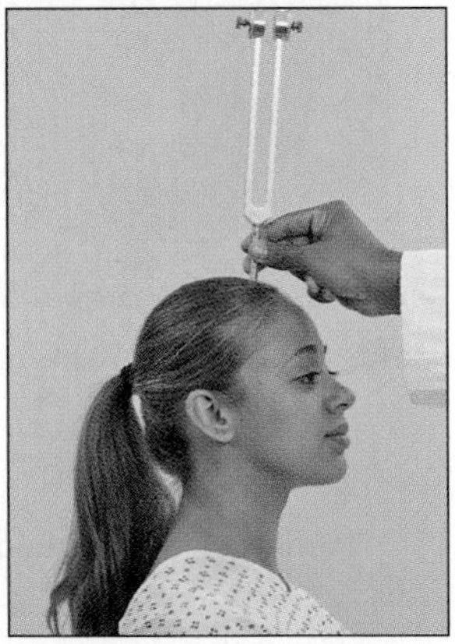

❺ Placing the base of a tuning fork on the client's skull (Weber's test)

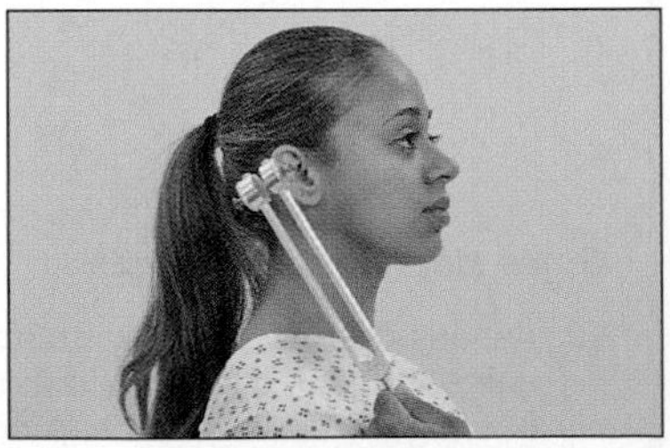

❼ Tuning fork prongs placed in front of the client's ear (Rinne test)

11. Document findings in the client record by using forms or checklists supplemented by narrative notes when appropriate.

EVALUATION

- Perform a detailed follow-up examination of neurological and other systems based on findings that deviated from expected or normal for the client.
- Report significant deviations from normal to the appropriate members of the health-care team.

Lifespan Considerations

Assessing the Ears and Hearing

INFANTS

- To assess gross hearing, ring a bell from behind the infant or have the parent call the child's name to check for a response. Newborns will quiet to the sound and may open their eyes wider. By 3 to 4 months of age, the child will turn head and eyes toward the sound.
- All newborns should be assessed for hearing by using auditory brain response testing before being discharged from the hospital.

CHILDREN

- To inspect the external canal and tympanic membrane in children younger than 3 years old, pull the pinna down and back. Insert the speculum only 0.5 cm to 1 cm.
- Hearing loss is becoming more common in adolescents and young adults, probably as a result of exposure to loud music and prolonged use of headsets at loud volumes.

OLDER ADULTS

- The skin of the ear may appear dry and be less resilient because of the loss of connective tissue.
- Increased coarse and wirelike hair growth occurs along the pinna, antihelix, and tragus.
- The tympanic membrane is more translucent and less flexible.
- Earwax is drier.
- The pinna increases in both width and length, and the earlobe elongates.
- Sensorineural hearing loss occurs.
- **Presbycusis** (generalized hearing loss) occurs in all frequencies, although the first symptom is the loss of high-frequency sounds: the *f, s, sh,* and *ph* sounds. To such persons, conversation can be distorted and result in what appears to be inappropriate or confused behaviour.

Nose and Sinuses

The nasal passages can be inspected very simply with a flashlight. However, a nasal *speculum* and a penlight or an otoscope with a nasal attachment facilitates examination of the nasal attachment.

Assessment of the nose includes inspection and palpation of the external nose (the upper third of the nose is bone; the remainder is cartilage); determination of patency of the nasal cavities; and inspection of the nasal cavities.

If the client reports difficulty or abnormality in smell, the nurse may test the client's olfactory sense by asking the client to identify common odours, such as coffee or mint. This is done by asking the client to close the eyes and then placing vials containing the scent under the client's nose.

The nurse inspects, palpates, and percusses the facial sinuses (Figure 27.16). Skill 27.8 describes how to assess the nose and sinuses.

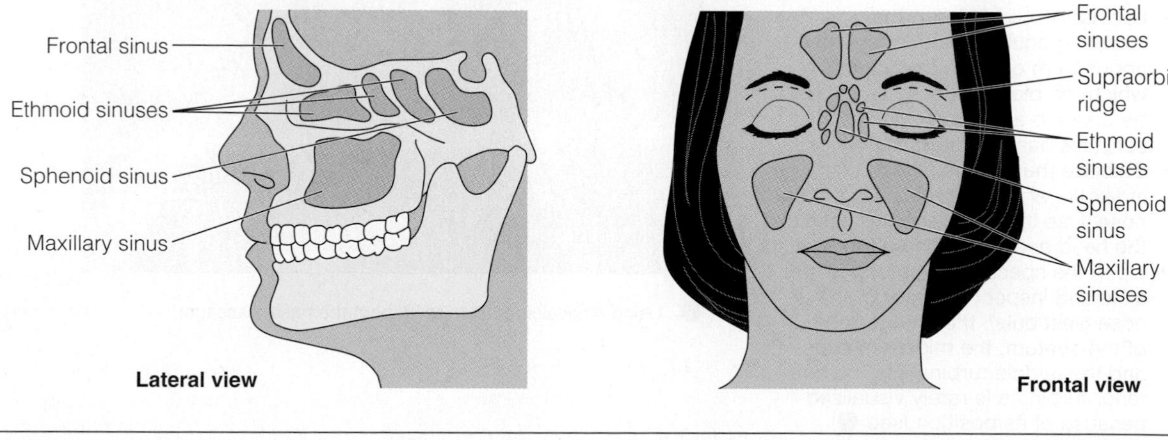

FIGURE 27.16 The facial sinuses

SKILL 27.8

ASSESSING THE NOSE AND SINUSES

Equipment

- Nasal speculum
- Flashlight or penlight

IMPLEMENTATION

Performance

1. Before performing the procedure, introduce yourself and verify the client's identity by using agency protocol. Explain to the client what you are going to do, why it is necessary, and how he or she can cooperate. Discuss how the results will be used in planning further care or treatments.
2. Perform hand hygiene and observe other appropriate infection prevention and control procedures.
3. Provide for client privacy.
4. Inquire whether the client has a history of allergies, difficulty breathing through the nose, sinus infections, injuries to nose or face, nosebleeds; any medications taken; any changes in sense of smell; any facial or nasal surgery.
5. Position the client comfortably, seated if possible.

ASSESSMENT	NORMAL FINDINGS	DEVIATIONS FROM NORMAL
Nose		
6. Inspect the external nose for any deviations in shape, size, or colour and flaring or discharge from the nares.	Symmetric and straight; no discharge or flaring; uniform colour	Asymmetric; discharge from nares; localized areas of redness or presence of skin lesions
7. Lightly palpate the external nose to determine any areas of tenderness, masses, and displacements of bone and cartilage.	Not tender; no lesions	Tenderness on palpation; presence of lesions
8. Determine patency of both nasal cavities. Ask the client to close the mouth, exert pressure on one nares, and breathe through the opposite nares. Repeat the procedure to assess patency of the opposite nares.	Air moves freely as the client breathes through the nares	Air movement is restricted in one or both nares
9. Inspect the nasal cavities by using a flashlight or a nasal speculum. • Hold the speculum in your right hand to inspect the client's left nostril and your left hand to inspect the client's right nostril. • Tip the client's head back. • Facing the client, insert the tip of the closed speculum (blades together) about 1 cm or up to the point at which the blade widens. Care must be taken to avoid pressure on the sensitive nasal septum (see ❶). • Stabilize the speculum with your index finger against the side of the nose. Use the other hand to position the head and then to hold the light. • Open the speculum as much as possible and inspect the floor of the nose (vestibule), the anterior portion of the septum, the middle meatus, and the middle turbinates. The posterior turbinate is rarely visualized because of its position (see ❷). • Inspect the lining of the nares and the integrity and the position of the nasal septum.		
10. Observe for the presence of redness, swelling, growths, and discharge.	Mucosa pink; clear, watery discharge; no lesions	Mucosa red, edematous; abnormal discharge (e.g., pus); presence of lesions (e.g., polyps)

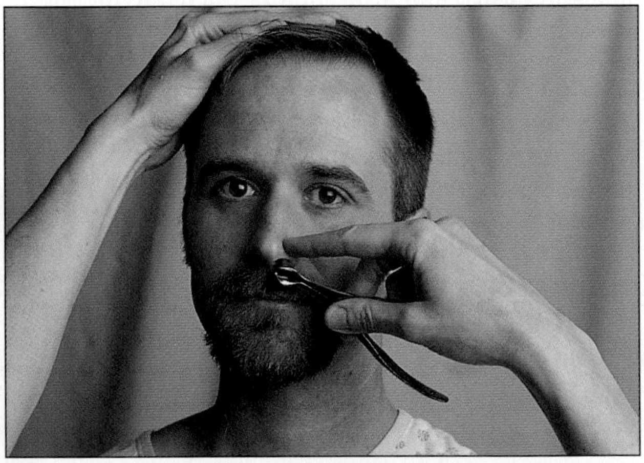

❶ Using a nasal speculum to inspect the nasal passages

(continued)

SKILL 27.8

ASSESSING THE NOSE AND SINUSES *(continued)*

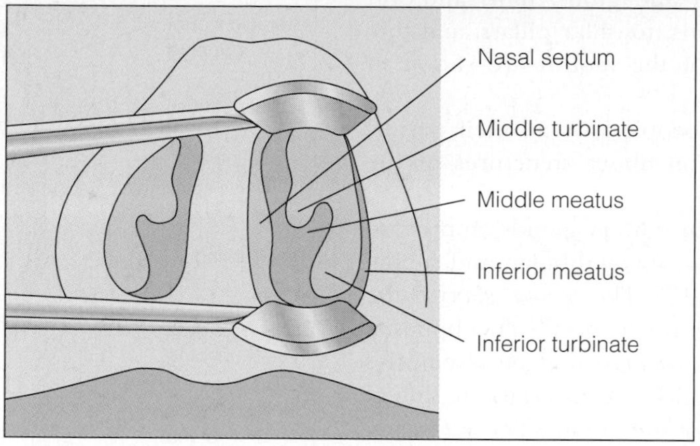

❷ The inferior and middle turbinates of the nasal passage

ASSESSMENT	NORMAL FINDINGS	DEVIATIONS FROM NORMAL
11. Inspect the nasal septum between the nasal chambers.	Nasal septum intact and in midline	Septum deviated to the right or to the left.
Facial Sinuses		
12. Palpate the maxillary and frontal sinuses for tenderness.	Not tender	Tenderness in one or more sinuses

13. Document findings in the client record by using forms or checklists supplemented by narrative notes when appropriate.

EVALUATION

- Perform a detailed follow-up examination of other systems based on findings that deviated from expected or normal for the client.
- Report significant deviations from normal to the appropriate members of the health-care team.

Lifespan Consideration

Assessing the Nose and Sinuses

INFANTS

- A speculum is usually not necessary to examine the septum, turbinates, and vestibule. Instead, push the tip of the nose upward with the thumb and shine a light into the nares.
- Ethmoid and maxillary sinuses are present at birth; frontal sinuses begin to develop by 1 to 2 years of age; and sphenoid sinuses develop later in childhood. Infants and young children have fewer sinus problems than older children and adolescents.

CHILDREN

- A speculum is usually not necessary to examine the septum, turbinates, and vestibule. It might cause the child to be apprehensive. Instead, push the tip of the nose upward with the thumb and shine a light into the nares.
- Ethmoid sinuses develop by age 6. Sinus problems in children younger than 6 are rare.
- Cough and runny nose are the most common signs of sinusitis in preadolescent children.
- Adolescents may have headaches, facial tenderness, and swelling, similar to the signs seen in adults.

OLDER ADULTS

- The sense of smell diminishes markedly because of a decrease in the number of olfactory nerve fibres and atrophy of the remaining fibres. Older persons are less able to identify and discriminate odours.
- Nosebleeds can result from hypertensive disease or other arterial vessel changes in older adults.

Mouth and Oropharynx

The mouth and pharynx are composed of a number of structures: lips, inner and buccal mucosa, the tongue, floor of the mouth, teeth and gums, hard and soft palates, uvula, salivary glands, tonsillar pillars, and tonsils. Anatomic structures of the mouth are shown in Figure 27.17.

By age 25 years, most people have all their permanent teeth. For information about structures of the teeth, see Chapter 29.

Normally, three pairs of salivary glands empty into the oral cavity: the parotid, submandibular, and sublingual glands (see Figure 27.17). The *parotid gland* is the largest and empties through the Stensen's duct opposite the second molar. The *submandibular gland* empties through Wharton's duct, which is situated at the side of the frenulum on the floor of the mouth. The *sublingual salivary gland* lies in the floor of the mouth and has numerous openings.

Dental **caries** (cavities) and **pyorrhea** (periodontal disease) are the two problems that most frequently affect the teeth. Both problems are commonly associated with plaque and tartar deposits. **Plaque** is an *invisible* soft film that adheres to the enamel surface of teeth; it consists of bacteria, molecules of saliva, and remnants of epithelial cells and leukocytes. When plaque accumulates on the teeth, dental calculus (tartar) forms. **Tartar** is a visible, hard deposit of plaque and dead bacteria that forms at the gum line. Tartar buildup can alter the fibres that attach the teeth to the gum and eventually disrupt bone tissue. Periodontal disease is characterized by **gingivitis** (inflamed gums), bleeding, receding gum lines, and the formation of pockets between the teeth and gums. In advanced periodontal disease, the teeth are loose, and pus is evident when the gums are pressed.

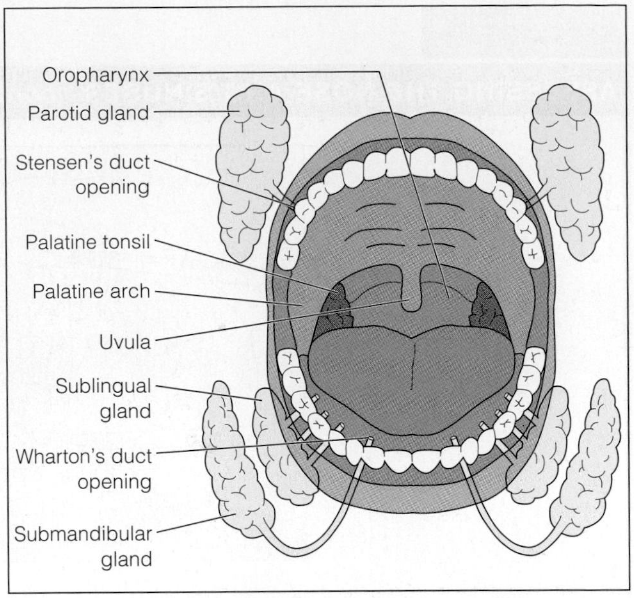

FIGURE 27.17 Anatomic structures of the mouth

Other problems nurses may see are **glossitis** (inflammation of the tongue), **stomatitis** (inflammation of the oral mucosa), and **parotitis** (inflammation of the parotid salivary gland). The accumulation of foul matter (food, microorganisms, and epithelial elements) on the teeth and gums is referred to as **sordes.**

Skill 27.9 describes assessment of the mouth and oropharynx.

SKILL 27.9

ASSESSING THE MOUTH AND OROPHARYNX

PLANNING

If possible, arrange for the client to sit with his or her head against a firm surface, such as a headrest or an examination table. This makes it easier for the client to hold the head still during the examination.

Equipment

- Clean gloves
- Tongue depressor
- 5 cm × 5 cm gauze pads
- Penlight

IMPLEMENTATION

Performance

1. Before performing the procedure, introduce yourself and verify the client's identity by using agency protocol. Explain to the client what you are going to do, why it is necessary, and how he or she can cooperate. Discuss how the results will be used in planning further care or treatments.
2. Perform hand hygiene and observe other appropriate infection prevention and control procedures.
3. Provide for client privacy.
4. Inquire whether the client has any history of the following: routine pattern of dental care, last visit to dentist; length of time ulcers or other lesions have been present; any denture discomfort; any medications the client is receiving.
5. Position the client comfortably, seated if possible.

(continued)

SKILL 27.9

ASSESSING THE MOUTH AND OROPHARYNX (*continued*)

ASSESSMENT	NORMAL FINDINGS	DEVIATIONS FROM NORMAL
Lips and Buccal Mucosa		
6. Inspect the outer lips for symmetry of contour, colour, and texture. Ask the client to purse the lips as if to whistle.	Uniform pink colour (darker, e.g., bluish hue, in Mediterranean groups and dark-skinned clients); soft, moist, smooth texture; symmetry of contour; ability to purse lips	Pallor; cyanosis; blisters; generalized or localized swelling; fissures, crusts, or scales (may result from excessive moisture, nutritional deficiency, or fluid deficit); inability to purse lips (may indicate facial nerve damage)
7. Inspect and palpate the inner lips and buccal mucosa for colour, moisture, texture, and the presence of lesions. • Apply clean gloves. • Ask the client to relax the mouth, and, for better visualization, pull the lip outward and away from the teeth. • Grasp the lip on each side between the thumb and index finger (see ❶). • Palpate any lesions for size, tenderness, and consistency. • Inspect the front teeth and gums.	Uniform pink colour (freckled brown pigmentation in dark-skinned clients); moist, smooth, soft, glistening, and elastic texture (drier oral mucosa in elderly clients because of decreased salivation)	Pallor; **leukoplakia** (white patches or spots on mucous membranes), red, bleeding; excessive dryness; mucosal cysts; irritations from dentures; abrasions, ulcerations; nodules

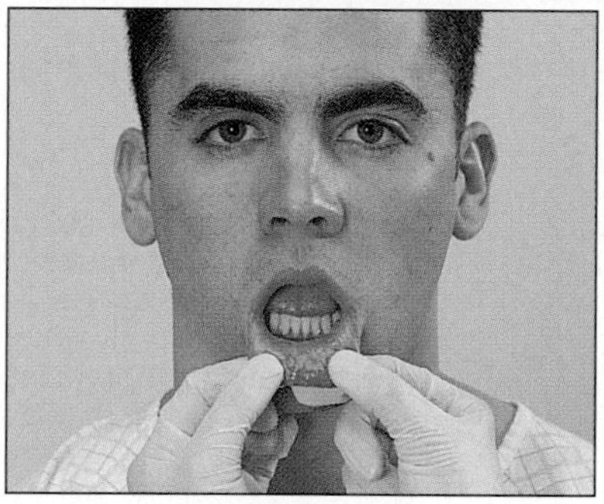

❶ Inspecting the mucosa of the lower lip

ASSESSMENT	NORMAL FINDINGS	DEVIATIONS FROM NORMAL
Teeth and Gums		
8. Inspect the teeth and gums while examining the inner lips and buccal mucosa. • Ask the client to open his or her mouth. Use a tongue depressor to retract the cheek (see ❷). View the surface buccal mucosa from top to bottom and back to front. A flashlight or penlight will help illuminate the surface. Repeat the procedure for the other side. • Ask the client to open his or her mouth again. Use a penlight to assist visualization, and move a finger along the inside cheek. Another finger may be moved outside the cheek. • Examine the back teeth. For proper vision of the molars, use the index fingers of both hands to retract the cheek (see ❸). Ask the client to relax his or her lips and first close, then open the jaw. **Rationale: Closing the jaw assists in observation of tooth alignment and loss of teeth; opening the jaw assists in observation of dental fillings and caries.** • Observe the number of teeth, tooth colour, the state of fillings, dental caries, and tartar along the base of the teeth. Note the presence and fit of partial or complete dentures.	32 adult teeth; smooth, white, shiny tooth enamel; pink gums (bluish or brown patches in dark-skinned clients); moist, firm texture to gums; no retraction of gums (pulling away from the teeth)	Missing teeth; ill-fitting dentures; brown or black discolouration of the enamel (may indicate staining or the presence of caries); excessively red gums; spongy texture; bleeding; tenderness (may indicate periodontal disease); receding, atrophied gums; swelling that partially covers the teeth

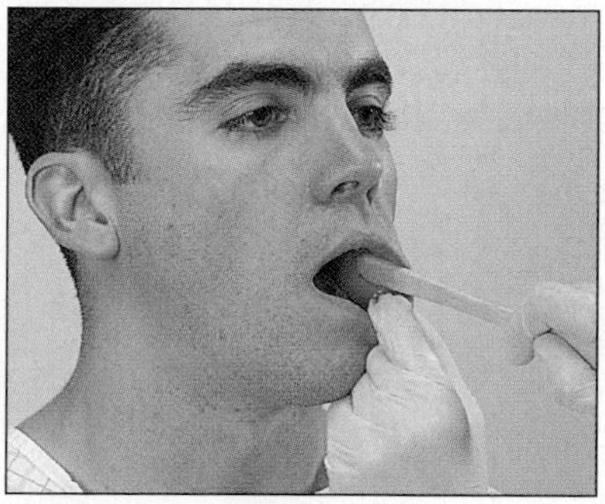

❷ Inspecting the buccal mucosa by using a tongue depressor

(continued)

SKILL 27.9

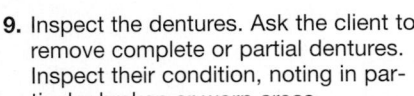

ASSESSING THE MOUTH AND OROPHARYNX (*continued*)

ASSESSMENT	NORMAL FINDINGS	DEVIATIONS FROM NORMAL
Gums • Inspect the gums around the molars. Observe for bleeding, colour, retraction (pulling away from the teeth), edema, and lesions. • Assess the texture of the gums by gently pressing the gum tissue with a tongue depressor.	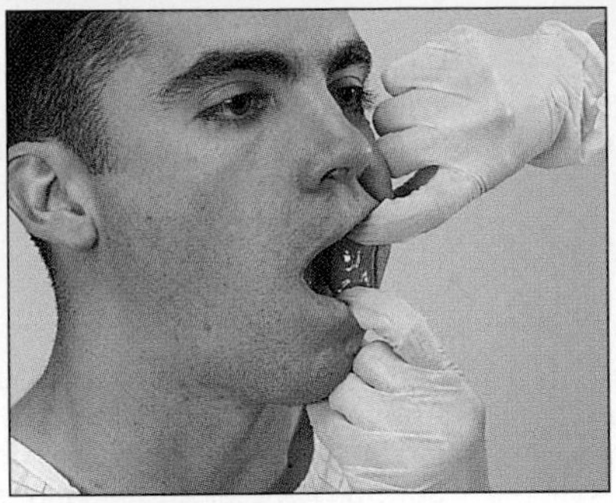	❸ Inspecting the back teeth
9. Inspect the dentures. Ask the client to remove complete or partial dentures. Inspect their condition, noting in particular broken or worn areas.	Smooth, intact dentures	Ill-fitting dentures; irritated and excoriated area under dentures
Tongue/Floor of the Mouth		
10. Inspect the surface of the tongue for position, colour, and texture. Ask the client to protrude the tongue.	Central position; pink colour (some brown pigmentation on tongue borders in dark-skinned clients); moist; slightly rough; thin whitish coating; smooth, lateral margins; no lesions; raised papillae (taste buds)	Deviated from centre, which may indicate damage to the hypoglossal (12th cranial) nerve; excessive trembling; smooth, red tongue (may indicate iron, vitamin B_{12}, or vitamin B_3 deficiency); dry, furry tongue (associated with fluid deficit); white coating (may be oral yeast infection); nodes, ulcerations, discolourations (white or red areas); areas of tenderness
11. Inspect tongue movement. Ask the client to roll the tongue upward and move it from side to side.	Moves freely; no tenderness	Restricted mobility
12. Inspect the base of the tongue, the mouth floor, and the frenulum. Ask the client to place the tip of the tongue against the roof of the mouth.	Smooth tongue base with prominent veins	Swelling, ulceration
13. Palpate the tongue and floor of the mouth for any nodules, lumps, or excoriated areas. To palpate the tongue, use a piece of gauze to grasp its tip (stabilize it), and with the index finger of your other hand, palpate the back of the tongue, its borders, and its base (see ❹). To assess function of the glossopharyngeal and hypoglossal nerves, see the neurological assessment, later in this chapter.	Smooth with no palpable nodules 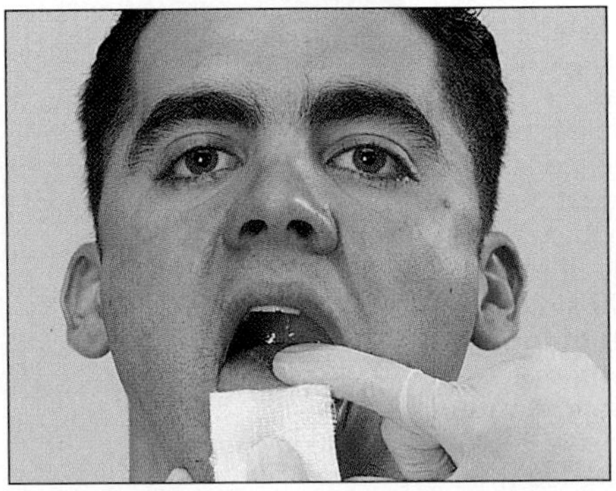 ❹ Palpating the tongue	Swelling, nodules
Salivary Glands		
14. Inspect salivary duct openings for any swelling or redness.	Same as colour of buccal mucosa and floor of mouth	Inflammation (redness and swelling)

(continued)

SKILL 27.9

ASSESSING THE MOUTH AND OROPHARYNX (*continued*)

ASSESSMENT	NORMAL FINDINGS	DEVIATIONS FROM NORMAL
Palates and Uvula		
15. Inspect the hard and soft palate for colour, shape, texture, and the presence of bony prominences. Ask the client to open the mouth wide and tilt his or her head backward. Then, depress the tongue with a tongue blade as necessary, and use a penlight for appropriate visualization.	Light pink, smooth, soft palate; lighter pink hard palate, more irregular texture	Discolouration (e.g., jaundice or pallor); palates the same colour; irritations; exostoses (bony growths) growing from the hard palate
16. Inspect the uvula for position and mobility while examining the palates. To observe the uvula, ask the client to say "ah" so that the soft palate rises.	Positioned in midline of soft palate	Deviation to one side from tumour or trauma; immobility, which may indicate damage to trigeminal (fifth cranial) nerve or vagus (tenth cranial) nerve
Oropharynx and Tonsils		
17. Inspect the oropharynx for colour and texture. Inspect one side at a time to avoid eliciting the gag reflex. To expose one side of the oropharynx, press a tongue blade against the tongue on the same side about halfway back while the client tilts the head back and opens his or her mouth wide. Use a penlight for illumination, if needed.	Pink and smooth posterior wall	Reddened or edematous; presence of lesions, plaques, or drainage
18. Inspect the tonsils (behind the fauces) for colour, discharge, and size.	Pink and smooth; no discharge; of normal size or not visible • *Grade 1 (normal):* The tonsils are behind the tonsillar pillars (the soft structures supporting the soft palate).	Inflamed; presence of discharge; swollen • *Grade 2:* The tonsils are between the pillars and the uvula. • *Grade 3:* The tonsils touch the uvula. • *Grade 4:* One or both tonsils extend to the midline of the oropharynx.
19. Elicit the gag reflex by pressing the posterior tongue with a tongue blade.	Present	Absent, which may indicate problems with glossopharyngeal (ninth cranial) or vagus (tenth cranial) nerves

20. Document findings in the client record by using forms or checklists supplemented by narrative notes when appropriate.

EVALUATION

- Perform a detailed follow-up examination of neurological and other systems based on findings that deviated from expected or normal for the client. Relate findings to previous assessment data if available.
- Report significant deviations from normal to the appropriate members of the health-care team.

Lifespan Considerations

Assessing the Mouth and Oropharynx

INFANTS

- Inspect the palate and uvula for a cleft. A bifid (forked) uvula may indicate an unsuspected cleft palate (i.e., a cleft in the cartilage that is covered by skin).
- Newborns may have a pearly white nodule on their gums, which resolves without treatment.
- The first teeth erupt at about 6 to 7 months of age. Assess for dental hygiene; parents should cleanse the infant's teeth daily with a soft cloth or soft toothbrush.
- Children should see a dentist by 1 year of age.

CHILDREN

- Tooth development should be appropriate for age. See Chapter 29. Permanent teeth are darker than deciduous teeth.
- White spots on teeth may indicate excessive fluoride ingestion.
- Drooling is normal up to 2 years of age.
- The tonsils are normally larger in children than in adults and usually extend beyond the palatine arch until the age of 11 or 12 years.
- Inspect the palate for a cleft.

OLDER ADULTS

- The oral mucosa may be drier than that of younger persons because of decreased salivary gland activity. Decreased salivation occurs in older adults who are taking prescribed medications, such as antidepressants, antihistamines, decongestants, diuretics, antihypertensives, tranquilizers, antispasmodics, and antineoplastics. Extreme dryness is associated with dehydration.
- Some receding of the gums occurs, giving an appearance of increased toothiness.
- There may be a brownish pigmentation to the gums, especially in Black persons.
- Taste sensations diminish. Diminished taste sensation is due to atrophy of the taste buds and a decreased sense of smell. It indicates diminished function of the fifth and seventh cranial nerves.
- Tiny purple or bluish-black swollen areas (varicosities) under the tongue, known as caviar spots, are not uncommon.
- The teeth may show signs of staining, erosion, chipping, and abrasions because of loss of dentin. Tooth loss occurs as a result of gum disease but is preventable with good dental hygiene.
- Older adults who are homebound or are in long-term-care facilities often have teeth or dentures in need of repair because of the difficulty of obtaining dental care in these situations. Do a thorough assessment of missing teeth and those in need of repair, whether they are natural teeth or dentures.

The Neck

Examination of the neck includes the muscles, lymph nodes, trachea, thyroid gland, carotid arteries, and jugular veins. Areas of the neck are defined by the sternocleidomastoid muscles, which divide each side of the neck into two triangles: the anterior and posterior (Figure 27.18). The trachea, thyroid gland, anterior cervical nodes, and carotid artery lie within the anterior triangle (Figure 27.19); the carotid artery runs parallel and anterior to the sternocleidomastoid muscle. The posterior lymph nodes lie within the posterior triangle (Figure 27.20).

Each sternocleidomastoid muscle extends from the upper sternum and the medial third of the clavicle to the mastoid process of the temporal bone behind the ear. These muscles turn and laterally flex the head. Each trapezius muscle extends from the occipital bone of the skull to the lateral third of the clavicle. These muscles draw the head to the side and back, elevate the chin, and elevate the shoulders to shrug them.

Lymph nodes in the neck that collect lymph from the head and neck structures are grouped serially and referred to as *chains*. See Figure 27.20 and Table 27.6.

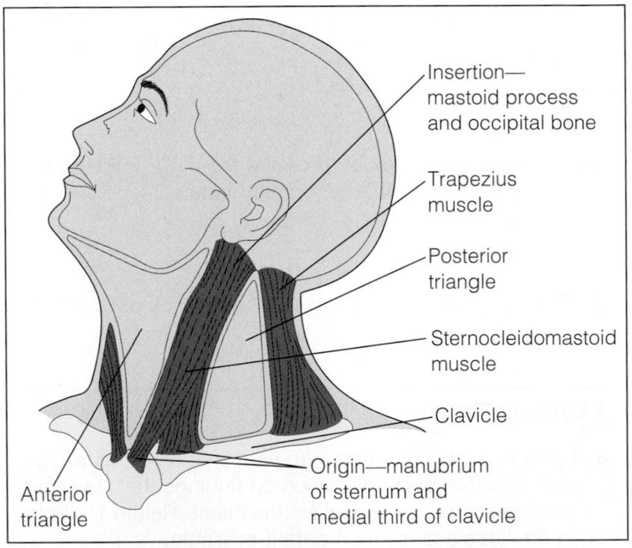

FIGURE 27.18 Major muscles of the neck

The deep cervical chain is not shown in Figure 27.20 because it lies beneath the sternocleidomastoid muscle.

Skill 27.10 describes how to assess the neck.

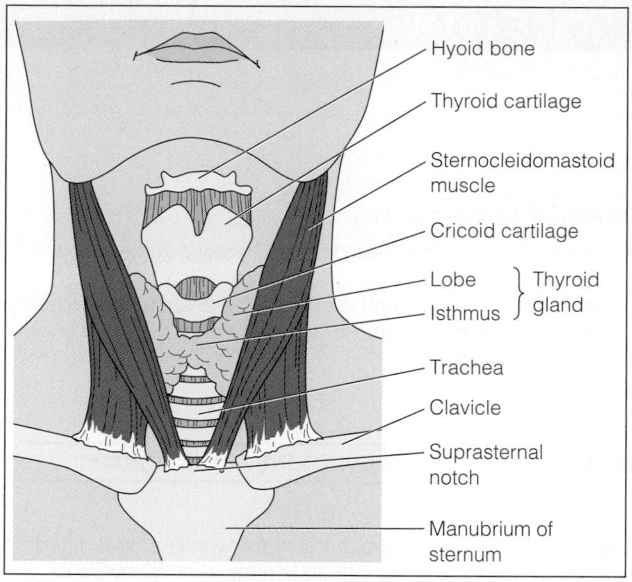

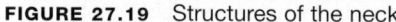

FIGURE 27.19 Structures of the neck

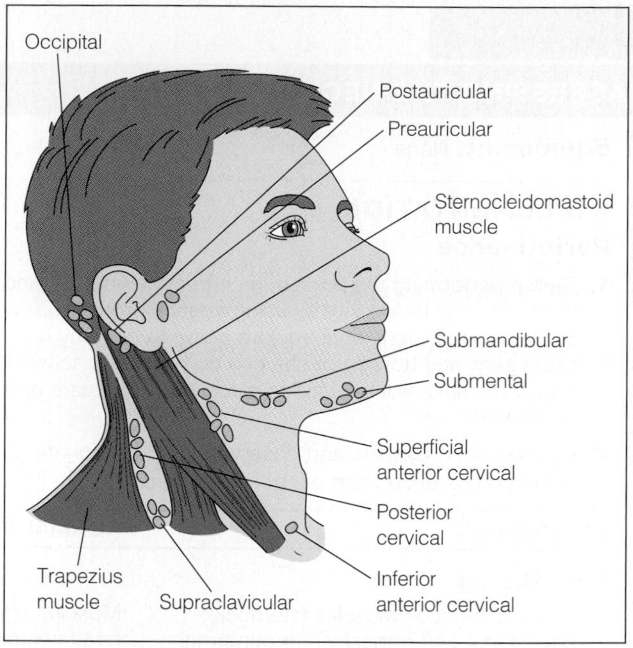

FIGURE 27.20 Lymph nodes of the neck

TABLE 27.6 Lymph Nodes of the Head and Neck

Node Centre	Location	Area Drained
Head		
Occipital	At the posterior base of the skull	The occipital region of the scalp and the deep structures of the back of the neck
Postauricular (mastoid)	Behind the auricle of the ear or in front of the mastoid process	The parietal region of the head and part of the ear
Preauricular	In front of the tragus of the ear	The forehead and upper face
Floor of Mouth		
Submandibular (submaxillary)	Along the medial border of the lower jaw, halfway between the angle of the jaw and the chin	The chin, upper lip, cheek, nose, teeth, eyelids, part of the tongue, and part of the floor of the mouth
Submental	Behind the tip of the mandible, in the midline, under the chin	The anterior third of the tongue, gums, and floor of the mouth
Neck		
Superficial (anterior) cervical chain	Along the anterior to the sternocleidomastoid muscle	The skin and neck
Posterior cervical chain	Along the anterior aspect of the trapezius muscle	The posterior and lateral regions of the neck, occiput, and mastoid
Deep cervical chain	Under the sternocleidomastoid muscle	The larynx, thyroid gland, trachea, and upper part of the esophagus
Supraclavicular	Above the clavicle, in the angle between the clavicle and the sternocleidomastoid muscle	The lateral regions of the neck and lungs

SKILL 27.10

ASSESSING THE NECK

Equipment: None

IMPLEMENTATION

Performance

1. Before performing the procedure, introduce yourself and verify the client's identity by using agency protocol. Explain to the client what you are going to do, why it is necessary, and how he or she can cooperate. Discuss how the results will be used in planning further care or treatments.
2. Perform hand hygiene and observe other appropriate infection prevention and control procedures.
3. Provide for client privacy.
4. Inquire whether the client has any history of the following: problems with neck lumps; neck pain or stiffness; when and how any lumps occurred; previous diagnoses of thyroid problems; and other treatments provided (e.g., surgery, radiation).

ASSESSMENT	NORMAL FINDINGS	DEVIATIONS FROM NORMAL
Neck Muscles		
5. Inspect the neck muscles (sternocleidomastoid and trapezius) for abnormal swellings or masses. Ask the client to hold the head erect.	Muscles equal in size; head centred	Unilateral neck swelling; head tilted to one side (indicates presence of masses, injury, muscle weakness, shortening of sternocleidomastoid muscle, scars)
6. Observe head movement. Ask client to	Coordinated, smooth movements with no discomfort	Muscle tremor, spasm, or stiffness
• Move the chin to the chest. **Rationale: This determines function of the sternocleidomastoid muscle.**	Head flexes 45°	Limited range of motion; painful movements; involuntary movements (e.g., up-and-down nodding movements associated with Parkinson's disease)
• Move the head back so that the chin points upward. **Rationale: This determines function of the trapezius muscle.**	Head hyperextends 60°	Head hyperextends less than 60°
• Move the head so that the ear is moved toward the shoulder on each side. **Rationale: This determines function of the sternocleidomastoid muscle.**	Head laterally flexes 40°	Head laterally flexes less than 40°
• Turn the head to the right and to the left. **Rationale: This determines function of the sternocleidomastoid muscle.**	Head laterally rotates 70°	Head laterally rotates less than 70°
7. Assess muscle strength. Ask the client to turn the head to one side against the resistance of your hand. Repeat with the other side. **Rationale: This determines the strength of the sternocleidomastoid muscle.**	Equal strength	Unequal strength
• Ask the client to shrug the shoulders against the resistance of your hands. **Rationale: This determines the strength of the trapezius muscles.**	Equal strength	Unequal strength
Lymph Nodes		
8. Palpate the entire neck for enlarged lymph nodes.	Not palpable	Enlarged, palpable, possibly tender (associated with infection and tumours)
• Face the client, and bend the client's head forward slightly or toward the side being examined. **Rationale: This relaxes the soft tissue and muscles.**		

(continued)

SKILL 27.10

ASSESSING THE NECK (*continued*)

ASSESSMENT	NORMAL FINDINGS	DEVIATIONS FROM NORMAL
• Palpate the nodes by using the pads of the fingers. Move the fingertips in a gentle rotating motion.		
• When examining the submental and submandibular nodes, place the fingertips under the mandible on the side nearest the palpating hand, and pull the skin and subcutaneous tissue laterally over the mandibular surface so that the tissue rolls over the nodes.		
• When palpating the supraclavicular nodes, have the client bend the head forward to relax the tissues of the anterior neck and to relax the shoulders so that the clavicles drop. Use your hand nearest the side to be examined when facing the client (i.e., your left hand for the client's right nodes). Use your free hand to flex the client's head forward if necessary. Hook your index and third fingers over the clavicle lateral to the sternocleidomastoid muscle (see ❶).		
• When palpating the anterior cervical nodes and posterior cervical nodes, move your fingertips slowly in a forward circular motion against the sternocleidomastoid and trapezius muscles, respectively.		
• To palpate the deep cervical nodes, bend or hook your fingers around the sternocleidomastoid muscle.		

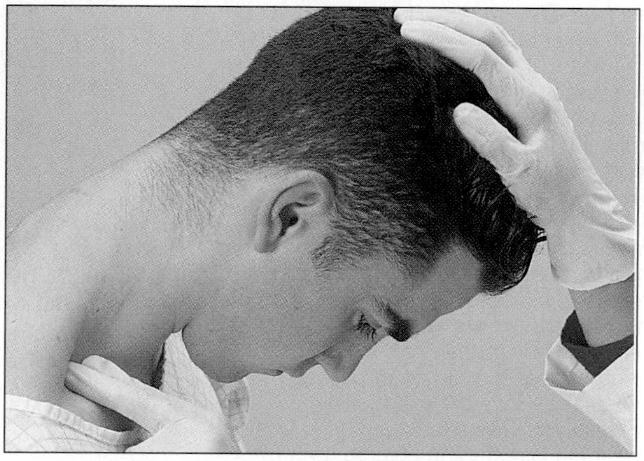

❶ Palpating the supraclavicular lymph nodes

ASSESSMENT	NORMAL FINDINGS	DEVIATIONS FROM NORMAL
Trachea		
9. Palpate the trachea for lateral deviation. Place your fingertip or thumb on the trachea in the suprasternal notch (see Figure 27.19, p. 595), and then move your finger laterally to the left and the right in spaces bordered by the clavicle, the anterior aspect of the sternocleidomastoid muscle, and the trachea.	Central placement in midline of neck; spaces equal on both sides	Deviation to one side, indicating possible neck tumour; thyroid enlargement; enlarged lymph nodes
Thyroid Gland		
10. Inspect the thyroid gland. Stand in front of the client. Observe the lower half of the neck overlying the thyroid gland for symmetry and visible masses.	Not visible on inspection	Visible diffuseness or local enlargement
• Ask the client to hyperextend the head and swallow. If necessary, offer a glass of water to make it easier for the client to swallow. **Rationale: This action determines how the thyroid and cricoid cartilages move and whether swallowing causes a bulging of the gland.**	Gland ascends during swallowing but is not visible	Gland is not fully moveable with swallowing

(*continued*)

SKILL 27.10

ASSESSING THE NECK (*continued*)

ASSESSMENT	NORMAL FINDINGS	DEVIATIONS FROM NORMAL
11. Palpate the thyroid gland for smoothness. Note any areas of enlargement, masses, or nodules. Stand in front of or behind the client, and ask the client to lower the chin slightly. **Rationale: Lowering the chin relaxes the neck muscles, facilitating palpation.**	Lobes may not be palpated; if palpated, lobes are small, smooth, centrally located, painless, and rise freely with swallowing	Solitary nodules

Posterior Approach

- Place your hands around the client's neck, with your fingertips on the lower half of the neck over the trachea (see ❷).
- Ask the client to swallow (taking a sip of water, if necessary). Feel for any enlargement of the thyroid isthmus as it rises. The isthmus lies across the trachea, below the cricoid cartilage. See Figure 27.19 (p. 595).
- To examine the right thyroid lobe, have the client lower the chin slightly and turn the head slightly to the right (the side being examined). With your left fingers, displace the trachea slightly to the right. With your right fingers, palpate the right thyroid lobe. Have the client swallow while you are palpating.
- Repeat the last step, in reverse, to examine the left thyroid lobe.

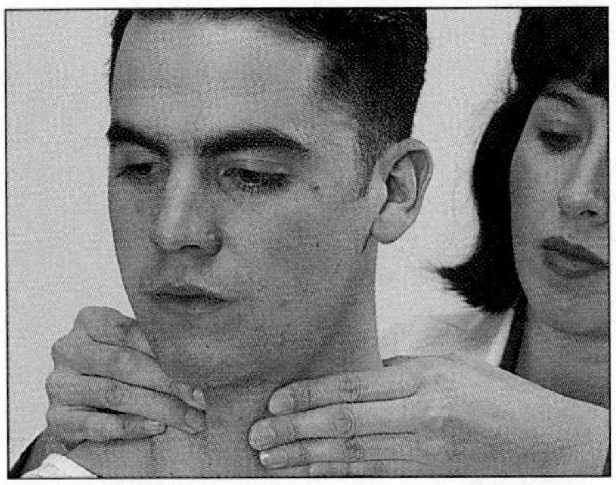

❷ Placement of the fingertips over the trachea to begin palpation of the thyroid gland (posterior approach)

Anterior Approach

- Place the tips of your index and middle fingers over the trachea, and palpate the thyroid isthmus as the client swallows.
- To examine the right thyroid lobe, have the client lower the chin slightly and turn the head slightly to the right. With your right fingers, displace the trachea slightly to the client's right (your left). With your left fingers, palpate the right thyroid lobe (see ❸).
- To examine the left thyroid lobe, repeat the above step in reverse.

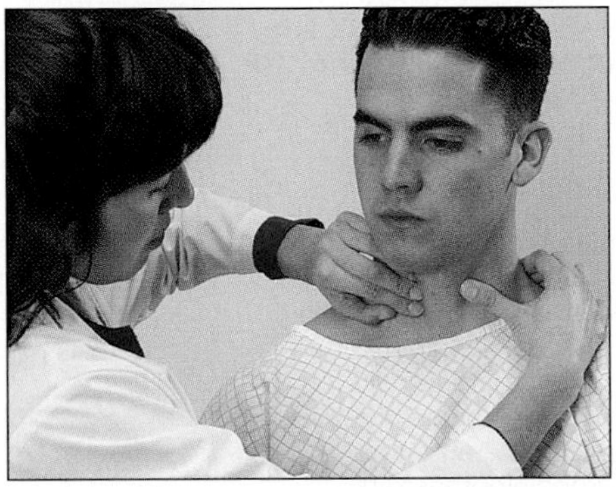

❸ Palpating the thyroid (anterior approach)

ASSESSMENT	NORMAL FINDINGS	DEVIATIONS FROM NORMAL
12. If enlargement of the gland is suspected, auscultate over the thyroid area for a bruit (a soft rushing sound created by turbulent blood flow). Use the bell of the stethoscope because it transmits this low frequency sound better than the diaphragm does.	Absence of bruit	Presence of bruit

(*continued*)

SKILL 27.10

ASSESSING THE NECK *(continued)*

13. Document findings in the client record by using forms or checklists supplemented by narrative notes when appropriate.

EVALUATION

- Perform a detailed follow-up examination of other systems based on findings that deviated from expected or normal for the client.
- Report significant deviations from normal to the appropriate members of the health-care team.

Lifespan Consideration

Assessing the Neck

INFANTS AND CHILDREN

- Examine the neck while the infant or child is lying supine. Lift the head and turn it from side to side to determine neck mobility.
- An infant's neck is normally short, lengthening by about age 3 years. This lack of length makes palpation of the trachea difficult.

Thorax and Lungs

Assessing the thorax and lungs is important in assessing the client's aeration status. Changes in the respiratory system can occur slowly or quickly. In clients with asthma or chronic obstructive pulmonary disease (COPD), such as chronic bronchitis and emphysema (a chronic pulmonary condition in which the air sacs, or alveoli, are dilated and distended), changes are frequently gradual. The onset of such conditions as pneumonia or pulmonary embolus (a blockage of an artery in the lungs by fat, air, tumour tissue, or a blood clot) is generally more acute or sudden.

Chest Landmarks

Before beginning the assessment, the nurse must be familiar with a series of imaginary lines on the chest wall and be able to locate the position of each rib and some spinous processes. These landmarks help the nurse to identify the position of underlying organs (e.g., lobes of the lung) and to record abnormal assessment findings. Figure 27.21 shows the anterior, lateral, and posterior series of lines. The *midsternal line* is a vertical line running through the centre of the sternum. The *midclavicular lines* (right and left) are vertical lines from the midpoints of the clavicles. The *anterior axillary lines* (right and left) are vertical lines from the anterior axillary folds (Figure 27.21A). Figure 27.21B shows the three imaginary lines of the lateral chest. The *posterior axillary line* is a vertical line from the posterior axillary fold. The *midaxillary line* is a vertical line from the apex of the axilla. The anterior axillary line is as described for part A. Figure 27.21C shows the posterior chest landmarks. The *vertebral line* is a vertical line along the spinous processes. The *scapular lines* (right and left) are vertical lines from the inferior angles of the scapulae.

Locating the position of each rib and certain spinous processes is essential for identifying underlying lobes of the lung. Figure 27.22A shows an anterior view of the chest and underlying lungs; Figure 27.22B, a posterior view; and Figure 27.22C, right and left lateral views. Each lung is first divided into the upper and lower lobes by an oblique fissure that runs from the level of the spinous process of the third thoracic vertebra (T-3) to the level of the sixth rib at the midclavicular line (MCL). The right upper lobe is abbreviated RUL; the right lower lobe, RLL. Similarly, the left upper lobe is abbreviated LUL; the left lower lobe, LLL. The right lung is further divided by a minor fissure into the right upper lobe and right middle lobe (RML). This fissure runs anteriorly from the right midaxillary line at the level of the fifth rib to the level of the fourth rib.

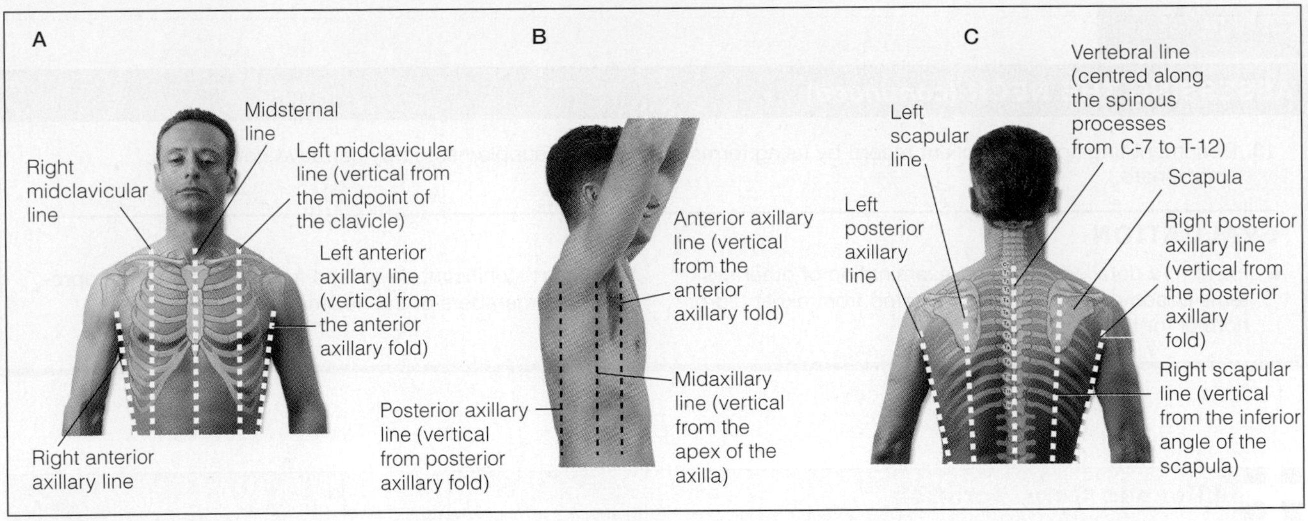

FIGURE 27.21 Chest wall landmarks: **A:** anterior chest; **B:** lateral chest; **C:** posterior chest

These specific landmarks, that is, T-3 and the fourth, fifth, and sixth ribs, are located as follows. The starting point for locating the ribs anteriorly is the **angle of Louis**, the junction between the body of the **sternum** (breastbone) and the **manubrium** (the handlelike superior part of the sternum that joins with the clavicles). The superior border of the second rib attaches to the sternum at this manubriosternal junction (Figure 27.23). The nurse can identify the manubrium by first palpating the clavicle and following its course to its attachment at the manubrium. The nurse then palpates and counts distal ribs and intercostal spaces from the second rib. It is important to note that an intercostal space is numbered according to the number of the rib immediately *above* the space. When palpating for rib identification, the nurse should palpate along the midclavicular line rather than the sternal border because the rib cartilages are very close at the sternum. Only the first seven ribs attach directly to the sternum.

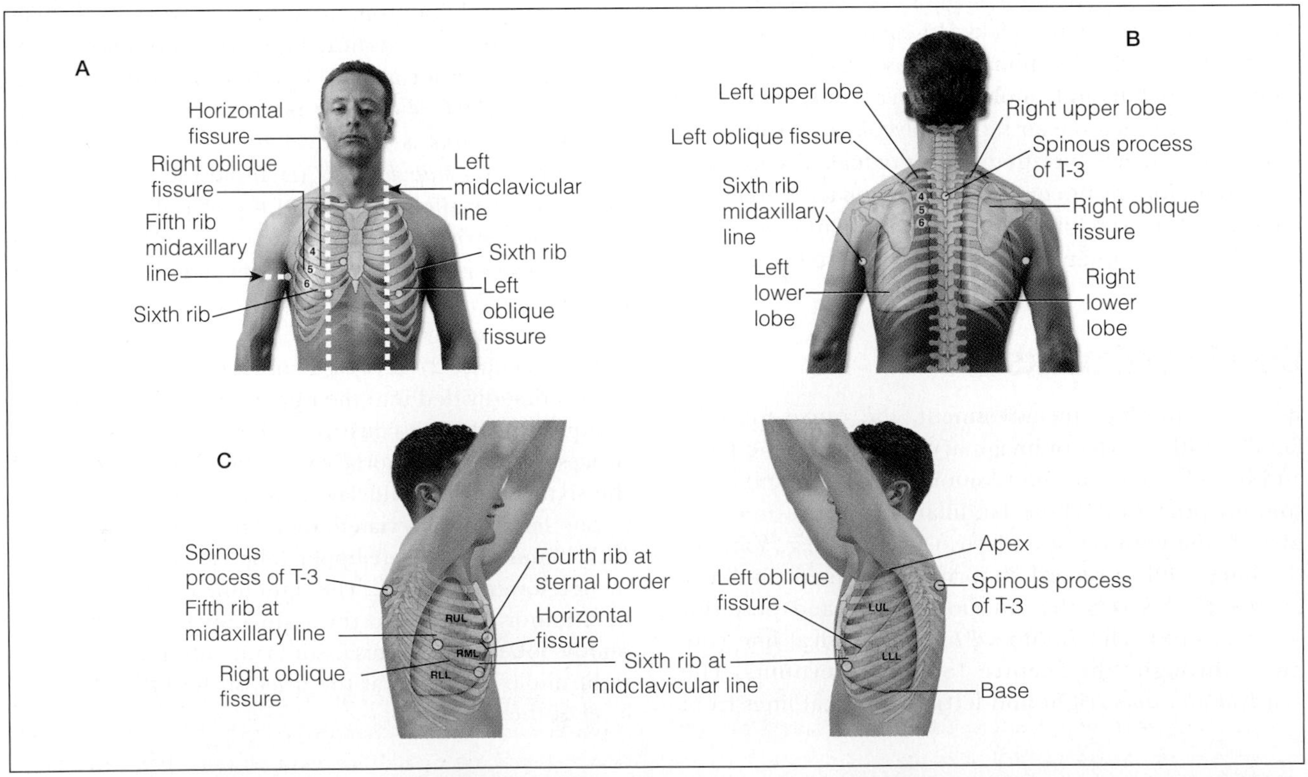

FIGURE 27.22 Chest landmarks: **A:** anterior chest landmarks and underlying lungs; **B:** posterior chest landmarks and underlying lungs; **C:** lateral chest landmarks and underlying lungs

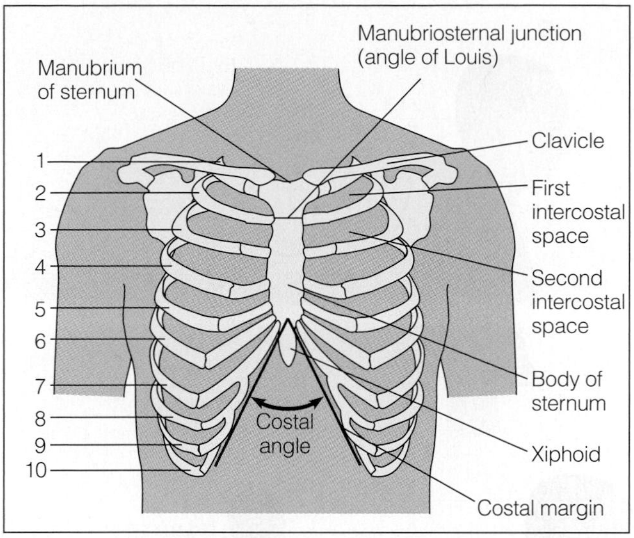

FIGURE 27.23 Location of the anterior ribs in relation to the angle of Louis and the sternum

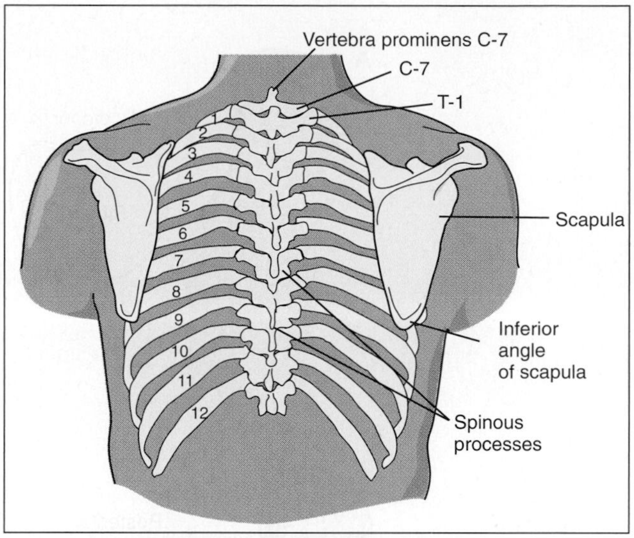

FIGURE 27.24 Location of the posterior ribs in relation to the spinous processes

The counting of ribs is more difficult on the posterior than on the anterior thorax. For identifying underlying lung lobes, the pertinent landmark is T-3. The starting point for locating T-3 is the spinous process of the seventh cervical vertebra (C-7) (Figure 27.24). When the client flexes the neck anteriorly, a prominent process can be observed and palpated. This is the spinous process of the seventh cervical vertebra. If two spinous processes are observed, the superior one is C-7, and the inferior one is the spinous process of the first thoracic vertebra (T-1). The nurse then palpates and counts the spinous processes from C-7 to T-3. Each spinous process up to T-4 is adjacent to the corresponding rib number; e.g., T-3 is adjacent to the third rib. After T-4, however, the spinous processes project obliquely, causing the spinous process of the vertebra to lie not over its correspondingly numbered rib, but over the rib below. Thus, the spinous process of T-5 lies over the body of T-6 and is adjacent to the sixth rib.

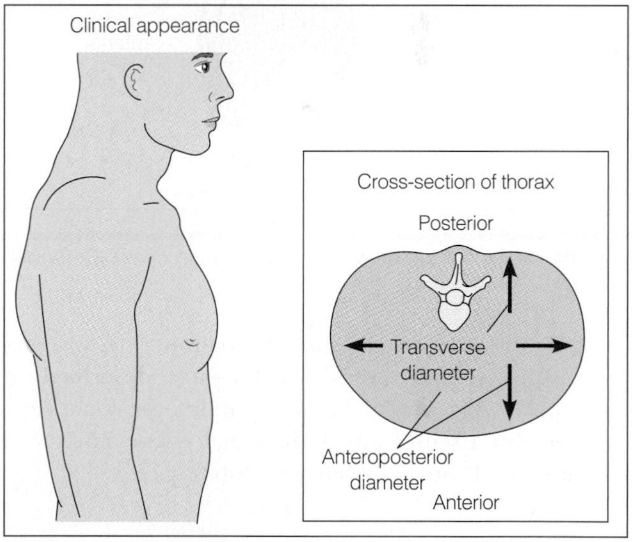

FIGURE 27.25 Configurations of the thorax showing anteroposterior diameter and transverse diameter

Chest Shape and Size

In adults, the thorax is oval. Its anteroposterior diameter is half its transverse diameter (Figure 27.25). The overall shape of the thorax is elliptical; that is, its diameter is smaller at the top than at the base. In older adults, kyphosis and osteoporosis alter the size of the chest cavity as the ribs move downward and forward.

The chest can acquire several deformities (Figure 27.26). *Pectus carinatum* (pigeon chest), a permanent deformity, can be caused by rickets. A narrow transverse diameter, an increased anteroposterior diameter, and a protruding sternum characterize pigeon chest. *Pectus excavatum* (a funnel chest), a congenital defect, is the opposite of pigeon chest in that the sternum is depressed, narrowing the anteroposterior diameter. Because the sternum points posteriorly in clients with a funnel chest, abnormal pressure on the heart can result in altered function. A barrel chest, in which the ratio of the anteroposterior to transverse diameter is 1 to 1, is seen in clients with thoracic kyphosis (excessive convex curvature of the thoracic spine) and emphysema. Scoliosis is a lateral deviation of the spine.

Breath Sounds

Abnormal breath sounds, called **adventitious breath sounds**, occur when air passes through narrowed airways or airways filled with fluid or mucus, or when pleural linings are inflamed. Table 27.7 describes normal breath sounds. Adventitious sounds are often superimposed over normal sounds. The main types of adventitious

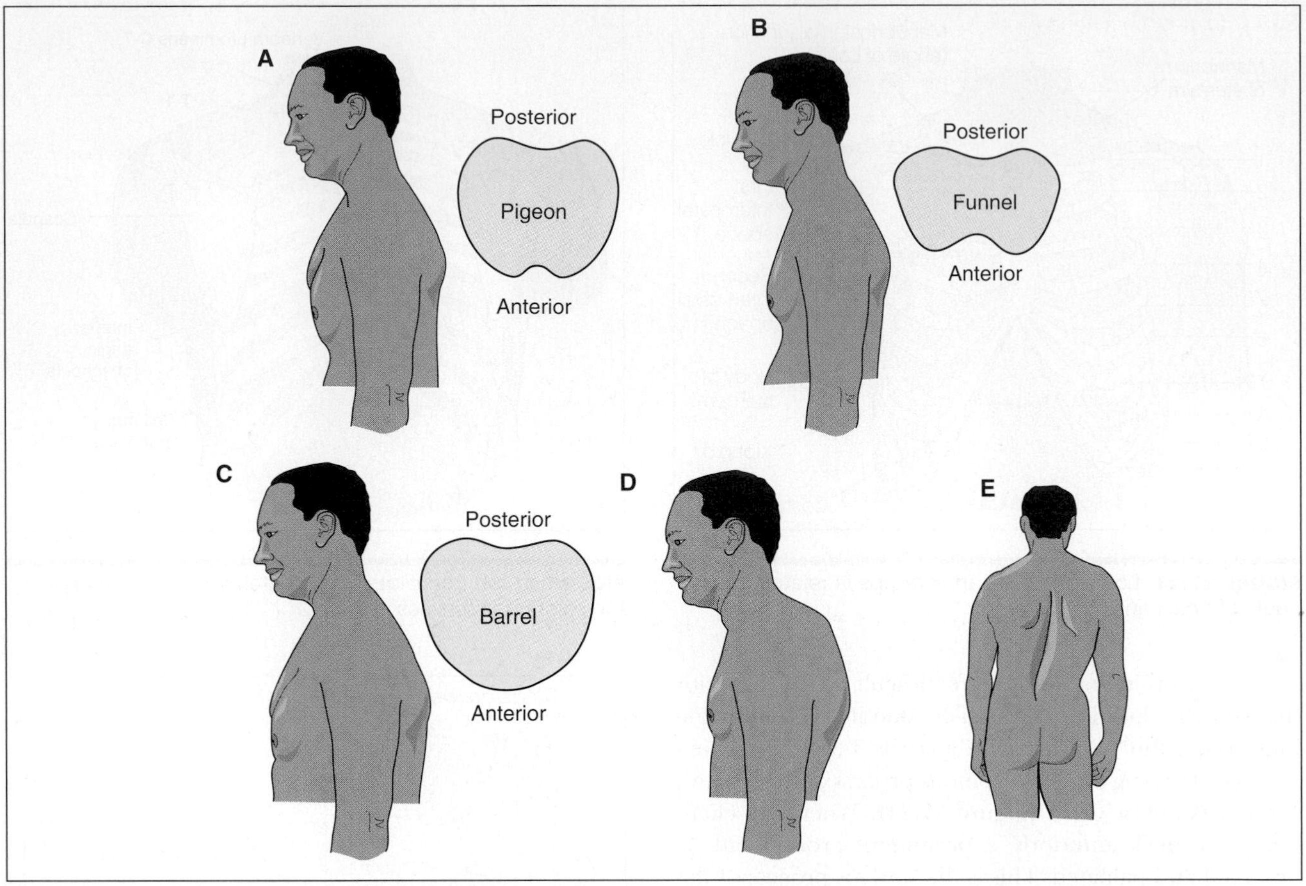

FIGURE 27.26 Chest deformities: **A:** pigeon chest; **B:** funnel chest; **C:** barrel chest; **D:** kyphosis; **E:** scoliosis

sounds—crackles (fine, coarse), friction rub, wheezes (sonorous, sibilant), and stridor—are described in Table 27.8. Absence of breath sounds over some lung areas is also a significant finding that is associated with collapsed and surgically removed lobes.

Assessment of the lungs and thorax includes all methods of examination: inspection, palpation, percussion, and auscultation. Skill 27.11 describes how to assess the thorax and lungs.

TABLE 27.7 Normal Breath Sounds

Type	Description	Location	Characteristics
Vesicular	Soft-intensity, low-pitched, "gentle sighing" sounds created by air moving through smaller airways (bronchioles and alveoli)	Over peripheral lung; best heard at base of lungs	Best heard on inspiration, which is about 2.5 times longer than the expiratory phase (5:2 ratio)
Bronchovesicular	Moderate-intensity and moderate-pitched "blowing" sounds created by air moving through larger airways (bronchi)	Between the scapulae and lateral to the sternum at the first and second intercostal spaces	Equal inspiratory and expiratory phases (1:1 ratio)
Bronchial (tubular)	High-pitched, loud, "harsh" sounds created by air moving through the trachea	Anteriorly over the trachea; not normally heard over lung tissue	Louder than vesicular sounds; have a short inspiratory phase and long expiratory phase (1:2 ratio)

TABLE 27.8 Adventitious Breath Sounds

Name	Description	Cause	Location
Fine crackles (formerly referred to as rales)	Dry, high-pitched, discontinuous crackling, popping. Sound can be simulated by rolling a lock of hair near the ear. Predominantly heard on inspiration but can be heard on both inspiration and expiration. May not be cleared by coughing.	Air passing through moisture (fluid or mucus) in small airways that suddenly reinflate	Most commonly heard in the bases of the lower lung lobes
Coarse crackles	Discontinuous, moist, low-pitched crackling, gurgling. Predominantly heard on inspiration but can be heard on both inspiration and expiration. May be altered by coughing.	Air passing through moisture (fluid or mucus) in large airways that suddenly reinflate	Loud sounds can be heard over most lung areas but predominate over the trachea and bronchi
Friction rub	Superficial grating or creaking sounds heard during inspiration and expiration. Not relieved by coughing.	Rubbing together of inflamed pleural surfaces	Heard most often in areas of greatest thoracic expansion (e.g., lower anterior and lateral chest)
Sonorous wheeze (formerly referred to as rhonchi)	Continuous, low-pitched snoring sound. Best heard on expiration. May be cleared by coughing.	Air passing through narrowing of large airways or obstruction of the bronchus	Heard over all lung fields
Sibilant wheeze	Continuous, high-pitched, musical sounds. Best heard on expiration. Not usually altered by coughing.	Air passing through narrowing of large airways or obstruction of the bronchus	Heard over all lung fields
Stridor	Continuous crowing sound, high pitched. Predominantly heard on inspiration.	Partial obstruction of larynx or trachea	Louder in neck than over chest wall

SKILL 27.11

ASSESSING THE THORAX AND LUNGS

PLANNING

For efficiency, the nurse usually examines the posterior chest first, then the anterior chest. For posterior and lateral chest examinations, the client is uncovered to the waist and in a sitting position. A sitting or lying position can be used for anterior chest examination. The sitting position is preferred because it maximizes chest expansion. Good lighting is essential, especially for chest inspection.

Equipment

- Stethoscope
- Skin marker or pencil
- Centimetre ruler

IMPLEMENTATION

Performance

1. Before performing the procedure, introduce yourself and verify the client's identity by using agency protocol. Explain to the client what you are going to do, why it is necessary, and how he or she can cooperate. Discuss how the results will be used in planning further care or treatments.
2. Perform hand hygiene and observe other appropriate infection prevention and control procedures.
3. Provide for client privacy. In women, drape the anterior chest when it is not being examined.
4. Inquire whether the client has any history of the following: family history of illness, including cancer, allergies, tuberculosis; lifestyle habits, such as smoking and occupational hazards (e.g., inhaling fumes); medications being taken; current problems (e.g., swellings, coughs, wheezing, pain).

(continued)

SKILL 27.11

ASSESSING THE THORAX AND LUNGS (*continued*)

ASSESSMENT	NORMAL FINDINGS	DEVIATIONS FROM NORMAL
Posterior Thorax		
5. Inspect the shape and symmetry of the thorax from the posterior and lateral views. Compare the anteroposterior diameter to the transverse diameter.	Anteroposterior to transverse diameter in ratio of 1:2; chest symmetric	Barrel chest; increased anteroposterior to transverse diameter; chest asymmetric
6. Inspect the spinal alignment for deformities. Have the client stand. From a lateral position, observe the three normal curvatures: cervical, thoracic, and lumbar.	Spine vertically aligned	Exaggerated spinal curvatures (kyphosis, lordosis)
• To assess for scoliosis, stand behind the client and have him or her stand. Observe the spinal alignment. Have the client bend forward at the waist and then observe the alignment again.	Spinal column is straight, right and left shoulders and hips are at same height.	Spinal column deviates to one side, often accentuated when bending over; shoulders or hips are not even
7. Palpate the posterior thorax.		
• For clients who have no respiratory complaints, rapidly assess the temperature and integrity of all chest skin.	Skin intact; uniform temperature	Skin lesions; areas of hyperthermia
• For clients who do have respiratory complaints, palpate all chest areas for bulges, tenderness, or abnormal movements. Avoid deep palpation for painful areas, especially if a fractured rib is suspected. In such a case, deep palpation could lead to displacement of the bone fragment against the lungs.	Chest wall intact; no tenderness; no masses	Lumps, bulges; depressions; areas of tenderness; moveable structures (e.g., rib)
8. Palpate the posterior chest for respiratory excursion (thoracic expansion). Place the palms of both your hands over the lower thorax with your thumbs adjacent to the spine and your fingers stretched laterally (see ❶). Ask the client to take a deep breath while you observe the movement of your hands and any lag in movement.	Full and symmetric chest expansion (i.e., when the client takes a deep breath, your thumbs should move apart an equal distance and at the same time; normally the thumbs separate 3 cm to 5 cm during deep inspiration)	Asymmetric or decreased chest expansion

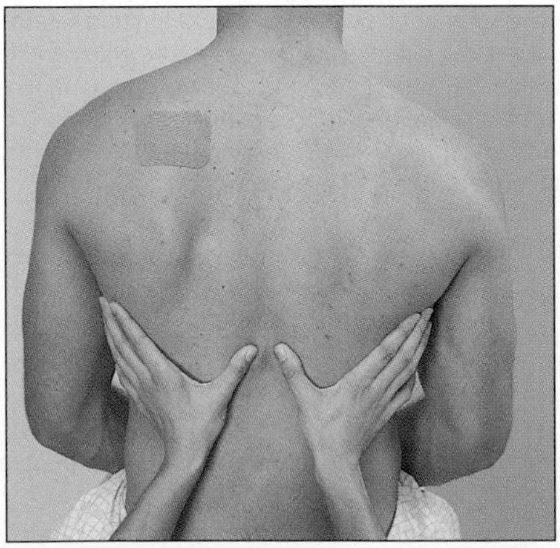

❶ Position of the nurse's hands when assessing respiratory excursion on the posterior thorax

(continued)

SKILL 27.11

ASSESSING THE THORAX AND LUNGS (*continued*)

ASSESSMENT	NORMAL FINDINGS	DEVIATIONS FROM NORMAL
9. Palpate the chest for vocal (tactile) fremitus, the faintly perceptible vibration felt through the chest wall when the client speaks. • Place the palmar surfaces of your fingertips or the ulnar aspect of your hand or closed fist on the posterior chest, starting near the apex of the lungs (see ❷, position A). • Ask the client to repeat such words as "blue moon" or "one, two, three." • Repeat the two steps, moving your hands sequentially to the base of the lungs, through positions B to E in ❷. • Compare the fremitus on both lungs and between the apex and the base of each lung, using either one hand and moving it from one side of the client to the corresponding area on the other side *or* using two hands that are placed simultaneously on the corresponding areas of each side of the chest.	Bilateral symmetry of vocal fremitus; fremitus is heard most clearly at the apex of the lungs Low-pitched voices of males are more readily palpated than higher-pitched voices of females	Decreased or absent fremitus (associated with pneumothorax); increased fremitus (associated with consolidated lung tissue, as in pneumonia)

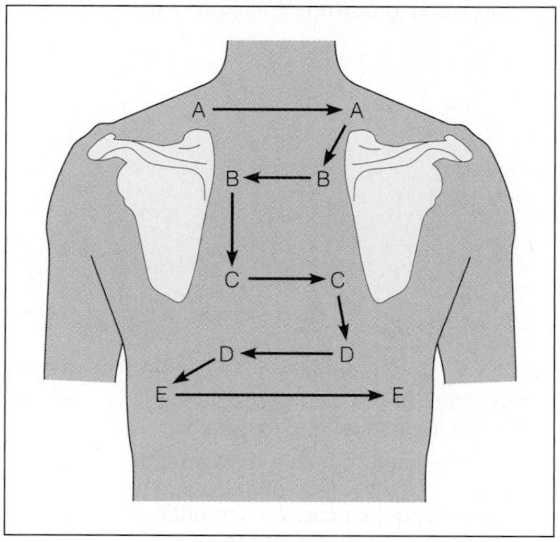

❷ Areas and sequence for palpating tactile fremitus on the posterior chest

ASSESSMENT	NORMAL FINDINGS	DEVIATIONS FROM NORMAL
10. Percuss the thorax. Percussion of the thorax is performed to determine whether underlying lung tissue is filled with air, liquid, or solid material and to determine the positions and boundaries of certain organs. Because percussion penetrates to a depth of 5 cm to 7 cm, it detects superficial rather than deep lesions. Percussion sounds and tones are described in Table 27.4 (p. 560). Normal percussion sounds in the posterior chest are shown in ❸. • Ask the client to bend the head and fold the arms forward across the chest. **Rationale: This separates the scapula and exposes more lung tissue to percussion.**	Percussion notes resonate, except over scapula; lowest point of resonance is at the diaphragm (i.e., at the level of the 8th to 10th rib posteriorly); *note:* percussion on a rib normally elicits dullness	Asymmetry in percussion; areas of dullness or flatness over lung tissue (associated with consolidation of lung tissue or a mass)

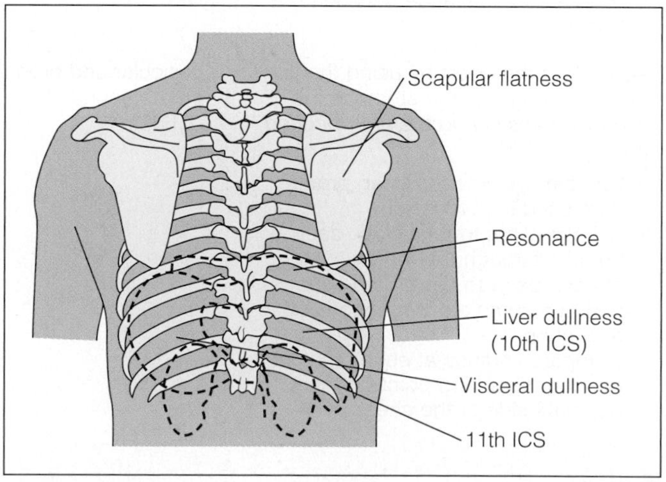

❸ Normal percussion sounds in the posterior chest

(continued)

SKILL 27.11

ASSESSING THE THORAX AND LUNGS (*continued*)

ASSESSMENT	NORMAL FINDINGS	DEVIATIONS FROM NORMAL
• Percuss in the intercostal spaces at about 5 cm intervals in a systematic sequence (see ❹). • Compare one side of the lung with the other. • Percuss the lateral thorax every few centimetres, starting at the axilla and working down to the eighth rib.		

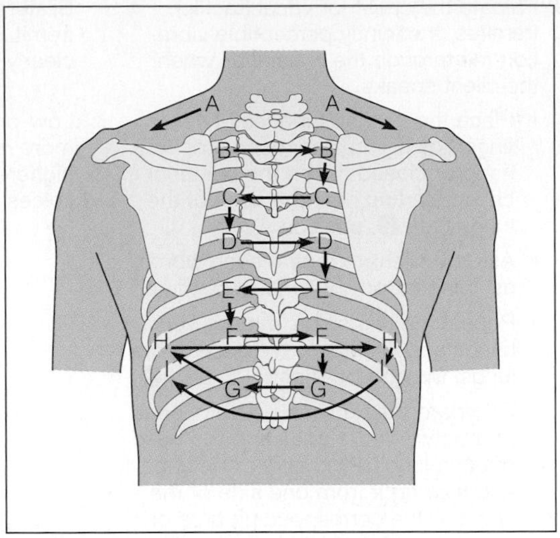

❹ Sequence for posterior chest percussion

ASSESSMENT	NORMAL FINDINGS	DEVIATIONS FROM NORMAL
11. Percuss for diaphragmatic excursion (movement of the diaphragm during maximal inspiration and expiration). • Ask the client to take a deep breath and hold it while you percuss downward along the scapular line until dullness is produced at the level of the diaphragm. Mark this point with a marking pencil, and repeat the procedure on the other side of the chest. • Ask the client to take a few normal breaths and then expel the last breath completely and hold it while you percuss upward from the marked point to assess and mark the diaphragmatic excursion during deep expiration on each side. • Measure the distance between the two marks.	Excursion is 3 cm to 5 cm bilaterally in women and 5 cm to 6 cm in men; diaphragm is usually slightly higher on the right side	Restricted excursion (associated with lung disorder)
12. Auscultate the chest by using the flat-disc diaphragm of the stethoscope (*best for transmitting the high-pitched breath sounds*). • Use the systematic zigzag procedure used in percussion. • Ask the client to take slow, deep breaths through the mouth. Listen at each point to the breath sounds during a complete inspiration and expiration. • Compare findings at each point with the corresponding point on the opposite side of the chest.	Vesicular and bronchovesicular breath sounds (see Table 27.7, p. 602.)	Adventitious breath sounds (e.g., crackles, wheezes, friction rub; see Table 27.8, p. 603) Absence of breath sounds

(continued)

SKILL 27.11

ASSESSING THE THORAX AND LUNGS (*continued*)

ASSESSMENT	NORMAL FINDINGS	DEVIATIONS FROM NORMAL
Anterior Thorax **13.** Inspect breathing patterns (e.g., respiratory rate and rhythm).	Quiet, rhythmic, and effortless respirations (see Chapter 28)	See Chapter 28, Box 28.4 (p. 684), for altered breathing patterns and sounds
14. Inspect the costal angle (angle formed by the intersection of the costal margins) and the angle at which the ribs enter the spine.	Costal angle is less than 90°, and the ribs insert into the spine at approximately a 45° angle (see Figure 27.23, p. 601)	Costal angle is widened (associated with chronic obstructive pulmonary disease)
15. Palpate the anterior chest (see posterior chest palpation).		
16. Palpate the anterior chest for respiratory excursion. • Place the palms of both your hands on the lower thorax, with your fingers laterally along the lower rib cage and your thumbs along the costal margins (see ❺). • Ask the client to take a deep breath while you observe the movement of your hands.	Full symmetric excursion; thumbs normally separate 3 cm to 5 cm	Asymmetric or decreased respiratory excursion

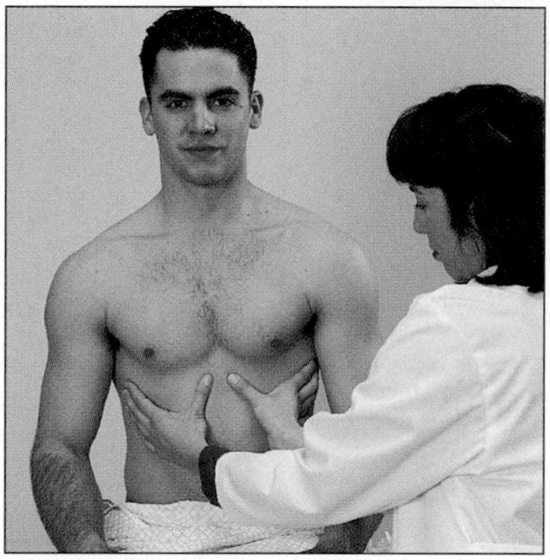

❺ Position of nurse's hands when assessing respiratory excursion on the anterior thorax

ASSESSMENT	NORMAL FINDINGS	DEVIATIONS FROM NORMAL
17. Palpate tactile fremitus in the same manner as for the posterior chest and by using the sequence shown in ❻. If the breasts are large and cannot be retracted adequately for palpation, this part of the examination is usually omitted.	Same as posterior vocal fremitus; fremitus is normally decreased over heart and breast tissue	Same as posterior fremitus

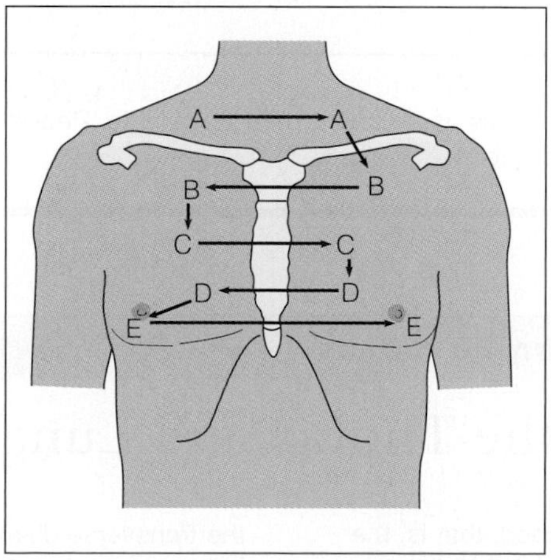

❻ Areas and sequence for palpating tactile fremitus on the anterior chest

(continued)

SKILL 27.11

ASSESSING THE THORAX AND LUNGS (*continued*)

ASSESSMENT	NORMAL FINDINGS	DEVIATIONS FROM NORMAL
18. Percuss the anterior chest systematically. • Begin above the clavicles in the supraclavicular space, and proceed downward to the diaphragm (see ❼). • Compare one side of the lung to the other. Displace female breasts for proper examination.	Percussion notes resonate down to the sixth rib at the level of the diaphragm but are flat over areas of heavy muscle and bone, dull on areas over the heart and the liver, and tympanic over the underlying stomach (see ❽).	Asymmetry in percussion notes; areas of dullness or flatness over lung tissue

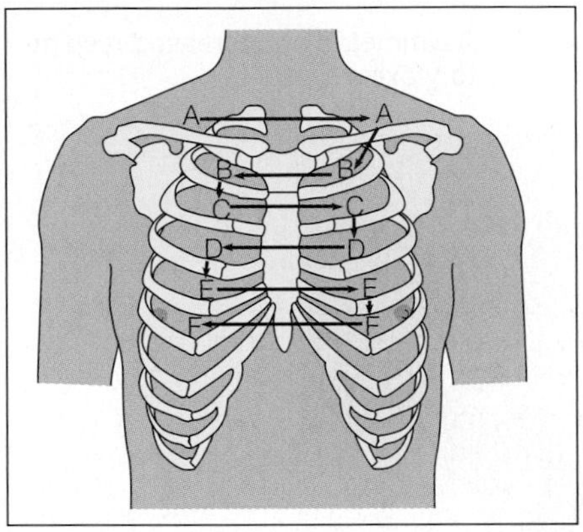

❼ Sequence for anterior chest percussion

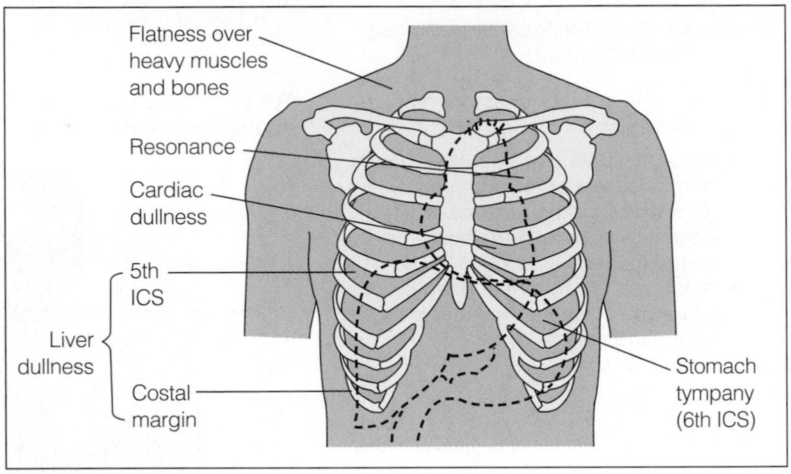

❽ Normal percussion sounds on the anterior thorax

19. Auscultate the trachea.	Bronchial and tubular breath sounds (see Table 27.7, p. 602)	Adventitious breath sounds (see Table 27.8, p. 603)
20. Auscultate the anterior chest. Use the sequence used in percussion (see ❼), beginning over the bronchi between the sternum and the clavicles.	Bronchovesicular and vesicular breath sounds (see Table 27.7, p. 602)	Adventitious breath sounds (see Table 27.8, p. 603)

21. Document findings in the client record by using forms or checklists supplemented by narrative notes when appropriate.

EVALUATION

Relate findings to previous assessment data if available. Report significant deviations from normal to the appropriate members of the health-care team.

Lifespan Considerations

Assessing the Thorax and Lungs

INFANTS

- The thorax is rounded; that is, the diameter from the front to the back (anteroposterior) is equal to the transverse diameter. See Figure 27.27. It is also cylindrical, having a nearly equal diameter at the top and the base. This makes it harder for infants to expand their thoracic space.

(continued)

Lifespan Considerations (*continued*)

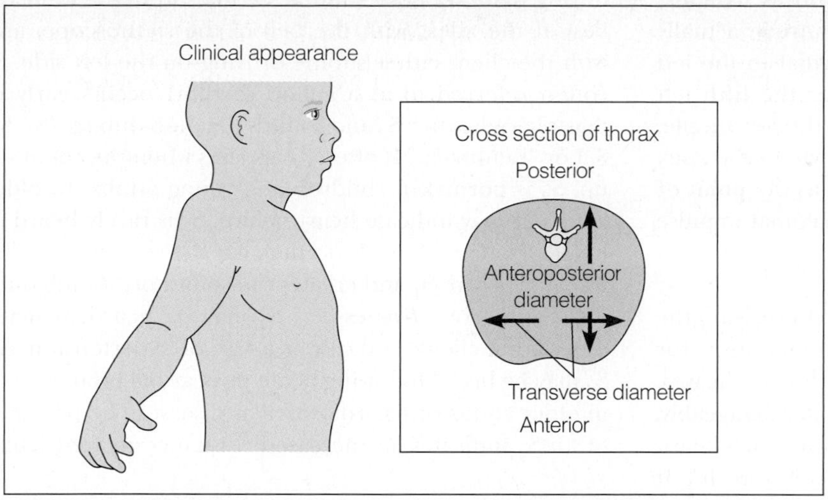

FIGURE 27.27 Configurations of the child's thorax showing anteroposterior diameter and transverse diameter

- To assess tactile fremitus, place the hand over the crying infant's chest.
- Infants tend to breathe by using their diaphragm; assess rate and rhythm by watching the abdomen, rather than the thorax, rise and fall.
- The right bronchial branch is short and angles down as it leaves the trachea, making it easy for small objects to be inhaled. Sudden onset of cough or other signs of respiratory distress may indicate the infant has inhaled a foreign object.

CHILDREN

- By about 6 years of age, the anteroposterior diameter has decreased in proportion to the transverse diameter, with a 1:2 ratio present.
- Children tend to breathe more abdominally than thoracically up to age 6.
- During the rapid growth spurts of adolescence, spinal curvature and rotation (scoliosis) may appear. Children should be assessed for scoliosis by age 12 and annually until their growth slows. Curvature greater than 10% should be referred for further medical evaluation.

OLDER ADULTS

- The thoracic curvature may be accentuated (kyphosis) because of osteoporosis and changes in cartilage resulting in collapse of the vertebrae.
- The anteroposterior diameter of the chest deepens, giving the person a barrel-chested appearance. This change is due to loss of skeletal muscle strength in the thorax and diaphragm and constant lung inflation from excessive expiratory pressure on the alveoli.
- Breathing rate and rhythm are unchanged at rest; the rate normally increases with activity but may take longer to return to the resting rate.
- Inspiratory muscles become less powerful, and the inspiration reserve volume decreases. A decrease in depth of respiration is therefore apparent.
- Expiration may require the use of accessory muscles. The expiratory reserve volume significantly increases because of the increased amount of air remaining in the lungs at the end of a normal breath.
- Small airways lose their cartilaginous support and elastic recoil; as a result, they tend to close, particularly in basal or dependent portions of the lung.
- Alveolar tissue loses its elasticity and changes to fibrous tissue. This thicker alveolar membrane decreases the pulmonary diffusion capacity. As a result, arterial oxyhemoglobin (a compound of oxygen and hemoglobin that transports oxygen) saturation and PaO_2 (partial pressure of oxygen) are slightly lower than those of young adults.
- Exertional capacity also decreases.
- Cilia in the airways decrease in number and are less effective in removing mucus; elderly clients are therefore at greater risk for pulmonary infections.

Cardiovascular and Peripheral Vascular Systems

Heart

Nurses assess the cardiovascular system through observations (inspection), palpation, and auscultation. The examination includes palpation of upper and lower extremity pulses; inspection of jugular venous distension; measurement of blood pressure bilaterally and while standing versus lying flat or sitting; and inspection, palpation, and auscultation of the heart. It is important to follow a systematic assessment of the cardiovascular system, starting with inspection and moving through to auscultation. Although heart examinations are initially performed while the client is in a semi-reclined position, other positions, such as left lateral recumbent, leaning forward, and standing, can also be used.

To assess the client's heart, the nurse must first determine its exact location. In the average adult, most of the heart lies behind and to the left of the sternum. A small portion (the right atrium) extends to the right of the sternum. The upper portion of the heart (both atria), referred to as its **base**, lies toward the back. The lower portion (the ventricles), referred to as its **apex**, points forward. The apex of the left ventricle actually touches the anterior chest wall at or medial to the left midclavicular line (MCL) and at or near the fifth left intercostal space, which is slightly below the left nipple. See Figure 28.13 (page 674). This point where the apex touches the anterior chest wall is known as the **point of maximal impulse (PMI)**. The point of maximal impulse refers to the point at which the apical impulse is most readily seen or felt.

The **precordium**, the area of the chest overlying the heart, is inspected and palpated simultaneously for the presence of abnormal pulsations or lifts or heaves. The terms **lift** and **heave**, often used interchangeably, refer to a rising along the sternal border with each heartbeat. A lift occurs when cardiac action is very forceful. It should be confirmed by palpation with the palm of the hand. Enlargement or overactivity of the left ventricle produces a heave lateral to the apex, whereas enlargement of the right ventricle produces a heave at or near the sternum.

Several heart sounds can be heard by auscultation. The normal first two heart sounds are produced by closure of the valves of the heart. The first heart sound, $\mathbf{S_1}$, occurs when the atrioventricular (A-V) valves close and is best heard at the apex. These valves close when the ventricles have been sufficiently filled. Although the right and left A-V valves do not close simultaneously, the closures occur closely enough to be heard as one sound (S_1), a dull, low-pitched sound described as "lub." After the ventricles empty their blood into the aorta and pulmonary arteries, the semilunar valves close, producing the second heart sound, $\mathbf{S_2}$, described as "dub." S_2 has a higher pitch than S_1 and is also shorter. The S_2 is best heard in the aortic and pulmonic areas. These two sounds, S_1 and S_2 ("lub-dub"), occur within one second or less, depending on the heart rate.

Heart sounds are audible anywhere on the precordial area, but they are best heard over the aortic, pulmonic, tricuspid, and apical areas (Figure 27.28). Each area is associated with the closure of heart valves: the aortic area with the aortic valve (inside the aorta as it arises from the left ventricle); the pulmonic area with the pulmonic valve (inside the pulmonary artery as it arises from the right ventricle); the tricuspid area with the tricuspid valve (between the right atrium and ventricle); and the apical (mitral) area with the mitral valve (between the left atrium and ventricle).

Associated with these sounds are systole and diastole. **Systole** is the period in which the ventricles contract. It begins with the first heart sound and ends at the second heart sound. Systole is normally shorter than diastole. **Diastole** is the period in which the ventricles relax. It starts with the second sound and ends at the subsequent first sound. Normally, no sounds are audible during these periods (Figure 27.29). The experienced nurse, however, may auscultate extra heart sounds (S_3 and S_4) during diastole. Both sounds are low in pitch and heard best at the apex, with the bell of the stethoscope, and with the client either supine or lying on the left side. S_3 (often referred to as a gallop rhythm) occurs early in diastole right after S_2 and sounds like "lub-dub-*ee*" (S_1, S_2, S_3) or "Kentuc-*ky*." It often disappears when the client sits up. S_3 is normal in children and young adults. In older adults, it may indicate heart failure. S_4 is rarely heard in healthy young adults. It occurs near the very end of diastole just before S_1 and creates the sound of "*dee*-lub-dub" (S_4, S_1, S_2) or "*Ten*-nessee." S_4 may be heard in many older adult clients and can be a sign of hypertension. An S_4 may be heard following acute myocardial infarction or in older adults with cardiovascular disease. The presence of an S_4 indicates an increased resistance to ventricular

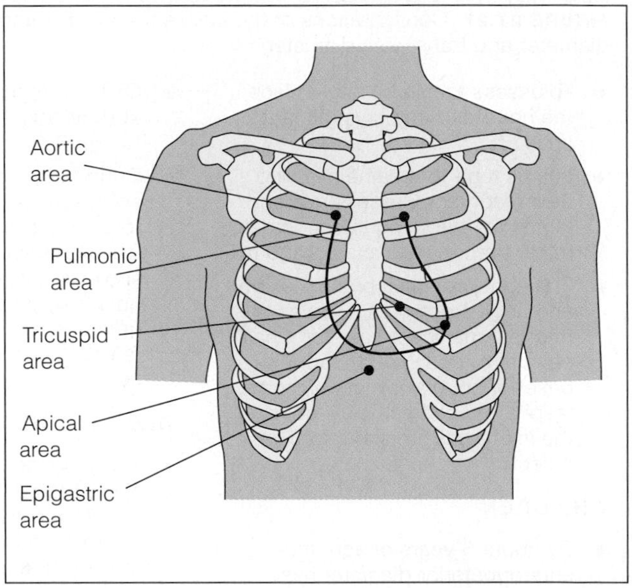

FIGURE 27.28 Anatomic sites of the precordium

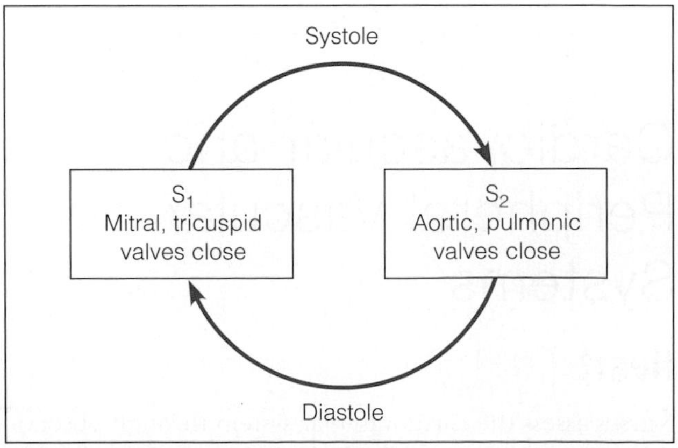

FIGURE 27.29 Relationship of heart sounds to systole and diastole

filling, which occurs because of a loss of compliance in the ventricular walls (e.g., hypertensive disease, coronary heart disease).

Normal heart sounds are summarized in Table 27.9. The nurse may also hear abnormal heart sounds, such as clicks, rubs, and murmurs. These are caused by valve disorders or impaired blood flow within the heart and require advanced training to diagnose.

Central Vessels

The *carotid arteries* supply oxygenated blood to the head and neck (Figure 27.30). Because they are the only source of blood to the brain, prolonged occlusion of one of these arteries can result in serious brain damage. The carotid pulses correlate with central aortic pressure, thus reflecting cardiac function better than the peripheral pulses. When cardiac output is diminished, the peripheral pulses may be difficult or impossible to feel, but the carotid pulse should be felt easily.

The carotid is also auscultated for a bruit, and if a bruit is found, the carotid artery is then palpated for a thrill. A **bruit** (a blowing or swishing sound), best heard with the diaphragm of the stethoscope, is created by turbulence of blood flow created by either a narrowed arterial lumen (a common development in older people) or to a condition, such as anemia or hyperthyroidism, that elevates cardiac output. A **thrill**, which frequently accompanies a bruit, is a vibrating sensation, like the purring of a cat or water running through a hose. It, too, indicates turbulent blood flow because of arterial obstruction.

The *jugular veins* drain blood from the head and neck directly into the superior vena cava and right side of the heart. The external jugular veins are superficial and may be visible above the clavicle. The internal jugular veins lie deeper along the carotid artery and may transmit pulsations onto the skin of the neck. Normally, external neck veins are distended and visible when a person lies down; they are flat and not as visible when a person stands up because gravity encourages venous drainage. By inspecting the jugular veins for pulsations and distension, the nurse can assess the adequacy of function of the right side of the heart and venous pressure. Bilateral jugular vein distension (JVD) may indicate right-sided heart failure.

Skill 27.12 describes how to assess the heart and central vessels.

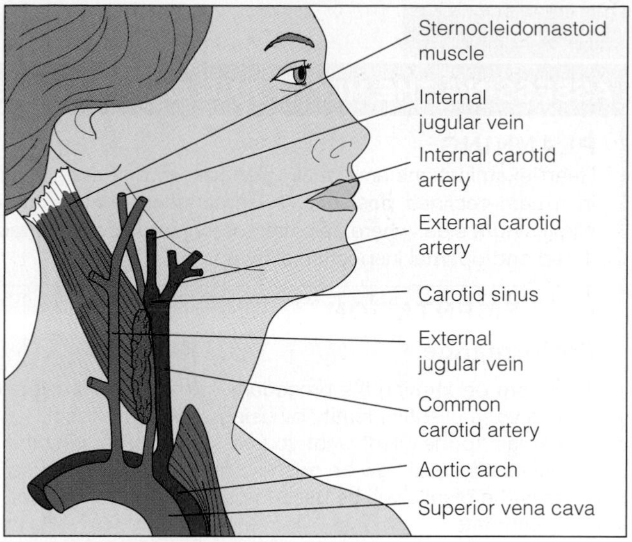

FIGURE 27.30 Arteries and veins of the right side of the neck

TABLE 27.9 Normal Heart Sounds

Sound or Phase	Description	Area: Aortic	Pulmonic	Tricuspid	Apical
S_1	Dull, low-pitched, and longer than S_2; sounds like "lub"	Less intensity than S_2	Less intensity than S_2	Louder than or equal to S_2	Louder than or equal to S_2
Systole	Normally silent interval between S_1 and S_2				
S_2	Higher pitch than S_1; sounds like "dub"	Louder than S_1	Louder than S_1; abnormal if louder than the aortic S_2 in adults more than 40 years of age	Less intensity than or equal to S_1	Less intensity than or equal to S_1
Diastole	Normally silent interval between S_2 and next S_1				

SKILL 27.12

ASSESSING THE HEART AND CENTRAL VESSELS

PLANNING

Heart examinations are usually performed while the client is in a semi-reclined position. The practitioner stands at the client's right side, where palpation of the cardiac area is facilitated and optimal inspection allowed.

Equipment

- Stethoscope
- Centimetre ruler

IMPLEMENTATION

Performance

1. Before performing the procedure, introduce yourself and verify the client's identity by using agency protocol. Explain to the client what you are going to do, why it is necessary, and how he or she can cooperate. Discuss how the results will be used in planning further care or treatments.
2. Perform hand hygiene and observe other appropriate infection prevention and control procedures.
3. Provide for client privacy.
4. Inquire whether the client has any history of the following: family history of incidence and age of heart disease, high cholesterol levels, hypertension, cerebrovascular accident (stroke), obesity, congenital heart disease, arterial disease, and rheumatic fever; client's past history of rheumatic fever, heart murmur, heart attack, varicosities, or heart failure; present signs or symptoms indicative of heart disease (e.g., fatigue, dyspnea, orthopnea, edema, cough, chest pain, palpitations, syncope, elevated blood pressure, wheezing, hemoptysis); presence of diseases that affect the heart (e.g., obesity, diabetes, lung disease, endocrine disorders); lifestyle habits that are risk factors for cardiac disease (e.g., smoking, excessive alcohol intake, eating and exercise patterns, areas and degree of stress perceived).

ASSESSMENT	NORMAL FINDINGS	DEVIATIONS FROM NORMAL
5. Simultaneously inspect and palpate the precordium for the presence of abnormal pulsations, lifts, or heaves. Locate the valve areas of the heart:		
• Locate the angle of Louis. It is felt as a prominence on the sternum.		
• Move your fingertips down each side of the angle until you can feel the second intercostal spaces. The client's right second intercostal space is the aortic area, and the left second intercostal space is the pulmonic area (see Figure 27.28, p. 610).		
• Inspect and palpate the aortic and pulmonic areas, observing them at an angle and to the side, to note the presence or absence of pulsations. *Observing these areas at an angle increases the likelihood of seeing pulsations.*	No pulsations	Pulsations
• From the pulmonic area, move your fingertips down three left intercostal spaces along the side of the sternum. The left fifth intercostal space close to the sternum is the tricuspid or right ventricular area.		
• Inspect and palpate the tricuspid area for pulsations and heaves or lifts.	No pulsations; no lift or heave	Pulsations; diffuse lift or heave, indicating enlarged or overactive right ventricle
• From the tricuspid area, move your fingertips laterally 5 cm to 7 cm to the left MCL. This is the apical or mitral area or PMI. If you have difficulty locating the PMI, have the client roll onto the left side to move the apex closer to the chest wall.		

(continued)

SKILL 27.12

ASSESSING THE HEART AND CENTRAL VESSELS *(continued)*

ASSESSMENT	NORMAL FINDINGS	DEVIATIONS FROM NORMAL
• Inspect and palpate the apical area for pulsation, noting its specific location (it may be displaced laterally or lower) and diameter. If displaced laterally, record the distance between the apex and the MCL in centimetres.	Pulsations visible in 50% of adults and palpable in most PMI in fifth left intercostal space at or medial to the MCL; diameter of 1 cm to 2 cm; no lift or heave	PMI displaced laterally or lower (indicates enlarged heart or aneurysm); diameter of more than 2 cm; diffuse lift or heave lateral to apex (indicates enlargement or overactivity of left ventricle)
• Inspect and palpate the epigastric area at the base of the sternum for abdominal aortic pulsations.	Aortic pulsations	Bounding abdominal pulsations (e.g., aortic aneurysm)
6. Auscultate the heart in all four anatomic sites: aortic, pulmonic, tricuspid, and apical (mitral). Auscultation need not be limited to these areas; however, the nurse may need to move the stethoscope to find the most audible sounds for each client. • Eliminate all sources of room noise. **Rationale: Heart sounds are of low intensity, and other noise hinders the nurse's ability to hear them.** • Keep the client in a supine position with head elevated 30° to 45°. • Use both the diaphragm and the bell to listen to all areas. • In every area of auscultation, distinguish both S_1 and S_2 sounds. • When auscultating, concentrate on one particular sound at a time in each area: the first heart sound, followed by systole, then the second heart sound, then diastole. Systole and diastole are normally silent intervals. • Later, re-examine the heart while the client is in the upright sitting position. **Rationale: Certain sounds are more audible in certain positions.**	S_1: usually heard at all sites, usually louder at apical area; S_2: usually heard at all sites, usually louder at base of heart; systole: silent interval, slightly shorter duration than diastole at normal heart rate (60 to 90 beats/min); diastole: silent interval, slightly longer duration than systole at normal heart rates; S_3 in children and young adults; S_4 in many older adults	Increased or decreased intensity; varying intensity with different beats; increased intensity at aortic area; increased intensity at pulmonic area; sharp-sounding ejection clicks; S_3 in older adults; S_4 may be a sign of hypertension
Carotid Arteries		
7. Palpate the carotid artery, using extreme caution (see Figure 27.30, p. 611). • Palpate only one carotid artery at a time. **Rationale: This ensures adequate blood flow through the other artery to the brain.** • Avoid exerting too much pressure and massaging the area. **Rationale: Pressure can occlude the artery and carotid sinus massage can precipitate bradycardia.** • The carotid sinus is a small dilation at the beginning of the internal carotid artery just above the bifurcation of the common carotid artery, in the upper third of the neck. • Ask the client to turn the head slightly toward the side being examined. This makes the carotid artery more accessible.	Symmetric pulse volumes; full pulsations, thrusting quality; quality remains same when client breathes, turns head, and changes from sitting to supine position; elastic arterial wall	Asymmetric volumes (possible stenosis or thrombosis); decreased pulsations (may indicate impaired left cardiac output); increased pulsations; thickening, hard, rigid, beaded, inelastic walls (indicate arteriosclerosis)

(continued)

SKILL 27.12

ASSESSING THE HEART AND CENTRAL VESSELS (*continued*)

ASSESSMENT	NORMAL FINDINGS	DEVIATIONS FROM NORMAL
8. Auscultate the carotid artery. • Turn the client's head slightly away from the side being examined. **Rationale: This facilitates the placement of the stethoscope.** • Auscultate the carotid artery on one side and then the other. • Listen for the presence of a bruit. If you hear a bruit, gently palpate the artery to determine the presence of a thrill.	No sound heard on auscultation	Presence of bruit in one or both arteries (suggests occlusive artery disease)
Jugular Veins		
9. Inspect the jugular veins for distension while the client is placed in a semi-Fowler's position (30° to 45° angle), with the head supported on a small pillow.	Veins not visible (indicating right side of heart is functioning normally)	Veins visibly distended (indicating advanced cardiopulmonary disease)
10. If jugular distension is present, assess the jugular venous pressure (JVP). • Locate the highest visible point of distension of the internal jugular vein. Although either the internal or the external jugular vein can be used, the internal jugular vein is more reliable. **Rationale: The external jugular vein is more easily affected by obstruction or kinking at the base of the neck.** • Measure the vertical height of this point in centimetres from the sternal angle, the point at which the clavicles meet (see ❶). • Repeat the preceding steps on the other side. Bilateral measurements of more than 3 cm to 4 cm are considered elevated (may indicate right-sided heart failure); unilateral distension (may be caused by local obstruction)		
11. Document findings in the client record by using forms or checklists supplemented by narrative notes when appropriate.		

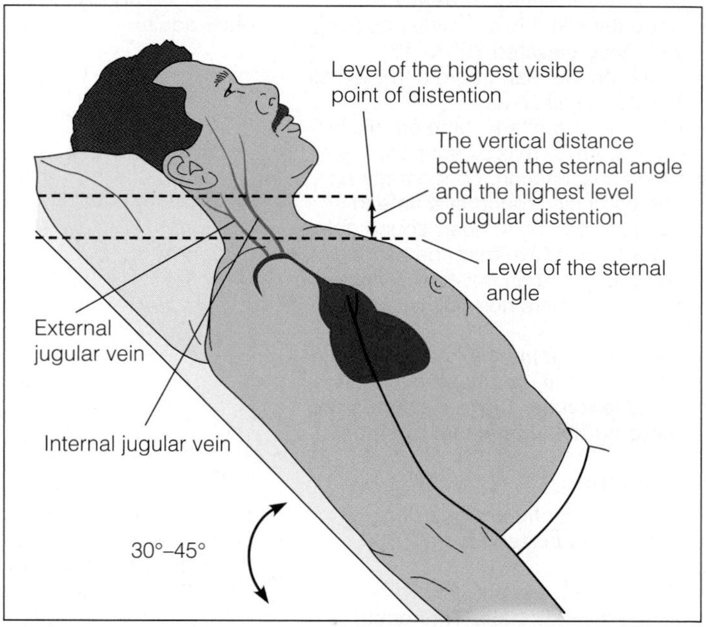

❶ Assessing the highest point of distension of the jugular vein

EVALUATION

- Perform a detailed follow-up examination based on findings that deviated from expected or normal for the client. Relate findings to previous assessment data if available.
- Report significant deviations from normal to the appropriate members of the health-care team.

Lifespan Considerations

Assessing the Heart and Central Vessels

INFANTS

- Physiological splitting of the second heart sound (S_2) may be heard when the child takes a deep breath and the aortic valve closes a split second before the pulmonic valve. If splitting of S_2 is heard during normal respirations, it is abnormal and may indicate an atrial-septal defect, pulmonary stenosis, or another heart problem.
- Infants may normally have sinus arrhythmia that is related to respiration. The heart rate slows during expiration and increases when the child breathes in.
- Murmurs may be heard in newborns as the structures of fetal circulation, especially the ductus arteriosus, close.

CHILDREN

- Heart sounds are louder because of the thinner chest wall.
- A third heart sound (S_3), caused as the ventricles fill, is best heard at the apex and is present in about one-third of all children
- The PMI is higher and more medial in children younger than 8 years old.

OLDER ADULTS

- If no disease is present, heart size remains the same throughout life.
- Cardiac output and strength of contraction decrease, thus lessening the older person's activity tolerance.
- The heart rate returns to its resting rate more slowly after exertion than it did when the individual was younger.
- S_4 heart sound is considered normal in older adults.
- Extra systoles commonly occur. Ten or more extra systoles per minute are considered abnormal.
- Sudden emotional and physical stresses can result in cardiac arrhythmias and heart failure.

Peripheral Vascular System

Assessing the peripheral vascular system includes measuring blood pressure; palpating peripheral pulses; inspecting, palpating, and auscultating the carotid pulse; inspecting the jugular and peripheral veins; and inspecting the skin and tissues to determine **perfusion** (blood supply to an area) to the extremities. Certain aspects of peripheral vascular assessment are often incorporated into other parts of the assessment procedure. For example, blood pressure is usually measured at the beginning of the physical examination (see the section on assessing blood pressure in Chapter 28). Pulse sites and pulse assessments are described in Chapter 28.

Skill 27.13 describes how to assess the peripheral vascular system.

SKILL 27.13

ASSESSING THE PERIPHERAL VASCULAR SYSTEM

Equipment: None

IMPLEMENTATION

Performance

1. Before performing the procedure, introduce yourself and verify the client's identity by using agency protocol. Explain to the client what you are going to do, why it is necessary, and how he or she can cooperate. Discuss how the results will be used in planning further care or treatments.
2. Perform hand hygiene and observe other appropriate infection prevention and control procedures.
3. Provide for client privacy.
4. Inquire whether the client has any history of the following: past history of heart disorders, varicosities, arterial disease, and hypertension; lifestyle habits, such as exercise patterns, activity patterns and tolerance, smoking, and use of alcohol.

ASSESSMENT	NORMAL FINDINGS	DEVIATIONS FROM NORMAL
5. Palpate the peripheral pulses individually and systematically on both sides of the client's body simultaneously (except the carotid pulse) to determine the symmetry of pulse volume. If you have difficulty palpating some of the peripheral pulses, use a Doppler ultrasound probe.	Symmetric pulse volumes; full pulsations	Asymmetric volumes (indicate impaired circulation); absence of pulsation (indicates arterial spasm or occlusion); decreased, weak, thready pulsations (indicate impaired cardiac output); increased pulse volume (may indicate hypertension, high cardiac output, or circulatory overload)

(continued)

SKILL 27.13

ASSESSING THE PERIPHERAL VASCULAR SYSTEM (*continued*)

ASSESSMENT	NORMAL FINDINGS	DEVIATIONS FROM NORMAL
Peripheral Veins		
6. Inspect the peripheral veins in the arms and legs for the presence or appearance of superficial veins when limbs are dependent and when limbs are elevated.	In dependent position, presence of distension and nodular bulges at calves; when limbs elevated, veins collapse (veins may appear tortuous or distended in older people)	Distended veins in the thigh or lower leg or on posterolateral part of calf from knee to ankle
7. Assess the peripheral leg veins for signs of phlebitis. • Inspect the calves for redness and swelling over vein sites. • Palpate the calves for firmness or tension of the muscles, the presence of edema over the dorsum of the foot, and areas of localized warmth. **Rationale: Palpation augments inspection findings, particularly in darker-pigmented people in whom redness may not be visible.** • Push the calves from side to side to test for tenderness. • Firmly dorsiflex the client's foot while supporting the entire leg in extension (Homans' test), or have the person stand or walk.	Limbs not tender; symmetric in size	Tenderness on palpation; pain in calf muscles with forceful dorsiflexion of the foot (positive Homans' test); warmth and redness over vein; swelling of one calf or leg
Peripheral Perfusion		
8. Inspect the skin of the hands and feet for colour, temperature, edema, and skin changes.	Skin colour pink; skin temperature not excessively warm or cold; no edema; skin texture resilient and moist	Cyanotic (venous insufficiency); pallor that increases with limb elevation; dependent rubor, a dusky red colour when limb is lowered (arterial insufficiency); brown pigmentation around ankles (arterial or chronic venous insufficiency); skin cool (arterial insufficiency); marked edema (venous insufficiency); mild edema (arterial insufficiency); skin thin and shiny or thick, waxy, shiny, and fragile, with reduced hair and ulceration (venous or arterial insufficiency)
9. Assess the adequacy of arterial flow if arterial insufficiency is suspected.		
Buerger's Test (Arterial Adequacy Test)		
• Assist the client to a supine position. Ask the client to raise one leg or one arm about 30 cm above heart level, move the foot or hand briskly up and down for about 1 minute, and then sit up and dangle the leg or arm. • Observe the time elapsed until return of original colour and vein filling.	Original colour returns in 10 seconds; veins in feet or hands fill in about 15 seconds	Delayed colour return or mottled appearance; delayed venous filling; marked redness of arms or legs (indicates arterial insufficiency)
Capillary Refill Test		
• Squeeze the client's fingernail and toenail between your fingers sufficiently to cause blanching (about 5 seconds). • Release the pressure, and observe how quickly normal colour returns.	Immediate return of colour (less than 2 to 3 seconds)	Delayed return of colour (arterial insufficiency)

(*continued*)

SKILL 27.13

ASSESSING THE PERIPHERAL VASCULAR SYSTEM (*continued*)

ASSESSMENT	NORMAL FINDINGS	DEVIATIONS FROM NORMAL
Other Assessments • Inspect the fingernails for changes indicative of circulatory impairment. See the section on assessment of nails earlier in this chapter (Skill 27.4, p. 571). • See also peripheral pulse assessment in Chapter 28 (Skill 28.2, p. 675).		

10. Document findings in the client record by using forms or checklists supplemented by narrative notes when appropriate.

EVALUATION

- Perform a detailed follow-up examination of the heart or central vessels, integument, or other systems based on findings that deviated from expected or normal for the client. Relate findings to previous assessment data if available.
- Report significant deviations from normal to the appropriate members of the health-care team.

Lifespan Considerations

Assessing the Peripheral Vascular System

INFANTS

- Screen for coarctation (narrowing) of the aorta by palpating the peripheral pulses and comparing the strength of the femoral pulses with the radial pulses and apical pulse. If coarctation is present, femoral pulses will be diminished and radial pulses will be stronger.

CHILDREN

- Palpation of pulses in the lower extremities (particularly the femoral pulses) is essential to screen for coarctation of the aorta.
- Changes in the peripheral vasculature, such as bruising, petechiae (small purple or red spots caused by a broken blood vessel), and purpura (larger red or purple spots caused by bleeding under the skin), can indicate serious systemic diseases in children (e.g., leukemia, meningococcemia).

OLDER ADULTS

- The overall effectiveness of blood vessels decreases as smooth muscle cells are replaced by connective tissue. The lower extremities are more likely to show signs of arterial and venous impairment because of the more distal and dependent position.
- Proximal arteries become thinner and dilate.
- Peripheral arteries become thicker and dilate less effectively because of arteriosclerotic changes in the vessel walls.
- Blood vessels lengthen and become more tortuous and prominent. Varicosities occur more frequently.
- In some instances, arteries may be palpated more easily because of the loss of supportive surrounding tissues. Often, however, the most distal pulses of the lower extremities are more difficult to palpate because of decreased arterial perfusion.
- Systolic and diastolic blood pressures may increase. See Chapter 28 for Canadian guidelines for measurement of blood pressure, follow-up, and lifestyle counselling.
- Peripheral edema is frequently observed and is most commonly the result of chronic venous insufficiency or low protein levels in the blood (hypoproteinemia).
- Carotid artery assessment is an essential aspect of peripheral vascular examination in the older adult.

The Breasts and Axillae

The breasts of men and women need to be inspected and palpated. Men have some glandular tissue beneath each nipple, a potential site for malignancy, whereas mature women have glandular tissue throughout the breast. In females, the largest portion of glandular breast tissue is located in the upper outer quadrant of each breast. From this quadrant, there is a projection of breast tissue into the axilla, called the **axillary tail of Spence** (Figure 27.31). The majority of breast tumours are located in this upper outer breast quadrant and in the tail of Spence. During assessment, the nurse can localize specific findings by using this division of the breast into quadrants and the axillary tail.

Skill 27.14 describes a nursing assessment of the breasts and axillae.

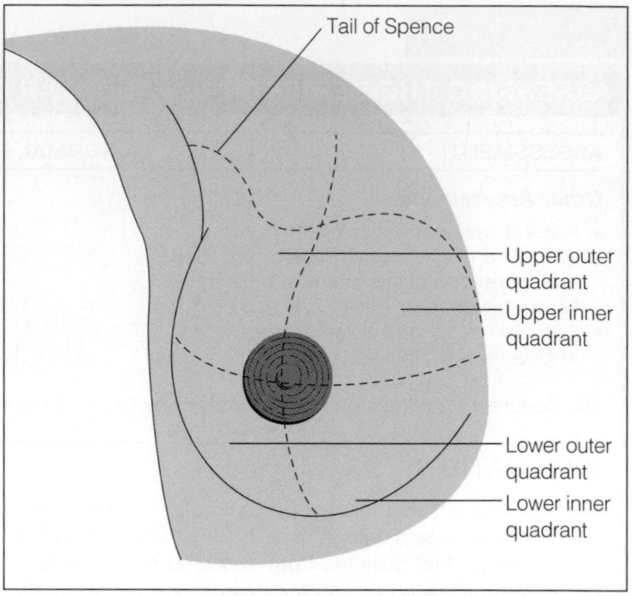

FIGURE 27.31 Four breast quadrants and the axillary tail of Spence

SKILL 27.14

ASSESSING THE BREASTS AND AXILLAE

Equipment: Centimetre ruler

IMPLEMENTATION

Performance

1. Before performing the procedure, introduce yourself and verify the client's identity by using agency protocol. Explain to the client what you are going to do, why it is necessary, and how he or she can cooperate. Inquire whether the client has ever had a clinical breast exam. Discuss how the results will be used in planning further care or treatments.
2. Perform hand hygiene and observe other appropriate infection prevention and control procedures.
3. Provide for client privacy.
4. Inquire whether the client has a history of breast masses and what was done about them; pain or tenderness in the breasts and relation to the woman's menstrual cycle; discharge from the nipple; medication history (some medications, e.g., oral contraceptives, steroids, digitalis, and diuretics, can cause nipple discharge; estrogen replacement therapy may be associated with the development of cysts or cancer); risk factors that may be associated with development of breast cancer (e.g., mother, sister, aunt with breast cancer; alcohol consumption, high-fat diet, obesity, use of oral contraceptives, menarche before age 12, menopause after age 55, age 30 or older at first pregnancy or never having been pregnant). Inquire whether the client monitors the look and feel of her breasts and notes the normal changes in relation to her menstrual cycle.

ASSESSMENT	NORMAL FINDINGS	DEVIATIONS FROM NORMAL
5. Inspect the breasts for size, symmetry, and contour or shape while the client is in a sitting position.	*Females:* Rounded shape; slightly unequal in size; generally symmetric *Males:* Breasts even with the chest wall; if obese, may be similar in shape to female breasts	Recent change in breast size; swellings; marked asymmetry
6. Inspect the skin of the breast for localized discolourations or hyperpigmentation, retraction or dimpling, localized hypervascular areas, swelling, or edema (see ❶).	Skin uniform in colour (same in appearance as skin of abdomen or back); skin smooth and intact; diffuse symmetric horizontal or vertical vascular pattern in light-skinned people; striae (stretch marks); moles and nevi	Localized discolourations or hyperpigmentation; retraction or dimpling (result of scar tissue or an invasive tumour); unilateral, localized hypervascular areas (associated with increased blood flow); swelling or edema appearing as pig skin or orange peel because of exaggeration of the pores

(continued)

SKILL 27.14

ASSESSING THE BREASTS AND AXILLAE (*continued*)

ASSESSMENT	NORMAL FINDINGS	DEVIATIONS FROM NORMAL
	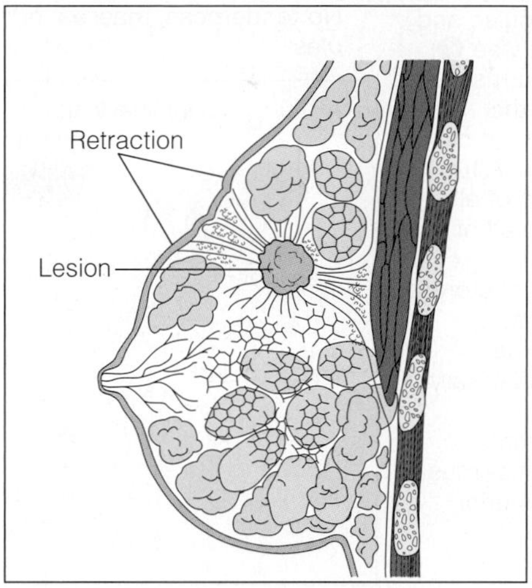 ❶ A lesion causing retraction of the skin	
7. Emphasize any retraction by having the client • Raise the arms above the head. • Push the hands together, with elbows flexed (see ❷). • Press the hands down on the hips (see ❸).	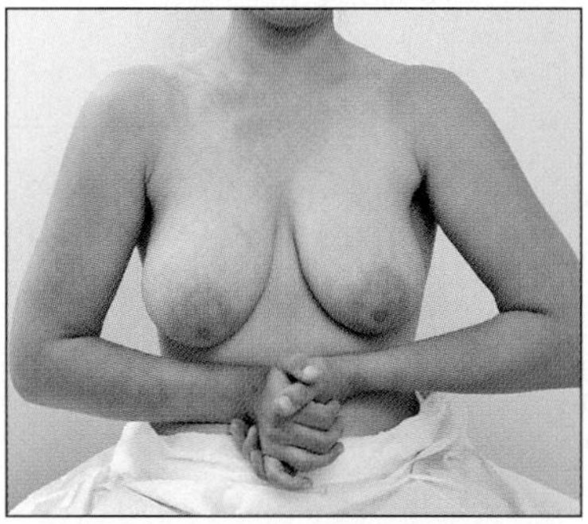 ❷ Pushing the hands together to accentuate retraction of breast tissues	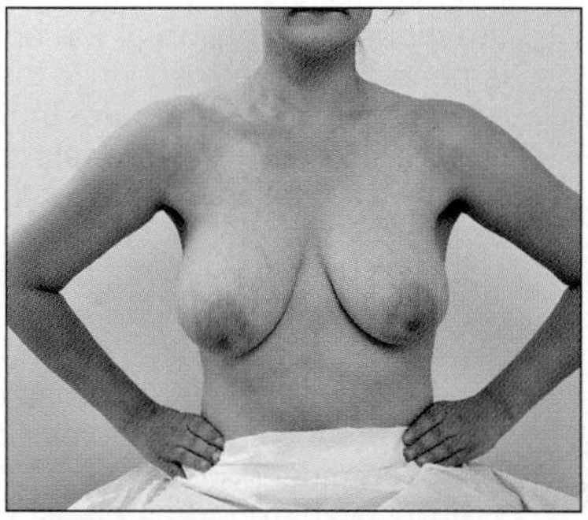 ❸ Pressing the hands down on the hips to accentuate retraction of breast tissue
8. Inspect the areola area for size, shape, symmetry, colour, surface characteristics, and any masses or lesions.	Round or oval and bilaterally the same; colour varies widely, from light pink to dark brown; irregular placement of sebaceous glands on the surface of the areola (Montgomery's tubercles)	Any asymmetry, mass, or lesion
9. Inspect the nipples for size, shape, position, colour, discharge, and lesions.	Round, everted, and equal in size; similar in colour; soft and smooth; both nipples point in same direction (out in young women and men, downward in older women); no discharge, except from pregnant or breastfeeding females; inversion of one or both nipples that is present from puberty	Asymmetrical size and colour; presence of discharge, crusts, or cracks; recent inversion of one or both nipples

(continued)

SKILL 27.14

ASSESSING THE BREASTS AND AXILLAE (*continued*)

ASSESSMENT	NORMAL FINDINGS	DEVIATIONS FROM NORMAL
10. Palpate the axillary, subclavicular, and supraclavicular lymph nodes (see ❹) while the client sits with the arms abducted and supported on the nurse's forearm. For palpation of clavicular lymph nodes, see Skill 27.10 (p. 596). Use the flat surfaces of all fingertips to palpate the four areas of the axilla: • The edge of the musculus pectoralis major (greater pectoral muscle) along the anterior axillary line • The thoracic wall in the midaxillary area • The upper part of the humerus • The anterior edge of the latissimus dorsi muscle along the posterior axillary line.	No tenderness, masses, or nodules	Tenderness, masses, or nodules

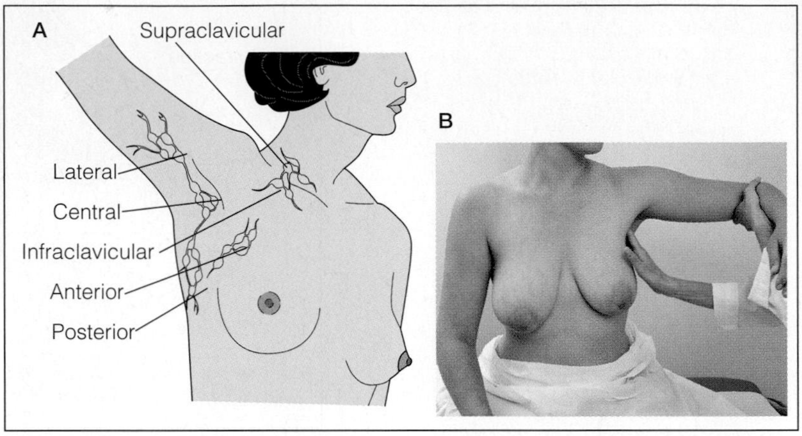

❹ Location and palpation of lymph nodes that drain the lateral breast: A: Lymph nodes; B: palpating the axilla

ASSESSMENT	NORMAL FINDINGS	DEVIATIONS FROM NORMAL
11. Palpate the breast for masses, tenderness, and any discharge from the nipples. Palpation of the breast is generally performed while the client is supine. **Rationale: In the supine position, the breasts flatten evenly against the chest wall, facilitating palpation.** • For clients who have a past history of breast masses, who are at high risk for breast cancer, or who have pendulous breasts, examination in both a supine and a sitting position is recommended. • If the client reports a breast lump, start with the rest of the breast to obtain baseline data that will serve as a comparison to the reportedly involved breast. • To enhance flattening of the breast, instruct the client to abduct the arm and place her hand behind her head. Then place a small pillow or rolled towel under the client's shoulder. • For palpation, use the palmar surface of the middle three fingertips (held together) and make a gentle rotary motion on the breast. • Choose one of three patterns for palpation: a. Hands of the clock or spokes on a wheel (see ❺) b. Concentric circles (see ❻)	No tenderness, masses, nodules, or nipple discharge	Tenderness, masses, nodules, or nipple discharge

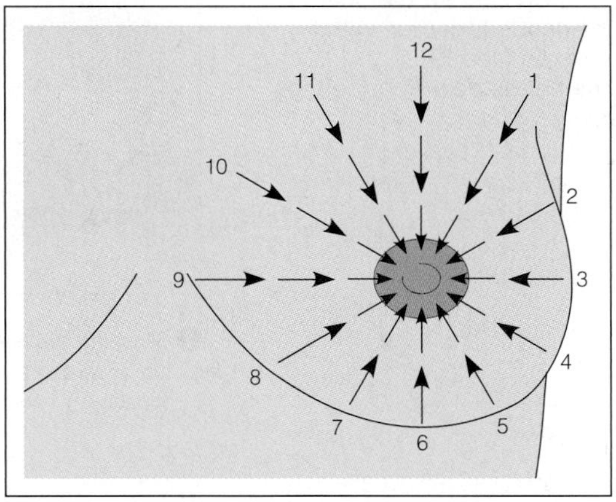

❺ Hands-of-the-clock or spokes-on-a-wheel pattern of breast palpation

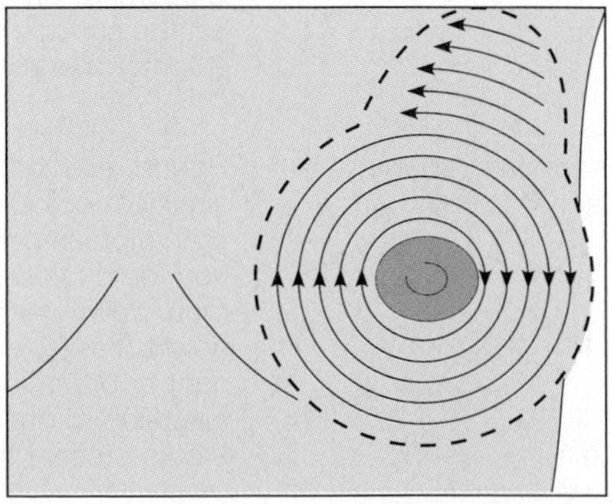

❻ Concentric circles pattern for breast palpation

(continued)

SKILL 27.14

ASSESSING THE BREASTS AND AXILLAE *(continued)*

ASSESSMENT	NORMAL FINDINGS	DEVIATIONS FROM NORMAL
c. Vertical strips pattern (see ❼) • Start at one point for palpation, and move systematically to the end point to ensure that all breast surfaces are assessed. • Pay particular attention to the upper outer quadrant area and the tail of Spence.		If you detect a mass, record the following data: a. *Location:* the exact location relative to the quadrants and axillary tail, or the clock (as in ❺), and the distance from the nipple in centimetres b. *Size*: the length, width, and thickness of the mass in centimetres. If you are able to determine the discrete edges, record this fact. c. *Shape:* whether the mass is round, oval, lobulated, indistinct, or irregular. d. *Consistency:* whether the mass is hard or soft. e. *Mobility:* whether the mass is moveable or fixed. f. *Skin over the lump:* whether it is reddened, dimpled, or retracted. g. *Nipple:* whether it is displaced or retracted. h. *Tenderness:* whether palpation is painful.
12. Palpate the areola and the nipples for masses. Compress each nipple to determine the presence of any discharge. If discharge is present, milk the breast along its radius to identify the discharge-producing lobe. Assess any discharge for amount, colour, consistency, and odour. Note also any tenderness on palpation.	No tenderness, masses, nodules, or nipple discharge	Tenderness, masses, nodules, or nipple discharge

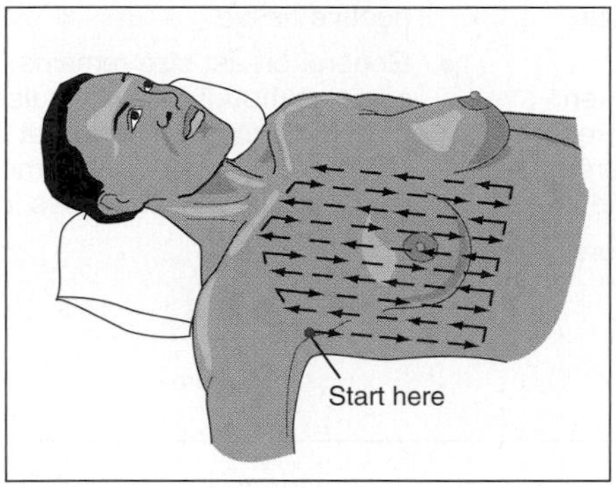

❼ Vertical strips pattern of breast palpation

13. Document findings in the client record by using forms or checklistssupplemented by narrative notes when appropriate.

EVALUATION

- Perform a detailed follow-up examination based on findings that deviated from expected or normal for the client. Relate findings to previous assessment data if available.
- Report significant deviations from normal to the appropriate members of the health-care team.

Lifespan Considerations

Assessing the Breasts and Axillae

INFANTS

- Newborns, both boys and girls, up to 2 weeks of age may have breast enlargement and galactorrhea (white discharge from the nipples or neonatal milk).
- Supernumerary (extra) nipples infrequently are present as small dimples along the mammary chain; these may be associated with renal anomalies.

(continued)

Lifespan Considerations (*continued*)

PREADOLESCENTS AND ADOLESCENTS

- Female breast development begins between 8 and 13 years of age and occurs in 5 stages. Development may be asymmetrical.

Stage 1 Prepubertal with no noticeable change

Stage 2 Breast bud with elevation of nipple and enlargement of the areola

Stage 3 Enlargement of the breast and areola; nipple flush with the breast surface

Stage 4 Projection of the areola and nipple forming a secondary mound over the breast

Stage 5 Recession of areola in most women by about age 14 or 15 years, leaving only the nipple projecting

- Boys can develop breast buds and have slight enlargement of the areola in early adolescence. Gynecomastia (further enlargement of breast tissue) can occur. This growth is transient, usually lasting about 2 years, resolving completely by late puberty.
- Axillary hair usually appears by age 13 and is related to adrenal rather than gonadal changes.

PREGNANT FEMALES

- Breast, areola, and nipple size increase.
- The areolae and nipples darken; nipples may become more erect; areolae contain small, scattered, elevated Montgomery's glands.
- Superficial veins become more prominent and jagged linear stretch marks may develop.
- Colostrum (a thick yellow fluid) may be expressed from the nipples after the first trimester.

OLDER ADULTS

- In the postmenopausal female, breasts change in shape and often appear pendulous or flaccid; they lack the firmness they had in younger years.
- The presence of breast lesions may be detected more readily because of the decrease in connective tissue.
- General breast size remains the same. Although glandular tissue atrophies, the amount of fat in breasts (predominantly in the lower quadrants) increases in most women.

Abdomen

The nurse locates and describes abdominal findings in a client by using two common methods of subdividing the abdomen: quadrants and regions. To divide the abdomen into quadrants, the nurse imagines two lines: a vertical line from the xyphoid process to the pubic symphysis, and a horizontal line across the umbilicus (Figure 27.32). These quadrants are labelled right upper quadrant (1), left upper quadrant (2), right lower quadrant (3), and left lower quadrant (4). Using the second method, division into nine regions, the nurse imagines two vertical lines that extend superiorly from the midpoints of the inguinal ligaments, and two horizontal lines, one at the level of the edge of the lower ribs and the other at the level of the iliac crests (Figure 27.33). Specific organs or parts of organs lie in each abdominal region. See Table 27.10 and Table 27.11.

In addition, practitioners often use certain landmarks to locate abdominal signs and symptoms. These are the xyphoid process of the sternum, the costal margins, the midline (a line drawn from the tip of the sternum through the umbilicus to the pubic symphysis), the anterosuperior iliac spine, the inguinal ligaments (Poupart's ligaments), and the superior margin of the pubic symphysis (Figure 27.34, p. 624).

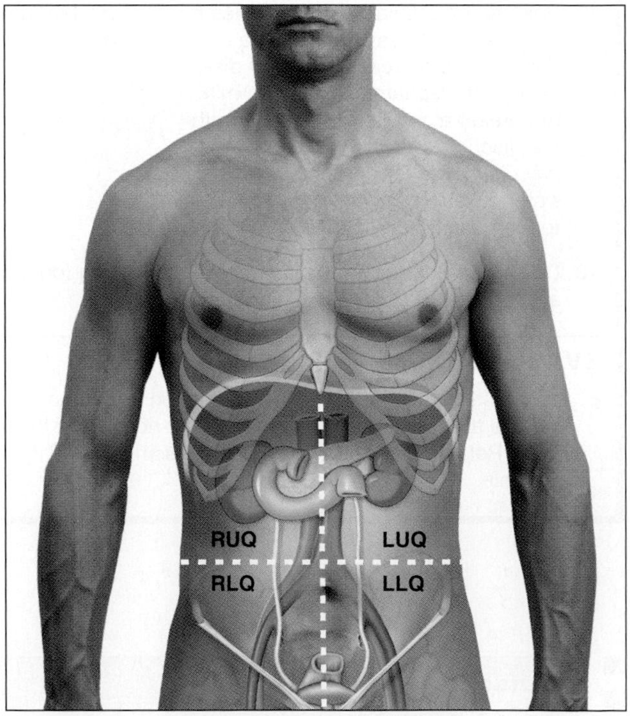

FIGURE 27.32 The four abdominal quadrants and the underlying organs: 1, right upper quadrant (RUQ); 2, left upper quadrant (LUQ); 3, right lower quadrant (RLQ); 4, left lower quadrant (LLQ)

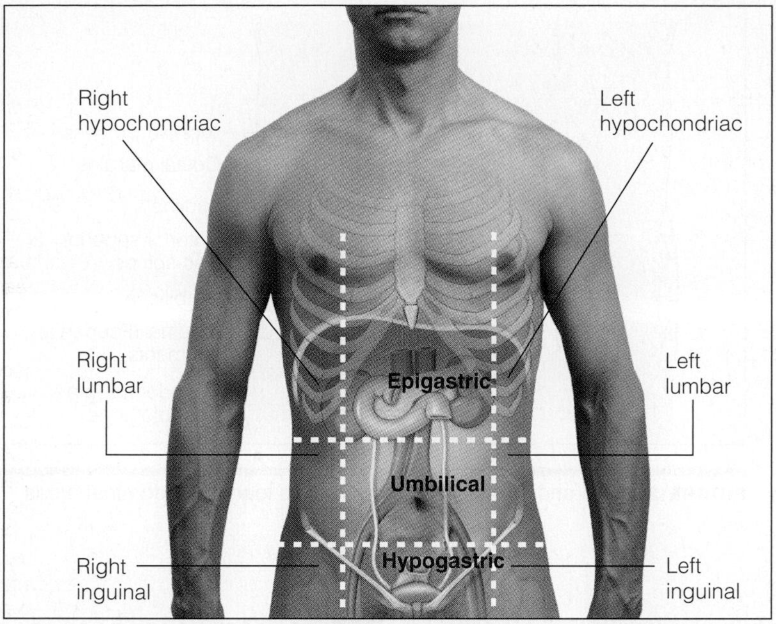

FIGURE 27.33 The nine abdominal regions: epigastric; left and right hypochondriac; umbilical; left and right lumbar; suprapubic and hypogastric; left and right inguinal or iliac

TABLE 27.10 Organs in the Four Abdominal Quadrants

Right Upper Quadrant	Left Upper Quadrant	Left Lower Quadrant	Right Lower Quadrant
Liver	Left lobe of liver	Lower lobe of left kidney	Lower lobe of right kidney
Gallbladder	Stomach	Sigmoid colon	Cecum
Duodenum	Spleen	Section of descending colon	Appendix
Head of pancreas	Upper lobe of left kidney	Left ovary	Section of ascending colon
Right adrenal gland	Pancreas	Left fallopian tube	Right ovary
Upper lobe of right kidney	Left adrenal gland	Left ureter	Right fallopian tube
Hepatic flexure of colon	Splenic flexure of colon	Left spermatic cord	Right ureter
Section of ascending colon	Section of transverse colon	Part of uterus	Right spermatic cord
Section of transverse colon	Section of descending colon		Part of uterus

TABLE 27.11 Organs in the Nine Abdominal Regions

Right Hypochondriac	Right Inguinal	Umbilical	
Right lobe of liver	Cecum	Omentum	Splenic flexure of colon
Gallbladder	Appendix	Mesentery	Upper half of left kidney
Part of duodenum	Lower end of ileum	Lower part of duodenum	Suprarenal gland
Hepatic flexure of colon	Right ureter	Part of jejunum and ileum	**Left Lumbar**
Upper half of right kidney	Right spermatic cord	**Hypogastric (Pubic)**	Descending colon
Suprarenal gland	Right ovary	Ileum	Lower half of left kidney
Right Lumbar	**Epigastric**	Bladder	Part of jejunum and ileum
Ascending colon	Aorta	Uterus	**Left Inguinal**
Lower half of right kidney	Pyloric end of stomach	**Left Hypochondriac**	Sigmoid colon
Part of duodenum and jejunum	Part of duodenum	Stomach	Left ureter
	Pancreas	Spleen	Left spermatic cord
	Part of liver	Tail of pancreas	Left ovary

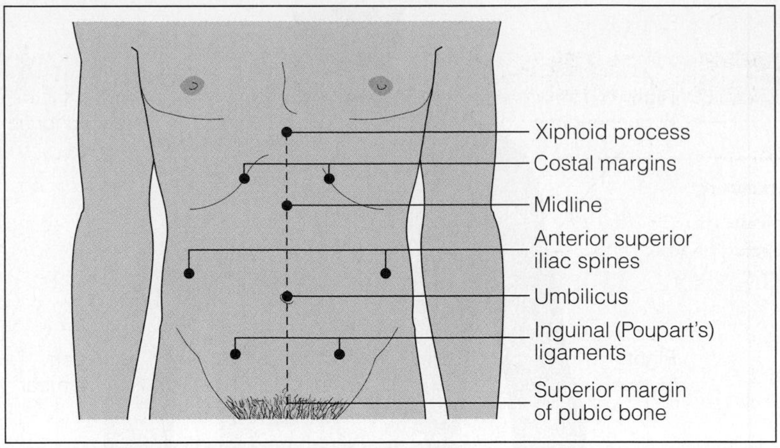

FIGURE 27.34 Landmarks commonly used to identify abdominal areas

Assessment of the abdomen involves all four methods of examination (inspection, auscultation, palpation, and percussion). When assessing the abdomen, the nurse performs inspection first, followed by auscultation, percussion, and palpation. Auscultation is done before these techniques because palpation and percussion cause movement or stimulation of the bowel, which can increase bowel motility and, thus, heighten bowel sounds, creating false results.

CLINICAL ALERT

If abdominal distension is observed on inspection, evaluation of the abdominal girth is necessary. Place a measuring tape around the abdomen at the level of the umbilicus. Mark the location of the measuring tape, so that additional measurement can be taken in the same location.

Skill 27.15 describes how to assess the abdomen.

SKILL 27.15

ASSESSING THE ABDOMEN

PLANNING

- Ask the client to urinate since an empty bladder makes the assessment more comfortable.
- Ensure that the room is warm since the client will be exposed.

Equipment

- Examining light
- Tape measure (metal or unstretchable cloth)
- Water-soluble skin-marking pencil
- Stethoscope

IMPLEMENTATION

Performance

1. Before performing the procedure, introduce yourself and verify the client's identity by using agency protocol. Explain to the client what you are going to do, why it is necessary, and how he or she can cooperate. Discuss how the results will be used in planning further care or treatments.
2. Perform hand hygiene and observe other appropriate infection prevention control procedures.
3. Provide for client privacy.
4. Inquire whether the client has any history of the following: incidence of abdominal pain; its location, onset, sequence, and chronology; its quality (description); its frequency; associated symptoms (e.g., nausea, vomiting, diarrhea); bowel habits; incidence of constipation or diarrhea (have client describe what client means by these terms); change in appetite, food intolerances, and foods ingested in last 24 hours; specific signs and symptoms (e.g., heartburn, flatulence, or belching, difficulty swallowing, hematemesis—vomiting blood—blood or mucus in stools, and aggravating and alleviating factors); previous problems and treatment (e.g., stomach ulcer, gallbladder surgery, history of jaundice).
5. Assist the client to a supine position, with the arms placed comfortably at the sides. Place small pillows beneath the knees and the head to reduce tension in the abdominal muscles. Expose only the client's abdomen from chest line to the pubic area to avoid chilling and shivering, which can tense the abdominal muscles.

(continued)

SKILL 27.15

ASSESSING THE ABDOMEN (*continued*)

ASSESSMENT	NORMAL FINDINGS	DEVIATIONS FROM NORMAL
Inspection of the Abdomen		
6. Inspect the abdomen for skin integrity (refer to the discussion of skin assessment, earlier in this chapter).	Unblemished skin; uniform colour; silver-white striae (stretch marks) or surgical scars	Presence of rash or other lesions; tense, glistening skin (may indicate ascites—an accumulation of fluid in the peritoneal cavity—edema); purple striae (associated with Cushing's disease or rapid weight gain and loss)
7. Inspect the abdomen for contour and symmetry:		
• Observe the abdominal contour (profile line from the rib margin to the pubic bone) while standing at the client's side when the client is supine.	Flat, rounded (convex), or scaphoid (concave)	Distended
• Ask the client to take a deep breath and to hold it. **Rationale: This makes an enlarged liver or spleen more obvious.**	No evidence of enlargement of liver or spleen	Evidence of enlargement of liver or spleen
• Assess the symmetry of contour while standing at the foot of the examination table.	Symmetric contour	Asymmetric contour (e.g., localized protrusions around umbilicus, inguinal ligaments, or scars, which can be a hernia or tumour)
• If distension is present, measure the abdominal girth by placing a tape around the abdomen at the level of the umbilicus (see ❶).		

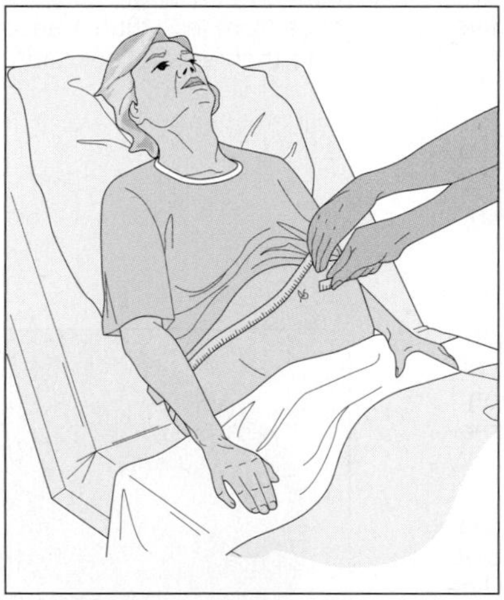

❶ Measuring abdominal girth

ASSESSMENT	NORMAL FINDINGS	DEVIATIONS FROM NORMAL
8. Observe abdominal movements associated with respiration, peristalsis, or aortic pulsations.	Symmetric movements caused by respiration; visible peristalsis in very lean people; aortic pulsations in thin persons at epigastric area	Limited movement because of pain or disease process; visible peristalsis in heavier clients (possible bowel obstruction); marked aortic pulsations
9. Observe the vascular pattern.	No visible vascular pattern	Visible venous pattern (dilated veins) is associated with liver disease, ascites and venocaval obstruction
Auscultation of the Abdomen		
10. Auscultate the abdomen for bowel sounds, vascular sounds, and peritoneal friction rubs. Warm the hands and the stethoscope diaphragms. **Rationale: Cold hands and a cold stethoscope may cause the client to contract the abdominal muscles, and these contractions may be heard during auscultation.**	Audible bowel sounds; absence of arterial bruits; absence of friction rub	Hypoactive (i.e., extremely soft and infrequent—one per minute), which can indicate decreased motility and are usually associated with manipulation of the bowel during surgery, inflammation, paralytic ileus, or late bowel obstruction; hyperactive or increased (i.e., high-pitched,

(continued)

SKILL 27.15

ASSESSING THE ABDOMEN (*continued*)

ASSESSMENT	NORMAL FINDINGS	DEVIATIONS FROM NORMAL
For Bowel Sounds • Use the flat-disc diaphragm. **Rationale: Intestinal sounds are relatively high pitched and best accentuated by the diaphragm. Light pressure with the stethoscope is adequate.** • Ask when the client last ate. **Rationale: Shortly after or long after eating, bowel sounds can normally increase. They are loudest when a meal is long overdue. Four to 7 hours after a meal, bowel sounds may be heard continuously over the ileocecal valve area while the digestive contents from the small intestine empty through the valve into the large intestine.** • Place diaphragm of the stethoscope in each of the four quadrants of the abdomen over all of the auscultatory sites shown in ❷. Listen for active bowel sounds.	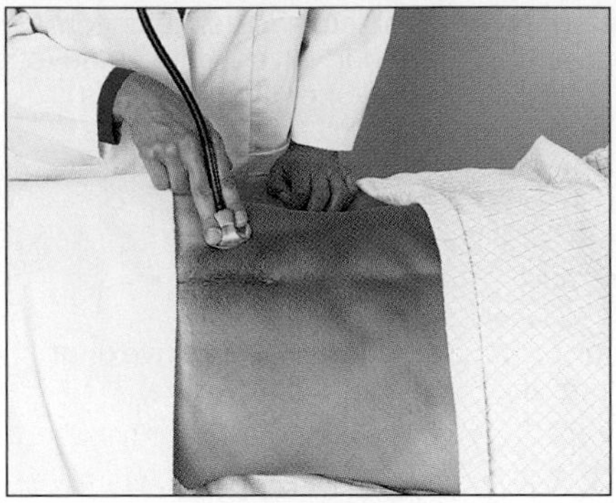 ❷ Auscultating the abdomen for bowel sounds Irregular gurgling noises occurring about every 5 to 20 seconds. The duration of a single sound may range from less than 1 second to more than several seconds	loud, rushing sounds that occur frequently—every 3 seconds), also known as borborygmi; hyperactive sounds indicate increased intestinal motility and are usually associated with diarrhea, an early bowel obstruction, or the use of laxatives; true absence of sounds (none heard in 3 to 5 minutes) indicates a cessation of intestinal motility; loud bruit over aortic area (possible aneurysm); bruit over renal or iliac arteries
For Vascular Sounds • Use the bell of the stethoscope over the aorta, renal arteries, iliac arteries, and femoral arteries (see ❸). • Listen for bruits.		
Peritoneal Friction Rubs • Peritoneal friction rubs are rough, grating sounds like two pieces of leather rubbing together. Friction rubs may be caused by inflammation, infections, or abnormal growths. • To auscultate the splenic site, place the stethoscope over the left lower rib cage in the anterior axillary line, and ask the client to take a deep breath. **Rationale: A deep breath may accentuate the sound of a friction rub area.** • To auscultate the liver site, place the stethoscope over the lower right rib cage. ❸ Sites for auscultating for vascular sounds	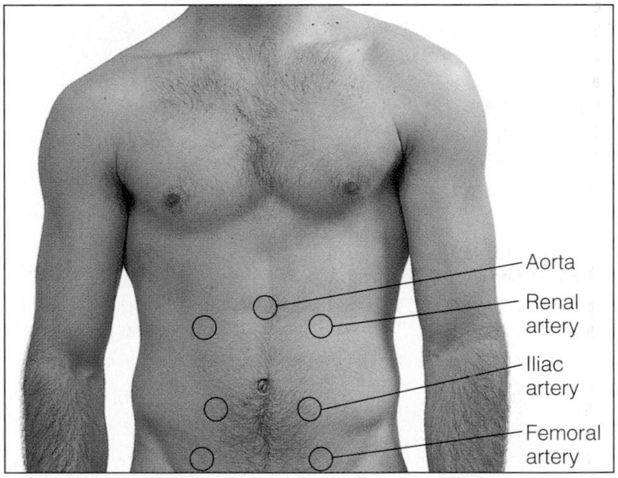	
Percussion of the Abdomen **11.** Percuss several areas in each of the four quadrants to determine presence of tympany (gas in stomach and intestines) and dullness (decrease, absence, or flatness of resonance over solid masses or fluid). Use a systematic pattern: begin in the lower left quadrant, proceed to the lower right quadrant, the upper right quadrant, and the upper left quadrant (see ❹).	Tympany over the stomach and gas-filled bowels; dullness, especially over the liver and spleen, or a full bladder	Large dull areas (associated with presence of fluid or a tumour)

(continued)

SKILL 27.15

ASSESSING THE ABDOMEN (*continued*)

ASSESSMENT	NORMAL FINDINGS	DEVIATIONS FROM NORMAL

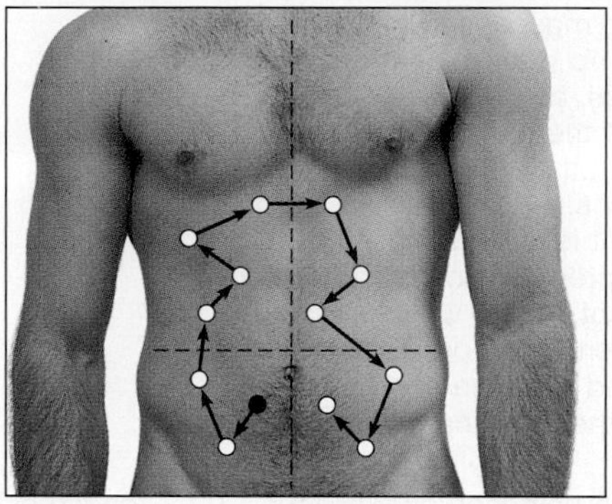

❹ Systematic percussion sites for all four quadrants

Percussion of the Liver

12. Percuss the liver to determine its size. Begin in the right MCL below the level of the umbilicus and proceed as follows:
    - Percuss upward over tympanic areas until a dull percussion sound indicates the lower liver border. Mark the site with a skin-marking pencil (see ❺).
    - Then percuss downward at the right MCL, beginning from an area of lung resonance and progressing downward until a dull percussion sound indicates the upper liver border (usually at the fifth to seventh interspace). Mark this site.
    - Measure the distance between the two marks (upper and lower liver border) in centimetres to establish the liver span or size.
    - Repeat these steps at the midsternal line.

Normal findings: 6 cm to 12 cm in the MCL 4 cm to 8 cm at the midsternal line

Deviations from normal: Enlarged size (associated with liver disease)

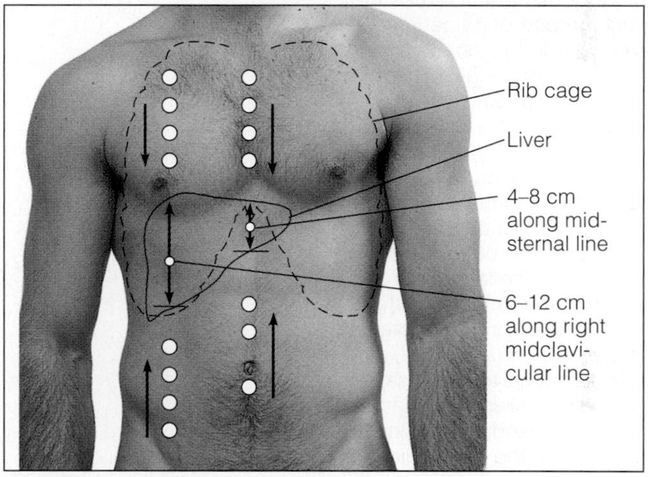

❺ Percussion pattern to determine liver size

Palpation of the Abdomen

13. Perform light palpation first to detect areas of tenderness or muscle guarding. Systematically explore all four quadrants. Ensure that the client's position is appropriate for relaxation of the abdominal muscles, and warm your hands. **Rationale: Cold hands can elicit muscle tension and thus impede palpatory evaluation.**

Normal findings: No tenderness; relaxed abdomen with smooth, consistent tension

Deviations from normal: Tenderness and hypersensitivity; superficial masses; localized areas of increased tension

Light Palpation

- Hold the palm of your hand slightly above the client's abdomen, with your fingers parallel to the abdomen.
- Depress the abdominal wall lightly, about 1 cm or to the depth of the subcutaneous tissue, with the pads of your fingers (see ❻).
- Move the finger pads in a slight circular motion.

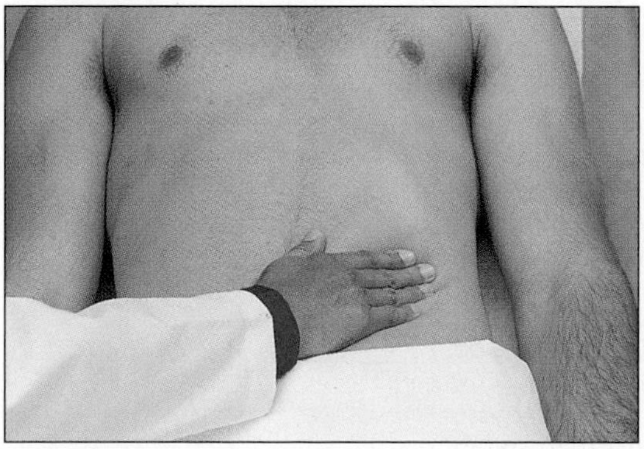

❻ Light palpation of the abdomen

(continued)

SKILL 27.15

ASSESSING THE ABDOMEN (*continued*)

ASSESSMENT	NORMAL FINDINGS	DEVIATIONS FROM NORMAL
• Note areas of tenderness or superficial pain, masses, and muscle guarding. To determine areas of tenderness, ask the client to tell you about them and watch for changes in the client's facial expressions. • If the client is excessively ticklish, begin by pressing your hand on top of the client's hand while pressing lightly. Then slide your hand off the client's and onto the abdomen to continue the examination.		
14. Perform deep palpation over all four quadrants. • Palpate sensitive areas last. • Press the distal half of the palmar surface of the fingers of one hand into the abdominal wall *or* use the bimanual method of palpation discussed earlier in this chapter. • Depress the abdominal wall about 4 cm to 5 cm (see ❼). • Note masses and the structure of underlying contents. If a mass is present, determine its size, location, mobility, contour, consistency, and tenderness. Normal abdominal structures that can be mistaken for masses include the lateral borders of the rectus abdominis muscles, the feces-filled colon, the aorta, and the uterus. • Check for rebound tenderness in areas where the client complains of pain. With one hand, press slowly and deeply over the area indicated and then lift the hand quickly. If the client does not complain of pain during the deep pressure but indicates pain at the release of the pressure, rebound tenderness is present. This can indicate peritoneal inflammation and should be reported to the health-care provider immediately.	Tenderness may be present near xyphoid process, over cecum, and over sigmoid colon	Generalized or localized areas of tenderness; mobile or fixed masses
Palpation of the Liver		
15. Palpate the liver to detect enlargement and tenderness. Two bimanual approaches are used in palpation of the liver. In using the first method, place one hand along the anterior rib cage and the other hand on the posterior rib cage. • Stand on the client's right side.	May not be palpable; border feels smooth	Enlarged (abnormal finding, even if liver is smooth and not tender); smooth but tender; nodular or hard

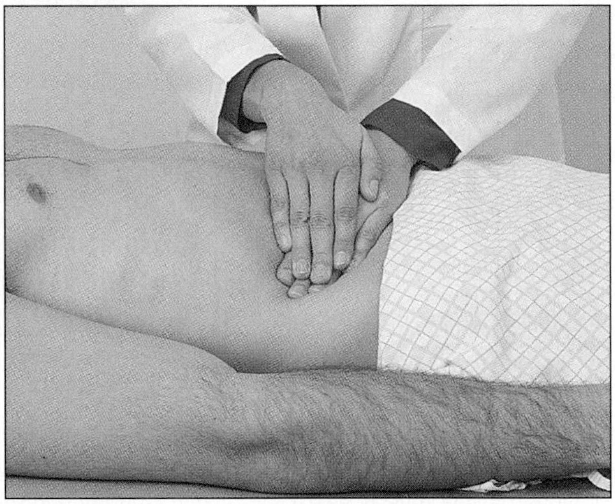

❼ Deep palpation of the abdomen

(continued)

SKILL 27.15

ASSESSING THE ABDOMEN (*continued*)

ASSESSMENT	NORMAL FINDINGS	DEVIATIONS FROM NORMAL
• Place your left hand on the posterior thorax at about the 11th or 12th rib. This hand is used to push upward and provide support of underlying structures for the subsequent anterior palpation. • Place your right hand along the rib cage at about a 45° angle to the right of the rectus abdominis muscle or parallel to the rectus muscle with the fingers pointing toward the rib cage (see 8). • While the client exhales, exert a gradual and gentle downward and forward pressure beneath the costal margin until you reach a depth of 4 cm to 5 cm. **Rationale: During expiration, the abdominal wall relaxes, facilitating deep palpation.** • Maintain your hand position, and ask the client to inhale deeply. **Rationale: This makes the liver border descend and moves the liver into a palpable position.** • While the client inhales, feel the liver border move against your hand. It should feel firm and have a regular contour. If you do not palpate the liver initially, ask the client to take two or three more deep breaths while you maintain or apply slightly more palpation pressure. Livers are harder to palpate in obese, tense, or very physically fit people. • If the liver is enlarged (i.e., palpable below the costal margin), measure the number of centimetres it extends below the costal region. A second method is the bimanual palpation method discussed previously, in which one hand is superimposed on the other (see Figure 27.2, p. 559). The techniques and principles used for palpating the liver with one hand apply to the two-hand method as well.	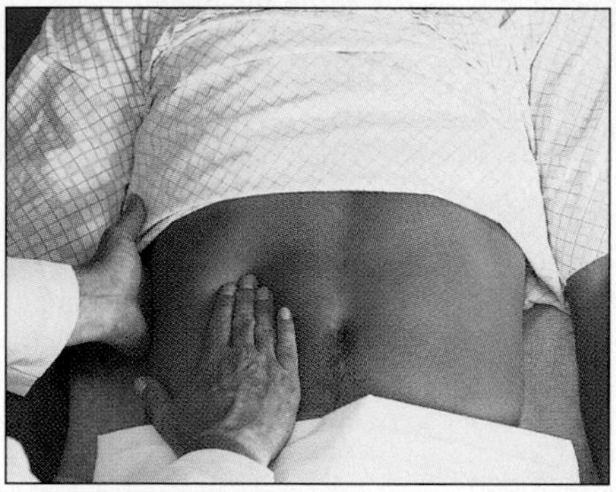 8 Palpating the liver 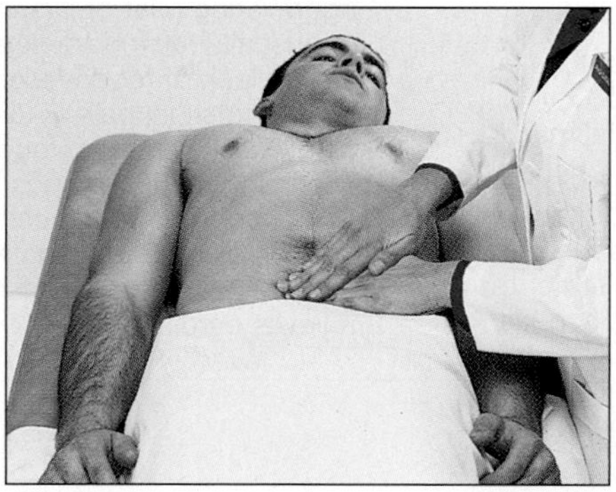 9 Palpating the bladder	
Palpation of the Bladder		
16. Palpate the area above the pubic symphysis if the client's history indicates possible urinary retention (see 9).	Not palpable	Distended and palpable as smooth, round, tense mass (indicates urinary retention)

17. Document findings in the client record by using forms or checklists supplemented by narrative notes when appropriate.

EVALUATION

- Perform a detailed follow-up examination of other systems based on findings that deviated from expected or normal for the client. Relate findings to previous assessment data if available.
- Report significant deviations from normal to the appropriate members of the health-care team.

Lifespan Considerations

Assessing the Abdomen

INFANTS

- Internal organs of newborns and infants are proportionately larger than those of older children and adults, so their abdomens are rounded and tend to protrude.
- The infant's liver may be palpable 1 cm to 2 cm below the right costal margin.
- Umbilical hernias may be present at birth.

CHILDREN

- Toddlers have a characteristic "pot belly" appearance, which can persist until age 3 to 4 years.
- Late-preschool-age and school-age children are leaner and have a flat abdomen.
- Peristaltic waves may be more visible than in adults.
- Children may not be able to pinpoint areas of tenderness; by observing facial expressions the examiner can determine areas of maximum tenderness.
- The liver is relatively larger than in adults. It can be palpated 1 cm to 2 cm below the right costal margin.
- If the child is ticklish, guarding, or fearful, use a task that requires concentration (such as squeezing the hands together) to distract the child, or have the child place his or her hands on yours as you palpate the abdomen, "helping" you to do the exam.

OLDER ADULTS

- The rounded abdomens of older adults are caused by an increase in adipose tissue and a decrease in muscle tone.
- The abdominal wall is slacker and thinner, making palpation easier and more accurate than in younger clients. Muscle wasting and loss of fibroconnective tissue occur.
- The pain threshold in older adults is often higher; major abdominal problems, such as appendicitis or other acute emergencies, may therefore go undetected.
- Gastrointestinal pain needs to be differentiated from cardiac pain. Gastrointestinal pain may be located in the chest or abdomen, whereas cardiac pain is usually located in the chest. Factors aggravating gastrointestinal pain are usually related to either ingestion or lack of food intake; gastrointestinal pain is usually relieved by antacids, food, or assuming an upright position. Common factors that can aggravate cardiac pain are activity or anxiety; rest or nitroglycerine relieves cardiac pain.
- Stool passes through the intestines at a slower rate in older adults, and the perception of stimuli that produce the urge to defecate often diminishes.
- Fecal incontinence can occur in confused or neurologically impaired older adults.
- Many older adults erroneously believe that the absence of a daily bowel movement signifies constipation. When assessing for constipation, the nurse must consider the client's diet, activity, medications, and characteristics and ease of passage of feces as well as the frequency of bowel movements.
- The incidence of colon cancer is higher among older than younger adults. Symptoms include a change in bowel function, rectal bleeding, and weight loss. Changes in bowel function, however, are associated with many factors, such as diet, exercise, and medications.
- Decreased absorption of oral medications often occurs with aging.
- In the liver, impaired metabolism of some drugs may occur with aging.

Musculoskeletal System

The musculoskeletal system encompasses the muscles, bones, and joints. The completeness of an assessment of this system depends largely on the needs and problems of the individual client. The nurse usually assesses the musculoskeletal system for muscle strength, tone, size, and symmetry of muscle development, fasciculations, and tremors. A **fasciculation** is an abnormal contraction (shortening) of a bundle of muscle fibres. A **tremor** is an involuntary trembling of a limb or body part. Tremors may involve large groups of muscle fibres or small bundles of muscle fibres. An **intention tremor** becomes more apparent when an individual attempts a voluntary movement, such as holding a cup of coffee. A **resting tremor** is more apparent when the client is at rest and it diminishes with activity.

Bones are assessed for normal form. Joints are assessed for tenderness, swelling, thickening, crepitation (the sound of bone grating on bone), presence of nodules, and range of motion. Body posture is assessed for normal standing and sitting positions. For information about body posture, see Chapter 38.

Skill 27.16 describes how to assess the musculoskeletal system.

SKILL 27.16

ASSESSING THE MUSCULOSKELETAL SYSTEM

Equipment: Goniometer

IMPLEMENTATION

Performance

1. Before performing the procedure, introduce yourself and verify the client's identity by using agency protocol. Explain to the client what you are going to do, why it is necessary, and how he or she can cooperate. Discuss how the results will be used in planning further care or treatments.
2. Perform hand hygiene and observe other appropriate infection prevention and control procedures.
3. Provide for client privacy.
4. Inquire whether the client has any history of the following: presence of muscle pain: onset, location, character, associated phenomena (e.g., redness and swelling of joints), and aggravating and alleviating factors; limitations to movement or inability to perform activities of daily living; previous sports injuries; loss of function without pain.

ASSESSMENT	NORMAL FINDINGS	DEVIATIONS FROM NORMAL
Muscles		
5. Inspect the muscles for size. Compare the muscles on one side of the body (e.g., of the arm, thigh, and calf) to the same muscle on the other side. For any discrepancies, measure the muscles with a tape.	Equal size on both sides of body	*Atrophy* (a decrease in size) or *hypertrophy* (an increase in size), asymmetry
6. Inspect the muscles and tendons for contractures (shortening).	No contractures	Malposition of body part, such as foot drop (foot flexed downward)
7. Inspect the muscles for tremors, for example, by having the client hold the arms out in front of the body.	No tremors	Presence of tremor
8. Palpate muscles at rest to determine muscle tonicity (the normal condition of tension, or tone, of a muscle at rest).	Normally firm	Atonic (lacking tone)
9. Palpate muscles while the client is active and passive for flaccidity, spasticity, and smoothness of movement.	Smooth coordinated movements	*Flaccidity* (weakness or laxness) or spasticity (sudden involuntary muscle contraction)
10. Test muscle strength. Compare the right side with the left side. *Sternocleidomastoid:* Client turns the head to one side against the resistance of your hand. Repeat with the other side. *Trapezius:* Client shrugs the shoulders against the resistance of your hands. *Deltoid:* Client holds arm up and resists while you try to push it down. *Biceps:* Client fully extends each arm and tries to flex it while you attempt to hold arm in extension. *Triceps:* Client flexes each arm and then tries to extend it against your attempt to keep arm in flexion. *Wrist and finger muscles:* Client spreads the fingers and resists as you attempt to push the fingers together. *Grip strength:* Client grasps your index and middle fingers while the you try to pull the fingers out.	Equal strength on each body side	25% or less of normal strength **Grading Muscle Strength** 0: 0% of normal strength; complete paralysis 1: 10% of normal strength; no movement, contraction of muscle is palpable or visible 2: 25% of normal strength; full muscle movement against gravity, with support 3: 50% of normal strength; normal movement against gravity 4: 75% of normal strength; normal full movement against gravity and against minimal resistance 5: 100% of normal strength; normal full movement against gravity and against full resistance

(continued)

SKILL 27.16

ASSESSING THE MUSCULOSKELETAL SYSTEM (*continued*)

ASSESSMENT	NORMAL FINDINGS	DEVIATIONS FROM NORMAL
Hip muscles: Client is supine, both legs extended; client raises one leg at a time while you attempt to hold it down.		
Hip abduction: Client is supine, both legs extended. Place your hands on the lateral surface of each knee; client spreads the legs apart against your resistance.		
Hip adduction: Client is in same position as for hip abduction. Place your hands between the knees; client brings the legs together against your resistance.		
Hamstrings: Client is supine, both knees bent. Client resists while you attempt to straighten the legs.		
Quadriceps: Client is supine, knee partially extended; client resists while you attempt to flex the knee.		
Muscles of the ankles and feet: Client resists while you attempt to dorsiflex the foot and again resists while you attempt to flex the foot.		
Bones		
11. Inspect the skeleton for structure.	No deformities	Bones misaligned
12. Palpate the bones to locate any areas of edema or tenderness.	No tenderness or swelling	Presence of tenderness or swelling (may indicate fracture, neoplasms, or osteoporosis)
Joints		
13. Inspect the joints for swelling. Palpate each joint for tenderness, smoothness of movement, swelling, crepitation, and presence of nodules.	No swelling; no tenderness, swelling, crepitation, or nodules; joints move smoothly	One or more swollen joints; presence of tenderness, swelling, crepitation, or nodules
14. Assess joint range of motion. See Chapter 38 for the types of joint movements. • Ask the client to move selected body parts. The amount of joint movement can be measured by a goniometer, a device that measures the angle of the joint in degrees (see ❶).	Varies to some degree in accordance with person's genetic makeup and degree of physical activity	Limited range of motion in one or more joints

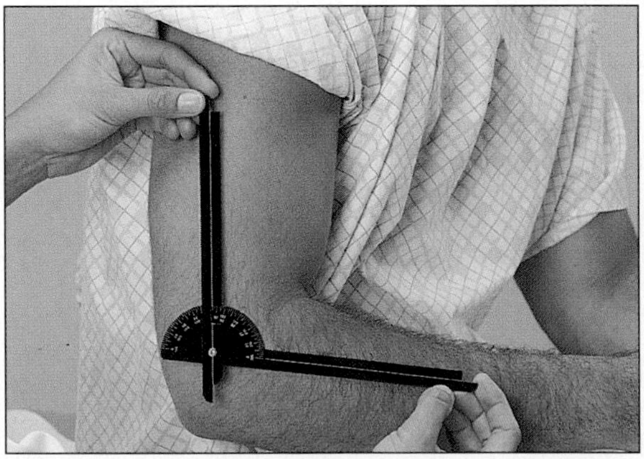

❶ A goniometer is used to measure range of motion

(continued)

SKILL 27.16

ASSESSING THE MUSCULOSKELETAL SYSTEM (*continued*)

15. Document findings in the client record by using forms or checklists supplemented by narrative notes when appropriate.

EVALUATION

- Perform a detailed follow-up examination of other systems based on findings that deviated from expected or normal for the client. Relate findings to previous assessment data if available.
- Report significant deviations from normal to the appropriate members of the health-care team.

Lifespan Considerations

Assessing the Musculoskeletal System

INFANTS

- Palpate the clavicles of newborns. A mass and crepitus may indicate a fracture experienced during vaginal delivery. The newborn may also have limited movement of the arm and shoulder on the affected side.
- When the arms and legs of newborns are pulled to extension and released, newborns naturally return to the flexed fetal position.
- Check muscle strength by holding the infant lightly under the arms with feet placed lightly on a table. Infants should not fall through the hands and should be able to bear body weight on their legs if normal muscle strength is present.
- Check infants for developmental dysplasia of the hip (congenital dislocation) by examining for asymmetric gluteal folds, asymmetric abduction of the legs (Ortolani and Barlow tests), or apparent shortening of the femur.
- Infants should be able to sit without support by 8 months of age, crawl by 7 to 10 months, and walk by 12 to 15 months.
- Observe for symmetry of muscle mass, strength, and function.

CHILDREN

- Pronation and "toeing in" of the feet is common in children between 12 and 30 months of age.
- Genu varum (bowleg) is normal in children for about 1 year after beginning to walk.
- Genu valgus (knock-knee) is normal in preschool and young school-age children.
- Lordosis (swayback) is common in children before age 5.
- Observe the child in normal activities to determine motor function.
- During the rapid growth spurts of adolescence, spinal curvature and rotation (scoliosis) may appear. Children should be assessed for scoliosis by age 12 and annually until their growth slows. Curvature greater than 10% should be referred for further medical evaluation.
- Muscle mass increases in adolescence, especially as children engage in strenuous physical activity, and requires increased nutritional intake.
- Children are at risk for injury related to physical activity and should be assessed for nutritional status, physical conditioning, and safety precautions in order to prevent injury.
- Adolescent girls who participate in strenuous athletic activities are at risk for delayed menses, osteoporosis, and eating disorders; assessment should include a history of these factors.

OLDER ADULTS

- Muscle mass decreases progressively with age, but wide variations exist among different individuals.
- The decrease in speed, strength, resistance to fatigue, reaction time, and coordination in the older person is due to a decrease in nerve conduction and muscle tone.
- The bones can become more fragile, and osteoporosis (if present) leads to a loss of total bone mass. As a result, some older adults are predisposed to fractures and compressed vertebrae.
- In most older adults, osteoarthritic changes in the joints can be observed.
- Note any surgical scars from joint replacement surgeries.

Neurological System

A thorough neurological examination can take 1 to 3 hours; however, routine screening tests are usually done first. If the results of these tests raise questions, more extensive evaluations are made. Three major considerations determine the extent of a neurological exam: (1) the client's chief complaints, (2) the client's physical condition (i.e., level of consciousness and ability to ambulate), because many parts of the examination require movement

Evidence-Informed Practice

Do Routine Screening Programs Have a Positive or Negative Psychological Impact?

Although screening for pathology in asymptomatic people is viewed as a means for early detection and treatment as well as being reassuring for many people, Doust, Mannes, Bastian, and Edwards (2007) hypothesize that a screening program might cause harm because of the physical and psychological effects of the screening process itself, the psychological effects that arise when there is a false positive result (i.e., the original screening indicates a problem but more detailed screening shows that there is no problem); any delay in diagnosis related to a false negative result (i.e., the screening test is negative but there is actually a problem); and the psychological effects of learning about a diagnosis earlier when nothing can be done to influence the pathology. This systematic review protocol outlines how these researchers will attempt to answer the hypotheses they have identified.

NURSING IMPLICATIONS: Most Canadians are aware of the many benefits of early detection of illness. However, as much as many people look forward to their annual checkup to make sure they receive the screening they need, others dread their periodic health assessment for fear that pathology will be detected. Nurses must be sensitive to the meaning that people attribute to the health-screening process and be aware of how positive or negative this can be for each client. Those who are stressed by the periodic health-screening process may need support before, during, and after the screening to ensure that the minimum harmful effects (if any) occur.

Source: Based on "Interventions for Improving Understanding and Minimising the Psychological Impact of Screening (Protocol)," by J. Doust, P. Mannes, H. Bastian, and A. Edwards, 2007, *Cochrane Database of Systematic Reviews 2007, 4.*

and coordination of the extremities, and (3) the client's willingness to participate and cooperate.

Examination of the neurological system includes assessment of (1) mental status, including level of consciousness, (2) the cranial nerves, (3) reflexes, (4) motor function, and (5) sensory function. Parts of the neurological assessment are performed throughout the health examination. For example, the nurse performs a large part of the mental status assessment during the taking of the history and when observing the client's general appearance. Also, the nurse assesses the function of many cranial nerves. The second, third, fourth, fifth, and sixth cranial nerves (ophthalmic branch) are assessed with the eyes and vision, and the eighth cranial nerve (cochlear branch) is assessed with the ears and hearing.

Mental Status

Assessment of mental status reveals the client's general cerebral function. These functions include intellectual (cognitive) and emotional (affective) functions.

If problems with the use of language, memory, concentration, or thought processes are noted during the nursing history, a more extensive examination is required during neurological assessment. Major areas of mental status assessment include language, orientation, memory, and attention span and calculation.

LANGUAGE Any defects in or loss of the power to express the self through speech, writing, or sign language, or to comprehend spoken or written language because of disease or injury of the cerebral cortex, is called **aphasia**. Aphasias can be categorized as sensory or receptive aphasia and motor or expressive aphasia.

Sensory or *receptive aphasia* is the loss of the ability to comprehend written or spoken words. Two types of sensory aphasia are auditory (or acoustic) aphasia and visual aphasia. Clients with *auditory aphasia* have lost the ability to understand the symbolic content associated with sounds. Clients with *visual aphasia* have lost the ability to understand printed or written letters and numbers.

Motor or *expressive aphasia* involves loss of the power to express the self through writing, making signs, or speaking. Clients may find that even though they can recall words, they have lost the ability to combine speech sounds into words.

ORIENTATION This aspect of the assessment determines the client's ability to recognize other persons (*person*), awareness of when and where they presently are (*time* and *place*), and who they are (*self*).

CLINICAL ALERT

Nurses often chart that the client is "awake, alert, and oriented ×3 [or times three]." This refers to accurate awareness of persons, time, and place. Remember, "person" indicates that the client recognizes others, not that the client can state what his or her own name is.

MEMORY The nurse assesses the client's recall of information presented seconds previously (immediate recall), events or information from earlier in the day or examination (recent memory), and knowledge recalled from months or years back (remote or long-term memory).

ATTENTION SPAN AND CALCULATION This component determines the client's ability to focus on a mental task that is expected to be able to be performed by persons of normal intelligence.

Level of Consciousness

Level of consciousness can lie anywhere along a continuum from a state of alertness to coma. A fully alert client responds to questions spontaneously; a comatose client may not respond to verbal stimuli. The Glasgow Coma Scale was originally developed to predict recovery from a head injury; however, it is used by many professionals to assess level of consciousness. It tests three major areas: eye response, motor response, and verbal response. An assessment totalling 15 points indicates the client is alert and completely oriented. A comatose client scores 7 or fewer points. See Table 27.12.

Cranial Nerves

The nurse needs to be aware of nerve functions to detect abnormalities (see Table 27.13). In some cases, each nerve is assessed; in other cases only selected nerve functions are evaluated.

Reflexes

A **reflex** is an automatic response of the body to a stimulus. It is not voluntarily learned or conscious. The deep tendon reflex is activated when a tendon is stimulated (tapped) and its associated muscle contracts. The quality of a reflex response varies among individuals and by age. As a person ages, reflex responses may become less intense.

TABLE 27.12 Levels of Consciousness: Glasgow Coma Scale

Faculty Measured	Response	Score
Eye opening	Spontaneous	4
	To verbal command	3
	To pain	2
	No response	1
Motor response	To verbal command	6
	To localized pain	5
	Flexes and withdraws	4
	Flexes abnormally	3
	Extends abnormally	2
	No response	1
Verbal response	Oriented, converses	5
	Disoriented, converses	4
	Uses inappropriate words	3
	Makes incomprehensible sounds	2
	No response	1
Glasgow Coma Scale Score		/15

CLINICAL ALERT

All questions and tests used in a neurological examination must be age, language, education level, and culturally appropriate. Individualize questions and tests before using them.

Reflexes are tested by using a percussion hammer. The response is described on a scale of 0 to 4. Experience is necessary to determine the appropriate scoring for an individual. When assessing reflexes, it is important for the nurse to compare one side of the body with the other to evaluate the symmetry of response. Several reflexes are normally tested during the physical examination: (1) the biceps reflex, (2) the triceps reflex, (3) the brachioradialis reflex, (4) the patellar reflex, (5) the Achilles reflex, and (6) the plantar (Babinski) reflex.

Motor Function

Neurological assessment of the motor system evaluates proprioception and cerebellar function. Structures involved in proprioception are the proprioceptors, the posterior columns of the spinal cord, the cerebellum, and the vestibular apparatus (which is innervated by the eighth cranial nerve) in the labyrinth of the internal ear.

Proprioceptors are sensory nerve terminals, occurring chiefly in the muscles, tendons, joints, and internal ear, that give information about movements and the position of the body. Stimuli from the proprioceptors travel through the posterior columns of the spinal cord. Deficits of function of the posterior columns of the spinal cord result in impairment of muscle and position sense. Clients with such an impairment often must watch their own arm and leg movements to ascertain the position of the limbs.

The cerebellum (1) helps to control posture; (2) acts with the cerebral cortex to make body movements smooth and coordinated; and (3) controls skeletal muscles to maintain equilibrium.

Sensory Function

Sensory functions include touch, pain, temperature, position, and tactile discrimination. The first three are routinely tested. The spinothalamic tract conducts sensations of superficial pain and temperature to the sensory cortex. The posterior column conducts the sensation of position. Generally, the face, arms, legs, hands, and feet are tested for touch and pain, although all parts of the body can be tested. If the client complains of numbness, peculiar sensations, or paralysis, the nurse should check sensation more carefully over flexor and extensor surfaces of limbs, mapping out clearly any abnormality of touch or pain by examining responses in the area about every 2.5 cm. This is

TABLE 27.13 Cranial Nerve Functions and Assessment Methods

Cranial Nerve	Name (Mnemonic)*	Type	Function	Assessment Method
I	Olfactory (On)	Sensory	Smell	Ask client to close eyes and identify different mild aromas, such as coffee, vanilla, orange, lemon, lime, chocolate.
II	Optic (Old)	Sensory	Vision and visual fields	Ask client to read Snellen chart, check visual fields by confrontation, and conduct an ophthalmoscopic examination.
III	Oculomotor (Olympus's)	Motor	Extraocular eye movement (EOM); movement of sphincter of pupil; movement of ciliary muscles of lens; opening of upper eyelid	Assess six ocular movements and pupil reaction.
IV	Trochlear (Towering)	Motor	EOM; specifically moves eyeball downward and laterally	Assess six ocular movements.
V	Trigeminal (Tops)			
	Ophthalmic branch	Sensory	Sensation of cornea, skin of face, and nasal mucosa	While client looks upward, lightly touch lateral sclera of eye to elicit blink reflex. To test light-touch sensation, have client close eyes, wipe a wisp of cotton (formed by twirling together a few fibres of cotton from a cotton ball or Q-Tip) over client's forehead and paranasal sinuses. To test deep sensation, use alternating blunt and sharp ends of a safety pin over same areas.
	Maxillary branch	Sensory	Sensation of skin of face and anterior oral cavity (tongue and teeth)	Assess skin sensation as for ophthalmic branch above.
	Mandibular branch	Sensory	Muscles of mastication; sensation of skin of face	Ask client to clench teeth.
VI	Abducens (A)	Motor	EOM; moves eyeball laterally	Assess directions of gaze.
VII	Facial (Finn)	Motor and sensory	Facial expression; taste (anterior two-thirds of tongue); closing of eyelid	Ask client to smile, raise the eyebrows, frown, puff out cheeks, close eyes tightly. Ask client to identify various tastes placed on tip and sides of tongue: sugar (sweet), salt, lemon juice (sour), and quinine (bitter); identify areas of taste.
VIII	Auditory (And)			
	Vestibular branch	Sensory	Equilibrium	Assessment methods are discussed with cerebellar functions (in next section).
	Cochlear branch	Sensory	Hearing	Assess client's ability to hear spoken word and vibrations of tuning fork.
IX	Glosso-pharyngeal (German)	Motor and sensory	Swallowing ability; tongue movement; taste (posterior tongue)	Apply tastes on posterior tongue for identification. Ask client to move tongue from side to side and up and down.
X	Vagus (Viewed)	Motor and sensory	Sensation of pharynx and larynx; swallowing; vocal cord movement	Assessed with cranial nerve IX; assess client's speech for hoarseness.
XI	Spinal accessory (Some)	Motor	Head movement; shrugging of shoulders	Ask client to shrug shoulders against resistance from your hands and turn head to side against resistance from your hand (repeat for other side).
XII	Hypoglossal (Hops)	Motor	Protrusion of tongue; moves tongue up and down and side to side	Ask client to protrude tongue at midline, then move it side to side.

**Mnemonic: On Old Olympus's Towering Tops A Finn And German Viewed Some Hops.*

a lengthy procedure. Abnormal responses to touch stimuli include loss of sensation **(anaesthesia)**; more than normal sensation **(hyperesthesia)**; less than normal sensation **(hypoesthesia)**; or an abnormal sensation, such as numbness and prickling as in "pins and needles" (**paresthesia**).

A more detailed neurological examination includes position sense, temperature sense, and tactile discrimination.

Three types of tactile discrimination are generally tested: **one-** and **two-point discrimination**, the ability to sense whether one or two areas of the skin are being stimulated by pressure; **stereognosis**, the act of recognizing objects by touching and manipulating them; and **extinction**, the failure to perceive touch on one side of the body when two symmetric areas of the body are touched simultaneously.

Skill 27.17 describes how to assess the neurological system.

SKILL 27.17

ASSESSING THE NEUROLOGICAL SYSTEM

PLANNING

If possible, determine whether a screening or full neurological examination is indicated. This will affect the preparation of the client, equipment, and timing.

Equipment (Depending on Components of Examination)

- Sugar, salt, lemon juice, quinine
- Percussion hammer
- Tongue depressors (one broken diagonally for testing pain sensation)
- Wisps of cotton wool to assess light-touch sensation
- Test tubes of hot and cold water for skin temperature assessment (optional)
- Pins or needles for tactile discrimination

IMPLEMENTATION

Performance

1. Before performing the procedure, introduce yourself and verify the client's identity by using agency protocol. Explain to the client what you are going to do, why it is necessary, and how he or she can cooperate. Discuss how the results will be used in planning further care or treatments.
2. Perform hand hygiene and observe other appropriate infection prevention and control procedures.
3. Provide for client privacy.
4. Inquire whether the client has any history of the following: presence of pain in the head, back, or extremities, as well as onset and aggravating and alleviating factors; disorientation to time, place, or person; speech disorder; history of loss of consciousness, fainting, convulsions, trauma, tingling or numbness, tremors or tics, limping, paralysis, uncontrolled muscle movements, loss of memory, mood swings, or problems with smell, vision, taste, touch, or hearing.

Language

5. If the client displays difficulty speaking,
   - Point to common objects, and ask the client to name them.
   - Ask the client to read some words and to match the printed and written words with pictures.
   - Ask the client to respond to simple verbal and written commands (e.g., "point to your toes" or "raise your left arm").

Orientation

6. Determine the client's orientation to *person, time, and place* by tactful questioning. Ask the client the city and province or territory of residence, time of day, date, day of the week, duration of illness, and names of family members. To evaluate the response, you must know the correct answer. More direct questioning may be necessary for some people (e.g., "Where are you now?" "What day is it today?"). Most people readily accept these questions if initially the nurse asks, "Do you get confused at times?" If the client cannot answer these questions accurately, also include assessment of the *self* by asking the client to state his or her full name.

Memory

7. Listen for lapses in memory. Ask the client about difficulty with memory. If problems are apparent, three categories of memory are tested: immediate recall, recent memory, and remote memory.

To assess immediate recall:

- Ask the client to repeat a series of three digits (e.g., 7, 4, 3), spoken slowly.
- Gradually increase the number of digits (e.g., 7, 4, 3, 5; then 7, 4, 3, 5, 6; and 7, 4, 3, 5, 6, 7, 2), until the client fails to repeat the series correctly.
- Start again with a series of three digits, but this time ask the client to repeat them backward. The average person can repeat a series of five to eight digits in sequence and four to six digits in reverse order.

To assess recent memory:

- Ask the client to recall the recent events of the day, such as how the client got to the clinic. This information must be validated.
- Ask the client to recall information given early in the interview (e.g., the name of a doctor or nurse).
- Provide the client with three facts to recall (e.g., a colour, an object, and an address), or a three-digit number, and ask the client to repeat all three. Later in the interview, ask the client to recall all three items.

(continued)

SKILL 27.17

ASSESSING THE NEUROLOGICAL SYSTEM *(continued)*

To assess remote memory, ask the client to describe a previous illness or surgery (e.g., 5 years ago), or a birthday or an anniversary.

Attention Span and Calculation

8. Test the ability to concentrate or maintain *attention span* by asking the client to recite the alphabet or to count backward from 100. Test the ability to calculate by asking the client to subtract 7 or 3 progressively from 100 (i.e., 100, 93, 86, 79, or 100, 97, 94, 91), referred to as *serial sevens* or *serial threes*. Normally, an adult can complete serial sevens test in about 90 seconds with three or fewer errors. Because educational level, language, or cultural differences affect calculating ability, this test may be inappropriate for some people.

Level of Consciousness

9. Apply the Glasgow Coma Scale: eye response, motor response, and verbal response. An assessment totalling 15 points indicates the client is alert and completely oriented. A comatose client scores 7 or fewer points (see Table 27.12, p. 635).

Cranial Nerves

10. For the specific functions and assessment methods of each cranial nerve, see Table 27.13 (p. 636). Test each nerve not already evaluated in another component of the health assessment.

Reflexes

11. Test reflexes by using a percussion hammer, comparing one side of the body with the other to evaluate the symmetry of response:
    0 No reflex response
    1 Minimal activity (hypoactive)
    2 Normal response
    3 More active than normal
    4 Maximal activity (hyperactive)

Biceps Reflex The biceps reflex tests the spinal cord level C-5 and C-6.

- Partially flex the client's arm at the elbow, and rest the forearm over the thighs, placing the palm of the hand down.
- Place the thumb of your nondominant hand horizontally over the biceps tendon.
- Deliver a blow (slight downward thrust) with the percussion hammer to your thumb (see ❶).
- Observe the normal slight flexion of the elbow, and feel the bicep's contraction through your thumb.

Triceps Reflex The triceps reflex tests the spinal cord level C-7 and C-8.

- Flex the client's arm at the elbow, and support it in the palm of your nondominant hand (see ❷).
- Palpate the triceps tendon about 2 cm to 5 cm above the elbow.
- Deliver a blow with the percussion hammer directly to the tendon.
- Observe the normal slight extension of the elbow.

Brachioradialis Reflex The brachioradialis reflex tests the spinal cord level C-3 and C-6.

- Rest the client's forearm in a relaxed position externally rotated on a firm surface.
- Deliver a blow with the percussion hammer directly on the radius 2 cm to 5 cm above the wrist or the styloid process, the bony prominence on the thumb side of the wrist (see ❸).
- Observe the normal flexion and supination of the forearm. The fingers of the hand may also extend slightly.

Patellar Reflex The patellar reflex tests the spinal cord level L-2, L-3, and L-4.

- Ask the client to sit on the edge of the examining table so that the legs hang freely.
- Locate the patellar tendon directly below the patella (kneecap).
- Deliver a blow with the percussion hammer directly to the tendon (see ❹).
- Observe the normal extension or kicking out of the leg as the quadriceps muscle contracts.
- If no response occurs and you suspect the client is not relaxed, ask the client to interlock the fingers and pull. **Rationale: This action often enhances relaxation so that a more accurate response is obtained.**

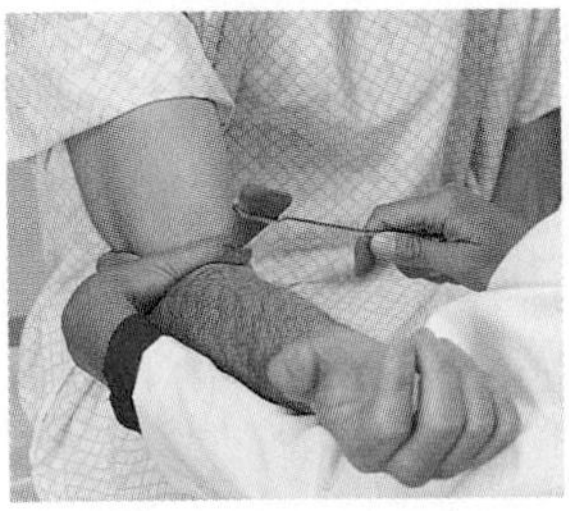

❶ The biceps reflex

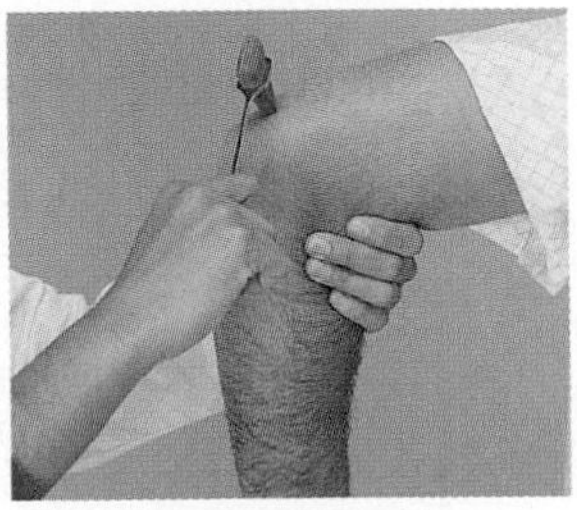

❷ The triceps reflex

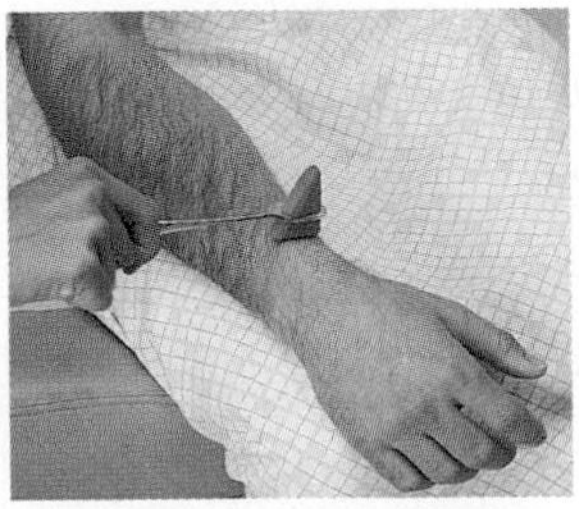

❸ The brachioradialis reflex

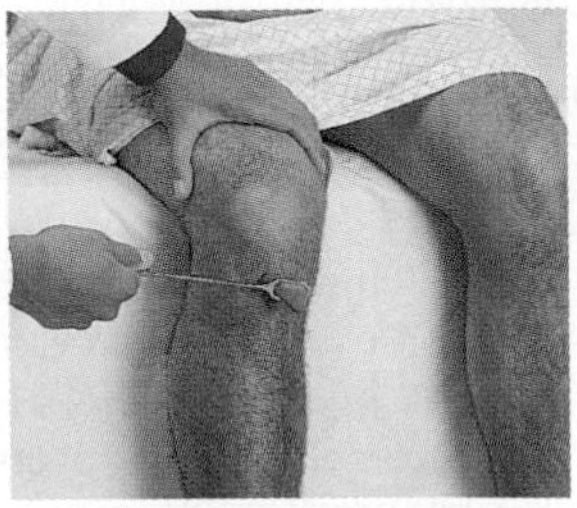

❹ The patellar reflex

(continued)

SKILL 27.17

ASSESSING THE NEUROLOGICAL SYSTEM *(continued)*

Achilles Reflex The Achilles reflex tests the spinal cord level S-1 and S-2.

- With the client in the same position as for the patellar reflex, slightly dorsiflex the client's ankle by supporting the ball of the foot lightly in the hand.
- Deliver a blow with the percussion hammer directly to the Achilles tendon just above the heel (see ❺).
- Observe and feel the normal plantar flexion (downward jerk) of the foot.

Plantar (Babinski) Reflex The planter, or Babinski, reflex is superficial. It may be absent in adults without pathology or overridden by voluntary control.

- Use a moderately sharp object, such as the handle of the percussion hammer, a key, or an applicator stick.
- Stroke the lateral border of the sole of the client's foot, starting at the heel, continuing to the ball of the foot, and then proceeding across the ball of the foot toward the big toe (see ❻).
- Observe the response. Normally, all five toes bend downward; this reaction is negative Babinski. In an abnormal (positive) Babinski response the toes spread outward and the big toe moves upward.

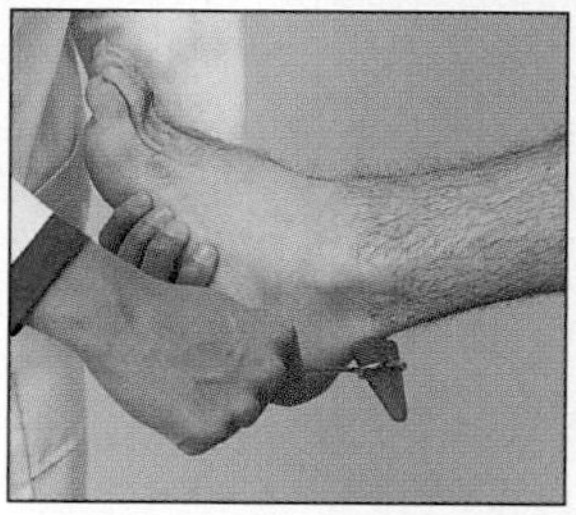

❺ The Achilles reflex

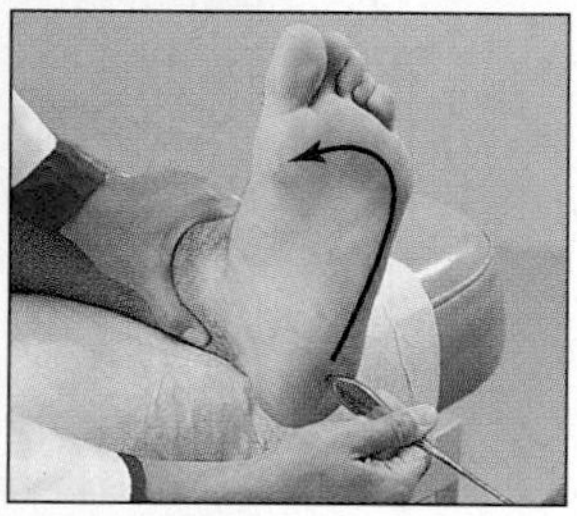

❻ The plantar (Babinski) reflex

ASSESSMENT	NORMAL FINDINGS	DEVIATIONS FROM NORMAL
Motor Function		
12. *Gross Motor and Balance Tests* Generally, the Romberg test and one other gross motor function and balance tests are used.		
Walking Gait Ask the client to walk across the room and back, and assess the client's gait.	Has upright posture and steady gait with opposing arm swing; walks unaided, maintaining balance	Has poor posture and unsteady, irregular, staggering gait with wide stance; bends legs only from hips; has rigid or no arm movements
Romberg Test Ask the client to stand with feet together and arms resting at the sides, first with eyes open, then closed. Stand close during this test. **Rationale: You may need to prevent the client from falling.**	Negative Romberg: may sway slightly but is able to maintain upright posture and foot stance	Positive Romberg: cannot maintain foot stance; moves the feet apart to maintain stance; if client cannot maintain balance with the eyes shut, client may have sensory ataxia (lack of coordination of the voluntary muscles); if balance cannot be maintained whether the eyes are open or shut, client may have cerebellar ataxia
Standing on One Foot with Eyes Closed Ask the client to close the eyes and stand on one foot. Repeat on the other foot. Stand close to the client during this test.	Maintains stance for at least 5 seconds	Cannot maintain stance for 5 seconds

(continued)

SKILL 27.17

ASSESSING THE NEUROLOGICAL SYSTEM (*continued*)

ASSESSMENT	NORMAL FINDINGS	DEVIATIONS FROM NORMAL
Heel-Toe Walking Ask the client to walk a straight line, placing the heel of one foot directly in front of the toes of the other foot (see ❼).	Maintains heel-toe walking along a straight line	Assumes a wider foot gait to stay upright

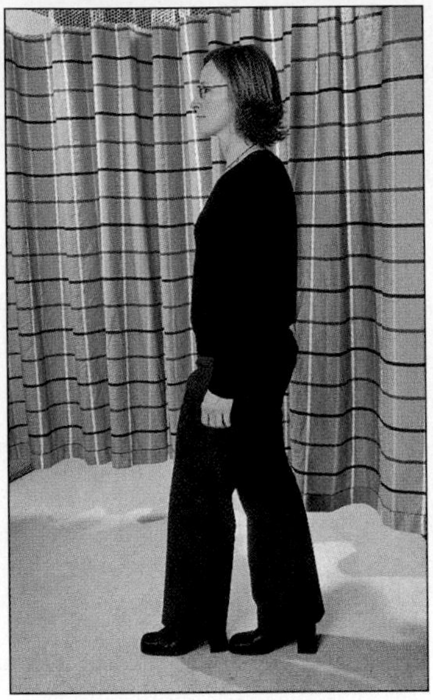

❼ Heel-toe walking

ASSESSMENT	NORMAL FINDINGS	DEVIATIONS FROM NORMAL
Toe or Heel Walking Ask the client to walk several steps on the toes and then on the heels.	Able to walk several steps on toes or heels	Cannot maintain balance on toes and heels
13. *Fine Motor Tests for the Upper Extremities*		
Finger-to-Nose Test Ask the client to abduct and extend the arms at shoulder height and then rapidly touch the nose alternately with one index finger and then the other. The client repeats the test with the eyes closed if the test is performed easily (see ❽).	Repeatedly and rhythmically touches the nose	Misses the nose or gives slow response

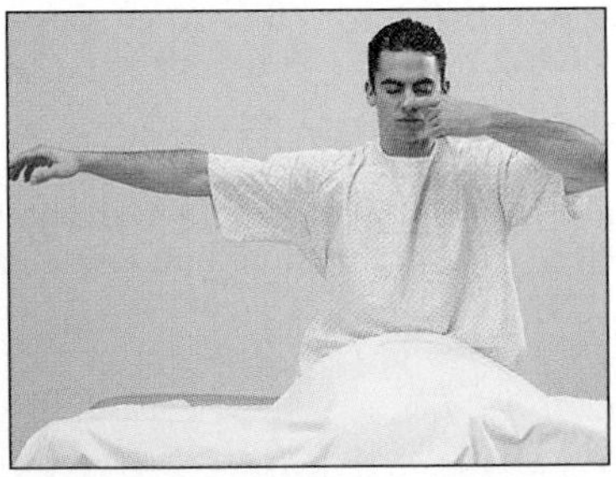

❽ Finger-to-nose test

ASSESSMENT	NORMAL FINDINGS	DEVIATIONS FROM NORMAL
Alternating Supination and Pronation of Hands on Knees Ask the client to pat both knees with the palms of both hands and then with the backs of the hands alternately at an ever-increasing rate (see ❾).	Can alternately supinate and pronate hands at rapid pace	Performs with slow, clumsy movements and irregular timing; has difficulty alternating from supination to pronation

(continued)

SKILL 27.17

ASSESSING THE NEUROLOGICAL SYSTEM (*continued*)

ASSESSMENT	NORMAL FINDINGS	DEVIATIONS FROM NORMAL

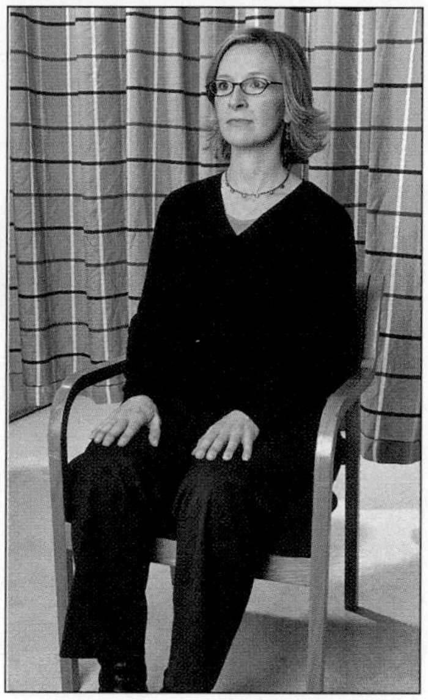

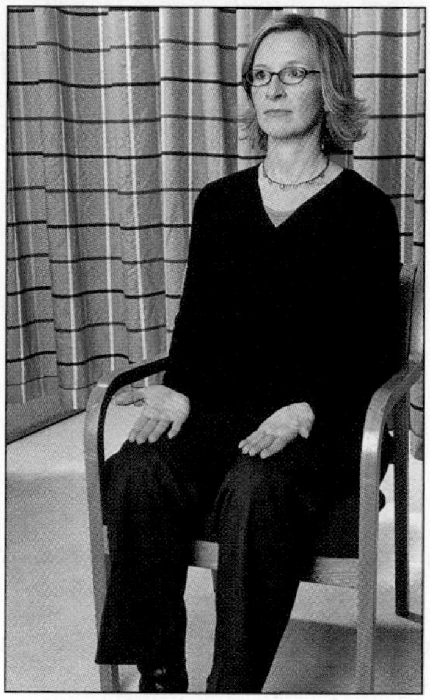

⑨ Alternating supination and pronation of hands on knees test

Finger to Nose and to the Nurse's Finger

Ask the client to touch the nose and then your index finger, held at a distance of about 45 cm, at a rapid and increasing rate (see ⑩).

Performs with coordination and rapidity

Misses the finger and moves slowly

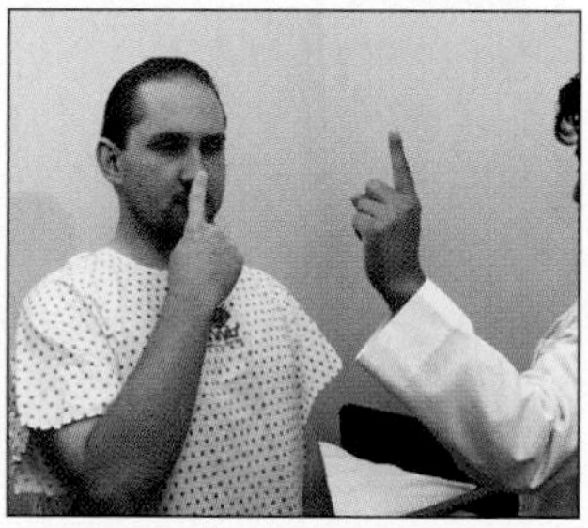

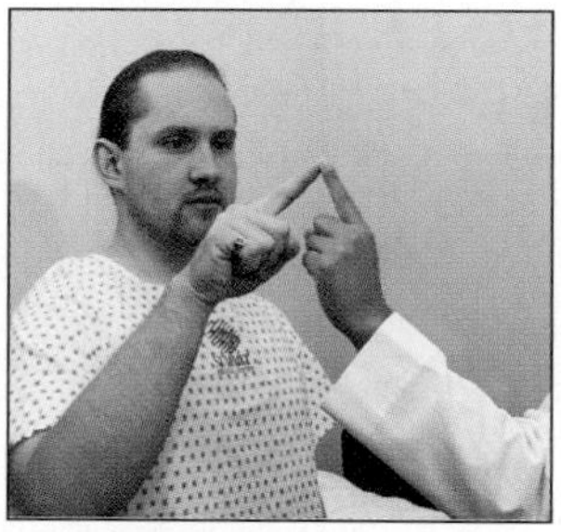

⑩ Finger-to-nose and to the nurse's finger test

Fingers to Fingers

Ask the client to spread the arms broadly at shoulder height and then bring the fingers together at the midline, first with the eyes open and then closed, first slowly and then rapidly (see ⑪).

Performs with accuracy and rapidity

Moves slowly and is unable to touch fingers consistently

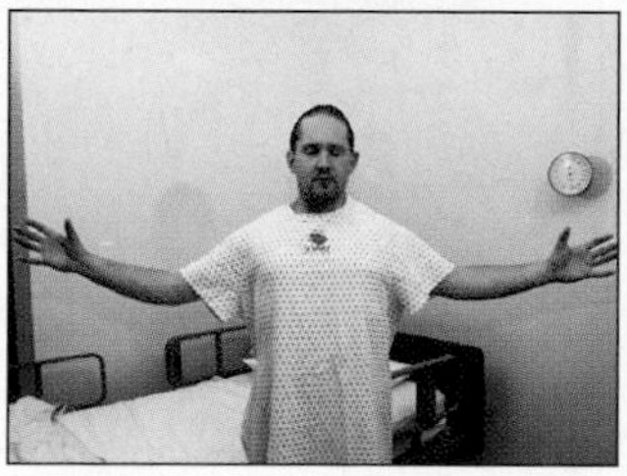

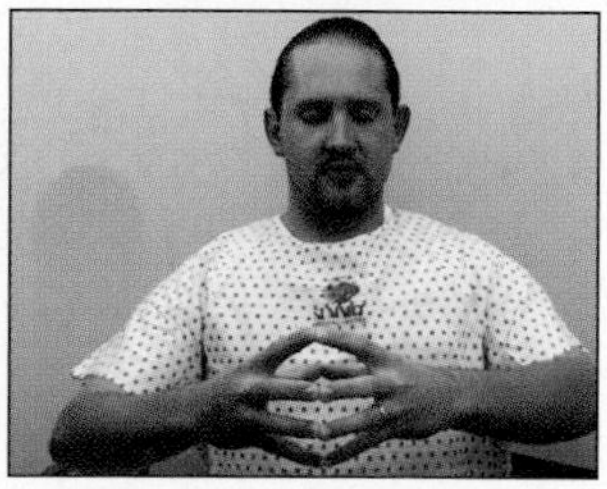

⑪ Fingers-to-fingers test

(continued)

SKILL 27.17

ASSESSING THE NEUROLOGICAL SYSTEM *(continued)*

ASSESSMENT	NORMAL FINDINGS	DEVIATIONS FROM NORMAL
Fingers to Thumb (Same Hand) Ask the client to touch each finger of one hand to the thumb of the same hand as rapidly as possible (see ⓬).	Rapidly touches each finger to thumb with each hand.	Cannot coordinate this fine discrete movement with either one or both hands

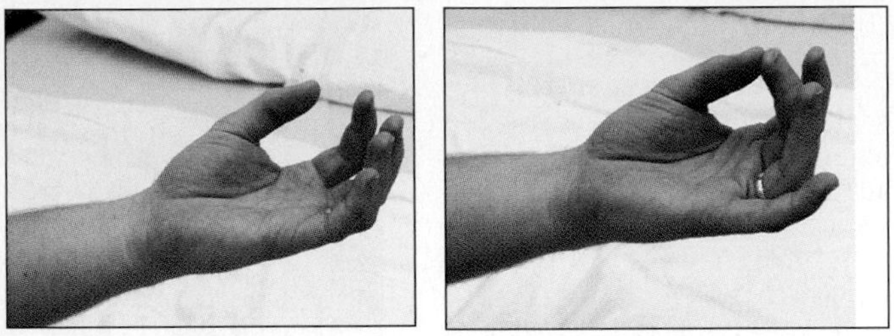

⓬ Fingers-to-thumb (same hand) test

ASSESSMENT	NORMAL FINDINGS	DEVIATIONS FROM NORMAL
14. *Fine Motor Tests for the Lower Extremities* Ask the client to lie supine and to perform these tests.		
Heel Down Opposite Shin Ask the client to place the heel of one foot just below the opposite knee and run the heel down the shin to the foot. Repeat with the other foot. The client may also use a sitting position for this test (see ⓭).	Demonstrates bilateral equal coordination	Has tremors or is awkward; heel moves off shin

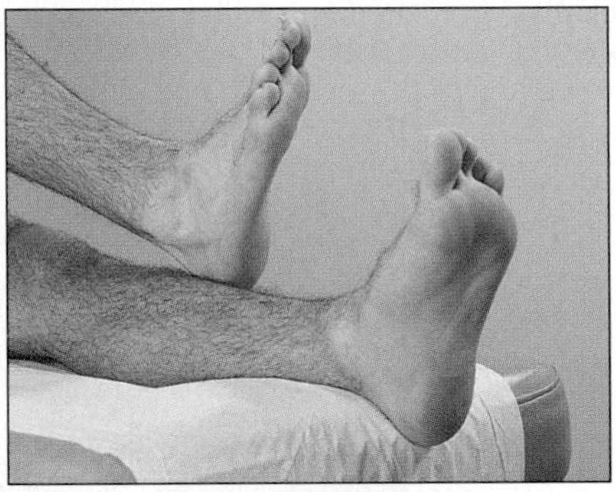

⓭ Heel down opposite shin

ASSESSMENT	NORMAL FINDINGS	DEVIATIONS FROM NORMAL
Toe or Ball of Foot to the Nurse's Finger Ask the client to touch your finger with the large toe of each foot (see ⓮).	Moves smoothly, with coordination	Misses your finger; cannot coordinate movement

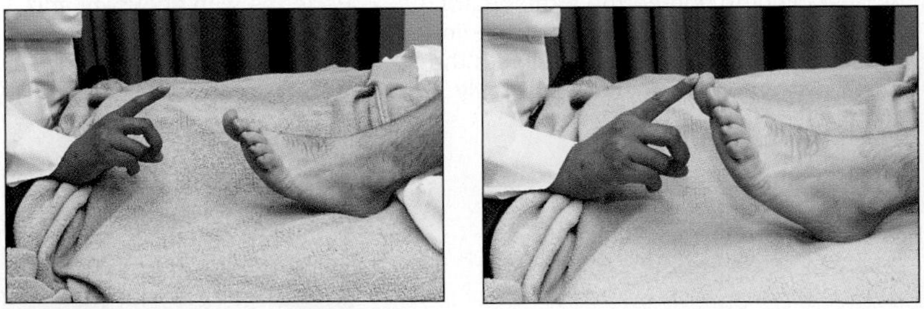

⓮ Toe or ball of foot to the nurse's finger test

15. *Light-Touch Sensation*

Compare the light-touch sensation of symmetric areas of the body. **Rationale: Sensitivity to touch varies among different skin areas.**

(continued)

SKILL 27.17

ASSESSING THE NEUROLOGICAL SYSTEM (*continued*)

ASSESSMENT	NORMAL FINDINGS	DEVIATIONS FROM NORMAL
• Ask the client to close the eyes and to respond by saying "yes" or "now" whenever the client feels the cotton wool wisp touching the skin. With a cotton wool wisp , lightly touch one specific spot and then the same spot on the other side of the body (see ⓯). Test areas on the forehead, cheek, hand, lower arm, abdomen, foot, and lower leg. Check a distal area of the limb first (i.e., the hand before the arm and the foot before the leg). **Rationale: The sensory nerve may be assumed to be intact if sensation is felt at its most distal part.** • Ask the client to point to the spot where the touch was felt. **Rationale: This demonstrates whether the client is able to determine tactile location (point localization); that is, the client can accurately perceive where he or she was touched. If areas of sensory dysfunction are found, determine the boundaries of sensation by testing responses about every 2.5 cm in the area. Make a sketch of the sensory loss area for recording purposes.**	Light tickling or touch sensation 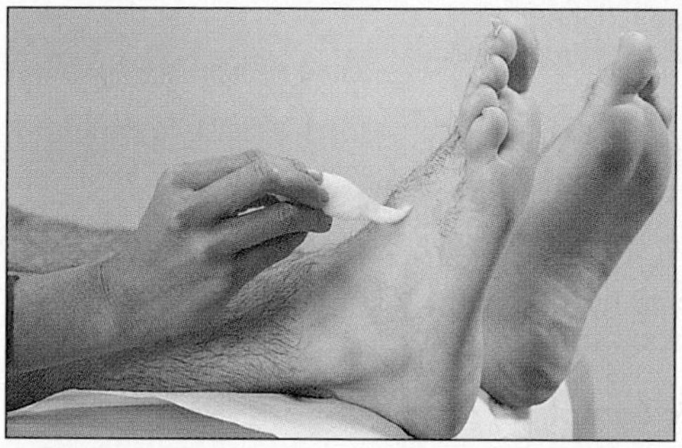 ⓯ Assessing light-touch sensation	Anaesthesia, hyperesthesia, hypoesthesia, or paresthesia
16. ***Pain Sensation*** Assess pain sensation as follows: • Ask the client to close the eyes and to say "sharp," "dull," or "don't know" when the sharp or dull end of the broken tongue depressor is felt. • Alternately, use the sharp and dull end to lightly prick designated anatomic areas at random (e.g., hand, forearm, foot, lower leg, abdomen) (see ⓰). The face is not tested in this manner. • Allow at least 2 seconds between each test to prevent summation effects of stimuli (i.e., several successive stimuli perceived as one stimulus).	Able to discriminate "sharp" and "dull" sensations 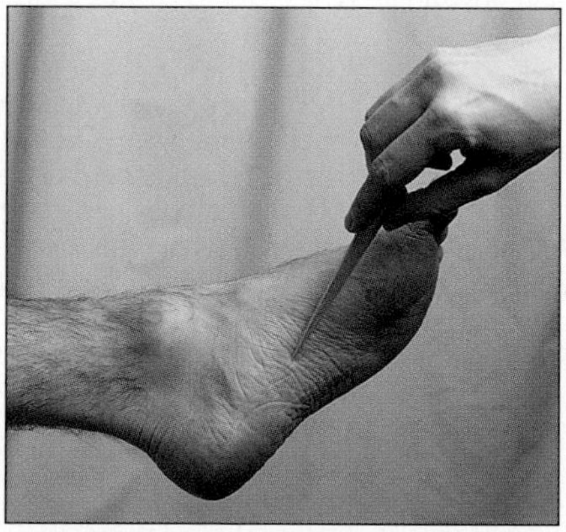 ⓰ Assessing pain sensation by using a broken tongue depressor	Areas of reduced, heightened, or absent sensation (map them out for recording purposes)

(continued)

SKILL 27.17

ASSESSING THE NEUROLOGICAL SYSTEM (*continued*)

ASSESSMENT	NORMAL FINDINGS	DEVIATIONS FROM NORMAL
17. *Temperature Sensation* Temperature sensation is not routinely tested if pain sensation is found to be within normal limits. If pain sensation is not normal or is absent, testing sensitivity to temperature may prove more reliable. • Touch skin areas with test tubes, one filled with warm water (40°C to 45°C) and one with cold water (5°C to 10°C). • Have the client respond by saying "warm," "cold," or "don't know."	Able to discriminate between "warm" and "cold" sensations	Areas of dulled or lost sensation (when sensations of pain are dulled, temperature sense is usually also impaired because distribution of these nerves over the body is similar)
18. *Position or Kinesthetic Sensation* Commonly, the middle fingers and the large toes are tested for the kinesthetic sensation (sense of position). • To test the fingers, support the client's arm and hand with one hand. To test the toes, place the client's heels on the examining table. • Ask the client to close his or her eyes. • Grasp a middle finger or a big toe firmly between your thumb and index finger, and exert the same pressure on both sides of the finger or toe while moving it (see ⑰). • Move the finger or toe until it is up, down, or straight out, and ask the client to identify the position. • Use a series of brisk up-and-down movements before bringing the finger or toe suddenly to rest in one of the three positions.	Can readily determine the position of fingers and toes	Unable to determine the position of one or more fingers or toes
19. *Tactile Discrimination* For all tests, the client's eyes need to be closed. ***One- and Two-Point Discrimination*** Alternately stimulate the skin with two pins simultaneously and then with one pin. Ask whether the client feels one or two pinpricks.	Perception varies widely in adults over different parts of the body; normally, a person can distinguish between a one- and two-point stimulus within the following minimum distances: Fingertips, 2.8 mm; Palms of hands, 8–12 mm; Chest, forearm, 40 mm; Back, 50–70 mm; Upper arm, thigh, 75 mm; Toes, 3–8 mm	Unable to sense whether one or two areas of the skin are being stimulated by pressure
Stereognosis Place a series of familiar objects, such as a key, paper clip, or coin, in the client's hand, and ask the client to identify each one.	Recognizes common objects	Unable to recognize common objects
If the client has a motor impairment of the hand and is unable to manipulate an object, write a number or letter on the client's palm, using a blunt instrument, and ask the client to identify it.	Able to identify numbers or letters written on palm (graphesthesia)	Unable to identify numbers or letters written on palm

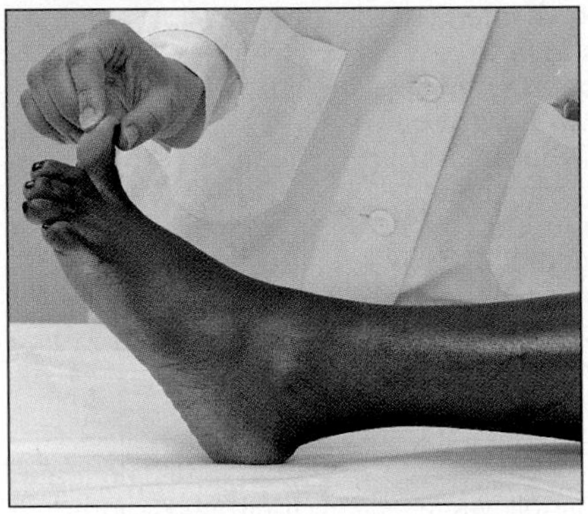

⑰ Position or kinesthetic sensation

(continued)

SKILL 27.17

ASSESSING THE NEUROLOGICAL SYSTEM (*continued*)

ASSESSMENT	NORMAL FINDINGS	DEVIATIONS FROM NORMAL
Extinction Phenomenon Simultaneously stimulate two symmetric areas of the body, such as the thighs, the cheeks, or the hands.	Both points of stimulus are felt	Failure to perceive touch on one side of the body when two symmetric areas of the body are touched simultaneously (frequently noted in clients with lesions of the sensory cortex)

20. Document findings in the client record by using forms or checklists supplemented by narrative notes when appropriate. Describe any abnormal findings in objective terms (e.g., "When asked to count backwards by threes, client made 7 errors and completed the task in 4 minutes").

EVALUATION

- Perform a detailed follow-up examination of other systems based on findings that deviated from expected or normal for the client. Relate findings to previous assessment data if available.
- Report significant deviations from normal to the appropriate members of the health-care team.

Lifespan Considerations

Assessing the Neurological System

INFANTS

- Reflexes commonly tested in newborns include the following:
  - *Rooting:* Stroke the side of the face near mouth; infant opens mouth and turns to the side that is stroked.
  - *Sucking:* Place finger 3 cm to 4 cm into mouth or have the mother place her nipple in the infant's mouth; infant sucks vigorously.
  - *Tonic neck:* Place infant supine, turn head to one side; arm on side to which head is turned extends; on opposite side, arm curls up (fencer's pose).
  - *Palmar grasp:* Place finger in infant's palm and press; infant curls fingers around it.
  - *Stepping:* Hold infant as if weight bearing on surface; infant steps along, one foot at a time.
  - *Moro:* Present loud noise or unexpected movement; infant spreads arms and legs, extends fingers, then flexes and brings hands together; infant may cry.
- Most of these reflexes disappear between 4 and 6 months of age.

CHILDREN

- Present the procedures as games whenever possible.
- A positive Babinski reflex is abnormal after the child ambulates or at age 2.
- For children younger than age 5, the Denver Developmental Screening Test II provides a comprehensive neurological evaluation, particularly for motor function.
- Note the child's ability to understand and follow directions.
- Assess immediate recall or recent memory by using names of cartoon characters. Normal recall in children is one item fewer than their age in years (e.g., a 4-year-old should be able to recall three items).
- Assess for signs of hyperactivity or abnormally short attention span.
- Children should be able to walk backward by age 2, balance on one foot for 5 seconds by age 4, heel-toe walk by age 5, and heel-toe walk backward by age 6.
- Romberg test is appropriate over age 3.

OLDER ADULTS

- A full neurological assessment can be lengthy. Conduct it in several sessions if indicated, and stop the tests if the client is noticeably fatigued.
- A decline in mental status is not a normal result of aging. Changes are more likely the result of physical or psychological disorders (e.g., fever, fluid and electrolyte imbalances, medications). Acute, abrupt-onset mental status changes are usually caused by delirium. These changes are often reversible with treatment. Chronic subtle insidious mental health changes are usually caused by dementia and are usually irreversible.
- Intelligence and learning ability are unaltered with age. Many factors, however, inhibit learning (e.g., anxiety, illness, pain, cultural barrier).
- Short-term memory is often less efficient. Long-term memory is usually unaltered.
- Because aging is often associated with loss of support persons, depression is a common disorder. Mood changes, weight loss, anorexia, constipation, and early morning awakening may be symptoms of depression.

(*continued*)

Lifespan Considerations (*continued*)

- The stress of being in unfamiliar situations can cause confusion in older adults.
- As a person ages, reflex responses may become less intense.
- Because older adults tire more easily than younger clients, a total neurological assessment is often done at a different time than the other parts of the physical assessment.
- Although there is a progressive decrease in the number of functioning neurons in the central nervous system and in the sense organs, older adults usually function well because of the abundant reserves in the number of brain cells.
- Impulse transmission and reaction to stimuli are slower.
- Many older adults have some impairment of hearing, vision, smell, temperature and pain sensation, memory, and mental endurance.
- Coordination changes, including a reduced speed of fine finger movements. Standing balance remains intact, and Romberg's test remains negative.
- Reflex responses may slightly increase or decrease. Many show loss of Achilles reflex, and the plantar reflex may be difficult to elicit.
- When testing sensory function, the nurse needs to give older adults time to respond. Normally, older adults have unaltered perception of light touch and superficial pain, decreased perception of deep pain, and decreased perception of temperature stimuli. Many also reveal a decrease or absence of position sense in the large toes.

The Female Genitals and Inguinal Lymph Nodes

The examination of the genitals and reproductive tract of women includes assessment of the inguinal lymph nodes and inspection and palpation of the external genitals. Completeness of the assessment of the genitals and reproductive tract depends on the needs and problems of the individual client. In most practice settings, generalist nurses perform only inspection of the external genitals and palpation of the inguinal lymph nodes.

Assessment of adolescent girls is limited to an inspection of the external genitals. For sexually active adolescents and adult women, an annual Papanicolaou test (Pap test) is advised for detecting cancer of the cervix. If an increased or abnormal vaginal discharge is present, specimens should be taken to check for sexually transmitted disease.

Examination of the genitals usually creates uncertainty and apprehension in females, and the lithotomy position required can cause embarrassment. The nurse must explain each part of the examination in advance and perform the examination in an objective and efficient manner. Appropriate draping is essential to prevent undue exposure of the client, and good lighting is required for the nurse to ensure accuracy of inspection.

Skill 27.18 describes how to assess the female genitals and inguinal lymph nodes.

SKILL 27.18

ASSESSING THE FEMALE GENITALS AND INGUINAL LYMPH NODES

Equipment

- Clean gloves
- Drape
- Supplemental lighting, if needed

IMPLEMENTATION

Performance

1. Before performing the procedure, introduce yourself and verify the client's identity by using agency protocol. Explain to the client what you are going to do, why it is necessary, and how she can cooperate. Discuss how the results will be used in planning further care or treatments.
2. Perform hand hygiene, apply gloves, and observe other appropriate infection prevention and control procedures.
3. Provide for client privacy. Request the presence of another woman if desired, required by agency policy, or requested by the client.
4. Inquire regarding the following: age of onset of menstruation, last menstrual period (LMP), regularity of cycle, duration, amount of daily flow, and whether menstruation is painful; incidence of pain during intercourse; vaginal discharge; number of pregnancies, number of live births, labour or delivery complications; urgency and frequency of urination at night; blood in urine, painful urination, incontinence; history of sexually transmitted disease, past and present.
5. Cover the pelvic area with a sheet or drape at all times when it is not actually being examined. Position the client supine with feet elevated on the stirrups of an examination table. Alternatively, assist the client into the dorsal recumbent position with knees flexed and thighs externally rotated.

(continued)

SKILL 27.18

ASSESSING THE FEMALE GENITALS AND INGUINAL LYMPH NODES (*continued*)

ASSESSMENT	NORMAL FINDINGS	DEVIATIONS FROM NORMAL
6. Inspect the distribution, amount, and characteristics of pubic hair.	There are wide variations; generally kinky in the menstruating adult, thinner and straighter after menopause; distributed in the shape of an inverse triangle	Scant pubic hair (may indicate hormonal problem); hair growth should not extend over the abdomen
7. Inspect the skin of the pubic area for parasites, inflammation, swelling, and lesions. To assess pubic skin adequately, separate the labia majora and labia minora.	Pubic skin intact, no lesions; skin of vulva area slightly darker than the rest of the body; labia round, full, and relatively symmetric in adult females	Lice, lesions, scars, fissures, swelling, erythema, excoriations (abrasions from scratching), varicosities (swollen and twisted veins), or leukoplakia
8. Inspect the clitoris, urethral orifice, and vaginal orifice when separating the labia minora.	Clitoris does not exceed 1 cm in width and 2 cm in length; urethral orifice appears as a small slit and is the same colour as surrounding tissues; no inflammation, swelling, or discharge	Presence of lesions; presence of inflammation, swelling, or discharge
9. Palpate the inguinal lymph nodes (see ❶). Use the pads of the fingers in a rotary motion, noting any enlargement or tenderness.	No enlargement or tenderness	Enlargement and tenderness

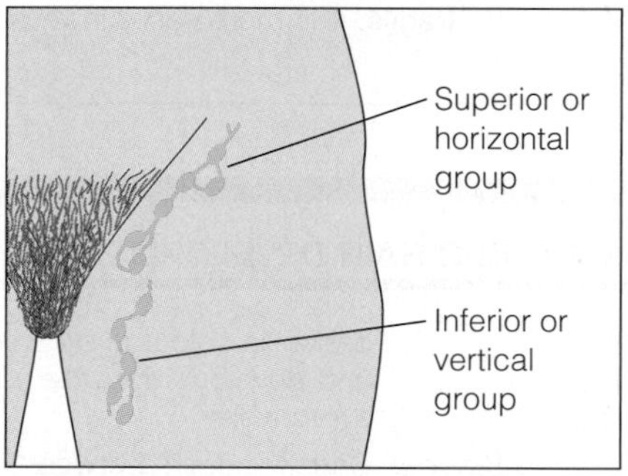

❶ Lymph nodes of the groin area

10. Document findings in the client record by using forms or checklists supplemented by narrative notes when appropriate.

EVALUATION

- Perform a detailed follow-up examination based on findings that deviated from expected or normal for the client. Relate findings to previous assessment data if available.
- Significant deviations from normal indicate the need for an internal vaginal examination.

Lifespan Considerations

Assessing the Female Genitals and Inguinal Lymph Nodes

INFANTS

- Infants can be held in a supine position on the parent's lap with the knees supported in a flexed position and separated.
- In newborns, because of maternal estrogen, the labia and clitoris may be edematous and enlarged, and newborns may have a small amount of white or bloody vaginal discharge.

(continued)

Lifespan Considerations (*continued*)

- Assess the mons and inguinal area for swelling or tenderness that may indicate presence of an inguinal hernia.

CHILDREN

- Ensure that you have the parent or guardian's approval to perform the examination and then tell the child what you are going to do. Preschool children are taught not to allow others to touch their "private parts."
- Assessment of adolescent girls is limited to inspection of the external genitals, unless the girl is sexually active. The presence of the parent during the exam will depend on the nature of the clinical situation and the provincial or territorial age of consent for medical investigation (e.g., some provinces require that the adolescent be at least 14 before being examined without parental presence or permission).
- Girls should be assessed for Tanner staging of pubertal development (see Box 27.7).
- Girls should have a Papanicolaou (Pap) test done if sexually active, or by age 18 years.
- Sexually active girls with abnormal vaginal discharge should be tested for a sexually transmitted infection.
- The clitoris is a common site for syphilitic chancres in younger females.

OLDER ADULTS

- Loss of pubic hair and a flattening of the labia occur.
- The clitoris is a potential site for cancerous lesions in older females.
- The vulva atrophies as a result of a reduction in vascularity, elasticity, adipose tissue, and estrogen levels. Because the vulva is more fragile, it is more easily irritated.
- The vaginal environment becomes drier and more alkaline, resulting in an alteration of the type of flora present and a predisposition to vaginitis. Dyspareunia (difficult or painful coitus) is also a common occurrence.
- The cervix and uterus decrease in size.
- The fallopian tubes and ovaries atrophy.
- Ovulation and estrogen production cease.
- Vaginal bleeding unrelated to estrogen therapy is abnormal in older women.
- Prolapse of the uterus can occur in older females, especially those who have had multiple pregnancies.
- Older females may be arthritic and find the lithotomy position uncomfortable. A semi-lithotomy position may be necessary.

BOX 27.7 TANNER STAGES OF PUBIC HAIR DEVELOPMENT IN FEMALES

Stage 1 Preadolescence. No pubic hair except for fine body hair.

Stage 2 Usually occurs at ages 11 and 12 years. Sparse, long, slightly pigmented curly hair develops along the labia.

Stage 3 Usually occurs at ages 12 and 13 years. Hair becomes darker in colour and curlier and develops over the pubic symphysis.

Stage 4 Usually occurs between ages 13 and 14 years. Hair assumes the texture and curl of the adult but is not as thick and does not appear on the thighs.

Stage 5 Sexual maturity. Hair assumes adult appearance and appears on the inner aspect of the upper thigh (see Figure 27.35).

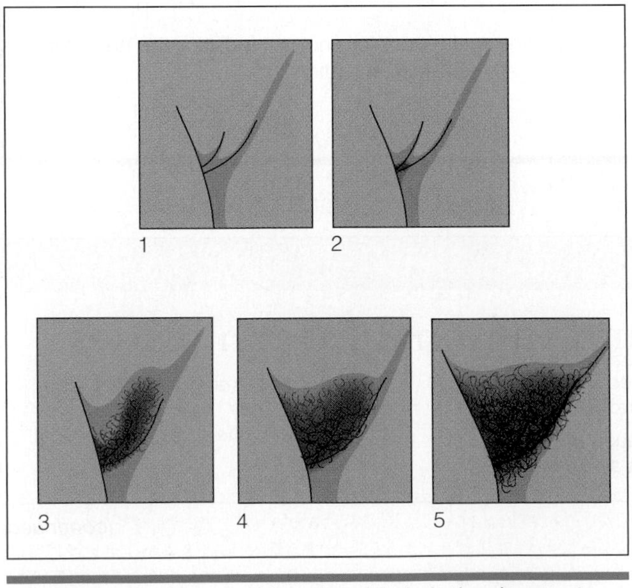

FIGURE 27.35 Stages of female pubic hair development

In many agencies, only midwives, labour and delivery nurses, and nurse practitioners examine the internal genitals. However, generalist nurses often assist with this examination and need to be familiar with the procedure. Examination of the internal genitals involves (1) palpating Skene's and Bartholin's glands; (2) assessing the pelvic musculature; (3) inserting a vaginal speculum to inspect the cervix and vagina; and (4) obtaining a Pap smear.

Palpation of *Skene's (paraurethral) glands* (Figure 27.36) is performed by inserting a gloved index finger palm upward into the vagina about 2.5 cm and milking the glands by pressing gently upward and outward. Discharge and tenderness are abnormal. If discharge is present, specimens are taken and gloves are changed before proceeding with further examination.

Bartholin's glands are located on the posterior aspect of the vaginal orifice. These are palpated as shown in Figure 27.37. Normally, Bartholin's glands are not tender or palpable.

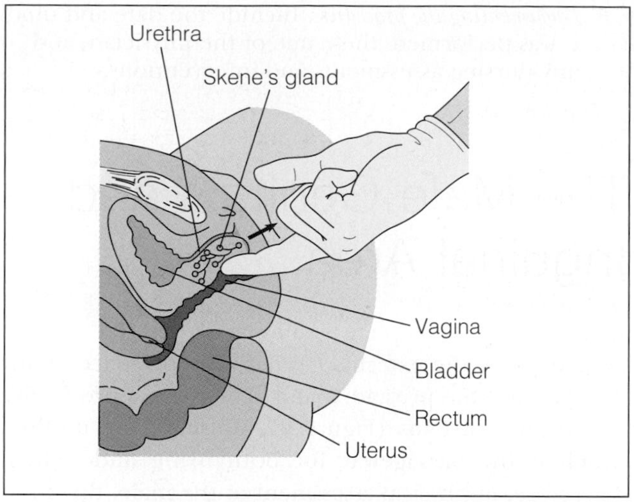

FIGURE 27.36 Palpating Skene's glands

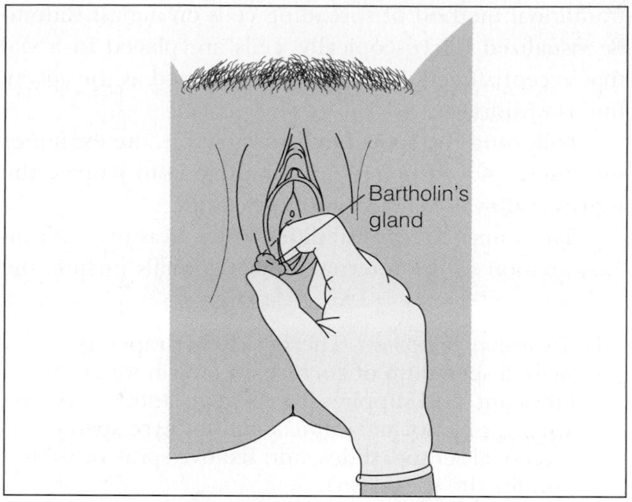

FIGURE 27.37 Palpating Bartholin's gland

To assess the *pelvic musculature,* the examiner (1) places two gloved fingers (index and middle finger) into the vagina, (2) asks the client to constrict her vaginal orifice, (3) asks the client to bear down while the fingers spread the vaginal wall laterally, and (4) observes the vaginal wall for bulges. Normally, a **nulliparous** woman (one who has never had a child) will have a high degree of muscle tone, whereas a **multiparous** woman (one who has had two or more pregnancies resulting in viable offspring by vaginal delivery) will have less tone. The walls should be intact with no bulges. Deviations from normal include a **cystocele** (bulging of the anterior wall and the bladder) and a **rectocele** (bulging of the posterior wall as a result of a prolapse of the posterior wall and the rectum).

The *speculum examination* of the vagina involves the insertion of a plastic or metal speculum that consists of two blades and an adjustable thumb screw (Figure 27.38). Various sizes are available (small, medium, and large); the appropriate size needs to be selected for each client. The speculum can be lubricated with water-soluble lubricant if specimens are *not* being collected. Most examiners lubricate the speculum with warm water. After visualizing the cervix, the examiner takes Pap smear specimens from one or more of the sites shown in Figure 27.39. Liquid-based cervical cytology is a new approach to analyzing cervical cells: instead of the

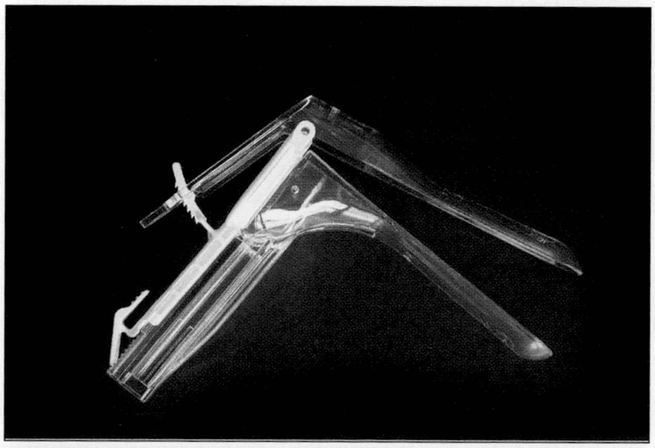

FIGURE 27.38 A vaginal speculum

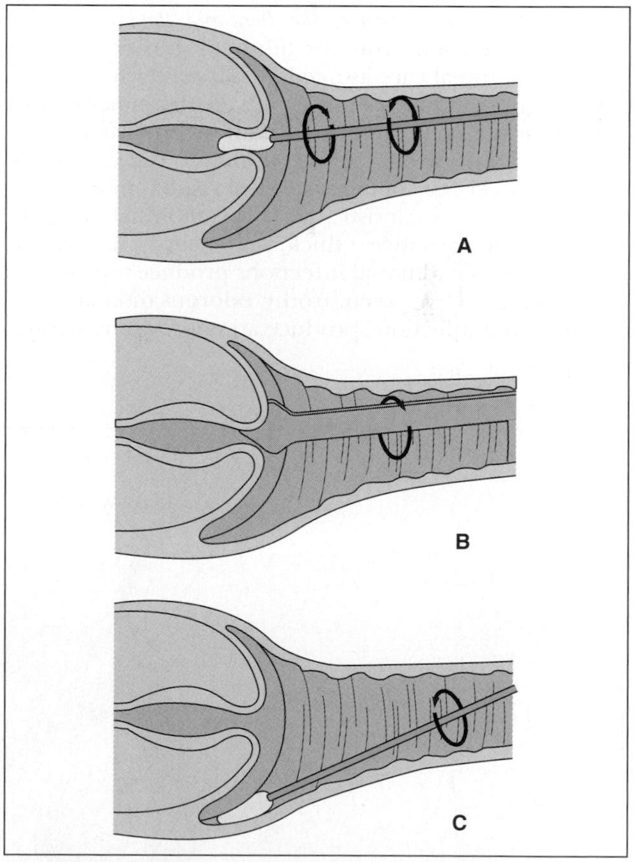

FIGURE 27.39 Methods of obtaining Pap smears:
A: Endocervical: a cotton swab is inserted into the cervical os and rotated clockwise and counterclockwise in the os; **B:** cervical scrape: an Ayre spatula with the longer end inserted into the cervical os is rotated to scrape cells from the outer surface; **C:** vaginal smear or pool: a cotton-tipped applicator or elongated spatula is inserted along the vaginal floor.

traditional method of spreading cells on a glass slide to be visualized microscopically, cells are placed in a vial that is centrifuged. The vagina is observed as the speculum is withdrawn.

Following the speculum examination, the examiner may insert gloved fingers into the vagina to palpate the uterus and ovaries for any abnormalities.

The nurse's responsibilities when assisting with an examination of the internal female genitals include the following:

1. *Assembling equipment.* These include drapes, gloves, vaginal speculum of correct size, warm water or lubricant, and supplies for cytology studies (cotton applicators, normal saline solution, Ayre spatula for a cervical scrape, slides, and fixative spray or solution for the specimen).
2. *Preparing the client.* Advise the client not to douche before the procedure. Explain the procedure. It should take only 5 minutes and is normally not painful. Assist the client to a lithotomy position as needed, and drape her appropriately.
3. *Supporting the client during the procedure.* This involves explaining the procedure as needed, and encouraging the client to take deep breaths that will help the pelvic muscles relax.
4. *Monitoring and assisting the client after the procedure.* Assist the client from the lithotomy position and with perineal care as needed. Observe any discharge from the vagina. Normally, characteristics of cervical mucus vary throughout the menstrual cycle from clear to white and from thin to thick, even stringy. Three common types of vaginal infections produce characteristic discharge: monilial or yeast infections produce a thick, white, curdy, patchy discharge; trichomonal infections produce a profuse, watery, grey or green, frothy, odorous discharge; bacterial infections produce an odorous discharge.
5. *Documenting the procedure.* Include the date and time it was performed, the name of the physician, and any nursing assessments and interventions.

The Male Genitals and Inguinal Area

In adult men, complete examination should include assessment of the external genitals, the presence of any hernias, and the prostate gland. The male reproductive and urinary systems (Figure 27.40) share the urethra, which is the passageway for both urine and semen. Therefore, in physical assessment of the male, these two systems are frequently assessed together.

Development of secondary sex characteristics is assessed in relationship to the client's age. See Table 27.14 for the five stages of the development of pubic hair, the penis, the testes, and the scrotum during puberty.

All male clients should be screened for the presence of inguinal or femoral hernias. A **hernia** is a protrusion of the intestine through the inguinal wall or canal. Cancer of the prostate gland is the most common cancer in adult men and occurs primarily in men over age 50. Examination of the prostate gland is performed with the examination of the rectum and anus.

Testicular cancer is much rarer than prostate cancer and occurs primarily in young men aged 15 to 35 years. Testicular cancer is most commonly found on the anterior and lateral surfaces of the testes. **Testicular self-examination** should be conducted monthly. See Chapter 45.

Skill 27.19 describes how the nurse can conduct an assessment of the male genitals and inguinal area.

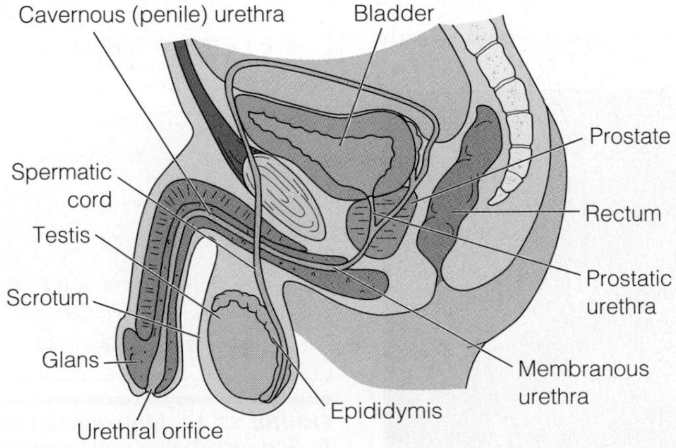

FIGURE 27.40 The male urogenital tract

TABLE 27.14 Tanner Stages of Development of Pubic Hair, Penis, and Testes/Scrotum (12 to 16 Years)

Stage	Pubic Hair	Penis	Testes/Scrotum
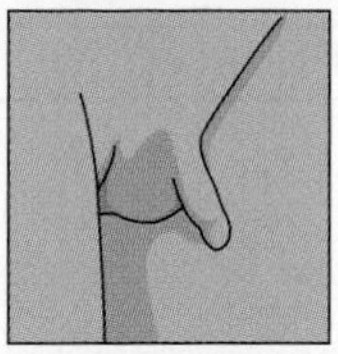 1	None, except for body hair like that on the abdomen	Size is relative to body size, as in childhood	Size is relative to body size, as in childhood
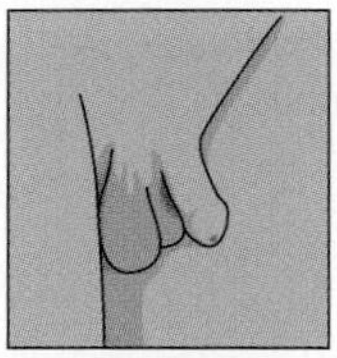 2	Scant, long, slightly pigmented at base of penis	Slight enlargement occurs	Becomes reddened in colour and enlarged
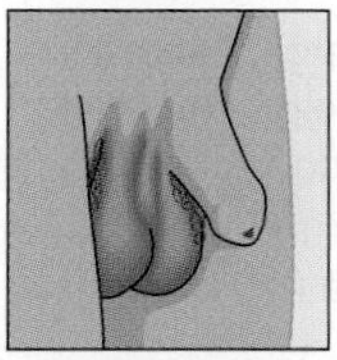 3	Darker, begins to curl and becomes more coarse; extends over pubic symphysis	Elongation occurs	Continuing enlargement
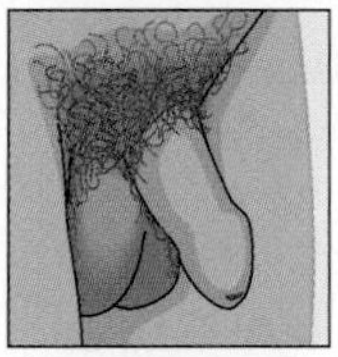 4	Continues to darken and thicken; extends on the sides, above, and below	Increase in both breadth and length; glans develops	Continuing enlargement; colour darkens
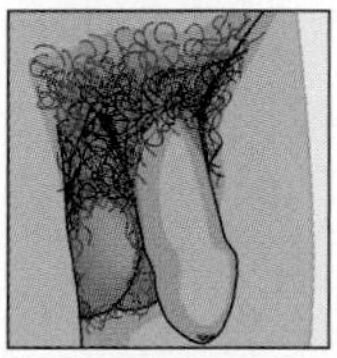 5	Adult distribution that extends to inner thighs, umbilicus, and anus	Adult appearance	Adult appearance

SKILL 27.19

ASSESSING THE MALE GENITALS AND INGUINAL AREA

Equipment: Clean gloves

IMPLEMENTATION

Performance

1. Before performing the procedure, introduce yourself and verify the client's identity by using agency protocol. Explain to the client what you are going to do, why it is necessary, and how he can cooperate. Discuss how the results will be used in planning further care or treatments.
2. Perform hand hygiene, apply gloves, and observe other appropriate infection prevention and control procedures.
3. Provide for client privacy. Request the presence of another person if desired, required by agency policy, or requested by the client.
4. Inquire whether the client has any history of the following: urinary incontinence, frequency, urgency, abdominal pain; symptoms of sexually transmitted disease; swellings that could indicate presence of hernia; family history of nephritis, malignancy of the prostate, or malignancy of the kidney. Inquire about usual voiding patterns and changes, and bladder control.
5. Cover the pelvic area with a sheet or drape at all times when it is not actually being examined.

(continued)

SKILL 27.19

ASSESSING THE MALE GENITALS AND INGUINAL AREA *(continued)*

ASSESSMENT	NORMAL FINDINGS	DEVIATIONS FROM NORMAL
Pubic Hair		
6. Inspect the distribution, amount, and characteristics of pubic hair.	Triangular distribution, often spreading up the abdomen	Scant amount or absence of hair
Penis		
7. Inspect the penile shaft and glans penis for lesions, nodules, swellings, and inflammation.	Penile skin intact; appears slightly wrinkled and varies in colour as widely as other body skin; foreskin easily retractable from the glans penis; small amount of thick white smegma between the glans and foreskin	Presence of lesions, nodules, swellings, or inflammation
8. Inspect the urethral meatus for swelling, inflammation, and discharge. • Compress or ask the client to compress the glans slightly to open the urethral meatus to inspect it for discharge.	Pink and slit-like appearance; positioned at the tip of the penis	Inflammation; discharge; variation in meatal locations (e.g., hypospadias, on the underside of the penile shaft, and epispadias, on the upper side of the penile shaft)
9. Palpate the penis for tenderness, thickening, and nodules. Use your thumb and first two fingers.	Smooth and semi-firm; is slightly moveable over the underlying structures	Presence of tenderness, thickening, or nodules; immobility
Scrotum		
10. Inspect the scrotum for appearance, general size, and symmetry. • To facilitate inspection of the scrotum during a physical examination, ask the client to hold the penis out of the way. • Inspect all skin surfaces by spreading the rugated surface skin and lifting the scrotum as needed to observe posterior surfaces.	Scrotal skin is darker in colour than that of the rest of the body and is loose Size varies with temperature changes (the dartos muscles contract when the area is cold and relax when the area is warm) Scrotum appears asymmetric (left testis is usually lower than right testis)	Discolourations; any tightening of skin (may indicate edema or mass)
11. Palpate the scrotum to assess status of underlying testes, epididymis (the narrow tube connecting the back of each testicle to its vas deferens), and spermatic cord. Palpate both testes simultaneously for comparative purposes. • Using your first two fingers and thumb, palpate each testis for size, consistency, shape, smoothness, and presence of masses. During assessment of male adolescents, establish the descent of the testicles into the scrotum; note undescended testes. • Palpate the epididymis between your thumb and index finger. It is located at the top of the testis and extends behind it.	Testicles are rubbery, smooth, and free of nodules and masses; testis is about 2 cm × 4 cm; epididymis is resilient, normally tender, and softer than the spermatic cord; spermatic cord is firm	Testicles are enlarged, with uneven surface (possible tumour); epididymis is nonresilient and painful

(continued)

SKILL 27.19

ASSESSING THE MALE GENITALS AND INGUINAL AREA *(continued)*

ASSESSMENT	NORMAL FINDINGS	DEVIATIONS FROM NORMAL
• Palpate the spermatic cord between thumb and index finger. It is usually found at the top lateral portion of the scrotum and feels firm. • If swelling, irregularities, or nodules are detected during the scrotal examination, attempt to transilluminate the lesion. This is done by darkening the room and shining a flashlight behind the scrotum through the mass. **Rationale: Serous fluid causes the light to show with a red glow; tissue or blood does not transilluminate.** • Describe all scrotal masses in terms of their size, shape, placement, consistency, tenderness, and presence of transillumination.		
Inguinal Area		
12. Inspect both inguinal areas for bulges while the client is standing, if possible. • First, have the client remain at rest. • Next, have the client hold his breath and strain or bear down as though having a bowel movement. Bearing down may make the hernia more visible.	No swelling or bulges	Swelling or bulge (possible inguinal or femoral hernia)

13. Document findings in the client record by using forms or checklists supplemented by narrative notes when appropriate.

EVALUATION

- Perform a detailed follow-up examination based on findings that deviated from expected or normal for the client. Relate findings to previous assessment data if available.
- Report significant deviations from normal to the appropriate members of the health-care team.

Lifespan Considerations

Assessing the Male Genitals and Inguinal Area

INFANTS

- The foreskin of the uncircumcised infant is normally tight at birth and should not be retracted. It will gradually loosen as the baby grows and is usually fully retractable by 2 to 3 years of age. Assess for cleanliness, redness, or irritation.
- Assess for placement of the urethral meatus.
- Palpate the scrotum to determine if the testes are descended; in the newborn and infant, the testes may retract into the inguinal canal, especially with stimulation of the cremasteric reflex (lightly stroking the superior and medial part of the thigh causes the cremaster muscle to pull up the scrotum and testis on that side).
- Assess the inguinal area for swelling or tenderness that may indicate presence of an inguinal hernia.

(continued)

Lifespan Considerations (*continued*)

CHILDREN

- Ensure that you have the parent or guardian's approval to perform the examination and then tell the child what you are going to do. Preschool children are taught to not allow others to touch their "private parts."
- In young boys, the cremasteric reflex can cause the testes to ascend into the inguinal canal. If possible, have the boy sit cross-legged, which stretches the muscle and decreases the reflex.

OLDER ADULTS

- The penis decreases in size with age; the size and firmness of the testes decrease.
- Testosterone is produced in smaller amounts.
- More time and direct physical stimulation are required for an older man to achieve an erection, but the patient can maintain the erection for a longer period before ejaculation than he could at a younger age.
- Seminal fluid is reduced in amount and viscosity.
- Urinary frequency, nocturia, dribbling, and problems with beginning and ending the stream are usually the result of prostatic enlargement.

The Anus and Rectum

Rectal examination, an essential part of every *comprehensive* physical examination, involves inspection and palpation (digital examination). The extent of the assessment of the rectum and anus depends on the rectal problems stated by the client in the nursing history.

Skill 27.20 describes how to assess the rectum and anus.

SKILL 27.20

ASSESSING THE ANUS AND RECTUM

Equipment

- Clean gloves
- Water-soluble lubricant

IMPLEMENTATION

Performance

1. Before performing the procedure, introduce yourself and verify the client's identity by using agency protocol. Explain to the client what you are going to do, why it is necessary, and how he or she can cooperate. Discuss how the results will be used in planning further care or treatments. Because digital examination can cause apprehension and embarrassment in the client, it is important that the nurse help the client relax by encouraging the client to take slow, deep breaths (tension can cause spasms of the anal sphincters, making the examination uncomfortable) and inform the client about potential sensations, such as feelings of defecation or passing gas.
2. Perform hand hygiene, apply gloves, and observe other appropriate infection prevention and control procedures for all anal and rectal examinations.
3. Provide for client privacy. Drape the client appropriately to prevent undue exposure of body parts.
4. Inquire whether the client has any history of the following: bright blood in stools, tarry black stools, diarrhea, constipation, abdominal pain, excessive gas, hemorrhoids, or rectal pain; family history of colorectal cancer; when last stool specimen for occult blood was performed and the results; and for males, if not obtained during the genitourinary examination, signs or symptoms of prostate enlargement (e.g., slow urinary stream, hesitance, frequency, dribbling, and nocturia).
5. Position the client. In adults, a left lateral or Sims' position with the upper leg acutely flexed is required for the examination. For females, a dorsal recumbent position with hips externally rotated and knees flexed or a lithotomy position may be used (see ❶). For males, a standing position while the client bends over the examining table may also be used. This position is commonly used to examine the prostate gland.

(continued)

SKILL 27.20

ASSESSING THE ANUS AND RECTUM *(continued)*

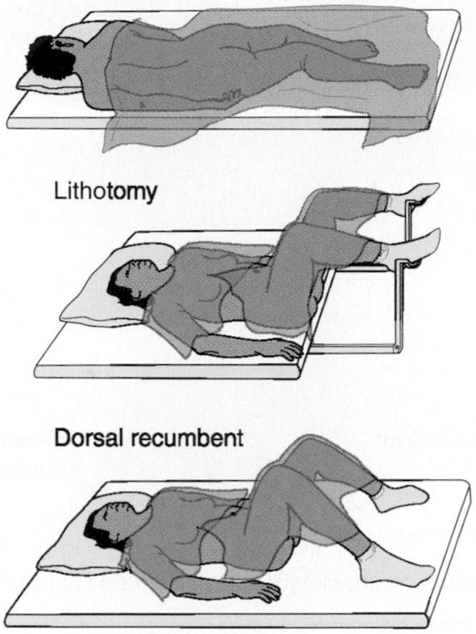

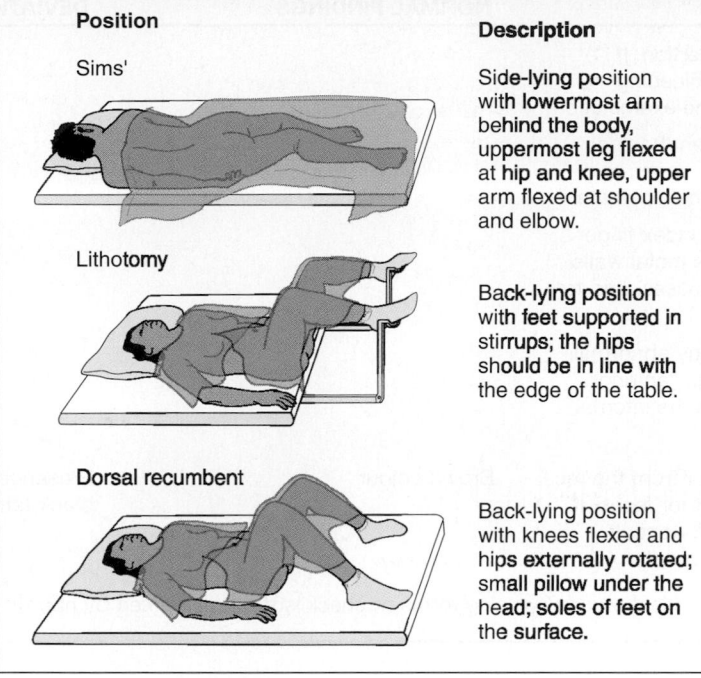

Position	Description
Sims'	Side-lying position with lowermost arm behind the body, uppermost leg flexed at hip and knee, upper arm flexed at shoulder and elbow.
Lithotomy	Back-lying position with feet supported in stirrups; the hips should be in line with the edge of the table.
Dorsal recumbent	Back-lying position with knees flexed and hips externally rotated; small pillow under the head; soles of feet on the surface.

❶ Left Sims', lithotomy, and dorsal recumbent positions

ASSESSMENT	NORMAL FINDINGS	DEVIATIONS FROM NORMAL
6. Inspect the anus and surrounding tissue for colour, integrity, and skin lesions. Then, ask the client to bear down as though defecating. Bearing down creates slight pressure on the skin that may accentuate rectal fissures, rectal prolapse, polyps, or internal hemorrhoids. Describe the location of all abnormal findings in terms of a clock, with the 12 o'clock position toward the pubic symphysis.	Intact perianal skin; usually slightly more pigmented than the skin of the buttocks; anal skin is normally more pigmented, coarser, and moister than perianal skin and is usually hairless	Presence of fissures (cracks), ulcers, excoriations, inflammations, abscesses, protruding hemorrhoids (dilated veins seen as reddened protrusions of the skin), lumps or tumours, fistula openings, or rectal prolapse (varying degrees of protrusion of the rectal mucous membrane through the anus)
7. Palpate the rectum for anal sphincter tonicity, nodules, masses, and tenderness. • Lubricate your gloved index finger, and instruct the client to bear downward as though having a bowel movement. **Rationale: This relaxes the anal sphincter.** • Slowly insert your finger into the anus and into the rectum in the direction of the umbilicus. The anal canal (distance from the anal opening to the anorectal junction) is short (less than 3 cm). The posterior wall of the rectum follows the curve of the coccyx and sacrum. The nurse's finger is usually able to palpate a distance of 6 cm to 10 cm.	Anal sphincter has good tone; rectal wall is smooth and not tender	Hypertonicity of the anal sphincter (may occur in the presence of an anal fissure or other lesion that causes contraction); hypotonicity of anal sphincter (may occur after rectal surgery or result from a neurological deficiency); rectal wall is tender and nodular

(continued)

SKILL 27.20

ASSESSING THE ANUS AND RECTUM (*continued*)

ASSESSMENT	NORMAL FINDINGS	DEVIATIONS FROM NORMAL
• Never force digital insertion. If lesions are painful or bleeding occurs, discontinue the examination. • Ask the client to tighten the anal sphincter around your finger, and note the tone of the anal sphincter. • Rotate the pad of the index finger along the anal and the rectal walls, feeling for nodules, masses, and tenderness. • Note the location of any abnormalities of the rectum (e.g., "anterior wall, 2 cm proximal to the internal anal sphincter").		
8. On withdrawing the finger from the rectum and anus, observe it for feces. If ordered, perform a test for occult blood on the stool (see Chapter 40).	Brown colour	Presence of mucus, blood, or black tarry stool

9. Document findings in the client record by using forms or checklists supplemented by narrative notes when appropriate.

EVALUATION

- Perform a detailed follow-up examination based on findings that deviated from expected or normal for the client. Relate findings to previous assessment data if available.
- Report significant deviations from normal to the appropriate members of the health-care team.

Lifespan Considerations

Assessing the Rectum and Anus

INFANTS

- Lightly touching the anus should result in a brief anal contraction ("wink" reflex).
- If the infant has normal bowel function, a rectal examination is not routinely performed.

CHILDREN

- Erythema and scratch marks around the anus may indicate a pinworm parasite. Children with this condition may be disturbed by itching during sleep.
- A rectal examination is not routinely performed on children.

OLDER ADULTS

- Chronic constipation and straining at stool cause an increase in the frequency of hemorrhoids and rectal prolapse.

Case Study 27

Mrs. J., a 32-year-old Inuit woman, comes to the clinic because she felt a lump in her breast. When you begin the breast examination, the patient shrieks and asks, "What do you think you are doing?"

Critical Thinking Questions

1. How would you respond to this patient?
2. How would you develop nursing interventions to help put patients at ease for an invasive procedure that has a vital role in physical assessment?

3. How will you address patients in a manner likely to gain their trust and cooperation?

After working through these questions, go to the MyNursingLab at **http://www.mynursinglab.com** to check your answers.

KEY TERMS

inspection
palpation
percussion
pleximeter
plexor
flatness
dullness
resonance
hyperresonance
tympany
auscultation
pitch
intensity
duration
quality
hyperhidrosis
bromhidrosis
pallor
cyanosis
jaundice
erythema
melanin
vitiligo
albinism
edema
primary skin lesions
secondary skin lesions
alopecia
hirsutism
koilonychia
clubbing
paronychia
blanch test
normocephalic
visual acuity
visual fields
myopia
hyperopia
presbyopia
astigmatism
conjunctivitis
dacryocystitis
hordeolum (sty)
cataracts
glaucoma
mydriasis
miosis
anisocoria
nystagmus
arcus senilis
otoscope
auricle
pinna
tympanic membrane
lobule
helix
antihelix
tragus
triangular fossa
external auditory meatus
mastoid
cerumen
ossicles
malleus
incus
stapes
eustachian tube
cochlea
vestibule
semicircular canals
conduction hearing loss
sensorineural hearing loss
mixed hearing loss
presbycusis
caries
pyorrhea
plaque
tartar
gingivitis
glossitis
stomatitis
parotitis
sordes
leukoplakia
angle of Louis
sternum
manubrium
adventitious breath sounds
base
apex
point of maximal impulse (PMI)
precordium
lift
heave
S_1
S_2
systole
diastole
bruit
thrill
perfusion
axillary tail of Spence
fasciculation
tremor
intention tremor
resting tremor
aphasia
reflex
proprioceptors
anaesthesia
hyperesthesia
hypoesthesia
paresthesia
one-point discrimination
two-point discrimination
stereognosis
extinction
nulliparous
multiparous
cystocele
rectocele
hernia
testicular self-examination

CHAPTER HIGHLIGHTS

- The health examination is conducted to assess the function and integrity of the client's body parts.
- The health examination may entail a complete head-to-toe assessment or individual assessment of a body system or body part.
- The health assessment is conducted in a systematic manner that requires the fewest position changes for the client.
- Aspects of the physical assessment procedures should be incorporated in the assessment, intervention, and evaluation phases of the nursing process.
- Data obtained in the physical health examination supplement, confirm, or refute data obtained during the nursing history.
- Nursing history data help the nurse focus on specific aspects of the physical health examination.
- Data obtained in the physical health examination help the nurse establish nursing diagnoses, plan the client's care, and evaluate the outcomes of nursing care.
- Initial assessment findings provide baseline data about the client's functional abilities against which subsequent assessment findings are compared.
- Skills in inspection, palpation, percussion, and auscultation are required for the physical health examination; these skills are used in that order throughout the examination except during abdominal assessment, when the order is inspection, auscultation, percussion, and palpation.
- Knowledge of the normal structure and function of body parts and systems is a prerequisite to conducting physical assessment.

ASSESS YOUR LEARNING

1. The nurse documents the patient's complaints of numbness and tingling in the right arm and right leg as which of the following?

a. Hyperesthesia
b. Hypoesthesia
c. Paresthesia
d. Extinction

2. The nurse positions the client sitting upright during palpation of which of the following areas?

a. Abdomen
b. Genitals
c. Breast
d. Head and neck

3. Which of the following is the correct order to conduct the assessment of the abdomen?

a. Inspection, palpation, percussion, auscultation
b. Inspection, percussion, palpation, auscultation
c. Auscultation, inspection, palpation, percussion
d. Inspection, auscultation, palpation, percussion

4. In older adults, the nurse must remember which of the following while conducting the health assessment?

a. The vital organs are in different locations because of aging.
b. This population fatigues easily and the exam must be tailored to best support the client.
c. Members of this population usually have memory lapses.
d. The nurse should always help the client off the examination table.

5. When the nurse is broaching sensitive topics, it is best to do which of the following?

a. Clearly state any personal feelings on the topic of discussion.
b. Be vague with the questions to make sure the patient is not embarrassed.
c. Be nonjudgmental.
d. Omit this kind of assessment so that neither the nurse nor the patient will feel uncomfortable.

6. After auscultating the abdomen, the nurse should report which of the following for further follow-up?

a. Bruit over the aorta
b. Absence of bowel sounds for 60 seconds
c. Continuous bowel sounds over the ileocecal valve
d. An irregular pattern of bowel sounds

7. If unable to locate the client's popliteal pulse during a routine examination, the nurse should perform which of the following next?

a. Check for a pedal pulse.
b. Check for a femoral pulse.
c. Take the client's blood pressure on that thigh.
d. Ask another nurse to try to locate the pulse.

8. Which of the following techniques should the nurse use to palpate the lymph nodes?

a. Use the flat of all four fingers in a vertical and then side-to-side motion.
b. Use the back of the hand and feel for temperature variation between the right and left sides.

c. Use the pads and tips of your index and middle fingers in a circular motion.

d. Compress the nodes between the index fingers of both hands.

9. If the client complains of loss of short-term memory, the nurse would assess this by doing which of the following?

a. Have the client repeat a series of three numbers, increasing to eight if possible.

b. Have the client describe his or her childhood illnesses.

c. Ask the client to describe how he or she arrived at your location.

d. Ask the client to count backward from 100 subtracting 7 each time.

10. Which of the following indicates a normal finding on general percussion of the lungs?

a. Tympany over the right upper lobe

b. Resonance over the left upper lobe

c. Hyperresonance over the left lower lobe

d. Dullness above the left 10th intercostal space

After working through these questions, go to the MyNursingLab at ***http://www.mynursinglab.com*** *to check your answers and see explanations.*

SUGGESTED READINGS

Manser, R. L., Irving, L. B., Stone, C., Byrnes, G., Abramson, M., & Campbell, D. (2004). Screening for lung cancer. *Cochrane Database of Systematic Reviews, 2004,* 3. Art. No.: CD001991.

Lung cancer is the leading cause of cancer deaths in Canada, but there is no evidence that routine screening by using chest X-ray or sputum samples is warranted. This review found that "early detection methods such as chest x-ray, testing sputum or CT scan do not appear to have much impact on either treatment or number of deaths from lung cancer. The review found frequent chest x-rays may cause harm."

Tingley, D. H. (2007). Vision screening essentials: Screening today for eye disorders in the pediatric patient. *Pediatrics in Review, 28,* 54–61.

This article provides an interesting overview of the visual screening requirements in children. The excellent photos are an added bonus to this research-based article.

WEBLINKS

Canadian Cancer Society

http://www.cancer.ca

This site provides educational resources related to cancer, including risk reduction.

McGill University Virtual Stethoscope

http://sprojects.mmi.mcgill.ca/dir/mvs.html

This site allows listeners to hear normal and adventitious lung sounds. Links are made with pathophysiology.

REFERENCES CONSULTED

Bickley, L., & Szilagyi, P. (2007). *Bates' guide to physical examination and history taking* (9th ed.). Philadelphia, PA: Lippincott Williams & Wilkins.

Boulware, L. E., Marinopoulos, S., Phillips, K. A., Hwang, C. W, Maynor, K., Merenstein, D., et al. (2007). Systematic review: The value of the periodic health evaluation. *Annals of Internal Medicine, 146,* 289–300.

Canadian Cancer Society & National Cancer Institute of Canada. (2007). *Canadian cancer statistics 2007.* Toronto: Canadian Cancer Society.

D'Amico, D., & Barbarito, C. (2007). *Health and physical assessment in nursing.* Upper Saddle, NJ: Pearson Education.

Dubey, V., & Glazier, R. (2006). Preventive care checklist form: Evidence-based tool to improve preventive health care during complete health assessment of adults. *Canadian Family Physician, 52*(1), 48–55.

Estes, M. E., & Buck, M. (2008). *Health assessment and physical examination.* Toronto: Nelson.

Kösters, J. P., & Gøtzsche, P. C. (2003). Regular self-examination or clinical examination for early detection of breast cancer. *The Cochrane Database of Systematic Reviews, 2.* Art. No.: CD003373.

Leddin, D., Hunt, R., Champion, M., Cockeram, A., Flook, N., Gould, et al. (2004). Guidelines on colon cancer screening. *Canadian Journal of Gastroenterology, 18*(2), 93–99.

Peacock, S. (2004). Systematic health assessment: A case study. *Practice Nursing, 15*(6), 270, 271–274.

Public Health Agency of Canada. (2002). *Technical report for the national committee on colorectal cancer screening.* Ottawa: Health Canada.

Pullen, R. L. (2004). Clinical do's & don'ts. Neurological assessment for pronator drift. *Nursing, 34*(3), 22.

Pullen, R. L. (2005). Clinical do's & don'ts. Testing the corneal reflex. *Nursing, 35*(11), 68.

Rushing, J. (2005). Clinical do's & don'ts. Assessing for ascites. *Nursing, 35*(2), 68.

Ringash, J., & the Canadian Task Force on Preventive Health Care. (2001). Preventive health care, 2001 update: Screening mammography among women aged 40–49 years at average risk of breast cancer. *Canadian Medical Association Journal, 164*(4), 469–476.

Seidel, H., Ball, J., Dains, J., & Benedict, G. (2006). *Mosby's guide to physical examination* (6th ed.). St. Louis, MO: Mosby Elsevier.

Sin, D. D., Spier, S., Svenson, L. W., Schopflocher, D. P., Senthilselvan, A., Cowie, R. L., et al. (2004). The relationship between birth weight and childhood asthma. *Archives of Pediatric and Adolescent Medicine, 158*, 60–64.

Thomas Hess, C. (2008). *Clinical guide: Skin and wound care* (6th ed.). Philadelphia, PA: Lippincott, Williams & Wilkins.

Chapter 28

Vital Signs

The **vital signs** are body temperature, pulse, respirations, and blood pressure. Recently, many agencies have designated pain as the fifth vital sign, to be assessed at the same time as each of the other four. Pain assessment is covered in Chapter 34. Pulse oximetry is also commonly measured at the same time as the traditional vital signs. These signs, which should be looked at in total, are checked to monitor the functions of the body. Vital signs reflect changes in function that otherwise might not be observed. Monitoring a client's vital signs should not be an automatic or routine procedure; it should be a thoughtful, scientific assessment. Vital signs, which should be evaluated with reference to the client's present and prior health status, are compared with accepted normal standards.

When and how often to assess a specific client's vital signs are chiefly nursing judgments, depending on the client's health status. Some agencies have policies about taking clients' vital signs, and physicians may specify frequency (e.g., "blood pressure q2h"). Ordered assessments, however, should be considered the minimum; a nurse should measure vital signs more often if the client's health status requires it. Examples of times to assess vital signs are listed in Box 28.1.

OBJECTIVES

After studying this chapter, you should be able to

1. Describe factors that affect the vital signs and accurate measurement of them
2. Identify the normal range variations in body temperature, pulse, respirations, and blood pressure that occur across the lifespan
3. Explain the body's system of thermoregulation and identify factors influencing the body's heat production.
4. Explain and compare oral, rectal, axillary, tympanic membrane, and temporal artery methods of measuring body temperature
5. Describe appropriate nursing care for alterations in body temperature
6. Identify nine sites commonly used to assess the pulse and state the reasons for use of each
7. Explain the characteristics that should be included when assessing pulses
8. Explain how to measure the apical pulse and apical-radial pulse
9. Describe the mechanics of breathing and the mechanisms that control respirations
10. Identify the components of a respiratory assessment
11. Identify noninvasive methods for measuring blood pressure, and differentiate between systolic and diastolic blood pressure, including the five phases of Korotkoff's sounds
12. Discuss measurement of blood oxygenation by using pulse oximetry

BOX 28.1 TIMES TO ASSESS VITAL SIGNS

Vital signs should be assessed at these times:

- On admission to a health-care agency to obtain baseline data
- When a client has a change in health status or reports symptoms, such as chest pain or feeling hot or faint
- Before and after surgery or an invasive procedure
- Before or after the administration of a medication that could affect the respiratory or cardiovascular systems, (e.g., before giving a digitalis preparation, before and after the administration of an opioid)
- Before and after any nursing intervention that could affect the vital signs (e.g., ambulating a client who has been on bed rest)

Body Temperature

Body temperature reflects the balance between heat produced and heat lost from the body, and it is measured in units called degrees. The body has two kinds of temperatures: core temperature and surface temperature. **Core temperature** is the temperature of the deep tissues of the body, such as the cranium, thorax, abdominal cavity, and pelvic cavity. It remains relatively constant. The **surface temperature** is the temperature of the skin, subcutaneous tissue, and fat. It, by contrast, fluctuates in response to the environment.

The normal core body temperature is a range of temperatures (Figure 28.1). When measured orally, the average body temperature of an adult is between 36.7°C and 37°C, with a normal range of 36°C to 38°C.

The body continually produces heat as a byproduct of metabolism. When the amount of heat produced by the body exactly equals the amount of heat lost, the person is in **heat balance** (Figure 28.2).

A number of factors affect the body's heat production. The most important are these five:

1. *Basal metabolic rate.* The **basal metabolic rate (BMR)** is the rate of energy utilization in the body required to maintain essential activities, such as breathing. Metabolic rates decrease with age. In general, the younger the person, the higher is the BMR.
2. *Muscle activity.* Muscle activity, including shivering, increases the BMR.
3. *Thyroxine output.* Increased thyroxine output increases the rate of cellular metabolism throughout the body. This effect is called **chemical thermogenesis**, the stimulation of heat production in the body through increased cellular metabolism.
4. *Sympathetic stimulation, including release of epinephrine and norepinephrine.* Sympathetic stimulation of the autonomic nervous system (such as during stress) causes the release of epinephrine and norepinephrine. These hormones directly affect liver and muscle cells, thereby increasing cellular metabolism and heat production.
5. *Fever.* Fever increases the cellular metabolic rate and thus further increases the body's temperature.

Heat is lost from the body through radiation, conduction, convection, and vaporization. **Radiation** is the transfer of heat from the surface of one object to the surface of another without contact between the two objects, mostly in the form of infrared rays. **Conduction** is the transfer of heat from one molecule to a molecule of lower temperature. Conductive transfer cannot take

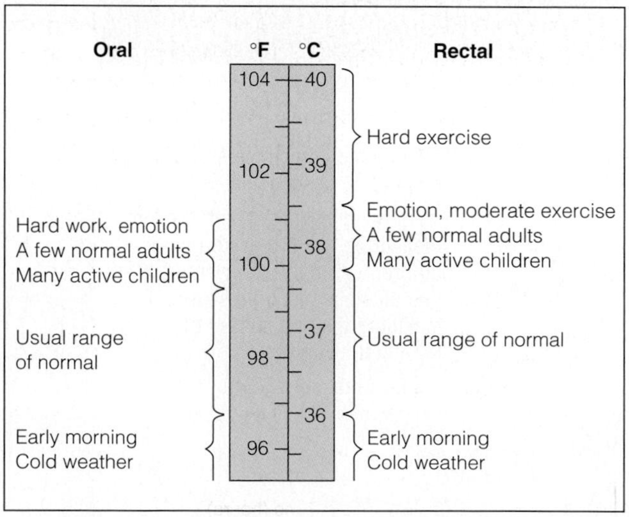

FIGURE 28.1 Estimated ranges of body temperature in normal persons

(From **Fever and the Regulation of Body Temperature,** *by E. F. Dubois, 1948, Springfield, IL: Charles C. Thomas. Reprinted with permission.)*

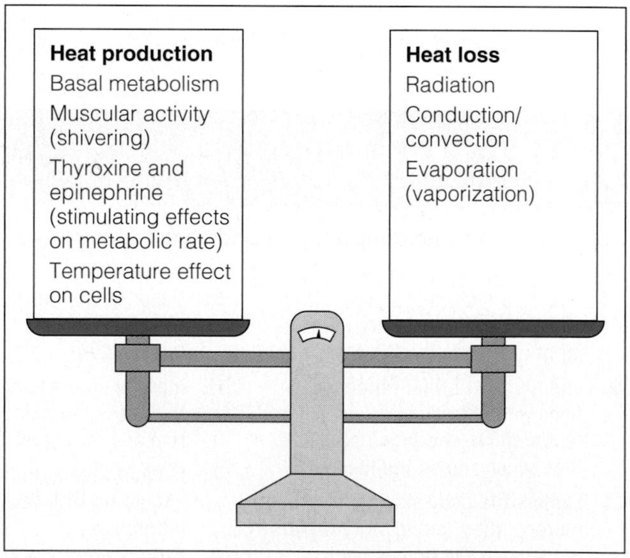

FIGURE 28.2 As long as heat production and heat loss are properly balanced, body temperature remains constant. Factors contributing to heat production (and temperature rise) are shown on the left side of the scale; those contributing to heat loss (and temperature drop) are shown on the right side.

(Adapted from **Human Anatomy and Physiology,** *4th ed. (p. 953), by E. N. Marieb, 1998, Menlo Parks, CA: Benjamin/Cummings. Adapted with permission.)*

place without contact between the molecules and normally accounts for minimal heat loss, except, for example, when a body is immersed in cold water. The amount of heat transferred depends on the temperature difference and the amount and duration of the contact.

Convection is the dispersion of heat by air currents. The body usually has a small amount of warm air adjacent to it. This warm air rises and is replaced by cooler air, and so people always lose a small amount of heat through convection.

Vaporization is continuous evaporation of moisture from the respiratory tract, from the mucosa of the mouth, and from the skin. This continuous and unnoticed water loss is called **insensible water loss**, and the accompanying heat loss is called **insensible heat loss**. Insensible heat loss accounts for about 10% of basal heat loss. When the body temperature increases, vaporization accounts for greater heat loss.

Regulation of Body Temperature

The system that regulates body temperature has three main parts: (1) sensors on the skin and in the core, (2) an integrator in the hypothalamus, and (3) an effector system that adjusts the production and loss of heat. Most *sensors* or *sensory receptors* are in the skin. The skin has more receptors for cold than for warmth. Therefore, skin sensors detect cold more efficiently than warmth.

When the skin becomes chilled over the entire body, three physiological processes take place to increase the body temperature:

1. Shivering increases heat production.
2. Sweating is inhibited to decrease heat loss.
3. Vasoconstriction decreases heat loss.

The **hypothalamic integrator**, the centre that controls the core temperature, is located in the preoptic area of the hypothalamus. When the sensors in the hypothalamus detect heat, they send out signals intended to reduce the temperature, that is, to decrease heat production and increase heat loss. When the cold sensors are stimulated, signals are sent out to increase heat production and decrease heat loss.

The signals from the cold-sensitive receptors of the hypothalamus initiate *effectors,* such as vasoconstriction, shivering, and the release of epinephrine, which increases cellular metabolism and, hence, heat production. When the warmth-sensitive receptors in the hypothalamus are stimulated, the effector system sends out signals that initiate sweating and peripheral vasodilation. Also, when this system is stimulated, the person consciously makes appropriate adjustments, such as putting on additional clothing in response to cold or turning on a fan in response to heat.

Factors Affecting Body Temperature

Nurses should be aware of the factors that can affect a client's body temperature in order to recognize normal temperature variations and understand the significance of body temperature measurements that deviate from normal. Among the factors that affect body temperature are the following:

1. *Age.* The infant is greatly influenced by the temperature of the environment and must be protected from extreme changes. Until puberty, children's temperatures continue to be more labile (changeable) than those of adults. Many older people, particularly those older than 75 years, are at risk of hypothermia (temperatures below 36°C) for a variety of reasons, such as inadequate diet, loss of subcutaneous fat, lack of activity, and reduced thermoregulatory efficiency. Older people are also particularly sensitive to extremes in the environmental temperature because of decreased thermoregulatory controls.
2. *Diurnal variations (circadian rhythms).* Body temperatures normally change throughout the day, varying as much as 1°C between the early morning and the late afternoon. The point of highest body temperature is usually reached between 1600 and 1800 hours (4 p.m. and 6 p.m.), and the lowest point is reached during sleep between 0400 and 0600 hours (4 a.m. and 6 a.m.). See Figure 28.3.
3. *Exercise.* Hard work or strenuous exercise can increase body temperature to as high as 38.3°C to 40°C when measured rectally.
4. *Hormones.* Women usually experience more hormone fluctuations than men do. In women, progesterone secretion at the time of ovulation raises body temperature by about 0.3°C to 0.6°C above basal temperature.
5. *Stress.* Stimulation of the sympathetic nervous system can increase the production of epinephrine and norepinephrine, thereby increasing metabolic activity and heat production. Nurses can anticipate that a highly stressed or anxious client could have an elevated body temperature for that reason.
6. *Environment.* Extremes in environmental temperatures can affect a person's temperature regulatory

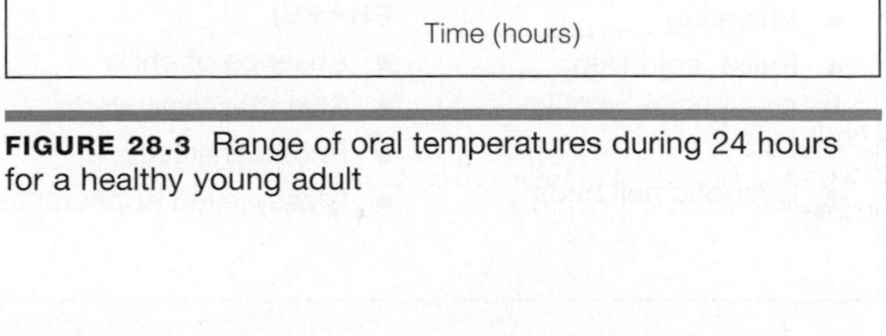

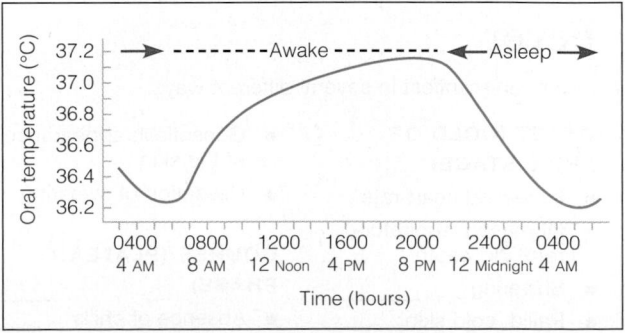

FIGURE 28.3 Range of oral temperatures during 24 hours for a healthy young adult

systems. If the temperature is assessed in a very warm room and the body temperature cannot be modified by convection, conduction, or radiation, the temperature will be elevated. Similarly, if the client has been outside in extremely cold weather without suitable clothing, the body temperature may be low.

Alterations in Body Temperature

Two primary alterations in body temperature occur: pyrexia (hyperthermia, fever) and hypothermia

PYREXIA A body temperature above the usual range is called **pyrexia**, **hyperthermia**, or (in lay terms) **fever**. A very high fever, such as 41°C, is called **hyperpyrexia** (Figure 28.4). The client who has a fever is referred to as **febrile**; the one who does not have a fever is **afebrile.**

Four common types of fevers are intermittent, remittent, relapsing, and constant. During an **intermittent fever**, the body temperature alternates at regular intervals between periods of fever and periods of normal or subnormal temperatures. This occurs, for example, with the disease malaria. During a **remittent fever**, such as with a cold or influenza, a wide range of temperature fluctuations (more than 2°C) occurs in 24 hours, all of which are above normal. In a **relapsing fever**, short febrile periods of a few days are interspersed with periods of 1 or 2 days of normal temperature. During a **constant fever**, the body temperature fluctuates minimally but always remains above normal. This can occur with typhoid fever. A temperature that rises to fever level rapidly following a normal temperature and then returns to normal within a few hours is called a **fever spike**. Bacterial blood infections often cause fever spikes.

In some conditions, an elevated temperature is not a true fever. Two examples are heat exhaustion and heat stroke. **Heat exhaustion** is a result of excessive heat and dehydration. Signs of heat exhaustion include pallor, dizziness, nausea, vomiting, fainting, and a moderately increased temperature (38.5°C to 39°C). Persons experiencing **heat stroke** generally have been exercising in hot weather, have warm, flushed skin, and often do not sweat. They usually have a temperature of 41°C or higher and may be delirious, unconscious, or having seizures.

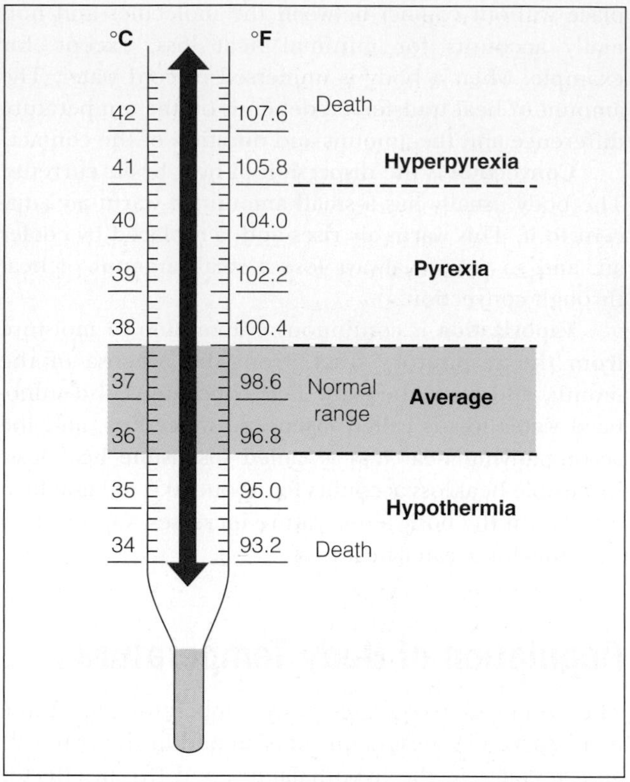

FIGURE 28.4 Terms used to describe alterations in body temperature (oral measurements) and ranges in Celsius and Fahrenheit scales

The clinical signs of fever vary with the onset, course, and abatement stages of the fever (see the Clinical Manifestations box).

These signs occur as a result of changes in the *set point* of the temperature control mechanism regulated by the hypothalamus. Under normal conditions, whenever the core temperature rises above 37°C, the rate of heat

Clinical Manifestations

Fever

Fever can manifest in several different ways:

ONSET (COLD OR CHILL STAGE)

- Increased heart rate
- Increased respiratory rate and depth
- Shivering
- Pallid, cold skin
- Complaints of feeling cold
- Cyanotic nail beds
- Gooseflesh appearance of the skin
- Cessation of sweating

COURSE (PLATEAU PHASE)

- Absence of chills
- Skin that feels warm
- Photosensitivity
- Glassy-eyed appearance
- Increased pulse and respiratory rates
- Increased thirst
- Mild to severe dehydration
- Drowsiness, restlessness, delirium, or convulsions
- Herpetic lesions of the mouth
- Loss of appetite (if the fever is prolonged)
- Malaise, weakness, and aching muscles

DEFERVESCENCE (FEVER ABATEMENT OR FLUSH PHASE)

- Skin that appears flushed and feels warm
- Sweating
- Decreased shivering
- Possible dehydration

loss becomes greater than heat production, resulting in a fall in temperature toward the set point level. Conversely, when the core temperature falls below 37°C, the rate of heat production becomes greater than heat loss, resulting in a rise in temperature toward the set point.

In a fever, however, the set point of the hypothalamic thermostat changes suddenly from the normal level to a higher than normal value (e.g., 39.5°C) as a result of the effects of tissue destruction, pyrogenic substances, or dehydration on the hypothalamus. Although the set point changes rapidly, the core body temperature (i.e., the blood temperature) reaches this new set point only after several hours. During this interval, the usual heat production responses that cause elevation of the body temperature occur: chills, feeling of coldness, cold skin because of vasoconstriction, and shivering. This is called the *chill phase*.

When the core temperature reaches the new set point, the person feels neither cold nor hot and no longer experiences chills (the *plateau phase*). Depending on the degree of temperature elevation, various other signs may occur at this stage. Very high temperatures, such as 41°C to 42°C, damage the parenchyma (the key elements essential to functioning) of cells throughout the body, particularly in the brain, where destruction of neuronal cells is irreversible. Damage to the liver, kidneys, and other body organs can also be great enough to disrupt functioning and eventually cause death.

When the cause of the high temperature is suddenly removed, the set point of the hypothalamic thermostat is suddenly reduced to a lower value, perhaps even back to the original normal level. In this instance, the hypothalamus now attempts to lower the temperature to 37°C, and the usual heat loss responses causing a reduction of the body temperature occur: excessive sweating and a hot, flushed skin because of sudden vasodilation. This sudden change of events is known as the *flush* or *defervescent stage* of a pyrexic condition.

Nursing interventions for a client who has a fever are designed to support the body's normal physiological processes, provide comfort, and prevent complications. During the course of the fever, the nurse must monitor the client's vital signs closely.

Nursing measures during the chill phase are designed to help the client decrease heat loss. At this time, the body's physiological processes are attempting to raise the core temperature to the new set point temperature. During the flush or crisis phase, the body processes are attempting to lower the core temperature to the reduced or normal set point temperature. At this time, the nurse takes measures to increase heat loss and decrease heat production. Nursing interventions for a client with fever are shown in Box 28.2. See the Teaching: Clinical box for an explanation of why people experience fevers.

HYPOTHERMIA **Hypothermia** is a core body temperature below the lower limit of normal. The three physiological mechanisms of hypothermia are (1) excessive heat loss, (2) inadequate heat production to

BOX 28.2 NURSING INTERVENTIONS FOR CLIENTS WITH FEVER

Nurses can do several things to help a client through each stage of a fever:

- Monitor vital signs.
- Assess skin colour and temperature.
- Monitor white blood cell count, hematocrit value, and other pertinent laboratory reports for indications of infection or dehydration.
- Remove excess blankets when the client feels warm, but provide extra warmth when the client feels chilled.
- Provide adequate nutrition and fluids (e.g., 2500 mL to 3000 mL per day if not contraindicated) to meet the increased metabolic demands and prevent dehydration.
- Measure intake and output.
- Reduce physical activity to limit heat production, especially during the flush stage.
- Administer antipyretics (drugs that reduce the level of fever), as ordered.
- Provide oral hygiene to keep the mucous membranes moist. They can become dry and cracked as a result of excessive fluid loss.
- Provide a tepid sponge bath to increase heat loss through conduction (the patient must not shiver during this bath or else the fever will rise).
- Provide dry clothing and bed linens.

TEACHING: CLINICAL

Why do people have fevers?

Fever is not an illness but a sign of other problems within the body. The fever triggers the immune system to release chemicals (pyrogens) that cause the body's temperature to rise (reset the set point).This activation of the immune system is a protective mechanism of the body.

Clinical Manifestations

Hypothermia

Hypothermia typically manifests in the following ways:

- Decreased body temperature, pulse, and respirations
- Severe shivering (initially)
- Feelings of cold and chills
- Pale, cool, waxy skin
- Frostbite (nose, fingers, toes)
- Hypotension
- Decreased urinary output
- Lack of muscle coordination
- Disorientation
- Drowsiness progressing to coma

counteract the heat loss, and (3) impaired hypothalamic thermoregulation. The clinical signs of hypothermia are given in the Clinical Manifestations box.

Hypothermia can be induced or accidental. *Induced hypothermia* is the deliberate lowering of the body temperature to decrease the need for oxygen by the body tissues. Induced hypothermia can involve the whole body or a body part. It may be indicated for certain surgical cases (e.g., cardiac and brain surgery) but remains controversial. *Accidental hypothermia* can occur as a result of (1) exposure to a cold environment (i.e., below 16°C), (2) immersion in cold water, and (3) lack of adequate clothing, shelter, or heat. In older people, the problem can be compounded by a decreased metabolic rate and the use of sedatives, which depress the metabolic rate. If skin and underlying tissues are damaged by freezing cold, this results in frostbite. Frostbite most commonly occurs in hands, feet, nose, and ears.

Managing hypothermia involves removing the client from the cold and warming the client's body. For the client with mild hypothermia, the body is warmed by applying blankets; for the client with severe hypothermia, a hyperthermia blanket (an electrically controlled blanket that provides a specified temperature) is applied, and warm intravenous fluids are given. Wet clothing, which increases heat loss because of the high conductivity of water, should be replaced with dry clothing. See Box 28.3 for nursing interventions for clients who have hypothermia.

BOX 28.3 NURSING INTERVENTIONS FOR CLIENTS WITH HYPOTHERMIA

Nurses can do the following things to help a client who has hypothermia:

- Provide a warm environment (room temperature).
- Provide dry clothing.
- Apply warm blankets.
- Keep limbs close to the body.
- Cover the client's scalp with a cap or turban.
- Supply warm oral or intravenous fluids.
- Apply warming pads.

Assessing Body Temperature

The most common sites for measuring body temperature are oral, rectal, axillary, and tympanic membrane, and skin or temporal artery. Each of the sites has advantages and disadvantages (see Table 28.1).

The body temperature is frequently measured *orally*. If a client has ingested hot food or fluids or has been smoking, the nurse should wait 30 minutes before taking the temperature orally to ensure that the temperature of the mouth has not been affected by the temperature of the food, fluid, or warm smoke.

Rectal temperature readings are considered to be very accurate. Because inserting a rectal thermometer can pro-

TABLE 28.1 Advantages and Disadvantages of Five Sites for Body Temperature Measurement

Site	Advantages	Disadvantages
Oral	Accessible and convenient	Thermometers can break if bitten. Inaccurate if client has just ingested hot or cold food or fluid or smoked. Could injure the mouth following oral surgery.
Rectal	Reliable measurement	Inconvenient and more unpleasant for clients; difficult for client who cannot turn to the side. Could injure the rectum following rectal surgery. Presence of stool may interfere with thermometer placement. If the stool is soft, the thermometer may be embedded in stool rather than against the mucosal wall of the rectum. If the stool is impacted, the depth of thermometer insertion may be insufficient. May stimulate a vagal reaction leading to bradycardia. In newborns and infants, insertion or rectal thermometer has caused ulcerations and rectal perforations.
Axillary	Safe and noninvasive	The thermometer must be left in place a long time to obtain an accurate measurement.
Tympanic membrane	Readily accessible; reflects the core temperature. Very fast.	Can be uncomfortable and involves risk of injuring the membrane if the probe is inserted too far. Repeated measurements may vary. Right and left measurements can differ. Presence of cerumen can affect the reading.
Temporal artery	Safe and noninvasive; very fast.	Requires electronic equipment that may be expensive or unavailable; variation in technique needed if the client has perspiration on the forehead.

Evidence-Informed Practice

How Do Beverages and Respiratory Rates Affect Oral Temperature Readings?

Quatrara and colleagues (2007) used a randomized control study to examine how the consumption of hot and cold beverages and the respiratory rate affected oral thermometer measurements when using an electric thermometer. Although a lot of research has previously been done by using glass mercury thermometers, there has been a lack of research on factors that influence temperature when measured with an electronic thermometer. The researchers found that the long-standing recommendation to wait at least 30 minutes following drinking a hot or cold beverage was supported when using electronic thermometers. Patients who had bradypnea had higher temperature elevations than patients with a normal respiratory rate.

NURSING IMPLICATIONS: Nurses must continue to make sure that patients have not ingested hot or cold beverages to ensure accurate temperature recordings when measuring oral temperature by using an electronic thermometer. Patients who have lower respiratory rates, such as those on opioids, can have slightly higher temperature readings as a result of their slowed respirations.

Source: Based on "The Effect of Respiratory Rate and Ingestion of Hot and Cold Beverages on the Accuracy of Oral Temperatures Measured by Electronic Thermometers," by B. Quatrara, J. Coffman, T. Jenkins, K. Mann, K. McGough, M. Conaway, and S. Burns, 2007, *Medsurg Nursing, 16*(2), pp. 105–108.

duce vagal stimulation, which can cause bradycardia, taking rectal temperatures is generally contraindicated for clients with cardiac arrhythmias or recovering from a myocardial infarction. Rectal temperatures are usually contraindicated in clients who are undergoing rectal surgery, have diarrhea or diseases of the rectum, are immunosuppressed, have a clotting disorder, or have significant hemorrhoids.

The *axilla* is the preferred site for measuring temperature in newborns because it is accessible and offers no possibility of rectal perforation. However, research indicates that the axillary method is inaccurate when assessing a fever (Ball & Bindler, 2008). Nurses should check agency protocol when taking the temperature of newborns, infants, toddlers, and children. The axillary method of temperature assessment is appropriate for adult clients with oral inflammation or wired jaws, for clients recovering from oral surgery, clients who are breathing through their mouths (e.g., following nasal surgery), irrational clients, and clients for whom other temperature sites are contraindicated.

The *tympanic membrane,* or nearby tissue in the ear canal, is a frequent site for estimating core body temperature. Like the sublingual oral site, the tympanic membrane has an abundant arterial blood supply, primarily from branches of the external carotid artery. Because temperature sensors applied directly to the tympanic membrane can be uncomfortable and involve risk of membrane injury or perforation, noninvasive *infrared thermometers* are used.

The temperature can also be measured on the forehead by using a chemical thermometer or a temporal artery thermometer. Forehead temperature measurements are most useful for infants and children on occasions when a more invasive measurement is not necessary.

TYPES OF THERMOMETERS Traditionally, body temperatures have been measured by using mercury-in-glass thermometers. Glass thermometers can be hazardous because of exposure to mercury, which is toxic to humans, and broken glass if the thermometer cracks or breaks. In 1999, the Canadian Environmental Protection Act listed mercury as a toxic substance and identified the goal of eliminating mercury from our environments. Hospitals should no longer use mercury-in-glass thermometers. However, the general population may not be aware of the risks associated with mercury-in-glass thermometers and may still have them in their homes. Nurses should advocate for the safe disposal of mercury thermometers and guide clients to purchase safer alternatives.

If the nurse is present when a client is using a mercury thermometer and it breaks, the nurse should follow Environment Canada's (2004) recommendations for cleaning up small mercury spills. These precautions are necessary because unsealed mercury slowly vaporizes into the air and these vapours are toxic. The highlights of the procedure include opening windows to increase ventilation; keeping children and pets away from the area; wearing rubber gloves and using stiff paper to slide the mercury beads onto a plastic dustpan; using a flashlight to search for the beads since the light will reflect off the mercury; pouring the mercury into a large-mouthed container; closing the container with an air-tight lid and sealing the lid with masking or duct tape; placing the container in a sealable bag and sealing it; contacting the municipal waste department for further disposal instructions; and thoroughly washing and rinsing any body part that has come in contact with the mercury. Do not use any type of vacuum cleaner or broom since these will disperse the mercury and be contaminated. Do not pour the mercury down a toilet or drain, and do not wash or reuse contaminated materials. Disposal instructions vary with the extent of the spill and whether the spill occurs on porous material (e.g., a carpet). *It is recommended that Environment Canada be consulted for detailed instructions.*

CLINICAL ALERT

Whenever mercury-in-glass thermometers are encountered, the nurse should recommend their immediate replacement with less hazardous thermometers and their safe disposal.

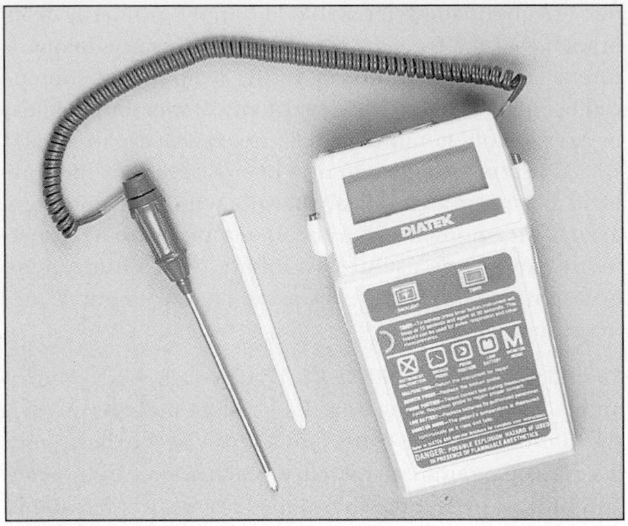

FIGURE 28.5 An electronic thermometer. Note the probe and probe cover.

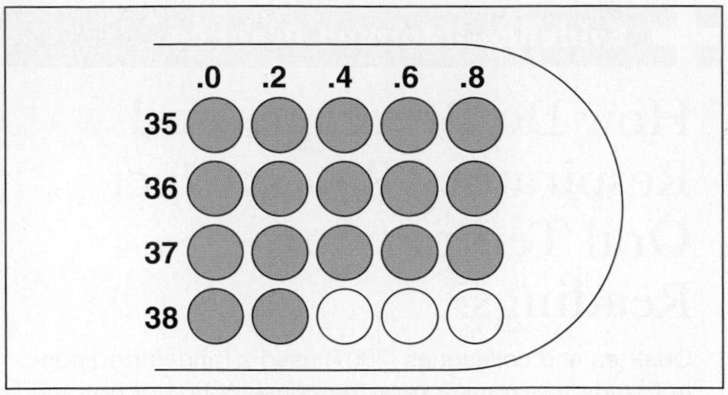

FIGURE 28.6 A chemical thermometer showing a reading of 38.2°C.

Electronic thermometers can provide a reading in only 2 to 60 seconds, depending on the model. The equipment consists of a battery-operated portable electronic unit, a probe that the nurse attaches to the unit, and a probe cover, which is usually disposable (Figure 28.5). Some models have a different circuit and probe for each method of measurement.

Chemical disposable thermometers are also used to measure body temperatures. Chemical thermometers that use liquid crystal dots or bars, heat-sensitive tape, or patches applied to the forehead change colour to indicate temperature. Some of these are single use and others can be reused. One type that has small chemical dots at one end is shown in Figure 28.6. To read the temperature, the nurse notes the highest reading among the dots that have changed colour.

Temperature-sensitive tape can also be used to obtain a general indication of body surface temperature. It does not indicate the core temperature. The tape contains liquid crystals that change colour according to temperature. When applied to the skin, usually on the forehead or abdomen, the temperature digits on the tape respond by changing colour (Figure 28.7). The skin area should be dry. After the length of time specified by the manufacturer (e.g., 15 seconds), a colour appears on the tape. The tape is removed and discarded after the colour has been compared with the scale provided by the manufacturer. This method is particularly useful at home and for infants whose temperatures are to be monitored.

Infrared thermometers sense body heat in the form of infrared energy given off by a heat source, which, in the ear canal, is primarily the tympanic membrane (Figure 28.8). The infrared thermometer makes no contact with the tympanic membrane.

Temporal artery (TA) thermometers determine temperature by using a scanning infrared thermometer that compares arterial temperature in the temporal artery of the forehead to the temperature in the room and calculates the heat balance to approximate the core temperature of the blood in the pulmonary artery (Roy, Powell, & Gerson, 2003). The probe is placed in the middle of the forehead and then drawn laterally to the hairline. If the client has perspiration on the forehead, the

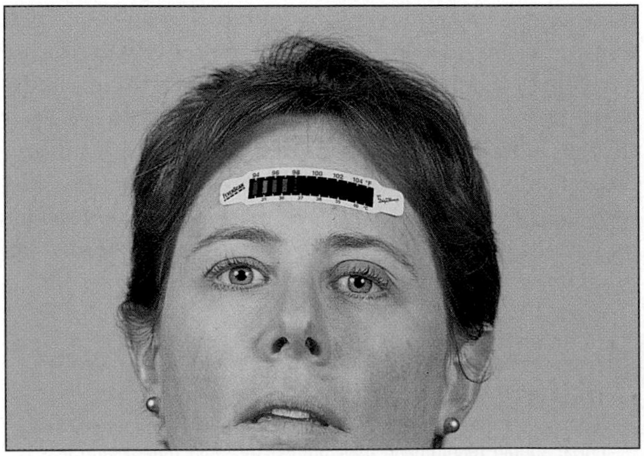

FIGURE 28.7 A temperature-sensitive skin tape

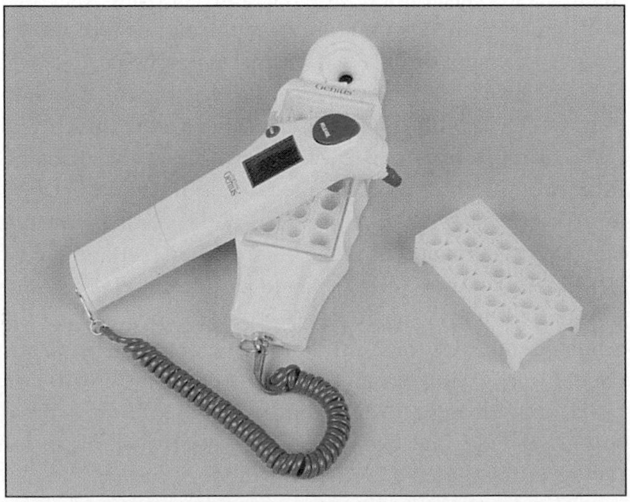

FIGURE 28.8 An infrared (tympanic) thermometer used to measure the tympanic membrane temperature.

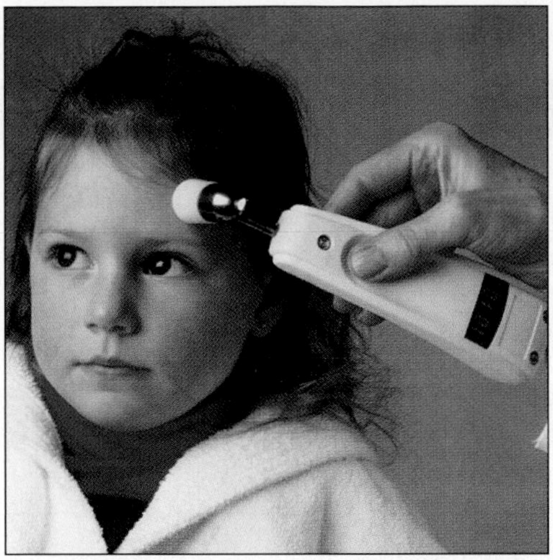

FIGURE 28.9 A temporal artery thermometer

probe is also touched behind the earlobe so the thermometer can compensate for evaporative cooling (Figure 28.9).

TEMPERATURE SCALES The body temperature is measured in degrees on the Celsius scale in keeping with Canada's adoption of the Système Internationale d'Unités (metric system) as the national standard of measurement in 1971.

Sometimes, however, a nurse needs to convert a Fahrenheit reading to Celsius, or vice versa. Although the conversion can be accomplished by using several different formulas, the most common is described here. To convert from Fahrenheit to Celsius, deduct 32 from the Fahrenheit reading and then multiply by 5/9:

$$°C = (\text{Fahrenheit temperature} - 32) \times 5/9$$

For example, when the Fahrenheit reading is 100:

$$°C = (100 - 32) \times 5/9 = 68 \times 5/9 = 37.8$$

To convert from Celsius to Fahrenheit, multiply the Celsius reading by 9/5 and then add 32:

$$°F = (\text{Celsius temperature} \times 9/5) + 32$$

For example, when the Celsius reading is 40:

$$°F = (40 \times 9/5) + 32 = 72 + 32 = 104$$

Clients may need to be taught how to use and read a thermometer properly when they are sent home. See the Teaching: Home Care box.

Skill 28.1 explains how to measure body temperature.

TEACHING: HOME CARE

Temperature

Being able to take their temperature at home is an important skill for clients to have:

- Teach the client accurate use and reading of the type of thermometer to be used. Examine the thermometer used by the client in the home for safety and proper functioning. Facilitate the replacement of mercury thermometers with nonmercury ones. See the section on types of thermometers earlier in the chapter for instructions regarding management of a broken mercury thermometer.
- Observe the client or caregiver taking and reading a temperature. Reinforce the importance of reporting the site and type of thermometer used and the value of using one consistently.
- Discuss means of keeping the thermometer clean, such as warm water and soap, and avoiding cross-contamination.
- Ensure that the client has water-soluble lubricant if using a rectal thermometer.
- Instruct the client or family member to notify the health-care provider if the temperature is 38°C or higher.
- When making a home visit, take a thermometer with you in case the clients do not have a functional thermometer of their own.
- Check that the client knows how to record the temperature. Provide a recording chart or table if indicated.
- Discuss environmental control modifications that should be taken during illness or extreme climate conditions (e.g., heating, air conditioning, appropriate clothing and bedding).

SKILL 28.1

ASSESSING BODY TEMPERATURE

PURPOSE

- To establish baseline data for subsequent evaluation
- To identify whether the core temperature is within normal range
- To determine changes in the core temperature in response to specific therapies (e.g., antipyretic medication, immunosuppressive therapy, invasive procedure)
- To monitor clients at risk for alterations in temperature (e.g., clients at risk for infection or diagnosis of infection; those who have been exposed to temperature extremes)

(continued)

SKILL 28.1

ASSESSING BODY TEMPERATURE (*continued*)

ASSESSMENT

Assess

- Clinical signs of fever
- Clinical signs of hypothermia
- Site most appropriate for measurement
- Factors that can alter core body temperature

Equipment

- Thermometer
- Thermometer sheath or cover
- Towel, if the axillary site is used
- Water-soluble lubricant and tissue, if the rectal site is used
- Disposable gloves
- Tissues or wipes

IMPLEMENTATION

Preparation

Check that all equipment is functioning normally.

Performance

1. Before performing the procedure, introduce yourself and verify the client's identity by using agency protocol. Explain to the client what you are going to do, why it is necessary, and how he or she can cooperate.
2. Perform hand hygiene and observe other appropriate infection prevention and control procedures. Don gloves if performing a rectal temperature.
3. Provide for client privacy.
4. Place the client in the appropriate position (e.g., lateral or Sims' position for inserting a rectal thermometer).
5. Place the thermometer (see ❶ through ❺).
   - Apply a protective sheath or probe cover if appropriate.
   - Lubricate a rectal thermometer.
6. Wait the appropriate amount of time. Electronic and tympanic thermometers will indicate that the reading is complete through a light or tone. Check package instructions for length of time to wait before reading chemical dot or tape thermometers.
7. Remove the thermometer and discard the cover or wipe with a tissue if necessary.
8. Read the temperature and record it on your worksheet. If the temperature is obviously too high, too low, or inconsistent with the client's condition, recheck it with a thermometer known to be functioning properly.
9. Wash the thermometer if necessary and return it to the storage location.
10. Document the temperature in the client record. A rectal temperature may be recorded with an R next to the value or with the mark on a graphic sheet circled. An axillary temperature may be recorded with AX or marked on a graphic sheet with an X.

EVALUATION

- Compare the temperature measurement to baseline data, the normal range for the age of the client, and the client's previous temperatures. Analyze by considering the time of day and any additional influencing factors and other vital signs.
- Conduct appropriate follow-up, such as notifying the appropriate members of the health-care team, giving a medication, or altering the client's environment. This includes teaching the client how to lower an elevated temperature through such actions as increasing fluid intake, coughing and deep breathing, or removing heavy coverings.

Thermometer Placement

Oral Place the bulb on either side of the frenulum (see ❶).

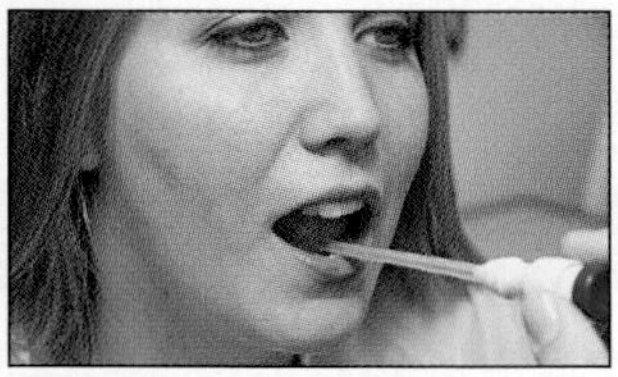

❶ Oral thermometer placement

Rectal Apply clean gloves.
Instruct the client to take a slow deep breath during insertion (see ❷).
Never force the thermometer if resistance is felt.
Insert 3.5 cm in adults.

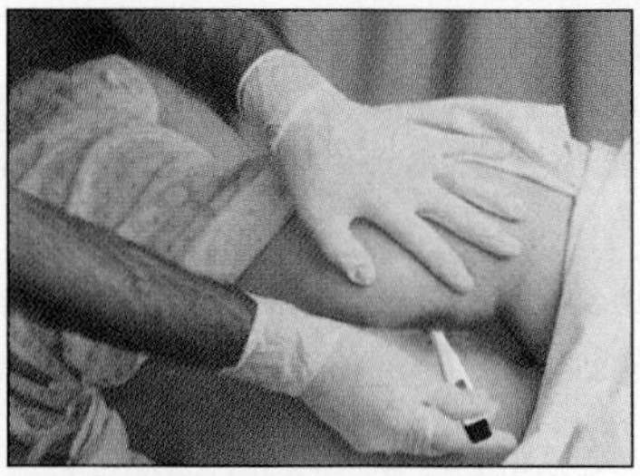

❷ Inserting a rectal thermometer

(continued)

SKILL 28.1

ASSESSING BODY TEMPERATURE (*continued*)

Axillary Pat the axilla dry if very moist.
Place the bulb in the centre of the axilla (see ❸).

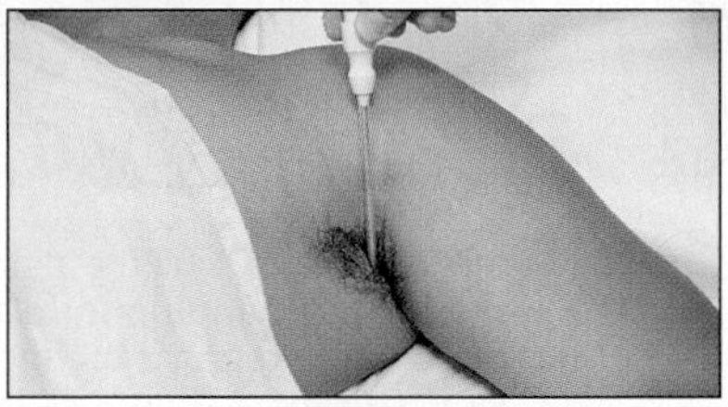

❸ Placing the thermometer in the centre of the axilla

Tympanic Pull the pinna slightly upward and backward (see ❹).

Point the probe slightly anteriorly, toward the eardrum.

Insert the probe slowly by using a circular motion until snug.

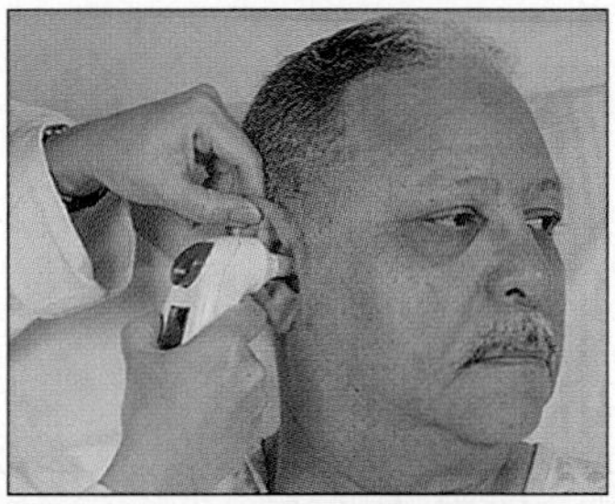

❹ Inserting a tympanic thermometer

Temporal Artery Brush hair aside if covering the TA area. With the probe flush on the centre of forehead, depress the red button and keep it depressed. Slowly slide the probe midline across the forehead to the hairline, not down the side of the face (see ❺). Lift the probe from forehead and touch it on the neck, just behind the earlobe (❺ B). Release the button.

CLINICAL ALERT

Be sure to record the temperature from an electronic thermometer before replacing the probe into the charging unit. With many models, replacing the probe erases the temperature from the display.

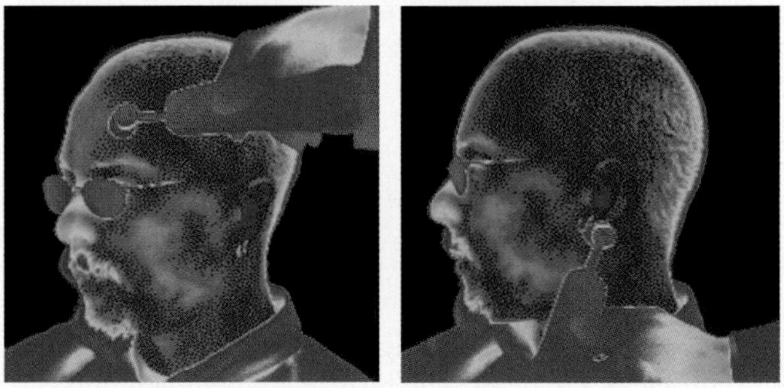

A B

❺ A and B Positioning the temporal artery thermometer

Lifespan Considerations

INFANTS

- The body temperature of newborns is extremely labile, and newborns must be kept warm and dry to prevent hypothermia.
- When using the axillary site, you need to hold the infant's arm against the chest (see Figure 28.10).
- The axillary route may not be as accurate as other routes for detecting fevers in children (Ball & Bindler, 2008).
- The tympanic route is fast and convenient. Place the infant supine and stabilize the head.

Pull the pinna straight back and slightly downward. Direct the probe tip anteriorly and insert far enough to seal the canal. The tip will not touch the tympanic membrane.

- Avoid the tympanic route in a child with active ear infections or tympanic membrane drainage tubes.
- The tympanic membrane route may be more accurate in determining temperature in febrile infants (Liu, Chang, & Chang, 2004; Nimah, Bshesh, Callahan, & Jacobs, 2006).

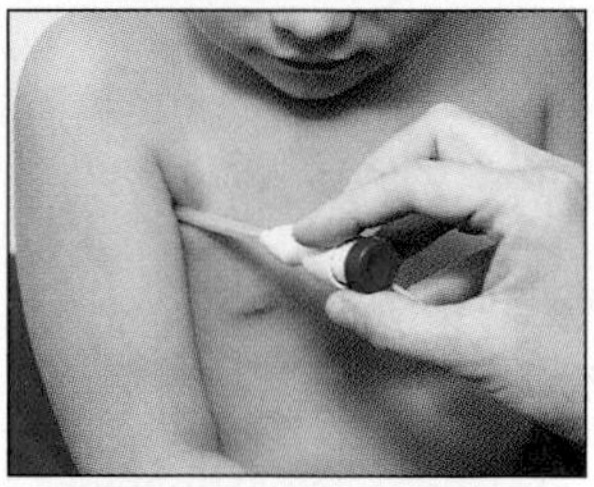

FIGURE 28.10 Axillary thermometer placement

(continued)

Lifespan Considerations (*continued*)

- When using a temporal artery thermometer, touching only the forehead or behind the ear is needed.
- The rectal route is least desirable in infants.

CHILDREN

- Tympanic or temporal artery sites are preferred.
- For the tympanic route, have the child held on an adult's lap with the child's head held gently against the adult for support. Pull the pinna straight back and upward for children over age 3 (see Figure 28.11).
- Avoid the tympanic route in a child with active ear infections or tympanic membrane drainage tubes.
- The oral route can be used for children over age 3, but unbreakable electronic thermometers are recommended.
- For a rectal temperature, place the child prone across your lap or in a side-lying position with the knees flexed. Insert the thermometer 2.5 cm into the rectum.

OLDER ADULTS

- Older adults' temperatures tend to be lower than those of middle-aged adults.
- Their temperatures are strongly influenced by both environmental and internal temperature changes. Their thermoregulation control processes are not as efficient as when they were younger, and they are at higher risk for both hypothermia and hyperthermia.
- Older adults can develop significant buildup of ear cerumen that may interfere with tympanic thermometer readings.
- Older adults are more likely to have hemorrhoids. Inspect the anus before taking a rectal temperature.

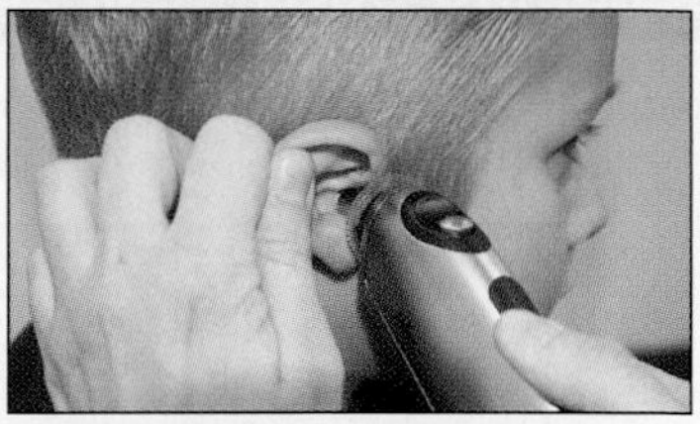

FIGURE 28.11 Pull the pinna of the ear back and up for placement of a tympanic thermometer in a child more than 3 years old; pull it back and down for children younger than 3.

- Older adults' temperatures may not be a valid indication of the seriousness of the pathology of a disease. They can have pneumonia or a urinary tract infection and have only a slight temperature elevation. Other symptoms, such as confusion and restlessness, may be displayed and need follow-up to determine whether there is an underlying process.

Pulse

The **pulse** is a wave of blood created by contraction of the left ventricle of the heart. The heart is a pulsating pump, and blood enters the arteries with each contraction, causing pressure pulses or pulse waves. Generally, the pulse wave represents the stroke volume output and the amount of blood that enters the arteries with each ventricular contraction. **Compliance** of the arteries is their ability to contract and expand. When a person's arteries lose their distensibility, as can happen in old age, greater pressure is required to pump the blood into the arteries.

Cardiac output is the volume of blood pumped into the arteries by the heart and equals the result of the stroke volume (SV) times the heart rate (HR) per minute. For example, 65 mL × 70 beats per minute = 4.55 L per minute. When an adult is resting, the heart pumps about 5 L of blood each minute.

In a healthy person, the pulse reflects the heartbeat; that is, the pulse rate is the same as the rate of the ventricular contractions of the heart. However, in some types of cardiovascular disease, the heartbeat and pulse rates can differ. For example, a client's heart may produce very weak or small pulse waves that are not detectable in a peripheral pulse distal to the heart. In these instances, the nurse should assess the heartbeat *and* the peripheral pulse. See the section on assessing the apical pulse later in this chapter. A **peripheral pulse** is located in the periphery of the body, for example, in the foot, hand, or neck. The **apical pulse**, in contrast, is a central pulse; that is, it is located at the apex of the heart. It is also referred to as the **point of maximal impulse (PMI)**.

Factors Affecting Pulse Rate

The rate of the pulse is expressed in beats per minute (bpm). A pulse rate varies according to a number of factors. The nurse should consider each of the following factors when assessing a client's pulse:

- *Age.* As age increases, the pulse rate gradually decreases. See Table 28.2 for specific variations in pulse rates from birth to adulthood.
- *Gender.* After puberty, the average male's pulse rate is slightly lower than the average female's.
- *Exercise.* The pulse rate normally increases with activity. The rate of increase in the professional athlete is often less than in the average person because of greater cardiac size, strength, and efficiency.
- *Fever.* The pulse rate increases (1) in response to the lowered blood pressure that results from peripheral vasodilation associated with elevated body temperature, and (2) with an increased metabolic rate.
- *Medications and other ingestants.* Many substances affect the heart rate and pulse. For example, cardiotonics (e.g., digitalis preparations) and beta blockers decrease the heart rate, whereas caffeine, nicotine, and epinephrine increase the heart rate.

- *Hypovolemia.* Loss of blood from the vascular system (hemorrhage) normally increases pulse rate. In adults, the loss of a small amount of blood (e.g., 500 mL, the amount lost after a blood donation) results in a temporary adjustment of the heart rate as the body compensates for the lost blood volume. An adult has about 5 L of blood in the system and can usually lose up to 10% without adverse effects. Fluid volume deficits caused by extensive diarrhea and vomiting or prolonged lack of fluid intake can also cause increased pulse rate.
- *Stress.* In response to stress, sympathetic nervous stimulation increases the overall activity of the heart. Stress increases the rate as well as the force of the heartbeat. Fear and anxiety, as well as the perception of severe pain, stimulate the sympathetic system.
- *Position changes.* When a person assumes a sitting or standing position, blood usually pools in dependent vessels of the venous system. Pooling results in a transient decrease in the venous blood return to the heart and a subsequent reduction in blood pressure and increase in heart rate.
- *Pathology.* Certain diseases, such as some heart conditions or those that impair oxygenation, can alter the resting pulse rate.

Pulse Sites

A pulse can be measured in nine sites (Figure 28.12):

1. *Temporal,* where the temporal artery passes over the temporal bone of the head. The site is superior (above) and lateral to (away from the midline of) the eye.
2. *Carotid,* at the side of the neck where the carotid artery runs between the trachea and the sternocleidomastoid muscle.

CLINICAL ALERT
Never press both carotid arteries at the same time as this can cause a reflex drop in blood pressure or pulse rate.

TABLE 28.2 Variations in Pulse and Respirations by Age

Age	Pulse Average (and Ranges)	Respirations Average (and Ranges)
Newborn (0–4 weeks)	130 (80–180)	35 (30–80)
< 1 year	120 (80–140)	30 (20–40)
1–4 years	110 (80–120)	25 (20–50)
5–8 years	100 (75–120)	20 (15–25)
9–10 years	70 (50–90)	19 (15–25)
11–19 years	75 (50–90)	18 (15–20)
20–64 years	80 (60–100)	16 (12–20)
> 65	70 (60–100)	16 (15–20)

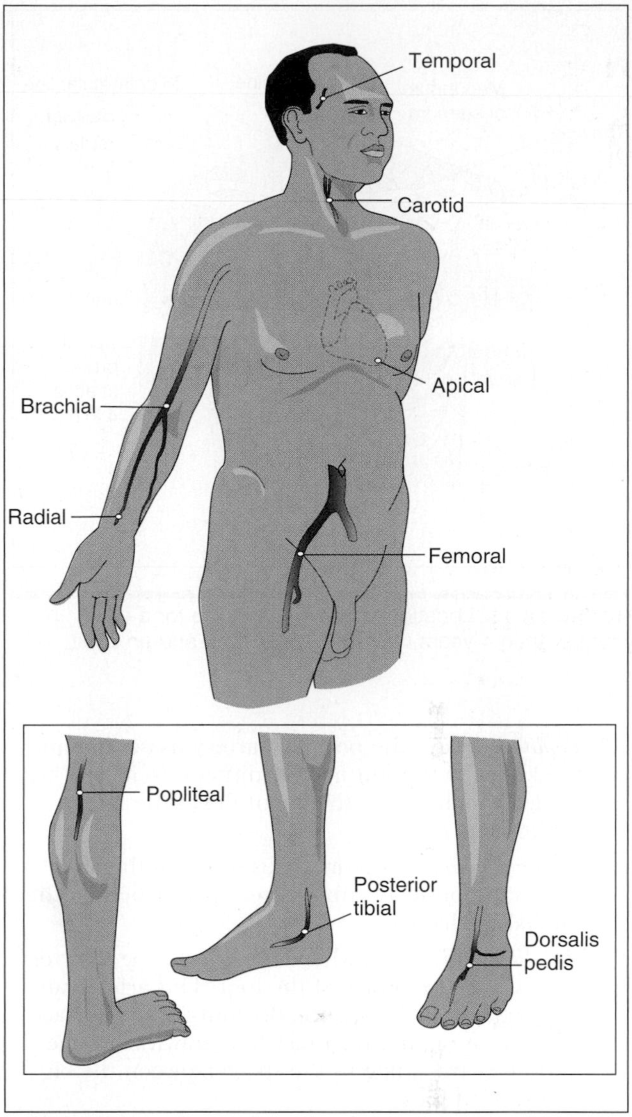

FIGURE 28.12 Nine sites commonly used for assessing a pulse

3. *Apical,* at the apex of the heart. In an adult, this is located on the left side of the chest, no more than 8 cm to the left of the sternum (breastbone) and at the fourth, fifth, or sixth intercostal space (area between the ribs). In older adults, the apex may be further left if there are conditions that have led to an enlarged heart. Before 4 years of age, the apex is left of the midclavicular line (MCL); between 4 and 6 years, it is at the MCL (see Figure 28.13). For a child 7 to 9 years of age, the apical pulse is located at the fourth or fifth intercostal space.
4. *Brachial,* at the inner aspect of the biceps muscle of the arm (especially in infants) or medially in the antecubital space.
5. *Radial,* where the radial artery runs along the radial bone, on the thumb side of the inner aspect of the wrist.
6. *Femoral,* where the femoral artery passes alongside the inguinal ligament.

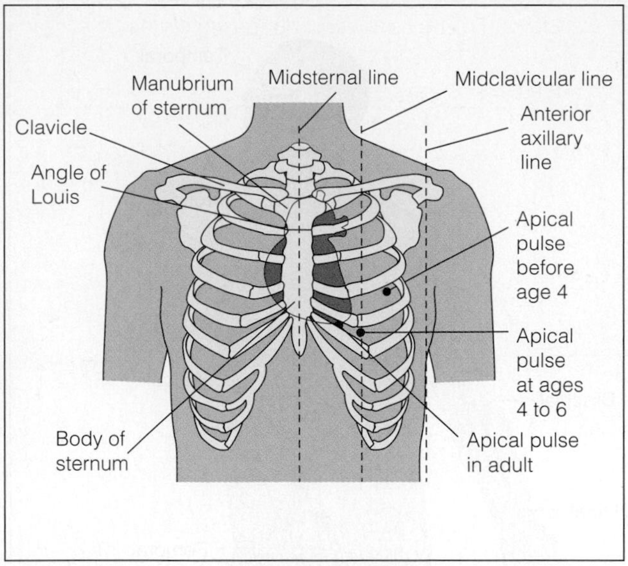

FIGURE 28.13 Location of the apical pulse for a child younger than 4 years, a child 4 to 6 years, and an adult

7. *Popliteal,* where the popliteal artery passes behind the knee. This point may be difficult to locate, but it can be palpated if the client flexes the knee slightly.
8. *Posterior tibial,* on the medial surface of the ankle, where the posterior tibial artery passes behind the medial malleolus.
9. *Pedal (dorsalis pedis),* where the dorsalis pedis artery passes over the bones of the foot. This artery can be palpated by feeling the dorsum (upper surface) of the foot on an imaginary line drawn from the middle of the ankle to the space between the big and second toes.

The radial site is most commonly used. It is easily detected in most people and readily accessible. The reasons for use of each site are given in Table 28.3.

Assessing the Pulse

A pulse is commonly assessed by palpation (feeling) or auscultation (hearing). The middle three fingertips are used for palpating all pulse sites except the apex of the heart. A stethoscope is used for assessing apical pulses and fetal heart tones. A Doppler ultrasound stethoscope (DUS; see Figure 28.14) is used for pulses that are difficult to assess. The DUS headset has earpieces similar to standard stethoscope earpieces, but it has a long cord attached to a volume-controlled audio unit and an ultrasound transducer. The DUS detects movement of red blood cells through a blood vessel, magnifying the sound. In contrast to the conventional stethoscope, it excludes environmental sounds. It cannot detect blood flow in deep vessels or in blood vessels underlying bone, such as the vessels in the abdomen, thorax, or skull.

TABLE 28.3 Reasons for Using Specific Pulse Site

Pulse Site	Reasons for Use
Radial	Readily accessible
Temporal	Used when radial pulse is not accessible
Carotid	Used during cardiac arrest or shock in adults Used to determine circulation to the brain
Apical	Routinely used in infants and children up to 3 years of age Used to determine discrepancies with radial pulse Used to monitor some medication effects
Brachial	Used to measure blood pressure Used during cardiac arrest in infants
Femoral	Used in cases of cardiac arrest or shock Used to determine circulation to the leg
Popliteal	Used to determine circulation to the lower leg
Posterior tibial	Used to determine circulation to the foot
Pedal	Used to determine circulation to the foot

A pulse is normally palpated by applying moderate pressure with the three middle fingers of the hand. The pads on the most distal aspects of the finger are the most sensitive areas for detecting a pulse. Excessive pressure can obliterate a pulse, whereas too little pressure may make it undetectable. Before the nurse assesses the *resting* pulse, the client should assume a comfortable position. The nurse should also be aware of the following:

- Any medication that could affect the heart rate
- Whether the client has been physically active; if so, wait 10 to 15 minutes until the client has rested and the pulse has returned to its usual rate
- Any baseline data about the normal heart rate for the client; for example, a physically fit athlete may have a heart rate below 60 bpm
- Whether the client should assume a particular position (e.g., sitting); in some clients, the rate changes with the position because of changes in blood flow volume and autonomic nervous system activity

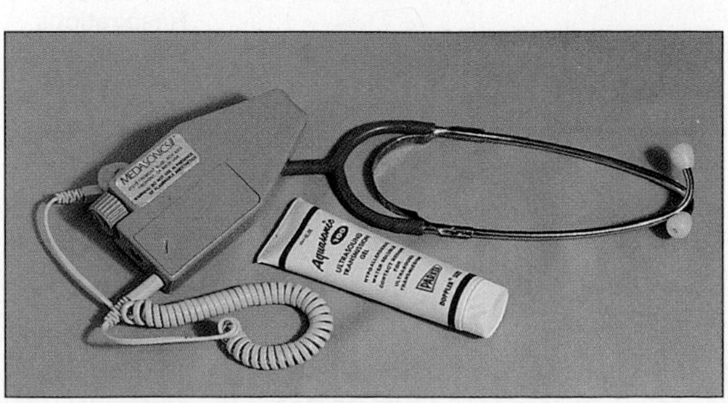

FIGURE 28.14 An ultrasound (Doppler) stethoscope

When assessing the pulse, the nurse collects the following data: the rate, rhythm, volume, arterial wall elasticity, and presence or absence of bilateral equality. An excessively fast heart rate (e.g., more than 100 bpm in an adult) is referred to as **tachycardia**. A heart rate in an adult of 60 bpm or fewer is called **bradycardia**. If a client has tachycardia or bradycardia, the apical pulse should be assessed.

The **pulse rhythm** is the pattern of the beats and the intervals between the beats. Equal time elapses between beats of a normal pulse. A pulse with an irregular rhythm is referred to as a **dysrhythmia** or **arrhythmia**. It may consist of random, irregular beats or a predictable pattern of irregular beats referred to as regular irregular arrhythmia. When a dysrhythmia is detected, the apical pulse should be assessed. An electrocardiogram (ECG) is necessary to further define the dysrhythmia.

Pulse volume, also called the pulse strength or amplitude, refers to the force of blood with each beat. Usually, the pulse volume is the same with each beat. It can range from absent to bounding. A normal pulse can be felt with moderate pressure of the fingers and can be obliterated with greater pressure. A forceful or full blood volume that is obliterated only with difficulty is called a *full* or *bounding* pulse. A pulse that is readily obliterated with pressure from the fingers is referred to as *weak, feeble*, or *thready*. A pulse volume can be measured on a scale of 0 to 3 (indicated by *x*/3) or 0 to 4 (indicated by *x*/4), depending on the agency (see Table 28.4).

The **elasticity of the arterial wall** reflects its expansibility or its deformities. A healthy, normal artery feels straight, smooth, soft, and pliable. Older people often have inelastic arteries that feel twisted (tortuous) and irregular on palpation.

When assessing a peripheral pulse to determine the adequacy of blood flow to a particular area of the body, the nurse should also assess the corresponding pulse on the other side of the body. The second assessment gives the nurse data to compare the pulses. For example, when assessing the blood flow to the right foot, the nurse assesses the right dorsalis pedis pulse and then the left dorsalis pedis pulse. If the client's right and left pulses are the same, the client's dorsalis pedis pulses are *bilaterally equal*. The pulse rate does not need to be counted when assessing for perfusion and equality.

When a peripheral pulse is located, it indicates that pulses more proximal to that location will also be present. For example, if the dorsalis pedis, the most distal pulse of the lower extremity, cannot be felt, the nurse next palpates for the posterior tibial pulse. If it is not felt, the popliteal pulse must be assessed. If the popliteal pulse is found, it is not necessary to assess the femoral pulse since it must also be present in order for the more distal pulse to exist.

Skill 28.2 provides guidelines for assessing a peripheral pulse.

TABLE 28.4 Scales for Measuring Pulse Volume

3-Point Scale	Description of Pulse
0	Absent, not discernible
+1	Thready or weak, difficult to feel
+2	Normal, detected readily, obliterated by strong pressure
+3	Bounding, difficult to obliterate
4-Point Scale	**Description of Pulse**
0	Absent, not discernible
+1	Thready or weak, difficult to feel
+2	Normal, detected readily, obliterated by strong pressure
+3	Increased
+4	Bounding

SKILL 28.2

ASSESSING A PERIPHERAL PULSE

PURPOSES

- To establish baseline data for subsequent evaluation
- To identify whether the pulse rate is within normal range
- To determine whether the pulse rhythm is regular and the pulse volume is appropriate
- To compare the equality of corresponding peripheral pulses bilaterally
- To monitor and assess changes in the client's health status
- To monitor clients at risk for pulse alterations (e.g., those with a history of heart disease or experiencing cardiac arrhythmias, hemorrhage, acute pain, infusion of large volumes of fluids, fever)
- To evaluate blood perfusion to the extremities

ASSESSMENT

Assess

- Clinical signs of cardiovascular alterations, such as dyspnea (difficult respirations), fatigue, pallor, cyanosis (bluish discolouration of skin and mucous membranes), palpitations, syncope (fainting), or impaired peripheral tissue perfusion as evidenced by skin discolouration and cool temperature
- Factors that may alter pulse rate (e.g., emotional status and activity level)
- Which site is most appropriate for assessment based on the purpose

(continued)

SKILL 28.2

ASSESSING A PERIPHERAL PULSE (*continued*)

Equipment

- Watch with a second hand or indicator
- If using a DUS: transducer probe, stethoscope headset, transmission gel, and tissues or wipes

IMPLEMENTATION

Preparation

If using a DUS, check that the equipment is functioning normally.

Performance

1. Before performing the procedure, introduce yourself and verify the client's identity by using agency protocol. Explain to the client what you are going to do, why it is necessary, and how he or she can cooperate.
2. Perform hand hygiene and observe other appropriate infection prevention and control procedures.
3. Provide for client privacy.
4. Select the pulse point. Normally, the radial pulse is taken, unless it cannot be exposed or circulation to another body area is to be assessed.
5. Assist the client to a comfortable resting position. When the radial pulse is assessed, with the palm facing downward, the client's arm can rest alongside the body or the forearm can rest at a 90-degree angle across the chest. For the client who can sit, the forearm can rest across the thigh, with the palm of the hand facing downward or inward.
6. Palpate and count the pulse. Place two or three middle fingertips lightly and squarely over the pulse point (see ❶). **Rationale: Using the thumb is contraindicated because the nurse's thumb has a pulse that could be mistaken for the client's pulse.**
   - Count for 15 seconds and multiply by 4. Record the pulse in beats per minute on your worksheet. If taking a client's pulse for the first time, when obtaining baseline data, or if the pulse is irregular, count for a full minute. If an irregular pulse is found, also take the apical pulse.

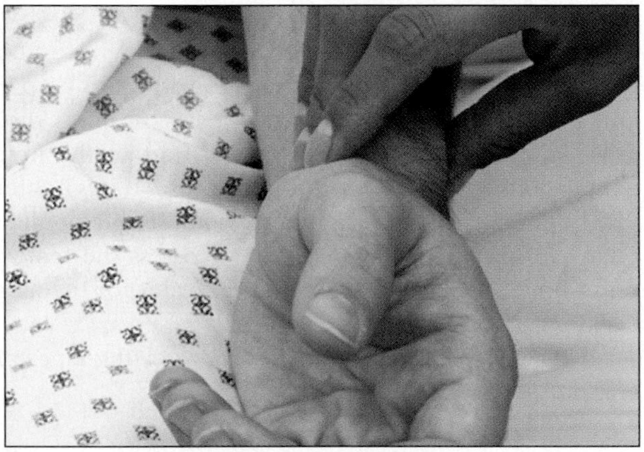

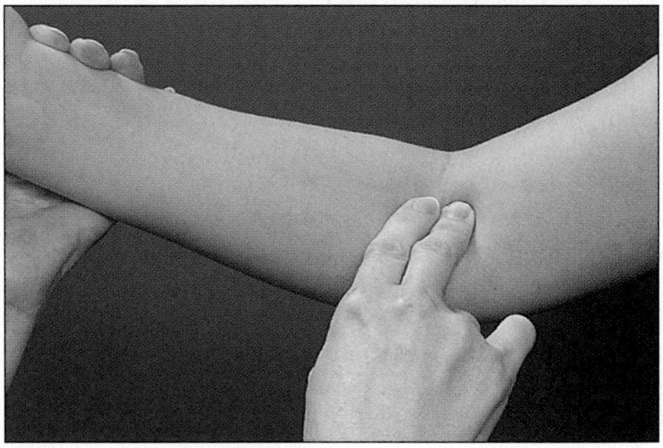

❶ Assessing the pulses

A Radial

B Brachial

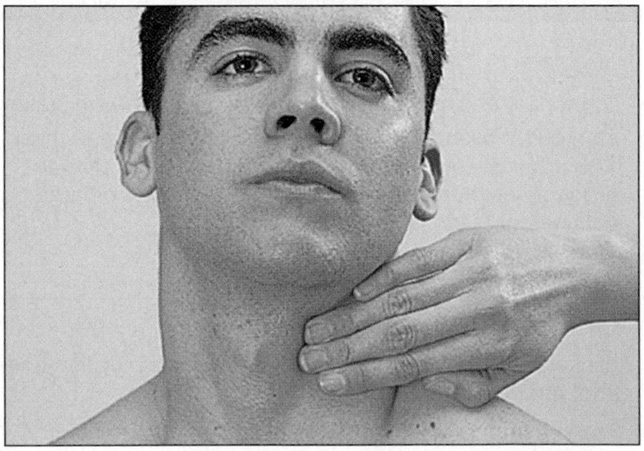

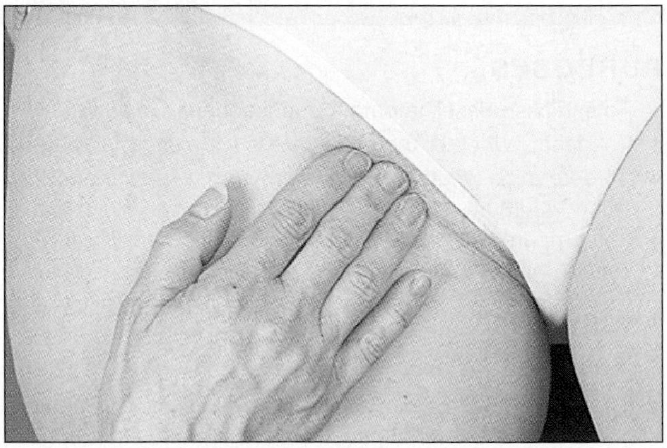

C Carotid

D Femoral

(*continued*)

SKILL 28.2

ASSESSING A PERIPHERAL PULSE (*continued*)

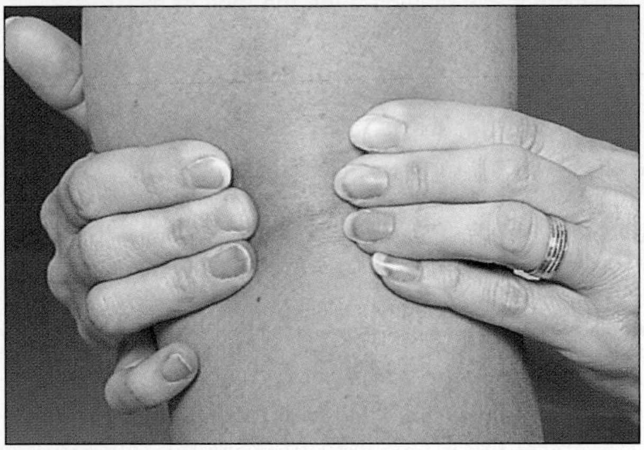

E Popliteal

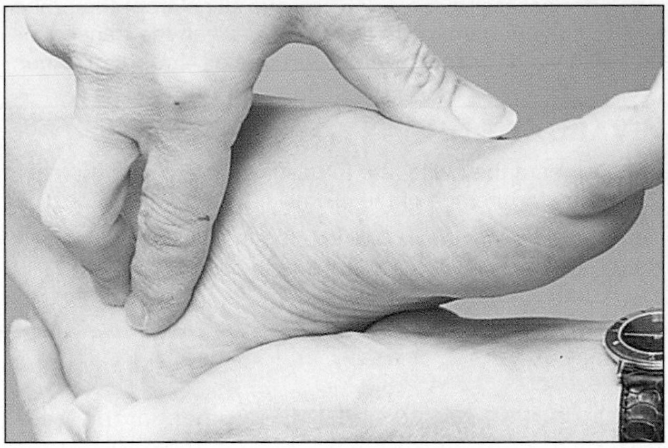

F Posterior tibial

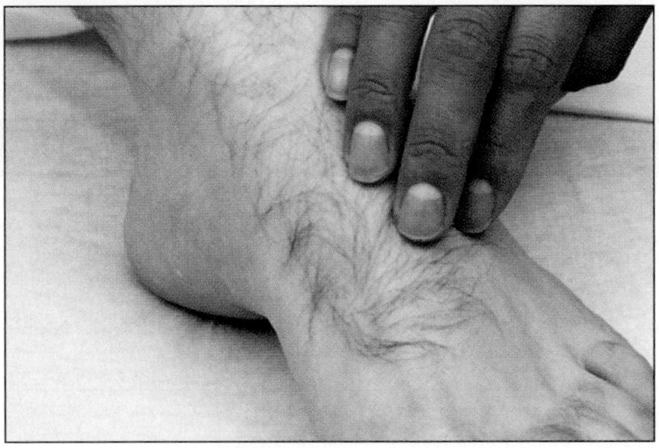

G Pedal (dorsalis pedis)

7. Assess the pulse rhythm and volume.
   - Assess the pulse rhythm by noting the pattern of the intervals between the beats. A normal pulse has equal periods between beats. If this is an initial assessment, assess for 1 minute.
   - Assess the pulse volume. A normal pulse can be felt with moderate pressure, and the pressure is equal with each beat. A forceful pulse volume is full; an easily obliterated pulse is weak. Record the rhythm and volume on your worksheet.
8. Document the pulse rate, rhythm, and volume (see Table 28.4, p. 675) and your actions in the client record. Also record pertinent related data, such as variation in pulse rate compared with normal for the client and abnormal skin colour and skin temperature, in the nurse's notes.

Variation: Using a DUS

- If using a DUS, plug the stethoscope headset into one of the two output jacks located next to the volume control. DUS units may have two jacks so that a second person can listen to the signals.
- Apply transmission gel either to the probe at the narrow end of the plastic case housing the transducer, or to the client's skin. **Rationale: Ultrasound beams do not travel well through air. The gel makes an airtight seal, which then promotes optimal ultrasound wave transmission.**
- Press the On button.
- Hold the probe against the skin over the pulse site. Use a light pressure, and keep the probe in contact with the skin (see ❷). **Rationale: Too much pressure can stop the blood flow and obliterate the signal.**
- Adjust the volume if necessary. Distinguish artery sounds from vein sounds. The artery sound (signal) is distinctively pulsating and has a pumping quality. The venous sound is intermittent and varies with respirations. Both artery and vein sounds are heard simultaneously through the DUS because major arteries and veins are situated close together throughout the body. If arterial sounds cannot be easily heard, reposition the probe.

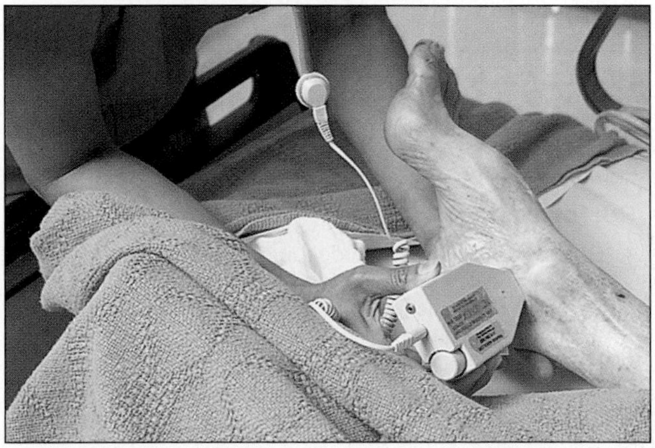

❷ Using a (Doppler) ultrasound stethoscope to assess the posterior tibial pulse

(continued)

SKILL 28.2

ASSESSING A PERIPHERAL PULSE (*continued*)

- After assessing the pulse, remove all gel from the probe to prevent damage to the surface. Clean the transducer with water-based solution. **Rationale: Alcohol or other disinfectants may damage the face of the transducer**. Remove all gel from the client.

EVALUATION

- Compare the pulse rate to baseline data or the normal range for the age of the client.
- Relate pulse rate and volume to other vital signs, and relate pulse rhythm and volume to baseline data and health status.
- If assessing peripheral pulses, evaluate equality, rate, and volume in corresponding extremities.
- Conduct appropriate follow-up, such as notifying the appropriate members of the health-care team or giving medication.

APICAL PULSE ASSESSMENT Assessment of the apical pulse is indicated for clients whose peripheral pulse is irregular, as well as for clients with known cardiovascular, pulmonary, and renal diseases. It is commonly assessed before administering medications that affect heart rate. The apical site is also used to assess the pulse for newborns, infants, and children up to 2 to 3 years old. Skill 28.3 presents guidelines for assessing the apical pulse.

SKILL 28.3

ASSESSING AN APICAL PULSE

PURPOSES

- To obtain the heart rate of newborns, infants, and children 2 to 3 years old or of an adult with an irregular peripheral pulse
- To establish baseline data for subsequent evaluation
- To determine whether the cardiac rate is within normal range and the rhythm is regular
- To monitor clients with cardiac disease and those receiving medications to improve heart action

ASSESSMENT

Assess

- Clinical signs of cardiovascular alterations (e.g., dyspnea, fatigue or weakness, pallor, cyanosis, syncope)
- Factors that may alter pulse rate (e.g., emotional status, activity level, and medications that affect heart rate, such as digoxin, beta blockers, or calcium channel blockers)

Equipment

- Watch with a second hand or indicator
- Stethoscope
- Antiseptic wipes
- If using a DUS: the transducer probe, the stethoscope headset, transmission gel, and tissues or wipes

IMPLEMENTATION

Preparation

If using a DUS, check that the equipment is functioning normally.

Performance

1. Before performing the procedure, introduce yourself and verify the client's identity by using agency protocol. Explain to the client what you are going to do, why it is necessary, and how he or she can cooperate.
2. Perform hand hygiene and observe other appropriate infection prevention and control procedures.
3. Provide for client privacy.
4. Position the client appropriately in a comfortable supine position or in a sitting position. Expose the area of the chest over the apex of the heart.
5. Locate the apical impulse. This is the point over the apex of the heart where the apical pulse can be most clearly heard.
   - Palpate the angle of Louis (the angle between the manubrium, the top of the sternum, and the body of the sternum). It is palpated just below the suprasternal notch and is felt as a prominence (see Figure 28.13, p. 674).
   - Slide your index finger just to the left of the sternum, and palpate the second intercostal space (see ❶).
   - Place your middle or next finger in the third intercostal space, and continue palpating downward until you locate the fifth intercostal space (see ❷).
   - Move your index finger laterally along the fifth intercostal space toward the MCL (see ❸). Normally, the apical impulse is palpable at or just medial to the MCL.

(continued)

SKILL 28.3

ASSESSING AN APICAL PULSE (*continued*)

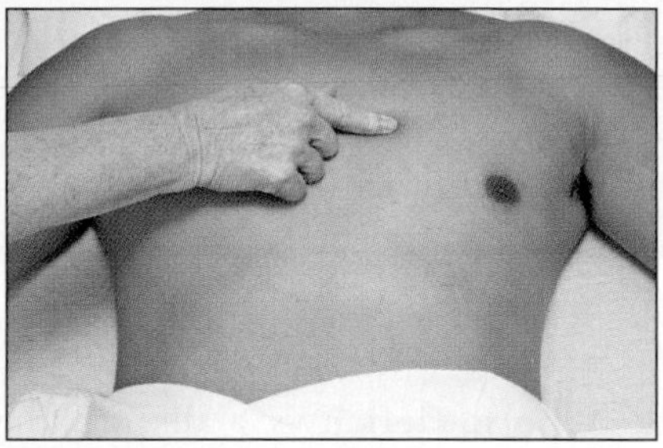

❶ Second intercostal space

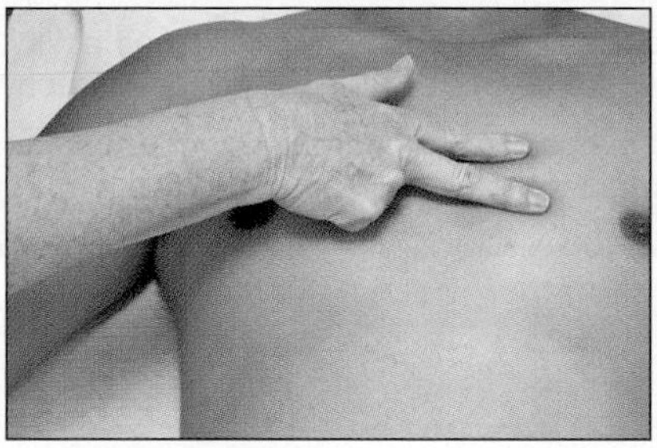

❷ Third intercostal space

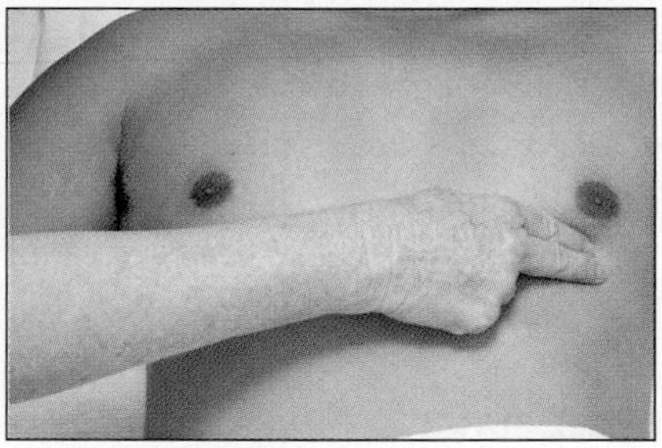

❸ Fifth intercostal space, MCL

6. Auscultate and count heartbeats.
   - Use antiseptic wipes to clean the earpieces and diaphragm of the stethoscope if their cleanliness is in doubt. **Rationale: The diaphragm needs to be cleaned and disinfected if soiled with body substances.**
   - Warm the diaphragm of the stethoscope by holding it in the palm of the hand for a moment. **Rationale: The metal of the diaphragm is usually cold and can startle the client when placed immediately on the chest.**
   - Insert the earpieces of the stethoscope into your ears in the direction of the ear canals, or slightly forward. **Rationale: This facilitates hearing.**
   - Tap your finger lightly on the diaphragm *to be sure it is the active side of the head*. If necessary, rotate the head to select the diaphragm side (see ❹).
   - Place the diaphragm of the stethoscope over the apical impulse and listen for the normal S_1 and S_2 heart sounds, which are heard as "lub-dub" (see ❺). **Rationale: The heartbeat is normally loudest over the apex of the heart**. Each lub-dub is counted as one heartbeat. **Rationale: The two heart sounds are produced by closure of the heart valves. The S_1 heart sound (lub) occurs when the atrioventricular valves close after the ventricles have been sufficiently filled. The S_2 heart sound (dub) occurs when the semilunar valves close after the ventricles empty.**
   - If you have difficulty hearing the apical pulse, ask the supine client to roll onto his or her left side or the sitting client to lean slightly forward. **Rationale: This positioning moves the apex of the heart closer to the chest wall.**
   - If the rhythm is regular, count the heartbeats for 30 seconds and multiply by 2. If the rhythm is irregular or for giving certain medications, such as digoxin, count the beats for 60 seconds. **Rationale: A 60-second count provides a more accurate assessment of an irregular pulse than a 30-second count.**
7. Assess the rhythm and the strength of the heartbeat.
   - Assess the rhythm of the heartbeat by noting the pattern of intervals between the beats. A normal pulse has equal time periods between beats.
   - Assess the strength (volume) of the heartbeat. Normally, the heartbeats are equal in strength and can be described as strong or weak.
8. Document the pulse site, rate, rhythm, and volume (see Table 28.4, p. 675) and nursing actions in the client record. Also record pertinent related data, such as variation in pulse rate compared with normal for the client and abnormal skin colour and skin temperature.

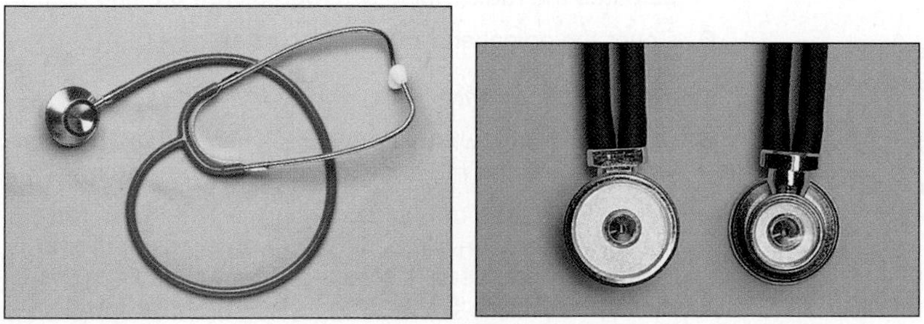

A B

❹ A: Stethoscope with both a bell-shaped and flat-disc amplifier; B: closeup of a flat-disc amplifier (left) and a bell amplifier (right)

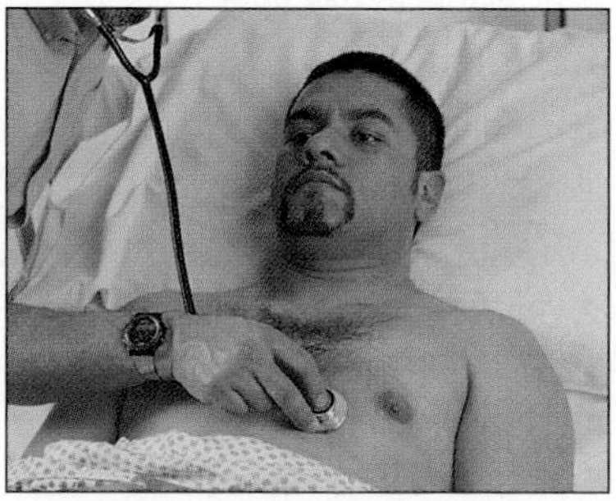

❺ Taking an apical pulse by using the flat disc of the stethoscope. Note how the amplifier is held against the chest.

(continued)

SKILL 28.3

ASSESSING AN APICAL PULSE (*continued*)

EVALUATION

- Relate the pulse rate to other vital signs. Relate the pulse rhythm to baseline data and health status.
- Report to the appropriate members of the health-care team any abnormal findings, such as irregular rhythm, reduced ability to hear the heartbeat, pallor, cyanosis, dyspnea, tachycardia, or bradycardia.
- Conduct appropriate follow-up, such as administering medication ordered based on apical heart rate.

APICAL-RADIAL PULSE ASSESSMENT An **apical-radial pulse** may need to be assessed for clients with certain cardiovascular disorders. Normally, the apical and radial rates are identical. An apical pulse rate greater than a radial pulse rate can indicate that the thrust of the blood from the heart is too weak for the wave to be felt at the peripheral pulse site, or it can indicate that vascular disease is preventing impulses from being transmitted. A **pulse deficit** is a discrepancy between the two pulse rates and needs to be reported promptly. In no instance is the radial pulse greater than the apical pulse.

An apical-radial pulse can be taken by two nurses or one nurse, although the two-nurse technique is more accurate. Skill 28.4 outlines the steps for assessing an apical-radial pulse.

SKILL 28.4

ASSESSING AN APICAL-RADIAL PULSE

PURPOSE

- To determine adequacy of peripheral circulation or presence of pulse deficit

ASSESSMENT

Assess

- Clinical signs of hypovolemic shock (hypotension, pallor, cyanosis, and cold, clammy skin)

Equipment

- Watch with a second hand or indicator
- Stethoscope
- Antiseptic wipes

IMPLEMENTATION

Preparation

If using the two-nurse technique, ensure that the other nurse is available at this time.

Performance

1. Before performing the procedure, introduce yourself and verify the client's identity by using agency protocol. Explain to the client what you are going to do, why it is necessary, and how he or she can cooperate.
2. Perform hand hygiene and observe other appropriate infection prevention and control procedures.
3. Provide for client privacy.
4. Position the client appropriately. Assist the client to a comfortable supine or sitting position. Expose the area of the chest over the apex of the heart. If previous measurements were taken, determine what position the client assumed, and use the same position. **Rationale: This ensures an accurate comparative measurement.**
5. Locate the apical and radial pulse sites. In the two-nurse technique, one nurse locates the apical impulse by palpation or with the stethoscope while the other nurse palpates the radial pulse site (See Skills 28.2 and 28.3.)
6. Count the apical and radial pulse rates.

Two-Nurse Technique

- Place the watch where both nurses can see it. The nurse who is taking the radial pulse may hold the watch.
- Decide on a time to begin counting. A time when the second hand is on 12, 3, 6, or 9 or an even number on digital clocks is usually selected. The nurse taking the radial pulse says "Start" at the same time. **Rationale: This ensures that simultaneous counts are taken.**
- Each nurse counts the pulse rate for 60 seconds. Both nurses end the count when the nurse taking the radial pulse says "Stop." **Rationale: A full 60-second count is necessary for accurate assessment of any discrepancies between the two pulse sites.**

(continued)

SKILL 28.4

ASSESSING AN APICAL-RADIAL PULSE (*continued*)

- The nurse who assesses the apical rate also assesses the apical pulse rhythm and volume (i.e., whether the heartbeat is strong or weak). If the pulse is irregular, note whether the irregular beats come at random or at predictable times.
- The nurse assessing the radial pulse rate also assesses the radial pulse rhythm and volume.

One-Nurse Technique

- Assess the apical pulse for 60 seconds.
- Assess the radial pulse for 60 seconds.

7. Document the apical and radial pulse rates, rhythm, volume, and any pulse deficit in the client record. Also record related data, such as variation in pulse rate compared with normal for the client and other pertinent observations, such as pallor, cyanosis, or dyspnea.

EVALUATION

- Relate pulse rate and rhythm to other vital signs, to baseline data, and to general health status.
- Report to the appropriate members of the health-care team any changes from previous measurements or any discrepancy between the two pulses.
- Conduct appropriate follow-up, such as administering medication or other actions to be taken for a discrepancy in the apical and radial pulse rates.

Lifespan Considerations

INFANTS

- Use the apical pulse for the heart rate of newborns, infants, and children 2 to 3 years old to establish baseline data for subsequent evaluation, to determine whether the cardiac rate is within normal range, and to determine whether the rhythm is regular.
- The radial pulse is not used for children younger than 2 years of age.
- Place a baby in a supine position, and offer a pacifier if the baby is crying or restless. Crying and physical activity will increase the pulse rate. For this reason, take the apical pulse rate of infants and small children before assessing body temperatures.
- Locate the apical pulse in the fourth intercostal space, lateral to the midclavicular line during infancy.
- Brachial, popliteal, and femoral pulses may be palpated. Because of a normally low blood pressure and rapid heart rate, infants' other distal pulses may be hard to feel.
- Newborn infants may have heart murmurs that are not pathological but reflect functional incomplete closure of fetal heart structures (ductus arteriosus or foramen ovale).

CHILDREN

- To take a peripheral pulse, position the child comfortably in the adult's arms, or have the adult remain close by. This may decrease anxiety and yield more accurate results.
- To assess the apical pulse, assist a young child to a comfortable supine or sitting position.
- Demonstrate the procedure to the child by using a stuffed animal or doll, and allow the child to handle the stethoscope before beginning the procedure. This will decrease anxiety and promote cooperation.
- The apex of the heart is normally located in the fourth intercostal space in young children and in the fifth intercostal space in children 7 years of age and older.
- Locate the apical impulse along the fourth intercostal space, between the MCL and the anterior axillary line (see Figure 28.13, p. 674).
- Count the pulse before performing other uncomfortable procedures so that the rate is not artificially elevated by the discomfort.

OLDER ADULTS

- If the client has severe hand or arm tremors, the radial pulse may be difficult to count.
- Cardiac changes in older adults, such as a decrease in cardiac output, sclerotic changes to heart valves, and dysrhythmias, often indicate that obtaining an apical pulse will be more accurate.
- Older adults often have decreased peripheral circulation, so pedal pulses should also be checked for regularity, volume, and symmetry.
- The pulse returns to baseline after exercise more slowly than with other age groups.

Home Care Considerations

- If appropriate, teach the client or family member to take a pulse. Ensure correct technique by having them demonstrate.
- Assist in obtaining and using an electronic pulse device if indicated.
- Teach the client to monitor the pulse before taking medications that affect the heart rate. Tell the client to report any notable changes in heart rate or rhythm (regularity) to the appropriate member of the health-care team.

Respirations

Respiration is the act of breathing. **External respiration** refers to the interchange of oxygen and carbon dioxide between the alveoli of the lungs and the pulmonary blood. **Internal respiration**, by contrast, takes place throughout the body; it is the interchange of these same gases between the circulating blood and the cells of the body tissues.

Inhalation or **inspiration** refers to the intake of air into the lungs. **Exhalation** or **expiration** refers to breathing out or the movement of gases from the lungs to the atmosphere. **Ventilation** is also used to refer to the movement of air in and out of the lungs.

Breathing is of basically two types: **costal (thoracic) breathing** and **diaphragmatic (abdominal) breathing**. Costal breathing involves the external intercostal muscles and other accessory muscles, such as the sternocleidomastoid muscles. It can be observed by the movement of the chest upward and outward. By contrast, diaphragmatic breathing involves the contraction and relaxation of the diaphragm, and it is observed by the movement of the abdomen, which occurs as a result of the diaphragm's contraction and downward movement.

Mechanics and Regulation of Breathing

During *inhalation,* the following processes normally occur (Figure 28.15): the diaphragm contracts (flattens), the ribs move upward and outward, and the sternum moves outward, thus enlarging the thorax and permitting the lungs to expand. During *exhalation* (Figure 28.16), the diaphragm relaxes, the ribs move downward and inward, and the sternum moves inward, thus decreasing the size of the thorax as the lungs are compressed. Normally, breathing is carried out automatically and effortlessly. An inspiration lasts 1 to 1.5 seconds, and an expiration lasts 2 to 3 seconds.

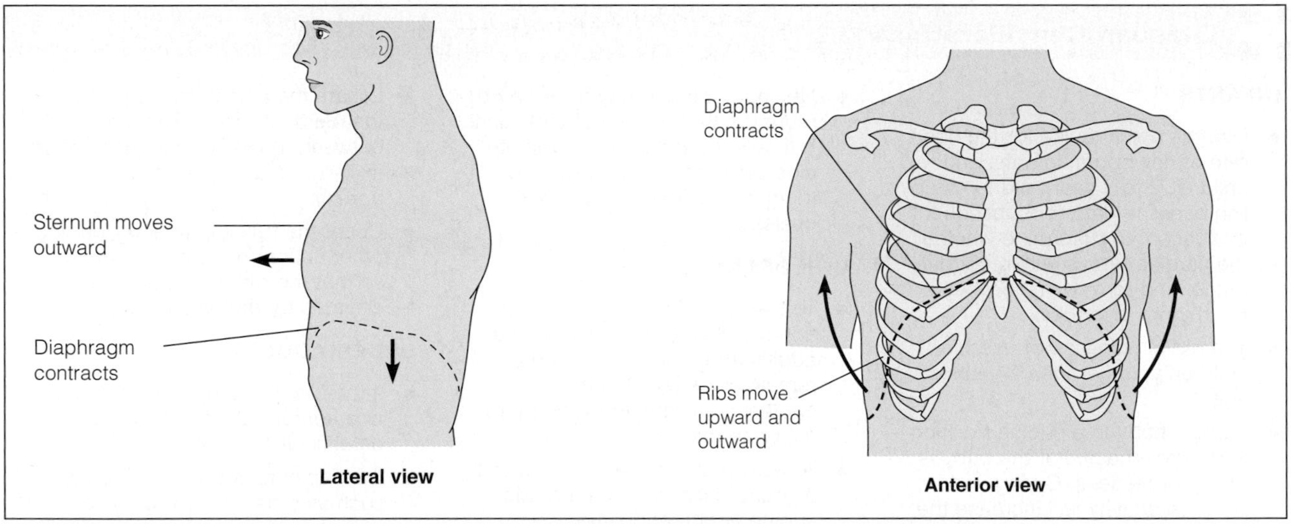

FIGURE 28.15 Respiratory inhalation: *Left,* lateral view; *Right,* anterior view

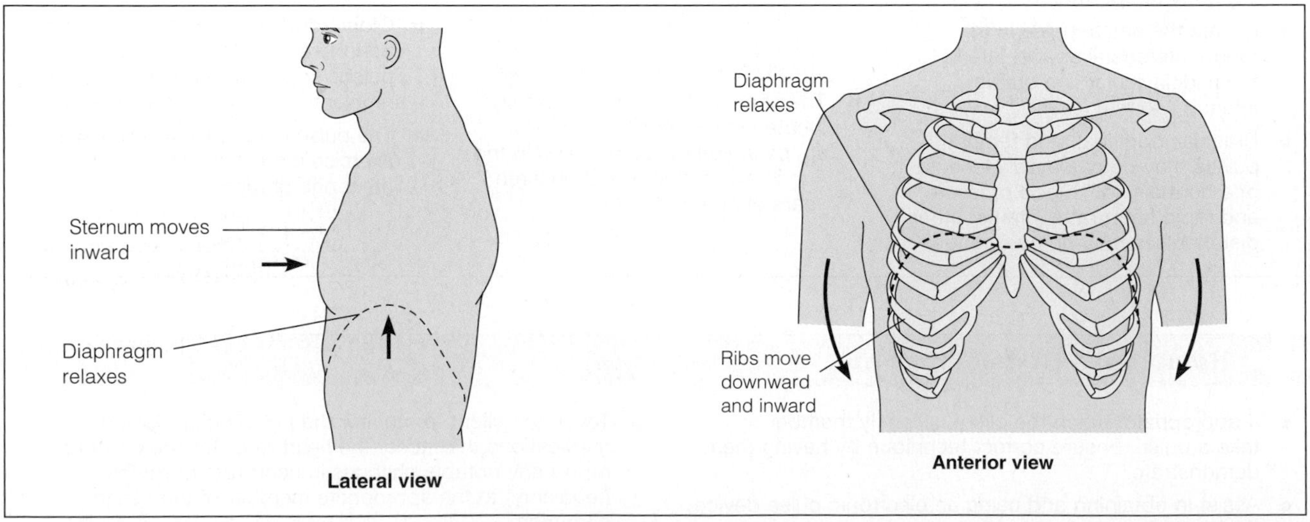

FIGURE 28.16 Respiratory exhalation: *Left,* lateral view; *Right,* anterior view

Respiration is controlled by (1) respiratory centres in the medulla oblongata and the pons of the brain, and (2) by chemoreceptors located centrally in the medulla and peripherally in the carotid and aortic bodies. These centres and receptors respond to changes in the concentrations of oxygen (O_2), carbon dioxide (CO_2), and hydrogen (H^+) in the arterial blood. See Chapter 42 for details.

Assessing Respirations

Respirations should be assessed when the client is relaxed because exercise affects respirations, increasing their rate and depth. Anxiety is likely to affect respiratory rate and depth as well. Respirations may also need to be assessed after exercise to identify the client's tolerance to activity. Before assessing a client's respirations, a nurse should be aware of

- The client's normal breathing pattern
- The influence of the client's health problems on respirations
- Any medications or therapies that might affect respirations
- The relationship of the client's respirations to cardiovascular function

The rate, depth, rhythm, and special characteristics of respirations should be assessed. The *respiratory rate* is normally described in breaths per minute. Breathing that is normal in rate and depth is called **eupnea**. Abnormally slow respirations are referred to as **bradypnea**, and abnormally fast respirations are called **tachypnea**. **Apnea** is the absence of breathing. For the respiratory rates for different age groups, see Table 28.2 (page 673).

Factors Affecting Respirations

Several factors influence respiratory rate. Those that increase the rate include exercise (increases metabolism), stress (readies the body for "fight or flight"), increased environmental temperature, and lowered oxygen concentration at increased altitudes. Factors that may decrease the respiratory rate include decreased environmental temperature, certain medications (e.g., opioids), and increased intracranial pressure.

The *depth* of a person's respirations can be established by watching the movement of the chest. Respiratory depth is generally described as normal, deep, or shallow. *Deep respirations* are those in which a large volume of air is inhaled and exhaled, inflating most of the lungs. *Shallow respirations* involve the exchange of a small volume of air and often the minimal use of lung tissue. During a normal inspiration and expiration, an adult takes in about 500 mL of air. This volume is called the **tidal volume**. For further information about pulmonary volumes and pulmonary capacities, see Chapter 42.

Body position also affects the amount of air that can be inhaled. People in a supine position experience two physiological processes that suppress respiration: an increase in the volume of blood inside the thoracic cavity and compression of the chest. Consequently, clients lying on their back have poorer lung aeration which predisposes them to the stasis of fluids and subsequent infection.

Certain medications also affect the respiratory depth. For example, when taken in large doses, opioids, such as morphine, and barbiturates, such as secobarbital sodium, depress the respiratory centres in the brain, thereby depressing the respiratory rate and depth. **Hyperventilation** refers to very deep, rapid respirations; **hypoventilation** refers to very shallow, slow respirations.

Respiratory rhythm or **pattern** refers to the regularity of the expirations and the inspirations. Normally, respirations are evenly spaced. Respiratory rhythm can be described as *regular* or *irregular.* An infant's respiratory rhythm may be less regular than an adult's. See Chapter 42 for details about abnormal respiratory rhythms.

Respiratory quality or **character** refers to those aspects of breathing that are different from normal, effortless breathing. Two of these are the amount of effort a client must exert to breathe and the sound of breathing. Usually, breathing does not require noticeable effort; some clients, however, breathe only with decided effort, referred to as *laboured breathing.*

The *sound* of breathing is also significant. Normal breathing is silent, but a number of abnormal sounds, such as a wheeze, are obvious to the nurse's ear. Many sounds occur as a result of the presence of fluid in the lungs and are most clearly heard with a stethoscope. See Chapter 27 for methods used to assess lung sounds. For details about altered breathing patterns and terms used to describe various patterns and sounds, see Box 28.4.

The effectiveness of respirations is measured in part by the uptake of oxygen from the air into the blood and the release of carbon dioxide from the blood into expired air. The amount of hemoglobin in arterial blood that is saturated with oxygen can be measured indirectly through pulse oximetry. A pulse oximeter provides a digital readout of both the client's pulse rate and the oxygen saturation (see Skill 28.7, page 697).

Skill 28.5 provides guidelines for assessing respirations.

BOX 28.4 ALTERED BREATHING PATTERNS AND SOUNDS

The following lists describe altered breathing patterns and sounds:

BREATHING PATTERNS

Rate

- *Tachypnea*: rapid respiration marked by quick, shallow breaths
- *Bradypnea*: abnormally slow breathing
- *Apnea*: cessation of breathing

Volume

- *Hyperventilation*: an increase in the amount of air in the lungs, characterized by increased rate and depth of breaths
- *Hypoventilation*: a reduction in the amount of air in the lungs, characterized by shallow respirations
- *Kussmaul's respiration*: abnormally deep, very rapid sighing respirations characteristic of diabetic ketoacidosis

Rhythm

- *Cheyne-Stokes respiration*: rhythmic waxing and waning of respirations, from very deep to very shallow breathing and temporary apnea; often associated with cardiac failure, increased intracranial pressure, or brain damage

Ease or Effort

- *Dyspnea*: the subjective sensation of difficult or uncomfortable breathing or breathlessness (shortness of breath) the individual has a persistent, unsatisfied need for air and feels distressed
- *Orthopnea*: ability to breathe only in upright sitting or standing positions

BREATH SOUNDS

Audible without Amplification

- *Stridor*: a shrill, harsh sound heard during inspiration with laryngeal obstruction
- *Stertor*: snoring or sonorous respiration, usually caused by a partial obstruction of the upper airway
- *Wheeze*: continuous, high-pitched musical squeak or whistling sound occurring on expiration and sometimes on inspiration when air moves through a narrowed or partially obstructed airway
- *Bubbling sounds:* heard as air passes through moist secretions in the respiratory tract

CHEST MOVEMENTS

- *Intercostal retraction*: indrawing between the ribs
- *Substernal retraction*: indrawing beneath the breastbone
- *Suprasternal retraction*: indrawing above the clavicles
- *Flail chest*: the ballooning out of the chest wall through injured rib spaces; results in *paradoxical breathing,* during which the chest wall balloons on expiration but is depressed or sucked inward on inspiration
- *Tracheal tugging:* downward tugging of the trachea with each heart contraction as an effect of an aortic aneurysm

SECRETIONS AND COUGHING

- *Hemoptysis:* the presence of blood in the sputum
- *Productive cough:* a cough accompanied by expectorated secretions
- *Nonproductive cough:* a dry, harsh cough without secretions

SKILL 28.5

ASSESSING RESPIRATIONS

PURPOSES

- To acquire baseline data against which future measurements can be compared
- To monitor abnormal respirations and respiratory patterns and identify changes
- To assess respirations before the administration of a medication, such as morphine (an abnormally slow respiratory rate may warrant withholding the medication)
- To monitor respirations following the administration of a general anaesthetic or any medication that influences respirations
- To monitor clients at risk for respiratory alterations (e.g., those with fever, pain, acute anxiety, chronic obstructive pulmonary disease, respiratory infection, pulmonary edema or emboli, chest trauma or constriction, brain stem injury)

ASSESSMENT

Assess

- Skin and mucous membrane colour (e.g., cyanosis or pallor)
- Position assumed for breathing (e.g., use of orthopneic [upright] position)
- Signs of cerebral anoxia (e.g., irritability, restlessness, drowsiness, or loss of consciousness)
- Chest movements (e.g., retractions between the ribs or above or below the sternum)
- Activity tolerance
- Chest pain
- Dyspnea
- Medications affecting respiratory rate

Equipment

- Watch with a second hand or indicator

(continued)

SKILL 28.5

ASSESSING RESPIRATIONS (*continued*)

IMPLEMENTATION

Preparation

For a routine assessment of respirations, determine the client's activity schedule and choose a suitable time to monitor the respirations. A client who has been exercising will need to rest for a few minutes to permit the accelerated respiratory rate to return to normal.

Performance

1. Before performing the procedure, introduce yourself and verify the client's identity by using agency protocol. Explain to the client what you are going to do, why it is necessary, and how he or she can cooperate.
2. Perform hand hygiene and observe other appropriate infection prevention and control procedures.
3. Provide for client privacy.
4. Observe or palpate and count the respiratory rate.
   - The client's awareness that the nurse is counting the respiratory rate could cause the client to purposefully alter the respiratory pattern. If you anticipate this, place a hand against the client's chest to feel the chest movements with breathing, or place the client's arm across the chest and observe the chest movements while supposedly taking the radial pulse.
   - Count the respiratory rate for 30 seconds if the respirations are regular. Count for 60 seconds if they are irregular. An inhalation and an exhalation count as one respiration.
5. Observe the depth, rhythm, and character of respirations.
   - Observe the respirations for depth by watching the movement of the chest. **Rationale: During deep respirations, a large volume of air is exchanged; during shallow respirations, a small volume is exchanged.**
   - Observe the respirations for regular or irregular rhythm. **Rationale: Normally, respirations are evenly spaced.**
   - Observe the character of respirations—the sound they produce and the effort they require. **Rationale: Normally, respirations are silent and effortless.**
6. Document the respiratory rate, depth, rhythm, and character on the appropriate record.

CLINICAL ALERT

An adult sleeping client's respirations can fall to fewer than 10 shallow breaths per minute. Use other vital signs to validate the client's condition.

EVALUATION

- Relate respiratory rate to other vital signs, in particular, pulse rate; relate respiratory rhythm and depth to baseline data and health status.
- Report to the appropriate members of the health-care team any respiratory rate significantly above or below the normal range and any notable change in respirations from previous assessments; irregular respiratory rhythm; inadequate respiratory depth; abnormal character of breathing (orthopnea, wheezing, stridor, or bubbling); and any complaints of dyspnea.
- Conduct appropriate follow-up, such as administering oxygen or other appropriate medications, treatments, or positioning the client to ease breathing, and requesting involvement of other members of the health-care team, such as the respiratory therapist.

Lifespan Considerations

INFANTS

- An infant or a child who is crying will have an abnormal respiratory rate and rhythm and needs to be quieted before respirations can be accurately assessed.
- Infants and young children use their diaphragms for inhalation and exhalation. If necessary, place your hand gently on the infant's abdomen to feel the rapid rise and fall during respirations.
- Most newborns are complete nose breathers, and nasal obstruction can be lifethreatening.
- Some newborns display periodic breathing, in which they pause for a few seconds between respirations. This condition can be normal, but parents should be alert to prolonged or frequent pauses (apnea) that require medical attention.
- Compared with adults, infants have fewer alveoli and their airways have a smaller diameter. As a result, infants' respiratory rate and effort of breathing will increase with respiratory infections.

CHILDREN

- Because young children are diaphragmatic breathers, observe the rise and fall of the abdomen. If necessary, place your hand gently on the abdomen to feel the rapid rise and fall during respirations.
- Count respirations before performing other uncomfortable procedures so that the respiratory rate is not artificially elevated by the discomfort.

OLDER ADULTS

- Ask the client to remain quiet, or count respirations after taking the pulse.
- Older adults experience anatomical and physiological changes that cause the respiratory system to be less efficient. Any changes in rate or type of breathing should be reported immediately.

Home Care Considerations

- Monitor respiratory rate following the administration of respiratory depressants, such as morphine.
- Assess the home setting for factors that could interfere with breathing, such as exhaust, gas, paint fumes, or persons who smoke.
- If the client has just come in from another room, allow the client to rest a minute or two before counting respirations.
- Have an adult hold a child gently to reduce movement while counting respirations.

Blood Pressure

Blood pressure is a measurement of the pressure exerted by the blood on the vessel walls as it flows through the arteries. Because the blood moves in waves, two blood pressure measures exist. The **systolic pressure** is the pressure of the blood exerted on the artery wall as a result of contraction of the maximum left ventricle, that is, the pressure of the height of the blood wave. The **diastolic pressure** is the pressure when the ventricles are at rest. Diastolic pressure is the lower pressure present at all times within the arteries. The difference between the systolic and the diastolic pressures is called the **pulse pressure**. A normal pulse pressure is about 40 mm Hg but can be as high as 100 mm Hg during exercise. A consistently elevated pulse pressure occurs in arteriosclerosis. A low pulse pressure (e.g., less than 25 mm Hg) occurs in such conditions as severe heart failure.

Blood pressure is measured in millimetres of mercury (mm Hg) and recorded as a fraction: the systolic pressure over the diastolic pressure. The average blood pressure of a healthy adult is 120/80 mm Hg (pulse pressure of 40). The Canadian Hypertension Education Program (2008) considers adult blood pressure measurements between 130 mm Hg and 139 mm Hg systolic or 85 mm Hg and 89 mm Hg diastolic as high normal.

A number of health conditions can be indicated by changes observed in blood pressure recordings among individuals. It is important for the nurse to know a specific client's baseline blood pressure as blood pressure can vary considerably. For example, if a client's usual blood pressure is 120/80 mm Hg and it is assessed following surgery to be 80/20 mm Hg, this significant drop in measure may indicate complications and the physician needs to be informed. The trend or pattern of blood pressure readings is usually of greater significance than a single result.

Determinants of Blood Pressure

Arterial blood pressure is determined by blood flow and the resistance to blood flow as indicated in the following formula: MAP = CO × SVR, where MAP refers to mean arterial pressure (the pressure in the arteries throughout the cardiac cycle), CO refers to cardiac output, and SVR refers to systemic vascular resistance.

CARDIAC OUTPUT *Cardiac output* is the volume of blood pumped into the arteries by the heart. It is seen as an indicator of the pumping action of the heart. When the pumping action of the heart is weak, less blood is pumped into arteries, and the blood pressure decreases. When the heart's pumping action is strong and the volume of blood pumped into the circulation increases, the blood pressure increases.

SYSTEMIC VASCULAR RESISTANCE **Systemic vascular resistance (SVR)**, which is the resistance against which the heart must pump to eject the blood into the systemic circulation (excluding the pulmonary vasculature), is influenced by the size of the arterioles and capillaries, the compliance of the arteries, the blood volume, and the blood viscosity. Increased SVR leads to an increased blood pressure; decreased SVR leads to a decreased blood pressure. The diastolic pressure is especially affected by the resistance in the peripheral vasculature.

The internal diameter or capacity of the arterioles and the capillaries influences SVR in that the smaller the lumen of a vessel, the greater the resistance. Normally, the arterioles are in a state of partial constriction. Increased vasoconstriction, such as occurs with smoking, raises the SVR and, hence, the blood pressure; vasodilation, such as occurs during a long and hot shower, lowers the SVR (leading to lower blood pressure).

If the normal elastic and muscular tissues of the arteries are replaced with fibrous tissue, such as occurs in arteriosclerosis, their compliance (distensibility, elasticity) is decreased. The arteries account for most of the systemic resistance. Chapter 42 discusses arteriosclerosis in detail.

When the blood volume decreases (for example, as a result of a hemorrhage or dehydration), the blood pressure decreases because of decreased fluid exerting pressure on the arteries. Conversely, when the volume increases (for example, as a result of a rapid intravenous infusion), the blood pressure increases because of the greater fluid volume within the circulatory system.

Viscosity is a physical property that results from friction of molecules in a fluid. A viscous (or thick) fluid has a great deal of friction among the molecules as they slide by one another. The viscosity of blood is mostly determined by **hematocrit** (the proportion of red blood cells to the blood plasma). Blood pressure is higher when the blood is highly viscous (i.e., when the hematocrit is more than 0.6 to 0.65).

Factors Affecting Blood Pressure

Age, exercise, stress, race, obesity, gender, medications, sodium intake, diurnal variations, and disease processes are factors influencing blood pressure.

- *Age.* Newborns have a mean systolic pressure of about 75 mm Hg. The pressure rises with age, reaching a peak at the onset of puberty, and then tends to decline somewhat. It rises again in older adults, with half of Canadians over age 65 having hypertension and an estimated 90% of those with normal blood pressure at 55 who will go on to develop hypertension at some later point (Canadian Hypertension Education Program [CHEP], 2008). In older adults, elasticity of the arteries is decreased—the arteries are more rigid and less yielding to the pressure of the blood. This produces an elevated systolic pressure. Because the walls no longer retract as flexibly with decreased pressure, the diastolic pressure may also be high.
- *Exercise.* Physical activity increases the cardiac output and hence the blood pressure; thus, 20 to 30 minutes of rest following exercise is indicated before the resting blood pressure can be reliably assessed.
- *Stress.* Stimulation of the sympathetic nervous system increases cardiac output and vasoconstriction of the arterioles, thus increasing the blood pressure reading. The *white coat effect* describes the elevation in blood pressure that occurs by virtue of the stress generated by going to a hospital or clinic for assessment. Severe pain, however, can decrease blood pressure greatly and cause shock by inhibiting the vasomotor centre and producing vasodilation.
- *Race.* Black males over 35 years usually exhibit higher blood pressures than other males of the same age.
- *Obesity.* Generally, overweight and obese people have higher blood pressure than people of normal weight. Both childhood and adult obesity predispose people to hypertension.
- *Gender.* After puberty, females usually have lower blood pressures than males of the same age; this difference is thought to be due to hormonal variations. Women generally have higher blood pressure following menopause.
- *Prescription drugs and other substances.* Many products can increase or decrease the blood pressure (e.g., sympathomimetic decongestants, caffeine, and liquorice increase blood pressure; diuretics and beta blockers lower blood pressure); nurses should be aware of prescribed medications and other substances that a client is taking and consider their possible impact when interpreting blood pressure readings.
- *Sodium intake.* A high sodium intake can increase the release of natriuretic hormone, which indirectly contributes to hypertension. Additionally, sodium stimulates vasopressor mechanisms, which cause vasoconstriction. A sodium intake of less than 100 mmol/day (2300 mg) is recommended for prevention of hypertension. People with hypertension should limit their dietary sodium intake to between 65 mmol/day and 100 mmol/day (1495 mg and 2300 mg) (CHEP, 2008). Health Canada (2008) recommends 1200 mg to 1500 mg as adequate sodium intake to meet daily requirements.
- *Diurnal variations.* Blood pressure is usually lowest early in the morning, when the metabolic rate is lowest, then rises throughout the day and peaks in the late afternoon or early evening.
- *Disease process.* Any condition affecting the cardiac output, blood volume, blood viscosity, or compliance of the arteries has a direct effect on the blood pressure.

The Teaching: Wellness box identifies several strategies to maintain a healthy blood pressure.

TEACHING: WELLNESS

Maintaining a Healthy Blood Pressure

The following are some ways clients can maintain a healthy blood pressure:

1. Maintain a healthy diet: high in fresh fruits, vegetables, low-fat dairy products, dietary fibre, whole grains, nonanimal protein (e.g., soy), and low in saturated fat and cholesterol, in keeping with Health Canada's (2007) *Eating Well with Canada's Food Guide*.
2. Reduce sodium intake to less than 100 mmol/day (2300 mg/day); ideally to 1500 mg/day.
3. Take part in regular physical activity: in addition to routine activities of daily living, accumulate 30 to 60 minutes of moderate intensity dynamic exercise 4 to 7 days per week (e.g., walking, swimming, cycling).
4. Reduce alcohol consumption to ≤ 2 standard drinks per day and ≤ 14/week for men and ≤ 9/week for women.
5. Attain and maintain a healthy BMI (18.5 to 24.9 kg/m^2) and a waist circumference < 102 cm for men and < 88 cm for women.
6. Abstain from smoking and maintain a smoke-free environment.
7. Practise stress management.

Source: Summarized with permission from CHEP (2008).

Hypertension

A blood pressure that is persistently above normal is called **hypertension**. A single elevated blood pressure reading indicates the need for reassessment. Blood pressure that is consistently more than 140/90 mm Hg is considered high and diagnostic of hypertension. Hypertension is a widespread health problem that affects more than 5 million Canadians, with many people not even knowing they have it (CHEP, 2008). Usually asymptomatic, hypertension—sometimes called the silent killer—is the number-one risk factor for strokes and a major risk factor for myocardial infarctions (heart attacks), heart failure, peripheral vascular disease, and blindness.

CHEP (2008) has developed an evidence-based algorithm (Figure 28.17) to ensure that screening and follow-up of blood pressure takes place so that the diagnosis of hypertension is made in the most expedited manner (e.g., a person who has blood pressure assessments of 140–179/90–109 and diabetes mellitus will receive a diagnosis of hypertension and the necessary treatment after only two assessments within 1 month). The algorithm includes the option of ambulatory and home assessment of blood pressure if these are available. The latter is particularly useful for monitoring clients with diabetes, chronic renal disease, white coat effect, or masked hypertension (blood pressure controlled at clinic visits but not at home). Nurses must be aware of these protocols as they play an important role in ensuring the appropriate assessment and follow-up of people with hypertension (McLean, Kingsbury, Costello, Cloutier, & Matheson, 2007).

An elevated blood pressure of unknown cause is called primary hypertension. An elevated blood pressure of known cause is called secondary hypertension. The majority (90%) of hypertension diagnoses are of the primary type. Factors associated with primary hypertension include thickening of the arterial walls, which reduces the size of the arterial lumen, loss of elasticity of the arteries, as well as lifestyle factors, such as cigarette smoking, obesity, heavy alcohol consumption, caffeine consumption, lack of physical exercise, high blood cholesterol levels, and continued exposure to stress. Follow-up care should include counselling for lifestyle changes as well as monitoring the blood pressure itself. Secondary hypertension causes include renal failure and tumours of the adrenal medulla.

Hypotension

Hypotension is a blood pressure that is below normal, that is, a systolic reading consistently between 85 mm Hg and 110 mm Hg in an adult. **Orthostatic hypotension** is a blood pressure that falls when the client sits or stands. It is usually the result of peripheral vasodilation in which the blood leaves the central body organs, especially the brain, and moves to the periphery, often causing the person to feel faint. Hypotension can also be caused by opioids, such as morphine, bleeding, severe burns, and prolonged diarrhea and vomiting. It is important to monitor hypotensive clients carefully to prevent falls. When assessing for orthostatic hypotension, follows these steps:

- Place the client in a supine position for at least 5 minutes to allow the blood pressure and pulse to stabilize in this position.
- Record the client's pulse and blood pressure.
- Assist the client to slowly sit or stand. Support the client in case of faintness.
- After 1 to 3 minutes in the upright position, recheck the pulse and blood pressure in the same sites as previously.
- Record the results. A rise in pulse of 20 bpm *or* a decrease in systolic or diastolic blood pressure of 10 mm Hg indicates orthostatic hypotension. However, interpret these changes with caution as wide discrepancies exist in the literature about the magnitude of the orthostatic response and its correlation with intravascular volume status (e.g., a healthy individual can have a drop in blood pressure despite normal vascular volume; a person with significantly low vascular volume may not have a postural drop) (Estes & Buck, 2008).

CLINICAL ALERT

CHEP (2008) advocates a "treat to target" approach to hypertension management as a means of reducing the many negative consequences of hypertension. The target is < 140/90 mm Hg or < 130/80 if the person has diabetes or chronic kidney disease.

Assessing Blood Pressure

EQUIPMENT Blood pressure is measured with a *blood pressure cuff*, a *sphygmomanometer,* and a *stethoscope.* The traditional blood pressure cuff consists of a rubber bladder that can be inflated with air (Figure 28.18). The bladder is covered with cloth and has two tubes attached to it. One tube connects to a bulb that inflates the bladder. A small valve on the side of this bulb releases the air from the bladder. When the valve is closed, air pumped into the bladder remains there.

The other tube is attached to a sphygmomanometer. The sphygmomanometer indicates the pressure of the air within the bladder. Sphygmomanometers come in two types: *aneroid* and *digital.* The aneroid sphygmomanometer is a calibrated dial with a needle that points to markings that correlate with BP values (Figure 28.19). Most agencies use digital (electronic) sphygmomanometers (Figure 28.20), which eliminate the need to listen to the sounds of the client's systolic and diastolic blood pressures through a stethoscope. Electronic blood pressure devices should be calibrated against an aneroid sphygmomanometer to check accuracy.

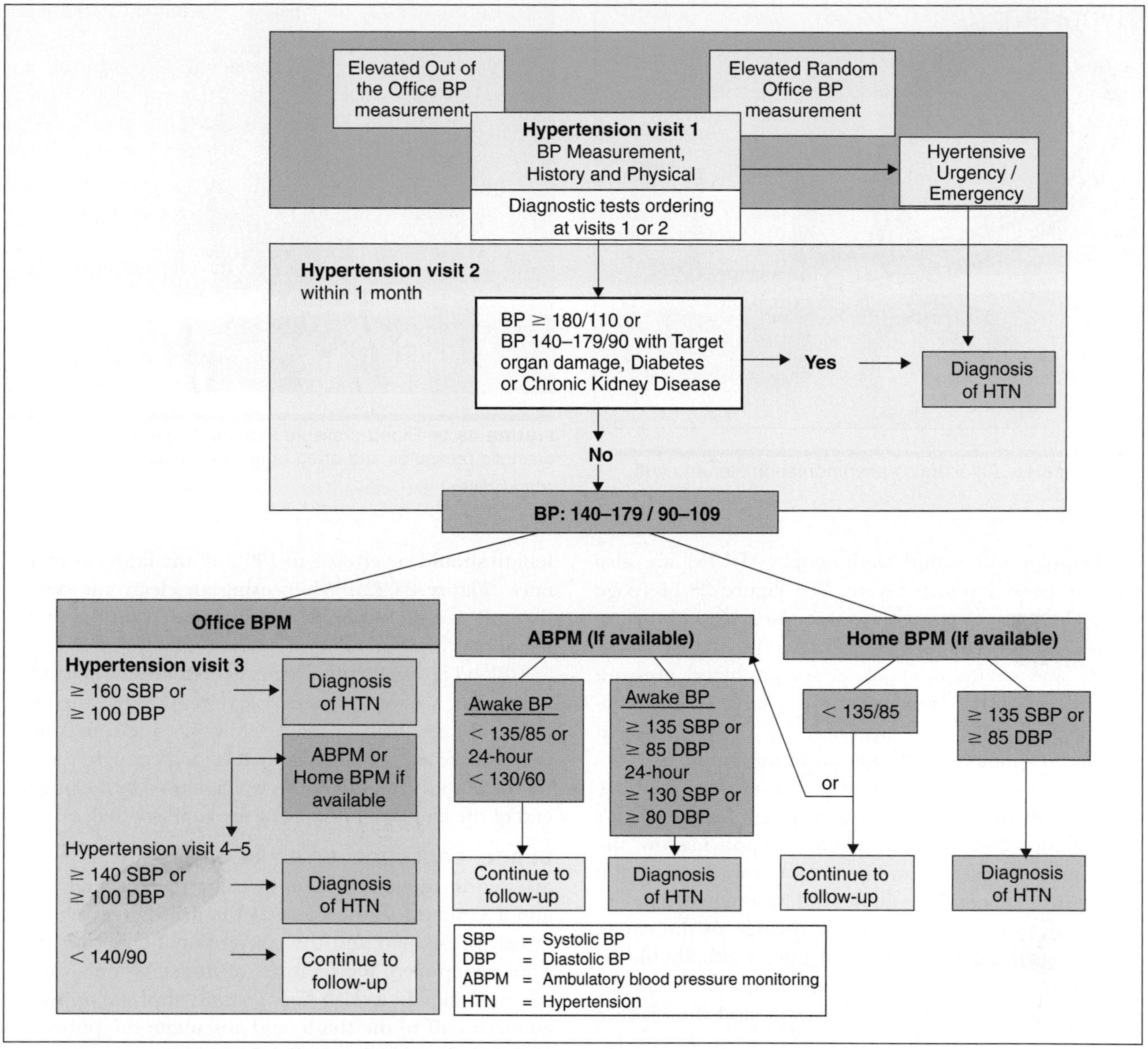

FIGURE 28.17 CHEP 2007 expedited assessment and diagnosis of patients with hypertension. The 2008 version remains unchanged.

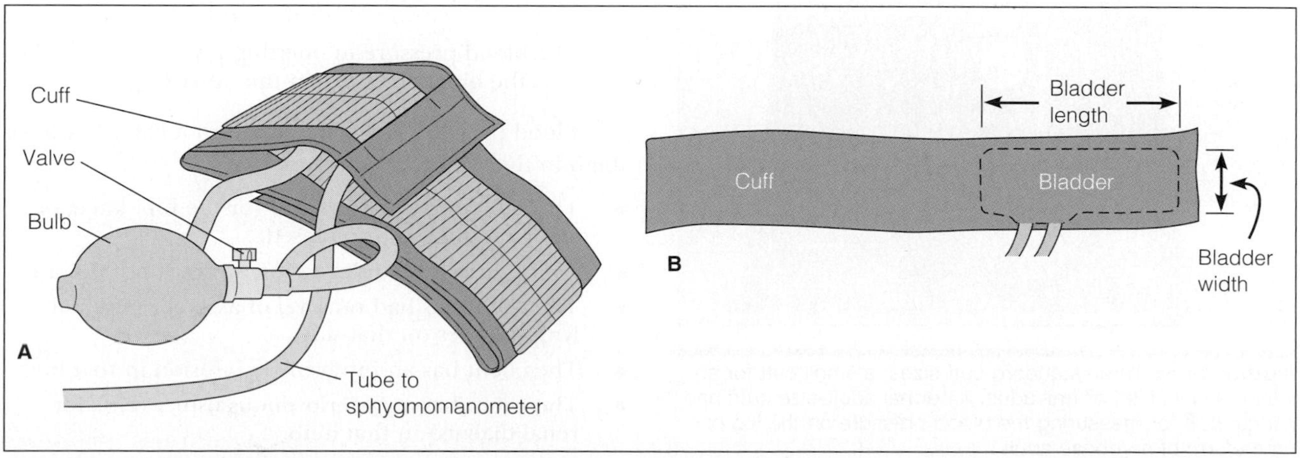

FIGURE 28.18 A: A blood pressure cuff and bulb; B: the bladder inside the cuff

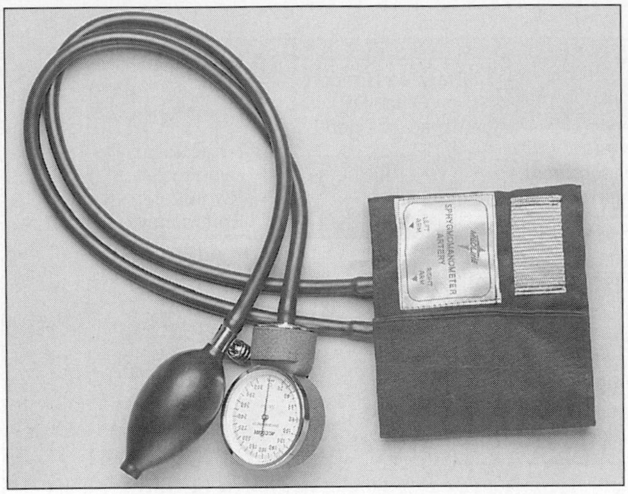

FIGURE 28.19 An aneroid sphygmomanometer and cuff

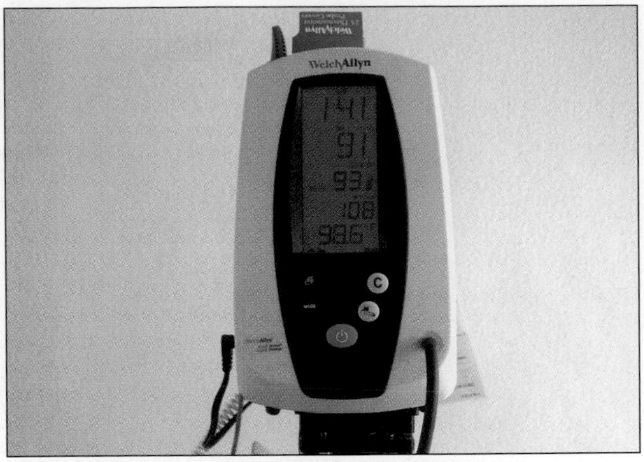

FIGURE 28.20 Blood pressure monitors register systolic and diastolic pressures and often other vital signs.
(Patrick Watson)

Doppler ultrasound stethoscopes (DUSs) are also used to assess blood pressure. See Figure 28.14 (page 674). These are of particular value when blood pressure sounds are difficult to hear, such as in infants, obese clients, and clients in shock. A systolic blood pressure assessed with a DUS is recorded with a large D, for example, 85D. Systolic pressure may be the only blood pressure obtainable with some ultrasound models.

Blood pressure cuffs come in various sizes; the bladder must be the correct width and length for the client's arm (Figure 28.21). If the bladder is too narrow, the blood pressure reading will be erroneously elevated; if it is too wide, the reading will be underestimated. The circumference of the limb, and *not* the age of the client, determines the cuff size. The bladder width should be 40% of the limb circumference or 20% wider than the diameter of the midpoint of the limb, and the bladder length should cover 80% to 100% of the limb circumference (Figure 28.22). When using an electronic device, the cuff size should be determined based on the manufacturer's recommendations (CHEP, 2008).

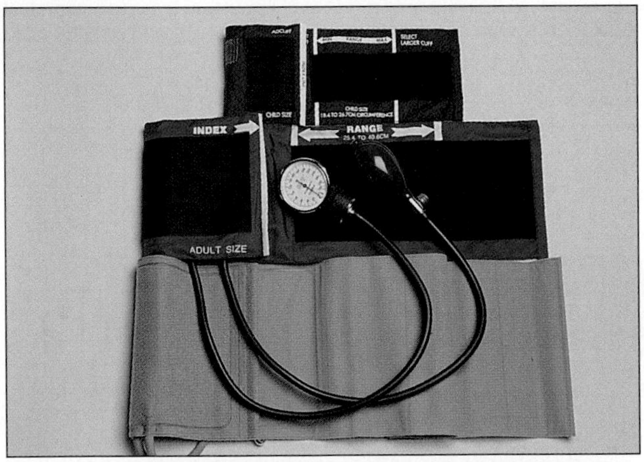

FIGURE 28.21 Three standard cuff sizes: a small cuff for an infant, small child, or frail adult; a normal adult-size cuff; and a large cuff for measuring the blood pressure on the leg or on the arm of an obese adult

Blood pressure cuffs are made of nondistensible material so that an even pressure is exerted around the limb. Most cuffs are held in place by hooks, snaps, or Velcro. Others have a cloth bandage that is long enough to encircle the limb several times; this type is closed by tucking the end of the bandage into one of the bandage folds.

BLOOD PRESSURE SITES Blood pressure is usually assessed in the client's arm by using the brachial artery and a standard stethoscope. If the arm is very large or grossly misshapen and the conventional cuff cannot be properly applied, leg or forearm measurements can be taken. To obtain a *thigh blood pressure,* apply an appropriate-sized cuff to the thigh, and auscultate the pulsations of the blood over the popliteal artery.

Assessing the blood pressure on a client's thigh is usually indicated in these situations:

- The blood pressure cannot be measured on either arm (e.g., because of burns or other trauma).
- The blood pressure in one thigh is to be compared with the blood pressure in the other thigh.

Blood pressure is *not* measured on a client's arm or thigh in the following situations:

- The shoulder, arm, or hand (or the hip, knee, or ankle) is injured or diseased.
- A cast or bulky bandage is on any part of the limb.
- The client has had removal of axilla or inguinal lymph nodes on that side.
- The client has an intravenous infusion in that limb.
- The client has an arteriovenous fistula (e.g., for renal dialysis) in that limb.

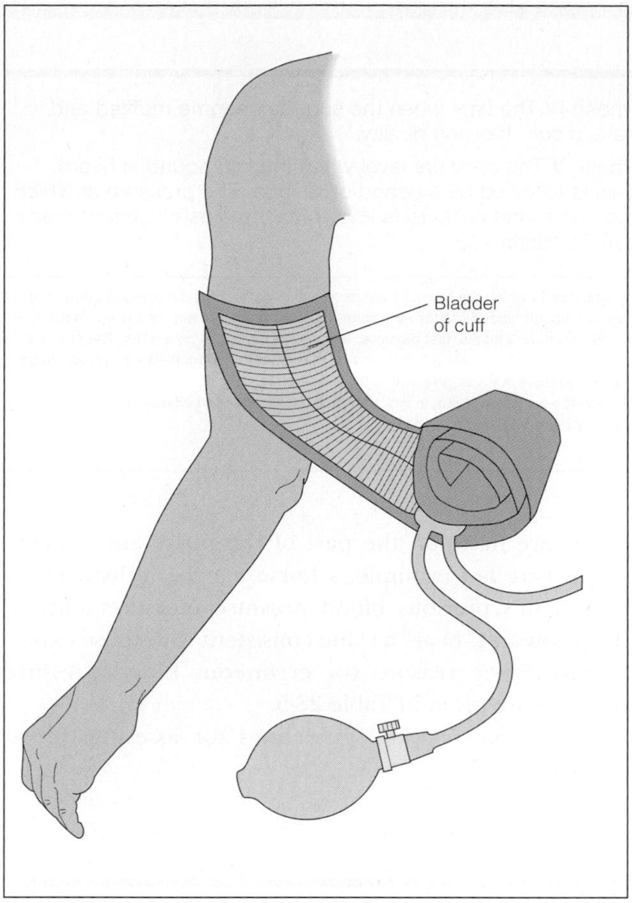

FIGURE 28.22 Determining that the bladder of a blood pressure cuff is 40% of the arm circumference or 20% wider than the diameter of the midpoint of the limb

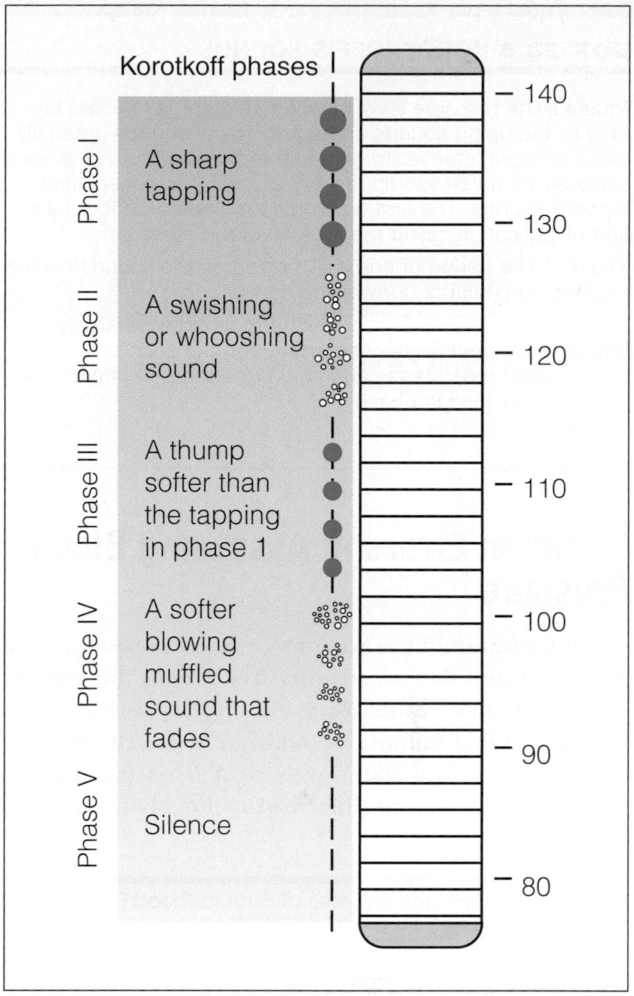

FIGURE 28.23 Korotkoff's sounds can be differentiated into five phases. In the illustration, the blood pressure is 138/90 or 138/102/90.

METHODS Blood pressure can be assessed directly or indirectly. *Direct (invasive monitoring) measurement* involves the insertion of a catheter into the brachial, radial, or femoral artery. Arterial pressure is represented as wave-like forms displayed on an oscilloscope. With correct placement, this pressure reading is highly accurate.

Two *noninvasive indirect methods* of measuring blood pressure are the auscultatory and palpatory methods. The *auscultatory method* is most commonly used in hospitals, clinics, and homes. Required equipment is a sphygmomanometer, a cuff, and a stethoscope. When carried out correctly, the auscultatory method is relatively accurate.

When taking a blood pressure by using a stethoscope, the nurse identifies the five phases in the series of sounds called **Korotkoff's sounds** (Figure 28.23). First the nurse pumps the cuff up to about 30 mm Hg above the palpatory systolic pressure (when the pulse is no longer felt—this is the point when the blood flow in the artery is stopped). Pressure is released slowly (2 mm Hg/beat), while the nurse observes the readings on the manometer and relates them to the sounds heard through the stethoscope. Five phases occur but may not always be audible (see Box 28.5).

The *palpatory method* is sometimes used when Korotkoff's sounds cannot be heard and electronic equipment to amplify the sounds is not available, or when an auscultatory gap occurs. An **auscultatory gap**, which occurs particularly in hypertensive clients, is the temporary disappearance of sounds normally heard over the brachial artery when the cuff pressure is high, followed by the reappearance of the sounds at a lower level. This temporary disappearance of sounds occurs in the latter part of phase I and phase II and may cover a range of 40 mm Hg. Instead of listening for the blood flow sounds, the nurse palpates the pulsations of the artery as the pressure in the cuff is released. The systolic pressure is read from the sphygmomanometer when the first pulsation is felt. A single whip-like vibration, felt in addition to the pulsations, identifies the point at which the pressure in the cuff nears the diastolic pressure. This vibration is no longer felt when the cuff pressure is below the diastolic pressure. To palpate the diastolic pressure, the nurse applies light to moderate pressure over the pulse point.

BOX 28.5 KOROTKOFF'S SOUNDS

Phase I The pressure level at which the first faint, clear tapping or thumping sounds are heard. These sounds gradually become more intense. To ensure that they are not extraneous sounds, the nurse should identify at least two consecutive tapping sounds. The first tapping sound heard during deflation of the cuff is called the systolic blood pressure.

Phase II The period during deflation when the sounds have a muffled, whooshing, or swishing quality.

Phase III The period during which the blood flows freely through an increasingly open artery and the sounds become crisper and more intense and again assume a thumping quality but softer than in phase I.

Phase IV The time when the sounds become muffled and have a soft, blowing quality.

Phase V The pressure level when the last sound is heard. This is followed by a period of silence. The pressure at which the last sound is heard is known as the diastolic blood pressure in adults.*

*In agencies in which the fourth phase is considered the diastolic pressure, three measures are recommended (systolic pressure, diastolic pressure, and phase V). These may be referred to as systolic, first diastolic, and second diastolic pressures. The phase V (second diastolic pressure) reading may be zero; that is, the muffled sounds are heard even when there is no air pressure in the blood pressure cuff. In some instances, muffled sounds are never heard, in which case a dash is inserted where the reading would normally be recorded (e.g., /–/110).

Common Errors in Assessing Blood Pressure

The importance of the accuracy of blood pressure assessments cannot be overemphasized. Many judgments about a client's health are made on the basis of blood pressure. It is an important indicator of the client's condition and is used extensively as a basis for nursing interventions. Two possible reasons for blood pressure errors are haste on the part of the nurse and subconscious bias. For example, a nurse may be influenced by the client's previous blood pressure measurements or diagnosis and "hear" a value consistent with those expectations. Some reasons for erroneous blood pressure readings are given in Table 28.5.

Skill 28.6 provides guidelines for assessing blood pressure.

TABLE 28.5 Selected Sources of Error in Blood Pressure Assessment

Error	Effect
Bladder cuff too narrow	Erroneously high
Bladder cuff too wide	Erroneously low
Arm unsupported	Erroneously high
Insufficient rest before the assessment	Erroneously high
Repeating assessment too quickly	Erroneously high systolic or low diastolic readings
Cuff wrapped too loosely or unevenly	Erroneously high
Deflating cuff too quickly	Erroneously low systolic and high diastolic readings
Deflating cuff too slowly	Erroneously high diastolic readings
Failure to use the same arm consistently	Inconsistent measurements
Arm above level of the heart	Erroneously low
Assessing immediately after a client eats a meal, smokes a cigarette, consumes alcohol, or is having pain	Erroneously high
Failure to identify auscultatory gap	Erroneously low systolic pressure and erroneously low diastolic pressure

SKILL 28.6

ASSESSING BLOOD PRESSURE

PURPOSES

- To obtain a baseline measure of arterial blood pressure for subsequent evaluation
- To determine the client's hemodynamic status (e.g., stroke volume of the heart and blood vessel resistance)
- To identify and monitor changes in blood pressure resulting from a disease process and medical therapy (e.g., presence or history of cardiovascular disease, renal disease, circulatory shock, or acute pain; rapid infusion of fluids or blood products)

(continued)

SKILL 28.6

ASSESSING BLOOD PRESSURE (*continued*)

ASSESSMENT

Assess

- Signs and symptoms of hypertension (e.g., headache, ringing in the ears, flushing of face, nosebleeds, fatigue)
- Signs and symptoms of hypotension (e.g., tachycardia, dizziness, mental confusion, restlessness, cool and clammy skin, pale or cyanotic skin)
- Factors affecting blood pressure (e.g., activity, emotional stress, pain, and time the client last smoked or ingested caffeine)
- Some blood pressure cuffs contain latex, so assess the client for latex allergy and obtain a latex-free cuff if indicated

PLANNING

Equipment

- Stethoscope or DUS
- Blood pressure cuff of the appropriate size (newborn, infant, child, small adult, adult, large adult, thigh)
- Sphygmomanometer

IMPLEMENTATION

Preparation

1. Ensure that the equipment is intact and functioning properly. Check for leaks in the tubing of the sphygmomanometer.
2. Make sure that the client has not smoked or ingested caffeine within 30 minutes before measurement. **Rationale: Smoking constricts blood vessels and caffeine increases the pulse rate. Both of these cause a temporary increase in blood pressure.**
3. The patient should be seated comfortably with back support for at least 5 minutes before commencing the blood pressure assessment (CHEP, 2008).

Performance

1. Before performing the procedure, introduce yourself and verify the client's identity by using agency protocol. Explain to the client what you are going to do, why it is necessary, and how he or she can cooperate. Discuss how the results will be used in planning further care or treatments.
2. Perform hand hygiene and observe other appropriate infection prevention and control procedures.
3. Provide for client privacy.
4. Position the client appropriately.
   - The adult client should be sitting with back support unless otherwise specified. Both feet should be flat on the floor (CHEP, 2008). **Rationale: Legs crossed at the knee result in elevated systolic and diastolic blood pressures**).
   - The elbow should be slightly flexed with the palm of the hand facing up and the forearm supported at heart level. Readings in any other position should be specified. The blood pressure is normally similar in sitting, standing, and lying positions, but it can vary significantly by position in certain persons. **Rationale: The blood pressure increases when the arm is below heart level and decreases when the arm is above heart level.**
   - Expose the upper arm.
5. Wrap the deflated cuff evenly around the bare upper arm. Locate the brachial artery (see ❶). Apply the centre of the bladder directly over the artery. **Rationale: The bladder inside the cuff must be directly over the artery to be compressed if the reading is to be accurate.**
   - For an adult, place the lower border of the cuff 3 cm above the antecubital space (CHEP, 2008).
6. If this is the client's initial examination, perform a preliminary palpatory determination of systolic pressure. **Rationale: The initial estimate tells the nurse the maximal pressure to which the manometer needs to**

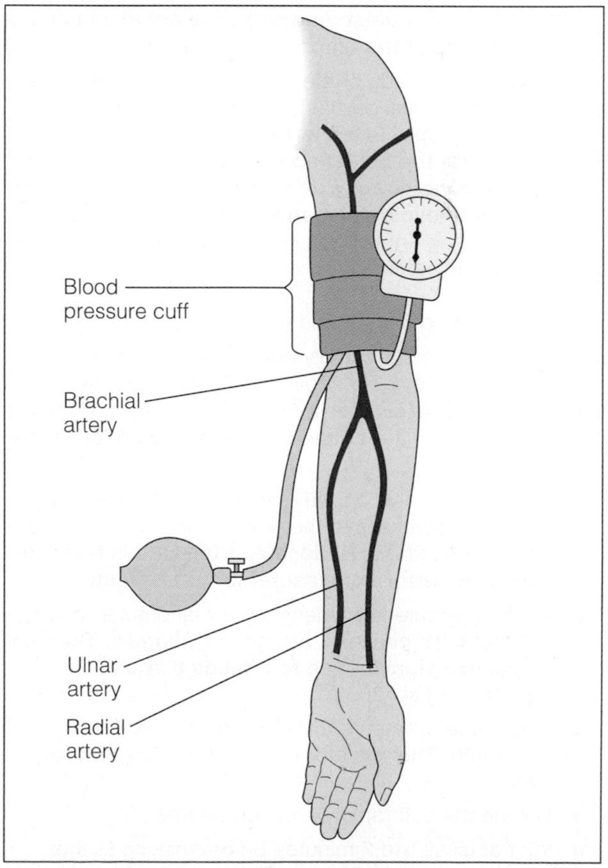

❶ Location of the brachial artery and application of the cuff

(continued)

SKILL 28.6

ASSESSING BLOOD PRESSURE (*continued*)

be elevated in subsequent determinations. It also prevents underestimation of the systolic pressure or overestimation of the diastolic pressure should an auscultatory gap occur.

- Palpate the brachial artery with the fingertips.
- Close the valve on the bulb.
- Pump up the cuff until you no longer feel the brachial pulse. At that pressure the blood cannot flow through the artery. Note the pressure on the sphygmomanometer at which the pulse is no longer felt. **Rationale: This gives an estimate of the systolic pressure.**
- Release the pressure completely in the cuff, and wait 1 to 2 minutes before making further measurements. **Rationale: A waiting period gives the blood trapped in the veins time to be released. Otherwise, false high systolic readings will occur.**

7. Position the stethoscope appropriately.
   - Cleanse the earpieces with antiseptic wipe.
   - Insert the ear attachments of the stethoscope in your ears so that they tilt slightly forward. **Rationale: Sounds are heard more clearly when the ear attachments follow the direction of the ear canal.**
   - Ensure that the stethoscope hangs freely from the ears to the diaphragm. **Rationale: If the stethoscope tubing rubs against an object, the noise can block the sounds of the blood within the artery.**
   - Place the bell side of the amplifier of the stethoscope over the brachial pulse site. **Rationale: Because the blood pressure is a low-frequency sound, it is best heard with the bell-shaped diaphragm. Place the stethoscope directly on skin, not on clothing over the site to avoid noise made from rubbing the amplifier against cloth.** Hold the diaphragm with the thumb and index finger.
8. Auscultate the client's blood pressure.
   - Pump up the cuff rapidly until the sphygmomanometer reads 30 mm Hg above the point where the brachial pulse disappeared (CHEP, 2008). **Rationale: This reduces the chance of a systolic auscultatory gap.**
   - Release the valve on the cuff carefully so that the pressure decreases at the rate of 2 mm Hg per heart beat (CHEP, 2008). **Rationale: If the rate is faster or slower, an error in measurement may occur.**
   - As the pressure falls, identify the manometer reading at Korotkoff's phases I, IV, and V. **Rationale: There is no clinical significance to phases II and III** (Pickering et al., 2005).
   - Auscultate at least 10 mm Hg below phase V. **Rationale: This excludes a diastolic auscultatory gap.**
   - Deflate the cuff rapidly and completely.
   - Wait at least 1 to 2 minutes before making further determinations. **Rationale: This permits blood trapped in the veins to be released.**
   - Repeat the above steps two more times to confirm the accuracy of the reading. Reject the first reading and average the next two (CHEP, 2008). These additional steps are especially important if the blood pressure reading falls outside of the normal range (although this may not be routine procedure for hospitalized or well clients). If there is > 5 mm Hg difference between the two readings, additional measurements may be taken and the results averaged (Pickering et al., 2005).
9. If this is the client's initial examination, repeat the procedure on the client's other arm and in the standing position (arm must be supported). The difference between the arms should be no more than 10 mm Hg. The arm found to have the higher pressure should be used for subsequent examinations.

Variation: Obtaining a Blood Pressure by the Palpation Method

If it is not possible to use a stethoscope to obtain the blood pressure or if the Korotkoff's sounds cannot be heard, palpate the radial or brachial pulse site as the cuff pressure is released. The manometer reading at the point where the pulse reappears represents a value between auscultated systolic and diastolic values.

Variation: Taking a Thigh Blood Pressure

- Help the client to assume a prone position. If the client cannot assume this position, measure the blood pressure while the client is in a supine position with the knee slightly flexed. Slight flexing of the knee will facilitate placing the stethoscope on the popliteal space (see ❷).
- Expose the thigh, taking care not to expose the client unduly.
- Locate the popliteal artery (Figure 28.12, p. 673).
- Wrap the cuff evenly around the mid-thigh with the compression bladder over the posterior aspect of the

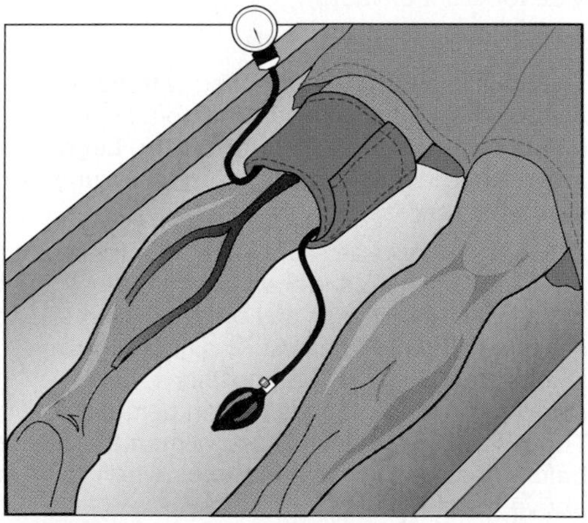

❷ Measuring blood pressure in the client's thigh: location of the popliteal artery and application of the pulse

(continued)

SKILL 28.6

ASSESSING BLOOD PRESSURE (*continued*)

thigh and the bottom edge above the knee. **Rationale: The bladder must be directly over the posterior popliteal artery for the reading to be accurate.**

- If this is the client's initial examination, perform a preliminary palpatory determination of systolic pressure by palpating the popliteal artery.
- In adults, the systolic pressure in the popliteal artery is usually 20 mm Hg to 30 mm Hg higher than that in the brachial artery because of use of a larger bladder; the diastolic pressure is usually the same.

Variation: Using an Electronic Indirect Blood Pressure Monitoring Device.

- Place the blood pressure cuff on the extremity according to the manufacturer's guidelines.
- Turn on the blood pressure switch.
- If appropriate, set the device for the desired number of minutes between blood pressure determinations.
- When the device has determined the blood pressure reading, note the digital results.

10. Remove the cuff.
11. Wipe the cuff with an approved disinfectant. **Rationale: Cuffs can become significantly contaminated.** Many institutions use disposable blood pressure cuffs. The client uses it for the length of stay and then it is discarded. This decreases the risk of spreading infection by sharing cuffs.
12. Document and report pertinent assessment data according to agency policy. Record the blood pressure to the nearest 2 mm Hg (or 1 mm Hg on electronic devices). Record two pressures in the form "130/80" where "130" is the systolic (phase 1) and "80" is the diastolic (phase V) pressure. Record three pressures in the form "130/90/0," where "130" is the systolic, "90" is the first diastolic (phase IV), and sounds are audible even after the cuff is completely deflated (Pickering et al., 2005). Use the abbreviations RA or RL for right arm or right leg and LA or LL for left arm or left leg. Record a difference of greater than 10 mm Hg between the two arms or legs.

CLINICAL ALERT

An electronic or automatic blood pressure cuff can be left in place for many hours. Remove the cuff and check skin condition periodically.

EVALUATION

- Relate blood pressure to other vital signs, to baseline data, and to health status.
- Report any significant change in the client's blood pressure. Also report these findings:
  - Systolic blood pressure (of an adult) above 130 mm Hg
  - Diastolic blood pressure (of an adult) above 85 mm Hg
  - Systolic blood pressure (of an adult) below 100 mm Hg
- Conduct appropriate follow-up, such as administration of medication. If the blood pressure is significantly higher or lower than usual, implement appropriate safety precautions.

Lifespan Considerations

Blood Pressure

INFANTS

- Use a pediatric stethoscope with small diaphragm.
- The lower edge of the blood pressure cuff can be closer to the antecubital space of an infant.
- Use the palpation method if auscultation with a stethoscope or DUS is unsuccessful.
- Arm and thigh pressures are equivalent in children less than 1 year of age.
- One quick way to determine the normal systolic blood pressure of a child is to use the following formula: Normal systolic BP $= 80 + (2 \times$ child's age in years)

CHILDREN

- Blood pressure should be measured in all children more than 3 years of age and in children less than 3 years of age with certain medical conditions (e.g., congenital heart disease, renal malformation, medications that affect blood pressure).

(continued)

Lifespan Considerations (continued)

- Explain each step of the process and what it will feel like. Demonstrate on a doll.
- Use the palpation technique for children less than 3 years old.
- Cuff bladder width should be 40% and length should be 80% to 100% of the arm circumference (Figure 28.24).
- Take the blood pressure before performing other uncomfortable procedures so that the blood pressure is not artificially elevated by the discomfort.
- In children, the diastolic pressure is considered to be the onset of phase IV, where the sounds become muffled.
- In children, the thigh pressure is about 10 mm Hg higher than the arm.

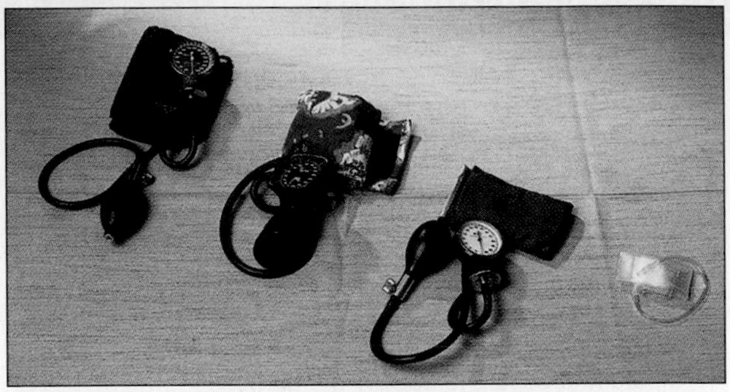

FIGURE 28.24 Pediatric blood pressure cuffs (with manometers)

OLDER ADULTS

- Skin may be very fragile. Do not allow cuff pressure to remain high any longer than necessary.
- Determine whether the client is taking antihypertensives and, if so, when the last dose was taken.
- Medications that cause vasodilation (antihypertensive medications) along with the loss of baroreceptor efficiency in older adults place them at increased risk for having orthostatic hypotension. Measuring blood pressure while the client is in the lying, sitting, and standing positions and noting any changes can determine this.
- If the client has arm contractures, assess the blood pressure by palpation, with the arm in a relaxed position. If this is not possible, take a thigh blood pressure.

Home Care Considerations

Blood Pressure

If taught properly, clients can take blood pressure readings at home:

- Home blood pressure measurement done by the client or family can detect elevated pressures not identified when the client is seen in a medical office, which is of special importance for people with diabetes, chronic renal disease, or demonstrated white coat effect. Home blood pressure readings can be used in the diagnosis of hypertension (CHEP, 2008).
- Observe the client or family member taking the blood pressure and provide feedback if further instruction is needed.
- Clients should purchase home BP monitoring devices, preferably with data-recording capabilities, that have "Recommended by the Canadian Hypertension Society" noted on the packaging. (Visit the CHEP website for photos of approved equipment.)
- If the client takes blood pressure readings at home, use the same equipment or calibrate it against a system known to be accurate.
- If the client is in a chair or low bed, position yourself so that you maintain the client's arm at heart level and you can read the sphygmomanometer at eye level.

Oxygen Saturation

A **pulse oximeter** is a noninvasive device that estimates a client's arterial blood oxygen saturation (SpO_2) by means of a sensor attached to the client's finger (Figure 28.25), toe, nose, earlobe, or forehead (or around the hand or foot of a neonate). Pulse oximetry is often used instead of the riskier, more painful, and invasive arterial blood gas measurement of blood oxygen saturation (SaO_2). The pulse oximeter can detect hypoxemia (low blood oxygen) before clinical signs and symptoms, such as dusky skin colour and dusky nail bed colour, develop.

The pulse oximeter's sensor has two parts: (1) two light-emitting diodes (LEDs)—one red, the other infrared—that transmit light through nails, tissue, venous blood, and arterial blood; and (2) a photodetector placed directly opposite the LEDs (e.g., the other side of the finger, toe, or nose). The photodetector measures the amount of red and infrared light absorbed by oxygenated and deoxygenated hemoglobin in peripheral arterial blood and reports it as SpO_2. Normal SpO_2 as measured by pulse oximetry is 95% to 100%, and an SpO_2 below 70% is life threatening.

Pulse oximeters with various types of sensors are available from several manufacturers. The oximeter unit

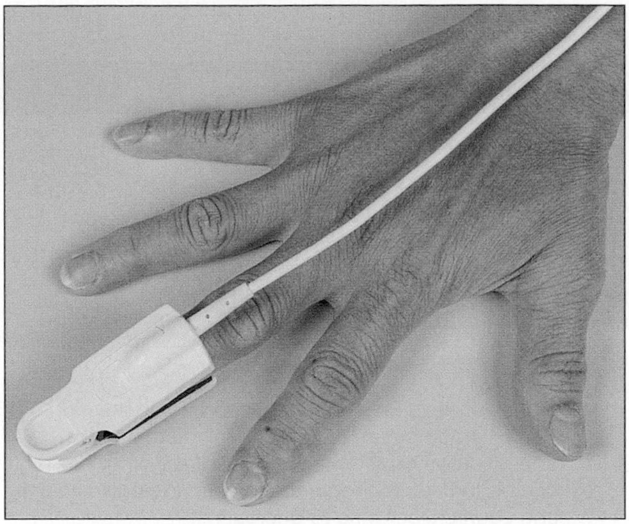

FIGURE 28.25 Fingertip oximeter sensor (adult)

consists of an inlet connection for the sensor cable and a faceplate that indicates (1) the oxygen saturation measurement (expressed as a percentage) and (2) the pulse rate. Cordless units are also available (Figure 28.26). A preset alarm system signals high and low SpO_2 measurements and a high and low pulse rate. The high and low SpO_2 levels are generally preset at 100% and 85%, respectively, for adults. The high and low pulse rate alarms are usually preset at 140 and 50 bpm for adults. These alarm limits can, however, be changed according to the manufacturer's directions.

Factors Affecting Oxygen Saturation Readings

Several factors can affect oxygen saturation readings:

- *Hemoglobin.* If the hemoglobin is fully saturated with oxygen, the SpO_2 will appear normal even if the total hemoglobin level is low. Thus, the client could be severely anemic and have inadequate oxygen to supply the tissues but the pulse oximeter would return a normal value.
- *Circulation.* The oximeter will not return an accurate reading if the area under the sensor has impaired circulation.
- *Activity.* Shivering or excessive movement of the sensor site can interfere with accurate readings.
- *Carbon monoxide poisoning.* Pulse oximeters cannot discriminate between hemoglobin saturated with carbon monoxide versus oxygen. In this case, other measures of oxygenation are needed.

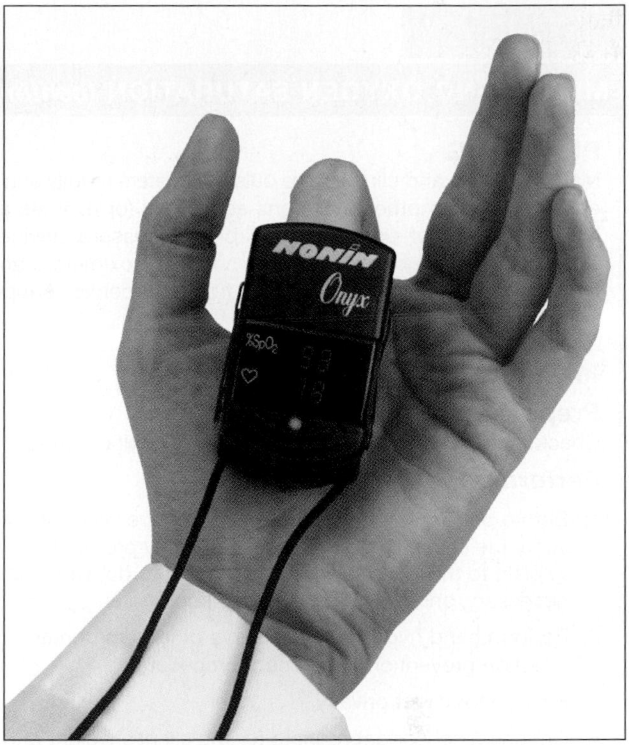

FIGURE 28.26 Fingertip oximeter sensor (cordless)

Skill 28.7 outlines the steps in measuring oxygen saturation. See Chapter 42 for a more extensive discussion of oxygenation.

SKILL 28.7

MEASURING OXYGEN SATURATION

PURPOSES

- To estimate the arterial blood oxygen saturation (SaO_2)
- To detect the presence of hypoxemia before visible signs develop

ASSESSMENT

Assess

- The best location for a pulse oximeter sensor, based on the client's age and physical condition; unless contraindicated, the finger is usually selected for adults
- The client's overall condition, including risk factors for development of hypoxemia (e.g., respiratory or cardiac disease) and hemoglobin level
- Vital signs, skin colour and temperature, nail bed colour, and tissue perfusion of extremities as baseline data
- Adhesive allergy

(continued)

SKILL 28.7

MEASURING OXYGEN SATURATION (*continued*)

PLANNING

Many hospitals and clinics have pulse oximeters readily available for use with other vital signs equipment (or even as an integrated part of the electronic blood pressure device). Other facilities may have a limited supply of oximeters and the nurse may need to request it from the central supply department.

Equipment

- Nail polish remover as needed
- Alcohol wipe
- Sheet or towel
- Pulse oximeter

IMPLEMENTATION

Preparation

Check that the oximeter equipment is functioning normally.

Performance

1. Before performing the procedure, introduce yourself and verify the client's identity by using agency protocol. Explain to the client what you are going to do, why it is necessary, and how he or she can cooperate.
2. Perform hand hygiene and observe other appropriate infection prevention and control procedures.
3. Provide for client privacy.
4. Choose a sensor appropriate for the client's weight and size, and the desired location. Because weight limits of sensors overlap, a pediatric sensor could be used for a small adult.
   - If the client is allergic to adhesive, use a clip or sensor without adhesive. If using an extremity, assess the proximal pulse and capillary refill at the point closest to the site.
   - If the client has low tissue perfusion because of peripheral vascular disease or therapy that uses vasoconstrictive medications, use a nasal sensor or a reflectance sensor on the forehead. Avoid using lower extremities that have a compromised circulation and extremities that are used for infusions or other invasive monitoring.
5. Prepare the site.
   - Clean the site with an alcohol wipe before applying the sensor.
   - It may be necessary to remove a female client's dark nail polish. **Rationale: It can interfere with accurate measurements**. Alternately, position the sensor on the side of the finger rather than perpendicular to the nail bed (Chan, Chan, & Chan, 2003).
6. Apply the sensor, and connect it to the pulse oximeter.
   - Make sure the LED and photodetector are accurately aligned, that is, opposite each other on either side of the finger, toe, nose, or earlobe. Many sensors have markings to facilitate correct alignment of the LEDs and photodetector.
   - Attach the sensor cable to the connection outlet on the oximeter. Turn on the machine according to the manufacturer's directions. Appropriate connection will be confirmed by an audible beep indicating each arterial pulsation. Some devices have a wheel that can be turned clockwise to increase the pulse volume and counterclockwise to decrease it.
   - Ensure that the bar of light or waveform on the face of the oximeter fluctuates with each pulsation.
7. Set and turn on the alarm when using continuous monitoring.
   - Check the preset alarm limits for high and low oxygen saturation and high and low pulse rates. Change these alarm limits according to the manufacturer's directions as indicated. Ensure that the audio and visual alarms are on before you leave the client. A tone will be heard and a number will blink on the faceplate.
8. Ensure client safety.
   - Inspect and move or change the location of an adhesive toe or finger sensor every 4 hours and a spring-tension sensor every 2 hours.
   - Inspect the sensor site tissues for irritation from adhesive sensors.
9. Ensure the accuracy of measurement.
   - Minimize motion artifacts by using an adhesive sensor, or immobilize the client's monitoring site. **Rationale: Movement of the client's finger or toe may be misinterpreted by the oximeter as arterial pulsations**.
   - If indicated, cover the sensor with a sheet or towel to block large amounts of light from external sources (e.g., sunlight, procedure lamps, or bilirubin lights in the nursery). **Rationale: Bright room light may be sensed by the photodetector and alter the SpO_2 value** (Popovich, Richiuso, & Danek, 2004).
   - Compare the pulse rate indicated by the oximeter to the radial pulse periodically. **Rationale: A large discrepancy between the two values may indicate oximeter malfunction**.
10. Document the oxygen saturation (SpO_2) as measured by pulse oximetry on the appropriate record at designated intervals.

EVALUATION

- Compare the oxygen saturation as measured with the pulse oximeter (SpO_2) with the client's previous oxygen saturation level, including any invasive SaO_2 measurements. Relate to the pulse rate and other vital signs.
- Conduct appropriate follow-up, such as notifying the appropriate members of the health-care team, adjusting oxygen therapy, or providing breathing treatments.

Lifespan Considerations

Pulse Oximetry

INFANTS

- If an appropriate-sized finger or toe sensor (Figure 28.27) is not available, consider using an earlobe or forehead sensor.
- The high and low SpO_2 levels are generally preset at 95% and 80% for neonates.
- The high and low pulse rate alarms are usually preset at 200 and 100 for neonates.
- The oximeter may need to be taped, wrapped with an elastic bandage, or covered by a stocking to keep it in place.

CHILDREN

- Instruct the child that the sensor does not hurt. Disconnect the probe whenever possible to allow for movement.

OLDER ADULTS

- Use of vasoconstrictive medications, poor circulation, or thickened nails in older adults may make finger or toe sensors inaccurate.

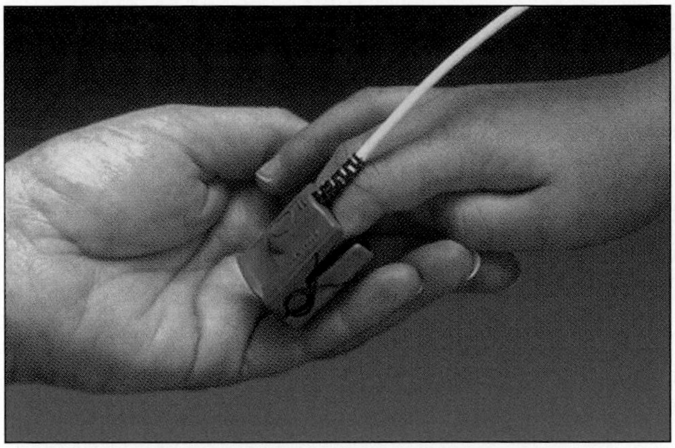

FIGURE 28.27 Fingertip oximeter sensor (child)

Home Care Considerations

Pulse Oximetry

Pulse oximetry can be used in a home setting:

- Pulse oximetry is a quick, inexpensive, noninvasive method of assessing oxygenation. Like an automatic blood pressure cuff, it also provides a pulse rate reading. Use in the ambulatory or home setting whenever indicated.
- If the client requires frequent or continuous home monitoring, teach the client and family how to apply and maintain the equipment. Remind them to rotate the site periodically and assess for skin trauma.

Case Study 28

Mrs. Burne, 75 years old, has just been transferred to her own bed from the postanaesthetic care unit stretcher, following a total hip replacement for osteoarthritis. After a verbal report from the registered nurse, you assess her vital signs. On taking her blood pressure, you are unable to hear any Korotkoff's sounds during release of the valve. You repeat the procedure after 3 minutes and obtain a reading of 180/110 LA supine. Her temperature (tympanic) is 35.8°C and pulse (radial) is 90 bpm, regular, 2+/4 amplitude. Her respirations are 28 and shallow. The pulse oximeter indicates an SpO_2 of 95%. Mrs. Burne is awake and oriented. Her skin is warm and has normal colour.

Critical Thinking Questions

1. What would you say to her when you were unable to hear the Korotkoff's sounds?
2. What is your analysis of the blood pressure reading of 180/110? What further data do you need to collect?
3. How do you interpret her temperature, pulse, and respiratory rate?

After working through these questions, go to the MyNursingLab at **http://www.mynursinglab.com** to check your answers.

KEY TERMS

vital signs
body temperature
core temperature
surface temperature
heat balance
basal metabolic rate (BMR)
chemical thermogenesis
radiation
conduction
convection
vaporization
insensible water loss
insensible heat loss
hypothalamic integrator
pyrexia
hyperthermia
fever
hyperpyrexia
febrile
afebrile
intermittent fever
remittent fever
relapsing fever
constant fever
fever spike
heat exhaustion
heat stroke
hypothermia
pulse
compliance
cardiac output
peripheral pulse
apical pulse
point of maximal impulse (PMI)
tachycardia
bradycardia
pulse rhythm
dysrhythmia
arrhythmia
pulse volume
elasticity of the arterial wall
apical-radial pulse
pulse deficit
respiration
external respiration
internal respiration
inhalation
inspiration
exhalation
expiration
ventilation
costal (thoracic) breathing
diaphragmatic (abdominal) breathing
eupnea
bradypnea
tachypnea
apnea
tidal volume
hyperventilation
hypoventilation
respiratory rhythm or pattern
respiratory quality or character
blood pressure
systolic pressure
diastolic pressure
pulse pressure
systematic vascular resistance (SVR)
hematocrit
hypertension
hypotension
orthostatic hypotension
Korotkoff's sounds
auscultatory gap
pulse oximeter

CHAPTER HIGHLIGHTS

- Vital signs reflect changes in body function that otherwise might not be observed.
- Body temperature is the balance between heat produced by the body and heat lost from the body.
- Factors affecting body temperature include age, diurnal variations, exercise, hormones, stress, and environmental temperatures.
- Four common types of fever are intermittent, remittent, relapsing, and constant.
- During a fever, the set point of the hypothalamic thermostat changes suddenly from the normal level to a higher than normal level, but several hours elapse before the core temperature reaches the new set point.
- Hypothermia involves three mechanisms: excessive heat loss, inadequate heat production by body cells, and increasing impairment of hypothalamic thermoregulation.
- The nurse selects the most appropriate site to measure temperature according to the client's age and condition.
- Pulse rate and volume reflect the stroke volume output, the compliance of the client's arteries, and the adequacy of blood flow.
- Normally a peripheral pulse reflects the client's heartbeat, but it may differ from the heartbeat in clients with certain cardiovascular diseases; in these instances, the nurse takes an apical pulse and compares it with the peripheral pulse.
- Many factors may affect a person's pulse rate: age, gender, exercise, presence of fever, certain medications, hypovolemia, stress, position changes (in some situations), and pathology.
- Although the radial pulse is the site most commonly used, eight other sites can be used in certain situations.
- The difference between the apical and radial pulses is called pulse deficit.
- Respirations are normally quiet, effortless, and automatic and are assessed by observing respiratory rate, depth, rhythm, quality, and effectiveness.

- Blood pressure reflects cardiac output and peripheral vascular resistance.
- Among the factors influencing blood pressure are age, exercise, stress, race, gender, medications, obesity, diurnal variations, and disease processes.
- Orthostatic hypotension occurs when blood pressure falls as the client assumes an upright position.
- A blood pressure cuff too large or too small will give false readings.
- During blood pressure measurement, the artery must be held at heart level.
- Pulse oximetry is a noninvasive means of measuring the percentage of hemoglobin saturated with oxygen. A normal SpO_2 result is 95% to 100%.
- Pulse oximeter sensors can be placed on the finger, hand, foot, or nose.

ASSESS YOUR LEARNING

1. The client's temperature at 8:00 a.m. taken by using an oral electronic thermometer is 36.1°C. All other vital signs are within normal range. What would the nurse do next?
   - **a.** Wait 15 minutes and retake it.
   - **b.** Check what the client's temperature was the last time.
   - **c.** Retake it by using a different thermometer.
   - **d.** Chart the temperature; it is normal.

2. For which of the following clients would the nurse take an apical pulse rather than a radial pulse?
   - **a.** A client in shock
   - **b.** A client for whom the nurse is checking the response to changing from a lying to a sitting position
   - **c.** A client with an arrhythmia
   - **d.** A client less than 24 hours postoperative

3. For a client with a previous blood pressure of 138/74 and pulse of 64, approximately how long should the nurse take to release the blood pressure cuff in order to obtain an accurate reading?
   - **a.** 20 seconds
   - **b.** 45 seconds
   - **c.** 60 seconds
   - **d.** 120 seconds

4. An 85-year-old client has had a cerebrovascular accident (stroke) resulting in right-sided facial drooping and difficulty swallowing. The client is unable to move or maintain a position unaided. Which of the following would be appropriate site(s) for taking the temperature?
   - **a.** Oral
   - **b.** Rectal
   - **c.** Axillary, oral, or temporal artery
   - **d.** Axillary, tympanic, or temporal artery

5. A client with *Ineffective Peripheral Tissue Perfusion* would be expected to have which of the following findings?
   - **a.** Bounding radial pulse
   - **b.** Irregular apical pulse
   - **c.** Carotid pulse stronger on the left side than the right
   - **d.** Absent posterior tibial and pedal pulses

6. The proper assessment of the respiratory rate should include which of the following?
   - **a.** Measurement of oxygen saturation by using pulse oximetry
   - **b.** Asking the patient to take 5 deep breaths before you start
   - **c.** Counting the respiration for 15 seconds and multiplying by 4
   - **d.** Counting the respirations for a full minute.

7. A client states, "I feel so breathless all the time." The nurse documents that the patient is experiencing which of the following?
   - **a.** Hypoventilation
   - **b.** Laboured breathing
   - **c.** Dyspnea
   - **d.** Orthopnea

8. When auscultating the blood pressure, you hear the following:

   At 180 mm Hg: thumping continuing down to

   150 mm Hg: muffled sounds continuing down to

   130 mm Hg: soft thumping sounds continuing down to 105 mm Hg: muffled sounds continuing down to

   95 mm Hg: silence

   You record the blood pressure as which of the following?
   - **a.** 180/95
   - **b.** 180/105/95
   - **c.** 180/150/95
   - **d.** 130/195

9. The nurse is participating in a blood pressure screening clinic. One client's blood pressure is 160/94. On two repeat measures at the same screening clinic, his blood pressure remains the same. The client states that he feels well, takes insulin, but takes no medication for blood pressure. Based on the CHEP (2008) algorithm, the nurse would recommend which of the following?
   - **a.** The client should return in 1 month for a repeat blood pressure assessment.
   - **b.** The client should be referred to a physician for diagnosis and treatment of hypertension.
   - **c.** The client should be told to go to a local pharmacy once a week for 4 weeks to have his blood pressure checked.
   - **d.** The client should focus on regulating his blood glucose, remaining physically active, reducing the salt in his diet, and avoiding smoking.

10. The nurse obtains an oxygen saturation value (SpO_2) of 70% by pulse oximeter in a client who is alert and oriented and who has come to an ambulatory clinic because of feeling short of breath. The client's respiratory rate is 16/minute; her heart rate is 74 bpm, regular and +2/4 amplitude. What is the first thing the nurse should do in this situation?
    - **a.** Seek help.
    - **b.** Administer oxygen therapy.
    - **c.** Auscultate the lungs.
    - **d.** Retake the oxygen saturation.

After working through these questions, go to the MyNursingLab at ***http://www.mynursinglab.com*** *to check your answers and see explanations.*

SUGGESTED READINGS

Canadian Hypertension Education Program. (2008). *2008 CHEP recommendations for the management of hypertension.* Ottawa: Author. Retrieved May 19, 2008, from http://hypertension.ca/chep/wp-content/uploads/2008/03/2008-chepspiral-booklet-final_jan28.pdf

This document is extremely relevant to Canadian nurses. Given the prevalence of hypertension in Canadian society, all nurses, regardless of place of employment, must be aware of the most current assessment and treatment guidelines for this silent killer. The CHEP recommendations generally change from year to year, so checking the general website of http://hypertension.ca will yield annual updates as they appear.

McLean, D., Kingsbury, K., Costello, J., Cloutier, L., & Matheson, S. (2007). 2007 Hypertension Education Program (CHEP) recommendations: Management of hypertension by nurses. *Canadian Journal of Cardiovascular Nursing, 17*(2), 10–16.

The authors discuss the important role of the nurse in the assessment and follow-up of people with normal, high normal, and high blood pressure (hypertension).

National High Blood Pressure Education Program Working Group on High Blood Pressure in Children and Adolescents. (2004). The fourth report on the diagnosis, evaluation and treatment of high blood pressure in children and adolescents. *Pediatrics, 114*, 555–576.

The assessment and management of hypertension in pediatrics requires specialized knowledge. This report provides a comprehensive summary of recommendations for health-care professionals working in this area.

Smith, L. S. (2004). Temperature measurement in critical care adults: A comparison of thermometry and measurement routes. *Biological Research for Nursing, 6*(2), 117–125.

This article provides an interesting review of literature on the various methods of assessing temperature.

WEBLINKS

Blood Pressure Canada

http://www.hypertension.ca/bpc/

This site provides the general population and health-care professionals with up-to-date information on blood pressure assessment, management, and the effects of uncontrolled blood pressure.

Canadian Heart and Stroke Foundation

http://www.heartandstroke.ca

The website of the Heart and Stroke Foundation of Canada is a reliable source of information on heart disease and stroke. The foundation's mission is to improve the health of Canadians by preventing and reducing disability and death from heart disease and stroke through research, health promotion, and advocacy.

Canadian Council of Cardiovascular Nurses

http://www.cardiovascularnurse.com

The Canadian Council of Cardiovascular Nurses maintains this site for its members and others interested in the specialty. Their mission is to advance the profession and the cardiovascular health of Canadians through education, standards, research, and health promotion. Information includes future conferences, news, journals, standards, national and provincial and territorial committee links, and employment opportunities.

Canadian Coalition for High Blood Pressure Prevention and Control

http://www.canadianbpcoalition.org

This group seeks to increase public knowledge of cardiovascular diseases and high blood pressure. The site provides a variety of educational resources, including an emphasis on teaching correct blood pressure measurement by health-care professionals.

Canadian Hypertension Society

http://www.hypertension.ca

This site offers a wealth of information about healthy blood pressure management. It is useful for lay Canadians as well as health professionals.

Canadian Hypertension Education Program

http://www.hypertension.ca/chep/

A subset of the Canadian Hypertension Society's website, this link provides the most up-to-date, evidence-based recommendations for the assessment and management of hypertension.

REFERENCES

Ball, J. W., & Bindler, R. C. (2008). *Pediatric nursing: Caring for children* (4th ed.). Upper Saddle River, NJ: Prentice Hall Health.

Canadian Hypertension Education Program. (2008). *2008 CHEP recommendations for the management of hypertension.* Ottawa: Author. Retrieved May 19, 2008 from http://hypertension.ca/chep/wp-content/uploads/2008/03/2008-chepspiral-booklet-final_jan28.pdf

Chan, M. M., Chan, M. D., & Chan, E. D. (2003). What is the effect of nail polish on pulse oximetry? *Chest, 123,* 2163–2164.

Environment Canada. (2004). *Mercury and the environment: Cleaning up small mercury spills.* Retrieved May 19, 2008, from http://www.ec.gc.ca/MERCURY/EN/cu.cfm

Estes, M. E., & Buck, M. (2008). *Health assessment and physical examination.* Toronto: Nelson.

Health Canada. (2007). *Eating well with Canada's food guide.* Retrieved January 8, 2008, from http://www.hc-sc.gc.ca/fn-an/food-guide-aliment/index_e.html

Health Canada. (2008). *Healthy living: Sodium.* Retrieved June 12, 2008, from http://www.hc-sc.gc.ca/hl-vs/iyh-vsv/food-aliment/sodium-eng.php

Liu, C. C., Chang, R. E., & Chang, W. C. (2004). Limitations of forehead infrared body temperature detection for fever screening for severe acute respiratory syndrome. *Infection Control Hospital Epidemiology, 25,* 1109–1111.

McLean, D., Kingsbury, K., Costello, J., Cloutier, L., & Matheson, S. (2007). 2007 Hypertension Education Program (CHEP) recommendations: Management of hypertension by nurses. *Canadian Journal of Cardiovascular Nursing, 17*(2), 10–16.

Nimah, M. M., Bshesh, K., Callahan, J., & Jacobs, B. R. (2006). Infrared tympanic thermometry in comparison with other temperature measurement techniques in febrile children. *Pediatric Critical Care Medicine, 7,* 48–55.

Pickering, T. G., Hall, J. E., Appel, L. J., Falkner, B. E., Graves, J., Hill, M. N., et al. (2005). Recommendations for blood pressure measurement in humans and experimental animals: Part 1: Blood pressure measurement in humans: A statement for professionals from the subcommittee of professional and public education of the American Heart Association council on high blood pressure research. *Circulation, 111,* 697–716.

Popovich, D. M., Richiuso, N., & Danek, G. (2004). Pediatric health care providers' knowledge of pulse oximetry. *Pediatric Nursing, 30*(1), 14–20.

Roy, S., Powell, K., & Gerson, L. W. (2003). Temporal artery temperature measurements in healthy infants, children, and adolescents. *Clinical Pediatrics, 42,* 433–437.

Chapter 29

Hygiene

Hygiene is the science of health and its maintenance. It is a highly personal matter determined by individual values and practices. It involves care of the skin, hair, nails, teeth, oral and nasal cavities, eyes, ears, and perineal and genital care. **Personal hygiene** is self-care that includes bathing, toileting, general body cleaning, and grooming. Individuals engage in personal hygiene activities to fulfill the need for physical, social, and emotional comfort, as well as for safety.

Nurses frequently encounter people who require varying degrees of assistance, from minimal intervention to complete care, to attain their optimal hygiene needs. Responsibility for assisting clients to meet their hygiene needs encompasses not only the *activities* related to hygiene but also comprehensive assessment, mutual goal setting and planning, interventions, and evaluation of the extent to which the hygiene needs are met. This approach is based on thorough knowledge of relevant anatomy and physiology, developmental considerations, factors affecting hygiene practices, and knowledge of current research regarding these practices and the determinants of health (see Table 29.1 and the Lifespan Considerations box for bathing on page 706).

OBJECTIVES

After studying this chapter, you should be able to

1. Explain the main purpose of hygiene
2. Relate determinants of health to the practice of personal hygiene
3. Discuss comprehensive assessment related to hygiene
4. Discuss common conditions affecting clients' hygiene needs
5. Apply the nursing process to caring for common hygiene problems related to the skin, feet, nails, mouth, hair, eyes, ears, and nose
6. Describe hygiene care for various types of baths, oral hygiene, perineal care, contact lenses, artificial eyes, and hearing aids
7. Identify safety and comfort measures underlying bed-making procedures

Skin

The skin is the largest organ of the body. It serves five major functions:

1. It protects underlying tissues from injury by preventing the passage of microorganisms. The skin and mucous membranes are considered the body's first line of defence.
2. It regulates the body temperature. Cooling the body occurs through the heat loss processes of evaporation of perspiration, and by radiation and conduction of heat from the body when the blood vessels of the skin are vasodilated. Body heat is conserved through lack of perspiration and by vasoconstriction. See Chapter 28 for a detailed discussion of body heat losses and gains.
3. It secretes **sebum**, an oily substance that softens and lubricates the hair and skin, prevents the hair from becoming brittle, and decreases water loss from the skin when the external humidity is low. Because fat is a poor conductor of heat, sebum lessens the amount of heat lost from the skin. Sebum also has a **bactericidal** (bacteria-killing) action.
4. It transmits sensations through nerve receptors, which are sensitive to pain, temperature, touch, and pressure.
5. It produces and absorbs vitamin D in conjunction with ultraviolet rays from the sun, which activate a vitamin D precursor present in the skin.

The normal skin of a healthy person has transient and resident microorganisms that are not usually harmful. See Table 32.1 (page 878) for some common resident organisms.

Sudoriferous (sweat) glands are on all body surfaces, except the lips and parts of the genitals. The body has 2 to 5 million of these glands, which are all present at birth. They are most numerous on the palms of the hands and the soles of the feet. Sweat glands are classified as apocrine and eccrine. The **apocrine glands**, located largely in the axillae and anogenital areas, begin to function at puberty under the influence of androgens. Although their secretion is produced almost constantly, apocrine glands are of little use in thermoregulation. The secretion of these glands is odourless, but when decomposed or acted on by bacteria on the skin, it takes on a musky, unpleasant odour. The **eccrine glands** are important physiologically. They are more numerous than the apocrine glands and are found chiefly on the palms of the hands, the soles of the feet, and the forehead. The sweat they produce cools the body through evaporation. Sweat is made up of water, sodium, potassium, chloride, glucose, urea, and lactate.

Assessing

Assessment of the client's ability to engage in self-care activities includes a nursing history to determine the client's usual hygiene practices and self-care abilities, and the existence of any problems or potential problems associated with the skin, oral cavity, hair, nails, and other structures requiring hygiene. Important considerations include the client's balance, ability to sit unsupported, activity tolerance, coordination, strength, range of motion, and vision and hearing. Difficulties the client may encounter in performing activities related to

TABLE 29.1 Determinants of Health Influencing Individual Hygiene Practices

Determinant of Health	Influence on Hygiene Practices
Culture	Body odour is offensive in some cultures and not in others. Culture affects health-related choices and strongly influences choices regarding frequency and type of bathing, privacy during personal hygiene, and acceptability of body odour. Certain foods, such as garlic and spicy foods typically consumed in some cultures, also contribute to noticeable body odour.
Religion	Ceremonial washing is practised in some religions.
Income and Social Status	Finances can affect the availability of resources for maintaining hygiene practices. This may include the client's inability to purchase cleansing products, such as soap and shampoo. Some individuals may also lack privacy in which to bathe, if privacy is a cultural norm.
Physical Environment	The availability of facilities may be limited (e.g., to homeless clients) and access to devices (e.g., tub, chairs, and lifts) to ensure safety may be limited.
Developmental Level	Hygiene needs depend on age and stage of development. Particular considerations need to be given to infants and older adults (see the Lifespan Considerations box on bathing).
Personal Health Practices	Individual preferences regarding when and how to perform personal hygiene give the nurse an opportunity to individualize care. However, particular considerations should be given to individuals who are unable to completely meet their own needs for hygiene because of illness. Compromised physical or emotional health (e.g., in neuromuscular diseases) may lead to lack of motivation or energy to engage in personal hygiene practices. Individual preferences regarding evening or morning tub bath, showers, or other must be considered. Choice of products, preferred activities (e.g., washing hair, trimming nails, dental and oral hygiene) are individual.

Lifespan Considerations

Bathing

NEWBORNS

Newborns do not need to be bathed daily, and they do not need tub baths. Sponge baths are recommended. The diaper area is cleansed with each diaper change and any milk that remains on the face or in neck creases can be wiped away by using water and a mild soap.

After the bath, the infant should be immediately dried and wrapped. Parents need to be advised that the infant's ability to regulate body temperature is not fully developed so babies tend to cool more quickly than older children and adults. Furthermore, the body surface area is large compared to body mass, so the infant's body loses heat readily if the baby is exposed for any length of time. The use of lotions, baby oil, and powders is not recommended because they can cause skin irritation and rashes (Scott Ricci, 2007).

OLDER ADULTS

As an activity of daily living (ADL), bathing has cultural, social, and epidemiological implications. However, because of a possible range of disabilities affecting the ability of the older adult to meet the need for hygiene, the hygienic and therapeutic aspects of hygiene can be compromised. In a recent study of bathing disabilities, Naik, Concato, and Gill (2004) reported a range of concerns. These varied from inability to adjust water temperature and flow to "complete dependence with transferring to and from the bathing position" (p. 1808). The combination of postures, grips, and actions required to accomplish the tasks of bathing are complex and challenging for some individuals. Compromised balance, which occurs in virtually all people over the age of 80 years, further affects the ability to complete ADLs. Additional factors, such as arthritis, fatigue, weakness, effects of stroke (brain attack), dyspnea, and generalized lack of wellness, compromise the older person's ability further. The challenge for the nurse is to complete a comprehensive assessment not only of the individual client but also of the facilities available in the home.

Naik and Gill (2005) reported that the environment can be modified to promote the safety and well-being of older clients during personal hygiene. Common devices include the use of nonskid mats and abrasive bathtub strips, tub or shower seats (see Figure 29.1), and hand bars (see Figure 29.2). Nurses in home care settings must thoroughly assess the environment and the capability of older adult clients and implement strategies to further promote their safety while meeting their personal hygiene needs.

In addition to environmental and health concerns, the normal growth and development of older adults involves changes to the resiliency, texture, and sensitivity of their skin (Ebersole, Hess, Touhy, & Jett, 2005). Important considerations are presented in Table 29.2.

hygiene include the inability to wash any or all of the body, to obtain or get to a source of water, to regulate the temperature or flow of the water, to unfasten or remove clothing, and to get dressed again following bathing. Clients who have difficulty with elimination may also have difficulties associated with removing or unfastening clothing to access the toilet or commode.

Assessment data about the client's skin care practices enable the nurse to incorporate the client's preferences into an overall plan of care designed to meet the need for hygiene. Clients whose cognitive function is impaired or whose illness alters energy levels and motivation will require assistance. It is important for the nurse to determine the client's functional level to maintain and promote as much client independence as possible and as safely as

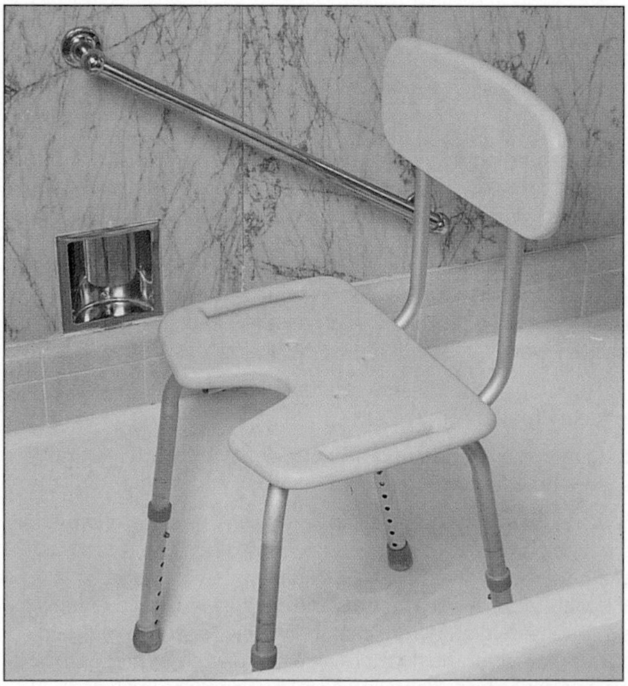

FIGURE 29.1 Tub or shower seat

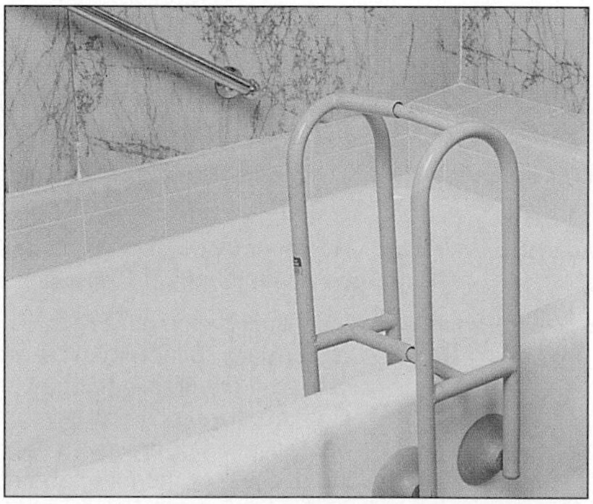

FIGURE 29.2 Hand bars on the side of a bathtub

TABLE 29.2 Developmental Consideration: Assessment of Skin in Older Adults

Skin Alterations Due to Aging	Implications for the Older Adult
Subcutaneous and dermal tissue become thin	Increased risk of skin tears, less capacity to insulate
Decreased activity of sebaceous and sweat glands	Decreased perspiration, dryer skin, and increased incidence of pruritus
Decreased vascularity to the skin	Skin temperature is cooler, and pallor may be apparent
Loss of subcutaneous tissue	Skin tends to wrinkle and sag
Decreased rate of nail growth	Nails become softer and may tear more easily
Melanocytes (cells that make the pigment that colours hair and skin) decrease in number	Hair turns grey, pigmented spots on the skin become more apparent

Source: Adapted from *Health Assessment in Nursing* (pp. 145, 147, 149, 150), by L. Sims, D. D'Amico, L. Stiesmeyer, and I. Webster, 1995), Redwood City, CA: Addison Wesley Nursing.

possible. When working with clients who have skin conditions, the nurse must attend to the client's self-concept (see Chapter 44). Some skin conditions present clients with physical challenges and concerns, and they may experience psychological and social ramifications as well.

Questions to elicit data about hygiene practices are shown in the Assessment: Interview box.

The *presence of past, current, or potential skin problems* alerts the nurse to specific nursing interventions or referrals the client may require. The client may provide descriptions of these problems during the nursing history, or the nurse may observe deviations from normal during the physical examination. Common skin problems and implications for nursing interventions are summarized in Table 29.3.

ASSESSMENT IN THE COMMUNITY OR HOME CARE SETTING To meet the hygiene needs of clients living in the community, the nurse must consider the client's environment, the family or caregiver, and the community. See the Assessment: Home Care box on hygiene.

Diagnosing

Nursing diagnoses that are generally considered applicable to hygiene include *Self-Care Deficit* and possibly *Deficient Knowledge. Self-Care Deficit* is defined as "impaired ability to perform or complete bathing/hygiene activities for oneself" (NANDA International, 2007, p. 183). Factors related to *Self-Care Deficit* include weakness, fatigue, neuromuscular and musculoskeletal problems, environmental barriers, perceptual or cognitive impairment, pain, inability to perceive body parts, inability to transfer or mobilize effectively and safely, and emotional states, such as severe anxiety (see Boxes 29.1 and 29.2). The diagnoses *Risk for Impaired Skin Integrity* and *Impaired Skin Integrity* are discussed in Chapter 33.

ASSESSMENT: INTERVIEW

Data Collection for Hygiene Practices

The following questions can help the nurse learn about the client's hygiene practices:

SKIN CARE PRACTICES

- What is your usual time to shower or bathe?
- What products, such as soap, shampoo, deodorant, do you prefer to use?
- What products do you prefer to use on your face?
- How frequently do you clean or discard applicators or puffs that you use on your face?
- Are there any products or practices that you avoid because of how they affect your skin?

SELF-CARE ABILITIES

- Do you have any problems managing your own hygiene?
- What assistance can the nurse give you to help you meet your need for hygiene?

SKIN PROBLEMS

- Do you have any tendency toward dry skin, acne, itchiness, rashes, bruising, excessive perspiration, or lack of perspiration?
- Do you have any allergies? If so, to what?

TABLE 29.3 Common Problems Affecting the Skin

Problem and Appearance	Nursing Implications
Abrasion Superficial layers of the skin are scraped or rubbed away. Area is reddened and may have localized bleeding or serous weeping.	1. Prone to infection; therefore, wound should be kept clean and dry. 2. Do not wear rings or jewellery when providing care to avoid causing abrasions to clients. 3. Lift, do not pull, a client across a bed. See Chapter 38.
Excessive Dryness Skin can appear flaky and rough.	1. Prone to infection if the skin cracks; therefore, provide alcohol-free lotions to moisturize the skin and prevent cracking. 2. Bathe client less frequently; do not use soap, or limit use of nonirritating soap. Rinse skin thoroughly because soap can be irritating and drying. 3. Encourage increased fluid intake, if health permits, to prevent dehydration.
Ammonia Dermatitis (Diaper Rash) Caused by skin bacteria reacting with urea in the urine. The skin becomes reddened and sore.	1. Keep skin dry and clean by applying protective ointments containing zinc oxide to areas at risk (e.g., buttocks and perineum). 2. Boil an infant's diapers or wash them with an antibacterial detergent to prevent infection. Rinse diapers well because detergent is irritating to an infant's skin.
Acne Inflammatory condition with papules and pustules.	1. Keep the skin clean to prevent secondary infection. 2. Treatment varies widely so integrate prescribed or recommended approaches into care.
Erythema Redness associated with a variety of conditions, such as rashes, exposure to sun, elevated body temperature.	1. Wash area carefully to remove excess microorganisms. 2. Apply antiseptic spray or lotion to prevent itching, promote healing, and prevent skin breakdown.
Hirsutism Excessive hair on a person's body and face, particularly in women.	1. Remove unwanted hair by using depilatories, shaving, electrolysis, or tweezing. 2. Enhance client's self-concept. See Chapter 44.

ASSESSMENT: HOME CARE

Hygiene

Nurses need to consider all the following elements in meeting the hygiene needs of clients living in the community:

CLIENT AND ENVIRONMENT

- *Self-care abilities for hygiene:* Assess the client's ability to bathe, to manipulate water taps, to dress and undress, to groom, and to use the toilet.
- *Self-care aids required:* Determine whether the client needs a shower seat (Figure 29.3), a hand shower, a nonskid surface or mat in the tub or shower, hand bars on the sides of the tub, or a raised toilet seat.
- *Facilities:* Check for the presence of laundry facilities and running water.
- *Mechanical barriers:* Note furniture that obstructs access to the bathroom and toilet, or a doorway too narrow for a wheelchair.

FAMILY

- *Caregiver availability, skills, and responses:* Determine whether individuals are available and able to assist with bathing, dressing, toileting, nail care, shampooing, shopping for hygienic or grooming aids, and so on.
- *Education needs:* Assess whether the caregiver needs instructions in how to assist the client in and out of the tub, on and off the toilet, and so on.
- *Family role changes and coping:* Assess the effects of client's illness on financial status, parenting, spousal roles, sexuality, and social roles.

COMMUNITY

- Explore resources that will provide assistance with bathing, laundry, and foot care (e.g., home health aid, podiatrist).
- Consult a social worker or a home care nurse as needed to coordinate placement of a client unable to remain in the home or to identify community resources that will help the client stay in the home.
- Consider consulting with (1) a physical therapist to assess, develop, and improve the client's motor function, (2) a home care nurse to provide follow-up for care, teaching, and support, and (3) an occupational therapist to assess and develop the client's abilities to perform activities of daily living.

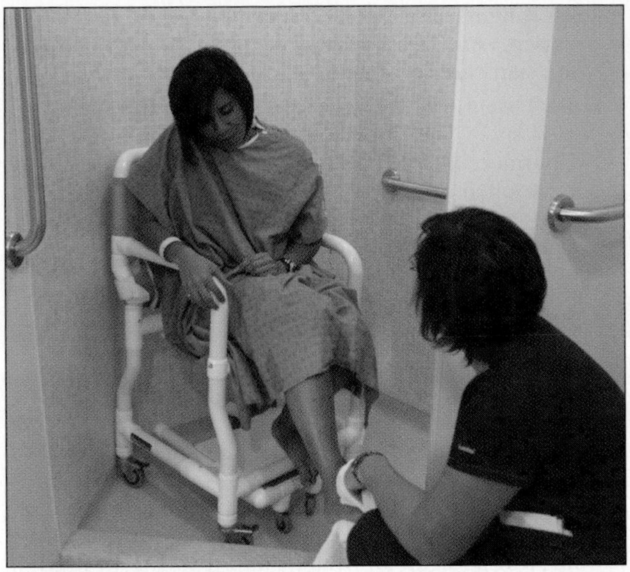

FIGURE 29.3 Using a tub or shower seat

Planning

Planning activities can include assisting dependent clients with bathing, skin care, and perineal care, providing back massages to promote circulation, and instructing clients about appropriate hygiene practices and therapies to prevent skin lesions. Consider the client's personal preferences, health, and limitations (Evans-Smith, 2005); the best time to give the care; and the equipment, facilities, and personnel available. A

BOX 29.2 ETIOLOGIES OF SELF-CARE DEFICITS

Deficits in self-care can have different causes:

- Visual impairment
- Activity intolerance or weakness
- Pain or discomfort
- Mental impairment
- Neuromuscular or skeletal impairment
- Psychological or motivational impairment
- Medically prescribed restriction
- Therapeutic procedure restraining mobility (e.g., intravenous infusion, cast)
- Environmental barriers

REFLECT ON PRIMARY HEALTH CARE

Nurses engage in health-promotion activities to fulfill clients' basic needs for cleanliness and comfort and to prevent infections. They seek opportunities to assess, diagnose, plan, implement, and evaluate clients' hygiene needs, such as bathing, nails, hair, and skin care. As well, they work with interdisciplinary teams to coordinate the type and level of hygiene care to be provided to clients in both home and hospital settings. Consider how you can engage in health promotion and intersectional collaboration activities in your nursing care planning process.

BOX 29.1 PRACTICE APPLICATION: ASSESSMENT DATA CLUSTERS AND RELATED NURSING DIAGNOSES FOR CLIENTS WITH SKIN PROBLEMS

	Nursing Diagnosis	Associated Diagnoses
Case Situation 1 Jayashekar Singh, 75 years old, suffered a stroke 2 weeks ago that resulted in paralysis of his left side. He states, "I don't want a bath. I can wash myself. I just want to be left alone." He is withdrawn and uncommunicative.	*Self-Care Deficit:* Bathing/Hygiene related to paralyzed left upper and lower limbs and lack of motivation	*Deficient Knowledge* related to • Lack of experience in providing hygiene care to dependent persons • Unfamiliarity with devices available to facilitate sitting on or rising from toilet • Self-Esteem, Situational Low related to body odours
Case Situation 2 Brian Yellowbird, a 15-year-old, has facial pustules and papules. Facial skin is inflamed. He states, "I hate going to school or anywhere looking like this. I don't think any girl wants to go out with me. Can you do something to get rid of this?"	*Self-Esteem Disturbance* related to facial pustules and papules	*Deficient Knowledge* related to • Lack of experience with skin condition (acne) and need to prevent secondary infection • New therapeutic regimen to manage skin problems • Self-Esteem, Situational Low related to visible skin problem, acne

client's personal preferences—about when and how to bathe, for example—should be followed as long as they are compatible with the client's health and the equipment available. Nurses need to provide whatever assistance the client requires, either directly or by delegating this task to other nursing personnel.

PLANNING FOR HOME CARE To provide for continuity of care, the nurse must assess the client's and family's abilities for care (see the Reflect on Primary Health Care box on the previous page) and the need for referrals and home health services. In addition, the nurse needs to determine the client's learning needs.

Implementing

Nursing interventions discussed in this chapter focus on hygiene measures; the etiology of the nursing diagnoses established may point to other interventions that promote circulation, promote self-esteem, restore nutritional status, correct fluid deficits or excesses, or prevent problems associated with immobility. Nursing strategies that deal with these etiologies are provided in other chapters.

The classes of interventions according to the Nursing Interventions Classification (NIC) include interventions to promote comfort, to provide or assist with activities of daily living, to maintain or restore tissue integrity, and to optimize circulation to the tissue (Bulechek, Butcher, & Dochterman, 2008).

GENERAL PRINCIPLES OF SKIN CARE

1. *An intact, healthy skin is the body's first line of defence.* Nurses need to ensure that all skin care measures prevent injury and irritation. Scratching the skin with jewellery or long or sharp fingernails must be avoided. Harsh rubbing or use of rough towels and washcloths can cause tissue damage, particularly when the skin is irritated or when circulation or sensation is diminished. Bottom bed sheets are kept taut and free from wrinkles to reduce friction and abrasion to the skin. Top bed linens are arranged to prevent undue pressure on the toes. When necessary, bed cradles or footboards are used to keep bedclothes off the feet.
2. *The degree to which the skin protects the underlying tissues from injury depends on the general health of the cells, the amount of subcutaneous tissue, and the dryness of the skin.* Skin that is poorly nourished and dry is less easily protected and more vulnerable to injury. When the skin is dry, lotions or creams with lanolin can be applied, and bathing is limited to once or twice a week.
3. *Moisture in contact with the skin for more than a short time can result in increased bacterial growth and irritation.* After a bath, the client's skin is dried carefully. Particular attention is paid to such areas as the axillae, the groin, beneath the breasts, and between the toes, where the potential for irritation is greatest. Clients who are incontinent of urine or feces or who perspire excessively are provided with immediate skin care to prevent skin irritation.
4. *Body odours are caused by skin bacteria acting on body secretions.* Cleanliness is the best deodorant. Commercial deodorants and antiperspirants should be applied only after the skin is cleaned. Deodorants diminish odours, whereas antiperspirants reduce the amount of perspiration. Neither is applied immediately after shaving because of the possibility of skin irritation, and they are not used on skin that is already irritated.
5. *Skin sensitivity to irritation and injury varies among individuals and in accordance with their health.* Skin sensitivity is generally greater in infants, very young children, and older people. A person's nutritional status also affects sensitivity. Emaciated or obese persons tend to experience more skin irritation and injury. The same tendency is seen in individuals with poor dietary habits and insufficient fluid intake. Even in healthy persons, skin sensitivity is highly variable. Some people's skin is sensitive to the chemicals in skin care agents and cosmetics. Hypoallergenic cosmetics and soaps or soap substitutes are available. The nurse needs to ascertain whether the client has any sensitivities and what agents are appropriate to use.
6. *Agents used for skin care have selective actions and purposes.* Commonly used agents are described in Table 29.4.

BATHING Bathing removes accumulated oil, perspiration, dead skin cells, and some bacteria. The nurse can appreciate the quantity of oil and dead skin cells produced when observing a person after the removal of a cast that has been on for 6 weeks. The skin is crusty, flaky, and dry underneath the cast. Applications of oil over several days are usually necessary to remove the debris.

Excessive bathing, however, can interfere with the intended lubricating effect of the sebum, causing dryness of the skin. This is an important consideration, especially for older adults, who produce less sebum.

In addition to cleaning the skin, bathing also stimulates circulation. A warm bath dilates superficial arterioles, bringing more blood and nourishment to the skin. Massaging the skin has the same effect. Rubbing with long smooth strokes from the distal to proximal parts of extremities (from the point farthest from the body to the point closest) is particularly effective in facilitating venous blood flow.

Bathing also produces a sense of well-being. It is refreshing and relaxing and frequently improves morale, appearance, and self-respect. Some people take a morning shower for its refreshing, stimulating effect. Others prefer an evening bath because it is relaxing. These effects are more evident when a person is ill. For example, it is not uncommon for clients who have had a restless or sleepless night to feel relaxed, comfortable, and sleepy after a morning bath.

TABLE 29.4 Agents Commonly Used on the Skin

Type	Description
Soap	Lowers surface tension and, thus, helps in cleaning. Some soaps contain antibacterial agents that can change the natural flora of the skin.
Detergent	Used instead of soap for cleaning. Some people who are allergic to soaps may not be allergic to detergents and vice versa. Do not use on older adult clients.
Bath oil	Used in bathwater; provides an oily film on the skin that softens and prevents chapping. Oils can make the tub surface slippery, and clients should be instructed about safety measures (e.g., using nonskid tub surface or mat).
Skin cream/lotion	Provides a film on the skin that prevents evaporation and, therefore, chapping.
Powder	Although not generally recommended because of a risk of clumping of the product, powder can be used to absorb water and prevent friction. For example, powder under the breasts can prevent skin irritation. Some powders are antibacterial.
Deodorant	Masks or diminishes body odours.
Antiperspirant	Reduces the amount of perspiration.

Bathing offers an excellent opportunity for the nurse to assess ill clients. The nurse can observe for such conditions as edema or rashes. While assisting a client with a bath, the nurse can also assess the client's psychosocial needs, such as orientation to time and ability to cope with the illness. Learning needs, such as a diabetic client's need to learn foot care, can also be assessed.

Caution is needed when bathing clients who are receiving intravenous therapy. Easy-to-remove gowns that have Velcro or snap fasteners along the sleeves may be used. If a special gown is not available, the nurse needs to pay particular attention when changing the client's gown after the bath or whenever the gown becomes soiled. General guidelines are provided in Box 29.3. These guidelines do not apply if the client has an IV pump. In this situation, use a special gown or do not put the sleeve of the gown over the client's involved arm.

BOX 29.3 CHANGING A HOSPITAL GOWN FOR A CLIENT WITH AN INTRAVENOUS INFUSION WITHOUT A PUMP

Changing a gown for a client receiving intravenous therapy requires special attention:

- Slip the gown completely off the arm without the infusion and onto the tubing connected to the arm with the infusion.
- Holding the container above the client's arm, slide the sleeve up over the container to remove the used gown.
- Place the clean gown sleeve for the arm with the infusion over the container as if it were an extension of the client's arm, from the inside of the gown to the sleeve cuff.
- Re-hang the container. Slide the gown carefully over the tubing toward the client's hand.
- Guide the client's arm and tubing into the sleeve, taking care not to pull on the tubing or IV site.
- Assist the client to put the other arm into the second sleeve of the gown, and fasten as usual.
- Count the rate of flow of the infusion to make sure it is correct before leaving the bedside.

CATEGORIES OF BATHS Two categories of baths are given to clients: cleansing and therapeutic. **Cleansing baths** are given chiefly for hygiene purposes and include the following:

- *Complete bed bath.* The nurse washes the entire body of an individual who needs total assistance.
- *Self-help bed bath.* Clients confined to bed are able to bathe themselves with assistance from the nurse for washing the back and perhaps the feet.
- *Partial bath.* Only the parts of the client's body that might cause discomfort or odour are washed: the face, hands, axillae, perineal area, and back. The arms, chest, abdomen, legs, and feet are omitted. The nurse provides this bath for clients who need total assistance, and assists self-sufficient clients confined to bed by washing their backs. Some ambulatory clients prefer to take a partial bath at the sink with the nurse assisting as needed, particularly with their backs.
- *Bag bath.* The bag bath is a packaged disposable bathing system that contains 8 to 12 no-rinse cleansing washcloths with emollients and moisturizers to protect the skin. The solution and washcloths are warmed in a microwave. The warming time is about 1 minute, but to ensure the safety of the client, the nurse needs to determine how long it takes to attain a desirable temperature. Each area of the body is cleaned with a different cloth and then air dried. Bag baths save time and are easy to perform.
- *Disposable bed bath.* For very ill or debilitated clients, disposable bed baths have been reported to save time and be comfortable for clients (Larson et al., 2004). The costs for individual disposable baths are

higher than traditional baths, but costs are offset through the use of fewer products because of the no-rinse cleansers.

- *Tub bath*. Tub baths are preferred to bed baths because it is easier to wash and rinse the entire body in a tub. Tubs are also used for therapeutic baths. The amount of assistance the nurse offers depends on the abilities of the client. Specially designed tubs are available for those needing total assistance. These tubs greatly reduce the work of the nurse in lifting clients in and out of the tub and offer greater benefits than a sponge bath in bed. See Figures 29.4 and 29.5 for using a bath lift to assist the client into a raised tub.
- *Shower.* Many ambulatory clients are able to use shower facilities and require only minimal assistance from the nurse.

The water for a bath should feel comfortably warm to the client. People vary in their sensitivity to heat; generally, the temperature should be 43°C to 46°C. Most clients will verify a suitable temperature. The water for a bed bath should be changed when cleansing from a dirtier to a cleaner area, or when bath water becomes dirty or cool. Bath water becomes contaminated with skin flora during bathing and can become a reservoir for recontamination or for moving bacteria from one part of the client's body to another (Larson et al., 2004).

Therapeutic baths are given for physical effects, such as to soothe irritated skin or to treat a specific area, such as the perineum. Medications can be placed in the water. A therapeutic bath is generally taken in a tub one-third or one-half full. The client remains in the bath for a designated time, often 20 to 30 minutes. If the client's back, chest, and arms are to be treated, these areas need to be immersed in the solution. The bath temperature is generally included in the order; 37.7°C to 46°C may be ordered for adults and 40.5°C is usually ordered for infants.

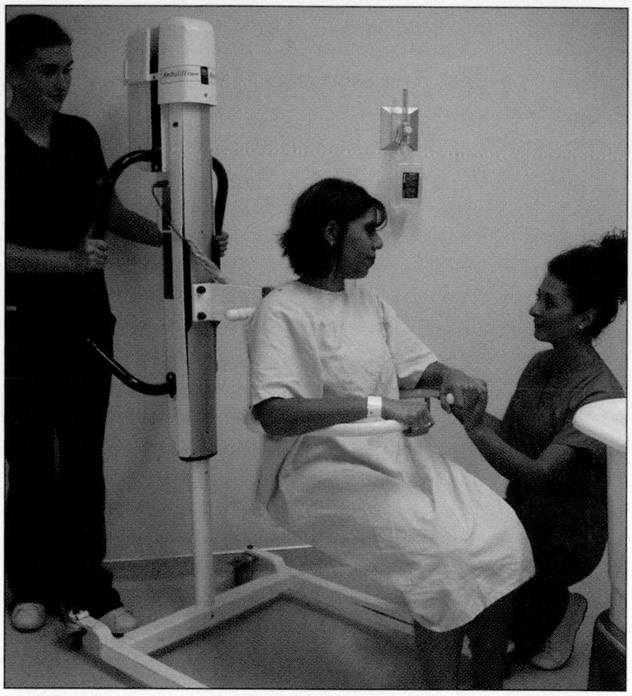

FIGURE 29.4 Using a bath lift

Before bathing a client, determine (1) the type of bath needed and what assistance is required (Evans-Smith, 2005); (2) other care the client is receiving, such as X-rays or physiotherapy, so that the bath can be coordinated with those activities to prevent undue fatigue; and (3) the bed linen required. The caregiver should wear gloves when body fluids or open lesions are present. Skill 29.1 provides guidelines for bathing an adult or a pediatric client.

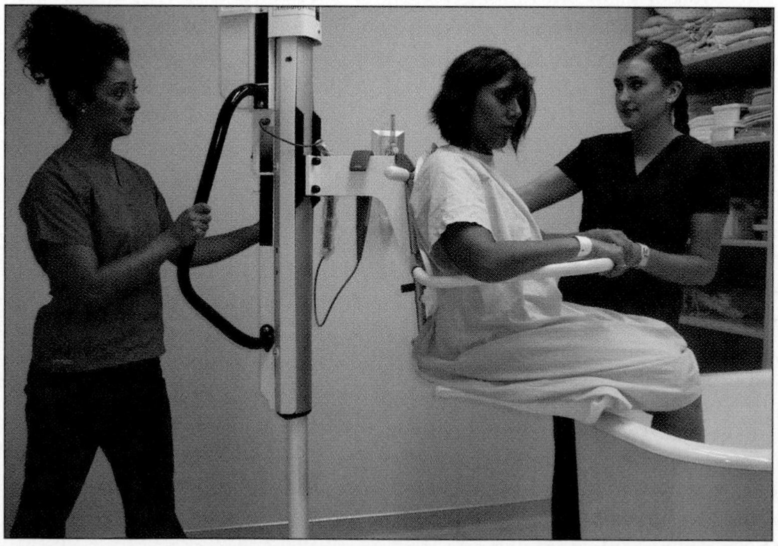

FIGURE 29.5 Using a bath lift to assist the client into a raised tub

SKILL 29.1

BATHING AN ADULT OR A PEDIATRIC CLIENT

PURPOSES

- To remove transient microorganisms, body secretions and excretions, and dead skin cells
- To stimulate circulation to the skin
- To promote a sense of well-being
- To produce relaxation and comfort
- To prevent and eliminate unpleasant body odours

ASSESSMENT

Assess

- Condition of the skin (colour, texture, and turgor; presence of pigmented spots; temperature; lesions; excoriations, abrasions, and bruises)
- Physical or emotional factors (e.g., fatigue, sensitivity to cold, need for control, anxiety or fear)
- Presence of pain and need for adjunctive measures (e.g., an analgesic) before the bath
- Range of motion of the joints
- Any other aspect of health that may affect the client's bathing process (e.g., mobility, strength, cognition)
- Need for use of clean gloves during the bath

Equipment

- Basin or sink with warm water (between 43°C and 46°C)
- Soap and soap dish
- Linens: bath blanket, two bath towels, washcloth, clean gown or pyjamas or clothes as needed, additional bed linen and towels, if required
- Gloves, if appropriate (e.g., presence of body fluids or open lesions)
- Personal hygiene articles (e.g., deodorant, powder, lotions)
- Shaving equipment
- Table for bathing equipment
- Laundry hamper

IMPLEMENTATION

Preparation

Before bathing a client, determine (1) the purpose and type of bath the client needs; (2) the self-care ability of the client; (3) any movement or positioning precautions specific to the client; (4) other care the client may be receiving, such as physical therapy or X-rays, in order to coordinate all aspects of health care and prevent unnecessary fatigue; (5) the client's comfort level with being bathed by someone else; and (6) the necessary bath equipment and linens.

Performance

1. Before performing the procedure, introduce yourself and verify the client's identity by using agency protocol. Explain to the client what you are going to do, why it is necessary, and how he or she can cooperate. Discuss with the client the plan for bathing and explain any unfamiliar procedures to the client.
2. Perform hand hygiene and observe other appropriate infection prevention and control procedures.
3. Provide for client privacy by drawing the curtains around the bed or closing the door to the room. Some agencies provide signs indicating the need for privacy. **Rationale: Hygiene is a personal matter.**
4. Prepare the client and the environment.
   - Invite a family member or significant other to participate if the client prefers it.
   - Close windows and doors to ensure the room is a comfortable temperature. **Rationale: Air currents increase loss of heat from the body by convection.**
   - Offer the client a bedpan or urinal or ask whether the client wants to use the toilet or commode. **Rationale: Warm water and activity can stimulate the need to void. The client will be more comfortable after voiding, and voiding before cleaning the perineum is advisable.**
   - Encourage the client to perform as much personal self-care as possible. **Rationale: This promotes independence, exercise, and self-esteem.**
   - During the bath, assess each area of the skin carefully.

For a Bed Bath

5. Prepare the bed and position the client appropriately.
   - Position the bed at a comfortable working height. Lower the side rail on the side closest to you. Keep the other side rail *up*. Help the client to move near you. **Rationale: This avoids undue reaching and straining and promotes good body mechanics.**
   - Place a bath blanket over the top sheet. Remove the top sheet from under the bath blanket by starting at the client's shoulders and moving the linen down toward the client's feet (see ❶). Ask the client to grasp and hold the top of the bath blanket while you pull the linen to the foot of the bed.

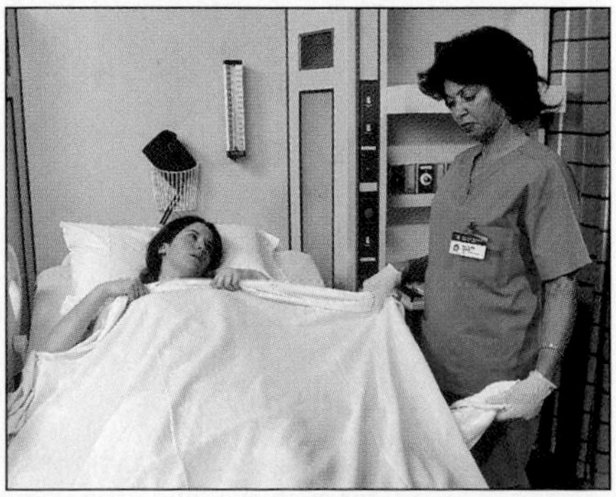

❶ Remove the top sheet from under the bath blanket.

(continued)

SKILL 29.1

BATHING AN ADULT OR A PEDIATRIC CLIENT (*continued*)

Rationale: The bath blanket provides comfort, warmth, and privacy. *Note:* If the bed linen is to be reused, place it over the bedside chair. If it is to be changed, place it in the linen hamper, not on the floor.

- Remove client's gown while keeping the client covered with the bath blanket. Place the gown in the linen hamper. If a client has an intravenous infusion, follow the procedures in Box 29.3 (page 711) regarding changing the hospital gown.

6. Make a bath mitt with the washcloth. **Rationale: A bath mitt retains water and heat better than a cloth loosely held and prevents the ends of the washcloth from dragging across the skin.** See ❷ for the triangular method and ❸ for the rectangular method.
7. Wash the face. **Rationale: Begin the bath at the cleanest area and work downward toward the feet.**
   - Place the towel under the client's head.
   - Wash the client's eyes with water only and dry them well. Use a separate corner of the washcloth for each eye. **Rationale: The use of separate corners prevents the transmission of microorganisms from one eye to the other.** Wipe from the inner to the outer canthus (see ❹). **Rationale: This prevents secretions from entering the nasolacrimal ducts.**

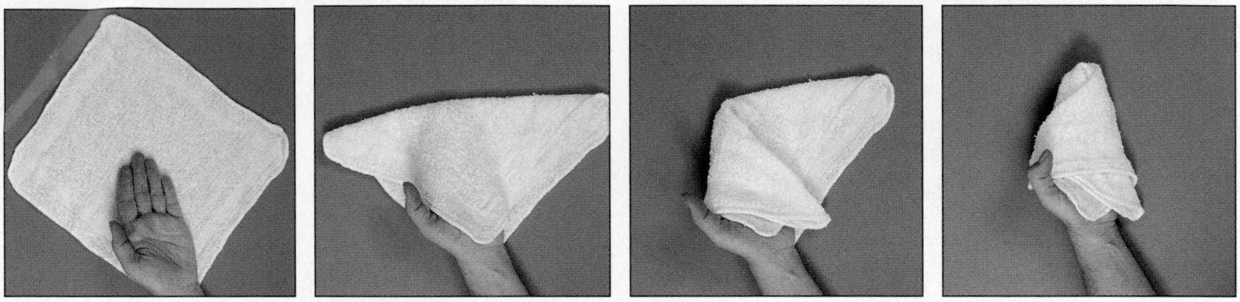

A B C D

❷ Making a bath mitt, triangular method. **A:** Lay the back of your hand on the washcloth; **B:** fold the top corner over your hand; **C:** fold the side corners over your hand; **D:** tuck the second corner under the cloth on the palm side to secure the mitt.

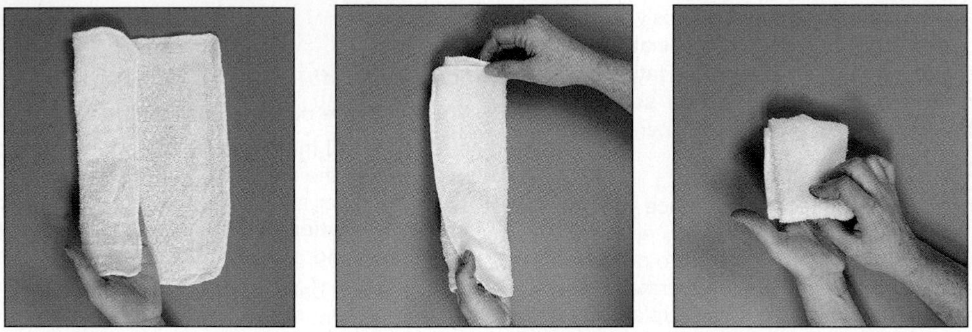

A B C

❸ Making a bath mitt, rectangular method. **A:** Lay the back of your hand on the washcloth and fold one side over your hand; **B:** fold the second side over your hand; **C:** fold the top of the cloth down and tuck it under the folded side against your palm to secure the mitt.

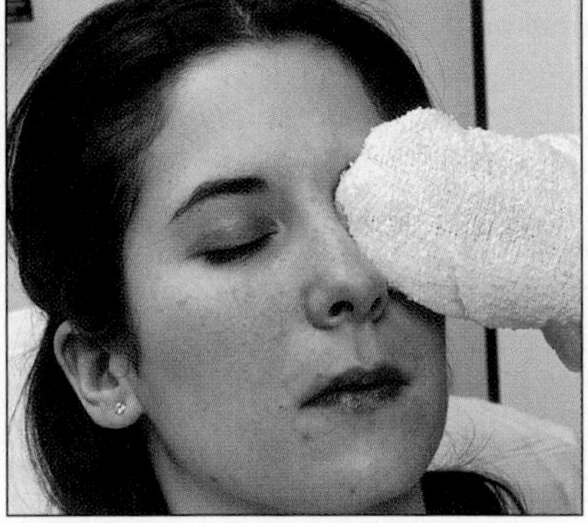

❹ Use a separate corner of the washcloth for each eye, and wipe from the inner to the outer canthus.

(*continued*)

SKILL 29.1

BATHING AN ADULT OR A PEDIATRIC CLIENT (*continued*)

- Ask whether the client wants soap used on the face. **Rationale: Soap has a drying effect, and the face, which is exposed to the air more than other body parts, tends to be drier.**
- Wash, rinse, and dry the client's face, ears, and neck.
- Remove the towel from under the client's head.

8. Wash the arms and hands. Omit the arms for a partial bath.
   - Place a towel lengthwise under the arm away from you. **Rationale: It protects the bed from becoming wet.**
   - Wash, rinse, and dry the arm by elevating the client's arm and supporting the client's wrist and elbow (see ❺). Use long, firm strokes from wrist to shoulder, including the axillary area. **Rationale: Firm strokes from distal to proximal areas promote circulation by increasing venous blood return.**
   - Apply deodorant or powder if desired.
   - (Optional) Place a towel on the bed and put a wash-basin on it. Place the client's hands in the basin. **Rationale: Many clients enjoy immersing their hands in the basin and washing themselves. Soaking loosens dirt under the nails.** Assist the client as needed to wash, rinse, and dry the hands, paying particular attention to the spaces between the fingers.
   - Repeat for the hand and arm nearest you. Exercise caution if an intravenous infusion is present, and check its flow after moving the arm.
9. Wash the chest and abdomen. Omit the chest and abdomen for a partial bath. However, the areas under a woman's breast may require bathing if this area is irritated or if the client has significant perspiration under the breasts.
   - Place the bath towel lengthwise over the chest. Fold the bath blanket down to the client's pubic area. **Rationale: This keeps the client warm while preventing unnecessary exposure of the chest.**
   - Lift the bath towel off the chest, and bathe the chest and abdomen with your mitted hand by using long, firm strokes (see ❻). Give special attention to the skin under the breasts and any other skin folds, particularly if the client is overweight. Rinse and dry well.
   - Replace the bath blanket when the areas have been dried.
10. Wash the legs and feet. Omit legs and feet for a partial bath.
    - Expose the leg farthest from you by folding the bath blanket toward the other leg, being careful to keep the perineum covered. **Rationale: Covering the perineum promotes privacy and maintains the client's dignity.**
    - Lift the leg and place the bath towel lengthwise under the leg. Wash, rinse, and dry the leg by using long, smooth, firm strokes from the ankle to the knee to the thigh (see ❼). **Rationale: Washing from the distal to proximal areas promotes circulation by stimulating venous blood flow.**

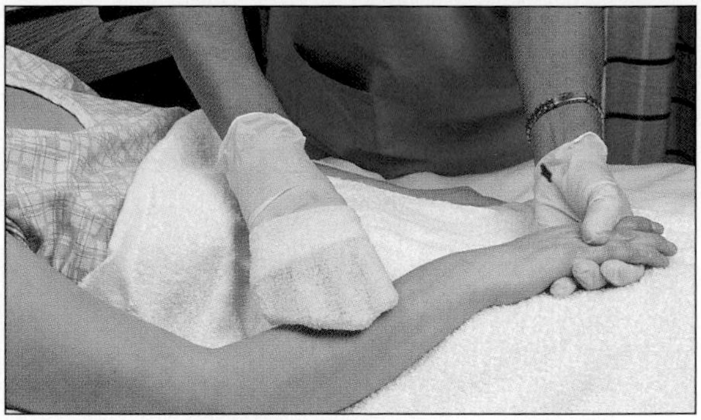

❺ Washing the far arm by using long, firm strokes from wrist to shoulder area

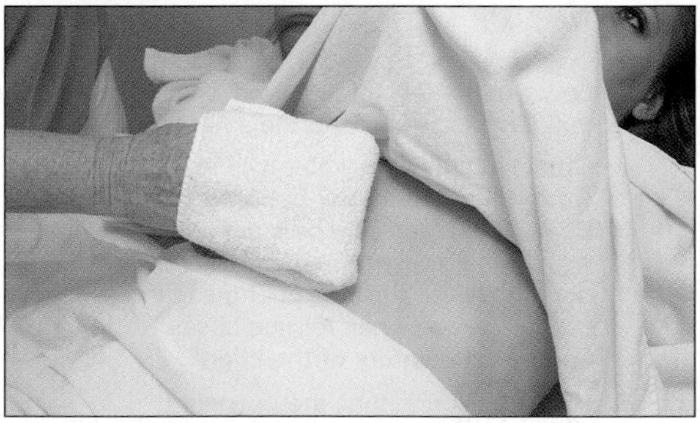

❻ Washing the chest and abdomen

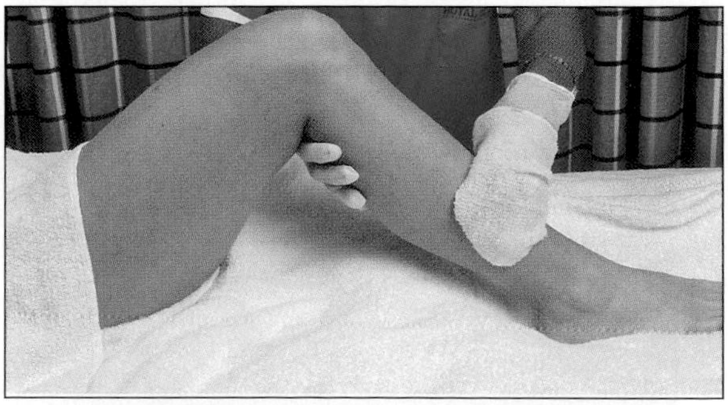

❼ Washing far leg

(*continued*)

SKILL 29.1

BATHING AN ADULT OR A PEDIATRIC CLIENT (*continued*)

- Reverse the coverings and repeat for the other leg.
- Wash the feet by placing them in the basin of water (see ❽).

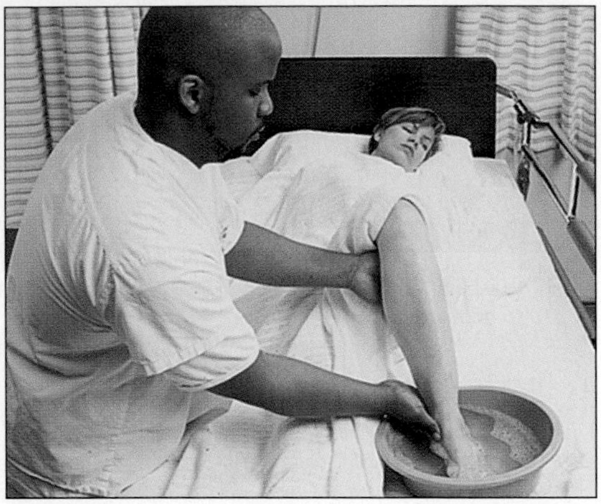

❽ Soaking a foot in a basin

- Dry each foot. Pay particular attention to the spaces between the toes. If preferred, wash one foot after that leg before washing the other leg.
- Obtain fresh, warm water whenever necessary. **Rationale: Water may become dirty or cold.** Because surface skin cells are removed with washing, the bathwater from dark-skinned clients may be dark, however, this does not mean the client is dirty. Lower the bed when refilling basin. **Rationale: This ensures the safety of the client.**

11. Wash the back and then the perineum.

- Assist the client into a prone or side-lying position facing away from you. Place the bath towel lengthwise alongside the back and buttocks while keeping the client covered with the bath blanket as much as possible. **Rationale: This provides warmth and prevents undue exposure.**
- Wash and dry the client's back, moving from the shoulders to the buttocks and upper thighs, paying attention to the gluteal folds (see ❾).

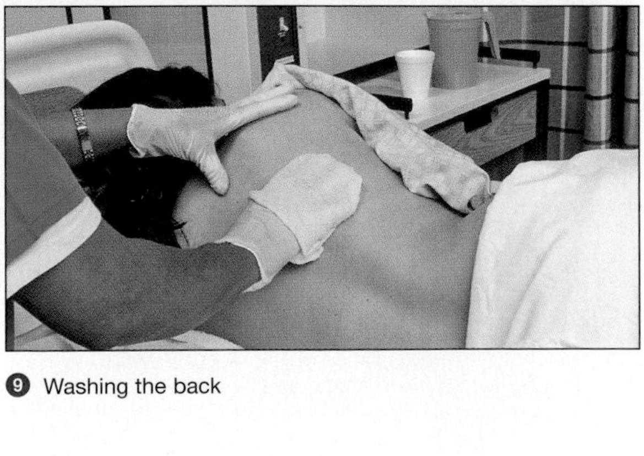

❾ Washing the back

- Perform a back massage now or after completion of the bath.
- Assist the client to the supine position and determine whether the client can wash the perineal area independently. If the client cannot do so, drape the client and wash the area.

12. Assist the client with grooming aids, such as powder, lotion, or deodorant.

- Use powder sparingly. Release as little as possible into the air. **Rationale: This will avoid irritation of the respiratory tract by powder inhalation. Excessive powder can cause caking, which leads to skin irritation.**
- Help the client put on a clean gown or pyjamas.
- Assist the client to care for hair, mouth, and nails. Some people prefer or need mouth care before their bath.

For a Tub Bath or Shower

13. Prepare the client and the tub.

- Fill the tub about one-third to one-half full of water at 43°C to 46°C. **Rationale: Sufficient water is needed to cover the perineal area.**
- Cover all intravenous catheters or wound dressings with plastic coverings, and instruct the client to prevent wetting these areas if possible.
- Put a rubber bath mat or towel on the floor of the tub if safety strips are not on the tub floor. **Rationale: These prevent slipping during the bath or shower.**

14. Assist the client into the shower or tub.

- Assist the client taking a standing shower with the initial adjustment of the water temperature and water flow pressure, as needed. Some clients need a chair to sit on in the shower because of weakness. Hot water can cause older adults to feel faint.
- If the client requires considerable assistance with a tub bath, a hydraulic bathtub chair may be required (see "Variation").
- Explain how the client can signal for help, leave the client for 2 to 5 minutes, and place an "occupied" sign on the door. For safety reasons, do not leave a client with decreased cognition or clients who may be at risk (e.g., history of seizures, syncope).

15. Assist the client with washing and then getting out of the tub.

- Wash the client's back, lower legs, and feet, if necessary.
- Assist the client out of the tub. If the client is unsteady, place a bath towel over the client's shoulders and drain the tub of water before the client attempts to get out of it. **Rationale: Draining the water first lessens the likelihood of a fall. The towel prevents chilling.**

(continued)

SKILL 29.1

BATHING AN ADULT OR A PEDIATRIC CLIENT (*continued*)

16. Dry the client, and assist with follow-up care.
- Follow step 12.
- Assist the client back to his or her bed.
- Clean the tub or shower in accordance with agency practice, discard the used linen in the laundry hamper, and place the "unoccupied" sign on the door.

17. Document the following:
- The type of bath given (i.e., complete, partial, or self-help); this is usually recorded on a flowsheet
- Skin assessment, such as excoriation, erythema, exudates, rashes, drainage, or skin breakdown
- Nursing interventions related to skin integrity
- The ability of the client to assist or cooperate with bathing
- The client's response to bathing
- Educational needs regarding hygiene
- Information or teaching shared with the client or the family

Variation: Bathing by Using a Hydraulic Bathtub Chair
A hydraulic lift, often used in long-term-care or rehabilitation settings, can facilitate the safe transfer of a client who is unable to ambulate to a tub. The lift also helps eliminate strain on the nurse's back.
- Bring the client to the tub room in a wheelchair or shower chair.
- Fill the tub and check the water temperature *to avoid thermal injury to the client.*
- Lower the hydraulic chair lift to its lowest point, outside the tub.
- Transfer the client to the chair lift and secure the seat belt (see ⑩).
- Raise the chair lift above the tub.
- Support the client's legs as the chair is moved over the tub *to avoid injury to the legs.*
- Position the client's legs down into the water and slowly lower the chair lift into the tub.
- Assist in bathing the client, if appropriate.
- Reverse the procedure when taking the client out of the tub.
- Dry the client and transport him or her to the room.

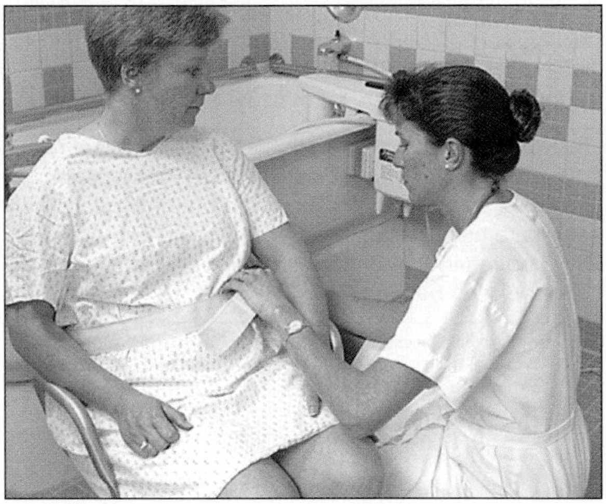

⑩ Secure the seat belt before moving the client in a hydraulic bathtub chair.

EVALUATION

- Note the client's tolerance of the procedure (e.g., respiratory rate and effort, pulse rate, behaviours of acceptance or resistance, statements regarding comfort).
- Conduct appropriate follow-up:
  - Condition and integrity of skin (dryness, turgor, redness, lesions, and so on)
  - Client's strength
  - Percentage of bath done without assistance
- Relate to prior assessment data, if appropriate.

TEACHING: HOME CARE

Hygiene

Suggest the client or family do the following:
- Consider purchasing a bath seat that fits in the tub or shower.
- Install a hand shower for use with a bath seat and shampooing.
- Use a nonskid surface on the tub or shower floor.
- Install hand bars on both sides of the tub or shower to facilitate transfers in and out of the tub or shower.
- Carefully monitor the temperature of the bathwater.
- Apply lotion *after* the client is out of the tub or shower since lotions may make the tub surface or shower floor slippery.

Evidence-Informed Practice

Does Bath Grab Bar Placement Matter for Older Adults?

Bathroom falls are a significant health hazard among older adults. Sveistrup, Lockett, Edwards, and Aminzedeh's (2006) Canadian study involved 103 community-living older adults responding to questions related to their current bathing practices, fall history, sociodemographic characteristics, balance measures, and details about the home bathing environment in relation to the bath tub grab bar configurations. They were then videotaped using the configurations when entering and exiting the tub. The participants' profile did not relate to the configurations or patterns of grab bar use. The likelihood of using the grab bar was determined by the safety, comfort, and ease of use.

NURSING IMPLICATIONS: Nurses have a critical role to play in health promotion. Assessment of bathroom facilities and education about the optimum placement and safe use of assistive devices could contribute to a reduction in the number and severity of falls that occur during bathing

Source: Based on "Evaluation of Bath Grab Bar Placement for Older Adults," by H. Sveistrup, D. Lockett, N. Edwards, and F. Aminzedeh, 2006, *Technology and Disability, 18*(2), pp. 45–55.

PERINEAL-GENITAL CARE Perineal-genital care is also called *perineal care* or *peri-care.* Perineal care as part of the bed bath can be embarrassing for many clients. Nurses also may find it embarrassing initially, particularly with clients of the opposite sex (Grant, Giddings, & Beale, 2005). However, most clients who require a bed bath from the nurse are able to clean their own genital areas with minimal assistance. The nurse may need to hand a moistened washcloth to the client, rinse the washcloth, and provide a towel.

Because some clients are unfamiliar with terminology for the genitals and perineum, it may be difficult for nurses to explain what is expected. Most clients, however, understand what is meant if the nurse simply says, "I'll give you a washcloth to finish your bath." Older clients may use the term *private parts.* Whatever expression the nurse uses, it needs to be one that the client understands and one that is comfortable for the nurse to use.

The nurse needs to provide perineal care efficiently and matter-of-factly. Nurses should wear gloves while providing this care for the comfort of the client and to protect themselves. Skill 29.2 explains how to provide perineal-genital care.

SKILL 29.2

PROVIDING PERINEAL-GENITAL CARE

PURPOSES

- To remove normal perineal secretions and odours
- To promote client comfort

ASSESSMENT

Assess for the presence of

- Irritation, excoriation, inflammation, swelling
- Excessive discharge
- Odour, pain, or discomfort
- Urinary or fecal incontinence
- Recent rectal or perineal surgery
- Indwelling catheter

Determine

- Perineal-genital hygiene practices
- Self-care abilities

Equipment

Perineal-genital care provided in conjunction with the bed bath:

- Bath towel
- Bath blanket
- Clean gloves
- Bath basin with water at 43°C to 46°C
- Soap
- Washcloth

Special perineal-genital care:

- Bath towel
- Bath blanket
- Clean gloves
- Cotton balls or swabs
- Solution bottle, pitcher, or container filled with warm water or a prescribed solution
- Bedpan to receive rinse water
- Moisture-resistant bag or receptacle for used cotton swabs
- Perineal pad

(continued)

SKILL 29.2

PROVIDING PERINEAL-GENITAL CARE (*continued*)

IMPLEMENTATION

Preparation

- Determine whether the client is experiencing any discomfort in the perineal-genital area.
- Obtain and prepare the necessary equipment and supplies.

Performance

1. Before performing the procedure, introduce yourself and verify the client's identity by using agency protocol. Explain to the client what you are going to do, why it is necessary, and how he or she can cooperate, being particularly sensitive to any embarrassment felt by the client.
2. Perform hand hygiene and observe other appropriate infection prevention and control procedures (e.g., clean gloves).
3. Provide for client privacy by drawing the curtains around the bed or closing the door to the room. Some agencies provide signs indicating the need for privacy. **Rationale: Hygiene is a personal matter.**
4. Prepare the client:
   - Fold the top bed linen to the foot of the bed and fold the gown up to expose the genital area.
   - Place a bath towel under the client's hips. **Rationale: The bath towel prevents the bed from becoming soiled.**
5. Position and drape the client and clean the upper inner thighs.

For Females

- Position the female in a back-lying position with the knees flexed and spread well apart.
- Cover her body and legs with the bath blanket positioned so a corner is at her chin, the opposite corner at her feet, and the other two on the sides. Drape the legs by tucking the bottom corners of the bath blanket under the inner sides of the legs (see ❶). **Rationale: Minimum exposure lessens embarrassment and helps to provide warmth.** Bring the middle portion of the base of the blanket up over the pubic area.
- Put on gloves; wash and dry the upper inner thighs.

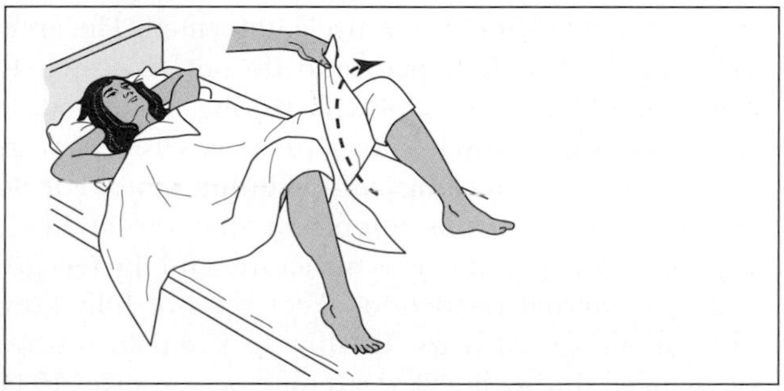

❶ Draping the client for perineal-genital care

For Males

- Position the male client in a supine position with knees slightly flexed and hips slightly externally rotated.
- Put on gloves; wash and dry the upper inner thighs.

6. Inspect the perineal area.
   - Note areas of inflammation, excoriation, or swelling, especially between the labia in females and the scrotal folds in males.
   - Also note excessive discharge or secretions from the orifices and the presence of odours.
7. Wash and dry the perineal-genital area.

For Females

- Clean the labia majora. Then spread the labia to wash the folds between the labia majora and the labia minora (see ❷). **Rationale: Secretions that tend to collect around the labia minora facilitate bacterial growth.**

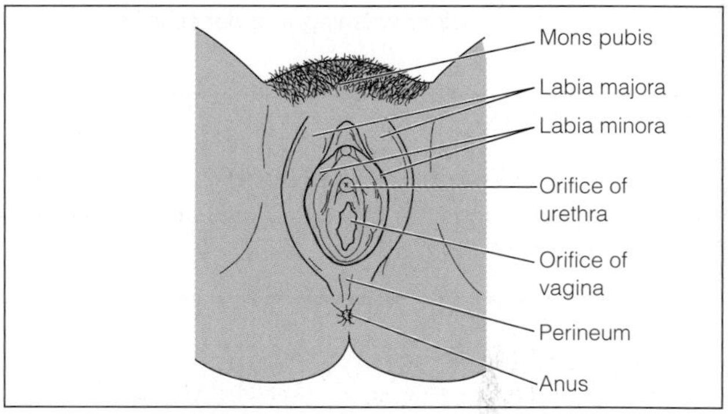

❷ Female genitals

- Use separate quarters of the washcloth for each stroke, and wipe from the pubis to the rectum. For menstruating women and clients with indwelling catheters, use clean wipes. Take a clean wipe for each stroke. **Rationale: Using separate quarters of the washcloth or new wipes prevents the transmission of microorganisms from one area to the other. Wipe from the area of least contamination (the pubis) to that of greatest (the rectum).**
- Rinse the area well. You may place the client on a bedpan and use a periwash or solution bottle to pour warm water over the area. Dry the perineum thoroughly, paying particular attention to the folds between the labia. **Rationale: Moisture supports the growth of many microorganisms.**

For Males

- Wash and dry the penis, using firm strokes.
- If the client is uncircumcised, retract the prepuce (foreskin) to expose the glans penis (the tip of the penis) for cleaning. Replace the foreskin after

(continued)

SKILL 29.2

PROVIDING PERINEAL-GENITAL CARE (*continued*)

cleaning the glans penis (see ❸). **Rationale: Retracting the foreskin is necessary to remove the smegma (thick, cheesy secretion) that collects under the foreskin and facilitates bacterial growth. Replacing the foreskin prevents constriction of the penis, which may cause edema.**

- Wash and dry the scrotum. The posterior folds of the scrotum may need to be cleaned when the buttocks are cleaned (see step 9). **Rationale: The scrotum tends to be more soiled than the penis because of its proximity to the rectum; thus, it is usually cleaned after the penis.**

8. Inspect perineal orifices for intactness.

- Inspect particularly around the urethra in clients with indwelling catheters. **Rationale: A catheter can cause excoriation around the urethra.**

9. Clean between the buttocks.

- Assist the client to turn onto the side facing away from you.
- Pay particular attention to the anal area and posterior folds of the scrotum in males. Clean the anus with toilet tissue before washing it, if necessary.

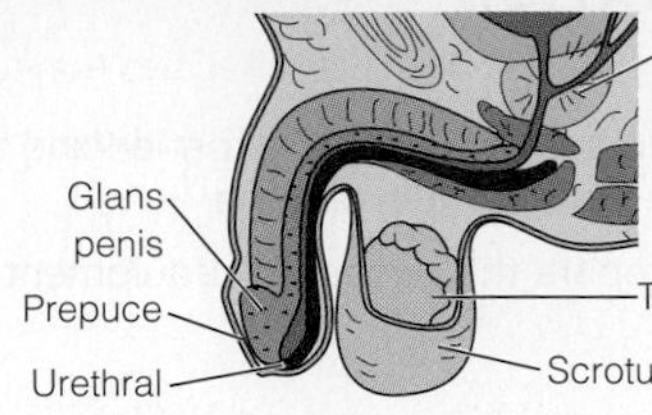

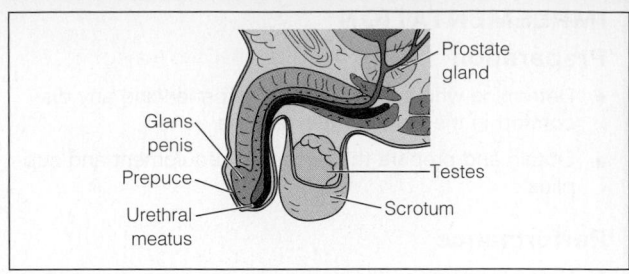

❸ Male genitals

- Dry the area well.
- For postdelivery or menstruating females, apply a perineal pad as needed from front to back. **Rationale: This prevents contamination of the vagina and urethra from the anal area.**

10. Document any unusual findings, such as redness, excoriation, skin breakdown, discharge or drainage, and any localized areas of tenderness.

EVALUATION

- Relate current assessments to previous assessments.
- Conduct appropriate follow-up, such as prescribed ointment for excoriation.
- Report any deviation from normal to the appropriate members of the health-care team.

Evaluating

By using data collected during care, the nurse judges whether desired outcomes have been achieved. Examples of client goals and related outcomes are shown in Table 29.5.

If the outcomes are not achieved, the nurse explores reasons why:

- Did the nurse overestimate the client's functional abilities (physical, mental, emotional) for self-care?
- Were clear instructions provided to the client?
- Were appropriate assistive devices or supplies available to the client?
- Did the client's condition change?
- Were required analgesics provided before hygiene care?
- What currently prescribed medications and therapies could affect the client's abilities or tissue integrity?

Feet

Proper assessment and care of feet is important at any age. This care becomes even more important with aging clients and when such conditions as circulatory disturbances or diabetes mellitus are present.

Developmental Variations

At birth, a baby's foot is relatively unformed. The arches are supported by fatty pads and do not take their full shape until 5 to 6 years of age. During childhood, the bones and small muscles of the feet are easily damaged by tight, binding stockings and ill-fitting shoes. For normal development, it is important that the arches be supported and that the bony structures and the feet grow with no external restrictions. Feet are not fully grown until about age 20 years. Healthy feet remain relatively unchanged during life. The average person takes 10 000 steps per day. Each step places 2 to 3 times the force of

TABLE 29.5 Evaluating Goals and Outcomes: Self-Care, Bathing, Dressing, and Grooming

Goal	Examples of Desired Outcomes
Maintains skin cleanliness	Obtains bath supplies Regulates water flow and temperature Bathes in tub twice weekly with assistance Washes and dries body with direction Gets in and out of tub with assistance
Maintains clean-clothed appearance	Chooses and obtains clean clothing from closet and drawers Puts on and removes clothing Fastens clothing with assistance Ties shoes with assistance
Maintains well-groomed appearance	Applies make-up Shaves self Cares for nails Combs or brushes hair Uses caregiver help for shampoo
Maintains sense of well-being	Reports satisfaction with appearance Reports satisfaction with level of dependence

the body weight on the feet. This repetitive use leads to normal changes associated with aging. These include wider and longer feet, mild settling of the arches, and loss of natural padding on the bottom of the heels. The cartilage around the joints also deteriorates, producing loss of normal range of motion of the foot and ankle. Older adult clients often require special attention for their feet. For example, reduced blood supply and accompanying arteriosclerosis can make a foot prone to infection following trauma.

Assessing

NURSING HISTORY The nurse determines the client's history of (1) normal nail and foot care practices, (2) type of footwear worn, (3) self-care abilities, (4) presence of factors that place the client at risk for foot problems, (5) any foot discomfort, and (6) any perceived problems with foot mobility (see the Assessment: Interview box on foot hygiene).

PHYSICAL ASSESSMENT Each foot and toe is inspected for shape, size, and presence of lesions and is palpated to assess areas of tenderness, edema, and circulatory status. Normally, the toes are straight and flat. See Table 29.6 for physical assessment methods for the feet. Common foot problems include calluses, corns, unpleasant odours, plantar warts, fissures between the toes, and fungal infections, such as athlete's foot.

ASSESSMENT: INTERVIEW

Foot Hygiene

FOOT CARE PRACTICES

- How often do you wash your feet and cut your toenails?
- What hygiene products do you usually use on your feet (cleanser, foot powder or deodorant, lotion, or cream)?
- What type of shoes and socks do you wear?
- How often do you change your socks or put on clean socks?
- Do you ever go barefoot? If so, when, where, and how often?

SELF-CARE ABILITIES

- Do you have any problems managing your foot care? If so, what are these?
- How can the nurses best help you?

FOOT PROBLEMS AND RISK FACTORS

- Do you have any problems with foot odour?
- Do you have any foot discomfort? If so, where? When does this occur? What do you do to relieve the discomfort? Does this discomfort affect how you walk?
- Have you noticed any problems with foot mobility (e.g., joint stiffness)?
- Do you have diabetes, any circulatory problems affecting your feet (e.g., swelling, changes in skin colour, arthritis), or any instances of prolonged exposure to chemicals or water?

A **callus** is a thickened portion of epidermis, a mass of keratotic material. Most calluses are painless and flat and are found on the bottom or side of the foot over a bony prominence. Calluses are usually caused by pressure from shoes. They can be softened by soaking the foot in warm water with Epsom salts. Creams with lanolin help to keep the skin soft and prevent the formation of calluses.

A **corn** is a keratosis caused by friction and pressure from a shoe. It commonly occurs on the fourth or fifth toe, usually over a bony prominence, such as a joint. Corns are usually conical (circular and raised). The base is the surface of the corn and the apex is in deeper tissues, sometimes even attached to bone. Corns are generally removed surgically. They are prevented from reforming by relieving the pressure on the area (generally by wearing properly fitting shoes) and massaging the tissue to promote circulation. The use of oval corn pads should be avoided because they increase pressure and decrease circulation.

Unpleasant odours occur as a result of perspiration and its interaction with microorganisms. Regular and frequent washing of the feet and wearing clean hosiery help

TABLE 29.6 Assessment of the Feet

Method	Normal Findings	Deviations from Normal
Inspect all skin surfaces, particularly between the toes, for cleanliness, odour, dryness, inflammation, swelling, abrasions, or other lesions.	Intact skin Absence of swelling or inflammation	Excessive dryness Areas of inflammation or swelling (e.g., corns, calluses) Fissures Scaling and cracking of skin (e.g., athlete's foot) Plantar warts
Palpate anterior and posterior surfaces of ankles and feet for edema.	No swelling	Swelling or pitting edema
Palpate dorsalis pedis pulse on dorsal surface of foot and posterior tibial pulse behind the medial malledus.	Strong, regular pulses in both feet	Weak or absent pulses in one foot or both feet
Compare skin temperatures of the two feet.	Warm skin	Cool skin temperature in one or both feet
Assess sensation of touch.	Sensation of touch	Absence of sensation
Assess movement.	Movement of feet or toes	Decreased movement of feet or toes

minimize odour. Medicated foot powders and deodorants also help prevent this problem.

Plantar warts appear on the sole of the foot. These warts are caused by the virus *Papovavirus hominis* (human papillomavirus). They are moderately contagious. The warts are frequently painful and often make walking difficult. A physician may curettage the warts (scrape them out), use a carbon dioxide laser to excise them, or freeze them with liquid nitrogen several times.

Fissures, or deep grooves, frequently occur between the toes as a result of dryness and cracking of the skin. The treatment of choice is good foot hygiene and application of an antiseptic to prevent infection. Often, a small piece of gauze is inserted between the toes in applying the antiseptic and is left in place to assist healing by allowing air to reach the area.

Tinea pedis (athlete's foot or ringworm of the foot) is caused by a fungus. The symptoms are scaling and cracking of the skin, particularly between the toes. Sometimes, small blisters form, containing a thin fluid. In severe cases, the lesions can also appear on other parts of the body, particularly the hands. Treatments usually involve the application of commercial antifungal ointments or powders. Prevention is important. Common preventive measures are keeping the feet well ventilated, drying the feet well after bathing, wearing clean socks or stockings, and not going barefoot in public showers.

An **ingrown nail**, the growing inward of the nail into the soft tissues around it, most often results from improper nail trimming. Pressure applied to the area causes localized pain. Treatment involves frequent, hot antiseptic soaks and, possibly, surgical removal of the portion of nail embedded in the skin. Preventing recurrence involves appropriate instruction and adherence to proper nail-trimming techniques.

Diagnosing

A number of nursing diagnoses can apply to clients with foot or foot care problems. The most common diagnostic labels, along with possible contributing factors, are as follows:

- *Self-Care Deficit* (foot care) related to
  - **a.** Visual impairment
  - **b.** Impaired hand coordination
  - **c.** Other contributing factors (see Box 29.2, page 709).
- *Risk for Impaired Skin Integrity* related to
  - **a.** Altered tissue perfusion: peripheral (associated with edema, inadequate arterial circulation)
  - **b.** Poorly fitting shoes
- *Risk for Infection* related to
  - **a.** Impaired skin integrity (ingrown toenail, corn, trauma)
  - **b.** Deficient nail or foot care
- *Deficient Knowledge* (diabetic foot care) related to
  - **a.** Lack of information
  - **b.** Newly established medical diagnosis (diabetes) and necessary foot hygiene practices

Examples of assessment data clusters and related nursing diagnoses are shown in Table 29.7.

TABLE 29.7 Clients with Foot Problems

Data Cluster Sally Brown, an 83-year-old widow, lives alone, has home-maker services twice a week and Meals on Wheels service daily, and manages to shower once a week with daughter's help. Has pronounced hand tremors and obvious cataracts. States, "I can't see well enough to cut my nails and even if I could see, my hands shake so badly."

Nursing Diagnosis/ Definition	Sample Desired Outcome*/ Definition	Indicators	Selected Interventions*/ Definition	Sample NIC Activities
Self-Care Deficit: Hygiene (Foot Care) related to impaired hand coordination and visual impairment/*Impaired ability to perform or complete bathing/hygiene activities for oneself*	Self-Care: Hygiene *Ability to maintain own personal cleanliness and kempt appearance independently with or without assistive device*	Severely compromised: • Cares for nails	Foot Care *Cleansing and inspecting the feet for the purposes of relaxation, cleanliness, and healthy skin*	• Inspect skin for irritation, cracking, lesions, corns, calluses, or edema • Instruct family on the importance of foot care • Cut normal-thickness toenails when soft by using a toenail clipper and the curve of the toe as a guide • Refer to podiatrist for trimming of thickened nails, as appropriate

Data Cluster Kyle Stevens, 14 years old, lives with his mother and eight sisters and brothers in a three-room walk-up. Bathroom down the hall is shared with other tenants in the building. Shoes are ragged and fit poorly. States, "I can't get new ones."

Risk for Impaired Skin Integrity related to poorly fitting shoes and limited access to bathing facilities/*At risk for skin being adversely altered*	Tissue Integrity: Skin & Mucous Membranes *Structural intactness and normal physiological function of skin and mucous membranes*	Not compromised • Skin intactness	Skin Surveillance *Collection and analysis of client data to maintain skin and mucous membrane integrity*	• Monitor skin for areas of redness and breakdown • Monitor skin for excessive dryness and moisture • Institute measures to prevent deterioration of skin • Instruct client and family about signs of skin breakdown

Data Cluster Jim Wakefield, 64 years old, was recently diagnosed with diabetes mellitus. States he has heard of "diabetes" and is worried because a friend of his father's had diabetes and, after cutting his foot, he eventually had his leg amputated.

Deficient Knowledge (Diabetic Foot Care) related to misinterpretation of information/ *Absence or deficiency of cognitive information related to a specific topic*	Knowledge: Diabetes Management *Extent of understanding conveyed about diabetes mellitus and the precaution of complications*	Substantial knowledge • Description of preventive foot care practices	Teaching: Disease *Assisting the client to understand information related to a specific disease process*	• Appraise the client's current level of knowledge related to diabetes • Provide information to the client about diabetes, as appropriate • Discuss lifestyle changes that may be required to prevent future complications or control the disease process • Describe rationale behind foot care management • Instruct the client on which signs and symptoms to report to health-care provider, as appropriate

Planning

Planning involves (1) identifying nursing interventions that will help the client maintain or restore healthy foot care practices, and (2) establishing desired outcomes for each client. Interventions may include teaching the client about correct nail and foot care, proper footwear, and ways to prevent potential foot problems (e.g., infection, injury, and decreased circulation). For clients with self-care difficulties, the nurse plans a schedule for soaking the client's feet and assisting with regular cleaning and trimming of nails if not contraindicated. Foot and nail care is often provided during the client's bath but can be provided at any time in the day to accommodate the client's preference or schedule. The frequency of foot care is determined by the nurse and client and is based on objective assessment data and the client's specific problems. For some clients, the feet need to be bathed daily; for those whose feet perspire excessively, bathing more than once a day may be necessary.

Examples of desired health outcomes to evaluate the achievement of goals and the effectiveness of the nursing interventions include the client doing the following:

- Participates in self-care (foot hygiene) at optimal level of capacity
- Describes hygiene and other interventions (e.g., proper footwear) to maintain skin integrity, prevent infection, and maintain peripheral tissue perfusion
- Demonstrates optimal hygiene, as evidenced by
  - Intact, smooth, pink, soft, hydrated, and warm skin
  - Intact cuticles and skin surrounding nails
  - Correct foot care and nail care practices

Implementing

Skill 29.3 describes how to provide foot care.

SKILL 29.3

PROVIDING FOOT CARE

PURPOSES

- To maintain the skin integrity of the feet
- To prevent foot infections
- To prevent foot odours
- To assess or monitor foot problems

ASSESSMENT

Determine

- History of any problems with foot discomfort, foot odour, foot mobility, circulatory problems (e.g., swelling, changes in skin colour or temperature, and pain), structural problems (e.g., bunion, hammer toe, or overlapping digits)
- Usual foot care practices (e.g., frequency of washing feet and cutting nails, foot hygiene products used, how often socks are changed, whether the client ever goes barefoot, whether the client sees a podiatrist)

Assess

- Skin surfaces for cleanliness, odour, dryness, and intactness
- Each foot and toe for shape, size, presence of lesions (e.g., corn, callus, wart, or rash), and areas of tenderness, ankle edema
- Skin temperatures of both feet to assess circulatory status
- Pedal pulses: dorsalis pedis and posterior tibialis
- Self-care abilities (e.g., any problems managing foot care)

Equipment

- Washbasin containing warm water
- Pillow
- Moisture-resistant disposable pad
- Towels
- Soap
- Washcloth
- Toenail cleaning and trimming equipment, if agency policy permits
- Lotion or foot powder

IMPLEMENTATION

Performance

1. Before performing the procedure, introduce yourself and verify the client's identity by using agency protocol. Explain to the client what you are going to do, why it is necessary, and how he or she can cooperate.
2. Perform hand hygiene and observe other appropriate infection prevention and control procedures.
3. Provide for client privacy by drawing the curtains around the bed or closing the door to the room. Some agencies provide signs indicating the need for privacy. **Rationale: Hygiene is a personal matter.**
4. Prepare the equipment and the client.
   - Fill the washbasin with warm water at about 40°C to 43°C. **Rationale: Warm water promotes circulation, comforts, and refreshes.**

(continued)

SKILL 29.3

PROVIDING FOOT CARE (*continued*)

- Assist the ambulatory client to a sitting position in a chair, or the bed client to a supine or semi-Fowler's position.
- Place a pillow under the bed client's knees. **Rationale: This provides support and prevents muscle fatigue.**
- Place the washbasin on the moisture-resistant pad at the foot of the bed for a bed client or on the floor in front of the chair for an ambulatory client.
- For a bed client, pad the rim of the washbasin with a towel. **Rationale: The towel prevents undue pressure on the skin.**

5. Wash the foot and soak it.
   - Place one of the client's feet in the basin and wash it with soap, paying particular attention to the interdigital areas. Prolonged soaking is generally not recommended for diabetic clients or individuals with peripheral vascular disease. **Rationale: Prolonged soaking may remove natural skin oils, thus drying the skin and making it more susceptible to cracking and injury.**
   - Rinse the foot well to remove soap. **Rationale: Soap irritates the skin if not completely removed.**
   - Rub callused areas of the foot with the washcloth. **Rationale: This helps remove dead skin layers.**
   - If the nails are brittle or thick and require trimming, replace the water and allow the foot to soak for 10 to 20 minutes. **Rationale: Soaking softens the nails and loosens debris under them.**
   - Clean the nails as required with an orange stick. **Rationale: This removes excess debris that harbours microorganisms.**
   - Remove the foot from the basin and place it on the towel.
6. Dry the foot thoroughly and apply lotion or foot powder.
   - Blot the foot gently with the towel to dry it thoroughly, particularly between the toes. **Rationale: Harsh rubbing can damage the skin. Thorough drying reduces the risk of infection.**
   - Apply lotion or lanolin cream to the foot but not between the toes. **Rationale: This lubricates dry skin and keeps the area between the toes dry.**
   - *Or* apply a foot powder containing a nonirritating deodorant if the feet tend to perspire excessively. **Rationale: Foot powders have greater absorbent properties than regular bath powders; some also contain menthol, which makes the feet feel cool.**
7. If agency policy permits, trim the nails of the first foot while the second foot is soaking.
   - See the discussion on nails for the appropriate method to trim nails. Note that in many agencies, toenail trimming requires a physician's order or is contraindicated for clients with diabetes mellitus, toe infections, and peripheral vascular disease, unless performed by a podiatrist, general practice physician, or advanced practice provider, such as a nurse practitioner.
8. Document any foot problems observed.
   - Foot care is not generally recorded unless problems are noted.
   - Record any signs of inflammation, infection, breaks in the skin, corns, troublesome calluses, bunions, and pressure areas. This is of particular importance for clients with peripheral vascular disease and diabetes.

EVALUATION

- Inspect nails and skin after the soak.
- Compare to prior assessment data.
- Report any abnormalities to the appropriate members of the health-care team.

TEACHING: CLINICAL

Foot Care

- Wash the feet daily, and dry them well, especially between the toes.
- When washing, inspect the skin of the feet for breaks or red or swollen areas. Use a mirror, if needed, to visualize all areas.
- To prevent burns, check the water temperature before immersing the feet or stepping into the bathwater.
- Use creams or lotions to moisten the skin, or soak the feet in warm water with Epsom salts to avoid excessive drying of the skin of the feet. Lotion will also soften calluses. A lotion that reduces dryness effectively is a mixture of lanolin and mineral oil.
- To prevent or control an unpleasant odour caused by excessive foot perspiration, wash the feet frequently

(continued)

TEACHING: CLINICAL (*continued*)

and change socks and shoes at least daily. Special deodorant sprays or absorbent foot powders are also helpful.

- File the toenails, rather than cutting them, to avoid skin injury. File the nails straight across the ends of the toes. If the nails are too thick or misshapen to file, consult a podiatrist.
- Wear clean stockings or socks daily. Avoid socks with holes or darns that can cause pressure areas.
- Wear correctly fitting shoes that neither restrict the foot nor rub on any area; rubbing can cause corns and calluses. Check worn shoes for rough spots in the lining. Break in new shoes gradually by increasing the wearing time by 30 to 60 minutes each day.
- Avoid walking barefoot because injury and infection may result. Wear footwear (for example, shower sandals) in public showers and in change areas to avoid contracting athlete's foot or other infections.
- Several times each day, exercise the feet to promote circulation. Point the feet upward, point them downward, and move them in circles.
- Avoid wearing constricting garments, such as knee-high stockings, and avoid sitting with the legs crossed at the knees or ankles, which may decrease circulation.
- When the feet are cold, use extra blankets and wear warm socks rather than using heating pads or hot water bottles, which may cause burns.
- Wash any cut on the foot thoroughly, apply a mild antiseptic, and notify the health-care provider if indicated.
- Avoid self-treatment for corns or calluses. Pumice stones and some callus and corn applications are injurious to the skin. Consult a podiatrist or the health-care provider first.
- Notify the health-care provider if you notice abnormal sores or drainage, pain, or changes in temperature, colour, and sensation of the foot.

Evaluating

See examples of desired health outcomes earlier in the Planning section.

Nails

Nails are normally present at birth. They continue to grow throughout life and change very little until people are much older. At that time, the nails tend to be tougher, more brittle, and, in some cases, thicker. The nails of an older person normally grow less quickly than those of a younger person and may be ridged and grooved.

Assessing

During the nursing history, the nurse explores the client's usual nail care practices, self-care abilities, and any problems associated with them. See the Assessment: Interview box. Physical assessment involves inspection of the nails (see Chapter 27).

ASSESSMENT: INTERVIEW

Nail Hygiene

Ask about your client's nail care practices:

- What are your usual nail care practices?
- Do you have any problems managing your nail care? If so, what are these?
- Have you had any problems associated with your nails (e.g., inflammation of the tissue surrounding the nail, injury, prolonged exposure to water or chemicals, circulatory problems)?

Diagnosing

Nursing diagnoses related to nail care and nail problems include *Self-Care Deficit* and *Risk for Infection.* Below are examples of these nursing diagnoses and contributing factors:

- *Self-Care Deficit: Grooming* related to
  a. Impaired vision
  b. Impaired hand coordination
- *Risk for Infection* around the nail bed related to
  a. Impaired skin integrity of cuticles
  b. Altered peripheral circulation

Planning

The nurse identifies measures that will assist the client to develop or maintain healthy nail care practices. A schedule of nail care needs to be established. The following are examples of desired client outcomes used to evaluate the effectiveness of nursing interventions:

- Demonstrates healthy nail care practices as shown by
  a. Clean, short nails with smooth edges
  b. Intact cuticles and hydrated surrounding skin

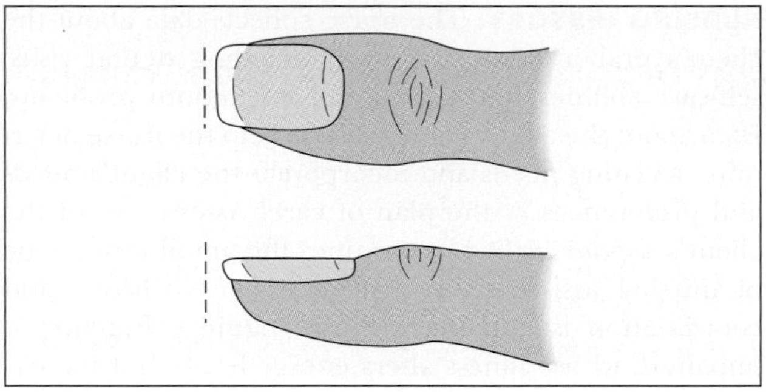

FIGURE 29.6 Fingernails are trimmed straight across

- Describes factors contributing to the nail problem
- Describes preventive interventions for the specific nail problem
- Demonstrates nail care as instructed
- Has pink nail beds and quick return of nail bed colour after blanch test

Implementing

To provide nail care, the nurse needs a nail cutter or sharp scissors, a nail file, an orange stick to push back the cuticle, hand lotion or mineral oil to lubricate any dry tissue around the nails, and a basin of water to soak the nails if they are particularly thick or hard.

Hands or feet are soaked, if needed, and dried; then the nail is cut or filed straight across beyond the end of the finger or toe. See Figure 29.6. Avoid trimming or digging into nails at the lateral corners. This predisposes the client to ingrown toenails. Clients who have diabetes or circulatory problems should have their nails filed, rather than cut; inadvertent injury to tissues can occur if scissors are used. After the initial cut or filing, the nail is filed to round the corners, and the nurse cleans under the nail. The nurse then gently pushes back the cuticle, taking care not to injure it. The next finger or toe is cared for in the same manner. Any abnormalities, such as an infected cuticle or inflammation of the tissue around the nail, are recorded and reported.

Evaluating

See examples of desired health outcomes earlier in the Planning section.

Mouth

Developmental Variations

Teeth usually appear 5 to 8 months after birth. Each tooth has three parts: the crown, the root, and the pulp cavity (Figure 29.7). The **crown** is the exposed part of the tooth that is outside the gum. It is covered with a hard substance called **enamel**. The ivory-coloured internal part of the crown below the enamel is the **dentin**. The root of a tooth is embedded in the jaw and covered by a bony tissue called **cementum**. The **pulp cavity** in the centre of the tooth contains the blood vessels and nerves.

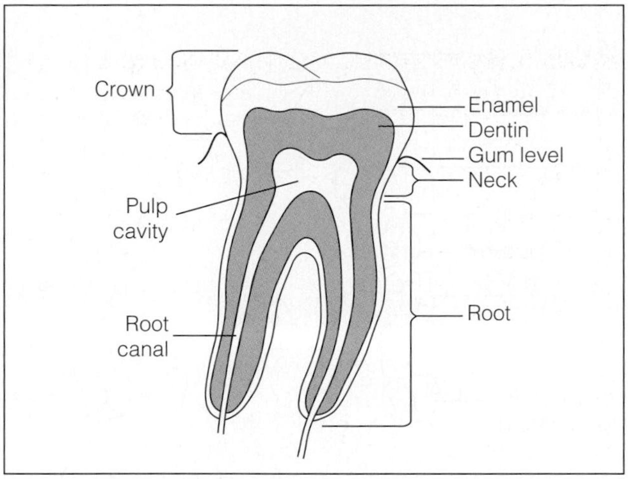

FIGURE 29.7 The anatomy of a tooth

By the time children are 2 years old, they usually have all 20 of their temporary teeth (Figure 29.8). At about age 6 or 7 years, children start losing their deciduous teeth, and these are gradually replaced by the 32 permanent teeth (Figure 29.9). By age 25 years, most people have all their permanent teeth.

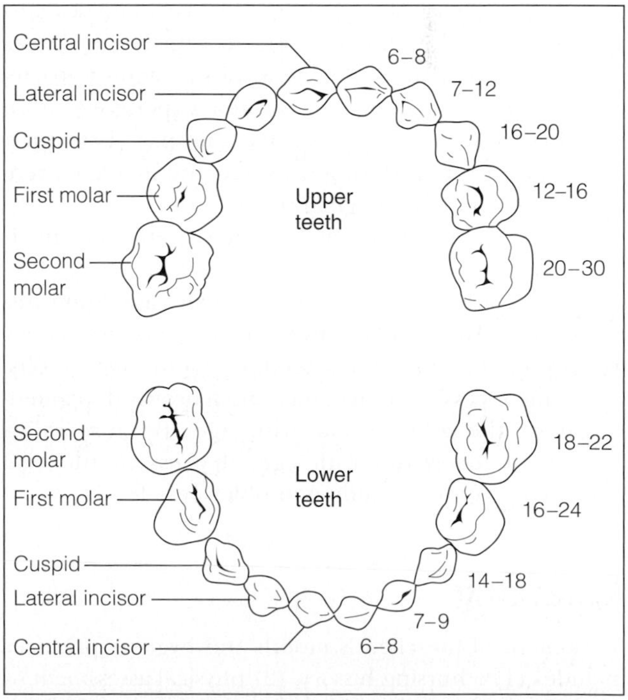

FIGURE 29.8 Temporary teeth and their times of eruption (stated in months)

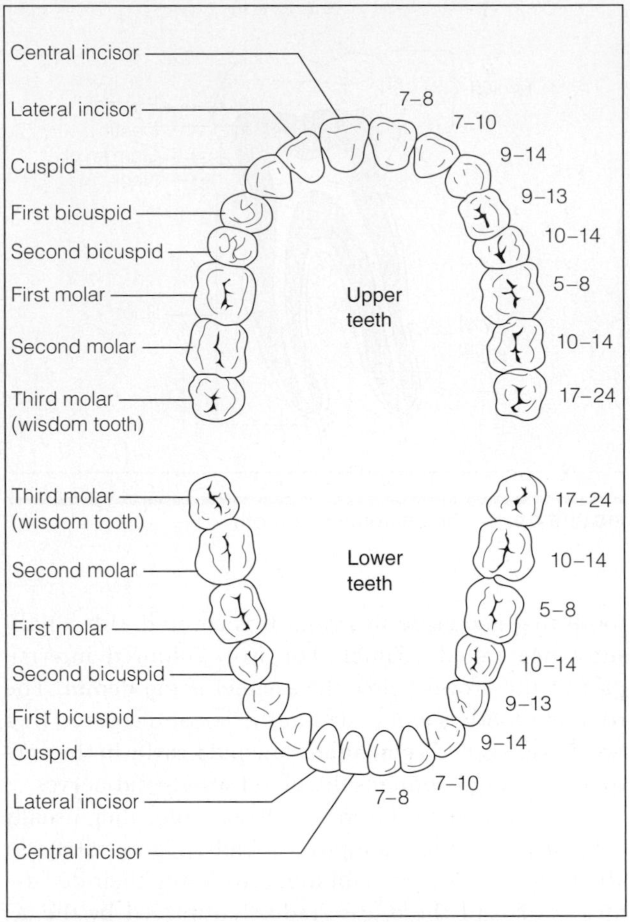

FIGURE 29.9 Permanent teeth and their times of eruption (stated in years)

The incidence of periodontal disease increases during pregnancy because the rise in female hormones affects gingival tissue and increases its reaction to bacterial plaque. Many pregnant women experience more bleeding from the gingival sulcus (the space between a tooth and the gum) during brushing and increased redness and swelling of the **gingiva** (the gum).

Some older adults may have few permanent teeth left, and some have dentures. Older individuals may lose teeth mainly because of **periodontal disease** (gum disease), rather than **dental caries** (cavities); however, caries can also be the cause of lost teeth in middle-aged adults.

Some recession of the gums and a brownish pigmentation of the gums occur with age. Because saliva production decreases with age, dryness of the oral mucosa is a common finding in older people.

Assessing

Assessment of the client's mouth and hygiene practices includes (1) a nursing history, (2) physical assessment of the mouth, and (3) identification of clients at risk for developing oral problems.

NURSING HISTORY The nurse collects data about the client's oral hygiene practices, including dental visits, self-care abilities, and past or current mouth problems. Data about the client's oral hygiene help the nurse determine learning needs and incorporate the client's needs and preferences in the plan of care. Assessment of the client's *self-care abilities* determines the amount and type of nursing assistance to provide. Clients whose hand coordination is impaired, whose cognitive function is impaired, whose illness alters energy levels and motivation, or whose therapy imposes restrictions on activities will need assistance from the nurse. Information about *past or current problems* alerts the nurse to specific interventions or referrals that may be necessary. Questions to elicit oral hygiene information are shown in the Assessment: Interview box.

PHYSICAL ASSESSMENT For information about mouth assessment, see Chapter 27. Dental caries and periodontal disease are the two problems that most frequently affect the teeth. Both problems are commonly associated with plaque and tartar deposits. **Plaque** is an *invisible* soft film that adheres to the enamel surface of teeth; it consists of bacteria, molecules of saliva, and remnants of epithelial cells and leukocytes. **Tartar** (dental calculus) is a visible, hard deposit of plaque and dead bacteria that forms at the gum lines. Tartar buildup can alter the fibres that attach the teeth to the gum and eventually disrupt bone tissue. Periodontal disease is characterized by **gingivitis** (red, swollen gingiva), bleeding, receding gum lines, and the formation of pockets between the teeth and gums. In advanced periodontal disease (**pyorrhea**), the teeth are loose and pus is evident when the gums are pressed. See Table 29.8 for additional problems of the mouth.

ASSESSMENT: INTERVIEW

Oral Hygiene

Ask about your client's oral hygiene prcatices:

ORAL HYGIENE PRACTICES

- What are your usual mouth care or denture care practices?
- What oral hygiene products do you routinely use (e.g., mouthwash, type of toothpaste, dental floss, denture cleaner)?
- When was your last dental examination, and how often do you see your dentist?

SELF-CARE ABILITIES

- Do you have any problems managing your mouth care?

PAST OR CURRENT MOUTH PROBLEMS

- Have you had or do you have any problems, such as bleeding, swollen or reddened gums, ulcerations, lumps, or tooth pain?

TABLE 29.8 Common Problems of the Mouth

Problem	Description	Nursing Implications
Halitosis	Bad breath	Teach or provide regular oral hygiene.
Glossitis	Inflammation of the tongue	As above
Gingivitis	Inflammation of the gums	As above
Periodontal disease	Gums that appear spongy and bleeding	As above
Reddened or excoriated mucosa		Check for ill-fitting dentures.
Excessive dryness of the buccal mucosa (inside of cheek)		Advise increased fluid intake, as client's health permits.
Cheilosis	Cracking of lips	Advise client to lubricate lips; use antimicrobial ointment to prevent infection.
Dental caries	Teeth have darkened areas, may be painful	Advise client to see a dentist.
Sordes	Accumulation of foul matter (food, microorganisms, and epithelial elements) in the mouth	Teach or provide regular cleaning.
Stomatitis	Inflammation of the oral mucosa	Teach or provide regular cleaning.
Parotitis	Inflammation of the parotid salivary glands	Teach or provide regular oral hygiene.

IDENTIFYING CLIENTS AT RISK Certain clients are prone to oral problems because of lack of knowledge or the inability to maintain oral hygiene. Among these are seriously ill, confused, comatose, depressed, and dehydrated clients. In addition, people with nasogastric tubes or those receiving oxygen are likely to develop dry oral mucous membranes, especially if they breathe through their mouths. Clients who have had oral or jaw surgery must have meticulous oral hygiene care to prevent the development of infections.

Healthy-appearing individuals, too, may be at risk (Kwan, Petersen, Pine, & Borutta, 2005; Watt, 2005). High-risk variables, such as inadequate nutrition, excessive intake of refined sugars, and family history of periodontal disease, also need to be identified. Some older people may also be at risk, for example, those who choose salty or enamel-eroding sugary foods because of a decline in their number of taste buds. The decreased saliva production in older adults, which produces a dry mouth and thinning of the oral mucosa, is another factor.

A dry mouth can be aggravated by poor fluid intake, heavy smoking, alcohol use, high salt intake, anxiety, and many medications. Medications that can cause dryness of the mouth include diuretics; laxatives, if used excessively; and tranquilizers, such as chlorpromazine (Thorazine) and diazepam (Valium). Some chemotherapeutic agents used to treat cancer also cause oral dryness and lesions.

Diagnosing

Three nursing diagnoses related to problems with oral hygiene and the oral cavity are *Self-Care Deficit, Altered Oral Mucous Membrane,* and *Deficient Knowledge.* NANDA International (2007) includes oral hygiene in the diagnostic label *Self-Care Deficit: Bathing/Hygiene.* In this chapter, the diagnosis *Self-Care Deficit: Oral Hygiene* will be used for clients unable to perform oral care independently. This includes the inability to brush or floss teeth or clean dentures.

The diagnosis *Altered Oral Mucous Membrane* refers to the state in which an individual experiences "disruptions of the lips and/or soft tissue of the oral cavity" (NANDA International, 2007, p. 152). Manifestations include a coated tongue; dry mouth; dental caries; halitosis; gingivitis; oral plaque, pain, discomfort, erythema, lesions, or ulcers; and lack of or decreased salivation. These may be the result of inadequate oral hygiene; physical injury or drying effect (e.g., mouth breathing, oxygen therapy, decreased salivation, temperature extreme, NPO); mechanical trauma (e.g., surgery, injury from oral tube, broken teeth or ill-fitting dentures); chemical trauma (e.g., side-effects of medications); or radiation injury.

See examples of assessment data clusters and related nursing diagnoses in Table 29.9.

TABLE 29.9 Clinical Application: Assessment Data Clusters and Related Nursing Diagnoses for Clients with Oral Cavity Problems

Data Cluster	Nursing Diagnosis
Aaliya Ahmed, 77 years old, suffered a cerebrovascular accident (stroke). She is unconscious and breathing through the mouth via O_2 facemask. 2500 mL of intravenous fluid ordered daily.	*Self-Care Deficit: Oral Hygiene* related to cognitive inability (unconsciousness)
Sein Win, 46 years old, was admitted with a fractured femur. His teeth are stained from heavy smoking. One large cavity is evident in second lower left molar. He has tartar buildup along gum margins and pronounced halitosis. Gums are reddened in some areas and bleed when flossed. He states, "I can't remember when I last saw a dentist."	*Altered Oral Mucous Membrane* related to ineffective oral hygiene

Planning

The goals for clients with oral hygiene or oral problems are as follows:

- To maintain or improve oral hygiene practices
- To maintain or restore the integrity of the oral tissues
- To prevent associated risks, such as dental caries and inflammation or injury of the gums, tongue, or oral mucosa

Implementing

Good oral hygiene includes daily stimulation of the gums, mechanical brushing and flossing of the teeth, and flushing of the mouth. The nurse has various opportunities to teach good oral hygiene by inspecting whether clients (especially children) have brushed their teeth or by actually providing mouth care to clients who are ill or incapacitated. The nurse can also be instrumental in identifying problems that require the intervention of a dentist or an oral surgeon and arranging a referral.

PROMOTING ORAL HEALTH THROUGH THE LIFESPAN

A major role of the nurse in promoting oral health is to teach clients about specific oral hygienic measures.

Infants and Toddlers Most dentists recommend that dental hygiene should begin when the first tooth erupts and be practised after each feeding. Cleaning can be accomplished by using a wet washcloth or a cotton ball or small piece of gauze moistened with water.

Dental caries occur frequently during the toddler period, often as a result of the excessive intake of sweets or a prolonged use of a bottle during naps and at bedtime. The nurse should provide parents the following instructions to promote and maintain dental health:

- Beginning at about 18 months of age, brush the child's teeth with a soft toothbrush. Use only a toothbrush moistened with water. Introduce toothpaste later; use one that contains fluoride.
- Give a fluoride supplement daily or as recommended by the physician or dentist, unless the drinking water is fluoridated.
- Schedule an initial dental visit for the child at about 2 or 3 years of age, as soon as all 20 primary teeth have erupted.
- Some dentists recommend an inspection type of visit when the child is about 18 months old to provide an early pleasant introduction to the dental examination.
- Seek professional dental attention for any problems, such as discolouring of the teeth, chipping, or signs of infection, such as redness and swelling.

Preschoolers and School-Age Children Because deciduous teeth guide the entrance of permanent teeth, dental care is essential to keep these teeth in good repair. Abnormally placed or lost deciduous teeth can cause misalignment of permanent teeth. Fluoride is essential to prevent dental caries. Preschoolers need to be taught to brush their teeth after eating and to limit their intake of refined sugars. Parental supervision may be needed to ensure the completion of these self-care activities.

TEACHING: WELLNESS

Measures to Prevent Tooth Decay

Several oral hygiene practices can help prevent tooth decay:

- Brush the teeth thoroughly after meals and at bedtime. Assist children or inspect their mouths to be sure the teeth are clean. If the teeth cannot be brushed after meals, vigorous rinsing of the mouth with water is recommended.
- Floss the teeth daily.
- Ensure an adequate intake of nutrients, particularly calcium, phosphorus, vitamins A, C, and D, and fluoride.
- Avoid sweet foods and drinks between meals. Take them in moderation at meals.
- Eat coarse, fibrous foods (cleansing foods), such as fresh fruits and raw vegetables.
- Have topical fluoride applications as prescribed by the dentist in locales where fluoridated water is not available.
- Have a checkup by a dentist every 6 to 9 months.

Regular dental checkups are required during these years when permanent teeth appear.

Adolescents and Adults Proper diet and tooth and mouth care should be taught to adolescents and adults. See specific measures to prevent tooth decay in the Teaching: Wellness box.

CARE OF TEETH

Brushing and Flossing the Teeth Thorough brushing of the teeth is important in preventing tooth decay. The mechanical action of brushing removes food particles that can harbour and incubate bacteria. It also stimulates circulation in the gums, thus maintaining their healthy firmness. One of the techniques recommended for brushing teeth is called the **sulcular technique**, which removes plaque and cleans under the gingival margins. Fluoride toothpaste is recommended because of its antibacterial protection. An effective dentifrice (toothpaste) can also be made by using baking soda.

Caring for Dentures Some people have artificial teeth or dentures. A plate or denture is a complete set of teeth. Some clients may have a bridge, which is a partial set of artificial teeth. Artificial teeth either are fixed and cannot be removed or are removable. People who wear dentures or other types of oral prostheses should be encouraged to use them. Those who do not wear their prostheses are prone to shrinkage of the gums, which results in further tooth loss.

Like natural teeth, artificial dentures collect microorganisms and food. They need to be cleaned regularly, at least once a day. They can be removed from the mouth, scrubbed with a toothbrush, rinsed, and reinserted. Some people use a dentifrice for cleaning teeth, and others use commercial cleaning compounds for plates.

ASSISTING CLIENTS WITH ORAL CARE When providing mouth care for partially or completely dependent clients, the nurse should wear gloves to guard against infections. Other required equipment includes a curved basin that fits snugly under the client's chin (e.g., a kidney basin or emesis basin) to receive the rinse water and a towel to protect the client and the bedclothes. See Skill 29.4. When providing care of dentures, it is important to assess the client's need for privacy when dentures are removed and cleaned.

SKILL 29.4

BRUSHING AND FLOSSING THE TEETH

PURPOSES

- To remove food particles from around and between the teeth
- To remove dental plaque
- To promote the client's feelings of well-being
- To prevent sores and infection of the oral tissues

ASSESSMENT

- Determine the extent of the client's self-care abilities.
- Assess the client's usual mouth care practices.
- Inspect lips, gums, oral mucosa, and tongue for deviations from normal.
- Identify the presence of oral problems, such as tooth caries, halitosis, gingivitis, and loose or broken teeth.
- Check whether the client has bridgework or wears dentures. If the client has dentures, ask if any tenderness or soreness is present and, if so, the location of the areas for ongoing assessment.

Equipment

For Brushing and Flossing

- Towel
- Disposable gloves
- Curved basin
- Toothbrush (soft bristle)
- Cup of tepid water
- Dentifrice
- Mouthwash
- Dental floss, at least two pieces 20 cm long
- Floss holder (optional)

For Cleaning Artificial Dentures

- Disposable gloves
- Tissue or piece of gauze
- Denture container
- Clean washcloth
- Toothbrush or stiff-bristled brush
- Dentifrice or denture cleaner
- Tepid water
- Container of mouthwash
- Curved basin
- Towel

(continued)

SKILL 29.4

BRUSHING AND FLOSSING THE TEETH (*continued*)

IMPLEMENTATION

Preparation

Assemble all the necessary equipment.

Performance

1. Before performing the procedure, introduce yourself and verify the client's identity by using agency protocol. Explain to the client what you are going to do, why it is necessary, and how he or she can cooperate.
2. Perform hand hygiene and observe other appropriate infection prevention and control procedures (e.g., disposable gloves). **Rationale: Wearing gloves while providing mouth care prevents the nurse from acquiring infections. Gloves also prevent transmission of microorganisms to the client.**
3. Provide for client privacy by drawing the curtains around the bed or closing the door to the room. Some agencies provide signs indicating the need for privacy. **Rationale: Hygiene is a personal matter.**
4. Prepare the client.
   - Assist the client to a sitting position in bed, if health permits. If not, assist the client to a side-lying position with the head turned *so liquid is prevented from draining down the client's throat.*
5. Prepare the equipment.
   - Place the towel under the client's chin.
   - Put on disposable gloves.
   - Moisten the bristles of the toothbrush with tepid water and apply the dentifrice to the toothbrush.
   - Use a soft toothbrush (a small one for a child) and the client's choice of dentifrice.
   - For the client who must remain in bed, place or hold the curved basin under the client's chin, fitting the small curve around the chin or neck.
   - Inspect the mouth and teeth.
6. Floss the teeth.
   - Assist the client to floss independently, or floss the teeth of an alert and cooperative client as follows. Waxed floss is less likely to fray than unwaxed floss; particles between the teeth attach more readily to unwaxed floss than to waxed floss.
     a. Wrap one end of the floss around the third finger of each hand (see ❶).
     b. To floss the upper teeth, use your thumb and index finger to stretch the floss. Move the floss up and down between the teeth. When the floss reaches the gum line, gently slide the floss into the space between the gum and the tooth. Gently move the floss away from the gum with up and down motions (Canadian Dental Association, 2005). Start at the back on the right side and work around to the back of the left side, or work from the centre teeth to the back of the jaw on either side.
     c. To floss the lower teeth, use your index fingers to stretch the floss (see ❷).

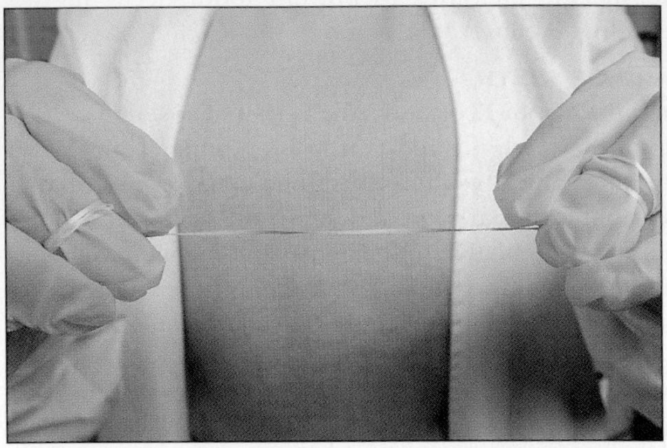

❶ Stretching the floss between the third finger of each hand

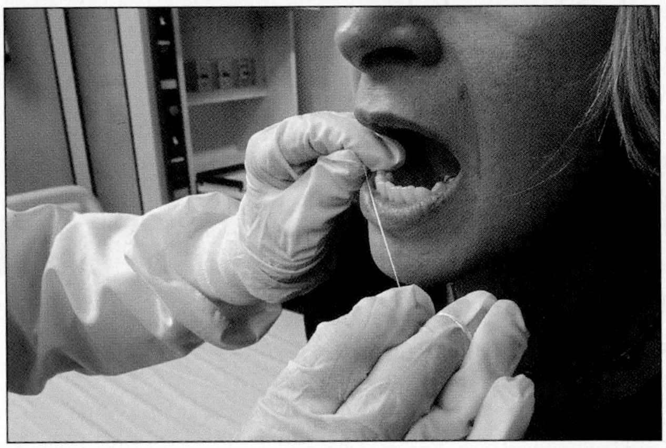

❷ Flossing the lower teeth by using the index fingers to stretch the floss

   - Give the client tepid water or mouthwash to rinse the mouth and a curved basin in which to spit the water.
   - Assist the client in wiping the mouth.
7. Brush the teeth.
   - Hand the toothbrush to the client, or brush the client's teeth as follows:
     a. Hold the brush against the teeth with the bristles at a 45-degree angle. The tips of the outer bristles should rest against and penetrate under the gingival sulcus (see ❸). The brush will clean under the sulcus of two or three teeth at one time. **Rationale: This sulcular technique removes plaque and cleans under the gingival margins.**
     b. Use a gentle, circular, massaging motion, and brush down from the gumline to the chewing surface of the teeth in short strokes (see ❹).
     c. Repeat until all outer and inner surfaces of the teeth and sulci of the gums are cleaned.

(continued)

SKILL 29.4

BRUSHING AND FLOSSING THE TEETH (*continued*)

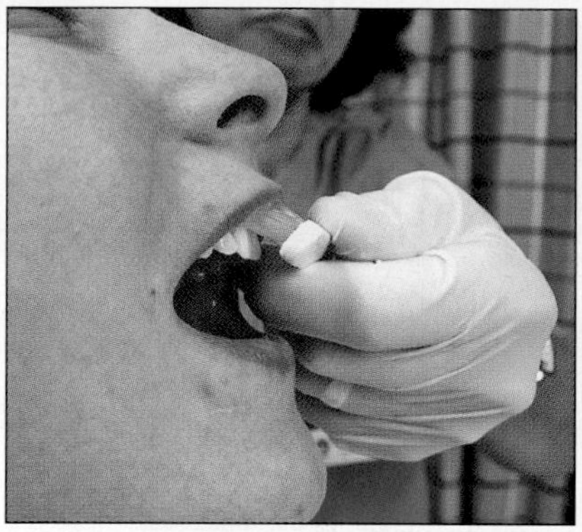

❸ The sulcular technique: Place the bristles at a 45-degree angle with the tips of the outer bristles under the gumline, where the gums and teeth meet.

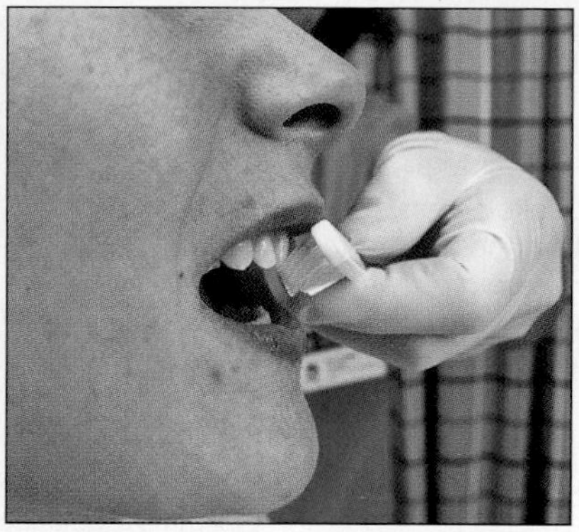

❹ Brushing from the sulcus to the crown of the teeth

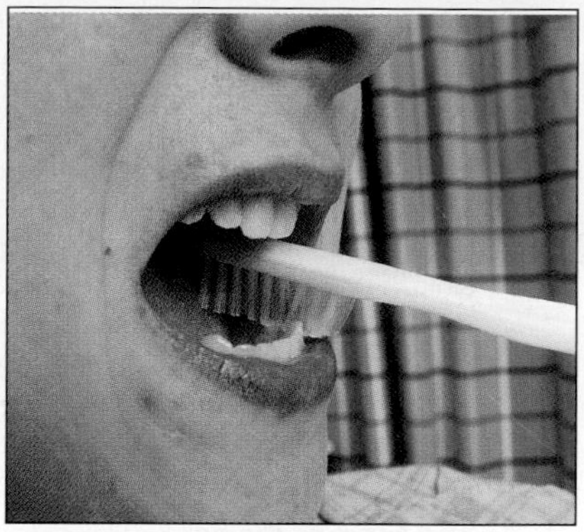

❺ Brushing the biting surfaces

d. Clean the biting surfaces by moving the brush back and forth over them in short strokes (see ❺).

e. Brush the tongue gently with the toothbrush. **Rationale: Brushing removes bacteria and freshens breath. A coated tongue may be caused by poor oral hygiene and low fluid intake. Brushing gently and carefully helps prevent gagging or vomiting.**

- Hand the client the water cup or mouthwash to rinse the mouth vigorously. Then ask the client to spit the water and excess dentifrice into the basin. Some agencies supply a standard mouthwash. Alternatively, a mouth rinse of normal saline can be an effective cleaner and moisturizer. **Rationale: Vigorous rinsing loosens food particles and washes out already loosened particles.**
- Repeat the preceding steps until the mouth is free of dentifrice and food particles.
- Remove the curved basin and help the client wipe the mouth.

8. Remove and dispose of equipment appropriately.
   - Remove and clean the curved basin.
   - Remove and discard the gloves.

EVALUATION

Document assessment of the teeth, tongue, gums, and oral mucosa. Include any problems, such as sores or inflammation, bleeding, and swelling of the gums. Brushing and flossing teeth are not usually recorded.

Variation: Artificial Dentures

1. Remove the dentures.
   - Put on gloves. **Rationale: Wearing gloves decreases the likelihood of spreading infection.**
   - If the client cannot remove the dentures, take the tissue or gauze, grasp the upper plate at the front teeth with your thumb and second finger, and move the denture up and down slightly (see ❻). **Rationale: The slight movement breaks the suction that holds the plate on the roof of the mouth.**
   - Lower the upper plate, move it out of the mouth, and place it in the denture container.
   - Lift the lower plate, turning it so that the left side, for example, is slightly lower than the right, to remove the plate from the mouth without stretching the lips. Place the lower plate in the denture container.

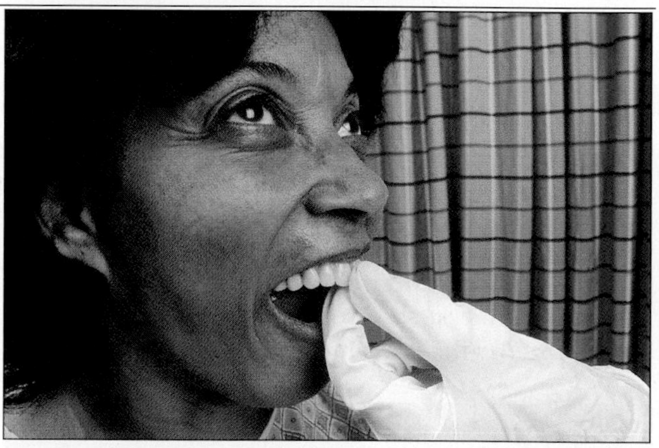

❻ Removing the top dentures by first breaking the suction

(*continued*)

SKILL 29.4

BRUSHING AND FLOSSING THE TEETH *(continued)*

- Remove a partial denture by exerting equal pressure on the border of each side of the denture, not on the clasps, which can bend or break.

2. Clean the dentures.
   - Take the denture container to a sink. Take care not to drop the dentures. Place a washcloth in the bowl of the sink *to prevent damage if the dentures are dropped.*
   - Use a toothbrush or special stiff-bristled brush to scrub the dentures with the cleaning agent and tepid water.
   - Rinse the dentures with tepid running water. **Rationale: Rinsing removes the cleaning agent and food particles**.
   - If the dentures are stained, soak them in a commercial cleaner. Be sure to follow the manufacturer's directions. To prevent corrosion, dentures with metal parts should not be soaked overnight.
3. Inspect the dentures and the mouth.
   - Observe the dentures for any rough, sharp, or worn areas that could irritate the tongue or mucous membranes of the mouth, lips, and gums.
   - Inspect the mouth for any redness, irritated areas, or indications of infection.
   - Assess the fit of the dentures. People who have dentures should see a dentist at least once a year to check the fit and the presence of any irritation to the soft tissues of the mouth. Clients who need repairs to their dentures or new dentures may need a referral for financial assistance.

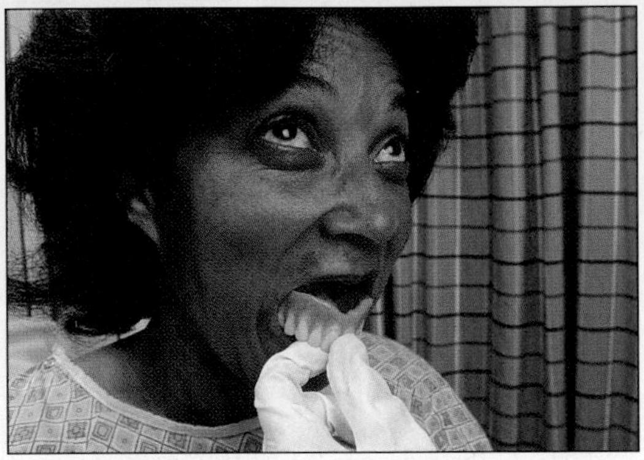

❼ Inserting the dentures at a slight angle

4. Return the dentures to the mouth.
   - Offer some mouthwash and a curved basin to rinse the mouth. If the client cannot insert the dentures independently, insert the plates one at a time. Hold each plate at a slight angle while inserting it, to avoid injuring the lips (see ❼).
5. Assist the client as needed.
   - Wipe the client's hands and mouth with the towel.
   - If the client does not want to or cannot wear the dentures, store them in a denture container with water. Label the container with the client's name and identification number.
6. Remove and discard gloves.

EVALUATION

Document and report all assessments including any problems, such as an irritated area on the mucous membrane.

Foam swabs (Figure 29.10) are often used in healthcare agencies to clean the mouths of dependent clients. These swabs are convenient and effective in removing excess debris from the teeth and mouth but should be used infrequently and for short periods (i.e., fewer than 3 days). Foam swabs are not as effective as a toothbrush in removing plaque from sheltered areas of the teeth and gingival crevices (Munro, Grap, & Kleinpell, 2004). Lemon-glycerine swabs are not recommended as they irritate and dry the oral mucosa and can decalcify teeth.

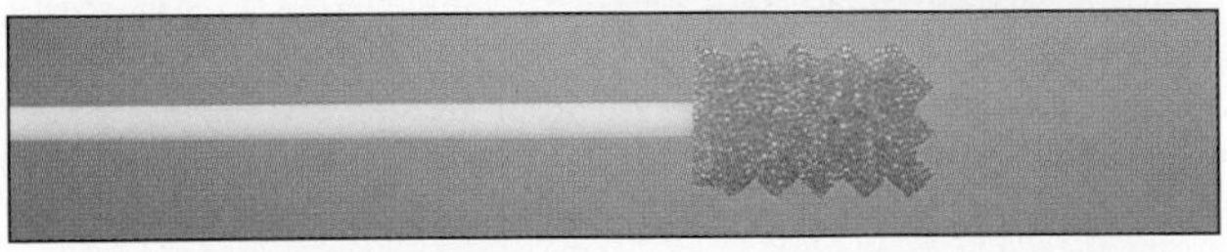

FIGURE 29.10 An example of a foam swab used to clean the mouth of a dependent client

Special Oral Hygiene For the client who is debilitated or unconscious or who has excessive dryness, sores, or irritations of the mouth, it may be necessary to clean the oral mucosa and tongue in addition to the teeth. Agency practices differ concerning special mouth care and the frequency with which it is provided. Depending on the health of the client's mouth, special care may be needed every 2 to 8 hours.

Mouth care for unconscious or debilitated clients is important because their mouths tend to become dry and consequently predisposed to infections. Dryness occurs because the client cannot take fluids by mouth, is often breathing through the mouth, or may be receiving oxygen, which tends to dry the mucous membranes. For clients with special oral hygiene needs, the nurse needs to focus on removal of plaque and microorganisms as well as to promote client comfort. If possible, a soft-bristled toothbrush should be used as it provides the best means of plaque removal. A sodium bicarbonate toothpaste will help dissolve mucus and reduce the saliva's acidity, which helps decrease bacteria (Nainar & Mohummed, 2004). If the client cannot tolerate the use of a toothbrush, the nurse can use a foam swab or gauze soaked with saline to swab the teeth and tongue.

The nurse can use commercially prepared mouthwashes, tepid water, or normal saline (according to agency policy) for oral hygiene. Long-term use of commercially prepared mouthwashes can lead to further dryness of the mucosa and changes in tooth enamel. Mineral oil is contraindicated because aspiration of it can initiate an infection (lipid pneumonia). Regular strength hydrogen peroxide is *not* recommended for use in oral care because it irritates healthy oral mucosa and may alter the microflora of the mouth. Skill 29.5 focuses on oral care for the unconscious person, but it can be adapted for conscious persons who are seriously ill or have mouth problems.

SKILL 29.5

PROVIDING ORAL CARE FOR AN UNCONSCIOUS CLIENT

PURPOSES

- To maintain the intactness and health of the lips, tongue, and mucous membranes of the mouth
- To prevent oral infections
- To clean and moisten the membranes of the mouth and lips

ASSESSMENT

- Inspect lips, gums, oral mucosa, and tongue for deviations from normal.
- Identify the presence of oral problems, such as tooth caries, halitosis, gingivitis, and loose or broken teeth.
- Assess for a gag reflex, when appropriate.

Equipment

- Towel
- Curved basin
- Disposable clean gloves
- Bite-block to hold the mouth open and teeth apart (optional)
- Toothbrush
- Cup of tepid water
- Dentifrice or denture cleaner
- Tissue or piece of gauze to remove dentures (optional)
- Denture container as needed
- Mouthwash
- Rubber-tipped bulb syringe
- Suction catheter with suction apparatus when aspiration is a concern
- Foam swabs and cleaning solution for cleaning the mucous membranes
- Water-soluble lip moisturizer

IMPLEMENTATION

Performance

1. Before performing the procedure, introduce yourself and verify the client's identity by using agency protocol. Explain to the client and the family what you are going to do and why it is necessary.
2. Perform hand hygiene and observe other appropriate infection prevention and control procedures (e.g., disposable gloves).
3. Provide for client privacy by drawing the curtains around the bed or closing the door to the room. Some agencies provide signs indicating the need for privacy. **Rationale: Hygiene is a personal matter.**
4. Prepare the client.
   - Position the unconscious client in a side-lying position, with the head of the bed lowered. **Rationale: In this position, the saliva automatically runs out by gravity rather than being aspirated into the lungs.** This position is chosen for the unconscious client receiving mouth care. If the client's head cannot be lowered, turn it to one side. **Rationale: The fluid will**

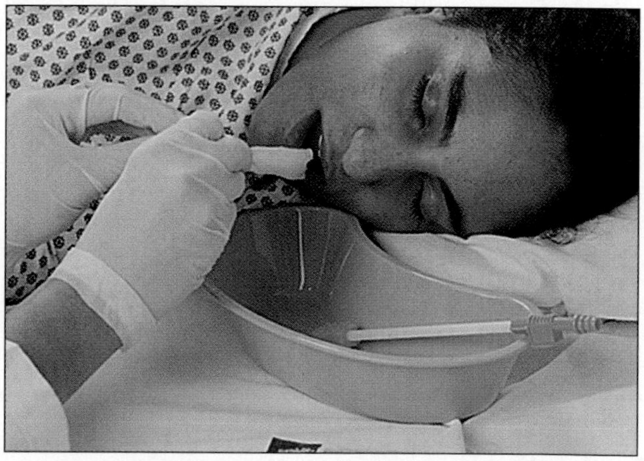

❶ Position of client and placement of curved basin when providing special mouth care

(continued)

SKILL 29.5

PROVIDING ORAL CARE FOR AN UNCONSCIOUS CLIENT (*continued*)

readily run out of the mouth or pool in the side of the mouth, where it can be suctioned.

- Place the towel under the client's chin.
- Place the curved basin against the client's chin and lower cheek to receive the fluid from the mouth (see ❶).
- Put on gloves.

5. Clean the teeth and rinse the mouth.
   - If the person has natural teeth, brush the teeth as described in Skill 29.4 (p. 732). Brush gently and carefully to avoid injuring the gums. If the client has artificial teeth, clean them as described in the "Variation" component of Skill 29.4 (p. 733).
   - Rinse the client's mouth by drawing about 10 mL of water or alcohol-free mouthwash into the syringe and injecting it gently into each side of the mouth. **Rationale: If the solution is injected with force, some of it may flow down the client's throat and be aspirated into the lungs.**
   - Watch carefully to make sure that all the rinsing solution has run out of the mouth into the basin. If not, suction the fluid from the mouth. **Rationale: Fluid remaining in the mouth can be aspirated into the lungs.**
   - Repeat rinsing until the mouth is free of dentifrice, if used.
6. Inspect and clean the oral tissues.
   - If the tissues appear dry or unclean, clean them with foam swabs or gauze and cleaning solution, following agency policy.
   - Picking up a moistened foam swab, wipe the mucous membrane of one cheek. Discard the swab in a waste container; use a fresh one to clean the next area. **Rationale: Using separate applicators for each area of the mouth prevents the transfer of microorganisms from one area to another.**
   - Clean all mouth tissues in an orderly progression, using separate applicators: the cheeks, roof of the mouth, base of the mouth, and tongue.
   - Observe the tissues closely for inflammation and dryness.
   - Rinse the client's mouth as described in step 5.
   - Remove and discard gloves.
7. Ensure client comfort.
   - Remove the basin, and dry around the client's mouth with the towel. Replace artificial dentures, if indicated.
   - Lubricate the client's lips with water-soluble moisturizer. **Rationale: Lubrication prevents cracking and subsequent infection.**
8. Document assessment of the teeth, tongue, gums, and oral mucosa. Include any problems, such as sores or inflammation and swelling of the gums.

EVALUATION

- Consider the client's medical diagnosis and treatment (e.g., chemotherapy, oxygen) and the necessary nursing interventions related to oral hygiene.
- Conduct an ongoing assessment, if appropriate, of the oral mucosa, gums, tongue, and lips.
- Report deviations from normal to the appropriate members of the health-care team.
- Conduct appropriate follow-up, such as a referral to a dentist for dental caries.

Special Consideration: Oral Care for a Client with Dementia Good oral hygiene is important for the client with dementia in order to meet the need for hygiene as well as to promote feelings of well-being. Poor oral health can contribute to pain, tooth loss, poor nutrition, and low self-esteem. Regardless of the extent of the dementia, it is important for the nurse to communicate in a quiet, assured manner.

Early Stages of Dementia In the early stages of dementia, clients will generally be able to clean their own teeth or dentures. Although they may require some assistance to complete the entire task, they may need only reminders and supervision. If help is required, preparing the toothbrush with a small amount of toothpaste, and either guiding the client's hand or showing the client what to do should suffice.

Later Stages of Dementia As the dementia progresses, the client will usually need increasing amounts of assistance in order to fully meet the need for hygiene. The caregiver may need to take over the task entirely. Assessment is essential since some clients will recall what is involved in dental care and may complete care with very little intervention. However, at times, the nurse will be required to assume complete responsibility for this care.

One approach that is safe for both the client and the nurse is to have the client sit in a straight-backed chair, such as a dining room or kitchen chair. The nurse then stands behind the client, supporting the client against the nurse's body, and gently cradling the client's head in the nurse's nondominant arm. The nurse can then brush the client's teeth.

Evaluating

By using data collected during care—status of oral mucosa, lips, tongue, teeth, and so on—the nurse judges whether desired outcomes have been achieved. Examples of client goals and related outcomes are shown in Table 29.10.

If outcomes are *not* achieved, the nurse and client need to explore the reasons before modifying the care plan. Examples of factors to consider are similar to those shown for *Self-Care Deficit* in Box 29.2 (page 709).

TABLE 29.10 Evaluation Goals and Outcomes: Oral Hygiene and Health

Goal	Desired Outcomes
Improves oral hygiene practices	Mucosa, tongue, and lips are pink, moist, and intact.
	Dental surfaces are free of debris and plaque.
	Breath is free of halitosis.
	Brushes teeth after meals and at bedtime.
	Flosses teeth daily.
	Obtains regular dental care.
	Uses fluoridation or fluoride supplements, as recommended.
Maintains integrity of oral tissues	Mucosa is intact, smooth, well hydrated, and uniform in colour.
	Gums are firm, well hydrated, not bleeding, and of uniform colour.
	Tongue is well hydrated.
	Lips are smooth and well hydrated.
	Oral tissues are free of inflammation and pain.

Hair Care

Developmental Variations

Newborns may have **lanugo** (the fine hair on the body of the fetus over their shoulders, back, and sacrum). This generally disappears, and the hair distribution on the eyebrows, head, and, eyelashes of young children subsequently becomes noticeable. Some newborns have hair on their scalps; others are free of hair at birth but grow hair over the scalp during the first year of life. Pubic hair usually appears in early puberty, followed, in about 6 months, by the growth of axillary hair. Boys develop facial hair in later puberty.

In adolescence, the sebaceous glands increase in activity as a result of increased hormone levels. As a result, hair follicle openings enlarge to accommodate the increased amount of sebum, which can make the adolescent's hair oilier.

In older adults, the hair is generally thinner, grows more slowly, and loses its colour as a result of aging tissues and diminishing circulation. Men often lose their scalp hair and may become completely bald. This phenomenon can also occur when a man is relatively young. The older person's hair tends to be drier than normal. With age, axillary and pubic hair becomes finer and more scant, in contrast to the eyebrows, which become bristly and coarse. Many women develop hair on their faces, which may be a concern to them.

Assessing

NURSING HISTORY When taking the nursing history, the nurse elicits data about usual hair care, self-care abilities, history of hair or scalp problems, and conditions known to affect the hair. Chemotherapeutic agents and radiation of the head may cause alopecia (hair loss). Hypothyroidism may cause the hair to be thin, dry, and brittle. Use of some hair dyes and curling or straightening preparations can cause the hair to become dry and brittle. Questions to elicit these data are shown in the Assessment; Interview box for hair care.

PHYSICAL ASSESSMENT Physical assessment of the hair is discussed in Chapter 27. Problems include dandruff, hair loss, ticks, pediculosis, scabies, and hirsutism.

DANDRUFF Often accompanied by itching, dandruff appears as a diffuse scaling of the scalp. In severe cases, it involves the auditory canals and the eyebrows. Dandruff can usually be treated effectively with a commercial shampoo. In severe or persistent cases, the client may need the advice of a physician.

HAIR LOSS Hair loss and growth are continual processes. Some permanent thinning of hair normally occurs with aging. Baldness, common in men, is thought to be a hereditary condition for which there is no known remedy other than the wearing of a hairpiece or a costly surgical hair transplantation in which hair is taken from the back or the sides of the scalp and surgically moved to the hairless area. Although some medications are being developed, their long-term outcomes are unknown.

TICKS **Ticks** are small grey-brown parasites that bite into tissue and suck blood. Ticks can transmit several diseases to people, in particular Rocky Mountain spotted fever,

ASSESSMENT: INTERVIEW

Hair Care

Ask the client about hair care:

HAIR CARE PRACTICES

- How do you usually take care of your hair?
- What hair care products do you routinely use (e.g., hair spray, lubricant, shampoo, conditioners, hair dye, curling or straightening preparations)?

SELF-CARE ABILITIES

- Do you have any problems managing your hair?

PAST OR CURRENT HAIR PROBLEMS

- Have you had any of the following conditions or therapies: recent chemotherapy, hypothyroidism, radiation of the head, unexplained loss of hair, growth of excessive body hair?
- How do you manage these hair problems?

Lyme disease, and tularemia. Ticks should never be forcibly pulled from the skin because the sucking apparatus may remain and become infected. To ease removal, cover the tick with mineral oil or a lubricating jelly, such as petroleum jelly. This deprives the tick of oxygen, causing suffocation.

PEDICULOSIS (LICE) **Lice** are parasitic insects that infest mammals. Infestation with lice is called **pediculosis**. Hundreds of varieties of lice can infest humans. Three common kinds are *Pediculus capitis* (the head louse), *Pediculus corporis* (the body louse), and *Pediculus pubis* (the crab louse).

Head and pubic lice lay their eggs on the hairs; the eggs look like oval particles, similar to dandruff, clinging to the hair. Bites and pustular eruptions may also be noticed at the hairlines and behind the ears. Lice are very small, greyish white, and difficult to see. The crab louse in the pubic area has red legs. Lice can be contracted from infested clothes and direct contact with an infested person.

Pediculus capitis is found on the scalp and tends to stay hidden in the hairs; similarly, *Pediculus pubis* stays in pubic hair. *Pediculus corporis* tends to cling to clothing so that when a client undresses, the lice may not be evident on the body; these lice suck blood from the person and lay their eggs on the clothing. The nurse can suspect their presence in the clothing if (1) the person habitually scratches, (2) he or she has scratches on the skin, and (3) he or she has hemorrhagic spots on the skin where the lice have sucked blood.

Treatment consists of the application of pediculocides and manual removal of nits. The preferred drug for use on children is permethrin 1% cream rinse, which kills both adult lice and nits. The repeated use of stronger chemicals on children is not advised, so daily removal of nits from a child's hair, using a specifically designed nit or flea comb, is essential. See Box 29.4 for prevention of pediculosis.

SCABIES **Scabies** is a contagious skin infestation by the itch mite. The characteristic lesion is the burrow produced by the female mite as it penetrates into the upper layers of the skin. Burrows are short, wavy, brown or black threadlike lesions most commonly observed between the webs of the fingers and the folds of the wrists and elbows. The mites cause intense itching that is more pronounced at night because the increased warmth of the skin has a stimulating effect on the parasites. Secondary lesions caused by scratching include vesicles, papules, pustules, excoriations, and crusts. Treatment involves thorough cleansing of the body with soap and water to remove scales and debris from crusts, and followed by an application of a scabicide lotion. All bed linens and clothing should be washed in very hot or boiling water.

BOX 29.4 PREVENTING PEDICULOSIS

Clients can take steps to prevent pediculosis:

- Machine wash all washable clothing, toys, and linens in hot water, followed by drying in a dryer set at the highest temperature.
- Vacuum all upholstered furniture and carpets.
- Soak any items used in treatment in either the pediculocide or boiling water.
- Discourage sharing of headgear, brushes, and combs among all children.
- Conduct regular pediculosis screening in daycares and schools.
- Provide education for children and parents on preventative measures.

HIRSUTISM The growth of excessive body hair is called **hirsutism**. The acceptance of body hair in the axillae and on the legs is largely dictated by culture.

Diagnosing

Nursing diagnoses related to hair hygiene and hair and scalp problems include *Self-Care Deficit: Grooming, Impaired Skin Integrity, Risk for Infection,* and *Body Image, Disturbed.* Examples of these nursing diagnoses with contributing factors are the following:

- *Self-Care Deficit: Grooming* related to
  - **a.** Activity intolerance
  - **b.** Imposed immobility (bed rest)
  - **c.** Pain in upper extremities
  - **d.** Altered level of consciousness
  - **e.** Lack of motivation associated with depression
- *Impaired Skin Integrity* related to
  - **a.** Scalp laceration
  - **b.** Insect bite
- *Risk for Infection* related to
  - **a.** Scalp laceration
  - **b.** Insect bite
- *Body Image, Disturbed* related to
  - **a.** Alopecia
  - **b.** Hirsutism

Planning

In planning care, the nurse identifies nursing activities that will assist the client to achieve these goals:

- Maintain or improve hair care
- Maintain or improve a sense of well-being
- Prevent specific hair and scalp problems

Examples of desired health outcomes to evaluate the effectiveness of nursing interventions have the client doing the following:

- Performs hair grooming with assistance (specify)
- Has clean, well-groomed, resilient hair with a healthy sheen
- Has reduced or absent scalp lesions or infestations
- Describes contributing factors, interventions, and preventive measures for specific hair problem (e.g., dandruff)

Plans for assisting the client should take into account the client's personal preferences, health, and energy resources, as well as the time, equipment, and personnel available. Often, clients like to receive hair care after a bath, before receiving visitors, and before retiring. At some agencies, shampoos can be given to clients only after a physician's order.

Implementing

BRUSHING AND COMBING HAIR Long hair can present a problem for clients confined to bed as it may become matted. It should be combed and brushed at least once a day to prevent this. A brush with stiff bristles provides the best stimulation to blood circulation in the scalp. The bristles should not be so sharp that they injure the client's scalp, however. A comb with dull, even teeth is advisable. A comb with sharp teeth might injure the scalp; combs that are too fine can pull and break the hair. Some clients prefer to have their hair tied neatly in the back or braided until other assistance is available or until they feel better and can look after it themselves.

Dark-skinned people often have thicker, drier, curlier hair than light-skinned people. Spiralled or very curly hair may stand out from the scalp. Although the shafts of spiralled hair look strong and wiry, they have less strength than straight hair shafts and can break easily. Many Black people have hair that is naturally curly and may become matted easily. This type of hair tends to be dry, so shampooing is generally needed less often than with people of other ethnic origin. Skill 29.6 describes how to provide hair care for clients.

SKILL 29.6

PROVIDING HAIR CARE FOR CLIENTS

PURPOSES

- To increase the client's comfort
- To stimulate the blood circulation to the scalp
- To assess or monitor hair or scalp problems (e.g., matted hair or dandruff)
- To distribute hair oils and provide a healthy sheen

ASSESSMENT

Determine

- History of the following conditions or therapies: recent chemotherapy, hypothyroidism, radiation of the head, unexplained hair loss, and growth of excessive body hair
- Usual hair care practices and routinely used hair care products (e.g., hair spray, shampoo, conditioners, hair oil preparation, hair dye, curling or straightening preparations)
- Whether wetting the hair will make it easier to comb: kinky hair is easier to comb when wet and is very difficult to comb when it dries (Jackson, 1998, p. 102)

Assess

- Condition of the hair and scalp. Is the hair straight, curly, kinky? Is the hair matted or tangled? Is the scalp dry?
- Evenness of hair growth over the scalp, in particular, any patchy loss of hair; hair texture, oiliness, thickness, or thinness; presence of lesions, infections, or infestations on the scalp; presence of hirsutism.
- Self-care abilities (e.g., any problems managing hair care).

Planning

Brushing and combing hair, shampooing hair, and shaving facial hair can be delegated to another member of the health-care team unless the client has a condition in which the procedure would be contraindicated (e.g., cervical spinal injury or trauma). The nurse needs to assess the health-care team member's knowledge and experience of hair care for clients of other cultures, if appropriate.

Equipment

- Clean brush and comb
- A wide-toothed comb is usually used for Black people because finer combs pull the hair into knots and can also break the hair
- Towel
- Hair oil preparation, if appropriate

(continued)

SKILL 29.6

PROVIDING HAIR CARE FOR CLIENTS *(continued)*

IMPLEMENTATION

1. Before performing the procedure, introduce yourself and verify the client's identity by using agency protocol. Explain to the client what you are going to do, why it is necessary, and how he or she can cooperate.
2. Perform hand hygiene and observe other appropriate infection prevention and control procedures.
3. Provide for client privacy by drawing the curtains around the bed or closing the door to the room. Some agencies provide signs indicating the need for privacy. **Rationale: Hygiene is a personal matter.**
4. Position and prepare the client appropriately.
   - Assist the client who can sit to move to a chair. **Rationale: Hair is more easily brushed and combed when the client is sitting.** If health permits, assist a client confined to a bed to a sitting position by raising the head of the bed. Otherwise, assist the client to alternate side-lying positions, and do one side of the head at a time.
   - If the client remains in bed, place a clean towel over the pillow and the client's shoulders. Place a towel over the shoulders of the sitting client. **Rationale: The towel collects any removed hair, dirt, and scaly material.**
   - Remove any pins or ribbons in the hair.
5. Remove any mats or tangles gradually.
   - Mats can usually be pulled apart with fingers or worked out with repeated brushings.
   - If the hair is very tangled, rub alcohol or oil, such as mineral oil, on the strands to help loosen the tangles.
   - Comb out tangles in a small section of hair toward the ends. Stabilize the hair with one hand and comb toward the ends of the hair with the other hand. **Rationale: This avoids discomfort and scalp trauma.**
6. Brush and comb the hair.
   - For short hair, brush and comb one side at a time. Divide long hair into two sections by parting it down the middle from the front to the back. If the hair is very thick, divide each section into front and back subsections or into several layers.
7. Arrange the hair as neatly and attractively as possible, according to the individual's preferences.
   - Braiding long hair helps prevent tangles.
8. Document assessments and special nursing interventions. Daily combing and brushing of the hair are not normally recorded.

Variation: Hair Care for Black Clients

- Position and prepare the client.
- Separate the hair into four sections, proceeding from one section to the next.
- Untangle the hair first, if appropriate.
- Use fingers to reduce hair breakage and discomfort. Move fingers in a circular motion starting at the roots and gently moving up to the tip of the hair.
- Comb the hair.
- Dampen the hair with water or a leave-in conditioner. **Rationale: This will help loosen any tangles.**
- Apply hair oil preparation as the client indicates.
- Using a large and open-toothed comb, grasp a small section of hair and, holding the hair at the tip, start untangling at the tip and work down toward the scalp (Jackson, 1998).
- Ask the client if he or she would like the hair braided. **Rationale: Braiding will decrease tangling; however, the choice is the client's.**

EVALUATION

- Conduct ongoing assessments for problems, such as dandruff, alopecia, pediculosis, scalp lesions, or excessive dryness or matting.
- Evaluate effectiveness of medication (e.g., for treating pediculosis), if appropriate.

SHAMPOOING THE HAIR Hair should be washed as often as needed to keep it clean. There are several ways to shampoo clients' hair depending on their health, strength, and age. The client who is well enough to take a shower can shampoo while in the shower. The client who is unable to shower may be given a shampoo while sitting on a chair in front of a sink. The back-lying client who can move to a stretcher can be given a shampoo on a stretcher wheeled to a sink. The client who must remain in bed can be given a shampoo with water brought to the bedside.

Shampoo basins to catch the water and direct it to the washbasin or other receptacle are usually made of plastic or metal. A pail or large washbasin can be used as a receptacle for the shampoo water. If possible, the receptacle should be large enough to hold all the shampoo water so that it does not have to be emptied during the procedure.

Water used for the shampoo should be 40.5°C for an adult or child to be comfortable and not injure the scalp. A medicated shampoo may be used as prescribed by the physician in order to treat lice or other conditions of the scalp. Dry shampoos are also available. They will remove some of the dirt, odour, and oil. Their main disadvantage is that they dry the hair and scalp if used frequently. Another alternative is the shampoo cap, which is a comfortable and efficient alternative to shampooing. It is particularly suited to bedridden and very ill clients. See Figure 29.11.

How often a person needs a shampoo is highly individual, depending largely on the person's activities and the amount of sebum secreted by the scalp. Oily hair tends to look stringy and dirty, and it feels unclean to the person.

Skill 29.7 explains how to provide a shampoo for a client confined to bed.

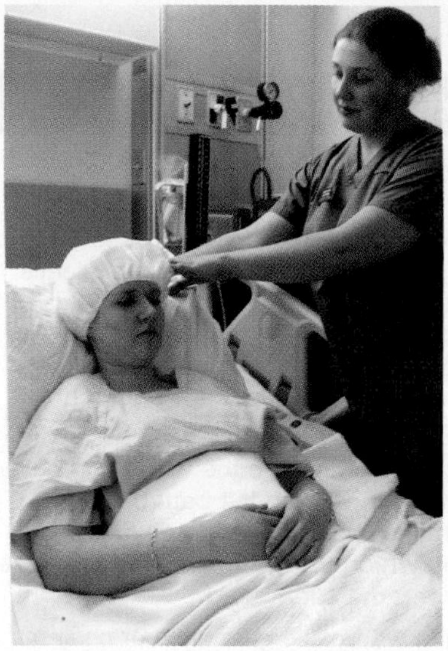

FIGURE 29.11 Using a shampoo cap to clean the hair of a client confined to bed

SKILL 29.7

SHAMPOOING THE HAIR OF A CLIENT CONFINED TO BED

PURPOSES

- To stimulate the blood circulation to the scalp through massage
- To clean the hair and increase the client's sense of well-being

ASSESSMENT

- Determine routinely used shampoo products

Assess

- Any scalp problems
- Activity tolerance of the client

Equipment

- Comb and brush
- Plastic sheet or pad
- Two bath towels
- Shampoo basin
- Washcloth or pad
- Bath blanket
- Receptacle for the shampoo water
- Pitcher of water
- Bath thermometer
- Liquid or cream shampoo
- Hair dryer

IMPLEMENTATION

Preparation

- Determine whether a physician's order is needed before a shampoo can be given. **Rationale: Some agencies require an order depending on the client's condition.**
- Determine the type of shampoo to be used (e.g., medicated shampoo).
- Determine the best time of day for the shampoo. Discuss this with the client. A person who must remain in bed may find the shampoo tiring. Choose a time when the client is rested and can rest after the procedure.

Performance

1. Before performing the procedure, introduce yourself and verify the client's identity by using agency protocol. Explain to the client what you are going to do, why it is necessary if appropriate, and how he or she can cooperate.
2. Perform hand hygiene and observe other appropriate infection prevention and control procedures as needed.
3. Provide for client privacy by drawing the curtains around the bed or closing the door to the room. Some agencies provide signs indicating the need for privacy. **Rationale: Hygiene is a personal matter.**
4. Position and prepare the client appropriately.
   - Assist the client to the side of the bed from which you will work.
   - Remove pins and ribbons from the hair, and brush and comb it to remove any tangles.
5. Arrange the equipment.
   - Put the plastic sheet or pad on the bed under the client's head. **Rationale: The plastic keeps the bedding dry.**
   - Remove the pillow from under the client's head, and place it under the shoulders unless there is some underlying condition (e.g., neck surgery, arthritis of the neck). **Rationale: This hyperextends the neck.**

(continued)

SKILL 29.7

SHAMPOOING THE HAIR OF A CLIENT CONFINED TO BED (*continued*)

- Tuck a bath towel around the client's shoulders. **Rationale: This keeps the shoulders dry.**
- Place the shampoo basin under the head (see ❶), putting a folded washcloth or pad where the client's neck rests on the edge of the basin. If the client is on a stretcher, the neck can rest on the edge of the sink with the washcloth as padding. **Rationale: Padding supports the muscles of the neck and prevents undue strain and discomfort.**
- Fanfold the top bedding down to the waist, and cover the upper part of the client with the bath blanket. **Rationale: The folded bedding will stay dry, and the bath blanket, which can be discarded after the shampoo, will keep the client warm.**
- Place the receiving receptacle on a table or chair at the bedside. Put the spout of the shampoo basin over the receptacle.

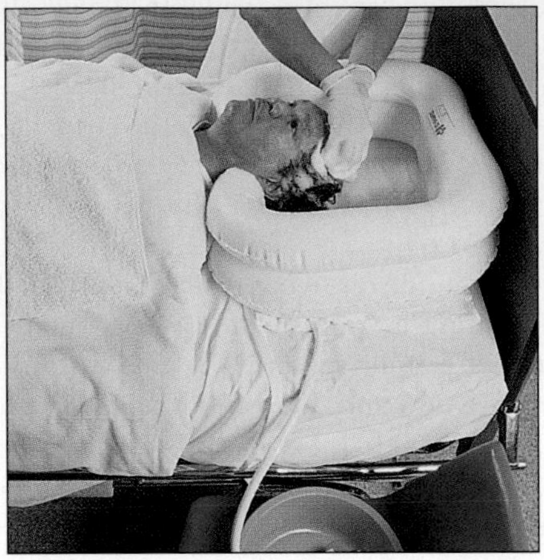

❶ Shampooing the hair of a client confined to bed (note the shampoo basin and the receptacle below)

6. Protect the client's eyes.
   - Place a damp washcloth over the client's eyes. **Rationale: The washcloth protects the eyes from soapy water. A damp washcloth will not slip.**
7. Shampoo the hair.
   - Wet the hair thoroughly with the water.
   - Apply shampoo to the scalp. Make a good lather with the shampoo while massaging the scalp with the pads of your fingertips. Massage all areas of the scalp systematically, for example, starting at the front and working toward the back of the head. **Rationale: Massaging stimulates the blood circulation in the scalp. The pads of the fingers are used so that the fingernails will not scratch the scalp.**
   - Rinse the hair briefly, and apply shampoo again.
   - Make a good lather and massage the scalp as before.
   - Rinse the hair thoroughly this time to remove all shampoo. **Rationale: Shampoo remaining in the hair may dry and irritate the hair and scalp.**
   - Squeeze as much water as possible out of the hair with your hands.
8. Dry the hair thoroughly.
   - Rub the client's hair with a heavy towel.
   - Dry the hair with the dryer. Set the temperature at "warm."
   - Continually move the dryer to prevent burning the client's scalp.
9. Ensure client comfort.
   - Assist the person confined to bed to a comfortable position.
   - Arrange the hair using a clean brush and comb.
10. Document the shampoo and any assessments.

EVALUATION

Conduct ongoing assessments, such as any scalp problems or intolerance to the procedure. Report any problems noted to the nurse in charge.

BEARD AND MOUSTACHE CARE Beards and moustaches also require daily care. The most important aspect of the care is to keep them clean. Food particles tend to collect in beards and moustaches, and they need washing and combing periodically. Clients may also want a beard or moustache trim to maintain a well-groomed appearance. A beard or moustache should not be shaved off without the client's consent.

Male clients often shave or are shaved after a bath. Frequently, clients supply their own electric or safety razors. See Box 29.5 for the steps involved in shaving facial hair with a safety razor.

Evaluating

See examples of desired health outcomes earlier in the Planning section.

BOX 29.5 USING A SAFETY RAZOR TO SHAVE FACIAL HAIR

Follow these steps when shaving a client by using a safety razor:

- When possible, it is preferable to shave a client by using an electric razor.
- Wear gloves in case there are facial nicks and contact with blood.
- Apply shaving cream or soap and water to soften the bristles and make the skin more pliable.
- Hold the skin taut, particularly around creases, to prevent cutting the skin.
- Hold the razor so that the blade is at a 45-degree angle to the skin, and shave in short, firm strokes in the direction of hair growth, being careful not to cut or nick the skin.
- After shaving the entire area, wipe the client's face with a wet washcloth to remove any remaining shaving cream and hair.
- Dry the face well, then apply aftershave lotion or powder as the client prefers.
- To prevent irritating the skin, pat on the lotion with the fingers and avoid rubbing the face.

Eyes

Normally, eyes require no special hygiene because lacrimal fluid continually washes the eyes, and the eyelids and lashes prevent the entrance of foreign particles. Special interventions are needed, however, for unconscious clients, for clients recovering from eye surgery, and for those with eye injuries, irritations, infections, or systemic diseases affecting the eyes. In unconscious clients, the blink reflex may be absent, and excessive drainage may accumulate along eyelid margins. In clients with eye trauma or eye infections, excessive discharge or drainage is common. Excessive secretions on the lashes need to be removed before they dry on the lashes as crusts. Clients who wear eyeglasses, contact lenses, or an artificial eye also may require instruction from and care by the nurse.

Assessing

NURSING HISTORY During the nursing history, the nurse obtains data about the client's eyeglasses or contact lenses, recent examination by an ophthalmologist, and any history of eye problems and related treatments. Questions to elicit these data are shown in the Assessment: Interview box.

ASSESSMENT: INTERVIEW

Eyes

Ask the client about eye care:

FOR CLIENTS WHO WEAR EYEGLASSES

- When do you use your glasses?
- What is your vision like with and without the glasses?

FOR CLIENTS WHO WEAR CONTACT LENSES

- How often do you wear lenses? daily? on special occasions?
- How long do you wear your lenses in a given day, including sleep time?
- Do you have any problems with the lenses (e.g., cleaning, insertion, removal, damage)?
- Do you carry an emergency identification label to alert others to remove the lenses and ensure appropriate care in an emergency? (If not, advise the client to acquire one.)
- What are your insertion and removal procedures?
- What are your cleaning and storage procedures?
- Have you had any problems with either or both eyes or eyelids, such as excessive tearing, burning, redness, discomfort, sensitivity to light, swelling, or feelings of dryness? Describe them.
- Are you using any eye drops or ointments? (These medications can combine chemically with *soft* lenses and cause lens damage and eye irritation.)

FOR CLIENTS WHO HAVE A PROSTHESIS

- How long have you worn a prosthesis?
- How do you care for your prosthesis?
- Do you have any discharge or redness around the orbital cavity?
- Do you have any periorbital pain or swelling?

FOR ALL CLIENTS

- When did you last have your eyesight tested?
- Are you currently taking any eye medication? If so, provide name, dosage, and frequency.
- Do you have any of the following eye problems: difficulty reading or seeing objects, blurring of vision, tearing, spots or floaters, photophobia (sensitivity to light), burning, itching, dryness, pain, double vision, flashing lights, or halos around lights?

PHYSICAL ASSESSMENT In physical assessment, all external eye structures are inspected for signs of inflammation, excessive drainage, encrustations, or other obvious abnormalities. Inspection of the external eye structures is discussed in Chapter 27.

Diagnosing

Nursing diagnoses related to eye problems include *Self-Care Deficit, Risk for Infection,* and *Risk for Injury.* Examples of these diagnoses and possible contributing factors are as follows:

- *Self-Care Deficit* (contact lens insertion, removal, and cleaning) related to
  - a. Deficient knowledge
  - b. Impaired vision associated with cataracts
- *Risk for Infection* related to
  - a. Improper contact lens hygiene
  - b. Accumulation of secretions on eyelids
- *Risk for Injury* related to
  - a. Prolonged wearing of contact lenses
  - b. Absence of blink reflex associated with unconsciousness
  - c. Falls, especially in older adults

Planning

In planning care, the nurse identifies nursing activities that will assist the client to maintain the integrity of the eye structures or a prosthesis and to prevent eye injury and infection. Nursing activities may include teaching clients about how to insert, clean, and remove contact lenses or a prosthesis and ways to protect the eyes from injury and strain. Examples of desired outcomes to evaluate the effectiveness of nursing interventions include

- Conjunctiva and sclera free of inflammation
- Eyelids free of secretions
- No tearing
- No eye discomfort
- Demonstration of appropriate methods of caring for contact lenses
- Description of interventions to prevent eye injury and infection

Implementing

EYE CARE Dried secretions that have accumulated on the lashes need to be softened and wiped away. Soften dried secretions by placing a sterile cotton ball moistened with sterile water or normal saline over the lid margins. Wipe the loosened secretions from the inner canthus of the eye to the outer canthus to prevent the particles and fluid from draining into the lacrimal sac and nasolacrimal duct.

BOX 29.6 EYE CARE FOR THE COMATOSE CLIENT

When a comatose client's corneal reflex is impaired, eye care is essential to keep moist the areas of the cornea that are exposed to air:

- Administer moist compresses to cover the eyes every 2 to 4 hours.
- Clean the eyes with saline solution and cotton balls. Wipe from the inner to outer canthus. This method prevents debris from being washed into the nasolacrimal duct.
- Use a new cotton ball for each wipe to prevent extending infection in one eye or to the other eye.
- Instill ophthalmic ointment or artificial tears into the lower lids as ordered. This keeps the eyes moist.
- If the client's corneal reflex is absent, keep the eyes moist with artificial tears and protect the eye with a protective shield. These interventions should be ordered by a physician.
- Monitor the eyes for redness, exudate, or ulceration.

If the client is unconscious and lacks a blink reflex or cannot close the eyelids completely, drying and irritation of the cornea must be prevented. Lubricating eye drops may be ordered. See Box 29.6 for providing eye care for the comatose client.

EYE SAFETY Eye safety is also an important consideration of eye care. The body's natural eye defences can be augmented by instructing the client to wear safety lenses, goggles, or shields for high-risk activities.

EYEGLASS CARE It is essential that the nurse exercise caution when cleaning eyeglasses to prevent breaking or scratching the lenses. Glass lenses can be cleaned with warm water and dried with a soft cloth that will not scratch the lenses. Plastic lenses are easily scratched and may require special cleaning solutions and drying cloths. When not being worn, all glasses should be placed in a case, labelled appropriately, and stored in the client's bedside table drawer.

CONTACT LENS CARE Most contact lenses, hard or soft, are used to replace eyeglasses for full-time wear. The most commonly used kind is soft lenses, which can be clear or coloured, conventional or disposable, daily wear or extended wear, and with or without correction for astigmatism (toric lenses). Disposable contact lenses are worn one time only and then disposed. Some disposable lenses are designed to be changed every 2 weeks.

Some people require bifocals and may be fitted with contact lenses by using a monovision strategy, in which the correction in one eye is for best distance vision, while the correction in the other eye is adjusted to allow comfortable reading vision. Bifocal soft contact lenses are also available in either conventional or disposable options.

Rigid gas-permeable contact lenses, either in spherical or in a variety of toric designs, are also used to replace glasses. A rigid contact lens may restore much vision if the person has significant corneal damage. In a disfigured eye, a custom-designed soft masking contact lens with as close a colour match to the uninjured eye as possible can produce marked cosmetic effect rather than use of a full prosthesis.

Most clients normally care for their own contact lenses. In general, lens manufacturers provide detailed cleaning instructions. Depending on the type of lens and cleaning method used, warm tap water, normal saline, or special rinsing or soaking solutions may be used.

All contact lens users should have a special container for their lenses. Some contain a solution so that the lenses are stored wet; in others, the lenses are dry. Each lens container has a label indicating whether it is for the right or left lens. It is essential that the correct lens be stored in the appropriate cup so that it can be worn in the correct eye. Clean gloves should be worn when removing or inserting contact lenses.

Removing Contact Lenses Hard contact lenses must be positioned directly over the cornea for proper removal. If the lens is displaced, the nurse asks the client to look straight ahead and gently exerts pressure on the upper and lower lids to move the lens back onto the cornea. Figure 29.12 shows the steps needed to remove a hard lens. To avoid lens mixups, the nurse places the first lens in its designated cup in the storage base before removing the second lens (Figure 29.13).

Removal of soft lenses differs in two ways. First, have the client look forward. Retract the lower lid with one hand. Using the pad of the index finger of the other hand, move the lens down to the inferior part of the sclera. This reduces the risk of damage to the cornea. Second, remove the lens by gently pinching the lens between the pads of the thumb and index finger. Pinching causes the lens to double up, so that air enters underneath the lens, overcoming the suction and allowing removal. Use the pads of the fingers to prevent scratching the eye or the lens with the fingernails.

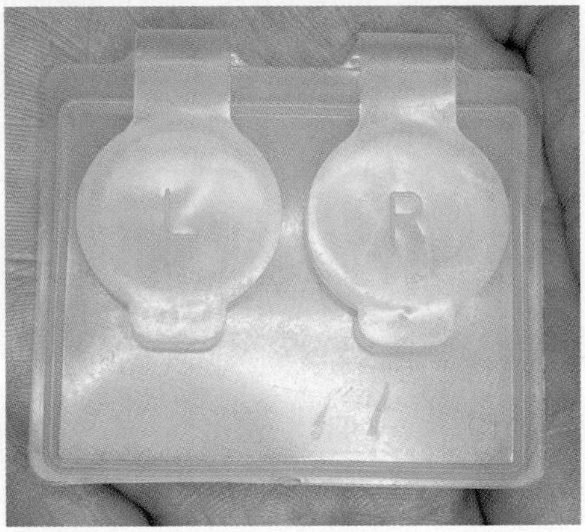

FIGURE 29.13 Storing lenses

Figure 29.14 shows a client removing her own contact lens by using the method described. Note that a nurse would need to wear gloves.

Inserting Contact Lenses Seriously ill clients whose contact lenses have been removed will not need them reinserted until they become more active in their care and require the lenses to see properly. Contact lenses need to be lubricated in a sterile, nonirritating wetting solution (usually a saline solution) before they are inserted. The wetting solution helps the lens glide over the cornea, thus reducing the risk of injury. Most clients, when well, will reinsert the lenses independently.

ARTIFICIAL EYES (PROSTHESIS) Artificial eyes are usually made of plastic instead of glass. Some are permanently implanted; others are removed regularly for cleaning as required. Most clients who wear a removable artificial eye follow their own care regimen.

To remove an artificial eye, the nurse dons clean gloves and uses the dominant thumb to pull the client's lower eye-

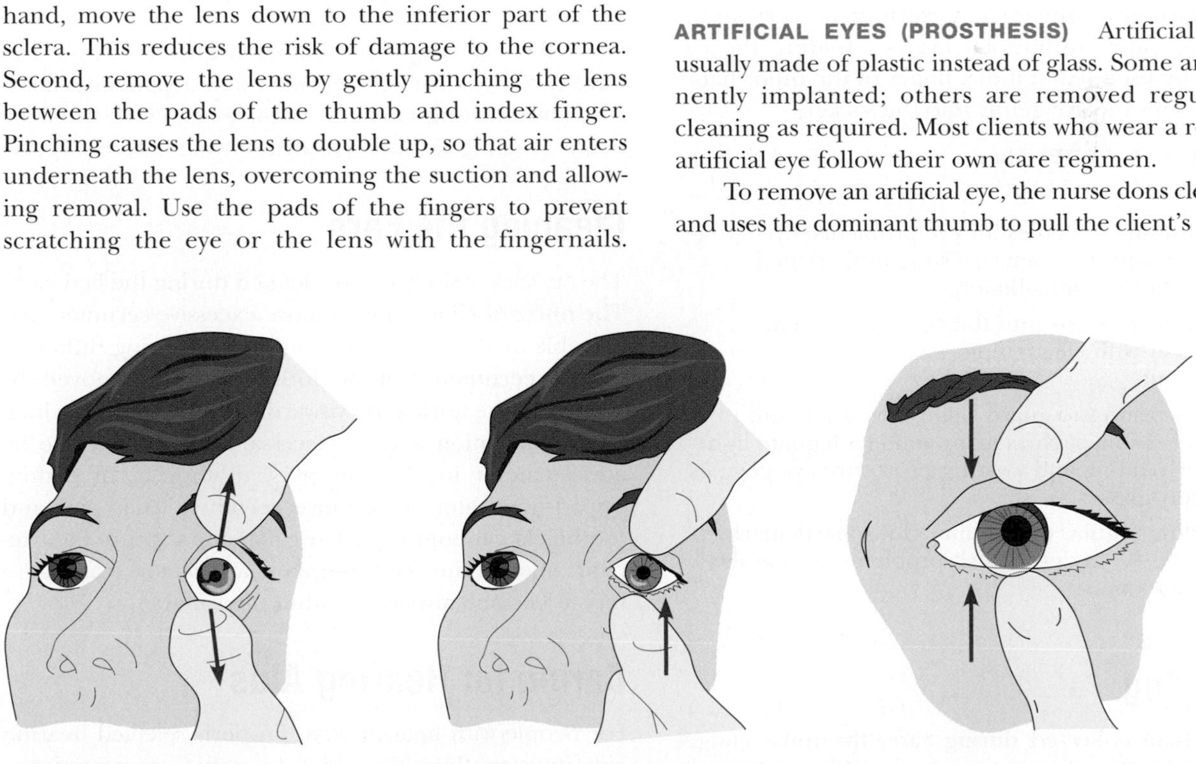

A B C

FIGURE 29.12 Removing hard contact lenses

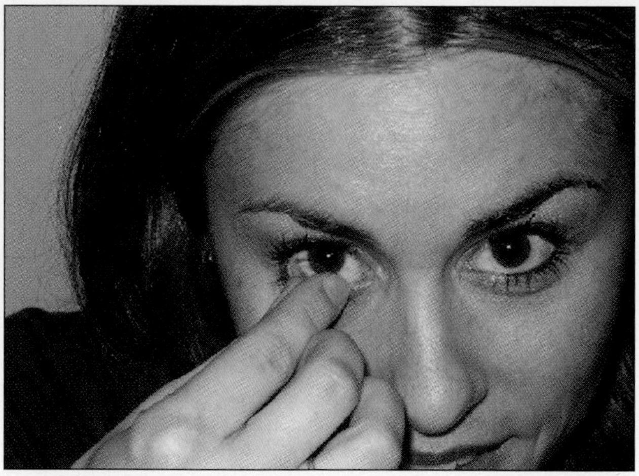

FIGURE 29.14 Removing a soft lens by pinching between the pads of the thumb and index finger

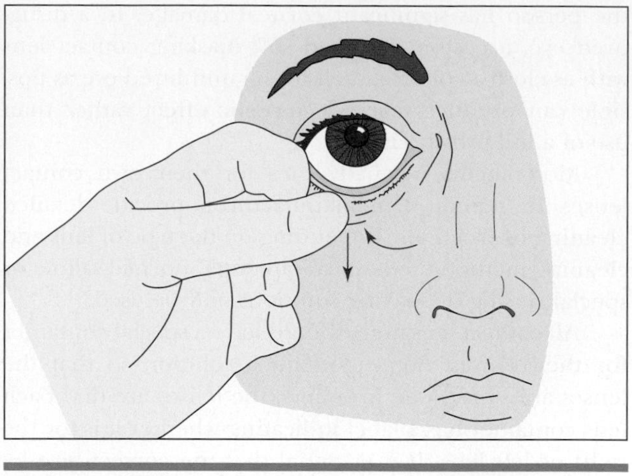

FIGURE 29.15 Removing an artificial eye by retracting the lower eyelid and exerting slight pressure below the eyelid

lid down over the infraorbital bone, exerting slight pressure below the eyelid to overcome the suction (Figure 29.15). An alternative method is to compress a small rubber bulb and apply the tip directly to the eye. As the nurse gradually releases the finger pressure on the bulb, the suction of the bulb counteracts the suction holding the eye in the socket and draws the prosthesis out of the socket.

The artificial eye is cleaned with warm normal saline and placed in a container filled with water or saline solution. The socket and tissues around the eye are usually cleaned with cotton wipes and normal saline. To reinsert the eye, the nurse uses the thumb and index finger of one hand to retract the eyelids, exerting pressure on the supraorbital and infraorbital bones. Holding the eye between the thumb and index finger of the other hand, the nurse slips the eye gently into the socket.

GENERAL EYE CARE Many clients may need to learn specific information about care of the eyes:

- Avoid home remedies for eye problems. Eye irritations or injuries at any age should be treated medically and immediately.
- If dirt or dust gets into the eyes, clean them copiously with clean, tepid water as an emergency treatment.
- Take measures to guard against eyestrain and to protect vision, such as maintaining adequate lighting for reading and wearing protective eye goggles or safety glasses.
- Schedule regular eye examinations, particularly after age 40, to detect such problems as cataracts and glaucoma.

Evaluating

By using data collected during care, the nurse judges whether desired outcomes have been achieved. The following are examples of desired outcomes to evaluate the effectiveness of nursing interventions:

- Conjunctiva and sclera free of inflammation
- Eyelids free of secretions
- No tearing
- No eye discomfort
- Demonstration of appropriate methods of caring for contact lenses
- Description of interventions to prevent eye injury and infection

Ears

Normally, ears require minimal hygiene. Clients who have excessive cerumen (earwax) and dependent clients who have hearing aids may require assistance from the nurse. Hearing aids are usually removed before surgery.

Cleaning the Ears

The auricles of the ears are cleaned during the bed bath. The nurse or client must remove excessive cerumen that is visible or that causes discomfort or hearing difficulty. Visible cerumen can be loosened and removed by retracting the auricle downward. If this measure is ineffective, irrigation may be necessary. Clients need to be advised never to use hair pins, toothpicks, or cotton-tipped applicators to remove cerumen. Hair pins and toothpicks can injure the ear canal and rupture the tympanic membrane; cotton-tipped applicators can cause wax to become impacted within the canal.

Caring for Hearing Aids

For people with hearing loss, properly selected hearing aids improve the ability to hear and to communicate. The basic intent of older hearing aids is simply to amplify sound. However, newer programmable hearing aids in

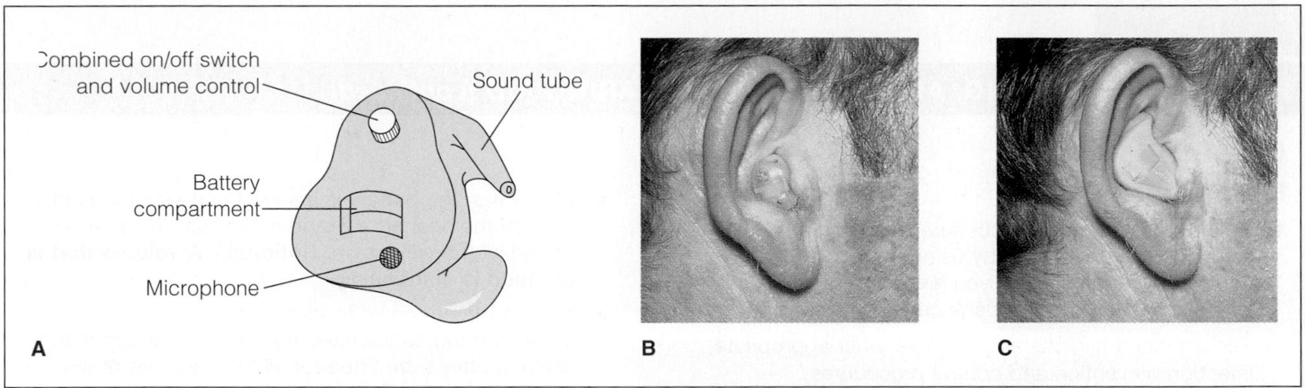

FIGURE 29.16 **A:** An in-the-ear hearing aid; **B:** small hearing aid in ear canal; **C:** large hearing aid in ear canal.

analog and digital types do not operate by amplifying sound; rather, they input auditory signals, and these signals are translated via a computer chip specific to the individual client.

Hearing aids consist of a microphone that picks up sound and converts it to electric energy, an amplifier that magnifies the electric energy electronically, a receiver that converts the amplified energy back to sound energy, and an earmould that directs the sound into the ear. Hearing aids have several types:

- *In-the-ear aid (ITE, or intra-aural).* This one-piece aid has all its components housed in the earmould (Figure 29.16).
- *In-the-canal (ITC) aid.* This is the most compact and least visible aid, fitting completely inside the ear canal. In addition to having cosmetic appeal, the ITC does not interfere with telephone use or the wearing of eyeglasses. However, it is not suitable for clients with progressive hearing loss; it requires adequate ear canal diameter and length for a good fit; and it tends to plug with cerumen more than other aids.

Hearing aids containing microcomputers are very sensitive to the effects of moisture and impact, both of which can cause extensive and often costly damage to the aid. Care must be taken to avoid exposing these aids to either source of damage.

For correct functioning, hearing aids require appropriate handling during insertion and removal, regular cleaning of the earmould, and replacement of dead batteries. With proper care, hearing aids generally last 5 to 10 years. Earmoulds generally need readjustment every 2 to 3 years. See the Home Care Considerations box and Skill 29.8 for hearing aid care.

Home Care Considerations

Hearing Aids

Clients may need to learn about their hearing aids:

- People who need a hearing aid may not wear one because they view the hearing aid as a stigma of old age.
- It is important for the client who just purchased a hearing aid to know that it often takes weeks or even months to adjust to the hearing aid. At first, sounds will seem shrill as they start hearing high-frequency sounds they had forgotten. Remind them that it is a hearing aid, not a hearing cure. Encourage them to not give up.
- The client needs to adjust to the hearing aid gradually by increasing the amount of time each day until the aid can be worn for a full day (Anderson, 1998).
- Encourage clients to purchase their hearing aids from a company that has a minimum warranty of a 30-day return policy.
- Emphasize the importance of maintaining the hearing aid by having it cleaned and checked regularly.

SKILL 29.8

REMOVING, CLEANING, AND INSERTING A HEARING AID

PURPOSE

- To maintain proper hearing aid function

ASSESSMENT

Determine whether the client has experienced any problems with the hearing aid and hearing aid practices. Assess for the presence of inflammation, excessive wax, drainage, or discomfort in the external ear.

Equipment

- Client's hearing aid
- Soap, water, and towels or a damp cloth
- Pipe cleaner or toothpick (optional)
- New battery (if needed)

(continued)

SKILL 29.8

REMOVING, CLEANING, AND INSERTING A HEARING AID *(continued)*

IMPLEMENTATION

Performance

1. Before performing the procedure, introduce yourself and verify the client's identity by using agency protocol. Explain to the client what you are going to do, why it is necessary, and how he or she can cooperate.
2. Perform hand hygiene and observe other appropriate infection prevention and control procedures.
3. Provide for client privacy by drawing the curtains around the bed or closing the door to the room. Some agencies provide signs indicating the need for privacy. **Rationale: Hygiene is a personal matter.**
4. Remove the hearing aid.
   - Turn the hearing aid off and lower the volume. The on/off switch may be labelled O (off), M (microphone), T (telephone), or TM (telephone/microphone). **Rationale: The batteries continue to run if the hearing aid is not turned off.**
   - Remove the earmould by rotating it slightly forward and pulling it outward.
   - If the hearing aid will not to be used for several days, remove the battery. **Rationale: Removal prevents corrosion of the hearing aid from battery leakage.**
   - Store the hearing aid in a safe place and label with client's name. Avoid exposure to heat and moisture. **Rationale: Proper storage prevents loss or damage.**
5. Clean the earmould.
   - Detach the earmould if possible. Disconnect the earmould from the receiver of a body hearing aid or from the hearing aid case of behind-the-ear and eyeglass hearing aids, where the tubing meets the hook of the case. Do not remove the earmould if it is glued or secured by a small metal ring. **Rationale: Removal facilitates cleaning and prevents inadvertent damage to the other parts.**
   - If the earmould is detachable, soak it in a mild soapy solution. Rinse and dry it well. Do not use isopropyl alcohol. **Rationale: Alcohol can damage the hearing aid.**
   - If the earmould is not detachable or is for an in-the-ear aid, wipe the earmould with a damp cloth.
   - Check that the earmould opening is patent. Remove any excess moisture through the opening or remove debris (e.g., earwax) with a pipe cleaner or toothpick.
   - Reattach the earmould if it was detached from the rest of the hearing aid.
6. Insert the hearing aid.
   - Determine from the client whether the earmould is for the left or the right ear.
   - Check that the battery is inserted in the hearing aid. Turn off the hearing aid, and make sure the volume is turned all the way down. **Rationale: A volume that is too loud is distressing.**
   - Inspect the earmould to identify the ear canal portion. Some earmoulds are fitted for only the ear canal and concha; others are fitted for all the contours of the ear. The canal portion, common to all, can be used as a guide for correct insertion.
   - Line up the parts of the earmould with the corresponding parts of the client's ear.
   - Rotate the earmould slightly forward, and insert the ear canal portion.
   - Gently press the earmould into the ear while rotating it backward.
   - Check that the earmould fits snugly by asking the client if it feels secure and comfortable.
   - Adjust the other components of a behind-the-ear or body hearing aid.
   - Turn the hearing aid on, and adjust the volume according to the client's preferences.
7. Correct problems associated with improper functioning.
   - If the sound is weak or there is no sound,
     a. Ensure that the volume is turned high enough.
     b. Ensure that the earmould opening is not clogged.
     c. Check the battery by turning the hearing aid on, turning up the volume, cupping your hand over the earmould, and listening. A constant whistling sound indicates the battery is functioning. If necessary, replace the battery. Be sure that the negative (–) and positive (+) signs on the battery match those where indicated on the hearing aid.
     d. Ensure that the ear canal is not blocked with wax, which can obstruct sound waves.
   - If the client reports a whistling sound or squeal after insertion,
     a. Turn the volume down.
     b. Ensure that the earmould is properly attached to the receiver.
     c. Reinsert the earmould.
8. Document pertinent data.
   - Removal and insertion of a hearing aid are not normally recorded.
   - Report and record any problems the client has with the hearing aid.

EVALUATION

- Speak to the client in a normal conversational tone and observe client behaviours.
- Compare the client's hearing ability to previous assessments.
- Report any deviations from normal for the client to the appropriate members of the health-care team.

Nose

Nurses usually need not provide special care for the nose, because clients can ordinarily clear nasal secretions by blowing gently into a soft tissue. When the external nares are encrusted with dried secretions, they should be cleaned with a cotton-tipped applicator or moistened with saline or water. The applicator should not be inserted beyond the length of the cotton tip; inserting it farther can cause injury to the mucosa.

Supporting a Hygienic Environment

Because people are usually confined to bed when ill, often for long periods, the bed becomes an important element in the client's life. A place that is clean, safe, and comfortable contributes to the client's ability to rest and sleep and to a sense of well-being. Basic furniture in a health-care facility includes the bed, bedside table, overbed table, one or more chairs, and a storage space for the client's clothing and other personal items. Most bed units also have a nurse call system, light fixtures, electric outlets, and hygienic equipment in the bedside table. Four types of equipment often installed in an acute-care facility are a *suction outlet* for several kinds of suction, an *oxygen outlet* for most oxygen equipment, an air outlet for nebulizers and humidifiers, and a *sphygmomanometer* to measure the client's blood pressure. Some long-term-care agencies also permit clients to have *personal furniture,* such as a television, a chair, and lamps, at the bedside. In the home, a client often has both personal and medical equipment.

Environment

When providing a comfortable environment, it is important to consider the client's age, severity of illness, and level of activity.

TEMPERATURE The very young, the very old, and the acutely ill frequently need a room temperature higher than normal. A room temperature between 20°C and 23°C is comfortable for most clients.

VENTILATION Good ventilation is important to remove unpleasant odours and stale air. Odours caused by urine, draining wounds, or vomitus, for example, can be offensive. Room deodorizers can help eliminate odours. However, good hygienic practices are the best way to prevent offensive body and breath odours. Hospitals are required to monitor smoking. Hospitals frequently no longer have smoking areas and prohibit smoking in any patient/client areas.

NOISE Ill persons are usually sensitive to noise, such as clanging of metal equipment, loud talking, and laughter. Nurses should try to control noise in health-care settings.

Hospital Beds

The frame of a hospital bed is divided into three sections. This permits the head and the foot to be elevated separately. Most hospital beds have electric motors to operate the moveable joints. The motor is activated by pressing a button or moving a small lever, located either at the side of the bed or on a small panel separate from the bed but attached to it by a cable, which the patient can readily use. See Table 29.11 for common bed positions.

Hospital beds are usually 65 cm high and 1 m wide, narrower than the usual bed so that the nurse can reach the patient from either side of the bed without undue stretching. The length is usually 2 m. Some beds can be extended in length to accommodate very tall patents. Long-term-care facilities for ambulatory residents usually have low beds to facilitate safe movement in and out of bed. Most hospital beds have high and low positions that can be adjusted either mechanically or electrically by a button or lever. The high position permits the nurse to reach the patient without undue stretching or stooping. The low position allows the patient to step easily to the floor.

MATTRESSES Mattresses are usually covered with a water-repellent material that resists soiling and can be cleaned easily. Most mattresses have handles on the sides called lugs by which the mattress can be moved.

Many special mattresses are also used in hospitals to relieve pressure on the body's bony prominences, such as the sacrum and heels. They are particularly helpful for clients confined to bed for long periods of time. For additional information about mattresses, see Chapter 33, Table 33.3 (page 949).

SIDE RAILS Side rails, or safety sides, are used on both hospital beds and stretchers. They are of various shapes and sizes and are usually made of metal or high-density plastic. Devices to raise and lower them differ. Often, one or two knobs are pulled to release the side and permit it to be moved. When side rails are being used, it is important that the nurse *never* leave the bedside while the rail or rails are lowered. Some side rails have two positions: up and down. Others have three: high, intermediate, and low.

For decades, the use of side rails was routine practice, with the rationale that the side rails serve as a safe and effective means of preventing clients from falling out of bed. Research, however, has not validated this assumption. Several studies have shown that raised side rails do not deter older clients from getting out of bed unassisted and can lead to more serious falls, injuries, and even death (Capezuti, 2004; Talerico & Capezuti, 2001). The move in an organization toward using evidence-based decision making for patient safety must be reinforced (O'Connor,

TABLE 29.11 Common Bed Positions

Flat 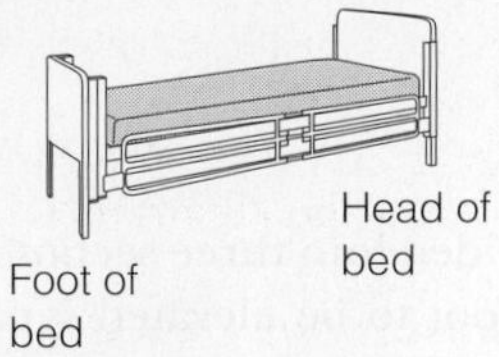	Mattress is completely horizontal.	Client sleeping in a variety of bed positions, such as back-lying, side-lying, and prone (face down) To maintain spinal alignment for clients with spinal injuries To assist clients to move and turn in bed Bed-making by nurse
Fowler's position 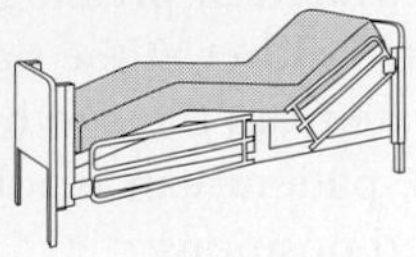	Semisitting position in which head of bed is raised to angle of at least 45°. Knees may be flexed or horizontal.	Convenient for eating, reading, visiting, watching TV Relief from lying positions To promote lung expansion for clients with respiratory problems To assist a client to a sitting position on the edge of the bed
Semi-Fowler's position 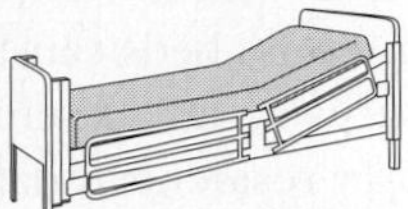	Head of bed is raised only to 30° angle.	Relief from lying position To promote lung expansion
Trendelenburg's position 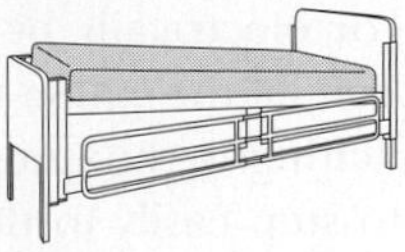	Head of bed is lowered and the foot is raised in a straight incline.	To promote venous circulation in certain clients To provide postural drainage of basal lung lobes
Reverse Trendelenburg's position 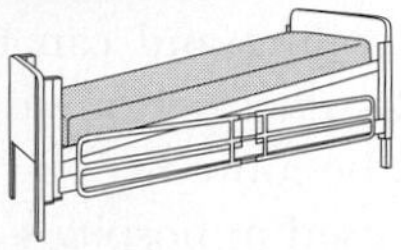	Head of bed raised and the foot lowered. Straight tilt in direction opposite to Trendelenburg's position.	To promote stomach emptying and prevent esophageal reflux in clients with hiatal hernias

Creager, Mooney, Laizner, & Ritchie, 2006). The routine use of side rails in both acute-care and long-term-care settings is now decreasing. Alternatives to side rails do exist and can include a low-height bed, bedrail bumper pads, motion sensors, bed alarms, use of nonskid socks, and clearing of clutter in the room (see Chapter 30, the section on "Safety in the Health-Care Settings").

FOOTBOARD OR FOOT BOOT The footboard or foot boot is used to support the immobilized client's foot in a normal right angle to the legs to prevent plantar flexion contractures. See Chapter 38, the section "Positioning Clients."

BED CRADLES A bed cradle, sometimes called an *Anderson frame,* is a device designed to keep the top bedclothes off the feet, legs, and even abdomen of a patient. The bedclothes are arranged over the device and may be pinned or tucked in place. Bed cradles come in several types. One of the most common is a curved metal rod that fits over the bed. Part of the cradle fits under the mattress, and small metal brackets press down on each side of the mattress to keep the cradle in place. The frame of some cradles extends over half of the width of the bed, above one leg.

INTRAVENOUS POLES Intravenous poles, usually made of metal, support intravenous (IV) infusion containers while fluid is being administered to a patient. These rods were traditionally freestanding on the floor beside the bed. Intravenous rods may also be attached to the hospital beds. Some hospital units have overhead hanging rods on a track for IVs.

MAKING BEDS Nurses need to be able to prepare hospital beds in different ways for specific purposes. In most instances, beds are made after the client receives certain care and when beds are unoccupied. At times, however, nurses need to make an occupied bed or prepare a bed for a client who is having surgery (an anaesthetic, postoperative, or surgical bed).

Regardless of what type of bed equipment is available, whether the bed is occupied or unoccupied, or the purpose for which the bed is being prepared, certain guidelines pertain to all bed-making. See Box 29.7.

BOX 29.7 BED-MAKING

The following guidelines apply to any bed-making:

- Wash hands thoroughly after handling a client's bed linen. Linens and equipment that have been soiled with secretions and excretions harbour microorganisms that can be transmitted to others directly or by the nurse's hands or uniform.
- Hold soiled linen away from uniform.
- Linen for one client is *never* (even momentarily) placed on another client's bed or furniture.
- Place soiled linen directly in a portable linen hamper or tucked into a pillow case at the end of the bed before it is gathered up for disposal. For esthetic purposes as well as to reduce transfer of microorganisms, placing soiled or dirty linens on the floor is to be avoided.
- Do not shake soiled linen in the air because shaking can disseminate secretions and excretions and the microorganisms they contain.
- When stripping and making a bed, conserve time and energy by stripping and making up one side as much as possible before working on the other side.
- To avoid unnecessary trips to the linen supply area, gather all linen before starting to strip a bed.

An *unoccupied bed* can be either closed or open. Generally, the top covers of an open bed are folded back (thus the term *open bed*) to make it easier for a client to get in. Open and closed beds are made the same way, except that the top sheet, blanket, and bedspread of a *closed bed* are drawn up to the top of the bed and under the pillows.

Bed sheets are often changed after bed baths. The linen can be collected before the bath. The linen is not usually changed unless it is soiled. Check the policy at each health agency. Unfitted sheets, blankets, and bedspreads are mitred at the corners of the bed. The purpose of mitring is to secure the bedclothes while the bed is occupied. Figure 29.17 shows how to mitre the corner of a bed. Skill 29.9 explains how to change an unoccupied bed.

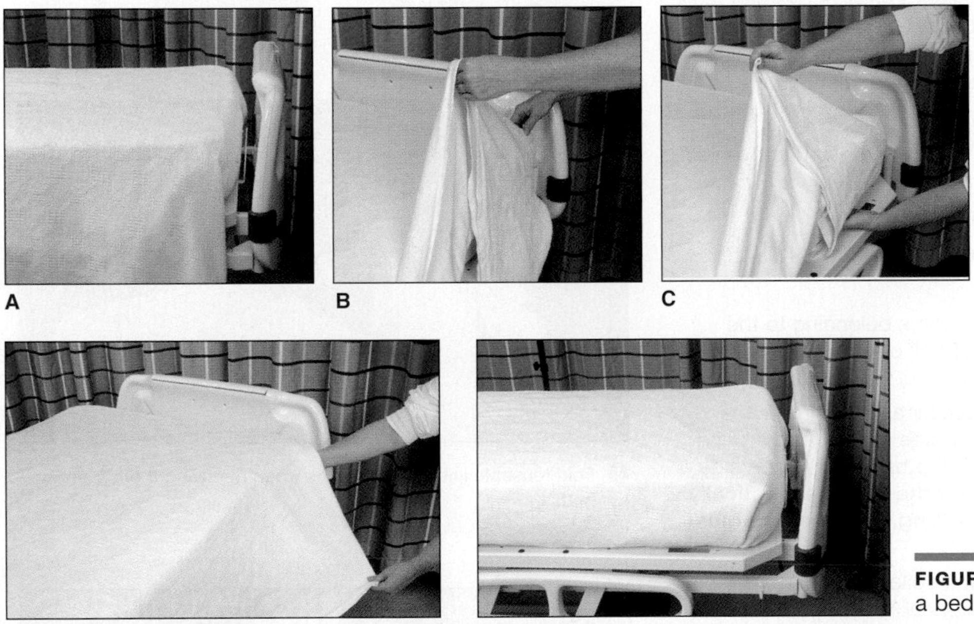

A B C D E

FIGURE 29.17 Mitring the corner of a bed

SKILL 29.9

CHANGING AN UNOCCUPIED BED

PURPOSES

- To promote the client's comfort
- To provide a clean, neat environment for the client
- To provide a smooth, wrinkle-free bed foundation, thus minimizing sources of skin irritation

ASSESSMENT

- Assess the client's health status to determine whether the person can safely get out of bed. In some hospitals/health-care facilities it is necessary to have a written order if the client has been in bed continuously.

(continued)

SKILL 29.9

CHANGING AN UNOCCUPIED BED *(continued)*

- Assess the client's pulse and respirations if indicated.
- Note all the tubes and equipment connected to the client. **Rationale: These may influence the need for additional linens or waterproof pads, or asssistance.**

Equipment

- Two flat sheets or one fitted and one flat sheet
- Cloth drawsheet (optional)
- One blanket
- One bedspread
- Waterproof pads (optional)
- Pillowcase for the head pillow
- Plastic laundry bag or portable linen hamper, if available

IMPLEMENTATION

Preparation

Determine what linens the client already has in the room *to avoid stockpiling of unnecessary extra linens.*

Performance

1. Before performing the procedure, introduce yourself and verify the client's identity by using agency protocol. Explain to the client what you are going to do, why it is necessary, and how he or she can cooperate.
2. Perform hand hygiene and observe other appropriate infection prevention and control procedures.
3. Provide for client privacy.
4. Place the fresh linen on the client's chair or overbed table; do not use another client's bed. **Rationale: This prevents cross-contamination (the movement of microorganisms from one client to another) via soiled linen.**
5. Assess and assist the client out of bed.
   - Make sure that this is an appropriate and convenient time for the client to be out of bed.
   - Assist the client to a comfortable chair.
6. Raise the bed to a comfortable working height.
7. Strip the bed.
   - Check bed linens for any items belonging to the client, and detach the call bell or any drainage tubes from the bed linen.
   - Loosen all bedding systematically, starting at the head of the bed on the far side and moving around the bed up to the head of the bed on the near side. **Rationale: Moving around the bed systematically prevents stretching, reaching, and possible muscle strain.**
   - Remove the pillowcases, if soiled, and place the pillows on the bedside chair near the foot of the bed.
   - Fold reusable linens, such as the bedspread and top sheet on the bed, into fourths. First, fold the linen in half by bringing the top edge even with the bottom edge, and then grasp it at the centre of the middle fold and bottom edges (see ❶). **Rationale: Folding linens saves time and energy when reapplying the linens on the bed and keeps them clean.**
   - Remove the waterproof pad and discard it if soiled.
   - Roll all soiled linen inside the bottom sheet, hold it away from your uniform, and place it directly in the linen hamper, not on the floor (see ❷). **Rationale: These actions are essential to prevent the transmission of microorganisms to the nurse, clients, and others.**
   - Grasp the mattress securely, using the lugs if present, and move the mattress up to the head of the bed.
8. Apply the bottom sheet and drawsheet.
   - Place the folded bottom sheet with its centre fold on the centre of the bed. Make sure the sheet is hem-side down for a smooth foundation. Spread the sheet out over the mattress, and allow a sufficient amount of sheet at the top to tuck under the mattress (see ❸). **Rationale: The top of the sheet needs to be well tucked under to remain securely in place, especially when the head of the bed is elevated.** Place the sheet along the edge of the mattress at the foot of the bed and do not tuck it in (unless it is a contour or fitted sheet).

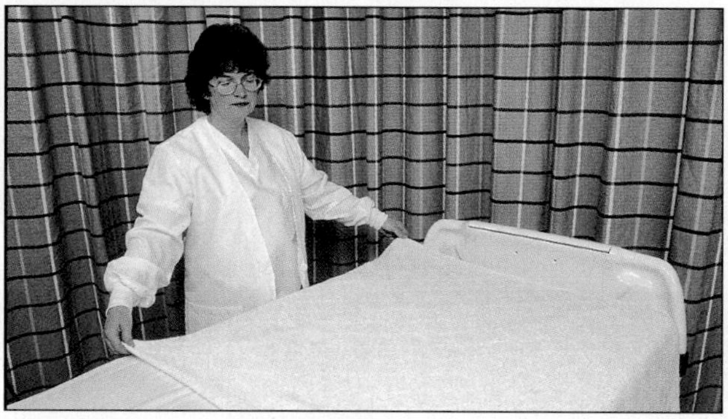

❶ Fold reusable linens into fourths when removing them from the bed.

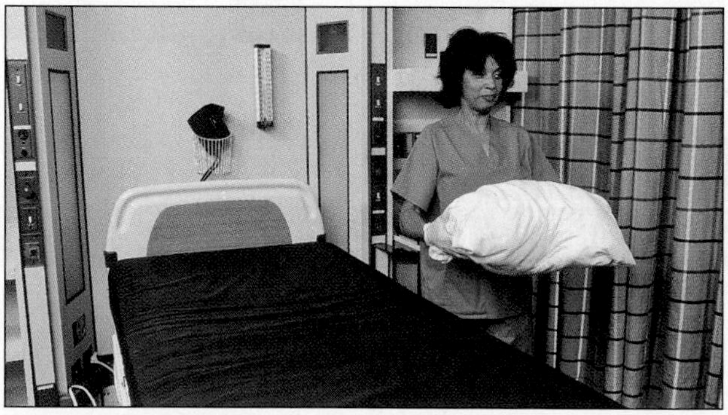

❷ Roll soiled linen inside the bottom sheet and hold away from the body.

(continued)

SKILL 29.9

CHANGING AN UNOCCUPIED BED *(continued)*

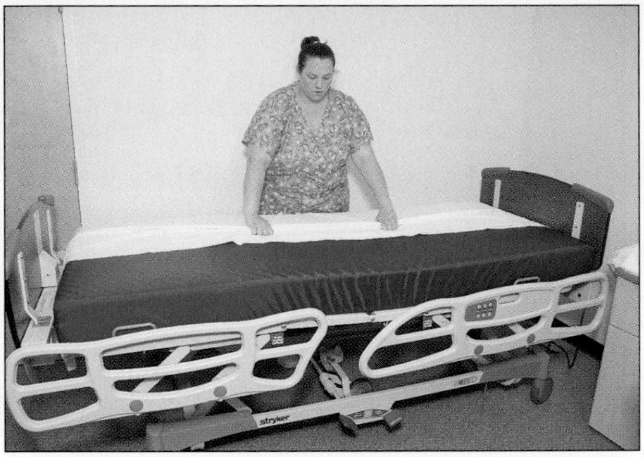

❸ Placing a bottom sheet on the bed

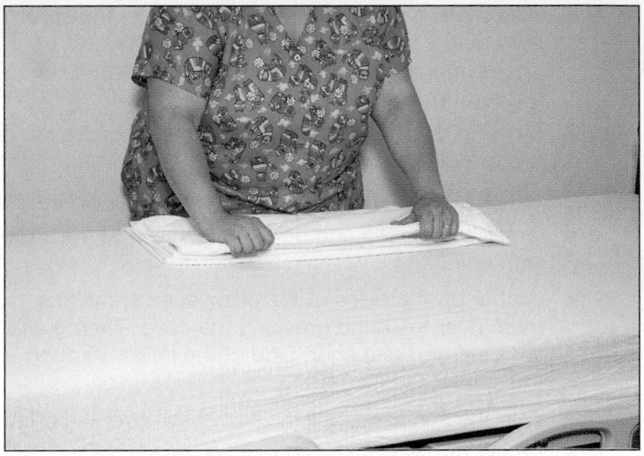

❹ Placing a clean drawsheet on the bed

- Mitre the sheet at the top corner on the near side (see Figure 29.17, p. 751) and tuck the sheet under the mattress, working from the head of the bed to the foot.
- If a waterproof drawsheet is used, place it over the bottom sheet so that the centrefold is at the centre-line of the bed and the top and bottom edges extend from the middle of the client's back to the area of the mid thigh or knee. Fanfold the uppermost half of the folded drawsheet at the centre or far edge of the bed and tuck in the near edge (see ❹).
- Lay the cloth drawsheet over the waterproof sheet in the same manner.
- *Optional:* Before moving to the other side of the bed, place the top linens on the bed hem-side up, unfold them, tuck them in, and mitre the bottom corners. **Rationale: Completing one entire side of the bed at a time saves time and energy.**

9. Move to the other side and secure the bottom linens.
   - Tuck the bottom sheet under the head of the mattress, pull the sheet firmly, and mitre the corner of the sheet.
   - Pull the remainder of the sheet firmly so that there are no wrinkles. **Rationale: Wrinkles can cause discomfort for the client and breakdown of skin.** Tuck in the sheet at the side.
   - Complete this same process for the drawsheet.

10. Apply or complete the top sheet, blanket, and spread.
    - Place the top sheet, hem-side up, on the bed so that its centrefold is at the centre of the bed and the top edge is even with the top edge of the mattress.
    - Unfold the sheet over the bed.
    - *Optional:* Make a vertical or a horizontal toe pleat in the sheet to provide additional room for the client's feet.

      a. *Vertical toe pleat:* Make a fold in the sheet 5 cm to 10 cm perpendicular to the foot of the bed (see ❺).

      b. *Horizontal toe pleat:* Make a fold in the sheet 5 cm to 10 cm across the bed near the foot (see ❻).

      Loosening the top covers around the feet after the client is in bed is another way to provide additional space.
    - Follow the same procedure for the blanket and the spread, but place the top edges about 15 cm from the head of the bed to allow a cuff of sheet to be folded over them.
    - Tuck in the sheet, blanket, and spread at the foot of the bed, and mitre the corner, using all three layers of linen. Leave the sides of the top sheet, blanket, and spread hanging freely unless toe pleats were provided.

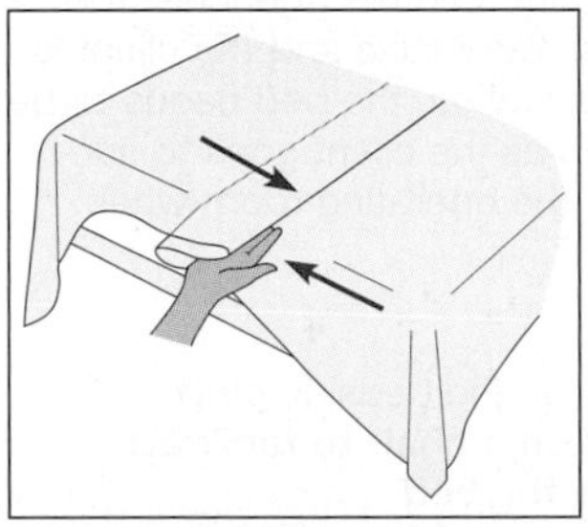

❺ A vertical toe pleat

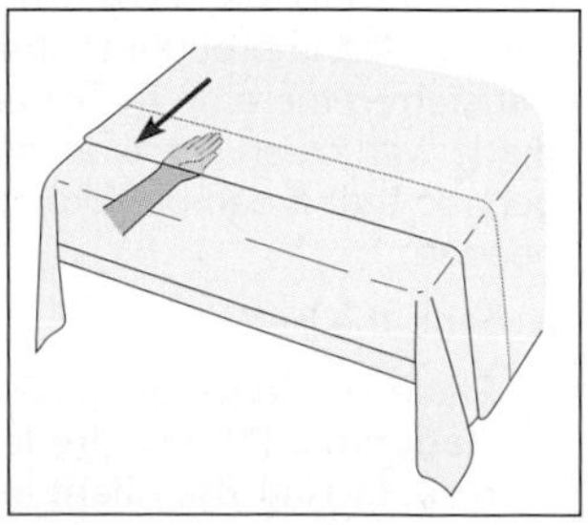

❻ A horizontal toe pleat

(continued)

SKILL 29.9

CHANGING AN UNOCCUPIED BED *(continued)*

- Fold the top of the top sheet down over the spread, providing a cuff (see ❼). **Rationale: The cuff of sheet makes it easier for the client to pull the covers up**.
- Move to the other side of the bed and secure the top bedding in the same manner.

11. Put clean pillowcases on the pillows as required.
    - Grasp the closed end of the pillowcase at the centre with one hand.
    - Gather up the sides of the pillowcase and place them over the hand grasping the case. Then grasp the centre of one short side of the pillow through the pillowcase (see ❽).
    - With the free hand, pull the pillowcase over the pillow.
    - Adjust the pillowcase so that the pillow fits into the corners of the case and the seams are straight. **Rationale: A smoothly fitting pillowcase is more comfortable than a wrinkled one**.
    - Place the pillows appropriately at the head of the bed.
12. Provide for client comfort and safety.
    - Attach the signal cord so that the client can conveniently reach it. Some cords have clamps that attach to the sheet or pillowcase. Others are attached by a safety pin.
    - If the bed is currently being used by a client, either fold back the top covers at one side or fanfold them down to the centre of the bed. **Rationale: This makes it easier for the client to get into the bed**.
    - Place the bedside table and the overbed table so that they are available to the client.
    - Leave the bed in the high position if the client is returning by stretcher, or place in the low position if the client is returning to bed after being up.
13. Document and report pertinent data.
    - Bed-making is not normally recorded.
    - Record any nursing assessments, such as the client's physical status and pulse and respiratory rates before and after being out of bed, as indicated.

Variation: Surgical Bed

While the client is in the operating room, the client's bed is prepared for the postoperative phase. In some agencies, the client is brought back to the unit on a stretcher and transferred to the bed in the room. In other agencies, the client's bed is brought to the surgery suite and the client is transferred there. In the latter situation, the bed needs to be made with clean linens as soon as the client goes to surgery so that it can be taken to the operating room when needed.

- Strip the bed.
- Place and leave the pillows on the bedside chair. **Rationale: Pillows are left on a chair to facilitate transferring the client into the bed**.
- Apply the bottom linens as for an unoccupied bed. Place a bath blanket on the foundation of the bed if this is agency practice. **Rationale: A flannel bath blanket provides additional warmth**.
- Place the top covers (sheet, blanket, and bedspread) on the bed as you would for an unoccupied bed. Do not tuck them in, mitre the corners, or make a toe pleat.
- Make a cuff at the top of the bed as you would for an unoccupied bed. Fold the top linens up from the bottom.
- On the side of the bed where the client will be transferred, fold up the two outer corners of the top linens so they meet in the middle of the bed, forming a triangle (see ❾).
- Pick up the apex of the triangle and fanfold the top linens lengthwise to the other side of the bed *to facilitate the client's transfer into the bed* (see ❿).
- Leave the bed in high position with the side rails down. **Rationale: The high position facilitates the transfer of the client**.
- Lock the wheels of the bed if the bed is not to be moved. **Rationale: Locking the wheels keeps the bed from rolling when the client is transferred from the stretcher to the bed**.

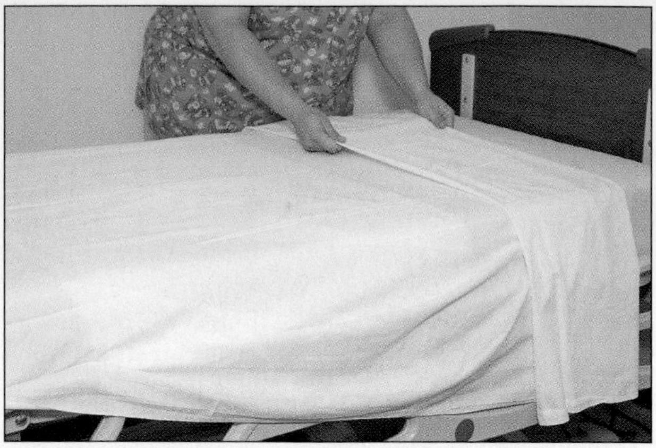

❼ Making a cuff of the top linens

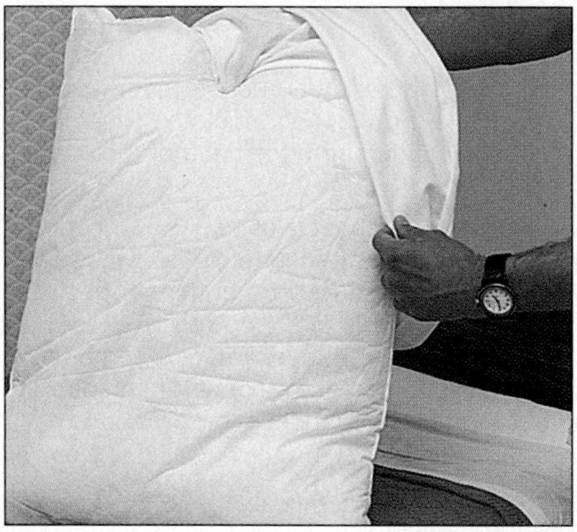

❽ Method for putting a clean pillowcase on a pillow

(continued)

SKILL 29.9

CHANGING AN UNOCCUPIED BED *(continued)*

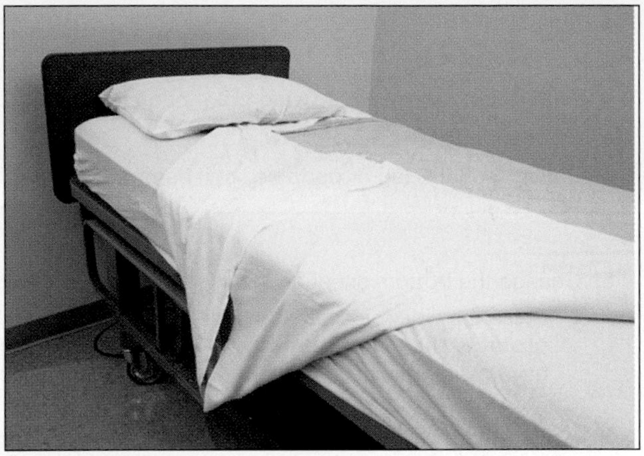

❾ Fold up the two outer corners of the top linens, forming a triangle.

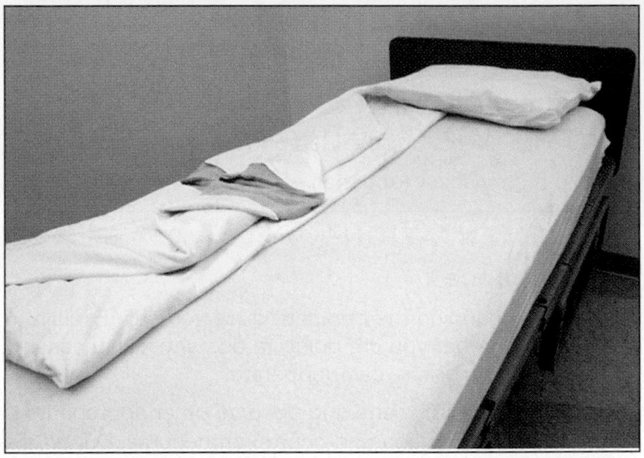

❿ Surgical bed: the linens are horizontally fanfolded to the other side of the bed to facilitate transfer of the client into the bed.

EVALUATION

- Make sure the call bell is accessible to the client.
- Relate client parameters of activity (e.g., pulse and respirations) to previous assessment data, particularly if the client has been on bed rest for an extended time or if it is the first time that the client is getting out of bed after surgery.

CHANGING AN OCCUPIED BED Some clients may be too weak to get out of bed. Either the nature of their illness may contraindicate their sitting out of bed, or they may be restricted in bed by the presence of traction or other therapies. When changing an *occupied bed,* the nurse works quickly, disturbs the client as little as possible to conserve the client's energy, and uses the following guidelines:

- Maintain the client in good body alignment. Never move or position a client in a manner that is contraindicated by the client's health. Obtain help, if necessary, to ensure the client's safety.
- Move the client gently and smoothly. Rough handling can cause the client discomfort and abrade the skin.
- Explain to the client what you plan to do throughout the procedure before you do it. Use terms that the client can understand.
- Use the bed-making time to assess and meet the client's needs.

Skill 29.10 describes how to change an occupied bed.

SKILL 29.10

CHANGING AN OCCUPIED BED

PURPOSES

- To conserve the client's energy
- To promote client comfort
- To provide a clean, neat environment for the client
- To provide a smooth, wrinkle-free bed foundation, thus minimizing sources of skin irritation

ASSESSMENT

- Note specific orders or precautions for moving and positioning the client.
- Determine the presence of incontinence or excessive drainage from other sources, indicating the need for protective waterproof pads.

(continued)

SKILL 29.10

CHANGING AN OCCUPIED BED *(continued)*

- Assess skin condition and the need for a special mattress (e.g., egg crate), footboard, or heel protectors.

Equipment

- Two flat sheets or one fitted and one flat sheet
- Cloth drawsheet (optional)
- One blanket
- One bedspread
- Waterproof drawsheet or waterproof pads (optional)
- Pillowcase for the head pillow
- Plastic laundry bag or portable linen hamper, if available

IMPLEMENTATION

Performance

1. Before changing the bed, introduce yourself. Explain to the client what you are going to do, why it is necessary, and how he or she can cooperate.
2. Perform hand hygiene and observe other appropriate infection prevention and control procedures. Put on disposable gloves if linen is soiled with body fluids.
3. Provide for client privacy.
4. Remove the top bedding.
   - Remove any equipment attached to the bed linen, such as a call light.
   - Loosen all the top linen at the foot of the bed, and remove the spread and the blanket.
   - Leave the top sheet over the client (the top sheet can remain over the client if it is being changed and if it will provide sufficient warmth), or replace it with a bath blanket as follows:
     a. Spread the bath blanket over the top sheet.
     b. Ask the client to hold the top edge of the blanket.
     c. Reaching under the blanket from the side, grasp the top edge of the sheet and draw it down to the foot of the bed, leaving the blanket in place (see ❶).
     d. Remove the sheet from the bed and place it in the soiled linen hamper.
5. Change the bottom sheet and drawsheet.
   - Raise the side rail nearest the client. **Rationale: This protects the client from falling**. If the bed does not have a side rail, have another nurse support the client at the edge of the bed.
   - Assist the client to turn on the side facing away from the side where the clean linen is.
   - Loosen the foundation of the linen on the side of the bed near the linen supply.
   - Fanfold the drawsheet and the bottom sheet at the centre of the bed (see ❷), as close to and under the client as possible. **Rationale: Doing this leaves the near half of the bed free to be changed**.
   - Place the clean bottom sheet on the bed, and vertically fanfold the half to be used on the far side of the bed as close to the client as possible (see ❸). Tuck the sheet under the near half of the bed and mitre the corner if a contour sheet is not being used.
   - Place the clean drawsheet on the bed with the centrefold at the centre of the bed. Fanfold the uppermost half vertically at the centre of the bed and tuck the near side edge under the side of the mattress (see ❹).
   - Assist the client to roll over toward you onto the clean side of the bed. The client rolls over the fanfolded linen at the centre of the bed.
   - Move the pillows to the clean side for the client's use. Raise the side rail before leaving the side of the bed.

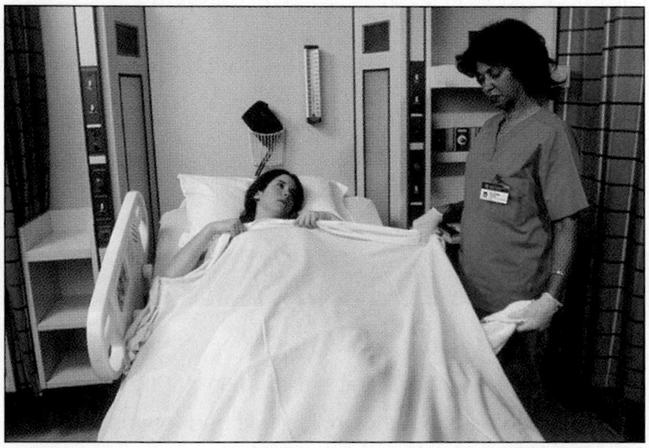

❶ Removing top linens under a bath blanket

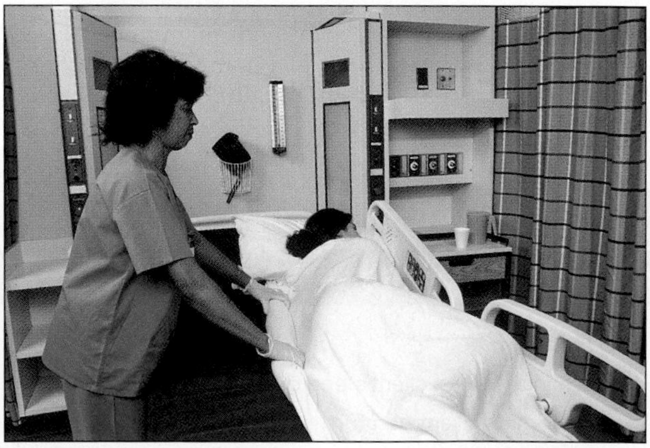

❷ Moving soiled linen as close to the client as possible

(continued)

SKILL 29.10

CHANGING AN OCCUPIED BED *(continued)*

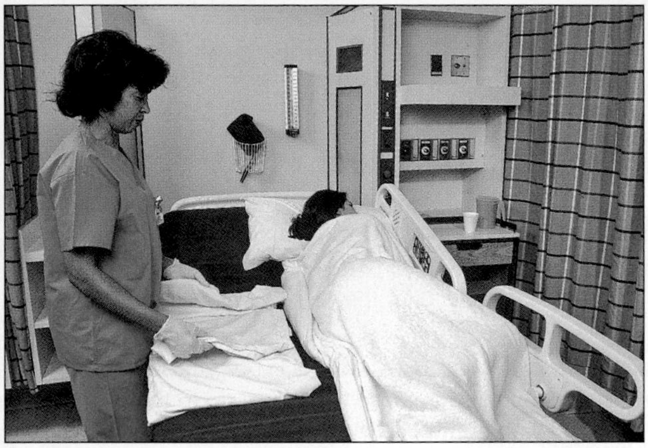

❸ Placing a clean bottom sheet on half of the bed

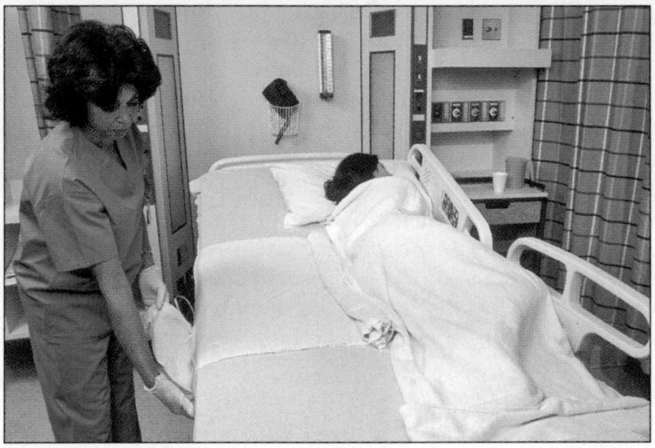

❹ Placing a clean drawsheet on the bed

- Move to the other side of the bed and lower the side rail.
- Remove the used linen and place it in the portable hamper.
- Unfold the fanfolded bottom sheet from the centre of the bed.
- Facing the side of the bed, use both hands to pull the bottom sheet so that it is smooth and tuck the excess under the side of the mattress.
- Unfold the drawsheet fanfolded at the centre of the bed and pull it tightly with both hands. Pull the sheet in three sections: (a) Face the side of the bed to pull the middle section, (b) face the far top corner to pull the bottom section, and (c) face the far bottom corner to pull the top section.
- Tuck the excess drawsheet under the side of the mattress.

6. Reposition the client in the centre of the bed.
   - Reposition the pillows at the centre of the bed.
   - Assist the client to the centre of the bed. Determine what position the client requires or prefers and assist the client to that position.
7. Apply or complete the top bedding.
   - Spread the top sheet over the client and either ask the client to hold the top edge of the sheet or tuck it under the shoulders. The sheet should remain over the client when the bath blanket or used sheet is removed (see ❺).
   - Complete the top of the bed.
8. Ensure the continued safety of the client.
   - Raise the side rails. Place the bed in the low position before leaving the bedside.
   - Attach the call bell to the bed linen within the client's reach.
   - Put items used by the client within easy reach.
9. Bed-making is not normally recorded.

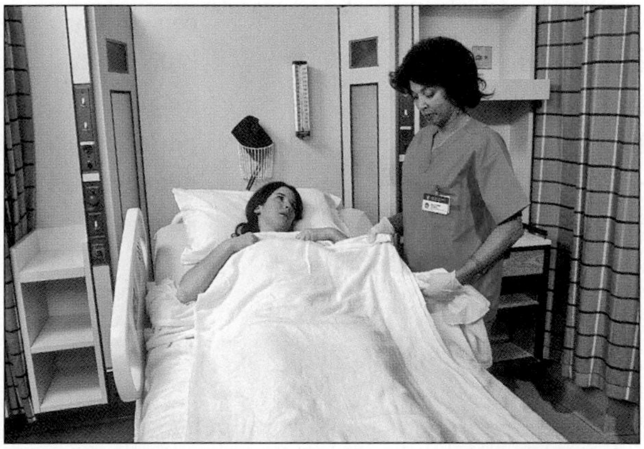

❺ Client holds top edge of sheet while nurse removes bath blanket

EVALUATION

Conduct appropriate follow-up, such as determining the client's comfort and safety, the patency of all drainage tubes, and the client's access to call bell to summon help when needed.

Case Study 29

It is the fourth day following Mrs. Pavica Perinic's abdominal surgery. She is progressing well, is ambulating several times each day, has been providing for her own hygienic needs, and is planning to go home tomorrow. During your early morning assessment, you note that Mrs. Perinic's hair is oily and she has an unpleasant body odour. Her dentures in a container at the bedside are in need of cleaning. You check her abdominal incision and verify that there is no drainage, redness, or signs of infection. You inquire about her ability to take care of her own bath and personal needs, and offer to assist her with her bath. She replies that she had a bath yesterday, doesn't feel that she needs another one today, and requests to omit her personal care for the day.

Critical Thinking Questions

1. Support or contradict the use of the nursing diagnosis *Self-Care Deficit: Bathing/Hygiene* as an appropriate nursing diagnosis for Mrs. Perinic.
2. Explain why it would be in Mrs. Perinic's best interests for you to assist her with hygienic care, even though she doesn't feel she needs a bath.
3. What factors should you consider before you attempt to encourage Mrs. Perinic to attend to her personal care?
4. What approaches might you use if you feel that Mrs. Perinic does need her hair shampooed and needs to have her personal care attended to?
5. What advantages does performing baths and personal hygiene for clients offer the nurse?

After working through these questions, go to the MyNursingLab at **http://www.mynursinglab.com** to check your answers.

KEY TERMS

hygiene
personal hygiene
sebum
bactericidal
sudoriferous (sweat) glands
apocrine glands
eccrine glands
cleansing bath
therapeutic bath
callus
corn
plantar warts
fissures
tinea pedis
ingrown toenail
crown
enamel
dentin
cementum
pulp cavity
gingiva
periodontal disease
dental caries
plaque
tartar
gingivitis
pyorrhea
sulcular technique
foam swabs
lanugo
ticks
lice
pediculosis
scabies
hirsutism

CHAPTER HIGHLIGHTS

- Clients' hygiene practices are influenced, to a large degree, by relevant health determinants.
- When clients cannot meet their own hygiene needs, the nurse assists them.
- The major functions of the skin are to help regulate body temperature, to protect underlying tissues, to secrete sebum, and to contain nerve receptors that act in sensory perception.
- The nurse considers clients' preferences when planning for their hygiene care.
- Nurses provide perineal-genital care for clients who are unable to care for themselves.
- Nurses can often teach clients how to prevent foot problems.
- Oral hygiene should include daily dental flossing and mechanical brushing of the teeth.
- Regular dental checkups and fluoride supplements are recommended to maintain healthy teeth.
- Nurses provide special oral care to clients who are unable to manage their own care (e.g., they are unconscious) and who have oral problems.
- Hair care includes daily combing and brushing and regular shampooing.
- Nurses may need to assist clients with their artificial eyes, eyeglasses, and contact lenses.

- Clients with hearing aids may require nursing assistance with the devices.
- Changing bed linens is a part of maintaining hygiene.
- It is important to keep beds clean and comfortable for clients.

ASSESS YOUR LEARNING

1. Mrs. Ouellette, 49 years old, is receiving intravenous antibiotic treatment. What should the nurse do with regards to the intravenous equipment?

a. Change the tubing at the first signs of discolouration.

b. Clean the insertion site for the antibiotic treatment every day with a physiological solution.

c. Reinforce the dressing to the intravenous site by adding extra adhesive tape every day.

d. Wash hands before and after handling the intravenous equipment.

2. The client is unresponsive and requires complete care. Before proceeding with mouth care on an unconscious client, the nurse will assess for which of the following?

a. Presence of any pain

b. Condition of the skin

c. Condition of the mouth

d. Presence of a gag reflex

3. A client with diabetes has very dry skin on her feet. To promote skin integrity of this client's feet, the nurse will suggest that the client do which of the following?

a. Soak her feet frequently.

b. Apply foot powder daily.

c. Use nonperfumed lotion.

d. Avoid knee-high stockings.

4. Appropriate treatment for an adolescent client with acne includes which of the following?

a. Frequent washing with very warm water and a mild commercial soap

b. Soaking with warm water, followed by gentle squeezing of pustules

c. Washing with medicated soap daily, with active abrading once a week

d. Washing with medicated soap, followed by application of medicated cream

5. Which of the following is a treatment for pediculosis in a child?

a. Melatonin 3.5% lotion and daily scalp massage while wearing gloves

b. Permethrin 1% cream rinse and use of a fine-toothed comb

c. Paraffin 2% solution left on scalp for 6 hours and then washed out

d. Peroxide 1% and baking soda in a paste that is brushed out when dried

6. In planning foot care for an older adult, which of the following is the correct rationale on which to base decisions about the care?

a. Use of lotion is avoided as this creates a moist environment for growth of bacteria.

b. It is sometimes necessary to extend the cutting of a nail into the sulcus (nail groove).

c. Painless calluses should not be removed as they provide protection for underlying tissue.

d. Unpleasant foot odours in older adults are usually the result of poor hygiene practices.

The next four questions are related to this scenario:

Tal Chakar-Aimaq is a 77-year-old man who had a cerebrovascular accident (stroke) 2 weeks ago. Although he has made a remarkable recovery, he has residual right-sided weakness and requires assistance to meet his hygiene needs.

7. The most relevant nursing diagnosis for this client is which of the following?

a. *Deficient Knowledge* related to not understanding how to manage his own care

b. *Potential for Altered Self-Esteem* related to inability to complete his own care

c. *Self-Care Deficit* related to inability to complete care independently

d. *Altered Skin Integrity* related to his not completing half of his hygiene

8. In considering hygiene care for Mr. Chakar-Aimaq, the nurse will adhere to which of the following principles?

a. The level of independence before illness is generally quite different from the present level.

b. If the nurse is doing the care, it is not necessary to assess the environment for safety.

c. To prevent frustration for the client, the nurse should recognize the client's limits.

d. Allow the client to do what he can or wants to do to, regardless of the time it takes.

9. Mr. Chakar-Aimaq tends to remain positioned on either his left side or on his back, and he moves very little without assistance. Which of the following is the priority nursing action intended to reduce the risk of skin breakdown?

a. Keep his skin dry and clean, and the bed linens free of wrinkles.

b. Ensure adequate hydration, and mobilize him frequently.

c. Use powder on his back, and change the bed linens twice a day.

d. Use pillows to prop him in his preferred position, and rub his back.

10. In planning hair care for Mr. Chakar-Aimaq, which of the following principles is a priority for the nurse to consider at this point in his recovery?

a. Shampooing should be done daily to maintain hygiene.

b. Brushing the hair improves circulation to the scalp.

c. Neglecting hair care is culturally unacceptable to him.

d. Asking Mr. Chakar-Aimaq what he prefers is inappropriate.

*After working though these questions, go to the MyNursingLab at **http://www.mynursinglab.com** to check your answers and see explanations.*

SUGGESTED READINGS

Kwan, S. Y. L., Petersen, P. E., Pine, C. M., & Borutta, A. (2005). Health-promoting schools: An opportunity for oral health promotion. *Bulletin of the World Health Organization, 83*(9), 677–695.

Schools provide an excellent opportunity for health promotion among students and, through teaching students, may possibly influence the health behaviours in families and communities. Poor oral health can affect children's quality of life, their performance at school, and their success in later life. The World Health Organization Global Health School Initiative is addressed, as well as some of the challenges in promoting health in developing and developed countries.

Subramanyan, K. (2004). Role of mild cleansing in the management of client skin. *Dermatology Therapy, 17,* 26–29.

Routine daily skin care is an essential part of comprehensive, holistic management of clients. Cleansing plays a role in removing unwanted dirt, soil, and bacteria from the skin as well as in removing dead surface cells, which prepares the skin to absorb any medicated creams or lotions. Cleansers based on mild synthetic surfactants or emollients cause minimal disturbance to the skin barrier, resulting in effective cleansing.

Turabelidze, G., Lin, M., Wolkoff, B., Dodson, B., Gladbach, S., & Zhu, B. P. (2006). Personal hygiene and methicillin-resistant staphylococcus aureus infection. *Emerging Infectious Diseases, 12*(3), 422–427.

This article concludes that improving hygiene practices and environmental conditions may help prevent methicillin-resistant staphylococcus aureus outbreaks in institutions, such as prison settings.

WEBLINKS

Centers for Disease Control and Prevention

http://www.cdc.gov/handhygiene/

This site provides guidelines and interactive training for hand hygiene in health-care settings.

Health Nexus

http://www.healthnexus.ca/events/upstream/speakers.htm

This bilingual website provides health promoters with a wide range of resources in an easy-to-use format.

REFERENCES

Anderson, E. G. (1998). Deafness is a scourge and you can say that again. *Geriatrics, 53*(8), 65–69.

Bulechek, G. M., Butcher, H. K., & Dochterman, J. C. (Eds.). (2008). *Nursing interventions classification (NIC).* St. Louis, MO: Mosby Elsevier.

Canadian Dental Association. (2005). *Flossing and brushing.* Retrieved on October 1, 2008, from http://www.cda-adc.ca/en/oral_health/cfyt/dental_care/flossing_brushing.asp

Capezuti, E. (2004). Guidelines address side rail entrapment. *American Journal of Nursing, 104*(5), 74.

Ebersole, P., Hess, P., Touhy, T., & Jett, K. (2005). *Gerontological nursing & healthy aging* (2nd ed.). Toronto: Elsevier (Mosby).

Evans-Smith, P. (2005). *Taylor's clinical nursing skills: A nursing process approach.* Philadelphia, PA: Lippincott Williams.

Grant, B. M., Giddings, L. S., & Beale, J. E. (2005). Vulnerable bodies: Competing discourses of intimate bodily care. *Journal of Nursing Education, 44*(11), 498–504.

Jackson, F. (1998). The ABC's of black hair and skin care. *ABNF Journal, 9*(5), 100–104.

Kwan, S. Y. L., Petersen, P. E., Pine, C. M., & Borutta, A. (2005). Health-promoting schools: An opportunity for oral health promotion. *Bulletin of the World Health Organization, 83*(9), 677–695.

Larson, E. L., Ciliberti, T., Chantler, C., Abraham, J., Lazaro, E. M., Venturanza, M., et al. (2004). Comparison of traditional and disposable bed baths in critically ill patients. *American Journal of Critical Care, 13*(3), 235–241.

Munro, C. L., Grap, M. J., & Kleinpell, R. (2004). Oral health and care in the intensive care unit: State of the science. *American Journal of Critical Care, 13*(1), 25–34.

Naik, A. D., Concato, J., & Gill, T. M. (2004). Bathing disability in community-living older persons: Common, consequential, and complex. *Journal of the American Geriatric Society, 52*(11), 1805–1810.

Naik, A. D., & Gill, T. M. (2005). Underutilization of environmental adaptations for bathing in community-living older persons. *Journal of the American Geriatric Society, 53*(9), 1497–1503.

Nainar, S. M., & Mohummed, S. (2004). Role of infant feeding practices on the dental health of children. *Clinical Pediatrics, 43*(2), 129–133.

NANDA International. (2007). *Nursing diagnoses: Definitions and classification, 2007–2008.* Philadelphia, PA: Author.

O'Connor, P., Creager, J., Mooney, S., Laizner, A. M., & Ritchie, J. A. (2006). Taking aim at fall injury adverse events: Best practices and organizational change. *Healthcare Quarterly, 9*(Sp), 43–49.

Scott Ricci, S. (2007). *Essentials of maternity, newborn, and women's health nursing.* Philadelphia, PA: Lippincott Williams & Wilkins.

Talerico, K. A., & Capezuti, E. (2001). Myths and facts about side rails. *American Journal of Nursing, 101*(7), 43–48.

Watt, R. C. (2005). Strategies and approaches in oral disease prevention and health promotion. *Public Health Reviews, 83*(9), 711–718.

Chapter 30

Safety

Patient safety is fundamental to nursing care and health care across all settings. It is not merely a mandate; it is a moral and ethical imperative in caring for others (Canadian Nurses Association [CNA], 2003). Because nurses work with individuals, families, groups, and communities in a range of settings (e.g., the home, schools, acute-care and long-term-care facilities, and community clinics) and with people across all points in the lifespan in both health and illness situations, they can play a major role in promoting the safety of the Canadian population. Through their vigilance, nurses act to keep patients safe, identify areas of risk, and recognize situations in need of improvement (Canadian Nurses Association & University of Toronto Faculty of Nursing, 2004; Nicklin, 2003).

Promoting safety includes preventing injury across all stages of the lifespan. The U.S. National Safety Council defines **injury** as "physical harm or damage to the body resulting from an exchange, usually acute, of mechanical, chemical, thermal, or other environmental energy that exceeds the body's tolerance" (Canada Injury, 2007). Injury may also result from lack of essential energy such as oxygen (e.g., asphyxiation) or heat (e.g., hypothermia) (Baker, O'Neill, Ginsburg, & Guohua, 1992). Although the terms *injury* and *accident* are sometimes used interchangeably, safety experts indicate that most injuries are predictable and therefore preventable, unlike **accidents**, which are random or chance events that are not preventable (Pless & Hagel, 2005). Injury can be differentiated by intent: **unintentional injuries** result from unplanned events, such as motor vehicle collisions, falls, drowning,

OBJECTIVES

After studying this chapter, you should be able to

1. Discuss nine factors that affect people's ability to protect themselves from unintentional injury
2. Describe the five parts to assessing clients at risk for unintentional injury
3. List the seven patient safety goals of the Canadian Council on Health Services Accreditation
4. Identify common potential hazards throughout the lifespan
5. Give examples of nursing diagnoses, outcomes, and interventions for clients at risk for unintentional injury
6. Plan strategies to maintain safety in the home, community, and health-care setting, including prevention strategies across the lifespan for motor vehicle accidents, thermal injury, falls, poisoning, suffocation or choking, excessive noise, electric hazards, and firearms
7. Explain measures to prevent falls
8. Discuss implementation of seizure precautions
9. Describe 12 alternatives to restraints
10. Describe the procedural steps in applying restraints and discuss the use and legal implications of restraints
11. List seven desired health outcomes to use in evaluating the selected strategies for injury prevention

fire, or the ingestion of foreign objects; **intentional injuries** are the result of purposeful harm, such as in the case of child abuse, assault, or homicide.

As a result of an increased awareness of the frequency and significance of adverse events, patient safety has become a key priority for all stakeholders. **Adverse events** are unintended injuries or complications that result in death, disability, or prolonged hospital stays and that are the result of health-care management (Royal College of Physicians and Surgeons, 2003). Specific to the health-care system, efforts are aimed at the reduction and mitigation of unsafe acts and at the use of evidence-informed practices that lead to optimal patient outcomes. Nurses themselves have their own safety concerns, owing to the nature of risks in the workplace setting. Providing a safe work environment for nurses so that they, in turn, can ensure the safety of the patients they work with has emerged as another priority in the health-care setting. See the Nursing and Canadian Society box for some facts on safety research and improvements and their implications for nursing practice.

Nursing and Canadian Society

Fact	Implications for Nursing Practice
Safer Healthcare Now! is a grassroots organization that was launched in 2005. It offers Canadian health-care organizations the opportunity to participate in and support a campaign dedicated to improving patient safety through the implementation of targeted interventions in patient care.	Nurses must be prepared to be challenged by all stakeholders when safety is an issue. Many Canadians are concerned and nurses must be aware that they are taking action. The interventions (e.g., preventing hospital-acquired infections; treating acute myocardial infarction) are of interest to nurses.
Safe Kids Canada is working toward a 25% reduction in preventable injuries by 2016. Its report *Child & Youth Unintentional Injury, 1994–2003: 10 Years in Review* (2006) indicates that Canadians have made progress in child safety, with overall death rates from childhood injury and hospitalization rates dropping by 37% and 34%, respectively.	Nurses can take advantage of the many safety initiatives of Safe Kids Canada, especially during Safe Kids Week. This organization advocates for the three E's in preventing childhood injuries: educate, engineer, enforce.
The Registered Nurses' Association of Ontario (RNAO) released its *Prevention of Falls and Fall Injuries in the Older Adult* best practice guideline in 2005.	Nurses require more evidence to inform their practice, particularly in such nurse-sensitive areas as fall prevention.
The *Canadian Patient Safety Dictionary* (Royal College of Physicians and Surgeons, 2003) provides definitions of several terms used in the area of patient safety. It provides a discussion on how recommended definitions were determined.	This dictionary helps to ensure that nurses and other members of the health-care team use a common language when assessing, monitoring, and evaluating patient safety issues.
The Canadian Patient Safety Institute (CPSI) was established in 2004 to provide a forum in which knowledge and information about optimal patient safety practices can be shared.	Nurses need the most up-to-date knowledge to guide their practice. The CPSI provides a forum in which key stakeholders can identify issues and evolve research programs to enhance patient safety.
The article "Safety in Home Care: A Broadened Perspective of Patient Safety" (Lang, Edwards, & Fleiszer, 2008) highlights key issues in understanding safety in home care settings.	As the trend toward home-based care continues, nurses must be aware of the safety issues in this setting; findings from this document have helped to establish research and care priorities.
The release of *Building a Safer System: National Integrated Strategy for Improving Patient Safety in Canadian Health Care* (Leonard, Hoffman, & the National Steering Committee on Patient Safety, 2002) was pivotal in establishing safety priorities within governmental and health-care systems, including a call to adopt a nonpunitive approach to errors in health care.	This report supported the need for system changes to enable nurses to provide safe care and advocated for a culture of safety in which nurses could feel "safe and supported" rather than "shamed and blamed" when they reported errors.

Factors Affecting Safety

People's ability to protect themselves from injury is affected by such factors as age and development, lifestyle, mobility and health status, sensory-perceptual alterations, cognitive awareness, emotional state, ability to communicate, safety awareness, and environmental factors. Nurses need to assess each of these factors when they plan care or help clients learn to protect themselves.

Age and Development

The age-dependent cognitive, psychological, language, and physical changes that occur across the lifespan influence an individual's ability to identify, anticipate, prevent, and recover from a range of health risks. Unfortunately, unintentional injury is the leading cause of death and hospitalization for children 1 to 14 years of age (Canadian Institute of Child Health, 2002). Canada ranks 22nd out of 29 Organisation for Economic Co-operation and Development (OECD) countries when it comes to preventable childhood injuries and deaths (Leitch, 2007).

Consider the following examples. Toddlers and preschool-age children are attracted to the water but generally lack a sense of danger. This is compounded by the fact that a top-heavy build makes them more vulnerable to falling into the water, and their relatively small lungs fill quickly with water. This age group has the highest incidence of drowning (Safe Kids Canada, 2006). The adolescent, whose thoughts usually include the *personal fable,* may believe he or she is immune to adverse outcomes when engaging in risky behaviour. In older adults, the combination of reduced reflex activity and diminished sensory acuity can lead to increased risk of falling. Box 30.1 summarizes selected safety hazards throughout the lifespan.

BOX 30.1 SELECTED SAFETY HAZARDS THROUGHOUT THE LIFESPAN

The following, organized by age groups most affected, are some important safety hazards. Preventive measures are discussed later in this chapter.

- *Developing fetus:* Exposure to teratogens (maternal smoking, alcohol, certain medications, radiation)
- *0–14 years*: The three leading causes of injury-related death are motor vehicle collisions (17%), drowning (15%), and threats to breathing (11%); almost half (44%) of injury-related hospitalizations are due to falls (Safe Kids Canada, 2006)
- *Newborns and infants:* Drowning; motor vehicle collisions (passenger); burns (e.g., spilled hot liquids, bath water), threats to breathing (choking, suffocation, strangulation), falls, electric shock, poisoning
- *Toddlers and preschoolers:* motor vehicle collisions (passenger and pedestrian or cyclist), drowning, falling, threats to breathing (choking, suffocation, strangulation), lacerations, burns, poisoning, electric shock, harm from other people or animals
- *School-age children:* Motor vehicle collisions (passenger and pedestrian or cyclist), drowning, all-terrain vehicle and snowmobile accidents, burns
- *Adolescents:* Motor vehicle collisions (passenger and pedestrian or cyclist), all-terrain vehicle and snowmobile accidents, falls, drowning, cycling accidents, problematic substance use
- *Older adults:* Falls, burns, and motor vehicle collisions (passenger and pedestrian)

Lifestyle

Lifestyle factors that place people at risk include unsafe work environments, residence in neighbourhoods with high crime rates, access to guns and ammunition, abuse of alcohol and street drugs, and lack of income to buy safety equipment or make necessary repairs. Risk-taking behaviour is a factor in some accidents.

Mobility and Health Status

People with impaired mobility because of paralysis, muscle weakness, or poor balance or coordination are at increased risk of injury. Clients with paraplegia may be unable to move even when they perceive discomfort. Hemiplegic clients or clients with leg casts often have poor balance and fall easily. Clients weakened by illness or surgery may not be fully aware of their limitations.

Sensory-Perceptual Alterations

Accurate sensory perception of environmental stimuli is vital to safety. People with impaired touch perception, hearing, taste, smell, and vision are highly susceptible to injury. A person who does not see well may trip over an object; a deaf person will not hear a siren in traffic; and people with anosmia (impaired olfactory sense) may not smell burning food or the sulphur aroma of a natural gas leak.

Cognitive Awareness

Awareness is the ability to perceive environmental stimuli and body reactions and to respond appropriately through thought and action. Clients with impaired awareness include people lacking sleep, unconscious or semiconscious persons, disoriented people who may not understand where they are or what to do to protect themselves, people who perceive stimuli that do not exist, and people whose judgment is altered by disease or medications (e.g., opioids, tranquilizers, hypnotics, and sedatives).

Emotional State

Extreme emotional states can alter the ability to perceive environmental hazards. Stressful situations can reduce a person's level of concentration, cause errors of judgment, and decrease awareness of external stimuli. People with depression may think and react to environmental stimuli more slowly than usual.

Ability to Communicate

Individuals with diminished ability to receive and convey information are at risk for injury. They include aphasic clients, people with language barriers, and those unable to read. For example, the person unable to interpret the sign "No smoking: oxygen in use" could cause a fire or an explosion.

Safety Awareness

Information about water safety, car safety, fire prevention, and the many age-specific hazards and their preventive measures is crucial to safety. Clients in unfamiliar environments (e.g., hospital) or dealing with new treatments (e.g., oxygen therapy, hot packs) frequently need specific safety information. The Reflect on Primary Health Care box describes how public participation can also raise safety awareness.

Environmental Factors

Depending on the client's situation, the nurse may need to assess the environment of the home, workplace, or community. Client safety is affected by the health-care setting. Bioterrorism has become a safety concern related to the environment.

HOME A safe home requires, among many things, well-maintained flooring and carpets, a nonskid bathtub or shower surface, strategically placed and functioning smoke alarms and carbon monoxide detectors, and knowledge of fire escape routes. Outdoor areas, such as swimming pools, need to be safely secured and maintained. Adequate lighting, both inside and out, will minimize the potential for accidents.

WORKPLACE A range of chemical, biological, physical, ergonomic, and psychosocial hazards exist in the workplace. Workers exposed to temperature extremes, those who lack adequate training on the use of mechanical equipment, or those who are the victims of sexual harassment or discrimination in the workplace are all at risk for ill health. The work environment of the nurse includes such risks to safety as exposure to viral or bacterial agents and potentially aggressive clients.

COMMUNITY Adequate street lighting; safe water and sewage treatment; restrictions on pollution, including smoke-free environments; and regulation of consumer products and sanitation in food buying and handling all contribute to a healthy, hazard-free community. A safe and secure community strives to be free of excess noise, crime, traffic congestion, dilapidated housing, or unprotected creeks and landfills.

HEALTH-CARE SETTING, INCLUDING HOME CARE Safety issues within the Canadian health-care setting have come to the forefront since the release of the *Canadian Adverse Events Study* (Baker et al., 2004) indicating that as many as 1 in 13 hospitalized patients can experience adverse events, including death, with as many as 3.9% of these events deemed preventable.

Safety problems arise from *acts of omission* (failure to institute the appropriate therapeutic intervention), such as lack of assessment to predict risk of falls, lack of discharge teaching; or *acts of commission* (incorrect diagnosis or treatment, or poor performance), such as errors in medication dosage, wrong-site surgery, restraint-related injuries or death, burns, mistaken identity, and hospital-acquired infection. The National Steering Committee on Patient Safety (Leonard et al., 2002) links errors, in part, to the gap between the increased complexity of care that has resulted from advances in diagnostic and treatment options, and outdated communication systems and poor product design. A shortage of qualified health-care personnel, the quality of communication patterns among health professionals, and the quality of the nursing practice environment have also been identified as influencing patient safety outcomes (Tourangeau, Cranley, & Jeffs, 2006). Patient safety is viewed as going beyond the blaming of individual professionals to looking at the multiple system factors whose complex interplay ultimately influences whether safety is assured.

Patient safety concerns also occur in home care situations. Family members, friends, and informal caregivers under the indirect supervision of medically trained personnel are taking on complex care, from administering intravenous antibiotics, through caring for a partner who is paralyzed, to caring for a child who is ventilator

REFLECT ON PRIMARY HEALTH CARE

Mothers Against Drunk Driving (MADD) is an example of how *public participation* can raise awareness about the role of alcohol and risk-taking behaviours in many unintentional injuries caused by motor vehicle collisions. Reflect on the benefits of *intersectoral cooperation*, such as a nurse and parent who has lost a child to drunk driving speaking at a high school preparing for its graduation dance or a rally to raise the minimum age for obtaining a driver's licence, in reducing the incidence of drunk driving.

dependent. Family members' safety may also be at risk as they take on such activities as lifting heavy equipment or moving their family member in and out of bed or a bath. Research is needed on the impact of home care on the physical, emotional, and functional safety of the patient, family, and other caregivers (Lang et al., 2008).

BIOTERRORISM When anthrax paralyzed the United States postal system after the September 11, 2001, terrorist attacks on the Twin Towers of New York City, awareness of bioterrorism as a threat to safety emerged. Terrorism includes chemical, biological, or nuclear weapons, but **bioterrorism** is the use of a microorganism with the deliberate intent of causing infection in order to achieve certain goals (Public Health Agency of Canada, 2001). Bioterrorism is of concern because it has potentially far-reaching effects because of easy transmission, high mortality rates, and public panic.

Assessing

Assessing clients at risk for unintentional injury involves (1) noting pertinent indicators in the nursing history and physical examination, (2) using specifically developed risk-assessment tools, (3) evaluating the client's home environment, (4) assessing standards related to patient safety goals in hospitals, and (5) addressing bioterrorism.

Nursing History and Physical Examination

The nursing history and physical examination can reveal considerable data about the client's safety practices and risks for injury. Data include age and developmental level; general health status; mobility status; presence of physiological or perceptual deficits, such as olfactory, visual, tactile, taste, or other sensory impairments; altered thought processes or impaired cognitive or emotional capabilities; problematic substance use; indications of abuse or neglect; and a history of unintentional injury. A safety history also includes the client's awareness of hazards, knowledge of safety precautions at home and at work, and any perceived threats to safety (Figure 30.1).

Risk-Assessment Tools

Risk-assessment tools are available to determine which clients are at risk for specific kinds of injury, such as falls, or for the general assessment necessary to keep clients safe in their homes and in health-care settings. In general, these tools direct the nurse to appraise multiple factors affecting safety. The tools summarize specific data contained in the client's nursing history and physical examination. Client risk factors and environmental hazards for falls are discussed later in this chapter.

Home Hazard Appraisal

Hazards in the home are major causes of falls, fire, poisoning, suffocation, and other accidents, such as those caused by improper use of household equipment, tools, and cooking utensils. See Chapter 13, Box 13.7 (page 247), for a summary of specific data necessary for a home hazard appraisal.

National Patient Safety Goals

The Canadian Council on Health Services Accreditation (CCHSA) augmented the assessment standards related to patient and client safety after the release of the *Canadian Adverse Events Study* (Baker et al., 2004). CCHSA (2007, 2008) identifies seven patient and client safety goals:

1. *Creating a culture of safety within the organization,* as evidenced by such indicators as a formal policy and process of disclosure of adverse events to patients or families; support mechanisms for patients, family, and care or service providers to help them recover from the emotional reactions that occur when receiving or being implicated in unintentional harm.
2. *Improving the effectiveness of coordination of communication among care and service providers and with the recipients of care or services across the continuum,* as evidenced by such indicators as patients or clients or the family being informed about their role in patient safety and staff taking seriously patient or family questions or comments about potential error (e.g., a patient who is surprised that he is being sent for a test may indicate that the wrong patient is being solicited); effective mechanisms for transfer of information at handoff points, such as change of shift, transfer between units or institutions, and discharge home; processes for verifying such high-risk care and service activities as the receiving of test results and the administration of surgical or other invasive procedures (e.g., how are the right patient and right operative site safely identified?).
3. *Ensuring the safe use of high-risk medications,* as evidenced by such indicators as the absence of concentrated electrolytes (e.g., potassium chloride) from care units; a limited number of drug concentrations being available on the care unit (multiple strengths of the same medication can contribute to overdosing or underdosing of the medication); and staff receiving adequate training on all infusion pumps to ensure the safe administration of parenteral drugs.
4. *Creating a work life and physical environment that supports the safe delivery of care and service,* as evidenced by training on patient safety to all staff; staff having a clear understanding of the roles, responsibilities,

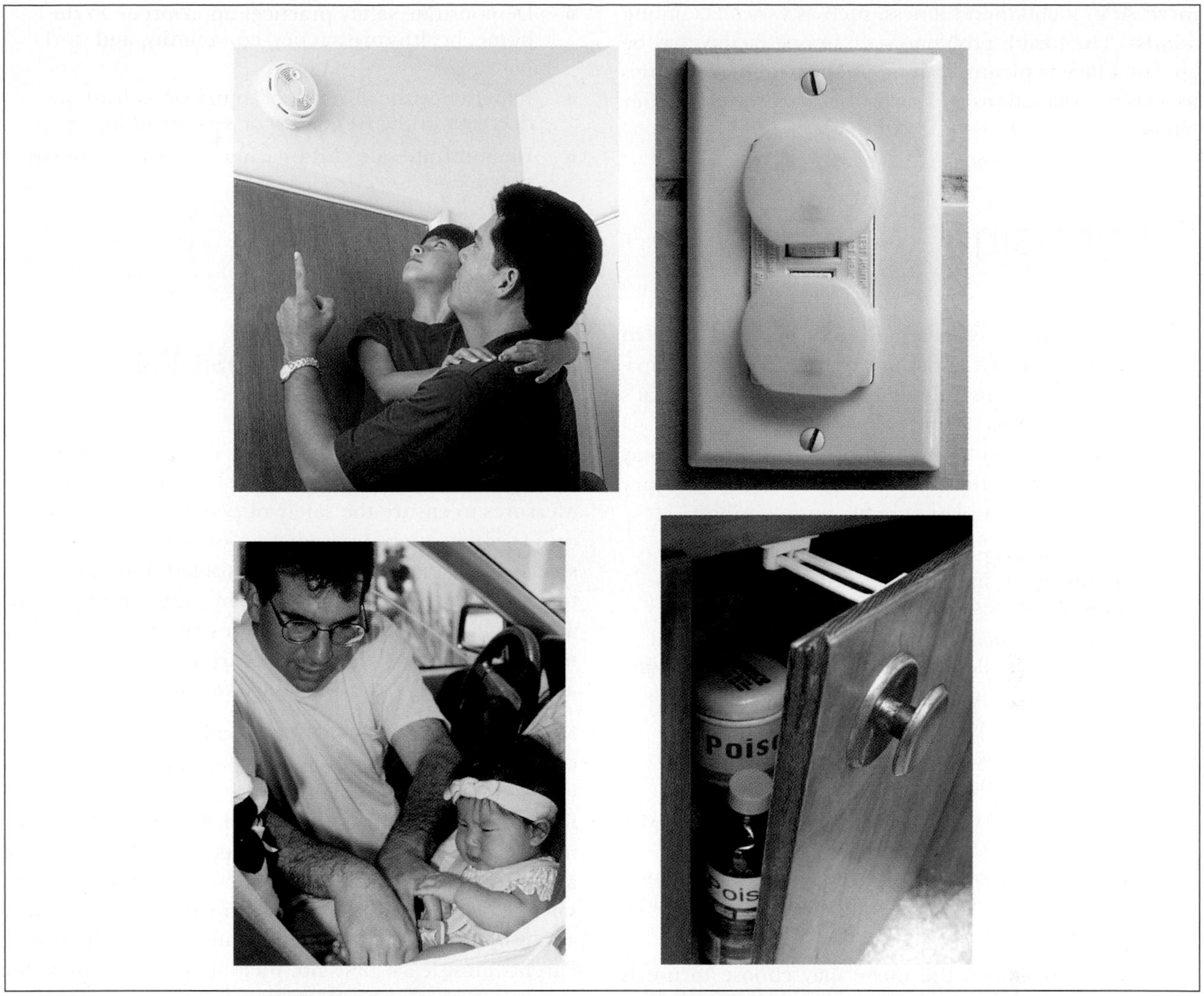

FIGURE 30.1 Nurses need to teach clients about safety and how to prevent accidents, such as by using smoke detectors, safety covers for electrical outlets, childproof locks on drawers and cabinets, and infant car seats.

and accountabilities of health-team members in relation to patient and client care and safety; and defective equipment not being used until adequately prepared.

5. *Reducing the risk of health services organization–acquired infections and their impact across the continuum of care and service,* as evidenced by adherence to federal and provincial or territorial infection control guidelines and implementation of protocols to ensure the administration of pneumococcal and influenza vaccines in at-risk populations (including health-care professionals).
6. *Reducing the risk of injuries resulting from patient falls,* as evidenced by implementing fall-prevention programs, identifying at-risk populations, and addressing their specific needs.
7. *Risk assessment in high-risk populations,* as evidenced by procedures for identifying those at risk for pressure ulcers or suicide.

The CCHSA assessment focuses on system-wide indicators of safety, marking a shift from the method of finding out who made the error (e.g., creating an environment of fear and scapegoating) to analyzing the system to find out why the error occurred (e.g., creating an environment of learning and improvement).

Bioterrorism

Health-care workers, especially emergency medical responders and front-line workers, many of whom are nurses, need to be alert to circumstances or patterns that can indicate bioterrorism, such as an unusual geographic clustering of illness (e.g., persons who attended the same public event), the hospital or community clinic receiving an increase of patients with similar symptoms, or an unusual age distribution for common diseases (e.g., an increase in a childhood illness, such as varicella, among adults). The health problems seen in one facility may be part of a bigger picture; calling public health authorities to report observations and suspicions may reveal a larger pattern.

Diagnosing

NANDA International (2007) offers a broad diagnostic label related to safety issues: *Risk for Injury:* A state in which the individual is at risk for injury as a result of environmental conditions interacting with the individual's adaptive and defence resources.

This broad label consists of subcategories that may be preferred when the nurse wants to describe injury more specifically or isolate suitable interventions:

- *Risk for Poisoning:* Accentuated risk of accidental exposure to, or ingestion of, drugs or dangerous products in doses sufficient to cause poisoning
- *Risk for Suffocation:* Accentuated risk of accidental suffocation (inadequate air available for inhalation)
- *Risk for Trauma:* Accentuated risk of accidental tissue injury (e.g., wound, burn, or fracture)
- *Latex Allergy Response:* A hypersensitive reaction to natural latex rubber products
- *Risk for Latex Allergy Response:* Risk of hypersensitivity to natural latex rubber products
- *Risk for Aspiration:* At risk for the entry of gastrointestinal secretions, oropharyngeal secretions, solids, or fluids into tracheobronchial passages

Another diagnosis the nurse may choose to use is *Deficient Knowledge (Accident Prevention):* Inability to state or explain information or demonstrate a required skill related to safety of self and others.

Planning

Nurses must use knowledge about the predictable and contributing factors related to unintentional injury as they plan their care. Nurses can help people understand that most *accidents* are not devoid of explanation; rather, they have one or more factors that could have been anticipated, predicted, and, most importantly, eliminated. The major goal for clients with safety risks is to prevent unintentional injury.

Nursing interventions to meet desired outcomes are largely directed toward helping the client and family to do the following:

- Identify and remove or reduce environmental hazards in the home, workplace, community, and health agency
- Demonstrate safety practices appropriate to the home, health-care agency, community, and workplace
- Experience the absence of injury or, at least, a decrease in the frequency or severity of injury
- Demonstrate safe childrearing practices or lifestyle practices

Implementing

Promoting Safety across the Lifespan

Hazards to safety occur at all ages and vary according to the age and development level of the individual. Measures to ensure the safety of people of all ages focus on (1) observation or prediction of potentially harmful situations so that harm can be avoided and (2) health teaching that promotes wellness by empowering clients and families to protect themselves from injury. Safety measures covering the lifespan from infancy to older adults are listed in the Teaching: Wellness box.

NEWBORNS AND INFANTS Accidents are a leading cause of death during infancy, especially during the first year of life. Infants are completely dependent on others for care and are oblivious to such dangers as falling or ingesting harmful substances. Parents need to learn the amount of observation necessary to maintain infant safety. They must continually anticipate risks and identify and remove common hazards in and around the home. Parents must learn first aid, including interventions for airway obstruction and cardiopulmonary resuscitation. Common accidents during infancy include drowning, motor vehicle collisions, burns, choking, suffocation or strangulation, falls, and poisoning. Education and support of parents can help them become knowledgeable and better prepared to protect their children.

TODDLERS Toddlers are curious and like to feel and taste everything. Their rapidly changing mobility skills, from crawling to walking to running, mean they can gain access to physical locations they were not able to reach as infants. They are fascinated by potential dangers, such as pools and busy streets, so they need constant supervision and protection (Figure 30.2, page 771). Parents can prevent many accidents by toddler-proofing the child's environment. This practice extends to using proper car restraints, promoting a safe environment to avoid falls, and removing or securing all items that can pose a safety hazard to the child.

PRESCHOOLERS Preschool-age children are active and can be clumsy, making them susceptible to injury. Environmental control continues, keeping hazards, such as matches, medicines, and other potential poisons, out of sight and reach. Safety education includes learning

TEACHING: WELLNESS

Safety Measures throughout the Lifespan

Across the lifespan, several measures can help promote safety:

NEWBORNS AND INFANTS

- Infant car seats must meet Canadian motor vehicle safety standards and be used correctly at all times. A rear-facing infant seat, properly secured in the back seat of the vehicle, is recommended from birth to about 1 year old. Check seat labels for specific weight and height limits and detailed installation instructions for particular models.
- Bath safety includes constant supervision and checking the water temperature before placing the child in the bath; turn cold water off last to avoid a burn if tap is inadvertently turned on.
- Hold the infant upright during feeding and do not prop the bottle if the infant is bottle fed. Bottle nipples displaying signs of wear and tear should be discarded. Cut food in small pieces, and do not feed the infant foods that could be choked on, such as peanuts, raisins, or popcorn. Hotdogs and gluey foods, such as white bread with peanut butter, can occlude an airway; cutting a wiener down the middle and then into small bits, and toasting the bread and spreading only a thin layer of peanut butter are safer alternatives.
- Health Canada (2004, 2007) indicated that cribs manufactured only after 1986 meet Canadian safety standards; the space between slats can be no more than 6 cm apart; no more than a 3 cm gap on any side is allowed when the mattress is pushed into one of the corners of the crib. *Bumper pads are not recommended.* To prevent strangulation, babies should never be harnessed or tied in a crib or placed near window blind or electric cords. Unless otherwise contraindicated, place the baby on his or her back to reduce the risk of sudden infant death syndrome.
- Use a playpen with sides made of small-size netting. Only playpens whose upper perimeter has protrusions (e.g., rivets, plastic knobs, bolts) that are less than half a centimetre are safe.
- Provide large soft toys with no small detachable or sharp-edged parts.
- To avoid strangulation, never tie or hang pacifiers or any other objects around the neck of a baby or a young child; Health Canada (2006) recommends that pacifiers be replaced at least every two months.
- Use guard gates on stairs and screens on windows. Gates that have large diamond-shaped or large V-shaped openings at the top are not allowed to be sold in Canada. Supervise the infant in swings and highchairs.
- Cover electrical outlets and keep cords out of reach.
- Place plants, household cleaners, and other potentially poisonous substances out of reach.
- Baby walkers have been banned from sale in Canada since 2004. Anyone with a hand-me-down baby walker is advised to destroy it.

TODDLERS AND PRESCHOOLERS

- A properly installed, forward-facing Canadian motor vehicle safety approved car seat is used with children who are between 10 kg and 18 kg, generally from about age 1 to 4 1/2 years (Transport Canada, 2006).
- Provide constant supervision when in or near water, including pools, baths, beaches, ditches, and wells. Safe Kids Canada recommends that adults remain within arms' reach if the child does not swim well. Fence-in pools according to provincial, territorial, or municipal standards. Safe Kids Canada (2007) recommends fences be at least 1.2 m high, enclosing all four sides of the pool and with a self-closing gate. Properly secured life jackets must be worn when boating.
- Avoid choking by not allowing children to run with anything in the mouth; teach children not to put small objects in their mouth or nose; ensure food is chewed properly: nuts, carrots, hard fruits, popcorn, and large pieces of hotdog are leading causes of choking in this age group; supervise balloon use: latex balloons are not recommended for play.
- To avoid strangulation, keep blind and curtain cords out of reach, remove drawstrings or cords on the child's clothing, avoid long scarves in winter (they can become snagged on play equipment). To avoid asphyxiation, remove doors from unused equipment, such as refrigerators.
- Children under 6 years of age should not be allowed to use a trampoline, even when supervised (Health Canada, 2006).
- Keep sharp objects (such as knives and scissors) out of children's reach.
- On the stove, place hot pots on back burners with the handles turned inward. Cover electrical outlets with plugs.
- Teach children about the dangers of playing with matches, fire, and heating appliances.
- Keep cleaning solutions, insecticides, medications, and other poisons in locked cupboards.
- Keep windows and balconies screened.
- Teach children not to run or ride into the street and supervise street crossing, including teaching about traffic lights and the importance of looking both ways.
- Obtain a low bed when the child begins to climb.
- Teach children to play in safe areas, not on streets and railroad tracks, and to avoid strangers.

(continued)

TEACHING: WELLNESS (*continued*)

SCHOOL-AGE CHILDREN

- A booster seat properly secured in the rear seat of a car is used from 18 kg until at least 36 kg, generally from age 4 1/2 to 8 years. Between approximately 9 and 14 years, children are secured in the rear seat with the seat belt (ideally with a shoulder belt). Front-seat airbags can be dangerous for children 12 or younger (Transport Canada, 2006).
- Teach children safety rules for recreational and sports activities: never swim alone, always wear a life jacket when in a boat, and wear protective gear (e.g., helmet, knee and elbow pads) when engaging in risky activities (e.g., hockey, skateboarding, inline skating, using a scooter).
- Supervise contact sports and activities in which children aim at a target.
- Teach children to obey all traffic and safety rules for bicycling, skateboarding, inline skating, and so on.
- Help children learn safe ways to use the stove, garden tools, and other equipment.
- Supervise children when they use saws, electric appliances, tools, and other potentially dangerous equipment.
- Teach children not to play with fireworks, gunpowder, or firearms. Keep firearms unloaded, locked up, and out of reach.
- Teach children to avoid excavation sites, quarries, vacant buildings, and playing around heavy machinery.
- Teach children the health hazards of smoking. If you smoke, stop.
- Teach children the effects of drugs and alcohol on judgment and coordination.

ADOLESCENTS

- Have adolescents complete a drivers' education course, and take practice drives with them in various kinds of weather.
- Set firm limits on automobile use (including all-terrain vehicles and snowmobiles): never drive after drinking or using drugs, always use seatbelts, and never ride with a driver who is under the influence of alcohol or drugs. Encourage adolescents to call home for a ride if they have been drinking, assuring them they can do so without a reprimand.
- Allow only adolescents over age 16 to drive an all-terrain (four-wheeled) vehicle or snowmobile (Canadian Paediatric Society, 2007; Safe Kids Canada, 2006). Safe Kids Canada recognizes that in some regions of Canada, all-terrain vehicles are the only means of transportation; it recommends safe, workable solutions to transportation, such as the child being accompanied by an adult.
- Teach adolescents to wear proper safety equipment (e.g., helmet, padding) when participating in sports (e.g., inline skating, hockey, football) or when riding scooters and other sports vehicles.
- Encourage adolescents to swim, jog, and go boating (always wearing a life jacket) in groups so they can get help in an emergency.
- Inform the adolescent of the dangers of alcohol, other drugs, and unprotected sex. Include teaching about date rape prevention and defence.
- Teach about the dangers of sunbathing and tanning beds. Encourage them to use sun block and wear protective clothing when doing outdoor activities.
- Be alert to changes in the adolescent's mood and behaviour. Listen to and maintain open communication with the adolescent. Open communication is a powerful preventive measure.
- Set a good example of behaviour that the adolescent can follow.

YOUNG ADULTS

- Reinforce motor vehicle safety: Use designated drivers or public transport if alcohol is consumed, routinely check brakes and tires, and use seat and shoulder belts or car seats for all passengers.
- Remind the young adult to repair potential fire hazards, such as electric wiring.
- Reinforce water safety: Know the depth of a pool or lake before diving; supervise backyard pools and other water activities; wear a life jacket when in a boat.
- Discuss evaluating the potential for workplace injuries or death when making decisions about a career or an occupation. Encourage the young adult to participate actively in programs that reduce occupational hazards.
- Reinforce the importance of limiting sun exposure, using sunblocking agents, and wearing protective clothing.
- Encourage young adults who are having trouble coping with the pressures, responsibilities, and expectations of adulthood to seek counselling.

MIDDLE-AGED ADULTS

- Reinforce motor vehicle safety: Use seat belts and drive within the speed limit, especially at night. Test visual acuity periodically.
- Make certain stairways are well lit and uncluttered.
- Equip bathrooms with hand grasps and nonskid bath mats.
- Test smoke detectors, fire alarms, and carbon monoxide detectors regularly.
- Keep all machines and tools in good working condition at work and at home. Follow safety precautions when using machinery.
- Reinforce safety measures taught earlier in life, such as the hazards of excessive sun exposure.

(continued)

TEACHING: WELLNESS (*continued*)

OLDER ADULTS

- Encourage the client to have regular vision and hearing tests.
- Assist the client to have a home hazard appraisal.
- Encourage the client to keep as active as possible.
- Ensure appropriate lighting and mark doorways and edges of steps as needed.
- Keep the environment tidy and uncluttered, and securely fasten rugs.
- Wear shoes or well-fitting slippers with nonskid soles.
- Use ambulatory devices as necessary (cane, crutches, walker, braces, wheelchair).
- Monitor gait and balance.
- Adapt living arrangements to one floor if necessary.
- Encourage exercise and activity as tolerated to maintain muscle strength, joint flexibility, and balance.
- Encourage the client to request assistance rather than take a risk.
- Keep the bed in the low position.
- Install grab bars in bathrooms and set the hot water tank at no more than 49°C.
- Instruct the client to rise slowly from a lying to a sitting to a standing position, and to stand in place for several seconds before walking.
- Encourage annual or more frequent review of all medications prescribed.

such things as how to cross streets or how to ride bicycles safely. Children must be cautioned to avoid known hazards, such as swimming without adult supervision. Parents must maintain careful surveillance as the developmental level of the preschooler does not allow for self-reliance in matters of safety. For example, telling a preschooler to stay away from the pool when no one is around *cannot replace* a latched enclosure in promoting the child's safety. The preschool-age child's cognitive and motor skills increase quickly; hence, safety measures must keep up with the acquisition of new skills.

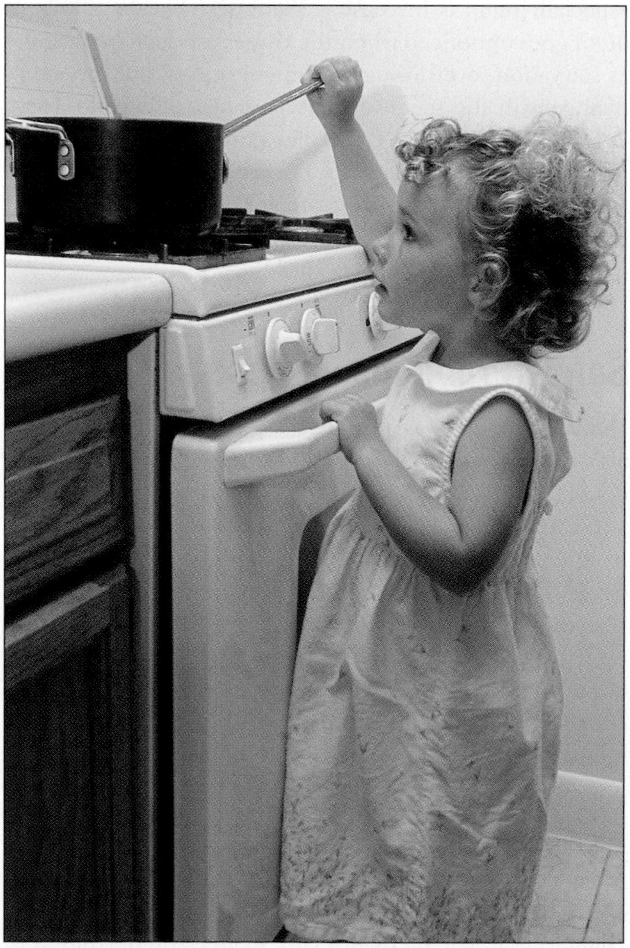

FIGURE 30.2 Promoting safety (e.g., by placing hot pots on back burners with handles turned inward) is required to keep children from injury.

SCHOOL-AGE CHILDREN By the time children attend school, they are learning to think before they act and must make safety decisions on their own as they are away from the constant supervision of parents and caregivers. They want to play with other children in such activities as bicycling, swimming, and skating. Although sensitive to peer pressure, the school-age child generally responds to rules. Accidents are the leading cause of death in school-age children, with the most frequent causes being motor vehicle collisions (including all-terrain vehicles and snowmobiles), drownings, and burns. School-age children often sustain unintentional injury during outdoor activities, such as bicycling, skateboarding, and inline skating, as well playing in playgrounds.

ADOLESCENTS Obtaining a driver's licence can be an important event in the life of an adolescent, but the privilege comes with many risks: motor vehicle collisions remain the leading cause of death and disability in Canadian teenagers. Because teens lack driving experience and may use driving as an outlet for stress, as a way to assert independence, or as a way to impress peers, parents need to assess the teenager's level of responsibility, problem solving, and ability to resist peer pressure as they determine driving privileges. The age of the teenager alone does not determine readiness to handle this responsibility.

Adolescents are at risk for sports injuries because their coordination skills are not fully developed. However, sports activities are important to the adolescent's self-esteem and overall development so all efforts must be made to provide protective equipment and foster safe play. Young workers have been identified as a particularly high-risk group for traumatic occupational injuries in Canada. Part-time employment status, lack of preparation and education in workplace risks, an eagerness to please, and viewing aches or pain simply as part of the job can all contribute to occupational injuries (Breslin, Polzer, MacEachen, Morrongiello, & Shannon, 2006). Parents can coach their adolescents to ensure that they get the necessary safety training specific for their job.

The adolescent's mental health may give rise to safety concerns related to suicide risk. Suicide, a form of intentional injury, is the second leading cause of death among teenagers, especially boys, and families need to be aware of the signs of suicidal ideation. Economic deprivation, family breakup, depression, and access to firearms are key factors influencing the high suicide rate in this age group, and family and friends can monitor those risks. Concerns about potential suicidal risk should be referred to a mental health professional or a crisis centre.

YOUNG ADULTS Motor vehicle collisions are the leading cause of mortality for this group; other causes of accidental death include drowning (especially men), burns, and firearms. Exposure to natural radiation from sunbathing or outdoor activities is a safety hazard for many young adults. Suicide is another leading cause of death in this age group, and it is thought that many suicides are mistaken for accidental death (e.g., automobile accidents, drug overdoses). As during adolescence, the prevention of suicide includes identifying behaviours that indicate potential problems: depression, decreased interest in previously pleasurable activities, and an increase in isolation. A young adult identified as being at risk for suicide should be referred to a mental health professional or a crisis centre.

MIDDLE-AGED ADULTS Changing physiological factors, as well as preoccupations with personal, family, and work-related responsibilities, may contribute to the accident rate of middle-aged persons. Motor vehicle collisions are the most common cause of accidental death in this age group. Decreased reaction times and decreased visual acuity can make the middle-aged adult prone to accidents. Other accidental causes of death in this age group include falls, burns, poisonings, and drownings. Occupational accidents continue to be a significant safety hazard during the middle years.

OLDER ADULTS Accident prevention is a major concern for older adults. For some, because vision is limited, reflexes are slowed, or bones are brittle, climbing stairs, driving a car, and even walking require caution. Driving, particularly at night, requires caution because the accommodation of the eye to light is impaired and the peripheral vision is diminished. Older adults need to learn to turn their head before changing lanes and should not rely on side vision, for example, when crossing a street or changing lanes.

Fires are a hazard if memory problems are present; appliances may be left on or cigarettes may not be extinguished. Because of reduced sensitivity to pain and heat, care must be taken to prevent burns when the person bathes or uses heating devices. People at risk for wandering because of organic brain syndromes need to wear identification devices. They can also be registered with the local Alzheimer Society of Canada's Safely Home program.

Decrease in temperature regulation in the older adult can increase the risk of hypothermia and hyperthermia. Reduced renal function increases the risk of toxicity from medications (e.g., the older adult who takes analgesics or sedatives may become lethargic or confused). The nurse teaches the importance of taking only prescribed medications and that over-the-counter medications must be reported because they can influence the pharmacokinetics or pharmacodynamics of prescribed medications.

A home environment that was previously safe may need modifications for older adults to decrease the risk of injury. A plan and telephone numbers of those to call should be available for emergency situations.

Unfortunately, the incidence of suicide in older adults, especially men, is increasing (Statistics Canada, 2007). It often goes unnoticed when the causes are such behaviours as starvation, overdosing with medications, and noncompliance with the medical treatment plan. Ebersole, Hess, Touhy, Jett, & Luggen (2008) list important factors linked to suicide risk in older adults: uncontrollable pain, loss of a loved one, major life changes, major depression, and social isolation. Unlike other age groups, older adults rarely threaten suicide; they just do it.

Safety Problems across the Lifespan

Domestic violence is a safety concern involving individuals of all ages. It includes child abuse, intimate partner abuse, and abuse of older adults, and it affects the health and safety of families and the community. Statistics are likely inaccurate because of the underreporting of incidents. Nurses should be involved in working with all phases of domestic violence: prevention, screening, referrals for treatment, and follow-up care. Situations of domestic violence usually necessitate interprofessional collaboration among the health-care team, law enforcement agencies, and other community agencies.

Safety in the Health-Care Setting

Since the release of the *Canadian Adverse Events Study* (Baker et al., 2004), health-care agencies have rallied to address patient safety. The basis for the provision of safe nursing care is addressed throughout a range of chapters in this book, for example, Chapter 31 addresses safe medication administration practices, and Chapter 32 focuses on nursing care to minimize health-care associated infection. Leonard et al. (2004) and Kohn, Corrigan, and Donaldson (2000) suggest that beyond learning specific details of direct nursing care and knowing the CCHSA safety goals, nurses need to work toward building new systems to improve patient safety by doing the following:

- Creating a culture of safety in which human error is viewed as inevitable and, subject to limited qualifications, no blame is assigned when adverse events are reported. Disclosures of errors and near-miss situations are encouraged so that in-depth analysis can take place to minimize risks of subsequent similar events.
- Conducting a comprehensive assessment of known and potential safety issues and providing education, anticipatory guidance, and learning opportunities, such as the use of simulated high-risk scenarios to rehearse or learn skills that are essential to patient safety.
- Promoting effective teamwork and communication. Client safety may be at risk if critical, relevant information is not communicated appropriately between and among members of the health-care team.
- Involving health-care workers in the design of work processes and workspaces to promote efficiency and safety.

Preventing Specific Hazards

Implementing measures to prevent specific hazards or unintentional injuries, such as scalds and burns, fires, falls, poisoning, suffocation, electrocution, and so on are critical aspects of nursing care. Nurses have many opportunities and responsibilities to implement health teaching about a range of known safety hazards.

SCALDS AND BURNS A **scald** is a burn from a hot liquid or vapour, such as steam. A **burn** results from excessive exposure to thermal (scald, flame, contact), chemical, electric, or radioactive agents.

Examples of home hazards that can cause scalds include pot handles that protrude over the edge of a stove, electric appliances (used to heat liquids or oils) with dangling cords, and excessively hot bath water. Although Safe Kids Canada (2005) recommends that hot water tanks be set at *no more than 49°C,* the majority of water tanks in Canadian homes are set at 60°C, the temperature at which a person can sustain a third-degree burn within 1 to 5 seconds!

Touching a stovetop element can cause a contact burn; accidental ingestion of a caustic cleaning product can cause a chemical burn. The risk of scalds and burns is greater for clients whose skin sensitivity to temperature is impaired, such as a patient with peripheral neuropathy who cannot sense that a heat pack is too hot. The nurse must assess how well clients can protect themselves and what special precautions, if any, need to be taken.

FIRES Fires continue to be a constant risk in both health-care settings and homes. Agency fires usually result from malfunctioning electrical equipment or combustion of anaesthetic gas. Home fires most frequently result from careless disposal of burning cigarettes or matches, from grease, or from faulty electrical wiring.

AGENCY FIRES In health-care agencies, fire is particularly hazardous when people are incapacitated and unable to leave the building without assistance. It is extremely important for nurses to be aware of the fire safety regulations and fire-prevention practices of the agency in which they work. When a fire occurs, the nurse follows four sequential priorities that can easily be remembered using the RACE mnemonic:

R **R**escue and **R**emove persons who are in immediate danger.
A **A**ctivate the fire alarm and call for help.
C **C**ontain or **C**onfine the fire and smoke (e.g., close doors).
E **E**xtinguish the fire if possible; otherwise **E**vacuate.

Extinguishing the fire requires knowledge of three categories of fire, classified according to the type of material that is burning:

- *Class A:* Paper, wood, upholstery, rags, ordinary rubbish
- *Class B:* Flammable liquids and gases
- *Class C:* Electrical

The right type of extinguisher must be used to fight the fire. Extinguishers have picture symbols showing the type of fire for which they are to be used. Nurses and clients should ensure they know how the extinguishers in their settings function so that they can be ready to use them in case of an emergency.

HOME FIRES Nursing interventions for home fires focus on teaching fire safety, including the following:

- Keep lighters and matches out of sight and reach of children, have regular inspections of electrical systems, and adopt a no smoking policy (especially in bed or on the couch).
- Keep emergency numbers near the telephone, or stored for speed dialling.
- Ensure that smoke alarms, fire extinguishers, and carbon monoxide detectors are operable and appropriately located.
- Test smoke alarms and carbon monoxide detectors monthly and change batteries twice a year (if not hard-wired). Choosing special days, such as birthdays, January 1 and June 1, or the days the clocks change for daylight savings time, can help people remember this important safety detail.
- Have a family fire drill plan. Every member needs to know the nearest exit from different locations of the home.
- In the event of a fire, close the windows and doors if possible; cover your mouth and nose with a damp

cloth when exiting through a smoke-filled area; and avoid heavy smoke by assuming a bent position with the head as close to the floor as possible.

FALLS People of any age can fall, but infants, toddlers, and older adults are particularly at risk for falls causing serious injury. Falls are the leading cause of unintentional injuries among older adults, with upward of 58% of seniors seen in emergency rooms being there because of falls (Canadian Hospitals Injury Reporting and Prevention Program, 2002). Falls in older adults are linked to multiple modifiable and nonmodifiable biological or medical, behavioural, environmental, and socioeconomic factors (Public Health Agency of Canada, 2005; RNAO, 2005).

Biological or medical factors include gait instability and lower-limb weakness; reduced general physical fitness; impaired balance and/or gait; vision problems, such as reduced acuity, difficulty accommodating to light and darkness; cognitive impairment; chronic illness, in particular arthritis, stroke, and Parkinson's disease; and acute illness events.

Behavioural factors include a positive fall history; a fear of falling, which can lead to tension and stiffness, making the person more susceptible; risk-taking behaviour, such as not heeding warnings of risk; taking culprit medications, such as antihypertensive agents or diuretics, that can lead to orthostatic hypotension or cardiac syncope, and benzodiazepines, such as alprazolam (Xanax) or diazepam (Valium); polypharmacy (taking five or more medications); excessive alcohol intake; and footwear (poor fitting; slippery footing), clothing (can cause tripping or can get caught on objects or in doorways), and handbags (can cause imbalance or get caught in doorways).

Environmental factors include stairs, in-home features like lack of grab bars, inadequate lighting, clutter, and scatter rugs. Socioeconomic factors include low income, poor housing, and reduced sense of connectedness (which links to going out unassisted).

Although hip and femur fractures are the most frequent complication of falls in older adults (followed by wrist facture) (Public Health Agency of Canada, 2005), a hip fracture may actually *precede* a fall, thus *causing* it. In fact, it is estimated that 40% of falls leading to hospitalization are the *result* of hip fractures and that the number of hip fractures will increase dramatically from 23 375 in 1993 to more than 88 000 cases by the year 2041, as the Canadian population ages (Smartrisk, 1998).

Most falls occur in the home and usually involve falling down stairs and in the bedroom or bathroom. Fear of falling is common in older adults, especially those who live alone and who anticipate being helpless and unable to summon help after a fall. For these individuals the nurse should encourage daily or more frequent contact with a friend or family member, installation of a personal emergency response system, and measures to maintain a physical environment that prevents falls. Selected risk factors and associated preventive measures for falls are shown in Table 30.1.

Evidence-Informed Practice

What Safety Hazards Do Older Adults Deal with When Attempting to Maintain Their Health by Regular Walking?

Physical activity in the form of walking enhances physiological, psychological, and social health. However, walking is also associated with falls in older adults, particularly when they encounter environmental hazards. So, it becomes a paradox: seniors are at risk from inactivity (e.g., reduced muscle mass, osteoporosis, social isolation), yet active seniors are at risk from being active (e.g., falls).

Lockett, Willis, and Edwards (2006) asked a group of 13 seniors living in an urban centre to take pictures (a research method called photovoice) of barriers to and facilitators of walking in their Ottawa neighbourhoods. The photos and focus group discussions about their experiences revealed that *safety* was the main consideration for deciding whether and where to walk. Fall hazards predominated, with concerns and visual documentation of poorly maintained sidewalks, uneven surfaces, and lack of rest stops. Participants who used assistive devices, like a walker, reported "insurmountable" risks during the winter. The article provides a series of photos to illustrate important risks of one woman's trip to the shopping mall.

NURSING IMPLICATIONS: Nurses must be aware that walking on a daily or thrice weekly basis can be almost impossible for many older clients. Nurses should ask clients how easy or difficult it is to perform this activity and look for alternative solutions when the barriers pose a risk. Community nurses can establish intersectoral collaborations to address the range of hazards, such as lobbying for safer sidewalks. The use of photos (photovoice) is an interesting strategy to enhance the quality and quantity of relevant data that the nurse can collect—the photos provide details and insights that would otherwise be missed. These client-specific data can help nurses develop more accurate assessment and analysis of health issues, as well as ensuring more relevant goals and interventions.

Source: Based on "Through Seniors' Eyes: An Exploratory Qualitative Study to Identify Environmental Barriers to and Facilitators of Walking," by D. Lockett, A. Willis, and N. Edwards, 2006, *Canadian Journal of Nursing Research, 3*(3), pp. 48–65.

TABLE 30.1 Risk Factors and Preventive Measures for Falls

Risk Factors	Preventive Measures
History of falling	Conduct a detailed analysis of the reasons underlying any previous falls to determine modifiable factors or circumstances that can become preventive measures. Protective measures (such as hip pads and kneepads) should be considered if previous preventive measures have not been successful.
Poor vision	Ensure eyeglasses are functional. Encourage the client to allow time for visual adjustment if wearing bifocals. Ensure lighting is appropriate, including having a light switch at the top and bottom of stairs. Night lighting of stairs and hallways that does not need to be switched on is also recommended (Public Health Agency of Canada, 2006). Mark doorways and stair edgings as needed. Encourage the client to keep the environment tidy.
Presence of stairs, in particular if stair geometry is non-uniform, steep, winding, or curved	Look for securely attached handrails on each side of the stairway; handrails should extend, without a break, the full length of the stairs as well as beyond the bottom and top of the stairs with a tactile indicator (i.e., slight bend) to indicate the stair is coming to an end. If the stairs are problematic, ask the client to consider renovating them to Canada Mortgage and Housing Corporation (2003) recommendations (rise no higher than 178 mm, with a run not shorter than 279 mm).
Cognitive dysfunction (confusion, disorientation, impaired memory, or judgment)	Set safe limits to activities. Remove unsafe objects. Consider the need for constant surveillance.
Gait instability (impaired gait or balance) or lower-limb weakness or dysfunction	Ask the client to wear shoes or well-fitting slippers with nonskid soles. Have the client use ambulatory devices as necessary (cane, crutches, walker, braces, wheelchair). Ensure the environment is uncluttered and rugs are securely fastened. Suggest the client adapt living arrangements to one floor, if feasible. It may require installing an additional phone or bathroom, and having frequently used items nearby. Encourage exercise and activity as tolerated to maintain muscle strength and joint flexibility. Tai Chi exercises can enhance balance (Li et al., 2005; RNAO, 2005). Suggest the client wear hip protectors (underwear types exist) or elbow and knee protectors as protective measures.
Difficulty getting in and out of a chair or bed	Encourage the client to request assistance. Keep the bed in the low position. Install a side rail on the bed to provide grip. Install grab bars in bathrooms and raised toilet seats.
Orthostatic hypotension	Instruct the client to rise slowly from a lying to a sitting to a standing position and to stand in place for several seconds before walking.
Urinary frequency, nocturia (having to get up in the night to urinate), receiving diuretics	Provide a bedside commode (without wheels). Assist with voiding on a frequent and scheduled basis.
Weakness from disease process or therapy	Encourage the client to summon help. Monitor activity tolerance.
Polypharmacy (clients taking more than five medications) or those prescribed benzodiazepines, tricyclic antidepressants, selective serotonin-reuptake inhibitors, trazodone	Monitor orientation and alertness status. Discuss how alcohol contributes to fall-related injuries and encourage the client not to mix alcohol and medications or avoid alcohol if necessary. Encourage annual or more frequent review of all medications prescribed. Discuss alternative solutions to such symptoms as anxiety and insomnia other than benzodiazepines.

CLINICAL ALERT

Although falls can break bones, broken bones can cause falls. When a client is brought to hospital for treatment of a bone fracture, it is important to determine if a fracture caused the fall or if the fall caused the fracture. The health history of the former scenario generally reveals pain or a "cracking noise" before the fall. Falls in older adults may be due to arrhythmias, problems with the vestibular apparatus, hypoglycemic episodes, hypotensive episodes, or being pushed (in the case of abuse).

The nurse can use an assessment tool, called the Get Up and Go (GUG) Test, in a hospital, subacute, or home setting. Kimbell (2002) describes the following steps of the test:

1. Observe the client's posture while he or she sits in a straight-backed chair.
2. Ask the client to rise from the chair into a standing position. Observe whether the client stands by using only the leg muscles or if the client needs to push himself or herself up with the hands.
3. Once the client is comfortably standing, ask him or her to close the eyes. Does the client sway?
4. Ask the client to open his or her eyes, walk 3 metres, turn around, and return to the chair. Observe gait, balance, speed, and stability. How smoothly does the client turn?
5. When the client gets to the chair, ask him or her to turn and sit down. Observe how smoothly the client performs this motion.

The GUG score ranges from 0 to 4. The client who is able to perform all five steps with ease receives a score of 0; the score is 1 if the client must use his or her hands to get out of the chair; the client who is able to stand but requires multiple pushes to get up scores a 3; and the client who is unable to get up without assistance receives a 4. This quick assessment, along with an assessment of the client's environment, can help the nurse recommend safety measures to the client and family.

Prevention of falls in health-care agencies is an ongoing concern. Other than the illness process that necessitates hospitalization, being in a hospital poses additional fall risks (e.g., an unfamiliar environment, reluctance to ask for help for fear of being a burden, and a lack of usual safety reminders). Health-care environments are designed with many safety features to reduce the risk of falls, such as railings along corridors; call bells at each bedside; safety bars in toilet areas; locks on bed, wheelchair, and stretcher wheels; side rails on beds; and night-lights. In addition, nurses can implement measures to decrease the incidence of falls (see Practice Guidelines 30.1).

PRACTICE GUIDELINES 30.1

Preventing Falls in Health-Care Agencies

Guidelines	Rationales
On admission, orient clients to their surroundings and explain the call system. Encourage the client to use the call bell to request assistance. Ensure that the bell is within easy reach.	Familiarity with surroundings increases awareness of risks and resources; access to help when required is important to ensure safety. Informing clients that help is eagerly available will help reduce reluctance to ask for assistance.
Perform a fall-risk assessment by using a standardized tool, such as the Morse Fall Scale or STRATIFY (St. Thomas Risk Assessment Tool in Falling Elderly Inpatients) (Oliver, Britton, Seed, Martin, & Hopper, 1997).	Previous history of falls is predictive of future falls; risk assessment can identify modifiable factors that will determine relevant, client-specific fall-prevention strategies.
Assess the client's ability to ambulate and transfer. Provide walking aids and assistance as required. Consult with other members of the health-care team, such as physical and occupational therapists, to help address mobility issues.	Mobility risks increase the risk of falls. Environmental resources can buffer client deficits, such as a walker providing stability. Interprofessional collaboration results in a sharing of expertise to augment the quality of patient care.
Closely supervise clients at risk for falls, especially at night.	Clients are at increased risk of falling at night because of possible disorientation, poor lighting, and effects of sleeping aids.
Place bedside tables and overbed tables near the bed or chair (but avoid obstructing movement). Keep the environment tidy; in particular, keep light cords from underfoot and furniture out of the way.	Easy access to personal supplies will prevent the client from overreaching, which can cause loss of balance with a resultant fall. Any clutter can cause imbalance and a possible fall.
Always keep hospital beds in the low position and the wheels locked when not providing care.	Clients can move in or out of bed easily. If a fall occurs, it will be from the lowest height.

(continued)

PRACTICE GUIDELINES 30.1

Preventing Falls in Health-Care Agencies *(continued)*

Guidelines	Rationales
Use beds designed to promote patient safety (Figure 30.3).	Equipment that is designed with patient safety in mind (e.g., low height, easy-grip rails, smaller openings in side rails, automatic night-light) can augment the safety repertoire.

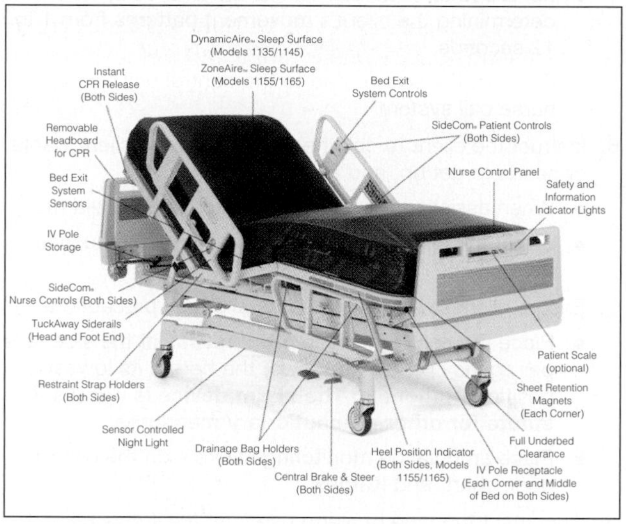

FIGURE 30.3 The Advanta Bed is designed for improved patient safety.

Guidelines	Rationales
Bed rails should not be raised routinely for the purpose of reducing falls. Use individualized interventions (e.g., an alarm sensitive to client position, a bed-exit alarm) rather than side rails for confused clients. If side rails are used to help with movement, consider half or three-quarter side rails in the event the client will attempt to crawl around or over full-length side rails.	People with memory impairment, altered mobility, nocturia, and other sleep disorders can become entrapped in side rails and many, in fact, are more likely to fall trying to get out around or over the raised rails. Alternative technology is available to alert the team when the client attempts to crawl out of bed. The half or three-quarter rail provides a movement aid while giving the patient who is trying to get up a safer way out than over or between full-length rails.

Electronic devices are available to detect when clients are attempting to get out of bed. A bed or chair safety monitoring device has a position-sensitive switch that triggers an audio alarm when the client attempts to get out of the bed or chair. Skill 30.1 describes how to use these devices.

SKILL 30.1

USING A BED OR CHAIR EXIT SAFETY MONITORING DEVICE

PURPOSES

- To alert the nurse that the client is attempting to get out of bed
- To help decrease the risk of client falls

ASSESSMENT

Assess

- Mobility status
- Judgment about ability to get out of bed safely
- Proximity of client's room to nurses' station
- Position of side rails
- Functioning status of call light

PLANNING

Determine the appropriate location for the device. If the device will be applied to a thigh, ensure that the location has intact skin.

Equipment

- Alarm and control device
- Sensor device
- Connection to nurse call system

(continued)

SKILL 30.1

USING A BED OR CHAIR EXIT SAFETY MONITORING DEVICE *(continued)*

IMPLEMENTATION

Performance

1. Before performing the procedure, introduce yourself and verify the client's identity by using agency protocol. Explain to the client and family the purpose and procedure of using a safety monitoring device.
   - Explain that the device does not limit mobility in any manner; rather, it alerts the staff when the client is about to get out of bed.
   - Explain that the nurse must be called when the client needs to get out of bed.
2. Perform hand hygiene and observe other appropriate infection prevention and control procedures.
3. Provide for client privacy.
4. Test the battery device and alarm sound. **Rationale: Testing ensures that the device is functioning properly before use.**
5. Apply the sensor pad or leg band.
   - Place the leg band according to the manufacturer's recommendation (see ❶). Place the client's leg in a straight horizontal position. **Rationale: The alarm device is position sensitive; that is, when it approaches a near-vertical position (such as in walking, crawling, or kneeling as the client attempts to get out of bed), the audio alarm will be triggered.**

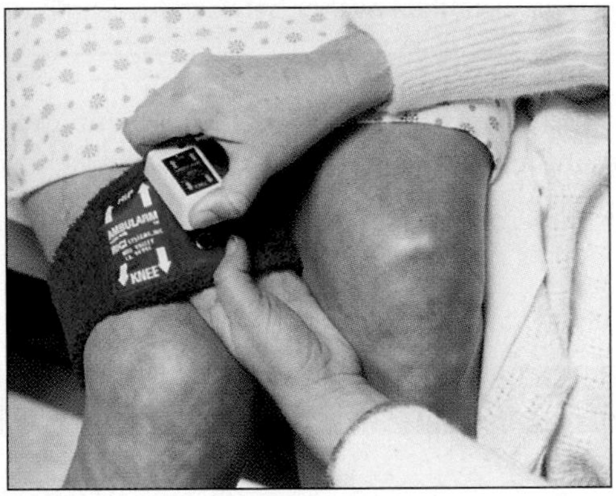

❶ Placing the leg band alarm

   - For the bed or chair device, the sensor is usually placed under the buttocks area (see ❷).
   - For a bed or chair device, set the time delay for determining the client's movement patterns from 1 to 12 seconds.
   - Connect the sensor pad to the control unit and the nurse call system.
6. Instruct the client to call the nurse when the client wants or needs to get up, and assist as required.
   - When assisting the client up, deactivate the alarm.
   - Assist the client back to bed, and reattach the alarm device.
7. Ensure client safety with additional safety precautions.
   - Place the call light within client reach, lift the side rails per agency policy, and lower the bed to its lowest position. **Rationale: The alarm device is not a substitute for other precautionary measures.**
   - Place ambulation monitoring stickers on the client's door, chart, and Kardex.
8. Document the type of alarm used, where it was placed, and its effectiveness in the client record by using forms or checklists supplemented by narrative notes when appropriate. Record all additional safety precautions and interventions discussed and employed.

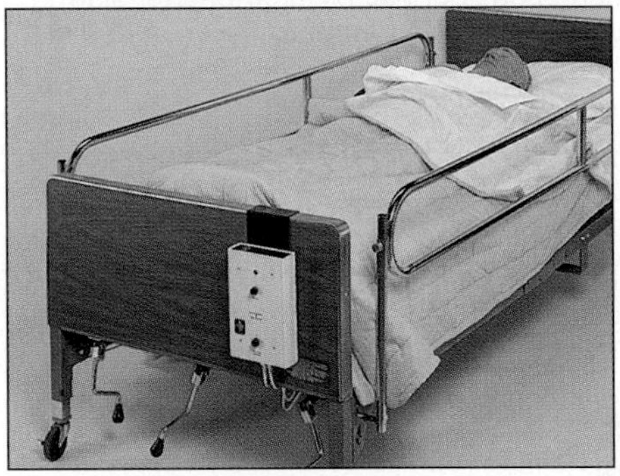

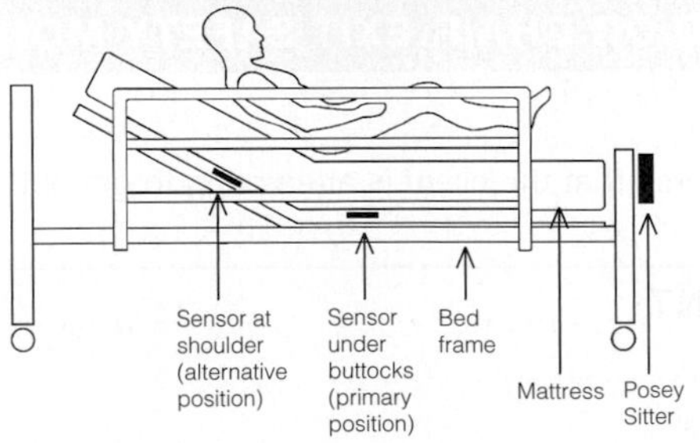

❷ Placement of a bed exit-monitoring device

EVALUATION

- If the alarm is too sensitive to client movements that are not an attempt to move from the bed or chair, reassess and modify alarm controls accordingly.
- Conduct appropriate follow-up relating to effectiveness of the safety precautions.
- Report any difficulties in using the device or any falls to the appropriate members of the health-care team.

Home Care Considerations

Using a Bed or Chair Exit Safety Monitoring Device

If the device is used in the home, instruct caregivers to do the following:

- Test the monitoring device every 12 to 24 hours to ensure that it is working.
- Check the volume of the alarm to be certain they can hear it.

Use of the device does not take the place of proper supervision of clients at risk for falling. Assessment of the reasons for falling, especially among older adults, can lead to effective prevention.

CLINICAL ALERT

Fall-risk prediction (identifying the fall-prone client) *must* be paired with fall-intervention strategies that prevent falls and protect the patient from injury in the event that a fall occurs (Morse, 2006). Assessing for risk does not prevent falls unless the data obtained from the assessment are used to guide the planning and implementation phases of the nursing care plan.

Although fall prevention is important, nurses may also need to implement fall-protective strategies so that if the individual at risk does fall, he or she will not be injured. Examples of fall-protection strategies include hip pads, kneepads, helmets, and padding on furniture.

SEIZURES A **seizure** is a sudden onset of excessive electrical discharges in one or more areas of the brain. Seizures can develop at any time during a person's life and can occur at any time. Clients may be prone to seizures because of permanent or temporary medical conditions, such as drug reactions, epilepsy, or extreme fever; seizures can occur with no known cause.

Seizures are classified into two categories: partial and generalized. Partial seizures (also called focal) involve electrical discharges from one area of the brain. In contrast, generalized seizures affect the whole brain. Each of these seizure categories includes different types of seizure depending on the characteristics of the seizure activity (e.g., loss of consciousness or no impairment to consciousness). Thus, it is important for the nurse to thoroughly describe the observations before, during, and after a client's seizure episode. Clients are at risk for injury if they experience seizures that involve the entire body, such as *grand mal* (tonic-clonic) seizures or any seizure that includes loss of consciousness. **Seizure precautions** are safety measures taken by the nurse to protect clients from injury should they have a seizure. Skill 30.2 describes how to implement seizure precautions.

SKILL 30.2

IMPLEMENTING SEIZURE PRECAUTIONS

PURPOSE

- Protect the client from injury

ASSESSMENT

Assess the history of seizures during the admission assessment. If the client has experienced a seizure previously, ask for detailed information, including characteristics of an aura or warning symptoms that indicate the seizure is beginning, duration and frequency of the seizures, consequences of the seizures (e.g., incontinence or difficulty breathing), and actions that should be taken to prevent or reduce seizure activity.

PLANNING

Review emergency procedures: a respiratory arrest or other injury can result from a seizure.

Equipment

- Blankets or other linens to pad side rails
- Oral suction equipment
- Oxygen equipment

IMPLEMENTATION

Performance

1. Before performing the procedure, introduce yourself and verify the patient's identity by using agency protocol. Explain to the patient what you are going to do, why it is necessary, and how he or she can cooperate.
2. Perform hand hygiene and observe other appropriate infection prevention and control procedures. If the patient is actively seizing, apply clean gloves in preparation for performing respiratory care measures.

(continued)

SKILL 30.2

IMPLEMENTING SEIZURE PRECAUTIONS (*continued*)

3. Provide for patient privacy.
4. Pad the bed of any patient who might have a seizure. Secure blankets or other linens around the head, foot, and side rails of the bed (see ❶).
5. Put oral suction equipment in place and test to ensure that it is functional. **Rationale: Suctioning may be needed to prevent aspiration of oral secretions.**
6. If a seizure occurs,
   - Remain with the patient and call for assistance. Do not restrain the patient.
   - If the client is not in bed, assist to the floor and protect the patient's head in your lap or on a pillow. Loosen any clothing around the patient's neck and chest.
   - Turn the patient to a lateral position if possible. **Rationale: Turning to the side allows secretions to drain out of the mouth, decreasing the risk of aspiration, and helps keep the tongue from occluding the airway.**
   - Move items in the environment to ensure the patient does not experience an injury.
   - Do not insert anything into the patient's mouth.
   - Time the seizure duration.
   - Observe the progression of the seizure, noting the sequence and type of limb involvement. Observe skin colour. When the seizure allows, check pulse and respirations.
   - Apply oxygen according to agency policy.
   - Use equipment to suction the oral airway if the client vomits or has excessive oral secretions.

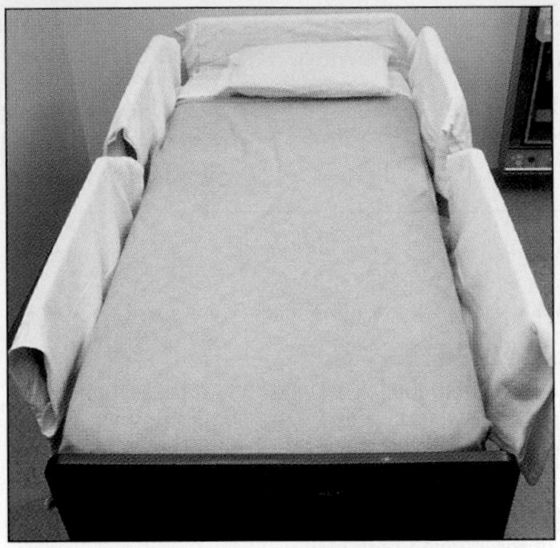

❶ Padding a bed for seizure precautions

   - Administer anticonvulsant medications, as prescribed.
   - When the seizure has subsided, assist the patient to a comfortable position. Reorient. Explain what happened. Reassure the patient. Provide hygiene as necessary. Allow the patient to verbalize feelings about the seizure.
7. Document the event in the patient record by using forms or checklists supplemented by narrative notes when appropriate.

EVALUATION

- Perform a detailed follow-up examination of the patient. Administer medications if indicated and prescribed.
- Report significant deviations from normal to the appropriate members of the health-care team.

Lifespan Considerations

Implementing Seizure Precautions

INFANTS

- About 24% of children experience seizures, most during infancy (Ball & Bindler, 2008).

CHILDREN

- Febrile seizures occur more commonly than in adults and are usually preventable through antipyretics and tepid baths.
- Determine oxygenation. Apply oxygen if pulse oximetry reading is less than 95%.
- Children who have frequent seizures may need to wear helmets for protection.
- Children taking anticonvulsant medications should wear a medical identification tag (bracelet or necklace).

Home Care Considerations

Implementing Seizure Precautions

- If clients have frequent or recurrent seizures or take anticonvulsant medications, they should wear a medical identification tag (bracelet or necklace) and carry a card listing any medications they take.
- When making home visits, inspect anticonvulsant medications and confirm that clients are taking them correctly. Blood-level measurements may be required periodically.
- Assist the client in determining which persons in the community should or must be informed of their seizure disorder (e.g., employers, health-care providers such as dentists, motor vehicle department if driving, companions).
- Discuss safety precautions for inside and out of the home. If seizures are not well controlled, activities that may require restriction or direct supervision by others include tub bathing, swimming, cooking, using electric equipment or machinery, and driving.
- Discuss with the client and family factors that may precipitate a seizure.

POISONING Nearly two-thirds (64%) of poisoning incidents occur in children 1 to 4 years old (Safe Kids Canada, 2006). Inadequate supervision and improper storage of medications (including vitamin and iron supplements) and household products (e.g., cleaning products, alcohol, paint thinner, pesticides) are the major reasons for poisoning in children. Implementing poison prevention for children is focused on childproofing the environment, including disposing of unused medications by returning them to a pharmacy and properly storing risky products.

Adolescent and adult poisonings are usually caused by excess intake of drugs used for recreation or in suicide attempts. Implementing poison prevention in these age groups focuses on providing information and counselling. Poisoning in the older adult usually results from accidental ingestion of a toxic substance (e.g., because of failing eyesight) or an overdose of prescription or over-the-counter medications. People with altered mental status, such as dementia, are at risk for poisoning as they may lack judgment or memory about risky substances. Poison prevention focuses on safeguarding the environment, monitoring the underlying problems, and regularly reviewing prescription and over-the-counter medications. A telephone number for the nearest poison control centre should be readily available so that accurate, up-to-date information about potential hazards and recommended treatment can be obtained as needed.

Nurses intervene in community settings by educating the public about what to do in the event of poisoning. Identify the specific poison by searching for an opened container, empty bottle, or other evidence. Contact the poison control centre, indicate the exact quantity of poison the person ingested, and state the person's age and apparent symptoms. Keep the person as quiet as possible and lying on his or her side or sitting with his or her head placed between the legs to prevent aspiration of vomitus. The Teaching: Wellness box provides additional guidelines for helping clients to prevent poisoning.

TEACHING: WELLNESS

Preventing Poisoning

Clients can take steps to help prevent poisonings:

- Lock potentially toxic products, including prescription and over-the-counter drugs and cleaning agents, in a cupboard, or attach special plastic hooks to the insides of cabinet doors to keep them securely closed. Unlatching these hooks requires firmer thumb pressure than small children can usually exert. Don't let children watch you open the latches. Kids learn fast!
- Avoid storing toxic liquids or solids in food containers, such as soft drink bottles, peanut butter jars, or milk cartons.
- Keep medications and potential poisons in their original containers so that warning labels and child-resistant packaging remain intact. Do not reuse empty containers to store different substances. The labels of poisons usually specify first aid and precautionary measures.
- Do not rely on cooking to destroy toxic chemicals in plants. Never use anything prepared from nature as a medicine or tea.
- Teach children never to eat any part of an unknown plant or mushroom and not to put leaves, stems, bark, seeds, nuts, or berries from any plant into their mouths.
- Place poison warning stickers designed for children on containers of bleach, lye, kerosene, solvent, and other toxic substances.
- Do not refer to medicine as candy or pretend false enjoyment when taking medications in front of children; allow them to see the necessity of the medicine without glamorizing it.
- Read and follow label directions on all products before using them.
- Remove poisonous plants from the home, and avoid planting poisonous plants in the yard.
- Be aware of the local Poison Control emergency phone number, and display it near or on all telephones in the home so that it is available to babysitters, family, and friends.

CARBON MONOXIDE POISONING **Carbon monoxide** (CO) is a colourless, odourless, toxic gas that is a product of incomplete combustion. Exposure to CO can cause symptoms of headaches, dizziness, weakness, nausea, vomiting, and loss of muscle control. Prolonged exposure can lead to unconsciousness, brain damage, and death. Learning how to prevent CO exposure is important because all gasoline-powered vehicles or generators; lawn mowers; kerosene lanterns, heaters, and stoves; propane stoves; charcoal barbecues; and burning wood emit CO.

People are at risk for CO poisoning any time they use an appliance in which incomplete combustion of its fuel can occur. Sources of CO include malfunctioning furnaces, exhaust vents for gas appliances, wood-burning fireplaces that are not properly vented, exhaust fumes from idling cars, and charcoal briquettes (Health Canada, 2008). A significant cluster of CO poisoning occurred during the 1998 ice storm in Eastern Canada. One person died and 27 were hospitalized as a result of CO poisoning. CO detectors are available for the home and are mandatory in some Canadian cities.

CHOKING OR SUFFOCATION **Choking**, when a person's trachea is obstructed by either a foreign body, such as a chunk of food, or a liquid, such as vomitus, leads to suffocation. The universal sign of distress for a choking victim is the grasping of the anterior neck and being unable to speak or cough. The emergency response is the **Heimlich manoeuvre**, or abdominal thrust, which can dislodge the foreign object and re-establish an airway. See Figure 30.4.

Suffocation, also referred to as **asphyxiation**, is lack of oxygen intake that can ultimately lead to unconsciousness and death. Suffocation occurs in situations of crush injuries to the chest, drowning, CO poisoning, or smothering (such as when a child covers his or her face with a plastic bag).

Other causes of suffocation are drowning, gas or smoke inhalation, accidental strangulation by the shoulder harness of a seat belt, and being trapped in a confined space (e.g., a discarded refrigerator). If a person does not receive immediate relief from suffocation, the interrupted breathing leads to respiratory and cardiac arrest and death. Any obstruction to the air passages must be immediately removed and life support measures instituted when an arrest occurs.

EXCESSIVE NOISE Excessive noise is a health hazard that can cause hearing loss, depending on the overall level of noise, the frequency range of the noise, and the duration of exposure and individual susceptibility. Sound levels above 120 decibels (dB) are painful and may cause hearing damage even if a person is exposed for only a short period. Exposure to 85 dB to 95 dB for several hours a day can lead to progressive or permanent hearing loss. No known risk of hearing loss is associated with sound levels below 70 dB.

When ill or injured, people can become sensitive to noises that normally would not disturb them. Loud voices, the clatter of dishes, and even a nearby television can disturb clients, some of whom react angrily. Noise in hospital can be one of several factors contributing to sensory overload. Physiological effects of noise include increased heart and respiratory rates, increased muscular activity, nausea, and hearing loss (if the noise is sufficiently loud).

Noise can be minimized by acoustic tile on ceilings, walls, and floors; drapes and carpeting to absorb sound; background music to mask noise and have a calming effect (on some people); keeping your voice down while giving care or talking in the background; and appropriate alarm settings to reduce false alarms.

ELECTRICAL HAZARDS All electric equipment must be properly grounded. The electric plug of grounded equipment has three prongs. The two short prongs transmit the power to the equipment. The third, longer prong is the grounding device, which carries short circuits or stray electric current to the ground (Figure 30.5). Grounding prongs offer a path of least resistance to stray electric currents.

Faulty equipment, such as equipment with a frayed cord, presents a danger of electric shock or may start a fire. For example, an electric spark near certain anaesthetic gases or a high concentration of oxygen can cause a fire or explosion. Actions to reduce electrical hazards are described in the Teaching: Wellness box.

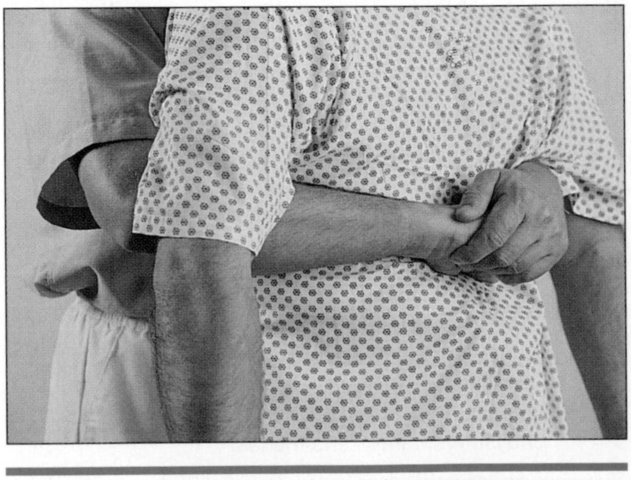

FIGURE 30.4 Performing the Heimlich manoeuvre

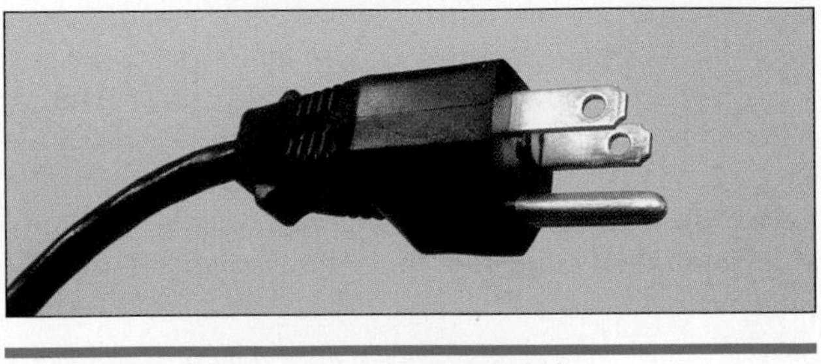

FIGURE 30.5 Three-pronged grounded plug

TEACHING: WELLNESS

Reducing Electrical Hazards

Take steps to reduce electrical hazards:

- Check cords for fraying or other signs of damage before using an appliance. Do not use it if the cord is damaged.
- Avoid overloading outlets and fuse boxes with too many appliances; use grounded outlets and plugs.
- Always pull a plug from the wall outlet by firmly grasping the plug and pulling it straight out. Pulling a plug by its cord can damage the cord and plug unit.
- Ensure that ground fault circuit interrupters (GFCIs) have been installed wherever electrical appliances or equipment can inadvertently come in contact with water, such as near sinks, bathtubs, or showers, or outdoors.
- Keep electric cords and appliances out of the reach of children, and place protective covers over wall outlets to protect young children.
- Carefully read instructions before operating electric equipment.
- Always disconnect appliances before cleaning or repairing them.
- Unplug any appliance that has given a tingling sensation or shock and have an electrician evaluate it.
- Keep electric cords coiled or taped to the ground away from areas of traffic to prevent people from damaging the cords or tripping over them.

When major electrical injury does occur, such as macroshock, when the current finds a pathway through the body, the victim may sustain both superficial and deep burns, muscle contractions, and cardiac and respiratory arrest, necessitating cardiopulmonary resuscitation and life support. Small currents can cause microshock when the current flows through a direct pathway to the heart, such as during intracardiac catheterization. Using machines in good repair, wearing shoes with rubber soles, standing on a nonconductive floor, and using nonconductive gloves can prevent shock. Rescuers must not touch the victim until the electricity is shut off or the victim has been removed from contact with the electric current; otherwise, the rescuer can also receive electrical injury.

CLINICAL ALERT

Reconsider keeping firearms in the home if a family member is at risk for suicide or if children are found playing with the firearms. Any victim of domestic violence whose aggressor has access to a firearm can contact police to report the concern.

FIREARMS Canadian regulations about firearm ownership are very strict and gun registration is required. Any gun owner is required to follow a range of safety precautions to ensure that no harm or injury results from improper gun use or storage. Access to firearms is a serious concern in homes with children and in situations of suicidal ideation or domestic violence. Members of any household in which guns are present must take full responsibility for following basic firearm safety rules: store all guns in sturdy locked cabinets and make sure the keys are inaccessible to children; store bullets in a different location from the gun; and don't use firearms while affected by alcohol or other drugs of any kind, including over-the-counter medications that can change sensorium.

RADIATION Radiation injury can occur from overexposure to radioactive materials used in diagnostic and therapeutic procedures. Clients being examined by using radiography or fluoroscopy generally receive minimal exposure and few precautions are necessary. Nurses need to protect themselves, however, from radiation when some clients are receiving radiation therapy. Exposure to radiation can be minimized by (1) limiting the time near the source, (2) providing as much distance as possible from the source, and (3) using shielding devices, such as lead aprons, when near the source. Nurses need to become familiar with agency protocols related to radiation therapy.

Procedure-Related and Equipment-Related Accidents

Risk assessment in the health-care setting must include risks related to procedures and equipment. Whether giving a medication or assisting a patient out of bed, nurses need to follow safeguards to prevent errors or unintentional injury. Nurses must be aware of and adhere to provincial or territorial regulations of occupational health and safety. The Workplace Hazardous Materials Information System (WHMIS) is an example of a legislated mechanism to ensure safety when using a range of risky products (Figure 30.6).

When an accident or error does occur, most agencies require that the incident be reported. The nurse completes the report immediately after taking whatever action is required to safeguard the patient and notifying the appropriate superior. For additional information about incident reports, see Chapter 6.

Restraining Clients

Restraints are physical, chemical, or environmental measures used to control the physical or behavioural activity of a person or a portion of his or her body (College of Nurses of

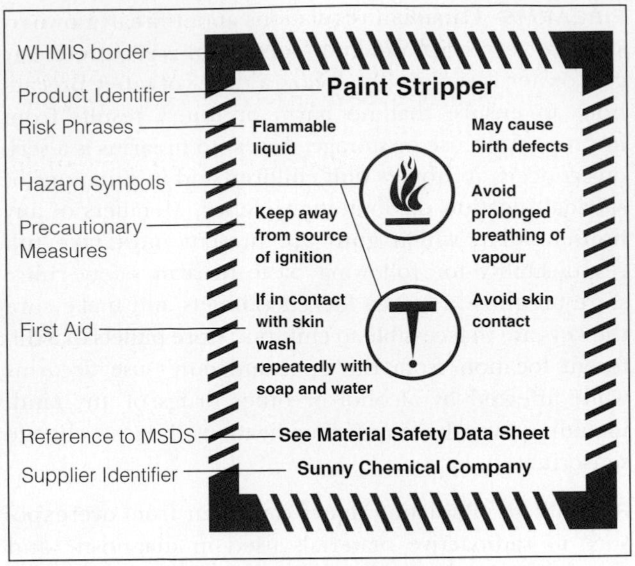

FIGURE 30.6 WHMIS system of labelling

Ontario, 2005). **Physical restraints** are any manual method or physical or mechanical device, material, or equipment attached to the client's body (e.g., vest or wrist restraint); they cannot be removed easily, and they restrict the client's movement. **Environmental restraints** control a person's mobility (e.g., a secured unit or raised bed rails). **Chemical restraints** are medications, such as neuroleptics, anxiolytics, sedatives, and psychotropic agents, used to control disruptive behaviour. The purpose of restraints is to prevent the client from injuring himself or herself or others *only* after every other means of ensuring safety has been unsuccessful and documented. If restraints are deemed necessary, then a policy of **least restraint** should be enacted: use the minimum amount of restraint needed to ensure safety (e.g., by securing one hand rather than both). See the alternatives to the use of restraints in Box 30.2.

Restraints can contribute to muscle atrophy, skin deterioration, urinary incontinence, constipation, and respiratory infection because the patient is more likely to remain recumbent or bedridden when restrained. Coroners' reports have linked restraints to deaths, such as suffocation from becoming trapped between bedrails when trying to climb out of bed, strangulation when the ties of a restraint vest encircle the neck, or aspiration from vomitus when protective movements are limited by restraints. In addition to the physical safety concerns, many consider restraints to be demeaning and to limit a client's autonomy. They can be harmful psychologically, such as by making a client feel ashamed or guilty. For clients with a history of sexual abuse, being placed in restraints has been linked to flashbacks and potential exacerbation of post-traumatic stress disorder symptoms (Mohr, Petti, & Mohr, 2003). The focus in health care is to explore ways to prevent, reduce, and eliminate the use of restraints while protecting a client's safety, rights, and dignity.

BOX 30.2 ALTERNATIVES TO RESTRAINTS

Some alternatives to restraints are as follows:

- Assign the care of a client to a team who can share in providing continuous or periodic surveillance and monitoring.
- Place the client in an area that is constantly or closely supervised; prepare the client if relocation is required to limit possible confusion or anxiety.
- Stay with a client who is using a bedside commode or the bathroom if the client is confused or sedated or has a gait disturbance or a high-risk score for falling.
- Monitor all medications and, if possible, lower or eliminate dosages of sedatives or psychotropics.
- Position beds at their lowest level to facilitate getting in and out of bed.
- Replace full-length side rails with half- or three-quarter-length rails to prevent confused clients from climbing over rails or falling from the end of the bed.
- Wedge pillows or pads against the sides of a wheelchair to keep a client well positioned.
- Place a removable lap tray on a wheelchair to provide support and help keep the client in place.
- To quiet agitated clients, try a warm beverage, soft lights, a back rub, or a walk.
- Use environmental restraints, such as pieces of furniture or large plants, as barriers to keep clients from wandering beyond appropriate areas.
- Try to determine the causes of a client's sundowner syndrome (nocturnal wandering and disorientation as darkness falls, associated with dementia). Possible causes include poor hearing, poor eyesight, or pain.
- Regularly monitor clients for changes in physical and cognitive functional abilities and risk factors.

LEGAL IMPLICATIONS OF RESTRAINTS Because restraints restrict the individual's freedom, their use has legal implications. Nurses need to know agency policies and provincial or territorial laws about restraining clients. A clear understanding of what constitutes a restraint is important. For example, if a patient has the side rails up to help with side-to-side movement in the bed, then this situation is not one of restraint; if, however, the side rails are up to confine the patient, then the use of side rails is considered an environmental restraint. Most agencies and provincial or territorial legislation require informed consent of the patient or legal representative before implementing restraints in non-emergency situations. A collective prescription or policy will generally identify the steps to be followed before using restraints. Some institutions allow for individual decision making in emergency situations, but the trend is toward documented interdisciplinary and patient or family dialogue *before* their use. Continued use of restraints must also be addressed, often within specific time frames (e.g., involuntary restraint may require reassessment every 2 to 4 hours, voluntary restraint is generally reviewed every 8 or 24 hours). Most agencies require visual or auditory supervision of any client in restraint so that any safety issues can be quickly addressed.

CLINICAL ALERT

Restrained clients may become more restless and anxious as a result of the loss of self-control. The nurse *must* keep in mind that such behaviours may be the result of pain or hypoxia from improper restraint application. A patient who was agitated and suddenly becomes quiet must be assessed to ensure that the change in behaviour is the result of calmness rather than a hypoxic or other physiological event.

Clients have the right to be free from restraints that are not necessary. As a result, there must be justification that the use of restraints will protect the client and that less restrictive measures were attempted and found ineffective. Restraints *cannot* be used for staff convenience or client punishment. Given that the above conditions are met and restraints are needed, it is important for the nurse to be able to correctly apply restraints without endangering client safety.

SELECTING A RESTRAINT Before selecting a restraint, nurses need to understand its purpose clearly and measure it against the following five criteria:

1. It restricts the client's movement as little as possible. If a client needs to have one arm restrained, do not restrain the entire body.
2. It does not interfere with the client's treatment or health problem. If a client has poor blood circulation to the hands, apply a restraint that will not aggravate that circulatory problem.
3. It is readily changeable. Restraints need to be changed frequently, especially if they become soiled. Keeping other guidelines in mind, choose a restraint that can be changed with minimal disturbance to the client.
4. It is safe for the particular client. Choose a restraint with which the client cannot self-inflict injury. For example, a physically restrained person could be injured trying to climb out of bed if one wrist is tied to the bed frame. A jacket restraint would restrain the person more safely.
5. It is the least obvious to others. Clients and visitors can be embarrassed by a restraint, even though they understand why it is being used. The less obvious the restraint, the more comfortable people feel.

KINDS OF RESTRAINTS The most common types of restraints for adults are jacket or vest restraints, belt restraints, mitt or hand restraints, and limb restraints. Although bed rails can be used to aid in turning or repositioning and reduce the risk of patients falling out of bed during transport, they are also seen as restraints in that they can limit purposeful movement. Geri-chairs and wheelchairs with lap trays are also classified as forms of restraints. Restraints for infants and children include mummy restraints, elbow restraints, and crib nets. When using restraints, the nurse will find Practice Guidelines 30.2 helpful.

Several types of vest restraints are used, but all are essentially sleeveless jackets or vests with straps (tails)

PRACTICE GUIDELINES 30.2

Applying Restraints

Guidelines	Rationales
Ensure that all alternative measures other than restraints have been exhausted and that the *least* restraint option is being used. Assure the client and the family that the restraint is temporary and protective.	Underlying reasons for restraints must be addressed and corrected if possible as their use is associated with psychological (guilt, anger, shame, feeling punished) and physiological (strangulation, skin breakdown, constipation) risks.
Obtain consent from the client or guardian and ensure that necessary collective or physician prescriptions are in order.	Legal and ethical considerations require informed consent, unless in an emergency situation. Health agencies generally have specific protocols and lines of authority to ensure practices are consistent and safe.
If restraints are applied, ensure the following:	
• Apply the restraint so that the client can move as freely as possible without defeating the purpose of the restraint.	Inability to move can cause anxiety and agitation, and enhance the risk of physiological complications, such as aspiration if vomiting.
• Apply a restraint so it can be released quickly in case of an emergency and supports the normal anatomy of the body part.	Time is of the essence in emergency situations; contractures and discomfort can arise from poor body alignment.
• Limb restraints are applied securely but not tightly. Always tie a limb restraint with a knot (e.g., a clove hitch) that will not tighten when pulled.	Tight restraints can impede blood circulation and are uncomfortable.
• Pad bony prominences (e.g., wrists, ankles) before applying a restraint over them. Immediately report and document any persistent reddened or broken skin areas under the restraint.	The movement of a restraint without padding over bony prominences can abrade the skin. Any sign of skin breakdown or poor circulation may mean restraints are improperly attached or contraindicated.

(continued)

PRACTICE GUIDELINES 30.2

Applying Restraints (*continued*)

Guidelines	Rationales
At the first indication of cyanosis or pallor, coldness of a skin area, or a client's complaint of tingling, pain, or numbness, loosen the restraint and exercise the limb.	Poor circulation must be corrected immediately to avoid tissue or neurological damage.
Tie the ends of a body restraint to the part of the bed that moves to elevate the head.	Tying the ends to a side rail or to the fixed frame of the bed will cause injury if the bed position is changed.
Assess the response to restraints per agency protocol and time frame, generally at least once an hour. Assessment must include determining a continued need for the restraints.	Regular assessment is necessary to ensure safety and that the underlying cause of the behaviour necessitating the original use of the restraints persists or no longer exists.
Provide range-of-motion (ROM) exercises and skin care, and assist with basic needs: hygiene, positioning, nutrition, hydration, elimination.	Maintenance of general health needs must be met to prevent further deterioration.
Provide emotional support throughout and after restraints are removed.	Psychological trauma must be avoided; some patients can feel isolated, become panicky if left alone, and become fearful, especially if they have claustrophobic tendencies. Patients can have negative emotions even when restraints are no longer being used.

that can be tied to the bed frame under the mattress These body restraints are used to ensure the safety of confused or sedated clients in beds or wheelchairs. "Front" and "back" labels on vest restraints ensure that they are applied correctly and safely.

Belt or safety strap body restraints (Figure 30.7) are used to ensure the safety of all clients who are being moved on stretchers or in wheelchairs. Some wheelchairs have a soft, padded safety bar that attaches to side brackets that are installed under the armrests. To prevent the person from slumping forward, the nurse then attaches a shoulder Y strap to the bar and over the client's shoulders to the rear handles. Other safety belt models have a three-loop design. One loop surrounds the person's waist and the other two attach to the rear handles. If such restraints are unavailable, the nurse can place a folded towel or small sheet around the client's waist and fasten it at the back of the wheelchair. Belt restraints can also be used for certain clients confined to bed or to chairs.

A mitt or hand restraint (Figure 30.8) is used to prevent confused clients from using their hands or fingers to scratch and injure themselves. For example, a confused client may need to be prevented from pulling at intravenous tubing or at a head bandage following neurosurgery. Hand or mitt restraints allow the client to

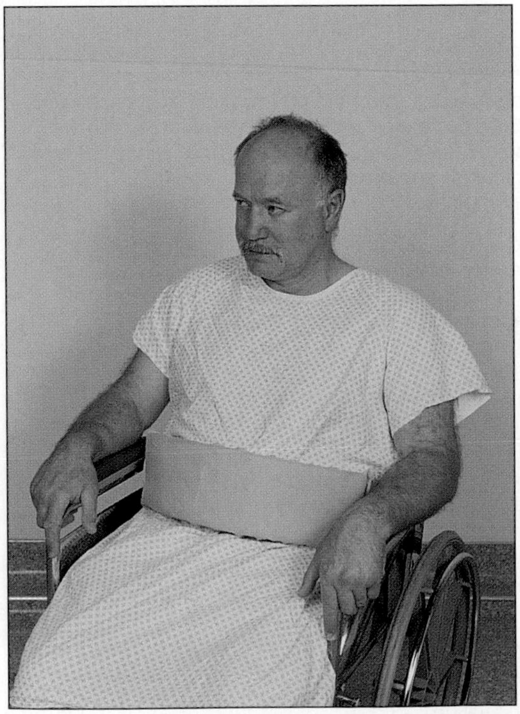

FIGURE 30.7 A belt restraint

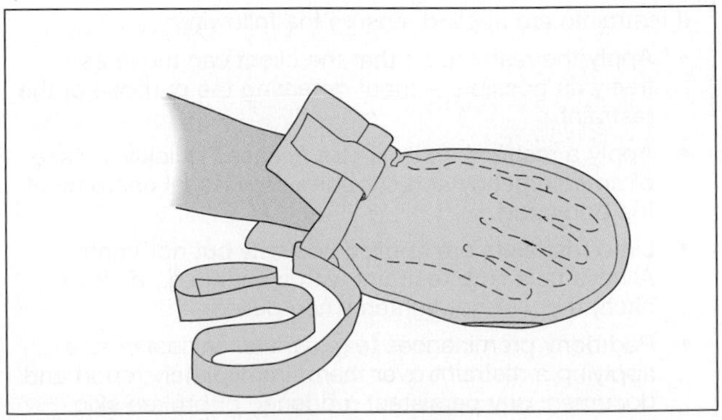

FIGURE 30.8 A mitt restraint

be ambulatory and to move the arm freely rather than be confined to a bed or a chair. Mittens need to be removed on a regular basis to permit the client to wash and exercise the hands. The nurse also needs to take off the mitten to check the circulation to the hand.

Limb restraints (Figure 30.9) can be used to immobilize a limb, primarily for therapeutic reasons (e.g., to maintain an intravenous infusion). See Skill 30.3 for applying restraints.

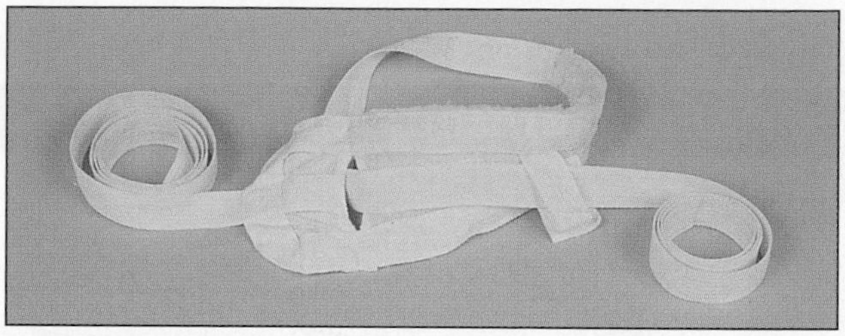

FIGURE 30.9 A limb restraint

SKILL 30.3

APPLYING RESTRAINTS

PURPOSES

- To promote safety and prevent injury *only when all other less restrictive measures have been exhausted*
- To allow a medical or surgical treatment to proceed without client interference (e.g., to prevent movements that would disrupt therapy to a limb connected to tubes or an appliance)

ASSESSMENT

Assess

- The behaviour indicating the possible need for a restraint
- Underlying causes for the assessed behaviour
- What other protective measures can be implemented before applying a restraint
- The status of skin to which restraint is to be applied
- The circulatory status distal to restraints and of extremities
- The effectiveness of other available safety precautions

PLANNING

Review institutional policy for restraints and seek consultation as appropriate before independently deciding to apply a restraint. *Many Canadian institutions require interdisciplinary discussions and informed patient or legal guardian consent before instituting restraints.*

Equipment

- Appropriate type and size of restraint

IMPLEMENTATION

Performance

1. Before performing the procedure, introduce yourself and verify the patient's identity by using agency protocol. Explain to the patient and family what you are going to do, why it is necessary, and how they can cooperate. Discuss how the results will be used in planning further care or treatments. Allow time for the patient to express feelings about being restrained. Provide needed emotional reassurance that the restraints will be used only when absolutely necessary and that there will be close contact with the client in case assistance is required.
2. Perform hand hygiene and observe other appropriate infection prevention and control procedures.
3. Provide for patient privacy if indicated.
4. Apply the selected restraint.

Belt Restraint (Safety Belt)

- Determine that the safety belt is in good order. If a Velcro safety belt is to be used, make sure that both pieces of Velcro are intact.
- If the belt has a long portion and a shorter portion, place the long portion of the belt behind (under) the bedridden client and secure it to the moveable part of the bed frame. **Rationale: The long attached portion will then move up when the head of the bed is elevated and will not tighten around the client.**
- Place the shorter portion of the belt around the patent's waist, over the gown. There should be a finger's width between the belt and the client.
- *Or* attach the belt around the patient's waist, and fasten it at the back of the chair.
- *Or* if the belt is attached to a stretcher, secure the belt firmly over the patient's hips or abdomen. **Rationale: Belt restraints must be applied to all patients on stretchers even when the side rails are up.**

Jacket Restraint

- Place the vest on the patient, with opening at the front or the back, depending on the vest type.
- Pull the tie on the end of the vest flap across the chest, and place it through the slit in the opposite side of the chest.
- Repeat for the other tie.
- Use a half-bow knot to secure each tie around the moveable bed frame or behind the chair to a chair leg (see ❶ and ❷). **Rationale: A half-bow knot does not tighten or slip when the attached end is pulled but unties easily when the loose end is pulled.**

(continued)

SKILL 30.3

APPLYING RESTRAINTS *(continued)*

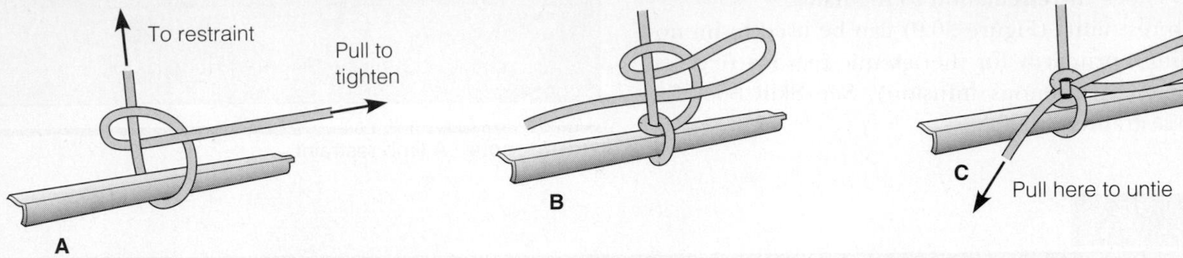

❶ To make a half-bow knot (quick-release knot), first place the restraint tie under the side frame of the bed (or around a chair leg). **A:** Bring the free end up, around, under, and over the attached end of the tie and pull it tight. **B:** Again take the free end over and under the attached end of the tie, but this time make a half-bow loop. **C:** Tighten the free end of the tie and the bow until the knot is secure. To untie the knot, pull the end of the tie and then loosen the first cross over the tie.

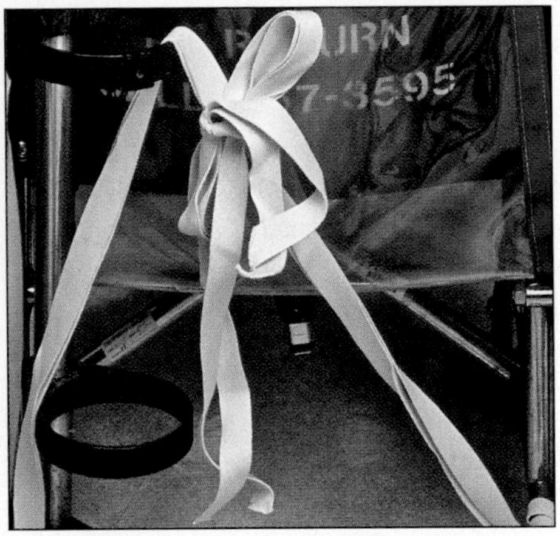

❷ Half-bow (quick-release) knot

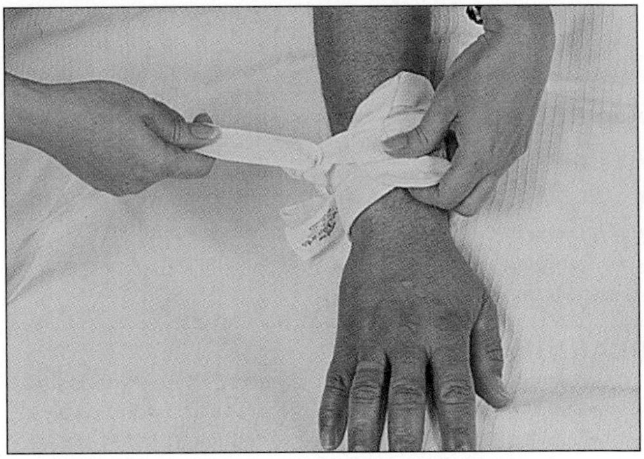

❸ Ensure that two fingers can be inserted between the restraint and the wrist or ankle.

- *Or* fasten the ties together behind the chair by using a slip or quick-release knot.
- Ensure that the client is positioned appropriately to enable maximum chest expansion for breathing.

Mitt Restraint

- Apply the commercial thumbless mitt (Figure 30.8) to the hand to be restrained. Make sure the fingers can be slightly flexed and are not caught under the hand.
- Follow the manufacturer's directions for securing the mitt.
- If a mitt is to be worn for several days, remove it at regular intervals per agency protocol. Wash and exercise the patient's hand, then reapply the mitt. Check agency practices about recommended intervals for removal.
- Assess the patient's circulation to the hands shortly after the mitt is applied and at regular intervals. **Rationale: Client complaints of numbness, discomfort, or inability to move the fingers could indicate impaired circulation to the hand.**

Wrist or Ankle Restraint

- Pad bony prominences on the wrist or ankle if needed to prevent skin breakdown.
- Apply the padded portion of the restraint around the ankle or wrist.
- Pull the tie of the restraint through the slit in the wrist portion or through the buckle (see ❸).
- By using a half-bow knot (quick-release knot), attach the other end of the restraint to the moveable portion of the bed frame. **Rationale: If the ties are attached to the movable portion, the wrist or ankle will not be pulled when the bed position is changed.**

5. Adjust the plan of care as required, for example, to include releasing the restraint, providing skin care, helping with range-of-motion exercises, and attending to the patent's physical needs by providing fluids, nutrition, and toileting.
6. Record on the patient's chart the behaviours indicating the need for the restraint, all other interventions implemented in attempt to avoid the use of restraints and their outcomes, and the time the physician was notified of the need for restraint. Also record the following:
   - The type of restraint applied, the time it was applied, and the goal for its application
   - The patient's response to the restraint
   - The times that the restraints were removed and skin care given
   - Any other assessments and interventions
   - Explanations given to the patient and significant others

(continued)

SKILL 30.3

APPLYING RESTRAINTS (*continued*)

EVALUATION

- Perform a detailed follow-up of the need for the restraints and the patient's physical and emotional response. Relate these findings to previous data if available.
- Evaluate circulatory status of restrained limbs at least on an hourly basis.
- Evaluate skin status beneath restraints at least on an hourly basis.
- Remove the restraints as soon as they are no longer needed and document the removal.
- Report significant deviations from normal to the appropriate members of the health-care team.

Lifespan Considerations

Restraints

INFANTS

Elbow restraints (Figure 30.10) are used to prevent infants or small children from flexing their elbows to touch or reach their face or head, especially after surgery. Ready-made elbow restraints are available commercially.

A mummy restraint (Figure 30.11) is a folding of a blanket or sheet around the infant to prevent movement during a procedure, such as eye irrigation or collection of a blood specimen.

- Obtain a blanket or sheet large enough so that the distance between opposite corners is about twice the length of the infant's body. Lay the blanket or sheet on a flat, dry surface.
- Fold down one corner, and place the baby on it in the supine position.
- Fold the right side of the blanket over the infant's body, leaving the left arm free (Figure 30.11A). The right arm is in a natural position at the side.
- Fold the excess blanket at the bottom up under the infant (Figure 30.11B, 2).
- With the left arm in a natural position at the baby's side, fold the left side of the blanket over the infant, including the arm, and tuck the blanket under the body (Figure 30.11B, 3).
- Remain with the infant who is in a mummy restraint until the specific procedure is completed.

CHILDREN

A crib net is simply a device placed over the top of a crib to prevent active young children from climbing out of the crib. At the same time, it allows them freedom to move about in the crib. The crib net or dome is not attached to the movable parts of the crib so that the caregiver can have access to the child without removing the dome or net.

- Place the net over the sides and ends of the crib.
- Secure the ties to the springs or frame of the crib. The crib sides can then be freely lowered without removing the net.
- Test with your hand that the net will stretch if the child stands against it in the crib.

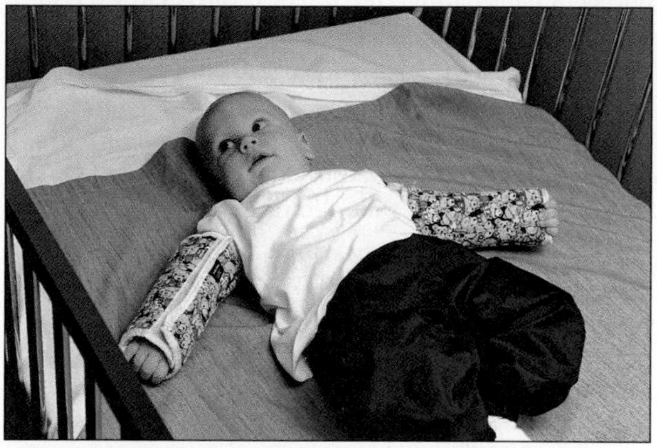

FIGURE 30.10 Infant with elbow restraints

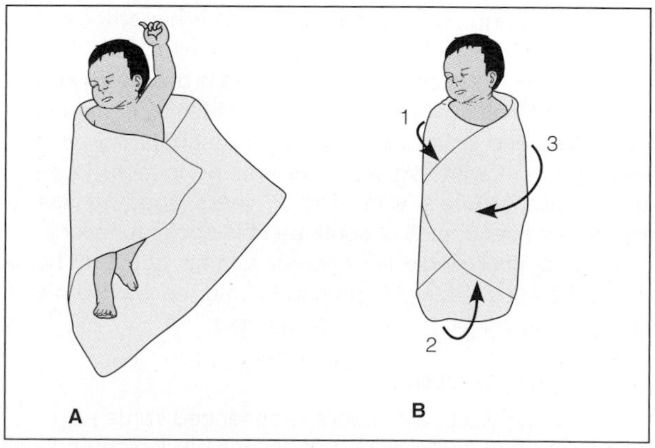

FIGURE 30.11 Making a mummy restraint

Home Care Considerations

Applying Restraints

Restraints may be necessary for clients in wheelchairs or in the home. Safety guidelines apply in all cases. Assess the knowledge and skill of all caregivers in the use of restraints and educate as indicated.

- Use means other than restraints as much as possible, and stay with the client.
- Pad bony prominences, such as wrists and ankles, if needed before applying a restraint over them.
- Tie restraints with knots that will not tighten when pulled, and tie them to parts of the wheelchair that do not move. Release the knots quickly in case of emergency.
- Assess restrained limbs for signs of impaired blood circulation.
- Always stay with a client whose restraint is temporarily removed.

Evaluating

To prevent client injury, the nurse's role is largely educative, and desired outcomes reflect the client's acquisition of knowledge of hazards, behaviours that incorporate safety practices, and skills to perform in the event of certain emergencies. The nurse needs to individualize these for clients. Examples of desired outcomes include the client being able to do the following:

- Describe methods to prevent specific hazards (e.g., falls, suffocation, choking, fires, drowning, electric shock)
- Report use of home safety measures (e.g., fire safety measures, smoke detector and CO detector maintenance, fall-prevention strategies, burn-prevention measures, poison-prevention measures, safe storage of hazardous materials, firearm safety precautions, electrocution prevention, water safety precautions, motor vehicle safety)
- Alter home physical environment to reduce the risk of injury
- Describe emergency procedures for poisoning and fire
- Describe age-specific risks, work safety risks, or community safety risks
- Demonstrate correct use of child safety seats
- Demonstrate correct administration of cardiopulmonary resuscitation

Case Study 30

Mr. Moore is a 72-year-old widower who is recovering from a fall in which he fractured his hip and underwent surgical repair 1 week ago. He will be staying with his son for 2 weeks after he is discharged from the hospital, but he is eager to return to his own home. Once he is home, his son will visit nightly after work, he will receive Meals on Wheels once a day, and a home health-care attendant will visit weekly to assist with hygienic care until he is more independent. Mr. Moore's wife died 3 years ago; he has remained independent and continued his social functions. He lives in a small single-level house with his dog, and he enjoys gardening. Before fracturing his hip, he walked his dog daily. You will be his home care nurse.

Critical Thinking Questions

1. While hospitalized, Mr. Moore experienced some mild confusion during the night, but his nurses decided not to restrain him. What are the best reasons for avoiding the use of restraints for such clients as Mr. Moore?
2. What are some of the factors that may affect Mr. Moore's safety as he returns home?
3. What do you need to assess concerning Mr. Moore's safety, and what suggestions can you make for enhancing his safety?
4. What strengths do you note about Mr. Moore that may protect him from injury when he returns home?

After working through these questions, go to the MyNursingLab at **http://www.mynursinglab.com** to check your answers.

KEY TERMS

injury
accidents
unintentional injuries
intentional injuries
adverse event
bioterrorism
scald
burn
seizure
seizure precautions
carbon monoxide
choking
Heimlich manoeuvre
suffocation
asphyxiation
restraints
physical restraints
environmental restraints
chemical restraints
least restraint

CHAPTER HIGHLIGHTS

- Unintentional injuries are a major cause of death among Canadians.
- Nurses need to be aware of what constitutes a safe environment for specific individuals and for groups of people in the home, community, health-care agency, and workplace.
- Hazards to safety occur at all ages and vary according to the age and development of the individual.
- Nursing assessment of safety includes assessing factors that can affect safety: age and development, lifestyle, mobility and health status, sensory-perceptual alterations, cognitive awareness, emotional state, ability to communicate, safety awareness, and environmental factors.
- Nurses assess clients at risk for injury through such methods as taking a nursing history and conducting a physical examination, using risk assessment tools, evaluating the home environment, assessing standards of safety in the health-care setting, and addressing bioterrorism.
- Studies and reports (e.g., *Canadian Adverse Events Study*) indicate that the incidence of medical errors in hospitals is too high and many are preventable. Patient safety goals focus on system-wide issues and solutions.
- Major nursing diagnoses for clients at risk for unintentional injury can be categorized as *Risk for Injury,* with six subcategories: *Risk for Poisoning, Risk for Suffocation, Risk for Trauma, Latex Allergy Response, Risk for Latex Allergy Response,* and *Risk for Aspiration.*
- When planning for safety needs of clients, nurses need to consider physical factors in the environment and the psychological and physiological state of the individual. Clients often need to change their health behaviour and may need to modify the environment.
- Measures to ensure the safety of people of all ages focus on (1) observation or prediction of situations that are potentially harmful and (2) client education that empowers clients to safeguard themselves and their families from injury. Education is a major health-protection strategy in preventing unintentional injury.
- Nurses must be familiar with fire procedures in their health-care agency. In the event of a fire, the nurse must RACE: **R**escue or **R**emove persons who are in immediate danger; **A**ctivate the alarm and call for help; **C**ontain or **C**onfine the fire and smoke; **E**xtinguish the fire if possible; otherwise **E**vacuate.
- Falls are a common cause of injury among older adults. Prevention of falls in the home and health-care setting is a continuous concern. Fall-risk assessment, fall-prevention, and fall-protection strategies are numerous. Side rails do not protect hospitalized clients from falls; it is more likely the client will fall trying to get around or over the side rail.
- Seizure precautions are safety measures taken by the nurse to protect clients from injury should the client have a seziure.
- Major reasons for poisoning in children are inadequate supervision and improper storage of medications and household toxic substances.
- Suffocation can occur when foreign objects are swallowed or inhaled, cutting off the person's oxygen supply.
- Prolonged exposure to excessive noise can produce hearing loss.
- Faulty electric equipment and improper grounding pose health hazards in the hospital and at home. Accidents can be prevented by using grounded outlets and plugs, putting protective covers over outlets, keeping appliances in good repair, and making sure that electric wiring and circuits meet safety standards.
- Firearms pose a risk to individuals of all ages. Adults must take full responsibility for following safety procedures when keeping firearms in the home, including storage of ammunition in a separate location.
- Various alternatives to restraints must be considered before a restraint is applied.
- Because restraints restrict a client's basic freedom to move, careful assessment and accurate, complete documentation are important when restraints are used.

ASSESS YOUR LEARNING

1. What is the correct sequence of the following nursing priorities if a fire occurs in a health-care setting?
   1 Pull the fire alarm
   2 Extinguish the fire
   3 Remove clients from the site of danger
   4 Contain the fire
   a. 3, 1, 4, 2
   b. 1, 4, 3, 2
   c. 3, 1, 2, 4
   d. 1, 4, 2, 3

2. A hospitalized 90-year-old woman who uses a walker is receiving diuretic medication and must use the bathroom several times each night. To promote safety, which of the following should the nurse do?
   a. Leave the bathroom light on.
   b. Withhold her diuretic medication.
   c. Provide a bedside commode.
   d. Keep the side rails up.

3. A 75-year-old man is hospitalized with a cerebrovascular accident (stroke). He is unable to ambulate without help but becomes disoriented at times and tries to get out of bed. What is the most appropriate safety measure for this patient?
   a. Restrain him in bed.
   b. Ask a family member to stay with him.
   c. Check the patient every 15 minutes.
   d. Use a bed exit safety-monitoring device.

4. Which of the following nursing interventions is the highest in priority for a client at risk for falls in a hospital setting?
   a. Keep all the side rails up.
   b. Review prescribed medications.
   c. Complete the Get Up and Go test.
   d. Place the bed in the lowest position.

5. The Canadian Council on Health Services Accreditation's patient safety goals address the need to decrease the number of errors in hospitals. Which of the following practices will help increase client safety?
   a. Improve the nurse's ability to multitask.
   b. Identify the health-care practitioners who are incompetent.
   c. Establish strict policies and procedures.
   d. Create a culture of safety.

6. The nurse, at the change-of-shift report, learns that one of the patients in his care has bilateral soft wrist restraints. The patient is confused, has been trying to get out of bed, and had pulled out the IV line, which was subsequently reinserted. Which of the following actions by the nurse is inappropriate?
   a. Document the behaviours that require continued use of the restraints.
   b. Ensure that the restraints are tied to the side rails.
   c. Provide range-of-motion exercises when the restraints are removed.
   d. Orient the patient.

7. A client is being admitted to the hospital because of a seizure that occurred at home. The client has no previous history of seizures. In planning the client's nursing care, which of the following measures is the most essential at this time of admission?
   a. Place a padded tongue depressor at the head of the bed.
   b. Pad the bed with blankets.
   c. Inform the client about the importance of wearing a medical identification tag.
   d. Teach the client about epilepsy.

8. Marcel, 8 years old, is admitted to the pediatric unit following a convulsive (i.e., seizure) episode at home. When entering Marcel's room, the nurse notes that he is having a convulsion. What should the nurse do as a priority in this situation?
   a. Draw the curtains to provide Marcel with privacy.
   b. Place a pillow under Marcel's head to prevent trauma.
   c. Reassure Marcel by talking to him gently.
   d. Ensure airway patency for Marcel.

9. Mr. Taylor, 85 years old, has a history of dementia. He is known to strike out during personal care. What is the best way to minimize risk to the nurse when giving Mr. Taylor a tub bath?
   a. Encourage the client to remain calm.
   b. Ask a colleague for assistance.
   c. Give him a shower instead.
   d. Administer a sedative prior to his bath.

10. Mr. Sanders has had Alzheimer's disease for 3 years. He is 75 years old and lives with his 72-year-old wife. He takes little part in his care and is confused at times. The nurse suggests prevention strategies to Mrs. Sanders, who is worried about her husband roaming at night. Which of the following suggestions by the nurse would reduce the risk of unintentional injury?
    a. Install an alarm bell on the bedroom door.
    b. Ensure adequate lighting in the house.
    c. Administer sleeping medication to Mr. Sanders before he retires.
    d. Ensure that someone stays with him.

After working through these questions, go to the MyNursingLab at **http://www.mynursinglab.com** *to check your answers and see explanations.*

SUGGESTED READINGS

Howe, T. E., Rochester, L., Jackson, A., Banks, P. M., & Blair, V. A. (2007). Exercise for improving balance in older people. *Cochrane Database of Systematic Reviews, 4,* Art. No.: CD004963.

This systematic review provides an excellent analysis of the benefits of exercise in improving balance, which ultimately reduces the number of falls.

Kendrick, D., Coupland, C., Mulvaney, C., Simpson, J., Smith, S. J., Sutton, A., et al. (2007). Home safety education and provision of safety equipment for injury prevention. *Cochrane Database of Systematic Reviews, 1,* Art. No.: CD005014.

This systematic review looked at 80 research papers on home safety education programs. The authors of this review conclude that these programs are effective in increasing home safety practices, such as installing fire alarms, ensuring safe hot water tank temperature, using electrical socket covers, and storing unsafe objects out of the reach of children. The review provides an excellent overview of how effective one-on-one education influences safety practices.

Morse, J. M. (2006). The safety of safety research: The case of patient fall research. *Canadian Journal of Nursing Research, 38*(2), 74–88; Commentary by Oliver, D. (2006). Assessing the risk of falls in hospitals: Time for a rethink? *Canadian Journal of Nursing Research, 38*(2), 89–94; Morse, J. M. (2006). Response. *Canadian Journal of Nursing Research, 38*(2), 95–96.

In this triad of articles, Morse and Oliver, leaders in fall research, debate the discrepancies between predicting and preventing falls. The articles provide updates on safety issues and offer insight into the academic discussion on the range of issues.

WEBLINKS

Canadian Nurses Association's Patient Safety Resource Guide

http://www.cna-nurses.ca/cna/practice/environment/safety/guide/default_e.aspx

This site offers a searchable database containing references related to all aspects of patient safety.

Canadian Patient Safety Institute

http://www.patientsafetyinstitute.ca/index.html

This resource provides a range of information about a variety of safety issues in Canada. It offers an electronic newsletter, research updates, safety resources, and relevant links to other websites.

Canada Safety Council

http://www.safety-council.org/index.html

This site offers a range of tips on safety for all age groups. It addresses topical safety issues, such as minimum alcohol level standards and internet safety.

Public Health Agency of Canada: Injury Surveillance On-Line

http://dsol-smed.phac-aspc.gc.ca/dsol-smed/is-sb/index_e.html

Injuries treated in the emergency departments of the Canadian Hospitals Injury Reporting and Prevention Program (CHIRPP) are summarized at this site. Nurses can monitor trends so that relevant health-promotion and injury-prevention programs can be developed.

Safe Kids Canada

http://www.sickkids.ca/safekidscanada/

Parents, children, and health professionals can all benefit from this site, which offers practical, fun, and up-to-date material on injury prevention for all childhood age groups.

Smartrisk

http://www.smartrisk.ca

Smartrisk is a Canadian nonprofit organization dedicated to preventing injuries and saving lives. This site provides a range of creative and educational safety learning opportunities.

REFERENCES

Baker, G. R., Norton, P. G., Flintoft, V., Blais, R., Brown, A., Cox, J., et al. (2004). The Canadian adverse event study: The incidence of adverse events among hospital patients in Canada. *Canadian Medical Association Journal, 170*(11), 1678–1686.

Baker, S. P., O'Neill, B., Ginsburg, M. J., & Guohua, L. (1992). *The injury fact book.* New York: Oxford University Press.

Ball, J., & Bindler, R. (2008). *Pediatric nursing: Caring for children* (4th ed.). Upper Saddle River, NJ: Prentice Hall Health.

Breslin, F. C., Polzer, J., MacEachen, E., Morrongiello, B., & Shannon, H. (2006). Workplace Injury or "part of the job"? Towards a gendered understanding of injuries and complaints among young workers. *Social Science & Medicine, 64,* 782–793.

Canada Injury. (2007). *What is injury?* Retrieved May 21, 2008, from http://www.canadainjury.com/node/2

Canada Mortgage and Housing Corporation. (2003). *About your house: Preventing falls on stairs.* Ottawa: Author.

Canadian Council on Health Services Accreditation. (2007). *CCHSA patient/client safety goals and required organizational practices (ROPs): Evaluation of implementation and evidence of compliance for 2007.* Retrieved May 24, 2008, from http://www.cchsa.ca/upload/files/pdf/Patient%20Safety/PS%20ROP%20version%202%201%20for%202007%20E.pdf

Canadian Council on Health Services Accreditation. (2008). *CCHSA patient safety required organizational practices (ROPs): New ROPs for 2008 accreditation surveys.* Retrieved May 31, 2008, from http://www.cchsa.ca/upload/files/pdf/Patient%20Safety/new%20PS%20ROP%202008%20E.pdf

Canadian Hospitals Injury Reporting and Prevention Program. (2002). *Summary statistics CHIRP database.*

Retrieved May 31, 2008, from http://www.phac-aspc.gc.ca/injury-bles/

Canadian Institute of Child Health. (2002). *The health of Canada's children* (3rd ed.). Ottawa: Author.

Canadian Nurses Association. (2003). *Position statement: Patient safety.* Ottawa: Author.

Canadian Nurses Association & University of Toronto Faculty of Nursing. (2004). *Nurses and patient safety: A discussion paper.* Ottawa: Author.

Canadian Paediatric Society. (2007). *Are we doing enough? A status report on Canadian public policy and child and youth health.* Retrieved May 24, 2008, from http://www.voicesforchildren.ca/documents/CPSreport.pdf

College of Nurses of Ontario. (2005). *Practice standard: Restraints.* Toronto: Author.

Ebersole, P., Hess, P., Touhy, T., Jett, K., & Luggen, A. (2008). *Toward healthy aging: Human needs and nursing response* (7th ed.). St. Louis, MO: Mosby/Elsevier.

Health Canada. (2004). *Crib safety.* Ottawa: Health Canada.

Health Canada. (2005). *Reducing fire risk from cigarettes.* Retrieved May 29, 2008, from http://www.hc-sc.gc.ca/hl-vs/tobac-tabac/res/news-nouvelles/fs-if/fire-incendie_html

Health Canada. (2006). *Is your child safe?* Ottawa: Author.

Health Canada. (2007). *Crib safety fact sheet.* Ottawa: Health Canada.

Health Canada. (2008). *Smoke detectors, carbon monoxide detectors, and charcoal.* Retrieved May 30, 2008, from http://www.hc-sc.gc.ca/cps-spc/house-domes/fire-feu/detect_e.html.

Kimbell, S. (2002). Breaking the fall factor. *Nursing Management, 33*(9), 22–26.

Kohn, L. T., Corrigan, J. M., & Donaldson, M. S. (Eds.). (2000) *To err is human. Building a safer health system.* Washington, DC: National Academy Press.

Lang, A., Edwards, N., & Fleiszer, A. (2008). Safety in home care: A broadened perspective of patient safety. *International Journal for Quality in Health Care, 20*(2), 130–135.

Leitch, K. (2007). *Reaching for the top: A report by the advisor on healthy children and youth.* Ottawa: Health Canada.

Leonard, P., Hoffman, C., & the National Steering Committee on Patient Safety. (2002). *Building a safer system: A national integrated strategy for improving patient safety in Canadian health care.* Retrieved May 31, 2008, from http://rcpsc.medical.org/publications/building_a_safer_system_e.pdf

Li, F., Harmer, P, Fisher, J., McAuley, E., Chaumeton, N., Eckstrom, E., et al. (2005). Tai Chi and fall reductions in older adults: A randomized controlled trial. *Journal of Gerontology, 60*(2), 187–194.

Mohr, W. K., Petti, T. A., & Mohr, B. D. (2003). Adverse effects associated with physical restraint. *Canadian Journal of Psychiatry, 48*(5), 330–337.

Morse, J. M. (2006). The safety of safety research: The case of patient fall research. *Canadian Journal of Nursing Research, 38*(2), 74–88.

NANDA International. (2007). *Nursing diagnoses: Definitions and classification, 2007–2008.* Philadelphia, PA: Author.

Nicklin, W. (2003). Patient safety: Springboard to nursing accountability. *Canadian Journal of Nursing Leadership, 16*(4), 66–68.

Oliver, D., Britton, M., Seed, P., Martin, F. C., & Hopper, A. H. (1997). Development and evaluation of evidence based risk assessment tool (STRATIFY) to predict which elderly inpatients will fall: Case-control and cohort studies. *British Medical Journal, 315,* 1049–1053.

Pless, I. B., & Hagel, B.E. (2005). Injury prevention: A glossary of terms. *Journal of Epidemiology and Community Health, 59,* 182–185.

Public Health Agency of Canada. (2001). Bioterrorism and public health. *Canada Communicable Disease Report, 27*(4), 29–31.

Public Health Agency of Canada. (2005). *Report on seniors' falls in Canada: Chapter 3 Risk factors for falls and fall-related injuries in seniors. Technical Report.* Ottawa: Minister of Public Works and Government Services.

Public Health Agency of Canada. (2006). *The safe living guide: A guide to home safety for seniors.* Retrieved May 24, 2008, from http://www.phac-aspc.gc.ca/seniors-aines/pubs/safelive/slg02_e.htm

Registered Nurses' Association of Ontario. (2005). *Prevention of falls and fall injuries in the older adult.* Toronto: Author.

Royal College of Physicians and Surgeons. (2003). *Canadian patient safety dictionary.* Retrieved May 24, 2008, from http://rcpsc.medical.org/publications/PatientSafetyDictionary_e.pdf

Safe Kids Canada. (2005). *Hot water burns like fire: Discussion paper on tap water scalds prevention.* Retrieved May 29, 2008, from http://www.sickkids.ca/SKCPublicPolicyAdvocacy/custom/TapwaterscaldsDISCUSSIONPAPERrevised2005.pdf

Safe Kids Canada. (2006). *Child & youth unintentional injury, 1994–2003: 10 years in review.* Retrieved May 24, 2008, from http://www.sickkids.ca/SKCForPartners/custom/SKW06NationalReportENG.pdf

Safe Kids Canada. (2007). *Position statement: Pool drowning and the need for safer pool fencing.* Retrieved January 30, 2008, from http://www.sickkids.ca/SKCPublicPolicyAdvocacy/custom/SKC_PoolFencingPositionStatementENG.pdf

Smartrisk. (1998). *The economic burden of unintentional injury in Canada.* Toronto: Author.

Statistics Canada. (2007). *Mortality: Summary list of causes, 2002, 2003, 2004.* Ottawa: Author.

Tourangeau, A. E., Cranley, L. A., & Jeffs, L. (2006). Impact of nursing on hospital patient mortality: A focused review and related policy implications. *Quality and Safety in Health Care, 15,* 4–8.

Transport Canada. (2006). *Keep kids safe: Car time 1-2-3-4.* TP #13511. Retrieved May 21, 2008, from http://www.tc.gc.ca/roadsafety/tp/tp13511/pdf/tp13511e.pdf

Chapter 31

Medication Administration

Pharmacology is the science concerned with drugs and their actions on living organisms. Strictly speaking, a drug is any chemical substance that can have an effect on living organisms. A **medication** is a substance administered for the diagnosis, treatment, or prevention of a health condition or disease. In the health-care context, the words *medication* and *drug* are used interchangeably. Over the centuries, the number of drugs available has dramatically increased, and knowledge about these drugs has become more comprehensive. As nurses are the health-care professionals primarily responsible for the calculation, administration, and evaluation of the effects of drugs, it is essential that they are knowledgeable about pharmacokinetics (action of the body on the drug) and pharmacodynamics (action of the drug on the body).

OBJECTIVES

After studying this chapter, you should be able to

1. Define selected terms related to the administration of medications
2. Identify physiological factors and individual variables affecting medication action
3. Distinguish among the enteral, parenteral, and topical routes of medication administration
4. Identify the nine essential parts of a medication prescription
5. Recognize common abbreviations used in prescriptions
6. List six essential steps to follow when administering medications
7. State the 10 rights in accurate medication administration
8. Describe the physiological changes in older adults that alter medication administration and effectiveness
9. Describe the essential steps in safely administering enteral medications by oral, sublingual, buccal routes, or through nasogastric or gastrostomy tubes
10. Describe the essential steps in safely administering parenteral medications by subcutaneous, intramuscular, intradermal, and intravenous routes
11. Describe the essential steps in safely administering topical medications: dermatological, ophthalmic, otic, nasal, rectal, vaginal, and respiratory inhalation preparations

Key Concepts in Pharmacology

In Canada, medications are usually dispensed on the order of physicians, dentists, chiropodists, midwives, and nurse practitioners (also called registered nurses in the extended class [RNEC] in Ontario) for therapeutic use. The written direction for the preparation and administration of a drug is called a **prescription**. One drug can have as many as four kinds of names: its generic name, official name, chemical name, and trademark or brand name. The **generic name** is given before a drug becomes official. The generic name is approved by Health Canada under the Food and Drug Regulations. The **official name** is the name under which the drug is listed in one of the official publications (e.g., the *Compendium of Pharmaceuticals and Specialties*, the *Canadian Formulary*, the *United States Pharmacopeia*) and is often the same as the generic name. The **chemical name** describes the chemical constituents and molecular structure of the drug precisely. The chemical name of Aspirin, for example, is acetylsalicylic acid. The **trademark**, or **brand name**, is the name given by the drug manufacturer, which means that the drug has a registered trademark and patent. A patent gives the manufacturing company the exclusive right to sell the drug for 20 years in Canada. The trade name is identified by manufacturers with the symbol ™ or ® in the upper right corner of the name (for example, Aspirin®). Once the patent period ends, other companies can produce the same drug. As a result, the same drug manufactured by several companies will have several trade names. For example, the drug Aspirin (official name) is known by the trade names Bayer and Entrophen.

Each drug evaluated by Health Canada Therapeutic Products Directorate and approved for sale in Canada receives an eight-digit Drug Identification Number. This number is found on the label of all prescription and over-the-counter drugs (OTCs) as well as natural health products. See Figure 31.1.

Hepatitis B Vaccine

DIN: 02243576
Pedriatic Presentation
(thimerosal-free)

DIN: 00749486
Adult Presentation

DIN: 02243676
Adult Presentation
(thimerosal-free)

DIN: 02245977
Adult Dialysis Presentation
(thimerosal-free)

FIGURE 31.1 Drug Identification Number

Look-Alike and Sound-Alike Health Product Names

Many marketed brand drugs sound similar in name (sound-alike), are labelled and packaged in similar ways (look-alike), and can be easily confused when written or spoken. Examples of look-alike and sound-alike trade names are Celebrex, Celexa, and Cerebyx. It is easy to comprehend how these drugs sound similar when pronounced or look alike when written. Medication errors are one of the most common adverse events that occur in health care. The recommendations of the Institute for Safe Medication Practices Canada (2006) to prevent errors are to use tall-man lettering (DOBUTamine and DOPamine), to ensure that both generic and brand names are used when ordering a prescription, and to include the reason that the medication is being used. It is imperative that nurses are meticulous and check and double check to ensure the medication administered is the one prescribed.

Drug Classifications

Medications are usually classed according to the action on the organ or system in the body, therapeutic use or relief of symptoms, and the desired effect. For example, the classification of all drugs used for hypertension is antihypertensive agents and includes diuretics, angiotensin-converting-enzyme (ACE) inhibitors, and calcium channel blockers. Each of the classes can also be used to treat other conditions (e.g., diuretics are used to manage heart failure).

Medication Forms

Medications are available in a variety of forms. See Table 31.1. The route of administration is determined by the physical and chemical properties of the drug, the condition of the patient, the desired action of the drug, its speed of absorption, and how quickly a response is required.

Drug Legislation

The administration of drugs in Canada is controlled by law. Canadians proposed legislation concerning the sale of drugs, cosmetics, and medical devices quite some time

TABLE 31.1 Types of Drug Preparations

Type	Description
Aerosol spray or foam	A liquid, powder, or foam deposited in a thin layer on the skin by air pressure
Aqueous solution	One or more drugs dissolved in water
Aqueous suspension	One or more drugs dispersed in a liquid, such as water
Caplet	A solid form, shaped like a capsule, coated and easily swallowed
Capsule	A gelatinous container to hold a drug in powder, liquid, or oil form
Cream	A nongreasy, semisolid preparation used on the skin
Elixir	A sweetened and aromatic solution of alcohol used as a vehicle for medicinal agents
Extract	A concentrated form of a drug made from vegetables or animals
Enteric coated	A tablet or capsule coated with an insoluable substance that will not dissolve until it reaches the small intestine; drugs that are not enteric coated usually are rendered ineffective in the acidic juices of the stomach
Gel or jelly	A clear or translucent semisolid that liquefies when applied to the skin
Inhalation	A solution of a drug, or a combination of drugs, administered as a nebulized mist
Liniment	A medication mixed with alcohol, oil, or soapy emollient and applied to the skin
Lotion	A medication in a liquid suspension applied to the skin
Lozenge (troche)	A flat, round, or oval preparation that dissolves and releases a drug when held in the mouth
Ointment (salve, unction)	A semisolid preparation of one or more drugs used for application to the skin and mucous membrane
Paste	A preparation like an ointment, but thicker and stiff, that penetrates the skin less than an ointment
Pessary	A type of medicated suppository that is normally inserted into the vagina
Pill	One or more drugs mixed with a cohesive material, in oval, round, or flattened shapes
Powder	A finely ground drug or drugs; some are used internally, others externally
Suppository	One or several drugs mixed with a firm base such as gelatin and shaped for insertion into the body (e.g., the rectum); the base dissolves gradually at body temperature, releasing the drug
Syrup	An aqueous solution of sugar often used to disguise unpleasant-tasting drugs
Tablet	A powdered drug compressed into a hard small disc; some are readily broken along a scored line; others are enteric coated to prevent them from dissolving in the stomach
Tincture	An alcoholic or water-and-alcohol solution prepared from drugs derived from plants
Transdermal disk or patch	A semipermeable membrane shaped in the form of a disc or patch that contains a drug to be absorbed through the skin over a long period of time

before these concerns became evident in the United States. For example, in 1875, the Parliament of Canada passed an act to prevent the sale of contaminated food, alcohol, and drugs (both controlled and restricted). By the early part of the twentieth century, a legal framework was established in Canada for drug control. By 1908, all medicines, as well as tobacco and alcohol, had some regulations.

The Canadian Food and Drugs Act, enacted in 1953 with amendments since, is the major piece of legislation that was responsible for the regulation of drugs in Canada. The Food and Drug Regulations prescribe

- Standards of composition
- Strength
- Potency
- Purity
- Safety
- Efficacy
- Quality or other property of the article of food or drug to which they refer

The second purpose of the Canadian Food and Drugs Act is to address the purchasing and advertising of drugs, cosmetics, foods, and medical devices, and enforce regulations. For example, no one is allowed to "sell any drug that was manufactured, prepared, preserved, packaged, or stored under unsanitary conditions" (Department of Justice, 1985, p. 2).

Drug Standards

Many drugs have natural (e.g., plant, mineral, and animal) sources, and others are synthesized in the laboratory. For example, digitalis and opium are plant derived, iron and sodium chloride are minerals, insulin and vaccines can have animal or human sources, and the sulphonamides and propoxyphene hydrochloride (the analgesic Darvon) are the products of laboratory synthesis. Early drugs were derived from the three natural sources only. During the past 45 years, however, more and more drugs have been produced synthetically.

Drugs vary in strength and activity. Drugs derived from plants, for example, vary in strength according to the age of the plant, the variety, the place in which it is grown, and the method by which it is preserved. Drugs must be pure and of uniform strength if drug dosages are to be predictable in their effect. Drug standards have therefore been developed to ensure uniform quality. In North America, official drugs are designated by the Canadian Federal Food, Drug, and Cosmetic Act and the American Federal Food, Drug, and Cosmetic Act. In Canada, drugs are listed in the *British Pharmacopoeia*. Drugs on the list are described according to a variety of properties including their specific chemical and physical properties, where and how they are produced, identity and purity, method of storage, category, and normal dosages. In the United States, the *United States Pharmacopeia* (*USP*) is used to identify the drugs.

A **pharmacopoeia** (also spelled *pharmacopeia*) is a book containing a list of products used in medicine, with descriptions of the product, chemical tests for determining identity and purity, and formulas and prescriptions. The *Canadian Formulary* lists drugs used extensively in Canada but not necessarily listed in the *British Pharmacopoeia*. The United States' *National Formulary* lists drugs and their therapeutic value and can include drugs that may still be used but are not listed in the *USP*.

Pharmacopoeias and formularies are invaluable references for nurses and nursing students. Nurses not only administer thousands of medications but also are responsible for assessing their effectiveness and recognizing unfavourable reactions to drugs. Since it is impossible to commit to memory all pertinent information about a very large number of drugs, nurses must have a reliable reference readily available.

The Controlled Drugs and Substances Act

The Controlled Drugs and Substances Act, passed in 1996, replaced the former Canadian Narcotic Control Act, which had replaced the Canadian Opium and Narcotic Act of 1952. Regulations regarding possession, sale, manufacture, production, and distribution of opioids are all covered in the Controlled Drugs and Substances Act. Health Canada is responsible for the administration of policies, while the Royal Canadian Mounted Police are responsible for the enforcement of the act.

Marijuana is effective in relieving nausea in chemotherapy, controlling epileptic seizures, treating glaucoma, and easing the pain of individuals with AIDS. In 2001, Health Canada implemented the Marihuana Medical Access Regulations (MMAR), effectively making Canada the first country in the world to allow its citizens to legally access cannabis for medicinal purposes. In 2005, Canada was the first country to approve Sativex for the use of neuropathic pain in multiple sclerosis. Since 2005, selected Canadian pharmacies have been allowed to distribute medicinal marijuana for use by MMAR authorized clients. This initiative makes Canada the second country in the world (after the Netherlands) to allow access to medical marijuana in pharmacies. Concerns about the quality and safety of natural health products led to the development of the Natural Health Products Regulations under the Food and Drugs Act of 2004. Table 31.2 provides a summary of Canadian and U.S. drug legislation.

Application to Nursing Practice

In Canada, nursing practice is regulated under federal and provincial or territorial legislation. The administration of medications is included within these regulations. Laws and policies for medication administration differ across the country (i.e., the prescription domain of advanced practice nurses will vary across provinces and territories). Nurses need to know how nursing practice acts in their jurisdictions define and limit their functions and be able to recognize the limits of their own knowledge and skill in the administration of medications. To function beyond the limits of nursing practice acts or beyond their ability endangers clients' lives and leaves nurses open to malpractice suits. Under the law, nurses are responsible for their own actions, regardless of whether there is a written order. If a health-care provider writes an incorrect order (e.g., digoxin 25 mg, instead of digoxin 0.25 mg), a nurse who administers the written incorrect dosage can be held responsible for the error. Therefore, nurses should question any order that appears unreasonable and not administer the medication until the prescription is clarified.

TABLE 31.2 Canadian and U.S. Drug Legislation

Canadian Drug Legislation		United States Drug Legislation	
Legislation	**Content**	**Legislation**	**Content**
Proprietary or Patent Medicine Act (1908)	Protects the public against unsafe and ineffective over-the-counter drugs.	Food, Drug, and Cosmetic Act (1938)	Implemented by the Food and Drug Administration (FDA); requires that labels be accurate and that all drugs be tested for harmful effects.
Canada Food and Drugs Act (1953)	Prohibits advertising any food, drug, cosmetic, or device as a cure for certain specified diseases. Sets standards for manufacture, distribution, and sale of all drugs, with the exception of opioids.	Durkham-Humphrey Amendment (1952)	Clearly differentiates drugs that can be sold only with a prescription, those that can be sold without a prescription, and those that should not be refilled without a new prescription.
Canadian Narcotic Control Act (1961)	Allows only authorized people to possess opioids. Specifies records about opioids that must be kept.	Kefauver-Harris Amendment (1962)	Requires proof of safety and efficacy of a drug for approval.
Controlled Drugs and Substances Act (1996)	Canadian Narcotic Control Act is subsumed under this act.	Comprehensive Drug Abuse Prevention and Control Act (1970) (Controlled Substances Act)	Categorizes controlled substances and limits how often a prescription can be filled; established government-funded programs to prevent and treat drug dependence.
Marijuana Medical Access Regulations (2001)	Allows for special access to marijuana for medical purposes.		
Natural Health Products Regulations (2004)	Ensures that natural health products are safe, effective, and of high quality.		

Another aspect of nursing practice governed by law is the use of controlled substances. In hospitals, controlled substances are kept in a locked drawer, cupboard, medication cart, or computer-controlled dispensing system. Agencies have special inventory forms for recording the use of controlled substances (for example, a restricted drug administration form). The information required usually includes the name of the patient, the date and time of administration, the name of the drug, the dosage, and the signature of the person who prepared and gave the drug. The name of the individual who ordered the drug may also be part of the record. Included on the record are details of the controlled substances wasted during the drug preparation. When a portion or all of a controlled substance dose is discarded, the nurse must ask a second nurse to witness the discarding. Both nurses must sign the control inventory form.

Before removing a controlled substance, the nurse verifies the number actually available with the number indicated on the opioid or controlled substance inventory record. In most agencies, counts of controlled substances are also taken at the end of each shift. The count total should tally with the total at the end of the last shift minus the number used. If the totals do not tally at any time and the discrepancy cannot be resolved, it must be reported immediately to the nurse manager, nursing supervisor, and pharmacy, according to agency policy. In facilities that use a computerized dispensing system, manual counts are not required because the dispensing system runs a continuous count; however, discrepancies must be accounted for. Most health-care agencies maintain a list of high-alert medications, including controlled substances, which require the verification of two registered nurses.

Effects of Drugs

The **therapeutic effect** or **desired effect** of a drug relates to the reason the drug is prescribed. The therapeutic effect is also known as the *primary effect.* For example, the therapeutic effect of morphine sulphate is analgesia, and the therapeutic effect of diazepam is relief of anxiety. See Table 31.3 for kinds of therapeutic actions.

A **side effect**, or *secondary effect,* of a drug is one that is unintended. Side effects are usually predictable and are either harmless or potentially harmful. For example, digitalis (digoxin) increases the strength of myocardial contractions (desired effect), but it can have the side effect of causing bradycardia (decreasing the heart rate too much). Some side effects are tolerated for the drug's therapeutic effect; undesired and unplanned side effects, also called *adverse effects,* may justify the discontinuation of a drug.

Drug toxicity (deleterious effects of a drug on an organism or a tissue) results from overdosage, ingestion of a drug intended for external use, and buildup of the drug in the blood because of impaired metabolism or excretion (a cumulative effect). Some toxic effects are apparent immediately; some are not apparent for weeks

TABLE 31.3 Therapeutic Actions of Drugs

Drug Type	Description	Examples
Curative	Cures a disease or condition	Penicillin for infection
Chemotherapeutic	Destroys malignant cells	Methotrexate for leukemia
Palliative	Relieves the symptoms of a disease but does not affect the disease itself	Morphine sulphate, acetaminophen for pain
Restorative	Returns the body to health	Vitamin, mineral supplements
Supportive	Supports body function until other treatments or the body's response can take over	Norepinephrine bitartrate for low blood pressure; acetaminophen for high body temperature
Substitutive	Replaces body fluids or substances	Thyroxine for hypothyroidism, insulin for diabetes mellitus

or months. Fortunately, most drug toxicity can be avoided if careful attention is paid to dosage and if patients are monitored for toxicity. An example of a toxic effect is liver failure caused by the cumulative effect of methotrexate (an anti-metabolite that is used to treat rheumatoid arthritis and certain types of cancer).

A **drug allergy** is an immunological reaction to a drug. When a patient is first exposed to an antigen (foreign substance), the body may react by producing antibodies. A drug can be antigenic and induce an allergic reaction. Allergic reactions can be either mild or severe. A mild reaction has a variety of symptoms, from skin rashes to diarrhea. See Table 31.4. An allergic reaction can occur anytime from a few minutes to 2 weeks after the administration of the drug. An **anaphylactic reaction** (a severe allergic reaction) usually occurs immediately after the administration of the drug. Common symptoms of an anaphylactic reaction (also known as anaphylactic shock) include bronchospasm, laryngeal edema, acute hypotension, and tachycardia. This response can be fatal unless the symptoms are noticed immediately and treatment is obtained promptly.

TABLE 31.4 Common Mild Allergic Responses

Symptom	Description/Rationale
Skin rash	Either an intraepidermal vesicle rash or a rash typified by an urticarial wheal or macular eruption; rash is usually generalized over the body
Pruritus	Itching of the skin with or without a rash
Angioedema	Edema caused by increased permeability of the blood capillaries
Rhinitis	Excessive watery discharge from the nose
Lacrimal tearing	Excessive tearing
Nausea, vomiting	Stimulation of these centres in the brain
Wheezing and dyspnea	Shortness of breath and wheezing on inhalation and exhalation caused by accumulated fluids and swelling of the respiratory tissues
Diarrhea	Irritation of the mucosa of the large intestine

Drug tolerance exists in a person who has unusually low physiological activity in response to a drug and who requires increases in the dosage to maintain a given therapeutic effect. Drugs that commonly produce tolerance are opiates, barbiturates, ethyl alcohol, and tobacco. A **cumulative effect** is the increasing response to repeated doses of a drug that occurs when the rate of administration exceeds the rate of metabolism or excretion. As a result, the amount of the drug builds up in the patient's body unless the dosage is adjusted. Toxic symptoms can occur. An **idiosyncratic effect** occurs when an individual's response to a drug is extreme sensitivity in low dosage or extreme sensitivity in high dosage, or a response that is quite different from the usual response expected.

A **drug interaction** occurs when the administration of one drug before, at the same time as, or after another drug alters the effect of one or both drugs. The effect of one or both drugs can be either increased (**potentiating effect**) or decreased (**inhibiting effect**). Potentiating effects can be additive or synergistic. When two of the same types of drug increase the action of each other, it is known as additive. A **synergistic effect** occurs when two different drugs given together increase the action of one of the drugs. Drug interactions can be beneficial or harmful. For example, probenecid, which blocks the excretion of penicillin, can be given with penicillin to increase blood levels of the penicillin for longer periods (synergistic effect). Two analgesics, such as acetaminophen and codeine, are often given together because together they provide greater pain relief (additive effect). In addition, certain foods can adversely interact with a medication and potentiate or inhibit its effect. For example, large amounts of leafy, green vegetables may inhibit the anticoagulant effect of warfarin.

Certain conditions can be unintentionally caused by therapy. This is referred to as **iatrogenic disease**. Some examples of iatrogenic disease as a result of drug therapy are liver damage, renal failure, and fetal abnormalities.

Problematic Substance Use

Although no universal definition of **problematic substance use** exists, it is present when a disruption occurs in any area of an individual's life (medical, physical, financial, occupational, family, interpersonal, social, legal, or academic) because of the inappropriate intake of a substance, either continually or periodically. **Drug misuse** is the improper use of common medications in ways that can lead to acute and chronic toxicity. Both OTC drugs and prescription drugs can be problematic when misused. Laxatives, antacids, vitamins, headache remedies, and cough and cold medications are often self-prescribed and overused.

The *Diagnostic and Statistical Manual of Mental Disorders* (*DSM-IV-TR*) identifies specific criteria for the diagnosis of problematic substance use and substance dependence. **Drug dependence** is a person's reliance on or need to take a drug or substance. Drug dependence comes in two types: psychological and physical. Psychological dependence is emotional reliance on a drug to maintain a sense of well-being, accompanied by feelings of need or cravings for that drug. For example, an individual may come to depend on a drug to reduce anxiety or feel happy. Psychological dependence has various degrees, ranging from mild desire to craving and compulsive use of the drug.

Physical dependence is associated with an altered physiological state in which there may be biochemical changes in body tissues, especially the nervous system. A person dependent on a drug who then stops using the medication will experience withdrawal symptoms.

Illicit drugs, also called *street drugs,* are those sold illegally. Illicit drugs are of two types: (1) drugs unavailable for purchase under any circumstances, such as heroin (in North America), and (2) drugs normally available with a prescription that are being obtained through illegal channels (for example, oxycodone). Illicit drugs often are taken because of their mood-altering effect; that is, they make the person feel happy or relaxed.

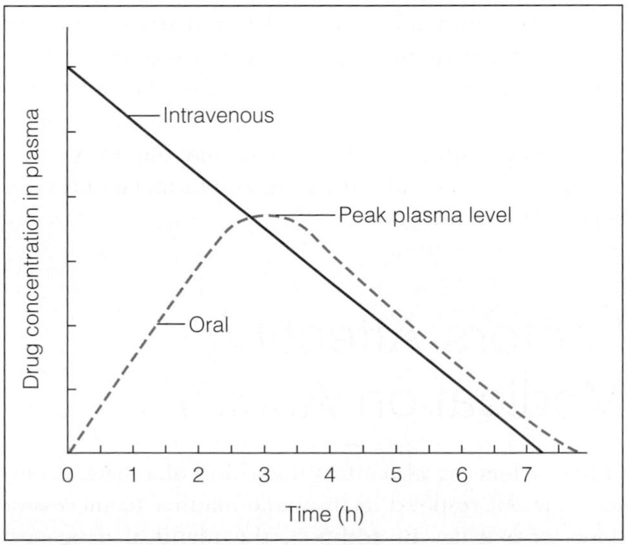

FIGURE 31.2 A graphic plot of drug concentration in the blood plasma following a single dose

Actions of Drugs in the Body

The action of a drug in the body can be described in terms of its **half-life (elimination half-life)**, the time interval required for the body's elimination processes to reduce the concentration of the drug in the body by one half. For example, if a drug's half-life is 8 hours, then the amount of drug in the body is as follows:

- Initially: 100%
- After 8 hours: 50%
- After 16 hours: 25%
- After 24 hours: 12.5%
- After 32 hours: 6.25%

Because the purpose of most drug therapy is to maintain a constant drug level in the body, repeated doses are required to maintain that level. When an orally administered drug is absorbed from the gastrointestinal tract into the blood plasma, its concentration in the plasma increases until the elimination rate equals the rate of absorption. This point is known as the **peak plasma level** (Figure 31.2). Unless the patient receives another dose of the drug, the concentration steadily decreases. The following key terms are related to drug action:

- ***Onset of action:*** The time after administration until the body initially responds to the drug
- *Peak plasma level:* The highest plasma level achieved by a single dose, when the elimination rate of a drug equals the absorption rate
- *Drug half-life:* The time required for the elimination process to reduce the concentration of the drug to one half what it was at initial administration
- ***Plateau:*** A maintained concentration of a drug in the plasma during a series of scheduled doses

Pharmacodynamics

Pharmacodynamics is the process by which a drug alters cell physiology. Drugs act on cellular structures known as receptors. Any drug that has a direct action on a receptor and alters its functional properties is known as an **agonist**. A drug that interacts with a cell receptor without stimulating it and blocks the action of the agonist is known as an **antagonist**. Drugs that have a synergistic effect produce a response by stimulating enzyme activity or hormone production.

Pharmacokinetics

Pharmacokinetics is the study of the absorption, distribution, biotransformation, and excretion of drugs.

ABSORPTION **Absorption** is the process by which a drug passes into the bloodstream. Unless the drug is administered directly into the bloodstream, absorption is the first step in the movement of the drug through the body. For absorption to occur, the correct form of the drug must be given by the route intended. Drugs may be absorbed into the body by various routes, such as through the skin, through the mucous membranes, by inhalation, by injection, or by oral ingestion.

The rate of absorption of a drug in the stomach is variable. Food, for example, can delay the dissolution and absorption of some drugs as well as their passage into the small intestine, where most drug absorption occurs. Food can also combine with molecules of certain drugs, thereby changing the drugs' molecular structure and inhibiting or preventing their absorption. Another factor that affects the absorption of some drugs is the acid medium in the stomach. Acidity can vary according to the time of day, the foods ingested, and the age of the patient. Some drugs do not dissolve or have limited ability to dissolve in the gastrointestinal fluids, decreasing the drugs' absorption into the bloodstream. Some drugs are absorbed by tissues before they reach the stomach. For example, nitroglycerine is administered under the tongue or as a buccal spray because it is absorbed into the blood vessels that carry it directly to the heart, the intended site of action. If swallowed, this drug will be absorbed into the bloodstream and carried to the liver, where it will be metabolized. Some drugs are extensively metabolized in the liver and only a small amount of drug enters the systemic circulation and reaches the target organ, a result known as the **first-pass effect**.

A drug administered directly into the bloodstream (i.e., injection or intravenous) is immediately absorbed in the vascular system. This route is preferred for rapid action. Because subcutaneous tissue has a poorer blood supply than muscle tissue does, absorption from subcutaneous tissue is slower. The rate of absorption of a drug can be accelerated by the application of heat. Heat increases blood flow to the area. Conversely, cold decreases blood flow to the area and decreases the rate of absorption. Some drugs intended to be absorbed slowly are suspended in a low-solubility medium, such as oil. The absorption of drugs from the rectum into the bloodstream tends to be unpredictable. Therefore, this route is normally used when other routes are unavailable or when the intended action is localized to the rectum or sigmoid colon.

DISTRIBUTION **Distribution** is the transportation of a drug from its site of absorption to its site of action. When a drug enters the bloodstream, it is carried to the most vascular organs—that is, liver, kidneys, and brain. Body areas with lower blood supply—that is, skin and muscles—receive the drug later. The chemical and physical properties of a drug largely determine the area of the body to which the drug will be attracted. For example, fat-soluble drugs accumulate in fatty tissue, whereas other drugs bind with plasma proteins.

BIOTRANSFORMATION **Biotransformation**, also called **detoxification** or **metabolism**, is a process by which a drug is converted to a less active form. Most biotransformation takes place in the liver, where many drug-metabolizing enzymes in the cells detoxify the drugs. The products of this process are called **metabolites**. There are two types of metabolites: active and inactive. An *active metabolite* has a pharmacological action itself, whereas an *inactive metabolite* does not.

Biotransformation can be altered if a person is young, is older, or has an unhealthy liver. Nurses must be alert to the accumulation of the active drug in these clients and to subsequent toxicity.

EXCRETION **Excretion** is the process by which metabolites and drugs are eliminated from the body. Most metabolites are eliminated by the kidneys in the urine; however, some are excreted in feces, breath, perspiration, saliva, and breast milk. Certain drugs, such as general anaesthetic agents, are excreted in an unchanged form via the respiratory tract. The efficiency with which the kidneys excrete drugs and metabolites diminishes with age. Older people may require smaller doses of a drug because the drug and its metabolites can accumulate in the body.

Factors Affecting Medication Action

Other factors can also affect the action of a drug. A person may not respond in the same manner to successive doses of a drug. In addition, the identical drug and dosage can affect individuals differently.

Developmental Factors

During pregnancy, women must be cautious about taking medications. Most drugs are contraindicated because of the possible adverse effects on the fetus.

Infants usually require smaller dosages because of their body size and the immaturity of their organs, especially the liver and kidneys. Infants often do not have all the enzymes required for drug metabolism and, therefore, may require different medications from those for adults. In adolescence or adulthood, allergic reactions can occur to drugs formerly tolerated.

Older adults have different responses to medications because of physiological changes that accompany aging. These changes include decreased liver and kidney function, which can result in the accumulation of the drug in the body. In addition, the older person may be on multiple drugs, and incompatibilities can occur.

Older adults often experience decreased gastric mobility, gastric acid production, and blood flow, all of which can impair drug absorption. Increased adipose tissue and decreased total body fluid proportionate to the body mass can increase the possibility of drug toxicity. Older adults may have a decreased number of protein-binding sites and changes in the blood-brain barrier. The latter permits fat-soluble drugs to move readily to the brain, often resulting in dizziness and confusion.

Gender

Differences in the way men and women respond to drugs are chiefly related to the distribution of body fat and fluid and to hormonal differences. Historically, most drug research was conducted on men. Now, drug researchers include both women and men in their studies, when appropriate.

Cultural, Ethnic, and Genetic Factors

A client's response to a drug is influenced by genetic variations, such as gender, size, and body composition. This variation in response is called **pharmacogenetics.**

According to Lea (2005), drug metabolism and variations in enzymes are genetically determined and, as a result, can affect a drug response. For example, the genes that control liver metabolism vary. Some clients may have slow liver metabolism and not achieve an adequate response to a medication, whereas others are rapid metabolizers and may require lower doses of a medication to avoid adverse reactions. A new genetic blood test, approved in 2004, analyzes genes in a client's blood for variations that could cause variations in the metabolism of certain drugs. This information can help health-care providers to individualize medication treatment and avoid adverse reactions.

A new field of study, **ethnopharmacology**, is the study of the effect of ethnicity on responses to prescribed mediation (Munoz & Hilgenberg, 2005). Research has shown that certain medications can work well at usual therapeutic dosages for certain ethnic groups but be toxic for others.

Cultural factors and practices (e.g., values and beliefs) can also affect a drug's action. For example, a natural health product herbal remedy (e.g., ginseng) may speed up or slow down the metabolism of prescribed medications. Guidelines for nurses who care for clients from varied cultures are provided in Box 31.1.

Diet

Nutrients can affect the action of a medication. For example, vitamin K, found in green leafy vegetables, can counteract the effect of an anticoagulant, such as warfarin. Grapefruit juice is well known to affect the absorption of many medications. It inhibits an intestinal enzyme, CYP3A, which normally prevents drugs from being used properly as it partially destroys medications before they can be absorbed. Refer to Table 39.2 (page 1175) for a list of nutrients that can affect the pharmacodynamics and pharmacokinetics of medications.

Environment

The patient's environment can affect the action of drugs, particularly those used to alter behaviour and mood. Therefore, nurses assessing the effects of a drug need to consider the drug in the context of the patient's personality.

Environmental temperature can also affect drug activity. When environmental temperature is high, the peripheral blood vessels dilate, which can intensify the action of vasodilators. In contrast, a cold environment and consequent vasoconstriction can inhibit the action of vasodilators but enhance the action of vasoconstrictors. A patient who takes a sedative or analgesic in a busy, noisy environment may have less benefit than if the environment is quiet and peaceful.

Psychological Factors

A patient's expectations of the effects of a drug can affect the response to the drug. For example, a patient who believes that codeine is ineffective as an analgesic may experience no relief from pain after it is given.

Illness and Disease

Illness and disease can also affect the action of drugs. For example, acetaminophen can reduce the body temperature of a feverish patient but has no effect on the body temperature of a patient without fever. Drug action is altered in patients with circulatory, liver, or kidney dysfunction.

BOX 31.1 ETHNOPHARMACOLOGY

Knowing that ethnicity can affect drug response helps the nurse provide culturally competent care. In the past, clinical drug research was conducted on Caucasian males, even when the health disorder being studied was prevalent in other ethnic groups. Ethnopharmacological research has focused on two major classifications: psychotropic and antihypertensive medications.

PSYCHOTROPIC MEDICATIONS

Research has found that Black people experience faster therapeutic responses, higher serum concentrations, and more adverse reactions than Caucasian clients taking tricyclic antidepressants. Black patients may require lower doses of lithium than Caucasian patients do.

ANTIHYPERTENSIVE MEDICATIONS

Studies have shown that the antihypertensive medications angiotensin-converting enzyme (ACE) inhibitors (e.g., captopril and enalapril) and angiotensin II receptor antagonists (e.g., losartan) were found to be less effective in Blacks than in Caucasians. Thiazide diuretics appear to be more effective antihypertensives in Blacks than Caucasians. The efficacy of beta blockers can vary among ethnic groups. Blacks may require higher dosages than Caucasians, and Asians usually require lower doses than Caucasians.

IMPLICATIONS FOR NURSING INTERVENTIONS

Remember that differences in medication responses are possible among different ethnic groups as are differences *within* ethnic groups:

- Ask about health beliefs, values, and customs or practices.
- Conduct a cultural assessment with each patient.
- Learn about drugs that are likely to elicit varied responses in people from different ethnic groups, as well as the potential for adverse effects.
- Ask the patient direct, specific questions to reveal the presence or absence of potential adverse effects of medications.
- Monitor the patient and document findings carefully as it may be possible to maintain therapeutic benefit at a lower dosage of a given drug.
- Keep cultural context in mind when planning education for patients and families.

Source: From "Ethnopharmacology," by C. Munoz and C. Hilgenberg, 2005, *American Journal of Nursing, 105*(8), pp. 40–48. Adapted with permission.

Time of Administration

The time of administration of oral medications affects the relative speed with which they act. Orally administered medications are absorbed more quickly if the stomach is empty. Thus, oral medications taken 2 hours before meals act faster than those taken after meals. However, some medications, for example, iron preparations, irritate the gastrointestinal tract and need to be given after a meal, when they will be better tolerated.

Routes of Administration

The route of drug administration is associated with the extent of the therapeutic response that occurs, as well as with the specific rate of the action. Therefore, the route chosen (see Table 31.5) needs to be determined on the basis of the individual client. For example, a patient who is vomiting will not have good absorption of the drug from the gastrointestinal system when the drug is administered orally. The patient may not be able to retain the drug in the stomach long enough for the drug to take effect. The route of administration should be indicated when the drug is ordered. The most common routes of administration of medications are via the gastrointestinal tract (enteral) or by injection (parenteral). Medications can also be applied to a circumscribed surface area as in topical applications.

Enteral

The **enteral** route is defined as through the gastrointestinal tract. **Oral** administration is the most common, least expensive, and most convenient enteral route for most clients. In oral administration, the drug is swallowed. Oral administration is considered to be the safest method of medication administration. The major disadvantages of oral administration are the possibly unpleasant taste of the drugs, irritation of the gastric mucosa, irregular absorption from the gastrointestinal tract, slow absorption, and, in some cases, harm to the patient's teeth. For example, ferrous sulphate can stain the teeth.

In **sublingual** administration, a drug is placed under the tongue where it dissolves (Figure 31.3). In a relatively short time, the drug is largely absorbed into the blood vessels on the underside of the tongue in the salivary secretions. The medication should not be swallowed. The medication, once absorbed in the mucosal membranes, enters the systemic circulation without first passing through the liver. Nitroglycerine is one example of a drug commonly given in this manner.

Buccal means "pertaining to the cheek." In buccal administration, a medication (e.g., a tablet) is held in the mouth between the gum and mucous membrane of the cheek until the drug dissolves (Figure 31.4). The drug may act locally on the mucous membranes of the mouth or systemically when it is swallowed in the saliva.

TABLE 31.5 Routes of Administration

Route	Advantages	Disadvantages
Oral	Most convenient Usually least expensive Safe, does not break skin barrier Administration usually does not cause stress	Inappropriate for clients with nausea or vomiting Drug may have unpleasant taste or odour Inappropriate when gastrointestinal tract has reduced motility Inappropriate if client cannot swallow or is unconscious Cannot be used before certain diagnostic tests or surgical procedures Drug may discolour teeth, harm tooth enamel Drug may irritate gastric mucosa Drug can be aspirated by seriously ill clients
Sublingual	Same as for oral, *plus* Drug can be administered for local effect Drug is rapidly absorbed into the bloodstream More potent than oral route because drug directly enters the blood and bypasses the liver	If swallowed, drug may be inactivated by gastric juice Drug must remain under tongue until dissolved and absorbed
Buccal	Same as for sublingual, *plus* Drug must remain against the cheek until dissolved and absorbed	Drug must remain against the cheek until dissolved and absorbed
Subcutaneous	Onset of drug action is faster than oral	Must involve sterile technique because it breaks skin barrier More expensive than oral Can administer only small volume Slower absorption than intramuscular administration Some drugs can irritate tissues and cause pain Can be anxiety producing
Intramuscular	Pain from irritating drugs is minimized Can administer larger volume than subcutaneous Drug is rapidly absorbed	Breaks skin barrier Can be anxiety producing Can cause discomfort Obese patients may receive subcutaneous injection if needle is not long enough (Nisbet, 2006)
Intradermal	Absorption is slow (this is an advantage in testing for allergies)	Amount of drug administered must be small Breaks skin barrier
Intravenous	Rapid effect	Limited to highly soluble drugs Drug distribution inhibited by poor circulation
Rectal	Can be used when drug has objectionable taste or odour Drug released at slow, steady rate	Dose absorbed is unpredictable May be perceived as unpleasant by client
Vaginal	Provides local therapeutic effect	Limited use
Topical	Provides a local effect Few side effects	May be messy and may soil clothes Drug can enter body through abrasions and cause systemic effects
Transdermal	Prolonged systemic effect Few side effects Avoids gastrointestinal absorption problems	Leaves residue on the skin that may soil clothes
Inhalation	Introduces drug throughout respiratory tract Rapid localized relief Drug can be administered to unconscious client	Drug intended for localized effect can have systemic effect Of use only for the respiratory system

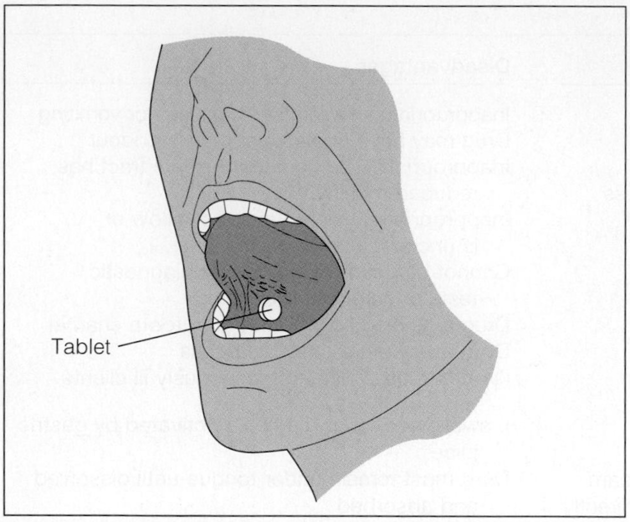

FIGURE 31.3 Sublingual administration of a tablet

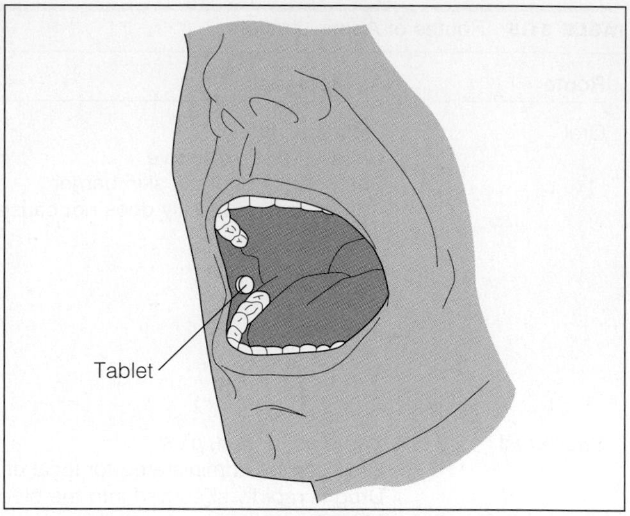

FIGURE 31.4 Buccal administration of a tablet

Parenteral

The **parenteral** route is defined as other than through the alimentary or respiratory tract; that is, by injection. The following are some of the more common routes for parenteral administration:

- **Subcutaneous** (**hypodermic**): into the subcutaneous (connective) tissue, just below the skin
- **Intramuscular**: into a muscle
- **Intradermal**: under the epidermis (into the dermis)
- **Intravenous**: into a vein

Some of the less commonly used routes for parenteral administration are **intra-arterial** (into an artery), **intracardiac** (into the heart muscle), **intraosseous** (into a bone), **intrathecal** or **intraspinal** (into the spinal canal), **intrapleural** (into the pleural space), **epidural** (into the epidural space), and **intra-articular** (into a joint). Sterile equipment and sterile drug solution are essential for all parenteral therapy. The main advantage of parenteral administration is fast absorption.

Topical

Topical applications are those applied to a circumscribed surface area of the body. They affect only the area to which they are applied. Topical applications include the following:

- *Dermatological preparations:* applied to the skin
- *Instillations and irrigations:* applied into body cavities or orifices, such as the urinary bladder, eyes, ears, nose, rectum, or vagina
- *Inhalations:* administered into the respiratory tract by a nebulizer or positive pressure breathing apparatus; air, oxygen, and vapour are generally used to carry the drug into the lungs

Medication Prescription

A physician usually determines the patient's medication needs and prescribes medications, although in some settings, nurse practitioners prescribe drugs. Each health-care agency will have its own policies. Medication orders can be written, verbal, or telephoned. Nurses need to know the agency policies about medication prescriptions (e.g., who is permitted to accept telephone and verbal orders).

Policies about prescriptions vary considerably from agency to agency. For example, a patient's medications are frequently automatically cancelled after surgery or an examination involving an anaesthetic agent. A new prescription following the procedure or surgery must then be written. Most agencies have a list of abbreviations that are acceptable to use within that agency to avoid confusion and error. The Institute for Safe Medication Practices Canada (ISMP Canada) has generated a list of potentially dangerous abbreviations, symbols, and dose designations that are frequently associated with harmful medication errors. Many institutions in Canada are implementing ISMP Canada's recommendations. Table 31.6 summarizes ISMP Canada's recommendations (2006). ISMP (US) (2006) has a more extensive list of abbreviations, symbols, and dose designations that are frequently misinterpreted and often associated with harmful medication errors, which is available on the IMSP (US) website.

Most agencies also have lists of abbreviations officially accepted for use in the agency. See Table 31.7 on page 808 for a list of some accepted abbreviations.

TABLE 31.6 Do Not Use: Dangerous Abbreviations, Symbols, and Dose Designations

Abbreviation	Intended Meaning	Potential Problem	Correction
U IU	unit international unit	Mistaken for "0"(zero), "4" (four), or cc Mistaken for "IV" (intravenous) or "10" (ten)	Use "unit". Use "unit".
Abbreviations for drug names		Misinterpreted because of similar abbreviations of multiple drugs; e.g., MS, MSO_4 (morphine sulphate), $MgSO_4$ (magnesium sulphate) may be confused for one another	Do not abbreviate drug names.
QD QOD	Every day Every other day	QD and QOD have been mistaken for each other, or as "qid"; the Q has also been misinterpreted as "2" (two)	Use "daily" and "every other day".
OD	Every day	Mistaken for "right eye" (OD = oculus dexter).	Use "daily".
OS, OD, OU	Left eye, right eye, both eyes	May be confused with one another.	Use "left eye," "right eye" or "both eyes".
D/C	Discharge	Interpreted as "discontinue whatever medications follow" (typically discharge medications).	Use "discharge".
cc	cubic centimetre	Mistaken for "u" (units).	Use "mL" or "millilitre".
µg	microgram	Mistaken for "mg" (milligram) resulting in one thousand-fold overdose.	Use "mcg".
Symbol	**Intended Meaning**	**Potential Problem**	**Correction**
@	at	Mistaken for "2" (two) or "5" (five).	Use "at".
> <	Greater than Less than	Mistaken for "7" (seven) or the letter "L". Confused with each other.	Use "greater than"/ "more than" or "less than"/"lower than".
Dose Designation	**Intended Meaning**	**Potential Problem**	**Correction**
Trailing zero	*x*.0 mg	Decimal point is overlooked resulting in a 10-fold dose error. (e.g., 3.0 mg is interpreted as 30 mg)	Never use a zero by itself after a decimal point. Use "*x* mg".
Lack of leading zero,	.*x* mg	Decimal point is overlooked resulting in a 10-fold dose error. (e.g., .3 is interpreted as 3 mg)	Always use a zero before a decimal point. Use "0.*x* mg".

Source: Reprinted with permission from ISMP Canada.

Types of Medication Prescriptions

Common medication prescriptions include the standing order, the single order, the stat order, the prn order, and the protocol order (sometimes referred to as a collective prescription).

1. The **standing order** (routine order) is the most common type of order that indicates a drug is to be given regularly for a set time or until a specified termination date is reached. A standing order may be carried out indefinitely (e.g., multiple vitamins daily) until an order is written to cancel it, or it may be carried out for a specified number of days (e.g., erythromycin 500 mg PO q6h for 7 days). In some agencies, standing orders are automatically cancelled after a specified number of days and must be then reordered.
2. The **single order** or one-time order is for medication to be given once at a specified time (e.g., lorazepam 1 mg po hs the evening before surgery).
3. A **stat order** is a single order of medication that is to be administered immediately (e.g., furosemide 80 mg po stat).
4. A **prn order**, as needed order, permits the nurse to give a medication when, in the nurse's judgment, the patient requires it (e.g., acetaminophen 325–650 mg po q4h prn). The nurse must use good judgment about when the medication is needed and when it can be safely administered.

TABLE 31.7 Common Abbreviations Used in Medication Orders

Abbreviation	Explanation
ac (*ante cibum*)	before meals
ad lib	freely, as desired
bid	twice a day
cap	capsules
hs	at bedtime
IM	intramuscular
IV	intravenous
pc (*post cibum*)	after meals
po or PO (*per os*)	by mouth
prn	when needed
q2h	every 2 hours
q4h	every 4 hours
q6h	every 6 hours
q8h	every 8 hours
stat	at once

5. A **protocol order** or **collective prescription** is a set of criteria and orders under which a medication is to be administered. For example, heparin protocols and insulin protocols are often used in hospital settings for a variety of patients.

Essential Parts of a Drug Order

The drug order has seven essential parts, as listed in Box 31.2. In addition, unless it is a standing order, it should state the number of doses or the number of days the drug is to be administered.

The *patient's full name,* that is, the first and last names and middle initials or names, should always be used to avoid confusion between two patients who have the same last name. In health-care agencies, an identifying wristband must be on all patients and used to compare the information that accompanies each dose of medication. In some agencies, the patient's identification number and physician's name are put on the order as further identification. Some hospitals imprint the patient's name, identification number, and room number on all forms.

BOX 31.2 ESSENTIAL PARTS OF A DRUG ORDER

A drug order has the following essential parts:

- Full name of the client
- Date and time the order is written
- Generic and trade name of the drug to be administered
- Dosage of the drug
- Route of administration
- Frequency of administration
- Signature of the person writing the order

In addition to *the day, the month, and the year* the order was written, some agencies also require that the *time of day* be written. Writing the time of day on the order can eliminate errors when the nursing shifts change and makes clear when certain orders automatically terminate. For example, in some settings, opioids can be ordered only for 48 hours after surgery. Therefore, a drug that is ordered at 1600 hours November 1, 2009, is automatically cancelled at 1600 November 3, 2009. Many health agencies use the 24-hour clock, which eliminates confusion between morning and afternoon times. The 24-hour clock begins at midnight, which is 00:00 hours.

The *name of the drug to be administered* must be clearly written—the recommendation is for both generic and trade name form to be written. In some settings, only generic names are permitted; however, trade names are widely used in hospitals and other health-care settings.

The *dosage of the drug* includes the amount, the times or *frequency of administration,* and, in many instances, the strength; for example, tetracycline *250 mg* (amount) *4 times a day* (frequency); potassium chloride *10%* (strength) *5 mL* (amount) *3 times a day with meals* (time and frequency). Dosages should be written in the metric system.

Also included in the order is the *route of administration* of the drug. It is not unusual for a drug to have several possible routes of administration; therefore, it is essential that the route be included in the order.

The *signature* of the ordering physician or nurse makes the drug order a legal request. An unsigned order has no validity, and the ordering physician or nurse needs to be notified if the order is unsigned.

When a health-care provider writes a prescription for a patient, the prescription includes information for the pharmacist. Therefore, a prescription's content differs from that of a medication order in a hospital. Compare the parts of a prescription listed in Box 31.3 with those shown in Figure 31.5.

Communicating a Medication Order

A drug order is written on the patient's chart by a physician or by a registered nurse receiving a telephone or verbal order from a physician. Most agencies have a specified time frame (e.g., 24 or 48 hours) in which the physician issuing the telephone or verbal order must cosign the order written by the nurse. Because of the risk of error that can arise from telephone communication, some agencies require that two nurses listen to the verbal order; other agencies do not permit such orders. The medication order is then copied by a nurse or clerk to a Kardex or medication administration record (MAR). Increasingly, nurses are being provided with computer printouts of a patient's medications instead of copying

BOX 31.3 PARTS OF A PRESCRIPTION

A prescription has the following important parts:

- Descriptive information about the client: name, address, and sometimes age, health insurance number (or identification number)
- Date on which the prescription was written
- The Rx symbol (based on the Latin word *recipere*, meaning "take thou")
- Medication name, dosage, and strength
- Route of administration
- Dispensing instructions for the pharmacist, for example, "Dispense 30 capsules"
- Directions for administration to be given to the client, for example, "Sig. Tab 1 with meals"
- Refill or special labelling, for example, "Refill × 1"
- Prescriber's signature

the physician's order. This method avoids errors of copying and saves nursing time.

Medication administration records (Figure 31.6 is an example of a computerized medication form) vary in form according to agency, but all include the patient's name, room, and bed number; drug name and dose; and times and method of administration. In some agencies, the date the order was prescribed and the date the order expires are also included.

The nurse should always question the physician about any order that is ambiguous, unusual (e.g., an abnormally high dosage of a medication), or contraindicated. When the nurse believes that a medication prescription is inappropriate, the following actions are required:

- Contact the physician and discuss the rationale for believing the medication or dosage to be inappropriate.
- Document in the notes when the physician was notified, what was conveyed to the physician, and how the physician responded.
- If the physician cannot be reached, document all attempts to contact the physician and the reason for withholding the medication.
- If someone else gives the medication, document data about the patient's condition before and after the medication.
- If a report is indicated, clearly document factual information.

Systems of Measurement

Two systems of measurement are used in Canada: the metric system and the household system, which is similar to the apothecaries' system.

Name Jane Cleary Age 36

Address 3376 W. 141st St., Regina SK Date Nov 1, 2009

This prescription will be filled generically unless physician signs on line stating "Dispense as written."

℞

Tetracycline 250 mg po

Disp. #30

Sig. 1 qid take on an empty stomach

F. March

Dispense as Written — Substitution Permissible

Frances March, M.D. 120 Madison Road Regina, SK

Ph. No. 685-9533

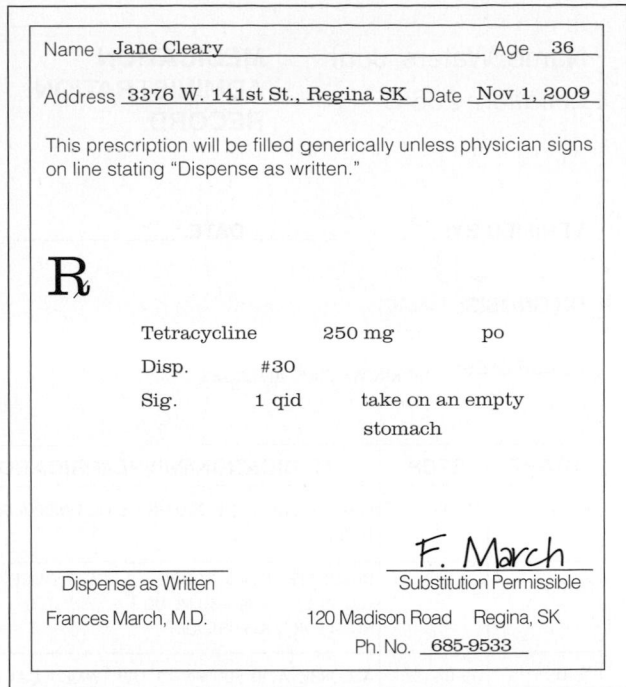

FIGURE 31.5 A prescription filled out by a physician

Metric System

The metric system, devised by the French in the latter part of the eighteenth century, is the standard system of measurement in Canada and most European countries. In the metric system, the basic unit of length is the metre, the basic unit of mass is the gram, and the basic unit of volume is the litre. The system is based on a decimal system (i.e., powers of 10).

Prefixes derived from Latin designate subdivisions of the basic unit: *deci* (1/10 or 0.1), *centi* (1/100 or 0.01), and *milli* (1/1000 or 0.001). Multiples of the basic units are designated by prefixes derived from Greek: *deca* (10), *hecto* (100), and *kilo* (1000). Only the measurements of volume (the litre) and of weight (the gram) are discussed in this chapter. These are the measures used in medication administration (Figure 31.7). The kilogram (kg) is a multiple of the gram (g), and the milligram (mg) and microgram (mcg or μg) are subdivisions. Fractional parts of the litre (L) are usually expressed in millilitres (mL), for example, one half of a litre is 500 mL; multiples of the litre are usually expressed as litres or millilitres, for example, 2.5 litres or 2500 mL.

Household System

Many people are more familiar with household measures. Household measures can be used when more accurate systems of measure are not required. Included in household measures are drops, teaspoons, tablespoons, cups, and glasses. Equivalent units of the household system are listed in Table 31.8.

Name: Waters, Juni
Location: 236 B

MEDICATION ADMINISTRATION RECORD

PAGE 1 OF 1

PRN#:
MRN#: **AGE:**
ADM: 08-04-09 **SEX:**
DOB: **HT:**
DR. **WT:**

VERIFIED BY: ______________ **DATE:** ______________

DIAGNOSIS: ALOC
PNEUMONIA

ALLERGIES: NO KNOWN DRUG ALLERGIES

GENERATED: 08-07-09 07:32
FOR PERIOD: 08-07-09 08:00
THROUGH: 08-08-09 07:59

START	STOP	MEDICATION/IV/IVPB/IRRIGATION		0800–1559	1600–2359	0000–0759
08-06	09-05	FERROUS SULPHATE 300 MG = 5 ML TWICE A DAY PO (FES04)	(973539)	09	17	
08-06	09-05	DOCUSATE SODIUM 100 MG = 1 UDCUP TWICE A DAY PO (COLACE) 100 MG/30 ML UD HOLD FOR LOOSE STOOL	(973532)	09	17	
08-05	09-04	ASCORBIC ACID 500 MG = 1 TAB TWICE A DAY PO (VITAMIN C) 500 MG TAB	(972096)	09	17	
08-05	09-04	LEVOTHYROXINE 0.05 MG = 1 TAB DAILY PO (SYNTHROID) 0.05 MG TAB	(972095)	09		
08-05	09-04	ASPIRIN 325 MG = 1 TAB DAILY PO (ASPIRIN) 325 MG TAB *W/FOOD TO AVOID GI UPSET	(972094)	09		
08-04	08-14	CEF ROXIME ADDV. 1.500 G =1 VIAL EVERY 8 HOURS IV (KEFUROX) 1.5 G ADDV *ATTACH TO D_5W 50 ML ADDV BAG *ACTIVATE BEFORE INFUSION* * INFUSE OVER 30 MIN*	(971776)	14	22	06
		PRN ORDERS				
08-04	09-03	ACETAMINOPHEN 650 MG = 1SUPP EVERY 4 HOURS AS NEEDED PR (TYLENOL) 650 MG SUPP	(971779)			

INITIALS	SIGNATURE	SHIFT	INITIALS	SIGNATURE	SHIFT	INITIALS	SIGNATURE	SHIFT

SITE CODES: **A. Right Upper Outer Quadrant Gluteus** **B. Left Upper Outer Quadrant Gluteus** **C. Right Outer Aspect Arm** **D. Left Outer Aspect Arm** **E. RIght Ventrogluteal** **F. Left Ventrogluteal** **G. Abdomen** **H. Right Thigh** **I. Left Thigh**

FIGURE 31.6 Medication administration record (MAR)

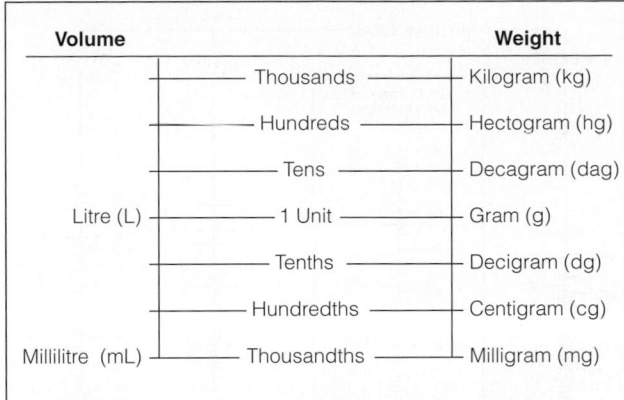

Volume		Weight
	Thousands	Kilogram (kg)
	Hundreds	Hectogram (hg)
	Tens	Decagram (dag)
Litre (L)	1 Unit	Gram (g)
	Tenths	Decigram (dg)
	Hundredths	Centigram (cg)
Millilitre (mL)	Thousandths	Milligram (mg)

FIGURE 31.7 Basic metric measurements of volume and weight and their symbols

Apothecaries' System

A system that is much older than the metric system, known as the apothecaries' system, was brought to North America from Britain during the Colonial period. Some of the units of mass used in the apothecaries' system include the scruple, the dram, the ounce, and the pound. Units of volume are the fluid dram, the fluid ounce, the pint, the quart, and the gallon.

It is important to emphasize that although the pound and the fluid ounce may be seen in clinical practice, the standard units of measurement used should be the metric system.

CONVERTING UNITS OF WEIGHT WITHIN THE METRIC SYSTEM It is relatively simple to arrive at equivalent units of weight within the metric system because the system is based on units of 10. Only three metric units of weight are used for drug dosages: the gram (g), milligram (mg), and microgram (mcg or μg); 1000 mg or 1 000 000 mcg equals 1 g. Equivalents are computed by dividing or multiplying; for example, to change milligrams to grams, the nurse divides the number of milligrams by 1000. The simplest way to divide by 1000 is to move the decimal point three places to the left:

500 mg = ? g

Move the decimal point three places to the *left:*

Answer = 0.5 g

Conversely, to convert grams to milligrams, multiply the number of grams by 1000, or move the decimal point three places to the right:

0.006 g = ? mg

Move the decimal point three places to the *right:*

Answer = 6 mg

CONVERTING WEIGHTS AND MEASURES BETWEEN SYSTEMS When preparing patient medications, a nurse may need to convert weights or volumes from one system to another. For example, a patient may know his weight in pounds, yet the amount of drug to be given is based on mg/kg of body weight (1 kg = 2.2 lb). To prepare the correct dose, the nurse must convert from the apothecaries' (pounds) to the metric system (kilograms):

$$2.2 \text{ lb} = 1 \text{ kg}$$
$$110 \text{ lb} = x \text{ kg}$$
$$x = \frac{110 \times 1}{2.2}$$
$$= 50 \text{ kg}$$

TABLE 31.8 Approximate Volume and Weight Equivalents: Metric, Apothecaries', and Household Systems

Metric	Apothecaries'	Household
1 mL	= 15 minims (min or m)	= 15 drops (gtt)
5 mL	= 1 fluid dram	= 1 teaspoon (tsp)
15 mL	= 3 fluid drams	= 1 tablespoon (Tbsp)
30 mL	= 1 fluid ounce	= 30 mL
500 mL	= 1 pint (pt)	= 500 mL
1000 mL (1 L)	= 1 quart (qt)	= 1000 mL
4000 mL	= 1 gallon (gal)	= 4000 mL
30 g	= 1 ounce (oz)	= 30 g
1000 g (1 kg)	= 2.2 pounds (lb)	= 1000 g

- Millilitres are commonly used in prescribing liquid medications, such as cough syrups, laxatives, antacids, and antibiotics for children.
- Litres and millilitres are the volumes commonly used in preparing solutions for enemas, irrigating solutions for douches, bladder irrigations, and solutions for cleaning open wounds.

The conversion of milligrams to grams was previously discussed. The decimal point is moved three spaces to the left: 3000 mg = 3 g.

Calculating Dosages

Several formulas can be used to calculate drug dosages. One formula uses ratios:

$$\frac{\text{Dose on hand}}{\text{Quantity on hand}} = \frac{\text{Desired dose}}{\text{Quantity desired } (x)}$$

For example, clarithromycin 250 mg is ordered. It is supplied in a liquid form containing 125 mg in 5 mL. To calculate the dosage, the nurse uses the following formula:

$$\frac{\text{Dose on hand (125 mg)}}{\text{Quantity on hand (5 mL)}} = \frac{\text{Desired dose (250 mg)}}{\text{Quantity desired } (x)}$$

Then, the nurse cross-multiplies:

$$125\,x = 5 \text{ mL} \times 250 \text{ mg}$$
$$x = \frac{5 \text{ mL} \times 250 \text{ mg}}{125 \text{ mg}}$$
$$x = 10 \text{ mL}$$

Therefore, the dose ordered is 10 mL.

The nurse can also use this formula to calculate dosages:

$$\text{Amount to administer } (x) = \frac{\text{Desired dose}}{\text{Dose on hand}} \times \text{Quantity on hand}$$

For example, heparin is often distributed in large vials in prepared dilutions of 10 000 units per mL. If the order calls for 5000 units, the nurse can use the preceding formula to calculate:

$$x = \frac{5000 \text{ units}}{10\,000 \text{ units}} \times 1 \text{ mL}$$

$$x = 0.5 \text{ mL}$$

Therefore, the nurse injects 0.5 mL for a 5000-unit dose.

DOSAGES FOR CHILDREN Although dosage is stated in the medication order, nurses must understand safe dosage for children. Unlike adult dosages, children's dosages are not always standard. Because body size significantly affects dosage, pediatric medications will often be prescribed based on weight (e.g., *x* mg per kg body weight) or based on body surface area.

A child prescribed a medication based on his or her *weight* should be weighed daily to ensure accuracy. An example of a medication prescribed by weight is cloxacillin 55 mg/kg q6h. If the child weighs 20 kg, the dosage will be 1100 mg of cloxacillin (55 mg/kg × 20 kg) every 6 hours.

Body surface area is determined by using a nomogram and the child's height and weight. This is considered to be the most accurate method of calculating a child's dose. Standard nomograms give a child's body surface area according to weight and height (Figure 31.8). The formula is the ratio of the child's body surface area to the surface area of an average adult (1.7 square metres, or 1.7 m^2), multiplied by the normal adult dose of the drug:

$$\text{Child's dose} = \frac{\text{Surface area of child } (m^2)}{1.7 \text{ m}^2} \times \text{Normal adult dose}$$

For example, a child who weighs 10 kg and is 50 cm tall has a body surface area of 0.4 m^2. Therefore, the child's dose of tetracycline, corresponding to an adult dose of 250 mg, would be as follows:

$$\text{Child's dose} = \frac{0.4 \text{ m}^2}{1.7 \text{ m}^2} \times 250 \text{ mg}$$

$$= 0.23 \times 250 = 58.82 \text{ mg}$$

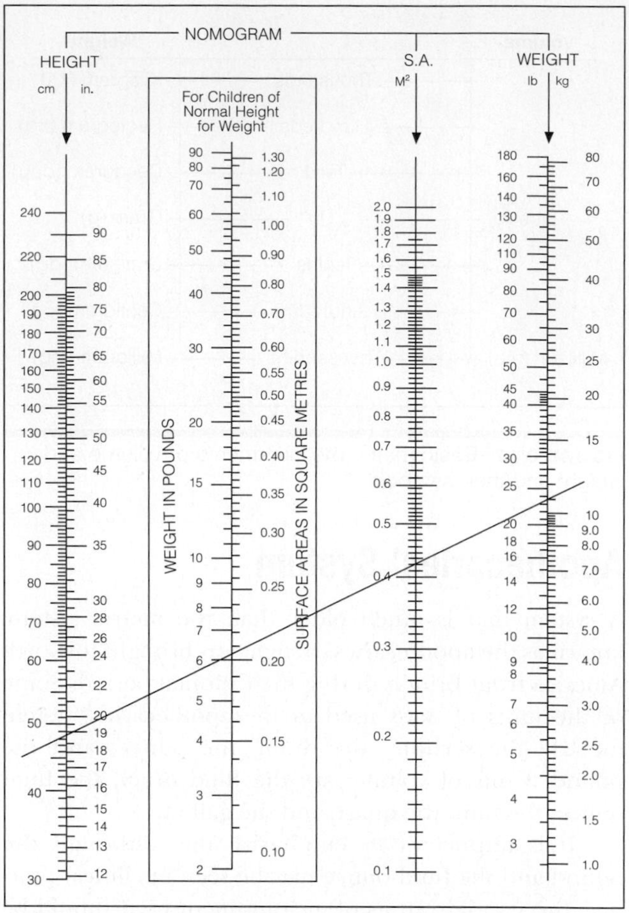

FIGURE 31.8 A nomogram with estimated body surface area. A straight line is drawn between the child's height (on the left) and the child's weight (on the right). The point at which the line intersects the surface area column is the estimated body surface area.

Administering Medications Safely

The nurse should always assess a patient's health status and obtain a medication history *before* administering any medication to obtain baseline data by which to evaluate the effectiveness of the medication. The extent of the assessment depends on the patient's illness or current condition, the intended drug, and the route of administration. For example, if a patient is experiencing dyspnea, the nurse assesses respirations carefully before administering any medication that might affect breathing. It is important to determine whether the route of administration is suitable. For example, a patient who is nauseated may not be able to retain in the stomach a drug taken orally.

The **medication history** includes information about the drugs the patient is taking currently or has taken recently. This includes prescription drugs; over-the-counter drugs, such as antacids, alcohol, and tobacco; vitamins and natural health products, including herbal remedies; and illicit drugs, such as marijuana. Sometimes, an incompatibility with one or more of these drugs affects the choice of a new medication.

Older adults often take vitamins, herbs, and food supplements, or use folk remedies that they do not list in their medication history. Because many of these have unknown or unpredictable actions and side effects, they need to be noted, with attention paid to possible incompatibilities with other prescribed medications.

An important part of the history is patients' knowledge of their drug allergies. Some clients can tell a nurse, "I am allergic to penicillin, adhesive tape, and curry." The nurse should clarify with the patient any side effects, adverse reactions, or allergic responses to medications. Other patients may not be sure about allergic reactions. An illness occurring after a drug was taken may not be identified as an allergy, but the patient may associate the drug with an illness or unusual reaction. The patient's health-care provider can often give information about allergies. During the history, the nurse tries to elicit information about drug dependencies. How often drugs are taken and the patient's perceived need for them are measures of dependence.

Also included in the patient history are the patient's normal eating habits. Sometimes, the medication schedule needs to be coordinated with mealtimes or the ingestion of foods. When a medication must be taken with food on a specified schedule, patients can often adjust their mealtime or have a snack (e.g., with a bedtime medication). In addition, certain foods are incompatible with certain medications, for example, milk is incompatible with tetracycline.

It is also important for the nurse to identify any problems the patient may have in self-administering a medication. A patient with poor eyesight, for example, may require special labels for the medication container; older adult patients with unsteady hands may not be able to hold a syringe or to inject themselves or another person. Obtaining information as to how and where patients store their medications is also important. If patients have difficulty opening certain containers, they may change containers but leave old labels on, which increases the risk of medication errors.

The nurse needs to consider socioeconomic factors for all patients, but especially for older adults. Two common problems are lack of transportation to obtain medications and inadequate finances to purchase medications. When aware of these problems, the nurse can refer proper resources for the patient.

It is essential that the effect or response of the patient to the drug be documented. Positive, negative, and neutral effects need to be noted as these can affect the need for a dosage change, maintenance, or a change in medication.

Medication Reconciliation

Another safety issue that affects the nurse is ensuring that patients receive the appropriate medications and dosages on admission, during transfer, and at discharge. According to the *Canadian Adverse Events Study* (Baker et al., 2004), one out of nine drugs administered to adults in hospitals and skilled nursing facilities is in error, and nearly 24% of preventable adverse drug events are related to medication error. As a result, the Medication Reconciliation Project was one of six evidence-based, system-wide national interventions promoted and coordinated by the Canadian Patient Safety Institute as part of its Safer Healthcare Now! initiative, aimed at reducing preventable complications and deaths in Canadian hospitals. Six interventions were targeted. One was the reduction of adverse drug events through medication reconciliation. Medication reconciliation is designed to reduce medication errors and involves the creation of a list of all medications that a patient is currently taking, including drug name, dosage, frequency, and route, and comparing them with all medications that have been prescribed during admission, transfer, and discharge. Over-the-counter medicines, natural health products, and other herbal products are also considered in medication reconciliation.

The Canadian Council on Health Services Accreditation (CCHSA) has made patient safety a crucial component of the accreditation process. Since 2006, it has required that protocols and processes for medication reconciliation be in place, particularly in transition areas, such as on admission, during transfer between units, and at discharge.

Medication Dispensing Systems

Medical facilities vary in their medication dispensing systems. The systems can include the following:

- *Medication cart.* The medication cart is on wheels, allowing the nurse to move the cart to outside the patient's room. The cart contains small numbered drawers that correlate to the room numbers on the nursing unit. The small drawer is labelled with the name of the patient currently in that room and holds the patient's medications for the shift or 24 hours (Figure 31.9). The medication is usually in unit-dose packaging; that is, the individual drug

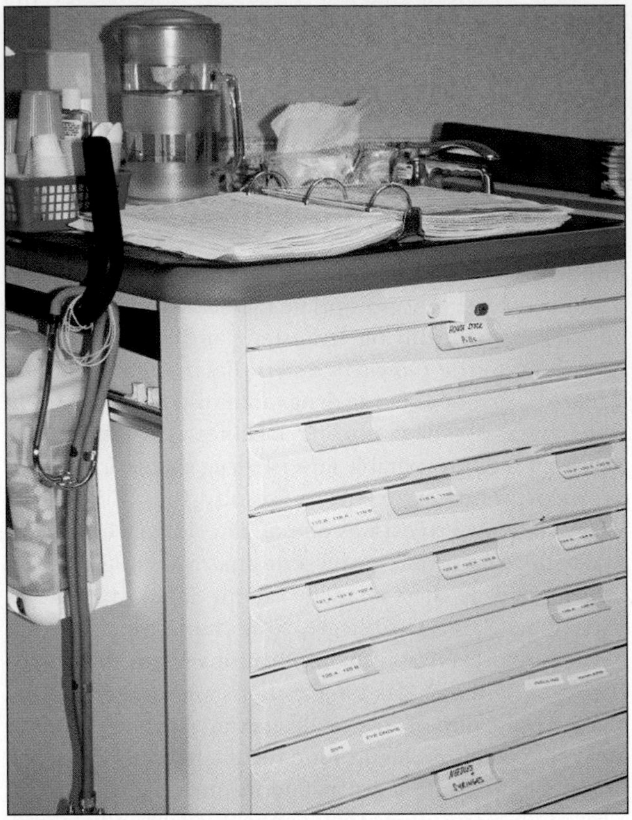

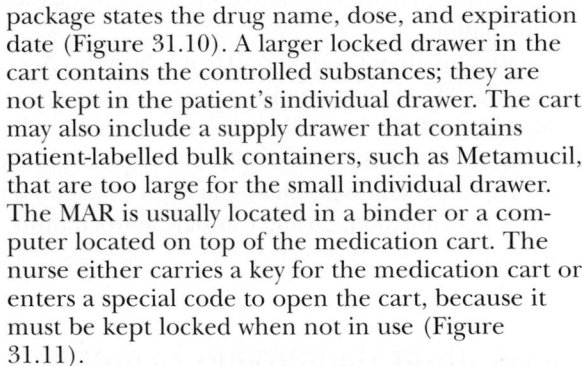

FIGURE 31.9 Medication cart

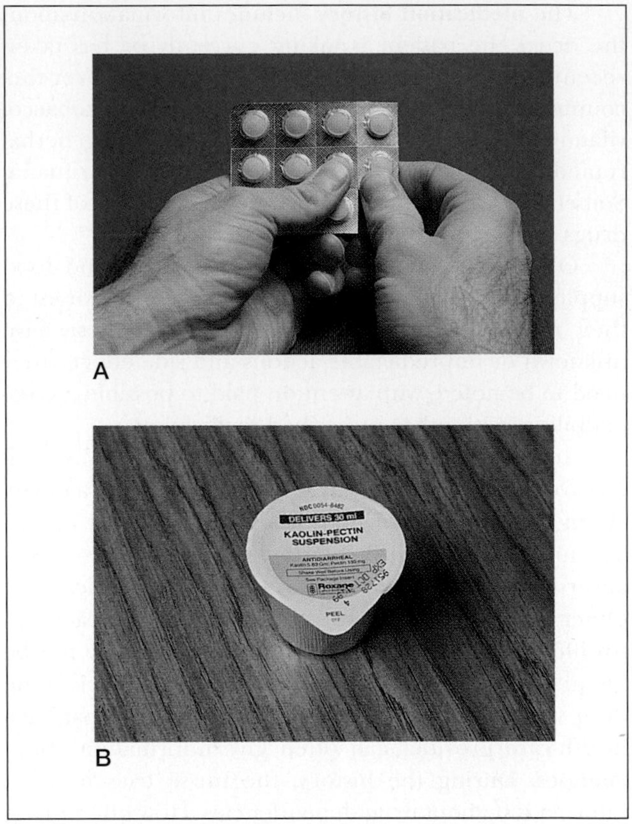

FIGURE 31.10 Unit-dose packages: A: tablets; B: liquid medications

package states the drug name, dose, and expiration date (Figure 31.10). A larger locked drawer in the cart contains the controlled substances; they are not kept in the patient's individual drawer. The cart may also include a supply drawer that contains patient-labelled bulk containers, such as Metamucil, that are too large for the small individual drawer. The MAR is usually located in a binder or a computer located on top of the medication cart. The nurse either carries a key for the medication cart or enters a special code to open the cart, because it must be kept locked when not in use (Figure 31.11).

- *Medication cabinet.* Some facilities have a locked cabinet in the patient's room. This cabinet holds the patient's unit-dose medications and MAR. Controlled substances are not kept in this cabinet but at another location on the nursing unit. The nurse uses either a key or a special code for opening the patient's medication cabinet, because it must be locked when not in use.
- *Medication room.* Depending on the facility, a medication room may be used for a variety of purposes. For example, the medication carts, when not in use, may be placed in this room. The medication room may also be the central location for stock medications, controlled medications, or drugs used for emergencies. The medication room may have a refrigerator for intravenous and other medications needing a cold environment. The room may also contain other medication administration supplies (syringes, needles, etc.). Nurses access the medication room by either a key or a special code as the room is often kept locked. Check agency policy.
- *Automated dispensing cabinet (ADC).* This computerized access system (Figure 31.12) automates the distribution, management, and control of medications. Similar to automated teller machines, these cabinets require the nurse to use a password to access the system, select the patient's name from an onscreen list, and select the medications.

Process of Administering Medications

When administering any drug, regardless of the route of administration, the nurse must do the following:

1. *Identify the patient.* Errors can and do occur, often because one patient gets a drug intended for another. In hospitals, most patients wear some sort of identification, such as a wristband with their

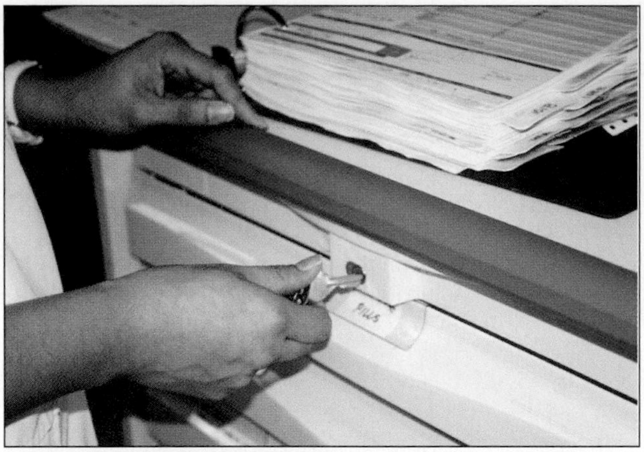

FIGURE 31.11 The medication cart is kept locked when not in use. The nurse is using a key to access client medications.

name and hospital identification number. Before giving the patient any drug, check the identification band with the MAR (see Figure 31.6). Some hospitals use barcode technology for medication administration. A nurse preparing to administer a medication by using barcode technology scans or enters the nurse's own ID, the patient's wristband, and each package of medication to be administered. Barcoding often includes two or more person-specific identifiers, which meets the identifier requirement (see Figure 31.13). As a double-check, if unsure, or if the patient has no wristband (e.g., in a community setting), ask the patient's name, have the family identify the patient, or ask another nurse to identify the patient before administering any medication.

CLINICAL ALERT

Do not ask, "Are you Derek James?" because the patient may answer "yes" to the wrong name. It is better to ask, "What is your name?"

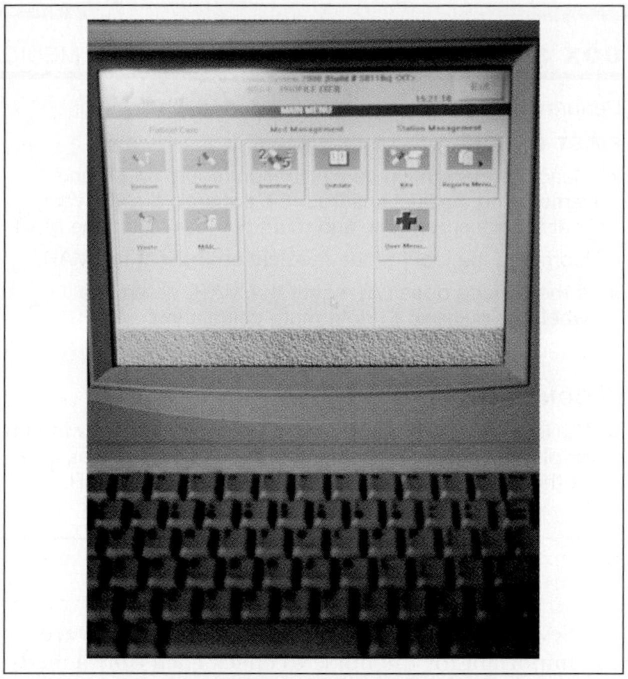

FIGURE 31.12 Computerized medication access system

2. *Inform the patient.* If the patient is unfamiliar with the medication, the nurse should explain the intended action and any side effects or adverse effects that might occur. Listen to the patient. It is easy for a nurse to be so focused on the task of timely medication administration that he or she misses relevant information provided by the patient. For example, if the patient says that he doesn't take a pill for high blood pressure, this should be an alert for the nurse to stop and check whether this is the correct medication for that patient.
3. *Administer the drug.* Read medication orders and records carefully and perform three checks against the labelled medications (see Box 31.4). Then administer the medication in the prescribed dosage, by the route ordered, at the correct time.

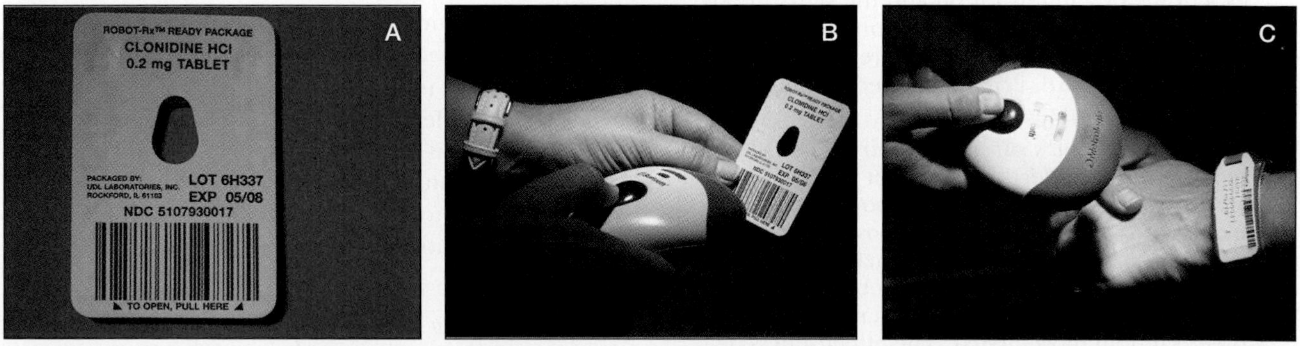

FIGURE 31.13 A: A sample barcode; **B:** the nurse scans the barcode on the medication package and **C:** the barcode on the client's wristband before administering the medication.

(Shirlee Snyder)

BOX 31.4 CHECK THREE TIMES FOR SAFE MEDICATION ADMINISTRATION

Perform three checks against the labelled medication:

FIRST CHECK

- Read the medication administration record (MAR) and remove the medications from the patient's drawer. Verify that the patient's name and room number match the MAR.
- Compare the label of the medication against the MAR.
- If the dosage does not match the MAR, determine whether you need to do a math calculation.
- Check the expiration date of the medication.

SECOND CHECK

- While preparing the medication (e.g., pouring, drawing up, or placing unopened package in a medication cup), look at the medication label and check against the MAR.

THIRD CHECK

- Recheck the label on the container (e.g., vial, bottle, or unused unit-dose medications) before returning it to its storage place.
- *Or* check the label on the medication against the MAR before opening the package at the bedside.

Source: From *Safe Meds,* by P. Przybycien, 2005, St. Louis, MO: Mosby. Adapted with permission.

Several aspects of medication administration are important for the nurse to check each time a medication is administered. These are referred to as the "rights." Traditionally, there were five rights to medication administration. More rights have been added over the last few years, with the latest total being 10 rights (see Box 31.5).

4. *Provide adjunctive interventions as indicated.* Patients may need help when receiving medications. They may require physical assistance, for instance, in assuming positions for intramuscular injections, or they may need guidance about measures, such as drinking fluids, to enhance drug effectiveness and prevent complications. Nurses must anticipate questions, comments, and fears from patients about their medications. The nurse can allay fears by listening carefully to patients' concerns and giving correct information.
5. *Record the drug administered.* The facts recorded in the chart, in ink or by computer printout, are the name of the drug, the dosage, the method of administration, any specific relevant data, such as pulse rate (taken in most settings before the administration of digitalis), and any other pertinent information. The record should also include the exact time of administration and the signature of the nurse providing the medication. Often, medications that are given regularly are recorded on a special flow record. Prn or stat medications are recorded separately.
6. *Evaluate the patient's response to the drug.* The kinds of behaviour that reflect the action or lack of action of a drug and its untoward effects (both minor and major) are as variable as the purposes of the drugs themselves. The anxious patient may show the desired effects of a tranquilizer by behaviour that reflects a lowered stress level (e.g., slower speech or fewer random movements). The effectiveness of a sedative can often be measured by how well a patient slept; the effectiveness of an antispasmodic, by how much pain the patient feels. In all nursing activities, nurses need to be aware of the medications that a patient is taking and record their effectiveness on the patient's chart, as assessed by the patient and the nurse, and report the patient's response to the relevant health-care team members.

Developmental Considerations

It is important for the nurse to be aware of how growth and development affects administration of medications for all age groups, particularly infants and the older population.

INFANTS AND CHILDREN Knowledge of growth and development is essential for the nurse administering medications to children. Oral medications for children are often prepared in sweetened liquid form to make them more palatable. The parents may provide suggestions about what method is best for their child. Necessary foods, such as milk or orange juice, should not be used to mask the taste of medications because the child may develop unpleasant associations and refuse that food in the future.

Children tend to fear any procedure in which a needle is used because they anticipate pain or because the procedure is unfamiliar and threatening. The nurse needs to acknowledge that the child will feel some pain, since denying this fact only deepens the child's distrust. After the injection, the nurse (or the parent) can cuddle and speak softly to the infant and give the child a toy to dispel the association of the nurse only with pain.

OLDER ADULTS Older adults can present special problems, most of which are related to physiological changes, to past experiences, and to established attitudes toward medications. Altered pharmacokinetics in older adults includes changes in absorption, distribution, metabo-

BOX 31.5 TEN "RIGHTS" OF MEDICATION ADMINISTRATION

These 10 rights must be checked every time:

1. RIGHT MEDICATION

- Ensure the medication given is the medication ordered.

2. RIGHT DOSE

- Ensure the dose ordered is appropriate for the patient.
- Give special attention if the calculation indicates multiple pills or tablets or a large quantity of a liquid medication. This can be a cue that the math calculation may be incorrect.
- Double-check calculations that appear questionable.
- Know the usual dosage range of the medication.
- Question a dosage outside of the usual dosage range.

3. RIGHT TIME

- Give the medication at the right frequency and at the time ordered, according to agency policy.
- Know that medications given within 30 minutes before or after the scheduled time are considered to meet the right time standard.

4. RIGHT ROUTE

- Give the medication by the ordered route.
- Make certain that the route is safe and appropriate for the patient.

5. RIGHT PATIENT

- Ensure the medication is given to the intended patient.
- Check the patient's identification band with each administration of a medication.
- Know the agency's name alert procedure when patients with the same or similar last names are on the nursing unit.

6. RIGHT PATIENT EDUCATION

- Explain information about the medication to the patient (e.g., why receiving, what to expect, any precautions).

7. RIGHT DOCUMENTATION

- Document medication administration after giving it, not before.
- If the time of administration differs from prescribed time, note the time on the MAR and explain the reason and follow-through activities (e.g., pharmacy states medication will be available in 2 hours) in nursing notes.
- If a medication is not given, follow the agency's policy for documenting the reason.

8. RIGHT TO REFUSE

- Adult patients have the right to refuse any medication.
- The nurse's role is to ensure that the patient is fully informed of the potential consequences of refusal and to communicate the patient's refusal to the appropriate member of the health-care team.

9. RIGHT ASSESSMENT

- Know which medications require specific assessments before administration (e.g., apical pulse, blood pressure, laboratory results).
- Understand medication orders that include specific parameters for administration (e.g., do not give if pulse less than 60 bpm or systolic blood pressure less than 100 mm Hg).

10. RIGHT EVALUATION

- Conduct appropriate follow-up (e.g., was the desired effect achieved or not? Did the patient experience any side effects or adverse reactions?).

Evidence-Informed Practice

Do Look-Alike Vials Lead to Significant Errors in Heparin Administration?

Anticoagulants are among the top 10 drugs reported as causing harm when an error in administration occurs. The most prevalent heparin error is incorrect dosage—usually too much—which places the patient at risk for coagulation problems. Koczmara, Cheng, and Hyland (2008) summarized key results of the Institute for Safe Medication Practices's pan-Canadian Anticoagulant Safety Survey. Despite evidence that look-alike vials of heparin 10 000 units/mL and heparin 1000 units/mL are often mistaken, the majority of respondents (55%) indicated that they did not use any safeguards to avoid mixups. The authors provided qualitative data from several incident reports documenting errors of heparin administration. One report discusses how several children received 1000 times more heparin than ordered because a 10 000 units/mL heparin vial was used instead of a 10 units/mL vial.

NURSING IMPLICATIONS: **Ensuring that the patient receives the correct dosage of medication as prescribed is a key nursing responsibility. Although the Institute for Safe Medication Practices has been telling health professionals about the risks of look-alike preparations for several years, this article is a reminder of how important these recommendations are and how many institutions have still not adopted them.**

Source: Based on "Preventing Substitution Errors Involving High-Concentration Heparin Products," by C. Koczmara, R. Cheng, and S. Hyland, 2008, *Dynamics*, *19*(1), pp. 32–34.

lism, and excretion. Box 31.6 summarizes the physiological changes that can affect the administration and effectiveness of medications in older adults.

Some pharmacokinetic changes enhance the possibility of cumulative effects and toxicity. For example, impaired circulation delays the action of medications given intramuscularly or subcutaneously. Digitalis, which is frequently taken by older adults, can accumulate to toxic levels and be lethal.

The possibility of error increases with the number of medications taken, whether self-administered at home or administered in a hospital. The greater number of medications also compounds the problem of drug interactions. Careful routine review of patient medications, potential effects and adverse side effects, drug and food interactions, and patient's response to the drug is imperative.

Older adults usually require smaller dosages of drugs, especially sedatives and other central nervous system depressants. Reactions of older adults to medications, particularly sedatives, are unpredictable and often bizarre. It is not uncommon to see irritability, confusion, disorientation, restlessness, and incontinence as a result of sedatives. Nurses, therefore, need to observe patients carefully for untoward reactions. Prescribers often follow the unwritten rule to "start low and go slow" when prescribing medications for the older population. The initial prescribed dosage will often be low and then gradually increased, with careful monitoring of actions and side effects of the drug.

BOX 31.6 PHYSIOLOGICAL CHANGES ASSOCIATED WITH AGING THAT INFLUENCE MEDICATION ADMINISTRATION AND EFFECTIVENESS

Some physiological changes that occur as people get older can affect both the administration and the effectiveness of medications:

- Altered memory
- Decreased visual acuity
- Decreased renal function, resulting in slower elimination of drugs and higher drug concentrations in the bloodstream for longer periods
- Less complete and slower absorption from the gastrointestinal tract
- Increased proportion of fat to lean body mass, which facilitates retention of fat-soluble drugs and increases potential for toxicity
- Decreased liver function, which hinders biotransformation of drugs
- Decreased organ sensitivity, which means that the response to the same drug concentration in the vicinity of the target organ is less in older adults than in younger people
- Altered quality of organ responsiveness, resulting in adverse effects becoming pronounced before therapeutic effects are achieved
- Decreased manual dexterity because of arthritis or decreased flexibility

The attitudes of older adults toward medical care and medications vary. Older adults tend to believe in the wisdom of the physician more readily than do younger people. Some seniors are bewildered by the prescription of several medications and may passively accept their medications from nurses but not swallow them, spitting them out after the nurse leaves the room. For this reason, the nurse is advised to stay with clients until they have swallowed the medications. Other clients may be suspicious of medications and actively refuse them.

Seniors are mature adults capable of reasoning. Therefore, the nurse needs to explain the reasons for and the effects of medications. This education can prevent clients from continuing to take a medication long after there is a need for it or from discontinuing a drug too quickly. For example, clients should know that diuretics will cause them to urinate more frequently and may reduce ankle edema. Instructions about medications need to be given to all clients. These instructions should include when to take the drug, what effects to expect, and when to consult a health-care provider.

Because some clients are required to take several medications daily and because visual acuity and memory may be impaired, the nurse needs to develop simple, realistic plans for clients to follow at home. For example, medications that are scheduled to be taken with meals or at bedtime help clients to remember to take their medications. Some clients may take their medications and then 1 hour later may not remember whether they took them. One solution to forgetfulness is to use a special container or glass strictly for medications. An empty glass or container indicates that the person took the pills. Loss of visual acuity presents problems that can be overcome by writing out the plan in block letters large enough to be read. In some situations, the help of a spouse, son, or daughter can be helpful.

Older adults can have a decrease in dexterity because of arthritis or stiffness of their hands and fingers, causing difficulty in opening medication containers or in self-administration of other medications, such as eye drops, eardrops, insulin injections, and inhalers. Nurses can help clients make the necessary changes or enlist the assistance of another person to help them administer their medications.

Administering Enteral Medications

Oral Medications

The oral route is the most common route by which medications are given. This is the route of choice as long as a patient is able to swallow and retain the drug in the stomach. See Skill 31.1. Oral medications are contraindicated when a patient is vomiting, has diarrhea, has continuous gastric or intestinal suction, or is unconscious and unable to swallow. Generally these patients have the order "nothing by mouth" (Latin is *nil per os:* NPO).

SKILL 31.1

ADMINISTERING ORAL MEDICATIONS

PURPOSE

To provide a medication that has systemic effects or local effects on the gastrointestinal tract or both (see specific drug action)

ASSESSMENT

Assess the following:

- Allergies to medications
- Client's ability to swallow the medication
- Presence of vomiting or diarrhea that would interfere with the ability to absorb the medication
- Specific drug action, side effects, interactions, and adverse reactions
- Patient's knowledge of and learning needs about the medication
- Perform appropriate assessments (e.g., vital signs, laboratory results) specific to the medication.
- Determine if the assessment data influence administration of the medication (i.e., is it appropriate to administer the medication or does the medication need to be held and the prescriber notified?).

Equipment

- Dispensing system
- Disposable medication cups: small paper or plastic cups for tablets and capsules, waxed or plastic calibrated medication cups for liquids
- Medication administration record (MAR) or computer printout
- Pill crusher or cutter
- Straws to administer medications that may discolour the teeth or to facilitate the ingestion of liquid medication for certain patients
- Drinking glass and water or juice
- Applesauce or pudding to use for crushed medications for patients who may choke on liquids

IMPLEMENTATION

Preparation

1. Know the reason why the patient is receiving the medication and the drug classification, action, contraindications, usual dosage range, side effects, and special nursing considerations. **Rationale: A thorough knowledge of the medication to be administered assists in evaluating its therapeutic effect. The nurse can also use this knowledge to educate the patient**.
2. Check the MAR.
   - Check the MAR for the drug name, dosage, frequency, route of administration, and expiration date for administering the medication, if appropriate. **Rationale: Certain medications (e.g., opioids, antibiotics) have a specified time frame at which they expire and need to be reordered**.
   - If the MAR is unclear or pertinent information is missing, compare the MAR with the prescriber's most recent written order.
   - Report any discrepancies to the charge nurse or the prescriber, as agency policy dictates.
3. Verify the patient's ability to take medication orally. Determine whether the patient can swallow, is NPO, is nauseated or vomiting, has gastric suction, or has diminished or absent bowel sounds.
4. Organize the supplies. Assemble the MAR(s) for each patient together so that medications can be prepared for one patient at a time. **Rationale: Organization of supplies saves time and reduces the chance of error**.

Performance

1. Perform hand hygiene and observe other appropriate infection prevention and control procedures.
2. Unlock the dispensing system (if applicable).
3. Obtain appropriate medication.
   - Read the MAR and take the appropriate medication from the shelf, drawer, or refrigerator. The medication may be dispensed in a bottle, box, or unit-dose package.
   - Compare the label of the medication container or unit-dose package against the order on the MAR or computer printout. See ❶. **Rationale: This is a**

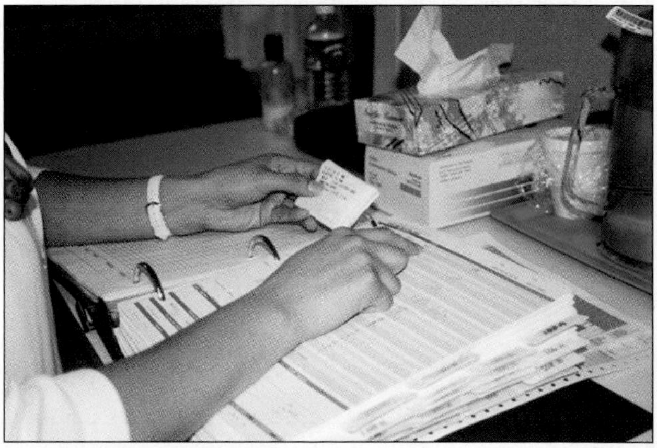

❶ Compare the medication label to the MAR

(continued)

SKILL 31.1

ADMINISTERING ORAL MEDICATIONS (*continued*)

safety check to ensure that the right medication is given. If these are not identical, recheck the prescriber's written order in the patient's chart. If there is still a discrepancy, check with the nurse in charge or the pharmacist.

- Check the expiration date of the medication. **Rationale: Return expired medications to the pharmacy. Outdated medications are not safe to administer.**
- Use only medications that have clear, legible labels *to ensure accuracy.*

4. Prepare the medication.
   - Calculate the medication dosage accurately.
   - Prepare the correct amount of medication for the required dose, without contaminating the medication. **Rationale: Aseptic technique maintains drug cleanliness.**
   - While preparing the medication, recheck each prepared drug and container with the MAR again. **Rationale: This second safety check reduces the chance of error.**

Tablets or Capsules

- Place packaged unit-dose capsules or tablets directly into the medicine container. See Figure 31.10A. Do not remove the medication from the package until at the bedside. **Rationale: The wrapper keeps the medication clean. Not removing the medication facilitates identification of the medication in the event the patient refuses the drug or assessment data indicate to hold the medication. Unopened unit-dose packages can usually be returned to the medication cart.**
- If using a stock container, pour the required number into the bottle cap, and then transfer the medication to the disposable cup without touching the tablets (see ❷).
- Keep opioids and medications that require specific assessments, such as pulse measurements, respiratory rate or depth, or blood pressure, separate from the others. **Rationale: This reminds the nurse to complete the needed assessments in order to decide whether to give the medication if indicated.**
- Break only scored tablets if necessary to obtain the correct dosage. Use a cutting or splitting device if needed (see ❸). Check the agency policy as to whether unused portions of a medication can be discarded and, if so, how they are to be discarded.

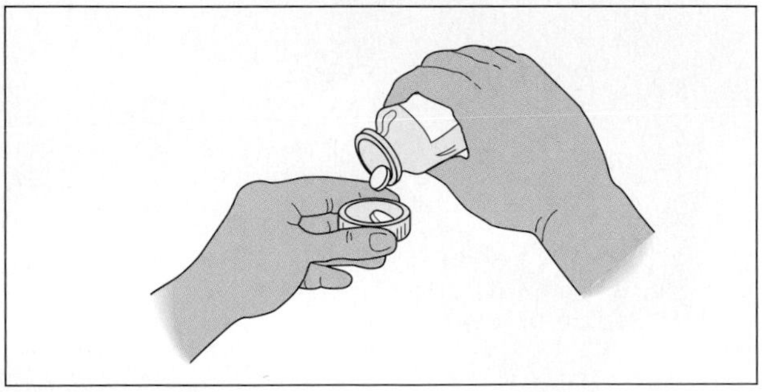

❷ Pouring a tablet into the bottle cap

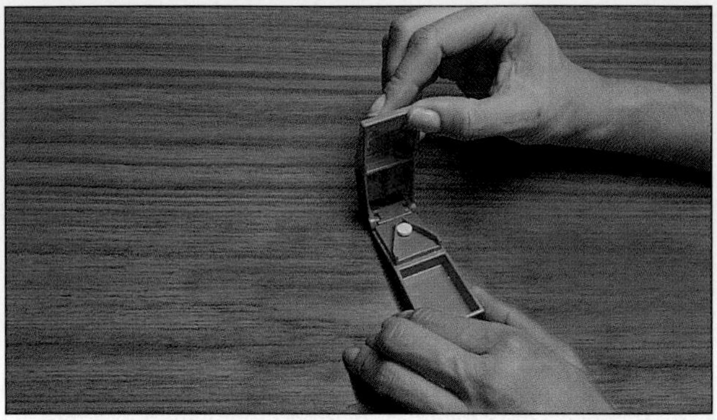

❸ A cutting device can be used to divide tablets.

- If the patient has difficulty swallowing, crush the tablets to a fine powder with a pill crusher or between two medication cups. Then, mix the powder with a small amount of soft food (e.g., custard, applesauce). Some medications should not be crushed (e.g., time-released and enteric coated). An example of tablets that should not be crushed is oxycodone, a long-acting opioid that normally lasts 12 hours after administration. If the tablet is crushed, the patient gets a surge of relief in the first 2 hours and then may start having severe pain again in 4 to 6 hours, as the effects wear off too soon. The crushing of these tablets causes an uneven effect, and the long-acting action of the medication is lost.

Liquid Medication

- Thoroughly mix the medication before pouring. Discard any medication that has changed colour or turned cloudy.
- Remove the cap and place it upside down on the countertop *to avoid contaminating the inside of the cap.*
- Hold the bottle so the label is next to your palm and pour the medication away from the label (see ❹).

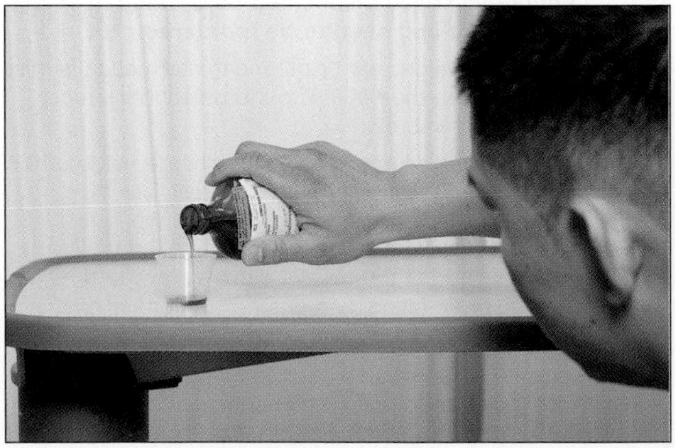

❹ Pouring a liquid medication from a bottle

(*continued*)

SKILL 31.1

ADMINISTERING ORAL MEDICATIONS (*continued*)

Rationale: This prevents the label from becoming soiled and illegible as a result of spilled liquid.

- Place the medication cup on a flat surface at eye level and fill it to the desired level, using the *bottom* of the **meniscus** (crescent-shaped upper surface of a column of liquid) to align with the container scale (see ❺). **Rationale: This method ensures accuracy of measurement.**
- Before capping the bottle, wipe the lip with a paper towel. **Rationale: This prevents the cap from sticking.**
- When giving small amounts of liquids (e.g., < 5 mL), prepare the medication in a sterile syringe without the needle or in a specially designed oral syringe. Label the syringe with the name of the medication and the route (PO). **Rationale: Any oral solutions removed from their original container and placed into a syringe should be labelled to avoid medications being given by the wrong route (e.g., IV). This practice facilitates client safety and avoids tragic errors.**
- Keep unit-dose liquids in their package and open them at the bedside.

Oral Opioids

- If an agency uses a manual recording system for controlled substances, check the opioid record for the previous drug count and compare it with the supply available. Some medications, including opioids, are kept in plastic containers that are sectioned and numbered (see ❻).
- Remove the next available tablet and drop it in the medicine cup.
- After removing a tablet, record the necessary information on the appropriate opioid control record and sign it.
- *Note:* Computer-controlled dispensing systems allow access only to the selected drug and automatically record its use.

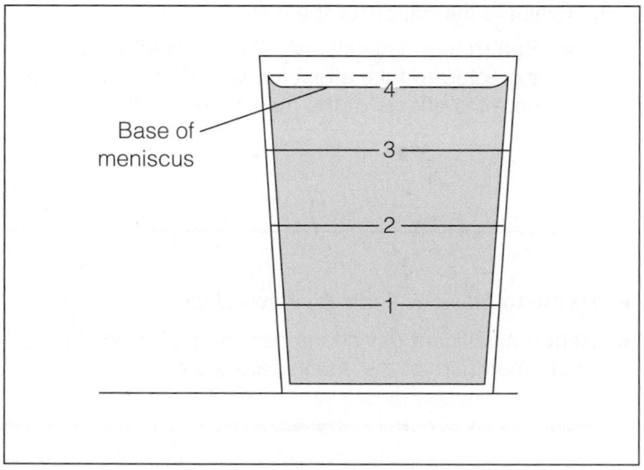

❺ The base of the meniscus is the measuring guide.

All Medications

- Place the prepared medication and MAR together on the medication cart.
- Recheck the label on the container before returning the bottle, box, or envelope to its storage place. **Rationale: This third check further reduces the risk of error.**
- Avoid leaving prepared medications unattended. **Rationale: This precaution prevents potential mishandling errors.**
- Lock the medication cart before entering the client's room. This is a *safety measure because medication carts are not to be left open when unattended.*
- Check the room number against the MAR if agency policy does not allow the MAR to be removed from the medication cart. **Rationale: This is another safety measure to ensure that the nurse is entering the correct client room.**

5. Provide for client privacy.

6. Prepare the client.

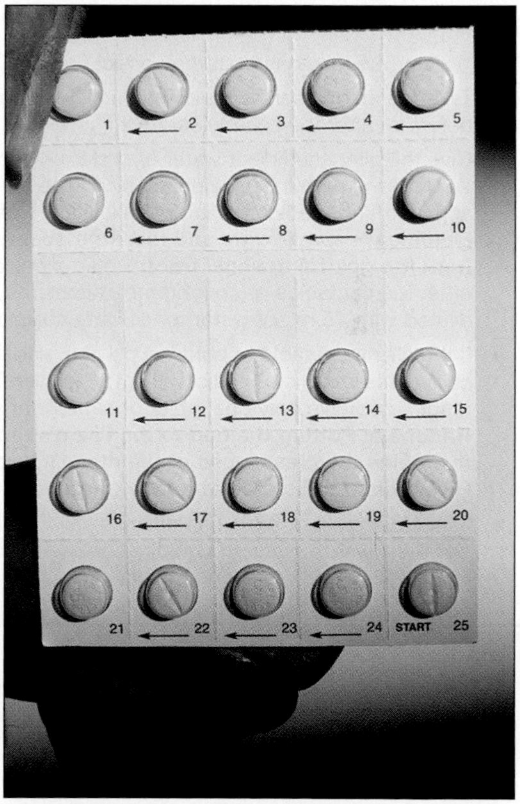

❻ Some opioids are kept in specially designed packages or plastic containers that are sectioned and numbered.

(continued)

SKILL 31.1

ADMINISTERING ORAL MEDICATIONS (*continued*)

- Check the client's identification band. **Rationale: This ensures that the right client receives the medication.**
- Assist the client to a sitting position or, if not possible, to a side-lying position. **Rationale: These positions facilitate swallowing and prevent aspiration.**
- If not previously assessed, take the required assessment measures, such as pulse and respiratory rates or blood pressure. Take the apical pulse rate before administering digitalis preparations. Take blood pressure before giving antihypertensive drugs. Take the respiratory rate before administering opioids. **Rationale: Opioids depress the respiratory centre.** If any of the findings are above or below the predetermined parameters, consult the appropriate member of the health-care team before administering the medication.

7. Explain the purpose of the medication and how it will help, using language that the client can understand. Include relevant information about effects; for example, tell the client receiving a diuretic to expect an increase in urine output. **Rationale: Information can facilitate acceptance of and compliance with the therapy.**
8. Administer the medication at the correct time.
   - Take the medication to the client within 30 minutes before or after the scheduled time.
   - Give the client sufficient water or preferred juice to swallow the medication. Before using juice, check for any food and medication incompatibilities. **Rationale: Fluids ease swallowing and facilitate absorption from the gastrointestinal tract.** Liquid medications other than antacids or cough preparations may be diluted with 15 mL of water to facilitate absorption.
   - If the client is unable to hold the pill cup, use the pill cup to introduce the medication into the client's mouth, and give only one tablet or capsule at a time. **Rationale: Putting the cup to the client's mouth maintains the cleanliness of the nurse's hands. Giving one medication at a time eases swallowing.**
   - If an older child or adult has difficulty swallowing, ask the client to place the medication on the back of the tongue before taking the water. **Rationale: Stimulation of the back of the tongue produces the swallowing reflex.**
   - If the medication has an objectionable taste, ask the client to suck a few ice chips beforehand, or give the medication with juice, applesauce, or bread if there are no contraindications. **Rationale: The cold of the ice chips will desensitize the taste buds, and juices or bread can mask the taste of the medication.**
   - If the client says that the medication you are about to give is different from what the client has been receiving, do not give the medication without first checking the original order. **Rationale: Most clients are familiar with the appearance of medications taken previously. Unfamiliar medications may signal a possible error.**
   - Stay with the client until all medications have been swallowed. **Rationale: The nurse must see the client swallow the medication before the drug administration can be recorded.** The nurse may need to check the client's mouth to ensure that the medication was swallowed and not hidden inside the cheek. A physician's order or agency policy is required for medications left at the bedside.
9. Document each medication given.
   - Record the medication given, dosage, time, any complaints or assessments of the client, and your signature.
   - If medication was refused or omitted, record this fact on the appropriate record; document the reason, when possible, and the nurse's actions according to agency policy.
10. Dispose of all supplies appropriately.
    - Replenish stock (e.g., medication cups) and return the cart to the appropriate place.
    - Discard used disposable supplies.
11. Evaluate the effects of the medication.
    - Return to the client when the medication is expected to take effect (usually 30 minutes) to evaluate the effects of the medication on the client.

EVALUATION

- Conduct appropriate follow-up: desired effect (e.g., relief of pain or decrease in body temperature), any adverse effects or side effects (e.g., nausea, vomiting, skin rash, change in vital signs).
- Relate to previous findings, if available.
- Report significant deviations from normal to the appropriate members of the health-care team.

Lifespan Considerations

Administering Oral Medications

Knowledge of growth and development is essential for the nurse administering medications to infants and children.

- Nurses must know the range of safe medication dosages for infants and children.

INFANTS

- Oral medications can be effectively administered in several ways:
    - A syringe or dropper
    - A medication nipple, which allows the infant to suck the medication
    - Mixed in small amounts of food
    - A spoon or medication cup, for older children
- Never mix medications into foods that are essential, since the infant may associate the food with an unpleasant taste and refuse that food in the future. Never mix medications with formula.
- Place a small amount of liquid medication along the inside of the baby's cheek and wait for the infant to swallow before giving more to prevent aspiration or spitting out.
- When using a spoon, retrieve and refeed medication that is thrust outward by the infant's tongue.

CHILDREN

- Whenever possible, give children a choice between the use of a spoon, dropper, or syringe.
- Dilute the oral medication, if indicated, with a small amount of water. Many oral medications are readily swallowed if they are diluted. If large quantities of water are used, the child may refuse to drink the entire amount and receive only a portion of the medication.
- Oral medications for children are usually prepared in sweetened liquid form to make them more palatable. Crush medications that are not supplied in liquid form and mix them with substances available on most pediatric units, such as honey, flavoured syrup, jam, or a fruit puree.
- Necessary foods, such as milk or orange juice, should not be used to mask the taste of medications because the child may develop unpleasant associations and refuse that food in the future.
- Disguise disagreeable-tasting medications with sweet-tasting substances mentioned previously. However, present any altered medication to the child honestly and not as a food or treat.
- Place the young child or toddler on your lap or a parent's lap in a sitting position.
- Administer the medication slowly with a measuring spoon, plastic syringe, or medicine cup.
- To prevent nausea, pour a carbonated beverage over finely crushed ice, and give it before or immediately after the medication is administered.
- Follow medication with a drink of water or juice or a frozen juice bar to remove any unpleasant aftertaste.
- For children who take sweetened medications on a long-term basis, follow the medication administration with oral hygiene. These children are at high risk for dental caries.

OLDER ADULTS

- The physiological changes associated with aging influence medication administration and effectiveness. Examples include altered memory, less acute vision, decreased renal function, less complete and slower absorption from the gastrointestinal tract, and decreased liver function. Many of these changes enhance the possibility of cumulative effects and toxicity.
- Older adults usually require smaller dosages of drugs, especially sedatives and other central nervous system depressants.
- Older adults are mature adults capable of reasoning. The nurse, therefore, needs to explain the reasons for and the effects of the patient's medications.
- Socioeconomic factors, such as lack of transportation and decreased finances, may influence obtaining medications when needed.
- An increase in marketing and availability of vitamins, herbs, and supplements alerts the nurse to include this information in a medication history.

Home Care Considerations

Administering Medication

Instruct the patient to do the following:

- Learn the names of the medications, their actions, and possible adverse effects. Carry a complete list of all prescriptions, OTC medications, and home remedies at all times.
- Keep all medications out of reach of children and pets.
- If using a syringe to administer the medication to an infant or child, remove and dispose of the plastic cap that fits on the end of the syringe. Infants and small children have been known to choke on these caps.
- Take medications only as prescribed. Know which medications need to be taken on an empty stomach and which can be taken with food or meals. Immediately consult the nurse, pharmacist, or physician about any problems with the medication.
- Always check the medication label to make sure the correct medication is being taken.

(continued)

Home Care Considerations (*continued*)

- Request labels printed with larger type on medication containers if there is difficulty reading the label.
- Check the expiration date and discard outdated medications. Health Canada (2005) advises against flushing medications down the toilet or throwing them in the garbage. Instead, bring them to a municipal waste site or a pharmacy that participates in a disposal program for environmentally safe disposal.
- If a dose or more is missed, do not take two or more doses; ask the pharmacist or health-care provider for instructions.
- Do not crush or cut a tablet or capsule without first checking with the physician or pharmacist. Doing so may affect the medication's absorption.
- Always check with the pharmacist before taking any nonprescription medications. Some OTC medications can interact with the prescribed medication.
- Ask the pharmacist to substitute childproof caps with ones that are more easily opened, if necessary.
- Never stop taking the medication without first discussing with the health-care provider.
- Additionally, the nurse can set up a medication plan to assist patients and family members to remember a schedule. Weekly pill containers (available at pharmacies) or a written plan may be helpful.

Nasogastric and Gastrostomy Medications

For clients who cannot take anything by mouth (NPO) and have a **nasogastric tube** or a **gastrostomy tube** in place, an alternative route for administering medications is through the nasogastric or gastrostomy tube. A nasogastric (NG) tube is inserted by way of the nasopharynx and is placed into the patient's stomach for the purpose of feeding the patient or to remove gastric secretions. A gastrostomy tube is surgically placed directly into the patient's stomach and provides another route for administering nutrition and medications. See Chapter 39 for further discussion of nasogastric and gastrostomy tubes. Practice guidelines for administering medications by nasogastric tubes and gastrostomy tubes are shown in Practice Guidelines 31.1.

PRACTICE GUIDELINES 31.1

Administering Medications by Nasogastric or Gastrostomy Tube

Guidelines	Rationales
Always check with the pharmacist to see whether the patient's medications come in a liquid form.	This form is less likely to cause tube obstruction.
If medications do not come in liquid form, check to see whether they may be crushed. Crush the tablet into a fine powder and dissolve in at least 30 mL of warm water. Use only water for mixing and flushing. Nurses are encouraged to consult with a pharmacist.	Crushing enteric-coated, sustained-action, enzyme-specific, buccal, and sublingual tablets affects pharmacokinetics or causes gastric irritation. Cold liquids can cause patient discomfort and may not dissolve medication. Some medications are mixed with other fluids, such as normal saline, in order to maximize dissolution. Whole or undissolved medications will clog the tube.
If the nasogastric or gastrostomy tube is also being used for enteral feeding, then ensure that the medication is compatible with the feeding solution.	A physical incompatibility can exist, leading to precipitation that can occlude the tube (e.g., ferrous sulphate and potassium chloride liquids are incompatible with most enteral formulae).
If bulk-forming laxatives (e.g., Metamucil) are prescribed, consult the appropriate member of the health-care team for an alternative prescription.	These medication preparations form a semisolid mass and can occlude the tube.
Read medication labels carefully before opening a capsule. Open capsules and mix the contents with water *only* with the pharmacist's advice.	The pellets inside some capsules (e.g., Effexor XR) can be poured down the tube, provided they are not crushed. Manufacturer's instructions may indicate drug-specific information that is relevant.

(continued)

PRACTICE GUIDELINES 31.1

Administering Medications by Nasogastric or Gastrostomy Tube *(continued)*

Guidelines	Rationales
Assess the tube placement (see Chapter 39 for methods to assess tube placement). Before giving the medication, aspirate all the stomach contents and measure the residual volume. Check agency policy if the residual volume is greater than 100 mL.	Displacement of the tube can lead to inadvertently administering medications outside the gastrointestinal tract (e.g., into the lungs). Excess residual volume may mean that peristalsis is not effective in moving stomach contents forward. Adding medication to a high residual volume can lead to poor absorption.
When administering a medication, remove the plunger from the syringe and connect the syringe to a pinched or kinked tube.	Pinching or kinking the tube prevents excess air from entering the stomach and causing distension.
Put 15 mL to 30 mL (5 mL to 10 mL for children) of water into the syringe barrel to flush the tube before administering the first medication. Raise or lower the barrel of the syringe to adjust the flow as needed. Pinch or clamp the tubing before all the water is instilled.	Flushing ensures that the medication does not come in contact with any other substance; clamping will prevent excess air from entering the stomach.
Pour liquid or dissolved medication into the syringe barrel and allow to flow by gravity into the enteral tube.	This avoids any trauma.
If you are giving several medications, administer each one separately and flush with at least 15 mL to 30 mL (5 mL for children) of tap water between each medication. Consult the appropriate health-care professional if the patient is on fluid restriction.	This will avoid any possible interactions between the medications. The flush volume may put some clients at risk for fluid volume overload.
When you have finished administering all medications, flush with another 15 mL to 30 mL (5 mL to 10 mL for children) of warm water.	Flushing with water clears the tube and ensures that the patient has received all of the medication.
If the tube is connected to suction, disconnect the suction and keep the tube clamped for a minimum of 20 to 30 minutes after giving the medication; some agencies recommend 1 to 2 hours.	This process enhances absorption of the medication.

Parenteral Medications

Parenteral administration of medications is a common nursing procedure. Nurses give parenteral medications intradermally (ID), subcutaneously (SC, SQ), intramuscularly (IM), or intravenously (IV). Because these medications are absorbed more quickly than oral medications and are irretrievable once injected, the nurse must prepare and administer them carefully and accurately. Administering parenteral drugs requires the same nursing knowledge as for oral and topical drugs; however, because injections are invasive procedures, aseptic technique must be used to minimize the risk of infection.

Equipment

To administer parenteral medications, nurses use syringes and needles to withdraw medication from ampules and vials.

SYRINGES Syringes have three parts: the tip, which connects with the needle; the barrel, or outside part, on which the scales are printed; and the plunger, which fits inside the barrel (Figure 31.14). When handling a

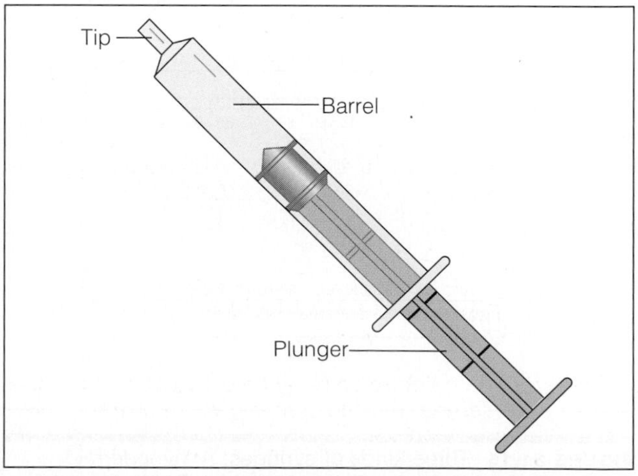

FIGURE 31.14 The three parts of a syringe

syringe, the nurse may touch the outside of the barrel and the handle of the plunger; however, the nurse must *avoid letting any unsterile object contact the tip or inside of the barrel, the shaft of the plunger, or the shaft or tip of the needle.*

Several kinds of syringes are available, differing in size, shape, and material. The three most commonly used types are the standard hypodermic syringe, the insulin syringe, and the tuberculin syringe (Figure 31.15). A *hypodermic syringe* comes in 2 mL, 2.5 mL, 3 mL, and 5 mL sizes. A scale on the syringe marks off gradations (e.g., 0.1 mL) to allow for fractions of a millilitre to be administered.

Insulin syringes are similar to hypodermic syringes, but they have a scale specially designed for insulin: a 100-unit calibrated scale intended for use with 100-unit insulin. All insulin syringes are calibrated on the 100-unit scale in North America. This is the only syringe that should be used to administer insulin. Several low-dose insulin syringes are available but they often have a non-removable needle. The correct choice of syringe is based on the amount of insulin required (Figure 31.16).

The *tuberculin syringe* was originally designed to administer tuberculin. It is a narrow syringe calibrated in tenths and hundredths of a millilitre (up to 1 mL) on one scale and, depending on where the syringe was manufactured, in sixteenths of a minim (up to 1 minim) on the other scale. This type of syringe can also be useful in administering other drugs, particularly when small or precise measurement is indicated (e.g., pediatric dosages).

Syringes are made in other sizes as well (e.g., 5 mL, 10 mL, 20 mL, and 50 mL). These are not generally used to administer drugs directly but can be useful for adding medications to intravenous solutions or for irrigating wounds. The tip of a syringe varies and is classified as either a Luer-Lok or non-Luer-Lok. A Luer-Lok syringe has a tip that requires the needle to be twisted onto it to avoid accidental removal of the needle (see Figure 31.17). The non-Luer-Lok syringe has a smooth graduated tip, and needles are slipped onto it. The larger 50 mL non-Luer-Lok syringe is often used for irrigation purposes (e.g., wounds, tubes) (see Figure 31.18).

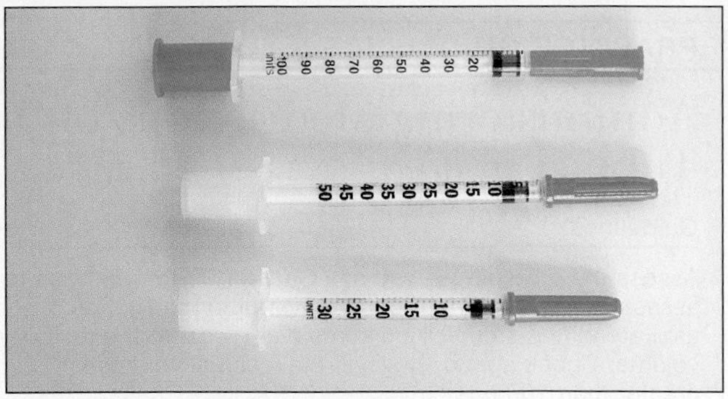

FIGURE 31.16 Different insulin syringes based on the amount of insulin required

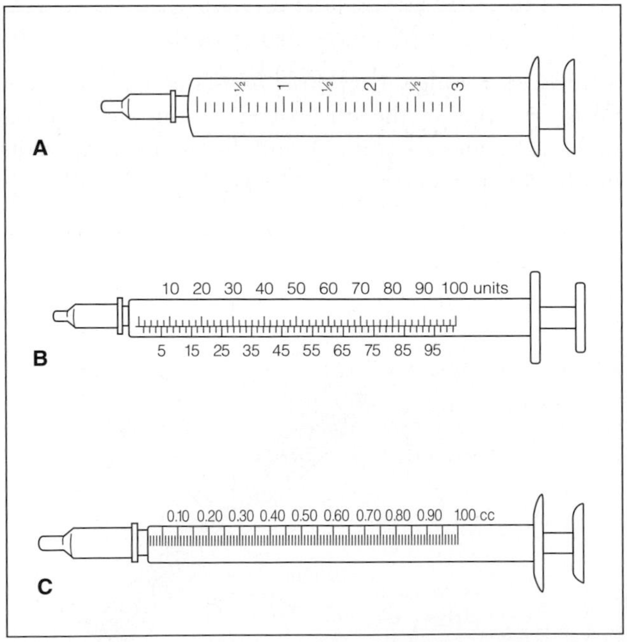

FIGURE 31.15 Three kinds of syringes: A: hypodermic syringe marked in tenths (0.1) of millilitres; B: insulin syringe marked in 100 units; C: tuberculin syringe marked in tenths and hundredths (0.01) of cubic millimetres

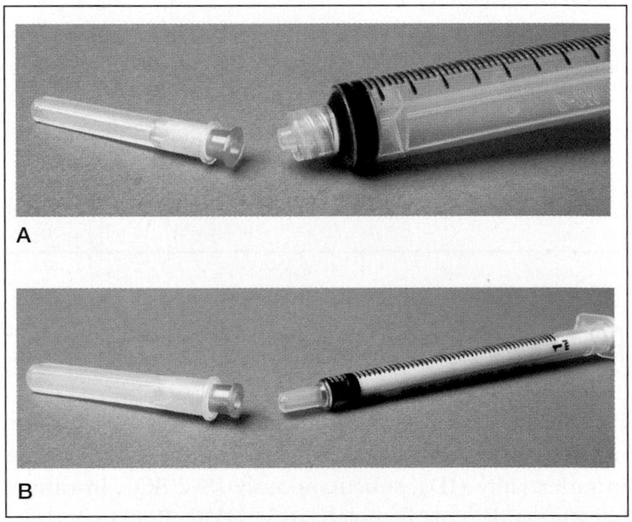

FIGURE 31.17 Tips of syringes: A: Luer-Lok (note threaded tip); B: non-Luer-Lok syringe (note the smooth graduated tip)

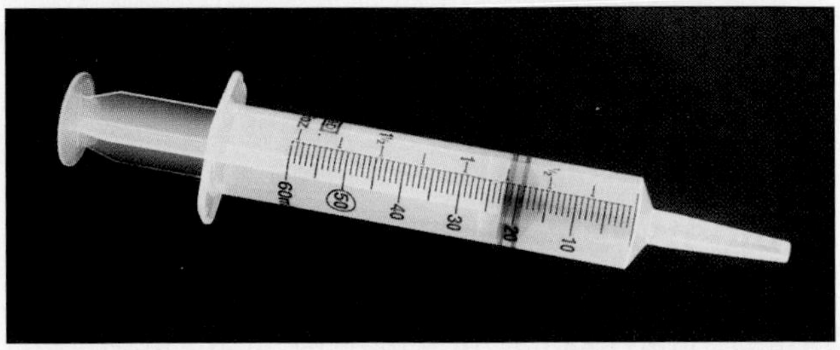

FIGURE 31.18 A 50 mL non-Luer-Lok syringe, which can be used for irrigation of tubes or wounds

Most syringes used today are made of plastic, are individually packaged for sterility in a paper wrapper or a rigid plastic container (Figure 31.19), and are disposable. The syringe and needle may be packaged together or separately. Needleless systems are also available in which the needle is replaced by a plastic cannula.

Injectable medications are frequently supplied in disposable **prefilled unit-dose systems**. These are available as prefilled syringes ready for use or prefilled sterile cartridges and needles that require the attachment of a reusable holder (injection system) before use (Figure 31.20). Examples of the latter system are the Tubex and Carpuject injection systems. The manufacturers provide specific directions for use. Because most prefilled cartridges are overfilled, excess medication must be ejected before the injection to ensure the right dosage. As the needle is fused to the syringe, the nurse is unable to change the gauge or length of the needle. The nurse, however, can transfer the medication into a regular syringe if the assessment of the patient necessitates a different needle gauge or length.

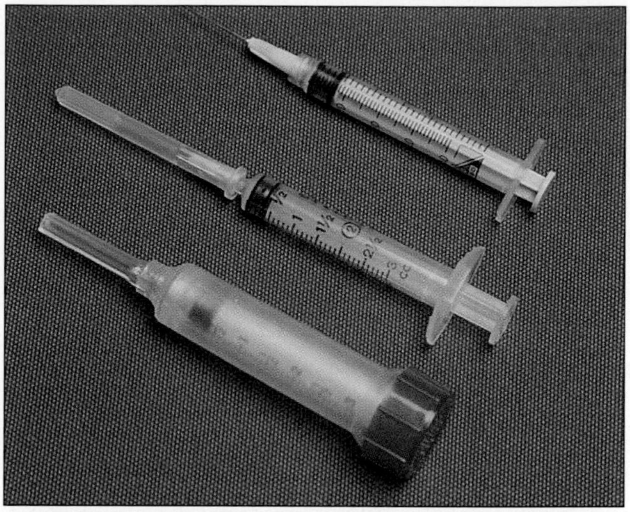

FIGURE 31.19 Disposable plastic syringes and needles: **top:** with syringe and needle exposed; **middle:** with plastic cap over the needle; **bottom:** with plastic case over the needle and syringe

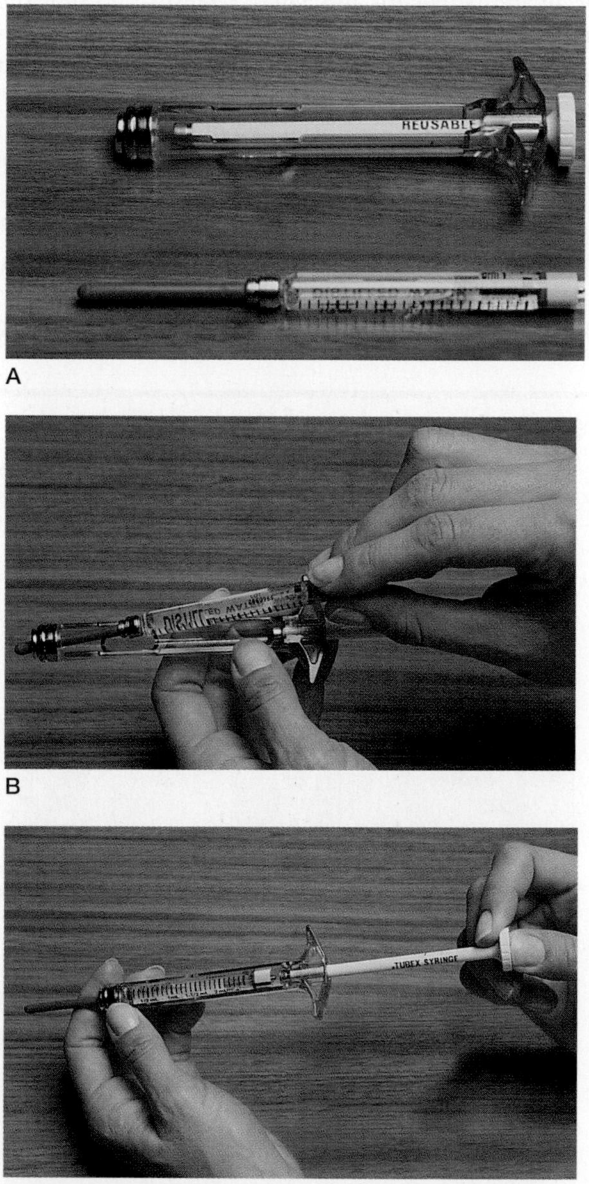

A

B

C

FIGURE 31.20 **A:** Syringe and prefilled sterile cartridge with needle; **B:** assembling the device; **C:** the cartridge slides into the syringe barrel, turns, and locks at the needle end. The plunger then screws into the cartridge end.

NEEDLES Needles are made of stainless steel, and most are disposable. Reusable needles (e.g., for special procedures) need to be sharpened periodically before resterilization because the points become dull with use and are occasionally damaged or acquire burrs on the tips. A dull or damaged needle should *never* be used.

A needle has three discernible parts: the **hub**, which fits onto the syringe; the **cannula**, or **shaft**, which is attached to the hub; and the **bevel**, which is the slanted part at the tip of the needle (Figure 31.21). A disposable needle has a plastic hub. Needles used for injections have three variable characteristics:

1. *Slant or length of the bevel.* The bevel of the needle may be short or long. Longer bevels provide the sharpest needles, cause less discomfort, and are commonly used for subcutaneous and

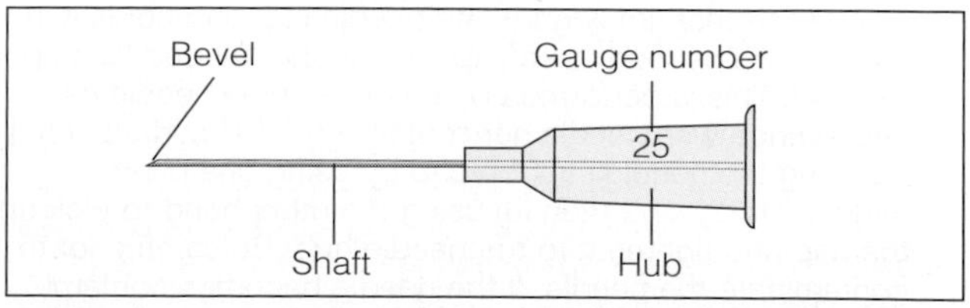

FIGURE 31.21 The parts of a needle

intramuscular injections. Short bevels are used for intradermal and intravenous injections because a long bevel can become occluded if it rests against the side of a blood vessel.

2. *Length of the shaft.* The shaft length of commonly used needles varies from 10 mm to 5 cm. The appropriate needle length is chosen according to the patient's muscle development, the patient's weight, and the type of injection.
3. ***Gauge** (or **diameter**) of the shaft.* The gauge of needles used for humans varies from 16 (1.651 mm in diameter) to 28 (0.356 mm in diameter). The larger the gauge number, the smaller the diameter of the shaft. Smaller gauges cause less tissue trauma and are ideal for daily subcutaneous injections, such as insulin; larger gauges are necessary for viscous medications, such as penicillin.

For an adult requiring a subcutaneous injection, it is appropriate to use a needle of 24 gauge to 26 gauge and 8 mm to 16 mm long. Slender adults and children may require a 7 mm needle, while obese clients may require a 12 mm or 12.7 mm needle. For an intradermal injection, choose a 26-gauge or 27-gauge needle. For intramuscular injections, a longer needle (e.g., 2.5 cm to 3.8 cm) with a larger gauge (e.g., 20 gauge to 22 gauge) is used. Slender adults and children usually require a shorter needle. The nurse must assess the patient to determine the appropriate needle length.

Preventing Needle-Stick Injuries

One of the most potentially hazardous procedures that health-care personnel face involves using and disposing of needles and sharps. Needle-stick injuries (i.e., puncture injuries) present a major risk for infection with hepatitis B virus, HIV, and many other pathogens. Standards have been set by the Canadian Centre for Occupational Health and Safety (2005) to prevent such injuries. Some of these are summarized in Box 31.7. If an accidental needle-stick injury occurs, the nurse needs to follow specific steps outlined by the agency.

Safety syringes have been designed in recent years to protect health-care workers. Safety devices are categorized as either *passive* or *active.* The nurse does not need to activate the passive safety device. For example, for some syringes, after injection, the needle retracts imme-

BOX 31.7 AVOIDING PUNCTURE INJURIES

Preventing needle-stick injuries is extremely important. Nurses should pay close attention to the following standards:

- Use appropriate puncture-proof disposal containers to dispose of *uncapped* needles and sharps. These are provided in all patient areas (Figure 31.22). Never throw sharps in wastebaskets. Sharps include any items that can cut or puncture skin, such as the following:
  - Needles
  - Surgical blades
  - Lancets
  - Razors
  - Broken glass
  - Broken capillary pipettes
  - Exposed dental wires
  - Reusable items (e.g., large-bore needles, hooks, rasps, drill points)
  - Any sharp instrument
- Never bend or break needles before disposal.
- Never recap used needles (e.g., that have been inserted into a patient) except under specified circumstances (e.g., when transporting a syringe to the laboratory for an arterial blood gas or blood culture).
- When recapping a needle (e. g., drawing up a medication into a syringe before administration), use a safety mechanical device that firmly grips the needle cap and holds it in place until it is ready to recap. Use a one-handed "scoop" method. This is performed by (1) placing the needle cap and syringe with needle horizontally on a flat surface, (2) inserting the needle into the cap by using one hand (Figure 31.23), and then (3) using the other hand to pick up the cap and tighten it to the needle hub. Be careful not to contaminate the needle. If the needle becomes contaminated, replace the needle with a new one.

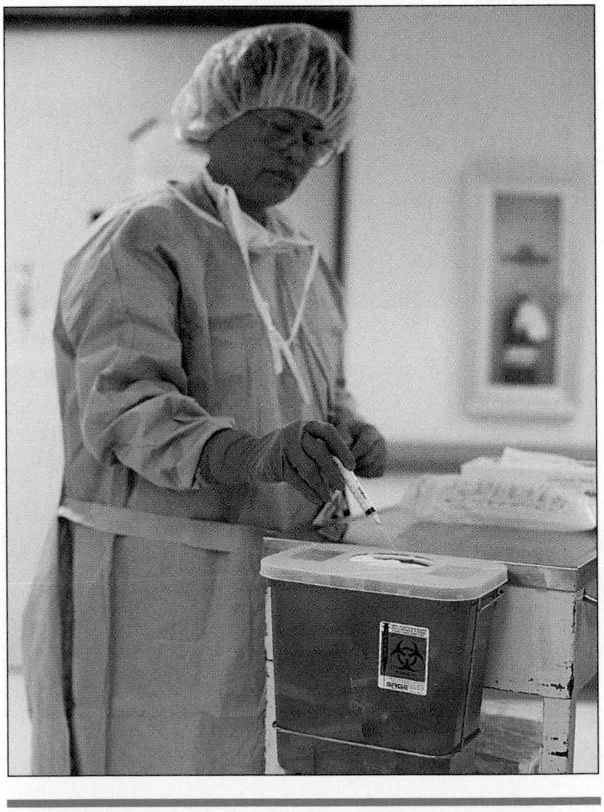

FIGURE 31.22 A disposal container for contaminated needles and other sharps

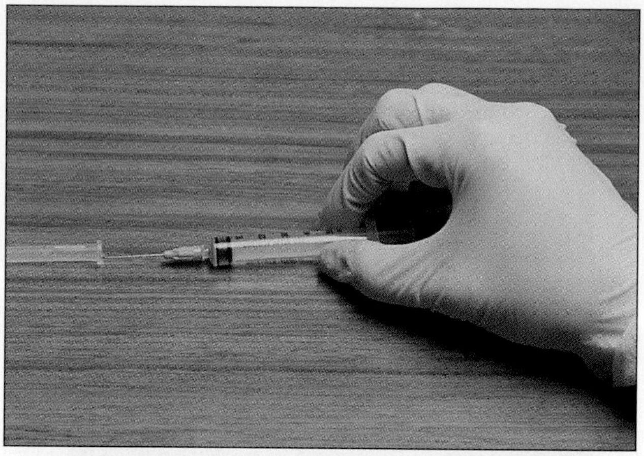

FIGURE 31.23 Recapping a used needle by using the scoop method

diately into the barrel (see Figure 31.24). In contrast, the active safety device requires the nurse to manually activate the safety feature. For example, the nurse activates a mechanism to retract the needle into the syringe barrel, or the nurse, after injection, manually pulls a plastic sheath or guard over the needle (see Figure 31.25).

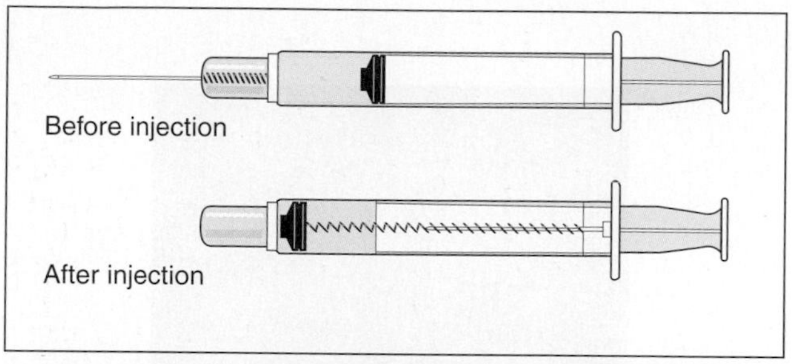

FIGURE 31.24 Passive safety device: the needle retracts immediately into the barrel after injection

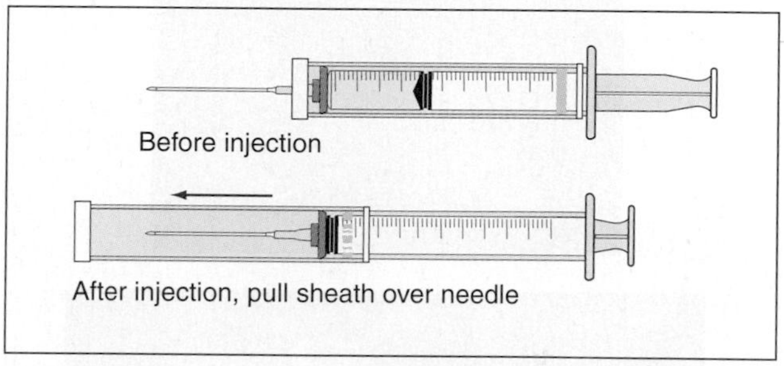

FIGURE 31.25 Active safety device: the nurse manually pulls the sheath or guard over the needle after injection

Preparing Injectable Medications

Injectable medications can be prepared by withdrawing the medication from an ampule or a vial into a sterile syringe, by using prefilled syringes, or by using needleless injection systems. Figure 31.26 shows an example of a needleless system used to access medication from a vial.

AMPULES AND VIALS *Ampules* and *vials* (Figure 31.27) are frequently used to package sterile parenteral medications. An **ampule** is a glass container usually designed to hold a single dose of a drug. It is made of clear glass and has a distinctive shape with a constricted neck. Ampules vary in size, ranging from 1 mL to 10 mL or more. Most ampule necks have coloured marks around them, indicating where they are scored for easy opening.

To access the medication in an ampule, the ampule must be broken at its constricted neck. Traditionally, files have been used to score the ampule. Today, plastic ampule openers are available that prevent injury from broken glass. The device consists of a plastic cap that fits over the top of an ampule. The head of the ampule, when broken, remains inside the cap (Figure 31.28) and is placed into a sharps container (Figure 31.22). If an ampule opener is not available, the neck should be filed with a small file, and then broken off at that point. Once the ampule is broken, the fluid is aspirated into a syringe by using a filter needle. This prevents aspiration of any glass particles.

A **vial** is a small glass bottle with a sealed rubber cap. Vials come in different sizes, from single to multidose vials. They usually have a metal or plastic cap that protects the rubber seal and must be removed to access the medication. To access the medication in a vial, the vial must be pierced with a needle. In addition, air must be injected into a vial before the medication can be withdrawn. Failure to inject air before withdrawing the medication leaves a vacuum within the vial that makes withdrawal difficult.

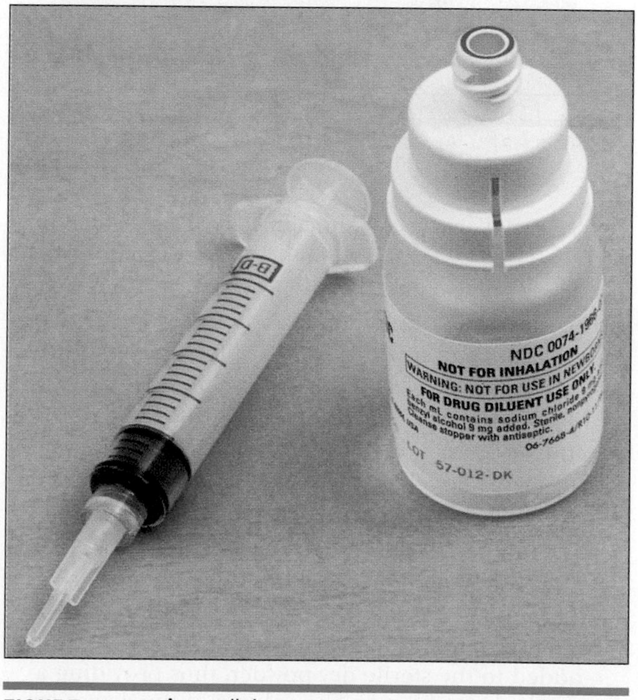

FIGURE 31.26 A needleless system can extract medication from a vial.

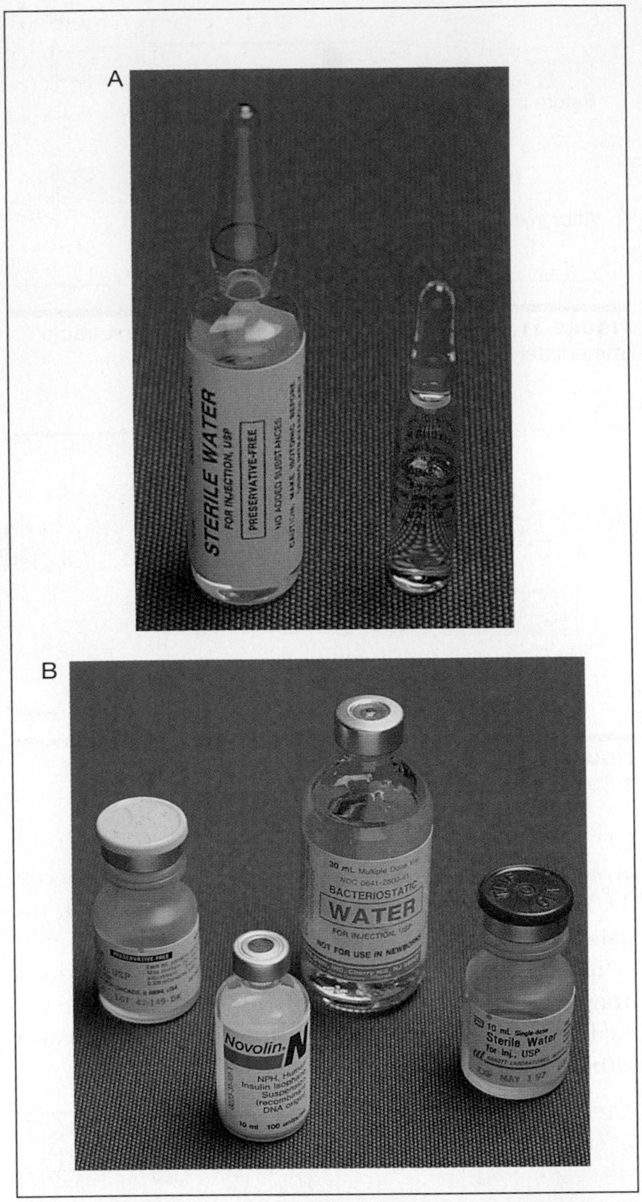

FIGURE 31.27 A: Ampules; B: vials

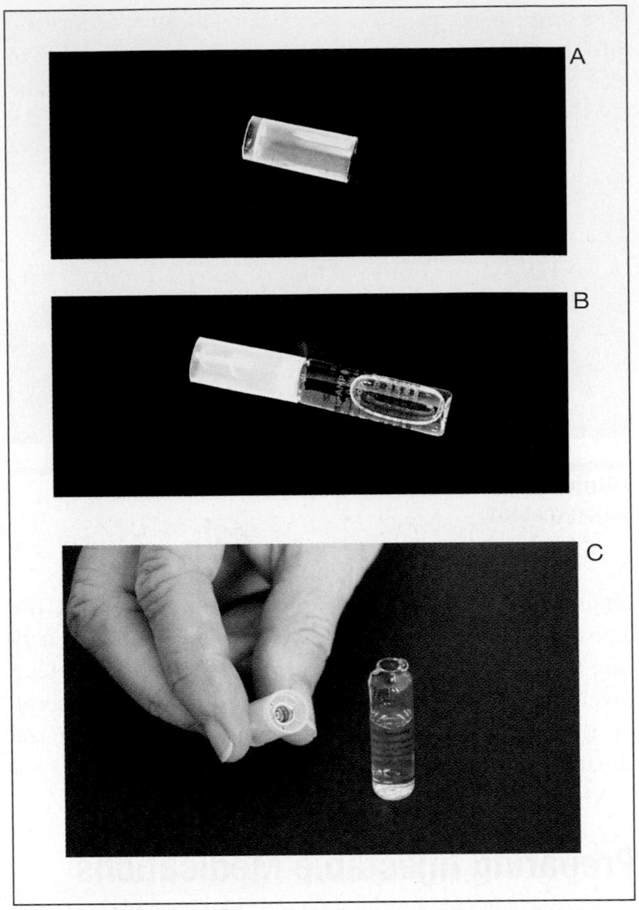

FIGURE 31.28 A: Ampule opener; B: plastic opener is placed over top of ampule; C: top of ampule remains in opener after ampule is broken

Several drugs (e.g., penicillin) are dispensed as powders in vials. A liquid (diluent) must be added to a powdered medication before it can be injected. The technique of adding a diluent to a powdered drug to prepare it for administration is called **reconstitution**. Powdered drugs usually have printed instructions enclosed with each packaged vial that describe the amount and kind of diluent to be added. Commonly used diluents are sterile water or sterile normal saline. Some preparations are supplied in individual-dose vials; others come in multidose vials. The following are two examples of the preparation of powdered drugs:

1. *Single-dose vial*: The instructions for preparing a single-dose vial specify that 1.5 mL of sterile water be added to the sterile dry powder, thus providing a single dose of 2 mL. The volume of the drug powder was 0.5 mL. Therefore, the 1.5 mL of water plus the 0.5 mL of powder results in 2 mL of solution. In other instances, the addition of a solution does not increase the volume. Therefore, it is important to follow the manufacturer's directions.
2. *Multidose vial*: A dose of 750 mg of a drug is ordered for a patient. On hand is a 10 g multidose vial. The directions for preparation read: "Add 8.5 mL of sterile water, and each millilitre will contain 1 g or 1000 mg." To determine the amount to inject, the nurse calculates as follows:

$$1 \text{ mL} = 1000 \text{ mg}$$
$$x \text{ mL} = 750 \text{ mg}$$
$$\text{(cross multiply)}$$
$$x = \frac{750 \text{ mg} \times 1 \text{ mL}}{1000 \text{ mg}}$$
$$x = 0.75 \text{ mL}$$

The nurse will give 0.75 mL of the medication.

Glass and rubber particulate have been found in medications withdrawn from ampules and vials by using a regular needle. As a result, it is strongly recommended that the nurse use a filter needle when withdrawing medications from ampules and vials to prevent withdrawing glass and rubber particles. After drawing the medication into the syringe, the filter needle is replaced with the regular needle for injection. This prevents tracking of the medication through the patient's tissues during the insertion of the needle, which, in turn, minimizes discomfort. Research validates this practice, especially in clients receiving intramuscular injections on a repeated basis or with injections that use larger bore needles.

Precautions must also be taken with patients who have latex allergies. Multidose vials with rubber stoppers may contain latex; therefore, strict policies and procedures are in place to prevent cross-contamination and an allergic reaction in the patient. Agencies may require the removal of the rubber stopper before drawing up of medications. Individual hospital policies are adhered to.

Skill 31.2 and Skill 31.3 describe how to prepare medications from ampules and vials, respectively. In addition, it is important to remember that when powdered drugs have been reconstituted, the date and time should be written on the label of the vial. Many of these drugs have to be used within a certain time period following reconstitution, so nurses need to know the expiration time after it has been reconstituted.

SKILL 31.2

PREPARING MEDICATIONS FROM AMPULES

Equipment

- MAR or computer printout
- Ampule of sterile medication
- File (if ampule is not scored) and small gauze square, or ampule opener
- Antiseptic swabs
- Syringe
- Needle for administering medication
- Filter needle for withdrawing medication from the ampule

IMPLEMENTATION

Preparation

1. Check the label on the ampule carefully against the MAR to make sure that the correct medication is being prepared.
2. Follow the three checks for administering medications. Read the label on the medication (1) when it is taken from the medication cart, (2) before withdrawing the medication, and (3) after withdrawing the medication.
3. Organize the equipment.

Performance

1. Perform hand hygiene and observe other appropriate infection prevention and control procedures.
2. Prepare the medication ampule for drug withdrawal.
   - Flick the upper stem of the ampule several times with a fingernail or, holding the upper stem of the ampule, make a large circle with the arm extended. **Rationale: This will bring all medication down to the main portion of the ampule.**
   - Use an ampule opener or place a piece of sterile gauze or antiseptic wipe between your thumb and the ampule neck or around the ampule neck, and break off the top by *bending* it toward you to ensure the ampule is broken away from you and away from others (see ❶). **Rationale: The sterile gauze protects the fingers from the broken glass, and any glass fragments will spray away from the nurse.**
   - *Or* place the antiseptic wipe packet over the top of the ampule before breaking off the top. **Rationale: This method ensures that all glass fragments fall into the packet and reduces the risk of cuts.**
   - Dispose of the top of the ampule in the sharps container.
3. Withdraw the medication.
   - Place the ampule on a flat surface.
   - Attach the filter needle to the syringe. **Rationale: The filter needle prevents glass particles from being withdrawn with the medication.**
   - Remove the cap from the filter needle and insert the needle into the centre of the ampule. Do not touch the rim of the ampule with the needle tip or shaft. **Rationale: This will keep the needle sterile.**
   - Withdraw the amount of drug required for the dosage.

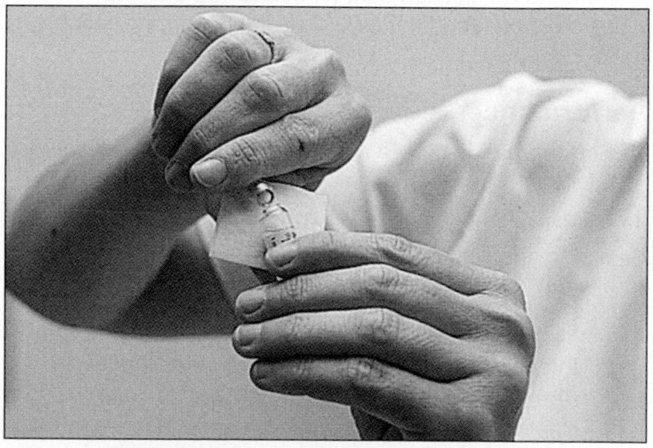

❶ Breaking the neck of an ampule

(continued)

SKILL 31.2

PREPARING MEDICATIONS FROM AMPULES (*continued*)

- With a single-dose ampule, hold the ampule slightly on its side, if necessary, to obtain more than the ordered amount of medication (see ❷).
- Dispose of the filter needle by placing in a sharps container.
- If giving an injection, replace the filter needle with a regular needle, tighten the cap at the hub of the needle, and push solution into the needle, to the prescribed amount.

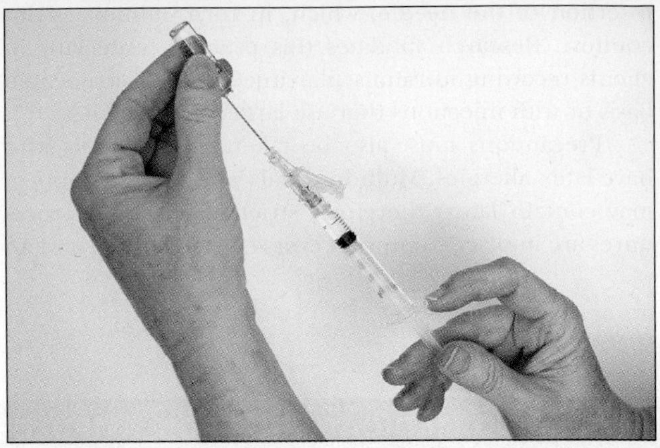

❷ Withdrawing a medication from an ampule

SKILL 31.3

PREPARING MEDICATIONS FROM VIALS

Equipment

- MAR or computer printout
- Vial of sterile medication
- Antiseptic swabs
- Safety needle and syringe
- Filter needle (check agency policy)
- Sterile water or normal saline, if drug is in powdered form

IMPLEMENTATION

Preparation

1. Check the label on the vial carefully against the MAR to make sure that the correct medication is being prepared.
2. Follow the three checks for administering medications. Read the label on the medication (1) when it is taken from the medication cart, (2) before withdrawing the medication, and (3) after withdrawing the medication.
3. Organize the equipment.

Performance

1. Perform hand hygiene and observe other appropriate infection prevention and control procedures.
2. Prepare the medication vial for drug withdrawal.
   - Mix the solution, if necessary, by rotating the vial between the palms of the hands, not by shaking. **Rationale: Some vials contain aqueous suspensions, which settle when they stand. In some instances, shaking is contraindicated because it may cause the mixture to foam.**
   - Remove the protective cap, or use an antiseptic wipe and rub in a circular motion to clean the rubber cap of a previously opened vial. **Rationale: The antiseptic cleans the cap and reduces the number of microorganisms.**
3. Withdraw the medication.
   - Attach a filter needle as agency practice dictates to draw up premixed liquid medications from multidose vials. **Rationale: The filter prevents any solid particles from being drawn up through the needle.**
   - Ensure that the needle is firmly attached to the syringe.
   - Remove the cap from the needle; then draw up into the syringe the volume of air equal to the volume of the medication to be withdrawn.
   - Carefully insert the needle into the upright vial through the centre of the rubber cap, maintaining the sterility of the needle.
   - Inject the air into the vial, keeping the bevel of the needle above the surface of the medication (see ❶). **Rationale: The air will allow the medication to be drawn out easily because it prevents negative pressure from being created inside the vial. The bevel is kept above the medication to avoid creating bubbles in the medication.**

(*continued*)

SKILL 31.3

PREPARING MEDICATIONS FROM VIALS (*continued*)

- Withdraw the prescribed amount of medication by using one of the following methods:
  - a. Hold the vial down (i.e., with the base lower than the top), move the needle tip so that it is below the fluid level, and withdraw the medication. Avoid drawing up the last drops of the vial (see ❷). **Rationale: Proponents of this method indicate that keeping the vial in the upright position while withdrawing the medication allows particulate matter to precipitate out of the solution. Leaving the last few drops reduces the chance of withdrawing foreign particles.**
  - b. *Or* invert the vial and ensure the needle tip is below the fluid level; gradually withdraw the medication (see ❸). **Rationale: Keeping the tip of the needle below the liquid level prevents air from being drawn into the syringe.**
- Hold the syringe and vial at eye level to determine that the correct dosage of drug is drawn into the syringe. Eject air remaining at the top of the syringe into the vial.
- When the correct volume of medication plus a little more (e.g., 0.25 mL) is obtained, withdraw the needle from the vial, and replace the cap over the needle by using the scoop method, thus maintaining its sterility.
- If necessary, tap the syringe barrel to dislodge any air bubbles present in the syringe. **Rationale: The tapping motion will cause the air bubbles to rise to the top of the syringe where they can be ejected out of the syringe.**
- If giving an injection, replace the filter needle, if used, with a regular or safety needle of the correct gauge and length. Eject air from the new needle and verify the correct medication volume before injecting the patient.

Variation: Preparing and Using Multidose Vials

- Read the manufacturer's directions.
- Withdraw an equivalent amount of air from the vial before adding the diluent, unless otherwise indicated by the directions.
- Add the amount of sterile water or saline indicated in the directions.
- If a multidose vial is reconstituted, label the vial with the date and time it was prepared, the amount of drug contained in each millilitre of solution, and your initials. **Rationale: Time is an important factor to consider in the expiration of medications.**
- Once the medication is reconstituted, store it in a refrigerator or as recommended by the manufacturer.

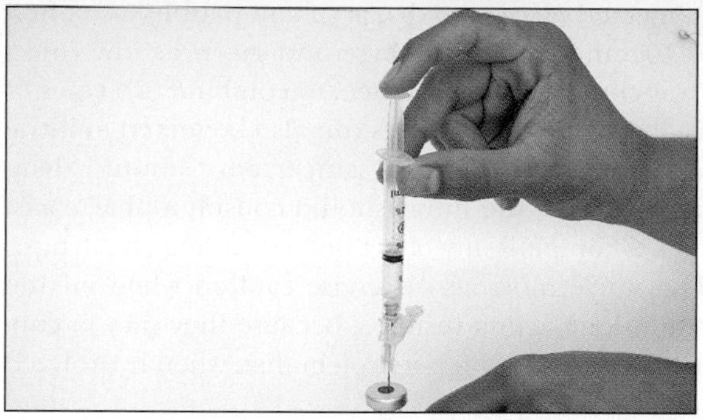

❶ Injecting air into a vial

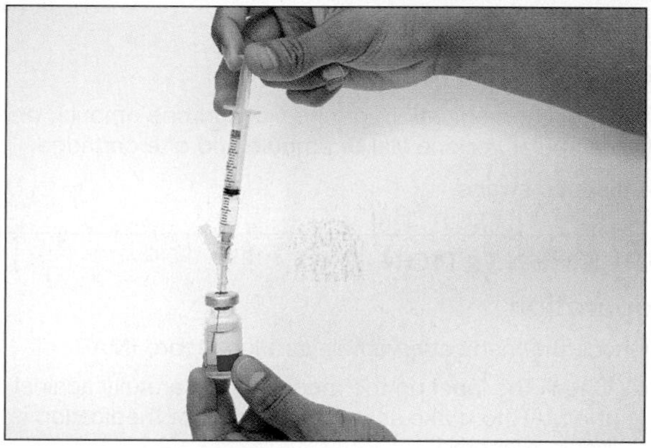

❷ Withdrawing a medication from a vial that is held with the base down

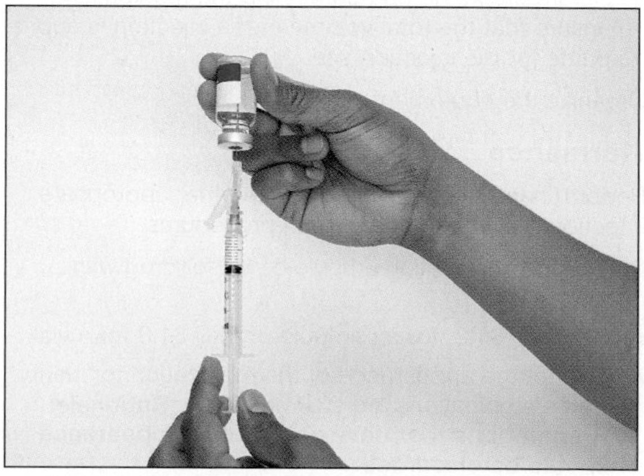

❸ Withdrawing a medication from an inverted vial

Mixing Medications in One Syringe

Frequently, patients need more than one drug injected at the same time. To spare the patient the experience of being injected twice, two drugs (if compatible) are often mixed together in one syringe and given as one injection. It is common, for instance, to combine two types of insulin in this manner. Drugs can also be mixed in intravenous solutions. When uncertain about drug incompatibilities, the nurse should consult a pharmacist or check a compatibility chart before mixing the drugs.

The nurse must also exercise caution when mixing short- and long-acting insulins, because they vary in content. Chemically, insulin is a protein that, when hydrolyzed in the body, yields a number of amino acids. Some insulin preparations contain an additional modifying protein, such as globulin or protamine, which slows absorption. This fact is particularly relevant to mixing two insulin preparations for injection because many insulin syringes have needles that cannot be changed. A vial of insulin that does not have the added protein (e.g., regular insulin) should never be contaminated with insulin that does have the added protein (e.g., Lente or NPH insulin). Premixed formulations of insulin are becoming more popular as they bypass the mixing procedure, which can be cumbersome for certain clients, especially those who have problems with vision or dexterity. Skill 31.4 describes how to mix medications in one syringe.

SKILL 31.4

MIXING MEDICATIONS BY USING ONE SYRINGE

Equipment

- MAR or computer printout
- Two vials of medication, or one vial and one ampule, or two ampules, or one vial or ampule and one cartridge
- Antiseptic swabs
- Sterile syringe and safety needle or insulin syringe (if insulin is being given, use a small-gauge hypodermic needle, such as a 26 gauge)
- Additional sterile subcutaneous or intramuscular needle (optional)

IMPLEMENTATION

Preparation

1. Check the medication administration record (MAR).
   - Check the label on the medications carefully against the MAR to make sure that the correct medication is being prepared.
   - Follow the three checks for administering medications. Read the label on the medication (1) when it is taken from the medication cart, (2) before withdrawing the medication, and (3) after withdrawing the medication.
   - Before preparing and combining the medications, ensure that the total volume of the injection is appropriate for the injection site.
2. Organize the equipment.

Performance

1. Perform hand hygiene and observe other appropriate infection prevention and control procedures.
2. Prepare the medication ampule or vial for drug withdrawal.
   - See Skill 31.2, for an ampule or Skill 31.3 for a vial.
   - Inspect the appearance of the medication for clarity. Some medications are always cloudy. **Rationale: Preparations that have changed in appearance should be discarded.**
   - If using insulin, thoroughly mix the solution in each vial before administration. Rotate the vials between the palms of the hands and invert the vials. **Rationale: Mixing ensures an adequate concentration and thus an accurate dose. Shaking insulin vials can make the medication frothy, making precise measurement difficult.**
   - Clean the tops of the vials with antiseptic swabs.
3. Withdraw the medications.

Mixing Medications from Two Vials

- Take the syringe and draw up a volume of air equal to the volume of medications to be withdrawn from both vials A *and* B.
- Inject a volume of air equal to the volume of medication to be withdrawn into vial A. Make sure the needle does not touch the solution. **Rationale: This prevents cross-contamination of the medications.**
- Withdraw the needle from vial A and inject the remaining air into vial B.
- Withdraw the required amount of medication from vial B. **Rationale: The same needle is used to inject air into and withdraw medication from the second vial. It must not be contaminated with the medication in vial A.**
- By using a newly attached sterile needle, withdraw the required amount of medication from vial A. Avoid pushing the plunger as that will introduce medication B into vial A. If using a syringe with a fused needle, withdraw the medication from vial A. The syringe now contains a mixture of medications from vials A and B. **Rationale: With this method, neither vial is contaminated by microorganisms or by medication from the other vial.** Be careful to withdraw only the ordered amount and to not create air bubbles. **Rationale: The syringe now contains two medications and an excess amount cannot be returned to the vial.**

See also the Variation later in this Skill box.

(continued)

SKILL 31.4

MIXING MEDICATIONS BY USING ONE SYRINGE *(continued)*

Mixing Medications from One Vial and One Ampule

- First prepare and withdraw the medication from the vial. **Rationale: Ampules do not require the addition of air before withdrawal of the drug.**
- Then withdraw the required amount of medication from the ampule.

Mixing Medications from One Cartridge and One Vial or Ampule

- First ensure that the correct dose of the medication is in the cartridge. Discard any excess medication and air.
- Draw up the required medication from a vial or an ampule into the cartridge. Note that when withdrawing medication from a vial, an equal amount of air must first be injected into the vial.
- If the total volume to be injected exceeds the capacity of the cartridge, use a syringe with sufficient capacity to withdraw the desired amount of medication from the vial or ampule, and transfer the required amount from the cartridge to the syringe.

Variation: Mixing Insulins

If premixed insulin preparations are not available, then mixing two insulins in a syringe is required. The following is an example of mixing 10 units of regular insulin and 30 units of neutral protamine Hagedorn (NPH) insulin.

- Inject 30 units of air into the NPH vial (N) and withdraw the needle. (There should be no insulin in the needle.) The needle should not touch the insulin (see ❶).
- Inject 10 units of air into the regular insulin vial (R) and immediately withdraw 10 units of regular insulin (see ❷ and ❸). **Rationale: Withdrawing the regular insulin first will minimize the possibility of the regular insulin becoming contaminated with the additional protein in the NPH.**
- Reinsert the needle into the NPH insulin vial and withdraw 30 units of NPH insulin (see ❹). (The air was previously injected into the vial.) Be careful to withdraw only the ordered amount and to not create air bubbles. If excess medication has been drawn up, discard the syringe and begin the procedure over again. **Rationale: The syringe now contains two medications, and an excess amount cannot be returned to the vial because the syringe contains regular insulin, which, if returned to the NPH vial, would dilute the NPH with regular insulin. The NPH vial would not provide accurate future dosages of NPH insulin.**

By using this method, you avoid adding NPH insulin to the regular insulin.

New extended long-acting insulins, glargine (Lantus) and detemir (Levemir) are also clear and colourless and should not be confused with rapid or short-acting insulins. These insulins are not to be mixed with any other insulin or mixed in a solution, such as an intravenous solution.

CLINICAL ALERT

One way to determine which insulin to withdraw first is to remember the saying "Clear before cloudy." Regular insulin is clear and NPH is cloudy because of the proteins in the insulin.

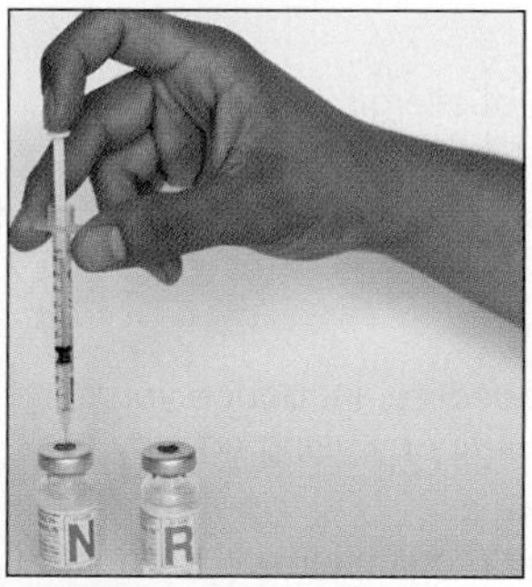

❶ Mixing intermediate- and short-acting insulin together: step 1

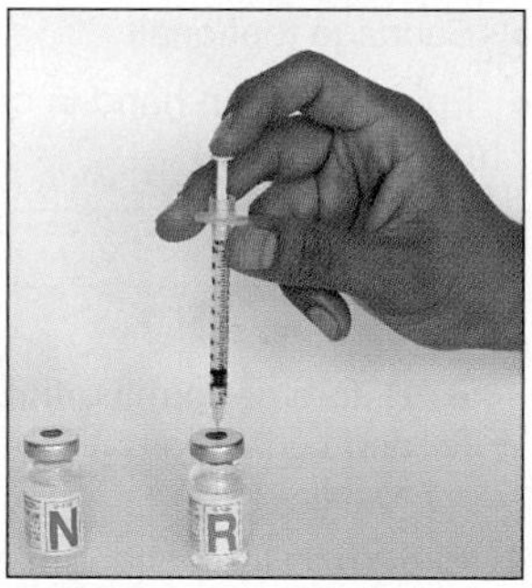

❷ Step 2

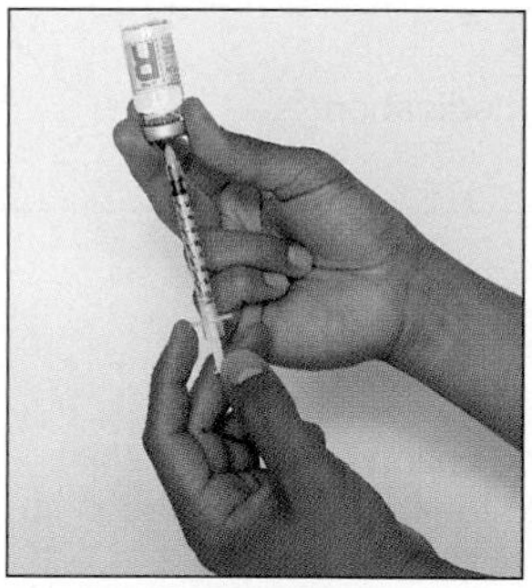

❸ Step 3

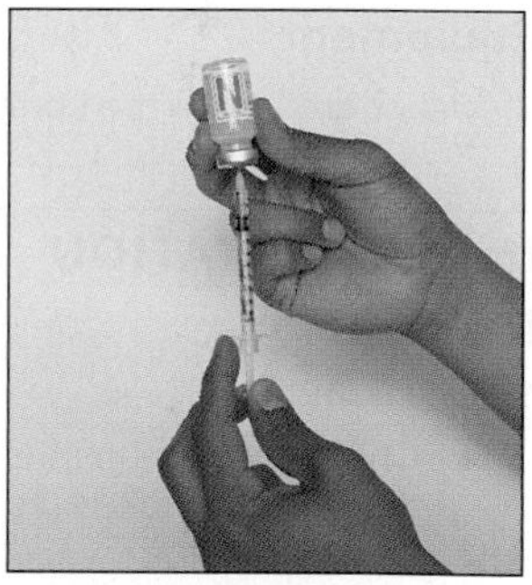

❹ Step 4

Intradermal Injections

An intradermal (ID) injection is the administration of a drug into the dermal layer of the skin, just beneath the epidermis. Usually, only a small amount of drug is injected (e.g., 0.1 mL). This method of administration is frequently indicated for allergy testing and tuberculosis (TB) screening. Common sites for intradermal injections are the flexor aspect of the forearm, the upper chest, and the back, beneath the scapulae (Figure 31.29). The left arm is commonly used for TB screening and the right arm is used for all other tests. The steps for administering an intradermal are described in Skill 31.5.

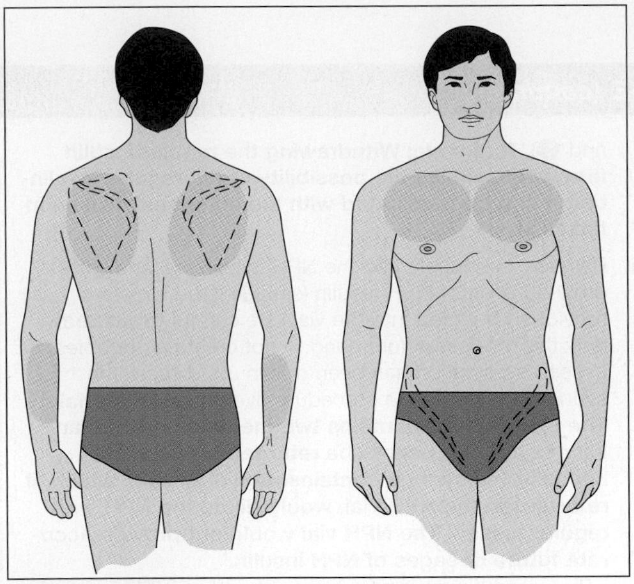

FIGURE 31.29 Body sites commonly used for intradermal injections

SKILL 31.5

ADMINISTERING AN INTRADERMAL INJECTION FOR SKIN TESTS

PURPOSE

To provide a medication that the patient requires for allergy testing and tuberculosis screening

ASSESSMENT

Assess

- Appearance of injection site
- Specific drug action and expected response
- Patient's knowledge of drug action and response

Check agency protocol about sites to use for skin tests.

Equipment

- Vial or ampule of the correct medication
- Sterile 1 mL syringe calibrated into hundredths of a millilitre (i.e., tuberculin syringe) and a 26-gauge to 27-gauge safety needle that is 12 mm to 16 mm long
- Antiseptic swabs
- 10 cm sterile gauze square (optional)
- Clean gloves (according to agency protocol)
- Bandage (optional)
- Epinephrine on hand in case of allergic anaphylactic reaction

IMPLEMENTATION

Preparation

1. Check the MAR.
   - Check the label on the medication carefully against the MAR to make sure that the correct medication is being prepared.
   - Follow the three checks for administering medications. Read the label on the medication (1) when it is taken from the medication cart, (2) before withdrawing the medication, and (3) after withdrawing the medication.
2. Organize the equipment.
3. Prepare the patient
   - Before performing the procedure, introduce yourself and verify the patient's identity by using agency protocol.
4. Explain to the patient that the medication will produce a small wheal, sometimes called a *bleb.* A *wheal* is a small raised area, like a blister. The patient will feel a slight prick as the needle enters the skin. Some medications are absorbed slowly through the capillaries into the general circulation, and the bleb gradually disappears. Other drugs remain in the area and interact with the body tissues to produce redness and induration (hardening), which will need to be interpreted at a particular time (e.g., in 24 or 48 hours). This reaction will also gradually disappear. **Rationale: Information can facilitate acceptance of and compliance with the therapy.**
5. Provide for patient privacy.
6. Select and clean the site.

Performance

1. Perform hand hygiene and observe other appropriate infection prevention and control procedures (e.g., clean gloves).
2. Prepare the medication from the vial or ampule for drug withdrawal.
   - See Skills 31.2 and 31.3.

(continued)

SKILL 31.5

ADMINISTERING AN INTRADERMAL INJECTION FOR SKIN TESTS *(continued)*

- Select a site (e.g., the forearm about a hand's width above the wrist and three or four finger widths below the antecubital space).
- Avoid using sites that are tender, inflamed, or swollen and those that have lesions.
- Put on gloves as indicated by agency policy.
- Cleanse the skin at the site by using a firm circular motion, starting at the centre and widening the circle outward. Allow the area to dry thoroughly.

7. Prepare the syringe for the injection.
   - Remove the needle cap while waiting for the antiseptic to dry.
   - Expel any air bubbles from the syringe. Small bubbles that adhere to the plunger are of no consequence. **Rationale: A small amount of air will not harm the tissue.**
   - Grasp the syringe in your dominant hand, close to the hub, holding it between thumb and forefinger. Hold the needle almost parallel to the skin surface, with the bevel of the needle up. **Rationale: The possibility of the medication entering the subcutaneous tissue increases when using an angle greater than 15 degrees. The bevel up position provides more comfort for the nurse and is faster to administer (Tarnow & King, 2004).**
8. Inject the fluid.
   - With the nondominant hand, pull the skin at the site until it is taut. For example, if using the ventral forearm, grasp the patient's dorsal forearm and gently pull it to tighten the ventral skin (see ❶A). **Rationale: Taut skin allows for easier entry of the needle and less discomfort for the client.**
   - Insert the tip of the needle far enough to place the bevel through the epidermis into the dermis. The outline for the bevel should be visible under the skin surface (see ❶B).
   - Stabilize the syringe and needle. Inject the medication carefully and slowly so that it produces a small wheal on the skin (see ❶C). **Rationale: This verifies that the medication entered the dermis.**
   - Withdraw the needle quickly at the same angle at which it was inserted. Activate the needle safety device. Apply a bandage if indicated.
   - Do not massage the area. **Rationale: Massage can dispense the medication into the tissue or out through the needle insertion site.**
   - Dispose of the syringe and needle into the sharps container. **Rationale: To prevent needle-stick injuries, do not recap the needle.**
   - Remove gloves.

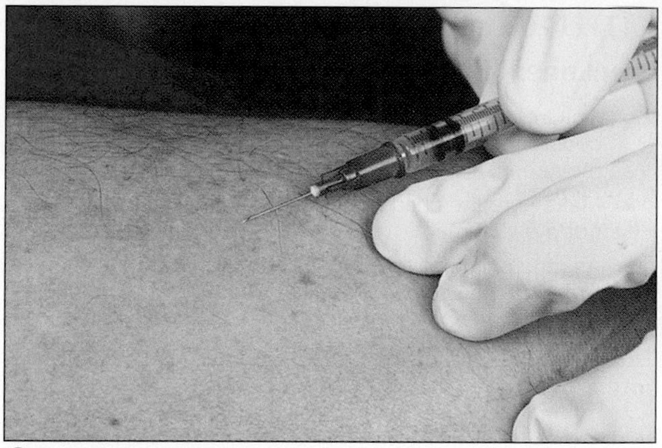

❶ A An intradermal injection

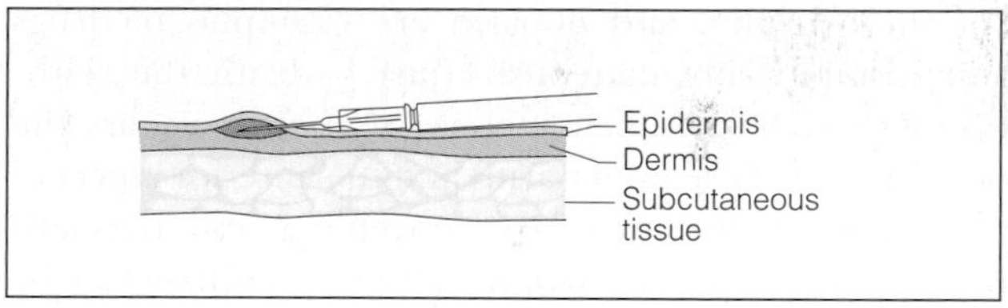

❶ B

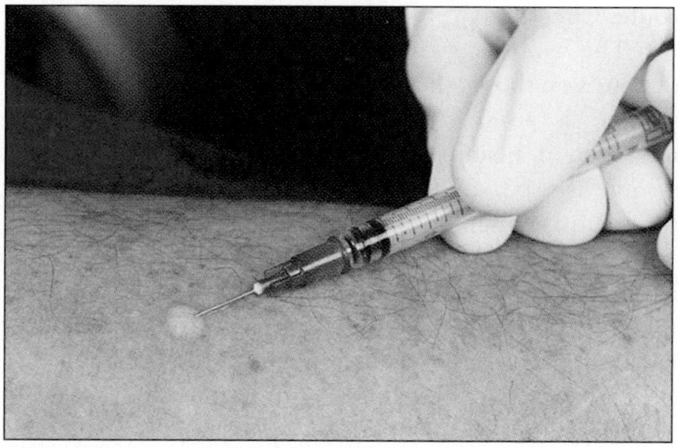

❶ C

   - Circle the injection site with ink to observe for redness or induration (hardening), per agency policy.
9. Document all relevant information.
   - Record the testing material given, time, dosage, route, site, and nursing assessments.

EVALUATION

- Evaluate the patient's response to the testing substance. **Rationale: Some medications used in testing can cause allergic reactions. It may be necessary to use epinephrine.**
- Evaluate the condition of the site in 24 or 48 hours, depending on the test. Measure the area of redness and induration in millimetres at the largest diameter and document findings.

Lifespan Considerations

Administering an Intradermal Injection

CHILDREN

- Children should be gently restrained during the procedure in order to prevent injury from a sudden movement.
- Make sure the child understands that the injection is not a punishment.
- Ask the child not to rub or scratch the injection site. *Rubbing the site can interfere with test results by irritating the underlying tissue.*

Home Care Considerations

Administering an Intradermal Injection

- Assess the patient's knowledge about the intradermal injection and the reason for follow-up with the health-care professional. Set up an appointment for the visit.
- Instruct and explain why the injection site should not be washed, rubbed, or scratched.

Subcutaneous Injections

Vaccines, insulin, and heparin are examples of drugs administered subcutaneously (just beneath the skin). Common sites for subcutaneous (SC) injections are the outer aspect of the upper arms and the anterior aspect of the thighs. These areas are convenient and normally have good blood circulation. Other areas that can be used are the abdomen, the scapular areas of the upper back, and the upper ventrogluteal and dorsogluteal areas (see Figure 31.30). Only small doses (0.5 mL to 1 mL) of medication are usually injected via the subcutaneous route. Check agency policy.

The type of syringe for subcutaneous injections depends on the medication to be given. Generally a 2 mL syringe is used for most subcutaneous injections. However, if insulin is being administered, an insulin syringe is used; and if heparin is being administered, a tuberculin syringe or prefilled cartridge may be used.

Needle sizes and lengths are selected based on the patient's body mass, the intended angle of insertion, and the planned site. Generally, a 25-gauge, 16 mm needle is used for adults of normal weight and the needle is inserted at a 45-degree angle; a 10 mm needle is used at a 90-degree angle. A child may need a 13 mm needle inserted at a 45-degree angle.

One method nurses use to determine length of needle is to pinch the tissue at the site and select a needle length that is half the width of the skin fold. To determine the angle of insertion, a general rule to follow relates to the amount of tissue that can be bunched or grasped at the site. A 45-degree angle is used when 2.5 cm of tissue can be grasped at the site; a 90-degree angle is used when 5 cm of tissue can be grasped.

For administering insulin to adults, the Canadian Diabetes Association recommends that a small-gauge needle is used (e.g., 28 gauge) to minimize tissue injury and subcutaneous leakage. Unless otherwise indicated, the insulin should be injected at a 90-degree angle.

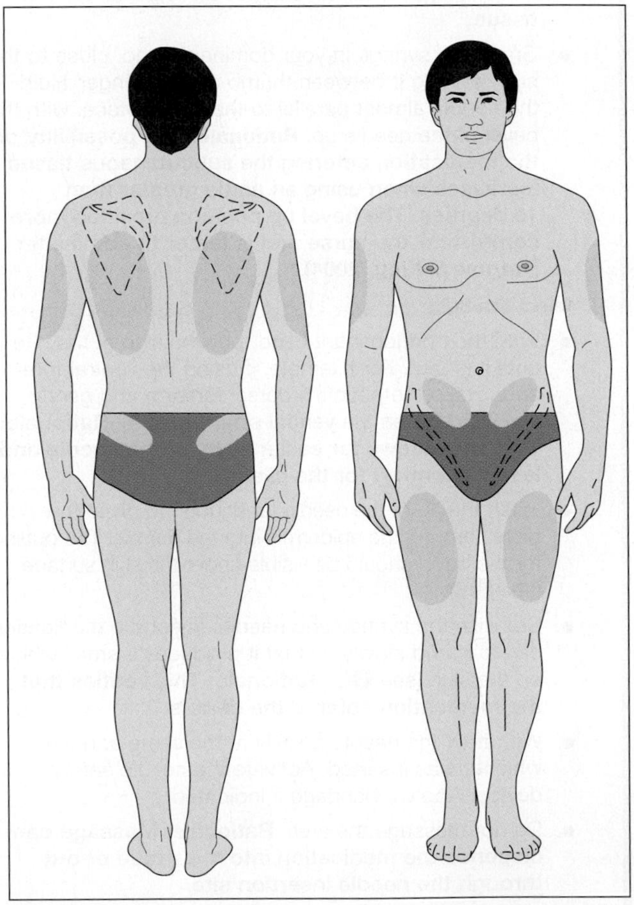

FIGURE 31.30 Body sites commonly used for subcutaneous injections

Insulin syringes are smaller, have fine needles, and also have special coatings on the needles to allow for an injection that is as pain free as possible. Insulin pens (similar in appearance to a writing pen) are another delivery system for insulin that is available to clients. Insulin is supplied in 1.5 mL or 3.0 mL cartridges containing 300 units of insulin. The cartridge is inserted into the pen and remains there until all the insulin is used. A short needle is attached to the end of the pen and changed for each injection or cleaned and reused two or three times. The cartridges may contain a variety of different types of insulin, such as Humulin-N or Humulin-R, and premixed formulations with a fixed ratio of insulin, such as Humulin-30/70 (30% regular insulin and 70% NPH insulin). Disposable pens are also now available that are discarded once the insulin is finished.

Subcutaneous injection sites need to be rotated in an orderly fashion to minimize tissue damage, aid absorption, and avoid discomfort. This is especially important for clients who must receive repeated injections, such as diabetics. Many factors influence insulin absorption, especially the choice of injection site. Insulin is absorbed most quickly when injected into the abdomen and almost as quickly when injected into the arms. It is absorbed most slowly when injected into the thighs or buttocks. Varying injection sites within the same anatomical site (approximately 2.5 cm apart) rather than between sites is recommended to limit variations in blood glucose levels (e.g., rotate sites for 1 to 2 weeks within one anatomical area, such as the right abdomen, then move to another anatomical area such as the left abdomen) (Registered Nurses' Association of Ontario, 2004).

Nurses have traditionally been taught to aspirate by pulling back on the plunger after inserting the needle and before injecting the medication. Absence of blood was believed to indicate that the needle was in subcutaneous tissue and not in the more vascular muscular tissue. According to the Canadian Diabetes Association, routine aspiration is no longer recommended with insulin administration. It is likely that students will observe that the practice of aspirating subcutaneous injections will vary among nurses.

Alcohol has also been traditionally used to cleanse the injection site before injecting the medication. While swabbing the area for 5 seconds may result in reduced bacteria, no prevention of infection occurs. Infection from injections is more likely related to contaminated syringes or needles rather than lack of cleansing of the skin site. *Cleansing of the injection site is now considered an optional step for home injection of insulin.*

The steps for administering a subcutaneous injection are described in Skill 31.6.

SKILL 31.6

ADMINISTERING A SUBCUTANEOUS INJECTION

PURPOSE

- To provide a medication the patient requires (see specific drug action)
- To allow slower absorption of a medication compared with either the intramuscular or intravenous route

ASSESSMENT

Assess

- Allergies to medication
- Specific drug action, side effects, and adverse reactions
- Client's knowledge and learning needs about the medication
- Status and appearance of subcutaneous site for lesions, erythema, swelling, ecchymosis, inflammation, and tissue damage from previous injections
- Ability to cooperate during the injection
- Previous injection sites used

Equipment

- Patient's MAR or computer printout
- Vial or ampule of the correct sterile medication
- Syringe and needle (e.g., 1 mL or 2 mL syringe, 25-gauge needle, 10 mm to 16 mm long)
- Antiseptic swabs
- Dry sterile gauze for opening an ampule (optional)
- Clean gloves

IMPLEMENTATION

Preparation

1. Check the MAR.
   - Check the label on the medication carefully against the MAR to make sure that the correct medication is being prepared.
   - Follow the three checks for administering medications. Read the label on the medication (1) when it is taken from the medication cart, (2) before withdrawing the medication, and (3) after withdrawing the medication.
2. Organize the equipment.

Performance

1. Perform hand hygiene and observe other appropriate infection prevention and control procedures (e.g., clean gloves).
2. Prepare the medication from the ampule or vial for drug withdrawal.
   - See Skill 31.2 (ampule) or Skill 31.3 (vial).
3. Provide for patient privacy.
4. Prepare the patient.

(continued)

SKILL 31.6

ADMINISTERING A SUBCUTANEOUS INJECTION (*continued*)

- Before performing the procedure, introduce yourself and verify the patient's identity by using agency protocol.
- Assist the patient to a position in which the arm, leg, or abdomen can be relaxed, depending on the site to be used. **Rationale: A relaxed position of the site minimizes discomfort.**
- Obtain assistance in holding an uncooperative patient. **Rationale: This prevents injury caused by sudden movement after needle insertion.**

5. Explain the purpose of the medication and how it will help, using language that the patient can understand. Include relevant information about effects of the medication. **Rationale: Information can facilitate acceptance of and compliance with therapy.**
6. Select and clean the site.
   - Select a site free of tenderness, hardness, swelling, scarring, itching, burning, or localized inflammation. Select a site that has not been used frequently. **Rationale: These conditions could hinder the absorption of the medication and may also increase the likelihood of injury and discomfort at the injection site.**
   - Put on clean gloves.
   - As agency protocol indicates, clean the site with an antiseptic swab. Start at the centre of the site and clean in a widening circle to about 5 cm. Allow the area to dry thoroughly. **Rationale: The mechanical action of swabbing removes skin secretions, which contain microorganisms.**
   - Place and hold the swab between the third and fourth fingers of the nondominant hand, or position the swab on the patient's skin above the intended site. **Rationale: Using this technique keeps the swab readily accessible when the needle is withdrawn.**
7. Prepare the syringe for injection.
   - Remove the needle cap while waiting for the antiseptic to dry. Pull the cap straight off to avoid contaminating the needle by the outside edge of the cap. **Rationale: The needle will become contaminated if it touches anything but the inside of the cap, which is sterile.**
   - Dispose of the needle cap.
8. Inject the medication.
   - Grasp the syringe in your dominant hand by holding it between your thumb and fingers. With your palm facing to the side or upward for a 45-degree angle insertion, or with your palm downward for a 90-degree angle insertion, prepare to inject (see ❶).
   - By using the nondominant hand, pinch or spread the skin at the site, and insert the needle by using the dominant hand and a firm steady push. Recommendations vary about whether to pinch or spread the skin and at what angle to administer subcutaneous injections. The most important consideration is the depth of the subcutaneous tissue in the area to be injected. If the patient has more than 1.25 cm of adipose tissue in the injection site, it would be safe to administer the injection at a 90-degree angle with the skin spread. If the patient is thin or lean and lacks adipose tissue, the subcutaneous injection should be given with the skin pinched and at a 45- to 60-degree angle. One way to check whether the pinch of skin is subcutaneous tissue is to ask the patient to flex and extend the elbow. If any muscle is being held in the pinch, you will feel it contract and relax. If so, release the pinch and try again (see ❷).

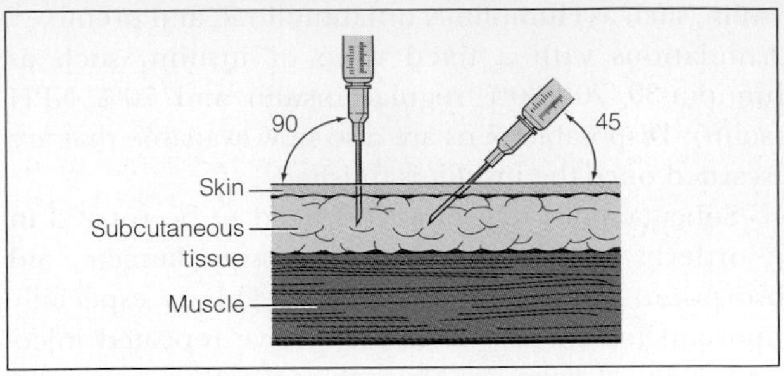

❶ Inserting a needle into the subcutaneous tissue by using 90- and 45-degree angles

   - When the needle is inserted, move your nondominant hand to the end of the plunger. Some nurses find it easier to move the nondominant hand to the barrel of the syringe and the dominant hand to the end of the plunger.
   - Inject the medication by holding the syringe steady, with a slow, even pressure. **Rationale: Holding the syringe steady and injecting the medication at an even pressure minimizes discomfort for the client.**
   - It is recommended with many subcutaneous injections, especially insulin, to wait 10 seconds or count slowly to 10 before withdrawing the needle. **Rationale: This ensures that the medication dissipates into the tissue.**

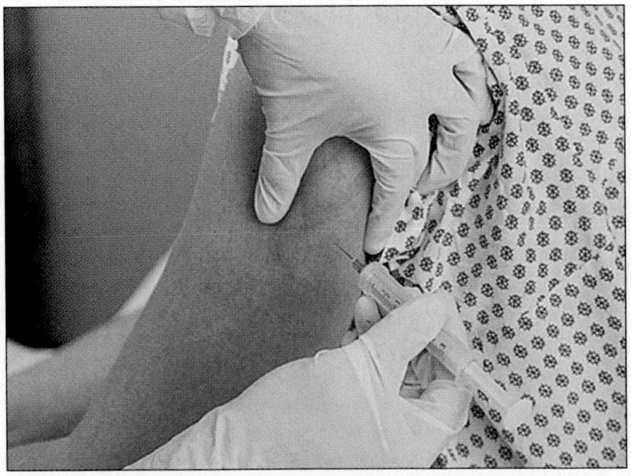

❷ Administering a subcutaneous injection into pinched tissue

(continued)

SKILL 31.6

ADMINISTERING A SUBCUTANEOUS INJECTION *(continued)*

9. Remove the needle.
   - Remove the needle smoothly, pulling along the same angle as the needle was inserted while depressing the skin with your nondominant hand. **Rationale: Depressing the skin places countertraction on it and minimizes the client's discomfort when the needle is withdrawn.**
   - If bleeding occurs, apply pressure to the site with dry sterile gauze until it stops. *Bleeding rarely occurs after subcutaneous injection.*
10. Dispose of supplies appropriately.
    - Activate the needle safety device or discard the uncapped needle and attached syringe into designated receptacles. **Rationale: Proper disposal protects the nurse and others from injury and contamination.**
    - Remove gloves and perform hand hygiene.
11. Document all relevant information.
    - Document the medication given, dosage, time, route, and any assessments.
    - Many agencies prefer that medication administration be recorded on the medication record. The progress notes are used when prn medications are given or when there is a special problem.
12. Assess the effectiveness of the medication at the time it is expected to act and document it.

Variation: Administering a Heparin Injection

The subcutaneous administration of heparin and low-molecular-weight heparin (e.g., enoxaparin [Lovenox]) requires special precautions because of the drug's anticoagulant properties.

- Select a site on the abdomen at least 10 cm *away* from the umbilicus and above the level of the iliac crests. Some agencies support the practice of subcutaneous injection of heparin in the thighs or arms as alternative sites to the abdomen.
- Use a 10 mm 25-gauge or 26-gauge needle or smaller, and insert it at a 90-degree angle. If a patient is very lean or wasted, use a needle longer than 10 mm and insert it at a 45-degree angle. The arms or thighs may be used as alternative sites.
- Do *not* aspirate when giving heparin by subcutaneous injection. **Rationale: Aspiration can possibly damage the surrounding tissue and cause bleeding as well as bruising.**
- Do not massage the site after the injection. **Rationale: Massaging could cause bleeding and ecchymoses (bruises) and hasten drug absorption.**
- Alternate the sites of subsequent injections.

EVALUATION

- Conduct appropriate follow-up, such as desired effect (e.g., relief of pain, sedation, lowered blood sugar, a prothrombin time within established limits), any adverse effects (e.g., nausea, vomiting, skin rash), and clinical signs of side effects.
- Relate to previous findings, if available.
- Report deviations from normal to the appropriate members of the health-care team.

Home Care Considerations

Subcutaneous Injections

- If the patient has impaired vision, consider filling syringes and storing them in an appropriate environment (e.g., the refrigerator) or obtaining prefilled medication syringes.
- For frequent injections, develop a plan with the patient for site rotation and explain the rationale for injection site rotation.
- For cost-saving measures, only in cases where alternate solutions cannot be found, teach able clients to safely reuse disposable syringes. Clients with diabetes can be taught to use the same syringe two to three times. They should be instructed to change syringes when the needle appears dull. Patients should be encouraged to maintain needle asepsis, practise safe recapping, and assess for needle dullness with each injection. However, patients with poor personal hygiene, acute concurrent illness, open wounds on the hands, or reduced resistance to infection should be discouraged from reusing syringes.
- Some clients may request an inhaled version of insulin (e.g., Exubera). Insulin that is inhaled through the mouth remains controversial, as some patients developed primary lung cancer during clinical trials (Canadian Medical Association, 2008). Inhaled insulin is not yet available in Canada.
- For clients who use insulin, ensure that at least one knowledgeable support person can correctly inject insulin in an emergency situation and recognize and treat hypoglycemia.

Intramuscular Injections

Injections into muscle tissue, called intramuscular (IM) injections, are absorbed more quickly than subcutaneous injections because of increased blood supply to the body tissues. Muscles can also take a larger volume of fluid without discomfort than subcutaneous tissues can, although the amount varies among individuals, chiefly with muscle size and condition and with the site used. An adult with well-developed muscles can usually safely tolerate up to 3 mL (some references cite up to 5 mL can be tolerated, but it is essential to check agency policy for recommended amounts) of medication in the gluteus medius and gluteus maximus muscles (Figure 31.31). A volume of 1 mL to 2 mL is usually recommended for adults with less developed muscles. A volume of 0.5 mL to 1 mL is recommended for the deltoid muscle.

Usually a 2 mL, 3 mL, or 5 mL syringe is used. The size of syringe used depends on the amount of medication being administered. The standard prepackaged intramuscular needle is 3.8 cm and 21 gauge or 22 gauge. Several factors dictate the size and length of the needle to be used:

- The muscle
- The type of solution
- The amount of adipose tissue covering the muscle
- The age of the patient

For example, a smaller needle, such as a 23-gauge to 25-gauge needle 2.5 cm long, is commonly used for the deltoid muscle. More viscous solutions require a larger gauge (e.g., 20 gauge). Obese clients may require a needle longer than 3.8 cm (e.g., 5 cm), and emaciated clients may require a shorter needle (e.g., 2.5 cm). Canada's *Immunization Guide* (Minister of Public Works and Government Services Canada, 2006) notes that for intramuscular injection of vaccines, a 22-gauge to 25-gauge needle that is long enough to reach muscle is recommended. Generally, this means 2.2 cm to 2.5 cm for infants, 2.2 cm to 2.5 cm for toddlers and older children, and 2.5 cm to 3.8 cm for adolescents and adults.

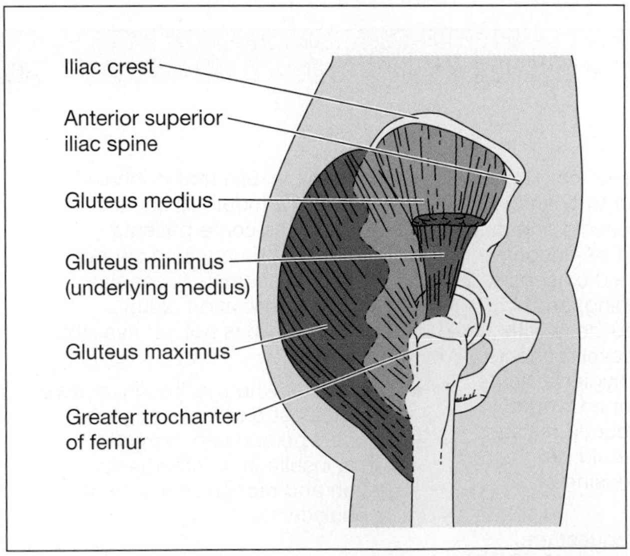

FIGURE 31.31 Lateral view of the right buttock showing the three gluteal muscles used for intramuscular injections

A major consideration in the administration of intramuscular injections is the selection of a safe site located away from large blood vessels, nerves, and bone. Several body sites can be used for intramuscular injections. These sites are discussed in detail next. Contraindications for using a specific site include tissue injury and the presence of nodules, lumps, abscesses, tenderness, or other pathology. Canada's *Immunization Guide* (Minister of Public Works and Government Services Canada, 2006) recommends that the muscles of the buttock *not* be used for active immunization because the presence of adipose tissue in this area makes absorption of vaccines variable (i.e., fat tissue makes it difficult to ensure that the needle length choice is accurate so the risk is that a subcutaneous rather than an intramuscular injection is given).

VENTROGLUTEAL SITE The ventrogluteal site is in the gluteus medius muscle, which lies over the gluteus minimus (see Figure 31.31). The ventrogluteal site is the *preferred* site for intramuscular injections in the buttock area for the following reasons:

- The area contains no large nerves or blood vessels.
- It provides the greatest thickness of gluteal muscle, consisting of both the gluteus medius and the gluteus minimus.
- The area is sealed off by bone.
- It contains consistently less fat than the buttock area, thus eliminating the need to determine the depth of subcutaneous fat.

The ventrogluteal site is suitable for children older than 1 year and for adults (note: some references cite 7 months as the age when this site can be used; this text opts for the conservative 1 year). The client position for the injection can be a supine, prone, or side-lying position. The side-lying position, however, helps locate the ventrogluteal site more easily. Position the patient on the appropriate side with the knee bent and raised slightly toward the chest. The trochanter will protrude, which facilitates locating the ventrogluteal site. To establish the exact site, the nurse places the heel of the hand on the patient's greater trochanter, with the fingers pointing toward the patient's head. The right hand is used for the left hip, and the left hand for the right hip. With the index finger on the patient's anterior superior iliac spine, the nurse stretches the middle finger dorsally (toward the buttocks), palpating the crest of the ilium and then pressing below it. The triangle formed by the index finger, the third finger, and the crest of the ilium is the injection site (see Figures 31.32 and 31.33).

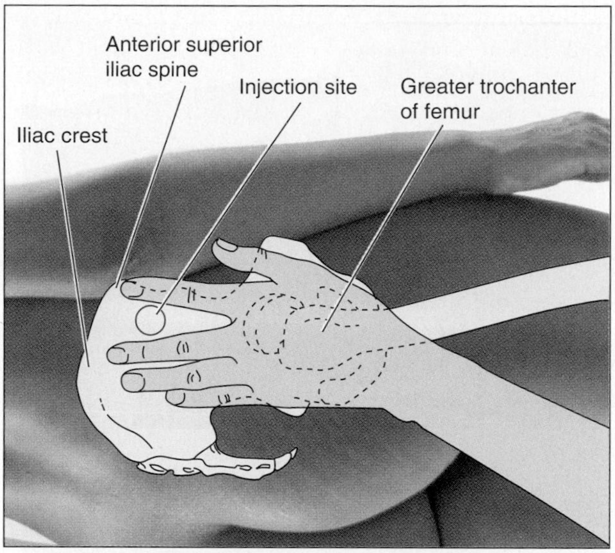

FIGURE 31.32 Landmarks for the ventrogluteal site of an intramuscular injection

DORSOGLUTEAL SITE The dorsogluteal site is composed of the thick gluteal muscles of the buttocks (see Figure 31.31). The dorsogluteal site can be used for adults and for children with well-developed gluteal muscles. Because these muscles are developed by walking, this site should not be used for children younger than 3 years unless the child has been walking for at least 1 year. While the use of the dorsogluteal is limited, if it is used the nurse must choose the injection site carefully to avoid striking the sciatic nerve, major blood vessels, or bone.

The nurse palpates the posterior superior iliac spine and then draws an imaginary line to the greater trochanter of the femur. This line is lateral to and parallel to the sciatic nerve. The injection site is lateral and superior to this line (Figure 31.34). Palpating the ilium and the trochanter is important; visual calculations alone can result in an injection that is placed too low and injures other structures.

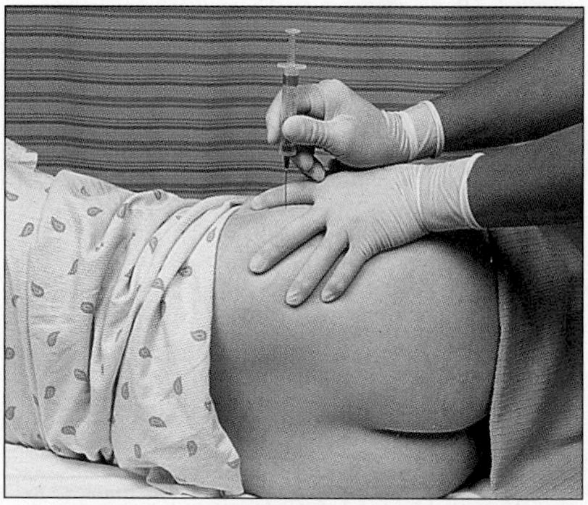

FIGURE 31.33 Administering an intramuscular injection into the ventrogluteal muscle

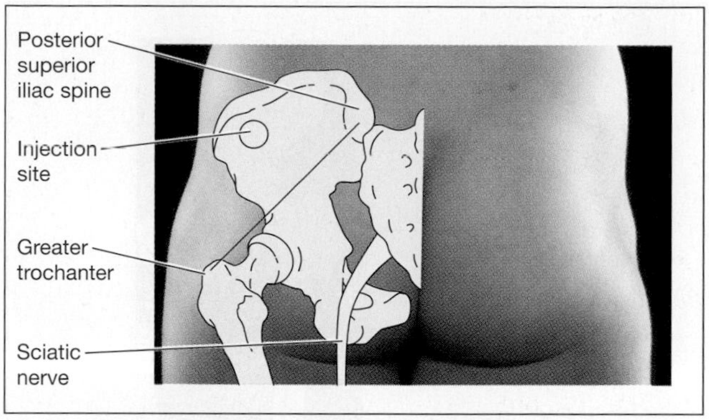

FIGURE 31.34 Landmarks for the dorsogluteal site for an intramuscular injection

The patient needs to assume a prone position with the toes pointed inward or a side-lying position with the upper knee flexed and in front of the lower leg. These positions promote muscle relaxation and, therefore, minimize discomfort from the injection.

This site has the most variable absorption in obese clients when the needle length is not adequate to reach muscle tissue (i.e., what is thought to be an intramuscular injection is, in fact, a subcutaneous injection).

VASTUS LATERALIS SITE The vastus lateralis muscle is usually thick and well developed in both adults and children. It is recommended as the site of choice for intramuscular injections for infants 1 year and younger (Minister of Public Works and Government Services Canada, 2006). Because the area has no major blood vessels or nerves, it is desirable for infants whose gluteal muscles are poorly developed. It is situated on the anterior lateral aspect of the infant's thigh (Figure 31.35). The middle third of the muscle is suggested as the site. It is established by dividing the area between the greater trochanter of the femur and the lateral femoral condyle

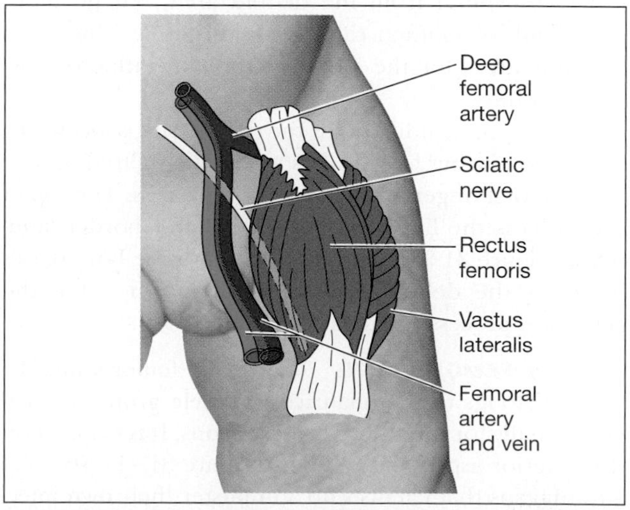

FIGURE 31.35 The vastus lateralis muscle of the infant's upper thigh, used for intramuscular injections

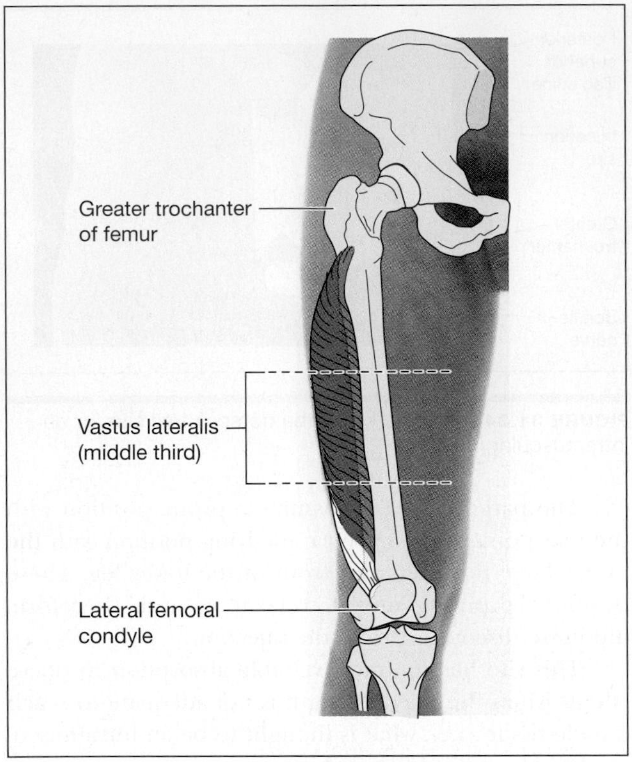

FIGURE 31.36 Landmarks of the vastus lateralis site of an adult's right thigh, used for an intramuscular injection

into thirds and selecting the middle third (Figure 31.36 and 31.37). The patient can assume a supine or a sitting position for an injection into this site.

DELTOID SITE The deltoid muscle is found on the lateral aspect of the upper arm. It is not used often for intramuscular injections because it is a relatively small muscle and is close to the radial nerve and radial artery. It is sometimes considered for use in adults because of rapid absorption from the deltoid area, but no more than 1 mL of solution can be administered. This site is recommended for the administration of influenza vaccine in adults.

The upper landmark for the deltoid site is located by the nurse placing four fingers across the deltoid muscle with the first finger on the acromion process. The top of the axilla is the line that marks the lower border landmark (Figure 31.38). A triangle within these boundaries indicates the deltoid muscle, about 5 cm below the acromion process (Figures 31.39 and 31.40).

RECTUS FEMORIS SITE The rectus femoris muscle, which belongs to the quadriceps muscle group, is used occasionally for intramuscular injections. It is situated on the anterior aspect of the thigh (Figure 31.41). Its chief advantage is that clients who administer their own injections can reach this site easily. Its main disadvantage is

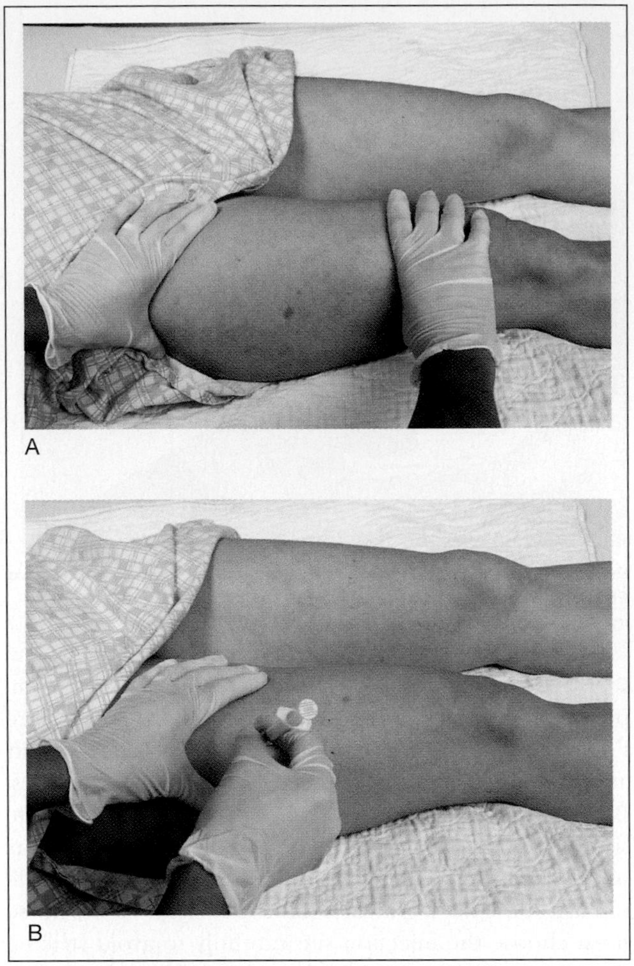

FIGURE 31.37 A: Determining landmarks; **B:** administering an intramuscular injection into the vastus lateralis site

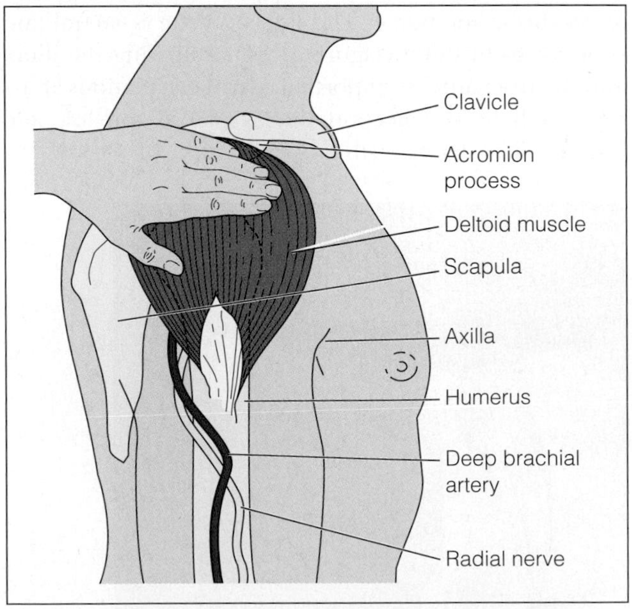

FIGURE 31.38 A method of establishing the deltoid muscle site for an intramuscular injection

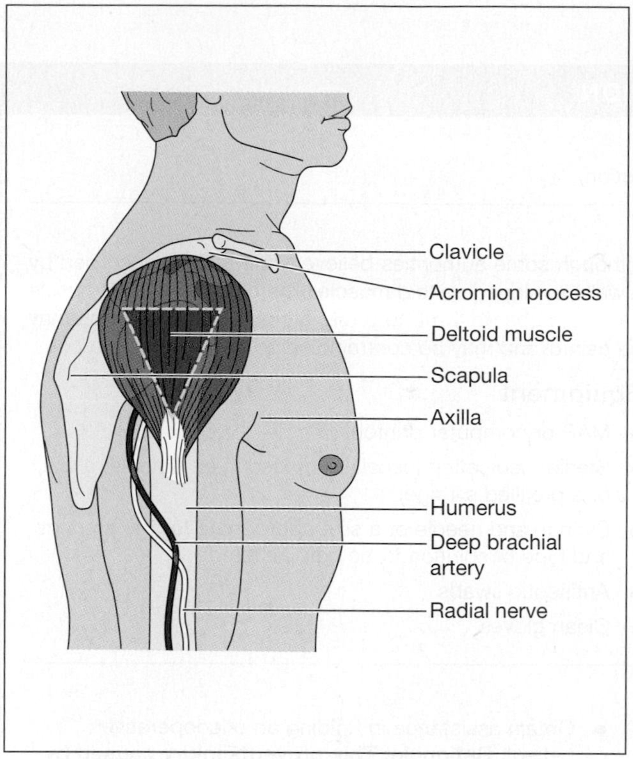

FIGURE 31.39 Landmarks for the deltoid muscle of the upper arm, used for intramuscular injection

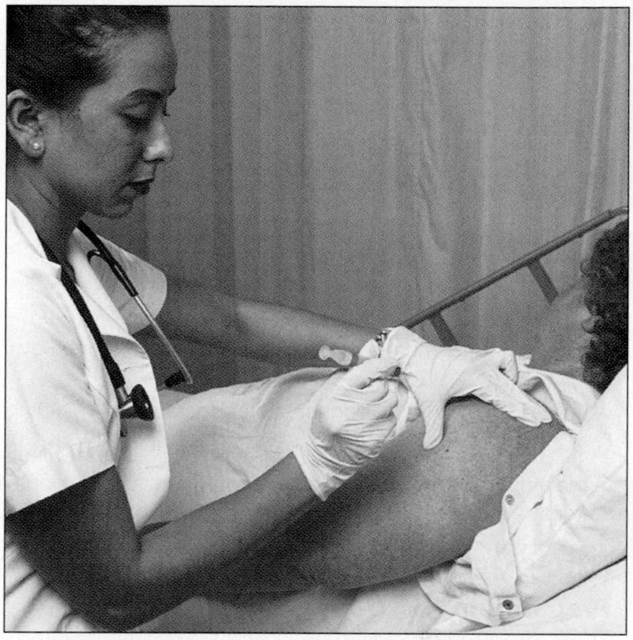

FIGURE 31.40 Administering an intramuscular injection into the deltoid site

that an injection here can cause considerable discomfort for some people.

IM INJECTION TECHNIQUE Skill 31.7 describes how to administer an intramuscular injection by using the Z-track technique, which is recommended for intramuscular injections (Nicoll & Hesby, 2002, p. 157). The Z-track method has been found to be less painful than the traditional injection technique and decreases leakage of irritating and discolouring medications into the subcutaneous tissue (Nicoll & Hesby, 2002; Pullen, 2005). Although the Z-track technique is not always used in practice, research evidence does support its effectiveness and recommends its routine use.

Nicoll and Hesby (2002) reported that researchers found that "applying pressure to the site for ten seconds before injection reduced injection pain" (p. 158). Further research is needed to determine additional techniques that will minimize the degree of pain at the time of injection.

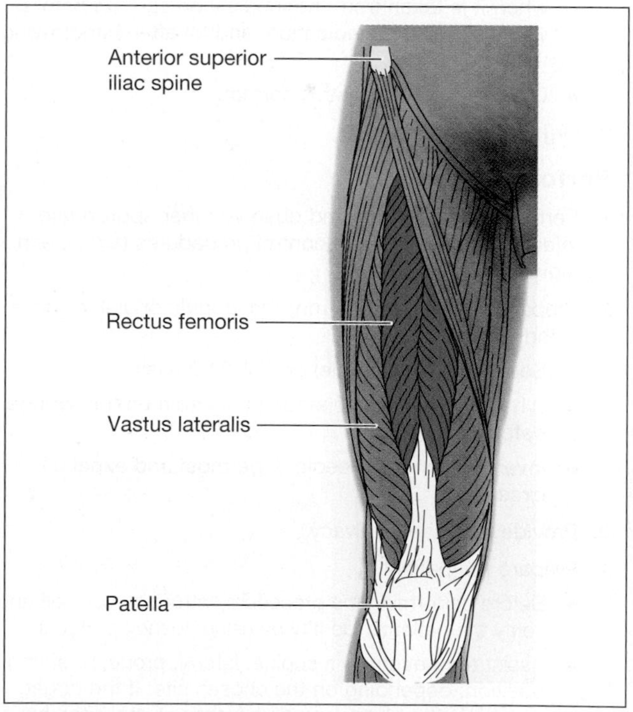

FIGURE 31.41 Landmarks for the rectus femoris muscle of the upper right thigh, used for intramuscular injections

SKILL 31.7

ADMINISTERING AN INTRAMUSCULAR INJECTION

PURPOSE

To provide a medication the patient requires (see specific drug action)

ASSESSMENT

Assess

- Patient allergies to medications
- Specific drug action, side effects, and adverse reactions
- Patient's knowledge of and learning needs about the medication
- Tissue integrity of the selected site
- Patient's age and weight to determine site and needle size
- Patient's ability or willingness to cooperate

Determine whether the size of the muscle is appropriate to the amount of medication to be injected. An average adult's deltoid muscle can usually absorb 0.5 mL of medication, although some authorities believe 1 mL can be absorbed by a well-developed deltoid muscle. The gluteus medius muscle can often absorb 1 mL to 5 mL, although 4 mL to 5 mL may be painful and may be contraindicated by agency protocol.

Equipment

- MAR or computer printout
- Sterile medication (usually provided in an ampule, a vial, or a prefilled syringe)
- Syringe and needle of a size appropriate for the amount and type of solution to be administered
- Antiseptic swabs
- Clean gloves

IMPLEMENTATION

Preparation

1. Check the MAR.
   - Check the label on the medication carefully against the MAR to make sure that the correct medication is being prepared.
   - Follow the three checks for administering the medication and dose. Read the label on the medication (1) when it is taken from the medication cart, (2) before withdrawing the medication, and (3) after withdrawing the medication.
   - Confirm that the dose is correct.
2. Organize the equipment.

Performance

1. Perform hand hygiene and observe other appropriate infection prevention and control procedures (e.g., clean gloves).
2. Prepare the medication from the ampule or vial for drug withdrawal.
   - See Skill 31.2 (ampule) or Skill 31.3 (vial).
   - Whenever feasible, change the needle on the syringe before the injection.
   - Invert the syringe needle uppermost and expel all excess air.
3. Provide for patient privacy.
4. Prepare the patient.
   - Before performing the procedure, introduce yourself and verify the patient's identity by using agency protocol.
   - Assist the patient to a supine, lateral, prone, or sitting position, depending on the chosen site. If the target muscle is the gluteus medius (ventrogluteal site), have the patient in the supine position, flex the knees; in the lateral position, flex the upper leg; and in the prone position, toe in. **Rationale: Appropriate positioning promotes relaxation of the target muscle.**
   - Obtain assistance in holding an uncooperative patient. **Rationale: This prevents injury caused by sudden movement after needle insertion.**
5. Explain the purpose of the medication and how it will help, using language that the patient can understand. Include relevant information about effects of the medication. **Rationale: Information can facilitate acceptance of and compliance with therapy.**
6. Select, locate, and clean the site.
   - Select a site free of skin lesions, tenderness, swelling, hardness, or localized inflammation and one that has not been used frequently.
   - If injections are to be frequent, alternate sites. Avoid using the same site twice in a row. **Rationale: This is to reduce the discomfort of intramuscular injections.**
   - Locate the exact site for the injection. See the discussion of sites earlier in this chapter.
   - Put on clean gloves.
   - Clean the site with an antiseptic swab. Use a circular motion, start at the centre, and move outward about 5 cm.
   - Transfer and hold the swab between the third and fourth fingers of your nondominant hand in readiness for needle withdrawal, or position the swab on the patient's skin above the intended site. Allow skin to dry before injecting medication. **Rationale: This will help reduce the discomfort of the injection.**
7. Prepare the syringe for injection.
   - Remove the needle cover and discard without contaminating the needle.
   - If using a prefilled unit-dose medication, take caution to avoid dripping medication on the needle before injection. If this does occur, wipe the medication off the needle with sterile gauze. Some sources recommend changing the needle if possible. **Rationale: Medication left on the needle can cause pain when it is tracked through the subcutaneous tissue.**

(continued)

SKILL 31.7

ADMINISTERING AN INTRAMUSCULAR INJECTION (*continued*)

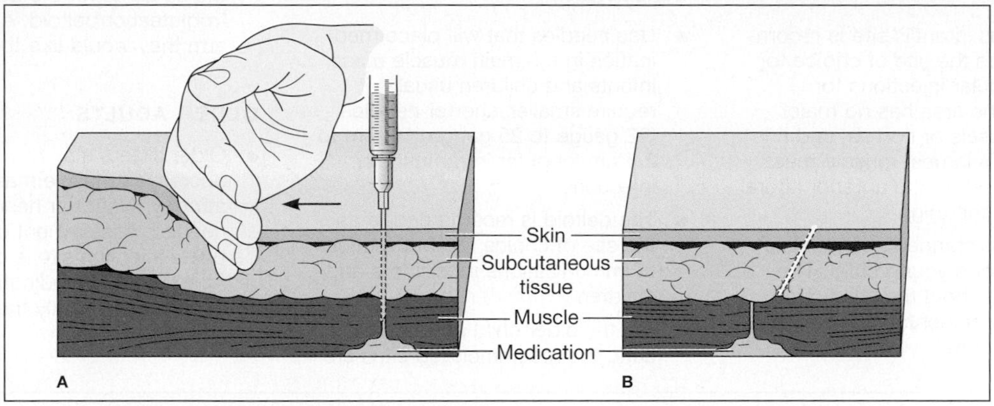

❶ Inserting an intramuscular needle at a 90-degree angle by using the Z-track method; **A:** skin pulled to the side; **B:** skin released. Note: when the skin returns to its normal position after the needle is withdrawn, a seal is formed over the intramuscular site. This prevents seepage of the medication into the subcutaneous tissues and subsequent discomfort.

8. Inject the medication by using a Z-track technique.
   - Use the ulnar side of the nondominant hand to pull the skin approximately 2.5 cm to the side. Under some circumstances, such as for an emaciated patient or an infant, the muscle may be pinched (see ❶). **Rationale: Pulling the skin and subcutaneous tissue or pinching the muscle makes it firmer and facilitates needle insertion.**
   - Holding the syringe between the thumb and forefinger (as if holding a pencil), pierce the skin quickly and smoothly at a 90-degree angle (see ❶), and insert the needle into the muscle. **Rationale: Using a quick motion lessens the client's discomfort.**
   - Hold the barrel of the syringe steady with your nondominant hand and aspirate by pulling back on the plunger with your dominant hand (if injecting a vaccination, skip this step). Aspirate for 5 to 10 seconds. **Rationale: If the needle is in a small blood vessel, it takes time for the blood to appear.** If blood appears in the syringe, withdraw the needle, discard the syringe, and prepare a new injection. **Rationale: This step determines whether the needle has been inserted into a blood vessel.** Although some controversy exists with subcutaneous aspiration practices, aspiration continues to be recommended with IM injection to avoid medication injection into the bloodstream (Barr & Thomas, 2005). "There are no studies that have assessed the need for aspiration before IM injection of vaccines in relation to vaccine safety" (Minister of Public Works and Government Services Canada, 2006).
   - If blood does not appear, inject the medication steadily and slowly (approximately 10 seconds per millilitre) while holding the syringe steady. **Rationale: Injecting medication slowly promotes comfort and allows time for tissue to expand and begin absorption of the medication (Nicoll & Hesby, 2002). Holding the syringe steady minimizes discomfort.**
   - After injection, wait 10 seconds. **Rationale: This permits the medication to disperse into the muscle tissue, thus decreasing the client's discomfort.**
9. Withdraw the needle.
   - Withdraw the needle smoothly at the same angle of insertion. **Rationale: This minimizes tissue injury.** Release the skin.
   - Apply gentle pressure at the site with a dry sponge. **Rationale: Use of an alcohol swab may cause pain or a burning sensation.**
   - If bleeding occurs, apply pressure with a dry sterile gauze until it stops.
10. Activate the needle safety device or discard the uncapped needle and attached syringe into the proper receptacle.
    - Remove gloves. Perform hand hygiene.
11. Document all relevant information.
    - Include the time of administration, drug name, dose, route, and the patient's reactions.
12. Assess effectiveness of the medication at the time it is expected to act.

EVALUATION

- Conduct appropriate follow-up, such as the following:
  - Desired effect (e.g., relief of pain or vomiting)
  - Any adverse reactions or side effects
  - Local skin or tissue reactions at injection site (e.g., redness, swelling, pain, or other evidence of tissue damage)
- Relate to previous findings, if available.
- Report significant deviations from normal to the appropriate members of the health-care team.

Lifespan Considerations

Intramuscular Injections

INFANTS

- The vastus lateralis site is recommended as the site of choice for intramuscular injections for infants. The area has no major blood vessels or nerves, and it is the infant's largest muscle mass. It is situated on the anterior lateral aspect of the thigh.
- Obtain assistance to immobilize an infant or a young child. The parent may hold the child. This prevents accidental injury during the procedure.

CHILDREN

- Use needles that will place medication in the main muscle mass; infants and children usually require smaller, shorter needles (22 gauge to 25 gauge, 16 mm to 2.5 cm long) for intramuscular injections.
- The deltoid is recommended as the site of choice for IM injection of immunizations in toddlers and children.
- For the older child and adolescent, the recommended sites are the same as for the adult: ventrogluteal or deltoid. Ask which arm they would like the injection in.

OLDER ADULTS

- Older clients may have a decreased muscle mass or muscle atrophy. A shorter needle may be needed. Assessment of the appropriate injection site is critical. Absorption of medication may occur more quickly than expected.

Intravenous Medications

Medications administered intravenously (IV) enter the bloodstream directly through a vein and are appropriate when a rapid effect is required. This route is also appropriate when medications are too irritating to tissues to be given by other routes. When an intravenous line is already established, this route is desirable because it avoids the discomfort of other parenteral routes. Medications administered intravenously use the following methods:

- Large-volume infusion of intravenous fluid
- Intermittent intravenous infusion (piggyback or tandem setups)
- Volume-controlled infusion (often used for children)
- Intravenous push or bolus
- Intermittent injection ports (device)

In all these methods, the patient has an existing intravenous line or an IV access site, such as a saline or heparin lock. Most agencies have procedures and policies about who may administer an IV medication. Chapter 43 (Skill 43.1, page 1407) describes the technique for performing a venipuncture and establishing an IV line.

The potential hazards in administering intravenous medications include rapid, severe reactions to the medication, infection, and fluid volume overload. With all IV medication administration, it is important to observe clients closely for signs of adverse reactions. Once the drug enters the bloodstream directly and acts immediately, there is no way it can be withdrawn or its action terminated. Therefore, the nurse must take special care to avoid any errors in the preparation of the drug and the calculation of the dosage. When the drug being administered is particularly potent, an antidote to the drug should be available. In addition, the vital signs are assessed before, during, and after infusion of the drug.

Before adding any medications to an existing intravenous infusion, the nurse must check for the "ten rights" and check compatibility of the drug and the existing intravenous fluid. Be aware of any incompatibilities of the drug and the fluid that is infusing. For example, the drug phenytoin (Dilantin) is incompatible with glucose and will form a precipitate if injected through a port in an intravenous line with glucose or dextrose infusing.

LARGE VOLUME INFUSIONS Mixing a medication into a large-volume IV container is the safest and easiest way to administer a drug intravenously. The drugs are diluted in volumes of 500 mL or 1000 mL of compatible fluids. It may be necessary to consult a pharmacist to confirm compatibility. Fluids such as IV normal saline or Ringer's lactate are frequently used. Commonly added drugs are potassium chloride and vitamins. It may also be necessary to ensure the compatibility of some drugs with the plastic IV bag and tubing. A glass IV bottle and special tubing may be used in special situations. See Skill 31.8.

The main danger of infusing a large volume of fluid is circulatory overload (hypervolemia). See Chapter 43.

The nurse adds the medication to the infusing fluid container or before it is hung. In some hospitals, the pharmacist adds the medication to the container, or premixed fluid solutions, such as potassium chloride (KCl) in 1000 mL of 5% dextrose in water (D_5W), prepared by the manufacturer are used.

SKILL 31.8

ADDING MEDICATIONS TO INTRAVENOUS FLUID CONTAINERS

PURPOSE

- To provide and maintain a constant level of a medication in the blood
- To administer well-diluted medications at a continuous and slow rate

ASSESSMENT

- Inspect and palpate the intravenous insertion site for signs of infection, infiltration, or a dislocated catheter.
- Inspect the surrounding skin for redness, pallor, or swelling.
- Palpate the surrounding tissues for coldness and the presence of edema, which could indicate leakage of the IV fluid into the tissues.
- Take vital signs for baseline data for medication that is particularly potent.
- Determine whether the patient has allergies to the medication.
- Check the compatibility of the medication and IV fluid.

Equipment

- MAR or computer printout
- Correct sterile medication
- Diluent for medication in powdered form (see manufacturer's instructions)
- Correct solution container
- Antiseptic swabs
- Sterile syringe of appropriate size (e.g., 5 mL or 10 mL) and a 2.5 cm or 3.8 cm, 20-gauge or 21-gauge sterile needle or equivalent needleless system
- IV additive label

IMPLEMENTATION

Preparation

1. Check the MAR.
   - Check the label on the medication carefully against the MAR.
   - Follow the three checks for administering medications. Read the label on the medication (1) when it is taken from the medication cart, (2) before withdrawing the medication, and (3) after withdrawing the medication.
   - Confirm that the dosage and route are correct.
   - Verify which infusion solution is to be used with the medication.
   - Consult a pharmacist, if required, to confirm compatibility of the drugs and solutions being mixed.
2. Organize the equipment.

Performance

1. Perform hand hygiene and observe other appropriate infection prevention and control procedures.
2. Prepare the medication ampule or vial for drug withdrawal.
   - See Skill 31.2 (ampule) or Skill 31.3 (vial).
   - Check the agency's practice for using a filter needle to withdraw premixed liquid medications from multidose vials or from ampules.
3. Add the medication.

To a New IV Container

- Locate the injection port. Clean the port with the antiseptic or alcohol swab. **Rationale: This reduces the risk of introducing microorganisms into the container when the needle is inserted.**
- Remove the needle cap from the syringe, insert the needle through the centre of the injection port, and inject the medication into the bag. Activate the needle safety device (see ❶).
- Mix the medication and solution by gently rotating the bag or bottle (see ❷). **Rationale: This should disperse the medication throughout the solution.**

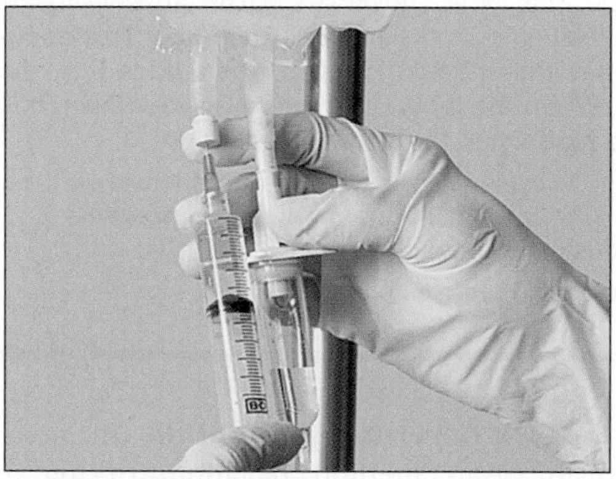

❶ Inserting a medication through the injection port of a fluid container

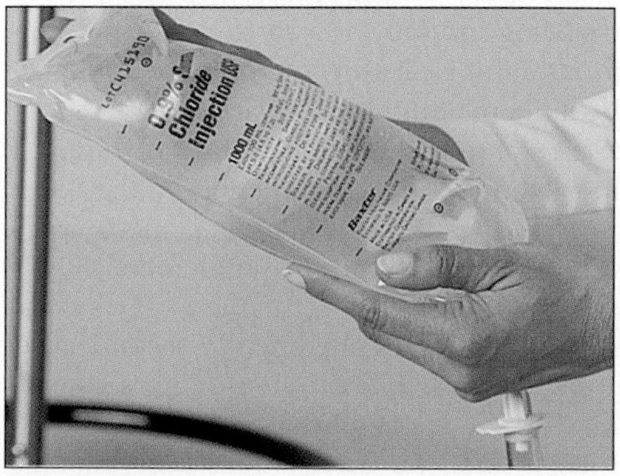

❷ Rotating an intravenous bag to distribute a medication

(continued)

SKILL 31.8

ADDING MEDICATIONS TO INTRAVENOUS FLUID CONTAINERS (*continued*)

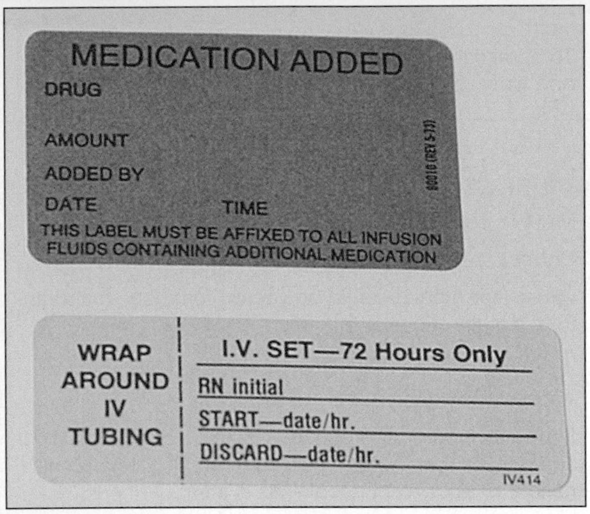

MEDICATION ADDED
DRUG
AMOUNT
ADDED BY
DATE
TIME
THIS LABEL MUST BE AFFIXED TO ALL INFUSION FLUIDS CONTAINING ADDITIONAL MEDICATION
WRAP AROUND IV TUBING
I.V. SET—72 Hours Only
RN initial
START—date/hr.
DISCARD—date/hr.
IV414

❸ **Top:** Label indicating a medication added to an IV infusion; **Bottom:** label indicating time for IV tubing change

- Complete the IV additive label with the name and dose of medication, date, time, and nurse's initials. Attach it upside down on the bag or bottle (see ❸). **Rationale: This documents that the medication has been added to the solution. When the label is attached upside down, it is easier to read when the bag is hanging up.**
- Clamp the IV tubing. Spike the bag or bottle with IV tubing and hang the IV. **Rationale: Clamping prevents rapid infusion of the solution.**
- Regulate infusion rate as ordered.

To an Existing Infusion

- Determine that the IV solution in the container is sufficient for adding the medication. **Rationale: Sufficient volume is necessary to dilute the medication adequately.**
- Confirm the desired dilution of the medication, that is, the amount of medication per millilitre of solution.
- Close the infusion clamp. **Rationale: This prevents the medication from infusing directly into the client as it is injected into the bag or bottle.**
- Wipe the medication port with the alcohol or disinfectant swab. **Rationale: This reduces the risk of introducing microorganisms into the container when the needle is inserted.** Remove the needle cover from the medication syringe.
- While supporting and stabilizing the bag with your thumb and forefinger, carefully insert the syringe needle through the port and inject the medication. **Rationale: The bag is supported during the injection of the medication to avoid punctures.** If the bag is too high to reach easily, lower it from the IV pole. Activate the needle safety device.
- Remove the bag from the pole and gently rotate the bag. **Rationale: This will mix the medication and solution.**
- Rehang the container and regulate the flow rate. **Rationale: This establishes the correct flow rate.**
- Complete the medication label and apply it to the IV container.

4. Dispose of the equipment and supplies according to agency practice. **Rationale: This prevents inadvertent injury to others and the spread of microorganisms.**
5. Document the medication on the appropriate form in the patient's record.

INTERMITTENT INTRAVENOUS INFUSIONS An intermittent infusion is a method of administering a medication mixed in a small amount of IV solution, such as 50 mL or 100 mL (see Figure 31.42). The drug is administered at regular intervals, such as every 4 hours, with the drug being infused for a short period of time, such as 30 to 60 minutes. Two commonly used additive setups are the tandem and the piggyback.

In a **tandem** setup or alignment, a second container is attached to the line of the first container at the lower, secondary port (Figure 31.43A). It permits medications to be administered intermittently or simultaneously with the primary solution.

In the **piggyback** setup or alignment, a secondary set connects the second container to the tubing of the primary container at the upper port (see Figure 31.43B). This setup is used solely for intermittent drug administration. Various manufacturers' designs may vary, so the nurse must check the manufacturer's labelling and directions carefully. Traditionally, the tubing of the secondary

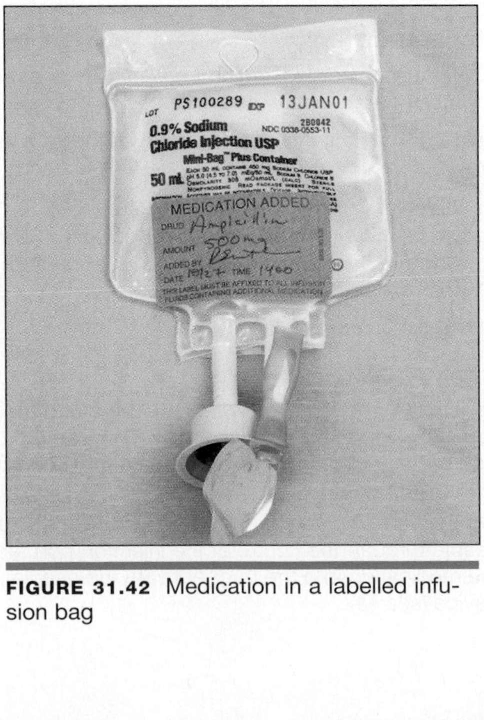

FIGURE 31.42 Medication in a labelled infusion bag

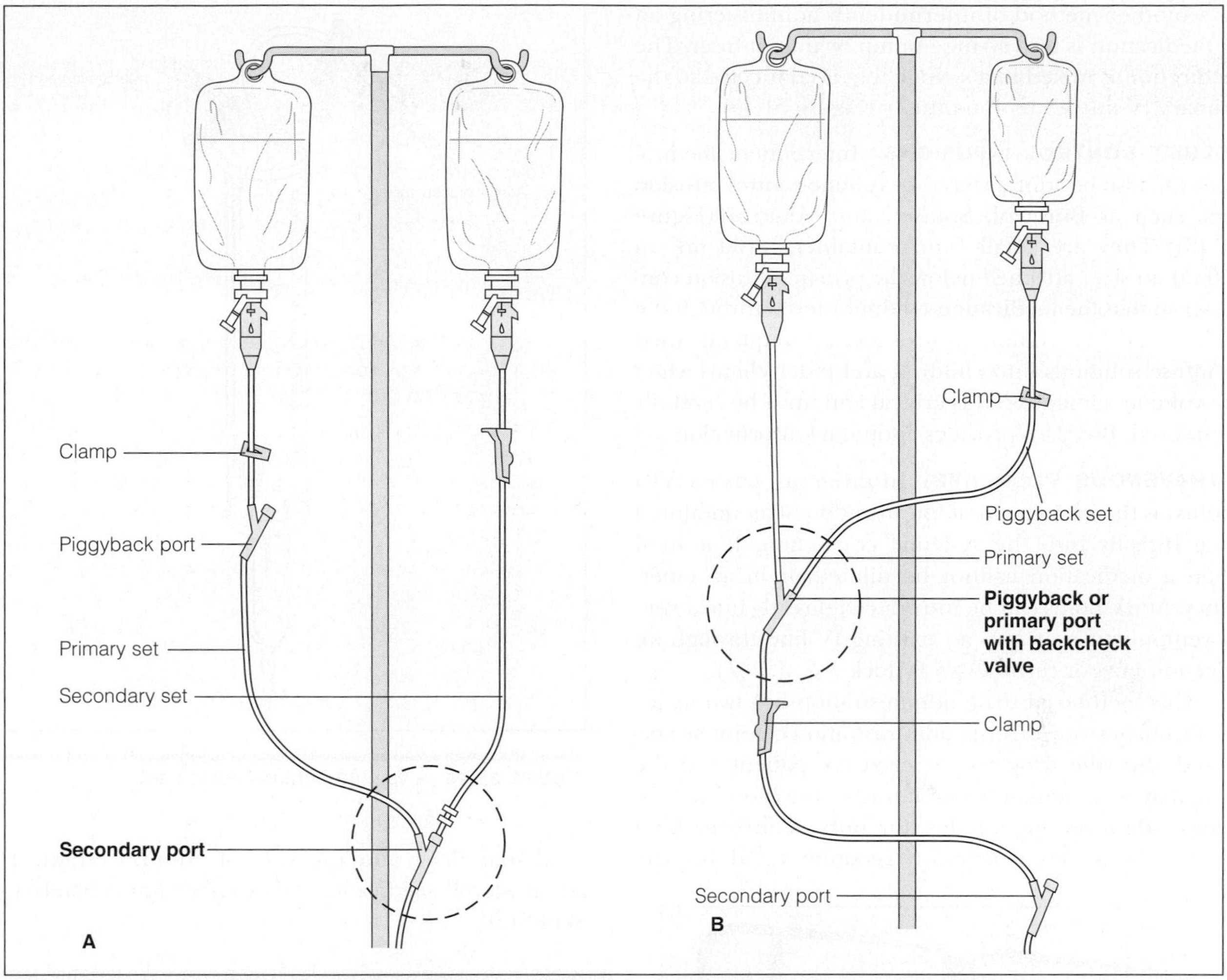

FIGURE 31.43 Secondary intravenous lines: A: a tandem intravenous alignment; B: an intravenous piggyback (IVPB) alignment

set has been attached to ports of the primary infusion by inserting a needle through the port and taping it in place. Needleless systems are now available. The needleless systems can use threaded-lock or lever-lock cannulae to connect the secondary set to the ports of the primary infusion (Figure 31.44). This system prevents needlestick injuries as well as touch contamination at the IV connection site.

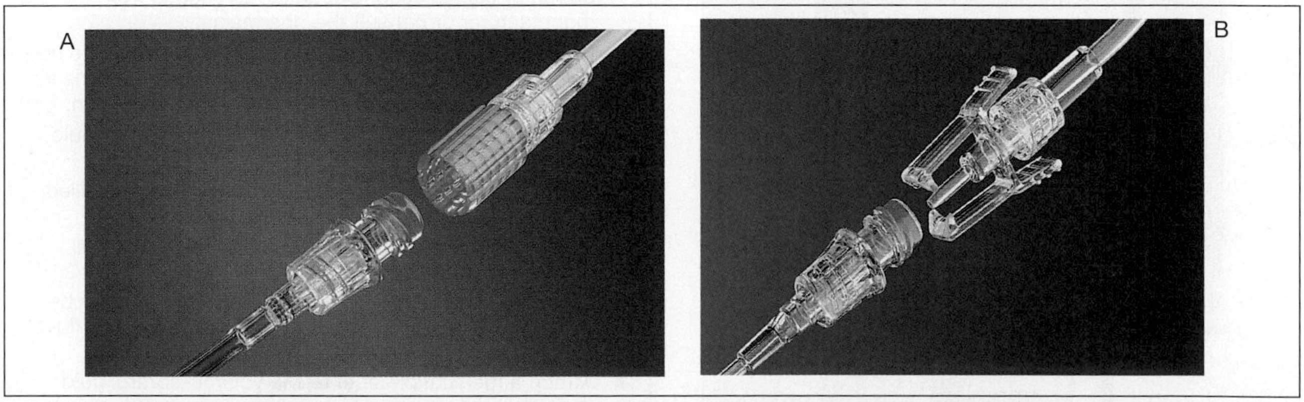

FIGURE 31.44 Needleless cannulae used to connect the tubing of secondary sets to primary infusions: A: threaded-lock cannula; B: lever-lock cannula

Another method of intermittently administering an IV medication is by a syringe pump or mini-infuser. The medication is mixed in a syringe that is connected to the primary IV line via a mini-infuser (Figure 31.45).

VOLUME-CONTROL INFUSIONS Intermittent medications can also be administered by **volume-control infusion sets**, such as Buretrol, Soluset, and Volutrol (Figure 31.46). They are small fluid containers (100 mL to 150 mL in size) attached below the primary infusion container so that the medication is administered through the patient's IV line. Volume-control sets are frequently used to infuse solutions into children and older clients when the volume administered is critical and must be carefully monitored. Box 31.8 provides additional information.

INTRAVENOUS PUSH (IVP) Intravenous push (IVP) (bolus) is the intravenous administration of an undiluted drug directly into the systemic circulation. It is used when a medication cannot be diluted or in an emergency. An IV bolus can be introduced directly into a vein by venipuncture or into an existing IV line through an injection port or through an IV lock.

This method of drug administration has two major disadvantages: any error in administration cannot be corrected after the drug has entered the patient and the drug may be irritating to the lining of the blood vessels. Before administering a bolus, the nurse should look up the maximum concentration recommended for the particular drug and the rate of administration. The administered medication takes effect immediately (see Skill 31.9).

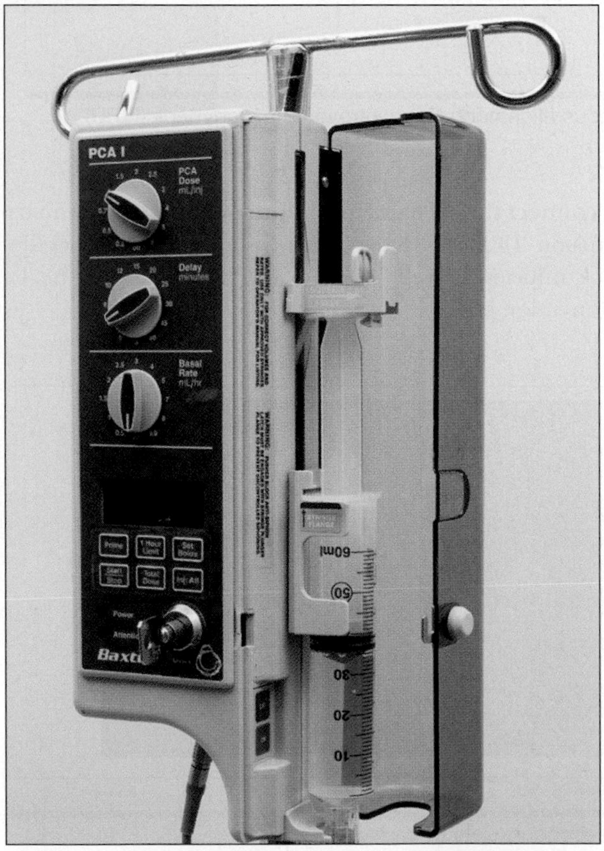

FIGURE 31.45 Syringe pump or mini-infuser for administration of IV medications

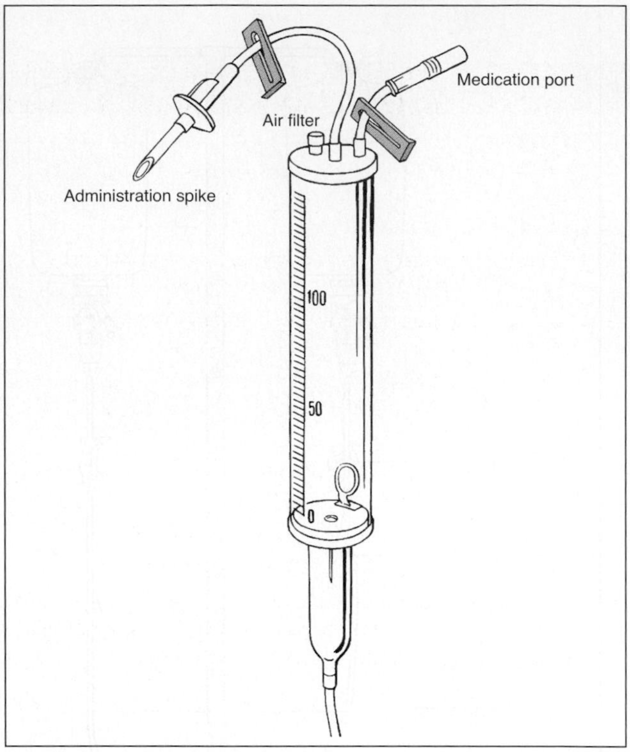

FIGURE 31.46 A volume-control infusion set

BOX 31.8 ADDING A MEDICATION TO A VOLUME-CONTROL INFUSION

The following steps are necessary when adding a medication to a volume-control infusion:

- Withdraw the required dose of the medication into a syringe.
- Ensure that there is sufficient fluid in the volume-control fluid chamber to dilute the medication. Generally, at least 50 mL of fluid is used. Check the directions from the drug manufacturer or consult the pharmacist.
- Close the inflow to the fluid chamber by adjusting the upper roller or slide clamp above the fluid chamber; also ensure that the clamp on the air vent of the chamber is open.
- Clean the medication port on the volume-control fluid chamber with an antiseptic swab.
- Inject the medication into the port of the partially filled volume-control set.
- Gently rotate the fluid chamber until the fluid is well mixed.
- Open the line's upper clamp, and regulate the flow by adjusting the lower roller or slide clamp below the fluid chamber.
- Attach a medication label to the volume-control fluid chamber.
- Document relevant data, and monitor the patient and the infusion.

SKILL 31.9

ADMINISTERING INTRAVENOUS MEDICATIONS USING IV PUSH

PURPOSE

To achieve immediate and maximum effects of a medication

ASSESSMENT

- Inspect and palpate the IV insertion site for signs of infection, infiltration, or a dislocated catheter.
- Inspect the surrounding skin for redness, pallor, or swelling.
- Palpate the surrounding tissues for coldness and the presence of edema, which could indicate leakage of the IV fluid into the tissues.
- Take vital signs for baseline data if the medication being administered is particularly potent.
- Determine if the patient has allergies to the medication.
- Check the compatibility of the medication and IV fluid.
- Determine specific drug action, side effects, normal dosage, recommended administration time, and peak action time.
- Check patency of IV.

Equipment

IV Push for an Existing Line

- Medication in a vial or an ampule
- Sterile syringe (3 mL to 5 mL) to prepare the medication
- Sterile needles 21 gauge to 25 gauge, 2.5 cm (unnecessary if using a needleless system)
- Antiseptic swabs
- Watch with a digital readout or second hand
- Clean gloves

IV Push for an IV Lock

- Medication in a vial or an ampule
- Sterile syringe (3 mL to 5 mL) to prepare the medication
- Sterile syringe (3 mL) for the saline or heparin flush
- Vial of normal saline to flush the IV catheter or vial of heparin flush solution or both, depending on agency practice. This maintains the patency of the heparin or saline lock. Saline is frequently used for peripheral locks.
- Sterile needles (21 gauge) (unnecessary if using a needleless system)
- Antiseptic swabs
- Watch with a digital readout or second hand
- Disposable gloves

IMPLEMENTATION

Preparation

1. Check the MAR.
   - Check the label on the medication carefully against the MAR to make sure that the correct medication is being prepared.
   - Follow the three checks for correct medication and dose. Read the label on the medication (1) when it is taken from the medication cart, (2) before withdrawing the medication, and (3) after withdrawing the medication.
   - Calculate medication dosage accurately.
   - Confirm that the route is correct.
2. Organize the equipment.

Performance

1. Perform hand hygiene and observe other appropriate infection prevention and control procedures.
2. Prepare the medication.

Existing Line

- Prepare the medication according to the manufacturer's direction.

IV Lock

a. Flushing with saline
   - Prepare two syringes, each with 1 mL of sterile normal saline.

b. Flushing with heparin (if indicated by agency policy) and saline
   - Prepare one syringe with 1 mL of heparin flush solution (if indicated by agency policy).
   - Prepare two syringes with 1 mL each of sterile normal saline.
   - Draw up the medication into a syringe.

3. Put a small-gauge needle on the syringe if using a needle system.
4. Perform hand hygiene and put on clean gloves. **Rationale: This reduces the transmission of microorganisms and reduces the likelihood of the nurse's hands contacting the client's blood**.
5. Provide for client privacy.
6. Prepare the client.
   - Before performing the procedure, introduce yourself and verify the client's identity by using agency protocol.
   - If not previously assessed, take the appropriate assessment measures necessary for the medication. If any of the findings are above or below the predetermined parameters, consult the appropriate member of the health-care team before administering the medication.
7. Explain the purpose of the medication and how it will help, using language that the client can understand. Include relevant information about the effects of the medication.
8. Administer the medication by IV push. Bunce (2003) reported that the use of the "push-stop-push-stop" technique is helpful, especially for central venous

(continued)

SKILL 31.9

ADMINISTERING INTRAVENOUS MEDICATIONS USING IV PUSH (*continued*)

catheters. **Rationale: This creates turbulence in the flow through the catheter, which reduces the residue buildup in the line and the potential for occlusion.**

IV Lock with Needle

- Clean the diaphragm of the IV lock with the antiseptic swab. **Rationale: This prevents microorganisms from entering the circulatory system during the needle insertion.**
- Insert the needle of the syringe containing normal saline through the centre of the diaphragm (see ❶) and aspirate for blood. **Rationale: The presence of blood confirms that the catheter or needle is in the vein. In some situations, blood will not return even though the lock is patent.**

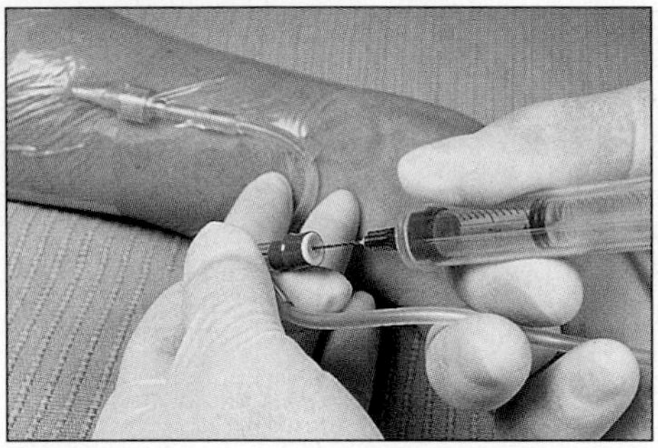

❶ Inserting a needle through the diaphragm of an IV lock

- Flush the lock by injecting 1 mL of saline slowly. **Rationale: This removes blood and heparin (if present) from the needle and the lock.**
- Remove the needle and syringe. Activate the needle safety device.
- Clean the lock's diaphragm with an antiseptic swab. **Rationale: This prevents the transfer of microorganisms.**
- Insert the needle of the syringe containing the prepared medication through the centre of the diaphragm.
- Inject the medication slowly at the recommended rate of infusion. Use a watch or digital readout to time the injection. Observe the client closely for adverse reactions. Remove the needle and syringe when all medication is administered. **Rationale: Injecting the drug too rapidly can have a serious untoward reaction.**
- Activate the needle safety device.
- Clean the diaphragm of the lock.
- Attach the second saline syringe, and inject 1 mL of saline. **Rationale: The saline injection flushes the medication through the catheter and prepares the lock for heparin if this medication is used. Heparin is incompatible with many medications.**
- If heparin is to be used, insert the heparin syringe and inject the heparin slowly into the lock.

IV Lock with Needleless System

- Remove the protective cap from the needleless port.
- Insert syringe containing normal saline into the lock.
- Flush the lock with 1 mL sterile saline. **Rationale: This clears the lock of blood.**
- Remove the syringe.
- Insert the syringe containing the medication into the valve (see ❷).
- Inject the medication, following the precautions described previously.
- Withdraw the syringe.
- Repeat injection of 1 mL of saline.
- Place a new sterile cap over the lock.

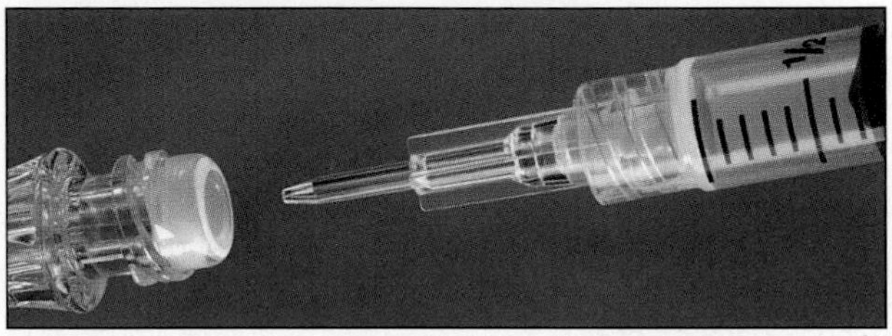

❷ A blunt plastic cannula replaces the sharp steel needle

Existing Line

- Identify the injection port closest to the client. Some ports have a circle indicating the site for the needle insertion. **Rationale: An injection port must be used because it is self-sealing. Any puncture to the plastic tubing will leak.**
- Clean the port with an antiseptic swab.
- Stop the IV flow by closing the clamp or pinching the tubing above the injection port.
- Connect the syringe to the IV system.

  a. Needle system
  - Hold the port steady.
  - Insert the needle of the syringe that contains the medication through the centre of the port (see ❸). **Rationale: This prevents damage to the IV line and to the diaphragm of the port.**

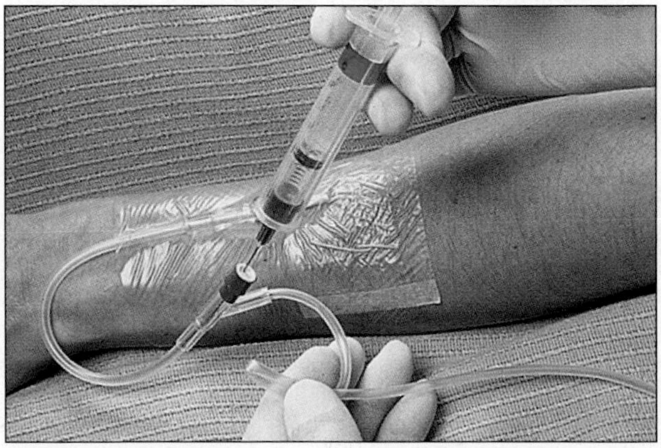

❸ Injecting a medication by IV push to an existing IV by using a needle system

(continued)

SKILL 31.9

ADMINISTERING INTRAVENOUS MEDICATIONS USING IV PUSH (*continued*)

b. Needleless system
   - Remove the cap from the needleless injection port. Connect the tip of the syringe directly to the port (see ❹).

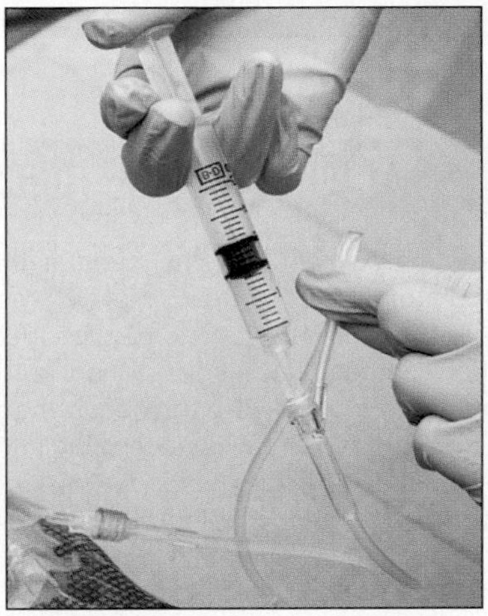

❹ Injecting a medication by IV push to an existing IV by using a needleless system

   - Inject the medication at the ordered rate. Use the watch or digital readout to time the medication administration. **Rationale: This ensures safe drug administration because a too rapid injection could be dangerous.**
   - Release the clamp or tubing.
   - After injecting the medication, withdraw the needle and activate the needle safety device. For a needleless system, detach the syringe and attach a new sterile cap to the port.

9. Dispose of equipment according to agency practice. **Rationale: This reduces needle-stick injuries and the spread of microorganisms.**
10. Remove and dispose of gloves. Perform hand hygiene.
11. Observe the client closely for adverse reactions.
12. Determine agency practice about recommended times for changing the IV lock. Some agencies advocate a change every 48 to 72 hours for peripheral IV devices.
13. Document all relevant information.
    - Record the date, time, drug, dose, and route; client response; and assessments of infusion or heparin lock site, if appropriate.

EVALUATION

- Conduct appropriate follow-up, such as desired effect of medication, any adverse reactions or side effects, or change in vital signs.
- Reassess the status of IV lock site and patency of the IV infusion, if running.
- Relate to previous findings, if available.
- Report significant deviations from normal to the appropriate members of the health-care team.

Home Care Considerations

Administering IV Antibiotics

Shortened hospital stays and the need to cut costs have led to clients or their caregivers being taught to administer IV antibiotics at home by intravenous push, by continuous ambulatory drug delivery (CADD) pump mechanisms, or by positive pressure elastomeric technologies (e.g., Intermate infusion pump). These clients generally have an indwelling peripheral venous catheter or a central venous access device, such as a peripherally inserted central catheter (see Chapter 43). The venous access device must be flushed before and after administration to maintain patency, to ensure that no drug-drug interaction occurs within the tubing, and to administer the complete prescribed dosage.

The nurse must:

- Know the adverse side effects of the medication and the delivery system:
  - Allergic reaction
  - Phlebitis (pain and tenderness over the vein, erythema, swelling, and warmth)
  - Speed shock (systemic reaction when a drug is given too rapidly)
  - Venous spasm (cramping and pain above infusion site)
  - Infiltration
  - Line blockage
- Assess the caregiver or client's eyesight, manual dexterity, general ability to use the technology, and ability to monitor the response to the medication delivery. All are needed for safe administration of the antibiotic.

(*continued*)

Home Care Considerations (*continued*)

- Provide thorough teaching about the following:
  - Venous access device
  - Administration rate (minutes/dose)
  - Functioning of the technology (when applicable)
- Schedule for medication administration
- Flushing technique
- Adverse reactions
- Signs that indicate an emergency and the need to call 911
- Proper storage of medication an care of equipment
- Inspect the appearance of the medication and check the expiration date.

INTERMITTENT INFUSION DEVICES *Intermittent infusion devices* (see Figure 31.47) can be attached to an intravenous catheter or needle to allow medications to be administered intravenously without requiring repeated needle sticks or a continuous intravenous infusion. Intermittent injection ports have either a resealable latex injection site for needle access or a port that allows a syringe or a needleless adapter to be connected for administering medications. Needleless systems are preferred; they significantly reduce the risk of needle-stick injuries among health-care professionals. Skill 43.5 (page 1419) describes how to convert an intravenous infusion to an intermittent injection port. With the needleless system, the injection adapter can be attached at the time of intravenous catheter placement, allowing a closed system to be maintained.

Intermittent injection ports may be flushed with sterile saline before and after medication administration. Most agencies use saline flushes with medication administration through peripheral IV lines. When administering a medication through a central venous access device (CVAD), some agencies use the mnemonic SASH (saline, administer drug, saline, heparin) for the flushing procedure (Bunce, 2003). Flushing the port maintains patency of the intravenous catheter and port, and reduces the risks of mixing incompatible medications within the system (see Skill 31.9).

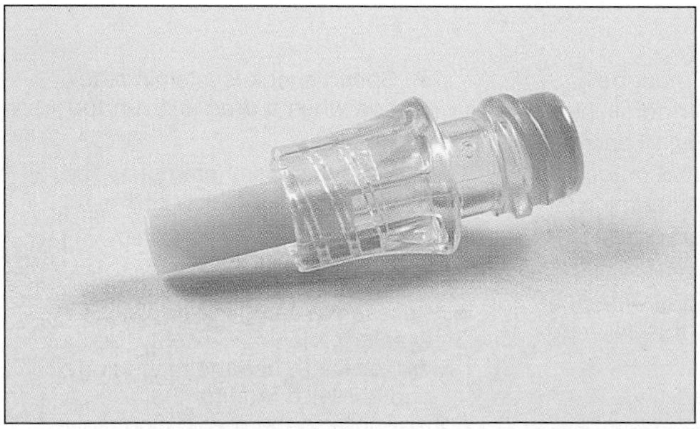

FIGURE 31.47 Intermittent infusion device with injection port

REFLECT ON PRIMARY HEALTH CARE

New medication delivery systems, such as the continuous ambulatory drug delivery (CADD) pump and Intermate positive pressure system, allow people who would otherwise require hospitalization to remain in their homes as they receive intravenous therapy. Find out if this form of *technology* is accessible in your institution or community. If it is, find out how accessible care is for the home care client who has problems with his or her medication delivery system.

Clients who require long-term venous access for administering medications (e.g., people receiving chemotherapy for cancer treatment) may have a specialized catheter or port to allow central venous access (see the Reflect on Primary Health Care box). The catheter may be tunnelled subcutaneously and accessed through an intermittent injection port attached to the distal end of the venous catheter. Other devices have an *implantable port* or *vascular access port* surgically inserted under the skin so that no portion of the device exits the body. To administer medications, the port is accessed by using a specialized needle through the skin. See Chapter 43 for more information about central venous lines.

Topical Medications

A topical medication is applied locally to the skin or to mucous membranes in such areas as the eye, external ear canal, nose, vagina, and rectum. Most topical applications used therapeutically are not absorbed well, completely, or predictably when applied to intact skin because the skin's thick outer layer serves as a natural barrier to drug diffusion. This route of absorption through the skin, called **percutaneous**, can be increased if the skin is altered by a laceration, burn, or some other problem. However, if high concentrations or large amounts of a topical medication are applied to the skin, especially if it is done repeatedly, sufficient amounts of the drug can enter the bloodstream to cause systemic effects, usually undesirable ones.

Skin Applications

Topical skin or *dermatological* preparations include ointments, pastes, creams, lotions, powders, sprays, and patches. See Table 31.1 earlier in this chapter (page 797). See Practice Guidelines 31.2. Before applying a dermatological preparation, thoroughly clean the area with soap and water and dry the area by using a patting motion. Skin encrustations harbour microorganisms and these as well as previously applied applications can prevent the medication from coming in contact with the area to be treated. Nurses should wear gloves when administering skin applications and always use surgical asepsis when an open wound is present.

One type of topical or dermatological medication delivery system is the **transdermal patch**. This system administers sustained-action medications (e.g., nitroglycerine, estrogen, and nicotine) via multilayered films containing the drug and an adhesive layer. The rate of delivery of the drug is controlled and varies with each product (e.g., from 12 hours to 1 week). Generally, the patch is applied to a hairless, clean area of skin that is not subject to excessive movement or wrinkling (e.g., the trunk or lower abdomen). It may also be applied on the side, lower back, or buttocks. Patches should not be applied to areas with cuts, burns, or abrasions, or on distal parts of extremities (e.g., the forearms). If hair is likely to interfere with patch adhesion or removal, clipping (not shaving) may be necessary before application (Figure 31.48).

Reddening of the skin with or without mild local itching or burning, as well as allergic contact dermatitis, can occasionally occur. On removal of the patch, any slight reddening of the skin usually disappears within a few hours. All applications should be changed regularly to prevent local irritation, and each successive application should be placed on a different site. All clients need to be assessed for allergies to the drug and to materials in the patch before the patch is applied. If a patient has a transdermal patch on and develops a fever, the medication may be absorbed and metabolize at a faster rate than normal. The patient will need to be monitored for changes in effects of the medication.

When transdermal patches are removed, care needs to be taken as to how and where they are discarded. In the home environment, if they are simply discarded into a trash can, pets or children can be exposed to them, causing effects from any drug remaining on the patch. When removed, they should be folded with the medication side to the inside, put into a closed container, and kept out of reach of children and pets. The container can be brought to a pharmacy that participates in a disposal program or to a municipal waste site for proper disposal.

CLINICAL ALERT

Gloves should be worn by the nurse when applying a transdermal patch to avoid getting any medication on the hands, which can result in the nurse receiving the effect of the medication.

CLINICAL ALERT

It is important to keep track of the transdermal patches. Some patches are clear and may be difficult to see and, as a result, be overlooked. If the patient is obese, patches may be difficult to find in the skin folds. Duplication of patches may cause adverse reactions. Remove the old patch before applying a new one.

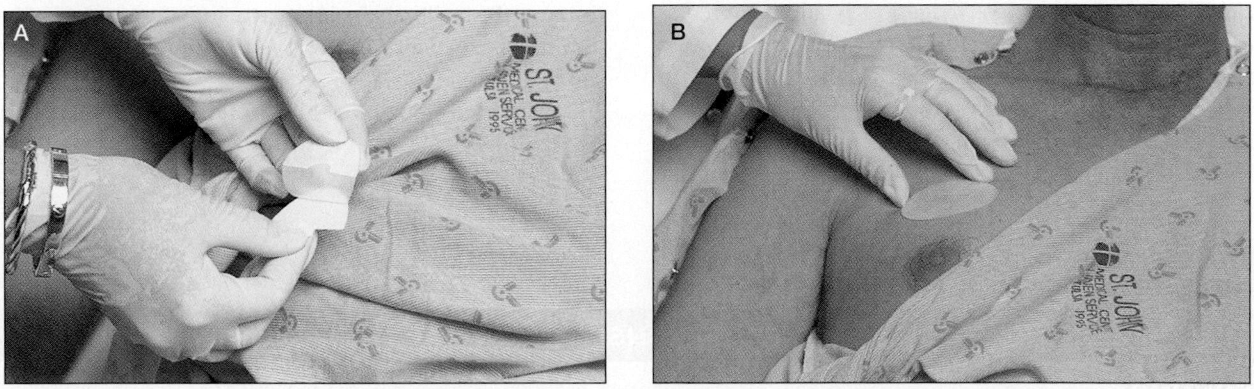

FIGURE 31.48 Transdermal patch administration: A: protective coating removed from patch; B: patch immediately applied to clean, dry, hairless skin and labelled with date, time, and initials

(From Pharmacology for Nurses: A Pathophysiologic Approach *(p. 38), by Michael Patrick Adams, Dianne L. Josephson, and Leland Norman Holland Jr., 2005, Upper Saddle River, NJ: Pearson Education.)*

PRACTICE GUIDELINES 31.2

Applying Skin Preparations

Guidelines	Rationales
Powder	
Make sure the skin surface is dry. Spread apart any skin folds, and sprinkle the site until the area is covered with a fine thin layer. Cover the site with a dressing, if ordered.	Applying powder to a damp or moist area gives rise to clumping; powder can be easily brushed off if not protected.
Suspension-Based Lotion	
Shake the container before use. Put a little lotion on a small gauze dressing or pad, and apply the lotion to the skin by stroking it evenly in the direction of the hair growth.	Shaking distributes suspended particles; using a gauze or pad will avoid hand absorption.
Creams, Ointments, Pastes, and Oil-Based Lotions	
Warm and soften the preparation in the gloved hands. Smear it evenly over the skin by using long strokes that follow the direction of the hair growth. Explain that the skin may feel somewhat greasy after application. Apply a sterile dressing if ordered by the health-care provider.	Warming the preparation makes it easier to apply and to prevent chilling (if a large area is to be treated).
Aerosol Spray	
Shake the container well to mix the contents. Hold the spray container at the recommended distance from the area (usually about 15 cm to 30 cm, but check the label). Cover the patient's face with a towel if the upper chest or neck is to be sprayed. Have patient wear goggles if indicated. Spray the medication over the specified area.	The patient must not inhale the aerosol.
Transdermal Patches	
Ensure that all previous patches have been removed. Select a clean, dry area that is free of hair and matches the manufacturer's recommendations. Remove the patch from its protective covering, holding it without touching the adhesive edges, and apply it by pressing firmly with the palm of the hand for about 10 seconds. Advise the patient to avoid using a heating pad over the area.	The presence of multiple patches leads to increased dosage of medication than that prescribed. The hand provides heat that can cause an increase in circulation and the rate of absorption. Remove the patch at the appropriate time, folding it so that the medicated side is covered.

Ophthalmic Instillations

Medications can be administered to the eyes by using irrigations or instillations. Eye irrigation is administered to wash out the conjunctival sac to remove secretions or foreign bodies or to remove chemicals that can injure the eye. Medications for the eyes, called **ophthalmic** medications, are instilled in the form of liquids or ointments. Eye drops are packaged in monodrip plastic containers that are used to administer the preparation. Ointments are usually supplied in small tubes. All containers must state that the medication is for ophthalmic use. Sterile preparations and sterile technique are indicated. Prescribed liquids are usually dilute, for example, less than 1% strength.

Skill 31.10 illustrates how to administer ophthalmic instillations.

SKILL 31.10

ADMINISTERING OPHTHALMIC INSTILLATIONS

PURPOSE

To provide an eye medication the patient requires (e.g., an antibiotic) to treat an infection or for other reasons (see specific drug action)

ASSESSMENT

In addition to the assessment performed by the nurse related to the administration of any medication, before applying ophthalmic medications, assess:

- The appearance of eye and surrounding structures for lesions, exudate, erythema, or swelling

(continued)

SKILL 31.10

ADMINISTERING OPHTHALMIC INSTILLATIONS (*continued*)

- The location and nature of any discharge, lacrimation, and swelling of the eyelids or of the lacrimal gland
- Patient complaints (e.g., itching, burning pain, blurred vision, and photophobia)
- Patient behaviour (e.g., squinting, blinking excessively, frowning, or rubbing the eyes)

Determine whether assessment data influence administration of the medication (i.e., is it appropriate to administer the medication or does the medication need to be held and the appropriate member of the health-care team notified?).

Equipment

- Clean gloves
- Sterile absorbent sponges soaked in sterile normal saline
- Medication
- Dry sterile absorbent sponges
- Sterile eye dressing (pad) as needed and paper eye tape to secure it

For an irrigation add the following:

- Irrigating solution (e.g., normal saline) and irrigating syringe or tubing
- Dry sterile absorbent sponges
- Moisture-resistant towel
- Basin (e.g., emesis basin)

IMPLEMENTATION

Preparation

1. Check the MAR.
   - Check the MAR for the drug name, dose, and strength. Also confirm the prescribed frequency of the instillation and which eye is to be treated.
   - If the MAR is unclear or pertinent information is missing, compare it with the most recent written order.
   - Report any discrepancies to the appropriate member of the health-care team, as agency policy dictates.
2. Know the reason that the patient is receiving the medication, drug classification, contraindications, usual dose range, side effects, and nursing considerations for administering and evaluating the intended outcomes of the medication.

Performance

1. Compare the label on the medication tube or bottle with the medication record and check the expiration date.
2. If necessary, calculate the medication dosage.
3. Introduce yourself and explain to the patient what you are going to do, why it is necessary, and how he or she can cooperate. The administration of an ophthalmic medication is not usually painful. Ointments are often soothing to the eye, but some liquid preparations may sting initially. Discuss how the results will be used in planning further care or treatments.
4. Perform hand hygiene and observe other appropriate infection prevention and control procedures.
5. Provide for patient privacy.
6. Prepare the patient.
   - Before performing the procedure, verify the patient's identity using agency protocol.
   - Assist the patient to a comfortable position, either sitting or lying.
7. Clean the eyelid and the eyelashes.
   - Put on clean gloves.
   - Use sterile cotton balls moistened with sterile irrigating solution or sterile normal saline, and wipe from the inner canthus to the outer canthus. **Rationale: If not removed, material on the eyelid and lashes can be washed into the eye. Cleaning toward the outer canthus prevents contamination of the other eye and the lacrimal duct.**
8. Administer the eye medication.
   - Check the ophthalmic preparation for the name, strength, and number of drops if a liquid is used. **Rationale: Checking medication data is essential to prevent a medication error**.
   - Draw the correct number of drops into the shaft of the dropper if a dropper is used. If ointment is used, discard the first bead. **Rationale: The first bead of ointment from a tube is considered to be contaminated**.
   - Instruct the patient to look up to the ceiling. Give the patient a dry sterile absorbent sponge. **Rationale: The person is less likely to blink if looking up. While the patient looks up, the cornea is partially protected by the upper eyelid. A sponge is needed to press on the nasolacrimal duct after a liquid instillation to prevent systemic absorption or to wipe excess ointment from the eyelashes after an ointment is instilled**.
   - Expose the lower conjunctival sac by placing the thumb or fingers of your nondominant hand on the patient's cheekbone just below the eye and gently drawing down the skin on the cheek. If the tissues are edematous, handle the tissues carefully to avoid damaging them. **Rationale: Placing the fingers on the cheekbone minimizes the possibility of touching the cornea, avoids putting any pressure on the eyeball, and prevents the person from blinking or squinting**.
   - Holding the medication in the dominant hand, place hand on patient's forehead to stabilize head. Approach the eye from the side and instill the correct number of drops onto the outer third of the lower conjunctival sac. Hold the dropper 1 cm to 2 cm

(*continued*)

SKILL 31.10

ADMINISTERING OPHTHALMIC INSTILLATIONS (*continued*)

above the sac (see ❶). **Rationale: The patient is less likely to blink if a side approach is used. When instilled into the conjunctival sac, drops will not harm the cornea as they might if dropped directly on it. The dropper must not touch the sac or the cornea.**

- *Or* holding the tube above the lower conjunctival sac, squeeze 2 cm of ointment from the tube into the lower conjunctival sac from the inner canthus outward (see ❷).
- Instruct the patient to close the eyelids but not to squeeze them shut. **Rationale: Closing the eye spreads the medication over the eyeball. Squeezing can injure the eye and push out the medication.**
- For liquid medications, press firmly or have the patient press firmly on the nasolacrimal duct for at least 30 seconds (see ❸). **Rationale: Pressing on the nasolacrimal duct prevents the medication from running out of the eye and down the duct, preventing systemic absorption.**

Variation: Irrigation

- Place absorbent pads under the head, neck, and shoulders. Place an emesis basin next to the eye to catch drainage. Some eye medications cause systemic reactions, such as confusion or a decrease in heart rate and blood pressure, if the eye drops go down the nasolacrimal duct and get into the systemic circulation.
- Expose the lower conjunctival sac. Or, to irrigate in stages, first hold the lower lid down, then hold the upper lid up. Exert pressure on the bony prominences of the cheekbone and beneath the eyebrow when holding the eyelids. **Rationale: Separating the lids prevents reflex blinking. Exerting pressure on the bony prominences minimizes the possibility of pressing the eyeball and causing discomfort.**
- Fill and hold the eye irrigator about 2.5 cm above the eye. **Rationale: At this height the pressure of the solution will not damage the eye tissue, and the irrigator will not touch the eye.**
- Irrigate the eye, directing the solution onto the lower conjunctival sac and from the inner canthus to the outer canthus. **Rationale: Directing the solution in this way prevents possible injury to the cornea and prevents fluid and contaminants from flowing down the nasolacrimal duct.**
- Irrigate until the solution leaving the eye is clear (no discharge is present) or until all the solution has been used.
- Instruct the patient to close and move the eye periodically. **Rationale: Eye closure and movement help to move secretions from the upper to the lower conjunctival sac.**

9. Clean and dry the eyelids as needed. Wipe the eyelids gently from the inner to the outer canthus to collect excess medication.

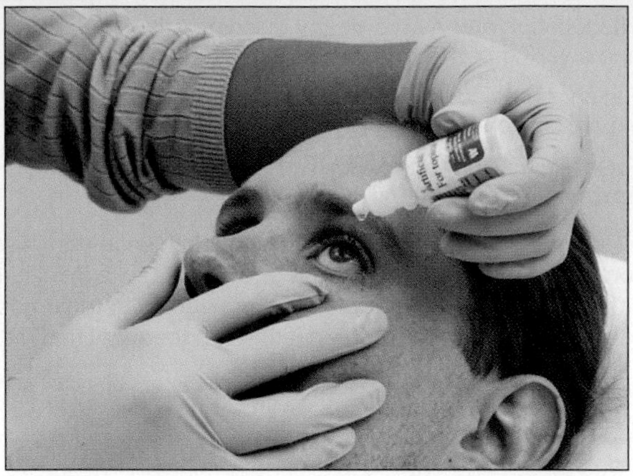

❶ Instilling an eye drop into the lower conjunctival sac

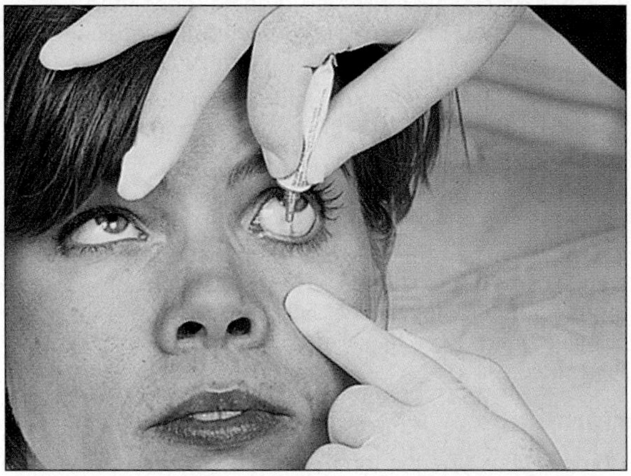

❷ Ilnstilling an eye ointment into the lower conjunctival sac

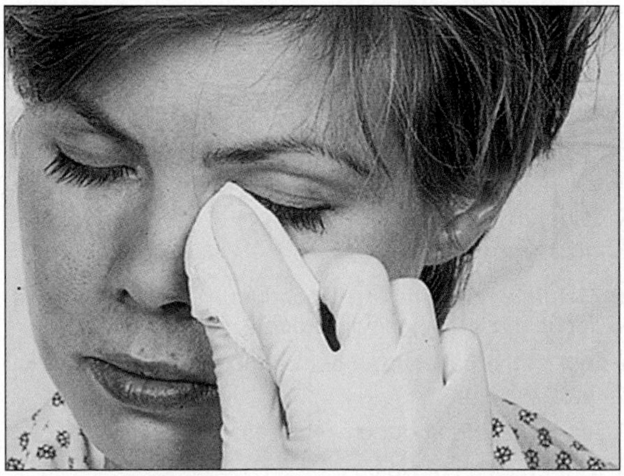

❸ Pressing on the nasolacrimal duct

(continued)

SKILL 31.10

ADMINISTERING OPHTHALMIC INSTILLATIONS (*continued*)

10. Apply an eye pad if needed, and secure it with paper eye tape. '
11. Assess the patient's response immediately after the instillation or irrigation and again after the medication should have acted.
12. Document all relevant assessments and interventions. Include the name of the drug or irrigating solution, the strength, the number of drops if a liquid medication, the time, and the response of the patient.

EVALUATION

- Perform follow-up based on findings of the effectiveness of the administration or outcomes that deviated from expected or normal for the patient. Relate findings to previous data, if available.
- Report significant deviations from normal to the appropriate members of the health-care team.

Lifespan Considerations

Administering Ophthalmic Medications

INFANTS AND CHILDREN

- Explain the technique to the parents of an infant or a child.
- For a young child or an infant, obtain assistance to immobilize the arms and head. The parent may hold the infant or young child. *This prevents accidental injury during medication administration.*
- For a young child, use a doll to demonstrate the procedure. *This facilitates cooperation and decreases anxiety.*
- Drops may be tolerated better by children than ointment since drops are less likely to cause blurred vision.
- An intravenous (IV) bag and tubing may be used to deliver irrigating fluid to the eye (Figure 31.49).

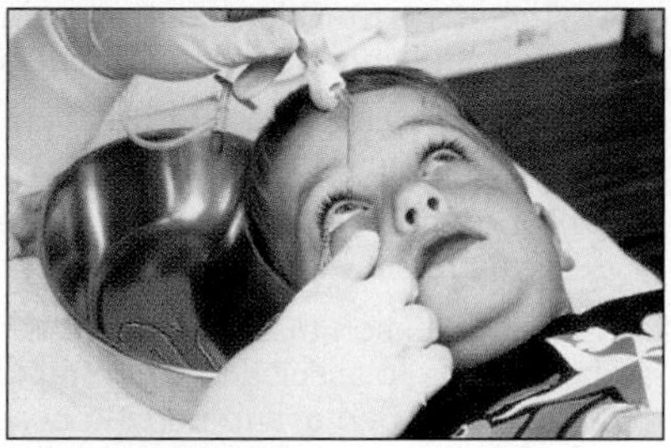

FIGURE 31.49 Eye irrigation by using IV tubing

Otic Instillations

Instillations or irrigations of the external auditory canal are referred to as **otic** and are generally carried out for cleaning purposes. Sometimes applications of heat and antiseptic solutions are prescribed. Irrigations performed in a hospital require aseptic technique so that microorganisms are not introduced into the ear. Sterile technique is used if the eardrum is perforated. The position of the external auditory canal varies with age. In the child younger than 3 years of age, it is directed upward. In the adult, the external auditory canal is an S-shaped structure about 2.5 cm long. Skill 31.11 explains the technique used to administer otic instillations.

SKILL 31.11

ADMINISTERING OTIC INSTILLATIONS

PURPOSE

- To soften earwax so that it can be readily removed at a later time
- To provide local therapy to reduce inflammation, destroy infective organisms in the external ear canal, or both
- To relieve pain

ASSESSMENT

In addition to the assessment performed by the nurse related to the administration of any medications, before applying otic medications, assess:

- The appearance of the pinna of the ear and meatus for signs of redness and abrasions
- The type and amount of any discharge

(continued)

SKILL 31.11

ADMINISTERING OTIC INSTILLATIONS (*continued*)

Determine whether assessment data influence administration of the medication (i.e., is it appropriate to administer the medication or does the medication need to be held and the appropriate member of the health-care team notified?).

Equipment

- Clean gloves
- Cotton-tipped applicator
- Correct medication bottle with a dropper
- Flexible rubber tip (optional) for the end of the dropper, which prevents injury from sudden motion, for example, by a child or disoriented patient
- Cotton fluff

For irrigation, add

- Moisture-resistant towel
- Basin (e.g., emesis basin)
- Irrigating solution at the appropriate temperature, about 500 mL (16 oz) or as ordered
- Container for the irrigating solution
- Syringe (rubber bulb or Asepto syringe is frequently used)

IMPLEMENTATION

Preparation

1. Check the MAR.
   - Check the MAR for the drug name, strength, number of drops, and prescribed frequency.
   - If the MAR is unclear or pertinent information is missing, compare it with the most recent written order.
   - Report any discrepancies to the appropriate member of the health-care team, as agency policy dictates.
2. Know the reason that the patient is receiving the medication, drug classification, contraindications, usual dose range, side effects, and nursing considerations for administering and evaluating the intended outcomes of the medication.

Performance

1. Compare the label on the medication container with the medication record and check the expiration date.
2. If necessary, calculate the medication dosage.
3. Explain to the patient what you are going to do, why it is necessary, and how he or she can cooperate. The administration of an otic medication is not usually painful. Discuss how the results will be used in planning further care or treatments.
4. Perform hand hygiene and observe other appropriate infection prevention and control procedures.
5. Provide for patient privacy.
6. Prepare the patient.
   - Before performing the procedure, introduce yourself and verify the patient's identity by using agency protocol.
   - Assist the patient to a comfortable position for eardrops, lying with the ear being treated uppermost.
7. Clean the pinna of the ear and the meatus of the ear canal.
   - Put on gloves if infection is suspected.
   - Use cotton-tipped applicators and solution to wipe the pinna and auditory meatus. **Rationale: This removes any discharge present before the instillation so that it won't be washed into the ear canal.**
8. Administer the ear medication.
   - Warm the medication container in your hand, or place it in warm water for a short time. **Rationale: This promotes client comfort.**
   - Partially fill the ear dropper with medication.
   - Straighten the ear canal by pulling pinna upward and backward for clients older than 3 years of age (see ❶). **Rationale: The auditory canal is straightened so that the solution can flow the entire length of the canal.**
   - Instill the correct number of drops along the side of the ear canal (see ❷).

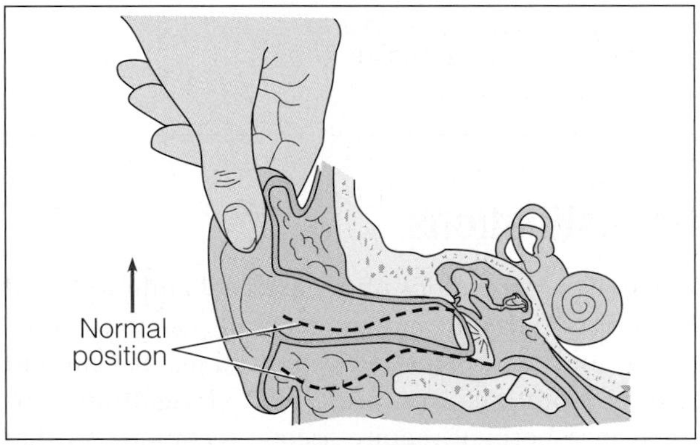

❶ Straightening the adult ear canal by pulling pinna upward and backward

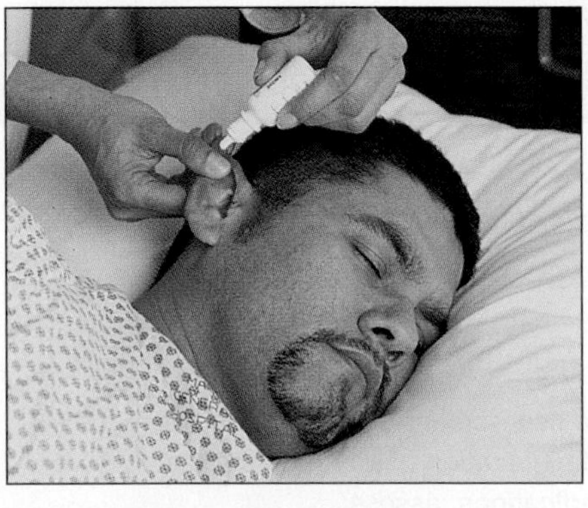

❷ Instilling ear drops

(continued)

SKILL 31.11

ADMINISTERING OTIC INSTILLATIONS *(continued)*

- Press gently but firmly a few times on the tragus of the ear (the cartilaginous projection in front of the exterior meatus of the ear). **Rationale: Pressing on the tragus assists the flow of medication into the ear canal.**
- Ask the patient to remain in the side-lying position for about 5 minutes. **Rationale: This prevents the drops from escaping and allows the medication to reach all sides of the canal cavity.**
- Insert a small piece of cotton fluff loosely at the meatus of the auditory canal for 15 to 20 minutes. Do not press it into the canal. **Rationale: The cotton helps retain the medication when the client is up. If pressed tightly into the canal, the cotton would interfere with the action of the drug and the outward movement of normal secretions.**

Variation: Ear Irrigation

- Explain that the patient may experience a feeling of fullness, warmth, and, occasionally, discomfort when the fluid comes in contact with the tympanic membrane.
- Assist the patient to a sitting or lying position, with head tilted toward the affected ear (see ❸). **Rationale: The solution can then flow from the ear canal to a basin.**
- Place the moisture-resistant towel around the patient's shoulder under the ear to be irrigated, and place the basin under the ear to be irrigated.
- Fill the syringe with solution.
- *Or* hang up the irrigating container, and run solution through the tubing and the nozzle. **Rationale: Solution is run through to remove air from the tubing and nozzle.**
- Straighten the ear canal.
- Insert the tip of the syringe into the auditory meatus, and direct the solution gently upward against the top of the canal. **Rationale: The solution will flow around the entire canal and out at the bottom. The solution is instilled gently because strong pressure from the fluid can cause discomfort and damage the tympanic membranes.**

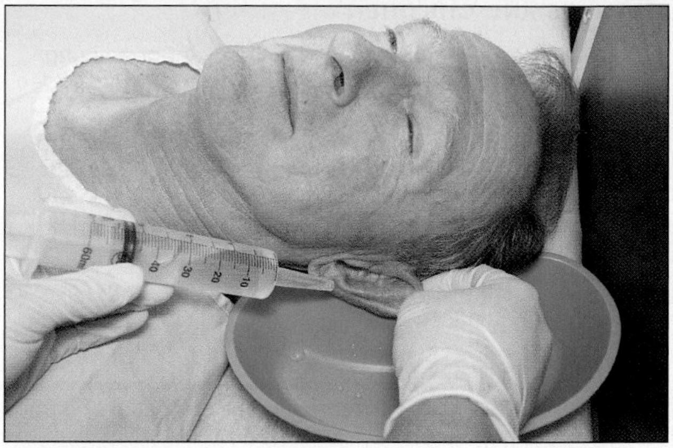

❸ Ear irrigation

- Continue instilling the fluid until all the solution is used or until the canal is cleaned, depending on the purpose of the irrigation. Take care not to block the outward flow of the solution with the syringe.
- Assist the patient to a side-lying position on the affected side. **Rationale: Lying with the affected side down helps drain the excess fluid by gravity.**
- Place a cotton ball in the auditory meatus to absorb the excess fluid.

9. Assess the patient's response and the character and amount of discharge, appearance of the canal, discomfort, and so on, immediately after the instillation and again when the medication is expected to act. Inspect the cotton for any drainage.
10. Document all nursing assessments and interventions relative to the procedure. Include the name of the drug or irrigating solution, the strength, the number of drops if a liquid medication, the time, and the response of the patient.

EVALUATION

- Perform follow-up based on findings of the effectiveness of the administration or outcomes that deviated from expected or normal for the patient. Relate findings to previous data, if available.
- Report significant deviations from normal to the appropriate members of the health-care team.

Lifespan Considerations

Administering Otic Medications

INFANTS AND CHILDREN

- Obtain assistance to immobilize an infant or a young child. *This prevents accidental injury caused by sudden movement during the procedure.*
- Because in infants and children younger than 3 years of age, the ear canal is directed upward, to administer medication, gently pull the pinna down and back (Figure 31.50). For a child *older* than 3 years of age, pull the pinna upward and backward.

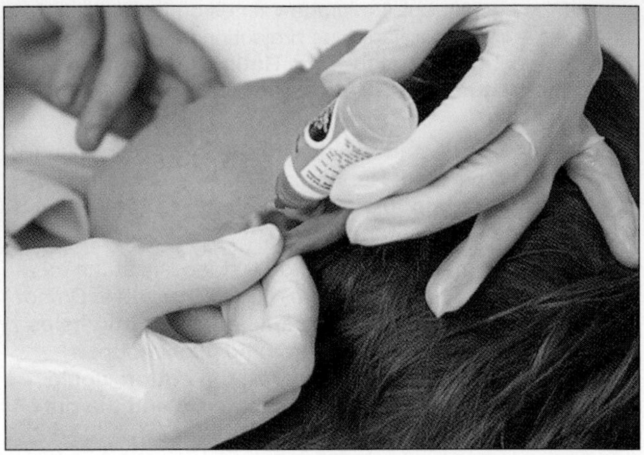

FIGURE 31.50 Straightening the ear canal of a child by pulling the pinna down and back

Nasal Instillations

Nasal instillations (nose drops and sprays) are usually instilled for their astringent effect (to shrink swollen mucous membranes), to loosen secretions and facilitate drainage, or to treat infections of the nasal cavity or sinuses. Nasal decongestants are the most common nasal instillations. Many of these products are available without a prescription. Clients need to be taught to use these agents with caution. Chronic use of nasal decongestants can lead to a rebound effect, that is, an increase in nasal congestion. If excess decongestant solution is swallowed, serious systemic effects may also develop, especially in children. Saline drops are safer as a decongestant for children.

Usually, clients self-administer nasal sprays. In the supine position with the head tilted back, the patient holds the tip of the container just inside the nares and inhales as the spray enters the nasal passages. For clients who use nasal sprays repeatedly, the nares need to be assessed for irritation. In children, nasal sprays are given with the head in an upright position to prevent excess spray from being swallowed.

Nasal drops may be used to treat sinus infections. Clients need to learn ways to position themselves to effectively treat the affected sinus:

- To treat the ethmoid and sphenoid sinuses, instruct the patient to lie back with the head over the edge of the bed or a pillow under the shoulders so that the head is tipped backward (Figure 31.51).
- To treat the maxillary and frontal sinuses, instruct the patient to assume the same back-lying position, with the head turned toward the side to be treated (Figure 31.52). The patient should also be instructed to (1) breathe through the mouth to prevent aspiration of

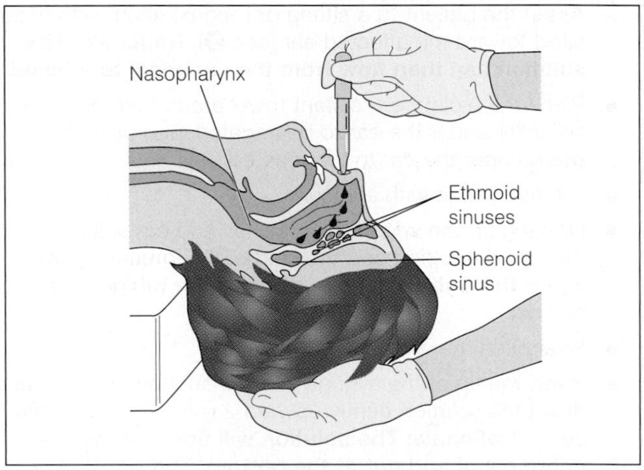

FIGURE 31.51 Position of the head to instill drops into the ethmoid and sphenoid sinuses

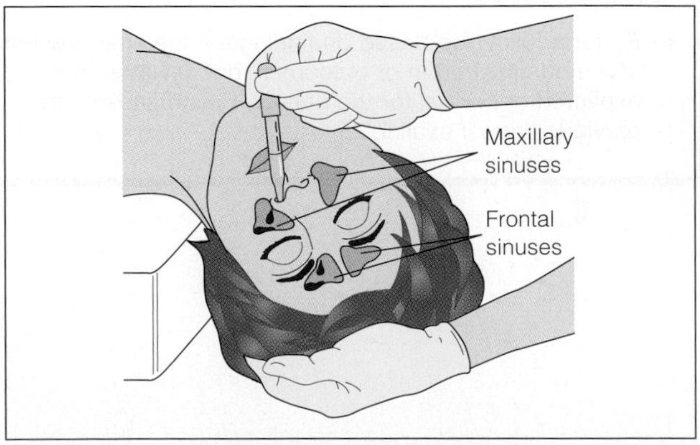

FIGURE 31.52 Position of the head to instill drops into the maxillary and frontal sinuses

medication into the trachea and bronchi, (2) remain in a back-lying position for at least 1 minute so that the solution will come into contact with all of the nasal surface, and (3) avoid blowing the nose for several minutes.

Vaginal Instillations

Vaginal medications, or instillations, are inserted as creams, jellies, foams, or suppositories to treat infection or to relieve vaginal discomfort (e.g., itching or pain). Medical aseptic technique is usually used. Vaginal creams, jellies, and foams are applied by using a tubular applicator with a plunger. Suppositories are inserted with the index finger of a gloved hand. Suppositories are designed to melt at body temperature, so they are generally stored in the refrigerator to keep them firm for insertion. See Skill 31.12 for administering vaginal instillations.

A vaginal irrigation (douche) is the washing of the vagina by a liquid at a low pressure. Vaginal irrigations are not necessary for ordinary female hygiene but are used to prevent infection by applying an antimicrobial solution that discourages the growth of microorganisms, to remove an offensive or irritating discharge, and to reduce inflammation or prevent hemorrhage by the application of heat or cold. In hospitals, sterile supplies and equipment are used; in a home, sterility is not usually necessary because people are accustomed to the microorganisms in their environments. Sterile technique, however, is indicated if there is an open wound.

SKILL 31.12

ADMINISTERING VAGINAL INSTILLATIONS

PURPOSE

- To treat or prevent infection
- To reduce inflammation
- To relieve vaginal discomfort

ASSESSMENT

Assess

In addition to the assessment performed by the nurse related to the administration of any medications, before applying vaginal medications, assess:

- The vaginal orifice for inflammation and the amount, character, and odour of vaginal discharge
- For complaints of vaginal discomfort (e.g., burning or itching)

Determine if assessment data influence administration of the medication (i.e., is it appropriate to administer the medication or does the medication need to be held and the appropriate member of the health-care team notified?).

Equipment

- Drape
- Correct vaginal suppository or cream
- Applicator for vaginal cream
- Clean gloves
- Lubricant for a suppository
- Disposable towel
- Clean perineal pad

For an irrigation, add

- Moisture-proof pad
- Vaginal irrigation set (these are often disposable) containing a nozzle, tubing and a clamp, and a container for the solution
- Irrigating solution

IMPLEMENTATION

Preparation

1. Check the MAR.
   - Check the MAR for the drug name, strength, and prescribed frequency.
   - If the MAR is unclear or pertinent information is missing, compare it with the most recent written order.
   - Report any discrepancies to the appropriate member of the health-care team, as agency policy dictates.
2. Know the reason that the patient is receiving the medication, drug classification, contraindications, usual dose range, side effects, and nursing considerations for administering and evaluating the intended outcomes of the medication.

Performance

1. Compare the label on the medication container with the medication record and check the expiration date.
2. If necessary, calculate the medication dosage.
3. Explain to the patient what you are going to do, why it is necessary, and how she can cooperate. Explain to the patient that a vaginal instillation is normally a painless procedure and, in fact, may bring relief from itching and burning if an infection is present. Many people feel embarrassed about this procedure, and some may prefer to perform the procedure themselves if instruction is provided. Discuss how the results will be used in planning further care or treatments.

(continued)

SKILL 31.12

ADMINISTERING VAGINAL INSTILLATIONS (*continued*)

4. Perform hand hygiene and observe other appropriate infection prevention and control procedures.
5. Provide for patient privacy.
6. Prepare the patient.
   - Before performing the procedure, introduce yourself and verify the patient's identity by using agency protocol.
   - Ask the patient to void. **Rationale: If the bladder is empty, the patient will have less discomfort during the treatment, and the possibility of injuring the vaginal lining is decreased.**
   - Assist the patient to a back-lying position with the knees flexed and the hips rotated laterally.
   - Drape the patient appropriately so that only the perineal area is exposed.
7. Prepare the equipment.
   - Unwrap the suppository, and put it on the opened wrapper.
   - *Or* fill the applicator with the prescribed cream, jelly, or foam. Directions are provided with the manufacturer's applicator.
8. Assess and clean the perineal area.
   - Put on gloves. **Rationale: Gloves prevent contamination of the nurse's hands from vaginal and perineal microorganisms.**
   - Inspect the vaginal orifice, note any odour of discharge from the vagina, and ask about any vaginal discomfort.
   - Provide perineal care to remove microorganisms. **Rationale: This decreases the chance of moving microorganisms into the vagina.**
9. Administer the vaginal suppository, cream, foam, jelly, or irrigation.

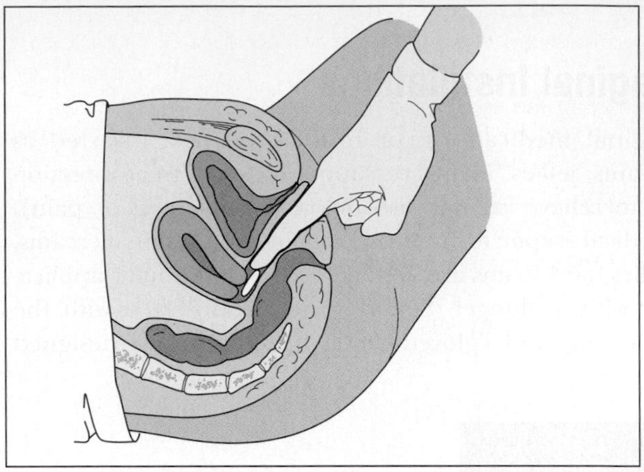

❶ Instilling a vaginal suppository

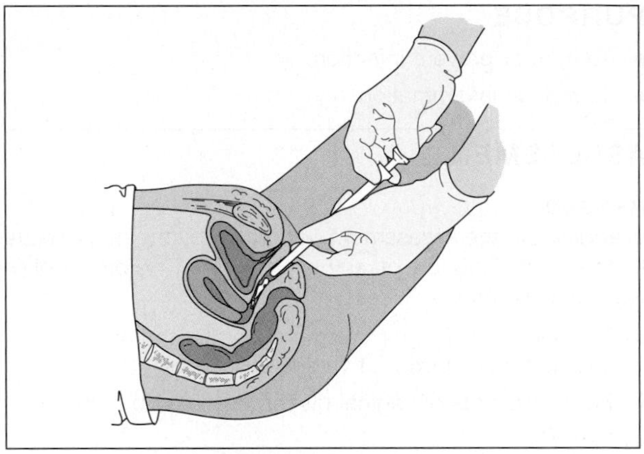

❷ Using an applicator to instill a vaginal cream

Suppository

- Lubricate the rounded (smooth) end of the suppository, which is inserted first. **Rationale: Lubrication facilitates insertion.**
- Lubricate your gloved index finger.
- Expose the vaginal orifice by separating the labia with your nondominant hand.
- Insert the suppository about 8 cm to 10 cm along the posterior wall of the vagina, or as far as it will go (see ❶). **Rationale: The posterior wall of the vagina is about 2.5 cm longer than the anterior wall because the cervix protrudes into the uppermost portion of the anterior wall.**
- Ask the patient to remain lying in the supine position for 5 to 10 minutes following insertion. The hips may also be elevated on a pillow. **Rationale: This position allows the medication to flow into the posterior fornix after it has melted.**

Vaginal Cream, Jelly, or Foam

- Gently insert the applicator about 5 cm.
- Slowly push the plunger until the applicator is empty (see ❷).
- Remove the applicator and place it on the towel. **Rationale: The applicator is put on the towel to prevent the spread of microorganisms.**
- Discard the applicator if disposable or clean it according to the manufacturer's directions.
- Ask the patient to remain lying in the supine position for 5 to 10 minutes following the insertion.

Irrigation

- Place the patient on a bedpan.
- Clamp the tubing. Hold the irrigating container about 30 cm above the vagina. **Rationale: At this height, the pressure of the solution should not be great enough to injure the vaginal lining.**
- Run fluid through the tubing and nozzle into the bedpan. **Rationale: Fluid is run through the tubing to remove air and to moisten the nozzle.**

(continued)

SKILL 31.12

ADMINISTERING VAGINAL INSTILLATIONS (*continued*)

- Insert the nozzle carefully into the vagina. Direct the nozzle toward the sacrum, following the direction of the vagina.
- Insert the nozzle about 7 cm to 10 cm, start the flow, and rotate the nozzle several times. **Rationale: Rotating the nozzle irrigates all parts of the vagina.**
- Use all of the irrigating solution, permitting it to flow out freely into the bedpan.
- Remove the nozzle from the vagina.
- Assist the patient to a sitting position on the bedpan. **Rationale: Sitting on the bedpan will help drain the remaining fluid by gravity.**

10. Ensure patient comfort.
- Dry the perineum with tissues as required.
- Apply a clean perineal pad if there is excessive drainage.

11. Document all nursing assessments and interventions relative to the procedure. Include the name of the drug or irrigating solution, the strength, the time, and the response of the patient.

EVALUATION

- Perform follow-up based on findings of the effectiveness of the administration or outcomes that deviated from expected or normal for the patient. Relate findings to previous data, if available.
- Report significant deviations from normal to the appropriate members of the health-care team.

Rectal Instillations

Insertion of medications into the rectum in the form of suppositories is a frequent practice. Rectal administration is a convenient and safe method of giving certain medications. Advantages include the following:

- It avoids irritation of the upper gastrointestinal tract in clients who encounter this problem (e.g., in clients who are nauseated or vomiting).
- It is advantageous when the medication has an objectionable taste or odour.
- The drug is released at a slow but steady rate.
- Rectal suppositories are thought to provide higher levels of medication in the bloodstream (titres) because the venous blood from the lower rectum is not transported through the liver.

To insert a rectal suppository,

- Assist the patient to a left lateral or left Sims' position, with the upper leg flexed.
- Fold back the top bedclothes to expose the buttocks.
- Put a glove on the hand that will be used to insert the suppository.
- Unwrap the suppository and lubricate the smooth rounded end, or see the manufacturer's instructions. The rounded end is usually inserted first and the lubricant reduces irritation of the mucosa.
- Lubricate the gloved index finger.
- Encourage the patient to relax by breathing through the mouth. This usually relaxes the external anal sphincter.
- Insert the suppository gently into the anal canal, rounded end first (or according to manufacturer's instructions), along the rectal wall using the gloved index finger. For an adult, insert the suppository beyond the internal sphincter (i.e., 10 cm) (see Figure 31.53).
- Avoid embedding the suppository in feces in order for the suppository to be absorbed effectively.
- Press the patient's buttocks together for a few minutes.
- Ask the patient to remain in the left lateral or supine position for at least 5 minutes to help retain the suppository. The suppository should be retained varying lengths of time according to manufacturer's instructions.

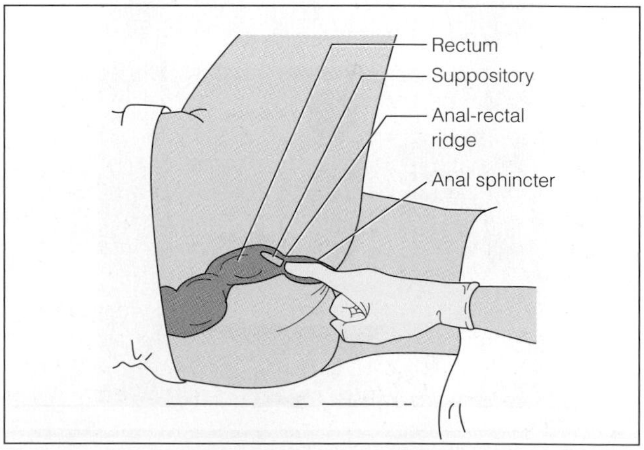

FIGURE 31.53 Inserting a rectal suppository beyond the internal sphincter along the rectal wall

See the Lifespan Considerations box for guidelines on using rectal instillations in infants and children.

Respiratory Inhalation

Nebulizers deliver most medications administered through the inhaled route. A nebulizer is used to deliver a fine spray (fog or mist) of medication or moisture to a patient. There are two kinds of nebulization: *atomization* and *aerosolization*. In atomization, a device called an *atomizer* produces rather large droplets for inhalation. In aerosolization, the droplets are suspended in a gas, such as oxygen. The smaller the droplets, the farther they can be inhaled into the respiratory tract. When a medication is intended for the nasal mucosa, it is inhaled through the nose; when it is intended for the trachea, bronchi, or lungs, it is inhaled through the mouth.

A large-volume nebulizer can provide a heated or cool mist. It is used for long-term therapy, such as that following a tracheostomy. The ultrasonic nebulizer (Figure 31.54) provides 100% humidity and can provide particles small enough to be inhaled deeply into the respiratory tract.

The **metered-dose inhaler (MDI)**, a handheld nebulizer (Figure 31.55), is a pressurized container of medication that can be used by the patient to release the medication through a nosepiece or mouthpiece. The force with which the air moves through the nebulizer causes the large particles of medicated solution to break up into finer particles, forming a mist or fine spray. According to Bower (2005), metered-dose inhalers can deliver accurate doses, provide for target action at the needed sites, and cause fewer systemic effects than medication delivered by other routes.

To ensure correct delivery of the prescribed medication by MDIs, nurses need to instruct clients to use aerosol inhalers properly. The patient compresses the medication canister by hand to release medication through a mouthpiece. An extender or spacer can be attached to the mouthpiece to facilitate medication absorption for better results (Figure 31.56). Spacers are holding chambers into which the medication is fired and from which the patient inhales, so that the dose is not lost by exhalation. The Teaching: Clinical box provides instructions for clients about using an MDI (see also the Home Care Considerations box). Newer breath-activated MDIs are being produced in which inhalation triggers the release of a measured dose of medication.

Lifespan Considerations

Administering Rectal Medications

INFANTS AND CHILDREN

Use the following guidelines when administering rectal medications to infants or children:

- Obtain assistance to immobilize an infant or a young child. This prevents accidental injury caused by sudden movement during the procedure.
- For a child younger than 3 years, the nurse should use the gloved fifth finger for insertion. After this age, the index finger can usually be used.
- For a child or an infant, insert a suppository 5 cm or less.

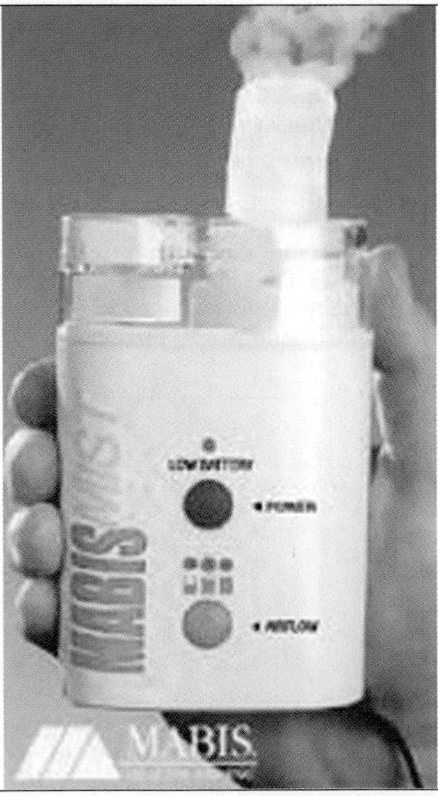

FIGURE 31.54 Ultrasonic nebulizer

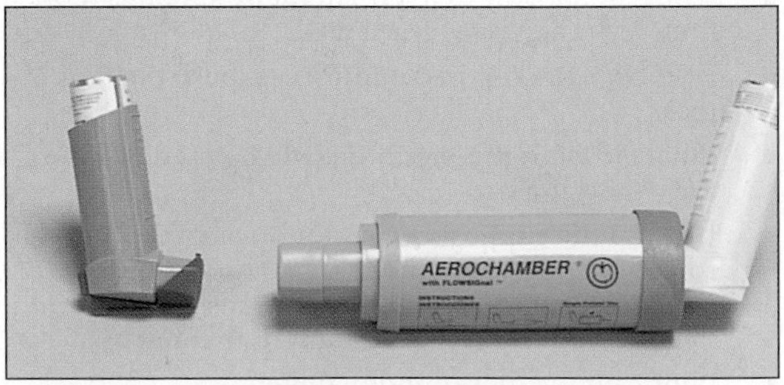

FIGURE 31.55 Metered-dose inhaler

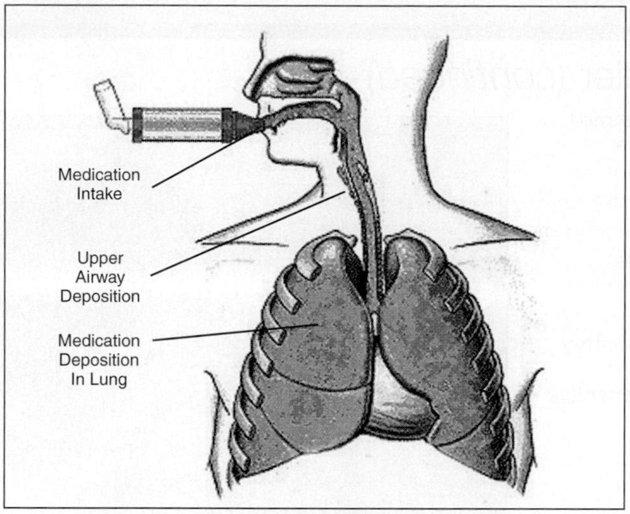

FIGURE 31.56 Delivery of medication to the lungs by using a metered-dose inhaler extender

TEACHING: CLINICAL

Using a Metered-Dose Inhaler

- Ensure that the canister is firmly and fully inserted into the inhaler.
- Remove the mouthpiece cap and shake the inhaler vigorously for 3 to 5 seconds to mix the medication evenly.
- Exhale comfortably (as in a normal full breath).
- Hold the canister with the mouthpiece down, as illustrated in Figure 31.57.
  a. Hold the MDI 2 cm to 4 cm from the open mouth (Figure 31.57).
  b. *Or* put the mouthpiece far enough into the mouth with its opening toward the throat such that the lips can tightly close around the mouthpiece. An MDI with a spacer or extender is always placed in the mouth (Figure 31.58). This method should not be used for steroid medications via an MDI because it is not considered as efficient in delivery of the medication (Bower, 2005).

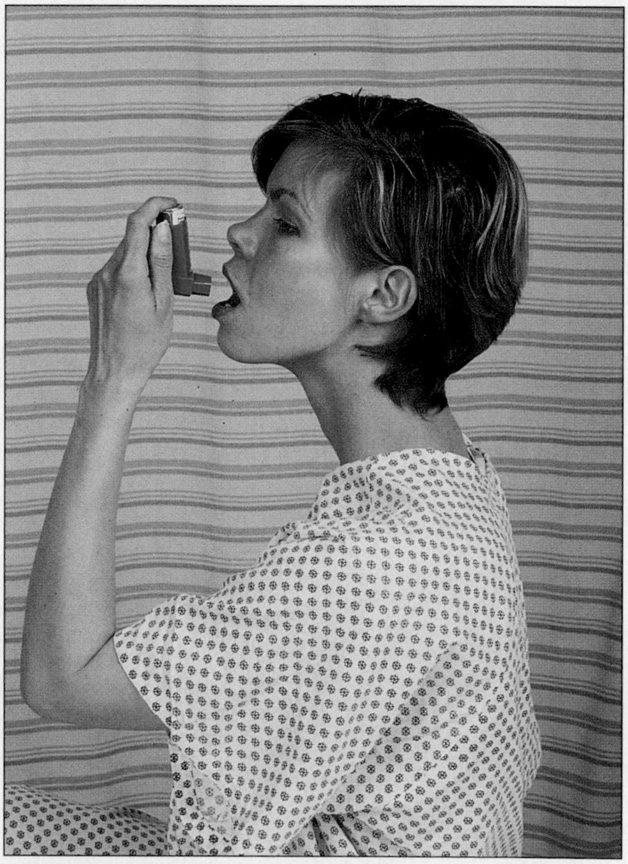

FIGURE 31.57 Inhaler positioned away from the open mouth

ADMINISTERING THE MEDICATION

- Press down *once* on the MDI canister (which releases the dose) and inhale slowly (for 3 to 5 seconds) and deeply through the mouth.
- Hold your breath for 10 seconds or as long as possible. *This allows the aerosol to reach deeper airways.*
- Remove the inhaler from or away from the mouth.
- Exhale slowly through *pursed* lips. Controlled exhalation keeps the small airways open during exhalation.
- Repeat the inhalation if ordered. Wait 20 to 30 seconds between inhalations of bronchodilator medications. Waiting allows the first inhalation to work, enabling the subsequent dose to reach deeper into the lungs.
- Following use of the inhaler, rinse mouth with tap water to remove any remaining medication and reduce irritation and risk of infection.

(continued)

TEACHING: CLINICAL

Using a Metered-Dose Inhaler (*continued*)

- Clean the MDI mouthpiece after each use. Use mild soap and water, rinse it, and let it air dry before replacing it on the device.
- Store the canister at room temperature. Avoid extremes of temperature.
- Report adverse reactions, such as restlessness, palpitations, nervousness, or rash to the appropriate member of the health-care team.
- Many MDIs contain steroids for an anti-inflammatory effect. Prolonged use increases the risk of fungal infections in the mouth, indicating a need for attentive mouth care.

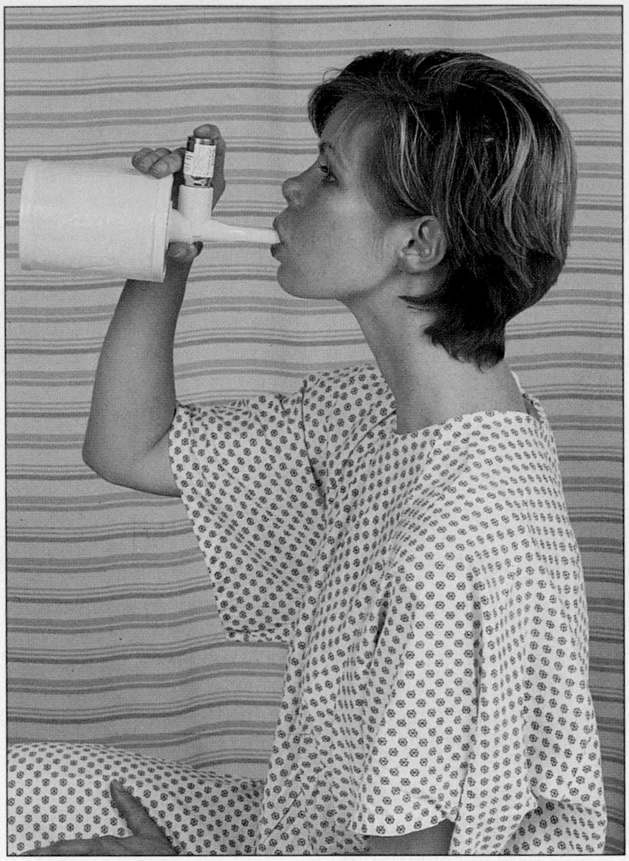

FIGURE 31.58 An extender spacer attached to a mouthpiece placed in the mouth

Home Care Considerations

Metered-Dose Inhalers

- Cleaning the metered-dose inhaler mouthpiece at least once a week is recommended, though some manufacturers indicate more frequent cleaning. Depending on the manufacturer's instructions, some mouthpieces are simply wiped with a wet cloth, while others require that the canister be removed from the mouthpiece with the mouthpiece then either washed with warm, soapy water or soaked in a solution, such as 500 mL of water with 60 mL of vinegar added.
- Teach clients how to determine the amount of medication remaining in a metered-dose inhaler canister:
  - Calculate the number of days' doses in a canister. Divide the number of doses (puffs) in the canister (on the label) by the number of puffs taken per day (Bower, 2005). Newer inhalers (e.g., Advair) come with a dose-counting mechanism. A previous method of floating the canister in water is not considered accurate because some of the propellant may remain (even after the medication is gone), which leads the client to incorrectly believe medication is being received.
- Review instructions and periodically assess the client's techniques for using an inhaler spacer or chamber correctly. Research shows that these devices assist in delivering the medication deeply into the lungs rather than only to the oropharynx.

If two inhalers are to be used, the bronchodilator medication (which opens the airways) should be given before other medications. Bower (2005) recommends the use of the mnemonic *B before C* to remember bronchodilator before corticosteroid.

Inhaled steroids may not be correctly used by clients because they do not associate these medications with immediate symptom relief. The bronchodilators act to open the airways in the short term. However, it is the inhaled steroids that act to keep airway inflammation under control. See the Lifespan Considerations box for information on administering inhalers to children.

Irrigations

An **irrigation (lavage)** is the washing out of a body cavity by a stream of water or other fluid that may or may not be medicated. Irrigation is performed for one or more of the following reasons:

- To clean the area (i.e., to remove a foreign object or excessive secretions or discharge)
- To apply heat or cold
- To apply a medication, such as an antiseptic
- To reduce inflammation
- To relieve discomfort

Asepsis is required when there is a break in the skin (e.g., in a wound irrigation) or whenever a sterile body cavity (e.g., the bladder) is entered. Some irrigations (e.g., a vaginal, rectal, or gastric irrigation) are often safely conducted by using medical asepsis.

Different kinds of syringes are used for irrigations. The most common are the Asepto and the rubber bulb (Figure 31.59). The syringes are often calibrated, permit-

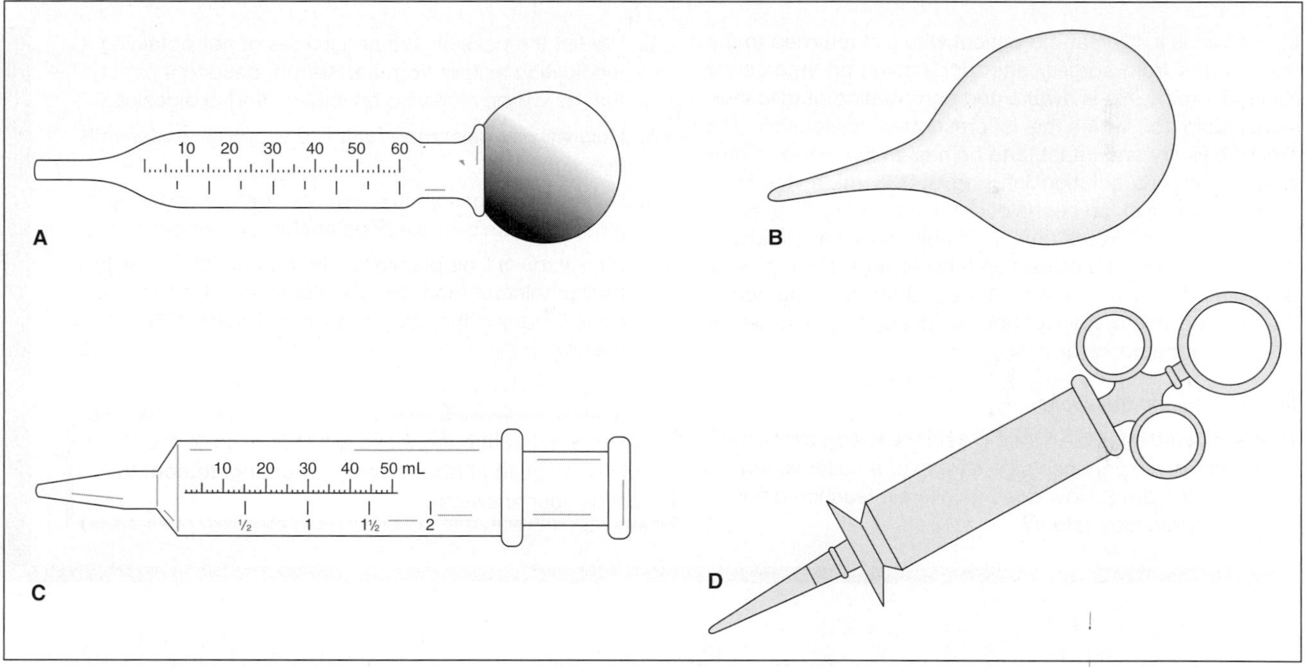

FIGURE 31.59 Four types of syringes commonly used for irrigations: **A:** Asepto; **B:** rubber bulb; **C:** piston syringe; **D:** Pomeroy

Lifespan Considerations

Administering Metered-Dose Inhalers and Nebulizers

CHILDREN

- Spacers hold a medication in suspension and provide the child an opportunity to take several deep breaths in order to inhale all the medication.
- A mask is used for nebulizer treatments, allowing the child to breathe naturally. Some infants and children may be frightened or uncomfortable with the mask and become resistant. Use a doll or stuffed animal to demonstrate the use of the mask, and allow the child to play with the equipment before putting it in place. Having the child sit in the parent's lap during the procedure can help the child relax and be more cooperative.

ting the nurse to determine the amount of irrigant being delivered at any given time.

The *Asepto syringe* is a plastic (or glass) syringe with a rubber bulb. Squeezing the air out of the bulb produces negative pressure, and fluid can be sucked into the syringe. When the bulb is squeezed again, the fluid is ejected from the syringe. Asepto syringes come in several sizes ranging from 30 mL to 120 mL.

The *rubber bulb syringe* is often used for irrigating the ears. Like the Asepto syringe, the rubber bulb syringe comes in a range of sizes.

Other syringes that can be used are the piston syringe, which has a tip to which a catheter can be attached, and the Pomeroy syringe. Catheters can be used for deep-wound irrigations and for some types of bladder irrigations. The Pomeroy syringe is a metal syringe commonly used for ear irrigations. A shield near the tip prevents the solution from spraying outward. Plastic squeezable bottles are also available for irrigations. These are commonly used for perineal irrigations and some wound irrigations.

The type, amount, temperature, and strength of the solution and the frequency of the irrigation are ordered by the physician. Generally, normal saline at body temperature (37°C) is used unless specified otherwise. The amount of solution used varies with the site and purpose of the irrigation. Guidelines for administering eye and ear irrigations are given in Skill 31.10 (eye) and Skill 31.11 (ear).

Case Study 31

Mr. Ketron is a 40-year-old patient who just returned to the nursing unit from surgery after undergoing an emergency appendectomy. He is awake and complaining of mild incisional pain for which he is prescribed analgesics. His dressing is dry and intact, and he has an intravenous infusion of Ringer's solution infusing at 125 mL/h. He is to receive cefazolin (a cephalosporin antibiotic) 1 g intravenously every 4 hours until he is able to tolerate fluids, at which time he will be placed on oral cefixime 200 mg twice daily until discharged and for 1 week after returning home. Because of a history of alcoholism, he also has an order for vitamin K intramuscular.

Critical Thinking Questions

1. It is always possible that a person receiving antibiotic drugs may experience side effects or an allergic reaction to the drug. How does an allergic reaction differ from a drug side effect?
2. Predict the possible consequences of not obtaining a medication history from Mr. Ketron, despite the fact that he will be receiving antibiotics and analgesics.
3. How will you select the best site to give the vitamin K injection?
4. What precautions should you take before administering Mr. Ketron's intravenous antibiotic medication?
5. Mr. Ketron will be placed on the oral antibiotic when he can tolerate food and oral fluids. What difference does it make if this drug is given before or after meals?

After working through these questions, go to the MyNursingLab at **http://www.mynursinglab.com** to check your answers.

KEY TERMS

pharmacology
medication
prescription
generic name
official name
chemical name
trademark (brand name)
pharmacopoeia
therapeutic effect (desired effect)
side effect
drug toxicity
drug allergy
anaphylactic reaction
drug tolerance
cumulative effect
idiosyncratic effect
drug interaction
potentiating effect
inhibiting effect
synergistic effect
iatrogenic disease
problematic substance use
drug misuse
drug dependence
illicit drugs
half-life (elimination half-life)
peak plasma level

onset of action
plateau
pharmacodynamics
agonist
antagonist
pharmacokinetics
absorption
first-pass effect
distribution
biotransformation (detoxification, metabolism)
metabolites
excretion
pharmacogenetics
ethnopharmacology
enteral
oral
sublingual
buccal
parenteral
subcutaneous (hypodermic)
intramuscular
intradermal
intravenous
intra-arterial
intracardiac
intraosseous
intrathecal (intraspinal)
intrapleural
epidural
intra-articular
topical
standing order
single order
stat order
prn order
protocol order (collective prescription)
medication history
nasogastric tube
gastrostomy tube
prefilled unit-dose system
hub
cannula (shaft)
bevel
gauge (diameter)
ampule
vial
reconstitution
tandem
piggyback
volume-control infusion set
percutaneous
transdermal patch
ophthalmic
otic
metered-dose inhaler (MDI)
irrigation (lavage)

CHAPTER HIGHLIGHTS

- Federal drug legislation in Canada regulates the production, prescription, distribution, and administration of drugs.
- Nursing practice acts define limits on the nurse's responsibilities regarding medications.
- Medications have several names. Nurses need to know the *generic* and *trade* names of a medication and be aware of its therapeutic and side effects.
- Adverse effects of medications include drug toxicity, drug allergy, drug tolerance, idiosyncratic effect, and drug interactions.
- Several factors other than the drug itself can affect its action. These include pregnancy; age; gender; cultural, ethnic, and genetic factors; diet; client environment; psychological factors; illness and disease; and time of administration.
- Various routes are used to administer medications: oral, sublingual, buccal, parenteral, topical, or via a nasogastric or gastrostomy tube. When administering a medication, the nurse must ensure that it is appropriate for the route specified.
- Medication orders must include the patient name, date and time the order is written, name of the medication, dosage, route, frequency of administration, and signature of the person writing the order. Nurses must question any unclear orders before implementing the order.
- Telephone or verbal orders must be cosigned by the physician within a time specified by agency policy (usually 24 to 48 hours). Some agencies require that two nurses listen to a telephone order.
- Three systems of measurement are used in North America: the metric system, the apothecaries' system, and the household system. Weights and measures may need to be converted by the nurse within these three systems.
- Several formulas can be used to calculate dosages. Pediatric dosages are often calculated by incorporating the child's weight or body surface area.
- Nurses must always assess a patient's physical status before giving any medication and obtain a medication history.
- Medication reconciliation is another method that the nurse uses to ensure that clients receive the appropriate medications and dosages. Three important areas for medication reconciliation to occur are (1) on admission, (2) during shift reports and transfers, and with new medication orders, and (3) on discharge.
- When administering medications, the nurse observes *specified ten rights* to ensure accurate administration. When preparing medications, the nurse checks the medication container label against the medication administration record (MAR) or printout *three* times.
- The nurse who prepares the medication administers it and must never leave a prepared medication unattended.

- The nurse always identifies the patient appropriately before administering a medication and stays with the patient until the medication is taken.
- Medications, once given, are documented as soon as possible after administration.
- Medications given parenterally act more quickly than those given orally or topically and must be prepared using aseptic technique.
- When preparing two insulins to be mixed in the same syringe, a vial of unmodified insulin should never be contaminated with modified insulin.
- Proper site selection is essential for an intramuscular injection to prevent tissue, blood vessel, bone, and nerve damage. The nurse should always palpate anatomic landmarks when selecting a site.
- The Z-track method for intramuscular injection is recommended to prevent discomfort caused by leakage of irritating or staining medication into subcutaneous tissues.
- Clients receiving a series of injections should have the injection sites rotated.
- After use, needles should not be recapped but must be placed in puncture-resistant containers.
- Intravenous medications can be administered by various methods: in a large-volume infusion of intravenous fluid; by intermittent intravenous infusion; by volume-controlled infusion; by intravenous push (IVP) or bolus; or by intermittent venous access. In all these methods, the patient has an existing intravenous line or an IV access site, such as a heparin or saline lock.
- Topical medications are applied to the skin and mucous membranes primarily for their local effects, although some systemic effects may occur.
- A metered-dose inhaler (MDI) is a handheld nebulizer that can be used by clients to self-administer measured doses of an aerosol medication. To ensure correct delivery of the prescribed medication by MDIs, nurses need to instruct clients to use aerosol inhalers correctly.
- Irrigations of body cavities may be performed (1) to remove a foreign object or excessive secretions or discharge, (2) to apply heat or cold, (3) to apply a medication, such as an antiseptic, (4) to reduce inflammation, or (5) to relieve discomfort.
- Asepsis for an irrigation is required when there is a break in the skin (e.g., in a wound irrigation) or whenever a sterile body cavity (e.g., the bladder) is entered.

ASSESS YOUR LEARNING

1. A patient tells the nurse, "This pill is a different colour from the one that I usually take at home." Which of the following is the best response by the nurse?

a. "Go ahead and take your medicine."
b. "I will recheck your medication orders."
c. "Maybe the doctor ordered a different medication."
d. "I'll leave the pill here while I check with the doctor."

2. Which of the following medications listed on a patient's medication administration record (MAR) should the nurse question?

a. Furosemide 40 mg, po, STAT
b. Ampicillin 500 mg, q6h, IV
c. Humulin-R insulin 30 units, sc, every am, ac
d. Codeine q4–6h, po, prn for pain

3. The physician prescribed 4 mL of immunoglobulin to be given IM to a 40-year-old female rape victim who is 170 cm tall and weighs 61 kg. Which of the following is the most appropriate method of administration?

a. Tuberculin syringe, 25 gauge to 27 gauge, 6 mm to 16 mm needle
b. Two 3 mL syringes, 20 gauge to 23 gauge, 3.8 cm needle
c. Two 2 mL syringes, 25 gauge, 16 mm needle
d. Two 2 mL syringes, 20 gauge to 23 gauge, 2.5 cm needle

4. The nurse is to administer 0.8 mL of medication subcutaneously in the upper arm to a 50-year-old patient who weighs 180 kg. The nurse can grasp approximately 10 cm of the patient's tissue at the upper arm. Which of the following is the most appropriate syringe for the nurse to use?

a. Tuberculin syringe, 25 gauge to 27 gauge, 6 mm to 16 mm needle
b. Two 3 mL syringes, 20 gauge to 23 gauge, 3.8 cm needle
c. 2 mL syringe, 25 gauge, 16 mm needle
d. 2 mL syringe, 20 gauge to 23 gauge, 2.5 cm needle

5. The nurse is to administer an intradermal tuberculin test to a 22-year-old male who is 182 cm tall and weighs 82 kg. Which of the following is the most appropriate for the nurse to use?

a. A tuberculin syringe, 25 gauge to 27 gauge, 6 mm to 16 mm needle
b. Two 3 mL syringes, 20 gauge to 23 gauge, 3.8 cm needle
c. 2 mL syringe, 25 gauge, 16 mm needle
d. 2 mL syringe, 20 gauge to 23 gauge, 2.5 cm needle

6. The nurse calculates that 93.75% of a medication with a half-life of 12 hours will be eliminated from a patient's body in how many hours following administration?

a. 24 hours

b. 36 hours
c. 48 hours
d. 60 hours

7. Which of the following dosages is most appropriate for the nurse to administer to an older adult patient with renal insufficiency about to receive a cardiac medication?
   a. A decreased dosage
   b. A standard dosage
   c. An increased dosage
   d. A divided dosage

8. Which of the following is the correct method when administering an otic medication to a 2-year-old patient?
   a. Pull the ear straight back.
   b. Pull the ear down and back.
   c. Pull the ear up and back.
   d. Pull the ear straight upward.

9. A physician writes a prescription for 0.16 mg of digoxin intravenously every day. The medication is available in a concentration of 400 mcg per mL. How many mL will the nurse administer?
   a. 0.4 mL
   b. 0.04 mL
   c. 0.16 mL
   d. 4 mL

10. Christian, 4 years old and weighing 15 kg, has been admitted for a bacterial respiratory infection. The pediatrician orders cefotaxime sodium (Claforan) 60 mg/kg/day, I.V. What amount of medication should the nurse administer every 6 hours?
   a. 175 mg
   b. 200 mg
   c. 225 mg
   d. 250 mg

After working through these questions, go to the MyNursingLab at ***http://www.mynursinglab.com*** *to check your answers and see explanations.*

SUGGESTED READINGS

Audrain-McGovern, J., Al Koudsi, N., Rodriguez, D., Wileyto, E. P., Shields, P. G., & Tyndale, R. F. (2007). The Role of CYP2A6 in the emergence of nicotine dependence in adolescents. *Pediatrics, 119*(1), 264–274.

This article is a good example of the role of pharmacogenetics in influencing nicotine dependence. Dr. Rachel Tyndale is the Canada Research Chair in Pharmacogenetics.

Farrar, D., Tuffnell, D. J., & West, J. (2007). Continuous subcutaneous insulin infusion versus multiple daily injections of insulin for pregnant women with diabetes. *Cochrane Database of Systematic Reviews, 3,* Art. No.: CD005542.

Medication administration in pregnancy requires specialized knowledge. This systematic review provides an interesting summary of the research on insulin regulation of blood glucose during pregnancy.

WEBLINKS

Canadian Centre on Substance Abuse

http://www.ccsa.ca

This nonprofit organization has a mission "to provide objective, evidence-based information and advice that will help reduce the health, social and economic harm associated with substance abuse and addictions."

Canadian Network of Substance Abuse and Allied Professionals

http://www.cnsaap.ca/cnsaap/

This website provides extensive resources for nurses and other health professionals working with clients who have problematic substance use issues. Provincial and territorial resources are listed. The site was developed specifically to inform, educate, and support Canada's problematic substance use workforce.

The Centre for Addiction and Mental Health (CAMH)

http://www.camh.net

The centre is Canada's leading addiction and mental health teaching hospital, providing direct care for people with mental health and addiction problems, a research facility, an education and training institute, and a community-based organization providing health-promotion services across Ontario.

Canadian Pharmacists Association

http://www.pharmacists.ca/flash.cfm

The association is the national organization for pharmacists. Its website provides a source for drug information, pharmacy practices, and patient information.

Health Canada Therapeutic Drugs Database

http://www.hc-sc.gc.ca/dhp-mps/prodpharma/databasdon/index_e.html

The Drug Product Database (DPD) contains product-specific information on drugs approved for use in Canada.

REFERENCES

Baker, G. R., Norton, P. G., Flintoft, V., Blais, R., Brown, A., Cox, J., et al. (2004). The Canadian adverse events study: The incidence of adverse events among hospital patients in Canada. *Canadian Medical Association Journal, 170*(11), 1678–1686.

Barr, D. H., & Thomas, C. H. (2005). Is aspiration necessary during intramuscular injection? *Advance Online Editions for Nurses, 7*(18), 27.

Bower, L. M. (2005). Is your patient's metered-dose inhaler technique up to snuff? *Nursing 2005, 35*(8), 50–51.

Bunce, M. (2003). Troubleshooting central lines. *RN, 66*(12), 28–34.

Canadian Centre for Occupational Health and Safety. (2005). *Needle stick injuries.* Retrieved June 5, 2008, from http://www.ccohs.ca/oshanswers/diseases/needlestick_injuries.html

Canadian Medical Association. 2008. *Drug advisories.* Retrieved June 3, 2008, from http://www.cmaj.ca/misc/advisories.shtml

Department of Justice Canada. (1985). *Food and drugs act: Food and drug regulations.* Retrieved June 2, 2008, from http://laws.justice.gc.ca/en/F-27/C.R.C.-c.870/115860.html

Health Canada. (2005). *Proper use and disposal of medication.* Retrieved June 3, 2008, from http://www.hc-sc.gc.ca/hl-vs/iyh-vsv/med/disposal-defaire-eng.php#pr

Institute for Safe Medication Practices. (2006). *ISMP's list of error-prone abbreviations, symbols, and dose designations.* Retrieved June 4, 2008, from http://www.ismp.org/Tools/errorproneabbreviations.pdf

Institute for Safe Medication Practices Canada. (2006). Eliminate use of dangerous abbreviations, symbols, and dose designations. *ISMP Canada Safety Bulletin, 6*(4), 1–4.

Lea, D. H. (2005). Tailoring drug therapy with pharmacogenetics. *Nursing, 35*(4), 22–23.

Minister of Public Works and Government Services Canada. (2006). *Canadian immunization guide* (7th ed.). Ottawa: Government of Canada.

Munoz, C., & Hilgenberg, C. (2005). Ethnopharmacology. *American Journal of Nursing, 105*(8), 40–48.

Nicoll, L. H., & Hesby, A. (2002). Intramuscular injection: An integrative research review and guideline for evidence-based practice. *Applied Nursing Research, 16*(2), 149–162.

Nisbet, A. C. (2006). Intramuscular gluteal injections in the increasingly obese population. *British Medical Journal, 332,* 637–638.

Pullen, R. L. (2005). Administering medication by the Z-track method. *Nursing 35*(7), 24.

Registered Nurses' Association of Ontario. (2004). *Nursing best practice guideline: Subcutaneous administration of insulin in adults with Type 2 Diabetes.* Toronto: Author.

Tarnow, K., & King, N. (2004). Intradermal injections: Traditional bevel up versus bevel down. *Applied Nursing Research, 17*(4), 275–282.

Chapter 32

Infection Prevention and Control

Nurses are directly involved in providing a biologically safe environment. Microorganisms exist everywhere in the environment: in air, in water, in soil, and on body surfaces. The skin, intestinal tract, and mucous membranes lining other areas open to the outside (e.g., mouth, upper respiratory tract, vagina, and lower urinary tract) have different types of **normal** or **resident flora** (the collective bacteria in a given area). See Table 32.1 for common resident organisms. Most microorganisms are harmless, and some are even beneficial. An important role of resident flora, for example, is to prevent a potential **pathogen**, a microorganism with the potential to cause disease, from taking up residence. Bacteria on the skin or mucous membranes produce toxic metabolites, or alter local pH, thus repressing the growth of other species. Some microorganisms found in the intestines (e.g., enterobacteria) produce substances that are lethal to related strains of bacteria. Other gut flora produce B vitamins and vitamin K.

OBJECTIVES

After studying this chapter, you should be able to

1. Identify risks for health-care-associated infections
2. Describe the specific and nonspecific body defences against microorganisms
3. Outline the pathophysiology of infection and describe the characteristics of the five major types of microorganisms that can cause an infection
4. Describe the six links in the chain of infection and identify measures that break each link
5. Describe the six routes of transmission of microorganisms
6. Describe factors that place people at risk for developing an infection
7. List indications for hand hygiene and describe cough etiquette
8. Correctly perform aseptic practices, including performing hand hygiene, donning and removing a face mask, gowning, donning and removing disposable gloves (clean versus sterile), bagging articles, and managing equipment used for clients
9. Describe the system of routine practices and additional precautions, and compare these with other systems
10. Identify nursing responsibilities in infection prevention and control
11. Outline relevant nursing diagnoses and contributing factors for clients at risk for infection and those who have an infection
12. Explain the measures to take to prevent or manage a potential exposure to a blood-borne pathogen

TABLE 32.1 Examples of Common Resident Organisms

Body Area	Organisms
Skin	Coagulase-negative staphylococci *Propionibacterium acnes* *Staphylococcus aureus* *Corynebacterium xerosis* *Pityrosporum ovale* (yeast)
Nasal passages	*Staphylococcus aureus* Coagulase-negative staphylococci
Oropharynx	*Streptococcus pneumoniae*
Bronchi, lungs	None
Mouth	*Streptococcus mutans* *Lactobacillus* *Bacteroides* *Actinomyces* None
Stomach	None
Esophagus	*Bacteroides*
Intestine	*Fusobacterium* *Eubacterium* *Lactobacillus* *Streptococcus* *Enterobacteriaceae* *Shigella* *Escherichia coli*
Urethral orifice	Coagulase-negative staphylococci
Urethra (lower)	*Proteus*
Bladder, ureters, kidneys	None
Vagina	*Lactobacillus* *Bacteroides* *Clostridium* *Candida albicans*
Blood, lymph system	None

An **infection** is an invasion of body tissue by microorganisms and their subsequent proliferation there, with damage to host tissue. Such a microorganism is called an **infectious agent**. Some infections are caused by normal resident flora when they move to a different part of the body. For example, *Escherichia coli* is a normal inhabitant of the large intestine but a common cause of infection of the urinary tract. Other infections are caused by microorganisms that are acquired from the environment or from another person.

Infectious diseases are a major cause of death worldwide and a leading cause of illness in Canada. The control of the spread of microorganisms and the protection of people from communicable diseases and infections are carried out on international, national, provincial or territorial, community, and individual levels. The World Health Organization (WHO) is the major regulatory agency at the international level. In Canada, the Public Health Agency of Canada (PHAC) is the principal public health agency at the national level, with its Nosocomial and Occupational Infections section concerned with infection prevention and control. At the provincial and territorial level, health departments track epidemics and illnesses as reports are made throughout a particular area. At the local level, hospitals and continuing-care facilities have infection-control practitioners who are responsible for monitoring infection rates and implementing appropriate education, prevention and control strategies, or other programs.

The Community and Hospital Infection Control Association—Canada (CHICA-Canada) has articulated core competencies in infection prevention and control for health-care workers (Henderson and CHICA-Canada, Education Committee, 2006). Required knowledge and skills relate to the transmission of microorganisms, hand hygiene, routine practices and additional precautions, personal protective equipment, personal safety, sterilization and disinfection, and critical assessment of risk. Key strategies for the prevention and control of infections involve eliminating microorganisms, reducing transmission of organisms to an individual, and reducing the susceptibility of that individual. **Asepsis** is freedom from disease-causing microorganisms. To decrease the possibility of transferring microorganisms from one place to another, aseptic technique is used in such procedures as dressing changes and insertion of intravenous lines. Handwashing is another method used to reduce transmission of organisms.

Health-Care-Associated Infections

Infections that are associated with the delivery of health-care services in a health-care facility were traditionally called **nosocomial infections**. Nosocomial infections can either develop during a client's stay in a facility or manifest after discharge. Standard definitions are available for different sites of infection (e.g., pneumonia, surgical site infection). The broader term of **health-care-associated infections** is now preferred as it includes infections in all settings, including hospitals, long-term-care or continuing-care facilities, community, home care, health-care professionals' offices, or test centres. Health-care-associated infections are not limited to clients; microorganisms may also be acquired by health-care personnel working in

Evidence-Informed Practice

How Well Do Health-Care Workers Wash Their Hands?

In this study, Raboud and colleagues (2004) assessed the handwashing behaviour of nurses. A research assistant observed seven nurses for one shift each (day or night) on a medical ward in a tertiary care hospital in a large Canadian city, for a total of 379 client visits. In 24% of the visits, the nurse had no direct contact with the clients or their immediate environment; handwashing occurred in 4% of these visits. Eleven percent of the visits involved contact with body fluids; handwashing occurred in 81% of these visits and the nurse wore gloves 86% of the time. Forty percent of the visits involved contact with skin; handwashing occurred after 61% of these visits and the nurse wore gloves 33% of the time. Twenty-four percent of the visits involved contact with environment; handwashing occurred for 38% of these visits and the nurse wore gloves 15% of the time.

The key limitation of the study is the small number of observations over a short time in a single setting. However, these results are consistent with other similar studies.

NURSING IMPLICATIONS: Hand hygiene after higher-risk situations (e.g., exposure to body fluids or skin contact) should be reinforced. More importantly, the role of the environment in transmission and the need for hand hygiene after contact with the client's immediate environment need to be emphasized. Besides education about when and how to perform hand hygiene, work environments need to be structured so as to facilitate hand hygiene (e.g., easy access to sinks or alcohol-based hand rub).

Source: "Patterns of Handwashing Behavior and Visits to Patients on a General Medical Ward of Health-Care Workers," by J. Raboud, R. Saskin, K. Wong, C. Moore, G. Parucha, J. Bennett, K. Green, D. Low, M. Leob, A. Simor, and A. McGeer, 2004, *Infection Control and Hospital Epidemiology, 25*(3), pp. 198–202.

the facility (e.g., hepatitis B infection and HIV infection) and can cause significant illness and time lost from work.

Health-care-associated infections are receiving increasing attention. The most common settings in which health-care-associated infections develop are surgical or medical intensive care units in hospitals. Infections of the urinary tract, surgical site, and lower respiratory tract are the most common types of health-care-associated infections. Although less common, line-associated bacteremias, infections with antibiotic-resistant organisms, and *Clostridium difficile*–associated diarrhea are associated with higher mortality and health-care costs.

The microorganisms that cause health-care-associated infections can originate from an endogenous (internal) source or from an exogenous (external) source. Most health-care-associated infections appear to have endogenous sources, and many factors contribute to health-care-associated infections. A number of infections are the direct result of diagnostic or therapeutic procedures. One example of such an infection is **bacteremia** (bacteria in the bloodstream) that results from contamination of an intravascular line. Not all health-care-associated infections are procedure-related, and not all infections are preventable. A key factor contributing to the development of health-care-associated infections is the *presence of compromised hosts,* that is, clients whose normal defences have been lowered by surgery or illness. The hands of personnel serve as a common vehicle for the spread of microorganisms. *Insufficient hand hygiene* is thus an important factor contributing to the spread of organisms in health-care settings.

A point prevalence study conducted by the Canadian Nosocomial Infection Surveillance Program (2002) found that 10.5% of hospitalized adults and 9.1% of children had a health-care-associated infection. The cost of health-care-associated infections to the client, the facility, and the funding sources (e.g., insurance companies and federal, provincial and territorial, or local governments) is great. These infections extend hospitalization time, increase clients' time away from work, cause disability and discomfort, and even result in loss of life. See Table 32.2 for common health-care-associated infections.

TABLE 32.2 Health-Care-Associated Infections

Most Common Microorganisms	Causes
Urinary Tract	
Escherichia coli	Catheterization technique
Enterococcus species	Contamination of closed drainage system
Pseudomonas aeruginosa	Inadequate hand hygiene
Surgical Sites	
Staphylococcus aureus (including methicillin-resistant strains [MRSA])	Inadequate hand hygiene
Enterococcus species (including vancomycin-resistant strains [VRE])	Inadequate preparative skin preparation or antibiotic prophylaxis
Pseudomonas aeruginosa	Contaminated water
Bloodstream	
Coagulase-negative staphylococci	Inadequate hand hygiene
Staphylococcus aureus	Improper intravenous fluid, tubing, and site care technique
Enterococcus species	Inadequate hand hygiene, contamination from feces
Hepatitis B	Needle puncture
Pneumonia	
Staphylococcus aureus	Inadequate hand hygiene
Pseudomonas aeruginosa	Improper suctioning technique
Enterobacter species	
Gastrointestrial	
Norovirus	Inadequate hand hygiene

Types of Organisms Causing Infections

Five major categories of microorganisms cause infection in humans: bacteria, viruses, fungi, protozoa, and helminths. **Bacteria**, by far the most common infection-causing microorganisms, are large enough to be seen with a light microscope, can replicate outside of host cells, and are fairly easily grown in a laboratory. Several hundred species can cause disease in humans and can live and be transported through air, water, food, soil, body tissues and fluids, and inanimate objects. Most of the organisms in Table 32.2 are bacteria.

Viruses consist primarily of nucleic acid and lipoproteins and therefore must enter living cells in order to reproduce. They can be seen only with an electron microscope and cannot easily be grown in most hospital laboratories. Common viruses include rhinoviruses (which cause the common cold), influenza, hepatitis, herpes, and human immunodeficiency virus (HIV). **Fungi** include yeasts and moulds. *Candida albicans* is a yeast considered to be normal flora in the human vagina.

Protozoa are single-celled organisms, while **helminths** (worms) are multicelled organisms. Both are classified as **parasites** as they live on other living organisms with benefit only to themselves. Few cause health-care-associated infections, although some, such as the protozoa that cause malaria, present enormous public health challenges.

Bacteria, some fungi, and some protozoa are susceptible to antibiotics, while viruses are not. A limited number of available antiviral drugs are effective for certain viral infections. Other classes of drugs are used to treat infections caused by protozoa and helminths.

Some microorganisms affect only specific tissues, resulting in a predictable clinical picture. For example, rhinoviruses infect the nasopharynx causing signs and symptoms of the common cold, while the hepatitis B virus infects only the liver, resulting in the jaundice of hepatitis. Other microorganisms can infect a variety of tissues. For example, *Staphylococcus* species can cause skin infections, pneumonia, and gastroenteritis. Many different microorganisms can therefore cause a similar disease, such as pneumonia or diarrhea. Health assessment and laboratory testing are necessary to determine the exact infectious agent in any particular case of infection.

Microorganisms also vary in the severity of the diseases they produce and their degree of **communicability**, that is, their ability to be spread from one person to another. For example, the common cold virus is more readily transmitted than the bacillus that causes leprosy (*Mycobacterium leprae*). If the infectious agent can be transmitted to an individual by direct or indirect contact, through a vector or vehicle, or as an airborne infection, as described later in the chapter, the resulting condition is called a **communicable disease**.

Pathogenicity is the ability to produce disease. Many microorganisms that are normally harmless can cause disease under certain circumstances. A *true pathogen* causes disease or infection in a healthy individual. An **opportunistic pathogen** causes disease only in a susceptible individual. Pathogens vary in their **virulence**, that is, their power to overcome the host's defences. Different species have different **virulence factors** or evasion mechanisms, such as proteins that strengthen adherence to target cells, affect motility, or promote resistance to acid, enzymes, or antibiotics. Bacteria that acquire resistance to certain antibiotics frequently become resistant to many classes of antibiotics, reducing treatment options and effectiveness. Some microorganisms, such as the measles virus, have the ability to infect almost all susceptible people after exposure. By contrast, such microorganisms as the tuberculosis bacillus infect a relatively small number of the population who are susceptible and exposed, usually people who are poorly nourished or immunocompromised.

Body Defences against Infection

Individuals normally have defences that protect the body from infection when exposed to an infectious agent. These defences can be categorized as nonspecific and specific. **Nonspecific defences** protect the person against all microorganisms, regardless of prior exposure. The **specific defences** of the immune system, by contrast, are directed against identifiable bacteria, viruses, fungi, or other infectious agents recognized by the host from prior exposure.

Nonspecific Defences

Nonspecific body defences include anatomical and physiological barriers and the inflammatory response.

ANATOMICAL AND PHYSIOLOGICAL BARRIERS

Intact skin and mucous membranes are the body's first line of defence against microorganisms. Unless the skin and mucosa become cracked and broken, they are effective barriers against bacteria. Fungi can live on the skin, but they cannot penetrate it. The dryness of the skin also acts as a deterrent to bacteria, which are most plentiful in moist areas of the body, such as the perineum and axillae. Resident bacteria of the skin also prevent other bacteria from multiplying. They use up the available nourishment, and the end products of their metabolism inhibit other bacteria. Normal secretions make the skin slightly acidic; acidity also inhibits bacterial growth.

The nasal passages have a defensive function. As entering air follows the tortuous route of the passage, it comes in contact with moist mucous membranes and *cilia* (tiny hairs). These trap microorganisms, dust, and foreign materials. The *lungs* have alveolar **macrophages** (large phagocytes). **Phagocytes** are cells that ingest microorganisms, other cells, and foreign particles.

Each body orifice also has protective mechanisms. The oral cavity regularly sheds mucosal epithelium to rid the mouth of colonizers. The flow of saliva and its partial buffering action help prevent infections. Saliva contains microbial inhibitors, such as lactoferrin, lysozyme, and secretory IgA.

The *eye* is protected from infection by tears, which continually wash microorganisms away and contain inhibiting lysozyme. The gastrointestinal tract also has defences against infection. The high acidity of the stomach normally prevents microbial growth. The resident flora of the large intestine helps prevent the establishment of disease-producing microorganisms. Peristalsis also tends to move microbes out of the body.

The *vagina* also has natural defences against infection. When a girl reaches puberty, lactobacilli ferment sugars in the vaginal secretions, creating a vaginal pH of 3.5 to 4.5. This low pH inhibits the growth of many disease-producing microorganisms. The entrance to the urethra normally harbours many microorganisms. These include coagulase-negative staphylococci (from the skin) and *Escherichia coli* (from feces). It is believed that the urine flow has a flushing and bacteriostatic action that keeps the bacteria from ascending the urethra. An intact mucosal surface also acts as a barrier.

INFLAMMATORY RESPONSE **Inflammation** is a local and nonspecific defensive response of the tissues to injury or infection. It is an adaptive mechanism that destroys or dilutes the injurious agent, prevents further spread of the injury, and promotes the repair of damaged tissue. Five signs characterize inflammation: (1) pain, (2) swelling, (3) redness, (4) heat, and (5) impaired function of the body part, if the injury is severe. Commonly, words with the suffix *-itis* describe an inflammatory process. For example, *appendicitis* means inflammation of the appendix; *gastritis* means inflammation of the stomach lining.

Injurious stressors to body tissues can be categorized as physical agents, chemical agents, and microorganisms. *Physical agents* include mechanical objects causing trauma to tissues, excessive heat or cold, and radiation. *Chemical agents* include external irritants (e.g., strong acids, alkalis, poisons, and irritating gases) and internal irritants (substances manufactured within the body, such as excessive hydrochloric acid in the stomach). *Microorganisms* include the broad groups of bacteria, viruses, fungi, protozoa, and helminths.

The inflammatory response involves a series of dynamic events commonly referred to as the three stages of the inflammatory response:

1. *First stage:* Vascular and cellular responses
2. *Second stage:* Exudate production
3. *Third stage:* Reparative phase

VASCULAR AND CELLULAR RESPONSES At the start of the first stage of inflammation, the damage to tissue cells caused by the infectious agent leads to synthesis of prostaglandins and leukotrienes from the damaged cell membranes, release of serotonin and histamine from platelets and mast cells or basophils, respectively, and activation of bradykinin. These chemical mediators cause constriction of the blood vessels at the site of injury, lasting only a few moments. This initial vasoconstriction is rapidly followed by dilation of small blood vessels, caused by the same chemical mediators. Thus, more blood flows to the injured area. This marked increase in blood supply is referred to as **hyperemia** and is responsible for the characteristic signs of redness and heat as warm blood flows to the surface.

Most of these chemical mediators also cause increased vascular permeability at the injured site. The result of this altered permeability is an outpouring of fluid, proteins, and leukocytes into the interstitial spaces, clinically manifested by the characteristic inflammatory signs of edema (swelling) and pain. The pain is caused by the pressure of accumulating fluid on local nerve endings and by stimulation of pain receptors by the chemical mediators. Too much fluid pouring into such areas as the pleural or pericardial cavity can seriously affect organ function. In other areas, such as joints, mobility is impaired. Chemical mediators will also stimulate mucous production if the site of infection involves a mucous membrane (e.g., infection of the bronchi) or stimulate smooth muscle contraction if the site of infection has smooth muscle. For example, in the lung, smooth muscle contraction leads to bronchospasm, while in the gastrointestinal tract, smooth muscle contraction leads to increased peristalsis and thus diarrhea.

Blood flow slows in the dilated vessels, allowing more **leukocytes** (white blood cells) to arrive at the injured tissues. When the blood flow slows, leukocytes aggregate or line up along this inner surface of the blood vessels. This process is known as **margination**. Leukocytes then move between the cells of the now permeable blood vessel wall into the affected tissue spaces, a process called **emigration.**

The actual passage of blood corpuscles through the blood vessel wall is referred to as **diapedesis**. Leukocytes are attracted to injured cells by **chemotaxis.**

In response to the exit of leukocytes from the blood vessels, the bone marrow produces large numbers of leukocytes and releases them into the bloodstream (**leukocytosis**). A number of **cytokines** (chemical mediators) produced by the leukocytes are responsible for stimulating this increase. An increase in white blood cell count is a sign associated with inflammation. A normal leukocyte count of 4.5×10^9/L to 11×10^9/L of blood can rise to 20×10^9/L or more when extensive inflammation occurs. Cytokines released from the leukocytes or molecules associated with bacterial cell walls also act as **pyrogens**, stimulating the production of fever.

Exudate Production In the second stage of inflammation, the inflammatory **exudate** is produced, consisting of fluid that escaped from the blood vessels, dead phagocytic cells, dead bacteria and dead tissue cells, and the products that they release. Exudate that contains leukocytes is called **pus**; it is frequently yellow because of the colour of the cells as they age. The nature and amount of exudate vary according to the tissue involved and the intensity and duration of the inflammation. The major types of exudate are *serous* (clear, containing serum but no cells), *sanguinous* (containing red blood cells), and *purulent* (containing pus).

Thromboplastin (a product released by injured tissue cells) initiates the coagulation pathway, resulting in a plasma protein called **fibrinogen** being converted to fibrin. Threads of fibrin and platelets together form an interlacing network to make a barrier, wall off the area, and prevent spread of the injurious agent. During the second stage, the injurious agent is destroyed by leukocytes, and the exudate is cleared away by lymphatic drainage.

Reparative Phase The third stage of the inflammatory response involves the repair of injured tissues by regeneration or replacement with fibrous tissue (scar) formation. **Regeneration** is the replacement of destroyed tissue cells by cells that are identical or similar in structure and function. It involves not only replacement of damaged cells one by one but also organization of these cells so that the architectural pattern and function of the tissue are restored. The ability to reproduce cells varies considerably from one type of tissue to another. For example, epithelial tissues of the skin and of the digestive and respiratory tracts have a good regenerative capacity, provided that their underlying support structures are intact. The same holds true for osseous, lymphoid, and bone marrow tissues. Tissues that have little regenerative capacity include nervous, muscular, and elastic tissues.

When regeneration is not possible, repair occurs by *fibrous tissue formation*. **Fibrous (scar) tissue** has the capacity to proliferate under the unusual conditions of ischemia and altered pH. The inflammatory exudate with its interlacing network of fibrin provides the framework for this tissue to develop. Damaged tissues are replaced with the connective tissue elements of collagen, blood capillaries, lymphatics, and other tissue-bound substances. In the early stages of this process, the tissue is called **granulation tissue**. It is a fragile, gelatinous tissue, appearing pink or red because of the many newly formed capillaries. Later in the process, the tissue shrinks (the capillaries are constricted, even obliterated) and the collagen fibres contract so that a firmer fibrous tissue remains. This is called **cicatrix** or scar.

Specific Defences

Specific defences of the body involve the immune system, which responds to foreign proteins in the body (e.g., bacteria or transplanted tissues). In some cases, the immune system even responds to the body's own proteins. Foreign proteins in the body are called **antigens** and are considered invaders. If the proteins originate in a person's own body, the antigen is called an **autoantigen**. Immunity is the specific resistance of the body to infection (pathogens or their toxins). Acquired immunity has two major types: active and passive. See Table 32.3. In **active immunity**, the host produces its own antibodies in response to natural antigens (e.g., infection) or artificial antigens (e.g., vaccines). With **passive immunity**, the host receives antibodies produced by another source, either natural (e.g., from a nursing mother) or artificial (e.g., from an injection of immune serum).

ANTIBODY-MEDIATED DEFENCES Another name for the *antibody-mediated defences* is **humoral (circulating) immunity**. **Antibodies**, also called **immunoglobulins**, are

TABLE 32.3 Types of Acquired Immunity

Type	Antigen or Antibody Source	Duration
1. Active	Antibodies are produced by the body in response to an antigen.	Long
a. Natural	Antibodies are formed in the presence of active infection in the body.	Lifelong
b. Artificial	Antigens (vaccines or toxoids) are administered to stimulate antibody production.	Many years: the immunity must be reinforced by booster inoculations
2. Passive	Antibodies are produced by another source, animal or human.	Short
a. Natural	Antibodies are transferred naturally from an immune mother to her baby through the placenta or in colostrum.	6 months to 1 year
b. Artificial	Immune serum (antibody) from an animal or another human is injected.	2 to 3 weeks

part of the body's plasma proteins. B lymphocytes are activated when they recognize a foreign invader, an antigen. They then differentiate into plasma cells, which secrete antibodies that bind specifically to the foreign antigen. This results in *neutralization* of a virus or toxin so it cannot enter or injure the target host cell, or *opsonization* (coating) of a bacterial cell to make it more attractive to leukocytes. The antigen-antibody complex also activates the complement system, which initiates inflammation and further helps eliminate the foreign invader. The antibody-mediated responses defend primarily against bacterial infection by opsonizing bacteria that are replicating in tissue and against viral infection by neutralizing viruses in the bloodstream before they enter host cells (i.e., in the extracellular phase).

Immunoglobulins (Ig) are divided into five classes, written as follows: IgM, IgG, IgA, IgD, and IgE. IgM, IgG, and IgA act in the protective function just described. They differ in that IgM and IgG are found in the bloodstream, while IgA is generally found in mucous membrane secretions. IgM is produced early and lasts only a short time; IgM to measles virus infection, for example, lasts about 1 month after the infection. The presence of IgM in a laboratory analysis therefore shows current or very recent infection. IgG or IgA are produced later and can last a very long time (years or decades for some infectious agents). On second or subsequent exposure to the same antigen, only IgG or IgA are produced, at a much faster rate than occurs after the initial infection.

IgD has no direct protective function. It acts as an antigen receptor for B lymphocytes. IgE is also not involved in the protective response to infectious agents. It is the key mediator in allergic reactions.

CELL-MEDIATED DEFENCES The **cell-mediated defences**, or **cellular immunity**, occur through the T-cell system. On exposure to an antigen, the lymphoid tissues release large numbers of activated T cells into the lymph system. These T cells pass into the general circulation. T cells come in three main groups: (1) *helper T cells*, which help in the activation of both B cells and cytotoxic T cells; (2) *cytotoxic T cells*, which attack and kill microorganisms and sometimes the body's own cells; and (3) *suppressor T cells*, which can suppress the functions of the helper T cells and the cytotoxic T cells. The cytotoxic T cells act against their specific antigen, which may be a part of a bacterial cell wall or an altered host cell (e.g., virus-infected host cell). Prostaglandins are synthesized from the cell membrane damaged by the cytotoxic T cells, initiating inflammation. The cytotoxic T-cell mediated response defends against bacterial infections and against the intracellular phases of viral infections. When cell-mediated immunity is lost, as occurs with HIV infection, an individual is defenceless against most viral, bacterial, and fungal infections.

Pathophysiology of Infection

When an infection occurs, the infectious agent enters the host body, moves to its preferred target site, and overcomes the host defences. It will encounter defences at the site of entry as well as when moving to its target site (e.g., moving in the bloodstream to the liver in the case of hepatitis B virus). At the site of infection, the infectious agent multiplies, causing physical damage to the host cells. Bacteria replicate outside host cells within the tissue, taking up space and putting physical pressure on host cells, thereby damaging them. Some bacteria also produce a toxin that gets absorbed into the bloodstream and moves to other cells, damaging them. Viruses enter host cells and take over their protein-synthesizing machinery (ribosomes) so that the host cell then produces **virions** (new virus particles). The virions exit the host cell through *exocytosis* (budding from the cell membrane) or by causing *lysis* (destruction) of the host cell. The virions move into neighbouring cells to infect them, repeating the cycle.

Damage to the host cell initiates the inflammatory response, while recognition of the infectious agent by the immune system leads to antibody-mediated or cytotoxic T-cell-mediated immune responses, both of which ultimately also promote inflammation. The white blood cells called in by the inflammatory and immune responses destroy the infectious agents and initiate phagocytosis and repair of the damaged tissue.

Clinical manifestations of infection result from both altered function of the damaged tissue and from the inflammatory response that is initiated in defence. Classic signs and symptoms of infection related to inflammation are redness and swelling at the site of infection, local pain, presence of purulent exudate, fever, and elevated leukocyte count. The clinical manifestations associated with altered tissue function depend on the tissue involved. For example, mucous production and edema of the airways with pneumonia lead to altered gas exchange and thus hypoxia, while with hepatitis, the damage that occurs to the ability of liver cells to conjugate bilirubin leads to the accumulation of bilirubin and results in jaundice.

The Clinical Spectrum of Infection

Colonization is the process by which strains of microorganisms become resident flora. In this state, the microorganisms may grow and multiply but do not cause physiological changes in host tissue. The presence of colonizing bacteria does not mean the person has an infection. Infection occurs when newly introduced or resident microorganisms succeed in invading a part of the body in which the host's defence mechanisms are ineffective and the pathogen causes tissue damage. If tissue damage is localized to a few cells or a small part of the tissue, then changes may not be noticeable unless they are looked for specifically with relevant types of testing. When this occurs and there is no clinical evidence of disease, the infection is called *asymptomatic* or *subclinical*. Some subclinical infections can cause significant damage, however. For example, cytomegalovirus infection in a pregnant woman can lead to significant disease in the unborn child. When a detectable alteration in normal tissue function occurs, the infection is called *overt* and presents as disease.

Infections can be local or systemic. A **local infection** is limited to the specific part of the body in which the microorganisms remain. If the microorganisms spread and damage different parts of the body, it is a **systemic infection**. When a culture of the person's blood reveals microorganisms, the condition is called *bacteremia*. When bacteremia results in systemic infection, it is referred to as **septicemia.**

Infections are also acute or chronic. Acute infections generally appear suddenly or last a short time. A chronic infection may occur slowly, over a very long period, and can last months or years.

A **carrier** is a person or an animal that harbours a specific infectious agent and serves as a potential source of infection yet does not manifest any clinical signs of disease. The carrier state can also exist in the incubation period, convalescence, and post-convalescence of an individual with a clinically recognizable disease. This type of carrier is referred to as an *incubatory* or *convalescent carrier.* Under either circumstance, the carrier state can be of short duration (*temporary* or *transient carrier*) or long duration (*chronic carrier*).

Infection: An Imbalance between Microorganisms and Defences

Given the defence mechanisms available, it should be clear that the very presence of a microorganism entering the body is not enough to determine that an infection will occur. For an infection to occur, the microorganisms have to overcome the defences. This defeat can occur in the following cases:

- The microorganisms are highly virulent (even if present in small numbers) and so are able to overcome normal defence mechanisms.
- The **microbial load** (number of infectious agents present) is greater than the number that the available defence mechanisms can handle quickly, so the microorganisms are able to proliferate.
- Defence mechanisms are reduced or compromised, and thus host resistance is low, so that the host cannot overcome a microbial load that he or she would be expected to normally be able to handle.

Reducing the risk of infection therefore involves ensuring that defences are greater than the microorganisms' ability to overcome them. This goal can be accomplished by either reducing microbial load or strengthening host resistance. Both can be accomplished in clinical practice, while it is not possible to directly affect virulence.

The chain of infection is an important framework for understanding how microorganisms enter a host or move from one to another. Breaking any link in the chain is the key to infection prevention and control.

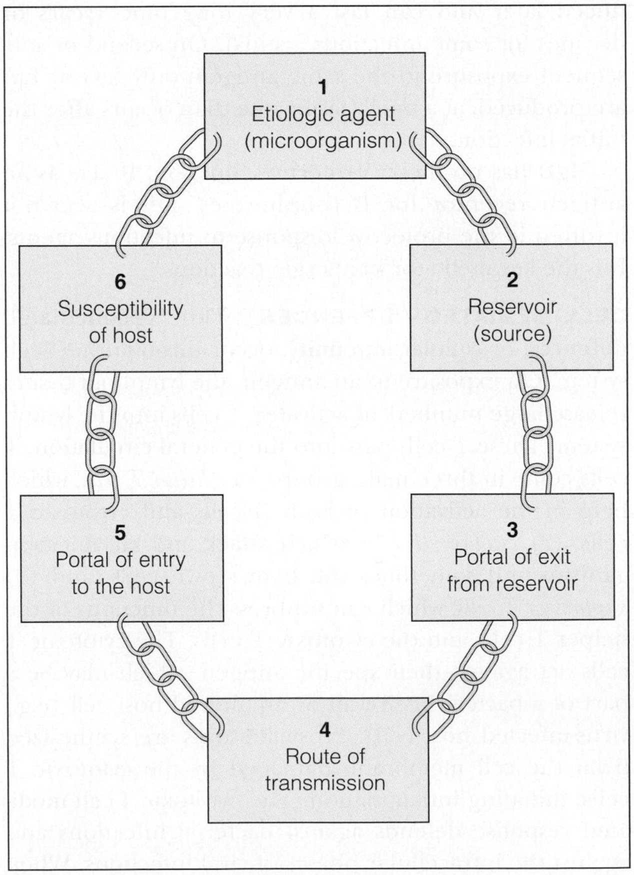

FIGURE 32.1 The chain of infection

The Chain of Infection

Six links make up the chain of infection (Figure 32.1): (1) the etiological agent or microorganism, (2) the place in which the organism naturally resides (reservoir), (3) a portal of exit from the reservoir, (4) a route (mode) of transmission, (5) a portal of entry into a host, and (6) the susceptibility of the host.

Etiological Agent

The extent to which any microorganism is capable of producing an infectious process depends on the number of organisms present, the virulence and pathogenicity of the organisms, the ability of the organisms to enter the body, the susceptibility of the host, and the ability of the organisms to live in the host's body. The presence of an infectious agent is a necessary condition for an infection to occur, but alone, the mere presence of an infectious agent is insufficient to ensure that an infection will develop.

Reservoir

Many **reservoirs**, or sources of microorganisms, exist. Common sources are other humans, the client's own microorganisms, plants, animals, or the general environment. People are the most common source of infection for others and for themselves. For example, the person with an influenza virus frequently spreads it to others. When resistance is lowered by fatigue and other factors, an infection may develop.

Insects, birds, and other animals are common reservoirs of infection. For example, the *Anopheles* mosquito carries the malaria parasite. Food, water, milk, and feces also can be reservoirs. In hospitals, urinary catheters, wound dressings contaminated with purulent exudates, oxygen humidity canisters, and contaminated bedside surfaces are all examples of reservoirs.

Portal of Exit from Reservoir

Before an infection can establish itself in a host, the microorganisms must leave the reservoir. Common human reservoirs and their associated portals of exit are summarized in Table 32.4.

Route of Transmission

After a microorganism leaves its source or reservoir, it requires a route of transmission to reach another person or host through a *receptive portal of entry*. There are six possible routes: (1) direct contact, (2) indirect contact,

TABLE 32.4 Human Reservoirs, Common Infectious Microorganisms, and Portals of Exit

Body Area (Source)	Common Infectious Organisms	Portals of Exit
Respiratory tract	Parainfluenza virus *Mycobacterium tuberculosis* *Staphylococcus aureus*	Nose or mouth through sneezing, coughing, breathing, or talking; endotracheal tubes or tracheostomies
Gastrointestinal tract	Hepatitis A virus *Salmonella* species	Mouth: saliva, vomitus; anus: feces; ostomies; drainage tubes (e.g., nasogastric or T-tubes)
Urinary tract	*Escherichia coli* enterococci Enterococci *Pseudomonas aeruginosa*	Urethral meatus and urinary diversion ostomies
Reproductive tract (including genitals)	*Neisseria gonorrhoeae* *Treponema pallidum* Herpes simplex virus type 2 Hepatitis B virus	Vagina: vaginal discharge; urinary meatus: semen, urine; urethral discharge; contaminated urine
Blood	Hepatitis B virus Human immunodeficiency virus (HIV) *Staphylococcus aureus* Coagulase-negative staphylococci	Open wound, needle puncture site, any disruption of intact skin or mucous membrane surfaces
Tissue	*Staphylococcus aureus* *Escherichia coli* *Proteus* species Beta-hemolytic *streptococcus* group A or B	Drainage from cut or wound

(3) droplet transmission, (4) airborne transmission, (5) vehicle-borne transmission, and (6) vector-borne transmission.

DIRECT CONTACT TRANSMISSION **Direct contact transmission** involves immediate and direct transfer of microorganisms from person to person through touching, biting, kissing, or sexual intercourse, that is, body surface to body surface.

INDIRECT CONTACT TRANSMISSION **Indirect contact transmission** involves passive transfer from the reservoir to an intermediate inanimate object in the recipient's immediate environment and then to the recipient (e.g., hands touch a contaminated doorknob, pick up microorganisms, and transfer them to the recipient's mucous membrane). The length of time that the microorganism remains infectious on inanimate surfaces depends on the microorganism and the relative humidity and temperature of the environment.

DROPLET TRANSMISSION **Droplet transmission** is also a form of direct contact but is usually considered separately as it requires different interventions. Droplets are large droplets of respiratory secretions, larger than 5 microns in diameter. They are generated from sneezing (see Figure 32.2), coughing, spitting, singing, talking, or procedures, such as suctioning. Droplets can be projected a short distance but do not remain suspended in air for long. The larger the particle, the faster it falls. About 85% of the droplets generated by an average sneeze or closed-mouth cough, and 92% of those generated by an open-mouth cough, are larger than 20 microns and will take less than 4 minutes to fall 3 metres (Evans, 2000). If the source and the recipient are within this distance of each other, the droplet spray can be deposited into the conjunctiva or onto the mucous membranes of the eye, nose, or mouth of the recipient. This route transmits the majority of agents causing respiratory infections. Droplets also contaminate the local environment, contributing to indirect contact transmission.

AIRBORNE TRANSMISSION **Airborne transmission** can involve droplet nuclei, which have an average size of less than 5 microns, or dust. **Droplet nuclei**, the residue of evaporated droplets emitted from an infected host, such as someone with tuberculosis, can remain in the air for long periods. Dust particles containing an infectious agent (e.g., varicella virus) can also become airborne. The material is transmitted by air currents to a suitable portal of entry, usually the respiratory tract, of another person. The droplet nuclei are inhaled into the lower respiratory tract and are also deposited on the person's mucous membranes. Very few infectious agents are spread by airborne transmission: tuberculosis, varicella, measles, and smallpox.

VEHICLE-BORNE TRANSMISSION In **vehicle-borne transmission**, a *vehicle* is any substance that serves as an intermediate means to transport and introduce an infectious agent into a susceptible host through a suitable portal of entry. *Fomites* (inanimate materials or objects), such as handkerchiefs, toys, soiled clothes, cooking or eating utensils, and surgical instruments or dressings, can act as vehicles. Water, food, milk, blood, serum, and plasma are other vehicles. For example, a food handler who carries the hepatitis A virus may contaminate food or water with fecal particles. A susceptible host then ingests the food. This is called the **fecal-oral route** of transmission, with the contaminated food acting as the vehicle.

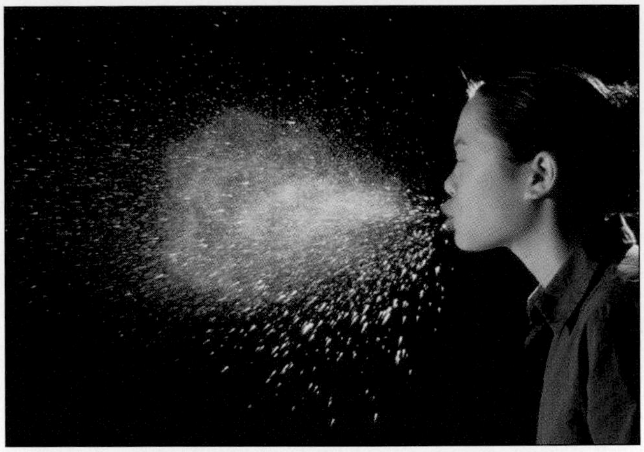

FIGURE 32.2 Droplet dispersion from a sneeze

VECTOR-BORNE TRANSMISSION A *vector* is an animal or insect that serves as an intermediate means of transporting the infectious agent. **Vector-borne transmission** can occur when salivary fluid is injected during biting or when feces or other materials are deposited on the skin through the bite wound or a traumatized skin area.

Portal of Entry to the Host

Before a person can become infected, microorganisms must enter the body. The skin is a barrier to infectious agents; however, any break in the skin can readily serve as a portal of entry. Other examples of portals of entry are the mucous membranes of the eyes, the respiratory tract, the gastrointestinal tract, or the bloodstream (e.g., with intravenous administration). Often, microorganisms enter the body of the host by the same route they used to leave the source.

Susceptibility of the Host

A **susceptible host** is any person who is at risk for infection. **Compromised hosts** are persons at increased risk, individuals who, for one or more reasons, are more likely than others to develop an infection. Impairment of the body's natural defences and a number of other factors can affect susceptibility to infection.

FACTORS INCREASING SUSCEPTIBILITY TO INFECTION Whether a microorganism causes an infection depends on a number of factors previously mentioned. One of the most important factors is host susceptibility, which is affected by age, immune status, heredity, level of stress, nutritional status, current medical therapy, obesity, smoking, existing disease processes, and some past or recent surgical interventions.

Age influences the risk of infection (see the Lifespan Considerations box). Newborns and older adults have reduced defences against infection. Infections are a major cause of death among newborns, who have immature immune systems and are protected only for the first 2 or 3 months by immunoglobulins passively received from the mother. Between 1 and 3 months of age, infants begin to synthesize their own immunoglobulins. Immunizations against diphtheria, tetanus, pertussis, and polio are usually started at 2 months, when the infant's immune system can respond. Immunizations are discussed later in the chapter.

Lifespan Considerations

Infections

CHILDREN

Infections are an expected part of childhood, with most children experiencing some kind of infection from time to time. The majority of these infections are caused by viruses and, for the most part, are transient, relatively benign, and overcome by the body's natural defences and supportive care. In some cases, severe, even life-threatening, infections occur. Considerations related to children include the following:

- Newborns may not be able to respond to infections because of an underdeveloped immune system. As a result, in the first few months of life, infections may not be associated with typical signs and symptoms (e.g., an infant with an infection may not have a fever).
- Newborns have some naturally acquired immunity transferred from the mother across the placenta.
- Breastfed infants enjoy higher levels of immunity against infections than formula-fed infants do.
- Fevers lower than 39°C in children should not be treated, except for comfort of the child.
- Children between 6 months and 5 years are at higher risk for febrile (fever-induced) seizures. Febrile seizures are not associated with neurological seizure disorders (e.g., epilepsy).
- Children who are immune compromised (e.g., leukemia, HIV) or have a chronic health condition (e.g., cystic fibrosis, sickle-cell anemia, congenital heart disease) need extra precautions to prevent exposure to infectious agents.
- Hand hygiene, comprehensive immunizations, good nutrition, adequate hydration, and appropriate rest are essential to preventing and treating infections in children.
- Handwashing and good hygiene in daycare and schools are important to prevent the spread of infections.
- Adolescents are at high risk for sexually transmitted infections and should be well educated about how to prevent infections.

OLDER ADULTS

Normal aging may predispose older adults to increased risk of infection and delayed healing. Anatomical and physiological agents that are protective when a person is younger often change in structure and function with increasing age, and the protective ability of those agents decreases. Changes take place in the skin, respiratory tract, gastrointestinal system, kidneys, and immune system. If unchallenged, these systems work well to maintain homeostasis for the individual, but if compromised by stress, illness, infections, treatments, or surgeries, they often cannot keep up and therefore are not able to provide adequate protection. Special considerations for older adults are as follows:

- Nutrition can be poor in older adults and certain components, especially adequate protein, are necessary to build up and maintain the immune system.
- Diabetes mellitus, which occurs more frequently in older adults, increases the risk of infection and delayed healing by causing an alteration in nutrition and impaired peripheral circulation, which decrease the oxygen transport to the tissues.
- The immune system reacts slowly to the introduction of antigens, allowing the antigen to reproduce itself several times before it is recognized by the immune system. T-cell effectiveness is often decreased because of immaturity.
- The normal inflammatory response is delayed. This delay often causes atypical responses to infections with unusual presentations. Instead of displaying redness, swelling, and fever usually associated with infections, atypical symptoms, such as confusion and disorientation, agitation, incontinence, falls, lethargy, and general fatigue, are often seen first.

Recognizing these changes in older adults is important in early detection and treatment of infections and to avoid delayed healing. The following nursing interventions promote prevention:

- Provide and teach ways to improve nutritional status.
- Use strict aseptic technique to decrease chance of infections (especially health-care-associated infections in health-care facilities).
- Encourage older adults to have regular immunizations for influenza and pneumonia.
- Be alert to subtle atypical signs of infection and act quickly to diagnose and treat.

With advancing age, the immune responses again weaken. Although much is still to be learned about aging, it is known that immunity to infection decreases with age. Because of the prevalence of influenza and pneumonia and their potential for causing death, the National Advisory Committee on Immunization (2007a) recommends annual immunization against influenza for older adults, for the very young, and for persons with chronic cardiac, respiratory, metabolic, and renal diseases, and those capable of transmitting influenza to these individuals.

Immune status is an important factor for host susceptibility or resistance to a specific infectious agent. The presence of antibodies from prior exposure, either by natural infection or vaccination, will act to destroy the infectious agent when encountered again before it can lead to infection. **Immunization** or **vaccination** is therefore an important strategy for decreasing host susceptibility, although not all infections are vaccine preventable.

Heredity influences the development of infection in that some people have a genetic susceptibility to certain infections. For example, some may be deficient in serum immunoglobulins, which play a significant role in the internal defence mechanisms of the body.

The nature, number, and duration of physical and emotional *stressors* can influence susceptibility to infection. Stressors elevate blood cortisol. Prolonged elevation of blood cortisol decreases inflammatory and immune responses, depletes energy stores, leads to a state of exhaustion, and decreases resistance to infection. For example, a person recovering from a major operation or injury is more likely to develop an infection than is a healthy person.

Resistance to infection depends on adequate *nutritional status.* Because antibodies are proteins, the ability to synthesize antibodies can be impaired by inadequate nutrition, especially when protein reserves are depleted (e.g., as a result of injury, surgery, or debilitating diseases, such as cancer).

Some *medical therapies* predispose a person to infection. Radiation treatments for cancer destroy not only cancerous cells but also some normal cells, thereby damaging normal defences or barriers. Some *diagnostic procedures* can also predispose the client to an infection, especially when the skin is broken or sterile body cavities are penetrated during the procedure. Certain *medications* also increase susceptibility to infection. Antineoplastic (anticancer) medications can depress bone marrow function, resulting in inadequate production of white blood cells necessary to combat infections. Anti-inflammatory medications, such as corticosteroids, inhibit the inflammatory response that is an essential defence against infection. Even some antibiotics that are used to treat infections can have adverse effects. Antibiotics may kill resident flora, allowing the proliferation of strains that would not grow and multiply in the body under normal conditions. *Clostridium difficile* infection, for example, is associated with antibiotic use. Certain antibiotics can also induce antibiotic resistance in some strains of organisms, making such infections difficult to treat.

Obesity contributes to infection because it is associated with decreased blood flow to skin and underlying tissue. Delivery of oxygen, nutrients, and leukocytes is therefore compromised, interfering with both rapid elimination of infectious agents and tissue repair.

Smoking increases susceptibility to infection by damaging respiratory defences and by impairing tissue oxygenation. Oxygen is important to tissue maintenance and repair, and to the energy production required for the inflammatory and immune responses. Any situation that leads to tissue hypoxia, such as smoking, compromised blood flow, or *anemia,* will increase susceptibility to infection.

Any *disease* that lessens the body's defences against infection places the client at risk. Examples are chronic pulmonary disease, which impairs ciliary action and weakens the mucous barrier; peripheral vascular disease, which restricts blood flow; burns, which impair skin integrity; chronic or debilitating diseases, which deplete protein reserves; and such immune system diseases as leukemia and aplastic anemia, which alter the production of white blood cells. *Diabetes mellitus* is a major underlying disease predisposing clients to infection for a number of reasons. For example, glycosylation of hemoglobin and other proteins impairs oxygenation of tissues and disrupts leukocyte function (critical to phagocytosis). Increased serum glucose levels also provide a source of energy that will support bacterial growth.

Previous surgery at the same site can increase risk of infection because scar tissue has reduced blood supply, interfering with delivery of leukocytes, oxygen, and nutrients.

Breaking the Chain: Prevention and Control of Health-Care-Associated Infections

The key to the prevention and control of infection is breaking one of the links in the chain of infection. Doing so can either prevent a new infection from occurring or realign an imbalance between the numbers of microorganisms and the host defence mechanisms to promote more rapid recovery from an existing infection. Many health-care-associated infections can be disrupted by (1) eliminating microorganisms and their reservoirs; (2) reducing transmission through the use of proper hand hygiene, the use of personal protective equipment to protect portals of entry, and the use of aseptic and sterile technique when warranted; and (3) supporting host defences or reducing susceptibility. Identification of clients at risk and implementation of appropriate strategies are essential aspects of infection prevention and control. Tables 32.5 and 32.6 summarize nursing interventions that break the chain of infection.

Elimination of Microorganisms and Reservoirs

The first links in the chain, the etiological agent (i.e., microorganism) and the reservoir, are interrupted by a variety of strategies. Some reservoirs can be physically eliminated or reduced, for example, through removal and proper disposal of contaminated dressings, frequent emptying of catheter bags, or replacement of contaminated oxygen equipment. Other reservoirs can be affected through decontamination or antimicrobial agents.

DECONTAMINATION Decontamination has three levels: cleaning, disinfecting, and sterilizing. These are important for reducing infections caused by exogenous flora from the environment or transmitted through equipment or other materials. Items usually should be cleaned before being disinfected or sterilized. Items intended for single-use should be discarded and not processed for reuse.

CLEANING Cleaning physically removes contaminants (e.g., fluids and microorganisms) with detergent and mechanical removal. Cleaning is the lowest level of decontamination and is appropriate for items used on intact skin. When cleaning visibly soiled objects, nurses must always wear gloves to avoid direct contact with infectious microorganisms. Most objects used in the care of clients, whether forceps or draw sheets, can be cleaned by rinsing them in cold water to remove any organic material, washing them with hot soapy water, then rinsing them again to remove the soap. The following steps should be followed when cleaning objects in a hospital or in a home:

1. Rinse the article with cold water to remove organic material. Hot water coagulates the protein of organic material and tends to make it adhere. Examples of organic material are blood, pus, and respiratory secretions.

TABLE 32.5 Nursing Interventions That Break the Chain of Infection: Infectious Agent and Reservoir

Link	Interventions	Rationale
Etiologic agent (microorganism)	Ensure that articles are correctly cleaned and disinfected or sterilized before use.	Correct cleaning, disinfecting, and sterilizing reduce or eliminate microorganisms.
	Educate clients and support persons about appropriate methods to clean, disinfect, and sterilize articles.	Knowledge of ways to reduce or eliminate microorganisms is a step in the direction of gaining compliance with aseptic practices.
Reservoir (source)	Change dressings and bandages when they are soiled or wet.	Moist dressings are ideal environments for microorganisms to grow and multiply.
	Assist clients to carry out appropriate skin and oral hygiene.	Hygiene measures reduce the numbers of resident and transient microorganisms and the likelihood of infection.
	Dispose of damp, soiled linens appropriately.	Damp, soiled linens provide an environment for microorganism growth.
	Dispose of feces and urine in appropriate receptacles.	Urine and feces contain many microorganisms. Feces may also be the source of certain microorganisms, such as the hepatitis A virus, in asymptomatic carriers.
	Ensure that all fluid containers, such as bedside water jugs and suction and drainage bottles, are covered or capped.	Prolonged exposure increases the risk of contamination by airborne pathogens.
	Empty suction and drainage bottles at the end of each shift or before they become full or according to agency policy.	Drainage harbours microorganisms that, if left for long periods, proliferate and are at risk for transmission to others.
Portal of exit from the reservoir	Avoid talking, coughing, or sneezing over open wounds or sterile fields, and cover the mouth and nose when coughing and sneezing.	These measures limit the number of microorganisms that escape from the respiratory tract.

TABLE 32.6 Nursing Interventions That Break the Chain of Infection: Transmission and Susceptible Host

Link	Interventions	Rationale
Route of transmission	Perform hand hygiene as per guidelines, for example, between client contacts; after touching blood, any body fluids, or contaminated items; and before performing invasive procedures or touching open wounds. Instruct clients and support persons to perform hand hygiene before handling food or eating, after eliminating, and after touching infectious material.	Hand hygiene is an important means of controlling and preventing the transmission of microorganisms.
	Place discarded soiled materials in moistureproof refuse bags.	Moistureproof bags prevent the spread of microorganisms by capillary action.
	Steadily hold used bedpans away from clothing to prevent spillage, and dispose of urine and feces in appropriate receptacles.	Feces in particular contain many microorganisms.
	Place used bedpans on disposable bed pad, not directly on patient-use surfaces (e.g., overbed table). Avoid splashing when emptying.	Preventing contamination of the patients' environment can reduce transmission of organisms.
	Use routine practice for *all* clients at *all* times, regardless of their diagnosis or presumed infection status.	All clients can harbour potentially infectious microorganisms that can be transmitted to others.
	Wear masks and eye protection when in close contact with clients who have infections transmitted by droplets from the respiratory tract.	Masks and eyewear reduce the spread of droplet-transmitted microorganisms.
	Wear masks and eye protection when sprays of body fluid are possible (e.g., during irrigation procedures).	Masks and eye protection provide protection from microorganisms in clients' blood, body fluids, nonintact skin, and mucous membranes.
	Wear gloves when handling secretions and excretions. Wear gowns if there is danger of soiling clothing with blood, any body fluids, nonintact skin, and mucous membranes.	Gloves and gowns prevent soiling of the hands and clothing.
	Use sterile technique (see p. 898) for invasive procedures (e.g., injections, catheterizations).	Invasive procedures penetrate the body's natural protective barriers to microorganisms.
Portal of entry to the susceptible host	Use sterile technique when exposing open wounds or handling dressings.	Open wounds are vulnerable to microbial infection.
	Place used disposable needles and syringes in puncture-resistant containers for disposal.	Injuries from needles contaminated by blood or body fluids from an infected client or carrier are a primary cause of hepatitis B virus (HBV) and HIV transmission to health-care workers.
	Provide all clients with their own personal care items.	People have less resistance to another person's microorganisms than to their own.
Susceptible host	Maintain the integrity of the client's skin and mucous membranes.	Intact skin and mucous membranes protect against invasion by microorganisms.
	Ensure that the client receives a balanced diet.	A balanced diet supplies proteins and vitamins necessary to build or maintain body tissues.
	Educate the public about the importance of immunizations.	Immunizations protect people against some infectious diseases.

2. Wash the article in hot water and soap. The emulsifying action of soap reduces surface tension and facilitates the removal of dirt. Washing dislodges the emulsified dirt.
3. Use an abrasive, such as a stiff-bristled brush, to clean equipment with grooves and corners. Friction helps dislodge foreign material.
4. Rinse the article well with warm to hot water.
5. Dry the article. It is now considered clean.
6. Clean the brush and sink. These are considered soiled until they are cleaned appropriately, usually with a disinfectant.

DISINFECTING **Disinfection** reduces the number of microorganisms but will not eliminate them all, and it does not kill most spores. It provides a medium level of decontamination and is appropriate for items that have contact with mucous membranes or are contaminated by microorganisms that are easily transmitted. A **disinfectant** is a chemical preparation, such as phenol or iodine compounds, used on inanimate objects. In comparison, an antiseptic is a chemical preparation used on skin or tissue. Disinfectants are frequently caustic and toxic to tissues. Disinfectants and antiseptics often have similar chemical components, but the disinfectant is a more concentrated solution. Disinfectants are able to destroy a variety of pathogens but are ineffective against spores. Table 32.7 lists commonly used antiseptics and disinfectants.

Both antiseptics and disinfectants are said to have bactericidal or bacteriostatic properties. A *bactericidal* preparation destroys bacteria, whereas a *bacteriostatic* preparation prevents the growth and reproduction of some bacteria.

When disinfecting articles, nurses need to follow agency protocols and manufacturer recommendations and consider the following:

1. The type and number of infectious organisms. Some microorganisms are readily destroyed, whereas others require longer contact with the disinfectant.
2. The recommended concentration of the disinfectant and the duration of contact.
3. The temperature of the environment. Most disinfectants are intended for use at room temperature.
4. The presence of soap. Some disinfectants are ineffective in the presence of soap or detergent.
5. The presence of organic materials. The presence of saliva, blood, pus, or excretions can readily inactivate many disinfectants.
6. The surface areas to be treated. The disinfecting agent must come into contact with all surfaces and areas.

STERILIZING **Sterilization** is a process that destroys *all* microorganisms, including spores and viruses. It provides the highest level of decontamination and is indicated for items that penetrate skin or mucous membranes, or enter sterile body areas. Four commonly used methods of sterilization are moist heat, gas, boiling water, and radiation.

Moist Heat For sterilizing, moist heat (steam) can be employed in two ways: as steam under pressure or as free steam. Steam under pressure (autoclave) attains temperatures higher than the boiling point. The time required to sterilize an item relates to how long it takes to destroy spores at the temperature of the autoclave, which varies from 15 minutes at 121°C to 3 minutes at 134°C.

Free steam, 100°C, is used to sterilize objects that would be destroyed at the higher temperature and pressure of the autoclave. Usually, it is necessary to steam the article for 30 minutes on three consecutive days. The intervals are required so that unkilled spores will return to their vegetative state and again become vulnerable to the heat.

Gas Ethylene oxide gas destroys microorganisms by interfering with their metabolic processes. It is also effective against spores. Its advantages are good penetration and effectiveness for heat-sensitive items. Its major disadvantage is its toxicity to humans.

Boiling Water Boiling water is the most practical and inexpensive method for sterilizing in the home. The main disadvantage is that spores and some viruses are not killed by this method. The water temperature rises no higher than 100°C. Boiling a minimum of 15 minutes is advised for disinfection of articles in the home.

TABLE 32.7 Commonly Used Antiseptics and Disinfectants, Effectiveness, and Use

	Effective Against					
Agent	**Bacteria**	**Tuberculosis**	**Spores**	**Fungi**	**Viruses**	**Use on**
Isopropyl and ethyl alcohol	X	X		X	X	Hands, vial stoppers
Chlorine (bleach)	X	X	X	X	X	Blood spills
Hydrogen peroxide	X	X	X	X	X	Surfaces
Iodophors	X	X	X	X	X	Equipment; intact skin and tissues if diluted
Phenol	X	X		X	X	Surfaces
Chlorhexidine gluconate (Hibiclens)	X				X	Hands
Triclosan (Bacti-Stat)	X					Hands, intact skin

Radiation Both ionizing and nonionizing radiation can be used for disinfection and sterilization. Ultraviolet light, a type of nonionizing radiation, can be used for disinfection. Its main drawback is that the ultraviolet rays do not penetrate deeply. Ionizing radiation is used effectively in industry to sterilize foods, drugs, and other items that are sensitive to heat. Its main advantage is that it is effective for items that are difficult to sterilize; its chief disadvantage is that the equipment is very expensive.

Nurses should be familiar with the cleaning, disinfecting, and sterilizing protocols of the agency in which they practise.

ANTIMICROBIAL AGENTS **Antimicrobial agents** kill or slow the growth of infectious agents. Antibiotics or antiviral drugs can reduce the number of infectious agents present in the host, allowing the body's defences to eliminate them. Antibiotics, for example, are given at the start of surgery to reduce the number of bacteria at the surgical site at the time of the incision, thereby reducing surgical site infection. **Antiseptics**, antimicrobial agents that remove both transient and resident flora on living tissue (e.g., skin), are also used to reduce the number of infectious agents present near the site of a surgical incision or insertion point (e.g., for an intravenous line or chest tube). Their use reduces the number of infections caused by the client's endogenous flora.

Reduction of Transmission

The transmission of microorganisms can be reduced through the use of proper hand hygiene, the use of personal protective equipment to protect portals of entry, and the use of aseptic technique when warranted.

HAND HYGIENE The importance of hand hygiene in every setting, including hospitals, cannot be overemphasized. It is considered the single most effective infection prevention and control measure. Any person can harbour microorganisms that are currently harmless yet potentially harmful to that person or to others *if they find a portal of entry*. As a health-care worker's hands are in continuous contact with patients and their environments, those hands are most at risk for contamination with organisms. Subsequent transfer of the organisms to other patients and health-care personnel, to the environment, or to the health-care worker involved might then occur. It is critical that hands be cleaned frequently and correctly. The term **hand hygiene** refers to both handwashing and the use of hand sanitizers.

Handwashing with soap and water physically removes transient microorganisms carried on the hands but not resident flora. Skill 32.1 describes correct handwashing techniques. Using an adequate amount of soap, rubbing the hands together to create friction, covering all surfaces of the hand, ensuring that rinsing occurs under running water, and turning off the tap with a paper towel are essential components of a handwashing procedure. Plain soap will successfully remove most transient microbial flora, whereas antimicrobial (antiseptic) soap is designed for use under conditions of heavy microbial soiling or if antimicrobial-resistant organisms are a factor or a possibility. Soap and sink manufacturers' recommendations should be adhered to for proper use.

SKILL 32.1

HANDWASHING

PURPOSES

- To reduce the number of microorganisms on the hands
- To reduce the risk of cross-contamination among clients
- To reduce the risk of transmission of microorganisms to clients
- To reduce the risk of transmission of infectious organisms to oneself

ASSESSMENT

Determine the client's

- Presence of factors increasing susceptibility to infection and possibility of undiagnosed infection (e.g., HIV)
- Use of immunosuppressive medications
- Recent diagnostic procedures or treatments that penetrated the skin or a body cavity
- Current nutritional status
- Signs and symptoms indicating the presence of an infection:
  - Localized signs, such as swelling, redness, pain or tenderness with palpation or movement, palpable heat at site, loss of function of affected body part, presence of exudate
  - Systemic indications, such as fever, increased pulse and respiratory rates, lack of energy, anorexia, enlarged lymph nodes

Planning

Determine the location of running water and soap or soap substitutes.

Equipment

- Soap
- Warm running water
- Disposable or sanitized towels
- Hand brush (if necessary)

(continued)

SKILL 32.1

HANDWASHING (*continued*)

IMPLEMENTATION

Preparation

Assess the hands.

- Nails should be kept short. **Rationale: Short, natural nails are less likely to harbour microorganisms, scratch a client, or puncture gloves.**
- Remove all jewellery. Some nurses prefer to slide their watches up above their elbows. Others pin the watch to the uniform. **Rationale: Microorganisms can lodge in the settings of jewellery and under rings on fingers. Removal facilitates proper cleaning of the hands and arms.** The jewellery itself also needs to be washed. It is better to not wear it at all.
- Check hands for breaks in the skin, such as hangnails or cuts. Use lotions to prevent hangnails and cracked, dry skin. **Rationale: A nurse who has broken skin areas may have to change work assignments with decreased risk for transmission of infectious organisms or wear gloves for protection.**
- Do not apply fingernail polish or artificial nails. **Rationale: Both can harbour microorganisms.**

Performance

1. If you are washing your hands where the client can observe you, introduce yourself and explain to the client what you are going to do and why it is necessary.
2. Turn on the water, and adjust the flow.
   - Faucet controls have five common types:
     a. Hand-operated handles
     b. Knee levers. Move these with the knee to regulate flow and temperature (see ❶).
     c. Foot pedals. Press these with the foot to regulate flow and temperature (see ❷).
     d. Elbow controls. Move these with the elbows instead of the hands.
     e. Infrared controls. The water runs when motion is detected at a preset distance.
   - Adjust the flow so that the water is warm. **Rationale: Warm water removes less of the protective oil of the skin than does hot water.**
3. Wet the hands thoroughly by holding them under the running water, and apply soap to the hands. Hold the hands lower than the elbows so that the water flows from the arms to the fingertips. **Rationale: The water should flow from the least contaminated to the most contaminated area; the hands are generally considered more contaminated than the lower arms.**
   - If the soap is liquid, apply 2 mL to 5 mL. If it is bar soap, rub it firmly between the hands.
4. Thoroughly wash and rinse the hands.
   - Using firm, rubbing, and circular movements, wash the palm, back, and wrist of each hand. Interlace the fingers and thumbs and move the hands back and forth (see ❸), continuing this motion for *at least* 15 seconds. **Rationale: Friction and brisk action help remove microorganisms mechanically. Interlacing the fingers and thumbs cleans the interdigital spaces.**
   - Rub the fingertips against the palm of the opposite hand. **Rationale: The nails and fingertips are commonly missed during handwashing.**
   - Rinse the hands for at least 10 seconds by using a rubbing motion. **Rationale: This ensures removal of microorganisms.**
5. Thoroughly pat dry the hands and arms.
   - Dry hands and arms thoroughly from fingertips to wrist, without scrubbing, by using a separate paper towel for each arm. **Rationale: Moist skin becomes chapped readily, as does dry skin that is rubbed vigorously; chapping produces lesions.**
   - Discard each paper towel in the appropriate container.

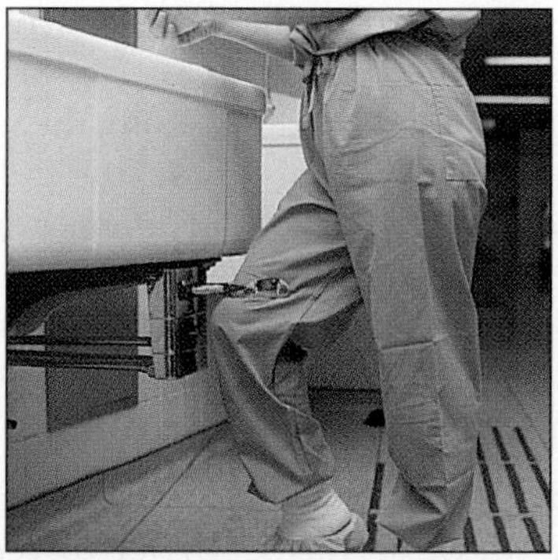

❶ A knee-lever faucet control

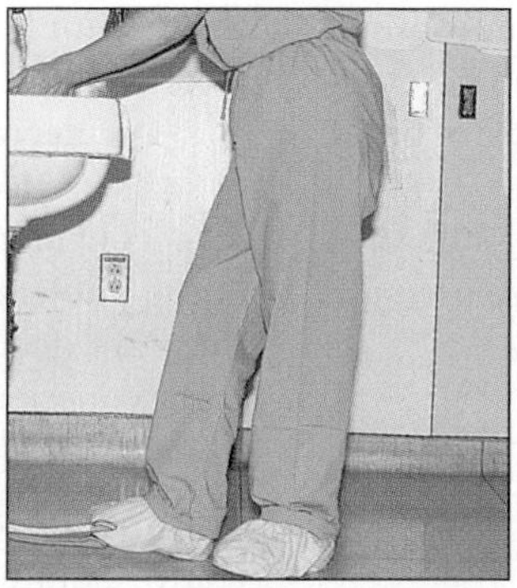

❷ A foot-pedal faucet control

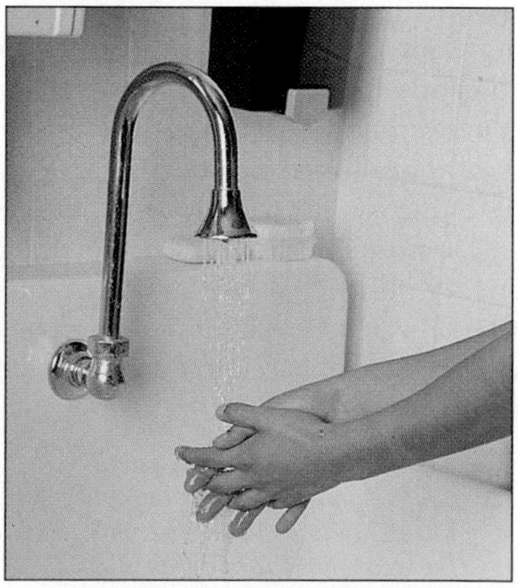

❸ Interlacing the fingers during handwashing

(continued)

SKILL 32.1

HANDWASHING (continued)

6. Turn off the water.
   - Use a dry, clean paper towel to grasp a hand-operated control (see ❹). **Rationale: This prevents the nurse from picking up microorganisms from the faucet handles.**

Variation: Handwashing before Sterile Techniques

- Apply the soap and wash as described in steps 3 and 4, but hold the hands higher than the elbows during this hand wash. Wet the hands and forearms under the running water, letting it run from the fingertips to the elbows so that the hands become cleaner than the elbows (see ❺). Ensure that at least 2 minutes of friction is used for surgical handwashing. **Rationale: In this way, the water runs from the area with the fewest microorganisms to areas with a relatively greater number.**
- After washing and rinsing, use a towel to dry one hand thoroughly in an encircling motion from the fingers to the elbow. Use a clean towel to dry the other hand and arm. **Rationale: A clean towel prevents the transfer of microorganisms from one elbow (least clean area) to the other hand (cleanest area).**

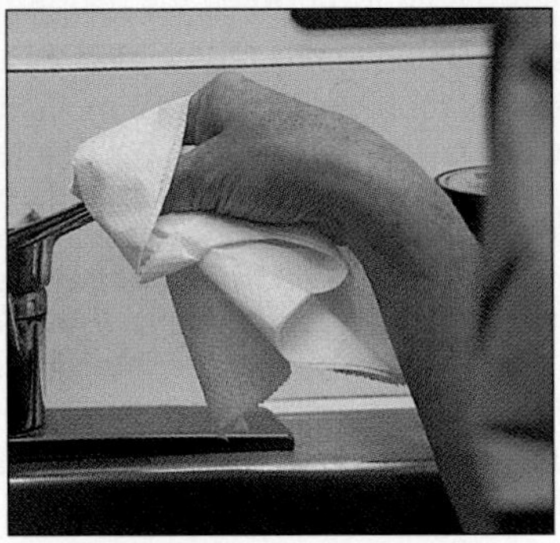

❹ Using a paper towel to grasp the handle of a hand-operated faucet

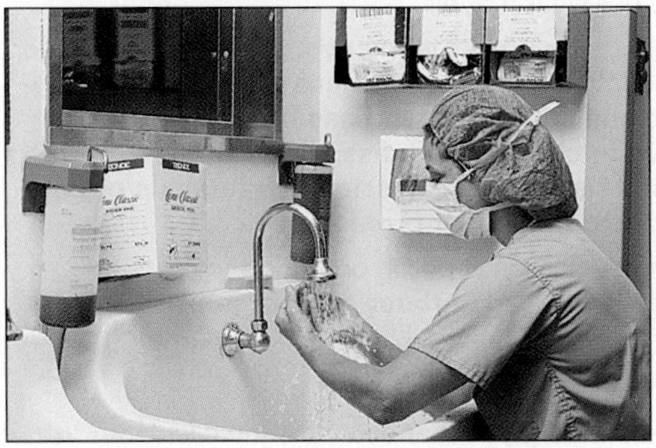

❺ The hands are held higher than the elbows during a handwash before sterile technique.

EVALUATION

No traditional evaluation exists for the effectiveness of the individual nurse's handwashing. Institutional quality control departments monitor the occurrence of client infections and investigate those situations in which health-care providers are implicated in the transmission of infectious organisms.

Waterless *alcohol-based hand rubs* kill microorganisms on the hands and are more effective than soap and water in reducing hand contamination. They facilitate hand hygiene compliance because of ease of accessibility, reduced time required to perform, and reduced skin irritation. They are therefore the preferred method of hand hygiene.

CHICA-Canada (2008) recommends the following steps when alcohol-based hand rub products are used for hand hygiene:

1. *Remove hand and arm jewellery.*
2. *Apply enough product to cover all surfaces of the hands; follow manufacturer's instructions for the amount of product to use.*
3. *Use a rubbing motion to evenly distribute the antiseptic product over all surfaces of the hands, particularly between fingers, fingertips, back of hands and base of thumbs.*
4. *Rub hands until your hands feel dry (minimum 15 to 30 seconds). Do not use paper towels.*

However, alcohol-based hand rubs have reduced effectiveness when there is physical material on the hands, such as secretions. When there is visible soiling, hands should be washed before or instead of using an alcohol-based hand rub.

The decisions as to what product to use, the amount of soap or alcohol-based hand rub to use, the frequency of performing hand hygiene, as well as the actual technique implemented remain with the health-care worker. They are decisions that must be made with an unrelentingly conscientious attitude. The indications for hand hygiene are shown in Box 32.1.

PERSONAL PROTECTIVE EQUIPMENT Personal protective equipment (PPE) acts as a barrier to reduce a health-care worker's exposure to microorganisms and reduce carriage of microorganisms by the health-care worker. PPE includes gloves, gowns, face masks, respirators, and eyewear.

BOX 32.1 RECOMMENDATIONS FOR HAND HYGIENE

Indications for the frequency of hand hygiene depend on the following:

- The type, intensity, duration, and sequence of activity
- The degree of contamination associated with the contact
- The susceptibility to infection of the health-care recipient

Hand hygiene must be performed at these times:

- Between direct contact with individual patients, residents, or clients
- Before performing invasive procedures
- Before caring for patients in intensive care units and immunocompromised patients
- After contact with blood or body fluids, or items known or considered likely to be contaminated with blood, body fluids, secretions, or excretions
- Between certain procedures on the same patient where soiling of hands is likely, to avoid cross-contamination of body sites
- After situations or procedures in which microbial or blood contamination of hands is likely
- Immediately after removing gloves
- Before preparing, handling, serving, or eating food, and before feeding a patient when hands are soiled after personal body functions (e.g., using the toilet, blowing the nose)
- Whenever the health-care provider is in doubt about the necessity for doing so
- Before entering the unit or agency at the beginning of a work period and when leaving at the end of a work period

GLOVES Gloves are worn for three reasons. First, they protect the hands when the nurse is likely to handle any body substances, for example, blood, urine, feces, sputum, mucous, and nonintact skin. Second, gloves reduce the likelihood of nurses transmitting their own endogenous microorganisms to individuals receiving care. Nurses who have open sores or cuts on the hands must wear gloves for protection. Third, gloves reduce the chance that the nurse's hands will transmit microorganisms from one client or a fomite to another client. In all situations, gloves are changed between client contacts. The hands are washed each time gloves are removed for two primary reasons: (1) the gloves may have imperfections or be damaged during wearing so that they could allow microorganisms to pass through to the skin and (2) the hands may become contaminated during glove removal. For most activities, disposable *clean* gloves are used. No special technique is required to don clean disposable gloves.

If a gown is worn, the nurse pulls up the gloves to cover the cuffs of the gown. If a gown is not worn, the nurse pulls up the cuffs to cover the wrists. Sterile gloves are used when the hands will come in contact with an open wound or when the hands might introduce microorganisms into a body orifice that is normally considered sterile.

Many of the gloves used in infection control are made of latex rubber, as are various other items used in health care (e.g., catheters, blood pressure cuffs, rubber sheets, intravenous tubing, stockings and binders, adhesive bandages, and dental dams). As a result of the frequent use of gloves, health-care workers and clients with chronic illnesses have increasingly reported allergic reactions to latex. In addition, latex gloves lubricated by powder or cornstarch are particularly allergenic because the latex allergen adheres to the powder, which is aerosolized during glove use and inhaled by the user. Latex gloves that are labelled *hypoallergenic* still contain measurable latex and should not be used by or on persons with known latex sensitivity. The people at greatest risk for developing latex allergies are those with other allergic conditions and those who have had frequent or long-term exposure to latex.

Latex allergies can be either local or systemic and may take the form of dermatitis, urticaria (hives), bronchospasm, or anaphylaxis. Clients and health-care workers should be assessed for possible allergies by taking a thorough history. Clients should be asked if they have had any adverse reactions to such items as balloons, condoms, and dishwashing or utility gloves. Strategies to avoid sensitization or exposure to latex include use of nonlatex products, nonlatex barriers between latex products and the skin, and gloves that are unpowdered. People with significant allergies should have no contact with latex products. Health-care agencies are striving to provide alternatives to latex equipment and supplies.

Skill 32.2 describes application and removal of nonsterile gloves.

GOWNS Clean or disposable impervious (water-resistant) gowns or plastic aprons are worn during procedures when the nurse's uniform is likely to become soiled. *Single use of a gown* (using a gown only once before it is discarded or laundered) is the usual practice in health-care agencies. After the gown is worn, the nurse discards it (if it is paper) or places it in a laundry hamper. Before leaving the client's room, the nurse makes sure that hands are washed.

Sterile gowns may be indicated when the nurse changes the dressings of a client with extensive wounds (e.g., burns).

A gown worn for protection is always assumed to have become contaminated during use. Skill 32.2 provides guidelines for donning and removing a gown.

FACE MASKS AND RESPIRATORS During certain techniques requiring sterile technique, masks are worn to prevent droplet contact transmission of exhaled microorganisms to the sterile field or to a client's open wound. Masks are also worn as part of routine practices to protect the nurse from splashes of body substances from the client. Surgical and procedure masks protect the

SKILL 32.2

DONNING AND REMOVING PERSONAL PROTECTIVE EQUIPMENT (GLOVES, GOWN, MASK, EYEWEAR)

PURPOSES

- To protect health-care workers and clients from transmission of potentially infective materials

ASSESSMENT

Consider which activities will be required while the nurse is in the patient's room.

Planning

- Application and removal of personal protective equipment (PPE) can be time-consuming. Prioritize care and arrange for personnel to care for your other clients if indicated.
- Determine which supplies are present within the patient's room and which must be brought to the room.
- Consider whether special handling is indicated for removal of any specimens or other materials from the room.

Equipment

As indicated, according to which activities will be performed. Ensure that extra supplies are easily available.

- Gown
- Mask
- Eyewear
- Clean gloves

IMPLEMENTATION

Preparation

Remove and secure all loose items, such as name tags or jewellery.

Performance

1. Before performing the procedure, introduce yourself and verify the client's identity by using agency protocol. Explain to the client what you are going to do, why it is necessary, and how he or she can cooperate.
2. Perform proper hand hygiene.
3. Don a clean gown.
   - Pick up a clean gown, and allow it to unfold in front of you without allowing it to touch any area soiled with body substances.
   - Slide the arms and the hands through the sleeves.
   - Fasten the ties at the neck to keep the gown in place.
   - Overlap the gown at the back as much as possible, and fasten the waist ties or belt (see ❶). **Rationale: Overlapping securely covers the uniform at the back. Waist ties keep the gown from falling away from the body, which can cause inadvertent soiling of the uniform.**
4. Don the face mask.
   - Locate the top edge of the mask. The mask usually has a narrow metal strip along the edge.
   - Hold the mask by the top two strings or loops.
   - Place the upper edge of the mask over the bridge of the nose, and tie the upper ties at the back of the head or secure the loops around the ears. If glasses are worn, fit the upper edge of the mask under the glasses. **Rationale: With the edge of the mask under the glasses, clouding of the glasses is less likely to occur.**
   - Secure the lower edge of the mask under the chin, and tie the lower ties at the nape of the neck (see ❷). **Rationale: To be effective, a mask must cover both**

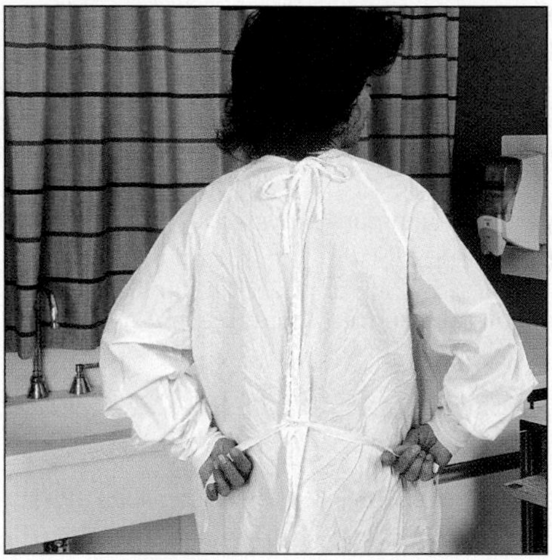

❶ Overlapping the gown at the back to cover the nurse's uniform

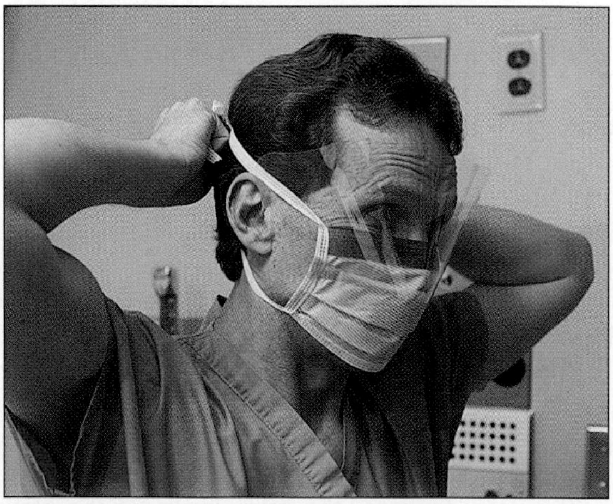

❷ A face mask and eye protection covering the nose, mouth, and eyes

(continued)

SKILL 32.2

DONNING AND REMOVING PERSONAL PROTECTIVE EQUIPMENT (GLOVES, GOWN, MASK, EYEWEAR) *(continued)*

the nose and the mouth, because air moves in and out of both.

- If the mask has a metal strip, adjust this firmly over the bridge of the nose. **Rationale: A secure fit prevents both the escape and the inhalation of microorganisms around the edges of the mask and the fogging of eyeglasses.**
- Wear the mask only once, and do not wear any mask longer than the manufacturer recommends or once it becomes wet. **Rationale: A mask should be used only once because it becomes ineffective when moist.**
- Do not leave a used face mask hanging around the neck.

5. Don protective eyewear if it is not combined with the face mask.
6. Don clean disposable gloves.
   - No special technique is required.
   - If wearing a gown, pull up the gloves to cover the cuffs of the gown. If not wearing a gown, pull up the gloves to cover the wrists.
7. To remove soiled PPE, remove the gloves first since they are the most soiled.
   - If wearing a gown that is tied at the waist in front, undo the ties before removing gloves.
   - Remove the first glove by grasping it on its palmar surface, taking care to touch only glove to glove (see ❸). **Rationale: This keeps the soiled parts of the used gloves from touching the skin of the wrist or hand.**
   - Pull off the first glove completely by inverting or rolling the glove inside out.
   - Continue to hold the inverted removed glove by the fingers of the remaining gloved hand. Place the first two fingers of the bare hand inside the cuff of the second glove (see ❹). **Rationale: Touching the outside of the second soiled glove with the bare hand is avoided.**
   - Pull off the second glove to the fingers by turning it inside out. This pulls the first glove inside the second glove. **Rationale: The soiled part of the glove is folded to the inside to reduce the chance of transferring any microorganisms by direct contact.**
   - By using the bare hand, continue to remove the gloves, which are now inside out, and dispose of them in the refuse container (see ❺).
8. Perform proper hand hygiene.
9. Remove protective eyewear and dispose of properly or place in the appropriate receptacle for cleaning.
10. Remove the gown when preparing to leave the room. Unless a gown is grossly soiled with body substances, no special precautions are needed to remove it. If a gown is grossly soiled,

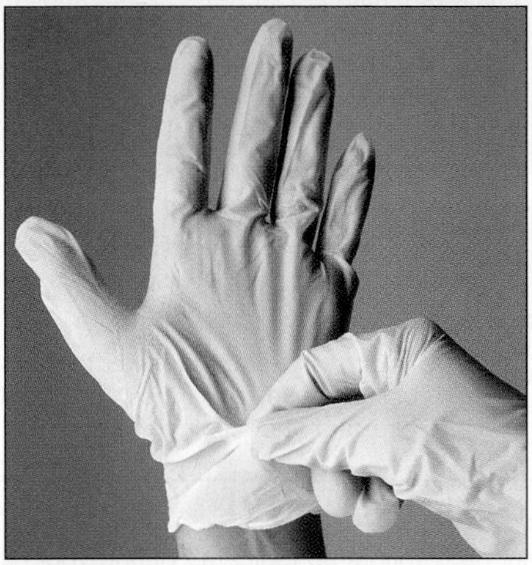

❸ Plucking the palmar surface below the cuff of a contaminated glove

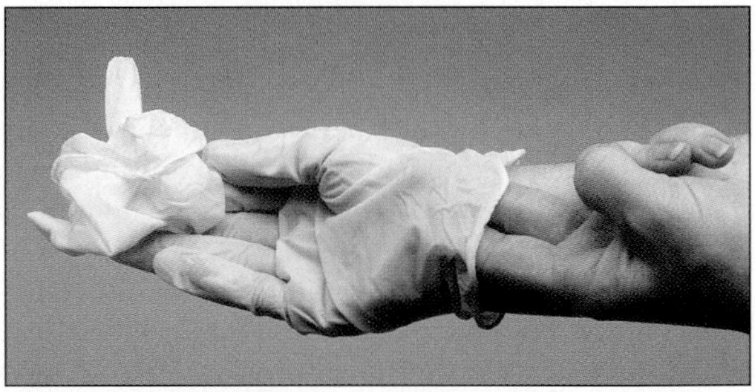

❹ Inserting fingers to remove the second contaminated glove

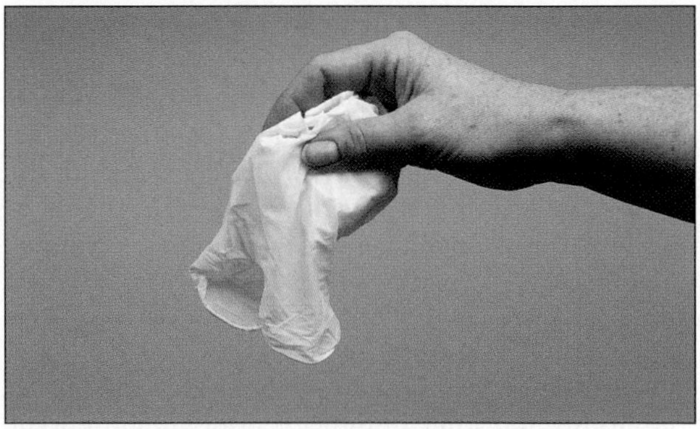

❺ Holding contaminated gloves, which are inside out

(continued)

SKILL 32.2

DONNING AND REMOVING PERSONAL PROTECTIVE EQUIPMENT (GLOVES, GOWN, MASK, EYEWEAR) (*continued*)

- Avoid touching soiled parts on the outside of the gown, if possible. **Rationale: The top part of the gown may be soiled, for example, if you have been holding an infant who has a respiratory infection.**
- Grasp the gown along the inside of the neck and pull down over the shoulders.
- Roll up the gown with the soiled part inside, and discard it in the appropriate container.

11. Remove the mask.
    - Remove the mask at the doorway to the client's room. If using a respirator mask, remove it after leaving the room and closing the door.
    - If using a mask with strings, first untie the *lower* strings of the mask. **Rationale: This prevents the top part of the mask from falling onto the chest.**
    - Untie the top strings and, while holding the ties securely, remove the mask from the face. If side loops are present, lift the side loops up and away from the ears and face. Do not touch the front of the mask. **Rationale: The front of the mask through which the nurse has been breathing is contaminated.**
    - Discard a disposable mask in the waste container.
    - Perform proper hand hygiene again.

EVALUATION

- Conduct any follow-up indicated during your care of the client. If any failure of the equipment has occurred and exposure to potentially infective materials is suspected, follow the steps in Box 32.4 later in this chapter (p. 921).
- Ensure that an adequate supply of equipment is available for the next health-care provider.

wearer's mouth and nose and thus are worn to reduce the risk for transmission of organisms by droplet contact and by splatters of body substances. In addition to health-care personnel, family members and others who are close to the client should wear masks if the infection (e.g., mumps or acute respiratory diseases in children) is transmitted by droplet transmission.

Various types of masks differ in their filtration effectiveness and fit. Single-use disposable surgical masks are effective for use when the nurse provides care to most clients but should be changed if they become wet or soiled. These masks are discarded in the waste container after use.

Surgical masks do not create a tight seal around the mouth and nose so that not all of the air breathed by the wearer is filtered through the mask itself. They are therefore not considered effective against smaller droplets and droplet nuclei. Disposable particulate **respirators** are masks made of a high-filtration material and are designed to create a tight seal around the mouth and nose. An N95-level respirator filters out at least 95% of airborne particles under standard conditions, excluding oil particles (the *N* of N95 stands for *not resistant to oil*). Respirators need to be fitted—health-care providers need to choose a size and style of respirator mask that allows a good seal. Most institutions provide a selection of respirators; assessing an individual for an appropriate respirator is called **fit testing.**

Fit testing is done by an appropriately trained individual. While done in some places on an annual basis, regulations vary by jurisdiction as to the frequency with which fit testing must occur. *Fit checking* means assessing the adequacy of the seal and should be done each time a respirator is worn (Public Health Agency of Canada, 2003).

Respirators should be worn by all persons entering the room when the infection (e.g., pulmonary tuberculosis) is transmitted by the airborne route. Respirators should also be worn during aerosol-generating procedures (e.g., bronchoscopy or suctioning).

Guidelines for donning and removing a facemask are found in Skill 32.2. Special care must be taken to avoid self-contamination when removing the mask or respirator.

EYEWEAR Protective eyewear (goggles, glasses, or face shields) and masks may be indicated in situations in which body substances may splatter the face, thereby allowing entry of microorganisms through the eyes or respiratory tract. If the nurse wears prescription eyeglasses, goggles must still be worn over the glasses because the protection must extend around the sides of the glasses. Guidelines for donning and removing eyewear are found in Skill 32.2.

ASEPTIC AND STERILE TECHNIQUE *Asepsis* means "without infection" and implies the absence of disease-causing microorganisms. To decrease the possibility of transferring microorganisms from one place to another, aseptic technique or sterile technique is used. The two terms are not the same. **Aseptic technique** is sometimes referred to as **clean technique**, where clean denotes the absence of almost all, but not all, microorganisms. While efforts are made to reduce transfer of microorganisms, items in use may not be sterile (e.g., use of clean forceps) and activity occurs outside of a sterile field (e.g., a wound during a dressing change). **Sterile technique** employs stricter measures to maintain sterility throughout the procedure. It refers to using sterile items within a sterile field, such as an operative site in an operating room, or in an intensive care unit when a sterile drape is applied for insertion of a central venous access device.

Approaches to asepsis will vary, depending on the procedure and setting. For example, before an operating room procedure, the scrub nurse generally puts on a mask and cap, performs a surgical hand scrub, and then dons a sterile gown and gloves. In a general care area, the nurse may only perform a handwash and don sterile gloves. In both areas, the nurse works with sterile equipment and a sterile field. The basic principles of sterile technique appear in Table 32.8, with examples from nursing practice that relate to each principle.

TABLE 32.8 Principles and Practices of Establishing and Maintaining a Sterile Field

Principle	Practices
All objects used in a sterile field must be sterile.	All articles are sterilized appropriately by dry or moist heat, chemicals, or radiation before use.
	Sterile articles can be stored for only a prescribed time; after that, they are considered unsterile.
	Always check a package containing a sterile object for intactness, dryness, and expiration date. Any package that appears open, torn, punctured, or wet is considered unsterile. Never assume an item is sterile; if in doubt, consider the item unsterile.
	Storage areas should be clean, dry, off the floor, and away from sinks.
	Always check chemical indicators of sterilization before using a package. The indicator is often a tape used to fasten the package or contained inside the package. The indicator changes colour during sterilization, indicating that the contents have undergone a sterilization procedure. If the colour change is not evident, the package is considered unsterile. Commercially prepared sterile packages may not have indicators but are marked with the word *sterile*.
Sterile objects become unsterile when touched by unsterile objects.	Handle sterile objects that will touch open wounds or enter body cavities only with sterile forceps or sterile gloved hands.
	Discard or resterilize objects that come into contact with unsterile objects.
	Whenever the sterility of an object is questionable, assume the article is unsterile.
Sterile items that are out of vision or below the waist level of the nurse are considered unsterile.	Once left unattended, a sterile field is considered unsterile.
	Sterile objects are always kept in view. Nurses should not turn their backs on a sterile field.
	Only the front part of a sterile gown (from the waist to the shoulder) and 5 cm above the elbows to the cuff of the sleeves are considered sterile.
	Always keep sterile gloved hands in sight and above waist level; touch only objects that are sterile.
	Sterile draped tables are considered sterile only at surface level.
	Once a sterile field becomes unsterile, it must be set up again before proceeding.
Sterile objects can become unsterile by prolonged exposure to airborne microorganisms.	Keep doors closed and traffic to a minimum in areas where a sterile procedure is being performed; moving air can carry dust and microorganisms.
	Keep areas in which sterile procedures are carried out as clean as possible by frequent damp cleaning with detergent germicides to minimize contaminants in the area.
	Keep hair clean and short, tied back, or enclosed in a net to prevent hair from falling on sterile objects. Microorganisms on the hair can make a sterile field unsterile.
	Wear surgical caps in operating rooms, delivery rooms, and burn units.
	Refrain from sneezing or coughing over a sterile field. This can render the field unsterile because of the spray of droplets containing microorganisms from the respiratory tract. Some nurses recommend that masks covering the mouth and the nose be worn when working over a sterile field or an open wound.
	Nurses with mild upper respiratory tract infections should refrain from carrying out sterile procedures, or should wear masks.
	When working over a sterile field, talking should be kept to a minimum. Turn the head from the field if talking is necessary.
	To prevent microorganisms from falling over a sterile field, refrain from reaching over a sterile field, unless sterile gloves are worn, and refrain from moving unsterile objects over a sterile field.

(continued)

TABLE 32.8 Principles and Practices of Establishing and Maintaining a Sterile Field (*continued*)

Principle	Practices
Fluids flow in the direction of gravity.	Hold instruments with the tips below the handles. When the tips are held higher than the handles, fluid can flow onto the handle and become contaminated by the hands. When the forceps are again pointed downward, the fluid flows back down and contaminates the tips. During a surgical handwash, hold the hands higher than the elbows to prevent contaminants from the forearms from reaching the hands.
Moisture that passes through a sterile object draws microorganisms from unsterile surfaces above or below to the sterile surface by capillary action.	Sterile moistureproof barriers are used beneath sterile objects. Liquids (sterile saline or antiseptics) are frequently poured into containers on a sterile field. If they are spilled onto the sterile field, the barrier keeps the liquid from seeping beneath it. Keep the sterile covers on sterile equipment dry. Damp surfaces can attract microorganisms in the air. Replace sterile drapes that do not have a sterile barrier underneath when they become moist.
The edges of a sterile field are considered unsterile.	A 2.5 cm margin at each edge of an opened drape is considered unsterile because the edges are in contact with unsterile surfaces. Place all sterile objects more than 2.5 cm inside the edges of a sterile field. Any article that falls outside the edges of a sterile field is considered unsterile.
The skin is unsterile and cannot be sterilized.	Use sterile gloves or sterile forceps to handle sterile items. Prior to a surgical aseptic procedure, wash the hands to reduce the number of microorganisms on them.
Conscientiousness, alertness, and honesty are essential qualities in maintaining surgical asepsis.	When a sterile object becomes unsterile, it does not necessarily change in appearance. The person who sees a sterile object become contaminated must correct or report the situation. Do not set up a sterile field ahead of time for future use.

STERILE FIELD A **sterile field** is a microorganism-free area. Nurses often establish a sterile field by using the innermost side of a sterile wrapper or by using a sterile drape. When the field is established, sterile supplies and sterile solutions can be placed on it. Sterile forceps are used in many instances to handle and transfer the sterile supplies.

So that their sterility can be maintained, supplies are wrapped in a variety of materials. Commercially prepared items are frequently wrapped in plastic, paper, or glass. In the past, it was not unusual for sterile liquids (e.g., sterile water for irrigations) to be supplied in large containers. This practice is considered undesirable today because once a container has been opened, there can be no guarantee that it is sterile. Liquids are preferably packaged in amounts adequate for single use only; leftover liquid is discarded.

The Home Care Considerations box contains information that the nurse should teach the client to maintain a sterile field at home.

Skill 32.3 describes how to establish and maintain a sterile field.

Home Care Considerations

Sterile Field

Creating a sterile field is essential in many procedures conducted in the home:

- Clean and wipe dry a flat surface for the sterile field.
- Keep pets and uninvolved small children out of the area when setting up for and performing sterile procedures.
- Dispose of all soiled materials in a waterproof bag. Check with the agency as to how to dispose of medical refuse.
- Remove all instruments from the home or other setting in which others might accidentally find them. *New or used instruments can be sharp or capable of causing injury. Used instruments may transmit infection.* Check with the agency for instructions on the cleansing of reusable supplies and disposal of single-use instruments.
- If appropriate, teach the client and family members the principles and rationale underlying use of a sterile field.

SKILL 32.3

ESTABLISHING AND MAINTAINING A STERILE FIELD

PURPOSE

- To maintain the sterility of supplies and equipment

ASSESSMENT

Review the client's record or discuss with the client or other health-care team members exactly what procedure will be performed that requires a sterile field. Determine the client's presence or risk for infection and ability to cope with the procedure.

Determine, if possible, what supplies and techniques have been used in the past to perform the procedures for this client. Attempt to determine if the procedure will be performed again in the future, so appropriate client teaching can be done and adequate supplies will be available.

Schedule the procedure at a time consistent with the order, the need for the procedure, and the client's other activities.

Equipment

- Package containing a sterile drape
- Sterile equipment as needed (e.g., packaged gauze, wrapped sterile bowl, antiseptic solution, sterile forceps)

IMPLEMENTATION

Preparation

- Ensure that the package is clean and dry; if moisture is noted on the inside of a plastic-wrapped package or the outside of a cloth-wrapped package, it is considered contaminated and must be discarded.
- Check the sterilization expiration dates on the package, and look for any indications that it has been previously opened. Spots or stains on cloth-wrapped or paper-wrapped objects may indicated contamination and should not be used.
- Follow agency practice for disposal of possibly contaminated packages.

Performance

1. Before performing the procedure, introduce yourself and verify the client's identity by using agency protocol. Explain to the client what you are going to do, why it is necessary, and how he or she can cooperate.
2. Observe other appropriate infection prevention and control procedures (see Skills 32.1 and 32.2).
3. Provide for client privacy.
4. Open the package. If the package is inside a plastic cover, remove the cover.

To Open a Wrapped Package on a Clean Surface

- Place the package in the centre of the work area so that the top flap of the wrapper opens away from you. **Rationale: This position prevents the nurse from reaching directly over the exposed sterile contents, which could contaminate them.**
- Reaching from the side of the package (not over it), pinch the first flap on the outside of the wrapper between the thumb and index finger (see ❶). **Rationale: Touching only the outside of the wrapper maintains the sterility of the inside of the wrapper.** Pull the flap open, laying it flat on the far surface.
- Repeat for the side flaps, opening the top one first. Use the right hand for the right flap, and the left hand for the left flap (see ❷). **Rationale: By using both hands, the nurse avoids reaching over the sterile contents.**
- Pull the fourth flap toward you by grasping the corner that is turned down (see ❸). Make sure that the flap does not touch any object. **Rationale: If the inner surface touches any unsterile article, it is contaminated.**

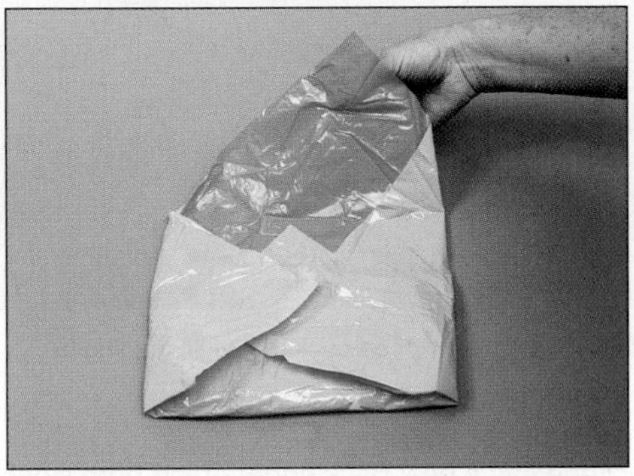

❶ Opening the first flap of a sterile wrapped package

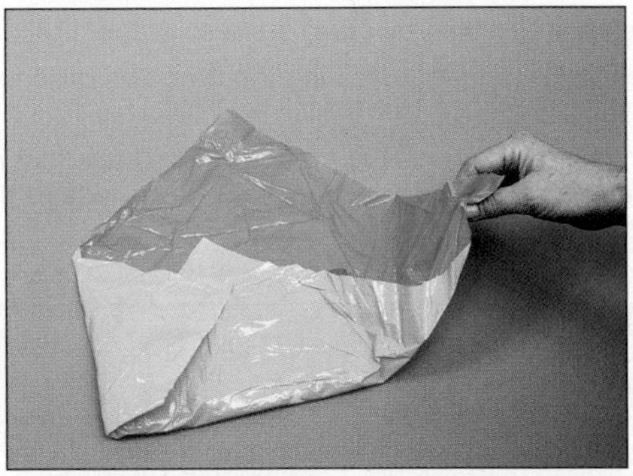

❷ Opening the second flap to the side

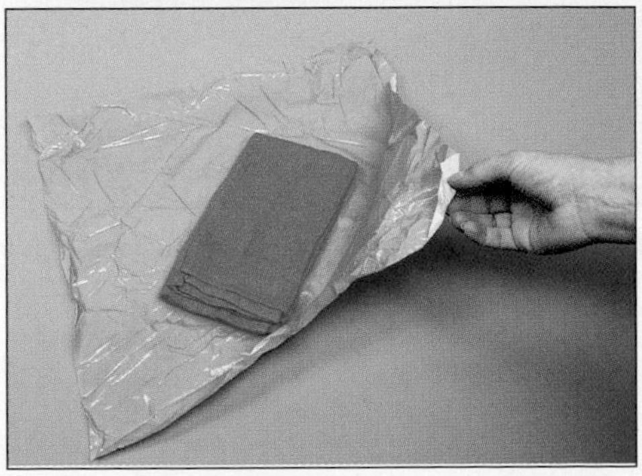

❸ Pulling the last flap toward you by grasping the corner

(continued)

SKILL 32.3

ESTABLISHING AND MAINTAINING A STERILE FIELD *(continued)*

Variation: Opening a Wrapped Package while Holding It

- Hold the package in one hand with the top flap opening away from you.
- By using the other hand, open the package as described above, pulling the corners of the flaps well back and not reaching across the contents of the package (see ❹). **Rationale: The hands are considered contaminated, and at no time should they touch the contents of the package.**

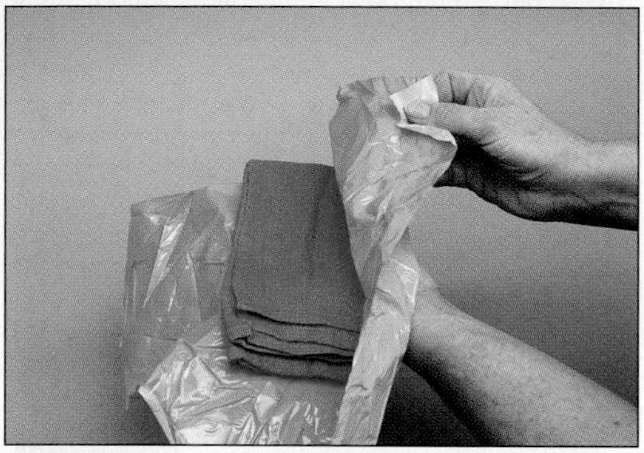

❹ Opening a wrapped package while holding it

- If the package has a peel back edge, grasp both sides of the edge, one with each hand, and pull apart gently (see ❻).

5. Establish a sterile field by using a sterile drape.
   - Open the package containing the drape as described above.
   - With one hand, pluck the corner of the drape that is folded back on the top touching only one side of the drape.

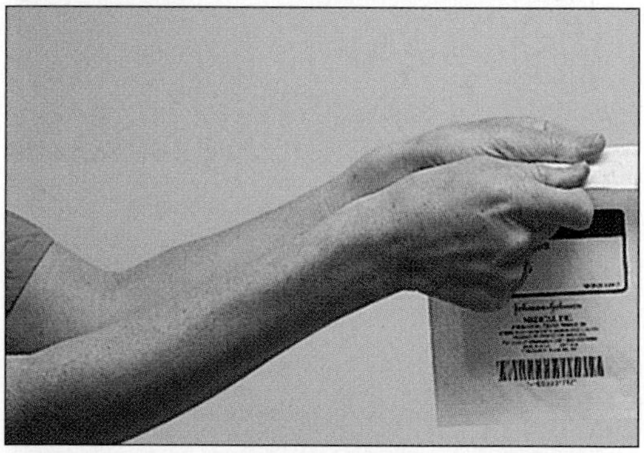

❻ Opening a sterile package that has a partially sealed edge

Variation: Opening Commercially Prepared Packages

Commercially prepared sterile packages and containers usually have manufacturer's directions for opening.

- If the flap of the package has a peel back corner, hold the container in one hand and pull back on the flap with the other hand (see ❺).

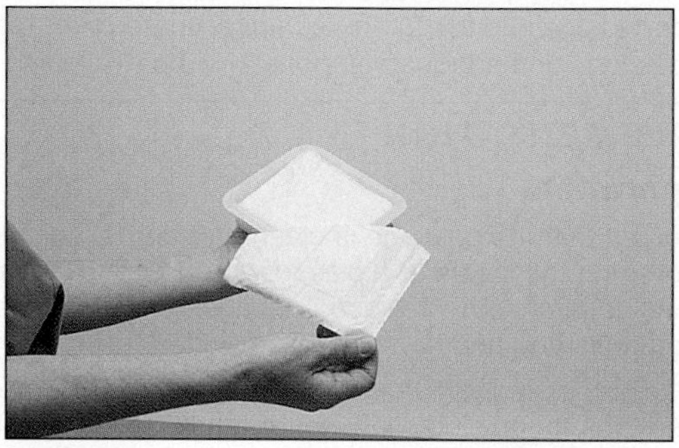

❺ Opening a sterile package that has a peel back corner

- Lift the drape out of the cover and allow it to open freely without touching any objects (see ❼). **Rationale: If the drape touches the outside of the package or any unsterile surface or object, it is considered contaminated.**
- Discard the cover.
- With the other hand, carefully pick up another corner of the drape, holding it well away from you, and again, touching only the same side of the drape as the first hand.

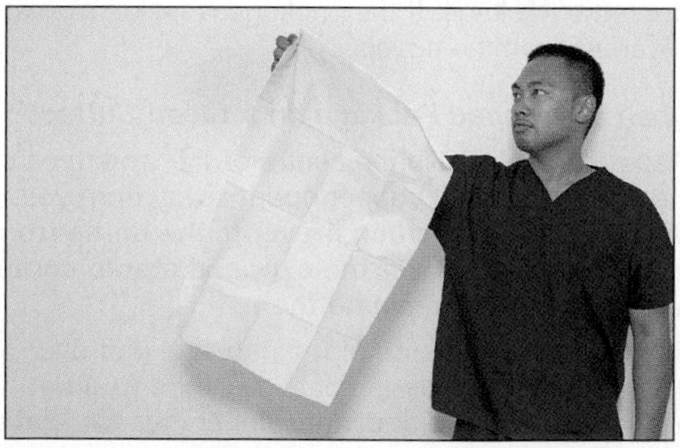

❼ Allowing a drape to open freely without touching any objects

(continued)

SKILL 32.3

ESTABLISHING AND MAINTAINING A STERILE FIELD (*continued*)

- Lay the drape on a clean and dry surface, placing the bottom (i.e., the freely hanging side) farthest from you (see ❽). **Rationale: By placing the lowermost side farthest away, the nurse avoids leaning over the sterile field and contaminating it.**

6. Add necessary sterile supplies, being careful not to touch the drape with the hands.

To Add Wrapped Supplies to a Sterile Field

- Open each wrapped package as described in the preceding steps.
- With the free hand, grasp the corners of the wrapper and hold them against the wrist of the other hand (see ❾). **Rationale: The unsterile hand is now covered by the sterile wrapper.**
- Place the sterile bowl, drape, or other supply on the sterile field by approaching from an angle, rather than holding the arm over the field.
- Discard the wrapper.

Variation: Adding Commercially Packaged Supplies to a Sterile Field

- Open each package as previously described.
- Hold the package 15 cm above the field, and allow the contents to drop on the field (see ❿). Keep in mind that 2.5 cm around the edge of the field is considered contaminated. **Rationale: At a height of 15 cm, the outside of the package is not likely to touch and contaminate the sterile fields.**

Adding Solution to a Sterile Container

Liquids (e.g., normal saline) may need to be poured into containers within a sterile field. Unwrapped bottles or flasks that contain sterile solution are considered sterile on the inside and contaminated on the outside because the bottle has been handled. Bottles used in an operating room may be sterilized on the outside as well as the inside, however, and these are handled with sterile gloves.

- Before pouring any liquid, read the label three times to ensure you have the correct solution and concentration (strength).
- Obtain the exact amount of solution, if possible. **Rationale: Once a sterile container has been opened, its sterility cannot be ensured for future use unless it is used again immediately.**
- Remove the lid or cap from the bottle and invert the lid before placing it on a surface that is not sterile. **Rationale: Inverting the lid maintains the sterility of the inside surface because it is not allowed to touch an unsterile surface.**

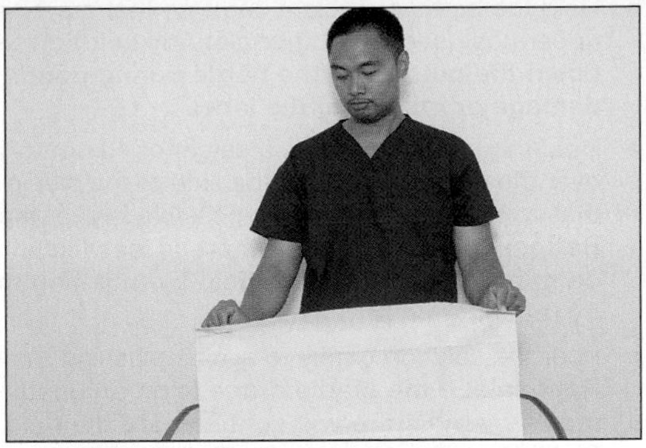

❽ Placing a drape on a surface

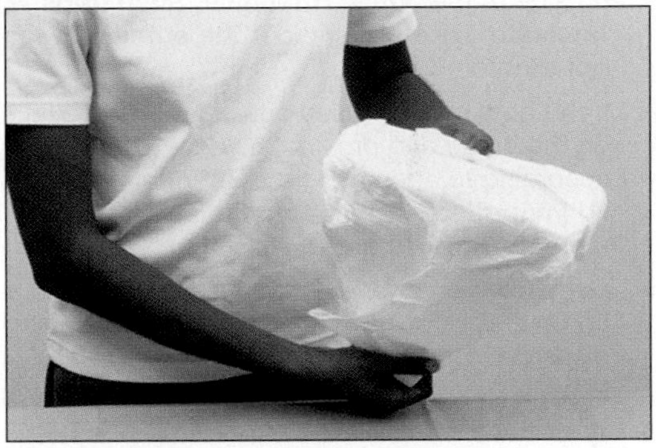

❾ Adding wrapped sterile supplies to a sterile field

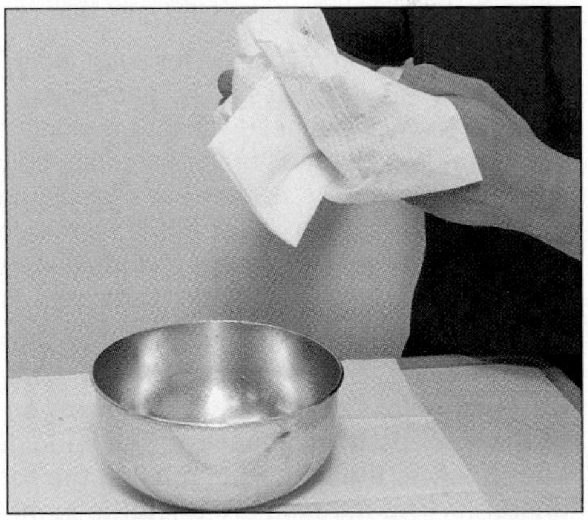

❿ Adding commercially packaged gauze to a sterile filed

(continued)

SKILL 32.3

ESTABLISHING AND MAINTAINING A STERILE FIELD (*continued*)

- Hold the bottle at a slight angle so that the label is uppermost (see ⓫). **Rationale: Any solution that flows down the outside of the bottle during pouring will not damage or obliterate the label.**
- Hold the bottle of fluid at a height of 10 cm to 15 cm over the container and to the side of the sterile field so that as little of the bottle as possible is over the field. **Rationale: At this height, there is less likelihood of contaminating the sterile field by touching the field or by reaching an arm over it.**
- Pour the solution gently to avoid splashing the liquid. **Rationale: If the sterile drape is on an unsterile surface, any moisture will contaminate the field by facilitating the movement of microorganisms through the drape.**
- Tilt the neck of the bottle back to vertical quickly when done pouring so that none of the liquid flows down the outside of the bottle. **Rationale: Such drips would contaminate the sterile field if the outside of the bottle is not sterile.**
- If the bottle will be used again, replace the lid securely on the bottle and provide the date and time of opening according to agency policy. **Rationale: Replacing the lid immediately maintains the sterility of the inner aspect of the lid and the solution.**
- Depending on agency policy, a sterile container of solution that is opened may be used only once and then discarded (such as in the operating room). In other settings, policy may permit recapped bottles to be reused within 24 hours.
- If the bottle of solution is used again, the lip of the container should be cleansed by pouring a small amount of solution (and then discarding) before pouring solution into the sterile container.

8. Use sterile forceps to handle certain sterile supplies.
   - Forceps are commonly used for such techniques as changing a sterile dressing and shortening a drain. Transfer forceps are used to move a sterile article from one place to another, for example, transferring sterile gauze from its package to a sterile dressing tray. Forceps may be discarded or resterilized after use. Commonly used forceps include hemostats, or artery forceps (see ⓬), and tissue forceps (see ⓭).
   - Keep the tips of wet forceps lower than the wrist at all times unless you are wearing sterile gloves (see ⓮). **Rationale: Gravity prevents liquids on the tips of the forceps from flowing to the handles and later back to the tips, thus making the forceps unsterile. The handles are unsterile once they are held by the bare hand.**
   - Hold sterile forceps above waist level. **Rationale: Items held below waist level are considered contaminated.**
   - Hold sterile forceps within your visual field. **Rationale: While out of sight, forceps may, unknown to the user, become contaminated. Any forceps that go out of sight should be considered unsterile.**

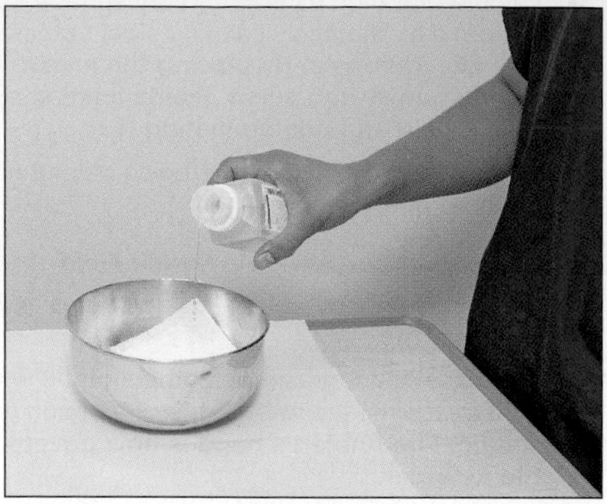

⓫ Adding liquid to a sterile bowl

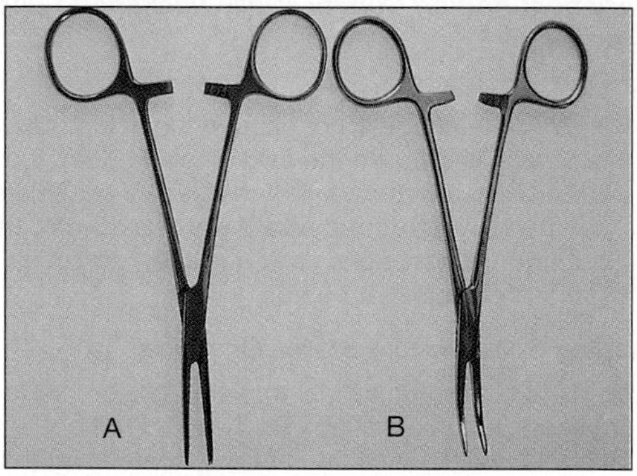

⓬ Hemostats: **A:** straight; **B:** curved

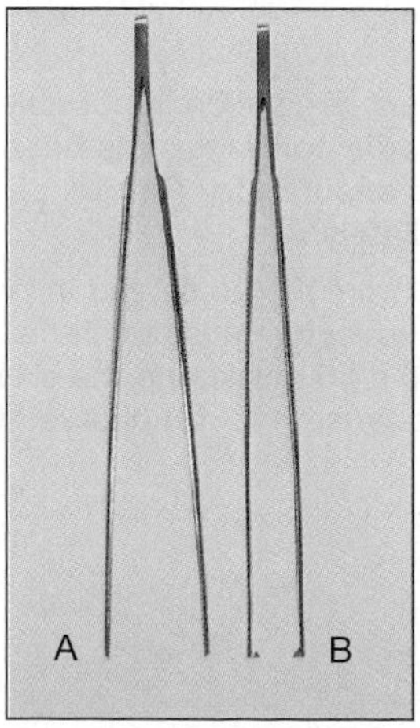

⓭ Tissue forceps: **A:** plain; **B:** toothed

(*continued*)

SKILL 32.3

ESTABLISHING AND MAINTAINING A STERILE FIELD (*continued*)

- When using forceps to lift sterile supplies out of a commercially prepared package, be sure that the forceps do not touch the edges or outside of the wrapper. **Rationale: The edges and outside of the package are exposed to the air and are handled and are, thus, unsterile.**
- Deposit a sterile item on a sterile field without permitting moist forceps to touch the sterile field when the surface under the sterile field is unsterile and a barrier drape is not used. A *barrier drape* is resistant to moisture and should be used whenever a procedure involves moisture. **Rationale: Made of chemically treated cotton or synthetic materials, barrier drapes prevent a sterile field from becoming contaminated when the drape becomes wet. It is known that a sterile cloth becomes unsterile when dampened (even with sterile water) if it is on an unsterile surface or has contact with any unsterile object. Microorganisms can move through a damp sterile cloth from an unsterile surface by capillary action.**
- When placing forceps whose handles were in contact with the bare hand, position the handles outside the sterile area. **Rationale: The handles of these forceps harbour microorganisms from the bare hand.**

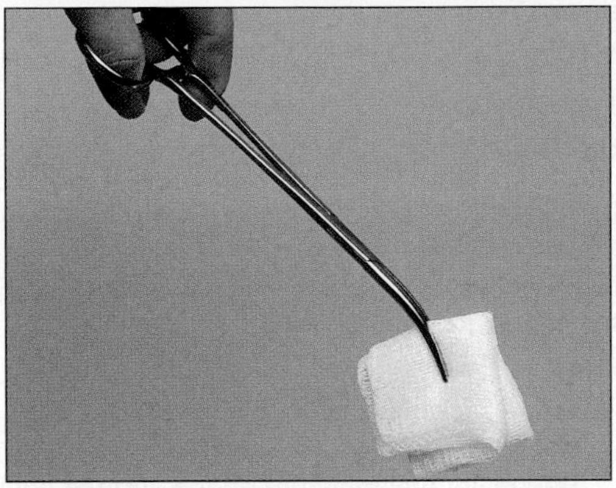

⓮ Holding forceps with an ungloved hand, keeping the tips pointing downward

EVALUATION

Conduct any follow-up indicated during your care of the client. Ensure that adequate numbers and types of sterile supplies are available for the next health-care provider.

Sterile Gloves Sterile gloves are worn during many procedures to maintain the sterility of equipment and protect the client. Sterile gloves are packaged with a cuff of about 5 cm and with the palms facing upward when the package is opened. The package usually indicates the size of the glove (e.g., size 6 or 7 1/2).

Sterile gloves can be donned by the open or the closed method. The open method is most frequently used outside the operating room because the closed method requires that the nurse wear a sterile gown. Skill 32.4 describes how to don and remove sterile gloves by using the open method.

SKILL 32.4

DONNING AND REMOVING STERILE GLOVES (OPEN METHOD)

PURPOSES

- To enable the nurse to handle sterile objects freely
- To prevent clients at risk (e.g., those with open wounds) from becoming infected by microorganisms on the nurse's hands

ASSESSMENT

Review the client's record and orders to determine exactly what procedure will be performed that requires sterile gloves. Check the client record and ask about latex allergies. Use nonlatex gloves whenever possible.

Planning

Think through the procedure, planning which steps need to be completed before the gloves can be applied. Determine what additional supplies are needed to perform the procedure for this client. Always have an extra pair of sterile gloves available.

Equipment

- Package of sterile gloves

(continued)

SKILL 32.4

DONNING AND REMOVING STERILE GLOVES (OPEN METHOD) (*continued*)

IMPLEMENTATION

Preparation

Ensure the sterility of the package of gloves.

Performance

1. Before performing the procedure, introduce yourself and verify the client's identity by using agency protocol. Explain to the client what you are going to do, why it is necessary, and how he or she can cooperate.
2. Observe other appropriate infection prevention and control procedures (see Skills 32.1, 32.2, and 32.3).
3. Provide for client privacy.
4. Open the package of sterile gloves.
   - Place the package of gloves on a clean, dry surface. **Rationale: Any moisture on the surface could contaminate the gloves.**
   - Some gloves are packed in an inner as well as an outer package. Open the outer package without contaminating the gloves or the inner package. See Skill 32.3.
   - Remove the inner package from the outer package.
   - Open the inner package as in step 4 of Skill 32.3 or according to the manufacturer's directions. Some manufacturers provide a numbered sequence for opening the flaps and folded tabs to grasp for opening the flaps. If no tabs are provided, pluck the flap so that the fingers do not touch the inner surfaces. **Rationale: The inner surfaces, which are next to the sterile gloves, will remain sterile.**
5. Put the first glove on the dominant hand.
   - If the gloves are packaged so that they lie side by side, grasp the glove for the dominant hand by its cuff (on the palmar side) with the thumb and first finger of the nondominant hand. Touch only the inside of the cuff (see ❶). **Rationale: The hands are not sterile. By touching only the inside of the glove, the nurse avoids contaminating the outside.**
   - *Or* if the gloves are packaged one on top of the other, grasp the cuff of the top glove as above, using the opposite hand.
   - Insert the dominant hand into the glove and pull the glove on. Keep the thumb of the inserted hand against the palm of the hand during insertion (see ❷). **Rationale: If the thumb is kept against the palm, it is less likely to contaminate the outside of the glove.**
   - Leave the cuff turned down. **Rationale: Attempting to further unfold the cuff is likely to contaminate the gloves.**
6. Put the second glove on the nondominant hand.
   - Pick up the other glove with the sterile gloved hand, inserting the gloved fingers under the cuff and holding the gloved thumb close to the gloved palm (see ❸). **Rationale: This helps prevent accidental contamination of the glove by the bare hand.**

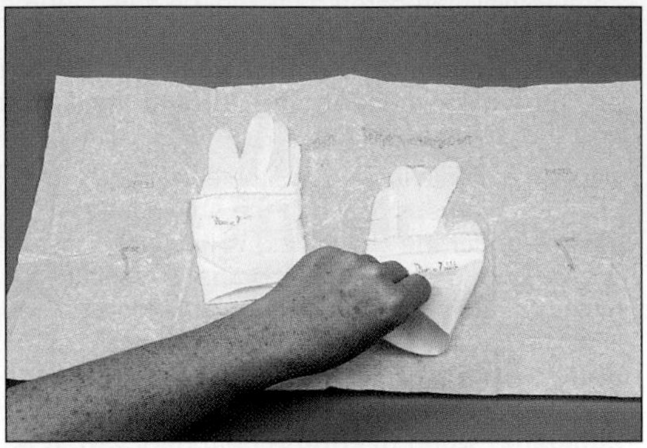

❶ Picking up the first sterile glove

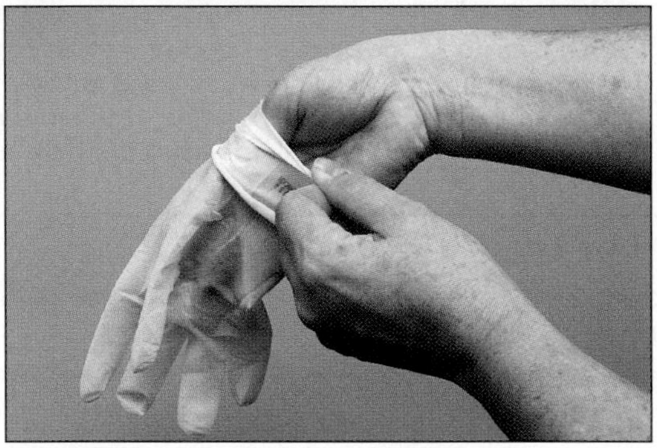

❷ Putting on the first sterile glove

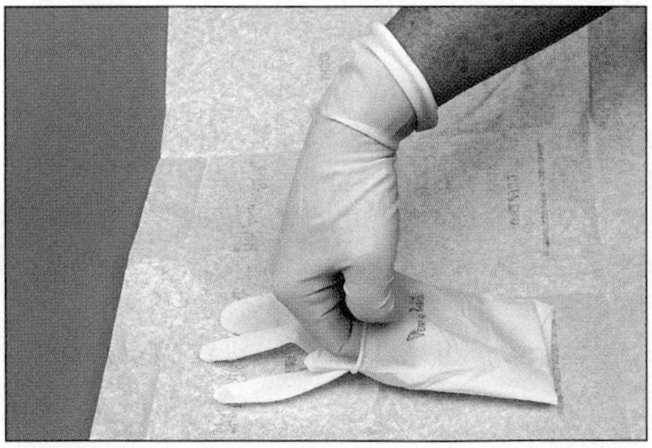

❸ Picking up the second sterile glove

(continued)

SKILL 32.4

DONNING AND REMOVING STERILE GLOVES (OPEN METHOD) *(continued)*

- Pull on the second glove carefully. Hold the thumb of the gloved first hand as far as possible from the palm (see ❹). **Rationale: In this position, the thumb is less likely to touch the arm and become contaminated.**
- Adjust each glove so that it fits smoothly, and carefully pull up the cuffs by sliding the fingers under the cuffs.

7. Remove and dispose of used gloves.
   - Remove them by turning them inside out. See Skill 32.2.

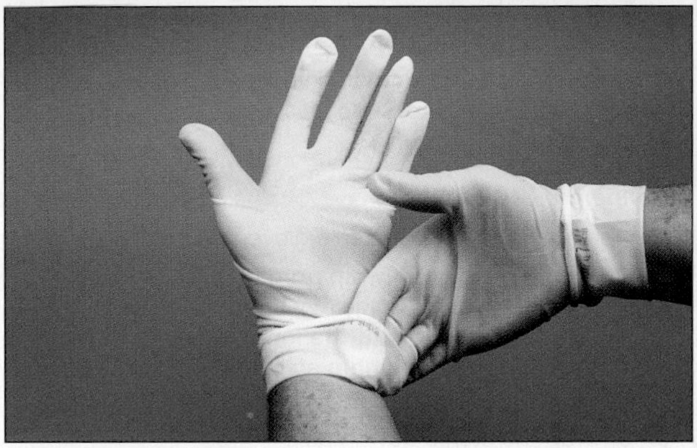

❹ Putting on the second sterile glove

EVALUATION

Conduct any follow-up indicated during your care of the client. Ensure that adequate numbers and types of sterile supplies are available for the next health-care provider.

Latex and latex-free (e.g., nitrile and vinyl) sterile gloves are available to protect the nurse from contact with blood and body fluids. Latex and nitrile are more flexible than vinyl, mould to the wearer's hands, allow freedom of movement, and have the added feature of resealing tiny punctures automatically. Therefore, wear latex or nitrile gloves when performing tasks (1) that demand flexibility, (2) that place stress on the material (e.g., turning stopcocks, handling sharp instruments or tape), and (3) that involve a high risk of exposure to pathogens. Vinyl gloves should be chosen for tasks unlikely to stress the glove material, requiring minimal precision, or with minimal risk of exposure to pathogens.

Sterile Gowns Sterile gowning and closed gloving are chiefly carried out in operating or delivery rooms. The closed method of gloving can be used only when a sterile gown is worn because the gloves are handled through the sleeves of the gown. Before these procedures, the nurse dons a hair cover and a mask, and performs a surgical handwash.

Skill 32.5 describes the steps in donning a sterile gown and sterile gloves by the closed method.

SKILL 32.5

DONNING A STERILE GOWN AND STERILE GLOVES (CLOSED METHOD)

PURPOSES

- To enable the nurse to work close to a sterile field and handle sterile objects freely
- To protect clients from becoming contaminated with microorganisms on the nurse's hands, arms, and clothing

ASSESSMENT

Review the client's record and orders to determine exactly what procedure will be performed that requires sterile gloves. Check the client record and ask about latex allergies. Use nonlatex gloves whenever possible.

Planning

Think through the procedure, planning which steps need to be completed before the gown and gloves can be applied.

Determine what additional supplies are needed to perform the procedure for this client. Always have an extra pair of sterile gloves and an extra sterile gown available.

Equipment

- Sterile pack containing a sterile gown
- Sterile gloves

IMPLEMENTATION

Ensure the sterility of the gown and gloves.

Performance

1. Before performing the procedure, introduce yourself and verify the client's identity by using agency protocol.

(continued)

SKILL 32.5

DONNING A STERILE GOWN AND STERILE GLOVES (CLOSED METHOD) *(continued)*

Explain to the client what you are going to do, why it is necessary, and how he or she can cooperate.

2. Observe other appropriate infection prevention and control procedures (see Skills 32.1, 32.2, and 32.3).
3. Provide for client privacy.

Donning a Sterile Gown

4. Open the package of sterile gloves.
   - Remove the outer wrap from the sterile gloves and leave the gloves in their inner sterile wrap on the sterile field. **Rationale: If the inner wrapper is not touched, it will remain sterile**. See Skill 32.3, step 4 (p. 901).
5. Unwrap the sterile gown pack.
6. Perform proper hand hygiene. (See "Variation" at the end of Skill 32.1 and review agency practice.)
7. Put on the sterile gown.
   - Grasp the sterile gown at the neck, hold it away from you, and permit it to unfold freely without touching anything, including the uniform. **Rationale: The gown will be unsterile if its outer surface touches any unsterile objects**.
   - Put the hands inside the shoulders of the gown, and work the arms partway into the sleeves without touching the outside of the gown (see ❶).
   - If donning sterile gloves by using the *closed* method (see below), work the hands down the sleeves only to the proximal edge of the cuffs.
   - *Or* if donning sterile gloves by using the *open* method, work the hands down the sleeves and through the cuffs.
   - Have a co-worker wearing a hair cover and mask grasp the neck ties without touching the outside of the gown and pull the gown upward to cover the neckline of your uniform in front and back. The co-worker ties the neck ties. Gowning continues at step 11.

Donning Sterile Gloves (Closed Method)

8. Open the sterile glove wrapper while the hands are still covered by the sleeves (see ❷).
9. Put the glove on the nondominant hand (see ❸).
   - With the *dominant* hand, pick up the *opposite* glove with the thumb and index finger, handling it through the sleeve.
   - Lay the glove on the opposite gown cuff, thumb side down, with the glove opening pointed toward the fingers. Position the dominant hand palm upward inside the sleeve.

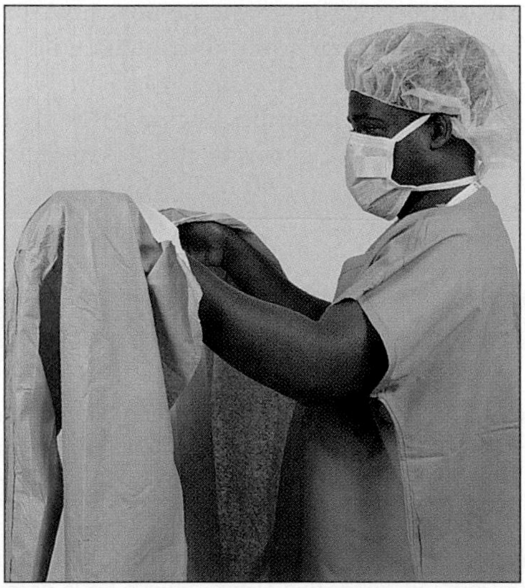

❶ Putting on a sterile gown

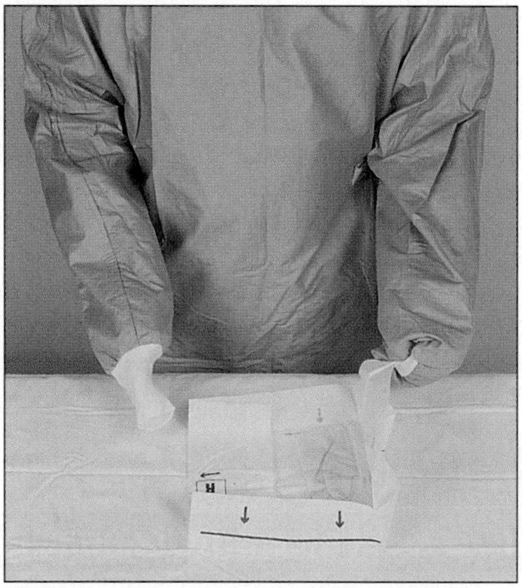

❷ Opening the sterile glove wrapper

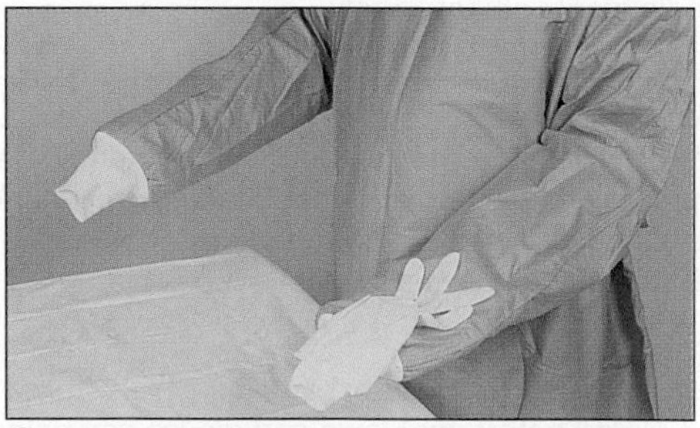

❸ Positioning the first sterile glove for the nondominant hand

(continued)

SKILL 32.5

DONNING A STERILE GOWN AND STERILE GLOVES (CLOSED METHOD) (*continued*)

- Use the nondominant hand to grasp the cuff of the glove through the gown cuff, and firmly anchor it.
- With the dominant hand working through its sleeve, grasp the upper side of the glove's cuff, and stretch it over the cuff of the gown.
- Pull the sleeve up to draw the cuff over the wrist as you extend the fingers of the nondominant hand into the glove's fingers (see ❹).

10. Put the glove on the dominant hand.
    - Place the fingers of the gloved hand under the cuff of the remaining glove.
    - Place the glove over the cuff of the second sleeve.
    - Extend the fingers into the glove as you pull the glove up over the gown cuff (see ❺).

Completion of Gowning

11. Complete gowning as follows:
    - Have a co-worker wearing a hair cover and mask hold the waist tie of your gown by using sterile gloves or a sterile forcep or drape. **Rationale: This approach keeps the ties sterile.**
    - Make a three-quarter turn, then take the tie from the co-worker and secure it in front of the gown.
    - *Or* have a co-worker wearing sterile gloves take the two ties at each side of the gown and tie them at the back of the gown, making sure that your uniform is completely covered. **Rationale: Both methods ensure that the back of the gown remains sterile.**
    - When worn, sterile gowns should be considered *sterile* only in front from the waist to the shoulder. The sleeves should be considered sterile from the cuff to 5 cm above the elbow, since the arms of a scrubbed person must move across a sterile field. Moisture collection and friction areas, such as the neckline, shoulders, underarms and back, should be considered unsterile.
12. Remove and dispose of used gown and gloves.
    - If soiled, remove the attire by turning it inside out. See removal of disposable gowns and gloves in Skill 32.2 for the sequence of removing the gown.

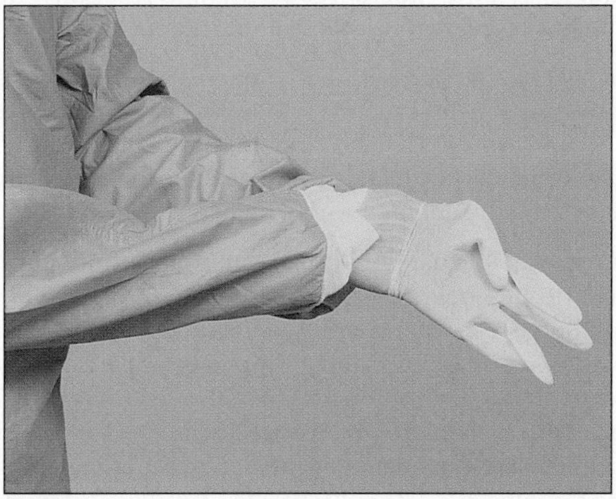

❹ Pulling on the first sterile glove

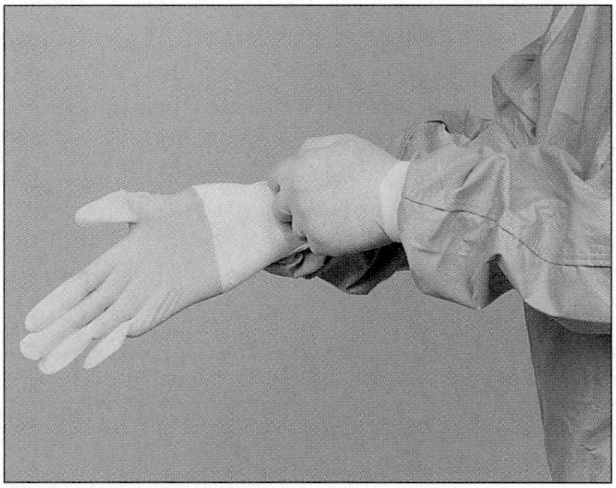

❺ Extending the fingers into the second glove of the dominant hand

EVALUATION

- Conduct any follow-up indicated during your care of the client. Ensure that adequate numbers and types of sterile supplies are available for the next health-care provider.

Support of the Defences of a Susceptible Host

People are constantly in contact with microorganisms in the environment. Normally, a person's natural defences ward off the development of an infection. *Susceptibility* is the degree to which an individual can be affected, that is, the likelihood of an organism causing an infection in that person. Factors affecting a person's susceptibility have previously been identified. Although it is not possible to specifically manipulate age or heredity as risk factors, a number of strategies can support host defences.

CLINICAL ALERT

A person does not need to have an identified infection in order to pass potentially infective microorganisms to another person. Even normal microorganisms for one person can infect another person.

HYGIENE Maintaining the intactness of the skin and mucous membranes retains a barrier against microorganisms entering the body. In addition, oral care, including flossing the teeth, reduces the likelihood of an oral infection. Regular and thorough bathing and shampooing remove microorganisms, and the dirt that contains them, that can cause an infection.

NUTRITION A balanced diet enhances the health of all body tissues, helps keep the skin intact, and promotes the skin's ability to repel microorganisms. Adequate nutrition enables tissues to maintain and rebuild themselves and helps keep the immune system functioning well.

FLUID An adequate fluid intake permits a fluid output that flushes out the bladder and urethra, removing microorganisms that could cause an infection. Adequate hydration also helps maintain the natural barriers since dehydrated skin or mucous membranes have breaks through which microorganisms can enter. Adequate rest and sleep are essential to health and to renewing energy. See Chapter 37.

STRESS Excessive stress predisposes people to infections. Nurses can assist clients to learn stress-reducing techniques. See Chapter 47.

OPTIMIZING TISSUE OXYGENATION AND BLOOD FLOW Optimizing blood flow allows sufficient numbers of leukocytes to reach a given tissue; these are key cells for reducing the number of microorganisms locally. Adequate tissue oxygenation will promote production of ATP (adenosine triphosphate) for use by the leukocytes and either replacement or strengthening of the tissue. Reducing smoking, ensuring adequate hydration, managing pain, reducing stress, reducing obesity, and correcting anemia are all strategies that promote blood flow and tissue oxygenation.

GLYCEMIC CONTROL Uncontrolled diabetes is a major risk factor for a variety of infections. Maintaining glycemic control can reduce the physiological changes that increase risk. Studies have shown that hemoglobin A1C levels of less than 7%, the target indicator of glycemic control, are significantly associated with lower rates of infection in surgical patients (Dronge et al., 2006). Diabetic clients need to be taught to monitor their blood glucose levels and appropriate diet, exercise, and medication strategies for controlling them.

IMMUNIZATIONS Immunizations have dramatically decreased the incidence of infectious diseases. It is recommended that immunizations begin shortly after birth and be completed in early childhood, except for boosters (see Table 32.9 for recommended immunizations for Canadian children). Immunizations are frequently given in combination to minimize multiple injections. Because immunization schedules change frequently, it is advisable to update immunization schedules yearly. The information can be obtained from the Public Health Agency of Canada National Advisory Committee on Immunization. Similar committees exist in other countries, including the United States, Australia, and the United Kingdom, and as part of the World Health Organization.

All adults should ensure they are adequately immunized, by completion of childhood vaccination or by booster doses, as appropriate, against the following diseases: diphtheria, tetanus, pertussis, polio, measles, mumps, and rubella (see Table 32.10). Immunization

TABLE 32.9 Routine Immunization Schedules for Infants and Children

Age at vaccination	DTaP-IPV	Hib	MMR	Var	HB	Pneu-C-7	Men-C	Tdap	Inf
Birth					Infancy 3 doses ★				
2 months	⊖	✦				⧓	⊙		
4 months	⊖	✦				⧓	(⊙)		
6 months	⊖	✦				⧓	⊙ or		6–23 months ⊗ 1–2 doses
12 months			■	●		⧓ 12–15 months	⊙ if not yet given		
18 months	⊖	✦	■						
4–6 years	⊖		or ■						
14–15 years					Pre-teen/teen 2–3 doses		⊙ if not yet given	▲	

⊖ Diphtheria, tetanus, acellular pertussis and inactivated polio virus vaccine (DTaP-IPV)

✦ *Haemophilus influenzae* type b conjugate vaccine (Hib)

■ Measles, mumps, and rubella vaccine (MMR)

● Varicella vaccine (Var)

★ Hepatitis B vaccine (HB)

⧓ Pneumococcal conjugate vaccine: 7-valent (Pneu-C-7)

⊙ Meningococcal C conjugate vaccine (Men-C)

▲ Diphtheria, tetanus, acellular pertussis vaccine: adult/adolescent formulation (Tdap)

⊗ Influenza vaccine (Flu)

Source: *Canadian Immunization Guide* (7th ed.) 2006, by the Public Health Agency of Canada, Ottawa: Minister of Public Works and Government Services Canada, 2006.

Notes: There are provincial and territorial variations to this immunization schedule.

TABLE 32.10 Adult Immunization Schedule: Routine and Specific Risk Situations

Vaccine or Toxoid	Dosing Schedule If No Record or Unclear History of Immunization	Booster Schedule if Primary Series Completed
Tetanus and diphtheria given as Td; and pertussis given as Tdap	Doses 1 and 2, 4 to 8 weeks apart and dose 3 at 6 to 12 months later; one of the doses should be given as Tdap for pertussis protection	Td every 10 years; 1 dose should be given as Tdap if not previously given in adulthood
Measles, mumps, and rubella given as MMR	1 dose for adults born in or after 1970 without a history of measles or those individuals without evidence of immunity to rubella or mumps; second dose for selected groups	Not routinely required
Varicella	Doses 1 and 2 at least 4 weeks apart for susceptible adults (no history of natural disease or seronegativity)	Not currently recommended
Influenza	Adults ≥ 65 years; adults < 65 years at high risk of influenza-related complications, their household contacts, health-care workers, and all those wanting to be protected against influenza	Every autumn by using current recommended vaccine formulation
Pneumococcal polysaccharide	Adults ≥ 65 years; adults < 65 who have conditions putting them at increased risk of pneumococcal disease	1 dose

Source: *Canadian Immunization Guide* (7th ed.) 2006, by the Public Health Agency of Canada, Ottawa: Minister of Public Works and Government Services Canada.

programs are also available for high-risk groups, such as health-care personnel, people who have had a splenectomy, and people travelling, each of which require individual assessment. In view of the increased risk of exposure to communicable diseases, the following vaccines are also recommended for all health-care workers and others providing personal care: hepatitis B, influenza, and varicella if seronegative.

New vaccines are reviewed as they appear and may be recommended for very specific populations. For example, Gardasil, a vaccine against the human papillomavirus (HPV), is recommended for girls 9 to 13, before they commence sexual intercourse, and females between 14 and 26 years of age, even if they are already sexually active, have had previous Pap abnormalities, or have had a previous HPV infection (National Advisory Committee on Immunization, 2007b).

Routine Practices and Additional Precautions

History of Isolation Precautions

Isolation precautions refer to measures designed to prevent the spread of infections or potentially infectious microorganisms to health-care personnel, clients, and visitors. A variety of infection prevention and control measures are used to decrease the risk of transmission of microorganisms in hospitals.

The history of Canada's isolation guidelines, under the guidance of the Laboratory Centre for Disease Control (LCDC), which has been replaced by the Public Health Agency of Canada, parallels that of the United States' Centers for Disease Control and Prevention (CDC).

Historically, health-care workers applied PPE and other measures when a client or resident was known to have or suspected of having an infection or communicable disease. To facilitate implementation, recommendations were written as systems of either category-specific or disease-specific isolation.

Category-specific isolation precautions were based on the presumed major mechanism of transmission and included seven categories: (1) strict isolation, (2) contact isolation, (3) respiratory isolation, (4) tuberculosis isolation, (5) enteric precautions, (6) drainage or secretions precautions, and (7) blood or body fluid precautions.

Disease-specific isolation precautions provided precautions for specific diseases. These precautions delineated using private rooms with special ventilation, having the client share a room with other clients infected with the same organism, and gowning to prevent gross soiling of clothes for specific infectious diseases.

In the 1980s, it became increasingly recognized that a number of people carried blood-borne infectious agents without being identified as carriers. In 1987, the CDC and LCDC therefore presented recommendations (revised in 1988) for *universal precautions* (*UP*) on *all clients* to decrease the risk of transmitting unidentified pathogens. Universal precautions applied to those body fluids associated with *blood-borne pathogens,* namely, hepatitis B virus, hepatitis C virus, and HIV. This included blood and other body fluids containing visible blood. The recommendation did not imply that universal precautions replaced disease-specific or category-specific precautions but that they should be used in conjunction with them.

The *body substance isolation* (BSI) system, introduced in the early 1990s, employed generic infection prevention and control precautions for *all* clients, except those with the few diseases transmitted through the airborne route. This system was based on three premises:

1. All people have an increased risk for infection from microorganisms placed on their mucous membranes and nonintact skin.
2. All people are likely to have potentially infectious microorganisms in all of their moist body sites and substances.
3. An unknown portion of clients and health-care workers will always be colonized or infected with potentially infectious microorganisms in their blood and other moist body sites and substances.

The term *body substance* included blood and some body fluids but also urine, feces, wound drainage, oral secretions, and any other body substance. Barrier precautions addressed the activity performed as opposed to the diagnosis.

Recommendations evolved further in the mid-1990s, with selection of the best recommendations from all previous work being merged into standard precautions and three categories of transmission-based precautions. This framework was directed at acute-care facilities and did not address specific needs of long-term-care, ambulatory care, and home care agencies. To this end, Canadian authorities advocated the terms *routine practices* and *additional precautions* in place of *standard precautions* and *transmission-based precautions,* to emphasize the need to apply precautions to all patients, no matter the venue of health care. This system of routine practices and additional precautions, first published in 1999 (Health Canada, 1999), remains current today and provides recommendations that include these settings, as well as include special considerations for the prevention of transmission of tuberculosis, blood-borne pathogens, hemorrhagic fevers, and certain multidrug-resistant organisms, such as vancomycin-resistant enterococci (VRE).

Routine Practices

Routine practices are used in the care of all clients regardless of their diagnosis or possible infection status. They apply to blood, all body fluids, secretions, and excretions (*except sweat*), nonintact skin, and mucous membranes whether or not blood is present or visible. Routine practices combine the major features of universal precautions and body substance isolation. Recommended practices for routine practices are shown in Box 32.2.

BOX 32.2 RECOMMENDED ROUTINE PRACTICES

- These recommendations are designed for *all* clients (i.e., in hospital, long-term-care facilities, community, and any other care setting).
- These precautions apply to blood; all body fluids, excretions, and secretions except sweat; nonintact (broken) skin; and mucous membranes.
- They are designed to reduce risk of transmission of microorganisms from recognized and unrecognized sources.

1. Wash hands after contact with blood, body fluids, secretions, excretions, nonintact skin, mucous membranes, and contaminated objects whether or not gloves are worn. If hands are not visibly soiled, then hand hygiene may be performed with an alcohol-based hand rub. Hand hygiene is performed between client contacts.
   a. Perform hand hygiene immediately after removing gloves.
   b. Use a plain soap for routine handwashing.
   c. Use an antimicrobial agent or an antiseptic agent for the control of specific outbreaks of infection.
2. Wear clean gloves when touching blood, body fluids, secretions, excretions, nonintact skin and mucous membranes, and contaminated items (e.g., soiled gowns).
   a. Clean gloves can be unsterile unless their use is intended to prevent the entrance of microorganisms into the body. See the discussion of sterile gloves in this chapter.
   b. Remove gloves before touching uncontaminated items and surfaces.
   c. Perform hand hygiene immediately after removing gloves.
3. Wear a mask, eye protection, or a face shield if splashes or sprays of blood, body fluids, secretions, or excretions can be expected.
4. Wear a clean, nonsterile gown if client care is likely to result in splashes or sprays of blood, body fluids, secretions, or excretions. The gown is intended to protect clothing.
   a. Remove a soiled gown carefully to avoid the transfer of microorganisms to others (i.e., clients, other health-care workers, or yourself).
   b. Perform hand hygiene after removing gown.

(continued)

BOX 32.2 RECOMMENDED PRACTICES FOR ROUTINE PRACTICES (*continued*)

5. Handle client care equipment that is soiled with blood, body fluids, secretions, or excretions carefully to prevent the transfer of microorganisms to others and to the environment.
   a. Make sure reusable equipment is cleaned and reprocessed correctly.
   b. Dispose of single-use equipment correctly.
6. Handle, transport, and process linen that is soiled with blood, body fluids, secretions, or excretions in a manner to prevent contamination of clothing and the transfer of microorganisms to others and to the environment.
7. Prevent injuries from used scalpels, needles, or other equipment, and place in puncture-resistant containers.

Additional Precautions

Additional precautions are used in addition to routine practices for clients with *known* or *suspected* infections that are spread in one of three ways: by airborne transmission, by droplet transmission, or by contact (direct or indirect). The three types of additional precautions can be used alone or in combination with each other but they are always used *in addition* to routine practices. They encompass all the conditions or diseases previously listed in the category-specific or disease-specific classifications. Recommended practices for additional precautions are shown in Box 32.3.

BOX 32.3 RECOMMENDED ADDITIONAL PRECAUTIONS

The following are additional precautions:

AIRBORNE PRECAUTIONS

Use the routine practices as well as the following:

1. Place the client in a private room that has negative air pressure, six to nine air changes per hour, and either discharge of air to the outside or a filtration system for the room air. Keep doors closed.
2. If a private room is not available, place the client with another client who is infected with the same microorganism.
3. Wear a respirator (e.g., N95) when entering the room of a client who is known or suspected of having primary tuberculosis.
4. Susceptible people should not enter the room of a client who has rubella (measles) or varicella (chickenpox). If they must enter, they should wear a respirator.
5. Limit movement of client outside the room to essential purposes. Place a surgical mask on the client during transport.
6. Perform hand hygiene after removing a respirator.

DROPLET PRECAUTIONS

Use the routine practices as well as the following:

1. Place the client in a private room.
2. If a private room is not available, place the client with another client who is infected with the same microorganism.
3. Wear a mask if working within 1 to 2 metres of the client.
4. Limit movement of the client outside the room to essential purposes. Place a surgical mask on the client during transport.
5. Perform hand hygiene after removing mask.

CONTACT PRECAUTIONS

Use the routine practices as well as the following:

1. Place the client in a private room.
2. If a private room is not available, place the client with another client who is infected with the same microorganism.
3. Wear gloves on entering the client's room.
   a. Change gloves after contact with infectious material.
   b. Remove gloves before leaving the client's room.
   c. Perform hand hygiene immediately after removing gloves.
   d. After handwashing, do not touch possibly contaminated surfaces or items in the room.
4. Wear a gown when entering a room if there is a possibility of contact with infected surfaces or items, or if the client is incontinent, or has diarrhea, a colostomy, or wound drainage not contained by a dressing.
   a. Remove gown in the client's room.
   b. Make sure uniform does not contact possible contaminated surfaces.
5. Limit movement of the client outside the room.
6. Dedicate the use of noncritical client care equipment to a single client or to clients with the same infecting microorganisms.

Source: Summarized from "Routine Practices and Additional Precautions for Preventing the Transmission of Infection in Health Care," by Health Canada, 1999, *Canada Communicable Disease Report, 25S4* (July), pp. 1–155. © Minister of Public Works and Government Services Canada, 2002.

Airborne precautions are used for clients known or suspected to have serious illnesses transmitted by airborne droplet nuclei smaller than 5 microns. Examples of such illnesses include measles, rubeola, varicella (including disseminated zoster), and tuberculosis.

Droplet precautions are used for clients known or suspected to have serious illnesses transmitted by particle droplets larger than 5 microns. Examples of such illnesses are diphtheria (pharyngeal); pertussis (whooping cough); mumps; rubella; influenza, pneumonia, scarlet fever in infants and young children; and pneumonic plague.

Contact precautions are used for clients known or suspected to have serious illnesses easily transmitted by direct client contact or by contact with items in the client's environment. Such illnesses include gastrointestinal, respiratory, skin, or wound infections or colonization with multidrug-resistant bacteria; specific enteric infections, such as *Clostridium difficile,* enterohemorrhagic *Escherichia coli* O157:H7, *Shigella,* and hepatitis A in diapered or incontinent clients; respiratory syncytial virus, parainfluenza virus, or enteroviral infections in infants and young children; and highly contagious skin infections, such as herpes simplex virus, impetigo, pediculosis, and scabies.

SPECIAL CONSIDERATIONS: COUGH ETIQUETTE To further reduce transmission by droplets, respiratory secretions should be contained as much as possible. **Cough etiquette** involves coughing or sneezing into tissues or cloth (e.g., sleeves) rather than hands, which become contaminated. Used tissues should be immediately discarded, not saved for reuse, and hands washed or decontaminated with an alcohol-based hand rub. Further containment of infection can be achieved by recognizing when you pose a risk to others and staying home from work and not socializing.

SPECIAL CONSIDERATIONS: MULTIDRUG-RESISTANT ORGANISMS AND EMERGING PATHOGENS In addition to the preceding precautions, additional measures can be used for specific communicable diseases caused by multidrug or antibiotic-resistant organisms, such as vancomycin-resistant enterococci (VRE) or methicillin-resistant *Staphylococcus aureus* (MRSA). Nurses should follow their agency's guidelines with respect to these pathogens, as protocols vary by jurisdiction. Additional precautions may also be warranted for newly emerging infectious agents, such as severe acute respiratory syndrome (SARS), or microorganisms that are difficult to eliminate from the environment, such as *Clostridium difficile* or norovirus.

SPECIAL CONSIDERATIONS: IMMUNOCOMPROMISED CLIENTS Compromised clients are those who are highly susceptible to infection, such as those who

- Have diseases (e.g., leukemia) or have received treatments (e.g., cancer chemotherapy) that depress the resistance to infectious organisms
- Have extensive skin impairments, such as severe dermatitis or major burns that cannot be effectively covered with dressings

Such clients are often infected by their own microorganisms (endogenous source), but they can also be infected by microorganisms carried on the inadequately washed hands of health-care personnel, and by nonsterile items (food, water, air, and client care equipment). Guidelines for severely compromised (immunocompromised) clients include the use of routine practices and additional precautions appropriate to their condition. Additional cleaning and use of protective clothing are not necessary beyond routine practices. The need for a single room depends on the extent to which the individual is compromised. Handwashing by health-care workers and visitors, and protection from those with infection, are essential to reducing transmission of organisms.

Practical Issues for Implementation of Precautions

Disposal of Soiled Equipment and Supplies

Many pieces of equipment are supplied for single use only and are disposed of after use. Some items, however, are reusable. Agencies have specific policies and procedures for handling soiled equipment (e.g., disposal, cleaning, disinfecting, and sterilizing); the nurse needs to be familiar with these practices and with what items can be reused. Appropriate handling of soiled equipment and supplies is essential for these reasons:

- To prevent inadvertent exposure of health-care workers to articles contaminated with body substances
- To prevent contamination of the environment

See Skill 32.2 for removing soiled PPE. Information about cleaning, disinfecting, and sterilizing is presented earlier in this chapter.

BAGGING Most articles do not need to be placed in bags unless they are contaminated, or likely to have been contaminated, with infective material, such as pus, blood, body fluids, feces, or respiratory secretions. Contaminated articles need to be enclosed in a sturdy bag impervious to microorganisms before removal from the client's room. Some agencies use labels or bags of a particular colour that designate them as infective wastes.

Follow agency protocol, or use the following guidelines to handle and bag soiled items:

- Use a single bag if it is sturdy and impervious to microorganisms, and if the contaminated articles can be placed in the bag without soiling or contaminating its outside.
- Double-bag if the above conditions are not met.
- Place garbage and soiled *disposable* equipment, including dressings and tissues, in the plastic bag that lines the waste container. Some agencies separate dry and wet waste material and incinerate dry items, such as paper towels and disposable items. No special precautions are required for disposable equipment that is not contaminated.
- Place *nondisposable* or *reusable* equipment that is visibly soiled in a labelled bag before removing it from the client's room or cubicle, and send it to a central processing area for decontamination. Some agencies may require that glass and metal items be placed in separate bags from rubber and plastic items. Glass and metal can be sterilized in an autoclave, but rubber and plastic are damaged by this process and must be cleaned by other methods, such as gas sterilization.
- Disassemble *special procedure trays* into component parts. Some components are disposable; others need to be sent to the laundry or central services for cleaning and decontaminating.
- Bag soiled *clothing* before sending it home or to the agency laundry.

LINENS Handle soiled linen as little as possible and with minimal manipulation before placing it in the laundry hamper. This prevents gross microbial contamination of the air and persons handling the linen. Close the bag before sending it to the laundry, in accordance with agency protocol.

LABORATORY SPECIMENS Laboratory specimens, if placed in a leakproof container with a secure lid, need no special precautions. Use care when collecting specimens to avoid contaminating the outside of the container. Containers that are visibly contaminated on the outside should be placed inside a sealable plastic bag before sending them to the laboratory. This prevents personnel from having hand contact with potentially infective material.

DISHES Dishes require no special precautions. Soiling of dishes can largely be prevented by encouraging clients to wash their hands before eating. Some agencies use paper dishes for convenience, which are disposed of in the refuse container.

BLOOD PRESSURE EQUIPMENT Other than routine cleaning, blood pressure equipment needs no special precautions unless it becomes contaminated with infective material. If it does become contaminated, follow agency practice. Cleaning procedures vary according to whether it is a wall or portable unit.

THERMOMETERS Nondisposable used thermometers are generally disinfected after use. Check agency practice.

DISPOSABLE NEEDLES, SYRINGES, AND SHARPS Place needles, syringes, and sharps (e.g., lancets, scalpels, and broken glass) into a puncture-resistant container. To avoid puncture wounds, do not detach needles from the syringe or recap the needle before disposal. See Chapter 31 for preventing needle-stick injuries.

TOYS Personal toys that are visibly contaminated are bagged and sent home. Agency toys, if visibly soiled, may require cleaning. Check agency practice. Depending on the type of microorganism, its transmission, and the child's hygiene behaviours, special precautions may be required. For example, a child who has an enteric infection that can be spread by contact transmission or by fomites may not be allowed to share toys with others.

HAZARDOUS MATERIAL In addition to precautions discussed in this chapter, significant emphasis is placed on avoiding injury caused by sharp instruments, measures to be taken in case of exposure to blood-borne pathogens, and communication of biohazards to employees. Health Canada (2008) requires that Workplace Hazardous Materials Information System (WHMIS) labels be affixed to containers of regulated waste and to refrigerators and freezers containing blood or other potentially infectious materials. The labels required are fluorescent orange or orange-red and feature the biohazard symbol shown in Figure 32.3.

Transporting Clients with Infections

Transporting clients with infections outside their own rooms is avoided unless absolutely necessary. If a client

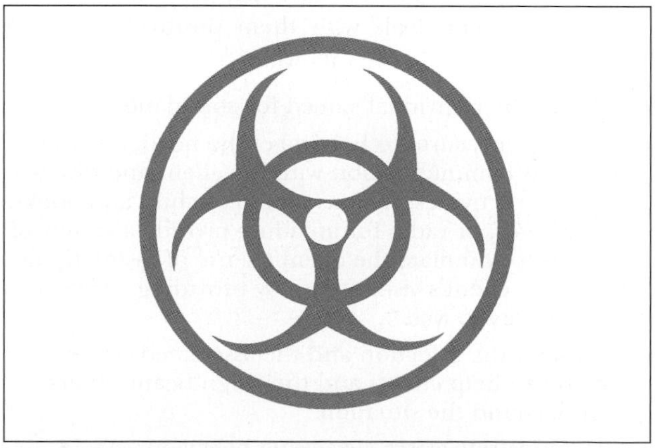

FIGURE 32.3 Biohazard infectious materials

(From Health Canada. Workplace Hazardous Materials Information System. http://www.hc-sc.gc.ca/hecs-sesc/whmis/whmis_symbols.htm)

must be moved, the nurse implements appropriate measures to prevent soilage of the environment. For example, the nurse ensures that any draining wound is securely covered or places a surgical mask on the client who has an airborne infection. In addition, the nurse notifies personnel at the receiving area of any infection risk so that they can maintain necessary precautions. Follow agency protocol.

Psychosocial Needs of Clients Requiring Isolation Precautions

Clients requiring isolation precautions can develop several problems as a result of the separation from others and of the special precautions taken in their care. Two of the most common are sensory deprivation and feelings of inferiority. *Sensory deprivation* occurs when the environment lacks normal stimuli for the client, for example, communication with others. Nurses should, therefore, be alert to common clinical signs of sensory deprivation: boredom, inactivity, slowness of thought, daydreaming, increased sleeping, thought disorganization, anxiety, hallucinations, and panic. Furthermore, nurses should be aware that staff members might contribute to sensory deprivation by spending less time with the client than might otherwise occur, especially if the client is in a single room, or if gowns and masks are required. Since the latter require additional time for client care, nurses may not be able to frequently or quickly check on a client.

A client's *feeling of inferiority* can be due to the perception of the infection itself or to the required precautions. In North America, many people place a high value on cleanliness, and the idea of being "soiled," "contaminated," or "dirty" can give clients the feeling that they are at fault and are substandard. Although this is inaccurate, the infected persons may feel they are not as good as others and blame themselves.

Nurses need to provide care that prevents these two problems or that deals with them positively. Nursing interventions include the following:

- Assess the individual's need for stimulation.
- Initiate measures to help meet the need, including regular communication with the client and diversionary activities, such as toys for a child and books, television, or radio for an adult; provide a variety of foods to stimulate the client's sense of taste; stimulate the client's visual sense by providing a view or an activity to watch.
- Explain the infection and the associated procedures to help clients and their significant others understand the situation.
- Demonstrate warm, accepting behaviour. Avoid conveying to the client any sense of annoyance about the precautions or any feelings of revulsion about the infection.
- Do not use stricter precautions than are indicated by the diagnosis or the client's condition.

Nursing Responsibility for Infection Prevention and Control

Initiation of practices to prevent the transmission of microorganisms is generally a nursing responsibility and is based on a comprehensive assessment of the client. This assessment takes into account the status of the client's normal defence mechanisms, the client's ability to implement necessary precautions, and the source and mode of transmission of the infectious agent. The nurse then decides whether to wear gloves, gowns, masks, or protective eyewear. In all client situations, nurses must *perform appropriate hand hygiene.* Nurses should be aware of resources in their practice setting, such as an infection prevention and control policy and procedure manuals or infection-control practitioners, and refer to these resources for guidance when necessary.

Besides initiating and maintaining routine practices and additional precautions, nurses have a responsibility for evaluating changes in the client's condition that could indicate a need for further precautions, or indicate that additional precautions are no longer warranted. In some agencies or practice settings, especially community health, nurses are responsible for notifying the local public health officials about notifiable diseases so that accurate incidence rates can be calculated and contacts managed, as appropriate. Nurses might also be responsible for alerting infection-control practitioners about incidence or clusters of infections, or situations that might increase risk of infection. Nurses share responsibility for ensuring visitors wash their hands and follow posted instructions, and for assisting clients to clean their hands after using the toilet and before eating (see the Reflect on Primary Health Care box). Furthermore, nurses can demonstrate prevention behaviours by updating their immunizations and not reporting to work when ill.

In addition to the precautions cited within this chapter, the nurse implements specific actions relevant to infection prevention and control when performing many

REFLECT ON PRIMARY HEALTH CARE

Canadians have become increasingly aware of the importance of hand hygiene in the prevention and control of infection. Consider the role of *intersectoral collaboration* the next time you see a sign in a washroom reminding you to wash your hands. Automated wall mounted alcohol-based hand rub dispensers at entrance ways to public facilities and automatic sensor water faucets are examples of *appropriate technology* to limit the spread of infection. The next time a client or patient asks, "have you washed your hands?" consider that this person is a true *participant* in his or her health care.

specific therapies discussed throughout this book. The following are some examples:

- Use strict aseptic technique when performing any invasive procedure (e.g., inserting an intravenous needle or catheter, suctioning an airway, and inserting a urinary catheter) and when changing surgical dressings.
- Handle needles and syringes carefully to avoid needle-stick injuries. See Chapter 31.
- Change intravenous cannulae, tubing, and solution containers according to agency policy. See Chapter 43.
- Check all sterile supplies for expiry date and intact packaging before use.
- Prevent urinary infections by maintaining a closed urinary drainage system with a downward flow of urine. Do not irrigate a catheter unless ordered to do so. Provide regular catheter and perineal care. Keep the drainage bag and spout off the floor. See Chapter 41.
- Implement measures to prevent impaired skin integrity and to prevent accumulation of secretions in the lungs (for example, encourage the client to move, breathe deeply, and cough at least every two hours).

Assessing

NURSING HISTORY During the nursing history, the nurse assesses (1) the degree to which a client is at risk for developing an infection, and (2) any client complaints suggesting the presence of an infection. To identify clients at risk, the nurse reviews the client's chart and structures the nursing interview to collect data regarding the factors influencing the development of infection, especially existing disease process, history of recurrent infections, current medications and therapeutic measures, current emotional stressors, nutritional status, and history of immunizations. To obtain subjective data that may indicate the presence of an infection, the nurse asks whether the client has experienced loss of energy, loss of appetite, nausea, headache, or other signs associated with specific body systems (e.g., difficulty urinating, urinary frequency, or a sore throat). Specific questions to be asked depend on the clinical situation and should be directly related to what the suspected infection might be or the type of infection for which the client is likely at risk. See the Assessment: Interview box for sample assessment questions.

PHYSICAL ASSESSMENT Signs and symptoms of an infection vary according to the body area involved. For example, sneezing, watery or mucoid discharge from the nose, and nasal stuffiness commonly occur with an infection of the nose and sinuses; urinary frequency and sometimes cloudy or discoloured urine often occur with a urinary infection. Signs and symptoms of *localized infection* include the following:

- Localized swelling
- Localized redness
- Pain or tenderness with palpation or movement
- Palpable heat at the infected area
- Loss of function of the body part affected, depending on the site and extent of involvement
- Drainage from open wounds; exudate may be of various colours

Signs and symptoms of *systemic infection* are as follows:

- Fever
- Increased pulse and respiratory rate, if the fever is high
- Lassitude, malaise, and loss of energy
- Anorexia and, in some situations, nausea and vomiting
- Enlargement and tenderness of lymph nodes that drain the area of infection

LABORATORY DATA Laboratory data that indicate the presence of an infection include the following:

- Elevated leukocyte (white blood cell or WBC) count, if it is higher than 11×10^9/L.
- Increases in specific types of leukocytes as revealed in the differential white blood cell count. Specific

ASSESSMENT: INTERVIEW

Clients at Risk for Infections

The questions a nurse needs to ask will depend on the client, but the following provide a good guideline:

- When were you last immunized for diphtheria, tetanus, poliomyelitis, rubella, measles, influenza, hepatitis, and pneumococcal pneumonia?*
- When did you last have a tuberculin skin test?*
- What infections have you had in the past, and how were these treated?
- Have any of these infections recurred?
- Are you taking any antineoplastic, anti-inflammatory, or antibiotic medications?
- Do you smoke?
- Are you overweight?
- Do you have diabetes? If yes, how well controlled is it?
- Have you recently been exposed to someone with an infection?
- Have you had any recent diagnostic procedure or therapy that penetrated your skin or a body cavity?*
- What past surgeries have you had?
- How would you describe your nutritional status in terms of a well-balanced diet?
- On a scale of 0 to 10, how would you rate the stress you have experienced in the last 6 months?

* These questions would be tailored according to the nature of the infection the person is at risk for or suspected of having.

types of white blood cells are increased or decreased in certain infections.

- Urine, blood, sputum, or other drainage *cultures* that indicate the presence of pathogenic microorganisms. Culture and sensitivity testing involves laboratory cultivation of bacteria or yeast in a special growth medium. Laboratories report the specific species as well as its sensitivity or resistance to specific antibiotics. A Gram stain smear is also done, to identify the presence of bacteria, white blood cells, and epithelial cells in the original specimen. The presence of numerous white blood cells is indicative of infection, whereas the presence of numerous epithelial cells is indicative of a poor-quality specimen (e.g., sputum may be contaminated with saliva). Collecting a good specimen is important if results are to be credible and useful. See also Skill 33.1 (page 944), "Obtaining a Wound Drainage Specimen for Culture."

Diagnosing

The NANDA International (2007) nursing diagnostic labels for problems associated with the transmission of microorganisms are (1) *Risk for Infection:* the state in which an individual is at risk for being invaded by an opportunistic or pathogenic microorganism from endogenous or exogenous sources; and (2) *Risk for Transmission of Infection*: the state in which an individual is at risk for transferring an opportunistic or pathogenic agent to others. Related factors may be pathophysiological in nature, treatment related, situational, or maturational.

Clients who have, or are at risk for, an infection are prime candidates for other physical and psychological problems. Examples of nursing diagnoses or collaborative problems that can arise from the actual presence of an infection include the following:

- *Potential Complication of Infection: Fever*
- *Imbalanced Nutrition Less Than Body Requirements* if the client is too ill to eat adequately
- *Acute Pain* if the client is experiencing tissue damage and discomfort
- *Impaired Social Interaction* or *Social Isolation* if the client is required to be separated from others during a contagious episode
- *Anxiety* if the client is apprehensive regarding changes in life activities resulting from the infection or its treatment, such as absence from work or inability to perform usual functions

Planning

The major goals for clients susceptible to infection are to

- Maintain or restore defences
- Avoid the spread of infectious organisms
- Reduce or alleviate problems associated with the infection

Desired health outcomes depend on the individual client's condition. Examples of desired health outcomes, although established in the planning phase, are provided in Table 32.11 in the "Evaluating" section later in this chapter (page 920).

Nursing strategies to meet the three broad goals stated above generally include the measures previously described for breaking the chain of infection, such as using meticulous hand hygiene and aseptic techniques to prevent the spread of potentially infectious microorganisms, implementing measures to support the defences of a susceptible host, and teaching clients about protective measures to prevent infections and the spread of infectious agents when an infection is present.

Examples of interventions related to clients at risk for infection include the following:

- Environmental management
- Infection prevention and control (e.g., minimizing the acquisition and transmission of infectious agents)
- Risk identification
- Teaching of individuals
- Wound care

Specific nursing activities associated with each of these interventions can be selected to meet the individual needs of the client.

PLANNING FOR HOME CARE Clients being discharged following hospital care for an infection often require continued care to completely eliminate the infection or to adapt to a chronic state. In addition, such clients may be at increased risk for reinfection or development of an opportunistic infection following therapy for existing pathogens.

In preparation for discharge, the nurse needs to know the clients and family's risks, needs, strengths, and resources. The nurse tailors the teaching plan for the client and family (see the Teaching: Home Care box).

Implementing

Whenever possible, the nurse invokes strategies to prevent infection. If infection cannot be prevented, the nurse works to prevent the spread of the infection within and between persons and to treat the existing infection. In the previous sections, specific nursing activities were described that interfere with the chain of infection to prevent and control transmission of infectious organisms and that promote care of the infected client. These activities were summarized earlier in Tables 32.5 and 32.6.

Evaluating

By using data collected during care—vital signs, breath sounds, skin status, characteristics of urine or other

TEACHING: HOME CARE

Environmental Management

The way the client takes care of an infection after going home is important. The nurse can help by teaching the client how to do it correctly:

- Discuss injury proofing the home to prevent the possibility of further tissue injury (e.g., use of padding, handrails, removal of hazards).
- Explore ways to control the environmental temperature and airflow (especially if the client has an airborne pathogen).
- Determine the advisability of visitors and family members in close proximity to the client.
- Describe ways to manipulate the bed, the room, and other household facilities.

INFECTION CONTROL

- Based on assessment of client and family knowledge, teach proper hand hygiene (e.g. before handling foods, before eating, after toileting, before and after any required home care treatment, and after touching any body substances, such as wound drainage) and related hygiene measures to all family members.
- Promote nail care: keep fingernails short, clean, and well manicured to eliminate rough edges or hangnails, which can harbour microorganisms.
- Instruct not to share personal care items, such as toothbrush, washcloths, and towels, and describe the rationale of how infections can be transmitted from shared personal items.
- Discuss antimicrobial soaps and effective disinfectants.
- Ensure access to and proper use of gloves and other barriers as indicated by the type of infection or risk.
- Discuss the relationship among hygiene, rest, activity, and nutrition in the chain of infection.
- Instruct about proper administration of medication.
- Instruct about cleaning reusable equipment and supplies. Use soap and water, and disinfect with a chlorine bleach solution.

INFECTION PREVENTION

- Teach the client and family members how to avoid infections.
- Suggest techniques for safe food preservation and preparation (e.g., wash raw fruits and vegetables before eating them, refrigerate all opened and unpackaged foods).
- Remind to avoid coughing, sneezing, or breathing directly on others. Cover the mouth and nose with a tissue or the sleeve to prevent the transmission of airborne microorganisms.
- Inform of the importance of maintaining sufficient fluid intake to promote urine production and output. This helps flush the bladder and urethra of microorganisms.
- Emphasize the need for proper immunizations of all family members.

WOUND CARE

- Teach the client and family the signs of wound healing and of wound infection and why monitoring of the wound is important.
- Delineate the factors that promote wound healing.
- Explain the proper technique for changing the dressing and disposing of the soiled one. Reinforce the need to place contaminated dressings and other disposable items containing body fluids in moistureproof plastic bags.
- Advise to put used needles in a puncture-resistant container with a screw-top lid. Label so as not to discard in the garbage.

REFERRALS

- Provide appropriate information regarding how to access community resources, home care agencies, sources of supplies, and community or public health departments for immunizations.

drainage, laboratory blood values, and so on—the nurse judges whether client health outcomes have been achieved. Examples of client goals and related health outcomes are shown in Table 32.11.

If outcomes are not achieved, the nurse may need to consider such questions as the following:

- Were appropriate measures implemented to prevent skin breakdown and lung infection?
- Was strict aseptic technique implemented for invasive procedures?
- Are prescribed medications affecting the immune system?
- Is client placement appropriate to reduce the risk of transmission of microorganisms?
- Did the client and family misunderstand or fail to comply with necessary instructions?

Occupational Health Issues Related to Infection

The Public Health Agency of Canada provides guidelines to protect health-care workers from occupational exposure to blood-borne pathogens in the workplace. **Occupational exposure** is defined as reasonably anticipated skin, eye, mucous membrane, or parenteral contact with blood or other potentially infectious materials that may result from the performance of an employee's duties.

The transmission of infectious fluids in the clinical setting has three major modes:

TABLE 32.11 Evaluation of Goals and Health Outcomes: Risk for Infection

Goal	Examples of Desired Health Outcomes	Goal	Examples of Desired Health Outcomes
Maintain body defences	Skin integrity intact Mucous membranes intact WBC values within normal range T-cell levels within normal range Respiratory assessment findings within normal range (e.g., respiratory rate, rhythm, depth, and breath sounds) Urinary tract assessment findings within normal range (e.g., urine colour, clarity, odour, and consistency)	Avoid spread of microorganisms	Gastrointestinal tract assessment findings within normal range (e.g., stool colour, odour, and consistency, and emesis is absent) Immunizations recommended for age are current Describes mode of transmission of microorganism Demonstrates infection prevention and control practices that reduce transmission Follows prescribed treatment for diagnosed infection

1. *Puncture wounds* from contaminated needles or other sharps, commonly referred to as needle-stick injuries
2. *Skin contact,* which allows infectious fluids to enter through wounds and broken or damaged skin
3. *Mucous membrane* contact, which allows infectious fluids to enter through mucous membranes of the eyes, mouth, and nose

Conscientious use of routine precautions, appropriately using PPE (gloves, masks, gowns, goggles, face shields, shoe covers, special resuscitative equipment), and avoiding carelessness in the clinical area will reduce the risk of injury to the caregiver. Used needles and sharp items should be disposed of immediately after use, without recapping of needles. Puncture resistant containers need to be placed for easy access in areas where the items are used. Measures to be taken in case of possible exposure to blood-borne pathogens are outlined in Box 32.4. Nurses should follow their agency's specific protocols for managing exposure and for handling blood or body fluid spills.

Nurses who themselves are infected with a blood-borne pathogen must ensure that they practise in a manner that does not put their clients at risk (Canadian Nurses Association, 2006). Most health-care agencies and some nursing regulatory bodies have expert panels to advise nurses and other health-care professionals in these situations.

The *Canadian Immunization Guide* (Minister of Public Works and Government Services Canada, 2006) recommends that health-care employers make the hepatitis B vaccine and vaccination series available to all employees. Other vaccinations may also be made available (e.g., nurses working in an obstetric area should be vaccinated against rubella to protect pregnant clients and their fetuses).

Roles of the Infection-Control Practitioner

Infection-control practitioners (ICPs) are important in both acute-care and continuing-care facilities. Many organizations, however, do not meet the recommendation of one ICP per 100 to 150 beds for acute care, and one per 100 to 250 beds for long-term care (Dougherty, 2001; O'Boyle, Jackson, & Henley, 2002; Zoutman et al., 2003). The role of the ICP is less developed in community health settings, outside of control of communicable diseases. The majority of ICPs come from a nursing background, though some may have a background in microbiology or epidemiology.

Key roles and activities of ICPs relate to the following:

- Surveillance of infections to monitor rates and trends in order to identify problems or affirm success of interventions
- Outbreak identification and management
- Staff education related to infection prevention and control, for example, with respect to using routine practices and additional precautions, promoting hand hygiene, or addressing and preventing specific problems
- Consultation with staff on individual client management
- Development, implementation, and evaluation of policies and procedures with specific implications

BOX 32.4 STEPS TO FOLLOW AFTER EXPOSURE TO BLOOD-BORNE PATHOGENS

The following are important steps to follow after exposure to blood-borne pathogens:

- Report the incident immediately to appropriate personnel within the agency.
- Complete an injury report.
- Seek appropriate evaluation and follow-up. This includes the following:
  - Identification and documentation of the source individual when feasible and legal
  - Testing of the source individual's blood when feasible and consent is given
  - Making results of the test available to the source individual's health-care provider
  - Testing of blood of the exposed health-care personnel (with consent)
  - Postexposure prophylaxis if medically indicated (e.g., hepatitis B vaccine for hepatitis B virus, or recommended agents for HIV)
  - Medical counselling regarding personal risk of infection or risk of infecting others
- For a puncture or laceration,
  - Encourage bleeding.
  - Clean the area with soap and water.
  - Initiate first aid and seek treatment, if indicated.
- For a mucous membrane exposure (eyes, nose, mouth), flush with saline solution or water for 5 to 10 minutes.

HIV POSTEXPOSURE PROTOCOL (PEP)

- Treatment should be started as soon as possible, preferably within hours after exposure. Treatment may be less effective when started more than 24 hours after exposure. Starting treatment after a longer period (e.g., 1 week) should be considered for high-risk exposures previously untreated.
- For high-risk exposure (high blood volume *and* source with a high HIV titre), three-drug treatment is recommended.
- For increased risk exposure (high blood volume *or* source with a high HIV titre), three-drug treatment is recommended.
- For low-risk exposure (neither high blood volume nor source with a high HIV titre), two-drug treatment is considered.
- Drug prophylaxis continues for 4 weeks.
- Drug regimens vary and new drugs and regimens are continually being developed.
- HIV antibody tests are done shortly after exposure (baseline), and 6 weeks, 3 months, and 6 months thereafter.

HEPATITIS B

- Anti-HBs testing 1 to 2 months after last vaccine dose
- Hepatitis B immunoglobulin (HBIg) or hepatitis B vaccine (or both) within 1 to 7 days following exposure for nonimmunue workers

HEPATITIS C

- Anti-HCV and ALT (alanine aminotransferase) at baseline and 4 to 6 months after exposure

for infection prevention and control (e.g., IV insertion or maintenance, O.R. procedures, infection prevention and control manual)

- Acting as consultants to a variety of committees on issues related to, or that may have an impact on, infection prevention and control (e.g., policy and procedure committee, selection of products for purchase)

ICPs also collaborate with occupational health and safety staff on specific issues, such as prevention and management of sharps injuries, or annual influenza immunization campaigns. Finally, ICPs are an integral part of infection prevention and control committees, which all health-care organizations must have. Such committees are multidisciplinary, including representatives from the clinical laboratory, housekeeping, maintenance, dietary, pharmacy, nursing, medicine, and client care areas. Their mandate is to monitor the infection prevention and control programs, advise ICPs on direction, and facilitate consultation between key groups.

Infection Prevention and Control Is a Shared Responsibility

Nurses are key players in preventing and controlling infections, given the nature and extent of their contact with clients. Their focus is most commonly on individuals and small groups (e.g., by identifying risks, performing hand hygiene, minimizing exposure of portals of entry to microorganisms, and using routine practices and additional precautions). They also contribute to promoting a safe work environment. Administrators share responsibility in promoting a safe work environment by ensuring appropriate staffing (in numbers and skills), implementing evidence-informed guidelines, and advocating for adequate supplies and structures (e.g., ventilation or environmental controls). Use of PPE alone is insufficient for preventing and controlling infections in the absence of administrative supports and engineering controls. Infection-control practitioners focus on larger groups and institutions, both helping to identify problems and intervening to resolve them. Together health-care providers, clients and families, administrators, and infection-control practitioners can reduce the incidence of infections and their impact.

Case Study 32

Mrs. Cortez is a 76-year-old woman who is independent, lives alone, and prefers not to rely on others unless absolutely necessary. She was active and healthy until about 6 months ago, at which time she developed a persistent upper respiratory tract infection. Because she was unable to obtain or prepare food, she lost weight and became very weak. She finally sought medical attention, but she has not yet fully recovered. Mrs. Cortez was admitted to the acute-care facility for fever, shortness of breath, productive cough, dehydration, and nutritional deficiency. An initial Gram stain of a sputum specimen suggests that she does not have tuberculosis but may have pneumococcal pneumonia.

Critical Thinking Questions

1. Mrs. Cortez's physician suspects that she has pneumonia, a serious lower respiratory tract infection. Identify factors that increase Mrs. Cortez's risk for such an infection, and explain how each factor contributes to the risk.
2. What assessment data would be helpful to the nurse when planning care for Mrs. Cortez?
3. What routine practices and additional precautions should be instituted for Mrs. Cortez? Explain your reasoning in terms of the chain of infection.
4. What should the nurse teach Mrs. Cortez and her visitors with respect to preventing infection?
5. The nurse notes that the housekeeping aide is leaving Mrs. Cortez's room. The aide stops to wash her hands, soaping them and rubbing them together under running water for about 5 seconds. She then turns off the water before reaching for the paper towels to dry her hands. Should the nurse intervene, and if so, in what way?

After working through these questions, go to the MyNursingLab at **http://www.mynursinglab.com** to check your answers.

KEY TERMS

normal flora
resident flora
pathogen
infection
infectious agent
asepsis
nosocomial infections
health-care-associated infections
bacteremia
bacteria
viruses
fungi
protozoa
helminths
parasites
communicability
communicable disease
pathogenicity
opportunistic pathogen
virulence
virulence factors
nonspecific defences
specific defences
macrophages
phagocytes
inflammation
hyperemia
leukocytes
margination
emigration
diapedesis
chemotaxis
leukocytosis
cytokine
pryogen
exudate
pus
fibrinogen
regeneration
fibrous (scar) tissue
granulation tissue
cicatrix
antigens
autoantigens
active immunity
passive immunity
humoral (circulating) immunity
antibody (immunoglobulin)
cell-mediated defences (cellular immunity)
virions
colonization
local infection
systemic infection
septicemia
carrier
microbial load
reservoir
direct contact transmission
indirect contact transmission
droplet transmission
airborne transmission
droplet nuclei

vehicle-borne transmission
fecal-oral route
vector-borne transmission
susceptible host
compromised host
immunization (vaccination)
disinfection
disinfectant
sterilization
antimicrobial agent
antiseptic
hand hygiene
respirator
fit testing
aseptic technique
clean technique
sterile technique
sterile field
isolation precautions
routine practices
additional precautions
airborne precautions
droplet precautions
contact precautions
cough etiquette
occupational exposure

CHAPTER HIGHLIGHTS

- Microorganisms are everywhere. Most are harmless and some are beneficial; however, many can cause infection in susceptible persons.
- Some normal body flora produce toxic metabolites, alter local pH, or physically compete for space, thereby inhibiting growth of foreign bacteria.
- Effective control of infectious disease is an international, national, community, and individual responsibility.
- Health-care-associated infections have significant impact on morbidity, mortality, quality of life, and health-care costs. Major sites for these infections are the respiratory and urinary tracts, the bloodstream, and surgical or open wounds.
- Bacteria and viruses are responsible for most health-care-associated infections. They differ in their ability to be spread from individual to individual, and in their ability to produce disease.
- Humans have both specific and nonspecific defences that combat infectious agents.
- Intact skin and mucous membranes are the body's first line of defence against microorganisms.
- Some body secretions (e.g., saliva and tears) contain enzymes that act as antibacterial agents.
- The inflammatory response limits physical, chemical, and microbial injury and promotes repair of injured tissue.
- Immunity is the specific resistance of the body to infectious agents. Antibodies neutralize viruses or toxins so that they cannot enter or damage cells, while cytotoxic T cells target and kill specific bacteria or virus-infected cells.
- Acquired immunity is active or passive and, in either case, can be naturally or artificially induced.
- Clinical manifestations of infection result from both altered function of the damaged tissue and from the inflammatory response that is initiated in defence.
- In colonization, microorganisms grow and multiply but do not cause physiologic changes in host tissue. In infection, microorganisms cause tissue damage.
- Infection occurs when there is an imbalance between microorganisms and host defences (e.g., high microbial load or low resistance).
- An infection can develop if the six links in the chain of infection—infectious agent, reservoir, portal of exit, mode of transmission, portal of entry, and susceptible host—are not interrupted.
- The six routes of transmission are direct contact, indirect contact, droplet, airborne, vehicle-borne, and vector-borne.
- Factors that contribute to nosocomial infection risks are invasive procedures, medical therapies, the existence of susceptible persons, inappropriate use of antibiotics, and insufficient hand hygiene after client contact and after contact with body substances.
- Especially at risk of acquiring an infection are the very young or old; those with poor nutritional status, a deficiency of serum immunoglobulins, multiple stressors, insufficient immunizations, obesity, anemia, poorly controlled diabetes, or an existing disease process; those who smoke; and those receiving certain medical therapies.
- Infectious agents can be eliminated by physically removing reservoirs, by using antimicrobial drugs to kill microorganisms or slow their growth, by physically cleaning materials, by disinfecting, or by sterilizing.
- Hand hygiene, considered to be the single most effective infection control measure, includes both handwashing (to physically remove transient microorganisms) and use of an alcohol-based hand rub (to kill microorganisms), done correctly and at indicated times to reduce hand carriage of microorganisms.
- Personal protective equipment (gloves, gowns, face masks, respirators, and eyewear) disrupts transmission of microorganisms from patient to caregiver and from client to client via the caregiver.
- Surgical masks protect against infections transmitted via the droplet route, while respirators, if properly fitted and used, protect against infections transmitted by both the airborne and the droplet routes.
- Asepsis is the freedom from infection or infectious material.
- Clean technique keeps the area free from most microorganisms, whereas sterile technique refers to working within a sterile field, using sterile items,

and keeping an area or objects free of all microorganisms.

- Supporting host defences by addressing individual risk factors for infection is important in breaking the chain of infection.
- Routine practices rely on hand hygiene and use of appropriate personal protective equipment, and they are used to protect against exposure to all blood and body fluids from all clients, regardless of infection status.
- Additional precautions are used in addition to routine practices when clients have infections that are transmitted through the airborne, droplet, and contact routes.
- Cough etiquette involves containing respiratory secretions by coughing or sneezing into a tissue (which is then discarded) or cloth (e.g., sleeve), accompanied by hand hygiene.
- Additional protocols may be in effect, depending on the practice setting, for clients who are immunocompromised or who have infections caused by multidrug-resistant organisms.
- Clients requiring isolation precautions are susceptible to sensory deprivation and decreased self-esteem.
- Nursing responsibilities for infection prevention and control include assessing clients' risks for infection or status of an infection and problems or complications associated with the infection; implementing routine practices and additional precautions and other interventions appropriate to the client's needs and situation; evaluating outcomes; and preventing the transmission of microorganisms from infected clients to others.
- The nurse must be knowledgeable about sources and modes of transmission of microorganisms.
- Nurses must also take measures to protect themselves and others from sharps injuries.
- Infection-control practitioners are key personnel for infection prevention and control, helping to identify problems and intervene to resolve them. They are an excellent resource for nurses.
- Infection prevention and control is a shared responsibility.

ASSESS YOUR LEARNING

1. A patient is a chronic carrier of an infection. To prevent the spread of the infection to other patients or health-care providers, the nurse emphasizes interventions that do which of the following?
   - **a.** Eliminate the reservoir.
   - **b.** Block the portal of exit from the reservoir.
   - **c.** Block the portal of entry into the host.
   - **d.** Decrease the susceptibility of the host.
2. The most effective nursing action for controlling the spread of infection includes which of the following?
   - **a.** Performing hand hygiene before and after client contact
   - **b.** Wearing gloves and masks for all client care
   - **c.** Implementing isolation precautions
   - **d.** Administering broad-spectrum prophylactic antibiotics
3. In caring for a patient on contact precautions for a draining infected foot ulcer, the nurse should perform which of the following?
   - **a.** Wear a mask during dressing changes.
   - **b.** Provide disposable meal trays and silverware.
   - **c.** Follow routine practices in all interactions with the patient.
   - **d.** Use aseptic technique for all direct contact with the patient.
4. When caring for a single patient during one shift, it is appropriate for the nurse to reuse which of the following personal protective equipment?
   - **a.** Goggles
   - **b.** Gown
   - **c.** Surgical mask
   - **d.** Clean gloves
5. While donning sterile gloves (open method), the cuff of the first glove rolls under itself about 0.5 cm. Which is the best action for the nurse?
   - **a.** Remove the glove and start over with a new pair.
   - **b.** Wait until the second glove is in place and then unroll the cuff with the other sterile hand.
   - **c.** Ask a colleague to assist by unrolling the cuff.
   - **d.** Leave the cuff rolled under.
6. After evaluating a 69-year-old patient's chart, the nurse concludes that this patient's immunizations are up-to-date. What evidence supports this conclusion?
   - **a.** Had a tetanus booster at age 65
   - **b.** Receives the influenza vaccine every second year
   - **c.** Seeks a second dose of pneumococcal vaccine
   - **d.** Has not received the hepatitis B vaccine
7. The nurse has taught a client and family general infection prevention strategies. Which of the following statements by the client indicates effective learning has occurred?
   - **a.** "We will use antimicrobial soap and hot water to wash our hands at least three times per day."
   - **b.** "We must wash or peel all raw fruits and vegetables before eating."
   - **c.** "A wound or sore is not infected unless we see it draining pus."
   - **d.** "We should not share toothbrushes but it is OK to share towels and washcloths."
8. Which of the numbered areas in the following figure are considered sterile on a person in the operating room? Assume that all articles were sterile when applied.

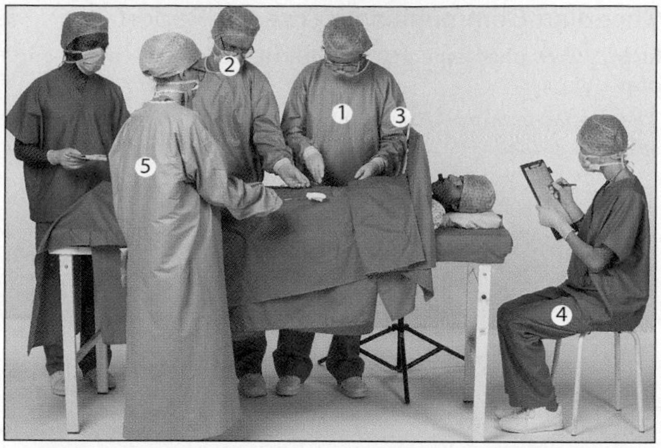

9. The nurse determines that a field remains sterile if which of the following conditions exist?
   a. The tips of wet forceps are held upward when held in ungloved hands.
   b. The field was set up 1 hour before the procedure.
   c. Sterile items are kept at least 5 cm from the edge of the field.
   d. The nurse reaches over the field rather than around the edges.
10. Sue and Mary are co-workers who have desks beside each other and share a telephone. Sue comes to work with a cold. She is tired, has a low-grade fever, and is sneezing frequently. What can Sue do to minimize the risk that Mary will develop the same respiratory infection?
   a. She should stay a minimum of 0.5 metres from Mary.
   b. She should take an antipyretic agent to lower her fever.
   c. She should sneeze into a tissue or her sleeve.
   d. She should not come to work if the symptoms do not subside within 2 days.

After working through these questions, go to the MyNursingLab at ***http://www.mynursinglab.com*** *to check your answers and see explanations.*

SUGGESTED READINGS

Goering, R. V., Dockrell, H. M., Zuckerman, M., Wakelin, D., Roitt, I., Mims, C., & Chiodini, P. L. (2008). *Mims' medical microbiology* (4th ed.). Edinburgh, UK: Elsevier.

This text summarizes, in a reader friendly way, key details about microorganisms and the infections they cause.

Mayhall, C. G. (Ed.). (2004). *Hospital epidemiology and infection control.* Philadelphia, PA: Lippincott Williams & Wilkins.

This is a key reference text used by infection-control practitioners. It provides details on epidemiology, surveillance, common infections, and recommended practices for a variety of settings.

Phillips, N. (2007). *Berry & Kohn's operating room technique* (11th ed.). St Louis, MO: Mosby.

This text summarizes principles and procedures related to establishing, maintaining, and working within sterile fields.

Wilson J. (2006). *Infection control in clinical practice* (3rd ed.). Edinburgh, UK: Baillière Tindall Elsevier.

This text is targeted toward clinicians rather than infection-control practitioners. It covers key points related to basic principles and to specific practices for common sites of infection.

WEBLINKS

Public Health Agency of Canada: Nosocomial and Occupational Infections

http://www.phac-aspc.gc.ca/nois-sinp/index.html

This site has links to the Infection Control Guidelines Series as well as to the Canadian Nosocomial Infection Surveillance Program.

Public Health Agency of Canada: Canadian Nosocomial Infection Surveillance Program

http://www.phac-aspc.gc.ca/nois-sinp/survprog_e.html

This site has links to the Canadian Nosocomial Infection Surveillance Program surveillance projects and publications.

Public Health Agency of Canada: Canadian Immunization Guide

http://www.phac-aspc.gc.ca/publicat/cig-gci/index.html

This site provides the most up-to-date recommendations for immunizing Canadians.

Public Health Agency of Canada

http://www.phac-aspc.gc.ca/new_e.html

This is the main website for the Public Health Agency of Canada. It includes links to a number of topics, including information about chronic diseases, emergency preparedness, health promotion, immunization and vaccines, infectious diseases, injury prevention, public health practice, surveillance, and travel health.

Community and Hospital Infection Control Association—Canada (CHICA-Canada)

http://www.chica.org

This website, while targeted primarily to infection-control practitioners, has links to information useful for education about infection control issues.

Centers for Disease Control and Prevention

http://www.cdc.gov

CDC is the American equivalent of the Public Health Agency of Canada.

Canadian Communicable Disease Report

http://www.phac-aspc.gc.ca/publicat/ccdr-rmtc/index-eng.php

The website contains this publication of the Public Health Branch of Health Canada.

REFERENCES

Canadian Nosocomial Infection Surveillance Program. (2002). *Point prevalence study.* Retrieved January 2, 2008, from http://www.phac-aspc.gc.ca/nois-sinp/projects/pps_e.html

Canadian Nurses Association. (2006). *Blood-borne pathogens: Registered nurses and their ethical obligations.* Ottawa: Author. Retrieved May 26, 2008, from http://www.cna-aiic.ca/CNA/documents/pdf/publications/PS86_Blood_Borne_Pathogen_e.pdf

Community and Hospital Infection Control Association—Canada. (2008). *Hand hygiene procedures.* Retrieved May 26, 2008, from http://www.chica.org/links_handhygiene.html#PROCEDURES

Dougherty, J. (2001). Development of a resource model for infection prevention and control programs in acute, long term, and home care settings: Conference proceedings of the Infection Prevention and Control Alliance. *Canadian Journal of Infection Control, 16*(2), 35–39.

Dronge, A. S., Perkal, M. F., Kancir, S., Concato, J., Asian, M., & Rosenthal, R. A. (2006). Long-term glycemic control and postoperative infectious complications. *Archives of Surgery, 141*(4), 365–380.

Evans, D. (2000). Epidemiology and etiology of occupational infectious diseases. In A. Couturier (Ed.), *Occupational and environmental infectious diseases: Epidemiology, prevention and clinical management* (pp. 37–132). Beverly, MA: Occupational and Environmental Medicine Press.

Health Canada. (1999). Routine practices and additional precautions for preventing the transmission of infection in health care. *Canada Communicable Disease Report, 25S4*(July), 1–155.

Health Canada. (2008). *Workplace Hazardous Materials Information System: Official national site.* Retrieved July 4, 2008, from http://www.hc-sc.gc.ca/ewh-semt/occup-travail/whmis-simdut/index_e.html

Henderson, E., & Community and Hospital Infection Control Association—Canada, Education Committee. (2006). Infection prevention and control core competencies for health care workers: A consensus document. *Canadian Journal of Infection Control, 21*(1), 62–67.

Minister of Public Works and Government Services Canada. (2006). *Canadian immunization guide* (7th ed.). Ottawa: Government of Canada.

NANDA International. (2007). *Nursing diagnoses: Definitions and classification, 2007–2008.* Philadelphia, PA: Author.

National Advisory Committee on Immunization. (2007a). Statement on influenza vaccination for the 2007–2008 season. *Canada Communicable Disease Report, 33 ACS-7*(July), 1–38.

National Advisory Committee on Immunization. (2007b). Statement on human papillomavirus vaccine. *Canada Communicable Disease Report, 33 ACS-2* (February), 1–32.

O'Boyle, C., Jackson, M., & Henley, S. J. (2002). Staffing requirements for infection control programs in US health care facilities: Delphi project. *American Journal of Infection Control, 30*(6), 321–333.

Public Health Agency of Canada. (2003). *Infection control guidance for respirators (masks) worn by health care workers.* Retrieved May 26, 2008, from http://www.phac-aspc.gc.ca/sars-sras/pdf/sars-respiratormasks-0606_e.pdf

Zoutman, D. E., Ford, B. D., Bryce, E., Goudeau, M., Hebert, G., Henderson, E., Paton, S., et. al. (2003). The state of infection surveillance and control in Canadian acute care hospitals. *American Journal of Infection Control, 31*(5), 266–272; discussion: 272–273.

Chapter 33

Skin Integrity and Wound Care

The skin, or integument, is the largest organ in the body and serves a variety of important functions in maintaining health and protecting the individual from harm. Although impaired skin integrity is uncommon in most healthy individuals, it poses a particular threat to vulnerable populations (e.g., older adults) as well as those experiencing a health crisis or an invasive procedure.

The prevention of breakdown should be the essential goal of any skin care program (Registered Nurses' Association of Ontario [RNAO], 2005) and nurses must routinely encourage health-promotion practices to maintain their clients' skin integrity. When disruptions occur, however, effective wound management requires a comprehensive knowledge of the wound healing process, sensitivity to the experience of the client, and excellent care informed by the most recent and valid evidence.

OBJECTIVES

After studying this chapter, you should be able to

1. Discuss factors affecting skin integrity and develop an appropriate, evidence-informed plan for maintaining skin integrity
2. Classify wounds according to depth, chronicity, and level of contamination
3. Identify 10 risk factors for pressure ulcer development
4. Compare and contrast the six stages of pressure ulcer classification
5. Describe the process of wound healing and five factors that can affect healing
6. Differentiate among wound colonization, contamination, and infection
7. Identify assessment data pertinent to the integument
8. Describe special considerations associated with lower limb ulcers
9. List the essential steps of obtaining wound specimens, selecting and applying dressings, and irrigating a wound
10. Contrast the indications and contraindications of commonly used dressing materials and supportive or immobilizing devices
11. List adjunctive therapies that are used to promote wound healing
12. Explain physiological responses to heat and cold and describe the methods of applying dry and moist heat and cold

Skin Function and Integrity

Intact skin refers to surface skin and skin layers that are free of disruption or alteration. See Chapter 27 for details regarding physical examination of the integument. The skin provides a protective interface between the environment and the internal organs of the body. It also plays a major role in thermoregulation, vitamin D synthesis, immune function, and the transmission of the sensory impulses of touch, pain, pressure, vibration, and temperature. As an organ of communication, the appearance of the skin is closely linked with self-perception. When the integrity of the skin is damaged or scarred, changes may occur in self-esteem, body image, and social interactions (Pellard, 2006).

Skin integrity is influenced by factors intrinsic to the individual, such as age, genetics, and general health, as well as extrinsic factors, such as hygiene, living conditions, and mechanical forces, such as shear. Genetics and heredity determine many aspects of a person's skin, including skin colour, sensitivity to sunlight, and allergies. Age influences skin integrity in that the skin of both the very young and the very old is more fragile and susceptible to injury than that of most adults. Sensory or cognitive impairments, poor nutrition, obesity, infection, medications (e.g., corticosteroids), and many chronic illnesses and their treatment can also interfere with the appearance and function of the integument. People with impaired peripheral circulation may have skin on the legs that appears shiny, has lost its hair distribution, and damages easily. Some medications, corticosteroids for example, cause thinning of the skin and allow it to be much more readily harmed. Many medications increase sensitivity to sunlight and can predispose the person to severe sunburns. Some of the most common ones that cause this damage are certain antibiotics, chemotherapy drugs for cancer, and some psychotherapeutic drugs. Poor nutrition alone can interfere with the appearance and function of normal skin.

Skin integrity must be viewed in the context of the whole person. A history and focused physical assessment provide invaluable data about skin integrity problems. Psychosocial assessments are equally important in order to determine the client's ability and motivation to understand and adhere to any treatment program (RNAO, 2005).

Types of Wounds

Body wounds are either intentional or unintentional. *Intentional* trauma occurs during therapy. Examples are operations or venipunctures. Although removing a tumour is therapeutic, skin integrity is traumatized. *Unintentional* wounds are accidental; for example, a person may fracture an arm in a motor vehicle collision. If the tissues are traumatized without a break in the skin, the wound is *closed*. The wound is *open* when the skin or mucous membrane surface is broken.

BOX 33.1 CLASSIFYING WOUNDS BY DEPTH

Wounds can be classified by depth:

- **Partial-thickness wound:** Confined to the skin, that is, the dermis and epidermis; heals by regeneration
- **Full-thickness wound:** Involving the dermis, epidermis, subcutaneous tissue, and possibly muscle and bone; requires connective tissue repair

Wounds can be described according to how they are acquired (see Table 33.1). They also can be described according to the likelihood and degree of contamination:

- **Clean wounds** are uninfected operative wounds without inflammation. Surgery does not involve entering the respiratory, alimentary, genital, or uninfected urinary tract. The wound is closed by the surgeon and, if necessary, drained with a closed drainage system.
- **Clean-contaminated wounds** are surgical wounds in which the respiratory, alimentary, genital, or urinary tract has been entered under controlled conditions and without unusual contamination.
- **Contaminated wounds** include open, fresh, accidental wounds, surgical wounds that involve a major break in sterile technique or gross spillage from the gastrointestinal tract, and incisions in which acute, nonpurulent inflammation is visible.
- **Dirty or infected wounds** include old traumatic wounds with retained dead tissue and wounds that involve existing clinical infection or perforated viscera.

Wounds, excluding pressure ulcers and burns, can also be classified by depth, that is, the tissue layers involved in the wound (see Box 33.1).

Wounds are considered to be *acute* or *chronic,* depending on the healing process and the inflammatory response to trauma. An **acute wound** is one that heals within an expected time frame, while a **chronic wound** describes any break or alteration in the skin that is of long duration (often 3 months or more) or recurs frequently.

Pressure Ulcers

Pressure ulcers are a serious, costly, and, unfortunately, common problem in many health-care settings. Pressure ulcers are also called *decubitus ulcers, pressure sores,* and *distortion sores,* although the preferred term is *pressure ulcers.*

TABLE 33.1 Types of Wounds

Type	Cause	Description and Characteristics
Incision	Sharp instrument (e.g., knife or scalpel), usually intentional	Open wound; painful; deep or shallow
Contusion	Blow from a blunt instrument	Closed wound, skin appears ecchymotic (bruised) because of damaged blood vessels
Abrasion	Surface scrape, either unintentional (e.g., scraped knee from a fall) or intentional (e.g., dermal abrasion to remove pockmarks)	Open wound involving the skin; painful
Puncture	Penetration of the skin and often the underlying tissues by a sharp instrument, either intentional or unintentional	Open wound
Laceration	Tissues torn apart, often from accidents (e.g., with machinery)	Open wound; edges are often jagged
Penetrating wound	Penetration of the skin and the underlying tissues, usually unintentional (e.g., from a bullet or metal fragments)	Open wound

Note that use of the term *bedsores* has fallen out of practice, as pressure ulcers can develop even in the patient who is not bedridden. According the National Pressure Ulcer Advisory Panel (NPUAP) (2007), a **pressure ulcer** is "localized injury to the skin and/or underlying tissue, usually over a bony prominence, as a result of pressure, or pressure in combination with shear and/or friction."

The incidence and prevalence of pressure ulcers in various health-care settings can vary widely. In hospitals, incidence rates of between 1% and 30% have been reported, with higher rates reported in intensive care units, where patients are less mobile and are critically ill. In Canada, estimates of pressure ulcer prevalence across various settings are 25.1% for acute-care settings, 29.9% for non-acute-care settings, 22.1% in mixed health-care settings, and 15.1% in community care. The overall estimate of prevalence in all health-care institutions in Canada is 26.0% (Woodbury & Houghton, 2004). The Canadian Association of Wound Care (2004) estimated the cost of treating a patient with a pressure ulcer in a long-term-care setting to be an average of $24 050 for 3 months of treatment.

In this chapter, we use pressure ulcers as an example in order to identify healing strategies for chronic wounds, recognizing, however, that chronic ulcers have many causes. Venous leg ulcers and diabetic foot ulcers are other common types of chronic ulcers that will be discussed briefly. The Canadian Association of Wound Care (2006) has published a *Quick Reference Guide* summarizing best practice recommendations for wound bed preparation, as well as for the prevention and treatment of pressure ulcers, venous leg ulcers, and diabetic foot ulcers (see Box 33.2).

Etiology of Pressure Ulcers

Pressure ulcers are the result of localized **ischemia**, a deficiency in the blood supply to the tissue. External pressure (such as compression between the surface of the bed and the bony skeleton) that exceeds capillary closing pressure causes occlusion of blood vessels, decreased tissue perfusion, and, possibly, tissue necrosis. Blood cannot reach the tissue, the cells are deprived of oxygen and nutrients, the waste products of metabolism accumulate in the cells, and the tissue consequently dies.

After the skin has been compressed, blood flow is interrupted, and the skin becomes pale. When pressure is relieved, the skin takes on a bright-red flush called **reactive hyperemia**, which is the body's way of quickly restoring blood flow to an area. The flush is due to vasodilation, a process in which extra blood floods the area to compensate for the preceding period of impeded blood flow. Reactive hyperemia usually lasts one-half to three-quarters as long as the duration of impeded blood flow to the area. If the redness disappears in that time, no tissue damage is likely. If, however, the redness does not disappear, then tissue damage (abnormal reactive hyperemia) has already occurred.

Risk Factors

Key contributors to the development of pressure ulcers include mechanical loads (e.g., pressure, friction, and shear), immobility, inadequate nutrition, fecal and urinary incontinence, decreased mental status, diminished sensation, excessive body heat, advanced age, and the presence of certain chronic medical conditions.

MECHANICAL LOADS **Mechanical loads** are extrinsic forces, such as pressure, friction, and shear, that cause soft tissue damage and potentially lead to blood flow impedance, tissue necrosis, and pressure ulcer development (RNAO, 2005). **Friction** is a mechanical force that occurs when two surfaces move across each other and often results in damage to the superficial layers of skin (RNAO, 2005). Poor lifting techniques and voluntary or involuntary movements by the client are common causes of friction injuries. **Shearing** is a combination of friction and pressure that typically results when the skin

BOX 33.2 CANADIAN ASSOCIATION OF WOUND CARE QUICK REFERENCE GUIDE RECOMMENDATIONS FOR PRACTICE

QRG
Quick Reference Guide
RECOMMENDATIONS FOR PRACTICE

CAWC·ACSP

1 PREPARING THE WOUND BED

R. Gary Sibbald, BSc MD FRCPC (Med) FRCPC (Derm); Heather L. Orsted, RN BN ET MSc; Patricia M. Coutts, RN; David H. Keast, MSc MD FCFP

No.	Recommendations
Identify and Treat the Cause	
1.	Assess the patient's ability to heal. Adequate blood supply must be present as well as the correction of other important host factors to support healing.
2.	Diagnose and correct or modify treatable causes of tissue damage.
Address Patient-centred Concerns	
3.	Assess and support the management of patient-centred concerns (pain and quality of life) to enable healing.
4.	Provide patient education and support to increase adherence to treatment plan.
Provide Local Wound Care	
5.	Assess and monitor the wound history and physical characteristics (location + MEASURE*).
6.	Debride healable wounds by removing non-viable, contaminated or infected tissue (through surgical, autolytic, enzymatic, mechanical or larval [biologic] methods). Non-healable wounds should have only non-viable tissue removed; active debridement to bleeding tissue is contraindicated.
7.	Cleanse wounds with low toxicity solutions (such as normal saline or water). Topical antiseptic solutions should be reserved for wounds that are non-healable or those in which the local bacterial burden is of greater concern than the stimulation of healing.
8.	Assess and treat the wound for increased bacterial burden or infection (distinguish from persistent inflammation of non-bacterial origin).
9.	Select a dressing that is appropriate for the needs of the wound, the patient and the caregiver or clinical setting.
10.	Evaluate expected rate of wound healing. If suboptimal, reassess recommendations 1 to 9.
11.	Use active wound therapies (biological agents, skin grafts, adjunctive therapies) when other factors have been corrected and healing still does not progress.
Provide Organizational Support	
12.	For improved outcomes, education and evidence base must be tied to interprofessional teams with the co-operation of health-care systems.

* MEASURE is an acronym for **M**easure, **E**xudate, **A**ppearance, **S**uffering, **U**ndermining, **R**e-evaluate and **E**dge.

2 PREVENTION & TREATMENT OF PRESSURE ULCERS

David H. Keast, MSc MD FCFP; Nancy Parslow, RN ET; Pamela E. Houghton, BScPT PhD; Linda Norton, OT Reg (Ont); Chris Fraser, BSc RD

No.	Recommendation
Identify and Treat the Cause	
1.	Complete a patient history and a targeted physical examination to determine general health and risk factors that may lead to pressure ulcer formation or that may affect healing of existing ulcers.
2.	Assess and modify situations where pressure may be increased.
3.	Maximize nutritional status.
4.	Manage moisture and incontinence.
5.	Maximize activity and mobility, reducing or eliminating friction and shear.
Address Patient-centred Concerns	
6.	Assess and control pain.
7.	Assess and assist with psychosocial needs.
Provide Local Wound Care	
8.	Stage, assess and treat the wound. Provide an optimal wound environment consistent with the principles of *Preparing the Wound Bed*.
9.	Introduce adjunctive modalities or biologically active dressings where appropriate.
10.	Consider surgical intervention for deep non-healing ulcers (Stage III and Stage IV).
Provide Organizational Support	
11.	Develop an interdisciplinary team specific to the needs of the patient.
12.	Educate patients, caregivers, and healthcare providers on the prevention and treatment of pressure ulcers.

and superficial tissues remain stationary, while the deeper tissues attached to bone move downward. Shearing between two tissue layers leads to stretching, kinking, and tearing of the vessels at a subcutaneous level, resulting in ischemia, endothelial damage, and, possibly, cell death (RNAO, 2005). Dragging patients up in bed or allowing them to slide down in the bed are common sources of shearing injury.

IMMOBILITY Although pressure is the major cause of pressure ulcers, immobility and inactivity are also important risk factors. Immobility refers to a reduction in the amount and control of movement a person has. Normally, people move when they experience discomfort caused by pressure on an area of the body. Healthy people rarely exceed their tolerance for pressure. However, paralysis, extreme weakness, immobility, or any cause of decreased activity can hinder a person's ability to change positions independently and relieve the pressure, even if the person can perceive the pressure.

INADEQUATE NUTRITION Nutritional factors are crucial in the development of pressure ulcers. Generally, prolonged inadequate nutrition causes weight loss, muscle atrophy, and the loss of subcutaneous tissue. These three changes reduce the amount of padding between the skin and the bones and increase the risk of pressure ulcer development. Nutritional risk factors for pressure ulcer development include low prealbumin levels, low serum transferrin levels, low hemoglobin, low lymphocyte counts, dehydration, poor food or fluid intake, and unintentional weight loss (Langemo et al., 2006). Among older adult patients, malnutrition is a particularly significant problem, with poor nutritional status being found to increase the risk of death in residents of long-term-care facilities in Canada (Allard et al., 2004).

Hypoproteinemia (abnormally low protein content in the blood), caused by either inadequate intake or abnormal loss, predisposes the client to dependent edema. Edema (the presence of excess fluid in the tissues) makes skin more prone to injury by decreasing its elasticity, resilience, and vitality. Edema increases the distance between the capillaries and the cells, thereby slowing the diffusion of oxygen to the tissue cells and of metabolites away from the cells.

CAWC Quick Reference Guide

PROVIDES RECOMMENDATIONS FOR BEST PRACTICES

The directors and members of the Canadian Association of Wound Care have updated the four articles covering the recommendations for best practice in the areas of (1) Preparing the Wound Bed, (2) Pressure Ulcers, (3) Venous Leg Ulcers, and (4) Diabetic Foot Ulcers.

These quick reference guides (QRGs) are excerpts from the articles published in *Wound Care Canada* and reprinted here with the permission. The complete articles can be accessed through the CAWC Web site at **www.cawc.net**.

The QRGs are not intended to be complete protocols in themselves but aids in the diagnosis, prevention and treatment of specific wounds.

3 PREVENTION & TREATMENT OF VENOUS LEG ULCERS

Cathy Burrows, RN BScN; Rob Miller, MD FRCP (c); Debbie Townsend, RN; Ritchie Bellefontaine, BSc RVT; Gerald MacKean, MD FRCS (c); Heather L. Orsted, RN BN ET MSc; David H. Keast, MSc MD FCFP

No.	Recommendations
	Identify and Treat the Cause
1.	Obtain a careful history to determine the venous characteristics and to rule out other diagnoses: assess pain and identify the systemic and local factors that may impair wound healing.
2.	Perform a physical assessment. This will include a bilateral lower limb assessment as well as an ankle-brachial pressure index (ABPI) test on all patients with venous ulcers to help rule out the presence of arterial disease.
3.	Determine the cause(s) of chronic venous insufficiency based on etiology: abnormal valves (reflux), obstruction, or calf-muscle-pump failure.
4.	Implement appropriate compression therapy.
5.	Implement medical therapy if indicated for chronic venous insufficiency (superficial and deep thrombosis, woody fibrosis).
6.	Consider surgical management if significant superficial or perforator vein disease exists in the absence of extensive deep disease.
	Address Patient-centred Concerns
7.	Communicate with the patients, the family and the caregivers to establish realistic expectations for healing and provide information for care and management of venous disease. The presence or absence of a social support system is important for treatment and prevention of venous leg ulcers.
	Provide Local Wound Care
8.	Assess the wound.
9.	Provide local wound care. Optimize the local wound healing environment through debridement, bacterial balance, and moisture balance. Consider appropriate adjunctive therapies.
	Provide Organizational Support
10.	Consult appropriate disciplines to maximize and individualize the treatment plan to address factors and co-factors that may affect healing (e.g., mobility and nutrition).

4 PREVENTION, DIAGNOSIS & TREATMENT OF DIABETIC FOOT ULCERS

Heather L. Orsted, RN BN ET MSc; Gordon E. Searles, OD MD MSc FRCPC FACP CCI; Heather Trowell, BSc OT (c); Leah Shapera, RN MSN; Pat Miller, RN ET; John Rahman, CO

No.	Recommendations
	Identify and Treat the Cause
1.	Take a careful history to determine general health, diabetic control, complications and co-factors that may cause skin breakdown or affect the healing of an ulcer.
2.	Complete a physical assessment that includes vascular status, bony/structural deformities (and footwear), and sensation.
3.	Classify persons with diabetes into a risk category to support co-ordination of care.
4.	Modify factors that cause skin breakdown and/or influence healing and make referral(s) to the team to ensure comprehensive care.
5.	Provide pressure downloading if there is loss of protective sensation.
	Address Patient-centred Concerns
6.	Provide individualized education as indicated by patient need and by risk category.
	Provide Local Wound Care
7.	Assess diabetic foot ulceration(s).
8.	Provide an optimum wound environment: debridement, moisture balance, infection control.
9.	Determine effectiveness of interventions, reassess if healing is not occurring at expected rate.
10.	Consider the use of biological agents and adjunctive therapies.
	Provide Organizational Support
11.	Establish, train and empower a team to work with patients with diabetes.

www.cawc.net

Canadian Association of Wound Care — Association canadienne du soin des plaies

Source: *Quick Reference Guide: Recommendations for Practice,* 2006, by the Canadian Association of Wound Care, Toronto: Author. Retrieved July 5, 2008, from http://www.cawc.net/open/library/clinical/QRG2006E.pdf.

FECAL AND URINARY INCONTINENCE Moisture, particularly from incontinence, promotes skin **maceration** (tissue softened by prolonged wetting or soaking) and causes the epidermis to be more easily eroded and susceptible to injury. Digestive enzymes in feces also contribute to skin excoriation. Any accumulation of secretions or excretions is irritating to the skin, harbours microorganisms, and makes an individual prone to skin breakdown and infection.

DECREASED MENTAL STATUS Individuals with a reduced level of awareness, for example, those who are unconscious or heavily sedated, are at risk for pressure ulcers because they are less able to recognize and respond to the pain associated with prolonged pressure.

DIMINISHED SENSATION Paralysis, stroke, or other neurological disease may cause loss of sensation in a body area. Loss of sensation reduces a person's ability to respond to injurious heat and cold and to feel the tingling (pins and needles) that signals loss of circulation.

EXCESSIVE BODY HEAT Body heat is another factor in the development of pressure ulcers. An elevated body temperature increases the body's metabolic rate, thus increasing the need of the cells for oxygen. This increased need is particularly severe in the cells of an area under pressure, which are already oxygen deficient. Therefore, severe infections with accompanying elevated body temperatures can affect the body's ability to deal with the effects of tissue compression.

ADVANCED AGE The aging process brings about several changes in the skin and its supporting structures, making the older person more prone to impaired skin integrity and altered wound healing. These changes include the following:

- Loss of lean body mass
- Generalized thinning of the epidermis
- Decreased strength and elasticity of the skin because of changes in the collagen fibres of the dermis

- Increased dryness because of a decrease in the amount of oil produced by the sebaceous glands
- Diminished pain perception because of a reduction in the number of cutaneous end organs responsible for the sensation of pressure and light touch
- Diminished venous and arterial flow because of aging vascular walls

CHRONIC MEDICAL CONDITIONS The presence of certain chronic conditions, such as diabetes mellitus and cardiovascular disease, place individuals at particular risk for developing pressure ulcers. These conditions result in poor perfusion, compromising oxygen and nutrient delivery to the tissues.

OTHER FACTORS Other factors contributing to the formation of pressure ulcers are poor lifting techniques, incorrect positioning, repeated injections in the same area, hard support surfaces, and incorrect application of pressure-relieving devices.

CLINICAL ALERT
Although much effort goes into treating a pressure, arterial, or venous ulcer, keep in mind that, unless the cause is identified and treated, the ulcer might never be cured.

Classification of Pressure Ulcers

The most widely accepted system for classifying the degree of observed tissue damage is NPUAP's updated staging system (Wound, Ostomy and Continence Nurses Society [WOCN], 2007). In 2007, the original I to IV stage classification (Figure 33.1) was augmented by two stages, one on deep tissue injury, and one on unstageable pressure ulcers:

- *Suspected deep tissue injury:* Purple or maroon localized area of discoloured intact skin or blood-filled blister caused by damage of underlying soft tissue from pressure or shear (Figure 33.2, page 934). The discolouration may be preceded by tissue that is painful, firm, mushy, boggy, warmer, or cooler as compared with adjacent tissue.
- *Stage I:* Intact skin with nonblanchable redness of a localized area, usually over a bony prominence. Darkly pigmented skin may not have visible blanching; its colour may differ from the surrounding area.
- *Stage II:* Partial-thickness skin loss presenting as a shallow open ulcer with a red-pink wound bed, without slough. It may also present as an intact or open or ruptured serum-filled blister.
- *Stage III:* Full-thickness tissue loss. Subcutaneous fat may be visible but bone, tendon, or muscle is not exposed. Slough may be present but does not obscure the depth of tissue loss. It may include undermining and tunnelling.
- *Stage IV:* Full-thickness tissue loss with exposed bone, tendon, or muscle. Slough or **eschar** (a covering of dried plasma proteins and dead cells) may be present on some parts of the wound bed. It often includes undermining and tunnelling.
- *Unstageable:* Full-thickness tissue loss in which the base of the ulcer is covered by slough (yellow, tan, grey, green, or brown) or eschar (tan, brown, or black) in the wound bed.

REVERSE (DOWN) STAGING Clinical studies indicate that as deep ulcers heal, the lost muscle, fat, and dermis is *not* replaced. Instead, granulation tissue fills the defect before epithelialization occurs. Given this information, it is not appropriate to reverse or *down* stage a healing ulcer. For example, a stage III pressure ulcer does not become a stage II or a stage I in your documentation during healing. Instead, a granulating stage III wound is classified as "granulating stage III." Progress is documented by noting an improvement in the actual characteristics: size, depth, amount of necrotic tissue, amount of exudate, and so on (WOCN, 2007).

Risk-Assessment Tools

Although clients may be at risk for developing a number of different alterations in skin integrity, the most common and most preventable are pressure ulcers. The RNAO *Nursing Best Practice Guideline: Risk Assessment and Prevention of Pressure Ulcers* (2005) notes that the client's risk is determined by a combination of clinical judgment and the use of a reliable risk-assessment tool. Several risk-assessment tools are available that provide the nurse with systematic means of identifying clients at high risk for pressure ulcer development.

The Braden scale for predicting pressure ulcer risk (Figure 33.3, page 935) is frequently used in practice settings. This scale consists of six subscales: sensory perception, moisture, activity, mobility, nutrition, and friction and shear. A total of 23 points is possible. Clients with scores between 15 and 18 are considered at risk; those with scores of 13 to 14 are considered at moderate risk; and those with scores of 10 to 12 are considered at high risk (Braden, 2001).

Widely accepted clinical standards for the frequency of risk assessments are based on research findings that suggest the majority of pressure ulcers develop within the first 2 to 3 weeks after admission to a facility (RNAO, 2005). The frequency of risk assessments should be based on the findings of the initial admission assessment and the frequency of changes in the client's health status. Braden (2001) suggests the following risk-assessment schedule for different health-care settings:

- Long-term-care facilities: on admission, then every week for 4 weeks and quarterly thereafter
- Intensive care units: daily
- General medical or surgical units: every other day
- Community: every home visit

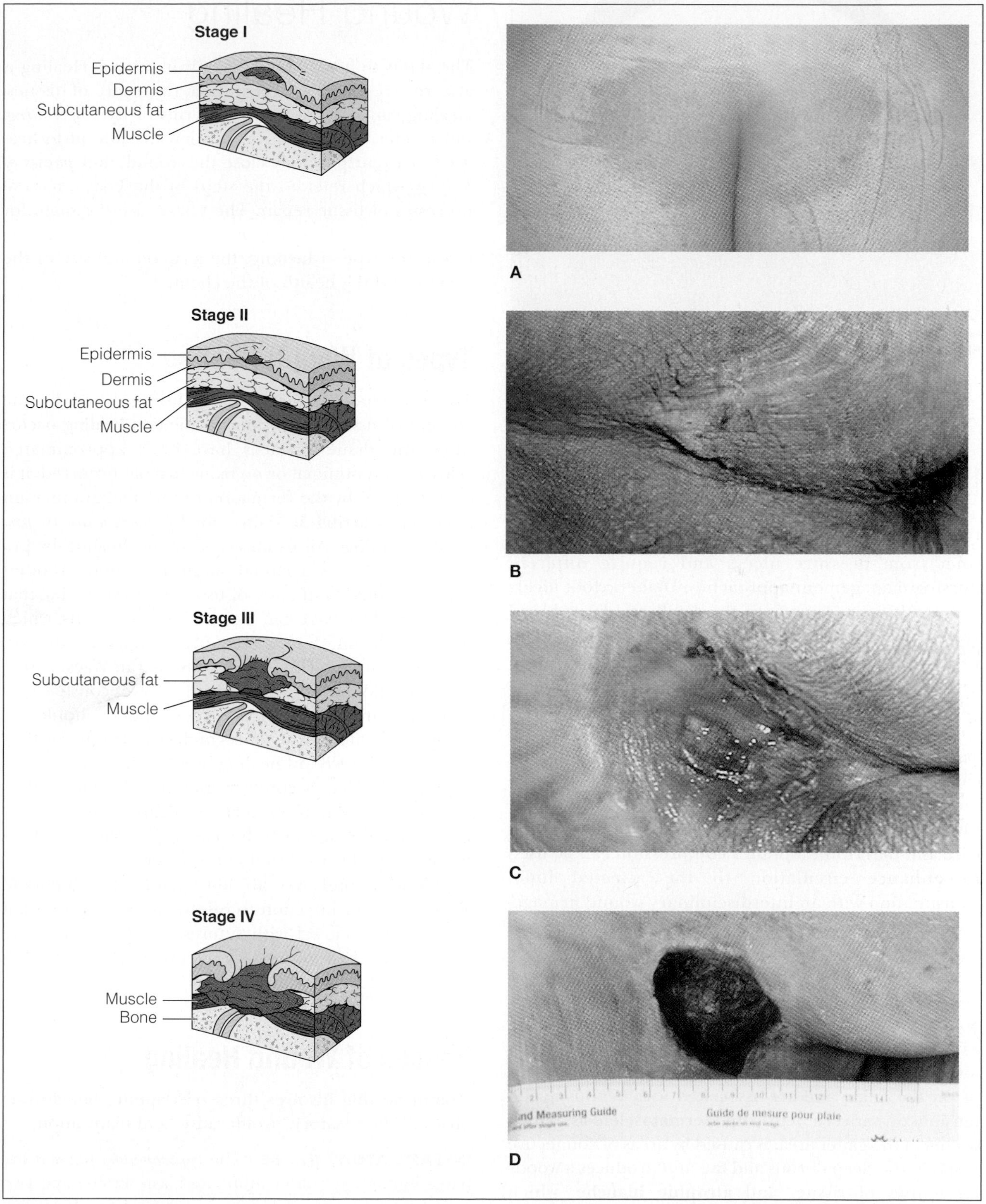

FIGURE 33.1 Stages I to IV of pressure ulcers. **A:** stage I: a defined area of persistent redness signalling potential ulceration; **B:** stage II: partial-thickness skin loss (abrasion, blister, or shallow crater) involving the epidermis and possibly the dermis; **C:** stage III: full-thickness skin loss involving damage or necrosis of subcutaneous tissue that may extend down to, but not through, underlying fascia; **D:** stage IV: full-thickness skin loss with extensive destruction, tissue necrosis, or damage to muscle, bone, or supporting structures, such as a tendon or joint capsule. Undermining and sinus tract may also be present.

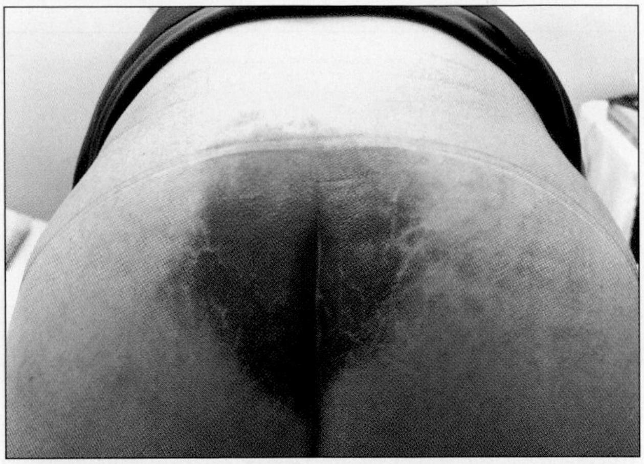

FIGURE 33.2 Suspected deep tissue injury

Lower Extremity Ulcers

Ulcers of the lower extremities are etiologically distinct from pressure ulcers and require different nursing management approaches. Diabetic foot ulcers can result from damage to the small and large blood vessels and nerve of the foot. Diabetes is the leading cause of nontraumatic lower extremity amputations, with most amputations preceded by foot ulcers (RNAO, 2005). Because arterial or venous insufficiency is another major cause of leg ulcers, careful assessment of the patient is essential to appropriate care. For example, special blood pressure measurements (ankle-brachial index) that use Doppler ultrasound readings are taken to rule out arterial disease and determine whether compression can be used to enhance circulation to the affected limb. Consultation with an interdisciplinary wound management team is critical when caring for patients with any type of lower extremity ulcer.

Table 33.2 describes the differences in limb appearance between patients with arterial and venous ulcers. Some common ulcers include those on the **gaiter area**, which extends from 2.5 cm below the malleolus to the lower third of the calf; **ankle flares**, which appear near or on the ankle and are associated with venous hypertension or varicose veins; **lipodermatosclerosis**, which occurs in the gaiter area, is caused by areas of connective tissue in the deep dermis and fat, and produces a woody hardening of tissue; and **atrophie blanche**, which appears as white atrophic lesions and is often associated with venous disease.

Wound Healing

The ability to heal is a quality of living tissue. Healing is also referred to as **regeneration** (renewal) of tissues. Healing can be considered in terms of *types of healing*, which refer to the decision to allow the wound to heal itself or to purposefully close the wound, and *phases of healing*, which refer to the steps in the body's natural processes of tissue repair. The phases are the same for all wounds, but the rate of healing depends on such factors as the type of healing, the location and size of the wound, and the health of the client.

Types of Wound Healing

The two types of healing are distinguished by the amount of tissue loss. **Primary intention healing** occurs when the tissue surfaces have been approximated (closed) and minimal or no tissue loss has occurred; it is characterized by the formation of minimal granulation tissue and scarring. It is also called *primary union* or *first intention healing*. An example of wound healing by primary intention is a closed surgical incision. Another example would be the use of tissue adhesive, a glue that can be used to seal clean lacerations or incisions, which may result in better looking scars (Coulthard, Worthington, Esposito, van der Elst, & van Waes, 2005).

A wound that is extensive and involves considerable tissue loss, and in which the edges cannot or should not be approximated, heals by **secondary intention healing**. An example of wound healing by secondary intention is a pressure ulcer. Secondary intention healing differs from primary intention healing in three ways: (1) the repair time is longer; (2) the scarring is greater; and (3) the susceptibility to infection is greater.

Those wounds that are left open for 3 to 5 days to allow edema or infection to resolve or exudate to drain and are then closed with sutures, staples, or adhesive skin closures heal by **tertiary intention**. This method is also called **delayed primary intention healing.**

Phases of Wound Healing

Wound healing involves three overlapping but distinct phases: inflammatory, proliferative, and maturation.

INFLAMMATORY PHASE The *inflammatory phase* is initiated immediately after injury and lasts 3 to 6 days. Two major processes occur during this phase: hemostasis and phagocytosis.

Hemostasis (the cessation of bleeding) results from vasoconstriction of the larger blood vessels in the affected area, retraction (drawing back) of injured blood vessels, the deposition of **fibrin** (connective tissue), and the formation of blood clots in the area. The blood clots,

BRADEN SCALE FOR PREDICTING PRESSURE SORE RISK

Patient's Name ______________________ Evaluator's Name ______________________ Date of Assessment

SENSORY PERCEPTION Ability to respond meaningfully to pressure-related discomfort	**1. Completely Limited:** Unresponsive (does not moan, flinch, or grasp) to painful stimuli, due to diminished level of consciousness or sedation, OR limited ability to feel pain over most of body surface.	**2. Very Limited:** Responds only to painful stimuli. Cannot communicate discomfort except by moaning or restlessness, OR has a sensory impairment which limits the ability to feel pain or discomfort over 1/2 of body.	**3. Slightly Limited:** Responds to verbal commands but cannot always communicate discomfort or need to be turned, OR has some sensory impairment which limits ability to feel pain or discomfort in 1 or 2 extremities.	**4. No Impairment:** Responds to verbal commands. Has no sensory deficit which would limit ability to feel or voice pain or discomfort.				
MOISTURE Degree to which skin is exposed to moisture	**1. Constantly Moist:** Skin is kept moist almost constantly by perspiration, urine, etc. Dampness is detected every time patient is moved or turned.	**2. Moist:** Skin is often but not always moist. Linen must be changed at least once a shift.	**3. Occasionally Moist:** Skin is occasionally moist, requiring an extra linen change approximately once a day.	**4. Rarely Moist:** Skin is usually dry; linen requires changing only at routine intervals.				
ACTIVITY Degree of physical activity	**1. Bedfast:** Confined to bed.	**2. Chairfast:** Ability to walk severely limited or nonexistent. Cannot bear own weight and/or must be assisted into chair or wheelchair.	**3. Walks Occasionally:** Walks occasionally during day but for very short distances, with or without assistance. Spends majority of each shift in bed or chair.	**4. Walks Frequently:** Walks outside the room at least twice a day and inside room at least once every 2 hours during waking hours.				
MOBILITY Ability to change and control body position	**1. Completely Immobile:** Does not make even slight changes in body or extremity position without assistance.	**2. Very Limited:** Makes occasional slight changes in body or extremity position but unable to make frequent or significant changes independently.	**3. Slightly Limited:** Makes frequent though slight changes in body or extremity position independently.	**4. No Limitations:** Makes major and frequent changes in position without assistance.				
NUTRITION Usual food intake pattern	**1. Very Poor:** Never eats a complete meal. Rarely eats more than 1/3 of any food offered. Eats 2 servings or less of protein (meat or dairy products) per day. Takes fluids poorly. Does not take a liquid dietary supplement, OR is NPO and/or maintained on clear liquids or IV's for more than 5 days.	**2. Probably Inadequate:** Rarely eats a complete meal and generally eats only about 1/2 of any food offered. Protein intake includes only 3 servings of meat or dairy products per day. Occasionally will take a dietary supplement, OR receives less than optimum amount of liquid diet or tube feeding.	**3. Adequate:** Eats over half of most meals. Eats a total of 4 servings of protein (meat, dairy products) each day. Occasionally will refuse a meal, but will usually take a supplement if offered, OR is on a tube feeding or TPN regimen, which probably meets most of nutritional needs.	**4. Excellent:** Eats most of every meal. Never refuses a meal. Usually eats a total of 4 or more servings of meat and dairy products. Occasionally eats between meals. Does not require supplementation.				
FRICTION AND SHEAR	**1. Problem:** Requires moderate to maximum assistance in moving. Complete lifting without sliding against sheets is impossible. Frequently slides down in bed or chair, requiring frequent repositioning with maximum assistance. Spasticity, contractures, or agitation leads to almost constant friction.	**2. Potential Problem:** Moves feebly or requires minimum assistance. During a move skin probably slides to some extent against sheets, chair, restraints, or other devices. Maintains relatively good position in chair or bed most of the time but occasionally slides down.	**3. No Apparent Problem:** Moves in bed and in chair independently and has sufficient muscle strength to lift up completely during move. Maintains good position in bed or chair at all times.					
				Total Score				

FIGURE 33.3 Braden scale for predicting pressure ulcer risk

(Clinical Practice Guideline, Pressure Ulcers in Adults: Prediction and Prevention (pp. 16–17), by U.S. Department of Health and Human Services, PPPPUA Pub. No. 92-0047, 1992, Rockville, MD: Public Health Service. Copyright © Barbara Braden and Nancy Bergstrom, 1988. Reprinted with permission.)

TABLE 33.2 Comparison of the Manifestations of Arterial and Venous Disease in the Lower Limbs

Arterial Disease	Venous Disease
Ulcers with a "punched out" appearance	Usually shallow, moist ulcers
Base of wound poorly perfused, pale, dry	Situated on the gaiter area of the leg (the gaiter area is 2.5 cm below the malleolus to the lower one-third of the calf)
Cold legs/feet in a warm environment	Edema
Shiny, taut skin	Eczema
Dependent rubour	Ankle flare (the characteristic clinical sign evident in the region of the ankle associated with venous hypertension or varicose veins as a result of a number of engorged veins in the area)
Pale or blue feet	Lipodermatosclerosis (deposit of fibrin in the deep dermis and fat, resulting in a woody induration of the gaiter area of the calf)
Gangrenous toes	Hyperpigmentation
	Atrophie blanche (white atrophic lesions often associated with venous disease). Tiny visible blood vessels, called teleangiectasia, are often seen in the centre

Source: From *Nursing Best Practice Guideline: Assessment and Management of Venous Leg Ulcers,* by the Registered Nurses' Association of Ontario, 2004, Toronto: Author.

formed from blood platelets, provide a matrix of fibrin that becomes the framework for cell repair. A scab also forms on the surface of the wound. Consisting of clots and dead and dying tissue, this scab serves to aid hemostasis and inhibit contamination of the wound by microorganisms. Below the scab, epithelial cells migrate into the wound from the edges. The epithelial cells serve as a barrier between the body and the environment, preventing the entry of microorganisms.

The inflammatory phase also involves vascular and cellular responses intended to remove any foreign substances and dead and dying tissues. The blood supply to the wound increases, bringing with it substances and nutrients needed in the healing process. The area appears reddened and edematous as a result. Exudate of fluid and cell debris is a normal accumulation and helps cleanse the wound.

During cell migration, leukocytes (specifically, neutrophils) move into the interstitial space. These are replaced about 24 hours after injury by macrophages, which arise from the blood monocytes. These macrophages engulf microorganisms and cellular debris by a process known as phagocytosis. The macrophages also secrete an angiogenesis factor (AGF), which stimulates the formation of epithelial buds at the end of injured blood vessels. The microcirculatory network that results sustains the healing process and the wound during its life. This inflammatory response is essential to healing, and measures that impair inflammation, such as steroid medications, can place the healing process at risk.

PROLIFERATIVE PHASE The *proliferative phase,* the second phase in healing, extends from day 3 or 4 to about day 21 after injury. Fibroblasts (connective tissue cells), which migrate into the wound starting about 24 hours after injury, begin to synthesize collagen and a substance called proteoglycan about day 5 after injury. **Collagen** is a whitish protein substance that adds tensile strength to the wound. As the amount of collagen increases, so does the strength of the wound; thus, the chance that the wound will open decreases progressively. If the wound is sutured, a raised healing ridge appears under the intact suture line. In a wound that is not sutured, the new collagen is often visible.

Capillaries grow across the wound, increasing the blood supply, which brings with it oxygen and nutrients needed for healing. Fibroblasts move from the bloodstream into the wound, depositing fibrin. As the capillary network develops, the tissue becomes a translucent red colour. This tissue, called **granulation tissue**, is fragile and bleeds easily.

When the skin edges of a wound are not sutured, the area fills in with granulation tissue. When the granulation tissue matures, marginal epithelial cells migrate to it, proliferating over this connective tissue base to fill the wound. If the wound does not close by epithelialization, the area becomes covered with dried plasma proteins and dead cells, called *eschar.* Initially, wounds healing by secondary intention ooze blood-tinged drainage. Later, if they are not covered by epithelial cells, they become covered with thick, grey, fibrinous tissue that is eventually converted into dense scar tissue.

MATURATION PHASE The *maturation phase* begins about day 21 and healing can extend 1 or 2 years after the injury. Fibroblasts continue to synthesize collagen. The collagen fibres themselves, which were initially laid in a haphazard fashion, reorganize into a more orderly structure. During maturation, the wound is remodelled and contracted. The scar becomes stronger but the repaired area is never as strong as the original tissue. Scar tissue is at increased risk of re-ulceration because it will not achieve more than 80% of the tissue's pre-injury tensile strength (Health Quality Council, 2006). In some individuals, particularly dark-skinned persons, an abnormal amount of collagen is laid down. This can result in a hypertrophic scar, or **keloid.**

One method of documenting the progress of healing in pressure ulcers is to use the pressure ulcer scale for healing (PUSH) tool (Berlowitz, Ratliff, Cuddigan, Rodeheaver, & National Pressure Ulcer Advisory Panel, 2005). This validated tool (Figure 33.4) assigns scores to the ulcer length, width, amount of exudate, and tissue type. The change in the total score over time can be used as an indication of healing.

Types of Wound Drainage

Exudate is material, such as fluid and cells, that escapes from blood vessels during the inflammatory process and is deposited in tissue or on tissue surfaces. The nature and amount of exudate vary according to the tissue involved, the intensity and duration of the inflammation, and the presence of microorganisms.

Exudate has three major types: serous, purulent, and sanguineous (hemorrhagic). A **serous exudate** consists chiefly of serum (the clear portion of the blood) derived from blood and the serous membranes of the body, such as the peritoneum. It looks watery and has few cells. An example is the fluid in a blister from a burn.

A **purulent exudate** is thicker than serous exudate because of the presence of pus, which consists of leukocytes, liquefied dead tissue debris, and dead and living bacteria. The process of pus formation is referred to as **suppuration**, and the bacteria that produce pus are called **pyogenic bacteria**. Not all microorganisms are pyogenic. Purulent exudates vary in colour, some acquiring tinges of blue, green, or yellow. The colour may depend on the causative organism.

A **sanguineous (hemorrhagic) exudate** consists of large amounts of red blood cells, indicating damage to capillaries that is severe enough to allow the escape of red blood cells from plasma. This type of exudate is frequently seen in open wounds. Nurses often need to distinguish whether the sanguineous exudate is dark or bright. A bright sanguineous exudate indicates fresh bleeding, whereas dark sanguineous exudate denotes older bleeding.

Mixed types of exudates are often observed. A **serosanguineous** (consisting of clear and blood-tinged drainage) **exudate** is commonly seen in surgical incisions. A *purosanguineous* discharge (consisting of pus and blood) is often seen in a new wound that is infected.

CLINICAL ALERT

A bright sanguineous exudate indicates fresh bleeding, whereas dark sanguineous exudate denotes older bleeding.

Complications Relating to Wound Healing

HEMORRHAGE Some escape of blood from a wound is normal. **Hemorrhage** (persistent bleeding), however, is abnormal. It may be caused by a dislodged clot, a slipped ligature, or erosion of a blood vessel, for example.

Internal hemorrhage can often be detected by swelling or distension in the area of the wound and, possibly, sanguineous drainage from a surgical drain. Some clients will have a **hematoma**, a localized collection of blood underneath the skin that may appear as a reddish-blue swelling. A large hematoma can be dangerous in that it places pressure on blood vessels and can, thus, obstruct blood flow.

External hemorrhage is often easily identified from the blood that either appears under a dressing or escapes from the dressing and pools under the client. The risk of hemorrhage is greatest during the first 48 hours after surgery. Hemorrhage is an emergency; the nurse should apply extra sterile pressure dressings to the area and monitor the client's vital signs. In many instances, the client must be taken to the operating room for surgical intervention.

INFECTION A wound can be infected with microorganisms at the time of injury, during surgery, or postoperatively, that is, during open wound healing. An **infection** is the disease process produced by those microorganisms.

Wounds that occur as a result of injury (e.g., bullet and knife wounds) are most likely to be contaminated at the time of injury. Surgical site infections (SSIs) account for about 40% of all hospital-associated infections among surgical patients (Odom-Forren, 2006). Most SSIs are caused when the patient's own flora enters the body through the incision, but outside sources of contamination also pose significant risk. Hyperglycemia, smoking, prolonged preoperative hospital stay, and postoperative hypothermia all increase a patient's risk of developing an SSI (Odom-Forren, 2006). Surgical infection is most likely to become apparent 2 to 11 days postoperatively.

DEHISCENCE WITH POSSIBLE EVISCERATION **Dehiscence** is the partial or total rupturing of a sutured wound. Dehiscence usually involves an abdominal wound in which the layers below the skin also separate. **Evisceration** is the protrusion of the internal viscera through an incision. A number of factors, including obesity, smoking, poor nutrition, multiple traumas, failure of suturing, excessive coughing, vomiting, and dehydration,

NATIONAL PRESSURE ULCER ADVISORY PANEL

Pressure Ulcer Scale for Healing (PUSH)
PUSH Tool 3.0

Patient Name____________________ Patient ID#____________

Ulcer Location ____________________ Date ____________

Directions:

Observe and measure the pressure ulcer. Categorize the ulcer with respect to surface area, exudate, and type of wound tissue. Record a sub-score for each of these ulcer characteristics. Add the sub-scores to obtain the total score. A comparison of total scores measured over time provides an indication of the improvement or deterioration in pressure ulcer healing.

LENGTH X WIDTH (in cm^2)	**0** 0	**1** < 0.3	**2** 0.3 – 0.6	**3** 0.7 – 1.0	**4** 1.1 – 2.0	**5** 2.1 – 3.0	**Sub-score**
		6 3.1 – 4.0	**7** 4.1 – 8.0	**8** 8.1 – 12.0	**9** 12.1 – 24.0	**10** > 24.0	
EXUDATE AMOUNT	**0** None	**1** Light	**2** Moderate	**3** Heavy			**Sub-score**
TISSUE TYPE	**0** Closed	**1** Epithelial Tissue	**2** Granulation Tissue	**3** Slough	**4** Necrotic Tissue		**Sub-score**
							TOTAL SCORE

Length x Width: Measure the greatest length (head to toe) and the greatest width (side to side) using a centimeter ruler. Multiply these two measurements (length x width) to obtain an estimate of surface area in square centimeters (cm2). Caveat: Do not guess! Always use a centimeter ruler and always use the same method each time the ulcer is measured.

Exudate Amount: Estimate the amount of exudate (drainage) present after removal of the dressing and before applying any topical agent to the ulcer. Estimate the exudate (drainage) as none, light, moderate, or heavy.

Tissue Type: This refers to the types of tissue that are present in the wound (ulcer) bed. Score as a "4" if there is any necrotic tissue present. Score as a "3" if there is any amount of slough present and necrotic tissue is absent. Score as a "2" if the wound is clean and contains granulation tissue. A superficial wound that is reepithelializing is scored as a "1." When the wound is closed, score as a "0."

4 – Necrotic Tissue (Eschar): black, brown, or tan tissue that adheres firmly to the wound bed or ulcer edges and may be either firmer or softer than surrounding skin.

3 – Slough: yellow or white tissue that adheres to the ulcer bed in strings or thick clumps, or is mucinous.

2 – Granulation Tissue: pink or beefy red tissue with a shiny, moist, granular appearance.

1 – Epithelial Tissue: for superficial ulcers, new pink or shiny tissue (skin) that grows in from the edges or as islands on the ulcer surface.

0 – Closed/Resurfaced: the wound is completely covered with epithelium (new skin).

www.npuap.org
11F

PUSH Tool Version 3.0:9/15/98

FIGURE 33.4 Pressure ulcer scale for healing (PUSH) tool

heighten a client's risk of wound dehiscence. Wound dehiscence is more likely to occur 4 to 5 days postoperatively before extensive collagen is deposited in the wound. Clients at risk for dehiscence may be prescribed an abdominal binder for support.

An increase in the flow of serosanguineous drainage into the wound dressing can indicate an impending dehiscence. Dehiscence may also be preceded by sudden straining, and it is not unusual for a client to feel that something has given way. When dehiscence or evisceration occurs, the wound should be quickly supported by large sterile dressings soaked in sterile normal saline. The client is placed in bed with knees bent to decrease pull on the incision and emotional support is provided. The surgeon should be notified, as immediate surgical repair of the area may be necessary.

Factors Affecting Wound Healing

Characteristics of the individual, such as age, nutritional status, lifestyle, and medications, influence the speed of wound healing.

LIFESPAN CONSIDERATIONS Healthy children and adults often heal more quickly than older adults, who are at higher risk of having chronic diseases that hinder healing. For example, impaired liver function can impair the synthesis of blood clotting factors. Box 33.3 lists factors inhibiting wound healing in older adults.

NUTRITION Wound healing increases the body's energy and protein needs. Clients require a diet rich in protein, carbohydrates, lipids, vitamins A and C, and minerals, such as zinc (Langemo et al., 2006). Malnourished clients may require time to improve their nutritional status before surgery, if this is possible. Obese clients are at increased risk of wound infection and slower healing because adipose tissue usually has a minimal blood supply.

LIFESTYLE People who exercise regularly tend to have good circulation, and because blood brings oxygen and nourishment to the wound, they are more likely to heal quickly. Smoking constricts arterioles, and it reduces the amount of functional hemoglobin in the blood, thus limiting the oxygen-carrying capacity of the blood.

MEDICATIONS Anti-inflammatory drugs (e.g., steroids and Aspirin), heparin, and antineoplastic agents interfere with healing. Prolonged use of antibiotics can make a person susceptible to wound infection by resistant organisms.

CONTAMINATION, COLONIZATION, AND INFECTION Considerable debate has occurred about the influences of bacterial contamination, colonization, and infection on wound healing. All chronic wounds are presumed to be in a state of bacterial **contamination**, in which bacteria are present but are neither attached to the wound surface nor replicating (Dolynchuk et al., 2000), but not all chronic wounds become infected. This contrasts with **colonization**, in which bacteria are attached to the wound surface and are replicating. In neither contamination nor colonization, however, do bacteria interfere with wound healing. When bacteria become invasive and cause an inflammatory response, the wound may proceed to shows signs of local infection, which can progress to systemic infection. The most common microcolonies of bacteria in wounds are *Staphylococcus* and *Pseudomonas* (Fowler, Krasner, & Sibbald, 2002).

A number of factors predispose clients to wound infections (Vazquez & Keast, 2006). Systemic factors that increase the likelihood of a wound infection include vascular disease, edema, malnutrition, diabetes mellitus, alcoholism, prior surgery or radiation, drugs (e.g., corticosteroids), and inherited immune defects. Local factors that should be noted as increasing the chance of wound infection include a large wound area, increased wound depth, degree of chronicity, anatomic location (distal extremity, perineal), presence of foreign bodies, necrotic tissue, reduced perfusion, and degree of post-wound contamination. In addition to the classic signs of infection (erythema, induration, and increased pain), friable (jelly-like) granulation tissue, unstable epithelial bridges, or a failure to respond to therapy are subtle signs of infection (Dolynchuk et al., 2000). Clients who are immunosuppressed, such as those with human immunodeficiency virus (HIV) infection or receiving myelosuppressive treatment for cancer, are especially susceptible to wound infections.

Systemic antibiotics should not be routinely used for pressure ulcers with only clinical signs of local infec-

BOX 33.3 FACTORS INHIBITING WOUND HEALING IN OLDER ADULTS

Wounds in older adults can heal more slowly for several reasons:

- Vascular changes associated with aging, such as atherosclerosis and atrophy of capillaries in the skin, can impair blood flow to the wound.
- Collagen tissue is less flexible, which increases the risk of damage from pressure, friction, and shear.
- Scar tissue is less elastic.
- Changes in the immune system may reduce the formation of the antibodies and monocytes necessary for wound healing.
- Nutritional deficiencies may reduce the numbers of red blood cells and leukocytes, thus impeding the delivery of oxygen and the inflammatory response essential for wound healing. Oxygen is needed for the synthesis of collagen and the formation of new epithelial cells.
- Having diabetes or cardiovascular disease increases the risk of delayed healing because of impaired oxygen delivery to these tissues.
- Cell renewal is slower, leading to delayed healing.

tion, but they may be required when patients are diagnosed with (1) bacteremia, (2) sepsis, (3) advancing cellulitis, or (4) osteomyelitis. Topical antibiotics (effective for Gram negative, Gram positive, and anaerobic organisms) may be given a 2-week trial in the case of clean pressure ulcers that do not show evidence of healing or are continuing to produce exudate after 2 to 4 weeks of optimal treatment (RNAO, 2007).

Assessing

Assessment of Skin Integrity

In addition to the history and psychosocial assessment, the nurse conducts an examination of the integument as part of a routine assessment and during regular care. Removing barriers to assessment is very important. Antiembolism stockings, braces, or devices must be removed to assess the skin condition underneath.

NURSING HISTORY AND PHYSICAL EXAMINATION Completion of a patient history and targeted physical examination to determine general health and risk factors that may lead to impaired skin integrity is a key component of the nursing history. During the review of systems as part of the nursing history, information is collected regarding skin diseases, previous bruising, general skin condition, skin lesions, and usual healing of ulcers. Inspection and palpation of the skin focus on determination of skin colour, temperature, texture, turgor, presence of edema, vascularity, and characteristics of any lesions that are present. Particular attention is paid to skin condition in areas most likely to break down: in skin folds, such as under the breasts; in areas that are frequently moist, such as the perineum; and in areas that are subject to pressure, such as the temporal region and occiput of the skull, ears, scapulae, spinous processes, shoulders, elbows, sacrum, ischial tuberosities, trochanters, knees, malleoli, metatarsal areas, heels, and toes (RNAO, 2005).

Practice Guidelines 33.1 describes the principles of assessing common pressure sites.

Pain

Pain is a patient-centred concern that is all too often neglected in the provision of wound care. Patients with impaired skin integrity frequently experience pain occurring with dressing changes that is unfortunately undertreated or not treated at all (Shukla et al., 2005). The most severe pain is usually experienced during dressing changes and dressing removal (Moffatt, Franks, & Hollinworth, 2002). Best practice guidelines from the RNAO (2007) recommend that all patients receiving wound care should be routinely assessed for pain by using a validated assessment tool that is easy to use and appropriate for the cognitive ability of the client.

Assessment of Wounds

Nurses commonly assess both untreated and treated wounds. Although a pressure ulcer can be categorized as an untreated or a treated wound, the specific assessment of pressure ulcers is discussed separately.

UNTREATED WOUNDS Untreated wounds usually are seen shortly after an injury (e.g., at the scene of an accident). Assessment for these wounds is shown in Box 33.4. Guidelines for care follow:

- Control severe bleeding by (1) applying direct pressure over the wound, and (2) elevating the involved extremity.
- Prevent infection by (1) cleaning or flushing abrasions or lacerations with water and (2) covering the wound with a clean dressing, if possible (a sterile dressing is preferred). When applying a dressing, wrap the wound tightly enough to apply pressure and approximate the wound edges, if possible. If the first layer of dressing becomes saturated with blood, apply a second layer. Do so without removing the first layer of dressing because blood clots might be disturbed, resulting in more bleeding.
- Control swelling and pain by applying cold over the wound and surrounding tissues (see the section "Heat and Cold Applications" later in the chapter).
- If bleeding is severe, if internal bleeding is suspected, and if emergency equipment is available, assess the client for signs of shock (rapid, thready pulse; cold clammy skin; pallor; lowered blood pressure).

BOX 33.4 ASSESSING UNTREATED WOUNDS

INITIAL ASSESSMENT

Untreated wounds need to be assessed carefully:

- Assess the location and extent of tissue damage (e.g., partial thickness or full thickness). Measure the wound length, width, and depth.
- Inspect the wound for bleeding. The amount of bleeding varies according to the type of wound and location. Penetrating wounds may cause internal bleeding.
- Inspect the wound for foreign bodies (soil, broken glass, shreds of cloth, or other foreign substances).
- Assess associated injuries, such as fractures, internal bleeding, spinal cord injuries, or head trauma.
- If the wound is contaminated with foreign material, determine when the client last had a tetanus toxoid injection. A tetanus immunization or booster may be necessary.

PRACTICE GUIDELINES 33.1

Assessing Common Pressure Sites

Guidelines	Rationales
Ensure the lighting is good, preferably natural or fluorescent.	Incandescent lights can create a transilluminating effect.
Regulate the environment before beginning the assessment so that the room is neither too hot nor too cold.	Heat can cause the skin to flush; cold can cause the skin to blanch or become cyanotic.
Inspect pressure areas (see Figure 33.5) for discolouration, which can be caused by impaired blood circulation to the area. The pressure areas should a have brisk capillary refill or blanch response when gently palpated by using the end of a finger or thumb.	

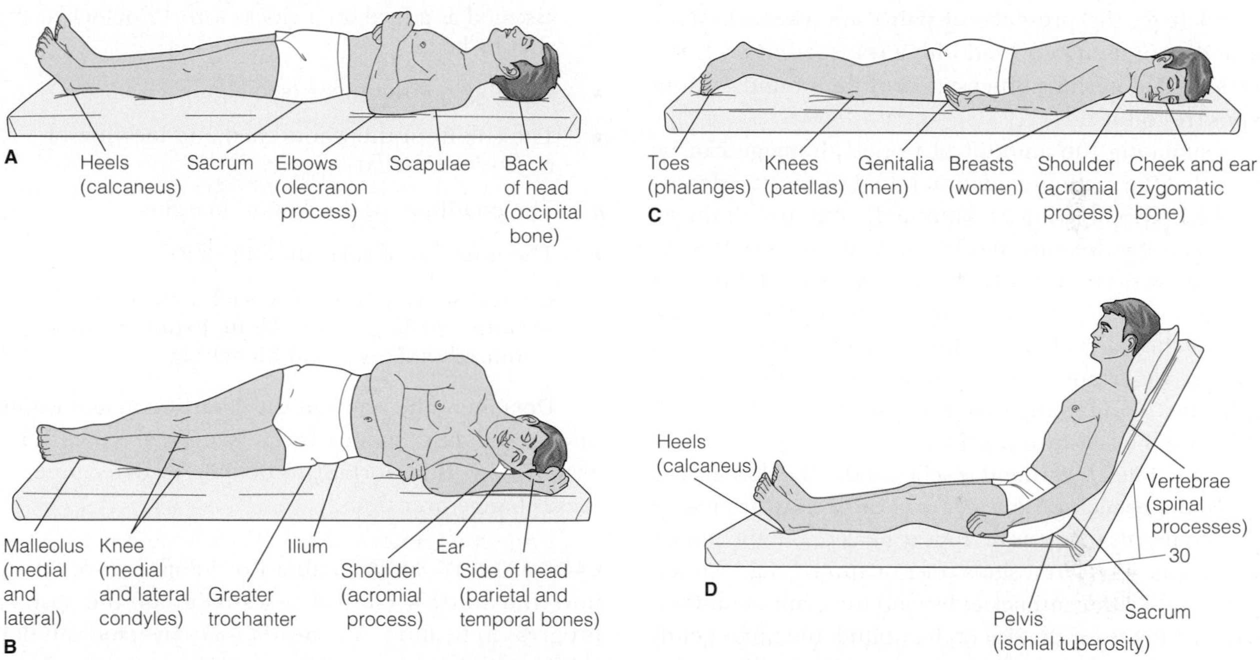

FIGURE 33.5 Body pressure areas in **A:** supine position; **B:** lateral position; **C:** prone position; **D:** Fowler's position.

Guidelines	Rationales
Inspect pressure areas for abrasions and excoriations. An abrasion can occur when skin rubs against a sheet (e.g., when the client is pulled).	Excoriations can occur when the skin has prolonged contact with body secretions or excretions or with dampness in skin folds.
Palpate the surface temperature of the skin over the pressure areas (warm your hands first). Normally, the temperature is the same as that of the surrounding skin.	Increased temperature is abnormal and may be due to inflammation or blood trapped in the area.
Palpate over bony prominences and dependent body areas for the presence of edema, which feels spongy or boggy.	Edema slows the diffusion of oxygen to the tissue cells and of metabolites away from the cells.

TREATED WOUNDS Treated wounds, or *sutured wounds* are regularly assessed to determine the progress of healing. Assessment of a treated wound involves observation of its size and location; the approximation of wound edges; the condition of the wound closure devices (e.g., sutures, staples), as well as the presence of any odour, swelling, redness, bruising, or pain. The status of any drains and the type and amount of drainage are also important to note. In some long-term facilities, home care situations, and outpatient clinics, photographs are taken weekly for a visual record of the progress of pressure ulcers and wounds. Other assessments are documented and dated along with the photograph.

If the wound itself cannot be directly inspected, the dressing is inspected and other data regarding the wound (e.g., the presence of pain) are assessed. Many treated wounds are covered with a transparent occlusive dressing that permits observation of the wound without exposure to the air.

Estimating the amount of wound drainage can be difficult. One recommendation is to describe the degree to which the dressing is saturated. Minimal drainage only stains the dressing, moderate drainage saturates the dressing without leakage before scheduled dressing changes, and heavy drainage overflows the dressing before scheduled changes (Brown, 2006). These terms, plus the description of the drainage and the amount and type of dressing material used, should be well understood by all care providers.

Sometimes, the wound reaches under the skin surface (called **undermining**). The edges of the wound around an open centre may be raw or appear healed, but the undermining can result in a sinus tract or tunnel that extends the wound many centimetres beyond the main wound surface. To fully assess the size of the wound, the nurse gently explores the undermined area with a thin, flexible probe. Do not use a cotton-tipped swab since it can leave behind fibres in the wound. Once the end of the tract is reached, gently raise the probe so that the bulge created by the end can be seen and its length measured on the skin surface. Sinus tracts are often caused by infection and have significant drainage. They may be treated by using antibiotics, irrigation, surgical incision to open and drain the tract, or vacuum therapy for large tracts.

Further details about surgical wound assessment are discussed in Chapter 35.

PRESSURE ULCERS When a pressure ulcer (or any chronic ulcer) is present, the nurse needs to use a tool that will accurately and consistently assess the wound and surrounding skin. The quantifiable tool should compare two or more measurements over time, be able to detect small changes in the wound, and be reproducible in a clinical setting. This assessment will provide baseline data to evaluate the repair process and be used to drive treatment decisions. An example is the PUSH tool, which was shown in Figure 33.4.

When a pressure ulcer is present, the nurse notes the following:

- The location of the ulcer in relation to a bony prominence
- The size of lesion in centimetres: measure length, width, and depth, beginning with length (head to toe) and then width (side to side); to measure depth, gently insert a sterile gloved finger at the deepest part of the wound, and then measure the finger against a measuring guide
- The presence of undermining or sinus tracts, assessed as a face on a clock, with 12'oclock at the client's head
- The stage of the ulcer (see Figure 33.1)
- The colour of the wound bed and location of necrosis or eschar
- The condition of the wound margins
- The integrity of surrounding skin
- Clinical signs of infection, such as redness, warmth, swelling, pain, odour, exudate (note colour of exudate), and blanching

Document the status of the client's skin and wounds on the standard agency form (see Figure 33.6 for an example). It is important to be able to determine how these change over time.

LABORATORY DATA Laboratory data can often support the nurse's clinical assessment of the wound's progress in healing. A *decreased leukocyte count* can delay healing and increase the possibility of infection. A *hemoglobin* level below normal range indicates poor oxygen delivery to the tissues. *Blood coagulation studies* are also significant. Prolonged coagulation times can result in excessive blood loss and prolonged clot absorption. Hypercoagulability can lead to intravascular clotting. Intra-arterial clotting can result in a deficient blood supply to the wound area. *Serum protein analysis,* including *albumin,* provides an indication of the body's nutritional reserves for rebuilding cells. *Wound cultures* can either confirm or rule out the presence of infection. Sensitivity studies are helpful in the selection of appropriate antibiotic therapy. The nurse obtains a wound culture whenever an infection is suspected.

Skill 33.1 provides guidelines on obtaining a specimen of wound drainage.

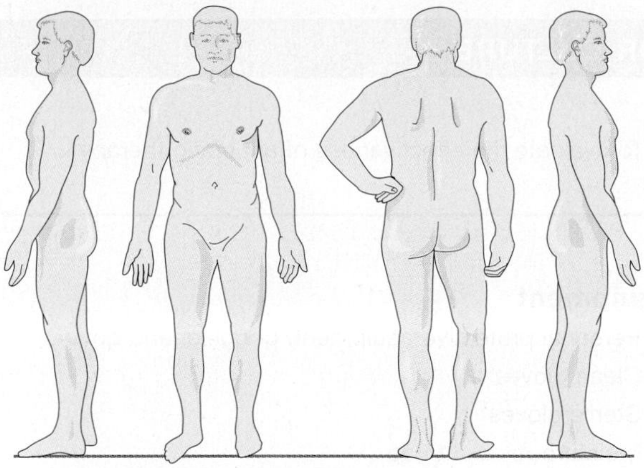

Description of Pressure Ulcers & Classification

Stage I: Characterized by erythema that does not resolve within minutes of pressure relief. Skin remains intact.

Stage II: Partial thickness loss of skin involving the epidermis or dermis or may involve both. The ulcer is superficial and may present as a blister, an abrasion, or a shallow crater. Free of eschar.

Stage III: Full thickness loss that goes through the dermis to the subcutaneous tissue but does not extend through the underlying fascia. Appears as a crater and may include undermining.

Stage IV: Full thickness skin loss with extensive damage through the subcutaneous tissue to the fascia and may involve muscle layers, joint, and bone.

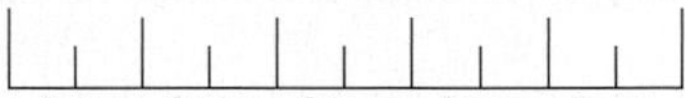

- IDENTIFY LOCATION OF ALL PRESSURE ULCERS ABOVE BY NUMBERING (1, 2, 3): IF MORE THAN 3, USE ADDITIONAL SHEET.
- COMPLETE CHART BELOW FOR SITE #1, USE REVERSE SIDE FOR SITES 2 & 3.

Patient Admitted On: ______________________

Date Sheet Initiated: ______________________

Pressure relief methods in use:

❑ Low Airloss Bed

❑ Low Airloss Mattress Overlay

❑ Turning q2h when pt. supine and q1h if HOB↑

❑ Pressure Reducing Mattress Overlay

❑ Other ______________________

Date MD notified of ulcer: ______________________

DOCUMENT WEEKLY AND PRN SIGNIFICANT CHANGE IN ULCER'S APPEARANCE

SITE #1: LOCATION		DESCRIBE TREATMENT:			FREQUENCY:	
DATE / TIME						
DIMENSIONS: (cm)	LENGTH					
	WIDTH					
	DEPTH					
ODOUR (none or foul)						
DESCRIBE DRAINAGE (purulent, serous, serosanguineous) and AMOUNT (scant, moderate, copious)						
STAGE (see above)						
COMMENTARY: (i.e., describe tissue surrounding ulcer: is there undermining? % necrotic vs % granular, etc.)						
NURSE						

WOUND/SKIN DOCUMENTATION SHEET

FIGURE 33.6 Wound and skin documentation sheet

SKILL 33.1

OBTAINING A WOUND DRAINAGE SPECIMEN FOR CULTURE

PURPOSES

- To identify the microorganisms potentially causing an infection and the antibiotics to which they are sensitive
- To evaluate the effectiveness of antibiotic therapy

ASSESSMENT

Assess

- Appearance of the wound and surrounding tissue; check the character and amount of wound drainage
- Client complaints of pain or discomfort at the wound site
- Signs of infection, such as fever, chills, or elevated white blood cell count (WBC)

Planning

Before obtaining a specimen of wound drainage, determine

- Whether agency policy suggests that the wound should be cleaned before obtaining the specimen
- Whether the site from which to take the specimen has been specified

Equipment

- Personal protective equipment, goggles, and gown
- Clean gloves
- Sterile gloves
- Moisture-resistant bag
- Sterile dressing set
- Normal saline and irrigating syringe
- Culture tube with swab and culture medium (aerobic and anaerobic tubes are available) or sterile syringe with needle for anaerobic culture
- Completed labels for each container
- Completed requisition to accompany the specimens to the laboratory

IMPLEMENTATION

Preparation

Check the medical orders to determine whether the specimen is to be collected for an *aerobic* (growing only in the presence of oxygen) or *anaerobic* (growing only in the absence of oxygen) culture. Aerobic organisms are generally found on the surface of the wound, whereas anaerobic organisms would be found in deep wounds, tunnels, and cavities. Administer an analgesic 30 minutes before the procedure if the client is complaining of pain at the wound site.

Performance

1. Before performing the procedure, introduce yourself and verify the client's identity by using agency protocol. Explain to the client what you are going to do, why it is necessary, and how he or she can cooperate. Discuss how the results will be used in planning further care or treatments.
2. Perform hand hygiene and observe other appropriate infection prevention and control procedures (e.g., gloves).
3. Provide for client privacy.
4. Remove any moist outer dressings that cover the wound.
   - Put on clean gloves.
   - Remove the outer dressing, and observe any drainage on the dressing. Hold the dressing so that the client does not see the drainage. **Rationale: The appearance of the drainage could upset the client.**
   - Determine the amount of the drainage, for example, "one 5 cm × 2 cm gauze saturated with pale yellow drainage."
   - Discard the dressing in the moisture-proof bag. Handle it carefully so that the dressing does not touch the outside of the bag. **Rationale: Touching the outside of the bag will contaminate it.**
   - Remove your gloves and dispose of them properly.
5. Open the sterile dressing set by using sterile technique (see Skill 32.3, page 901).
6. Assess the wound.
   - Put on sterile gloves (see Skill 32.4, page 905).
   - Assess the appearance of the tissues in and around the wound and the drainage. Infection can cause reddened tissues with a thick discharge, which may be foul smelling, whitish, or coloured.
7. Cleanse the wound.
   - By using gauze swabs or irrigation (see Skill 33.4 later in this chapter), cleanse the wound with normal saline until all exudate has been removed. **Rationale: This removes any debris so that any microorganisms that are actually a part of the wound are accurately determined, rather than any contamination.**
   - After cleansing, apply a sterile gauze pad to the wound. **Rationale: This absorbs excess cleansing solution.**
   - If a topical antimicrobial ointment or cream is being used to treat the wound, use a swab to remove it. **Rationale: Residual antiseptic must be removed before culture.**
   - Remove and discard sterile gloves.
8. Obtain the aerobic culture.
   - Open a specimen tube and place the cap upside down on a firm, dry surface so that the inside will not become contaminated or if the swab is attached to the lid, twist the cap to loosen the swab. Hold the tube in one hand and take out the swab in the other.
   - Rotate the swab over an area of tissue 1 cm^2. Apply sufficient pressure to express fluid from within the wound tissue (see ❶). **Rationale: Microorganisms**

(continued)

SKILL 33.1

OBTAINING A WOUND DRAINAGE SPECIMEN FOR CULTURE *(continued)*

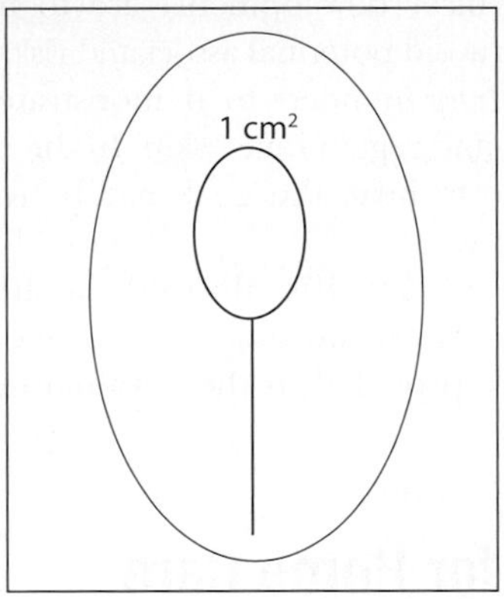

❶ Rotate the swab over an area of granulation tissue 1 cm^2.

that are most likely to be responsible for a wound infection reside in viable tissue.

- Do not use pus or pooled exudates to culture. **Rationale: These secretions contain a mixture of contaminants that are not the same as those causing the infection.**
- Avoid touching the swab to intact skin at the wound edges. **Rationale: This prevents the introduction of superficial skin organisms into the culture.**
- Return the swab to the culture tube, taking care not to touch the top or the outside of the tube. **Rationale: The outside of the container must remain free of pathogenic microorganisms to prevent their spread to others.**
- Crush the inner ampule containing the medium for organism growth at the bottom of the tube. **Rationale: This ensures that the swab with the specimen is surrounded by culture medium.**
- Twist the cap to secure.
- If a specimen is required from another site, repeat the steps. Specify the exact site (e.g., inferior drain site or lower aspect of incision) on the label of each container. Be sure to put each swab in the appropriately labelled tube.

9. Dress the wound.
- Apply any prescribed medication to the wound.
- Cover the wound with a sterile wound dressing. See Table 33.4 for selected types of wound dressings.

10. Arrange for the specimen to be transported to the laboratory immediately. Be sure to include the completed requisition.

11. Document all relevant information.
- Record on the client's chart the taking of the specimen and source.
- Include the date and time, the appearance of the wound, the colour, consistency, amount, and odour of any drainage, the type of culture collected, and any discomfort experienced by the client.

Variation: Obtaining a Specimen for Anaerobic Culture

- Insert a sterile 10 mL syringe (without needle) into the wound, and aspirate 1 mL to 5 mL of drainage into the syringe.
- Attach the needle to the syringe, and expel all air from the syringe and needle.
- Immediately inject the drainage into the anaerobic culture tube and cap the tube tightly.
- *Or* use an anaerobic culture swab system in which the swab is immediately placed into a tube filled with an oxygen-free gas or a gel environment.
- Label the tube or syringe appropriately.
- Send the tube or syringe of drainage to the laboratory immediately. Do not refrigerate the specimen.

EVALUATION

- Compare the findings of wound assessment and drainage to previous assessments to determine any changes.
- Report the culture results to the appropriate health-care team members.
- Conduct appropriate follow-up, such as administering antibiotics or modifying wound treatment as prescribed.

CLINICAL ALERT

Wound cleansing *must* be done before obtaining a specimen for culture. The goal of a culture is to evaluate the microorganisms present in the wound tissue. Failure to cleanse means that the results are indicative of contaminants, such as wound exudate, topical therapies, or nonviable tissue, which could lead to inappropriate or unnecessary treatment.

Diagnosing

The NANDA International (2007) nursing diagnoses that relate to clients who have skin wounds or who are at risk for skin breakdown are as follows:

- *Risk for Impaired Skin Integrity:* At risk for skin being adversely altered
- *Impaired Skin Integrity:* Altered epidermis and/or dermis

- *Impaired Tissue Integrity:* Damage to mucous membrane, corneal, integumentary, or subcutaneous tissues

Impaired Skin Integrity commonly applies to stage I and II (partial-thickness skin loss) pressure ulcers and to superficial wounds extending through the epidermis or the dermis. *Impaired Tissue Integrity* applies to stage III and IV (full-thickness skin loss) pressure ulcers and to wounds extending into subcutaneous tissue, muscle, or bone.

Additional nursing diagnoses may be appropriate for clients with existing impaired skin or tissue integrity. Examples of these diagnoses include the following:

- *Risk for Infection* if the skin impairment is severe, the client is immunosuppressed, or the wound is caused by trauma
- *Pain* related to nerve involvement within the tissue impairment or as a consequence of procedures used to treat the wound
- *Body Image, Disturbed* if the wound or dressing cause the client significant negative feelings about his or her appearance
- *Anxiety* if the client experiences apprehension related to care of the wound or the eventual outcome of the healing process

Planning

The major goals for clients at *Risk for Impaired Skin Integrity* (e.g., pressure ulcer development) are to maintain skin integrity and to avoid potential associated risks. Clients with *Impaired Skin Integrity* need to demonstrate progressive wound healing and regain intact skin. In the event that the client is unable to heal, the goal may be to palliate the wound.

Examples of specific desired health outcomes related to these goals, although established in the planning phase, are provided in the "Evaluating" section of this chapter.

Planning for Home Care

Increasingly, wound care is provided in the home rather than in health-care facilities. The client and family assume much of the responsibility for assessing and treating existing wounds and for helping to prevent pressure ulcers. The Assessment: Home Care box outlines appropriate assessment for clients who have wounds or pressure ulcers or who are at risk for develop-

ASSESSMENT: HOME CARE

Wound Care and Prevention of Pressure Ulcers

Assess the client's and the family's understanding of wounds and wound care:

CLIENT AND ENVIRONMENT

- *Current level of knowledge:* Understanding of the cause of the wound or risk for developing a pressure ulcer; prevention or treatment strategies
- *Self-care abilities for mobility:* Physical ability to change position, ambulate, and transfer, including the use of assistive devices
- *Self-care abilities for wound care:* Manual dexterity and visual acuity necessary to perform skin assessments and wound treatments
- *Facilities:* Presence of running water, garbage, and bathroom needed to perform wound care and contain potentially infectious materials
- *Current level of nutrition:* Eating habits and preferences, laboratory values indicating need for teaching or other intervention

FAMILY

- *Caregiver availability, skills, and responses:* Willingness to assist with wound care and actions to prevent pressure ulcers
- *Family role changes and coping:* Effect on financial status, parenting and spousal roles, sexuality, social roles
- *Alternative potential primary or respite caregivers:* For example, other family members, volunteers, church members, paid caregivers or housekeeping services, available community respite care (adult daycare, senior centres, and so on)

COMMUNITY

- *Resources:* Availability and familiarity with possible sources of assistance, such as equipment and supply companies, organizations that offer medical supplies or financial assistance, home care agencies

TEACHING: CLINICAL

Skin Integrity

Nurses must teach the client and family wound preventive and skin integrity care measures before discharge:

MAINTAINING INTACT SKIN

- Discuss the relationship between adequate nutrition (especially fluids, protein, vitamins B and C, iron, zinc, and calories) and healthy skin.
- Demonstrate appropriate positions for pressure relief.

(continued)

TEACHING: CLINICAL (*continued*)

- Establish a turning or repositioning schedule.
- Demonstrate the application of appropriate skin protection agents and devices.
- Instruct to report persistent reddened areas.
- Identify potential sources of skin trauma and means of avoidance.

PROMOTING WOUND HEALING

- Discuss the importance of adequate nutrition (especially fluids, protein, vitamins B and C, iron, zinc, and calories).
- Instruct in wound assessment and provide mechanism for documenting.
- Emphasize the principles of infection prevention and control, especially hand hygiene and the proper methods of handling used dressings.
- Provide information about signs of wound infection and other complications to report.
- Reinforce the appropriate aspects of pressure ulcer prevention.
- Demonstrate wound care techniques, such as wound cleansing and dressing change.
- Discuss pain control measures, if needed.

ing alterations in skin integrity. In planning for client discharge, nurses are accountable for teaching the client and family wound preventive and skin integrity care measures (see the Teaching: Clinical box).

Implementing

Many interventions exist to help preserve a client's skin and underlying tissues. An initial step involves identifying clients at risk for breakdown since risk factors provide the basis for prophylaxis (RNAO, 2005). Refer to the Braden scale in Figure 33.3 (page 935).

Nursing interventions for maintaining skin integrity and wound care involve supporting wound healing, preventing pressure ulcers, treating pressure ulcers, dressing and cleaning wounds, applying heat and cold, and supporting and immobilizing wounds. Wounds must be reassessed on a regular basis to determine the adequacy of the treatment plan.

Supporting Wound Healing

The four major areas in which nurses can help clients develop optimal conditions for wound healing are maintaining moist wound healing, providing sufficient nutrition and hydration, preventing wound infections, and using proper positioning.

MAINTAINING MOIST WOUND HEALING The frequency of dressing change should support moist wound bed conditions. Wound beds that are too dry or disturbed too often fail to heal.

PROVIDING NUTRITION AND FLUIDS Clients should be assisted to take in at least 2500 mL of fluids a day unless conditions contraindicate this amount. Although no evidence shows that excessive doses of vitamins or minerals enhance wound healing, adequate amounts are extremely important. The nurse should ensure that clients receive sufficient protein, vitamins C, A, B_1, and B_5, and zinc. Consultations with a registered dietitian or speech language pathologist (in the case of swallowing difficulties) may be very helpful (RNAO, 2005).

PREVENTING INFECTION Controlling wound infection has two main aspects: preventing microorganisms from entering the wound, and preventing the transmission of blood-borne pathogens to or from the client to others. See Box 33.5 and Chapter 32 for more information about infection prevention and control.

POSITIONING To promote wound healing, clients must be positioned to keep pressure off the wound (sometimes referred to as *offloading*). Changes of position and transfers can be accomplished without shear or friction damage. In addition to proper positioning, the client

BOX 33.5 GUIDELINES FOR PREVENTING INFECTION AND THE TRANSMISSION OF BLOOD-BORNE PATHOGENS

Preventing infection is an extremely important part of wound care:

- Perform hand hygiene before and after caring for wounds.
- Masks and protective eyewear (e.g., goggles, safety glasses) or face shields should be worn to protect mucous membranes, nonintact skin, and conjunctiva during procedures that are likely to generate splashes of blood or fluids capable of transmitting blood-borne pathogens. Wherever a possibility exists for exposure to blood or fluid capable of transmitting blood-borne pathogens, masks and protective eyewear should be worn.
- Touch an open or fresh surgical wound only when wearing sterile gloves or using sterile forceps.
- Remove, change, or reinforce dressings over closed wounds when they become wet.

Source: These recommendations are based on the principles outlined in "Prevention and Control of Occupational Infections in Health Care," by the Public Health Agency of Canada, 2002, *Canada Communicable Disease Report, 28S1*. Retrieved June 1, 2008, from http://www.phac-aspc.gc.ca/publicat/ccdr-rmtc/02vol28/28s1/index.html.

should be assisted to be as mobile as possible because activity enhances circulation. If the client cannot move independently, range-of-motion exercises and a turning schedule are implemented.

Preventing Pressure Ulcers

To reduce the likelihood of pressure ulcer development in all clients, the nurse employs a variety of preventive measures (i.e., skin hygiene and pressure relief devices) to maintain the skin integrity and instructs the client, support people, and caregivers in how to prevent pressure ulcers.

PROVIDING NUTRITION Optimal nutrition promotes wound healing, maintains immune competence, and decreases the risk of infection (RNAO, 2007). Because an inadequate intake of calories, protein, vitamins, and iron is believed to be a risk factor for pressure ulcer development, nutritional supplements should be considered for nutritionally compromised clients. The diet should be similar to one that supports wound healing, as discussed earlier. Monitor weight regularly to help assess nutritional status. Pertinent lab work should also be monitored, including lymphocyte count, protein (especially albumin), and hemoglobin.

MAINTAINING SKIN HYGIENE Obtain baseline data by using an established tool and then reassess the skin at least daily in the hospital and weekly at home. When bathing the client, the nurse should minimize the force and friction applied to the skin and use mild cleansing agents that minimize irritation and dryness and that do not disrupt the skin's natural barriers. Also, the nurse should avoid using hot water, which increases skin dryness and irritation. Nurses can minimize skin dryness by avoiding exposure to cold and low humidity. Dry skin is best treated with moisturizing lotions applied while the skin is moist after bathing. The client's skin should be kept clean and dry and free of irritation and maceration by urine, feces, sweat, and incomplete drying after a bath. Apply skin protection if indicated. Dimethicone-based creams or alcohol-free barrier films are available in liquid, spray, and moist wipe format and are very effective in preventing moisture or drainage from collecting on the skin. In most cases, the nurse can apply these without a physician's prescription. Petroleum-based creams and ointments are no longer advised because of poor overall skin protection and interference with diaper or incontinence product absorption.

AVOIDING SKIN TRAUMA Massage over bony prominences should be avoided. Traditionally, nurses have used massage to stimulate blood circulation, with the intention of preventing pressure ulcers. Scientific evidence does not support this belief and, in fact, suggests that massage may lead to deep tissue trauma (RNAO, 2005).

Appropriate positioning is critical in addressing issues related to pressure (RNAO, 2007). Providing the client with a smooth, firm, and wrinkle-free foundation on which to sit or lie helps prevent skin trauma. To prevent injury caused by friction and shear, clients must be positioned, transferred, and turned correctly. For bedridden clients, shear force can be reduced by elevating the head of the bed to no more than 30 degrees, if this position is not contraindicated by the client's condition (RNAO, 2007). (For example, clients with respiratory disorders may find it easier to breathe in Fowler's position.) When the head of the bed is raised, the skin and superficial fascia stick to the bed linen while the deep fascia and skeleton slide down toward the bottom of the bed. As a result, blood vessels in the sacral area become twisted, and the tissues in the area can become ischemic and necrotic. Baby powder and cornstarch are never used as friction or moisture prevention. These powders create harmful abrasive grit damaging to tissues and are considered a respiratory hazard when airborne.

Frequent shifts in position, even if only slight, effectively change pressure points. The client should shift weight 10 to 15 degrees every 15 to 30 minutes and, whenever possible, exercise or ambulate to stimulate blood circulation.

When lifting a client to change position, nurses should use a lifting device, such as a trapeze, rather than dragging the client across or up in bed. The friction that results from dragging the skin against a sheet can cause blisters and abrasions, which may contribute to more extensive tissue damage. Therefore, the use of devices that lift the client's weight off the bed surface is the method of choice.

A client who has a pressure ulcer on a seating surface should be discouraged from sitting, when possible. It is important to obtain a seating assessment if a client has a pressure ulcer on a sitting surface that requires relief from pressure (RNAO, 2007). Any at-risk client confined to bed—even when a special support mattress is used—should be repositioned at least every 2 hours, depending on the client's need, to allow another body surface to bear the weight. Six body positions can usually be used: prone, supine, right and left lateral (side lying), and right and left Sims' positions. When a lateral position is used, the nurse should avoid positioning the client directly on the trochanter and instead position the client on a 30-degree angle (RNAO, 2007). A written schedule should be established for turning and repositioning.

PROVIDING SUPPORTIVE DEVICES For circulation to remain uncompromised, pressure on the bony prominences should remain below capillary pressure for as much time as possible through a combination of turning, positioning, and using pressure-relieving surfaces. Mean capillary pressure can be estimated at 20 mm Hg. Although some research has been conducted evaluating the effectiveness of pressure-reducing support surfaces in preventing pressure ulcers in clients at low, intermediate, or high risk, the results are often inconclusive. The nurse should review the manufacturer's product descriptions that report the amount of time that the pressure between the surface and the bony prominence is above or below specified levels and determine whether this is adequate to protect a particular client.

For clients confined to bed, three types of support surfaces can be used to relieve pressure. The overlay mattress is applied on top of the standard bed mattress. A replacement mattress is used instead of the standard mattress; most are made of foam and gel combinations. Clients who have an existing pressure ulcer and remain at risk should have a high-specification foam mattress in place of the regular mattress (RNAO, 2007). Specialty beds replace hospital beds. They provide pressure relief, eliminate shear and friction, and decrease moisture. Examples are high-air-loss beds, low-air-loss beds, and beds that provide kinetic therapy. Such dynamic support surfaces should be used in cases in which the client cannot assume a variety of positions without bearing weight on the ulcer or is functionally dependent and has large, deep, or multiple ulcers (RNAO, 2007). Kinetic therapy air-loss beds turn the patient automatically 200 times per day and are designed for total pressure relief. These beds eliminate friction, shear, and maceration. However, these specialty beds are costly to rent and may place small-framed patients at risk of falls. Table 33.3 lists selected mechanical devices for reducing pressure on body parts.

TABLE 33.3 Mechanical Devices for Reducing Pressure on Body Parts

Device	Description and Comments
Gel flotation pads	Polyvinyl, silicone, or Silastic pads filled with a gelatinous substance similar to fat.
Pillows and wedges (foam, gel, air, fluid)	Supports positioning and offloads bone on bone contact.
Heel protectors (sheepskin boots, padded splints, off-loading inflatable boots, foam blocks)	Can raise or "float" a body part (e.g., heels) off of surface. Prevent shearing and limit pressure on heel area (see Figure 33.7).
Memory foam mattress or chair pad	Polyurethane foam mattress distributes weight over bony areas evenly. Foam moulds to the body.
Alternating pressure mattress	Composed of a number of cells in which the pressure alternately increases and decreases; uses a pump (see Figure 33.8).
Water bed	Support surface filled with water. Water temperature can be controlled.
Static low-air-loss (LAL) bed	Consists of many air-filled cushions divided into four or five sections. Separate controls permit each section to be inflated to a different level of firmness; thus pressure can be reduced on bony prominences but increased under other body areas for support (see Figure 33.9).
Active or second-generation LAL bed	Like the static LAL, but in addition gently pulsates or rotates from side to side, thus stimulating capillary blood flow and facilitating movement of pulmonary secretions.

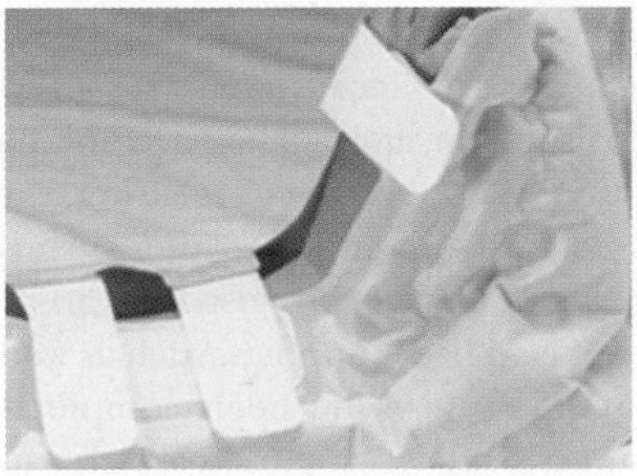

FIGURE 33.7 Heel protector

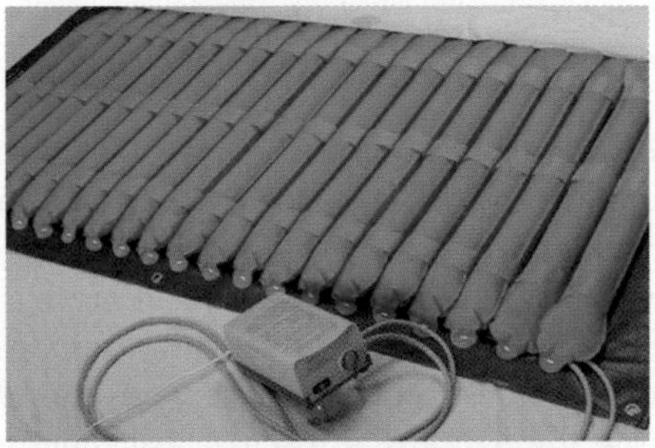

FIGURE 33.8 Alternating pressure mattress

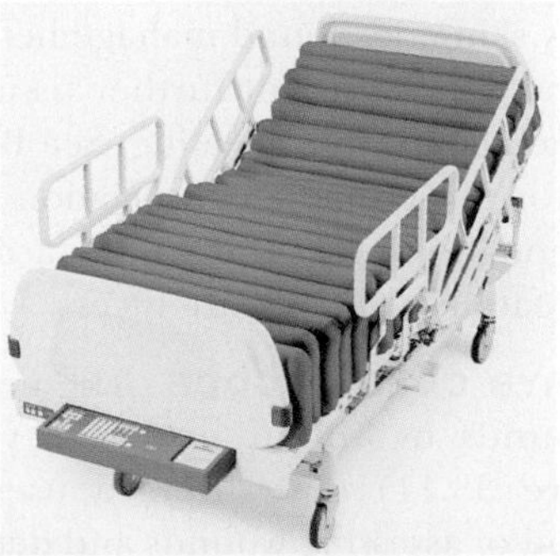

FIGURE 33.9 Low-air-loss bed

(continued)

TABLE 33.3 Mechanical Devices for Reducing Pressure on Body Parts (*continued*)

Air-fluidized (AF) bed (static high-air-loss bed)	Forced temperature-controlled air is circulated around millions of tiny silicone-coated beads, producing a fluidlike movement. Provides uniform support to body contours. Decreases skin maceration by its drying effect. Moisture from the client penetrates the linens and soaks the beads. Airflow forces the beads away from the client and rapidly dries the sheet. A major disadvantage is that the head of the bed cannot be elevated. Some beds are a unique combination of air fluidized therapy and low-air-loss therapy on an articulating frame. These are used with patients who require head elevation (see Figure 33.10).

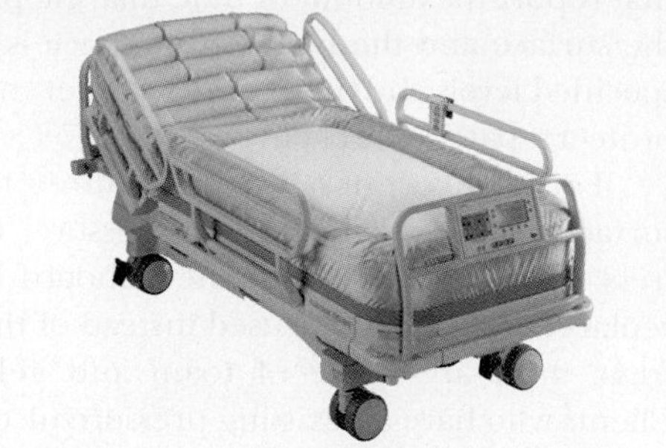

FIGURE 33.10 Low-air-loss and air-fluidized combo bed (Clinitron/Rite Hite)

When a client is confined to bed or to a chair, pressure-reducing devices, such as pillows made of high-density foam, gel, air, or a combination of these, can be used. When the client is sitting, weight should be distributed over the entire seating surface so that pressure does not centre on just one area. To protect a client's heels in bed, supports, such as wedges or pillows, can be used to raise the heels completely off the bed. Doughnut-type devices should not be used since they limit blood flow and can cause tissue damage to the areas in direct contact with the device (RNAO, 2005).

Treating Pressure Ulcers

Pressure ulcers are a challenge for nurses because of the number of variables involved (e.g., risk factors, types of ulcers, and degrees of impairment) and the numerous treatment measures advocated. Existing and potential infections are the most serious complications of pressure ulcers. For clients with compromised skin integrity of the lower limbs, a vascular assessment is essential to rule out arterial disease and to determine appropriate therapy (RNAO, 2007).

In treating pressure ulcers, nurses should follow the agency skin and wound management protocols. Prompt treatment can prevent further tissue damage and pain and facilitate wound healing. See Box 33.2 (pages 930–931) for the Canadian Association of Wound Care recommendations for practice regarding the prevention and treatment of pressure ulcers.

R	**Red wounds** may vary from pale pink to a beefy red with the colour indicating the presence and depth of granulation tissue. Red wounds can be in the inflammatory or proliferative phase of wound healing. There is a need to cover a red wound for protection and to keep it moist. Both protection from trauma and a moist wound bed enhance wound healing.
Y	**Yellow wounds** vary in colour from pale ivory to various shades of yellow, green, and brown. The yellow/green/brown colour indicates the presence of slough (dead but moist tissue). Yellow wounds actively generate wound fluid and need to be debrided to remove the slough and reduce the bacterial load.
B	**Black wounds** are covered with tissue that is a black/brown, or tan. The colour indicates the presence of dead tissue that is dehydrated to various degrees. Often black wounds are referred to as being covered with eschar, a thick hard leathery appearing material. When eschar is covering a wound, the depth cannot be accurately assessed until the eschar is removed. In most cases, eschar provides an excellent medium for bacterial proliferation and needs to be removed to prevent infection and promote wound healing. In patients with diabetes with inadequate blood supply, dry eschar is kept intact until a thorough vascular exam has been completed.

FIGURE 33.11 RYB colour wound classification system

THE RYB COLOUR CODE The universal classification of wounds by colour uses red, yellow, black (RYB) (Figure 33.11) and offers a user-friendly, practical method of assessing wounds and determining treatment options (Fowler et al., 2003). The colour classification describes the wound in terms of its surface appearance (Cuzzell, 1988). The red denotes granulation tissue; the yellow indicates slough; and the black, necrotic tissue. Some authors suggest that the colour reflects the phase of healing (inflammatory or proliferative) of the open wound (Krasner, 1995). The goals of wound care by using this system are to *protect* (cover) red, *cleanse* yellow, and *debride* black.

Wounds that are red are usually in the late regeneration phase of tissue repair (i.e., developing granulation tissue). They need to be protected to avoid disturbance to regenerating tissue. The nurse protects red wounds by (1) gentle cleansing (i.e., use of a noncytotoxic wound cleanser applied without pressure), (2) protecting periwound skin with an alcohol-free barrier film, (3) filling dead space with hydrogel or alginate, (4) covering with an appropriate dressing, such as transparent film, hydrocolloid dressing, or a clear absorbent acrylic dressing, and (5) changing the dressing as infrequently as possible.

Yellow wounds are characterized primarily by liquid to semi-liquid slough that is often accompanied by purulent drainage. The nurse *cleanses* yellow wounds to remove nonviable tissue. Methods used include applying wet-to-damp dressings; irrigating the wound; using absorbent dressing materials, such as impregnated nonadherent hydrogel dressings or other exudate absorbers; and consulting with the physician about the need for a topical antimicrobial to minimize bacterial growth.

Black wounds are covered with thick necrotic tissue or eschar. Black wounds require **debridement** (removal of necrotic or devitalized tissue that interferes with wound healing), except in cases of foot ulcers with dry eschar (RNAO, 2007). Removal of nonviable tissue from a wound must occur before the wound can heal.

Debridement can be achieved in four different ways: sharp, mechanical, chemical, and autolytic. The method of debridement will depend on (1) the client's condition and goals of treatment; (2) the type, quantity, and location of necrotic tissue; and (3) the depth and amount of fluid (RNAO, 2007). Refer to Box 33.2 for the Canadian Association of Wound Care's recommendations for preparing the wound bed.

In *sharp debridement,* a sharp instrument (scalpel or scissors) is used to separate and remove dead tissue. Generally, this high-risk procedure is performed only by specially trained health professionals (e.g., wound, ostomy, and continence nurses [WOCNs]; qualified physical therapists). Sharp debridement should be used if there is urgent need for debridement, such as advancing cellulitis or sepsis (RNAO, 2007). Sharp debridement entails a serious risk of bleeding, may require an anaesthetic, and has the potential to cause injury to nervous or other viable tissue (RNAO, 2007).

Mechanical debridement refers to the removal of foreign material and devitalized or contaminated tissue from a wound by physical forces. Wet-to-dry dressing, whirlpool baths, dextranomers, and wound irrigations are examples of mechanical debridement. This treatment may be used as a preparation for sharp debridement. Mechanical debridement has a number of important disadvantages. It is a slow and often painful process that must be discontinued once the necrotic tissue has been removed. Pain management should be an integral part of nursing care for the client undergoing mechanical debridement.

Chemical or *enzymatic debridement* is the topical application of proteolytic substances (enzymes) to break down devitalized tissues. Collagenase enzyme agents, such as papain-urea, are currently most recommended for this use. This method is relatively slow, but it can be helpful for clients who are not candidates for sharp debridement, clients in long-term care or home care, and clients in whom ulcer infection is not present (RNAO, 2007).

In *autolytic debridement,* synthetic dressings are used to cover a wound and allow eschar to self-digest by the action of enzymes present in wound fluids. Although this method takes longer than the other three, it is the most selective and therefore causes the least damage to healthy surrounding and healing tissues. Because occlusive synthetic dressings create an anaerobic environment, they should never be used if an infection in the wound is suspected. Recently, the use of fly larvae (maggots, *Phaenicia sericata*) has received increased attention. Larval therapy can be extremely effective in cleansing chronic wounds because the maggots secrete enzymes that break down necrotic tissue (while leaving healthy tissue untouched), ingest bacteria, and decrease bacterial growth through the rise in surface pH that results from their presence (Sosin, 2005).

Most wounds display a combination of colours and are called mixed-colour wounds. In these wounds, care is planned to address the most serious problem first (Fowler et al., 2003). Thus, the highest priority is to address the black, then the yellow, and finally the red. Black and yellow wounds need to be debrided and both types kept moist. The appearance of the wound is documented by percentage (e.g., 50% red, 25% yellow, and 25% black).

The RYB system is an excellent conceptual framework for guiding the local treatment of the wound, although its use has limitations (Fowler et al., 2003). This system does not address the underlying pathology and treatment needed for specific pathologies, such as the compression that would be needed to treat a venous ulcer. Consultation with a wound care specialist is important in determining appropriate therapies, particularly when the ulcer is a manifestation of a systemic disease.

Dressing Wounds

Dressings are applied for the following purposes:

- To protect the wound from mechanical injury
- To protect the wound from microbial contamination
- To provide or maintain humidity of the wound
- To provide thermal insulation
- To absorb drainage or debride a wound, or both
- To prevent hemorrhage (when applied as a pressure dressing or with elastic bandages)
- To splint or immobilize the wound site and thereby facilitate healing and prevent injury
- To provide psychological (aesthetic) comfort

The development of interactive wound dressings has produced dressings that work with the environment of the wound to promote wound healing. Moisture-retentive dressings promote wound healing by optimizing the local wound environment (RNAO, 2007).

TYPES OF DRESSING A wide, and sometimes confusing, array of dressings are available for wound management. Table 33.4 provides a summary of selected types of wound dressings. A number of factors influence the type of dressing that is appropriate for any given wound. Box 33.6 lists RNAO guidelines (2007) regarding factors to consider when selecting a dressing for local wound care.

In many settings, dressing cost is also a concern, particularly if extended treatment is required. A wound management consultant can help to select the dressing that best meets both the needs of the client and the need for cost containment.

Common gauze dressings can be applied in several ways to achieve different goals (see Table 33.5).

MOISTURE RETENTIVE: TRANSPARENT FILMS Transparent films are often applied to superficial wounds and skin breaks with minimal damage (Figure 33.12).

TABLE 33.4 Selected Types of Wound Care Products

Product Type	Description	Purpose	Examples
Wound cleansers	Noncytotoxic liquids. *Must not be confused with skin cleansers, which are meant for intact skin only.*	Normal saline in the preferred cleanser, although commercial products containing surfactants may be helpful with removal of debris.	Normal saline, Shur-Clens, Safe-Clens, Restore
Moisture retentive dressings: Transparent films	Adhesive moisture vapour permeable polyurethane or other synthetic films are *nonabsorbent* dressings that allow exchange of oxygen and moisture vapour between the atmosphere and wound bed. They are impermeable to bacteria and water.	To provide protection against contamination and friction; to maintain a clean moist surface that facilitates cellular migration; to provide insulation by preventing fluid evaporation; and to facilitate wound assessment	Op-Site, Tegaderm, Biocclusive, Flexifix
Moisture retentive: Nonadherents (impregnated or nonimpregnated)	Woven or nonwoven cotton or synthetic materials that may be impregnated with medicated or unmedicated ointments. Require secondary dressings to secure them in place.	Designed to provide a contact dressing of low adherence and support the delivery of topical antibacterials and antibiotics	Nonimpregnated: Mepore, ETE, Mepitel, Primapore, Alldress Impregnated: Xeroform, Adaptic, Jelonet, Bactigras, Sofratulle, Viscopaste
Wound hydration: Hydrocolloids	Waterproof adhesive wafers, pastes, or powders. Wafers, designed to be worn for up to 7 days, consist of two layers. The inner adhesive layer has particles that absorb exudate and form a hydrated gel over the wound; the outer film provides a seal; wear time of 3 to 7 days	To absorb light to moderate exudate; to produce a moist environment that facilitates debridement and healing but does not cause maceration of surrounding skin; to protect the wound from bacterial contamination, foreign debris, and urine or feces	DuoDERM, Comfeel, Tegasorb, Restore, SignaDress
Wound hydration: Hydrogels	Hydrophilic moisture-donating polymers prepared in sheets or gels for use in granulating wounds, minimally exudating wounds, or wounds requiring debridement; can be used in combination with transparent films, foams, hydrocolloids or other nonadherent cover dressings; wear time varies from 1 to 3 days.	To assist with the liquefaction of necrotic tissue or slough; rehydrate the wound bed; and fill in dead space	IntraSite, Vigilon, Normlgel, Hypergel, DuoDERM Hydroactive Gel, Tegagel

(continued)

TABLE 33.4 Selected Types of Wound Care Products (*continued*)

Product Type	Description	Purpose	Examples
Absorbent dressings: Foams	Sheet or cavity dressings of non-adherent polyurethane foams used for wound with moderate to copious amounts of drainage; maintain autolytic debridement during wound cleansing phase; reduces dressing bulk; wear time can be extended as volume of drainage decreases to a maximum of 4 to 7 days	To absorb moderate amounts of exudate	Lyofoam, Allevyn, Biatain, Mepilex, Hydrasorb
Absorbent dressings: Alginates	Nonadherent sheets or ropes that absorb moderate to large amounts of exudate; many products have hemostatic properties; require a secondary dressing; remove residue by flushing wound with saline; maximum wear time of 4 days.	To absorb exudate and facilitate hemostasis	Algisite, Kaltostat, Tegagen, Fibracol
Absorbent dressings: Hydrofibre, hypertonic gauze	Nonadherent sheets or ribbon gauze used for copiously draining wounds; promote comfort by decreasing dressing bulk; requires a moisture retentive cover dressing; layering dressing increases absorption capacity; wear time of 1 to 4 days	To provide a moist wound surface by interacting with exudate; to form a gelatinous mass; to absorb exudate; to eliminate dead space or pack wounds; and to support debridement	Aquacel, Mesalt
Antimicrobials	Topical antimicrobial agents reduce bacterial burden in wounds	To decrease surface bacteria without excessive toxicity to the cells in the wound base	Iodosorb, Acticoat, Aquacel Ag. silver sulfadiazine, metronidazole gel, polymyxin B sulphate—Bacitracin zinc
Skin barriers	Liquids, creams, pastes, ointments or solids; products containing alcohol can cause burning if skin is not intact; liquid product must be dry before dressing is applied	To protect periwound skin from exudate and stripping by adhesives	Skin Prep, Skin Gel, Sween, Calmoseptine, Triple Care, Critic-Aid, Coloplast

BOX 33.6 FACTORS TO CONSIDER IN LOCAL WOUND CARE

When choosing a wound dressing, the nurse should consider the following issues:

- Etiology of the wound
- Client's general health status, preference, goals of care, and environment
- Location of the wound
- Size of the wound, including depth and undermining
- A dressing sufficient in size to loosely fill the wound cavity
- Type and amount of exudate
- Risk of infection
- Risk of recurrence
- Type of tissue involved
- Phase of the wound healing process
- Frequency of dressing change
- Comfort and cosmetic appearance
- Where and by whom the dressing will be changed (e.g., caregiver expertise)
- Product availability
- Does not cause trauma to wound bed on removal

Source: *Assessment and Management of Stage I to IV Pressure Ulcers*, by the Registered Nurses' Association of Ontario, 2007, Toronto: Author.

TABLE 33.5 Modes of Applying Gauze Dressings

Dressing	Description	Purpose
Dry-to-dry	A layer of wide-mesh cotton gauze lies next to the wound surface. A second layer of dry absorbent cotton or Dacron is on top.	Protect the wound. If the wound is open or draining, necrotic debris and exudate are trapped in the interstices of the gauze layer and are removed when the dressing is removed.
Wet-to-dry	Next to the wound surface is a layer of wide-mesh cotton gauze saturated with saline or an antimicrobial solution. This layer is covered by a moist absorbent material that is moistened with the same solution.	Debride the wound. Necrotic debris is softened by the solution and then adheres to the mesh gauze as it dries. It is removed when the dressing is removed. Also, moisture helps dilute viscous exudate.
Wet-to-damp	A variation of the wet-to-dry dressing, this dressing is removed before it has completely dried	The wound is debrided when the gauze is removed.
Wet-to-wet	A layer of wide-mesh gauze saturated with saline lies next to the wound surface. Above is a second layer of absorbent material saturated with the same solution. The entire dressing is kept moist with a wetting agent.	The wound surface is continually bathed. Moisture dilutes viscous exudate.

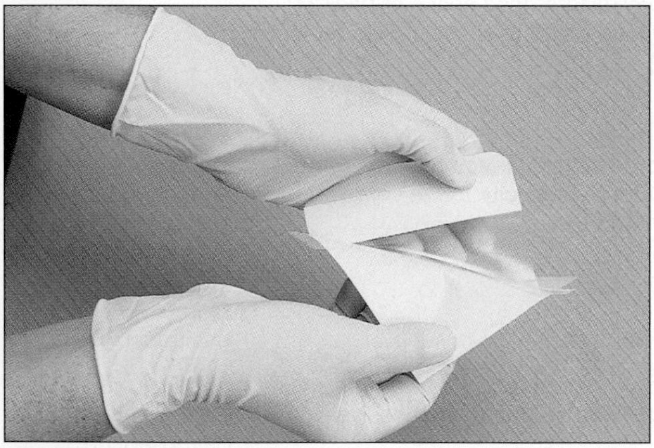

FIGURE 33.12 A transparent wound dressing

The following considerations are important when using transparent films:

- Transparent films are nonporous, self-adhesive dressings that are often left in place for up to 7 days.
- Because they are transparent, the wound can be assessed through them.
- Because they are semi-occlusive, the wound remains moist and retains the serous exudate, which promotes epithelial growth, supports autolytic debridement, and reduces the risk of infection. They should not be used if there is evidence of a yeast infection as this condition may be exacerbated.
- Because they are elastic, they can be placed over a joint without disrupting the client's mobility.
- They adhere only to the skin area around the wound and not to the wound itself because they keep the wound moist. The use of a liquid skin barrier on the periwound skin can increase adhesion and wear time.
- They allow the client to shower or bathe without removing the dressing.
- They can be removed without damaging wound tissues, although caution must be used if the client has fragile periwound skin.

Skill 33.2 describes how to apply a moist transparent wound barrier.

Hydrocolloid Dressings Hydrocolloid dressings (see Table 33.4) are frequently used in wounds with minimal drainage and those requiring debridement (see the Reflect on Primary Health Care box on page 956). The following considerations are important when using hydrocolloid dressings:

- Dressing sheets can be cut to fit difficult areas, but the dressing must always extend at least 2.5 cm to 5 cm beyond the wound margins to promote adherence and extend wear time. Taping the edges with a paper tape may improve wear time.
- Hydrocolloids do not need a cover dressing and are water resistant, so the client can shower or bathe.
- Hydrocolloid dressings can remain in place for 3 to 7 days, with the frequency of dressing changes dependent on the amount of drainage. The dressing should be changed before leakage occurs.

SKILL 33.2

APPLYING AND REMOVING A MOIST TRANSPARENT WOUND BARRIER DRESSING

PURPOSES

- To provide a moist wound environment and promote wound healing
- To protect the wound from trauma and infectious agents
- To facilitate assessment of wound healing

ASSESSMENT

Assess

- Appearance and size of the wound
- Amount and character of exudate
- Complaints of discomfort
- Signs of systemic infection (e.g., elevated body temperature, diaphoresis, malaise, leukocytosis)

Planning

- Before applying or changing a moist transparent wound barrier, determine agency protocol about solutions used to clean the wound and whether clean or sterile technique is to be used. Many agencies recommend clean rather than sterile technique for chronic wounds, such as a pressure ulcer.
- Obtain assistance as needed. If the size of the wound necessitates it, acquire the assistance of a co-worker to help apply the dressing.

Equipment

- Disposable gloves
- Hair scissors or clippers
- Alcohol or acetone
- Moisture-proof bag
- Sterile gloves (optional)
- Sterile gauze and the wound-cleaning agents specified by the physician or agency (e.g., sterile saline)
- Wound barrier dressing
- Scissors
- Paper tape

IMPLEMENTATION

Performance

1. Before performing the procedure, introduce yourself and verify the client's identity by using agency protocol. Explain to the client what you are going to do, why it is necessary, and how he or she can cooperate. Discuss how the results will be used in planning further care or treatments.
2. Perform hand hygiene and observe other appropriate infection prevention and control procedures.
3. Thoroughly clean the skin area around the wound. Put on disposable gloves.
   - Clean the skin around the wound well with normal saline or a nonirritating wound cleansing agent. Always rinse and dry the adjacent skin completely before applying a dressing.
   - Clip the hair about 5 cm around the wound area, if indicated.
   - If adherence of the dressing is a concern, clean the area adjacent to the wound with alcohol or acetone, and allow it to dry. **Rationale: Alcohol or acetone defats the skin. Defatted, clean, dry skin ensures better adhesion of the dressing.**
   - Remove gloves, and dispose of them in the moisture-proof bag.
4. Clean the wound, if indicated.
   - Put on clean disposable or sterile gloves in accordance with agency practice.
   - Clean the wound with the prescribed solution. Either (a) pour the sterile solution directly on the wound and collect drainage with an emesis basin, or (b) with forceps, use a moist sterile gauze to clean the wound.
   - Dry the surrounding skin with a dry gauze.
5. Assess the wound.
   - See "Assessment" earlier in the procedure.
6. Apply the wound barrier.
   - Some agencies require transparent dressings be dated to ensure timeliness of dressing changes. If this is required, write the date and time of application on the dressing with ballpoint pen.
   - Remove part of the paper backing on the dressing. If you have an assistant, remove all of the paper backing; the two of you should hold the coloured tabs attached to the dressing.
   - Apply the dressing at one edge of the wound site, allowing at least 2.5 cm coverage of the skin surrounding the wound.
   - Gently lay or press the barrier over the wound. Keep it free of wrinkles, but avoid stretching it too tightly. **Rationale: A stretched dressing restricts mobility.**
   - Cut off the coloured tabs after the wound is completely covered.
   - Remove and dispose of gloves appropriately.
7. Reinforce the dressing only if absolutely needed.
   - Apply paper or other porous tape to the edges of the dressing.
8. Assess the wound area at least daily.
   - Determine the extent of serous fluid accumulation under the dressing, wound healing, and the need to repair the dressing.
   - If excessive serum has accumulated, consider replacing the transparent wound barrier with a more absorbent type of dressing, such as hydrocolloid.
   - If the dressing is leaking, remove it and apply another dressing.
9. Document the procedure and all nursing assessments.
10. To remove the dressing, stretch the product to break the adhesive bond and prevent skin stripping.

(continued)

SKILL 33.2

APPLYING AND REMOVING A MOIST TRANSPARENT WOUND BARRIER DRESSING (*continued*)

EVALUATION

Perform follow-up based on findings in relation to the amount of granulation tissue or degree of healing; amount of serous fluid under dressing; and discomfort associated with wound care.

These dressings should not be used for wounds with copious drainage but are suitable for wounds with small amounts of drainage.

- Hydrocolloids have a characteristic odour that is often mistaken for a sign of wound infection. Clinical judgment must be used in assessing for the presence of an infection.
- Although hydrocolloids provide an effective bacterial barrier, they should *not* be used when infection is suspected. If signs and symptoms of a clinical infection occur (uncharacteristic odour, changes in colour of exudate, fever, or cellulitis), a bacterial culture should be taken and medical treatment initiated.
- Hydrocolloids decrease pain and, thus, reduce the need for analgesics.

REFLECT ON PRIMARY HEALTH CARE

Appropriate use of technology in wound care, particularly in the case of chronic wounds, has meant an increase in quality of life for many patients. For example, helping a home care client learn how to use hydrocolloid or hydrogel products can mean a reduction in dressing changes from two or three times a day to once every 1, 2, or even 7 days. This type of intervention also reduces the costs to the health-care system. Because the nurse is not spending as much time performing wound care, he or she can address other aspects of the client's health.

Skill 33.3 describes how to apply hydrocolloid dressings.

SKILL 33.3

APPLYING A HYDROCOLLOID DRESSING

PURPOSES

- To maintain a moist wound surface and promote healing
- To prevent the entrance of microorganisms into the wound
- To minimize wound discomfort
- To promote autolysis of necrotic material by white blood cells
- To decrease the frequency of dressing changes

ASSESSMENT

Assess

- Appearance and size of the wound
- Amount and character of exudate
- Complaints of discomfort
- Signs of systemic infection (e.g., elevated body temperature, diaphoresis, malaise, leukocytosis)

Planning

A hydrocolloid dressing should be changed whenever it becomes dislodged, leaks, or develops an odour. If the wound has substantial drainage or yellow slough, the dressing may need to be changed every 24 to 72 hours. When drainage subsides, the dressing can be left in place for 3 to 7 days. The procedure may be clean or sterile depending on agency policy.

Equipment

- Clean disposable gloves
- Moisture-proof bag
- Dressing set
- Sterile normal saline or other cleaning agent used by the agency
- Sterile gloves (optional)
- Hydrocolloid dressing at least 2.5 cm to 5 cm larger than wound on all four sides
- Paper tape

IMPLEMENTATION

Performance

1. Before performing the procedure, introduce yourself and verify the client's identity by using agency protocol. Explain to the client what you are going to do, why it is necessary, and how he or she can cooperate. Discuss how the results will be used in planning further care or treatments.

(continued)

SKILL 33.3

APPLYING A HYDROCOLLOID DRESSING *(continued)*

2. Perform hand hygiene and observe other appropriate infection prevention and control procedures.
3. Remove the old dressing.
   - Put on disposable gloves.
   - Pull the dressing off gradually in the direction of hair growth. **Rationale: This minimizes skin irritation.**
   - Dispose of the soiled dressing in the moisture-proof bag.
4. Clean the skin area around the wound.
   - Gently wash the skin surrounding the wound with a mild cleansing agent or with normal saline, and dry it thoroughly with gauze squares.
   - Leave the residue that is difficult to remove on the skin. It will wear off in time. **Rationale: Attempts to remove residue can irritate the surrounding skin.**
   - Remove gloves and dispose of them in the moisture-proof bag.
5. Clean the wound, if indicated.
   - Open the sterile dressing supplies.
   - Pour saline or other cleaning agent into the sterile container.
   - Put on disposable or sterile gloves in accordance with agency protocol.
   - With forceps, clean the wound with the prescribed solution.
6. Assess the wound.
   - Observe the appearance and the size of the wound and the amount and character of exudate.
   - Determine presence of pain.
7. Apply the dressing.
   - Follow the manufacturer's instructions.
   - Remove and dispose of the gloves.
   - Optional: Tape all four sides of the dressing as required or according to agency protocol. **Rationale: Taping prevents the dressing from adhering to bed linens and the edges from lifting.**
8. Assess and change the dressing, as indicated.
   - Inspect the dressing at least daily for leakage, dislodgement, odour, and wrinkling.
   - Change the dressing if any of these signs are present.
9. Document the technique and all nursing assessments.

EVALUATION

Perform follow-up based on findings in relation to the amount of granulation tissue or degree of healing; amount of serous fluid under dressing; and discomfort associated with wound care.

SECURING DRESSINGS The nurse tapes the dressing over the wound, ensuring that it covers the entire wound and does not become dislodged. The correct type of tape should be selected and, ideally, the ends of the tape should be folded over slightly in advance of securing to aid ease of removal. Elastic tape can provide pressure; hypoallergenic tape is used when a client is allergic to other tape. The nurse follows these steps:

1. Place the tape so that the dressing cannot be folded back to expose the wound. Place strips at the ends of the dressing, and space tapes evenly in the middle (Figure 33.13A).
2. Ensure that the tape is long and wide enough to adhere to several centimetres of skin on each side of the dressing, but not so long or wide that the tape loosens with activity (Figure 33.13B).
3. Place the tape in the opposite direction from the body action, for example, across a body joint or crease, not lengthwise (Figure 33.14).

Montgomery straps (*tie tapes*) are commonly used for wounds requiring frequent dressing changes (Figure 33.15). These straps prevent skin irritation and the discomfort caused by removing the adhesive each time the dressing is changed. Medical tapes can cause injuries if used incorrectly. Blisters will form when too much tension is applied while placing the tape, when edema has collected after the tape was placed, and when alcohol or benzoic-based prep solutions are used under the tape. Medical tape manufacturers issue safety guidelines for specific taper products. Before using medical tapes read the safety guidelines for indications of use and safe application and removal.

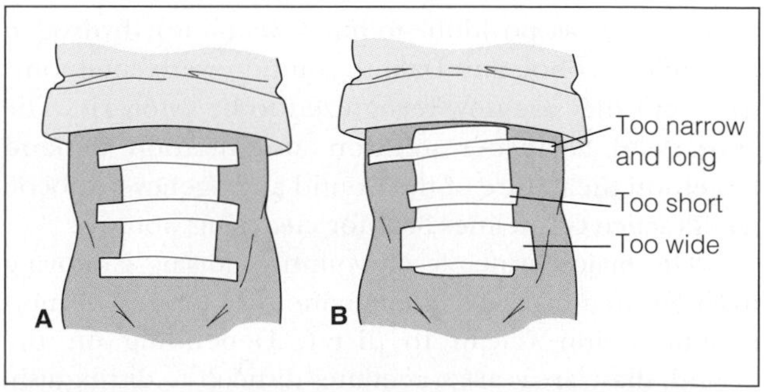

FIGURE 33.13 The strips of tape should be placed at the ends of the dressing and must be sufficiently long and wide to secure the dressing. The tape should adhere to intact skin.

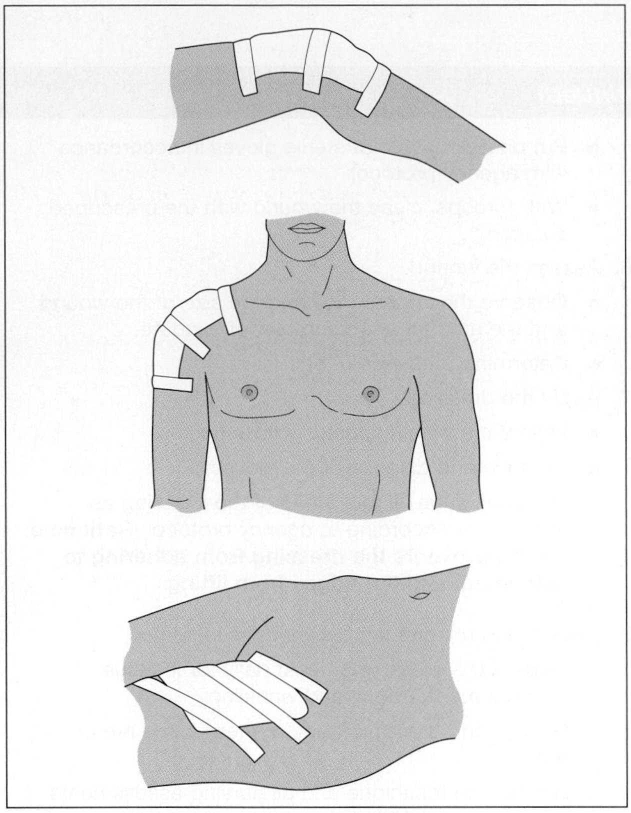

FIGURE 33.14 Dressings over moving parts must remain secure in spite of the movement. Place the tape over a joint at a right angle to the direction the joint moves.

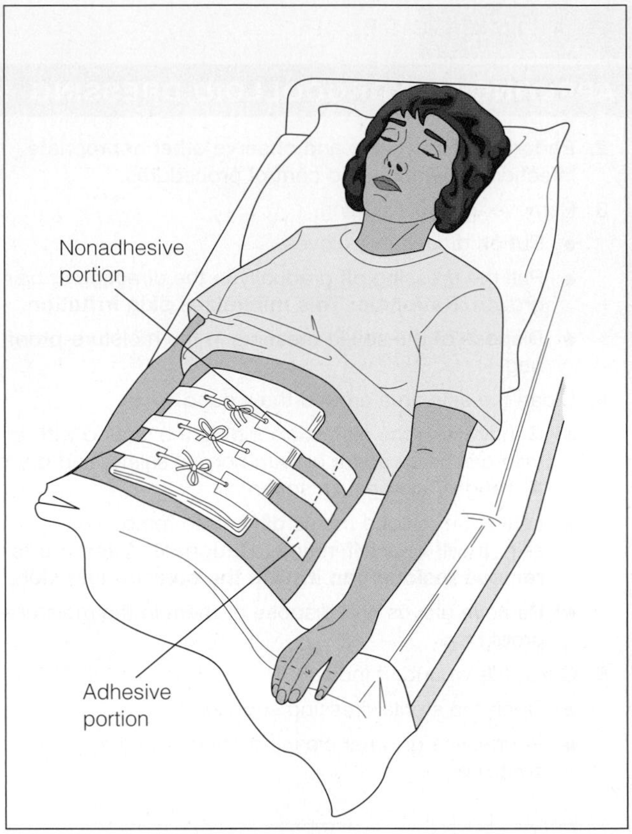

FIGURE 33.15 Montgomery straps, or tie tapes, are used to secure large dressings that require frequent changing.

Cleansing Wounds

Wound cleansing is a critical aspect of wound management and forms the basis for good healing. Wound cleansing is the process of using noncytotoxic fluids to reduce the bacterial burden and to remove devitalized tissue, metabolic wastes, and topical agents that can inhibit wound healing (Consortium for Spinal Cord Medicine, 2000). The goal of routine wound cleansing is to minimize chemical and mechanical trauma while providing a clean wound bed. In the past, antimicrobial agents, such as povidone-iodine (Betadine), hydrogen peroxide, alcohol, and Dakin's solution were commonly used, but they are now recognized to be cytotoxic. The choices of cleansing solution and method depend largely on the nature of the wound and agency protocol. See Practice Guidelines 33.2 for cleansing wounds.

The major principle of wound cleansing is moving from an area of least contamination to an area of most contamination (clean to dirty). Depending on the wound, these areas are sometimes difficult to distinguish.

Commonly used methods to clean a surgical wound and drain site are outlined in Chapter 35.

WOUND IRRIGATION AND PACKING Preparing the wound bed for healing is an essential component of any wound management strategy. The goal of preparation is to optimize the wound bed to ensure unimpeded tissue repair and regeneration (Sibbald, Mahoney, & the V.A.C. Therapy Canadian Consensus Group, 2003). The wound bed preparation paradigm advocated by the Canadian Association of Wound Care (2006) urges clinicians to first address patient-centred concerns and the etiology of the wound before tackling local wound healing strategies.

Irrigation (lavage) is the washing or flushing out of an area. It is a means of cleansing the wound. Sterile technique is required for wound irrigation because there is a break in the skin integrity.

The use of piston syringes instead of bulb syringes to irrigate a wound reduces the risk of aspirating drainage and provides safe, effective pressure. For deep wounds with small openings, a sterile straight catheter may also be necessary. Irrigation pressures should range from 4 psi to 15 psi (pounds per square inch). Below 4 psi, the irrigation may not be effective, and above 15 psi it may damage tissues. A 35 mL syringe with a 19-gauge needle or catheter or a 30 mL syringe with an 18-gauge needle or catheter provide approximately 8 psi (Bergstrom, Braden, Laguzza, & Holman, 1994). Some providers advocate the use of a commercial oral water jet for wound cleansing. This device can be effective if kept at the lowest setting that provides the desired pressure. Frequently used irrigation solutions are sterile normal saline, lactated Ringer's solution, and antibiotic solutions.

Skill 33.4 details the steps involved in irrigating a wound.

PRACTICE GUIDELINES 33.2

Cleansing Wounds

Guidelines	Rationales
Follow routine practices and additional precautions for personal protection, wear gloves, gown, goggles, and mask as indicated.	The patient and the health-care practitioner require protection from pathogens.
Use physiological solutions, such as isotonic saline or lactated Ringer's solution, to clean or irrigate wounds. Commercial wound cleansers often contain surfactants that help to remove debris and may be helpful in some circumstances. Do not use skin cleansers or antiseptic agents (e.g., povidone-iodine, iodophor, sodium hypochlorite [Dakin's] solution, hydrogen peroxide, acetic acid) to clean wounds (RNAO, 2007). When possible, warm the solution to body temperature just before use. Microwave heating is not recommended.	Warming the solution prevents lowering of the wound temperature, which slows the healing process. Microwave heating could cause the solution to become too hot.
Cleanse wounds at each dressing change. To reduce surface bacteria and tissue trauma, the wound should be gently irrigated with 100 mL of solution (RNAO, 2007).	Foreign bodies and devitalized tissue act as a focus for infection and can delay healing; too much pressure can lead to trauma.
Use sufficient irrigation pressure to enhance wound cleansing. Effective and safe ulcer irrigation pressure ranges from 4 psi to 15 psi (pounds per square inch). Pressures in this range can be generated by using either (1) a 35 mL syringe with a 19-gauge angiocath or (2) a single-use 100 mL squeeze bottle (RNAO, 2007).	Wound cleansing must not cause trauma to the wound bed.
If a wound is clean, has little exudate, and reveals healthy granulation tissue, avoid repeated cleaning.	Unnecessary cleaning can delay wound healing by traumatizing newly produced, delicate tissues, reducing the surface temperature of the wound, and removing exudate, which itself may have bactericidal properties.
Use gauze squares. Avoid using cotton balls and other products that shed fibres onto the wound surface.	The fibres become embedded in granulation tissue and can act as foci for infection. They may also stimulate foreign body reactions, prolonging the inflammatory phase of healing and delaying the healing process.
Avoid drying a wound after cleansing it. Dry the skin around the wound only.	Healing is improved when a wound is moist; healing is deterred in dry wounds.
Clean the wound in an outward direction.	Cleaning in this direction avoids transferring organisms from the surrounding skin into the wound.

Evidence-Informed Practice

How Are Skin Tears Best Prevented and Treated?

Skin tears that result from trauma to the skin can be extremely difficult to manage. Although they have traditionally been seen as less significant when compared with pressure ulcers or arterial and venous ulcers, skin tears can be equally difficult to manage and can lead to such complications as pain and wound infection. Leblanc, Christensen, Orsted, and Keast (2008) reviewed the current literature, including the Registered Nurses' Association of Ontario's and the National Guideline Clearinghouse's guidelines for preventing and treating skin tears.

Based on this review, the authors developed a set of best practice recommendations for the prevention and treatment of skin tears. Examples of recommendations include identifying risk factors (e.g., being older than 85 years, removing tape, seeing ecchymoses (bruising), and using corticosteroids for a long time); supporting the prevention of skin tears through skin hygiene and hydration, the use of appropriate clothing (e.g., long sleeves, long pants); and the removal of environmental risk factors (e.g., by padding sharp corners on furniture). The authors support the use of the Payne-Martin classification for skin tears, categories I through III, to develop treatment goals and interventions. Colour photos are used throughout the article to illustrate the skin tear categories. A quick reference guide and table summarizing skin tear care relative to the category of injury are provided.

NURSING IMPLICATIONS: Until a more formal evaluation of the literature can provide nurses with best practice guidelines in the prevention and treatment of skin tears, this article's recommendations are useful when nurses are working with clients at risk for skin tears. The quick reference guide and table outlining recommendations for dressing selection based on category of skin tear are the only ones of their kind in the literature.

Source: Based on "Best Practice Recommendations for the Prevention and Treatment of Skin Tears," by K. Leblanc, D. Christensen, H. Orsted, and D. H. Keast, 2008, *Wound Care Canada, 6*(1), pp. 14–30.

SKILL 33.4

IRRIGATING A WOUND

PURPOSES

- To clean the area
- To apply heat and hasten the healing process
- To apply an antimicrobial solution

ASSESSMENT

Assess

- The client's record to determine previous appearance and size of the wound
- The character of the exudate
- The presence of pain and the time of the last analgesia
- Clinical signs of systemic infection
- Allergies to the wound irrigation agent or tape

Planning

- Before irrigating a wound, determine (1) the type of irrigating solution to be used, (2) the frequency of irrigations, and (3) the temperature of the solution.
- If possible, schedule the irrigation at a time convenient for the client. Some irrigations require only a few minutes and others can take much longer.

Equipment

- Sterile dressing equipment and dressing materials
- Sterile irrigating syringes (e.g., a 30 mL to 60 mL syringe) with a #19 angiocath attached or a 100 mL squeezable bottle with irrigating tip
- Sterile graduated container for the irrigating solution
- Moisture-proof bag
- Irrigating solution, usually 100 mL to 150 mL of solution, warmed to body temperature, according to agency policy
- Goggles, gown, and mask
- Clean gloves
- Sterile gloves
- Moisture-proof sterile drape

Although a wound may already be contaminated, sterile equipment is usually used during irrigation to prevent the possibility of adding new nonresident microorganisms to the site. In settings outside of hospitals, some reusable supplies, such as irrigating syringes or basins, may be cleaned and used again for a specific wound.

IMPLEMENTATION

Performance

1. Before performing the procedure, introduce yourself and verify the client's identity by using agency protocol. Explain to the client what you are going to do, why it is necessary, and how he or she can cooperate. Discuss how the results will be used in planning further care or treatments.
2. Perform hand hygiene and observe other appropriate infection prevention and control procedures (e.g., goggles).
3. Provide for client privacy.
4. Prepare the client.
   - Assist the client to a position in which the irrigating solution will flow by gravity from the upper end of the wound to the lower end and then into the basin.
   - Place the waterproof drape over the client and the bed.
   - Put on clean gloves and remove and discard the old dressing.
   - If indicated, clean the wound from the centre of the wound outward, using circular strokes.
   - Use a separate swab for each stroke, and discard each swab after use. **Rationale: This prevents the introduction of microorganisms to other wound areas.**
   - Assess the wound and drainage.
   - Remove and discard gloves.
5. Prepare the equipment.
   - Open the sterile dressing set and supplies.
   - Pour the ordered solution into the solution container.
   - Position the basin below the wound to receive the irrigating fluid.
   - Put on sterile gloves
6. Irrigate the wound.
   - Instill a steady stream of irrigating solution into the wound. Make sure all areas of the wound are irrigated.
   - Use either a syringe with a catheter attached or with an irrigating tip to flush the wound (see ❶), or a 100 mL squeezable bottle with irrigating tip.

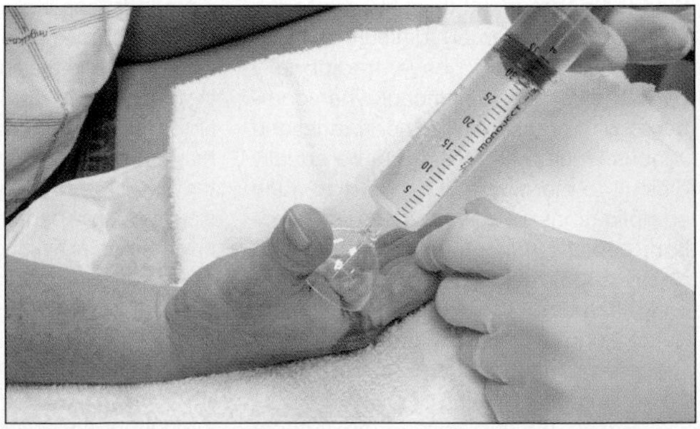

❶ Irrigating an open wound

(continued)

SKILL 33.4

IRRIGATING A WOUND (*continued*)

- If you are using a catheter to reach tracks or crevices, insert the catheter into the wound until resistance is met. Do not force the catheter. **Rationale: Forcing the catheter can cause tissue damage.**
- Continue irrigating until the solution becomes clear (no exudate is present).
- Dry the area around the wound. **Rationale: Moisture left on the skin promotes the growth of microorganisms and can cause skin irritation and breakdown.**

7. Assess and dress the wound.
   - Assess the appearance of the wound again, noting in particular the type and amount of exudate still present and the presence and extent of granulation tissue.
   - Using sterile technique, apply a dressing to the wound based on the amount of drainage expected (see Table 33.4).
8. Document the irrigation and the client's response in the client record by using forms or checklists supplemented by narrative notes when appropriate. Many agencies use a designated wound and skin documentation sheet (see Figure 33.6, p. 943).

EVALUATION

- Perform follow-up based on findings that deviate from expected or normal for the client. Relate findings to previous assessment data if available.
- Report significant deviations from normal to the appropriate health-care team members.

Lifespan Considerations

Pressure Ulcer and Wound Care

INFANTS

- The skin of infants is more fragile than that of older children and adults, and it is more susceptible to infection, shear, and burns.

CHILDREN

- *Staphylococcus* and fungus are two major infectious agents affecting the skin of children. Abrasions or small lacerations, commonly experienced by children, provide an entry in the skin for these organisms. Minor wounds should be cleansed with warm, soapy water, and covered with a sterile bandage. Children should be instructed not to touch the wound.
- With more serious skin lesions, remind the child not to touch the wound, drains, or dressing. Cover with an appropriate bandage that will remain intact during the child's usual activities. Cover a transparent dressing with opaque material if viewing the site is distressing to the child. Restrain only when all alternatives have been tried and when absolutely necessary.
- For younger children, demonstrate wound care on a doll. Reassure that the wound will not be permanent and that nothing will fall out of the body.

OLDER ADULTS

- Hold wrinkled skin taut during application of a transparent dressing. Obtain assistance if needed.
- Skin is more fragile and can easily tear with removal of tape (especially adhesive tape). Use paper tape and tape remover as indicated, keeping tape use to the minimum required. Use extreme caution during tape removal.
- Older adults who are in long-term-care facilities often have immobility, malnutrition, and incontinence, all of which increase the risk for development of skin breakdown.
- Skin breakdown can occur as quickly as within 2 hours, and so assessments should be done with each repositioning of the client.
- A thorough assessment of a client's heels should be done every shift. The skin can break down quickly from friction of movement in bed.

Home Care Considerations

Wound Care

- Perform appropriate client teaching for promoting wound healing and maintenance of healthy skin.
- Instruct family about hygiene and asepsis; hand hygiene before and after dressing changes; and the use of a clean area for storage of dressing supplies.
- Instruct the client and family on where to obtain needed supplies. Be sensitive to the cost of dressings (e.g., transparent barriers are costly) and suggest less expensive alternatives if necessary. Be

(*continued*)

Home Care Considerations (*continued*)

creative in the use of household items for padding pressure areas.

- Instruct the client and family in proper disposal of contaminated dressings. All contaminated items should be double bagged in moisture-proof bags.
- Verify how the client can bathe with the wound (i.e., does the wound need to be covered with a waterproof barrier or should it be cleansed in the shower?).
- Potable tap water can be used to cleanse wounds instead of normal saline (Fernandez & Griffiths, 2008).

Gauze packing by using the wet-to-damp technique has been used to pack wounds that require debridement. In this technique, moist 10 cm × 10 cm non-cotton-filled gauzes are packed in the wound to absorb exudate but they are not allowed to dry before removal. However, newer advanced dressing materials have significant advantages over the use of gauze. Box 33.7 summarizes issues related to using damp gauze versus advanced dressings.

Adjunctive Therapies

Many of the techniques described here for dressing and cleansing wounds can be combined, depending on the specific type of wound. In addition, a number of adjunctive therapies can be used to facilitate wound healing. Electrical stimulation, therapeutic ultrasound, ultraviolet light, pulsed electromagnetic fields, and surgery may be helpful for some clients.

Vacuum-assisted closure (VAC) is a commonly used adjunctive therapy that employs negative pressure (vacuum) to remove fluid from difficult-to-heal wounds (Sibbald et al., 2003). The fluid passes through a sealed dressing and tubing connected to a collection container (see Figure 33.16). To implement VAC therapy, it is important for the wound to have been thoroughly debrided, to be free of active untreated infection (e.g., cellulitis), and to not involve fistulae to internal organs or cavities. VAC dressings are changed three times per week or when the seal has broken. VAC removes exudate to help optimize fluid balance. VAC is not usually initiated until the more conventional treatments, such as dressings, have proven ineffective because of the significant financial costs and the mobility limitations imposed on the client by the VAC equipment. Contraindications to the use of VAC include intracutaneous fistulae, necrotic tissue, untreated ostemyelitis, and malignancy (Sibbald et al., 2003).

Supporting and Immobilizing Wounds

Bandages and binders serve various purposes:

- Supporting a wound (e.g., a fractured bone)
- Immobilizing a wound (e.g., a strained shoulder)
- Applying pressure (e.g., elastic bandages on the lower extremities to improve venous blood flow)

BOX 33.7 ISSUES RELATED TO THE USE OF DAMP GAUZE VERSUS ADVANCED DRESSINGS

The nurse should be aware of the following issues in choosing a wound dressing:

- To keep the gauze damp, change or remoisten with saline frequently. *If the gauze is allowed to dry out, removal results in pain and disruption of wound healing through drying of the surface and tissue adherence to the gauze.*
- A wound requires moisture and warmth for optimal healing. Evaporation of the saline causes wound cooling, vasoconstriction, and dehydration.
- Moistened gauze cannot prevent introduction of bacteria into the wound.
- Gauze is easy to use and can be manipulated to fit almost any wound.
- The diversity of advanced dressings may be confusing for clients and health-care providers.
- Although gauze is much less expensive than advanced dressings (e.g., polymers, alginates, collagens), the cost per week can be higher because of the number of dressing changes required. Including the price of the dressing, gloves, saline, and tape, the materials cost for a gauze dressing change twice per day versus an advanced dressing three times per week is very similar. However, when taking into account the cost per nurse home visit, the gauze dressing is almost five times as expensive.
- Wounds have been shown to heal twice as quickly with advanced dressings compared with gauze.

Practitioners should become familiar with the range and uses of advanced dressing materials. The selection of dressing materials must consider time, material cost, client comfort, and speed of wound healing.

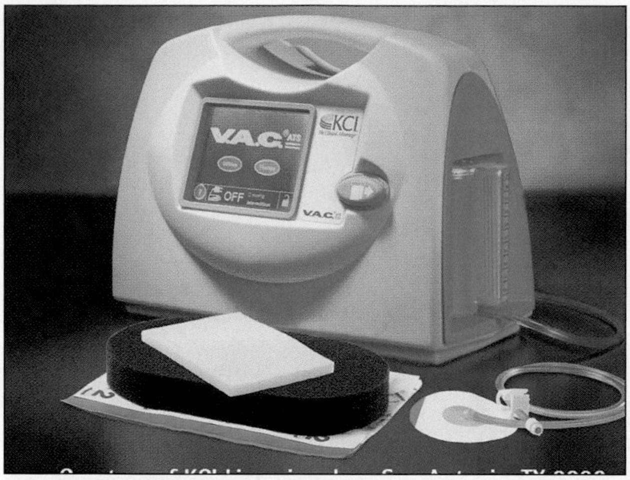

FIGURE 33.16 Vacuum-assisted closure (VAC) system for wounds

- Securing a dressing (e.g., for an extensive abdominal surgical wound)
- Retaining warmth (e.g., a flannel bandage on a rheumatoid joint)

Bandages and binders come in several different types and have several ways in which they are applied. When correctly applied, they promote healing, provide comfort, and can prevent injury. Practice Guidelines 33.3 focuses on bandaging.

BANDAGES A **bandage** is a strip of cloth used to wrap some part of the body. Bandages are available in various widths, most commonly 1.5 cm to 7.5 cm, and are usually supplied in rolls for easy application to a body part.

Many types of materials are used for bandages. Gauze is one of the most commonly used; it is light and porous and readily moulds to the body. It is also relatively inexpensive, so it is generally discarded when soiled. Gauze is frequently used to retain dressings on wounds and to bandage the fingers, hands, toes, and feet. It supports dressings and, at the same time, permits air to circulate; it can also be impregnated with gels or other medications for application to wounds.

Many kinds of elasticized bandages are applied to provide pressure to an area. They are commonly used as tensor bandages or as partial stockings to provide support and improve the venous circulation in the legs.

The width of the bandage used depends on the size of the body part to be bandaged. For example, a 2.5 cm bandage is used for a finger, a 5 cm bandage for an arm, and a 7.5 cm or 10 cm bandage for a leg. The larger the circumference of a part, the wider the bandage. Padding (e.g., abdominal pads and gauze squares) is frequently used to cover bony prominences (e.g., the elbow) or to separate skin surfaces (e.g., the fingers).

Before applying a bandage, the nurse needs to know its purpose and assess the area requiring support (see Box 33.8). When bandages are used to secure dressings, the nurse wears gloves to prevent contact with body fluids.

Basic Turns for Roller Bandages Applying bandages to various parts of the body involves one or more of five basic bandaging turns: circular, spiral, spiral reverse, recurrent, and figure eight. *Circular* turns are used to anchor bandages and to terminate them. Circular turns usually are not applied directly over a wound because of the discomfort the bandage would cause.

PRACTICE GUIDELINES 33.3

Bandaging

Guidelines	Rationales
Whenever possible, bandage the part in its normal position, with the joint slightly flexed.	The use of this position avoids putting strain on the ligaments and the muscles of the joint.
Pad between skin surfaces and over bony prominences.	Pads prevent friction from the bandage and consequent abrasion of the skin.
Always bandage body parts by working from the distal to the proximal end.	This method aids the return flow of venous blood.
Bandage with even pressure.	Even pressure prevents interference with blood circulation.
Whenever possible, leave the end of the body part (e.g., the toes) exposed.	This exposure allows for the adequacy of the blood circulation to the extremity to be determined.
Cover dressings with bandages at least 5 cm beyond the edges of the dressing.	This covering prevents the dressing and wound from becoming contaminated.
Face the client when applying a bandage.	This position maintains uniform tension and the appropriate direction of the bandage.

BOX 33.8 ASSESSING BEFORE APPLYING BANDAGES OR BINDERS

The nurse must assess a wound or an injury before applying bandages or binders:

- Inspect and palpate the area for swelling.
- Inspect for the presence of and status of wounds (open wounds will require a dressing before a bandage or binder is applied).
- Note the presence of drainage (amount, colour, odour, viscosity).
- Inspect and palpate for adequacy of circulation: skin temperature, blanching (capillary refill), peripheral pulses, colour, and sensation. Pale or cyanotic skin, cool temperature, tingling, and numbness can indicate impaired circulation.
- Ask the client about any pain experienced (location, intensity, onset, quality).
- Assess the ability of the client to reapply the bandage or binder, when needed (home care).
- Assess the capabilities of the client regarding activities of daily living (e.g., to eat, dress, comb hair, bathe), and assess the assistance required during the convalescence period.

Spiral turns are used to bandage parts of the body that are fairly uniform in circumference, for example, the upper arm or upper leg. *Spiral reverse* turns are used to bandage cylindrical parts of the body that are not uniform in circumference, for example, the lower leg or forearm. *Recurrent* turns are used to cover distal parts of the body, for example, the end of a finger, the skull, or the stump of an amputation. *Figure-eight* turns are used to bandage an elbow, knee, or ankle, because they permit some movement after application.

Circular Turns

- Hold the bandage in your dominant hand, keeping the roll uppermost, and unroll the bandage about 8 cm. This length of unrolled bandage allows good control for placement and tension.
- Apply the end of the bandage to the part of the body to be bandaged. Hold the end down with the thumb of the other hand (Figure 33.17).
- Encircle the body part a few times or as often as needed, making sure that each layer overlaps one-half to two-thirds of the previous layer. This provides even support to the area.
- The bandage should be firm, but not too tight. Ask the client if the bandage feels comfortable. A tight bandage can interfere with blood circulation, whereas a loose bandage does not provide adequate protection.
- Secure the end of the bandage with tape or a safety pin over an uninjured area. Pins can cause discomfort when situated over an injured area.

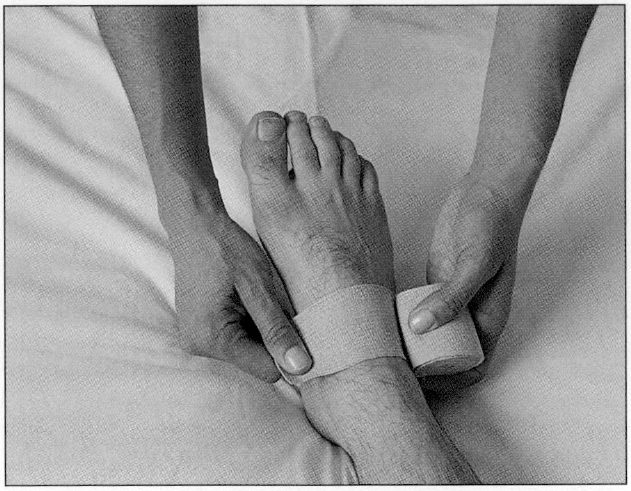

FIGURE 33.17 Starting a bandage with two circular turns

Spiral Turns

- Make two circular turns. Two circular turns anchor the bandage.
- Continue spiral turns at about a 30-degree angle, each turn overlapping the preceding one by two-thirds the width of the bandage (Figure 33.18).
- Terminate the bandage with two circular turns, and secure the end of the bandage with tape or a safety pin over an uninjured area.

Spiral Reverse Turns

- Anchor the bandage with two circular turns, and bring the bandage upward at about a 30-degree angle.
- Place the thumb of your free hand on the upper edge of the bandage (Figure 33.19A). The thumb will hold the bandage while it is folded on itself.

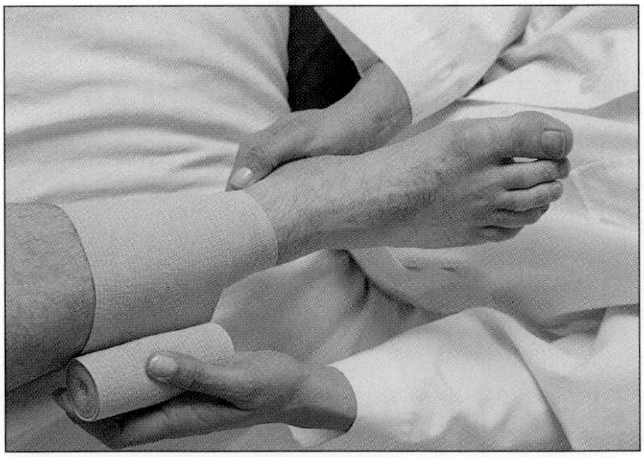

FIGURE 33.18 Applying spiral turns

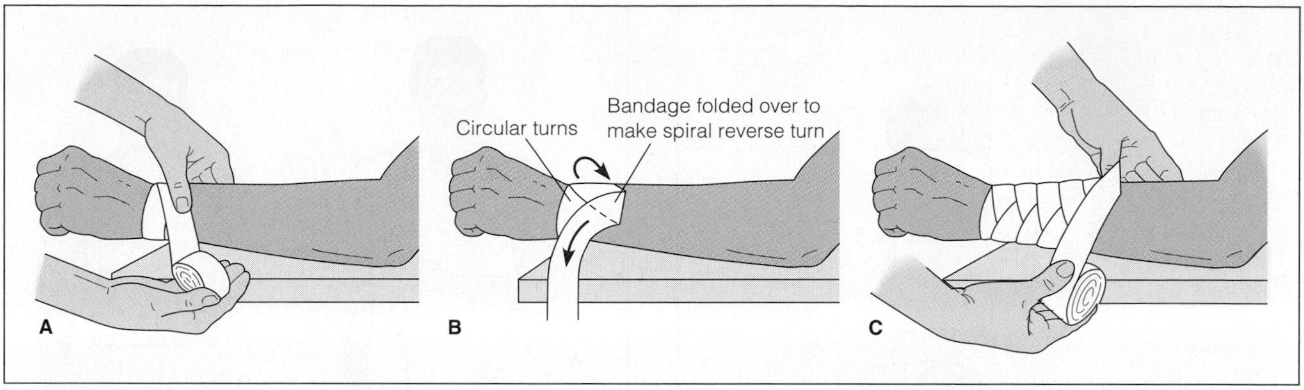

FIGURE 33.19 Applying spiral reverse turns

- Unroll the bandage about 15 cm, and then turn your hand so that the bandage falls over itself (Figure 33.19B).
- Continue the bandage around the limb, overlapping each previous turn by two-thirds the width of the bandage. Make each bandage turn at the same position on the limb so that the turns of the bandage will be aligned (Figure 33.19C).
- Terminate the bandage with two circular turns, and secure the end of the bandage with tape or a safety pin over an uninjured area.

Recurrent Turns

- Anchor the bandage with two circular turns.
- Fold the bandage back on itself, and bring it centrally over the distal end to be bandaged (Figure 33.20).
- Holding it with the other hand, bring the bandage back over the end to the right of the centre bandage but overlapping it by two-thirds the width of the bandage.
- Bring the bandage back on the left side, also overlapping the first turn by two-thirds the width of the bandage.
- Continue this pattern of alternating right and left until the area is covered. Overlap the preceding turn by two-thirds the bandage width each time.
- Terminate the bandage with two circular turns (Figure 33.21). Secure the end with tape or a safety pin over an uninjured area.

Figure-Eight Turns

- Anchor the bandage with two circular turns.
- Carry the bandage above the joint, around it, and then below it, making a figure eight (Figure 33.22).
- Continue above and below the joint, overlapping the previous turn by two-thirds the width of the bandage.
- Terminate the bandage above the joint with two circular turns, and then secure the end with tape or a safety pin over an uninjured area.

BINDERS A binder is a type of bandage designed for a specific body part, for example, the triangular binder (sling) fits the arm. Binders are used to support large areas of the body, such as the abdomen, arm, or chest. Binders can be simple, inexpensive, and customizable by using plain material, such as the triangular sling described below. Or they can be of commercial design, which are often more expensive and slightly less

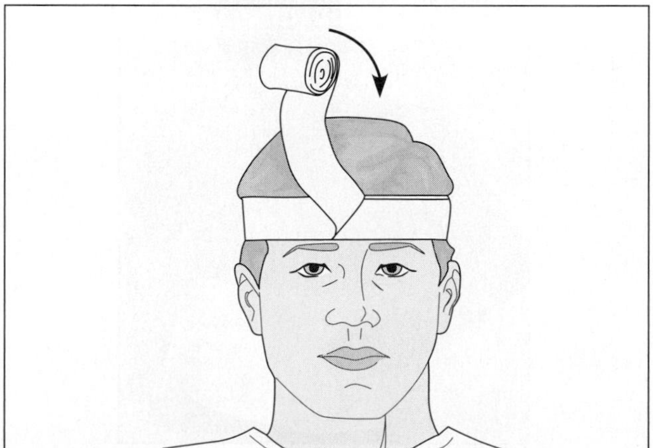

FIGURE 33.20 Starting a recurrent bandage

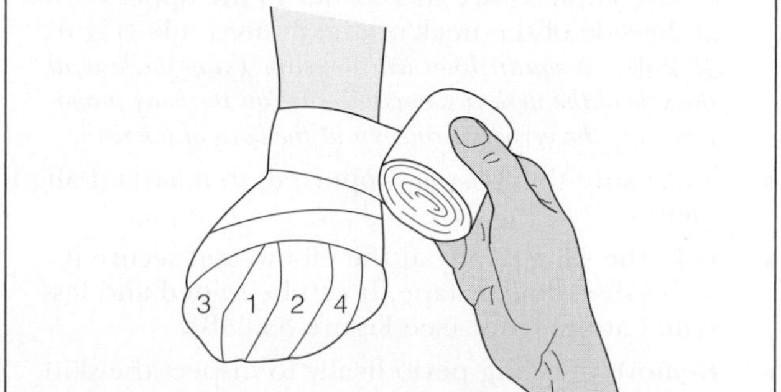

FIGURE 33.21 Completing a recurrent bandage

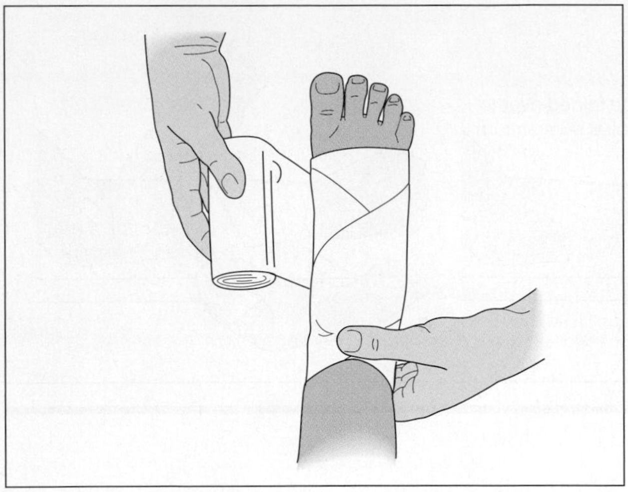

FIGURE 33.22 Applying a figure-eight bandage

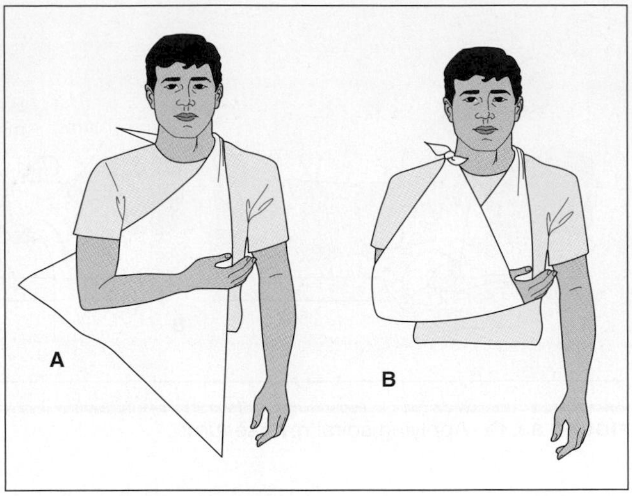

FIGURE 33.23 Large arm sling

modifiable, such as the hook-and-loop (Velcro) binder described below.

Triangular Arm Sling

- Ask the client to flex the elbow to an 80-degree angle or less, depending on the purpose. The thumb should be facing upward or inward toward the body. *An 80-degree angle is sufficient to support the forearm, to prevent swelling of the hand, and to relieve pressure on the shoulder joint (e.g., to support the paralyzed arm of a stroke client whose shoulder might otherwise become dislocated).* A more acute angle is preferred if there is swelling of the hand (see how to apply a sling for maximum hand elevation, below).
- Place one end of the unfolded triangular binder over the shoulder of the uninjured side so that the binder falls down the front of the chest of the client with the point of the triangle (apex) under the elbow of the injured side (see Figure 33.23A).
- Take the upper corner, and carry it around the neck until it hangs over the shoulder on the injured side.
- Bring the lower corner of the binder up over the arm to the shoulder of the injured side. By using a square knot, secure this corner to the upper corner at the side of the neck on the injured side (Figure 33.23B). *A square knot will not slip. Tying the knot at the side of the neck prevents pressure on the bony prominences of the vertebral column at the back of the neck.*
- Make sure the wrist is supported, to maintain alignment.
- Fold the sling neatly at the elbow, and secure it with safety pins or tape. It can be folded and fastened at the front (see Figure 33.23B).
- Remove the sling periodically to inspect the skin for indications of irritation, especially around the site of the knot.

Straight Abdominal Binder

- With the client in a supine position, place the binder smoothly under the body, with the upper border of the binder at the waist and the lower border at the level of the gluteal fold. *A binder placed over the waist interferes with respiration; one placed too low interferes with elimination and walking.*
- Apply padding over the iliac crests if the client is thin.
- Bring the ends around the client, overlap them, and secure them with pins or Velcro (Figure 33.24). Place the top pin horizontally at the waist to allow for comfort when moving.

Securing Peritoneal Dressings Previously, T-binders were used to secure dressings to the peritoneal area. T-binders have been replaced with sanitary disposable garments that fit like underwear. Placing an appropriately

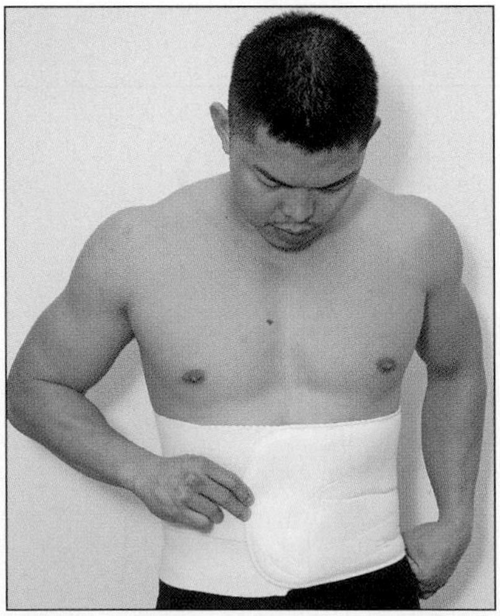

FIGURE 33.24 A straight abdominal binder

Lifespan Considerations

Applying Bandages and Binders

Children and older adults need special considerations when the nurse is applying a bandage or binder:

CHILDREN

- Allow the child to help with the procedure by holding supplies, opening boxes, counting turns, and so on.
- If a young client is apprehensive, demonstrate the procedure on a doll or stuffed animal.
- Encourage the child to decorate the bandage.
- Teach the caregivers to apply bandages and binders safely.

OLDER ADULTS

- Older clients may need extra support during the procedure, especially if arthritis, contractures, or tremors are present.
- Avoid constricting the client's circulation with a tight bandage or binder. Observe skin and bony prominences frequently for signs of impaired circulation. The risk for skin breakdown increases with age.

Home Care Considerations

Applying Bandages and Binders

Before a client is discharged, he or she will need to understand the bandage or binder:

- Assess the client's or caregiver's knowledge level of the reason for bandages or binders, and ability and willingness to perform the bandaging procedure.
- Ensure that the client has the proper supplies; assess for adequate and safe storage of supplies in the home, and ensure the client knows how to obtain replacement supplies.
- The client should have two binders so that he or she has one to wear while the other is being washed. Bandages and binders should be washed inside a mesh laundry bag to keep them from becoming twisted and to prevent Velcro or hooks from catching on other laundry.
- Instruct the client's caregiver on the importance of and how to do the following:

  a. Perform hand hygiene thoroughly before handling dressing supplies and applying the bandage.
  b. Report skin breakdown and redness, pain, or pallor of the affected area.
  c. Check for adequate peripheral circulation after applying the bandage.

sized abdominal pad or sanitary napkin in the garment allows the wound to be protected and drainage to be collected for either males or females.

See the Lifespan Considerations box for guidelines on applying bandages and binders to children and older adults, and the Home Care Considerations box for information that clients will need when discharged with a bandage or binder.

Evaluating

The goals established during the planning phase are evaluated according to specific desired health outcomes also established in that phase. Examples of these are shown in Table 33.6.

To judge whether client outcomes have been achieved, the nurse uses data collected during care, such as skin status over bony prominences and perineal area, nutritional and fluid intake, mental status, signs of healing if an ulcer is present, and so on. If outcomes are *not* achieved, the nurse should explore the reasons why:

- Has the client's physical condition changed?
- Were risk factors correctly identified?
- Were appropriate lifting devices and techniques used?
- Did the client fail to comply with instructions about moving and turning? Why?
- Were appropriate pressure-relieving devices used, and were they applied correctly?
- Was the repositioning schedule adhered to?
- Are the client's nutritional and fluid intake adequate?
- Were appropriate measures used to control incontinence and protect the client's skin?
- Was the wound supported and immobilized effectively?
- Were stringent infection prevention and control practices implemented when cleaning and changing dressings to prevent infection?

TABLE 33.6 Evaluation Goals and Outcomes: Skin Integrity and Wound Healing

Goal	Examples of Desired Outcomes
Maintain skin integrity	Skin intact over bony prominences Skin is supple without signs of edema or dehydration Skin colour in expected range (e.g., no redness, or redness that blanches and returns to normal within a few minutes) Skin temperature within normal range
Promote primary intention wound healing	Wound edges are approximated Decrease (or absence) of serosanguineous drainage Decrease in surrounding skin inflammation Absence of purulent drainage Absence of wound odour
Promote secondary intention wound healing	Decrease in length, width, and depth of wound Presence of and increase in granulation tissue Intact skin surrounding wound Decrease (or absence) of drainage
Support the nonhealing wound (palliation)	Pain control Infection control Odour control Absence of further breakdown

- Was the client receiving anti-inflammatory medications that interfere with healing?
- Was the appropriate dressing applied to keep the wound moist or absorb exudate, or both, as needed?

Heat and Cold Applications

Heat and cold are applied to the body for local and systemic effects. Table 33.7 lists the physiological effects of heat and cold.

Physiological Responses

LOCAL EFFECTS OF HEAT Heat is an old remedy for aches and pains, and people often equate heat with comfort and relief. Heat causes vasodilation and increases blood flow to the affected area, bringing oxygen, nutrients, antibodies, and leukocytes.

TABLE 33.7 Physiological Effects of Heat and Cold

Heat	Cold
Vasodilation	Vasoconstriction
Increases capillary permeability	Decreases capillary permeability
Increases cellular metabolism	Decreases cellular metabolism
Increases inflammation	Slows bacterial growth, decreases inflammation
Sedative effect	Local anaesthetic effect

Application of heat promotes soft tissue healing and increases suppuration. A possible disadvantage of heat is that it increases capillary permeability, which allows extracellular fluid and substances, such as plasma proteins, to pass through the capillary walls and can result in edema or an increase in preexisting edema. Heat is often used for clients with musculoskeletal problems, such as low back pain, contractures, and joint stiffness from arthritis.

LOCAL EFFECTS OF COLD Generally, the physiologic effects of cold are opposite to the effects of heat. Cold lowers the temperature of the skin and underlying tissues and causes vasoconstriction. Vasoconstriction reduces blood flow to the affected area and thus reduces the supply of oxygen and metabolites, decreases the removal of wastes, and produces skin pallor and coolness. Prolonged exposure to cold results in impaired circulation, cell deprivation, and subsequent damage to the tissues from lack of oxygen and nourishment. The signs of tissue damage caused by cold are a bluish-purple mottled appearance of the skin, numbness, and sometimes blisters and pain. Cold is most often used for sports injuries (e.g., sprains, strains, fractures) to limit post-injury swelling and bleeding.

SYSTEMIC EFFECTS OF HEAT AND COLD Heat applied to a localized body area, particularly a large body area, can cause excessive peripheral vasodilation, which produces a drop in blood pressure. A significant drop in blood pressure can cause fainting. Clients who have heart or pulmonary disease and who have circulatory disturbances, such as arteriosclerosis, are more prone to this effect than healthy people are. With extensive cold applications and vasoconstriction, a client's blood pressure can increase because blood is shunted from the cutaneous circulation to the internal blood vessels. Shivering, a generalized effect of prolonged cold, is a normal response as the body attempts to warm itself.

THERMAL TOLERANCE Various parts of the body differ in tolerance to heat and cold. The physiological tolerance of individuals also varies (see Box 33.9).

Specific conditions necessitate precautions in the use of hot or cold applications:

BOX 33.9 VARIABLES AFFECTING PHYSIOLOGICAL TOLERANCE TO HEAT AND COLD

Different parts of the body react in different ways to heat and cold:

- *Body part.* The back of the hand and foot are not very temperature sensitive. In contrast, the inner aspect of the wrist and forearm, the neck, and the perineal area are temperature sensitive.
- *Size of the exposed body part.* The larger the area exposed to heat and cold, the lower the tolerance.
- *Individual tolerance.* The very young and the very old generally have the lowest tolerance. Persons who have neurosensory impairments may have a high tolerance, but the risk of injury is greater.
- *Length of exposure.* People feel hot and cold applications most while the temperature is changing. After a period of time, tolerance increases.
- *Intactness of skin.* Injured skin areas are more sensitive to temperature variations.

- *Neurosensory impairment.* People with sensory impairments are unable to perceive that heat is damaging the tissues and are at risk for burns or are unable to perceive discomfort from cold and prevent tissue injury.
- *Impaired mental status.* People who are confused or have an altered level of consciousness need monitoring during applications to ensure safe therapy.
- *Impaired circulation.* People with peripheral vascular disease, diabetes, or congestive heart failure lack the normal ability to dissipate heat via the blood circulation, which puts them at risk for tissue damage with heat and cold applications.
- *Immediately after injury or surgery.* Heat increases bleeding and swelling.
- *Open wounds.* Cold can decrease blood flow to the wound, thereby inhibiting healing.

ADAPTATION OF THERMAL RECEPTORS Heat and cold receptors adapt to temperature changes. When they are subjected to an abrupt change in temperature, the receptors are strongly stimulated initially. This strong stimulation declines rapidly during the first few seconds and then more slowly during the next half hour or more as the receptors adapt to the new temperature.

Nurses and clients need to understand this adaptive response when applying heat and cold. Clients may be tempted to change the temperature of a thermal application because of the change in thermal sensation following adaptation. Increasing the temperature of a hot application after adaptation can result in serious burns. Decreasing the temperature of a cold application can result in pain and serious impairment of circulation to the body part. Table 33.8 lists temperatures of hot and cold applications.

REBOUND PHENOMENON The rebound phenomenon occurs at the time the maximum therapeutic effect of the hot or cold application is achieved and the opposite effect begins. For example, heat produces maximum vasodilation in 20 to 30 minutes; continuation of the application beyond 30 to 45 minutes brings tissue congestion, and the blood vessels then constrict for reasons unknown. If the heat application is continued, the client is at risk for burns because the constricted blood vessels are unable to dissipate the heat adequately via the blood circulation.

With cold applications, maximum vasoconstriction occurs when the involved skin reaches a temperature of 15°C. Below 15°C, vasodilation begins. This mechanism is protective: It helps to prevent freezing of body tissues normally exposed to cold, such as the nose and ears. It also explains the ruddiness of the skin of a person who has been walking in cold weather.

An understanding of the rebound phenomenon is essential for the nurse and client. *Thermal applications must be halted before the rebound phenomenon begins.*

TABLE 33.8 Temperatures for Hot and Cold Applications

Description	Temperature	Application
Very Cold	Less than 15°C	Ice bags
Cold	15°C–18°C	Cold pack
Cool	18°C–27°C	Cool compresses
Tepid	27°C–37°C	Sponge bath
Warm	37°C–40°C	Warm bath, aquathermia pads
Hot	40°C–46°C	Hot soak, irrigations, hot compresses
Very hot	More than 46°C	Hot water bag for adults

Applying Heat and Cold

Heat can be applied to the body in both dry and moist forms. Dry heat is applied locally by means of a hot water bottle, aquathermia pad, disposable heat pack, or electric pad. Moist heat can be provided by compress, hot pack, soak, or sitz bath. Selected indications for the use of heat and cold are found in Table 33.9.

TABLE 33.9 Selected Indications of Heat and Cold

Indication	Effect of Heat	Effect of Cold
Muscle spasm	Relaxes muscles and increases their contractility	Relaxes muscles and decreases muscle contractility
Inflammation	Increases blood flow, softens exudates	Vasoconstriction decreases capillary permeability, decreases blood flow, slows cellular metabolism
Pain	Relieves pain, possibly by promoting muscle relaxation, increasing circulation, and promoting psychological relaxation and a feeling of comfort; acts as a counter-irritant	Decreases pain by slowing nerve conduction rate and blocking nerve impulses; produces numbness, acts as a counter-irritant, increases pain threshold
Contracture	Reduces contracture and increases joint range of motion by allowing greater distension of muscles and connective tissue	
Joint stiffness	Reduces joint stiffness by decreasing viscosity of synovial fluid and increasing tissue distensibility	
Traumatic injury		Decreases bleeding by constricting blood vessels; decreases edema by reducing capillary permeability

Dry cold is generally applied locally by means of a cold pack, ice bag, ice glove, or ice collar. Moist cold can be provided by compress or a cooling sponge bath.

For all local applications of heat or cold, the nurse needs to follow these guidelines:

- Determine the client's ability to tolerate the therapy.
- Identify conditions that might contraindicate treatment (e.g., bleeding, circulatory impairment).
- Explain the application to the client.
- Assess the skin area to which the heat or cold will be applied.
- Ask the client to report any discomfort.
- Return to the client 15 minutes after starting the heat or cold, and observe the local skin area for any untoward signs (e.g., redness). Stop the application if any problems occur.
- Remove the equipment at the designated time, and dispose of it appropriately.
- Examine the area to which the heat or cold was applied, and record the client's response.

For contraindications to the use of heat or cold, see Box 33.10.

BOX 33.10 CONTRAINDICATIONS TO THE USE OF HEAT AND COLD

Determine the presence of any conditions contraindicating the use of heat:

- *The first 24 hours after traumatic injury.* Heat increases bleeding and swelling.
- *Active hemorrhage.* Heat causes vasodilation and increases bleeding.
- *Noninflammatory edema.* Heat increases capillary permeability and edema.
- *Localized malignant tumour.* Because heat accelerates cell metabolism and cell growth and increases circulation, it may accelerate metastases (secondary tumours).
- *Skin disorder that causes redness or blisters.* Heat can burn or cause further damage to the skin.

Determine the presence of any conditions contraindicating the use of cold:

- *Open wounds.* Cold can increase tissue damage by decreasing blood flow to an open wound.
- *Impaired circulation.* Cold can further impair nourishment of the tissues and cause tissue damage. In clients with Raynaud's disease, cold increases arterial spasm.
- *Allergy or hypersensitivity to cold.* Some clients have an allergy to cold that may be manifested by an inflammatory response, for example, erythema, hives, swelling, joint pain, and occasional muscle spasm. Some react with a sudden increase in blood pressure, which can be hazardous if the person is hypertensive.

Determine the presence of any conditions indicating the need for special precautions during heat and cold therapy:

- *Neurosensory impairment.* Persons with sensory impairments are unable to perceive that heat is damaging the tissues and are at risk for burns, or they are unable to perceive discomfort from cold and are unable to prevent tissue injury.
- *Impaired mental status.* Persons who are confused or have an altered level of consciousness need monitoring and supervision during applications to ensure safe therapy.
- *Impaired circulation.* Persons with peripheral vascular disease, diabetes, or congestive heart failure lack the normal ability to dissipate heat via the blood circulation, which puts them at risk for tissue damage with heat applications. Cold applications are contraindicated for these people.
- *Open wounds.* Tissues around an open wound are more sensitive to heat and cold.

HOT WATER BAG A hot water bag or bottle is a common source of dry heat used in the home. It is convenient and relatively inexpensive. However, because of the danger of burning from improper use, many agencies use other means.

The following temperatures of the water in the bag are considered safe in most situations and provide the desired effect: normal adult and child over 2 years, 46°C to 52°C, debilitated or unconscious adult, or child under 2 years, 40.5°C to 46°C.

To apply a hot water bag, the nurse should do the following:

- Measure the temperature of the water by using a bath thermometer.
- Fill the bag about two-thirds full.
- Expel the remaining air and secure the top. With the air removed, the bag can be moulded to the body part.
- Dry the bag and hold it upside down to test for leakage.
- Wrap the bag in a towel or cover and place it on the body site.
- Remove after 30 minutes or in accordance with agency protocol.

AQUATHERMIA PAD The aquathermia or aquamatic pad (also referred to as a K-pad) is a pad constructed with tubes containing water. The pad is attached by tubing to an electrically powered control unit that has an opening for water and a temperature gauge (Figure 33.25). Some aquathermia pads have an absorbent surface through which moist heat can be applied. The other surface of the pad is waterproof. These pads are disposable.

To apply an aquathermia pad, the nurse carries out the following steps:

- Fill the reservoir of the unit two-thirds full of distilled water.
- Set the desired temperature. Check the manufacturer's instructions. Most units are set at 40.5°C for adults.
- Cover the pad and plug in the unit. Some manufacturers suggest warming the pad before applying it.
- Apply the pad to the body part. The treatment is usually continued for 30 minutes. Check orders and agency protocol.

HOT AND COLD PACKS Commercially prepared hot and cold packs (Figure 33.26) provide heat or cold for a designated time. Directions on the package tell how to initiate the heating or cooling process, for example, by striking, squeezing, or kneading the pack.

ELECTRIC PADS Electric pads provide a constant, even heat, are lightweight, and can be moulded to a body part. Electric pads, however, can burn if the setting is too high. Some models have waterproof covers for use when the pad is placed over a moist dressing.

In applying electric pads, the nurse follows these guidelines:

- Do not insert sharp objects (e.g., pins) into the pad. The pin could damage a wire and cause an electric shock.
- Ensure that the body area is dry unless the pad has a waterproof cover on the pad. Electricity in the presence of water can cause a shock.
- Use pads with a preset heating switch so a client cannot increase the heat.
- Do not place the pad under the client. Heat will not dissipate, and the client may be burned.

ICE BAGS, ICE GLOVES, AND ICE COLLARS Ice bags, ice gloves, and ice collars are filled either with ice chips or with an alcohol-based solution. They are applied to the body to provide cold to a localized area (e.g., a collar is often applied to the throat following a tonsillectomy). Always wrap the container in a towel or cover.

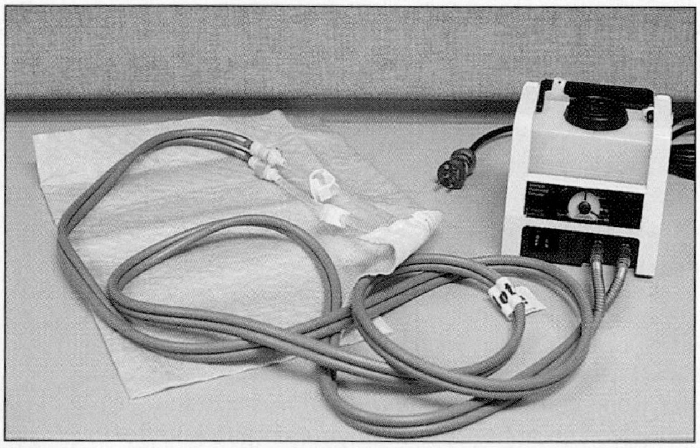

FIGURE 33.25 An aquathermia unit

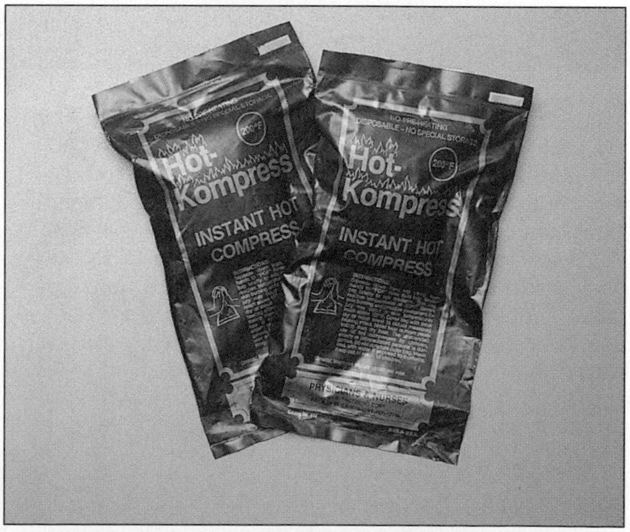

FIGURE 33.26 Commercially prepared disposable hot packs

COMPRESSES Compresses can be either warm or cold. A **compress** is a moist gauze dressing applied to a wound. When hot compresses are ordered, the solution is heated to the temperature indicated by the order or according to agency protocol, for example, 40.5°C. When there is a break in the skin or when the body part (e.g., an eye) is vulnerable to microbial invasion, sterile technique is necessary; therefore, sterile gloves are needed to apply the compress and all materials must be sterile.

SOAK A soak refers to immersing a body part (e.g., an arm) in a solution or to wrapping a part in gauze dressings and then saturating the dressing with a solution. Sterile technique is generally indicated for open wounds, such as a burn or an unhealed surgical incision. Determine agency protocol regarding the temperature of the solution. Hot soaks are frequently done to soften and remove encrusted secretions and dead tissue.

SITZ BATH A **sitz bath**, or hip bath, is used to soak a client's pelvic area. The client sits in a special tub or chair and is usually immersed from the mid-thighs to the iliac crests or umbilicus. Special tubs or chairs are preferred because when the legs are also immersed, as in a regular bathtub, blood circulation to the perineum or pelvic area is decreased. Disposable sitz baths are also available.

The temperature of the water should be from 40°C to 43°C, unless the client is unable to tolerate the heat. Determine agency protocol. Some sitz tubs have temperature indicators attached to the water taps. The duration of the bath is generally 15 to 20 minutes, depending on the client's health. Follow these steps to provide a sitz bath:

- Assist the client into the tub. Provide support for the client's feet; a footstool can prevent pressure on the backs of the thighs.
- Provide a bath blanket for the client's shoulders and eliminate drafts to prevent chilling.
- Observe the client closely during the bath for signs of faintness, dizziness, weakness, accelerated pulse rate, and pallor.
- Maintain the water temperature.
- Following the sitz bath, assist the client out of the tub. Help the client to dry.

COOLING SPONGE BATH The purpose of a cooling sponge bath is to reduce a client's fever by promoting heat loss through conduction and vaporization. Cool sponge baths are used with extreme caution and only for clients with very high temperatures, such as over 40°C, because rapid skin temperature drop can cause chills that actually increase heat production. The bath is accompanied by antipyretic medication that acts to reset the hypothalamus set point. The temperatures for cooling sponge baths range from 18°C to 32°C.

To provide a cooling sponge bath, the nurse should do the following:

- Sponge the face, arms, legs, back, and buttocks. The chest and abdomen are not usually sponged. Each area is sponged slowly and gently. Rubbing may increase heat production.
- Leave each area wet and cover with a damp towel.
- Place ice bags and cold packs, if used, or a cool cloth on the forehead for comfort and in each axilla and at the groin. These areas contain large superficial blood vessels that help the transfer of heat.
- Sponge one body part and then another. The sponge bath should take about 30 minutes. A bath given more quickly tends to increase the body's heat production by causing shivering.
- Discontinue the bath if the client becomes pale or cyanotic or shivers, or if the pulse becomes rapid or irregular.
- Reassess the vital signs at 15 minutes and after completing the sponge bath.

Case Study 33

You have been assigned to care for Mr. Johns, a 74-year-old client being treated for a urinary tract disorder. Mr. Johns suffered a cerebrovascular accident (stroke) 6 months ago and has had difficulty ambulating and attending to his own needs because of right-sided weakness. While assessing Mr. Johns, you note that he is thin for his height, is incontinent of foul-smelling urine, and has deeply reddened areas on his right hip, coccyx, and entire peritoneal area. Mr. Johns is alert and oriented to person, place, and time, but he has decreased sensation on his entire right side. He spends most of his time in bed or sitting at his bedside in a chair because of his difficulty with ambulation.

Critical Thinking Questions

1. What data suggest that Mr. Johns is particularly vulnerable to pressure ulcer development?
2. What additional information do you need in order to use the Braden scale to determine Mr. Johns's potential for pressure ulcer development?
3. What independent measures can you take to protect Mr. Johns's skin from further breakdown?
4. Considering that Mr. Johns does have impaired skin integrity, why is it important to institute treatment for pressure ulcers at this time?

After working through these questions, go to the MyNursingLab at **http://www.mynursinglab.com** to check your answers.

KEY TERMS

clean wound
clean-contaminated wound
contaminated wound
dirty (infected) wound
partial-thickness wound
full-thickness wound
acute wound
chronic wound
pressure ulcers
ischemia
reactive hyperemia
mechanical load
friction
shear
maceration
eschar
gaiter area
ankle flare
lipodermatosclerosis
atrophie blanche
regeneration
primary intention healing
secondary intention healing
tertiary intention healing
delayed primary intention healing
hemostasis
fibrin
collagen
granulation tissue
keloid
exudate
serous exudate
purulent exudate
suppuration
pyogenic bacteria
sanguineous (hemorrhagic) exudate
serosanguineous exudate
hemorrhage
hematoma
infection
dehiscence
evisceration
contamination
colonization
undermining
debridement
vacuum-assisted closure
bandage
compress
sitz bath

CHAPTER HIGHLIGHTS

- Maintaining skin integrity is an important independent function of nursing.
- Wounds are described as acute or chronic; closed or open; and clean, clean-contaminated, contaminated, or dirty (infected). Wounds are also classified by depth as partial thickness or full thickness. In addition, wounds are classified according to how they are acquired, as incisions, contusions, abrasions, punctures, lacerations, and penetrating wounds.
- Pressure ulcers are areas of localized damage to the skin and underlying tissue and are usually the result of external forces, such as pressure, friction, and shear.
- Mechanical loads are extrinsic forces, such as pressure, friction, and shear, that cause soft tissue damage and potentially lead to blood flow impedance, tissue necrosis, and pressure ulcer development.
- Factors increasing the risk for the development of pressure ulcers include immobility and inactivity, inadequate nutrition, fecal and urinary incontinence, decreased mental status, diminished sensation, excessive body heat, advanced age, and certain chronic medical conditions.
- Pressure ulcers have six recognized stages, which reflect the degree of tissue damage, suspected deep tissue injury, and unstageable wounds.
- Two types of wound healing are distinguished by the amount of tissue loss: primary intention healing and secondary intention healing. Tertiary intention healing is delayed primary intention healing.
- The wound-healing process has three phases: inflammatory, proliferative, and maturation.
- Major types of wound exudate are serous, purulent, and sanguineous (hemorrhagic). Exudate can be a combination of two or three (e.g., serosanguineous). The process of pus formation is referred to as suppuration.
- The main complications of wound healing are hemorrhage, infection, dehiscence, and evisceration, each of which is identifiable by specific clinical signs and symptoms.
- Although all chronic wounds are presumed to be bacterially contaminated (a state in which bacteria are not attached or replicating), colonization refers to the state in which bacteria are attached to the wound surface and replicating. When bacteria become invasive and cause an inflammatory response, the wound may proceed to shows signs of local infection, which can itself progress to systemic infection.
- Factors affecting wound healing include developmental stage, nutritional status, lifestyle, medications, the presence of infection, and the presence of chronic medical conditions.
- Risk-assessment tools are available to identify clients at risk for pressure ulcer development. These should be used on a regular basis.
- Meticulous skin examination of common pressure points by the nurse is an important ongoing assessment activity for clients at risk.
- When a pressure ulcer is present, the nurse describes the ulcer in terms of location, size, depth, stage, colour, status of wound margins and

surrounding skin, and specific signs of infection, if present.

- Wound assessment is an ongoing process to evaluate healing; the nurse assesses wounds by visual inspection, palpation, and the sense of smell. Essential data for wounds include wound appearance, size, drainage, swelling, pain, and the presence of tubes and drains.
- Laboratory data that can be used to assess the progress of wound healing include leukocyte count, blood coagulation studies, serum protein analysis, and wound cultures. Nurses are usually responsible for obtaining specimens of wound drainage for culture.
- The NANDA International (2007) nursing diagnoses *Risk for Impaired Skin Integrity, Impaired Skin Integrity,* and *Impaired Tissue Integrity* apply to clients who have skin wounds or who are at risk for skin breakdown.
- Nursing diagnoses related to clients with existing impaired skin or tissue integrity may include *Risk for Infection, Pain, Anxiety,* and *Body Image, Disturbed.*
- Major goals for clients at risk for skin impairments are to maintain skin integrity and avoid potential associated risks.
- Nursing interventions aimed at preventing skin disruptions include conducting ongoing assessment of risk factors and skin status; providing skin care to maintain skin integrity; ensuring adequate nutrition; implementing measures to avoid skin trauma; providing supportive devices; and teaching the client.
- Treatment for pressure ulcers varies according to the stage of the ulcer and agency protocol.
- Major nursing responsibilities related to wound care include preventing infection, preventing further tissue damage, preventing hemorrhage, promoting healing, and preventing skin excoriation around draining wounds.
- Wound care may involve cleaning wounds, changing dressings, maintaining drains, irrigating, inserting packing, and applying bandages and binders.
- The RYB colour code of wounds can assist nurses to provide appropriate nursing interventions for wounds that heal by secondary intention. In this scheme, the nurse protects *red,* cleanses *yellow,* and debrides *black* according to agency policy and physician's orders.
- Various dressing materials are available to protect wounds and to keep the wound bed moist, thus facilitating healing.
- Dressings have been developed for use with specific types of wounds. These include transparent adhesive films, impregnated nonadherent dressings, hydrocolloids, hydrogels, polyurethane foams, and exudate absorbers. The nurse must be aware of the specific indications and contraindications for use.
- The type of dressing used depends on (1) location, size, and type of the wound; (2) amount of exudate; (3) whether or not the wound requires debridement, is infected, or has sinus tracts; and (4) such considerations as frequency of dressing change, ease or difficulty of dressing applications, and cost.
- Heat and cold produce specific local physiological and systemic responses that account for their therapeutic effects.
- Various parts of the body differ in tolerance to heat and cold. The physiological tolerance of individuals also varies. Specific conditions, such as neurosensory and circulatory impairments, necessitate precautions when applying heat or cold.
- When applying heat and cold, clients and nurses need to be aware of the effects of thermal receptor adaptation and the rebound phenomenon.

ASSESS YOUR LEARNING

1. Your client has a Braden scale score of 17. What is the appropriate nursing action?
   - **a.** Assess the client again in 24 hours; the score is within normal limits.
   - **b.** Implement a turning schedule; the client is at an increased risk of skin breakdown.
   - **c.** Apply a transparent wound barrier to major pressure sites; the client is at a moderate risk of skin breakdown.
   - **d.** Request a prescription for a special low-air-loss bed; the client is at a very high risk of skin breakdown.
2. Proper technique for performing a wound culture includes which of the following?
   - **a.** Cleansing the wound before obtaining the specimen
   - **b.** Swabbing for the specimen in the area with the largest collection of drainage
   - **c.** Removing crusts or scabs with sterile forceps and then culturing the site beneath
   - **d.** Waiting 8 hours following a dose of antibiotic to obtain the specimen
3. A client has a pressure ulcer with a shallow partial-skin-thickness eroded area but no necrotic areas. The nurse would treat the area with which of the following dressings?
   - **a.** Alginate
   - **b.** Dry gauze
   - **c.** Hydrocolloid
   - **d.** No dressing is indicated.

4. Thirty minutes after the application of a heating pad is initiated, the client requests that the nurse leave it in place. What should the nurse explain to the client?

a. Heat application for longer than 30 minutes can actually cause the opposite effect (constriction) of the one desired (dilation).

b. It will be acceptable to leave the pad in place if the temperature is reduced.

c. It will be acceptable to leave the pad in place for another 30 minutes if the site appears satisfactory when assessed.

d. It will be acceptable to leave the pad in place as long as it is moist heat.

5. Which statement, if made by the client or family member, would indicate the need for further teaching?

a. "If a skin area gets red but then the red goes away after turning, I should report it to the nurse."

b. "Putting foam pads under the heels or other bony areas can help decrease pressure."

c. "If a person cannot turn himself or herself in bed, someone should help the person change position every 4 hours."

d. "The skin should be washed with only warm water (not hot) and lotion put on while the skin is still a little wet."

6. Your client has a pressure ulcer on his heel. It is 3 cm deep and 2 cm wide, and is covered with black eschar. According to the NPUAP (2007) updated staging system, how would this wound be classified?

a. Stage III

b. Stage IV

c. Suspected deep tissue injury

d. Unstageable

7. Which of the following is an appropriate nursing diagnosis for a client with large areas of skin excoriation resulting from scratching an allergic rash?

a. Risk for Impaired Skin Integrity

b. Impaired Skin Integrity

c. Impaired Tissue Integrity

d. Risk for Infection

8. Mr. Boyle, 55 years old, smoked a pack of cigarettes each day. Two weeks ago, he experienced a stroke. Mr. Boyle has left hemiplegia and will be transferred to a rehabilitation hospital within the week. How would the nurse best prevent the development of a pressure ulcer for Mr. Boyle?

a. Encourage Mr. Boyle to re-position himself as necessary.

b. Turn Mr. Boyle q. 1–2h or as necessary, depending on his needs.

c. Massage bony prominences with moisturizing cream.

d. Place Mr. Boyle in a semi-Fowler's position.

9. Which of the following items are used to perform wound irrigation? Select all that apply.

a. Clean gloves

b. Sterile gloves

c. Refrigerated irrigating solution

d. 60 mL syringe

10. Which of the following indicates proper use of a triangle arm sling?

a. The elbow is kept flexed at 90 degrees or more.

b. The knot is placed on either side of the vertebrae of the neck.

c. The sling extends to just proximal of the hand.

d. The sling is removed every 2 hours to check for circulation and skin integrity.

After working through these questions, go to the MyNursingLab at ***http://www.mynursinglab.com*** *to check your answers and see explanations.*

SUGGESTED READINGS

O'Meara, S., Al-Kurdi, D., & Ovington, L. G. (2008). Antibiotics and antiseptics for venous leg ulcers. *Cochrane Database of Systematic Reviews, 1,* Art. No.: CD003557.

This systematic review provides a relevant and comprehensive summary of 22 studies on the use of antibiotics and antiseptics in the treatment of venous leg ulcers. The authors indicate a lack of quality research in this area on which to develop practice guidelines.

Rose, P., Cohen, R., & Amsel, R. (2006). Development of a scale to measure the risk of skin breakdown in critically ill patients. *American Journal of Critical Care, 15*(3), 337.

This Canadian study investigated how the unique aspects of the critically ill patient influence the frequency and nature of screening for risk of skin breakdown. This article is of special interest to nurses working in critical care settings.

Van Rijswijk, L. (2004). Bridging the gap between research and practice: Moist dressings are better than dry ones. *American Journal of Nursing, 104*(2), 28–30.

This article describes several practices still common in nursing that are contrary to the research on effective wound care strategies. The author cites the abundance of different products available for wound care as one obstacle to evidence-based practice. The author also suggests the use of a multidisciplinary wound care protocol review committee as a strategy for overcoming the obstacle.

Woo, K. Y., & Sibbald, R. G. (2008). Chronic wound pain: A conceptual model. *Advances in Skin and Wound Care, 21*(4), 175–188.

These Canadian authors discuss the complexities of chronic wound pain, including the fact that unrelenting pain from a nonhealing wound contributes to further delays in the wound-healing processes. They provide an excellent overview of the etiology, the epidemiology, patient concerns, and treatment approaches related to chronic wound pain.

WEBLINKS

Canadian Association of Enterostomal Therapists

http://www.caet.ca

The Canadian Association of Enterostomal Therapists (CAET) is a professional nursing organization that focuses on the nursing specialty of enterostomal therapy, which explores ostomy, wound, and continence issues. The CAET believes that all persons with the following conditions are entitled to the comprehensive services of an enterostomal therapy nurse: abdominal stomata, fistulae, draining wounds, and selected disorders of the integumentary, gastrointestinal, and genitourinary systems. The CAET promotes education, research, and standards for enterostomal therapy nursing practice.

Canadian Association of Wound Care

http://www.cawc.net

The Canadian Association of Wound Care (CAWC) is Canada's only interdisciplinary organization dedicated to the advancement of wound care practice. The CAWC facilitates best practice through excellence in education, clinical practice, public policy, research, and international partnerships.

National Pressure Ulcer Advisory Panel

http://www.npuap.org

This U.S. organization provides multidisciplinary leadership for improved patient outcomes in pressure ulcer prevention and management through education, public policy, and research.

European Pressure Ulcer Advisory Panel

http://www.epuap.com

The mission of this European organization is to provide relief to persons suffering from or at risk of pressure ulcers, in particular through research and the education of the public.

Wound Healing Society

http://www.woundheal.org

The Wound Healing Society is a nonprofit, international organization that provides a forum for discussions among scientists, physicians, licensed practitioners, industrial representatives, and others with interest in the field of wound healing.

Wound, Ostomy and Continence Nurses Society

http://www.wocn.org

Based in the United States, this international society brings together nurses who are experts in the care of patients with wound, ostomy, and continence problems.

REFERENCES

Allard, J. P., Aghdassi E., McArthur, M., McGeer, A., Simor, A., Abdolell, M., et al. (2004). Nutrition risk factors for survival in the elderly living in Canadian long-term care facilities. *Journal of the American Geriatrics Society, 52,* 59–65.

Berlowitz, D. R., Ratliff, C., Cuddigan, J., Rodeheaver, G. T., & National Pressure Ulcer Advisory Panel. (2005). The PUSH tool: A survey to determine its perceived usefulness. *Advances in Skin & Wound Care, 18*(9), 480–483.

Bergstrom, N., Braden, B. J., Laguzza, A., & Holman, V. (1994). The Braden scale for predicting pressure sore risk. *Nursing Research, 36,* 205–210.

Braden, B. J. (2001). Risk assessment in pressure ulcer prevention. In D. Krasner, G. Rodeheaver, & R. G. Sibbald (Eds.), *Chronic wound care: A clinical source book for health care professionals* (3rd ed.) (pp. 641–651). Wayne, PA: HMP Communications.

Brown, G. (2006). Wound documentation: Managing risk. *Advances in Skin and Wound Care, 19,* 155–165.

Canadian Association of Wound Care. (2004). *Prevalence of chronic wounds in Canada.* Retrieved June 2, 2008, from http://www.cawc.net/open/library/research/pandi

Canadian Association of Wound Care. (2006). *Quick reference guide: Recommendations for practice.* Toronto: Author. Retrieved July 5, 2008, from http://www.cawc.net/open/library/clinical/QRG2006E.pdf

Consortium for Spinal Cord Medicine. (2000). *Pressure ulcer prevention and treatment following spinal cord injury: A clinical practice guideline for health-care professionals.* Washington, DC: Paralyzed Veterans of America.

Coulthard, P., Worthington, H., Esposito, M., van der Elst, M., & van Waes, O. J. F. (2005). Tissue adhesives for closure of surgical incisions. *The Cochrane Library* (ID #CD004287).

Cuzzell, J. (1988). Wound care forum: The new RYB color code. *American Journal of Nursing, 88* (10), 1342–1346.

Dolynchuk K., Keast, D., Campbell, K., Houghton, P., Orsted, H., Sibbald, G., et al. (2000). Best practices for the prevention and treatment of pressure ulcers. *Ostomy Wound Management, 46*(11), 38–52.

Fernandez, R., & Griffiths, R. (2008). Water for wound cleansing. *Cochrane Database of Systematic Reviews* 2008, Issue 1. Art. No.: CD003861. DOI: 10.1002/14651858.CD003861.pub2

Fowler, E., Krasner, D., & Sibbald, G. (2002). Healing environments for chronic wound care: Optimizing local wound management as a component of holistic interdisciplinary patient care. *Curative Health Services,* pp. 5–6.

Fowler, E., Vesely, N., Johnson, V., Harwood, J., Tran, J., & Amberry, T. (2003). Wound care for persons with diabetes. *Home Healthcare Nurse, 21*(8), 531–540.

Health Quality Council. (2006). *Saskatchewan Skin and Wound Care Guidelines.* Saskatoon, SK: Health Quality Council.

Krasner, D. (1995). Wound care: How to use the red-yellow-black system. *American Journal of Nursing, 95*(5), 44–47.

Langemo, D., Anderson, J., Hanson, D., Hunter, S., Thompson, P., & Posthauer, M. E. (2006). Nutritional considerations in wound care. *Advances in Skin and Wound Care, 19*(6), 197–303.

Moffat C. J., Franks P. J., & Hollinworth, H. (2002). Understanding wound pain and trauma: An international perspective. *European Wound Management Association Position Document, 2,* 2–7.

NANDA International. (2007). *Nursing diagnoses: Definitions and classification, 2007–2008.* Philadelphia, PA: Author.

National Pressure Ulcer Advisory Panel. (2007). *Updated staging system.* Retrieved June 1, 2008, from http://www.npuap.org/pr2.htm

Odom-Forren, J. (2006). Preventing surgical site infections. *Nursing 2006, 36*(6), 59–63.

Pellard, S. (2006). Body image and acute burn injuries: A literature review. *Journal of Wound Care, 15*(3), 129–132.

Registered Nurses' Association of Ontario. (2004). *Nursing best practice guideline: Assessment and management of venous leg ulcers.* Toronto: Author.

Registered Nurses' Association of Ontario. (2005). *Nursing best practice guideline: Risk assessment and prevention of pressure ulcers* (Rev. ed.). Toronto: Author.

Registered Nurses' Association of Ontario. (2007). *Assessment and management of stage I to IV pressure ulcers* (Revised). Toronto: Author.

Shukla, D., Tripathi, A. K., Agrawal, S., Ansari, M. A., Rastogi, A., & Shukla, V. K. (2005). Pain in acute and chronic wounds: A descriptive study. *Ostomy/Wound Management, 51*(11), 47–51.

Sibbald R. G., Mahoney, J., & the V.A.C. Therapy Canadian Consensus Group. (2003). A consensus report on the use of vacuum-assisted closure in chronic, difficult to heal wounds. *Ostomy/Wound Management, 49*(11), 52–66.

Sosin, J. (2005). Ancient remedy heals today's wounds. *Nursing Spectrum, 14*(6), 32–33.

Vazquez, J. A., & Keast, D. H. (2006). Contemporary issue in wound infection: Managing the risks, treating the problem. Supplement to the November 2006 issue of *Wounds,* 1–17.

Wound, Ostomy and Continence Nurses Society. (2007). *New position statement on pressure ulcer staging.* Retrieved December 20, 2007, from http://www.wocn.org/pdfs/WOCN_Library/Position_Statements/PressureUlcerStaging.pdf

Woodbury, M. G., & Houghton, P. E. (2004). Prevalence of pressure ulcers in Canadian health care settings. *Ostomy/Wound Management, 50*(1), 22–38.

Chapter 34

Pain Management

Canada has a rich history in the interprofessional study and treatment of pain. Seminal work by Melzack and Wall (1965), in addition to their strong humanitarian commitment to caring for clients suffering from pain, paved the way for other exceptional Canadian researchers to understand pain mechanisms and their implications for effective pain management. Pain is an unpleasant, multidimensional, and subjective experience; only the person experiencing the pain can describe it (if he or she is verbal). No two people experience pain the same way; the experience of pain and its related responses are unique to each client and are influenced by the person's context and past pain experiences. Therefore, effective pain management requires skillful communication and assessment on the part of the nurse.

Despite great advancements in pain research over the past five decades, unrelieved acute pain remains a ubiquitous problem with numerous physiological, psychological, and economic consequences (Dahl et al., 2003; McGillion, Watt-Watson, LeFort, & Stevens, 2007; O'Gara, 1988; Watt-Watson, Chung, Chan, & McGillion, 2004; Watt-Watson & Graydon, 1995; Watt-Watson & Stevens, 1998). Significant numbers of hospitalized clients unnecessarily experience moderate to severe pain after surgery or interventional procedures, which can delay recovery and discharge from hospital (Morrison et al., 2003). Major contributors to unrelieved pain are knowledge gaps and pain-related misbeliefs among health professional groups, clients, and families.

OBJECTIVES

After studying this chapter, you should be able to

1. Identify types and categories of pain according to duration, origin, location, etiology, and intensity
2. Differentiate pain threshold from pain tolerance
3. Describe pain transduction, transmission, modulation, and perception
4. Discuss pain theory, nervous system plasticity, and their application to nursing care
5. Outline subjective and objective data to collect and analyze when assessing pain
6. List examples of nursing diagnoses for clients with pain
7. State outcome criteria by which to evaluate a client's response to interventions for pain
8. Identify barriers to effective pain management
9. Discuss pharmacological and nonpharmacological interventions for pain
10. Define tolerance, physical dependence, and addiction
11. Identify rationales for using various analgesic delivery routes

Despite advancements in the understanding of pain and its consequences among scientists, health professional groups, and client advocacy organizations in Canada, pain management practices generally need improvement. Until recently, poor pain relief has been tolerated as the norm and unrelieved pain has not been a priority. Historically, many health professionals have not asked clients about their pain and major discrepancies have been noted between patients' pain experiences and priorities, and health professionals' pain assessments (McGillion, Watt-Watson, Kim, & Graham, 2004). The problem has been compounded by the fact that many clients expect to have pain while in hospital, do not admit to having pain, and are reluctant to ask for help.

A major priority for nurses is the development of in-depth knowledge about pain mechanisms, assessment, and pharmacological and nonpharmacological management strategies. The Canadian Pain Society (CPS) emphasizes that clients have a right to the best pain relief possible (Watt-Watson, Clark, Finley, & Watson, 1999) and that nurses should be familiar with the following principles:

1. Unrelieved acute pain complicates recovery.
2. Routine assessment is essential for effective pain management, including patients' self-reports, where possible, to minimize or prevent pain.
3. The best pain management involves patients, families, and health professionals, where patients and families are encouraged to communicate the severity of pain and health professionals are knowledgeable about pain relief options.

The Nature of Pain

An earlier definition of pain by McCaffery and Pasero (1999, p. 11), defines pain as "whatever the experiencing person says it is, existing whenever he (or she) says it does." This definition helped to change practice by emphasizing that health-care professionals must believe clients with respect to their experience of pain and must pay particular attention to the client's subjective experience of pain, as pain self-reports are key to effective pain assessment and management.

Although this definition made a major positive impact on pain management, it is now viewed as too simplistic as clients do not always admit to pain and may not know how, or be able, to tell someone else that they are experiencing pain. Moreover, clients are not always able to distinguish their pain from what their pain may mean to them, that is, how they may be suffering (McGillion, Watt-Watson, Kim, & Graham, 2004; McGillion et al., 2007). The current well-accepted definition of **pain** by the International Association for the Study of Pain is the unpleasant sensory and emotional experience associated with actual or potential damage, or described in terms of such damage (Merskey & Bogduk, 1994). This definition accounts for the highly subjective and multidimensional nature of pain, with sensory-discriminative, cognitive-evaluative, and motivational-affective components. Many clients need encouragement or help to communicate their pain experience, with respect in particular to its intensity, duration, qualities, and related individual responses.

Types of Pain

Pain can be described in terms of the duration, origin, etiology, location, intensity, and quality. When pain lasts only through the expected recovery period, it is described as **acute pain**. Acute pain is purposeful, informing the person that something is wrong. Typically the onset of acute pain is sudden because of a noxious stimulus, such as trauma, and the location of the pain can usually be easily identified.

Chronic pain lasts beyond the usual course for recovery (Bonica, 1990; Merskey & Bogduk, 1994) and has no purpose. Many clinicians use the interval of 3 to 6 months' duration to define pain as chronic. Chronic pain can be further classified as chronic cancer pain or noncancer pain. When chronic pain is extremely difficult to relieve, as with some cancers, it can be classified as intractable (Salerno & Willens, 1996); because its onset can be subtle, it may be difficult for the client to determine when their chronic pain started. It can also often be difficult to pinpoint the location of chronic pain as it is typically more diffuse than acute pain. Chronic pain is complex and can become all-consuming, causing irritability, insomnia, and withdrawal from family, friends, and interests (Watt-Watson, Evans, & Watson, 1988).

Health-care professionals need to recognize that individual and family responses to chronic pain vary widely. For many, achieving adequate chronic pain relief is a constant struggle characterized by exhaustion, financial drain, and concern that there may not be anyone who can help. Clients and families need encouragement

TABLE 34.1 Comparison of Acute and Chronic Pain

Acute Pain	Chronic Pain
Usually sudden onset	Onset may be sudden or gradual
Duration usually transient (up to 3 months)	Duration prolonged (months to years)
Mild to severe	Mild to severe
Sympathetic nervous system responses: Increased pulse rate Increased respiratory rate Elevated blood pressure Diaphoresis Dilated pupils	Parasympathetic nervous system responses: Vital signs normal (because of adaptation) Dry, warm skin Pupils normal or dilated
Purposeful warning/ related to tissue injury; resolves with healing	No purpose; continues beyond healing
Client may appear restless and anxious	Client may appear depressed and withdrawn
Client commonly exhibits behaviour indicative of pain: crying, rubbing area, holding area	Behaviour indicative of obvious pain often absent

REFLECT ON PRIMARY HEALTH CARE

Intersectoral collaboration is essential in the assessment, treatment, and follow-up of a person experiencing pain. Find out whether any pain clinics or networks are available in your region. In pain clinics, professionals, such as physicians, nurses, social workers, physiotherapists, psychologists, pharmacologists, and chaplains, work together to treat the client dealing with chronic pain.

and support to express the impact of chronic pain on their lives. Continuity among health-care professionals involved in the care of those with chronic pain is critical to achieving safe and optimal pain relief (see the Reflect on Primary Health Care box).

Table 34.1 outlines some common differences in physiological and behavioural responses to acute and chronic pain.

Pain can also be categorized according to its origin as somatic or visceral. **Somatic pain** originates in the skin, muscles, bone, or connective tissue. The sharp sensation of a paper cut or aching of a sprained ankle are examples of somatic pain. **Visceral pain** results from stimulation of pain receptors in the organs. Visceral pain tends to be diffuse and often feels like deep somatic pain, that is, burning, aching, or a feeling of pressure. Visceral pain is frequently caused by stretching of the tissues, ischemia, or muscle spasms. For example, an obstructed bowel or blocked coronary artery will result in visceral pain.

Neuropathic pain is the result of injury to the peripheral or central nervous system that frequently results in a persistent pain problem. The nerves may be abnormal because of illness (e.g., postherpetic neuralgia, diabetic peripheral neuropathy), injury (e.g., phantom limb pain, spinal cord injury pain), or undetermined reasons. Subtypes of neuropathic pain are being developed based on the part of the nervous system believed to be damaged. **Peripheral neuropathic pain** (e.g., phantom limb pain, postherpetic neuralgia, carpal tunnel syndrome) follows damage or sensitization of peripheral nerves. **Central neuropathic pain** (e.g., spinal cord injury pain, post-stroke pain, multiple sclerosis pain) results from malfunctioning nerves in the central nervous system. **Sympathetically maintained pain** occurs occasionally when abnormal connections between pain fibres and the sympathetic nervous system perpetuate problems with both the pain and the sympathetically controlled functions (e.g., edema, temperature and blood flow regulation). Neuropathic pain is typically chronic; described as burning, an electric shock, or tingling, dull, and aching; episodes of sharp, shooting pain can also be experienced (Herr, 2002) and tends to be difficult to treat. Unfortunately, evidence suggests that in some instances, neuropathic pain results from a failure to treat pain effectively during the perioperative period (Manias, Bucknall, & Botti, 2005).

Pain can also be described according to where it is experienced in the body. **Radiating pain** is perceived at the source of the pain and extends to nearby tissues. For example, cardiac pain may be felt not only in the chest but also along the left shoulder and down the arm. **Referred pain** is pain felt in a part of the body that is considerably removed from the tissues causing the pain. For example, pain from one part of the abdominal viscera may be perceived in an area of the skin remote from the organ causing the pain (Figure 34.1). Referred pain is complex and occurs most often with damage to visceral organs. The mechanisms of referred pain relate to the spatial organization of the grey matter of the spinal cord into five distinct laminae (I to V) or layers. It is thought that noxious stimuli from both somatic and visceral structures may converge via lamina V neurons, making it difficult for higher brain centres to discriminate the original sources of these noxious inputs (Basbaum & Jessell, 2000).

Intractable pain is pain that is highly resistant to relief. One example is the pain from an advanced cancer. Often, health-care professionals must employ a number of nonpharmacological and pharmacological approaches, such as imagery and patient-controlled analgesia (PCA), to provide a client with adequate pain relief.

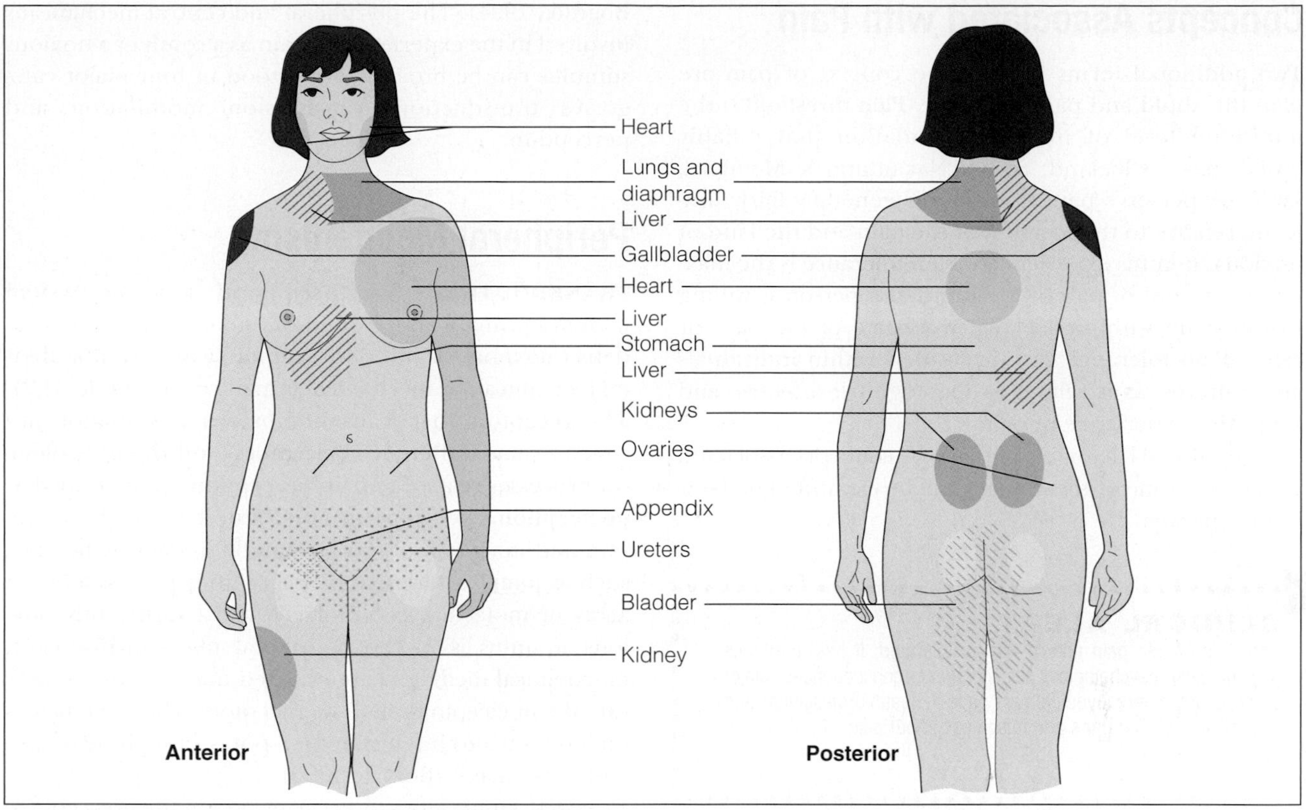

FIGURE 34.1 Common sites of referred pain from various body organs

The intensity of pain is generally rated by using a numerical scale from 0 (no pain) to 10 (pain as bad as you can imagine). Linking the rating to health and functioning scores, pain in the 1 to 3 ranges is deemed *mild pain*, a rating of 4 to 6 is *moderate pain*, and pain reaching 7 to 10 is ranked *severe pain*. The quality of pain is described by using adjectives, such as *stabbing* or *throbbing*.

Common pain syndromes are briefly described in the Clinical Manifestations box.

Clinical Manifestations

The following are some common pain syndromes:

- *Postherpetic neuralgia.* An episode of herpes zoster (shingles) has two phases: a vesicular eruption and neurological pain that often encircles the body. The pain ranges from mild to severe. In the postherpetic syndrome, severe pain persists for months or years with burning or electric-shock pain in the area of the original eruption.
- *Phantom pain.* Phantom sensation, the feeling that a lost body part is present, occurs in most people after amputation. For many, this sensation is painful; it may occur spontaneously or be evoked (e.g., by using a poorly fitting prosthesis). When the amputation involves a limb, it is termed *phantom limb pain*, whereas following breast removal, it is called *post-mastectomy pain*. Phantom pain varies and may be burning, severe, crushing, or a cramping sensation. This pain is neuropathic in nature and is complex because of the loss of sensory input into the central nervous system from the amputated region.
- *Trigeminal neuralgia.* Trigeminal neuralgia is an intense stabbing pain that is distributed by one or more branches of the trigeminal (fifth cranial) nerve. The pain is usually experienced in parts of the face and head, for example, gums, cheek, and surface of the head.
- *Headache.* Headache is a common somatic pain that can be caused by either intracranial or extracranial problems. To establish a plan to prevent or treat headache, the nurse needs to assess the quality, location, onset, duration, and frequency of the pain, as well as any signs and symptoms that precede the headache.
- *Fibromyalgia*. Fibromyalgia is a chronic disorder that is characterized by widespread musculoskeletal pain, fatigue, and multiple tender points. A *tender point* is tenderness that occurs in a precise, localized area, particularly in the neck, spine, shoulders, and hips. People with this syndrome can also experience sleep disturbances, morning stiffness, irritable bowel syndrome, anxiety, and other symptoms. Although the symptoms present as muscle pain, stiffness, and weakness, it is considered by many to be a problem of abnormal CNS functioning, particularly as it relates to the way nerves process pain.

Concepts Associated with Pain

Two additional terms used in the context of pain are pain threshold and pain tolerance. **Pain threshold** is the minimum level of noxious stimulation that reliably evokes pain (Cleeland, Serlin, Nakamura, & Mendoza, 1997). A person's pain threshold is generally fairly uniform, relative to the location of the pain and the kind of noxious stimulus experienced. **Pain tolerance** is the maximum amount of painful stimuli that a person is willing to withstand without seeking avoidance of the pain or relief. Pain tolerance can vary widely within individuals and cultures, as it relates to the cognitive-affective and subjective experience of pain.

See Box 34.1 for a summary of concepts associated with pain. Some of these terms will be expanded on later in the chapter.

CLINICAL ALERT

Unrelieved acute pain should not be tolerated; it has numerous physiological, psychological, and economic consequences. Major contributors to unrelieved pain are patient, health professional, and societal knowledge gaps and misbeliefs about pain.

Pain Mechanisms

The experience of pain is complex and multidimensional, with sensory-discriminative, cognitive-evaluative, and motivational-affective components (Merskey & Bogduk, 1994). The peripheral and central mechanisms involved in the experience of pain as a result of a noxious stimulus can be broadly understood in four major categories: transduction, transmission, modulation, and perception.

Peripheral Mechanisms

TRANSDUCTION The peripheral nervous system includes primary afferent sensory neurons specialized to detect **noxious**, or injurious, stimuli, which can be thermal, chemical, or mechanical in nature (see Table 34.2). The receptors that transmit noxious information are called primary afferent **nociceptors**, and the physiological processes related to pain perception are described as **nociception**. Nociceptors are located throughout the skin and mucosa and less frequently in deep structures, such as joints, arteries, and viscera; they possess a broad array of molecular receptors. When a sufficiently noxious stimulus is in the peripheral microenvironment, biochemical mediators are released that sensitize or activate the nociceptors via these receptors. These mediators include serotonin, histamine, potassium, bradykinin, and substance P (Bonica, 1990).

Bradykinin causes direct activation of the nociceptors, the release of inflammatory chemicals, such as histamine, and vasodilation and increased capillary permeability, resulting in reddened and tender tissue. Bradykinin also stimulates the release of prostaglandins. These compounds further excite nociceptors and enhance the effect of bradykinin and histamine. Substance P acts on blood vessels in the damaged area to release chemicals that con-

BOX 34.1 CONCEPTS ASSOCIATED WITH PAIN

The following are terms used in the study of pain and pain management:

- *Acute pain:* Pain that is directly related to tissue injury and resolves when tissue heals
- *Cancer pain:* Pain associated with the disease, treatment, or some other factor in individuals with cancer
- *Chronic pain:* Pain that persists beyond 6 months secondary to chronic disorders or nerve malfunctions that produce ongoing pain after healing is complete
- *Intractable pain:* A pain state (generally severe) for which no cure is possible after accepted medical evaluation and treatments have been implemented; focus of treatment turns from cure to pain reduction, functional improvement, and the enhancement of quality of life
- *Neuropathic pain:* Pain that is related to damaged or malfunctioning nervous tissue in the peripheral or central nervous system
- *Nociceptive pain:* Pain that is directly related to tissue damage; may be somatic (e.g., damage to skin, muscle, bone) or visceral (e.g., damage to organs)
- *Pain threshold:* The process of recognizing, defining, and responding to pain
- *Pain tolerance:* The most pain an individual is willing or able to tolerate before taking evasive actions
- *Phantom pain:* Painful sensations felt from a part of the body that has been amputated; can arise from the residual limb (e.g., stump pain) or nerves that lost communication with the missing part

The following states indicate abnormal nerve functioning, and the associated cause needs to be identified or treated (as possible) before irreversible damage occurs:

- **Allodynia**: Sensation of pain from a stimulus that normally does not produce pain (e.g., light touch)
- **Dysesthesia**: An unpleasant abnormal sensation that can be either spontaneous or evoked
- **Hyperalgesia**: Increased sensation of pain in response to a normally painful stimulus

TABLE 34.2 Types of Noxious Stimuli

Stimulus Type	Physiological Basis of Pain
Mechanical	
1. Trauma to body tissues (e.g., surgery)	Tissue damage; direct irritation of the pain receptors; inflammation
2. Alterations in body tissues (e.g., edema)	Pressure on pain receptors
3. Blockage of a body duct	Distension of the lumen of the duct
4. Tumour	Pressure on pain receptors; irritation of nerve endings
5. Muscle spasm	Stimulation of pain receptors (also see chemical stimuli)
Thermal	
Extreme heat or cold (e.g., burns)	Tissue destruction; stimulation of thermosensitive pain receptors
Chemical	
1. Tissue ischemia (e.g., blocked coronary artery)	Stimulation of pain receptors because of accumulated lactic acid (and other chemicals, such as bradykinin and enzymes) in tissues
2. Muscle spasm	Tissue ischemia secondary to mechanical stimulation (see above)

tribute to the conduction of nociception and, like prostaglandins, it increases the inflammatory response. Substance P also serves as a neurotransmitter, enhancing the movement of impulses across the nerve synapse from the primary afferent neuron to the second-order neuron in the dorsal horn of the spinal cord (see Figure 34.2). **Transduction** occurs when the excited nociceptor converts the surrounding noxious stimulus into an action potential (i.e., electrochemical impulse) that is then carried to the central nervous system (CNS).

TRANSMISSION **Transmission** occurs when noxious information is conducted via two types of nociceptive fibres: A-delta and C fibres. The A-delta fibres have a relatively large diameter, are myelinated, and rapidly conduct the impulse. These fibres are associated with the sensation of sharp, pricking pain. The other set of nociceptive fibres is the small-diameter, unmyelinated C fibres. The C fibres transmit the impulse more slowly and mediate long-lasting, burning pain.

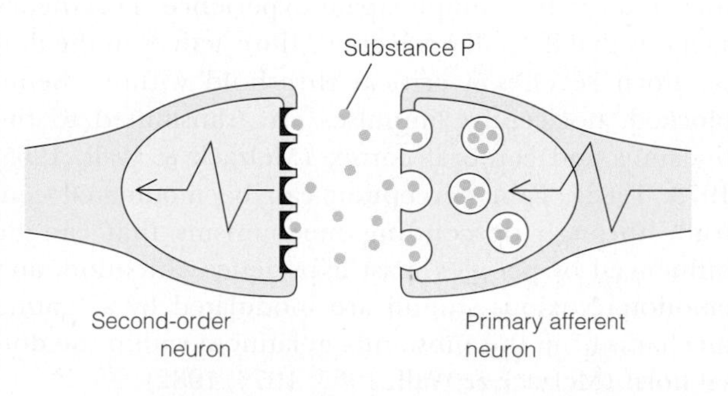

FIGURE 34.2 Substance P assists the transmission of impulses across the synapse from the primary afferent neuron to a second-order neuron.

Central Mechanisms

The terminals of nociceptors enter the dorsal horn of the spinal cord through the dorsal root and synapse onto second-order neurons (Figure 34.3). The fast A-delta fibres primarily conduct impulses from mechanical and thermal pain. They synapse with second-order neurons (long fibres) that cross immediately to the opposite side of the spinal cord and enter the lateral spinothalamic tract and ascend to the brain.

A few fibres terminate in the reticular areas of the brain stem, but most terminate in the thalamus. From there, signals are sent to the basal areas of the brain and to the somatic sensory cortex (Figure 34.4). The slow, C fibres conduct impulses from mechanical, thermal, and chemical stimuli. These impulses often pass through one or more additional short neurons before travelling up to the brain by the spinothalamic tract.

MODULATION In **modulation**, noxious impulses stimulate regions of the midbrain. Descending spinal fibres, from the thalamus through the midbrain and medulla to the dorsal horn, conduct nociceptive inhibitory impulses and release endogenous opioids to inhibit the release of neurotransmitters and the noxious stimuli presynaptically. Endogenous opioids are naturally occurring morphine-like pentapeptides that exist in three general classes: enkephalins, dynorphins, and beta endorphins. These substances bind to opiate receptor sites in the central and peripheral nervous system, blocking or modulating noxious impulses (Melzack & Wall, 1996). The opiate-binding receptor sites are identified as mu, kappa, and delta and are the same sites to which exogenous opioid analgesics (e.g., oxycodone) bind to provide pain relief.

PERCEPTION The final process, **perception**, occurs when the client becomes conscious of the pain. Four key

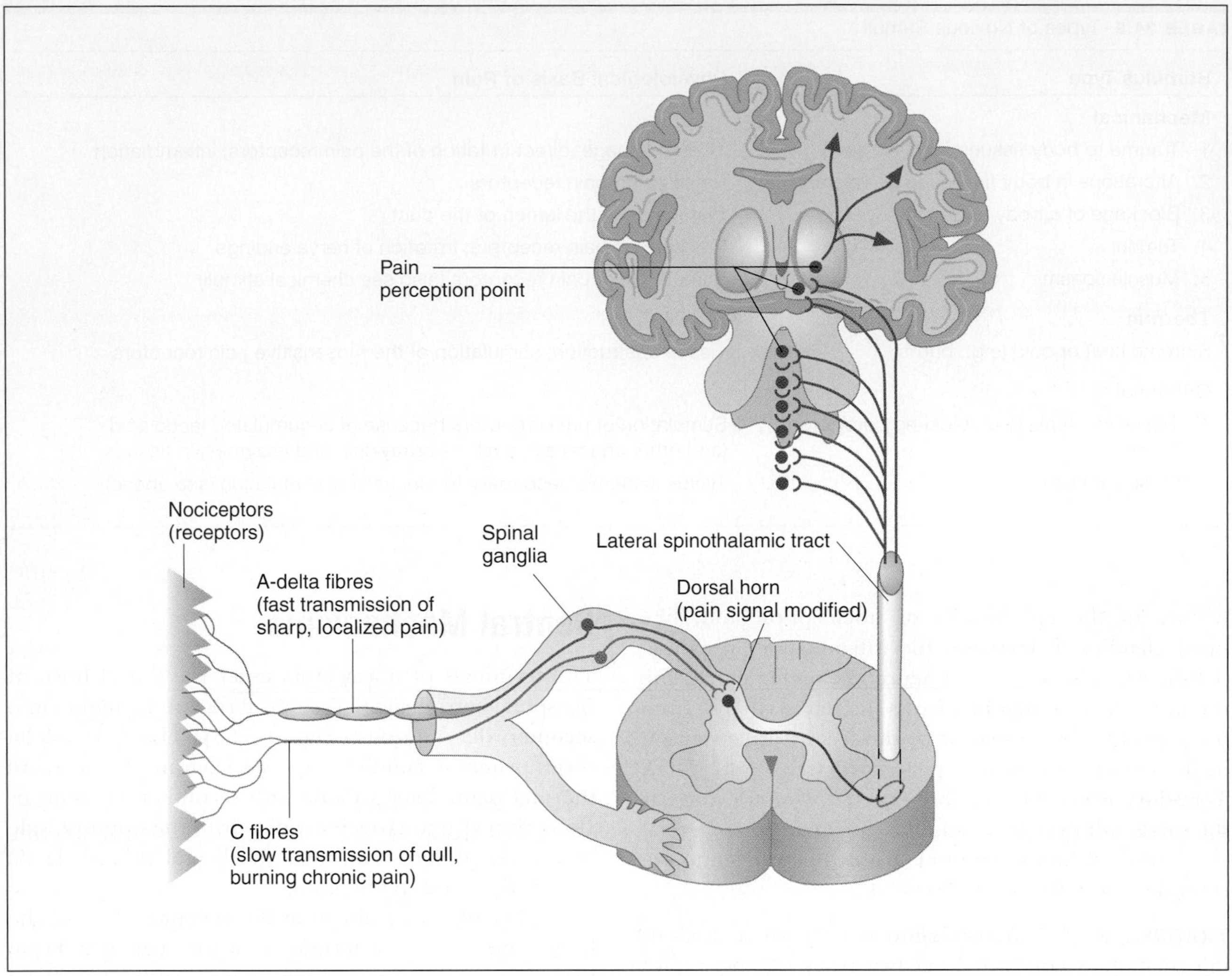

FIGURE 34.3 Peripheral and central pain mechanisms

regions of the cerebral cortex are thought to be activated by noxious stimuli via the ascending pathways: the insular cortex, the anterior cingulate cortex, and the primary and secondary somatosensory cortices (Craig & Sorkin, 2004). These regions, together with other areas of the forebrain, produce the sensory-discriminative, motivational-affective, and cognitive-evaluative aspects of the pain experience, as well as motoric integration of noxious stimuli and pain memory (Basbaum & Bushnell, 2002; Basbaum & Jessell, 2000; Craig & Sorkin, 2004). The insular cortex in particular is understood as being critical to the integration of the multidimensional aspects of pain.

Gate Control Theory

In 1965, Melzack and Wall proposed the gate control theory (GCT). GCT (Melzack, 1990; Melzack & Wall, 1965, 1973, 1982) proposed that interneurons of the substantia gelatinosa act as a gate, regulating the input of large and small fibres to lamina V cells (Figure 34.5).

According to GCT, pain is not a simple sensory experience but one that involves central mechanisms that result in the complex pain experience. This theory suggests that if small nociceptive fibre activity in the dorsal horn reaches a critical threshold without being blocked, nociceptive impulses are transmitted to the thalamus and cerebral cortex (Melzack & Wall, 1965, 1973, 1982). Pain perception can be modulated centrally through descending mechanisms that can be influenced by peoples' past experience, attention, and emotion. Noxious stimuli are modulated by a "gating mechanism" in the substantia gelatinosa within the dorsal horn (Melzack & Wall, 1965, 1973, 1982).

This gating mechanism can be open, partially open, or closed. The position of the gate is influenced by the relative amounts of activity in large non-nociceptive (A-beta) and small nociceptive (A-delta and C) fibres. Increased activity in the large fibres closes the gate or

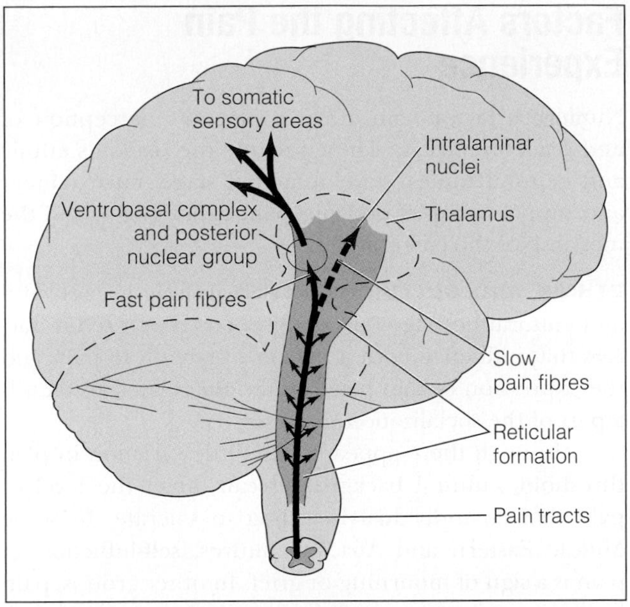

FIGURE 34.4 The transmission of nociceptive information to higher brain centres

inhibits transmission of noxious messages carried by the small fibres to transmission cells (T cells) in the substantia gelatinosa (Melzack & Wall, 1965, 1973, 1982). However, if noxious impulses are not blocked by large fibre activity (i.e., the gate is open or partially open) and reach a critical level, they will be transmitted to second-order neurons in the substantia gelatinosa. The noxious impulse is then transmitted to the thalamus and cerebral cortex, via ascending nociceptive second-order neurons. As previously discussed, specialized large-diameter fibres activate selective cognitive processes that influence, by way of descending fibres, the modulating properties of the gating mechanism (Basbaum & Jessell, 2000).

Since GCT was developed, pain knowledge has greatly evolved. Cumulative research has led to more advanced understanding of the nature of pain and pain mechanisms, including sensitization, cortical processing, and spinal and supraspinal mechanisms of pain control, beyond Melzack and Wall's original theory. Although GCT greatly enhanced understanding of the complexity of the pain experience and the potential consequences of unrelieved pain, it is largely a theory of acute pain. GCT cannot, for example, explain why a person develops chronic pain long after the original injury has healed.

Nervous System Plasticity: Peripheral and Central Sensitization

The role of plasticity of the nervous system in *peripheral and central sensitization* is now being recognized, along with the individuality of pain perception and response (Basbaum & Jessell, 2000). Noxious stimuli are transmitted by C-fibre nociceptors with slow conducting unmyelinated axons and by A-delta nociceptors with thinly myelinated axons. In the context of pain, **nervous system plasticity** refers to the fact that pain mechanisms in the peripheral and central nervous systems can change in response to continued noxious stimulation, a process known as sensitization (Basbaum & Jessell). For example, **peripheral sensitization** of peripheral nociceptors can occur after injury, surgery, or inflammation because of chemicals released from damaged cells, such as bradykinin, histamine, and prostaglandins. Peripheral sensitization can change nociceptors so that they transmit spontaneous discharges and respond at a lowered threshold to both nociceptive and non-nociceptive stimuli (Basbaum & Jesell). Moreover, prolonged firing of nociceptors with severe and persistent injury, such as surgery, causes dorsal horn spinal cord neurons to become more responsive to all inputs, resulting in a phenomenon known as **central sensitization.** Central sensitization can result in abnormal interpretation of normal stimuli and chronic pain that lasts long after the original trauma. Central sensitization may cause persistent pain after the injured tissue has healed because of changes within the CNS (Basbaum & Jessell).

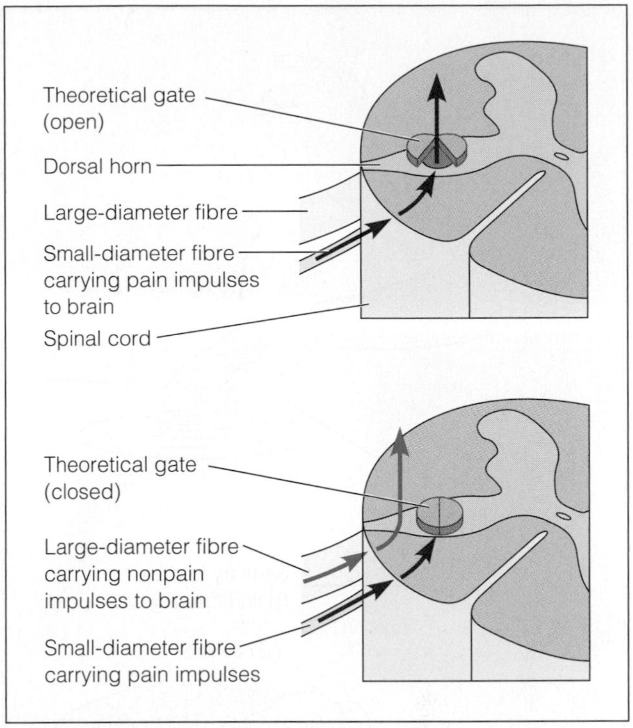

FIGURE 34.5 A schematic illustration of the gate control theory

Responses to Pain

The body's response to pain is a complex process rather than a specific action. It involves physiological and psychosocial aspects. Initially, the sympathetic nervous system responds, resulting in the fight-or-flight response.

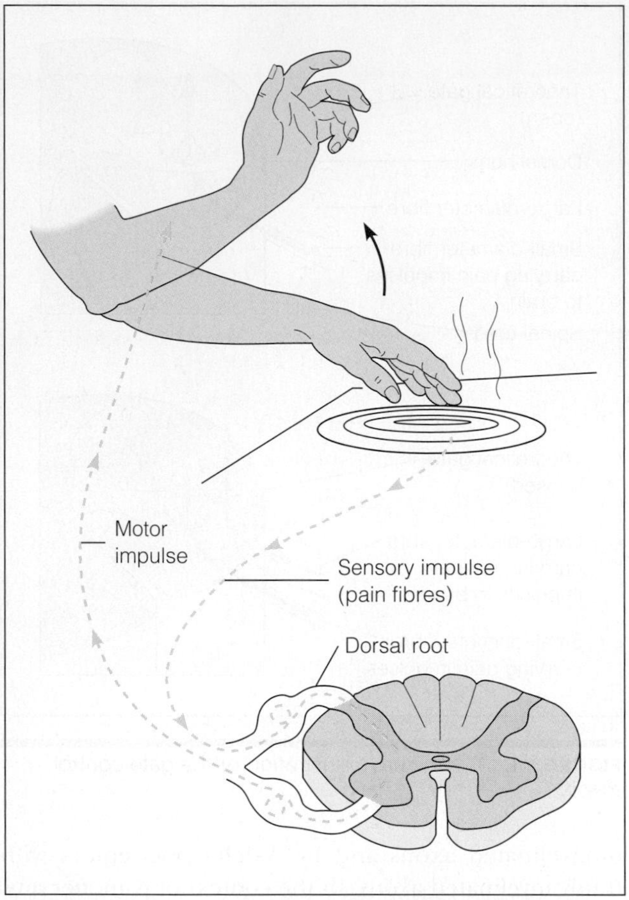

FIGURE 34.6 Proprioceptive reflex to a noxious stimulus

As pain continues, the body adapts as the parasympathetic nervous system takes over, reversing many of the initial physiological responses. This adaptation to the pain occurs after several hours or days of pain. The actual pain receptors adapt very little and continue to transmit the pain message. This serves the purpose of keeping the person continually aware of the damaging stimuli causing the pain (Guyton & Hall, 2006). The person may learn to cope with the pain through cognitive and behavioural activities, such as diversions, imagery, and excessive sleeping. The individual may respond to pain by seeking out physical interventions to manage the pain, such as analgesics, massage, and exercise.

A proprioceptive reflex also occurs with the stimulation of pain receptors. Impulses travel along sensory pain fibres to the spinal cord. There, they synapse with motor neurons, and the impulses travel back via motor fibres to a muscle near the site of the pain (Figure 34.6). The muscle then contracts in a protective action. For example, when a person touches a hot stove, the hand reflexively draws back from the heat even before the person is aware of the pain.

Factors Affecting the Pain Experience

Numerous factors can affect a person's perception of and reaction to pain. These include the person's ethnic and cultural values, developmental stage, environment and support people, previous pain experiences, and the meaning of the current pain.

ETHNIC AND CULTURAL VALUES Ethnic background and cultural heritage have long been recognized as factors that influence both a person's reaction to pain and the expression of that pain. Behaviour related to pain is a part of the socialization process.

Although there appears to be little variation in pain threshold, cultural background can affect the level of pain that an individual is willing to tolerate. In some Middle Eastern and African cultures, self-infliction of pain is a sign of mourning or grief. In other groups, pain is anticipated as part of the ritualistic practices and, therefore, tolerance of pain signifies strength and endurance. Additionally, the expression of pain varies widely. Studies have shown that individuals of northern European descent tend to be more stoic and less expressive of their pain than individuals from southern European backgrounds.

Nurses must realize they have their own attitudes and expectations about pain. For example, nurses may place a higher value on silent suffering or self-control in response to pain. Nurses expect people to be objective about pain and to be able to provide a detailed description of the pain. Nurses who deny, refute, or downplay the pain they observe in others may be culturally incompetent (unaware and emotionally apathetic toward others' viewpoints). To become culturally competent, nurses must become knowledgeable about differences in the meaning of and appropriate responses to pain while being sympathetic to concerns and developing the skills needed to address pain in a culturally sensitive way.

DEVELOPMENTAL STAGE The ages and developmental levels of clients are important factors that will influence their reactions to and expressions of pain. Some age variations and related nursing interventions are presented in Table 34.3.

The field of pain management for infants and children has grown significantly. Research indicates that term and preterm neonates have the anatomical, physiological, and biochemical elements necessary for pain transmission (Johnston, Stevens, Yang, & Horton, 1995). Moreover, neonates as young as 25 weeks gestational age are capable of processing pain at a cortical level, which highlights the potential for higher-level pain processing in infants (Bartocci, Bergqvist, Lagercrantz, & Anand, 2006; Slater et al., 2006). However, children's pain is often undertreated

TABLE 34.3 Age Variations in the Pain Experience

Age Group	Pain Perception and Behaviour	Selected Nursing Interventions
Infant	Perceives pain	Give a glucose pacifier.
	Responds to pain with increased sensitivity	Use tactile stimulation (e.g. gently rub other side of affected area).
	Older infant tries to avoid pain; for example, turns away and physically resists	Play music or tapes of a heartbeat.
Toddler and preschooler	Develops the ability to describe pain and its intensity and location	Distract the child with toys, books, pictures. Involve the child in blowing bubbles as a way of "blowing away the pain."
	Often responds with crying and anger because child perceives pain as a threat to security	Appeal to the child's belief in magic by using a "magic" blanket or glove to take away pain.
	Reasoning with child at this stage is not always successful	Hold the child to provide comfort.
	May consider pain a punishment	Explore misconceptions about pain.
	Feels sad	
	May learn there are gender differences in pain expression	
	Tends to hold someone accountable for the pain	
School-age child	Tries to be brave when facing pain	Use imagery to turn off "pain switches."
	Rationalizes in an attempt to explain the pain	Provide a behavioural rehearsal of what to expect and how it will look and feel.
	Responsive to explanations	
	Can usually identify the location and describe the pain	
	With persistent pain, may regress to an earlier stage of development	Provide support and nurturing.
Adolescent	May be slow to acknowledge pain	Provide opportunities to discuss pain.
	Recognizing pain or "giving in" may be considered weakness	Provide privacy.
	Wants to appear brave in front of peers and not report pain	Present choices for dealing with pain. Encourage music or TV for distraction.
Adult	Behaviours exhibited when experiencing pain may be gender-based behaviours learned as a child	Deal with any misbeliefs about pain.
	May ignore pain because to admit it is perceived as a sign of weakness or failure	Focus on the client's control in dealing with the pain.
	May use pain for secondary gain, for example, to get attention	
	Fear of what pain means may prevent some adults from taking action	Allay fears and anxiety, when possible.
Older adult	May perceive pain as part of the aging process	Spend time with the client, and listen carefully.
	May have decreased sensations or perceptions of the pain	
	Lethargy, anorexia, and fatigue may be indicators of pain	
	May withhold complaints of pain because of fear of the treatment, of any lifestyle changes that may be involved, or of becoming dependent	Clarify misbeliefs. Encourage independence, whenever possible.
	May describe pain differently, that is, as "ache," "hurt," or "discomfort"	
	May consider it unacceptable to admit to or show pain	

because they may be less able to articulate their pain experience and needs compared with adults (Stevens, 1999). Pain in children can be assessed by using self-report, observational or behavioural, and physiological measures. Ideally, the nurse should use a composite measure that includes self-report and one or more of the other indicators (Champion, Goodenough, von Baeyer, & Thomas, 1998). When self-report is not applicable (e.g., infants, preverbal children, cognitively impaired children), behavioural observation should be the primary source for pain assessment (von Baeyer & Spagrud, 2007).

Pain is generally more prevalent in the older population because of the presence of acute and chronic disease. Although pain threshold does not appear to change with aging, the effect of analgesics may increase because of physiological changes related to drug metabolism and excretion.

ENVIRONMENT AND SUPPORT PEOPLE A strange environment, such as a hospital with its noises, lights, and activity, can compound pain. In addition, the lonely person who is without a support network may perceive pain as severe, whereas the person who has supportive people around may perceive less pain. Some people prefer to withdraw when they are in pain, whereas others prefer the distraction of people and activity around them. Family caregivers can be a significant support for a person in pain. With the increase in outpatient and home care, families are assuming an increased responsibility for the management of pain. Education related to the assessment and management of pain can positively affect the perceived quality of life for both clients and their caregivers (McCaffery & Pasero, 1999).

Some clients use pain to acquire secondary gains, that is, special attention from support people and nurses. If the situation becomes difficult for the support people, the nurse can intervene and discuss the problem before the support people become angry and avoid the client.

Expectations of significant others can affect a person's perceptions of and responses to pain. In some situations, for example, girls may be permitted to express pain more openly than boys. Family role can also affect how a person perceives or responds to pain. For instance, a single mother supporting three children may ignore pain because of her need to stay on the job. The presence of support people often changes a client's reaction to pain. For example, toddlers often tolerate pain more readily when supportive parents or nurses are nearby.

PAST PAIN EXPERIENCES Previous pain experiences can influence a client's response to pain. People who have personally experienced pain or who have been exposed to the suffering of someone close are often more threatened by anticipated pain than are people without a pain experience. In addition, the success or lack of success of pain relief measures influences a person's expectations for relief. For example, a person who has tried several pain relief measures without success may have little hope about the helpfulness of nursing interventions.

MEANING OF PAIN The meaning of the pain can contribute to the overall pain experience (Arntz & Claassens, 2004; McGillion et al., 2007). Some clients may accept pain more readily than others, depending on the circumstances and the client's interpretation of its significance. A client who associates the pain with a positive outcome may withstand the pain amazingly well. For example, a woman giving birth to a child or an athlete undergoing knee surgery to prolong his career may tolerate pain better because of the benefit associated with it. These clients may view the pain as a temporary inconvenience rather than a potential threat or disruption to daily life.

By contrast, clients with unrelenting chronic pain may suffer more intensely. Chronic pain affects the body, mind, spirit, and social relationships in an undesirable way. Physically, the pain limits functioning and contributes to disuse or deconditioning. For many, the changes in activities of daily living (e.g., eating, sleeping, toileting) also take a toll. The side effects of the many medications used to try to control the pain also place a heavy burden on the sufferer's body.

Mentally, individuals with chronic pain change their outlook, becoming more pessimistic, often to the point of helplessness and hopelessness. Mood often becomes impaired when pain persists: the sadness of being unable to do important or enjoyable activities, combined with self-doubts and learned helplessness, can contribute to depression. The anxiety surrounding the timing of pain flares, the worry about the physical ability to do what is needed, and the uncertainty about coping with multiple competing demands (including pain control) can escalate emotionally, to the point of panic.

Spiritually, pain can be viewed in a variety of ways. It may be perceived as a punishment for wrongdoing, a betrayal by a higher power, a test of fortitude, or a threat to the essence of who the person is. As such, pain can be a source of spiritual distress or be a source of strength and enlightenment. Socially, pain often strains valued relationships, in part because of the impaired ability to fulfill role expectations.

Assessing

Accurate pain assessment is essential for effective pain management. In fact, many health facilities are making pain assessment the **fifth vital sign**. Because pain is a complex, subjective, and multidimensional experience, no simple method can objectively determine how much pain an individual experiences. Therefore, nurses need to assess all factors affecting the pain experience, including physiological, psychological, behavioural, emotional, and sociocultural factors. Nurses should also tailor pain assessments to the unique developmental levels, communication capabilities, and cultural needs of their clients.

In general, pain should be assessed on hospital admission and routinely thereafter, as well as before, during, and after therapeutic interventions (Canadian Pain Society, 2005). However, the extent and frequency of the pain assessment will vary according to the situation. For clients experiencing acute or severe pain, the nurse may focus only on location, quality, severity, and early intervention. Clients with less severe or chronic pain can usually provide a more detailed description of the experience. Frequency of pain assessment usually depends on the pain management intervention being used and the clinical circumstances. For example, in the initial postoperative period, pain is often assessed whenever vital signs are taken, which may be as often as every 15 minutes and then extended to every 2 to 4 hours. Following pain management interventions, pain intensity should be reassessed at an interval appropriate for the intervention. For example, following the intravenous administration of morphine, the severity of pain should be reassessed in 20 to 30 minutes.

Because it has been found that many people will not voice their pain unless asked about it, pain assessments *must* be initiated by the nurse. Some of the many reasons clients may be reluctant to report pain are listed in Box 34.2. Knowledge deficits and problematic beliefs may underlie some of these reasons, especially those regarding pharmacological pain management interventions. When conducting pain assessments, it is essential that nurses listen to and rely on the client's perceptions of pain because pain is a subjective experience. Believing the person who is conveying their perceptions of and experiencing the pain is crucial to establishing a sense of trust.

Comprehensive pain assessments consist of two major components: (1) a history of the client's current pain experience, and (2) direct observation of the behavioural and physiological responses of the client. The goal of assessment is to gain an objective understanding of a subjective experience.

History of the Current Pain Experience

When taking histories of current pain experiences, the nurse must provide an opportunity for clients to express, in their own words, how they view the pain and the situation. This will help the nurse understand what the pain means to the client and how the client is coping. Remember that each person's pain experience is unique and that the client is the best interpreter of the pain experience. Questions regarding the client's current pain experience should be specific and individualized. For example, questions asked of an accident victim would be different from those asked of a postoperative client or one suffering from chronic pain. The initial pain assessment for someone in *severe acute pain* may consist of only a few questions before intervention occurs. In addition, the nurse may focus on the following:

BOX 34.2 REASONS THAT CLIENTS MAY BE RELUCTANT TO REPORT PAIN

Some clients are hesitant to report pain for a number of reasons:

- Unwillingness to trouble staff who are perceived as busy
- Concern about being labelled as a *complainer* or *bad patient*
- Fear of the injectable route of analgesic administration—children in particular
- Belief that pain is to be expected as part of the recovery process
- Belief that pain is a normal part of aging or a necessary part of life—older adults in particular
- Belief that expressions of pain reveal weakness
- Difficulty expressing personal discomfort
- Concern about potential risks associated with opioid drugs (e.g., addiction)
- Fear about the cause of pain or that reporting pain will lead to further tests and expenses
- Concern about the possibility of unwanted side effects, especially of opioid drugs
- Concern that use of drugs now will render the drug inefficient if or when the pain becomes worse

- Previous pain management strategies used (pharmacological and nonpharmacological) and their effectiveness
- When and what analgesics were last taken
- Other medications being taken
- Allergies to medications

For the person with *chronic pain,* the nurse may focus on the client's coping mechanisms, the effectiveness of current pain management, and the ways in which the pain has affected activities of daily living (ADLs).

Data that should be obtained in a comprehensive history of a client's current pain experience include pain location, intensity, quality, patterns, precipitating factors, alleviating factors, associated symptoms, effect on ADLs, past pain experiences, meaning of the pain to the person, coping resources, and affective responses. Questions to elicit this data are shown in the Assessment: Interview box.

LOCATION To ascertain the specific location of the pain, ask the individual to point to the site of the discomfort. It is also important to determine whether the pain radiates from the indicated site. A body outline can assist in identifying pain locations. The client marks the location of pain on the body outline. This tool can be especially effective with clients who have more than one source of pain.

When assessing the location of a child's pain, the nurse needs to understand the child's vocabulary. For example, *tummy* might refer either to the abdomen or to part of the chest. Asking the child to point to the pain helps clarify the child's word usage to identify location. Again, the use of body outlines can assist in identifying

ASSESSMENT: INTERVIEW

History of the Current Pain Experience

It is important for the nurse to obtain accurate data on a client's pain:

- *Location:* Where is your pain?
- *Intensity:* On a scale of 0 to 10 (with 0 meaning "No pain" and 10 meaning "Pain as bad as you can imagine"), how would you rate the degree of pain you are having?
- *Quality:* Tell me what your pain feels like.
- *Pattern*
  a. *Time of onset:* When did or does the pain start?
  b. *Duration:* How long have you had it or how long does it usually last?
  c. *Constancy:* Do you have pain-free periods? When? For how long?
- *Precipitating factors:* What triggers the pain or makes it worse?
- *Alleviating factors:* What have you found helpful for lessening or relieving the pain (i.e., pharmacological and nonpharmacological interventions)? What pain medications do you use? Have you experienced any side effects?
- *Associated symptoms:* Do you have any other symptoms (e.g., nausea, dizziness, blurred vision, shortness of breath) before, during, or after your pain?
- *Effects on activities of daily living:* How does the pain affect your daily activities (e.g., eating, working, sleeping, and social and recreational activities)?
- *Past pain experiences:* Tell me about past pain experiences you have had and the effectiveness of pain relief measures.
- *Meaning of pain:* How do you interpret your pain? What outcomes (implications) do you anticipate from this pain? What do you fear most about your pain?
- *Coping resources:* What do you usually do to help cope with pain?
- *Affective response:* How does the pain make you feel (e.g., anxious, depressed, frightened, tired)?

pain locations. Parents can also be helpful in interpreting the meaning of a child's words.

When documenting pain location, the nurse can use various body landmarks. Further clarification is possible with the use of such terms as *proximal, distal, medial, lateral,* and *diffuse.*

PAIN INTENSITY The client's self-report is the single most important indicator of pain intensity. Studies have shown that health-care providers tend to underestimate clients' pain intensity (Guru & Dubinsky, 2000; Trentin, Visentin, de Marco, & Zanolin, 2001), which compromises their pain management. Self-report pain intensity measures provide an easy method to determine how much pain a client is experiencing. Valid and reliable self-report measures that are commonly used with adults include numerical rating scales (NRSs), visual analogue scales (VASs), and verbal rating scales (VRSs). Such scales provide consistency for nurses to communicate with the client and other health-care providers. NRSs are commonly used in clinical practice and recommended as a core outcome measure of pain intensity for clinical pain trials in adults because they are easy to administer and score, and are preferred by and useful with a diversity of clients (Jensen & Karoly, 2001). An 11-point NRS (Cleeland, 1991) is shown in Figure 34.7. Using an 11-point NRS involves asking clients to rate their pain from 0 to 10, with 0 meaning "No pain" and 10 meaning "Pain as bad as you can imagine." Verbal NRSs do not require paper and pencil; however, the nurse should document the score reported by the client.

When noting pain intensity, it is important to determine any related factors that may be affecting the pain. Possible causes need to be assessed when the intensity changes. For example, the abrupt cessation of acute abdominal pain may indicate a ruptured appendix. Several factors can affect the client's perception of pain intensity: (1) the amount of distraction or the client's concentration on another event, (2) the client's state of consciousness, (3) the level of activity, and (4) the client's expectations.

Not all clients can understand or relate to NRSs. These include children who are unable to verbally communicate their discomfort and clients with impairments in cognition or communication. Faces scales may be easier to use for these clients (Jensen & Karoly, 2001). Faces scales use photographs or line drawings that illustrate facial expressions of individuals experiencing different levels of pain severity. Each face has a number so that the pain intensity can be documented. For example, the Faces Pain Scale—Revised (Hicks, von Baeyer, Spafford, van Korlaar, & Goodenough, 2001), shown in Figure 34.8, is a valid and reliable faces scale that can be used with school-age children and is recommended for use in pediatric pain clinical trials (Stinson, Kavanagh, Yamada, Gill, & Stevens, 2006). When measuring pain intensity in children, it is critical that the nurse uses a self-report measure recommended for the child's age and developmental level.

For effective use of self-report pain intensity measures, clients need to be educated about how to use the scale, as well as how the information will be used to determine changes in their condition and the effectiveness of pain management interventions. Clients should also be asked to indicate what level of comfort is acceptable to them so that

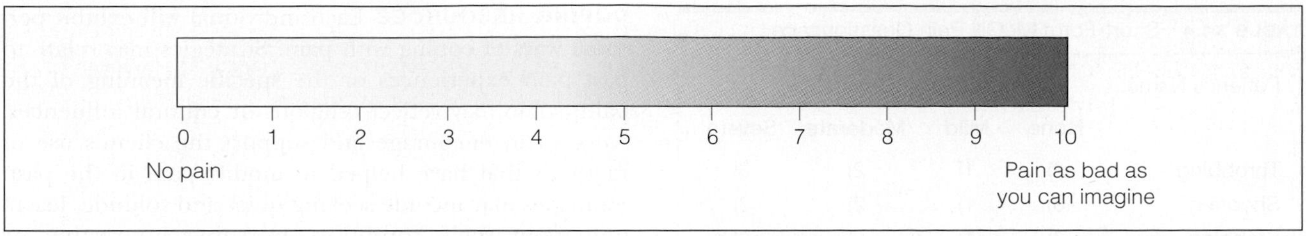

FIGURE 34.7 An 11-point numerical rating scale

they can perform specific activities. This will ensure that adequate pain management is achieved (Pasero, 1997).

When it is not possible to use a self-report measure with a client, the nurse must rely on observation of behaviour and the physiological cues discussed later in this section. The input of the client's significant others, such as parents or caregivers, can assist the nurse in interpreting the observations. An objective description of the behaviour and physiological data is then documented.

PAIN QUALITY Descriptive adjectives help people communicate the quality of their pain, which can provide information on the nature of the pain (i.e., nociceptive, neuropathic, or a combination of both). A headache may be described as "hammerlike" or an abdominal pain as "piercing, like a knife." Sometimes, clients have difficulty describing their pain because they have never experienced any sensation like it. This is particularly true of children and of adults who have neuropathic pain. The McGill pain questionnaire (MPQ) (Melzack, 1975) and its short-form (Melzack, 1987) are reliable and valid measures of pain quality for different types of pain in adults. Some of the terms commonly used to describe pain, as listed in the short-form MPQ, are shown in Table 34.4.

Nurses need to record the exact words clients use to describe pain. Exact information can be significant in both the diagnosis of the pain etiology and the treatment choices. For example, key descriptors, such as "burning" and "electrical" may help the nurse to identify neuropathic pain.

PATTERN The pattern of pain includes time of onset, duration, and recurrence or intervals without pain. The nurse therefore determines when the pain began; how long the pain lasts; whether it recurs and, if so, the length of the interval without pain; and when the pain last occurred.

PRECIPITATING FACTORS Certain activities sometimes precede pain. For example, physical exertion may precede chest pain, or abdominal pain may occur after eating. These observations can help prevent pain and determine its cause. Environmental factors, such as extreme cold or heat, can affect some types of pain. For example, sudden exercise on a hot day can cause muscle spasm. Physical and emotional stressors can also precipitate pain. Strong emotions can trigger a migraine headache or an episode of angina. Extreme physical exertion can precipitate muscle spasms in the neck, shoulders, or back.

ALLEVIATING FACTORS Nurses must ask clients to describe anything that they have done to help alleviate the pain (e.g., home remedies, such as herbal teas, or medications, rest, applications of heat or cold, prayer, or distractions like watching TV). It is important to explore the effect that both pharmacological and nonpharmacological interventions had on the pain, including whether or not relief was obtained or whether the pain became worse. Any side effects of pain-relieving interventions should also be documented.

ASSOCIATED SYMPTOMS Also included in a comprehensive pain assessment are other associated symptoms,

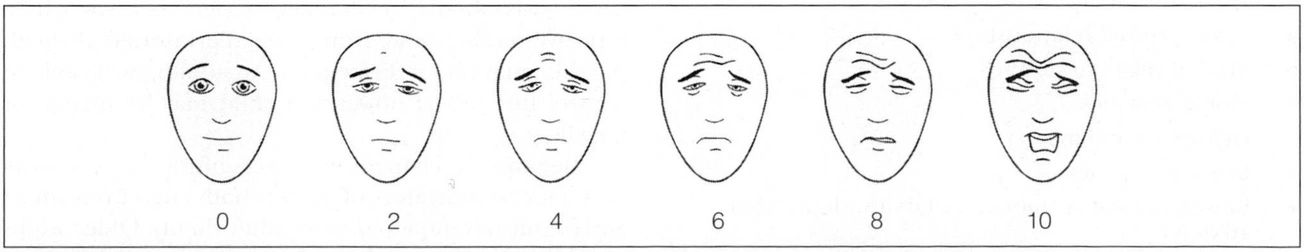

FIGURE 34.8 The Faces Pain Scale—Revised. The left-most face shows no pain, while the right-most face shows very much pain. Clients are asked to point to the face that shows how much they hurt right now. The numbers are not shown to the client, but are used by the nurse to score the indicated level of pain intensity.

Source: From "The Faces Pain Scale—Revised: Toward a Common Metric In Pediatric Pain Measurement," by C. L. Hicks, C. L. von Baeyer, P. A. Spafford, I. van Korlaar, and B. Goodenough, 2001, **Pain**, *93(2), pp. 173–183. Reprinted with permission of the International Association for the Study of Pain. Available online at http://www.painsourcebook.ca*

TABLE 34.4 Short-Form McGill Pain Questionnaire

Patient's Name: Date:

	None	Mild	Moderate	Severe
Throbbing	0)	1)	2)	3)
Shooting	0)	1)	2)	3)
Stabbing	0)	1)	2)	3)
Sharp	0)	1)	2)	3)
Cramping	0)	1)	2)	3)
Gnawing	0)	1)	2)	3)
Hot-Burning	0)	1)	2)	3)
Aching	0)	1)	2)	3)
Heavy	0)	1)	2)	3)
Tender	0)	1)	2)	3)
Splitting	0)	1)	2)	3)
Tiring-Exhausting	0)	1)	2)	3)
Sickening	0)	1)	2)	3)
Fearful	0)	1)	2)	3)
Punishing-Cruel	0)	1)	2)	3)

No pain — Worst Possible Pain

PPI (Point Pain Intensity)

0 No Pain	4 Horrible
1 Mild	5 Excruciating
2 Discomforting	
3 Distressing	

Source: "McGill Pain Questionnaire," by R. Melzack, 1975, *Pain, 1*, 277–299. Reproduced with permission.

such as nausea, vomiting, dizziness, and diarrhea. These symptoms may relate to the onset of the pain or they may result from the presence of the pain.

EFFECT ON ACTIVITIES OF DAILY LIVING Knowing how ADLs are affected by pain helps the nurse understand the client's perspective on the pain's severity. The nurse asks the client to describe how the pain has affected the following aspects of life:

- Sleep
- Appetite
- Concentration
- Work or school
- Interpersonal relationships
- Marital relations and sex
- Home activities
- Driving or walking
- Leisure activities
- Emotional status (mood, irritability, depression, anxiety)

A rating scale of none, a little, or a great deal, or another range, can be used to determine the degree of alteration.

COPING RESOURCES Each individual will exhibit personal ways of coping with pain. Strategies may relate to past pain experiences or the specific meaning of the pain; some may reflect religious or cultural influences. Nurses can encourage and support the client's use of methods that have helped to modify pain in the past. Strategies may include seeking quiet and solitude, learning about their condition, pursuing interesting or exciting activities (for distraction), prayer (or other meaningful rituals), or social support (from family, friends, support groups, etc.).

AFFECTIVE RESPONSES Affective responses vary according to the situation, the degree and duration of pain, the interpretation of it, and many other factors. The nurse needs to explore the client's feelings, such as anxiety, fear, exhaustion, depression, or a sense of failure. Pain affect can be measured by using the "Affective" subscale of the MPQ (Melzack, 1975). Because many people with chronic pain become depressed and potentially suicidal, it may also be necessary to assess the client's suicide risk. In such situations, the nurse needs to ask the client, "Do you ever feel so bad that you want to die? Do you feel that way now?"

Observation of Behavioural and Physiological Responses

People show wide variations in *behavioural responses* to pain. For clients who are very young, aphasic, confused, or disoriented, nonverbal expressions may be the only means of communicating pain. Facial expression is often the first indication of pain, and it may be the only one. Clenched teeth, tightly shut eyes, open sombre eyes, biting of the lower lip, and other facial grimaces may be indicative of pain. Vocalizations like moaning and groaning or crying and screaming are also associated with pain.

Immobilization of the body or a part of the body may also indicate pain. The client with chest pain often holds the left arm across the chest. A person with abdominal pain may assume the position of greatest comfort, often flexing the knees and hips and moving reluctantly.

Purposeless body movements can also indicate pain. For example, clients may toss and turn in bed or fling their arms about. Involuntary movements, such as a reflexive jerking away from a needle inserted through the skin, may also indicate pain. An adult may be able to control this reflex; however, a child may be unable or unwilling to do so.

Behavioural changes, such as confusion and restlessness, may be indicators of pain in both cognitively intact and cognitively impaired older adult clients. Older adults with chronic pain may become hostile or aggressive.

Rhythmic body movements or rubbing may indicate pain. An adult or child may assume a fetal position and rock back and forth when experiencing abdominal pain. During labour, a woman may massage her abdomen rhythmically with her hands.

It is important to note that behavioural responses can be controlled and therefore may not be very revealing. Also, many behavioural responses (e.g., crying) are not unique to pain. When pain is chronic, overt behavioural responses are rare as pain behaviours habituate over time and the individual develops personal coping styles for dealing with the pain.

Physiological responses vary with the origin and duration of the pain. Early in the onset of acute pain, the sympathetic nervous system is stimulated, resulting in increased blood pressure, pulse rate, respiratory rate, pallor, diaphoresis, and pupil dilation. Although the nociceptors do not adapt to painful stimuli, the sympathetic nervous system does adapt, making the physiological responses less evident or even absent. With visceral pain, signs of parasympathetic stimulation may be observed, such as decreased blood pressure and pulse rate, pupil constriction, and warm dry skin. Physiological responses are likely to be absent in people with chronic pain because of CNS adaptation.

Valid and reliable instruments can be used to measure a client's behavioural and physiological responses to pain. For example, the premature infant pain profile (PIPP) (Stevens, Johnston, Petryshen, & Taddio, 1996) is a composite pain instrument that can be used to measure behavioural, physiological, and contextual indicators of pain in neonates.

Daily Pain Diary

For clients who experience chronic pain, a daily diary may help the client and the nurse identify pain patterns and factors that exacerbate or mediate the pain experience. In home care, the family or other caregiver can be taught to complete the diary. The record can include time or onset of pain, activity before pain, pain-related positions or behaviours, pain intensity level, duration of pain, and the use of pharmacological and nonpharmacological pain management strategies. Recorded data can provide the basis for developing or modifying the plan for care. For this tool to be effective, it is important that the client uses it routinely. Therefore, the nurse should educate the client and family about the value and use of the diary in achieving effective pain control. Determining the client's abilities to use the diary is essential.

Diagnosing

NANDA International (2007) includes the following diagnostic labels for clients experiencing pain or discomfort:

- *Acute Pain:* Unpleasant sensory and emotional experience arising from actual or potential tissue damage or described in terms of such damage; sudden or slow onset of any intensity from mild to severe with an anticipated or predictable end and duration of less than 6 months.
- *Chronic Pain:* Unpleasant sensory and emotional experience arising from actual or potential tissue damage; sudden or slow onset of any intensity from mild to severe, constant or recurring without an anticipated or predictable end and a duration of greater than 6 months.

When writing the diagnostic statement, the nurse should specify the location (e.g., right ankle pain, or left frontal headache). Etiological factors and precipitating factors, when known, must also be part of the diagnostic statement and can include both physiological and psychological factors. For example, in addition to the injurious agent, related factors may include knowledge deficit of pain management techniques or fear of drug tolerance or addiction. Clinical examples of assessment data clusters and associated nursing diagnoses are shown in Table 34.5.

Because the presence of pain can affect so many facets of a person's functioning, pain may be the etiology of other nursing diagnoses. Examples of such nursing diagnoses follow:

- *Ineffective Airway Clearance* related to weak cough secondary to postoperative incisional abdominal pain
- *Anxiety* related to past experiences of poor control of pain and to anticipation of pain

TABLE 34.5 Clinical Application: Assessment Data and Related Nursing Diagnoses for a Client Experiencing Pain

Data Cluster	Nursing Diagnosis
Mary Anderson, 75, fell and broke her right hip while shopping. She had surgery yesterday to repair the fracture. She rates her pain in the surgical site as 6 on a 0–10 scale and states the pain goes up to 9 when she is repositioned in bed. Morphine 10 mg q4h prn is ordered. She received a dose 5 hours ago. States, "I try to hold out as long as I can before asking for a pain killer."	*Acute Pain* related to surgical repair of right hip fracture and movement *Deficient Knowledge* related to lack of information or misinformation regarding pain treatment strategies
Lan Nguyen, 51, was diagnosed with breast cancer 3 years ago and had a metastatic lung tumour removed 6 months ago. She describes prolonged post-thoracotomy pain as "hot, stabbing, and unbearable." Lan states that although she loves sewing and needlepoint, she is unable to participate in these activities currently because of the pain.	*Chronic Pain* related to nerve damage and sustained pain sensation *Self-Concept Disturbance* related to inability to participate in sewing and needlepoint

- *Ineffective Coping* related to prolonged continuous back pain, ineffective pain management, and inadequate support systems
- *Ineffective Health Maintenance* related to chronic pain and fatigue
- *Deficient Knowledge* (pain control measures) related to lack of exposure to information resources
- *Impaired Physical Mobility* related to arthritic pain in knee and ankle joints
- *Insomnia* related to increased pain perception at night

Planning

Although the established goals will vary according to the diagnosis and its defining characteristics, individual examples include the following:

- Modify or minimize pain to enable partial or complete resumption of daily activities
- Enhance abilities to control pain
- Demonstrate actions to control pain and associated symptoms

Examples of desired outcomes for each of these goals, although established in the planning phase, are provided in Table 34.10 (page 1010) in the "Evaluating" section of this chapter.

Examples of nursing interventions to assist clients experiencing pain include specific nursing activities associated with each of these interventions, which can be selected to meet the individual needs of the client. See the "Implementing" section of this chapter for details. A Sample Nursing Care Plan is provided.

When planning, nurses need to choose pain relief measures appropriate for the client based on the assessment data and input from the client or support persons.

Sample Care Plan for Acute Pain

ASSESSMENT DATA

Nursing Assessment

Mr. Lee Chin is a 57-year-old Chinese-Canadian businessman who was admitted to the surgical unit of an urban hospital for treatment of a possible strangulated inguinal hernia. Two days ago, he had a partial bowel resection. Postoperative orders include NPO, intravenous infusion of 5% dextrose in 0.45% sodium chloride (D5 1/2NS) at 125 mL/h left arm, nasogastric tube to low intermittent suction. Mr. Chin is in a dorsal recumbent (supine) position and is attempting to draw up his legs. He appears restless and is complaining of pain (7 on a scale of 0 to 10).

Physical Examination

Height: 188 cm

Weight: 90 kg

BMI: 25.5

Temperature: 37°C

Pulse: 90 bpm, 2+ amplitude, regular

Respirations: 24/min

Blood pressure: 158/82 mm Hg

Skin pale and moist, pupils dilated; midline abdominal incision, sutures dry and intact

Diagnostic Data

Chest X-ray and urinalysis negative, WBC 12.0×10^9/L

Nursing Diagnosis

Acute severe pain related to surgical incision stimulation of mechanosensitive receptors (as evidenced by restlessness; pallor; elevated pulse, respirations, and systolic blood pressure; and dilated pupils)

Client Goal

The client will experience minimal abdominal pain and discomfort.

Desired Health Outcomes

1. Pain control as evidenced by demonstrating ability to use analgesics appropriately, use nonpharmacological relief measures, and report uncontrolled symptoms to the health-care team.
2. Pain level controlled as evidenced by no or mild reported pain; protective body positioning; restlessness; perspiration; change in BP, HR, R from normal baseline data.

NURSING INTERVENTIONS AND SELECTED ACTIVITIES WITH RATIONALES [*IN ITALICS*]*

Pain Management

• Perform a comprehensive assessment of pain to include location, characteristics, onset, duration, frequency, quality, intensity or severity, and precipitating factors of pain.	*Pain is a subjective experience and must be described by the client in order to plan effective treatment.*
• Consider cultural influences on Mr. Chin's pain response (e.g., cultural beliefs about pain can result in a stoic attitude).	*Each person experiences and expresses pain in an individual manner by using a variety of sociocultural adaptation techniques.*
• Reduce or eliminate factors that precipitate or increase Mr. Chin's pain experience (e.g., fear, fatigue, monotony, and lack of knowledge).	*Personal factors can influence pain and pain tolerance. Those factors that may be precipitating or augmenting pain should be reduced or eliminated to enhance the overall pain management program.*

(continued)

Sample Care Plan for Acute Pain (*continued*)

• Teach the use of nonpharmacological techniques (e.g., relaxation, guided imagery, music therapy, distraction, and massage) before, after, and, if possible, during painful activities; before pain occurs or increases; and along with other pain relief measures.	*The use of noninvasive pain relief measures can increase the release of endorphins and enhance the therapeutic effects of analgesics.*
• Provide Mr. Chin with optimal pain relief with prescribed analgesics.	*Each client has a right to expect maximum pain relief. Optimal pain relief by using analgesics includes determining the preferred route, drug, dosage, and frequency for each individual.*
• Medicate before an activity to increase participation, but evaluate the hazard of sedation.	*Turning and ambulation activities will be enhanced if pain is controlled.*
• Evaluate the effectiveness of the pain control measures used through ongoing assessment of Mr. Chin's pain experience.	*Research shows that the most common reason for unrelieved pain is failure to routinely assess pain and pain relief. Many clients silently tolerate pain if not specifically asked about it.*
Analgesic Administration	
• Check the prescription for drug, dose, and frequency of analgesic prescribed.	*Ensures that the nurse has the right drug, right route, right dosage, right client, and right frequency.*
• Determine analgesic selections (opioid or non-opioid) based on type and severity of pain.	*Various types of pain (e.g., acute, chronic, neuropathic, arthritic) require different analgesic approaches. Some types of pain respond to non-opioid drugs alone, while others can be relieved by combining a low-dose opioid with the non-opioid.*
• Institute regular dosing and monitoring, as appropriate, if Mr. Chin receives opioid analgesics.	*Side effects of opioid narcotics include drowsiness and sedation.*
• Encourage Mr. Chin to communicate when his pain is at a 4/10 or greater and request prn pain medication for breakthrough pain.	*Severe pain is more difficult to control and increases the client's anxiety and fatigue. The preventive approach to pain management can reduce the total 24-hour analgesic dose.*
• Evaluate the effectiveness of the analgesic at regular, frequent intervals after each administration and especially after the initial doses, also observing for any signs and symptoms of untoward effects (e.g., respiratory depression, nausea and vomiting, dry mouth, and constipation).	*The analgesic dose may not be adequate to raise the client's pain threshold or may be causing intolerable or dangerous side effects or both. Ongoing evaluation will assist in making necessary adjustments for effective pain management.*
• Document Mr. Chin's response to analgesics and any untoward effects.	*Documentation facilitates pain management by communicating effective and ineffective pain management strategies to the entire health-care team.*
• Implement actions to decrease untoward effects of analgesics (e.g., constipation and gastric irritation).	*Constipation is a common side effect of opioid narcotics and a treatment plan to prevent occurrence should be instituted at the beginning of analgesic therapy. For Mr. Chin, constipation could result from his primary condition or his analgesia. Assess for overall gastrointestinal (GI) functioning, possible complications of surgery, as well as opioid-induced constipation or gastritis caused by non-steroidal anti-inflammatory drugs (NSAIDs).*
Simple Relaxation Therapy	
• Consider Mr. Chin's willingness and ability to participate, preference, past experiences, and contraindications before selecting a specific relaxation strategy.	*The client must feel comfortable trying a different approach to pain management. To avoid ineffective strategies, the client should be involved in the planning process.*
• Elicit behaviours that are conditioned to produce relaxation, such as deep breathing, yawning, abdominal breathing, or peaceful imaging.	*Relaxation techniques help reduce skeletal muscle tension, which will reduce the intensity of the pain.*

(continued)

Sample Care Plan for Acute Pain (*continued*)

• Create a quiet, nondisruptive environment with dim lights and comfortable temperature, when possible.	*Comfort and a quiet atmosphere promote a relaxed feeling and permit the client to focus on the relaxation technique, rather than on external distraction.*
• Individualize the content of the relaxation intervention (e.g., by asking for suggestions about what Mr. Chin enjoys or finds relaxing).	*Each person may find different images or approaches to relaxation more helpful than others.*
• Demonstrate and practise the relaxation technique with Mr. Chin.	*Return demonstrations by the participant provide an opportunity for the nurse to evaluate the effectiveness of teaching sessions.*
• Evaluate and document his response to relaxation therapy.	*Conveys to the health-care team effective strategies in reducing or eliminating pain.*

EVALUATION

Outcomes partially met. The client verbalizes pain and discomfort, requesting analgesics at onset of pain. States "the pain is a 2" (on a scale of 0 to 10) 30 minutes after parenteral analgesic administration. Practises rhythmic breathing q3 to 4h during the day and requests analgesic 30 minutes before ambulation. Remains hesitant to cough and deep breathe even following analgesic administration on second postoperative day.

*Interventions and activities selected are only a sample of those suggested in the *Nursing Interventions Classification (NIC),* by G. M. Bulechek, H. K. Butcher, and J. C. Dochterman (Eds.), 2008, St. Louis, MO: Mosby Elsevier, and should be individualized for each client.

Nursing interventions can include a variety of pharmacological and nonpharmacological interventions. Developing a plan that incorporates a wide range of strategies is usually most effective. Whether in acute care or in home care, it is important for everyone involved in pain management to understand the plan of care. The plan should be documented in the client's record; in home care, a copy needs to be made available to the client, support persons, and caregivers. Involvement of the client and support persons is essential in pain management.

When the client's pattern and level of pain can be anticipated or is already known, regular or scheduled administration of analgesics can provide a therapeutic plasma level. The importance and meaning of a stable drug level in pain management should be explained to the patient. With acute pain, this may be possible in the first 24 to 48 hours following surgery, when the client is likely to have pain requiring opioid analgesics. Frequency of administration can be adjusted to prevent pain from recurring. When persistent cancer-related pain exists, analgesics should be given around the clock (ATC) with additional breakthrough (as needed: prn) doses available. Nonpharmacological interventions should also be regularly scheduled. The additional advantage of scheduling measures is that the client spends less time in pain and does not experience the anxiety or fear of the pain recurring.

Planning for Home Care

In preparation for discharge, the nurse needs to determine the client's and family's needs, strengths, and resources. The Assessment: Home Care box describes the specific assessment data required when establishing a discharge plan. By using the assessment data, the nurse tailors a teaching plan for the client and family (see the Teaching: Home Care box on monitoring pain).

Implementing

Pain management is the alleviation of pain or a reduction in pain to a level of comfort that is acceptable to the client. It includes two basic types of nursing interventions: pharmacological and nonpharmacological interventions. Nursing management of pain consists of both independent and collaborative nursing actions. In general, noninvasive measures can be performed as an independent nursing function, whereas administration of analgesic medications requires a physician's prescription. However, the decision to administer the prescribed medication is frequently the nurse's, often requiring judgment as to the dose to be given and the time of administration.

ASSESSMENT: HOME CARE

Pain

The nurse needs to determine the client's and family's ability to effectively cope with pain once the client is discharged:

CLIENT

- *Level of knowledge:* Pharmacological and non-pharmacological pain relief measures selected; adverse effects and measures to counteract these effects; warning signs to report to health-care provider
- *Self-care abilities for analgesic administration:* Ability to use analgesics appropriately (e.g., to prepare correct dosages of analgesics and adhere to scheduled administration); physical dexterity to take pills or to administer intravenous medications and to store medications safely; and ability to obtain prescriptions or over-the-counter medications at the pharmacy

FAMILY

- *Caregiver availability, skills, and willingness:* Primary and secondary persons able and willing to assist with pain management; shopping if the client has restricted activity; ability to comprehend selected therapies (e.g., infusion pumps, imagery, massage, positioning, and relaxation techniques) and perform them or assist the client with them, as needed
- *Family role changes and coping:* Effect on financial status, parenting and spousal roles, sexuality, social roles

COMMUNITY

- *Resources:* Availability of and familiarity with resources, such as supplies, home care aid, or financial assistance

TEACHING: HOME CARE

Monitoring Pain

Understanding pain and monitoring it for changes are important tasks when a client returns home:

- Teach client to keep a pain diary to monitor pain onset, activity before pain, pain intensity, aggravating and alleviating factors, use of analgesics or other relief measures.
- Instruct client to contact a health-care professional if planned pain control measures are ineffective or adverse effects arise and are problematic.

PAIN CONTROL

- Teach the use of selected nonpharmacological techniques, such as relaxation, guided imagery, distraction, music therapy, massage, and so on.
- Discuss the actions, potential adverse effects, dosages, frequency, and route of administration of prescribed analgesics.
- Suggest ways to handle adverse effects of medications.
- Provide accurate information about tolerance, physical dependence, and addiction if opioid analgesics are prescribed and these topics are of concern.
- Instruct the client to use pain control measures *before* the pain becomes moderate to severe.
- Inform the client of the consequences of untreated pain.
- Demonstrate and have the client or caregiver redemonstrate appropriate skills to administer analgesics (e.g., skin patches, injections, infusion pumps, or patient-controlled analgesia) when appropriate. If a home infusion pump is being used, caregivers need to be able to do the following:
  - **a.** Demonstrate stopping and starting the pump
  - **b.** Change the medication cartridge and tubing
  - **c.** Adjust the delivery dose
  - **d** Demonstrate site care
  - **e.** Identify signs indicating the need to change an infusion site
  - **f.** Describe care of the pump and insertion site when the client is ambulatory, bathing, sleeping, or travelling
  - **g.** Perform problem solving for pumps when alarms are activated
  - **h.** Change the battery

RESOURCES

Nurses should provide appropriate information about how to access community resources, home care agencies, and associations that offer self-help strategies and educational materials. Examples of these are the Canadian Pain Coalition, Victorian Order of Nurses, Canadian Cancer Society, and the Chronic Pain Association of Canada (see the Weblinks section of this chapter for websites).

Generally speaking, a combination of strategies is best for the client in pain. Sometimes strategies need to be tried and changed until the client obtains effective pain relief.

Barriers to Pain Management

Misbeliefs and knowledge deficits of nurses, other health professionals, and clients can interfere with effective pain management. Some of these involve attitudes of the nurse or the client as well as knowledge deficits. Clients respond to pain experiences on the basis of their culture, personal experiences, and the meaning the pain has for them. For many people, pain is expected and accepted as a normal aspect of illness and treatments, such as surgery. Clients and families may lack knowledge of the adverse effects of pain and may have misinformation and fears regarding the use of analgesics. Clients may not report pain because they expect nothing can be done, they think it is not severe enough, or they feel it would distract or prejudice the health care provided. Other common misbeliefs are shown in Table 34.6.

Key Strategies in Pain Management

ACKNOWLEDGING AND ACCEPTING Basic to effective pain management is comprehensive pain assessment (see the "Assessing" section), which begins with believing the client. Four ways of communicating this belief follow:

1. Verbally acknowledge the presence of the pain and use standardized measures to clarify pain intensity, quality, and impact.
2. Listen attentively to what the client says about the pain, restating your understanding of the reported discomfort. Use empathetic statements, such as "I'm sorry you are hurting. It must be upsetting. I want to help you feel better."
3. Convey that you need to understand the client's pain experience and whether pain treatments are effective or not. Ask, for example, "Has the pain treatment reduced the intensity of your pain?"
4. Attend to the client's needs for pain relief promptly. It is unconscionable to believe the patient's report of pain and then do nothing!

TABLE 34.6 Common Misbeliefs about Pain

Misbelief	Correction
Clients experience severe pain only when they have had major surgery.	Even after minor surgery, clients can experience intense pain.
The nurse or other health-care professionals are the authorities on a client's pain.	The person who experiences the pain is the only authority on its existence and nature.
Administering analgesics regularly for pain will lead to addiction.	Clients are unlikely to become addicted to an analgesic provided to treat pain.
The amount of tissue damage is directly related to the amount of pain.	Pain is a subjective experience, and the intensity and duration of pain vary considerably among individuals.
Visible physiological or behavioural signs accompany pain and can be used to verify its existence.	Even with severe pain, periods of physiological and behavioural adaptation can occur.

ASSISTING SUPPORT PERSONS Support persons often need assistance to respond positively to the client experiencing pain. Nurses can help by giving them accurate information about the pain and providing opportunities for them to discuss their emotional reactions, which may include anger, fear, frustration, and feelings of inadequacy. Enlisting the aid of support persons in the provision of pain relief to the client, such as by massaging the client's back, may diminish their feelings of helplessness and foster a more positive attitude toward the client's pain experience. Support persons also may need the nurse's understanding and reassurance, and perhaps access to resources that will help them cope as they add the caregiver role to an already stressful life circumstance.

REDUCING MISBELIEFS ABOUT PAIN Misbeliefs refer to incorrect beliefs that are thought to be true despite evidence to the contrary. It is important to recognize that people's beliefs about pain and their related responses to pain and treatments can be deeply entrenched and a function of a complex array of contextual and societal factors. Reducing a client's misbeliefs about the pain and its treatment will help to guard against inadequate pain management. The nurse should explain to clients that pain is a highly individualized experience and that they need to help clinicians understand their pain experience. Misbeliefs are also dealt with when nurses and clients have comprehensive discussions about the client's pain experience, including the intensity and quality of the pain, the impact of the pain, its aggravating and alleviating factors, and any fears and concerns the client may be struggling with, such as fears of opioid addiction or common opioid adverse effects, such as constipation (Watt-Watson, 1992; Watt-Watson et al., 2001).

REDUCING FEAR AND ANXIETY It is important to address the meaning of pain, along with emotional components, such as anxiety or fear, associated with the pain experience. When clients have no opportunity to talk about the pain and associated fears, their perceptions and reactions to the pain can intensify; in particular, the meaning of pain can affect pain intensity (Arntz & Claassens, 2004). If the nurse establishes an effective pattern of assessment and communication and promptly attends to the client's pain-related needs, effective pain relief is more likely. By providing accurate information, the nurse can also reduce many of the client's fears, such as a fear of addiction or a fear that the pain will always be present.

PREVENTING PAIN A preventive approach to pain relief involves the provision of measures to treat the pain before it occurs or before it becomes moderate to severe. **Preemptive analgesia** is the administration of analgesics before an invasive or operative procedure in order to treat pain before it occurs. For example, evidence suggests that treating clients perioperatively with local infiltration of an anaesthetic or parenteral administration of an opioid can reduce postoperative pain and decrease the potential for the development of chronic pain (Katz, 2003). Intra-operative and postoperative administration of analgesics is also important for optimal pain relief. Nurses can use a preemptive approach by providing analgesic as prescribed ATC, rather than prn.

Pharmacological Pain Management

Pharmacological pain management involves the use of opioids, nonsteroidal anti-inflammatory drugs (NSAIDs), and coanalgesics (see Box 34.3).

OPIOID ANALGESICS Opioid analgesics include naturally occurring and synthetic opium derivatives, such as morphine and codeine. Opioids were commonly referred to in clinical settings as *narcotics*; this language is not appropriate as narcotics include drugs not used for pain treatment. Opioids relieve pain by binding to opiate receptors and activating endogenous pain modulation in the CNS. Opiate receptors are of several different types, including mu, delta, and kappa receptors. The mu receptor is most commonly associated with pain relief. These drugs are prescribed by a physician or nurse practitioner practising under medical directive. The nurse requires knowledge of appropriate dose, duration of effect, time to onset, and strategies to manage adverse effects.

Opioids come in three primary types:

1. *Full agonists.* **Full agonists** bind to opioid receptors, mimicking the effects of endogenous opioids, or endorphins. Examples of full agonists include morphine, codeine, and hydromorphone (Dilaudid). Meperidine (Demerol) is also a full agonist, but is *not recommended* (see the Clinical Alert). Full agonists have no **ceiling dose**, the level at which increasing the dose results in no further increase in analgesia. Hence, their dose can be steadily increased to relieve pain.
2. *Mixed agonists-antagonists.* **Agonist-antagonist analgesic** drugs can act like opioids and relieve pain (agonist effect) when given to a client who has not taken any pure opioids. However, they can block or inactivate other opioid analgesics when given to a client who has been taking pure opioids (antagonist effect). These drugs include dezocine (Dalgan), pentazocine hydrochloride (Talwin), butorphanol tartrate (Stadol), and nalbuphine hydrochloride (Nubain). They block the mu receptor site and activate a kappa receptor site. If a client has been receiving a mu agonist (e.g., morphine) daily for more than a couple of weeks, the administration of a mixed agonist-antagonist may result in the inactivation of the morphine effect and increase pain. These drugs have a **ceiling effect** (larger doses of a medication have progressively smaller incremental effects) that limits the dose. They are not recommended for use in terminally ill clients.
3. *Partial agonists.* **Partial agonists** have a ceiling effect. These drugs, such as buprenorphine (Buprenex), block the mu receptors or are neutral at that receptor but bind at a kappa receptor site. Buprenorphine has good analgesic potency and is emerging as an alternative to methadone for opioid maintenance treatment programs.

BOX 34.3 CATEGORIES AND EXAMPLES OF ANALGESICS

The following are just some of the analgesics available:

OPIOID ANALGESICS

- Fentanyl citrate (Duragesic)
- Oxycodone (OxyContin)
- Hydromorphone hydrochloride (Dilaudid)
- Morphine sulphate (morphine)
- Codeine (Tylenol No. 3)

NON-OPIOID ANALGESICS

- Acetaminophen (Tylenol)
- Acetylsalicylic acid (Aspirin)
- Diclofenac sodium (Voltaren)
- Ibuprofen (Motrin, Advil)
- Indomethacin sodium trihydrate (Indocid)
- Naprosyn (Naproxen)
- Piroxicam (Feldene)
- Tolmetin sodium (Tolectin)
- Celecoxib (Celebrex)

COANALGESICS

- Antidepressants (amitriptyline [Elavil] nortriptyline [Aventyl])
- Anticonvulsants (carbamazepine [Tegretol], gabapentin [Neurontin])

CLINICAL ALERT

Nurses must challenge the general use of meperidine (i.e., Demerol) in the clinical setting. This drug has a short duration (2 to 3 hours), and its toxic metabolite, normeperidine, accumulates with repetitive dosing, causing CNS excitability and possibly seizures.

Opioids are the most effective analgesic for the relief of moderate to severe pain and must be given on a regular basis to prevent pain from recurring. Acetaminophen is thought to work on the CNS and is commonly used in combination with a number of opioids, such as oxycodone (e.g., Percocet), codeine (e.g., Tylenol No. 1, Tylenol No. 2, Tylenol No. 3, Tylenol No. 4).

Adverse effects of opioids vary with the physiological state of the patient. Constipation is the most common side effect. **Opioid antagonists**, such as naloxone hydrochloride (Narcan), bind to opioid receptors but do not activate them, effectively blocking the action of opioids. Opioid antagonists hydrochloride will reverse any depressive effect.

Box 34.4 provides suggested measures to prevent side effects of opioid analgesics. As sedation can occur in some instances, nurses should assess and document the client's level of sedation. If sedation is a problem, respiratory status must also be frequently monitored. Early recognition of an increasing level of sedation or respiratory depression will enable the nurse to implement appropriate measures promptly.

When administering opioids, it is important to distinguish among the effects of *tolerance, physical dependence,* and *addiction.* With **tolerance**, progressively larger doses are needed to produce the same analgesic effects; with **physical dependence**, people experience a need to continue to use the drug to prevent symptoms of withdrawal; with **addiction**, adverse behaviour is present that features a compulsion for the drug and a preoccupation with drug use predominantly for psychological effect, despite actual or potential harm.

Drug tolerance can occur for some clients with some conditions, usually when pain is first being controlled or when the pain increases. The need for dose escalation can often be disease or pain progression, rather than tolerance. Drug tolerance is a physiological response to opioids and requires increasing the dose until pain relief is attained. Because full agonist opioids do not have a ceiling or maximum amount, drug tolerance should not preclude achievement of adequate analgesia, with incremental dosage increases, as ordered. Physical dependence is characterized by withdrawal symptoms concomitant with sudden decrease or abrupt termination of opioid use, or administration of an opioid antagonist. Withdrawal symptoms can include vomiting, diarrhea, abdominal cramping, tremors, chills, diaphoresis, myalgia, arthralgia (joint pain not caused by inflammation), and coryza (inflammation of the mucous membranes of the nose). Physical dependence and drug tolerance are involuntary behaviours and are the physiological result of frequent ongoing opioid administration. Although physical dependence and tolerance develop, symptoms of withdrawal rarely occur because, as pain decreases, the dosage is gradually tapered and no symptoms are experienced. *Physical dependence and drug tolerance do not represent addiction.* Determination of opioid addiction requires expert assessment of client history and risks factors for addiction and potential biopsychological factors that may be involved. Clinicians should not presume that patients' persistence or expression of the urgent need for pain relief is drug seeking or addictive behaviour. True opioid addiction is rare if opioids are prescribed and monitored appropriately. It is important to note that opioids can be effective for those with a

BOX 34.4 OPIOID ADVERSE EFFECTS: PREVENTIVE AND TREATMENT MEASURES

Opioids can have a number of side effects that nurses can help to alleviate:

CONSTIPATION

- Increase fluid intake (e.g., 6 to 8 glasses daily).
- Add more fibre and bulk-forming agents to the diet (e.g., fresh fruits and vegetables). Increased exercise is often ineffective in controlling this type of constipation.
- Administer daily stool softeners combined with a mild laxative (e.g., Senokot-S) as a first line of prevention against constipation for clients on opioid maintenance therapy.
- Stimulants (e.g., bisacodyl), osmotic laxatives (e.g., lactulose, sorbitol, and polyethylene glycol), enemas (e.g., tap water and sodium phosphate), and even prokinetic agents (e.g., metoclopramide) can be needed for refractory cases of constipation.

NAUSEA AND VOMITING

- Inform the client that tolerance to this emetic effect generally develops after several days of opioid therapy.
- Provide an antiemetic, as required.
- Change the dose or analgesic agent, as indicated.

SEDATION

- Inform the client that tolerance usually develops over several days.
- Observe the client for evidence of respiratory depression that may occur with sedation.

RESPIRATORY DEPRESSION

- If the client is receiving intravenous patient-controlled analgesia (PCA), stop, change, or slow the infusion and continually reassess.
- Administer an opioid antagonist, such as naloxone (Narcan), until respirations return to an acceptable rate. Follow agency policy for administration and monitoring.

PRURITUS

- Apply cool packs and lotion, and provide a diversional activity.
- Administer an antihistamine (e.g., diphenhydramine hydrochloride [Benadryl]) as ordered.
- Inform the client that tolerance also develops to pruritus.

URINARY RETENTION

- The nurse may need to catheterize the client or change or lower the opioid dose.
- Administer narcotic antagonist (naloxone [Narcan]) as ordered, according to agency policy.

history of chemical dependency on opioids; this requires prescription, supervision, and support by clinicians with expertise in pain management and chemical dependency. Guidelines for safe administration of opioids are available from a number of pain societies, such as the Canadian Pain Society and the International Association for the Study of Pain (see the Weblinks section of this chapter for websites).

EQUIANALGESIC DOSING As nurses are responsible for evaluating the effectiveness of analgesics, monitoring for adverse effects, and advocating for change when an analgesic in not effective, it is important to understand the concept of **equianalgesia**, which refers to the relative potency of various opioid analgesics compared with a standard dose of parenteral morphine. An equianalgesic dose is the dose of one analgesic that has the same pain-relieving effect as another drug. This concept makes it possible to change one analgesic for another or to change the route of administration, for example, from parenteral to oral opioid doses. Equianalgesic dosing also allows comparisons to be made between weak analgesics, such as codeine, for mild pain, and stronger analgesics, such as morphine, for moderate to severe pain.

The two basic techniques for calculating doses based on equianalgesic equivalents are the ratio and cross-multiplication methods. For example, with the ratio technique, it is known that the oral:IV morphine ratio is 3:1, meaning IV morphine is 3 times as potent as oral morphine. Thus, a client who has required 100 mg of IV morphine per day will require 300 mg of oral morphine per day to control the same level of pain. If a different client who had an opioid requirement of 40 mg IV morphine per day were to be switched to oral Dilaudid, the equianalgesia chart informs the nurse that 10 mg IV morphine is equivalent to 7.5 mg hydromorphone (Dilaudid). By using the cross-multiplication technique (x represents the unknown dose), the following steps are calculated:

10 mg IV morphine = 7.5 mg oral hydromorphone
40 mg IV morphine = x mg hydromorphone
Cross-multiply:

$$10x = 7.5 \times 40$$
$$10x = 300$$
$$x = 30 \text{ mg hydromorphone}$$

Thus, 30 mg oral hydromorphone per day would provide equivalent analgesia to 40 mg of parenteral morphine per day. The hydromorphone dose is then divided based on the duration of action of the available preparations (e.g., Dilaudid every 4 hours).

NONSTEROIDAL ANTI-INFLAMMATORY DRUGS (NSAIDS) **Nonsteroidal anti-inflammatory drugs (NSAIDs)**, sometimes referred to as non-opioids, include such drugs as Aspirin and ibuprofen. These analgesics have anti-inflammatory, analgesic, and antipyretic effects. They relieve pain by mainly inhibiting the synthesis of prostaglandins, which sensitize nerve endings and trigger pain. Individual drugs in this category vary widely in their analgesic properties, metabolism, excretion, and adverse effects. In addition, the analgesic activity of these drugs has a ceiling effect.

The most common adverse effect of NSAIDs is dyspepsia, which can be minimized by taking the medication with food. Stomach ulcers and gastric bleeding have also been reported; those on longer-term NSAID therapy may be prescribed proton-pump inhibitors to preserve the gastric mucosa. NSAIDs may be contraindicated for those with impaired blood clotting, gastrointestinal bleeding or ulcer risk, renal disease, thrombocytopenia (low platelet levels), Aspirin triad (i.e., bronchial asthma, Aspirin intolerance, and rhinitis), and possible infection. Many NSAIDs require a prescription and all have a maximum daily dose limit. Depending on the nature of the pain problem, NSAIDs may be prescribed in combination with opioids or coanalgesics.

Evidence-Informed Practice

Can a Self-Management Program Help Clients Cope with Chronic Cardiac Pain?

McGillion, Watt-Watson, Lefort, and Stevens (2007) conducted a qualitative study that followed a group of people suffering from chronic cardiac pain to evaluate whether feelings of control and self-efficacy could be increased, and feelings of anger and frustration could be reduced, by using a nurse-led standardized angina psychoeducation program called the Chronic Angina Self-Management Program. The participants and interested family members shared coping strategies, clarified misbeliefs about their pain, discussed angina-management strategies, learned about lifestyle factors influencing their pain, and practised stress reduction and relaxation techniques. At the end of the program "participants experienced positive shifts in the meaning of their cardiac pain" (p. 61): although they knew their chronic pain experience would not go away, they felt better able to manage it and maintain a satisfying quality of life.

NURSING IMPLICATIONS: Coping with chronic pain can be debilitating, both psychologically and physically. The relatively short nursing intervention using the Chronic Angina Self-Management Program provides nurses with an alternative resource to help clients deal with their potentially debilitating situation.

Source: Based on "Positive Shifts in the Perceived Meaning of Cardiac Pain Following a Psychoeducation Program for Chronic Stable Angina," by M. McGillion, J. Watt-Watson, S. LeFort, and B. Stevens, 2007, *Canadian Journal of Nursing Research, 39*(2), pp. 48–65.

Acetaminophen (Tylenol) has a different mechanism of action and side effect or toxicity profile. It does not affect platelet function and rarely causes GI distress, ulcers, or skin or cardiovascular problems. Hepatotoxicity, and possibly renal toxicity, does occur with higher doses or with long-term use. Generally, 10 g of acetaminophen is considered a lethal dose, with 6 g per day causing measurable liver damage. It is recommended that otherwise young and healthy people limit acetaminophen consumption to less than 4 g/day, with susceptible individuals (e.g., older adults, those with a history of alcoholism, those with liver disease) limiting their consumption to 2.4 g/day or less.

Misbeliefs about non-opioids are presented in Table 34.7.

COANALGESICS A **coanalgesic** agent (formerly known as an adjuvant) is a medication that is not classified as a pain medication but that has properties that can reduce pain, alone or in combination with other analgesics; relieve other discomforts; potentiate the effect of pain medications; or reduce the pain medication's side effects. Examples of coanalgesics are antidepressants, such as amitriptyline (Elavil) or nortriptyline (Aventyl), which interfere with the reuptake of epinephrine and serotonin, leading to reduced pain perception when given in low doses.

Anticonvulsants, such as carbamazepine (Tegretol), stabilize nerve membranes, reducing excitability and spontaneous firing. Anxiolytics, sedatives, and antispasmotics are examples of medicines that relieve other discomforts but do not alleviate pain and thus should be used in addition to, rather than instead of, analgesics. Examples of medications used to reduce the side effects of analgesics include stimulants, laxatives, and antiemetics.

Coanalgesics appear to be particularly beneficial for the management of neuropathic pain. Tricyclic antidepressant drugs seem to be particularly useful for central neuropathic pain, which often manifests as pain with a burning, unusual, or stinging quality. Anticonvulsant drugs, like gabapentin (Neurontin), seem particularly useful for peripheral neuropathic conditions that often present with a stabbing, shooting, or electrical-shock quality. There is a growing scientific and clinical basis for the use of these medications in relieving pain, especially for persistent pain that is not relieved by the analgesic classes of medication alone.

Placebo Response

The **placebo response** occurs when people experience pain relief from an intervention that may not be directly related to the actual pain relief method employed.

TABLE 34.7 Misbeliefs about Non-opioids

Misbelief	Correction
Regular daily use of NSAIDs is much safer than taking opioids.	Side effects from long-term use of NSAIDs are considerably more severe and life threatening than the side effects from daily doses of oral morphine or other opioids. The most common side effect from long-term use of opioids is constipation, whereas NSAIDs can cause gastric ulcers, increased bleeding time, and renal insufficiency. Acetaminophen can cause hepatotoxicity.
A non-opioid should not be given at the same time as an opioid.	It is safe to administer a non-opioid and opioid at the same time. Giving a dose of non-opioid at the same time as a dose of opioid poses no more danger than giving the doses at different times. In fact, many opioids are compounded with a non-opioid (e.g., Percocet [oxycodone and acetaminophen]).
Administering antacids with NSAIDs is an effective method of reducing gastric distress.	Administering antacids with NSAIDs can lessen distress but may be counterproductive. Antacids reduce the absorption and therefore the effectiveness of the NSAID by releasing the drug in the stomach rather than in the small intestine where absorption occurs.
Non-opioids are not useful analgesics for severe pain.	Non-opioids alone are rarely sufficient to relieve severe pain, but they are an important part in the total analgesic plan. One of the basic principles of analgesic therapy is: Whenever pain is severe enough to require an opioid, adding a non-opioid should be considered.
Gastric distress (e.g., abdominal pain) is indicative of NSAID-induced gastric ulceration.	Most clients with gastric lesions have no symptoms until bleeding or perforation occurs.

Source: From *Pain: Clinical Manual*, 2nd ed., by M. McCaffery and C. Pasero, 1999, St. Louis, MO: Mosby. Reprinted with permission from Elsevier Science.

Health professionals can cause a positive placebo response by the ways they interact with patients. The nurse's empathic approach toward the patient, such as listening without judgment, giving opportunities to express pain and permission to do so, and recognizing the person's unique responses help to facilitate pain relief. Medication placebos, such as giving a saline injection instead of an opioid, are unethical.

Routes for Opioid Delivery

Opioids have traditionally been administered by oral routes, subcutaneous routes and continuous subcutaneous infusions, intramuscular routes, and intravenous routes. In addition, newer methods of delivering opioids have been developed where these routes are not feasible; examples are transnasal, transdermal, and rectal drug therapy, and intraspinal infusion.

ORAL Oral administration of opioids remains the preferred route of delivery because of ease of administration. Because the duration of action of most immediate release (IR) opioids is approximately 4 hours, people with chronic pain have had to awaken several times during the night to medicate themselves for pain. To circumvent this problem, *long-acting* or slow-release forms of opioids with a duration of 8 to 12 hours have been developed. Examples of long-acting preparations are MS Contin, OxyContin, and Hydromorph Contin. Clients receiving long-acting preparations also need prn doses of immediate-release analgesics (e.g., short-acting morphine, Percocet) for acute breakthrough pain.

SUBCUTANEOUS The subcutaneous (SC) route has been used extensively to deliver opioids, and another technique uses subcutaneous catheters and infusion pumps to provide *continuous subcutaneous infusion* (CSCI). The SC route is helpful for people who need long-term use of parenteral opioids and are unable to take opioids orally over the long-term, such as those experiencing dysphagia or gastrointestinal obstruction. CSCI involves the use of a small, light, battery-operated pump that administers the drug through a 23- or 25-gauge butterfly needle. The needle should be rotated between sites on the abdomen and thigh areas every 3 to 7 days. Patient mobility can be maintained by attaching the pump to a belt, or using a shoulder bag or holster to hold the pump (Figure 34.9).

Because the client or the caregivers must operate the pump and change and care for the injection site, the nurse needs to provide appropriate instruction on assessment of pump functioning and care. Clients or their caregivers need to be able to do the following:

- Describe the basic parts and symbols of the system
- Identify ways to determine whether the pump is working

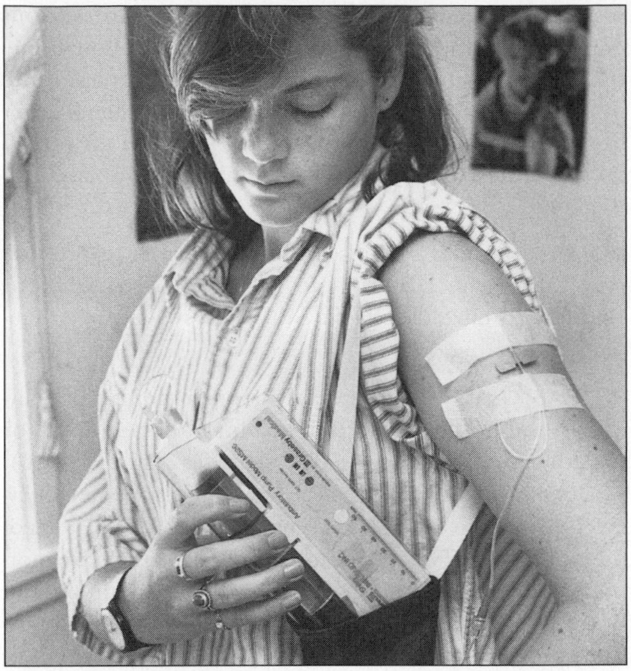

FIGURE 34.9 A continuous subcutaneous infusion device

- Change the battery
- Change the medication
- Demonstrate stopping and starting the pump
- Demonstrate tubing care, site care, and changing of the injection site
- Identify signs indicating the need to change an injection site
- Describe general care of the pump when the client is ambulatory, bathing, sleeping, or travelling
- Identify ways to solve problems when the alarm signals or when the pump is not working

INTRAMUSCULAR The intramuscular (IM) route should not be used; it is the least desirable route for opioid administration because of variable absorption, pain involved with administration, and the need to repeat administration every 3 to 4 hours.

INTRAVENOUS The intravenous (IV) route provides rapid and effective relief of acute pain. The analgesic can be administered by continuous IV infusion, or by patient-controlled analgesia (PCA) (see the discussion on PCA later in this chapter).

TRANSNASAL Transnasal administration has the advantage of rapid action of the medication because of direct absorption through the vascular nasal mucosa. A commonly used agent is the mixed agonist-antagonist butorphanol (Stadol) for acute headaches.

TRANSDERMAL Transdermal drug therapy is advantageous in that it delivers a relatively stable plasma drug level and is noninvasive. Fentanyl (Duragesic) is an opioid currently available as a skin patch with various dosages. It provides drug delivery for up to 72 hours. The transdermal route is distinguished from the topical route in that the effects of the medications are systemic after the medication is absorbed; topical medications placed on the skin work locally at the point they are placed on the body.

RECTAL Several opioids are now available in suppository form. The rectal route is particularly useful for clients who have dysphagia (difficulty swallowing), nausea, or vomiting.

INTRASPINAL An increasingly popular method of delivery is the infusion of opioids into the epidural or intrathecal (subarachnoid) space (Figure 34.10). Analgesics administered via the intraspinal route are delivered adjacent to the opioid receptors in the dorsal horn of the spinal cord. Two commonly used medications are morphine sulphate and fentanyl. All medicines administered by the intraspinal route need to be sterile and preservative free (preservatives are neurotoxic). The major benefit of intraspinal drug therapy is superior analgesia with less medication used. The epidural space is most commonly used because the dura mater acts as a protective barrier against infection, including meningitis, and there is less risk of developing a spinal headache. Intraspinal catheters are not in constant contact with blood, and thus an infusion can be stopped and restarted later without concern that the catheter has become clotted off.

Intrathecal administration delivers medication directly into the cerebrospinal fluid (CSF) that bathes and nourishes the spinal cord. Medicines quickly and efficiently bind to the opioid receptor sites in the dorsal horn when administered in this way, speeding the onset and peak effect, while prolonging the duration of action of the analgesic. An example of how the route of administration affects the relative potency of opioids is as follows. A client who needs 300 mg of oral morphine per day to control pain will need 100 mg of parenteral morphine, 10 mg of epidural morphine, and only 1 mg of intrathecal morphine in a 24-hour period. Very little drug is absorbed by blood vessels into the systemic circulation. In fact, the drug must circulate through the CSF to be excreted. As a result, onset of respiratory depression can be delayed (24 hours after the administration) as medication that has left the spinal opioid sites travels through the brain to be eliminated.

In contrast, the epidural space is separated from the spinal cord by the dura mater, which acts as a barrier to drug diffusion. In addition, it is filled with fatty tissue and an extensive venous system. With this diffusion delay, some medications (especially fat-soluble medications like fentanyl) from the epidural space enter the systemic circulation via the venous plexus. Thus, a higher dose of opiate is required to create the desired effect, which can produce side effects of itching, urinary retention, and respiratory depression. Often, a mixture of an opioid (e.g., fentanyl) and a local anaesthetic (e.g., bupivacaine) are combined to lower the dose of opioid needed. As a result, there may be an increase in fall risk for some clients who develop muscular weakness in their legs or orthostatic hypotension in response to the local anaesthetic.

Intraspinal analgesia can be administered by three modes of operation:

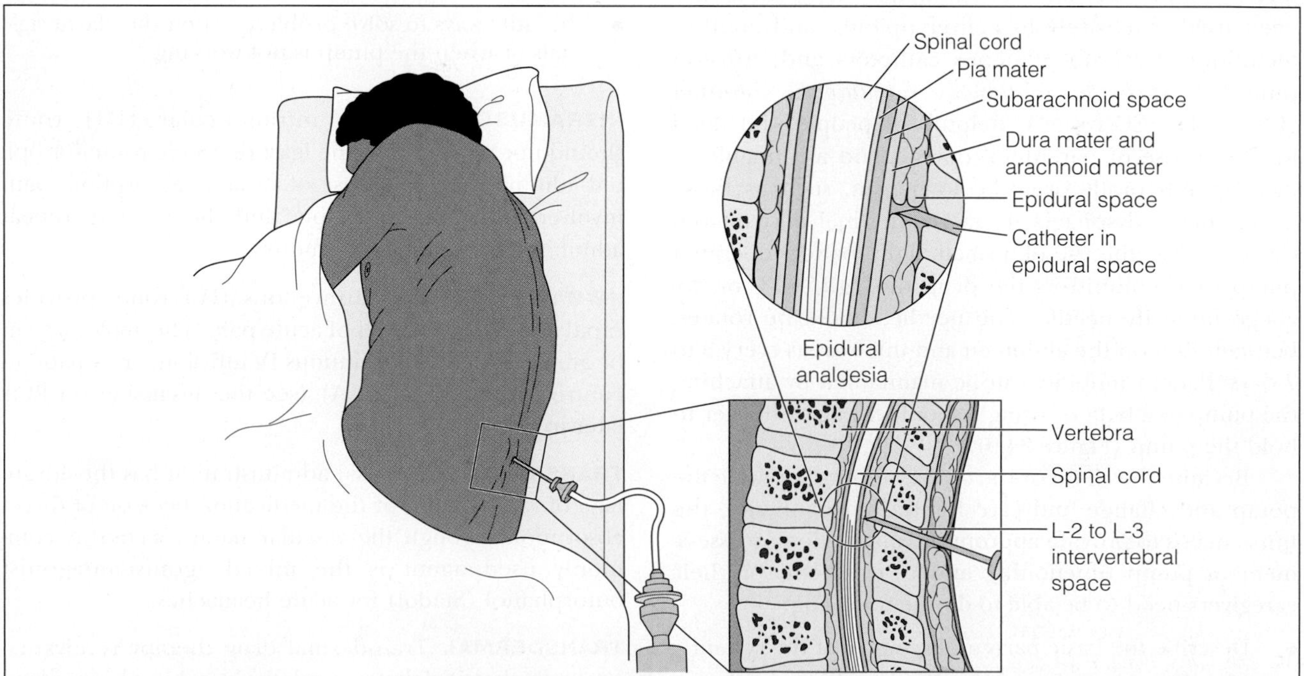

FIGURE 34.10 Placement of intraspinal catheter in the epidural space

1. *Bolus.* A single dose, or repeated bolus doses, can be provided. When clients have spinal anaesthesia (e.g., during a caesarean section), a bolus of 1 mg intrathecal morphine can provide significant pain control for up to 24 hours. For shorter-acting medications, an epidural catheter may be intact and accessed by a qualified health professional (e.g., anaesthesiologist) to administer bolus doses on an as needed basis. Check agency policy regarding who can provide these bolus doses, how they are documented, and the post-bolus monitoring procedures.
2. *Continuous infusion administered by pump.* The pump can be external (for acute or chronic pain) or surgically implanted (for chronic pain) to provide a continuous infusion of pain relievers into the epidural or intrathecal space.
3. *Continuous plus intermittent bolus.* With this mode of operation, the client receives a continuous infusion, with bolus rescue doses administered for breakthrough pain. Often a pump with *patient-controlled epidural analgesia (PCEA)* capabilities is used for this mode of operation. This is similar to patient-controlled analgesia (detailed later) in which a basal rate may or may not be used to meet the client's anticipated analgesic need, with the client's ability to request an incremental dose by pressing a button set at intervals. PCEA is often used to manage acute postoperative pain, chronic pain, and intractable cancer pain. The so-called walking epidurals used for women in labour are typically PCEA devices that are programmed in the bolus mode without a continuous infusion (basal rate) set.

The needle is inserted into the intrathecal or epidural space (typically in the lumbar region) and a catheter is threaded through the needle to the desired level. The catheter is connected to tubing that is then positioned along the spine and over the client's shoulder for the nurse to access. The entire catheter and tubing are taped securely to prevent dislodgement. Often an occlusive transparent dressing is placed over the insertion site for easy identification of catheter displacement or local inflammation. Temporary catheters, used for short-term acute pain management, are usually placed at the lumbar or thoracic vertebral level and often removed after 2 to 4 days. Permanent catheters, for clients with chronic pain, may be tunnelled subcutaneously through the skin and exit at the client's side, or be connected to a pump implanted in the abdomen. Tunnelling of the catheter reduces the risk of infection and displacement of the catheter. After the catheter is inserted, the nurse is responsible for monitoring the infusion and assessing the client per institutional policy. Nursing care of clients with intraspinal infusions is summarized in Table 34.8.

There are misconceptions that either overstate or ignore the risks of spinal analgesia. This is, in part, due to the importance of the technique of the professional inserting the catheter, which varies considerably. In general, clients receiving epidural analgesia do not need to be monitored in an intensive care setting, but they do need vigilant assessment of their pain, neurological and respiratory status, and the insertion site frequently during the course of therapy.

Patient-Controlled Analgesia

Patient-controlled analgesia (PCA) is a method that allows patients to self-administer their own opioids whenever they feel it is necessary. PCA may involve oral medications or an infusion system with a pump. With a PCA pump, the patient pushes a button to release a set amount of opioid by bolus via the intravenous, subcutaneous, or epidural route. PCA pumps usually have a chamber or cartridge that contains the analgesic, a mechanism for setting the ordered dose, and a control for client activation (see Figure 34.11). When patients want a dose of analgesic, they can push a button attached to the infusion pump and the preset dose is delivered. A programmable lockout interval (usually 10 to 15 minutes) follows the dose, when an additional dose cannot be given even if the client activates the button. It is also possible to program the maximum dose that can be delivered over a period of hours (usually 4). Many pumps are capable of delivering a low continuous infusion, or basal rate, to provide sustained analgesia during times of rest and sleep. Older children can be taught to use PCAs (see Figure 34.12 and the Lifespan Considerations box).

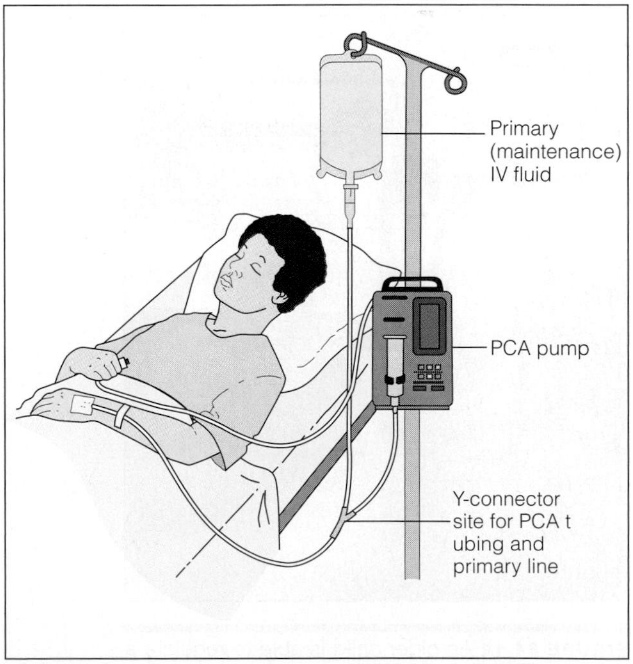

FIGURE 34.11 PCA pump setup with line introduced into the injection port of a primary line

TABLE 34.8 Nursing Interventions for Clients Receiving Analgesics through an Epidural Catheter

Nursing Goal	Interventions
Maintain client safety	Label the tubing, the infusion bag, and the front of the pump with tape marked EPIDURAL to prevent confusion with similar looking IV lines. Post sign above client's bed indicating epidural is in place. Secure all connections with tape. If there is no continuous infusion, apply tape over all injection ports on the epidural line to avoid the injection of substances intended for IV administration into the epidural catheter. Do not use alcohol in any care of catheter or insertion site as it can be neurotoxic.
Maintain catheter placement	Secure temporary catheters with tape. When bolus doses are used, gently aspirate before medication administration to determine that the catheter has not migrated into the subarachnoid space. (Expect < 1 mL of fluid return in syringe.) Assist client in repositioning or moving out of bed. Assess insertion site for leakage with each bolus dose or at least every 8–12 hours.
Prevent infection	Use strict aseptic techniques with all epidural-related procedures. Maintain a sterile occlusive dressing over insertion site. Assess insertion site for signs of infection.
Maintain urinary and bowel function	Monitor intake and output. Assess for bowel and bladder distension.
Prevent respiratory depression	Assess sedation level and respiratory status q1h for the first 24 hours and q4h thereafter. Do not administer other opioids or central nervous system depressants, unless ordered. Keep a 0.4 mg ampule of naloxone hydrochloride (Narcan) at the bedside. Notify the clinician in charge if the respiratory rate falls below 8 per minute or if the client is difficult to rouse.

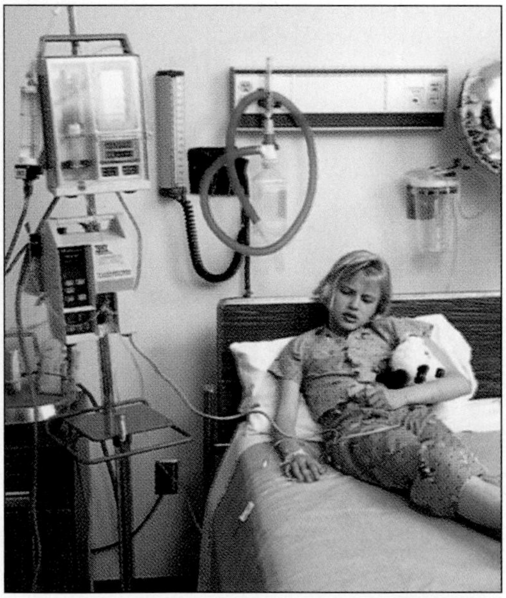

FIGURE 34.12 An older child is able to regulate a PCA pump.

Lifespan Considerations

PCA Pump

CHILDREN

- Include the parents in the teaching.
- Assess the child's ability to use the client control button.

OLDER ADULTS

- Carefully monitor older adults for medication side effects.
- Use cautiously in individuals with impaired pulmonary or renal function.
- Assess the client's cognitive and physical ability to use the client control button.

People using PCA tend to take less total analgesia than those receiving intermittent injections (McCaffery & Pasero, 1999). PCA is used for the management of postoperative pain; for other types of acute pain, such as sickle-cell crisis; and for cancer pain. A major advantage to PCA is that it can meet pain relief needs of clients in a flexible manner relative to conventional analgesic methods (McIntyre, 2001). Whether in an acute-care hospital setting, an ambulatory clinic, or home care, the nurse is responsible for the initial instruction regarding the use of the PCA and for the ongoing monitoring of the therapy (see the Teaching: Clinical box and the Teaching: Home Care box). The client's pain must be assessed at regular intervals and analgesic use documented in the patient's record. Client concerns about addiction and adverse effects also need to be assessed and addressed.

TEACHING: HOME CARE

PCA Pump

- Monitor for signs and symptoms of oversedation, such as excessive drowsiness, slowed respiratory rate, or change in mental state.
- Do not adjust settings without consulting with the appropriate health-care provider.
- Tape to the back of the pump appropriate emergency contact numbers (i.e., ambulance, home care agency, and pump manufacturer).

Nonpharmacological Pain Management

Nonpharmacological pain management consists of a variety of physical, cognitive-behavioural, and lifestyle pain management strategies that target the body, mind, spirit, and social interactions (see Table 34.9). Physical modalities include cutaneous stimulation, immobilization or therapeutic exercises, transcutaneous electrical nerve stimulation (TENS), and acupuncture. Mind-body (cognitive-behavioural) interventions include distracting activities, relaxation techniques, imagery, meditation, biofeedback, hypnosis, cognitive reframing, emotional counselling, and spiritually directed approaches, like therapeutic touch or reiki. Lifestyle management approaches include symptom monitoring, stress management, exercise, nutrition, pacing activities, disability management, and other approaches needed by many clients with persistent pain that has drastically changed their life. Further information on selected mind-body interventions are detailed in Chapter 15. The discussion here is limited to selected physical and cognitive-behavioural interventions.

TEACHING: CLINICAL

Client Self-Management of Pain by Using a PCA Pump

Choose a time to teach the client about pain management when the pain is controlled so that the client is able to focus on the teaching.

Teaching the client about self-management of pain can include the following:

- Demonstrate the operation of the PCA pump and explain that the client can safely push the button without fear of overmedicating. Sometimes it helps clients who are reluctant to repeatedly push the button to know that they must dose themselves (i.e., push the button) 5 to 10 times to receive the same amount of medication (10 mg morphine equivalent) they would receive in a standard injection.
- Describe the use of the pain scale and encourage the client to respond in order to demonstrate understanding.
- Explore a variety of nondrug pain relief techniques that the client is willing to learn and use to promote pain relief and optimize functioning.
- Explain to the client the need to notify staff when ambulation is desired (e.g., for bathroom use) if applicable.

PHYSICAL INTERVENTIONS The goals of physical intervention include providing comfort, altering physiological responses to reduce pain perception, and optimizing functioning.

CUTANEOUS STIMULATION Cutaneous stimulation can provide effective temporary pain relief. It distracts the client and focuses attention on the tactile stimuli, away from the painful sensations, thus reducing pain perception. Cutaneous stimulation is also believed to create the release of endorphins that block pain stimuli transmission and stimulate large-diameter A-beta sensory nerve fibres, thus decreasing the transmission of pain impulses through the smaller A-delta and C fibres. Cutaneous stimulation techniques include the following:

- Massage
- Application of heat or cold
- Acupressure
- Contralateral stimulation

Cutaneous stimulation can be applied directly to the painful area, proximal to the pain, distal to the pain (along the nerve path or dermatome), and contralateral (exact location, opposite side of the body) to the pain. Cutaneous stimulation is contraindicated in areas of skin breakdown and for those clients with impaired neurological functioning.

MASSAGE Massage is a comfort measure that can aid relaxation and decrease muscle tension and may ease anxiety as the physical contact communicates caring. Massage can also decrease pain intensity by increasing superficial circulation to the area. Massage can involve the back and neck, hands and arms, or feet (see Chapter 37 for back massage).

Heat and Cold Applications A warm bath, warm pads, ice bags, ice massage, warm or cold compresses, and warm or cold sitz baths, in general, relieve pain and promote healing of injured tissues (see Chapter 33).

Acupressure Acupressure developed from the ancient Chinese healing system of acupuncture. The therapist applies finger pressure to points that correspond to many of the points used in acupuncture (see Chapter 15).

TABLE 34.9 Nonpharmacological Interventions for Pain Control

Target Domain of Pain Control	Intervention
Body	Reducing pain triggers, promoting comfort
	Massage
	Applying heat or ice
	Electric stimulation (TENS)
	Positioning, bracing (selective immobilization)
	Acupressure
	Diet, nutritional supplements
	Exercise, pacing activities
	Invasive interventions (e.g., blocks)
	Sleep hygiene
Mind	Relaxation, imagery
	Self-hypnosis
	Pain diary, journal writing
	Distracting attention
	Repatterning thinking
	Attitude adjustment
	Reducing fear, anxiety, stress
	Reducing sadness, helplessness
	Information about pain
Spirit	Prayer, meditation
	Self-reflection about life and pain
	Meaningful rituals
	Energy work (e.g., therapeutic touch, reiki)
	Spiritual healing
Social interactions	Functional restoration
	Improved communication
	Family therapy
	Problem solving
	Vocational training
	Volunteering
	Support groups

Contralateral Stimulation Contralateral stimulation can be accomplished by stimulating the skin in an area opposite to the painful area (e.g., stimulating the left knee if the pain is in the right knee). The contralateral area may be scratched for itching, massaged for cramps, if appropriate, or treated with cold packs or analgesic ointments. This method is particularly useful when the painful area cannot be touched because it is hypersensitive, when it is inaccessible by a cast or bandages, or when the pain is felt in a missing part (phantom pain).

IMMOBILIZATION AND BRACING Immobilizing or restricting the movement of a painful body part (e.g., arthritic joint, traumatized limb) may help to manage episodes of acute pain. Splints or supportive devices should hold joints in the position of optimal function and should be removed regularly in accordance with agency protocol to provide range-of-motion (ROM) exercises, if not contraindicated. Prolonged immobilization can result in joint contracture, muscle atrophy, and cardiovascular problems. Therefore, clients should be encouraged to participate in self-care activities and remain as active as possible, with frequent ROM exercises.

TRANSCUTANEOUS ELECTRICAL NERVE STIMULATION **Transcutaneous electrical nerve stimulation (TENS)** is a method of applying low-voltage electrical stimulation directly over identified pain areas, at an acupressure point, along peripheral nerve areas that innervate the pain area, or along the spinal column. The TENS unit consists of a portable, battery-operated device with lead wire and electrode pads that are applied to the chosen area of skin (Figure 34.13). Cutaneous stimulation from the TENS unit is thought to activate large-diameter fibres that modulate the transmission of the nociceptive impulse in the peripheral nervous system and CNS (closing the pain gate), resulting in pain relief. This stimulation may also cause a release of endorphins from the CNS centres.

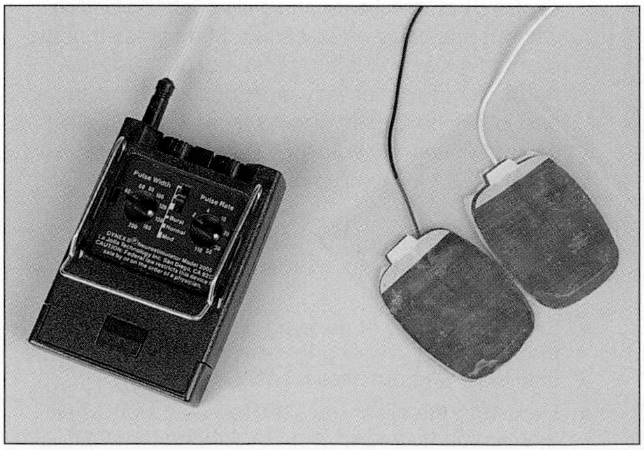

FIGURE 34.13 A transcutaneous electrical nerve stimulator (TENS)

ACUPUNCTURE Acupuncture, a form of traditional Chinese medicine, involves the insertion of thin sterile needles into specific points of the skin with the goal of relieving pain (see Chapter 15).

Cognitive-Behavioural Interventions

The goals of cognitive-behavioural interventions include providing comfort, altering psychological responses to reduce pain perception, and optimizing functioning. Selected cognitive-behavioural interventions include distraction, elicitation of the relaxation response, and psychoeducation.

DISTRACTION Distraction draws the person's attention away from the pain and lessens the perception of pain. In some instances, distraction can make a client completely unaware of pain. For example, a client recovering from surgery may feel no pain while watching a football game on television, yet feel pain again when the game is over. Different types of distractions are shown in Box 34.5.

ELICITATION OF THE RELAXATION RESPONSE Stress increases pain, in part by increasing muscle tension, activating the sympathetic nervous system, and putting the client at risk for stress-related types of pain (e.g., tension headaches). The relaxation response decreases and counteracts the harmful effects of stress, including the effect it has on physical, cognitive, and emotional functioning. Eliciting this response requires more than simply helping a person to relax; rather it involves a structured technique designed to focus the mind and relax muscle groups. Basic techniques with helpful scripts are detailed by McCaffery and Pasero (1999), with common techniques including progressive relaxation, breath-focus relaxation, and meditation. The nurse can coach the client, urge self-directed meditation, or provide an audiotaped guide to help elicit the relaxation response. Many clients can achieve the desired state after a few attempts, but mastery of this skill requires daily practice over a few weeks. In general, relaxation techniques by themselves do not have remarkable pain-relieving properties; however, they can reduce pain that may have been exacerbated by stress. Some clients may become more consciously aware of their pain while practising relaxation techniques before they have mastered controlling mind chatter and remaining mentally focused.

BOX 34.5 TYPES OF DISTRACTION

In some cases, using the following distractions lessen a client's pain:

VISUAL DISTRACTION

- Reading or watching TV
- Watching a baseball game
- Guided imagery

AUDITORY DISTRACTION

- Humour
- Listening to music

TACTILE DISTRACTION

- Slow, rhythmic breathing
- Massage
- Holding or stroking a pet or toy

INTELLECTUAL DISTRACTION

- Crossword puzzles
- Card games (e.g., bridge)
- Hobbies (e.g., stamp collecting, writing a story)

PSYCHOEDUCATION Once the client has mastered the basic skills for eliciting the relaxation response, techniques of imagery or self-hypnosis can be used. Both imagery and hypnosis begin with attaining a deep state of relaxation and are capable of altering the experience of pain, for example, by having the client replace their pain with a feeling of pleasant numbness (Arnstein, 2004). Additional posthypnotic suggestions can then be made, linking these pleasant numb sensations to coping efforts used during the day (e.g., "every time you stop to take a slow, deep, diaphragmatic breath, you will feel this pleasant numbness instead of pain").

Psychoeducation is increasingly being used as an adjunctive means of managing the impact of chronic pain on health-related quality of life and disability (Lefort, Gray-Donald, Rowat, & Jeans, 1998; McGillion, Watt-Watson, Kim, & Yamada, 2004; McGillion et al., 2007). Psychoeducational interventions are group self-management education programs delivered by a trained facilitator; clients can be accompanied by family members or friends if they want. The focus is to provide participants with an opportunity to enhance their skills for self-care. Through rehearsal and application of various cognitive and behavioural self-management techniques, participants learn to set realistic self-management goals in relation to their chronic pain. The goal-setting process allows for the self-attribution of success, thereby improving perceived self-efficacy in managing symptoms. Nurses facilitating psychoeducation programs require expertise in psychoeducational techniques, group process, and assessment of participants' readiness to engage in self-management.

Nonpharmacological Invasive Therapies

A **nerve block** is a chemical interruption of a nerve pathway, created by injecting a local anaesthetic into the nerve. Nerve blocks are widely used during dental work.

The injected drug blocks nerve pathways from the painful tooth, thus stopping the transmission of pain impulses to the brain. Nerve blocks are often used to relieve the pain of whiplash injury, lower-back disorders, bursitis, and cancer. Sometimes, alcohol blocks are used. These, however, destroy nerve fibres and, as a result, are generally used only for peripheral blocks because peripheral nerve fibres regenerate.

Pain-conduction pathways can be interrupted surgically. Because this disruption is permanent, surgery is performed only as a last resort, generally for intractable pain. Several surgical procedures may be performed. A **cordotomy** obliterates pain and temperature sensation below the level of the spinothalamic portion of the anterolateral tract severed and is usually done for pain in the legs and trunk. A **rhizotomy** interrupts the anterior or posterior nerve root between the ganglion and the cord. Interruption of anterior *motor* nerve roots stops spasmodic movements that accompany paraplegia. Interruption of posterior *sensory* nerve roots eliminates pain in areas innervated by that specific nerve root. Rhizotomies are generally performed on cervical nerve roots to alleviate pain of the head and neck from cancer or neuralgia.

In **neurectomy**, peripheral or cranial nerves are interrupted to alleviate localized pain, such as pain in the lower leg or foot arising from a vascular occlusion. In a **sympathectomy**, pathways of the sympathetic division of the autonomic nervous system are severed. This procedure eliminates vasospasm, improves peripheral blood supply, and, thus, is effective in treating painful vascular disorders, such as angina and Raynaud's disease.

Spinal cord stimulation (SCS) is used with nonmalignant pain that has not been controlled with less invasive therapies. SCS involves the insertion of an electrode adjacent to the spinal cord in the epidural space. The electrode is attached to an impulse generator (external or implanted) that sends electric impulses to the spinal cord to control pain.

See the Lifespan Considerations box for age-specific ways to manage pain.

Evaluating

By using the desired outcomes established during the planning stage as a guide, the nurse and client determine whether client goals and outcomes have been achieved. Examples of client goals and related outcomes are shown in Table 34.10.

To assist in the evaluation process, a flowsheet or a client diary may be helpful. Columns for day, time, onset of pain, activity before pain, pain-relief measure, and duration of pain can be devised to help the client and nurse determine the effectiveness of pain-relief strategies.

If desired health outcomes are *not* achieved, the nurse and client need to explore the reasons before

TABLE 34.10 Evaluation Goals and Outcomes: Pain

Goal	Examples of Desired Health Outcomes
Modify or minimize pain to enable partial or complete resumption of daily activities	Reports pain relief at level of (specify) or less, on a scale of 0 to 10; or expresses feelings of reasonable comfort
	Reports decreased frequency and length of pain episodes or decreased fear and anxiety
	Absence of nonverbal pain responses, such as restlessness, muscle tension, protective body position, facial grimacing (specify)
	Reports increase in mobility and physical activity, in hours of uninterrupted sleep at night, and in quality of life
Enhance abilities to control pain	Identifies factors that precipitate or intensify the pain experience
	Identifies both pharmacological and nonpharmacological pain management techniques
	Identifies ways to prevent side effects of drugs
Demonstrate actions to control pain and associated symptoms	Reduces or eliminates factors that precipitate or intensify the pain experience
	Uses a pain diary to monitor pain pattern and effectiveness of pain measures
	Uses planned nonpharmacological pain relief measures (specify)
	Uses analgesics appropriately

Lifespan Considerations

Pain Management

INFANTS

- Giving an infant, particularly a very low-birth-weight infant, a water and sucrose solution administered through a pacifier provides some evidence of pain reduction during procedures that may be painful, but it should not be a substitute for anaesthetic or analgesic medications.

CHILDREN

- Distract the child with toys, books, or pictures.
- Hold the child to console him or her and provide comfort.
- Explore misbeliefs about pain and correct them in understandable concrete terms. Be aware of how your explanations may be misunderstood. For example, telling a child he or she won't hurt during surgery because they will be "put to sleep" will be very upsetting to a child who knows of an animal that was "put to sleep."
- Children can use their imagination during guided imagery. To use the pain switch, ask the child to imagine a pain switch (even give it a colour) and tell him or her to visualize turning the switch off in the area where he or she has pain. A "magic glove" or "magic blanket" is an imaginary object that the child applies on areas of the body (e.g., hand, thigh, back, hip) to lessen discomfort.

OLDER ADULTS

- Promote the client's use of pain-control measures that have worked in the past.
- Spend time with the client and listen carefully.
- Clarify misbeliefs. Encourage independence whenever possible.
- Carefully review the treatment plan to avoid drug-drug, food-drug, or disease-drug interactions.

modifying the care plan. The following are some questions the nurse might consider:

- Is adequate analgesic being given? Would the client benefit from a change in dose or in the time interval between doses?
- Were the client's beliefs and values about pain therapy considered?
- Did the client understate the pain experience for some reason?
- Were appropriate instructions provided to allay misbeliefs about pain management?
- Did the client and support people understand the instructions about pain management techniques?
- Is the client receiving adequate support from significant others?
- Has the client's physical condition changed, necessitating modifications in interventions?
- Should selected intervention strategies be re-evaluated?

Case Study 34

Mrs. Lundahl, 45 years old, underwent an emergency anterior bowel resection approximately 6 hours ago. She has a 15 cm midline incision that is covered with a dry and intact surgical dressing. On assessing Mrs. Lundahl, you note that she is perspiring, lying in a rigid position, holding her abdomen, and grimacing. Her blood pressure is 150/90; heart rate, 100; and respiratory rate, 32. She rates her pain as 8 on a scale of 0 to 10.

Critical Thinking Questions

1. What conclusions, if any, can be drawn about Mrs. Lundahl's pain status?
2. Does Mrs. Lundahl's rating of her pain as 8 mean that she is not experiencing pain severe enough to warrant intervention?
3. What type of pain is Mrs. Lundahl experiencing?
4. What interventions, in addition to pain medication, may be useful in reducing Mrs. Lundahl's pain?
5. How will you know if your interventions have been effective in reducing Mrs. Lundahl's pain?

After working through these questions, go to the MyNursingLab at **http://www.mynursinglab.com** to check your answers.

KEY TERMS

pain
acute pain
chronic pain
somatic pain
visceral pain
neuropathic pain
peripheral neuropathic pain
central neuropathic pain
sympathetically maintained pain
radiating pain
referred pain
intractable pain
pain threshold
pain tolerance
allodynia
dysesthesia
hyperalgesia
noxious
nociceptors
nociception
transduction
transmission
modulation
perception
nervous system plasticity
peripheral sensitization
central sensitization
fifth vital sign
pain management
preemptive analgesia
full agonist
ceiling dose
agonist-antagonist analgesic
ceiling effect
partial agonist
opioid antagonist
tolerance
physical dependence
addiction
equianalgesia
nonsteroidal anti-inflammatory drug (NSAID)
coanalgesic
placebo response
patient-controlled analgesia (PCA)
transcutaneous electrical nerve stimulation (TENS)
nerve block
cordotomy
rhizotomy
neurectomy
sympathectomy
spinal cord stimulation (SCS)

CHAPTER HIGHLIGHTS

- Pain is a subjective, multidimensional experience with sensory-discriminative, cognitive-evaluative, and motivational-affective components; many clients need encouragement or help to communicate their pain experience with respect to, in particular, its intensity, duration, qualities, and related individual responses.
- Unrelieved pain has multiple serious consequences and can prolong recovery from surgery, disease, and trauma.
- Pain can be categorized according to its origin as cutaneous, deep somatic, or visceral, or according to its cause as acute pain, chronic cancer pain, or chronic noncancer pain.
- Pain threshold is relatively similar in all people and changes little in the same individual over time; conversely, pain tolerance and response vary considerably from person to person *and* in the same person at different times and in different circumstances.
- For pain to be experienced, primary afferent nociceptors must be stimulated. Three types of pain stimuli are mechanical, thermal, and chemical.
- The pain process involves transduction, transmission, modulation, and perception.
- Endogenous opioids, critical to pain modulation, include enkephalins, endorphins, and dynorphins.
- Gate control theory is the basis of many pain-intervention strategies and explains the multidimensional nature of pain; yet it is a theory of acute pain, and it cannot account for nervous system plasticity.
- Numerous factors influence a person's perception and reaction to pain: ethnic and cultural values, developmental stage, environment and support people, past pain experiences, and meaning of pain.
- Pain is subjective, and the most reliable indicator of the presence or intensity of pain is the client's self-report. Assessment of a client who is experiencing pain should include a comprehensive pain history.
- Although the nursing diagnosis given to clients suffering pain is *Acute Pain* or *Chronic Pain,* the pain itself may be the etiology of many other nursing diagnoses.
- Overall client goals include preventing, modifying, or eliminating pain so that the client is able to partially or completely resume usual daily activities and to cope more effectively with the pain experience.
- When planning, nurses need to choose pain-relief measures appropriate for the client. Nursing interventions should include a variety of pharmacological and nonpharmacological interventions. Selecting several strategies from both broad categories is usually most effective.
- Scheduling the measures to *prevent* pain is far more supportive of the client than trying to deal with pain once it is established.
- Pain management includes two basic types of nursing interventions: pharmacological and nonpharmacological.
- Major nursing functions for all clients are to acknowledge and convey belief in the client's pain, assist support people, reduce misbeliefs about pain, and reduce fear and anxiety associated with the pain.
- Pharmacological interventions, prescribed by the physician or nurse practitioner under medical

directives, include the use of opioids, non-opioids or NSAIDs, and coanalgesics.

- The nurse assesses the client's pain needs, administers the prescribed analgesics, and evaluates the client's response to analgesics provided.
- Analgesic medication can be delivered through a variety of routes and methods to meet the specific needs of the client. These routes include oral, subcutaneous with a continuous infusion, intravenous, transnasal, transdermal or topical, rectal, and intraspinal.
- Patient-controlled analgesia (PCA) enables the client to exercise control and minimize feelings of helplessness.
- Physical nonpharmacological pain interventions include such cutaneous stimulation as warm and cold applications, massage, acupressure, and contralateral stimulation; transcutaneous electrical nerve stimulation (TENS); and immobilization or bracing.
- Examples of cognitive-behavioural interventions include distraction techniques and psychoeducation.
- Evaluation of the client's pain therapy includes the response of the client, the changes in the pain, and the client's perceptions of the effectiveness of the therapy. Ongoing verbal or written feedback from the client and family is integral to this process.

ASSESS YOUR LEARNING

1. When an excited nociceptor converts a noxious stimulus into an action potential, this is referred to as which of the following?

a. Modulation
b. Perception
c. Transduction
d. Transmission

2. Which of the following is the definition of the placebo response?

a. The person's pain is not real.
b. Inflammation has subsided.
c. Endogenous opioids have been released.
d. The client has failed to respond to opioids.

3. Which of the following will the nurse perform to check for the presence of the most common adverse effect of opioids?

a. A respiratory assessment
b. A bladder scan or palpation
c. An assessment of the level of pruritus
d. An assessment of the patient's bowel function

4. A patient admitted for treatment of unmanaged chronic pain is prescribed morphine and nortriptyline, an antidepressant. The patient states, "I'm here for pain, not depression! Give me the morphine but I refuse the other pill!" The nurse responds with which of the following statements about the antidepressant?

a. "This pill is meant to prevent you from getting depressed because of the pain you have been experiencing."
b. "This pill will help reduce any inflammation that you might have."
c. "This pill will help your nervous system by increasing your body's own pain-reducing substances."
d. "This pill helps to block the pain signals from going up your spinal cord."

5. A patient recovering from a surgical intervention requires increasing doses of analgesia in the post-operative period to control pain. Of the following possibilities, which is the most likely hypothesis to explain this pattern?

a. Tolerance to the analgesia has occurred.
b. Dependence on the analgesia has occurred.
c. Addiction to the analgesia has occurred.
d. Compulsive drug abuse has been established.

6. The patient is prescribed morphine 2.5 mg to 5.0 mg IV every 4 hours. He received 2.5 mg IV 4 hours ago for pain rated at 3 on a scale of 0 to 10. He is now watching TV and visiting with family members. When asked about his pain, he rates it as a 5. His vital signs (VS) are stable. What nursing intervention is the most appropriate?

a. Give morphine 3.5 mg IV and inform him to continue watching TV because it is a distraction from the pain.
b. Give 2.5 mg of morphine IV to avoid the client becoming addicted.
c. Give nothing at this time because he is not exhibiting any signs of pain.
d. Give morphine 5.0 mg IV and reassess in 20 minutes.

7. During an admission nursing assessment, a patient with diabetes describes his leg pain as a "dull, burning sensation." The nurse recognizes this description as characteristic of which type of pain?

a. Referred
b. Somatic
c. Visceral
d. Neuropathic

8. Which of the following is the need to continue the use of an opioid to prevent the symptoms of withdrawal?

a. A psychological response
b. A physiological response
c. A threshold response
d. An addictive response

9. Ms. Aitken, 45 years old, has acute pain following a fractured ankle. The physician's order is acetaminophen (Tylenol #3) 30 mg of codeine one to two tablets, q. 3–4h. p.r.n. Although the last dose given was one hour ago, she reports severe pain. What nursing action is most appropriate?

a. Consult the nurse-in-charge.

b. Reassess Ms. Aitken's pain in 15 minutes.

c. Notify the physician of Ms. Aitken's pain level.

d. Administer an additional dose while awaiting a new order.

10. A patient who has been receiving 100 mg IV morphine per day is now being prescribed oral hydromorphone (Dilaudid). The equianalgesia chart indicates that 10 mg IV morphine is equivalent to 7.5 mg hydromorphone. The equianalgesic dose of hydromorphone in this case is ______ mg.

After working through these questions, go to the MyNursingLab at ***http://www.mynursinglab.com*** *to check your answers and see explanations.*

SUGGESTED READINGS

Jovey, R. D. (2002). *Managing pain: The Canadian healthcare professional's reference.* Toronto: Rogers Media.

This book is a Canadian practical guide to acute and chronic pain management.

McMahon, S. B., & Koltzenburg, M. (2006). *Wall and Melzack's textbook of pain* (5th ed.). Philadelphia, PA: Elsevier Limited.

This text provides a comprehensive overview of pain theory, assessment, and management.

Merskey, H., Loeser, J. D., & Dubner, R. (2005). *The paths of pain: 1975–2005.* Seattle: IASP Press.

This text provides an overview of the science of pain theory and mechanisms, from 1975 to 2005.

Turk, D. C., & Melzack, R. (2001). *The handbook of pain assessment.* New York: Guilford Press.

This text provides an overview of key principles in pain assessment and measurement, and up-to-date information on the psychometric properties of key pain measures.

WEBLINKS

The Canadian Pain Society

http://www.canadianpainsociety.ca

The Canadian Pain Society is a chapter of the International Association for the Study of Pain. The site provides information on research opportunities, conferences, interest groups, and news about pain practices.

International Association for the Study of Pain

http://www.iasp-pain.org

This association is the largest multidisciplinary nonprofit international association in the field of pain. Its goal is to advance research on pain and improve the care of clients with pain. The site provides an overview of the association and its activities, as well as links to publications and continuing education initiatives.

University of Toronto Centre for the Study of Pain

http://www.utoronto.ca/pain

Described on the site is the Centre for the Study of Pain, which is a partnership involving the Faculties of Dentistry, Medicine, and Nursing.

Institute for the Study and Treatment of Pain

http://www.istop.org

A Canadian nonprofit society dedicated to research, treatment, training, and education in chronic pain. Information about the society and treatment options for people with chronic pain is available at this site.

Canadian Pain Coalition

http://www.canadianpaincoalition.ca

The Canadian Pain Coalition is "a partnership of patient pain groups, health professionals who care for people in pain, and scientists studying better ways of treating pain."

Canadian Cancer Society

http://www.cancer.ca

The Canadian Cancer Society's website offers information on coping with pain. Click on Treatment, and then Managing Pain. It emphasizes that pain treatments are available and that the way each person feels pain is unique.

Chronic Pain Association of Canada

http://www.chronicpaincanada.com

The Chronic Pain Association of Canada is a nonprofit group that focuses on treatments and the management of chronic intractable pain.

REFERENCES

Arnstein, P. M. (2004). Chronic neuropathic pain: Issues in patient education. *Pain Management Nursing, 5*(4), 34–41.

Arntz, A., & Claassens, L. (2004). The meaning of pain influences its experienced intensity. *Pain, 109,* 20–25.

Bartocci, M., Bergqvist, L. L., Lagercrantz, H., & Anand, K. J. S. (2006). Pain activates cortical areas in the preterm newborn brain. *Pain, 122,* 109–117.

Basbaum, A., & Bushnell, M. C. (2002). Pain: Basic mechanisms. In M. A. Giamberardino (Ed.), *Pain 2002, an updated review: Refresher course and syllabus* (pp. 3–9). Seattle: IASP Press.

Basbaum, A. I., & Jessell, T. M. (2000). Perception of pain. In E. Kandel, J. Schurtz, & T. M. Jessell (Eds.), *Principles of neuroscience* (4th ed.) (pp. 472–490). New York: McGraw-Hill.

Bonica, J. J. (1990). *The management of pain* (2nd ed.). Philadelphia, PA: Lea & Febiger.

Canadian Pain Society. (2005). *Accreditation pain standard: Making it happen!* Retrieved December 14, 2007, from http://www.canadianpainsociety.ca/accreditation_manual.pdf

Champion, G. D., Goodenough, B., von Baeyer, C. L., & Thomas, W. (1998). Measurement of pain by self-report. In G. A. Finley & P. J. McGrath (Eds.), *Measurement of Pain in Infants and Children. Progress in Pain Research and Management, Vol. 10* (pp. 123–160). Seattle: IASP Press.

Cleeland, C. S. (1991). Pain assessment in cancer. In D. Osoba (Ed.), *Effect of cancer on quality of life* (pp. 293–305). Boca Raton, FL: CRC Press.

Cleeland S., Serlin, R., Nakamura, Y., & Mendoza, T. (1997). Effects of culture and language on ratings of cancer pain and patterns of functional interference. In T. Jensen, J. Turner, & Z. Wiesenfeld-Hallin (Eds.), *Proceedings of the 8th World Congress on Pain, Vol. 8* (pp. 35–52). Seattle: IASP Press.

Craig, A. D., & Sorkin, L. S. (2004). *Encyclopedia of life sciences: Pain and analgesia.* Retrieved October 19, 2007, from http://www.els.net

Dahl, J. L., Gordon, D., Ward, S., Skemp, M., Wochos, S., & Schurr, M. (2003). Institutionalizing pain management: The post-operative pain management quality improvement project. *Journal of Pain, 4,* 361–371.

Guru, V., & Dubinsky, I. (2000). The patient vs. caregiver perception of acute pain in the emergency department. *Journal of Emergency Medicine, 18*(1), 7–12.

Guyton, A., & Hall, J. E. (2006). *Textbook of medical physiology* (11th ed.). Philadelphia, PA: Saunders.

Herr, K. (2002). Chronic pain: Challenges and assessment strategies. *Journal of Gerontological Nursing, 28*(1), 20–27.

Hicks, C. L., von Baeyer, C. L., Spafford, P. A., van Korlaar, I., & Goodenough, B. (2001). The Faces Pain Scale—Revised: Toward a common metric in pediatric pain measurement. *Pain, 93*(2), 173–183.

Jensen, M. P., & Karoly, P. (2001). Self-report scales and procedures for assessing pain in adults. In D. C. Turk & R. Melzack (Eds.), *Handbook of Pain Assessment* (pp. 15–33). New York: Guilford Press.

Johnston, C. C., Stevens, B. J., Yang, F., & Horton, L. (1995). Differential response to pain by very premature neonates. *Pain, 61,* 471–479.

Katz, J. (2003). Timing of treatment and preemptive analgesia. In D. J. Rowbotham & P. E. Macintyre (Eds.), *Clinical pain management: Acute pain* (pp. 113–163). London, UK: Arnold.

LeFort, S., Gray-Donald, K., Rowat, K. M., & Jeans, M. E. (1998). Randomised controlled trial of a community based psychoeducation program for the self-management of chronic pain. *Pain, 74,* 297–306.

Manias, E., Bucknall, T., & Botti, M. (2005). Nurses' strategies for managing pain in the postoperative setting. *Pain Management Nursing, 6,* 18–29.

McCaffery, M., & Pasero, C. (1999). *Pain: Clinical manual* (2nd ed.). St. Louis, MO: Mosby.

McGillion, M. H., Watt-Watson, J. H., Kim, J., & Graham, A. (2004). Learning by heart: A focused group study to determine the self-management learning needs of chronic stable angina patients. *Canadian Journal of Cardiovascular Nursing, 14,* 12–22.

McGillion, M. H., Watt-Watson, J. H., Kim, J., & Yamada, J. (2004). A systematic review of psychoeducational interventions for the management of chronic stable angina. *Journal of Nursing Management, 12,* 1–9.

McGillion, M., Watt-Watson, J., LeFort, S., & Stevens, B. (2007). Positive shifts in the perceived meaning of cardiac pain following a psychoeducation program for chronic stable angina, *Canadian Journal of Nursing Research, 39*(2), 48–65.

McIntyre, P. E. (2001). Safety and efficacy of patient controlled analgesia. *British Journal of Anaesthesia, 87,* 36–46.

Melzack, R. (1975). The McGill pain questionnaire: Major properties and scoring methods. *Pain, 1,* 277–299.

Melzack, R. (1987). The short-form McGill pain questionnaire. *Pain, 30,* 191–197

Melzack, R. (1990). The tragedy of needless pain. *Scientific American, 262,* 27–33.

Melzack, R., & Wall, P. D. (1965). Pain mechanisms: A new theory. *Science, 150*(November), 971–979.

Melzack, R., & Wall, P. (1973). *The puzzle of pain.* London: Basic Books.

Melzack, R., & Wall, P. (1982). *The challenge of pain.* (2nd ed.). New York: Penguin Books.

Melzack, R., & Wall, P. D. (1996). *The challenge of pain,* New York: Penguin Books.

Merskey, H., & Bogduk, N. (Eds.). (1994). *Classification of chronic pain: Descriptions of chronic pain syndromes and definitions of pain terms* (2nd ed.). Seattle: IASP Press.

Morrison, R. S., Magazinger, J., McLaughlin, M. A., Orosz, G., Silberzweig, S. B., Koval, K. J., et al. (2003). The impact of post-operative pain on outcomes following hip fracture. *Pain, 103,* 303–311.

NANDA International. (2007). *Nursing diagnoses: Definitions and classification, 2007–2008.* Philadelphia, PA: Author.

O'Gara, P. (1988). The hemodynamic consequences of pain and its management. *Journal of Intensive Care Medicine, 3,* 3.

Pasero, C. (1997). Pain ratings: The fifth vital sign. *American Journal of Nursing, 97*(2), 15–16.

Salerno, E., & Willens, J. (1996). *Pain management handbook: An interdisciplinary approach.* St. Louis, MO: Mosby.

Slater, R., Cantarella, A., Gallella, S., Worley, A., Boyd, S., Meek, J., et al. (2006). Cortical pain responses in human infants. *Journal of Neuroscience, 26*(14), 3662–3666.

Stevens, B. (1999). Pain in infants. In M. McCaffery & C. Pasero (Eds.), *Pain: Clinical Manual* (pp. 626–673). St. Louis, MO: Mosby.

Stevens, B., Johnston, C., Petryshen, P., & Taddio, A. (1996). Premature Infant Pain Profile: Development and initial validation. *Clinical Journal of Pain, 12*(1), 13–22.

Stinson, J., Kavanagh, T., Yamada, J., Gill, N., & Stevens, B. (2006). Systematic review of the psychometric properties, interpretability and feasibility of self-report pain intensity measures of use in clinical trials in children and adolescents. *Pain, 125*(1–2), 143–157.

Trentin, L., Visentin, M., de Marco, R., & Zanolin, E. (2001). Prevalence of pain in a public hospital: Correlation between patients and caregivers. *Journal of Headache Pain, 2,* 73–78.

von Baeyer, C. L., & Spagrud, L. J. (2007). Systematic review of observational (behavioral) measures of pain for children and adolescents aged 3 to 18 years. *Pain, 127*(1–2), 140–150.

Watt-Watson, J. (1992). Misbeliefs about pain. In J. Watt-Watson & M. Donovan (Eds.), *Pain management: Nursing perspective* (pp. 36–58), St. Louis, MO: Mosby Yearbook.

Watt-Watson, J., Chung, F., Chan, V. W. S., & McGillion, M. (2004). Pain management following discharge after ambulatory same-day surgery. *Journal of Nursing Management, 12,* 153–161.

Watt-Watson, J. Clark, A. J., Finley, A., & Watson, P. (1999). Canadian Pain Society position statement on pain relief. *Pain Research and Management, 4,* 75.

Watt-Watson, J., Evans, R., & Watson, C. P. (1988). Relationships among coping responses and perceptions of pain intensity, depression and family functioning. *Clinical Journal of Pain, 4,* 101.

Watt-Watson, J., & Graydon, J. (1995). Impact of surgery on head and neck cancer patients and their caregivers. *Nursing Clinics of North America, 30,* 659.

Watt-Watson, J., & Stevens, B. (1998). Managing pain after coronary artery bypass surgery. *Journal of Cardiovascular Nursing, 12,* 39–51.

Watt-Watson, J., Stevens, B., Streiner, D., Garfinkel, P., & Gallop, R. (2001). Relationship between pain knowledge and pain management outcomes for their postoperative cardiac patients. *Journal of Advanced Nursing, 36,* 535–545.

Chapter 35

Caring for Perioperative Clients

Surgery is a unique experience of a planned physical alteration encompassing three phases: preoperative, intraoperative, and postoperative. These three phases are together referred to as the **perioperative period**.

The **preoperative phase** begins when the decision to have surgery is made and ends when the client is transferred to the operating table. The nursing activities associated with this phase include assessing the client, identifying potential or actual health problems, planning specific care based on the individual's needs, and providing preoperative teaching for the client, the family, and significant others. Efforts are being made nationally to reduce the wait time (preoperative phase) for cancer, cardiac, hip and knee replacement, and cataract surgeries (see the Reflect on Primary Health Care box).

OBJECTIVES

After studying this chapter, you should be able to

1. Describe the three phases of the perioperative period
2. Discuss types of surgery according to purpose, degree of urgency, invasiveness, and degree of risk
3. Identify the nursing history, physical assessment, and screening tests essential to a thorough preoperative assessment
4. Outline nursing responsibilities in planning perioperative nursing care
5. Describe essential preoperative teaching, including pain control, moving, leg exercises, and deep-breathing and coughing exercises
6. Outline the physical preparation needs for a client having surgery, including nutrition and fluids, elimination, hygiene, medications, rest, care of valuables and prostheses, special orders, and surgical skin preparation
7. Compare three types of anaesthesia and techniques for administering local and regional anaesthesia
8. Identify essential nursing assessments and interventions during the immediate postanaesthetic phase
9. Demonstrate ongoing nursing assessments and interventions for the postoperative client
10. Discuss potential postoperative complications and describe ten nursing interventions to prevent them
11. Identify the essential aspects of managing gastrointestinal suction
12. Describe appropriate wound care for a postoperative client

REFLECT ON PRIMARY HEALTH CARE

Find out how *accessible* operative care is in your community. Are relatively common surgeries, such as joint replacement surgery, sight restoration (e.g., cataract surgery), or cardiac surgery, available in your region? If so, how long do people wait for such procedures? Consider the impact on the client and family if people need to travel a distance or wait several weeks or months to have one of these interventions.

The **intraoperative phase** begins when the client is transferred to the operating suite and ends when the client is admitted to the postanaesthesia care unit (PACU), also called the postanaesthetic recovery room (PARR) or recovery room (RR). The nursing activities related to this phase include a variety of specialized procedures designed to create and maintain a safe therapeutic environment for the client and the health-care personnel.

The **postoperative phase** begins with the admission of the client to the postanaesthesia area and ends when healing is complete. During the postoperative phase, nursing activities include assessing the client's response (physiological and psychological) to surgery, performing interventions to facilitate healing and prevent complications, teaching and providing support to the client and support people, and planning for home care. The goal is to assist the client to achieve the most optimal health status possible.

Perioperative nursing is practised in hospital-based inpatient or outpatient surgical, laser, or endoscopic suites and freestanding outpatient or ambulatory surgical centres. Outpatient procedures do not require an overnight stay. The client goes to the outpatient site the day of surgery, has the operation, and leaves the same day. In these instances, the three phases of the perioperative period are shortened, and the postoperative phase continues at home. The nurse's role in assessing, teaching, and following up is vital to successful outcomes for clients who undergo day surgery.

Types of Surgery

Surgical procedures are commonly grouped according to (1) purpose, (2) degree of urgency, (3) level of invasiveness, and (4) degree of risk.

Purpose

Surgical procedures can be categorized according to their purpose (see Box 35.1).

Degree of Urgency

Surgery is classified by its urgency and necessity to preserve the client's life, body part, or body function. **Emergency surgery** is performed immediately to preserve function or the life of the client. Surgeries to control internal hemorrhage, trauma, or ruptured aneurysm are examples of emergency surgeries. **Urgent surgery** occurs when the surgical problem requires attention within 24 to 48 hours, such as surgery to remove a kidney stone that is not likely to be passed naturally by the individual. **Elective surgery** is performed when surgical intervention is the preferred treatment for a condition that is not imminently life threatening (but may ultimately threaten life or well-being) or to improve the client's life. Examples of elective surgeries include laparoscopic techniques (used either as a diagnostic tool or therapeutic access method), which are among the most common procedures in surgery worldwide, such as laparoscopic cholecystectomy for chronic gallbladder disease. Further elective surgeries include hip replacement surgery and plastic surgery procedures, such as breast reduction surgery.

Level of Invasiveness

Surgery is also classified based on how invasive the procedure is with respect to the body. **Invasive (open) surgery** involves large incisions made to visualize and provide direct access to the area requiring surgery. Cardiac and abdominal surgeries are often invasive in nature. **Minimally invasive surgery** (sometimes referred to as laparoscopic, closed, or keyhole surgery) involves multiple small incisions through which specialized telescopic equipment is inserted to provide indirect visualization and manipulation of a specific body site or organ. Cholecystectomy (gallbladder removal) and arthroscopy (examination or repair of a joint) are examples of procedures commonly performed by using

BOX 35.1 PURPOSES OF SURGICAL PROCEDURES

Surgery is performed for various reasons:

- *Diagnostic:* Confirms or establishes a diagnosis (e.g., biopsy of a mass in a breast)
- *Palliative:* Relieves or reduces pain or symptoms of a disease but does not cure (e.g., resection of nerve roots)
- *Ablative or curative:* Removes a diseased body part (e.g., removal of a gallbladder: cholecystectomy)
- *Constructive:* Restores function or appearance that has been lost or reduced (e.g., breast implant)
- *Transplant:* Replaces malfunctioning structures (e.g., kidney transplant)

minimally invasive approaches. Some agencies perform cardiac and neurosurgery by using minimally invasive techniques. Generally the patient experiences less trauma, pain, and scarring with minimally invasive techniques compared with more invasive approaches. However, both approaches can involve complications, such as infection, bleeding, and internal organ damage. Minimally invasive procedures are not necessarily minor surgery in that general anaesthesia can be required.

Degree of Risk

Surgery is also classified as major or minor according to the degree of risk to the client. **Major surgery** involves a high degree of risk, for a variety of reasons: it may be complicated or prolonged, large losses of blood may occur, vital organs may be involved, or postoperative complications may be likely. Examples are an organ transplant, open heart surgery, and the removal of a kidney. In contrast, **minor surgery** normally involves little risk, produces few complications, and is often performed in a day surgery. Examples are a breast biopsy, the removal of tonsils, and knee surgery.

The degree of risk involved in a surgical procedure is affected by the individual's age, general health, nutritional status, use of medications, and mental health.

AGE Neonates or infants and older adults are greater surgical risks than children and adults. Age and developmental status affect children's ability to cope with the physiological and psychological stresses of surgery. Neonates and infants have a higher metabolic rate and a different physiological makeup than adults. For example, the blood volume in an infant is small, and its fluid reserves are limited, which increase the risk of volume depletion during surgery, resulting in inadequate oxygenation of body tissues. Because of the infant's relatively large body surface area and immature temperature regulatory mechanisms, the risk of hypothermia during surgery is significant. Other organ systems, such as the kidneys, liver, and immune system, have not achieved maturity in infants, affecting their ability to metabolize and eliminate drugs and resist infection.

Toddlers and older children are better able to withstand surgery physiologically, but they often fear separation from their parents, painful events (e.g., injections), strangers, bodily injury or mutilation, and death. The child's developmental level and age-appropriate communication are important in implementing the pediatric plan of care. The parent-child relationship, the parents' coping abilities, and the preoperative teaching and support will affect how well the child is able to deal with these surgical fears and the level of anxiety experienced.

The older adult often has fewer physiological reserves to meet the extra demands caused by surgery. The physiological deficits of aging increase the surgical risk for the older adult. For example, because of a lower percentage of body water, decreased kidney function, and a decreased thirst response, older adults are at greater risk for fluid and electrolyte imbalances.

Many older adults demonstrate changes in liver and kidney function, both of which can affect response to anaesthesia and other medications that may be administered during the perioperative period. The older adult may be poorly nourished, which can impair healing. Declines in sensory function (hearing in particular) or the presence of dementia make it more difficult to understand directions and teaching. In addition, the older adult is more likely to have a chronic disease, such as cardiovascular disease, chronic lung disease, or diabetes, that affects healing and responses to medication and surgery.

GENERAL HEALTH Surgery is least risky when the client's general health is good. Any infection or pathophysiology increases the risk. Of particular concern are upper respiratory tract infections, which, together with a general anaesthetic, can adversely affect respiratory function. Where the risk of infection is high, antibiotics may be administered parenterally within 1 hour of surgery and continued for 24 to 72 hours. This practice allows time for drugs to reach therapeutic levels in the tissues but does not permit bacterial resistance to develop. Common health problems that increase surgical risk and may lead to the decision to postpone or cancel surgery are listed in Box 35.2.

NUTRITIONAL STATUS Adequate nutrition is required for normal tissue repair. Surgery increases the body's need for nutrients for the needed tissue healing and prevention of infection required during the postoperative period. Obesity and malnutrition increase surgical risk.

Obesity contributes to postoperative complications, such as pneumonia, wound infections, and wound separation. Both obese and underweight clients are vulnerable to pressure ulcer formation because of positioning required for surgery. The perioperative nurse provides padding and other measures to protect the client's skin over pressure points during surgery.

Protein, vitamins, and minerals are essential for healthy wound healing (see Chapter 33). A malnourished client is at risk for delayed wound healing, wound infection, and fluid and electrolyte alterations. If a client has serious malnutrition, the surgery may be postponed to improve the client's nutritional status. If the surgery cannot be delayed, parenteral or enteral nutrition may be initiated.

MEDICATION HISTORY The regular use of certain prescribed and over-the-counter (OTC) medications can increase surgical risk. The following medications have the potential to affect physiological functions of the body and interact with anaesthesia, causing serious problems.

- Medications that *potentiate bleeding* increase the risk of hemorrhaging. Patients receiving *anticoagulants,* such as warfarin (Coumadin) or heparin, must be assessed by the health team and have a risk-benefit

BOX 35.2 HEALTH PROBLEMS THAT INCREASE SURGICAL RISK

These health problems can cause surgery to be delayed or cancelled:

- Malnutrition can lead to delayed wound healing, infection, and reduced energy. Protein and vitamins are needed for wound healing; vitamin K is essential for blood clotting.
- Obesity can lead to hypertension, impaired cardiac function, and impaired respiratory ventilation. Obese clients are also more likely to have delayed wound healing and wound infection because adipose tissue impedes blood circulation and its delivery of the nutrients, antibodies, and enzymes required for wound healing.
- Cardiac conditions, such as angina pectoris, recent myocardial infarction, hypertension, and heart failure, weaken the heart. Well-controlled cardiac problems generally pose minimal operative risk.
- Blood coagulation disorders can lead to severe bleeding, hemorrhage, and subsequent shock.
- Upper respiratory tract infections or chronic obstructive lung diseases, such as emphysema, adversely affect pulmonary function, especially when exacerbated by the effects of general anaesthesia. They also predispose the client to postoperative lung infections.
- Renal disease impairs regulation of the body's fluids and electrolytes and excretion of drugs and other toxins.
- Diabetes mellitus predisposes the client to wound infection and delayed healing.
- Liver disease (e.g., cirrhosis) impairs the liver's abilities to detoxify medications used during surgery, produce the prothrombin necessary for blood clotting, and metabolize nutrients essential for healing.
- Uncontrolled neurological disease, such as epilepsy, can result in seizures during surgery or recovery.

Evidence-Informed Practice

When Should Feeding Be Resumed Following Surgery?

The systematic review conducted by Anderson, Lewis, and Thomas (2006) examined the benefits and risks of enteral feeding within 24 hours following colorectal surgery. Their conclusions indicate that there is no advantage to the postoperative recovery by keeping the patient in a fasting state or giving fluids only. In fact, there was a trend toward a reduction in mortality and earlier discharge in patients given early feeding.

NURSING IMPLICATIONS: The guidelines for the introduction of food following surgery and, in particular, following gastrointestinal surgery have traditionally focused on nil per os (nothing by mouth) for upward of several days following surgery. Nurses should question traditional practices if the standard approach to postoperative resumption of liquids and food are not current and based on evidence.

Source: Based on "Early Enteral Nutrition within 24h of Colorectal Surgery versus Later Commencement of Feeding for Postoperative Complications," by H. K. Andersen, S. J. Lewis, and S. Thomas, 2006, *Cochrane Database of Systematic Reviews*, *4*, Art. No.: CD004080.

analysis conducted (Lecompte & Hardy, 2006). For people taking *antiplatelet agents,* such as acetylsalicylic acid (Aspirin), if the risk of bleeding exceeds the risk associated with thrombosis, it will generally be recommended that they discontinue the therapy for 7 to 10 days before the surgery. Unlike acetylsalicylic acid, the effects of which are irreversible, the antiplatelet effects of nonsteroidal anti-inflammatory drugs (e.g., ibuprofen) last only hours so preoperative cessation is of shorter duration, generally 24 to 48 hours.

- *Antidepressants,* particularly monoamine oxidase inhibitors (MAOs) and St. John's wort, a herbal product, increase the hypotensive action of anaesthesia.
- *Antihypertensives* interact with anaesthetic agents and can cause bradycardia, hypotension, and impaired circulation.
- *Tranquilizers* can interact with anaesthetics, increasing the risk of respiratory depression.
- *Insulin* may need to be adjusted in the perioperative period to account for the fasting or altered nutritional intake of the client; the stress of surgery can cause a rise in blood glucose.
- *Diuretics,* particularly thiazides, can affect fluid and electrolyte balance (particularly potassium) after surgery.
- *Corticosteroids,* with prolonged use, decrease the anti-inflammatory effect and can interfere with wound healing and increase the risk of infection.
- *Herbal medications,* such as garlic, ginkgo, and ginseng can affect bleeding time; ephedra can cause cardiovascular instability; ginseng can cause hypoglycemia; kava and valerian can potentiate the sedative effect of anaesthetics.

Clients may be unaware of the potential adverse interactions of medications and fail to report the use of medications for conditions unrelated to the indication for surgery. The nurse who collects a preoperative history should ask the client and family about the use of commonly prescribed medications and OTC preparations that the client takes.

MENTAL HEALTH STATUS Alterations in cognitive function (e.g., dementia or a developmental disability) or presence of a mental health problem (e.g., panic disorder or schizophrenia) can affect the client's ability to understand and cope with the stresses of surgery. Symptoms of confusion, disorientation, and agitation can be aggravated by the change of environment in the hospital, interfering with the client's ability to cooperate with preoperative and postoperative care.

Extreme anxiety increases surgical risk and interferes with the client's ability to process information and respond appropriately to instructions. In some instances, professional counselling is indicated before surgery. It is also important to determine whether clients have coping skills and support systems to help them.

Preoperative Phase

Preoperative Consent

Before any surgical procedure, clients must sign a consent form, which is generally supplied by the agency. This requirement protects the individual's autonomy and ensures that they have a clear understanding about the surgery, the benefits, and the risks. It also protects the hospital and the health personnel from a claim by the client or family that permission was not granted. The consent form becomes a part of the client's record and goes to the operating room with the client.

The surgeon maintains legal responsibility for ensuring that the patient is giving *informed* consent and ensuring that the client understands the procedure to be performed. If it is not clear that the client understands and consents to the surgery, the nurse has the responsibility of contacting the surgeon before surgery proceeds.

Preoperative informed consent should include the following:

- Nature and intention of the surgery
- Name and qualifications of the person performing the surgery
- Risks, including tissue damage, disfigurement, or even death
- Chances of success
- Possible alternative measures
- The right of the client to refuse consent or later withdraw consent

Informed consent is possible only when the patient understands the information being provided, that is, speaks the language and is conscious, mentally competent, and not under the influence of sedatives. The patient must also be legally capable. In Canada, depending on the laws of the province or territory, a minor under a certain age cannot legally give consent or can give consent only for certain procedures (e.g., in some provinces, a 14-year-old can give consent for an abortion but not cardiac surgery). Nurses must be aware of their responsibilities regarding consents and of the particular hospital policies. See Chapter 6 for further information about informed consent.

Assessing

Preoperative assessment includes collecting and reviewing specific client data to determine the client's needs throughout the perioperative experience.

NURSING HISTORY The nursing history obtained before surgery provides client data that help the nurse plan preoperative and postoperative care. The nurse completes a history according to agency form or policy. The Assessment: Interview box summarizes essential preoperative information that should be collected in the nursing history. It is also important that the nursing history include an assessment of any preoperative concerns of the patient or the family.

PHYSICAL ASSESSMENT Preoperatively, the nurse performs a brief but complete physical assessment, paying particular attention to systems that could affect the client's response to anaesthesia or surgery. A brief or mini mental status examination provides valuable baseline data for evaluating the client's mental status and alertness after surgery. It is also important to evaluate the client's ability to understand what is happening. For example, assessment of hearing and vision help guide perioperative teaching. Respiratory and cardiovascular assessment not only provides baseline data for evaluating the client's perioperative status but also can alert caregivers to a problem (e.g., respiratory infection or irregular pulse rate) that can affect the client's response to surgery and anaesthesia. Other systems (e.g., gastrointestinal, genitourinary, and musculoskeletal) are examined to provide baseline data (see Chapter 27).

SCREENING TESTS The surgeon or anaesthesiologist orders preoperative diagnostic tests. Abnormalities may warrant treatment before surgery. The nurse's responsibility is to check the orders carefully, to see that they are carried out, and to ensure that the results are obtained and entered into the client's record before surgery. Table 35.1 lists preoperative screening tests that may be prescribed based on Canadian Anesthesiologists' Society recommendations (2007).

Diagnosing

NANDA International (2007) nursing diagnoses that may be appropriate for the preoperative client include the following:

- *Deficient Knowledge* related to
  - A lack of education about the perioperative process
  - A lack of exposure to the specific perioperative experience
- *Anxiety* related to
  - Effects of surgery on ability to function in usual roles

ASSESSMENT: INTERVIEW

Preoperative Assessment Data

The following information must be gathered in the nursing history before surgery:

- *Current health status.* Essential information includes general health status and the presence of any chronic diseases, such as diabetes or asthma, that may affect the client's response to surgery or anaesthesia. Note any physical limitations that may affect the client's mobility or ability to communicate after surgery, as well as any prostheses, such as hearing aids or contact lenses.
- *Allergies.* Include allergies to prescription and nonprescription drugs, food allergies, and allergies to tape, latex, soaps, or antiseptic agents. Some food allergies indicate a potential reaction to drugs or substances used during surgery or diagnostic procedures; for example, an allergy to seafood alerts the nurse to a potential allergy to iodine-based dyes or soaps commonly used in hospitals; people who are allergic to foods, such as kiwi, banana, avocados, and chestnuts, may also have an allergy to latex in what is called latex-food syndrome.
- *Medications.* List all current medications (prescribed and OTC). It may be vital to maintain a blood level of some medications (e.g., anticonvulsants) throughout the surgical experience; others, such as anticoagulants or Aspirin, increase the risks of surgery and anaesthesia and need to be discontinued several days before surgery. It is important to include in the list any herbal remedies the client currently takes.
- *Previous surgeries and anaesthetic history.* Previous surgical and anaesthetic (general and local) experiences can influence the client's physical and psychological responses to surgery or may reveal unexpected responses to anaesthesia, such as cardiac arrest or malignant hyperthermia crisis.
- *Mental status.* The client's mental status and ability to understand and respond appropriately can affect the entire perioperative experience. Note any developmental disabilities, mental health problems, history of dementia, or excessive anxiety related to the procedure.
- *Understanding of the surgical procedure and anaesthesia.* The client should have a good understanding of the planned procedure and what to expect during and after surgery, as well as the expected outcome of the procedure.
- *Smoking.* Smokers may have more difficulty clearing respiratory secretions after surgery, increasing the risk of postoperative complications, such as pneumonia and atelectasis. Smoking also results in reduced oxygen-carrying capacity, increasing the risk of hypoxemia and delayed wound healing. Nicotine stimulates the surgical stress response, leading to increased workload for the heart.
- *Alcohol and other mind-altering substances.* Use of substances that affect the central nervous system, liver, or other body systems can affect the client's response to anaesthesia, surgery, and postoperative recovery.
- *Coping.* Clients with a healthy self-concept who have successfully employed appropriate coping mechanisms in the past are better able to deal with the stressors associated with surgery.
- *Social resources.* Determine the availability of family or other caregivers as well as the client's social support network. These resources are important to the client's recovery, particularly for the client undergoing same-day or short-stay surgery.
- *Cultural and spiritual considerations.* Culture and spirituality influence the client's response to surgery; respecting cultural and spiritual beliefs and practices can reduce preoperative anxiety and improve recovery.

  - Outcome of exploratory surgery for malignancy
  - Risk of death
  - Loss of control during anaesthesia or waking up during anaesthesia
  - Perceived inadequate postoperative analgesia
  - Change in health status or body image
- *Disturbed Sleep Pattern* related to
  - Hospital routines
  - Psychological stress
- *Anticipatory Grieving* related to
  - Perceived loss of body part associated with planned surgery

Planning

The overall goal in the preoperative period is to ensure that the client is mentally and physically prepared for surgery. Examples of nursing activities to meet this goal are discussed in the "Implementing" section that follows.

Planning should involve the client, family, and significant others. Preoperative care planning and teaching interventions are usually done on an outpatient basis, either in person or via a telephone interview by the perioperative nurse.

PLANNING FOR HOME CARE For the perioperative client, discharge planning begins before admission for the planned procedure. Early planning to meet the discharge needs of the client is particularly important for outpatient procedures, as generally these clients are discharged within hours after the procedure is performed.

Discharge planning incorporates an assessment of the client's, and his or her family's or significant other's abilities and resources for care, financial resources, and the need for referrals and home health services. However, the extent of discharge planning and home care will vary significantly for clients having different types of surgery.

TABLE 35.1 Preoperative Screening Tests

Test	Rationale
Complete blood count (CBC)	RBCs, hemoglobin (Hgb), and hematocrit (Hct) are important to the oxygen-carrying capacity of the blood; WBCs are an indicator of immune function; generally required for patients with chronic cardiovascular, pulmonary, renal, or hepatic disease; malignancy; and those undergoing major open surgery
Blood grouping and cross-matching	Determined in case blood transfusion is required during or after surgery
Serum electrolytes (Na^+, K^+, Ca^{2+}, Mg^{2+}, Cl^-, HCO_3^-)	To evaluate fluid and electrolyte status; generally required in any patient at risk of imbalance (e.g., chronic illness, digoxin or diuretic therapy)
Fasting blood glucose	High levels may indicate undiagnosed diabetes mellitus
Blood urea nitrogen (BUN) and creatinine	To evaluate renal function
Alanine aminotransferase (ALT), aspartate aminotransferase (AST), and bilirubin	To evaluate liver function
Serum albumin and total protein	To evaluate nutritional status; generally only in high-risk patients
International normalized ratio (INR) and activated partial thromboplastin time (APTT)	To evaluate coagulation; generally recommended for patients with liver disease or taking anticoagulent therapy
Urinalysis	To determine urine composition and possible abnormal components (e.g., protein or glucose) or infection
Chest X-ray	To evaluate respiratory status and heart size
Electrocardiogram (ECG)	To identify preexisting cardiac problems or disease
Pregnancy test (serum β-HCG)	To identify whether the client is pregnant; generally recommended in all females of childbearing age

Implementing

The major nursing activity to ensure that the client is prepared for surgery is preoperative teaching.

PREOPERATIVE TEACHING Preoperative teaching is a vital part of nursing care. Studies have shown that preoperative teaching reduces clients' anxiety and postoperative complications, as well as increasing their satisfaction with the surgical experience. Good preoperative teaching also facilitates the client's return to work and other activities of daily living (ADLs). Four dimensions of preoperative teaching have been identified as important to clients:

1. *Information, including what will happen to the client, when, and what the client will experience, such as expected sensations and discomfort.* The nurse needs to listen carefully and attentively to the client to identify specific concerns and fears. Typical questions include the following: What will happen during surgery? How will I feel after the operation? What will the surgeon find? How long will I be in the hospital?
2. *Psychosocial support to reduce anxiety.* The nurse provides support by actively listening and providing accurate information. It is important to rectify any misbeliefs the client may have.
3. *The roles of the client and support people in preoperative preparation, the surgical procedure, and during the postoperative phase.* Understanding his or her role during the perioperative experience increases the client's sense of control and reduces anxiety. This includes what will be expected of the client, desired behaviours, self-care activities, and what the client can do to facilitate recovery.
4. *Skills training.* These skills include moving, breathing deeply, coughing, splinting incisions with the hands or a pillow, and using an incentive spirometer.

If the client is scheduled for outpatient surgery, preoperative teaching is often provided before the day of surgery by using some combination of videos and verbal and written instructions. The client may have an appointment with the outpatient surgery staff (usually scheduled to coincide with preoperative diagnostic testing) to discuss preoperative concerns and implement the teaching plan. Written instructions are always provided to reinforce verbal teaching. Teaching is further reinforced on admission the day of surgery and before discharge from the postanaesthesia unit. Preoperative instructions are summarized in the Teaching: Clinical box.

When the client is a child, addressing the fears and anxieties of both the child and the family is vital. Parents

TEACHING: CLINICAL

Preoperative Instructions

Clients need to understand the preoperative instructions they are given and what to expect immediately after surgery:

PREOPERATIVE REGIMEN

- Explain the need for preoperative tests (e.g., laboratory, X-ray, ECG).
- Discuss bowel preparation, if required.
- Discuss skin preparation, including operative area and preoperative bath or shower.
- Discuss preoperative medications, if prescribed.
- Explain the need to avoid smoking and alcohol consumption 24 to 48 hours preoperatively. Encouragement and support for smoke cessation are generally effective for short-term smoke cessation (Møller & Villebro, 2005).
- Explain individual therapies ordered by the physician, such as intravenous therapy, the insertion of a urinary catheter or nasogastric tube, use of a spirometer, or antiembolism stockings.
- Discuss the visit by the anaesthetist.
- Explain the need to restrict or eliminate food and oral fluid intake before surgery. Follow the institution's or the Canadian Anesthesiologists' Society's (2007) guidelines, discussed later.
- Provide a general timetable for perioperative events, including the time of surgery.
- Discuss the need to remove jewellery (including all body piercings), makeup, and all prostheses (e.g., eyeglasses, hearing aids, complete or partial dentures, wigs) immediately before surgery. In some cases, the surgeon may leave instructions for the client to leave hearing aids and eyeglasses on to enable better communication.
- Inform the client about the preoperative holding area, and give the location of the waiting room for support people (a surgical liaison nurse may visit support people intraoperatively to update them on the condition of the surgical patient).
- Teach deep-breathing and coughing exercises, leg exercises, ways to turn and move (see Skill 35.1), and splinting techniques.
- Complete the preoperative checklist.

POSTOPERATIVE REGIMEN

- Discuss the postanaesthesia recovery room's routines and emergency equipment.
- Review type and frequency of assessment activities.
- Discuss pain management.
- Explain usual activity restrictions and precautions related to getting up for the first time postoperatively.
- Describe usual dietary alterations.
- Discuss postoperative dressings and drains.
- Provide an explanation and tour of the intensive care unit if the client is to be transferred there postoperatively.

OUTPATIENT SURGICAL CLIENTS

- Confirm the place and time of surgery, including when to arrive (e.g., 1 to 1.5 hours before scheduled surgery) and where to register (e.g., reception desk).
- Discuss what to wear (e.g., clients having hand surgery should wear a garment with large sleeve openings to fit over a bulky dressing; all clients need to leave valuables at home).
- Explain the need for a responsible adult to drive or accompany the client home, and arrange a place for them to meet. Discuss discharge criteria and how long the client should expect to stay postoperatively.
- Discuss medications, including specific preoperative medications and the client's current medication regimen.
- Provide anticipatory guidance about the expected recovery trajectory so that the client can make necessary plans (e.g., childcare may need to be arranged; special dietary foods may need to be purchased).
- Communicate by telephone the evening before surgery to confirm time of surgery and arrival time, and call again the evening after surgery to assess progress.

need to know what to expect and to be able to express their concerns. Parents should be considered members of the perioperative team and be allowed to participate in providing as much care as possible.

Skill 35.1 provides guidelines for teaching clients about moving, leg exercises, deep breathing, and coughing.

SKILL 35.1

TEACHING MOVING, LEG EXERCISES, DEEP BREATHING, AND COUGHING

PURPOSES

Moving

- To promote venous return
- To enhance lung expansion and mobilize secretions
- To stimulate gastrointestinal mobility
- To facilitate early ambulation

Leg Exercises

- To promote venous return, thereby preventing thrombophlebitis and thrombus formation

Deep Breathing and Coughing

- To enhance lung expansion and mobilize secretions, thereby preventing atelectasis and pneumonia

(continued)

SKILL 35.1

TEACHING MOVING, LEG EXERCISES, DEEP BREATHING, AND COUGHING *(continued)*

ASSESSMENT
Assess the following:
- Vital signs
- Discomfort
- Temperature and colour of feet and legs
- Breath sounds
- Presence of dyspnea or cough
- Learning needs of the client
- Anxiety level of the client
- The client's experience with previous surgeries and anaesthesia

Planning
Before commencing to teach moving, leg exercises, deep-breathing exercises, and coughing, determine (1) the type of surgery, (2) the time of the surgery, (3) the name of the surgeon, (4) the preoperative orders, (5) the agency's policies for preoperative care, and (6) the learning needs of the client. Also, verify that the physician has completed the medical history and physical examination and that the consent form has been signed by the client or the family or substitute decision maker.

Equipment
- Pillow
- Teaching materials (e.g., videotape, written materials) if available at the agency

IMPLEMENTATION
Preparation
Ensure that potential distracters (e.g., pain, TV, visitors) to teaching are not present. Family and significant others should be included in the teaching plan, if appropriate.

Performance
1. Before performing the procedure, introduce yourself and verify the client's identity by using agency protocol. Explain to the client what you are going to teach and the importance of the client's participation in the exercises he or she is going to be taught.
2. Perform hand hygiene and observe other appropriate infection prevention and control procedures.
3. Provide for client privacy.
4. Show the client ways to turn in bed and to get out of bed.
   - Instruct a client who will have a right abdominal incision or a right-sided chest incision to turn to the left side of the bed and sit up as follows:
     a. Flex the knees.
     b. Splint the wound by holding the left arm and hand or a small pillow against the incision.
     c. Turn to the left while pushing with the right foot and grasping a partial side rail on the left side of the bed with the right hand.
     d. Come to a sitting position on the side of the bed by using the right arm and hand to push down against the mattress and swinging the feet over the edge of the bed.
   - Teach a client with a left abdominal or left-sided chest incision to perform the same procedure but splint with the right arm and turn to the right.
   - For clients with orthopedic surgery (e.g., hip surgery), use special aids, such as a trapeze, to assist with movement.
5. Teach the client the following three leg exercises:
   - Alternate dorsiflexion and plantar flexion of the feet. **Rationale: This exercise is sometimes referred to as calf pumping because it alternately contracts and relaxes the calf muscles, including the gastrocnemius muscles.** See ❶.

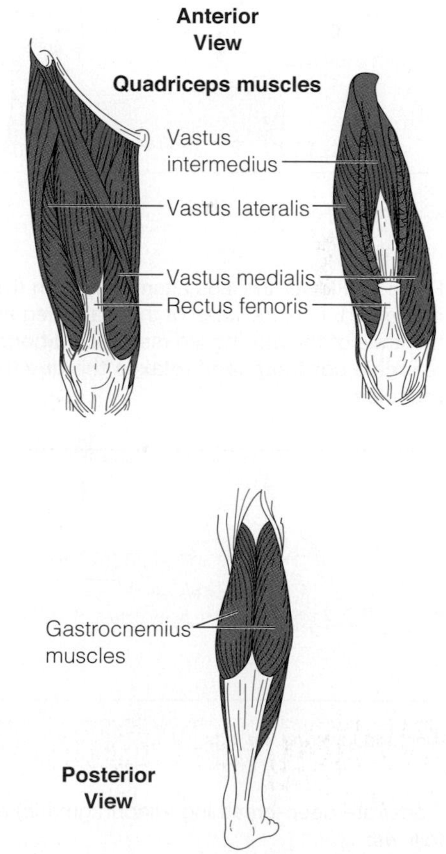

❶ Leg muscles: anterior and posterior views

(continued)

SKILL 35.1

TEACHING MOVING, LEG EXERCISES, DEEP BREATHING, AND COUGHING (*continued*)

- Flex and extend the knees, and press the backs of the knees into the bed while dorsiflexing the feet (see ❷). Instruct clients who cannot raise their legs to do isometric exercises that contract and relax the muscles.

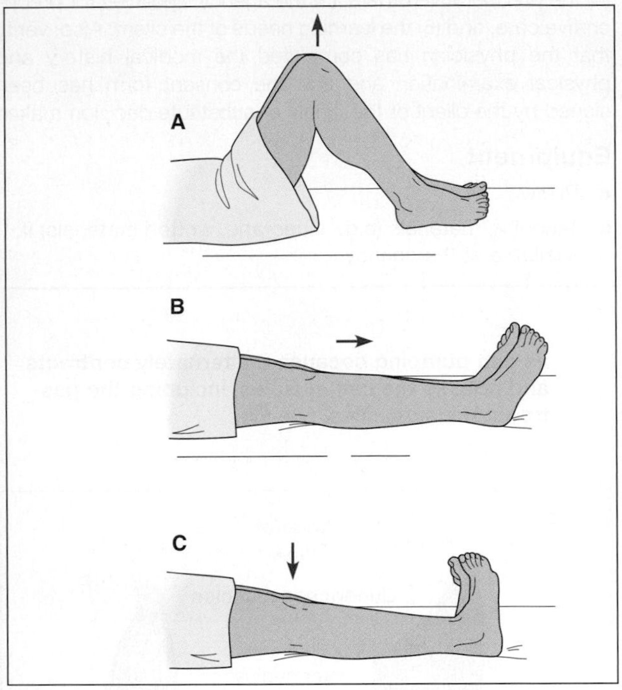

❷ Flexing and extending the knees

- Raise and lower the legs alternately from the surface of the bed. Flex the knee of the stable leg and extend the knee of the moving leg (see ❸). **Rationale: This exercise contracts and relaxes the quadriceps muscles**.

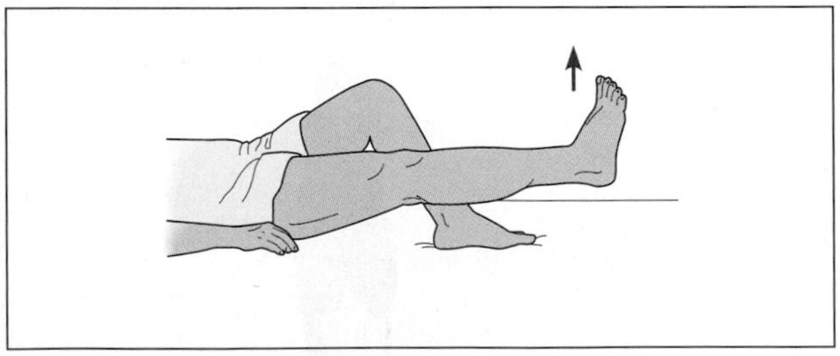

❸ Raising and lowering the legs

6. Demonstrate deep-breathing (diaphragmatic) exercises as follows:
   - Place your hands palms down on the border of your rib cage, and inhale slowly and evenly through the nose until the greatest chest expansion is achieved (see ❹).
   - Hold your breath for two to three seconds.
   - Then, exhale slowly through the mouth.
   - Continue exhalation until maximum chest contraction has been achieved.

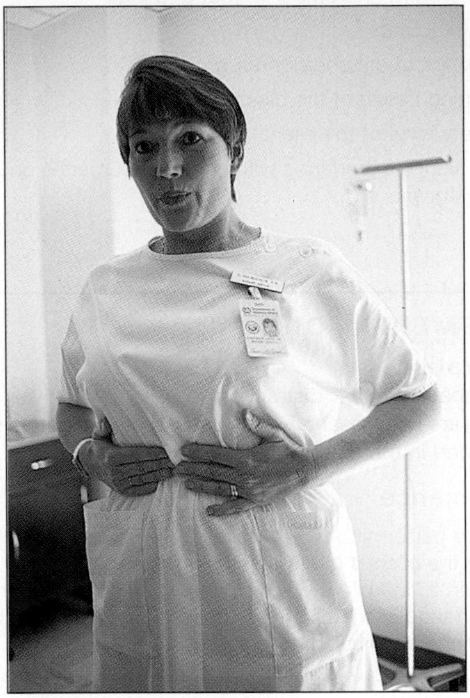

❹ Demonstrating deep breathing

7. Help the client perform deep-breathing exercises.
   - Ask the client to assume a sitting position.
   - Place the palms of your hands on the border of the client's rib cage to assess respiratory depth.
   - Ask the client to perform deep breathing, as described in step 6.
8. Instruct the client to cough voluntarily after five deep inhalations.
   - Ask the client to inhale deeply, hold the breath for a few seconds, and then cough once or twice.
   - Ensure that the client coughs deeply and does not just clear the throat.
9. If the incision will be painful when the client coughs, demonstrate techniques to splint the abdomen.
   - Show the client how to support the incision by placing the palms of the hands on either side of the incision site or directly over the incision site, holding the palm of one hand over the other. **Rationale: Coughing uses the abdominal and other accessory respiratory muscles. Splinting the incision can reduce pain while coughing if the incision is near any of these muscles.**

(continued)

SKILL 35.1

TEACHING MOVING, LEG EXERCISES, DEEP BREATHING, AND COUGHING *(continued)*

- Show the client how to splint the abdomen with clasped hands and a firmly rolled pillow held against the client's abdomen (see ❺).

10. Inform the client about the expected frequency of these exercises.
    - Instruct the client to start the exercises as soon after surgery as possible.
    - Encourage clients with abdominal or chest surgery to carry out deep breathing and coughing at least every 2 hours, taking a minimum of five breaths at each session. Note, however, that the number of breaths and frequency of deep breathing varies with the client's condition. People who are susceptible to pulmonary problems may need deep-breathing exercises every hour. People with chronic respiratory disease may need special breathing exercises (e.g., pursed-lip breathing, abdominal breathing, exercises using various kinds of incentive spirometers). See Chapter 42.
11. Document the teaching and all assessments.

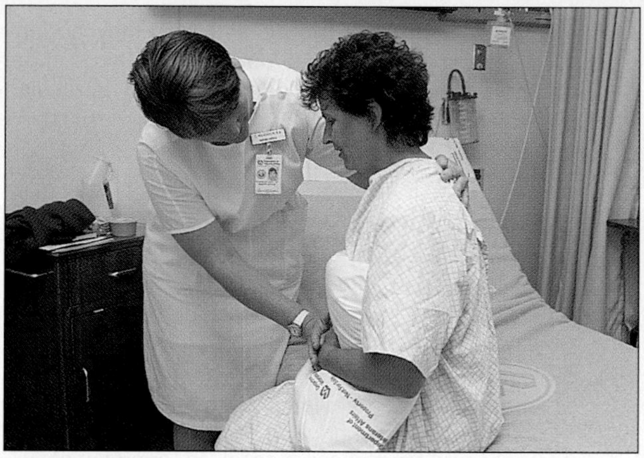

❺ Splinting an incision with a pillow while coughing

EVALUATION

Document the outcome of the teaching plan, such as the following:

- Client's demonstrated ability to perform moving, leg exercises, deep-breathing, and coughing exercises
- Client's verbalization of key information presented

Lifespan Considerations

Preoperative Teaching

CHILDREN

- Parents need to know what to expect and to be able to express their concerns.
- Separation from parents often is the child's greatest fear; the time of separation should be minimized and parents allowed to interact with the child both immediately preceding and following the surgery.
- Teaching and communicating with children (both timing and content) should be geared to the child's developmental level and cognitive abilities (e.g., "You will have a sore tummy").
- Play is an effective teaching tool with children (e.g., the child can put a bandage on an incision on a doll).

OLDER ADULTS

- Assess hearing ability to ensure the older client hears the necessary information.
- Assess short-term memory. Presenting one focused idea at a time and repeating or reinforcing information may be necessary.
- Older adults are at greater risk for postoperative complications, such as pneumonia. Reinforce moving and deep-breathing and coughing exercises.
- Assess potential postoperative needs at this time. Arrangements can be made preoperatively to obtain necessary items. Examples are medical equipment, such as walkers, raised toilet seats, bed trapezes, Meals on Wheels, and help with transportation.
- If the older client will need to be in extended care for a period of time after surgery, this is the time to initiate these plans.
- Assess the client for risk of pressure ulcer development postoperatively and be extra attentive to use of proper paddings and support devices to prevent injury during positioning and transfers in the operating room. Risks for pressure ulcers include the following:
    - Older age
    - Poor nutritional status
    - History of diabetes or cardiovascular problems
    - History of taking steroids, which cause increased bruising and skin breakdown

TEACHING: HOME CARE

Postoperative Instructions

Adults want information about activities they normally perform while they are recovering at home. This is important information for all surgical clients and particularly clients having the surgery as outpatients. Discuss the following areas:

- *Food.* Eat small portions at first because anaesthesia and certain analgesics slow gastric emptying.
- *Bowel movements.* Constipation occurs frequently because of decreased gastrointestinal mobility with different causes (e.g., anaesthesia, decreased activity, opioids). Discuss strategies to prevent constipation.
- *Sexual activity.* Intimacy, such as gentle hugging and kissing, is allowed for clients when they feel like it. Full sexual intercourse cannot be resumed until wound soreness and tenderness is resolved, approximately 2 to 4 weeks. Check with the surgeon for gynecological procedures.
- *Wound care.* Discuss wound strength and care, including the signs and symptoms of infection and when to notify the surgeon.
- *Lifting.* Be specific about weight limits, if appropriate. Relate the weight limit to everyday items (e.g., 4 litres of milk weighs 4 kilograms).
- *Pain.* Provide information about the client's analgesia. Ask the client to describe his or her daily activities and discuss ways to avoid or reduce painful activities.
- *Bathing.* Check with the surgeon because some prefer the wound to be kept dry. If allowed, tell the client to shower, letting the warm water wash over the incision and gently pat the incision dry.
- *Activities.* Advise the client that he or she will tire easily and to plan short activities with frequent rest breaks.

PHYSICAL PREPARATION Preoperative preparation includes the following areas: nutrition and fluids, elimination, hygiene, medications, rest, care of valuables and prostheses, special orders, and surgical skin preparation. In many agencies, a preoperative checklist is used on the day of surgery. The nurse checks the agency's forms and follows appropriate documenting procedures. It is essential that all pertinent records (laboratory records, X-ray films, consents) be available for perioperative personnel to refer to and that all physical preparation be completed to ensure client safety.

NUTRITION AND FLUIDS Adequate hydration and nutrition promote healing. Nurses need to identify and record any signs of malnutrition or fluid imbalance. If the client is receiving intravenous fluids or is on measured fluid intake and output, nurses must ensure that the fluids are carefully measured. The order "NPO after midnight" has been a long-standing tradition because it was believed that anaesthetics depress gastrointestinal functioning and there was a danger the client would vomit and aspirate during the administration of a general anaesthetic. Re-evaluation and research, however, do not support this tradition for patients at normal risk of aspiration or regurgitation. Drinking clear fluids up to a few hours before surgery does not increase the risk of regurgitation during or after surgery (Brady, Kinn, & Stuart, 2003) and leads to improved comfort and behaviour in the postoperative period (Brady, Kinn, O'Rourke, Randhawa, & Stuart, 2005). Box 35.3 summarizes the Canadian Anesthesiologists' Society (2007) guidelines for minimum fasting times before elective surgical procedures. Emergent or urgent procedures should be undertaken after considering the risk of delaying surgery versus the risk of aspiration of gastric contents.

BOX 35.3 MINIMUM FASTING GUIDELINES FOR ELECTIVE SURGICAL PROCEDURES

Before elective surgery, these fasting times should be followed:

- 8 hours after a meal that includes meat, fried food, or fatty foods
- 6 hours after a light meal (such as toast and a clear fluid)
- 6 hours after ingestion of infant formula or nonhuman milk
- 4 hours after ingestion of breast milk
- 2 hours after clear fluids

Source: Based on *Guidelines: The Preanaesthetic Period*, by the Canadian Anesthesiologists' Society, 2007, retrieved June 19, 2008, from http://www.cas.ca/members/sign_in/guidelines/preanaesthetic/

ELIMINATION Enemas before surgery are no longer routine, but cleansing enemas may be ordered if bowel surgery is planned. The enemas help prevent postoperative constipation and contamination of the surgical area by feces. After surgery involving the intestines, peristalsis often doesn't return for 24 to 48 hours.

Before surgery, a retention catheter may be ordered to ensure that the bladder remains empty. This helps prevent inadvertent injury to the bladder, particularly during pelvic surgery. If the client does not have a catheter, it is important to empty the bladder before receiving preoperative medications. The bladder must be empty during the operation.

HYGIENE In some settings, clients are asked to bathe or shower the evening or morning of surgery (or both). The purpose of hygiene measures is to reduce the risk of wound infection. The bath includes a shampoo, whenever possible.

The client's nails should be trimmed and free of polish and all cosmetics should be removed so that the nail beds, skin, and lips are visible when circulation is assessed during the perioperative phases.

Intraoperatively the client may be required to wear a surgical cap to contain the client's hair and any microorganisms on the hair and scalp.

Before going into the operating room the client should remove all hairpins and clips as they may cause pressure or accidental damage to the scalp when the client is unconscious. The client also removes personal clothing and puts on a hospital gown.

Medications The anaesthetist may temporarily discontinue routinely taken medications the day of surgery. In some settings, preoperative medications are given to the client before going to the operating room. Common preoperative medications include the following:

- *Sedatives and tranquilizers,* such as lorazepam (Ativan) and diazepam (Valium), to reduce anxiety and ease anaesthetic induction
- *Opioids,* such as morphine, to provide client sedation and reduce the required amount of anaesthetic
- *Anticholinergics,* such as atropine, scopolamine, and glycopyrrolate (Robinul), to reduce oral and pulmonary secretions and prevent laryngospasm
- *Histamine-receptor antagonists,* such as cimetidine (Tagamet) and ranitidine (Zantac), to reduce gastric fluid volume and gastric acidity
- *Neuroleptanalgesic agents,* such as Innovar (droperidol and fentanyl), to induce general calmness and sleepiness
- *Antibiotics,* such as cephalosporins administered 1 to 2 hours before surgery for prophylaxis against operative site infection.

Preoperative medications must be given at a scheduled time or *on call,* that is, when the operating room notifies the nurse to give the medication.

Rest and Sleep Nurses should do everything to help the client sleep the night before surgery. Often, a sedative is ordered. Adequate rest helps the client manage the stress of surgery and helps healing.

Care of Valuables Valuables, such as jewellery and money, should be labelled and placed in safekeeping if the client's support people cannot take them home. Removing jewellery also includes body-piercing jewellery; there is a risk of injury from burns if an electrosurgical unit is used. If a client cannot or does not want to remove a wedding band, the nurse can tape it in place. Wedding bands must be removed, however, if there is danger of the fingers swelling after surgery. Situations warranting removal include surgery on or cast application to an arm and a mastectomy that involves removal of the lymph nodes. (Mastectomies may cause edema of the arm and hand.)

Care of Prostheses All prostheses (artificial body parts, such as partial or complete dentures, contact lenses, artificial eyes, and artificial limbs), as well as eyeglasses, wigs, and false eyelashes, must be removed before surgery. Hearing aids are often left in place and the operating room personnel notified.

In some hospitals, dentures are placed in a locked storage area; in others, they are placed in labelled containers and kept at the client's bedside. Partial dentures can become dislodged and obstruct an unconscious client's breathing. The nurse also checks for the presence of chewing gum or loose teeth, a common problem with five- or six-year-olds undergoing tonsillectomy. Loose teeth can become dislodged and be aspirated during anaesthesia.

Special Orders The nurse checks the surgeon's orders for special requirements (e.g., the insertion of a nasogastric tube before surgery, the administration of medications, such as insulin, the application of antiembolism stockings).

CLINICAL ALERT

Multiple safety checks are recommended before and during surgery to ensure that the *correct patient* receives the *correct procedure* and, in such surgeries as hip replacement, lung lobectomy, or mastectomy, that the *correct side* is operated on. To minimize wrong-sided surgery, the Canadian Orthopedic Association (2005) recommends a standardized procedure for limb identification by using a permanent marking pen to initial the operative site.

Preoperative Skin Preparation The Operating Room Nurses Association of Canada (2006) recommends the following skin preparation practices to reduce the risk of postoperative wound infections: the client is encouraged to shower and shampoo or wash the surgical site before arriving in the surgical setting; the nurse assesses the surgical site for moles, warts, rashes, or other skin conditions, such as pustules, abrasions, or exudate, and documents their presence before skin preparation.

In the past, hair around the surgical site was removed by shaving. It is now known that shaving causes microscopic skin abrasions that provide a portal of entry for microorganisms, so shaving around the surgical site is *not* recommended. Safer Healthcare Now! (2007) recommends that if surgical site hair removal is needed, it should be done by using hair clippers or depilatory. The Safer Healthcare Now! national campaign to reduce surgical site infections also recommends that razors be removed entirely from hospital stock and that patients be educated not to shave themselves.

SAFETY PROTOCOLS Protocols to ensure correct patient, correct site, and correct procedure were developed after sentinel events involving wrong person, wrong site, and wrong procedure surgical errors. Three key steps ensure patient safety throughout the surgical procedure. The first step requires preoperative verification. Although client verification used to be a one-time procedure, newer protocols require client verification at the time surgery is scheduled, during admission, and whenever the patient is transferred to another caregiver. The second step involves marking of the operative site in an unambiguous manner. Although the type of mark may vary across institutions, the surgical site marking method *must* be consistent throughout the facility. The facility chooses its own surgical site marking method (e.g., the client's initials, surgeon's initials, the word *YES*). An X is considered ambiguous (e.g., some people may interpret it as "X marks the spot," while others may interpret the X as "this is *not* the site") and cannot be used for marking the site. The mark must be permanent and visible after the client has been prepped and draped for surgery.

The third step is called time-out. Before surgery begins, the surgical team takes a time-out to conduct a final verification of the correct client, procedure, and site. Any questions or concerns must be resolved before the procedure can begin.

VITAL SIGNS Preoperatively assess and document vital signs for baseline data. Report any abnormal findings, such as elevated blood pressure or elevated temperature.

ANTIEMBOLISM STOCKINGS Antiembolism stockings are firm elastic hose that compress the veins of the legs and thereby facilitate the return of venous blood to the heart. They also improve arterial circulation to the feet and prevent edema of the legs and feet. These stockings are frequently applied to surgical clients.

The stockings come in several types. One type extends from the foot to the knee and another from the foot to midthigh. These stockings usually have a partial foot that exposes the heel or toes so that extremity circulation can be assessed. Elastic stockings usually come in small, medium, and large sizes. Skill 35.2 details the steps required to apply antiembolism stockings.

SKILL 35.2

APPLYING ANTIEMBOLISM STOCKINGS

PURPOSES

- To facilitate venous return from the lower extremities
- To prevent venous stasis and venous thrombosis
- To reduce peripheral edema

ASSESSMENT

Assess both lower extremities for the following:

- Rates, volumes, and rhythms of posterior tibial and dorsalis pedis pulses
- Skin colour (note pallor, cyanosis, or other pigmentation)
- Skin temperature
- Presence of distended veins or edema
- Skin condition (e.g., thickened, shiny, taut)
- Homans' sign (pain in calf with passive dorsiflexion)
- Pressure zones
- Decreased circulation (numbness, tingling, pain)

Planning

Before applying antiembolism stockings, determine any potential or present circulatory problems and the surgeon's orders involving the lower extremities.

Equipment

- Tape measure
- Clean antiembolism stockings of appropriate size and type ordered

IMPLEMENTATION

Preparation

Take measurements as needed to obtain the appropriate size stockings:

- Measure the length of both legs from the heel to the gluteal fold (for thigh-length stockings) or from the heel to the popliteal space (for knee-length stockings).
- Measure the circumference of each calf and each thigh at the widest point.
- Compare the measurements to the size chart to obtain stockings of correct size. Obtain two sizes if there is a significant difference. **Rationale: Stockings that are too large for the client do not place adequate pressure on the legs to facilitate venous return and may bunch, increasing the risk of pressure and skin irritation. Stockings that are too small may impede blood flow to the feet and cause discomfort.**

Performance

1. Before performing the procedure, introduce yourself and verify the client's identity by using agency protocol. Explain to the client what you are going to do, why it is necessary, and how he or she can cooperate.
2. Perform hand hygiene and observe other appropriate infection prevention and control procedures.
3. Provide for client privacy.

(continued)

SKILL 35.2

APPLYING ANTIEMBOLISM STOCKINGS (*continued*)

4. Select an appropriate time to apply the stockings.
   - Apply stockings in the morning, if possible, before the client rises. **Rationale: In sitting and standing positions, the veins can become distended so that edema occurs; the stockings should be applied before this happens.**
   - Assist the client who has been ambulating to lie down and elevate the legs for 15 to 30 minutes before applying the stockings. **Rationale: This facilitates venous return and reduces swelling.**
5. Prepare the client.
   - Assist the client to a lying position in bed.
   - Wash and dry the legs, as needed.
6. Apply the stockings.
   - Reach inside the stocking from the top, and grasping the heel, turn the upper portion of the stocking inside out over the foot portion. **Rationale: Firm elastic stockings are easier to fit over the foot and calf when inverted in this manner, rather than bunching the stocking up.**
   - Ask the client to point the toes, and position the stocking on the client's foot, taking care to place the toe and heel portions of the stocking appropriately (see ❶) **Rationale: Pointing the toes makes application easier.**
   - Grasp the upper edge of the stocking and gently pull the stocking over the leg, turning it right side out in the process (see ❷).
   - Inspect the client's leg and stocking, smoothing any folds or creases. Ensure that the stocking is not rolled down or bunched at the top or ankle. **Rationale: Folds and creases can cause skin irritation under the stocking; bunching of the stocking can further impair venous return.**
   - Remove the stockings for 30 minutes every 8 hours, inspecting the legs and skin while the stockings are off.
   - Soiled stockings can be laundered by hand with warm water and mild soap. Hang to dry.
7. Document the procedure. Record the procedure, your assessment data, and when the stockings are removed and reapplied.

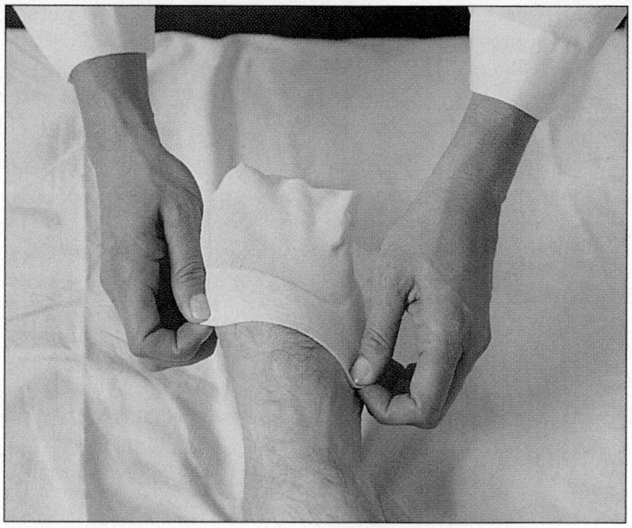

❶ Applying the inverted stocking over the toes

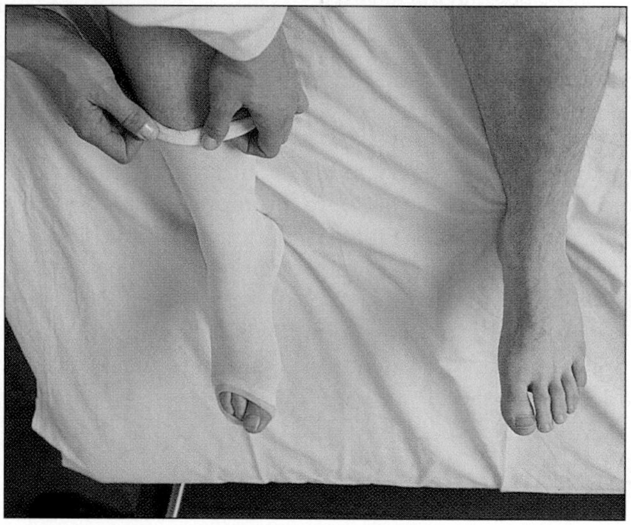

❷ Pulling the stocking snugly over the leg

EVALUATION

- Remove antiembolism stockings one to three times a day for 30 minutes for skin care and inspection.
- Note the appearance of the legs and skin integrity, any edema, peripheral pulses, skin colour and temperature, and compare with previous assessment data.
- If complications occur, remove the stockings and report findings to the appropriate members of the health-care team.

Lifespan Considerations

Antiembolism Stockings

CHILDREN

- Antiembolism stockings are not frequently used on children.

OLDER ADULTS

- Because the elastic is quite strong in antiembolism stockings, older adults may need assistance with putting on the stockings. Clients with arthritis may need to have another person put the stockings on for them.
- Many older adults have circulation problems and wear antiembolism stockings. It is important to check for wrinkles in the stockings and to see if the stocking has rolled down or twisted. If so, correct immediately because the stockings must be evenly distributed over the limb to promote rather than hinder circulation.
- Stockings should be removed once each shift so that a thorough assessment can be made of legs and feet. Redness and skin breakdown on the heels can occur quickly and go undetected if not thoroughly assessed on a regular basis.

Home Care Considerations

Antiembolism Stockings

- Teach the client or caregiver how to apply the antiembolism stockings.
- Stress the importance of no wrinkles or rolling down of the stockings and the rationale.
- Instruct the client or caregiver to remove the stockings daily and inspect the skin on the legs.
- Provide instructions about the following:
  - Laundering the stockings
- The need for two pairs of stockings to allow for one pair to be worn while the other is being laundered
- Replacing the stockings when they lose their elasticity

SEQUENTIAL COMPRESSION DEVICES Clients who are undergoing surgery may benefit from a sequential compression device (SCD) to promote venous return from the legs. SCDs inflate and deflate plastic sleeves wrapped around the legs to promote venous flow. SCDs are discussed in Chapter 42. Skill 42.6 (page 1359) outlines how to apply a sequential compression device. Application for SCDs needs to follow physician's orders and agency policy.

Evaluating

The goals established during the planning phase are evaluated according to specific desired health outcomes, also established in that phase.

Intraoperative Phase

The intraoperative nurse is a vital member of the surgical team, advocating for the client, maintaining safety, and continually assessing the needs of the client and the team.

Types of Anaesthesia

Anaesthesia is classified as *general* or *regional* or *local.* Anaesthetic agents are administered by an anaesthesiologist. **General anaesthesia** is the loss of all sensation and consciousness. Under general anaesthesia, protective reflexes, such as cough and gag reflexes, are lost. A general anaesthetic acts by blocking awareness centres in the brain so that amnesia (loss of memory), analgesia (insensibility to pain), hypnosis (artificial sleep), and relaxation (rendering a part of the body less tense) occur. General anaesthetics are usually administered by intravenous infusion or by inhalation of gases through a mask or through an endotracheal tube inserted into the trachea.

General anaesthesia has certain advantages. Because the client is unconscious, rather than awake and anxious, respiration and cardiac function are readily regulated. Also, the anaesthesia can be adjusted to the length of the operation and the client's age and physical status. Its chief disadvantage is that it depresses the respiratory and circulatory systems. Some clients become more anxious about a general anaesthetic than about the surgery itself. Often, this is because they fear losing the capacity to control their own bodies.

Local anaesthesia interrupts the transmission of nerve impulses to a specific small area (e.g., index finger). Local anaesthesia is used for minor surgical procedures, such as suturing a small wound, performing a biopsy, or during tooth extraction. **Regional anaesthesia** is the temporary interruption of the transmission of nerve impulses to and from a specific area or region of the body (e.g., an arm). In both local and regional anaesthesia, the client loses sensation in an area of the body but remains conscious.

Local anaesthesia can be given in the following ways:

- **Topical (surface) anaesthesia** can be applied directly to the skin and mucous membranes, open skin surfaces, wounds, and burns. The most commonly used topical agents are lidocaine (Xylocaine) and benzocaine. A topical patch, such as a eutectic mixture of local anaesthetics (or the EMLA patch), can be applied before injection or intravenous insertion. Topical anaesthetics are readily absorbed and act rapidly.
- In **local infiltration**, an anaesthetic agent is injected into a specific area. Lidocaine is used most commonly.

Several techniques are used in regional anaesthesia:

- A **nerve block** is a technique in which the anaesthetic agent is injected into and around a nerve or small nerve group that supplies sensation to a small area of the body. Major blocks involve multiple nerves or a *plexus* (e.g., the brachial plexus anaesthetizes the arm); minor blocks involve a single nerve (e.g., a facial nerve).
- An **intravenous block (Bier block)** is used most often for procedures involving the arm, wrist, and hand. An occlusion tourniquet is applied to the extremity to prevent infiltration and absorption of the injected intravenous agent beyond the involved extremity.
- **Spinal anaesthesia** is also referred to as a **subarachnoid block (SAB)**. It requires a lumbar puncture through one of the interspaces between lumbar disc 2 (L-2) and the sacrum (S-1). An anaesthetic agent is injected into the subarachnoid space surrounding the spinal cord. Spinal anaesthesia is often categorized as a low, mid, or high spinal. *Low spinals* (saddle or caudal blocks) are primarily used for surgeries involving the perineal or rectal areas. *Mid spinals* (below the level of the umbilicus—T-10) can be used for hernia repairs or appendectomies, and *high spinals* (reaching the nipple line—T-4) can be used for surgeries, such as cesarean sections.
- **Epidural (peridural) anaesthesia** is an injection of an anaesthetic agent into the epidural space, the area inside the spinal column but outside the dura mater.

Conscious sedation may be used alone or in conjunction with regional anaesthesia for some diagnostic tests and surgical procedures. **Conscious sedation** is defined as minimal depression of the level of consciousness in which the client retains the ability to consciously maintain a patent airway and respond appropriately to commands. Intravenous opioids, such as morphine or fentanyl (Sublimaze), and antianxiety agents, such as diazepam (Valium) or midazolam (Versed), are commonly used to induce and maintain conscious sedation. Conscious sedation increases the client's pain threshold and induces a degree of amnesia but allows for prompt reversal of its effects and a rapid return to normal ADLs. Such procedures as endoscopies, incision and drainage of abscesses, and even balloon angioplasty can be performed under conscious sedation.

Assessing

On the client's admission to the surgical suite or procedure room, the perioperative nurse confirms the client's identity and assesses the client's physical and emotional status. The nurse verifies the information on the preoperative checklist and evaluates the client's knowledge about the surgery and events to follow. The client's response to preoperative medications is assessed, as well as the placement and patency of tubes, such as IV lines, nasogastric tubes, and urinary catheters.

Assessment continues throughout surgery as the nurse and the anaesthetist continuously monitor the client's vital signs (including blood pressure, heart rate, respiratory rate, and temperature), ECG, and oxygen saturation. Fluid intake and urinary output are monitored throughout surgery, and blood loss is estimated. In addition, arterial and venous pressures, pulmonary artery pressures, and laboratory values, such as blood glucose, hemoglobin, hematocrit, serum electrolytes, and arterial blood gases, may be evaluated during surgery. Continual assessment is necessary to rapidly identify adverse responses to surgery or anaesthesia and intervene promptly to prevent complications.

During the intraoperative period, the nurse is aware of potential problems that could occur. These problems are likely related to the position of the patient, the effects of the anaesthesia, equipment used and potential hazards, disruption of tissue perfusion during surgery, and the incision. The nurse also considers that complications that can occur are hemorrhage, surgical site infection, and neuromuscular injury.

Diagnosing

NANDA International (2007) nursing diagnoses that may be appropriate for the intraoperative client include the following:

- *Risk for Aspiration*
- *Ineffective Protection*
- *Impaired Skin Integrity*
- *Risk for Perioperative-Positioning Injury*
- *Risk for Imbalanced Body Temperature*
- *Ineffective Tissue Perfusion*
- *Risk for Deficient Fluid Volume*

Planning

The overall goals of care in the intraoperative period are to maintain the client's safety and to maintain homeostasis. Examples of nursing practices to achieve these goals include the following:

- Position the client appropriately for surgery
- Perform preoperative skin preparation

- Assist in preparing and maintaining the sterile field
- Open and dispense sterile supplies during surgery
- Provide medications and solutions for the sterile field
- Monitor and maintain a safe, aseptic environment
- Manage catheters, tubes, drains, and specimens
- Perform sponge, sharp, and instrument counts
- Document nursing care provided and the client's response to interventions

Implementing

Intraoperative interventions are carried out by the circulating nurse and the scrub nurse. The **circulating nurse** coordinates activities and manages client care by continually assessing client safety, aseptic practice, and the environment (e.g., temperature, humidity, and lighting). The **scrub nurse** assists the surgeon. A scrub nurse wears a sterile gown, gloves, a cap, and eye protection. His or her responsibilities include draping the client with sterile drapes and handling sterile instruments and supplies. The circulating nurse and scrub nurse are responsible for accounting for all sponges, needles, and instruments at the close of the surgery. This precaution avoids leaving any supplies inside the client.

SURGICAL SKIN PREPARATION Surgical skin preparation involves cleaning the surgical site, removing hair *only* if necessary, and applying an antimicrobial agent. In most surgery centres, skin preparation is done by surgery personnel close to the time of surgery. The Safer Healthcare Now! (2007) campaign to reduce surgical site infections indicates that *no* surgical site hair removal should be performed by shaving with a razor. In cases when surgical site hair removal is required, then it is to be done with clippers or depilatory. In such situations, hair is to be removed as close to the time of surgery as possible and not near the sterile field, to avoid dispersal of loose hair and potential contamination of the sterile field. If a depilatory is used, hypersensitivity testing is performed before applying it to the surgical site.

The surgical site and surrounding area is prepared with an antimicrobial agent when indicated. A nontoxic antimicrobial agent with a broad range of germicidal action is used to remove transient microbes from the skin, reduce the resident microbial count to subpathogenic amounts, and inhibit rapid rebound growth of microbes.

POSITIONING Proper positioning of the client during surgery is an important responsibility shared by the nurse, surgeon, and anaesthetist. The ideal intraoperative client position provides the following:

- Optimal visualization of and access to the surgical site.
- Optimal access for assessing and maintaining anaesthesia and vital functions (vital signs, respirations, cardiovascular function).
- Protection of the client from harm (anatomical and physiological considerations).

Positioning is performed after anaesthesia is induced and before surgical draping of the client. The client is lifted into position to prevent shearing forces on the skin from sliding or rolling. The exact position for the client depends on the operation, that is, the surgical approach. For example, a lithotomy position is usually used for vaginal surgery.

Positions on the operating table are maintained by straps, and body prominences are frequently padded. The position should consider normal joint range of motion and good body alignment, thereby avoiding strain or injury to muscles, bones, and ligaments.

CLINICAL ALERT

Be especially aware of the intraoperative position required for older adults. Because older adults are vulnerable to pressure ulcer formation, check the appropriate pressure points of that surgical position on the client.

Evaluating

The intraoperative nurse uses the goals developed during the planning stage (e.g., maintain client safety) and collects data to evaluate whether the desired outcomes have been achieved.

DOCUMENTATION Throughout the intraoperative phase, the nurse documents client care activities, such as IV fluid infusions, positioning, gastric suction, and urinary catheterization.

Postoperative Phase

Nursing during the postoperative phase is especially important for the client's recovery. Anaesthesia impairs the ability of clients to respond to environmental stimuli and to help themselves, although the degree of consciousness of clients will vary. Moreover, surgery itself traumatizes the body by disrupting protective mechanisms and homeostasis.

Immediate Postanaesthetic Phase

Recovery or PACU nurses have specialized skills to care for clients recovering from anaesthesia and surgery (Figure 35.1). Once the health status has stabilized, the

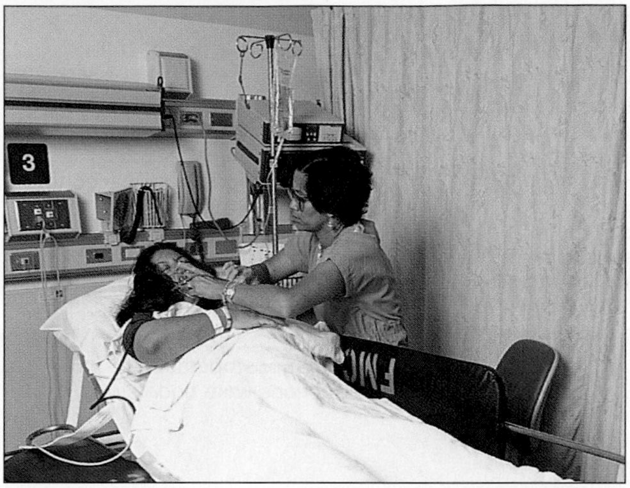

FIGURE 35.1 PACU nurse provides constant assessment and care for clients recovering from anaesthesia and surgery.

client is returned to the nursing unit or, in the case of an outpatient-surgery client, to the outpatient-surgery area before discharge. Clinical assessment of the client in the immediate postanaesthetic period is summarized in Box 35.4.

PREPARING FOR ONGOING CARE OF THE POSTOPERATIVE CLIENT While the client is in the operating room, the client's bed and room are prepared for the postoperative phase. In some agencies, the client is brought back to the unit on a stretcher and transferred to the bed in the room. In other agencies, the client's bed is brought to the surgery suite, and the client is transferred there. In the latter situation, the bed needs to be made with clean linens as soon as the client goes to surgery so that it can be taken to the operating room when needed. In addition, the nurse must obtain and set up any special equipment, such as an intravenous pole, suction, oxygen equipment, and orthopedic appliances (e.g., traction). If these are not requested on the client's record, the nurse should consult with the perioperative nurse or surgeon. See the Lifespan Considerations box for important postoperative issues for children and older adults.

BOX 35.4 IMMEDIATE POSTANAESTHETIC PHASE

PACU nurses assess the following right after surgery:

- Adequacy of airway
- Oxygen saturation
- Adequacy of ventilation
- Respiratory rate, rhythm, and depth
- Use of accessory muscles
- Breath sounds
- Cardiovascular status
- Heart rate and rhythm
- Peripheral pulse amplitude and equality
- Blood pressure
- Capillary filling
- Level of consciousness
- Arousable with verbal stimuli
- Fully awake
- Oriented to time, person, and place
- Temperature
- Presence of protective reflexes (e.g., gag, cough)
- Activity, ability to move extremities
- Skin colour (pink, pale, dusky, blotchy, cyanotic, jaundiced)
- Fluid status
- Intake and output
- Status of IV infusions (type of fluid, rate, amount in container, patency of tubing)
- Signs of dehydration or fluid overload (see Chapter 43)
- Condition of operative site
- Status of dressing
- Drainage (amount, type, and colour)
- Patency of and character and amount of drainage from catheters, tubes, and drains
- Discomfort (i.e., pain) (type, location, and severity), nausea, vomiting
- Safety (i.e., necessity for side rails, call bell within reach)

Lifespan Considerations

Postoperative Care

Postoperative care of children and older adults requires some special considerations:

CHILDREN

- Infants and young children may not be able to state their level of pain postoperatively, may be physically active, and may appear not to have much pain. Use nonverbal signs, such as crying, fussiness, refusal to eat, disturbed sleep, increased heart rate, increased blood pressure, and agitation, to assess pain.
- Children are often undermedicated for pain postoperatively. Nurses should be alert to subtle signs of pain and provide medication in a timely manner. Well-controlled pain levels facilitate the healing process in children.
- Some recovery rooms or PACUs encourage parents to be present when their child wakes from surgery.

(continued)

Lifespan Considerations (*continued*)

Having the parent at the bedside has been shown to calm the child and reduce parental anxiety.

OLDER ADULTS

- Older adults have less efficient reserves and may take longer to recover postoperatively. Be attentive to vital signs, intake and output, and mental status, and note significant changes.
- Clients with dementia often experience an increase in confusion and agitation from the medications and anaesthesia used during surgery. This poses a safety risk during the postoperative period and requires nursing staff to monitor these clients more frequently. It is important to maintain a calm, reassuring attitude. These changes are often long lasting, taking days or weeks to return to the preoperative level of cognition.
- Older adults may experience more fatigue and weakness after surgery. Encouraging activity is crucial but needs to be paced to prevent exhaustion.
- When surgery is done on an outpatient basis, nurses should follow up with phone calls that evening and the next day to check on the client's condition and make sure that postoperative instructions were understood.

Assessing

As soon as the client returns to the nursing unit, the nurse conducts an initial assessment. The sequence of these activities varies with the situation. For example, the nurse may need to check the physician's stat orders before conducting the initial assessment; in such a case, nursing interventions to implement the orders can be carried out at the same time as the assessment.

The nurse consults the surgeon's postoperative orders to learn the following:

- Food and fluids permitted by mouth
- Intravenous solutions and intravenous medications
- Position in bed
- Medications ordered (e.g., analgesics, antibiotics)
- Laboratory tests
- Intake and output, which in some agencies are monitored for all postoperative clients
- Activity permitted, including ambulation

The nurse also checks the PACU record for the following data:

- Operation performed
- Presence and location of any drains
- Anaesthetic used
- Postoperative diagnosis
- Estimated blood loss
- Medications administered in the recovery room

Many hospitals have postoperative protocols for regular assessment of clients. In some agencies, assessments are made every 15 minutes until vital signs stabilize, every hour for the next 4 hours, then every 4 hours for the next 2 days. It is important that the assessments be made as often as the client's condition requires. The nurse assesses the following:

- *Level of consciousness.* Assess orientation to time, place, and person. Most clients are fully conscious but drowsy when returned to their unit. Assess reaction to verbal stimuli and ability to move extremities.
- *Vital signs.* Take the client's vital signs (including pain level) every 15 minutes until stable or in accordance with agency protocol. Vital signs may need to be taken more frequently based on the client's condition. Compare initial findings with PACU data. In addition, assess the client's lung sounds and assess for signs of common circulatory problems, such as postoperative hypotension, hemorrhage, or shock. Hypovolemia from fluid losses during surgery is a common cause of postoperative hypotension. Hemorrhage can result from insecure ligation of blood vessels or disruption of sutures or staples used to close a wound. Massive hemorrhage or cardiac insufficiency can lead to shock postoperatively. Potential postoperative complications with their manifestations and preventive measures are listed in Table 35.2.
- *Skin colour and temperature,* particularly that of the lips and nail beds. The colour of the lips and nail beds is an indicator of tissue perfusion. Pale, cyanotic, cool, and moist skin may be a sign of circulatory problems.
- *Comfort.* Assess pain with the client's vital signs and, as needed, between vital sign measurements. Assess the location, type, and intensity of the pain. Do not assume that reported pain is incisional; other causes can include muscle strains, flatus, and angina. Shoulder pain following minimally invasive abdominal surgery can result from residual carbon dioxide gas remaining in the abdominal cavity and causing referred pain. Ask the client to rate the pain on a scale of 0 to 10, with 0 being *no pain* and 10 being *pain as bad as you can imagine.* Evaluate the client for objective indicators of pain: pallor, perspiration, muscle tension, and reluctance to cough, move, or ambulate. Determine when and what analgesics were last administered, and assess the client for any side effects of medication, such as nausea and vomiting.
- *Fluid balance.* Assess the type and amount of intravenous fluids, flow rate, and infusion site. Monitor the client's fluid intake and output. In addition to watching for shock, assess the client for signs of

TABLE 35.2 Potential Postoperative Problems

Problem	Description	Cause	Clinical Signs	Preventative Interventions
Respiratory				
Pneumonia	Inflammation of the alveoli	Infection, toxins, or irritants causing inflammatory process; immobility and impaired ventilation result in atelectasis and promote growth of pathogens	Elevated temperature, cough, expectoration of blood-tinged or purulent sputum, dyspnea, chest pain	Deep-breathing exercises and coughing, moving in bed, early ambulation
Atelectasis	A condition in which alveoli collapse and are not ventilated	Mucous plugs blocking bronchial passageways, inadequate lung expansion, analgesics, immobility	Dyspnea, tachypnea, tachycardia; diaphoresis, anxiety; pleural pain, decreased chest wall movement; dull or absent breath sounds; decreased oxygen saturation	Deep-breathing exercises and coughing, moving in bed, early ambulation
Pulmonary embolism	Blood clot that has moved to the lungs and blocks a pulmonary artery, thus obstructing blood flow to a portion of the lung	Stasis of venous blood from immobility, venous injury from fractures or during surgery, use of oral contraceptives high in estrogen, preexisting coagulation or circulatory disorder	Sudden chest pain, shortness of breath, cyanosis, shock (tachycardia, low blood pressure)	Turning, ambulation, antiembolism stockings, sequential compression devices
Circulatory				
Hypovolemia	Inadequate circulating blood volume	Fluid deficit, hemorrhage	Tachycardia, decreased urine output, decreased blood pressure	Early detection of signs; fluid or blood replacement
Hemorrhage	Internal or external bleeding	Disruption of sutures, insecure ligation of blood vessels	Overt bleeding (dressings saturated with bright blood; bright, free-flowing blood in drains or chest tubes), increased pain, increasing abdominal girth, swelling or bruising around incision	Early detection of signs
Hypovolemic shock	Inadequate tissue perfusion resulting from markedly reduced circulating blood volume	Severe hypovolemia from fluid deficit or hemorrhage	Rapid weak pulse, dyspnea, tachypnea; restlessness and anxiety; urine output less than 30 mL/h; decreased blood pressure; cool, clammy skin, thirst, pallor	Maintain blood volume through adequate fluid replacement, prevent hemorrhage; early detection of signs
Thrombophlebitis	Inflammation of the veins, usually of the legs and associated with a blood clot	Slowed venous blood flow caused by immobility or prolonged sitting; trauma to vein, resulting in inflammation and increased blood coagulability	Aching, cramping pain; affected area is swollen, red, and hot to touch; vein feels hard; discomfort in calf when foot is dorsiflexed or when client walks (Homans' sign)	Early ambulation, leg exercises, antiembolism stockings, SCDs, adequate fluid intake
Thrombus	Blood clot attached to wall of vein or artery (most commonly the leg veins)	As for thrombophlebitis for venous thrombi; disruption or inflammation of arterial wall for arterial thrombi	*Venous:* same as thrombophlebitis *Arterial:* pain and pallor of affected extremity; decreased or absent peripheral pulses	*Venous:* same as thrombophlebitis *Arterial:* maintain prescribed position; early detection of signs

(continued)

TABLE 35.2 Potential Postoperative Problems (*continued*)

Problem	Description	Cause	Clinical Signs	Preventative Interventions
Embolus	Foreign body or clot that has moved from its site of formation to another area of the body (e.g., the lungs, heart, or brain)	Venous or arterial thrombus; broken intravenous catheter, fat, or amniotic fluid	In venous system, usually becomes a pulmonary embolus (see pulmonary embolism); signs of arterial emboli may depend on the location	Turning, ambulation, leg exercises, sequential compression devices; careful maintenance of IV catheters
Urinary				
Urinary retention	Inability to empty the bladder, with excessive accumulation of urine in the bladder	Depressed bladder muscle tone from narcotics and anaesthetics; handling of tissues during surgery on adjacent organs (rectum, vagina)	Fluid intake larger than output; inability to void or frequent voiding of small amounts, bladder distention, suprapubic discomfort, restlessness	Monitoring of fluid intake and output, interventions to facilitate voiding, urinary catheterization as needed
Urinary tract infection	Inflammation of the bladder, ureters, or urethra	Immobilization and limited fluid intake, instrumentation of the urinary tract	Burning sensation when voiding, urgency, cloudy urine, lower abdominal pain	Adequate fluid intake, early ambulation, aseptic straight catheterization only as necessary, good perineal hygiene
Gastrointestinal				
Nausea and vomiting		Pain, abdominal distension, ingesting food or fluids before return of peristalsis, certain medications, anxiety	Complaints of feeling sick to the stomach, retching, or gagging	IV fluids until peristalsis returns; then clear fluids, full fluids, and regular diet; antiemetic drugs if ordered; analgesics for pain
Constipation	Infrequent or no stool passage for abnormal length of time (e.g., within 48 hours after solid diet started)	Lack of dietary roughage, analgesics (decreased intestinal motility), immobility	Absence of stool elimination, abdominal distension, and discomfort	Adequate fluid intake, high-fibre diet, early ambulation
Tympanites	Retention of gases within the intestines	Slowed motility of the intestines caused by handling of the bowel during surgery and the effects of anaesthesia	Obvious abdominal distension, abdominal discomfort (gas pains), absence of bowel sounds	Early ambulation; avoid using a straw, provide ice chips or water at room temperature
Postoperative ileus	Intestinal obstruction characterized by lack of peristaltic activity	Handling the bowel during surgery, anaesthesia, electrolyte imbalance, wound infection	Abdominal pain and distension; constipation; absent bowel sounds; vomiting	
Wound				
Wound infection	Inflammation and infection of incision or drain site	Poor aseptic technique; laboratory analysis of wound swab identifies causative microorganism	Purulent exudate, redness, tenderness, elevated body temperature, wound odour	Keep wound clean and dry, use surgical aseptic technique when changing dressings
Wound dehiscence	Separation of a suture line before the incision heals	Malnutrition (emaciation, obesity), poor circulation, excessive strain on suture line	Increased incision drainage, tissues underlying skin become visible along parts of the incision	Adequate nutrition, appropriate incisional support and avoidance of strain
Wound evisceration	Extrusion of internal organs and tissues through the incision	Same as for wound dehiscence	Opening of incision and visible protrusion of organs	Same as for wound dehiscence

(*continued*)

TABLE 35.2 Potential Postoperative Problems (*continued*)

Problem	Description	Cause	Clinical Signs	Preventative Interventions
Psychological				
Postoperative depression	Mental disorder characterized by altered mood	Weakness, surprise nature of emergency surgery, news of malignancy, severely altered body image, other personal matter; may be a physiological response to some surgeries	Anorexia, tearfulness, loss of ambition, withdrawal, rejection of others, feelings of dejection, sleep disturbances (insomnia or excessive sleeping)	Adequate rest, physical activity, opportunity to express anger and other negative feelings

circulatory overload, and monitor serum electrolytes. Anaesthetics and surgery affect the hormones regulating fluid and electrolyte balance (aldosterone and ADH in particular), placing the client at risk for decreased urine output and fluid and electrolyte imbalances. Assess for the presence of nausea and vomiting.

- *Dressings and bedclothes.* Inspect the client's dressings and the bedclothes underneath the client. Excessive sanguineous drainage on dressings or bedclothes, often appearing underneath the client, can indicate hemorrhage. The amount of drainage on dressings is recorded by describing the diameter of the stains or by denoting the number and type of dressings saturated with drainage.
- *Drains and tubes.* Determine colour, consistency, and amount of drainage from all tubes and drains. All tubes should be patent, and tubes and suction equipment should be functioning. Drainage bags must be hanging properly.

Document the client's time of arrival and all assessments. Many agencies have progress flow records for this purpose. Alter the frequency, parameters, and priorities to meet the individual needs of the client.

Diagnosing

Because surgery can involve many body systems, both directly and indirectly, and is a complex experience for the client, the nursing diagnoses focus on a wide variety of actual, potential, and collaborative problems.

ASSESSMENT: HOME CARE

Surgical Clients

The following are guidelines for assessing home care for surgical clients before discharge:

CLIENT

- *Self-care abilities:* Ability to manage hygiene and other self-care, to perform wound care, as needed, to manage tubes and stomas, and to manage prescribed medications
- *Supplies required:* Wound care supplies, such as dressings, hypoallergenic tape, cleansing solutions, binders or slings, elastic wraps, irrigating syringe and solution
- *Assistive devices required:* Walker, cane, raised toilet seat, commode, overhead trapeze, grab bars
- *Current level of knowledge:* Postoperative pain management, wound care, dressing changes, urinary catheters or other drains, activity restrictions, dietary prescriptions, prescribed exercises (e.g., range-of-motion, postmastectomy exercises), infection prevention and control measures, such as hand hygiene

FAMILY

- *Caregiver availability, skills, and responses:* Willingness and ability to assume responsibility for care, as needed (e.g., wound care, catheter and tube management, meal preparation, assistance with ADLs, shopping, transportation to and from appointments), other available caregivers
- *Family role changes and coping:* Effect on parenting and spousal roles, sexuality, social roles, financial status
- *Financial resources:* Ability to purchase necessary supplies and equipment; other sources of funding or financial assistance (e.g., private insurance)

HOME

- Elicit information from the client, family, or significant other regarding the physical environment of the home and potential issues postoperatively, which may include the presence of stairs, access to the home, and accessibility of the kitchen, bathroom, and bedroom

COMMUNITY

- Available community resources, such as equipment and supply companies, support and educational organizations and groups (e.g., ostomy clubs and Reach for Recovery), home health-care agencies or providers, access to pharmacy services, transportation services for medical care, Meals on Wheels, and other support organizations

Actual and potential NANDA International (2007) diagnoses for the postoperative client include the following:

- *Acute Pain*
- *Risk for Infection*
- *Risk for Injury*
- *Risk for Deficient Fluid Volume*
- *Ineffective Airway Clearance*
- *Ineffective Breathing Pattern*
- *Self-Care Deficit: Bathing/Hygiene, Dressing/Grooming, Toileting*
- *Ineffective Health Maintenance*
- *Disturbed Body Image*

Planning

Postoperative care planning and discharge planning begin in the preoperative phase when preoperative teaching is implemented. Client goals during the postoperative period include the following:

- Maintain comfort
- Promote healing
- Prevent associated risks, such as respiratory or cardiovascular complications, infection, and other common problems associated with surgery
- Restore the highest possible level of wellness

PLANNING FOR HOME CARE To provide for continuity of care for the surgical client after discharge, the nurse needs to consider the client's needs for assistance with care in the home setting. Discharge planning for both the outpatient-surgery client and the client who has been hospitalized for several days following surgery incorporates an assessment of the client's and family's abilities for self-care, financial resources, and the need for referrals and home health services. The accompanying Assessment: Home Care box on the previous page outlines the assessment for a surgical client; however, it is important to remember that surgical clients have diverse needs and additional assessment data may be required.

HOME CARE TEACHING Once the home care assessment is complete, nurses must meet the learning needs of clients and their support people to ensure continuity of care and restoration of the client's health. Teaching should focus on actions to maintain comfort, to promote healing and restore wellness, and to make use of appropriate community agencies and other sources of help.

Maintaining Comfort

- Instruct the client to use analgesics as ordered, not allowing pain to become severe before taking the prescribed dose.
- If not contraindicated, discuss the use of OTC analgesics, such as acetaminophen, as postoperative pain becomes less severe or if the client is reluctant to use prescription drugs because of side effects.
- Teach the client to avoid using alcohol or other central nervous system depressants while taking opioids.
- Discuss the importance of gradually resuming activities and avoiding overexertion.
- Emphasize the importance of paying attention to increasing pain or discomfort. Instruct the client to contact the physician if pain increases after a period of decreasing discomfort.
- Teach the client to use nonpharmacological measures, such as conscious relaxation, distraction, meditation, or visualization, to help manage pain.

Promoting Healing

- If indicated, teach the client how to change wound dressings and perform wound care.
- Emphasize the importance of hygiene and handwashing to prevent infections.
- Instruct the client to report promptly to the appropriate member of the health-care team any increasing redness, swelling, pain, or discharge from the incision or drain sites.
- Discuss any prescribed activity restrictions, such as avoiding lifting.
- Discuss the importance of keeping follow-up appointments to monitor healing and recovery after surgery.

Restoring Wellness

- Discuss the relationship of increasing activities to restoring wellness and promoting a sense of well-being.
- Teach the client that surgery and stressors can depress immune function and to avoid exposure to illness (e.g., crowded areas and people with upper respiratory illnesses) whenever possible.
- Emphasize the importance of adequate rest for healing and immune function.
- If appropriate, discuss lifestyle changes to promote wellness, such as stopping smoking, increasing activity level, reducing stress, and consuming a healthy diet high in fruits, vegetables, and whole grains with adequate protein to promote healing.

Using Community Agencies and Other Sources of Help

- Provide information about where durable medical equipment can be purchased, rented, or obtained free of charge; how to access home health care and other services; and where to obtain supplies, such as dressings or nutritional supplements.
- Suggest additional sources of information, such as the Canadian Association of Wound Care, Reach to Recovery, United Ostomy Association of Canada, and so on.

Making Referrals The nurse needs to consider appropriate referrals for the client, such as the following:

- Home health agencies for wound care and assessment and for assistance with ADLs, if necessary

- Community social services for assistance in obtaining medical and assistive equipment
- Respiratory, physical, or occupational therapy services, as indicated

Implementing

Nursing interventions designed to promote client recovery and prevent complications include (1) pain management, (2) appropriate positioning, (3) incentive spirometry and deep-breathing and coughing exercises, (4) leg exercises, (5) early ambulation, (6) adequate hydration, (7) proper diet, (8) promotion of urinary elimination, (9) suction maintenance, and (10) wound care.

PAIN MANAGEMENT Although pain is a sensory and emotional experience that serves to alert people to harm and initiate responses to avoid or minimize harm, pain in the surgical client has little protective value. It can, in fact, have detrimental effects, leading to stimulation of the sympathetic nervous system, tachycardia, shallow breathing, atelectasis, altered gas exchange, immobility, and immunosuppression. See Chapter 34 for an in-depth discussion of pain and pain management.

Pain is usually greatest 12 to 36 hours after surgery, decreasing after the second or third postoperative day. During the initial postoperative period, patient-controlled analgesia (PCA) or continuous analgesic administration through an intravenous catheter is often prescribed. The nurse monitors the infusion or amount of analgesic administered by PCA, assesses the client's pain relief, and notifies the physician if the client is experiencing unacceptable side effects or inadequate pain relief. Around-the-clock parenteral or oral analgesics should be administered on a routine basis (the timing will vary depending on the medication, route, and dose) for the first 24 to 36 hours according to the physician's prescription. Additional as needed (prn) analgesia should be administered for breakthrough pain. When routine analgesic administration is no longer necessary, the prescribed analgesic is generally given before scheduled activities and rest periods.

An anti-inflammatory agent, such as ibuprofen, is often administered as a coanalgesic with opioids. This combination enhances pain relief. Clients need to be reminded that analgesics are most effective when taken on a regular basis or before pain becomes severe. Because muscle tension increases pain perception and responses, nurses need to use nonpharmacological measures in addition to prescribed analgesia. These include ensuring that the client is warm and providing back rubs, position changes, diversional activities, and adjunctive measures, such as imagery.

POSITIONING Position the client as ordered. Clients who have had spinal anaesthetics usually lie flat for 8 to 12 hours. An unconscious or semiconscious client is placed on the side with no pillow and no elevation of the head, in a position that allows fluids to drain from the mouth. Unless contraindicated, elevation of affected extremities (e.g., following foot surgery) with the distal extremity higher than the heart promotes venous drainage and reduces swelling.

DEEP-BREATHING AND COUGHING EXERCISES Deep-breathing exercises help remove mucus, which can form and remain in the lungs because of the effects of general anaesthetic and analgesics. These drugs depress the action of both the cilia of the mucous membranes lining the respiratory tract and the respiratory centre in the brain. By increasing lung expansion and preventing the accumulation of secretions, deep breathing helps prevent pneumonia and **atelectasis** (collapse of the alveoli), which can result from stagnation of fluid in the lungs.

An incentive spirometer is often ordered for the postoperative client to encourage deep breathing. This device measures the flow of air inhaled through a mouthpiece (see Chapter 42). The client is instructed to breathe in through the mouthpiece until a certain level is achieved (usually measured by a ball within an enclosed chamber). Inhalation and ventilation are enhanced by using the incentive spirometer.

Deep breathing frequently initiates the coughing reflex. Voluntary coughing in conjunction with deep breathing facilitates the movement and expectoration of respiratory tract secretions. Coughing may be contraindicated postoperatively, depending on the type of surgery (e.g., craniotomy, eye surgery).

Encourage the client to do deep-breathing and coughing exercises hourly, or at least every 2 hours, during waking hours for the first few days. Assist the client to a sitting position in bed or on the side of the bed. The client can splint the incision with a pillow when coughing, or the nurse can splint the incision for the client to reduce discomfort.

LEG EXERCISES Encourage the client to do leg exercises taught in the preoperative period every 1 to 2 hours during waking hours. Muscle contractions compress the veins, preventing the stasis of blood in the veins, a cause of **thrombus** (stationary clot adhered to the wall of a vessel) formation and subsequent **thrombophlebitis** (inflammation of a vein followed by formation of a blood clot) and **emboli** (blood clots that have moved). Contractions also promote arterial blood flow.

MOVING AND AMBULATION Encourage and assist the client to turn from side to side at least every 2 hours. Turning alternates which lung can achieve maximum expansion because it is uppermost. Avoid placing pillows or rolls under the client's knees because pressure on the popliteal blood vessels can interfere with blood circulation to and from the lower extremities. Clients who practise turning before surgery usually find it easier to do after surgery.

The client should ambulate as soon as possible after surgery in accordance with the surgeon's orders.

Generally, clients begin ambulation the evening of the day of surgery or the first day after surgery unless contraindicated. Early ambulation prevents respiratory, circulatory, urinary, and gastrointestinal complications. It also prevents general muscle weakness. Schedule ambulation for periods after the client has taken an analgesic or when the client is comfortable. Ambulation should be gradual, starting with the client sitting on the bed and dangling the feet over the side. A client who cannot ambulate is periodically assisted to a sitting position in bed, if allowed, and turned frequently. The sitting position permits the greatest lung expansion.

HYDRATION Maintain intravenous infusions, as ordered, to replace body fluids lost either before or during surgery. When oral intake is permitted, initially offer only small sips of water. Large amounts of water can induce vomiting because anaesthetics and opioid analgesics temporarily inhibit the motility of the stomach. The patient who cannot take fluids by mouth *may* be allowed by the surgeon's orders to suck ice chips. Provide mouth care and place a mouthwash at the client's bedside. Postoperative clients often complain of thirst and a dry, sticky mouth. These discomforts are a result of the preoperative fasting period, preoperative medications (such as atropine), and loss of body fluid.

Measure the patient's fluid intake and output for at least two days or until fluid balance is stable without an intravenous infusion. Ensuring adequate fluid balance is important. Sufficient fluids keep the respiratory mucous membranes and secretions moist, thus facilitating the expectoration of mucus during coughing. Also, an adequate fluid balance is important to maintain renal and cardiovascular function.

PROPER DIET The surgeon orders the client's postoperative diet. Depending on the extent of surgery and the organs involved, the client may be allowed nothing by mouth for several days or may be able to resume oral intake when nausea is no longer present. When "diet as tolerated" is ordered, offer clear liquids initially. If the client tolerates these with no nausea or vomiting, the diet can often progress to full liquids and then to a regular diet, provided that gastrointestinal functioning is normal. Assess the return of peristalsis by auscultating the abdomen (see Chapter 27). Gurgling and rumbling sounds indicate peristalsis, as does passing of flatulence. Anaesthetic agents, opioids, handling of the intestines during abdominal surgery, fasting, and inactivity all inhibit peristalsis. Therefore, bowel sounds should be carefully assessed every 4 to 6 hours. Although in the past, oral fluids and food were started only after the return of peristalsis, more recent evidence indicates that fluids and food actually assist in the return of peristalsis (Anderson et al., 2006).

Observe the client's tolerance of the food and fluids ingested and note and report the passage of flatus, abdominal distension, bowel movements, and eructation (burping).

URINARY ELIMINATION Provide measures that promote urinary elimination. For example, help male clients stand at the bedside, or female clients to a bedside commode, if allowed, and ensure that fluid intake is adequate. Determine whether the client has any difficulties voiding and assess the client for bladder distension. Report to the surgeon if a client does not void within 8 hours following surgery, unless another time frame is specified.

Anaesthetic agents temporarily depress urinary bladder tone, which usually returns within 6 to 8 hours after surgery. Surgery in the pubic area, vagina, or rectum, during which the surgeon may manipulate the bladder, often causes urinary retention. If all measures to promote voiding fail, a urinary catheterization is often ordered (see Chapter 41). Measure the fluid intake and output (I & O) of all new postoperative clients. Generally, I & O records are kept for at least 2 days or until the client re-establishes fluid balance without an IV or a catheter in place.

SUCTION Some patients return from surgery with a gastric or intestinal tube in place and orders to connect the tube to suction. For more information about gastrointestinal tubes, see Chapter 39. The suction ordered can be continuous or intermittent. Intermittent suction is applied when a single-lumen gastric tube is used to reduce the risk of damaging the mucous membrane near the distal port of the tube. Continuous suction may be applied if a double-lumen tube is in place (Figure 35.2). Fluids and electrolytes must be replaced intravenously when gastric suction or continuous drainage is ordered. Nasogastric tubes can be irrigated if the lumen becomes clogged. They are generally irrigated before and after tube feedings or the instillation of medications. Nasogastric irrigation may require a physician's order, particularly following gastrointestinal surgery. Agency policy for irrigations must be followed. Skill 35.3 describes the management of gastrointestinal suction.

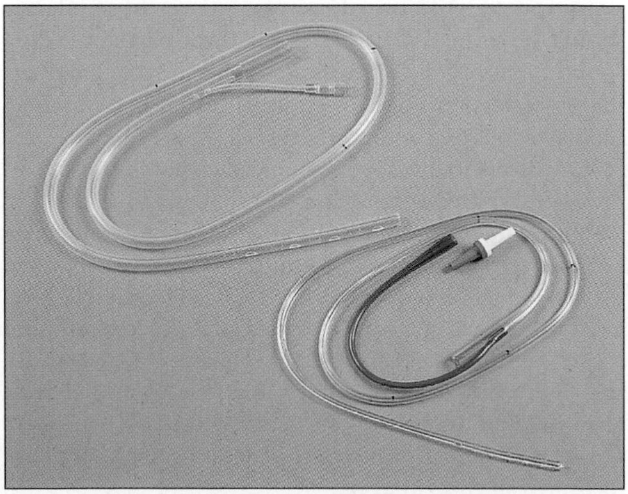

FIGURE 35.2 Nasogastric tubes used for gastric decompression: **Top left:** Levin (single-lumen) tube; **lower right:** Salem sump (double-lumen) tube with antireflux valve

SKILL 35.3

MANAGING GASTROINTESTINAL SUCTION

PURPOSES

- To relieve abdominal distension
- To maintain gastric decompression after surgery
- To remove blood and secretions from the gastrointestinal tract
- To relieve discomfort (e.g., when a client has a bowel obstruction)
- To maintain the patency of the nasogastric tube

ASSESSMENT

Assess the following:

- Presence of abdominal distension on palpation
- Bowel sounds
- Abdominal discomfort
- Vital signs for baseline data
- Amount and characteristics of drainage
- Nausea, vomiting

Planning

Before initiating gastric suction, determine (1) whether the suction is continuous or intermittent; (2) the ordered suction pressure (a low suction pressure is between 80 mm Hg and 100 mm Hg, and a high pressure is between 100 mm Hg and 120 mm Hg); (3) whether there is an order to irrigate the gastrointestinal tube, and if so, the type of solution to use; and (4) agency policy and physician's orders.

Equipment

Initiating Suction

- Gastrointestinal tube in place in the client
- Basin
- 50 mL syringe with an adapter
- Stethoscope
- Suction device for either continuous or intermittent suction
- Connector and connecting tubing
- Clean gloves

Maintaining Suction

- Graduated container as required to measure gastric drainage
- Basin of water
- Cotton-tipped applicators
- Ointment or lubricant
- Clean gloves

Irrigation

- Stethoscope
- Disposable irrigating set containing a sterile 50 mL syringe, moisture-resistant pad, basin, and graduated container
- Sterile normal saline (500 mL) or the ordered solution

IMPLEMENTATION

Performance

1. Before performing the procedure, introduce yourself and verify the client's identity by using agency protocol. Explain to the client what you are going to do, why it is necessary, and how he or she can cooperate. Discuss the purpose for the gastrointestinal suction.
2. Perform hand hygiene and observe other appropriate infection prevention and control procedures (e.g., clean gloves).
3. Provide for client privacy.

Initiating Suction

4. Position the client appropriately.
   - Assist the client to a semi-Fowler's position if it is not contraindicated. **Rationale: In semi-Fowler's position, the tube is not as likely to lie against the wall of the stomach and will, therefore, suction most efficiently. Semi-Fowler's position also prevents reflux of gastric contents, which could lead to aspiration.**
5. Confirm that the tube is in the stomach.
   - Put on clean gloves.
   - Aspirate stomach contents and check their acidity by using a pH test strip.
   - Insert air into the tube with the syringe, and listen with a stethoscope over the stomach (just below the xiphoid process) for a swish of air.
   - Use other methods in accordance with agency protocol. See Chapter 39, Skill 39.2 (page 1205).
6. Set and check the suction.
   - Connect the appropriate suction regulator to the wall suction outlet and the collection device to the regulator. *Intermittent suction regulators* generally are used with single-lumen tubes and apply suction for a set interval (15 to 60 seconds), followed by an interval of no suction. Intermittent suction is set at 80 mm Hg to 100 mm Hg (check agency policy) or as ordered by the physician. Check the suction level by occluding the drainage tube and observing the regulator dial during a suction cycle. *Continuous suction regulators* are used with double-lumen (e.g., Salem sump) nasogastric tubes. Set continuous suction as ordered by the physician, or at 60 mm Hg to 120 mm Hg (check agency policy).
   - If using a portable suction machine, turn on the machine and regulate the suction as above. The Gomco pump has two settings: low intermittent for single-lumen tubes, and high for double-lumen tubes.
   - Test for proper suctioning by occluding the tube.

(continued)

SKILL 35.3

MANAGING GASTROINTESTINAL SUCTION (*continued*)

7. Establish gastric suction.
   - Connect the gastrointestinal tube to the suction tubing by using the connector.
   - If a Salem sump tube is in place, connect the larger lumen to the suction equipment. This double-lumen tube has a smaller tube running inside the primary suction tube. **Rationale: The smaller tube provides a continuous flow of atmospheric air through the drainage tube at its distal end and prevents excessive suction force on the gastric mucosa at the drainage outlets. Damage to the gastric mucosa is thus avoided.**
   - Always keep the air vent tube of a Salem sump tube open and above the level of the stomach when suction is applied. **Rationale: Closing the vent would stop the sump action and cause mucosal damage. Keeping the end of the air vent tube higher than the stomach prevents reflux of gastric contents into the air lumen of the tube.**
   - After suction is applied, watch the tubing for a few minutes until the gastric contents appear to be running through the tubing into the receptacle. A Salem sump tube makes a soft, hissing sound when it is functioning correctly.
   - If the suction is not working properly, check that all connections are tight and that the tubing is not kinked.
   - Anchor the tubing to the patient's gown so that it does not loop below the suction bottle. **Rationale: If the tubing falls below the suction bottle, the suction may be obstructed because of the pressure required to push the fluid against gravity.**
8. Assess the drainage.
   - Observe the amount, colour, odour, and consistency of the drainage. Normal gastric drainage has a mucoid consistency and is either colourless or yellow-green because of the presence of bile. A coffee-grounds colour and consistency may indicate bleeding.
   - Test the gastric drainage for pH and blood (by using Hematest), when indicated. A person who has had gastrointestinal surgery can be expected to have some blood in the drainage.

Maintaining Suction

9. Assess the client and the suction system regularly.
   - Assess the client every 30 minutes until the system is running effectively and then every two hours, or as the client's health indicates, to ensure that the suction is functioning properly. If the client complains of fullness, nausea, or epigastric pain, or if the flow of gastric secretions is absent in the tubing or in the collection bottle, ineffective suctioning or blockage of the nasogastric tube is likely.
   - Inspect the suction system for patency of the system (e.g., kinks or blockages in the tubing) and tightness of the connections. **Rationale: Loose connections can permit air to enter and thus decrease the effectiveness of the suction by decreasing the negative pressure.**
10. Relieve blockages, if present.
    - Put on clean gloves.
    - Check the suction equipment. To do this, disconnect the nasogastric tube from the suction over a collecting basin (to collect gastric drainage), and then, with the suction on, place the end of the suction tubing in a basin of water. If water is drawn into the drainage bottle, the suction equipment is functioning properly, but the nasogastric tube is either blocked or positioned incorrectly.
    - Reposition the client (e.g., to the other side) if permitted. **Rationale: This may facilitate drainage.**
    - Rotate the nasogastric tube, and reposition it. This step is contraindicated for clients with gastric surgery. **Rationale: Moving the tube may interfere with gastric sutures.**
    - Irrigate the nasogastric tube as agency protocol states or on the order of the physician (see steps 14 to 16).
11. Prevent reflux into the vent lumen of a Salem sump tube. **Rationale: Reflux of gastric contents into the vent lumen can occur when stomach pressure exceeds atmospheric pressure. In this situation, gastric contents follow the path of least resistance and flow out the vent lumen rather than the drainage lumen.**

    To prevent reflux
    - Place the vent tubing higher than the client's stomach to prevent gastric fluid backup into the blue lumen air vent.
    - Keep the drainage lumen free of particulate matter that may obstruct the lumen (see steps 14 to 16 for irrigating a nasogastric tube).
12. Ensure client comfort.
    - Clean the client's nostrils, as needed, using the cotton-tipped applicators and water. Apply a water-soluble lubricant or ointment.
    - Provide mouth care every 2 hours and as needed. Some postoperative clients are permitted to suck ice chips or a moist cloth to maintain the moisture of the oral mucous membranes. A physician's order is required.
13. Empty the drainage receptacle according to agency policy or physician's order.
    - Clamp the nasogastric tube, and turn off the suction.
    - Put on clean gloves.
    - If the receptacle is graduated, determine the amount of drainage.
    - Disconnect the receptacle.
    - If the receptacle is not graduated, empty the contents into a graduated container and measure.
    - Inspect the drainage carefully for colour, consistency, and presence of substances (e.g., blood clots).
    - Discard and replace receptacle, *or* rinse the receptacle with cool water and reattach it to the suction. Check agency policy.

(continued)

SKILL 35.3

MANAGING GASTROINTESTINAL SUCTION (*continued*)

- Turn on the suction, and unclamp the nasogastric tube.
- Observe the system for several minutes to make sure function is re-established.
- Go to step 17.

Irrigating a Gastrointestinal Tube

14. Prepare the client and the equipment.
- Verify physician's orders and agency policy.
- Place the moisture-resistant pad under the end of the gastrointestinal tube.
- Turn off the suction.
- Put on clean gloves.
- Disconnect the gastrointestinal tube from the connector.
- Determine that the tube is in the stomach. See step 5. **Rationale: This ensures that the irrigating solution enters the client's stomach.**

15. Irrigate the tube.
- Draw up the ordered volume of irrigating solution into the syringe; 30 mL of solution per instillation is usual, but up to 60 mL may be given per instillation, if ordered.
- Attach the syringe to the nasogastric tube, and slowly inject the solution.
- Gently aspirate the solution if indicated by agency policy. **Rationale: Forceful withdrawal could damage the gastric mucosa.**
- If you encounter difficulty in withdrawing the solution, inject 20 mL of air and aspirate again, or reposition the client or the nasogastric tube. **Rationale: Air and repositioning may move the end of the tube away from the stomach wall.** If the aspirating difficulty continues, reattach the tube in intermittent low suction, and notify the nurse in charge or the physician.
- Repeat the preceding steps until the ordered amount of solution is used.
- Note: A Salem sump tube can also be irrigated through the vent lumen without interrupting suction. However, only small quantities of irrigant can be injected via this lumen compared with the drainage lumen.
- After irrigating a Salem sump tube, inject 10 mL to 20 mL of air into the vent lumen while applying suction to the drainage lumen. **Rationale: This tests the patency of the vent and ensures sump functioning.**

16. Re-establish suction.
- Reconnect the nasogastric tube to suction.
- If a Salem sump tube is used, inject the air vent lumen with 10 mL to 20 mL of air after reconnecting the tube to suction.
- Observe the system for several minutes to make sure it is functioning.

17. Document all relevant information.
- Record the time suction was started. Also, record the pressure established, the colour and consistency of the drainage, and nursing assessments.
- During maintenance, record assessments, supportive nursing measures, and data about the suction system.
- When irrigating the tube, record verification of tube placement; the time of the irrigation; the amount and type of irrigating solution used; the number of times irrigated; the amount, colour, and consistency of the returns; the patency of the system following the irrigation; and nursing assessments.
- Record client response and teaching.

EVALUATION

- Conduct appropriate follow-up, such as relief of abdominal distension or discomfort, bowel sounds, character and amount of gastric drainage, integrity of nares; hydration of oral mucous membranes, patency of the tube, system functioning, and relief of nausea and vomiting.
- Compare with previous findings if available.
- Report significant deviations from normal to the appropriate members of the health-care team.

TEACHING: HOME CARE

Gastrointestinal Suction

Instruct the caregiver to do the following:

- Maintain suction, as ordered; do *not* increase or decrease the suction without instructions from the nurse or the physician.
- Offer mouth care every 2 hours.
- Avoid tension and pulling on the tube by securing it to the gown.
- Check the patency of the tube if nausea or vomiting occur.
- Report an increasing amount of drainage or bloody drainage.

Suction can also be applied to other drainage tubes, such as chest tubes or a wound drain. The type and amount of suction is ordered by the physician. Most agencies have *wall suction units* available (Figure 35.3). A suction regulator with a drainage receptacle connects to a wall outlet that provides negative pressure. Check the receptacle frequently to prevent excess drainage from interfering with the suction apparatus; empty or change the receptacle according to agency policy. *Portable electric suction units* or *pumps* (e.g., the Gomco pump) can be used in the home or when wall suction is not available.

WOUND CARE Most clients return from surgery with a wound that has been closed with sutures, staples, or fibrin sealant and covered by a dressing, although in some cases, such as when there is an infection, the wound is left open. Dressings are inspected regularly to ensure that they are clean, dry, and intact. Excessive drainage may indicate hemorrhage, infection, or an open wound.

When dressings are changed, the nurse assesses the wound for appearance, size, drainage, swelling, pain, and the status of drains or tubes (see Box 35.5).

For surgical incisions healing by primary intention, the nurse can expect the following sequential signs of healing:

1. *Absence of bleeding and the appearance of a clot binding the wound edges.* The wound edges are well approximated and bound by fibrin in the clot within the first few hours after surgical closure.
2. *Inflammation (redness and swelling) at the wound edges for one to three days.*
3. *Reduction in inflammation when the clot diminishes,* as granulation tissue starts to bridge the area. The wound is bridged and closed within 7 to 10 days. Increased inflammation associated with fever and drainage is indicative of wound infection; the wound edges then appear brightly inflamed and swollen.
4. *Scar formation.* Collagen synthesis starts 4 days after injury and continues for 6 months or longer.
5. *Diminished scar size* over a period of months or years. An increase in scar size indicates keloid formation.

See Chapter 33 for information about wound healing, wound drainage, cleaning wounds, wound irrigation, hot and cold applications, and supporting and immobilizing wounds.

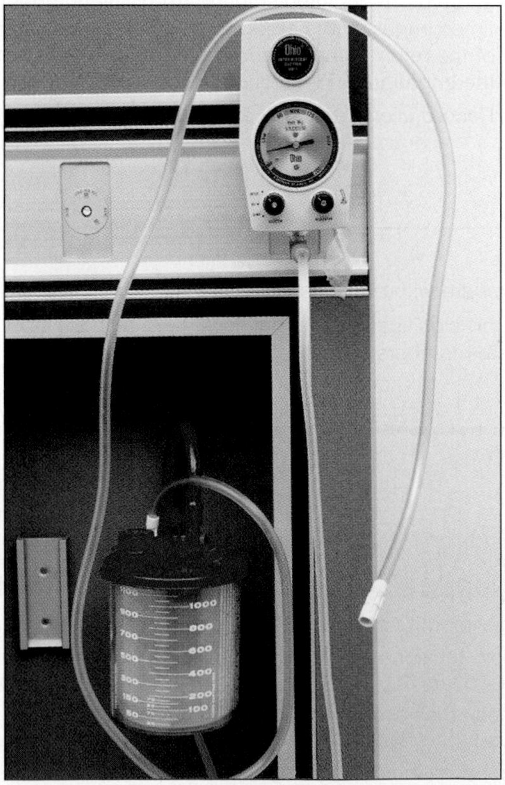

FIGURE 35.3 Wall suction unit for generating negative pressure for nasogastric suction

BOX 35.5 ASSESSING SURGICAL WOUNDS

Assess surgical wounds for the following:

APPEARANCE

- Inspect the colour of the wound (e.g., for bruising and redness) and surrounding area and the approximation of wound edges. If present, note the security of the sutures or staples.

SIZE

- Note the size and location of dehiscence, if present.

DRAINAGE

- Observe the location, colour, consistency, odour, and degree of saturation of dressings. Note the number of gauzes saturated or the diameter of drainage on the gauze.

EDEMA

- Observe the amount of swelling; minimal to moderate swelling is normal in early stages of wound healing.

PAIN

- Expect severe to moderate postoperative pain for 3 to 5 days; persistent severe pain or sudden onset of severe pain may indicate internal hemorrhaging or infection. Note specific areas of incision that cause pain when cleansed or dressed.

DRAINS OR TUBES

- Inspect drain security and placement, amount and character of drainage, and functioning of collecting apparatus, if present. Note the method of security (e.g., sutures, safety pin).

CLINICAL ALERT

Assess the client immediately if she or he reports a *giving* or *popping* sensation in the incisional area. The client may be experiencing dehiscence or evisceration of the wound.

SURGICAL DRESSINGS Not all surgical dressings require changing. Sometimes, surgeons in the operating room apply a dressing that remains in place until the sutures or staples are removed, and no further dressings are required. In many situations, however, surgical dressings are changed regularly to prevent the growth of microorganisms.

In some instances, a client may have a Penrose drain inserted (see page 1050). In this situation, the main surgical incision is considered cleaner than the surgical stab wound made for the drain insertion because the drainage is usually considerable. The main incision is, therefore, cleaned first, and *under no circumstances are materials that were used to clean the stab wound used* subsequently to clean the main incision. In this way, the main incision is kept free of the microorganisms around the stab wound. Box 35.5 summarizes important data to be collected in assessing surgical wounds. Cleaning a wound and applying a sterile dressing are detailed in Skill 35.4.

SKILL 35.4

CLEANING A CLOSED WOUND AND APPLYING A STERILE DRESSING

PURPOSES

- To promote wound healing by primary intention
- To prevent infection
- To assess the healing process
- To protect the wound from mechanical trauma

ASSESSMENT

Assess the following:

- Client allergies to wound cleaning agents
- The appearance and size of the wound
- The amount and character of exudates
- Client complaints of discomfort
- The time of the last analgesia
- Signs of systemic infection (e.g., elevated body temperature, diaphoresis, malaise, leukocytosis)
- Presence of sutures or staples, drains, and materials used to dress the wound previously
- Client response to postoperative recovery

Planning

Before changing a dressing, determine any specific orders about the wound or dressing.

Equipment

- Bath blanket (if necessary)
- Moisture-proof bag
- Mask (optional)
- Acetone or another solution (if necessary, to loosen adhesive)
- Clean gloves
- Sterile gloves
- Sterile dressing set; if none is available, gather the following sterile items from a central supply cart:
  - Drape or towel
  - Sterile gauze squares
  - Container for the cleaning solution
  - Cleaning solution (e.g., normal saline)
  - Antiseptic solution for cleansing table surface
  - Two pairs of sterile forceps (thumb or artery)
  - Sterile gauze dressings and surgipads
  - Additional supplies required for the particular dressing (e.g., extra gauze dressings and ointment, if ordered)
  - Tape, tie tapes, or binder

IMPLEMENTATION

Preparation

- Validate the physician's order and check agency policy.
- Acquire assistance for changing a dressing on a restless or confused adult. **Rationale: The person might move and contaminate the sterile field or the wound.**
- Assist the client to a comfortable position in which the wound can be readily exposed. Expose only the wound area by using a bath blanket to cover the client, if necessary. **Rationale: Undue exposure is physically and psychologically distressing to most people.**
- Make a cuff on the moisture-proof bag for disposal of the soiled dressings, and place the bag within reach. It can be taped to the bedclothes away from the sterile field. **Rationale: Making a cuff helps keep the outside of the bag free from contamination by the soiled dressings and prevents subsequent contamination of the nurse's hands or of sterile instrument tips when discarding dressings or sponges. Placing the bag within reach prevents the nurse from reaching across the sterile field and the wound and potentially contaminating these areas.**
- Clean the table surface for the sterile field with antiseptic solution.
- Put on a mask, if required. **Rationale: Some agencies require that a mask be worn for surgical dressing changes to prevent contamination of the wound by droplet spray from the nurse's respiratory tract.**

Performance

1. Before performing the procedure, introduce yourself and verify the client's identity by using agency protocol. Explain to the client what you are going to do, why it is necessary, and how he or she can cooperate. Discuss how the results will be used in planning further care or treatments.

(continued)

SKILL 35.4

CLEANING A CLOSED WOUND AND APPLYING A STERILE DRESSING (*continued*)

2. Perform hand hygiene and observe other appropriate infection prevention and control procedures.
3. Provide for client privacy.
4. Remove binders and tape.
   - Remove binders, if used, and place them aside. Untie tie tapes, if used. Montgomery straps (tie tapes) are commonly used for wounds requiring frequent dressing changes (see ❶). **Rationale: These straps prevent skin irritation and discomfort caused by removing the adhesive each time the dressing is changed.**
   - If adhesive tape was used, remove it by holding down the skin and pulling parallel to the skin and toward the dressing. **Rationale: Pressing down on the skin provides countertraction against the pulling motion. Tape is pulled toward the incision to prevent strain on the wound.**
   - Use a solvent to loosen tape, if required. **Rationale: Moistening the tape with acetone or a similar solvent lessens the discomfort of removal, particularly from hairy surfaces.**
5. Remove and dispose of soiled dressings appropriately.

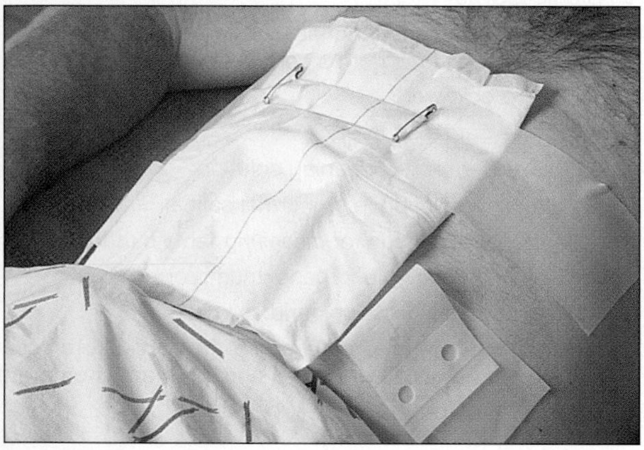

❶ Montgomery tapes holding dressing

   - Put on clean disposable gloves, and remove the outer abdominal dressing or surgipad.
   - Lift the outer dressing so that the underside is away from the client's face. **Rationale: The appearance and odour of the drainage may be upsetting to the client.** Note any drainage.
   - Place the soiled dressing in the moisture-proof bag without touching the outside of the bag. **Rationale: Contamination of the outside of the bag is avoided to prevent the spread of microorganisms to the nurse and subsequently to others.**
   - Remove the *under* dressings with a sterile forceps, taking care not to dislodge any drains. If the gauze sticks to the drain, support the drain with one hand and remove the gauze with the other.
   - Assess the location, type (colour, consistency), and odour of wound drainage and the number of gauzes saturated or the diameter of drainage collected on the dressings.
   - Discard the soiled dressings in the bag as before.
   - Remove gloves, dispose of them in the moisture-proof bag, and perform hand hygiene.
6. Set up the sterile supplies by using aseptic technique.
   - Open the sterile dressing set by using surgical aseptic technique.
   - Place the sterile drape beside the wound.
   - Open the sterile cleaning solution, and pour it over the gauze sponges in the plastic container.
7. Clean the wound, if indicated.
   - Clean the wound by using your gloved hands, or forceps and gauze swabs moistened with cleaning solution.
   - If using forceps, keep the forceps tips lower than the handles at all times. **Rationale: This prevents contamination by fluid travelling up to the handle and nurse's wrist and back to the tips.**
   - Use the cleaning methods illustrated and described in ❷ or one recommended by agency protocol.

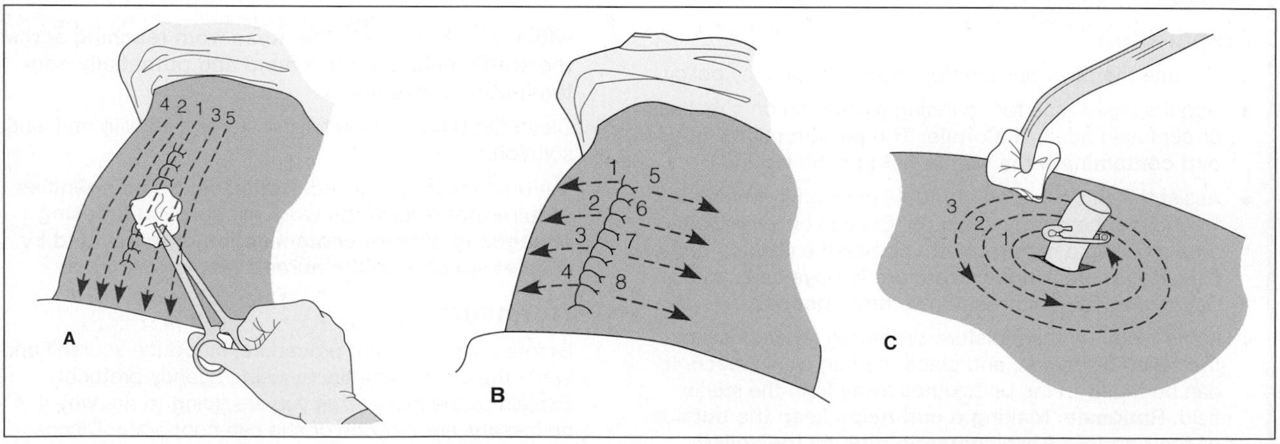

❷ Methods of cleaning surgical wounds: **A:** cleaning the wound from top to bottom, starting at the centre; **B:** cleaning a wound outward from the incision; **C:** cleaning around a drain site. For all methods, a clean sterile swab is used for each stroke.

(continued)

SKILL 35.4

CLEANING A CLOSED WOUND AND APPLYING A STERILE DRESSING (*continued*)

- Use a separate swab for each stroke, and discard each swab after use. **Rationale: This prevents the introduction of microorganisms to other wound areas.**
- If a drain is present, clean it next, taking care to avoid reaching across the cleaned incision. Clean the skin around the drain site by swabbing in half or full circles from around the drain site outward, using separate swabs for each wipe (see ❷C).
- Support and hold the drain erect while cleaning around it. Clean as many times as necessary to remove the drainage. Clean the drain, cleansing at the stab wound and then up the drain away from skin.
- Dry the drain area with dry gauze swabs, as required. Do not dry the incision or wound itself. **Rationale: Moisture facilitates wound healing.**

8. Apply dressings to the drain site and the incision.
   - Place a precut 10 cm × 10 cm gauze snugly around the drain (see ❸). **Rationale: This dressing absorbs the drainage and helps prevent it from excoriating the skin. Using precut gauze instead of cutting the gauze prevents any threads from coming loose and getting into the wound where they could cause inflammation and provide a site for infection.**
   - Apply the sterile dressings one at a time over the drain site. Place the bulk of the dressings over the drain area and below the drain, depending on the client's usual position. **Rationale: Layers of dressings are placed for best absorption of drainage, which flows by gravity.**
   - Apply the final surgipad or abdominal pad over the entire site. Secure the dressing with tape or ties.
9. Document the procedure and all nursing assessments.

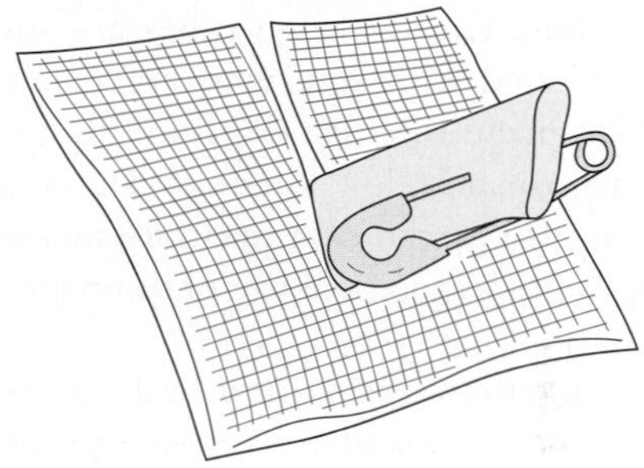

❸ Precut gauze in place around a drain

EVALUATION

- Conduct appropriate follow-up, such as amount of granulation tissue or degree of healing; amount of drainage and its colour, consistency, and odour; presence of inflammation; and degree of discomfort associated with the incision or drain site.
- Compare with previous findings, if available.
- Report significant deviations from normal to the appropriate members of the health-care team.

TEACHING: HOME CARE

Cleaning a Closed Wound

Instruct caregivers to do the following:

- Provide analgesics approximately 30 minutes before the procedure if the wound care causes pain or discomfort.
- Perform hand hygiene and dry before handling wound care supplies and providing wound care.
- Clean and wipe dry a flat surface for the sterile field.
- Keep pets out of the area when setting up for and performing sterile procedures.
- Acquire all needed supplies before starting a *sterile* procedure.
- Maintain sterile or clean technique, as instructed.
- Handle all *sterile* supplies from the outside of the wrapper or the edges.
- Do not touch the parts of supplies or equipment that will touch the patient.
- Avoid skin injury by using paper tape or Montgomery tie tapes instead of adhesive tape.
- Report any increasing wound drainage, pain, redness, increasing swelling, or opening or gaping of wound edges.
- Place any soiled dressing materials in a waterproof bag and dispose of it according to public health recommendations.

Wound Drains and Suction Surgical drains, for example a **Penrose drain**, are inserted to permit the drainage of excessive serosanguineous fluid and purulent material and to promote healing of underlying tissues. These drains may be inserted and sutured through the incision line, but they are most commonly inserted through stab wounds a few centimetres away from the incision line so that the incision itself can be kept dry. Without a drain, some wounds would heal on the surface and trap the discharge inside, and an abscess might form.

A **closed-wound drainage system** consists of a drain connected to either an electric suction or a portable drainage suction, such as a Hemovac (Figure 35.4) or Jackson-Pratt (Figure 35.5). The closed system reduces the possible entry of microorganisms into the wound through the drain. The drainage tubes are sutured in place and connected to a reservoir. For example, the Jackson-Pratt drainage tube is connected to a reservoir that maintains constant low suction. These portable wound suctions also provide for accurate measurement of the drainage and prevent leakage of drainage over the incision site.

The surgeon inserts the wound drainage tube during surgery. Generally, the suction is discontinued from 3 to 5 days postoperatively or when the drainage is minimal. Nurses are responsible for maintaining the wound suction, which hastens the healing process by draining excess exudate that might otherwise interfere with the formation of granulation tissue.

Closed-wound drainage systems have directions for use printed on the drainage container. When emptying the container, the nurse should wear gloves and avoid touching the drainage port (Figure 35.6). To re-establish suction, the nurse places the container on a solid, flat surface with the port open. The palm of one hand presses the top and bottom together while the other hand cleanses the opening and plug with an alcohol swab (Figure 35.7). Replace the drainage plug before releasing hand pressure to re-establish the vacuum necessary for the closed drainage system to work.

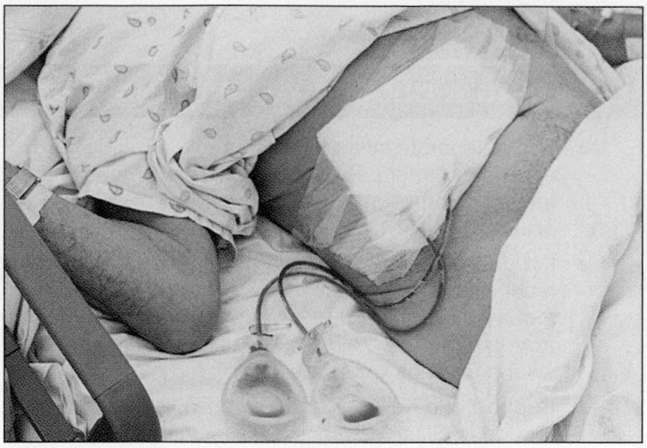

FIGURE 35.5 Two Jackson-Pratt devices compressed to facilitate collection of exudates

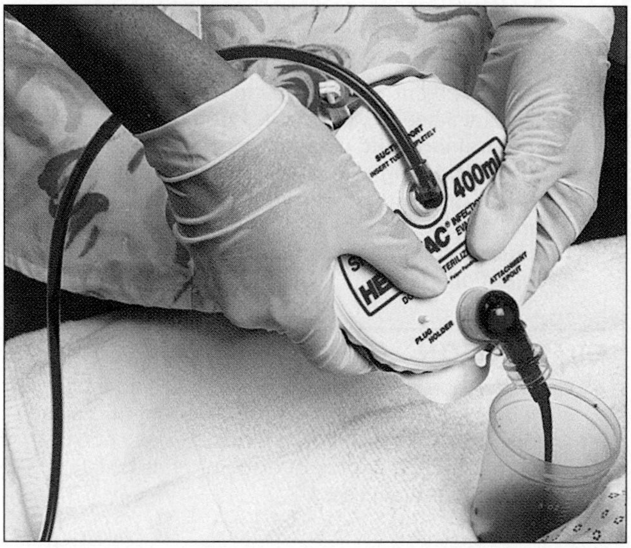

FIGURE 35.6 Emptying drainage from Hemovac drainage system

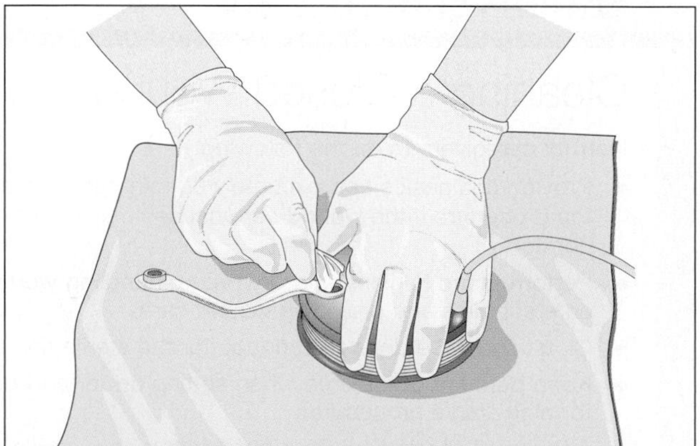

FIGURE 35.7 With one hand, press the top and bottom together. With the other hand, clean the opening and plug with an alcohol swab. Replace the plug before releasing hand.

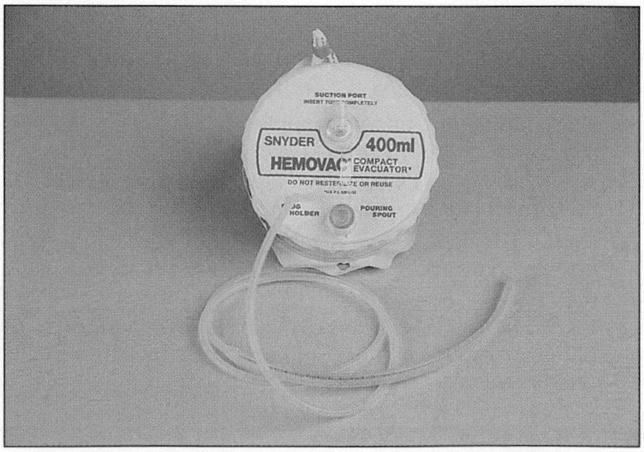

FIGURE 35.4 Hemovac closed-wound drainage system

SUTURES A **suture** is a thread used to sew body tissues together. Sutures used to attach tissues beneath the skin are often made of an absorbable material that disappears in several days. Skin sutures, by contrast, are made of a variety of nonabsorbable materials, such as silk, cotton, linen, wire, nylon, and Dacron (polyester fibre). Silver wire clips or staples are also available. Usually, skin sutures are removed 7 to 10 days after surgery.

Suturing can be done by using various methods. Skin sutures can be broadly categorized as either *interrupted* (each stitch is tied and knotted separately) or *continuous* (one thread runs in a series of stitches and is tied only at the beginning and at the end of the run). Common methods of suturing are illustrated in Figure 35.8.

Retention sutures are very large sutures used in addition to skin sutures for some incisions (Figure 35.9). They attach underlying tissues of fat and muscle as well as skin and are used to support incisions in obese individuals or when healing may be prolonged. They are frequently left in place longer than skin sutures (14 to 21 days) but, in some instances, are removed at the same time as the skin sutures. To prevent these large sutures from irritating the incision, the surgeon may place rubber tubing over them or a roll of gauze under them extending down the incision line.

The physician orders the removal of sutures. In some agencies, only physicians remove sutures; in others, registered nurses and nursing students with appropriate supervision can do so. Agency policies about removal of retention sutures vary. The nurse should verify whether they are to be removed and who can remove them.

Sterile technique and special suture scissors are used in suture removal. The scissors have a short, curved cutting tip that readily slides under the suture (Figure 35.10).

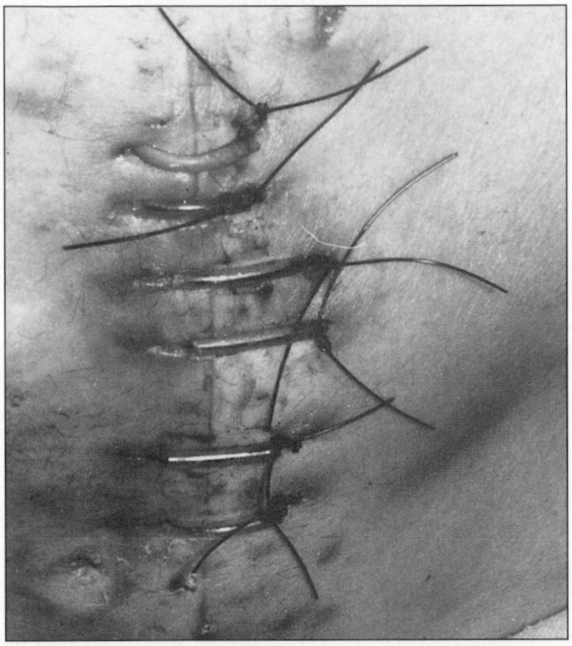

FIGURE 35.9 A surgical incision with retention sutures

Wire clips or staples are removed with a special instrument that squeezes the centre of the clip to remove it from the skin (Figure 35.11).

Guidelines for removing sutures follow:

- Before removing skin sutures, verify (1) the orders for suture removal (in many instances, only *alternate* interrupted sutures are removed one day, and the remaining sutures are removed a day or two later), and (2) whether a dressing is to be applied following the suture removal. Some physicians prefer no dressing; others prefer a small, light gauze dressing to prevent friction by clothing.

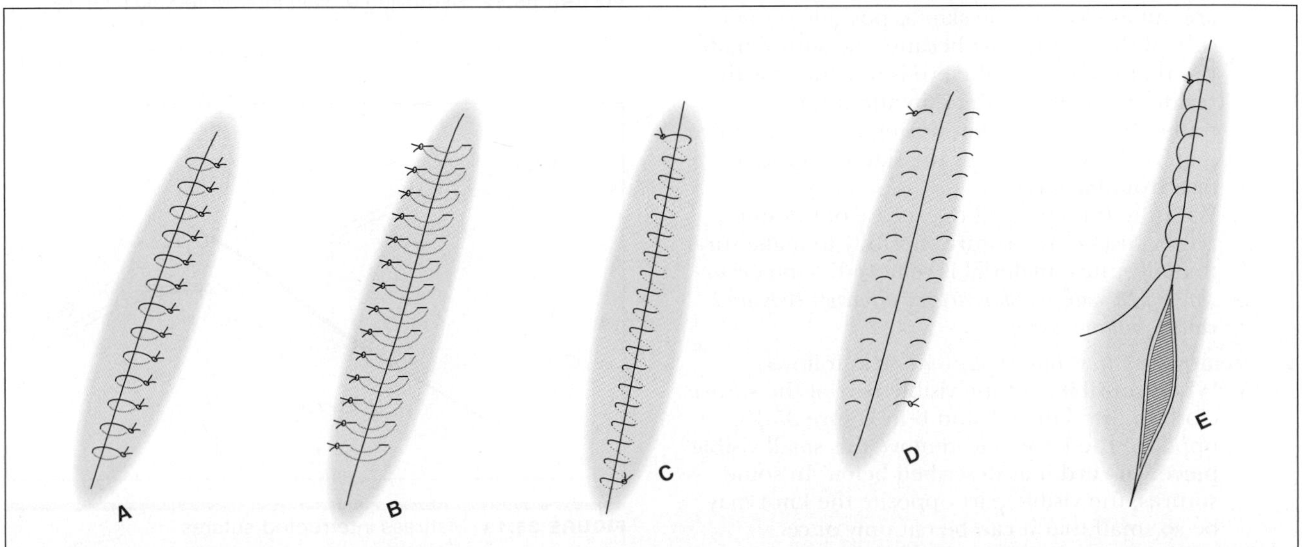

FIGURE 35.8 Common sutures: **A:** plain interrupted; **B:** mattress interrupted; **C:** plain continuous; **D:** mattress continuous; **E:** blanket continuous

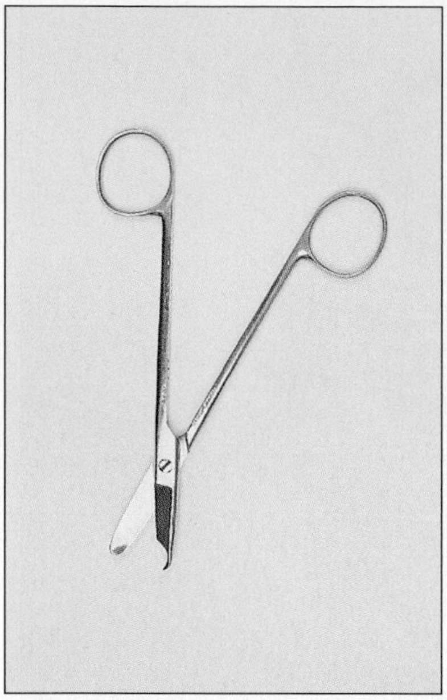

FIGURE 35.10 Suture scissors

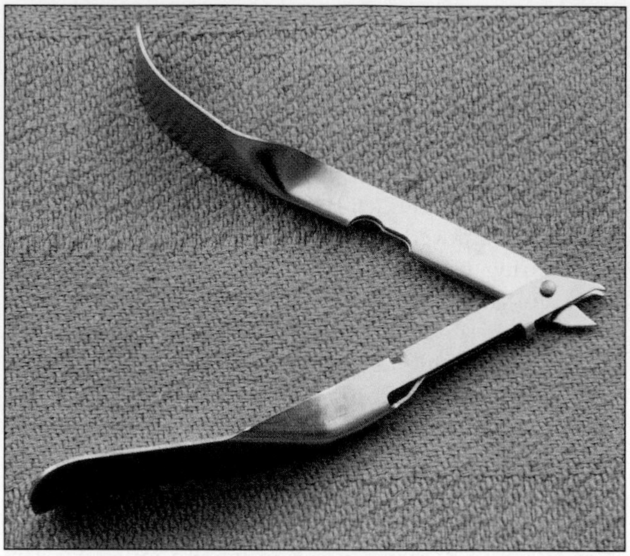

FIGURE 35.11 Staple remover

- Inform the client that suture removal may produce slight discomfort, such as a pulling or stinging sensation, but it should not be painful.
- Remove dressings and clean the incision in accordance with agency protocol. Cleaning the suture line with normal saline before and after suture removal may help prevent infection.
- Put on sterile gloves.
- Remove *plain interrupted sutures* as follows:
  a. Grasp the suture at the knot with a pair of forceps.
  b. Place the curved tip of the suture scissors under the suture as close to the skin as possible, either on the side opposite the knot (Figure 35.12) or directly under the knot. Cut the suture. Sutures are cut as close to the skin as possible on one side of the visible part because the suture material that is visible to the eye is in contact with resident bacteria of the skin and must not be pulled beneath the skin during removal. Suture material that is beneath the skin is considered free from bacteria.
  c. With the forceps, pull the suture out in one piece. Inspect the suture carefully to make sure that all suture material is removed. *Suture material left beneath the skin acts as a foreign body and causes inflammation.*
- Remove *mattress interrupted sutures* as follows:
  a. When possible, cut the visible part of the suture close to the skin at A and B in Figure 35.13, opposite the knot, and remove this small visible piece. Discard it as described below. In some sutures, the visible part opposite the knot may be so small that it can be cut only once.
  b. Grasp the knot (Figure 35.13C) with forceps. Remove the remainder of the suture beneath the skin by pulling out in the direction of the knot.

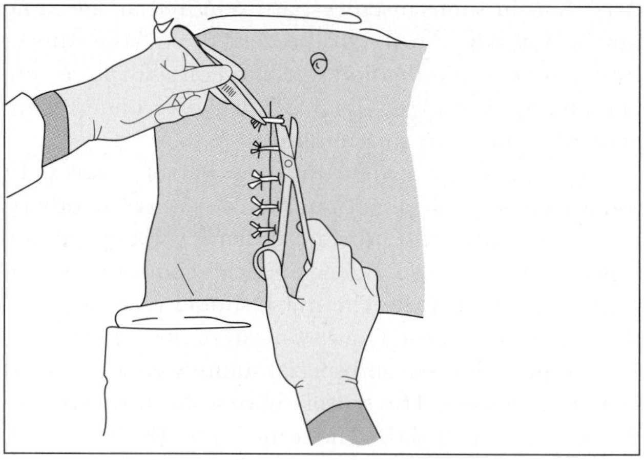

FIGURE 35.12 Removing a plain interrupted skin suture

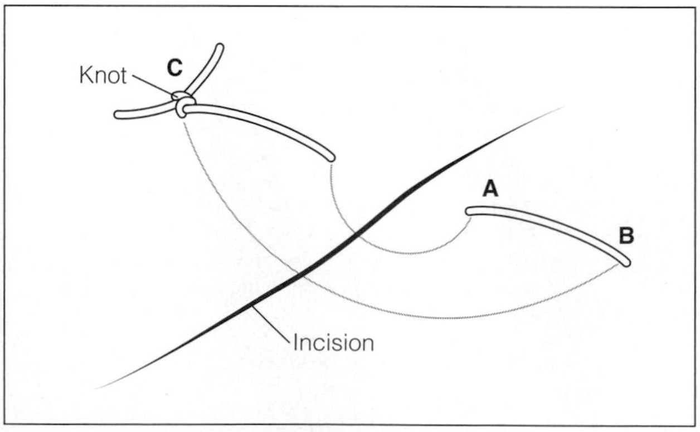

FIGURE 35.13 Mattress interrupted sutures

- Discard the suture onto a piece of sterile gauze or into the moisture-proof bag, being careful not to contaminate the forceps tips.

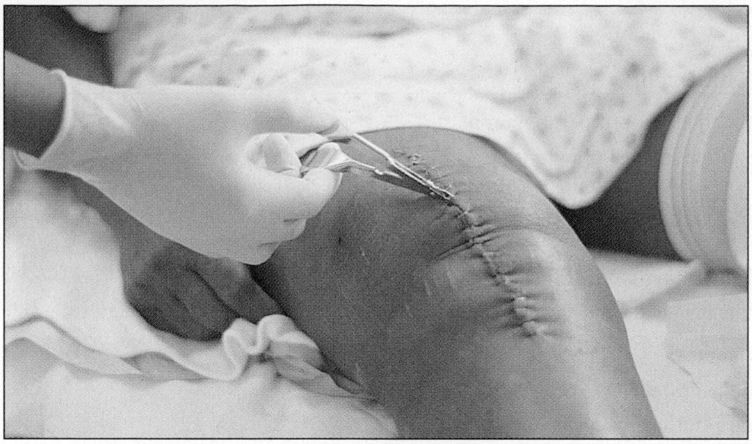

FIGURE 35.14 Removing surgical clips or staples

- Continue to remove *alternate* sutures (except for continuous sutures in which all sutures are removed), that is, the third, fifth, seventh, and so forth, if no dehiscence occurs. *Alternate sutures are removed first so that remaining sutures keep the skin edges in close approximation and prevent any dehiscence from becoming large.*
- If no dehiscence occurs, remove the remaining sutures. If dehiscence does occur, do not remove the remaining sutures, and report the dehiscence to the nurse in charge.
- If Steri-Strips are ordered by the physician, apply them to the wound after removing the sutures or clips. Some physicians order Steri-Strip application to provide additional support to the healing wound.
- Reapply a dressing, if indicated.
- Document the suture removal; number of sutures removed; appearance of the incision; application of a dressing, Steri-Strips, or butterfly tapes (if appropriate); client teaching; and client tolerance of the procedure.
- Remove staples as follows:
  a. Remove dressings and clean the incision in accordance with agency protocol.
  b. Place the lower tips of a sterile staple remover under the staple.
  c. Squeeze the handles together until they are completely closed (Figure 35.14). Pressing the handles together causes the staple to bend in the middle and pulls the edges of the staple out of the skin. Do not lift the staple remover when squeezing the handles.
  d. When both ends of the staple are visible, gently move the staple away from the incision site.
  e. Hold the staple remover over a disposable container, release the staple remover handles and release the staple.

If the sutures are to be removed outside a clinical setting, sterile technique is used (see the Home Care Considerations box for client information).

Home Care Considerations

Removing Sutures or Staples

Perform the procedure in a well-lighted, private area of the home and give the client the following information:

- Instruct the client to observe the incision daily and call the appropriate member of the health-care team if increased redness, drainage, or open areas are observed.
- Provide instructions and supplies for care of the incision, and tell the client when to shower for the first time.
- Assess the client's ability to keep the incision clean and protected at home.

Evaluating

By using the goals developed during the planning stage—maintaining comfort, promoting healing, restoring wellness, and preventing risks associated with surgery—the nurse collects data to evaluate whether the identified goals and desired outcomes have been achieved. Examples of client goals and related outcomes are shown in Table 35.3.

If the desired outcomes are not achieved, the nurse, client, and support people need to explore the reasons why before modifying the care plan. For example, if the goal "Maintain comfort" is *not* met, questions to be considered include the following:

- What is the client's perception of the problem?
- Does the client understand how to use PCA?
- Is the prescribed analgesic dose adequate for the client?
- Is the client allowing pain to become intense before requesting medication or using PCA?
- Where is the client's pain? Could it be due to a problem unrelated to surgery (e.g., chronic arthritis, anginal pain)?
- Is there evidence of a complication that could cause increased pain (an infection, abscess, or hematoma)?

TABLE 35.3 Evaluation Goals and Outcomes: Postoperative Clients

Goal	Examples of Desired Outcomes
Maintain comfort	Verbalizes satisfaction with pain control measures Absence of nonverbal indications of pain (e.g., protective body position, restlessness, facial expressions of pain) Absence of physiological indications of pain (e.g., muscle tension; perspiration; change in blood pressure, heart rate, respiratory rate, and pupil size; loss of appetite) Moves and ambulates with minimal difficulty Rests for extended periods
Promote healing	Incision clean, dry, and intact Wound edges approximated well Balanced fluid intake and output Tolerating diet rich in fibre, protein, and vitamins A and C Active bowel sounds within 48 hours Normal defecation within 3 days following ingestion of food Hemoglobin, hematocrit, and serum electrolytes within normal limits
Prevent risks associated with surgery	Performs deep breathing, coughing, and incentive spirometry, as instructed Normal auscultated breath sounds Adequate respiratory excursion (depth) Performs leg exercises, as instructed Walks increasing distances (specify) each day Stable vital signs Strong and equal peripheral pulses in all four extremities
Restore highest possible level of wellness	Increasingly participates in self-care activities (specify) Asks pertinent questions concerning ongoing care Seeks help, as appropriate Demonstrates ability to care for incision Reports ability to manage ongoing care

Case Study 35

Mr. Teng is a 77-year-old client with a history of chronic obstructive pulmonary disease. Currently, his respiratory condition is being controlled with medications, and he is free of infection. He has just been transferred to the postanaesthesia care unit following a hernia repair performed under spinal anaesthesia. His blood pressure is 132/88, pulse 84, respirations 28, and tympanic temperature is 36.8°C. He is awake and stable.

Critical Thinking Questions

1. What factors place Mr. Teng at increased risk for the development of complications during and after surgery?
2. Speculate about why Mr. Teng's surgeon and anaesthetist decided to perform Mr. Teng's surgery under regional anaesthesia as opposed to general anaesthesia.
3. What preparations were taken during the preoperative period to protect Mr. Teng from possible complications during and after his surgery?
4. How will Mr. Teng's postoperative assessments differ from those of a person who received general anaesthesia?
5. What postoperative precautions are especially important to Mr. Teng in view of his chronic lung condition?

After working through these questions, go to the MyNursingLab at **http://www.mynursinglab.com** to check your answers.

KEY TERMS

perioperative period
preoperative phase
intraoperative phase
postoperative phase
emergency surgery
urgent surgery
elective surgery
invasive (open) surgery
minimally invasive surgery
major surgery
minor surgery
general anaesthesia
local anaesthesia
regional anaesthesia
topical (surface) anaesthesia
local infiltration
nerve block
intravenous block (Bier block)
spinal anaesthesia (subarachnoid block)
epidural (peridural) anaesthesia
conscious sedation
circulating nurse
scrub nurse
atelectasis
thrombus
thrombophlebitis
emboli
Penrose drain
closed-wound drainage system
suture

CHAPTER HIGHLIGHTS

- Surgery is a unique experience that creates stress and necessitates physical and psychological changes.
- The perioperative period includes three phases: preoperative, intraoperative, and postoperative.
- Surgical procedures are categorized by degree of urgency, purpose, invasiveness, and degree of risk.
- Such factors as age, general health, nutritional status, medication history, and mental status affect a client's risk during surgery.
- Clients must agree to surgery and sign an informed consent.
- Nursing history and physical assessment data are important sources for planning preoperative and postoperative care.
- The overall goal of nursing care during the preoperative phase is to prepare the client mentally and physically for surgery.
- Preoperative teaching includes situational information and psychosocial support, the role of the client throughout the perioperative period, expected sensations and discomfort, and training for the postoperative period.
- Preoperative teaching should include moving, leg exercises, and coughing and deep-breathing exercises. Many aspects of preoperative teaching are intended to prevent postoperative complications.
- Physical preparation includes the following areas: nutrition and fluids, elimination, hygiene, rest, medications, care of valuables and prostheses, special orders, and surgical skin preparation.
- Antiembolism stockings or sequential compression devices may be ordered for some clients to facilitate venous return.
- A preoperative checklist provides a guide to and documentation of a client's preparation before surgery.
- Maintaining the client's safety is the overall goal of nursing care during the intraoperative phase.
- Anaesthesia is general, local, or regional. General anaesthesia involves the loss of all sensation and consciousness. Local anaesthesia techniques include topical anaesthesia and local infiltration; regional anaesthesia techniques include nerve block, intravenous block, spinal anaesthesia (subarachnoid block), and epidural. Conscious sedation is used as an adjunctive.
- Surgical skin preparation should be carried out as close to the time of surgery as possible and is commonly performed during the intraoperative phase.
- Positioning of the client during surgery is important to reduce the risk of tissue and nerve damage.
- Immediate postanaesthetic care focuses on assessment and monitoring parameters to prevent complications from anaesthesia or surgery.
- Initial and ongoing assessment of the postoperative client includes level of consciousness, vital signs, oxygen saturation, skin colour and temperature, comfort, fluid balance, dressings, drains, and tubes.
- The overall goals of nursing care during the postoperative period are to promote comfort and healing, restore the highest possible level of wellness, and prevent associated risks, such as infection or respiratory and cardiovascular complications.
- Ongoing postoperative nursing interventions include (1) managing pain, (2) positioning appropriately, (3) encouraging incentive spirometry and deep-breathing and coughing exercises, (4) promoting leg exercises, (5) encouraging early ambulation, (6) maintaining adequate hydration, (7) promoting a proper diet, (8) promoting urinary elimination, (9) continuing gastrointestinal suction, and (10) providing wound care.
- Sterile technique is used when changing dressings on surgical wounds to promote healing and reduce the risk of infection.
- Penrose drains and Hemovac drainage systems are examples of drains that may be placed in or near surgical wounds to promote drainage of excess serosanguineous or purulent exudate.
- Sutures, wire clips, or staples are used to approximate skin and underlying tissues after surgery. These are generally removed 7 to 10 days after surgery.

ASSESS YOUR LEARNING

1. Which of the following tests is the best for determining the status of a client's preoperative liver function?
   a. Serum electrolytes
   b. Blood urea nitrogen (BUN), creatinine
   c. Alanine aminotransferase (ALT), aspirate aminotransferase (AST), bilirubin
   d. Serum albumin

2. A client who is having a mastectomy expresses sadness about losing her breast. Based on this information, the nurse would identify that the client is at risk for which nursing diagnosis?
   a. *Body Image Disturbance*
   b. *Anticipatory Grieving*
   c. *Fear*
   d. *Ineffective Coping*

3. Which of the following statements by the client indicates that the preoperative teaching regarding elective abdominal surgery has been effective?
   a. "I cannot eat or drink anything after midnight."
   b. "I'm not going to cough after surgery because it might open my incision."
   c. "I might have a stroke if I stop taking my anticoagulant."
   d. "The nurse showed me how to contract and relax my calf muscles."

4. The nurse assesses a postoperative client who has a rapid and weak pulse, urine output of less than 30 mL/h, and decreased blood pressure. The client's skin is cool and clammy. What complication should the nurse suspect?
   a. Thrombophlebitis
   b. Hypovolemic shock
   c. Aspiration pneumonia
   d. Wound dehiscence

5. The client is most likely to require the greatest amount of analgesia for pain during which of the following times?
   a. Immediately after surgery
   b. 4 hours after surgery
   c. 12 to 36 hours after surgery
   d. 48 to 60 hours after surgery

6. Ms. Johnson, 28 years old, returns to the unit after a large bowel resection and creation of a colostomy with a Hemovac in place. Which of the following nursing assessments should be included in the initial postoperative documentation?
   a. Vital signs and status of the stoma.
   b. Ability to perform deep breathing and coughing exercises.
   c. Position of the client postoperatively.
   d. Amount of drainage in the Hemovac.

7. A semiconscious client in the postanaesthesia care unit (PACU) is experiencing dyspnea. Which of the following actions should the nurse perform first?
   a. Place a pillow under the client's head.
   b. Remove the oropharyngeal airway.
   c. Apply oxygen by mask.
   d. Reposition the client to keep the tongue forward.

8. The client's postoperative orders state "diet as tolerated." The client has been NPO. The nurse will advance the client's diet to clear liquids based on which of the following assessments? Select all that apply.
   a. No complaints of nausea or vomiting
   b. Pain level is maintained at a rating of 2 to 3 out of 10
   c. Ambulates with minimal assistance
   d. Presence of bowel sounds

9. Which of the following is the overall goal of nursing care during the intraoperative phase?
   a. The client's safety
   b. The client's informed consent
   c. The client's quality of life
   d. The client's coping abilities

10. The nurse plans to remove the client's sutures. Which of the following actions demonstrates appropriate standards of care?
    a. Use clean technique.
    b. Remove sutures one after the other along the length of the incision line.
    c. Place the curved tip of the suture scissors under the suture as close to the skin as possible.
    d. Pull the suture material that is visible beneath the skin during removal.

After working through these questions, go to the MyNursingLab at ***http://www.mynursinglab.com*** *to check your answers and see explanations.*

SUGGESTED READINGS

Glover, D. E. (2006). Perioperative clinical nurse specialist role delineation: A systematic review. *AORN Journal, 84*(6), 1017–1030.

This article summarizes the benefits of a CNS in perioperative care but indicates that this role is not well established. The article provides interesting ideas on how the role can be developed.

Hasankhani H., Mohammadi, E., Moazzami, F., Mokhtari, F., & Naghgizadh. M. (2007). The effects of intravenous fluids temperature on perioperative hemodynamic situation, post-operative shivering, and recovery in orthopaedic surgery. *Canadian Operating Room Nursing Journal, 25*(1), 20–24, 26–27.

This article discusses the benefits of warming intravenous fluids rather than infusing them at room temperature in promoting postoperative recovery.

Lipp, A., & Edwards, P. (2002). Disposable surgical face masks for preventing surgical wound infection in clean surgery. *Cochrane Database of Systematic Reviews,* 1, Art. No.: CD002929.

This systematic review provides an excellent discussion on the effectiveness of masks in preventing wound infections during surgery.

Operating Room Nurses Association of Canada. (2006). *Recommended standards, guidelines and position statements for perioperative nursing practice.* Vancouver: Author.

This document provides an overview of knowledge of surgical principles and methods to improve the care of surgical clients. The standards outline the scope of responsibility of the perioperative nurse.

WEBLINKS

The Canadian Anesthesiologists' Society

http://www.cas.ca

This not-for-profit voluntary organization's website provides current information and guidelines for the practice of anaesthesia and patient information about anaesthesia.

Operating Room Nurses Association of Canada

http://www.ornac.ca

This website provides information related to the history, mission, values, and standards of practice of operating room nurses.

REFERENCES

Anderson, H. K., Lewis, S. J., & Thomas, S. (2006). Early enteral nutrition within 24h of colorectal surgery versus later commencement of feeding for postoperative complications. *Cochrane Database of Systematic Reviews, 4,* Art. No.: CD004080.

Brady, M., Kinn, S., O'Rourke, K., Randhawa, N., & Stuart, P. (2005). Preoperative fasting for preventing perioperative complications in children. *Cochrane Database of Systematic Review, 2,* Art. No.: CD005285.

Brady, M., Kinn, S., & Stuart, P. (2003). Preoperative fasting for adults to prevent perioperative complications. *Cochrane Database of Systematic Reviews, 4,* Art. No.: CD004423.

Canadian Anesthesiologists' Society. (2007). *Guidelines: The preanaesthetic period.* Retrieved June 19, 2008, from http://www.cas.ca/members/sign_in/guidelines/preanaesthetic/

Canadian Orthopedic Association. (2005). Wrong sided surgery in orthopaedics. Retrieved June 22, 2008, from http://www.coa-aco.org/library/health_policy/wrong_sided_surgery_in_orthopaedics.html

Lecompte, T., & Hardy, J. F. (2006). Antiplatelet agents and perioperative bleeding. *Canadian Journal of Anaesthesia, 53,* S103–S112.

Møller, A., & Villebro, N. (2005). Interventions for preoperative smoking cessation. *Cochrane Database of Systematic Reviews, 3,* Art. No.: CD002294.

NANDA International. (2007). *Nursing diagnoses: Definitions and classification, 2007–2008.* Philadelphia, PA: Author.

Operating Room Nurses Association of Canada. (2006). *Recommended standards, guidelines and position statements for perioperative nursing practice.* Vancouver: Author.

Safer Healthcare Now! (2007). *Prevent surgical site infections: How-to guide.* Retrieved June 22, 2008, from http://www.saferhealthcarenow.ca/Default.aspx?folderId=82&contentId=182

UNIT 6

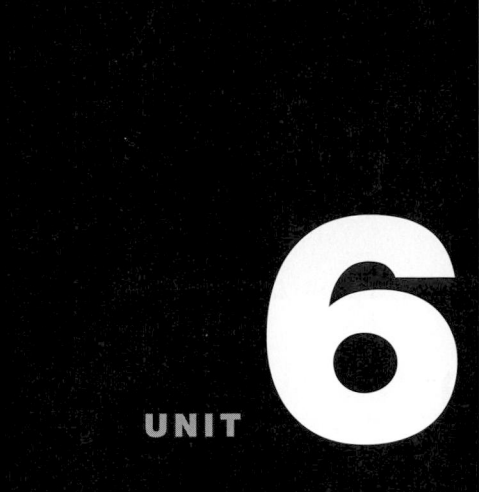

Promoting Physiological Health

CHAPTER 36
Sensory Perception

CHAPTER 37
Rest and Sleep

CHAPTER 38
Activity and Exercise

CHAPTER 39
Nutrition

CHAPTER 40
Fecal Elimination

CHAPTER 41
Urinary Elimination

CHAPTER 42
Oxygenation and Circulation

CHAPTER 43
Fluid, Electrolyte, and Acid-Base Balance

Chapter 36

Sensory Perception

An individual's senses are essential for growth, development, and survival. Sensory stimuli give meaning to events in the environment. Any alteration in people's sensory functions can affect their ability to function within the environment. Nurses can help them find ways to function safely in this often confusing environment.

OBJECTIVES

After studying this chapter, you should be able to

1. Discuss anatomical and physiological components of the sensory-perceptual process
2. Describe three factors that affect a client's sensory functioning
3. Outline six essential components in assessing a client's sensory-perceptual function
4. Identify the clinical signs and symptoms of sensory overload and deprivation
5. Develop nursing diagnoses and outcome criteria for clients with impaired sensory function
6. Discuss nursing interventions to promote and maintain sensory function
7. Contrast the characteristics of delirium with the characteristics of dementia
8. Describe nursing strategies to promote and maintain orientation to person, place, time, and situation for the client who is disoriented

Components of the Sensory-Perceptual Process

Reception and Perception

The sensory process involves two components: reception and perception. **Sensory reception** is the process of receiving stimuli or data. These stimuli are either external or internal to the body. **External stimuli** are *visual* (sight), *auditory* (hearing), *olfactory* (smell), *tactile* (touch), and *gustatory* (taste). **Internal stimuli** are kinesthetic or visceral. **Kinesthetic** refers to awareness of the position and movement of body parts. For example, a person walking is aware of which leg is forward. A related sense is **stereognosis**, the awareness of an object's size, shape, and texture by touch. For example, a person holding a tennis ball is aware of its size, round shape, and soft surface without seeing it. **Visceral** refers to any large organ within the body. Visceral organs can produce stimuli that make a person aware of them (e.g., a full stomach). **Sensory perception** involves the conscious organization and translation of the data or stimuli into meaningful information.

For an individual to be aware of the surroundings, four aspects of the sensory process must be present: a stimulus, a receptor, impulse conduction, and perception.

- **Stimulus**. A stimulus is an agent or act that stimulates a nerve receptor (e.g., a sound wave that produces vibrations on your tympanic membrane).
- **Receptor**. A nerve cell acts as a receptor by converting the stimulus to a nerve impulse. Most receptors are specific, that is, sensitive to only one type of stimulus, such as visual, auditory, or touch. Sound waves create vibrations that are carried through the ear to the receptor hairs of the organ of Corti.
- **Impulse conduction**. The impulse travels along nerve pathways to the spinal cord or directly to the brain (Figure 36.1). The vibrations received in the organ of Corti in the inner ear are translated into electric impulses, which travel along the acoustic nerve to the brain.
- **Perception**. Perception, or awareness and interpretation of stimuli, takes place in the brain where specialized brain cells interpret the nature and the quality of the sensory stimuli. The level of consciousness affects the perception of the stimuli. The cerebral cortex of the brain then interprets the meaning of sound and initiates the appropriate response.

Arousal Mechanism

For a person to receive and interpret stimuli, the brain must be alert. The **reticular activating system (RAS)** in the brain stem acts to mediate the arousal mechanism. The RAS has two components: the *reticular excitatory area* (REA) and the *reticular inhibitory area* (RIA). The REA is responsible for stimulus arousal and wakefulness, and the RIA has the opposite function.

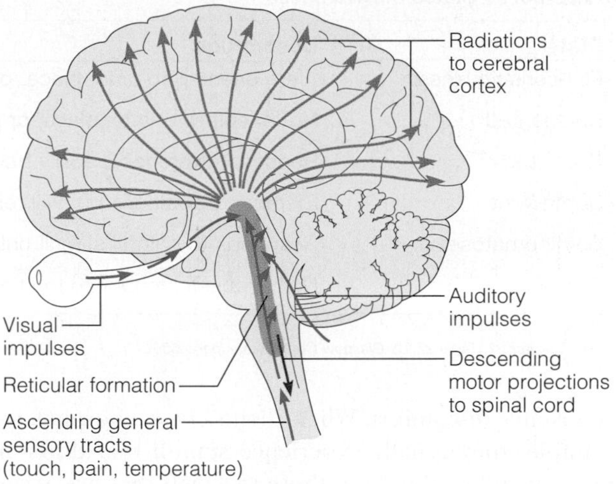

FIGURE 36.1 Nerve impulses run along the ascending sensory tracts to reach the reticular activating system (RAS); when certain impulses reach the cerebral cortex, they are perceived.

Source: From **Human Anatomy & Physiology**, *6th ed., by Elaine N. Marieb. Copyright © 2004 (p. 456) by Benjamin Cummings Publishing Company. Reprinted with permission.*

People have their own zone of optimum arousal, the level at which the person feels comfortable. **Sensoristasis** is the term used to describe optimum arousal for an individual. Beyond this comfort zone, people must adapt to increased or decreased sensory stimuli. An absence of stimuli from the RAS to the cerebrum results in the brain becoming inactive or useless.

The brain has the capacity to adapt to most sensory stimuli. For example, a person living in a city may not notice traffic noises that someone from a rural area finds loud and disturbing. Not all sensory stimuli are acted on; some are stored by the memory to be used at a later date. Cognition is cerebral functioning. It involves such processes as conscious thought, reality orientation, problem solving, judgment, and comprehension.

Awareness is the ability to perceive environmental stimuli and body reactions and to respond appropriately through thought and action. The normal, alert person can assimilate many kinds of information at one time. Awareness exists in several states (see Table 36.1).

Sensory Alterations

People become accustomed to certain sensory stimuli, and when these change markedly, the individual may

TABLE 36.1 States of Awareness

State	Description
Full consciousness	Alert; oriented to time, place, person; understands verbal and written words
Disoriented	Not oriented to time, place, or person
Confused	Reduced awareness, easily bewildered; poor memory, misinterprets stimuli; impaired judgment
Somnolent	Extreme drowsiness but will respond to stimuli
Semicomatose	Responds to painful stimuli only
Coma*	No purposeful response to stimuli; may still react to deep pain but only with atypical posturing

See Chapter 27, Table 27.12: Glasgow Coma Scale (page 635).

experience discomfort. When clients enter a hospital, for example, they usually experience stimuli that differ in quantity and quality from those to which they are accustomed. These changes can cause clients to become confused and disoriented.

Nurses should be aware of the behaviours that often result from different stimuli. Colour, sound, privacy, and social interaction for clients can be modified to more closely resemble those in their home environment. Factors that contribute to alterations in behaviour include sensory deprivation, sensory overload, and sensory deficits.

Sensory Deprivation

Sensory deprivation is generally thought of as a decrease in or lack of meaningful stimuli. When a person experiences sensory deprivation, the balance in the RAS is disturbed. The RAS is unable to maintain normal stimulation to the cerebral cortex. This reduced stimulation causes the person to become more acutely aware of the remaining stimuli and often perceive these in a distorted manner. Thus, the person often experiences alterations in perception, cognition, and emotion. See the Clinical Manifestations box on sensory deprivation.

Clinical Manifestations

Sensory Deprivation

Sensory deprivation can manifest in several ways:

- Excessive yawning, drowsiness, sleeping
- Decreased attention span, difficulty concentrating, decreased problem solving
- Impaired memory
- Periodic disorientation, general confusion, or nocturnal confusion
- Preoccupation with somatic complaints, such as palpitations
- Hallucinations or delusions
- Crying, annoyance over small matters, depression
- Apathy, emotional lability

Sensory Overload

Sensory overload generally occurs when a person is unable to process or manage the amount or intensity of sensory stimuli. Three factors contribute to sensory overload:

1. Increased quantity or quality of internal stimuli, such as pain, dyspnea, anxiety
2. Increased quantity or quality of external stimuli, such as a noisy health-care setting, intrusive diagnostic studies, contact with many strangers
3. Inability to disregard stimuli selectively, perhaps as a result of nervous system disturbances or medications that stimulate the arousal mechanism

Sensory overload can limit the brain's capability to filter or respond to specific stimuli. The individual may experience difficulty perceiving the environment in a way that makes sense; their thoughts race in many directions and restlessness occurs. The person may feel overwhelmed and out of control. The nurse must recognize that the sights and sounds that are familiar to them often represent overload to clients. Such factors as pain, lack of sleep, and worry can also contribute to sensory overload. People who have sensory overload may appear fatigued and may not be able to internalize new information. See the Clinical Manifestations box on sensory overload.

Sensory Deficits

A **sensory deficit** is impaired reception, perception, or both of one or more of the senses. Blindness and deaf-

Clinical Manifestations

Sensory Overload

Sensory overload can manifest in several ways:

- Complaints of fatigue, sleeplessness
- Irritability, anxiety, restlessness
- Periodic or general disorientation
- Reduced problem-solving ability and task performance
- Increased muscle tension
- Scattered attention and racing thoughts

ness are sensory deficits. When only one sense is affected, other senses may become more acute. However, sudden loss of eyesight can result in disorientation.

With a gradual loss of sensory function, individuals often develop behaviours to compensate for the loss; sometimes, these behaviours are unconscious. For example, a person with gradual hearing loss in the right ear may unconsciously turn the left ear toward a speaker. Some neurological diseases cause changes in the kinesthetic sense and tactile perception. Diseases of the inner ear, for example Meniere's disease, can cause loss of kinesthetic sense so that standing or walking is impossible.

Clients with sensory deficits are at risk of both sensory deprivation and sensory overload. Persons with vision problems may be unable to read, watch television, or recognize persons by sight. An unfamiliar environment can add to their confusion. Blind people often have highly structured home environments; the diversity and unfamiliarity of the hospital environment can create sensory overload. Impaired vision limits the person's ability to move around readily or socialize with others.

Factors Affecting Sensory Function

A number of factors affect the amount and quality of sensory stimulation, including a person's developmental stage, culture, level of stress, medications and illness, and lifestyle and personality.

Developmental Stage

Perception of sensation is critical to the intellectual, social, and physical development of infants and children. Newborns should be screened for hearing deficits before hospital discharge. If a hearing loss is detected, treatment can begin early and complications, such as speech loss, can be prevented.

Infants learn to recognize the face of the mother or caregiver and establish bonding essential to later emotional development. Young children respond to music by singing and dancing as they begin to interact with their peers. As children grow, they learn to interpret visual and auditory signals when preparing to cross the street. Adults have many learned responses to sensory cues. The sudden loss or impairment of any sense can have profound effects on both children and adults.

Normal changes of aging often result in varying degrees of impairments in sensory perception of the senses: hearing, vision, smell, taste, and touch. These physiologic changes in older adults put them at higher risk for altered sensory function. While accurate figures are very difficult to obtain, "there are approximately 310 000 profoundly deaf and deafened Canadians and possibly 2.8 million hard of hearing Canadians" (Canadian Association of the Deaf, 2007, p. 1). Hearing loss is one of the most common health complaints reported by older adults. The diminishing of sensory perception that can come with aging or chronic disease (e.g., diabetes, strokes, and other neurologic disorders, such as Parkinson's disease) is generally gradual. *Presbycusis,* a type of inner ear hearing loss, is common with aging. The ability to hear high-frequency sounds and distinguish from background sounds is most affected. People with sensory impairments, such as hearing loss, tend to experience isolation and increased life stresses (Gibson & Gibson, 2004).

Culture

An individual's culture often determines the amount of stimulation that a person considers usual or "normal." For example, a child raised in a large, active Italian family may be accustomed to more stimulation than an only child raised in an English-Canadian family. In addition, the normal amount of stimulation associated with ethnic origin, religious affiliation, or income level may also affect the amount of stimulation an individual desires and believes to be meaningful. The sudden change in cultural surroundings experienced by immigrants or visitors to a new country, in which differences in language, dress, and cultural behaviours abound, can result in sensory overload or culture shock.

Cultural deprivation or **cultural care deprivation** is a lack of culturally assistive, supportive, or facilitative acts. Nurses must be aware of and sensitive to what stimulation is culturally acceptable to a client. In some cultures, touching is comforting and acceptable, whereas in others, it may be offensive. Some clients find the presence of cultural or religious symbols reassuring (see Chapter 46, the section "Spiritual Symbols"). Nurses should accommodate clients' needs, provided these practices do not endanger health.

Stress

During times of increased stress, people may find their senses already overloaded and seek to decrease sensory stimulation. For example, people dealing with physical illness, pain, hospitalization, and diagnostic tests may want to have only close support people visit. They may also need the nurse's help to decrease unnecessary stimuli (e.g., noise) as much as possible. Alternatively, clients may seek sensory stimulation during times of low stress.

Medications and Illness

Certain medications can alter an individual's awareness of environmental stimuli. Opiates, antidepressants, and sedatives, for example, can decrease awareness or alter perception of stimuli.

Anyone taking several medications concurrently may show alterations in sensory function; older adults are especially at risk and need to be monitored carefully. Certain medications (e.g., ASA, furosemide, aminoglycosides, and certain chemotherapeutic agents), if taken for a long time, become adversely toxic to the auditory nerve, impairing hearing and causing tinnitus or balance disturbances.

Certain diseases or trauma affect sensory reception or perception. Direct sensory organ damage can occur as a result of the following:

- Diabetic retinopathy is a complication of diabetes mellitus in which tiny retinal hemorrhages can lead to blindness.
- Glaucoma, characterized by increased intraocular pressure that causes visual changes, eventually leads to permanent damage to the optic nerve.
- Cataracts, an opacity of the lens of the eye, blurs vision.
- Recurrent ear infections may damage the tympanic membrane and contribute to hearing loss.
- Atherosclerosis restricts blood flow to the receptor organs and the brain, decreasing awareness and slowing responses.
- Multiple sclerosis, a central nervous system disease, is characterized by varying degrees of sensory loss and paralysis.

Lifestyle and Personality

Lifestyle influences the quality and quantity of stimulation to which an individual is accustomed. A client who is employed in a large company may be accustomed to many diverse stimuli, whereas a client who is self-employed and works in the home is exposed to fewer, less diverse stimuli. People's personalities also differ in terms of the quantity and quality of stimuli they are comfortable with. Some people delight in constantly changing stimuli and excitement, whereas others prefer a more structured life with few changes.

Assessing

Nursing assessment of sensory-perceptual functioning includes six components: (1) a nursing history, (2) a mental status examination, (3) a physical examination, (4) the identification of clients at risk, (5) an evaluation of the client's environment, and (6) an assessment of the social support network.

Nursing History

The nurse assesses present sensory perceptions, usual functioning, sensory deficits, and potential problems. In some instances, significant others can provide data the client cannot. For example, support people may reveal signs of recent changes in the client's hearing ability, such as inattention to others, recent mood swings, difficulty following clear instructions, frequent requests to have something repeated, and unusually loud radio or television volumes. To assess for risk of sensory loss, the nurse should also inquire about family history (e.g., glaucoma, diabetes), occupational or recreational exposures (e.g., noise level), and self-care practices (e.g., ear wax removal). Examples of interview questions to elicit data about the client's sensory-perceptual functioning are shown in the Assessment: Interview box.

Mental Status Examination

Mental status is critical to any evaluation of the sensory-perceptual process. Usually, data on mental status, including level of consciousness, orientation, memory, and attention span, can be obtained during nursing history (see Chapter 27). It is important to note that sensory alterations can cause changes in cognitive functioning (Wahl & Heyl, 2003).

Physical Examination

Physical assessment determines whether the senses are impaired. During the physical examination, the nurse assesses vision and hearing, olfactory, gustatory, tactile, and kinesthetic senses. The examination should reveal the client's specific vision and hearing abilities; perception of heat, cold, light touch, and pain in the limbs; and awareness of the position of the body parts. Specific sensory tests include the following:

- *Visual acuity* and *visual fields,* by using a Snellen chart or other reading material (e.g., a newspaper)
- *Hearing acuity,* by observing the client's conversation with others and by performing the whisper test, and Weber and Rinne tuning fork tests
- *Olfactory sense,* by having the client identify specific aromas
- *Gustatory sense,* by identifying three tastes, such as lemon, salt, and sugar
- *Tactile sense,* by testing light touch, sharp and dull sensation, two-point discrimination, hot and cold sensation, vibration sense, position sense, and stereognosis

These tests are described in detail in Chapter 27. The nurse should also determine whether sensory adaptive devices that the client uses, such as eyeglasses or hearing aids, function properly.

ASSESSMENT: INTERVIEW

Sensory-Perceptual Functioning

The following questions can be used to find out more information about a client's sensory-perceptual functioning:

VISUAL

- How would you rate your vision (excellent, good, fair, or poor)?
- Do you wear eyeglasses or contact lenses?
- Describe any recent changes in your vision.
- Do you have any difficulty seeing near or far objects?
- Have you ever experienced blurred vision, double vision, spots moving in front of your eyes, blind spots, light sensitivity, flashing lights, halos around objects or difficulty seeing at night?
- When did you last visit an eye doctor?

AUDITORY

- How would you rate your hearing (excellent, good, fair, or poor)?
- Do you wear a hearing aid?
- Describe any recent changes in your hearing.
- Can you locate the direction of sounds and distinguish various voices?
- Do you experience any ringing, buzzing, humming, crackling noises, fullness in the ears, dizziness, or vertigo?

GUSTATORY

- Have you experienced any changes in taste (e.g., difficulty in differentiating sweet, sour, salty, and bitter tastes)?
- Do you enjoy the taste of foods as you did previously?

OLFACTORY

- Have you experienced any changes in your ability to smell?
- Do things (e.g., foods, flowers, and perfumes) smell the same as previously?
- Can you distinguish foods by their odours or tell when something is burning?
- Have you experienced any changes in appetite? (Changes in appetite may be related to an impaired sense of smell.)

TACTILE

- Are you experiencing any pain or discomfort?
- Have you experienced any decrease in your ability to perceive heat, cold, or pain in your limbs?
- Do you have any numbness or tingling in your extremities?

KINESTHETIC

- Have you noticed any difficulty in perceiving the position of parts of your body?

Identification of Clients at Risk for Sensory Deprivation or Overload

Clients at risk for sensory-perceptual alterations need to be identified to ensure that preventive measures can be initiated. Box 36.1 describes clients at risk for sensory alterations.

Client Environment

The nurse assesses the client's environment for quantity, quality, and type of stimuli. The client's environment may produce insufficient stimuli, placing the client at risk for sensory deprivation, or excessive stimuli, placing the client at risk for sensory overload. Nonstimulating environments include those that (1) severely restrict physical activity and (2) limit social contact with family and friends. Because appropriate or meaningful stimuli decrease the incidence of sensory deprivation, the nurse must consider the client's health-care environment for the presence of the following stimuli:

- Television, radio, or other auditory device (e.g., MP3 or CD players)
- Clock or calendar
- Reading material (age and language appropriate)
- Toys or activities for children (age appropriate)
- Number and compatibility of roommates
- Number of visitors in home or care facility

To assess a health-care or home environment that produces excessive stimuli, the nurse considers, where appropriate, bright light, noise, therapeutic measures, frequency of assessments and procedures, the presence of a TV, pets, bright colours, adequacy of lighting, and so on.

CLINICAL ALERT

Are you aware of the noise level around you or the noise level you create while providing nursing care? The standard of 45 decibels (dB) for rest and sleep is often not met. Sounds in critical care units range from 60 dB to 83 dB, contributing to sensory overload.

Social Support Network

The degree of isolation a person feels is significantly influenced by the level of support from family members and friends. The nurse assesses (1) whether the client lives alone, (2) who visits and when, and (3) any signs

BOX 36.1 CLIENTS AT RISK FOR SENSORY DEPRIVATION AND OVERLOAD

Some clients are at risk for sensory deprivation:

- Clients who are confined to a nonstimulating, monotonous environment in the home or health-care agency
- Clients who have impaired vision or hearing
- Clients who have mobility restrictions (e.g., quadriplegia, paraplegia, on bed rest, or in a traction apparatus)
- Clients who are unable to process stimuli (e.g., clients who have brain damage or who are taking medications that affect the central nervous system)
- Clients who have emotional disorders (e.g., depression) and withdraw within themselves
- Clients who have limited social contact with family and friends (e.g., clients from a different culture)

Others are at risk for sensory overload:

- Clients who have pain or discomfort
- Clients who are acutely ill and have been admitted to an acute-care facility
- Clients who are being closely monitored in an intensive care unit (ICU) (see Figure 36.2) and have intrusive tubes (e.g., IVs, catheters, nasogastric or endotracheal tubes)
- Clients who have decreased cognitive ability (e.g., head injury)

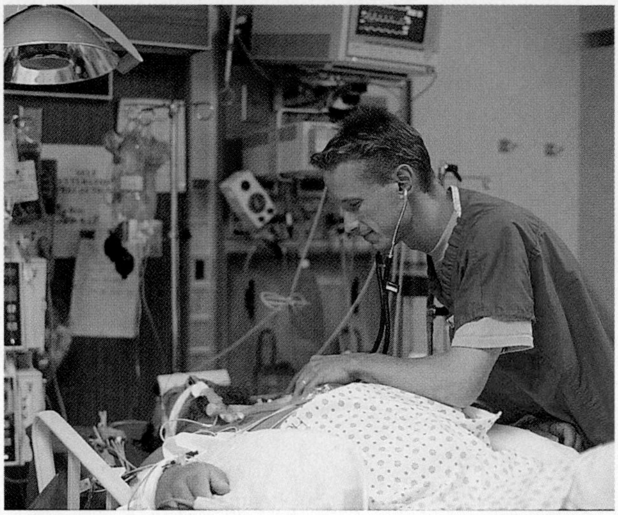

FIGURE 36.2 A patient in an ICU may experience sensory overload.

indicating social deprivation, such as withdrawal from contact with others to avoid embarrassment or dependence on others, negative self-image, reports of lack of meaningful communication with others, and absence of opportunities to discuss fears or concerns.

Diagnosing

NANDA International (2007) includes the following diagnostic labels for sensory perception alterations:

- *Disturbed Sensory Perception (Specify: Visual, Auditory, Kinesthetic, Gustatory, Tactile, Olfactory):* Change in the amount or patterning of incoming stimuli accompanied by an impaired, distorted, diminished, or exaggerated response to such stimuli (NANDA International, 2007, p. 195). This diagnostic label is used to describe clients whose perception has been altered by physiological factors, such as pain, sleep deprivation, immobility, and excessive or decreased meaningful environmental stimuli (Carpenito-Moyet, 2008, p. 415).
- *Acute Confusion:* Abrupt onset of a cluster of reversible disturbances of attention, cognition, consciousness, and perception that develop over a short period of time (NANDA International, 2007, p. 41).
- *Chronic Confusion:* Irreversible, long-standing, or progressive deterioration of intellect and personality characterized by decreased capacity for intellectual thought processes and decreased ability to interpret environmental stimuli, manifested by disturbances of behaviour, orientation, and memory (NANDA International, 2007, p. 42).
- *Impaired Memory:* Inability to remember or recall behaviour skills or bits of information. This may be attributed to pathophysiological or situational causes that are either temporary or permanent (NANDA International, 2007, p. 135).

CLINICAL ALERT

It is easy to confuse the two nursing diagnoses *Disturbed Sensory Perception* and *Disturbed Thought Processes. Disturbed Sensory Perception* refers to sensory input—the person's ability to accurately interpret stimuli. In contrast, when a person's cognitive abilities interfere with the ability to interpret stimuli accurately (because of mental disorders, like dementia), the diagnosis is more likely *Disturbed Thought Processes.* Verify your assessment data to distinguish whether the primary problem is one of sensory input or of cognitive ability.

Sensory-Perceptual Problem as the Etiology

Depending on the data obtained, alterations in sensory-perceptual function can affect other areas of human functioning and indicate other diagnoses. In these instances, the sensory-perceptual problem becomes the etiology.

Examples of nursing diagnoses for which sensory-perceptual alterations are the etiology include the following:

- *Risk for Injury* related to sensory-perceptual alterations (specify). For example,
  a. Visual impairment (e.g., decreased depth perception)
  b. Reduced tactile sensation secondary to neurological or circulatory alterations
  c. Decreased sense of smell
  d. Hearing impairment
  e. Decreased kinesthetic sense
- *Impaired Home Maintenance* related to sensory-perceptual alterations (declining visual abilities)
- *Risk for Impaired Skin Integrity* related to sensory-perceptual alterations (reduced tactile sensation)
- *Impaired Verbal Communication* related to sensory-perceptual alterations (specify). For example,
  a. Altered level of consciousness
  b. Hearing impairment
  c. Sensory overload
  d. Sensory deprivation
- *Self-Care Deficit: Bathing/Hygiene* related to sensory-perceptual alterations (specify). For example,
  a. Visual impairment
  b. Diminished kinesthetic sense
  c. Inability to perceive body parts or spatial relationship
- *Social Isolation* related to sensory-perceptual alterations (specify). For example,
  a. Impaired vision
  b. Impaired hearing

Planning

Planning includes goals associated with the care of clients *independent of setting* and those specific to the home environment. The overall outcome criteria for clients with sensory-perception alterations include the following:

- Prevent injury
- Maintain the function of existing senses
- Develop an effective communication mechanism
- Prevent sensory overload or deprivation
- Reduce social isolation
- Perform activities of daily living independently and safely

Examples of desired outcomes related to these goals are described in Table 36.3 in the "Evaluating" section later in this chapter (page 1074).

Appropriate nursing activities may include the following interventions:

- Cognitive stimulation
- Communication enhancement: hearing deficit
- Communication enhancement: visual deficit
- Nutrition management
- Environmental management
- Fall prevention
- Body mechanics promotion
- Peripheral sensation management
- Emotional support
- Surveillance: safety

Planning for Continuity of Care

The nurse should also consider the client's needs for assistance with care in the home or residential treatment setting. Some clients with severe alterations in sensory-perceptual functioning may be discharged to an assisted-living facility that provides the specific support the client requires. Discharge planning incorporates a reassessment of the client's abilities for self-care, the availability and skills of support people, financial resources, and the need for referrals and home health services. A major aspect of discharge planning involves the instructional needs of the client and family. The Assessment: Home Care box for sensory-perception alterations outlines major needs of the clients and families.

Implementing

Nurses can assist clients with sensory alterations by promoting healthy sensory function, by adjusting environmental stimuli, and by helping clients to manage acute sensory deficits.

ASSESSMENT: HOME CARE

Sensory-Perception Disturbances

Clients with sensory-perception alterations usually have the following needs:

CLIENT AND ENVIRONMENT

- *Self-care abilities:* Ability to care for self while adapting to sensory impairment
- *Safety:* Physical safety of client's environment, including lighting, noise, access, lack of clutter or obstructions, use of stairs, assistive devices with respect to sensory impairment, such as flashing fire alarms or telephones for those with hearing impairments
- *Level of knowledge:* Assistive devices that are available; ways to maximize the use of other senses; local, regional, or national organizations that provide education, training, support, or other assistance (e.g., Canadian National Institute for the Blind, the Canadian Hearing Society)
- *Resources:* Availability of family, friends, community assistance, such as senior centres, transportation, and religious or cultural organizations

Promoting Healthy Sensory Function

The arousal mechanism for sensation is normally present at birth; however, it is undifferentiated. All senses are also present at birth, although some changes in function occur during the growth process. Early screening to detect problems in the visual and hearing functions is essential and key to prevent serious problems. For example, periodic vision screening of all newborns and children is recommended to detect congenital blindness, strabismus, and refractive errors. Children with chronic ear infections and people who live or work in an environment where there is a high noise level should undergo routine auditory testing. Women who are considering pregnancy should be advised of the importance of testing for syphilis and rubella, which may cause hearing impairments in newborns.

Healthy sensory function can be promoted with environmental stimuli that provide appropriate sensory input. This input should vary and be neither excessive nor too limited. As many senses as possible should be stimulated. Various colours, sounds, textures, smells, and body positions can provide various sensations. Nurses can teach parents and family members ways to stimulate infants and children. Social activities often help stimulate the mind and the senses in older adults.

Nurses should also teach clients at risk of sensory loss how to prevent the loss and should discuss preventive health measures, such as getting regular eye examinations and controlling chronic diseases (e.g., diabetes). See the Teaching: Wellness box on preventing sensory impairments.

TEACHING: WELLNESS

Preventing Sensory Impairments

Clients can take some steps to prevent sensory impairments:

- Have regular health examinations.
- Have regular eye examinations to screen for eye problems. For clients age 40 and older, a medical eye examination is generally recommended every 3 to 5 years, or every 1 to 2 years with diabetes or a family history of glaucoma.
- Seek early medical attention (1) if signs suggesting visual impairment arise, for example, failure to react to light or reduced eye contact from an infant; (2) if the child complains of an earache or has an ear infection; and (3) for persistent eye redness, discharge, or increased tearing; growths on or near the eye; pupil asymmetry or other irregularity; or any pain or discomfort.
- Obtain regular childhood immunizations against diseases capable of causing hearing loss (e.g., rubella, mumps, and measles).
- Avoid giving infants and toddlers toys with pointed handles. Keep pointed instruments out of reach and supervise preschoolers when they use scissors.
- Supervise and teach toddlers and preschoolers not to walk or run with a pointed object in their hands.
- Teach children and adolescents the proper use of sports equipment (e.g., hockey sticks).
- Wear protective eye goggles when using power tools, riding motorcycles, or spraying chemicals.
- Wear ear protectors when working in an environment with high noise levels or brief loud impulse noises (e.g., blasting).
- Wear glasses with UV protection to avoid damage from ultraviolet rays; never look directly at the sun.

Ensuring Client Safety

Nurses must implement safety precautions in health-care settings for clients with sensory deficits. Examples of precautions include keeping the bed in the lowest position and placing the call light within reach.

Adjusting Environmental Stimuli

The client functions best when the environment is somewhat similar to that of the individual's ordinary daily life. Sometimes nurses need to take steps to adjust the client's environment to prevent either sensory overload or sensory deprivation.

PREVENTING SENSORY OVERLOAD For clients who are at risk of overstimulation, nurses should reduce the number and type of environmental stimuli. The nurse can counteract sensory overload by blocking stimuli and by helping the client organize the stimuli and alter responses to the stimuli.

Dark glasses can partially block light rays, and a window shade or drape can reduce visual stimulation. Earplugs reduce auditory stimuli, as do soft background music and earphones. The odour from a draining wound can be minimized by keeping the dressing dry and clean and using a room deodorizer.

Another method of blocking stimuli is to reduce novelty and surprise and provide rest intervals free of interruptions. Sometimes, the number of visitors and the length of visits must be restricted. Also, carrying out several nursing measures together allows the client an uninterrupted period of rest before the next activity.

By explaining sounds in the environment, the nurse can help the client organize them mentally (e.g., a buzzer signals the need to change an IV). When clients understand their meaning, stimuli are frequently less confusing and more easily ignored. People can also learn to alter their responses to the stimuli. Clients can employ relaxation techniques to reduce anxiety and stress, despite continual sensory stimulation. See Box 36.2.

PREVENTING SENSORY DEPRIVATION For clients who are at risk for sensory deprivation, nurses can increase environmental stimuli in a number of ways. For example, newspapers, books, and television can stimulate the visual and auditory senses. Providing objects that are pleasant to touch, such as a pet to stroke, can provide tactile and interactive stimulation. Clocks that differentiate night from day by colour can help orient a client to time. The olfactory sense can be stimulated by the presence of fresh flowers or plants.

Arrangements should also be made for people to visit and talk with the client regularly. Many church and community groups provide visitors to shut-ins, that is, people who are confined to their homes or who reside in nursing homes. See Box 36.3 for measures to prevent sensory deprivation.

Managing Acute Sensory Deficits

When assisting clients who have a sensory deficit, the nurse needs to (1) encourage the use of sensory aids to support residual sensory function, (2) promote the use of other senses, (3) communicate effectively, and (4) ensure client safety. See the Reflect on Primary Health Care box.

BOX 36.2 PREVENTING SENSORY OVERLOAD

The following steps can help prevent sensory overload in clients:

- Minimize unnecessary light, noise, and distraction. Provide dark glasses and earplugs, as needed.
- Control pain, as indicated.
- Introduce yourself by name, and address the client by name.
- Provide orienting cues, such as clocks, calendars, equipment, and furniture in the room.
- Limit visitors.
- Plan care to allow for uninterrupted periods of rest, at least 2 hours at a time if possible.
- Schedule a routine of care so the client knows when and what to expect (post a schedule for the client wherever possible).
- Speak in a low tone of voice and in an unhurried manner.
- Provide new information gradually to enable the client to process the meaning. When providing information, ask the client to repeat it so that there are no misunderstandings.
- Describe any tests and procedures to the client beforehand.
- Reduce noxious odours. Empty a commode or bedpan immediately after use; keep wounds clean and covered; use a room deodorizer when indicated; and provide good ventilation.
- Take time to discuss the client's problems and to correct misinterpretations.
- Assist the client with stress-reducing techniques.

BOX 36.3 PREVENTING SENSORY DEPRIVATION

The following steps can help prevent sensory deprivation in clients:

- Encourage the client to use eyeglasses and hearing aids.
- Address the client by name and touch the client while speaking, if this is not culturally offensive.
- Communicate frequently with the client, and maintain meaningful interactions (e.g., discuss current events).
- Provide a telephone, radio or TV, clock, and calendar.
- Provide murals, pictures, sculptures, and wall hangings. Many libraries and museums will lend artwork free of charge, or a local school may provide art projects developed by the students.
- Have family and friends bring freshly cut flowers and plants.
- Consider having a resident pet (e.g., a fish, a cat, or a bird), or make arrangements for pets to visit on a regular basis.
- Include different textured objects to feel (e.g., a sheepskin pillow, a silk scarf, or a soft blanket).
- Increase tactile stimulation through physical care measures (e.g., back massages, hair care, or foot soaks).
- Encourage social interaction through activity groups or visits by family and friends.
- Encourage the use of crossword puzzles or games to stimulate mental function.
- Encourage environment changes, such as a walk through a mall or, for an immobilized client, sitting near a window or at a place on the nursing unit where the client can watch local traffic.
- Encourage the use of self-stimulation techniques, such as singing, humming, whistling, or reciting.

ENCOURAGING THE USE OF SENSORY AIDS Many sensory aids are available for clients who have visual and hearing deficits. See examples in Box 36.4. Whether in the health-care or home setting, the assistance of support people needs to be enlisted, whenever possible, to help the client deal with the deficit.

PROMOTING THE USE OF OTHER SENSES When one sense is lost, the nurse can teach the client to use other senses to compensate the loss. This stimulation is similar to that provided to prevent sensory deprivation discussed earlier. However, the type of stimulation needs to be adapted to the client's specific deficit. For example, for the visually impaired client, stimulation of hearing, taste,

REFLECT ON PRIMARY HEALTH CARE

When working with patients who have sensory alterations, the principles of accessibility and appropriate technology can be used. Significant advances in technology have been made to assist persons with sensory deficits and their families. Ensuring acceptance and accessibility of the technological advances is an important nursing contribution to health promotion, another principle of primary health care.

BOX 36.4 SENSORY AIDS FOR VISUAL AND HEARING DEFICITS

Sensory aids can help clients with vision and hearing deficits:

VISION

- Eyeglasses of the correct prescription that are clean and in good repair
- Adequate room lighting, including night-lights
- Sunglasses or shades on windows to reduce glare
- Bright contrasting colours in the environment
- A magnifying glass
- A phone dialler with large numbers
- A clock and wristwatch with large numbers
- Colour code or texture code on stoves, washer, medicine containers, and so on
- Coloured or raised rims on dishes
- Reading material with large print
- A wristwatch that allows touch to determine time or gives audible time
- Braille or recorded books
- A seeing-eye dog

HEARING

- Hearing aid and battery in good order
- Lip reading
- Sign language
- Amplified telephones
- Teletypewriter communication device for the deaf (TTY)
- Amplified telephone ringers and doorbells
- Flashing alarm clocks
- Flashing smoke detectors
- Pen and paper available

smell, and touch can be encouraged. A radio, audiotapes of music or books, clocks that chime, music boxes, and wind chimes can be used for auditory stimulation. Diets that include a variety of flavours, temperatures, and textures can be planned to stimulate the taste buds. Taking sips of water between foods and eating foods separately can emphasize the taste sensation. Fresh flowers, room fragrances, brewing coffee, and baking can stimulate the sense of smell. Measures, such as providing a hug, massage, hair brushing, grooming, different textures in clothing and upholstery fabrics, and pets, can be used to stimulate touch receptors.

COMMUNICATING EFFECTIVELY Communication with clients who have sensory deficits should convey respect, enhance the person's self-esteem, and ensure the exchange of correct information. A person with a hearing impairment has to concentrate more than other people and, therefore, tires more readily. Fatigue compounded by an illness can further reduce the person's ability to hear. A person with a visual impairment is unable to observe most nonverbal cues during communication and relies largely on the spoken word and tone of voice. Guidelines for communicating with people who are visually or hearing impaired are shown in Box 36.5.

ENSURING CLIENT SAFETY Nurses should implement safety precautions in health-care settings for clients with sensory deficits and teach them special precautions to ensure their safety at home.

IMPAIRED VISION For clients with vision impairments who are in a health-care setting, nurses should do the following:

- Orient the client to the arrangement of room furnishings and maintain an uncluttered environment.
- Keep pathways clear.

BOX 36.5 COMMUNICATING WITH CLIENTS WHO HAVE A VISION OR HEARING DEFICIT

Some accommodations must be made for clients who have vision or hearing deficits:

VISION DEFICIT

- Always announce your presence and identify yourself by name.
- Stay in the client's field of vision.
- Speak in a warm and pleasant tone of voice; avoid speaking louder than necessary.
- Always explain what you are about to do before touching the person.
- Explain the sounds in the environment.
- Indicate when the conversation has ended and when you are leaving the room.

HEARING DEFICIT

- Before initiating conversation, move to a position where the person can see you.
- Decrease background noises (e.g., radio) before speaking.
- Talk at a moderate rate and in a normal tone of voice.
- Address the person directly. Do not turn away in the middle of the conversation. Make sure the person can see your face easily and that it is in good light.
- Avoid covering up your mouth or talking when you have something in your mouth, such as chewing gum.
- Keep your voice at the same volume throughout each sentence, without dropping your voice at the end of each sentence.
- Always speak as clearly and accurately as possible. Articulate consonants with particular care. Use other words when the client has difficulty hearing phrases.
- Do not overarticulate: mouthing or overdoing articulation is just as troublesome as mumbling. Pantomime, write ideas, or use sign language, if necessary.
- Use simple words and short sentences.
- Pronounce every name with care. Make a reference to the name for easier understanding, for example, "Joan, the girl from the office" or "Sears, the big downtown store."
- Change to a new subject at a slower rate, making sure that the person follows the change to the new subject. A key word or two at the beginning of a new topic is a good indicator.

- Do not rearrange furniture without orienting the client. Ensure that housekeeping personnel are informed about this.
- Organize self-care articles within the client's reach, and orient the client to their location.
- Keep the call light within easy reach, and place the bed in the low position.
- Assist with ambulation by standing to the client's side, walking about 30 cm ahead, and allowing the person to grasp your arm. Confirm whether the client prefers grasping your arm with their dominant or nondominant hand.

Research has established an association between vision impairment and greater disability in activities of daily living (e.g., bathing, dressing, eating) and instrumental tasks (e.g., shopping, housekeeping) (Horowitz, 2004). Visual impairment can challenge a client's adherence to a medication regimen. It creates difficulty in reading labels and can lead to taking the incorrect amount of a medication or the incorrect medication. Studies have also shown that visual impairment increases the risk of depression among older adults living in the community (Horowitz, 2003, 2004). Explanations for this relationship vary. One explanation is that vision loss leads to increased disability, which leads to depression. Another explanation states that loss of vision causes fear—a fear of losing autonomy and becoming dependent on others. Vision loss also affects how a person obtains information (e.g., reading the newspaper). In addition, reading is often a leisure activity and its loss can affect a person's quality of life. It is important for the nurse to be aware of and assess for signs of depression. Intervene as appropriate if an older adult is experiencing depression as a result of vision impairment.

Impaired Hearing Clients with hearing impairments who are unable to hear the alarms of IV pumps and cardiac monitors need to be assessed frequently. They can be taught to use their visual sense to identify kinks in the IV tubing or a loose ECG lead. For home safety, clients with impaired hearing need to obtain devices that either amplify sounds or respond with flashing lights to such sounds as a doorbell or smoke detectors, a baby crying, or a burglar alarm. The sounds of doorbells and alarm clocks may be amplified or changed to a lower frequency or buzzer-like sound. These devices can be obtained from hearing aid dealers, telephone companies, and appliance stores.

An important consequence of a decline in hearing as a person ages is the person having difficulty understanding speech. Factors that influence this difficulty are the environment, rate of speech, and presence of an accent. Environments that are noisy and reverberant (echoing, hollow sounds) cause difficulty for older adult listeners. Older adults with a hearing loss have difficulty understanding fast speech. Research indicates that the older adult's ability to process fast verbal information is slower and that rapid speech allows for less time for the older adult to recognize the acoustic or auditory cues of the speech (Gordon-Salant, 2005). A person who speaks with an accent may vary their pronunciation of syllables or words, making it challenging for the older adult.

Impaired Olfactory Sense Clients with an impaired sense of smell need to be taught about the dangers of cleaning with chemicals, such as ammonia. Because a gas leak can go undetected, clients need to keep gas stoves and furnaces in good working order. Strong chemicals, such as ammonia, used in confined spaces, such as a bathroom, can affect the client before the client smells them. Food poisoning is a concern with clients who have difficulty detecting spoiled meat or dairy products. These clients need to carefully inspect food for freshness and check expiration dates on food packages. Installing a smoke detector near the stove is particularly important, as is taking care to not leave the stove unattended.

Impaired Tactile Sense Clients with an impaired sense of touch may not be aware of hot temperatures, which can cause burns, or pressure on bony prominences, which can produce pressure ulcers. Clients with decreased sensation to temperature should have the temperature adjusted on their hot water heater and test water temperature with a thermometer before bathing. Clients with decreased sensation to pressure must change their position frequently. Avoid use of heating pads and hot water bottles as burns may result (see Chapter 30, the section on older adults, under "Promoting Safety across the Lifespan").

Helping the Confused Client

Confusion can occur in clients of all ages, but it is more commonly seen in older people. The terms *acute confusion* and *delirium* are used interchangeably by most health professionals, with nurses tending to favour the use of *acute confusion* and physicians using the term *delirium* (McCurren & Cronin, 2003). Delirium occurs in 6% to 30% of the general hospital population and 7% to 52% of postsurgical clients (Edwards, 2003). Delirium in the intensive care unit (ICU) is a common problem and has been described as sundown syndrome, ICU psychosis, and ICU syndrome. Delirium is unrecognized or misdiagnosed by both the physician and the nurse in up to two-thirds of cases (Hanley, 2004, p. 218).

Older adults are at risk for delirium when hospitalized for numerous reasons. They often have other chronic medical problems (e.g., dementia, chronic obstructive pulmonary disease, hypertension, or stroke), and they are taking numerous medications, like anticholinergics, opiates, and sedatives, which may increase the risk for delirium. Many older adults have vision or hearing loss; the unfamiliarity of a hospital, possible sleep deprivation, stress, and sensory overload increase their risk for developing delirium.

Confusion often presents with subtle symptoms, but an attempt should be made to differentiate between *acute confusion (delirium)* and *chronic confusion (dementia)*. **Acute confusion** has an abrupt onset and a cause that, when treated, reverses the confusion. **Dementia** is often called chronic confusion with symptoms that are gradual and irreversible (e.g., Alzheimer's disease). It is often difficult to differentiate between the two conditions (see Table 36.2), but it is important to treat the causes, if possible, in order to reverse the condition. Clients who are confused often know something is wrong and want help. Box 36.6 lists nursing interventions to help promote a therapeutic environment for the client with acute confusion or delirium.

Helping the Unconscious Client

The number of people surviving with traumatic brain injury is increasing, and most experience some form of coma with significant deficits. According to Gerber (2005), **coma** is a deep state of unconsciousness that lasts for more than 2 to 4 weeks following a traumatic brain injury. Previously, the patient would be medically stabilized and approximately 6 months later transferred to a rehabilitation setting for coma stimulation. It is thought that unconscious patients suffered from sensory deprivation because they are in a cold, sterile environment, immobilized, and without the usual stimulation humans need. The current trend is to begin a coma stimulation program earlier, while the patient is in the acute-care setting.

Evidence-Informed Practice

Which Stroke Impairments Predict Discharge Function, Length of Stay, and Discharge Destination in Stroke Rehabilitation?

Wee and Hopman (2005) evaluated 313 stroke rehabilitation patients to examine the impact that various stroke impairments had on predicting discharge function, rehabilitation length of stay, and discharge destination after inpatient rehabilitation. The relationship between the number of stroke risk factors present and the recurrence of strokes during the rehabilitation period was also evaluated. The 313 subjects were consecutively enrolled. Information regarding the type of stroke and the individual's stroke-related impairments (e.g., balance, aphasia, body neglect) was collected. Other information regarding any recurrent strokes, the length of the inpatient rehabilitation stay, the discharge destination, the subject's function at discharge, and the availability of family support at discharge was also collected. Admission function, balance, the number of stroke-related impairments, and family support were found to be important factors in predicting a client's length of inpatient rehabilitation stay. The presence of body neglect, balance, and family support were predictive factors for determining the client's discharge destination.

NURSING IMPLICATIONS: When planning inpatient discharge for clients who have experienced a stroke, family support, along with individual stroke-related impairments, is an important consideration.

Source: "Stroke Impairment Predictors of Discharge Function, Length of Stay, and Discharge Destination in Stroke Rehabilitation," by J. Y. M. Wee and W. M. Hopman, 2005, *American Journal of Physical Medicine & Rehabilitation, 84*(4), pp. 604–612.

BOX 36.6 PROMOTING A THERAPEUTIC ENVIRONMENT FOR PERSONS WITH ACUTE CONFUSION

The following nursing interventions can help a client who has acute confusion or delirium:

- Wear a readable nametag.
- Address the client by name and introduce yourself frequently.
- Identify time and date: "Today is December 5, and it is 8 o'clock in the morning."
- Orient the client to place (e.g., home, hospital, nursing home), if indicated.
- Place a calendar and clock in the client's room. Provide a means of marking the current date or holidays.
- Speak clearly and calmly to the client, allowing time for your words to be processed and for the client to respond.
- Provide frequent face-to-face contact.
- Keep glasses and hearing aids within reach.
- Provide clear, concise explanations of each treatment procedure or task.
- Ensure adequate pain management.
- Reinforce reality by interpreting unfamiliar sounds, sights, and smells; correct any misconceptions of events or situations.
- Schedule activities (e.g., meals, bath, activity, treatments, and rest periods) at the same time each day to provide a sense of security. If possible, assign the same caregivers.
- Provide adequate rest.
- Keep familiar items in the client's environment (e.g., photographs), and keep the environment uncluttered. A disorganized, cluttered environment increases confusion.
- Encourage the client to wear familiar or personal clothing and to arrange personal hygiene articles in order of use.
- Encourage participation in familiar activities or hobbies to emphasize the client's strengths.
- Tell the client when you are leaving and when you will return.

TABLE 36.2 Differentiating between Delirium and Dementia

Characteristic	Delirium or Acute Confusion	Dementia
Distinguishing feature	Acute or abruptly fluctuating change in mental status.	Progressive memory impairment, irreversible.
Onset	Sudden, acute onset.	Slow, insidious.
Duration	Temporary. May last hours to less than 1 month.	Chronic, gradual, months to years.
Time of day	Worsens at twilight or at night.	Possible changes with time of day.
Sleep–wake cycles	Disturbed. Cycles often reversed.	Disturbed. Fragmented. Awakens often during the night.
Alertness	Fluctuates. May be alert and oriented during the day but become confused and disoriented at night.	Generally normal.
Thinking	Disorganized, distorted. Slow or accelerated. Incoherent.	Judgment impaired. Difficulty with abstraction and word finding.
Memory	Alterations in recent and immediate memory.	Alterations in recent and long-term memory.
Perecption	May have visual, auditory, and tactile hallucinations. Misinterpretation of real sensory experiences.	Delusions. Usually no hallucinations.
Causative and risk factors	Cerebral and cardiovascular disease, infections, reduced hearing and vision, environmental change, stress, sleep deprivation, polypharmacy, dehydration.	Alzheimer's disease. Multiple infarct dementia.

Sources: Adapted from *Screening for Delirium and Depression in Older Adults* (p. 26), by the Registered Nurses' Association of Ontario, 2003, Toronto: Author; and *Fundamentals of Nursing: Concepts, Process, and Practice,* 8th ed. (p. 994), by A. Berman, S. J. Snyder, B. Kozier, and G. Erb, 2008, Upper Saddle River, NJ: Pearson-Prentice Hall.

Coma stimulation consists of providing sensory stimulation to promote brain recovery by waking up the RAS. Box 36.7 provides examples of sensory stimulation that a nurse or family member can provide for the unconscious patient. It is important that the stimulation be delivered in a quiet environment (to prevent sensory overload) and done slowly to allow time for a response to occur. Sensory stimulation sessions are of a certain time duration (e.g., 30 to 45 minutes), and the number of sessions will vary in a 12-hour day. As well, the patient needs sleep and rest periods that alternate with the structured sensory stimulation sessions.

BOX 36.7 PROMOTING SENSORY STIMULATION FOR THE UNCONSCIOUS PATIENT

Unconscious patients can benefit from the following types of sensory stimulation:

AUDITORY

- Introduce yourself to the patient.
- Orient the patient to time, month, year, location, and what happened.
- Inform the patient beforehand about the care to be provided.
- Read literature aloud to the patient.
- Play a tape recording of a familiar voice.
- Talk directly to the patient.

VISUAL

- Safely support the patient in an upright position in bed (provides normal visual orientation).

OLFACTORY

- Provide aromatic stimuli that can include the patient's favourites (e.g., coffee, lemon, cologne or perfume).

GUSTATORY

- Provide mouth care by using a mint-flavoured cleaning agent.
- Place different tastes on tongue.

TACTILE

- Incorporate tactile stimulation during bath activities (e.g., temperature and texture of washcloth, back massage, brushing hair, rubbing lotion on extremities).

KINESTHETIC

- Perform range-of-motion exercises.
- Change the patient's position.

Source: From "Understanding and Managing Coma Stimulation: Are We Doing Everything We Can?" by C. Gerber, 2005, *Critical Care Nursing Quarterly, 28*(2), pp. 94–108. Adapted with permission.

Evaluating

By using the measurable desired outcomes developed during the planning stage, the nurse collects data needed to judge whether client goals and outcomes have been achieved. Examples of client goals and related outcomes are shown in Table 36.3. If outcomes are not achieved, the nurse and client, and support people, if appropriate, need to explore the reasons why before modifying the care plan. See the Sample Care Plan and the Concept Map for nursing management of clients with sensory perceptual impairments.

TABLE 36.3 Evaluation Goals and Outcomes: Sensory-Perceptual Alterations

Goal	Examples of Desired Outcomes
Maintain or promote sensory functioning	Uses protective devices (e.g., protective eyewear and ear protectors) appropriately Identifies hazards to sensory organs
or	Demonstrates effective use of assistive devices (specify)
Prevent sensory deprivation or overload	Experiences a 3- to 4-hour uninterrupted sleep period in 24 hours (sensory overload) Orients to time, place, and person Reports increased energy and reduced feelings of anxiety (sensory overload) Reports decreased boredom and depression (sensory deprivation) Demonstrates increased attention span (sensory deprivation)
Maintain or improve communication	Demonstrates appropriate emotional responses Uses assistive devices for communication (e.g., hearing aid, writing implements, large print) Expresses thoughts and feelings about sensory deficits or unusual sensory experiences
Prevent injury	Identifies factors that increase risk for injury Makes appropriate use of sensory aids Alters home environment and practices to prevent injury
Reduce social isolation	Identifies factors or behaviours that produce social isolation Formulates a plan to become more involved with others Identifies community resources that will assist in decreasing social isolation

Sample Care Plan for Sensory-Perceptual Alteration

ASSESSMENT DATA

Nursing Assessment

Sophia Demetrios is an 82-year-old widow who has recently become a resident of an extended-care facility. Just before her admission, she underwent hip replacement surgery and also experienced more difficulty with hearing. Her children were concerned about her physical safety and lack of socialization and urged her to enter a nursing home. Mrs. Demetrios had cared for herself independently for 15 years in her own home. Three days after admission, the nurse finds the client confused and disoriented to person, place, and time. She appears restless, withdrawn, and her syntax is sometimes inappropriate. She states, "I'm afraid of all of these strange creatures in this orphanage."

Physical Examination

Height: 160 cm
Weight: 55.3 kg
Temperature: 37°C
Pulse: 72 bpm
Respirations: 18/min
Blood Pressure: 128/74 mm Hg
Rinne Test: negative

Diagnostic Data

Chest X-ray, CBC, and urinalysis all within normal ranges

Nursing Diagnosis

Sensory-Perceptual Alterations (sensory overload) related to change in environment, hearing loss (as evidenced by disorientation to time, place, person; restlessness; and altered behaviour)

Client Goals

The client will demonstrate (1) decreased symptoms and increased level of orientation to reality; and (2) improved ability to communicate.

Desired Health Outcomes

1. Is oriented to place, month, and year when questioned by day 3
2. Identifies one or two caregivers by name by day 4
3. Communicates needs effectively with care provider by day 5

(continued)

Sample Care Plan for Sensory-Perceptual Alteration *(continued)*

NURSING INTERVENTIONS AND SELECTED ACTIVITIES WITH RATIONALES [*IN ITALICS*]*

Reality Orientation

Intervention	Rationale
• Provide a consistent physical environment and a daily routine.	*Routine eliminates the element of surprise, overstimulation, and further confusion.*
• Provide caregivers who are familiar to Mrs. Demetrios.	*Familiarity with caregivers helps reduce confusion and facilitates the establishment of rapport.*
• Provide a low-stimulation environment for Mrs. Demetrios because disorientation may be increased by overstimulation.	*A disruption in the quality or quantity of incoming stimuli can affect a person's cognitive status. Sensory overload blocks out meaningful stimuli.*
• Provide for adequate rest, sleep, and daytime naps.	*Rest reduces overstimulation and fatigue, which may be contributing factors to confusion.*
• Use a calm approach when interacting with Mrs. Demetrios.	*This method promotes communication that enhances the person's sense of dignity.*
• Speak to the client in a slow, distinct manner with appropriate volume.	*The client who has difficulty hearing will be better able to lip-read and comprehend speech.*
• Engage Mrs. Demetrios in concrete and reality-oriented activities, like ADLs, that focus on something outside the self.	*These activities assist the individual to differentiate between own thoughts and reality.*

Communication Enhancement: Hearing Deficit

Intervention	Rationale
• Facilitate the use of hearing aids.	*Hearing can be enhanced if the volume is appropriate and the hearing aid is consistently used.*
• Listen attentively.	*Effective listening is essential in a nurse–client relationship. Poor listening skills can undermine trust and block therapeutic communication.*
• Use simple words and short sentences.	*The use of simple terms and short sentences facilitates understanding and minimizes anxiety.*
• Obtain Mrs. Demetrios's attention through touch.	*Gaining the attention of a client with a hearing impairment is an essential first step toward effective communication. However, the client's personal space should be respected and permission to touch should be obtained.*

EVALUATION

Goal met. Mrs. Demetrios identifies her primary nurse by sight and name on the third day. She is aware that Christmas is 3 weeks away and is anxious to go shopping with the group. She bathes herself each morning and makes her own bed. Her daughter has brought new batteries for her hearing aid, which she wears during the day.

*Interventions and activities selected are only a sample of those suggested in the *Nursing Interventions Classification (NIC)*, by G. M. Bulechek, H. K. Butcher, and J. C. Dochterman (Eds.), 2008, St. Louis, MO: Mosby Elsevier, and should be individualized for each client.

CONCEPT MAP

Sensory-Perceptual Disturbances

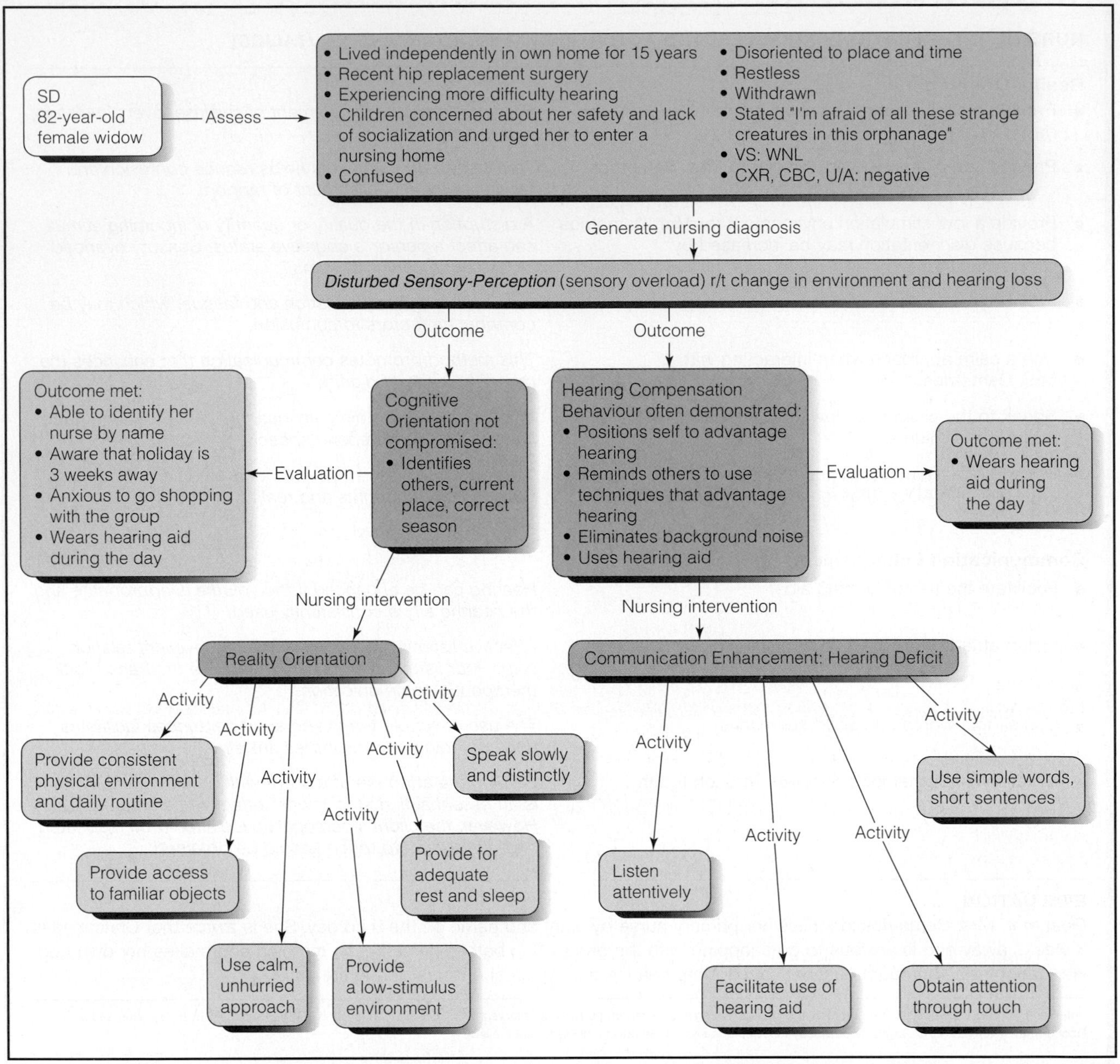

Case Study 36

Mrs. Donais is a 61-year-old client who is being cared for in the critical care unit following an automobile accident in which she suffered extensive traumatic injuries. Mrs. Donais is connected to several monitoring devices, has an intubation tube and ventilator to assist her with respirations, and is receiving various medications, including analgesics for pain.

Critical Thinking Questions

1. Identify factors that place Mrs. Donais at risk for the development of sensory deprivation or overload.
2. What assessment findings would suggest that Mrs. Donais is experiencing sensory overload as opposed to sensory deprivation?
3. How can you intervene to reduce Mrs. Donais's risk for disturbed sensory perception during this stressful event?
4. How might the care of a client in the home setting differ from the care of a client, such as Mrs. Donais, who is receiving care in a critical care unit?

After working through these questions, go to the MyNursingLab at **http://www.mynursinglab.com** to check your answers.

KEY TERMS

sensory reception
external stimuli
internal stimuli
kinesthetic
stereognosis
visceral
sensory perception
stimulus
receptor
impulse conduction
perception
reticular activating system (RAS)
sensoristasis
awareness
sensory deprivation
sensory overload
sensory deficit
cultural deprivation
cultural care deprivation
acute confusion
dementia
coma

CHAPTER HIGHLIGHTS

- The sensory experience consists of two components: sensory reception and sensory perception.
- Sensory stimuli can be either external or internal. Visual, auditory, olfactory, tactile, and gustatory stimuli orient a person to the *external* environment. Kinesthetic and visceral stimuli orient the person to the *internal* environment. Kinesthetic stimuli make the person aware of the position and movement of body parts.
- Sensory perception involves the awareness and interpretation of stimuli into meaningful information. This process occurs in the cerebral cortex.
- The reticular activating system (RAS), with its many ascending and descending connections to other areas of the brain, monitors and regulates incoming stimuli. The RAS maintains, enhances, or inhibits cortical arousal.
- The normal, alert person can assimilate many kinds of information at one time and respond appropriately through thought and action.
- Sensory deprivation occurs when a person receives decreased sensory input or monotonous or meaningless sensory input.
- Sensory overload occurs when a person experiences excessive sensory input and is unable to process or manage the stimuli. The person feels overwhelmed and not in control.
- Responses to both sensory deprivation and sensory overload include perceptual changes (e.g., mild distortions or hallucinations), cognitive changes (e.g., decreased concentration and problem-solving ability), and affective changes (e.g., apathy, anxiety, anger, depression, and rapid mood swings).
- Clients at risk for sensory deprivation include (1) those who are homebound or institutionalized, (2) those on bed rest or isolation precautions, (3) those with sensory deficits, (4) those who come from a different culture, (5) those with certain affective disorders or disturbances of the nervous system, and (6) those on certain medications that affect the central nervous system.
- Clients at risk for sensory overload include (1) those in pain, (2) those in intensive care units, (3) those with intrusive and uncomfortable monitoring or treatment equipment, and (4) those with disturbances of the nervous system.
- Factors affecting sensory stimulation include developmental stage, culture, level of stress, medications and illness, and lifestyle and personality.
- Assessment for sensory-perceptual alterations includes (1) a nursing history to identify sensory deficits, (2) a physical examination, (3) a mental status examination, (4) the identification of clients at risk, (5) an evaluation of immediate environment, and (6) an assessment of the social support network.
- NANDA International (2007) nursing diagnoses related to a client's sensory-perceptual impairments are *Sensory/Perceptual Disturbances: Visual, Auditory, Gustatory, Olfactory, Tactile, Kinesthetic; Acute Confusion; Risk for Acute Confusion; Chronic Confusion; Impaired Memory; Social Isolation; Impaired Verbal Communication; Risk for Impaired Skin Integrity; Self-Care Deficit: Bathing/Hygiene, Dressing/Grooming, Feeding and Toileting; Impaired Home Maintenance;* and *Risk for Injury.*
- Goals for persons with sensory-perceptual alterations include (1) maintaining or promoting the function of existing senses, (2) maintaining or improving communication, (3) preventing injury, (4) avoiding sensory deprivation or overload, (5) reducing social isolation, (6) maintaining or restoring ability to function safely in the environment and to perform self-care, and (7) reducing risk of damage to sensory organs.
- Interventions to prevent or modify sensory deprivation, sensory overload, and sensory deficits include promoting healthy sensory function, adjusting environmental stimuli, and managing sensory deficits.
- Clients with sensory deficits need instruction about sensory aids available to support residual sensory function, ways to promote the use of other senses, and methods to ensure safety from bodily harm.
- Nurses and support persons need to devise and implement effective communication mechanisms for clients who have visual and hearing impairments.
- Confused clients and unconscious clients need care that is directed to promoting their orientation to time, place, person, and situation.

ASSESS YOUR LEARNING

1. Mr. Jackson, 69 years old, had a recent right cerebrovascular accident with sensory-perceptual deficits. Which of the following nursing interventions is an appropriate strategy to address Mr. Jackman's deficits?
   - **a.** Identify Mr. Jackman's previous strengths.
   - **b.** Refer Mr. Jackman to a speech pathologist.
   - **c.** Approach Mr. Jackman from the unaffected side.
   - **d.** Minimize auditory sensory stimulation.

2. Which client is at greatest risk for experiencing sensory overload?
   - **a.** A 40-year-old client in isolation with no family
   - **b.** A 28-year-old quadriplegic client in a private room
   - **c.** A 16-year-old listening to loud music
   - **d.** An 80-year-old client admitted for emergency surgery

3. An alert 80-year-old client is transferred to a long-term-care facility. On the second night, he becomes confused and agitated. What is the most appropriate nursing diagnosis?
   - **a.** *Chronic Confusion*
   - **b.** *Impaired Memory*
   - **c.** *Disturbed Sensory Perception*
   - **d.** *Disturbed Thought Processes*

4. The nursing diagnosis *Risk for Impaired Skin Integrity* related to sensory-perception disturbance would best fit which of the following clients?
   - **a.** One who cut his foot by stepping on broken glass
   - **b.** One who uses a wheelchair because of paraplegia
   - **c.** One who wears glasses because of poor vision
   - **d.** One who is legally blind and smokes in bed

5. Which of the following statements indicates that the client needs a sensory aid in the home?
   - **a.** "I tripped over that rug again."
   - **b.** "I can't hear the doorbell."
   - **c.** "My eyesight is good if I wear my glasses."
   - **d.** "I can hear the TV if I turn it up high."

6. A hospitalized client is disoriented and believes she is in a train station. Which of the following is the most appropriate response by the nurse?
   - **a.** "You wouldn't be getting a bath at the train station."
   - **b.** "Let's finish your bath before the train arrives."
   - **c.** "Don't you know where you are?"
   - **d.** "It may seem like a train station sometimes, but this is Valley Hospital."

7. A client with impaired vision is admitted to the hospital. Which intervention is most appropriate to meet the client's needs?
   - **a.** Identify yourself by name.
   - **b.** Increase background noise.
   - **c.** Explain the sounds in the environment.
   - **d.** Keep your voice at the same level throughout the conversation.

8. A client is exhibiting signs and symptoms of acute confusion or delirium. The nurse implements which of the following strategies to promote a therapeutic environment?
   - **a.** Keep the lights in the room dimmed to reduce stimulation.
   - **b.** Keep the environmental noise level high to increase stimulation.
   - **c.** Keep the room organized and clean.
   - **d.** Use restraints for client safety.

9. Which of the following clinical signs are most likely to be present in a client at risk for sensory deprivation?
   - **a.** Sleeplessness
   - **b.** Increased muscle tension
   - **c.** Irritability
   - **d.** Crying

10. An 85-year-old client has impaired hearing. When creating his care plan, which of the following should have the highest priority?
    - **a.** Obtaining an amplified telephone
    - **b.** Teaching the importance of changing his position
    - **c.** Providing reading material with large print
    - **d.** Checking expiration dates on food packages

After working through these questions, go to the MyNursingLab at ***http://www.mynursinglab.com*** *to check your answers and see explanations.*

SUGGESTED READINGS

Reed, P., & Tilly, J. (2008). Dementia care practice recommendations for nursing homes and assisted living, Phase 2: Falls, wandering, and physical restraints. *Alzheimer's Care Today, 9*(1), 51–59.

This article presents evidence-based recommendations for the provision and improvement of person-centred care in assisted-living residences and nursing homes in the areas of resident wandering, resident falls, and physical-restraint-free care.

Wallhagen, M., Pettengill, E., & Whiteside, M. (2006). Sensory impairment in older adults: Part 1: Hearing loss. *American Journal of Nursing, 106*(10), 40–48.

This article describes hearing impairment as a debilitating problem for many older adults. It presents assessment and intervention strategies for nurses to assist their aging clients to maintain optimal communication functioning.

WEBLINKS

Canadian National Institute for the Blind

http://www.cnib.ca

This site provides information related to vision impairments.

Canadian Association of the Deaf

http://www.cad.ca

This site provides information related to the deaf and hearing impaired in Canada.

Canadian Hard of Hearing Association

http://www.chha.ca

A nonprofit association that is operated by those with hearing deficits; its role is to promote the interests of its members and to inform.

The Canadian Hearing Society

http://www.chs.ca

The society provides services that augment the independence of deaf, deafened, and hard of hearing people and that encourage prevention of hearing loss.

Alzheimer Society of Canada

http://www.alzheimer.ca

The Alzheimer Society of Canada identifies, develops, and facilitates national priorities that enable its members to effectively alleviate the personal and social consequences of Alzheimer's disease and related disorders. It also promotes research and leads the search for a cure.

REFERENCES

Canadian Association of the Deaf. (2007). Statistics on deaf Canadians. Retrieved November 2, 2008, from http://www.cad.ca/en/issues/statistics_on_deaf_canadians.asp

Carpenito-Moyet, L. J. (2008). *Nursing diagnosis: Application to clinical practice* (12th ed.). Philadelphia, PA: Lippincott Williams & Wilkins.

Edwards, N. (2003). Differentiating the three D's: Delirium, dementia, and depression. *Medsurg Nursing, 12*(6), 347–357.

Gerber, C. (2005). Understanding and managing coma stimulation: Are we doing everything we can? *Critical Care Nursing Quarterly, 28*(2), 94–108.

Gibson, J., & Gibson, C. (2004). Researching the impact. *Listen/Écoute, 13*(3), 8.

Gordon-Salant, S. (2005). Hearing loss and aging: New research findings and clinical implications. *Journal of Rehabilitation Research & Development, 42*(4), 9–24.

Hanley, C. (2004). Delirium in the acute care setting. *Medsurg Nursing, 13*(4), 217–225.

Horowitz, A. (2003). Depression and vision and hearing impairment in later life. *Generations, 27*(1), 32–38.

Horowitz, A. (2004). The prevalence and consequences of vision impairment in later life. *Topics in Geriatric Rehabilitation, 20*(3), 185–195.

McCurren, C., & Cronin, S. N. (2003). Delirium: Elders tell their stories and guide nursing practice. *Medsurg Nursing, 12*(5), 318–323.

NANDA International. (2007). *Nursing diagnoses: Definitions and classification, 2007–2008.* Philadelphia, PA: Author.

Wahl, H., & Heyl, V. (2003). Connection between vision, hearing, and cognitive function, *Generations, 27*(1), 39–47.

Chapter 37

Rest and Sleep

Rest and sleep are essential for health. People who are ill or injured frequently require more rest and sleep than normal. Debilitated individuals expend considerable energy to regain health or maintain activities of daily living, leading to increased and frequent fatigue and a greater need for more rest and sleep than usual. Providing patients with an environment that supports both rest and sleep is an important nursing function.

The meaning of rest and the need for rest vary among individuals. **Rest** implies calmness, relaxation without emotional stress, refreshment, and a recovery of strength. Rest does not always mean complete inactivity; some people find certain behaviours, such as walking outdoors, restful. When rest is prescribed for a client, both nurse and client must know whether the client is to be inactive and whether that inactivity involves the whole body or a body part (e.g., an arm). Balanced rest and activity contribute to improved concentration and a sense of physical and mental well-being.

Sleep is a basic human need. Historically, sleep was viewed as a state of unconsciousness. More recently, **sleep** has come to be considered an altered state of consciousness in which the individual's perception of and reaction to the environment are decreased. Sleep is characterized by minimal physical activity, variable levels of consciousness, changes in the body's physiological processes, and decreased responsiveness to external stimuli. Some environmental stimuli, such as a smoke detector alarm, will usually awaken a sleeper, whereas other nonmeaningful noises will be selectively disregarded.

Sleep is critical for normal development, health, function, and healing. Despite sleep's pivotal role in health, many Canadians receive less sleep than they need. Polls by the U.S.-based National

OBJECTIVES

After studying this chapter, you should be able to

1. Explain the physiology and the functions of sleep
2. Identify the characteristics of NREM and REM sleep
3. Describe variations in sleep patterns throughout the lifespan
4. Explain nine factors that affect normal sleep
5. Describe six common sleep disorders
6. Outline the four components of a sleep pattern assessment
7. Develop nursing diagnoses, outcomes, and nursing interventions related to sleep problems
8. Describe five interventions that promote normal sleep

Sleep Foundation (NSF) support a sleep deficit spanning all ages, from infants to the oldest adults. The prevalence of sleep disorders and sleep insufficiency is significant and has serious consequences. For example, almost 20% of all serious car crash injuries are associated with driver sleepiness (Institute of Medicine [IOM], 2006, p. 25). Sleepiness at work has been reported to impair concentration, reduce the amount and quality of work completed, and lead to injury, lateness, and increased sick time (National Sleep Foundation, 2000). Each year US$50 billion is reported to be lost in workplace productivity because of sleep deprivation (Carmona, 2004). Despite the efforts of a growing number of sleep clinicians, researchers, and national organizations, such as the Canadian Sleep Society, and international organizations, such as the Associated Professional Sleep Society, many members of the general public and health professions are unaware of the consequences of chronic sleep loss (e.g., increased risk of hypertension, diabetes, obesity, depression, heart attack, and stroke).

Physiology of Sleep

Three major processes interact to shape sleep and wake patterns: a homeostatic function or drive, circadian rhythms, and ultradian or sleep state and stage processes. The cyclic nature of sleep is thought to be controlled by centres located in the lower part of the brain. Neurons within the reticular formation, located in the brain stem, integrate sensory information from the peripheral nervous system and relay the information to the cerebral cortex. The upper part of the reticular formation consists of a network of ascending nerve fibres called the reticular activating system (RAS), which is involved with the sleep-wake cycle. An intact cerebral cortex and reticular formation are necessary for the regulation of sleep and waking states.

Neurotransmitters, located within neurons in the brain, affect the sleep-wake cycles. For example, serotonin is thought to lessen the response to sensory stimulation and gamma-aminobutyric acid (GABA) to shut off the activity in the neurons of the RAS. Another key factor to sleep is exposure to darkness. Darkness and the reduced mental and physical activity associated with sleep preparation cause a decrease in stimulation of the RAS. During this time, the pineal gland in the brain begins to actively secrete the natural hormone melatonin, and the person feels less alert. During sleep, growth hormone is secreted and cortisol, a stimulating hormone, is inhibited.

With the beginning of daylight, melatonin is at its lowest level in the body and cortisol is at its peak. Wakefulness is also associated with high levels of acetylcholine, dopamine, and noradrenaline. Acetylcholine is released in the reticular formation, dopamine in the midbrain, and noradrenaline in the pons. These neurotransmitters are localized within the reticular formation and influence cerebral cortical arousal.

Homeostatic Function of Sleep

Patterns of sleep and wake are dependent on complex homeostatic factors. Although the effects of sleep on the body are not completely understood, we do know that sleep exerts physiological effects on the nervous system and other body structures. Sleep seems to have a homeostatic role, restoring normal levels of activity and normal balance among parts of the nervous system, including the autonomic nervous system. This **homeostatic function** or **homeostatic drive** of sleep is linked to a powerful mechanism that increases the likelihood of falling asleep as the length of time awake increases, and, conversely, that stimulates wakefulness following a period of restful sleep.

Circadian Rhythms

Biological rhythms exist in plants, animals, and humans. In humans, these are controlled from within the body and are synchronized with environmental factors, such as light and dark. The most familiar biological rhythm, the **circadian rhythm**, or sleep-wake cycle, is regulated in all mammals by the suprachiasmatic nuclei of the hypothalamus. The term *circadian* is from the Latin *circa dies*, meaning "about a day." The human circadian cycle is actually closer to 25 hours, rather than 24 hours, making it relatively easy to get off schedule by staying up late.

Sleep is a complex biological rhythm. When a person's biological clock coincides with sleep-wake patterns and light-dark cycles, the person is said to be in circadian synchronization; that is, the person is awake when the physiological and psychological rhythms are most active and is asleep when the physiological and psychological rhythms are most inactive. Circadian regularity begins to develop by the sixth week of life, and by 3 to 6 months most infants have a regular sleep-wake cycle.

CLINICAL ALERT

Given Canada's northern latitudes, daylight length varies markedly across the year. The farther north, the more variation there is. The prolonged darkness of northern winters and the frequently cloudy fall and winter days of coastal regions contribute to sleep disturbances associated with seasonal affective disorders. Conversely, the long daylight in the summer evenings promotes late-night activity, making it especially challenging to obtain sufficient amounts of sleep and to keep to regular sleep and wake schedules.

Homeostatic Drive

The underlying basis for the homeostatic drive is not completely understood, although it is known that wakefulness is associated with energy loss, fatigue, and a buildup of metabolites, including adenosine. The temporary effectiveness of caffeine, an adenosine antagonist, as a stimulant to combat sleepiness has grown dramatically in popularity, although paradoxically often itself contributing to sleep problems. The homeostatic drive is extremely powerful and is the reason that individuals will fall asleep while driving, despite certain injury or death. Conversely, a nap that lasts too long or is taken late in the day can reduce this drive, making it difficult to fall asleep at the normal bedtime.

States and Stages of Sleep

Sleep architecture refers to the basic organization of normal sleep. People have two sleep states: **NREM (non-rapid-eye-movement) sleep** and **REM (rapid-eye-movement) sleep**. During sleep, NREM and REM sleep alternate in cycles. Irregular cycling or absent sleep stages are associated with sleep disorders (IOM, 2006, p. 42).

NREM SLEEP NREM sleep occurs when activity in the RAS is inhibited. About 75% to 80% of sleep during a night is NREM sleep. NREM sleep is divided into four stages, each associated with distinct brain activity and physiology. *Stage I* is the stage of very light sleep and lasts only a few minutes. During this stage, the person feels drowsy and relaxed, the eyes roll from side to side, and the heart and respiratory rates drop slightly. The sleeper can be readily awakened and may deny that he or she was sleeping.

Stage II is the stage of light sleep during which body processes continue to slow down. The eyes are generally still, the heart and respiratory rates decrease slightly, and body temperature falls. Stage II lasts only about 10 to 15 minutes but constitutes 44% to 55% of total sleep (IOM, 2006, p. 44). An individual in stage II requires more intense stimuli than in stage I to awaken.

Stages III and IV are the deepest stages of sleep, differing only in the percentage of delta waves recorded during a 30-second period. During *deep sleep* or **slow-wave sleep (SWS)**, the sleeper's heart and respiratory rates drop 20% to 30% below those exhibited during waking hours. The sleeper is difficult to arouse. The person is not disturbed by sensory stimuli, the skeletal muscles are very relaxed, reflexes are diminished, and snoring is most likely to occur. These stages are essential for restoring energy and releasing important growth hormones. See Box 37.1. Recently, the American Academy of Sleep Medicine has revised their scoring protocols for sleep, including sleep stages. One of the changes is to consider all stage 3 and stage 4 sleep as just stage 3 sleep, or more precisely, "Stage N3."

REM SLEEP REM sleep usually recurs about every 90 minutes and lasts 5 to 30 minutes. Most dreams take place during REM sleep but usually will not be remembered unless the person arouses briefly at the end of the REM period.

During REM sleep, the brain is highly active, and brain metabolism can increase as much as 20%. For example, during REM sleep, levels of acetylcholine and dopamine increase, with the highest levels of acetylcholine release occurring during REM sleep (see Box 37.2). Since both of these neurotransmitters are associated with cortical activation, it makes sense that their levels would be high during dreaming sleep. This type of sleep is also called paradoxical sleep because electroencephalogram (EEG) activity resembles that of wakefulness. Distinctive eye movements occur, voluntary muscle tone is dramatically decreased, and deep tendon reflexes are absent. In this phase, the sleeper may be difficult to arouse or may wake spontaneously, gastric secretions increase, and heart and respiratory rates often are irregular. It is thought that the regions of the brain that are used in learning, thinking, and organizing information are stimulated during REM sleep.

Sleep Cycles

During a sleep cycle, a sleeper passes from stage I NREM sleep through stages II and III to stage IV in about 20 to 30 minutes. Stage IV may last about 30 minutes. These

BOX 37.1 PHYSIOLOGICAL CHANGES DURING NREM SLEEP

In the four stages of NREM sleep, some essential changes occur:

- Arterial blood pressure falls.
- Pulse rate decreases.
- Peripheral blood vessels dilate.
- Cardiac output decreases.
- Skeletal muscles relax.
- Basal metabolic rate decreases 10% to 30%.
- Growth hormone levels peak.
- Intracranial pressure decreases.

BOX 37.2 PHYSIOLOGICAL CHANGES DURING REM SLEEP

Although REM sleep likely stimulates the brain, other physiological changes occur:

- Voluntary muscle tone is depressed.
- Heart and respiratory rate are often irregular.
- Blood pressure surges can occur.
- Temperature regulation is minimal or absent.

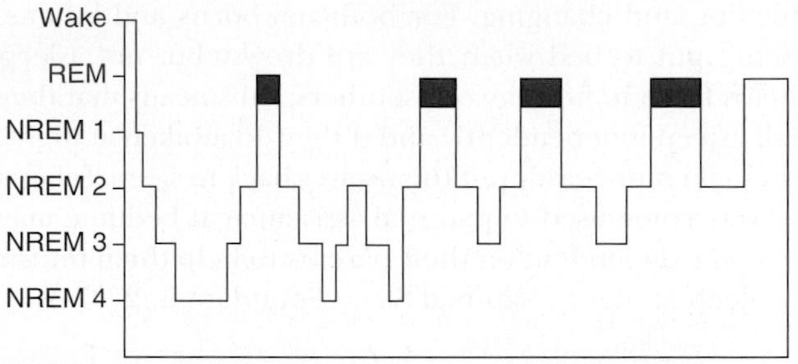

FIGURE 37.1 Time spent in REM and NREM stages of sleep by an adult

stages are then followed by stages III and II, in that order. Thereafter, the first REM stage occurs, lasting about 10 minutes. This sequence completes the first sleep cycle. The healthy adult sleeper usually experiences four to six cycles of sleep during 7 to 8 hours (see Figure 37.1). Each cycle lasts about 90 minutes. The sleeper who is awakened during any stage begins anew at stage I NREM sleep and proceeds through all the stages to REM sleep.

The duration of NREM stages and REM sleep varies throughout the sleep period. As the night progresses, the sleeper spends less time in stages III and IV of NREM sleep. REM sleep increases, and dreams tend to lengthen. If the sleeper is very tired, REM cycles are often short. Before sleep ends, periods of near-wakefulness occur, and stages I and II NREM sleep and REM sleep predominate. The ratio of NREM to REM sleep varies with age.

Recent research has shown that sleep deprivation is associated with significant cognitive and health problems. Therefore, although re-establishing the sleep-wake rhythm (e.g., after the disruption of surgery) is important for healthy sleep, it is not appropriate to restrict daytime napping in hospitalized clients as their sleep needs are often increased.

CLINICAL ALERT

Sudden infant death syndrome (SIDS) continues to be the leading cause of death in babies 1 month to 1 year of age. The Back to Sleep campaign has been successful in reducing deaths attributed to SIDS. Bed sharing remains controversial and may be a contributing factor to infant deaths during sleep. Parents who want to bed share need to made aware of the risks, and the Canadian Medical Association recommends that the safest approach is to offer infants a pacifier and have them sleep in a separate crib in the parent's room (Hunt & Hauck, 2006).

The birth of a baby is often an exciting but exhausting time for parents. Nurses should encourage parents to set realistic goals, seek and accept help with other duties, and nap when possible. Performing nighttime feeds and changes quietly and with lowered lights can also help begin to establish day and night rhythms in babies and foster a more rapid return to sleep for the parent.

Normal Sleep Patterns and Requirements

Newborns

Newborns sleep 16 to 18 hours a day, on an irregular schedule with periods of 1 to 3 hours of wake. Unlike older children and adults, newborns enter REM sleep (called active sleep in the newborn) immediately. Rapid eye movements are observable through closed lids, and body movements and irregular respirations may be seen. Quiet sleep (NREM with not yet fully differentiated sleep stages) is characterized by regular respirations, closed eyes, and the absence of body and eye movements. Premature babies spend nearly 80% of the time in REM sleep and this amount decreases to 50% at term. Cycles of active and quiet sleep last about 50 minutes.

Infants

At first, infants awaken every 3 or 4 hours, eat, and then go back to sleep. Periods of wakefulness gradually increase during the first months. By 6 months, most infants sleep through the night (from midnight to 5 a.m.) and begin to establish a pattern of daytime naps. At the end of the first year, an infant usually takes two naps per day and should get about 14 to 15 hours of sleep in 24 hours.

CLINICAL ALERT

A nursing intervention providing infant sleep education and sleep strategy classes, sleep charts, and biweekly telephone calls for 2 weeks to parents with healthy 6- to 12-month-old infants was tested on 70 parents by using a one-group, pretest, posttest design. The findings supported that sleep interventions can significantly improve parents' sleep quality, understanding of their infant's sleep behaviours, and parental fatigue and mood (Hall, Clauson, Carty, Janssen, & Saunders, 2006).

Much of the infant's sleep time is spent in light sleep. During light sleep, the infant may exhibit movement, gurgles, and coughing. Parents should check that infants are truly awake before picking them up for feeding and changing. For both newborns and infants, being put to bed when they are drowsy but not asleep helps them to become self-soothers; this means that they fall asleep independently and if they do awaken at night, they can more easily put themselves back to sleep. Infants who become used to parental assistance at bedtime may become dependent on their parents to help them return to sleep at night (National Sleep Foundation, 2007a).

Toddlers

Between 12 and 14 hours of sleep are recommended for children 1 to 3 years of age. About 30% is REM sleep. Most still need an afternoon nap, but the need for mid-morning naps gradually decreases. The toddler may exhibit a great deal of resistance to going to bed and may awaken during the night. Nighttime fears and nightmares are common. A security object, such as a blanket or stuffed animal, may help. Parents need assurance that maintaining a daily sleep or rest schedule and a consistent, relaxing, and positive bedtime routine will promote good sleep habits for the entire family.

Preschoolers

The preschool child (3 to 5 years of age) requires 11 to 13 hours of sleep per night, particularly if the child is in preschool. Sleep needs fluctuate in relation to activity and growth spurts. Many children of this age dislike bedtime and resist by requesting another story or television program. The 4- to 5-year-old may become restless and irritable if sleep requirements are not met. A nap or quiet time during the day may be needed to restore energy levels.

Children in this age group benefit from bedtime rituals. Parents can help children by cueing them that bedtime is approaching and by continuing to use the same positive, clear, and consistent approach suggested for the toddler. Preschool children wake up frequently at night and they may be afraid of the dark or experience night terrors or nightmares. A relaxing bedtime story and discussion and problem solving of fears can help reduce the number of nightmares. Night terrors, often accompanied by loud screaming and thrashing, are usually not recalled by the child, but are alarming and disrupting to the parent. Children usually outgrow these sleep disturbances. If night terrors occur regularly, frequency may be reduced by briefly waking and resettling the child 15 to 20 minutes before usual onset.

School-Age Children

The school-age child (5 to 12 years of age) needs between 10 to 12 hours of sleep, but most receive less because of increasing demands (e.g., homework, sports, social activities). They may also be spending more time at the computer and watching television. Some may be drinking caffeinated beverages or eating foods containing chocolate and sugar. All these activities can lead to difficulty falling asleep and insufficient sleep. Nurses can teach parents and school-age children about healthy sleep habits. A healthy diet, a consistent sleep schedule, and a bedtime routine need to be continued.

CLINICAL ALERT

Children who have a television or computer in their bedroom are more likely to get less sleep than needed.

Adolescents

Adolescents (12 to 18 years of age) require 8.5 to 10 hours of sleep each night, however, few actually get that much sleep. According to a Canadian-based study of high school students (N = 3235), 70% of students are sleep deprived (Gibson et al., 2006). Lack of sleep can lead to significant sleepiness at school and negatively affect grades, attendance, sports, extracurricular activities, and work. Fatigue contributes to negative moods (e.g., unhappiness, irritability) and poorer coping. Sleepy teens are also at greater risk for car accidents. Nurses can educate parents, teens, and teachers about sleep and the reasons why sleep health needs to be a priority.

As children reach adolescence, their circadian rhythms tend to shift. Research in the 1990s found that later sleep and later wake patterns among adolescents are biologically determined (National Sleep Foundation, 2007b). This shift is often in contrast to the early hours demanded by school and work routines, making adolescents especially vulnerable to receiving insufficient amounts of sleep.

During adolescence, boys begin to experience **nocturnal emissions** (orgasm and emission of semen during sleep), known as *wet dreams*, several times each month. Boys need to be informed about this normal development to prevent embarrassment and fear.

Adults

The sleep-wake cycle remains very important to health throughout life. Most adults in their early to middle adult years (19 to 64 years of age) require 7 to 9 hours of sleep each night. About 20% of time is spent in REM sleep. During adulthood, most individuals experience a slight but steady increase in arousals over time and between the fourth and fifth decade, the amount of SWS begins to decrease. Shift work, school, and childcare or eldercare (or both) often lead to irregular sleep schedules. Late-night social and sports activities, alcohol, caffeine, nicotine, computer, and television are other factors contributing to the sleep deprivation and sleep disturbances experienced by many adult Canadians.

Older Adults

The older adult (ages 65 years and over) sleeps between 7 and 9 hours per night. SWS is markedly decreased with increased age and may be absent entirely. A hallmark change with age is a tendency toward earlier bedtime and wake times. Older adults usually awaken 1.3 hours earlier and go to bed approximately 1 hour earlier than younger adults. Older adults may show an increase in disturbed sleep (lighter sleep, more awakenings, difficulty falling back to sleep) that can have a negative effect on their quality of life, mood, and alertness. Although the ability to sleep becomes more difficult, the need to sleep does not decrease with age (IOM, 2006, pp. 57–59). Many older adults compensate with a daytime nap.

A strong relationship exists among sleep, health, and aging. Healthy older adults are more likely to sleep well, whereas as the number of medical conditions experienced increases, so does the likelihood of sleep problems (Nagel, Markie, Richards, & Taylor, 2003). Nurses should assess routinely for sleep problems and be aware that sleep disorders can exacerbate other health conditions and complicate their treatment. Many older adults with dementia experience *sundown syndrome*. Although not a primary sleep disorder, the late afternoon onset of agitation, anxiety, and confusion associated with the disorder can last throughout the night, further disturbing sleep and the sleep of those nearby.

Factors Affecting Sleep

Both the quality and the quantity of sleep are affected by a number of factors. *Sleep quality* is a subjective characteristic and is often determined by whether a person wakes up feeling energetic or not. *Quantity of sleep* is the total time the individual sleeps.

Health and Illness

Normal states of health, such as rapid growth, menstruation, perimenopause, pregnancy, and parenthood, can temporarily alter sleep patterns. Nurses should reassure parents that young children and teens sleep more during periods of rapid growth and that this additional sleep is normal, needed, and temporary. For women, sleep quality is reported to be poorer 3 to 6 days before menstruation and during the first 4 days of menstruation. Disruptions in menstrual function are linked to circadian rhythm disturbances (Baker & Driver, 2007). Hot flashes, common to perimenopause, can be especially sleep disturbing. Wearing breathable nightwear and layering bedcovers can help to support a faster return to sleep. Pregnancy is associated with sleep pattern change. Women are sleepier than usual early in pregnancy because of increased levels of circulating progesterone; they often experience nocturia (the need to urinate during the night) in the first and third trimesters because of pressure on the bladder from the growing fetus; and they experience increasing sleep disturbance in the third trimester in the form of more nighttime awakenings, lighter sleep, and less total sleep time. Postpartum recovery and the sleep-disrupting care demands of a newborn and infant make parenthood, and the early months of childcare, especially tiring for parents.

Illness that causes pain or physical distress can result in sleep problems. People who are ill require more sleep than normal, and the normal rhythm of sleep and wakefulness is often disturbed. For example, patients with cancer and their caregivers both frequently suffer disturbed sleep-wake patterns related to symptoms or their management (Berger et al., 2005).

Respiratory conditions can disturb an individual's sleep. Shortness of breath makes sleep difficult, and people who have nasal congestion or sinus drainage may have trouble breathing and hence difficulty sleeping.

People who have gastric or duodenal ulcers may find their sleep disturbed because of pain, often a result of the increased gastric secretions that occur during REM sleep. Certain endocrine disturbances can also affect sleep. Hyperthyroidism lengthens presleep time, often making it difficult for a client to fall asleep. Hypothyroidism, conversely, decreases stage IV sleep. Women with low levels of estrogen often report excessive fatigue. In addition, they may experience sleep disruptions, in part, because of the discomfort associated with hot flashes or night sweats that can occur with reduced estrogen levels. Elevated body temperatures can cause some reduction in SWS and REM sleep.

Nocturia disrupts sleep and is a common problem for individuals with urinary tract infection or irritation, with bladder emptying difficulties (e.g., prostate hypertrophy), or in the early and late stages of pregnancy, as previously described. Individuals may waken several times through the night to urinate and may have difficulty getting back to sleep.

Emotional Stress

Anxiety and depression frequently disturb sleep. A person preoccupied with personal problems may be unable to relax sufficiently to get to sleep. Anxiety increases the norepinephrine levels in the blood through stimulation of the sympathetic nervous system. This chemical change results in less stage IV NREM and REM sleep and more stage changes and awakenings.

People who are depressed typically have disturbed sleep, manifested either as insomnia or excessive sleeping. They may report difficulty getting to sleep, frequent awakenings and the inability to get back to sleep, or early morning wakening. Sleep disturbance may precede the onset of other symptoms of depression (Voyer, Verreault, Cappeliez, Holmes, & Nkogho Mengue, 2005). This association may be physiological, through neurotransmitter imbalance, as well as psychological, through worry and negative thoughts.

Environment

Environment can promote or hinder sleep. The absence of usual stimuli or the presence of unfamiliar stimuli can prevent people from sleeping, and nurses may overestimate the amount of sleep patients are receiving (Nicolàs et al., 2008). Hospital and long-term-care environments can be quite noisy, and special care needs to be taken to reduce noise in the hallways and nursing care units. A balance between daytime activity and quiet periods, and the delivery of only prioritized nighttime nursing care, can promote sleep health in long-term-care residents (Koch, Haesler, Tiziani, & Wilson, 2006).

Discomfort from environmental temperature (e.g., too hot or cold) and poor or excessive ventilation can also affect sleep. Light levels can be another factor. A person accustomed to darkness while sleeping may find it difficult to sleep in the light. Another influence includes the comfort and size of the bed and firmness of the pillow. A person's partner who has different sleep habits, who snores, or who has other sleep difficulties, such as periodic limb movement, can cause sleep problems. Pets can also significantly disrupt sleep.

Homelessness is a growing problem in all major Canadian cities (Laird, 2007). One immediate and major health consequence of this social housing crisis is chronic, severe sleep disturbance and deprivation—if you are cold, hungry, wet, in pain, or do not feel safe, you do not sleep well, if at all.

> **Evidence-Informed Practice**
>
> ### How Does Violence against Women Affect Their Sleep?
>
> In this study, Rasmussen (2007) asked 30 women who were dealing with violence in their relationships about their dreams, nightmares, and sleep patterns. The women came from transition centres and a family counselling centre. Half the women reported having weekly nightmares, with half indicating it was a recurring dream. In addition, the majority of the participants reported getting approximately 6 hours of sleep per night, with difficulty falling asleep.
>
> **NURSING IMPLICATIONS:** **Reported sleep difficulties may well be symptomatic of many other things in people's lives. Through trust and communication, nurses can sometimes assess some of the factors contributing to the sleep difficulty.**
>
> Source: Based on "No Refuge: An Exploratory Survey of Nightmares, Dreams, and Sleep Patterns in Women Dealing with Relationship Violence," by B. Rasmussen, 2007, *Violence Against Women, 13*(3), pp. 314–322.

Lifestyle

People who have an irregular sleep-wake schedule are more likely to experience poor quality sleep. Moderate exercise in the morning or early afternoon is conducive to sleep, but vigorous exercise late in the day can delay sleep onset. The person's ability to relax before retiring is an important factor affecting the ability to fall asleep. It is best, therefore, to avoid doing homework or office work before or after getting into bed.

Shift work and travel across time zones disrupt the normal circadian rhythm. Night-shift workers frequently obtain less sleep than other workers and have difficulty falling asleep after getting off work. Wearing dark wraparound sunglasses during the drive home and using light-blocking shades can minimize the alerting effects of exposure to daylight, thus making it easier to fall asleep when body temperature is rising. Nurses who work extended shifts and night shifts were found to be at significant risk for drowsiness on the drive home from work (Scott et al., 2007). Nurses working extended shifts (more than 12.5 hours) were found to be at greater risk for decreased vigilance, work injuries, and medical errors (Lockely et al., 2007).

Stimulants and Alcohol

Caffeine-containing beverages act as stimulants of the central nervous system. Drinking caffeinated beverages in the afternoon or evening can interfere with sleep. People who drink an excessive amount of alcohol often find their sleep disturbed. Excessive alcohol disrupts REM sleep although it may initially hasten sleep onset. While making up for lost REM sleep after some of the effects of the alcohol have worn off, people often experience nightmares. Tolerance to alcohol also affects sleep; the alcohol-tolerant person may be unable to sleep well and may become irritable as a result.

Diet

Weight gain has been associated with reduced total sleep time, fragmented sleep, and earlier awakening. During periods of sleep deprivation, ghrelin, a hormone that stimulates hunger, is oversecreted, while leptin, a satiety hormone, is suppressed, contributing to junk food cravings when staying up late at night. Conversely, weight loss is associated with an increase in total sleep time and less fragmented sleep. L-tryptophan—found, for example, in turkey and milk—may induce sleep. Although typical dietary levels of these foods may not have a strong impact, warm milk does help some people get to sleep.

Smoking

Nicotine has a stimulating effect on the body, and smokers often have more difficulty falling asleep and staying asleep than nonsmokers. Heavy smokers often awaken early, because of nicotine withdrawal. By reducing daily intake and refraining from smoking after the evening meal, the person usually sleeps better (Jefferson et al., 2005; Ohida et al., 2007; Wetter & Young, 1994). Although the immediate withdrawal period when stopping smoking can result in disturbed sleep related to the nicotine withdrawal, sleeping patterns often improve once people are past the withdrawal period.

Motivation

Motivation can increase alertness in some situations (e.g., a moderately tired person may be able to stay alert while attending an interesting concert or surfing the internet late at night). Motivation alone, however, is usually not sufficient to overcome the normal circadian drive to sleep during the night. Neither is motivation sufficient to overcome sleepiness caused by insufficient sleep. Boredom alone is not sufficient to cause sleepiness, but when insufficient sleep combines with boredom, sleep is more likely to occur.

Medications

Some medications affect the quality of sleep. Hypnotics can interfere with SWS and suppress REM sleep. Beta blockers and steroids have been known to cause insomnia and nightmares. Opioids, such as meperidine hydrochloride (Demerol) and morphine, are known to suppress REM sleep and to cause frequent awakenings and drowsiness. Tranquilizers interfere with REM sleep. Although antidepressants suppress REM sleep, this effect is considered a therapeutic action; selectively depriving a depressed client of REM sleep will result in an immediate but transient improvement in mood. Clients accustomed to taking hypnotic medications and antidepressants may experience a REM rebound (increased REM sleep) when these medications are discontinued. Warning clients to expect a period of more intense dreams when these medications are discontinued may reduce their anxiety about this symptom. See Box 37.3 for drugs that can affect sleep.

BOX 37.3 DRUGS THAT AFFECT SLEEP AND WAKE

These drugs can disrupt REM sleep, delay sleep onset, decrease sleep time, cause nightmares, or increase daytime drowsiness:

- Alcohol
- Amphetamines
- Antidepressants
- Antihistamines
- Beta blockers
- Bronchodilators
- Caffeine
- Decongestants
- Opioids
- Steroids
- Thyroid supplements

Common Sleep Disorders

Knowledge of common sleep disorders helps nurses obtain and recognize pertinent data. Sleep disorders can be categorized as primary disorders, secondary disorders, and parasomnias. **Primary sleep disorders** are those in which the person's sleep problem is the main disorder. These disorders include insomnia, hypersomnia, narcolepsy, sleep apnea, and periodic limb movements. **Secondary sleep disorders** are sleep disturbances caused by another clinical disorder, such as thyroid dysfunction, depression, or alcoholism. **Parasomnias**, such as somnambulism or bruxism (teeth grinding), are described as unwanted behaviours or experiences occurring during sleep onset, within sleep, or during arousal from sleep.

Insomnia

Insomnia, the most common sleep problem, is the inability to obtain an adequate amount or quality of sleep. People suffering from insomnia do not feel refreshed on arising. Insomnia has three types:

1. Difficulty in falling asleep (initial or onset insomnia)
2. Difficulty in staying asleep because of frequent or prolonged waking (intermittent or maintenance insomnia)
3. Early morning or premature waking (terminal insomnia)

Some insomniacs have been observed to fall asleep and obtain more sleep than they perceive they do. This type of insomnia is referred to as *sleep state misperception*.

Such a condition is no less distressing than the other types of insomnia and can lead to increased wakefulness.

Insomnia can result from physical discomfort but, more often, is a result of mental overstimulation caused by anxiety. People sometimes become anxious because they think they might not be able to sleep. People who become habituated to drugs or who drink large quantities of alcohol are likely to have insomnia.

Insomnia is often characterized by predisposing, precipitating, and perpetuating factors. *Predisposing* factors include hyperarousal, predisposition to depression, and tendency to be a night owl. *Precipitating* factors can include periods of stress or grief, the loss of a loved one, a new job, a new child, or a perceived need for increased vigilance. *Perpetuating* factors include fear of not being able to sleep, irregular sleeping patterns to try to catch up, and association of the bedroom with the struggle to sleep. Treatment for insomnia frequently requires the client to develop new behaviour patterns that induce sleep. Short-term use of hypnotics during periods of stress may be helpful in reducing the impact of a precipitating event, but they should not be relied on for long-term use. Psychological and behavioural therapies alone, or in combination with short-acting hypnotics, are recommended for the management of chronic insomnia (Morgenthaler et al., 2006)

Hypersomnia

Hypersomnia, the opposite of insomnia, is excessive sleep, particularly in the daytime. The afflicted person often sleeps until noon and takes many naps during the day. Hypersomnia can be caused by medical conditions, for example, central nervous system damage and certain kidney, liver, or metabolic disorders, such as diabetic acidosis and hypothyroidism. In some instances, a person uses hypersomnia as a coping mechanism to avoid facing the responsibilities of the day.

Narcolepsy

Narcolepsy is a disorder of sleep-wake instability caused by the lack of the chemical hypocretin in the area of the central nervous system that regulates sleep. Patients with narcolepsy have sleep attacks or excessive daytime sleepiness, and their sleep at night usually begins with a sleep-onset REM period. The majority of patients also have cataplexy, or the sudden onset of muscle weakness or paralysis in association with strong emotion; sleep paralysis (transient paralysis when falling asleep or waking up); hypnagogic hallucinations (visual, auditory, or tactile hallucinations at sleep onset or when waking up); and fragmented nighttime sleep. Their fragmented nocturnal sleep is not the cause of their excessive daytime sleepiness; many clients, particularly younger clients, have sound restorative nocturnal sleep but still cannot stay awake during the daytime. Onset of symptoms tends to occur between ages 15 and 30, and symptom severity usually stabilizes within the first 5 years of onset. Central nervous system stimulants, such as methylphenidate (Ritalin), or amphetamines have been used to reduce daytime sleepiness.

Sleep Apnea

Sleep apnea is characterized by frequent periodic cessation of breathing during sleep. This disorder needs to be assessed by a sleep specialist, but it is often suspected when the person has loud snoring, frequent nocturnal awakenings, excessive daytime sleepiness, morning headaches, memory and cognitive problems, irritability or other personality changes, and physiological changes, such as hypertension, cardiac arrhythmias, and metabolic syndrome (Caples, Garcia-Touchard, & Somers, 2007; Parish, Adam, & Facchiano, 2007). Although sleep apnea is most frequently diagnosed in men and postmenopausal women, it can occur during childhood.

The periods of apnea, which last from 10 seconds to 2 minutes, occur during REM or NREM sleep. Frequency of episodes ranges from 50 to 600 per night.

Three common types of sleep apnea are obstructive apnea, central apnea, and mixed apnea. *Obstructive apnea* occurs when the structures of the pharynx or oral cavity block the flow of air. The person continues to try to breathe; that is, the chest and abdominal muscles move. Increased carbon dioxide levels lead to partial arousal, thus opening the airway. Obesity, enlarged tonsils, a deviated nasal septum, nasal polyps, or reduced muscle tone predispose the client to obstructive apnea. Patients with Down syndrome are an underrecognized but high-risk group for this sleep disorder (Shott et al., 2006).

Central apnea is thought to involve a defect in the respiratory centre of the brain. All actions involved in breathing, such as chest movement and airflow, cease. Clients who have brain stem injuries and muscular dystrophy, for example, often have central sleep apnea. *Mixed apnea* is a combination of central apnea and obstructive apnea.

The use of a nasal continuous positive airway pressure (CPAP) device at night is effective as it helps keep the upper airway open. Surgical procedures to remove tonsils, realign the mandible, or open the upper airway are effective for some people. Oral appliances may also be used.

Periodic Limb Movements of Sleep and Restless Legs Syndrome

Periodic limb movements of sleep (PLMS) are repetitive, jerky movements, usually of the lower limbs, during sleep that can contribute to frequent partial arousals and excessive daytime sleepiness. People who experience periodic limb movements during sleep often experience **restless legs syndrome (RLS)** (crawling, aching sensations) when they are resting or trying to fall asleep. RLS can severely disturb the sleep of both the individual with it and his or her bed partner. Although the underlying cause is usually not serious, RLS can accompany other conditions, such as peripheral neuropathy, iron deficiency, or kidney failure. Many drugs, such as antidepressants, antihistamines, caffeine, alcohol, and nicotine, can make PLMS worse. Opioids, muscle relaxants, sedatives, certain medications for epilepsy, and medications similar to those used in treating Parkinson's disease can bring relief in severe cases. Good sleep health practices, regular moderate exercise, stress reduction, warm baths, and massage are effective self-care strategies for RLS treatment.

Parasomnias

Parasomnia is a kind of behaviour that may interfere with sleep. Box 37.4 describes four kinds of parasomnia, all of which are typically more frequent during times of stress.

Sleep Deprivation

A prolonged disturbance results in decreases in amount, quality, and consistency of sleep and can lead to a syndrome referred to as **sleep deprivation**. This is not a sleep disorder in itself but a result of sleep disturbances. It produces a variety of physiological and behavioural symptoms, the severity of which depends on the degree of the deprivation. The prevalence of chronic sleep deprivation is a growing concern in this 24-hour society.

BOX 37.4 PARASOMNIAS

- *Somnambulism:* Somnambulism (sleepwalking) occurs during stages III and IV of NREM sleep. It is episodic and usually occurs 1 to 2 hours after falling asleep. Sleepwalkers tend not to notice dangers (e.g., stairs) and often need to be protected from injury.
- *Sleeptalking:* Talking during sleep occurs during NREM sleep before REM sleep. It rarely presents a problem to the person unless it becomes troublesome to others.
- *Nocturnal enuresis:* Bed wetting that occurs during sleep in children more than 3 years old is called nocturnal enuresis. More males than females are affected. It often occurs 1 to 2 hours after falling asleep when rousing from NREM stages III to IV.
- *Bruxism:* Usually occurring during stage II NREM sleep, this clenching and grinding of the teeth can eventually erode dental crowns, cause teeth to come loose, and lead to temperomandibular joint pain.

Assessing

In addition to a comprehensive health history, the assessment of a client's sleep and rest includes a sleep and rest history, a sleep diary, a physical examination, and a review of diagnostic studies.

Sleep and Rest History

A brief general sleep and rest history should be obtained for all clients entering a health-care facility or being seen in the community. This enables the nurse to incorporate the client's needs and preferences in the plan of care. Although sleep is a health priority, many patients will not report sleep problems unless specifically asked, assuming that sleep is not that important or that little can be done to improve it. A general sleep and rest history should include the following:

- Usual sleeping pattern, specifically sleeping and waking times; length of time to fall asleep; hours of undisturbed sleep; number and reason for sleep interruptions; quality of or satisfaction with sleep; and time and length of naps and rest periods
- Usual sleeping environment, including whether single or shared sleep space, location (e.g., bed, couch, floor, outdoors, single or shared room); safety, comfort level, noise level, pets
- Bedtime rituals performed to help the person fall asleep (e.g., a glass of hot milk, reading or other method of relaxing, and special equipment or positioning aids)
- Use of sleep medication, other drugs, and other stimulants (e.g., prescription, over the counter, herbal, recreational, dietary)
- Preferred sleep environment (e.g., room temperature, noise level, night-light)
- Preferred ways to rest, including amount, type, and timing of exercise
- Recent changes in sleep and rest patterns or difficulties in sleeping, including the number of awakenings

If the client indicates a recent pattern change or difficulties in sleeping, a more detailed history is required. This detailed history should explore the exact nature of the problem and its cause, when it first began and its frequency, how it affects daily living, what the client is doing to cope with the problem, and whether these methods have been effective. Questions the nurse might ask the client with a sleeping disturbance are shown in the Assessment: Interview box. Information from the bed partner on snoring, breathing patterns, leg movements, sleeptalking, and sleepwalking is also important in detecting sleep disorders.

ASSESSMENT: INTERVIEW

Sleep Disturbances

Questions	Comments
A. Understanding the problem from the client's perspective	
• What is the biggest problem with your sleep at this time?	Helps client focus
• When did you first notice this problem?	Determine whether acute or chronic, may probe as to what was happening in the client's life about the time the problem started (e.g., change in job, weight gain)
• How often does it occur?	(e.g., every night, only when overtired)
• What makes it worse?	(e.g., alcohol makes sleep apnea worse)
• What have you found that helps deal with this sleep problem?	(e.g., sleeping in front of the television or away from home suggests the bedroom has become associated with the struggle to sleep)
• What do you think might be causing or contributing to the problem?	Clients often aware of probable etiologies
• How is this problem affecting you? others in your family and workplace?	Sleep disorders often affect others (e.g., snoring, worry about safety)
B. Understanding the problem from the bed partner's perspective	
• What concerns do you have about your partner's sleep?	The bed partner can provide valuable information about behaviours during sleep as well as waking hours
• What have you noticed that seems to make it better? worse?	
C. Screening questions to assist in planning care and determining need for referral	
• What do you do to prepare for sleep?	Listen for rituals, tendency to be busy right up to bedtime
• Do you have difficulty getting to sleep?	Probe as to length of time to go to sleep (10 to 30 minutes is within normal range)
• Do you have difficulty with wakening during the night and being unable to get back to sleep?	If yes, probe as to what the client does if awake for long periods (e.g., racing thoughts)
• Do you waken earlier in the morning than you would like?	Particularly common with depression
• How do you feel when you wake up in the morning?	Morning headaches and feeling unrefreshed are common symptoms of sleep apnea
• Do you sleep more than usual? less than usual?	Inquire regarding family or work pressures, fatigue
• Do you have periods of overwhelming tiredness? If yes, when does this happen? Do you ever feel suddenly weak when laughing or upset?	A positive response may suggest narcolepsy, especially if the client also has symptoms of cataplexy
• Has anyone ever told you that you snore? stop breathing in your sleep? sleepwalk? sleeptalk?	Snoring and apneas suggest sleep apnea; parasomnias, such as somnambulism, are uncommon in adults and can be worsened by stress
D. Additional Information	
• Collect data on current medications (include over-the-counter and street drugs), time and amount of caffeine use, and smoking.	Many medications and other substances affect sleep
• Explore lifestyle regarding shift work or frequent travel across time zones.	Note circadian effects

Sleep Diary

Sometimes, clients with a sleeping problem can provide more precise information if they keep a written record of their sleep pattern and the habits associated with it. Such a sleep diary or log can be kept by clients who are sleeping at home and should be maintained for at least 1 week. A sleep diary may include all of the following information or selected aspects of it that pertain to the client's specific problem:

- Total number of sleep hours per night
- Number, length, and timing of naps
- Activities performed 2 to 3 hours before bedtime (type, duration, and time)

- Bedtime rituals (e.g., ingestion of food, fluid, or medication) before going to bed
- (1) Time of going to bed, (2) approximate time to fall asleep after lights out, (3) any instances of waking up and duration of these periods, (4) final time of waking during the night, and (5) time out of bed
- How rested the patient feels on awakening; (e.g., 0 "not rested at all" to 10 "completely rested")
- Worries that the client believes may affect sleep
- Factors that the client believes have a positive or negative effect on sleep

From the sleep diary, the nurse can help the client detect such patterns as an irregular sleep schedule and the effect of napping on nighttime sleep. Sleep efficiency can be calculated by dividing the actual time spent asleep by the total time in bed multiplied by 100. Clients who have a sleep efficiency of less than 85 percent should be encouraged to reduce their time in bed by not going to bed until sleepy and getting up at the same time every morning.

Physical Examination

Examination of the client includes observation of the client's body structure, facial appearance, behaviour, and energy level. Obesity, enlarged tongue or tonsils, obstructed nares, and such conditions as Down syndrome all increase the risk of obstructive sleep apnea. Darkened areas around the eyes, puffy eyelids, reddened conjunctiva, glazed or dull-appearing eyes, and limited facial expression are indicative of sleep insufficiency. Such behaviours as irritability, restlessness, inattentiveness, slowed speech, slumped posture, hand tremor, yawning, rubbing the eyes, withdrawal, confusion, and poor coordination are also suggestive of sleep problems. Lack of energy may be noted by observing whether the client appears physically weak, lethargic, or fatigued. A recent injury or fall should alert staff to assess for potential sleep problems: injuries, across the developmental spectrum, are strongly linked to insufficient or disturbed sleep (Fletcher & Hirdes, 2005).

Diagnostic Studies

Sleep is measured objectively by **polysomnography**, in which an electroencephalogram (EEG), electromyogram (EMG), and electro-oculogram (EOG) are recorded simultaneously. This simultaneous recording divides sleep into REM and NREM sleep. Electrodes are placed on the scalp to record brain waves (EEG), on the outer canthus of each eye to record eye movement (EOG), and on the chin muscles to record the structural electromyogram (EMG). The following may also be monitored, depending on findings of the initial interview: respiratory effort and airflow, ECG, leg movements, and oxygen saturation. Oxygen saturation is determined by monitoring arterial blood or with an *oximeter,* a light-sensitive electric cell that attaches to the ear or a finger. Oxygen saturation and ECG assessments are of particular importance if sleep apnea is suspected. Through polysomnography, the client's activity (movements, struggling, noisy respirations) during sleep can be assessed. Activity the client is unaware of may be the cause of arousal during sleep. A less invasive, objective, proxy assessment of sleep and wake can be achieved by using actigraphy. A watch-sized motion sensor, called an accelerometer, is worn on the nondominant wrist or ankle and provides a measure of rest and activity.

Diagnosing

Insomnia, the NANDA International (2007) diagnosis given to clients with sleep problems, is usually made more explicit with descriptions, such as "difficulty falling asleep" or "difficulty staying asleep." For example, *Insomnia (delayed onset of sleep)* related to overstimulation before bedtime.

Various factors or etiologies may be involved and should be specified for the individual. These include physical discomfort or pain; anxiety about actual or anticipated loss of a loved one, loss of a job, or worry about a family member's behaviour or illness; frequent changes in sleep time because of shift work or overtime; and changes in sleep environment or bedtime rituals (e.g., noise or overstimulation of hospital environment; alcohol or other drug dependency; drug withdrawal; misuse of sedatives prescribed for insomnia; and effects of medications, such as steroids or stimulants).

Examples of assessment data clusters and related nursing diagnoses for sleep pattern disturbances are shown in Table 37.1

Sleep pattern disturbances can also be stated as the etiology of another diagnosis, in which case the nursing interventions are directed toward the sleep disturbance itself. Examples include the following:

- *Risk for Injury* related to somnambulism
- *Ineffective Individual Coping* related to insufficient quality and quantity of sleep
- *Fatigue* related to insomnia
- *Risk for Impaired Gas Exchange* related to sleep apnea
- *Disturbed Thought Processes* related to chronic insomnia
- *Activity Intolerance* related to sleep deprivation

Planning

The major goal for clients with sleep disturbances is to maintain (or develop) a sleeping pattern that provides sufficient energy for daily activities. The nurse plans specific nursing interventions based on the etiology of each

TABLE 37.1 Clinical Application: Assessment Data Clusters and Related Nursing Diagnoses for Clients with Sleep Problems

Data Cluster	Nursing Diagnosis
Francine Leduc, 51, states she has had a problem falling asleep since her mastectomy 2 months ago. She says fears of prognosis become prominent when she is not active and busy. She has tried reading or watching TV, but neither make her sleepy or relaxed. She appears agitated and restless.	*Insomnia (delayed sleep onset)* related to fear of prognosis and difficulty relaxing
Joseph Nitchke, 83, was admitted to a four-bed room in the extended-care unit 3 days ago. He states he falls asleep about 10 p.m. but is awakened by roommate's snoring. He states, "At home I used to have a hot cup of Ovaltine whenever I awakened."	*Insomnia (sleep maintenance)* related to change in sleep environment and sleep-time rituals
Tim Mulroney states he was fired from his job because of problematic alcohol abuse. He joined Alcoholics Anonymous but has been unable to get any work for the past 2 years. He states, "Every day I wake up at 4 a.m. (full of self-reproach and self-punitive thinking) and can't get back to sleep."	*Insomnia (terminal early morning waking)* related to low self-esteem secondary to loss of job and inability to obtain employment
Lourdes Cabrera, a high school student whose parents recently divorced, broke up with her boyfriend 2 weeks ago. She states she does not have the energy to get up in the morning and just wants to sleep all the time. She has Grade 12 examinations next week.	*Insomnia* related to inability to cope with multiple stresses
Tom Longboat states that recent shortage of firefighters has resulted in extensive overtime and frequent "double shifts" and rotations from his usual two-week 7–3 and 3–7 shifts. He states, "All I want to do is go to sleep when I get home, but I can't. I guess I'm too riled up."	*Sleep Pattern Disturbance* (*altered sleep-wake pattern*) related to frequent changes in sleep time

nursing diagnosis. These interventions may include reducing environmental distractions; promoting bedtime rituals; providing comfort measures; scheduling nursing care to provide for uninterrupted sleep periods; and teaching stress reduction, relaxation techniques, or ways to develop good sleep habits. If the sleep disturbance is the etiology of the nursing diagnosis, the nurse plans specific strategies to relieve insomnia and deal with sleep deprivation.

The Iowa Intervention Projects Nursing Interventions Classification (NIC) system is a tool for planning nursing interventions (Bulechek, Butcher, & Dochterman, 2008). Examples of NIC interventions to assist clients with sleep disturbances include the following:

- Anxiety reduction
- Environmental management: comfort
- Sleep enhancement
- Simple massage
- Simple relaxation therapy

Specific nursing activities associated with each of these interventions can be selected to meet the individual needs of the client. See the accompanying Sample Care Plan, which uses NIC interventions and selected activities.

Sample Care Plan for Rest and Sleep

ASSESSMENT DATA

Nursing Assessment

Jack Harrison is a 36-year-old police officer assigned to a high-crime police precinct. One week ago, he received a surface bullet wound to his arm. Today, he arrives at the outpatient clinic to have the wound redressed. While speaking with the nurse, Mr. Harrison mentions that he has recently been promoted to the rank of detective and has assumed new responsibilities. He states that since his promotion, he has experienced increasing difficulty falling asleep and sometimes staying asleep. He expresses concern over the danger of his occupation and his desire to do well in his new position. He complains of waking up feeling tired and irritable.

Physical Examination

Height: 185.4 cm

Weight: 85.7 kg

Temperature: 37°C

Pulse: 80 bpm

Respirations: 18/minute

Blood pressure: 144/88 mm Hg

Pale, drawn, with dark circles under eyes

Diagnostic Data

X-ray left arm: evidence of superficial soft tissue injury

Nursing Diagnosis

Sleep Pattern Disturbance related to anxiety and overstimulation (as evidenced by difficulty falling and remaining asleep, fatigue, irritability, drawn facial appearance, dark circles under eyes)

Client Goals

The client will (1) establish a satisfactory sleep and rest pattern and awaken feeling rested and (2) identify sources of anxiety and coping strategies.

(continued)

Sample Care Plan for Rest and Sleep *(continued)*

Desired Health Outcomes

1. Describes one or two factors that contribute to insomnia
2. Identifies two or three measures that induce sleep
3. Verbalizes decreased irritability and a greater sense of well-being by day 21
4. Recognizes his coping patterns by day 7
5. Identifies effective new and old coping strategies by day 10

NURSING INTERVENTIONS AND SELECTED ACTIVITIES WITH RATIONALES* *[IN ITALICS]*

Sleep Enhancement

- Determine the client's sleep and activity pattern. — *The amount of sleep an individual needs varies with lifestyle, health, and age.*
- Encourage Mr. Harrison to establish a bedtime routine to facilitate transition from wakefulness to sleep. — *Rituals and routines induce comfort, relaxation, and sleep.*
- Encourage him to stop working on projects or other stressful activities at least 1 hour before bedtime. — *Stress interferes with a person's ability to relax, rest, and sleep.*
- Teach Mr. Harrison and significant others about factors (e.g., physiological, psychological, lifestyle, frequent work shift changes, excessively long work hours, and other environmental factors) that contribute to sleep pattern disturbances. — *Knowledge of predisposing factors can enable the client to begin to control factors that inhibit sleep.*
- Discuss with Mr. Harrison and his family comfort measures, sleep-promoting techniques, and lifestyle changes that can contribute to optimal sleep. — *Knowledge of factors that affect sleep enables the client to implement changes in lifestyle and before bedtime activities.*
- Monitor bedtime food and beverage intake for items that facilitate or interfere with sleep. — *Milk and protein foods contain L-tryptophan, a precursor of serotonin, which is thought to induce and maintain sleep. Stimulants should be avoided because they inhibit sleep.*

Security Enhancement

- Discuss specific situations or individuals that threaten Mr. Harrison or his family. — *Fear is reduced when the reality of a situation is confronted in a safe environment. Awareness of factors that intensify fears enhances control.*
- Help Mr. Harrison and his family identify what factors increase their sense of security. — *Stress and anxiety can increase a person's risk of stress-related illness. If unable to remove the stressor, the individual can be taught to change ways of responding.*
- Assist him to use coping responses that have been successful in the past. — *Feelings of safety and security increase when an individual identifies previously successful ways of dealing with anxiety-provoking or fearful situations.*

Anxiety Reduction

- Create an atmosphere that facilitates trust. — *Trust is an essential first step in the therapeutic relationship.*
- Seek to understand Mr. Harrison's perspective of a stressful situation. — *Anxiety is a feeling aroused by a vague, nonspecific threat. Identifying the client's perspective will facilitate planning for the best approach to anxiety reduction.*
- Encourage verbalization of feelings, perceptions, and fears. — *Open expression of feelings facilitates identification of specific emotions, such as anger or helplessness, distorted perceptions, and unrealistic fears.*
- Help Mr. Harrison identify situations that precipitate anxiety. — *Describing what the person experienced immediately before feeling anxious, and identifying associated events, will enable the client to prevent or recognize his anxiety in order to initiate problem solving.*
- Determine the client's decision-making ability. — *Maladaptive coping mechanisms are characterized by an inability to make decisions and choices.*

EVALUATION

Goal met. Mr. Harrison acknowledges his insomnia is a somatic expression of his anxiety regarding job promotion and fear of failing. He states that talking with the police department counsellor has been helpful. He is practising relaxation techniques each night and sleeps an average of 7 hours a night. Mr. Harrison expresses a greater sense of well-being.

*Interventions and activities selected are only a sample of those suggested in the *Nursing Interventions Classification (NIC)*, by G. M. Bulechek, H. K. Butcher, and J. C. Dochterman (Eds.), 2008, St. Louis, MO: Mosby Elsevier, and should be individualized for each client.

Implementing

Nursing interventions to enhance the quantity and quality of clients' sleep involve largely nonpharmacological measures. These involve health teaching about sleep habits; support of bedtime rituals; the provision of a restful environment; specific measures to promote comfort and relaxation; and essential considerations about the use of sleep medications.

For hospitalized patients, sleep problems are often related to the hospital environment or their illness. Assisting the client to sleep in such instances can be challenging to a nurse, often involving scheduling activities, administering analgesics, and providing a supportive environment. Some interventions to reduce environmental distractions are listed in Box 37.5.

Teaching Clients about Sleep Habits

Healthy individuals need to learn the importance of rest and sleep in maintaining active and productive lifestyles. They need to learn (1) the conditions that promote sleep and those that interfere with sleep, (2) the safe use of sleep medications, (3) the effects of other prescribed medications on sleep, and (4) the effects of their disease states on sleep. See the Teaching: Wellness box for ways to promote sleep and rest.

BOX 37.5 REDUCING ENVIRONMENTAL DISTRACTIONS IN HOSPITALS

Many patients have trouble sleeping in a hospital. The nurse can try the following interventions to help:

- Close the window curtains if street lights shine through.
- Close the curtains between clients in semiprivate and larger rooms.
- Reduce or eliminate overhead lighting; provide a night-light at the bedside or in the bathroom.
- Close the door of the patient's room.
- Adhere to agency policy about times to turn off communal televisions or radios.
- Lower the ring tone of nearby telephones.
- Discontinue use of the paging system after a certain hour (e.g., 2100 hours), or reduce its volume.
- Keep required staff conversations at low levels; conduct nursing reports or other discussions in a separate area away from patient rooms.
- Wear rubber-soled shoes.
- Ensure that all cart wheels are well oiled.
- Perform only essential nursing tasks during sleeping hours.
- Pair patients with frequent nocturnal needs in the same room to minimize disturbances for other patients.

Supporting Bedtime Rituals

Most people are accustomed to bedtime rituals or presleep routines that are conducive to comfort and relaxation. Altering or eliminating such routines can affect a client's sleep. Common pre-bedtime activities of adults include taking an evening stroll, listening to music, watching television, taking a soothing bath, and praying. Children, too, are socialized into presleep routines, such as hearing a bedtime story, holding onto a favourite toy or blanket, and kissing everyone goodnight. Sleep is also usually preceded by hygiene routines, such as washing the face and hands (or bathing), brushing the teeth, and voiding.

In institutional settings, nurses can provide similar bedtime rituals—assisting with a hand and face wash, providing a massage or hot drink, plumping pillows, and providing extra blankets, as needed. Conversing about accomplishments of the day or enjoyable events, such as visits from friends, can also help relax clients and bring peace of mind.

Creating a Restful Environment

To create a restful environment, the nurse needs to reduce environmental distractions, reduce sleep interruptions, ensure a safe environment, and provide a room temperature that is satisfactory to the client.

The environment must also be safe so that the client can relax. People who are unaccustomed to narrow hospital beds may feel more secure with side rails. Additional safety measures include the following:

- Placing beds in low positions
- Using night-lights
- Placing call bells within easy reach

Promoting Comfort and Relaxation

Comfort measures are essential to help the client fall asleep and stay asleep, especially if the effects of the person's illness interfere with sleep. A concerned, caring attitude, along with the following interventions, can significantly promote client comfort and sleep:

- Provide loose-fitting cotton or flannel nightwear.
- Assist patients with hygiene routines.
- Make sure the bed linen is smooth, clean, and dry.
- Assist or encourage the patient to void before bedtime.
- Offer to provide a back massage before sleep (see Skill 37.1).
- Position dependent patients appropriately to aid muscle relaxation, and provide supportive devices to protect pressure areas.
- Schedule medications, especially diuretics, to prevent nocturnal awakenings.

TEACHING: WELLNESS

Promoting Rest and Sleep

SLEEP PATTERN

- Establish a regular bedtime and wake-up time for all days of the week to prevent disruptions in your biological rhythm. Eliminate lengthy naps or, if a daytime nap is necessary, take it at the same time each day and limit the time to 30 minutes, preferably once a day.
- Get adequate exercise during the day to reduce stress, but avoid excessive physical exertion 2 hours before bedtime.
- Avoid dealing with office work or family problems before bedtime.
- Establish a regular routine before sleep, such as reading, listening to soft music, taking a warm bath, or doing some other quiet activity you enjoy.
- When you are unable to sleep, pursue some relaxing activity until you feel drowsy.
- If you have trouble falling asleep, get up and pursue nonstrenuous activity until you feel sleepy.
- Use the bed mainly for sleep so that you associate it with sleep.

ENVIRONMENT

- Ensure appropriate lighting, temperature, and ventilation.
- Keep noise to a minimum; block out extraneous noise, as necessary, with soft music.

DIET

- Avoid heavy meals 3 hours before bedtime.
- Avoid alcohol and caffeine-containing foods and beverages (coffee, tea, chocolate) at least 4 hours before bedtime.
- Decrease fluid intake 2 to 4 hours before sleep, if necessary, to avoid the need to use the bathroom during sleeping hours.
- If a bedtime snack is necessary, consume only light carbohydrates or a milk drink. Heavy or spicy foods can cause gastrointestinal upsets that disturb sleep.

MEDICATIONS

- Use sleeping medications only as a last resort. Take them judiciously (e.g., 3 times a week at most). Use over-the-counter medications sparingly because many contain antihistamines that cause daytime drowsiness.
- Take analgesics 30 minutes before bedtime to relieve aches and pains, if necessary.
- Consult with your health-care provider about adjusting other medications that may cause insomnia.
- Take diuretics and stimulating medications early in the day.

- For patients who have pain, administer analgesics 30 minutes before sleep, or apply warm or cool applications or supportive dressings or splints to painful areas.
- For patients who have breathing problems, administer prescribed medications, such as bronchodilators, before bedtime, and position clients appropriately (e.g., semi-Fowler's position) to facilitate breathing.
- Listen to the patient's concerns, and deal with problems as they arise.

SKILL 37.1

PROVIDING A BACK MASSAGE

PURPOSES

- To relieve muscle tension
- To promote physical and mental relaxation
- To relieve insomnia

ASSESSMENT

Assess the following:

- Behaviours indicating the potential need for a back massage, such as difficulty sleeping related to tenseness or anxiety
- Whether the client wants a massage; some individuals do not enjoy a massage
- Contraindications for back massage (e.g., impaired skin integrity, neck or spinal trauma)

Planning

Ensure that you have the full amount of time available for the massage. Although the actual technique may require only about 5 minutes, the entire process should be conducted in a calm and unhurried manner.

Equipment

- Lotion or oil
- Towel for excess lotion

(continued)

SKILL 37.1

PROVIDING A BACK MASSAGE *(continued)*

IMPLEMENTATION

Preparation

Determine (1) previous assessments of the skin, (2) special lotions to be used, and (3) positions contraindicated for the client. Arrange for a quiet environment with no interruptions to promote maximum effect of the back massage.

Performance

1. Before performing the procedure, introduce yourself and verify the client's identity by using agency protocol. Explain to the client what you are going to do, why it is necessary, and how he or she can cooperate. Encourage the client to give you feedback as to the amount of pressure you are using during the back rub.
2. Perform hand hygiene.
3. Provide for client privacy.
4. Prepare the client
   - Assist the client to move to the near side of the bed within your reach and adjust the bed to a comfortable working height. **Rationale: This prevents back strain**.
   - Establish which position the client prefers. The prone position is recommended for a back rub. The side-lying position can be used if a client cannot assume the prone position.
   - Expose the back from the shoulders to the inferior sacral area. Cover the remainder of the body. **Rationale: This will prevent chilling and minimize exposure**.
5. Massage the back.
   - Pour a small amount of lotion onto the palms of your hands and hold it for a minute. The lotion bottle can also be placed in a bath basin filled with warm water. **Rationale: Back rub preparations tend to feel uncomfortably cold to people. Warming the solution facilitates client comfort**.
   - Use your palm and begin in the sacral area, using smooth, circular strokes (referred to as effleurage).
   - Move your hands up the centre of the back and then over both scapulae.
   - Massage in a circular motion over the scapulae.
   - Move your hands down the sides of the back.
   - Massage the areas over the right and left iliac crests (see ❶).
   - Apply firm, continuous pressure without breaking contact with the client's skin.

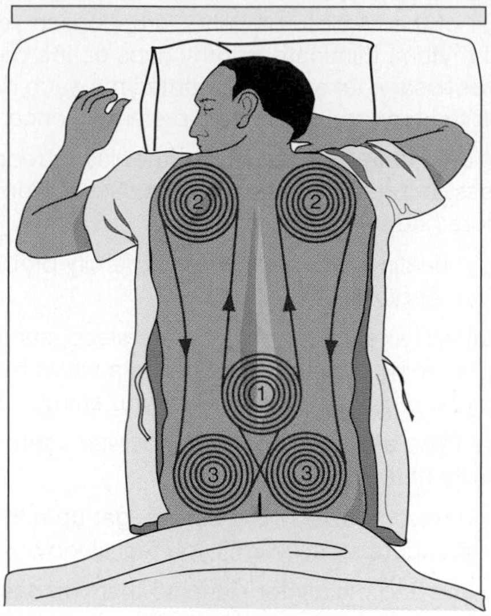

❶ A back rub pattern

   - Repeat above for 3 to 5 minutes obtaining more lotion as necessary.
   - While massaging the back, assess for skin redness and areas of decreased circulation.
   - Pat dry any excess lotion with a towel.

Variation: Petrissage

Petrissage (kneading or gently grasping tissues of the skin, subcutaneous tissue, and muscle between the fingers) of the back and shoulders of the client. Use with caution with clients who have bleeding disorders or who are on anticoagulant therapy.

- Petrissage first up the vertebral column and then over the entire back. *Petrissage is stimulating, especially if done quickly and with firm pressure.*
- Observe the client carefully to ensure that petrissage does not cause pain or discomfort. If the client grimaces or withdraws from the touch, ease the kneading pressure.
- End the massage with long movements, and tell the client you are finishing.

Variation: Effleurage and petrissage of the upper back and shoulders.

This area often experiences the most tension.

6. Document the massage and your observations.

EVALUATION

Compare the client's current response to his or her previous response. Is there a positive client outcome, such as increased relaxation because of the back massage?

People of any age, but especially older adults, are unable to sleep well if they feel cold. Changes in circulation, metabolism, and body tissue density reduce the older person's ability to generate and conserve heat. To compound this problem, hospital gowns have short sleeves and are made of thin fabric. Sheets also are often made of polyester, rather than a warm fabric, such as cotton flannel. Interventions to keep older adult clients warm during sleep are shown in Box 37.6.

Emotional stress obviously interferes with a person's ability to relax, rest, and sleep, and inability to sleep further aggravates feelings of tension. Sleep rarely occurs until a person is relaxed. Relaxation techniques can be encouraged as part of the nightly routine. Slow, deep breathing for a few minutes followed by slow, rhythmic contraction and relaxation of muscles can alleviate tension and induce calm. Imagery, meditation, and yoga can also be taught. These techniques are discussed in Chapters 15 and 47.

BOX 37.6 HELPING OLDER PATIENTS KEEP WARM IN BED

Try these suggestions to help older adults stay warm while sleeping:

- Provide a warmed bath blanket, if possible.
- Use cotton flannel sheets, if possible, for warmth. Alternatively, apply thermal blankets between the sheet and bedspread.
- Encourage the patient to wear his or her own clothing, such as a flannel nightgown or pyjamas, a loose-fitting jogging suit, nonconstricting thermal socks, leg warmers, long underwear, sleeping cap, or a sweater, or to use a favourite quilt or blanket.

Safely Enhancing Sleep with Medications

Sleep medications often prescribed on a prn (as needed) basis for clients include the sedative-hypnotics, which induce sleep, and antianxiety drugs or tranquilizers (benzodiazepines), which decrease anxiety and tension. When prn sleep medications are ordered in institutional settings, the nurse is responsible for making decisions with the client about when to administer them. These medications should be administered only with complete knowledge of their actions and effects and only when indicated. These medications are contraindicated in pregnant women because of their associated risk of congenital anomalies and in nursing mothers because the medication could be excreted in breast milk. New, shorter-acting benzodiazepines should be considered if a medication is needed because they cause less daytime sedation. Drug hangover is particularly problematic in older adults or those with reduced clearance capacity. Whenever possible, nonpharmacological interventions to induce and maintain sleep, discussed earlier, are the preferred interventions.

Both nurses and clients need to be aware of the actions, effects, and risks of the specific medication prescribed. Although medications vary in their activity and effects, considerations include the following:

- Sedative-hypnotic medications produce a general central nervous system (CNS) depression and an unnatural sleep; REM or NREM sleep is altered to some extent and daytime drowsiness and a morning hangover effect may occur.
- Antianxiety medications decrease levels of arousal by facilitating the action of neurons in the central nervous system that suppress responsiveness to stimulation.
- Sleep medications vary in their onset and duration of action and will impair waking function as long as they are chemically active. Some medication effects can last many hours beyond the time that the client's perception of daytime drowsiness and impaired psychomotor skills have disappeared. Clients need to be cautioned about such effects and about driving or handling machinery while the drug is in their system.
- Sleep medications affect REM sleep more than NREM sleep. Clients need to be informed that 1 or 2 nights of increased dreaming (REM rebound) is usual after the drug is discontinued.
- Initial doses of medications should be low and increases added gradually, depending on the client's response. Older adults, in particular, are susceptible to side effects because of metabolic changes; they need to be closely monitored for changes in mental alertness and coordination. Clients need to be instructed to take the smallest effective dose and then only for a few nights or intermittently as required.
- Regular use of any sleep medication can lead to tolerance over time (e.g., 4 weeks) and rebound insomnia. In some instances, this may lead clients to increase the dosage or complement the drug with alcohol. Clients must be cautioned about developing a pattern of drug dependency.
- Abrupt cessation of *barbiturate* sedative-hypnotics can create withdrawal symptoms, such as restlessness, tremors, weakness, insomnia, increased heart rate, seizures, convulsions, and even death. Long-term users need to taper withdrawal under the supervision of a specialist.

Evaluating

Using data collected during care and the desired outcomes developed during the planning stage as a guide, the nurse judges whether client goals and outcomes have been achieved. Data collection may include (1) observations of the duration of the client's sleep and the presence

TABLE 37.2 Evaluation Goals and Outcomes: Sleep Pattern Disturbances

Goal	Examples of Desired Outcomes
Develop a sleep-wake pattern that ensures sufficient energy for daily activities	Identifies possible causes of sleeping problem
	Identifies stress-relieving measures that enhance ability to fall asleep
	Uses planned relaxation techniques before bedtime
	Falls asleep within 20 to 30 minutes of going to bed
	Sleeps specified number of hours per night or for longer intervals between nursing care functions
	Reports feelings of being rested or refreshed after waking
Decrease signs of sleep deprivation	Absence of signs of sleep deprivation, such as excessive yawning, circles under eyes, and slow responses
	Demonstrates more motivation for activity and animation in activity
Increase physical and psychological comfort level before and during sleep	Reports satisfaction with pain control measures and positioning techniques
	Reports satisfaction with physical surroundings
	Reports effectiveness of bedtime rituals and relaxation techniques (e.g., backrubs, soft music, warm soothing bath) in reducing anxiety

of signs of REM and NREM sleep, and (2) questions about how the client feels on awakening or about the effectiveness of specific interventions, such as the use of relaxation techniques, adherence to a consistent sleep-wake cycle, or the ingestion of milk products before bedtime. Examples of client goals and related outcomes are shown in Table 37.2.

If the desired outcomes are *not* achieved, the nurse, client, and support people, if appropriate, should explore the reasons why, which may include answers to the following questions:

- Were etiological factors correctly identified?
- Has the client's physical condition or medication therapy changed?
- Did the client comply with instructions about establishing a regular sleep-wake pattern?
- Did the client avoid ingesting caffeine?
- Were all possible measures taken to provide a restful environment for the client?
- Were bedtime rituals supported?
- Were the comfort and relaxation measures effective?

Case Study 37

While making rounds at 1:00 a.m., you note that Jo Su-Mi, a 23-year-old woman recovering from surgery, is awake and watching television. Concerned that Ms. Su-Mi may be experiencing too much pain to sleep, you question her about how she is feeling. She states that she is not having pain; she just cannot sleep. On further questioning, you learn that she has a pattern of sleepless nights. She explains that she usually goes to bed by 11:00 p.m. after exercising but frequently has difficulty falling asleep. Sometimes, she listens to the radio or watches TV until she is able to sleep. She usually has a soft drink at bedtime but avoids coffee or tea because it keeps her awake. Ms. Su-Mi admits that she is frequently sleepy during the day and has considered getting a prescription for a sleeping pill from her doctor so that she can develop a better sleep routine.

Critical Thinking Questions

1. Explain why keeping a sleep diary might be beneficial for Ms. Su-Mi.
2. What further information would be helpful to obtain from her about her sleep problem?
3. What suggestions can you make that may help her develop better sleep habits when she returns home?
4. What are the most common problems that interfere with clients' ability to sleep while hospitalized?

After working through these questions, go to the MyNursingLab at **http://www.mynursinglab.com** to check your answers.

KEY TERMS

rest
sleep
homeostatic function (homeostatic drive)
circadian rhythm
sleep architecture
NREM sleep
REM sleep
slow-wave sleep (SWS)
nocturnal emissions
primary sleep disorders
secondary sleep disorders
parasomnias
insomnia
hypersomnia
narcolepsy
sleep apnea
periodic limb movements of sleep
restless legs syndrome
sleep deprivation
polysomnography

CHAPTER HIGHLIGHTS

- Sleep is a naturally occurring altered-consciousness state in which a person's perception of and reaction to the environment are decreased.
- The sleep cycle is controlled by specialized areas in the brain stem and is affected by the individual's circadian rhythm.
- Rest and sleep are restorative, protective, and energy conserving.
- During a normal night's sleep, an adult has four to six sleep cycles, each with NREM (quiet) and REM (rapid-eye-movement) sleep.
- NREM sleep consists of four stages, progressing from stage I, very light sleep, to stage IV, deep sleep. NREM sleep constitutes most of a sleep cycle.
- REM sleep recurs about every 90 minutes and is often associated with dreaming.
- The ratio of NREM to REM sleep varies with age.
- Many factors can affect sleep, including health and illness, environment, lifestyle, emotional stress, alcohol and stimulants, diet, smoking, motivation, and medications.
- Common sleep disorders include insomnia, hypersomnia, narcolepsy, sleep apnea, periodic limb movements, and parasomnias, such as somnambulism, talking during sleep, nocturnal enuresis, and bruxism.
- Assessment of a client's sleep includes obtaining a sleep history, reviewing a sleep diary, conducting a physical examination to detect signs of sleep deprivation, and reviewing diagnostic studies.
- Nursing responsibilities to help clients sleep include (1) teaching clients ways to enhance sleep and rest, (2) supporting bedtime rituals, (3) creating a restful environment, (4) promoting comfort and relaxation, and (5) using prescribed sleep medications.
- Nonpharmacological interventions to induce and maintain sleep are the preferred interventions.

ASSESS YOUR LEARNING

1. Mr. Janssen is 34 years old, married with two children, and has been diagnosed with multiple sclerosis. The reason for his hospitalization is an acute exacerbation-remitting episode. Mr. Janssen has been up in his chair visiting with his family for 3 hours and is visibly fatigued. How can the nurse promote a balance between rest and activity for Mr. Janssen?

a. Inform the family when the unit rest periods are scheduled.
b. Insist that Mr. Janssen abide by the scheduled rest periods.
c. Wait until Mr. Janssen's family leaves the unit to discuss rest periods with him.
d. Discuss the importance of rest periods with Mr. Janssen and his family.

2. Gamma-aminobutyric acid (GABA) is believed to have what role in sleep-wake cycles?

a. It lessens the response to sensory stimulation.
b. It deactivates the neurons of the reticular activating system.
c. It triggers the release of melatonin, a sleep-inducing hormone.
d. It stimulates the brain at the end of the sleep period, causing the person to awaken.

3. Sarah Horowitz, 35 years old and 16 weeks pregnant, was admitted to emergency with vaginal bleeding. She has been in the observation area and has been sleeping for the past hour and a half. Her vital signs have been stable, and the bleeding has stopped. When you check in on Sarah, you notice that her eyes are closed but moving in short, sharp bursts; her respiratory rate is 14 breaths/min but irregular; the monitor shows that her heart rate is fluctuating between 64 and 82 bpm. What should you do next?

a. Gently rouse the patient and assess vital signs.
b. Prepare the emergency cart and alert the medical team.
c. Immediately wake the patient fully and assess vital signs.
d. Do not disturb the patient and continue with observations and vital signs q1 to q2h.

4. A 74-year-old male patient is postop day 1 for prostate surgery. At 2 p.m., you notice that he is having his second nap of the day. You allow the patient to continue to sleep for which of the following reasons?
   a. Individuals need more total sleep as they age.
   b. Older patients who nap are usually depressed.
   c. Patients need more sleep than normal following surgery.
   d. The patient will need to be given a sleeping medication at night.

5. Emily Bruin, aged 15 years, has come to your health-care centre. She is in Grade 10, has a full course load, enjoys volunteer work, and is on the school hockey team. She looks pale, has dark circles under her eyes, and states that she feels exhausted and irritable most of the time. Which factor is likely contributing most to Emily's sleep disturbance?
   a. She is a straight A student.
   b. She has hockey practice Mondays and Thursdays from 8 p.m. to 9 p.m.
   c. She is a regular Saturday morning volunteer at the local Humane Society.
   d. She drinks two large coffees with double sugar, double cream every morning.

6. Kaki Ashoona, a 68-year-old Inuit woman, has been flown in from Cape Dorset to undergo a hysterectomy to treat a localized uterine cancer. Following surgery, Kaki is assigned to a four-bed room. The interpreter relays that Kaki is having considerable difficulty falling asleep at night. The nurse recognizes that further teaching to enhance optimal sleep health is needed when Kaki does which of the following?
   a. Takes an analgesic if the pain is "really bad"
   b. Confirms her discharge plans with the interpreter
   c. Asks for an extra blanket and wears a wool cap at night
   d. Has a cranberry bun and a small cup of wintergreen tea at bedtime

7. Pritam Singh Sageer is attending an evening concert at the Sikh Pavilion at Winnipeg's Folklorama. The lights lower and within minutes, he is snoring loudly. He snorts, gasps, and then awakens when shaken by his wife. Mr. Sageer is 54 years old, is 173 cm tall, and weighs 95 kg. You suspect that Mr. Sageer may have obstructive sleep apnea. Which one of the following health assessments would support this condition?
   a. A short, thick neck and a history of hypertension
   b. Difficulty falling asleep and a history of rheumatic fever
   c. Sudden loss of muscle tone when emotional and a history of sleepwalking
   d. Frequent evening migraine headaches and a history of irritable bowel syndrome

8. Laura DeLaat is a 40-year-old surgical nurse who has come to your sleep centre because of difficulty with her sleep-wake patterns. Laura works rotating day and night shifts, is a single parent of two teenage girls, and has an ailing mother who lives with their family. Following your assessment, you discuss several sleep health practices with Laura. Which statement suggests that Laura needs additional sleep health education?
   a. "I will take the bus home when I work nights."
   b. "If I work overtime, I can make up the sleep on my days off."
   c. "Regular daytime exercise will help reduce stress and make it easier for me to sleep."
   d. "I need to forward my phone to the answering machine and turn down the ring tone when I sleep days."

9. Canming Ma is a 79-year-old man who attended the Ottawa Valley Seniors' Health information session. He says that he has been taking the muscle relaxants that the doctor prescribed for his restless legs and asks you if there is anything else that he can do to help himself sleep. Which of the following is your best response?
   a. "Regular medication is the only treatment for RLS at this time."
   b. "Exercise, of any type, should be avoided to minimize strain on the leg muscles."
   c. "Caffeine can exacerbate RLS and should be reduced or eliminated from the diet."
   d. "Sleeping with the head of the bed raised will enhance blood flow to the feet and reduce symptoms."

10. Rachel and Justin Peters are the exhausted parents of Grace, a 7-month-old baby girl. Grace is healthy and is gaining weight as expected. Rachel gets up four times each night to briefly breastfeed the baby, and then Justin changes the baby and walks her to sleep. Rachel is pale and teary, and Justin admits that he is irritable and that he has difficulty concentrating at work. The nurse should advise the couple to do which of the following?
    a. Take turns sleeping with Grace to allow each to get more rest.
    b. Put Grace in her crib at bedtime when she is drowsy but not asleep.
    c. Provide Grace with a bottle of formula at night to drink if she awakens.
    d. Seek psychiatric counselling immediately as Rachel is suffering from postpartum depression.

After working through these questions, go to the MyNursingLab at ***http://www.mynursinglab.com*** *to check your answers and see explanations.*

SUGGESTED READINGS

Cuellar, N. G., Rogers, A., Hisghman, V., & Volpe, S. L. (2007). Assessment and treatment of sleep disorders in the older adult. *Geriatric Nursing, 28*(4), 254–264.

The authors provide an overview of three common sleep disorders (insomnia, sleep apnea, restless legs syndrome) in the older adult, discuss the impact on sleep for frequently prescribed medications and treatment options, and identify useful tools for sleep assessment.

Kamel, N. S., & Gammack, J. K. (2006). Insomnia in the elderly: Cause, approach, and treatment. *American Journal of Medicine, 119,* 463–469.

The authors review common causes of insomnia in the older adult and provide a detailed discussion of pharmacological and nonpharmacological treatment options for this disorder.

Kryger, M. H., Roth, T., & Dement, W. C. (Eds.). (2005). *Principle and practice of sleep medicine* (4th ed.). Philadelphia, PA: ElsevierSaunders.

This multi-authored, internationally recognized clinical resource provides a comprehensive overview of all aspects of sleep, sleep-wake disorders, diagnostic and measurement approaches, and pharmacological and nonpharmacological treatments.

Lower, J., Bonsack, C., & Guion, J. (2003). Peace and quiet. *Nursing Management, 34*(4), 40A–40D.

The authors reviewed factors that make it difficult for clients to rest in hospitals and steps that are needed to help provide a healing environment (e.g., uninterrupted sleep, massage, music). They describe their vision, implementation, and outcomes of providing quiet time between 2 p.m. and 4 p.m. for clients in two ICUs.

Ward, T. M., Rankin, S., & Lee, K. A. (2007). Caring for children with sleep problems. *Journal of Pediatric Nursing, 22*(4), 283–296.

The importance of sleep to the health and well-being of the child and family are described. Specific sleep problems common in children are discussed and screening tools and healthy sleep guidelines are identified.

WEBLINKS

Canadian Sleep Society

http://www.css.to/sleep/index.htm

This is an organization for health-care professionals and researchers in sleep and circadian rhythms. It also contains some information for lay people, including downloadable brochures and a list of sleep specialists willing to answer questions.

Canadian Lung Association

http://www.lung.ca/diseases-maladies/apnea-apnee_e.php

This website provides an interesting section on sleep apnea.

Alberta Sleep Apnea Society

http://www.sleep-apnea.ab.ca

This is a site for people wanting to learn more about sleep apnea and to join a support or advocacy group.

National Sleep Foundation

http://www.sleepfoundation.org

The U.S. foundation's website includes general sleep information for the lay public, such as self-assessment guides.

Mayo Clinic

http://www.mayoclinic.com

This informative site provides reputable and lay-friendly descriptions of symptoms, diagnostics, medical treatments, and self-care practices for a variety of sleep-related and other health conditions.

REFERENCES

Baker, F. C., & Driver, H. S. (2007). Circadian rhythms, sleep, and the menstrual cycle. *Sleep Medicine, 8,* 613–622.

Berger, A. M., Parker, K. P., Young-McCaughan, S., Mallory, G. A., Barsevick, A. M., Beck, S. L., et al. (2005). Sleep wake disturbances in people with cancer and their caregivers: State of the science. *Oncology Nursing Forum, 32*(6), E98–E26.

Bulechek, G. M., Butcher, H. K., & Dochterman, J. C. (Eds.). (2008). *Nursing interventions classification (NIC).* St. Louis, MO: Mosby Elsevier.

Caples, S. M., Garcia-Touchard, A., & Somers, V. K. (2007). Sleep-disordered breathing and cardiovascular risk. *Sleep, 30*(3), 291–303.

Carmona, R. H. (2004). *Text of remarks. Opening remarks presented at the Frontiers of Knowledge in Sleep & Sleep Disorders: Opportunities for improving health and quality of life.* National Institutes of Health, Bethesda, MD. Retrieved November 8, 2006, from http://www.nhlbi.nih.gov/meetings/slp_front.htm

Fletcher, P. C., & Hirdes, J. P. (2005). Risk factor for accidental injuries within senior citizens' homes: Analysis of the Canadian Survey on Ageing and Independence. *Journal of Gerontological Nursing, 31*(2), 49–57.

Gibson, E. S., Powles, A. C. P., Thabane, L., O'Brien, S., Molnar, D. S., Trajanovic, N., et al. (2006). "Sleepiness" is serious in adolescence: Two surveys of 3235 Canadian students. *BMC Public Health, 6,* 116. Retrieved July 6, 2008, from http://www.biomedcentral.com/1471-2458/6/116

Hall, W. A., Clauson, M., Carty, E. M., Janssen, P. A., & Saunders, R. A. (2006). Effects on parents of an intervention to resolve infant behavioral sleep problems. *Pediatric Nursing, 32*(3), 243–250.

Hunt, C. E., & Hauck, F. R. (2006). Sudden infant death syndrome. *Canadian Medical Association Journal, 174*(13), 1861–1868.

Institute of Medicine. (2006). *Sleep disorders and sleep deprivation: An unmet public health problem.* Washington, DC: Author.

Jefferson, C. D, Drake, C. L., Scofield, H. M., Myers, E., McClure, T., Roehrs, T., et al. (2005). Sleep hygiene practices in a population-based sample of insomniacs, *Sleep, 28*(5), 611–615.

Koch, S., Haesler, E. Tiziani, A., & Wilson, J. (2006). Effectiveness of sleep management strategies for residents of aged care facilities: Findings of a systematic review. *Journal of Clinical Nursing, 15*(10), 1267–1275.

Laird, G. (2007). *Shelter. Homelessness in a growth economy: Canada's 21st-century paradox.* Calgary: Sheldon Chumir Foundation for Ethics in Leadership.

Lockley, S. W., Berger, L. K., Ayas, N. T., Rothschild, J. M., Czeisler, C. A., Landrigan, C. P., et al. (2007). Effects of health care provider work hours and sleep deprivation on safety and performance. *Joint Commission Journal on Quality and Patient Safety, 33*(Suppl.), 7–18.

Morgenthaler, T., Kramer, M., Alessi, C., Friedman, L., Boehlecke, B., Brown, T., et al. (2006). Practice parameters for the psychological and behavioral treatment of insomnia: An update. An American Academy of Sleep medicine report. *Sleep, 29*(11), 1415–1419.

Nagel, C. L., Markie, M. G., Richards, K. C., & Taylor, J. L. (2003). Sleep promotion in hospitalized elderly. *Medsurg Nursing, 12*(5), 279–290.

NANDA International. (2007). *Nursing diagnoses: Definitions and classification, 2007–2008.* Philadelphia, PA: Author.

National Sleep Foundation. (2000). *2000 sleep in America poll.* Retrieved February 11, 2008, from http://www.sleepfoundation.org/NSF

National Sleep Foundation. (2007a). *Children and sleep.* Retrieved May 5, 2007, from http://www.sleepfoundation.org/site/c.huIXKjM0IxF/b.2418873/k.B9AD/Children_and_Sleep.htm

National Sleep Foundation. (2007b). *Teens and sleep.* Retrieved May 5, 2007, from http://www.sleepfoundation.org/site/c.huIXKjM0IxF/b.2418863/k.94BD/Teens_and_Sleep.htm

Nicolàs, A., Aizipitarte, E, Iruarrizaga, A., Vàzquez, M., Margall, A., & Asiain, C. (2008). Perceptions of night-time sleep by surgical patients in an intensive care unit. *Nursing in Critical Care, 13*(1), 25–33.

Ohida, T., Kaneita, Y., Osaki, Y., Harano, S., Tanihata, T., Takemura, S., et al. (2007). Is passive smoking associated with sleep disturbance among pregnant women? *Sleep, 30*(9), 1155–1161.

Parish, J. M., Adam, T., & Facchiano, L. (2007). Relationship of metabolic syndrome and obstructive sleep apnea. *Journal of Clinical Sleep Medicine, 3*(5), 467–472.

Scott, L. D., Hwang, W. T., Rogers, A. E., Nysse, T., Dean, G. E., & Dinges, D. F. (2007). The relationship between nurse work schedules, sleep duration, and drowsy driving. *Sleep, 30*(12), 1801–1807.

Shott, S. R., Amin, R., Chini, B., Heubi, C., Hotze, S., & Askers, R. (2006). Obstructive sleep apnea: Should all children with Down syndrome be tested? *Archives of Otolaryngology, Head and Neck Surgery, 132*(4), 432–436.

Voyer, P., Verreault, R., Cappeliez, P., Holmes, D., & Nkogho Mengue, P. (2005). Symptoms of psychological distress among older adults in Canadian long-term care centres. *Aging & Mental Health, 9*(6), 542–554.

Wetter, D. W., & Young, T. B. (1994). The relation between cigarette smoking and sleep disturbance. *Preventive Medicine, 23*(3), 328–334.

Chapter 38

Activity and Exercise

A strong, well-developed body of literature supports the benefits of activity and exercise in maintaining health status and in preventing the development of such illnesses as type 2 diabetes, heart disease, cancer, and respiratory illnesses. Canadians who are physically active report less chronic illness, improved mental health, greater life satisfaction, and less stress both at home and at work (Canadian Fitness and Lifestyle Research Institute [CFLRI], 2006). Unfortunately, only about half of Canadians perform regular daily activity, and those who are sedentary, especially men, are more likely to be obese (Statistics Canada, 2005). It is estimated that inactivity costs the health-care system at least $2.1 billion a year in direct health-care costs and leads to an economic drain of approximately $5.3 billion a year (Katzmarzyk & Janssen, 2004). Although the majority of Canadians know about the benefits of activity, such barriers as work commitments and tight deadlines and lack of safe roads or sidewalks to perform physical activity, such as walking or bicycling, are cited (CFLRI, 2006). See the Reflect on Primary Health Care for a creative solution.

OBJECTIVES

After studying this chapter, you should be able to

1. Identify benefits of general fitness and exercise
2. Describe four basic elements of normal movement
3. Differentiate isotonic, isometric, isokinetic, aerobic, and anaerobic exercises
4. Compare the effects of exercise and immobility on body systems
5. Identify seven factors influencing a person's body alignment and activity
6. Assess activity-exercise patterns, alignment, mobility capabilities and limitations, activity tolerance, and potential problems related to immobility
7. Develop nursing diagnoses and outcomes related to activity, exercise, and mobility problems
8. Use safe practices when positioning, moving, lifting, and ambulating clients

REFLECT ON PRIMARY HEALTH CARE

A nurse and a psychologist demonstrated *intersectoral collaboration* when they worked with the management of a local shopping mall in an urban centre. They offered a walkabout program three times a week to older adults, people with physical disabilities, and new parents as a way of socializing, staying fit, and getting support during winter months, when many would otherwise be isolated or lack any physical activity because of a fear of falling on the slippery sidewalks. Find out whether any creative programs are available to people in your community. If not, what *health-promotion* activities related to physical activity and exercise are available? Do these resources address the special needs of the very young, the older adult, or the person with a physical disability?

In 2005, the Integrated Pan-Canadian Healthy Living Strategy set the goal of increasing by 20% the proportion of Canadians who participate in regular physical activity based on 30 minutes/day of moderate to vigorous activity. The simple messages, such as *Every Day for Life! Be Active, Your Way*, or *Age Is No Barrier*, espoused by the Public Health Agency of Canada say that becoming active can be relatively easy and incorporated into everyone's daily lifestyle.

An **activity-exercise pattern** refers to a person's routine of exercise, activity, leisure, and recreation. It includes (1) activities of daily living (ADLs) that require energy expenditure, such as hygiene, cooking, shopping, eating, working, and maintaining the home; and (2) the type, quality, and quantity of exercise, including sports. The *Handbook for Canada's Physical Activity Guide to Healthy Active Living* (Public Health Agency of Canada, 2003) recommends building physical activity into all aspects of daily life. **Active living** refers to adding physical activity to the time spent at home, at work, at school, at play.

Mobility, the ability to move freely, easily, rhythmically, and purposefully in the environment, is an essential part of living. People must move to protect themselves from trauma and to meet their basic needs. Mobility is vital to independence; a fully immobilized person is vulnerable and dependent physically on others.

People often define their health and physical fitness by their activity because mental well-being and the effectiveness of body functioning depend largely on their mobility status. For example, when a person is upright, the lungs expand more easily, peristalsis (intestinal activity) is more effective, and the kidneys are able to empty completely. In addition, motion is essential for the proper functioning of bones and muscles.

The ability to move also influences self-esteem and body image, both components of self-concept. For most people, self-esteem depends on a sense of independence and a feeling of usefulness or being needed. People with mobility impairments may feel helpless and burdensome to others, and their ability to work and earn a living may be compromised. Body image can be altered by paralysis, amputations, or any motor impairment. The reaction of others to impaired mobility can also alter self-esteem and body image significantly.

Normal Movement

Normal movement and stability are the result of an intact musculoskeletal system, an intact nervous system, and intact inner ear structures responsible for equilibrium. Body movement requires coordinated muscle activity and neurological integration. It involves four basic elements: body alignment (posture), joint mobility, balance (stability), and coordinated movement.

Alignment and Posture

Proper body alignment and posture bring body parts into line in a manner that promotes optimal balance and maximal body function in whatever position the client assumes: standing, sitting, or lying down. The line of gravity and the body's centre of gravity influence standing alignment and balance. A person maintains balance as long as the **line of gravity** (an imaginary vertical line drawn through the body's centre of gravity) passes through the **centre of gravity** (the point at which all of the body's mass is centred) and the **base of support** (the foundation on which the body rests). In humans, the usual line of gravity begins at the top of the head and falls between the shoulders, through the trunk, slightly anterior to the sacrum, and between the weight-bearing joints and base of support (Figure 38.1). For a person in the upright position, the centre of gravity is located in the centre of the pelvis, approximately midway between the umbilicus and the symphysis pubis. For greatest balance and stability, a standing adult must centre body weight symmetrically along the line of gravity. Greater stability and balance are provided in the sitting or lying position than in the standing position. The feet of the chair or bed form a considerably wider base of support, the centre of gravity is lower, and the line of gravity is less mobile.

When the body is well aligned, strain on the joints, muscles, tendons, or ligaments is minimized and the internal structures and organs are supported. People are usually unaware of the functions of the abdominal and skeletal muscles that function almost continuously, making tiny adjustments that enable an erect or seated posture despite the endless downward pull of gravity. Sustained contraction of the muscles supporting this upright position is called **postural tonus**. The extensor muscles, often referred to as the *antigravity* muscles, carry the major load.

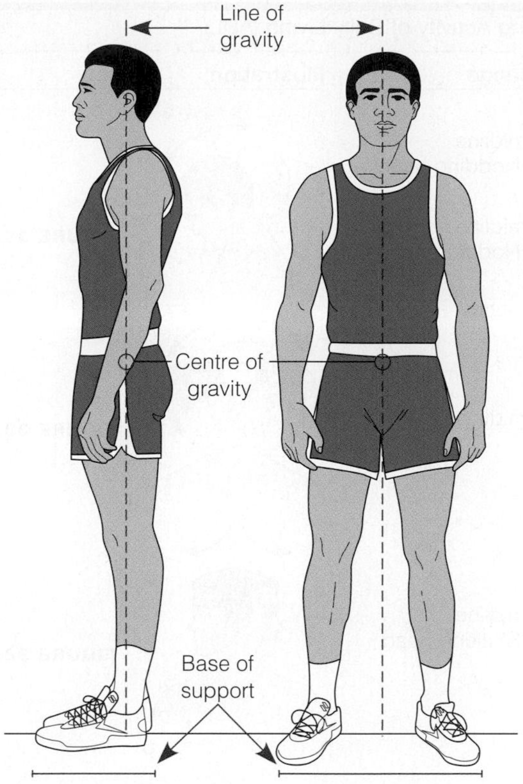

FIGURE 38.1 The centre of gravity and the line of gravity influence standing alignment.

Proper body alignment enhances lung expansion and promotes efficient circulatory, respiratory, renal, and gastrointestinal functions. Conversely, poor body alignment detracts from a pleasing appearance and affects an individual's health adversely. A person's posture is one criterion for assessing general health, physical fitness, and attractiveness. Posture reflects the mood, self-esteem, and personality of an individual.

Joint Mobility

Joints are the functional units of the musculoskeletal system. The bones of the skeleton articulate at the joints and most of the skeletal muscles attach to the bones at the joint. Muscles are categorized according to the type of joint movement they produce on contraction. Muscles are, therefore, called flexors, extensors, internal rotators, and the like. The flexor muscles are stronger than the extensor muscles. Thus, when a person is inactive, the joints are pulled into a flexed (bent) position. If this tendency is not counteracted with exercise and position changes, the muscles permanently shorten, and the joint becomes fixed in a flexed position (contracture). The types of joint movement are shown in Table 38.1.

The **range of motion (ROM)** of a joint is the maximum movement that is possible for that joint. Joint ROM varies from individual to individual and is determined by genetic makeup, developmental patterns, the presence or absence of disease, and the amount of physical activity in which the person normally engages. Table 38.2 shows the various joint movements and the usual ROMs.

Balance

The mechanisms involved in maintaining balance and posture are complex and beyond the scope of this book. Mechanisms of equilibrium (sense of balance) respond, frequently without our awareness, to various head movements. The equilibrium sense depends on informational

TABLE 38.1 Types of Joint Movements

Movement	Action	Movement	Action
Flexion	Decreasing the angle of the joint (e.g., bending the elbow)	Eversion	Turning the sole of the foot outward by moving the ankle joint
Extension	Increasing the angle of the joint (e.g., straightening the arm at the elbow)	Inversion	Turning the sole of the foot inward by moving the ankle joint
Hyperextension	Overextension or straightening of a joint (e.g., bending the head backward)	Pronation	Moving the bones of the forearm so that the palm of the hand faces downward when held in front of the body
Abduction	Movement of the bone away from the midline of the body	Supination	Moving the bones of the forearm so that the palm of the hand faces upward when held in front of the body
Adduction	Movement of the bone toward the midline of the body	Protraction	Moving a part of the body forward in the same plane parallel to the ground
Rotation	Movement of the bone around its central axis	Retraction	Moving a part of the body backward in the same plane parallel to the ground
Circumduction	Movement of the distal part of the bone in a circle while the proximal end remains fixed		

TABLE 38.2 Selected Joint Movements and Examples of Corresponding Activity of Daily Living (ADL)

Body Part—Type of Joint/Movement	Normal Range	Illustration
Neck—Pivot Joint		
Flexion. Move the head from the upright midline position forward so that the chin rests on the chest (Figure 38.2).	45° from midline Example: Nodding head "yes"	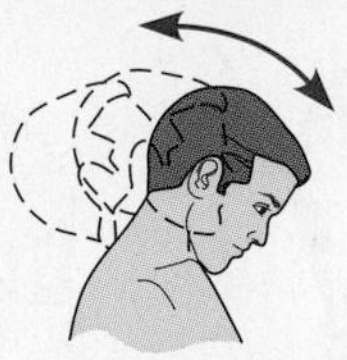 **FIGURE 38.2**
Extension. Move the head from the flexed position to the upright position (Figure 38.2).	45° from midline Example: Nodding head "yes"	
Hyperextension. Move the head from the upright position back as far as possible.	45° from midline	
Lateral flexion. Move the head laterally to the right and left shoulders (Figure 38.3).	40° from midline	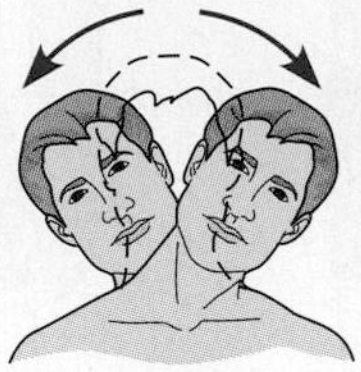 **FIGURE 38.3**
Rotation. Turn the face as far as possible to the right and left (Figure 38.4).	70° from midline Example: Shaking head "no"	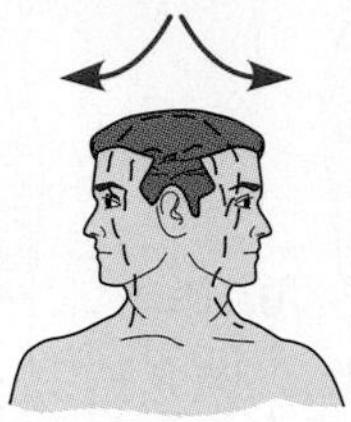 **FIGURE 38.4**
Shoulder—Ball-and-Socket Joint		
Flexion. Raise each arm from a position by the side forward and upward to a position beside the head (Figure 38.5).	180° from the side Example: Reaching to turn on overhead light	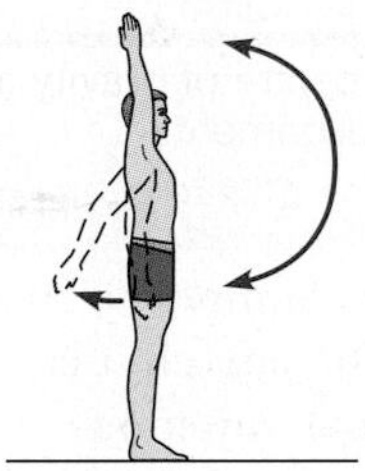 **FIGURE 38.5**
Extension. Move each arm from a vertical position beside the head forward and down to a resting position at the side of the body (Figure 38.5).	180° from vertical position beside the head	
Hyperextension. Move each arm from a resting side position to behind the body (Figure 38.5).	50° from side position	
Abduction. Move each arm laterally from a resting position at the sides to a side position above the head, palm of the hand away from the head (Figure 38.6).	180° Example: Reaching to bedside stand on same side of bed as arm	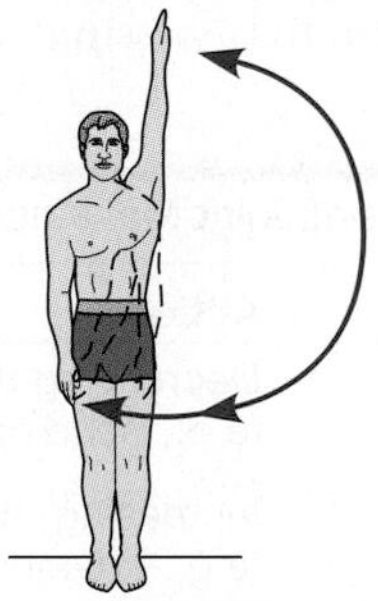 **FIGURE 38.6**
Adduction (anterior). Move each arm from a position beside the head downward laterally and across the front of the body as far as possible (Figure 38.6).	50° Example: Reaching across body toward opposite side of bed	
Circumduction. Move each arm forward, up, back, and down in a full circle (Figure 38.7).	360°	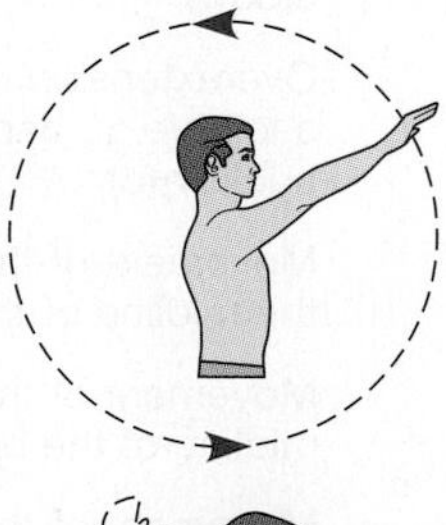 **FIGURE 38.7**
External rotation. With each arm held out to the side at shoulder level and the elbow bent to a right angle, fingers pointing down, move the arm upward so that the fingers point up (Figure 38.8).	90° Example: Reaching over opposite shoulder to scratch upper back	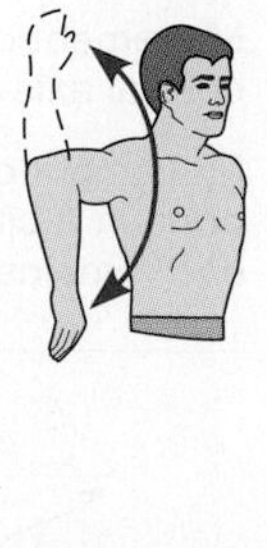 **Figure 38.8**
Internal rotation. With each arm held out to the side at shoulder level and the elbow bent to a right angle, fingers pointing up, bring the arm forward and down so that the fingers point down (Figure 38.8).	90° Example: Reaching to scratch same side lower back	

(continued)

TABLE 38.2 Selected Joint Movements and Examples of Corresponding Activity of Daily Living (ADL) *(continued)*

Body Part—Type of Joint/Movement	Normal Range	Illustration
Elbow—Hinge Joint		
Flexion. Bring each lower arm forward and upward so that the hand is at the shoulder (Figure 38.9).	150° Example: Eating, bathing, shaving	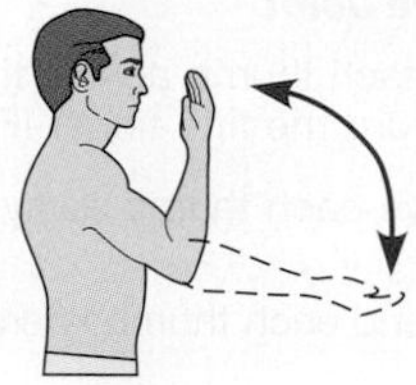 **Figure 38.9**
Extension. Bring each lower arm forward and downward, straightening the arm (Figure 38.9).	150° Example: Eating, bathing, shaving	
Rotation for supination. Turn each hand and forearm so that the palm is facing upward (Figure 38.10).	70° to 90°	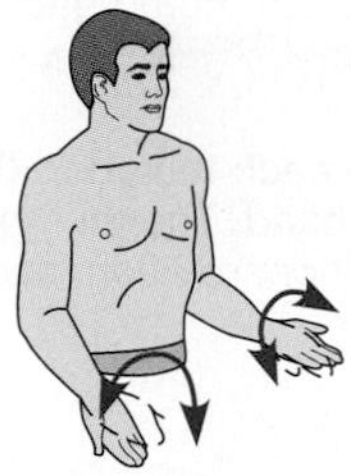 **Figure 38.10**
Rotation for pronation. Turn each hand and forearm so that the palm is facing downward (Figure 38.10).	70° to 90°	
Wrist—Condyloid Joint		
Flexion. Bring the fingers of each hand toward the inner aspect of the forearm (Figure 38.11).	80° to 90° Example: Eating, bathing, shaving, writing	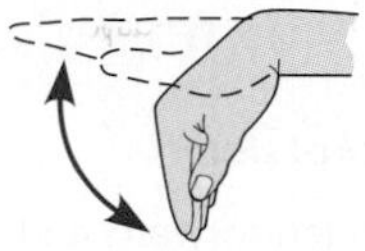 **Figure 38.11**
Extension. Straighten each hand to the same plane as the arm (Figure 38.11).	80° to 90° Example: Eating, bathing, shaving	
Hyperextension. Bend the fingers of each hand back as far as possible (Figure 38.12).	70° to 90°	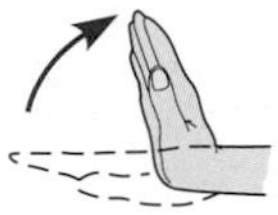 **Figure 38.12**
Radial flexion (abduction). Bend each wrist laterally toward the thumb side with hand supinated (Figure 38.13).	0° to 20°	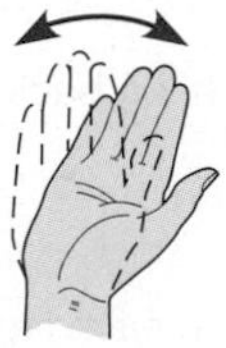 **Figure 38.13**
Ulnar flexion (adduction). Bend each wrist laterally toward the fifth finger with the hand supinated (Figure 38.13).	30° to 50°	
Hand and Fingers: Metacarpophalangeal Joints—Condyloid; Interphalangeal Joints—Hinge		
Flexion. Make a fist with each hand (Figure 38.14).	90° Example: Squeezing, gripping, writing	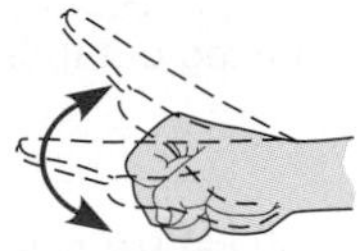 **Figure 38.14**
Extension. Straighten the fingers of each hand (Figure 38.14).	30°	
Hyperextension. Bend the fingers of each hand back as far as possible.	30°	
Abduction. Spread the fingers of each hand apart (Figure 38.15).	20°	
Adduction. Bring the fingers of each hand together (Figure 38.15).	20° Example: Writing, gripping, eating, many hobbies involving fine motor coordination (e.g., art, music)	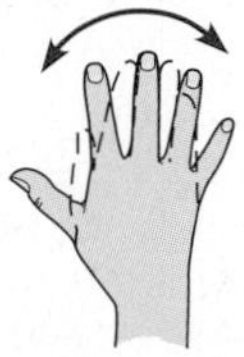 **Figure 38.15**

(continued)

TABLE 38.2 Selected Joint Movements and Examples of Corresponding Activity of Daily Living (ADL) *(continued)*

Body Part—Type of Joint/Movement	Normal Range	Illustration
Thumb—Saddle Joint		
Flexion. Move each thumb across the palmar surface of the hand toward the fifth finger (Figure 38.16).	90°	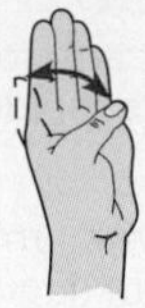 Figure 38.16
Extension. Move each thumb away from the hand.	90°	
Abduction. Extend each thumb laterally (Figure 38.17).	30°	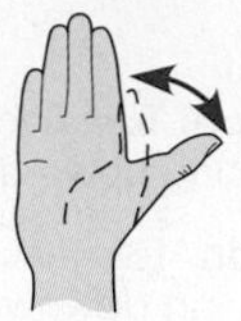 Figure 38.17
Adduction. Move each thumb back to the hand (Figure 38.17).	30°	
Opposition. Touch each thumb to the top of each finger of the same hand. The thumb joint movements involved are abduction, rotation, and flexion (Figure 38.18).		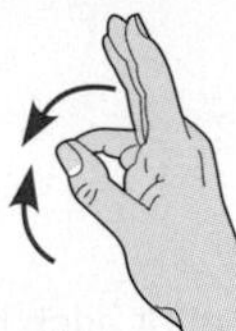 Figure 38.18
Hip—Ball-and-Socket Joint		
Flexion. Move each leg forward and upward. The knee may be extended or flexed (Figure 38.19).	Knee extended, 90°; knee flexed, 120° Example: Walking, leg lifts in front of body	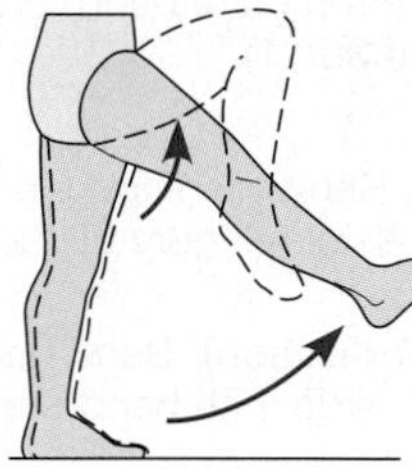 Figure 38.19
Extension. Move each leg back beside the other (Figure 38.20).	90° to 120° Example: Walking, lining the leg up with the body	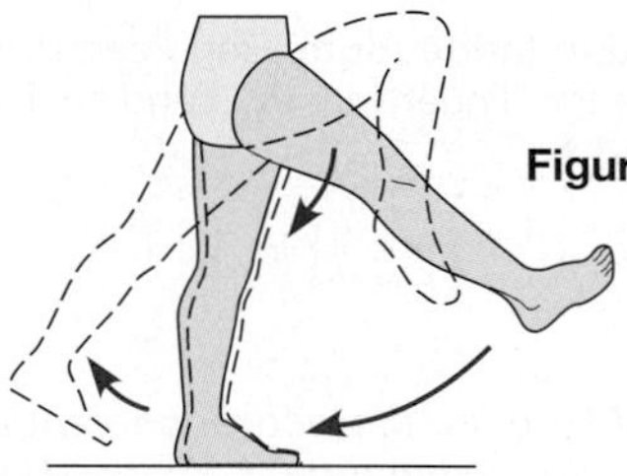 Figure 38.20
Hyperextension. Move each leg back behind the body (Figure 38.20).	30° to 50° Example: Walking, lying on side and reaching leg behind body	
Abduction. Move each leg out to the side (Figure 38.21).	45° to 50° Example: Moving leg away from body	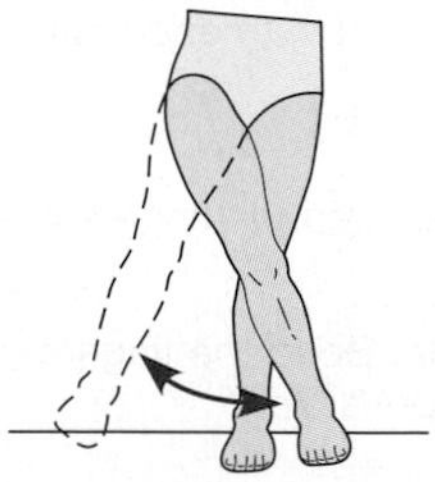 Figure 38.21
Adduction. Move each leg back to the other leg and beyond in front of it (Figure 38.21).	20° to 30° beyond other leg Example: Moving leg over the other leg toward the middle of the body	
Circumduction. Move each leg backward, up, to the side, and down in a circle (Figure 38.22).	360° Example: Leg circles clockwise and counter-clockwise	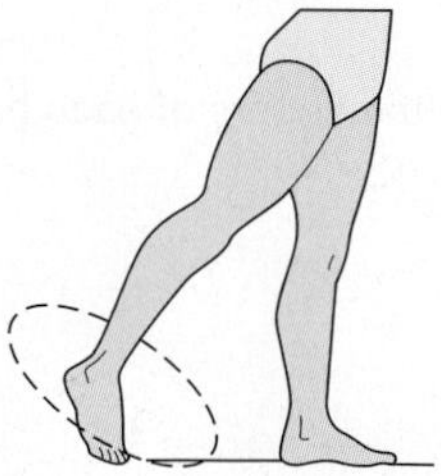 Figure 38.22

(continued)

TABLE 38.2 Selected Joint Movements and Examples of Corresponding Activity of Daily Living (ADL) *(continued)*

Body Part—Type of Joint/Movement	Normal Range	Illustration
Internal rotation. Turn each foot and leg inward so that the toes point as far as possible toward the other leg (Figure 38.23).	45°	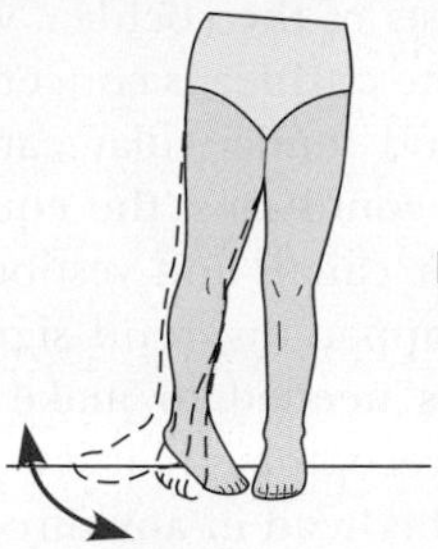 **Figure 38.23**
External rotation. Turn each foot and leg outward so that the toes point as far as possible away from the other leg (Figure 38.23).	45°	
Knee—Hinge Joint		
Flexion. Bend each leg, bringing the heel toward the back of the thigh (Figure 38.24).	120° to 130° Example: Knee bends, walking	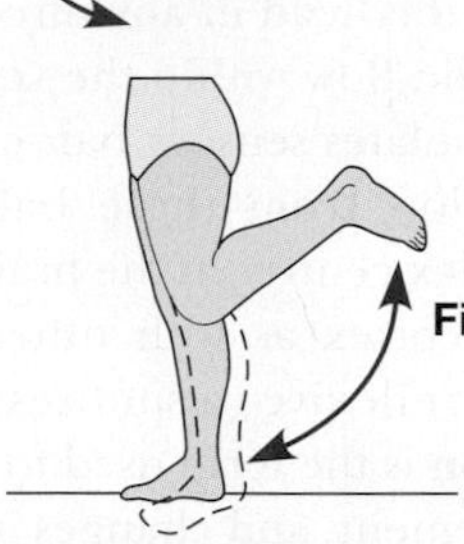 **Figure 38.24**
Extension. Straighten each leg, returning the foot to its position beside the other foot (Figure 38.24).	120° to 130° Example: Straightening leg from bent position, walking	
Ankle—Hinge Joint		
Extension (plantar flexion). Point the toes of each foot downward (Figure 38.25).	45° to 50° Example: Pressing toes away from face, walking	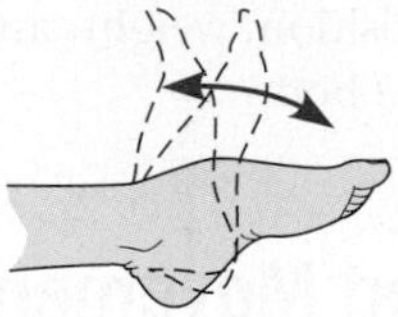 **Figure 38.25**
Flexion (dorsiflexion). Point the toes of each foot upward (Figure 38.25).	20° Example: Pulling toes toward face, walking	
Foot—Gliding		
Eversion. Turn the sole of each foot laterally (Figure 38.26).	5° Example: Foot circles clockwise and counter-clockwise	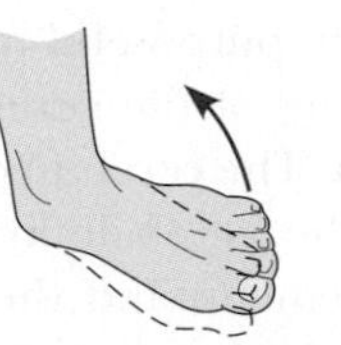 **Figure 38.26**
Inversion. Turn the sole of each foot medially.		
Toes: Interphalangeal Joints—Hinge; Metatarsophalangeal Joints—Hinge; Intertarsal Joints—Gliding		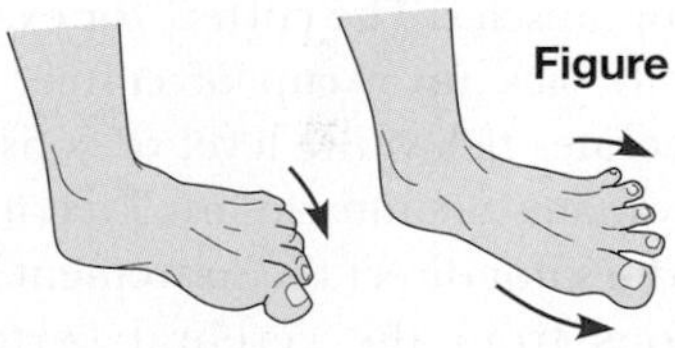 **Figure 38.27**
Flexion. Curl the toe joints of each foot downward (Figure 38.27).	35° to 60°	
Extension. Straighten the toes of each foot (Figure 38.27).	35° to 60°	
Trunk—Gliding Joint		
Flexion. Bend the trunk toward the toes (Figure 38.28).	70° to 90° Example: Touching toes	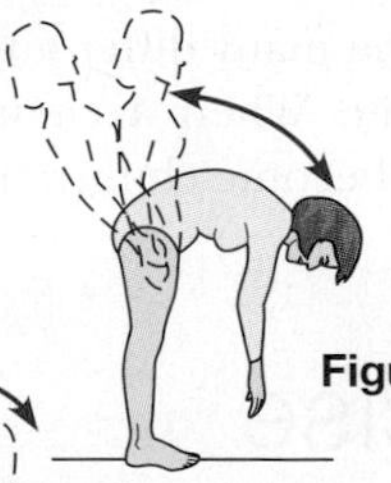 **Figure 38.28**
Extension. Straighten the trunk from a flexed position (Figure 38.28).	70° to 90°	
Hyperextension. Bend the trunk backward.	20° to 30° Example: Gentle supported back bend with hands on buttocks	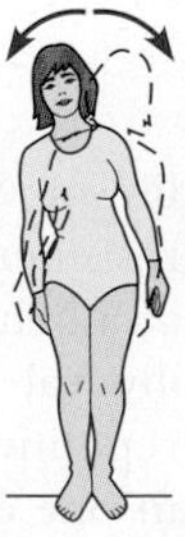 **Figure 38.29**
Lateral flexion. Bend the trunk to the right and to the left (Figure 38.29).	35° on each side Example: Gently allow right hand to slide down right side of thigh; repeat on left side	
Rotation. Turn the upper part of the body from side to side (Figure 38.30).	30° to 45° Example: Gently swing torso right and left, maintaining forward hip alignment	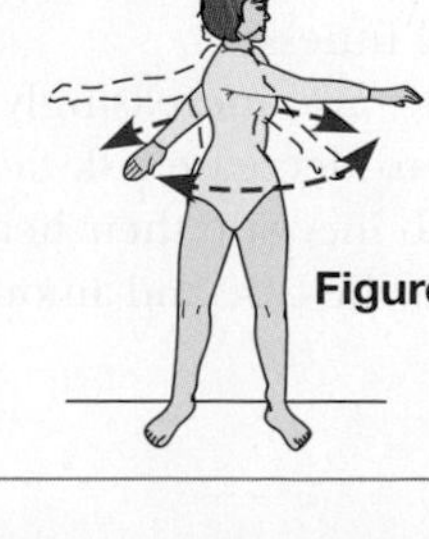 **Figure 38.30**

inputs from the labyrinth (inner ear), vision (vestibulo-ocular input), and stretch receptors of muscles and tendons (proprioceptors and vestibulospinal input). The labyrinth consists of the cochlea, vestibule, and semicircular canals. The cochlea is concerned with hearing and the vestibule and semicircular canals with equilibrium. Under normal conditions, the equilibrium receptors in the semicircular canals and vestibule, collectively called the vestibular apparatus, send signals to the brain that initiate reflexes needed to make required changes in position. The receptors (hairlike cells) respond to displacement of the head in any direction. When the head moves, the fluid flow within the vestibule and semicircular canals stimulates sensory hair cells.

Information from these balance receptors goes directly to reflex centres in the brain stem, rather than to the cerebral cortex as with other special senses. This enables fast reflexive responses to body imbalance. **Proprioception** is the term used to describe awareness of posture, movement, and changes in equilibrium and the knowledge of position, weight, and resistance of objects in relation to the body.

Coordinated Movement

Balanced, smooth, purposeful movement is the result of proper functioning of the cerebral cortex, cerebellum, and basal ganglia. The cerebral cortex initiates voluntary motor activity; the cerebellum coordinates the motor activities of movement; and the basal ganglia maintain posture. The cerebral cortex operates in terms of movements, not muscles. The cortex, for example, may direct the arm to pick up a cup of coffee. The cerebellum, which operates below the level of consciousness, blends and coordinates the muscles involved in voluntary movement. It does not direct the movement but translates the instructions from the cerebral cortex into detailed actions by the many different muscles in the hand, arm, and shoulder. When a client's cerebellum is injured, movements become clumsy, unsure, and uncoordinated.

Exercise

Physical activity is the bodily movement produced by skeletal muscles that requires energy expenditure and can produce progressive health benefits.

Exercise is a type of physical activity defined as a planned, structured, and repetitive bodily movement done to improve or maintain one or more components of physical fitness.

People are increasingly participating in exercise programs to decrease risk factors for cardiovascular disease and to increase their health and well-being. **Activity tolerance** is the type and amount of exercise or daily living activities an individual is able to perform without experiencing adverse effects. **Functional strength** is another goal of exercise and is defined as the ability of the body to perform work.

Types of Exercise

Exercise involves the active contraction and relaxation of muscles. Exercises can be classified according to the type of muscle contraction (isotonic, isometric, or isokinetic) and according to the source of energy (aerobic or anaerobic).

Isotonic (dynamic) exercises are those in which the muscle shortens to produce muscle contraction and active movement. Most physical conditioning exercises—running, walking, swimming, cycling, and other such activities—are isotonic, as are ADLs and *active* ROM exercises (those initiated by the client). Examples of isotonic *bed* exercises are pushing or pulling against a stationary object, using a trapeze to lift the body off the bed, lifting

Evidence-Informed Practice

Does Stretching before Exercise Reduce Muscle Soreness?

Many Canadians believe that performing stretching exercises before physical activity is beneficial in promoting agility during exercise and limiting sore muscles after exercise. Herbert and de Noronha (2007) sought to answer the question of whether stretching prevents or reduces muscle soreness after exercise. Having reviewed more than 50 years of literature, the only quality research studies that were included for review were conducted on young, healthy adults under age 40. The systematic review concluded that "muscle stretching does not reduce delayed-onset muscle soreness in young healthy adults."

NURSING IMPLICATIONS: Nurses can help young adults seeking to improve their fitness level to understand that warmup stretching will not guarantee that they don't develop muscle soreness following exercise. For some, this may be important information so that they will not have false expectations of this strategy. Anyone who lacks motivation to exercise may be disappointed when warmups don't have the outcomes expected. These findings support the fact that nurses must emphasize the general guidelines outlined in the *Handbook for Canada's Physical Activity Guide to Healthy Active Living* (Public Health Agency of Canada, 2003, p. 2) to "start slowly and build up."

Source: Based on "Stretching to Prevent or Reduce Muscle Soreness after Exercise," by R. D. Herbert and M. de Noronha, 2007, *Cochrane Database of Systematic Reviews, 4*, Art. No.: CD004577.

the buttocks off the bed by pushing with the hands against the mattress, and pushing the body to a sitting position.

Isotonic exercises increase muscle tone, mass, and strength and maintain joint flexibility and circulation. During isotonic exercise, both heart rate and cardiac output quicken to increase blood flow to all parts of the body. Little or no change in blood pressure occurs.

Isometric (static or setting) exercises are those in which a change in muscle tension occurs but no change in muscle length and no muscle or joint movement takes place. These exercises are useful for strengthening abdominal, gluteal, and quadriceps muscles used in ambulation; for maintaining strength in immobilized muscles in casts or traction; and for endurance training. An example of isometric bed exercise would be squeezing a towel or pillow between the knees while at the same time tightening the muscles in the fronts of the thighs by pressing the knees downward (see Figure 38.31) and holding for 10 seconds. These are often called *quad sets.* Isometric exercises produce a moderate increase in heart rate and cardiac output but no appreciable increase in blood flow to other parts of the body.

Isokinetic (resistive) exercises involve muscle contraction or tension against resistance; thus, they can be either isotonic or isometric. During isokinetic exercises, the person moves (isotonic) or tenses (isometric) against resistance. Special machines or devices provide the resistance to the movement. These exercises are used in physical conditioning and are often done to build certain muscle groups; for example, the pectorals (chest muscles) may be increased in size and strength by lifting weights. An increase in blood pressure and blood flow to muscles occurs with resistance training.

Aerobic exercise is an activity in which the amount of oxygen taken into the body is greater than or equal to the amount the body requires. Aerobic exercises use large muscle groups, are performed continuously, and are rhythmic in nature. Examples are walking, jogging, running, bicycling, dancing, cross-country skiing, jumping rope, rowing, swimming, and skating. Aerobic exercises improve cardiovascular conditioning and physical fitness.

The *intensity* of exercise can be measured in three ways:

1. *Target heart rate.* The goal is to work up to and sustain a target heart rate during exercise, based on the person's age. To determine the target heart rate, first calculate the person's maximum heart rate by subtracting her or his current age in years from 220. Then, obtain the target heart rate by taking 60% to 85% of the maximum. Because heart rates vary among individuals, the tests that follow are replacing this measure.
2. *Talk test.* This test is easier to implement and keeps most people at 60% of maximum heart rate or more. When exercising, the person should experience laboured breathing, yet still be able to carry on a conversation.

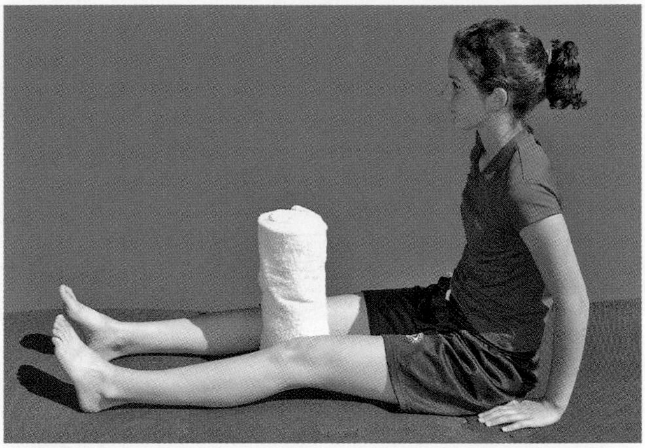

FIGURE 38.31 Example of an isometric exercise for the legs: the client sits or lies on a flat surface with the legs straight out. With a rolled towel between the knees, the client pushes the knees together and tightens the muscles in the front of the thighs by forcing the knees downward and holding for 10 seconds.

3. *Borg scale of perceived exertion* (Borg, 1998). This scale measures how difficult the exercise feels to the person in terms of heart and lung exertion. The scale progresses from 1 to 20 with the following markers: 7 = very, very light; 9 = very light; 11 = fairly light; 13 = somewhat hard; 15 = hard; 17 = very hard; and 19 = very, very hard.

"Very, very hard" corresponds closely to 100% of maximum heart rate. "Very light" is close to 40%. Most people need to strive for the "somewhat hard" level (13/20), which corresponds to 75% of maximum heart rate.

Anaerobic exercise involves activity in which the muscles cannot draw out enough oxygen from the bloodstream, and anaerobic pathways are used to provide additional energy for a short time. This type of exercise, such as weight lifting and sprinting, is used in endurance training for athletes.

The *Handbook for Canada's Physical Activity Guide to Healthy Living* (Public Health Agency of Canada, 2003) (Figure 38.32) identifies activities that increase strength, endurance, and flexibility. Box 38.1 describes the benefit, frequency, and type of exercise recommended. A reduction in sedentary activities is also important.

Benefits of Exercise

Regular exercise is essential for healthy functioning of major body systems. The benefits of exercise on these systems follow.

MUSCULOSKELETAL SYSTEM The size, shape, tone, and strength of skeletal and cardiac muscles are maintained with mild exercise and increased with strenuous exercise. With strenuous exercise, muscles **hypertrophy**

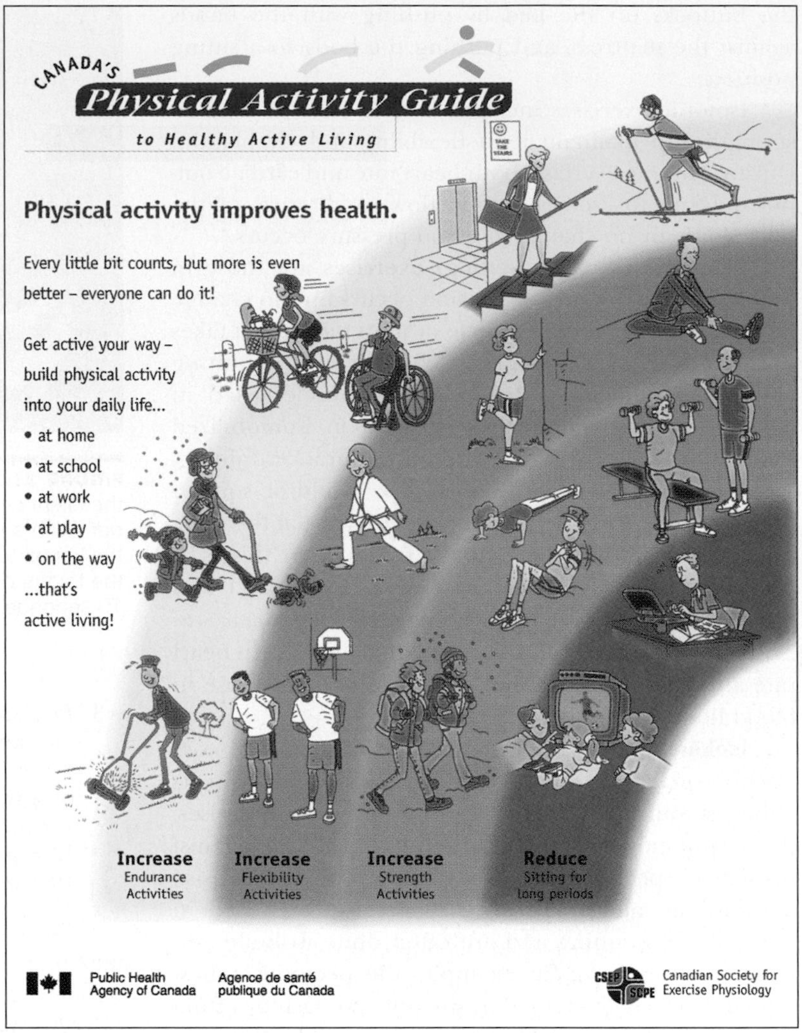

FIGURE 38.32 *Handbook for Canada's Physical Activity Guide to Healthy Active Living*

(From Handbook for Canada's Physical Activity Guide to Healthy Active Living, by the Public Health Agency of Canada, 2003, Ottawa: Author.)

(enlarge), and the efficiency of muscular contraction increases. Hypertrophy is commonly seen in the arm muscles of a tennis player, the leg muscles of a skater, the arm and hand muscles of a carpenter, and the body muscles of weight lifters.

Exercise can increase balance, a key determinant in older adults' risk of falling (Howe, Rochester, Jackson, Banks, & Blair, 2007), reduce pain (Busch, Barber, Overend, Peloso, & Schachter, 2007), and improve joint flexibility and ROM (Han et al., 2004). Aquatic exercise can improve functioning of some people with osteoarthritis (Bartels et al., 2007).

Bone density is maintained through weight bearing by maintaining a balance between *osteoblasts* (bone-building cells) and *osteoclasts* (bone-resorption and breakdown cells). Weight-bearing exercise (e.g., walking)

BOX 38.1 GUIDELINES FOR PHYSICAL ACTIVITY

Activity Group	Benefit	Frequency	Type of Exercise
Endurance	Endurance activities help the heart, lungs, and circulatory system	4–7 days a week	Continuous activities such as walking, cycling, tennis, swimming
Flexibility	Flexibility activities help with easy movement, keeping muscles relaxed and joints mobile	4–7 days a week	Gentle bending, reaching, and stretching such as gardening, mopping the floor, yard work, stretching exercises
Strength	Strength activities help bones and muscles stay strong, improve posture, and prevent some diseases	2–4 days a week	Activities against resistance such as heavy yard work, climbing stairs, weight training routines

Source: Information from *Handbook for Canada's Physical Activity Guide to Healthy Active Living* (pp. 5–7), by the Public Health Agency of Canada, 2003, Ottawa: Author.

can be effective in enhancing lumbar spine and hip density in women at risk, such as postmenopausal women (Bonaiuti et al., 2002).

CARDIOVASCULAR SYSTEM The Heart and Stroke Foundation of Canada (2008) guidelines for primary prevention of stroke and heart disease place great emphasis on physical activity as a means of promoting cardiovascular health and of reducing important risk factors, such as high blood cholesterol, hypertension, and obesity.

Adequate moderate-intensity exercise (40% to 60% of maximum capacity, such as walking 1.6 km in 15 to 20 minutes) increases the heart rate, the strength of heart muscle contraction, and the blood supply to the heart and muscles through increased cardiac output. High-density lipoprotein levels can be increased with regular endurance-type exercise. Exercise promotes heart health by mediating the harmful effects of stress. It can also improve the quality of life for people who already have heart disease, such as clients with mild to moderate heart failure (Rees, Taylor, Singh, Coats, & Ebrahim, 2004).

RESPIRATORY SYSTEM Ventilation (air circulation into and out of the lungs) and oxygen intake increases during exercise, thereby improving gas exchange. Adequate exercise also prevents pooling of secretions in the bronchi and bronchioles, decreasing breathing effort and risk of infection. Attention to exercising muscles of respiration (by deep breathing) throughout activity as well as rest enhances oxygenation (improving stamina) and circulation of lymph (improving immune function). A strong body of evidence supports the use of lower extremity exercise forms (e.g., walking, treadmill, stationary bike, stair climbing) for treating individuals with chronic obstructive pulmonary disease (Freeman, 2004). Research reports citing the benefits of yogic breathing and postures for asthmatics are increasing in the literature (Freeman, 2004; Micozzi, 2006).

GASTROINTESTINAL SYSTEM Exercise improves the appetite and increases gastrointestinal tract tone, improving digestion and elimination. Such activities as rowing, swimming, walking, and doing situps work the abdominal muscles and can help relieve constipation (Fontaine, 2005). Abdominal compressive exercise, such as with twisting and forward-bending yoga postures, has been shown to improve symptoms of irritable bowel syndrome (Fontaine, 2005; Micozzi, 2006).

METABOLIC SYSTEM Exercise elevates the metabolic rate, thus increasing the production of body heat and waste products. During strenuous exercise, the metabolic rate can increase to as much as 20 times the normal rate. This elevation lasts after exercise is completed. Exercise increases the use of triglycerides and fatty acids, resulting in a reduced level of serum triglycerides and cholesterol. Weight loss and exercise stabilize blood glucose and make cells more responsive to insulin. The Canadian Diabetes Association (n.d.) recommends at least 150 minutes of moderate-intensity aerobic exercise at least three times a week on nonconsecutive days for enhanced blood glucose control in people with type 2 diabetes mellitus.

URINARY SYSTEM As adequate exercise promotes efficient blood flow, the body excretes wastes more effectively. In addition, urinary stasis (stagnation) is usually prevented.

IMMUNE SYSTEM As respiratory and musculoskeletal effort increase with exercise and as gravity is enlisted with postural changes, lymph fluid is more efficiently pumped from tissues into lymph capillaries and vessels throughout the body. Circulation through the lymph nodes, where the destruction of pathogens and the removal of foreign antigens can occur, is also improved. Research in older adults has shown the benefits of moderate exercise on natural killer cell function, circulating T-cell function, and cytokine production, potentially increasing resistance to viral infections and preventing formation of malignant cells (Freeman, 2004).

Although moderate exercise seems to enhance immunity, strenuous exercise may reduce immune function, leaving a window of opportunity for infection during the recovery phase. Adequate rest is important after vigorous training to allow the body to recover (Edelman & Mandle, 2006).

PSYCHONEUROLOGICAL SYSTEM Mental or affective disorders, such as depression or chronic stress, can affect a person's desire to move. The depressed person may lack enthusiasm for taking part in any activity and may even lack energy for usual hygiene practices. Lack of visible energy is seen in a slumped posture with head bowed. Chronic stress can deplete the body's energy reserves to the point that fatigue discourages the desire to exercise, even though exercise can energize the person and facilitate coping. By contrast, individuals with eating disorders may exercise excessively in an effort to prevent weight gain.

A strong and growing body of evidence supports the role of exercise in elevating mood and relieving stress and anxiety across the lifespan (Larun, Nordheim, Ekeland, Hagen, & Heian, 2006). Solid data examining relationships between aerobic and nonaerobic styles of exercise support the use of this modality to relieve symptoms of depression. The mechanism of action is thought to be a result of one or more of the following: exercise increases levels of metabolites for neurotransmitters, such as norepinephrine and serotonin; exercise releases endogenous opioids, thus increasing levels of endorphins; exercise increases levels of oxygen to the brain and other body systems, inducing euphoria; and through muscular exertion (especially with movement modalities, such as yoga and Tai Chi) the body releases stored stress associated with accumulated emotional demands. Regular exercise also improves quality of sleep for most individuals (Freeman, 2004).

By eliciting the **relaxation response (RR)**, exercise is beneficial for counteracting some of the harmful effects of stress on the body and mind. First described by Dr. Herbert Benson, the RR is a healthful physiological state that can be elicited through deep relaxation breathing with emphasis on a prolonged exhalation phase (Edelman & Mandle, 2006). Emphasis on the exhalation recruits the parasympathetic nervous system response, the "rest and digest" reflex. Progressive muscle relaxation techniques involve contracting and then releasing groups of muscles throughout the body until all parts of the body feel relaxed. These movements are subtle and, along with relaxation breathing, can be done by almost anyone at any time, regardless of mobility or fitness status, providing potent stress relief and neurocardiovascular health benefits.

Factors Affecting Body Alignment and Activity

A number of factors affect an individual's body alignment, mobility, and daily activity level. These include growth and development, nutrition, personal values and attitudes, certain external factors, prescribed limitations, physical health, and mental health.

Growth and Development

A person's age and musculoskeletal and nervous system development affect posture, body proportions, body mass, body movements, and reflexes. Newborns' movements are reflexive and random. All extremities are generally flexed but can be passively moved through a full ROM. As the neurological system matures, control over movement progresses during the first year. Gross motor development precedes fine motor skills. Gross motor development occurs in a head-to-toe fashion, that is, it progresses from head control, to crawling, to pulling up to a standing position, to standing, and to walking, usually after the first birthday. Initially, walking involves a wide stance and unsteady gait, thus the term *toddler*. From ages 1 to 5 years, both gross and fine motor skills are refined. For example, preschoolers master riding a tricycle, dancing, running, jumping, using crayons to draw, fastening or using zippers, and brushing their teeth.

From 6 to 12 years, refinement of motor skills continues and exercise patterns for later life are generally determined. Many schools provide some physical education and competitive sports programs to enhance physical activity. Posture in school-age children is usually excellent. In adolescence, growth spurts and such behaviours as carrying heavy book bags on one shoulder and extended computer use can result in poor postural changes that often persist into adulthood.

Adults between 20 and 40 years of age generally have few physical changes affecting mobility if they have no significant weight gain, with the exception of pregnant women. Pregnancy alters the centre of gravity and affects balance so that activities in which the body is supported (e.g., swimming and cycling) are favoured. Evidence shows that pregnant women who engage in aerobic exercise can improve their physical fitness (Kramer & McDonald, 2006). Exercise can also help pregnant women avoid excess weight gain, thus preventing long-term obesity after delivery. Leaner babies may also be at a lower risk for obesity later in life.

As age advances, muscle tone and bone density decrease, joints lose flexibility, reaction time slows, and bone mass decreases, particularly in women who have osteoporosis. **Osteoporosis** is a condition in which the bones become brittle and fragile because of calcium depletion. Osteoporosis is common in older women and primarily affects the weight-bearing joints of the lower extremities and anterior aspects of spinal bones, causing compression fractures of the vertebrae and hip fractures. All these changes affect older adults' posture, gait, and balance. Posture becomes forward leaning and stooped, which shifts the centre of gravity forward. To compensate for this shift, the knees flex slightly for support and the base of support is widened. Gait becomes wide-based, short-stepped, and shuffling. A strong body of research supports the benefits of regular activity for older adults to maintain and regain strength, flexibility, cardiovascular fitness, and bone density.

Nutrition

Both undernutrition and overnutrition can influence body alignment and mobility. Poorly nourished people may have muscle weakness and fatigue. Vitamin D deficiency causes bone deformity during growth. Inadequate calcium intake and vitamin D synthesis increase the risk of osteoporosis. Obesity can distort movement and stress joints, adversely affecting posture, balance, and joint health.

Personal Values and Attitudes

Whether people value regular exercise is often the result of family influences. In families that incorporate regular exercise in their daily routine or spend time together in physical endeavours (baseball, hiking, swimming), children learn to value physical activity. Sedentary families, conversely, participate in sports only as spectators, watching the ball game or hockey game on television, and this lifestyle is often transmitted to their children. With the increase in TV, computer, and video activities, youth are increasingly sedentary, with attendant declines in health.

Values about physical appearance also influence some people's participation in regular exercise. People who value a muscular build or physical attractiveness may participate in regular exercise programs to produce the appearance they desire. The choice of physical activity or type of exercise is also influenced by values. Choices may be influenced by geographic location and cultural role expectations.

External Factors

Many external factors affect a person's mobility. Excessively high temperature and high humidity discourage activity, whereas comfortable temperature and humidity are conducive to activity, such as a brisk walk or a game of tennis. The availability of recreational facilities also influences activity; for example, lack of money may prohibit a client from joining an exercise group or swimming in an indoor pool. Neighbourhood safety promotes outdoor activity, whereas an unsafe environment discourages people from going outdoors.

Prescribed Limitations

Limitations to movement are medically prescribed for some health problems. To promote healing, such devices as casts, braces, splints, and traction are often used to immobilize body parts. Clients who are short of breath may be advised not to walk up stairs. Bed rest may be the therapeutic choice for certain clients, for example, to relieve edema, to reduce metabolic and oxygen needs, to promote tissue repair, or to decrease pain.

The term **bed rest** varies in meaning to some extent. In some agencies, bed rest means strict confinement to bed or *complete bed rest.* Others allow the client to use a bedside commode. Nurses need to familiarize themselves with the meaning of the term *bed rest* in their practice setting. In any case, the effects of limiting activity are immediate and negative. For example, muscle strength atrophies at approximately 3% per day with complete bed rest.

Physical Health

Mobility and activity tolerance are affected by any disorder that impairs the ability of the nervous system, musculoskeletal system, cardiovascular system, respiratory system, and vestibular apparatus. Congenital problems, such as hip dysplasia, spina bifida, cerebral palsy, and the muscular dystrophies, affect motor functioning. Disorders of the nervous system, such as Parkinson's disease, multiple sclerosis, central nervous system tumours, cerebrovascular accidents (strokes), infectious processes (e.g., meningitis), and head and spinal cord injuries, can leave muscle groups weakened, **spastic** (with too much muscle tone), **flaccid** (without muscle tone), or with **paresis** (partial paralysis). Musculoskeletal disorders affecting mobility include strains, sprains, fractures, joint dislocations, amputations, and joint replacements. Inner ear infections and dizziness can impair balance. Many other acute and chronic illnesses that limit the supply of oxygen and nutrients needed for muscle contraction and movement can seriously affect activity tolerance. Examples include chronic obstructive lung disease, anemia, congestive heart failure, and angina.

Mental Health

Mental or affective disorders, such as depression or chronic stress, can affect a person's desire to move. The depressed person may lack enthusiasm for taking part in any activity and may even lack energy for usual hygiene practices. Lack of visible energy is seen in a slumped posture with head bowed. By contrast, happy, confident people usually stand erect. Chronic stress can deplete the body's energy reserves to the point that fatigue discourages the desire to exercise even though exercise can energize the person and facilitate coping.

Effects of Immobility

Individuals who have inactive lifestyles or who are faced with inactivity because of illness or injury are at risk for many problems that can affect major body systems. Whether immobility causes problems often depends on the duration of the inactivity, the client's health status, and the client's sensory awareness. The most obvious signs of prolonged immobility are often manifested in the musculoskeletal system, and the deconditioning effects can be observed even after a few days. Clients experience a significant decrease in muscular strength and agility whenever they do not maintain a moderate amount of physical activity. In addition, immobility adversely affects the cardiovascular, respiratory, metabolic, urinary, and psychoneurological systems. Nurses need to understand these effects and encourage client movement as much as possible. Early ambulation after illness or surgery is an essential measure to prevent complications. See Table 38.3 for desired outcomes and nursing interventions to prevent problems of immobility.

Musculoskeletal System

Prolonged immobility often affects the musculoskeletal system first, sometimes within days:

- *Disuse osteoporosis.* Without the stress of weight-bearing activity, the bones demineralize. They are depleted chiefly of calcium, which gives the bones strength and density. Regardless of the amount of calcium in a person's diet, the demineralization process, known as osteoporosis, continues with

TABLE 38.3 Desired Outcomes and Nursing Interventions to Prevent the Problems of Immobility (Disuse Syndrome)

Desired Health Outcome	Nursing Interventions	Rationale
Maintains **normal musculoskeletal function**, as evidenced by usual range of motion in all body joints and maintenance of baseline muscle mass and strength	Implement appropriate exercise program (isometric, isotonic, or passive exercises) at least every two hours as indicated.	Isotonic exercises prevent contractures and muscle atrophy. Isometric exercises maintain muscle tone. Passive exercises maintain joint mobility.
	Encourage active participation in self-care activities.	Self-care activities involve active movement of joints and muscles.
	Compare muscle size and strength to baseline data and on each side of the body daily. See Skill 27.16 (p. 631) for details about testing and grading muscle strength.	Early detection of muscle atrophy or decreased strength facilitates early intervention to correct the problem.
	Position clients in good alignment.	Good alignment prevents contractures and maintains structural integrity of muscles and joints.
	Ambulate client, as tolerated, or assist to stand at bedside.	Weight bearing prevents disuse osteoporosis.
Experiences **minimal cardiovascular alterations**, as evidenced by maintenance of baseline vital signs and signs of adequate venous blood flow (absence of edema, calf pain, inflammation, venous distention, skin changes)	Monitor vital signs according to client needs and agency protocol (e.g., bid or tid).	Regular monitoring enables the nurse to detect alterations early.
	Instruct client how and when to avoid the Valsalva manoeuvre.	The Valsalva manoeuvre increases the stress on the heart.
	Apply antiembolism stockings as indicated (see Skill 35.2, p. 1030).	Use of antiembolism stockings prevents thrombus formation, venous engorgement, dependent edema, and orthostatic hypotension.
	Elevate legs several times each day for 20 minutes.	Elevation increases peripheral venous circulation.
	Implement measures to prevent postural hypotension.	
	Assess skin of lower limbs and measure calf circumferences, as indicated.	Regular inspection and measurement enable the nurse to detect changes.
	See also interventions for musculoskeletal function.	These interventions also stimulate blood circulation and prevent cardiovascular complications.
Maintains **normal respiratory function**, as evidenced by normal breath sounds during auscultation; normal chest expansion; and absence of chest pain, fever, or other respiratory signs indicative of pulmonary infarction, emboli, or atelectasis	Assess breath sounds and chest expansion at least every 4 hours.	This allows the nurse to detect onset of abnormal breath sounds and inadequate chest expansion.
	Teach clients to take five deep breaths and to cough every waking hour.	Deep breaths and coughing increase alveolar expansion, prevent stasis of secretions, promote adequate gaseous exchange, and maintain a patent airway.
	Establish a position schedule, and alter client's position at least every 2 hours. Ambulate client, if possible, or place client in chair.	Changes in position allow previously dependent lung areas to expand and promote movement and subsequent removal of secretions by coughing.

(continued)

immobility. The bones become spongy and may gradually deform and fracture easily.

- *Disuse atrophy.* Unused muscles **atrophy** (decrease in size), losing most of their strength and normal function.
- *Contractures.* When the muscle fibres are not moved, eventually a **contracture** (permanent shortening of the muscle) forms, limiting joint mobility. This process eventually involves the tendons, ligaments, and joint capsules; it is often irreversible except by surgical intervention. Joint deformities, such as plantar flexion contracture (foot drop) (Figure 38.33), wrist drop, and external hip rotation, occur when a stronger muscle dominates the opposite muscle.
- *Stiffness and pain in the joints.* Without movement, the collagen (connective) tissues at the joint become ankylosed (permanently immobile). In addition, as the bones demineralize, excess calcium may deposit in the joints, contributing to stiffness and pain.

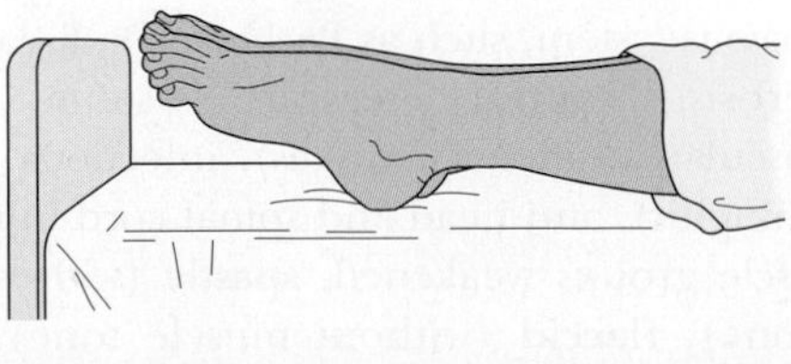

FIGURE 38.33 Plantar flexion contracture (foot drop)

TABLE 38.3 Desired Outcomes and Nursing Interventions to Prevent the Problems of Immobility (Disuse Syndrome) *(continued)*

Desired Health Outcome	Nursing Interventions	Rationale
Maintains **normal elimination pattern**, as evidenced by clear amber urinary output of at least 1500 mL per day; urine specific gravity of 1.010 to 1.030; an acidic urine; absence of signs of urinary retention, calculi, or infection; and excretion of formed semisolid stool at least every 2 or 3 days	Monitor colour, clarity, amount, acidity, and specific gravity of urine; colour and characteristics of feces; and frequency of defecation. Ask whether client has pain when urinating.	Decreased urinary output, cloudy urine, and painful urination are indicative of urinary retention and infection. Alkaline urine increases the risk for calculi. Constipation is associated with immobility. Increase fluid to increase urinary output to decrease incidence of renal calculi.
	Refer to Chapter 40 for interventions to prevent constipation. Teach clients to select high-fibre foods.	High-fibre foods promote intestinal peristalsis and defecation. See Chapter 39 for foods high in fibre.
Maintains **intact integument**, as evidenced by clean, intact, well-hydrated skin and absence of pressure signs (pallor, redness, increased warmth, or tenderness) over pressure areas	See "Preventing Pressure Ulcers" in Chapter 33.	Preventing skin breakdown is imperative to promote recovery and optimize quality of life
Maintains **social, emotional, and intellectual well-being**, as evidenced by actively participating in and making decisions about care, verbalizing concerns, maintaining positive relationships with others, and performing satisfying activities	Encourage the client to make as many decisions as possible, such as placement of personal items, daily plan of activities, clothes to wear.	Decision making enhances self-esteem.
	Plan time to be available to the client other than task-oriented time.	Being available for the client may encourage open expression of feelings.
	Explore diversional activities of interest to the client, and develop a daily activity plan.	A satisfying daily activity prevents boredom and gives the client something to look forward to.

Cardiovascular System

The cardiovascular system also shows the deconditioning effects of immobility:

- *Diminished cardiac reserve.* Decreased mobility creates an imbalance in the autonomic nervous system, resulting in a preponderance of sympathetic activity over cholinergic activity that increases heart rate. A rapid heart rate reduces diastolic pressure, coronary blood flow, and the capacity of the heart to respond to any metabolic demands above the basal levels. Because of this diminished cardiac reserve, the immobilized person may experience tachycardia with even minimal exertion.
- *Increased use of Valsalva manoeuvre.* The **Valsalva manoeuvre** refers to holding the breath and straining against a closed glottis. For example, clients tend to hold their breath when attempting to move up in a bed or sit on a bedpan. This builds up sufficient pressure on the large veins in the thorax to interfere with the return blood flow to the heart and coronary arteries. When the client exhales and the glottis again opens, pressure is suddenly released, and a surge of blood flows to the heart. Cardiac arrhythmias can result if the client has cardiac disease.
- *Orthostatic (postural) hypotension.* **Orthostatic hypotension** is a common result of immobilization. Under normal conditions, sympathetic nervous system activity causes automatic vasoconstriction in the blood vessels in the lower half of the body when a mobile person changes from a horizontal to a vertical posture. Vasoconstriction prevents pooling of the blood in the legs and effectively maintains central blood pressure to ensure adequate perfusion of the heart and brain. During any prolonged immobility, this reflex becomes dormant. When the immobile person attempts to sit or stand, this reconstricting mechanism fails to function properly in spite of increased adrenalin output. The blood pools in the lower extremities, and central blood pressure drops. Cerebral perfusion is seriously compromised, and the person feels dizzy or lightheaded and may even faint. This sequence is usually accompanied by a sudden and marked increase in heart rate, the body's effort to protect the brain from an inadequate blood supply.
- *Venous vasodilation and stasis.* The skeletal muscles of an active person contract with each movement, compressing the blood vessels in those muscles and helping to pump the blood back to the heart against gravity. The tiny valves in the leg veins aid in venous return to the heart by preventing backward flow of blood and pooling. In an immobile person, the skeletal muscles do not contract sufficiently, and the muscles atrophy. The skeletal muscles can no longer assist in pumping blood back to the heart against gravity. Blood pools in the leg veins, causing vasodilation and engorgement. The valves in the veins can no longer work effectively to prevent

backward flow of blood and pooling (Figure 38.34). This phenomenon is known as incompetent valves. As the blood continues to pool in the veins, its greater volume increases venous blood pressure, which can become much higher than that exerted by the tissues surrounding the vessel.

- *Dependent edema.* When the venous pressure is sufficiently great, some of the serous part of the blood is forced out of the blood vessel into the interstitial spaces surrounding the blood vessel, causing edema. Edema is most common in parts of the body positioned below heart level and maintained in that position. Dependent edema is most likely to occur around the sacrum or heels of a client who sits up in bed or in the feet and lower legs of a client who sits on the side of the bed. Edema further impedes venous return of blood to the heart, causing more pooling and more edema. Edematous tissue is uncomfortable and more susceptible to injury than normal tissue.
- *Thrombus formation.* Three factors, known as *Virchow's triad,* collectively predispose a client to the formation of a **thrombophlebitis** (a clot that is loosely attached to an inflamed vein wall): impaired venous return to the heart, hypercoagulability of the blood, and injury to a vessel wall. A **thrombus** (clot) is particularly dangerous if it breaks loose from the vein wall and enters the general circulation as an **embolus** (a clot that has moved from its place of origin, causing obstruction to circulation elsewhere). Large emboli that enter the pulmonary circulation may occlude the vessels that nourish the lungs and cause an infarcted (dead) area of the lung. If the infarcted area is large, pulmonary function is seriously compromised, and death may ensue. Emboli travelling to the coronary vessels or brain can produce a similarly dangerous outcome.

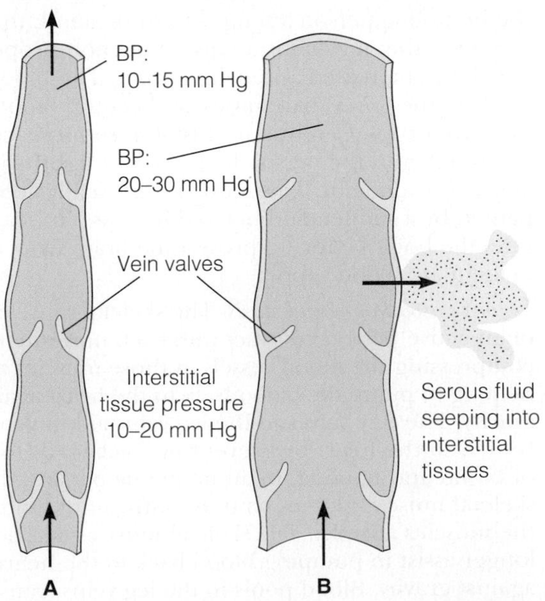

FIGURE 38.34 Leg veins: **A:** in a mobile person; **B:** in an immobile person

Respiratory System

Prolonged immobility can harm the respiratory system:

- *Decreased respiratory movement.* In a recumbent, immobile client, ventilation of the lungs is passively altered. The body presses against the rigid bed and curtails chest movement. The abdominal organs push against the diaphragm, further restricting lung movement and making it difficult to expand the lungs fully. An immobile recumbent person rarely sighs, partly because overall muscle atrophy also affects the respiratory muscles and partly because he or she has no need to do so without the stimulus of activity. Without these periodic stretching movements, the cartilaginous intercostal joints may become fixed in an expiratory phase of respiration, further restricting the potential for maximal ventilation. These changes produce shallow respirations and reduce vital capacity significantly. **Vital capacity** is the maximum amount of air that can be exhaled after a maximum inhalation.
- *Pooling of respiratory secretions.* Secretions of the respiratory tract are normally expelled by changing posture and by coughing. Inactivity allows secretions to pool by gravity (Figure 38.35), interfering with the normal diffusion of oxygen and carbon dioxide in the alveoli. The ability to cough up secretions can also be hindered by loss of respiratory muscle tone, dehydration (which thickens secretions), or sedatives that depress the cough reflex. Poor oxygenation and retention of carbon dioxide in the blood can result in respiratory acidosis, a potentially lethal disorder.

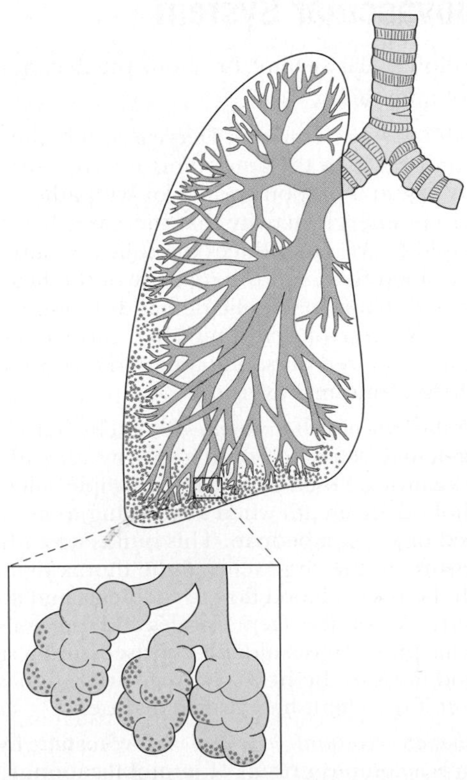

FIGURE 38.35 Pooling of secretions in the lungs of an immobile person

- *Atelectasis.* When ventilation is decreased, pooled secretions can accumulate in a dependent area of a bronchiole and effectively block it. Because of changes in regional blood flow, bed rest decreases the amount of surfactant produced. (Surfactant enables the alveoli to remain open.) The combination of decreased surfactant and blockage of a bronchiole with mucous can cause atelectasis (the collapse of a lobe or of an entire lung) distal to the mucous blockage. Immobile, older adult, postoperative clients are at greatest risk of atelectasis.
- *Hypostatic pneumonia.* Pooled secretions provide excellent media for bacterial growth. Under these conditions, a minor upper respiratory infection can evolve rapidly into a severe infection of the lower respiratory tract. Hypostatic pneumonia caused by static respiratory secretions can severely impair oxygen–carbon dioxide exchange in the alveoli and is a fairly common cause of death among weakened, immobile persons, especially heavy smokers.

Metabolic System

The metabolic system suffers when a person is immobile as well:

- *Decreased metabolic rate.* **Metabolism** refers to the sum of all the physical and chemical processes by which living substance is formed and maintained and by which energy is made available for use by the body. **Basal metabolism** is the minimal energy expended for the maintenance of these processes. The metabolic rate is the rate of basal metabolism expressed in calories per hour per square metre of body surface. In immobile clients, the basal metabolic rate and gastrointestinal motility and secretions of various digestive glands decrease as the energy requirements of the body decrease.
- *Negative nitrogen balance.* An active person's body maintains a balance between **anabolism** (protein synthesis) and **catabolism** (protein breakdown). Immobility creates a marked imbalance, and the catabolic processes exceed the anabolic processes. Catabolized muscle mass releases nitrogen. Over time, more nitrogen is excreted than is ingested, producing negative nitrogen balance. The negative nitrogen balance represents a depletion of protein stores that are essential for building muscle tissue and for wound healing.
- *Anorexia.* **Anorexia** (loss of appetite) occurs as a result of the decreased metabolic rate and the increased catabolism that accompany immobility. Reduced caloric intake is usually a response to the decreased energy requirements of the inactive person. If protein intake is reduced, the nitrogen imbalance may become more pronounced, sometimes so severely that malnutrition ensues.
- *Negative calcium balance.* A negative calcium balance occurs as a direct result of immobility. Greater amounts of calcium are extracted from bone than can be replaced. The absence of weight bearing and of stress on the musculoskeletal structures is the direct cause of the calcium loss from bones. Weight bearing and stress are also required for calcium to be replaced in bone. A similar process occurs with the body's stores of phosphate, causing a negative phosphate balance during immobility.

Urinary System

When a person is immobile, the urinary system is impaired:

- *Urinary stasis.* In a mobile person, gravity plays an important role in the emptying of the kidneys and the bladder. The shape and position of the kidneys and active kidney contractions are important in completely emptying the urine from the calyces, renal pelvis, and ureters (Figure 38.36A). The shape and position of the urinary bladder (the detrusor muscle) and active bladder contractions are also important in achieving complete emptying (Figure 38.37A). When the person remains in a horizontal position, gravity impedes the emptying of urine from the kidneys and the urinary bladder. To urinate, the person who is supine (in a back-lying position) must push upward, against gravity (Figure 38.36B and Figure 38.37B). The renal pelvis may fill with urine before it is pushed into the ureters. Emptying is not as complete, and **urinary stasis** (stoppage or slowdown of flow) occurs after a few days of bed rest. Because of the overall decrease in muscle tone during immobilization, including the tone of the detrusor muscle, bladder emptying is further compromised.
- *Renal calculi.* In a mobile person, calcium in the urine remains dissolved because calcium and citric acid are balanced in appropriately acidic urine. With immobility and the resulting excessive amounts of calcium (and phosphate) in the urine, this balance is no longer maintained. The urine becomes more alkaline, and the calcium salts precipitate out as crystals to form renal calculi (stones). In an immobile person in a horizontal position, the renal pelvis filled with stagnant, alkaline urine is an ideal location for calculi to form. The stones usually develop in the renal pelvis and pass through the ureters into the bladder. As the stones pass along the long, narrow ureters, they cause extreme pain and bleeding and can sometimes obstruct the urinary tract.

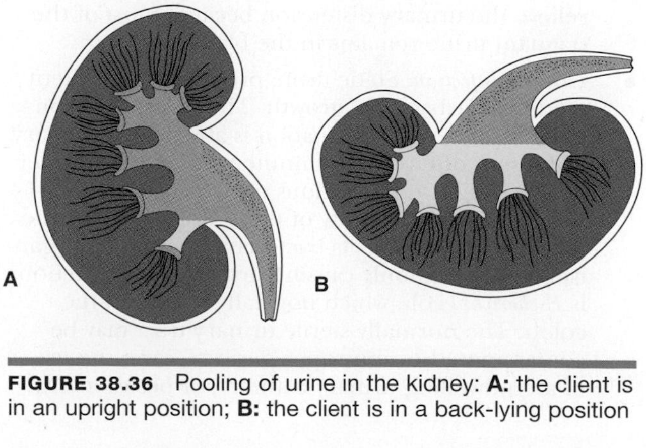

FIGURE 38.36 Pooling of urine in the kidney: **A:** the client is in an upright position; **B:** the client is in a back-lying position

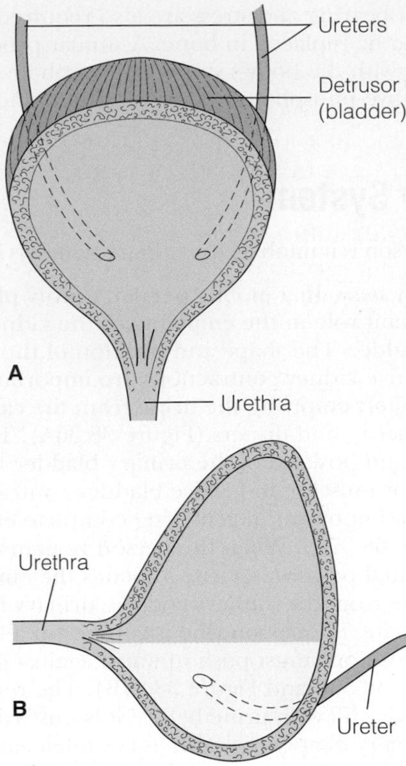

FIGURE 38.37 Pooling of urine in the urinary bladder: **A:** the client is in an upright position; **B:** the client is in a back-lying position

- *Urinary retention.* The immobile person may experience **urinary retention** (accumulation of urine in the bladder), bladder distension, and occasionally **urinary incontinence** (involuntary urination). The decreased muscle tone of the urinary bladder inhibits its ability to empty completely. In addition, the discomfort of using a bedpan or urinal, the embarrassment and lack of privacy associated with this function, and the unnatural position for urination combine to make it difficult for the client to relax the perineal muscles sufficiently to urinate while lying in bed. When urination is not possible, the bladder gradually becomes distended with urine. The bladder may stretch excessively, eventually inhibiting the urge to void. When bladder distension is considerable, some involuntary urinary "dribbling" may occur (retention with overflow). This does not relieve the urinary distension because most of the stagnant urine remains in the bladder.
- *Urinary infection.* Static urine provides an excellent medium for bacterial growth. The flushing action of normal, frequent urination is absent, and urinary distension often causes minute tears in the bladder mucosa, allowing infectious organisms to enter. The increased alkalinity of the urine caused by the hypercalcuria supports bacterial growth. The organism most commonly causing urinary tract infections is *Escherichia* coli, which normally resides in the colon. The normally sterile urinary tract may be contaminated by improper perineal care, the use of an indwelling urinary catheter, or occasionally, **urinary reflux** (backward flow). During reflux, contaminated urine from an overly distended bladder backs up into the renal pelvis to contaminate the kidney pelvis as well.

Gastrointestinal System

Prolonged immobility can affect the gastrointestinal system:

- *Constipation.* Constipation is a frequent problem for immobilized people because of decreased peristalsis and colon motility. The overall skeletal muscle weakness affects the abdominal and perineal muscles used in defecation. When the stool becomes very hard, more strength is required to expel it. The immobile person may lack this strength.
- *Weakened defecation reflex.* The bedfast person's unnatural and uncomfortable position on the bedpan does not facilitate elimination. The backward-leaning posture does not promote effective use of the muscles used in defecation. Some people are reluctant to use the bedpan in the presence of others. The embarrassment, lack of privacy, dependence on others to assist with the bedpan, and disruption of normal bowel habits may cause the individual to postpone or ignore the urge for elimination. Repeated postponement eventually suppresses the urge and weakens the defecation reflex.
- *Valsalva manoeuvre.* Some persons may make excessive use of the Valsalva manoeuvre by straining in an attempt to expel the hard stool. This effort dangerously increases intra-abdominal and intrathoracic pressures and places undue stress on the heart and circulatory system.

Integumentary System

Immobility can lead to changes in the integumentary system:

- *Reduced skin turgor.* The skin can atrophy as a result of prolonged immobility. Shifts in body fluids between the fluid compartments can affect the consistency and health of the dermis and subcutaneous tissues in dependent parts of the body, eventually causing a gradual loss in skin **turgor** (elasticity).
- *Skin breakdown.* Normal blood circulation relies on muscle activity. Immobility impedes circulation and diminishes the supply of nutrients to specific areas. As a result, skin breakdown and formation of pressure ulcers can occur.

Psychoneurological System

Immobility can affect a person's self-esteem and neurological functioning:

- *Lowered self-esteem.* Because of a decline in the production of mood-elevating substances, such as endorphins, people experience negative effects on mood when unable to engage in physical activity. People who are unable to carry out the usual activities related to their roles (e.g., as breadwinner, husband, mother, or athlete) become aware of an increased dependence on others. These factors lower the person's self-esteem. Frustration and the decrease in self-esteem may, in turn, provoke exaggerated emotional reactions. Emotional reactions vary considerably. Some individuals become apathetic and withdrawn, some regress, and some become angry and aggressive.

- *Reduced cognitive abilities.* Because the immobilized person's participation in life becomes much narrower and the variety of stimuli decreases, the person's perception of time intervals deteriorates. Problem-solving and decision-making abilities often decline as a result of the lack of intellectual stimulation and the stress of the illness and immobility. In addition, the loss of control over events can cause anxiety.

Assessing

Assessment relative to a client's activity and exercise includes a nursing history and a physical examination of body alignment, gait, appearance and movement of joints, capabilities and limitations for movement, muscle mass and strength, activity tolerance, problems related to immobility, and physical fitness.

The nurse collects information from the client, from other nurses, and from the client's records. The examination and history are important sources of information about disabilities affecting the client's mobility and activity status, such as contractures, edema, pain in the extremities, or generalized fatigue.

Nursing History

An activity and exercise history is usually part of the comprehensive nursing history form. Examples of interview questions to elicit these data are shown in the Assessment: Interview box. If the client indicates a recent pattern change or difficulties with mobility, a more detailed history is required. This detailed history should include the specific nature of the problem, when it first began, its frequency, its causes, if known, how the problem affects daily living, what the client is doing to cope with the problem, and whether these methods have been effective.

ASSESSMENT: INTERVIEW

Activity and Exercise

The nurse can use these questions to gather data about the client's activity and exercise:

DAILY ACTIVITY LEVEL

- What activities do you usually carry out during a routine day?
- Are you able to carry out the following tasks of daily life independently?
  a. Eating
  b. Dressing and grooming
  c. Bathing
  d. Toileting
  e. Ambulating
  f. Using a wheelchair
  g. Transferring in and out of bed, bath, and car
  h. Cooking
  i. Maintaining the home
  j. Shopping
- Where problems exist in your ability to carry out such tasks,
  a. What do you have to depend on family or friends to do for you?
  b. How is the task achieved (by family, friend, agency, or use of specialized equipment)?

ACTIVITY TOLERANCE

- How much and what types of activities make you tired?
- Do you ever experience dizziness, shortness of breath, marked increase in respiratory rate, or other problems following mild or moderate activity?

EXERCISE

- What type of exercise do you carry out to enhance your physical fitness?
- What is the frequency and length of this exercise session?
- Do you believe exercise is beneficial to health? Explain.

FACTORS AFFECTING MOBILITY

- *Environmental factors.* Do stairs, lack of railings or other assistive devices, or an unsafe neighbourhood impede your mobility or exercise regimen?
- *Health problems.* Do any of the following physical or mental health problems, past or current, affect your muscle strength or endurance: heart disease, lung disease, stroke, cancer, neuromuscular problems, musculoskeletal problems, visual or mental impairments, trauma, or pain?
- *Financial factors.* Are your finances adequate to obtain equipment or other aids that you require to enhance your mobility?
- *Lifestyle variables.* Do cultural, leisure, or employment practices influence activity and mobility patterns?

Physical Examination

BODY ALIGNMENT Assessment of body alignment includes an inspection of the client if the client is able to stand. The purpose of body alignment assessment is to identify the following:

- Normal developmental variations in posture
- Poor posture and learning needs to maintain good posture
- Factors contributing to poor posture, such as fatigue or low self-esteem
- Muscle weakness or other motor impairments

To assess alignment, the nurse views the client from lateral (Figure 38.38A), anterior, and posterior perspectives. From the anterior and posterior views, the nurse should observe the following:

- Whether the shoulders and hips are level
- Whether the toes point forward
- Whether the spine is straight, not curved to either side

The slumped posture (Figure 38.38B) is the most common problem that occurs when people stand. The neck is flexed far forward, the abdomen protrudes, the pelvis is thrust forward to create **lordosis** (an exaggerated curvature of the lumbar spine), and the knees are markedly hyperextended. Lower back pain and fatigue occur quickly in people with poor posture.

GAIT The characteristic pattern of a person's **gait** (walk) is assessed to determine the client's mobility and risk for injury through falling. Two phases of normal gait are stance and swing (Figure 38.39). In the *stance phase,* (1) the heel of the right foot strikes the ground, and (2) body weight is spread over the ball of the right foot, while the left heel pushes off and leaves the ground. In the *swing phase,* the leg from behind moves in front of the body. When one leg is in the swing phase, the other is in the stance phase.

The nurse assesses gait as the client walks into the room or asks the client to walk a distance of 3.5 m down a hallway and observes for the following:

- Chin is level, gaze is straight ahead, sternum is lifted, and shoulders are down and back, relaxed away from the ears.
- Heel strikes the ground before the toe.
- Feet are dorsiflexed in the swing phase.
- Arm opposite the swing-through foot moves forward at the same time.
- Gait is smooth, coordinated, and rhythmic, with even weight borne on each foot. Hips gently sway with spinal rotation; the body moves forward smoothly, stopping and starting with ease.

The nurse may also assess **pace** (the number of steps taken per minute). A normal walking pace is 70 to 100 steps per minute. The pace of an older person may slow to about 40 steps per minute.

The nurse should also note the client's need for a prosthesis or assistive device, such as a cane or walker. For a client who uses assistive aids, the nurse assesses gait without the device and compares the assisted and unassisted gaits.

APPEARANCE AND MOVEMENT OF JOINTS Physical examination of the joints involves inspection, palpation, assessment of range of active motion, and, if active

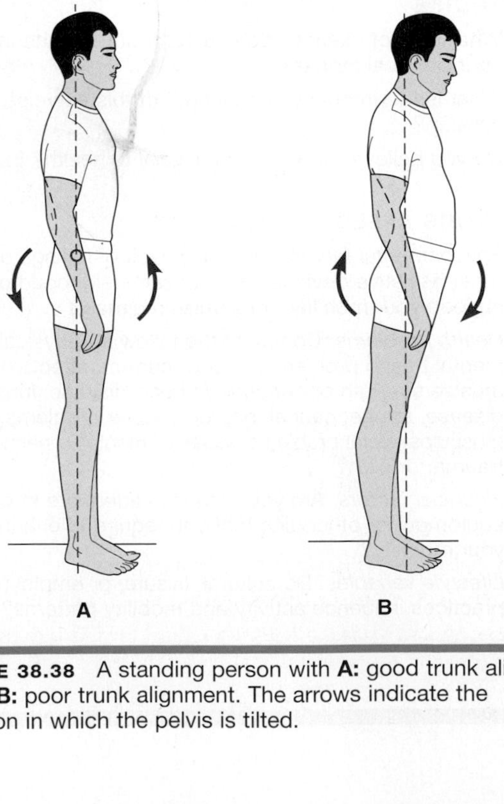

FIGURE 38.38 A standing person with **A:** good trunk alignment; **B:** poor trunk alignment. The arrows indicate the direction in which the pelvis is tilted.

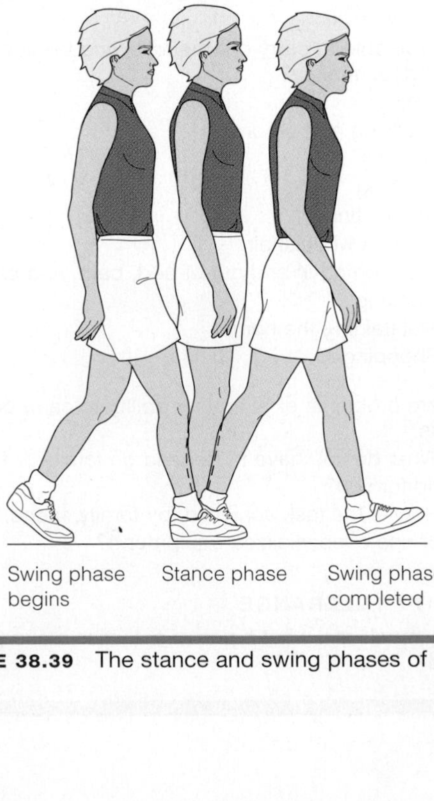

FIGURE 38.39 The stance and swing phases of a normal gait

motion is not possible, assessment of range of passive motion. The nurse should assess the following:

- Any joint swelling or redness, which could indicate the presence of an injury or inflammation
- Any deformity, such as a bony enlargement or contracture, and symmetry of involvement.
- The muscle development associated with each joint and the relative size and symmetry of the muscles on each side of the body.
- Any reported or palpable tenderness.
- **Crepitation**, which is a palpable or an audible crackling or grating sensation produced by joint motion and frequently experienced in joints that have suffered repeated trauma over time.
- Increased temperature over the joint. Palpate the joint by using the backs of the fingers and compare the temperature with that of the symmetric joint.
- The degree of joint movement. Ask the client to move selected body parts as shown in Table 38.2. If indicated, measure the amount of movement with a goniometer, a device that measures the angle of the joint in degrees (see Figure 1 in Skill 27.16, page 632).

Assessment of ROM should not be unduly fatiguing, and the joint movements need to be performed smoothly, slowly, and rhythmically. No joint should be forced. Uneven, jerky movement and forcing can injure the joint and its surrounding muscles and ligaments.

CAPABILITIES AND LIMITATIONS FOR MOVEMENT The nurse needs to obtain data that may indicate hindrances or restrictions to the client's movement and the need for assistance, including the following:

- How the client's illness influences the ability to move and whether the client's health contraindicates any exertion, position, or movement.
- Encumbrances to movement, such as an intravenous line in place or a heavy cast on one leg.
- Mental alertness and ability to follow directions. Check whether the client is receiving medications that hinder the ability to walk safely. Opioids, sedatives, tranquilizers, and some antihistamines cause drowsiness, dizziness, weakness, and orthostatic hypotension.
- Balance and coordination.
- The presence of orthostatic hypotension before transfers. Specifically, assess for any increase in pulse rate, marked fall in blood pressure, dizziness, lightheadedness, and dimming of vision when the client moves from a supine to a vertical posture.
- Degree of comfort. People who have pain may not want to move and require an analgesic before they are moved.
- Vision: Is it adequate to prevent falls?

The nurse also assesses the amount of assistance the client requires for the following:

- Moving in the bed. In particular, observe for the amount of assistance the client requires for turning
  a. From a supine position to a lateral position
  b. From a lateral position on one side to a lateral position on the other
  c. From a supine position to a sitting position in bed
- Rising from a lying position to a sitting position on the edge of the bed. Healthy people can normally rise without support from the arms.
- Rising from a chair to a standing position. Normally, this can be done without pushing with the arms.
- Coordination and balance. Determine the client's abilities to hold the body erect, to bear weight and keep balance in a standing position on one or both legs, to take steps, and to push off from a chair or bed.

MUSCLE MASS AND STRENGTH Before the client undertakes a change in position or attempts to ambulate, it is essential that the nurse assess the client's strength and ability to move. Providing appropriate assistance lowers the risk of muscle strain and body injury to both the client and nurse. Assessment of upper extremity strength is especially important for clients who use ambulation aids, such as walkers and crutches. For information on how to determine muscle mass and strength in lower and upper extremities, see Chapter 27.

ACTIVITY TOLERANCE By determining an appropriate activity level for a client, the nurse can predict whether the client has the strength and endurance to participate in activities that require similar expenditures of energy. This assessment is useful in encouraging increasing independence in people who (1) have a cardiovascular or respiratory disability, (2) have been completely immobilized for a prolonged period, (3) have decreased muscle mass or a musculoskeletal disorder, (4) have experienced inadequate sleep, (5) have experienced pain, or (6) are depressed, anxious, or unmotivated.

The most useful measures in predicting activity tolerance are heart rate, strength, and rhythm; respiratory rate, depth, and rhythm; and blood pressure. These data are obtained at the following times:

- Before the activity starts (baseline data) while the client is at rest
- During the activity
- Immediately after the activity stops
- Three minutes after the activity has stopped and the client has rested

The activity should be stopped immediately in the event of any physiological change indicating the activity is too strenuous or prolonged for the client. These changes include the following:

- Sudden facial pallor
- Feelings of dizziness or weakness
- Change in level of consciousness
- Heart rate or respiratory rate that significantly exceeds baseline or established levels
- Change in heart or respiratory rhythm from regular to irregular

- Weakening of the pulse
- Dyspnea, shortness of breath, or chest pain
- Diastolic blood pressure change of 10 mm Hg or more

If, however, the client tolerates the activity well, and if the client's heart rate returns to baseline levels within three minutes after the activity ceases, the activity is considered safe. This activity, then, can serve as a standard for predicting the client's tolerance for similar activities.

PROBLEMS RELATED TO IMMOBILITY When collecting data pertaining to the problems of immobility, the nurse uses the assessment methods of inspection, palpation, and auscultation; checks results of laboratory tests; and takes measurements, including body weight, fluid intake, and fluid output. Specific techniques for assessing immobility problems and abnormal assessment findings related to the complications of immobility are listed in Table 38.4.

It is extremely important to obtain and record baseline assessment data soon after the client first becomes immobile. These baseline data serve as the standard against which all data collected throughout the period of immobilization are compared.

Because a major nursing responsibility is to prevent the complications of immobility, the nurse needs to identify clients at risk of developing such complications before problems arise. Clients at risk include those who (1) are poorly nourished, (2) have decreased sensitivity to pain, temperature, or pressure, (3) have existing cardiovascular, pulmonary, or neuromuscular problems, or (4) have an altered level of consciousness.

Diagnosing

Mobility problems may be appropriate as the diagnostic label or as the etiology for other nursing diagnoses. NANDA International (2007) includes the following nursing diagnostic labels for activity and exercise problems:

- *Activity Intolerance* (specify level), insufficient physiological or psychological energy to endure or complete required or desired daily activities. Four levels that can be used after the diagnostic label are as follows:
  - *Level I:* Walk, regular pace, on level ground indefinitely; climb one flight of stairs or more but more short of breath than normal

TABLE 38.4 Assessing Problems of Immobility

Assessment	Problem
Musculoskeletal System	
Measure arm and leg circumferences	Decreased circumference caused by decreased muscle mass
Palpate and observe body joints	Stiffness or pain in joints
Take goniometric measurements of joint ROM	Decreased joint ROM, joint contractures
Cardiovascular System	
Auscultate the heart	Increased heart rate
Measure blood pressure	Orthostatic hypotension
Palpate and observe sacrum, legs, and feet	Peripheral dependent edema, increased peripheral vein engorgement
Palpate extremity pulses	Weak peripheral pulses
Check capillary refill	Decreased peripheral circulation
Measure calf muscle circumferences	Edema; thrombus formation
Observe calf muscle for redness, tenderness, and swelling	Thrombophlebitis
Respiratory System	
Observe chest movements	Asymmetric chest movements, dyspnea
Auscultate chest	Diminished breath sounds, crackles, wheezes, and increased respiratory rate
Metabolic System	
Measure height and weight	Weight loss caused by muscle atrophy and loss of subcutaneous fat
Take anthropometric measurements	Loss of body muscle and subcutaneous fat
Palpate body skin	Generalized edema caused by low blood protein levels
Urinary System	
Measure intake and output	Dehydration
Inspect urine output	Cloudy, dark urine, high specific gravity
Palpate urinary bladder	Distended urinary bladder caused by urinary retention
Gastrointestinal System	
Observe stool	Hard, dry, small stool
Auscultate bowel sounds	Decreased bowel sounds because of decreased intestinal motility
Integumentary System	
Observe skin for intactness, redness, pallor, warmth, tenderness	Break in skin integrity, pressure areas
Psychoneurological System	
Observe behaviours, affect, and cognition Monitor developmental skills in children	Anger, flat affect, confusion crying, anxiety, decline in cognitive function, or vegetative signs such as sleep and appetite disturbances that warrant further evaluation

    - *Level II:* Walk one city block 160 m on level ground; climb one flight slowly without stopping
    - *Level III:* Walk no more than 16 m on level ground without stopping; unable to climb one flight of stairs without stopping
    - *Level IV:* Dyspnea and fatigue at rest
- *Risk for Activity Intolerance:* Presence of risk factors for experiencing insufficient physiological or psychological energy to endure or complete required or desired daily activities
- *Impaired Physical Mobility:* Limitation in independent, purposeful physical movement of the body or of one or more extremities (more specific versions of this diagnosis are *Impaired Bed Mobility, Impaired Walking, Impaired Wheelchair Mobility,* and *Impaired Transfer Ability*)
- *Sedentary Lifestyle:* Reports a habit of life that is characterized by a low physical activity level
- *Risk for Disuse Syndrome:* Risk for deterioration of body systems as a result of prescribed or unavoidable musculoskeletal inactivity

Depending on the data obtained, problems with mobility often affect other areas of human functioning and indicate other diagnoses. In these instances, the mobility problem becomes the etiology. Examples in which *Impaired Physical Mobility* is the etiology follow. The etiology needs to be described more explicitly in such terms as reduced ROM, neuromuscular impairment or musculoskeletal impairment of upper and lower extremities, or joint pain.

- *Fear* (of falling)
- *Risk for Falls*
- *Powerlessness*
- *Self-Care Deficit*
- *Low Self-Esteem*
- *Ineffective Coping*

When problems associated with prolonged immobility arise, many other diagnoses may be necessary. Examples include, but are not limited to, the following:

- *Ineffective Airway Clearance* if there is stasis of pulmonary secretions
- *Risk for Infection* if there is stasis of urinary or pulmonary secretions
- *Risk for Injury* if orthostatic hypotension is present

Planning

Positioning, transferring, and ambulating clients are almost always independent nursing functions. The physician usually orders specific body positions only after surgery, anaesthesia, or trauma involving the nervous and musculoskeletal systems. All clients should have an activity order written by their physician when they are admitted to the agency for care and following surgery and invasive diagnostic procedures (e.g., an angiogram, a lumbar puncture).

As part of planning, the nurse is responsible for identifying those clients who need assistance with body alignment and determining the degree of assistance they need. The nurse must be sensitive to the client's need to function as independently as possible yet provide assistance when the client needs it.

Most clients require some nursing guidance and assistance to learn about, achieve, and maintain proper body mechanics. The nurse should also plan to teach clients applicable skills. For example, a client with a back injury needs to learn how to get out of bed safely and comfortably; a client with an injured leg needs to learn how to transfer from bed to wheelchair safely; and a client with a newly acquired walker needs to learn how to use it safely. Nurses often teach family members or caregivers safe moving, lifting, and transfer techniques in the home setting.

The goals established for clients vary according to the diagnosis and defining characteristics related to each individual. Examples of overall goals for clients with actual or potential problems related to mobility or activity follow:

- Increase tolerance for physical activity.
- Restore or improve the capability to ambulate or participate in ADLs.
- Avoid injury from falling or improper use of body mechanics.
- Improve physical fitness.
- Avoid any complications associated with immobility.
- Maintain or enhance social, emotional, and intellectual well-being.

Planning for Home Care

Clients who have been hospitalized for activity or mobility problems often need continued care in the home. In preparation for discharge, the nurse needs to determine the client's actual and potential health problems, strengths, and resources. The Assessment: Home Care box describes the specific assessment data required before establishing a discharge plan for clients with mobility or activity problems. A major aspect of discharge planning involves instructional needs of the client and family; see the Teaching: Home Care box.

Implementing

Nurses can initiate and apply a wide variety of exercise and activity interventions as needed to address a multitude of client concerns. Nursing interventions that pertain to exercise and activity include activity therapy;

ASSESSMENT: HOME CARE

Ability and Activity Problems

To create a discharge plan, the nurse needs to collect these data:

CLIENT AND ENVIRONMENT

- *Capabilities or tolerance for required and desired activities:* Self-care (feeding, bathing, toileting, dressing, grooming, home maintenance, shopping, cooking), recreational activities
- *Mobility aids required:* Cane, walker, crutches, wheelchair, transfer boards
- *Equipment required if immobilized:* Special bed, side rails, pressure-reducing mattress
- *Current level of knowledge:* Body mechanics for use of mobility aids; specific exercises prescribed
- *Home mobility hazard appraisal:* Adequacy of lighting; presence of handrails; safety of pathways and stairs; congested areas; unanchored rugs, mats, or electrical cords; and any other obstacles to safe movement; structural adjustments needed for wheelchair access

FAMILY OR CAREGIVER

- *Caregiver availability, skills, and willingness to assist:* Assess learning needs and develop appropriate teaching plan, primary people able to assist client with self-care, movement, shopping, and so on; physical and emotional status to assist with care
- *Family role changes and coping:* Effect on financial status, parenting and spousal roles, social roles
- *Availability of caregiver support:* Other support people available for occasional duties, such as shopping, transportation, housekeeping, cooking, budgeting, respite care

COMMUNITY

- *Resources:* Availability and familiarity with sources of medical equipment, financial assistance, homemaker services, hygiene care, and other services; Meals on Wheels; spiritual counsellors and visitors; sources of respite for caregiver

TEACHING: HOME CARE

Activity and Exercise

Discharge planning includes teaching the client and family about the following:

MAINTAINING MUSCULOSKELETAL FUNCTION

- Teach the systematic performance of passive or assistive ROM exercises to maintain joint mobility.
- As appropriate, demonstrate the proper way to perform isotonic, isometric, or isokinetic exercises to maintain muscle mass and tone (collaborate with the physician and physical therapist on these). Incorporate ADLs into exercise program, if appropriate.
- Provide a written schedule for the type, frequency, and duration of exercises; encourage the use of a progress graph or chart to facilitate adherence with the therapy.
- Offer an ambulation schedule, as appropriate.
- Instruct in the availability of assistive ambulatory devices and correct use of them.
- Discuss pain-control measures required before exercise, as appropriate.

PREVENTING INJURY

- Provide assistive devices for moving and transferring, whenever possible, and teach safe transfer and ambulation techniques.
- Discuss safety measures to avoid falls (e.g., locking wheelchairs, wearing appropriate footwear, using rubber tips on crutches, keeping the environment safe, and using mechanical aids, such as a raised toilet seat, grab bars, a urinal, a bedpan or commode, to facilitate toileting).
- Teach the use of proper body mechanics, especially for those times when assistive equipment is not used.
- Teach ways to prevent postural hypotension.

MANAGING ENERGY TO PREVENT FATIGUE

- Discuss activity and rest patterns and develop a plan, as indicated; intersperse rest periods with activity periods.
- Discuss ways to minimize fatigue, such as performing activities more slowly and for shorter periods, resting more often, and using more assistance, as required.
- Provide information about available resources to help with ADLs and home maintenance management.
- Teach ways to increase energy (e.g., increasing intake of high-energy foods, ensuring adequate rest and sleep, controlling pain).
- Teach techniques to monitor activity tolerance as appropriate.

REFERRALS

Provide appropriate information about accessing community resources: home care agencies, sources of adaptive equipment, and so on.

calming technique; cardiac care; rehabilitation; cognitive stimulation; constipation management; distraction; exercise promotion (strength and stretching); exercise therapy (ambulation, balance, joint mobility, muscle control); fall prevention; health education; infection prevention; memory training; mood management; pelvic muscle exercise; pressure ulcer prevention; progressive muscle relaxation; recreation therapy; religious ritual enhancement; self-care assistance; self-esteem enhancement; simple relaxation therapy; sleep enhancement; spiritual growth facilitation; sports-injury prevention; teaching: prescribed activity or exercise; therapeutic play; weight management and weight reduction.

Nursing strategies to maintain or promote body alignment and mobility involve positioning clients appropriately, moving and turning clients in bed, transferring clients, providing ROM exercises, ambulating clients with or without mechanical aids, and creating strategies to prevent the complications of immobility. Whenever positioning, moving, lifting, and ambulating clients, nurses must use proper body mechanics to avoid musculoskeletal strain and injury.

Using Body Mechanics

Body mechanics is the term used to describe the efficient, coordinated, and safe use of the body to move objects and carry out ADLs. The major purpose of body mechanics is to facilitate the safe and efficient use of appropriate muscle groups to maintain balance, reduce the energy required, reduce fatigue, and decrease the risk of injury. Although good body mechanics is essential for clients, it is of utmost concern for nurses who, even with careful attention to body mechanics, experience one of the highest incidences of work-related back injuries (Canadian Nurses Association, 2006; O'Brien-Pallas et al., 2004). Unfortunately, many nurses further contribute to their injuries by continuing to work despite the presence of significant musculoskeletal pain (O'Brien-Pallas et al., 2004). The aging of the nursing workforce poses challenges for ways to decrease musculoskeletal injury in nurses (Lavoie-Tremblay, O'Brien-Pallas, Viens, Hamelin Brabant, & Gelinas, 2006). Important evidence exists of the following:

- Training in body mechanics alone does not prevent job-related injury (Canadian Centre for Occupational Health and Safety [CCOHS], 2003).
- Health workers who wear back belts to protect themselves from back injury may not be reducing their risk at all. The use of back belts in preventing health-care-worker back injury remains controversial and may even give the worker a false sense of security, thus leading to lax body mechanics (Ammendolia, Kerr, Bombardier, & the Canadian Task Force on Preventive Health Care, 2003).
- Back injuries are more prevalent in 20- to 45-year-old health-care workers when compared with those over 45 who have developed expertise in relation to lifting and turning patients (CCOHS, 2003).
- The average person should lift no more than 20 kg (CCOHS, 2003).
- Although there is a risk of injury caused by peak forces during acute events, musculoskeletal injuries can also result from cumulative loading (Occupational Health and Safety Agency for Healthcare in British Columbia, 2006).
- Strained nurse–physician relationships are correlated with musculoskeletal injuries in nurses (O'Brien-Pallas et al., 2004).

Fortunately, the development of assistive client-handling equipment and devices has rendered strict manual patient handling unnecessary. The equipment is also thought to provide greater client safety, dignity, and comfort. Costs of equipment appear to be less than the costs of work-related injury (Nelson, 2007). The equipment recommendations include full sling mechanical lift devices for totally dependent or extensive assistance level clients; full sling stand assist lift or full sling mechanical lifts for dependent lifts from the floor; and transfer or gait belts for client-assisted lifts from the floor.

Until all work settings provide safe environments in which nurses have the equipment they need, content pertaining to body mechanics will be included in this chapter. Readers are encouraged to support "no manual lift" and "no solo lift" policies in their workplaces and to become involved in legislation and equipment-purchase initiatives. Nurses must participate in this shift in ergonomic awareness and are encouraged to visit the Canadian Nurses Association website to read about workplace initiatives to promote nurses' health.

When a person moves, the centre of gravity shifts continuously in the direction of the moving body parts. Balance depends on the interrelationship of the centre of gravity, the line of gravity, and the base of support. When a person moves, the closer the line of gravity is to the centre of the base of support, the greater the person's stability (Figure 38.40A). Conversely, the closer the line of gravity is to the edge of the base of support, the more precarious the balance (Figure 38.40B). If the line of gravity falls outside the base of support, the person falls (Figure 38.40C).

The broader the base of support and the lower the centre of gravity, the greater the stability and balance. Body balance, therefore, can be greatly enhanced by (1) widening the base of support, and (2) lowering the centre of gravity, bringing it closer to the base of support. The base of support is easily widened by spreading the feet farther apart. The centre of gravity is readily lowered by flexing the hips and knees until a squatting position is achieved. The importance of these alterations cannot be overemphasized for nurses.

Two movements to avoid because of their potential for causing back injury are twisting (rotation) of the thoracolumbar spine and acute flexion of the back with hips and knees straight (stooping). Undesirable twisting of the back can be prevented by squarely facing the direction of movement, whether pushing, pulling, or sliding, and moving the object directly toward or away from the centre of gravity.

LIFTING Because manual lifting of patients is a major factor in musculoskeletal and back injuries in nurses, it is important to remember that there are limits to the weight that nurses should lift without assistance from proper equipment or other persons. The CCOHS (2003) indicates that individuals should lift no more than 20 kg. Provincial and territorial standards may vary. The patient's weight, however, is not the only factor to consider when deciding whether lifting a patient is safe. For example, disoriented patients may initially be cooperative with movement but suddenly stop helping or become aggressive, putting the nurse at risk for injury. A patient with deformities or a high level of fatigue may add to the lifting challenge. Types of assistive equipment include partial standing lifts (Figure 38.41), permanently mounted ceiling lifts (Figure 38.42), and horizontal air-transfer mattresses (Figure 38.43).

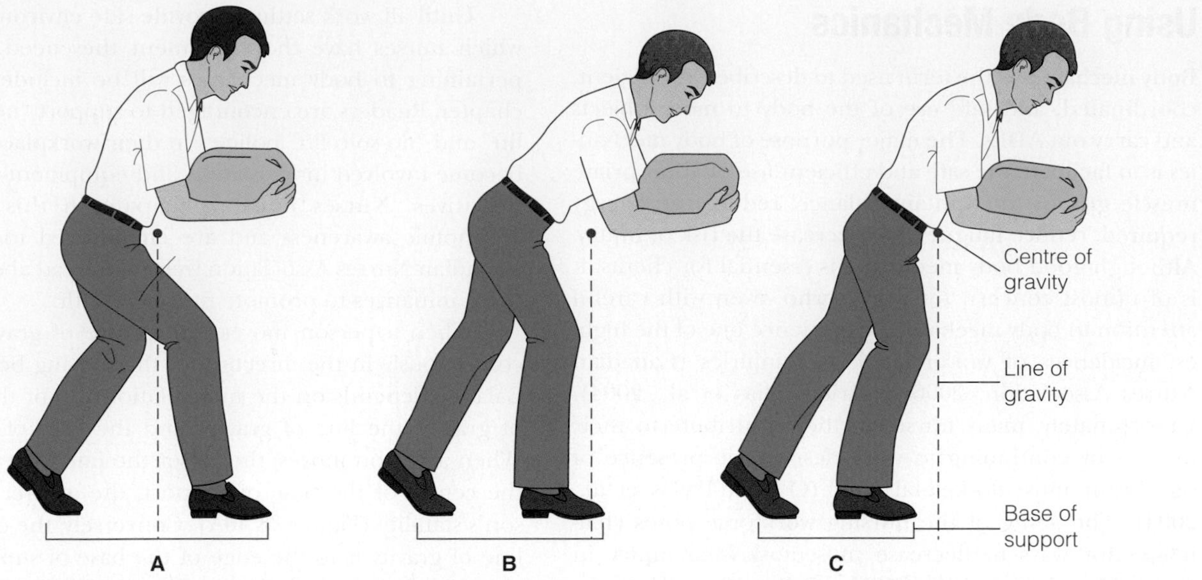

FIGURE 38.40 **A:** Balance is maintained when the line of gravity falls close to the base of support; **B:** balance is precarious when the line of gravity falls at the edge of the base of support; **C:** balance cannot be maintained when the line of gravity falls outside the base of support.

When a person lifts or carries an object, for example, a suitcase, the weight of the object becomes part of the person's body weight. This weight affects the location of the person's centre of gravity, which is displaced in the direction of the added weight. To counteract this potential imbalance, body parts (e.g., arm and trunk) move in a direction away from the weight. In this way, the centre of gravity is maintained over the same point in the base of support. By holding the lifted object as close as possible to the body's centre of gravity, the lifter avoids undue displacement of the centre of gravity and achieves greater stability.

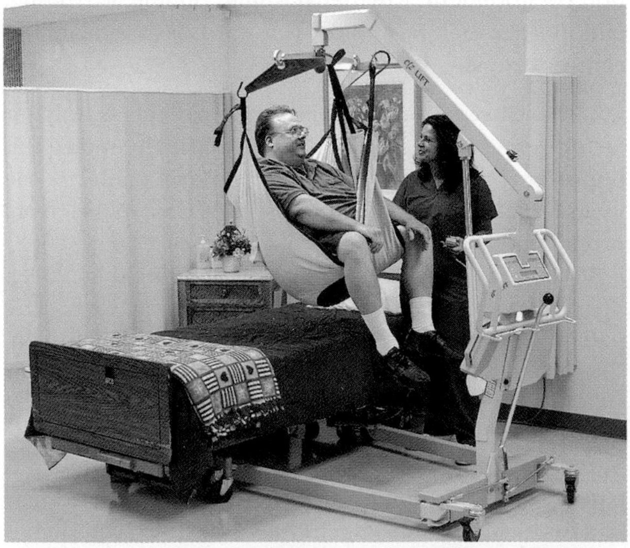

FIGURE 38.41 EZ Lift is an electric client lift that moves clients from a bed, a chair, a toilet, or the floor.

People can lift more weight when they use a lever than when they do not. In the body, the bones of the skeleton act as levers, a joint is a *fulcrum* (fixed point about which a lever moves), and the muscles exert the force (Figure 38.44). Use of the arms as levers is often applied in clinical practice when the nurse needs to raise a client's head off the bed, for example, or give back care to a client in traction.

Because lifting involves movement against gravity, the nurse must use major muscle groups of the thighs, knees, upper and lower arms, abdomen, and pelvis to prevent back strain. The nurse can increase overall muscle strength by synchronized use of as many muscle groups as possible during an activity. For instance, when the arms are used in an activity, dividing the work between the arms and legs helps prevent back strain.

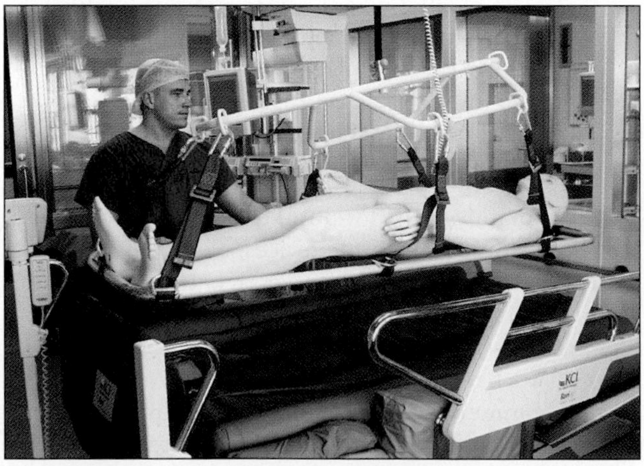

FIGURE 38.42 A permanently mounted ceiling lift with a mannequin being used for demonstration purposes

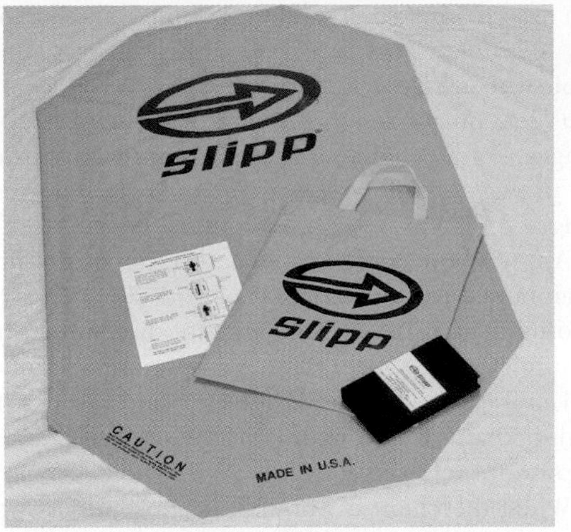

FIGURE 38.43 The Slipp Patient Mover is a client-moving device that reduces the nurse's exposure to back injuries and maximizes client comfort.

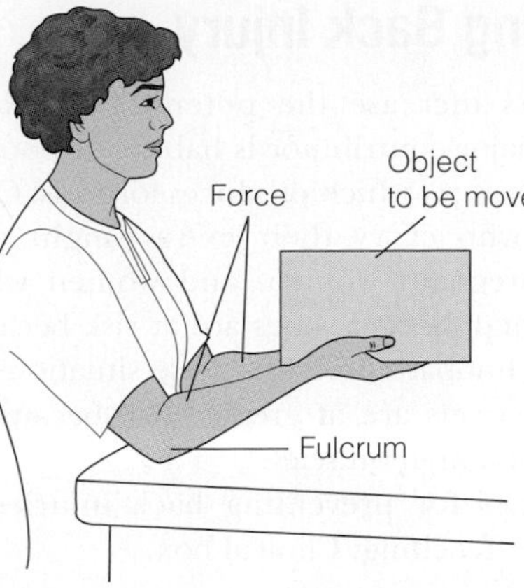

FIGURE 38.44 Using the arm as a lever

Another technique based on the principle of leverage can be used when lifting objects from the floor to waist level. In this technique, the back and knees are flexed until the load is at thigh level, at which point the knees remain flexed to provide thrust as the back begins to straighten (Figure 38.45). This technique provides for better balance, leverage, and synchronized use of muscles, which help avoid back pain and injury. When a nurse lifts an object to knee level, the shoulder and arm muscles pull, the abdominal and pelvic muscles contract for leverage and pull, and the thigh and leg muscles exert the upward thrust to bring the object off the floor. When one lifts an object from midthigh to waist level, force is provided essentially by the leg and thigh muscle groups, but the back and pelvic muscles remain contracted.

In all positions, it is important to maintain a distance of at least 30 cm (approximately shoulder width) between the feet and to keep the load close to the body, especially when it is at knee level). Before attempting the lift, the nurse must ensure that the floor is free of hazards, the path for moving the object is clear, and the nurse's base of support is secure.

PULLING AND PUSHING When pulling or pushing an object, a person maintains balance with least effort when the base of support is enlarged in the direction in which the movement is to be produced or opposed. For example, when pushing an object, a person can enlarge the base of support by moving the front foot forward. When pulling an object, a person can enlarge the base of support by (1) moving the rear leg back as the person is facing the object or (2) moving the front foot forward if the person is facing away from the object. It is easier and safer to pull an object toward the person's centre of gravity than to push it away, as the person can exert more control of the object's movement when pulling it.

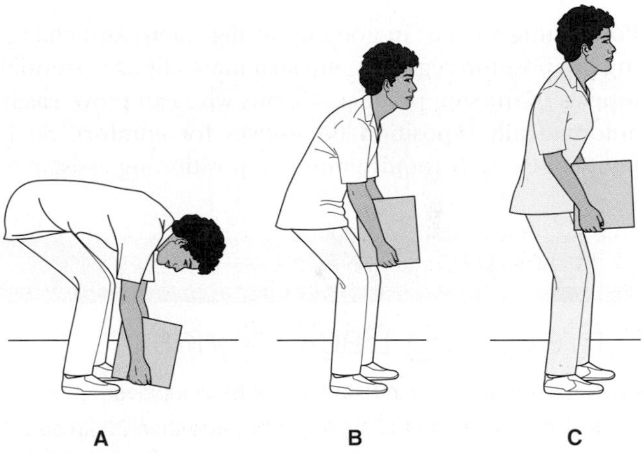

FIGURE 38.45 Lifting heavy objects from the floor to waist level. **A:** Stand close to the load and flex the back and, lowering the body to grasp the load, **B:** begin lifting with the back flexed, and gradually straighten the knees so that the leg muscles bear most of the burden; **C:** to hold or walk with the object, maintain a less flexed, but not completely straight, position.

PIVOTING Pivoting is a technique in which the body is turned in a way that avoids twisting of the spine. To pivot, place one foot ahead of the other, raise the heels very slightly, and put the body weight on the balls of the feet. When the weight is off the heels, the frictional surface is decreased and the knees are not twisted when turning. Keeping the body aligned, turn (pivot) about 90 degrees in the desired direction. The foot that was forward will now be behind.

CLINICAL ALERT

Lateral-assist devices, such as horizontal air-transfer mattresses and transfer chairs, are essential equipment for most client care areas to prevent acute and chronic back pain and disability. Observing principles of body mechanics is recommended even when using assistive equipment, as any lifting and forceful movement is potentially injurious, especially when repeated over time.

Preventing Back Injury

Many factors increase the potential for lower back injuries. A major contributor is habitually poor standing and sitting posture, which produces lordosis. Overweight individuals who carry their extra weight over their abdomen, pregnant women, and women who consistently wear high-heeled shoes are at risk because of the exaggerated lumbar curvature these situations produce. Sedentary persons are at greater risk because of weak back and abdominal muscles.

Guidelines for preventing back injuries are presented in the Teaching: Clinical box.

Positioning Clients

Positioning a client in good body alignment and changing the position regularly and systematically are essential aspects of nursing practice. Clients who can move easily automatically reposition themselves for comfort. Such people generally require minimal positioning assistance from nurses other than guidance about ways to maintain body alignment and to exercise their joints. However, people who are weak, frail, in pain, paralyzed, or unconscious rely on nurses to provide or assist with position changes. For all clients, it is important to assess the skin and provide skin care before and after a position change.

Any position, correct or incorrect, can be detrimental if maintained for a prolonged period. Frequent change of position helps to prevent muscle discomfort, undue pressure resulting in pressure ulcers, damage to superficial nerves and blood vessels, and contractures. Position changes also maintain muscle tone and stimulate postural reflexes.

When the client is not able to move independently or assist with moving, the *preferred method is to use appropriate assistive equipment, as well as to have two or more people move or turn the client.* Appropriate assistance reduces the risk of muscle strain and body injury to both the client and the nurse and is likely to protect the comfort and dignity of the client.

When positioning clients in bed, the nurse can do a number of things to ensure proper alignment and promote client comfort and safety:

- Make sure the mattress is firm and level yet has enough give to fill in and support natural body curvatures. A sagging mattress, a mattress that is too soft, or an underfilled waterbed used over a prolonged period can contribute to the development of hip flexion contractures and low back strain and pain. *Bed boards* made of plywood and placed beneath a sagging mattress are increasingly recommended for clients who have back problems or are prone to them. Some bed boards are hinged across the middle so that they will bend as the head of the bed is raised. It is particularly important in the home setting to inspect the mattress for support.
- Ensure that the bed is clean and dry. Wrinkled or damp sheets increase the risk of pressure ulcer formation. Make sure extremities can move freely, whenever possible. For example, the top bed sheets need to be loose enough for the client to move the feet.
- Place support devices in specified areas according to the client's position. See Box 38.2 for commonly used support devices. Use only those support devices needed to maintain alignment and to prevent stress on the client's muscles and joints. If the person is capable of movement, too many devices limit mobility and increase the potential for muscle weakness and atrophy.
- Avoid placing one body part, particularly one with bony prominences, directly on top of another body part. Excessive pressure can damage veins and predispose the client to thrombus formation and decubitus ulcers. Pressure against the popliteal space may damage nerves and blood vessels in this area. Pillows can provide needed cushioning.
- Plan a *systematic 24-hour schedule* for position changes.

TEACHING: CLINICAL

Preventing Back Injuries

These guidelines can help prevent back injuries:

- Understand that lifting loads of more than 20 kg can lead to back or musculoskeletal injury. Keep in mind that even lifting loads of less than this amount can cause injury if proper body mechanics are not used.
- Avoid lifting anything greater than 20 kg. Use assistive equipment, get help from co-workers, and participate in the purchasing or ordering process of appropriate assistive equipment for your work setting.
- Become consciously aware of your posture and body mechanics.
- When standing for a long time, periodically flex one hip and knee and rest your foot on an object, if possible.
- When sitting, keep your knees slightly higher than your hips.
- Use a firm mattress and soft pillow that provide good body support at natural body curvatures.
- Exercise regularly to maintain overall physical condition; include exercises that strengthen the pelvic, abdominal, and spinal muscles.
- Avoid exercises that cause pain or require spinal flexion with straight legs (e.g., toe touching and situps) or spinal rotation (twisting).
- When moving an object, spread your feet apart to provide a wide base of support.
- When lifting an object, distribute the weight between large muscles of the legs and arms.
- Wear clothing that allows you to use good body mechanics and comfortable low-heeled shoes that provide good foot support and will not cause you to slip, stumble, or turn your ankle.

BOX 38.2 SUPPORT DEVICES

The following are some commonly used support devices:

- *Pillows*. Different sizes are available. They are used for support or elevation of a body part (e.g., an arm). Specially designed dense pillows can be used to elevate the upper body.
- *Mattresses*. There are two types of mattresses: ones that fit on the bed frame (e.g., standard bed mattress) and those that fit *on* the standard bed mattress (e.g., egg-crate mattress). Mattresses should be evenly supportive.
- *Bed boards.* The boards are usually made of wood and are placed under the mattress to provide support.
- *Chair beds.* These beds can be placed into the position of a chair for clients who cannot move from the bed but require a sitting position.
- *Foot boot.* These are made of a variety of substances. They usually have a firm exterior and padding of foam to protect the skin. They provide support to the feet in a natural position and keep the weight of covers off the toes. Persons who are able to sit may benefit from high-top shoes to maintain foot alignment.
- *Footboard.* This is a flat panel often made of plastic or wood. It keeps the feet in dorsiflexion to prevent plantar flexion.

Sometimes, a person who appears well aligned may be experiencing real discomfort. Both appearance, in relation to alignment criteria, and comfort are important in achieving effective alignment.

FOWLER'S POSITION **Fowler's position**, or a semisitting position, is a bed position in which the head and trunk are raised 45 degrees. In **low-Fowler's**, or **semi-Fowler's position** (Figure 38.46), the head and trunk are raised 15 to 45 degrees; in **high-Fowler's position**, the head and trunk are raised 90 degrees (see Table 38.5). In this position, the knees may or may not be flexed.

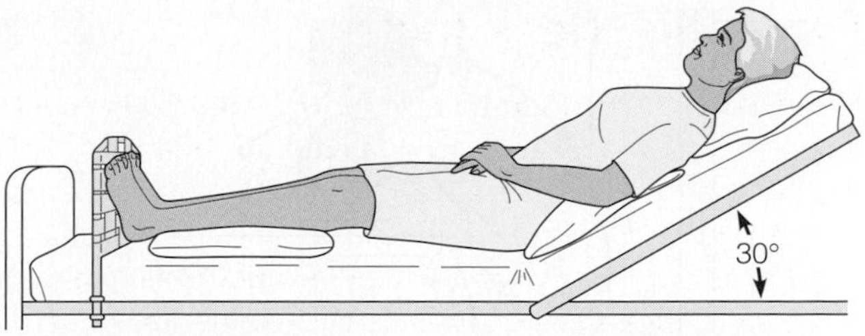

FIGURE 38.46 Low Fowler's or semi-Fowler's position (supported). Note that arm support is omitted in this instance. The amount of support depends on the needs of the client.

Fowler's position is the position of choice for people who have difficulty breathing and for some people with heart problems. When the client is in this position, gravity pulls the diaphragm downward, allowing greater chest expansion and lung ventilation. It is not the position of choice if the client is at risk for developing decubitus ulcers (because of the shearing force).

A common error nurses make when aligning clients in Fowler's position is placing an overly large pillow or more than one pillow behind the client's head. These errors promote the development of neck flexion contractures.

ORTHOPNEIC POSITION In the **orthopneic position**, the client sits in bed or on the side of the bed with an overbed table across the lap (Figure 38.47). This position facilitates respiration by allowing maximum chest expansion. It is particularly helpful to clients who have problems exhaling because they can press the lower part of the chest against the edge of the overbed table.

DORSAL RECUMBENT POSITION In the **dorsal recumbent** (back-lying) **position** (Figure 38.48), the client's head and shoulders are slightly elevated on a small pillow. In some agencies, the terms *dorsal recumbent* and *supine* are used interchangeably; strictly speaking, however, in

TABLE 38.5 Fowler's Position

Unsupported Position	Problem to Be Prevented	Corrective Measure*
Bed-sitting position with upper part of body elevated 30° to 90° commencing at hips	Posterior flexion of lumbar curvature	Pillow at lower back (lumbar region) to support lumbar region
Head rests on bed surface	Hyperextension of neck	Pillows to support head, neck, and upper back
Arms fall at sides	Shoulder muscle strain, possible dislocation of shoulders, edema of hands and arms with flaccid paralysis, flexion contracture of the wrist	Pillow under forearms to eliminate pull on shoulder and assist venous blood flow from hands and lower arms
Legs lie flat and straight on lower bed surface	Hyperextension of knees	Small pillow under thighs to flex knees
Heels rest on bed surface	Pressure on heels	Pillow under lower legs
Feet are in plantar flexion	Plantar flexion of feet (foot drop)	Footboard to provide support for dorsal flexion

**The amount of support depends on the needs of the individual client.*

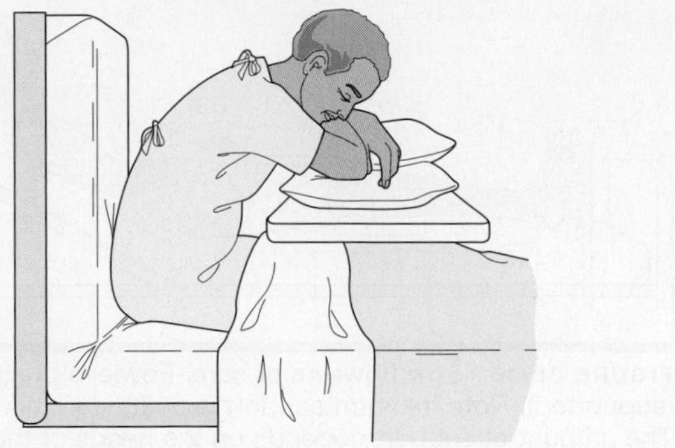

FIGURE 38.47 Orthopneic position

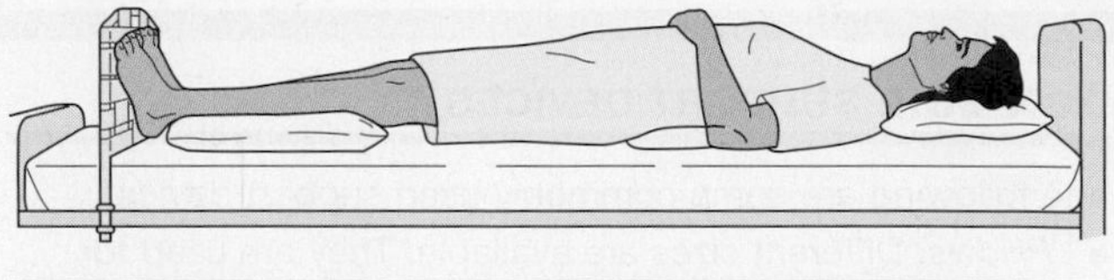

FIGURE 38.48 Dorsal recumbent position (supported)

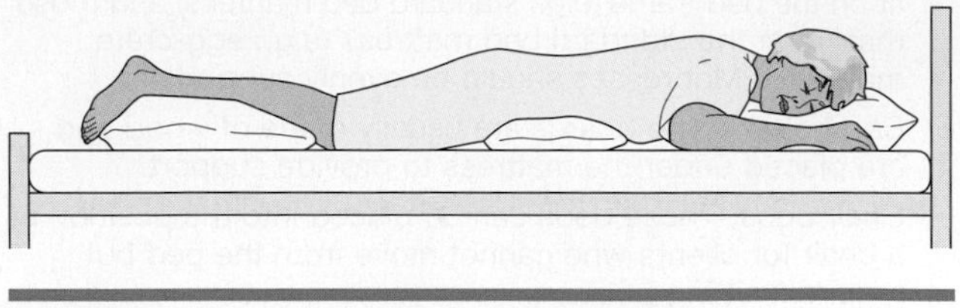

FIGURE 38.49 Prone position (supported)

the **supine** or **dorsal position** the head and shoulders are not elevated. In both positions, the client's forearms may be elevated on pillows or placed at the client's sides. Supports are similar in both positions, except for the head pillow. See Table 38.6. The dorsal recumbent position is used to provide comfort and to facilitate healing following certain surgeries or administration of anaesthetics (e.g., spinal).

PRONE POSITION In the **prone position**, the client lies on the abdomen with the head turned to one side (Figure 38.49). The hips are not flexed. Both children and adults often sleep in this position, sometimes with one or both arms flexed over their heads. This position has several advantages. It is the only bed position that allows full extension of the hip and knee joints. When used periodically, the prone position helps prevent flexion contractures of the hips and knees, thereby counteracting a problem caused by all other bed positions. The prone position also promotes drainage from the mouth and is especially useful for unconscious clients or those clients recovering from surgery of the mouth or throat. See Table 38.7.

The prone position poses some distinct disadvantages. The pull of gravity on the trunk produces a marked lordosis in most people, and the neck is rotated laterally to a significant degree. For this reason, the prone position may not be recommended for people with problems of the cervical or lumbar spine. This position also causes plantar flexion. Some clients with cardiac or respiratory problems find the prone position confining and suffocating because chest expansion is inhibited during respirations. The prone position should be used only when the client's back is correctly aligned, only for short periods, and only for people with no evidence of spinal abnormalities.

LATERAL POSITION In the **lateral** (side-lying) **position** (Figure 38.50), the person lies on one side of the body. Flexing the top hip and knee and placing this leg in front of the body creates a wider, triangular base of support and achieves greater stability. The greater the flexion of the top hip and knee, the greater the stability and balance in this position. This flexion reduces lordosis and promotes good back alignment. For this reason, the lateral position is good for resting and sleeping clients. The lateral position helps relieve pressure on the sacrum

TABLE 38.6 Dorsal Recumbent Position

Unsupported Position	Problem to Be Prevented	Corrective Measure*
Head is flat on bed surface	Hyperextension of neck in thick-chested person	Pillow of suitable thickness under head and shoulders if necessary for alignment
Lumbar curvature of spine is apparent	Posterior flexion of lumbar curvature	Roll or small pillow under lumbar curvature
Legs may be externally rotated	External rotation of legs	Roll or sandbag placed laterally to trochanter of femur (optional)
Legs are extended	Hyperextension of knees	Small pillow under thigh to flex knee slightly
Feet assume plantar flexion position	Plantar flexion (foot drop)	Footboard or rolled pillow to support feet in dorsal flexion
Heels on bed surface	Pressure on heels	Pillow under lower legs

**The amount of support depends on the needs of the individual client.*

TABLE 38.7 Prone Position

Unsupported Position	Problem to Be Prevented	Corrective Measure*
Head is turned to side and neck is slightly flexed	Flexion or hyperextension of neck	Small pillow under head unless contraindicated because of promotion of mucous drainage from mouth
Body lies flat on abdomen, accentuating lumbar curvature	Hyperextension of lumbar curvature; difficulty breathing; pressure on breasts (women); pressure on genitals (men)	Small pillow or roll under abdomen just below diaphragm
Toes rest on bed surface; feet are in plantar flexion	Plantar flexion (foot drop)	Allow feet to fall naturally over end of mattress, or support lower legs on a pillow so that toes do not touch the bed

The amount of support depends on the needs of the individual client.

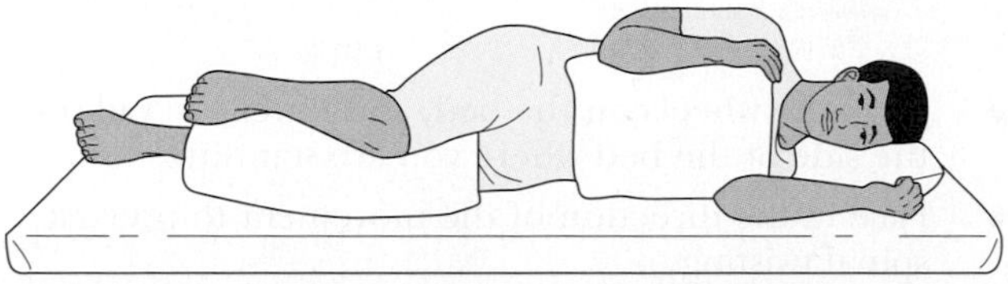

FIGURE 38.50 Lateral position (supported)

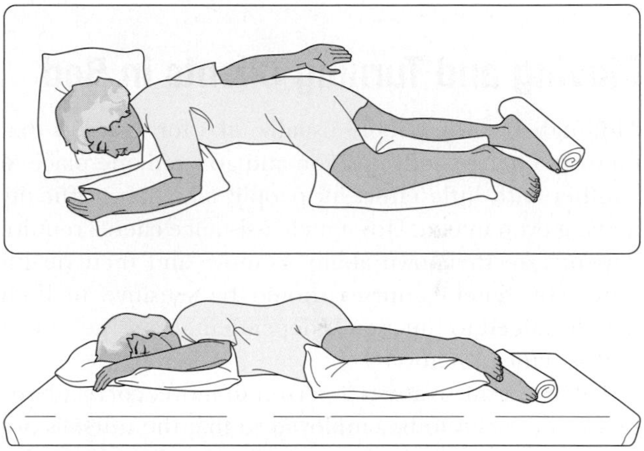

FIGURE 38.51 Sims' position (supported)

and heels in people who sit for much of the day or who are confined to bed and rest in Fowler's or dorsal recumbent positions much of the time. In the lateral position, most of the body's weight is borne by the lateral aspect of the lower scapula, the lateral aspect of the ilium, and the greater trochanter of the femur. People who have sensory or motor deficits on one side of the body usually find that lying on the uninvolved side is more comfortable (Table 38.8).

SIMS' POSITION In **Sims'** (semiprone) **position** (Figure 38.51), the client assumes a posture halfway between the lateral and the prone positions. The lower arm is positioned behind the client, and the upper arm is flexed at the shoulder and the elbow. Both legs are flexed in front of the client. The upper leg is more acutely flexed at both the hip and the knee than the lower one is.

Sims' position is occasionally used for unconscious clients because it facilitates drainage from the mouth and prevents aspiration of fluids. It is also used for paralyzed (paraplegic or hemiplegic) clients because it reduces pressure over the sacrum and greater trochanter of the hip. It can be used for clients undergoing examinations or treatments of the perineal area. Many people, especially pregnant women, find Sims' position comfortable for sleeping. People with sensory or motor deficits on one side of the body usually find that lying on the uninvolved side is more comfortable (see Table 38.9).

TABLE 38.8 Lateral Position

Unsupported Position	Problem to Be Prevented	Corrective Measure*
Body is turned to side, both arms in front of body, weight resting primarily on lateral aspects of scapula and ilium	Lateral flexion and fatigue of sternocleidomastoid muscles	Pillow under head and neck to provide good alignment
Upper arm and shoulder are rotated internally and adducted	Internal rotation and adduction of shoulder and subsequent limited function; impaired chest expansion	Pillow under upper arm to place it in good alignment; lower arm should be flexed comfortably
Upper thigh and leg are rotated internally and adducted	Internal rotation and adduction of femur; twisting of the spine	Pillow under leg and thigh to place them in good alignment; shoulders and hips should be aligned

The amount of support depends on the needs of the individual client.

TABLE 38.9 Sims' (Semiprone) Position

Unsupported Position	Problem to Be Prevented	Corrective Measure*
Head rests on bed surface; weight is borne by lateral aspects of cranial and facial bones	Lateral flexion of neck	Pillow supports head, maintaining it in good alignment unless drainage from the mouth is required
Upper shoulder and arm are internally rotated	Internal rotation of shoulder and arm; pressure on chest, restricting expansion during breathing	Pillow under upper arm to prevent internal rotation
Upper leg and thigh are adducted and internally rotated	Internal rotation and adduction of hip and leg	Pillow under upper leg to support it in alignment
Feet assume plantar flexion	Foot drop	Sandbags to support feet in dorsal flexion

**The amount of support depends on the needs of the individual client.*

Moving and Turning Clients in Bed

Although healthy people usually take for granted that they can change body position and go from one place to another with little effort, ill people may have difficulty moving even in bed. How much assistance clients require depends on their own ability to move and their health status. In general, nurses should be sensitive to both people's need to function independently and their need for assistance to move.

When a nurse assists a person to move, correct body mechanics need to be employed so that the nurse is not injured. Correct body alignment for the client must also be maintained so that undue stress is not placed on the musculoskeletal system.

Actions and rationales applicable to moving and positioning clients include these:

- Before moving a client, assess the degree of exertion permitted, the client's physical abilities (e.g., muscle strength, presence of paralysis), ability to assist with the move, ability to understand instructions, degree of comfort or discomfort when moving, weight, presence of orthostatic hypotension (particularly important when client will be standing), and your own strength and ability to move the client.
- If indicated, provide an analgesic before moving the client.
- Prepare any needed supportive devices and supportive equipment (e.g., pillows).
- Plan around encumbrances to movement, such as an IV or a heavy cast.
- Be alert to the effects of any medications the client takes that may impair alertness, balance, strength, or mobility.
- Explain the procedure to the client and listen to any suggestions the client or support people have.
- Provide privacy.
- Perform hand hygiene.
- Raise the height of the bed to bring the client close to your centre of gravity.
- Lock the wheels on the bed, and lower the rail on the side of the bed where you are standing.
- Face in the direction of the movement to prevent spinal twisting.
- Assume a broad stance to increase stability and provide balance.
- Lean your trunk slightly forward, and flex your hips, knees, and ankles to lower your centre of gravity, increase stability, and ensure use of large muscle groups during movements.
- Tighten your gluteal, abdominal, pelvic, leg, and arm muscles to prepare them for action and to prevent injury.
- Rock from the front leg to the back leg when pulling or from the back leg to the front leg when pushing to overcome inertia, counteract the client's weight, and help attain a balanced, smooth motion.
- After moving the client, determine the client's comfort, body alignment, tolerance of the activity (e.g., check pulse rate, respirations, oxygen saturation, blood pressure), and safety precautions required (e.g., side rails).

See Skill 38.1 on moving a client up in bed and Skill 38.2 on turning a client to a lateral or prone position in bed. Skill 38.3 describes how to logroll a client (**logrolling** is a technique used to turn a client whose body must at all times be kept in straight alignment, like a log). Skill 38.4 explains how to help a client to sit up on the edge of the bed.

Note: The Assessment, Planning, and Equipment sections as listed in Skill 38.1 are the same for each of these four procedures and are not repeated. The Evaluation section at the end of Skill 38.4 is also the same for all four procedures and, hence, is not repeated.

Transferring Clients

Many clients require some assistance in transferring between bed and chair or wheelchair, between wheelchair

SKILL 38.1

MOVING A CLIENT UP IN BED

Assessment

Before moving a client, assess the following:

- The client's physical abilities (e.g., muscle strength, presence of paralysis)
- Ability to understand instructions
- Degree of comfort or discomfort when moving (if needed, administer analgesics or perform other pain-relief measures; see Chapter 34)
- Client's weight
- The availability of equipment and other personnel to assist you

Planning

Review the client record to determine whether previous nurses have recorded information about the client's ability to move. Use proper assistive equipment and additional personnel whenever needed.

Equipment

- Assistive devices, such as overhead trapeze, pull or turn sheet, and transfer or sliding bar

PURPOSES

- Clients who have slid down in bed from the Fowler's position or have been pulled down by traction often need assistance to move up in bed.

IMPLEMENTATION

Preparation

Determine the following:

- Assistive devices that will be required
- Encumbrances to movement, such as an IV or a heavy cast on one leg
- Medications the client is receiving, because certain medications may hamper movement or alertness of the client
- Assistance required from other health-care personnel

Performance

1. Before performing the procedure, introduce yourself and verify the client's identity by using agency protocol. Explain to the client what you are going to do, why it is necessary, and how he or she can assist. Listen to any suggestions made by the client or support people.
2. Perform hand hygiene and observe other appropriate infection prevention and control procedures.
3. Provide for client privacy.
4. Adjust the bed and the client's position.
   - Adjust the head of the bed to a flat position or as low as the client can tolerate. Moving the client upward against gravity requires more force and can cause back strain.
   - Raise the bed to the height of your centre of gravity.
   - Lock the wheels on the bed and raise the rail on the side of the bed opposite you.
   - Remove all pillows, then place one against the head of the bed. **Rationale: This pillow protects the client's head from inadvertent injury against the top of the bed during the upward move.**
5. Elicit the client's help in lessening your workload.
   - Ask the client to flex the hips and knees and position the feet so that they can be used effectively for pushing. **Rationale: Flexing the hips and knees keeps the entire lower leg off the bed surface, preventing friction during movement, and ensures use of the large muscle groups in the client's legs when pushing, thus increasing the force of movement.**
   - Ask the client to
     a. Grasp the head of the bed with both hands and pull during the move.
     b. *Or* raise the upper part of the body on the elbows and push with the hands and forearms during the move.
     c. *Or* grasp the overhead trapeze with both hands and lift and pull during the move. **Rationale: Client assistance provides additional power to overcome inertia and friction during the move. These actions also keep the client's arms partially off the bed surface, reducing friction during movement, and make use of the large muscle groups of the client's arms to increase the force during movement.**
6. Position yourself appropriately, and move the client.
   - Face the direction of the movement, and then assume a broad stance with the foot nearest the bed behind the forward foot and weight on the forward foot. Lean your trunk forward from the hips. Flex hips, knees, and ankles.
   - Place your near arm under the client's thighs (see ❶). **Rationale: This supports the heaviest part of the body (the buttocks).** Push down on the mattress with the far arm. **Rationale: The far arm acts as a lever during the move.**
   - Tighten your gluteal, abdominal, leg, and arm muscles, and rock from the back leg to the front leg and back again. Then, shift your weight to the front leg as the client pushes with the heels and pulls with the arms so that the client moves toward the head of the bed.
7. Ensure client comfort.
   - Elevate the head of the bed and provide appropriate support devices for the client's new position.
   - See the sections on positioning clients earlier in this chapter.

(continued)

SKILL 38.1

MOVING A CLIENT UP IN BED (*continued*)

Variation: A Client Who Has Limited Strength of the Upper Extremities

- Assist the client to flex the hips and knees as in step 5. Place the client's arms across the chest. **Rationale: This keeps them off the bed surface and minimizes friction during movement**. Ask the client to flex the neck during the move and keep the head off the bed surface.
- Position yourself as in step 6, and place one arm under the client's back and shoulders and the other arm under the client's thighs. **Rationale: This placement of the arms distributes the client's weight and supports the heaviest part of the body (the buttocks)**. Shift your weight as in step 6.

Variation: Two Nurses Using a Hand–Forearm Interlock
Two people are required to move clients who are unable to assist because of their condition or weight. Using the technique described in step 6, with the second staff member on the opposite side of the bed, both of you interlock your forearms (see ❷) under the client's thighs and shoulders and lift the client up in bed.

Variation: Two Nurses Using a Turn Sheet
Two nurses can use a turn sheet to move a client up in bed. **Rationale: A turn sheet distributes the client's weight more evenly, decreases friction, and exerts a more even force on the client during the move. In addition, it prevents injury of the client's skin, because the friction created between two sheets when one is moved is less than that created by the client's body moving over the sheet**.

- Place a drawsheet or a full sheet folded in half under the client, extending from the shoulders to the thighs. Each person rolls up or fanfolds the turn sheet close to the client's body on either side.
- Both individuals grasp the sheet close to the shoulders and buttocks of the client. **Rationale: This draws the weight closer to the nurses' centre of gravity and increases the nurses' balance and stability, permitting a smoother movement**. Follow the method of moving clients with limited upper extremity strength as described earlier.

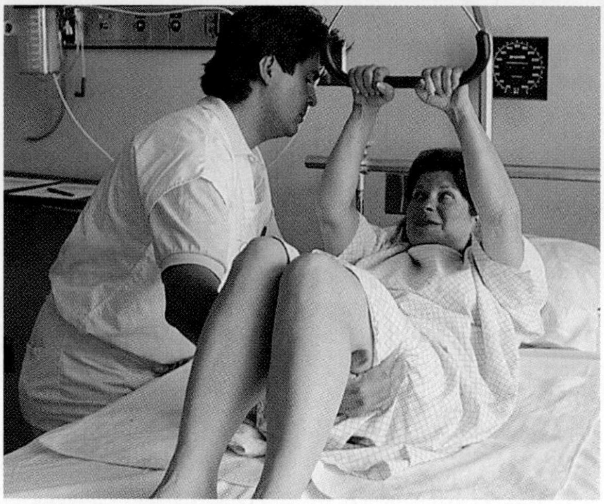

❶ Moving a client up in bed

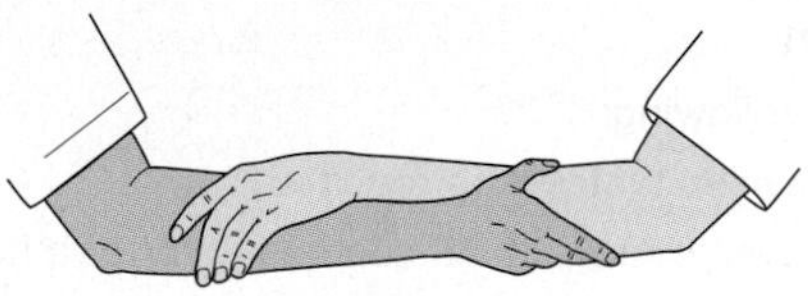

❷ Two nurses using the hand-forearm lock

8. Document all relevant information.

   Record the following:
   - Time and change of position moved from and position moved to
   - Any signs of pressure areas
   - Use of support devices
   - Ability of client to assist in moving and turning
   - Response of client to moving and turning (e.g., anxiety, discomfort, dizziness)

SKILL 38.2

TURNING A CLIENT TO A LATERAL OR PRONE POSITION IN BED

PURPOSES

- Movement to the lateral (side-lying) position may be necessary when placing a bedpan beneath the client, when changing the client's bed linen, or when repositioning the client.

IMPLEMENTATION

Preparation

Determine the following:

- Assistive devices that will be required
- Encumbrances to movement, such as an IV or a heavy cast on one leg
- Medications the client is receiving, because certain medications may hamper movement or alertness of the client
- Assistance required from other health-care personnel

(continued)

SKILL 38.2

TURNING A CLIENT TO A LATERAL OR PRONE POSITION IN BED *(continued)*

Performance

1. Before performing the procedure, introduce yourself and verify the client's identity by using agency protocol. Explain to the client what you are going to do, why it is necessary, and how he or she can assist.
2. Perform hand hygiene and observe other appropriate infection prevention and control procedures.
3. Provide for client privacy.
4. Position yourself and the client appropriately before performing the move.
   - Move the client closer to the side of the bed opposite the side the client will face when turned. **Rationale: This ensures that the client will be positioned safely in the centre of the bed after turning**. Use a pull sheet beneath the client's trunk and thighs to pull the client to the side of the bed. Roll up the sheet as close as possible to the client's body and pull the client to the side of the bed. Adjust the client's head and reposition the legs appropriately.
   - While standing on the side of the bed nearest the client, place the client's near arm across the chest. Abduct the client's far shoulder slightly from the side of the body and externally rotate the shoulder (Figure 38.8). **Rationale: Pulling the one arm forward facilitates the turning motion. Pulling the other arm away from the body and externally rotating the shoulder prevents that arm from being caught beneath the client's body during the roll**.
   - Place the client's near ankle and foot across the far ankle and foot. **Rationale: This facilitates the turning motion. Making these preparations on the side of the bed closest to the client helps prevent unnecessary reaching**.
   - Raise the side rail next to the client before going to the other side of the bed. **Rationale: This ensures that the client, who is close to the edge of the mattress, will not fall**.
   - Position yourself on the side of the bed toward which the client will turn, directly in line with the client's waistline and as close to the bed as possible.
   - Lean your trunk forward from the hips. Flex your hips, knees, and ankles. Assume a broad stance with one foot forward and the weight placed on this forward foot.
5. Pull or roll the client toward you to the lateral position.
   - Place one hand on the client's far hip and the other hand on the client's far shoulder (see ❶A). **Rationale: This position of the hands supports the client at the two heaviest parts of the body, providing greater control in movement during the roll**.
   - Tighten your gluteal, abdominal, leg, and arm muscles; rock backward, shifting your weight from the forward to the backward foot, and roll the client onto the side of the body to face you (see ❶B). **Rationale: Turning the client toward you promotes the client's sense of security**.

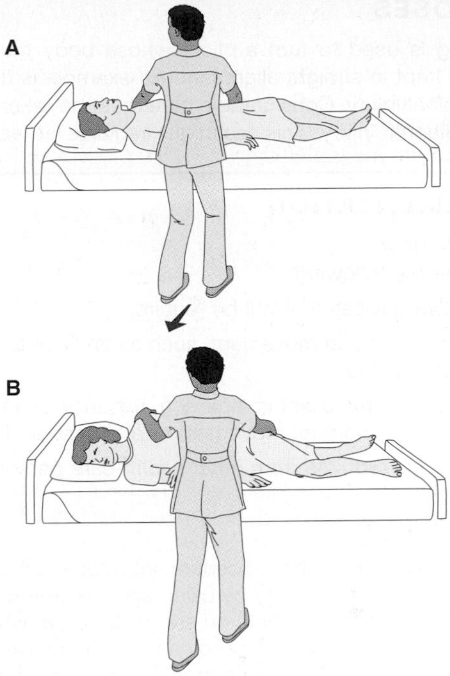

❶ Moving a client to a lateral position

   - Position the client on his or her side with arms and legs positioned and supported properly (see Table 38.8).

Variation: Turning the Client to a Prone Position
To turn a client to the prone position, follow the preceding steps, with two exceptions:

- Instead of abducting the far arm, keep the client's arm alongside the body for the client to roll over. **Rationale: Keeping the arm alongside the body prevents it from being pinned under the client when the client is rolled**.
- Roll the client completely onto the abdomen. **Rationale: It is essential to move the client as close as possible to the edge of the bed before the turn so that the client will be lying on the centre of the bed after rolling**. Never pull a client across the bed while the client is in the prone position. **Rationale: Doing so can injure a woman's breasts or a man's genitals.**

6. Document all relevant information.
   Record the following:
   - Time and change of position moved from and position moved to
   - Any signs of pressure areas
   - Use of support devices
   - Ability of client to assist in moving and turning
   - Response of client to moving and turning (e.g., anxiety, discomfort, dizziness)

SKILL 38.3

LOGROLLING A CLIENT

PURPOSES

Logrolling is used to turn a client whose body must at all times be kept in straight alignment. An example is the client with a spinal injury. Considerable care must be taken to prevent additional injury. This technique requires at least three nurses or, if the client is large, additional nurses are required. *For the client who has a cervical injury, one nurse must maintain the client's head and neck alignment.*

IMPLEMENTATION

Preparation

Determine the following:

- Assistive devices that will be required
- Encumbrances to movement, such as an IV or a heavy cast on one leg
- Medications the client is receiving, because certain medications may hamper movement or alertness of the client
- Assistance required from other health-care personnel

Performance

1. Before performing the procedure, introduce yourself and verify the client's identity by using agency protocol. Explain to the client what you are going to do, why it is necessary, and how he or she can cooperate. Discuss how the results will be used in planning further care or treatments.
2. Perform hand hygiene and observe other appropriate infection prevention and control procedures.
3. Provide for client privacy.
4. Position yourselves and the client appropriately before the move.
    - Raise height of bed to working height. Ensure that bed brakes are on.
    - Stand on the same side of the bed, and assume a broad stance with one foot ahead of the other.
    - Place the client's arms across the chest. **Rationale: Doing so maintains alignment during turn and ensures that the arms will not be injured or become trapped under the body when the body is turned.**
    - Incline your trunk, and flex your hips, knees, and ankles.
    - Place your arms under the client as shown in ❶ or ❷, depending on the client's size. **Rationale: Each staff member then has a major weight area of the client centred between the arms.**
    - Tighten your gluteal, pelvic, abdominal, leg, and arm muscles.
    - One nurse counts, "One, two, three, go." Then, at the same time, all staff members pull the client to the side of the bed by shifting weight to the back foot. **Rationale: Moving the client in unison maintains the client's body alignment.**
    - Elevate the side rail on this side of the bed. **Rationale: This prevents the client from falling while lying so close to the edge of the bed.**

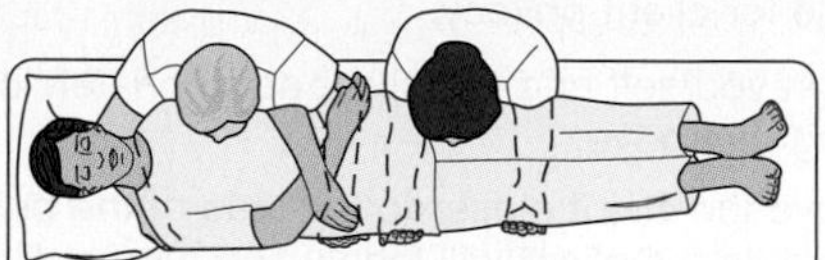

❶ Correct arm placement for moving a client to the side of the bed: two nurses

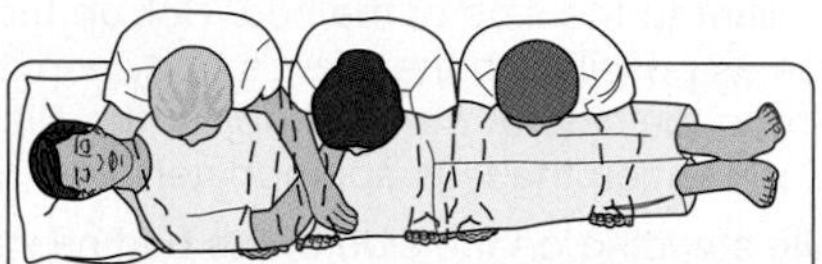

❷ Correct arm placement for moving a client to the side of the bed: three nurses

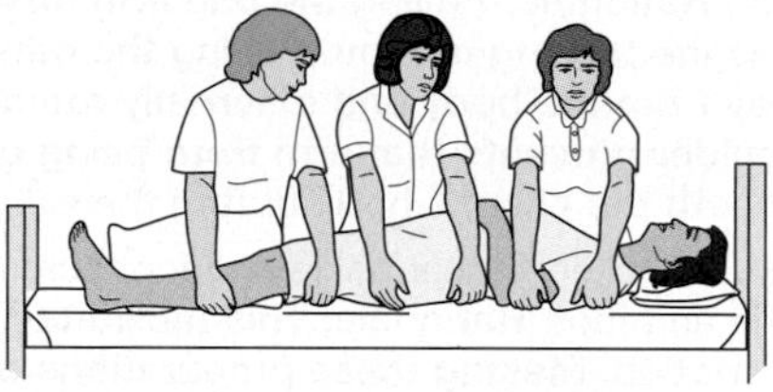

❸ Correct hand placement for logrolling a client

5. Move to the other side of the bed, and place supportive devices for the client when turned.
    - Place a pillow where it will support the client's head after the turn. **Rationale: The pillow prevents lateral flexion of the neck and ensures alignment of the cervical spine.**
    - Place one or two pillows between the client's legs to support the upper leg when the client is turned. **Rationale: This pillow prevents adduction of the upper leg, keeps the legs parallel and aligned, and prevents twisting of the spine.**
6. Roll and position the client in proper alignment.
    - All nurses flex the hips, knees, and ankles and assume a broad stance with one foot forward.
    - All nurses reach over the client and place hands as shown in ❸. **Rationale: Doing so centres a major weight area of the client between each nurse's arms.**
    - Tighten your gluteal, pelvic, abdominal, leg, and arm muscles.

(continued)

SKILL 38.3

LOGROLLING A CLIENT *(continued)*

- One nurse counts, "One, two, three, lift." Then, at the same time, all nurses roll the client to a lateral position.
- Support the client's head, back, and upper and lower extremities with pillows.

Variation: Using a Turn or Lift Sheet

- Use a turn sheet to facilitate logrolling. First, all staff members stand on the same side of the bed. Assume a broad stance with one foot forward, and grasp half of the fan-folded or rolled edge of the turn sheet. On a signal, pull the client toward both of you (see ❹).
- Before turning the client, place pillow supports for the head and legs, as described in step 5. This helps maintain the client's alignment when turning. Then, go to the other side of the bed (farthest from the client), and assume a stable stance. Reaching over the client, grasp the far edges of the turn sheet, and roll the client toward you (see ❺). The second nurse (behind the client) helps turn the client and provides pillow supports to ensure good alignment in the lateral position.

7. Document all relevant information.

   Record the following:

   - Time and change of position moved from and position moved to
   - Any signs of pressure areas
   - Use of support devices
   - Ability of client to assist in moving and turning
   - Response of client to moving and turning (e.g., anxiety, discomfort, dizziness)

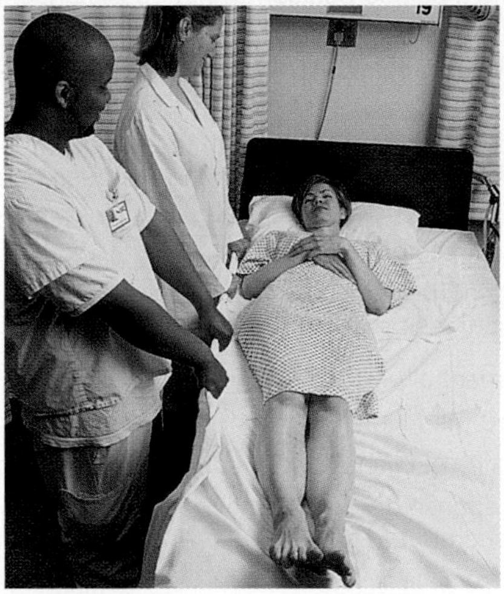

❹ By using a turn sheet, the nurses pull the sheet with the client on it to the edge of the bed.

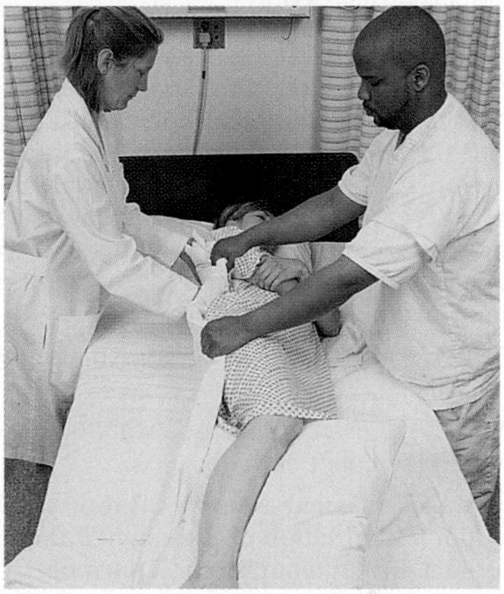

❺ The nurse on the right uses the far end of the sheet to roll the client toward him; the nurse on the left remains behind the client and helps with turning.

SKILL 38.4

ASSISTING THE CLIENT TO SIT ON THE SIDE OF THE BED

PURPOSES

The client assumes a sitting position on the edge of the bed before walking, moving to a chair or wheelchair, eating, or performing other activities.

IMPLEMENTATION

Preparation

Determine the following:

- Assistive devices that will be required
- Encumbrances to movement, such as an IV or a heavy cast on one leg
- Medications the client is receiving, because certain medications may hamper movement or alertness of the client
- Assistance required from other health-care personnel

Performance

1. Before performing the procedure, introduce yourself and verify the client's identity by using agency protocol. Explain to the client what you are going to do, why it is necessary, and how he or she can cooperate. Discuss how the results will be used in planning further care or treatments.
2. Perform hand hygiene and observe other appropriate infection prevention and control procedures.
3. Provide for client privacy.

(continued)

SKILL 38.4

ASSISTING THE CLIENT TO SIT ON THE SIDE OF THE BED *(continued)*

4. Position yourself and the client appropriately before performing the move.
   - Assist the client to a lateral position facing you.
   - Raise the head of the bed slowly to a low Fowler's position if not contraindicated. **Rationale: This decreases the distance that the client needs to move to sit up on the side of the bed.**
   - Position the client's feet and lower legs at the edge of the bed. **Rationale: This enables the client's feet to move easily off the bed during the movement, and the client is aided by gravity into a sitting position.**
   - Stand beside the client's hips and face the far corner of the bottom of the bed (the angle in which movement will occur). Assume a broad stance, placing the foot nearest the client forward. Incline your trunk slightly forward from the hips. Flex your hips, knees, and ankles (see ❶A).
5. Move the client to a sitting position.
   - Place one arm around the client's shoulders and the other arm beneath both of the client's thighs, near the knees. **Rationale: Supporting the client's shoulders prevents the client from falling backward during the movement. Supporting the client's thighs reduces friction of the thighs against the bed surface during the move and increases the force of the movement.**
   - Tighten your gluteal, pelvic, abdominal, leg, and arm muscles.
   - Instruct the client to push up with the hand closest to you on the count of three.
   - Lift the client's thighs slightly. **Rationale: This reduces the friction of the client's thighs and the nurse's arm against the bed surface.**
   - Pivot on the balls of your feet in the desired direction, facing the foot of the bed while pulling the client's feet and legs off the bed (see ❶B). **Rationale: Pivoting prevents twisting of the nurse's spine. The weight of the client's legs swinging downward increases downward movement of the lower body and helps make the client's upper body vertical.**
   - Keep supporting the client until the client is well balanced and comfortable. **Rationale: This movement may cause some clients to faint.**
   - Assess vital signs (e.g., pulse, respirations, and blood pressure) as indicated by the client's health status.

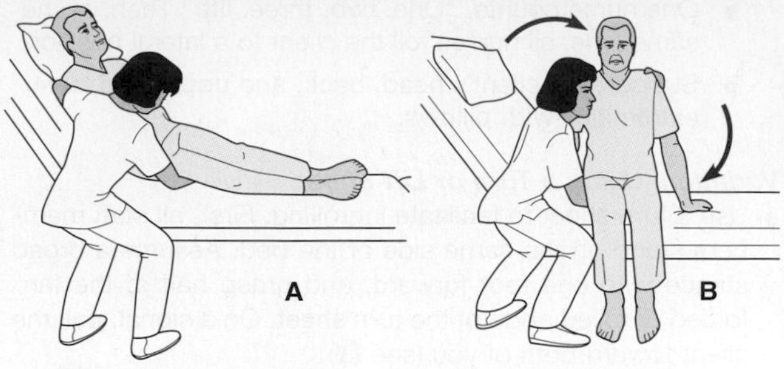

❶ Helping a client to a sitting position on the edge of the bed

Variation: Teaching a Client How to Sit on the Side of the Bed Independently

A client who has had recent abdominal surgery or who is weak may have too much abdominal pain or too little strength to sit straight up in bed. This person can be taught to assume a dangle position without assistance. Instruct the client to do the following:

- Roll to the side and lift the far leg over the near leg (see ❷A).
- Grasp the mattress edge with the lower arm and push the fist of the upper arm into the mattress (see ❷B).
- Push up with the arms as the heels and legs slide over the mattress edge (see ❷B).
- Maintain the sitting position by pushing both fists into the mattress behind and to the sides of the buttocks.

6. Document all relevant information.

   Record the following:
   - Ability of client to assist in moving and turning
   - Response of client to moving and turning (e.g., anxiety, discomfort, dizziness)

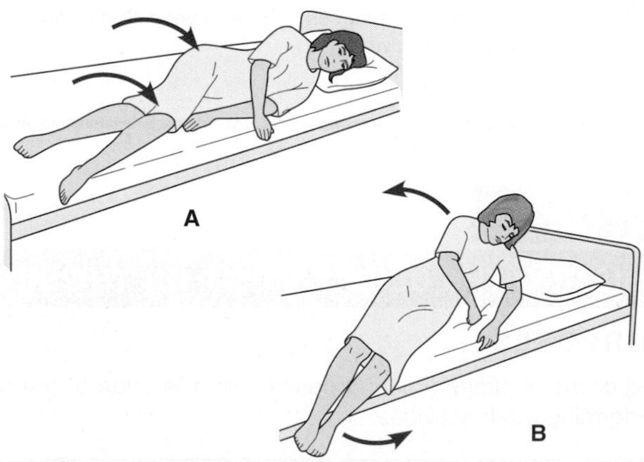

❷ Moving to a sitting position independently

EVALUATION

- Check the skin integrity of the pressure areas from the previous position.
- Conduct follow-up assessment for previous and new skin breakdown areas.
- Check for proper alignment after the position change. Do a visual check and ask the client for a comfort assessment.
- Determine that all required safety precautions (e.g., side rails) are in place.
- Determine client's tolerance of the activity (e.g., vital signs before and after dangling), particularly the first time the client changes position.
- Report significant changes to the appropriate member of the health-care team.

Lifespan Considerations

Positioning, Moving, and Turning Clients

INFANTS

- Position infants on their back for sleep, even after feeding. They have little risk of regurgitation and choking, and the rate of sudden infant death syndrome (SIDS) is significantly lower in infants who sleep on their backs.
- The skin of newborns can be fragile and may be abraded or torn (sheared) if the infant is pulled across a bed.

CHILDREN

- Carefully inspect at least three times in each 24-hour period the dependent skin surfaces of all infants and children confined to bed.

OLDER ADULTS

- Clients who have had cerebrovascular accidents (strokes) have a risk of shoulder displacement on the paralyzed side from improper moving or repositioning techniques. Use care when moving, positioning in bed, and transferring. Pillows or foam devices are helpful to support the affected arm and shoulder and prevent injury.
- Decreased subcutaneous fat and thinning of the skin place older adults at risk for skin breakdown. Repositioning approximately every 2 hours (more or less, depending on the unique needs of the individual client) helps reduce pressure on bony prominences and avoid tissue trauma.

and toilet, and between bed and stretcher. Before transferring any client, however, the nurse must determine the client's physical and mental capabilities to participate in the transfer technique. The client's weight must also be known to determine whether the transfer can be safely performed with one or more persons assisting or if a mechanical lift needs to be used. In addition, the nurse must analyze and organize the activity. General guidelines for transfer techniques include these:

- Plan what to do and how to do it. Determine the space in which the transfer is manoeuvred (bathrooms, for instance, are usually cramped); the number of assistants (one or two) needed to accomplish the transfer safely; the skill and strength of the nurse; whether a mechanical lift is required; and the client's capabilities.
- Check physician's orders and agency policies.
- Obtain essential equipment before starting (e.g., wheelchair), and check its function.
- Remove obstacles from the area used for the transfer.
- Explain the transfer to the client, including what the client should do.
- Explain the transfer to the nursing personnel who are helping; specify who will give directions (one person needs to be in charge).
- Place equipment to allow client to move toward stronger side.
- Always support or hold the client rather than the equipment and ensure the client's safety and dignity.
- During the transfer, explain step by step what the client should do, for example, "Move your right foot forward."
- Make a written plan of the transfer, including the client's tolerance (e.g., pulse and respiratory rates, blood pressure, and oxygen saturation).

Because wheelchairs and stretchers are unstable, they can cause falls and injury. Guidelines for the safe use of wheelchairs and stretchers are shown in Box 38.3.

Transfer (walking) belts provide the greatest safety. This belt may have a handle that allows the nurse to control movement of the client during the transfer. Most health-care agencies require personnel to use the transfer belt to ambulate or move clients. See Skill 38.5 for transferring a client between a bed and a chair and Skill 38.6 for transferring a client between a bed and a stretcher.

Home Care Considerations

Positioning, Moving, and Turning Clients

- Assess the height of the bed and the person's leg length to ensure that self-movement in and out of the bed are smooth.
- Inspect the client's mattress for support.
- Assess the caregivers' knowledge and application of body mechanics to prevent injury.
- Demonstrate how to turn and position the client in bed. Observe the caregiver performing a return demonstration. Re-evaluate this technique periodically to reinforce correct application of body mechanics.
- Teach caregivers the basic principles of body alignment and how to check for proper alignment after the client has been changed to a new position.
- Warn caregivers of the dangers of lifting and repositioning and encourage the use of assistive devices and a "no solo lift" policy.
- Teach the caregiver to check the client's skin for redness and integrity after repositioning the client. Stress the importance of informing the nurse about the length of time skin redness remains over pressure areas after the person has been repositioned. Emphasize that reddened areas should not be massaged as it may lead to tissue trauma.

BOX 38.3 WHEELCHAIR SAFETY AND THE SAFE USE OF STRETCHERS

Wheelchairs and stretchers are unsteady, and the nurse must take care when using them with clients:

WHEELCHAIRS

- Always lock the brakes on both wheels of the wheelchair when the client transfers in to or out of it. Locks should be used at all times, except when the client is being moved.
- Remove (if possible) or raise the footplates before transferring the client into the wheelchair.
- Lower the footplates after the transfer, and place the client's feet on them.
- Ensure the client is positioned well back in the seat of the wheelchair.
- Ensure body alignment is maintained. Protect extremities when transporting client (for example, through doorways).
- Use seat belts that fasten behind the wheelchair to protect confused clients from falls. *Note:* Seat belts are a form of restraint and must be used in accordance with policies and procedures that apply to the use of restraints (see Chapter 30).
- Back the wheelchair into or out of an elevator, rear large wheels first.
- Place your body between the wheelchair and the bottom of an incline.

STRETCHERS

- Lock the wheels of the bed and stretcher before the client transfers in to or out of them.
- Fasten safety straps across the client on a stretcher, and raise the side rails.
- Never leave a client unattended on a stretcher unless the wheels are locked and the side rails are raised on both sides or the safety straps are securely fastened across the client.
- Always push a stretcher from the end at which the client's head is positioned. This position protects the client's head in the event of a collision.
- If the stretcher has two swivel wheels and two stationary wheels,
  - **a.** Always position the client's head at the end with the stationary wheels.
  - **b.** Push the stretcher from the end with the stationary wheels. The stretcher is manoeuvred more easily when pushed from this end.
- Manoeuvre the stretcher when entering the elevator so that the client's head goes in first.

SKILL 38.5

TRANSFERRING BETWEEN BED AND CHAIR

PURPOSES

A client may need to be transferred between the bed and a wheelchair or chair, the bed and the commode, or a wheelchair and the toilet. This technique has numerous variations. Which variation the nurse selects depends on factors related to the client, the environment, and the health-care provider, which are assessed before beginning the transfer.

ASSESSMENT

Before transferring a client, assess the following:

- The client's body size
- The client's ability to follow instructions
- The client's activity tolerance
- The client's muscle strength
- The client's joint mobility
- The presence of paralysis
- The client's level of comfort
- The presence of orthostatic hypotension
- The technique with which the client is familiar
- The space in which the transfer will need to be manoeuvred (bathrooms, for example, are usually cramped)
- The number of assistants (one or two) needed to accomplish the transfer safely
- The skill and strength of the nurses

Planning

Review the client record to determine whether previous nurses have recorded information about the client's ability to transfer. Implement pain-relief measures so that they are effective when the transfer begins.

Equipment

- Robe or appropriate clothing
- Slippers or shoes with nonskid soles
- Transfer (walking) belt
- Chair, commode, wheelchair, or stretcher as appropriate to client need
- Sliding board

(continued)

SKILL 38.5

TRANSFERRING BETWEEN BED AND CHAIR (*continued*)

IMPLEMENTATION

Preparation

- Plan what to do and how to do it.
- Obtain essential equipment before starting (e.g., transfer belt, wheelchair), and check that it is functioning correctly.
- Remove obstacles from the area used for the transfer.

Performance

1. Before performing the procedure, introduce yourself and verify the client's identity by using agency protocol. Explain the transfer process to the client. During the transfer, explain step by step what the client should do, for example, "Move your right foot forward."
2. Perform hand hygiene and observe other appropriate infection prevention and control procedures.
3. Provide for client privacy.
4. Position the equipment appropriately.
   - Lower the bed to its lowest position so that the client's feet will rest flat on the floor. Lock the wheels of the bed.
   - Place the wheelchair parallel to the bed and as close to the bed as possible (see ❶). Put the wheelchair on the side of the bed that allows the client to move toward his or her stronger side. Lock the wheels of the wheelchair and remove, if possible, or raise the footplates.
5. Prepare and assess the client.
   - Assist the client to a sitting position on the side of the bed. See Skill 38.4.
   - Assess the client for orthostatic hypotension before moving the client from the bed.
   - Assist the client in putting on a bathrobe and nonskid slippers or shoes.
   - Place a transfer belt snugly around the client's waist. Check to be certain that the belt is securely fastened.

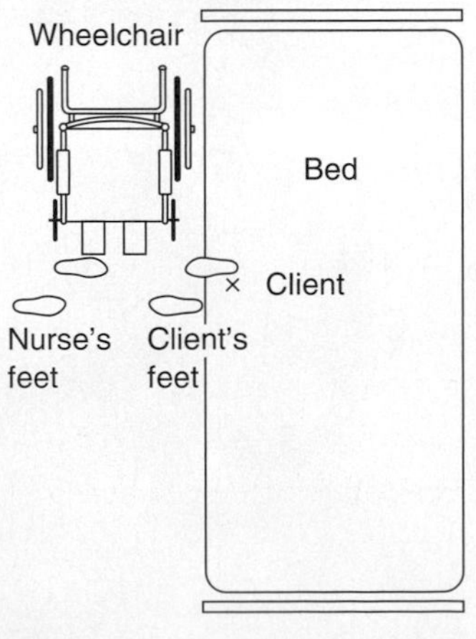

❶ The wheelchair is placed parallel to the bed as close to the bed as possible. Note that placement of the nurse's feet mirrors that of the client's feet.

6. Give explicit instructions to the client. Ask the client to do the following:
   - Move forward and sit on the edge of the bed. **Rationale: This brings the client's centre of gravity closer to the nurse's.**
   - Lean forward slightly from the hips. **Rationale: This brings the client's centre of gravity more directly over the base of support and positions the head and trunk in the direction of the movement.**
   - Place the foot of the stronger leg beneath the edge of the bed, and put the other foot forward. **Rationale: In this way, the client can use the stronger leg muscles to stand and power the movement. A broader base of support makes the client more stable during the transfer.**
   - Place the client's hands on the bed surface or on your waist so that the client can push while standing. **Rationale: This provides additional force for the movement and reduces the potential for strain on the nurse's back.** The client should not grasp your neck or shoulders for support. **Rationale: Doing so can injure the nurse.**
7. Position yourself correctly.
   - Stand directly in front of the client. Incline the trunk slightly forward from the hips. Flex the hips, knees, and ankles. Assume a broad stance, placing one foot forward and one back. Mirror the placement of the client's feet, if possible. **Rationale: This helps prevent loss of balance during the transfer.**
   - Encircle the client's waist with your arms, and grasp the transfer belt at the client's back (see ❷), with thumbs pointing downward. **Rationale: The belt provides a secure handle for holding onto the client and controlling the movement. Downward placement of the thumbs prevents potential wrist injury as the nurse lifts. By supporting the client in this**

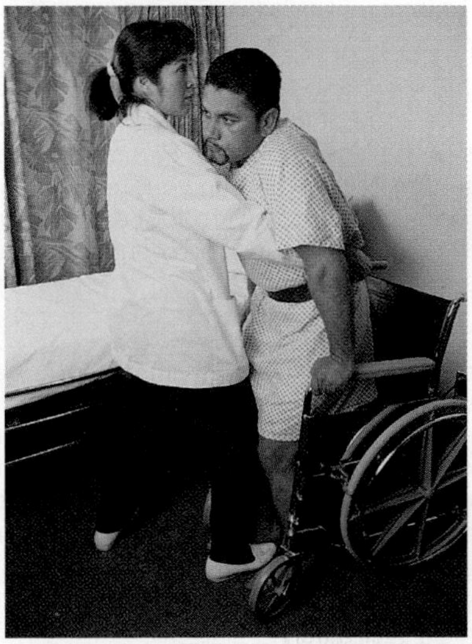

❷ Using a transfer (walking) belt

(continued)

SKILL 38.5

TRANSFERRING BETWEEN BED AND CHAIR *(continued)*

manner, you keep the client from tilting backward during the transfer.

- Tighten your gluteal, pelvic, abdominal, leg, and arm muscles.

8. Assist the client to stand, and then move together toward the wheelchair.
    - On the count of three, ask the client to push with the back foot, rock to the forward foot, and extend (straighten) the joints of the lower extremities. Push or pull up with the hands, while pushing with the forward foot, then rock to the back foot, extend the joints of the lower extremities, and pull the client (directly toward your centre of gravity) into a standing position.
    - Support the client in an upright standing position for a few moments. **Rationale: This allows the nurse and the client to extend the joints and provides the nurse with an opportunity to ensure that the client is all right before moving away from the bed.**
    - Together, pivot toward the wheelchair.
9. Assist the client to sit.
    - Ask the client to do the following:
        a. Back up to the wheelchair and place the legs against the seat. **Rationale: Having the client place the legs against the wheelchair seat minimizes the risk of the client's falling when sitting down.**
        b. Place the foot of the stronger leg slightly behind the other. **Rationale: This supports body weight during the movement.**
        c. Keep the other foot forward. **Rationale: This provides a broad base of support.**
        d. Place both hands on the wheelchair arms. **Rationale: This increases stability and lessens the strain on the nurse.**
    - Stand directly in front of the client. Place one foot forward and one back.
    - Tighten your grasp on the transfer belt, and tighten your gluteal, pelvic, abdominal, leg, and arm muscles.
    - On the count of three, have the client shift the body weight by rocking to the back foot. Lower the body onto the edge of the wheelchair seat by flexing the joints of the legs and arms. Place some body weight on the arms, while shifting your body weight by stepping back with the forward foot and pivoting toward the chair while lowering the client onto the wheelchair seat.
10. Ensure client safety.
    - Ask the client to push back into the wheelchair seat. **Rationale: Sitting well back on the seat provides a broader base of support and greater stability and minimizes the risk of falling from the wheelchair. A wheelchair can topple forward when the client sits on the edge of the seat and leans far forward.**
    - Lower the footplates, and place the client's feet on them.
    - Apply a seat belt as required.

Variation: Angling the Wheelchair

For clients who have difficulty walking, place the wheelchair at a 45-degree angle to the bed. **Rationale: This enables the client to pivot into the chair and lessens the amount of body rotation required.**

Variation: Transferring without a Belt

- For clients who need minimal assistance, place the hands against the sides of the client's chest (not at the axillae) during the transfer (see ❸). For clients who require more assistance, reach through the client's axillae and place the hands on the client's scapulae during the transfer. Avoid placing hands or pressure on the axillae, especially for clients who have upper extremity paralysis or paresis.
- Follow the steps described previously.

Variation: Transferring with a Belt and Two Nurses

- When the client is ready to stand, position yourselves on both sides of the client, facing the same direction as the client. Flex your hips, knees, and ankles; grasp the client's transfer belt at the back with the hand closest to the client, and with the other hand, support the client's elbows.
- Coordinating your efforts, all three of you stand simultaneously, pivot, and move to the wheelchair. Reverse the process to lower the client onto the wheelchair seat.

Variation: Transferring a Client with an Injured Lower Extremity or Hemiparesis

When the client has an injured lower extremity, movement should always occur toward the client's unaffected (strong) side. For example, if the client's right leg is injured and the client is sitting on the edge of bed preparing to transfer to a wheelchair, position the wheelchair on the client's left side. **Rationale: In this way, the client can use the unaffected leg most effectively and safely.**

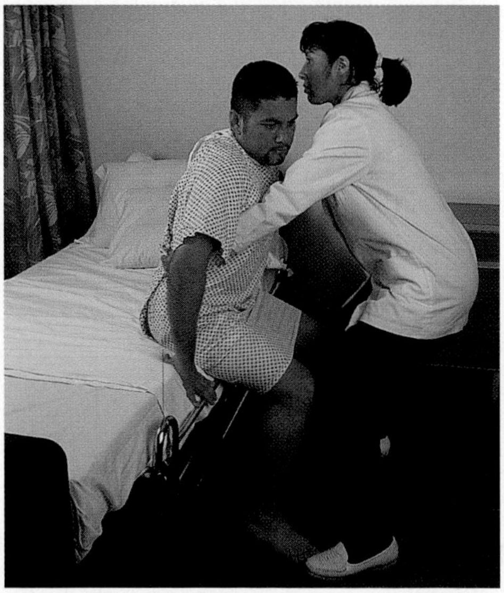

❸ Transferring without a belt

(continued)

SKILL 38.5

TRANSFERRING BETWEEN BED AND CHAIR *(continued)*

Variation: Using a Sliding Board

Have a client who cannot stand use a sliding board to move without nursing assistance. This method not only promotes the client's sense of independence but preserves your energy (see ❹).

11. Document relevant information:

- Client's ability to bear weight and pivot
- Number of staff needed for transfer
- Length of time up in chair
- Client response to transfer and being up in chair or wheelchair

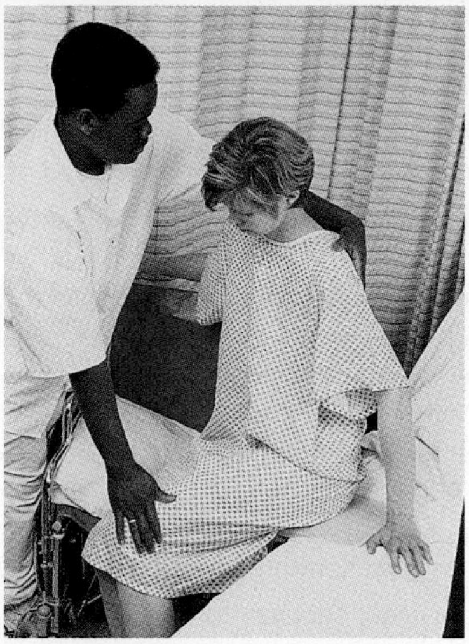

❹ Using a sliding board

SKILL 38.6

TRANSFERRING BETWEEN BED AND STRETCHER

PURPOSES

The stretcher, or gurney, is used to transfer supine clients from one location to another. Whenever the client is capable of accomplishing the transfer from bed to stretcher independently, either by lifting onto it or by rolling onto it, the client should be encouraged to do so. If the client cannot move onto the stretcher independently, at least two nurses are needed to assist with the transfer; more may be needed or a mechanical lift should be used if the weight being lifted exceeds agency policy for maximum lift weight.

ASSESSMENT

Before transferring a client, assess the following:

- The client's body size
- The client's ability to follow instructions
- The client's activity tolerance
- The client's level of comfort
- The space in which the transfer is manoeuvred
- The number of assistants (one or two others) needed to accomplish the transfer safely
- The skill and strength of the nurses

Planning

Review the client record to determine whether previous nurses have recorded information about how the client tolerated similar transfers. If indicated, implement pain-relief measures so that they are effective when the transfer begins.

Equipment

- Stretcher
- Optional: sliding board
- Mechanical lift may be required

IMPLEMENTATION

Preparation

Obtain the necessary equipment and nursing personnel to assist in the transfer.

Performance

1. Before performing the procedure, introduce yourself and verify the client's identity by using agency protocol. Explain to the client what you are going to do, why it is necessary, and how he or she can cooperate. Explain the transfer to the nursing personnel who are helping and specify who will give directions (one person needs to be in charge).
2. Perform hand hygiene and observe other appropriate infection prevention and control procedures.
3. Provide for client privacy.
4. Adjust the client's bed in preparation for the transfer.
   - Lower the head of the bed until it is flat or as low as the client can tolerate.

(continued)

SKILL 38.6

TRANSFERRING BETWEEN BED AND STRETCHER (*continued*)

- Raise the bed so that it is slightly higher than the surface of the stretcher. **Rationale: It is easier for the client to move down an incline.**
- Ensure that the wheels on the bed are locked.
- Pull the drawsheet out from both sides of the bed.

5. Move the client to the edge of the bed, and position the stretcher.
   - Roll the drawsheet as close to the client's side as possible.
   - Pull the client to the edge of the bed, and cover the client with a sheet or bath blanket to maintain comfort.
   - Place the stretcher parallel to the bed, next to the client, and lock its wheels.
   - Fill the gap that exists between the bed and the stretcher loosely with bath blankets or roller (optional).
6. Transfer the client securely to the stretcher.
   - Using the counting cadence in unison with the other staff members, press your body tightly against the stretcher. **Rationale: This prevents the stretcher from moving.**
   - Roll the pull sheet tightly against the client. **Rationale: This achieves better control over client movement.**
   - Flex your hips, and pull the client on the pull sheet in unison directly toward you and onto the stretcher. **Rationale: Pulling downward requires less force than pulling along a flat surface.**
   - Ask the client to flex the neck during the move, if possible, and place arms across the chest. **Rationale: This prevents injury to these body parts.**
   - A slider sheet may be used to decrease friction between the bed and client, facilitating easier movement.
7. Ensure client comfort and safety.
   - Make the client comfortable, unlock the stretcher wheels, and move the stretcher away from the bed.
   - Immediately raise the stretcher side rails and fasten the safety straps across the client. **Rationale: Because the stretcher is high and narrow, the client is in danger of falling unless these safety precautions are taken.**

Variation: Using a Transfer Board

The transfer board is a lacquered or smooth polyethylene board measuring 45 cm to 55 cm by 182 cm with handholds along its edges. Transfer mattresses are also available, as are mechanical assistive devices. It is imperative to have enough people assisting with the transfer to prevent injury to staff as well as patients. Turn the client to a lateral position away from you, position the board close to the client's back, and roll the client onto the board. Pull the client and board across the bed to the stretcher. Safety belts may be placed over the chest, abdomen, and legs.

8. Document relevant information:
   - Equipment used
   - Number of people needed for transfer
   - Destination if reason for transfer is transport from one location to another

EVALUATION

- Compare client capabilities, such as weight-bearing, pivoting ability, and strength and control to previous transfers.
- Report any significant deviations from normal to the appropriate members of the health-care team.

USING A HYDRAULIC LIFT Hydraulic lifts, such as the Hoyer lift, are an example of assistive equipment to take the place of manual lifts and transfers. The lift can be used in transferring the client between the bed and a wheelchair, the bed and the bathtub, and the bed and a stretcher. The Hoyer lift consists of a base on casters, a hydraulic mechanical pump, a mast boom, and a sling (Figure 38.52). The sling may consist of a one-piece or two-piece canvas seat. The one-piece seat stretches from the client's head to the knees. The two-piece seat has one canvas strap to support the client's buttocks and thighs and a second strap extending up to the axillae to support the back. It is important to be familiar with the model used and the practices that accompany use. Before using the lift, the nurse ensures that it is in working order and that the hooks, chains, straps, and canvas seat are in good repair. Most agencies recommend that two nurses operate a lift. Check agency policy.

Providing ROM Exercises

When people are ill, they often need to perform ROM exercises until they regain their normal activity levels. **Active ROM exercises** are isotonic exercises in which the client moves each joint in the body through its complete range of movement, maximally stretching all muscle groups within each plane over the joint. These exercises maintain or increase muscle strength, length, and endurance, and they help maintain cardiorespiratory function in an immobilized client. They also prevent deterioration of joint capsules, ankylosis, and contractures.

Full ROM does not occur spontaneously in the immobilized individual who independently achieves ADLs, independently moves about in bed, independently transfers between bed and wheelchair or chair, or independently ambulates a short distance because only a few muscle groups are maximally stretched during these

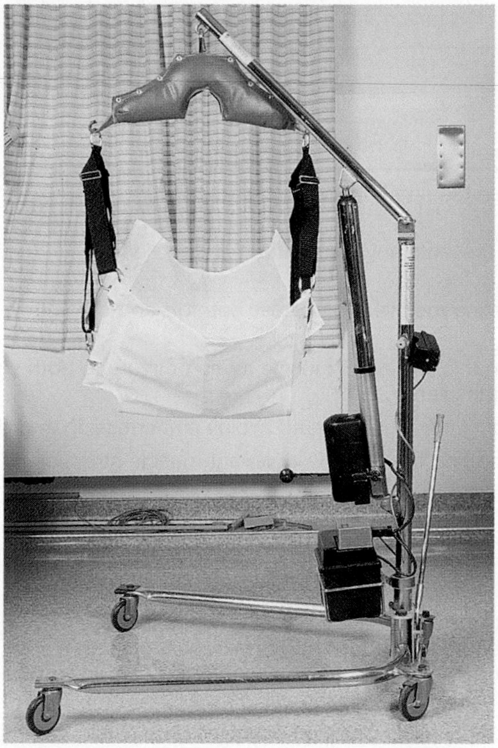

FIGURE 38.52 A one-piece seat hydraulic lift

activities. Although the client may successfully achieve some active ROM movements of the upper extremities while combing the hair, bathing, and dressing, the immobilized client is very unlikely to achieve any active ROM movements of the lower extremities when these are not used in the normal functions of standing and walking about. For this reason, most wheelchair and many ambulatory clients need active ROM exercises until they regain their normal activity levels.

At first, the nurse may need to teach the client to perform the needed ROM exercises; eventually, the client may be able to accomplish these independently. Instructions for the client performing active ROM exercises are shown in the accompanying Teaching: Clinical box.

During **passive ROM exercises**, another person moves each of the client's joints through its complete range of movement, maximally stretching all muscle groups within each plane over each joint. Because the client does not contract the muscles, passive ROM exercises are of no value in maintaining muscle strength but are useful in maintaining joint flexibility. For this reason, passive ROM exercises should be performed only when the client is unable to accomplish the movements actively.

Passive ROM exercises should be accomplished for each movement of the arms, legs, and neck *that the client is unable to achieve actively*. As with active ROM exercises, passive ROM exercises should be accomplished to the point of slight resistance, but not beyond, and never to the point of discomfort. The movements should be systematic, and the same sequence should be followed during each exercise session. Each exercise should consist of three repetitions, and the series of exercises should be done at least three times daily.

Performing one series of exercises along with the bath is helpful. Passive ROM exercises are accomplished most effectively when the client lies supine in bed. General guidelines for providing passive exercises are shown in Practice Guidelines 38.1.

During **active-assistive ROM exercises**, the client uses a stronger, opposite arm or leg to move each of the joints of a limb incapable of active motion. The client learns to support and move the weak arm or leg with the strong arm or leg as far as possible. Then, the nurse continues the movement passively to its maximal degree. This activity increases active movement on the strong side of the client's body and maintains joint flexibility on the weak side. Such exercise is especially useful for stroke victims who are hemiplegic (paralyzed on one half of the body).

TEACHING: CLINICAL

Active ROM Exercises

These instructions are for clients who need to perform ROM exercises:

- Perform each ROM exercise as taught to the point of slight resistance, but not beyond, and never to the point of discomfort.
- Perform the movements systematically by using the same sequence during each session.
- Perform each exercise three times.
- Perform each series of exercises at least three times daily.
- For older clients, it is not essential to achieve full ROM in all joints, Instead, emphasize that ROM exercise is also achieved while the client carries out ADLs, such as walking, dressing, combing hair, showering, and preparing a meal.

CLINICAL ALERT

Clients who require passive ROM exercises after a disability should have a goal of progressing to active-assistive ROM exercises and, finally, to active ROM exercises.

Ambulating Clients

Ambulation (the act of walking) is a function that most people take for granted. However, when people are ill, they are often confined to bed and are thus nonambulatory. The longer clients are in bed, the more difficulty they have walking.

PRACTICE GUIDELINES 38.1

Providing Passive ROM Exercises

Guidelines	Rationales
• Ensure that the client understands the reason for doing ROM exercises.	• Understanding improves collaboration.
• If there is a possibility of hand swelling, make sure rings are removed.	• This prevents any discomfort for the client.
• Clothe the client in a loose gown, and cover the body with a bath blanket.	• Covering the client promotes comfort and dignity.
• Use correct body mechanics when providing ROM exercise.	• Doing this will avoid muscle strain or injury to both you and the client.
• Expose only the limb being exercised.	• Keeping the client covered avoids embarrassing the client.
• Support the client's limbs above and below the joint as needed. (Figure 38.53). This may also be done by cupping joints in the palm of your hand or cradling limbs along your forearm (Figure 38.54). If a joint is painful (e.g., arthritic), support the limb in the muscular areas above and below the joint.	• Supporting the limbs will prevent muscle strain or injury.
• Use a firm, comfortable grip when handling the limb, and move the body parts smoothly, slowly, and rhythmically.	• Jerky movements cause discomfort and, possibly, injury. Fast movements can cause spasticity (sudden, prolonged involuntary muscle contraction) or rigidity (stiffness or inflexibility).
• Avoid moving or forcing a body part beyond the existing ROM. This is particularly important for people with flaccid (limp) paralysis, whose muscles can be stretched and joints dislocated without their awareness.	• Forcing a body part can cause muscle strain, pain, and injury.
• If muscle spasticity occurs during movement, stop the movement temporarily, but continue to apply slow, gentle pressure on the part until the muscle relaxes; then proceed with the motion.	• This process avoids any trauma to the muscle.
• If a contracture is present, apply slow firm pressure, without causing pain.	• This prevents injury yet increases the ROM of the joint.
• If rigidity occurs, apply slight pressure against the rigidity, and continue the exercise slowly, if possible.	• This helps muscles become slightly more relaxed, thus increasing the ROM.

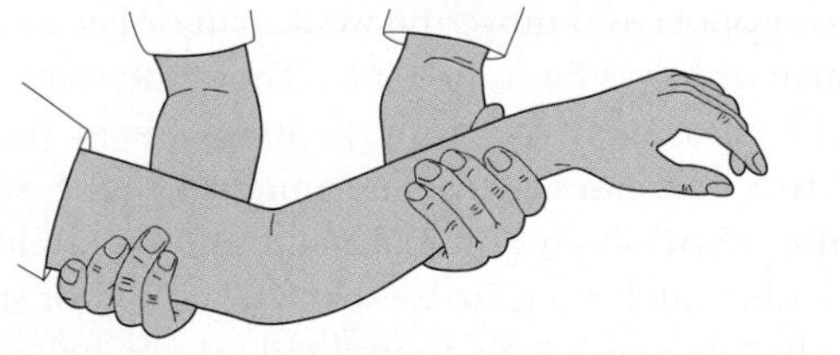

FIGURE 38.53 Supporting a limb above and below the joint for passive exercise

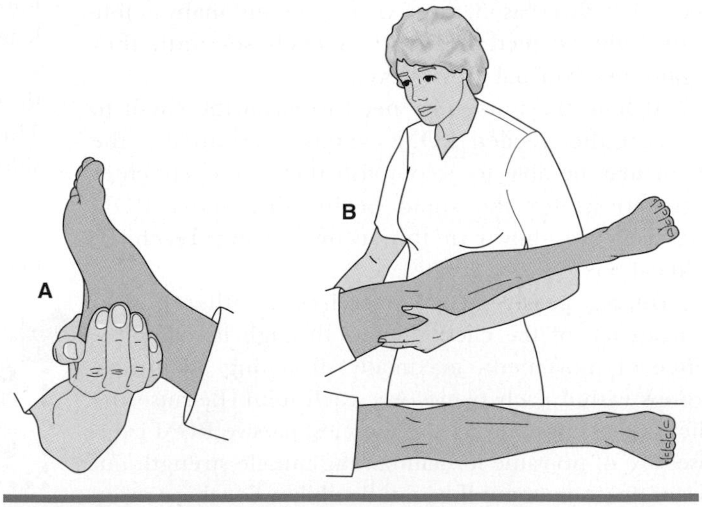

FIGURE 38.54 Holding limbs for support during passive exercise: **A:** cupping; **B:** cradling

Even one or two days of bed rest can make a person feel weak, unsteady, and shaky when first getting out of bed. A client who has had surgery, is older, or who has been immobilized for a longer time will feel more pronounced weakness. The potential problems of immobility are far less likely to occur when clients become ambulatory as soon as possible. The nurse can assist clients to prepare for ambulation by helping them become as independent as possible while in bed. Nurses should encourage clients to perform ADLs, maintain good body alignment, and carry out active ROM exercises to the maximum degree possible yet within the limitations imposed by their illness and recovery program.

PREAMBULATORY EXERCISES Clients who have been in bed for long periods often need a plan of isometric exercises to strengthen the muscles used for walking before attempting to walk. A physician's order may be required. One of the most important muscle groups is the quadriceps femoris, which extends the knee and flexes the thigh. This group is also important for elevating the legs, for example, for walking upstairs. These exercises are frequently called *quadriceps drills* or *sets.* To strengthen these muscles, the client consciously tenses them, drawing the kneecap upward and inward. The client pushes the popliteal space of the knee against the bed surface, relaxing the heels on the bed surface (Figure 38.55). On the count of 1, the muscles are tensed; they are held during the counts of 2, 3, 4; and they are relaxed at the count of 5. The exercise should be done within the client's tolerance, that is, without fatiguing the muscles. Carried out several times an hour during waking hours, this simple exercise significantly strengthens the muscles used for walking.

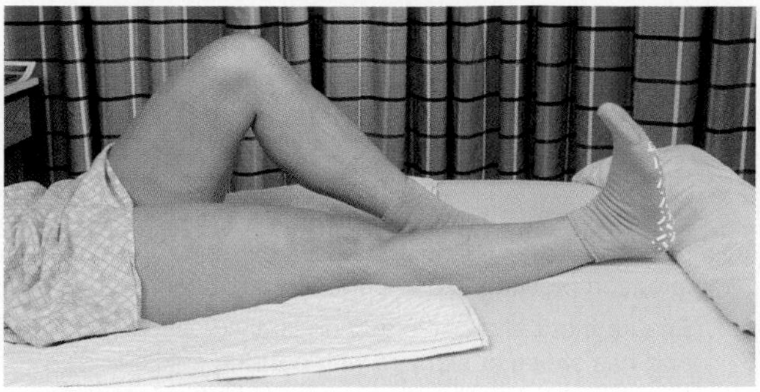

FIGURE 38.55 Tensing the quadriceps femoris muscles before ambulation

ASSISTING CLIENTS TO AMBULATE Clients who have been immobilized for even a few days may require assistance with ambulation. The amount of assistance will depend on the client's condition, including age, health status, cognition, and length of inactivity. Assistance may mean walking alongside the client while providing physical support (see Skill 38.7) or providing instruction to the client about the use of assistive devices, such as a cane, walker, or crutches (discussed later in this chapter).

SKILL 38.7

ASSISTING THE CLIENT TO AMBULATE

PURPOSES

- To provide a safe condition for the client to walk with whatever support is needed.

ASSESSMENT

Assess

- Length of time in bed and time up previously
- Baseline vital signs
- ROM of joints needed for ambulating (e.g., hips, knees, ankles)
- Muscle strength of lower extremities
- Need for ambulation aids (e.g., cane, walker, crutches)
- Client's intake of medications (e.g., opioids, sedatives, tranquilizers, and antihistamines) that may cause drowsiness, dizziness, weakness, and orthostatic hypotension and seriously hinder the client's ability to walk safely
- Presence of joint inflammation, fractures, muscle weakness, or other conditions that impair physical mobility
- Ability to understand directions
- Level of comfort

Planning

Implement pain-relief measures so that they are effective when the transfer begins.

The amount of assistance needed while ambulating will depend on the client's condition, for example, age, health status, length of inactivity, and emotional readiness. Review any previous experiences with ambulation and the success of such efforts. Plan the length of the walk with the client, in light of the nursing or physician's orders. Be prepared to shorten the walk according to the person's activity tolerance.

Equipment

- Transfer belt if the client is known to be unsteady
- Wheelchair for following client or chairs along the route if the client needs to rest

IMPLEMENTATION

Preparation

Be certain that others are available to assist you if needed. Also, plan the route of ambulation that has the fewest hazards.

Performance

1. Before performing the procedure, introduce yourself and verify the client's identity by using agency protocol. Explain to the client how you are going to assist, why ambulation is necessary, and how he or she can cooperate.

(continued)

SKILL 38.7

ASSISTING THE CLIENT TO AMBULATE *(continued)*

Discuss how this activity relates to the overall plan of care.

2. Perform hand hygiene and observe other appropriate infection prevention and control procedures.
3. Ensure that the client is appropriately dressed to walk and has shoes or slippers with nonskid soles.
4. Prepare the client for ambulation.
   - Apply elastic (antiembolism) stockings as required. See Skill 35.2 (page 1030).
   - Assist the client to sit on the edge of the bed.
   - Assess the client carefully for signs and symptoms of orthostatic hypotension (dizziness, light-headedness, pallor, or a sudden increase in blood pressure and heart rate) before leaving the bedside.
   - Ensure that the client is appropriately dressed to walk and wears shoes or slippers with nonskid soles. **Rationale: Proper attire and footwear prevent chilling and falling.**
   - Assist the client to stand by the side of the bed until the client feels secure.
5. Ensure client safety while assisting the client to ambulate.
   - Encourage the client to ambulate independently if the client is able, but walk beside the client's weak side and slightly behind, if appropriate.
   - Remain physically close to the client in case assistance is needed at any point.
   - Use a transfer or walking belt if the client is slightly weak and unstable. Make sure the belt is pulled snugly around the client's waist and fastened securely. Grasp the belt at the client's back, and walk behind and slightly to one side of the client (see ❶). The client's forearm can be supported with the other hand. If more support is needed, the nurse can grasp the transfer belt toward the front of the client with the other hand.
   - If it is the client's first time out of bed following surgery, injury, or an extended period of immobility, or if the client is quite weak or unstable, have an assistant follow you and the client with a wheelchair in case it is needed quickly.
   - If the client is moderately weak and unstable, walk on the client's weaker side and interlock your forearm with the client's closest forearm. Encourage the client to press the forearm against your hip or waist for stability, if desired. In addition, have the client wear a transfer or walking belt. **Rationale: You can quickly grab the belt and prevent a fall if the client feels faint.**
   - Encourage the client to assume a normal walking stance and gait as much as possible.
   - If the client is very weak and unstable, two people should assist with walking. **Rationale: The nurse and client are at risk of injury if the client is so compromised.**
6. Protect the client who begins to fall while ambulating.
   - If a client begins to experience the signs and symptoms of orthostatic hypotension or extreme weakness, quickly assist the client into a nearby wheelchair or other chair, and help the client to lower the head between the knees if not contraindicated. **Rationale: Lowering the head facilitates blood flow to the brain.**
   - Stay with the client. **Rationale: A client who faints while in this position could fall, head first, out of the chair.**
   - When the weakness subsides, assist the client back to bed.
   - If a chair is not close by, assist the client to a horizontal position on the floor before fainting occurs (see ❷).

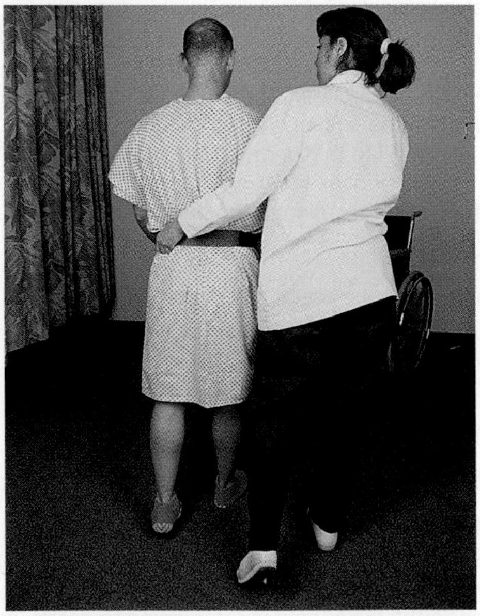

❶ Using a transfer (walking) belt to support the client

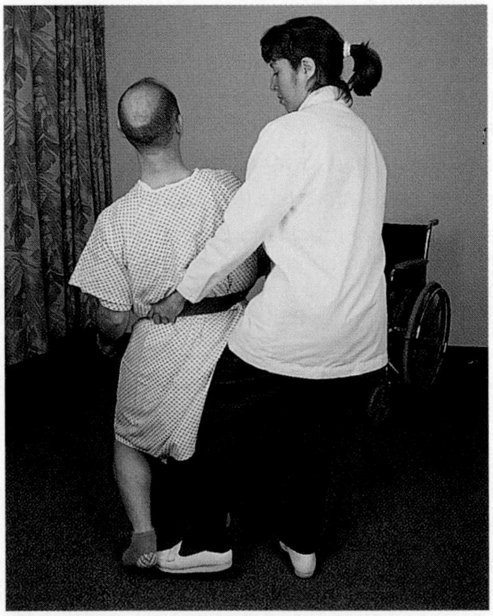

❷ Lowering a fainting client to the floor

(continued)

SKILL 38.7

ASSISTING THE CLIENT TO AMBULATE *(continued)*

Rationale: A vertical position may increase feelings of faintness.

a. Assume a broad stance with one foot in front of the other. **Rationale: A broad stance widens the nurse's base of support for stability. Placing one foot behind the other allows the nurse to rock backward and use the femoral muscles when supporting the client's weight and lowering the centre of gravity (see step b), thus preventing back strain.**

b. Bring the client backward so that your body supports the person. **Rationale: Clients who do faint or start to fall and cannot regain their strength or balance usually drop straight downward or pitch slightly forward because of the momentum of ambulating; thus, their head, hips, and knees are most vulnerable to injury. Bringing the client's weight backward against the nurse's body allows gradual movement to the floor without injury to the client.**

c. Allow the client to slide down your leg, and lower the person gently to the floor, making sure the client's head does not hit any objects.

Variation: Two Nurses

- After the client stands, assume a position with one nurse at either side. Grasp the inferior aspect of the client's upper arm with your nearest hand and the client's lower arm or hand with your other hand (see 3). **Rationale: This provides a secure grip for each nurse.**
- *Optional:* Place a walking belt around the client's waist. Each nurse grasps the side handle with the near hand and the lower aspect of the client's upper arm with the other hand.
- Walk in unison with the client, using a smooth, even gait, at the same speed and with steps the same size as the client's. **Rationale: This gives the client a greater feeling of security.**
- If the client starts to fall and cannot regain strength or balance, slip your arms under the client's axillae, grasp the client's hands, and lower the person gently to the floor or to a nearby chair (see 4). **Rationale: Placing the nurse's arms under the client's axillae evenly balances the client's weight between the two nurses, preventing injury to both the nurses and the client.**

7. Document the distance and duration of ambulation in the client record by using forms or checklists supplemented by narrative notes when appropriate. Include a description of the client's gait (including body alignment) when walking; pace; activity tolerance when walking (e.g., pulse rate, facial colour, any shortness of breath, feelings of dizziness, or weakness); degree of support required; and respiratory rate and blood pressure after initial ambulation to compare with baseline data.

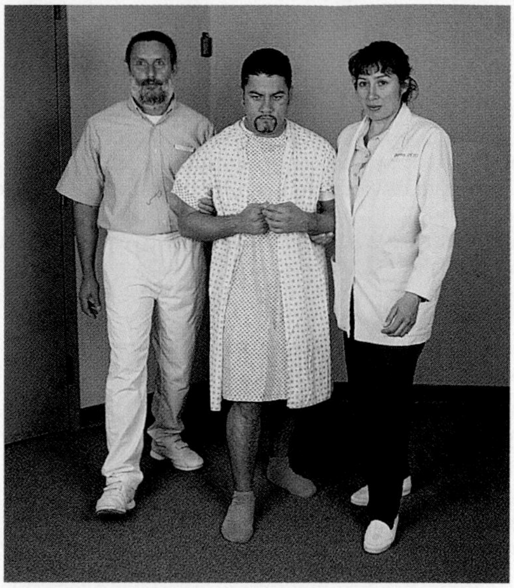

3 Two nurses supporting an ambulatory client

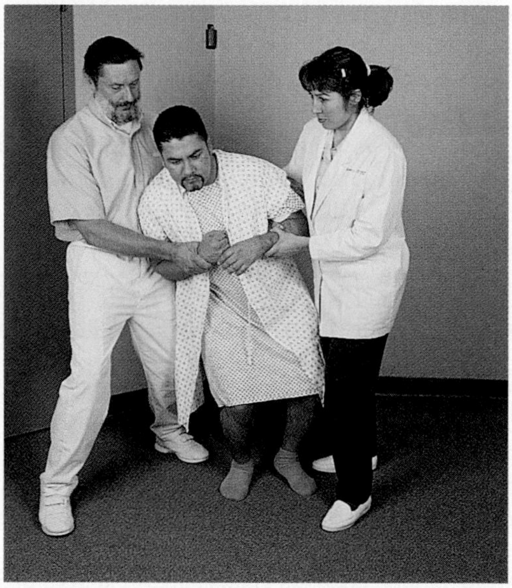

4 Two nurses lowering a fainting client to the floor

EVALUATION

Establish a plan for continued ambulation based on expected or normal ability for the client.

Lifespan Considerations

Assisting the Client to Ambulate

CHILDREN

- Children and adolescents who have suffered a sports injury (e.g., sprained ankle) may want to be more active than they should be. A cast, splint, or boot may be put in place to limit activity and assist in healing. Teach the child the importance of appropriate activity, and the use of assistive devices (e.g., crutches) if necessary. Help them focus on what they *can* do rather than what they cannot do (e.g., you can stand at the free-throw line and shoot baskets).

OLDER ADULTS

- Inquire how the client has ambulated previously and modify assistance accordingly.
- Take into account a decrease in speed, strength, resistance to fatigue, reaction time, and coordination because of a decrease in nerve conduction.
- Be cautious when using a transfer belt with a client with osteoporosis. Too much pressure from the belt can increase the risk of vertebral compression fractures.
- If assistive devices such as a walker or cane are used, make sure clients are supervised in the beginning to learn the proper method of using them. Crutches may be much more difficult for older adults because of decreased upper body strength.
- Be alert to signs of activity intolerance, especially in older adults with cardiac and lung problems.
- Set small goals and increase slowly to build endurance, strength, and flexibility.
- Be aware of any fall risks older adults may have, such as
  - Effects of medications
  - Neurological disorders
  - Environmental hazards
  - Orthostatic hypotension
- In older adults, the body's responses return to normal more slowly. For instance, an increase in heart rate from exercise may stay elevated for hours before returning to normal.

Some clients experience postural (orthostatic) hypotension on assuming a vertical position from a lying position and may need information about ways to control this problem (see the Teaching: Clinical box on controlling postural hypotension). The client may exhibit some or all of the following symptoms: pallor, diaphoresis, nausea, tachycardia, and dizziness. If any of these are present, the client should be assisted to a supine position in bed and closely assessed.

Using Mechanical Aids for Walking

Mechanical aids for ambulation include canes, walkers, and crutches.

CANES Three types of canes are used: the standard straight-legged cane; the tripod or crab cane, which has three feet; and the quad cane, which has four feet and provides the most support (Figure 38.56). Cane tips should

TEACHING: CLINICAL

Controlling Orthostatic Hypotension

Teach the client ways to control orthostatic (postural) hypotension:

- Rest with the head of the bed elevated 20 degrees to 30 degrees. This position makes the position change on rising less severe.
- Avoid sudden changes in position. Arise from bed in three stages:
  - **a.** Sit up in bed for at least 1 minute (or until symptoms subside).
  - **b.** Sit on the side of the bed with legs dangling for at least 1 minute.
  - **c.** Stand with care, holding onto the edge of the bed or another unmovable object for at least 1 minute. Gradual changes in position stimulate renin (a kidney enzyme that has a role in regulating blood pressure), which prevents a dramatic drop in pressure.
- Never bend down all the way to the floor or stand up too quickly after stooping. Baroreceptors (sensory nerve endings in the walls of blood vessels) cannot accommodate rapid change.
- Postpone activities, such as shaving and hair grooming, for at least 1 hour after rising. Baroreceptor reflexes are slow to respond after a night of recumbence during sleep.
- Wear elastic stockings at night to inhibit venous pooling in the legs.
- Be aware that the symptoms of hypotension are most severe at the following times:
  - **a.** 30 to 60 minutes after a heavy meal
  - **b.** 1 to 2 hours after taking an antihypertension medication
- Get out of a warm bath very slowly because warm temperatures can lead to venous pooling. Avoid hot water for bathing.
- Use a rocking chair to improve circulation in the lower extremities. Even mild leg exercises can strengthen muscle tone and enhance circulation.
- Refrain from any strenuous activity that results in holding the breath and bearing down. This Valsalva manoeuvre slows the heart rate, leading to subsequent lowering of blood pressure.

have rubber caps to improve traction and prevent slipping. The standard cane is 91 cm long; some aluminum canes can be adjusted from 56 cm to 97 cm. The length should permit the elbow to be slightly flexed. Clients may use either one or two canes depending on how much support they require. See the Teaching: Clinical box.

WALKERS Walkers are mechanical devices for ambulatory clients who need more support than a cane provides. See the Teaching: Clinical box on the next page.

Many types of walkers are available in different shapes and sizes, with devices suited to individual needs. The standard type is made of polished aluminum. It has four legs with rubber tips and plastic handgrips (Figure 38.59A). Many walkers have adjustable legs.

The standard walker needs to be picked up to be used. The client, therefore, requires partial strength in both hands and wrists; strong elbow extensors, such as triceps brachii; and strong shoulder depressors, such as the pectoralis minor. The client also needs the ability to bear at least partial weight on both legs.

Four-wheeled and two-wheeled models of walkers (roller walkers) (Figure 38.59B) do not need to be picked

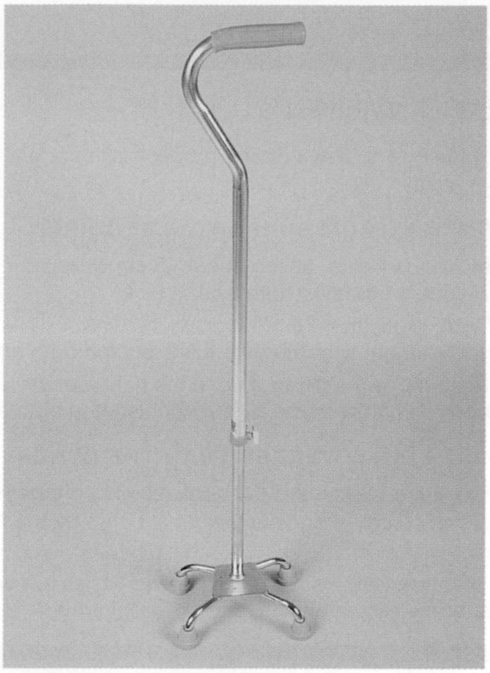

FIGURE 38.56 A quad cane

TEACHING: CLINICAL

Using Canes

Knowing how to use a cane properly is important for client safety:

- Hold the cane with the hand on the stronger side of the body to provide maximum support and appropriate body alignment when walking.
- Position the tip of a standard cane (and the nearest tip of other canes) about 15 cm to the side and 15 cm in front of the near foot, so that the elbow is slightly flexed.

WHEN MAXIMUM SUPPORT IS REQUIRED

- Move the cane forward about 30 cm, or a distance that is comfortable while the body weight is borne by both legs (Figure 38.57A).
- Then move the affected (weak) leg forward to the cane while the weight is borne by the cane and stronger leg (Figure 38.57B).
- Next, move the unaffected (stronger) leg forward ahead of the cane and weak leg while the weight is borne by the cane and weak leg (Figure 38.57C).
- Repeat the steps. This pattern of moving provides at least two points of support on the floor at all times.

AS YOU BECOME STRONGER AND REQUIRE LESS SUPPORT

- Move the cane and weak leg forward at the same time, while the weight is borne by the stronger leg (Figure 38.58A).
- Move the stronger leg forward, while the weight is borne by the cane and the weak leg (Figure 38.58B).

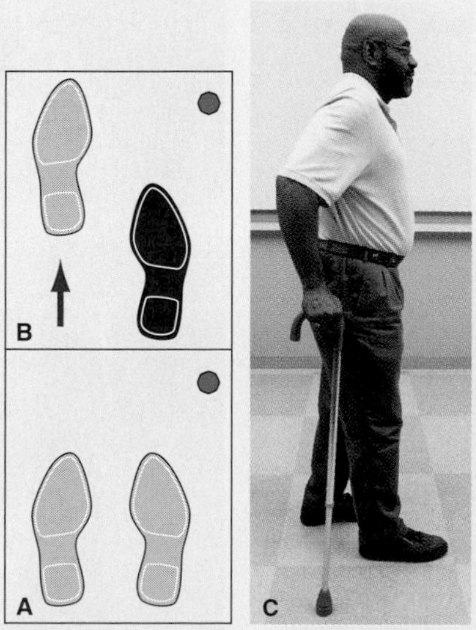

FIGURE 38.57 Steps involved in using a cane to provide maximum support

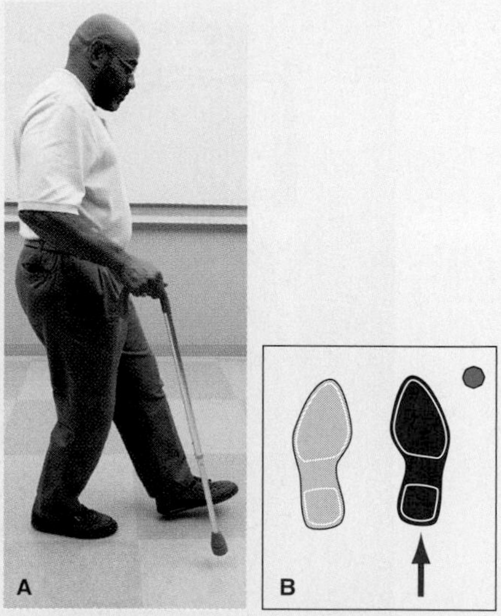

FIGURE 38.58 Steps involved in using a cane when less than maximum support is needed

TEACHING: CLINICAL

Using Walkers

Knowing how to use a walker properly is important for client safety:

WHEN MAXIMUM SUPPORT IS REQUIRED

- Move the walker ahead about 15 cm while your body weight is borne by both legs.
- Then, move the right foot up to the walker while your body weight is borne by the left leg and both arms.
- Next, move the left foot up to the right foot while your body weight is borne by the right leg and both arms.

IF ONE LEG IS WEAKER THAN THE OTHER

- Move the walker and the weak leg ahead together about 15 cm while your weight is borne by the stronger leg.
- Then, move the stronger leg ahead while your weight is borne by the affected leg and both arms.

up to be moved, but they are less stable than the standard walker. They are used by clients who are too weak or unstable to pick up and move the walker with each step. Some roller walkers have a seat at the back so the client can sit down to rest when desired. An adaptation of the standard and four-wheeled walker is one that has two tips and two wheels. This type provides more stability than the four-wheeled model yet still permits the client to keep the walker in contact with the ground at all times. The client tilts the walker forward, lifting the tips while the wheels remain on the ground, then pushes the walker forward.

The nurse may need to adjust the height of a client's walker so that the hand bar is just below the client's waist and the client's elbows are slightly flexed. This position helps the client assume a more normal stance. A walker that is too low causes the client to stoop; one that is too high makes the client stretch and reach.

CRUTCHES Crutches may be a temporary need for some people and a permanent one for others. Crutches should enable a person to ambulate independently; therefore, it is important to learn to use them properly. See the Teaching: Clinical box on the next page. Clients confined to bed are often unaware of weakness that becomes apparent when they try to stand or walk. Clients realize that they can no longer take balance for granted when they must cope with the weight of a heavy cast or a paralyzed limb. Frequently, progress is slower than the client anticipated. Encouragement from the nurse and the setting of realistic goals are especially important.

Several kinds of crutches are available. The most frequently used are the underarm crutch, or *axillary crutch,* with hand bars, and the *Lofstrand,* or *forearm crutch,* which extends only to the forearm (Figure 38.60). On the Lofstrand crutch, the metal forearm cuff and the metal bar stabilize the wrists and, thus, make walking safer and easier. The platform, or elbow extensor, crutch also has a cuff for the upper arm (Figure 38.60). This crutch is usually used by clients who require support for weak extensor muscles of the arm (e.g., weak triceps brachii). All crutches require suction tips, usually made of rubber,

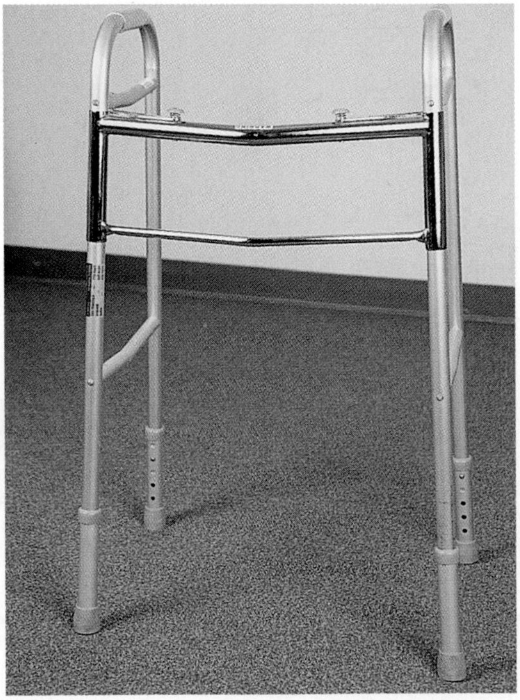
A

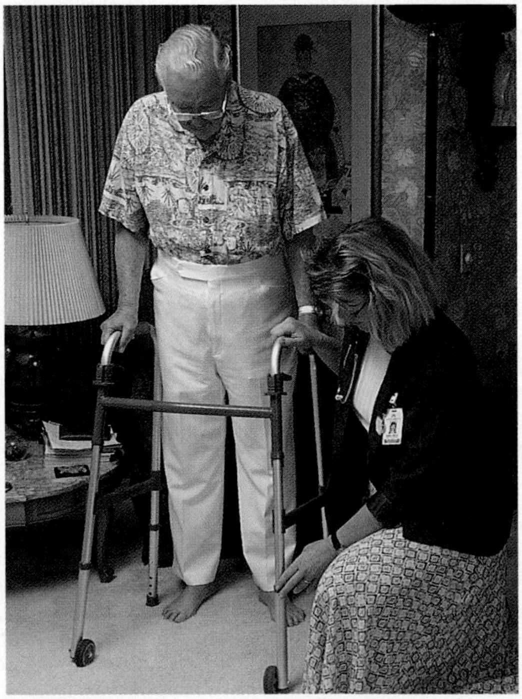
B

FIGURE 38.59 **A:** Standard walker; **B:** two-wheeled walker

TEACHING: CLINICAL

Using Crutches

Knowing how to use crutches properly is important for client safety:

- Follow the plan of exercises developed for you to strengthen your arm muscles before beginning crutch walking.
- Have a health-care professional establish the correct length for your crutches and the correct placement of the hand pieces. Crutches that are too long force your shoulders upward and make it difficult for you to push your body off the ground. Crutches that are too short will make you hunch over and develop an improper body stance.
- The weight of your body should be borne by the arms rather than the axillae (armpits). Continual pressure on the axillae can injure the radial nerve and eventually cause crutch palsy, a weakness of the muscles of the forearm, wrist, and hand.
- Maintain an erect posture as much as possible to prevent strain on muscles and joints and to maintain balance.
- Each step taken with crutches should be a comfortable distance for you. It is wise to start with a small rather than large step.
- Inspect the crutch tips regularly, and replace them if worn.
- Keep the crutch tips dry and clean to maintain their surface friction. If the tips become wet, dry them well before use.
- Wear a shoe with a low heel that grips the floor. Rubber soles decrease the chances of slipping. Adjust shoelaces so they cannot come untied or reach the floor where they might catch on the crutches. Consider shoes with alternative forms of closure (e.g., Velcro), especially if you cannot easily bend to tie laces. Slip-on shoes are acceptable only if they are snug and the heel does not come loose when the foot is bent.

which help prevent the crutches from slipping on a floor surface.

In crutch walking, the client's weight is borne by the muscles of the shoulder girdle and the upper extremities. Before beginning crutch walking, exercises that strengthen the upper arms and hands are recommended.

MEASURING CLIENTS FOR CRUTCHES When nurses measure clients for axillary crutches, it is most important to obtain the correct length for the crutches and the correct placement of the hand piece. Two methods of measuring crutch length are used:

1. The client stands erect and positions the crutch as shown in Figure 38.61. The nurse makes sure the axillary rest of the crutch is at least three finger widths, that is, 2.5 cm to 5 cm, below the axilla.
2. The client lies in a supine position and the nurse measures from the anterior fold of the axilla to the heel of the foot and adds 2.5 cm.

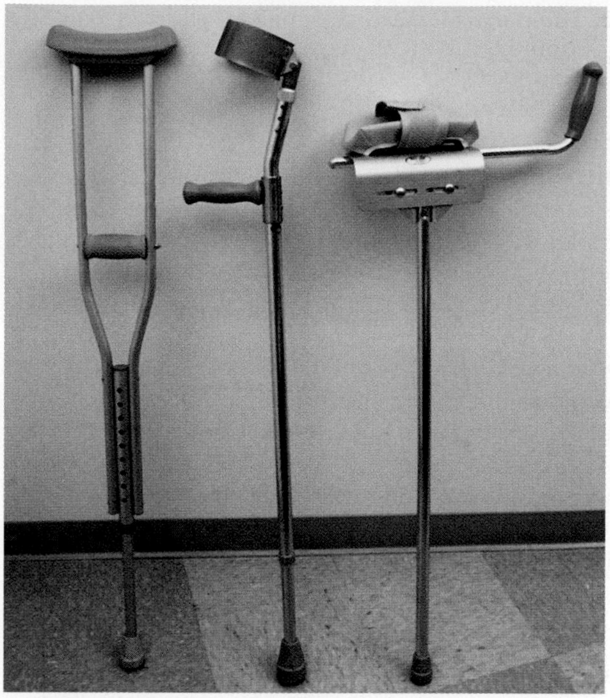

FIGURE 38.60 Types of crutches: axillary, Lofstrand, and platform

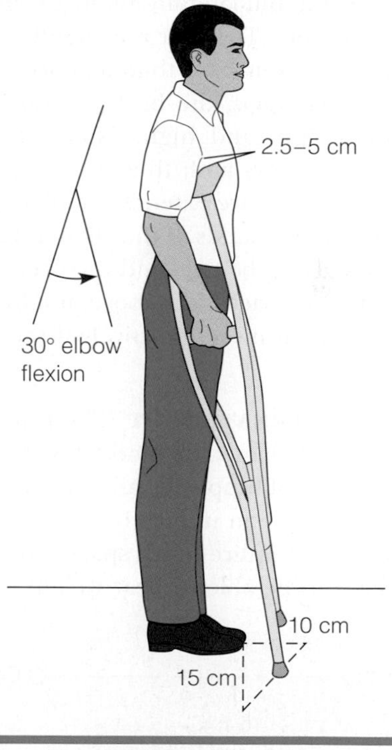

FIGURE 38.61 The standing position for measuring the correct length for crutches

The erect method is generally recommended over the supine measurement method. Note that to determine the correct placement of the hand bar:

1. The client stands upright and supports the body weight by the handgrips of the crutches.

2. The nurse measures the angle of elbow flexion. It should be about 30 degrees. A goniometer can be used to verify the correct angle or with the arm straight, the handgrip should be just above the wrist.

CRUTCH GAITS The crutch gait is the gait a person assumes on crutches by alternating body weight on one or both legs and the crutches. Five standard crutch gaits are the four-point gait, three-point gait, two-point gait, swing-to gait, and swing-through gait. The gait used depends on the following individual factors: (1) the ability to take steps, (2) the ability to bear weight and keep balance in a standing position on both legs or only one, and (3) the ability to hold the body erect.

Clients also need instruction about how to get into and out of chairs and go up and down stairs safely. All these crutch skills are best taught before the client is discharged and preferably before the client has surgery. The crutch gait may be ordered by the physician or physiotherapist.

CRUTCH STANCE (TRIPOD POSITION) Before crutch walking is attempted, the client needs to learn facts about posture and balance. The proper standing position with crutches is called the **tripod (triangle) position** (Figure 38.62). The crutches are placed about 15 cm in front of the feet and out laterally about 15 cm, creating a wide base of support. The feet are slightly apart. A tall person requires a wider base than a short person. Hips and knees are extended, the back is straight, and the head is held straight and high. There should be no hunch to the shoulders and, thus, no weight borne by the axillae. The elbows are extended sufficiently to allow weight bearing on the hands. If the client is unsteady, the nurse places a walking belt around the client's waist and grasps the belt at the back from above, not from below. A fall can be prevented more effectively if the belt is held from above.

FOUR-POINT ALTERNATE GAIT The **four-point alternate gait** is the most elementary and safest gait, providing at least three points of support at all times, but it requires coordination. Clients can use it when walking in crowds because it does not require much space. To use this gait, the client needs to be able to bear weight on both legs (Figure 38.63, reading from bottom to top). The nurse asks the client to do the following:

1. Move the right crutch ahead a suitable distance, such as 10 cm to 15 cm.

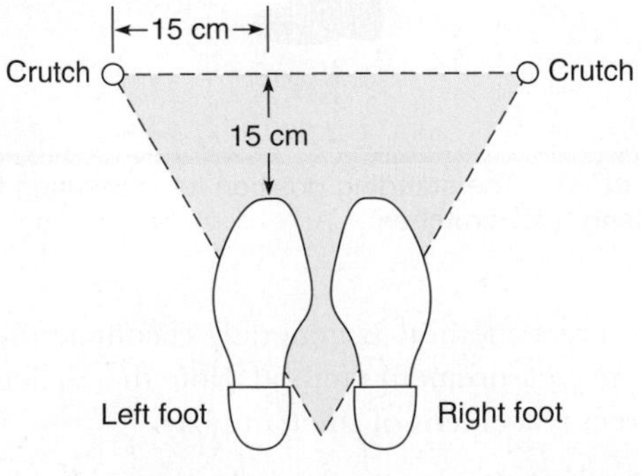

FIGURE 38.62 The tripod position

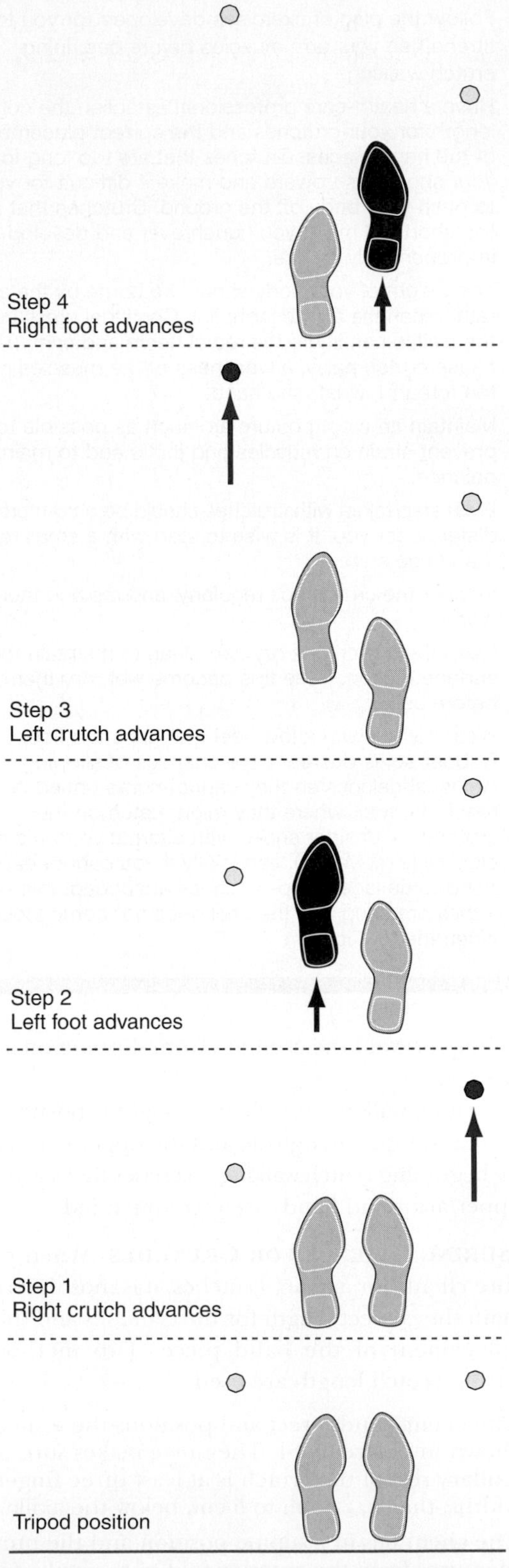

FIGURE 38.63 The four-point alternate crutch gait

2. Move the left foot forward, preferably to the level of the left crutch.
3. Move the left crutch forward.
4. Move the right foot forward.

THREE-POINT GAIT To use the **three-point gait**, the client must be able to bear the entire body weight on the unaffected leg. The two crutches and the unaffected leg bear weight alternately (Figure 38.64, reading from bottom to top). The nurse asks the client to do the following:

1. Move both crutches and the weaker leg forward.
2. Move the stronger leg forward.

TWO-POINT ALTERNATE GAIT The **two-point alternate gait** is faster than the four-point gait. It requires more balance because only two points support the body at any one time; it also requires at least partial weight bearing on each foot. In this gait, arm movements with the crutches are similar to the arm movements during normal walking (Figure 38.65, reading from bottom to top). The nurse asks the client to do the following:

1. Move the left crutch and the right foot forward together.
2. Move the right crutch and the left foot ahead together.

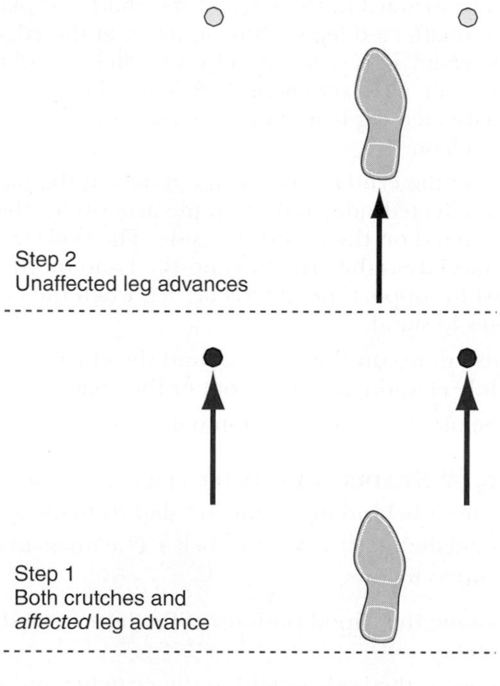

FIGURE 38.64 The three-point crutch gait

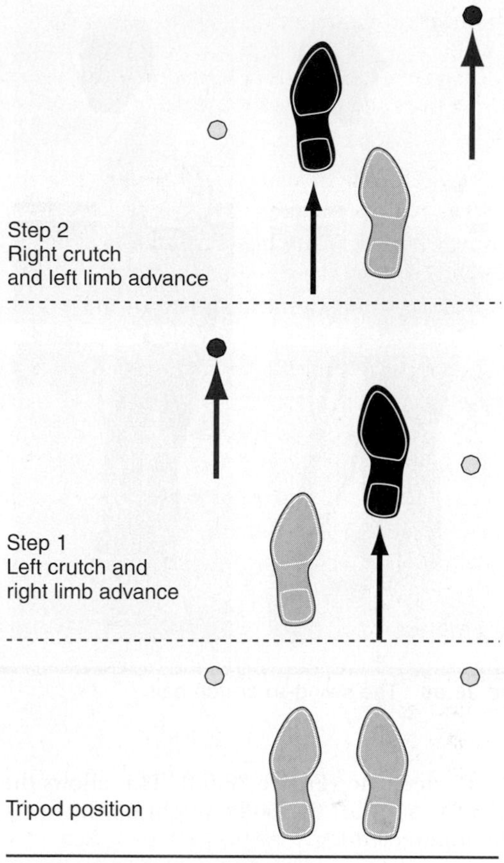

FIGURE 38.65 The two-point alternate crutch gait

SWING-TO GAIT The swing gaits are used by clients with paralysis of the legs and hips. Prolonged use of these gaits results in atrophy of the unused muscles. The **swing-to gait** is the easier of these two gaits. The nurse asks the client to do the following:

1. Move both crutches ahead together (Figure 38.66A).
2. Lift body weight by the arms and swing to the crutches (Figure 38.66B).

SWING-THROUGH GAIT The **swing-through gait** requires considerable skill, strength, and coordination. The nurse asks the client to do the following:

1. Move both crutches forward together (Figure 38.67A).
2. Lift body weight by the arms and *swing through and beyond* the crutch (Figure 38.67B).

GETTING INTO A CHAIR Chairs that have armrests and are secure or braced against a wall are essential for clients using crutches. For this procedure, the nurse instructs the client as follows:

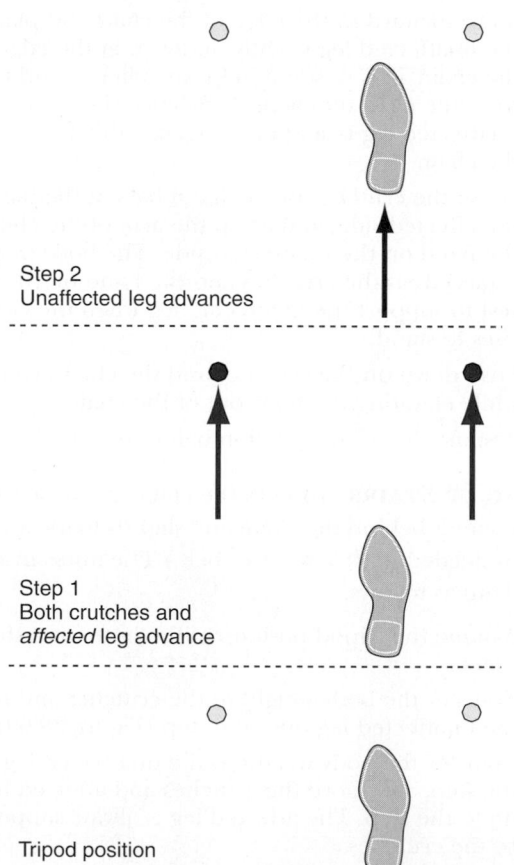

1. Stand with the back of the unaffected leg centred and against the chair. The chair helps support the client during the next steps.
2. Transfer the crutches to the hand on the affected side, and hold the crutches by the hand bars. Grasp the arm of the chair with the hand on the

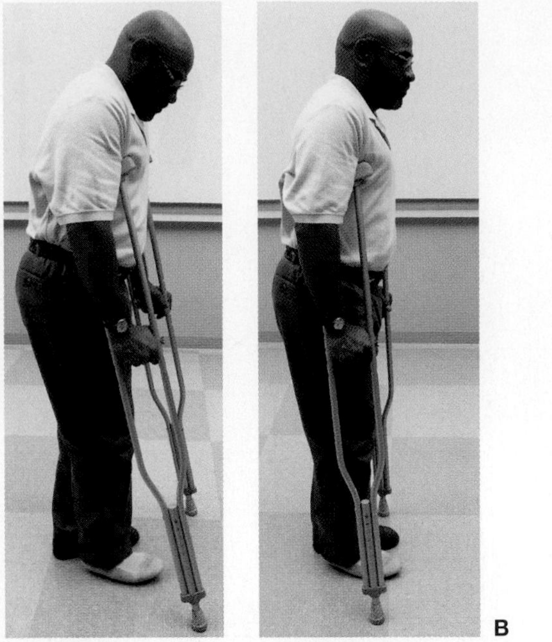

FIGURE 38.66 The swing-to crutch gait

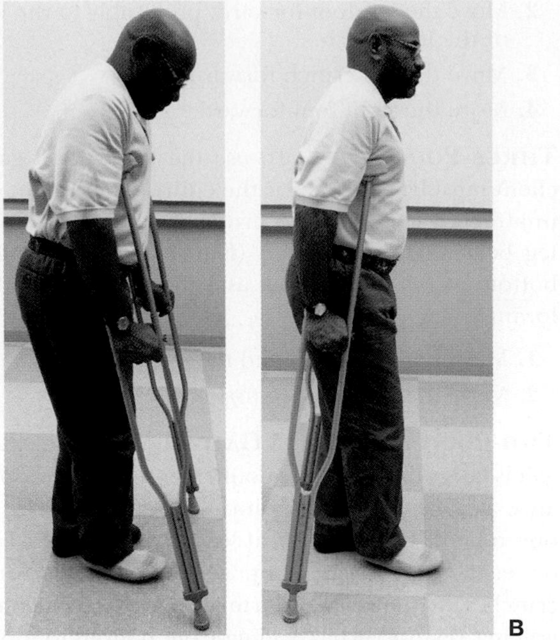

FIGURE 38.67 The swing-through crutch gait

unaffected side (Figure 38.68). This allows the client to support the body weight on the arms and the unaffected leg.

3. Lean forward, flex the knees and hips, and lower into the chair.

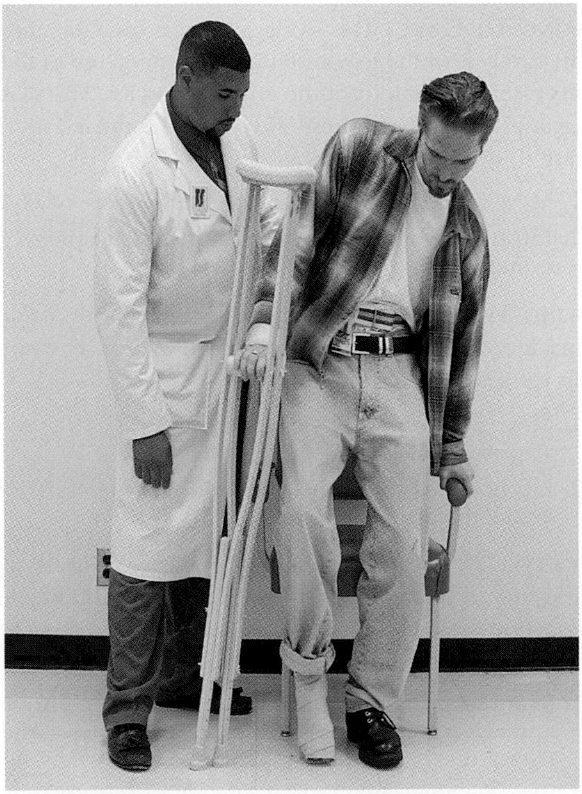

FIGURE 38.68 A client using crutches to get into a chair

Getting out of a Chair To guide a client in getting out of a chair, the nurse instructs the client to do the following:

1. Move forward to the edge of the chair and place the unaffected leg slightly under or at the edge of the chair. This position helps the client stand up from the chair and achieve balance since the unaffected leg is supported against the edge of the chair.
2. Grasp the crutches by the hand bars in the hand on the affected side, and grasp the arm of the chair by the hand on the unaffected side. The body weight is placed on the crutches and the hand on the armrest to support the unaffected leg when the client rises to stand.
3. Push down on the crutches and the chair armrest while elevating the body out of the chair.
4. Assume the tripod position before moving.

Going up Stairs To help the client go up stairs, the nurse stands behind the client and slightly to the affected side, if needed. (Use a transfer belt.) The nurse instructs the client as follows:

1. Assume the tripod position at the bottom of the stairs.
2. Transfer the body weight to the crutches and move the unaffected leg onto the step (Figure 38.69).
3. Transfer the body weight to the unaffected leg on the step, and move the crutches and affected leg up to the step. The affected leg is always supported by the crutches.
4. Repeat steps 2 and 3 until you reach the top of the stairs.

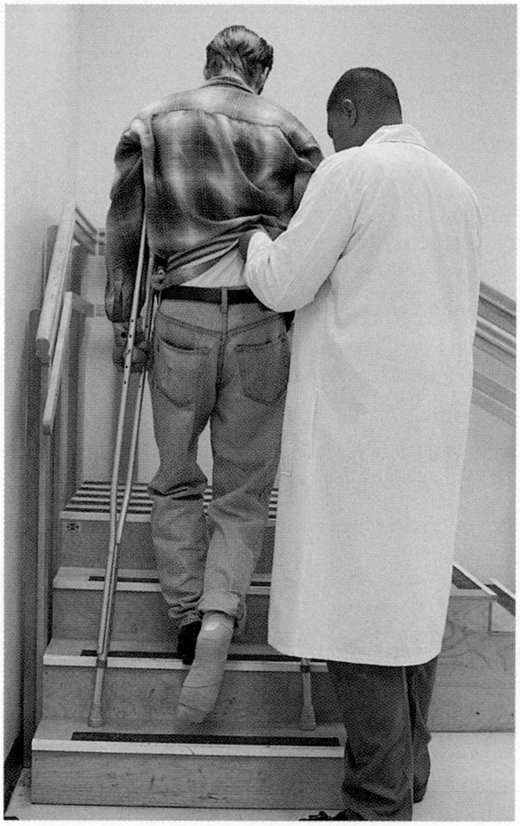

FIGURE 38.69 Climbing stairs: placing weight on the crutches while first moving the unaffected leg onto a step

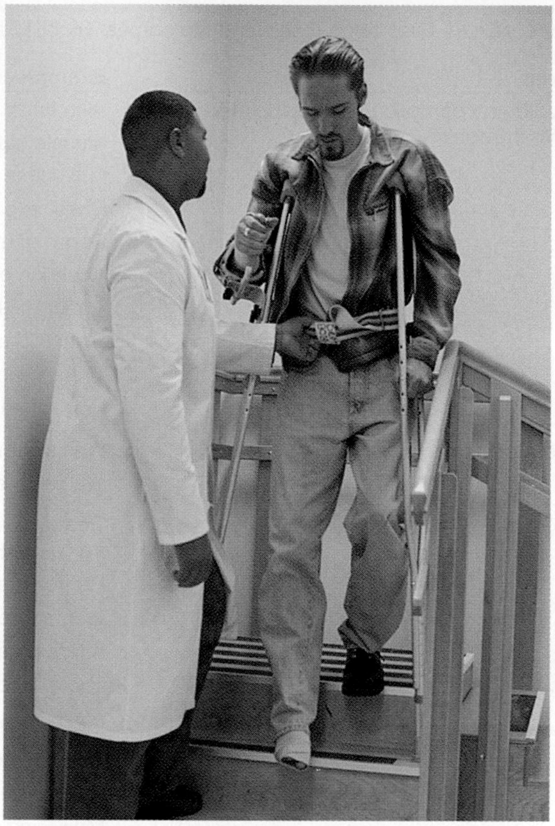

FIGURE 38.70 Descending stairs: moving the crutches and affected leg to the next step

GOING DOWN STAIRS To help the client go down stairs, the nurse stands one step below the client on the affected side, if needed. (Use a transfer belt.) The nurse instructs the client as follows:

1. Assume the tripod position at the top of the stairs.
2. Shift the body weight to the unaffected leg, and move the crutches and affected leg down onto the next step (Figure 38.70).
3. Transfer the body weight to the crutches, and move the unaffected leg to that step. The affected leg is always supported by the crutches.
4. Repeat steps 2 and 3 until you reach the bottom of the stairs.

Evaluating

The goals established during the planning phase are evaluated according to specific desired outcomes also established in that phase. Examples of these are shown in Table 38.10.

If outcomes are *not* achieved, the nurse, client, and support person, if appropriate, need to explore the reasons why before modifying the care plan. For example, the following questions may be considered if an immobilized client fails to maintain muscle mass and tone and joint mobility:

- Has the client's physical or mental condition changed motivation to perform required exercise?
- Were appropriate ROM exercises implemented?
- Was the client encouraged to participate in self-care activities as much as possible?
- Was the client encouraged to make as many decisions as possible when developing a daily activity plan and to express concerns?
- Did the nurse provide appropriate supervision and monitoring?
- Was the client's diet adequate to provide appropriate nourishment for energy requirements?

TABLE 38.10 Evaluation Goals and Outcomes: Mobility and Activity

Goal	Examples of Desired Outcomes
Avoid any complications associated with immobility	Skin intact
	Muscle size within preimmobility range
	Full active ROM of all joints
	Chest expansion symmetrical
	Depth of respirations within expected range
	Absence of adventitious breath sounds
	Abnormal heart rate, heart sounds, and dysrhythmia not present
	Skin-fold measurements within preimmobility range
	Urinary amount, colour, and odour within expected range
	Regular elimination
Restore ability to ambulate	Walks with effective gait with walker
	Walks up and down stairs with assistance of support person
Avoid injury from falling or improper use of body mechanics	Transfers safely to and from bed and chair and from chair to chair or to and from wheelchair
	Demonstrates use of good body mechanics when moving and lifting objects
	Wears appropriate footwear
	Alters home environment to eliminate hazards
	Implements measures to avoid postural hypotension
Increase tolerance for physical activity	Balances activity and rest periods
	Adapts lifestyle to energy level
	Recognizes energy limitation
	Maintains adequate nutrition

Case Study 38

Mrs. Gomez, 71, underwent surgery 2 days ago for repair of a fractured hip she suffered in a fall. She has an incision over her left hip area that is free of redness, with well-approximated edges. She experiences pain on movement even though she is receiving around-the-clock analgesia. The physician has ordered daily physical therapy and that Mrs. Gomez be ambulated three times daily. Mrs. Gomez does not want to get out of bed because she does not want to experience another fall.

Critical Thinking Questions

1. Why is it essential to maintain proper body alignment when turning Mrs. Gomez or helping her out of bed to ambulate?
2. What assessment findings would alert you that Mrs. Gomez is developing problems associated with her current state of decreased mobility?
3. Cite examples of exercises you can recommend for Mrs. Gomez that will reduce her risk for disuse syndrome during her recovery.
4. What are some of the factors you should consider before moving Mrs. Gomez to a sitting position on the edge of the bed in preparation for ambulation?
5. Mrs. Gomez will be using a walker to assist her with ambulation when she goes home. What teaching should be done before Mrs. Gomez's discharge from the hospital in regard to use of a walker?

After working through these questions, go to the MyNursingLab at **http://www.mynursinglab.com** to check your answers.

KEY TERMS

activity-exercise pattern
active living
mobility
line of gravity
centre of gravity
base of support
postural tonus
range of motion (ROM)
proprioception
physical activity
exercise
activity tolerance
functional strength
isotonic (dynamic) exercises
isometric (static or setting) exercises
isokinetic (resistive) exercises
aerobic exercise
anaerobic exercise
hypertrophy
relaxation response
osteoporosis
bed rest
spastic
flaccid
paresis
atrophy
contracture
Valsalva manoeuvre
orthostatic hypotension
thrombophlebitis
thrombus
embolus
vital capacity
metabolism
basal metabolism
anabolism
catabolism
anorexia
urinary stasis
urinary retention
urinary incontinence
urinary reflux
turgor
lordosis
gait
pace
crepitation
body mechanics
Fowler's position
low-Fowler's position
semi-Fowler's position
high-Fowler's position
orthopneic position
dorsal recumbent position
supine (dorsal) position
prone position
lateral position
Sims' position
logrolling
active ROM exercises
passive ROM exercises
active-assistive ROM exercises
ambulation
tripod (triangle) position
four-point alternate gait
three-point gait
two-point alternate gait
swing-to gait
swing-through gait

CHAPTER HIGHLIGHTS

- The ability to move freely, easily, and purposefully in the environment is essential for people to meet their basic needs.
- Exercise and activity are essential for maintaining and regaining health and wellness.
- Purposeful, coordinated movement of the body relies on the integrated functioning of the musculoskeletal system, the nervous system, and the vestibular apparatus of the inner ear.
- Body movement involves four basic elements: body alignment, joint mobility, balance, and coordinated movement.
- People maintain alignment and balance when the line of gravity passes through the centre of gravity and the base of support.
- The broader the base of support and the lower the centre of gravity, the greater is the stability and balance achieved.
- Exercise is physical activity performed to maintain muscle tone and joint mobility, to enhance physiological functioning of body systems, and to improve physical fitness. Activity tolerance is the type and amount of exercise or daily living activities an individual is able to perform without experiencing adverse effects. Functional strength is the ability to do work.
- Exercise is classified as isotonic, isometric, or isokinetic and aerobic or anaerobic. Isotonic exercises increase muscle mass, tone, and strength, joint flexibility, and body circulation. Isometric exercises increase muscle mass, tone, and strength, and circulation to the exercised part but do not involve joint mobility.
- Many factors influence body alignment and activity. These include growth and development, physical health, mental health, personal values and attitudes, and prescribed limitations to movement.
- Immobility affects almost every body organ and system adversely; complications also include psychosocial problems. Exercise, by contrast, provides many benefits to the same body organs and systems and can be used to prevent and treat many disease processes.
- Problems of immobility include disuse osteoporosis and atrophy; contractures; diminished cardiac reserve; orthostatic hypotension; venous stasis, edema, and thrombus formation; decreased respiratory movement and pooling of secretions; decreased metabolic rate and negative nitrogen

balance; urinary stasis, retention, and infection; constipation; and varying emotional reactions.

- Complete bed rest is almost never required, and it is usually dangerous because of the hazards of immobility. A risk-benefit assessment and ongoing assessment of rationale for complete bed rest is essential.
- The nurse has responsibilities (1) to determine root causes of immobility and address these whenever possible with the goal of getting the client moving as much and as soon as possible, (2) to prevent the complications of immobility and reduce the severity of any problems resulting from immobility, and (3) to partner with the client and appropriate support persons to design exercise programs that promote wellness in clients.
- Assessment relative to a client's activity and exercise includes a nursing history and physical examination of body alignment, gait, joint appearance and movement, capabilities and limitations for movement, muscle mass and strength, activity tolerance, and problems related to immobility.
- An activity and exercise history includes daily activity level, activity tolerance, type and frequency of exercise, and factors affecting mobility.
- NANDA International nursing diagnoses that relate to activity and mobility problems include *Activity Intolerance, Risk for Activity Intolerance, Impaired Physical Mobility,* and *Risk for Disuse Syndrome.* Other relevant diagnoses are *Self-Care Deficit, Risk for Injury, Fear* (of falling), *Powerlessness, Low Self-Esteem,* and, if the client is immobilized, many other potential problems, such as *Ineffective Airway Clearance* and *Risk for Infection.*
- *Body mechanics* is the efficient, coordinated, and safe use of the body to move objects and carry out the activities of daily living.
- Nurses must use good body mechanics in their daily work and especially when moving and turning clients in bed and assisting clients to make transfers. Proper body mechanics does not ensure protection from injury, however, and nurses and caregivers are encouraged to avoid manual lifting and repositioning of clients. At the very least, they should avoid solo lifting, repositioning, and transferring.
- Positioning a client in good body alignment and changing the position regularly and systematically are essential aspects of nursing practice.
- Before positioning dependent clients, the nurse should plan a systematic 24-hour schedule for position changes, including positions that provide for full extension of the neck, hips, and knees. The nurse also uses appropriate supportive devices to maintain alignment and prevent strain on the client's muscles and joints.
- Before moving, turning, or transferring a client, the nurse must consider the client's health status, degree of exertion permitted, physical ability to assist, ability to comprehend instruction, degree of discomfort, and weight, and whether to use assistive devices or another caregiver to assist.
- Assistance from others or the use of mechanical lifting aids is essential for most, if not all, nonpediatric clients.
- Safety measures must always be employed when the nurse uses a wheelchair or stretcher to move and transfer clients.
- Ambulating techniques that facilitate normal walking gait yet provide needed support are most effective. The nurse can assist clients to prepare for ambulation by helping them become as independent as possible while in bed.
- Preambulatory exercises that strengthen the muscles for walking are essential for clients who have been immobilized for a prolonged period.
- Clients need specific instructions about appropriate use of canes, walkers, and crutches.

ASSESS YOUR LEARNING

1. A client is concerned that because she has had a myocardial infarction (heart attack) she will not be able to enjoy active living in the future. Which of the following is the nurse's best response?

a. "People who have had a myocardial infarction should not start any physical activity program."

b. "Many risks and injuries can occur with exercise."

c. "To stay physically healthy after a myocardial infarction, a variety of activities are necessary but consult your physician before the exercise is begun."

d. "The older you are, the less active you need to be."

2. An 80-year-old male informs his nurse that he has "slowed down" since he had a mild cerebrovascular accident (stroke). He indicates that he has hired people to "look after everything so that all I have to do is watch TV." The nurse should explain which of the following?

a. Obesity will likely occur if he does not do 1 hour of exercise five times per week.

b. His strategy is a good one.

c. Adding physical activity within his tolerance level would help to decrease the risk of several serious diseases while improving a sense of well-being.

d. At 80 he should still be able to look after his home independently.

3. Knowing that the shoulder is a ball-and-socket joint, the nurse understands that a healthy shoulder can perform which of the following?

a. Circumduction

b. Supination

c. Inversion

d. Right-side flexion

4. The client is ambulating for the first time after surgery. She tells the nurse that she feels faint. Which of the following is the nurse's best action?

a. Find another nurse for help.

b. Return the client to her room as quickly as possible.

c. Tell the client to take rapid, shallow breaths.

d. Assist the client to a nearby chair.

5. A 58-year-old male is in hospital with a fractured right ankle. He was placed in a cast yesterday but is not to weight bear. You walk into the room to find him hopping on his left foot to the bathroom and he refuses to use a bedpan. What should you do?

a. Instruct the patient on using a cane in his right hand to assist with ambulation.

b. Instruct the patient on the use of the bedpan, and insist the he use it as this would be the simplest way to ensure his safety.

c. Instruct the patient on the use of crutches with a swing-thorough gait and urge him to use the call bell for assistance to use the washroom.

d. Instruct the patient on the use of a cane in his right hand to assist with ambulation.

6. During vigorous upper body exercises, which of the following would describe the reaction of the various body systems?

a. Musculoskeletal: increased blood flow to lower extremities
Cardiovascular: decreased heart rate with increased cardiac muscle perfusion
Respiratory: increased lung volume with increased fluid retention

b. Musculoskeletal: increased blood flow to upper and lower extremities
Cardiovascular: increased heart rate with increased cardiac muscle perfusion
Respiratory: increased lung expansion with increased respiratory rate

c. Musculoskeletal: increased blood flow to upper extremities
Cardiovascular: increased heart rate with decreased cardiac muscle perfusion
Respiratory: increased lung expansion with increased respiratory rate

d. Musculoskeletal: increased blood flow to upper and lower extremities
Cardiovascular: increased heart rate with decreased cardiac muscle perfusion
Respiratory: increased lung expansion with increased respiratory rate

7. Isotonic exercises are intended to achieve which of the following?

a. Strengthen immobilized muscles

b. Increase blood pressure

c. Increase muscle mass and strength

d. Decrease heart rate and cardiac output

8. To increase stability during patient transfer, the nurse increases the base of support by doing which of the following?

a. Leaning slightly backward

b. Spacing the feet further apart

c. Tensing the abdominal muscles

d. Bending the knees

9. The client weighs 110 kg. Which of the following statements by the nurse reflects an awareness of workplace injury prevention?

a. "The use of proper body mechanics will prevent me from injuring myself."

b. "I am physically fit so am at lesser risk for injury when transferring the client."

c. "I must use the mechanical lift and get another person to transfer the client from the bed to the chair."

d. "I will use the back belt to avoid hurting my back."

10. When assessing a client's gait, the nurse should look for and encourage which of the following?

a. The spine rotates, initiating locomotion.

b. The gaze is slightly downward.

c. The toes strike the ground before the heel.

d. The arm on the same side as the swing-through foot moves forward at the same time.

After working through these questions, go to the MyNursingLab at ***http://www.mynursinglab.com*** *to check your answers and see explanations.*

SUGGESTED READINGS

Herman, K. M., Ardern, C. I., Mason, C., Brien, S. E., & Katzmarzyk, P. T. (2007). Trends in physical activity research in Canada. *Applied Physiology, Nutrition, & Metabolism, 32*(3), 400–408.

The authors of this article have reviewed more than 5000 articles written on the topic of physical activity in Canadians. It is an interesting read to find out about the range of clinical and public health issues that Canadian researchers have addressed over the past 15 years.

Shaw, K., Gennat, H., O'Rourke, P., & Del Mar, C. (2006). Exercise for overweight or obesity. *Cochrane Database of Systematic Reviews, 4,* Art. No.: CD003817.

This systematic review draws important conclusions of interest to many Canadians. Although the review found support for exercise as a weight-loss strategy, it also found that cardiovascular benefits can be incurred through exercise, even if no weight loss occurs.

Waters, T. R. (2007). Patient handling tasks with high risk for musculoskeletal disorders in critical care. *Critical Care Nursing Clinics of North America, 19*(2), 131–143.

This article reviews a range of tasks, including positioning of patients and application of antiembolism stockings, that critical care nurses engage in as part of their day-to-day work. The authors summarize the risk evidence and offer interesting recommendations to minimize work-related injuries. Much of this article would be of interest to nurses in a range of acute-care settings.

WEBLINKS

Canadian Centre for Occupational Health and Safety (CCOHS)

http://www.ccohs.ca

This site offers information about general and specific occupational health and safety issues. Risks specific to registered nurses are identified.

Health Canada: Healthy Living—Physical Activity

http://www.hc-sc.gc.ca/hl-vs/physactiv/index_e.html

This site identifies the federal programs and initiatives related to fitness in Canada.

Canadian Fitness and Lifestyle Research Institute

http://www.cflri.ca/eng/

The mission of the institute is to enhance the well-being of Canadians through research and communication of information about physically active lifestyles to the public and private sectors.

Active Living Alliance for Canadians with a Disability

http://www.ala.ca

The alliance promotes inclusion and active living lifestyles for Canadians with disabilities by facilitating communication and collaboration among organizations, agencies, and individuals. The site provides provincial and territorial links to helpful local resources.

Public Health Agency of Canada: Healthy Living Unit

http://www.phac-aspc.gc.ca/pau-uap/fitness/

This site provides the physical activity guides for average Canadians, children and youth, and older adults. It offers a range of motivational posters and information to incorporate physical activity into daily life.

REFERENCES

Ammendolia C., Kerr, M. S., Bombardier, C., & the Canadian Task Force on Preventive Health Care. (2003). Use of back belts to prevent occupational low-back pain. Recommendation statement from the Canadian Task Force on Preventive Health Care. *Canadian Medical Association Journal, 169*(3), 213–214.

Bartels, E. M., Lund, H., Hagen, K. B., Dagfinrud, H., Christensen, R., & Danneskiold-Samsøe, B. (2007). Aquatic exercise for the treatment of knee and hip osteoarthritis. *Cochrane Database of Systematic Reviews, 4,* Art. No.: CD005523.

Bonaiuti, D., Shea, B., Iovine, R., Negrini, S., Robinson, V., Kemper, et al. (2002). Exercise for preventing and treating osteoporosis in postmenopausal women. *Cochrane Database of Systematic Reviews, 2,* Art. No.: CD000333.

Borg, G. (1998). *Borg's perceived exertion and pain scales.* Champaign, IL: Human Kinetics.

Busch, A. J., Barber, K. A. R., Overend, T. J., Peloso, P. M. J., & Schachter, C. L. (2007). Exercise for treating fibromyalgia syndrome. *Cochrane Database of Systematic Reviews, 4,* Art. No.: CD003786.

Canadian Centre for Occupational Health and Safety. (2003). *Occupations and workplaces: Registered nurses.* Retrieved June 6, 2008, from http://www.ccohs.ca/oshanswers/occup_workplace/nurse.html

Canadian Diabetes Association. (n.d.). *Physical activity and type 2 diabetes.* Retrieved June 5, 2008, from http://www.diabetes.ca/files/PhysicalActivity.pdf

Canadian Fitness and Lifestyle Research Institute. (2006). *2006 Physical activity and sport monitor.* Retrieved January 22, 2008, from http://www.cflri.ca/eng/statistics/surveys/pam2006.php

Canadian Nurses Association. (2006). *Trends in illness and injury-related absenteeism and overtime among publicly employed registered nurses.* Ottawa: Author.

Edelman, C., & Mandle, C. (2006). *Health promotion throughout the lifespan* (6th ed.). Philadelphia, PA: Mosby/Elsevier.

Fontaine, K. (2005). *Complementary and alternative therapies for nursing practice* (2nd ed.). Upper Saddle River, NJ: Pearson/Prentice Hall.

Freeman, L. (2004). *Mosby's complementary & alternative medicine: A research-based approach* (2nd ed.). St. Louis, MO: Mosby.

Han, A., Judd, M. G., Robinson, V. A., Taixiang, W., Tugwell, P., & Wells, G. (2004). Tai chi for treating rheumatoid arthritis. *Cochrane Database of Systematic Reviews, 3,* Art. No.: CD004849.

Heart and Stroke Foundation of Canada. (2008). *Physical inactivity.* Retrieved June 5, 2008, from http://www.heartandstroke.com/site/c.ikIQLcMWJtE/b.3484171/k.175/Physical_inactivity.htm

Howe, T. E., Rochester, L., Jackson, A., Banks, P. M. H., & Blair, V. A. (2007). Exercise for improving balance in older people. *Cochrane Database of Systematic Reviews, 4,* Art. No.: CD004963.

Katzmarzyk, P. T., & Janssen, I. (2004). The economic costs of physical inactivity and obesity in Canada: An update. *Canadian Journal of Applied Physiology, 29*(1), 90–115.

Kramer, M. S., & McDonald, S. W. (2006). Aerobic exercise for women during pregnancy. *Cochrane Database of Systematic Reviews, 3,* Art. No.: CD000180.

Larun, L., Nordheim, L. V., Ekeland, E., Hagen, K. B., & Heian, F. (2006). Exercise in prevention and treatment of anxiety and depression among children and young people. *Cochrane Database of Systematic Reviews, 3,* Art No.: CD004691.

Lavoie-Tremblay, M., O'Brien-Pallas, L., Viens, C., Hamelin Brabant, L., & Gelinas, C. (2006). Towards an integrated approach for the management of ageing nurses. *Journal of Nursing Management, 14,* 207–212.

Micozzi, M. (2006). *Fundamentals of complementary and alternative medicine* (3rd ed.). Philadelphia, PA: Mosby/Elsevier Publishers.

NANDA International. (2007). *Nursing diagnoses: Definitions and classification, 2007–2008.* Philadelphia, PA: Author.

Nelson, A. (2007). Update on evidence-based practices for safe patient handling and movement. *Orthopaedic Nursing, 25*(6), 367–368.

O'Brien-Pallas, L., Shamian, J., Thomson, D., Alksnis, C., Koehoorn, M., Kerr, M., et al. (2004). Work-related disability in Canadian nurses. *Journal of Nursing Scholarship, 36*(4), 352–357.

Occupational Health and Safety Agency for Healthcare in British Columbia. (2006). *Basic biomechanics literature review.* Retrieved June 5, 2008, from http://www.ohsah.bc.ca/462/2056/

Public Health Agency of Canada. (2003). *Handbook for Canada's physical activity guide to healthy active living.* Ottawa: Author. Retrieved July 6, 2008, from http://www.phac-aspc.gc.ca/pau-uap/fitness/pdf/handbook_e.pdf

Rees, K., Taylor, R. S., Singh, S., Coats, A. J. S., & Ebrahim, S. (2004). Exercise based rehabilitation for heart failure. *Cochrane Database of Systematic Reviews, 3,* Art. No.: CD003331.

Statistics Canada. (2005). Canadian community health survey: Obesity among children and adults. *The Daily,* July 6. Retrieved January 23, 2008, from http://www.statcan.ca/Daily/English/050706/d050706a.htm

Chapter 39

Nutrition

Nutrition is the sum of all the interactions between an organism and the food it consumes. In other words, nutrition is what a person eats and how the body uses it. **Nutrients** are organic, inorganic, and energy-producing substances found in foods and required for body functioning. People require the essential nutrients in food for the growth and maintenance of all body tissues and the normal functioning of all body processes. An adequate food intake consists of a balance of essential nutrients: water, carbohydrates, proteins, lipids, vitamins, and minerals. Foods differ greatly in their **nutritive value** (the nutrient content of a specified amount of food), and no one food provides all essential nutrients. In addition, the way in which foods are processed or cooked can make a difference in their nutritional value. Nutrients have three major functions: (1) providing energy for body processes and movement, (2) providing structural material for body tissues, and (3) regulating body processes.

Understanding how the body uses the nutrients that are ingested requires understanding the terms *metabolism, anabolism,* and *catabolism*. **Metabolism** refers to all biochemical and physiological processes by which the body grows and maintains itself. Energy metabolism refers to how the ingested nutrients are transformed into sources that can be used by the body as fuel. This process is continuous and includes **anabolism** (energy-using reactions that build) and **catabolism** (energy-producing reactions that break down).

Nurses can promote the health of Canadians by evaluating and facilitating adequate nutrition through the lifespan. Being well informed about the ever-changing topic of nutrition is a critical aspect of health promotion for nurses. It is essential that nurses' nutrition knowledge be based on

OBJECTIVES

After studying this chapter, you should be able to

1. Identify six essential nutrients and dietary sources of each
2. Describe normal digestion, absorption, and metabolism of carbohydrates, proteins, and lipids
3. Explain the essential aspects of energy balance
4. Discuss body weight and body mass standards
5. List 13 factors that influence nutrition
6. Outline developmental nutritional considerations
7. Evaluate a diet by using *Eating Well with Canada's Food Guide*
8. Discuss the essential components and purposes of nutritional screening and nutritional assessment
9. Outline nursing interventions to promote optimal nutrition
10. Identify risk factors for and clinical signs of malnutrition and plan, implement, and evaluate nursing care related to nutritional problems
11. Develop interventions to address the childhood obesity problem in Canada
12. Perform the skills of inserting enteral tubes, administering feedings and medications through enteral tubes, and removing enteral tubes

reliable science so that they can be critical consumers of available information and engage in evidence-informed practice.

The body's most basic nutrient need is water. (Body fluids are discussed in Chapter 43.) Because every cell requires a continuous supply of fuel, the most urgent nutritional need after water is for nutrients that provide fuel, or energy. The energy-providing nutrients are carbohydrates, proteins, and fats. These are called **macronutrients**. Hunger impels people to eat enough energy-providing nutrients to satisfy their energy needs, but no clear-cut body signals lead a person to ingest certain vitamins or minerals, both of which are often referred to as **micronutrients**.

Essential Nutrients: Macronutrients

Carbohydrates

Carbohydrates are composed of the elements carbon (C), hydrogen (H), and oxygen (O) and are of two basic kinds: (1) simple carbohydrates (sugars), and (2) complex carbohydrates (starches and fibre).

TYPES OF CARBOHYDRATES

SUGARS Sugars, the simplest of all carbohydrates, are water soluble and are produced naturally by both plants and animals. Sugars can be **monosaccharides** (single molecules) or **disaccharides** (double molecules). Of the three monosaccharides (glucose, fructose, and galactose), glucose is, by far, the most abundant.

Most sugars are produced naturally by plants, especially fruits, sugar cane, and sugar beet. However, lactose, a combination of glucose and galactose, is found in milk. Natural sources of carbohydrates also supply vital nutrients, such as protein, vitamins, and minerals, that are not found in processed foods. Processed or refined sugars (e.g., table sugar, molasses, and corn syrup) are those that have been extracted and concentrated from natural sources. Processed sugars are added to such foods as soft drinks, cookies, candy, ice cream, and some cereals. Processed carbohydrate foods are relatively low in nutrients in relation to the large number of calories they contain and thus are often referred to as *empty calories.* For example, alcoholic beverages can contain significant amounts of carbohydrate, but they are empty calories.

STARCHES Starches are the insoluble, nonsweet forms of carbohydrate. They are **polysaccharides**; that is, they are composed of branched chains of dozens, sometimes hundreds, of glucose molecules. Like sugars, nearly all starches exist naturally in plants, such as grains, legumes, and potatoes. Starches are processed in various ways, for example, in making such foods as cereals, breads, flour, and puddings.

FIBRE **Fibre**, another type of polysaccharide, is a complex carbohydrate derived from plants that cannot be digested by humans. Fibre comes in two forms: insoluble and soluble. **Insoluble fibre** acts as *roughage* and draws water into the colon, preventing constipation. Sources include wheat bran and the skins of some fruits and vegetables. This bulk satisfies the appetite and also helps the digestive tract to function effectively and to eliminate wastes. **Soluble fibre** is found in oats, legumes (peas, kidney beans, and lentils), some seeds, brown rice, barley, fruits (such as apples), some green vegetables (such as broccoli), and potatoes. As it passes through the digestive track, soluble fibre breaks down and forms a gel that is thought to reduce the amount of cholesterol that is absorbed. Soluble fibre delays gastric emptying and slows the entry of glucose into the bloodstream. Ultimately, this delay may prevent a rapid postprandial (post-meal) increase in blood glucose, improving glucose control for individuals with diabetes mellitus (Engel, 2007).

CARBOHYDRATE DIGESTION Through the digestive process, carbohydrates other than soluble and insoluble fibre are broken down into absorbable molecules. Most carbohydrate digestion occurs in the small intestine and occurs with the use of digestive enzyme. **Enzymes** are biological catalysts that speed up chemical reactions. Major enzymes of carbohydrate digestion include ptyalin (salivary amylase), pancreatic amylase, and the disaccharidases: maltase, sucrase, and lactase. The desired end products of carbohydrate digestion are monosaccharides. Some simple sugars are already monosaccharides and require no digestion. Essentially, all monosaccharides are absorbed by the small intestine in healthy people.

CARBOHYDRATE METABOLISM Monosaccharides, in the form of glucose, fructose, and galactose, arrive at the liver, where fructose and galactose are converted into glucose. The liver releases the glucose into the blood where the glucose levels are kept fairly constant by various hormones. After the ingestion of foods, the glucose levels are increased. Some glucose continues to circulate in the blood to maintain blood levels and to provide a readily available source of energy, while the remainder is either used as energy or stored. **Insulin**, a hormone secreted by the pancreas, enhances the transport of glucose into the cells.

STORAGE AND CONVERSION Carbohydrates are stored either as glycogen or as fat. **Glycogen** is a large polymer

Evidence-Informed Practice

How Can Nurses Use Nutrition to Prevent Constipation in Older Adults?

The Registered Nurses' Association of Ontario (2005) has developed a clinical guideline with practice recommendations for the prevention of constipation in the older adult. Recommendations that relate to nutrition include the following:

- Obtain information regarding:
  - Usual amount and type of daily fluid intake with particular attention to the amount of caffeine and alcohol consumed.
  - Usual dietary fibre and amount of food ingested.
- Fluid intake should be between 1500 and 2000 millilitres (mL) per day. Encourage client to take sips of fluid throughout the day and whenever possible minimize caffeinated and alcoholic beverages.
- Dietary fibre intake should be from 25 to 30 grams of dietary fibre per day. Dietary intake of fibre should be gradually increased once the client has a consistent fluid intake of 1500 mL per 24 hours. Consultation with a dietitian is highly recommended.

NURSING IMPLICATIONS: **The nurse plays a key role in preventing constipation in the older adult. Prevention of constipation through assessment and promotion of adequate fibre and fluids consumption should be a key component of interventions to promote healthy nutrition.**

Source: Bulleted list reproduced from *Prevention of Constipation in the Older Adult Population* (Rev. ed.), by the Registered Nurses' Association of Ontario, 2005, Toronto: Author.

(compound molecule) of glucose. The process of glycogen formation is called **glycogenesis**. Almost all body cells are capable of storing glycogen; however, most of it is stored in the liver and skeletal muscles, where it is available for conversion back to glucose. Only a limited supply of glycogen can be formed and glucose that cannot be stored as glycogen is converted to fat. When blood glucose levels fall below normal, the pancreas is stimulated to release **glucagon**, and this causes the liver to release glycogen. This process returns the blood glucose levels to normal. This simplified overview of carbohydrate metabolism describes how it occurs in healthy individuals; this process becomes much more complicated when abnormal nutritional states exist or when an underlying pathological condition is present.

Proteins

Proteins are organic substances composed of amino acids. Like carbohydrates, proteins contain carbon, hydrogen, and oxygen, but proteins also contain nitrogen. Every cell in the body contains some protein, and about three quarters of body solids are proteins.

Amino acids are categorized as essential or nonessential. **Essential amino acids** are those that cannot be manufactured in the body and must be supplied as part of the protein ingested in the diet. Nine essential amino acids—threonine, leucine, isoleucine, valine, lysine, methionine, phenylalanine, tryptophan, and histidine—are necessary for tissue growth and maintenance. A tenth essential amino acid, arginine, is required by the young but not by adults.

Nonessential amino acids are those that the body can manufacture. The body takes apart amino acids derived from the diet and reconstructs new ones from their basic elements (carbohydrates and nitrogen). Nonessential amino acids include glycine, alanine, aspartic acid, glutamic acid, proline, hydroxyproline, cystine, tyrosine, and serine.

Proteins can be complete or incomplete. **Complete proteins** contain all the essential amino acids plus many nonessential ones. Most animal proteins, including meats, poultry, fish, dairy products, and eggs, are complete proteins. Some animal proteins, however, contain less than the required amount of one or more essential amino acids and, therefore, cannot alone support continued growth. These proteins are sometimes referred to as **partially complete proteins**. Examples are some fish, which have small amounts of methionine, and the milk protein casein, which has little arginine.

Incomplete proteins lack one or more essential amino acids (most commonly lysine, methionine, or tryptophan) and are usually derived from vegetables. If, however, an appropriate mixture of plant proteins is provided in the diet, a balanced ration of essential amino acids can be achieved. For example, a combination of corn (low in tryptophan and lysine) and beans (low in methionine) is a complete protein. Such combinations of two or more vegetables are called **complementary proteins**. Another way to take full advantage of vegetable proteins is to eat them with a small amount of animal protein. Examples are spaghetti with cheese, rice with pork, noodles with tuna, and cereal with milk. See the discussion of vegetarian diets later in this chapter.

PROTEIN DIGESTION Digestion of protein foods begins in the stomach. However, most protein is digested in the small intestine, where enzymes break it down into successively smaller molecules and finally into amino acids, the end products of protein digestion. The pancreas secretes the proteolytic enzymes trypsin, chymotrypsin, and carboxypeptidase; glands in the intestinal wall secrete aminopeptidase and dipeptidase.

PROTEIN METABOLISM The liver coordinates the metabolism of amino acids and the creation of protein. Protein synthesis is a complicated process that assembles amino acids that are used to create proteins needed by the body. Protein metabolism includes three activities:

anabolism (building tissue), catabolism (breaking down tissue), and nitrogen balance.

ANABOLISM All body cells synthesize proteins from amino acids. The types of proteins formed depend on the characteristics of the cell and are controlled by its genes.

CATABOLISM Because a cell can accumulate only a limited amount of protein, excess amino acids are degraded for energy or converted to fat. Protein degradation occurs primarily in the liver.

NITROGEN BALANCE Because nitrogen is the element that distinguishes protein from lipids and carbohydrates, nitrogen balance reflects the status of protein nutrition in the body. **Nitrogen balance** is a measure of the degree of protein anabolism and catabolism; it is the net result of intake and loss of nitrogen. When nitrogen intake equals nitrogen output, a state of nitrogen balance exists. If the protein synthesis exceeds the protein breakdown, as in pregnancy, growth, and recovery from injury, then a positive nitrogen state exists. However, a negative nitrogen state occurs when the protein synthesis is less than the protein breakdown. This negative state could occur during starvation or malnutrition or in the catabolic phase of recovery.

PROTEIN STORAGE Amino acids are absorbed by active transport through the small intestine into the portal blood circulation. The liver uses some amino acids to synthesize specific proteins (e.g., liver cells and the plasma proteins albumin, globulin, and fibrinogen). Plasma proteins are a storage medium that can rapidly be converted back into amino acids.

Other amino acids are transported to tissues and cells throughout the body, where they are used to make protein for cell structures. In a sense, protein is stored as body tissue. The body cannot actually store excess amino acids for future use. However, a limited amount is available in the *metabolic pool* that exists because of the constant breakdown and buildup of the protein in body tissues.

Lipids

Lipids are organic substances that are greasy and insoluble in water but soluble in alcohol or ether. Lipids include triglycerides (fats and oils), phospholipids (lecithin), and sterols (cholesterols). Lipids have the same elements (carbon, hydrogen, and oxygen) as carbohydrates. Triglycerides have proportionally less oxygen and so provide more than double the amount of calories for an equivalent amount of carbohydrate.

Fatty acids, made up of carbon chains and hydrogen, are the basic structural units of most lipids. Fatty acids are described as saturated or unsaturated, according to the relative number of hydrogen atoms they contain. **Saturated fatty acids** are those in which all carbon atoms are filled to capacity (i.e., saturated) with hydrogen; an example is butyric acid, found in butter. An **unsaturated fatty acid** is one that could accommodate more hydrogen atoms than it currently does. It has at least two carbon atoms that are not attached to a hydrogen atom; instead, a double bond exists between the two carbon atoms. Fatty acids with one double bond are called **monounsaturated fatty acids**; those with more than one double bond (or many carbons not bonded to a hydrogen atom) are **polyunsaturated fatty acids**. An example of a polyunsaturated fatty acid is linoleic acid, found in vegetable oil.

Saturated fats are generally solid at room temperature. The exceptions are coconut and palm oils. Unsaturated fats have been hydrogenated by adding hydrogen to some of the double bonds to improve the stability and increase the function of the fat or oil. A consequence of hydrogenation is the alteration of the double hydrogen bonds, which results in a shift from the *cis* position to the *trans* position. The result is **transfats**, which are not normally found in nature. In the typical North American diet, 2% to 4% of total caloric intake comes from these fats. Transfats are reported to raise the "bad" cholesterol levels and lower "good" cholesterol. Transfats appear in hard margarine, fried foods, and many prepared bakery goods, such as doughnuts, cookies, muffins, croissants, and french fries. Health Canada recognized the risks of transfats and made changes to help Canadians make healthier choices. Canada was the first country in the world to introduce mandatory labelling of transfat: as of 2005, the transfat content of foods is required to be listed on most packaged foods.

Lipids that are required for normal growth and development but that cannot be synthesized by the body are called **essential fatty acids**. They also play a critical role in inflammation and the clotting mechanism. **Omega-3 fatty acids** and **omega-6 fatty acids** are essential fatty acids. Omega-3 fatty acids (e.g., alpha-linolenic acid) are polyunsaturated fats that have been shown to lower serum triglyceride levels, reduce blood pressure, and decrease factors contributing to blood clotting and strokes. Omega-3 fatty acids are found primarily in cold water fish (e.g., albacore, tuna, sardines, and lake trout), walnuts, flax, hemp, and canola oil.

Omega-6 fatty acids (e.g., linoleic acid, gamma-linolenic acid, arachidonic acid), also polyunsaturated fats, have anti-inflammatory, vasodilator, and antithrombotic properties; however, some evidence suggests that arachidonic acid, found in meat, poultry, and eggs, is associated with an increased risk of coronary artery disease, diabetes mellitus, osteoporosis, and some autoimmune disorders. Linoleic acid and gamma-linolenic acid can be found in cooking oils, including sunflower, safflower, corn, cottonseed, and soybean oils.

Some foods, such as milk and eggs, may have omega-3 and omega-6 fatty acids added to them. Linoleic acid and alpha-linolenic acid are essential for maintaining healthy skin and growth in children.

Based on their chemical structure, lipids are classified as simple or compound. Glycerides, the simple lipids, are the most common form of lipids. They consist of a glycerol molecule with up to three fatty acids attached. **Triglycerides** (which have three fatty acids) account for more than 90% of the lipids in food and in the body. Triglycerides can contain saturated or unsaturated fatty acids. Saturated triglycerides are found in animal products, such as butter, and are usually solid at room temperature. Unsaturated triglycerides are usually liquid at room temperature and are found in plant products, such as olive oil and corn oil.

Phospholipids contain a glycerol molecule and two fatty acids. They occur naturally in almost all foods. Rich sources include liver, eggs, wheat germ, and peanuts. They work as emulsifiers to keep fats suspended in the blood and other body fluids. They provide structure to the cell membrane and help in the transport of fat-soluble substances across that membrane. Lecithin is the best known phospholipid.

Sterols contain carbon, hydrogen, and oxygen arranged in rings. **Cholesterol**, a sterol, is a fatlike substance that is produced by the body and found in foods of animal origin. Most of the body's cholesterol is synthesized by the liver; however, some is absorbed from the diet.

Cholesterol is needed to create bile acids and to synthesize sex hormones and adrenocortical hormones. Cholesterol is found in all cell membranes. The cholesterol found in food is simply cholesterol—it is neither "good" nor "bad." The terms *good* and *bad* cholesterol are related to the **lipoprotein** (a group of compounds made by the body to move water-insoluble lipids) packages that transport the cholesterol through the blood. Two lipoproteins play a role in cholesterol levels: **low-density lipoproteins (LDLs)** and **high-density lipoproteins (HDLs)**. These endogenous lipoproteins carry fat and cholesterol to the tissues for use in energy production and for exchange with other products in cell metabolism. They are classified according to their ratio of fat to protein, and as their concentration of protein increases, their density increases. Because the LDLs carry cholesterol to the cells and deposit it there, they are considered to be the so-called *bad* cholesterol. The HDLs carry cholesterol from the tissues to the liver for catabolism and excretion and so are considered the *good* cholesterol.

LIPID DIGESTION Although the chemical digestion of fats begins in the stomach, fats are primarily digested in the small intestine, primarily by bile, pancreatic lipase, and enteric lipase, an intestinal enzyme. The end products of fat digestion are glycerol and fatty acids. Some fat is excreted in the feces.

LIPID METABOLISM Fatty acids and glycerol enter cells where they can be catabolized for energy or rebuilt and stored as triglycerides. Fat catabolism is regulated by adrenocorticotropin, epinephrine, glucagons, and glucocorticoids, whereas fat anabolism is stimulated by insulin.

LIPID STORAGE Lipids are stored in the liver, adipose tissue, and muscle tissue for release when needed for energy. Fat stored in subcutaneous tissue helps to provide insulation to the body. Fat that is stored in fatty tissue acts to protect vital organs by absorbing mechanical forces.

Essential Nutrients: Micronutrients

A **vitamin** is an organic compound that cannot be manufactured by the body and is needed in small quantities to catalyze metabolic processes. Thus, when vitamins are lacking in the diet, metabolic deficits result. Vitamins are generally classified as fat-soluble or water-soluble. **Water-soluble vitamins** include C and the B-complex vitamins: B_1 (thiamine), B_2 (riboflavin), B_3 (niacin or nicotinic acid), B_6 (pyridoxine), B_9 (folic acid), B_{12} (cobalamin), pantothenic acid, and biotin. The body cannot store water-soluble vitamins; thus, people must get a daily supply in the diet. Water-soluble vitamins can be affected by food processing, storage, and preparation.

Fat-soluble vitamins include vitamins A, D, E, and K. The body can store these vitamins, although the amounts of vitamins E and K the body can store are limited. Therefore, a daily supply of fat-soluble vitamins is not absolutely necessary. Vitamin content is highest in fresh foods that are consumed as soon as possible after harvest.

Minerals are found in organic compounds as inorganic compounds and as free ions. On oxidation, minerals leave an ash, which can be acidic or alkaline. Calcium and phosphorus make up 80% of all the mineral elements in the body. Minerals come in two categories: macrominerals and microminerals. **Macrominerals** are those that people require in daily amounts of more than 100 mg. They include calcium, phosphorus, sodium, potassium, magnesium, chloride, and sulphur. **Microminerals** are those that people require in daily amounts of less than 100 mg. They include iron, zinc, manganese, iodine, fluoride, copper, cobalt, chromium, and selenium.

Health Canada (2006) has developed recommendations for the daily intake of these key nutrients. These recommendations are based on sex and age, and whether a woman is pregnant or lactating. **Dietary reference intakes** are four reference values, *recommended dietary allowances, adequate intake, tolerable upper intake level,* and *estimated average requirement,* that are used for diet assessment and that form the basis of *Eating Well with Canada's Food Guide* (Health Canada, 2007a).

The **recommended dietary allowance** is the amount of a specific vitamin, micromineral, or macromineral that 97% to 98% of healthy individuals should consume based on their age and sex. These recommendations are available online (see the Weblinks section of this chapter for the website). **Adequate intake** is the recommended intake value when a recommended dietary allowance cannot be established; the **tolerable upper intake level** is the maximum amount of a nutrient that should be ingested to avoid any adverse effects (such as with the ingestion of fat-soluble vitamins); and the **estimated average requirement** is the nutrient intake that would meet the needs of 50% of a particular age and gender group.

Common problems associated with the lack of adequate mineral nutrients are iron deficiency resulting in anemia and osteoporosis resulting from loss of bone calcium. Additional information about major minerals associated with the body's fluid and electrolyte balance is found in Chapter 43.

Energy Balance

Energy balance is the relationship between the energy derived from food and the energy used by the body. The body uses energy for voluntary activities, such as walking and talking, and for involuntary activities, such as breathing and secreting enzymes. In theory, a person's energy balance should be determined by comparing his or her energy intake with his or her energy output. It is, however, more complex because each person metabolizes and stores nutrients in a unique way, although the process is the same.

Traditionally, a person's energy balance was determined by considering the caloric value of the nutrients ingested. Recently, the calorie theory has come into question because it does not fully explain the difficulty some individuals have in maintaining a normal weight. An alternative approach to energy balance is related to the glycemic potential of nutrients ingested.

The Caloric Theory Approach

The amount of energy that nutrients or foods supply to the body is their **caloric value**. A **calorie** is a unit of heat energy. A **small calorie** is the amount of heat required to raise the temperature of 1 gram of water 1°C. This unit of measure is used only in chemistry and physics. A **large calorie (Calorie, kilocalorie [kcal])** is the amount of heat required to raise the temperature of 1 gram of water from 15°C to 16°C and is the unit used in nutrition. It was recommended in 1970 that the unit kilojoule (kJ), a metric measurement, replace the kilocalorie. A **kilojoule** is the amount of energy required when a force of 1 newton (N) moves 1 kilogram of weight to a distance of 1 metre. However, to date, Canada and the United States have not made the change.

One calorie (kcal) equals 4.18 kJ. The energy liberated from the metabolism of food has been determined to be as follows:

- 4 calories/gram (about 16 kJ) of carbohydrates
- 4 calories/gram (about 16 kJ) of protein
- 9 calories/gram (about 37 kJ) of fat

The rate of metabolism, or metabolic rate, is normally expressed in terms of the rate of heat liberated during the biochemical and physiological processes by which the body grows and maintains itself. The **basal metabolic rate (BMR)** is the baseline number of calories required to support involuntary body functions at rest after a 12-hour fast. The **resting energy expenditure (REE)** is similar to the BMR, but with no 12-hour fasting period. The two terms are often used interchangeably. The REE of healthy persons is generally about 1 cal/kg of body weight/h for men and 0.9 cal/kg of body weight/h for women, although great variation exists among individuals. BMR is calculated by measuring the REE in the early morning, 12 hours after eating. The actual daily expenditure of energy depends on the individual's degree of activity.

Multiple factors influence a person's BMR. Lean body mass (muscle) requires more calories for maintenance than does adipose (fat) tissue. Thus, men and active children, who have a greater proportion of muscle mass, will have a higher BMR than women, who have a greater proportion of adipose tissue. BMR decreases as muscle mass is lost through the aging process, especially if the aging person is sedentary. The thyroid hormones (thyroxine, or T_4, and tri-iodothyronine, or T_3) regulate the BMR. Hyperthyroidism leads to increased BMR; hypothyroidism decreases BMR. Fever and disease states will increase the BMR. Every 0.83°C rise in body temperature will increase the BMR by about 7%. Increased cell activity associated with pathological conditions, such as cancer, head injury, or trauma, will increase the metabolic demand on the body. Pregnancy and lactation increase the metabolic needs of the body. Living in a very hot or very cold environment will increase the metabolic rate because the body uses more energy to regulate its temperature. During a stressful event, the release of stress hormones will raise the BMR. Ingestion of certain drugs can either increase (e.g., amphetamines) or decrease (e.g., opioids, muscle relaxants) the BMR. Some activities require many times the REE. Examples of approximate real caloric expenditures compared with the REE are as follows:

Light housework	210%
Walking steadily	350%
Heavy housework	400%
Labouring	500%
Average jogging/cycling/energetic swimming	700%

The Glycemic Index Approach

A food's **Glycemic Index (GI)** is determined by how quickly blood glucose levels rise after the food, a carbohydrate, is ingested. Understanding the tenets of this approach to energy balance requires understanding the metabolic process and the roles of glucagon and insulin. The primary function of carbohydrates is to provide fuel for energy production. After carbohydrates are ingested, they are broken down into glucose. If the glucose is not used immediately, it can be stored by the liver as glycogen. **Glycemic level** refers to the amount of glucose present in the blood. The glycemic peak, or maximum absorption level, occurs about 30 minutes after ingestion of the food.

If the glycemic level becomes low, a condition called **hypoglycemia**, the body is in need of fuel or glucose. The pancreas then secretes the hormone glucagon, which re-establishes the glycemic level. If the glycemic levels become high, following a glycemic peak, then the pancreas secretes another hormone, insulin. The role of insulin is to eliminate the excess glucose from the blood and facilitate its storage in the liver or muscles or as glycerides in the adipocytes (fat cells). If a carbohydrate has a high GI, then its ingestion will lead to a rapid increase in glucose in the blood—a condition referred to as **hyperglycemia**. The GI of a food can be altered by the way it is processed or prepared. For example, instant potatoes have a GI of 95; baked potatoes have a GI of 90; potatoes boiled without skin have a GI of 70; and potatoes boiled with skin have a GI of 65. Table 39.1 provides examples of foods with low, medium, and high Glycemic Index.

For some people, maintaining a balance between the blood glucose level and the insulin level is problematic. The result can be a state of **hyperinsulinemia**, meaning there is excess insulin present in the blood. If the state of hyperinsulinemia persists, glucose is stored in the adipocytes. In addition, this phenomenon is worsened by the development of **insulin resistance**, in which the sensitivity to insulin by the receptors on the cells is diminished. These two problems are classic hallmarks for the development of type 2 diabetes mellitus and **metabolic syndrome** (a constellation of central obesity, dyslipidemia, hypertension, and insulin resistance, leading to increased risk of type 2 diabetes mellitus and cardiovascular disease).

For people prone to weight gain, watching their caloric intake may not be sufficient. They may need to pay closer attention to the Glycemic Index of the carbohydrate than to its caloric value. The Canadian Diabetes Association (2008) advocates the use of the Glycemic Index for people with type 1 and type 2 diabetes mellitus.

Factors Affecting Nutrition

Although the nutritional content of food is important to consider in determining an eating plan, other major factors influence the selection and ingestion of food. For many Canadians, patterns of eating are influenced by stage of development, gender, ethnicity and culture, beliefs about food, personal preferences, religious practices, lifestyle, economics, medications or therapy, state of health, alcohol consumption, advertising, and psychological factors.

Stage of Development

People in rapid periods of growth (i.e., infancy and adolescence) have increased need for nutrients. Older people, on the other hand, need fewer calories and may need dietary changes in view of the risk of coronary

TABLE 39.1 Glycemic Indices of Selected Foods

Low GI (55 or less)	Medium GI (56–59)	High GI (70 or more)
100% stone ground whole wheat bread	Whole wheat bread	White bread
Heavy mixed grain bread	Rye bread	Kaiser roll
Pumpernickel bread	Pita	Bagel, white
Oat Bran™	Oatmeal	Bran flakes
All-Bran™	Grape Nuts™	Rice Krispies™
Converted or parboiled rice	Basmati rice	Corn Flakes™
Bulgar	Brown rice	Short-grain rice
Pasta/noodles	Couscous	Potato, baking (Russet)
Lentils/kidney/baked beans	Potato, new/white	Rice cakes
Chick peas	Popcorn	Pretzels
Sweet potato/yams	Black bean/green pea soup	French fries
	Ryvita™	

Source: *Glycemic Index,* by the Canadian Diabetes Association, 2008. Available online at http://www.diabetes.ca/files/Diabetes_GL_FINAL2_CPG03.pdf Reproduced with permission.

heart disease, osteoporosis, and hypertension. See the section "Nutritional Variations throughout the Lifespan."

Gender

Nutrient requirements are different for men and women because of body composition and reproductive functions. The larger muscle mass of men means a greater need for calories and proteins. Because of menstruation, women require more iron than men do. Pregnant and lactating women have increased caloric and fluid needs.

Ethnicity and Culture

The environment in which an individual is raised plays a major role in that person's food preferences and dietary habits. These dietary traditions have been passed on for generations. Dietary practices can include the way in which foods are prepared, what to eat or not to eat when a person is ill or pregnant, foods associated with rites of passage, and the variety of foods that are routinely included in the diet.

When a person is unwell or pregnant, it is important that the nurse understands the ramifications that person's culture will have on his or her overall nutritional state. For example, when giving information to a pregnant woman about her need for increased nutrients, the nurse must know whether the information is congruent with the client's ethnic background. If the information is incongruent, then equivalent food sources must be substituted. Teaching this client may also include discussing cultural myths about certain foods. The *Eating Well with Canada's Food Guide* takes into account the variety of foods that Canadians enjoy (Health Canada, 2007a).

Nurses should not use a *good food, bad food* approach but, rather, should realize that variations of intake are acceptable under different circumstances. The only universally accepted guidelines are (1) to eat a wide variety of foods to provide adequate nutrients and (2) to eat moderately to maintain correct body weight. Food preference probably differs as much among individuals of the same cultural background as it does generally between cultures. Not all Italians like pizza, for example, and many undoubtedly enjoy spicy Mexican food.

Beliefs about Food

Beliefs about effects of foods on health and well-being can affect food choices. Many people acquire their beliefs about food from television, magazines, and the internet.

Food fads that involve nontraditional food practices are relatively common. A **fad** is a widespread but short-lived interest or practice followed with considerable zeal. It may be based either on the belief that certain foods have special powers (e.g., large amounts of yogourt and vitamin E retard the aging process) or on the notion that certain foods are harmful (e.g., eating cabbage and onions sours breast milk). Many fad diets advocate certain eating patterns to stimulate rapid weight loss and are potentially dangerous. Often, such diets do not include the variety of foods necessary for good health. Proponents of the fad may also falsely claim that the body can be tricked into losing weight through the consumption of certain foods. Fad diet gurus often make unrealistic and unscientific claims about the rate of weight loss. It is important for nurses to recognize the popularity of fad diets so that they can promote balanced and nutritious food consumption.

Personal Preferences

People develop likes and dislikes based on associations with a typical food. Parents are key role models in their child's taste preferences. So, if a parent likes or dislikes certain foods, the child will probably have similar preferences. Also, the parents' eating patterns will be mimicked by the child. These preferences and habits are then carried into adulthood.

Individual likes and dislikes can also be related to familiarity. Children often say they dislike a food before they sample it. Some adults are very adventurous and eager to try new foods. Others prefer to eat the same foods over and over again. Preferences in the tastes, smells, flavours (blends of taste and smell), temperatures, colours, shapes, and sizes of food influence a person's food choices. For example, some people may prefer sweet and sour tastes to bitter or salty tastes. Textures play a great role in food preferences. Some people prefer crisp food to limp food, firm to soft, tender to tough, smooth to lumpy, or dry to soggy.

Religious Practices

Religious practice can influence the food selection and preparation. Some Protestant faiths prohibit consumption of meat, caffeine, or alcohol. Both Orthodox Judaism and Islam prohibit the consumption of pork or pork products. Some religions have strict guidelines for the preparation of foods or the combinations of foods that cannot be ingested at the same time (such as dairy and meat products in Judaism). The nurse must be sensitive to the client's religious beliefs when issues surrounding nutrition become paramount.

Lifestyle

A person's lifestyle is linked to his or her eating patterns. A less active person requires fewer nutrients than does a person who is engaged in heavy physical activity on a regular basis. For some individuals, meal preparation is either not important or not possible because of busy work schedules. These people often rely on restaurants and convenience foods to meet their nutritional needs. Others place a great deal of importance on what they ingest and how that food is produced and prepared.

Some Canadians may not have access to foods because of their physical state (e.g., cannot walk or drive to buy food). Other Canadians, including some Aboriginal people, may have difficulty accessing fresh fruit and vegetables at certain times of the year. Some people live in institutions and are totally dependent on caregivers to feed and nourish them. Whatever a person's lifestyle, the important consideration is to eat nourishing and well-balanced meals.

Economics

What, how much, and how often a person eats are frequently affected by socioeconomic status. For example, people with limited income may not be able to afford meat, milk, and fresh vegetables. In contrast, people with higher incomes may purchase more proteins and fats and fewer complex carbohydrates. Not all persons have the financial resources for extensive food preparation and storage. The nurse should not assume that clients have their own stove, refrigerator, or freezer. In some low-income areas or in remote villages, food costs at small local grocery stores can be significantly higher than at large chain stores farther away. It is estimated that 15% of Canadians experience food insecurity because of quantitative (insufficient intake, household food depletion) or qualitative (nutritional inadequacy, unsuitable food) factors resulting from economic issues (Statistics Canada, 2005).

Medications and Therapy

The relationship between drugs and nutrition is a critical consideration for nurses. Some drugs can alter appetite, disturb taste perception, or interfere with nutrient absorption or excretion. Clients should be encouraged to ask their pharmacist if there are known interactions between drugs and foods. For example, the calcium in milk hinders absorption of the antibiotic tetracycline but enhances the absorption of the antibiotic erythromycin. Selected drug and nutrient interactions are shown in Table 39.2.

It is important for the client to know whether the medications should be taken with food or on an empty stomach. Also, it is important for the clients to tell their pharmacist, physician, and nurse if they are taking any herbal remedies or over-the-counter medications. These nonprescription remedies and drugs can have a negative interaction with prescribed drugs or with foods they are eating. Older adults are at particular risk for drug–food interactions because of the number of medications they may take, age-related physiological changes affecting medication actions (e.g., a decrease in lean-to-fat ratio, a decrease in renal or hepatic function), and restricted diets. The nurse plays an important role in determining whether the client is knowledgeable about taking medication and in reinforcing correct information. See Chapter 31 for an extensive discussion of medications.

Therapies prescribed for certain diseases can also adversely affect eating patterns and nutrition. Certain antineoplastic agents (drugs that slow down and fight the development of tumours) can give rise to oral ulcers, intestinal bleeding, nausea and vomiting, or diarrhea, resulting in **anorexia** (reduced appetite) or diminished absorption of nutrients. Radiotherapy of the head and neck can cause decreased salivation, taste distortions, and swallowing difficulties; radiotherapy of the abdomen and pelvis can cause malabsorption, nausea, vomiting, and diarrhea.

Health

An individual's health status greatly affects eating habits and nutritional status. The lack of teeth, ill-fitting dentures, or a sore mouth makes chewing food difficult. **Dysphagia** (difficulty swallowing) because of a painfully inflamed throat, a cerebrovascular accident (stroke), or a stricture of the esophagus can prevent a person from obtaining adequate nourishment. Disease processes and surgery of the gastrointestinal tract can affect digestion, absorption, metabolism, and excretion of essential nutrients. Gastrointestinal and other diseases also create anorexia, nausea, vomiting, and diarrhea, all of which can adversely affect a person's appetite and nutritional status. Gallstones, which can block the flow of bile, are a common cause of impaired lipid digestion. Metabolic processes can be impaired by diseases of the liver. Diseases of the pancreas can affect glucose metabolism or fat digestion. Allergies to foods are a critical factor to consider.

Lactose intolerance or **lactose maldigestion** occurs when a person has a shortage of the enzyme lactase needed to breakdown lactose, a sugar in dairy products. Symptoms include abdominal pain, bloating, flatulence, cramping, nausea, and diarrhea. Certain people with lactose maldigestion can tolerate small quantities of dairy products, while others require lactase-enzyme supplementation or must avoid dairy products altogether. Lactose maldigestion is more common among adults of African, Asian, or Aboriginal descent (Dietitians of Canada, 2005).

Alcohol Consumption

The calories contained in alcoholic drinks include both those of the alcohol itself and of the juices or other beverages added to the drink. In total, these can constitute

TABLE 39.2 Selected Drug–Nutrient Interactions

Drug	Effect on Nutrition
Acetylsalicylic acid	Decreases serum folate and folacin nutrition Increases excretion of vitamin C, thiamine, potassium, amino acids, and glucose May cause nausea and gastritis
Antacids containing aluminum or magnesium hydroxide	Decrease absorption of phosphate and vitamin A Inactivate thiamine May cause deficiency of calcium and vitamin D Increase excretion of sodium, potassium, chloride, calcium, magnesium, zinc, and riboflavin
Thiazide diuretics	May cause anorexia, nausea, vomiting, diarrhea, or constipation Decrease absorption of vitamin B_{12}
Potassium chloride	Increases excretion of potassium, magnesium, and calcium May cause anorexia, nausea, or vomiting Is incompatible with protein hydrolysates
Laxatives	May cause calcium and potassium depletion Mineral oil and phenolphthalein (Ex-Lax) decrease absorption of vitamins A, D, E, and K
Antihypertensives	Hydralazine (Apresoline) may cause anorexia, vomiting, nausea, and constipation Methyldopa (Aldomet) increases need for vitamin B_{12} and folate May cause dry mouth, nausea, vomiting, diarrhea, and constipation
Anti-inflammatory agents	Colchicine decreases absorption of vitamin B_{12}, carotene, fat, lactose, sodium, potassium, protein, and cholesterol Prednisone decreases absorption of calcium and phosphorus
Antidepressants	Amitriptyline (Elavil) increases food intake (large amounts may suppress intake)
Antineoplastics	Can cause nausea, vomiting, anorexia, malabsorption, and diarrhea
Nutrient	**Effect on Drugs**
Grapefruit	Can cause toxicity when taken with a variety of medications including certain anti-arrhythmics (e.g., amiodarone), calcium channel blockers (e.g., nifedipine), statins (e.g., atorvastatin [Lipitor]), erectile dysfunction drugs (e.g., sildenafil), antiseizure agents (e.g., carbamazepine [Tegretol]), and immunosuppressants (e.g., cyclosporine).
Vitamin K	Can decrease the effectiveness of warfarin (Coumadin)
Tyramine (found in aged cheeses, tap beer, dried sausages, fermented soy, sauerkraut)	In combination with monoamine oxidase inhibitor (MAOI) medications e.g., phenelzine (Nardil), tranylcypromine (Parnate), isocarboxazid (Marplan), isoniazid, and linezolid, creates sudden increase in epinephrine, leading to headaches, increased pulse and blood pressure, and possible death
Milk	Interferes with absorption of tetracycline antibiotics

large numbers of calories, for example, 150 calories for a regular 341 mL beer, 160 calories for a screwdriver (45 mL vodka plus 120 mL orange juice). Drinking alcohol can lead to weight gain through the addition of these calories to the regular diet plus the effect of alcohol on fat metabolism. A small amount of the alcohol is converted directly to fat. However, the greater effect is that the remainder of the alcohol is converted into acetate by the liver. The acetate released to the bloodstream is used for energy instead of fat and the fat is then stored.

Excessive alcohol use contributes to nutritional deficiencies in a number of ways. Alcohol may replace food in a person's diet, and it can also depress the appetite. Excessive alcohol can have a toxic effect on the intestinal mucosa, thereby decreasing the absorption of nutrients. The need for vitamin B increases because it is used in alcohol metabolism. Alcohol can impair the storage of nutrients and increase nutrient catabolism and excretion.

A number of studies have shown some health benefits of moderate alcohol consumption. Examples include a reduced risk of cardiovascular disease. However, analysis of the literature indicates that the research has many flaws, and it is too early to make recommendations for clients (Masters, 2005). Pregnant women should avoid all alcohol consumption to prevent the development of fetal alcohol effects or fetal alcohol syndrome.

Advertising

Food producers try to persuade people to change from the product they currently use to the brand the producer is selling. Often, popular celebrities are used to influence television viewers' or radio listeners' choices. Advertising is thought to influence people's, particularly children's, food choices and eating patterns. Canada and a growing number of countries have adopted regulations prohibiting food advertising on programs targeting young children.

Think about how foods are laid out in a grocery store and what types of food are close at hand at the checkout counter. Such products as alcoholic beverages, cakes and other dessert mixes, soups, tea, coffee, frozen dinners, and soft drinks are more heavily advertised than products such as milk, canned seafood, bread, cheese, poultry, vegetables, and fruits.

Psychological Factors

A person's emotional state is a major factor in his or her eating pattern. The role of various neurotransmitters, such as serotonin, is important to consider in relation to mood and food ingestion. For example, through a complex process, the ingestion of carbohydrates boosts the release of serotonin in the brain. The release of serotonin leads to relaxation and a reduction in anxiety. For some people, being upset or distressed will cause them to eat very little. This reduction of food ingestion could be related to the release of increased amounts of epinephrine, which is a component of the stress-response syndrome. Anorexia and weight loss can indicate severe stress or depression. Anorexia nervosa and bulimia nervosa are severe psychophysiological conditions seen most frequently in female adolescents and are discussed later in this chapter.

Nutritional Variations throughout the Lifespan

Neonates to 1 Year

The neonate's fluid and nutritional needs are met by breast milk or formula. Fluid needs of infants are proportionately greater than those of adults because of a higher metabolic rate, immature kidneys, and greater water losses through the skin and the lungs. The latter is largely due to rapid respirations. Therefore, fluid balance is a critical factor in infants. Under normal environmental conditions, infants do not need additional water; however, neonates in very warm environments may require additional fluids. In these cases, water may be prescribed.

Breast milk should be the sole form of feeding for the first 6 months of life (Canadian Paediatric Society, Dietitians of Canada, & Health Canada, 2005) except in cases where the mother is HIV-positive or is taking certain medications (e.g., cyclophosphamide, Lithium), when alternatives to breastfeeding are advised (Health Canada, 2005). Breastfeeding can continue until 2 years of age or longer if the mother chooses. Health Canada (2004) recommends that all breastfed, healthy, term infants in Canada receive a daily vitamin D supplement of 10 mcg (400 IU). Supplementation should begin at birth and continue until the infant's diet includes at least 10 mcg (400 IU) per day of vitamin D from other dietary sources or until the breastfed infant reaches 1 year of age. If the mother chooses not to or cannot breastfeed, the infant should be fed iron-fortified commercial formulas until 9 to 12 months of age.

Demand feeding (i.e., feeding when the child is hungry) tends to decrease the problem of overfeeding or underfeeding the infant. The newborn who is hungry usually cries and exhibits tension in the entire body. The total daily nutritional requirement of the newborn is about 80 mL to 100 mL of breast milk or formula per kilogram of body weight. The newborn infant's stomach capacity is about 90 mL, and feedings are required every 2.5 to 4 hours. During feeding, the infant sucks readily and needs burping after each 30 mL of formula or after 5 minutes of breastfeeding. Burping is done by holding the infant in an upright position while gently patting the back. *Parents should be warned that infant bottles should never be propped up for feeding.* There is a real danger that aspiration or choking could result.

Infants demonstrate satisfaction by slowing their sucking activity or by falling asleep. Once satisfaction has been demonstrated, infants should not be coaxed into finishing the feeding. This could lead to discomfort or overfeeding. When feeding is completed, healthy infants can be placed in a lateral or supine position for sleep during the first 6 months of life to reduce the risk of sudden infant death syndrome (SIDS).

Regurgitation, or spitting up, of digested milk during or after a feeding is a common occurrence during the first year. Although this may be of concern to parents, it does not usually result in nutritional deficiency. Demonstration of adequate weight gain should reassure parents that the infant is receiving adequate nutrition.

The addition of solid food to the diet usually starts at 6 months of age. Six-month-old infants can consume solid food more readily because they can sit up and they have a decreased sucking reflex. Solid foods (strained or pureed) are generally introduced in the following order: iron-fortified cereals (e.g., rice), vegetables (yellow before green), fruits, egg yolks, and strained meats (see Box 39.1). Foods are introduced one at a time, usually with only one new food introduced every 5 days. With the eruption of teeth at about 7 to 9 months, the infant is ready to chew and can begin to experience different textures of food. At this time, the infant enjoys finger foods, such as pieces of skinless fruit, dry cereal, or toast.

At about 6 months of age, infants require iron supplementation to prevent iron-deficiency anemia. Iron can be obtained in fortified infant cereals. **Iron-deficiency anemia** is a form of anemia caused by inadequate supply of iron for synthesis of hemoglobin. Iron-fortified cereals are usually recommended by 6 months of age and are continued until the child reaches 18 months. As noted,

BOX 39.1 INFANT AND TODDLER FOOD SAFETY

Health Canada (2005) has made the following recommendations to ensure infant and toddler safety:

- Do not feed honey to infants less than 1 year of age. Honey can be a source of the *Clostridium botulinum* toxin.
- To prevent salmonella poisoning, cook all eggs well and do not feed products containing raw eggs to infants and toddlers.
- Do not feed hard, small and round, smooth, or sticky solid foods (such as candy, hotdogs, popcorn, and peanut butter). They can cause choking and aspiration.
- Always supervise infants and toddlers during feeding.
- Do not allow children to run around with food in their mouths.
- Do not prop up an infant's bottle.
- To prevent the development of food allergies, it is recommended that toddlers not be fed peanuts, nuts, or fish until 3 years of age. Egg whites can be offered after 1 year of age.

Canadian infants should continue to receive a daily 10 mcg (400 IU) vitamin D supplement until the age of 12 months (Health Canada, 2004).

Whole pasteurized cow's milk can be introduced between 9 and 12 months of age. Before this time, the digestive tract is immature and anemia can result, as cow's milk is a low source of iron and can cause microscopic gastrointestinal bleeding. Weaning from the breast or bottle to the cup takes place gradually and is usually achieved by age 1 year or later. Some infants have difficulty giving up the bottle, particularly at naptime or bedtime. Parents should be warned that having the bottle in bed can lead to **bottle-mouth syndrome**. The term describes decay of the teeth caused by constant contact with sweet liquid from the bottle. Dentists advocate brushing or cleaning the infant's teeth to prevent bottle-mouth syndrome, especially for the infant who requires a bottle only at naptime or bedtime. Weaning from the bottle can be facilitated by increasingly diluting the formula with water until the infant is drinking plain water; most infants do not like to drink plain water. By the age of 1 year, most infants can be completely fed on table food, and milk intake is about 600 mL per day.

Toddlers

Because of a maturing gastrointestinal tract, toddlers can eat most foods and adjust to three meals each day. In addition, by age 3 years, when most of the deciduous teeth have emerged, the toddler is able to bite and chew adult table food. Toddlers' manipulative skills are sufficiently well developed for them to learn how to feed themselves. Before the age of 20 months, most toddlers require help with glasses and cups because their wrist control is limited.

Developing independence may be exhibited through the toddler's refusal of certain foods. Meals should be short because of environmental distractions and the toddler's brief attention span. Often, toddlers display their liking of rituals by eating foods in a certain order, cutting foods a specific way, or accompanying certain foods with a particular drink.

The toddler is less likely to have fluid imbalances than the infant. The toddler's gastrointestinal function is more mature, and the percentage of fluid body weight is lower. A healthy toddler weighing 15 kg needs about 1250 mL of fluid per 24 hours.

During the toddler stage, the caloric requirement decreases to 1200 to 1800 kcal per day because of a decrease in the rate of growth. From 1 to 2 years of age, the toddler may be eating a combination of prepared toddler foods and some table foods. Parents should be instructed to read labels carefully and be aware that the table foods offer more variety, are less expensive, and are more nutritious than prepared toddler foods. Deficiencies of iron, calcium, and vitamins C and A, which are common toddler deficiencies, should also be discussed.

The following suggestions may help parents meet the child's nutritional needs and promote effective parent-child interactions: (1) make mealtime a pleasant time by avoiding tensions at the table and discussions of bad behaviour; (2) offer a variety of simple, attractive foods in small portions, and avoid meals that combine foods into one dish, such as a stew; (3) do not use food as a reward or punish a child who does not eat; (4) schedule meals, sleep, and snack times that will allow for optimum appetite and behaviour; and (5) avoid the routine use of sweet desserts.

Preschoolers

The preschooler eats adult foods and should have the required amounts from *Eating Well with Canada's Food Guide* (Health Canada, 2007a). The preschooler requires 1600 kcal per day. Parents should become informed about the diet of their child in daycare or preschool settings so that they can be sure of meeting the child's total nutritional needs. Children at this age are very active and may rush through the meal to return to playing. Parents need to teach the preschooler how to use utensils and should provide them with the opportunity to practise (e.g., spreading margarine on bread). Active children often require snacks between meals. Cheese, fruits, yogourt, raw vegetables, and milk are good choices. Children at this age may enjoy helping in the kitchen, and both girls and boys should be encouraged to do so.

The preschooler is even less susceptible than the toddler to fluid imbalances. The average 5-year-old weighing 20 kg requires at least 75 mL of liquid per kilogram of body weight per day, or 1500 mL every 24 hours.

School-Age Children

Nutrition continues to be a high priority for growing children. School-age children require a balanced diet, including 2400 kcal per day. School-age children eat three meals a day and one or two nutritious snacks. Children need a protein-rich food at breakfast to sustain the prolonged physical and mental effort required at school. Studies have shown that children who skip breakfast become inattentive and restless by late morning and have decreased problem-solving ability. Undernourished children become fatigued easily and face a greater risk of infection, resulting in frequent absences from school.

The average healthy 8-year-old weighing 30 kg requires about 1750 mL of fluid per day. Many school-age children have only one meal a day with their family, at dinner. Mealtime should be a social time enjoyed by all, and families should refrain from watching television or discussing a child's poor eating habits at this time. Parents should be aware that children learn many of their food habits by observing their parents. Eating a balanced diet should be the norm for both parents and children.

The school-age child generally eats lunch at school. The child may bring lunch from home or buy lunch at the school cafeteria. Many dietary problems stem from this independence in food choices. The children may trade their food, not eat lunch at all, or buy sweets or junk food with their lunch money. Parents should discuss with the child the foods that they should eat and continue to provide a balanced diet in the home setting. Strict rules have been enacted in certain provinces and territories to limit unhealthy food choices offered in the school environment (e.g., banning pop and chocolate bars from vending machines).

Obesity is increasingly a problem that begins in the preadolescent period and continues in adolescence and adulthood (see Box 39.2). Between 1981 and 1996, there was an alarming increase in the prevalence of overweight and obese children in Canada. Twenty-six percent of all boys and girls aged 2 to 18 were obese. Among Aboriginal children, the rates are two to three times as high. A 2000 study of an Ojibwa-Cree community found that 64% of girls and 60% of boys were overweight. From 1981 to 1996, the prevalence of overweight children aged 7 to 13 increased from 10.6% to 32.6% for boys and increased from 13.1% to 26.6% for girls (Cole, Bellizzi, Flegal, & Dietz, 2000; Shields, 2004). From 1978 to 2004 in Canada, the overweight or obesity rate of adolescents aged 12 to 17 more than doubled from 14% to 29%, while the obesity rate alone tripled from 3% to 9% (Shields, 2004).

Poor eating habits and a sedentary lifestyle contribute to obesity. For children, hours spent in front of the television and on the computer result in less physical activity. Obesity in school-age children tends to result in a further decrease in activity. In one study of Cree children in Northern Quebec, 100% of obese children had fitness scores below the 20th percentile for their age and gender (Ng, Marshall, & Willows, 2006). For adults, sedentary employment has replaced physical labour and regular physical activity, resulting in a chronic energy imbalance.

BOX 39.2 THE OBESITY EPIDEMIC

In the last 25 years, there has been an exponential increase in the number of overweight and obese Canadians. Given the clear relationship between excess weight and the development of chronic disease, this trend is very alarming. Nurses play a key role in health promotion and must become proactively involved in addressing this problem at the level of the individual, family, and community. The etiology of obesity is complex. At a basic level, it is caused by a chronic energy imbalance whereby the number of calories consumed exceeds the number of calories expended. However, obesity has many contributing factors, including economics, genetics, culture, media, and education (Public Health Agency of Canada, 2007a). It is estimated that in 2001, the direct and indirect costs associated with obesity in Canada exceeded \$4.3 billion (Katzmarzyk & Janssen, 2004). One in 10 premature deaths of adults between 20 and 64 years of age is attributable to obesity (Lau et al., 2007). The latest data from the Canadian Community Health Survey in 2004 reveals that 59% of Canadian adults are overweight with a body mass index greater than 25 kg/m^2 and 23% are obese with a body mass index greater than 30 kg/m^2 (Lau et al., 2007).

The health consequences of being overweight or obese are serious. Overweight and obese individuals are at increased risk of type 2 diabetes mellitus, hypertension, dyslipidemia, stroke, coronary artery disease, obstructive sleep apnea, osteoarthritis, and certain cancers (Lau et al., 2007). Obese and overweight surgical patients are at increased risk of atelectasis and urinary retention, poor wound healing, and wound dehiscence. The psychological ramifications can also be severe. Obese adolescents, for example, are frequently rejected by their peers, badgered by their parents, and ridiculed on television and in the movies. Many feel ugly and socially unacceptable. Depression and low self-esteem are common among obese individuals. Increasingly, the health consequences of excess weight, such as the development of type 2 diabetes mellitus, are being seen in childhood and adolescence.

Preventing obesity is key to avoiding lifelong health problems. Convincing evidence suggests that increasing total physical activity decreases the risk of overweight and obesity. Breastfeeding and diets high in whole-grain cereals and dietary fibre, fruit, and vegetables also decrease the risk. The consumption of large quantities of highly sugared beverages, such as cola, is linked to increased risk (Brown, Kelly, & Summerbell, 2007).

Treatment of obesity includes low-calorie diets in combination with physical activity. In some cases, medication is used. Lifestyle modification and behavioural interventions will work in combination with other approaches. For extreme obesity, bariatric surgery may be indicated. The treatment of excess weight must include education and regular screening and interventions for obesity-related conditions. Regular physical activity is key (Wilding, 2007).

Nurses are responsible for identifying individuals at risk and intervening with a family-centred approach. Nurses can work with adults and children to do the following:

- Review the individual's eating habits.
- Alter food choices to better follow *Eating Well with Canada's Food Guide.*
- Use rewards other than food for children.
- Offer water instead of sugary drinks such as sports drinks and cola.
- Follow *Handbook for Canada's Physical Activity Guide to Healthy Active Living* (Public Health Agency of Canada, 2003b) (see Chapter 38).

Adolescents

The adolescent's need for nutrients and calories increases, especially during the growth spurt. In particular, the need for protein, calcium, vitamin D, iron, and B vitamins increases during adolescence. An adequate diet for an adolescent is three to four servings of milk products daily as well as appropriate amounts of meat, vegetables, fruits, breads, and cereals (see the section on *Canada's Food Guide* for serving recommendations). Calcium intake during adolescent years (1200 mg/day to 1500 mg/day) may help decrease osteoporosis (a decrease in bone density) in later life (Schettler & Gustafson, 2004).

Many parents observe that teenagers, particularly boys, seem to be eating all the time. Teenagers have active lifestyles and irregular eating patterns. They tend to snack frequently, often eating high-calorie foods, such as doughnuts, soft drinks, ice cream, and fast foods. Parents and nurses can promote better lifelong eating habits by encouraging teenagers to eat healthy snacks. Parents can provide healthy snacks, such as fruits and cheese, and, at the same time, limit the amount of junk food available in the home. The teenager's food choices relate to physical, social, and emotional factors and impulses and may not be influenced by teaching. Nurses need to advise parents that adolescents must take responsibility for their decisions in many areas of life, and parents should try to avoid conflicts that relate to food.

Common problems related to nutrition and self-esteem among adolescents are anorexia nervosa and bulimia nervosa, in addition to obesity, as discussed in Box 39.2.

Under social pressure to be slim, some adolescents severely limit their food intake to a level significantly below that required to meet the demands of normal growth. In some instances, the adolescent may develop an eating disorder, such as anorexia nervosa or bulimia. Anorexia nervosa and bulimia are severe psychophysiological conditions usually seen in adolescent girls and young women. They also occur in adolescent boys and men. **Anorexia nervosa** is characterized by a prolonged inability or refusal to eat, rapid weight loss, and emaciation in persons who continue to believe they are fat. People with anorexia nervosa may also induce vomiting and use laxatives and diuretics to remain thin. **Bulimia nervosa** is an uncontrollable compulsion to consume enormous amounts of food and then expel it by self-induced vomiting or by taking laxatives. These illnesses are most effectively treated in the early stages by psychotherapy. Hospitalization may be necessary when the effects of malnutrition become life threatening.

Young Adults

The nutritional habits established during young adulthood often lay the foundation for the patterns maintained throughout a person's life. Many young adults are aware of the four food groups but may not be knowledgeable about how many servings of each group they need or how much constitutes a serving. The nurse should discuss Health Canada's (2007a) *Eating Well with Canada's Food Guide* (Figure 39.1) with the young adult client and review serving and portion sizes with them.

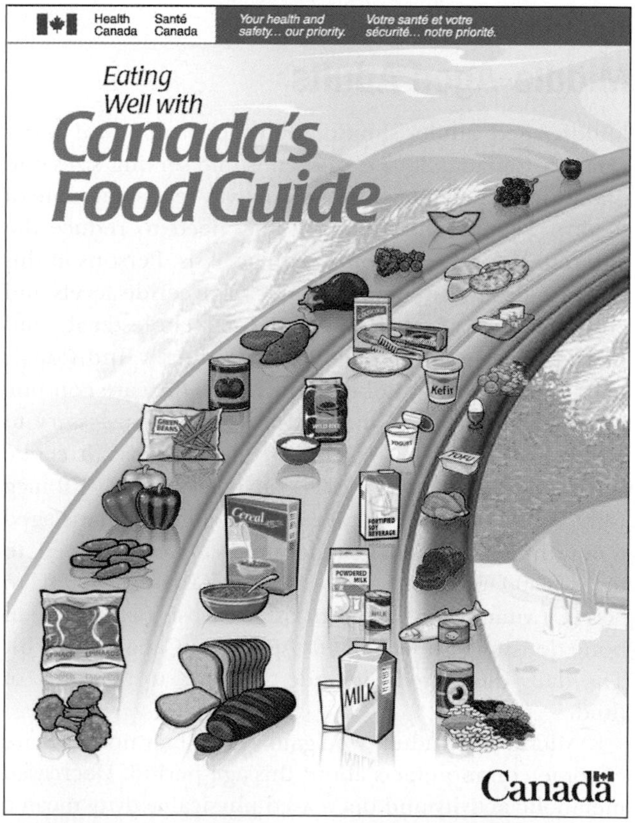

FIGURE 39.1 *Eating Well with Canada's Food Guide*
(Eating Well with Canada's Food Guide, ***by Health Canada, 2007, Ottawa: Author. Reproduced with the permission of the Minister of Public Works and Government Services Canada, 2007.)***

Young adult females are at risk for developing iron-deficiency anemia because of blood loss during their menstrual cycle. Therefore, they need to ensure that they are consuming adequate amounts of iron. Iron-rich foods include red meats, organ meats (liver and kidney), eggs, lentils, sole, cashews, molasses, broccoli, spinach, cooked oatmeal, raisins, and prune juice. Calcium is needed in young adulthood to maintain bones and help decrease the chances of developing osteoporosis in later life. Along with calcium, the person must have adequate vitamin D, which is necessary for the calcium to enter the bloodstream. Vitamin D is made in the skin on exposure to the sun. If the person does not get sufficient sun exposure (15 minutes three times each week), supplements may be indicated. Health Canada (2004) recommends that supplementation of vitamin D begin at age 50 but this may be started earlier if the client does not get adequate sun exposure or have enough dietary intake.

CLINICAL ALERT

The Public Health Agency of Canada (2003a) recommends that all women who are pregnant or who could become pregnant take a multivitamin with 400 mcg of folic acid (folate). Taking folic acid, a B vitamin, is thought to reduce the likelihood of neural tube defects (such as spina bifida) in the unborn child.

Middle-Aged Adults

Middle-aged adults should follow *Canada's Food Guide* (Health Canada, 2007a) and consume serving sizes and quantities congruent with their activity levels and state of health. This means that they may need to reduce the amount of food eaten on a regular basis. Persons in this group need to be aware of their triglyceride levels and cholesterol (LDLs, HDLs, and total cholesterol) and plan their nutritional intake accordingly. Individuals need to be cognizant of the type of fats they are consuming. In the case of some individuals, it is necessary to monitor the type of carbohydrate and its Glycemic Index. Health Canada (2004) advocates a daily 10 mcg (400 IU) vitamin D supplement for all Canadians aged more than 50 years. Postmenopausal women need to ingest 1500 mg calcium and 10 mcg to 20 mcg (400 IU to 800 IU) vitamin D to prevent osteoporosis (a decrease in bone density) (Public Health Agency of Canada, 2007b). The daily diet should include 2000 mL to 3000 mL of fluid.

Middle-aged adults who gain weight may not be aware of some common facts about this age period. Decreased metabolic activity and decreased physical activity mean a decrease in caloric need. The nurse's role in nutritional health promotion is to counsel clients to prevent obesity by reducing caloric intake and participating in 30 to 60 minutes of moderate physical activity per day. Referral to dietitians and weight-loss experts may be indicated in some cases.

Older Adults

Older adults should follow a meal plan congruent with their state of health, which may be deteriorating or may include one or more chronic conditions. Portion sizes may need to be reduced if the person is sedentary. Some older adults may need more carbohydrates for fibre and bulk, but most nutrient requirements remain relatively unchanged. Physical changes, such as tooth loss and impaired sense of taste and smell, can affect eating habits. Decreased saliva and gastric juice secretion can also affect a person's nutrition. Psychosocial factors can contribute to nutritional problems. Some older people who live alone may not want to cook for themselves or eat alone. As a result, they may adopt poor dietary habits. The death of the spouse, anxiety, depression, dependence on others, and lowered income all affect eating habits. Table 39.3 summarizes a range of problems associated with nutrition in the older adult.

Studies have shown that many older adults living in the community are at risk for malnutrition (see the Teaching: Wellness box for ways that nurses can help). A study by Krondl, Lau, Coleman, and Stocker (2003) found that older Canadians receiving meals delivered at home from nutrition support services were particularly at risk for deficiencies in magnesium, zinc, and folate. Nurses must be aware that the risk for malnutrition is still present even with support services. Among institutionalized older adults, the risk of malnutrition is particularly salient. One study of long-term-care facilities in Saskatchewan revealed that the menus did not offer the recommended number of servings of grains and vegetables and fruit identified by *Canada's Food Guide*. Residents were receiving only 88% of the recommended calories for males 50 to 74 years (Lengyel, Zello, Smith, & Whiting, 2003).

Standards for a Healthy Diet

Various daily food guides have been developed to help healthy people meet the daily requirements of essential nutrients and to facilitate meal planning. Food group plans emphasize the general types or groups of foods, rather than specific foods, because related foods are similar in composition and often have similar nutrient values. For example, all grains, whether wheat or oats, are significant sources of carbohydrate, iron, and the B vitamin thiamine. *Eating Well with Canada's Food Guide* (Health Canada, 2007a) provides recommendations for healthy nutrition for people aged 2 years and up.

TABLE 39.3 Problems Associated with Nutrition in Older Adults

Problem	Nursing Interventions
Difficulty chewing (may lead to a deficiency in vitamins A and C, minerals, and fibre)	Encourage regular visits to the dentist to have teeth and dentures repaired, refitted, or replaced. Chop fruits and vegetables finely; shred green, leafy vegetables; select ground meat, poultry, or fish.
Lowered glucose tolerance	Eat more carbohydrates (e.g., whole-wheat breads, cereals, brown rice, pasta, potatoes, and legumes) rather than sugar-rich foods.
Decreased social interaction, loneliness	Promote appropriate social interaction at meals, when possible. Encourage the client and spouse to take an interest in food preparation and serving, perhaps as an activity they can do together. If food preparation is not possible, suggest community resources, such as Meals on Wheels. Suggest having picnics in the yard or inviting friends over for meals.
Loss of appetite and senses of smell and taste	Eat essential, nutrient-dense foods first; follow with desserts and low-nutrient-density foods. Review dietary restrictions, and find ways to make meals appealing within these guidelines. Eat small meals frequently instead of three large meals a day.
Limited income	Suggest using generic brands and coupons. Substitute milk, dairy products, and beans for meat. Avoid convenience foods, if able to cook. Buy foods that are on sale and freeze for future use. Suggest community resources and nutrition programs.
Difficulty sleeping at night	Have the major meal at noon and a lighter meal in the evening. Avoid tea, coffee, or other stimulants in the late afternoon or evening.

TEACHING: WELLNESS

Nutrition for Older Adults

Teach clients to include at least the minimal number of servings from each of the following groups from *Eating Well with Canada's Food Guide* (Health Canada, 2007a):

Vegetables and fruits	7 servings
Grain products	6 servings (female) 7 servings (male)
Milk products	3 servings
Meat and alternatives	2 servings (female) 3 servings (male)

- *Reduce caloric intake.* Caloric needs generally decrease in older people, often because of decreased activity. Older adults need to consume nutrient-dense foods and avoid foods that are high in calories but have few nutrients (empty calorie foods).
- *Reduce fat consumption.* Use leaner cuts of meat, and limit portions to 100 g to 150 g per day. (But be sure intake of the meat group is sufficient, because older people often consume inadequate amounts of these foods.) Broil, boil, or bake foods instead of frying them. Use low-fat milk and cheese; limit intake of butter, margarine, and salad dressings.
- *Reduce consumption of empty calories.* Substitute fruit or puddings made with low-fat milk in place of pastries, cookies, and rich desserts.
- *Reduce sodium consumption.* Avoid canned soups, ketchup, mustard, and salted, smoked, cured, and pickled meats (e.g., ham and bacon) as they are generally high in sodium. Do not add salt when cooking foods or at the table. Avoid excess use of salt substitutes as they can contain sodium and potassium chloride. Use spices and herbs for seasoning foods.
- *Ensure adequate calcium intake to prevent bone loss.* Most older adults need at least 1000 mg of calcium; postmenopausal women need 1500 mg. Milk, cheese, yogourt, cream soups, puddings, and frozen milk products are good sources.
- *Ensure adequate vitamin D intake.* Vitamin D is essential to maintain calcium homeostasis. Include milk because other dairy products are not usually fortified with vitamin D. Because daily vitamin D intake requirements exceed that which can be provided by following the *Eating Well with Canada's Food Guide*, Health Canada (2007) recommends that all Canadians aged over 50 years take a 10 mcg (400 IU) vitamin D supplement.
- *Consume fibre-rich foods and ensure adequate fluid intake to prevent constipation and minimize use of laxatives.* See the Evidence-Informed Practice box (p. 1168).

Eating Well with Canada's Food Guide

The goal of *Eating Well with Canada's Food Guide* (Health Canada, 2007a; see Figure 39.1) is to recommend healthy eating patterns to promote and maintain health. Following the guide allows Canadians to meet their nutrient needs and reduce the risk of obesity, osteoporosis, type 2 diabetes mellitus, coronary artery disease, and some cancers. The 2007 edition of the Food Guide takes into consideration the varied ethnic cultures and cuisines in Canada. Indeed, a specific guide for First Nations, Inuit, and Metis peoples was also developed to account for the consumption of caribou, bannock, and other foods (Health Canada, 2007b). See Figure 39.2.

Eating Well with Canada's Food Guide emphasizes a global pattern of eating over time rather than focusing on any one particular food choice (Health Canada, 2007a). The Food Guide thus represents a total diet approach. Similar to the previous editions of the Food Guide, this guide depicts foods from all macronutrient groups in a rainbow with four arcs. The smallest arc represents meat and alternative protein sources because this category of foods should have the smallest number of portions per day. Milk products appear in the next larger arc, with more servings per day depending on the person's age. Grains are represented in the next larger arc. This placement is a change from the 1992 edition of *Canada's Food Guide for Healthy Eating* in which grains occupied the largest arc. The largest arc in the 2007 edition is for fruit and vegetable products because this is the category from which most food intake should be derived. The guidelines stress that people should choose a variety of foods from within each of the four groups. An adult who follows the Food Guide will consume between 1800 and 3200 calories. See Figure 39.3 for the recommended number of daily servings in each of the four food groups. Key directional statements about other nutrition recommendations for Canadians also accompany the guide.

Serving Sizes

Eating Well with Canada's Food Guide encourages Canadians to eat the recommended number of servings of each food group each day (Health Canada, 2007a). Rather than counting calories, the guide measures food consumption with portions. The portion size varies depending on the food item in question. My Food Guide is a web-based tool for Canadians interested in customizing the Food Guide to their age, sex, activity level, and dietary preferences.

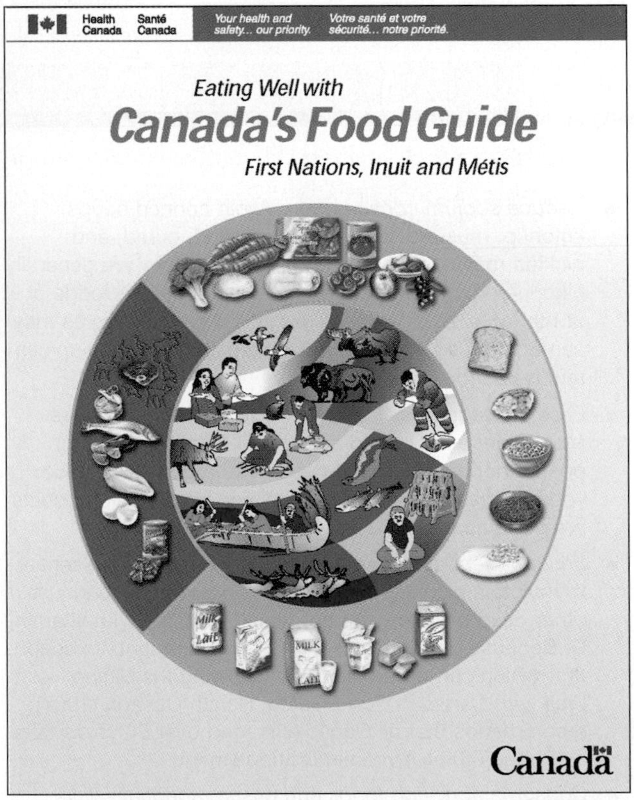

FIGURE 39.2 *Eating Well with Canada's Food Guide: First Nations, Inuit and Métis*

*(***Eating Well With Canada's Food Guide: First Nations, Inuit and Métis***, by Health Canada, 2007, Ottawa: Author. Reproduced with the Permission of the Minister of Public Works and Government Services Canada, 2007.)*

	Recommended Number of Food Guide Servings per day			
	Children 2–3 years old	Children 4–13 years old	Teens andAdults (Females)	(Males)
Vegetables and Fruit Fresh, frozen and canned.	4	5-6	7-8	7-10
Grain Products	3	4-6	6-7	7-8
Milk and Alternatives	2	2-4	Teens 3-4 Adults (19-50 years) 2 Adults (50+ years) 3	Teens 3-4 Adults (19-50 years) 2 Adults (50+ years) 3
Meat and Alternatives	1	1-2	2	3

FIGURE 39.3 Recommended number of food guide servings per day

(From **Eating Well with Canada's Food Guide***, by Health Canada, 2007, Ottawa: Author. Reproduced with the Permission of the Minister of Public Works and Government Services Canada, 2007.)*

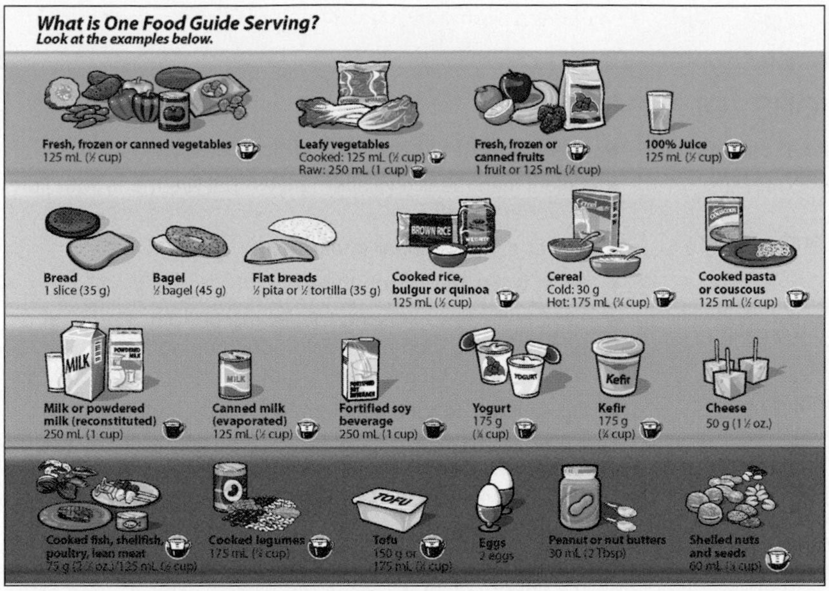

FIGURE 39.4 Portion grid to accompany *Eating Well with Canada's Food Guide*

(From **Eating Well with Canada's Food Guide**, *by Health Canada, 2007, Ottawa: Author. Reproduced with the Permission of the Minister of Public Works and Government Services Canada, 2007.)*

Figure 39.4 outlines sample portion sizes. It is important to note that many usual servings actually represent more than one portion. For example, a bagel is actually two servings of grains and 125 mL of juice is one serving of fruit and vegetables.

Food Labels

To be knowledgeable about food, it is helpful to read the food labels on packaged foods. Since 2003, Health Canada has stipulated that most food products must have clear nutrition labelling. Each label contains the ingredients in order of proportion and the number of calories supplied for each serving. The caloric content is further subdivided into proteins, carbohydrates, and fats. Fats are categorized further into saturated, monosaturated, or unsaturated and trans. Packages also list 13 nutrients and the percentage of their recommended daily intake contained in one serving. See Figure 39.5. The nurse can help clients learn how to read labels to achieve specific nutritional goals (e.g., lower sodium consumption).

Some of the nomenclature on the label may be unfamiliar to some clients. For example the salt content of foods is often listed as sodium. Clients with specific health conditions, such as diabetes mellitus, may be more concerned about the carbohydrate content of foods and may need guidance to identify sugars and fibre. As food purchasing is often a shared family responsibility, involving key family members and caregivers in the teaching may be appropriate. Children should be taught from an early age to read labels and to identify fat, sugar, and calorie content to empower them to make healthy food choices. The Teaching: Wellness box describes the facts that nurses should teach clients, based on Health Canada's (2007a) recommendations.

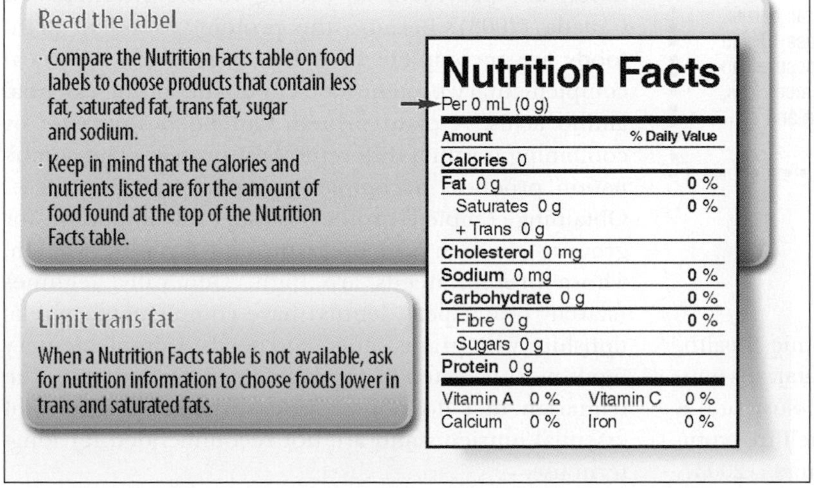

FIGURE 39.5 Nutrition facts table

(From **Eating Well with Canada's Food Guide**, *by Health Canada, 2007, Ottawa: Author. Reproduced with the Permission of the Minister of Public Works and Government Services Canada, 2007.)*

TEACHING: WELLNESS

Nutrition Recommendations for Canadians

The following recommendations can be found in *Eating Well with Canada's Food Guide* (Health Canada, 2007a) and Health Canada (2008) documentation:

- Every day, try to eat at least one orange and one dark green vegetable.
- Eat whole fruits and vegetables rather than drinking juice.
- Prepare vegetables and fruits with little or no added fat or sugar.
- Eat adequate amounts of sodium (52 mmol/day to 65 mmol/day or 1200 mg to 1500 mg) (Health Canada, 2008), but avoid sodium in excess of 100 mmol/day (2300 mg) per day (Canadian Hypertension Education Program, 2008). Prepare foods with little or no added salt. Look for foods that are *salt-free* (< 5 mg of sodium per serving), low in sodium (< 140 mg of sodium per serving), or reduced in sodium (at least 25% less sodium than the regular product) (Health Canada, 2008).
- Chose grain products that are lower in fat, sugar, and salt.
- Each day, make sure at least half of your grain products are whole grains.
- Drink lower fat milk (skim, 1%, or 2%) each day. Children younger than 2 years of age should drink whole milk.
- Select lower fat dairy products.
- Have meat alternatives, such as tofu, beans, and lentils, more often.
- Have at least two servings of fish per week.
- Select lean meat and alternatives that are made with little or no fat or salt.
- Lower salt and sugar intake.
- Drink water to quench thirst.
- Limit caffeine to 400 mg to 450 mg per day. Pregnant or breastfeeding women should consume no more than 300 mg per day. The average cup of coffee contains 200 mg.
- Consume alcohol in moderation, which is defined by Health Canada as fewer than 7 drinks per week. One drink is equivalent to 350 mL beer (5% alcohol), 150 mL wine (10% to 14% alcohol), or 50 mL hard liquor (40% alcohol).
- All women of childbearing age should consume 400 mcg (0.4 mg) of folic acid to prevent neural tube defects in the unborn child.
- All adults aged more than 50 years should take a 10 mcg (400 IU) vitamin D supplement.
- All adults should get between 30 and 60 minutes of moderate physical activity per day. Children and youth should aim for 90 minutes.

Source: Summarized from *Eating Well with Canada's Food Guide*, by Health Canada, 2007, Ottawa: Author.

CLINICAL ALERT

Health Canada (2007c) recommends that Canadians limit their consumption of fresh or frozen tuna, shark, swordfish, marlin, orange roughy, and escolar because of the presence of mercury in these fish. The general population should eat no more than 150 g per week. Pregnant and lactating women should eat only 150 g per *month*. Children aged 5 to 11 should eat only 125 g per month, and children 1 to 4 years should have only 75 g. This restriction does not apply to canned tuna. A serving of fish is 75 g or half a cup (125 mL). Organic mercury compounds, including methyl mercury, are harmful to the nervous system. The developing fetus is particularly at risk as mercury readily crosses the placental barrier. Mercury exposure, depending on the level, can decrease IQ and cause developmental delays. In an adult, high-level exposure can cause neurological impairment, including tremors, memory loss, intellectual impairment, and loss of muscle coordination and sensation (Health Canada, 2006).

Vegetarian Diets

People may become vegetarians for economic, health, religious, ethical, or ecological reasons. Vegetarians generally have lower cholesterol and blood pressure and a reduced occurrence of type 2 diabetes mellitus compared with nonvegetarians (Dietitians of Canada, 2003).

Vegetarian diets come in two basic types: those that use only plant foods and those that include milk, eggs, and dairy products. Some people eat fish and poultry but not beef, lamb, or pork; others eat only fresh fruit, juices, and nuts; and still others eat plant foods and dairy products but not eggs. See Box 39.3 for a summary of the types of vegetarians.

Vegetarian diets can be nutritionally sound if they include a wide variety of foods and if proper protein complementation and vitamin and mineral supplementation are provided, according to the Dietitians of Canada (2003). Because the proteins found in plant foods are incomplete proteins, vegetarians must eat complementary protein foods to obtain all the essential amino acids. A plant protein can be *complemented* by combining it with a different plant protein. The combination produces a complete protein (see Box 39.4). Obtaining complete proteins is especially important for growing children and pregnant and lactating women, whose protein needs are high. Generally, legumes (starchy beans, peas, lentils) have complementary relationships with grains, nuts, and seeds. Complementary foods must be eaten in the same meal. Such diets as the fruitarian diet do not provide sufficient amounts of essential nutrients and are not recommended for long-term use.

BOX 39.3 TYPES OF VEGETARIANS

Type	Description
Vegan	Strict vegetarian; avoids all foods of animal origin
Lacto-ovo vegetarian	Uses dairy products and eggs but avoids eating flesh
Lacto vegetarian	Uses dairy products but avoids eating flesh and eggs
Ovo vegetarian	Uses eggs but avoids dairy products and flesh
Pesco vegetarian	Uses dairy products, eggs, and fish but avoids all meat products
Partial vegetarian (semi-vegetarian)	Avoids selected meats (e.g., red meat)
Fruitarian	Uses only fresh (raw) fruits, juices, nuts, honey, and olive oil
Macrobiotic vegetarian	Progresses through 10 dietary stages from a widely inclusive selection to a restrictive selection

BOX 39.4 COMBINATIONS OF PLANT PROTEINS THAT PROVIDE COMPLETE PROTEINS

Grains plus legumes = complete protein
Legumes plus nuts or seeds = complete protein
Grains, legumes, nuts, or seeds plus milk or milk products (e.g., cheese) = complete protein

Grains	Legumes	Nuts and Seeds
Brown rice	Black beans	Almonds
Barley	Kidney beans	Brazil nuts
Corn meal	Lima beans	Cashews
Millet	Soybeans	Pecans
Oats/oatmeal	Lentils	Walnuts
Rye	Tofu	Pumpkin seeds
Whole wheat	Black-eyed peas	Sesame seeds
	Split peas	Sunflower seeds

Examples: Black-eyed peas and rice
Lentil soup and whole-wheat bread
Beans and tortillas
Lima beans and sesame seeds
Cereal with milk
Macaroni with cheese

Foods of animal origin are the best source of vitamin B_{12}. Therefore, vegans (strict vegetarians) need to obtain this vitamin from other sources: brewer's yeast, foods fortified with vitamin B_{12}, or a vitamin supplement. Because iron from plant sources (nonheme iron) is not absorbed as efficiently as is iron from meat (heme iron), vegans should eat iron-rich foods (e.g., green leafy vegetables, whole grains, raisins, and molasses) and iron-enriched foods. They should eat a food rich in vitamin C at each meal to enhance iron absorption. Calcium deficiency is a concern only for strict vegetarians. It can be prevented by including in the diet leafy green vegetables and soymilk and tofu (soybean curd) fortified with calcium. Thus, teaching clients to read food labels is essential to ensure that they consume foods that provide an adequate intake of vitamins and minerals.

Altered Nutrition

Malnutrition is commonly defined as the lack of necessary or appropriate food substances, but in practice malnutrition includes both undernutrition and overnutrition. In **undernutrition**, the person's caloric intake is less than the daily energy requirements, resulting in weight loss. **Overnutrition** refers to a caloric intake in excess of daily energy requirements, resulting in storage of energy in the form of adipose tissue. As the amount of stored fat increases, the individual becomes overweight or obese. A person is said to be **overweight** when his or her body mass index is between 25 kg/m^2 and 29.9 kg/m^2 and **obese** when the body mass index is more than 30 kg/m^2 (Health Canada, 2003). **Body mass index (BMI)** is a weight to height ratio, with weight (in kilograms) divided by the height (in metres) squared. (See later in the chapter for a discussion of BMI calculation.)

Excess body weight increases the stress on body organs and predisposes people to chronic health problems, such as hypertension and diabetes mellitus. Obesity that interferes with mobility or breathing is referred to as morbid obesity. Obese people may also manifest undernourishment in important nutrients (e.g., essential vitamins or minerals) even though excess calories are ingested.

Adipose tissue located in the visceral area of the abdomen is the most significant in the development of disease conditions. People with visceral fat are more prone to developing metabolic syndrome. In addition, fat located in the abdominal area is highly correlated with obstructive sleep apnea. Men are more likely to develop deposits of visceral fat, especially in midlife. In postmenopausal women, the likelihood of developing abdominal obesity also increases.

Adipose tissue located in the peripheral areas of the body does not place the individual at as high a risk for developing other health problems as does abdominal obesity, but it can lead to problems related to mobility and the development of varicose veins, and it increases the risk of developing osteoarthritis in weight-bearing joints. Peripheral obesity can also contribute to psychological problems associated with a person's attempts to achieve a more perfect body shape because reducing the size of the thighs, upper arms, or hips can be difficult.

Malnutrition occurs when the nutritional reserves are depleted and the nutrients being ingested are insufficient to meet day-to-day demands or the demands placed on the body by added metabolic stress. Malnutrition can occur even though the person is ingesting a large number of calories. For example, a person who primarily eats processed foods high in fats and carbohydrates may have a major deficiency of protein. Improper digestion and absorption of food may lead to malnutrition. An inadequate food intake may be caused by the inability to acquire and prepare food, inadequate knowledge about essential nutrients and a balanced diet, discomfort during or after eating, dysphagia (difficulty swallowing), anorexia (loss of appetite), or nausea or vomiting. Improper digestion and absorption of nutrients can be caused by an inadequate production of hormones or enzymes or by underlying pathological conditions resulting in inflammation or obstruction of the gastrointestinal tract.

A malnourished person may have greater than or less than *ideal body weight.* **Ideal body weight (IBW)** is the weight recommended for optimal health. To determine an individual's IBW, the nurse can quickly calculate an approximate body weight by using the rule of 5 for women and the rule of 6 for men. See Box 39.5. These approximate weights can be increased or decreased by 10% depending on the person's body frame.

Inadequate nutrition can be associated with weight loss, but not always. It is, however, associated with generalized weakness, altered functional ability, delayed wound healing, increased susceptibility to infection, decreased immunocompetence, and impaired pulmonary function. In the case of the hospitalized patient, malnutrition can prolong the length of time spent in the hospital. When a person is experiencing malnutrition, the stored glycogen is mobilized from the muscle and liver stores. These sources can last for only about 24 hours, and then the body fat stores are mobilized in the form of ketones, an alternative fuel to glucose.

Protein-calorie malnutrition, once associated with starvation in the developing countries, is now recognized as a significant problem for clients with long-term deficiencies in caloric intake (e.g., older adults, fad dieters, those with chronic diseases, those who live in institutions). Characteristics of protein-calorie malnutrition are weakness, apathy, increased risk of infection, poor drug tolerance, and poor wound healing.

BOX 39.5 APPROXIMATING IDEAL BODY WEIGHT

Rule of 5 for females:	*Rule of 6 for males:*
45 kg for 1.5 m of height	48 kg for 1.5 m of height
+ 2.3 kg for each 2.5 cm more than 1.5 m	+ 2.8 kg for each 2.5 cm more than 1.5 m
± 10% for body-frame size	± 10% for body-frame size

BOX 39.6 CALCULATING AND INTERPRETING PERCENTAGE OF IDEAL BODY WEIGHT (IBW)

> 120% of IBW	Obese
110%–119% of IBW	Overweight
90%–109% of IBW	IBW
80%–89% of IBW	Mildly underweight
70%–79% of IBW	Moderately underweight
< 69% of IBW	Severely underweight

To calculate an individual's percentage of ideal body weight use this formula:

$$\% \text{ IBW} = \frac{\text{Actual body weight (ABW)}}{\text{Ideal body weight (IBW)}} \times 100$$

Generally accepted standards for interpreting percentage of IBW are shown in Box 39.6.

Assessing

It is important that nurses consider the nutritional status of all the patients or clients in their care. Nutritional states are often overlooked until a major health problem is presented. Nutrition is one area that the nurse can focus on in the promotion of a healthy lifestyle and illness prevention. To assist a patient or client to improve an existing health problem or to achieve an optimal nutritional state, the nurse needs to conduct an assessment of the patient, develop and implement appropriate nursing interventions, and then evaluate the effectiveness of the intervention.

Nutritional Assessment

The purpose of a nutritional assessment is to gather and interpret data to determine the client's nutritional status and to identify problems. Components of a nutritional assessment are shown in Table 39.4 and can be remembered as ABCD data: anthropometric, biochemical, clinical, and dietary. A nutritional assessment is a collaborative endeavour. The nurse can conduct the initial nutritional assessment and, if necessary, additional in-depth screening can be performed by a nutritionist or dietitian and the physician. Nutritional assessment in children is complicated by the fact that children often eat at home, school, and at their friend's homes. Parents may not always be aware of their children's habits. As discussed, the lunch sent to school may not be the lunch the child actually eats. Including the child in the assessment process may increase the reliably of the report.

TABLE 39.4 Components of a Nutritional Assessment

	Screening Data	Additional In-Depth Data
Anthropometric Data	• Height • Weight • Weight change • Usual or ideal body weight • Body mass index	• Waist circumference • Waist-to-hip ratio • Skin-fold thickness (optional)
Biochemical Data	• Hemoglobin, hematocrit • Serum prealbumin, albumin • Total lymphocyte count • Total serum cholesterol • LDL, HDL • Fasting blood glucose	• Serum transferrin level • Urinary urea nitrogen (UUN), blood urea nitrogen (BUN) • Urinary creatinine excretion, serum creatinine • Thyroid stimulating hormone (THS)
Clinical Data	• Skin • Hair and nails • Mucous membranes • Activity level • History of current and past health issues • Drugs: prescribed and over the counter, herbal remedies, or recreational drugs	• Hair analysis • Neurological testing
Dietary Data	• Diet history • 24-hour food recall • Food frequency record • Food preferences • Ability to prepare food • Food allergies or intolerances	• Selective food frequency record • Food diary • Diet history

Nutritional Screening

Nurses carry out nutritional screening during routine nursing histories and physical examinations. Custom screening tools designed for a particular population (e.g., older adults or pregnant women) and specific disorders (e.g., cardiac disease) are available. Screening tools include the patient-generated subjective global assessment (PG-SGA). The PG-SGA is a method of classifying clients as either well nourished, moderately malnourished, or severely malnourished based on a dietary history and physical examination. It was established primarily for use with cancer patients but has been widely tested and is appropriate for both inpatient and outpatient clients with various diagnoses (Green & Watson, 2006). Clients who are found to be at moderate or high risk are followed up with a comprehensive assessment by a dietitian. Box 39.7 provides a summary of risk factors for nutritional problems.

The PG-SGA dietary history consists of five key components:

1. History of weight loss over the preceding 2 weeks and 6 months
2. Current pattern of dietary intake in comparison with the usual pattern
3. Presence of gastrointestinal symptoms that may reduce food intake
4. Functional capacity (ranging from bedridden to fully ambulatory)
5. Primary medical diagnosis and metabolic demands created by the underlying disease

The PG-SGA physical examination emphasizes three features:

1. Loss of subcutaneous fat
2. Muscle wasting
3. Presence of edema and ascites

These physical features are scored as normal (0), mild (1), moderate (2), and severe (3). The PG-SGA is able to provide approximately 80% positive identification of malnutrition when comparing the PG-SGA with traditional assessment methods that included anthropometrics and laboratory tests. Because the PG-SGA is a subjective assessment, the effectiveness of the tool depends largely on the experience of the health-care professional collecting and interpreting the data (Green & Watson, 2006).

Dietary Data

A dietary history includes data about the client's usual eating patterns and habits; allergies and food intolerances; frequency, types, and quantities of foods consumed; and social, economic, ethnic, or religious factors influencing nutrition. Specific factors to consider include, but are not limited to, living and eating alone, ability to purchase foods and prepare a meal, and the availability of refrigeration and cooking facilities.

Other information that is important addresses the client's appetite and hunger. These are two different aspects of eating and should not be considered the same.

BOX 39.7 SUMMARY OF RISK FACTORS FOR NUTRITIONAL PROBLEMS

Some factors can put clients at risk for nutritional problems:

DIET HISTORY

- Chewing or swallowing difficulties (because of ill-fitting dentures, dental caries, missing teeth, or cranial nerve deficits)
- Inadequate food intake
- Restricted or fad diets
- No nutrient intake for 10 or more days
- Intravenous fluids (other than total parenteral nutrition for 10 or more days)
- Inadequate food budget
- Inadequate food-preparation facilities
- Inadequate food-storage facilities
- Physical disabilities
- Living and eating alone

MEDICAL HISTORY

- Unintentional weight loss or gain of 10% within 6 months
- Fluid and electrolyte imbalance
- Oral and gastrointestinal surgery
- Dental problems: difficulty chewing, ill-fitting dentures
- Gastrointestinal problems: anorexia, dysphagia, nausea, vomiting, diarrhea, constipation
- Chronic illness: end-stage renal disease, liver disease, human immunodeficiency virus (HIV) infection, chronic obstructive pulmonary disease (COPD), cancer
- Alcohol or problematic substance use
- Neurological or cognitive impairment
- Psychiatric conditions: depression, anorexia nervosa, and bulimia nervosa
- Catabolic or hypermetabolic condition: burns, trauma
- Adolescent pregnancy or closely spaced pregnancies

MEDICATION HISTORY*

- Aspirin
- Antacid
- Antidepressants
- Antihypertensives
- Anti-inflammatory agents
- Antineoplastic agents
- Digitalis
- Laxatives
- Diuretics (thiazides)
- Hypoglycemic agents
- Glucocorticosteroids
- Potassium chloride

*The potential effects of some medications on nutrition are shown in Table 39.2.

A client may claim to have a good appetite and yet ingest very little food. Others may say they are never hungry, and yet they are observed to be eating frequently. For these reasons, keeping a food diary with associated mood states may help the person realize how much, in fact, is being consumed and why. It is important to know whether the client has eating binges. Does the client eat frequently in restaurants? What does the client know and understand about healthy nutrition and *Eating Well with Canada's Food Guide*?

Four possible methods for collecting dietary data are a 24-hour food recall, a food-frequency record, a food diary, and a diet history.

For a **24-hour food recall**, the nurse asks the client to recall all the food and beverages the client consumes during a typical 24-hour period. The data obtained is then generally evaluated according to *Canada's Food Guide* to judge overall adequacy.

A **food-frequency record** is a checklist that indicates how often general food groups or specific foods are eaten. Frequency may be categorized as times/day, times/week, times/month, or frequently, seldom, never. This record, like the 24-hour food recall, provides information about the types of foods eaten but not the quantities. When specific foods or nutrients are suspected of being deficient or excessive, the health-care professional may use a selective food-frequency record that focuses, for example, on fat, fruit, vegetable, and fibre intake.

A **food diary** is a detailed record of measured amounts (portion sizes) of all food and fluids a client consumes during a specified time, usually 3 to 7 days.

A **diet history** is a comprehensive, time-consuming assessment of a client's food intake that involves an extensive interview by a nutritionist or dietitian. It includes characteristics of foods usually eaten, as well as the frequency and amount of food consumed. Thus, it may include a 24-hour recall, a food-frequency record, and a food diary. Medical and psychosocial factors are also assessed to evaluate their impact on nutritional requirements, food habits, and choices. Data obtained are analyzed by computer and translated into caloric and nutrient intake. Results are compared with the recommended dietary allowances that are appropriate for the client's age, gender, and condition.

Health History

Information about the client's current health status and past health status needs to be obtained. This information should include medications, both prescribed and over-the-counter drugs (e.g., vitamins, herbal preparations) that the client is taking. The use and frequency of use of recreational drugs also need to be addressed. This may be the best time to find out what the client knows about the interactions between food and the drugs being taken. Information about the client's family history needs to be collected. Is there a history of heart disease, obesity, eating disorders, diabetes, and so on? Does the client exercise on a regular basis? Does the client use tobacco? If so, how much, how often, and for how long? Does the client consume alcohol? If so, how much, and how often? Does the client have any disabilities that may limit the ability to prepare food or eat? For example, if a person has advancing multiple sclerosis, he or she may have an intention tremor that causes the hands to shake so much that it is difficult to cook or use a regular fork or spoon. Does the client have difficulty swallowing? Does the client have a problem with choking or aspiration of food when eating?

Some of the health history information may have to be obtained from family members if the client has a cognitive impairment or speech disability. Also, some of this information may be obtained from other health professionals' histories if the nurse has access to such documentation.

Physical Examination

Physical examination reveals nutritional deficiencies and excesses in addition to obvious weight changes. Assessment focuses on rapidly proliferating tissues, such as skin, hair, nails, eyes, and mucosa, but also includes a systematic review comparable with any routine physical examination. See Box 39.8. The signs of malnutrition must be viewed as *suggestive* of malnutrition because the signs are nonspecific. For example, a red conjunctiva may indicate an infection, rather than a nutritional deficit, and dry, dull hair may be related to excessive exposure to the sun rather than kwashiorkor (severe protein depletion). To confirm malnutrition, clinical findings need to be substantiated with laboratory tests and dietary data.

BOX 39.8 CLINICAL SIGNS OF MALNUTRITION

Area of Examination	Signs Associated with Malnutrition
General appearance and vitality	Apathetic, listless, looks tired, easily fatigued
Weight	Overweight or underweight
Skin	Dry, flaky, or scaly; pale or pigmented; presence of petechiae or bruises; lack of subcutaneous fat
Nails	Brittle, pale, ridged, or spoon-shaped (iron)
Hair	Dry, dull, sparse, loss of colour, brittle (see Figure 39.6A)
Eyes	Pale or red conjunctiva, xerophthalmia (dryness), keratomalacia (soft cornea), dull cornea, night blindness (vitamin A deficiency)
Lips	Swollen, angular stomatitis (red cracks at side of mouth), cheilosis (vertical fissures caused by vitamin B deficiency) (see Figure 39.6B)
Tongue	Swollen; beefy red or magenta coloured (vitamin B deficiency); smooth appearance (vitamin B deficiency); decrease or increase in size (see Figure 39.6C)
Gums	Spongy, swollen, inflamed; bleed easily (vitamin C deficiency) (see Figure 39.6D)
Muscles	Underdeveloped, flaccid, wasted, soft
Gastrointestinal system	Anorexia, indigestion, diarrhea, constipation, enlarged liver, protruding abdomen
Nervous system	Decreased reflexes, sensory loss, paresthesias (burning and tingling of hands and feet caused by vitamin B deficiency), mental confusion or irritability

Anthropometric Measurements

Anthropometric measurements are noninvasive techniques that aim to quantify changes in body composition. The client's height and weight should be obtained. Self-reported data are often inaccurate, so accurate equipment and standardized procedures must be used to ensure accurate and precise readings. A beam-balance scale can be used to obtain weight and to measure the person's height. The person should not be wearing shoes and should have on only light clothing when stepping onto the scale. The client should be able to stand on the scale without any support, and should have voided before being weighed. If the patient is bedridden or unable to stand independently, a metabolic scale can be used, if available. A person should be weighed at the same time each day if repeated weight recordings are required. Bathroom scales are not always accurate, so they should only be used to obtain an approximation of the person's weight. The weight obtained should be compared with the client's usual and ideal body weights to determine weight change. Refer to Box 39.9.

CALCULATING PERCENTAGE OF WEIGHT GAIN OR LOSS Accurate assessment of the client's height, current body weight (CBW), and **usual body weight** (UBW) is essential. Although the client's CBW can be compared with an IBW discussed earlier, the IBW is based on healthy people and does not account for changes in the client's body composition that accompany illness or reflect any changes in weight. The client's UBW better

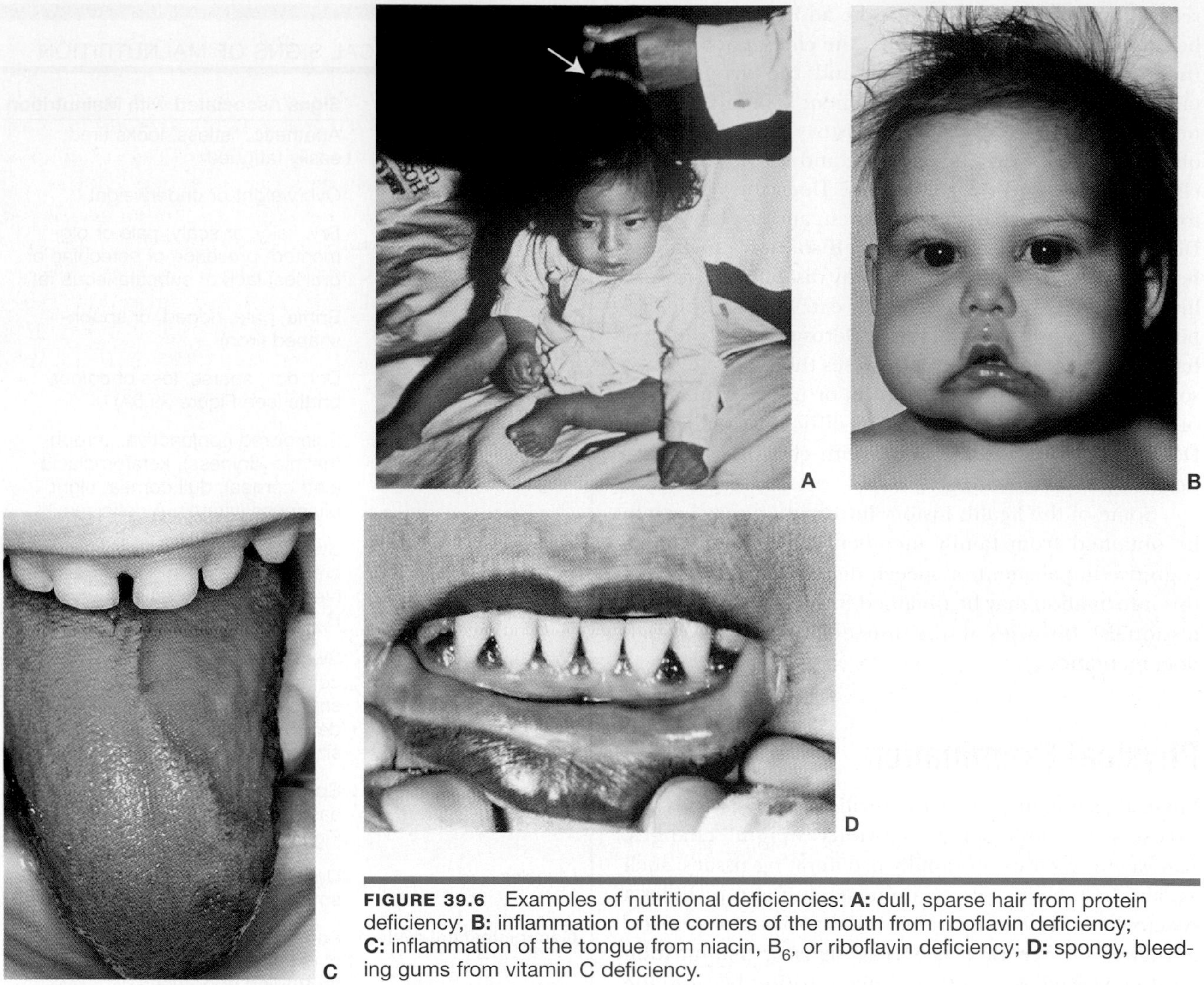

FIGURE 39.6 Examples of nutritional deficiencies: **A:** dull, sparse hair from protein deficiency; **B:** inflammation of the corners of the mouth from riboflavin deficiency; **C:** inflammation of the tongue from niacin, B_6, or riboflavin deficiency; **D:** spongy, bleeding gums from vitamin C deficiency.

BOX 39.9 CALCULATING AND INTERPRETING THE PERCENTAGE OF DEVIATION FROM USUAL BODY WEIGHT AND THE PERCENTAGE OF WEIGHT LOSS

Calculating Percentage of Usual Body Weight

$$\%\ \text{usual body weight} = \frac{\text{Current weight}}{\text{Usual body weight}} \times 100$$

Mild malnutrition	85%–90%
Moderate malnutrition	75%–84%
Severe malnutrition	less than 74%

Calculating Percentage of Weight Loss

$$\%\ \text{weight loss} = \frac{\text{Usual body weight} - \text{Current weight}}{\text{Usual weight}} \times 100$$

Significant weight loss	Severe weight loss
5% over 1 month	> 5% over 1 month
7.5% over 3 months	> 7.5% over 3 months
10% over 6 months	> 10% over 6 months

reflects weight change and the possibility of malnutrition. Calculation and interpretation of the percentage of deviation from UBW and the percentage of weight loss are shown in Box 39.9. An important aspect of weight assessment, obtained in the nursing history, is a description of **weight change**. The nurse should describe any weight loss or gain, the duration of the change, and whether the weight change was intentional or unintentional.

Increasingly, BMI is being used as an indicator of body composition. The BMI is an indicator of overall adiposity or obesity and can be used to determine whether an individual is at risk for developing serious health problems. A BMI, however, must be used with caution for certain individuals—for example, those who have a large lean body mass or who have ascites (peritoneal cavity fluid)—because their weight may not be attributable to adipose tissue. To calculate BMI, refer to the following steps or to the nomogram in Table 39.5.

1. Measure the person's height in metres (e.g., 1.5 m).
2. Measure the weight in kilograms (e.g., 60 kg).

3. Calculate the BMI by using the following formula:

$$\% \text{ BMI} = \frac{\text{Weight in kilograms}}{(\text{Height in metres})^2}$$

or

$$\frac{60 \text{ kg}}{(1.5 \text{ m})^2} = 26.6 \text{ kg/m}^2$$

Other important measures to obtain when determining degree of adiposity and location of adipose tissue are the **waist circumference** (WC) and the **hip circumference** (HC). The ratio of the waist circumference to the hip circumference is called the **waist-to-hip ratio** (WHR). These two measures can be used to ascertain where the adipose tissue is located. As discussed earlier in this chapter, adipose tissue located in the visceral area of the abdomen places the individual at risk for the development of metabolic syndrome and its comorbidities. To obtain a WC, have clients remove belts or tight-fitting clothing around the midsection of the body. Have them stand erect and breathe normally. Place the tape measure around the largest circumference of the waist area over the umbilicus (see Figure 39.7). An accurate assessment of this circumference can be a challenge when determining the WC in an individual with a very large abdominal pannus (skin fat fold). Table 39.6 summarizes risk categories associated with BMI and WC.

TABLE 39.5 Body Mass Index Nomogram

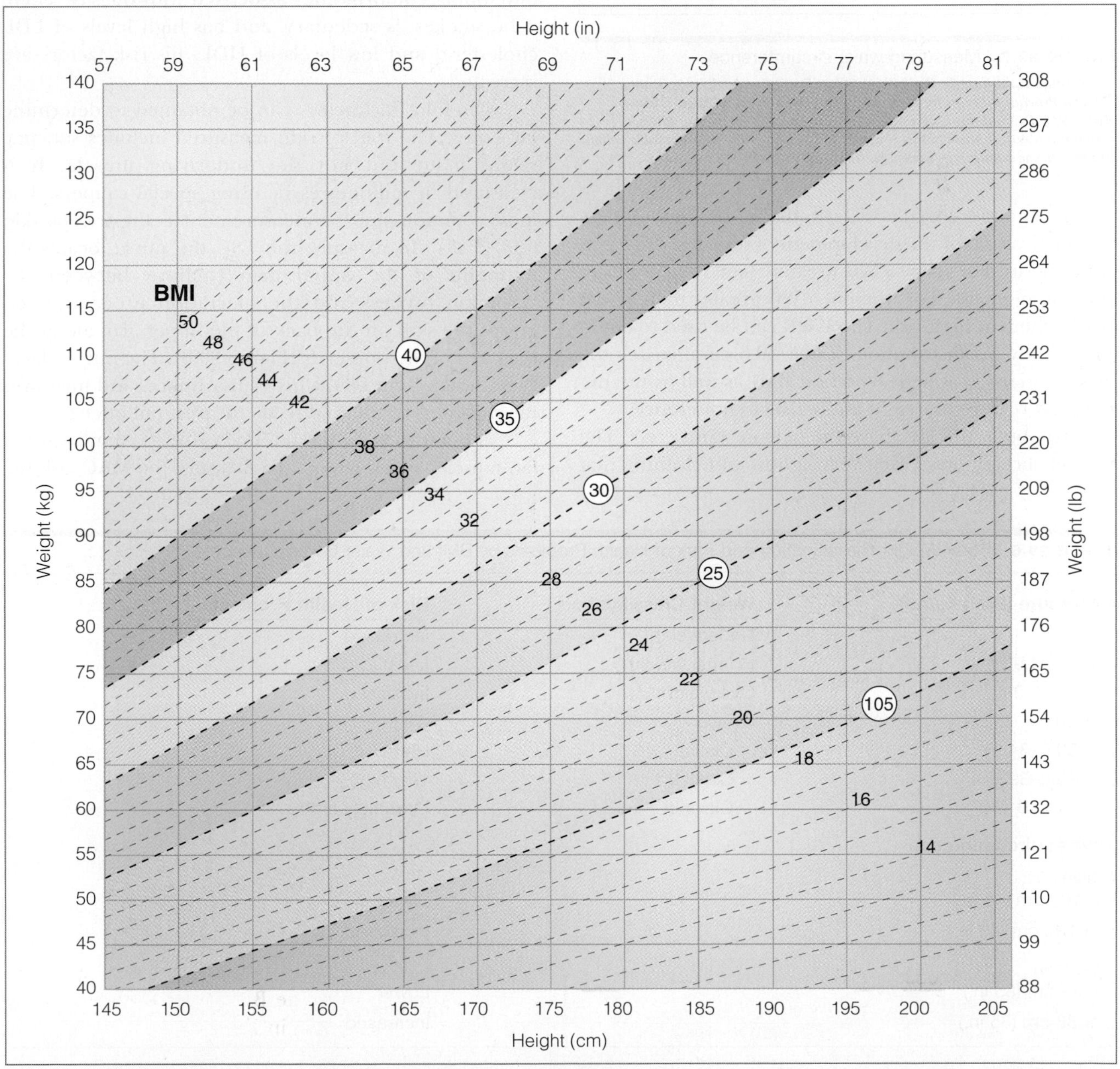

Source: *Body Mass Index (BMI) Nomogram,* by Health Canada, 2003, Ottawa: Author. Available online at http://www.hc-sc.gc.ca/fn-an/nutrition/weights-poids/guide-ld-adult/bmi_chart_java-graph_imc_java_e.html. Reproduced with the permission of the Minister of Public Works and Government Services Canada, 2003.

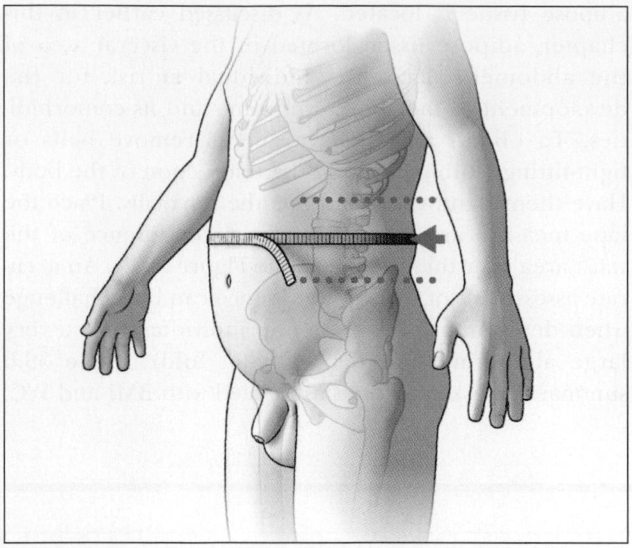

FIGURE 39.7 Measuring waist circumference

("Canadian Guidelines for Body Weight Classification in Adults: Application in Clinical Practice to Screen for Overweight and Obesity and to Assess Disease Risk," by J. D. Douketis, G. Paradis, H. Keller, and C. Martineau, 2005, **Canadian Medical Association Journal,** *172(8), pp. 995–998. Available online at http://www.cmaj.ca/cgi/content/full/172/8/995/F219)*

The gender-specific WC cutoffs can be used to identify relative risk for the development of diseases associated with obesity. For men, a WC greater than 102 cm places them at high risk. For women, a WC greater than 88 cm places them at high risk. The WHR can be used to determine body fat distribution. Table 39.6 summarizes the classifications of weight based on BMI as well as the disease risk relative to weight and waist circumference.

To obtain the HC, have the person stand erect. The person should be wearing very lightweight clothing that is not bulky around the hip area. The HC is taken around the largest part of the buttocks. If you have the client place the thumb on the top of the iliac crest and extend the hand open so that the small finger is reaching toward the hip joint, the tip of the small finger can be used to determine where to place the measuring tape. A WHR greater than 1 is indicative that a man has visceral fat accumulations. For a woman, a WHR greater than 0.8 is indicative of the presence of visceral fat deposits.

When interpreting the results of the BMI, WC, and WHR, the nurse must consider the relationship of these measures to one another. For example, a male client may have a BMI of 26, a WC of 103 cm, and a WHR of 1.2. The BMI would indicate that he is only slightly overweight, but his WC and WHR indicate that his fat is located in the visceral region, which places him at risk for developing comorbidities associated with obesity. Then, if he smokes, is sedentary, and has high levels of LDL cholesterol and low levels of HDL, his risk factors are increased.

Skin-fold thicknesses can be obtained to determine fat stores. The fold of skin measured includes subcutaneous tissue but not the underlying muscle. It is measured in millimetres by using special calipers. The most common site for measurement is the triceps skin fold (TSF). To measure the TSF, the nurse locates the midpoint of the upper arm (halfway between the acromion process and the olecranon process), then grasps the skin on the back of the upper arm along the long axis of the humerus (Figure 39.8). The nurse places the calipers 1 cm below his or her fingers and measures the thickness of the fold to the nearest millimetre.

The mid-arm circumference (MAC) is a measure of fat, muscle, and skeleton. To measure the MAC, ask the

TABLE 39.6 Body Weight Classification and Risk of Health Problems by BMI and Waist Circumference

Measure (BMI, kg/m^2)	Weight Classification	Risk of Health Problems
< 18.5	Underweight	Increased
18.5–24.9	Normal weight	Least
25.0–29.9	Overweight	Increased
≥ 30.0	Obese:	
30.0–34.9	Class I	High
35.0–39.9	Class II	Very high
≥ 40.0	Class III	Extremely high
Waist circumference		
Men		
< 102 cm (40 in.)		Lower
≥ 102 cm (40 in.)		Increased
Women		
< 88 cm (35 in.)		Lower
≥ 88 cm (35 in.)		Increased

Source: "Canadian Guidelines for Body Weight Classification in Adults: Application in Clinical Practice to Screen for Overweight and Obesity and to Assess Disease Risk," by J. D. Douketis, G. Paradis, H. Keller, and C. Martineau, 2005, *Canadian Medical Association Journal, 172*(8), pp. 995–998. Reprinted with permission of the publisher.

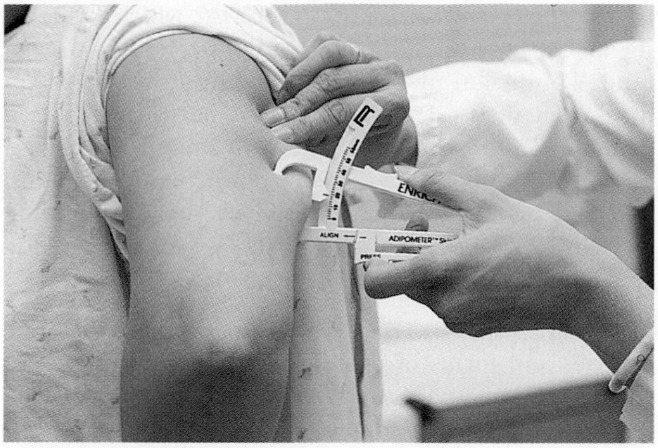

FIGURE 39.8 Measuring the triceps skin fold

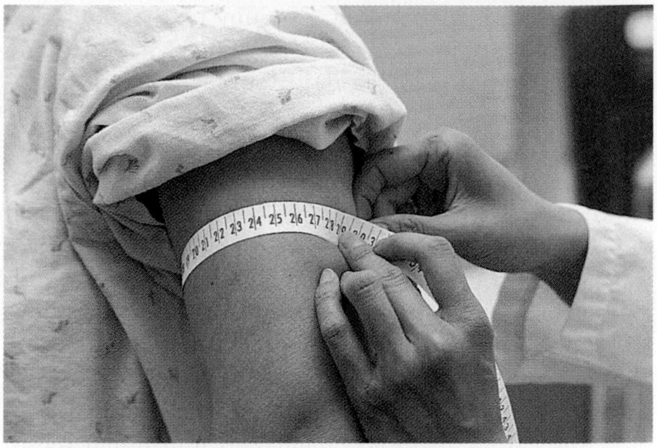

FIGURE 39.9 Measuring mid-upper-arm circumference

client to sit or stand with the arm hanging freely and the forearm flexed to horizontal. Measure the circumference at the midpoint of the arm, recording the measurement in centimetres, to the nearest millimetre (e.g., 24.6 cm) (Figure 39.9).

The mid-arm muscle circumference (MAMC) is then calculated by using reference tables or by using a formula that incorporates the TSF and the MAC. The MAMC is an estimate of lean body mass, or skeletal muscle reserves. If tables are not available, the nurse uses the following formula to calculate the MAMC from the triceps skin fold and MAC direct measurements:

$$\text{MAMC cm} = \text{MAC (cm)} - \frac{3.143 \text{ TSF (mm)}}{10}$$

Standard values for anthropometric measurements for adults are shown in Table 39.7.

Changes in anthropometric measurements often occur slowly and reflect chronic, rather than acute, changes in nutritional status. They are, therefore, used to monitor the client's progress over months to years, rather than days to weeks. Ideally, initial and subsequent measurements need to be taken by the same clinician. In addition, measurements obtained need to be interpreted with caution. Fluctuations in hydration status that often occur during illness can influence the accuracy of results. In addition, normal standards often do not account for normal changes in body composition, such as those that occur with aging.

Laboratory Tests

Laboratory tests provide objective data to the nutritional assessments, but because many factors can influence these tests, no single test specifically predicts nutritional risk or measures the presence or degree of a nutritional problem. The tests most commonly used are serum proteins (hemoglobin, albumin, prealbumin, transferrin), total lymphocyte count, total serum cholesterol, LDL, HDL, fasting blood glucose, thyroid stimulating hormone, and urinary urea nitrogen and creatinine.

BLOOD TESTS

SERUM PROTEINS *Serum protein* levels, as mentioned earlier, provide an estimate of visceral protein stores. Tests commonly include hemoglobin, albumin, transferrin, and total iron-binding capacity. A low *hemoglobin* level may be evidence of iron-deficiency anemia. However, abnormal blood loss or a pathological process, such as gastrointestinal cancer, must be ruled out before iron deficiency related to diet is confirmed.

Edema may be present if the client is experiencing malnutrition. When the serum protein is low, edema results because of the loss of colloidal osmotic pressure required to maintain the normal shift of fluid between the capillaries and the surrounding interstitial spaces. The edema may be present around the ankles or hands because of gravitational forces on the extremities, or it may affect the heart and lung actions in severe conditions.

Albumin, which accounts for more than 50% of the total serum proteins, is one of the most common visceral proteins evaluated as part of the nutritional assessment.

TABLE 39.7 Standard Values for Anthropometric Measurements for Adults

Measurement	Male	Female
Triceps skin fold (mm)	12	20
Mid-arm circumference (cm)	32	28
Mid-arm muscle circumference (cm)	54	30

Source: From *The Merck Manual of Diagnosis and Therapy*, 18th ed., by M. H. Beers and R. Berkow (Eds.), 2006. Copyright John Wiley & Sons. Reprinted with permission.

Because there is so much albumin in the body and because it is not broken down very quickly (i.e., it has a long half-life [18–20 days]), albumin concentrations change slowly. Thus, a low serum albumin level is a useful indicator of prolonged protein depletion rather than acute or short-term changes in nutritional status. However, many conditions besides malnutrition can depress albumin concentration, such as altered liver function, hydration status, and losses from open wounds and burns.

Prealbumin, also referred to as thyroxine-binding albumin and transthyretin, has the shortest half-life and smallest body pool, and is, therefore, the serum protein most responsive to rapid changes in nutritional status. Unfortunately, this assessment is very expensive. It may, however, be performed when initiating total parenteral nutrition for clients in their homes.

Transferrin is a protein that binds and carries iron from the intestine through the serum. Because it has a shorter half-life than albumin (8 to 9 days), transferrin is likely to respond more quickly to protein depletion than albumin. Serum transferrin can be measured directly or by a *total iron-binding capacity (TIBC) test,* which indicates the amount of iron in the blood to which transferrin can bind. Conversion of the TIBC reading to a transferrin measurement is calculated by a standard mathematical formula. Transferrin levels below normal indicate protein loss, iron-deficiency anemia, pregnancy, hepatitis, and liver dysfunction. An increase in total iron-binding capacity can indicate iron deficiency; a decrease can indicate anemia.

TOTAL LYMPHOCYTE COUNT Certain nutrient deficiencies and forms of protein-calorie malnutrition can depress the immune system. The total number of lymphocytes decreases as protein depletion occurs.

CHOLESTEROL TESTS Total serum cholesterol is a measure of all cholesterol (HDL, LDL, very-low density lipoprotein). It does not separate the HDL and the LDL, so they must be measured separately. High levels of total cholesterol are indicative of being at risk for cardiovascular disease. The levels of LDL and HDL more accurately reflect the risk factor for cardiovascular disease.

SKILL 39.1

OBTAINING A CAPILLARY BLOOD SPECIMEN TO MEASURE BLOOD GLUCOSE

PURPOSES

- To determine or monitor blood glucose levels of clients at risk for hyperglycemia or hypoglycemia
- To promote blood glucose regulation by the client
- To evaluate the effectiveness of insulin or oral hypoglycemic medication administration in the case of diabetes mellitus treatment

ASSESSMENT

- Before obtaining a capillary blood specimen, determine
  - The frequency and type of testing
  - The client's understanding of the procedure
  - The client's response to previous testing
- Assess the client's skin at the puncture site to determine that it is intact and the circulation is not compromised. Check colour, warmth, and capillary refill.
- Review the client's record for medications that may prolong bleeding, such as anticoagulants.
- Assess the client's self-care abilities that may affect accuracy of test results, such as visual impairment and finger dexterity.

Equipment

- Blood glucose meter (glucometer)
- Blood glucose reagent strip compatible with the meter
- 10 cm × 10 cm gauze
- Warm cloth or other warming device (optional)
- Antiseptic swab
- Disposable gloves
- Sterile lancet
- Lancet injector

IMPLEMENTATION

Preparation

Review the type of meter and manufacturer's instructions. Assemble the equipment at the bedside.

Performance

1. Before performing the procedure, introduce yourself and verify the client's identity by using agency protocol. Explain to the client what you are going to do, why it is necessary, and how he or she can cooperate. Discuss how the results will be used in planning further care or treatments.
2. Perform hand hygiene and observe other appropriate infection prevention and control procedures (e.g., gloves).
3. Provide for client privacy.
4. Prepare the equipment.
   - Calibrate the meter and run a control sample according to the manufacturer's instructions.
5. Select and prepare the vascular puncture site.
   - Choose a vascular puncture site (e.g., the side of an adult's finger). Avoid sites beside bone. Wrap the finger first in a warm cloth, *or* hold a finger in a dependent position. If the earlobe is used, rub it gently with a

(continued)

SKILL 39.1

OBTAINING A CAPILLARY BLOOD SPECIMEN TO MEASURE BLOOD GLUCOSE *(continued)*

small piece of gauze. **Rationale: These actions increase the blood flow to the area, ensure an adequate specimen, and reduce the need for a repeat puncture.**

- Clean the site with the antiseptic swab or soap and water and allow it to dry completely. **Rationale: Alcohol can affect accuracy and the site burns when punctured when wet with alcohol.**

6. Obtain the blood specimen.
   - Put on gloves.
   - Place the injector, if used, against the site, and release the needle, thus permitting it to pierce the skin. Make sure the lancet is perpendicular to the site (see ❶). **Rationale: The lancet is designed to pierce the skin at a specific depth when it is in a perpendicular position relative to the skin.**
   - *Or* prick the site with a lancet or needle by using a darting motion.
   - Gently squeeze (but do not touch) the puncture site until a large drop of blood forms. The size of the drop of blood can vary depending on the meter. Some meters require as little as 0.3 mL or not much larger than the period at the end of this sentence.
   - Hold the reagent strip under the puncture site until adequate blood covers the indicator square. The pad will absorb the blood and a chemical reaction will occur. Do not smear the blood (see ❷). **Rationale: This will cause an inaccurate reading.** Some meters wick the blood by just touching the puncture site with the edge of the strip.
   - Ask the client to apply pressure to the skin puncture site with gauze. **Rationale: Pressure will assist hemostasis.**
7. Expose the blood to the test strip for the period and the manner specified by the manufacturer. As soon as the blood is placed on the test strip:
   - Follow the manufacturer's recommendations on the glucose meter and monitor for the amount of time indicated by the manufacturer. **Rationale: The blood must remain in contact with the test pad for a prescribed time to obtain accurate results.** Some glucometers have the test strip placed in the machine before the specimen is obtained.
8. Measure the blood glucose.
   - Place the strip into the meter according to the manufacturer's instructions. Some devices require that the strip be wiped or blotted after a designated time before being inserted in the meter. Other strips do not require blotting or wiping. Refer to the manufacturer's recommendations for the specific procedure.
   - After the designated time, most glucose meters will display the glucose reading automatically. Correct timing ensures accurate results (see ❸).

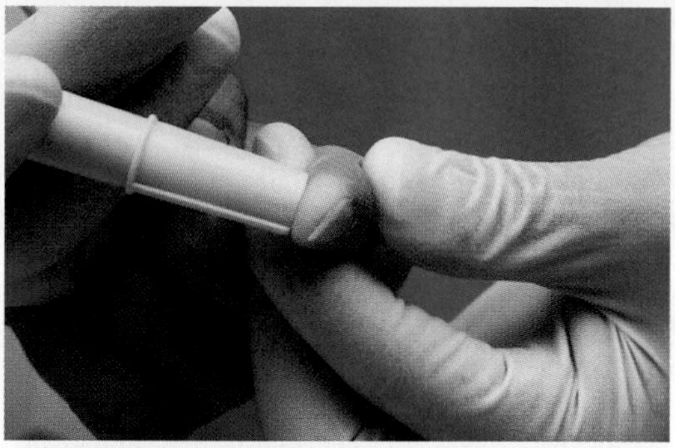

❶ Place the injector against the site.

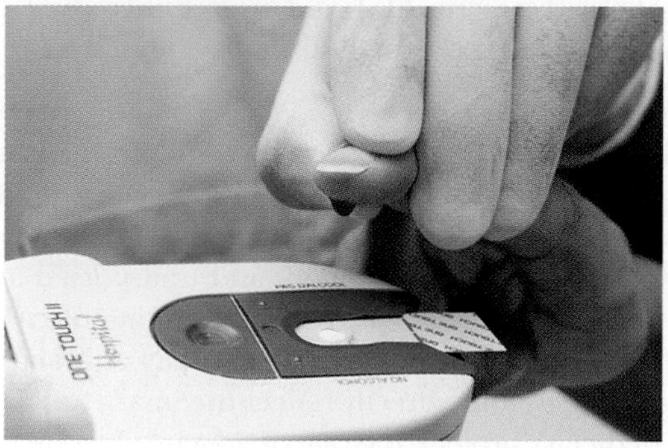

❷ Gently squeeze a drop of blood onto the reagent strip.

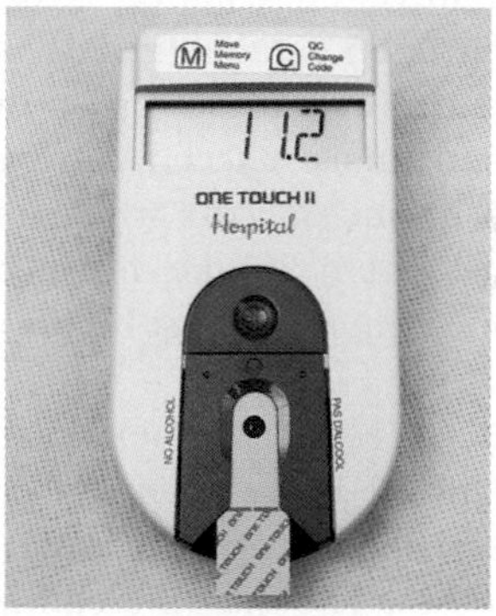

❸ The glucose meter will display the glucose reading.

   - Turn off the meter and discard the test strip and gauze in a biohazard container. Discard the lancet into a sharps container.

9. Document the method of testing and results on the client's record. If appropriate, record the client's understanding and ability to demonstrate the technique. The client's record may also include a flowsheet on which capillary blood glucose results and the amount, type, route, and time of insulin or hypoglycemic medication administration are recorded.

EVALUATION

- Compare glucose meter reading with normal blood glucose level, status of puncture site, and motivation of the client to perform the test independently.
- Report abnormal results to the appropriate member of the health-care team.

GLUCOSE TESTS Fasting blood glucose level is conducted to assess for type 2 diabetes mellitus and for hyperglycemic hyperosmolar nonketotic syndrome, a condition that develops mostly in older adults and people receiving total parenteral nutrition or peritoneal dialysis. Fasting blood glucose also is used to monitor glucose control in people with type 1 and type 2 diabetes as well. An elevated blood glucose level is an indicator of excess glucose in the blood. Skill 39.1 outlines how to obtain a capillary blood specimen to measure blood glucose by using a portable meter.

THYROID FUNCTION Assessing the function of a client's thyroid is important to determining whether his or her BMR is being regulated normally. If a client's thyroid stimulating hormone (TSH) levels are elevated, it is indicative that the thyroid is not producing adequate amounts of thyroxine (T_4) and tri-iodothyronine (T_3), and hence the rate of metabolism may be slowed.

URINARY TESTS *Urinary urea nitrogen* and *urinary creatinine* are measures of protein catabolism and the state of nitrogen balance. **Urea**, the chief end product of amino acid metabolism, is formed from ammonia detoxified by the liver, circulated in the blood, and transported to the kidneys for excretion. Urea concentrations in urine (UUG or urinary urea nitrogen) and blood (BUN or blood urea nitrogen), therefore, directly reflect the intake and breakdown of dietary protein, the rate of urea production in the liver, and the rate of urea removal by the kidneys.

The state of nitrogen balance is determined by comparing the nitrogen intake (grams of protein) to the nitrogen output over 24 hours. A positive nitrogen balance exists when intake exceeds nitrogen output; a negative nitrogen balance occurs when output exceeds nitrogen intake. Protein intake must be accurately recorded and kidney function must be normal to ensure the validity of a UUN.

Urinary creatinine reflects a person's total muscle mass because creatinine is the chief end product of the creatine produced when energy is released during skeletal muscle metabolism. The rate of creatinine formation is directly proportional to the total muscle mass. Creatinine is removed from the bloodstream by the kidneys and excreted in the urine at a rate that closely parallels its formation. The greater the muscle mass, the greater is the excretion of creatinine. As skeletal muscle atrophies during malnutrition, creatinine excretion decreases. Standards for creatinine excretion are developed on the basis of gender and height. Urinary creatinine is also influenced by protein intake, exercise, age, renal function, and thyroid function.

Diagnosing

NANDA International (2007) includes the following diagnostic labels for nutritional problems:

- *Imbalanced Nutrition: More Than Body Requirements*
- *Imbalanced Nutrition: Less Than Body Requirements*
- *Readiness for Enhanced Nutrition*
- *Risk for Imbalanced Nutrition: More Than Body Requirements*

Many other NANDA International (2007) nursing diagnoses may apply to certain individuals, because nutritional problems often affect other areas of human functioning. In this case, the nutritional diagnostic label may be used as the etiology of other diagnoses. Examples include the following:

- *Activity Intolerance* related to inadequate intake of iron-rich foods resulting in iron-deficiency anemia
- *Constipation* related to inadequate fluid intake and fibre intake
- *Low Self-Esteem* related to obesity
- *Risk for Infection* related to immunosuppression secondary to insufficient protein intake

Planning

Major goals for clients with or at risk for nutritional problems include the following:

- Maintain or restore optimal nutritional status
- Promote healthy nutritional practices
- Prevent complications associated with malnutrition
- Decrease weight
- Regain specified weight

Examples of desired outcomes related to some of these goals, although established in the planning phase, are provided in the Evaluating section of this chapter.

Examples of Nursing Intervention Classifications (NIC) interventions to enhance an individual's nutrition include the following:

- Nutritional counselling
- Nutrition management
- Nutritional monitoring
- Nutrition therapy
- Weight management
- Weight reduction assistance
- Weight gain assistance
- Energy management
- Exercise promotion
- Behaviour modification
- Enteral tube feeding
- Total parenteral nutrition (TPN) administration

Specific nursing activities associated with each of these interventions can be selected to meet the individual needs of the client. A Sample Care Plan that uses NIC interventions and selected activities is provided.

Sample Care Plan for Nutrition

ASSESSMENT DATA

Nursing Assessment

Mrs. Rose Santini, a 59-year-old homemaker from New Brunswick, attends a community hospital-sponsored health fair. She approaches the nutrition information booth, and the clinical specialist in nutritional support gathers a nutritional history. Mrs. Santini is very upset about her 9 kg weight gain. She relates to the nurse clinician that since the death of her husband 6 months ago, she has lost interest in many of her usual physical and social activities. She no longer attends exercise and swimming sessions and has lost contact with her couples' bridge group. Mrs. Santini states she is bored, depressed, and very unhappy about her appearance. She has a small frame and has always prided herself on her petite figure. She says her eating habits have changed considerably. She snacks while watching TV and rarely prepares a complete meal.

Physical Examination

Height: 162.6 cm

Weight: 63.6 kg

Temperature: 37°C

Pulse: 76 bpm

Respirations: 16/minute

Blood pressure: 144/84 mm Hg

Diagnostic Data

CBC normal, urinalysis normal, chest X-ray negative, thyroid profile within normal limits

Nursing Diagnosis

Imbalanced Nutrition: More than body requirements related to excess intake and decreased activity expenditure (as evidenced by weight gain of 9 kg, undesirable eating patterns).

Client Goals

The client will (1) change undesirable behaviours that contribute to weight gain, and (2) reach her ideal body weight for her height and frame.

Desired Health Outcomes

1. Plans three menus each day that result in a 500-calorie reduction in intake
2. Develops a physical exercise plan that engages her in 15 to 20 minutes of exercise each day
3. Identifies eating habits that contribute to weight gain by day 2

NURSING INTERVENTIONS AND SELECTED ACTIVITIES WITH RATIONALES* *[IN ITALICS]*

Weight-Reduction Assistance

- Determine current eating patterns by having Mrs. Santini keep a diary of what, when, and where she eats. *A diary increases the client's awareness of activities and foods that contribute to excessive intake.*
- Set a weekly goal for weight loss. *The desirable weight loss rate is 0.5 kg to 0.9 kg per week.*
- Encourage use of internal reward systems when goals are accomplished. *Goal setting provides motivation, which is essential for a successful weight-loss program.*
- Set a realistic plan with Mrs. Santini to include reduced food intake and increased energy expenditure. *A combined plan of calorie reduction and exercise can enhance weight loss since exercise increases caloric utilization.*
- Assist client to identify motivation for eating and internal and external cues associated with eating. *Awareness of factors that contribute to overeating will assist the individual in planning behaviour modification techniques to avoid situations that prompt excess food consumption.*
- Develop a daily meal plan with a well-balanced diet, reduced calories, and reduced fat. *Overweight people are often nutritionally deprived. Intake must be reduced by 500 calories per day to obtain a 0.5 kg per week weight loss.*
- Encourage attendance at support groups for weight loss or refer to a community weight control program. *Support groups can provide companionship, increase motivation, and offer practical solutions to problems associated with dieting.*

Nutritional Counselling

- Facilitate identification of eating behaviours to be changed. *This recognition increases the individual's awareness of those actions that contribute to excessive intake.*
- Use accepted nutritional standards to assist Mrs. Santini in evaluating adequacy of dietary intake. *Comparing the individual's dietary history with nutritional standards will facilitate identification of nutritional deficiencies and excesses.*
- Help Mrs. Santini to consider factors of age, past eating experiences, culture, and finances in planning ways to meet nutritional requirements. *Social, economic, physical, and psychological factors play a role in nutrition and malnutrition.*
- Discuss Mrs. Santini's knowledge of *Canada's Food Guide*, portion size, and perceptions of the needed diet modification. *This discussion helps determine the patient's knowledge base and identify misbeliefs or gaps in understanding.*

(continued)

Sample Care Plan for Nutrition *(continued)*

Nutritional Counselling *(continued)*

• Discuss food likes and dislikes.	*Incorporating Mrs. Santini's food preferences into the dietary plan will promote adherence to the weight-loss program.*
• Assist Mrs. Santini in stating her feelings and concerns about goal achievement.	*Fear of success, failure, or other concerns can block goal achievement.*
Behaviour Modification	
• Assist Mrs. Santini to identify strengths and reinforce these.	*Reinforcing strengths enhances self-esteem and encourages the individual to draw on these assets during the weight-loss program.*
• Encourage her to examine her own behaviour.	*Involving Mrs. Santini in self-appraisal will promote identification of behaviours that may be contributing to excessive caloric intake.*
• Identify the behaviour to be changed in specific, concrete terms (e.g., stop snacking in front of the TV).	*Identification of specific behaviours is essential for planning behaviour modification.*
• Consider that it is easier to increase a behaviour than to decrease a behaviour (e.g., increase activities or hobbies that involve the hands, such as sewing, versus decreasing TV snacking).	*Habitual behaviours are difficult to change. Breaking old habits may be easier if viewed from the standpoint of increasing an enjoyable, healthy activity.*
• Choose reinforcers that are meaningful to Mrs. Santini.	*Positive reinforcement is not likely to be an effective part of behaviour modification if the reinforcer is meaningless to the individual.*

EVALUATION

Goal met. Mrs. Santini kept a dietary log for 5 days and has planned balanced meals each day, resulting in a daily deficit of 400 to 500 calories. She is aware that she eats excessively because she is bored and depressed. She has re-established her former social contacts, including her church bridge club. Mrs. Santini has purchased a stationary bicycle and exercises 20 minutes daily. She enrolled in a knitting class that meets two nights per week. She has lost 0.7 kg in the past week. As a reward, Mrs. Santini renewed her membership to the YMCA.

*Interventions and activities selected are only a sample of those suggested in the *Nursing Interventions Classification (NIC)*, by G. M. Bulechek, H. K. Butcher, and J. C. Dochterman (Eds.), 2008, St. Louis, MO: Mosby Elsevier, and should be individualized for each client.

Planning for Home Care

To provide for continuity of care, the nurse must consider the client's need for assistance with nutrition. Some clients will need help with feeding, purchasing food, and preparing meals; others will need instructions about enteral and total parenteral nutrition therapy.

Home care planning incorporates an assessment of the client's and family's abilities for self-care, financial resources, and the need for referrals and home health services. The Assessment: Home Care box outlines a home care assessment for nutritional problems and needs. A major aspect of discharge planning involves instructional needs of the client and family. See the Teaching: Wellness box on healthy nutrition.

Implementing

Nursing interventions to promote optimal nutrition for hospitalized patients are often provided in collaboration with the physician, who writes the diet orders, and the dietitian, who informs patients about special diets and prepares feeding protocols. The nurse reinforces this instruction and, in addition, creates an atmosphere that encourages eating, provides assistance with eating, monitors the patient's appetite and food intake, administers enteral and parenteral feedings, and consults with the physician and dietitian about nutritional problems that arise.

In the community setting, the nurse's role is largely educational. For example, nurses promote optimal nutrition at health fairs, in schools, at prenatal classes, and with well or ill patients and support people in their homes. In the home setting, nurses also initiate nutritional screens, refer clients at risk to appropriate resources, instruct clients about enteral and parenteral feedings, and offer nutrition counselling as needed. Nutrition counselling involves more than simply providing information. The nurse must help clients integrate diet changes into their lifestyles and provide strategies to motivate them to change their eating habits. For children, the school setting is the ideal place to introduce

ASSESSMENT: HOME CARE

Nutrition

Before discharging clients, nurses need to assess their nutrition needs and any problems:

CLIENT AND ENVIRONMENT

- *Self-care abilities:* Assess the ability to feed self, to purchase food, and to prepare meals.
- *Adaptive feeding aids required:* Determine the need for special drinking cups, plates, or feeding utensils (see feeding aids later in this chapter).
- *Instructional needs:* Consider nutritional requirements (e.g., *Eating Well with Canada's Food Guide*, dietary guidelines, special diet); adaptive aids available; recommended lifestyle variations; and management of enteral or parenteral nutrition.
- *Physical environment:* Assess for the adequacy of water, electricity, refrigeration, and telephone facilities; and for the presence of a clean, secure area to store and set up enteral or parenteral equipment, as needed.
- *Abilities to manage enteral or parenteral nutrition* (discussed later in this chapter): Assess for the cognitive abilities to manage procedures and follow a prescribed schedule; the adequacy of manual dexterity to open sterile packages and handle equipment; the adequacy of visual acuity to read numbers on syringes and pumps; the ability to prepare formulas; and the ability to evaluate the status of the enteral or parenteral access device and report problems.

FAMILY

- *Caregiver availability, skills, and willingness:* Assess for primary and secondary persons able to assist with food purchase, meal preparation, and feeding and who are able to comprehend and administer special diets or the enteral or parenteral nutrition required.
- *Family role changes and coping*: Consider the effect on parenting and spousal roles, financial resources, and social roles.
- *Alternative potential primary or respite caregivers:* Assess, for example, other family members, volunteers, church members, paid caregivers, or housekeeping services, available community respite care (adult daycare, senior centres), and so on.

COMMUNITY

- *Current knowledge, use, and experience with community resources:* Determine the familiarity with nutritional counselling services; home health agencies for enteral or parenteral nutrition support; dietitian or nutritionist for planning appropriate meals for prescribed diet, planning ways to include ethnic food preferences into the diet, and providing written meal plans; medical equipment and supply sources; financial assistance services; support and educational services, such as the following:
  - Weight-management programs (e.g., Weight Watchers, Curves)
  - Dietitians of Canada for information on all nutrition topics
  - Health Canada
  - Meals on Wheels

TEACHING: WELLNESS

Healthy Nutrition

Discharge planning also includes teaching clients and their families about healthy nutrition:

- Instruct clients about the content of a healthy diet based on *Eating Well with Canada's Food Guide*.
- Encourage clients, particularly older clients, to reduce dietary fat.
- Instruct strict vegetarians, as needed, about proper protein complementation and additional vitamin and mineral supplementation.
- Discuss foods high in specific required nutrients, such as protein, iron, calcium, vitamin C, fibre, and so on.
- Discuss the importance of properly fitted dentures and dental care.
- Discuss safe food preparation and preservation techniques, as appropriate.

DIETARY ALTERATIONS

- Explain the purpose of the diet.
- Discuss allowed and excluded foods.
- Explain the importance of reading food labels when selecting foods.
- Include family or significant others as appropriate.
- Reinforce information provided by the dietitian or nutritionist as appropriate.
- Discuss herbs and spices as alternatives to salt, and discuss substitutes for sugar.

FOR OVERWEIGHT CLIENTS

- Discuss physiological, psychological, and lifestyle factors that predispose people to weight gain.
- Provide information about normal weight range and recommended calorie intake.
- Discuss principles of a well-balanced diet (see *Eating Well with Canada's Food Guide* or other food guidelines) and high- and low-calorie foods.
- Encourage intake of low-calorie caffeine-free beverages and plenty of water.
- Discuss ways to adapt eating practices by using smaller plates, smaller servings, chewing each bite a specified number of times, and putting the fork down between bites.
- Discuss ways to control the desire to eat by taking a walk, drinking a glass of water, or doing slow deep-breathing exercises.

(continued)

TEACHING: WELLNESS *(continued)*

- Discuss the importance of exercise and help the client plan an exercise program.
- Discuss stress-reduction techniques.
- Provide information about available community resources (e.g., weight-loss groups, dietary counselling, exercise programs, self-help groups).

FOR UNDERWEIGHT CLIENTS

- Discuss factors contributing to inadequate nutrition and weight loss.
- Discuss recommended calorie intake and normal weight range.
- Provide information about the content of a balanced diet based on *Canada's Food Guide*.
- Provide information about ways to increase calorie intake (e.g., high-protein or high-calorie foods and supplements).
- Discuss ways to manage, minimize, or alter the factors contributing to malnourishment.
- If appropriate, discuss ways to purchase low-cost nutritious foods.
- Provide information about community agencies that can assist in providing food (e.g., Meals on Wheels).

PREVENTING FOOD-BORNE ILLNESS

- Reinforce hygienic handling of food and dishes:
  - Wash hands before preparing foods.
  - Wash hands and all dishes and utensils with hot water and soap after contact with raw meats.
  - Defrost frozen foods in the refrigerator.
  - Cook beef, poultry, and eggs thoroughly. Use a cooking thermometer.
  - Refrigerate leftovers promptly (at 5°C or less) and keep no more than 3 to 5 days.
  - Wash or peel raw fruits and vegetables.
  - Do not use foods from containers that have been damaged or have opened seals.
  - Follow the rules "keep hot foods hot and cold foods cold" and "when in doubt, throw it out."
- Recommend the client consider a preventive vaccination for hepatitis A.
- Instruct clients to seek medical attention for prolonged vomiting, fever, abdominal pain, or severe diarrhea following a meal.

the concepts of healthy nutrition. *Canada's Food Guide* should play an essential part in the curriculum and cafeterias not selling junk food should be encouraged.

Assisting with Special Diets

Alterations in the client's diet are often needed to treat a disease process, such as diabetes mellitus, to prepare for a special examination or surgery, to increase or decrease weight, to restore nutritional deficits, or to allow an organ to rest and promote healing. Diets are modified in one or more of the following aspects: texture, kilocalories, specific nutrients, seasonings, or consistency.

Patients who do not have special needs eat the *regular* (standard or house) *diet,* a balanced diet that supplies the metabolic requirements of a sedentary person (about 2000 kcal). Most agencies offer patients a daily menu from which to select their meals for the next day; others provide standard meals to each patient on the general diet. Certain foods (e.g., cabbage, which tends to produce flatus, and highly seasoned and fried foods, which are difficult for some people to digest) are usually omitted from the regular diet.

TEMPORARY CONSISTENCY MODIFICATIONS Diets that are modified in consistency are often given to patients before and after surgery or to promote healing in patients with gastrointestinal distress. These diets include nothing by mouth or per ora, clear liquid, full liquid, soft, and diet as tolerated.

NOTHING PER ORA In **nothing per ora (NPO)**, food and fluid are prohibited, for example, before anaesthesia to prevent aspiration of stomach contents or after surgery until bowel sounds return. NPO status should be limited as much as possible to minimize nutritional and dehydration risks. Alternative methods of nutrition and hydration (e.g., intravenous therapy, enteral feeding) should be considered if the patient must remain without food or fluid.

CLEAR LIQUID DIET The **clear liquid diet** is limited to water, tea, coffee, clear broths, ginger ale or other carbonated beverages, strained and clear juices, and plain gelatin. This diet provides the patient with fluid and carbohydrate (in the form of sugar) but does not supply adequate protein, fat, vitamins, minerals, or calories (no more than 600 kcal/day). It is a short-term diet (24 to 36 hours) provided for patients after certain surgery or in the acute stages of infection, particularly of the gastrointestinal tract. The major objectives of this diet are to relieve thirst, prevent dehydration, and minimize stimulation of the gastrointestinal tract. Examples of foods allowed in clear diets are shown in Box 39.10.

FULL LIQUID DIET The **full liquid diet** contains only liquids or foods that turn to liquid at body temperature, such as ice cream (see Box 39.10). Full liquid diets are often eaten by patients who have gastrointestinal disturbances or are otherwise unable to tolerate solid or semisolid foods. This diet is not recommended for long-term use because it is low in iron, protein, and calories.

BOX 39.10 FOODS FOR CLEAR LIQUID, FULL LIQUID, AND SOFT DIETS

The following are some examples of allowed foods on clear liquid, full liquid, and soft diets:

CLEAR LIQUID	FULL LIQUID	SOFT
Coffee, regular and decaffeinated Tea (black, green, and white) Carbonated beverages Bouillon, fat-free broth Clear fruit juices (apple, cranberry, grape) Other fruit juices, strained Popsicles Gelatin Sugar, honey Hard candy	All foods on clear liquid diet, plus the following: Milk and milk drinks Puddings, custards Ice cream, sherbet Vegetable juices Refined or strained cereals (e.g., cream of rice) Cream, butter, margarine Eggs (in custard and pudding) Smooth peanut butter Yogourt	All foods on full and clear liquid diets, plus the following: *Meat:* All lean, tender meat, fish, or poultry (chopped, shredded); spaghetti sauce with ground meat, over pasta *Meat alternatives:* Scrambled eggs, omelette, poached eggs; cottage cheese and other mild cheese *Vegetables:* Mashed potatoes, sweet potatoes, or squash; vegetables in cream or cheese sauce; other cooked vegetables as tolerated (e.g., spinach, cauliflower, asparagus tips), chopped and mashed, as needed; avocado *Fruits:* Cooked or canned fruits; bananas; grapefruit and orange sections without membranes; applesauce *Breads and cereals:* Enriched rice, barley, pasta; all breads; cooked cereals (e.g., oatmeal) *Desserts:* Soft cake, bread pudding

In addition, its cholesterol content is high because of the amount of milk offered. Patients who must receive only liquids for long periods are usually given a nutritionally balanced oral supplement, such as Ensure or Boost. The full liquid diet is monotonous and difficult for patients to accept. Planning six or more feedings per day may encourage a more adequate intake.

SOFT DIET The **soft diet** is easily chewed and digested. It is often ordered for patients who have difficulty chewing and swallowing. It is a low-residue (low-fibre) diet containing very few uncooked foods; however, restrictions vary among agencies and according to individual tolerance. Examples of foods that can be included in a soft or semisoft diet are shown in Box 39.10. The **pureed diet** is a modification of the soft diet. Liquid can be added to the food, which is then blended to a semisolid consistency.

DIET AS TOLERATED **Diet as tolerated** is ordered when the patient's appetite, ability to eat, and tolerance for certain foods may change. For example, on the first postoperative day, a patient may be given a clear liquid diet. If no nausea occurs, normal intestinal motility has returned, and the patient feels like eating, the diet may be advanced to a full liquid, light, or regular diet.

MODIFICATION FOR DISEASE Many special diets are prescribed to meet the requirements for disease process or altered metabolism. For many medical conditions, specific diets may be prescribed. Patients with diabetes mellitus may be prescribed a diabetic diet that follows the Glycemic Index suggested by the Canadian Diabetes Association (2008). Patients with hypertension will need a sodium-reduced diet. Those with coronary artery disease or those at significant risk (e.g., because of family history of heart attack or stroke) may need a diet low in cholesterol and saturated fats. Patients with celiac disease who are intolerant to wheat gluten must avoid all gluten-containing products and may need to replace all grains with rice-based products. People with renal insufficiency need to limit the number of grams of protein they eat per day to protect their kidneys, and those with renal failure must avoid ingesting too much potassium because they cannot excrete it.

Patients with severe food allergies must take extreme precaution to avoid exposure to their triggers. It is recommended that these patients not eat anything unless they have their EpiPen nearby. In many cases, full-blown **anaphylaxis** can occur with hypotension, loss of consciousness, and, if not rapidly treated, death.

CLINICAL ALERT

In Canada, as many as 3% to 4% of the adult population and 6% of children are affected by food allergies, and the prevalence of such allergies is increasing (Health Canada, 2007d). Common food allergens include peanuts, tree nuts, sesame, soy, fish and seafood, wheat, eggs, and milk. When people are affected by food allergens, exposure to very tiny amounts of the food can trigger a reaction. Symptoms include difficulty breathing, facial swelling, itching, rash, cramps, and diarrhea. Full-blown *anaphylaxis* can occur. Patients who have food allergies must be taught how to avoid triggers, to use an EpiPen (epinephrine auto-injector), and what to do in the case of accidental exposure. These patients should wear a medical identification bracelet or necklace. Many schools now restrict certain foods to prevent accidental exposure.

Some patients must adapt their diets because of the medications they take. For example, patients who are taking antineoplastic medications and who have severely depressed immune systems (e.g., neutropenia) may need to eat only well-cooked foods to prevent the risk of infection. Glucocorticosteroid-dependent patients are encouraged to eat a low-carbohydrate, high-protein diet to prevent weight gain and muscle wasting.

Some clients must follow these diets (e.g., the diabetic diet) for a lifetime. If the diet is long term, the client must not only understand the diet but also develop a healthy, positive attitude toward it. Assisting clients and support persons with special diets is a function shared by the dietitian or nutritionist and the nurse. The dietitian informs the client and support persons about the specific foods allowed and not allowed and assists the client with meal planning. The nurse reinforces this instruction, assists the client to make changes, and evaluates the client's responses. All dietary instructions must be individually designed to meet the client's cognitive status, motivation level, lifestyle, culture, and economic status. Both nutritionists and dietitians help to adapt a diet to suit the client. Simple verbal instructions need to be given and reinforced with written material. Family and support persons must be included in the dietary instruction.

DYSPHAGIA Some clients may have no difficulty choosing a healthy diet but be at risk for nutritional problems because of dysphagia (difficulty swallowing). These clients may have inadequate solid or fluid intake, be unable to swallow their medications, or aspirate food or fluids into the lungs, causing pneumonia. Clients at risk for dysphagia include older adults, those who have experienced a stroke, cancer patients who have had radiation therapy to the head and neck, and others with cranial nerve dysfunction. Nurses may be the first persons to detect dysphagia and are in an excellent position to recommend further evaluation; implement specialized feeding techniques and diets; and work with clients, family members, and other health-care professionals to develop a plan to assist the client with difficulties. If the client's condition suggests dysphagia, the nurse should review the history in detail; interview the client or family; assess the mouth, throat, and chest; and observe the client swallowing. The presence of the gag reflex, often thought to indicate that the client can swallow safely, has not been shown to be a reliable indicator. Confirmation of the tendency for food to divert to the trachea is best done through X-ray.

A multidisciplinary group has developed the national dysphagia diet, which delineates standards of food textures (American Dietetic Association, 2003). The four levels of liquid foods are thin, nectar-like, honey-like, and spoon-thick liquids. The four levels of semisolid or solid foods are pureed, mechanically altered, advanced or mechanically soft, and regular or general. In consultation with the dietitian, occupational therapist, swallowing specialist, speech-language pathologist, or physician, these levels can be used to determine a consistent approach to a particular client's dysphagia. For example, a mechanically soft diet may result in lower pneumonia rates than a pureed diet in stroke patients with a history of aspiration pneumonia. Early detection and intervention can prevent the adverse outcomes of dysphagia in most clients.

Stimulating the Appetite

Physical illness, unfamiliar or unpalatable food, environmental and psychological factors, medications or therapies, and physical discomfort or pain may depress the appetites of many patients. A short-term decrease in food intake usually is not a problem for adults; over time, however, it leads to weight loss, decreased strength and stamina, and other nutritional problems. A decreased food intake is often accompanied by a decrease in fluid intake, which may cause fluid and electrolyte problems. Stimulating a person's appetite requires the nurse to determine the reason for the lack of appetite and then to deal with the problem. Some interventions for improving the client's appetite are summarized in Box 39.11.

Assisting Patients with Meals

Because patients in health-care agencies are frequently confined to their beds, meals are often brought to the

BOX 39.11 IMPROVING APPETITE

Nurses can try the following to help improve a client's appetite:

- Relieve illness symptoms that depress appetite before mealtime; for example, give an analgesic for pain, an antipyretic for fever, or allow rest for fatigue. Treat nausea well before the meal is presented to the patient.
- Provide familiar food that the person likes. Often, the relatives of patients are pleased to bring food from home but may need some guidance about special diet requirements.
- Select small portions so as not to discourage the anorexic patient.
- Avoid unpleasant or uncomfortable treatments immediately before or after a meal.
- Provide a tidy, clean environment that is free of unpleasant sights and odours. A soiled dressing, a used bedpan, an uncovered irrigation set, or even used dishes can negatively affect the appetite.
- Encourage or provide oral hygiene before mealtime. This improves the patient's ability to taste.
- Reduce psychological stress. A lack of understanding of therapy, the anticipation of an operation, and fear of the unknown can cause anorexia. Often, the nurse can help by discussing feelings with the patient, giving information and assistance, and allaying fears.
- Stimulate the patient's appetite by having the patient remember favourite foods and to think about those foods and their tastes. If possible, have family members supply these foods.

patient. The patient receives a tray that has been assembled in a central kitchen. Nursing personnel may be responsible for giving out and collecting the trays; however, in most settings, this is done by special dietary personnel. Long-term-care facilities and some hospitals serve meals to ambulatory patients in a special dining area. Other agencies have a coffee shop for food or machines from which patients can obtain sandwiches and beverages. Guidelines for providing meals to patients and residents are summarized in Box 39.12.

Two groups of people frequently require help with their meals: older adults who are weakened; and persons with disabilities, such as blind patients, those who must remain in a supine position, or those who cannot use their hands. The patient's nursing care plan will indicate that assistance is required with meals.

The nurse must be sensitive to patients' feelings of embarrassment, resentment, and loss of autonomy. Whenever possible, the nurse should help incapacitated patients feed themselves, rather than feed them. Some patients become depressed because they require help and because they believe they are burdensome to busy nursing personnel. Although feeding a patient is time-consuming, nurses should try to appear unhurried and convey that they have ample time. Sitting at the bedside is one way to convey this impression.

When feeding a patient, ask in which order the patient would like to eat the food. If the patient cannot see, tell the patient which food is being given. Always allow ample time for the patient to chew and swallow the food before offering more. Also, provide fluids as requested, or if the patient is unable to communicate, offer fluids after every three or four mouthfuls of solid food. It is important to make the time a pleasant one, choosing topics of conversation that are of interest to patients who want to talk.

Although normal utensils should be used whenever possible, special utensils may be needed to assist a patient to eat. For patients who have difficulty drinking from a cup or glass, a straw often permits them to obtain liquids with less effort and less spillage. Special drinking cups are also available. One model has a spout; another is specially designed to permit drinking with less tipping of the cup than is normally required.

Many adaptive feeding aids are available to help patients maintain independence. A standard eating utensil with a built-up or widened handle helps patients who cannot grasp objects easily. Utensils with wide handles can be purchased, or a regular eating utensil can be modified by taping foam around the handle. The foam increases friction and, thus, steadies the patient's grasp. Handles can be bent or angled to compensate for limited motion. Collars or bands that prevent the utensil from being dropped can be attached to the end of the handle and fit over the patient's hand.

BOX 39.12 PROVIDING MEALS TO PATIENTS

Nurses should observe the following guidelines when providing meals:

- Offer the patient assistance with hand hygiene and oral hygiene before a meal.
- Most people sit during a meal; if it is permitted, assist the patient to a comfortable position in bed or in a chair, whichever is appropriate.
- Clear the overbed table so that there is space for the tray. If the patient must remain in a lying position in bed, arrange the overbed table close to the bedside so that the patient can see and reach the food.
- Check each tray for the patient's name, the type of diet, and completeness. Do *not* leave an incorrect diet for a patient to eat.
- Assist the patient as required to remove the food covers, put spreads on the bread, pour the tea, and cut the meat.
- For a person who is blind, identify the placement of the food as you would describe the time on a clock (Figure 39.10). For instance, the nurse may say, "The potatoes are at 8 o'clock, the chicken at 12 o'clock, and the green beans at 4 o'clock."
- After the patient has completed the meal, observe how much and what the patient has eaten and the amount of fluid taken. Record fluid intake and calorie count, as required.
- If the patient is on a special diet or is having problems eating, record the amount of food eaten and any pain, fatigue, or nausea experienced.
- If the patient is not eating, document this so that changes can be made, such as rescheduling the meals, providing smaller, more frequent meals, or obtaining special self-feeding aids.

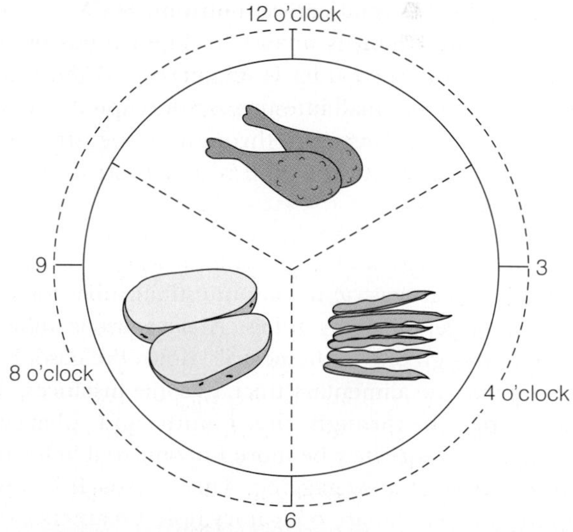

FIGURE 39.10 For a client who is blind, the nurse can use the clock system to describe the location of food on the plate.

Plates with rims and plastic or metal plate guards enable the patient to pick up the food by first pushing it against this raised edge. A suction cup or damp sponge or cloth can be placed under the dish to keep it from moving while the patient is eating. No-spill mugs and two-handled drinking cups are especially useful for persons with impaired hand coordination. Stretch terry cloth and knitted or crocheted glass covers enable the patient to keep a secure grasp on a glass. Lidded tip-proof glasses are also available. Figure 39.11 and Figure 39.12 show some of these aids.

Providing Special Community Nutritional Services

In many places, community programs have been developed to help special groups of the population meet their nutritional needs. For older people who cannot prepare meals or leave their homes, ready-to-eat meals or frozen dinners are delivered to the home by local organizations. Meals on Wheels is one such well-known organization. Online or telephone ordering with home delivery can be an option for people who can prepare meals but are unable to shop for groceries in person.

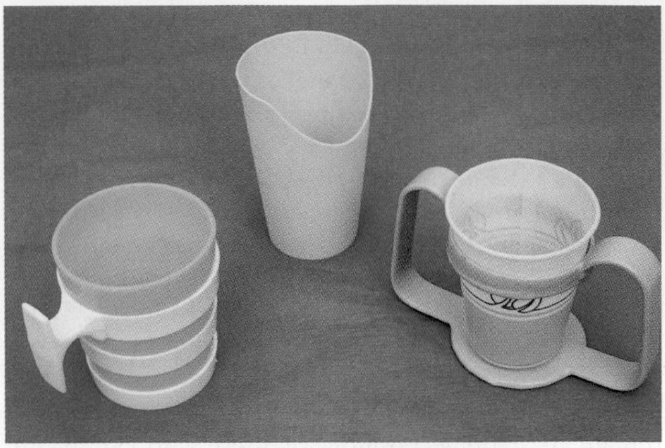

FIGURE 39.11 Left to right: glass holder, cup with hole for nose, two-handled cup holder

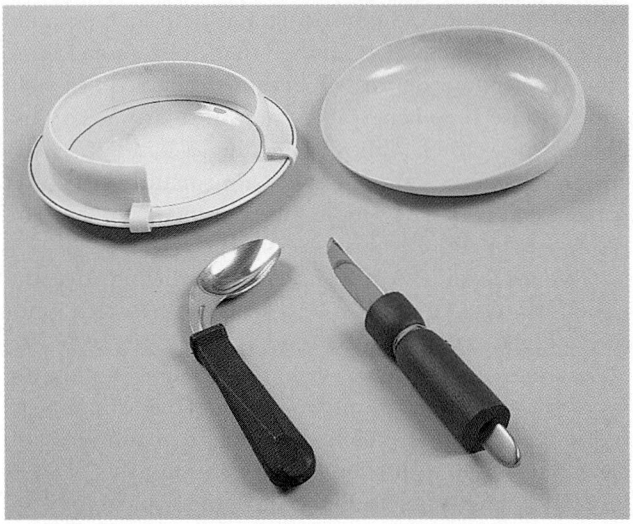

FIGURE 39.12 Dinner plate with guard attached and lip plate facilitate scooping; wide-handled spoon and knife facilitate grip

Providing Enteral Nutrition

Alternative feeding methods to ensure adequate nutrition include both enteral (through the gastrointestinal system) and parenteral (intravenous) methods. **Parenteral nutrition** involves the intravenous infusion of water, protein, carbohydrates, electrolytes, minerals, and vitamins through a central vein. **Enteral nutrition** (EN), also referred to as **total enteral nutrition** (TEN), is provided when the client is unable to ingest foods or the upper gastrointestinal tract is impaired and the transport of food to the small intestine is interrupted. Enteral feedings are administered through nasogastric and small-bore feeding tubes or through gastrostomy or jejunostomy tubes.

ENTERAL ACCESS DEVICES Enteral access is achieved by means of nasogastric or nasointestinal tubes, or gastrostomy or jejunostomy tubes. A **nasogastric tube** is inserted through one of the nostrils, down the nasopharynx, and into the alimentary tract. In some instances, the tube is passed through the mouth and pharynx, although this route may be more uncomfortable for the adult client and cause gagging. This approach is often used for infants who are obligatory nose breathers (who must breathe through the nose) and premature infants who have no gag reflex.

Traditional firm *large-bore* nasogastric tubes (i.e., those larger than 12 Fr in diameter) are placed in the stomach. Examples are the *Levin tube,* a flexible rubber or plastic single-lumen tube with holes near the tip, and the *Salem sump tube,* with a double lumen (Figure 39.13). The larger tube of the Salem sump allows delivery of liquids to the stomach or removal of gastric contents. When the Salem tube is used for suction of gastric contents, the smaller vent lumen (the proximal port is often referred to as the *blue pigtail*) allows for an inflow of atmospheric air, which prevents a vacuum if the gastric tube adheres to the wall of the stomach. Irritation of the gastric mucosa is thereby avoided. Softer, more flexible, and less irritating *small-bore nasoenteric tubes* (smaller than 12 Fr in diameter) are frequently used (Figure 39.14).

Nasogastric tubes are used for patients who have intact gag and cough reflexes, who have adequate gastric emptying, and who require short-term feedings. Skill 39.2 provides guidelines for inserting a nasogastric tube. Skill 39.3 outlines the steps for removing a nasogastric tube.

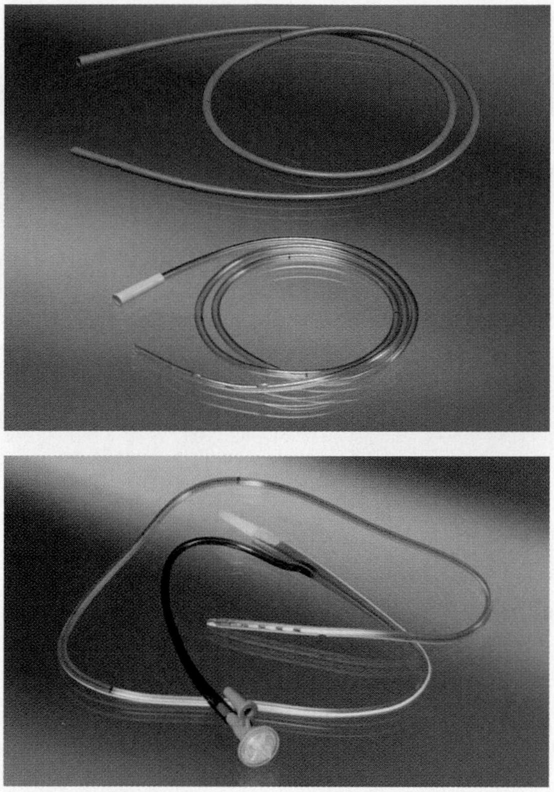

A

B

FIGURE 39.13 **A:** Single-lumen Levin tube; **B:** double-lumen Salem sump tube with filter on air vent port and connector on suction port

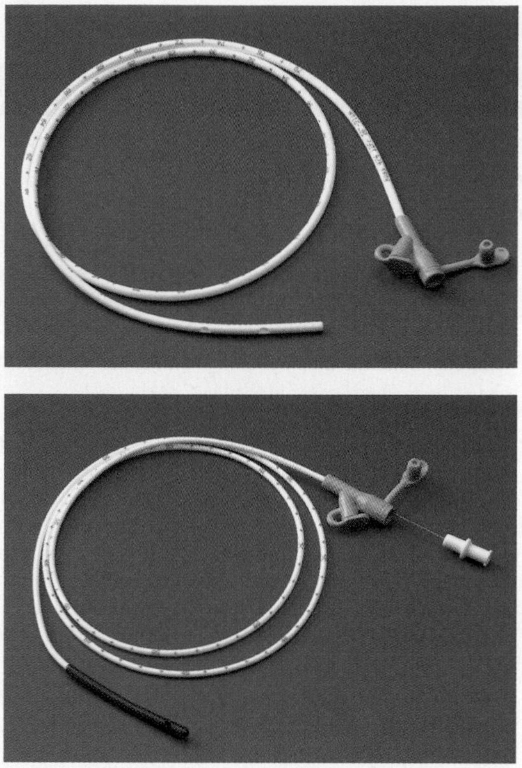

A

B

FIGURE 39.14 Nasoenteric feeding tubes: **A:** 12 Fr; **B:** 8 Fr. Opaque, stylet, weighted tip. Note that both have Y-port connector to permit irrigation and medication administration without disconnecting feeding device.

SKILL 39.2

INSERTING A NASOGASTRIC TUBE

PURPOSES

- To administer tube feedings and medications to patients unable to eat by mouth or swallow a sufficient diet without aspirating food or fluids into the lungs
- To establish a means for suctioning stomach contents to prevent gastric distension, nausea, and vomiting
- To remove stomach contents for laboratory analysis
- To lavage (wash) the stomach in case of poisoning or overdose of medications

ASSESSMENT

Assess the following:

- Check for a history of nasal surgery or deviated septum. Assess patency of nares.
- Determine presence of gag reflex.
- Assess mental status or ability to cooperate with the procedure.

Planning

Before inserting a nasogastric tube, determine the size of tube to be inserted and whether the tube is to be attached to suction.

Equipment

- Large- or small-bore tube (nonlatex preferred)
- Hypoallergenic adhesive tape, 2.5 cm wide
- Clean gloves
- Water-soluble lubricant
- Facial tissues
- Glass of water and drinking straw
- 20 mL to 50 mL syringe with an adapter
- Basin
- pH test strip or meter
- Bilirubin dipstick (optional)
- Stethoscope
- Disposable pad or towel
- Clamp or plug (optional)
- Antireflux valve for air vent if Salem sump tube is used
- Suction apparatus
- Safety pin and elastic band

(continued)

SKILL 39.2

INSERTING A NASOGASTRIC TUBE *(continued)*

IMPLEMENTATION

Preparation

- Assist the patient to a high-Fowler's position if his or her health condition permits, and support the head on a pillow. **Rationale: It is often easier to swallow in this position and gravity helps the passage of the tube.**
- Place a towel or disposable pad across the chest.

Performance

1. Before performing the insertion, introduce yourself and verify the patient's identity by using agency protocol. Explain to the patient what you are going to do, why it is necessary, and how he or she can cooperate. The passage of a gastric tube is unpleasant because the gag reflex is activated during insertion. Establish a method for the patient to indicate distress and a desire for you to pause the insertion. Raising a finger or hand is often used for this.
2. Perform hand hygiene and observe other appropriate infection prevention and control procedures (e.g., clean gloves).
3. Provide for patient privacy.
4. Assess the patient's nares.
    - Ask the patient to hyperextend the head, and, using a flashlight, observe the intactness of the tissues of the nostrils, including any irritations or abrasions.
    - Examine the nares for any obstructions or deformities by asking the patient to breathe through one nostril while occluding the other.
    - Select the nostril that has the greater airflow.
5. Prepare the tube.
    - If a small-bore tube is being used, ensure stylet or guide wire, if present, is secured in position. **Rationale: An improperly positioned stylet or guide wire can traumatize the nasopharynx, esophagus, and stomach.**
6. Determine how far to insert the tube.
    - Use the tube to mark off the distance from the tip of the patient's nose to the tip of the earlobe and then from the tip of the earlobe to the tip of the xyphoid (see ❶). **Rationale: This length approximates the distance from the nares to the stomach. This distance varies among individuals.**
    - Mark this length with adhesive tape if the tube does not have markings.
7. Insert the tube.
    - Put on gloves.
    - Lubricate the tip of the tube well with water-soluble lubricant or water to ease insertion. **Rationale: A water-soluble lubricant dissolves if the tube accidentally enters the lungs. An oil-based lubricant, such as petroleum jelly, will not dissolve and could cause respiratory complications if it enters the lungs.**

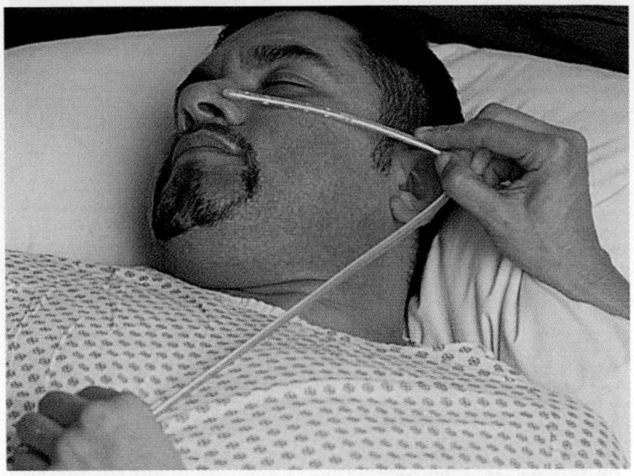

❶ Measuring the appropriate length to insert a nasogastric tube

    - Insert the tube, with its natural curve toward the patient, into the selected nostril. Ask the patient to hyperextend the neck, and gently advance the tube toward the nasopharynx. **Rationale: Hyperextension of the neck reduces the curvature of the nasopharyngeal junction.**
    - Direct the tube along the floor of the nostril and toward the ear on that side. **Rationale: Directing the tube along the floor avoids the turbinates (projections) along the lateral wall.**
    - Slight pressure and a twisting motion are sometimes required to pass the tube into the nasopharynx, and some patient's eyes may water at this point. **Rationale: Tears are a natural body response.** Provide the patient with tissues as needed.
    - If the tube meets resistance, withdraw it, relubricate it, and insert it in the other nostril. **Rationale: The tube should never be forced against resistance because of the danger of injury.**
    - Once the tube reaches the oropharynx (throat), the patient will feel the tube in the throat and may gag and retch. Ask the patient to tilt the head forward, and encourage the patient to drink and swallow (see ❷). **Rationale: Tilting the head forward facilitates passage of the tube into the posterior pharynx and esophagus rather than into the larynx; swallowing moves the epiglottis over the opening to the larynx.**
    - If the patient gags, stop passing the tube momentarily. Have the patient rest, take a few breaths, and take sips of water to calm the gag reflex.
    - In cooperation with the patient, pass the tube 5 cm to 10 cm with each swallow, until the indicated length is inserted.
    - If the patient continues to gag and the tube does not advance with each swallow, withdraw it slightly, and inspect the throat by looking through the mouth. **Rationale: The tube may be coiled in the throat.** If so, withdraw it until it is straight, and try again to insert it.

(continued)

SKILL 39.2

INSERTING A NASOGASTRIC TUBE (*continued*)

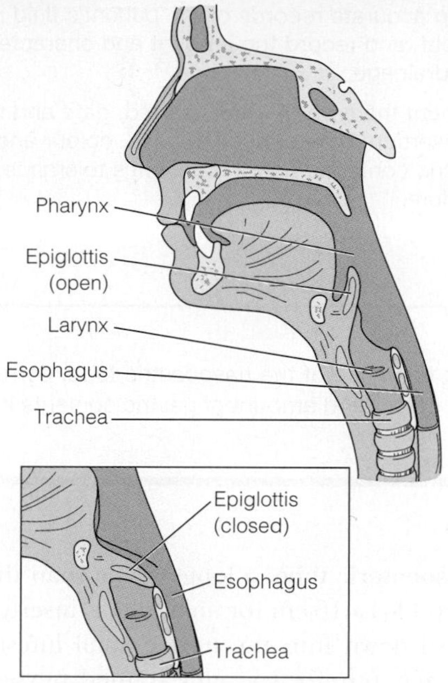

❷ Swallowing closes the epiglottis

8. Ascertain correct placement of the tube.
   - Aspirate stomach contents, and check the pH, which should be acidic. **Rationale: Testing pH is a reliable way to determine location of a feeding tube. Gastric contents are commonly pH 1 to 5; 6 or greater would indicate the contents are from lower in the intestinal tract or in the respiratory tract. Some researchers suggest that a pH of greater than 5 should be followed by further confirmation of tube location** (Huffman, Jarczyk, O'Brien, Pieper, & Bayne, 2004).
   - Aspirate can also optionally be tested for bilirubin. Bilirubin levels in the lungs should be almost zero, while levels in the stomach will be approximately 25.7 micromol/L and in the intestine over 171 micromol/L.
   - Almost all nasogastric tubes are radiopaque, and position can be confirmed by X-ray. Check agency policy. If a small-bore tube is used, leave the stylet or guide wire in place until correct position is verified by X-ray. If the stylet has been removed, never reinsert it while the tube is in place. **Rationale: The stylet is sharp and could pierce the tube and injure the patient or cut off the tube end.**
   - Place a stethoscope over the patient's epigastrium and inject 10 mL to 30 mL of air into the tube while listening for a whooshing sound. Although still one of the methods used, do not use this method as the *primary* method for determining placement of the feeding tube *because it does not guarantee tube position.*
   - If the signs indicate placement in the lungs, remove the tube and begin again.
   - If the signs do not indicate placement in the lung or stomach, advance the tube 5 cm, and repeat the tests.

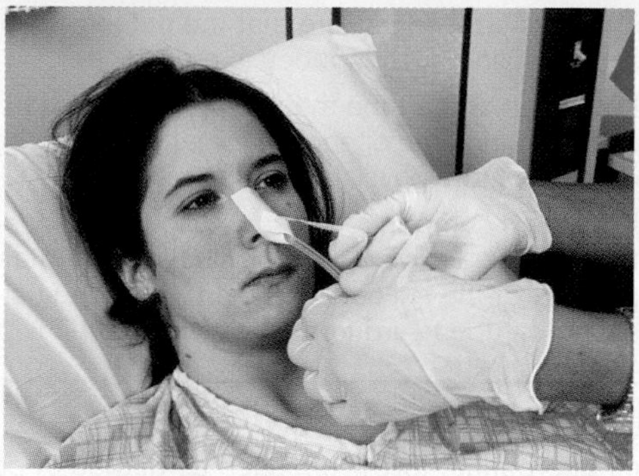

❸ Taping a nasogastric tube to the bridge of the nose

9. Secure the tube by taping it to the bridge of the patient's nose.
   - If the patient has oily skin, wipe the nose first with alcohol to defat the skin.
   - Cut 7.5 cm of tape, and split it lengthwise at one end, leaving a 2.5 cm tab at the end.
   - Place the tape over the bridge of the patient's nose, and bring the split ends either under and around the tubing, or under the tubing and back up over the nose (see ❸). **Rationale: Taping in this manner prevents the tube from pressing against and irritating the edge of the nostril.**
10. Once correct position has been determined, attach the tube to a suction source or feeding apparatus as ordered, or clamp the end of the tubing.
11. Secure the tube to the patient's gown.
    - Loop an elastic band around the end of the tubing, and attach the elastic band to the gown with a safety pin.
    - *Or* attach a piece of adhesive tape to the tube, and pin the tape to the gown. **Rationale: The tube is attached to prevent it from dangling and pulling.**
    - If a Salem sump tube is used, attach the antireflux valve to the vent port (if used) and position the port above the patient's waist. **Rationale: So that gastric contents do not flow into the vent lumen.**
12. Document relevant information: the insertion of the tube, the means by which correct placement was determined, and patient responses (e.g., discomfort or abdominal distension).
13. Establish a plan for providing daily nasogastric tube care.
    - Inspect the nostril for discharge and irritation.
    - Clean the nostril and tube with moistened, cotton-tipped applicators.
    - Apply water-soluble lubricant to the nostril if it appears dry or encrusted.
    - Change the adhesive tape as required.
    - Give frequent mouth care. Because of the presence of the tube, the patient may breathe through the mouth.

(*continued*)

SKILL 39.2

INSERTING A NASOGASTRIC TUBE *(continued)*

14. If suction is applied, ensure that the patency of both the nasogastric and suction tubes is maintained.
    - Irrigations of the tube may be required at regular intervals. In some agencies, irrigations must be ordered by the physician or dietitian.
    - If a Salem sump tube is used, follow agency policies for irrigating the vent lumen with air to maintain patency of the suctioning lumen. Often, a sucking sound can be heard from the vent port if it is patent.
    - Keep accurate records of the patient's fluid intake and output, and record the amount and characteristics of the drainage.
15. Document the type of tube inserted, date and time of tube insertion, type of suction used, colour and amount of gastric contents, and the patient's tolerance of the procedure.

EVALUATION

Conduct appropriate follow-up, such as degree of patient comfort, patient tolerance of the nasogastric tube, correct placement of nasogastric tube in stomach, patient understanding of restrictions, colour and amount of gastric contents if attached to suction, or stomach contents aspirated.

Lifespan Considerations

Inserting a Nasogastric Tube

INFANTS AND YOUNG CHILDREN

- Restraints may be necessary during tube insertion and throughout therapy. *Restraints will prevent accidental dislodging of the tube.*
- Place the infant in an infant seat, or position the infant with a rolled towel or pillow under the head and shoulders.
- When assessing the nares, obstruct one of the infant's nares, and feel for air passage from the other. If the nasal passageway is very small or is obstructed, an orogastric tube may be more appropriate.
- Measure appropriate nasogastric tube length from the nose to the tip of the earlobe and then to the point midway between the umbilicus and the xiphoid process.
- If an orogastric tube is used, measure from the tip of the earlobe to the corner of the mouth to the xiphoid process.
- Do not hyperextend or hyperflex an infant's neck. *Hyperextension or hyperflexion of the neck could occlude the airway.*

Although the focus of this chapter is nutrition, nasogastric tubes are inserted for reasons other than providing a route for feeding the patient. These include the following:

- To prevent nausea, vomiting, and gastric distension following surgery (in this case, the tube is attached to a suction source)
- To remove stomach contents for laboratory analysis
- To lavage (wash) the stomach in cases of poisoning or overdose of medications

A **nasoenteric tube**, a longer tube than the nasogastric tube (at least 16 cm for an adult) is inserted through one nostril down into the upper small intestine. Some agencies may require specially trained nurses or physicians for this procedure. Nasoenteric tubes are used for patients who are at risk for aspiration. Patients at risk for aspiration are those that manifest the following:

- Decreased level of consciousness
- Poor or absent cough or gag reflexes
- Endotracheal intubation
- Recent extubation
- Inability to cooperate with the procedure
- Restlessness or agitation

Gastrostomy and **jejunostomy** devices are used for long-term nutritional support, generally more than 6 to 8 weeks. Conventional tubes are placed surgically or by laparoscopy through the abdominal wall into the stomach (gastrostomy, Figure 39.15) or into the jejunum (jejunostomy, Figure 39.16). **Percutaneous endoscopic gastrostomy (PEG)** or **percutaneous endoscopic jejunostomy (PEJ)** is created by using an endoscope to visualize the inside of the stomach, making a puncture through the skin and subcutaneous tissues of the abdomen into the stomach, and inserting the PEG or PEJ catheter through the puncture.

The surgical opening is sutured tightly around the tube or catheter to prevent leakage. Care of this opening before it heals requires surgical asepsis. The catheter has an external bumper and an internal inflatable retention balloon to maintain placement. When the tract is established (about 1 month), the tube or catheter can be removed and reinserted for each feeding. Alternatively, a skin-level tube can be used that remains in place (Figure 39.17). A feeding set is attached when needed.

SKILL 39.3

REMOVING A NASOGASTRIC TUBE

ASSESSMENT

- Assess for the presence of bowel sounds.
- Assess for the absence of nausea or vomiting when tube is clamped.

Equipment

- Disposable pad or towel
- Tissues
- Clean gloves
- 50 mL syringe (optional)
- Plastic trash bag

IMPLEMENTATION

Preparation

- Confirm the physician's order to remove the tube.
- Assist the patient to a sitting position if health permits.
- Place the disposable pad or towel across the patient's chest to collect any spillage of secretions from the tube.
- Provide tissues to the patient to wipe the nose and mouth after tube removal.

Performance

1. Before performing the removal, introduce yourself and verify the patient's identity by using agency protocol. Explain to the patient what you are going to do, why it is necessary, and how he or she can cooperate. Discuss how the results will be used in planning further care or treatments.
2. Perform hand hygiene and observe other appropriate infection prevention and control procedures (e.g., clean gloves).
3. Provide for patient privacy.
4. Detach the tube.
   - Disconnect the nasogastric tube from the suction or feeding apparatus, if present.
   - Unpin the tube from the patient's gown.
   - Remove the adhesive tape securing the tube to the nose.
5. Remove the nasogastric tube.
   - Put on clean gloves.
   - (Optional) Instill 50 mL of air into the tube. **Rationale: This clears the tube of any contents such as feeding or gastric drainage.**
   - Ask the patient to take a deep breath and to hold it. **Rationale: This closes the glottis, thereby preventing accidental aspiration of any gastric contents.**
   - Pinch the tube with the gloved hand. **Rationale: Pinching the tube prevents any contents inside the tube from draining into the patient's throat.**
   - Smoothly, withdraw the tube.
   - Place the tube in the plastic bag. **Rationale: Placing the tube immediately into the bag prevents the transference of microorganisms from the tube to other articles or people.**
   - Observe the intactness of the tube.
6. Ensure patient comfort.
   - Provide mouth care if desired.
   - Assist the patient as required to blow the nose. **Rationale: Excessive secretions may have accumulated in the nasal passages.**
7. Dispose of the equipment appropriately.
   - Place the pad, bag with tube, and gloves in the receptacle designated by the agency. **Rationale: Correct disposal prevents the transmission of microorganisms.**
8. Document all relevant information.
   - Record the removal of the tube, the amount and appearance of any drainage if connected to suction, and any relevant assessments of the patient.

EVALUATION

- Perform a follow-up examination, such as presence of bowel sounds, absence of nausea or vomiting when tube is removed, and intactness of tissues of the nares.
- Relate findings to previous assessment data if available.
- Report significant deviations from normal to the appropriate members of the health-care team.

TESTING FEEDING TUBE PLACEMENT Before feedings are introduced, tube placement is confirmed by radiography if possible, particularly when a small-bore tube has been inserted or when the patient is at risk for aspiration. After placement is confirmed, the nurse marks the tube with indelible ink or tape at its exit point from the nose and documents the length of visible tubing for baseline data. The nurse is responsible, however, for verifying tube placement (i.e., gastrointestinal placement versus respiratory placement) before each intermittent feeding and at regular intervals (e.g., at least once per shift) when continuous feedings are being administered.

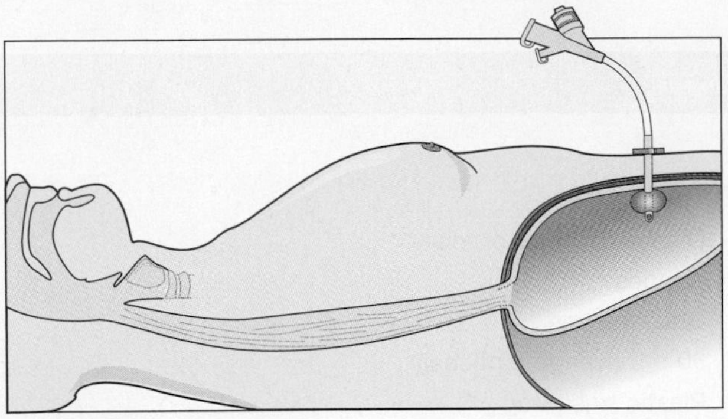

FIGURE 39.15 Percutaneous endoscopic gastrostomy (PEG) tube

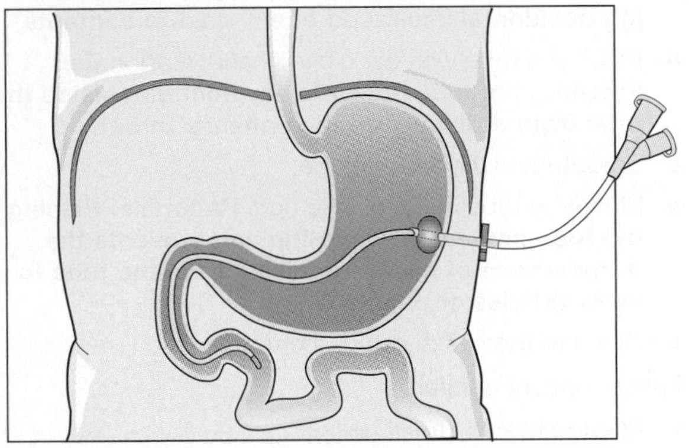

FIGURE 39.16 Percutaneous endoscopic jejunostomy (PEJ) tube

Methods nurses use to check tube placement include the following:

1. Aspirating gastrointestinal secretions. Small-bore tubes offer more resistance during aspirations than large-bore tubes and are more likely to collapse when negative pressure is applied. Gastric secretions tend to be grassy green, off white, or tan; intestinal fluid is stained with bile and is golden yellow or brownish green.
2. Measuring the pH of aspirated fluid. This is the recommended method to determine tube placement. Testing the pH of aspirates can help distinguish gastric from respiratory and intestinal placement (Metheny & Meert, 2004) as follows:
   - Gastric aspirates tend to be acidic and have a pH of 1 to 4 but may be as high as 6 if the patient is receiving medications that control gastric acid.
   - Small intestine aspirates generally have a pH equal to or higher than 6. Respiratory secretions are more alkaline, with values of 7 or higher. However, a slight possibility exists of respiratory placement when the pH reading is as low as 6. Therefore, when pH readings are 6 or higher, radiographic confirmation of tube location needs to be considered, especially in patients with diminished cough and gag reflexes.

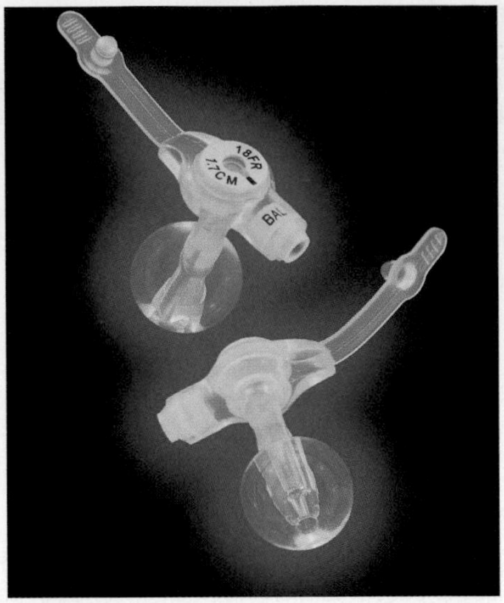

FIGURE 39.17 Low-profile gastrostomy feeding tube

3. Auscultating the epigastrium while injecting 5 mL to 20 mL of air. Air injected into the stomach produces whooshing, gurgling, or bubbling sounds over the epigastrium and the upper left quadrant. The accuracy of this method in confirming placement is less reliable than pH testing (American Association of Critical Care Nurses, 2005).
4. Confirming the length of tube insertion with the insertion mark. If more of the tube is now exposed, the position of the tip should be questioned.

Currently, the most effective method appears to be radiographic verification of tube placement. Repeated X-ray studies, however, are not feasible in terms of cost. More research is required to devise effective alternatives, especially for placement of small-bore tubes. In the meantime, nurses should (1) ensure initial radiographic verification of small-bore tubes, (2) aspirate contents when possible and check their acidity, (3) closely observe the patient for signs of obvious distress, and (4) consider tube dislodgment after episodes of coughing, sneezing, and vomiting.

ENTERAL FEEDINGS The type and frequency of feedings and amounts to be administered are ordered by the physician or the dietitian. Liquid feeding mixtures are available commercially or can be prepared by the dietary department in accordance with the physician's orders. A standard formula provides 1 kcal/mL of solution with protein, fat, carbohydrate, minerals, and vitamins in specified proportions.

Enteral feedings can be given intermittently or continuously. **Intermittent feedings** are the administration of 300 mL to 500 mL of enteral formula several times per day. The stomach is the preferred site for these feedings, which are usually administered over at least 30 minutes. Bolus intermittent feedings are those that use a syringe to deliver the formula into the stomach. Because the formula is delivered rapidly by this method, it is not usually recommended but can be used in long-term situations if the patient tolerates it. These feedings must be given only into the stomach; the patient must be monitored closely for distension and aspiration.

Continuous feedings are generally administered over 24 hours by using an infusion pump that guarantees a constant flow rate (Figure 39.18). Continuous feedings are essential when feedings are administered in the small bowel. They are also used when smaller-bore gastric tubes are in place or when gravity flow is insufficient to instill the feeding.

Cyclic feedings are continuous feedings that are administered in less than 24 hours (e.g., 12 to 16 hours). These feedings, often administered at night and referred to as nocturnal feedings, allow the patient to attempt to eat regular meals through the day. Because nocturnal feedings may use higher nutrient densities and faster infusion rates than the standard continuous feeding, particular attention needs to be given to monitoring fluid status and circulating volume overload.

Enteral feedings are administered to patients through open or closed systems. **Open systems** use an open-top container or a syringe (without plunger) for administration. Enteral feedings for use with open systems are provided in flip-top cans or powdered formulas that are reconstituted with sterile water. Sterile water, rather than tap water, is used to reduce the risk of microbial contamination. Open systems should have no more than 8 to 12 hours of formula poured into them. At the end of that time, the remaining formula should be discarded and the container rinsed before new formula is poured. In some institutions, the bag and tubing are discarded after 24 hours. **Closed systems** consist of a prefilled container that is spiked with enteral tubing and attached to the enteral access device. Prefilled containers generally have 1 L of formula and can hang safely for 24 to 48 hours if sterile technique is used.

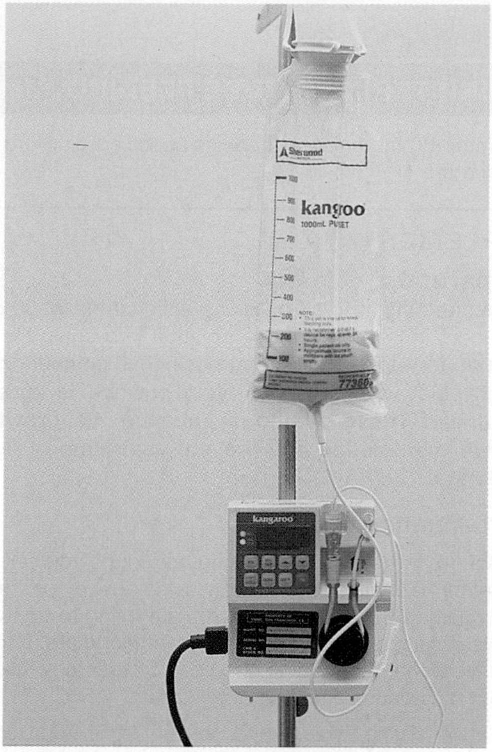

FIGURE 39.18 An enteric feeding pump

Skill 39.4 provides the essential steps involved in administering a tube feeding, and Skill 39.5 indicates the steps involved in administering a gastrostomy or jejunostomy tube feeding.

SKILL 39.4

ADMINISTERING A TUBE FEEDING

PURPOSES

- To restore or maintain nutritional status
- To administer medications

ASSESSMENT

Assess for the following:

- Any clinical signs of malnutrition or dehydration
- Allergies to any ingredient in the feeding; if the patient is lactose intolerant, check the tube feeding formula; notify the physician or dietitian if any incompatibilities exist
- The presence of bowel sounds
- Any problems that suggest lack of tolerance of previous feedings (e.g., delayed gastric emptying, abdominal distension, diarrhea, cramping, or constipation)

Planning

Before commencing a tube feeding, determine the type, amount, and frequency of feedings and tolerance of previous feedings.

Equipment

- Correct type and amount of feeding solution
- 60 mL catheter-tip syringe
- Emesis basin
- Clean gloves
- pH test strip or meter
- Large syringe or calibrated plastic feeding bag with label and tubing that can be attached to the feeding tube or prefilled bottle with a drip chamber, tubing, and a flow-regulator clamp
- Measuring container from which to pour the feeding (if using open system)

(continued)

SKILL 39.4

ADMINISTERING A TUBE FEEDING *(continued)*

- Water (60 mL unless otherwise specified) at room temperature
- Feeding pump as required

IMPLEMENTATION

Preparation

Assist the patient to a Fowler's position (at least 30 degrees elevation) in bed or a sitting position in a chair, the normal position for eating. If a sitting position is contraindicated, a slightly elevated right side-lying position is acceptable. **Rationale: These positions enhance the gravitational flow of the solution and prevent aspiration of fluid into the lungs.**

Performance

1. Before performing the feeding, introduce yourself and verify the patient's identity by using agency protocol. Explain to the patient what you are going to do, why it is necessary, and how he or she can cooperate. Inform the patient that the feeding should not cause any discomfort but may cause a feeling of fullness.
2. Perform hand hygiene and observe other appropriate infection prevention and control procedures (e.g., clean gloves).
3. Provide privacy for this procedure if the patient desires it. Tube feedings are embarrassing to some people.
4. Assess tube placement.
   - Attach the syringe to the open end of the tube and aspirate. Check the pH.
   - Allow 1 hour to elapse before testing the pH if the patient has received a medication.
   - Use a pH meter rather than pH paper if the patient is receiving a continuous feeding. Follow agency policy if the pH is greater than 6.
5. Assess residual feeding contents.
   - If the tube is placed in the stomach, aspirate all contents and measure the amount before administering the feeding. **Rationale: This is done to evaluate absorption of the last feeding; that is, whether undigested formula from a previous feeding remains. If the tube is in the small intestine, residual contents cannot be aspirated.**
   - If 100 mL (or more than half the last feeding) is withdrawn, check with the nurse in charge, or refer to agency policy before proceeding. The precise amount is usually determined by the physician's order or by agency policy. Recheck in 3 to 4 hours. **Rationale: At some agencies, a feeding is delayed when the specified amount or more of formula remains in the stomach. The feeding rate may need to be adjusted if gastric emptying is delayed.**
   - *Or* reinstill the gastric contents into the stomach if this is the agency policy or health-care provider's order. **Rationale: Removal of the contents could disturb the patient's electrolyte balance.**
   - If the patient is on a continuous feeding, check the gastric residual every 4 to 6 hours or according to agency protocol.
6. Administer the feeding.
   - Before administering the feeding, check the expiration date of the feeding. Warm the feeding to room temperature. **Rationale: An excessively cold feeding can cause abdominal cramps.**
   - When an open system is used, clean the top of the feeding container with alcohol before opening it. **Rationale: This minimizes the risk of contaminants entering the feeding syringe or feeding bag.**

Feeding Bag (Open System)

- Hang the labelled bag from an infusion pole about 30 cm above the tube's point of insertion into the patient.
- Clamp the tubing and add the formula to the bag.
- Open the clamp, run the formula through the tubing, and reclamp the tube. **Rationale: The formula will displace the air in the tubing, thus preventing the instillation of excess air into the patient's stomach or intestine.**
- Attach the bag to the feeding tube (see ❶) and regulate the drip by adjusting the clamp to the drop factor on the bag (e.g., 20 drops/mL) if not placed on a pump.

Syringe (Open System)

- Remove the plunger from the syringe and connect the syringe to a pinched or clamped nasogastric tube. **Rationale: Pinching or clamping the tube prevents excess air from entering the stomach and causing distension.**
- Add the feeding to the syringe barrel (see ❷).
- Permit the feeding to flow in slowly at the prescribed rate. Raise or lower the syringe to adjust the flow as needed. Pinch or clamp the tubing to stop the flow for a

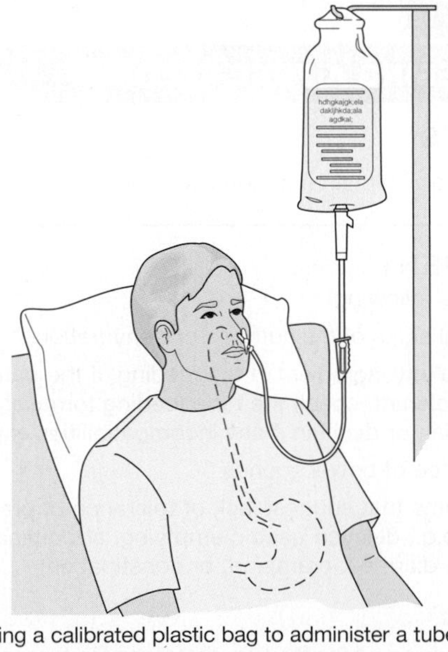

❶ Using a calibrated plastic bag to administer a tube feeding

(continued)

SKILL 39.4

ADMINISTERING A TUBE FEEDING (*continued*)

minute if the patient experiences discomfort. **Rationale: Quickly administered feedings can cause flatus, cramps, or vomiting.**

Prefilled Bottle with Drip Chamber (Closed System)

- Gently shake the prefilled bottle to ensure the contents have not separated. Remove the screw-on cap from the container and attach the administration set with the drip chamber and tubing (see ❸).
- Close the clamp on the tubing.
- Hang the container on an intravenous pole about 30 cm above the tube's insertion point into the patient. **Rationale: At this height, the formula should run at a safe rate into the stomach or intestine.**
- Squeeze the drip chamber to fill it to one-third to one-half of its capacity.
- Open the tubing clamp, run the formula through the tubing, and reclamp the tube. **Rationale: The formula will displace the air in the tubing, thus preventing the instillation of excess air.**
- Attach the feeding set tubing to the feeding tube and regulate the drip rate to deliver the feeding over the desired length of time, or attach to a feeding pump.

7. When the feeding is finished, and if another bottle is not to be immediately hung, flush the feeding tube before all the formula has run through the tubing.
  - Instill 50 mL to 100 mL of water through the feeding tube or medication port. **Rationale: Water flushes the lumen of the tube, preventing future blockage by sticky formula.**
  - Be sure to add the water before the feeding solution has drained from the neck of a syringe or from the tubing of an administration set. **Rationale: Adding the water before the syringe or tubing is empty prevents the instillation of air into the stomach or intestine and thus prevents unnecessary distension.**

8. Clamp the feeding tube. Remove the tubing of the administration set between feedings.
  - Clamp the feeding tube before all the water is instilled. **Rationale: Clamping prevents leakage and air from entering the tube if done before water is instilled.**

9. Ensure patient comfort and safety.
  - Secure the tubing to the patient's gown. **Rationale: This minimizes pulling of the tube, thus preventing discomfort and dislodgment.**
  - Ask the patient to remain sitting upright in Fowler's position or in a slightly elevated right lateral position for at least 30 minutes. **Rationale: These positions facilitate digestion and movement of the feeding from the stomach along the alimentary tract and prevent the potential aspiration of the feeding into the lungs.**
  - Check the agency's policy on the frequency of changing the nasogastric tube and the use of smaller lumen tubes if a large-bore tube is in place. **Rationale: These measures prevent irritation and erosion of the pharyngeal and esophageal mucous membranes.**

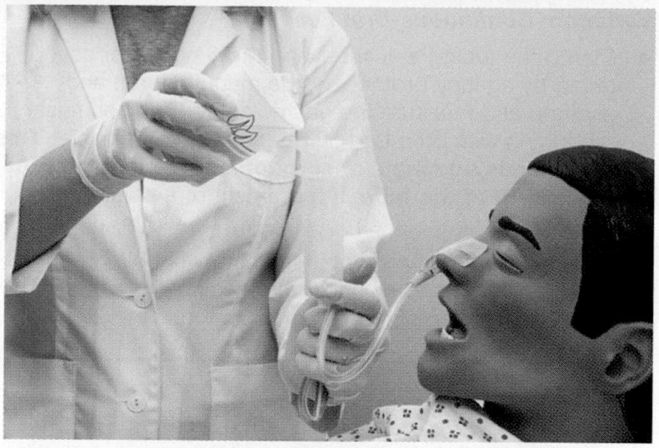

❷ Using the barrel of a syringe to administer a tube feeding

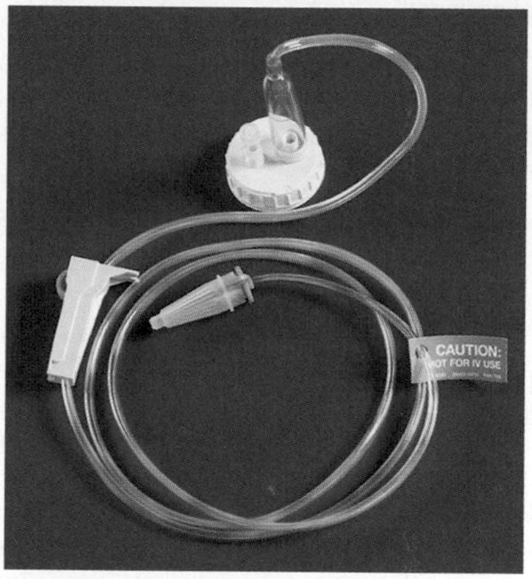

❸ Feeding set tubing with drip chamber

10. Dispose of equipment appropriately.
  - If the equipment is to be reused, wash it thoroughly with soap and water so that it is ready for reuse.
  - Change the equipment every 24 hours or according to agency policy.

11. Document all relevant information.
  - Document the feeding, including amount and kind of solution taken, duration of the feeding, and assessments of the patient.
  - Record the volume of the feeding and water administered on the patient's intake and output record.

12. Monitor the patient for possible problems.
  - Carefully assess patients receiving tube feedings for problems.
  - To prevent dehydration, give the patient supplemental water in addition to the prescribed tube feeding as ordered. The quantity of water to administer will be determined by physician or dietitian orders in some cases, or by agency policy.

(*continued*)

SKILL 39.4

ADMINISTERING A TUBE FEEDING (*continued*)

Variation: Continuous-Drip Feeding

- Clamp the tubing at least every 4 to 6 hours, or as indicated by agency protocol or the manufacturer, and aspirate and measure the gastric contents. Then flush the tubing with 30 mL to 50 mL of water. **Rationale: This determines adequate absorption and verifies correct placement of the tube.** If placement of a small-bore tube is questionable, a repeat X-ray should be done.
- Determine agency protocol regarding withholding a feeding. Many agencies withhold the feeding if more than 75 mL to 100 mL of feeding is aspirated.
- To prevent spoilage or bacterial contamination, do not allow a feeding solution in an open system to hang longer than 8 to 12 hours. A closed-bottle feeding may be able to hang for 24 to 48 hours. *Check agency policy or manufacturer's recommendations regarding time limits.*
- Follow agency policy regarding how frequently to change the feeding bag and tubing. Changing the feeding bag and tubing every 24 hours reduces the risk of contamination.

EVALUATION

Perform a follow-up examination of the following:

- Tolerance of feeding (e.g., nausea, cramping, gastric residual)
- Bowel sounds
- Regurgitation and feelings of fullness after feedings
- Weight gain or loss
- Fecal elimination pattern (e.g., diarrhea, flatulence, constipation)
- Skin turgor
- Urine output and specific gravity
- Glucose and acetone in urine
- Serum electrolytes, including potassium and sodium

Relate findings to previous assessment data if available. Report significant deviations from normal to the appropriate members of the health-care team.

CLINICAL ALERT

Do not add coloured food dye to tube feedings. Previously, blue dye was often added to assist in recognition of aspiration. However, Health Canada reports cases of adverse reactions to the dye, including toxicity and death.

SKILL 39.5

ADMINISTERING A GASTROSTOMY OR JEJUNOSTOMY FEEDING

PURPOSES

See Skill 39.4.

ASSESSMENT

See Skill 39.4

Planning

Before commencing a gastrostomy or jejunostomy feeding, determine the type and amount of feeding to be instilled, frequency of feedings, and any pertinent information about previous feedings (e.g., the position in which the patient best tolerates the feeding).

Equipment

- Correct amount of feeding solution
- Graduated container and tubing with clamp to hold the feeding
- 60 mL catheter-tip syringe

For a Tube That Remains in Place

- Mild soap and water
- Clean gloves
- Petrolatum, zinc oxide ointment, or other skin protectant
- Precut 10 cm × 10 cm gauze squares
- Uncut 10 cm × 10 cm gauze squares

For Tube Insertion

- Clean gloves
- Moisture-proof bag
- Water-soluble lubricant
- Feeding tube (if needed)

(continued)

SKILL 39.5

ADMINISTERING A GASTROSTOMY OR JEJUNOSTOMY FEEDING *(continued)*

IMPLEMENTATION

Preparation

See Skill 39.4.

Performance

1. Before performing the feeding, introduce yourself and verify the patient's identity by using agency protocol. Explain to the patient what you are going to do, why it is necessary, and how he or she can cooperate. Discuss how the results will be used in planning further care or treatments.
2. Perform hand hygiene and observe other appropriate infection prevention and control procedures (e.g., clean gloves).
3. Provide for patient privacy.
4. Assess and prepare the patient. See Skill 39.4.
5. Insert a feeding tube, if one is not already in place.
   - While wearing gloves, remove the dressing. Then discard the dressing and gloves in the moisture-proof bag.
   - Apply new clean gloves.
   - Lubricate the end of the tube, and insert it into the ostomy opening 10 cm to 15 cm.
6. Check the location and patency of a tube that is already in place.
   - Determine correct placement of the tube by aspirating secretions and checking the pH.
   - Follow agency policy for amount of residual formula. This may include withholding the feeding, rechecking in 3 to 4 hours, or notifying the health-care provider if a large residual remains.
   - For continuous feedings, check the residual every 4 to 6 hours and hold feedings according to agency policy.
   - Remove the syringe plunger. Pour 15 mL to 30 mL of water into the syringe, remove the tube clamp, and allow the water to flow into the tube. **Rationale: This determines the patency of the tube. If water flows freely, the tube is patent.**
   - If the water does not flow freely, notify the nurse in charge and the physician.
7. Administer the feeding.
   - Hold the barrel of the syringe 7 cm to 15 cm above the ostomy opening.
   - Slowly pour the solution into the syringe and allow it to flow through the tube by gravity.
   - Just before all the formula has run through and the syringe is empty, add 30 mL of water. **Rationale: Water flushes the tube and preserves its patency.**
   - If the tube is to remain in place, hold it upright, remove the syringe, and then clamp or plug the tube to prevent leakage.
   - If a catheter was inserted for the feeding, remove it.
8. Ensure patient comfort and safety.
   - After the feeding, ask the patient to remain in the sitting position or a slightly elevated right lateral position for at least 30 minutes. **Rationale: This minimizes the risk of aspiration.**
   - Assess status of peristomal skin. **Rationale: Gastric or jejunal drainage contains digestive enzymes that can irritate the skin. Document any redness and broken skin areas.**
   - Check orders about cleaning the peristomal skin, applying a skin protectant, and applying appropriate dressings. Generally, the peristomal skin is washed with mild soap and water at least once daily. The tube may be rotated between thumb and forefinger to release any sticking and promote tract formation. Petrolatum, zinc oxide ointment, or other skin protectant can be applied around the stoma, and precut 10 cm × 10 cm gauze squares can be placed around the tube. The precut squares are then covered with regular 10 cm × 10 cm gauze squares, and the tube is coiled over them.
   - Observe for common complications of enteral feedings: aspiration, hyperglycemia, abdominal distension, diarrhea, and fecal impaction. Report findings to the appropriate members of the health-care team. Often, a change in formula or rate of administration can correct problems.
   - When appropriate, teach the patient how to administer feedings and when to notify the health-care provider concerning problems.
9. Document all assessments and interventions.

Variation

The feeding can also be administered with a feeding bag or with a prefilled bottle with a drip chamber. See Skill 39.4.

EVALUATION

See Skill 39.4.

Before administering a tube feeding, the nurse must determine if the patient has any food allergies and assess tolerance to previous feedings. Table 39.8 lists essential assessments to conduct before administering tube feedings. The nurse must also check the expiration date on a commercially prepared formula or the preparation date and time of agency-prepared solution, discarding any formula that has passed the expiration date or that was prepared more than 24 hours previously.

Lifespan Considerations

Administering a Tube Feeding

INFANTS

- Feeding tubes may be reinserted at each feeding to prevent irritation of the mucous membrane, nasal airway obstruction, and stomach perforation, which can occur if the tube is left in place continuously. Check agency practice.

CHILDREN

- Position a small child or infant in your lap, provide a pacifier, and hold and cuddle the child during feedings. This promotes comfort, supports the normal sucking instinct of the infant, and facilitates digestion.

OLDER ADULTS

- Physiological changes associated with aging may make older adults more vulnerable to complications associated with enteral feedings. Decreased gastric emptying may necessitate checking frequently for gastric residual. Diarrhea from administering the feeding too fast or at too high a concentration can cause dehydration. If the feeding has a high concentration of glucose, assess for hyperglycemia. Because with aging, the body has a decreased ability to handle increased glucose levels.
- Such conditions as a hiatal hernia and diabetes mellitus may cause the stomach to empty more slowly. This delay increases the risk of aspiration in a patient receiving a tube feeding. Checking for gastric residual more frequently can help document this if it is an ongoing problem. Changing the formula or the rate of administration, repositioning the patient, or obtaining a physician's order for a medication to increase stomach emptying may resolve this problem.

Feedings are usually administered at room temperature unless the order specifies otherwise. The nurse warms the specified amount of solution in a basin of warm water or leaves it to stand until it reaches room temperature. Because a formula that is warmed can grow microorganisms, it should not hang longer than the manufacturer recommends. Continuous feeding should be kept cold; excessive heat coagulates feedings of milk and egg, and hot liquids can irritate the mucous membranes. However, excessively cold feedings can reduce the flow of digestive juices by causing vasoconstriction and may cause cramps.

Enteral feedings may be continued beyond hospital care in the client's home or may be initiated in the home. Guidelines for teaching clients and families about administration of tube feedings in the home are found in the Teaching: Home Care box. Box 39.13 summarizes the risks associated with enteral feeding.

ADMINISTERING MEDICATION THROUGH A FEEDING TUBE Medication that is normally taken by mouth may be administered via the nasoenteric tube if the patient cannot swallow. In most cases, medication in pill form will be crushed and mixed with a small amount of water and then inserted into the feeding tube. In other cases,

TABLE 39.8 Assessing Patients Receiving Tube Feedings

Assessment	Rationale
Allergies to any food in the feeding	Common allergenic foods include milk, eggs, and vegetable oil.
Bowel sounds before each feeding or, for continuous feedings, every 4 to 8 hours	To determine intestinal activity (peristalsis).
Abdominal distension; at least daily, measure abdominal girth at the umbilicus	Abdominal distension can indicate intolerance to a previous feeding.
Correct placement of tube, before feedings	To prevent aspiration of feedings.
Presence of regurgitation and feelings of fullness after feedings	May indicate delayed gastric emptying, need to decrease quantity or rate of the feeding, or high-fat content of the formula.
Dumping syndrome: nausea, vomiting, diarrhea, cramps, pallor, sweating, heart palpitations, increased pulse rate, and fainting after a feeding	Jejunostomy clients may experience these symptoms, which result when hypertonic foods and liquids suddenly distend the jejunum. To make the intestinal contents isotonic, body fluids shift rapidly from the client's vascular system.
Diarrhea, constipation, or flatulence	The lack of bulk in liquid feedings may cause constipation. The presence of hypertonic or concentrated ingredients may cause diarrhea and flatulence.
Urine for sugar and acetone	Hyperglycemia may occur if the sugar content is too high.
Hematocrit and urine specific gravity	Both increase as a result of dehydration.
Serum BUN and sodium levels	Feeding formula may have a high protein content. If a high protein intake is combined with an inadequate fluid intake, the kidneys may not be able to excrete nitrogenous wastes adequately.

TEACHING: HOME CARE

Tube Feedings

Clients and caregivers need guidance to manage these feedings in the home:

- *Preparation of the formula.* Include the name of the formula and how much and how often it is to be given; the need to inspect the formula for expiration date and leaks and cracks in bags or cans; how to mix or prepare the formula, if needed; and aseptic techniques, such as swabbing the container's top with alcohol before opening it, and changing the syringe administration set and reservoir every 24 hours.
- *Proper storage of the formula.* Include the need to refrigerate diluted or reconstituted formula and formula that contains additives.
- *Administration of the feeding.* Include proper hand hygiene and how to fill and hang the feeding bag. Discuss strategies for hanging formula containers if an IV pole is not available or is inconvenient. Review the operation of an infusion pump, if indicated; the feeding rate; and client positioning during and after the feeding. Plan for optimal timing of feedings to allow for daily activities. Many clients can tolerate having the majority of their feedings run during sleep so they are free from the equipment during the day.
- *Management of the enteral access device.* Teach and explain to the client or caregiver the rationale for how to assess for tube placement by using pH measurement before administering the feeding. Instruct regarding actions to take if the pH is greater than 6. Include site care, aseptic precautions, dressing change, as indicated, how the site should look normally, and flushing protocols (e.g., type of irrigant and schedule).
- *Daily monitoring needs.* Include temperature, weight, and intake and output.
- *Signs and symptoms of complications to report.* Include fever, increased respiratory rate, decrease in urine output, increased stool frequency, and altered level of consciousness.
- *Whom to contact regarding questions or problems.* Include emergency telephone numbers of home care agency, nursing clinician or physician, or other 24-hour on-call emergency number.

medication may be available in liquid form from the pharmacy. In all cases, it is important to flush the feeding tube with an adequate amount of water (at least 30 mL) after administration to prevent clogging (Dickerson, Tidwell, & Brown, 2003). When administering medication via a feeding tube, the nurse must take additional precautions to ensure patient safety:

- Ensure that the medication can be crushed. Enteric-coated extended-release formulations and cytotoxic drugs should not be crushed (Cornish, 2005). Consult the physician and pharmacist to determine whether an alternative formulation or administration route is available.
- Verify that the medication is compatible with the feeding solution. For example, Dilantin (phenytoin), an antiseizure medication, cannot be administered when a feeding solution is running, as absorption of the drug will be decreased. If the patient is on continuous feeds, an alternative route must be considered or the feed must be held for 1 to 2 hours before and after drug administration (Dickerson, Tidwell, & Brown, 2003).
- Use a clean mortar and pestle when crushing pills and ensure they are ground up to a fine powder so that larger pieces will not block the tube. Administer only one crushed pill at a time and flush with water between each one.
- Administer medication mixed only in water. Do not mix medication directly into feeding solution before administration.

MANAGING CLOGGED FEEDING TUBES Even if feeding tubes are flushed with water before and after feedings and medications, they can still become clogged. This blockage can occur when the feeding container runs dry, solid medication is not adequately crushed, or medications are mixed with formula. Even the important practice of aspirating to check residual volume increases the incidence of clogging (Reising & Neal, 2005). To avoid the necessity of removing the tube and reinserting

BOX 39.13 RISKS ASSOCIATED WITH ENTERAL FEEDINGS

Risk	Complication
Insertion of nasogastric tube	Damage to nose and sinuses, placement within intracranial space, bleeding of esophageal varices, bronchial/laryngeal placement, perforation of pharynx, esophagus
Insertion of PEG/PEJ	Perforation of colon or stomach, bleeding
Postinsertion complications	Pain, fistulae, erosion of nasal tissues, intestinal strictures
Reflux of gastrointestinal contents	Aspiration, gastroesophageal reflux
Displacement of tube	Patient removal of tube, tube falls out, bronchial or peritoneal administration of feeding
GI intolerance	Nausea, vomiting, diarrhea, abdominal distention
Metabolic complication	Hyperglycemia, electrolyte imbalance, fluid overload

Source: "Guidelines for Enteral Feeding in Adult Hospital Patients," by M. A. Stroud, H. Duncan, and J. Nightingale, 2003, *GUT, 52*(7), pp. vii1–vii12.

a new tube, both prevention and intervention strategies must be used.

To prevent clogged feeding tubes, flush liberally (at least 30 mL water) before, between, and after each separate medication is instilled, by using a 60 mL piston syringe. The larger the barrel of the syringe, the less the pressure exerted. Too great a pressure can rupture the tube, especially small-bore feeding tubes. Do not add medications to formula or to each other.

Many strategies have been used to try to unclog feeding tubes. Strategies that have shown inconsistent effectiveness include instilling meat tenderizer, carbonated beverages, or cranberry juice, or flushing with small barrel syringes with or without digestive enzymes, such as papain or chymotrypsin (Reising & Neal, 2005).

The first strategy that should be tried is to reposition the patient (this may allow a kink to straighten). Alternately flush and aspirate the tube with water. One institution has had success with a hollow catheter that allows unclogging solution to be delivered as the catheter is advanced down the clogged tube (Smith & Myers, 2005).

Providing Parenteral Nutrition

Parenteral nutrition (PN), also referred to as *total parenteral nutrition* (TPN) or *intravenous hyperalimentation* (IVH), is provided when the gastrointestinal tract is nonfunctional because of an interruption in its continuity or because its absorptive capacity is impaired. Parenteral nutrition is administered intravenously through a central venous catheter into the superior vena cava.

Parenteral feedings are solutions of dextrose, water, fat, proteins, electrolytes, vitamins, and trace elements; it is the provision of all needed calories. Because TPN solutions are *hypertonic* (highly concentrated in comparison to the solute concentration of blood), they are injected only into high-flow central veins, where they are diluted by the patient's blood.

TPN is a means of achieving an anabolic state in patients who are unable to maintain a normal nitrogen balance. Such patients may include those with severe malnutrition, severe burns, bowel disease disorders (e.g., ulcerative colitis or enteric fistula), acute renal failure, hepatic failure, metastatic cancer, or major surgeries in which nothing can be taken by mouth for more than 5 days.

TPN is not risk free. Infection prevention and control is of utmost importance during TPN therapy. The nurse must always observe surgical aseptic technique when changing solutions, tubing, dressings, and filters. Patients are at increased risk of fluid, electrolyte, and glucose imbalances and require frequent evaluation and modification of the TPN mixture.

TPN solutions are a mixture of 10% to 50% dextrose in water, amino acids, and special additives, such as vitamins (e.g., B complex, C, D, K), minerals (e.g., potassium, sodium, chloride, calcium, phosphate, magnesium), and trace elements (e.g., cobalt, zinc, manganese). Additives are adapted to each patient's nutritional needs. Fat emulsions may be given to provide essential fatty acids to correct or prevent essential fatty acid deficiency or to supplement the calories for patients who, for example, have high-calorie needs or cannot tolerate glucose as the only calorie source. Note that 1000 mL of 5% glucose or dextrose contains 50 grams of sugar. Thus, a litre of this solution provides fewer than 200 calories!

Because TPN solutions are high in glucose, infusions are started gradually to prevent hyperglycemia. The patient needs to adapt to TPN therapy by increasing insulin output from the pancreas. For example, an adult patient may be given 1 L (40 mL/h) of TPN solution the first day; if the infusion is tolerated, the amount may be increased to 2 L (80 mL/h) for 24 to 48 hours, and then to 3 L (120 mL/h) within 3 to 5 days. Glucose levels are monitored during the infusion.

When TPN therapy is to be discontinued, the TPN infusion rates are decreased slowly to prevent hyperinsulinemia and hypoglycemia. Weaning a patient from TPN can take up to 48 hours but can occur in 6 hours as long as the patient receives adequate carbohydrates either orally or intravenously.

Evaluating

The goals established in the planning phase are evaluated according to specific desired outcomes also established in that phase. Examples of these are shown in Table 39.9.

If the outcomes are *not* achieved, the nurse should explore the reasons why. The nurse might consider the following questions:

- Was the cause of the problem correctly identified?
- Was the family included in the teaching plan? Are they supportive?
- Is the client experiencing symptoms that cause loss of appetite (e.g., pain, nausea, fatigue)?
- Were the outcomes unrealistic for this person?
- Were the client's food preferences considered?
- Is anything interfering with digestion or absorption of nutrients (e.g., vomiting, diarrhea)?

TABLE 39.9 Evaluation Goals and Outcomes

Goal	Examples of Desired Health Outcomes
Maintain or improve nutritional status	• Weight within normal range for height and body frame • Body mass index within expected range • Ingests recommended servings from *Eating Well with Canada's Food Guide* • Uses fats sparingly • Uses salt, sodium, sugars, and alcohol in moderation
Decrease weight	• Identifies factors contributing to excess weight (or risk of excess weight) • Monitors eating habits for specified period (e.g., 1 week) and identifies behaviours that need to be modified to lose weight (or prevent weight gain) • Chooses and ingests a diet that reduces daily caloric intake (e.g., reduces calories by 500 per day for each 0.5 kg of weight loss desired per week) • Establishes a physical activity program of 20 to 30 minutes duration at least three times per week • Loses prescribed amount of weight (specify) • Verbalizes improvement in feelings about self and satisfaction with support provided
Regain specified weight	• Identifies factors contributing to inadequate nutritional intake • Identifies necessary dietary alterations and foods high in needed nutrients (e.g., calcium, iron, protein, total calories) • Consumes a well-balanced diet to restore deficient nutrients • Demonstrates decrease (or absence) of signs of malnutrition, as evidenced by: a. Weight gain of specified kilograms per week b. Skin-fold measurements or 80 percent of the standard measurement c. Reports of increased energy (specify) d. Hemoglobin, serum albumin or prealbumin, serum transferrin, and lymphocyte counts within normal ranges

Case Study 39

Mrs. Fai Lee, from Vancouver, is a 75-year-old woman who has recently been diagnosed with chronic lung disease, which has left her very susceptible to pneumonia. As a result, her physician has ordered three different oral medications that have resulted in her losing her appetite and suffering a 10-kilogram weight loss. Once overweight, Mrs. Lee is now within weight standards for her age and height. Mrs. Lee tells her visiting nurse, "Nothing sounds good and nothing tastes good. Meat is particularly distasteful to me right now." Mrs. Lee lives alone and is responsible for her own meal preparation.

Critical Thinking Skills

1. How do Mrs. Lee's age and health status affect her nutritional needs?
2. What further information do you need regarding Mrs. Lee's present diet?
3. What alternatives can you offer while Mrs. Lee is unable to tolerate meat?
4. Offer suggestions for ways to enhance Mrs. Lee's intake during this period of decreased appetite.
5. Do you think that Mrs. Lee is a good candidate for a feeding tube? Why, or why not?

After working through these questions, go to the MyNursingLab at http://www.mynursinglab.com to check your answers.

KEY TERMS

nutrition
nutrients
nutritive value
metabolism
anabolism
catabolism
macronutrients
micronutrients
monosaccharides
disaccharides
polysaccharides
fibre
insoluble fibre
soluble fibre
enzymes

insulin
glycogen
glucogenesis
glucagon
essential amino acids
nonessential amino acids
complete protein
partially complete protein
incomplete protein
complementary protein
nitrogen balance
lipids
fatty acids
saturated fatty acids
unsaturated fatty acids
monounsaturated fatty acids
polyunsaturated fatty acids
transfats
essential fatty acids
omega-3 fatty acids
omega-6 fatty acids
triglyceride
phospholipid
sterols
cholesterol
lipoprotein
low-density lipoprotein (LDL)
high-density lipoprotein (HDL)
vitamin
water-soluble vitamin
fat-soluble vitamin
mineral
macromineral
micromineral
dietary reference intakes
recommended dietary allowance
adequate intake
tolerable upper intake level
estimated average requirement
caloric value
calorie
small calorie
large calorie (kilocalorie)
kilojoule
basal metabolic rate (BMR)
resting energy expenditure (REE)
Glycemic Index (GI)
glycemic level
hypoglycemia
hyperglycemia
hyperinsulinemia
insulin resistance
metabolic syndrome
fad
anorexia
dysphagia
lactose intolerance (lactose maldigestion)
demand feeding
regurgitation
iron-deficiency anemia
bottle-mouth syndrome
anorexia nervosa
bulimia nervosa
malnutrition
undernutrition
overnutrition
overweight
obese
body mass index (BMI)
ideal body weight (IBW)
protein-calorie malnutrition
24-hour food recall
food frequency record
food diary
diet history
usual body weight
weight change
waist circumference
hip circumference
waist-to-hip ratio
urea
nothing per ora (NPO)
clear liquid diet
full liquid diet
soft diet
pureed diet
diet as tolerated
anaphylaxis
parenteral nutrition
enteral nutrition
total enteral nutrition
nasogastric tube
nasoenteric tube
gastrostomy
jejunostomy
percutaneous endoscopic gastrostomy (PEG)
percutaneous endoscopic jejunostomy (PEJ)
intermittent feeding
continuous feeding
cyclic feeding
open systems
closed systems

CHAPTER HIGHLIGHTS

- Although people are continually bombarded with information about what to eat and what not to eat, each person is responsible for selecting foods that provide essential nutrients. Nurses can assist people to evaluate the information they receive about nutrients.
- Essential nutrients are grouped into six categories: water, carbohydrates, fats, proteins, vitamins, and minerals.
- Nutrients serve three basic purposes: forming body structures (such as bones and blood), providing energy, and helping to regulate the body's biochemical reactions.
- Energy balance is the relationship between the energy derived from food and the energy used by the body.
- The amount of energy that nutrients or foods supply to the body is their caloric value. The amount of energy required to maintain basic body functions is referred to as the resting energy expenditure (REE). The basal metabolic rate (BMR) is the rate at which the body metabolizes food to maintain the energy and requirements of a person who is awake and at rest.
- A person's state of energy balance can be determined by comparing caloric intake with caloric expenditure.

- Ideal body weight (IBW) is the weight recommended for optimal health.
- Body mass index (BMI) is one indicator of changes in body fat stores and whether a person's weight is appropriate for height, and it may provide a useful estimate of nutrition.
- Factors influencing a person's nutrition include development, gender, ethnicity and culture, beliefs about foods, personal preferences, religious practices, lifestyle, economics, medications and medical therapy, health status, alcohol consumption, advertising, and psychological factors, such as stress, isolation, and depression.
- Nutritional needs vary considerably according to age, growth, and energy requirements. Adolescents have high energy requirements because of their rapid growth; a diet plentiful in milk, meats, green and yellow vegetables, and fresh fruits is required. Older adults often need to reduce their caloric intake because of decreases in metabolic rate and activity levels. Fats, sugary foods, and sodium must often be limited.
- The prevalence of obese and overweight Canadians of all ages is increasing dramatically. The long-term effects of certain nutrient excesses are among the many factors involved in certain diseases, such as coronary artery disease, diabetes mellitus, hypertension, and cancer. Canadian nurses must be proactive in the fight against obesity.
- Various daily food guides have been developed to help healthy people meet the daily requirements of essential nutrients and to facilitate meal planning. This includes *Eating Well with Canada's Food Guide* and *Eating Well with Canada's Food Guide: First Nations, Inuit and Métis.*
- Both inadequate and excessive intakes of nutrients result in malnutrition. The effects of malnutrition can be general or specific, depending on which nutrients and what level of deficiency or excess are involved.
- Assessment of nutritional status may involve all or some of the following: nursing history data, nutritional screening, physical examination, calculation of the percentage of weight loss, a dietary history, anthropometric measurements, and laboratory data.
- Major goals for clients with or at risk for nutritional problems include the following: maintaining or restoring optimal nutritional status, decreasing or regaining specified weight, promoting healthy nutritional practices, and preventing complications associated with malnutrition.
- Assisting patients and support persons with therapeutic diets is a function shared by the nurse and the dietitian. The nurse reinforces the dietitian's instructions, assists the patient to make beneficial changes, and evaluates the patient's response to planned changes.
- Because many hospitalized patients have poor appetites, a major responsibility of the nurse is to provide nursing interventions that stimulate their appetites.
- Whenever possible, the nurse should help incapacitated patients to feed themselves; a number of self-feeding aids can help patients who have difficulty handling regular utensils.
- The nurse can refer clients to various community programs that help meet nutritional needs.
- Enteral feedings, administered through nasogastric, nasoenteric, gastrostomy, or jejunostomy tubes, are provided when the patient is unable to ingest foods or the upper gastrointestinal tract is impaired.
- A nasogastric or nasoenteric tube is used to provide enteral nutrition for short-term use (less than 6 weeks), while a gastrostomy or jejunostomy tube can be used to supply nutrients via the enteral route for long-term use.
- The use of feeding tubes for the administration of medication must be done judiciously by the nurse to avoid drug interaction and inappropriate dosing when sustained-release medications are crushed.
- Total parenteral nutrition (TPN), provided when the gastrointestinal tract is nonfunctional (e.g., absorptive capacity impaired), is given intravenously into a large central vein (e.g., the superior vena cava).

ASSESS YOUR LEARNING

1. A 36-year-old adult male reports eating the following each day, on average: 2 servings of milk and alternatives, 2 servings of fruit, 3 serving of vegetables, 3 servings of meat and alternatives, and 8 servings of grain products. When following the recommendations of *Eating Well with Canada's Food Guide*, the nurse would counsel the client to do which of the following?

a. Maintain the diet; the servings are adequate.

b. Increase the number of servings of milk and alternatives.

c. Increase the number of servings of vegetables and fruits.

d. Decrease the number of servings of grain products.

2. Which of the following are allowed on a full liquid diet?

1. Scrambled eggs
2. Chocolate pudding
3. Tomato juice
4. Hard candy
5. Mashed potatoes
6. Cream of Wheat cereal
7. Oatmeal cereal
8. Fruit smoothies

a. 2, 3, 4, 6, 8

b. 1, 3, 8

c. 1, 5, 6, 7

d. 3, 6, 8

3. Which of the following is the best indication of proper placement of a nasogastric tube in the stomach?

a. The client is able to speak and is not coughing.

b. A radiograph confirms placement in the stomach.

c. The pH of the aspirate is less than 5.

d. A whooshing noise is heard when air is injected into the tube and a stethoscope is placed over the epigastric area.

4. What is the proper technique for gravity tube feeding?

a. Hang the feeding bag 30 cm higher than the tube's insertion point into the client.

b. Administer the next feeding only if there is less than 25 mL of residual volume from the previous feeding.

c. Place the client in the left lateral position.

d. Administer the feeding directly after removing it from the refrigerator.

5. A 55-year-old female is about 9 kg more than her desired weight. She has been on a low-calorie diet with no improvement. Which of the following statements reflects a healthy approach to the desired weight loss?

a. "I need to engage in 30 to 60 minutes of moderate physical activity most days of the week."

b. "I need to switch to a low-carbohydrate, low-fat diet."

c. "I need to keep a list of my forbidden foods on hand and write down what I eat."

d. "I need to buy more organic and fewer processed foods."

6. A resident of a long-term-care facility has mild dysphagia from a recent stroke. The nurse plans the client's meals based on which of the following?

a. The need to have at least one serving of thickened milk and alternatives (e.g., pudding, ice cream) per meal

b. The need to eliminate the beer occasionally ingested on weekends

c. The need to include as many of the client's favourite foods as possible

d. The need to increase the calories from lipids to 40%

7. Two months ago a client weighed 88.4 kg. The client now weighs 82.5 kg. Calculate the client's percentage weight loss and determine its significance.

a. 6.7% not significant weight loss

b. 6.7% significant weight loss

c. 13.4% severe weight loss

d. 3.3% not significant weight loss

8. A 52-year-old man has a waist circumference of 106 cm. He is 180 cm tall and weighs 98 kg. What is this individual's risk status with respect to the development of cardiovascular disease, type 2 diabetes, and hypertension, given his BMI and waist circumference?

a. No increased risk

b. High risk

c. Very high risk

d. Extremely high risk

9. A 4-month-old infant should consume which of the following each day?

a. Breast milk only

b. Breast milk at night and cow's milk in a bottle when the infant is at daycare

c. Iron-fortified cereal 4 times a day with breast milk when the infant is hungry between meals

d. Iron-fortified cereal makes up the bulk of the calories consumed; the infant is breastfed if the mother desires

10. Mrs. Hassan, 38 years old, has been sent home with a gastric feeding tube. Her husband will be administering a bolus feeding every 6 hours. What is the most important consideration the nurse should teach Mr. Hassan when administering gastric feedings?

a. Flush the tube with water before and after feedings.

b. Ensure Mrs. Hassan is supine with the head of her bed raised.

c. Place Mrs. Hassan in a side-lying position.

d. Administer Mrs. Hassan's feedings rapidly.

After working through these questions, go to the MyNursingLab at ***http://www.mynursinglab.com*** *to check your answers and see explanations.*

SUGGESTED READINGS

Douketis, J. D., Paradis, G., Keller, H., & Martineau, C. (2005). Canadian guidelines for body weight classification in adults: Application in clinical practice to screen for overweight and obesity and to assess disease risk. *Canadian Medical Association Journal, 172*(8), 995–998.

This article reviews the application of the Canadian guidelines for body weight classification in adults and how they can be used in clinical practice to identify clients at risk of obesity-related health complications.

Lau, D. C., Douketis, J. D., Morrison, K. M., Hramiak, I. M. Sharma, A. M., & Ur, E. (2007). 2006 Canadian clinical practice guidelines on the management and prevention of obesity in adults and children [summary]. *Canadian Medical Association Journal, 176*(8), s1–s13.

Evidence-based recommendations for use by health-care professionals in the screening, prevention, and treatment of obesity.

Payette, H., & Shatenstein. B. (2006). Determinants of healthy eating in community-dwelling elderly people. *Canadian Journal of Public Health, 96*(Supplement iii), s27–s31.

Multiple factors determine the eating habits of older people in Canada. A systematic literature review has identified a clear dichotomy between financially stable older people living independently and those in poor health with limited resources. Suggestions for future research are offered.

Registered Nurses' Association of Ontario. (2005). *Primary prevention of childhood obesity.* Toronto: Author.

This document contains specific recommendations for the prevention of obesity in childhood and assumes an ecological approach, with interventions targeted at the community, school, family, and individual.

WEBLINKS

Dietitians of Canada

http://www.dietitians.ca

This site introduces the Dietitians of Canada and the services that it provides to its members and the public.

Health Canada: Food and Nutrition

http://www.hc-sc.gc.ca/fn-an/index_e.html

This site is sponsored by Health Canada and provides an introduction to public information on food and nutrition. The site also has a search tool and permits access to Canadian legislative policy, allergy alerts, and other federal resources.

Healthy Canadians: A Source for a Healthier Lifestyle

http://www.healthycanadians.ca

This site is operated by the Government of Canada and provides information on health-related promotional campaigns supported by Health Canada and the Public Health Agency of Canada. Canadians can find information about physical activity, healthy eating, and smoking cessation here.

Health Canada: Office of Nutrition Policy and Promotion

http://www.hc-sc.gc.ca/ahc-asc/branch-dirgen/hpfb-dgpsa/onpp-bppn/index_e.html

This site is operated by Health Canada. The Office of Nutrition Policy and Promotion promotes the nutritional health and well-being of Canadians by acting as a central hub for current, reliable nutrition information available online.

Canadian Diabetes Association

http://www.diabetes.ca

Operated by the Canadian Diabetes Association, this site contains valuable information for health-care providers and patients. The latest clinical guidelines for diabetes care are contained on this site.

Health Canada: Dietary References Intake Tables and Recommended Dietary Allowances

http://www.hc-sc.gc.ca/fn-an/nutrition/reference/table/index_e.html

This site lists the daily recommended intakes for vitamins, microminerals, and macrominerals, divided by sex and age.

REFERENCES

American Association of Critical Care Nurses. (2005). *Verification of feeding tube placement.* Retrieved September 25, 2007, from http://www.aacn.org/AACN/practiceAlert.nsf/Files/VOFTP/$file/Verification%20of%20Feeding%20Tube%20Placement%2005-2005.pdf

American Dietetic Association. (2003). *National dysphagia diet: Standardization for optimal care.* Chicago: Author.

Brown, T., Kelly, S., & Summerbell, C. (2007). Prevention of obesity: A review of interventions. *Obesity Reviews, 8* (Suppl. 1), 127–130.

Canadian Diabetes Association. (2008). *The glycemic index.* Retrieved November 3, 2008, from http://www.diabetes.ca/files/Diabetes_GL_FINAL2_CPG03.pdf

Canadian Hypertension Education Program. (2008). *2008 CHEP recommendations for the management of hypertension.* Ottawa: Author. Retrieved June 9, 2008, from http://hypertension.ca/chep/wp-content/uploads/2008/03/2008-chepspiral-booklet-final_jan28.pdf

Canadian Paediatric Society, Dietitians of Canada, & Health Canada. (2005). *Nutrition for healthy term infants.* Ottawa: Minister of Public Works and Government Services. Retrieved January 3, 2008, from http://www.hc-sc.gc.ca/fn-an/pubs/infant-nourrisson/nut_infant_nourrisson_term_e.html

Cole, T. J., Bellizzi, M. C., Flegal, K. M., & Dietz, W. H. (2000). Establishing a standard definition for child overweight and obesity worldwide: International survey. *British Medical Journal, 320*(7244), 1240–1243.

Cornish, P. (2005). "Avoid the crush": Hazards of medication administration in patients with dysphagia or a feeding tube. *Canadian Medical Association Journal, 172*(7), 871–872.

Dickerson, R. N., Tidwell, A. C., & Brown, R. O. (2003). Adverse effects from inappropriate medication administration via a jejunostomy feeding tube. *Nutrition in Clinical Practice, 18*(5), 402–405.

Dietitians of Canada. (2003). A new food guide for North American vegetarians. *Canadian Journal of Dietetic Practice, 64*(2), 81–86.

Dietitians of Canada. (2005). *Milk matters.* Retrieved January 3, 2008, from http://www.dietitians.ca/public/content/eat_well_live_well/english/faqs_tips_facts/fact_sheets/index.asp?fn=view&id=1159&idstring=1159

Engel, J. V. (2007). *The benefits of eating fibre.* Retrieved June 10, 2008, from http://www.diabetes.ca/Section_About/fibre.asp

Green, S. M., & Watson, R. (2006). Nutritional screening and assessment tools for use by nurses: Literature review. *Journal of Advanced Nursing, 54*(4), 477–490.

Health Canada. (2003). *Canadian guidelines for body weight classification in adults.* Retrieved May 2, 2007, from http://www.hc-sc.gc.ca/fn-an/alt_formats/hpfb-dgpsa/pdf/nutrition/weight_book-livres_des_poids_e.pdf

Health Canada. (2004). *Vitamin D supplement for breastfed infants.* Retrieved January 3, 2008, from http://www.hc-sc.gc.ca/fn-an/alt_formats/hpfb-dgpsa/pdf/nutrition/vita_d_supp_e.pdf

Health Canada. (2005). *Nutrition for healthy term infants—Statement of the joint working group: Canadian Paediatric Society, Dietitians of Canada and Health Canada.* Retrieved May 3, 2007, from http://www.hc-sc.gc.ca/fn-an/pubs/infant-nourrisson/nut_infant_nourrisson_term_e.html

Health Canada. (2006). *Dietary reference intakes.* Retrieved June 10, 2008, from http://www.hc-sc.gc.ca/fn-an/nutrition/reference/table/index_e.html#rve

Health Canada. (2007a). *Eating Well with Canada's Food Guide.* Retrieved January 8, 2008, from http://www.hc-sc.gc.ca/fn-an/food-guide-aliment/index_e.html

Health Canada. (2007b). *Eating Well with Canada's Food Guide: First Nations, Inuit and Métis.* Retrieved June 2, 2008, from http://www.hc-sc.gc.ca/fn-an/pubs/fnim-pnim/index_e.html

Health Canada. (2007c). *Mercury in fish.* Retrieved January 2, 2008, from http://www.hc-sc.gc.ca/fn-an/securit/chem-chim/mercur/cons-adv-etud_e.html

Health Canada. (2007d). *Food allergies and intolerances.* Retrieved June 9, 2008, from http://www.hc-sc.gc.ca/fn-an/securit/allerg/index-eng.php

Health Canada. (2008). *Healthy living: Sodium.* Retrieved June 12, 2008, from http://www.hc-sc.gc.ca/hl-vs/iyh-vsv/food-aliment/sodium-eng.php

Huffman, S., Jarczyk, K. S., O'Brien, E., Pieper, P., & Bayne, A. (2004). Methods to confirm feeding tube placement: Application of research to practice. *Pediatric Nursing, 30,* 10–13.

Katzmarzyk, P. T., & Janssen, I. (2004). The economic costs associated with physical inactivity and obesity in Canada: An update. *Canadian Journal of Applied Psychology, 29*(1), 90–115.

Krondl, M., Lau, D., Coleman, P., & Stocker, G. (2003). Tailoring of nutritional support for older adults in the community. *Journal of Nutrition for the Elderly, 23,* 17–32.

Lau, D. C., Douketis, J. D., Morrison, K. M., Hramiak, I. M., Sharma, A. M., & Ur, E. (2007). 2006 Canadian clinical practice guidelines on the management and prevention of obesity in adults and children [summary]. *Canadian Medical Association Journal, 176(8),* s1–s13.

Lengyel, C. O., Zello, G. A., Smith, J. T., & Whiting, S. J. (2003). Evaluation of menu and food service practices of long-term care facilities of a health district in Canada. *Journal of Nutrition for the Elderly, 22,* 29–42.

Masters, J. A. (2005). Moderate drinking and cardiovascular disease. *Annual Review of Nursing Research, 23,* 65–97.

Metheny, N. A., & Meert, K. L. (2004). Monitoring feeding tube placement. *Nutrition in Clinical Practice, 19,* 487–495.

NANDA International. (2007). *Nursing diagnoses: Definitions and classification, 2007–2008.* Philadelphia, PA: Author.

Ng, C., Marshall, D., & Willows, N. (2006). Obesity, adiposity, physical fitness and activity levels in Cree children. *International Journal of Circumpolar Health, 65*(4), 322–330.

Public Health Agency of Canada. (2003a). *Folic acid.* Retrieved April 25, 2007, from http://www.phac-aspc.gc.ca/fa-af/index.html

Public Health Agency of Canada. (2003b). *Handbook for Canada's physical activity guide to healthy active living.* Ottawa: Author. Retrieved July 6, 2008, from http://www.phac-aspc.gc.ca/pau-uap/fitness/pdf/handbook_e.pdf

Public Health Agency of Canada. (2007a). *Childhood obesity and the role of the government of Canada.* Retrieved October 5, 2007, from http://www.phac-aspc.gc.ca/ch-se/obesity/obesity-eng.html

Public Health Agency of Canada. (2007b). *Osteoporosis—Info-Sheet for seniors.* Retrieved January 3, 2008, from http://www.phac-aspc.gc.ca/seniors-aines/pubs/info_sheets/osteoporosis/pdf/osteo_e.pdf

Reising, D. L., & Neal, R. S. (2005). Enteral tube flushing: What you think are the best practices may not be. *American Journal of Nursing, 105*(3), 58–64.

Schettler, A. E., & Gustafson, E. M. (2004). Osteoporosis prevention starts in adolescence. *Journal of the American Academy of Nurse Practitioners, 16,* 274–282.

Shields, M. (2004). *Nutrition: Findings from the Canadian health survey. Issue no. 1. Measured obesity: Overweight children and adolescents.* Ottawa: Statistics Canada. Retrieved May 27, 2006, from http://www.statcan.ca/english/research/82-620-MIE/2005001/pdf/cobesity.pdf

Smith, R., & Myers, S. A. (2005). Two devices that unclog feeding tubes. *RN, 68*(1), 36–42.

Statistics Canada. (2005). Food insecurity. *Health Reports, 16*(3).

Wilding, J. P. H. (2007). Treatment strategies for obesity. *Obesity Reviews, 8*(Suppl. 1), 137–144.

Chapter 40

Fecal Elimination

The elimination of feces is a prominent public topic in North America. Laxative advertisements describing such feelings as tiredness caused by irregularity keep the subject in the public consciousness. Some older adults are preoccupied with their bowels. People who have had a bowel movement once a day for 75 years can view missing 1 day as a serious problem, even though they may not have eaten anything for 2 days and, thus, have little fecal matter to eliminate.

Nurses frequently are consulted or involved in assisting clients with elimination problems. These problems can be embarrassing to clients and can cause considerable discomfort.

OBJECTIVES

After studying this chapter, you should be able to

1. Describe the functions of the lower intestinal tract
2. Identify 11 factors that influence fecal elimination and patterns of defecation
3. Distinguish normal from abnormal characteristics and constituents of feces
4. Conduct a thorough assessment of fecal elimination
5. Differentiate five common fecal elimination problems
6. Identify common causes and effects of selected fecal elimination problems
7. List examples of nursing diagnoses, outcomes, and interventions for clients with elimination problems
8. Discuss five measures that promote regular defecation
9. Relate common interventions to specific fecal elimination problems
10. Describe essentials of stoma care for clients with fecal ostomies
11. State desired health outcomes essential for evaluating the client's progress

Physiology of Defecation

Elimination of the waste products of digestion from the body is essential to health. The excreted waste products are referred to as **feces** or **stool.**

Large Intestine

The large intestine extends from the ileocecal (ileocolic) valve, which lies between the small and large intestines, to the anus. The colon (large intestine) in the adult is generally about 125 cm to 150 cm long. It has seven parts: the cecum; ascending, transverse, and descending colons; sigmoid colon; rectum; and anus or external orifice (Figure 40.1).

The large intestine is a muscular tube lined with mucous membrane (Figure 40.2). The muscle fibres are both circular and longitudinal, permitting the intestine to enlarge and contract in both width and length. The longitudinal muscles are shorter than the colon and, therefore, cause the large intestine to form pouches, or **haustra.**

The colon's main functions are absorption of water and nutrients, mucal protection of the intestinal wall, and fecal elimination. The contents of the colon normally represent foods ingested over the previous 4 days, although most of the waste products are excreted within 48 hours of **ingestion** (the act of taking food). The digested products leaving the stomach through the small intestine and then passing through the ileocecal valve are called **chyme**. The ileocecal valve, located at the junction of the ileum of the small intestine and the first part of the large intestine, regulates the flow of chyme into the large intestine and prevents backflow into the ileum. The colon absorbs water and significant amounts of sodium and chloride as food passes along it. As much as 1500 mL of chyme passes into the large intestine daily, and all but about 100 mL is absorbed in the proximal half of the colon. The 100 mL of fluid is excreted in the feces.

The colon also serves a protective function in that it secretes mucus. This mucus contains large amounts of bicarbonate ions. The mucus secretion is stimulated by excitation of parasympathetic nerves. During extreme stimulation—for example, as a result of emotions—large amounts of mucus are secreted, resulting in the passage of stringy mucus with little or no feces. Mucus serves to protect the wall of the large intestine from trauma by the acids formed in the feces, and it serves as an adherent for holding the fecal material together. Mucus also protects the intestinal wall from bacterial activity.

The colon acts to transport along its lumen the products of digestion (flatus and feces), which are eventually eliminated through the anal canal. **Flatus** is largely air

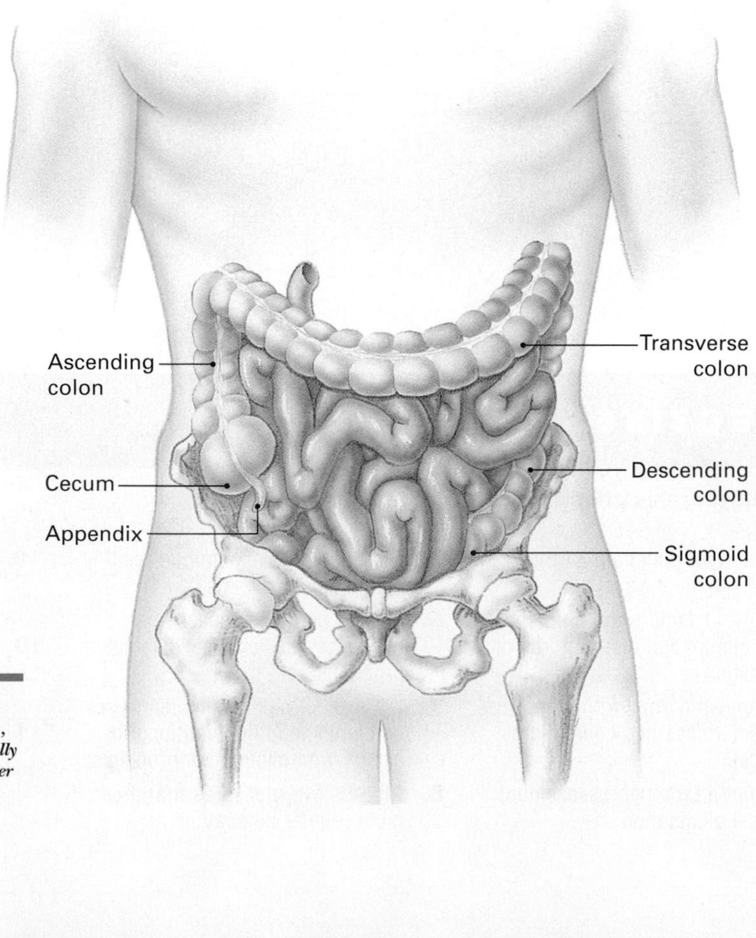

FIGURE 40.1 The large intestine

(From Medical Terminology: A Living Language, *3rd ed., by Bonnie F. Fremgan, Suzanne S. Frucht, 2005. Electronically reproduced with permission of Pearson Education Inc., Upper Saddle River, New Jersey.)*

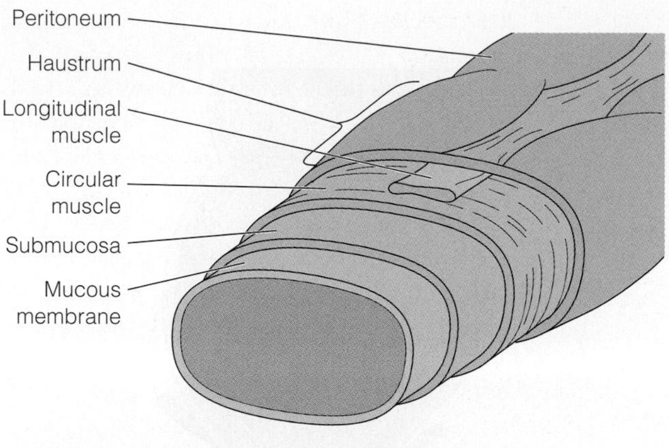

FIGURE 40.2 The layers of the wall of the large intestine

and the byproducts of the digestion of carbohydrates. Three types of movement occur in the large intestine: haustral churning, colon peristalsis, and mass peristalsis (Figure 40.3). **Haustral churning** or **haustral shuffling** involves movement of the chyme back and forth within the haustra. In addition to mixing the contents, this action aids in the absorption of water and moves the contents forward to the next haustrum. **Peristalsis** is wavelike movement produced by the circular and longitudinal muscle fibres of the intestinal walls; it propels the intestinal contents forward. Colon peristalsis is very sluggish and is thought to move the chyme very little along the large intestine. **Mass peristalsis**, the third type of colonic movement, involves a wave of powerful muscular contraction that moves over large areas of the colon. Usually, mass peristalsis occurs after eating, stimulated by the presence of food in the stomach and small intestine. In adults, mass peristaltic waves occur only a few times a day.

Rectum and Anal Canal

The rectum in the adult is usually 10 cm to 15 cm long; the most distal portion, 2.5 cm to 5 cm long, is the anal canal. In the rectum are three folds of tissue that extend across the rectum and several folds that extend vertically. Each vertical fold contains a vein and an artery. It is believed that these folds help retain feces within the rectum. When the veins become distended, as can occur with repeated pressure, a condition known as **hemorrhoids** occurs. Hemorrhoids can present internally or externally (Figure 40.4).

The anal canal is bounded by an internal and an external sphincter muscle (Figure 40.5). The *internal sphincter* is under involuntary control, and the *external sphincter* normally is voluntarily controlled. The external sphincter's action is augmented by the levator ani muscles of the pelvic floor. The internal sphincter muscle is innervated by the autonomic nervous system; the external sphincter is innervated by the somatic nervous system.

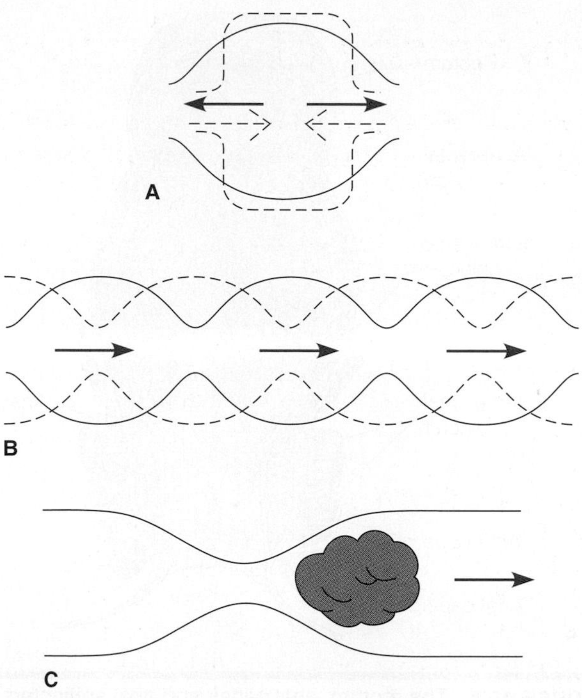

FIGURE 40.3 Three types of intestinal movements: **A:** haustral churning; **B:** peristalsis; **C:** mass peristalsis

Defecation

Defecation is the expulsion of feces from the anus and rectum. It is also called a *bowel movement*. The frequency of defecation is highly individual, varying from several times per day to two or three times per week. The amount defecated also varies from person to person. When peristaltic waves move the feces into the sigmoid colon and the rectum, the sensory nerves in the rectum are stimulated and the individual becomes aware of the need to defecate.

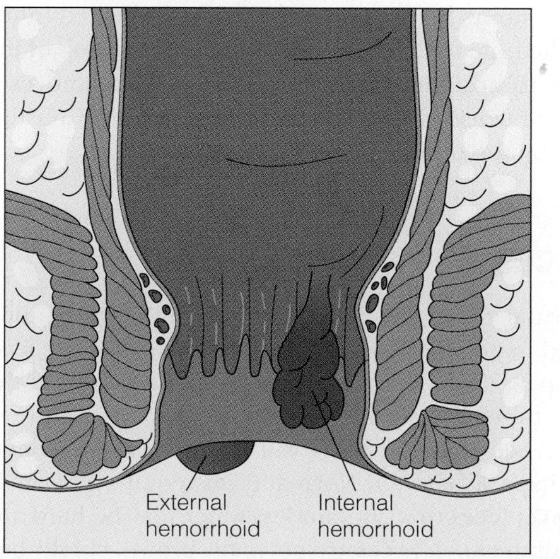

FIGURE 40.4 Internal and external hemorrhoids

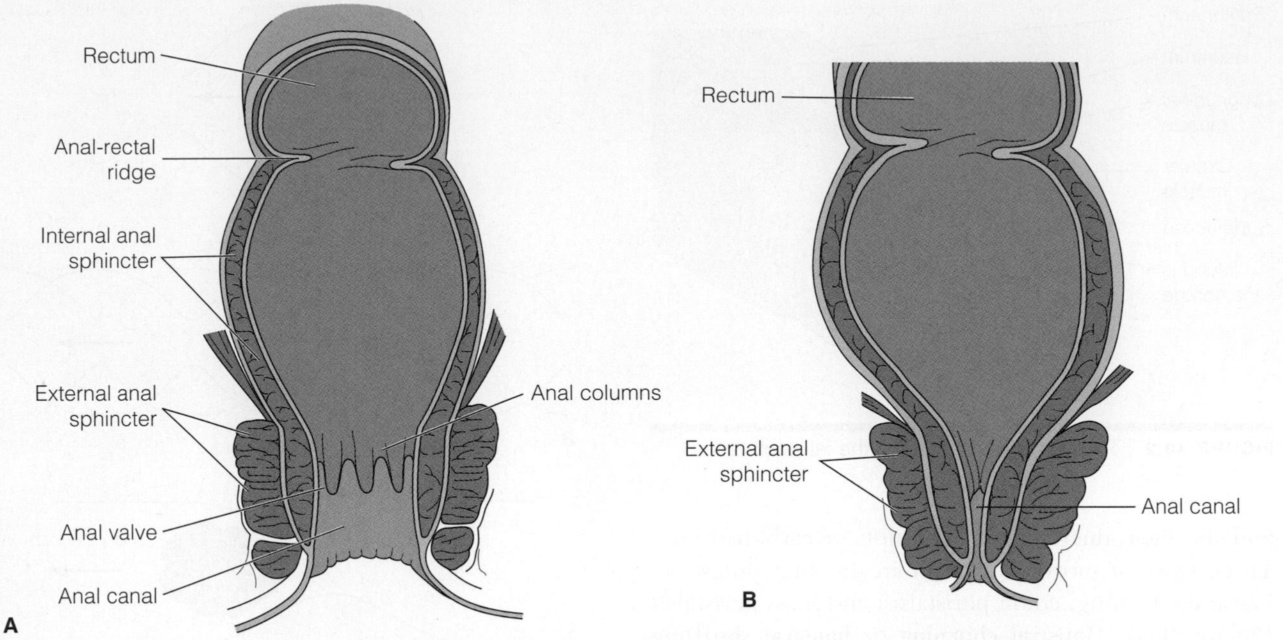

FIGURE 40.5 The rectum, anal canal, and anal sphincters: **A:** open; **B:** closed

When the *internal* anal sphincter relaxes, feces move into the anal canal. After the individual is seated on a toilet or bedpan, the *external* anal sphincter is relaxed voluntarily. Expulsion of the feces is assisted by contraction of the abdominal muscles and the diaphragm, which increases abdominal pressure, and by contraction of the levator ani muscles of the pelvic floor, which moves the feces through the anal canal. Normal defecation is facilitated by (1) thigh flexion, which increases the pressure within the abdomen, and (2) a sitting position, which increases the downward pressure on the rectum.

If the defecation reflex is ignored, or if defecation is consciously inhibited by contracting the external sphincter muscle, the urge to defecate normally disappears for a few hours before occurring again. Repeated inhibition of the urge to defecate can result in expansion of the rectum to accommodate accumulated feces and eventual loss of sensitivity to the need to defecate. Constipation can be the ultimate result.

Feces

Normal feces are made of about 75% water and 25% solid materials. They are soft but formed. If the feces are propelled very quickly along the large intestine, there is not time for most of the water in the chyme to be absorbed and the feces will be more fluid, containing perhaps 95% water. Normal feces require a normal fluid intake; feces that contain less water may be hard and difficult to expel. Feces are normally brown, chiefly because of the presence of stercobilin and urobilin, which are derived from **bilirubin** (a red pigment in bile). Another factor that affects fecal colour is the action of bacteria, such as *Escherichia coli* or staphylococci, which are normally present in the large intestine. The action of microorganisms on the chyme is also responsible for the odour of feces. See Table 40.1 for characteristics of normal and abnormal feces.

An adult usually forms 7 L to 10 L of flatus (gas) in the large intestine every 24 hours. The gases include carbon dioxide, methane, hydrogen, oxygen, and nitrogen. Some gases are swallowed with food and fluids taken by mouth; some are formed through the action of bacteria on the chyme in the large intestine; and other gas diffuses from the blood into the gastrointestinal tract.

Factors That Affect Defecation

Defecation patterns vary at different stages of life. Circumstances of development, diet, fluid intake and output, activity, psychological factors, habits, medications, diagnostic procedures, anaesthesia and surgery, pathological conditions, and pain also affect defecation.

Development

NEWBORNS AND INFANTS **Meconium** is the first fecal material passed by the newborn, normally up to 24 hours after birth. It is black, tarry, odourless, and sticky. Transitional stools, which follow for about a week, are

TABLE 40.1 Characteristics of Normal and Abnormal Feces

Characteristic	Normal	Abnormal	Possible Cause
Colour	Adult: brown Infant: yellow	Clay or white	Absence of bile pigment (bile obstruction); diagnostic study using barium
		Black or tarry	Drug (e.g., iron); bleeding from upper gastrointestinal tract (e.g., stomach, small intestine); diet high in red meat and dark green vegetables (e.g., spinach)
		Red	Bleeding from lower gastrointestinal tract (e.g., rectum); some foods (e.g., beets)
		Pale	Malabsorption of fats; diet high in milk and milk products and low in meat
		Orange or green	Intestinal infection
Consistency	Formed, soft, semisolid, moist	Hard, dry	Dehydration; decreased intestinal motility resulting from lack of fibre in diet, lack of exercise, emotional upset, laxative abuse
		Diarrhea	Increased intestinal motility (e.g., caused by irritation of the colon by bacteria)
Shape	Cylindrical (contour of rectum), about 2.5 cm in diameter in adults	Narrow, pencil-shaped, or stringlike stool	Obstructive condition of the rectum
Amount	Varies with diet (about 100 g to 400 g per day)		
Odour	Aromatic: affected by ingested food and person's own bacterial flora	Pungent	Infection, blood
Constituents	Small amounts of undigested roughage, sloughed dead bacteria and epithelial cells, fat, protein, dried constituents of digestive juices (e.g., bile pigments), inorganic matter (calcium, phosphates)	Pus	Bacterial infection
		Mucus	Inflammatory condition
		Parasites	
		Blood	Gastrointestinal bleeding
		Large quantities of fat	Malabsorption
		Foreign objects	Accidental ingestion

generally greenish yellow; they contain mucus and are loose.

Infants pass stool frequently, often after each feeding. Because the intestine is immature, water is not well absorbed and the stool is soft, liquid, and frequent. When the intestine matures, bacterial flora increase. After solid foods are introduced, the stool becomes less frequent and firmer.

Infants who are breastfed have bright yellow to golden feces, and infants who are taking formula will have dark yellow or tan stool that is more formed.

TODDLERS Some control of defecation starts at 1.5 to 2 years of age. By this time, children have learned to walk, and the nervous and muscular systems are sufficiently well developed to permit bowel control. A desire to control daytime bowel movements and to use the toilet generally starts when the child becomes aware of (1) the discomfort caused by a soiled diaper, and (2) the sensation that indicates the need for a bowel movement. Daytime control is normally attained by age 2.5 years after a process of toilet training.

SCHOOL-AGE CHILDREN AND ADOLESCENTS School-age children and adolescents have bowel habits similar to adults'. Patterns of defecation vary in frequency, quantity, and consistency. Some school-age children may voluntarily delay defecation (functional constipation) because of an activity, such as play. **Encopresis**, the passage or leakage of feces in children who are past the age of toilet training, generally after 4 years of age, can present as a bowel-management problem. Involuntary encopresis is frequently associated with constipation and can indicate fecal impaction. Voluntary soiling can indicate a developmental or emotional problem.

OLDER ADULTS Constipation is a common bowel-management problem in the older adult population. This experience is due, in part, to reduced activity levels, muscle weakness, and inadequate amounts of fluid and fibre intake. Physiologically, older adults secrete less mucus in the large intestine. Many older people believe that *regularity* means a bowel movement every day. Those who do not meet this criterion often seek over-the-counter preparations to relieve what they believe to be constipation. Older clients should be advised that normal patterns of bowel elimination vary considerably. For some, a normal pattern may be every other day; for others, twice a day. Adequate roughage in the diet, adequate exercise, and six to eight glasses of fluid daily are essential preventive measures for constipation. A cup of hot water or tea at a regular time in the morning is helpful for some. Responding to the **gastrocolic reflex** (increased peristalsis of the colon after food has entered the stomach) is also an important consideration. For example, toileting is recommended 5 to 15 minutes after meals, especially after breakfast when the gastrocolic reflex is strongest (Registered Nurses' Association of Ontario [RNAO], 2005).

The older adult should be warned that consistent use of laxatives inhibits natural defecation reflexes and is thought to cause, rather than cure, constipation. The habitual user of laxatives eventually requires larger or stronger doses because the effect is progressively reduced with continual use. Laxatives can also interfere with the body's electrolyte balance and decrease the absorption of certain vitamins. The reasons for constipation can range from lifestyle habits (e.g., lack of exercise) to serious malignant disorders. The nurse should evaluate any complaints of constipation carefully for each individual. A change in bowel habits over several weeks with or without weight loss, pain, or fever should be referred to a physician for a complete medical evaluation.

Diet

Sufficient bulk (cellulose, fibre) in the diet is necessary to provide fecal volume. Dietary fibre in the range of 25 g to 30 g per day is recommended (RNAO, 2005). However, high-fibre diets with insufficient amounts of fluids can cause constipation. Bland diets and low-fibre diets are lacking in bulk and, therefore, create insufficient residue of waste products to stimulate the reflex for defecation. Low-residue foods, such as rice, eggs, and lean meats, move more slowly through the intestinal tract. Increasing fluid intake with such foods increases their rate of movement.

Certain foods are difficult or impossible for some people to digest. This inability results in digestive upsets and, in some instances, the passage of watery stools. Irregular eating can also impair regular defecation. Individuals who eat at the same times every day usually have a regularly timed, physiological response to the food intake and a regular pattern of peristaltic activity in the colon.

Spicy foods can produce diarrhea and flatus in some individuals. Excessive sugar can also cause diarrhea. Other foods that can influence bowel elimination include the following:

- Gas-producing foods, such as cabbage, onions, cauliflower, bananas, and apples
- Laxative-producing foods, such as bran, prunes, figs, chocolate, and alcohol
- Constipation-producing foods, such as cheese, pasta, eggs, and lean meat

Fluid

When intake is inadequate or output (e.g., urine or vomitus) is excessive for any reason, the body continues to absorb fluid from the chyme as it passes along the colon. As a result, the chyme becomes drier than normal, resulting in hard feces. In addition, reduced fluid intake slows the chyme's passage along the intestines, further increasing the reabsorption of fluid from the chyme. Healthy fecal elimination usually requires a minimum daily fluid intake of 1500 mL to 2000 mL. Caffeine and alcoholic beverages should be limited because their diuretic properties result in a loss of fluid (RNAO, 2005). If chyme moves abnormally quickly through the large intestine, however, there is less time for fluid to be absorbed into the blood; as a result, the feces are soft or even watery.

Activity

Activity stimulates peristalsis, thus facilitating the movement of chyme along the colon. Weak abdominal and pelvic muscles are often ineffective in increasing the intra-abdominal pressure during defecation or in controlling defecation. Weak muscles can result from lack of exercise, immobility, or impaired neurological functioning. Walking 15 to 20 minutes a day can aid in fecal elimination. Clients confined to bed are often constipated. Bedridden clients can be given exercises to perform, such as pelvic tilts, low trunk rotation, and single leg lift exercises. Consultation with the appropriate members of the health-care team before beginning exercise programs is essential.

Psychological Factors

Some people who are anxious or angry experience increased peristaltic activity and subsequent diarrhea. In contrast, people who are depressed may experience slower intestinal motility, resulting in constipation. How a person responds to these emotional states is the result of individual differences in the response of the enteric nervous system to vagal stimulation from the brain.

Defecation Habits

Early bowel training can establish the habit of defecating at a regular time. Many people defecate after breakfast, when the gastrocolic reflex causes mass peristaltic waves in the large intestine. If a person ignores this urge to defecate, water continues to be absorbed, making the feces harder and more difficult to expel. When the normal defecation reflexes are inhibited or ignored, these conditioned reflexes tend to be progressively weakened. When habitually ignored, the urge to defecate is ultimately lost. Adults may ignore these reflexes because of the pressures of time or work. Hospitalized clients may suppress the urge because of embarrassment about using a bedpan, because of a lack of privacy, or because defecation is too uncomfortable.

CLINICAL ALERT

Individuals, especially children, may be reluctant to discuss elimination habits. Terms used to describe bowel movement or defecation can vary considerably. The nurse may need to try several different common words before finding one the client understands.

Medications

Some drugs have side effects that can interfere with normal elimination. Medications that have an anticholinergic effect (e.g., certain antihypertensive, antidepressant, and analgesic agents), antacids containing aluminum, iron supplements, opioids, antiparkinsonism drugs, and antihistamines are some of the common agents known to cause constipation.

Some medications directly affect elimination. **Laxatives** are medications that stimulate bowel activity and so assist fecal elimination. Other medications soften stool, facilitating defecation. Certain medications, such as dicyclomine hydrochloride (Bentyl), suppress peristaltic activity and sometimes are used to treat diarrhea.

Some medications affect the appearance of the feces. Any drug that causes gastrointestinal bleeding (e.g., acetylsalicylic products, such as Aspirin) can cause the stool to be red or black. Iron salts can cause the stool to be black because of the oxidation of the iron; antibiotics can cause a grey-green discolouration because of effects on digestion; and antacids can cause a whitish discolouration or white specks in the stool.

Diagnostic Procedures

Before certain diagnostic procedures, such as visualization of the sigmoid colon (sigmoidoscopy), the client is often restricted from ingesting food or fluid. The client may also be given a cleansing enema before the examination. In these instances, the client usually will not defecate normally until eating has resumed.

Anaesthesia and Surgery

General anaesthesia causes normal colonic movements to cease or slow down by blocking parasympathetic stimulation to the muscles of the colon. Clients who have regional or spinal anaesthesia are less likely to experience this problem.

Surgery that involves direct handling of the intestines can cause temporary cessation of intestinal movement. This condition, called **paralytic ileus**, usually lasts 24 to 48 hours. Listening for bowel sounds that reflect intestinal motility is an important nursing assessment following surgery. See Chapter 27 for assessment of bowel sounds.

Pathological Conditions

Spinal cord injuries and acquired head injuries can decrease the sensory stimulation for defecation. Impaired mobility may limit the client's ability to respond to the urge to defecate when the client is unable to reach a toilet or summon assistance. As a result, the client may experience *constipation* or *fecal incontinence.* Poorly functioning sphincters can also result in *fecal incontinence.*

Pain

Clients who experience discomfort when defecating (e.g., following hemorrhoid surgery) often suppress the urge to defecate to avoid the pain. Such clients can experience constipation as a result. Clients taking opioid analgesics for pain can also experience constipation as a side effect of the medication.

Common Fecal Elimination Problems

Five common problems are related to fecal elimination: constipation, fecal impaction, diarrhea, bowel incontinence, and flatulence.

Constipation

Constipation is defined as fewer than three bowel movements per week and the passage of small, dry, hard stool that is difficult to eliminate. It occurs when the movement of feces through the large intestine is slow, thus allowing time for additional absorption of fluid from the large intestine. Because of difficult evacuation of stool, there is increased effort or straining of the voluntary muscles of defecation. The person may also have a feeling of incomplete stool evacuation after defecation. It is important to define constipation in relation to the person's regular elimination pattern. Some people normally defecate only a few times a week; if their stool is soft in consistency, they are not considered to be constipated.

Chronic constipation exists when a client experiences two of the following for at least 25% of defecations in a 3-month period, with symptom onset at least 6 months before diagnosis: straining, passage of hard stool, sensation of incomplete evacuation, sensation of blockage in the rectum, fewer than 3 defecations a week, and the need for manual manoeuvres (e.g., digital stimulation) to prompt evacuation (Longstreth et al., 2006).

Careful assessment of the person's habits is necessary before a diagnosis of constipation is made. Box 40.1 lists the frequent defining characteristics of constipation.

Many causes and factors contribute to constipation. Among them are the following:

- Lifestyle related: insufficient fibre intake, insufficient fluid intake, insufficient activity or immobility, irregular defecation habits, changes in daily routine, lack of privacy
- Emotional disturbances, such as depression or mental confusion
- Medical conditions, such as diabetes mellitus (as a result of dysfunction of the autonomic nervous system), and other conditions with neurological effects, such as Parkinson's disease, stroke, spinal cord injury, acquired brain injury, or dementia
- Pelvic floor dysfunction or muscle damage
- Medications, such as opioids, iron supplements, antacids, antidepressants, antihistamines, anticholinergics, anaesthetics, calcium channel blockers, or chronic use of laxatives or enemas

Constipation can be hazardous to some clients. Straining associated with constipation often is accompanied by holding the breath. This Valsalva manoeuvre can present serious problems to people with heart disease, brain injuries, or respiratory disease. Holding the breath while bearing down increases intrathoracic and intracranial pressures. In addition, vagal tone is increased, resulting in a slowing of the heart rate (LeMone & Burke, 2008). To some degree, this pressure can be reduced if the person exhales through the mouth while straining. However, avoiding straining altogether is the best precaution. Hemorrhoids and anal fissures (narrow openings in the anus) are also complications of constipation (Singh et al., 2005).

BOX 40.1 DEFINING CHARACTERISTICS OF CONSTIPATION

The following are the characteristics of constipation:

- Decreased frequency of defecation
- Hard, dry, formed stools
- Straining at stool; painful defecation
- Reports of rectal fullness or pressure or incomplete bowel evacuation
- Abdominal pain, cramps, or distension
- Use of laxatives
- Anorexia, nausea

Fecal Impaction

Fecal impaction is a mass or collection of hardened, puttylike feces in the folds of the rectum. Impaction results from prolonged retention and accumulation of fecal material. In severe impactions, the feces accumulate and extend well up into the sigmoid colon and beyond. Fecal impaction is recognized by the passage of liquid fecal seepage (diarrhea) and no normal stool. The liquid portion of the feces seeps out around the impacted mass (Figure 40.6). Impaction can also be assessed by digital examination of the rectum, during which the hardened mass can often be palpated.

Along with fecal seepage and constipation, symptoms include frequent but nonproductive desire to defecate and rectal pain. A generalized feeling of illness results; the client becomes anorexic, the abdomen becomes distended, and nausea and vomiting may occur.

The causes of fecal impaction are usually poor defecation habits and constipation. The barium used in radiological examinations of the upper and lower gastrointestinal tracts can be a causative factor. Therefore, after these examinations, measures are usually taken to ensure removal of the barium.

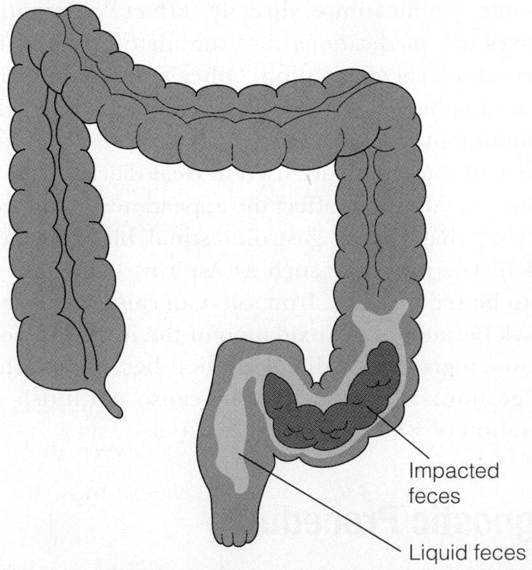

FIGURE 40.6 A fecal impaction with liquid feces passing around the impaction

An impaction can sometimes be palpated through the client's abdomen. Digital examination of the impaction through the rectum should be done gently and carefully because stimulation of the vagus nerve in the rectal wall can slow the client's heart.

Fecal impaction can generally be prevented; however, digital removal of impacted feces is sometimes necessary. Although digital rectal examination is within the scope of nursing practice, some agency policies require a physician's order for digital manipulation and removal of a fecal impaction.

When fecal impaction is suspected, the client, as prescribed by an appropriate member of the health-care team, is often given an oil retention enema, a cleansing enema 2 to 4 hours later, and daily additional cleansing enemas, suppositories, or stool softeners. If these measures fail, manual removal is often necessary.

Diarrhea

Diarrhea refers to the passage of liquid feces and an increased frequency of defecation. It is the opposite of constipation and results from rapid movement of fecal contents through the large intestine. Rapid passage of chyme reduces the time available for the large intestine to absorb water and electrolytes. Some people pass stool with increased frequency, but diarrhea is not present unless the stool is relatively unformed and excessively liquid. The person with diarrhea finds it difficult or impossible to control the urge to defecate for very long. Diarrhea and the threat of incontinence are sources of concern and embarrassment. Often, spasmodic cramps are associated with diarrhea. Bowel sounds are increased (see Chapter 27). Sometimes the client passes blood and excessive mucus; nausea and vomiting can also occur.

With persistent diarrhea, irritation of the anal region extending to the perineum and buttocks generally results. Fatigue, weakness, malaise, and emaciation are the results of prolonged diarrhea. The irritating effects of diarrhea stool increase the risk for skin breakdown. Therefore, the area around the anal region should be kept clean and dry and be protected with zinc oxide or other ointment. In addition, a fecal collector pouch can be used (see Figure 40.18, page 1252).

When the cause of diarrhea is irritants in the intestinal tract, diarrhea is thought to be a protective flushing mechanism. It can create serious fluid and electrolyte losses in the body, however, that can develop within a frighteningly short time, particularly in infants and small children. Antibiotic therapy can cause diarrhea because the balance of microbes in the gastrointestinal tract is altered. The development of *Clostridium difficile*–associated diarrhea (CDAD), the most common health-care-associated infectious diarrhea, carries a high risk because of the high mortality rate associated with this type of diarrhea (Poutanen & Simor, 2004). Unfortunately, the antibiotic treatment used for this diarrhea can lead to an exacerbation of the diarrhea itself (Nelson, 2007).

Table 40.2 lists some of the major causes of diarrhea and the physiological responses of the body.

Bowel Incontinence

Bowel incontinence, also called **fecal incontinence**, refers to the loss of voluntary ability to control fecal and gaseous discharges through the anal sphincter. The incontinence may occur at specific times, such as after meals, or it may occur irregularly. Two types of bowel incontinence are described: partial and major. *Partial incontinence* is the inability to control flatus or to prevent minor soiling. *Major incontinence* is the inability to control feces of normal consistency.

Fecal incontinence is generally associated with impaired functioning of the anal sphincter or its nerve supply, such as in some neuromuscular diseases, spinal cord trauma, and tumours of the external anal sphincter muscle.

TABLE 40.2 Major Causes of Diarrhea

Cause	Physiological Effect
Psychological stress (e.g., anxiety)	Increased intestinal motility and mucus secretion
Medications	
Antibiotics	Inflammation and infection of mucosa caused by overgrowth of pathogenic intestinal microorganisms
Iron	Irritation of intestinal mucosa
Cathartics	Irritation of intestinal mucosa
Allergy to food, fluid, drugs	Incomplete digestion of food or fluid
Intolerance of food or fluid	Increased intestinal motility and mucus secretion
Diseases of the colon such as	
Malabsorption syndrome	Reduced absorption of fluids
Crohn's disease	Inflammation of the mucosa often leading to ulcer formation

Fecal incontinence is an emotionally distressing problem that can ultimately lead to social isolation. Affected persons withdraw into their homes or, if in the hospital, the confines of their room to minimize the embarrassment associated with soiling. They may come to prefer easily washable night garments to street clothes. Incontinent feces are acidic and contain digestive enzymes that are highly irritating to skin. Therefore, as with diarrhea, the area around the anal region should be kept clean and dry and be protected with zinc oxide or other ointment. In addition, a rectal pouch can be used. Several surgical procedures are also used for the treatment of fecal incontinence. These include repair of the sphincter and fecal diversion or colostomy.

CLINICAL ALERT

The use of alcohol-based hand rub has been shown to be effective in decreasing the rates of acquired drug-resistant bacteria, such as vancomycin-resistant enterococcus (VRE) and clostridium difficile, common causes of diarrhea in hospitalized clients (Gordin, Schultz, Huber, & Gill, 2005). Nurses can aid in the reduction of these drug-resistant bacteria by promoting alcohol-based hand hygiene with visitors and staff members.

Flatulence

Flatus, air or gas in the gastrointestinal tract, has three primary causes: (1) action of bacteria on the chyme in the large intestine, (2) swallowed air, and (3) gas that diffuses from the bloodstream into the intestine.

Flatulence is the presence of *excessive* flatus in the intestines and leads to stretching and inflation of the intestines (*intestinal distension*). This condition is also referred to as *abdominal distension.* Large amounts of air and other gases can accumulate in the stomach, resulting in gastric distension.

Most gases that are swallowed are expelled through the mouth by **eructation** (belching). The gases formed in the large intestine are chiefly absorbed through the intestinal capillaries into the circulation. Flatulence can occur in the colon from a variety of causes, such as foods (e.g., cabbage, onions), abdominal surgery, or opioid analgesics. If the gas is propelled by increased colon activity before it can be absorbed, it may be expelled through the anus. If excessive gas cannot be expelled through the anus, it may be necessary to insert a rectal tube or provide a return flow enema to remove it.

Bowel Diversion Ostomies

An **ostomy** is an opening on the abdominal wall for the elimination of feces or urine. There are many types of ostomies. A **gastrostomy** is an opening through the abdominal wall into the stomach. A **jejunostomy** is an opening through the abdominal wall into the jejunum. An **ileostomy** is an opening into the ileum (small bowel). A **colostomy** is an opening into the colon (large bowel). A **ureterostomy** is an opening into the ureter. Gastrostomies and jejunostomies are generally performed to provide an alternative feeding route. The purpose of bowel and urinary ostomies is to divert and drain fecal or urinary material. Urinary diversion ostomies are discussed in Chapter 41. Bowel diversion ostomies are often classified according to (1) their status as permanent or temporary, (2) their anatomic location, and (3) the construction of the **stoma**, the opening created in the abdominal wall by the ostomy.

Permanence

Colostomies can be either temporary or permanent. Temporary colostomies are generally performed for traumatic injuries or inflammatory conditions of the bowel. They allow the distal diseased portion of the bowel to rest and heal. Permanent colostomies are performed to provide a means of elimination when the rectum or anus is nonfunctional as a result of a birth defect or a disease, such as cancer of the bowel. The diseased portion may or may not be removed.

Anatomic Location

An ileostomy generally empties from the distal end of the small intestine. A cecostomy empties from the cecum (the first part of the ascending colon). An ascending colostomy empties from the ascending colon. A transverse colostomy empties from the transverse colon. A descending colostomy empties from the descending colon. A sigmoidostomy empties from the sigmoid colon (Figure 40.7).

The location of the ostomy influences the character and management of the fecal drainage. The farther along the bowel, the more formed the stool is because the large bowel absorbs water from the fecal mass. In addition, more control over the frequency of stomal discharge can be established:

- An ileostomy produces liquid fecal drainage. Drainage is constant and cannot be regulated. Ileostomy drainage contains some digestive enzymes, which are damaging to the skin. For this reason, ileostomy clients must wear an appliance continuously and take special precautions to prevent skin breakdown. Compared with colostomies, however, odour is minimal because fewer bacteria are present.
- An ascending colostomy is similar to an ileostomy in that the drainage is liquid and cannot be regulated, and digestive enzymes are present. Odour, however,

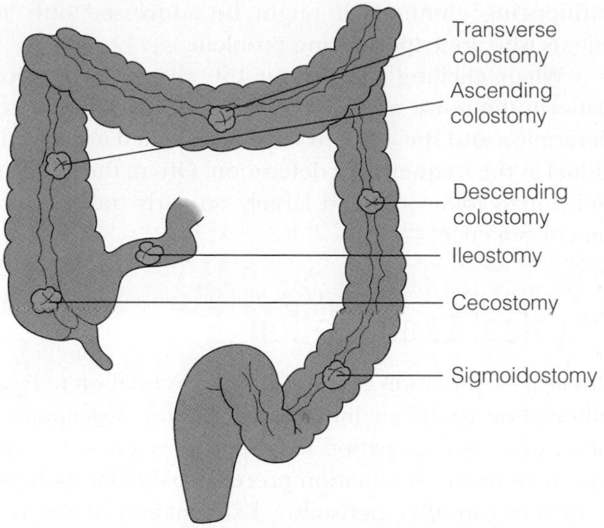

FIGURE 40.7 The locations of bowel diversion ostomies

is a problem requiring control (e.g., a deodorant inside the appliance).

- A transverse colostomy produces a malodorous, mushy drainage because some of the liquid has been absorbed. There is usually no control.
- A descending colostomy produces increasingly solid fecal drainage. Stools from a sigmoidostomy are of normal or formed consistency, and the frequency of discharge can be regulated. People with a sigmoidostomy may not have to wear an appliance at all times, and odours can usually be controlled.

The length of time that an ostomy is in place also helps determine the consistency of the stool, particularly with transverse and descending colostomies. Over time, the stool becomes more formed because the remaining functioning portions of the colon tend to compensate by increasing water absorption.

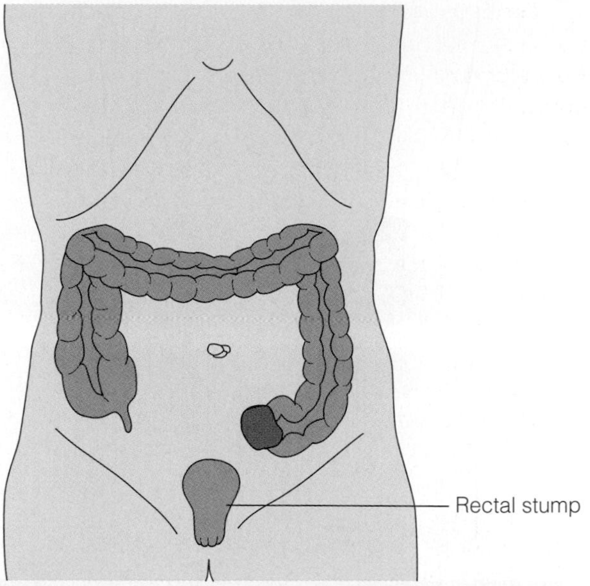

FIGURE 40.8 End colostomy; the diseased portion of bowel is removed and a rectal pouch remains.

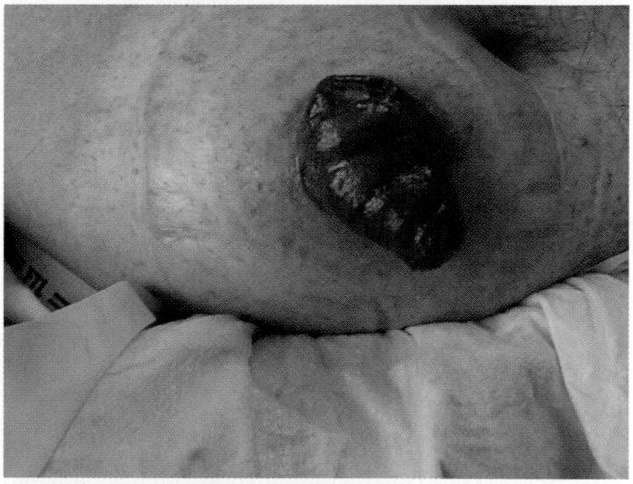

FIGURE 40.9 Loop colostomy

Construction of the Stoma

Surgical stoma constructions are described as single, loop, divided, or double-barrelled colostomies. The *single* stoma is created when one end of bowel is brought out through an opening onto the anterior abdominal wall. This is referred to as an *end* or *terminal* colostomy, and the stoma is permanent (Figure 40.8).

In the loop colostomy, a loop of bowel is brought out onto the abdominal wall and is supported by a plastic bridge, a glass rod, or a piece of rubber tubing (Figure 40.9). A loop stoma has two openings: (1) the proximal or afferent end, which is active, and (2) the distal or efferent end, which is inactive. The loop colostomy is usually performed as an emergency procedure and is often situated on the right transverse colon. It is a bulky stoma that is more difficult to manage than a single stoma.

The *divided colostomy* consists of two edges of bowel brought out onto the abdomen but separated from each other (Figure 40.10). The opening from the digestive or proximal end is the colostomy. The distal end in this situation is often referred to as a mucous fistula, since this section of bowel continues to secrete mucus. The divided colostomy is often used in situations where spillage of feces into the distal end of the bowel needs to be avoided.

The *double-barrelled colostomy* resembles a double-barrelled shotgun (Figure 40.11). In this type of colostomy, the proximal and distal loops of bowel are sutured together for about 10 cm and both ends are brought up onto the abdominal wall.

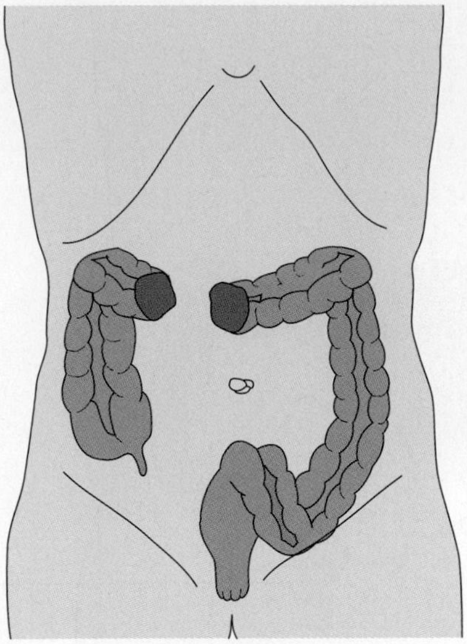

FIGURE 40.10 Divided colostomy with two separated stomas

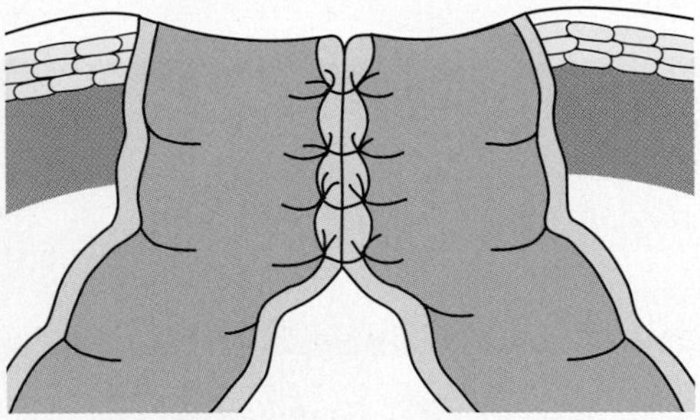

FIGURE 40.11 Double-barrelled colostomy

Assessing

Assessment of fecal elimination includes taking a nursing history; performing a physical examination of the abdomen, rectum, and anus; and inspecting the feces. The nurse also should review any data obtained from relevant diagnostic tests.

Nursing History

A nursing history for fecal elimination helps the nurse ascertain the client's normal pattern. The nurse elicits a description of usual feces and any recent changes and collects information about any past or current problems with elimination, the presence of an ostomy, and factors influencing the elimination pattern.

Examples of interview questions to elicit this information are shown in the Assessment: Interview box. The number of questions to ask is adapted to the individual client, according to the client's responses in the first three categories. For example, questions about factors influencing elimination might be addressed only to clients who are experiencing problems.

When eliciting data about the client's defecation pattern, the nurse needs to understand that the time of defecation and the amount of feces expelled are as individual as the frequency of defecation. Often, the patterns individuals follow depend largely on early training and on convenience.

Physical Examination

Physical examination of the abdomen in relation to fecal elimination problems includes inspection, auscultation, percussion, and palpation with specific reference to the intestinal tract. Auscultation precedes palpation because palpation can alter peristalsis. Examination of the rectum and anus includes inspection and palpation. Physical examination of the abdomen, rectum, and anus is discussed in Chapter 27.

Inspecting the Feces

The client's stool is inspected for colour, consistency, shape, amount, odour, and the presence of abnormal constituents. See Table 40.1 earlier in this chapter for a summary of normal and abnormal characteristics of stool and possible causes.

Diagnostic Studies

Diagnostic studies of the gastrointestinal tract include direct and indirect visualization techniques and laboratory tests for abnormal constituents.

VISUALIZATION TECHNIQUES *Direct visualization techniques* include **anoscopy**, the viewing of the anal canal; **proctoscopy**, the viewing of the rectum; **proctosigmoidoscopy**, the viewing of the rectum and sigmoid colon; and **colonoscopy**, the viewing of the large intestine. *Indirect visualization* of the gastrointestinal tract is achieved by roentgenography (X-ray). Radiographs of the gastrointestinal tract can detect strictures, obstructions, tumours, ulcers, inflammatory disease, or other structural changes, such as hiatal hernias. Visualization of the tract is enhanced by the introduction of a radiopaque substance, such as barium. For examination of the upper gastrointestinal tract or small bowel, the client drinks barium sulphate. This examination is often referred to as a *barium swallow.* For examination of the lower gastrointestinal tract, the client is given an enema containing barium. This examination is commonly referred to as a *barium enema.* These radiographs usually include *fluoroscopic examination,* that is, projection of the X-ray films onto a screen that permits continuous observation of the flow of barium.

ASSESSMENT: INTERVIEW

Fecal Elimination

The nurse can use these kinds of questions to gather information related to clients' fecal elimination:

DEFECATION PATTERN

- What is the frequency and time of day of defecation?
- Has this pattern changed recently?

DESCRIPTION OF FECES AND ANY CHANGES

- How would you describe your stool in terms of colour, texture (hard, soft, watery), shape, odour?
- Have you noticed any changes in your stool recently?

FECAL ELIMINATION PROBLEMS

- What problems have you had or do you now have with your bowel movements (constipation, diarrhea, excessive flatulence, seepage, or incontinence)?
- When and how often does it occur?
- What do you think causes it (food, fluids, exercise, emotions, medications, disease, surgery)?
- What have you done to try to solve the problem, and how effective was it?

FACTORS INFLUENCING ELIMINATION

- *Use of elimination aids.* What routines do you follow to maintain your usual defecation pattern? Do you use natural aids, such as specific foods or fluids (e.g., a glass of hot lemon juice before breakfast), laxatives, or enemas to maintain elimination?
- *Diet.* What foods do you believe affect defecation? What foods do you typically eat? What foods do you always avoid? Do you take meals at regular times?
- *Fluid.* What amount and kind of fluid do you take each day (e.g., six glasses of water, five cups of coffee)?
- *Exercise.* What is your usual daily exercise pattern? (Obtain specifics about exercise, rather than asking whether it is sufficient; ideas of what is sufficient vary among individuals.)
- *Medications.* Have you taken any medications that could affect the gastrointestinal tract (e.g., iron, antibiotics)?
- *Stress.* Are you experiencing any long-term or short-term stressors? If so, what are these? Do you think these affect your defecation pattern? How?

PRESENCE AND MANAGEMENT OF OSTOMY

- What is your usual routine with your colostomy or ileostomy?
- What type of appliance do you wear and did you bring a spare?
- What problems, if any, do you have with it?
- How can the nurses help you manage your colostomy or ileostomy?

LABORATORY TESTS

Collecting Stool Specimens The nurse is responsible for collecting stool specimens ordered for laboratory analysis. Before obtaining a specimen, the nurse needs to determine the reason for collecting the stool specimen and the correct method of obtaining and handling it (i.e., how much stool to obtain, whether a preservative needs to be added to the stool, and whether it needs to be sent immediately to the laboratory). It may be necessary to confirm this information by checking with the agency laboratory. In many situations, only a single specimen is required; in others, timed specimens are necessary, and every stool passed is collected within a designated time period.

Nurses need to give clients the following instructions:

- Defecate in a clean bedpan or bedside commode.
- If possible, do not contaminate the specimen with urine or menstrual discharge. Void before the specimen collection.
- Do not place toilet tissue in the bedpan after defecation. Contents of the paper can affect the laboratory analysis.
- Notify the nurse as soon as possible after defecation, particularly for specimens that need to be sent to the laboratory immediately.

To secure a stool specimen from a baby or young child who is not toilet trained, the nurse obtains newly passed feces from the diaper.

When obtaining stool samples, that is, when handling the client's bedpan, when transferring the stool sample to a specimen container, and when disposing of the bedpan contents, the nurse follows aseptic technique meticulously. Wear disposable gloves to prevent hand contamination, and take care not to contaminate the outside of the specimen container. Use one or two clean tongue blades to transfer the specimen to the container and then wrap them in a paper towel before disposing of them in the waste container. This practice lessens the chance of contact with other articles and the spread of microorganisms. The amount of stool to be sent depends on the purpose for which the specimen is collected. Usually about 2.5 cm of formed stool or 15 mL to 30 mL of liquid stool is adequate. For some timed specimens, however, the entire passed stool may need to be sent. Visible pus, mucus, or blood should be included in sample specimens. For a stool culture, the nurse dips a sterile swab into the specimen, preferably where purulent fecal matter is present and, by using sterile technique, places the swab in a sterile test tube.

Because fresh specimens provide the most accurate results, the nurse sends the specimen to the laboratory immediately. If this is not possible, the nurse follows the directions on the specimen container. In some instances, refrigeration is indicated because bacteriological changes take place in stool specimens left at room temperature.

Testing Feces for Occult Blood Stool is tested for **occult (hidden) blood** to detect gastrointestinal bleeding not visible to the eye. Bleeding can occur as a result of ulcers, inflammatory disease, or tumours. The test for occult blood, often referred to as the **guaiac test**, can be readily performed by the nurse in the clinical area or by the client at home. Guaiac paper used in the test is sensitive to fecal blood content.

A commonly used test product to measure occult blood is the *Hemoccult test,* which uses a chemical reagent to detect the presence of the enzyme peroxidase in the hemoglobin molecule (see the Reflect on Primary Health Care box).

To perform the test, the nurse or client uses a tongue blade to place a small amount of stool on a slide or card and then closes the card. The card is turned over and a few drops of the reagent are placed onto the smear on the back of the card. The nurse then observes for a colour change (Figure 40.12). A blue colour indicates a guaiac-positive result; that is, the presence of occult blood. No colour change or any colour other than blue is a negative finding, indicating the absence of blood in the stool. The Teaching: Clinical box has instructions for the client.

Certain foods, medications, and vitamin C can produce inaccurate test results. *False-positive results* can occur if the client has recently ingested (1) red meat (beef, lamb, liver, and processed meats); (2) raw vegetables or fruits, particularly radishes, turnips, horseradish, and melons; or (3) certain medications that irritate the gastric mucosa and cause bleeding, such as acetylsalicylic acid (e.g., Aspirin) or other nonsteroidal anti-inflammatory drugs, steroids, iron preparations, and anticoagulants. *False-negative results* can occur if the client has taken more than 250 mg per day of vitamin C from all sources (dietary and supplemental) up to 3 days before the test—even if bleeding is present.

REFLECT ON PRIMARY HEALTH CARE

Healthy fecal elimination requires a healthy diet that includes fresh fruits and vegetables to provide the recommended daily dietary fibre intake. Consider how this *health-promotion* strategy can be followed by members of your community whose income or accessibility to grocery stores is limited.

The *Hemoccult test* is used as an important screening tool for bowel cancer. Clients can test their feces at home and mail in the Hemoccult slide for analysis. Consider how this form of *technology* enables clients who have physical disabilities or who live in remote regions to obtain the recommended health screening.

Diagnosing

NANDA International (2007) includes the following diagnostic labels for fecal elimination problems:

- *Bowel Incontinence:* A change in usual bowel habits characterized by involuntary passage of stool
- *Constipation:* A change in usual bowel habits, characterized by a decrease in frequency or passage of hard, dry stools
- *Risk for Constipation:* Risk for a decrease in a person's normal frequency of defecation accompanied by difficult or incomplete passage of stool or passage of excessively hard, dry stool
- *Perceived Constipation:* A self-diagnosis of constipation; a daily bowel movement is ensured through abuse of laxatives, enemas, or suppositories
- *Diarrhea:* Passage of loose, unformed stools

Defining characteristics and etiologies of these diagnostic labels are discussed earlier (see the section

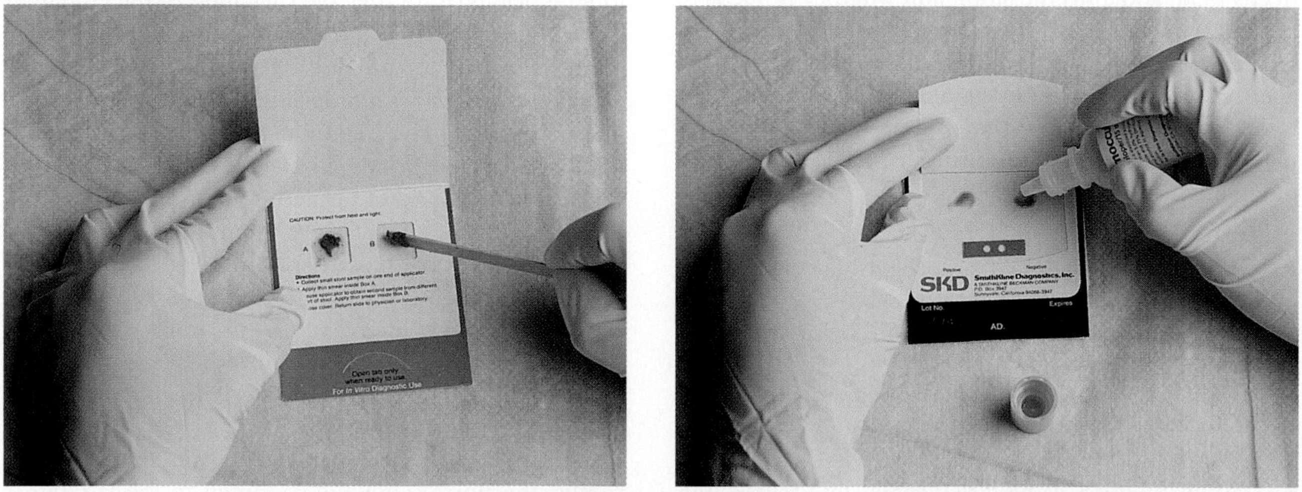

A

B

FIGURE 40.12 **A:** Opening the front cover of a Hemoccult slide and applying a thin smear of feces on the slide; **B:** opening the flap on the back of the slide and applying two drops of reagent over each smear.

TEACHING: CLINICAL

Assessing Stool for Occult Blood

The following are guidelines for clients to assess their stool for occult blood:

- Avoid restricted foods, medications, and vitamin C for the period recommended by the manufacturer and during the test. Usually, specified foods and vitamin C are restricted for 3 days before the test and specified medications for 7 days before the test, as recommended by the physician.
- Use a ballpoint pen to label the specimens with your name, address, age, and date of specimen. Usually, three specimens are collected from consecutive and different bowel movements. Each specimen must be dated accurately.
- Avoid collecting specimens during your menstrual period and for 3 days afterward or while you have bleeding hemorrhoids or blood in your urine.
- Remove toilet bowl cleaners from the toilet bowl. Flush the toilet twice before proceeding with the test.
- Avoid contaminating the specimen with urine or toilet tissue. Empty your bladder before the test. To facilitate specimen collection, transfer the stool to a clean, dry container. Wear disposable gloves.
- Use the tongue blade provided to transfer the specimen to the test folder or tape. Only a small amount of stool is required. Take the sample from the centre of a formed stool to ensure a uniform sample.
- Wrap the tongue blade in a paper towel and dispose of it in the waste receptacle. Do not flush the stick.
- Follow the manufacturer's directions explicitly for the test product being used. Test products vary. For example, for the *Hemoccult test,* a thin layer of feces is smeared over the boxes inside the envelope, and a drop of developing solution is applied on the opposite side of the specimen paper. For the *Hematest*, a thin layer of feces is smeared onto guaiac filter paper, a tablet is placed in the middle of the specimen, and two or three drops of water are added to the tablet.
- Consult your health-care provider if there is any problem understanding the instructions.
- Return completed specimens to your health-care provider or laboratory as instructed.

"Common Fecal Elimination Problems"). Clinical applications of these diagnoses are shown in Table 40.3.

Fecal elimination problems can affect many other areas of human functioning. Examples of possible nursing diagnoses include the following:

- *Risk for Deficient Fluid Volume* related to
  a. Prolonged diarrhea
  b. Abnormal fluid loss through ostomy
- *Risk for Impaired Skin Integrity* related to
  a. Prolonged diarrhea
  b. Bowel incontinence
  c. Bowel diversion ostomy
- *Disturbed Body Image* related to
  a. Ostomy
  b. Fecal incontinence
  c. Need for assistance with toileting
- *Deficient Knowledge* (bowel training, ostomy management) related to lack of previous experience

TABLE 40.3 Clinical Application: Assessment Data Clusters and Related Nursing Diagnoses

Data Cluster	Nursing Diagnosis
Mrs. Amy Ballaster states she feels fullness in her rectum and wants to move her bowels but cannot, even with straining. Her last bowel movement was 3 days ago. She lives alone and tends to eat only tea, toast, and noodle soup. Because of arthritis, her activities (gardening and walking) have decreased. Bowel sounds are decreased.	*Constipation* related to inadequate physical activity and insufficient fibre in diet
Marvin Lombardi reports having loose, liquid, light brown stools for two days. Passage of stools is associated with cramping abdominal pain. Bowel sounds are increased. Temperature is 38°C. He has not taken any medications but reports a feeling of general malaise. He states he "ate at a fast-food restaurant 2 nights ago."	*Diarrhea* of unknown etiology, possibly related to spoiled food
Mary Kuoko has had involuntary leakage of stool. She states her clothing is soiled several times a day. She says she is too embarrassed to go out with her friends because of the fecal odour. Last bowel movement was more than 3 days ago. Digital examination reveals impaction.	*Bowel Incontinence* related to fecal impaction
Mr. Dan Deer had a bowel diversion ostomy 2 days ago. Effluent is continuous and liquid. Peristomal skin is intact. Disposable colostomy device was applied.	*Risk for Impaired Skin Integrity* related to discharge from bowel diversion ostomy

- *Anxiety* related to
  - **a.** Lack of control of fecal elimination secondary to ostomy
  - **b.** Response of others to ostomy

Based on the assessment, a nurse may formulate other diagnoses independent of NANDA International (2007).

Planning

The major goals for clients with fecal elimination problems are to do the following:

- Maintain or restore normal bowel elimination pattern.
- Maintain or regain normal stool consistency.
- Prevent associated risks, such as fluid and electrolyte imbalance, skin breakdown, abdominal distension, and pain.

Examples of desired outcomes related to each of these goals, although established in the planning phase, are provided in Table 40.6 (page 1258) in the "Evaluating" section of this chapter.

Appropriate nursing interventions that relate to these broad goals must be identified. Preventive and corrective interventions to maintain or enhance fecal elimination include the following:

- Constipation or impaction management
- Bowel incontinence care
- Bowel management
- Bowel training
- Diarrhea management
- Coping enhancement
- Ostomy care

Specific nursing activities associated with each of these interventions can be selected to meet the client's individual needs. See the Sample Care Plan.

Sample Care Plan for Altered Bowel Elimination

ASSESSMENT DATA

Nursing Assessment

Mrs. Emma Brown is 78 years old. She has been a widow for 9 months. She lives alone in a low-income housing complex for older people. Her two children live with their families in a city approximately 240 km away. She always enjoyed cooking for her family; however, now that she is alone, she does not cook for herself. As a result, she has developed irregular eating patterns and tends to prepare soup-and-toast meals. She gets little exercise and has bouts of insomnia since her husband's death. For the past month, Mrs. Brown has been having a problem with constipation. She states she has a bowel movement about every 3 to 4 days and her stools are hard and painful to excrete. Mrs. Brown decides to attend the health fair sponsored by the housing complex and seeks assistance from the public health nurse.

Physical Examination

Height: 162 cm

Weight: 65 kg

Temperature: 36.2°C

Pulse: 82 bpm

Respirations: 20/min

Blood pressure: 128/74 mm Hg

Active bowel sounds, abdomen slightly distended

Diagnostic Data

CBC: Hgb 108 g/L

Urinalysis negative

Nursing Diagnosis

Constipation related to low-fibre diet and inactivity (as evidenced by infrequent, hard stools; painful defecation; abdominal distension)

Client Goals

Mrs. Brown will (1) establish a regular pattern of bowel elimination, (2) develop and maintain an exercise program, and (3) initiate nutritional alterations that will enhance regular bowel elimination.

Desired Health Outcomes

1. Increases daily fluid intake to 2000 mL unless contraindicated
2. Includes fibre in at least one meal per day
3. Walks for 20 minutes at least three times per week
4. Verbalizes relief of constipation by the second week

NURSING INTERVENTIONS AND SELECTED ACTIVITIES WITH RATIONALE* *[IN ITALICS]*

Constipation and Impaction Management

• Identify factors (e.g., medications, activity level, diet) that can cause or contribute to constipation.	*Assessing causative factors is an essential first step in teaching and planning for improved bowel elimination.*
• Encourage increased fluid intake, unless contraindicated.	*Sufficient fluid intake is necessary for the bowel to absorb sufficient amounts of liquid and promote proper stool consistency.*
• Evaluate her medication profile for gastrointestinal side effects.	*Constipation is a common side effect of many drugs, including opioid analgesics and antacids.*
• Teach Mrs. Brown how to keep a food diary.	*An appraisal of food intake will help identify whether Mrs. Brown is eating a well-balanced diet and consuming adequate amounts of fluid and fibre. Excessive meat or refined food intake will produce small, hard stools.*

(continued)

Sample Care Plan for Altered Bowel Elimination *(continued)*

Constipation and Impaction Management *(continued)*

• Instruct Mrs. Brown on a high-fibre diet, as appropriate.	*Fibre absorbs water, which adds bulk and softness to the stool and speeds up passage through the intestines.*
• Instruct her on the relationship of diet, exercise, and fluid intake to constipation and impaction.	*Fibre without adequate fluid can aggravate, not facilitate, bowel function.*
Exercise Promotion	
• Encourage verbalization of feelings about exercise or the need for exercise.	*Perceptions of the need for exercise can be influenced by misbeliefs, cultural and social beliefs, fears, or age.*
• Assist in identifying a positive role model for maintaining the exercise program.	*Individuals who have been successful in an exercise program can assist Mrs. Brown by providing incentive and enhancing motivation. For example, a walking partner may be beneficial.*
• Inform Mrs. Brown about the health benefits and physiological effects of exercise.	*Activity influences bowel elimination by improving muscle tone and stimulating peristalsis.*
• Instruct her about appropriate types of exercise for her level of health, in collaboration with a physician.	*Any individual beginning an exercise program should consult a physician primarily for a cardiac evaluation. Mrs. Brown's age and lack of activity should be considered in planning the level of activity.*
• Assist Mrs. Brown to set short-term and long-term goals for the exercise program.	*Realistic goal setting provides direction and motivation.*

EVALUATION

Goals not met. Mrs. Brown has kept a food diary and is able to identify the need for more fluid and fibre but has not consistently included fibre in her diet. She has started a walking program with a neighbour but is only able to walk for 10 minutes twice a week. She states her last bowel movement was 3 days ago.

*Interventions and activities selected are only a sample of those suggested in the *Nursing Interventions Classification (NIC)*, by G. M. Bulechek, H. K. Butcher, and J. C. Dochterman (Eds.), 2008, St. Louis, MO: Mosby Elsevier, and should be individualized for each client.

Planning for Home Care

Clients who have bowel diversion ostomies requiring fecal incontinence pouches, or who have other ongoing elimination problems, will need continuing care in the home setting. In preparation for discharge, the nurse needs to assess the client's and the family's abilities to meet specific care needs. The Assessment: Home Care box on fecal elimination outlines the specific assessment data required before developing a home care plan. By

ASSESSMENT: HOME CARE

Fecal Elimination

Assess the following to aid in developing a home care plan:

CLIENT AND ENVIRONMENT

- *Self-care abilities for toileting:* Ability to get to the toilet, to manipulate clothing for toileting, to perform toilet hygiene, and to flush the toilet
- *Mechanical aids required:* Walker, cane, wheelchair, raised toilet seat, grab bars, bedpan, commode
- *Mechanical barriers that limit access to the toilet or are unsafe:* Poor lighting, cluttered pathway to bathroom, narrow doorway for wheelchair, and so on
- *Bowel elimination problem:* Alterations in characteristics of feces, diarrhea, constipation, incontinence, presence of ostomy, and methods of handling these
- *Level of knowledge:* Planned bowel management or training program, prescribed medications, ostomy care, dietary alterations, and fluid and exercise requirements or restrictions
- *Facilities:* Adequacy of bathroom facilities to make possible toilet hygiene and ostomy care, and to contain potentially infectious fecal effluent or stool

FAMILY

- *Caregiver availability and skills:* People able to assist with toileting, medications, ostomy care, or other prescribed therapeutic measures
- *Family role changes and coping:* Effect on financial status, parenting and spousal roles, sexuality, social roles
- *Alternative potential primary or respite caregivers:* For example, other family members, volunteers, church members, paid caregivers or housekeeping services; available community respite care (adult day-care, senior centres)

COMMUNITY

- *Availability of and familiarity with possible sources of assistance:* Equipment and supply companies, financial assistance, home health-care agencies

TEACHING: HOME CARE

Fecal Elimination

The nurse uses the assessment data to create a teaching plan for the client and family:

FACILITATING TOILETING

- Ensure safe and easy access to the toilet. Make sure lighting is appropriate, scatter rugs are removed or securely fastened, and so on.
- Facilitate instruction, as needed, about transfer techniques. Contact a physical therapist or other appropriate health-care professional.
- Suggest ways that garments can be adjusted to make disrobing easier for toileting (e.g., Velcro closing on clothing).

MONITORING BOWEL ELIMINATION PATTERN

- If appropriate, instruct the client to keep a record of the time and frequency of stool passage, any associated pain, and colour and consistency of the stool.

DIETARY ALTERATIONS

- Provide information about required food and fluid alterations to promote defecation (see the Teaching: Wellness box on healthy defecation and Teaching: Clinical box on managing diarrhea).

MEDICATIONS

- Discuss problems associated with the overuse of laxatives, if appropriate, and the use of alternatives to laxatives, suppositories, and enemas.
- Discuss the addition of a fibre supplement if the client is taking a constipating medication (e.g., opioid analgesic),

MEASURES SPECIFIC TO ELIMINATION PROBLEM

- Provide instructions associated with specific elimination problems and treatment, such as
  a. Constipation
  b. Diarrhea
  c. Ostomy care
- See also bowel training programs later in the chapter.

COMMUNITY AGENCIES AND OTHER SOURCES OF HELP

- Make appropriate referrals to home care or community care for assistance with resources, such as installation of grab bars and raised toilet seats, structural alterations for wheelchair access, homemaker or home health-care aide services to assist with the activities of daily living (ADLs), and an enterostomal therapy nurse for assistance with stoma care and selection of ostomy appliances.
- Provide information about companies from which durable medical equipment (e.g., raised toilet seats, commodes, bedpans, urinals) can be purchased, rented, or obtained free, and where medical supplies, such as incontinence pads or ostomy irrigating supplies and appliances, can be obtained.
- Suggest additional sources of information and help, such as ostomy self-help and support groups or clubs.

using the assessment data, the nurse designs a teaching plan for the client and family (see the Teaching: Home Care box on fecal elimination).

Implementing

Promoting Regular Defecation

The nurse can help clients achieve regular defecation by attending to (1) the provision of privacy, (2) timing, (3) nutrition and fluids, (4) exercise, and (5) positioning. See also the Teaching: Wellness box on healthy defecation.

PRIVACY Privacy during defecation is extremely important to many people. The nurse should, therefore, provide as much privacy as possible to clients but may need to stay with clients who are too weak to be left alone. Some clients also prefer to wipe, wash, and dry themselves after defecating. A nurse may need to provide water and a washcloth and towel for this purpose. Clients should be assisted with hand hygiene following defecation.

TEACHING: WELLNESS

Healthy Defecation

Nurses should teach clients how to achieve regular defecation:

- Establish a regular exercise regimen.
- Include high-fibre foods (25 g to 30 g a day), such as vegetables, fruits, and whole grains, in the diet.
- Maintain fluid intake of at least 1500 mL to 2000 mL a day.
- Do not ignore the urge to defecate.
- Allow time to defecate, preferably at the same time each day.
- Avoid over-the-counter medications to treat constipation and diarrhea.

TIMING A client should be encouraged to defecate when the urge to defecate is recognized. To establish regular bowel elimination, the client and nurse can discuss when mass peristalsis normally occurs and provide time for defecation. Many people have well-established times and routines for defecation that should be part of the client's schedule. Other activities, such as bathing and ambulating, should not interfere with the defecation time. Also, clients should not be hurried and should be given adequate time to defecate.

NUTRITION AND FLUIDS The diet a client needs for regular normal elimination varies, depending on the kind of feces the client currently has, the frequency of defecation, and the types of foods that the client finds assist normal defecation.

CONSTIPATION Have the client increase daily fluid intake, and instruct the client to drink hot liquids and fruit juices, especially prune juice. Encourage the client to include fibre in the diet, that is, foods such as prunes, raw fruit, bran products, and whole-grain cereals and bread.

DIARRHEA Encourage oral intake of fluids and bland food. Eating small amounts of bland foods can be helpful because they are more easily absorbed. Diarrhea can lead to potassium loss. See the discussion of hypokalemia in Chapter 43. Excessively hot or cold fluids should be avoided because they stimulate peristalsis. In addition, highly spiced foods and high-fibre foods can aggravate diarrhea. Unfortunately, evidence that ingesting foods, such as yogourt, aged cheese, and buttermilk, that contain probiotics (bacteria and yeasts that resemble the normal bacteria found in the gastrointestinal tract) is effective in treating diarrhea is lacking (Allen, Okoko, Martinez, Gregorio, & Dans, 2003; Pillai & Nelson, 2008). See the Teaching: Clinical box on managing diarrhea.

EXERCISE Regular exercise helps clients develop a regular defecation pattern. A client with weak abdominal and pelvic muscles (which impede normal defecation) may be able to strengthen them with the following isometric exercises:

- In a supine position, the client tightens the abdominal muscles as though pulling them inward, holding them for about 10 seconds, and then relaxing them. This should be repeated 5 to 10 times, four times a day, depending on the client's health.
- Again in a supine position, the client can contract the thigh muscles and hold them contracted for about 10 seconds, repeating the exercise 5 to 10 times, four times a day. This helps the client confined to bed gain strength in the thigh muscles, thereby making it easier to use a bedpan.

POSITIONING Although the squatting position best facilitates defecation, on a toilet seat the best position for most people seems to be leaning forward.

For clients who have difficulty moving themselves to and from the toilet, an elevated toilet seat can be attached to a regular toilet. Clients then do not have to lower themselves far down onto the seat and do not have to lift as far off the seat. Elevated toilet seats can be purchased for use in the home.

TEACHING: CLINICAL

Managing Diarrhea

Ensure the client follows these guidelines in managing diarrhea:

- Drink at least 1.5 L to 2 L of water per day to prevent dehydration.
- Avoid alcohol, beverages with caffeine, and excessively hot or cold fluids, which aggravate the problem.
- Ingest foods with sodium and potassium. Most foods contain sodium. Potassium is found in dairy products, meats, and many vegetables and fruits, especially tomatoes, potatoes, bananas, cantaloupe, and apricots.
- Limit foods containing insoluble fibre, such as wholewheat and whole-grain breads and cereals, and raw fruits and vegetables.
- Increase foods containing soluble fibre, such as rice, oatmeal, and skinless fruits and potatoes.
- Limit fatty foods (e.g., dairy products and packaged processed meats).
- Thoroughly clean and dry the perianal area after passing stool to prevent skin irritation and breakdown. Use soft toilet tissue to clean and dry the area. Apply a moisture-barrier cream or ointment, such as zinc oxide or petrolatum, or an alcohol-free film barrier, as needed.
- Discontinue medications, as recommended by the physician, that cause diarrhea.
- When diarrhea has stopped, re-establish normal bowel flora by taking fermented dairy products containing probiotics, such as yogourt or buttermilk. Although probiotics are not effective in treating diarrhea, they seem to be useful after it has stopped.
- Consult a health-care provider immediately if weakness, dizziness, or loose stools persist more than 48 hours.

A bedside **commode**, a portable chair with a toilet seat and a receptacle beneath that can be emptied, is often used for the adult client who can get out of bed but is unable to walk to the bathroom. Some commodes can slide over the base of a regular toilet when the waste receptacle is removed, thus providing clients the privacy of a bathroom. Some commodes have a seat and can be used as a chair (Figure 40.13). Potty chairs are available for children.

Clients restricted to bed may need to use a **bedpan**, a receptacle for urine and feces. Female clients use a bedpan for both urine and feces; male clients use a bedpan for feces and a urinal for urine.

There are two main types of bedpans, the regular high-back pan and the slipper, or fracture, pan (Figure 40.14). The slipper pan has a low back and is used for clients unable to raise their buttocks because of physical problems or therapy that contraindicates such movement. Many older adults benefit from the use of a slipper pan. See Practice Guidelines 40.1 about giving and removing a bedpan.

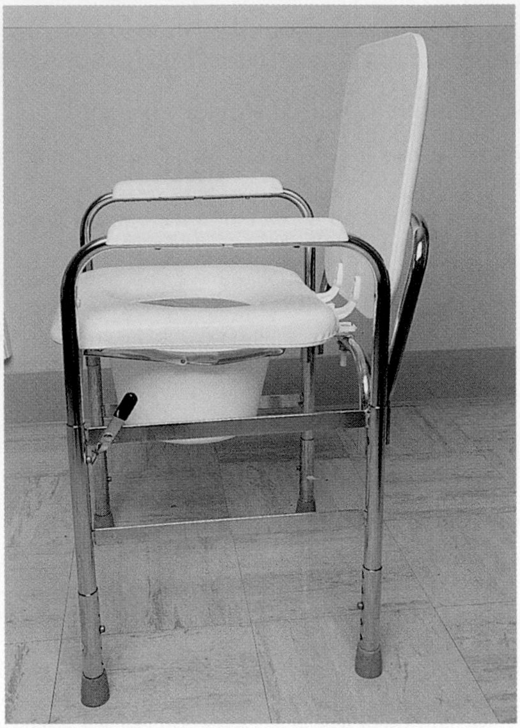

FIGURE 40.13 A commode with overlying seat

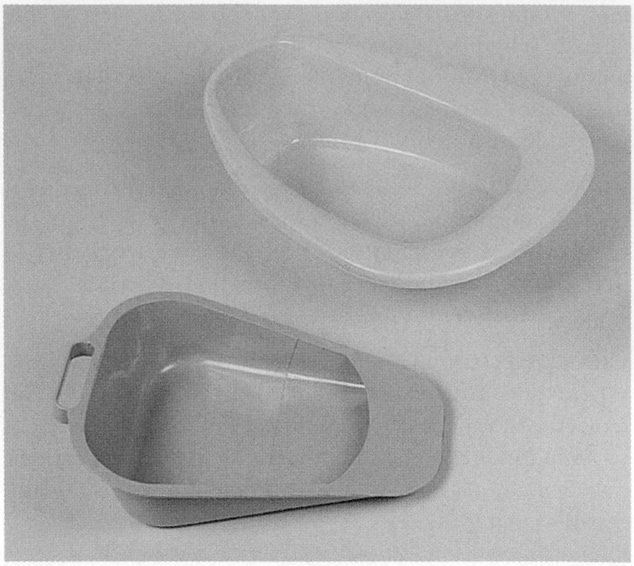

FIGURE 40.14 **Top:** the high-back or regular bedpan; **Bottom:** the slipper or fracture pan

PRACTICE GUIDELINES 40.1

Giving and Removing a Bedpan

Guidelines	Rationales
Perform hand hygiene and observe appropriate infection prevention and control procedures. Put on disposable gloves.	Routine practices and additional precautions prevent the spread of infection.
Provide privacy.	Procedures involving elimination are embarrassing to most clients.
If the bedpan is metal, warm it by rinsing it with warm water.	This facilitates patient comfort and sphincter relaxation.
Elevate the side rail on the opposite side to prevent the client from falling out of bed.	This is a patient safety measure.
Adjust the bed to a height appropriate to prevent back strain. Ask the client to assist by flexing the knees, resting the weight on the back and heels, and raising the buttocks, or by using a trapeze bar, if present.	The use of proper body mechanics decreases the risk of injury to the nurse. Encourage the patient to participate in self-care when able.
Help lift the client as needed by placing one hand under the lower back, resting your elbow on the mattress, and using your forearm as a lever.	The use of proper lifting techniques prevents injury to the nurse's back and increases the client's sense of security.
Place a regular bedpan so that the client's buttocks rest on the smooth, rounded rim. Place a slipper pan with the flat, low end under the client's buttocks (Figure 40.15).	Proper positioning of the bedpan promotes client comfort and avoids spillage.
For the client who cannot assist, obtain the assistance of another nurse to help place the client onto the bedpan. Turn the client on his or her side, place the bedpan against the buttocks (Figure 40.16), and roll the client back onto the bedpan.	Obtaining assistance ensures that the nurse does not sustain a back injury. The client movement to the side and then back ensures proper placement of the bedpan without having to lift the client.
To provide a more normal position for the client's lower back, elevate the client's bed to a semi-Fowler's position, if permitted. If elevation is contraindicated, support the client's back with pillows as needed.	Elevation of the bed or the use of pillows facilitates patient comfort and reduces the risk of hyperextension of the back.
Cover the client with bed linen.	This maintains client comfort and dignity.

(continued)

PRACTICE GUIDELINES 40.1

Giving and Removing a Bedpan *(continued)*

Provide toilet tissue, place the call light within reach, lower the bed to the low position, elevate the side rails, and leave the client alone, if not contraindicated.	Many clients find it difficult to have a bowel movement in the presence of another person. Allowing an able patient to wipe himself or herself promotes self-care and self-worth.
Answer the call bell promptly. Do not leave anyone on a bedpan longer than 15 minutes unless he or she is able to remove the pan by himself or herself.	Lengthy stays on a bedpan can cause pressure ulcers.
Put on gloves when removing the bedpan, hold the bedpan steady, cover the bedpan, and place it on a disposable pad on an adjacent chair. Return the bed to the position used when giving the bedpan.	This prevents spillage of the bedpan's contents, avoids contamination of patient-use surfaces (e.g., the chair), and maintains client dignity and comfort.
If the patient needs assistance, wipe perineal area with several layers of toilet tissue. If specimens are to be collected, discard the soiled tissue into a moisture-proof receptacle other than the bedpan. For female patients, wipe from the urethra toward the anus.	This prevents the transfer of rectal microorganisms into the urinary meatus.
Wash the perineal area of dependent clients with soap and water as indicated and thoroughly dry the area.	Cleansing prevents excoriation caused by stool left on the skin.
For all clients, offer warm water, soap, a washcloth, and a towel to wash the hands. Assist the client to a comfortable position, empty and clean the bedpan, and return it to the bedside.	These steps prevent infection and promote patient comfort.
Remove and discard your gloves and wash your hands.	Hand hygiene prevents cross-contamination.
Spray the room with air freshener, as needed, to control odour, unless contraindicated because of respiratory problems, allergies, or institutional policies.	Clients are often self-conscious about the odour.
Document colour, odour, amount, and consistency of urine and feces, and the condition of the perineal area.	Documentation is important to track changes and to prevent complications (e.g., constipation).

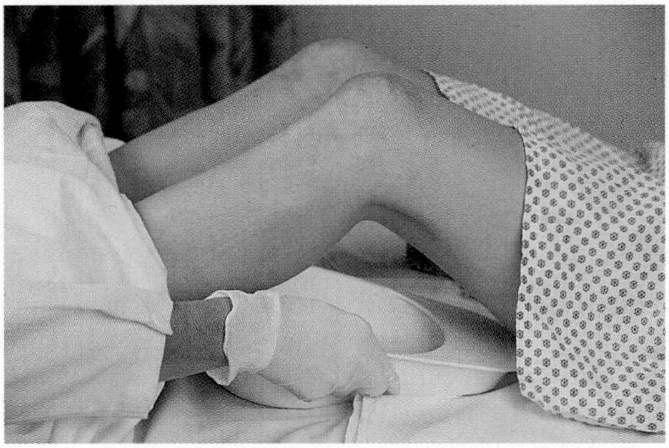

FIGURE 40.15 Placing a slipper pan under the buttocks

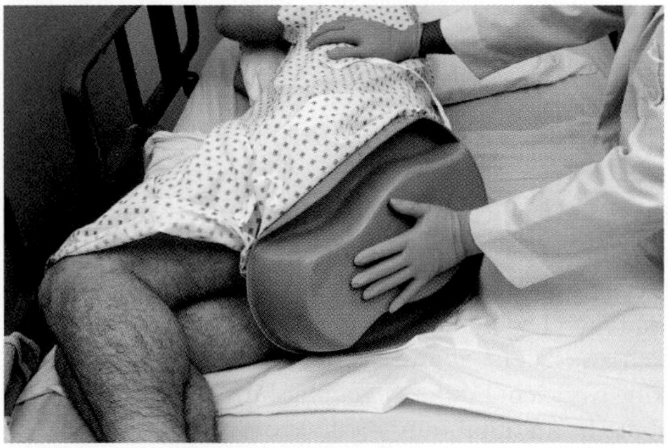

FIGURE 40.16 Placing a regular bedpan against the client's buttocks

Teaching about Medications

CATHARTICS AND LAXATIVES **Cathartics** are drugs that induce defecation. They can have a strong, purgative effect. A laxative is mild in comparison to a cathartic, and it produces frequent soft or liquid stools that are sometimes accompanied by abdominal cramps. Examples of cathartics are castor oil, cascara, phenolphthalein, and bisacodyl (Dulcolax). Table 40.4 describes the different types of laxatives.

Laxative abuse is believed to be a common problem. Older adults, in particular, often use laxatives improperly. Persistent self-administration of laxatives can result in chronic constipation. The trend now is toward the natural laxative approach, that is, increasing dietary fibre, such as that found in fruits and vegetables, to obtain a laxative effect.

Laxatives are contraindicated in the client who has nausea, cramps, colic, vomiting, or undiagnosed abdominal pain. Clients need to be informed about the dangers

TABLE 40.4 Types of Laxatives

Type	Action	Examples	Pertinent Teaching Information
Bulk-forming	Increases the fluid, gaseous, or solid bulk in the intestines	Psyllium hydrophilic mucilloid (Metamucil)	May take 12 or more hours to act. Sufficient fluid must be taken. Safe for long-term use.
Emollient or stool softener	Softens and delays the drying of the feces; permits fat and water to penetrate feces	Docusate sodium (Colace)	Slow-acting; may take several days.
Wetting agents	Lowers the surface tension of the feces, thus helping water to penetrate the feces	Docusate sodium (Colace)	Slow-acting; may take several days.
Stimulant or irritant	Irritates the intestinal mucosa or stimulates nerve endings in the wall of the intestine, causing rapid propulsion of the contents	Bisacodyl (Dulcolax), Senna (Senokot), sennoside (Ex-Lax), cascara	Acts more quickly than bulk-forming agents. Fluid is passed with the feces. May cause cramps. Prolonged use can cause fluid and electrolyte imbalance.
Lubricant	Lubricates the feces in the colon	Mineral oil	Prolonged use inhibits the absorption of some fat-soluble vitamins.
Saline or osmotic	Draws water into the intestine by osmosis, distends bowel, and stimulates peristalsis	Epsom salts, magnesium hydroxide (milk of magnesia), magnesium citrate, sodium phosphate (Fleet enema)	May be rapid acting. Can cause fluid and electrolyte imbalance, particularly in older adults and children with cardiac and renal diseases. Should not be used by elderly clients. Prolonged use inhibits the absorption of some fat-soluble vitamins.
		Electrolyte free polyethylene glycol (PEG3550) (Miralax)	A new laxative helpful in the treatment of constipation in children. Tasteless powder is mixed in flavoured liquid, such as juice.

of laxative use. Continual use of laxatives to encourage bowel evacuation weakens the bowel's natural responses to fecal distension, resulting in chronic constipation. To eliminate chronic laxative use, it is usually necessary to teach the client about dietary fibre, regular exercise, taking sufficient fluids, and establishing regular defecation habits. In addition, any medication regimen should be examined to see whether it could cause constipation.

Some laxatives are given in the form of a **suppository**, a solid, cone-shaped, medicated substance inserted into the rectum. Suppositories act in various ways: by softening the feces; by releasing gases, such as carbon dioxide, to distend the rectum; or by stimulating the nerve endings in the rectal mucosa. The best results can be obtained by inserting the suppository 30 minutes before the client's usual defecation time or when the peristaltic action is greatest, such as after breakfast.

ANTIFLATULENT MEDICATIONS Antiflatulent agents, such as simethicone, do not decrease the formation of flatus but they do coalesce the gas bubbles and facilitate their passage by belching through the mouth or expulsion through the anus. These agents are frequently combined with an antacid. Suppositories can also be given to relieve flatus by increasing intestinal motility.

ANTIDIARRHEAL MEDICATIONS These medications slow the motility of the intestine or absorb excess fluid in the intestine. See Practice Guidelines 40.2 on using antidiarrheals.

Administering Enemas

An **enema** is a solution introduced into the rectum and large intestine. An enema works by distending the intestine and sometimes irritating the intestinal mucosa, thereby increasing peristalsis and the excretion of feces and flatus.

TYPES OF ENEMAS Enemas are classified into four groups: cleansing, carminative, retention, and return flow.

CLEANSING ENEMAS Cleansing enemas are intended to remove feces. They are given chiefly to do the following:

- Prevent the escape of feces during surgery

PRACTICE GUIDELINES 40.2

Using Antidiarrheal Medications

Guidelines	Rationales
If the diarrhea persists for more than 3 or 4 days, determine the underlying cause.	Identifying the cause will ensure appropriate treatment. Using a medication, such as an opioid, when the cause is an infection, a toxin, or a poison may prolong diarrhea.
A complete review of the types of antidiarrheal agents being used is essential.	Long-term use of over-the-counter medications, such as loperamide hydrochloride (Imodium), can produce dependence. Some antidiarrheal agents, such as diphenoxylate hydrochloride (Lomotil), can cause drowsiness and should not be used when driving an automobile or running machinery. Kaolin-pectin preparations (e.g., Kaopectate) may absorb nutrients. Bismuth preparations (e.g., Pepto-Bismol), often used to treat travellers' diarrhea, may contain acetylsalicylic acid and should not be given to children or teens with varicella zoster (chickenpox), influenza, and other viral infections.

- Prepare the intestine for certain diagnostic tests, such as radiography or visualization tests (e.g., colonoscopy)
- Remove feces in instances of constipation or impaction
- Establish regular bowel function as part of a bowel training program

Cleansing enemas use a variety of solutions. See Table 40.5 for commonly used solutions.

Hypertonic solutions (e.g., sodium phosphate) exert osmotic pressure, which draws fluid from the interstitial space into the colon. The increased volume in the colon stimulates peristalsis and hence defecation. A commonly used hypertonic enema is the commercially prepared Fleet enema.

Hypotonic solutions (e.g., tap water) exert a lower osmotic pressure than the surrounding interstitial fluid, causing water to move from the colon into the interstitial space. Before the water moves from the colon, it stimulates peristalsis and defecation. Because the water moves out of the colon, the tap water enema should not be repeated because of the danger of circulatory overload when the water moves from the interstitial space into the circulatory system.

Isotonic solutions (e.g., physiological [normal] saline) are considered the safest enema solutions to use. They exert the same osmotic pressure as the interstitial fluid surrounding the colon. Therefore, there is no fluid movement into or out of the colon. The instilled volume of saline in the colon stimulates peristalsis.

Soapsuds enemas stimulate peristalsis by increasing the volume in the colon and irritating the mucosa. Only pure soap (e.g., castile soap) should be used in order to minimize mucosal irritation.

Some enemas are *large volume* (e.g., 500 mL to 1000 mL) for an adult and others are *small volume,* including hypertonic solutions. The latter, available commercially, act by drawing water into the colon, thus stimulating defecation. The amount of solution administered for a high-volume enema will depend on the age and medical condition of the individual. See Table 40.5 for approximate volumes of solutions.

TABLE 40.5 Commonly Used Enema Solutions

Solution	Constituents	Action	Time to Take Effect	Adverse Effects
Hypertonic	90 mL to 120 mL of solution (e.g., sodium phosphate)	Draws water into the colon	5 to 10 min	Retention of sodium
Hypotonic	500 mL to 1000 mL of tap water	Distends colon, stimulates peristalsis, and softens feces	15 to 20 min	Fluid and electrolyte imbalance; water intoxication
Isotonic	500 mL to 1000 mL of normal saline	Distends colon, stimulates peristalsis, and softens feces	15 to 20 min	Possible sodium retention
Soapsuds	500 mL to 1000 mL (3 mL to 5 mL soap to 1000 mL water)	Irritates mucosa, distends colon	10 to 15 min	Irritates and may damage mucosa
Oil (mineral, olive, cottonseed)	90 mL to 120 mL	Lubricates the feces and the colonic mucosa	1 to 3 hours	

Cleansing enemas can also be described as *high* or *low*. A *high enema* is given to cleanse as much of the colon as possible. The client changes from the left lateral position to the dorsal recumbent position and then to the right lateral position during administration so that the solution can follow the large intestine. See Figure 40.1 earlier. The low enema is used to clean the rectum and sigmoid colon only. The client maintains a left lateral position during administration. A medical prescription should specify when a high-enema technique is to be used.

The force of flow of the solution is governed by (1) the height of the solution container, (2) size of the tubing, (3) viscosity of the fluid, and (4) resistance of the rectum. The higher the solution container is held above the rectum, the faster is the flow and the greater is the force (pressure) in the rectum. During most adult enemas, the solution container should be no higher than 30 cm above the rectum. During a high cleansing enema, the solution container is usually held 30 cm to 45 cm above the rectum because the fluid is instilled farther to clean the entire bowel. For an infant, the solution container is held no more than 7.5 cm above the rectum.

CARMINATIVE ENEMA A *carminative enema* is given primarily to expel flatus. The solution instilled into the rectum releases gas, which, in turn, distends the rectum and the colon, thus stimulating peristalsis. For an adult, 60 mL to 80 mL of fluid is instilled.

RETENTION ENEMA A *retention enema* introduces oil or medication into the rectum and sigmoid colon. The oil is retained for a relatively long period (e.g., 1 to 3 hours). It acts to soften the feces and to lubricate the rectum and anal canal, thus facilitating passage of the feces.

RETURN-FLOW ENEMA A *return-flow enema* is used occasionally to expel flatus. Alternating flow of 100 mL to 200 mL of fluid into and out of the rectum and sigmoid colon stimulates peristalsis. This process is repeated five or six times until the flatus is expelled and abdominal distension is relieved.

Other types of enemas are also available; for example, medicated enemas, such as *antibiotic* enemas used to treat infections locally, *antihelmintic* enemas used to kill helminths, such as worms and intestinal parasites, and *nutritive* enemas used to administer fluids and nutrients to the rectum.

SKILL 40.1

ADMINISTERING AN ENEMA

PURPOSES

- To achieve one or more of the following actions: cleansing, carminative, retention, or return flow

ASSESSMENT

Assess the following:

- When the client last had a bowel movement and the amount, colour, and consistency of the feces
- Presence of abdominal distension (the distended abdomen appears swollen and feels firm, rather than soft, when palpated)
- Whether the client has sphincter control
- Whether the client can use a toilet or commode or must remain in bed and use a bedpan

Planning

Before administering an enema, determine whether a physician's order is required. At some agencies, a physician or other designated health-care professional must order the kind of enema and the time to give it, for example, the morning of the examination. When the client has rectal disease, the size of the rectal tube to use may be specified. At other agencies, enemas are given at the nurse's discretion (i.e., as necessary on a prn order). In addition, determine the presence of kidney or cardiac disease that contraindicates the use of a hypotonic solution.

Equipment

- Disposable linen-saver pad
- Bath blanket
- Bedpan or commode
- Disposable gloves
- Water-soluble lubricant, if tubing is not prelubricated
- Paper towel

Large-Volume Enema

- Solution container with tubing of correct size and tubing clamp
- Correct solution, amount, and temperature (37.7°C to 40°C for adults)

Small-Volume Enema

- Packaged container of enema solution with lubricated tip

IMPLEMENTATION

Preparation

- Lubricate about 5 cm of the rectal tube (some commercially prepared enema sets already have lubricated nozzles). **Rationale: Lubrication facilitates insertion through the sphincters and minimizes trauma.**

(continued)

SKILL 40.1

ADMINISTERING AN ENEMA (*continued*)

- Run some solution through the connecting tubing of a large-volume enema set and the rectal tube to expel any air in the tubing; then close the clamp. **Rationale: Air instilled into the rectum, although not harmful, causes unnecessary distension.**

Performance

1. Before performing the procedure, introduce yourself and verify the client's identity by using agency protocol. Explain to the client what you are going to do, why it is necessary, and how he or she can cooperate. Indicate that the client may experience a feeling of fullness while the solution is being administered.
2. Perform hand hygiene, apply clean gloves, and observe other appropriate infection prevention and control procedures.
3. Provide for client privacy.
4. Assist the adult client to a left lateral position, with the right leg as acutely flexed as possible (see ❶) and the linen-saver pad under the buttocks. **Rationale: This position facilitates the flow of solution by gravity into the sigmoid and descending colon, which are on the left side. Having the right leg acutely flexed provides for adequate exposure of the anus.**
5. Insert the enema tube.
   - For clients in the left lateral position, lift the upper buttock. **Rationale: To ensure good visualization of the anus.**
   - Insert the tube smoothly and slowly into the rectum, directing it toward the umbilicus (see ❷). **Rationale: The angle follows the normal contour of the rectum. Slow insertion prevents spasm of the sphincter.**
   - Insert the tube 7 cm to 10 cm. **Rationale: Because the anal canal is about 2.5 cm to 5 cm long in the adult, insertion to this point places the tip of the tube beyond the anal sphincter into the rectum.**
   - If resistance is encountered at the internal sphincter, ask the client to take a deep breath, then run a small amount of solution through the tube. **Rationale: This manoeuvre will help relax the internal anal sphincter.**
   - Never force tube or solution entry. If instilling a small amount of solution does not permit the tube to be advanced or the solution to freely flow, withdraw the tube. Check for any stool that may have blocked the tube during insertion. If present, flush it and retry the procedure. You may also perform a digital rectal examination to determine if there is an impaction or other mechanical blockage. If resistance persists, end the procedure and report the resistance to the health-care provider and nurse in charge.
6. Slowly administer the enema solution.
   - Raise the solution container, and open the clamp to allow fluid flow.
   - *Or* compress a pliable container by hand.
   - During most low enemas, hold or hang the solution container no higher than 30 cm above the rectum. **Rationale: The higher the solution container is held above the rectum, the faster the flow and the greater the force (pressure) in the rectum.** During a high enema, hang the solution container about 45 cm. **Rationale: The fluid must be instilled farther to clean the entire bowel. See agency protocol.**
   - Administer the fluid slowly. If the client complains of fullness or pain, lower the container or use the clamp to stop the flow for 30 seconds, and then restart the flow at a slower rate. **Rationale: Administering the enema slowly and stopping the flow momentarily decreases the likelihood of intestinal spasm and premature ejection of the solution.**
   - If using a plastic commercial container, roll it up as the fluid is instilled (see ❸).
   - After all the solution has been instilled or when the client cannot hold any more and feels the desire to defecate (the urge to defecate usually indicates that sufficient fluid has been administered), close the clamp, and remove the enema tube from the anus.
   - Place the enema tube in a disposable towel as you withdraw it.
7. Encourage the client to retain the enema.
   - Ask the client to remain lying down. It is easier for the client to retain the enema when lying down than when sitting or standing, because gravity promotes drainage and peristalsis.
   - Request that the client retain the solution for the appropriate amount of time, for example, 5 to 10 minutes for a cleansing enema or at least 30 minutes for a retention enema.

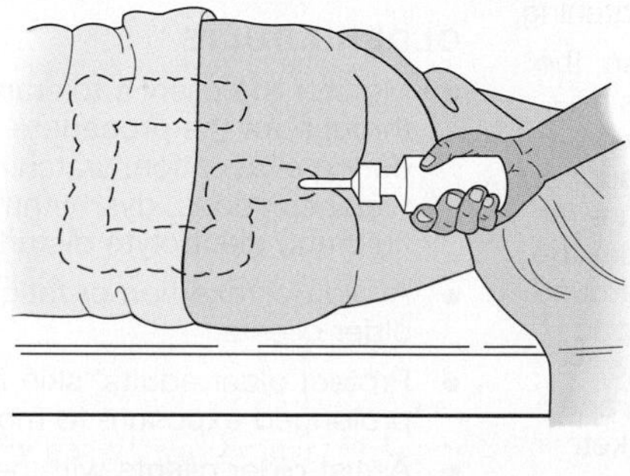

❶ Assuming a left lateral position for an enema. Note the commercially prepared enema.

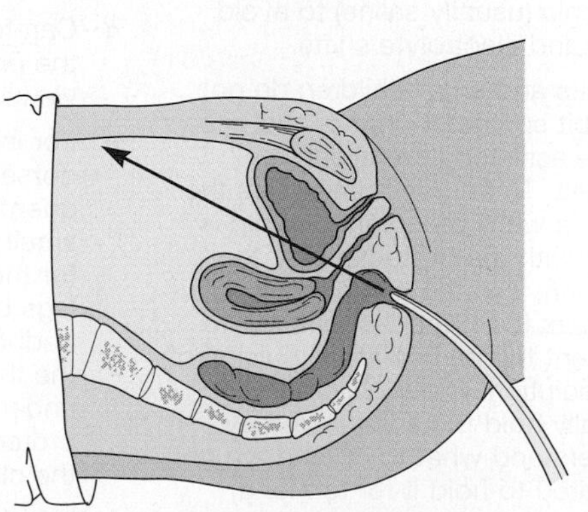

❷ Inserting the rectal tube following the direction of the rectum

(continued)

SKILL 40.1

ADMINISTERING AN ENEMA (*continued*)

8. Assist the client to defecate.
- Assist the client to a sitting position on the bedpan, commode, or toilet. A sitting position facilitates the act of defecation.
- Ask the client who is using the toilet not to flush it. The nurse needs to observe the feces.
- If a specimen of feces is required, ask the client to use a bedpan or commode.

9. Document the type and volume, if appropriate, of enema given. Describe the results.

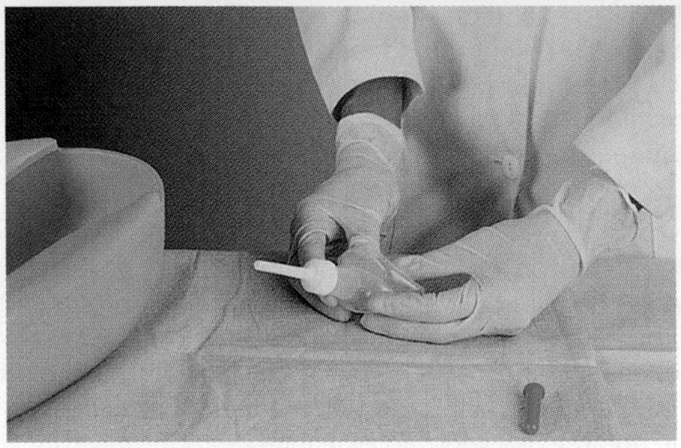

❸ Rolling up a commercial enema container

EVALUATION

Evaluate the amount, colour, and consistency of returns; relief of flatus or abdominal distension; and any problems encountered (e.g., resistance at the external or internal sphincter when inserting the rectal tube).

Home Care Considerations

Administering an Enema

Teach the caregiver or client the following:

- To make saline solution, mix one teaspoon of table salt to 500 mL of tap water.
- Use enemas only as directed. Do not rely on them for regular bowel evacuation.
- Before administration, make sure a bedpan, commode, or toilet is nearby.

EQUIPMENT Commercially prepared, low-volume, disposable enema kits are commonly used today. The kit includes a flexible bottle of solution with a prelubricated, firm tip.

Equipment for a large-volume enema is listed in Skill 40.1. A caregiver should wear disposable gloves during administration of an enema to prevent contact with body fluids, blood, and microorganisms. Skill 40.1 describes how to administer an enema.

Lifespan Considerations

Administering an Enema

INFANTS AND CHILDREN

- Provide a careful explanation to the parents and child before the procedure.
- The enema solution should be isotonic (usually saline) to avoid fluid and electrolyte shifts.
- Infants and small children do not exhibit sphincter control and need to be assisted in retaining the enema. The nurse administers the enema while the infant or child is lying with the buttocks over the bedpan, and the nurse firmly presses the buttocks together to prevent the immediate expulsion of the solution. Older children can usually hold the solution if they understand what to do and are not required to hold it for too long.
- Enema temperature should be 37.7°C unless otherwise ordered.
- Large-volume enemas consist of 50 mL to 200 mL in children younger than 18 months old; 200 mL to 300 mL in children 18 months to 5 years; and 300 mL to 500 mL in children 5 to 12 years old.
- Careful explanation is essential for the preschool child as the enema is viewed as intrusive and threatening.
- For infants and small children, the dorsal recumbent position is frequently used. Position them on a small padded bedpan with support for the back and head. Secure the legs by placing a diaper under the bedpan and then over and around the thighs. Place the under pad under the client's buttocks to protect the bed linen, and drape the client with the bath blanket.
- Insert the tube 5 cm to 7.5 cm in the child and only 2.5 cm to 3.75 cm in the infant.
- For children, lower the height of the solution container appropriately for the age of the child. See agency protocol.
- To assist a small child in retaining the solution apply firm pressure over the anus with tissue wipes, or firmly press the buttocks together.

OLDER ADULTS

- Monitor the client's tolerance throughout the procedure and during evacuation, watching for vagal episodes, dysrhythmias, and fluid and electrolyte disturbances.
- Avoid overexertion or fatigue for older clients.
- Protect older adults' skin from prolonged exposure to moisture.
- Assist older clients with perineal care as indicated.

Evidence-Informed Practice

Can Chronic Diarrhea in HIV Clients Be Controlled through a Behavioural and Dietary Intervention That Uses Normal Foods?

Diarrhea can be a chronic condition in HIV, reducing quality of life. The etiology of chronic diarrhea in this population is multifaceted and treatment is generally supportive. Anastasi, Capili, Kim, McMahon, and Heitkemper (2006) conducted a 24-week study evaluating the efficacy of implementing a dietary and behavioural intervention to decrease the frequency of diarrhea in this population. The treatment group consisted of 38 HIV-positive individuals with a mean age of 43.5 (13 females and 25 males). The control group was made up of 37 HIV-positive individuals (9 females and 28 males). The treatment group received personalized education regarding diet, nutrition, and diarrhea, in addition to behavioural skills training. The education was personalized following an analysis of individual food diaries. A brochure was used to guide the teaching.

Behavioural interventions included exploring attitudes toward following the diet and fostering beliefs that promoted following it. Barriers and strategies to overcome them were identified by the client. The nurse also provided strategies not identified by the client. In addition, skills for communicating and negotiating the importance of following the diet were practised.

Normal foods rather than formula preparations were chosen to promote long-term compliance and enable clients to live normally. The aim was to decrease the intake of insoluble fibre by 50% and totally eliminate caffeine. Although the intervention was based on food restriction, the goal was to empower clients through knowledge and decision making. By using the individualized food diaries, the participants decreased their fat, lactose, and insoluble fibre intake. Intake of soluble fibre was increased. The researchers reported that nutrition and behaviour skill building were effective in decreasing the frequency of diarrhea in the treatment group.

NURSING IMPLICATIONS: The life expectancy of clients with HIV has increased because of the availability of medications. These clients may be seen both in the community setting and in hospital settings. Nurses, as frontline staff, have the opportunity to identify clients in need of dietary modification. Providing individualized health teaching and behavioural interventions can assist these clients in improving their quality of life.

Source: Based on "Symptom Management of HIV-Related Diarrhea by Using Normal Foods: A Randomized Controlled Clinical Trial," by J. K. Anastasi, B. C. Capili, G. Kim, D. McMahon, and M. M. Heitkemper, 2006, *Journal of the Association of Nurses in AIDS Care, 17*(2), pp. 47–57.

Digitally Removing a Fecal Impaction

Digital removal involves breaking up the fecal mass digitally and removing it in portions. Because the bowel mucosa can be injured during this procedure, some agencies restrict and specify the personnel permitted to conduct digital disimpaction. Rectal stimulation is also contraindicated for some people because it may cause an excessive vagal response resulting in cardiac arrhythmias. Before disimpaction, it may be suggested that an oil retention enema be given and held for 30 minutes. (Check agency policy and physician's order.) After a disimpaction, the nurse can use various interventions to remove remaining feces, such as a cleansing enema or the insertion of a suppository as prescribed by the physician.

For digital removal of a fecal impaction, follow these steps:

1. Obtain assistance from a second person who can comfort the client during the procedure.
2. Ask the client to assume a left side-lying position, with the knees flexed and the back toward the nurse.
3. Place a bedpad under the client's buttocks and a bedpan nearby to receive stool.
4. Drape the client for comfort and to avoid unnecessary exposure of the body.

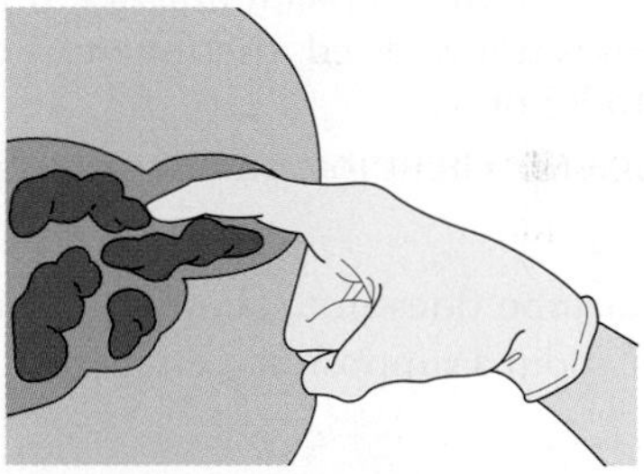

FIGURE 40.17 Digital removal of fecal impaction

5. Put on a pair of clean gloves, and liberally lubricate the index finger to be inserted.
6. Gently insert the index finger into the rectum, and move the finger toward the client's umbilicus along the length of the rectum.
7. Loosen and dislodge stool by gently massaging around it. Break up stool by working the finger into the hardened mass, taking care to avoid injury to the mucosa of the rectum (Figure 40.17).
8. Carefully work stool downward to the end of the rectum and remove it in small pieces. Continue to remove as much fecal material as possible. Periodically assess the client for signs of fatigue, such as facial pallor, diaphoresis, or change in pulse rate. Manual stimulation should be minimal.

9. Following disimpaction, assist the client to clean the anal area and buttocks. Then, assist the client onto a bedpan or commode for a short time because digital stimulation of the rectum often induces the urge to defecate.

Decreasing Flatulence

Flatus can be reduced or prevented in a number of ways, including getting exercise, moving in bed, ambulating, and avoiding gas-producing foods. Movement stimulates peristalsis, the escape of flatus, and the reabsorption of gases into the intestinal capillaries. One method of treating flatulence involves the insertion of a rectal tube:

1. Use a rectal tube 22 to 30 French for adults and a smaller size for children.
2. Have the client assume a side-lying position.
3. Lubricate the rectal tube to reduce mucous membrane irritation.
4. Expose the anus and insert the rectal tube into the rectum 7.5 cm to 10 cm. The rectal tube will stimulate peristalsis. Do not force the tube in if it does not insert easily. Secure the tube in place.
5. Wrap an abdominal or incontinence pad around the end of the rectal tube to catch any liquid that may be expelled. Some nurses suggest inserting the rectal tube and then placing the end into a receptacle filled with water. The passage of flatus will be seen as bubbles are produced.
6. Leave the tube in no longer than 30 minutes to avoid irritation of the rectal mucosa. If abdominal distension is not relieved, the tube can be inserted every 2 to 3 hours.
7. Encourage the client to assume various positions in bed.

If a rectal tube does not relieve flatus, consult with the physician about a suppository, enema, or medication.

Creating Bowel Training Programs

For clients who have chronic constipation, frequent impactions, or fecal incontinence, a *bowel training program* may be helpful. The program is based on factors within the client's control and is designed to help the client establish normal defecation. Such matters as food and fluid intake, exercise, and defecation habits are all considered. Before beginning such a program, clients must understand it and want to be involved. The major phases of the program are as follows:

- Determine the client's usual bowel habits and factors that help and hinder normal defecation.
- Design a plan with the client that includes the following:
  a. Fluid intake of at least 1500 mL to 2000 mL per day, unless contraindicated
  b. Increase in fibre in the diet
  c. Intake of hot drinks, especially just before the usual defecation time
  d. Increase in exercise
- Maintain the following daily routine for 2 to 3 weeks:
  a. Administer a cathartic suppository (e.g., bisacodyl [Dulcolax]) 30 minutes before the client's defecation time to stimulate peristalsis.
  b. When the client experiences the urge to defecate, assist the client to the toilet or commode or onto a bedpan. Note the length of time between the insertion of the suppository and the urge to defecate.
  c. Provide the client with privacy for defecation and a time limit; 15 minutes is usually sufficient to allow for defecation while minimizing the risk of skin breakdown.
  d. Teach the client to lean forward at the hips, to apply pressure on the abdomen with the hands, and to bear down for defecation. These measures increase pressure on the colon. Straining should be avoided because it can cause hemorrhoids.
- Provide positive feedback when the client successfully defecates. Refrain from negative feedback if the client fails to defecate.
- Offer encouragement to the client, and convey that patience is often required. Many clients require weeks or months of training to achieve success.

Using a Fecal Incontinence Pouch

To collect and contain large volumes of feces, the nurse may place a fecal incontinence collector pouch around the anal area (Figure 40.18). The purpose of the pouch is to prevent progressive perianal skin irritation and breakdown and frequent linen changes necessitated by incontinence.

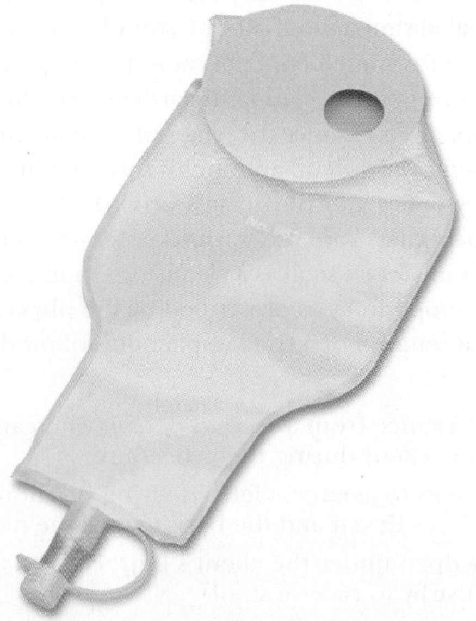

FIGURE 40.18 A drainable fecal collector pouch

A fecal collector is secured around the anal opening and may or may not be attached to drainage. Pouches are best applied before the perianal skin becomes excoriated. If perianal skin excoriation is present, the nurse either (1) applies a dimethicone-based moisture-barrier cream or alcohol-free barrier film to the skin to protect it from feces until it heals and then applies the pouch, or (2) applies a skin barrier or hydrocolloid barrier underneath the pouch to achieve the best possible seal.

Nursing responsibilities for clients with a rectal pouch include (1) regular assessment and documentation of the perianal skin status, (2) changing the bag every 72 hours or sooner if there is leakage, (3) maintaining the drainage system, and (4) providing explanations and support to the client.

Some clients (e.g., post-trauma, quadriplegic, paraplegic or post-stroke) may be treated for fecal incontinence with surgical repair of a damaged sphincter or with an artificial bowel sphincter. The artificial sphincter consists of three parts: a cuff around the anal canal, a pressure-regulating balloon, and a pump that inflates the cuff (Figure 40.19). The cuff is inflated to close the sphincter, maintaining continence. To have a bowel movement, the client deflates the cuff. The cuff automatically reinflates (generally in 10 minutes). Management of this device is usually specific to the device; contact the manufacturing company for details.

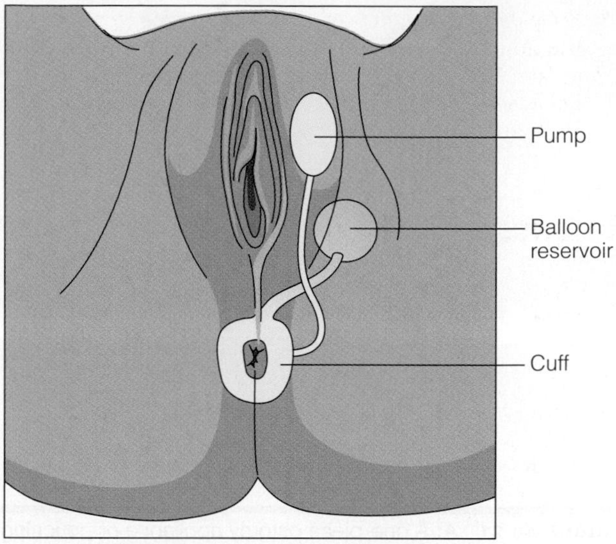

FIGURE 40.19 Inflatable artificial sphincter

Managing an Ostomy

Clients with fecal diversions need considerable psychological support, instruction, and physical care. This section is limited to the nurse's physical interventions of stoma assessment, application of an appliance to collect feces, and promotion of predictable evacuation with colostomy irrigation. Many agencies have enterostomal therapy nurses to assist these clients. National organizations (e.g., United Ostomy Association of Canada) aim to improve the quality of life of individuals who have or will require an ostomy. The United Ostomy Association of Canada is a volunteer-based organization, with chapters located across Canada. It provides emotional support, practical assistance, and informational services. Members of local chapters can meet and visit with a person who has a new ostomy. It is common for a client with a new ostomy to feel frightened and alone. Talking with another person who has gone through a similar experience may help the client realize that he or she is not alone and that others are willing to listen and help.

STOMA AND SKIN CARE Care of the stoma and skin is important for all clients who have ostomies. The fecal material from a colostomy or ileostomy is irritating to the peristomal skin. This is particularly true of stool from an ileostomy, which contains digestive enzymes. It is important to assess the peristomal skin for irritation each time the appliance is changed. Any irritation or skin breakdown needs to be treated immediately. The skin is kept clean by washing off any excretion and drying thoroughly.

An ostomy appliance should protect the skin, collect stool, and control odour. The appliance consists of a skin barrier and a pouch. Some clients may prefer to also wear an adjustable ostomy belt, which attaches to an ostomy pouch to hold the pouch firmly in place (Figure 40.20). Appliances can be one piece, in which the skin barrier is already attached to the pouch (Figure 40.21A), or an appliance can consist of two pieces: a separate pouch with a flange and a separate skin barrier with a flange where the pouch fastens to the barrier at the flange (Figure 40.21B). The pouch can be removed without removing the skin barrier when using a two-piece appliance. Pouches can be closed or drainable (Figure 40.22).

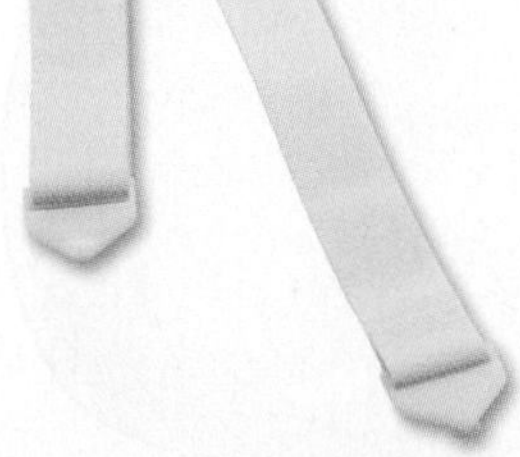

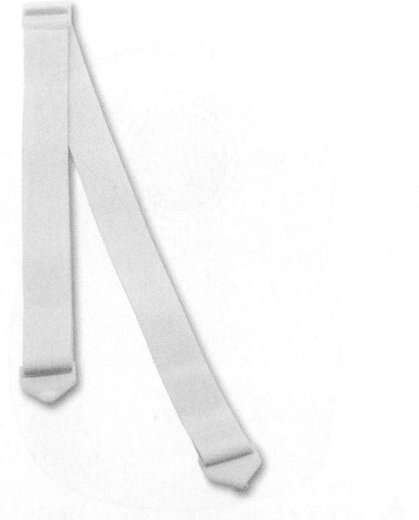

FIGURE 40.20 Adjustable ostomy belt

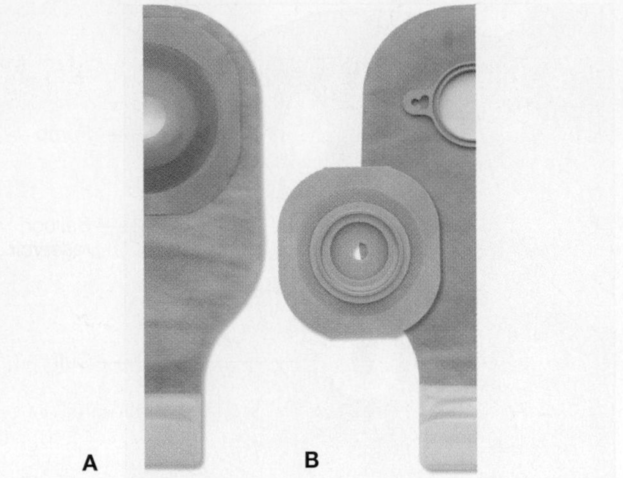

FIGURE 40.21 **A:** A one-piece ostomy appliance or pouching system; **B:** a two-piece ostomy appliance or pouching system

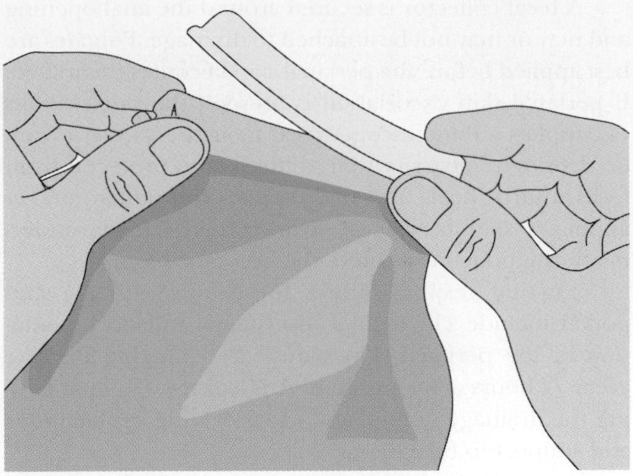

FIGURE 40.23 Applying a pouch clamp

A drainable pouch usually has a clip where the end of the pouch is folded over the clamp and clipped (Figure 40.23). Newer drainable pouches have an integrated closure system instead of a clamp. Drainable pouches are generally used by people who need to empty the pouch more than twice a day.

Closed pouches are often used by people who have a regular stoma discharge (e.g., sigmoid colostomy) and have to empty the pouch only one or two times a day. Some people find it easier to change a closed pouch than to empty a drainable pouch, which requires some dexterity.

Odour control is essential to clients' self-esteem. As soon as clients are ambulatory, they can learn to work with the ostomy in the bathroom to avoid odours at the bedside. Selecting the appropriate kind of appliance promotes odour control. An intact appliance contains odours. The appliance should be rinsed thoroughly when it is emptied. Deodorizers can be placed in the pouch of the appliance, or pouches with charcoal filter discs are available. In limited circumstances, oral preparations to control odour can be prescribed.

Ostomy appliances can be applied for up to 7 days. They need to be changed whenever the effluent leaks onto the peristomal skin or when it cannot be rinsed completely away. Many people prefer to change them daily or whenever they become soiled, but this practice can be detrimental to the integrity of the peristomal skin and is expensive. Check agency practice in this regard. Some people recommend removing the pouch and skin barrier twice a week to clean and inspect the peristomal skin. If the skin is erythematous, eroded, denuded, or ulcerated, the ostomy appliance should be changed every 24 to 48 hours to allow appropriate treatment of the skin. More frequent changes are recommended if the client complains of pain or discomfort.

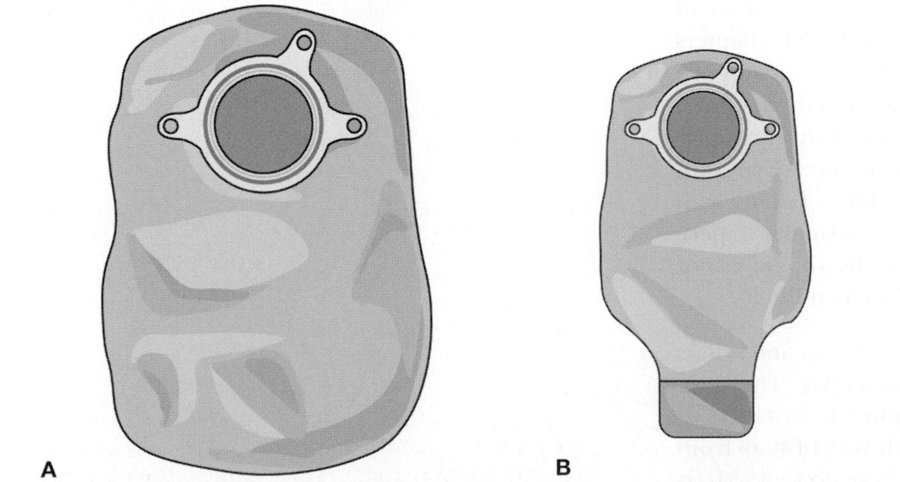

FIGURE 40.22 **A:** A closed pouch; **B:** a drainable pouch

SKILL 40.2

CHANGING A ONE-PIECE, DRAINABLE BOWEL DIVERSION OSTOMY APPLIANCE

Before changing a bowel diversion ostomy appliance, determine the kind of ostomy and its placement on the abdomen. It is important to confirm which is the functioning stoma and any orders about the care of the stomas.

PURPOSES

- To assess and care for the peristomal skin
- To collect effluent for assessment of the amount and type of output
- To minimize odours for the client's comfort and self-esteem

ASSESSMENT

Assess the following:

- *Stoma colour:* The stoma should appear red, similar in colour to the mucosal lining of the inner cheek. Very pale or darker-coloured stomas with a bluish or purplish hue indicate impaired blood circulation to the area.
- *Stoma size and shape:* Most stomas protrude slightly from the abdomen. New stomas normally appear swollen, but swelling generally decreases over 2 or 3 weeks or for as long as 6 weeks. Failure of swelling to recede may indicate a problem, such as blockage.
- *Stomal bleeding:* Slight bleeding initially when the stoma is touched is normal, but other bleeding should be reported.
- *Status of peristomal skin:* Any redness and irritation of the peristomal skin—the 5 cm to 12.5 cm of skin surrounding the stoma—should be noted. Transient redness after removal of adhesive is normal.
- *Amount and type of feces:* Assess the amount, colour, odour, and consistency. Inspect for abnormalities, such as pus or blood.
- *Symptoms:* Statements of burning sensation under the skin barrier may indicate skin breakdown. The presence of abdominal discomfort or distension also needs to be determined.
- The client's and the family members' learning needs regarding the ostomy and self-care.
- The client's emotional status, especially strategies used to cope with the body image changes and the ostomy.

Equipment

- Disposable gloves
- Bedpan
- Moisture-proof bag (for disposable pouches)
- Cleaning materials, including tissues, warm water, mild soap (optional), washcloth or cotton balls, towel
- Tissue or gauze pad
- Skin barrier (paste, powder, water, or liquid skin sealant)
- Stoma measuring guide
- Pen or pencil and scissors
- New ostomy appliance, with optional belt
- Tail closure clamp
- Deodorant for pouch (optional)

IMPLEMENTATION

Preparation

1. Determine the need for an appliance change.
   - Assess the used appliance for leakage of stool. **Rationale: Stool can irritate the peristomal skin.**
   - Ask the client about any discomfort at or around the stoma. **Rationale: A burning sensation may indicate breakdown beneath the faceplate of the pouch.**
   - Assess the fullness of the pouch. **Rationale: The weight of an overly full bag can loosen the skin barrier and separate it from the skin, causing the stool to leak and irritate the peristomal skin.**
2. If there is pouch leakage or discomfort at or around the stoma, change the appliance.
3. Select an appropriate time to change the appliance.
   - Avoid times close to meal or visiting hours. **Rationale: Ostomy odour and stool may reduce appetite or embarrass the client.**
   - Avoid times immediately after meals or the administration of any medications that may stimulate bowel evacuation. **Rationale: It is best to change the pouch when drainage is least likely to occur.**

Performance

1. Before performing the procedure, introduce yourself and verify the client's identity by using agency protocol. Explain to the client what you are going to do, why it is necessary, and how he or she can cooperate. Discuss how the results will be used in planning further care or treatments. Changing an ostomy appliance should not cause discomfort, but it may be distasteful to the client. Communicate acceptance and support to the client. It is important to change the appliance competently and quickly. Include support persons as appropriate.
2. Perform hand hygiene, apply clean gloves, and observe other appropriate infection prevention and control procedures.
3. Provide for client privacy, preferably in the bathroom, where clients can learn to deal with the ostomy as they would at home.
4. Assist the client to a comfortable sitting or lying position in bed or preferably a sitting or standing position in the bathroom. **Rationale: Lying or standing positions can facilitate smoother pouch application, that is, avoid wrinkles.**
5. Unfasten the belt if the client is wearing one.

(continued)

SKILL 40.2

CHANGING A ONE-PIECE, DRAINABLE BOWEL DIVERSION OSTOMY APPLIANCE *(continued)*

6. Empty the pouch and remove the ostomy skin barrier.
   - Empty the contents of a drainable pouch through the bottom opening into a bedpan or toilet. **Rationale: Emptying before removing the pouch prevents spillage of stool onto the client's skin**.
   - If the pouch uses a clamp, do not throw it away as it can be reused.
   - Assess the consistency, colour, and amount of stool.
   - Peel the skin barrier off slowly, beginning at the top and working downward, while holding the client's skin taut. **Rationale: Holding the skin taut minimizes client discomfort and prevents abrasion of the skin**.
   - Discard the disposable pouch in a moisture-proof bag.
7. Clean and dry the peristomal skin and stoma.
   - Use toilet tissue to remove excess stool.
   - Use warm water, mild soap (optional), and a washcloth to clean the skin and stoma (see ❶). Check agency practice on the use of soap. **Rationale: Soap is sometimes not advised because it can be irritating to the skin**. If soap is allowed, do not use deodorant or moisturizing soaps **Rationale: They may interfere with the adhesives in the skin barrier**.
   - Dry the area thoroughly by patting with a towel. **Rationale: Excess rubbing can abrade the skin**.
8. Assess the stoma and peristomal skin.
   - Inspect the stoma for colour, size, shape, and bleeding.
   - Inspect the peristomal skin for any redness, ulceration, or irritation. Transient redness after the removal of adhesive is normal.
9. Place a piece of tissue or gauze over the stoma, and change it as needed. **Rationale: This absorbs any seepage from the stoma while the ostomy appliance is being changed**.
10. Prepare and apply the skin barrier (peristomal seal).
    - Use the guide (see ❷) to measure the size of the stoma.
    - On the backing of the skin barrier, trace a circle the same size as the stomal opening.
    - Cut out the traced stoma pattern to make an opening in the skin barrier (see ❸). Make the opening no more than 0.3 cm to 0.4 cm larger than the stoma. **Rationale: This allows space for the stoma to expand slightly when functioning and minimizes the risk of stool contacting peristomal skin**.
    - Remove the backing to expose the sticky adhesive side. The backing can be saved and used as a pattern when making an opening for future skin barriers.

    For a one-piece pouching system:
    - Centre the skin barrier over the stoma (see ❹), and gently press it onto the client's skin for 30 seconds (see ❺). **Rationale: The heat and pressure help activate the adhesives in the skin barrier**.

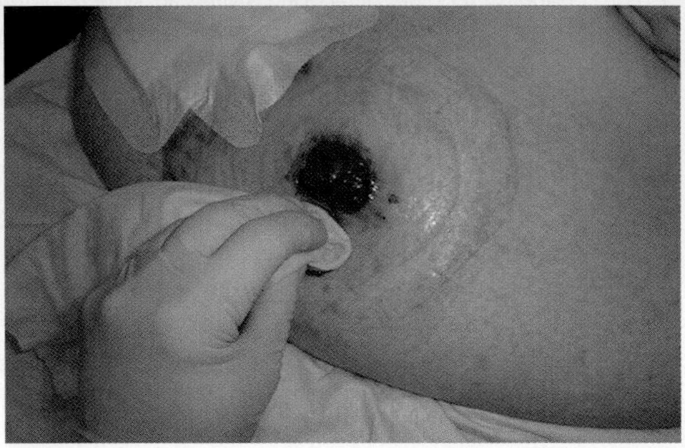

❶ Cleaning the skin

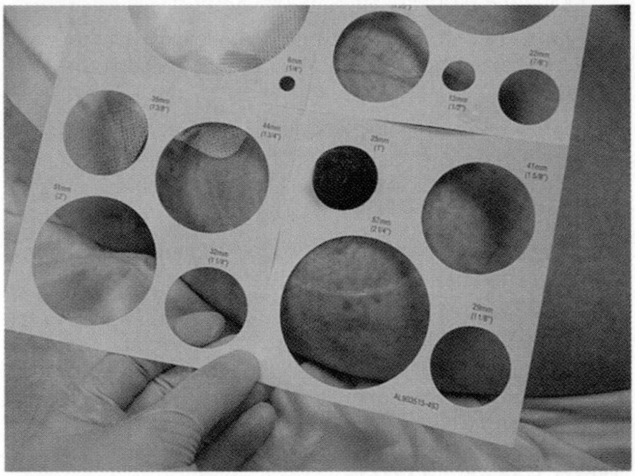

❷ A guide for measuring the stoma

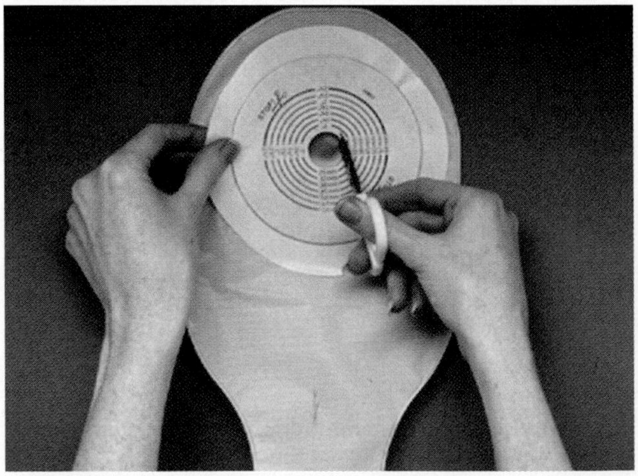

❸ The nurse is making a stoma opening on a disposable one-piece pouch.

(continued)

SKILL 40.2

CHANGING A ONE-PIECE, DRAINABLE BOWEL DIVERSION OSTOMY APPLIANCE *(continued)*

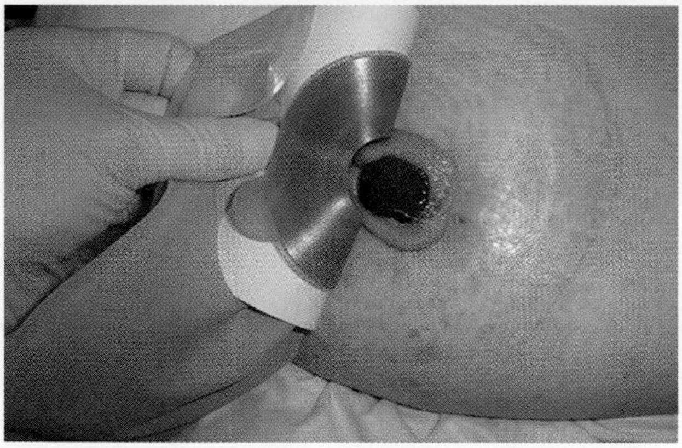

4 Centring the skin barrier over the stoma

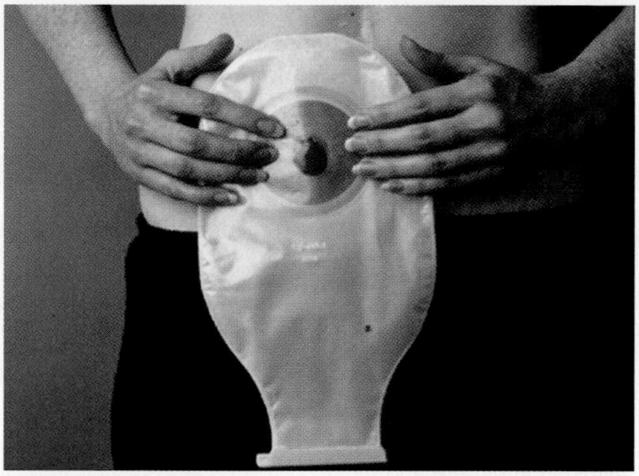

5 Pressing the skin barrier of a disposable one-piece pouch for 30 seconds to activate the adhesives in the skin barrier

For a two-piece pouching system:

- Centre the skin barrier over the stoma and gently press it onto the client's skin for 30 seconds.
- Remove the tissue over the stoma before applying the pouch.
- Snap the pouch onto the flange or skin barrier wafer.
- For drainable pouches, close the pouch according to the manufacturer's directions.

11. Document the procedure in the client record by using forms or checklists supplemented by narrative notes when appropriate. Report and record pertinent assessments and interventions. Report any increase in stoma size, change in colour indicative of circulatory impairment, and presence of skin irritation or erosion. Record on the client's chart any discolouration of the stoma, the appearance of the peristomal skin, the amount and type of drainage, the client's reaction to the procedure, the client's experience with the ostomy, and skills learned by the client.

EVALUATION

- Relate findings to previous data, if available. Adjust the teaching plan and nursing care plan as needed. Reinforce the teaching each time the care is performed.
- Perform detailed follow-up based on findings that deviated from expected for the client. Report such deviations to the appropriate member of the health-care team.

Home Care Considerations

Drainable Bowel Diversion Ostomy Appliances

- Provide the client with the names and phone numbers of an enterostomal therapist and a supply vendor.
- Suggest additional sources of information, such as the Crohn's and Colitis Foundation of Canada and the Canadian Association of Gastroenterology.
- Inform the client of signs to report to a health-care provider (e.g., peristomal redness, skin breakdown, and changes in stomal colour).

The type of ostomy and amount of output influences how often the pouch is emptied. The pouch is emptied when it is one-third to one-half full. If the pouch overfills, it can cause separation of the skin barrier from the skin and stool comes in contact with the skin. This results in the entire appliance needing to be removed and a new one applied.

Skill 40.2 explains how to change a bowel diversion ostomy appliance.

COLOSTOMY IRRIGATION A colostomy irrigation, similar to an enema, is a form of stoma management used only for clients who have a sigmoid or descending colostomy. It is not done for ileostomies because the feces are usually liquid. The purpose of irrigation is to distend the bowel sufficiently to stimulate peristalsis, which stimulates evacuation. When a regular evacuation pattern is achieved, the wearing of a colostomy pouch is unnecessary. Currently, colostomy irrigations are not routinely taught to most patients. Routine daily irrigations for control of the time of elimination ultimately become the client's decision. Some clients prefer to control the time of elimination through rigid dietary regulation and not be bothered with irrigations, which can take up to an hour to complete. When regulation by irrigation is chosen, it should be done at the same time each day. Control by irrigation also necessitates some control of the diet. For example, laxative foods that might cause an unexpected evacuation need to be avoided.

For most clients, a relatively small amount of fluid (300 mL to 500 mL) stimulates evacuation. For others, up to 1000 mL may be needed because a colostomy has no sphincter and the fluid tends to return as it is instilled. This problem is reduced by the use of a cone on the irrigating catheter. The cone helps hold the fluid within the bowel during the irrigation. Clients that have used irrigation for several years are more prone to peristomal hernias, bowel perforation, and electrolyte imbalance with large-volume irrigations (500 mL to 1000 mL). Careful observation and assessment of this practice may be required in older, more fragile clients.

TABLE 40.6 Evaluation Goals and Outcomes: Fecal Elimination

Elimination Problem and Goals	Examples of Desired Health Outcomes
Constipation	
Maintain or restore usual bowel elimination pattern and regain normal stool consistency	Identifies usual pattern of bowel elimination Identifies factors that alter bowel function Ingests adequate fluids (e.g., 1.5 L to 2 L of water daily) Ingests adequate amount of fibre (e.g., eats two high-fibre vegetables or fruits and at least one bran muffin or high-fibre bread or cereal daily) Walks for at least 20 minutes daily Reports: (a) bowel movement at least every 3 days, (b) regular time for defecation, (c) easy passage of stool Reports stool amount, colour, and consistency within normal limits Reports absence of distension, discomfort, and feeling of incomplete bowel evacuation
Perceived Constipation	
Restore normal bowel elimination pattern	Verbalizes understanding of need to decrease use of laxatives, enemas, and suppositories Accepts as normal an interval of 2 to 3 days between bowel movements Alters diet and exercise pattern to include adequate daily amounts of fibre, fluids, and exercise (see Constipation) Reports decreased use of laxative or suppository (e.g., only once per week) Reports stools of normal consistency and colour
Diarrhea	
Restore normal bowel elimination pattern	Reports stools of normal consistency and colour Reports decreased frequency of bowel evacuation (e.g., no more than 2 bowel movements per day) Reports absence of abdominal pain
Prevent potential problems associated with diarrhea	Maintains fluid and electrolyte balance, as evidenced by a. Serum electrolyte values of 135–145 mmol/L Potassium 3.5–5.0 mmol/L Chloride 95–105 mmol/L Bicarbonate 22–26 mmol/L b. Normal or baseline body weight or (specify weight gain) c. Normal skin turgor Maintains perianal skin integrity, as evidenced by absence of redness or breakdown
Bowel Incontinence	
Prevent potential problems associated with incontinence	Identifies factors causing incontinence Keeps a daily bowel evacuation diary that includes time, amount, and stool consistency Reports fewer episodes of incontinence and soiling Uses appropriate measures to maintain perianal skin integrity (e.g., hygiene measures and protective skin barriers) Demonstrates effective coping skills, as evidenced by a. Ability to meet self-care needs b. Participation in social activities once or twice per week

Evaluating

The goals established during the planning phase are evaluated according to specific desired outcomes also established in that phase. Examples of these are shown in Table 40.6.

If outcomes are not achieved, the nurse should explore the reasons why. The nurse might consider some or all of the following questions:

- Were the client's fluid intake and diet appropriate?
- Was the client's activity level appropriate?
- Are prescribed medications or other factors affecting the gastrointestinal function?
- Do the client and family understand the provided instructions well enough to comply with the required therapy?
- Were sufficient physical and emotional supports provided?

Case Study 40

Mr. Dubois is a 62-year-old man who suffered a cerebrovascular accident (stroke) about 3 months ago. He underwent aggressive medical management and extensive physical and occupational therapy, which improved his overall functioning. Currently, Mr. Dubois is able to provide much of his own care but must rely on an assistive device for safe ambulation. He is being followed on an outpatient basis by community health services. During your visit with Mr. Dubois at his home, you learn that he has been experiencing abdominal discomfort, increased flatulence, and intermittent diarrhea for the past several days. He states that he usually has a bowel movement every 1 to 2 days, and his last normal bowel movement was about 6 or 7 days ago. His wife says that he is not eating or drinking well because he feels bloated and uncomfortable much of the time.

Critical Thinking Questions

1. What conclusions, if any, can be drawn about Mr. Dubois's abdominal distress, diarrhea, and flatulence?
2. You learn that Mr. Dubois's stools have been liquid, in very small amounts, and at infrequent intervals, generally occurring when he feels the urge to defecate. What additional data are important to obtain from him?
3. What nursing intervention is most appropriate before making suggestions to correct the problem he is experiencing?
4. What suggestions can you give him about maintaining a regular bowel pattern?
5. Explain why cathartics and laxatives are generally contraindicated for people in Mr. Dubois's situation.

After working through these questions, go to the MyNursingLab at **http://www.mynursinglab.com** to check your answers.

KEY TERMS

feces
stool
haustra
ingestion
chyme
flatus
haustral churning
haustral shuffling
peristalsis
mass peristalsis
hemorrhoids
defecation
bilirubin
meconium
encopresis
gastrocolic reflex
laxatives
paralytic ileus
constipation
fecal impaction
diarrhea
bowel incontinence
fecal incontinence
flatulence
eructation
ostomy
gastrostomy
jejunostomy
ileostomy
colostomy
ureterostomy
stoma
anoscopy
proctoscopy
proctosigmoidoscopy
colonoscopy
occult blood
guaiac test
commode
bedpan
cathartics
suppository
enema

CHAPTER HIGHLIGHTS

- The primary functions of the large bowel are the excretion of digestive waste products and the maintenance of fluid balance.
- Patterns of fecal elimination vary greatly among people, but a regular pattern of fecal elimination with formed, soft stools is essential to health and a sense of well-being.
- A variety of factors affect defecation: developmental level, diet, fluid intake, activity and exercise, psychological factors, regular defecation, medications, diagnostic procedures, anaesthesia, pathological conditions, and pain.
- Common fecal elimination problems include constipation, fecal impaction, diarrhea, bowel incontinence, and flatulence. Each has specific defining characteristics and contributing causes that often relate to or are identical to the factors that affect defecation.
- Assessment relative to fecal elimination includes a nursing history; physical examination of the abdomen, rectum, and anus; and in some situations, visualization studies and inspection and analysis of stool for abnormal constituents, such as blood.
- A nursing history includes data about the client's defecation pattern, description of feces and any changes or problems associated with elimination, and data about possible factors altering bowel elimination.
- Physical examination of the abdomen includes methods of inspection, auscultation, percussion, and palpation. Physical examination of the rectum and anus includes inspection and palpation.
- When inspecting the client's stool, the nurse must observe its colour, consistency, shape, amount, and odour, and the presence of abnormal constituents.
- A function of the nurse is to assist clients with endoscopic and radiographic studies of the large intestine. Client assistance for visualization involves diet and bowel preparation before the study and appropriate follow-up care after the study.
- Clients also often need assistance to obtain stool specimens for laboratory analysis. In many agencies, nurses test the stool for occult blood.
- Lack of exercise, irregular defecation habits, stress, bland diets, and overuse of laxatives are all thought to contribute to constipation. Sufficient fluid and fibre intake are required to keep feces soft.
- An adverse effect of constipation is straining during defecation, during which the Valsalva manoeuvre may be used. Cardiac problems may ensue.
- An adverse effect of prolonged diarrhea is fluid and electrolyte imbalance.
- Digital removal of an impaction should be carried out gently because of vagal nerve stimulation and subsequent depressed cardiac rate. A physician's order is often necessary.
- Normal defecation is often facilitated in both well and ill clients by providing privacy, teaching clients to attend to defecation urges promptly, encouraging appropriate food and fluid intake, scheduling regular exercise, and assisting clients to normal sitting positions whenever possible.
- Additional nursing strategies include administering cathartics and antidiarrheals; administering cleansing, carminative, or retention enemas; removing an impaction digitally; inserting rectal tubes to decrease flatulence; applying protective skin agents; monitoring fluid and electrolyte balance; and instructing clients in ways to promote normal defecation.
- Clients who have bowel diversion ostomies require special care, with attention to psychological adjustment, diet, and stoma and skin care. A variety of stomal management methods are available to these clients, depending on the type and position of the ostomy.

ASSESS YOUR LEARNING

1. Clients should be taught that repeatedly ignoring the sensation of needing to defecate can result in which of the following?
   a. Constipation
   b. Diarrhea
   c. Incontinence
   d. Hemorrhoids
2. Mrs. Dejardin, a 45-year-old obese woman, presents to the emergency department with complaints of right-sided back pain. In removing her bedpan you note white, pasty stool. What would be the most appropriate action?
   a. Encourage Mrs. Dejardin to increase her fluid intake.
   b. Encourage Mrs. Dejardin to increase her fibre intake.
   c. Document the findings and notify the appropriate member of the health-care team.
   d. Obtain a thorough dietary history.
3. Jonathon O'Reilly has been ordered a barium swallow before a lower gastrointestinal CT scan. What action should the nurse take after the procedure?
   a. Maintain Jonathon NPO until the barium is expelled.
   b. Assess his abdomen for distension.
   c. Encourage fluids and ambulation.
   d. Use special precautions with his bodily waste.
4. What is a potential complication of a digital removal of a fecal impaction?
   a. Increased vagal tone
   b. Trauma to the rectum

c. Pain

d. Bowel perforation

5. In assessing a new colostomy, the nurse notes that the stoma is pale and grey. Which of the following actions is most appropriate?

a. Remove the appliance and examine the skin beneath the adhesive.

b. Notify the surgeon.

c. Document the findings and continue to monitor.

d. Irrigate the colostomy.

6. Mr. John is a 65-year-old man with chronic alcoholism. He is admitted with a peptic ulcer. On emptying Mr. John's bedpan, the nurse notes his stool is black and tarry. What is the most probable explanation?

a. The discolouration is a side effect of iron supplements.

b. He is experiencing an upper gastrointestinal bleed.

c. The discolouration is a side effect of taking ASA.

d. The discolouration is due to his ingestion of beets.

7. A young client with neutropenia (an abnormally low number of neutrophils in the blood), was recently discharged from hospital. She calls complaining of foul-smelling diarrhea occurring 5 to 6 times a day. What instructions should the nurse provide?

a. Increase fluid intake to prevent dehydration.

b. Take an over-the-counter antidiarrheal medication, such as Imodium.

c. Eat a bland diet until the frequency of loose stools decreases.

d. Obtain a stool sample and make an appointment with her family physician.

8. Jane is going to the operating room for bowel surgery. She has been prescribed an enema the evening before the procedure. What actions would the nurse would take in administering the enema?

a. Place the client in the left lateral position with the solution container at 25 cm above the rectum.

b. Place the client in the right lateral position with the solution container 25 cm above the rectum.

c. Place the client in the left lateral position with the solution container 45 cm above the rectum.

d. Place the client in the left lateral position with the solution container 45 cm above the rectum and reposition to the dorsal recumbent and right lateral positions.

9. Ann is a 50-year-old client admitted from the operating room following an ileostomy. When the nurse assesses Ann's ostomy, she notes that the adhesive backing has buckled. What is the nurse's immediate concern?

a. Skin breakdown

b. Infection

c. Swelling

d. Discomfort

10. A patient is prescribed morphine for pain associated with bladder cancer. What health teaching must be reinforced on discharge?

a. Morphine is addictive and should only be used when absolutely necessary.

b. Fluid and fibre intake should be increased.

c. Fluid and fibre intake should be decreased.

d. The patient's activity level should be reduced because of the sedation properties of morphine.

After working through these questions, go to the MyNursingLab at ***http://www.mynursinglab.com*** *to check your answers and see explanations.*

SUGGESTED READINGS

Bray, L., & Sanders, C. (2006). Preparing children and young people for stoma surgery. *Paediatric Nursing, 18*(4), 33–37.

Successful approaches employed in other forms of surgery are adapted to prepare the child for stoma surgery.

Johnson, J. Y. M., McMullen, L. M., Hasselback, P., Louie, M., & Duncan Saunders, L. (2006). Travelers' knowledge of prevention and treatment of travelers' diarrhea. *Journal of Travel Medicine, 13,* 351–355.

This study assesses the knowledge of travellers' diarrhea among a convenience sample of travellers heading to Mexico. Knowledge of this common affliction is key to prevention and treatment.

Johnston, B. C., Supina, A. L., Ospina, M., & Vohra, S. (2007). Probiotics for the prevention of pediatric antibiotic-associated diarrhea. *Cochrane Database of Systematic Reviews, Issue,* Art. No.: CD004827.

This systematic review evaluates the efficacy of probiotics in the prevention of antibiotic-induced diarrhea in children. The authors conclude that there is not enough evidence to support the routine use of probiotics to prevent pediatric antibiotic-associated diarrhea and provide an interesting review of literature.

Lefebvre, S. L., Waltner-Toews, D., Peregrine, A. S., Reid-Smith, R., Hodge, L., & Arroyo, L. G. (2006). Prevalence of zoonotic agents in dogs visiting hospitalized people in Ontario: Implications for infection control. *Journal of Hospital Infection, 62,* 454–466.

The authors of this study sought to determine the prevalence of visiting dogs carrying zoonotic infections so that infection control policies could be developed.

WEBLINKS

The Canadian Celiac Association

http://www.celiac.ca

This organization provides support and education for people who have celiac disease.

Crohn's and Colitis Foundation of Canada

http://www.ccfc.ca

This Canadian foundation is a national nonprofit organization committed to finding a cure for inflammatory bowel disease through raising funds for medical research. The website provides educational resources, including books, FAQs, and downloadable brochures.

Irritable Bowel Syndrome Self Help and Support Group

http://www.ibsgroup.org

The Irritable Bowel Syndrome (IBS) Self Help Group was formed in 1987 to provide support to those suffering from IBS, for those who are looking for support for someone who has IBS, and for medical professionals wanting to learn more about IBS. The website provides educational materials, including articles, videos, a newsletter, and up-to-date news on IBS.

The United Ostomy Association of Canada

http://www.ostomycanada.ca

The United Ostomy Association of Canada is dedicated to assisting all persons with gastrointestinal or urinary diversions. The website provides information about ostomies and support groups.

Colon Cancer Alliance

http://www.ccalliance.org

The Colon Cancer Alliance was founded in 1996 to provide support and education to individuals affected by colon cancer. The website provides educational materials, including downloadable fact sheets and brochures, current colorectal cancer news, and book reviews.

The Canadian Association for Enterostomal Therapy

http://www.caet.ca

The Canadian Association for Enterostomal Therapy is a nonprofit association specializing in the nursing care of patients with challenges in wound, ostomy, and continence. The website provides useful information and brochures for patients, families, and professionals dealing with clients who have ostomies.

REFERENCES

Allen, S. J., Okoko, B., Martinez, E., Gregorio, G., & Dans, L. F. (2003). Probiotics for treating infectious diarrhoea. *Cochrane Database of Systematic Reviews, 4,* Art. No.: CD003048.

Gordin, F. M., Schultz, M. E., Huber, R. A., & Gill, J. A. (2005). Reduction in nosocomial transmission of drug-resistant bacteria after introduction of an alcohol-based hand rub. *Infection Control and Hospital Epidemiology, 26*(7), 650–653.

LeMone, P., & Burke, K. M. (2008). *Medical surgical nursing: Critical thinking in client care* (4th ed.). Upper Saddle River, NJ: Prentice Hall.

Longstreth, G. F., Thompson, W. G., Chey, W. D., Houghton, L. A., Mearin, F., & Spiller, R. C. (2006). Functional bowel disorders. *Gastroenterology, 130*(5), 1480–1491.

NANDA International. (2007). *Nursing diagnoses: Definitions and classification, 2007–2008.* Philadelphia, PA: Author.

Nelson, R. (2007). Antibiotic treatment for *Clostridium difficile*–associated diarrhea in adults. *Cochrane Database of Systematic Reviews, 3,* Art. No.: CD004610.

Pillai, A., & Nelson, R. (2008). Probiotics for treatment of *Clostridium difficile*–associated colitis in adults. *Cochrane Database of Systematic Review, 1,* Art. No.: CD004611.

Poutanen, S. M., & Simor, A. E. (2004). *Clostridium difficile*–associated diarrhea in adults. *Canadian Medical Association Journal, 171*(1), 51–58.

Registered Nurses' Association of Ontario. (2005). *Best practice guideline: Prevention of constipation in the older adult population.* Toronto: Author.

Singh, G., Kahler, K., Bharathi, V., Mithal, A., Barghout, V., & Triadafilopoulos, G. (2005). Constipation in adults: Complications and comorbidities. *Gastroenterology, 128*(Suppl 2), A154.

Chapter 41

Urinary Elimination

Elimination from the urinary tract is usually taken for granted. Only when a problem arises do most people become aware of their urinary habits and any associated symptoms.

A person's urinary habits depend on physiological processes as well as sociocultural, familial, and personal norms and habits. In Canada, most people are accustomed to privacy and clean (even decorative) surroundings while they urinate. Personal habits regarding urination are affected by the social propriety of leaving to urinate, the availability of a private clean facility, and initial bladder training. The physiology of the urinary system is complex and is discussed in detail in this chapter.

OBJECTIVES

After studying this chapter, you should be able to

1. Describe the process of urination, from urine formation through micturition
2. Identify seven factors that influence urinary elimination
3. Discuss eight common alterations in urine production and elimination
4. List common causes of selected urinary problems
5. Describe nursing assessment of urinary function, including subjective and objective data
6. Outline normal and abnormal characteristics and constituents of urine
7. Explain how to collect urine specimens and conduct selected tests
8. Develop nursing diagnoses related to urinary elimination
9. List goals and desired health outcomes for clients with nursing diagnoses related to urinary elimination
10. Discuss interventions to maintain normal urinary elimination and to assist clients with altered urinary elimination
11. Identify strategies to prevent urinary tract infection
12. Identify interventions for clients with retention catheters or urinary diversions

Physiology of Urinary Elimination

Urinary elimination depends on effective functioning of the renal system, made up of the four urinary tract organs: kidneys, ureters, bladder, and urethra (Figure 41.1).

Kidneys

The paired kidneys are situated on either side of the spinal column, behind the peritoneal cavity. They are the primary regulators of fluid and acid-base balance in the body (see Chapter 43). The functional units of the kidneys, the nephrons, filter the blood and remove metabolic wastes. In the average adult, 1200 mL of blood, or about 21% of the cardiac output, passes through the kidneys every minute. Each kidney contains approximately 1 million nephrons. Each nephron has a **glomerulus**, a tuft of capillaries surrounded by **Bowman's capsule** (Figure 41.2). The endothelium of the glomerular capillaries is porous, allowing fluid and solutes to readily move across this membrane into the capsule. Plasma proteins and blood cells, however, are too large to cross the membrane normally. Glomerular filtrate is similar in composition to plasma, made up of water, electrolytes, glucose, amino acids, and metabolic wastes.

From Bowman's capsule, the filtrate moves into the tubule of the nephron. In the proximal convoluted tubule, most of the water and electrolytes are reabsorbed. Solutes, such as glucose, are reabsorbed in the loop of Henle, but in the same area, other substances are secreted into the filtrate, concentrating the urine. In the distal convoluted tubule, additional water and sodium are reabsorbed under the control of hormones, such as antidiuretic hormone (ADH) and aldosterone. This controlled reabsorption allows fine regulation of fluid and electrolyte balance in the body. When fluid intake is low or the concentration of solutes in the blood is high, ADH is released from the anterior pituitary, more water is reabsorbed in the distal tubule, and less urine is excreted. By contrast, when fluid intake is high or the blood solute concentration is low, ADH is suppressed. Without ADH, the distal tubule becomes impermeable to water, and more urine is excreted. Aldosterone also affects the tubule. When aldosterone is released from the adrenal cortex, sodium and water are reabsorbed in greater quantities, increasing the blood volume and decreasing urinary output.

Ureters

Once the urine is formed in the kidneys, it moves through the collecting ducts into the calyces of the renal pelvis and from there into the ureters. The ureters are

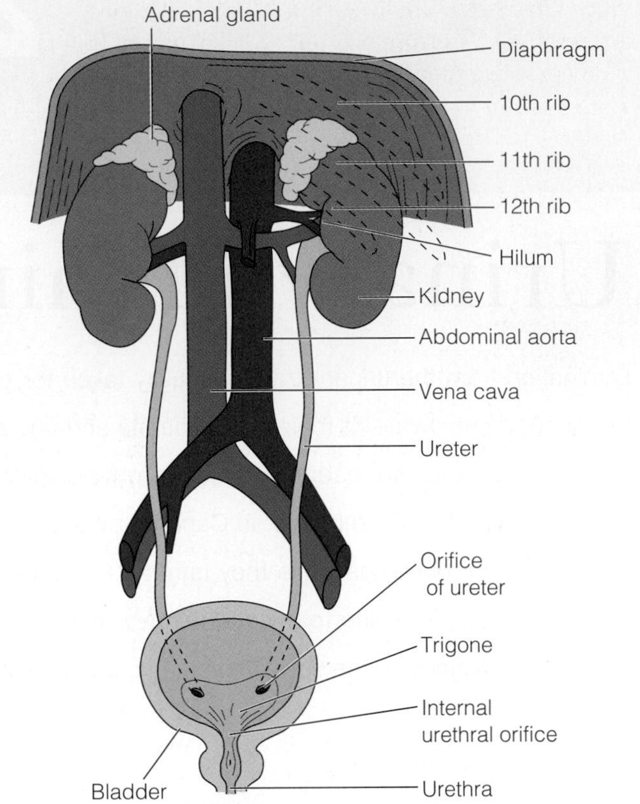

FIGURE 41.1 Anatomical structures of the urinary tract

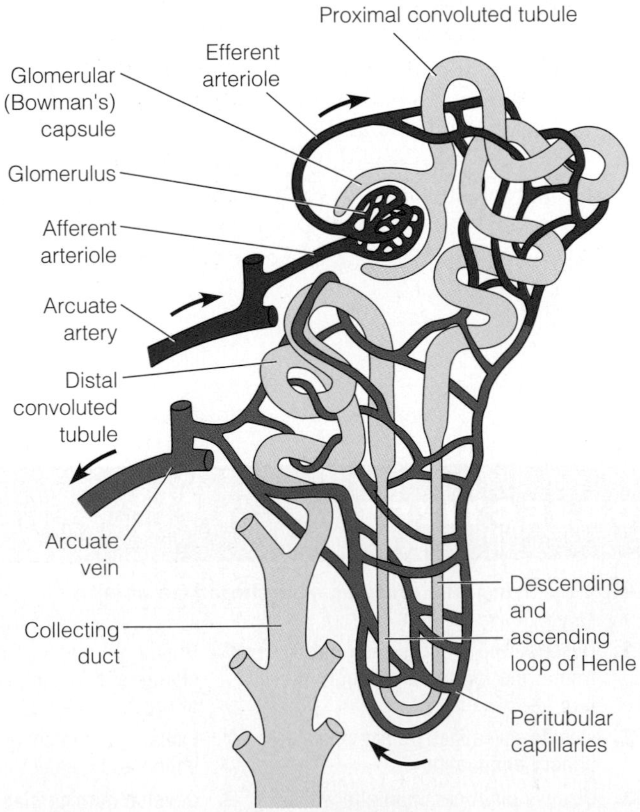

FIGURE 41.2 The nephrons of the kidney have six parts: the glomerulus, Bowman's capsule, proximal convoluted tubule, loop of Henle, distal convoluted tubule, and collecting duct

from 25 cm to 30 cm long in the adult and about 1.25 cm in diameter. The upper end of each ureter is funnel-shaped as it enters the kidney. The lower ends of the ureters enter the bladder at the posterior corners of the floor of the bladder (see Figure 41.1). At the junction between the ureter and the bladder, a flaplike fold of mucous membrane acts as a valve to prevent **reflux** (backflow) of urine up the ureters.

Bladder

The urinary bladder is a hollow, muscular organ that serves as a reservoir for urine and as the organ of excretion. When empty, it lies behind the symphysis pubis. In the male, the bladder lies in front of the rectum and above the prostate gland (see Figure 41.3); in the female, it lies in front of the uterus and vagina (see Figure 41.4). The wall of the bladder is made up of four layers: (1) an inner mucous layer, (2) a connective tissue layer, (3) three layers of smooth muscle fibres, some of which extend lengthwise, some obliquely, and some more or less circularly, and (4) an outer serous layer. The smooth muscle layers are collectively called the **detrusor muscle**. The detrusor muscle allows the bladder to expand as it fills with urine and to contract to release urine to the outside of the body during voiding (D'Amico & Barbarito, 2007). The **trigone** at the base of the bladder is a triangular area marked by the ureter openings at the posterior corners and the opening of the urethra at the anterior inferior corner. Urine exits the bladder through the urethra.

The bladder is capable of considerable distension because of *rugae* (folds) in the mucous membrane lining and because of the elasticity of its walls. When full, the dome of the bladder may extend above the symphysis pubis; in extreme situations, it may extend as high as the umbilicus. Normal bladder capacity is between 300 mL and 600 mL of urine.

Urethra

The urethra extends from the bladder to the urinary **meatus** (opening). In the adult female, the urethra lies directly behind the symphysis pubis, anterior to the vagina, and is about 4.0 cm long (see Figure 41.4). The urethra serves only as a passageway for the elimination of urine. The urinary meatus is located between the labia minora, in front of the vagina and below the clitoris. The male urethra is about 20 cm long and serves as a passageway for semen as well as urine (see Figure 41.3). The meatus is located at the distal end of the penis.

In both males and females, the urethra has a mucous membrane lining that is continuous with the bladder and the ureters. Thus, an infection of the urethra can extend through the urinary tract to the kidneys. Women are particularly prone to urinary tract infections because of their short urethra and the proximity of the urinary meatus to the vagina and anus.

Pelvic Floor

The vagina, the urethra, and the rectum pass through the pelvic floor, which consists of sheets of muscles and ligaments that provide support to the viscera of the pelvis (Figures 41.3 and 41.4). The floor extends from the symphysis pubis to the coccyx, forming a sling. Specific sphincter muscles contribute to the continence mechanism. The internal sphincter muscle situated in the proximal urethra and the bladder neck are composed of smooth muscle under *involuntary* control. It provides active tension designed to close the urethral lumen. The external sphincter muscle is composed of skeletal muscle under *voluntary* control, allowing the individual to choose when urine is eliminated.

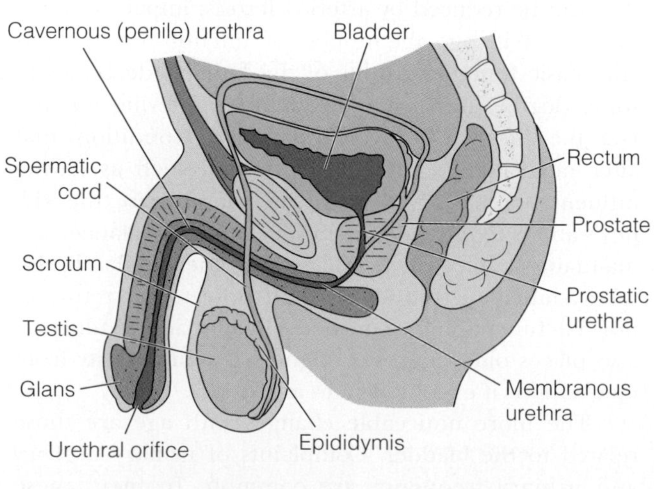

FIGURE 41.3 The male urogenital system

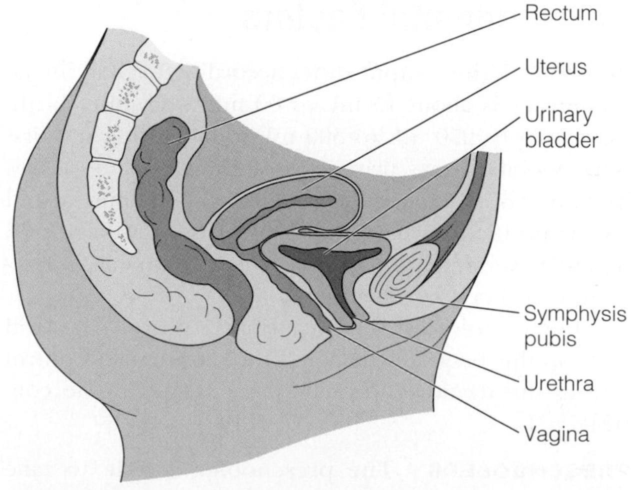

FIGURE 41.4 The female urogenital system

Urination

Micturition, **voiding**, and **urination** all refer to the process of emptying the urinary bladder. Urine collects in the bladder until pressure stimulates special sensory nerve endings in the bladder wall called *stretch receptors*. This occurs when the adult bladder contains between 250 mL and 450 mL of urine. In children, a considerably smaller volume, 50 mL to 200 mL, stimulates these nerves.

The stretch receptors transmit impulses to the spinal cord, specifically to the voiding reflex centre located at the level of the second to fourth sacral vertebrae, causing the internal sphincter to relax and stimulating the urge to void. If the time and place are appropriate for urination, the conscious portion of the brain relaxes the external urethral sphincter muscle and urination takes place. If the time and place are inappropriate, the micturition reflex usually subsides until the bladder becomes fuller and the reflex is stimulated again.

Voluntary control of urination is possible only if the nerves supplying the bladder and urethra, the neural tracts of the spinal cord and brain, and the motor area of the cerebrum are all intact. The individual must be able to sense that the bladder is full. Injury to any of these parts of the nervous system—for example, by a cerebral hemorrhage or spinal cord injury above the level of the sacral region—results in intermittent involuntary emptying of the bladder. Older people whose cognition is impaired may not be aware of the need to urinate or be able to respond to this urge by seeking toilet facilities.

Factors Affecting Voiding

Numerous factors affect the volume and characteristics of the urine produced and the manner in which it is excreted.

Developmental Factors

INFANTS Urine output varies according to fluid intake but usually is about 15 mL to 60 mL a day after birth, increasing to 250 mL to 500 mL a day during the first year. An infant may urinate as often as 20 times a day. The urine of the neonate is colourless and odourless and has a specific gravity of 1.008. Because newborns and infants have immature kidneys, they are unable to concentrate urine very effectively.

Infants are born without urinary control. Most will develop this between the ages of 2 and 5 years. Control during the daytime normally precedes nighttime control.

PRESCHOOLERS The preschooler is able to take responsibility for independent toileting. Parents need to realize that accidents do occur, and the child should never be punished or chastised for this. Children often forget to wash their hands or flush the toilet, and they need instruction in wiping themselves. Girls should be taught to wipe from front to back to prevent contamination of the urinary tract by feces.

SCHOOL-AGE CHILDREN The school-age child's elimination system reaches maturity during this period. The kidneys double in size between the ages of 5 and 10. During this period, the child urinates six to eight times a day and averages one to two bowel movements per day (see the Lifespan Considerations box). **Enuresis**, which is defined as the involuntary passing of urine after control should be established, can be a problem for some school-age children. It has many causes including failure to awaken, overproduction of urine at night, small nocturnal bladder capacity, or a combination of the three (Berry, 2006). About 10% of all 6-year-olds experience difficulty controlling the bladder.

Nocturnal enuresis, or bedwetting, is the involuntary passing of urine during sleep. Bedwetting should not be considered a problem until after the age of 6 years. The incidence of nocturnal enuresis declines as the child matures. About 75% of children with bedwetting experience this problem because of a small bladder capacity. Nocturnal enuresis is referred to as primary when the child has never achieved nighttime urinary control. The incidence of nocturnal enuresis declines as the child matures. Secondary enuresis appears after the child has achieved dryness for 6 consecutive months. It is often related to another problem, such as constipation, stress, or illness, and may resolve when the cause is eliminated. Recent research indicates that primary and secondary nocturnal enuresis may both be related to poor daytime voiding habits, and children should be taught to be aware of the sensation to void (Robson, Leung, & Van Howe, 2005).

OLDER ADULTS The excretory function of the kidney diminishes with age but usually not significantly below normal levels, unless a disease process intervenes. Blood flow can be reduced by arteriosclerosis, impairing renal function. With age, the number of functioning nephrons (the basic functional units of the kidney) decreases to some degree, impairing the kidney's filtering abilities (see the Lifespan Considerations box). Conditions that alter normal fluid intake and output, such as having influenza or having surgery, can compromise the kidney's ability to filter, maintain the acid-base balance, and maintain the electrolyte balance in older adults. It also takes a much longer time for these processes to return to normal functioning. The decrease in kidney function also places older adults at higher risk for toxicity from medications if excretion rates are longer.

The more noticeable changes with age are those related to the bladder. Complaints of urinary urgency and urinary frequency are common. In men, these changes are often due to an enlarged prostate gland; in

Lifespan Considerations

Factors Affecting Voiding

INFANTS AND CHILDREN

- Urinary tract infections (UTIs) are the second most common infection in children, after respiratory infections. They are seen more frequently in newborn and young infant boys than girls and are most often due to obstructions or malformations of the urinary system in these children (Ball & Bindler, 2008). In older infants and children, girls have more UTIs than boys do, usually caused by contamination of the urethra with stool (Cavagnaro, 2005).
- Teaching proper perineal hygiene can reduce infection. Girls should learn to wipe from front to back and wear cotton underwear.
- Teach children and parents that they should go to the bathroom as soon as the sensation to void is felt and not try to hold in the urine.

OLDER ADULTS

Many changes of aging cause specific problems in urinary elimination in the older adult. Many conditions can be treated and interventions can be used to either resolve or decrease the problem. Some of the following conditions are etiological factors in problems with urinary elimination:

- Many older men have enlarged prostate glands, which can inhibit complete emptying of the bladder. This results in urinary retention and urgency, which sometimes causes incontinence.
- Women past menopause have decreased estrogen, which results in a decrease in perineal tone and support of bladder, vagina, and supporting tissues. This often results in urgency and stress incontinence and can even increase the incidence of UTI.
- Increased stiffness and pain in joints, previous joint surgery, and neuromuscular problems can impair mobility and often make it difficult to get to the bathroom.
- Cognitive impairment, such as in dementia, often prevents the person from understanding the need to urinate and the actions needed to perform the activity.

Interventions that may improve these conditions are as follows:

- Medications or surgery to relieve obstructions in men and strengthen support in the urogenital area in women
- Behavioural training for better bladder control
- Safe, easy access to the bathroom or bedside commode, whether at home or in an institution, which includes a well-lit room, safe environment, and proper assistive devices within reach (such as walkers, canes)
- Habit training, such as taking the person to the bathroom at a regular, scheduled time can often work very well with people with cognitive impairments

women, they are often caused by weakened muscles supporting the bladder or weakness of the urethral sphincter. The capacity of the bladder and its ability to completely empty diminish with age. These factors explain the need for older adults to arise during the night to void (**nocturnal frequency**) and the failure to fully empty the bladder of residual urine (**retention**), predisposing the older adult to bladder infections.

See Table 41.1 for a summary of the developmental changes affecting urinary output.

Psychosocial Factors

For many people, a set of conditions helps stimulate the micturition reflex. These conditions include privacy, normal position, sufficient time, and occasionally, running water. Circumstances that counter the client's accustomed conditions can produce anxiety and muscle tension. As a result, the person is unable to relax the abdominal and perineal muscles and the external urethral sphincter, and voiding is inhibited. People may also voluntarily suppress urination (*voluntary urinary retention*) because of perceived time pressures; for example, nurses often ignore the urge to void until they are able to take a break. This behaviour can increase the risk of urinary tract infections (UTIs).

Fluid and Food Intake

The healthy body maintains a balance between the amount of fluid ingested and the amount of fluid eliminated. Therefore, when the amount of fluid intake increases, the output normally increases. Certain fluids, such as alcohol, increase fluid output by inhibiting the production of antidiuretic hormone. Fluids that contain caffeine (e.g., coffee, tea, and cola drinks) also increase urine production. By contrast, food and fluids high in sodium can cause fluid retention as water is retained to maintain the normal concentration of electrolytes.

Some foods and fluids can change the colour of urine. For example, beets and blackberries can cause urine to appear red; foods containing carotene can cause the urine to appear more yellow than usual.

TABLE 41.1 Changes in Urinary Elimination through the Lifespan

Stage	Variations
Fetus	The fetal kidney begins to excrete urine between the 11th and 12th weeks of development.
Infant	Ability to concentrate urine is minimal; therefore, urine appears light yellow.
	Because of neuromuscular immaturity, voluntary urinary control is absent.
Child	Kidney function reaches maturity between the first and second years of life; urine is concentrated effectively and appears a normal amber colour.
	Between 18 and 24 months of age, the child starts to recognize bladder fullness and is able to hold urine beyond the urge to void.
	At approximately 2.5 to 3 years of age, the child can perceive bladder fullness, hold urine after the urge to void, and communicate the need to urinate.
	Full urinary control usually occurs at age 4 or 5 years; daytime control is usually achieved by age 3 years.
	The kidneys grow in proportion to overall body growth.
Adult	The kidneys reach maximum size between 35 and 40 years of age.
	After 50 years, the kidneys begin to diminish in size and function. Most shrinkage occurs in the cortex of the kidney as individual nephrons are lost.
Older adult	An estimated 30% of nephrons are lost by age 80 years.
	Renal blood flow decreases because of vascular changes and a decrease in cardiac output.
	The ability to concentrate urine declines.
	Bladder muscle tone diminishes, causing increased frequency of urination and nocturia (awakening to urinate at night).
	Diminished bladder muscle tone and contractibility may lead to residual urine in the bladder after voiding, increasing the risk of bacterial growth and infection.
	Urinary incontinence may occur because of mobility problems or neurological impairments.

Medications

Many medications, particularly those affecting the autonomic nervous system, interfere with the normal urination process and may cause retention (see Box 41.1).

Diuretics (e.g., chlorothiazide, furosemide, and ethacrynic acid) increase urine formation by preventing the reabsorption of water and electrolytes from the tubules of the kidney into the bloodstream. Diuretics are commonly prescribed for hypertension and cardiac disease.

BOX 41.1 MEDICATIONS THAT MAY CAUSE URINARY RETENTION

The following medications can disrupt the normal urination process:

- Anticholinergic and antispasmodic medications, such as atropine, belladonna, Donnatal (containing atropine), and papaverine
- Antidepressant and antipsychotic agents, such as MAO inhibitors and phenothiazines
- Antiparkinsonism drugs, such as levodopa, trihexyphenidyl (Artane), and benztropine mesylate (Cogentin)
- Antihistamine preparations, such as Actifed and Sudafed
- Beta-adrenergic blockers, such as propranolol (Inderal)
- Antihypertensives, such as hydralazine (Apresoline) and methyldopate (Aldomet)
- Opioid analgesics, such as morphine and hydrocodone

Muscle Tone and Activity

Regular exercise increases muscle tone and the metabolic rate. Good muscle tone is important for maintaining the stretch and contractility of the detrusor muscle so the bladder can fill adequately and empty completely. Clients who require a retention catheter for a long period may have poor bladder muscle tone because continuous drainage of urine prevents the bladder from filling and emptying normally. Abdominal and pelvic floor muscle tone also contribute: abdominal muscle contraction assists in bladder emptying; pelvic floor muscle tone is a factor in being able to retain urine voluntarily once the urge to urinate is perceived.

Pathological Conditions

Some diseases and pathologies can affect the formation and excretion of urine. Diseases of the kidneys can affect the ability of the nephrons to produce urine. Abnormal amounts of protein or blood cells can be present in the urine, or the kidneys can virtually stop producing urine altogether, a condition known as renal failure. Heart and circulatory disorders, such as heart failure, shock, or hypertension, can affect blood flow to the kidneys, interfering with urine production. If abnormal amounts of fluid are lost through another route (e.g., vomiting or high fever), water is retained by the kidneys and urinary output falls.

Processes that interfere with the flow of urine from the kidneys to the urethra affect urinary excretion. A urinary stone (calculus) can obstruct a ureter, blocking urine flow from the kidney to the bladder. Hypertrophy (enlargement) of the prostate gland, a common condition affecting older men, can partially obstruct the urethra, impairing urination and bladder emptying.

Surgical and Diagnostic Procedures

Some surgical and diagnostic procedures can affect the passage of urine and the urine itself. The urethra can swell following a cystoscopy, and surgical procedures on any part of the urinary tract can result in some postoperative bleeding; as a result, the urine may be red- or pink-tinged for a time.

Spinal anaesthetics can affect the passage of urine because they decrease the client's awareness of the need to void. Surgery on structures adjacent to the urinary tract (e.g., the uterus) can also affect voiding because of swelling in the lower abdomen.

TABLE 41.2 Average Daily Urine Output by Age

Age	Amount (mL)
1 to 2 days	15 to 60
3 to 10 days	100 to 300
10 days to 2 months	250 to 450
2 months to 1 year	450 to 500
1 to 3 years	500 to 600
3 to 5 years	600 to 700
5 to 8 years	700 to 1000
8 to 14 years	800 to 1400
14 years through adulthood	1500
Older adulthood	1500 or less

Altered Urine Production

Although people's patterns of urination are highly individual, most people void about five to seven times a day. People usually void when they first awaken in the morning, before they go to bed, and around mealtimes. Table 41.2 shows the average urinary output per day at different ages. Altered urinary production includes polyuria, anuria, and oliguria. Selected factors associated with altered patterns of urine production are identified in Table 41.3.

Polyuria

Polyuria or *diuresis* refers to the production of abnormally large amounts of urine by the kidneys, often several litres more than the client's usual daily output. Polyuria can follow excessive fluid intake, a condition known as **polydipsia**, or can be associated with such diseases as diabetes mellitus, diabetes insipidus, or chronic nephritis. The term **diuresis** is often used when medications are given to promote urine output (diuretics) or to describe the effect of ingested substances, such as caffeine or alcohol, on urine production. Polyuria or diuresis can cause excessive fluid loss, leading to intense thirst, dehydration, and weight loss.

Oliguria and Anuria

The terms *oliguria* and *anuria* are used to describe decreased urinary output. **Oliguria** is low urine output, usually less than 500 mL a day or 30 mL an hour for an adult. Although oliguria can occur as a result of abnormal fluid losses or a lack of fluid intake, it often indicates impaired blood flow to the kidneys or impending renal failure and should be promptly reported to the healthcare provider. Restoring renal blood flow and urinary output promptly can prevent renal failure and its complications. **Anuria** refers to a lack of urine production.

Altered Urinary Elimination

Despite normal urine production, a number of factors or conditions can affect urinary elimination. Frequency, urgency, dysuria, and nocturia often are manifestations of underlying conditions, such as a UTI. Enuresis, incontinence, and retention, conversely, may be either a manifestation or the primary problem affecting urinary elimination. Selected factors associated with altered patterns of urine elimination are identified in Table 41.3.

Frequency and Nocturia

Urinary frequency is voiding at frequent intervals, that is, more often than usual. An increased intake of fluid causes some increase in the frequency of voiding. Such conditions as UTIs, stress, and pregnancy can cause frequent voiding of small quantities (50 mL to 100 mL) of urine. Total fluid intake and output may be normal. **Nocturia** is voiding two or more times at night. Like frequency, it is usually expressed in terms of the number of times the person gets out of bed to void, for example, "nocturia × 4."

Urgency

Urinary urgency is feeling the sudden *strong* desire to void. The bladder may or may not have a great deal of

TABLE 41.3 Selected Factors Associated with Altered Urinary Production and Elimination

Altered Production	Selected Associated Factors
Polyuria	Ingestion of fluids containing caffeine or alcohol Prescribed diuretic Presence of thirst, dehydration, and weight loss History of diabetes mellitus, diabetes insipidus, or kidney disease
Oliguria, anuria	Decrease in fluid intake Signs of dehydration Presence of hypotension, shock, or heart failure History of kidney disease Signs of renal failure, such as elevated blood urea nitrogen (BUN) and serum creatinine, edema, hypertension
Frequency or nocturia	Pregnancy Increase in fluid intake Urinary tract infection Any known contributing or initiating causes, such as stress
Urgency	Presence of psychological stress Urinary tract infection
Dysuria	Urinary tract inflammation, infection, or injury Presence of other signs that may accompany dysuria, such as hesitancy, hematuria, pyuria (pus in the urine) and frequency

Pattern	Selected Associated Factors
Enuresis	Family history of enuresis Difficult access to toilet facilities Home stresses
Incontinence	Bladder inflammation or other disease Difficulties in independent toileting (mobility impairment) Leakage when coughing, laughing, sneezing Cognitive impairment Constipation
Retention	Distended bladder on palpation and percussion Associated signs, such as pubic discomfort, restlessness, frequency, and small urine volume Recent anaesthesia Recent perineal surgery Presence of perineal swelling Medications prescribed Lack of privacy or other factors inhibiting micturition

urine, but the person feels a need to void immediately. Urgency accompanies psychological stress and irritation of the trigone and urethra. It is also common in young children and people who have poor external sphincter control and unstable bladder. It is an abnormal finding.

Dysuria

Dysuria means voiding that is either painful or difficult. It can accompany a stricture (decrease in calibre) of the urethra, urinary infections, and injury to the bladder and urethra. Often, clients will say they have to push to void or that burning accompanies or follows voiding. The burning may be described as severe, like a hot poker, or more subdued, like a sunburn. Often, **urinary hesitancy** (a delay and difficulty in initiating voiding) is associated with dysuria.

Enuresis

Enuresis is defined as involuntary urination in children beyond the age at which voluntary bladder control is normally acquired, usually 4 or 5 years of age. Nocturnal (nighttime) enuresis often is irregular in occurrence and affects boys more often than girls. **Diurnal (daytime) enuresis** may be persistent and pathological in origin. It affects women and girls more frequently.

Urinary Incontinence

Urinary incontinence (UI), or involuntary urination, is a symptom, not a disease. It can have a significant impact on the client's life, creating physical problems, such as skin breakdown, and possibly leading to psychosocial problems, such as embarrassment, isolation, and social withdrawal. According to the Canadian Urinary Bladder Survey (Herschorn, Corcos, Gajewski, Schulz, & Ciu, 2003), approximately 3% of Canadians experience some sort of urinary incontinence. The survey found that women experience more UI than men, with half of women older than 65 years experiencing UI. This experience is not unique to older clients: 10% of men and 16% of women aged 18 to 40 experience UI. Although incontinence is common in older adults, it is *not* a normal consequence of aging and can often be treated. Common causes of incontinence include UTIs, urethritis, pregnancy, hypercalcemia, volume overload, delirium, restricted mobility, stool impaction, and psychological causes (Morantz, 2005). Urinary incontinence can be transient or chronic.

The etiology of *transient incontinence* is generally from nonurinary system causes, such as infection, atrophic urethritis or vaginitis, restricted mobility, use of pharmaceuticals (e.g., diuretics), stool impaction or constipation, and delirium or acute confused state. Some of these factors are readily reversible, with a lessening of symptoms if not complete resolution of urinary incontinence.

Urinary incontinence may be a longstanding or chronic problem. Different types of chronic incontinence, each having a different etiology, include stress, urge, overflow, reflex, functional, and total incontinence (discussed later in the section "Diagnosing").

The preliminary assessment and identification of the symptom of urinary incontinence is truly within the scope of nursing practice. All clients should be asked about their voiding patterns. Older adults who are incontinent while in their home or who manage to contain or conceal their incontinence from others do not consider themselves incontinent. Therefore, when asked if they are incontinent, they may deny it. However, asking if they lose urine when they don't want to may provide more accurate information (Palmer & Newman, 2006). If incontinence is described, a thorough history and assessment is indicated. Treatment can include surgery, medication, or behavioural therapies. Nursing management of incontinence includes implementing individualized bladder programs, containment of urine, and meticulous skin care.

CLINICAL ALERT

The new onset of urinary incontinence in any client must be assessed thoroughly. Constipation, culprit medications (muscle relaxants, diuretics), fecal impaction, and infection are possible causes of acute urinary incontinence. The treatment of incontinence can be determined only after the cause is identified.

Urinary Retention

When the emptying of the bladder is impaired, urine accumulates and the bladder becomes overdistended, a condition known as **urinary retention**. Overdistension of the bladder causes poor contractility of the detrusor muscle, further impairing urination. Common causes of urinary retention include prostatic hypertrophy, surgery, and some medications (see Box 41.1).

Clients with urinary retention may experience overflow voiding or incontinence, eliminating 25 mL to 50 mL of urine at frequent intervals. The bladder is firm and distended on palpation and may be displaced to one side of midline.

Neurogenic Bladder

Impaired neurological function can interfere with the normal mechanisms of urine elimination, resulting in a **neurogenic bladder**. The client with a neurogenic bladder does not perceive bladder fullness and is unable to control the urinary sphincters. The bladder may become flaccid and distended or spastic, with frequent involuntary urination.

Assessing

A complete assessment of a client's urinary function includes the following:

- Collecting a nursing history
- Conducting a physical assessment of the genitourinary system, hydration status, and examination of the urine
- Relating the data obtained to the results of any diagnostic tests and procedures

NURSING HISTORY The nurse determines the client's normal voiding pattern and frequency, the appearance of the urine and any recent changes, any past or current problems with urination, the presence of an ostomy, and the factors influencing the elimination pattern.

Examples of questions to elicit this information are shown in the Assessment: Interview box. The number of questions asked depends on the individual and the responses to the first three categories.

PHYSICAL ASSESSMENT Complete physical assessment of the urinary tract usually includes percussion of the kidneys to detect areas of tenderness. Palpation and percussion of the bladder are also performed. See Chapter 27. If the client's history or current problems indicate a need for it, the urethral meatus of both male and female clients is inspected for swelling, discharge, and inflammation.

Because problems with urination can affect the elimination of wastes from the body, it is important that the nurse assess the skin for colour, texture, and tissue turgor as well as the presence of edema. If incontinence, dribbling, or dysuria is noted in the history, the skin of the perineum should be inspected for irritation because contact with urine can excoriate the skin.

ASSESSING URINE Normal urine consists of 96% water and 4% solutes. Organic solutes include urea, ammonia, creatinine, and uric acid. Urea is the chief organic solute. Inorganic solutes include sodium, chloride, potassium, sulphate, magnesium, and phosphorus. Sodium chloride is the most abundant inorganic salt. Characteristics of normal and abnormal urine are shown in Table 41.4.

MEASURING URINARY OUTPUT Normally, the kidneys produce urine at a rate of approximately 60 mL per hour or about 1500 mL per day. Urine output is affected by

ASSESSMENT: INTERVIEW

Urinary Elimination

The nurse can use the following questions to learn about the client's urinary elimination:

VOIDING PATTERN

- How many times do you void during a 24-hour period?
- Has this pattern changed recently?
- Do you need to get out of bed to void at night? How often?

DESCRIPTION OF URINE AND ANY CHANGES

- How would you describe your urine in terms of colour, clarity (clear, transparent, or cloudy), and odour (faint or strong)?

URINARY ELIMINATION PROBLEMS

- What problems have you had or do you now have with passing your urine?
  - Passage of small amounts of urine?
  - Voiding at more frequent intervals?
  - Trouble getting to the bathroom in time or feeling an urgent need to void?
  - Painful voiding?
  - Difficulty starting the urine stream?
- Frequent dribbling of urine or feeling of bladder fullness associated with voiding small amounts of urine?
- Reduced force of stream?
- Accidental leakage of urine? If so, when does this occur (e.g., when coughing, laughing, or sneezing; at night; during the day)?
- Past urinary tract illness, such as infection of the kidney, bladder, or urethra; urinary calculi; surgery of kidney, ureters, or bladder?

PRESENCE AND MANAGEMENT OF URINARY DIVERSION OSTOMY

- What is your usual routine with your ostomy?
- What problems, if any, do you have with it?
- How can the nurse help you manage it?

FACTORS INFLUENCING URINARY ELIMINATION

- *Medications*. Do you take any medications that could increase urinary output (e.g., diuretic) or cause retention of urine (e.g., anticholinergic-antispasmodic, antidepressant-antipsychotic, antiparkinsonism, antihistamines, antihypertensives)? Note specific medication, dosage, and frequency.
- *Fluid intake*. What amount and kind of fluid do you take each day (e.g., six glasses of water, five cups of coffee, three cola drinks with or without caffeine)?
- *Environmental factors*. Do you have any problems with toileting (mobility, removing clothing, toilet seat too low, facility without grab bar)?
- *Presence of long-term catheter*. How do you care for your catheter? Do you have any discomfort with it or other problems? How can the nurse help you manage it?
- *Stress*. Are you experiencing any long-term or short-term stress? If so, what are the stressors? Do you think these affect your urinary pattern?
- *Disease*. Have you had or do you have any illnesses that can affect urinary function, such as hypertension, heart disease, neurological disease (e.g., multiple sclerosis), cancer, prostatic enlargement, diabetes mellitus, or diabetes insipidus?
- *Diagnostic procedures*. Have you recently had a cystoscopy or spinal anaesthetic?

many factors, including fluid intake, body fluid losses through other routes, such as perspiration and breathing, and the cardiovascular and renal status of the individual.

Urine outputs of less than 30 mL per hour may indicate low blood volume or kidney malfunction and must be reported. In children, normal urine volume is 300 mL to 1500 mL per day (see Table 41.2).

To measure fluid output, the nurse follows these steps:

- Wear clean gloves to prevent contact with microorganisms or blood in the urine.
- Ask the client to void in a clean urinal, bedpan, commode, or toilet collection device (*urine hat*) (see Figure 41.5).
- Instruct the client to keep urine separate from feces and to avoid putting toilet paper in the urine collection container.
- Pour the voided urine into a calibrated container.
- Hold the container at eye level and read the amount in the container. Containers usually have a measuring scale on the inside.

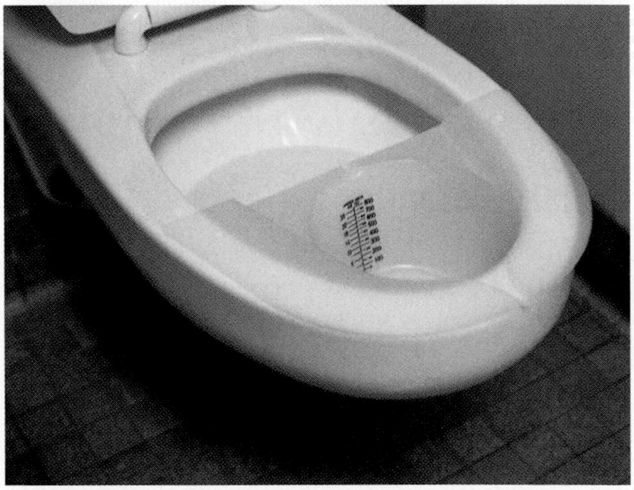

FIGURE 41.5 A urine hat: a urine collection device for the toilet

- If a clean specimen is required, pour some urine into the specimen container and discard the remainder, unless all urine is to be saved.

TABLE 41.4 Characteristics of Normal and Abnormal Urine

Characteristic	Normal	Abnormal	Nursing Considerations
Amount in 24 hours (adult)	1200 mL to 1500 mL	Less than 1200 mL More than 1500 mL A large amount more than intake	Urinary output normally is approximately equal to fluid intake. Output of less than 30 mL/h may indicate decreased blood flow to the kidneys and should be immediately reported.
Colour, clarity	Straw, amber Transparent	Dark amber Cloudy Dark orange Red or dark brown Mucus plugs, viscid, thick	Concentrated urine is darker in colour. Diluted urine can appear almost clear or very pale yellow. Some foods and drugs can colour urine (e.g., beets, phenazopyridine, phenytoin). Red blood cells in the urine (hematuria) may be evident as pink, bright red, or rusty brown urine. Menstrual bleeding can also colour urine but should not be confused with hematuria. White blood cells, bacteria, pus, or contaminants, such as prostatic fluid, sperm, or vaginal drainage, can cause cloudy urine.
Odour	Faint aromatic	Offensive	Some foods (e.g., asparagus) cause a musty odour; infected urine can have a fetid odour; urine high in glucose has a sweet odour.
Sterility	No microorganisms present	Microorganisms present	Urine specimens may be contaminated by bacteria from the perineum during collection.
pH	4.5 to 8	Less than 4.5 More than 8	Freshly voided urine is normally somewhat acidic. More acidic urine (low pH) is found in acidosis, starvation, diarrhea, or with a diet high in protein foods or cranberries. Alkaline urine may indicate a state of alkalosis, urinary tract infection, or a diet high in fruits and vegetables.
Specific gravity	1.010 to 1.025	Less than 1.010 More than 1.025	Diluted urine has a lower specific gravity; concentrated urine has a higher specific gravity.
Glucose	Not present	Present	Glucose in the urine indicates high blood glucose levels and may be indicative of undiagnosed or uncontrolled diabetes mellitus.
Ketone bodies (acetone)	Not present	Present	Ketones, the end product of the breakdown of fatty acids, are not normally present in the urine. They may be present in the urine of clients who have uncontrolled diabetes mellitus, are in a state of starvation, or who have ingested excessive amounts of acetylsalicylic acid (e.g., Aspirin).
Blood	Not present	Occult (microscopic) Bright red	Blood may be present in the urine of clients who have urinary tract infection, kidney disease, or bleeding from the urinary tract.

- Record the amount on the fluid intake and output sheet, which may be at the bedside or in the bathroom.
- Rinse the urine collection and measuring containers with cool water and store appropriately.
- Remove gloves and wash hands.
- Calculate and document the total output on the client's chart at the end of each shift and at the end of 24 hours.

Many clients can measure and record their own urine output when the procedure is explained to them.

When measuring urine from a client who has an indwelling catheter, the nurse follows these steps:

- Put on clean gloves.
- Take the clean calibrated container to the bedside.
- Place the container under the urine collection bag so that the spout of the bag is above the container but not touching it. The calibrated container is not sterile, but the inside of the collection bag is sterile (Figure 41.6).
- Open the spout and permit the urine to flow into the container.
- Close the spout, and then proceed as described in the previous list.

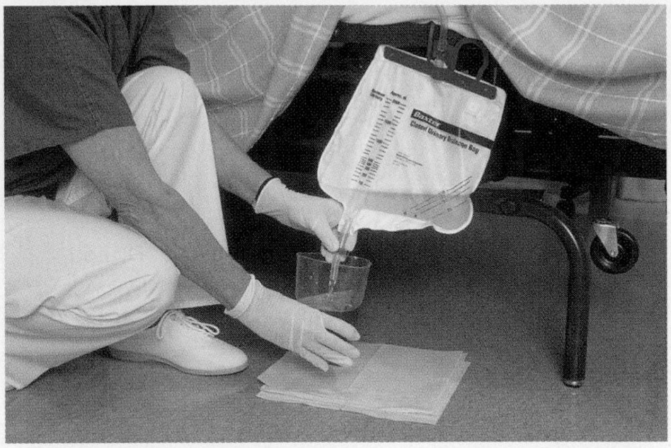

FIGURE 41.6 Urine being measured from a urine collection bag

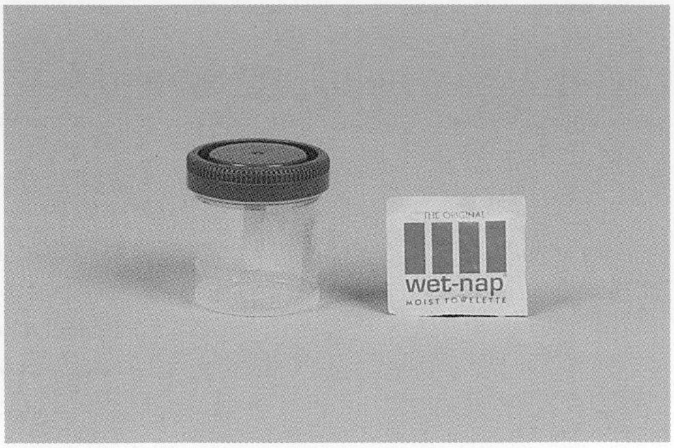

FIGURE 41.7 Disposable clean-catch specimen equipment

Measuring Residual Urine **Residual urine** (urine remaining in the bladder following the voiding) is normally 50 mL to 100 mL. However, a bladder outlet obstruction (e.g., enlargement of the prostate gland) or loss of bladder muscle tone can interfere with complete emptying of the bladder during urination. Manifestations of urine retention include frequent voiding of small amounts (e.g., less than 100 mL in an adult). Urinary stasis and UTIs are possible consequences of incomplete bladder emptying. Residual urine is measured to assess the amount of retained urine after voiding and determine the need for interventions (e.g., medications to promote detrusor muscle contraction).

To measure residual urine, the nurse performs a bladder scan or catheterizes the client immediately after the client has voided. The amount of urine voided and the amount obtained by catheterization are measured and recorded. An indwelling catheter may be inserted if the residual urine exceeds a specified amount.

COLLECTING URINE SPECIMENS The nurse is responsible for collecting urine specimens for a number of tests: clean voided specimens for routine urinalysis, *clean-catch* or *midstream urine specimens* for urine culture, and timed urine specimens for a variety of tests, depending on the client's specific health problem.

Clean Voided Urine Specimen Many clients are able to collect a clean voided specimen and provide the specimen independently, with minimal instructions. Male clients generally are able to void directly into the specimen container, and female clients usually sit or squat over the toilet, holding the container between their legs during voiding. About 120 mL of urine is generally required. Clients who are seriously ill, physically incapacitated, or disoriented may need to use a bedpan or urinal in bed; others may require supervision or assistance in the bathroom. Whatever the situation, explicit directions are required:

- The specimen must be free of fecal contamination, so urine must be kept separate from feces.
- Female clients should discard the toilet tissue in the toilet or in a waste bag, rather than in the bedpan, because tissue in the specimen makes laboratory analysis more difficult.
- The lid must be closed tightly on the container to prevent spillage of the urine and contamination of other objects.
- If the outside of the container has been contaminated by urine, clean it with a disinfectant and place in a clean plastic bag.

The nurse must (1) make sure that the specimen label and the laboratory requisition carry the correct information, and (2) attach them securely to the specimen. Inappropriate identification of the specimen can lead to errors of diagnosis or therapy for the client.

Clean-Catch or Midstream Urine Specimen Clean-catch or midstream voided specimens are collected when a urine culture is ordered to identify microorganisms causing UTIs. Although some contamination by skin bacteria can occur with a clean-catch specimen, the risk of introducing microorganisms into the urinary tract through catheterization is more significant. Care is taken to ensure that the specimen is as free as possible from contamination by microorganisms around the urinary meatus. Clean-catch specimens are collected into a sterile specimen container with a lid. Disposable clean-catch kits are available (Figure 41.7). Skill 41.1 explains how to collect a clean-catch urine specimen for culture.

Timed Urine Specimen Some urine examinations require collection of all urine produced and voided over a specific period of time, ranging from 1 to 2 hours to 24 hours (see the Home Care Considerations box on page 1276). Timed specimens generally either are refrigerated or contain a preservative to prevent bacterial growth or decomposition of urine components. Each voiding of urine is collected in a small, clean container and then emptied immediately into the large refrigerated bottle or carton.

SKILL 41.1

COLLECTING A URINE SPECIMEN FOR CULTURE AND SENSITIVITY BY CLEAN CATCH

PURPOSE

- To determine the presence of microorganisms, the type of organism(s), and the antibiotics to which the organisms are sensitive

ASSESSMENT

- Determine the ability of the client to provide the specimen.
- Assess the colour, odour, and consistency of the urine and the presence of clinical signs of urinary tract infection (e.g., frequency, urgency, dysuria, hematuria, flank pain, cloudy urine with foul odour).

Equipment

Equipment used varies from agency to agency. Some agencies use commercially prepared disposable clean-catch kits. Others are agency-prepared sterile trays. Both prepared trays and kits generally contain the following items:

- Clean gloves
- Antiseptic towelettes
- Sterile cotton balls or 5 cm × 5 cm gauze pads
- Sterile specimen container
- Specimen identification label

In addition the nurse needs to obtain the following:

- Completed laboratory requisition form
- Urine receptacle, if the client is not ambulatory
- Basin of warm water, soap, washcloth, and towel for the nonambulatory client

IMPLEMENTATION

Preparation

Gather the necessary equipment for the collection of the specimen. Use visual aids, if available, to assist the client to understand the midstream collection technique.

Performance

1. Before performing the procedure, introduce yourself and verify the client's identity by using agency protocol. Explain to the client that a urine specimen is required, give the reason, and explain the method to be used to collect it. Discuss how the results will be used in planning further care or treatments.
2. Perform hand hygiene and observe other appropriate infection prevention and control procedures.
3. Provide for client privacy.
4. For an ambulatory client who is able to follow directions, instruct the client on how to collect the specimen.
   - Direct or assist the client to the bathroom.
   - Ask the client to wash and dry the genitals and perineal area with soap and water. **Rationale: Washing the perineal area reduces the number of skin and transient bacteria, decreasing the risk of contaminating the urine specimen.**
   - Instruct the client on how to clean the urinary meatus with antiseptic towelettes. **Rationale: The antiseptic further reduces bacterial contamination of the urinary meatus and the risk of contaminating the specimen.**

For Female Clients

- Use each towelette only once. Clean the perineal area from front to back and discard the towelette. Use all towelettes provided (usually two or three) (see ❶). **Rationale: Cleaning from front to back cleans the area of least contamination to the area of greatest contamination.**

For Male Clients

- If uncircumcised, retract the foreskin slightly to expose the urinary meatus.
- Using a circular motion, clean the urinary meatus and the distal portion of the penis. Use each towelette only once, and then discard. Clean several centimetres down the shaft of the penis (see ❷). **Rationale: This cleans from the area of least contamination to the area of greatest contamination.**

5. For a client who requires assistance, prepare the client and equipment.
   - Wash the perineal area with soap and water, rinse, and dry.
   - Assist the client onto a clean commode or bedpan. If using a bedpan or urinal, position the client as upright as allowed or tolerated. **Rationale: Assuming**

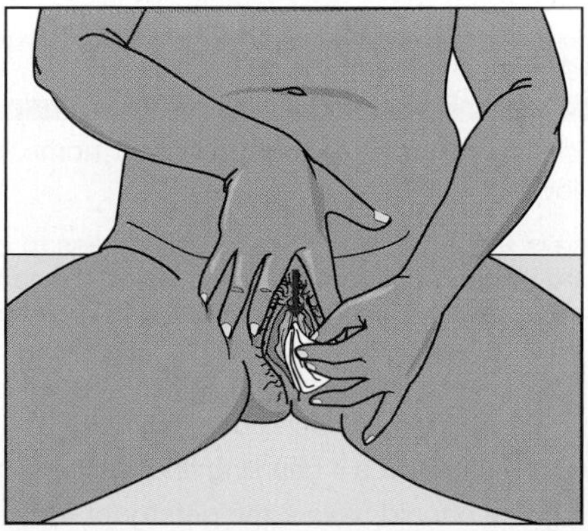

❶ Cleansing the female urinary meatus: spread the labia with one hand, and with the other hand, cleanse the perineal area from front to back.

(continued)

SKILL 41.1

COLLECTING A URINE SPECIMEN FOR CULTURE AND SENSITIVITY BY CLEAN CATCH (*continued*)

a normal anatomic position for voiding facilitates urination.

- Open the clean-catch kit, taking care not to contaminate the inside of the specimen container or lid. **Rationale: It is important to maintain sterility of the specimen container to prevent contamination of the specimen.**
- Put on clean gloves.
- Clean the urinary meatus and perineal area as described in step 4.

6. Collect the specimen from a nonambulatory client or instruct an ambulatory client on how to collect it.
   - Instruct the client to start voiding. **Rationale: Bacteria in the distal urethra and at the urinary meatus are cleared by the first few millilitres of urine expelled.**
   - Place the specimen container into the midstream of urine and collect the specimen, taking care not to touch the container to the perineum or penis. **Rationale: It is important to avoid contaminating the interior of the specimen container and the specimen itself.**
   - Collect urine in the container.
   - Cap the container tightly, touching only the outside of the container and the cap. **Rationale: This prevents contamination or spilling of the specimen.**
   - If necessary, clean the outside of the specimen container with disinfectant. **Rationale: This prevents transfer of microorganisms to others.**
7. Label the specimen and transport it to the laboratory.
   - Ensure that the specimen label is attached to the specimen cup, not the lid, and the laboratory requisition provides the correct information. Place the specimen in a plastic bag that has a biohazard label

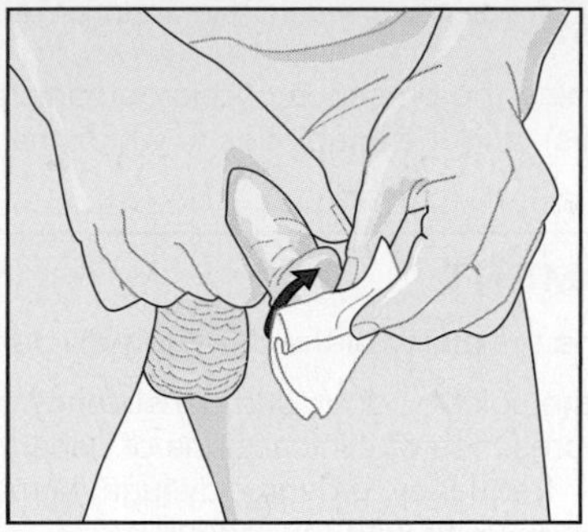

❷ Cleansing the male urinary meatus. Retract the foreskin if needed. Using a towelette, cleanse the urinary meatus by moving in a circular motion from the centre of the urethral opening, around the glans, and down the distal portion of the shaft of the penis.

   on it. Attach the requisition securely to the bag. **Rationale: Inaccurate identification or information on the specimen container risks errors in diagnosis or therapy.**
   - Arrange for the specimen to be sent to the laboratory immediately. **Rationale: Bacterial cultures must be started immediately before any contaminating organisms can grow, multiply, and produce false results.**
8. Document pertinent data.
   - Record collection of the specimen, any pertinent observations of the urine, such as colour, odour, or consistency, and any difficulty in voiding that the client experienced.
   - Indicate on the lab slip if the client is taking any current antibiotic therapy or if the client is menstruating.

EVALUATION

- Report and discuss lab results with the health-care team.
- Conduct appropriate follow-up nursing interventions as needed, such as administering prescribed medications and teaching the client.

Home Care Considerations

If the client will have to collect urine at home, consider the following:

- Assess the client's ability and willingness to collect a timed urine specimen. If poor eyesight or hand tremors are a problem, suggest using a clean funnel to pour the urine into the container.
- Always wash hands well with warm, soapy water before and after collecting urine samples.
- Always wear gloves if handling another person's urine.
- The home should have a refrigerator or other method for cooling the urine samples. Tell the client to keep the specimen container in plastic in the refrigerator, separate from other refrigerator contents. The client can also use a cooler with ice.

To collect a timed urine specimen, follow these steps:

- Obtain a specimen container with preservative (if indicated) from the laboratory. Label the container with identifying information for the client, the test to be performed, time started, and time of completion.
- Provide a clean receptacle to collect urine (bedpan, commode, or toilet collection device).
- Post signs in the client's chart, Kardex, room, and bathroom alerting personnel to save all urine during the specified time.
- At the start of the collection period, have the client void and discard this urine.
- Save all urine produced during the timed collection period in the container, refrigerating or placing the

container on ice as indicated. Avoid contaminating the urine with toilet paper or feces.

- At the end of the collection period, instruct the client to completely empty the bladder and save this voiding as part of the specimen. Take the entire amount of urine collected to the laboratory with the completed requisition.
- Record collection of the specimen, time started and completed, and any pertinent observations of the urine on appropriate records.

INDWELLING CATHETER SPECIMEN Sterile urine specimens can be obtained from closed drainage systems by inserting a sterile needle attached to a syringe through a drainage port in the tubing. Aspiration of urine from catheters can be done only with self-sealing rubber catheters—not plastic, silicone, or Silastic catheters. When self-sealing rubber catheters are used, the needle is inserted just above the place where the catheter is attached to the drainage tubing. The area from which to obtain urine may be marked by a patch on the catheter (Figure 41.8). Newer closed drainage urinary systems now have needleless ports, so a needle does not have to be used to obtain a sample. This protects the nurse from a needle-stick injury and maintains the integrity and sterility of the catheter system by eliminating the need to puncture the tubing (Davis, 2004). The needleless port accepts a Luer-Lok syringe (Figure 41.9). Position the syringe perpendicular to the centre of the port and insert, twist, and lock into the port. When the specimen is obtained and the syringe removed, the port seals itself.

To collect a specimen from a Foley (retention) catheter or a drainage tube, follow these steps:

- Put on disposable gloves.
- If there is no urine in the catheter, clamp the drainage tubing for about 15 to 20 minutes. This allows fresh urine to collect in the catheter.
- Wipe with a disinfectant swab the area in which the needle or Luer-Lok will be inserted. The site should be distal to the tube leading to the balloon to avoid puncturing this tube. Disinfecting the needle insertion site removes any microorganisms on the surface of the catheter, thereby avoiding contamination of the needle and the entrance of microorganisms into the catheter.
- Insert the needle at a 30- to 45-degree angle (Figure 41.8). This angle of entrance facilitates self-sealing of the rubber.
- Withdraw the required amount of urine, for example, 3 mL for a urine culture or 30 mL for a routine urinalysis.
- Transfer the urine to the specimen container. Make sure the needle does not touch the outside of the container if a sterile culture tube is used.
- Without recapping the needle, discard the syringe and needle in an appropriate sharps container.
- Cap the container.

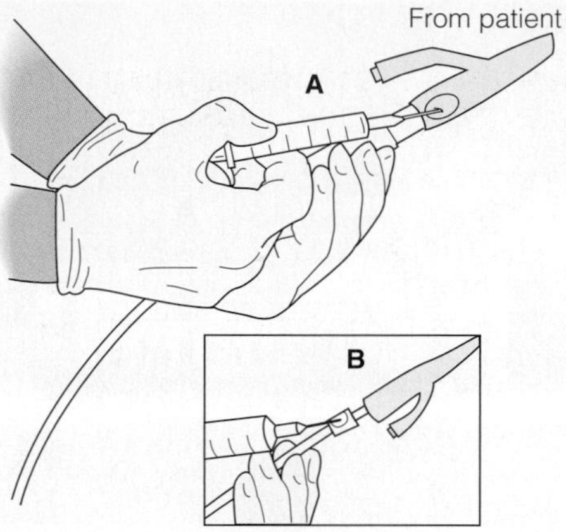

FIGURE 41.8 Obtaining a urine specimen from a retention catheter: **A:** from a specific area near the end of the catheter; **B:** from an access port in the tubing

- Unclamp the drainage tubing.
- Remove gloves and discard appropriately.
- Label the container, and send the urine to the laboratory immediately for analysis or refrigeration.
- Record collection of the specimen and any pertinent observations of the urine on the appropriate records.

URINE TESTING Several simple urine tests are often done by nurses on the nursing units. These include tests for specific gravity, pH, and the presence of abnormal constituents, such as glucose, ketones, protein, and occult blood.

Nurses in a health-care facility or clients in the home setting can use commercially prepared kits to test abnormal constituents in the urine. These kits contain the required equipment and an appropriate reagent, which may be in the form of a tablet, fluid, or paper test strip or dipstick. When the urine contacts the reagent, a chemical reaction occurs, causing a colour change that is then compared with a chart to interpret the significance of the colour (Figure 41.10). Specific directions for the amount

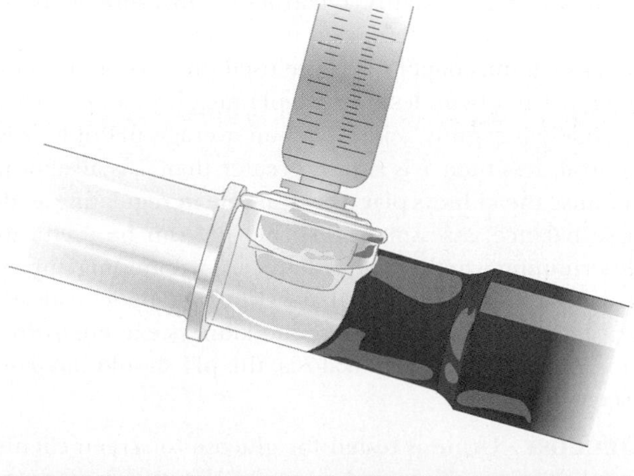

FIGURE 41.9 A needleless port that allows for needle-free aspiration of urine

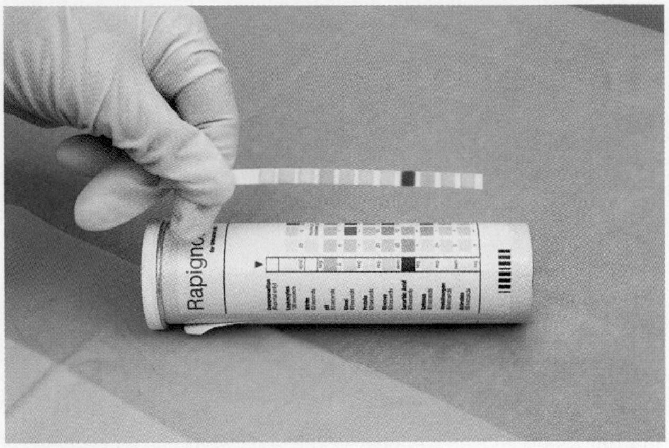

FIGURE 41.10 After dipping the reagent strip (dipstick) into fresh urine, wait the stated time and compare the results to the colour chart.

of urine needed, the time required for the chemical reaction, and the meaning of the colours produced vary among manufacturers. Thus, it is essential that nurses and clients read and follow directions supplied by each manufacturer. In addition, testing materials need to be checked to ascertain that they have not expired.

SPECIFIC GRAVITY The **specific gravity** is an indicator of urine concentration, or the amount of solutes (metabolic wastes and electrolytes) present in the urine. A *urinometer* or *hydrometer* in a cylinder of urine or a *spectrometer* or *refractometer* is used to measure the specific gravity. The specific gravity of distilled water is 1.000; the specific gravity of urine normally ranges from 1.010 to 1.025. As urine becomes more concentrated, its specific gravity increases. Excess fluid intake or diseases affecting the ability of the kidneys to concentrate urine can result in low specific gravity readings. A high specific gravity can indicate fluid deficit or dehydration, or excess solutes, such as glucose, in the urine.

URINARY PH **Urinary pH** is measured to determine the relative acidity or alkalinity of urine and assess the client's acid-base status. Quantitative measurements of urine pH can be performed in the laboratory, but dipsticks or litmus paper often are used on nursing units or in clinics to obtain less precise pH measurements. Urine normally is slightly acidic, with an average pH of 6 (7 is neutral, less than 7 is acidic, greater than 7 is alkaline). Because the kidneys play a critical role in regulating acid-base balance, assessment of urine pH can be useful in determining whether the kidneys are responding appropriately to acid-base imbalances. In metabolic acidosis, urine pH should decrease as the kidneys excrete hydrogen ions; in metabolic alkalosis, the pH should increase (see Chapter 43).

GLUCOSE Urine is tested for glucose to screen clients for diabetes mellitus and to assess clients during pregnancy for abnormal glucose tolerance. Normally, the amount of glucose in the urine is negligible, although individuals who have ingested large amounts of sugar may show small amounts of glucose in their urine.

KETONES Ketone bodies, a product of the breakdown of fatty acids, normally are not present in the urine. They may, however, be found in the urine of clients with poorly controlled diabetes. Urine ketone testing with reagent tablets or a dipstick also is used to evaluate ketoacidosis in clients with alcoholism, and those who are fasting, starving, or consuming high-protein diets.

PROTEIN Protein molecules normally are too large to escape from glomerular capillaries into the filtrate. If the glomerular membrane has been damaged, however (e.g., because of an inflammatory process, such as glomerulonephritis), it can become *leaky,* allowing proteins to escape. Urine testing for the presence of protein generally is done with a reagent strip, or dipstick.

OCCULT BLOOD Normal urine is free from blood. When blood is present, it may be clearly visible or not visible (**occult blood**). Commercial reagent strips are used to test for occult blood in the urine.

METABOLIC SUBSTANCES Blood levels of two metabolically produced substances, urea and creatinine, are routinely used to evaluate renal function. The kidneys, through filtration and tubular secretion, normally eliminate both. Urea, the end product of protein metabolism, is measured as **blood urea nitrogen (BUN)**. **Creatinine** is produced in relatively constant quantities by the muscles and is excreted by the kidneys. Thus, the amount of creatinine in the blood relates to renal excretory function. The **creatinine clearance** test uses 24-hour urine and serum creatinine levels to determine the glomerular filtration rate, a sensitive indicator of renal function.

VISUALIZATION PROCEDURES Visualization procedures also can be used to evaluate urinary function. An X-ray of the kidneys, ureters, and bladder is commonly referred to as KUB. **Intravenous pyelography (IVP)** and **retrograde pyelography** also are radiographic studies used to evaluate the urinary tract. In an intravenous pyelogram, contrast medium is injected intravenously; during retrograde pyelography, the contrast medium is instilled directly into the renal pelvis via the urethra, bladder, and ureters. Following injection or instillation of the contrast medium, radiographs are taken to evaluate urinary tract structures. **Renal ultrasonography** is a noninvasive test that uses reflected sound waves to visualize the kidneys. During a **cystoscopy**, the bladder, ureteral orifices, and urethra can be directly visualized using a **cystoscope,** a lighted instrument inserted through the urethra.

Nurses are responsible for preparing clients before these studies and for follow-up care.

Diagnosing

NANDA International (2007) includes one general diagnostic label for urinary elimination problems and several labels that are more specific:

- *Impaired Urinary Elimination:* Dysfunction in urine elimination.

Other NANDA International (2007) nursing diagnoses related to urinary elimination include the following:

- *Stress Incontinence:* Sudden leakage of urine occurring with activities that increase abdominal pressure (e.g., sneezing, coughing, laughing, lifting)
- *Reflex Urinary Incontinence:* Involuntary loss of urine at somewhat predictable intervals when a specific bladder volume is reached
- *Urge Urinary Incontinence:* Involuntary passage of urine occurring soon after a strong sense of urgency to void
- *Functional Urinary Incontinence:* Inability of usually continent person to reach the toilet in time to avoid unintentional loss of urine
- *Total Urinary Incontinence:* Continuous and unpredictable passage of urine
- *Urinary Retention:* Incomplete emptying of the bladder followed by overflow incontinence

Clinical examples of assessment data clusters and related nursing diagnoses are shown in Table 41.5.

Problems of urinary elimination can become the etiology for other problems experienced by the client. Examples include the following:

- *Risk for Infection* if the client has urinary retention or undergoes an invasive procedure, such as catheterization or cystoscopic examination.
- *Low Self-Esteem* or *Social Isolation* if the client is incontinent. Incontinence can be physically and emotionally distressing to clients because it is considered socially unacceptable. Often, the client is embarrassed about dribbling or having an accident and may restrict normal activities for this reason.
- *Risk for Impaired Skin Integrity* if the client is incontinent. Bed linens and clothes saturated with urine irritate and excoriate the skin. Prolonged skin dampness leads to dermatitis (inflammation of the skin) and subsequent formation of dermal ulcers.
- *Self-Care Deficit: Toileting* if the client has functional incontinence.
- *Risk for Deficient Fluid Volume* or *Excess Fluid Volume* if the client has impaired urinary function associated with a disease process.
- *Disturbed Body Image* if the client has a urinary diversion ostomy.
- *Risk for Caregiver Role Strain* if the client is incontinent and being cared for by a family member for extended periods.

Planning

The goals established will vary according to the diagnosis and defining characteristics. Examples of overall goals for clients with urinary elimination problems may include the following:

- Maintain or restore a normal voiding pattern
- Regain normal urine output
- Prevent associated risks, such as infection, skin breakdown, fluid and electrolyte imbalance, and lowered self-esteem
- Perform toilet activities independently with or without assistive devices

Examples of desired outcomes for each of these goals are provided in Table 41.6 in the "Evaluating" section (page 1303).

Selected nursing strategies to achieve the goals for problems of altered urinary elimination are discussed in the "Implementing" section. For example, for *urinary incontinence*, the following strategies may be considered: keeping a voiding record or diary; scheduled toileting; prompted voiding; Kegel (pelvic floor muscle) exercises;

TABLE 41.5 Assessment Data Clusters and Related Nursing Diagnoses

Data Cluster	Nursing Diagnosis
Mrs. Amy Brown, 75 years old, reports accidental loss of urine before she is able to reach the toilet. She is aware of the urge to void but states, "Because of my stroke, I sometimes can't get there soon enough."	*Functional Urinary Incontinence* related to mobility deficit
Anthony Cherry, a teenager with a spinal cord injury, has no awareness of bladder filling, the urge to void, or feelings of bladder fullness. He reports loss of urine at fairly regular intervals.	*Reflex, Urinary Incontinence* related to neurological impairment (spinal cord lesion)
Tammy Tyndale reports dribbling whenever she laughs, coughs, or sneezes. She is 8 months pregnant.	*Stress Urinary Incontinence* related to high intra-abdominal pressure associated with pregnancy
Mrs. Gail Brady reports urinary urgency, difficulty in getting to the bathroom in time, frequency (more often than every 2 hours), and leakage of urine when unable to reach the toilet in time.	*Urge Urinary Incontinence* related to unknown etiology

dietary and fluid intake alterations; assistive devices, such as a bedside commode, mobility aids, or a raised toilet seat; and incontinence aids, such as a condom drainage device for males, absorbent pads, and protective clothing.

For *urinary retention,* the nurse may consider such strategies as bladder training, positioning and relaxation techniques, Credé's manoeuvre, intermittent self-catheterization, and parasympathomimetic medications as indicated and prescribed.

Examples of interventions to manage urinary elimination problems include the following:

- Urinary elimination management
- Urinary incontinence care
- Prompted voiding
- Urinary habit training
- Urinary bladder training
- Urinary retention care
- Pelvic floor muscle exercise

Specific nursing activities associated with each of these interventions can be selected to meet the individual needs of the client. A Sample Care Plan for urinary elimination follows.

PLANNING FOR HOME CARE To provide for continuity of care, the nurse needs to consider the client's needs for teaching and assistance with care in the home. Discharge planning includes assessment of the client's and family's resources and abilities for self-care, available financial

Sample Care Plan for Urinary Elimination

ASSESSMENT DATA

Nursing Assessment

Mr. John Baker is a 68-year-old shopkeeper who was admitted to the hospital with urinary retention, hematuria, and fever. The admitting nurse gathers the following information when taking a nursing history. Mr. Baker states he has noticed urinary frequency during the day for the past 2 weeks and that he does not feel he has emptied his bladder after urinating. He also has to get up 2 or 3 times during the night to urinate. Over the past few days, he has had difficulty starting urination, and urine dribbles afterward. He verbalizes the embarrassment his urinary problems cause in his dealings with the public. Mr. Baker is concerned about the cause of this urinary problem. He is diagnosed with benign prostatic hypertrophy and referred to an urologist, who suggests a transurethral resection of the prostate (TURP) in several months. Mr. Baker is placed on antibiotic therapy.

Physical Examination

Height: 185.4 cm

Weight: 85.7 kg

Temperature: 38.1°C

Pulse: 88 bpm

Respirations: 20/minute

Blood pressure: 146/86 mm Hg

Catheterization for urinary retention yielded 300 mL amber urine. Foley left in place for 2 days.

Diagnostic Data

CBC normal; urinalysis: amber, clear, pH 6.5, specific gravity 1.025, negative for glucose, protein, ketone, RBCs, and bacteria; IVP: evidence of enlarged prostate gland

Nursing Diagnosis

Impaired Urinary Elimination (retention and overflow incontinence) related to bladder neck obstruction by enlarged prostate gland (as evidenced by dysuria, frequency, nocturia, dribbling, hesitancy, and bladder distension).

Client Goals

The client will demonstrate an understanding of prostatic hypertrophy and its treatment, and will improve urinary elimination patterns.

Desired Health Outcomes

1. Reports reduction of incontinent episodes
2. Monitors urinary output, recognizing that fluid intake should equal output
3. Verbalizes a state of dryness that is personally satisfactory
4. Describes how an enlarged prostate gland interferes with urination
5. Describes one or two aspects of treatment

NURSING INTERVENTIONS AND SELECTED ACTIVITIES WITH RATIONALES* *[IN ITALICS]*

Urinary Incontinence Care

• Monitor urinary elimination, including consistency, odour, volume, and colour.	*These parameters help determine adequacy of urinary tract function.*
• Help the client select an appropriate incontinence garment or a pad for short-term management while more definitive treatment is designed.	*Appropriate undergarments can help diminish the embarrassing aspects of urinary incontinence.*
• Instruct Mr. Baker to limit fluids for 2 to 3 hours before bedtime.	*Decreased fluid intake several hours before bedtime will decrease the incidence of urinary retention and overflow incontinence and promote rest.*
• Instruct him to drink a minimum of 1500 mL per day.	*Increased fluids during the day will increase urinary output and discourage bacterial growth.*
• Limit ingestion of bladder irritants (e.g., alcohol, colas, coffee, tea, and chocolate).	*Alcohol and caffeine have a natural diuretic effect and are bladder irritants.*

(continued)

Sample Care Plan for Urinary Elimination *(continued)*

Urinary Retention Care

• Instruct Mr. Baker or a family member to record urinary output.	*This serves as an indicator of urinary tract and renal function and of fluid balance.*
• Catheterize for residual urine, as ordered.	*An enlarged prostate compresses the urethra so that urine is retained. Checking for residual urine provides information about bladder emptying.*
• Implement intermittent catheterization, as ordered.	*This helps maintain tonicity of the bladder muscle by preventing overdistension and providing for complete emptying.*
• Provide enough time for bladder emptying (10 minutes).	*In addition to the effect of an enlarged prostate on the bladder, stress or anxiety can inhibit relaxation of the urinary sphincter. Sufficient time should be allowed for micturition.*
• Instruct the client in ways to avoid constipation or stool impaction.	*Impacted stool can place pressure on the bladder outlet, causing urinary retention.*

Teaching: Disease Process

• Appraise Mr. Baker's current level of knowledge about benign prostatic hypertrophy.	*Assessing the client's knowledge will provide a foundation for building a teaching plan based on his present understanding of his condition.*
• Explain the pathophysiology of the disease and how it relates to urinary anatomy and function.	*In this case, urinary retention and overflow incontinence are caused by obstruction of the bladder neck by an enlarged prostate gland.*
• Describe the rationale behind management, therapy, and treatment recommendations (e.g., TURP).	*Adequate information about treatment options is important to diminish anxiety, promote compliance, and enhance decision making.*
• Instruct Mr. Baker on which signs and symptoms to report to the health-care provider (e.g., burning on urination, hematuria, oliguria).	*In the individual with prostatic hypertrophy, urinary retention and an overdistended bladder reduce blood flow to the bladder wall, making it more susceptible to infection from bacterial growth. Monitoring for these manifestations of urinary tract infection is essential to prevent urosepsis.*

EVALUATION

Outcomes partially met. Following removal of the Foley catheter, Mr. Baker reported continued difficulty initiating a urinary stream but experienced less dribbling of urine. He and his wife selected an undergarment that was acceptable to Mr. Baker, and he reports that he feels more confident. Intake is approximately 200 mL in excess of output. He is able to discuss the correlation between his enlarged prostate and urinary difficulties. A transurethral resection of the prostate is scheduled in 2 weeks.

*Interventions and activities selected are only a sample of those suggested in the *Nursing Interventions Classification (NIC)*, by G. M. Bulechek, H. K. Butcher, and J. C. Dochterman (Eds.), 2008, St. Louis, MO: Mosby Elsevier, and should be individualized for each client.

resources, and the need for referrals and home care services. The Assessment: Home Care box outlines an assessment of home care capabilities related to urinary elimination problems and needs. The Teaching: Home Care box addresses the learning needs of the client and family in relation to urinary elimination.

Implementing

MAINTAINING NORMAL URINARY ELIMINATION Most interventions to maintain normal urinary elimination are independent nursing functions. These include promoting adequate fluid intake, maintaining normal voiding habits, and assisting with toileting.

PROMOTING FLUID INTAKE Increasing fluid intake increases urine production, which, in turn, stimulates the micturition reflex. A normal daily intake averaging 1500 mL of measurable fluids is adequate for most adult clients.

Many clients have increased fluid requirements, necessitating a higher daily fluid intake. For example, clients who have diaphoresis (are perspiring excessively) or who are experiencing abnormal fluid losses through vomiting, gastric suction, diarrhea, or wound drainage require fluid to replace these losses in addition to their normal daily intake requirements.

Clients who are at risk for UTIs or urinary calculi (stones) should consume 2000 mL to 3000 mL of fluid daily. Evidence suggests that ingesting cranberry juice

ASSESSMENT: HOME CARE

Urinary Elimination

Assess for the following:

CLIENT AND ENVIRONMENT

- *Self-care abilities:* Ability to consume adequate fluids, to perceive bladder fullness, to ambulate and get to the toilet, to manipulate clothing for toileting, and to perform hygiene measures after toileting
- *Assistive devices required:* Ambulatory aids, such as walker, cane, or wheelchair; safety devices, such as grab bars; toileting aids, such as raised toilet seat, urinal, commode, or bedpan; a urinary catheter
- *Home environment for factors that interfere with toileting:* Distance to the bathroom from living areas or bedrooms; barriers, such as stairways, scatter rugs, clutter, or narrow doorways that interfere with bathroom access; lighting (including night lighting that allows gradual transition from dark bedroom to light bathroom)
- *Urinary elimination problems:* Type of incontinence and precipitating factors; manifestations of UTIs, such as dysuria, frequency, urgency; evidence of prostatic hypertrophy and effect on urination; ability to perform self-catheterization and care for other urinary elimination devices, such as indwelling catheter, urinary diversion ostomy, or condom drainage
- *Current level of knowledge:* Fluid and dietary intake modifications to promote normal patterns of urinary elimination; bladder training methods and specific techniques to promote voiding; care for indwelling catheter or ostomy (if appropriate)

FAMILY

- *Caregiver availability, skills, and responses:* Ability and willingness to assume responsibilities for care, including assisting with toileting, intermittent catheterization, indwelling catheter care, urinary drainage devices or ostomy care; ready access to laundry facilities; access to and willingness to use respite or relief caregivers
- *Family role changes and coping:* Effect on spousal and family roles, sleep-rest patterns, sexuality, and social interactions
- *Financial resources:* Ability to purchase protective pads and garments, supplies for catheterization or ostomy care

COMMUNITY

- *Environment:* Access to public restrooms and sanitary facilities
- *Current knowledge of and experience with community resources:* Medical and assistive equipment, home care agencies, local pharmacies, available financial assistance, support, and educational organizations

TEACHING: HOME CARE

Urinary Elimination

Address the learning needs of the client and family in relation to urinary elimination:

FACILITATING URINARY ELIMINATION SELF-CARE

- Teach the client and family to maintain easy access to toilet facilities, including removing scatter rugs and ensuring that halls and doorways are free of clutter.
- Suggest graduated lighting for nighttime voiding: a dim night-light in the bedroom and low-wattage hallway lighting.
- Advise the client and family to install grab bars and elevated toilet seats, as needed.
- Provide for instruction in safe transfer techniques. Contact physical therapy to provide training, as needed.
- Suggest clothing that is easily removed for toileting, such as elastic-waist pants or Velcro closures.

PROMOTING URINARY ELIMINATION

- Instruct the client to respond to the urge to void as soon as possible; avoid voluntary urinary retention.
- Teach the client to empty the bladder completely at each voiding.
- Emphasize the importance of drinking eight to ten 250 mL glasses of water daily.
- Teach female clients about Kegel exercises to strengthen perineal muscles.
- Inform the client about the relationship between tobacco use and bladder cancer and provide information about smoking cessation programs, as indicated.
- Teach the client to promptly report any of the following to the health-care provider: pain or burning on urination, changes in urine colour or clarity (e.g., bright red, rusty, or cloudy urine), malodorous urine, or changes in voiding patterns (e.g., nocturia, frequency, dribbling).

INFECTION PREVENTION

- Teach the client to maintain perineal-genital cleanliness, washing with soap and water daily and cleansing the anal and perineal area after defecating.
- Instruct female clients to wipe from front to back (from the urinary meatus toward the anus) after voiding, and to discard toilet paper after each swipe.
- Provide information about products to protect the skin and clothing, and assistive devices for clients who are incontinent. Emphasize the importance of cleaning and drying the perineal area after incontinence episodes. Instruct in the use of protective skin barrier products, as needed.
- Teach clients with an indwelling catheter and their family about care measures, such as cleaning the urinary meatus, managing and emptying the collection device, maintaining a closed system, and bladder irrigation or flushing, if ordered.

(continued)

TEACHING: HOME CARE *(continued)*

- For clients with a urinary diversion, teach about care of the stoma, drainage devices, and surrounding skin. For continent diversions, teach the client how to catheterize the stoma to drain urine.
- For clients with an indwelling catheter or urinary diversion, emphasize the importance of maintaining a generous fluid intake (1500 mL) and of promptly reporting changes in urinary output; signs of urinary retention, such as abdominal pain and a palpable bladder; and manifestations of UTIs, such as malodorous urine, abdominal discomfort, fever, or confusion.

MEDICATIONS

- Emphasize the importance of taking medications as prescribed. Instruct the client to take the full course of antibiotics prescribed to treat a UTI, even though symptoms are relieved.
- Inform the client and family about any expected changes in urine colour or odour associated with prescribed medications.
- For clients with urinary retention, emphasize the need to contact the health-care provider before taking any medication (even over-the-counter medications, such as antihistamines) that may exacerbate symptoms (see Box 41.1).
- For clients taking medications that can damage the kidneys (e.g., aminoglycoside antibiotics), stress the importance of maintaining a generous fluid intake while taking the medication.
- Suggest measures to reduce anticipated side effects of prescribed medications, such as increasing intake of potassium-rich foods when taking a potassium-depleting diuretic, such as furosemide.

DIETARY ALTERATIONS

- Teach the client about dietary changes to promote urinary function, such as consuming foods that acidify the urine (e.g., eggs, chicken, peanuts, whole grains). It is thought that the fructose and flavanols found in cranberry juice prevent bacteria (particularly *Escherichia coli*) from adhering (sticking) to the wall of the bladder, especially in young women (Jepson & Craig, 2008). The actual amount of daily intake of such foods has not been determined.
- Instruct clients to limit their intake of caffeinated beverages (e.g., tea, coffee, cola drinks) and alcohol as these are bladder irritants that may increase incontinence. Also teach clients to limit their evening fluid intake to reduce the risk of nighttime incontinence episodes.

MEASURES SPECIFIC TO URINARY PROBLEMS

- Provide instructions for clients with specific urinary problems or treatments, such as
  - **a.** Timed urine specimens
  - **b.** Urinary incontinence
  - **c.** Urinary retention
  - **d.** Retention catheters

REFERRALS

- Make appropriate referrals to home care agencies, community agencies, or social services for assistance with resources, such as grab bars and raised toilet seats; providing wheelchair access to bathrooms; obtaining toileting aids, such as commodes, urinals, or bedpans; and services, such as home care aides, for assistance with activities of daily living.

COMMUNITY AGENCIES AND OTHER RESOURCES

- Provide information about resources for durable medical equipment, such as commodes or raised toilet seats; possible financial assistance; and medical supplies, such as drainage bags, incontinence briefs, or protective pads.
- Suggest additional sources of information and help, such as the United Ostomy Association of Canada, Canadian Continence Foundation, or the Kidney Foundation of Canada.

(or capsules) may prevent UTIs, especially in young women (Jepson & Craig, 2008). Dilute urine and frequent urination reduce the risk of UTIs and stone formation.

Increased fluid intake may be contraindicated for some clients, such as those with kidney failure or heart failure. For these clients, a fluid restriction may be necessary to prevent fluid overload and edema.

Maintaining Normal Voiding Habits Prescribed medical therapies often interfere with a client's normal voiding habits. When a client's urinary elimination pattern is adequate, the nurse helps the client adhere to normal voiding habits as much as possible. See Practice Guidelines 41.1.

Assisting with Toileting Clients who are weakened by a disease process or have a physical impairment may require assistance to toilet. The nurse should assist these clients to the bathroom and remain with them if the client is at risk for falling. The bathroom should contain an easily accessible call signal to summon help if needed. Clients also need to be encouraged to use handrails placed near the toilet.

For clients unable to use bathroom facilities, the nurse provides urinary equipment close to the bedside (e.g., urinal, bedpan, commode) and provides the necessary assistance to use them.

PREVENTING URINARY TRACT INFECTIONS The rate of urinary tract infection (UTI) is 50 times as prevalent in women as in men (Ross, 2006) because of the short urethra and its proximity to the anal and vaginal areas. UTIs are the most common type of health-care-associated infection found in long-term-care facilities (Midthun, 2004). Most UTIs are caused by bacteria common to the intestinal environment (e.g., *Escherichia coli*). These gastrointestinal bacteria can colonize the perineal area and move into the urethra, especially when there is urethral trauma, irritation, or manipulation. Women are particularly at risk.

PRACTICE GUIDELINES 41.1

Maintaining Normal Voiding Habits

Guidelines	Rationales
Positioning	
Assist the client to a normal position for voiding: standing for males; for females, squatting or leaning slightly forward when sitting. If the client is unable to ambulate to the lavatory, use a bedside commode for females and a urinal for males standing at the bedside, if possible.	These positions enhance movement of urine through the urinary tract by gravity.
Relaxation	
Provide privacy for the client, and allow the client sufficient time to void.	Many people cannot void in the presence of another person or in a rushed environment. Defecation will also be ensured, reducing the risk of constipation, which is a factor in the development of incontinence.
Suggest that the client read or listen to music. Provide sensory stimuli that may help the client relax.	These distractions help the client relax and not focus on voiding.
Pour warm water over the perineum of a female or have the client sit in a warm bath. Apply warmed blankets or towels to the lower abdomen of both men and women.	The warmth can promote relaxation.
Turn on running water within hearing distance of the client.	This aids in stimulating the voiding reflex and masks the sound of voiding for people who find this embarrassing.
Provide prescribed analgesics and emotional support.	This helps to relieve physical and emotional discomfort and decrease muscle tension.
Timing	
Assist clients who have the urge to void immediately. Offer toileting assistance to the client at usual times of voiding, for example, on awakening, before or after meals, and at bedtime.	Delays only increase the difficulty in starting to void, and the desire to void may pass.
For clients who are confined to bed	
Warm the bedpan.	A cold bedpan can prompt contraction of the perineal muscles and inhibit voiding.
Elevate the head of the client's bed to Fowler's position, place a small pillow or rolled towel at the small of the back, and have the client flex the hips and knees.	This position simulates the normal voiding position as closely as possible and increases physical support and comfort.

CLINICAL ALERT

UTIs are the most common problem associated with urinary catheterization and are the most common health-care-associated infection. Nurses should ensure urinary catheters are used *only* when absolutely necessary and removed as soon as possible. Routine cleaning of the perineal area and use of strict aseptic technique during insertion and manipulation of the catheter is critical in preventing infection.

For women who have experienced a UTI, nurses need to provide instructions about ways to prevent a recurrence. The following guidelines are useful for anyone:

- Drink eight 250 mL glasses of water per day to flush bacteria out of the urinary system. Avoid fluids that irritate the bladder, like alcohol and caffeine.
- Practise frequent voiding (every 2 to 4 hours) to flush bacteria out of the urethra and prevent organisms from ascending into the bladder. Do not hold urine; void when need arises. Void after sexual intercourse.
- Keep the genital area clean and dry. Avoid the use of harsh soaps, bubble bath, powder, or sprays in the perineal area. These substances can be irritating to the urethra and encourage inflammation and bacterial infection.
- Do not douche or use similar feminine hygiene products.
- Avoid tight-fitting pants or other clothing that creates irritation to the urethra and prevents ventilation of the perineal area.
- Wear cotton, rather than nylon, underclothes. Accumulation of perineal moisture facilitates bacterial growth and cotton enhances ventilation of the perineal area.
- Girls and women should always wipe the perineal area from front to back following urination or defecation in order to prevent introduction of gastrointestinal bacteria into the urethra.
- If recurrent urinary infections are a problem, take showers, rather than baths. Bacteria present in bathwater can readily enter the urethra.

MANAGING URINARY INCONTINENCE It is important to remember that urinary incontinence is *not* a normal part of aging and often is treatable. Independent nursing interventions for clients with urinary incontinence include (1) a behaviour-oriented continence training program that may consist of bladder training, habit training, prompted voiding, pelvic floor muscle exercises, and positive reinforcement; (2) meticulous skin care; and (3) for males, application of an external drainage device (condom).

CONTINENCE (BLADDER) TRAINING A continence training program requires the involvement of the nurse, the client, and support people. Clients must be alert and physically able to follow a program. Clients who are unable to remain continent for more than 2 hours may have difficulty in adhering to a continence training program (Registered Nurses' Association of Ontario [RNAO], 2005). The goal of training is to decrease the frequency of UI. A bladder training program may include the following (Roe, Ostaszkiewicz, Milne, & Wallace, 2007):

- **Bladder training**, which requires that the client postpone voiding, resist or inhibit the sensation of urgency, and void according to a timetable rather than according to the urge to void. The goals are to gradually lengthen the intervals between urination to correct the client's habit of frequent urination, to stabilize the bladder, and to diminish urgency. This form of training can be used for clients who have bladder instability and urge incontinence. Delayed voiding provides larger voided volumes and longer intervals between voiding. Initially, voiding may be encouraged every 2 to 3 hours. except during sleep, and then every 4 to 6 hours. A vital component of bladder training is inhibiting the urge-to-void sensation. To do this, the nurse instructs the client to practise deep, slow breathing until the urge diminishes or disappears. This breathing is performed every time the client has a premature urge to void. See Practice Guidelines 41.2.
- **Habit training**, also referred to as timed voiding or scheduled toileting, attempts to keep clients dry by having them void at *regular* intervals. With habit training, there is no attempt to motivate the client to delay voiding if the urge occurs. This approach can be effective in children who are experiencing urinary dysfunction. Biofeedback therapy in which the child is taught to relax the pelvic floor can also decrease incidents of wetting (Shei Dei Yang & Cheng Wang, 2005).
- **Prompted voiding** supplements habit training by encouraging the client to try to use the toilet (prompting) and reminding the client when to void (RNAO, 2005). This intervention is used for clients who need timely reminders from caregivers owing

Evidence-Informed Practice

What Self-Care Strategies Do Individuals with Urinary Incontinence Employ and What Factors Influence the Choice and Maintenance of Strategies?

Urinary incontinence affects 17% to 25% of all community-dwelling individuals. Conservative measures, such as dietary modification, bladder retraining, and pelvic floor muscle exercises (PFME), are generally recommended as first-line treatment. Milne and Moore (2006) conducted a qualitative study of adults with urinary incontinence to gain an understanding of the factors influencing motivation and maintenance of self-care in the home setting. The University of Alberta researchers recruited 33 females and 5 males to participate in individual interviews or focus groups. A loosely structured interview guide directed the focus groups.

The major self-care goal arising from analysis of the transcripts was the need to maintain a normal lifestyle. In an attempt to maintain normalcy, participants did not pursue dietary modifications, bladder retraining, or PFME. Participants reported that these strategies negatively affected their lifestyle. Not surprisingly none of the strategies were maintained for more than several days. Time restrictions and competing demands were identified as barriers to maintaining strategies. Barriers had an immediate and lingering effect on participants' rejection of the plan. The rejection of the strategies may have been influenced by a general lack of understanding of normal bladder function that was identified by many of the participants. A positive effect of the focus groups was the reports of perceived benefits of group support.

NURSING IMPLICATIONS: **The quality of life for incontinent adults in the community may be increased through dietary modification, bladder retraining, and PFME. In developing a plan of care it is paramount that the nurse engages the client in setting realistic goals and identifying barriers that may interfere with attainment of them. Teaching must be individualized, focusing on the client's daily routine and lifestyle. A thorough assessment of learning needs is critical. Follow-up of clients may facilitate discussion of previously unidentified barriers and alternative strategies. Client support may be enhanced through the introduction of group teaching sessions.**

Source: Based on "Factors Impacting Self-Care for Urinary Incontinence," by J. L. Milne and K. N. Moore, 2006, *Urologic Nursing, 26*(1), pp. 41–51.

to their physical or cognitive deficits. Caregivers using prompted voiding use three primary behaviours:

1. *Monitoring:* asking the incontinent person, at regular intervals, if he or she needs to use the toilet and taking the client to the toilet at regular intervals
2. *Prompting:* prompting the client to regularly use the toilet (e.g., "It is time to use the toilet. Do you need any help?") as well as encouraging toilet use between prompted voiding sessions
3. *Praising:* giving positive feedback for the maintenance of bladder control

Pelvic Floor Muscle Exercises Pelvic floor muscle exercises (PFME), or *Kegel exercises,* help to strengthen pelvic floor muscles and can reduce episodes of urinary incontinence (Hay-Smith & Dumoulin, 2006; Liao, Doughertya, Yuh-Shu Lioub, & Tsengb, 2006). The client can identify perineal muscles by stopping urination midstream or by tightening the anal sphincter as if to hold a bowel movement.

The following technique is sometimes used to teach PFME. Ask the client to think of her perineal muscles as an elevator. When the client relaxes, the elevator is on the first floor. To perform the exercise, contract the perineal muscles, bringing the elevator to the second, third, and fourth floors. Keep the elevator on the fourth floor for a few seconds, and then gradually relax the area. When the exercise is properly performed, contraction of the muscles of the buttocks and thighs is avoided. PFME can be performed anytime, anywhere, sitting or standing—

PRACTICE GUIDELINES 41.2

Bladder Training

Guidelines	Rationales
Determine the client's voiding pattern and encourage voiding at those times, or establish a regular voiding schedule. Help the client to maintain the schedule whether the client feels the urge or not (e.g., on awakening, every 1 or 2 hours during the day and evening, before retiring at night, and every 4 hours at night).	The stretching-relaxing sequence of such a schedule tends to increase bladder muscle tone and promote more voluntary control.
Encourage the client to inhibit the urge-to-void sensation when a premature urge to void is experienced. Instruct the client to practise slow, deep breathing until the urge diminishes or disappears.	Deep breathing aids in distracting the client from the urge to void.
When the client finds that voiding can be controlled, the intervals between voiding can be lengthened slightly without loss of continence.	This will help to increase muscle tone and decrease time spent in toileting.
Regulate fluid intake, particularly during evening hours.	This helps to reduce the need to void during the night.
Encourage fluids about half an hour before the voiding time between the hours of 0600 and 1800.	This aids in promoting voiding at the scheduled time.
Avoid excessive consumption of citrus juices, carbonated beverages (especially those containing artificial sweeteners), alcohol, and drinks containing caffeine.	These fluids irritate the bladder and tend to cause detrusor instability, increasing the risk of incontinence.
Schedule diuretics early in the morning.	This helps reduce the need to void during the night.
Explain to clients that adequate fluid intake is required to ensure adequate urine production, which stimulates the micturition reflex.	Clients may decrease fluid intake in an attempt to reduce episodes of incontinence.
Apply protector pads to keep the bed linen dry, and provide specially made waterproof underwear. Avoid using diapers, which are demeaning and also suggest that incontinence is permissible.	These measures aid in containing the urine and decrease the client's embarrassment.
Assist the client with an exercise program to increase the tone of abdominal and pelvic floor muscles.	Increasing tone of abdominal and pelvic floor muscles will foster continence through the voluntary control of voiding.
Provide positive reinforcements to encourage continence. Praise clients for attempting to go to the toilet and for maintaining continence.	Positive reinforcement will increase clients' self-esteem and promote compliance with the training program.
Maintain a voiding record to monitor the effectiveness of interventions; for example, a 3-day voiding record should be initiated at least 3 weeks and at most 8 weeks after a prompted voiding intervention is tested (RNAO, 2005).	Objective evidence provides evaluation feedback as to the effectiveness of the bladder training program.

even when voiding. Specific client instructions for performing PFME are summarized in the Teaching: Clinical box on pelvic floor muscle exercises (Kegels).

MAINTAINING SKIN INTEGRITY Skin that is continually moist becomes macerated. Urine that accumulates on the skin is converted to ammonia, which is very irritating to the skin. Because both skin irritation and maceration predispose the client to skin breakdown and ulceration, the incontinent person requires meticulous skin care. To maintain skin integrity, the nurse washes the client's perineal area with soap and water after episodes of incontinence, rinses it thoroughly, dries it thoroughly, and provides clean, dry clothing or bed linen. If the skin is irritated, the nurse applies barrier creams, such as zinc oxide ointment, to protect it from contact with urine. If it is necessary to pad the client's clothes for protection, the nurse should use products that absorb wetness and leave a dry surface in contact with the skin.

Specially designed *incontinence drawsheets* can be used that provide significant advantages over standard drawsheets for incontinent clients confined to bed. These sheets are like a drawsheet but are double layered, with a quilted upper nylon or polyester surface and an absorbent viscose rayon layer below. The rayon soaker layer generally has a waterproof backing on its underside. Fluid (i.e., urine) passes through the upper quilted layer and is absorbed and dispersed by the viscose rayon, leaving the quilted surface dry to the touch. This absorbent sheet helps maintain skin integrity: it does not stick to the skin when wet, it decreases the risk of bedsores, and it reduces odour.

APPLYING EXTERNAL URINARY DRAINAGE DEVICES The application of a condom or external catheter connected to a urinary drainage system is commonly prescribed for incontinent males. Use of a condom appliance is preferable to insertion of a retention catheter because the risk of UTIs is minimal.

TEACHING: CLINICAL

Pelvic Floor Muscle Exercises (Kegels)

Nurses can teach clients how to perform pelvic floor muscle exercises correctly:

- First, sit, lie or stand in a comfortable, relaxed position with legs apart.
- Contract your pelvic floor muscles whereby you pull your rectum, urethra, and vagina up inside, and hold for a count of 3 to 5 seconds. Then relax the same muscles for a count of 3 to 5 seconds.
- Initially perform each contraction 10 times, five times daily. Gradually increase the count to 10 seconds for both contraction and relaxation.
- Develop a schedule that will help remind you to do these exercises, for example, while driving to work, when working at the kitchen sink, or at scheduled times (e.g., 0700, 1000, 1300, 1600, and 1900 hours).
- Try to start and stop your stream of urine.
- To control episodes of stress incontinence, brace the muscles and use the Kegel manoeuvre when doing any activity that increases intra-abdominal pressure, such as coughing, laughing, sneezing, or lifting.

Methods of applying condoms vary according to how long the condom is to be worn. Condoms that are to be worn for a short period are generally applied with elastic tape only; if the condom is to be worn for a longer period (e.g., a few days), additional measures are required to protect the foreskin and to ensure secure attachment. The nurse needs to follow the manufacturer's instructions when applying a condom. First, the nurse determines when the client experiences incontinence. Some clients may require a condom appliance at night only, others continuously. Skill 41.2 describes how to apply a drainage condom.

SKILL 41.2

APPLYING AN EXTERNAL (CONDOM) CATHETER

PURPOSES

- To collect urine and control urinary incontinence
- To permit the client to engage in physical activity without fear of embarrassment because of leaking urine
- To prevent skin irritation as a result of urinary incontinence

ASSESSMENT

- Review the client record to determine a pattern of voiding and other pertinent data (e.g., times of urinary incontinence, amount of urine passed).
- Put on clean gloves and examine the client's penis for swelling or excoriation that would contraindicate the use of the condom catheter.

Planning

Determine whether the client has had an external catheter previously and any difficulties with it. Perform any procedures that are best completed without the catheter in place, for example, weighing the client would be easier without the tubing and bag.

(continued)

SKILL 41.2

APPLYING AN EXTERNAL (CONDOM) CATHETER *(continued)*

Equipment

- Leg drainage bag with tubing or urinary drainage bag with tubing
- Condom sheath
- Drape (e.g., sheet or bath blanket)
- Clean gloves
- Basin of warm water and soap
- Washcloth and towel
- Elastic tape or Velcro strap

IMPLEMENTATION

Preparation

- Assemble the leg drainage bag or urinary drainage bag for attachment to the condom sheath.
- Roll the condom outward onto itself to facilitate easier application (see ❶). On some models, an inner flap will be exposed. This flap is applied around the urinary meatus to prevent the reflux of urine.
- Position the client in either a supine or a sitting position.

Performance

1. Before performing the procedure, introduce yourself and verify the client's identity by using agency protocol. Explain to the client what you are going to do, why it is necessary, and how he can cooperate.
2. Perform hand hygiene, apply clean gloves, and observe other appropriate infection prevention and control procedures.
3. Provide for client privacy.
    - Drape the client appropriately with the bath blanket, exposing only the penis.
4. Inspect and clean the penis.
    - Clean the genital area and dry it thoroughly. **Rationale: This minimizes skin irritation and excoriation after the condom is applied.**
5. Apply and secure the condom.
    - Roll the condom smoothly over the penis, leaving 2.5 cm. between the end of the penis and the rubber or plastic connecting tube (see ❷). **Rationale: This space prevents irritation of the tip of the penis and provides for full drainage of urine.**
    - Secure the condom firmly, but not too tightly, to the penis. Some condoms have an adhesive inside the proximal end that adheres to the skin of the base of the penis. Many condoms are packaged with special tape. If neither is present, use a strip of elastic tape or Velcro around the base of the penis over the condom. Ordinary tape is contraindicated because it is not flexible and can stop blood flow.
6. Securely attach the urinary drainage system.
    - Make sure that the tip of the penis is not touching the condom and that the condom is not twisted. **Rationale: A twisted condom could obstruct the flow of urine.**
    - Attach the urinary drainage system to the condom.
    - Remove gloves and perform hand hygiene.
    - If the client is to remain in bed, attach the urinary drainage bag to the bed frame.
    - If the client is ambulatory, attach the bag to the client's leg (see ❸). **Rationale: Attaching the drainage bag to the leg helps control the movement of the tubing and prevents twisting of the thin material of the condom appliance at the tip of the penis.**
7. Teach the client about the drainage system.
    - Instruct the client to keep the drainage bag below the level of the condom and to avoid loops or kinks in the tubing.
8. Inspect the penis 30 minutes following the condom application, and check urine flow. Document these findings.
    - Assess the penis for swelling and discolouration, which indicates that the condom is too tight.

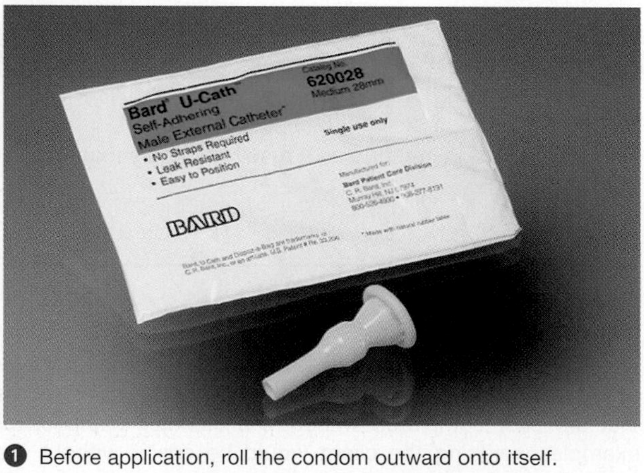

❶ Before application, roll the condom outward onto itself.

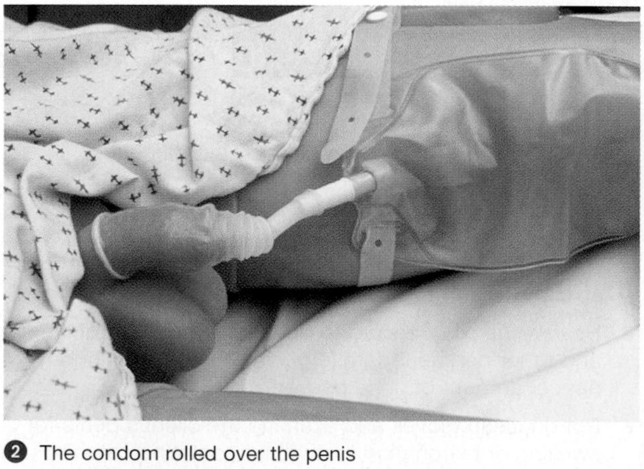

❷ The condom rolled over the penis

(continued)

SKILL 41.2

APPLYING AN EXTERNAL (CONDOM) CATHETER *(continued)*

- Assess urine flow if the client has voided. Normally, some urine is present in the tube if the flow is not obstructed.

9. Change the condom daily and provide skin care.
   - Remove the elastic or Velcro strip, apply clean gloves, and roll off the condom.
   - Wash the penis with soapy water, rinse, and dry it thoroughly.
   - Assess the foreskin for signs of irritation, swelling, and discolouration.
   - Reapply a new condom.
10. Document in the client record by using forms or checklists supplemented by narrative notes when appropriate. Record the application of the condom, the time, and pertinent observations, such as irritated areas on the penis.

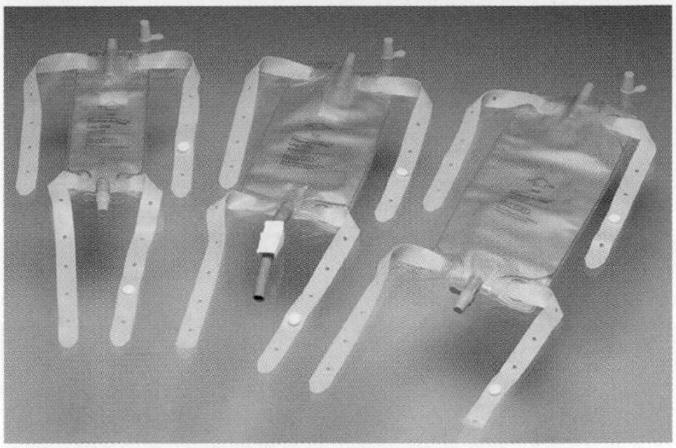
❸ Urinary drainage leg bags

EVALUATION

- Perform a detailed follow-up based on findings that deviated from expected or normal for the client. Relate findings to previous assessment data if available.
- Report significant deviations from normal to the appropriate member of the health-care team.

MANAGING URINARY RETENTION Interventions that assist the client to maintain a normal voiding pattern, discussed earlier, also apply when dealing with urinary retention. If these actions are unsuccessful, the health-care provider may order a cholinergic drug, such as bethanechol chloride (Urecholine) to stimulate bladder contraction and facilitate voiding. Clients who have a **flaccid** bladder (weak, soft, and lax bladder muscles) may use manual pressure on the bladder to promote bladder emptying. This is known as **Credé's manoeuvre** or *Credé's method.* It is not advised without a physician's order and is used only for clients who have lost and are not expected to regain voluntary bladder control. When all measures fail to initiate voiding, urinary catheterization may be necessary to empty the bladder completely. An indwelling Foley catheter may be inserted until the underlying cause is treated; alternatively, intermittent straight catheterization (every 3 to 4 hours) may be performed because the risk of UTIs is believed by some to be less than with an indwelling catheter.

URINARY CATHETERIZATION Urinary catheterization is the introduction of a catheter through the urethra into the urinary bladder. This is usually performed only when *absolutely necessary* because the procedure incurs certain hazards. Because the urinary structures are normally sterile, except at the end of the urethra, the danger exists of introducing microorganisms into the bladder. Clients who have lowered immune resistance are at the greatest risk. Once an infection is introduced into the bladder, it can ascend the ureters and eventually involve the kidneys. The hazard of infection remains after the catheter is in place because normal defence mechanisms, such as intermittent flushing of microorganisms from the urethra through voiding, are bypassed. Thus, strict sterile technique is used for catheterization.

Another hazard is trauma, particularly in the male client, whose urethra is longer and more tortuous. It is important to insert a catheter along the normal contour of the urethra. Damage to the urethra can occur if the catheter is forced through strictures or at an incorrect angle. In males, the urethra is normally curved, but it can be straightened by elevating the penis to a position perpendicular to the body.

Catheters are commonly made of rubber or plastics although they may be made from latex, silicone, or polyvinylchloride (PVC). Latex catheters are being withdrawn from most institutions because of the risk of allergies. They are sized by the diameter of the lumen by using the French (Fr) scale: the larger the number, the larger is the lumen. Either *straight catheters,* inserted to drain the bladder and then immediately removed, or *indwelling catheters,* which remain in the bladder to drain urine, can be used.

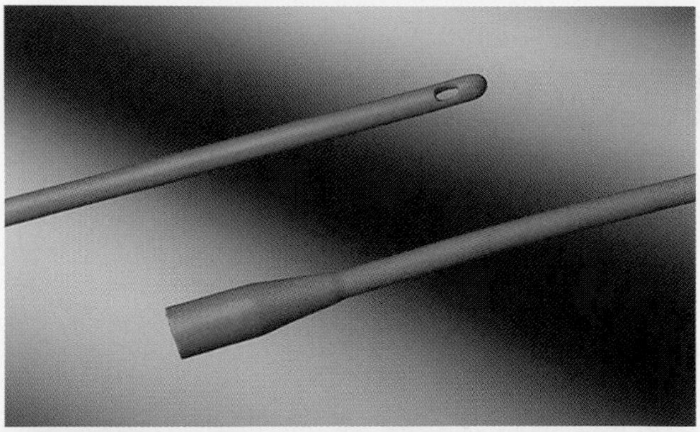

A

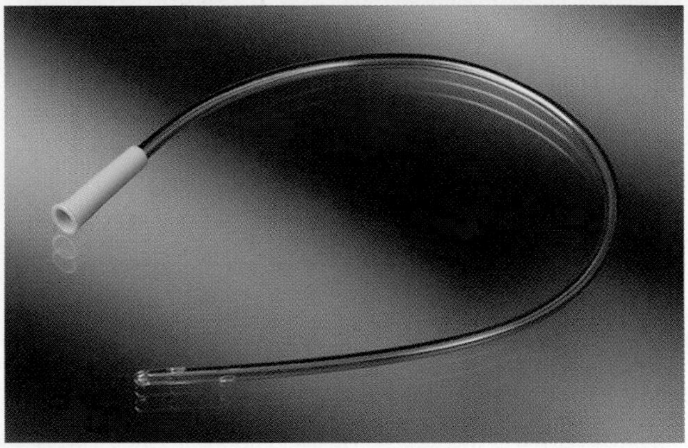

B

FIGURE 41.11 Straight catheters: **A:** red-rubber; **B:** Robinson

The straight catheter is a single-lumen tube with a small eye or opening about 1.25 cm from the insertion tip (Figure 41.11). The *coudé catheter* is a variation of the straight catheter. It is more rigid than other straight catheters and has a tapered, curved tip (Figure 41.12). This catheter may be used for men with prostatic hypertrophy as it is more easily controlled and less traumatic on insertion.

The *indwelling* (*retention*), or *Foley, catheter* is a double-lumen catheter. The larger lumen drains urine from the bladder. A second, smaller lumen is used to inflate a balloon near the tip of the catheter to hold the catheter in place within the bladder (Figure 41.13). Clients who require continuous or intermittent bladder irrigation may have a *three-way Foley catheter* (Figure 41.14). The three-way catheter has a third lumen through which sterile irrigating fluid can flow into the bladder. The fluid then exits the bladder through the drainage lumen along with the urine.

The balloons of indwelling catheters are sized by the volume of fluid used to inflate them. The three commonly used sizes are 5 mL, 10 mL, and 30 mL balloons. The size of the balloon is indicated on the catheter, along with the diameter, for example, "18 Fr—5 mL." Box 41.2 provides guidelines for catheter selection.

Indwelling catheters usually are connected to a *closed gravity drainage system.* This system consists of the catheter, drainage tubing, and a collecting bag for the urine. A closed system should not be opened anywhere along the system from catheter to collecting bag. Closed systems reduce the risk of microorganisms entering the system and infecting the urinary tract. Urinary drainage systems typically depend on the force of gravity to drain urine from the bladder to the collecting bag.

Skill 41.3 describes urethral urinary catheterization of females and males, using straight and indwelling catheters.

NURSING INTERVENTIONS FOR CLIENTS WITH INDWELLING CATHETERS Nursing care of the client with an indwelling catheter and continuous drainage is

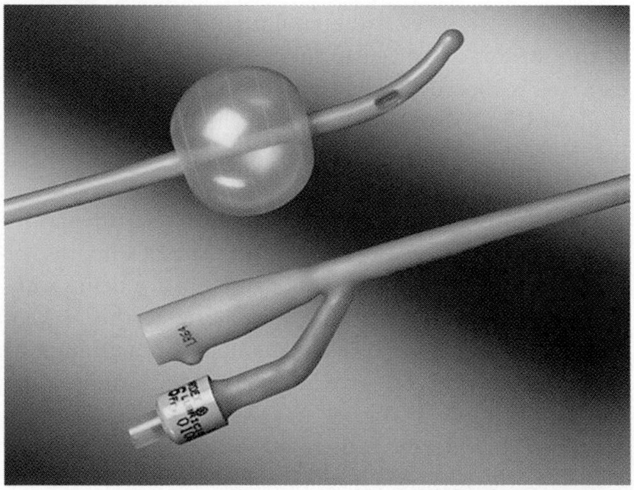

FIGURE 41.12 A coudé catheter

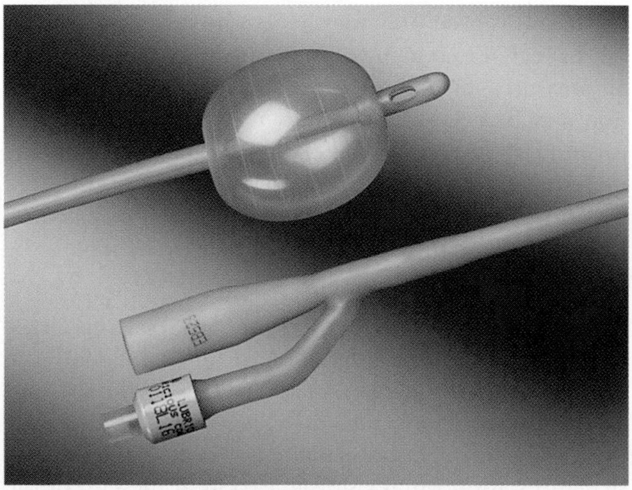

FIGURE 41.13 An indwelling or retention (Foley) catheter with balloon inflated

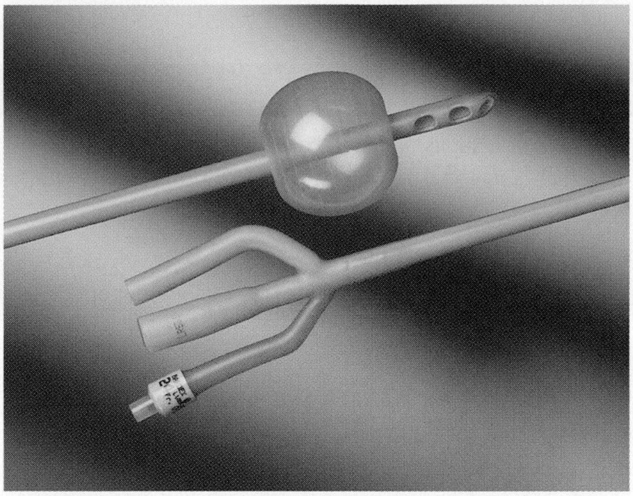

FIGURE 41.14 A three-way Foley catheter (often used for continuous bladder irrigation)

largely directed toward preventing infection of the urinary tract and encouraging urinary flow through the drainage system. It includes encouraging adequate amounts of fluid intake, accurately recording the fluid intake and output, changing the retention catheter and tubing, maintaining the patency of the drainage system,

BOX 41.2 SELECTING AN APPROPRIATE CATHETER

The following guidelines are used in choosing a catheter:

- Select the type of material in accordance with the estimated length of the catheterization period and the client's allergies.
  - **a.** Use *plastic* catheters for short periods only (e.g., 1 week or less) because they are inflexible.
  - **b.** Use a silicone or *rubber* catheter for periods of 2 or 3 weeks. Latex catheters are being withdrawn from most hospitals because of the risk of allergy.
  - **c.** Use *silicone* catheters for long-term use (e.g., 2 to 3 months) because they create less encrustation at the urethral meatus. However, they are expensive.
  - **d.** Use *PVC* catheters for 4- to 6-week periods. They soften at body temperature and conform to the urethra.
- Determine the appropriate catheter length by the client's gender. For adult females, use a 22 cm catheter; for adult males, a 40 cm catheter.
- Determine appropriate catheter size by the size of the urethral canal. Use sizes 8 Fr or 10 Fr for children and 14 Fr or 16 Fr for adults. Men frequently require a larger size than women do, for example, 18 Fr.
- Select the appropriate balloon size. For adults, use a 5 mL balloon to facilitate optimal urine drainage. The smaller balloons allow more complete bladder emptying because the catheter tip is closer to the urethral opening in the bladder. However, a 30 mL balloon or larger is commonly used to achieve hemostasis of the prostatic area following a prostatectomy. Use 3 mL balloons for children.

SKILL 41.3

PERFORMING URETHRAL URINARY CATHETERIZATION

PURPOSES

- To relieve discomfort from bladder distension or to provide gradual decompression of a distended bladder
- To assess the amount of residual urine if the bladder empties incompletely
- To obtain a sterile urine specimen
- To empty the bladder completely before surgery
- To facilitate accurate measurement of urinary output for critically ill clients whose output needs to be monitored hourly
- To provide for intermittent or continuous bladder drainage or irrigation
- To prevent urine from contacting an incision after perineal surgery
- To manage incontinence when other measures have failed

ASSESSMENT

- Determine the most appropriate method of catheterization based on the purpose and any criteria specified in the order, such as total amount of urine to be removed or size of catheter to be used.
- Use a straight catheter if only a spot urine specimen is needed, if the amount of residual urine is being measured, or if temporary decompression or emptying of the bladder is required.
- Use an indwelling or a retention catheter if the bladder must remain empty or continuous urine measurement or collection is needed.
- Assess the client's overall condition. Determine whether the client is able to cooperate and hold still during the procedure and whether the client can be positioned supine with head relatively flat.
- Determine when the client last voided or was last catheterized.
- Percuss the bladder to check for fullness or distension.
- When possible, complete a bladder scan to assess the amount of urine present in the bladder before performing a urethral catheterization.

(continued)

SKILL 41.3

PERFORMING URETHRAL URINARY CATHETERIZATION *(continued)*

Planning

Allow adequate time to perform the catheterization. Although the entire procedure can require as little as 15 minutes, several sources of difficulty could result in a much longer time.

Equipment

- Sterile catheter of appropriate size (an extra catheter should also be at hand)
- Catheterization kit (see ❶) or individual sterile items:
  - 1 to 2 pair sterile gloves
  - Waterproof drapes
  - Antiseptic solution
  - Cleansing balls
  - Forceps
  - Water-soluble lubricant
  - Urine receptacle
  - Specimen container
- For an indwelling catheter:
  - Syringe prefilled with sterile water in amount specified by catheter manufacturer
  - Collection bag and tubing
- 2% Xylocaine gel (if agency permits)
- Disposable clean gloves
- Supplies for performing perineal cleansing
- Bath blanket or sheet for draping the client
- Adequate lighting (use a flashlight or lamp if necessary)

IMPLEMENTATION

Preparation

If using a catheterization kit, read the label carefully to be sure all necessary items are included. Perform routine perineal care to cleanse the meatus from gross contamination. For women, use this time to locate the urinary meatus relative to surrounding structures (see ❷).

Performance

1. Before performing the procedure, introduce yourself and verify the client's identity by using agency protocol. Explain to the client what you are going to do, why it is necessary, and how he or she can cooperate.
2. Perform hand hygiene and observe other appropriate infection prevention and control procedures.
3. Provide for client privacy.
4. Place the client in the appropriate position and drape all areas except the perineum (see Skill 29.2, Figure 1, page 719).
   - Female: supine with knees flexed, feet about 50 cm apart, and hips slightly externally rotated, if possible
   - Male: supine, thighs slightly abducted or apart
5. Establish adequate lighting. Stand on the client's right if you are right-handed, on the client's left if you are left-handed.
6. If you are using a collecting bag and it is not contained within the catheterization kit, open the drainage package and place the end of the tubing within reach. **Rationale: Since one hand is needed to hold the catheter once it is in place, open the package while two hands are still available.**
7. If agency policy permits, apply clean gloves and inject 10 mL to 15 mL Xylocaine gel into the urethra of the male client. Wipe the underside of the shaft to distribute the gel up the urethra. Wait at least 5 minutes for the gel to take effect before inserting the catheter. Remove gloves.
8. Open the catheterization kit. Place a waterproof drape under the buttocks (female) or penis (male), without contaminating the centre of the drape with your hands.
9. Put on sterile gloves.
10. Organize the remaining supplies:
    - Saturate the cleansing balls with the antiseptic solution.
    - Open the lubricant package.
    - Remove the specimen container and place it nearby, with the lid loosely on top.

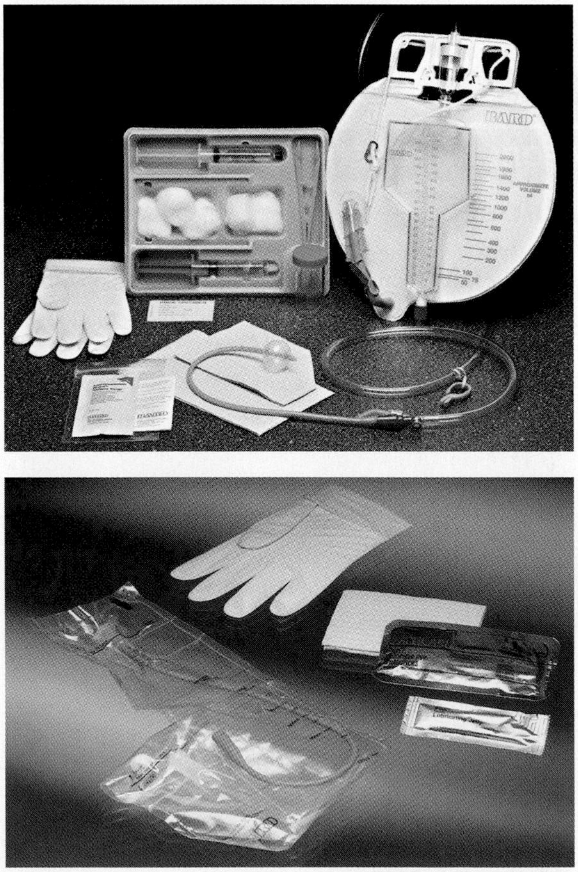

A

B

❶ Catheterization insertion kits: **A:** indwelling; **B:** straight

(continued)

SKILL 41.3

PERFORMING URETHRAL URINARY CATHETERIZATION (*continued*)

11. Attach the prefilled syringe to the indwelling catheter inflation hub and test the balloon. **Rationale: If the balloon malfunctions, it is important to replace it before use.**

12. Lubricate the catheter (2.5 cm to 5 cm for females, 5 cm to 15 cm for males) and place it with the drainage end inside the collection container.

13. If desired, place the fenestrated drape over the perineum, exposing the urinary meatus.

14. Cleanse the meatus. *Note:* The nondominant hand is considered contaminated once it touches the client's skin.

a. For women: Use your nondominant hand to spread the labia. Establish a firm but gentle position. The antiseptic may make the tissues slippery but the labia must not be allowed to return over the cleaned meatus. Pick up a cleansing ball with the forceps in your dominant hand and wipe one side of the labia majora in an anteroposterior direction (see ❸). Use great care that wiping the client does not contaminate this sterile hand. Use a new ball for the opposite side. Repeat for the labia minora. Use the last ball to cleanse directly over the meatus. *Note:* location of urethral meatus is best identified during the cleansing process.

b. For men: Use your nondominant hand to grasp the penis just below the glans. If necessary, retract the foreskin. Hold the penis firmly upright, with slight tension. **Rationale: Lifting the penis so that it is perpendicular to the body helps straighten the urethra.** Pick up a cleansing ball with the forceps in your dominant hand and wipe from the centre of the meatus in a circular motion around the glans. Use great care that wiping the client does not contaminate this sterile hand. Use a new ball and repeat three more times. The antiseptic may make the tissues slippery but the foreskin must not be allowed to return over the cleaned meatus or the penis be dropped.

15. Insert the catheter.

- Grasp the catheter firmly 8 cm to 10 cm from the tip. Ask the client to take a slow deep breath and insert the catheter as the client exhales. Slight resistance is expected as the catheter passes through the sphincters. If necessary, twist the catheter or hold pressure on the catheter until the sphincter relaxes.
- Advance the catheter 5 cm farther after the urine begins to flow through it. **Rationale: This ensures the catheter is fully in the bladder**. For male clients, some agency's policies and procedures indicate to advance the catheter to the Y bifurcation of the catheter.
- If the catheter accidentally contacts the labia or slips into the vagina, it is considered contaminated and a new, sterile catheter must be used. The contaminated catheter can be left in the vagina until the new catheter is inserted to avoid mistaking the vaginal opening for the urethral meatus.

16. Hold the catheter with the nondominant hand. In males, lay the penis down onto the drape, being careful that the catheter does not pull out.

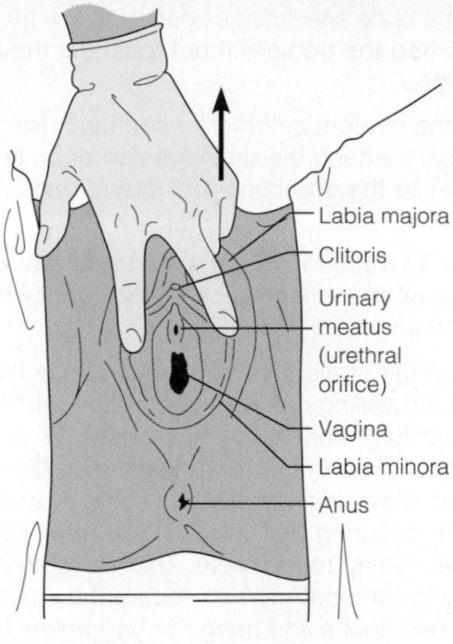

❷ To expose the urinary meatus, separate the labia minora and retract the tissue upward.

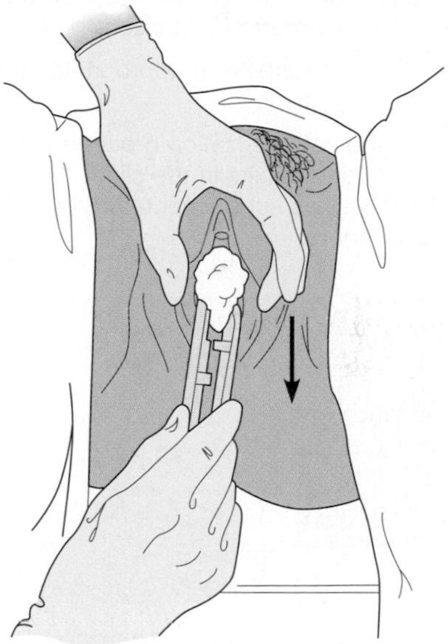

❸ When cleaning the urinary meatus, move the swab downward.

17. For an indwelling catheter, inflate the retention balloon with the designated volume.

- Without releasing the catheter, hold the inflation valve between two fingers of your nondominant hand while you attach the syringe (if not left attached earlier when testing the balloon) and inflate with your dominant hand. If the client complains of discomfort, immediately withdraw the instilled fluid, advance the catheter farther, and attempt to inflate the balloon again.
- Pull *gently* on the catheter until resistance is felt to ensure that the balloon has inflated and to place it in the trigone of the bladder (see ❹).

(continued)

SKILL 41.3

PERFORMING URETHRAL URINARY CATHETERIZATION (*continued*)

18. Collect a urine specimen if needed. Allow 20 mL to 30 mL to flow into the bottle without touching the catheter to the bottle.
19. Allow the straight catheter to continue draining. If necessary, attach the drainage end of an indwelling catheter to the collecting tubing and bag.
20. Examine and measure the urine. In some cases, only 750 mL to 1000 mL of urine are to be drained from the bladder at one time. Check agency policy for further instructions if this should occur.
21. Remove the straight catheter when urine flow stops. For an indwelling catheter, secure the catheter tubing to the inner thigh for female clients (see ❺) or the upper thigh or abdomen for male clients (see ❻) with enough slack to allow usual movement. Tape or a manufactured catheter-securing device should be used to secure the catheter tubing to the client. This prevents unnecessary trauma to the urethra. Also secure the collecting tubing to the bed linens and hang the bag below the level of the bladder. No tubing should fall below the top of the bag (see ❼).
22. Wipe the perineal area of any remaining antiseptic or lubricant. Replace the foreskin if retracted earlier. Return the client to a comfortable position.
23. Discard all used supplies in appropriate receptacles and perform hand hygiene.
24. Document the catheterization procedure, including catheter size and results in the client record by using forms or checklists supplemented by narrative notes when appropriate.

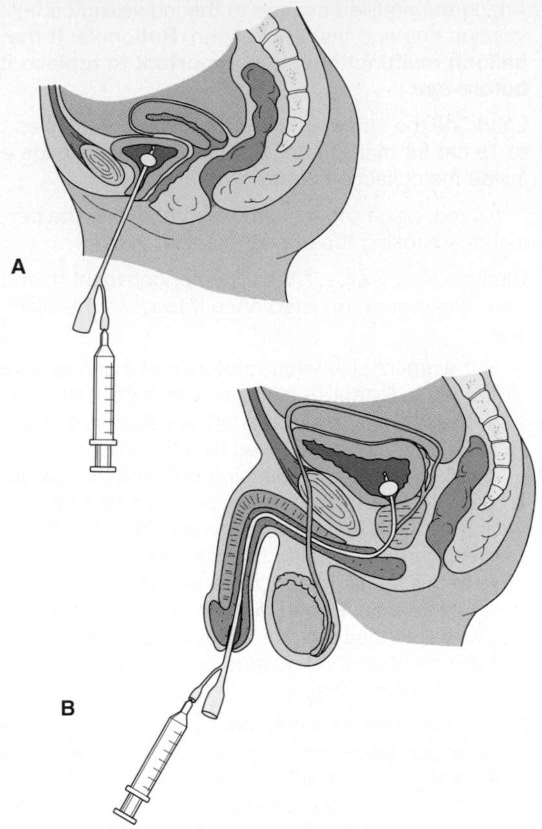

❹ Placement of indwelling catheter and inflated balloon: **A:** female client; **B:** male client

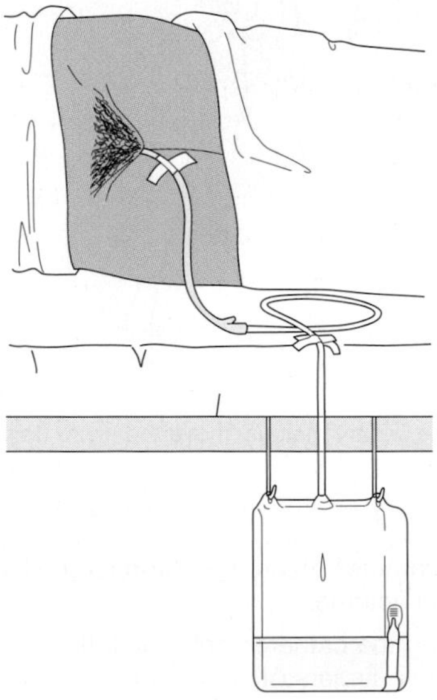

❺ Tape the catheter to the inside of a female's thigh.

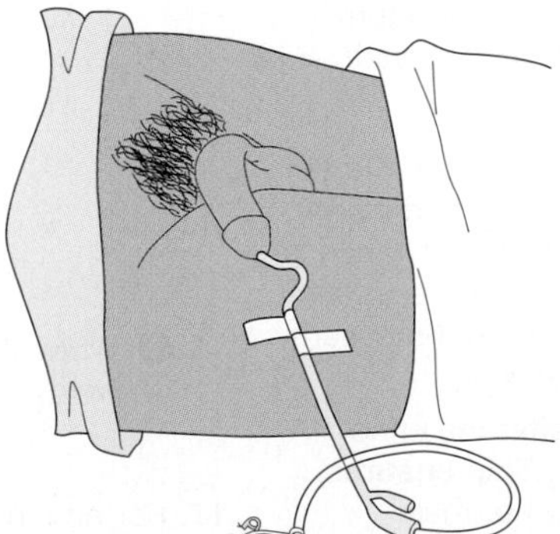

❻ Tape the catheter to the thigh or abdomen of a male client.

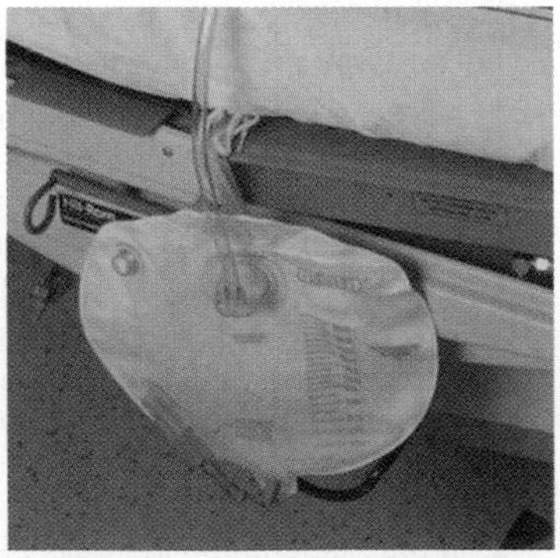

❼ Correct position for urine drainage bag and tubing

EVALUATION

Conduct appropriate follow-up, such as notifying the health-care team of the catheterization results. Perform a detailed follow-up based on findings that deviated from expected or normal for the client. Relate findings to previous assessment data if available. Teach the client how to care for the indwelling catheter, advise him or her to drink more fluids, and offer other appropriate instructions.

Home Care Considerations

Catheterization

For intermittent catheterization, instruct the client as follows:

- Follow instructions for clean technique.
- Wash hands well with warm water and soap before handling equipment or performing catheterization.
- Monitor for signs and symptoms of UTI, including burning, urgency, abdominal pain, and cloudy urine; in older adults, confusion may be an early sign.
- Ensure adequate oral intake of fluids.
- After each catheterization, assess the urine for colour, odour, clarity, and the presence of blood.
- Wash rubber catheters thoroughly with soap and water after use, dry, and store in a clean place.

For indwelling catheters, instruct the client as follows:

- Never pull on the catheter.
- Secure the catheter tubing to your leg by using a catheter-securing device.
- Ensure that there are no kinks or twists in the tubing.
- Keep the urine drainage bag below the level of the bladder (Figure 41.15). A leg bag can substitute for a hanging bag for those who are upright.
- Empty the drainage bag regularly.
- Take a shower rather than a tub bath; sitting in a tub allows bacteria easier access into the urinary tract.
- Monitor for signs and symptoms of UTI, including burning, urgency, abdominal pain, cloudy urine; in older adults confusion may be an early sign.

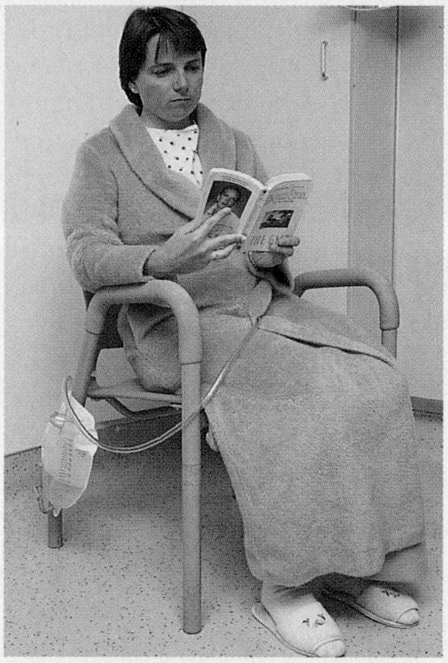

FIGURE 41.15 Positioning the collecting bag and tubing when sitting in a chair

- Ensure adequate oral intake of fluids.
- Clients who have indwelling catheters for lengthy periods need to have the catheter and bag changed at regular intervals. Changing equipment once a month is often the standard, although agency policy may differ.

Lifespan Considerations

Catheterization

INFANTS AND CHILDREN

- Adapt the size of the catheter for pediatric clients.
- Ask a family member to assist in holding the child during the catheterization, if appropriate.
- Explain the procedure to the family and the child in terms the child can understand.

OLDER ADULTS

- When catheterizing older adults, be very attentive to problems of limited movement, especially in the hips. Arthritis, or previous hip or knee surgery, can limit movement and cause discomfort. Modify the position (e.g., side lying) as needed to perform the procedure safely, and comfortably.
- For women, obtain the assistance of another nurse to flex and hold client's knees and hips as necessary or place her in a modified Sims' position.

preventing contamination of the drainage system, and teaching these measures to the client.

Fluids The client with an indwelling catheter should drink up to 3000 mL per day, if permitted. Increased fluid intake ensures an increased urine output, which keeps the bladder flushed out and decreases the likelihood of urinary stasis and subsequent infection. Large volumes of urine also minimize the risk of sediment or other particles obstructing the drainage tubing.

Dietary Measures Acidifying the urine of clients with a retention catheter may reduce the risk of UTI and calculus formation. Such foods as eggs, cheese, meat and poultry, whole grains, cranberries, plums and prunes, and tomatoes tend to increase the acidity of urine. Conversely, most fruits and vegetables, legumes, and milk and milk products result in alkaline urine.

Perineal Care Generally, no special cleaning other than routine hygienic care is necessary for clients with indwelling catheters, nor is special meatal care recommended. The retention catheter should be cleaned by swabbing down the tubing away from the meatus. Agency practices regarding catheter care vary considerably. The nurse should check agency practice in this regard.

Changing the Catheter and Tubing Indwelling catheters are used only when absolutely necessary and removed as soon as possible. However, some clients require long-term catheterization. Whenever possible, the closed catheter drainage system should be maintained, and the tubing not disconnected from the catheter for any reason. Routine changing of catheter and tubing is not recommended. Collection of sediment in the catheter or tubing or impaired urine drainage are indicators for changing the catheter and drainage system. When this occurs, the catheter and drainage system are removed and discarded, and a new sterile catheter with a closed drainage system is inserted.

Practice guidelines to prevent catheter-associated UTIs are given in Practice Guidelines 41.3. Ongoing assessment of clients with retention catheters is a high priority (see Box 41.3).

Removing Indwelling Catheters Indwelling catheters are removed after their purpose has been achieved, usually on the order of the physician. If the catheter has been in place for a short time (e.g., a few days), the client usually has little difficulty regaining normal urinary elimination patterns. Swelling of the urethra, however, may initially interfere with voiding, so the nurse should regularly assess the client for urinary retention until voiding is re-established.

Clients who have had an indwelling catheter for a prolonged period may require bladder retraining to regain bladder muscle tone. With an indwelling catheter in place, the bladder muscle does not stretch and contract regularly as it does when the bladder fills and empties by voiding. A few days before removal, the catheter may be clamped for specified periods of time (e.g., 2 to 4 hours), then released to allow the bladder to empty. This allows the bladder to distend and stimulates its musculature.

BOX 41.3 ONGOING ASSESSMENT OF CLIENTS WITH INDWELLING CATHETERS

It is essential that the nurse regularly assess clients with retention catheters:

- Ensure that there are no obstructions in the drainage tubing. Check that there are no kinks in the tubing, the client is not lying on the tubing, and the tubing is not clogged with mucus or blood.
- Check that there is no tension on the catheter or tubing, that the catheter is securely taped to the thigh or abdomen, and that the tubing is fastened appropriately to the bedclothes.
- Ensure that gravity drainage is maintained. Make sure there are no loops in the tubing below its entry to the drainage receptacle and that the drainage receptacle is below the level of the client's bladder.
- Ensure that the drainage system is well sealed or closed. Check that there are no leaks at the connection sites in open systems. Apply waterproof tape around the connection site of the catheter and tubing.
- Observe the flow of the urine every 2 or 3 hours, and note colour, odour, and any abnormal constituents. If sediment or blood clots are present, check the catheter more frequently to assess patency.

To remove an indwelling catheter, the nurse follows these steps:

- Obtain a receptacle for the catheter (e.g., a disposable basin), a clean towel, disposable gloves, and a sterile syringe to deflate the balloon. The syringe should be large enough to withdraw *all* the solution in the catheter balloon. The size of the balloon is indicated on the label at the end of the catheter.
- Before performing the procedure, introduce yourself and verify the client's identity. Perform hand hygiene and observe other appropriate infection prevention and control procedures.

PRACTICE GUIDELINES 41.3

Preventing Catheter-Associated Urinary Tract Infections

Guidelines	Rationales
Have an established infection prevention and control program.	Evidence-informed standards of practice that are used consistently across health-care professionals reduce the risk of infection.
Catheterize clients only when necessary, by using aseptic technique, sterile equipment, and trained personnel.	Aseptic technique eliminates the risk of introducing bacteria into the bladder.
Maintain a sterile closed-drainage system. Do not disconnect the catheter and drainage tubing unless absolutely necessary.	A closed system reduces the risk of bacteria entering the system.
Remove the catheter as soon as possible.	The risk of infection increases with the length of time the catheter is in situ.
Follow and reinforce good hand hygiene.	This prevents the introduction of bacteria.
Provide routine perineal hygiene, including cleansing with soap and water after defecation. Prevent contamination of the catheter with feces in the incontinent client.	Maintaining the catheter and perineal area clean prevents the migration of fecal bacteria into the bladder.

- Ask the client to assume a supine position as for a catheterization.
- Optional: Obtain a sterile specimen before removing the catheter. Check agency protocol.
- Remove the tape attaching the catheter to the client, don gloves, and then place the towel between the legs of the female client or over the thighs of the male.
- Insert the syringe into the injection port of the catheter, and withdraw the fluid from the balloon. If all the fluid cannot be removed, report this fact to the nurse in charge before proceeding.
- Do *not* pull the catheter while the balloon is inflated; doing so may injure the urethra.
- After all the fluid is withdrawn from the balloon, gently withdraw the catheter, and place it in the waste receptacle.
- Dry the perineal area with a towel.
- Remove gloves.
- Measure the urine in the drainage bag, and record the removal of the catheter. Include in the recording (1) the time the catheter was removed; (2) the amount, colour, and clarity of the urine; (3) the intactness of the catheter; and (4) instructions given to the client.
- Following removal of the catheter, determine the time of the first voiding and the amount voided during the first 24 hours. Compare this output to the client's intake.
- Observe for dysfunctional voiding behaviours (e.g., less than 100 mL per void), which might indicate urinary retention. If this occurs, perform an assessment of postvoid residuals by using a bladder scanner, if available. Generally postvoid residuals greater than 200 mL will require straight catheterization as needed.

CLEAN INTERMITTENT SELF-CATHETERIZATION

Clean intermittent self-catheterization (CISC) is performed by many clients who have some form of neurogenic bladder dysfunction, such as that caused by spinal cord injury. Aseptic technique is used. Clean intermittent self-catheterization does the following:

- Enables the client to retain independence and gain control of the bladder
- Reduces incidence of UTIs
- Protects the upper urinary tract from reflux
- Allows normal sexual relations without incontinence
- Reduces the use of aids and appliances
- Frees the client from embarrassing dribbling

The procedure for CISC is similar to that used by the nurse to catheterize a client. The steps are outlined in Teaching: Clinical box. Because the procedure requires great motivation and physical and mental preparation, client assessment is important.

TEACHING: CLINICAL

Clean Intermittent Self-Catheterization

It is essential the client understand how to perform self-catheterization properly:

- Catheterize as often as needed to maintain an acceptable residual urine volume. At first, catheterization may be necessary every 2 to 3 hours, decreasing to 4 to 6 hours.
- Attempt to void before catheterization; insert the catheter to remove residual urine if unable to void or if amount voided is insufficient (e.g., less than 100 mL).
- Assemble all needed supplies ahead of time. Good lighting is essential, especially for women.
- If female, remove a tampon before carrying out intermittent self-catheterization. A tampon can inhibit catheterization.
- Wash your hands.
- Clean the urinary meatus with either a towelette or soapy washcloth, and then rinse with a wet washcloth. If female, clean the area from front to back.
- Assume a position that is comfortable and that facilitates passage of the catheter, such as a semi-reclining position in bed or sitting on a chair or the toilet. Men may prefer to stand over the toilet; women may prefer to stand with one foot on the side of the bathtub.
- Apply lubricant to the catheter tip (2.5 cm to 5 cm for women; 5 cm to 15 cm for men).
- Insert the catheter until urine flows through.

  a. If a woman, locate the meatus by using a mirror or other aid, or use the touch technique as follows:
  - Place the index finger of your nondominant hand on your clitoris.
  - Place the third and fourth fingers at the vagina.
  - Locate the meatus between the index and third fingers.
  - Separate the labia with your dominant hand.
  - Direct the catheter through the meatus and then upward and forward toward the umbilicus.

  b. If a man, hold the penis with a slight upward tension at a 60- to 90-degree angle to insert the catheter. Return the penis to its natural position after catheter insertion when urine starts to flow.
- Hold the catheter in place until all urine is drained.
- Withdraw the catheter slowly to ensure complete drainage of urine.
- Wash the catheter with soap and water; store in a clean container. Replace the catheter when it becomes difficult to clean, or too soft or hard to insert easily.
- Contact your health-care provider if your urine appears cloudy or contains sediment; if you have bleeding, difficulty, or pain when passing the catheter; or if you have a fever.
- Drink at least 2000 mL to 2500 mL of fluid a day, unless contraindicated, to ensure adequate bladder filling and flushing.

The client should have the following:

- Sufficient manual dexterity to manipulate a catheter
- Sufficient mental ability
- Motivation and acceptance of the procedure
- For females, reasonable agility to access the urethra
- Bladder capacity not less than 100 mL

Before teaching CISC, the nurse should establish the client's voiding patterns, the volume voided, fluid intake, and residual amounts. Self-catheterization is easier to learn for males because of the visibility of the urinary meatus. Females need to learn initially with the aid of a mirror but eventually should perform the procedure by using only the sense of touch (see the Teaching: Clinical box on CISC).

URINARY IRRIGATIONS An **irrigation** is a flushing or washing out with a specified solution. *Bladder irrigation* is carried out on a physician's order, usually to wash out the bladder and sometimes to apply a medication to the bladder lining. *Catheter irrigations* may be performed to maintain or restore the patency of a catheter, for example, to remove pus or blood clots blocking the catheter.

The *closed method* is the preferred technique for catheter or bladder irrigation because it is associated with a lower risk of UTI. Closed catheter irrigations may be either continuous or intermittent. A three-way, or triple lumen, catheter generally is used for closed irrigations. The irrigating solution flows into the bladder through the irrigation port of the catheter and out through the urinary drainage lumen of the catheter.

Occasionally, an *open irrigation* may be necessary to restore catheter patency. The risk of injecting microorganisms into the urinary tract is greater with open irrigations as the connection between the indwelling catheter and the drainage tubing is broken. Strict precautions to maintain the sterility of the drainage tubing connector and interior of the indwelling catheter must be taken to minimize this risk. The type of irrigation (e.g., saline, water) and the volume required have not been definitively identified (Sinclair, Cross, Hagen, & Niël-Weise, 2006).

The open method of catheter or bladder irrigation is performed with double-lumen indwelling catheters; it may be necessary for clients who develop blood clots and mucus fragments that occlude the catheter and when it is undesirable to change the catheter. Techniques for catheter irrigation are outlined in Skill 41.4.

SKILL 41.4

PERFORMING BLADDER IRRIGATION

PURPOSES

- To maintain the patency of a urinary catheter and tubing (closed continuous irrigation)
- To free a blockage in a urinary catheter or tubing (open intermittent irrigation)

ASSESSMENT

- Determine the client's current urinary drainage system. Review the client record for recent intake and output and any difficulties the client has been experiencing with the system. Review the results of previous irrigations.
- Assess the client for any discomfort, bladder spasms, or distended bladder.

Planning

Before irrigating a catheter or bladder, check (1) the reason for the irrigation; (2) the prescription authorizing the continuous or intermittent irrigation (in most agencies, a physician or nurse practitioner's order is required); (3) the type of sterile solution, the amount and strength to be used, and the rate (if continuous); and (4) the type of catheter in place. If these are not specified on the client's chart, check agency protocol.

Equipment

- Clean gloves (2 pairs)
- Retention catheter in place
- Drainage tubing and bag (if not in place)
- Drainage tubing clamp
- Antiseptic swabs
- Sterile receptacle
- Sterile irrigating solution warmed or at room temperature (label the irrigant clearly with the words *Bladder Irrigation,* including the information about any medications that have been added to the original solution, and the date, time, and nurse's initials)
- Infusion tubing
- IV pole

IMPLEMENTATION

Performance

1. Introduce yourself and verify the client's identity by using agency protocol. Explain to the client what you are going to do, why it is necessary, and how he or she can cooperate. The irrigation should not be painful or uncomfortable. Discuss how the results will be used in planning further care or treatments.

(continued)

SKILL 41.4

PERFORMING BLADDER IRRIGATION (*continued*)

2. Perform hand hygiene and observe other appropriate infection prevention and control procedures.
3. Provide for client privacy.
4. Put on clean gloves.
5. Empty, measure, and record the amount and appearance of urine present in the drainage bag. Discard urine and gloves. **Rationale: Emptying the drainage bag allows more accurate measurement of urinary output after the irrigation is in place or completed. Assessing the character of the urine provides baseline data for later comparison.** Perform hand hygiene.
6. Prepare the equipment.
   - Connect the irrigation infusion tubing to the irrigating solution and flush the tubing with solution, keeping the tip sterile. **Rationale: Flushing the tubing removes air and prevents it from being instilled into the bladder.**
   - Apply clean gloves and cleanse the port with antiseptic swabs.
   - Connect the irrigation tubing to the input port of the three-way catheter.
   - Connect the drainage bag and tubing to the urinary drainage port if not already in place.
   - Remove gloves and perform hand hygiene.
7. Irrigate the bladder.
   a) For *closed continuous irrigation*, open the flow clamp on the urinary drainage tubing (if present). See ❶. **Rationale: This allows the irrigating solution to flow out of the bladder continuously.**
      - Open the regulating clamp on the irrigating tubing and adjust the flow rate as prescribed by the health-care provider or to 40 to 60 drops per minute if not specified.
      - Assess the drainage for amount, colour, and clarity. The amount of drainage should equal the amount of irrigant entering the bladder plus expected urine output.

   b) For *closed intermittent irrigation*, determine whether the solution is to remain in the bladder for a specified time.
      - If the solution is to remain in the bladder (a bladder irrigation or instillation), apply the flow clamp to the urinary drainage tubing. **Rationale: Closing the flow clamp allows the solution to be retained in the bladder and in contact with bladder walls.**
      - If the solution is being instilled to irrigate the catheter, open the flow clamp on the urinary drainage tubing. **Rationale: Irrigating solution will flow through the urinary drainage port and tubing, removing mucous shreds or clots.**
      - Open the flow clamp on the irrigating tubing, allowing the specified amount of solution to infuse. Clamp the tubing.
      - After the specified period for which the solution is to be retained, open the drainage tubing flow clamp and allow the bladder to empty.

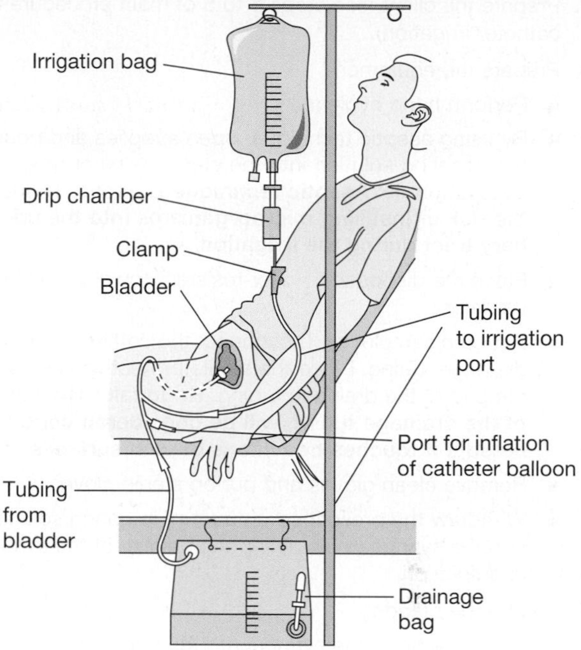

❶ A closed catheter or bladder irrigation system

      - Assess the drainage for amount, colour, and clarity. The amount of drainage should equal the amount of irrigant entering the bladder plus expected urine output.

8. Assess the client and the urinary output.
   - Assess the client's comfort.
   - Empty the drainage bag and measure the contents. Subtract the amount of irrigant instilled from the total volume of drainage to obtain the volume of urine output.
9. Document the procedure and results in the client record by using forms or checklists supplemented by narrative notes when appropriate.
   - Note any abnormal constituents, such as blood clots, pus, or mucous shreds.

Variation: Open Irrigation by Using a Two-Way Indwelling Catheter

1. Assemble the equipment. Use an irrigation set (see ❷) or assemble individual items, including
   - Clean gloves
   - Sterile gloves
   - Disposable water-resistant towel
   - Sterile irrigating solution
   - Sterile irrigation tray
   - Sterile basin
   - Sterile 50 mL Asepto syringe
   - Antiseptic swabs
   - Sterile protective cap (for catheter drainage tubing)

(continued)

SKILL 41.4

PERFORMING BLADDER IRRIGATION *(continued)*

2. Prepare the client (see steps 1 to 5 of main procedure for catheter irrigation).
3. Prepare the equipment.
   - Perform hand hygiene.
   - By using aseptic technique, open supplies and pour the irrigating solution into the sterile basin or receptacle. **Rationale: Aseptic technique is vital to reduce the risk of instilling microorganisms into the urinary tract during the irrigation.**
   - Place the disposable water-resistant towel under the catheter.
   - Put on clean gloves. Disconnect the catheter from the drainage tubing. Place the sterile protective cap over the end of the drainage tubing. **Rationale: The end of the drainage tubing will be considered contaminated if it touches bed linens or skin surfaces.**
   - Remove clean gloves and put on sterile gloves.
   - Withdraw the prescribed amount of irrigating solution into the syringe, maintaining the sterility of the syringe and solution.
4. Irrigate the bladder.
   - Insert the tip of the syringe into the catheter opening.
   - Gently and slowly inject the solution. In adults, about 30 mL to 40 mL generally is instilled for catheter irrigations; 100 mL to 200 mL may be instilled for bladder irrigation. **Rationale: Gentle instillation reduces the risks of injury to bladder mucosa and of bladder spasms.**
   - Remove the syringe and allow solution to drain into the basin.

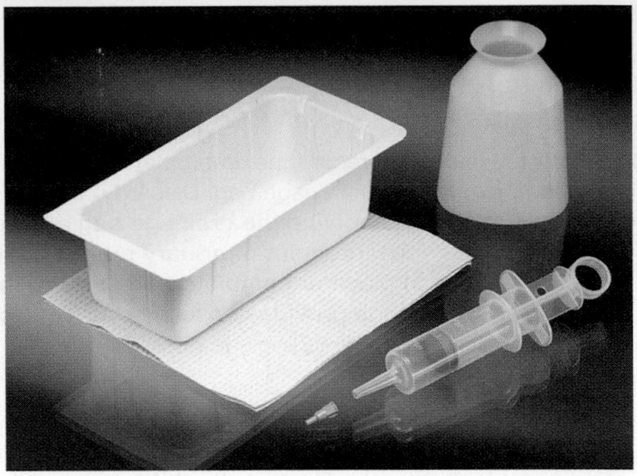

❷ An irrigation set

   - Continue to irrigate client's bladder until fluid returns are clear or clots are removed.
   - Remove the protective cap from the drainage tube and wipe with antiseptic swab or alcohol sponge.
   - Reconnect the catheter to drainage tubing.
   - Assess the drainage for amount, colour, and clarity. The amount of drainage should equal the amount of irrigant entering the bladder. Determine the amount of fluid used for the irrigation and subtract from total output on the client's I & O record.
5. Assess the client and the urinary output and document the procedure as in steps 8 and 9 above.

EVALUATION

- Perform detailed follow-up based on findings that deviated from expected or normal for the client. Relate findings to previous assessment data if available.
- Report significant deviations from normal to the health-care team.

SUPRAPUBIC CATHETER CARE A **suprapubic** catheter is inserted through the abdominal wall above the symphysis pubis into the urinary bladder (Figure 41.16). The physician inserts the catheter by using local anaesthesia or during bladder or vaginal surgery. The catheter may be secured in place with sutures, with a body seal, or with both sutures and a body seal. The catheter is then attached to a closed drainage system. Some evidence suggests that suprapubic catheters present lower risks of bacteriuria, less need for recatheterization, and less discomfort in comparison to indwelling or intermittent catheterization (Niël-Weise & van den Broek, 2005).

Care of clients with a suprapubic catheter includes regular assessments of the client's urine, fluid intake, and comfort; maintenance of a patent drainage system; skin care around the insertion site; periodic clamping of the catheter preparatory to removing it; and measurement of residual urine. Orders generally include leaving the catheter open to drainage for 48 to 72 hours, then clamping the catheter for 3- to 4-hour periods during the day until the client can void satisfactory amounts. Satisfactory voiding is determined by measuring the client's residual urine after voiding.

Care of the catheter insertion site involves sterile technique. Dressings around the suprapubic catheter are changed whenever they are soiled with drainage to prevent bacterial growth around the insertion site and reduce the potential for infection. Procedures for cleaning wounds and changing dressings are discussed in Chapter 33. Any redness and discharge at the skin around the insertion site must be reported.

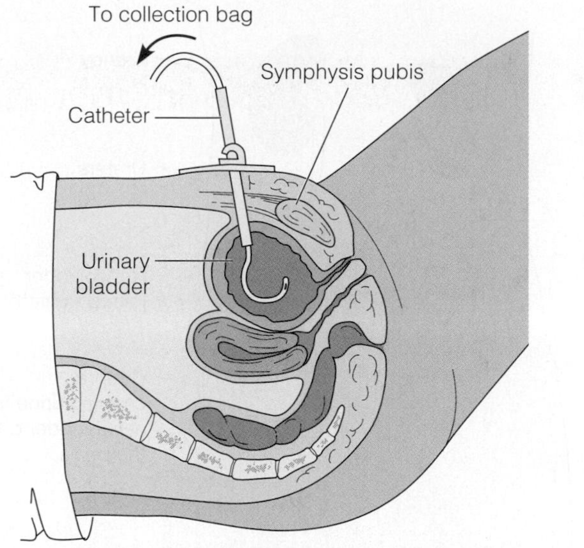

FIGURE 41.16 A suprapubic catheter in place

URINARY DIVERSIONS A urinary diversion is the surgical rerouting of urine from the kidneys to a site other than the bladder. Two categories of diversions are available: incontinent and continent.

INCONTINENT DIVERSIONS With incontinent diversions clients have no control over the passage of urine and require the use of an external ostomy appliance to contain the urine. Urinary diversions may or may not involve the removal of the bladder (cystectomy). Examples of incontinent diversions include ureterostomy, nephrostomy, vesicostomy, and ileal conduits. In a **ureterostomy**, one or both of the ureters is brought directly to the side of the abdomen to form small stomas. This procedure, however, has some disadvantages in that the stomas provide direct access for microorganisms from the skin to the kidneys, the small stomas are difficult to fit with an appliance to collect the urine, and they may narrow, impairing urine drainage. A **nephrostomy** diverts urine from the kidney to a stoma (Figure 41.17). A **vesicostomy** may be formed when the bladder is left intact but voiding through the urethra is not possible (e.g., because of an obstruction or a neurogenic bladder). The ureters remain connected to the bladder, and the bladder wall is surgically attached to an opening in the skin below the navel, forming an incontinent stoma.

The most common urinary diversion is the **ileal conduit** or ileal loop (Figure 41.18). In this procedure, a segment of the ileum is removed and the intestinal ends are reattached. One end of the portion removed is closed with sutures to create a pouch, and the other end is brought out through the abdominal wall to create a stoma. The ureters are implanted into the ileal pouch. The ileal stoma is more readily fitted with an appliance than are ureterostomies because of its larger size. The mucous membrane lining of the ileum also provides some protection from ascending infection. Urine drains continuously from the ileal pouch.

CONTINENT DIVERSIONS With continent diversions, a continence mechanism is created, giving clients control over the passage of urine, either by intermittent catheterization of the internal reservoir (e.g., *Kock pouch*) or by strained voiding (*neobladder*).

The **Kock** (pronounced "coke") **pouch**, or continent ileal bladder conduit, also uses a portion of the ileum to form a reservoir for urine (Figure 41.19). In this procedure, nipple valves are formed by doubling the tissue backward into the reservoir where the pouch connects to the skin and the ureters connect to the pouch. These valves close as the pouch fills with urine, preventing leakage and reflux of urine back toward the kidneys. The client empties the pouch by inserting a clean catheter approximately every 4 hours. Between catheterizations, a small dressing is worn to protect the stoma and clothing.

A **neobladder** replaces a diseased or damaged bladder with a piece of ileum, thus making a new bladder.

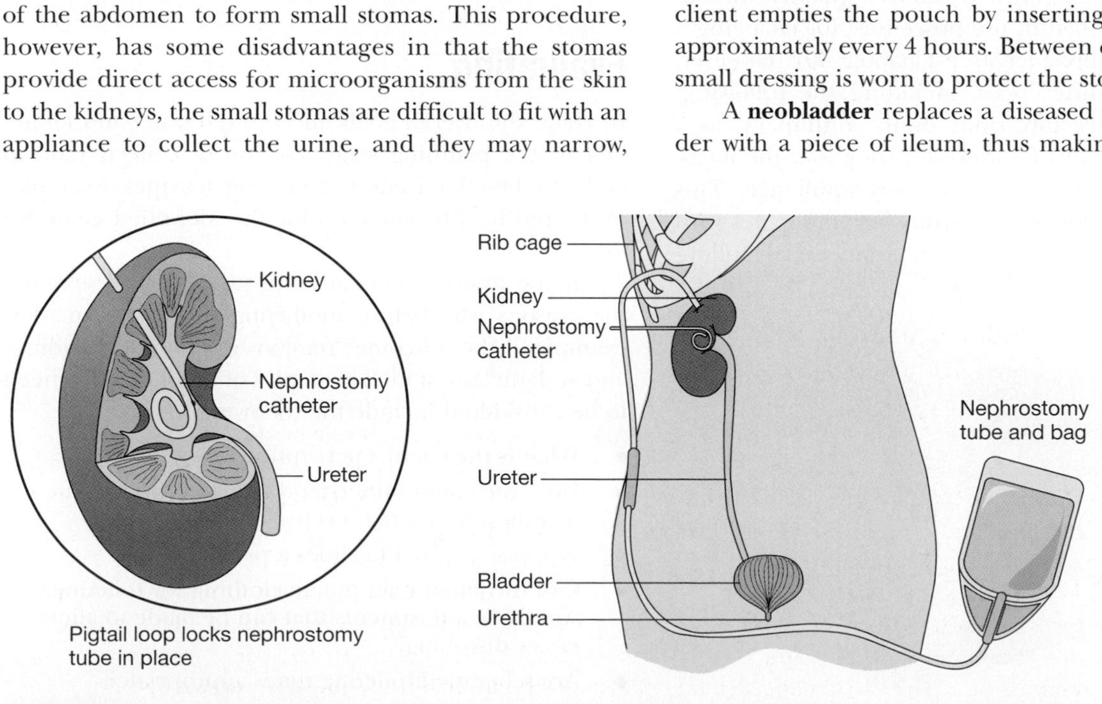

FIGURE 41.17 A nephrostomy

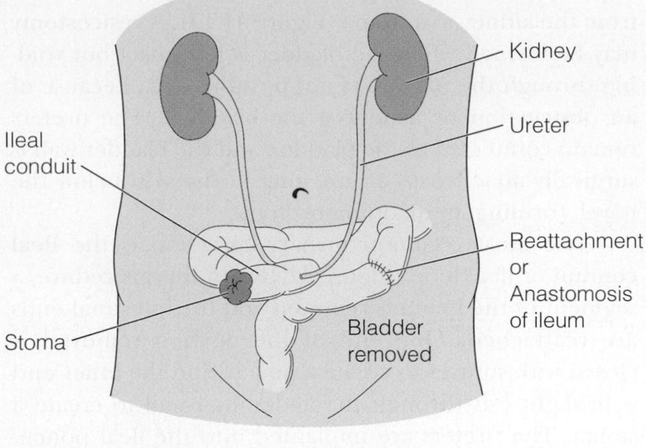

FIGURE 41.18 An incontinent urinary diversion (ileal conduit)

This new bladder is then sutured to the functional urethra. Clients with a neobladder can control voiding (Figure 41.20).

When caring for clients with a urinary diversion, the nurse must accurately assess intake and output, note any changes in urine colour, odour, or clarity (mucous shreds are commonly seen in the urine of clients with an ileal diversion), and frequently assess the condition of the stoma and surrounding skin. Clients who must wear a urine collection appliance are at risk for impaired skin integrity because of irritation by urine. Well-fitting appliances are vital. The nurse should consult with the enterostomal therapist to identify strategies for management of stoma and peristomal problems and the most appropriate appliance for the client's needs.

The steps of changing a urostomy appliance are similar to those described in the procedure for changing a bowel diversion appliance (see Chapter 40). However, there are some differences, including the following: incontinent urinary diversions drain continually; as a result, the stoma must be wicked throughout the measurement and change of the ostomy appliance. This prevents the peristomal skin from becoming wet with urine during the appliance change. Immediately following surgery, ureteral stents may be present and protruding from the stoma. They remain in place for 10 to 14 days postop and are removed, depending on institutional protocol, by either the surgeon or the nurse. Ureteral stents are used to maintain the patency of ureters at the anastomotic sites.

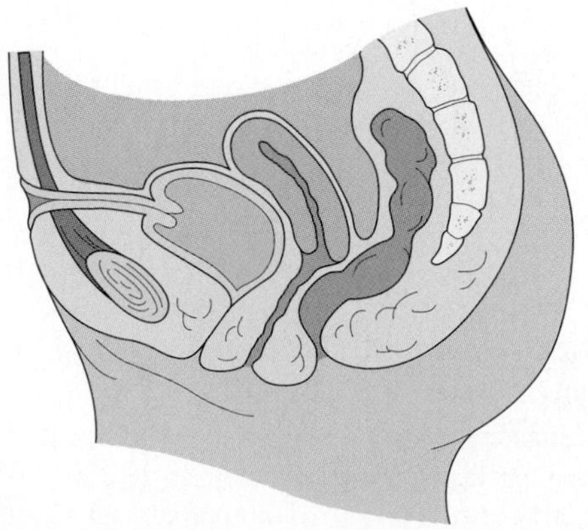

FIGURE 41.19 A continent urinary diversion (the Kock pouch)

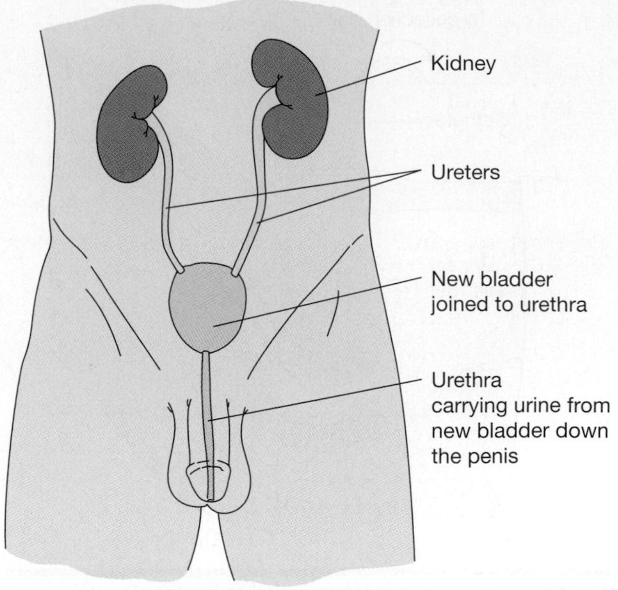

FIGURE 41.20 A neobladder

Clients with urinary diversions may experience problems with their body image and sexuality and may require assistance in coping with these changes and managing the stoma. Most clients are able to resume their normal activities and lifestyle.

Evaluating

By using the overall goals and desired outcomes identified in the planning stage, the nurse collects data to evaluate the effectiveness of nursing activities. Examples of desired health outcomes for the identified goals are listed in Table 41.6.

If the desired outcomes are not achieved, explore the reasons why before modifying the care plan. For example, if the outcome "remains dry between voidings and at night" is not met, examples of questions that need to be considered include the following:

- What is the client's perception of the problem?
- Does the client understand and comply with the health-care instructions provided?
- Is access to toilet facilities a problem?
- Can the client manipulate clothing for toileting? Are there adjustments that can be made to allow easier disrobing?
- Are scheduled toileting times appropriate?
- Is there adequate transition lighting for nighttime toileting?

TABLE 41.6 Evaluation Goals and Outcomes: Urinary Elimination

Goal	Examples of Desired Outcomes
Restore normal voiding pattern	Absence of pain, burning, hesitancy, or urgency with urination Voids at 3- to 4-hour intervals with no more than one voiding during the night Remains dry between voidings and at night Performs pelvic floor muscle exercises correctly at specified frequency
Perform toilet activities independently with or without assistive devices	Able to access toilet facilities or appropriate receptacle (urinal, commode) for voiding Able to manipulate clothing for voiding Able to get on and off toilet unassisted Cleans perineal area with tissue (and as necessary with soap and water) appropriately after voiding and defecating
Regain normal urine output	Quantity of urine at each voiding is within expected range (e.g., more than 150 mL) Bladder empties completely with each voiding (e.g., bladder is nonpalpable and postvoid residual is less than 100 mL) Urine colour, clarity, and odour are within normal limits Urinalysis values are within expected ranges (specific gravity, pH, protein, glucose, and ketones)
Avoid complications associated with altered urinary elimination (urinary tract infection, skin breakdown, fluid and electrolyte imbalance, body image disturbance, social isolation)	Absence of manifestations of UTI, such as dysuria, frequency, urgency, hematuria, or pyuria Identifies symptoms of and measures to prevent UTI Drinks at least 2000 mL to 2500 mL of fluid daily Fluid intake and output are balanced Serum electrolytes remain within expected values Skin of perineal area and over bony prominences (sacrum, hips), or around urinary stoma if client has one, remains intact Cares for urinary stoma and drainage collection devices as instructed Demonstrates appropriate technique in performing intermittent self-catheterization States or demonstrates acceptance of urinary diversion and ability to adjust to change in lifestyle Maintains or returns to previous social involvement

- Are mobility aids, such as a walker, elevated toilet seat, or grab bar, needed? If currently used, are they appropriate or adequate?
- Is the client performing pelvic floor muscle exercises appropriately as scheduled?
- Is the client's fluid intake adequate? Does the timing of fluid intake need to be adjusted (e.g., restricted after dinner)?
- Is the client restricting caffeine, citrus juice, carbonated beverages, and artificial sweetener intake?
- Is the client taking a diuretic? If so, when is the medication taken? Do the times need to be adjusted (e.g., taking second dose no later than 4 p.m.)?
- Should continence aids, such as a condom catheter or absorbent pads, be considered or used?

Case Study 41

Mrs. Gupta, 48 years old, is recovering from a motor vehicle collision on the TransCanada highway 4 days ago. In the collision, she sustained blunt trauma to her abdomen that necessitated the removal of her spleen. Additionally, she has a fractured femur and a mild concussion. She has an indwelling urinary catheter in place. On entering Mrs. Gupta's room to collect a urine specimen for culture and sensitivity, you note that Mrs. Gupta is restless and moaning. Her abdominal dressing is dry and intact and her urinary bag contains about 200 mL of golden-coloured urine. Her abdomen is tender and distended. When questioned, Mrs. Gupta is able to communicate that she is in pain but is unable to communicate the specifics of her pain.

Critical Thinking Questions

1. Is it correct to hypothesize that Mrs. Gupta's pain is due to her incision? Why, or why not?
2. What actions should be taken before administering analgesia to Mrs. Gutpa?
3. What precautions should be taken when collecting a urine sample from a person with an indwelling urinary catheter, and why?
4. What measures can be taken to prevent Mrs. Gupta from developing a urinary tract infection if it is not already present?
5. What interventions may be useful in helping Mrs. Gupta establish a normal urinary pattern following the removal of her catheter?

After working through these questions, go to the MyNursingLab at **http://www.mynursinglab.com** to check your answers.

KEY TERMS

glomerulus
Bowman's capsule
reflux
detrusor muscle
trigone
meatus
micturition
voiding
urination
enuresis
nocturnal enuresis
nocturnal frequency
retention
polyuria
polydipsia
diuresis
oliguria
anuria
urinary frequency
nocturia
urinary urgency
dysuria
urinary hesitancy
diurnal enuresis
urinary incontinence (UI)
urinary retention
neurogenic bladder
residual urine
specific gravity
urinary pH
occult blood
blood urea nitrogen (BUN)
creatinine
creatinine clearance
intravenous pyelography (IVP)
retrograde pyelography
renal ultrasonography
cystoscopy
cystoscope
bladder training
habit training
prompted voiding
flaccid
Credé's manoeuvre
irrigation
suprapubic
ureterostomy
nephrostomy
vesicostomy
ileal conduit
Kock pouch
neobladder

CHAPTER HIGHLIGHTS

- Urinary elimination depends on normal functioning of the urinary, cardiovascular, and nervous systems.
- Urine is formed in the nephron, the functional unit of the kidney, through a process of filtration, reabsorption, and secretion. Hormones, such as antidiuretic hormone (ADH) and aldosterone, affect the reabsorption of sodium and water, thus affecting the amount of urine formed.
- The normal process of urination is stimulated when sufficient urine collects in the bladder to stimulate stretch receptors. Impulses from stretch receptors are transmitted to the spinal cord and the brain, causing relaxation of the internal sphincter (unconscious control) and, if appropriate, relaxation of the external sphincter (conscious control).
- In the adult, urination generally occurs after 250 mL to 450 mL of urine has collected in the bladder.
- Many factors influence a person's urinary elimination, including growth and development, psychosocial factors, fluid and food intake, medications, muscle tone and activity, various diseases, and surgical and diagnostic procedures.
- Alterations in urine production and elimination include polyuria, oliguria and anuria, frequency or nocturia, urgency, dysuria, enuresis, incontinence, and retention. Each may have various influencing and associated factors that need to be identified.
- Assessment of a client's urinary function includes (1) a nursing history that identifies normal voiding patterns, usual urine and recent changes, past and current problems with urination, and factors influencing the elimination pattern; (2) a physical assessment of the genitourinary system; (3) inspection of the urine for amount, colour, clarity, and odour, and if indicated, (4) testing of urine for specific gravity, pH, and the presence of glucose, ketone bodies, protein, and occult blood.
- Incontinence can be physically and emotionally distressing to clients because it is considered socially unacceptable.
- Bladder training can often reduce episodes of incontinence.
- Clients with urinary retention not only experience discomfort but also are at risk of urinary tract infection.
- The most common cause of urinary tract infection is invasive procedures, such as catheterization and cystoscopic examination. Females, in particular, are prone to ascending urinary tract infections because of their short urethras.
- Goals for the client with problems with urinary elimination include maintaining or restoring normal elimination patterns and preventing associated risks, such as skin breakdown.
- In planning for home care, the nurse considers the client's needs for teaching and assistance or assistive devices in the home.
- Nursing interventions related to urinary elimination are generally directed toward facilitating the normal functioning of the urinary system or toward assisting the client with particular problems.
- Interventions include (1) assisting the client to maintain an appropriate fluid intake, (2) assisting

the client to maintain normal voiding patterns, (3) monitoring the client's daily fluid intake and output, and (4) maintaining cleanliness of the genital area.

- Urinary catheterization is frequently required for clients with urinary retention but is performed only after all other measures to facilitate voiding fail. Sterile technique is essential to prevent ascending urinary infections.
- Care of clients with indwelling catheters is directed toward preventing infection of the urinary tract and encouraging urinary flow through the drainage system.
- Clients with urinary retention can be taught to perform intermittent self-catheterization to enhance their independence, reduce the risk of infection, and eliminate incontinence.
- Bladder or catheter irrigations can be used to apply medication to bladder walls or maintain catheter patency.
- When the urinary bladder is removed, a urinary diversion is formed to allow urine to be eliminated from the body. The ileal conduit or ileal loop is the most common diversion and requires that the client wear a urine collection device continually over the stoma.

ASSESS YOUR LEARNING

1. Mr. Smith returns from the operating room with a three-way indwelling catheter following a prostatectomy. He suddenly complains of severe lower abdominal pain. What is the nurse's best first action?

a. Assess the patient for surgical pain and administer the prescribed analgesic.
b. Assess the patency of the catheter.
c. Palpate Mr. Smith's bladder.
d. Notify the surgeon.

2. Following the irrigation of an indwelling catheter, it is critical for the nurse to do which of the following?

a. Ensure the drainage tubing is not kinked.
b. Document findings in the chart.
c. Send a urine specimen.
d. Determine urine output.

3. Mrs. Chiu, an 80-year-old widow, is admitted to the ward with urinary retention. After inserting an indwelling catheter, the nurse notes a pungent odour and heavily sedimented urine with specks of blood. What is the nurse's most appropriate action?

a. Obtain a specimen for culture and sensitivity.
b. Notify the appropriate member of the health-care team about these findings.
c. Teach Mrs. Chiu the importance of adequate fluid intake.
d. Document the results and monitor.

4. Mr. Dupree is being discharged to his son's home following a stroke. He is incontinent of urine and feces and requires assistance with mobilization. Mr. Dupree's son is a busy executive and has hired a personal support worker to stay with his father during the day. What is an appropriate nursing diagnosis that may negatively affect the son's ability to care for his father?

a. *Deficient Knowledge* related to incontinence
b. *Social Isolation* related to his father's incontinence
c. *Risk for Infection*
d. *Risk for Caregiver Role Strain*

5. Sanjay Dhara was admitted to the ward following an all-terrain vehicle accident 2 weeks ago in which he suffered a moderate brain injury. Which of the following methods would be most appropriate for maintaining Sanjay's continence?

a. Bladder training
b. Prompted voiding
c. Habit training
d. Pelvic floor muscle exercises

6. Mr. Brown, 65 years old, underwent abdominal surgery 5 days ago. He is eating and drinking well, so his intravenous has been discontinued and his IV analgesic switched to morphine by mouth. His indwelling catheter was discontinued 24 hours ago. Mr. Brown has been incontinent of large of amounts of urine since the beginning of the shift. The most appropriate action would be which of the following?

a. Request a prescription to replace the indwelling catheter so as to prevent skin breakdown.
b. Apply an incontinence brief and provide frequent pericare.
c. Palpate Mr. Brown's bladder.
d. Request a prescription for insertion of a straight urinary catheter.

7. Which of the following behaviours indicates that the client on a bladder training program has met the expected outcomes?

a. Voids each time there is an urge
b. Practises slow, deep breathing until the urge decreases
c. Uses adult diapers, just in case
d. Drinks citrus juices and carbonated beverages

8. Melanie Borschnek, 32 years old, underwent surgery for an ileal conduit 4 days ago. She is currently refusing to participate in the care of her device. What is the most appropriate nursing diagnosis?

a. *Deficient Knowledge*
b. *Social Isolation*
c. *Low Self-Esteem*
d. *Disturbed Body Image*

9. June Foster, 45 years old, has her left leg in traction. She complains of the inability to void on the bed-pan. What actions can the nurse take that may help the client to void?

a. Close the bedside curtain.
b. Run warm water over the bedpan before positioning it under June.
c. Run water in the sink.
d. Place the bed in high-Fowler's position.

10. Elizabeth Newman underwent brain surgery for a tumour 2 days ago. Her urine output for the last 8 hours is 1200 mL (intake 600 mL). What is the most probable description for her output?

a. Polyuria
b. Dysuria
c. Diuresis
d. Enuresis

After working through these questions, go to the MyNursingLab at ***http://www.mynursinglab.com*** *to check your answers and see explanations.*

SUGGESTED READINGS

Canadian Continence Foundation. (2007). *Incontinence: A Canadian perspective.* Retrieved July 7, 2008, from http://www.continence-fdn.ca/pdf/Research_paper_August2007.pdf

This report provides an excellent review of the prevalence, burden, quality-of-life issues, and treatment options related to urinary incontinence in Canada. The document highlights the fact that many Canadians do not seek help with incontinence, likely because of the stigma associated with lack of bladder control.

Jepson, R. G., & Craig, J. (2008). Cranberries for preventing urinary tract infections. *Cochrane Database of Systematic Reviews, 1,* Art. No.: CD001321.

This systematic review provides an excellent summary of the studies addressing the use of cranberries (juice and capsule) in preventing UTIs. The authors conclude that cranberries are not a panacea for preventing UTIs in that they appear to be effective only in young women, with little evidence of effectiveness in older men and women or clients that need urinary catheterization. As well, there is no evidence to determine the amount of cranberries to be ingested. Those who drink cranberry juice tend not to continue, suggesting it is not a palatable drink for most people.

Lee, Y., Tsay, W., Lou, M., & Dai, Y. (2007). The effectiveness of implementing a bladder ultrasound programme in neurosurgical units. *Journal of Advanced Nursing, 57*(2), 192–200.

This quasi-experimental study examined the clinical benefits of using ultrasound bladder scanners as an alternative to determine the need for urethral catheterization. The results of the study indicate that the rate of clients in the control group who were unnecessarily catheterized was 34% in comparison to only 7% in the study group. The ultrasound shows promise as a noninvasive method of managing neurological patients with urination disorders.

MacDonald, C. D., & Butler, L. (2007). Clinical outlook. Silent no more: Elderly women's stories of living with urinary incontinence in long-term care. *Journal of Gerontological Nursing, 33*(1), 14–20.

Urinary incontinence (UI) is a prevalent health issue affecting the quality of life of many older adult women living in long-term care. This study explored older adult women's experiences with UI while living in long-term-care facilities. The results of this study provided information that could influence changes in nursing practice related to individualized UI care, empowering women experiencing UI and dispelling ageism in long-term care. The study also suggests opportunities for improving health-care education related to the quality of life for women who experience UI and the need to make the experience more visible and openly discussed as a health issue rather than a traditional condition of aging.

Milne, J. L., & Moore, K. N. (2006). Factors impacting self-care for urinary incontinence. *Urologic Nursing, 26*(1), 41–51.

The authors conducted a qualitative study to gain an understanding of strategies used by individuals to manage urinary incontinence at home. The focus of the study was to examine why some strategies were maintained and others were not. The results of this study provide insight into client motivation and are useful to planning educational programs for this population.

Smith, P. P., McCrery, R. J., & Appell, R. A. (2006). Current trends in the evaluation and management of female urinary incontinence. *Canadian Medical Association Journal, 175*(10), 1233–1240.

The authors review stress, urge, and mixed urinary incontinence. Effective treatment is based on the type of incontinence. Evaluation of the type of incontinence and the appropriate treatment is discussed.

WEBLINKS

Canadian Nurse Continence Advisors

http://www.cnca.ca

This national association, the Canadian Nursing Continence Advisor Association, promotes education, research, and clinical practice for the conservative management of incontinence.

The Canadian Continence Foundation

http://www.continence-fdn.ca

This nonprofit organization has as its focus the support of individuals with continence problems. The site provides fact sheets and information regarding incontinence. Free registration is required.

The Kidney Foundation of Canada

http://www.kidney.ca

The Kidney Foundation of Canada is a volunteer association that provides support to individuals with kidney disease. The site provides a variety of brochures pertaining to kidney disease.

The Canadian Association for Enterostomal Therapy

http://www.caet.ca

This nonprofit association specializes in the nursing care of patients with challenges in wound, ostomy, and continence. The website provides some useful information and brochures for patients, families, and professionals dealing with ostomies.

National Kidney and Urologic Diseases Information Clearinghouse

http://kidney.niddk.nih.gov/kudiseases/ez.asp

This excellent website provides information and online publications on all diseases and conditions affecting the kidneys and urological system.

REFERENCES

Ball, J., & Bindler, R. (2008). *Pediatric nursing: Caring for children* (4th ed.). Upper Saddle River, NJ: Prentice Hall Health.

Berry, A. K. (2006). Bladder matters. Helping children with nocturnal enuresis: The wait-and-see approach may not be in anyone's best interest. *American Journal of Nursing, 106*(8), 56–64.

Cavagnaro, S. M. F. (2005). Infección urinaria en la infancia. *Revista Chilena de Infectologia, 22*(2), 161–168.

D'Amico, D., & Barbarito, C. (2007). *Health & physical assessment in nursing.* Upper Saddle River, NJ: Pearson Education.

Davis, K. (2004). Need urine from a catheter system? Forget the needle! *Nursing, 34*(12), 64.

Hay-Smith, E. J. C., & Dumoulin, C. (2006). Pelvic floor muscle training versus no treatment, or inactive control treatments, for urinary incontinence in women. *The Cochrane Library, 4,* Art. No.: CD005654.

Herschorn, S., Corcos, J., Gajewski, J., Schulz, J., & Ciu, E. (2003). Canadian urinary bladder survey: Population-based study of symptoms and incontinence. *Neurology and Urodynamics, 22,* Part 5.

Jepson, R. G., & Craig, J. (2008). Cranberries for preventing urinary tract infections. *Cochrane Database of Systematic Reviews, 1,* Art. No.: CD001321.

Liao, Y. M., Doughertya, M. C., Yuh-Shu Lioub, Y., & Tsengb, I. (2006). Pelvic floor muscle training effect on urinary incontinence knowledge, attitudes, and severity: An experimental study. *International Journal of Nursing Studies, 43,* 29–37.

Midthun, S. J. (2004). Criteria for urinary tract infection in the elderly: Variables that challenge nursing assessment. *Urologic Nursing, 24*(3), 157–186.

Morantz, C. A. (2005). ACOG guidelines on urinary incontinence in women. *American Family Physician, 72*(1), 175–178.

NANDA International. (2007). *Nursing diagnoses: Definitions and classification, 2007–2008.* Philadelphia, PA: Author.

Niël-Weise, B. S., & van den Broek, P. J. (2005). Urinary catheter policies for short-term bladder drainage in adults. *Cochrane Database of Systematic Reviews, 3.* Art. No.: CD004203.

Palmer, M. H., & Newman, D. K. (2006). Bladder control: Educational needs of older adults. *Journal of Gerontological Nursing, 32*(1), 28–32.

Registered Nurses' Association of Ontario. (2005). *Promoting continence using prompted voiding* (Rev. ed.). Toronto: Author.

Robson, W. L. M., Leung, A. K. C., & Van Howe, R. (2005). Primary and secondary nocturnal enuresis: Similarities in presentation. *Pediatrics, 115,* 956–959.

Roe, B., Ostaszkiewicz, J., Milne, J., & Wallace, S. (2007). Systematic reviews of bladder training and voiding programmes in adults: A synopsis of findings from data analysis and outcomes using metastudy techniques. *Journal of Advanced Nursing 57*(1), 15–31.

Ross, S. M. (2006). Clinical applications of cranberry in urinary tract infections. *Holistic Nursing Practice, 20*(4), 213–214.

Shei Dei Yang, S., & Cheng Wang, C. (2005). Outpatient biofeedback relaxation of the pelvic floor in treating pediatric dysfunctional voiding: A short-course program is effective. *Urologia Internationalis, 74*(2), 118–122.

Sinclair, L., Cross, S., Hagen, S., & Niël-Weise, B. S. (2006). Washout policies for the management of long-term indwelling urinary catheterisation in adults (Protocol). *Cochrane Database of Systematic Reviews, 1,* Art. No.: CD004012.

Chapter 42

Oxygenation and Circulation

Oxygen (O_2) is a clear, odourless gas that constitutes approximately 21% of the air we breathe. Oxygen is necessary for all living cells and the absence of oxygen can lead to death. The transport of oxygen to body tissues and the removal of carbon dioxide (CO_2) and other byproducts is a complex process. The major systems involved in this process include the lungs, heart, and blood.

Although all systems in the body are indirectly involved in the oxygenation process, the respiratory system (lungs) and the cardiovascular system (heart and vasculature) are directly and interdependently involved. Impaired function of either system can negatively affect the other system. This impairment can cause significant changes in the ability to breathe, transport gases, and eliminate wastes, and can result in respiratory failure, cardiac dysfunction, and general inability to participate in the activities of daily living.

Respiration is the process of gas exchange between the individual and the environment. The process of respiration involves three components:

1. Pulmonary ventilation or breathing; the movement of air between the atmosphere and the alveoli of the lungs as we inhale and exhale
2. Gas exchange, which involves diffusion of oxygen and carbon dioxide between the alveoli and the pulmonary capillaries
3. Transport of oxygen from the lungs to the tissues, and carbon dioxide from the tissues to the lungs

OBJECTIVES

After studying this chapter, you should be able to

1. Outline the structure and function of the respiratory and cardiovascular systems
2. Describe the processes of breathing (ventilation) and gas exchange (respiration)
3. Identify seven factors that influence respiration and circulatory function
4. List the clinical manifestations of hypoxia
5. Identify 10 types of altered breathing patterns
6. Differentiate among the signs and symptoms of upper, lower, partial, and completely obstructed airways
7. Identify three major conditions that can alter respiratory function and three major conditions that can alter cardiovascular function
8. Describe the nurse's role in caring for clients undergoing diagnostic procedures related to cardiorespiratory function
9. Identify and describe nursing measures to promote cardiorespiratory function and oxygenation
10. Explain the use of therapeutic measures, such as artificial airways, medications, oxygen therapy, inhalation therapy, pharyngeal and tracheal suctioning, and chest drainage, to promote cardiorespiratory function
11. Describe the critical nature of cardiopulmonary resuscitation
12. State outcome criteria for evaluating client responses to measuring and promoting adequate oxygenation and circulation

The respiratory system has a major role in the first two components of respiration, while the cardiovascular system has a major role in the third component. Any impairment in gas transport caused by either a respiratory or a cardiovascular disease will lead to compromised gas exchange at the cellular level.

Physiology of the Respiratory System

The primary function of the respiratory system is gas exchange. Oxygen from inspired air diffuses from alveoli in the lungs into the blood in the pulmonary capillaries. Carbon dioxide, a waste product produced during cell metabolism, diffuses from the blood into the alveoli and is exhaled. Exchange of oxygen and carbon dioxide occurs at the alveolar-capillary membrane. The organs of the respiratory system facilitate this gas exchange and protect the body from foreign matter, such as particulates and pathogens.

Structure of the Respiratory System

The respiratory system (Figure 42.1) is divided structurally into the *upper airway* and the *lower airway*. The mouth, nose, and pharynx compose the upper airway. The larynx

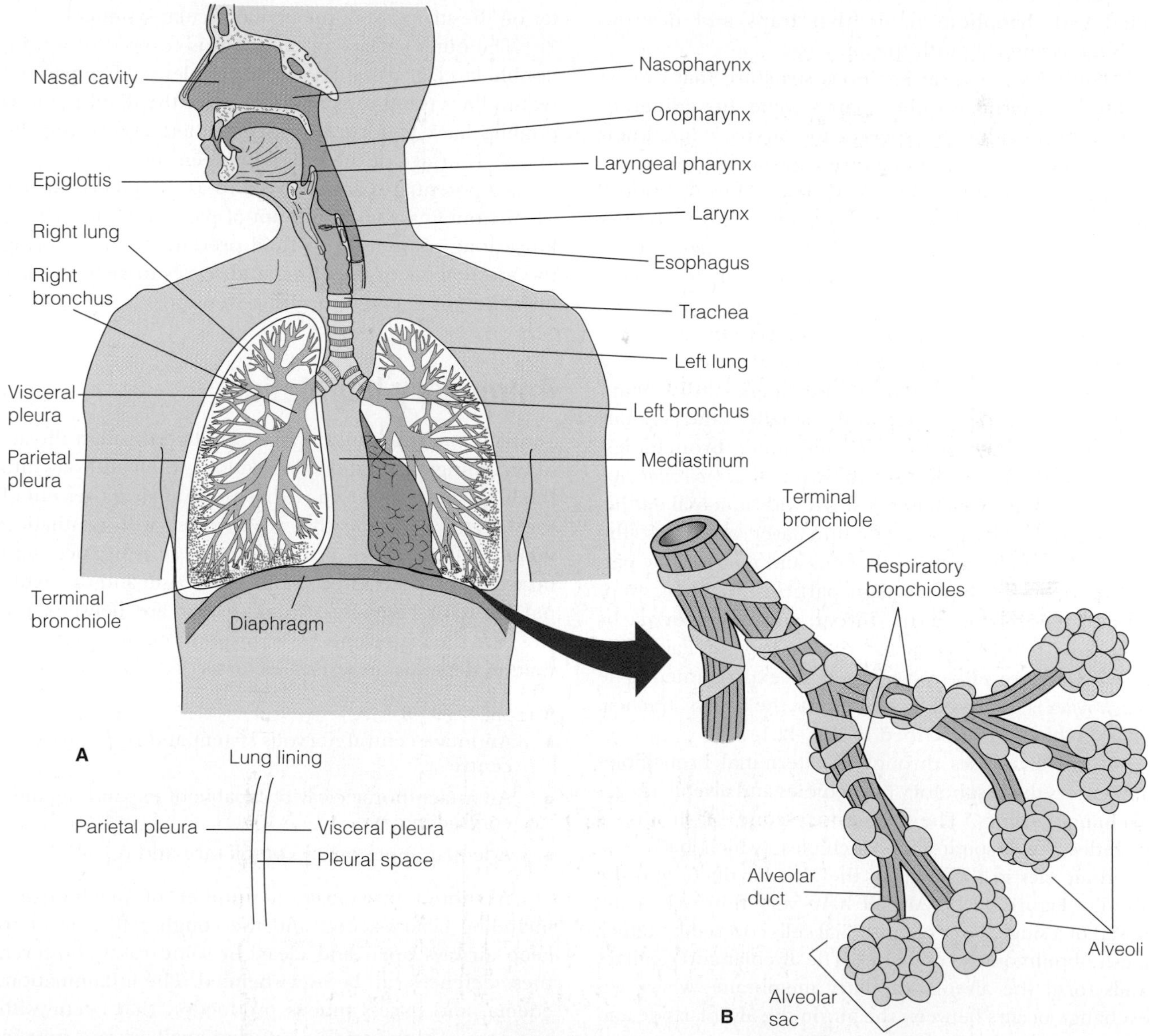

FIGURE 42.1 **A:** Organs of the respiratory tract; **B:** respiratory bronchioles, alveolar ducts, and alveoli

connects the upper and the lower airways. The lower airway includes the trachea and lungs, with the right and left mainstream bronchi, bronchioles, alveoli, pulmonary capillary network, and pleural membranes.

Air enters through the nose, where it is warmed, humidified, and filtered. Large particles in the air are trapped by the hairs at the entrance of the nares, and smaller particles are filtered and trapped as air changes direction on contact with the nasal turbinates and septum. The *sneeze reflex* is initiated by irritants in nasal passages, which stimulate the respiratory centre in the medulla by the trigeminal nerve (cranial nerve V). A large volume of air rapidly exits through the nose and mouth during a sneeze, helping clear nasal passages of foreign matter.

Inspired air passes from the nose through the pharynx, commonly known as the throat. The pharynx is a shared pathway for air and food. It includes both the nasopharynx and the oropharynx, which are richly supplied with lymphoid tissue that traps and destroys pathogens entering with the air.

The larynx is a cartilaginous structure that can be identified externally as the Adam's apple. In addition to its role in providing for speech, the larynx is important for maintaining airway patency and protecting the lower airways from swallowed food and fluids. During swallowing, the inlet to the larynx (the epiglottis) closes, routing food to the esophagus. The epiglottis is open during breathing, allowing air to move freely into the lower airways.

Below the larynx, the trachea leads to the right and left main bronchi (primary bronchi) and the conducting airways of the lungs. Within the lungs, the primary bronchi divide repeatedly into smaller and smaller bronchi, ending with the terminal bronchioles. Together, these airways are known as the *bronchial tree.* The trachea and bronchi are lined with mucosal epithelium. These cells produce a thin layer of mucus, the *mucus blanket,* that traps pathogens and microscopic particulate matter. These foreign particles are then swept upward toward the larynx, throat, and nasopharynx by cilia (tiny hairlike projections on the epithelial cells), where they are either swallowed or expectorated. The *cough reflex* is triggered by irritants in the larynx, trachea, or bronchi and is described in Box 42.1.

Until air passes through the terminal bronchioles and enters the respiratory bronchioles and alveoli, no gas exchange occurs. The respiratory zone of the lungs includes the respiratory bronchioles (which have scattered air sacs in their walls), the alveolar ducts, and the alveoli (Figure 42.1). Alveoli have very thin walls composed of a single layer of epithelial cells covered by a thick mesh of pulmonary capillaries. The alveolar and capillary walls form the alveolar-capillary membrane, where gas exchange occurs between the air on the alveolar side and the blood on the capillary side. The airways move air to and from the alveoli; the right ventricle and the pulmonary vascular system transport blood to the capillary side of the membrane. (See the section later in this chapter on the structure of the cardiovascular system.)

BOX 42.1 THE COUGH REFLEX

Irritants in the larynx, trachea, or bronchi can trigger the cough reflex:

- Nerve impulses are sent through the vagus nerve to the medulla.
- A large inspiration of approximately 2.5 L occurs.
- The epiglottis and glottis (vocal cords) close.
- A strong contraction of abdominal and internal intercostal muscles dramatically raises the pressure in the lungs.
- The epiglottis and glottis open suddenly.
- Air rushes outward with great velocity.
- Mucus and any foreign particles are dislodged from the lower respiratory tract and are propelled up and out.

The outer surface of the lungs is covered by a thin, double layer of tissue known as the pleura. The parietal pleura lines the thorax and surface of the diaphragm. It doubles back to form the visceral pleura, covering the external surface of the lungs. Between these pleural layers is a potential space referred to as the **pleural space**, which contains a small amount of pleural fluid, a serous lubricating solution. This fluid prevents friction during the movements of breathing and serves to keep the layers adherent through its surface tension.

Pulmonary Ventilation

Ventilation of the lungs is accomplished through the act of breathing: inspiration (inhalation) when air flows into the lung, and expiration (exhalation) as air moves out of the lungs. The forces that are involved with ventilation include elastic recoil properties, airway resistance, and inspiratory muscle efforts. The diaphragm and the external intercostal muscles (muscles that are between the ribs) are the major muscles of inspiration. Adequate ventilation depends on several factors:

- Clear airways
- An intact central nervous system and respiratory centre
- An intact thoracic cavity capable of expanding and contracting
- Adequate pulmonary compliance and recoil

As noted previously, a number of mechanisms, including ciliary action and the cough reflex, work to keep airways open and clear. In some cases, however, these defences can be overwhelmed. The inflammation, edema, and excess mucus production that occur with some types of pneumonia can clog small airways, impairing ventilation of the distal alveoli.

The respiratory centres of the medulla and pons in the brain stem control breathing. Severe head injury or drugs that depress the central nervous system (e.g., opioids, anaesthetics, or barbiturates) can affect the respiratory centres, impairing the drive to breathe.

Expansion and recoil of the lungs occurs passively in response to changes in pressures within the thoracic cavity and the lungs themselves. The **intrapleural pressure** (pressure in the pleural cavity surrounding the lungs) is always slightly negative in relation to atmospheric pressure. This negative or subatmospheric pressure is essential because it creates suction that holds the visceral pleura and the parietal pleura together as the chest cage expands and contracts. The recoil tendency of the lungs is a major factor in creating this negative pressure. The intrapleural fluid also contributes by causing the pleura to stick together, much like a film of water can cause two glass slides to adhere.

The **intrapulmonary pressure** (pressure within the lungs) always equalizes with atmospheric pressure. Inspiration occurs when the diaphragm and intercostal muscles contract, increasing the size of the thoracic cavity. The volume of the lungs increases, decreasing intrapulmonary pressure. Air then rushes into the lungs to equalize this pressure with atmospheric pressure. Conversely, when the diaphragm and intercostal muscles relax, the volume of the lungs decreases, intrapulmonary pressure rises, and air is expelled.

The degree of chest expansion during normal breathing is minimal, requiring little energy expenditure. In adults, approximately 500 mL of air is inspired and expired with each breath. This is known as **tidal volume**. Breathing during strenuous exercise or some types of heart disease requires greater chest expansion and effort. At this time, more than 1500 mL of air may be moved with each breath. *Accessory muscles of inspiration,* including the anterior neck muscles, sternocleidomastoid muscles, scalene muscles, intercostal muscles, and muscles of the abdomen, are employed. Active use of accessory muscles and noticeable increase in breathing effort are seen in clients with obstructive pulmonary disease.

Diseases, such as muscular dystrophy, or trauma, such as spinal cord injury, can affect the muscles of respiration, impairing the ability of the thoracic cavity to expand and contract. A gunshot wound or other trauma to the chest wall may allow intrapleural pressure to equalize with the atmosphere, causing the lung to collapse.

Lung compliance, the expansibility or stretchability of lung tissue, plays a significant role in the ease of ventilation. At birth, the fluid-filled lungs are stiff and resistant to expansion, similar to that of a new balloon that is difficult to inflate. With each subsequent breath, the alveoli become more compliant and easier to inflate, just as a balloon becomes easier to inflate after several tries. Lung compliance tends to decrease with aging, making it more difficult to expand the alveoli and increasing the risk of **atelectasis**, or collapse of a portion of the lung. The decreased compliance in older adults may be the result of chest wall rigidity from calcification of intercostal cartilage, decreased mobility of the ribs, or loss of elastic fibres in the lungs.

In contrast to lung compliance is **lung recoil** (elasticity), the continual tendency of the lungs to collapse away from the chest wall. Just as lung compliance is necessary for normal inspiration, lung recoil is necessary for normal expiration. Although elastic fibres in lung tissue contribute to lung recoil, the *surface tension* of fluid lining the alveoli has the greatest effect on recoil. Fluid molecules tend to draw together, reducing the size of the alveoli. **Surfactant**, a lipoprotein produced by specialized alveolar cells, acts like a detergent, reducing the surface tension of alveolar fluid. Without surfactant, lung expansion is exceedingly difficult and the lungs collapse. Premature infants whose lungs are not yet capable of producing adequate surfactant develop *respiratory distress syndrome* (*RDS*); adults can develop *adult respiratory distress syndrome* (*ARDS*), usually as a complication of serious illness or trauma.

Alveolar Gas Exchange

After the alveoli are ventilated, the second phase of the respiratory process—the diffusion of oxygen from the alveoli and into the pulmonary blood vessels—begins. **Diffusion** is the movement of gases or other particles from an area of greater pressure or concentration to an area of lower pressure or concentration.

Pressure differences in the gases on each side of the respiratory membrane obviously affect diffusion. When the pressure of oxygen is greater in the alveoli than in the blood, oxygen diffuses into the blood. The **partial pressure** (the pressure exerted by each individual gas in a mixture according to its concentration in the mixture) of oxygen (PaO_2) in the alveoli is about 100 mm Hg, whereas the PO_2 in the venous blood of the pulmonary arteries is about 60 mm Hg. These pressures rapidly equalize, however, so that the arterial oxygen pressure also reaches about 100 mm Hg. By contrast, carbon dioxide in the venous blood entering the pulmonary capillaries has a partial pressure of about 45 mm Hg (PCO_2), whereas that in the alveoli has a partial pressure of about 40 mm Hg. Therefore, carbon dioxide diffuses from the blood into the alveoli where it can be eliminated with expired air. When referring to the pressure of gas in the arterial blood, the abbreviation is PaO_2. When referring to partial pressure in venous blood, the abbreviation is PO_2.

Transport of Oxygen and Carbon Dioxide

The third part of the respiratory process involves the transport of respiratory gases. Oxygen needs to be transported from the lungs to the tissues, and carbon dioxide must be transported from the tissues back to the lungs. Normally, most of the oxygen (97%) combines loosely with **hemoglobin** (Hgb) (oxygen-carrying red pigment) in the **erythrocytes** (red blood cells [RBCs]) and is carried to the tissues as **oxyhemoglobin** (the compound of oxygen and hemoglobin). The remaining oxygen is dissolved and transported in the fluid of the plasma and cells.

Several factors affect the rate of oxygen transport from the lungs to the tissues:

1. Cardiac output
2. The number of erythrocytes and the blood hematocrit
3. Exercise

Normal **cardiac output** (the amount of blood pumped by the ventricles in 1 minute) is approximately 5 L per minute. Any pathological condition that decreases cardiac output (e.g., damage to the heart muscle, blood loss, or pooling of blood in the peripheral blood vessels) diminishes the amount of oxygen delivered to the tissues. The heart attempts to compensate for inadequate output by increasing its pumping rate (heart rate), but with severe damage or blood loss, this compensatory mechanism may not restore adequate blood flow and oxygen to the tissues.

The second factor influencing oxygen transport is the number of erythrocytes and the hematocrit. The **hematocrit** is the portion of the blood plasma that is made up of erythrocytes. In men, the number of circulating erythrocytes normally averages 4.5×10^{12} to 5.3×10^{12} cells per litre of blood, and in women, 4.1×10^{12} to 5.1×10^{12} cells per litre of blood. Normally, the hematocrit is 0.37 to 0.49 in men and 0.36 to 0.46 in women. Increasing the RBCs or decreasing the plasma component of the blood will result in an increased hematocrit (blood will be more viscous). An increased hematocrit results in more resistance and a slower blood flow, reducing the cardiac output and, therefore, reducing oxygen transport (e.g., dehydration—plasma content decreased; polycythemia—number of erythrocytes is increased).

Exercise also has a direct influence on oxygen transport. In well-trained athletes, oxygen transport can be increased up to 20 times the normal rate, in part because of an increased cardiac output and due to increased use of oxygen by the cells (utilization coefficient).

Carbon dioxide, continually produced in the processes of cell metabolism, is transported from the cells to the lungs in three ways: (1) the majority (about 65%) is carried inside the RBCs as bicarbonate (HCO_3^-) and is an important component of the bicarbonate buffer system (see Chapter 43); (2) a moderate amount of carbon dioxide (30%) combines with hemoglobin as *carbaminohemoglobin* for transport; and (3) smaller amounts (5%) are transported in solution in the plasma and as *carbonic acid* (the compound formed when carbon dioxide combines with water).

Respiratory Regulation

Respiratory regulation includes both neural and chemical controls to maintain the correct concentrations of oxygen, carbon dioxide, and hydrogen ions in body fluids. The nervous system adjusts the rate of alveolar ventilations to meet the needs of the body so that PaO_2 and $PaCO_2$ remain relatively constant. The body's respiratory centre consists of two groups of neurons located in the medulla oblongata and pons of the brain (dorsal respiratory group, pneumotaxic centre of upper and lower pons).

A chemosensitive centre in the medulla oblongata is highly responsive to increases in blood carbon dioxide and hydrogen ion concentration. By influencing other respiratory centres, this centre can increase the activity of the inspiratory centre and the rate and depth of respirations. In addition to this direct chemical stimulation of the respiratory centre in the brain, special neural receptors sensitive to decreases in O_2 concentration are located outside the central nervous system in the carotid bodies (just above the bifurcation of the common carotid arteries) and aortic bodies. Decreases in arterial oxygen concentrations stimulate these *chemoreceptors,* and they, in turn, stimulate the respiratory centre to increase ventilation. Of the three blood gases (hydrogen, oxygen, and carbon dioxide) that can trigger chemoreceptors, increased carbon dioxide concentration is the strongest stimulator of respiration.

However, in clients with certain lung ailments, such as emphysema, oxygen concentrations, *not carbon dioxide concentrations,* play a major role in regulating respiration. For such clients, decreased oxygen concentrations are the main stimuli for respiration. This is sometimes called the *hypoxic drive.* Increasing the concentration of oxygen can depress the respiratory rate, and, therefore, it is important that only low concentrations of supplemental oxygen be administered to these clients.

Physiology of the Cardiovascular System

The respiratory and cardiovascular systems are closely linked and dependent on each other to deliver oxygen to the tissues of the body. Alterations in function of either system can affect the other and lead to tissue **hypoxia**, or lack of oxygen.

The heart and the blood vessels make up the cardiovascular system. Together with blood, the cardiovascular system is the major transport system of the body, bringing oxygen and nutrients to the cells and removing wastes for disposal. The heart serves as the system pump, moving blood through the vessels to the tissues and then back to the heart.

The Heart

The heart (Figure 42.2) is a hollow, cone-shaped organ about the size of a fist. It is located in the mediastinum, between the lungs and underlying the sternum. It is enclosed by a double layer of fibroserous membrane known as the **pericardium**. The parietal, or outermost, pericardium protects the heart and anchors it to surrounding structures. The visceral pericardium adheres to the surface of the heart, forming the heart's outermost layer, the **epicardium**. A thin layer of serous fluid separates the parietal pericardium from the visceral pericardium. This arrangement prevents any friction rub between the two layers when the heart beats in the chest. The heart wall contains two additional layers: the **myocardium**, cardiac muscle cells that form the bulk of the heart and contract with each beat, and the **endocardium** lining the inside of the heart's chambers and great vessels.

Four hollow chambers within the heart, two upper **atria** and two lower **ventricles**, are separated longitudinally by the *interventricular septum,* forming two parallel pumps. The atria and ventricles are separated from each other by the *atrioventricular valves,* the *tricuspid valve* on the right and the *bicuspid* or *mitral valve* on the left. The ventricles, in turn, are separated from the great vessels (the pulmonary arteries and aorta) by the *semilunar valves:* the *pulmonic valve* on the right and the *aortic valve* on the left. The valves serve to direct the flow of blood, allowing it to move from the atria to the ventricles and from the ventricles to the great vessels, but preventing backflow.

Deoxygenated blood from the veins enters the right side of the heart through the superior (blood from head) and inferior (blood from body) venae cavae (singular is vena cava). Blood then flows into the right ventricle, which pumps it through the pulmonary artery into the lungs for gas exchange. Freshly oxygenated blood

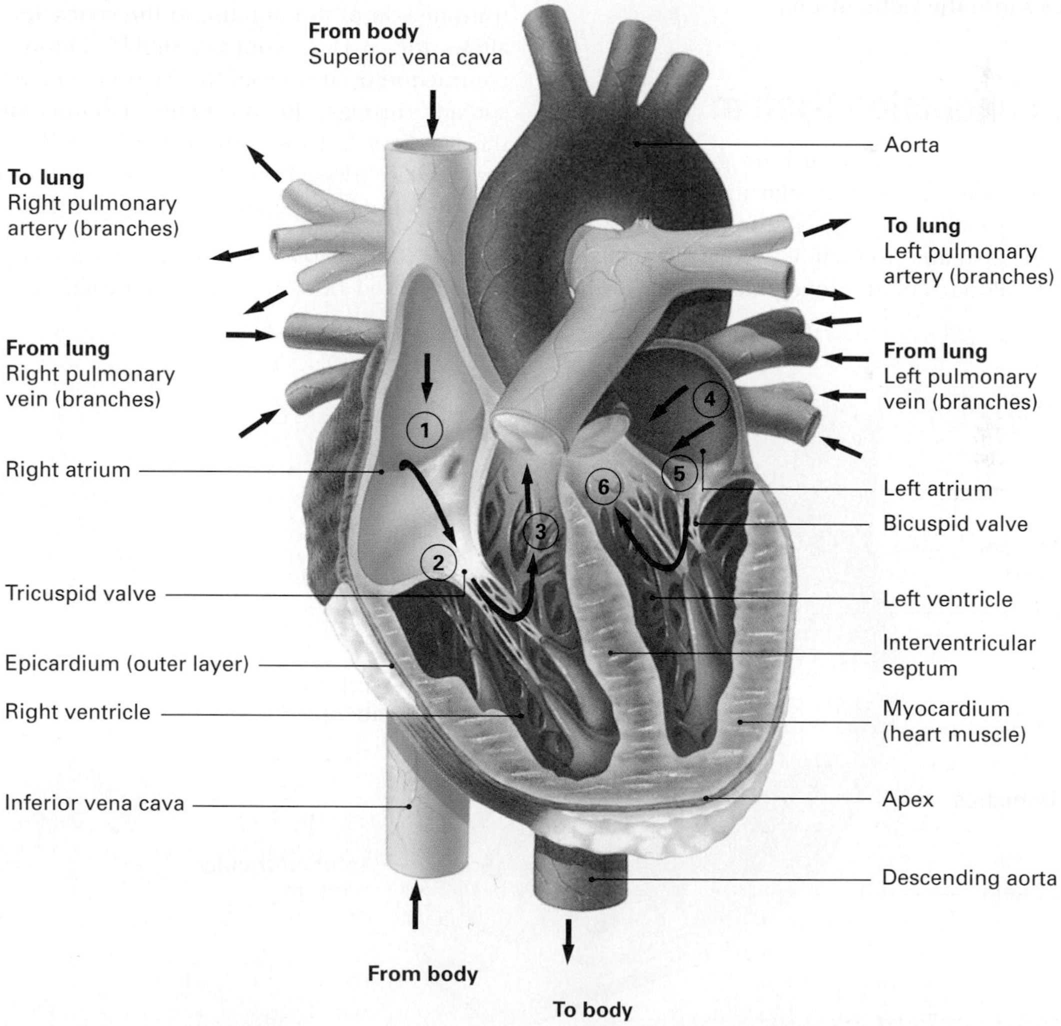

FIGURE 42.2 The heart: the diagram shows blood flow through the heart from the vena cava, right atrium (1), tricuspid valve (2), right ventricle (3), pulmonic valve, pulmonary arteries, pulmonary veins, left atrium (4), mitral valve (5), left ventricle (6), aortic valve, and the aorta

(From **Medical Terminology: A Living Language,** *3rd ed., by Bonnie F. Fremgen and Suzanne S. Frucht, 2005. Electronically reproduced by permission of Pearson Education, Inc., Upper Saddle River, New Jersey.)*

returns to the left atrium via the pulmonary veins. From the left atrium, the blood enters the left ventricle to be pumped out to the systemic circulation through the aorta.

CORONARY CIRCULATION The heart muscle moves blood to the lungs and peripheral tissues but receives no oxygen or nourishment from the blood within its chambers. Instead, it is supplied by a network of vessels known as the *coronary circulation.* The **coronary arteries** originate at the base of the aorta, branching out to encircle and penetrate the myocardium. The coronary arteries fill during ventricular relaxation, bringing oxygen-rich blood to the myocardium. If these arteries become clogged with atherosclerotic plaque or are obstructed by a blood clot, the myocardium area that is being supplied is deprived of oxygen, and the client may develop chest pain (angina) or experience a myocardial infarction (heart attack). The *cardiac veins* drain the deoxygenated blood from the myocardium into the *coronary sinus,* which empties into the right atrium.

Cardiac Conduction System

With each heartbeat, the myocardium goes through a cycle of contraction (*systole*) and relaxation (*diastole*). In **systole**, the heart ejects (propels) the blood into the pulmonary and systemic circulation. In **diastole**, the ventricles fill with blood. The diastolic phase of the cardiac cycle is twice as long as the systolic phase. This is important because diastole is largely a passive process.

Cardiac muscle contraction is a mechanical event that occurs in response to electrical stimulation. Cardiac muscle is unique in that, unlike skeletal muscle, it can generate electrical impulses and contractions independently of the nervous system. A network of specialized cells and pathways known as the *cardiac conduction system* normally controls the electrical activity and contraction of the heart.

The primary pacemaker of the heart is the **sinoatrial (SA or sinus) node**, located at the junction of the right atrium and superior vena cava. The SA node normally initiates electrical impulses that are conducted throughout the atria and result in atrial contraction. In adults, it usually fires at a regular rate of 60 to 100 times per minute, the "normal" heart rate. The impulse then spreads throughout the atria via the *interatrial pathways.* These conduction pathways converge and narrow through the **atrioventricular (AV) node**, slightly delaying transmission of the impulse to the ventricles. This delay allows the atria to contract slightly before ventricular contraction occurs. From the AV node, the impulse then spreads through the ventricular conduction pathways: the *bundle of His,* the right and left *bundle branches,* and the *Purkinje fibres.* These fibres terminate in ventricular muscle, stimulating contraction (Figure 42.3).

CARDIAC OUTPUT As the ventricles contract during systole, blood flows out of the ventricles into the great

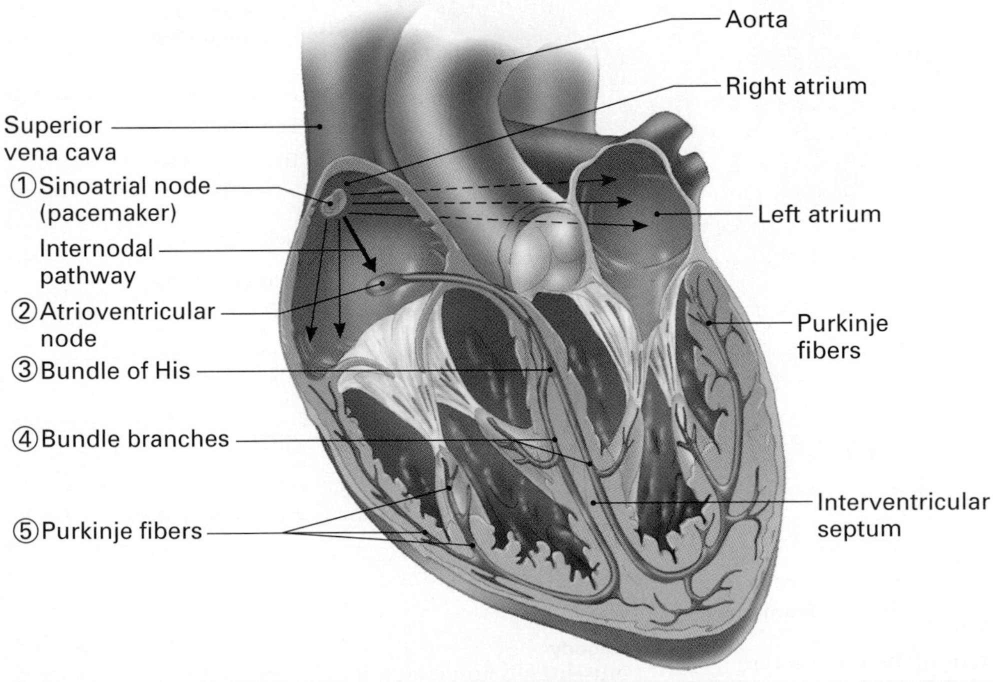

FIGURE 42.3 The electrical system of the heart. The impulse is initiated by the SA node, then travels to the AV node, the bundle of His, the bundle branches, and finally to the Purkinje fibres.

(From **Medical Terminology: A Living Language,** *3rd ed., by Bonnie F. Fremgen and Suzanne S. Frucht, 2005. Electronically reproduced by permission of Pearson Education, Inc., Upper Saddle River, New Jersey.)*

vessels and circulation. The heart muscle then relaxes, a phase known as diastole, allowing the ventricles to refill and the cardiac muscle to be perfused. This contraction and relaxation of the heart is known as the *cardiac cycle* or the heartbeat. The SA node stimulates the cardiac cycle to repeat between 60 and 100 times a minute in an adult.

With each contraction, a certain amount of blood, known as the **stroke volume (SV)**, is ejected from the ventricles into the circulation. In adults, the average stroke volume is about 70 mL per beat. Cardiac output (CO) is calculated by multiplying the stroke volume by the heart rate ($SV \times HR = CO$). The cardiac output is an important indicator of how well the heart is functioning as a pump. If the cardiac output is poor, tissue perfusion is decreased, and as a result, less oxygen and fewer nutrients reach the cells.

Cardiac output is affected by several factors:

- *Heart rate* is influenced by the autonomic nervous system; blood pressure; hormones, such as thyroid hormone; and some medications. An increased heart rate increases cardiac output even if the stroke volume does not change. However, heart rates that are very high or are sustained for a period can cause the cardiac output to drop. Very rapid heart rates, for example, more than 150 beats per minute, may not allow adequate time for the ventricles to fill, causing cardiac output to fall. Cardiac output decreases when the heart rate falls, if the stroke volume remains constant.
- **Preload** is the degree to which muscle fibres in the ventricle are stretched at the end of the relaxation period (diastole). It is sometimes referred to as the right or left ventricular end diastolic pressure (RVEDP or LVEDP). Preload largely depends on the amount of blood returning to the heart from the venous circulation. Increased volume causes increased stretch, leading to more forceful contraction of cardiac muscle fibres. For example, exercise increases venous return and the amount of blood in the ventricle before contraction; therefore, the heart contracts more forcefully, and stroke volume and cardiac output increase during exercise. Reduced venous return, such as when there is hemorrhage, results in a decrease in preload, leading to weaker contraction of cardiac muscle fibres.
- **Contractility** is the inherent ability of cardiac muscle fibres to shorten, or contract. Stroke volume decreases if contractility is poor, reducing cardiac output. Contractility also is affected by the autonomic nervous system and certain drugs. Positive inotropic drugs increase contractility, and negative inotropic drugs decrease the contractile strength.
- **Afterload** is the resistance against which the heart must pump to eject the blood into the circulation. Blood flows from an area of higher pressure to an area of lower pressure. To move blood into the circulatory system, the ventricles must generate sufficient pressure to overcome vascular resistance or the pressure within the arteries, known as afterload. The right ventricle pumps blood into the low-pressure, low-resistance pulmonary vascular system; therefore, the pressures generated by the right ventricle are fairly low. The left ventricle, by contrast, pumps blood into the higher-pressure systemic arterial system, generating much higher pressures and requiring more work. Systemic vasoconstriction and aortic valve stenosis (narrowing) lead to an increase afterload, increasing the cardiac workload; vasodilation, such as occurs with hydralazine therapy, in contrast, reduces afterload and the workload of the heart.

The Blood Vessels

With each cardiac contraction, blood is ejected into a closed system of blood vessels that transports blood to the tissues and returns it to the heart. The heart supports two circulatory systems: (1) the low-pressure pulmonary system, and (2) the higher-pressure systemic circulatory system.

Deoxygenated blood from the right ventricle enters the pulmonary vascular system through the pulmonary arteries. The pulmonary arteries subdivide into lobar arteries. These lobar arteries follow the main bronchi into the lungs and then branch out to form arterioles and the dense capillary networks that encompass the alveoli. Oxygen diffuses into the blood from the alveoli, and carbon dioxide diffuses into the alveoli from the blood. The blood then returns to the left side of the heart via the venules and the *pulmonary veins.* Note that the pulmonary vascular system is the only part of the circulatory system in which *arteries* (which transport blood away from the heart) carry deoxygenated blood and *veins* (which transport blood toward the heart) contain oxygenated blood.

The muscular left ventricle of the heart pumps oxygenated blood into the *aorta.* The blood then moves into major arteries that branch from the aorta into successively smaller arteries, *arterioles,* and, finally, the thin-walled *capillary beds* of organs and tissues. It is in the capillary beds that oxygen and nutrients are exchanged for metabolic waste products. The deoxygenated blood then returns to the heart through a series of *venules* and veins that become progressively larger until they empty into the right atrium via the superior and inferior venae cavae.

With the exception of capillaries, blood vessel walls have three distinct layers, or *tunics.* The innermost layer, the *tunica intima,* is smooth endothelium that facilitates blood flow. As individuals age, the intimal wall lining becomes less elastic and thicker and begins to degenerate and calcify. This does not allow adequate perfusion of nutrients into the cell, causing further degeneration. The *tunica media* is made up of elastic fibres and smooth muscle cells innervated by the autonomic nervous system. This allows vessels to constrict or dilate depending on the needs of the body. The tunica media is thicker and more muscular than in veins, a feature that helps maintain blood pressure and continuous circulation to the tissues. The outermost layer of blood vessels is the *tunica adventitia,* a layer of connective tissue that supports, protects, and anchors the vessel to surrounding tissues. Capillaries contain only one thin layer of tunica intima, allowing gases and molecules to diffuse between the blood and the tissues.

ARTERIAL CIRCULATION The arterial circulation moves blood pumped by the heart to the tissues by maintaining a constant flow to the capillary beds.

Blood flow—the volume of blood flowing through a given vessel, an organ, or the entire circulation over a specific time—is determined by *pressure differences* and *resistance.* Blood always moves from an area of higher pressure to an area of lower pressure. The greater the difference between pressures, the greater the blood flow. The **blood pressure** is the force exerted on arterial walls by the blood flowing within the vessel (see Chapter 28). The *mean arterial pressure* (*MAP*) is the pressure that maintains blood flow to the tissues throughout the cardiac cycle. It is a product of the cardiac output times the systemic vascular resistance (CO × SVR = MAP).

Resistance is the opposition to blood flow. An inverse relationship exists between the movement of blood through the vascular system and resistance (e.g., as blood flow decreases, resistance increases). **Systemic vascular resistance (SVR)** impedes or opposes blood flow to the tissues and is determined by the viscosity, or thickness, of the blood, blood vessel length, and blood vessel diameter.

VENOUS RETURN In contrast to the high-pressure arterial system, venous pressure is too low to adequately return blood from peripheral tissues to the heart without assistance. The fall in intrathoracic pressure that occurs with breathing draws blood upward toward the heart is an adaptation known as the *respiratory pump.* Skeletal muscle activity contributes to the *muscular pump,* as muscle contractions push blood toward the heart. Venous valves are vital in making these pumps work; once blood passes a valve, it cannot flow backward away from the heart. Figure 42.4 depicts the relationship between arteries and veins and the entire circulatory system.

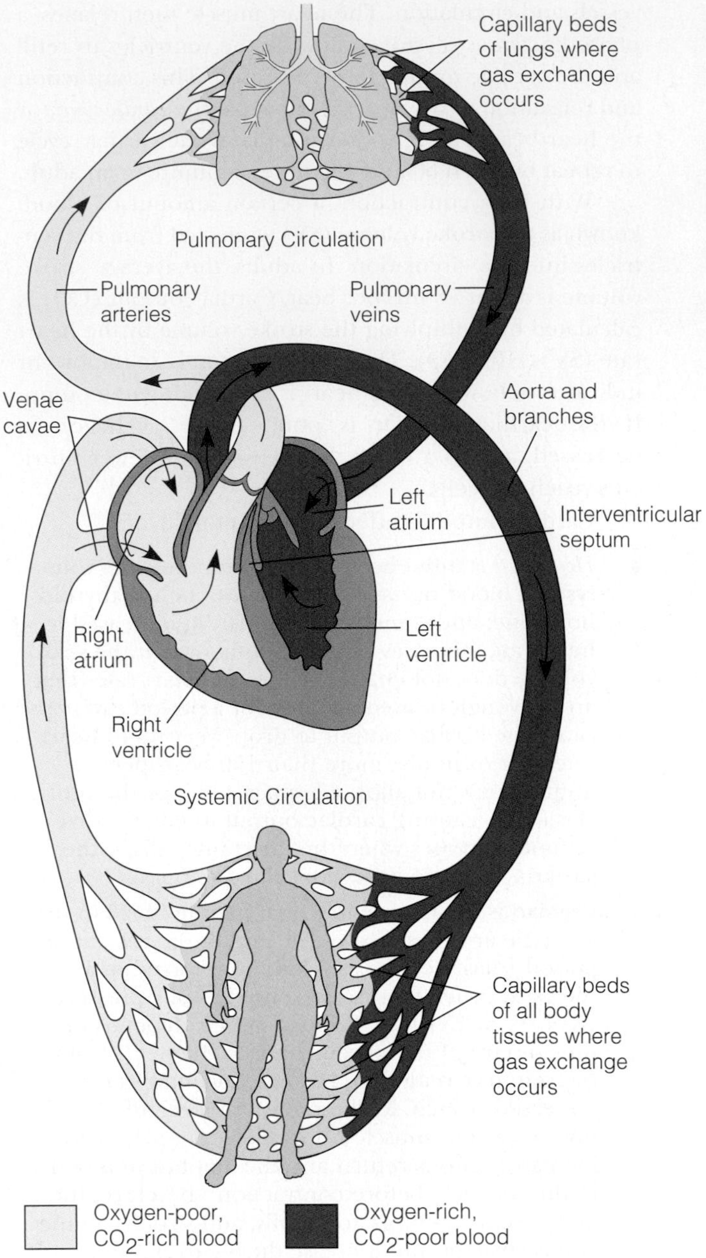

FIGURE 42.4 The heart and blood vessels: the left side of the heart pumps oxygenated blood into the arteries. Deoxygenated blood returns via the venous system into the right side of the heart.

Blood

Blood serves as the transport medium within the cardiovascular system, bringing oxygen and nutrients from the environment (via the lungs and gastrointestinal system) to the cells. Blood is a complex mixture of living formed elements (the blood cells) and proteins suspended in fluid (the plasma). Its primary functions are as follows:

- Transporting oxygen, nutrients, and hormones needed for cell metabolism to the cells, and metabolic wastes from the tissues for elimination
- Regulating acid-base balance, body temperature, pH, and fluid volume
- Preventing infection and blood loss

Most oxygen is transported bound to hemoglobin. Hemoglobin is a major component of erythrocytes, whose predominant responsibility is tissue oxygenation. Hemoglobin binds easily with oxygen, releasing it in the body tissues. When all four heme groups of the hemoglobin molecule are bound to oxygen, it is said to be *fully saturated.* Oxygen binding is affected by several factors, including the PO_2, temperature, pH, and PCO_2. Up to a certain point (about 70 mm Hg), the higher the PO_2, the greater the affinity of hemoglobin for oxygen and the more saturated the hemoglobin molecules. The relationship to temperature, pH, and PCO_2 are the opposite: at higher temperatures, greater hydrogen ion concentrations (lower pH), and higher PCO_2 levels, the affinity for oxygen decreases, and hemoglobin releases its oxygen molecules. *Anemia* (too few RBCs that contain too little or abnormal hemoglobin) interferes with oxygen delivery to the tissues, which often leads to fatigue and activity intolerance.

Factors Affecting Respiratory and Cardiovascular Function

Factors that influence oxygenation affect the cardiovascular system as well as the respiratory system. These factors include age and development, environment, lifestyle, health status, pharmacological agents, stress and coping, and gender.

Lifespan Considerations

At birth, profound changes occur in the respiratory and cardiovascular systems. The fluid-filled lungs drain, the PCO_2 rises, and the neonate takes the first breath. The lungs gradually expand with each subsequent breath, reaching full inflation by 2 weeks of age. As the lungs expand, pressures in the pulmonary vascular system fall, changing pressure relationships within the heart. The *foramen ovale* between the atria closes as pressures on the right side of the heart fall and pressures on the left side increase. Arterial PaO_2 rises and arterial $PaCO_2$ falls, prompting closure of the *ductus arteriosus* between the pulmonary artery and aorta.

Respiratory and pulse rates are highest and most variable in newborns. The respiratory rate of a neonate is 40 to 80 breaths per minute; in infancy, it averages about 30 per minute. The rate gradually decreases, averaging around 25 per minute in the preschooler and reaching the adult rate of 12 to 18 per minute by late adolescence. Because of their rib cage structure, infants rely almost exclusively on diaphragmatic movement for breathing. An infant's breathing pattern is primarily abdominal breathing, with the abdomen rising and falling with each breath.

The resting heart rate for a neonate ranges from 80 to 200 beats per minute, decreasing to 80 to 150 in infancy and early childhood, and reaching the adult rate of 60 to 100 by about age 10. Irregular heart rates are common in infants and young children, often increasing and decreasing with each breath. This pattern of irregularity is known as *sinus arrhythmia,* a normal variation of the heart rate.

As the conversion from fetal circulation takes place and pressures in the left side of the heart rise, the arterial blood pressure increases. Immediately after birth (1 to 3 days of age) the blood pressure averages about 65/40. By one month, the arterial pressure is about 90/55. It rises gradually to the adult norm of 120/80. With aging, blood pressure may again rise as arteriosclerosis affects the blood vessels, narrowing their lumen and decreasing their compliance (ability to distend). During middle adulthood, however, the incidence of *hypertension,* or an elevated blood pressure, increases significantly. Hypertension, known as the silent killer because of its lack of symptoms, is a major risk factor for cardiovascular disease. (See Chapter 28 for more discussion on hypertension.)

During infancy and childhood, upper respiratory infections are common and, fortunately, usually not serious. Infants and preschoolers also are at risk for airway obstruction by foreign objects, such as coins, peanuts, and small toys. *Cystic fibrosis* is a congenital disorder that affects the lungs, causing them to become congested with thick, tenacious (sticky) mucus. *Asthma* is another chronic disease often identified in childhood. The airways of the asthmatic child respond to such stimuli as allergens, exercise, or cold air by constricting, becoming edematous and producing excessive mucus. Airflow is impaired, and the child may wheeze as air moves through narrowed air passages.

As individuals age, the chest wall becomes more rigid and the lungs less elastic. More air is retained in the lungs at the end of each breath, and the **vital capacity**, or maximum amount of air that can be exchanged with each breath, decreases. The client with severe elasticity problems may have a *barrel chest,* with an anterior-posterior (AP) diameter approximately equal to the lateral diameter (normally, the AP diameter is about half the lateral diameter in adults). The older client is at increased risk for acute respiratory diseases, such as pneumonia, and chronic diseases, such as emphysema and chronic bronchitis. *Chronic obstructive pulmonary disease* (*COPD*) is seen more frequently in older adults, particularly after years of exposure to cigarette smoke or industrial pollutants.

Congenital heart defects may affect infants and children; however, acquired heart diseases are rare in childhood. *Rheumatic fever* is an inflammatory disorder that can occur following a streptococcal infection (e.g., strep throat). It can go on to damage the heart valves. For most people, the heart continues to function effectively well into older adulthood unless the blood supply to the heart muscle is impaired by blood vessel disease. *Cardiovascular disease* (*CVD*) is the leading cause of death in Canada and the United States. *Atherosclerosis,* the buildup of fatty plaque within the arteries, is the major contributor.

Although children are rarely affected by diseases of the blood vessels, both children and adults can have disorders of coagulation and platelets. Some disorders of coagulation are inherited (e.g., hemophilia), and in others, the etiology is unknown.

Environment

Altitude, heat, cold, and air pollution affect oxygenation. The higher the *altitude*, the lower the partial pressure of the oxygen (PO_2) an individual breathes. As a result, the person at high altitudes has increased respiratory and cardiac rates and increased respiratory depth, which usually become most apparent when the individual exercises.

The peripheral blood vessels dilate in response to *heat*, consequently, blood flows to the skin, increasing the amount of heat lost from the body surface. With vasodilation, the lumens of the blood vessels enlarge, thus decreasing the resistance to blood flow. In response, the heart rate and cardiac output increase to maintain blood pressure. The increased cardiac output requires additional oxygen, which causes increased rate and depth of breathing. In contrast, in a *cold* environment, the peripheral blood vessels constrict, raising the blood pressure, which, in turn, decreases cardiac action, thereby reducing the need for oxygen.

Healthy people exposed to *air pollution*, such as smog or second-hand smoke, may experience stinging of the eyes, headache, dizziness, coughing, and choking. People who have existing lung conditions or disease and altered respiratory function experience varying degrees of respiratory difficulty in a polluted environment. Some individuals are unable to maintain the activities of daily living (ADLs) in such an environment and require health-care assistance.

Lifestyle

Physical exercise or activity increases the rate and depth of respirations and the heart rate and hence the supply of oxygen in the body. With regular vigorous exercise, the heart muscle becomes more powerful and efficient. Aerobic exercise reduces the risk of cardiovascular disease by slowing the atherosclerotic process. Sedentary people, by contrast, have a higher risk of cardiovascular disease. They also lack the alveolar expansion and deep breathing patterns of people who participate in regular activity and they are less able to respond effectively to respiratory stressors.

Certain occupations can predispose an individual to lung disease. For example, silicosis is seen more often in sandstone blasters and potters than in the rest of the population; asbestosis is seen in asbestos workers; anthracosis affects coal miners; and organic dust disease occurs in farmers and agricultural employees who work with mouldy hay.

The cardiovascular and respiratory systems are affected by cigarette smoking. Nicotine increases the heart rate, blood pressure, and systemic vascular resistance, increasing the heart's workload. Smoking causes vasoconstriction of vessels, increased viscosity of the blood, and platelet adherence. Smoking can also potentiate further damage to the intimal wall lining of vessels, particularly if those vessels are already affected by athelerosclerosis, causing impairment of tissue oxygenation.

Evidence-Informed Practice

Do Nurses Implement Smoking Cessation Best Practice Guidelines?

Schultz, Johnson, and Bottorff (2006) surveyed 214 nurses from two British Columbia hospitals to determine the nurses' perception of and practice related to tobacco-reduction strategies with patients. The nurses agreed that they had a role to play in tobacco reduction; however, beyond assessment of smoking status, best practice guidelines related to tobacco reduction had not been integrated into the practice setting. The findings also suggested that nurses exposed to tobacco-reduction resources (in-hospital or community) were more likely to assess and document tobacco use and engage patients in tobacco-reduction strategies; that assisting with smoking cessation activities was restricted to nicotine replacement; and that arranging follow-up for interested patients was not a frequent activity. Nurses' perceptions of motivators to providing tobacco-reduction activities included administrative support and physician expectation of nurses' involvement in tobacco reduction. Barriers included lack of time, lack of preparedness, and lack of confidence in their ability to assist a patient with smoking cessation.

NURSING IMPLICATIONS: **Tobacco use is the leading cause of preventable mortality and morbidity (World Health Organization, 2000). Health-care providers, especially nurses, are encouraged to incorporate tobacco-reduction strategies into their practice. A Canadian initiative to prepare nurses to address tobacco use includes the dissemination of best practice guidelines for nurses (Registered Nurses' Association of Ontario [RNAO], 2003b) and an e-learning course related to the guidelines (RNAO, 2003a). Despite these resources, nurses feel unprepared to support tobacco reduction with patients. Consequently, researchers have suggested other strategies to facilitate the integration of these guidelines into practice, including providing nurses with relevant in-service education, along with clarification and standardization of which tobacco-reduction activities could reasonably be integrated into practice. As well, a commitment from health-care institutions and health-care systems to reducing tobacco use is required.**

Source: Based on "Registered Nurses' Perspectives on Tobacco Reduction: Views from Western Canada," by A. S. H. Schultz, J. L. Johnson, and J. I. Bottorff, 2006, *Canadian Journal of Nursing Research, 38*(4), 192–211.

Diet and other lifestyle factors also affect both cardiac and respiratory functions. A healthy diet with adequate calories, protein, and other nutrients is important to maintaining good immune function and increasing resistance to disease. Along with certain vitamins and minerals, dietary protein is important to preventing anemia. Similarly, a strong link exists between elevated serum lipid levels and the development of coronary heart disease. Lipoproteins circulate in the blood and are made up of cholesterol, triglycerides, and phospholipids. A high dietary intake of saturated fats is the most critical factor for the development of elevated serum lipids. In Canada, more than 40% of men and women have elevated total plasma cholesterol levels. The Heart and Stroke Foundation of Canada (2004) recommends that no more than 20% to 35% of total calories (about 45 g/day to 75 g/day for a woman and about 60 g/day to 105 g/day for a man) come from fats.

High salt intake (greater than 100 mmol/day [2300 mg/day]) can affect blood pressure and contribute to the development of hypertension (Canadian Hypertension Education Program, 2008). Although Health Canada (2008) indicates that adequate daily intake of sodium is between 1200 mg and 1500 mg (52 mmol/day to 65 mmol/day), most Canadians consume on average 3100 mg/day of sodium, excluding the salt added at the dinner table and in cooking (cited in Joffres, Campbell, Manns, & Tu, 2007). High intake of sodium can contribute to hypertension in two ways. First, it can increase the release of natriuretic hormone, which indirectly contributes to hypertension. Additionally, sodium stimulates vasopressor mechanisms, which cause vasoconstriction. Evidence suggests that other factors, such as low potassium, calcium, and magnesium intake, can contribute to vasoconstriction and the development of hypertension. High consumption of dairy products and dietary calcium has been found to reduce blood pressure levels (Ruidavets et al., 2006). (Chapter 28 discusses hypertension in more detail.)

Recent studies suggest that moderate alcohol use, in particular, red wine (no more than 120 mL of wine per day for women and 240 mL per day for men) may actually reduce the risk of heart disease; however, excessive alcohol intake negatively affects the body in several other ways (Saremi & Arora, 2008). Alcohol is a respiratory depressant, slowing respirations. Alcohol abusers often are malnourished, thereby increasing their risk of anemia and infections. Excess alcohol intake also increases the risk of hypertension, liver disease, and coagulation problems.

Health Status

In the healthy person, the cardiovascular and respiratory systems can provide sufficient oxygen to meet the body's needs. Diseases of the cardiovascular system often affect the delivery of oxygen to the cells of the body, while diseases of the respiratory system can adversely affect the oxygenation of the blood.

Numerous respiratory and cardiovascular diseases affect oxygenation. One cardiovascular condition that affects oxygenation but is often overlooked is anemia (described in the section "Cardiovascular Alterations" later in this chapter).

Pharmacological Agents

A variety of medications can decrease the rate and depth of respiration. The most common medications with this effect are the benzodiazepine sedative-hypnotics and antianxiety drugs, such as diazepam (Valium), flurazepam (Dalmane), and midazolam (Versed); barbiturates, such as phenobarbital; and opioids, such as morphine. Other pharmacological agents that can affect respiratory and cardiac function include bronchodilators and beta blockers. Bronchodilators, although given to improve oxygenation by dilating the bronchial tree, can also cause increased cardiac workload by increasing heart rate and blood pressure. Caution must be used when giving beta blockers to individuals with respiratory conditions because these medications can cause an increase in bronchoconstriction, thereby further compromising respiratory status. When administering bronchodilators, beta blockers, and opioids, the nurse must monitor ongoing respiratory status.

Stress and Coping

When stress and stressors are encountered, both psychological and physiological responses can affect oxygenation. Some people may hyperventilate in response to stress. When this occurs, PaO_2 rises and $PaCO_2$ falls. The person may experience light-headedness and numbness and tingling of the fingers, toes, and around the mouth as a result.

Physiologically, when an individual experiences stress, the sympathetic nervous system is stimulated and epinephrine and norepinephrine are released. Epinephrine causes the heart to contract more forcefully and the bronchioles to dilate, increasing blood flow and oxygen delivery to active muscles. Norepinephrine increases the blood pressure by causing vasoconstriction. Although these responses are adaptive in the short term, when stress continues, they can be destructive, increasing the risk of cardiovascular disease by increasing heart rate and blood pressure. See Chapter 47 for further discussion of stress and coping.

Other emotions, such as anger, may also be connected to heart disease. Recent studies indicate that people who repress their anger or become hostile appear to have a higher incidence of heart disease.

Gender

Through middle adulthood (until menopause), estrogen has a protective effect in women, slowing the progress of atherosclerosis and reducing the risk of cardiovascular disease. This effect is lost at menopause, but hormone replacement therapy may be beneficial in reducing this risk later in life. Possible benefits from HRT must be weighed against possible risks. This complex analysis requires thorough discussion between the woman and her health-care provider. Among people in their 40s and 50s, men also have a higher incidence of hypertension than women do.

Alterations in Function

Respiratory Alterations

Respiratory function can be altered by conditions that affect the following:

- The movement of air into or out of the lungs
- The diffusion of oxygen and carbon dioxide between the alveoli and the pulmonary capillaries
- The transport of oxygen and carbon dioxide via the blood to and from the tissue's cells

Three major alterations in respiration are hypoxia, altered breathing patterns, and obstructed or partially obstructed airway.

HYPOXIA Hypoxia is a condition of insufficient tissue oxygenation. Hypoxia can be further defined into four categories: anemic hypoxia, hypoxic hypoxia, circulatory hypoxia, and histotoxic hypoxia. Anemic hypoxia occurs when individuals have low hemoglobin and, therefore, have a decrease in the oxygen-carrying capacity of the cells. Hypoxic hypoxia results when oxygen levels remain low despite the body's ability to carry oxygen (e.g., occurs with high altitude, hypoventilation). Circulatory hypoxia refers to states in which cardiac output is decreased and, therefore, the oxygen-carrying ability is normal but the blood flow is decreased. Histotoxic hypoxia occurs as a result of the body's inability to adequately use available oxygen (e.g., cyanide poisoning). The Clinical Manifestations box lists signs of hypoxia.

Hypoventilation is a reduced rate and depth of respiration that can lead to hypoxia. It can also result in an increase in carbon dioxide levels in the blood, referred to as **hypercarbia** or **hypercapnia**. Hypoventilation can occur because of diseases of the respiratory muscles, drugs, or anaesthesia.

Hypoxia can also develop when the diffusion of oxygen from alveoli into the arterial blood decreases (e.g., pulmonary edema), or it can result from problems in the delivery of oxygen to the tissues (e.g., anemia, heart failure, and embolism). The term **hypoxemia** refers to reduced oxygen in the blood and is characterized by a low partial pressure of oxygen (PaO_2) in arterial blood or low hemoglobin saturation.

> **Clinical Manifestations**
>
> ### Hypoxia
>
> The following are all signs of hypoxia:
>
> - Rapid pulse
> - Rapid, shallow respirations and dyspnea
> - Increased restlessness or light-headedness
> - Flaring of the nares
> - Substernal or intercostal retractions or indrawing
> - Cyanosis

Cyanosis (bluish discolouration of the skin, nail beds, and mucous membranes caused by reduced hemoglobin-oxygen saturation) may be present with hypoxemia. Cyanosis requires two conditions: the blood must contain about 5 g or more of unoxygenated hemoglobin per 100 mL of blood, and the surface capillaries must be dilated. Factors that interfere with these conditions (e.g., severe anemia or the administration of epinephrine) will eliminate cyanosis as a sign even if the client is experiencing hypoxia.

Adequate oxygenation is essential for cerebral functioning. The cerebral cortex can tolerate hypoxia for only 3 to 5 minutes before permanent damage occurs. The face of the acutely hypoxic person usually appears anxious, tired, and drawn. The person usually assumes a sitting position, often leaning forward slightly to permit greater expansion of the thoracic cavity.

With *chronic* hypoxia, the client often appears fatigued and is lethargic. The client's fingers and toes may be clubbed as a result of long-term lack of oxygen in the arterial blood supply. With clubbing, the base of the nail becomes swollen and the ends of the fingers and toes increase in size. The angle between the nail and the base of the nail increases to more than 180 degrees (see Figure 27.10, page 571).

ALTERED BREATHING PATTERNS Breathing patterns refer to the rate, volume, rhythm, and relative ease or effort of respiration. Normal respiration (**eupnea**) is quiet, rhythmic, and effortless. **Tachypnea** (rapid respiratory rate) is seen with fevers, metabolic acidosis, pain, and hypoxemia. **Bradypnea** is an abnormally slow respiratory rate, which may be seen in clients who have been given anaesthetic gases (a respiratory depressant), who have metabolic alkalosis, or who have increased intracranial pressure (e.g., from brain injuries). **Apnea** is the cessation of breathing; *sleep apnea* is the cessation of breathing during sleep.

Hyperventilation, often called alveolar hyperventilation, is an increased movement of air into and out of the lungs. During hyperventilation, the rate and depth of respirations increase, and more CO_2 is eliminated than is produced. One particular type of hyperventilation that accompanies metabolic acidosis is **Kussmaul's respiration**, by which the body attempts to compensate (give off excess body acids) by blowing off the carbon dioxide through deep and rapid breathing. Hyperventilation can also occur in response to stress, as mentioned earlier.

Hypoventilation is inadequate alveolar ventilation, that is, ventilation that does not meet the body's requirements. As a result, carbon dioxide is retained in the bloodstream. Hypoventilation can occur as a result of collapse of the alveoli, leaving too few functioning alveoli to meet the body's ventilation needs, or it can result from airway obstruction or as the side effects of some drugs.

Abnormal respiratory *rhythms* create an irregular breathing pattern. Two abnormal respiratory rhythms follow:

- **Cheyne-Stokes respiration**. Marked rhythmic waxing and waning of respirations from very deep to very shallow breathing and temporary apnea; common causes include heart failure, increased intracranial pressure, and drug overdose
- **Biot's (cluster) respiration**. Shallow breaths interrupted by apnea; may be seen in clients with central nervous system disorders

The subjective sensation of difficult or uncomfortable breathing or breathlessness is called **dyspnea**. Because this experience is the most common disabling symptom of COPD, dyspnea is often considered the sixth vital sign in the assessment of people with COPD (RNAO, 2005). The dyspneic person often appears anxious and may describe their experience as shortness of breath (SOB) or a feeling of being unable to get enough air. Often, the nostrils are flared because of the increased effort of inspiration. The skin and mucous membranes may appear dusky and the heart rate is usually increased. **Orthopnea** is the inability to breathe except in an upright or a standing position.

OBSTRUCTED AIRWAY A completely or partially obstructed airway can occur anywhere along the upper or lower respiratory passageways. An upper airway obstruction—that is, in the nose, pharynx, or larynx—can be caused by a foreign object, such as food; by the tongue falling back into the oropharynx when a person is unconscious; or by secretions collecting in the passageways. In the last instance, the respirations will sound gurgly or bubbly as the air attempts to pass through the secretions. Lower airway obstruction involves partial or complete occlusion of the passageways in the bronchi and lungs, most often caused by increased accumulation of mucus or inflammatory exudate. *Obstructive sleep apnea* is repeated obstruction of the upper airway by the tongue or relaxed muscles of the pharynx for several seconds during sleep.

Assessing for and maintaining a patent (open) airway is a nursing responsibility, one that often requires immediate action. Partial obstruction of the upper airway passages is indicated by a low-pitched snoring sound during inhalation. Complete obstruction is indicated by extreme inspiratory effort that produces no chest movement. Such a client, in an effort to obtain air, may also exhibit marked sternal and intercostal retractions. Lower airway obstruction is not always as easy to observe. **Stridor**, a harsh, high-pitched sound, may be heard during inspiration. The client may have altered arterial blood gas levels, restlessness, anxiety, dyspnea, and **adventitious breath sounds** (abnormal breath sounds). See Table 27.8 (page 603) for details on adventitious breath sounds.

Cardiovascular Alterations

Cardiovascular function can be altered by conditions that affect the following:

1. The function of the heart as a pump
2. Blood flow to organs and peripheral tissues
3. The composition of the blood and its ability to transport oxygen and carbon dioxide

Three major alterations in cardiovascular function are (1) decreased cardiac output, (2) impaired tissue perfusion, and (3) disorders that affect the composition or amount of blood available for transport of gases.

DECREASED CARDIAC OUTPUT Although the heart normally is able to increase its rate and the force of its contraction to increase cardiac output during exercise, fever, or other times of need, some conditions interfere with these mechanisms.

The vessels that supply blood to the heart muscle can become occluded by atherosclerosis or a blood clot, shutting off the blood supply to a portion of the myocardium. When this happens, the tissue becomes *necrotic* and dies, a condition known as a **myocardial infarction (MI)** or heart attack. If a large portion of the heart muscle is affected, particularly in the left ventricle, cardiac output falls because the affected muscle no longer contracts. Signs and symptoms of myocardial infarction are variable and can include chest pain (substernal or radiating to the left arm or jaw), nausea, shortness of breath, and diaphoresis.

Heart failure can develop if the heart is not able to keep up with the body's need for oxygen and nutrients to the tissues. Heart failure can occur as a result of myocardial infarction, cardiomyopathy (disease of the myocardium—the heart muscle), and chronic overwork of the heart, such as in clients with uncontrolled hypertension or extensive arteriosclerosis. Systolic function in heart failure can either be preserved or be reduced, with the former having fewer complications than the latter. In *congestive heart failure* (CHF), the vessels of the pulmonary system become congested or engorged with blood. This may cause fluid to escape into the alveoli and interfere with gas exchange, a condition known as *pulmonary edema*. Signs of heart failure include pulmonary congestion, shortness of breath, tachycardia, tachypnea, peripheral vasoconstriction, and distended jugular veins. Other diseases, such as myocarditis (inflammation of the myocardium) and cardiomyopathy, also can affect the heart muscle, impairing its ability to contract and pump.

Very irregular or excessively rapid or slow heart rates can decrease cardiac output. With irregular or very rapid heart rates, the ventricles may not fill adequately between beats, so the stroke volume (amount pumped with each beat) falls. If the heart rate is too slow, the heart may not be able to increase its stroke volume enough to maintain the cardiac output. Abnormalities of the heart rate and rhythm are known as *dysrhythmias* and can be identified on the electrocardiogram (ECG).

Alterations in the structure of the heart can affect cardiac output. Congenital heart defects result in abnormal blood flow and may even allow venous and arterial blood to mix. The oxygen supply to the tissues is affected in this case. Acquired heart diseases, such as bacterial endocarditis (inflammation of the membrane lining the endocardium) and rheumatic fever, can damage the heart valves, affecting the flow of blood within the heart and to the great vessels. For example, if the mitral (bicuspid) valve becomes scarred and *stenotic* (constricted), it may not open fully, impairing filling of the left ventricle. Or if the mitral valve does not fully close (*mitral insufficiency*), blood may escape back or *regurgitate* into the left atrium instead of entering the aorta each time the ventricle contracts.

IMPAIRED TISSUE PERFUSION Atherosclerosis is, by far, the most common cause of impaired blood flow to organs and tissues. As vessels narrow and become obstructed, distal tissues receive less blood and oxygen, and fewer nutrients. **Ischemia** is a lack of blood supply caused by obstructed circulation. Any artery in the body can be affected by atherosclerosis, although the effects are often related to coronary arteries, vessels supplying blood to the brain, and arteries in peripheral tissues. Obstruction of the coronary arteries causes myocardial ischemia, often resulting in *angina pectoris* (chest pain caused by lack of blood flow to the heart). If the cerebral vessels are affected, the result may be a *transient ischemic attack* (*TIA*) or a *stroke*. Peripheral vascular disease leads to ischemia of distal tissues, such as the legs and feet, resulting in coagulation problems, gangrene, and amputation.

The major risk factors for atherosclerosis include cigarette smoking, high fat intake, obesity, and a sedentary lifestyle. Hypertension and diabetes also increase the risk for atherosclerosis, particularly if the blood pressure or blood glucose levels are not maintained at near-normal levels. Risk factors that can be modified include gender, age, race, and family history.

Although much less common, other disorders, such as vessel inflammation, arterial spasm, and blood clots, can occlude blood vessels, leading to ischemia. Tissue edema can impair flow through vessels and increases the distance oxygen and nutrients must diffuse to reach cells.

On the venous side, incompetent valves may allow blood to pool in the veins, causing edema and decreasing venous return to the heart (Figure 42.5). Veins also can become inflamed, reducing blood flow and increasing the risk of thrombus (clot) formation. Thrombi (the plural of thrombus) can then break loose, becoming emboli. These emboli tend to travel as far as the pulmonary circulation, where they become trapped in pulmonary vessels (*pulmonary emboli*), occluding blood supply to the capillary side of the alveolar-capillary membrane. Although alveolar ventilation to the affected area often remains adequate if the clots are relatively small, no gas exchange occurs because of impaired blood flow. Signs of acute pulmonary embolism can be nonspecific and variable but include sudden onset of shortness of breath and pleuritic pain (sharp pain in the chest that worsens with coughing and deep breathing).

BLOOD ALTERATIONS Because most oxygen is transported to the tissues in combination with hemoglobin, the problems of inadequate red blood cells (RBCs), low hemoglobin levels, or abnormal hemoglobin structure can affect tissue oxygenation. Anemia has several different causes: RBCs are lost along with other components because of acute or chronic bleeding; if the diet is deficient in iron or folic acid, hemoglobin and RBCs are not formed adequately; and some disorders cause RBCs to break down excessively. People with sickle-cell anemia produce an abnormal form of hemoglobin and can experience tissue ischemia during exacerbations of the disease.

Blood volume also affects tissue oxygenation. If the blood volume is inadequate, as in hemorrhage or severe dehydration, then blood pressure and cardiac output fall, and tissues may become ischemic. Conversely, clients

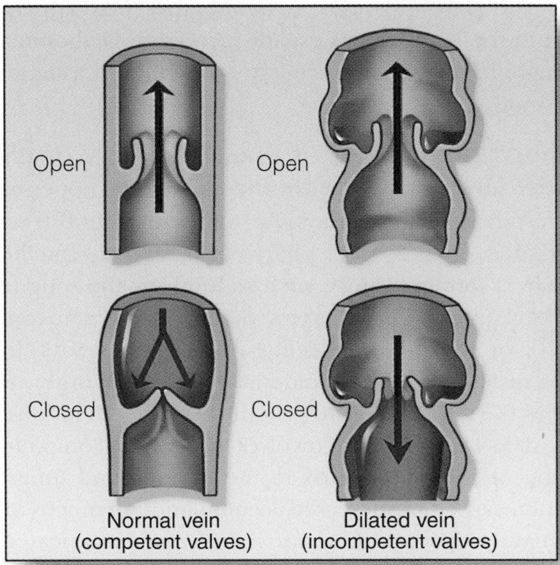

FIGURE 42.5 Vein with competent valve and vein with incompetent valve that allows blood to pool in the veins

(From **Medical Terminology: A Living Language,** *3rd ed., by Bonnie F. Fremgen and Suzanne S. Frucht, 2005. Electronically reproduced by permission of Pearson Education, Inc., Upper Saddle River, New Jersey.)*

with *hypervolemia* (excess blood volume), which can result from fluid retention or kidney failure, may develop heart failure and peripheral edema, leading to tissue ischemia.

Assessing

Nursing assessment of oxygenation and circulation status includes a history, physical examination, and review of relevant diagnostic data.

NURSING HISTORY A comprehensive nursing history status should include data about current and past respiratory and cardiovascular problems; lifestyle; the presence of cough, sputum, or pain; medications for heart, blood pressure, circulation, or breathing; and the presence of risk factors for impaired oxygenation or circulatory status. Examples of interview questions to elicit this information are shown in the Assessment: Interview box.

ASSESSMENT: INTERVIEW

Oxygenation and Circulation

The following questions can help the nurse obtain information about a client's respiratory and cardiovascular systems:

CURRENT RESPIRATORY PROBLEMS

- Have you noticed any changes in your breathing pattern (e.g., shortness of breath, difficulty breathing, need to be in upright position to breathe, or rapid and shallow breathing)?
- If so, which of your activities might cause these symptoms to occur?
- How many pillows do you use to sleep at night?

HISTORY OF RESPIRATORY DISEASE

- Have you had colds, the flu, allergies, croup, asthma, tuberculosis, bronchitis, pneumonia, or emphysema?
- How frequently have these occurred? How long did they last? And how were they treated?
- Have you been exposed to any pollutants?

CURRENT OR PAST CARDIOVASCULAR PROBLEMS

- Do you have high blood pressure?
- Do you have any history of heart disease, such as angina, heart attack, or heart failure? Have you ever had a cardiac catheterization, angiography, or angioplasty? Have you ever been diagnosed with rheumatic fever, endocarditis, pericarditis, or other diseases of the heart? If so, when?
- Have you ever been told that you have peripheral vascular disease? Do you ever develop pain in the calves of your legs when walking? How far can you walk before it occurs? What do you do to relieve it?
- Do you have pain in your lower limbs when resting? Does changing your position make the symptoms better or worse? Do you have pain, redness, or swelling in your calves?
- Do your feet and ankles ever swell or feel very cold, numb, or tingling?
- Do you become extremely fatigued with activity? Have you ever been told that you are anemic?

LIFESTYLE

- Do you smoke? If so, how much? Do you want to stop? If you don't smoke, did you smoke previously, and when did you stop?
- Does any member of your family smoke?
- Is there cigarette smoke or other pollutants (e.g., fumes, dust, coal, asbestos) in your workplace?
- Do you use alcohol? If so, how many drinks (mixed drinks, glasses of wine, or beers) do you usually have per day or per week?
- Describe your exercise patterns. What exercise (types) do you participate in? How often do you exercise, and for how long?

PRESENCE OF COUGH

- How often and how much do you cough?
- Is it *productive,* that is, accompanied by sputum, or *nonproductive,* that is, dry?
- Does the cough occur during certain activities or at certain times of the day?

DESCRIPTION OF SPUTUM

- When is the sputum produced?
- What is the amount, colour, thickness, and odour?
- Is it ever tinged with blood?

PRESENCE OF CHEST PAIN

- Do you experience any pain with breathing or activity?
- Where is the pain located?
- Describe the pain. How does it feel?
- Does it occur when you breathe in or out?
- How long does it last, and how does it affect your breathing?
- Do you experience any other symptoms when the pain occurs (e.g., nausea, shortness of breath or difficulty breathing, light-headedness, palpitations)?
- What activities precede your pain?
- What do you do to relieve the pain?

PRESENCE OF RISK FACTORS

- Do you have a family history of lung cancer, asthma, other respiratory diseases, cardiovascular disease (including strokes), or tuberculosis?

The nurse should also note the client's height, weight, body mass index, activity pattern, and dietary assessment. In addition to smoking, risk factors include obesity, sedentary lifestyle, and a diet high in saturated fats.

MEDICATION HISTORY

- Have you taken or do you take any medications for heart, blood pressure, or breathing (e.g., bronchodilator, inhalant, opioid)?
- If so, which ones? And what are the dosages, times taken, and results, including side effects?
- Do you use any herbal supplements? If so, which?

PHYSICAL EXAMINATION In assessing a client's oxygenation status, the nurse uses all four physical examination techniques: inspection, palpation, percussion, and auscultation. The nurse first observes the rate, depth, rhythm, and quality of respirations, noting the position the client assumes for breathing. Some clients with chronic respiratory problems prefer to bend forward at the waist to ease breathing or to sit leaning over a table because these positions permit greater lung expansion. Lying on the back or on either side restricts expansion of part of the thorax (the underlying portion). This relatively small increase in expansion may be important to a dyspneic client. Variations in the shape of the thorax may indicate adaptation to chronic respiratory conditions. For example, clients with emphysema frequently develop a barrel chest, in which the ratio of the anterior-posterior to lateral diameter is 1 to 1.

To examine the cardiovascular system, the nurse evaluates the blood pressure in both arms (the results should be within 10 mm Hg of each other) and palpates peripheral pulses for their strength and equality. Auscultation is done to determine the apical pulse rate, rhythm, and the quality of heart sounds, and carotid arteries are auscultated for bruits (the abnormal sound blood makes as it rushes past an obstruction). Information about the cardiovascular system is obtained by assessing the skin for colour, temperature, hair distribution, lesions, and peripheral edema. Clients with extensive peripheral vascular disease may have cool feet with weak pulses and shiny, nearly hairless shins. Pitting edema of the feet and ankles may be noted in clients with heart failure. The ankle-brachial index (ABI) and the toe brachial pressure index (TBPI) provide information about the arterial perfusion to the distal limbs (see Box 42.2). Chapter 27 provides detailed information on assessing the respiratory and cardiac systems.

DIAGNOSTIC STUDIES A range of diagnostic tests are available to assess respiratory and cardiac status, function, and level of oxygenation. Included are sputum samples, throat cultures, visualization procedures, venous and arterial blood specimens, pulmonary function tests, and cardiac monitoring.

Pulse oximetry is a noninvasive means of assessing the oxygen saturation (SpO_2) level, the percentage of hemoglobin that is combined with oxygen. Pulse oximetry is especially useful when invasive arterial blood gas sampling is not feasible to assess arterial oxygen saturation (SaO_2). Measuring oxygen saturation by using pulse oximetry is detailed in Skill 28.7 (page 697).

SPECIMENS **Sputum** is the mucus secretion from the lungs, bronchi, and trachea. It is important to differentiate it from *saliva,* the clear liquid secreted by the salivary glands in the mouth, sometimes referred to as *spit.* Healthy individuals do not produce sputum. Clients need to cough to bring sputum up from the lungs, bronchi, and trachea into the mouth in order to expectorate it into a collecting container. Sputum specimens are usually collected for one or more of the following reasons:

- For *culture and sensitivity,* to identify a specific microorganism and its drug sensitivities.
- For *cytology,* to identify the origin, structure, function, and pathology of cells. Specimens for cytology often require serial collection of three early-morning specimens that are tested to identify cancer in the lung and its specific cell type.
- For *acid-fast bacillus* (AFB), which also requires serial collection, often for 3 consecutive days, to identify the presence of tuberculosis (TB). Some agencies use a special glass container when the presence of AFB is suspected.
- To assess the *effectiveness of therapy.*

Sputum specimens are often collected in the morning. On awakening, the client can cough up the secretions that have accumulated during the night. Sometimes, specimens are collected during postural drainage, when the client can more readily produce sputum. When a client cannot cough, the nurse must sometimes use pharyngeal suctioning to obtain a specimen.

To collect a sputum specimen, the nurse follows these steps:

- Offer mouth care so that the specimen will not be contaminated with microorganisms from the mouth. Do not use mouthwash.
- Ask the client to breathe deeply and then cough up 15 mL to 30 mL of sputum.
- Wear gloves to avoid direct contact with the sputum. Follow special precautions if tuberculosis is suspected, obtaining the specimen in a room equipped with a special airflow system or ultraviolet light. If these options are not available, wear a mask capable of filtering droplet nuclei.
- Ask the client to expectorate (spit out) the sputum into the specimen container. Make sure the sputum does not contact the outside of the container (Figure 42.6). If the outside of the container does

BOX 42.2 CALCULATING AN ANKLE-BRACHIAL INDEX AND TOE BRACHIAL PRESSURE INDEX

Both assessments use a BP cuff and a Doppler ultrasound device to measure the systolic blood pressure using the client's brachial pulse and either the posterior tibial pulse and dorsalis pedis pulse (ABI) or the great toe's distal pulse (TBPI). The pressure index is calculated by dividing either the posterior tibial or dorsalis pedis (whichever is highest) in ABI or the toe's systolic pressure (TBPI) by the highest brachial systolic pressure. For example, for TBPI, the results consist of a right brachial pressure of 130 and a left brachial pressure of 128, along with a left great toe pressure of 130 and a right great toe pressure of 60. The left TBPI is 1 (130 divided by 130) and the right TBPI is 0.46 (60 divided by 130). A TBPI less than 0.64 warrants further evaluation and testing.

Source: From: "Determining the Toe Brachial Pressure Index," by P. A. Bonham, 2003, *Nursing, 33*(9), 54–55. Reprinted with permission.

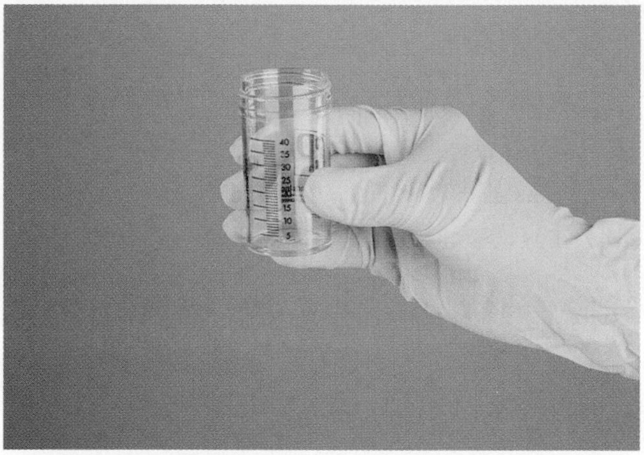

FIGURE 42.6 Sputum specimen container

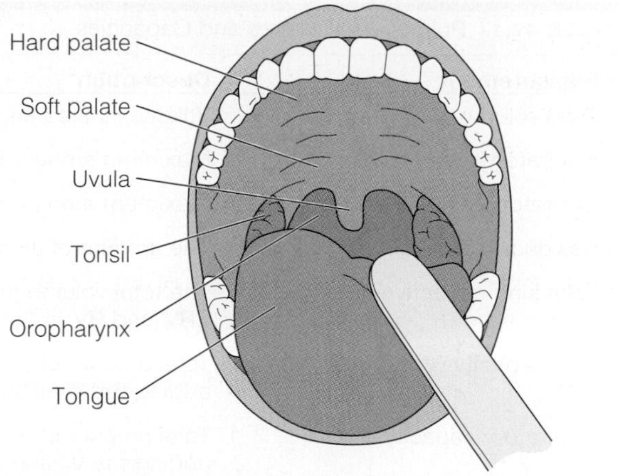

FIGURE 42.7 Depressing the tongue to view the pharynx

become contaminated, wash it with a disinfectant. Place the container in a plastic bag for transport to the lab.

- Label and arrange transport of the specimen to the laboratory. If transport cannot occur immediately, refrigerate the specimen. Bacterial cultures must be started immediately before any contaminating microorganisms can grow, multiply, and produce false results.
- Following sputum collection, offer mouthwash to remove any unpleasant taste.
- Document the amount of sputum collected, colour, odour, consistency (thick, tenacious, watery), and presence of **hemoptysis** (blood in the sputum).

A **throat culture** sample is collected from the mucosa of the oropharynx and tonsillar regions by using a culture swab. The sample is then cultured and examined for the presence of disease-producing microorganisms. To obtain a throat culture specimen, the nurse inserts the swab into the oropharynx and runs the swab along the tonsils and areas on the pharynx that are reddened or contain exudate. The gag reflex, active in some clients, may be decreased by having the client sit upright if health permits, open the mouth, extend the tongue, and say “ah,” and by taking the specimen quickly. The sitting position and extension of the tongue help expose the pharynx; saying “ah” relaxes the throat muscles and helps minimize contraction of the constrictor muscle of the pharynx (the gag reflex). If the posterior pharynx cannot be seen, use a light and depress the tongue with a tongue blade (Figure 42.7). See the Lifespan Considerations box for additional guidelines on taking specimens from infants, children, and older adults.

Lifespan Consideration

Sputum and Throat Specimens

INFANTS

- When taking a throat swab, avoid occluding an infant’s nose because infants normally breathe only through the nose.

CHILDREN

- Have a parent stand the young child between the parent’s legs, with the child’s back to the parent and the parent’s arms gently but firmly around the child. As the parent tips the child’s head back, ask the child to open wide and stick out his or her tongue. Assure the child that the procedure will be over quickly and may tickle but should not hurt.
- Cooperative children can be asked to put their hands under their buttocks, open their mouth, and laugh or pant like a dog (Ball & Bindler, 2008).

OLDER ADULTS

- Older adults may need encouragement to cough because a decreased cough reflex occurs with aging.
- Allow time for rest and recover between coughs when obtaining a sputum specimen.

PULMONARY FUNCTION TESTS *Pulmonary function tests* measure lung volume and capacity. Clients undergoing pulmonary function tests, which are usually carried out by a respiratory therapist, do not require an anaesthetic. The tests are painless, but the client’s cooperation is essential. Clients breathe into a machine and forcefully exhale all their breath and then inhale again. Pulmonary readings are recorded throughout the procedure and compared with any previous readings and with the baseline normal according to age, gender, height, and weight. Nurses need to explain the tests to people beforehand and help clients rest afterward because the tests are often tiring. Table 42.1 describes the measurements taken and Figure 42.8 shows their relationships and normal adult values.

BLOOD TESTS Specimens of venous blood are taken for a *complete blood count* (CBC), which includes hemoglobin and hematocrit measurements, erythrocyte (RBC)

TABLE 42.1 Pulmonary Volumes and Capacities

Measurement	Description
Tidal volume (V_T)	Volume inhaled and exhaled during normal quiet breathing
Inspiratory reserve volume (IRV)	Maximum amount of air that can be inhaled over and above a normal breath
Expiratory reserve volume (ERV)	Maximum amount of air that can be exhaled following a normal exhalation
Residual volume (RV)	The amount of air remaining in the lungs after maximal exhalation
Total lung capacity (TLC)	The total volume of the lungs at maximum inflation; calculated by adding the V_T, IRV, ERV, and RV
Vital capacity (VC)	Total amount of air that can be exhaled after a maximal inspiration; calculated by adding the V_T, IRV, and ERV
Inspiratory capacity (IC)	Total amount of air that can be inhaled following normal quiet exhalation; calculated by adding the V_T and IRV
Functional residual capacity (FRC)	The volume left in the lungs after normal exhalation; calculated by adding the ERV and RV
Minute volume (MV)	The total volume or amount of air breathed in 1 minute

count, leukocyte (white blood cell or WBC) count, RBC indices, and a differential white cell count.

The *hemoglobin* is a measure of the total amount of hemoglobin in the blood. The normal reference range for hemoglobin is 138 g/L to 180 g/L in men and 120 g/L to 160 g/L in women. The *hematocrit* measures the portion of erythrocytes (RBCs) in the plasma. The normal reference range for hematocrit is 0.37 to 0.49 of plasma in men and 0.36 to 0.46 of plasma in women. Hemoglobin and hematocrit increase with dehydration, as the blood becomes more concentrated, and decrease with hypervolemia and resulting hemodilution. Both the hemoglobin and the hematocrit are related to the erythrocyte count, the number of RBCs in whole blood. The normal reference range for RBCs is 4.5×10^{12}/L to 5.3×10^{12}/L in men and 4.1×10^{12}/L to 5.1×10^{12}/L in women. It also varies by age. Low RBC counts are indicative of anemia; clients with chronic hypoxia may develop higher than normal counts, a condition known as *polycythemia*. *RBC indices* may be performed as part of the CBC to evaluate the size, weight, and hemoglobin concentration of RBCs.

The *leukocyte* or *white blood cell* count determines the number of circulating WBCs in whole blood. The normal reference range for WBCs is 4.5×10^9/L to 11.0×10^9/L. High WBC counts are often seen in the presence of a bacterial infection; by contrast, WBC counts may be low if a viral infection is present. In the WBC differential, leukocytes are identified by type (e.g., neutrophil), and the percentage of each type is determined. This information is useful in diagnosing certain disorders that have characteristic patterns of distribution.

A number of other tests may be performed on blood plasma. These often are referred to as *blood chemistries*. Common chemistry examinations include determining

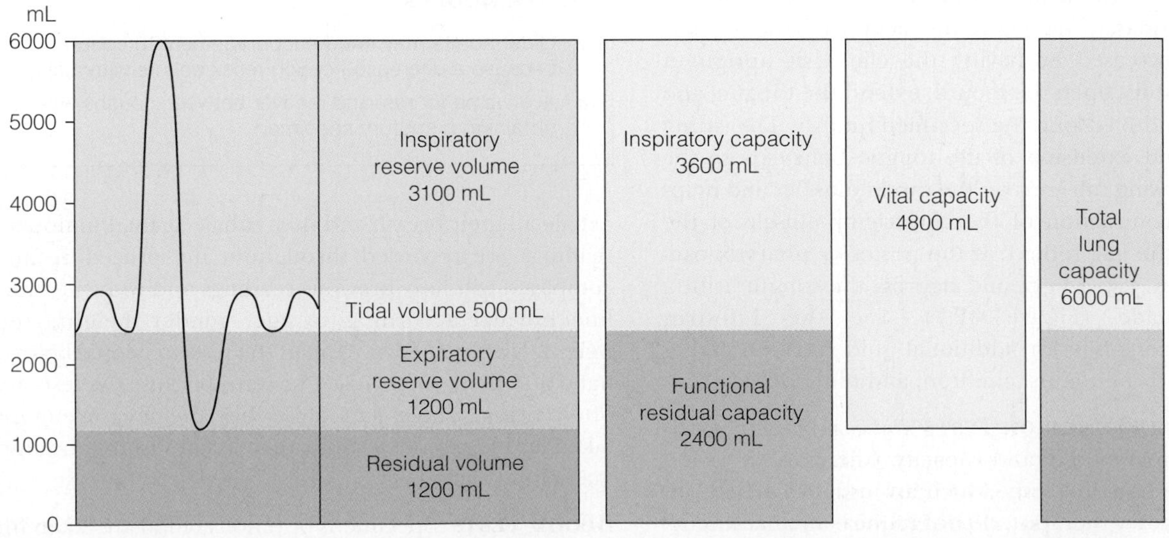

FIGURE 42.8 The relationship of lung volumes and capacities: volumes (mL) shown are for an average adult male; female volumes are 20% to 25% smaller.

serum electrolytes (sodium, potassium, chloride, calcium, and bicarbonate); certain enzymes, including lactic dehydrogenase (LDH), creatine kinase (CK), troponin, aspartate aminotransferase (AST), and alanine aminotransferase (ALT); serum glucose; hormones, such as thyroid hormone; metabolic waste products, such as creatinine and blood urea nitrogen (BUN); and other substances, such as cholesterol and triglycerides. These tests provide valuable diagnostic cues. For example, the enzymes **creatine kinase** and **troponin** are released into the blood during an MI. Elevated levels of these enzymes can help differentiate between an MI (when the cells actually die) and chest pain from a different cause, such as angina or pleuritic pain.

Measurement of *arterial blood gases* is another important diagnostic procedure (see Chapter 43). Specimens of arterial blood are normally taken by respiratory or specialty nurses or medical technicians. Blood for these tests is taken from the radial, brachial, or femoral arteries. Because of the relatively great pressure of the blood in these arteries, it is important to prevent hemorrhaging by applying pressure to the puncture site for at least 5 minutes after removing the needle.

CARDIAC MONITORING **Cardiac monitoring** allows for continuous observation of the client's cardiac rhythm. It is used in many instances: for clients who have known or suspected cardiovascular disease; during and after surgery; to monitor responses to drug therapy; and to monitor clients at risk for serious complications, such as shock. Electrodes placed on the client's chest can be attached to a bedside monitor (Figure 42.9). The monitor is equipped with alarms used to warn of potential problems, such as very fast or very slow heart rates and lethal arrhythmias. The alarm limits are set for 20 beats more and fewer than the client's baseline rate, often at 100 to 110 and 50 to 55, respectively, for adults.

For ambulatory clients (in the hospital or at home), the electrodes connect to a transmitter unit. This unit electronically sends the signal to a central monitor for display or may store the information to be retrieved later in the physician's office. The Holter monitor is a type of ambulatory monitoring. Electrodes are attached and the client wears the monitor for 24 hours. A continuous electrocardiogram is recorded and later analyzed for irregularities. Electrocardiography is most commonly a recording of 12 leads or 12 different views of the heart. In contrast, cardiac monitoring uses only one or two leads at a time.

ELECTROCARDIOGRAPHY Electrocardiography provides a graphic recording of the heart's electrical activity. Electrodes placed on the skin transmit the electrical impulses to an oscilloscope or graphic recorder. The wave forms recorded, the **electrocardiogram** or **ECG**, can then be examined to detect dysrhythmias and alterations in conduction indicative of myocardial ischemia or damage, enlargement of the heart, or drug effects.

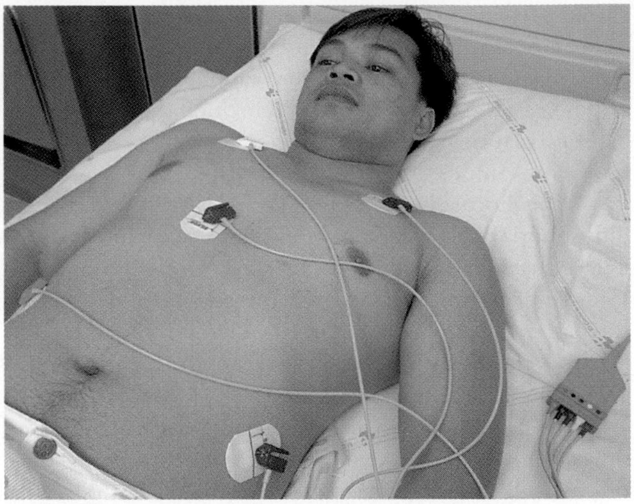

FIGURE 42.9 A client with cardiac monitoring

Stress electrocardiography uses ECGs to assess the client's response to an increased cardiac workload during exercise. As the body's demand for oxygen increases with exercise, the cardiac workload increases, as does the oxygen demand of the heart muscle itself. Clients with coronary artery disease may develop chest pain and characteristic ECG changes during exercise.

VISUALIZATION PROCEDURES A number of visualization procedures can be done to examine the respiratory tract and cardiovascular system. As these procedures are invasive, they require written informed consent. Roentgenography (X-ray), lung scan, endoscopy (bronchoscopy and laryngoscopy), angiography, and echocardiography are a few.

X-ray examination of the chest is done both to diagnose disease and to assess the progress of a disease. For an X-ray examination, the nurse needs to inform the client that jewellery and clothing from the waist up must be removed.

A **lung scan**, also known as a V/Q (ventilation/perfusion) scan, records the emissions from radioisotope-tagged albumin injected intravenously as it circulates through the lung. The *perfusion scan* (Q scan) is used to assess blood flow through the pulmonary vascular system. The *ventilation scan* (V scan), performed after the perfusion scan, detects ventilation abnormalities, particularly in clients with emphysema. For this scan, the client inhales a radioactive gas through a mask and then exhales it into room air. Radiation precautions are necessary only for mothers who are breastfeeding as the amount of radioactivity is very small. The scan takes 20 to 40 minutes.

Angiography is also an invasive procedure requiring informed consent of the client. A radiopaque dye is injected into the vessels to be examined. The flow of the dye through the vessels is assessed by using fluoroscopy and X-rays, and areas of narrowing or blockage can be observed. *Coronary angiography* is performed to evaluate the extent of coronary artery disease; *pulmonary angiography* may be performed to assess the pulmonary vascular system, particularly if pulmonary emboli are suspected. Other vessels that can be studied include the carotid and cerebral arteries, the renal arteries, and the vessels of the lower extremities.

An **echocardiogram** is a noninvasive test that uses ultrasound to visualize structures of the heart and evaluate left ventricular function. Images are produced as ultrasound waves reflect back to a transducer after striking cardiac structures. The client needs to be informed that this test causes no discomfort, although the conductive gel used may be cold.

Laryngoscopy and **bronchoscopy** are sterile procedures that use a laryngoscope and bronchoscope, respectively. During the procedure, tissue samples may be taken for biopsy. A local anaesthetic (e.g., xylocaine) and muscle relaxant (e.g., midazolam [Versed]) are usually given before the examination. The local anaesthetic is sprayed on the client's pharynx to prevent gagging; alternatively, the client gargles with the anaesthetic to anaesthetize the throat. The bronchoscope is then inserted to visualize the larynx or bronchi (Figure 42.10). Informed consent is required for these procedures. Food and fluids are withheld after the procedure until the gag reflex returns.

HEMODYNAMIC STUDIES **Hemodynamics** is the study of the forces or pressures involved in blood circulation. Hemodynamic studies or monitoring procedures may be performed to evaluate fluid status and cardiovascular function. Parameters evaluated in hemodynamic studies include heart rate, arterial blood pressure, central venous pressure, pressures in the pulmonary vascular system, and cardiac output. Some of these parameters—for example, heart rate, arterial blood pressure, and venous pressure—are measured directly by using an arterial, a central venous, or a pulmonary artery catheter; others, such as the stroke volume and cardiac output, are calculated. Hemodynamic studies are performed in a diagnostic cardiac laboratory and require written informed consent. Clients in intensive care and cardiac care units may undergo continuous hemodynamic monitoring to evaluate cardiovascular status and the effect of interventions. Nurses in these units are responsible for ongoing hemodynamic monitoring.

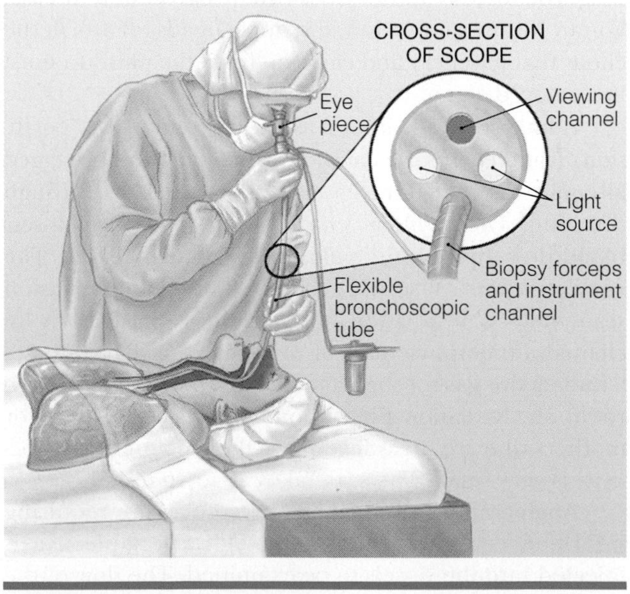

FIGURE 42.10 Bronchoscopy

(From **Medical Terminology: A Living Language,** *3rd ed., by Bonnie F. Fremgen and Suzanne S. Frucht, 2005. Electronically reproduced by permission of Pearson Education, Inc., Upper Saddle River, New Jersey.)*

Diagnosing

NANDA International (2007) includes the following diagnostic labels for clients with oxygenation and circulation problems:

- *Ineffective Airway Clearance:* Inability to clear secretions or obstructions from the respiratory tract to maintain a clear airway
- *Ineffective Breathing Pattern:* Inspiration, expiration, or both that does not provide adequate ventilation
- *Impaired Gas Exchange:* Excess or deficit in oxygenation or carbon dioxide elimination or both at the alveolar-capillary membrane
- *Ineffective Tissue Perfusion (Cardiopulmonary)*: Decrease in oxygen resulting in the failure to nourish the tissues at the capillary level
- *Decreased Cardiac Output:* Inadequate blood pumped by the heart to meet metabolic (demands) of the body
- *Activity Intolerance:* Insufficient physiological or psychological energy to complete required or desired daily activities

The preceding nursing diagnoses may also be the etiology of several other nursing diagnoses. Examples follow:

- *Anxiety* related to ineffective airway clearance and feeling of suffocation
- *Fatigue* related to ineffective breathing pattern
- *Fear* related to chronic disabling respiratory or cardiac illness
- *Powerlessness* related to inability to maintain independence in self-care activities because of altered cardiac tissue perfusion
- *Insomnia* related to orthopnea and required O_2 therapy
- *Social Isolation* related to activity intolerance and inability to travel to usual social activities

Planning

The overall goals for a client with oxygenation and circulation problems are as follows:

- Maintain a patent airway.
- Improve comfort and ease of breathing.

- Maintain or improve pulmonary ventilation and oxygenation.
- Maintain or improve tissue perfusion.
- Maintain or restore an adequate cardiac output.
- Improve ability to participate in physical activities.
- Prevent risks associated with oxygenation problems, such as skin and tissue breakdown, syncope, acid-base imbalances, and feelings of hopelessness and social isolation.

These desired health outcomes provide direction for planning interventions and as criteria for evaluating client progress. A clinical example of desired health outcomes, interventions, and activities is provided in the Sample Care Plan.

PLANNING FOR HOME CARE To provide for continuity of care, the nurse needs to consider the client's learning needs and needs for assistance with care in the home. Planning incorporates an assessment of the client's and family's knowledge and abilities for self-care, financial resources, and evaluation of the need for referrals and for home health services. The Assessment: Home Care box outlines issues related to the client's oxygenation problems and needs at home.

Sample Care Plan for Ineffective Airway Clearance

ASSESSMENT DATA

Nursing Assessment

Johti Singh is a 39-year-old secretary who was admitted to the hospital with an elevated temperature, fatigue, rapid and laboured respirations, and mild dehydration. The nursing history reveals that Ms. Singh has had a "bad cold" for several weeks that just would not go away. She has been dieting for several months and skipping meals. Ms. Singh mentions that in addition to her full-time job as a secretary, she is attending university classes 2 evenings a week. She has smoked one package of cigarettes per day since she was 18 years old. Chest X-ray confirms pneumonia.

Physical Examination

Height: 167.6 cm
Weight: 54.4 kg
Temperature: 39.4°C
Pulse: 116 bpm
Respirations: 24/minute
Blood Pressure: 118/70 mm Hg

Skin pale; cheeks flushed; chills; nasal flaring; use of accessory muscles; inspiratory crackles with diminished breath sounds right base; expectorating thick, yellow sputum

Diagnostic Data

Chest X-ray: right lobar infiltration
WBC: 14.0×10^9/L
pH: 7.49
(normal 7.35–7.45)
$PaCO_2$: 33 mm Hg
(normal 35–45 mm Hg)
HCO_3^-: 20 mmol/L
(normal 22–26 mmol/L)
PaO_2: 80 mm Hg
(normal 80–100 mm Hg)
SaO_2 88% (normal 95%–100%)

Nursing Diagnosis

Ineffective Airway Clearance related to thick sputum, secondary to pneumonia, and fatigue (as evidenced by rapid respirations, nasal flaring, adventitious breath sounds, and thick yellow sputum)

Client Goals

The client will demonstrate effective coughing and increased air exchange.

Desired Health Outcomes

1. Coughs and deep breathes q1h within first 24 h
2. Expectorates secretions from airway whenever necessary
3. Increases fluid intake to 3000 mL by day 2
4. Exhibits normal breath sounds throughout all lung fields

NURSING INTERVENTIONS AND SELECTED ACTIVITIES WITH RATIONALES* *[IN ITALICS]*

Cough Enhancement

- Assist Ms. Singh to a sitting position with head slightly flexed, shoulders relaxed, and knees flexed. *Lying flat causes the abdominal organs to shift toward the chest, crowding the lungs and making it more difficult to breathe.*
- Encourage her to take several deep breaths. *Deep breathing promotes oxygenation before controlled coughing.*
- Encourage her to take a deep breath, hold for 2 seconds, and cough two or three times in succession. *Controlled coughing is accomplished by closure of the glottis and the explosive expulsion of air from the lungs by the work of abdominal and chest muscles.*
- Encourage the use of incentive spirometry, as appropriate. *Breathing exercises help maximize ventilation.*
- Promote systemic fluid hydration, as appropriate. *Adequate fluid intake enhances liquefaction of pulmonary secretions and facilitates expectoration of mucus.*

(continued)

Sample Care Plan for Ineffective Airway Clearance *(continued)*

Respiratory Monitoring

• Monitor rate, rhythm, depth, and effort of respirations.	*This provides a basis for evaluating adequacy of ventilation.*
• Note chest movement, watching for symmetry, use of accessory muscles, and supraclavicular and intercostal muscle retractions.	*The presence of nasal flaring and the use of accessory muscles of respiration can occur in response to ineffective ventilation.*
• Auscultate breath sounds, noting areas of decreased or absent ventilation and presence of adventitious sounds.	*As fluid and mucus accumulate, abnormal breath sounds can be heard, including crackles and diminished breath sounds, owing to fluid-filled air spaces and diminished lung volume.*
• Auscultate lung sounds after treatments to note results.	*This assists in evaluating prescribed treatments and client outcomes.*
• Monitor the client's ability to cough effectively.	*Respiratory tract infections alter the amount and character of secretions. An ineffective cough compromises airway clearance and prevents mucus from being expelled.*
• Monitor client's respiratory secretions.	*People with pneumonia commonly produce rust-coloured, purulent sputum.*
• Institute respiratory therapy treatments (e.g., nebulizer), as needed.	*A variety of respiratory therapy treatments can be used to open constricted airways and liquefy secretions.*
• Monitor for increased restlessness, anxiety, and air hunger.	*These clinical manifestations are indicators of hypoxia.*
• Note changes in O_2 saturation, tidal CO_2, and changes in arterial blood gas values, as appropriate.	*This evaluates the status of oxygenation, ventilation, and acid-base balance.*

Oxygen Therapy

• Instruct Ms. Singh about the importance of leaving the oxygen delivery device on.	*Oxygen demand is greater during febrile illness and physical stress. At low PaO_2 levels in the atmosphere, oxygen saturation falls rapidly; therefore, oxygen should be maintained, especially during activity.*
• Periodically check the oxygen delivery device to ensure that the prescribed concentration is being delivered.	*Too much or too little oxygen can be detrimental, especially in the client with a history of smoking.*
• Observe for signs of oxygen-induced hypoventilation.	*In individuals with chronic lung disease, the stimulus for breathing is low oxygen levels rather than elevated carbon dioxide. This client is at risk for COPD because of smoking. Administration of high level of oxygen could lead to hypoventilation.*

EVALUATION

Goal partially met. Ms. Singh coughs and deep breathes purposefully q1–2h during the day. Her fluid intake is approximately 1500 mL each day. Cough continues to be productive of moderately thick, rust-coloured sputum. Inspiratory crackles continue to be present in right lower lobe. Her PaO_2 is 85 mm Hg and her SaO_2 is 95% on room air.

*Interventions and activities selected are only a sample of those suggested in the *Nursing Interventions Classification (NIC)*, by G. M. Bulechek, H. K. Butcher, and J. C. Dochterman (Eds.), 2008, St. Louis, MO: Mosby Elsevier, and should be individualized for each client.

Implementing

PROMOTING OXYGENATION Most people in good health give little thought to their respiratory and cardiovascular function. Changing position frequently, ambulating, and exercising usually maintain adequate ventilation, gas exchange, and cardiovascular function. The Teaching: Wellness boxes list other ways to promote healthy breathing and maintain a healthy heart.

When people become ill, their respiratory and cardiovascular functions may be inhibited for such reasons as pain and immobility. Shallow respirations inhibit both diaphragmatic excursion and lung distension. The result of inadequate chest expansion is stasis and pooling of respiratory secretions, which ultimately harbour microorganisms and promote infection.

Interventions by the nurse to maintain the normal respirations of clients include the following:

- Positioning the client to allow for maximum chest expansion
- Encouraging or providing frequent changes in position

ASSESSMENT: HOME CARE

Oxygenation

Assess the following areas related to the client's oxygenation problems and needs at home:

CLIENT

- *Self-care abilities:* Ability to ambulate and perform ADLs independently
- *Exercise and activity pattern:* Type and regularity of usual exercise, perceived and actual energy for desired and required leisure activities
- *Assistive devices required:* Supplemental oxygen, humidifier, nebulizer treatments or inhalers; walker, cane, or wheelchair; grab bars, shower chair, and other devices to promote safety and minimize energy expenditure; scale to monitor weight on a regular basis
- *Home environment* for factors that impair airway clearance, gas exchange, or activity tolerance: Indoor pollutants, such as cigarette smoke, dust; allergens, such as pets; dry air; and barriers, such as stairs
- *Current level of knowledge:* Importance of avoiding smoking and other pollutants; dietary salt and other restrictions (if appropriate); recommended activities; medications; need to limit exposure to respiratory infections; use of prescribed nebulizer, multidose inhaler, powdered dose inhaler, home oxygen; activity level

FAMILY

- *Caregiver availability, skills, and responses:* Ability and willingness to provide care as needed (helping with ADLs, providing meals, assisting with transportation and shopping, caring for dependants; performing treatments, such as percussion and postural drainage)
- *Family role changes and coping:* Effect on financial status, parenting and spousal roles, sexuality, social roles
- *Alternative potential primary or respite caregivers:* For example, other family members, volunteers, church members, paid caregivers or housekeeping services; available community respite care (e.g., adult daycare, senior centres)

COMMUNITY

- *Environment:* Usual temperature and humidity, presence of air pollutants, such as automobile exhaust, industrial smoke and pollutants, smoke from field burning
- *Current knowledge of and experience with community resources:* Medical and assistive equipment and supply companies, respiratory and physical therapy services, home health agencies, local pharmacies, available financial assistance, support and educational organizations such as the local lung association, COPD support groups

TEACHING: WELLNESS

Promoting Healthy Breathing

The nurse can teach clients the following ways to promote healthy breathing:

- Sit straight and stand erect to permit full lung expansion.
- Exercise regularly.
- Breathe through the nose.
- Breathe in so as to expand the chest fully.
- Do not smoke cigarettes, cigars, or pipes or use chewing tobacco.
- Eliminate or reduce the use of household pesticides and irritating chemical substances.
- Avoid exposure to second-hand smoke.
- Use building materials that do not emit vapours.
- Make sure furnaces, ovens, wood stoves, and fireplaces are correctly ventilated.
- Support a pollution-free environment.

TEACHING: WELLNESS

Promoting a Healthy Heart

The nurse can teach clients the following ways to keep their heart healthy:

- Exercise regularly, participating in at least 20 minutes (40 minutes is preferable) of vigorous exercise four to five times a week.
- Do not smoke.
- Maintain your ideal weight.
- Eat a diet low in total fat, saturated fats, and cholesterol and high in fibre.
- Drink alcohol in moderation, if at all, consuming no more than 30 mL of alcohol a day (one cocktail, one to one-and-a-half glasses of wine or beer).
- Reduce stress, and manage anger.
- Effectively manage diabetes and hypertension, maintaining blood glucose and blood pressure levels within normal limits.
- If female, consider hormone replacement therapy after menopause (or after a total hysterectomy).
- Consult your health-care provider about the advisability of low-dose Aspirin therapy to further reduce the risk of cardiovascular disease.

- Encouraging ambulation
- Implementing measures that promote comfort, such as giving analgesia
- Providing fluids and humidification
- Encouraging deep breathing and coughing

The semi-Fowler's or high-Fowler's position allows for maximum chest expansion in bed-confined clients, particularly dyspneic clients. The nurse also encourages clients to turn from side to side frequently so that alternate sides of the chest are permitted maximum expansion. Dyspneic clients often sit in bed and lean over their overbed tables (which are raised to a suitable height), usually with a pillow for support. This *orthopneic position* is an adaptation of the high-Fowler's position. It has a further advantage in that, unlike in high-Fowler's, the abdominal organs are not pressing on the diaphragm. Also, a client in the orthopneic position can press the lower part of the chest against the table to facilitate exhaling (Figure 42.11).

PROMOTING CIRCULATION Immobility is detrimental to cardiovascular function. Without exercise of the calf and leg muscles, blood pools in the veins of the lower extremities. This stagnant blood flow may allow clots to develop (*venous thrombosis*). With time, these clots can break loose and become emboli, eventually lodging in the small vessels of the pulmonary vascular system. Blood flow and gas exchange in the lungs are then impaired.

Many nursing interventions can help maintain cardiovascular function. They can be classified as vascular or cardiac.

VASCULAR Vascular nursing interventions to maintain cardiovascular function include the following:

- Position with the legs elevated to promote venous return to the heart. Although this intervention is important for people with venous dysfunction, care should be taken to avoid this position in clients with cardiac dysfunction because it will increase preload and may stress a dysfunctional heart.
- Avoid pillows under the knees or more than 15 degrees of knee flexion to improve blood flow to the lower extremities and reduce venous stagnation.
- Avoid crossing the legs or ankles.
- Encourage leg exercises, such as flexion and extension of the feet and active contraction and relaxation of calf muscles, for a client on bed rest, and promote ambulation as soon as possible.
- Encourage or provide frequent position changes.

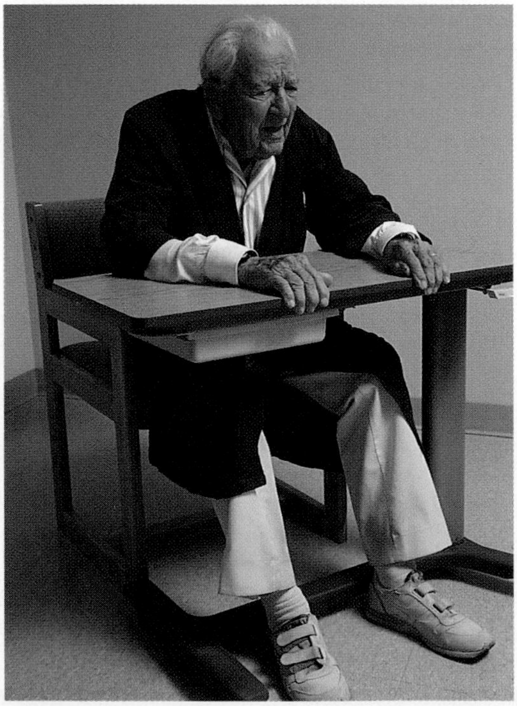

FIGURE 42.11 A client using the overbed table to assist with breathing

CARDIAC Cardiac nursing interventions to maintain cardiovascular function include the following:

- Position the client in high-Fowler's position to decrease preload and reduce pulmonary congestion.
- Monitor intake and output. Fluid restriction is not usually required for clients with mild to moderate cardiac dysfunction. With severe heart failure, fluid restriction may be required.

DEEP BREATHING AND COUGHING The nurse can facilitate respiratory functioning by encouraging deep-breathing exercises and coughing to remove secretions. Breathing exercises are frequently indicated for clients with restricted chest expansion, such as those with COPD or clients recovering from thoracic surgery and pneumonia.

A commonly employed breathing exercise is abdominal (diaphragmatic) and pursed-lip breathing. *Abdominal (diaphragmatic) breathing* permits deep full breaths with little effort. *Pursed-lip breathing* helps the client develop control over breathing. The pursed lips create a resistance to the air flowing out of the lungs, thereby prolonging exhalation and preventing airway collapse by maintaining positive airway pressure. The client purses the lips as if about to whistle and breathes out slowly and gently, tightening the abdominal muscles to exhale more effectively. The client usually inhales to a count of three and exhales to a count of seven.

Forceful coughing is often less effective than controlled or huff coughing techniques. Instructions for abdominal (diaphragmatic) and pursed-lip breathing and cough techniques are provided in the Teaching: Clinical boxes.

HYDRATION Adequate hydration maintains the moisture of the respiratory mucous membranes. Normally, respiratory tract secretions are thin and, therefore, are moved readily by ciliary action. However, when the client is dehydrated or when the environment has a low humidity, the respiratory secretions can become thick and tenacious. Fluid intake should be individually determined on the basis of respiratory and cardiovascular status. See Chapter 43 for normal daily fluid intake.

Humidifiers are devices that add water vapour to inspired air. Room humidifiers provide cool mist to room

TEACHING: CLINICAL

Abdominal (Diaphragmatic) and Pursed-Lip Breathing

The following are instructions for abdominal (diaphragmatic) and pursed-lip breathing:

- Assume a comfortable semisitting position in bed or a chair *or* a lying position in bed with one pillow.
- Flex your knees to relax the muscles of the abdomen.
- Place one or both hands on your abdomen, just below the ribs.
- Breathe in deeply through your nose, keeping your mouth closed.
- Concentrate on feeling your abdomen rise (expand) as far as possible; stay relaxed, and avoid arching your back. If you have difficulty raising your abdomen, take a quick, forceful breath through the nose.
- Then, purse your lips as if about to whistle, and breathe out slowly and gently, making a slow "whooshing" sound without puffing out the cheeks. This *pursed-lip breathing* creates a resistance to air flowing out of the lungs, increases pressure within the bronchi (main air passages), and minimizes collapse of smaller airways, a common problem for people with COPD.
- Concentrate on feeling the abdomen fall or sink, and tighten (contract) the abdominal muscles while breathing out to enhance effective exhalation. Count to seven during exhalation.
- Use this exercise every 2 hours and whenever you are feeling short of breath. Increase gradually to 5 to 10 minutes 4 times a day. Regular practice will help you do this type of breathing without conscious effort. The exercise, once learned, can be performed when sitting upright, standing, and walking.

air. Nebulizers are used to deliver humidity and medications. They may be used with oxygen delivery systems to provide moistened air directly to the client. Their purposes are to prevent mucous membranes from drying and becoming irritated and to loosen secretions for easier expectoration. It is important to follow the manufacturer's directions for cleaning and maintaining humidifiers to reduce potential sources of bacterial growth.

MEDICATIONS A number of types of medications can be used for clients with oxygenation problems. Bronchodilators, expectorants, and cough suppressants are some medications that are used to treat respiratory problems.

Bronchodilators, including sympathomimetic drugs and xanthines, reduce bronchospasm, opening tight or congested airways and facilitating ventilation. These drugs can be administered orally or intravenously, but the preferred route is by inhalation to prevent many systemic side effects. Since drugs used to dilate the bronchioles and improve breathing are usually drugs that enhance the sympathetic nervous system, clients must be monitored for side effects of increased heart rate, blood pressure, anxiety, and restlessness. This is especially important in older adults, who may also have cardiac problems. Another class of drugs used is the *anti-inflammatory drugs,* such as glucocorticoids. They can be given orally, intravenously, or by inhaler. They work by decreasing the edema and inflammation in the airways and allowing a better air exchange. If both bronchodilators and anti-inflammatory drugs are ordered by inhaler, the client should be instructed to use the bronchodilator inhaler first and then the anti-inflammatory. If the bronchioles are dilated first, more tissue is exposed for the anti-inflammatory drugs to act on.

TEACHING: CLINICAL

Controlled and Huff Coughing

Forceful coughing is often less effective than using controlled or huff coughing techniques:

- After using a bronchodilator treatment (if prescribed), inhale deeply, and hold your breath for a few seconds.
- Cough twice. The first cough loosens the mucus; the second expels secretions.
- For huff coughing, lean forward and exhale sharply with a "huff" sound. This technique helps keep your airways open while moving secretions up and out of the lungs.
- Inhale by taking rapid short breaths in succession ("sniffing") to prevent mucous from moving back into smaller airways.
- Rest.
- Try to avoid prolonged episodes of coughing as these may cause fatigue and hypoxia.

The *leukotriene modifiers* are relatively new medications that suppress the effects of leukotrienes on the smooth muscle of the respiratory tract. Leukotrienes cause bronchoconstriction, mucous production, and edema of the respiratory tract.

Expectorants help break up mucus, making it more liquid and easier to expectorate. Guaifenesin is a common expectorant found in many prescription and nonprescription cough syrups. When frequent or prolonged coughing interrupts sleep, a *cough suppressant,* such as codeine, may be prescribed. See the Teaching: Clinical box on using cough medications.

Other medications can be used to improve oxygenation by improving cardiovascular function. The *digitalis glycosides* act directly on the heart to improve the strength of contraction and slow the heart. The beta-adrenergic agonists, such as propranolol, affect the sympathetic nervous system to reduce the workload of the heart. These drugs can negatively affect people with asthma or COPD as they can constrict airways.

Other drugs, such as *nitrates, calcium channel blockers,* and *angiotensin-converting enzyme* (*ACE*) *inhibitors,* reduce

TEACHING: CLINICAL

Using Cough Medications

Teach clients to use these guidelines before starting a cough medication:

- Do not take cough medications in excessive amounts because of adverse side effects. Consult your nurse, pharmacist, or physician, as needed.
- If you have diabetes mellitus, avoid cough syrups that contain sugar or alcohol; these can disturb glucose metabolism.
- Be aware of side effects (e.g., drowsiness) that can make the operation of machinery dangerous.
- Be aware of interactions of cough medications with prescription and other nonprescription medications.

the workload of the heart and prevent vasoconstriction. In addition, various drugs are used to treat cardiac dysrhythmias. *Direct vasodilators* may be used for clients with peripheral vascular disease.

INCENTIVE SPIROMETRY **Incentive spirometers** (Figure 42.12), also referred to as *sustained maximal inspiration devices* (SMIs), measure the flow of air inhaled through a mouthpiece and are used to do the following:

- Maintain or improve pulmonary ventilation
- Counteract the effects of anaesthesia or hypoventilation
- Loosen respiratory secretions
- Facilitate respiratory gaseous exchange
- Expand collapsed alveoli

They offer an incentive to improve *inhalation*. When using an SMI, the client should be assisted into position, preferably an upright sitting position in bed or a chair, that facilitates maximum ventilation. The Teaching: Clinical box on using an incentive spirometer provides specific instructions for clients.

PERCUSSION, VIBRATION, AND POSTURAL DRAINAGE Percussion, vibration, and postural drainage (PVD) are dependent nursing functions performed according to a physician's order and agency policy. These procedures are contraindicated for some conditions (for example, rib fractures and bleeding disorders). Percussion, sometimes called *clapping*, is forceful striking of the skin with cupped hands. Mechanical percussion cups and vibrators are also available. When the hands are used, the fingers and thumb are held together and flexed slightly to form a cup, as if scooping up water. Percussion over congested lung areas can mechanically dislodge tenacious secretions from the bronchial walls. Cupped hands trap the air against the chest. The trapped air sets up vibrations through the chest wall.

To percuss a client's chest, the nurse follows these steps:

- Position the client (the lateral position is recommended if tolerated by client).
- Cover the area with a towel or gown to reduce discomfort.
- Ask the client to breathe slowly and deeply to promote relaxation.
- Alternately flex and extend the wrists rapidly to strike the chest (Figure 42.13).
- Percuss each affected lung segment for 1 to 2 minutes or according to agency policy.

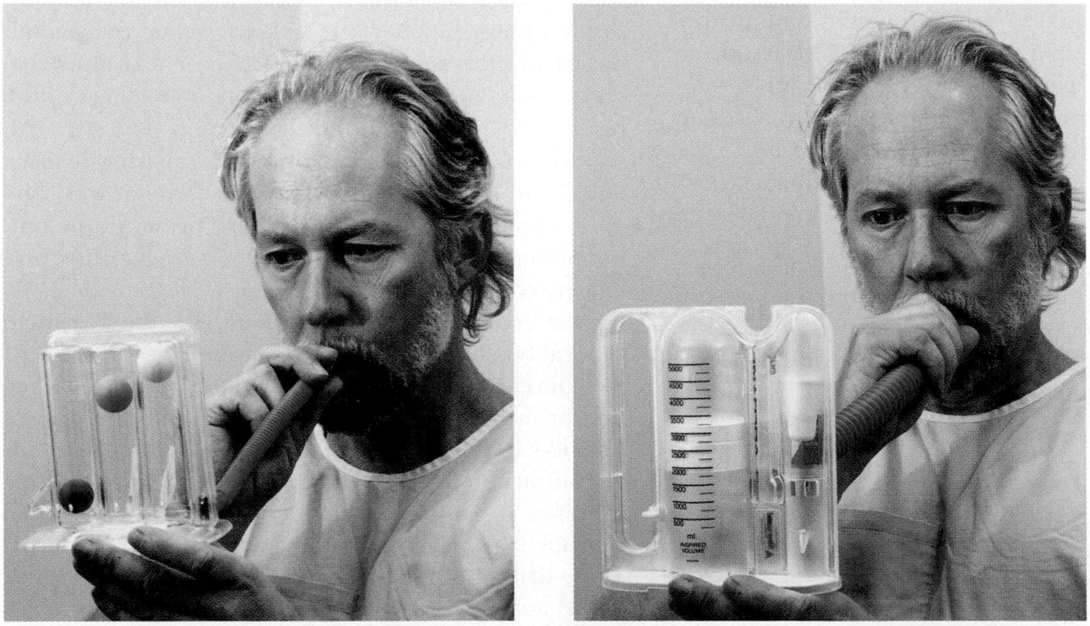

A B

FIGURE 42.12 **A:** Flow-oriented SMI; **B:** volume-oriented SMI

TEACHING: CLINICAL

Using an Incentive Spirometer

The following are guidelines for clients to use an incentive spirometer:

- Hold or place the spirometer in an upright position. A tilted *flow-oriented* device requires less effort to raise the balls or cylinder; a volume-oriented device will not function correctly unless upright.
- Exhale normally.
- Seal your lips tightly around the mouthpiece.
- Take in a *slow, deep breath* to elevate the balls or cylinder, and then hold the breath for 2 seconds initially, increasing to 6 seconds (optimum), to keep the balls or cylinder elevated, if possible.
- For a flow-oriented device, avoid brisk, low-volume breaths that snap the balls to the top of the chamber. Greater lung expansion is achieved with a very slow inspiration than with a brisk, shallow breath, even though it may not elevate the balls or keep them elevated while you hold your breath. Sustained elevation of the balls or cylinder ensures adequate ventilation of the alveoli (lung air sacs).
- If you have difficulty breathing only through your mouth, a nose clip can be used.
- Remove the mouthpiece, and exhale normally.
- Cough after the incentive effort. Deep ventilation can loosen secretions, and coughing can facilitate their removal.
- Relax, and take several normal breaths before using the spirometer again.
- Repeat the procedure several times and then four or five times hourly. Practice increases inspiratory volume, maintains alveolar ventilation, and prevents atelectasis (collapse of the air sacs).
- Clean the mouthpiece with water and shake it dry.

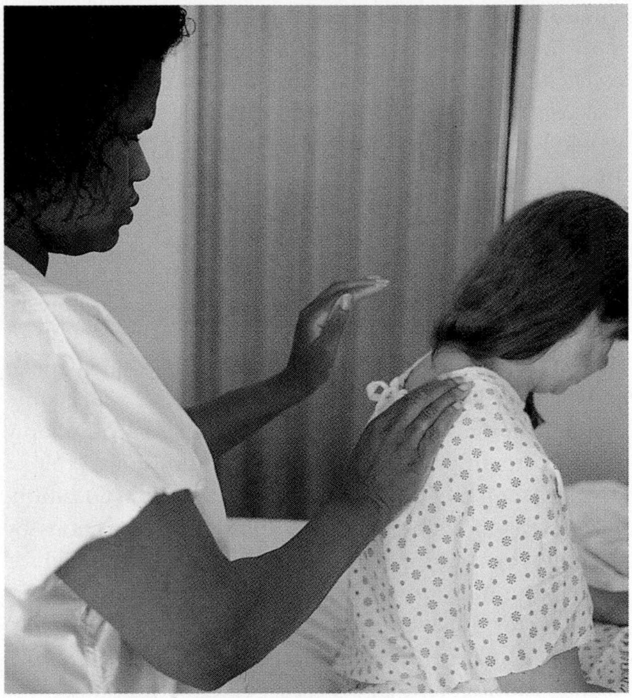

FIGURE 42.13 Percussing the upper posterior chest

When done correctly, the percussion action should produce a hollow, popping sound. Percussion is avoided over certain easily injured structures, such as the breasts, sternum, spinal column, and kidneys.

Vibration is a series of vigorous quiverings produced by hands that are placed flat against the client's chest wall (Figure 42.14). Vibration is used after percussion to increase the turbulence of the exhaled air and, thus, loosen thick secretions. It is often done alternately with percussion.

Postural drainage is the drainage by gravity of secretions from various lung segments. Secretions that remain in the lungs or respiratory airways promote bacterial growth and subsequent infection. They also can obstruct the smaller airways and cause atelectasis. Secretions in the major airways, such as the trachea and the right and left main bronchi, are usually coughed into the pharynx, where they can be expectorated, swallowed, or effectively removed by suctioning.

A wide variety of positions is necessary to drain all segments of the lungs, but not all positions are required for every client. Only those positions that drain specific affected areas are used. The lower lobes require drainage most frequently because the upper lobes drain during normal daily activities. Before postural drainage, the client may be given a bronchodilator medication or nebulization therapy to loosen secretions, as ordered by a physician. Frequently, postural drainage treatments are

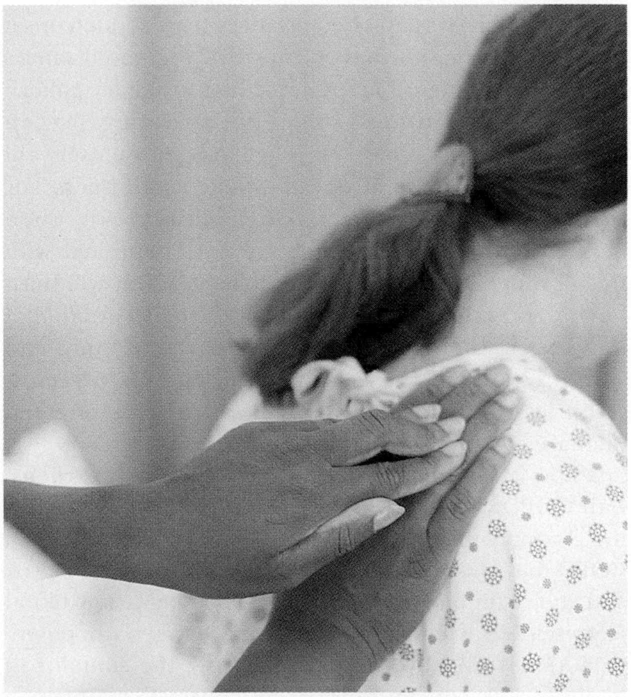

FIGURE 42.14 Vibrating the upper posterior chest

scheduled two or three times daily, as ordered by a physician, depending on the degree of lung congestion. Be aware of the client's exercise tolerance as postural drainage can be tiring. Postural drainage should also be avoided after meals as it puts the client at risk for vomiting and aspiration.

The nurse needs to evaluate the client's tolerance of postural drainage by assessing the stability of the client's vital signs, particularly the pulse and respiratory rates, and by noting signs of intolerance, such as pallor, diaphoresis, dyspnea, and fatigue. Some clients do not react well to certain drainage positions, and the nurse must make appropriate adjustments. For example, some become dyspneic in the Trendelenburg position and require only a moderate tilt or a shorter time in that position.

The sequence for PVD is usually as follows: positioning, percussion, vibration, and removal of secretions by coughing or suction. Each position is usually assumed for 10 to 15 minutes, although beginning treatments may start with shorter times that are gradually increased. Usually, the entire treatment, including preparatory nebulization, deep breathing, and all postures, takes 30 minutes.

Before and immediately after PVD, the nurse should auscultate the client's lungs and compare the findings with baseline data. Following PVD, document the amount, colour, and character of expectorated secretions, and note how well the client tolerated the procedure.

OXYGEN THERAPY Clients who have difficulty ventilating all areas of their lungs, those whose gas exchange is impaired, or people with heart failure may require oxygen therapy to prevent hypoxia. The concentration, method of delivery, and number of litres per minute of oxygen should be prescribed by a physician or nurse practitioner. In certain circumstances (e.g., sudden onset of chest pain or shortness of breath), registered nurses may initiate oxygen therapy according to agency policy.

Safety precautions are essential during oxygen therapy (see Box 42.3). Although oxygen by itself will not burn or explode, it does facilitate combustion. For example, a bed sheet ordinarily burns slowly when ignited in the atmosphere; however, if saturated with free-flowing oxygen and ignited by a spark, it will burn rapidly and explosively. The greater the concentration of the oxygen, the more rapidly fires start and burn, and such fires are difficult to extinguish. Because oxygen is colourless, odourless, and tasteless, people are often unaware of its presence.

Low oxygen concentrations are essential for clients with COPD. A high carbon dioxide level in the blood is the normal stimulus to breathe. However, people with COPD may chronically have a high carbon dioxide level, and their stimulus to breathe is hypoxemia (low blood oxygen level). High concentrations of oxygen can potentially relieve this hypoxemia, removing the stimulus to breathe; low concentrations, by contrast, maintain a slightly hypoxemia state, maintaining the respiratory drive.

BOX 42.3 OXYGEN THERAPY SAFETY PRECAUTIONS

Nurses should follow these guidelines when using oxygen therapy with clients:

- Place cautionary signs reading "No smoking: Oxygen in use" on the client's door, at the foot or head of the bed, and on the oxygen equipment.
- Instruct the client and visitors about the hazard of smoking with oxygen in use.
- For home oxygen use, teach family members and roommates to smoke only outside or in rooms well away from the client.
- Make sure that electric devices (such as razors, hearing aids, radios, televisions, and heating pads) are in good working order to prevent the occurrence of short-circuit sparks.
- Avoid materials that generate static electricity, such as woollen blankets and synthetic fabrics. Cotton blankets should be used, and clients and caregivers are advised to wear cotton fabrics.
- Avoid the use of volatile, flammable materials, such as oils, greases, alcohol, ether, and acetone (e.g., nail polish remover) near clients receiving oxygen.
- Ground electric monitoring equipment, suction machines, and portable diagnostic machines.
- Make known the location of fire extinguishers, and make sure personnel are trained in their use and in protocols associated with fire safety.

Oxygen is supplied in several different ways. In hospitals and long-term-care facilities, it is usually piped into wall outlets at the client's bedside, making it readily available for use at all times. Tanks or cylinders of oxygen under pressure are also frequently available for use when wall oxygen either is unavailable or is impractical (e.g., for transporting oxygen-dependent clients between treatment areas).

Clients who require oxygen therapy in the home can use small cylinders of oxygen, oxygen in liquid form, or an oxygen concentrator (see the Reflect on Primary Health Care box). Portable oxygen delivery systems are available to increase the client's independence. Home oxygen therapy services are readily available in most communities. These services generally supply the oxygen and delivery devices, training for the client and family, equipment maintenance, and emergency services should a problem occur.

REFLECT ON PRIMARY HEALTH CARE

The *appropriate use of technology* is evident when home oxygen therapy lets clients with severe cardiac or respiratory disease achieve their developmental and life goals. Consider how the legislation that requires cigarette products to be behind closed cabinets serves as a *health-promotion* strategy to ensure cardiac and respiratory health.

Oxygen administered from a cylinder or wall-outlet system is dry. Dry gases dehydrate the respiratory mucous membranes. Humidifying devices that add water vapour to inspired air are thus an essential adjunct of oxygen therapy, particularly for litre flows of more than 2 L per minute (Figure 42.15). These devices provide 20% to 40% humidity. The oxygen passes through sterile distilled water or tap water and then along a line to the device through which the moistened oxygen is inhaled (e.g., a cannula, nasal catheter, or oxygen mask).

Humidifiers prevent mucous membranes from drying and becoming irritated, and they loosen secretions for easier expectoration. Oxygen passing through water picks up water vapour before it reaches the client. The more bubbles created during this process, the more water vapour is produced. Very low litre flows (e.g., 1 L to 2 L per minute by nasal cannula) do not require humidification.

Oxygen cylinders need to be handled and stored with caution and strapped securely in wheeled transport devices or stands to prevent possible falls and outlet breakages. They should be placed away from traffic areas and heaters.

To use an oxygen wall outlet, the nurse carries out these steps:

- Attach the flow meter (Figure 42.16) to the wall outlet, exerting firm pressure. The flow meter should be in the off position.

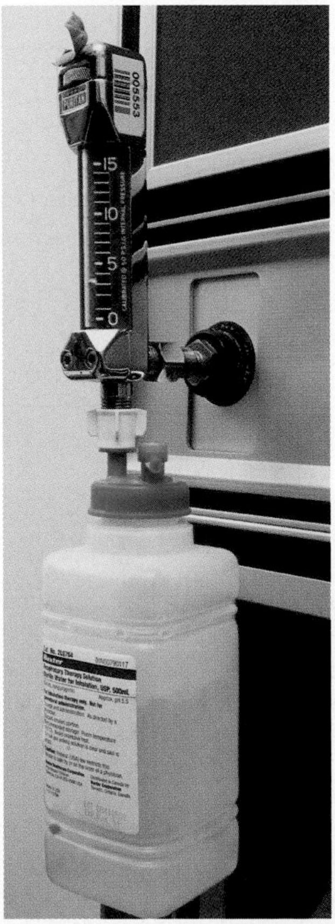

FIGURE 42.15 An oxygen humidifier attached to a wall outlet oxygen flow meter

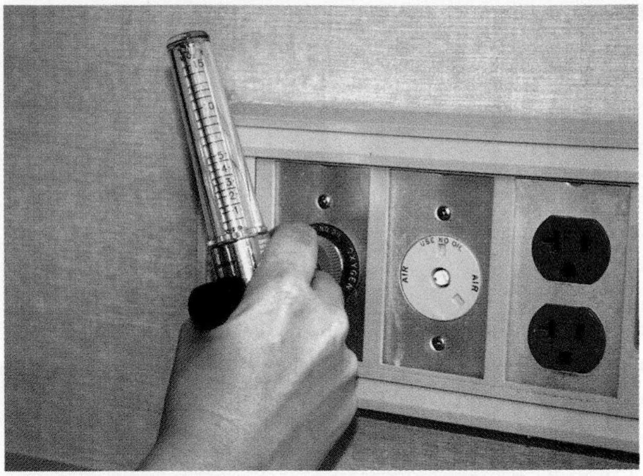

FIGURE 42.16 Insert flow meter into the wall unit.

- Fill the humidifier bottle with sterile distilled water in accordance with agency protocol. (This can be done before coming to the bedside.) The sterile distilled water should be changed every 24 hours or according to agency policy.
- Attach the humidifier bottle to the base of the flow meter.
- Attach the prescribed oxygen tubing and delivery device to the humidifier.
- Regulate the flow meter to the prescribed level. The line for the prescribed flow rate (e.g., 2 L/min) should be in the middle of the ball of the flow meter (Figure 42.17).

OXYGEN DELIVERY SYSTEMS A number of systems are available to deliver oxygen to the client. The choice of system depends on the client's oxygen needs, comfort, and developmental considerations, agency policy, and physician's orders. With many systems, the oxygen delivered mixes with room air before being inspired. The amount of oxygen delivered is determined by regulating its flow rate (e.g., 2 L to 6 L per minute). Precise regulation

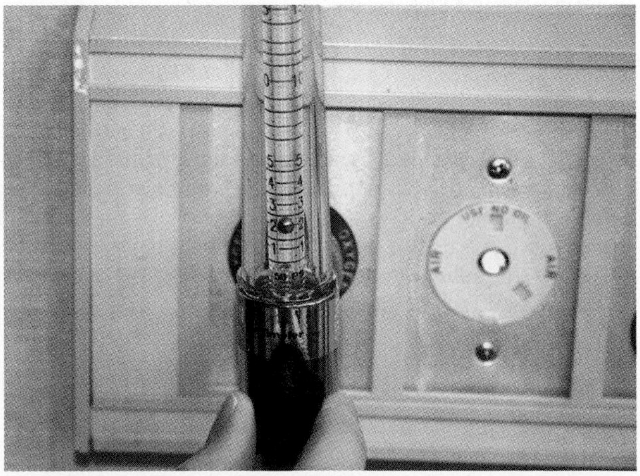

FIGURE 42.17 This flow meter is set to deliver 2 L/minute.

of the percentage of inspired oxygen, or fraction of inspired oxygen (FiO_2), is impossible. When it is important to regulate the percentage of oxygen received by the client more precisely, a device, such as a Venturi mask, can be used.

CANNULA The nasal cannula (nasal prongs) is the most common and inexpensive device used to administer oxygen (Figure 42.18). The nasal cannula is easy to apply and does not interfere with the client's ability to eat or talk. It is relatively comfortable, permits some freedom of movement, and is usually well tolerated by the client. It delivers a relatively low concentration of oxygen (24% to 45%) at flow rates of 2 L to 6 L per minute. At more than 6 L per minute, the client tends to swallow air, and the FiO_2 is *not* increased. Limitations to the cannula include its inability to deliver higher concentrations of oxygen and the fact that it can be drying and irritating to the mucous membranes. Administering oxygen by cannula is detailed in Skill 42.1.

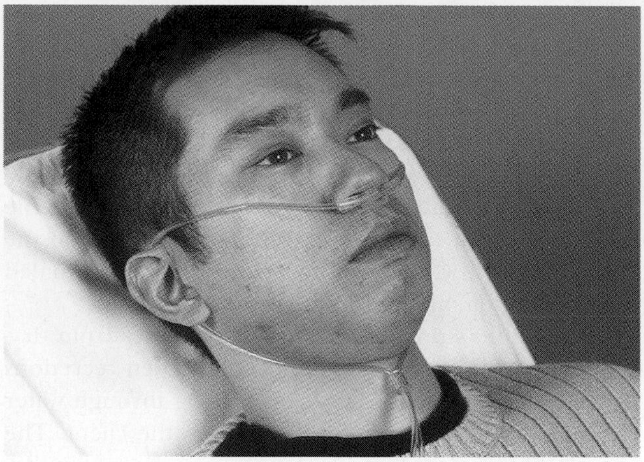

FIGURE 42.18 A nasal cannula

FACEMASK Facemasks that cover the client's nose and mouth can be used for oxygen inhalation. Exhalation

SKILL 42.1

ADMINISTERING OXYGEN BY CANNULA, FACEMASK, OR FACE TENT

Before administering oxygen, check (1) the prescription for oxygen, including the administering device and the litre flow rate (L/min) or the percentage of oxygen; (2) the levels of oxygen (PO_2) and carbon dioxide (PCO_2) in the client's arterial blood (PaO_2 is normally 80 mm Hg to 100 mm Hg; $PaCO_2$ is normally 35 mm Hg to 45 mm Hg); (3) whether the client has COPD; (4) the SaO_2; and (5) the hemoglobin.

PURPOSES

Cannula

- To deliver a relatively low concentration of oxygen when only minimal O_2 support is required
- To allow uninterrupted delivery of oxygen while the client ingests food or fluids

Facemask

- To provide moderate O_2 support and a higher concentration of oxygen or humidity than is provided by cannula

Face Tent

- To provide high humidity
- To provide oxygen when a mask is poorly tolerated
- To provide a high flow of O_2 when attached to a Venturi system

ASSESSMENT

See Chapter 27 for complete details on respiratory and cardiac assessment.

Assess vital signs; arterial blood gas levels; oxygen saturation levels (see Skill 28.7, p. 697); signs of hypoxia (e.g., tachycardia, tachypnea, dyspnea, pallor of mucous membranes); signs of hypercarbia (e.g., restlessness, hypertension, headache); lung sounds; patency of nares (if nasal cannula is to be used); mental status; signs of oxygen toxicity (e.g., tracheal irritation, cough, decreased pulmonary ventilation); and mouth breathing.

Equipment

Cannula

- Oxygen supply with a flow meter and adapter
- Humidifier with distilled water or tap water according to agency protocol
- Nasal cannula and tubing
- Gauze pads, tape

Facemask

- Oxygen supply with a flow meter and adapter
- Humidifier with sterile distilled or tap water according to agency policy
- Prescribed facemask of the appropriate size
- Padding for the elastic band

Face Tent

- Oxygen supply with a flow meter and adapter
- Humidifier with sterile distilled or tap water according to agency policy
- Face tent of the appropriate size
- Gauze pads, tape

(continued)

SKILL 42.1

ADMINISTERING OXYGEN BY CANNULA, FACEMASK, OR FACE TENT *(continued)*

IMPLEMENTATION

Preparation

1. Determine the need for oxygen therapy, and verify the prescription for the therapy.
   - In an emergency situation, provide the client with oxygen first before commencing a complete respiratory assessment.
   - Perform a respiratory assessment to determine the need for O_2 therapy and to develop baseline data if not already available.
2. Prepare the client and the support people.
   - Assist the client to a semi-Fowler's position, if possible. **Rationale: This position permits easier chest expansion and, hence, easier breathing**.
   - Explain that oxygen is not dangerous when safety precautions are observed and that it will ease the discomfort of dyspnea. Inform the client and support people about the safety precautions regarding oxygen use.

Performance

1. Before performing the procedure, introduce yourself and verify the client's identity by using agency protocol. Explain to the client what you are going to do, why it is necessary, and how he or she can cooperate. Discuss how the effects of the oxygen therapy will be used in planning further care or treatments.
2. Perform hand hygiene and observe other appropriate infection prevention and control procedures.
3. Provide for client privacy, if appropriate.
4. Set up the oxygen equipment and the humidifier.
   - Attach the flow meter to the wall outlet or tank. The flow meter should be in the off position.
   - If needed, fill the humidifier bottle. (This can be done before coming to the bedside.)
   - Attach the humidifier bottle to the base of the flow meter.
   - Attach the prescribed oxygen tubing and delivery device to the humidifier.
5. Turn on the oxygen at the prescribed rate, and ensure proper functioning.
   - Check that the oxygen is flowing freely through the tubing. There should be no kinks in the tubing, and the connections should be airtight. You should see bubbles in the humidifier as the oxygen flows through the water. You should feel the oxygen at the outlets of the cannula, mask, or tent.
   - Set the oxygen at the flow rate prescribed.
6. Apply the appropriate oxygen delivery device.

Cannula

- Put the cannula over the client's face, with the outlet prongs fitting into the nares and the elastic band around the head (Figure 42.18). Some models have a strap to adjust under the chin.
- If the cannula will not stay in place, tape it at the sides of the face.
- Pad the tubing and band over the ears and cheekbones, as needed.

Facemask

- Guide the mask toward the client's face, and apply it from the nose downward.
- Fit the mask to the contours of the client's face (see Figure 42.19). **Rationale: The mask should mould to the face so that very little oxygen escapes into the eyes or around the cheeks and chin**.
- Secure the elastic band around the client's head so that the mask is snug but comfortable.
- Pad the band behind the ears and over bony prominences. **Rationale: Padding will prevent irritation from the mask**.

Face Tent

- Place the tent over the client's face, and secure the ties around the head (see Figure 42.23). Assess the client regularly.
- Assess the client's vital signs, level of anxiety, colour, and ease of respirations, and provide support while the client adjusts to the device.
- Assess the client in 15 to 30 minutes, depending on the client's condition, and regularly thereafter.
- Assess the client regularly for clinical signs of hypoxia, tachycardia, confusion, dyspnea, restlessness, and cyanosis. Review oxygen saturation or arterial blood gas results if they are available.

Nasal Cannula

- Assess the client's nares for encrustations and irritation. Apply a water-soluble lubricant, as required, to soothe the mucous membranes.
- Assess the top of the patient's ears for any signs of irritation from the cannula strap. If present, padding with a gauze pad may relieve the discomfort.

Facemask or Tent

- Inspect the facial skin frequently for dampness or chafing, and dry and treat it as needed.
- Inspect the equipment on a regular basis.
- Check the litre flow and the level of water in the humidifier in 30 minutes and whenever providing care to the client.
- Maintain the level of water in the humidifier.
- Make sure that safety precautions are being followed.
- Document relevant data.
- Record the initiation of the therapy and all nursing assessments.

EVALUATION

- Perform follow-up based on findings that deviated from expected or normal for the client. Relate findings to previous data if available (e.g., check SaO_2 or SpO_2 to evaluate adequate oxygenation).
- Report significant deviations from normal to the appropriate members of the health-care team.

ports on the sides of the mask allow exhaled carbon dioxide to escape. A variety of oxygen masks are marketed:

- The *simple facemask* delivers oxygen concentrations from 40% to 60% at litre flows of 5 L to 8 L per minute, respectively (Figure 42.19).
- The *partial rebreather mask* delivers oxygen concentrations of 60% to 90% at litre flows of 6 L to 10 L per minute, respectively, depending on client respiratory rate and depth. The oxygen reservoir bag that is attached allows the client to rebreathe about the first third of the exhaled air in conjunction with oxygen (Figure 42.20). Thus, it increases the FiO_2 by recycling expired oxygen. The partial rebreather bag must not totally deflate during inspiration to avoid carbon dioxide buildup. If this problem occurs, the nurse increases the litre flow of oxygen.
- The *nonrebreather mask* delivers the highest oxygen concentration possible—that is, 95% to 100%—by means other than intubation or mechanical ventilation, depending on client respiratory rate and depth. One-way valves on the mask and between the reservoir bag and the mask prevent the room air and the client's exhaled air from entering the bag so that only the oxygen in the bag is inspired (Figure 42.21). To prevent carbon dioxide buildup, the nonrebreather bag must not totally deflate during inspiration. If it does, the nurse can correct this problem by increasing the litre flow of oxygen.
- The *Venturi mask* delivers oxygen concentrations varying from 24% to 50% at litre flows of 4 L to 10 L per minute (Figure 42.22). The Venturi mask has wide-bore tubing and colour-coded jet adapters that correspond to a precise oxygen concentration

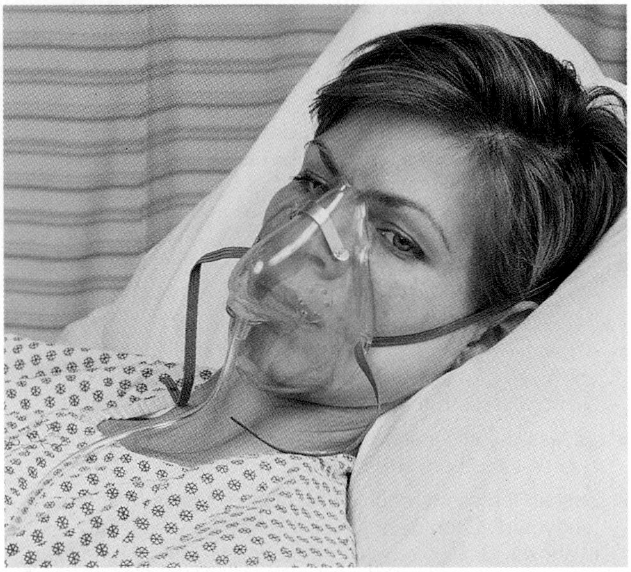

FIGURE 42.19 A simple facemask

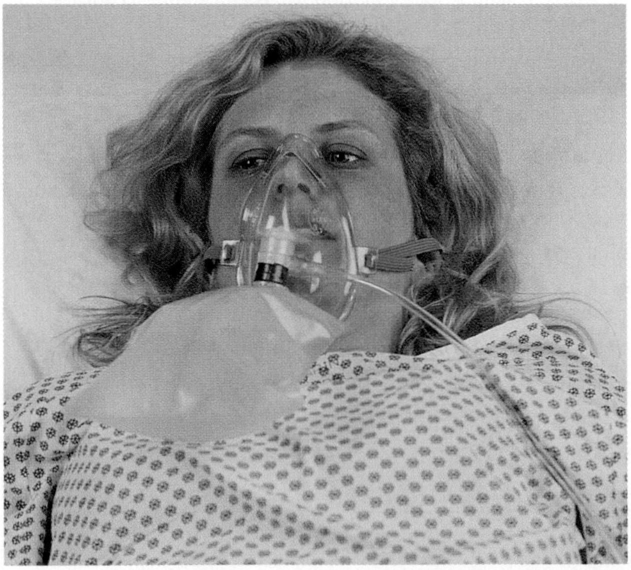

FIGURE 42.20 A partial rebreather mask

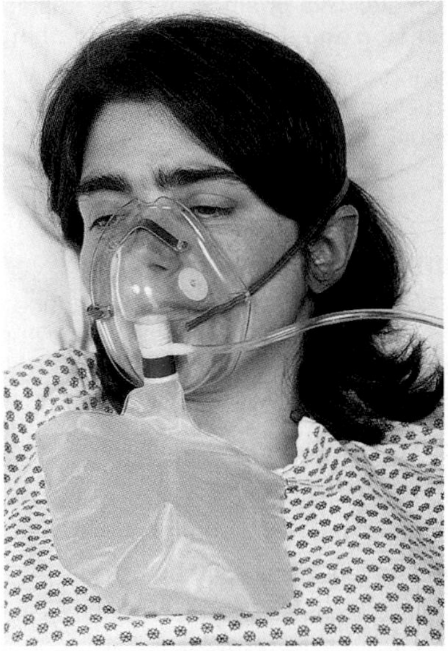

FIGURE 42.21 A nonrebreather mask

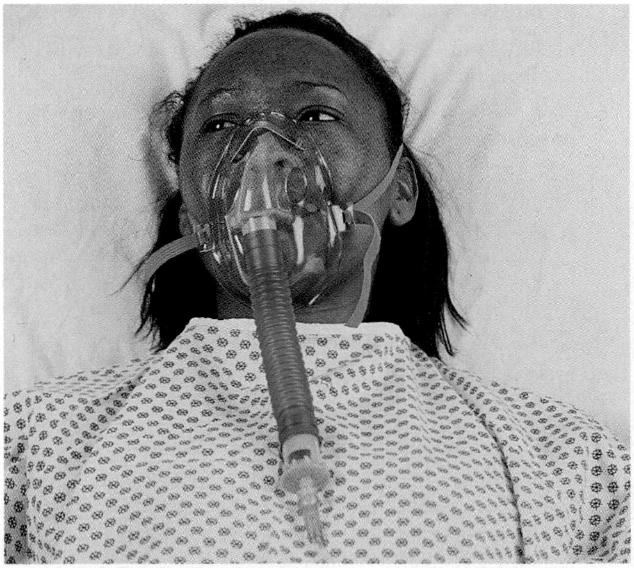

FIGURE 42.22 Venturi mask

and litre flow. For example, one colour-coded adapter delivers a 24% concentration of oxygen at 4 L per minute, and another colour-coded adapter delivers a 35% concentration of oxygen at 8 L per minute. The Venturi mask can be humidified through room air or additional humidification may be necessary. Follow the manufacturer's directions and agency policy for use of the Venturi mask.

Initiating oxygen by mask is much the same as initiating oxygen by cannula except that the nurse must find a mask of appropriate size. Smaller sizes are available for children. Administering oxygen by mask or face tent is detailed in Skill 42.1.

FACE TENT Face tents (Figure 42.23) can replace oxygen masks when masks are poorly tolerated by clients. Face tents provide varying concentrations of oxygen, for example, 30% to 50% concentration of oxygen at 4 L to 8 L per minute. Frequently inspect the client's facial skin for dampness or chafing, and dry and treat, as needed. As with facemasks, the client's facial skin must be kept dry.

When the client is an infant or a child, an oxygen hood or an oxygen tent (see Figure 42.24) can be used. See the Lifespan Considerations box. The Home Care Considerations box outlines three major oxygen systems for home care use.

CONTINUOUS POSITIVE AIRWAY PRESSURE THERAPY
Continuous positive airway pressure (CPAP) therapy provides a continuous flow of pressurized air to keep upper airway passages open. CPAP is often prescribed for the client experiencing obstructive sleep apnea (OSA). A CPAP machine keeps the upper airways open during sleep by delivering a continuous flow of pressurized air (Figure 42.27). The positive pressure delivered by a CPAP machine is constant and ranges from 4 cm H_2O to

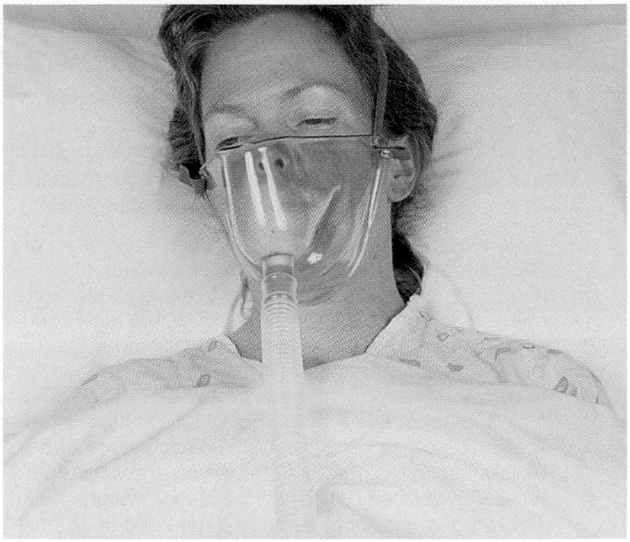

FIGURE 42.23 An oxygen face tent

Lifespan Considerations

Oxygen Delivery Equipment

Infants and children may cope better if an oxygen hood or an oxygen tent is used:

INFANTS

Oxygen Hood

- An oxygen hood is a rigid plastic dome that encloses an infant's head. It provides precise oxygen levels and high humidity.
- The gas should not be allowed to blow directly into the infant's face, and the hood should not rub against the infant's neck, chin, or shoulder.

CHILDREN

Oxygen Tent

- The tent consists of a rectangular, clear, plastic canopy with outlets that connect to an oxygen or compressed air source and to a humidifier that moisturizes the air or oxygen.
- Because the enclosed tent becomes very warm, some type of cooling mechanism, such as an ice chamber or a refrigeration unit, is provided to maintain the temperature at 20°C to 21°C.
- Cover the child with a gown or a cotton blanket. Some agencies provide gowns with hoods, or a small towel may be wrapped around the head. The child needs protection from chilling and from the dampness and condensation in the tent.

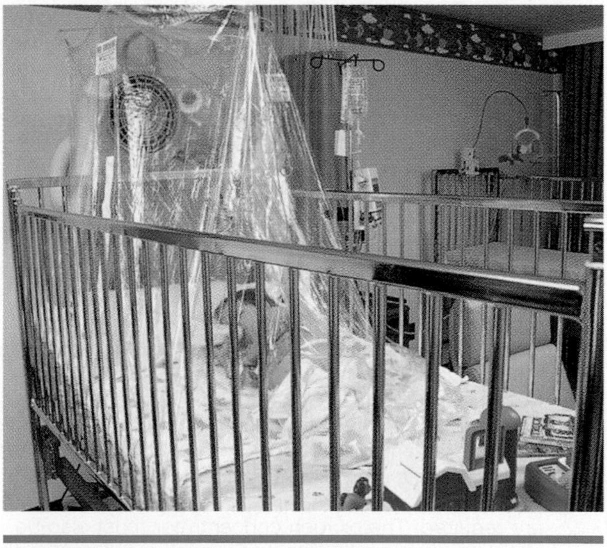

FIGURE 42.24 Pediatric oxygen tent

- Flood the tent with oxygen by setting the flow meter at 15 L/min for about 5 minutes. Then, adjust the flow meter according to orders (e.g., 10 L/min to 15 L/min). Flooding the tent quickly increases the oxygen to the desired level.
- The tent can deliver approximately 30% oxygen.

Home Care Considerations

Oxygen Equipment

Three major oxygen systems for home care use are available in most communities: cylinders or tanks of compressed gas, liquid (cryogenic) oxygen, and oxygen concentrators.

1. Cylinders (green tanks): Cylinders are the system of choice for clients who need oxygen episodically (e.g., on a prn basis). The advantages are that cylinders deliver all litre flows (1 L/min to 15 L/min), and oxygen evaporation does not occur during storage. The disadvantages are that the cylinders are heavy and awkward to move, the supply company must be notified when a refill is needed, and they are costly for the high-use client. A size D tank weighs about 3.5 kg and stores 425 L of oxygen; an E tank holds 680 L and is transported on wheels (Figure 42.25). The large H tank weighs 70 kg. The gauge on a full tank reads a pressure of at least 2000 pounds per square inch (psi), and a tank is considered empty when it reads less than 500 psi.
2. Liquid oxygen: Liquid systems have two parts: a large stationary container and a portable unit with a small lightweight tank that is refilled from the stationary unit. Liquid reservoirs store oxygen at –212°C in a smaller amount of space than for compressed gas. The advantages are that these reservoirs are lighter and cleaner than cylinders and they are easier to operate. The disadvantages of liquid oxygen are that many home care medical supply and service companies are not able to handle it, oxygen evaporation occurs when the unit is not used, only low flows (1 L/min to 4 L/min) can be used or freezing will occur, and the portable unit designed to be carried over the shoulder weighs 3.5 kg to 4 kg, a possible burden to the typical COPD client (Figure 42.26). A wheeled cart can be used to carry the unit but may be awkward.
3. Oxygen concentrators: Concentrators are electrically powered systems that manufacture oxygen from room air. At 1 L/min, such a system can deliver a concentration of about 95% oxygen, but the concentration drops when the flow rate increases (e.g., 75% concentration at 4 L/min). The advantages are that they look better, resembling furniture rather than medical equipment; they eliminate the need for regular delivery of oxygen or refilling of cylinders; they alleviate the client's anxiety about running out of oxygen because the supply of oxygen is constant; and they are the most economical system when continuous use is required. The major disadvantages of a concentrator are that it is expensive; lacks real portability (small units weigh 12 kg to 15 kg); tends to be noisy; is powered by electricity (an emergency backup unit, for example, an oxygen tank, must be provided for clients for whom a power failure could be life threatening); and heat produced by the concentrator motor is a problem for those who live in trailers, small houses, or warm climates where air conditioners are required. The oxygen concentrator must also be checked periodically with an O_2 analyzer to ensure that it is providing an adequate delivery of oxygen.

   Another type of oxygen concentrator is the *oxygen enricher.* It uses a plastic membrane that allows water vapour to pass through with the oxygen, thus eliminating the need for a humidifying device. It is also thought to filter out bacteria present in the air. The enricher provides an O_2 concentration of 40% at all flow rates, it tends to be quieter than the concentrator, it poses less risk of combustion (since the gas is only 40% oxygen), it has only two moving parts (thus decreasing the risk of something going wrong), and a nebulizer can be operated from the enricher because of the high flow rate.

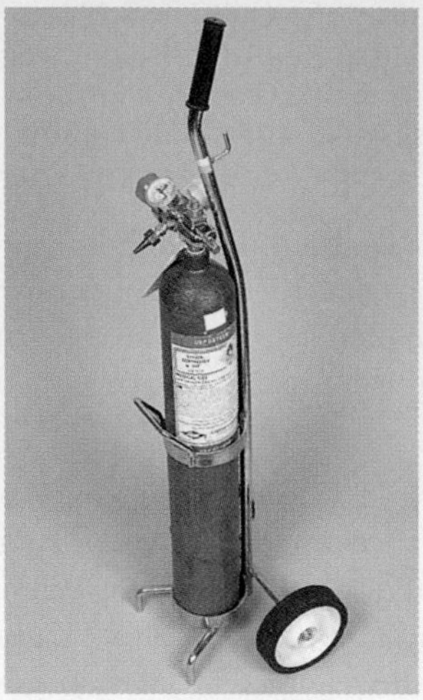

FIGURE 42.25 An E cylinder oxygen tank on a wheeled stand

Social services or the case manager needs to ensure that the client has appropriate help in choosing a reputable home oxygen vendor. Services furnished should include the following:

- Twenty-four-hour emergency service
- Trained personnel to make the initial delivery and instruct the client in safe and appropriate use of the oxygen and maintenance of the equipment
- At least monthly follow-up visits to check the equipment and reinstruct the client as necessary
- A regular cost review to ensure that the system is the most cost-effective one for that client, with routine notification of the physician or home care professional if it seems that another system is more appropriate

The nurse needs to also ensure that the client knows about the financial reimbursements available from insurance agencies.

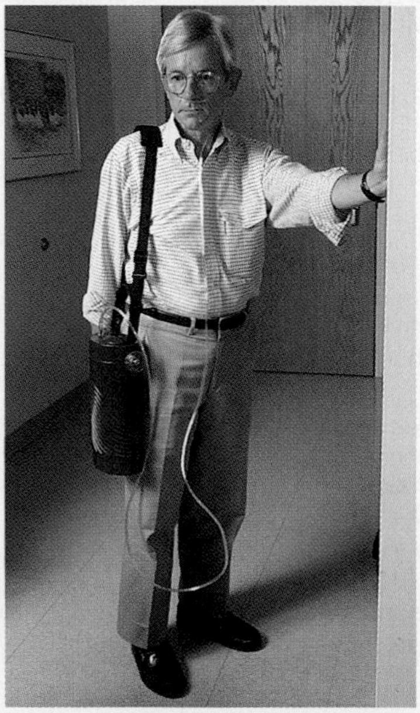

FIGURE 42.26 A portable liquid oxygen supply

20 cm H_2O (i.e., the amount of air pressure needed to move a column of water either 4 cm or 20 cm). The amount of pressure required to keep the airway open is individualized for each client, and is determined in a CPAP titration polysomnogram study. In cases of severe OSA, biphasic positive airway pressure (BiPAP) may be the recommended treatment. BiPAP is similar to CPAP, except the pressures differ on inhalation and exhalation with a higher pressure delivered on inhalation and a lower pressure on exhalation. Skill 42.2 describes how to use a CPAP machine.

ARTIFICIAL AIRWAYS Artificial airways are inserted to maintain a patent air passage for clients whose airway has become or may become obstructed. A patent airway is necessary so that air can flow to and from the lungs. Four of the more common types of airways are oropharyngeal, nasopharyngeal, endotracheal, and tracheostomy.

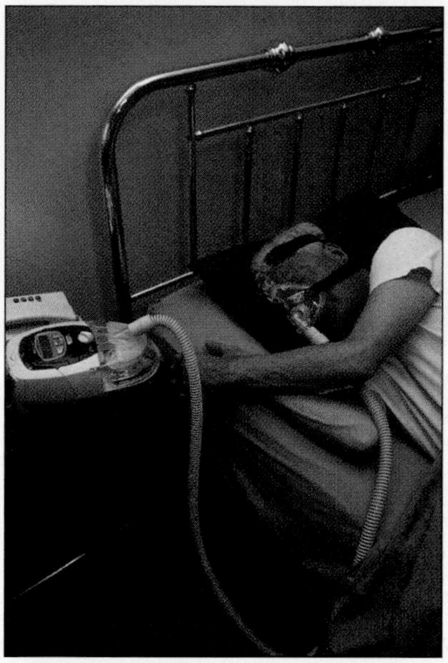

FIGURE 42.27 A CPAP mask is held in place by a headgear and tubing goes from the mask to the CPAP unit. The CPAP unit is plugged into an electrical outlet and provides a constant flow of air or oxygen to the mask.

SKILL 42.2

ADMINISTERING AIR BY CONTINUOUS POSITIVE AIRWAY PRESSURE (CPAP)

PURPOSES

- To deliver constant positive pressure air in a continuous flow to the upper respiratory airway to keep it open during sleep
- To maintain ventilation during sleep

ASSESSMENT

Assess respiratory status, including ease of breathing, rate, rhythm, depth, and SpO_2 (see Skill 28.7, p. 697) before and during sleep; dry nose, mouth, or throat; nasal congestion; epistaxis (nosebleed); and dry, irritated, or swollen eyes.

Planning

- Check the manufacturer's instructions for maintaining the CPAP machine.

Equipment

- Continuous positive airway pressure machine
- Corrugated tubing
- Prescribed face, nasal, or mouth mask of the appropriate size
- Headgear

IMPLEMENTATION

Preparation

1. Before performing the procedure, introduce yourself and verify the client's identity by using agency protocol.
2. Prepare the client.
   - Inform the client of the prescription of CPAP and the benefits of the intervention.
3. Choose an appropriate secure location close to where the client sleeps to install the CPAP machine. **Rationale: The equipment requires a physical location in proximity to the client and needs to be in a location where it will not fall.**

Performance

1. Perform hand hygiene and observe other appropriate infection prevention and control procedures.
2. Provide for client privacy, if appropriate.
3. Assess the client's nares for encrustations and irritation. Apply a water-soluble lubricant, as required, to soothe the mucous membranes.
4. Attach the corrugated tubing to the machine.
5. Attach the mask (nasal, mouth, or face) to the corrugated tubing.
6. Connect the headgear to the mask (follow the manufacturer's instructions).
7. Turn on the CPAP machine.
8. Position the headgear and mask on the client.
9. Document the initiation and duration of the therapy and all nursing assessments.

EVALUATION

Perform follow-up based on the client's response to the use of CPAP, for example, was the client comfortable during the night? Did the client experience any adverse outcomes, such as disrupted sleep?

OROPHARYNGEAL AND NASOPHARYNGEAL AIRWAYS Oropharyngeal and nasopharyngeal airways are used to keep the upper air passages open when they may become obstructed by secretions or the tongue. These airways are easy to insert and have a low risk of complications. Sizes vary and should be appropriate to the size and age of the client. The airway should be well lubricated with water or water-soluble gel before inserting.

Oropharyngeal airways (Figure 42.28) stimulate the gag reflex and are used only for clients with altered levels of consciousness (e.g., because of general anaesthesia, overdose, or head injury). To insert the airway, the nurse follows these steps:

- Place the client in supine or semi-Fowler's position.
- Perform hand hygiene and observe other appropriate infection prevention and control procedures.
- Put on gloves.
- Hold the lubricated airway by the outer flange, with the distal end pointing up.
- Open the client's mouth and insert the airway along the top of the tongue.
- When the distal end of the airway reaches the soft palate at the back of the mouth, rotate the airway 180 degrees downward, and slip it past the uvula into the oral pharynx.
- If not contraindicated, place the client in a side-lying position to allow secretions to drain out of the mouth.
- The oropharynx may be suctioned as needed by inserting the suction catheter alongside the airway.
- Do not tape the airway in place; remove it when the client begins to cough or gag.
- Provide mouth care at least every 2 hours, keeping suction available at the bedside.

As appropriate for the client's condition, remove the airway every 8 hours to assess the mouth and provide oral care. Reinsert the airway immediately.

Nasopharyngeal airways are tolerated better by alert clients. They are inserted through the nares, terminating in the oropharynx (Figure 42.29). When caring for a client with a nasopharyngeal airway, provide frequent oral and nares care, repositioning the airway in the other nare every 8 hours or as ordered to prevent necrosis of the mucosa.

ENDOTRACHEAL TUBES Endotracheal tubes are most commonly inserted for clients who have had general anaesthetics or for those in emergency situations where mechanical ventilation is required. An endotracheal tube can be inserted through either the mouth or the nose and into the trachea with the guide of a laryngoscope (Figure 42.30) by the physician or nurse with specialized education. The tube terminates just superior to the bifurcation of the trachea into the bronchi. The tube may have an air-filled cuff to prevent air leakage around it. Because an endotracheal tube passes through the epiglottis and glottis, the client is unable to speak while it is in place. Nursing interventions for clients with endotracheal tubes are shown in Box 42.4.

TRACHEOTOMY OR TRACHEOSTOMY Clients who need long-term airway support may have a **tracheotomy**, a surgical incision in the trachea just below the larynx. A **tracheostomy** is the opening made for the tube itself. A curved tracheostomy tube is inserted to extend through the stoma into the trachea (Figure 42.31). Tracheostomy tubes may be either plastic or metal and are available in different sizes.

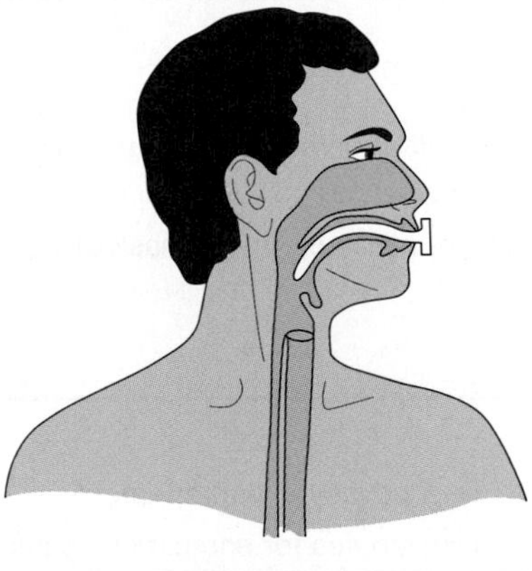

FIGURE 42.28 An oropharyngeal airway in place

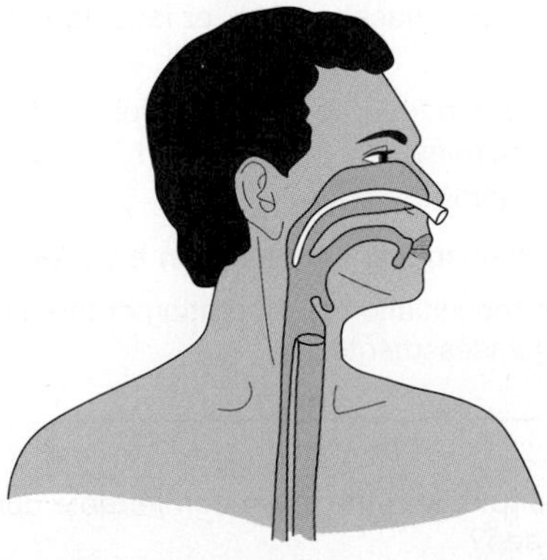

FIGURE 42.29 A nasopharyngeal airway in place

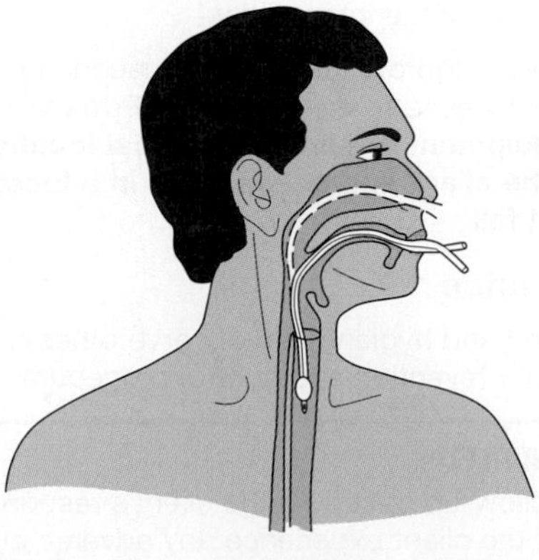

FIGURE 42.30 An endotracheal tube in place

BOX 42.4 NURSING INTERVENTIONS FOR CLIENTS WITH ENDOTRACHEAL TUBES

Nursing interventions for clients with endotracheal tubes are as follows:

- To prevent ventilator-associated pneumonia, Safer Healthcare Now! (2005) makes the following recommendations:
  - Keep the head of bed elevation between 30 and 45 degrees
  - Provide a daily break from sedation to assess the client's readiness for extubation by performing a spontaneous breathing trial
  - Use specially designed endotracheal evacuation tubes, called EVAC tubes, that have a separate lumen opening into the subglottic region from which contaminated oropharyngeal secretions that are above the endotracheal tube can be removed
- Assess the client's respiratory status at least every 1 to 2 hours, or more frequently if indicated. Include respiratory rate, rhythm, depth, equality of chest excursion, and lung sounds; level of consciousness; and colour of skin and mucous membranes in the assessment.
- Frequently assess nasal and oral mucosa for redness and irritation. Report any abnormal findings to the physician.
- Secure the endotracheal tube with tape to prevent accidental movement of the tube further into or out of the trachea. Assess the position of the tube frequently. Notify the physician immediately if the tube is dislodged out of the airway. If the tube advances into a main bronchus, it may need to be slightly withdrawn to ensure ventilation of both lungs.
- Use sterile or clean technique (depending on agency policy) to suction the endotracheal (or EVAC) tube as needed to remove excessive secretions. If an EVAC tube is not in place, suction the oropharynx as per agency policy.
- Closely monitor cuff pressure, maintaining a pressure of 20 mm Hg to 25 mm Hg (or as recommended by the tube manufacturer) to minimize the risk of tracheal tissue necrosis. If recommended, deflate the cuff periodically.
- Provide oral and nasal care every 2 to 4 hours. Use an oropharyngeal airway to prevent the client from biting down on an oral endotracheal tube. Move oral endotracheal tubes to the opposite side of the mouth every 8 hours or per agency protocol, taking care to maintain the position of the tube in the trachea.
- Provide humidified air or oxygen because the endotracheal tube bypasses the upper airways, which normally moisten the air.
- If the client is on mechanical ventilation, ensure that all alarms are enabled at all times as the client cannot call for help should an emergency occur.
- Communicate frequently with the client, providing a note pad or picture board for the client to use for communicating.
- Consider the use of a kinetic bed (rotational therapy) for the client who is at highest risk for atelectasis and pneumonia. These clients include those who are sedated and require a resuscitator for more than 3 to 4 days and those for whom manual turning and positioning is difficult, such as those who are morbidly obese, have a head injury, or are receiving traction.

Tracheostomy tubes (Figure 42.32) have an outer cannula that is inserted into the trachea and a flange that rests against the neck and allows the tube to be secured in place with tape or ties. All tubes also have an obturator, used to insert the outer cannula and then removed. The obturator is kept at the client's bedside in case the tube becomes dislodged and needs to be reinserted. Some tracheostomy tubes have an inner cannula that can be removed for periodic cleaning.

Cuffed tracheostomy tubes are surrounded by an inflatable cuff that produces an airtight seal between the tube and the trachea. This seal prevents aspiration of oropharyngeal secretions and air leakage between the tube and the trachea. Cuffed tubes are often used immediately after a tracheostomy and are essential when ventilating a tracheostomy client with a mechanical ventilator. Children do not require cuffed tubes because their tracheas are small enough to seal the air space around the tube.

Low-pressure cuffs (Figure 42.33) are commonly used to distribute a low, even pressure against the trachea, thus decreasing the risk of tracheal tissue necrosis. They do not need to be deflated periodically to reduce pressure on the tracheal wall. Foam cuffed tracheostomy tubes (Figure 42.34) do not require injected air; instead, when

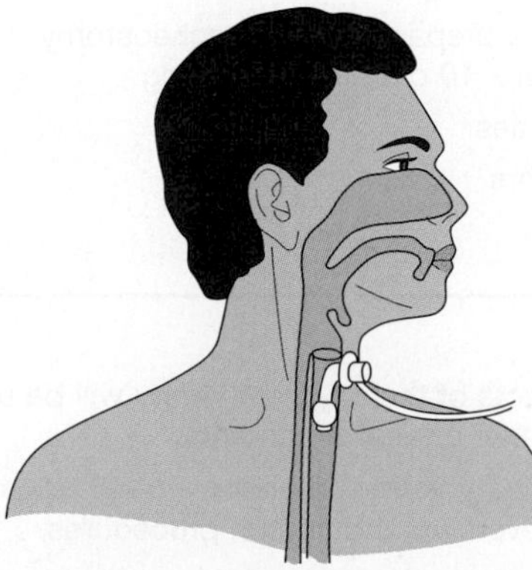

FIGURE 42.31 A tracheostomy tube in place

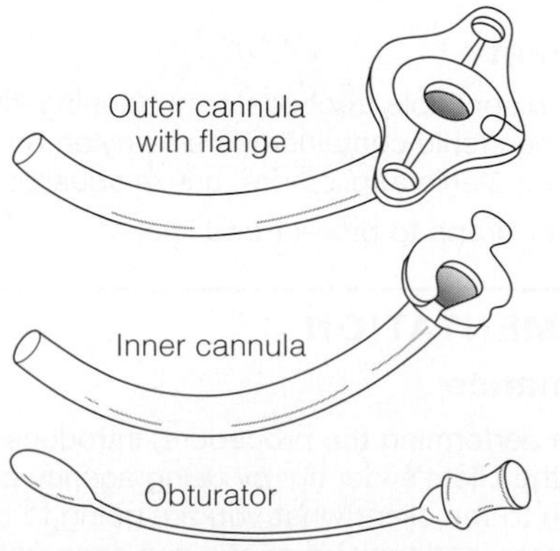

FIGURE 42.32 Components of a tracheostomy tube

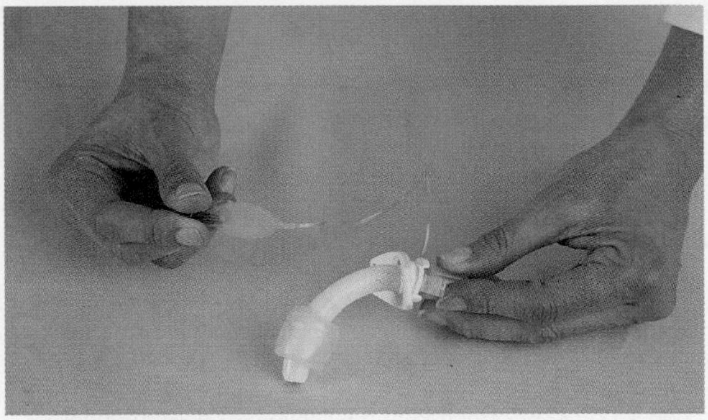

FIGURE 42.33 A tracheostomy tube with a low-pressure cuff

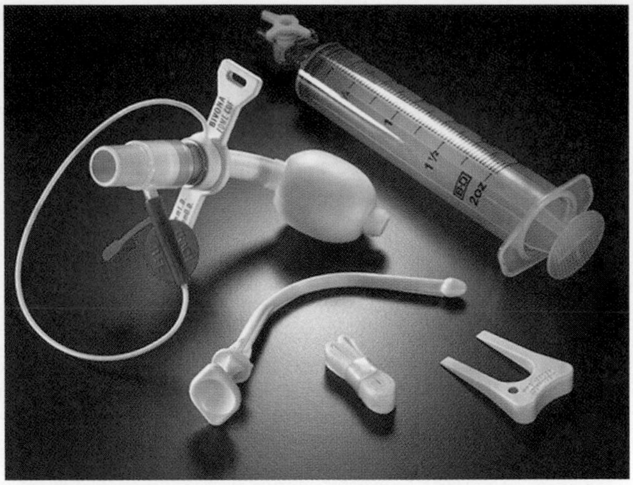

FIGURE 42.34 A tracheostomy tube with a foam cuff

the port is opened, ambient air enters the balloon, which then conforms to the client's trachea. Air is removed from the cuff before insertion or removal of the tube.

The nurse provides tracheostomy care for the client with a new or recent tracheostomy to maintain patency of the tube and reduce the risk of infection. Initially, a tracheostomy may need to be suctioned (see the section on suctioning that follows) and cleaned as often as every one to two hours. After the initial inflammatory response subsides, tracheostomy care may need to be done only once or twice a day, depending on the client. Skill 42.3 describes tracheostomy care.

SKILL 42.3

PROVIDING TRACHEOSTOMY CARE

PURPOSES

- To maintain airway patency
- To maintain cleanliness and prevent infection at the tracheostomy site
- To facilitate healing and prevent skin excoriation around the tracheostomy incision
- To promote comfort

ASSESSMENT

Assess the following:

- Respiratory status, including ease of breathing, rate, rhythm, depth, lung sounds, and oxygen saturation levels
- Pulse rate
- Character and amount of secretions from tracheostomy site
- Presence of drainage on tracheostomy dressing or ties
- Appearance of incision (note any redness, swelling, purulent discharge, or odour)

Equipment

- Sterile disposable tracheostomy cleaning kit or supplies, including sterile containers, sterile nylon brush or pipe cleaners, sterile applicators, gauze squares
- Towel or drape to protect bed linens
- Sterile suction catheter kit (suction catheter and sterile container for solution)
- Sterile normal saline (check agency policy for soaking solution)
- Sterile gloves (two pairs)
- Mask and goggles if required
- Recommended cleaning solution for cannula
- Clean gloves
- Moisture-proof bag
- Commercially prepared sterile tracheostomy dressing or sterile 10 cm × 10 cm gauze dressing
- Cotton twill ties
- Clean scissors

IMPLEMENTATION

Performance

1. Before performing the procedure, introduce yourself and verify the client's identity by using agency protocol. Explain to the client what you are going to do, why it is necessary, and how he or she can cooperate. Discuss how the effects of the oxygen therapy will be used in planning further care or treatments.
2. Perform hand hygiene and observe other appropriate infection prevention and control procedures.
3. Provide for client privacy.

(continued)

SKILL 42.3

PROVIDING TRACHEOSTOMY CARE (*continued*)

4. Prepare the client and the equipment.
   - Assist the client to a semi-Fowler's or Fowler's position. **Rationale: This promotes lung expansion.**
   - Explain the procedure to the client and provide for a means of communication, such as eye blinking or raising a finger to indicate pain or distress.
   - Open the tracheostomy kit or sterile basins. Pour the recommended cleaning solution into containers.
   - Establish a sterile field.
   - Open other sterile supplies, as needed, including sterile applicators, suction kit, and tracheostomy dressing.
5. Suction the tracheostomy tube.
   - Don sterile gloves and mask, goggles, and gown, if required.
   - Suction the full length of the tracheostomy tube to remove secretions and ensure a patent airway (see Skill 42.5).
   - Rinse the suction catheter and wrap the catheter around your hand. Peel off the glove so that it turns inside out over the catheter. Discard the glove and the catheter.
   - Using the gloved hand, unlock the inner cannula (if present) and remove it by gently pulling it out toward you in line with its curvature. Place the inner cannula in the soaking solution. **Rationale: This moistens and loosens dried secretions.**
   - Remove the soiled tracheostomy dressing. Place the soiled dressing in your gloved hand and peel the glove off so that it turns inside out over the dressing. Discard the glove and the dressing.
   - Put on sterile gloves. Keep your dominant hand sterile during the procedure.
6. Clean the inner cannula (see Variation for using a disposable cannula).
   - Remove the inner cannula from the soaking solution.
   - Clean the lumen and entire inner cannula thoroughly by using the brush or pipe cleaners moistened with sterile normal saline (see ❶). Inspect the cannula for cleanliness by holding it at eye level and looking through it into the light.
   - Rinse the inner cannula thoroughly in sterile normal saline. **Rationale: Thorough rinsing is important to remove the soaking or cleaning solution from the inner cannula.**
   - After rinsing, gently tap the cannula against the inside edge of the sterile saline container. Use a pipe cleaner folded in half to dry only the inside of the cannula; do not dry the outside. **Rationale: This removes excess liquid from the cannula and prevents possible aspiration by the client while leaving a film of moisture on the outer surface to lubricate the cannula for reinsertion.**
7. Replace the inner cannula, securing it in place.
   - Insert the inner cannula by grasping the outer flange and inserting the cannula in the direction of its curvature.
   - Lock the cannula in place by turning the lock (if present) into position to secure the flange of the inner cannula to the outer cannula.
8. Clean the incision site and tube flange.
   - Using sterile applicators or gauze dressings moistened with a normal saline, clean the incision site (see ❷). Use each applicator or gauze dressing only once and then discard. **Rationale: This avoids contaminating a clean area with a soiled gauze dressing or applicator.**
   - Hydrogen peroxide can be used (usually in half-strength solution mixed with sterile normal saline) to remove encrustations. Check agency policy. Thoroughly rinse the cleaned area by using gauze squares moistened with sterile normal saline. **Rationale: Hydrogen peroxide can be irritating to the skin and inhibits healing if not thoroughly removed.**
   - Clean the flange of the tube in the same manner.
   - Thoroughly dry the client's skin and tube flanges with dry gauze squares.
9. Apply a sterile dressing.
   - Use a commercially prepared tracheostomy dressing of nonravelling material, or open and refold a 10 cm × 10 cm gauze dressing into a V shape, as shown in ❸ A to ❸ D. Avoid using cotton-filled gauze squares or cutting the 10 × 10 gauze. **Rationale: Cotton lint or gauze fibres can be aspirated by the client, potentially creating a tracheal abscess.**

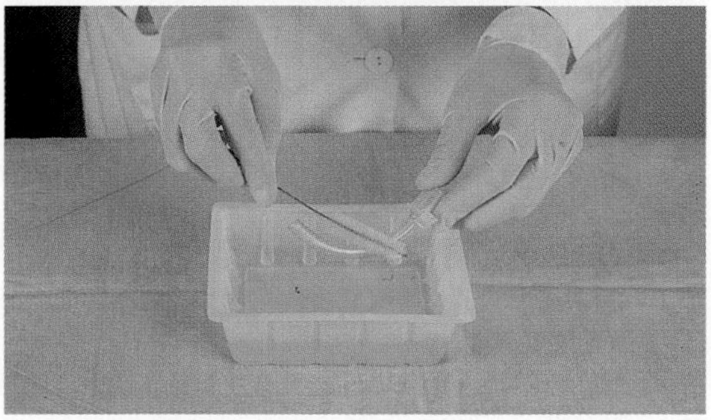

❶ Cleaning the inner cannula with a brush

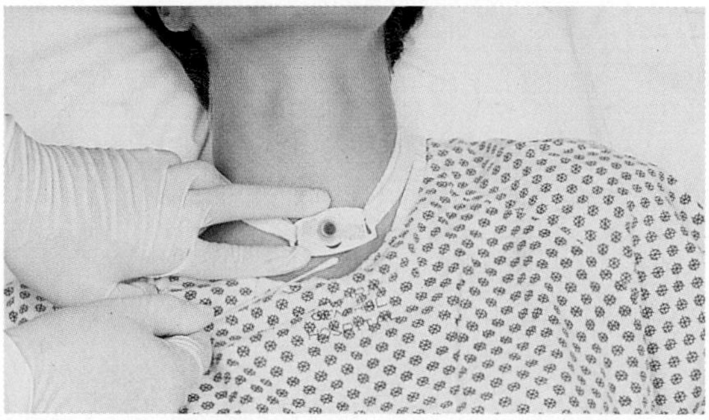

❷ Using an applicator stick to clean the tracheostomy site

(*continued*)

SKILL 42.3

PROVIDING TRACHEOSTOMY CARE (*continued*)

- Place the dressing under the flange of the tracheostomy tube as shown in ❸ E.
- While applying the dressing, ensure that the tracheostomy tube is securely supported. **Rationale: Excessive movement of the tracheostomy tube irritates the trachea.**

10. Change the tracheostomy ties.

- Change as needed to keep the skin clean and dry.
- Twill tape and specially manufactured Velcro ties are available. Twill tape is inexpensive and readily available, however, it is easily soiled and can trap moisture that leads to irritation of the skin of the neck. Velcro ties are becoming more commonly used (see ❹). They are wider and more comfortable and cause less skin abrasion.

Two-Strip Method

- Cut two unequal strips of twill tape, one approximately 25 cm long and the other about 50 cm long. **Rationale: Cutting one tape longer than the other allows them to be fastened at the side of the neck for easy access and to avoid the pressure of a knot on the skin at the back of the neck.**
- Cut a 1 cm lengthwise slit approximately 2.5 cm from one end of each strip. To do this, fold the end of the tape back onto itself about 2.5 cm, and then cut a slit in the middle of the tape from its folded edge.
- Leaving the old ties in place, thread the slit end of one clean tape through the eye of the tracheostomy flange from the bottom side; then thread the long end of the tape through the slit, pulling it taut until it is securely fastened to the flange. **Rationale: Leaving the old ties in place while securing the clean ties prevents inadvertent dislodging of the tracheostomy tube. Securing tapes in this manner avoids the use of knots, which can come untied or cause pressure and irritation.**
- If the old ties are very soiled or it is difficult to thread new ties onto the tracheostomy flange with old ties in place, have an assistant don a sterile glove and hold the tracheostomy in place while you replace the ties. This is very important because movement of the tube during this procedure can cause irritation and stimulate coughing. Coughing can dislodge the tube if the ties are undone.
- Repeat the process for the second tie.
- Ask the client to flex the neck. Slip the longer tape under the client's neck, place a finger between the tape and the client's neck (see ❺), and tie the tapes together at the side of the neck. **Rationale: Flexing the neck increases its circumference the way coughing does. Placing a finger under the ties prevents making the ties too tight, which could interfere with coughing or place pressure on the jugular veins.**
- Tie the ends of the tapes by using square knots. Cut off any long ends, leaving approximately 1 cm to 2 cm. **Rationale: Square knots prevent slippage and loosening. Adequate ends beyond the knot prevent the knot from inadvertently untying.**
- Once the clean ties are secured, remove the soiled ties and discard.

One-Strip Method (Twill Tape)

- Cut a length of twill tape 2.5 times the length needed to go around the client's neck from one tube flange to the other.
- Thread one end of the tape into the slot on one side of the flange.

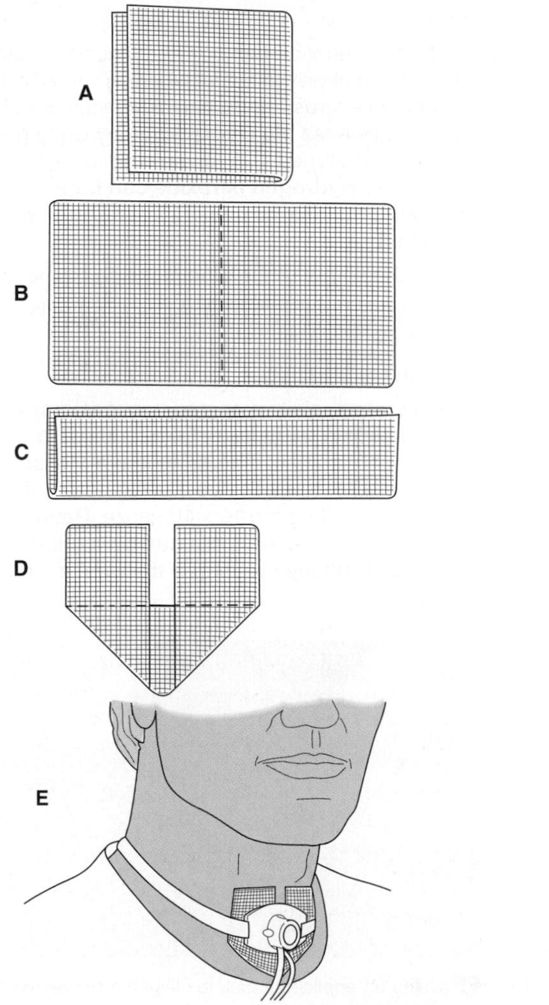

❸ Folding a 10 cm × 10 cm gauze to make a tracheostomy dressing

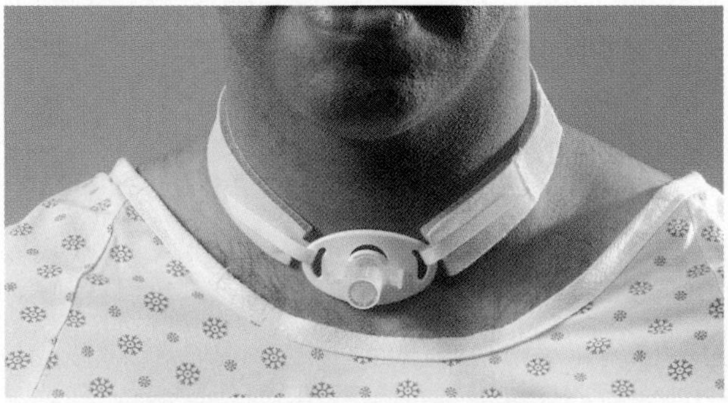

❹ A Velcro tracheostomy tie

(continued)

SKILL 42.3

PROVIDING TRACHEOSTOMY CARE *(continued)*

- Bring both ends of the tape together, and take them around the client's neck, keeping them flat and untwisted.
- Thread the end of the tape next to the client's neck through the other flange slot from the back to the front.
- Have the client flex the neck. Tie the loose ends with a square knot at the side of the client's neck, allowing for slack by placing a finger under the ties as with the two-strip method. Cut off long ends.

11. Tape and pad the knot.

- Place a folded 10 cm × 10 cm gauze square under the tie knot, and apply tape over the knot. **Rationale: This reduces skin irritation from the knot and prevents confusing the knot with the client's gown ties.**

12. Check the tightness of the ties.

- Frequently check the tightness of the tracheostomy ties and position of the tracheostomy tube. **Rationale: Swelling of the neck can cause the ties to become too taut, interfering with coughing and circulation. Ties can loosen in restless clients, allowing the tracheostomy tube to extrude from the stoma.**

13. Document all relevant information.

- Record suctioning, tracheostomy care, and the dressing change, noting your assessments.

Variation: Using a Disposable Inner Cannula

- Check policy for frequency of changing inner cannula because standards vary among institutions.

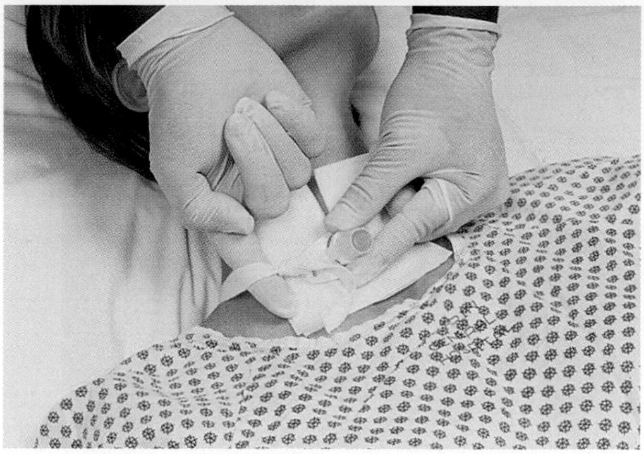

❺ Placing a finger underneath the tie tape before tying it

- Open a new cannula package.
- Using a gloved hand, unlock the current inner cannula (if present) and remove it by gently pulling it out toward you in line with its curvature.
- Check the cannula for amount and type of secretions and discard properly.
- Pick up the new inner cannula, touching only the outer locking portion.
- Insert the new inner cannula into the tracheostomy.
- Lock the cannula in place by turning the lock (if present).

EVALUATION

- Perform appropriate follow-up, such as determining character and amount of secretions, drainage from the tracheostomy, appearance of the tracheostomy incision, pulse rate, respiratory status compared with baseline data, and complaints of pain or discomfort at the tracheostomy site.
- Relate findings to previous assessment data if available.
- Report significant deviations from normal to the appropriate members of the health-care team.

When the client breathes through a tracheostomy, air is no longer filtered and humidified as it is when passing through the upper airways; therefore, special precautions are necessary. Humidity can be provided with a mist collar (Figure 42.35). Clients with long-term tracheostomies can wear a light scarf or a 10 cm × 10 cm gauze held in place with a cotton tie over the stoma to filter air as it enters the tracheostomy.

SUCTIONING When clients have difficulty handling their secretions or an airway is in place, suctioning may be necessary to clear air passages. **Suctioning** refers to the aspiration of secretions through a catheter connected to a suction machine or wall suction outlet. Even though the upper airways (the oropharynx and nasopharynx) are not sterile, sterile technique is recommended for all suctioning to avoid introducing pathogens into the airways.

Suction catheters are either open tipped or whistle tipped (Figure 42.36). The whistle-tipped catheter is less irritating to respiratory tissues, although the open-tipped catheter may be more effective for removing thick mucous plugs. An oral suction tube, or Yankauer device, is used to suction the oral cavity (Figure 42.37). Most suction catheters have a thumb port on the side to control the suction. The catheter is connected to suction tubing, which, in turn, is connected to a collection chamber and suction control gauge (Figure 42.38).

The nurse decides when suctioning is needed by assessing the client for signs of respiratory distress or evidence that the client is unable to cough up and expectorate secretions. Dyspnea, bubbling or rattling

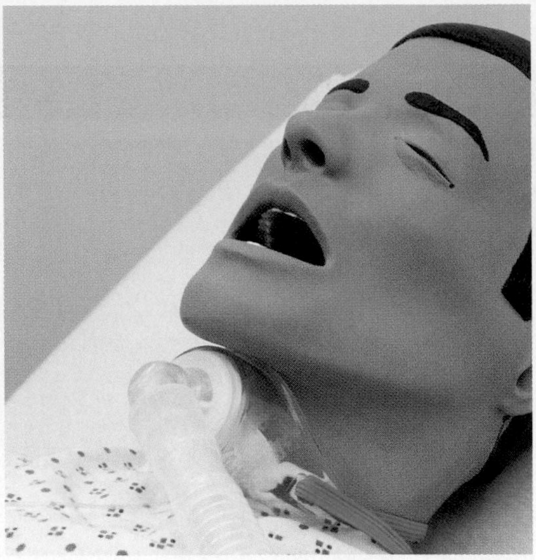

FIGURE 42.35 A tracheostomy mist collar

breath sounds, poor skin colour or cyanosis, or decreased SaO_2 may indicate the need for suctioning. Good nursing judgment is necessary, because suctioning irritates mucous membranes and can increase secretions if performed too frequently. In other words, suctioning is based on clinical need, not a fixed schedule.

Oral and nasopharyngeal suctioning removes secretions from the upper respiratory tract. Nasopharyngeal and nasotracheal suctioning provide closer access to the trachea and require sterile technique. Skill 42.4 outlines oropharyngeal and nasopharyngeal suctioning.

Following endotracheal intubation or a tracheotomy, the trachea and surrounding respiratory tissues are irritated and react by producing excessive secretions. Sterile suctioning is necessary to remove these secretions and maintain a patent airway. The frequency of suctioning depends on the client's assessment data and how recently the intubation was done. Additionally, suctioning may be necessary in clients who have increased secretions because of pneumonia or an inability to clear secretions because of an altered level of consciousness.

Suctioning is associated with several complications: hypoxemia, trauma to the airway, health-care-associated

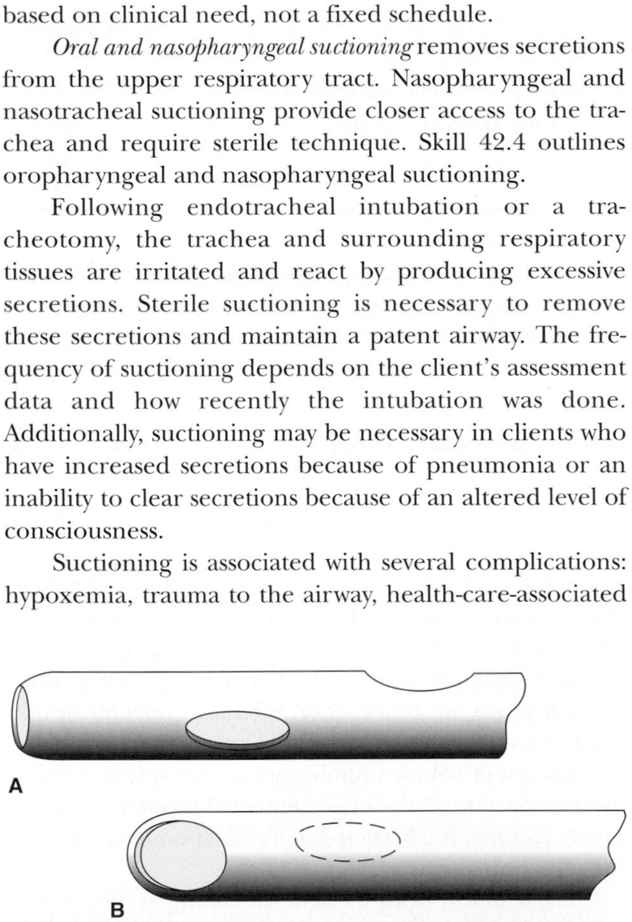

FIGURE 42.36 Types of suction catheters: **A:** open tipped; **B:** whistle tipped

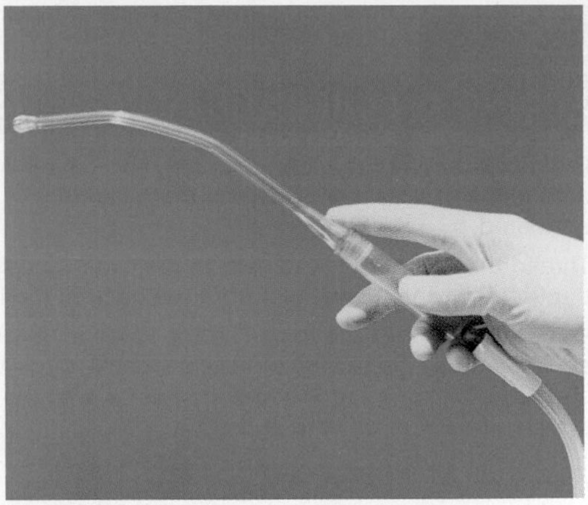

FIGURE 42.37 Oral (Yankauer) suction tube

infection, and cardiac dysrhythmias, which are related to the hypoxemia. Techniques to minimize or decrease these complications include the following (according to agency policy):

- *Hyperinflation.* This involves giving the client breaths that are 1 to 1.5 times the tidal volume set on the ventilator through the ventilator circuit or via a manual resuscitation bag. Three to five breaths are delivered before and after each pass of the suction catheter.
- *Hyperoxygenation.* This can be done with a manual resuscitation bag or through the ventilator and is performed by increasing the oxygen flow (usually to 100%) before suctioning and between suction attempts.

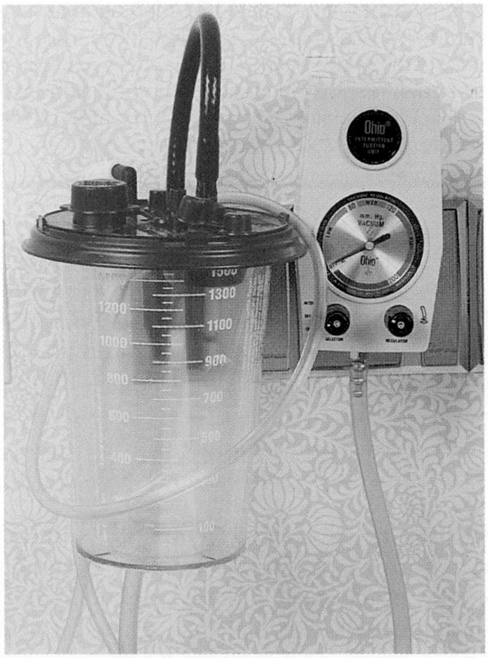

FIGURE 42.38 A wall suction unit

SKILL 42.4

OROPHARYNGEAL, NASOPHARYNGEAL, AND NASOTRACHEAL SUCTIONING

PURPOSES

- To remove secretions that obstruct the airway
- To facilitate ventilation
- To obtain secretions for diagnostic purposes
- To prevent infection that may result from accumulated secretions

ASSESSMENT

Assess for clinical signs indicating the need for suctioning:

- Restlessness
- Gurgling sounds during respiration
- Adventitious breath sounds when the chest is auscultated
- Change in mental status
- Colour of skin and mucous membranes
- Rate and pattern of respirations
- Pulse rate and rhythm
- Decreased oxygen saturation

Equipment

Oral and Nasopharyngeal or Nasotracheal Suctioning

- Towel or moisture-resistant pad
- Portable or wall suction machine with tubing and collection receptacle
- Sterile disposable container for fluids
- Sterile normal saline or water
- Goggles or face shield, if appropriate
- Moisture-resistant disposal bag
- Sputum trap, if specimen is to be collected

Oral and Oropharyngeal Suctioning

- Yankauer suction catheter or suction catheter kit
- Clean gloves

Nasopharyngeal or Nasotracheal Suctioning

- Sterile gloves
- Sterile suction catheter kit (12 Fr to 18 Fr for adults; 8 Fr to 10 Fr for children, and 5 Fr to 8 Fr for infants)
- Water-soluble lubricant
- Y-connector

IMPLEMENTATION

Performance

1. Before performing the procedure, introduce yourself and verify the client's identity by using agency protocol. Explain to the client what you are going to do, why it is necessary, and how he or she can cooperate. Inform the client that suctioning will relieve breathing difficulty and that the procedure is painless but may be uncomfortable and stimulate the cough, gag, or sneeze reflex. **Rationale: Knowing that the procedure will relieve breathing problems is often reassuring and enlists the client's cooperation.**
2. Perform hand hygiene and observe other appropriate infection prevention and control procedures.
3. Provide for client privacy.
4. Prepare the client.
   - Position a *conscious* person who has a functional gag reflex in the semi-Fowler's position with the head turned to one side for oral suctioning or with the neck hyperextended for nasal suctioning. **Rationale: These positions facilitate the insertion of the catheter and help prevent aspiration of secretions.**
   - Position an *unconscious* client in the lateral position, facing you. **Rationale: This position allows the tongue to fall forward so that it will not obstruct the catheter on insertion. Lateral position also facilitates drainage of secretions from the pharynx and prevents the possibility of aspiration.**
   - Place the towel or moisture-resistant pad over the pillow or under the chin.
5. Prepare the equipment.
   - Set the pressure on the suction gauge, and turn on the suction. Many suction devices are calibrated to three pressure ranges:
     - Wall Unit
       Adult: 100 mm Hg to 120 mm Hg
       Child: 95 mm Hg to 110 mm Hg
       Infant: 50 mm Hg to 95 mm Hg
     - Portable Unit
       Adult: 10 mm Hg to 15 mm Hg
       Child: 5 mm Hg to 10 mm Hg
       Infant: 2 mm Hg to 5 mm Hg

Oral and Oropharyngeal Suctioning

- Moisten the tip of the Yankauer or suction catheter with sterile water or saline. **Rationale: This reduces friction and eases insertion.**
- Pull the tongue forward, if necessary, using gauze.
- Do not apply suction (that is, leave your finger off the port) during insertion. **Rationale: Applying suction during insertion causes trauma to the mucous membrane.**
- Advance the catheter about 10 cm to 15 cm along one side of the mouth into the oropharynx. **Rationale: Directing the catheter along the side prevents gagging.**
- It may be necessary during oropharyngeal suctioning to apply suction to secretions that collect in the vestibule of the mouth and beneath the tongue.

(continued)

SKILL 42.4

OROPHARYNGEAL, NASOPHARYNGEAL, AND NASOTRACHEAL SUCTIONING *(continued)*

Nasopharyngeal and Nasotracheal Suctioning

- Open the lubricant if performing nasopharyngeal or nasotracheal suctioning
- Open the sterile suction package.
  - **a.** Set up the cup or container, touching only the outside.
  - **b.** Pour sterile water or saline into the container.
  - **c.** Put on the sterile gloves, or put a nonsterile glove on the nondominant hand and then a sterile glove on the dominant hand. **Rationale: The sterile gloved hand maintains the sterility of the suction catheter, and the unsterile glove prevents the transmission of microorganisms to the nurse.**
- With your sterile gloved hand, pick up the catheter and attach it to the suction unit (see ❶).

6. Make an approximate measure of the depth for the insertion of the catheter and test the equipment.
- Measure the distance between the tip of the client's nose and the earlobe, about 13 cm for an adult.
- Mark the position on the tube with the fingers of the sterile gloved hand.
- Test the pressure of the suction and the patency of the catheter by applying your sterile gloved finger or thumb to the port or open branch of the Y-connector (the suction control) to create suction.

7. Lubricate and introduce the catheter.
- Lubricate the catheter tip with sterile water, saline, or water-soluble lubricant. **Rationale: This reduces friction and eases insertion.**
- Remove oxygen with nondominant hand, if appropriate.
- *Without applying suction,* insert the catheter the premeasured or recommended distance into either nares and advance it along the floor of the nasal cavity. **Rationale: This avoids the nasal turbinates.**
- Never force the catheter against an obstruction. If one nostril is obstructed, try the other.

8. Perform suctioning.
- Apply your finger to the suction control port to start suction, and gently rotate the catheter. **Rationale: Gentle rotation of the catheter ensures that all surfaces are reached and prevents trauma to any one area of the respiratory mucosa because of prolonged suction.**
- Apply intermittent suction for 5 to 10 seconds while slowly withdrawing the catheter, then remove your finger from the control, and remove the catheter.
- A suction attempt should last only 10 to 15 seconds. During this time, the catheter is inserted, the suction applied and discontinued, and the catheter removed.

9. Rinse the catheter, and repeat suctioning as above.
- Rinse and flush the catheter with sterile water or saline.
- Relubricate the catheter, and repeat suctioning until the air passage is clear.
- Allow 30-second to 1-minute intervals between each suction, and limit suction attempts to two or three times. Assess cardiopulmonary status between each suctioning attempt. **Rationale: Applying suction for too long may cause secretions to increase or may decrease the client's oxygen supply.**
- Encourage the client to breathe deeply and to cough between suctions. Use supplemental oxygen, if appropriate. **Rationale: Coughing and deep breathing help carry secretions from the trachea and bronchi into the pharynx, where they can be reached with the suction catheter. Deep breathing and supplemental oxygen provide oxygen to the alveoli.**

10. Obtain a specimen if required.

Use a sputum trap (see ❷) as follows:
- Attach the suction catheter to the rubber tubing of the sputum trap.

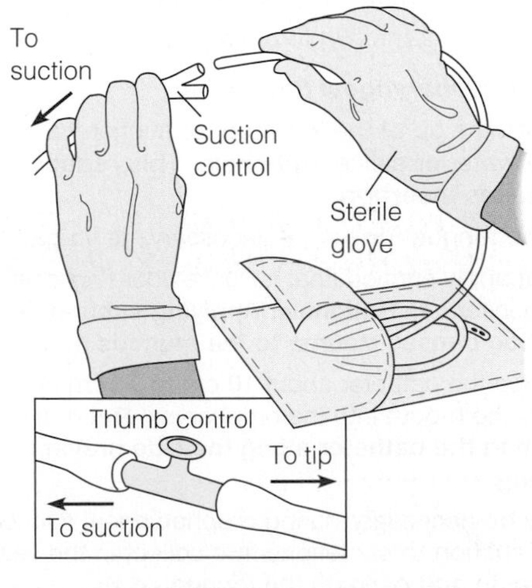

❶ Attaching the catheter to the suction unit

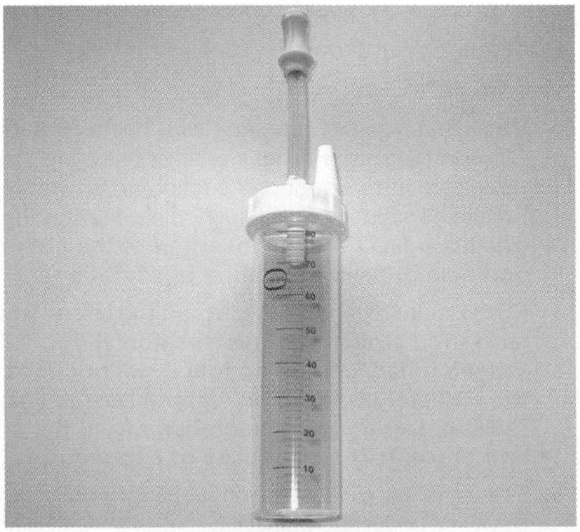
❷ A sputum collection trap

(continued)

SKILL 42.4

OROPHARYNGEAL, NASOPHARYNGEAL, AND NASOTRACHEAL SUCTIONING *(continued)*

- Attach the suction tubing to the sputum trap air vent.
- Suction the client's nasopharynx or oropharynx. The sputum trap will collect the mucus during suctioning.
- Remove the catheter from the client. Disconnect the sputum trap rubber tubing from the suction catheter. Remove the suction tubing from the trap air vent.
- Connect the rubber tubing of the sputum trap to the air vent. **Rationale: This retains any microorganisms in the sputum trap.**
- Connect the suction catheter to the tubing.
- Flush the catheter to remove secretions from the tubing.

11. Promote client comfort.
    - Offer to assist the client with oral or nasal hygiene.
    - Assist the client to a position that facilitates breathing.
12. Dispose of equipment and ensure availability for the next suction.
    - Dispose of the catheter, gloves, water, and waste container. Wrap the catheter around your sterile gloved hand, holding it as the glove is removed over it for disposal.
    - Rinse the suction tubing, as needed, by inserting the end of the tubing into the water container. Empty and rinse the suction collection container as needed or indicated by protocol. Change the suction tubing and container at least daily.
    - Ensure that supplies are available for the next suctioning (suction kit, gloves, water or normal saline).
13. Assess the effectiveness of suctioning.
    - Auscultate the client's breath sounds to ensure they are clear of secretions. Observe the client's skin colour and mucous membranes, dyspnea, level of anxiety, vital signs, and oxygen saturation level.
14. Document relevant data.
    - Record the procedure: the amount, consistency, colour, and odour of sputum (e.g., foamy, white mucus; thick, green-tinged mucus; or blood-flecked mucus), the number of suctioning attempts, and the client's breathing status before, during, and after the procedure. This may include lung sounds, rate and character of breathing, and oxygen saturation.

EVALUATION

- Conduct appropriate follow-up, such as appearance of secretions suctioned; breath sounds; respiratory rate, rhythm, and depth; pulse rate and rhythm; and skin colour.
- Compare findings with previous assessment data if available.
- Report significant deviations from normal to the appropriate members of the health-care team.

For tracheostomy and endotracheal suctioning, the diameter of the suction catheter should be about half the inside diameter of the tracheostomy or endotracheal tube so that hypoxia can be prevented. The nurse uses sterile techniques to prevent infection of the respiratory tract (see Skill 42.5). The traditional method of suctioning an endotracheal tube or tracheostomy is sometimes referred to as the *open method*. If a client is connected to a ventilator, the nurse disconnects the client from the ventilator, suctions the airway, reconnects the client to the ventilator, and discards the suction catheter. Drawbacks to the open airway suction system include the nurse needing to wear personal protective equipment (e.g., goggles or face shield, gown) to avoid exposure to the client's sputum and the potential cost of one-time catheter use, especially if the client requires frequent suctioning.

With the *closed airway/tracheal suction system* (*inline suctioning*) (Figure 42.39, page 1357), the suction

SKILL 42.5

SUCTIONING A TRACHEOSTOMY OR ENDOTRACHEAL TUBE

PURPOSES

- To maintain a patent airway and prevent airway obstructions
- To promote respiratory function (optimal exchange of oxygen and carbon dioxide into and out of the lungs)
- To prevent pneumonia that may result from accumulated secretions

ASSESSMENT

Assess the client for the presence of congestion on auscultation of the thorax. Note the client's inability to remove the secretions through coughing.

Equipment

- Resuscitation bag (Ambu bag) connected to 100% oxygen
- Sterile towel (optional)

(continued)

SKILL 42.5

SUCTIONING A TRACHEOSTOMY OR ENDOTRACHEAL TUBE *(continued)*

- Equipment for suctioning the oropharyngeal cavity (see Skill 42.4)
- Goggles and mask, if necessary
- Gown, if necessary
- Sterile gloves
- Moisture-resistant bag

IMPLEMENTATION

Performance

1. Before performing the procedure, introduce your self and verify the client's identity by using agency protocol. Explain to the client what you are going to do, why it is necessary, and how he or she can cooperate. Inform the client that suctioning usually causes some intermittent coughing and that this assists in removing secretions.
2. Perform hand hygiene and observe other appropriate infection prevention and control procedures.
3. Provide for client privacy.
4. Prepare the client.
   - If not contraindicated, place the client in semi-Fowler's position to promote deep breathing, maximum lung expansion, and productive coughing. **Rationale: Deep breathing oxygenates the lungs, counteracts the hypoxic effects of suctioning, and may induce coughing. Coughing helps loosen and move secretions.**
   - If necessary, provide analgesia as ordered by the physician before suctioning. **Rationale: Endotracheal suctioning stimulates the cough reflex, which can cause pain in clients who have had thoracic or abdominal surgery or who have experienced traumatic injury. Premedication can increase the client's comfort during the suctioning procedure.**
5. Prepare the equipment. Attach the resuscitation apparatus to the oxygen source (see ❶). Adjust the oxygen flow to 100%.
   - Open the sterile supplies in readiness for use.
   - Place the sterile towel, if used, across the client's chest below the tracheostomy.
   - Turn on the suction, and set the pressure in accordance with agency policy and manufacturer's recommendations.
   - Put on goggles, mask, and gown, if necessary.
   - Put on sterile gloves.
   - Holding the catheter in the dominant hand and the connector in the nondominant hand, attach the suction catheter to the suction tubing (see Skill 42.4, ❶).
6. Flush and lubricate the catheter.
   - Using the dominant hand, place the catheter tip in the sterile saline solution.
   - Using the thumb of the nondominant hand, occlude the thumb control, and suction a small amount of the sterile solution through the catheter. **Rationale: This determines that the suction equipment is working properly and lubricates the outside and the lumen of the catheter. Lubrication eases insertion and reduces tissue trauma during insertion. Lubricating the lumen also helps prevent secretions from sticking to the inside of the catheter.**
7. If the client does not have copious secretions, hyperventilate the lungs with a resuscitation bag before suctioning, as ordered by a physician and according to agency policy.
   - Summon an assistant, if one is available, for this step.
   - Using your nondominant hand, turn on the oxygen to 12 L/min to 15 L/min.
   - If the client is receiving oxygen, disconnect the oxygen source from the tracheostomy tube by using your nondominant hand.
   - Attach the resuscitator to the tracheostomy or endotracheal tube (see ❷).
   - Compress the Ambu bag three to five times as the client *inhales.* This is best done by a second person who can use both hands to compress the bag, providing a greater inflation volume.
   - Observe the rise and fall of the client's chest to assess the adequacy of each ventilation.
   - Remove the resuscitation device, and place it on the bed or the client's chest with the connector facing up.

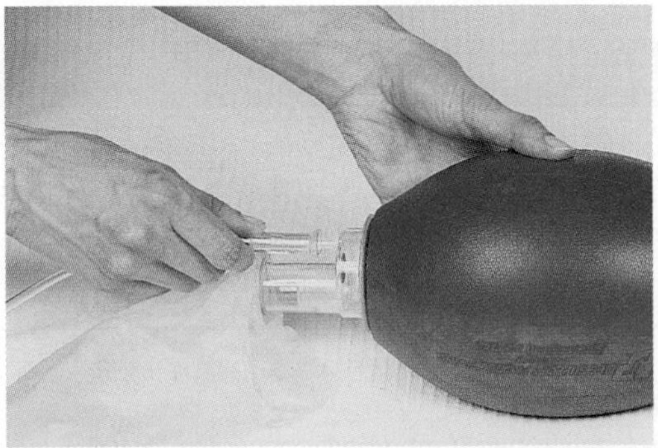

❶ Attaching the resuscitation apparatus to the oxygen source

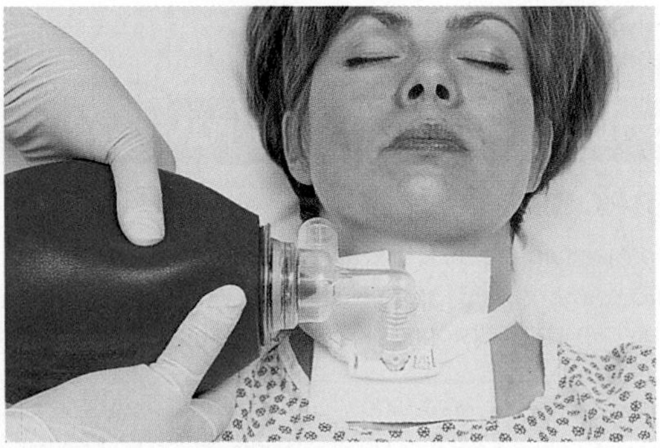

❷ Attaching the resuscitator to the tracheostomy

(continued)

SKILL 42.5

SUCTIONING A TRACHEOSTOMY OR ENDOTRACHEAL TUBE *(continued)*

Variation: Using a Ventilator to Provide Hyperventilation

- If the client is on a ventilator, use the ventilator for hyperventilation and hyperoxygenation. Newer models have a mode that provides 100% oxygen for 2 minutes and then switches back to the previous oxygen setting, as well as a manual breath or sigh button. **Rationale: The use of ventilator settings provides more consistent delivery of oxygenation and hyperinflation than does a resuscitation device.**

8. If the client has copious secretions, do not hyperventilate with a resuscitator. Instead, keep the regular oxygen delivery device on, and increase the litre flow or adjust the FiO_2 to 100% for several breaths before suctioning, according to agency policy. **Rationale: Hyperventilating a client who has copious secretions can force the secretions deeper into the respiratory tract.**

9. Quickly but gently insert the catheter *without* applying any suction.

- With your nondominant thumb off the suction port, quickly but gently insert the catheter into the trachea through the tracheostomy tube (see ❸). **Rationale: To prevent tissue trauma and oxygen loss, suction is not applied during insertion of the catheter.**
- Insert the catheter about 12.5 cm for adults, less for children, or less if the client coughs or you feel resistance. **Rationale: Resistance usually means that the catheter tip has reached the bifurcation of the trachea.** To prevent damaging the mucous membranes at the bifurcation, withdraw the catheter about 1 cm to 2 cm before applying suction.

10. Perform suctioning.

- Apply intermittent suction for 5 to 10 seconds by placing and removing the nondominant thumb over the thumb port. **Rationale: Suction time is restricted to 10 seconds or less to minimize oxygen loss.**
- Rotate the catheter by rolling it between your thumb and forefinger while slowly withdrawing it. **Rationale: This prevents tissue trauma by minimizing the suction time against any one part of the trachea.**
- Withdraw the catheter completely, and release the suction.
- Hyperventilate the client.
- Suction again, if needed.

11. Reassess the client's oxygenation status, and repeat suctioning.

- Observe the client's respirations and skin colour. Check the client's pulse, if necessary, by using your nondominant hand.
- Encourage the client to breathe deeply and to cough between suctions.
- Allow 2 to 3 minutes between suctions, when possible. **Rationale: This provides an opportunity for reoxygenation of the lungs.**

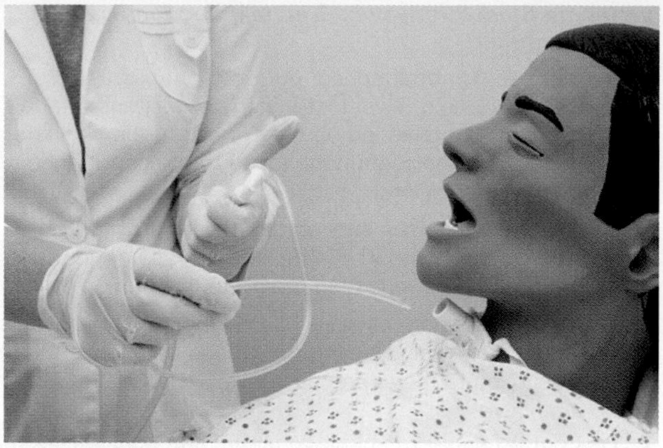

❸ Inserting the catheter into the trachea through the tracheostomy tube. *Note:* Suction is not applied while inserting the catheter.

- Flush the catheter, and repeat suctioning two or three times until the air passage is clear and the breathing is relatively effortless and quiet.
- After each suction, pick up the resuscitation bag with your nondominant hand and ventilate the client with no more than three breaths.

12. Dispose of equipment and ensure availability for the next suction.

- Flush the catheter and suction tubing.
- Turn off the suction, and disconnect the catheter from the suction tubing.
- Wrap the catheter around your sterile hand, and peel off the glove so that it turns inside out over the catheter.
- Discard the glove and the catheter in the moisture-resistant bag.
- Replenish the sterile fluid and supplies so that the suction is ready to be used again. **Rationale: Clients who require suctioning often require it quickly, so it is essential to leave the equipment at the bedside ready for use.**
- Be sure that the ventilator and oxygen settings are returned to pre-suctioning settings. **Rationale: On some ventilators this is automatic, but always check. It is very dangerous for clients to be left on 100% oxygen.**

13. Provide for client comfort and safety.

- Assist the client to a comfortable, safe position that aids breathing. If the person is conscious, a semi-Fowler's position is frequently indicated. If the person is unconscious, Sims' position aids in the drainage of secretions from the mouth.

14. Document relevant data.

- Record the suctioning procedure, including the amount and description of suction returns, cardiopulmonary assessment before and after suctioning, and client response.

(continued)

SKILL 42.5

SUCTIONING A TRACHEOSTOMY OR ENDOTRACHEAL TUBE (*continued*)

Variation: Closed Airway or Tracheal Suction System (Inline Catheter)

- If a catheter is not attached, put on clean gloves, aseptically open a new closed catheter set, and attach the ventilator connection on the T piece to the ventilator tubing. Attach the client connection to the endotracheal tube or tracheostomy.
- Attach one end of the suction connecting tubing to the suction connection port of the closed system and the other end of the connecting tubing to the suction device.
- Turn on the suction, occlude or kink tubing, and depress the suction control valve (on the closed catheter system) to set suction to the appropriate level. Release the suction control valve.
- Use the ventilator to hyperoxygenate and hyperinflate the client's lungs.
- Unlock the suction control mechanism if required by the manufacturer.
- Advance the suction catheter enclosed in its plastic sheath with the dominant hand. Steady the T piece with the nondominant hand.
- Depress the suction control valve and apply suction for no more than 10 seconds. Gently withdraw the catheter.
- Repeat as needed, remembering to provide hyperoxygenation and hyperinflation as needed.
- When completed suctioning, withdraw the catheter into its sleeve and close the access valve, if appropriate. **Rationale: If the system does not have an access valve on the client connector, the nurse needs to observe for the potential of the catheter migrating into the airway and partially obstructing the artificial airway.**
- Flush the catheter by instilling normal saline into the irrigation port and applying suction. Repeat until the catheter is clear.
- Close the irrigation port and close the suction valve.

EVALUATION

- Perform a follow-up examination of the client to determine the effectiveness of the suctioning (e.g., respiratory rate, depth, and character; breath sounds; colour of skin and nail beds; character and amount of secretions suctioned; changes in vital signs).
- Relate findings to previous assessment data if available.
- Report significant deviations from normal to the appropriate members of the health-care team.

Lifespan Considerations

Suctioning a Tracheostomy or Endotracheal Tube

INFANTS AND CHILDREN

- Have an assistant gently restrain the child to keep the child's hands out of the way. The assistant should maintain the child's head in the midline position.

OLDER ADULTS

- Do a thorough lung assessment before and after suctioning to determine effectiveness of suctioning and to be aware of any special problems.

catheter attaches to the ventilator tubing and the client does not need to be disconnected from the ventilator. The nurse is not exposed to any secretions because the suction catheter is enclosed in a plastic sheath. The catheter can be reused as many times as necessary until the system is changed. The nurse needs to inquire about the agency's policy for changing the closed suction system.

CHEST TUBES AND DRAINAGE SYSTEMS If the thin, double-layered pleural membrane is disrupted by lung disease, surgery, or trauma, the negative pressure between the pleural layers can be lost. The lung then collapses because it is no longer drawn outward as the diaphragm and intercostal muscles contract during inhalation. When air collects in the pleural space, it is known as a **pneumothorax**. A collection of blood in the

Home Care Considerations

Suctioning a Tracheostomy or Endotracheal Tube

- Whenever possible, the client should be encouraged to clear the airway by coughing.
- Clients may need to learn to suction their secretions if they cannot cough effectively.
- Clean gloves should be used when endotracheal suctioning is performed in the home environment.
- The nurse needs to instruct the caregiver on how to determine the need for suctioning and the correct process and rationale underlying the practice of suctioning, to avoid potential complications of suctioning.
- Stress the importance of adequate hydration as it thins secretions, which can aid in the removal of secretions by coughing or suctioning.

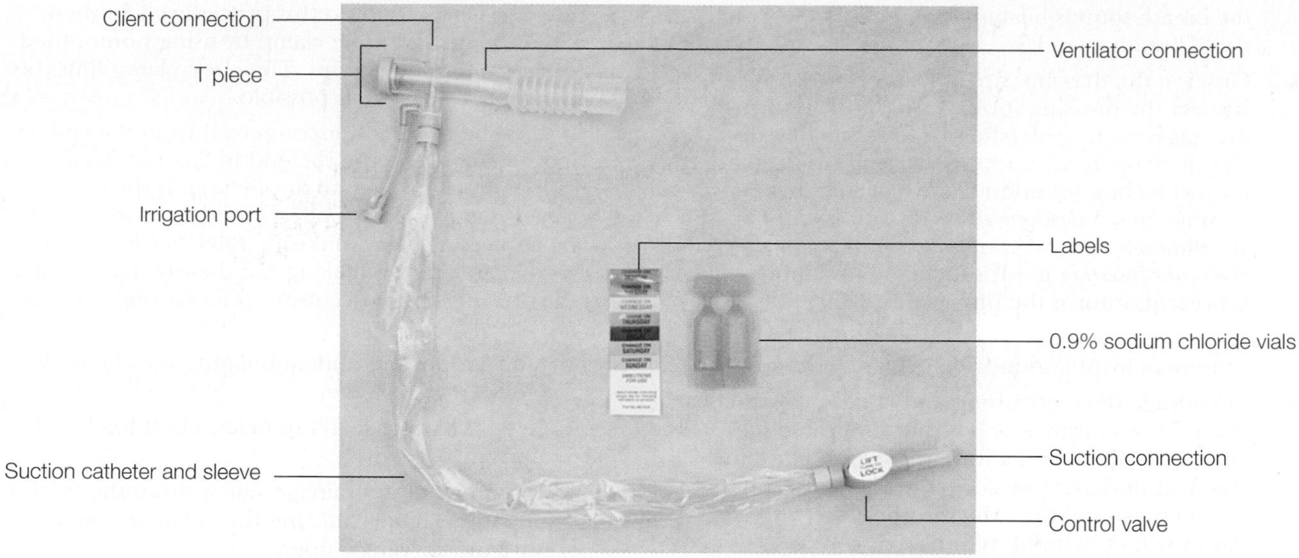

FIGURE 42.39 A closed airway suction (inline) system

pleural space, a **hemothorax,** or fluid, a pleural effusion, places pressure on lung tissue and interferes with lung expansion. Chest tubes can be inserted into the pleural cavity to restore negative pressure and drain collected fluid or blood. Because air rises, chest tubes for pneumothorax often are placed in the upper anterior thorax, whereas chest tubes used to drain fluid are generally placed in the lower lateral chest wall.

When chest tubes are inserted, they must be connected to a sealed drainage system or a one-way valve that allows air and fluid to be removed from the chest cavity but prevents air from entering from the outside. Water-seal drainage systems are used to prevent outside air from entering the chest tube. Sterile disposable systems commonly are used. These systems typically have a suction control chamber, a water seal chamber, and a closed collection chamber for drainage (Figure 42.40). With the water-seal system, when the client inhales, the water prevents air from entering the system from the atmosphere. During exhalation, however, air can exit the chest cavity, bubbling up through the water. Suction can be added to the system to facilitate removing air and secretions from the chest cavity. The drainage system should always be kept below the level of the client's chest to prevent fluid and drainage from being drawn back into the chest cavity.

A Heimlich valve or comparable system can be used for ambulatory clients (Figure 42.41). These valves allow air to escape from the chest cavity, but they close during inhalation to prevent air from entering.

Nursing responsibilities regarding drainage systems include the following:

- Monitor and maintain the patency and integrity of the drainage system.
- Assess the client's vital signs, oxygen saturation, cardiovascular status, and respiratory status. Check

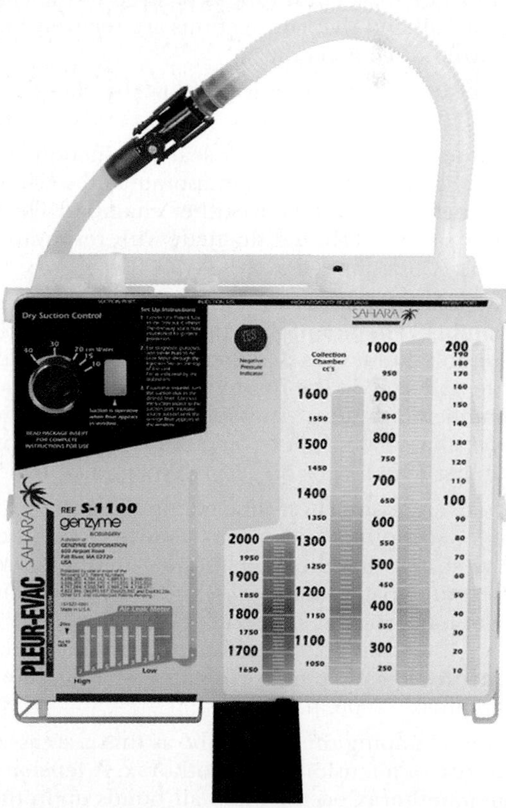

FIGURE 42.40 A disposable chest drainage system

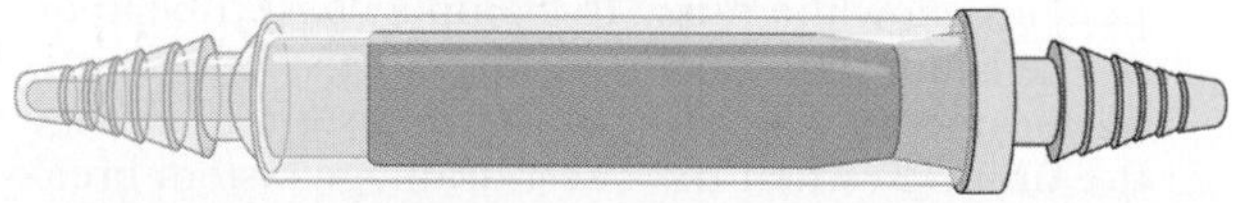

FIGURE 42.41 Heimlich chest drain valve

the breath sounds bilaterally and check for symmetry of breath sounds.

- Observe the dressing site at least every 4 hours. Inspect the dressing for excessive and abnormal drainage, such as bleeding or foul-smelling discharge. Palpate around the dressing site, and listen for a crackling sound indicative of subcutaneous emphysema. *Subcutaneous emphysema is air in the subcutaneous tissues and can result from a poor seal at the chest tube insertion site.* If subcutaneous emphysema is present, inform the physician.
- Determine the client's level of discomfort with and without activity, and medicate for pain if indicated.
- Encourage deep-breathing and coughing exercises every 2 hours (this may be contraindicated in clients who have had a lung removed). Have the client sit upright to perform the exercises, and splint the chest around the tube insertion site with a pillow or with a hand to minimize discomfort.
- Assist the client with range-of-motion exercises of the affected shoulder three times per day to maintain joint mobility.
- Ensure that the chest tube is secured to the client's chest wall and that connections are securely taped to avoid disconnection.
- Keep the collection devices below the client's chest level.
- Frequently check the water seal and suction control chambers. The water can evaporate and sterile water may need to be added to either chamber. The water seal level should fluctuate with respiratory effort (Coughlin & Parchinsky, 2006).
- Assess the drainage in the tubing and collection chamber. The drainage is measured at regularly scheduled times (as per agency policy). Mark the date and time at the fluid level on the drainage chamber. If drainage suddenly increases or if there is more than 100 mL/h of blood drainage (except for the first 3 hours postsurgery), inform the physician.
- Avoid aggressive chest tube manipulation (e.g., milking or stripping the tube) to remove clots. Studies have shown that these techniques do not improve chest tube patency. If necessary, however, a gentle technique, such as squeezing hand over hand along the tubing and releasing the tubing between squeezes may help improve patency (Coughlin & Parchinsky, 2006, p. 40).
- Avoid clamping the chest tube as this increases the risk of a tension pneumothorax. A **tension pneumothorax** occurs when air builds up in the pleural space and cannot escape, causing increased pressure. This pressure can eventually compromise cardiovascular function. A physician's order is required to clamp a chest tube. It is recommended that the nurse inquire about the reason for clamping the tube before carrying out the order. Some policies allow the nurse to clamp a chest tube in any of the following critical circumstances: (1) when disconnecting the chest drainage system to change the unit, (2) when the chest drainage system breaks or the integrity is disrupted for any reason, (3) when removing the chest tube. (Note that removing the chest tube is an advanced competency and the nurse must be certified to do this procedure.) In these circumstances, double clamp by using nontoothed or rubber-tipped clamps. The chest clamp must be unclamped as soon as possible.
- If the tube becomes disconnected from the collecting system, submerge the end in 2 cm of sterile saline or water to maintain the seal. If the chest tube is inadvertently pulled out, the wound should be immediately covered with a dry sterile dressing. If you can hear air leaking out the site, ensure that the dressing is not occlusive. *If the air cannot escape, this would lead to a tension pneumothorax.*
- When transporting and ambulating the client, do the following:
  - Keep the water-seal unit below chest level and upright.
  - Disconnect the drainage system from the suction apparatus before moving the client and make sure the air vent is open.
- Use routine practices and personal protective equipment while manipulating the system and assisting with insertion or removal.

Chest tube insertion and removal require sterile technique and must be done without introducing air or microorganisms into the pleural cavity. Removal of a chest tube is a brief but quite painful procedure. Medicate the client before the removal. Remove the dressing around the tube and prepare the dressing that will cover the insertion site. This will be an occlusive dressing if there is no purse-string suture around the insertion site to prevent air from entering the chest. Generally, the physician performs the removal but, in some areas, specially trained nurses may be permitted to do so.

PREVENTING VENOUS STASIS When clients have limited mobility or are confined to bed, venous return to the heart is impaired and the risk of venous stasis increases. Immobility is a problem not only for ill or debilitated clients but also for some travellers who sit with their legs dependent for long periods in a motor vehicle or an airplane. Venous stasis can lead to thrombus formation and edema of the extremities.

Preventing venous stasis is an important nursing intervention to reduce the risk of complications following surgery, trauma, or major medical problems. Prevention methods include pharmacological (e.g., unfractionated heparin or low molecular weight heparin) or mechanical (e.g., early mobilization, compression stockings, or intermittent pneumatic compression devices). Antiembolism stockings and sequential compression devices are additional measures to help prevent venous stasis.

ANTIEMBOLISM STOCKINGS Antiembolism stockings are firm elastic hosiery that provide varying degrees of leg compression. They are frequently used in clients with limited mobility, either because of restricted activities or because of prolonged standing (e.g., supermarket checkers and restaurant servers). Knee-high, thigh, and full stockings are available. Presized stockings are commonly used; some clients may require custom-made stockings. The length of the antiembolism stockings should be based on the individual client's condition (e.g., if a client has a history of popliteal clots, thigh-high or full stockings would be recommended to facilitate venous return throughout the leg).

When obtaining antiembolism stockings for a client, follow the manufacturer's recommendation for measuring and fitting the stockings. See Skill 35.2 (page 1030).

Sequential Compression or Pneumatic Pressure Devices Clients who are undergoing surgery or who are immobilized because of illness or injury may benefit from a sequential compression device (SCD) to promote venous return from the legs. SCDs inflate and deflate plastic sleeves wrapped around the legs to promote venous flow. The plastic sleeves are attached by tubing to an air pump that alternately inflates and deflates portions of the sleeve to a specified pressure. The ankle area inflates first, followed by the calf region, and then the thigh area. This sequential inflation and deflation assists the leg muscles in moving blood toward the heart.

Antiembolism stockings may be worn under the SCD to provide added support and protect the skin from irritation by the plastic. The SCD is removed for ambulation and is usually discontinued when the client resumes activities. SCDs are useful in *preventing* thrombi and edema from venous stasis, but they are not used for clients who have arterial insufficiency, cellulitis, infection of the extremity, or existing venous thrombosis. Pressure devices are available for rent or purchase for home use.

Skill 42.6 outlines how to apply a sequential compression device.

SKILL 42.6

APPLYING A SEQUENTIAL COMPRESSION DEVICE

PURPOSES

- To promote venous return from the legs
- To decrease the risk of deep vein thrombosis and pulmonary embolism

ASSESSMENT

Assess for baseline data:

- Cardiovascular status including heart rate and rhythm, peripheral pulses, and capillary refill
- Colour and temperature of extremities
- Movement and sensation of feet and lower extremities

Equipment

- Measuring tape
- Sequential compression device (SCD), including disposable sleeves, air pump, and tubing

IMPLEMENTATION

Performance

1. Before performing the procedure, introduce yourself and verify the client's identity by using agency protocol. Explain to the client what you are going to do, why it is necessary, and the procedure for applying the sequential compression device. **Rationale: The client's understanding and comfort will be increased by understanding the rationale for applying the SCD.**
2. Perform hand hygiene and observe other appropriate infection prevention and control procedures.
3. Provide for client privacy.
4. Prepare the client.
   - Place the client in a dorsal recumbent or semi-Fowler's position.
   - Measure the client's legs as recommended by the manufacturer if a thigh-length sleeve is required. **Rationale: Knee-length sleeves come in just one size; the thigh circumference determines the size needed for a thigh-length sleeve.**
5. Apply the sequential compression sleeves.
   - Place a sleeve under each leg with the opening at the knee.
   - Wrap the sleeve securely around the leg, securing the Velcro tabs (see ❶). Allow two fingers to fit between the leg and the sleeve. **Rationale: This amount of space ensures that the sleeve does not impair circulation when inflated.**
6. Connect the sleeves to the control unit and adjust the pressure, as recommended.
   - Connect the tubing to the sleeves and control unit, ensuring that arrows on the plug and the connector are in alignment and that the tubing is not kinked or twisted. **Rationale: Improper alignment or obstruction of the tubing by kinks or twists will interfere with operation of the SCD.**

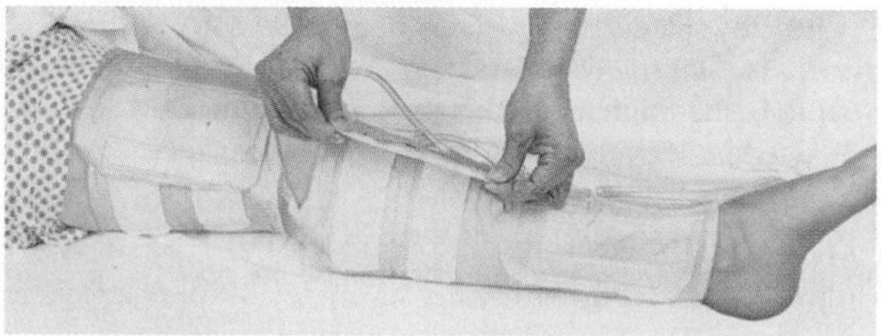

❶ Applying a sequential compression device to the leg

(continued)

SKILL 42.6

APPLYING A SEQUENTIAL COMPRESSION DEVICE *(continued)*

- Turn on the control unit, and adjust the alarms and pressures as needed. The sleeve cooling control and alarm should be on; ankle pressure should be set as recommended by the manufacturer. **Rationale: It is important to have the sleeve cooling control on for comfort and to reduce the risk of skin irritation from moisture under the sleeve. Alarms warn of possible control unit malfunctions.**

7. Document the procedure.
   - Record baseline assessment data and application of the SCD. Note control unit settings.
   - Assess and document skin integrity and neurovascular status regularly according to agency policy while the SCD is in place. Remove the unit and notify the physician if the client complains of numbness, tingling, or leg pain. **Rationale: These can be symptoms of nerve compression.**

EVALUATION

- Perform appropriate follow-up assessments, such as cardiovascular status, including pedal pulses, skin colour and temperature, skin integrity, and neurovascular status, including movement and sensation.
- Compare with baseline data if available.
- Report significant deviations from normal to the appropriate members of the health-care team.

CARDIOPULMONARY RESUSCITATION **Cardiopulmonary resuscitation (CPR)** is a combination of oral resuscitation (mouth-to-mouth breathing), which supplies oxygen to the lungs, and external cardiac massage (chest compression), which is intended to re-establish cardiac function and blood circulation. CPR is also referred to as basic life support (BLS).

A **cardiac arrest** is the cessation of cardiac function; the heart stops beating. Often, a cardiac arrest is unexpected and sudden. When it occurs, the heart no longer pumps blood to any of the organs of the body. Breathing then stops, and the person becomes unconscious and limp. Within 20 to 40 seconds of a cardiac arrest, the victim is clinically dead. After 4 to 6 minutes, the lack of oxygen supply to the brain causes permanent and extensive damage.

The three cardinal signs of a cardiac arrest are apnea, absence of a carotid or femoral pulse, and dilated pupils. The person's skin and mucous membranes appear pale or greyish and the skin feels cool. The pupils may be dilated. Cyanosis is evident when respiratory function fails before heart failure.

A **respiratory arrest** (pulmonary arrest) is the cessation of breathing. It often occurs as a result of a blocked airway, but it can occur following a cardiac arrest and for other reasons. A respiratory arrest may occur abruptly or be preceded by short, shallow breathing that becomes increasingly laboured.

It is vital that all nurses be trained to perform CPR so that resuscitation measures can be initiated immediately when a cardiac or respiratory arrest occurs. Nurses also can be instrumental in increasing community awareness of the need for CPR training and ensuring its availability. Most health-care agencies have established practices and policies regarding CPR.

Evaluating

By using the goals and desired health outcomes identified in the planning stage of the nursing process, the nurse collects data to evaluate the effectiveness of interventions. Examples of desired health outcomes for the goals identified for clients with oxygenation problems are found in Table 42.2.

If outcomes are *not* achieved, the nurse, client, and support person, if appropriate, need to explore the reasons why before modifying the care plan. For example, if the outcome "Respirations unlaboured and rate within expected range" is not met, examples of questions that need to be considered include the following:

- What is the client's perception of the problem?
- Is the client complaining of shortness of breath or difficulty breathing?
- Is the client taking medications or being treated with percussion, vibration, and postural drainage, as prescribed?
- Has the client been exposed to an upper respiratory infection that is affecting breathing?
- Is there a balance between factors that affect cardiac output, such as preload and afterload?
- Do other factors need to be considered, such as the client's psychological stress level?

Examples of questions to consider if the outcome "Able to complete ADLs without fatigue" is *not* met include the following:

- What other factors may be affecting the client's ability to complete ADLs?
- Is the client getting adequate sleep? If not, what is interfering with the client's rest?

TABLE 42.2 Evaluation Goals and Outcomes: Oxygenation and Circulation

Goal	Examples of Desired Health Outcomes
Maintain a patent airway	Unlaboured respirations and rate within expected range Clear lung sounds No stridor or wheezing Expels secretions effectively with coughing
Improve comfort and ease of breathing	Quiet, rhythmic, and effortless breathing pattern Respiratory rate, depth, and rhythm within expected range No dyspnea, shortness of breath (SOB), or orthopnea No restlessness or agitation Uses pursed-lip breathing, as needed
Maintain or improve pulmonary ventilation and oxygenation	Arterial blood gases within normal range SaO_2 is greater than 90% Respiratory rate, rhythm, and depth within expected range Symmetrical chest expansion No auscultated adventitious breath sounds No restlessness, agitation, cyanosis, or confusion
Maintain (or promote) cardiac function and output	Blood pressure (systolic and diastolic) within expected range Apical-radial heart rate and rhythm within expected range Heart and lung sounds normal Urinary output of 30 mL/h to 50 mL/h or greater No lethargy or extreme fatigue
Maintain or improve tissue perfusion	Capillary refill is brisk Strong and equal peripheral pulses Skin pink and warm, mucous membranes moist and pink; sensation intact No peripheral edema noted No localized extremity pain or pain with activity
Maintain (or improve) ability to participate in physical activities	Performs usual personal care activities (e.g., bathing, dressing, grooming, toileting) without shortness of breath or fatigue Food and fluid intake adequate to maintain energy level Blood tests within normal range (e.g., hemoglobin, blood gases) Balances rest and activity Adapts lifestyle to energy limitations
Avoid risks associated with oxygenation problems (acid-base imbalances, skin and tissue breakdown, syncope, hopelessness, social isolation)	Skin intact and adequate perfusion Serum electrolytes and blood gases within normal limits Neurological status within normal limits Cognitive status satisfactory (e.g., alert and oriented) Maintains participation in usual social activities Expresses positive future outlook and sense of inner peace

- Are there assistive devices (e.g., a shower chair, clothing that is easy to put on) that could help the client achieve this goal?
- Does the client need help with housework and other ADLs?
- Is the client's diet adequate to meet nutritional needs?

Case Study 42

Jerry Markert, 21, was admitted to the acute-care facility following a biking accident in which he received multiple injuries, including a hemothorax. He is receiving 6 L of oxygen, as ordered, by a nasal cannula, has a chest tube connected to a closed drainage system, and is attached to a pulse oximeter that indicates an oxygen saturation level of 98%. He is alert, stable, and progressing well.

Critical Thinking Skills

1. If Mr. Markert is stable and progressing well, why is his oxygen saturation being monitored?
2. Speculate about why Mr. Markert is receiving oxygen by a nasal cannula as opposed to a facemask.
3. Compare and contrast a hemothorax and a pneumothorax.
4. What precautions need to be taken when caring for Mr. Markert while his chest tube is in place?
5. Offer suggestions that would help Mr. Markert, or any person with a respiratory problem, to establish healthy breathing after his chest tube is removed.

After working through these questions, go to the MyNursingLab at **http://www.mynursinglab.com** to check your answers.

KEY TERMS

respiration
pleural space
intrapleural pressure
intrapulmonary pressure
tidal volume
lung compliance
atelectasis
lung recoil
surfactant
diffusion
partial pressure
hemoglobin
erythrocytes
oxyhemoglobin
cardiac output
hematocrit
hypoxia
pericardium
epicardium
myocardium
endocardium
atria
ventricles
coronary arteries
systole
diastole
sinoatrial (SA or sinus) node
atrioventricular (AV) node
stroke volume (SV)
preload
contractility
afterload
blood pressure
systemic vascular resistance (SVR)
vital capacity
hypercarbia
hypercapnia
hypoxemia
cyanosis
eupnea
tachypnea
bradypnea
apnea
hyperventilation
Kussmaul's respiration
hypoventilation
Cheyne-Stokes respiration
Biot's (cluster) respiration
dyspnea
orthopnea
stridor
adventitious breath sounds
myocardial infarction (MI)
heart failure
ischemia
sputum
hemoptysis
throat culture
creatine kinase
troponin
cardiac monitoring
electrocardiogram (ECG)
X-ray examination
lung scan
angiography
echocardiogram
laryngoscopy
bronchoscopy
hemodynamics
humidifiers
incentive spirometers
vibration
postural drainage
continuous positive airway pressure (CPAP)
tracheotomy
tracheostomy
suctioning
pneumothorax
hemothorax
tension pneumothorax
cardiopulmonary resuscitation (CPR)
cardiac arrest
respiratory arrest

CHAPTER HIGHLIGHTS

- Respiration is the process of gas exchange between the individual and the environment.
- The respiratory system contributes to effective respiration through pulmonary ventilation (the movement of air between the atmosphere and the lungs) and the diffusion of oxygen and carbon dioxide across the pulmonary membrane.
- The cardiovascular system transports these gases in the blood to and from the tissues and facilitates the diffusion of gases between the capillaries and body tissues.
- Alveoli and the capillaries that surround them form the respiratory membrane where gas exchange between the lungs and the blood occurs.
- Effective pulmonary ventilation, or breathing, requires clear airways, an intact central nervous system and respiratory centre, an intact thoracic cavity and musculature, and adequate pulmonary compliance (stretch) and recoil.
- Gas exchange occurs by diffusion as gas molecules move from an area of higher concentration to an area of lower concentration. At the respiratory membrane, oxygen moves from the alveolus into the blood, while carbon dioxide moves from the blood into the alveolus.
- Most oxygen (97%) is carried to the tissues loosely combined with hemoglobin in erythrocytes (red blood cells [RBCs]). Anemia, which is too few RBCs or low hemoglobin levels, impairs oxygen transportation.
- Carbon dioxide is transported within RBCs as bicarbonate or combined with hemoglobin, and in blood plasma as carbonic acid.
- The heart and the blood vessels make up the cardiovascular system, which, together with blood, is the major system for transporting oxygen and nutrients to the tissues and waste products away from the tissues for elimination.
- The right side of the heart receives deoxygenated blood from the body and pumps it to the lungs via the pulmonary arteries; the left side receives oxygenated blood from the lungs and pumps it out to the body via the aorta.
- Coronary arteries supply oxygen and nutrients to the heart muscle.
- The cardiac conduction system controls the electrical activity of the heart and the cardiac cycle: systole, contraction of the heart muscle and ejection of blood; and diastole, the relaxation period during which the heart fills with blood.
- Cardiac output depends on the stroke volume, or amount of blood ejected during systole, and the heart rate.
- The systemic blood vessels carry blood to the tissues through a system of arteries, arterioles, and capillaries and return it to the heart through the venules, veins, and venae cavae.
- Heart and respiratory rates normally are highest in neonates and infants, gradually slowing to adult ranges; the blood pressure rises gradually from birth to reach the adult range in adolescence.
- Aging affects both the respiratory and the cardiovascular systems: the chest wall becomes more rigid and lungs less elastic; atherosclerosis causes fatty plaque to develop within arteries.
- Other factors affecting oxygenation include the environment, lifestyle, health status, opioid analgesics, stress and coping, and gender.
- Hypoxia, insufficient oxygen in the tissues, can result from impaired ventilation (hypoventilation) or diffusion, or from impaired oxygen transportation to the tissues because of anemia or decreased cardiac output.
- Normal respirations are quiet and unlaboured; altered respiratory patterns include tachypnea, bradypnea, hyperventilation, hypoventilation, and dyspnea. Shortness of breath is a subjective sensation of not getting enough air.
- Airway obstruction interferes with ventilation. A low-pitched snoring sound, stridor, and abnormal breath sounds may accompany partial airway obstruction. Extreme inspiratory effort with no chest movement indicates complete upper airway obstruction.
- Decreased cardiac output, impaired tissue perfusion, and disorders affecting the blood are the major cardiovascular problems that can affect oxygenation.
- Cardiac output may fall with a myocardial infarction, heart failure, dysrhythmias, and structural alterations of the heart (e.g., valve deformities).
- The most common cause of impaired blood flow to tissues is atherosclerosis; this can lead to tissue ischemia and pain.
- To assess oxygenation, the nurse conducts a nursing history, performs a complete physical assessment of the client, and reviews relevant diagnostic data.
- The nursing history includes questions about current or past respiratory and cardiovascular problems, including hypertension; about lifestyle; presence of symptoms, such as cough or shortness of breath; smoking and other risk factors; and medications.
- Physical assessment should include a general assessment, as well as specific examination of the respiratory and cardiovascular systems.
- Cardiac monitoring is used for continuous observation of the heart rate and rhythm.
- Diagnostic tests that may be performed to assess oxygenation include sputum and throat culture specimens; blood tests, such as the CBC, hemoglobin, and hematocrit, blood chemistries, and arterial blood gases; electrocardiography (ECG) and stress electrocardiography; pulmonary function tests; visualization procedures, such as radiography, lung scans, angiography, echocardiography, laryngoscopy, and bronchoscopy; and hemodynamic studies.
- The nurse is responsible for obtaining specimens for diagnostic tests, preparing the client and the support people for diagnostic procedures, monitoring the

client's response to certain procedures, and reviewing records and reports of diagnostic tests.

- Nursing diagnoses for the client with problems of oxygenation include *Ineffective Airway Clearance, Ineffective Breathing Pattern, Impaired Gas Exchange, Altered Peripheral Tissue Perfusion, Decreased Cardiac Output,* and *Activity Intolerance.* These problems also may be the etiology for several other nursing diagnoses, including *Anxiety, Fatigue, Fear, Powerlessness, Sleep Pattern, Disturbed,* and *Social Isolation.*
- In planning care for clients with problems of oxygenation, the nurse establishes the following goals: maintain a patent airway; improve ease and comfort of breathing; maintain ventilation and oxygenation; ensure tissue perfusion; maintain cardiac output; improve the client's activity tolerance; and prevent risks, such as tissue breakdown and infection.
- In discharge and home care planning, the nurse assesses the client's self-care abilities and need for assistive devices, home environment, compliance with medical regimen, and knowledge level. The ability of the family or support people to provide assistance and financial support and to cope with the changes are also assessed, as are community factors, such as the environment and resources.
- The nurse teaches the client about home care activities to maintain a patent airway and gas exchange, to promote healthy breathing, and to maintain cardiac output and tissue perfusion. Dietary modifications, prescribed medications, and specific procedures also are taught, and the nurse makes referrals to community agencies as needed.
- Nursing interventions to promote oxygenation include promoting healthy breathing and a healthy heart, deep breathing and coughing, and hydration; administering medications; implementing measures to clear secretions (e.g., incentive spirometry, percussion, vibration, and postural drainage); initiating and monitoring oxygen therapy; initiating or assisting with procedures to maintain the airway (e.g., artificial airways, suctioning, and continuous positive airway pressure therapy); providing tracheostomy care; monitoring chest drainage systems; using antiembolism stockings and sequential compression devices to prevent venous stasis and edema; and administering cardiopulmonary resuscitation.
- The effectiveness of nursing interventions is evaluated by using the goals and desired health outcomes identified in the planning stage of the nursing process. If a goal is not met, the nurse asks pertinent questions to assess the reason for not meeting the goal.

ASSESS YOUR LEARNING

1. A client with chronic pulmonary disease has a bluish tinge around the lips. This would most accurately be documented as which of the following?

a. Hypoxia
b. Hypoxemia
c. Dyspnea
d. Cyanosis

2. A client with a chronic lung disorder requires some supplemental oxygen. Which of the following should the nurse consider as safe delivery?

a. Oxygen at 2 L/min per nasal cannula
b. Oxygen at 6 L/min per facemask
c. Oxygen at 8 L/min per partial rebreather mask
d. Oxygen at 10 L/min per nonrebreather mask

3. Which of the following represents proper nasopharyngeal or nasotracheal suction technique?

a. Lubricate the suction catheter with petroleum jelly (e.g., Vaseline) before and between insertions.
b. Apply suction intermittently while inserting the suction catheter.
c. Rotate the catheter while applying suction.
d. Hyperoxygenate the client with 100% oxygen for 30 minutes before and after suctioning.

4. Which of the following statements by the client indicates successful teaching regarding the proper use of an incentive spirometer?

a. "I should breathe out as fast and hard as possible into the device."
b. "I should inhale slowly and steadily to keep the balls up."
c. "I should use the device three times a day, after meals."
d. "The entire device should be washed thoroughly in sudsy water once a week."

5. The nurse is caring for a client with chest tubes. During ambulation, the connection between the tube and the water seal comes apart. Which of the following actions is most appropriate?

a. Assist the client with ambulation back to bed.
b. Reconnect the tube to the water seal.
c. Assess the client's lung sounds with a stethoscope.
d. Have the client cough forcibly several times.

6. Which of the following clients should be watched most closely for a problem with the transport of oxygen from the lungs to the tissues?

a. A client who has anemia
b. A client who has an infection
c. A client who has a fractured rib
d. A client who has a tumour of the medulla

7. The nurse is planning to perform percussion and postural drainage with a client. Which of the following is an important aspect of the planning?
   a. Percussion and postural drainage should be done before lunch.
   b. The order should be coughing, percussion, positioning, and then suctioning.
   c. A good time to perform percussion and postural drainage is in the morning after breakfast when the client is well rested.
   d. Percussion and postural drainage should always be preceded by 3 minutes of 100% oxygen.

8. Which of the following would most likely be included in the evaluation of the client goal of "demonstrate adequate tissue perfusion"?
   a. Symmetrical chest expansion
   b. Pursed-lip breathing
   c. Brisk capillary refill
   d. Activity intolerance

9. To prevent postoperative complications, the nurse assists the client with coughing and deep-breathing exercises. Which of the following would the nurse implementing this intervention recommend the patient?
   a. Perform coughing exercises 1 hour before meals and deep breathing 1 hour after meals.
   b. Cough forcefully as many times as tolerated.
   c. Perform huff coughing every 2 hours or as needed.
   d. Use diaphragmatic and pursed-lip breathing 5 to 10 times, four times a day.

10. Mr. Jacobs, 53 years old, was admitted to the hospital because of chest pain. His condition has deteriorated, and he develops crackles in his lower lobes of the lungs. He is feeling short of breath and anxious. The physician prescribes morphine sulphate (Morphine) 4 mg IV and furosemide (Lasix) 40 mg IV. Which of the following changes in condition best indicates that Mr. Jacobs is responding favourably to the medications?
    a. Decreased respiratory rate, decreased crackles.
    b. Decreased crackles, large diuresis.
    c. Increased pulse, increased respiratory rate.
    d. Decreased respiratory rate, decreased blood pressure.

After working through these questions, go to the MyNursingLab at ***http://www.mynursinglab.com*** *to check your answers and see explanations.*

SUGGESTED READINGS

Chin-Peukert, L. (2007). From the heart. *Canadian Medical Association Journal, 176*(5), 661–662.

The nurse-author of this touching article describes the range of emotions she and her family experience with heart surgery.

Thompson, T. L., & Dykeman, M. (2007). Nurse practitioners in Canadian heart failure clinics: Evidence to support their presence on health-care teams. *Canadian Journal of Nursing Leadership, 20*(2), 80–93.

This article describes the evidence that supports the role of nurses, in particular, nurse practitioners, in helping the growing number of Canadians who are coping with chronic heart failure.

Efre, A. J. (2004). Gender bias in acute myocardial infarction. *The Nurse Practitioner 29*(11), 42–55.

This article discusses the discrepancies in outcomes between men and women in the management of an acute myocardial infarction (AMI). The authors identify several reasons to explain the differences, and outline the steps to identification and treatment of an AMI.

Joffres, M. R., Campbell, N. R. C., Manns, B., & Tu, K. (2007). Estimate of the benefits of a population-based reduction in dietary sodium additives on hypertension and its related health care costs in Canada. *Canadian Journal of Cardiology, 23*(6), 437–443.

This interesting article identifies how reducing daily sodium intake by 30% can result in 1 million fewer hypertensive Canadians a year. Simple dietary measures had an even greater effect on blood pressure control in some patients than the antihypertensive therapy they were taking.

Morrison, R. (2006). Venous thromboembolism: Scope of the problem and the nurse's role in risk assessment and prevention. *Journal of Vascular Nursing, 24,* 82–90.

This article identifies risk factors and signs and symptoms associated with venous thromboembolism. Preventive measures and the nurse's role in prevention are discussed.

St. John, R. E., & J. F. Malen, (2004). Contemporary issues in adult tracheostomy management. *Critical Care Nursing Clinics of North America, 16,* 413–430.

This comprehensive article describes the process from tracheotomy and tube insertion, nursing care and management to prevent complications, decannulation, and so forth.

WEBLINKS

Canadian Lung Association

http://www.lung.ca

This is the umbrella association for the provincial and territorial groups; the website provides a variety of educational material for the public and health-care professionals. The Canadian Respiratory Health Professionals network offers a forum for dialogue at this site.

Public Health Agency of Canada: Centre for Chronic Disease Prevention and Control—Cardiovascular Disease

http://www.phac-aspc.gc.ca/ccdpc-cpcmc/cvd-mcv/index_e.html

The Cardiovascular Disease Division of the Public Health Agency of Canada provides facts about heart disease, health-promotion advice in the form of a Healthy Heart Kit, and links to heart-related associations. The website offers a range of resources and information.

Heart and Stroke Foundation of Canada

http://www.heartandstroke.ca

This national association provides information and support to the public and health-care professionals.

REFERENCES

Ball, J. W., & Bindler, R. C. (2008). *Pediatric nursing: Caring for children* (4th ed.). Upper Saddle River, NJ: Pearson/Prentice Hall.

Canadian Hypertension Education Program. (2008). *2008 CHEP recommendations for the management of hypertension.* Ottawa: Author. Retrieved July 1, 2008, from http://hypertension.ca/chep/wp-content/uploads/2008/03/2008-chepspiral-booklet-final_jan28.pdf

Coughlin, A. M., & Parchinsky, C. (2006). Go with the flow of chest tube therapy. *Nursing, 36*(3), 36–41.

Health Canada. (2008). *Healthy living: Sodium.* Retrieved June 30, 2008, from http://www.hc-sc.gc.ca/hl-vs/iyh-vsv/food-aliment/sodium-eng.php

Heart and Stroke Foundation of Canada. (2004). *Heart and Stroke Foundation of Canada position statement: Low-carbohydrate diets and heart disease and stroke.* Retrieved July 14, 2008, from http://www.heartandstroke.com/site/lpp.aspx?c= ikIQLcMWJtE&b=3799187&printmode=1

Joffres, M. R., Campbell, N. R. C., Manns, B., & Tu, K. (2007). Estimate of the benefits of a population-based reduction in dietary sodium additives on hypertension and its related health care costs in Canada. *Canadian Journal of Cardiology, 23*(6), 437–443.

NANDA International. (2007). *Nursing diagnoses: Definitions and classification, 2007–2008.* Philadelphia, PA: Author.

Registered Nurses' Association of Ontario. (2003a). *Helping people quit smoking: Nursing best practice guideline. Final report: Smoking cessation; e-learning for health professionals.* Toronto: Author.

Registered Nurses' Association of Ontario. (2003b). *Integrating smoking cessation into daily nursing practice.* Toronto: Author.

Registered Nurses' Association of Ontario. (2005). *Nursing care of dyspnea: The 6th vital sign in individuals with chronic obstructive pulmonary disease (COPD).* Toronto: Author.

Ruidavets, J., Bongard, V., Simon, C., Dallongeville, J., Ducimetiere, P., Arveiler, D., et al. (2006). Independent contribution of dairy products and calcium intake to blood pressure variations at a population level. *Journal of Hypertension, 24,* 671–681.

Safer Healthcare Now! (2005). *Prevent ventilator-associated pneumonia: Getting started kit.* Retrieved July 14, 2008, from http://www.saferhealthcarenow.ca/Default.aspx?folderId=82&contentId=180

Saremi, A., & Arora, R. (2008). The cardiovascular implications of alcohol and red wine. *American Journal of Therapeutics, 15,* 265–277.

World Health Organization. (2000). Tobacco-free initiative: Addressing the worldwide tobacco epidemic through effective, evidence-based treatment. Geneva, Switzerland: Author.

Chapter 43

Fluid, Electrolyte, and Acid-Base Balance

In good health, the body maintains a balance of fluids, electrolytes, and acids and bases. This balance, or physiological **homeostasis**, depends on multiple physiological processes that regulate fluid intake and output and the movement of water and the substances dissolved in it among the body compartments.

Almost every illness has the potential to threaten this balance. Even in normal daily living, excessive temperatures or vigorous activity can disturb the balance if adequate water and salt intakes are not maintained. Therapeutic measures, such as the use of diuretics or nasogastric suction, can also disturb the body's homeostasis unless water and electrolytes are replaced.

OBJECTIVES

After studying this chapter, you should be able to

1. Discuss the function, distribution, movement, and regulation of fluids and electrolytes in the body
2. Describe the regulation of acid-base balance in the body, including the roles of buffers, the lungs, and the kidneys
3. Identify factors affecting normal body fluid, electrolyte, and acid-base balance
4. Outline the risk factors for and the causes and effects of fluid, electrolyte, and acid-base imbalance
5. Collect assessment data related to the client's fluid, electrolyte, and acid-base balance
6. Select appropriate nursing diagnoses for clients with altered fluid, electrolyte, or acid-base balance
7. Teach clients ways to maintain fluid and electrolyte balance
8. Implement measures to correct imbalances of fluids and electrolytes or acids and bases, such as enteral or parenteral replacements and blood transfusions
9. Evaluate the effect of nursing and collaborative interventions on the client's fluid, electrolyte, or acid-base balance

Body Fluids and Electrolytes

In humans, the primary body fluid is water. Approximately 60% of the average healthy adult's weight is fluid. In good health, this volume of fluid remains relatively constant, and the individual's weight varies by less than 0.2 kg in 24 hours, regardless of the amount of fluid ingested.

Water, which is vital to health and normal cellular function, serves as:

- A medium for metabolic reactions within cells
- A transporter for nutrients, waste products, and other substances
- A lubricant
- An insulator and a shock absorber
- A means of regulating and maintaining body temperature

Age, gender, and body fat affect total body water. Infants have the highest proportion of water, accounting for 70% to 80% of their body weight. The proportion of body water decreases with age. In people older than 60 years of age, it represents about 50% of the total body weight. Women also have a lower percentage of body water than men do. Women and older adults have less body water because they generally have less muscle mass and a greater percentage of fat tissue than men and younger adults. Fat tissue is essentially free of water, whereas lean tissue contains a significant amount of water. Therefore, water makes up a greater percentage of a lean person's body weight than an obese person's.

Distribution of Body Fluids

The body's fluid is divided into two major components, intracellular and extracellular. **Intracellular fluid (ICF)** is found within the cells of the body. It constitutes approximately two-thirds of the total body fluid in adults. **Extracellular fluid (ECF)** is found outside the cells and accounts for about one-third of total body fluid. It is subdivided into three compartments: intravascular, interstitial, and transcellular fluid. **Intravascular fluid**, or **plasma**, accounts for approximately 20% of the ECF and is found within the vascular system. **Interstitial fluid**, accounting for approximately 75% of the ECF, surrounds the cells. The other 5% of the ECF includes lymph and transcellular fluids. **Transcellular fluid**, considered by some as distinct from intracellular and extracellular fluids, includes cerebrospinal, pericardial, pancreatic, pleural, peritoneal, intraocular, biliary, and synovial fluids (Figure 43.1).

Intracellular fluid is vital to normal cell functioning. It contains solutes, such as oxygen, electrolytes, and glucose, and it provides a medium in which metabolic processes of the cell take place.

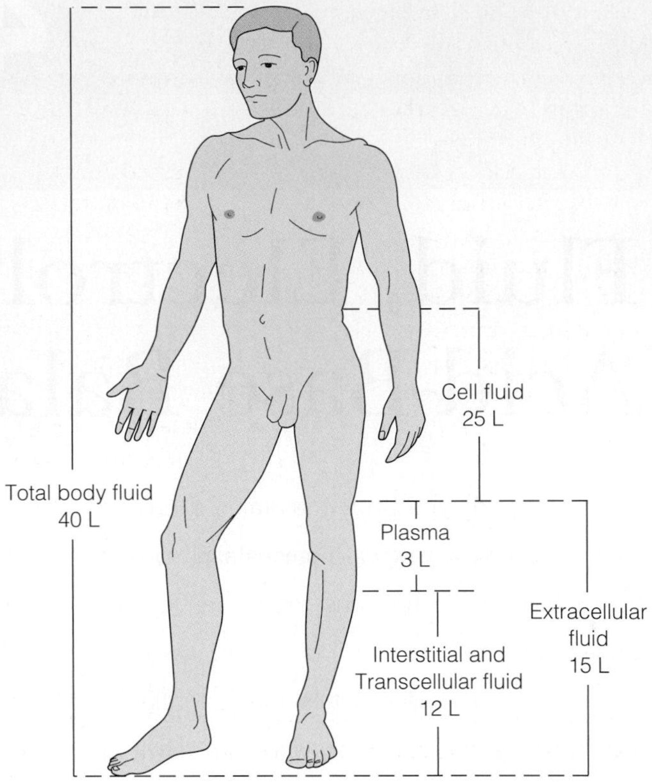

FIGURE 43.1 Total body fluid amounts to about 40 L in an adult male weighing 70 kg

Extracellular fluid provides the transport system that carries nutrients to, and waste products from, the cells. For example, plasma carries oxygen from the lungs and glucose from the gastrointestinal tract to the capillaries of the vascular system. From there, the oxygen and glucose move across the capillary membranes into the interstitial spaces and then across the cellular membranes into the cells. The opposite route is taken for waste products, such as carbon dioxide going from the cells to the lungs and metabolic acid wastes going eventually to the kidneys. Interstitial fluid, which composes three quarters of the ECF, transports wastes from the cells by way of the lymph system, as well as directly into the blood plasma through capillaries.

Composition of Body Fluids

Extracellular and intracellular fluids contain oxygen from the lungs, dissolved nutrients from the gastrointestinal tract, excretory products of metabolism, such as carbon dioxide, and electrically charged particles called **ions.**

Many salts dissociate in water, that is, break up into ions. The salt sodium chloride dissociates into one ion of sodium (Na^+) and one ion of chloride (Cl^-). These charged particles are called **electrolytes** because they are capable of conducting electricity. The number of ions that carry a positive charge, called **cations**, and ions that carry a negative charge, called **anions,** should be equal. Examples of cations are sodium (Na^+), potassium (K^+), calcium (Ca^{2+}), and magnesium (Mg^{2+}). Anions include chloride (Cl^-), bicarbonate (HCO_3^-), phosphate (PO_4^-), and sulphate (SO_4^{2-}).

For clinical purposes, the unit of measurement for electrolytes is the mole. A **mole** (mol) is defined as 6.02×10^{23} atoms, ions, or molecules of a substance (Silverthorn, 2006). One mole of a substance has the same number of atoms as any other substance. The *weight* of a mole is equal to the atomic mass or molecular weight of a particular substance expressed in grams (also known as the gram molecular weight). For example, the atomic mass of sodium is 23.0 and the atomic mass of potassium is 39.1; therefore, 1 mole of sodium weighs 23 g, whereas 1 mole of potassium (with the same number of atoms) weighs 39.1 g. The number of moles of a substance in a 1 L solution is known as the **molarity** (commonly abbreviated as mol/L). For example, dissolving 40.1 g of calcium (i.e., its gram molecular weight) in enough water to make 1 L would constitute a one molar solution of calcium. In humans, the solutes found in body fluids are usually so dilute that their concentrations are expressed in 1/1000th of a mole, that is, a millimole (mmol). In clinical practice, common laboratory values are reported in millimoles per litre (mmol/L). For example, the normal ranges for plasma sodium (Na^+) and chloride (Cl^-) are 135 mmol/L to 145 mmol/L and 95 mmol/L to 105 mmol/L, respectively. This system of measurement is known as Système Internationale d'Unités (the metric system) or SI units.

It is important to remember that laboratory tests are usually performed using blood plasma, an extracellular fluid. These results may show what is happening in the ECF. Normally, direct measurement of electrolyte concentration within the cell is not done.

The composition of fluids varies from one body compartment to another. In extracellular fluid, the principal electrolytes are sodium, chloride, and bicarbonate. Other electrolytes, such as potassium, calcium, and magnesium, are present in much smaller quantities. Plasma and interstitial fluid, the two primary components of ECF, contain similar electrolytes and solutes. Plasma is a protein-rich fluid containing large amounts of albumin; in contrast, interstitial fluid contains very little protein.

The composition of intracellular fluid differs significantly from that of ECF. Potassium and magnesium are the primary cations present in ICF, with phosphate and sulphate being the major anions. As in ECF, other electrolytes are present within the cell but in much smaller concentrations (Figure 43.2).

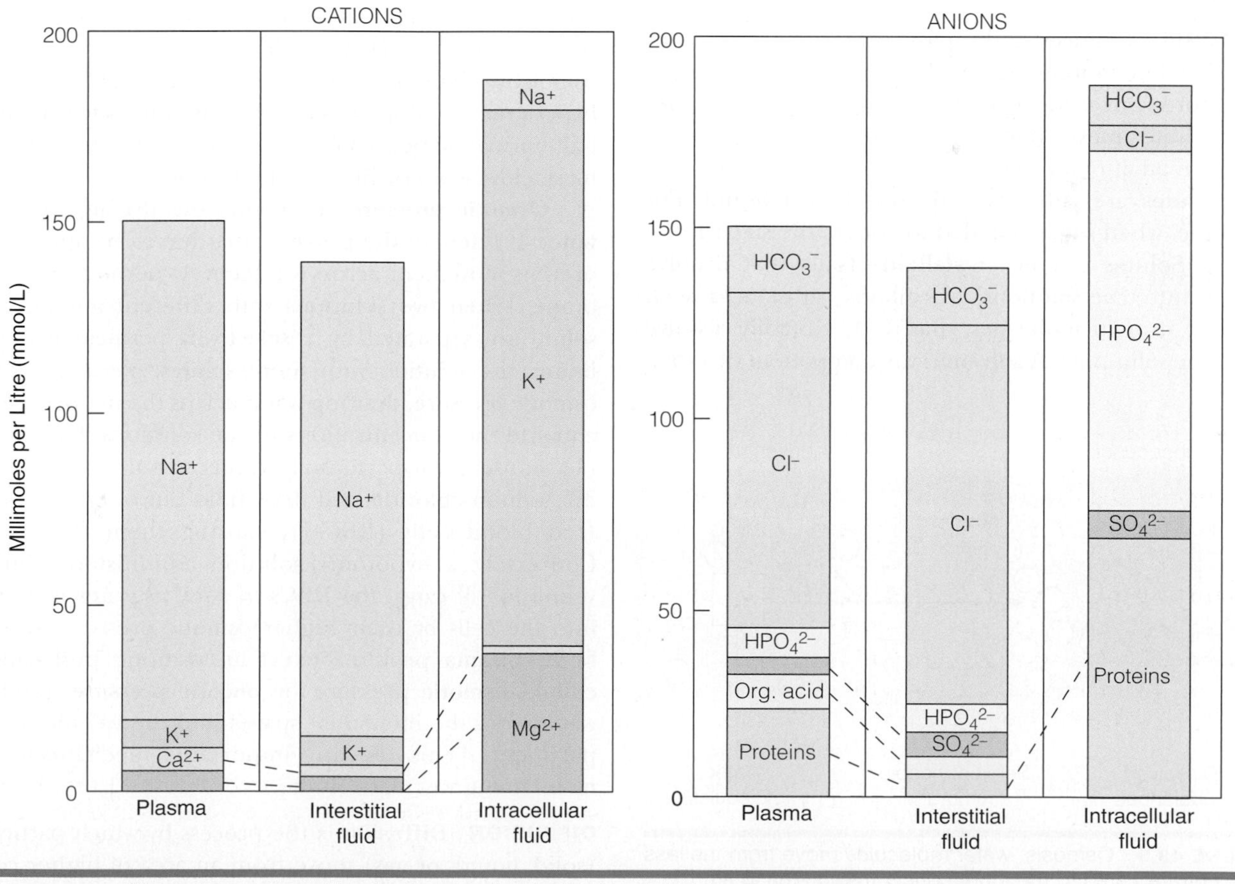

FIGURE 43.2 Electrolyte composition (cations and anions) of body fluid compartments

(From **Fundamentals of Anatomy and Physiology Interactive** *[Media ed.], 4th ed., by Fredric H. Martini and Rebecca H. Halyard, © 1998. Reproduced with permission of Pearson Education, Inc., Upper Saddle River, New Jersey.)*

Maintaining a balance of fluid volumes and electrolyte compositions in the fluid compartments of the body is essential to health. Normal and unusual fluid and electrolyte losses must be replaced if homeostasis is to be maintained.

Other body fluids, such as gastric and intestinal secretions, also contain electrolytes. Fluid and electrolyte imbalances can result from excessive loss of electrolytes from the gastrointestinal tract in severe vomiting, diarrhea, and suctioning of gastric secretions.

Movement of Body Fluids and Electrolytes

The body fluid compartments are separated from one another by cell membranes. Although these membranes are completely permeable to water, they are selectively permeable to solutes as substances move across them with varying degrees of ease. Small particles, such as ions, oxygen, and carbon dioxide, easily move across these membranes, but larger molecules, such as glucose and proteins, have more difficulty moving between fluid compartments.

The methods by which electrolytes and other solutes move are osmosis, diffusion, filtration, and active transport.

OSMOSIS **Osmosis** is the passive movement of water across cell membranes from a less concentrated solution to a more concentrated solution (Figure 43.3). In other words, water moves toward the higher concentration of solute in an attempt to equalize the concentrations.

Solutes are substances dissolved in a liquid. For example, when sugar is added to coffee, the sugar is the solute. Solutes can be **crystalloids** (salts that dissolve readily into true solutions) or **colloids** (substances, such as large protein molecules, that do not readily dissolve into true solutions). A **solvent** is the component of a solution that can dissolve a solute. In the previous example, coffee is the solvent for the sugar.

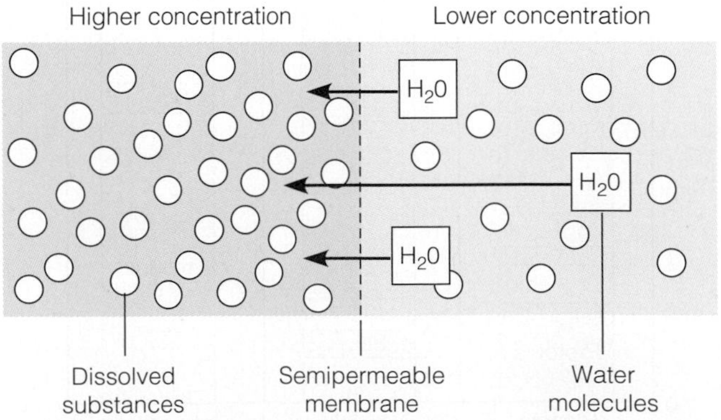

FIGURE 43.3 Osmosis: water molecules move from the less concentrated area to the more concentrated area in an attempt to equalize the concentration of solutions on two sides of a membrane.

In the body, water is the solvent; the solutes include electrolytes, oxygen, carbon dioxide, glucose, urea, amino acids, and proteins. Osmosis occurs when the concentration of solutes on one side of a selectively permeable membrane, such as the capillary membrane, is higher than on the other side. For example, a marathon runner loses a significant amount of water through perspiration, increasing the concentration of solutes in the plasma because of water loss. This higher solute concentration draws water from the interstitial spaces and cells into the vascular compartment to equalize the concentration of solutes in all fluid compartments. Osmosis is an important mechanism for maintaining homeostasis and fluid balance.

The concentration of solutes in body fluids is usually expressed as the **osmolality**. Osmolality is determined by the total solute concentration within a fluid compartment and is measured as parts of solute per kilogram of water. Osmolality is reported as milliosmoles per kilogram (mOsm/kg). Sodium is the greatest determinant of *serum osmolality,* with glucose and urea also contributing. Potassium, glucose, and urea are the primary contributors to the osmolality of intracellular fluid. The term *tonicity* can be used to refer to the osmolality of a solution. An **isotonic** solution has the same osmolality as body fluids. Normal saline, 0.9% sodium chloride, is an isotonic solution. **Hypertonic** solutions have a higher osmolality than body fluids; 3% sodium chloride is a hypertonic solution. **Hypotonic** solutions, such as one-half normal saline (0.45% sodium chloride), by contrast, have a lower osmolality than body fluids.

Osmotic pressure represents the driving force of water. It refers to the pressure that has to be applied to prevent movement across a selectively permeable membrane. When two solutions with different amounts of solute are separated by a selectively permeable membrane, the solution with more solutes exerts a higher osmotic pressure, drawing water across the membrane to equalize the concentrations of the solutions. For example, infusing a hypertonic intravenous solution, such as 3% sodium chloride, will draw fluid out of erythrocytes (red blood cells [RBCs]), causing them to shrink. Conversely, a hypotonic solution administered intravenously will cause the RBCs to swell as water is drawn into the cells by their higher osmotic pressure. In the body, plasma proteins exert an osmotic pull called **colloid osmotic pressure** or **oncotic pressure**, pulling water from the interstitial spaces into the vascular compartment. This is an important mechanism in maintaining vascular volume.

DIFFUSION **Diffusion** is the process by which particles (solid, liquid, or gas) move from an area of higher concentration to one of lower concentration (Chernecky, Macklin, & Murphy-Ende, 2006). For example, two gases become mixed by the constant motion of their molecules. In the body, diffusion of water, electrolytes, and other substances occurs through capillary membranes.

The rate of diffusion of substances varies according to (1) the size of the molecules, (2) the concentration of the solution, and (3) the temperature of the solution. Larger molecules move more slowly than smaller ones because large molecules require more energy to move. With diffusion, the molecules move from a solution of higher concentration to a solution of lower concentration (Figure 43.4). Increases in temperature increase the rate of motion of molecules and, therefore, the rate of diffusion.

FILTRATION **Filtration** is a process whereby fluid and solutes move together across a membrane from one compartment to another. The movement is from an area of higher liquid pressure to one of lower pressure. An example of filtration is the movement of fluid and nutrients from the capillaries of the arteries to the interstitial fluid around the cells. The pressure in the compartment that results in the movement of the fluid and substances dissolved in fluid out of the compartment is called **filtration pressure**. **Hydrostatic pressure** is the pressure exerted by a fluid within a closed system. The hydrostatic pressure of blood is the force exerted by blood against the vascular walls (e.g., the artery walls). The principle involved in hydrostatic pressure is that fluids move from the area of greater pressure to the area of lesser pressure. In the example of the blood vessels, the plasma proteins in the blood exert a colloid osmotic pressure or oncotic pressure that opposes the hydrostatic pressure and holds the fluid in the vascular compartment to maintain the vascular volume. Fluid filters out of the blood vessels when the hydrostatic pressure is greater than the osmotic pressure. The filtration pressure in this example is the difference between the hydrostatic pressure and the osmotic pressure (Figure 43.5).

ACTIVE TRANSPORT Substances can move across cell membranes from a less concentrated solution to a more concentrated one by **active transport** (Figure 43.6). This process differs from diffusion and osmosis in that metabolic energy is expended. In active transport, a substance combines with a carrier on the outside surface of the cell membrane, and they move to the inside surface of the cell membrane. Once inside, they separate, and the substance is released to the inside of the cell. A specific carrier is required for each substance, enzymes are required for active transport, and energy is expended.

This process is of particular importance in maintaining the differences in sodium and potassium ion concentrations of ECF and ICF. Under normal conditions, sodium concentrations are higher in the ECF, and potassium concentrations are higher inside the cells. To maintain these proportions, the active transport mechanism (the sodium-potassium pump) is activated, moving sodium from the cells and potassium into the cells.

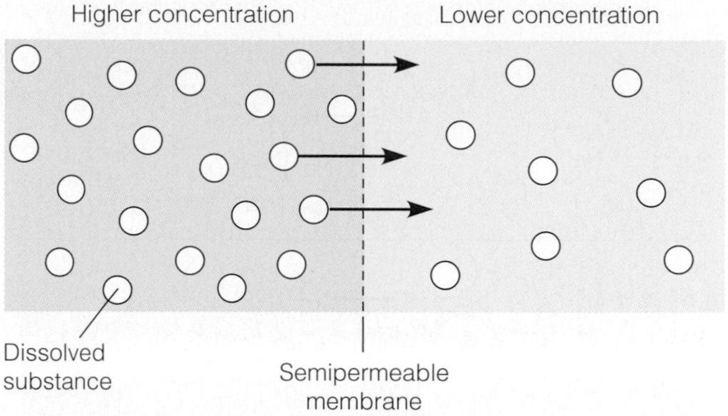

FIGURE 43.4 Diffusion: the movement of molecules through a semipermeable membrane from an area of higher concentration to an area of lower concentration

Regulating Body Fluids

In a healthy person the volumes and chemical composition of the fluid compartments stay within narrow limits.

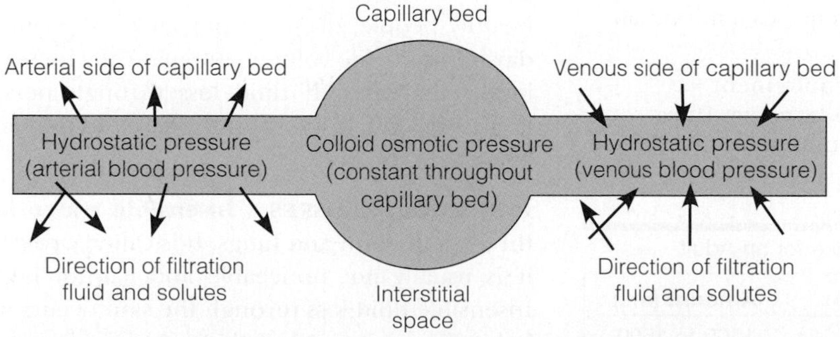

FIGURE 43.5 Schematic of filtration pressure changes within a capillary bed. On the arterial side, arterial blood pressure exceeds colloid osmotic pressure, so that water and dissolved substances move out of the capillary and into the interstitial space. On the venous side, venous blood pressure is less than colloid osmotic pressure, so that water and dissolved substances move into the capillary.

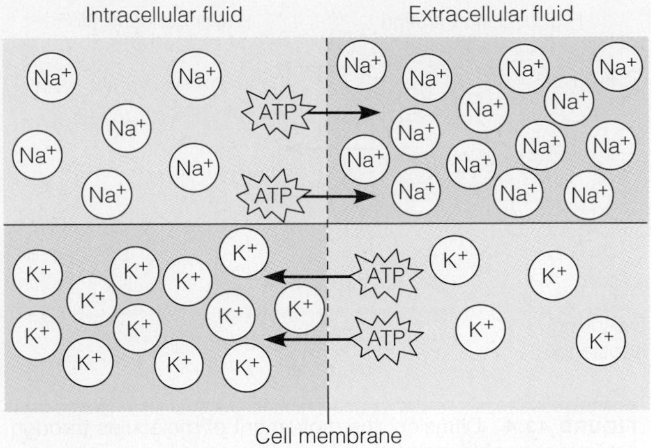

FIGURE 43.6 An example of active transport. Energy (adenosine triphosphate [ATP]) is used to move sodium molecules and potassium molecules across a semipermeable membrane against sodium's and potassium's concentration gradients (i.e., from areas of lesser concentration to areas of greater concentration).

Normally, fluid intake and fluid loss are balanced. Illness can upset this balance, causing the body to have too little or too much fluid.

FLUID INTAKE During periods of moderate activity at moderate temperature, the average adult requires a fluid intake of 30 mL/kg/day to 40 mL/kg/day. For an adult weighing 70 kg, the requirement would be 2100 mL to 2800 mL per day. Fluid intake comes from oral fluids as well as from solid foods that contain water. The oxidation of foods during metabolic processes produces approximately 200 mL per day. The water content of food is relatively high: fresh vegetables are approximately 90% water, fresh fruits, about 80%, and lean meats, around 60%. See Table 43.1.

Minimum daily fluid intake requirements for children are higher per kilogram of body weight owing to the greater proportion of body fluid, especially in newborns and infants. The following are formulae for minimum daily fluid requirements in children:

- Body weight 1 kg to 10 kg: requirement = 100 mL/kg (e.g., a baby weighing 5.5 kg requires a minimum of 550 mL fluid intake a day)
- Body weight 10 kg to 20 kg: requirement = 1000 mL + 50 mL/kg for each kg above 10 kg (e.g., a 15 kg child requires a minimum of 1250 mL fluid intake per day)
- Body weight more than 20 kg: requirement = 1500 + 20 mL/kg for each kg above 20 kg (e.g., a child weighing 22 kg requires a minimum of 1540 mL per day)

TABLE 43.1 Average Daily Fluid Intake for an Adult

Source	Amount (mL)
Oral fluids	1200 to 1500
Water in foods	1000 to 1100
Water as byproduct of food metabolism	200
Total	2400 to 2800

The thirst mechanism is the primary regulator of fluid intake. The thirst centre is located in the hypothalamus of the brain. A number of stimuli trigger this centre, including the osmotic pressure of body fluids, vascular volume, and angiotensin II (a hormone released in response to decreased blood flow to the kidneys). For example, a long-distance runner loses significant amounts of water through perspiration and rapid breathing during a race, increasing the concentration of solutes and the osmotic pressure of body fluids. This increased osmotic pressure stimulates the thirst centre, causing the runner to experience the sensation of thirst and the desire to drink to replace lost fluids.

Thirst is normally relieved immediately after drinking a small amount of fluid, even before it is absorbed from the gastrointestinal tract. However, this relief is only temporary, and the thirst returns in about 15 minutes. The thirst is again temporarily relieved after the ingested fluid distends the upper gastrointestinal tract. These mechanisms protect the individual from drinking too much because it takes from 30 minutes to 1 hour for the fluid to be absorbed and distributed throughout the body. See Figure 43.7

FLUID OUTPUT Fluid losses from the body counterbalance the adult's 2500 mL average daily intake of fluid, as shown in Table 43.2. Fluid output follows four routes:

1. Urine
2. Insensible (unmeasurable) loss through the apocrine glands of the skin as perspiration and through the lungs as water vapour in the expired air
3. Noticeable loss through the skin (from eccrine sweat glands)
4. Loss through the intestines in feces

URINE Urine formed by the kidneys and excreted from the urinary bladder is the major avenue of fluid output. Normal urine output for an adult is 1400 mL to 1500 mL per 24 hours, or at least 30 mL to 50 mL per hour. In healthy people, urine output may vary noticeably from day to day. Urine volume automatically increases as fluid intake increases. If fluid loss through perspiration is large, however, urine volume decreases to maintain fluid balance in the body.

INSENSIBLE LOSSES **Insensible water loss** occurs through the skin and lungs. It is called *insensible* because it is usually not noticeable and cannot be measured. Insensible fluid loss through the skin occurs in two ways. Solute-free water is lost through diffusion and through perspiration (which is noticeable but not measurable). Water losses through diffusion normally account for 350 mL to 400 mL per day. This transepidermal water loss is significantly increased if the protective layer of the

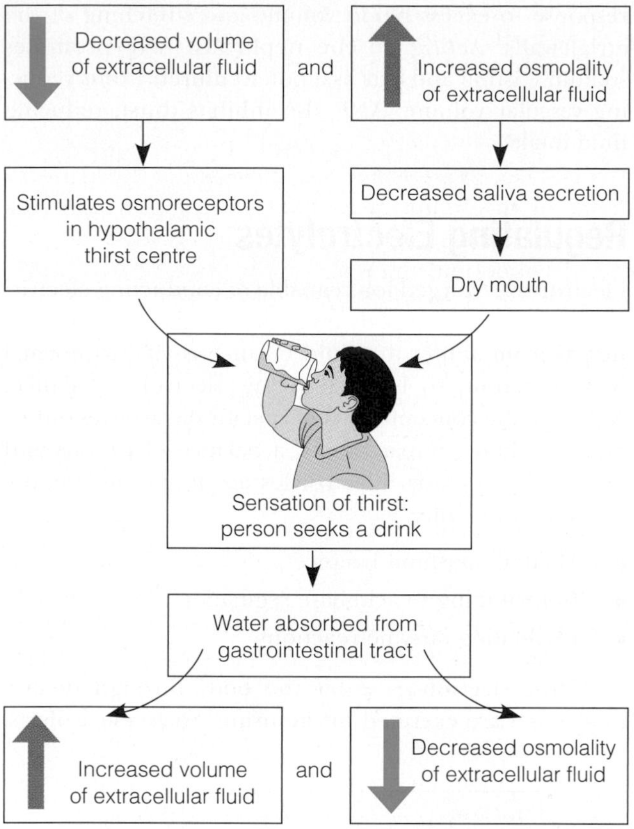

FIGURE 43.7 Factors stimulating water intake through the thirst mechanism

(From ***Medical Surgical Nursing: Critical Thinking in Client Care****, 3rd ed., by Priscilla LeMone and Karen M. Burke, © 2004. Reproduced with the permission of Pearson Education, Inc., Upper Saddle River, New Jersey.)*

skin is lost, as with burns or large abrasions. Perspiration varies depending on such factors as environmental temperature and metabolic activity. Fever and exercise increase metabolic activity and heat production, thereby increasing fluid losses through the skin.

Another type of insensible loss is the water in exhaled air. In an adult, this is normally 350 mL to 400 mL per day. When the respiratory rate accelerates, for example, with exercise or elevated body temperature, this loss increases.

SWEAT Sweat is produced by the eccrine sweat glands in response to the thermoregulatory centre in the hypothalamus and the sympathetic nervous system. Sweat is made up of water, sodium, potassium, and traces of urea. Excess sweat production can lead to both fluid and electrolyte imbalance.

FECES The chyme that passes from the small intestine into the large intestine contains water and electrolytes. The volume of chyme entering the large intestine in an adult is normally about 1500 mL per day. Of this amount, all but about 100 mL to 200 mL is reabsorbed in the proximal half of the large intestine.

Certain fluid losses are required to maintain normal body function. These are known as **obligatory losses.**

TABLE 43.2 Average Daily Fluid Output for an Adult

Route	Amount (mL)
Urine	1400 to 1500
Insensible losses	
Lungs	350 to 400
Skin	350 to 400
Sweat	100
Feces	100 to 200
Total	2200 to 2600

Approximately 500 mL of fluid *must* be excreted through the kidneys of an adult each day to eliminate metabolic waste products from the body. Water lost through respirations, through the skin, and in feces also are obligatory losses, necessary for temperature regulation and elimination of waste products. The total of all these losses is approximately 1400 mL to 1600 mL per day.

MAINTAINING HOMEOSTASIS The volume and composition of body fluids is regulated through several homeostatic mechanisms. Body systems contributing to this regulation include the kidneys, the endocrine system, the cardiovascular system, the lungs, and the gastrointestinal system. Hormones, such as antidiuretic hormone (also known as arginine vasopressin or AVP), the renin-angiotensin-aldosterone system, and atrial natriuretic factor are involved, as are mechanisms to monitor and maintain vascular volume.

KIDNEYS The kidneys are the primary regulator of body fluids and electrolyte balance. They regulate the volume and osmolality of extracellular fluids by regulating water and electrolyte excretion. The kidneys adjust the reabsorption of water from plasma filtrate and, ultimately, the amount excreted as urine. Although 135 L to 180 L of plasma per day is normally filtered in an adult, only about 1.5 L of urine is excreted. Electrolyte balance is maintained by selective retention and excretion by the kidneys. The kidneys also play a significant role in acid-base regulation, excreting hydrogen ions (H^+) and retaining bicarbonate.

Antidiuretic Hormone Antidiuretic hormone (ADH), which regulates water excretion from the kidney, is synthesized in the anterior portion of the hypothalamus, is secreted by the posterior pituitary, and acts on the collecting ducts of the nephrons. When serum osmolality rises, ADH is produced, causing the collecting ducts to become more permeable to water. This increased permeability allows more water to be reabsorbed into the blood. As more water is reabsorbed, urine output falls and serum osmolality decreases because the water dilutes body fluids. Conversely, if serum osmolality decreases, ADH secretion is suppressed, the collecting ducts become less permeable to water, and urine output increases. Excretion of excess water returns the serum osmolality to normal. Other factors also affect the production and release of ADH, including blood volume, temperature, pain, stress, and some drugs, such as opiates, barbiturates, alcohol, and nicotine. See Figure 43.8.

Renin-Angiotensin-Aldosterone System Specialized receptors in the juxtaglomerular apparatus of the kidney nephrons respond to changes in renal perfusion. This initiates the **renin-angiotensin-aldosterone system**. If blood flow or pressure to the kidney decreases, renin is released. Renin causes the conversion of angiotensinogen to angiotensin I, which is then converted to angiotensin II by angiotensin-converting enzyme. Angiotensin II acts directly on the nephrons to promote sodium and water retention. In addition, it stimulates the release of aldosterone from the adrenal cortex. Aldosterone also promotes sodium and, therefore, water retention in the distal nephron. The net effect of the renin-angiotensin-aldosterone system is to restore blood volume (and renal perfusion) through sodium and water retention.

Atrial Natriuretic Factor Arial natriuretic factor (ANF) is released from cells in the atrium of the heart in response to excess blood volume and stretching of the atrial walls. Acting on the nephrons, ANF promotes sodium wasting and acts as a potent diuretic, thus reducing vascular volume. ANF also inhibits thirst, reducing fluid intake.

Regulating Electrolytes

Electrolytes, charged ions capable of conducting electricity, are present in all body fluids and fluid compartments. Just as maintaining the fluid balance is vital to normal body function, so is maintaining electrolyte balance. Although the concentration of specific electrolytes differs between fluid compartments, a balance of cations and anions always exists. Electrolytes are important for the following functions:

- Maintaining fluid balance
- Contributing to acid-base regulation
- Facilitating enzyme reactions

Most electrolytes enter the body through dietary intake and are excreted in the urine. Some electrolytes,

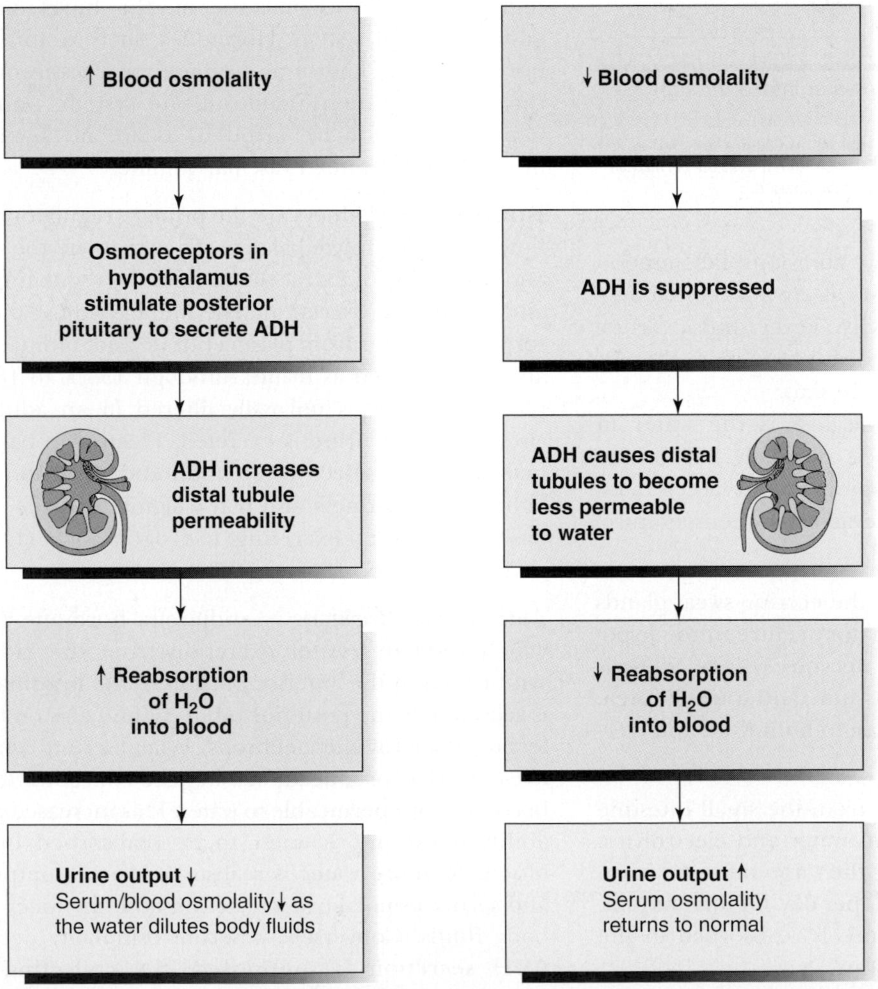

FIGURE 43.8 Antidiuretic hormone (ADH) regulates water excretion from the kidneys.

such as sodium and chloride, are not stored by the body and must be consumed daily to maintain normal levels. Potassium and calcium, conversely, are stored in the cells and bone, respectively. When serum levels drop, ions can shift out of the storage pool into the blood to maintain adequate serum levels for normal functioning. The regulatory mechanisms and functions of the major electrolytes are summarized in Table 43.3.

SODIUM (NA^+) Sodium is the most abundant cation in extracellular fluid and a major contributor to serum osmolality. Normal serum sodium levels are 135 mmol/L to 145 mmol/L. Sodium functions largely in controlling and regulating water balance. When sodium is reabsorbed from the kidney tubules, chloride and water are reabsorbed with it, thus maintaining ECF volume. Sodium is found in many foods, such as bacon, ham, processed cheese, and table salt.

POTASSIUM (K^+) Potassium is the major cation in ICF, with only a small amount found in plasma and interstitial fluid. ICF levels of potassium are usually 125 mmol/L to 140 mmol/L, while normal serum potassium levels are 3.5 mmol/L to 5.0 mmol/L. The ratio of intracellular to extracellular potassium must be maintained for neuromuscular response to stimuli. Potassium is a vital

TABLE 43.3 Regulation and Functions of Electrolytes

Electrolyte	Regulation	Function
Sodium (Na^+)	• Renal reabsorption or excretion • Aldosterone increases Na^+ reabsorption in collecting duct of nephrons	• Regulating ECF volume and distribution • Maintaining blood volume • Transmitting nerve impulses and contracting muscles
Potassium (K^+)	• Renal excretion and conservation • Aldosterone increases K^+ excretion • Movement into and out of cells • Insulin helps move K^+ into cells; tissue damage and acidosis shift K^+ out of cells into ECF	• Maintaining ICF osmolality • Transmitting nerve and other electrical impulses • Regulating cardiac impulse transmission and muscle contraction • Skeletal and smooth muscle function • Regulating acid-base balance
Calcium (Ca^{2+})	• Redistribution between bones and ECF • Parathyroid hormone and calcitriol increase serum Ca^{2+} levels; calcitonin decreases serum levels	• Forming bones and teeth • Transmitting nerve impulses • Regulating muscle contractions • Maintaining cardiac pacemaker (automaticity) • Blood clotting • Activating enzymes, such as pancreatic lipase and phospholipase
Magnesium (Mg^{2+})	• Conservation and excretion by kidneys • Intestinal absorption increased by vitamin D and parathyroid hormone	• Intracellular metabolism • Operating sodium-potassium pump • Relaxing muscle contractions • Transmitting nerve impulses • Regulating cardiac function
Chloride (Cl^-)	• Excreted and reabsorbed along with sodium in the kidneys • Aldosterone increases chloride reabsorption with sodium	• HCl production • Regulating ECF balance and vascular volume • Regulating acid-base balance • Buffer in oxygen–carbon dioxide exchange in RBCs
Phosphate (PO_4^-)	• Excretion and reabsorption by the kidneys • Parathyroid hormone decreases serum levels by increasing renal excretion • Reciprocal relationship with calcium: increasing serum calcium levels decreases phosphate levels; decreasing serum calcium increases phosphate	• Forming bones and teeth • Metabolizing carbohydrate, protein, and fat • Cellular metabolism; producing ATP and DNA • Muscle, nerve, and RBC function • Regulating acid-base balance • Regulating calcium levels
Bicarbonate (HCO_3^-)	• Excretion and reabsorption by the kidneys • Regeneration by kidneys	• Major body buffer involved in acid-base regulation

electrolyte for skeletal, cardiac, and smooth muscle activity. It is involved in maintaining acid-base balance as well, and it contributes to intracellular enzyme reactions. Many fruits and vegetables, meat, fish, and other foods contain potassium (see Box 43.1).

CALCIUM (CA^{2+}) The vast majority of calcium (99%) in the body is in the skeletal system, with a relatively small amount in extracellular fluid. Although this calcium outside the bones and teeth amounts to only about 1% of the total calcium in the body, it is vital in regulating muscle contraction and relaxation, neuromuscular function, coagulation, and cardiac function. ECF calcium is regulated by a complex interaction of parathyroid hormone, calcitonin, and calcitriol, a metabolite of vitamin D. When calcium levels in the ECF fall, parathyroid hormone and calcitriol cause calcium to be released from bones into the ECF and increase the absorption of calcium in the intestines, thus raising serum calcium levels. Conversely, calcitonin stimulates the deposition of calcium in bone, reducing the concentration of calcium ions in the blood.

With aging, the intestines absorb calcium less effectively and more calcium is excreted via the kidneys. Calcium shifts out of the bone to replace these ECF losses, increasing the risk of osteoporosis and fractures of the wrists, vertebrae, and hips. Lack of weight-bearing exercise (which helps keep calcium in the bones) and a vitamin D deficiency because of inadequate exposure to sunlight contribute to this risk.

Milk and milk products are the richest sources of calcium, with other foods, such as dark green leafy vegetables and canned salmon, containing smaller amounts. Calcium intake during adolescent years (1200 mg/day to 1500 mg/day) may help decrease osteoporosis (a decrease in bone density) in later life (Schettler & Gustafson, 2004). Postmenopausal women should ingest 1500 mg of calcium per day (Public Health Agency of Canada, 2007).

Serum calcium levels are often reported in two ways, based on the way calcium is circulating in the plasma. Approximately 50% of serum calcium circulates in a free, ionized, or unbound form. The other 50% circulates in the plasma, bound to either plasma proteins or other nonprotein ions. The normal total serum calcium level, which ranges from 2.2 mmol/L to 2.58 mmol/L, represents both bound and unbound calcium. The normal ionized serum calcium, which ranges from 1.0 mmol/L to 1.15 mmol/L, represents calcium circulating in the plasma in free, or unbound, form. It is not possible to measure bound calcium so it is deduced by subtracting the ionized serum calcium level from the total serum calcium level.

MAGNESIUM (MG^{2+}) Magnesium is primarily found in the skeleton and in ICF. It is the second most abundant intracellular cation, with normal serum levels of 0.65 mmol/L to 1.05 mmol/L. It is important for intracellular metabolism, being particularly involved in the production and use of ATP. Magnesium also is necessary for protein and DNA synthesis within the cells. Only about 1% of the body's magnesium is in ECF; here it is involved in regulating neuromuscular and cardiac function. Maintaining and ensuring adequate magnesium levels is an important part of care of clients with cardiac disorders. Cereal grains, nuts, dried fruit, legumes, and green leafy vegetables are good sources of magnesium in the diet, as are dairy products, meat, and fish.

CHLORIDE (CL^-) Chloride is the major anion of ECF, and normal serum levels are 95 mmol/L to 105 mmol/L. Chloride functions with sodium to regulate serum osmolality and blood volume. The concentration of chloride in ECF is regulated secondarily to sodium; when sodium is reabsorbed in the kidney, chloride usually follows. Chloride is a major component of gastric juice as hydrochloric acid (HCl) and is involved in regulating acid-base balance. It also acts as a buffer in the exchange of oxygen and carbon dioxide in RBCs. Chloride is found in the same foods as sodium.

PHOSPHATE (PO_4^-) Phosphate is the major anion of ICF. It also is found in ECF, bone, skeletal muscle, and nerve tissue. Normal serum levels of phosphate in adults range from 0.97 mmol/L to 1.45 mmol/L. Children have much higher phosphate levels than adults, with that of a newborn nearly twice that of an adult. Higher levels of growth hormone and a faster rate of skeletal growth probably account for this difference. Phosphate is essential for functioning of muscles, nerves, and RBCs. It is also involved in the metabolism of protein, fat, and carbohydrate. Phosphate is absorbed from the intestine and is found in many foods, such as meat, fish, poultry, milk products, and legumes.

BICARBONATE (HCO_3^-) Bicarbonate is present in both ICF and ECF. The normal serum bicarbonate level in adults is 22 mmol/L to 26 mmol/L. Its primary function is regulating acid-base balance as an essential component of the carbonic acid-bicarbonate buffering system.

BOX 43.1 POTASSIUM-RICH FOODS

VEGETABLES	FRUITS
Avocado	Dried fruits (e.g., raisins and dates)
Raw carrot	Banana
Baked potato	Apricot
Raw tomato	Cantaloupe
Spinach	Orange
MEATS AND FISH	**BEVERAGES**
Beef	Milk
Cod	Orange juice
Pork	Apricot nectar
Veal	

Extracellular bicarbonate levels are regulated by the kidneys. Bicarbonate is excreted when too much is present; if more is needed, the kidneys both produce and reabsorb bicarbonate ions. Unlike other electrolytes that must be consumed in the diet, adequate amounts of bicarbonate are produced through metabolic processes to meet the body's needs.

Acid-Base Balance and pH

An important part of regulating the chemical balance or homeostasis of body fluids is regulating their acidity or alkalinity. An **acid** is a substance that releases hydrogen ions (H^+) in solution. Strong acids, such as hydrochloric acid, release all or nearly all their hydrogen ions; weak acids, such as carbonic acid, release some hydrogen ions. **Bases**, or *alkalis*, have a low hydrogen ion concentration and can accept hydrogen ions in solution. The relative acidity or alkalinity of a solution is measured as **pH**. The pH reflects the hydrogen ion concentration of the solution: the higher the hydrogen ion concentration (and the more acidic the solution), the lower the pH. Water has a pH of 7 and is neutral; that is, it is neither acidic nor alkaline. Solutions with a pH lower than 7 are acidic; those with a pH higher than 7 are alkaline. The pH scale is logarithmic: a solution with a pH of 5 is 10 times as acidic as one with a pH of 6.

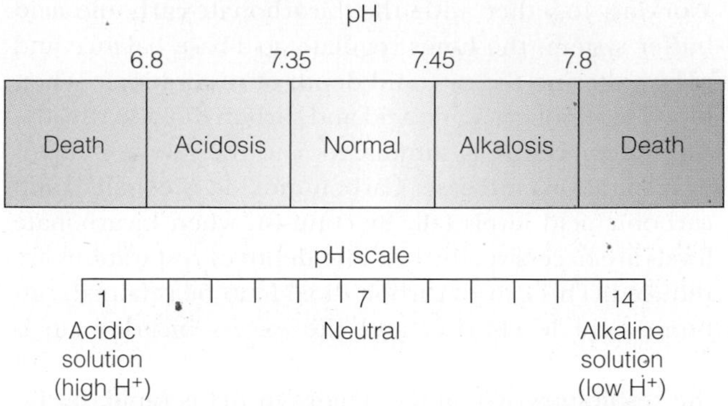

FIGURE 43.9 Body fluids are normally slightly alkaline, between a pH of 7.35 and 7.45.

Regulation of Acid-Base Balance

Body fluids are maintained within a narrow range that is slightly alkaline. The normal pH of arterial blood is between 7.35 and 7.45 (Figure 43.9). Acids are continually produced during metabolism. Several body systems, including buffers, the respiratory system, and the renal system, are actively involved in maintaining the narrow pH range necessary for optimal function. Buffers help maintain acid-base balance by neutralizing excess acids or bases. The lungs and the kidneys help maintain a normal pH by either excreting or retaining acids and bases.

BUFFERS **Buffers** prevent excessive changes in pH by removing or releasing hydrogen ions. If excess hydrogen ion is present in body fluids, buffers bind with the hydrogen ion, minimizing the change in pH. When body fluids become too alkaline, buffers can release hydrogen ion, again minimizing the change in pH. The action of a buffer is immediate but is limited in its capacity to maintain or restore normal acid-base balance.

The major buffer system in extracellular fluids is the bicarbonate (HCO_3^-) and carbonic acid (H_2CO_3) system. When a strong acid, such as hydrochloric acid (HCl), is added, it combines with bicarbonate and the pH drops only slightly. A strong base, such as sodium hydroxide, combines with carbonic acid, the weak acid of the buffer pair, and the pH remains within the narrow range of normal. The amounts of bicarbonate and carbonic acid in the body vary; however, as long as a ratio of 20 parts of bicarbonate to 1 part of carbonic acid is maintained, the pH remains within its normal range of 7.35 to 7.45 (Figure 43.10). Adding a strong acid to ECF can change this ratio, as bicarbonate is depleted in neutralizing the acid. When this happens, the pH drops, a condition called **acidosis.** The ratio can also be upset by adding a strong base to ECF, depleting carbonic acid as it combines with the base. In this case, the pH rises, and the client has **alkalosis.**

In addition to the bicarbonate-carbonic acid buffer system, plasma proteins, hemoglobin, and phosphates also function as buffers in body fluids.

RESPIRATORY REGULATION The lungs help regulate acid-base balance by eliminating or retaining carbon dioxide (CO_2), a potential acid. Combined with water, carbon dioxide forms carbonic acid ($CO_2 + H_2O = H_2CO_3$). This chemical reaction is reversible; carbonic acid breaks down into carbon dioxide and water.

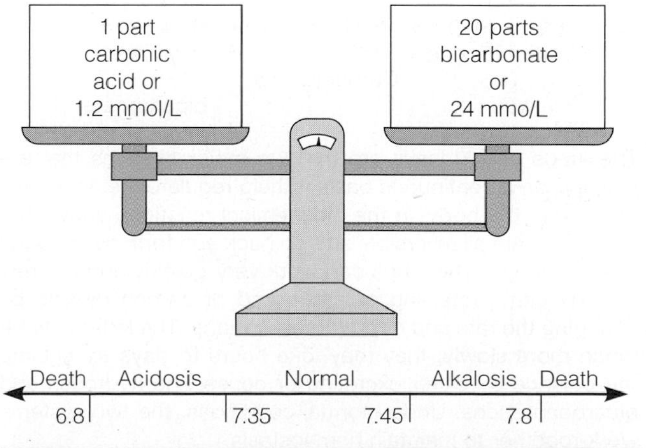

FIGURE 43.10 Carbonic acid-bicarbonate ratio and pH

Working together with the bicarbonate-carbonic acid buffer system, the lungs regulate acid-base balance and pH by altering the rate and depth of respirations. When blood levels of carbonic acid and carbon dioxide rise, the respiratory centre is stimulated, and the rate and depth of respirations increase. Carbon dioxide is exhaled, and carbonic acid levels fall. By contrast, when bicarbonate levels are excessive, the rate and depth of respirations are reduced. This causes carbon dioxide to be retained, carbonic acid levels rise, and the excess bicarbonate is neutralized. Although not instantaneous, the response of the respiratory system to changes in pH is rapid, occurring within minutes.

Carbon dioxide levels in the blood are measured as the partial pressure of the dissolved gas (PCO_2) in the blood. PCO_2 refers to the pressure of carbon dioxide in *venous* blood. $PaCO_2$ refers to the pressure of carbon dioxide in *arterial* blood. The normal $PaCO_2$ is 35 mm Hg to 45 mm Hg.

RENAL REGULATION Although buffers and the respiratory system can compensate for changes in pH, the kidneys are the ultimate long-term regulators of acid-base balance. They are slower to respond to changes, requiring hours to days to correct imbalances, but their response is more permanent and selective than those of the other systems.

The kidneys maintain acid-base balance by selectively excreting or conserving bicarbonate and hydrogen ions. When excess hydrogen ions are present and the pH falls (acidosis), the kidneys reabsorb and regenerate bicarbonate and excrete hydrogen ions. In the case of alkalosis and a high pH, excess bicarbonate is excreted, and hydrogen ions are retained. The relationship of the respiratory and renal regulation of acid-base balance is further explained in Box 43.2

BOX 43.2 PHYSIOLOGICAL REGULATION OF ACID-BASE BALANCE

Lungs		*Kidneys*
$CO_2 + H_2O$ ⟷	H_2CO_3 ⟷	$H^+ + HCO_3^-$
Carbon dioxide + water	Carbonic acid	Hydrogen + bicarbonate

The lungs and kidneys are the two major systems that are working on a continuous basis to help regulate the acid-base balance in the body. In the biochemical reactions above, the processes are all reversible and go back and forth as the body needs change. The lungs can work very quickly and do their part by either retaining or getting rid of carbon dioxide by changing the rate and depth of respirations. The kidneys work much more slowly; they may take hours to days to regulate the balance by either excreting or conserving hydrogen and bicarbonate ions. Under normal conditions, the two systems work together to maintain homeostasis.

Factors Affecting Body Fluid, Electrolytes, and the Acid-Base Balance

The ability of the body to adjust fluids, electrolytes, and acid-base balance is influenced by age, gender and body size, environmental temperature, and lifestyle.

Age

Infants and growing children have much greater fluid turnover than have adults because children's higher metabolic rate increases fluid loss. Infants lose more fluid through the kidneys because immature kidneys are less able to conserve water than are adult kidneys. The more rapid turnover of fluid plus the losses produced by disease can create critical fluid imbalances in children much more rapidly than in adults.

In older adults, the normal aging process can affect fluid balance (see the Lifespan Considerations box), increasing the risk of dehydration. When combined with the increased likelihood of heart disease, impaired renal function, and multiple drug regimens, the older adult's risk for fluid and electrolyte imbalance is significant. Additionally, it is important to consider that the older adult has thinner, more fragile skin and veins, which can make an intravenous insertion more difficult.

Gender and Body Size

Total body water also is affected by gender and body size. Because fat cells contain little or no water and lean tissue has a high water content, people with a higher percentage of body fat have less body fluid. Women have proportionately more body fat and less body water than men do. Water accounts for approximately 80% of a newborn's weight, 60% of an adult male's weight, but only 52% of an adult female's. In an obese individual, this percentage may be even smaller, with water responsible for only 30% to 40% of the person's weight.

Environmental Temperature

People with an illness and those participating in strenuous activity are at risk for fluid and electrolyte imbalances when the environmental temperature is high. Fluid losses through sweating are increased in hot environments as the body attempts to dissipate heat. These losses are even greater in people who have not been acclimatized to the environment.

Both salt and water are lost through sweating and both need to be replaced. When only water is replaced, salt depletion is a risk. The person who is salt depleted may

Lifespan Considerations

Fluid and Electrolyte Balance

INFANTS AND CHILDREN

Infants are at high risk for fluid and electrolyte imbalance for the following reasons:

- Their immature kidneys cannot concentrate urine.
- They have a rapid respiratory rate and proportionately larger body surface area than adults, leading to greater insensible fluid loss through the skin and respirations.
- They cannot express thirst or actively seek fluids.

Vomiting or diarrhea in infants and young children can lead quickly to electrolyte imbalance. Oral rehydration therapy (ORT) (e.g., electrolyte solutions, such as Pedialyte) should be used to restore fluid and electrolyte balance in mild to moderate dehydration (Canadian Paediatric Society Nutrition and Gastroenterology Committee, 2006). Prompt treatment with ORT can prevent the need for intravenous therapy and hospitalization. Even if the child is nauseated and vomiting, small sips of ORT can be helpful.

OLDER ADULTS

Certain changes related to aging place older adults at risk for serious problems with fluid and electrolyte imbalance, if homeostatic mechanisms are compromised. Some of the changes follow:

- A decrease in thirst sensation
- A decrease in the ability of the kidneys to concentrate urine
- A decrease in intracellular fluid and in total body water
- A decrease in response to body hormones that help regulate fluid and electrolytes

Other factors that may influence fluid and electrolyte balance in older adults include the following:

- Increased use of diuretics for hypertension and heart disease
- Decreased intake of food and water, especially in those with dementia or who are dependent on others to feed them and offer them fluids
- Preparations for certain diagnostic tests that have the client NPO for long periods or that cause diarrhea
- Clients with impaired renal function, such as those with diabetes
- Those having certain diagnostic procedures (dyes used for some procedures, such as arteriograms and cardiac catheterizations, can cause further renal problems; ensure the client is well hydrated before, during, and after the procedure to help in diluting and excreting the dye; if the client is NPO for the procedure, the nurse should check with the health-care provider to see whether IV fluids are needed)
- Any condition that can tax the normal compensatory mechanisms, such as a fever, influenza, surgery, or heat exposure

All these conditions increase older adults' risk for fluid and electrolyte imbalance. The change can happen quickly and become serious in a short time. Astute observations and quick actions by the nurse can help prevent serious consequences. A change in mental status may be the first symptom of impairment and must be further evaluated to determine the cause.

experience fatigue, weakness, headache, and gastrointestinal symptoms, such as anorexia and nausea. The risk of adverse effects is even greater if lost water is not replaced. Body temperature rises, and the person is at risk for heat exhaustion or heatstroke. Heatstroke can occur in older adults or ill people during prolonged periods of heat; it can also affect athletes and labourers when their heat production exceeds the body's ability to dissipate heat.

Consuming adequate amounts of cool liquids, particularly during strenuous activity, reduces the risk of adverse effects from heat. Balanced electrolyte solutions and carbohydrate-electrolyte solutions, such as sports drinks, are recommended because they replace both water and electrolytes lost through sweat.

Lifestyle

Other factors, such as diet, exercise, and stress, affect fluid, electrolyte, and acid-base balance. The intake of fluids and electrolytes is affected by diet. People with anorexia nervosa or bulimia are at risk for severe fluid and electrolyte imbalances because of inadequate intake or purging regimens (e.g., inducing vomiting, using diuretics and laxatives). Seriously malnourished people have decreased serum albumin levels and may develop edema because the osmotic draw of fluid into the vascular compartment is reduced. When calorie intake is not adequate to meet the body's needs, fat stores are broken down and fatty acids are released, increasing the risk of acidosis.

Regular weight-bearing physical exercise, such as walking, running, or bicycling, has a beneficial effect on calcium balance. The rate of bone loss that occurs in postmenopausal women and older men is slowed with regular exercise, reducing the risk of osteoporosis.

Stress can increase cellular metabolism, blood glucose concentration, and catecholamine levels. In addition, stress can increase production of ADH, which, in turn, decreases urine production. The overall response of the body to stress is to increase the blood volume.

Other lifestyle factors can also affect fluid, electrolyte, and acid-base balance. Heavy alcohol consumption affects electrolyte balance, increasing the risk of low calcium, magnesium, and phosphate levels. The risk of acidosis associated with breakdown of fat tissue also is greater in the person who drinks large amounts of alcohol.

Disturbances in Fluid, Electrolyte, and Acid-Base Balance

A number of factors, such as illness, trauma, surgery, and medications, can affect the body's ability to maintain fluid, electrolyte, and acid-base balance. The kidneys play a major role in maintaining fluid, electrolyte, and acid-base balance, and renal disease is a significant cause of imbalance. Clients who are confused or unable to communicate their needs are at risk for inadequate fluid intake. Vomiting, diarrhea, or nasogastric suction can cause significant fluid and electrolyte losses. Tissue trauma, such as burns, causes fluid and electrolytes to be lost from damaged cells. Decreased blood flow to the kidneys because of impaired cardiac function stimulates the renin-angiotensin-aldosterone system, causing sodium and water retention. Medications, such as diuretics or corticosteroids, can result in abnormal losses of electrolytes and fluid loss or retention. Diseases, such as diabetes mellitus or chronic obstructive pulmonary disease (COPD), can affect acid-base balance. Diabetic ketoacidosis, cancer, and head injury can also lead to electrolyte imbalances.

Fluid Imbalances

Fluid imbalances are of two basic types: isotonic and osmolar. Isotonic imbalances occur when water and electrolytes are lost or gained in equal proportions so that the osmolality of body fluids remains constant. Osmolar imbalances involve the loss or gain of *only* water so that the osmolality of the serum is altered. Thus, four categories of fluid imbalances can occur: (1) an isotonic loss of water and electrolytes, (2) an isotonic gain of water and electrolytes, (3) a hyperosmolar loss of only water, and (4) a hypo-osmolar gain of only water. These are referred to, respectively, as fluid volume deficit, fluid volume excess, dehydration (hyperosmolar imbalance), and overhydration (hypo-osmolar imbalance).

FLUID VOLUME DEFICIT Isotonic **fluid volume deficit (FVD)** occurs when the body loses both water and electrolytes from the ECF in similar proportions. Thus, the decreased volume of fluid remains isotonic. In FVD, fluid is initially lost from the intravascular compartment, so it often is called **hypovolemia**. FVD generally occurs as a result of (1) abnormal losses through the skin, gastrointestinal tract, or kidneys; (2) decreased intake of fluid; (3) bleeding; or (4) movement of fluid into a third space. See the section on third space syndrome that follows.

For the risk factors, clinical manifestations, and nursing interventions related to fluid volume deficit, see Table 43.4.

THIRD SPACE SYNDROME In **third space syndrome**, fluid shifts from the vascular space into an area where it is not readily accessible. This fluid remains in the body but is essentially unavailable for use, causing an isotonic fluid volume deficit. Fluid may be sequestered in the bowel, in the interstitial space as edema, in inflamed

TABLE 43.4 Isotonic Fluid Volume Deficit

Risk Factors	Clinical Manifestations	Nursing Interventions
Loss of water and electrolytes from • Vomiting • Diarrhea • Excessive sweating • Polyuria • Fever • Nasogastric suction • Abnormal drainage or wound losses • Bleeding Insufficient intake caused by • Anorexia • Nausea • Inability to access fluids • Impaired swallowing • Confusion, depression	Complaints of weakness and thirst Weight loss • 2% loss = mild FVD • 5% loss = moderate FVD • 8% loss = severe FVD Fluid intake less than output Decreased tissue turgor Dry mucous membranes, sunken eyeballs, decreased tearing Subnormal temperature Weak, rapid pulse Decreased blood pressure Postural (orthostatic) hypotension (significant drop in BP when moving from lying to sitting or standing position) Flat neck veins, decreased capillary refill Decreased central venous pressure (CVP) Decreased urine volume (< 30 mL/h) Increased specific gravity of urine (> 1.030) Increased hematocrit (HCT) Increased blood urea nitrogen (BUN)	Assess for clinical manifestations of FVD. Monitor weight and vital signs, including temperature. Assess tissue turgor. Assess breath sounds. Monitor fluid intake and output. Monitor laboratory findings. Administer oral and intravenous fluids, as indicated. Provide frequent mouth care. Implement measures to prevent skin breakdown. Provide for safety, for example, provide assistance to a client rising from bed.

tissue, or in potential spaces, such as the peritoneal or pleural cavities.

The client with third space syndrome has an isotonic fluid deficit but may not manifest apparent fluid loss or weight loss. Careful nursing assessment is vital to effectively identify and intervene for clients experiencing third spacing. Because the fluid shifts back into the vascular compartment after time, assessment for manifestations of fluid volume excess or hypervolemia is also vital.

FLUID VOLUME EXCESS **Fluid volume excess (FVE)** occurs when the body retains both water and sodium in similar proportions to normal ECF. This is commonly referred to as **hypervolemia** (increased blood volume). Because both water and sodium are retained, the serum sodium concentration remains essentially normal. FVE is always secondary to an increase in the total body sodium content, which leads to an increase in total body water. Because both water and sodium are retained, the serum sodium concentration remains essentially normal and the excess volume of fluid is isotonic. Specific causes of FVE include (1) excessive intake of sodium chloride; (2) the administration of sodium-containing infusions too rapidly, particularly to clients with impaired regulatory mechanisms; and (3) disease processes that alter regulatory mechanisms, such as heart failure, renal failure, cirrhosis of the liver, and Cushing's syndrome.

The risk factors, clinical manifestations, and nursing interventions for FVE are summarized in Table 43.5.

EDEMA In fluid volume excess, both intravascular and interstitial spaces have an increased water and sodium content. Excess interstitial fluid is known as **edema**. Edema typically is most apparent in areas where the tissue pressure is low, such as around the eyes, and in dependent tissues (known as *dependent edema*) where hydrostatic capillary pressure is high.

Edema can be caused by several different mechanisms. The three main mechanisms are increased capillary hydrostatic pressure, decreased plasma oncotic pressure, and increased capillary permeability. Edema may be due to FVE that increases capillary hydrostatic pressure, pushing fluid into the interstitial tissues. This type of edema is often seen in dependent tissues, such as the feet, hands, ankles, and sacrum, because of the effects of gravity. Low levels of plasma proteins from malnutrition or liver or kidney diseases can reduce the plasma oncotic pressure so that fluid is not drawn into the capillaries from interstitial tissues, causing edema. With tissue trauma and some disorders, such as allergic reactions, capillaries become more permeable, allowing fluid leaks from the capillaries. Obstructed lymph flow impairs the movement of fluid from interstitial tissues back into the vascular compartment, resulting in edema.

Pitting edema is edema that leaves a small depression or pit after finger pressure is applied to the swollen area. The pit is caused by movement of fluid to adjacent tissue, away from the point of pressure (Figure 43.11). The pit normally disappears within 10 to 30 seconds.

DEHYDRATION **Dehydration**, or *hyperosmolar imbalance*, occurs when water is lost from the body without significant loss of electrolytes. Because water is lost while electrolytes, particularly sodium, are retained, the serum osmolality and serum sodium levels increase. Water is drawn into the vascular compartment from the interstitial spaces and cells, resulting in cellular dehydration. Older adults are at particular risk for dehydration because of decreased thirst sensation. This type of water deficit also can affect clients who are hyperventilating, have a prolonged fever, are in diabetic ketoacidosis, or receiving enteral feedings with insufficient water intake.

TABLE 43.5 Isotonic Fluid Volume Excess

Risk Factors	Clinical Manifestations	Nursing Interventions
Excess intake of sodium-containing intravenous fluids	Weight gain • 2% gain = mild FVE • 5% gain = moderate FVE • 8% gain = severe FVE	Assess for clinical manifestations of FVE.
Excess ingestion of sodium in diet or medications (e.g., sodium bicarbonate antacids, such as Alka-Seltzer, or hypertonic enema solutions, such as Fleet)	Fluid intake greater than output	Monitor weight and vital signs.
Impaired fluid balance regulation related to • Heart failure • Renal failure • Cirrhosis of the liver	Moist mucous membranes	Assess for edema.
	Full, bounding pulse; tachycardia	Assess breath sounds, dyspnea.
	Increased blood pressure and central venous pressure (CVP)	Monitor fluid intake and output.
	Distended neck and peripheral veins; slow vein emptying	Monitor laboratory findings.
	Moist crackles in lungs; dyspnea, shortness of breath	Place client in Fowler's position.
	Mental confusion	Administer diuretics, as ordered.
	Peripheral edema	Restrict fluid intake, as ordered.
		Restrict dietary sodium, as ordered.
		Implement measures to prevent skin breakdown.

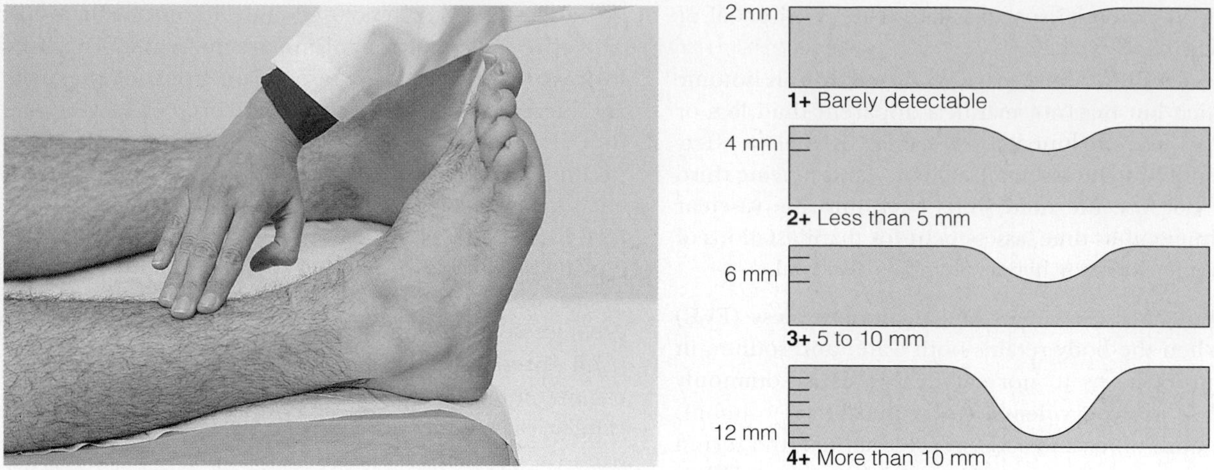

A B

FIGURE 43.11 Evaluation of edema: **A:** palpate for edema over the tibia, as shown here, and behind the medial malleolus and over the dorsum of each foot; **B:** four-point scale for grading edema

OVERHYDRATION **Overhydration**, also known as *hypo-osmolar imbalance* or *water excess,* occurs when water is gained in excess of electrolytes, resulting in low serum osmolality and low serum sodium levels. Water is drawn into the cells, causing them to swell. In the brain, this can lead to cerebral edema and impaired neurological function. Water intoxication often occurs when both fluid and electrolytes are lost, for example, through excessive sweating, but only water is replaced. It can also result from the syndrome of inappropriate antidiuretic hormone (SIADH), a disorder that can occur with malignant tumours, acquired immune deficiency syndrome (AIDS), head injury, or administration of certain drugs, such as barbiturates or anaesthetics. The characteristics of fluid volume gains and losses are noted in Table 43.6.

Electrolyte Imbalances

The most common and most significant electrolyte imbalances involve sodium, potassium, calcium, magnesium, chloride, and phosphate. Table 43.7 lists risk factors, clinical manifestations, and nursing interventions for several electrolyte imbalances.

SODIUM Sodium (Na^+), the most abundant cation in the ECF, not only moves into and out of the body but also moves in careful balance among the three fluid compartments. It is found in most body secretions, for example, saliva, gastric and intestinal secretions, bile, and pancreatic fluid. Therefore, continuous excretion of any of these fluids, such as via intestinal suction, can result in a sodium deficit. Because of its role in regulating water balance, sodium imbalances usually are accompanied by water imbalances.

TABLE 43.6 Comparison of Fluid Volume Gains and Fluid Volume Losses

Fluid Volume Gains	Etiology	Fluid Volume Losses	Etiology
Isotonic FVE (hypovolemia)	Excessive intake of sodium chloride Administration of sodium-containing infusions too rapidly Disease processes that alter regulatory mechanisms, such as heart failure, renal failure, cirrhosis of the liver, and Cushing's syndrome	Isotonic FVD (hypovolemia)	Increased losses through the skin, gastrointestinal tract, or kidney Decreased intake of fluid Bleeding Movement of fluid into a third space
Overhydration (hypo-osmolar imbalance or water excess)	Increased water, not sodium, as can occur with excess ADH, head injury, HIV, some drugs, water-only replacement	Dehydration (hyperosmolar imbalance)	Older adults with decreased thirst sensation Athletes with excessive sweating or hyperventilating Prolonged fever Diabetic ketoacidosis Enteral feedings with insufficient water intake

Hyponatremia is a sodium deficit, or serum sodium level of less than 135 mmol/L, and is, in acute-care settings, a common electrolyte imbalance. Because of sodium's role in determining the osmolality of ECF, hyponatremia typically results in a low serum osmolality. Water is drawn out of the vascular compartment into interstitial tissues and the cells (Figure 43.12A), causing the clinical manifestations associated with this disorder. As sodium levels decrease, the brain and nervous system are affected by cellular edema. Severe hyponatremia, a serum level below 110 mmol/L, is a medical emergency and can lead to permanent neurological damage (Astle, 2005).

Hypernatremia is excess sodium in ECF, or serum sodium of greater than 145 mmol/L. Because the osmotic pressure of extracellular fluid is increased, fluid moves out of the cells into the ECF (Figure 43.12B). As a result, the cells become dehydrated. Like hyponatremia, the primary manifestations of hypernatremia are neurological in nature.

It is important to note that a person's thirst mechanism protects against hypernatremia. For example, when an individual becomes thirsty, the body is stimulated to drink water, which helps correct the hypernatremia. Clients at risk for hypernatremia are those who are unable to access water (e.g., unconscious; unable to request fluids, such as infants or older adults with dementia; or ill clients with an impaired thirst mechanism).

POTASSIUM Although the amount of potassium (K^+) in extracellular fluid is small, it is vital to normal neuromuscular and cardiac function. Normal renal function is important for maintenance of potassium balance as 80% of potassium is excreted by the kidneys. Potassium must be replaced daily to maintain its balance. Normally, potassium is replaced through food. See Box 43.1 earlier to review foods high in potassium. Abnormalities in potassium balance represent the most common electrolyte imbalance in hospitalized patients.

Hypokalemia is a potassium deficit or a serum potassium level of less than 3.5 mmol/L. Gastrointestinal

TABLE 43.7 Electrolyte Imbalances

Risk Factors	Clinical Manifestations	Nursing Interventions
Hyponatremia		
Loss of sodium: • Gastrointestinal fluid loss • Sweating • Use of diuretics Gain of water: • Hypotonic tube feedings • Drinking water • Excess IV D5W (dextrose in water) administration Syndrome of inappropriate ADH (SIADH): • Head injury • AIDS • Malignant tumours	Lethargy, confusion, apprehension Muscle twitching Abdominal cramps Anorexia, nausea, vomiting Headache Seizures, coma *Laboratory findings:* Serum sodium below 135 mmol/L Serum osmolality below 280 mOsm/kg	Assess clinical manifestations. Monitor fluid intake and output. Monitor laboratory data (e.g., serum sodium). Assess client closely if administering hypertonic saline solutions. Encourage food and fluid high in sodium, if permitted (e.g., table salt, bacon, ham, processed cheese). Limit water intake, as indicated.
Hypernatremia		
Loss of fluids: • Insensible water loss (hyperventilation or fever) • Diarrhea • Water deprivation Excess salt intake: • Parenteral administration of saline solutions • Hypertonic tube feedings without adequate water • Excessive use of table salt (1 tsp or 5 mL contains 2300 mg of sodium) Conditions, such as: • Diabetes insipidus • Heatstroke	Thirst Dry, sticky mucous membranes Tongue red, dry, swollen Weakness Postural hypotension, dyspnea Severe hypernatremia: • Fatigue, restlessness • Decreasing level of consciousness • Disorientation • Convulsions *Laboratory findings:* Serum sodium above 145 mmol/L Serum osmolality above 300 mOsm/kg	Monitor fluid intake and output. Monitor behaviour changes (e.g., restlessness, disorientation). Monitor laboratory findings (e.g., serum sodium). Encourage fluids, as ordered. Monitor diet, as ordered (e.g., restrict intake of salt and foods high in sodium).

(continued)

TABLE 43.7 Electrolyte Imbalances *(continued)*

Risk Factors	Clinical Manifestations	Nursing Interventions
Hypokalemia		
Loss of potassium: • Vomiting and gastric suction • Diarrhea • Heavy perspiration Use of potassium-wasting drugs (e.g., diuretics) Poor intake of potassium (as with debilitated clients, clients with alcoholism, clients with anorexia) Hyperaldosteronism	Muscle weakness, leg cramps Fatigue, lethargy Anorexia, nausea, vomiting Decreased bowel sounds, decreased bowel motility Cardiac dysrhythmias Depressed deep-tendon reflexes *Laboratory findings:* Serum potassium below 3.5 mmol/L Arterial blood gases (ABGs) may show alkalosis T wave flattening and ST segment depression on ECG	Monitor heart rate and rhythm and ECG. Monitor clients receiving digitalis (e.g., digoxin) closely because hypokalemia increases risk of digitalis toxicity. Administer oral potassium, as ordered, with food or fluid to prevent gastric irritation. Administer diluted IV potassium solutions at a rate no faster than 10–20 mmol/h; never administer undiluted potassium intravenously. For clients receiving IV potassium, monitor for pain and inflammation at the injection site. Teach client about potassium-rich foods. Teach clients how to prevent excessive loss of potassium (e.g., through avoiding abuse of diuretics and laxatives).
Hyperkalemia		
Decreased potassium excretion: • Renal failure • Hypoaldosteronism • Potassium-conserving diuretics High potassium intake: • Excessive use of potassium-containing salt substitutes • Excessive or rapid IV infusion of potassium Potassium shift out of the tissue cells into the plasma (e.g., infections, burns, acidosis)	Gastrointestinal hyperactivity, diarrhea Irritability, apathy, confusion Cardiac dysrhythmias or arrest Muscle weakness, areflexia (absence of reflexes) Paresthesias and numbness in extremities *Laboratory findings:* Serum potassium above 5.0 mmol/L Peaked T wave, widened QRS on ECG	Closely monitor cardiac status and ECG. Administer diuretics and other medications, such as glucose and insulin, as ordered. Hold potassium supplements and potassium-conserving diuretics as ordered. Monitor serum K^+ levels carefully; a rapid drop can occur as potassium shifts into the cells. Teach clients to avoid foods high in potassium and salt substitutes.

(continued)

losses of potassium through vomiting and gastric suction are common causes of hypokalemia, as is the use of potassium-wasting diuretics, such as thiazide diuretics or loop diuretics (e.g., furosemide). Symptoms of hypokalemia are usually mild until the level drops below 3 mmol/L unless the decrease in potassium was rapid. When the decrease is gradual, the body compensates by shifting potassium from the intracellular environment into the serum.

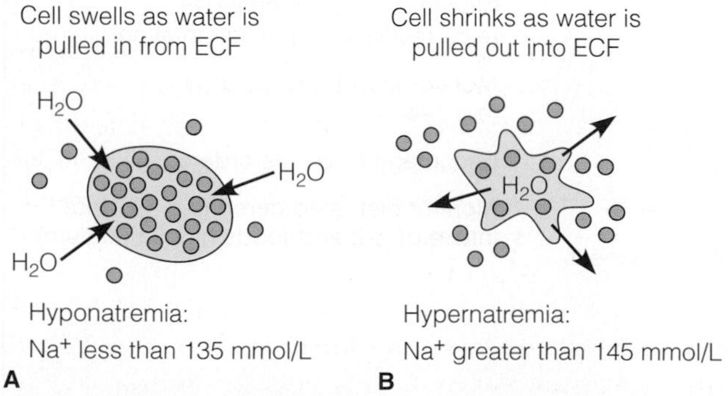

FIGURE 43.12 The extracellular sodium level affects cell size: **A:** in hyponatremia, cells swell; **B:** in hypernatremia, cells shrink.

Hyperkalemia is a potassium excess or a serum potassium level greater than 5.0 mmol/L. Hyperkalemia is less common than hypokalemia and rarely occurs in clients with normal renal function. It is, however, more dangerous than hypokalemia and can lead to cardiac arrest. As with hypokalemia, symptoms are more severe and occur at lower levels when the increase in potassium is abrupt.

CLINICAL ALERT

Potassium may be given intravenously for severe hypokalemia. It must *always* be diluted appropriately and *never* be given IV push. Potassium that is to be given IV should be mixed in the pharmacy and double checked by two nurses before administration. The usual concentration of IV potassium is 20 mmol/L to 40 mmol/L.

TABLE 43.7 Electrolyte Imbalances *(continued)*

Risk Factors	Clinical Manifestations	Nursing Interventions
Hypocalcemia		
Surgical removal of the parathyroid glands Conditions, such as: • Hypoparathyroidism • Acute pancreatitis • Hyperphosphatemia • Thyroid carcinoma Inadequate vitamin D intake Malabsorption Hypomagnesemia Alkalosis Sepsis Alcohol abuse	Numbness, tingling of the extremities and around the mouth Muscle tremors, cramps; if severe, can progress to tetany and convulsions Cardiac dysrhythmias; decreased cardiac output Positive Trousseau's and Chvostek's signs Confusion, anxiety, possible psychoses Dyspnea; laryngospasm Blood clots Bone fractures ECG changes *Laboratory findings:* Serum calcium less than 2.2 mmol/L (total) or 1.0 mmol/L (ionized)	Closely monitor respiratory and cardiovascular status. Take precautions to protect a confused client. Take seizure precautions. Have equipment for intubation available. Administer oral or parenteral calcium supplements as ordered. When administering intravenously, closely monitor cardiac status and ECG during infusion. Teach clients at high risk for osteoporosis about: • Dietary sources rich in calcium • Recommendation for 1500 mg of calcium per day • Calcium supplements as ordered • Regular exercise • Estrogen replacement therapy for postmenopausal women as ordered Monitor respiratory and cardiovascular status.
Hypercalcemia		
Prolonged immobilization Conditions, such as: • Hyperparathyroidism • Malignancy of the bone • Paget's disease	Lethargy, weakness Depressed deep-tendon reflexes Anorexia, nausea, vomiting Constipation Polyuria, hypercalciuria Flank pain secondary to urinary calculi Dysrhythmias, possible heart block Bone pain, fractures ECG changes *Laboratory findings:* Serum calcium greater than 2.58 mmol/L (total) or 1.15 mmol/L (ionized)	Increase client movement and exercise. Encourage oral fluids, as permitted, to maintain a dilute urine. Teach clients to limit intake of food and fluid high in calcium. Encourage ingestion of fibre to prevent constipation. Protect a confused client; monitor for pathological fractures in clients with long-term hypercalcemia. Encourage intake of acid-ash fluids (e.g., prune or cranberry juice) to counteract deposits of calcium salts in the urine.

(continued)

CALCIUM Levels of calcium (Ca^{2+}) in the body can be affected by many factors. **Hypocalcemia** is a calcium deficit, or a total serum calcium level of less than 2.2 mmol/L and an ionized calcium level of less than 1.0 mmol/L. Severe depletion of calcium can cause *tetany* (muscle spasms) and paresthesias (numbness and tingling around the mouth or in the hands and feet) and can lead to convulsions. Two signs indicate hypocalcemia: Chvostek's sign is contraction of the facial muscles that is produced by tapping the facial nerve in front of the ear (Figure 43.13A). Trousseau's sign is a carpal spasm that occurs by inflating a blood pressure cuff on the upper arm to 20 mm Hg greater than the systolic pressure for 2 to 5 minutes (Figure 43.13B). Clients at greatest risk for hypocalcemia are those whose parathyroid glands have been removed. Hypocalcemia is frequently associated with total thyroidectomy or bilateral neck surgery for cancer. Low serum magnesium levels (hypomagnesemia) and chronic alcoholism also increase the risk of hypocalcemia.

Hypercalcemia, or total serum calcium levels greater than 2.58 mmol/L, occurs when calcium is mobilized from the bony skeleton. This increase may be due to malignancy or prolonged immobilization.

MAGNESIUM The majority of magnesium (Mg^{2+}) is found intracellularly. Many organs, including nerves and

TABLE 43.7 Electrolyte Imbalances *(continued)*

Risk Factors	Clinical Manifestations	Nursing Interventions
Hypomagnesemia		
Excessive loss from the gastrointestinal tract (e.g., from nasogastric suction, diarrhea, fistula drainage) Long-term use of certain drugs (e.g., diuretics, aminoglycoside antibiotics) Conditions, such as: • Chronic alcoholism • Pancreatitis • Burns	Neuromuscular irritability with tremors Increased reflexes, tremors, convulsions Positive Chvostek's and Trousseau's signs Tachycardia, elevated blood pressure, dysrhythmias Disorientation and confusion Vertigo, anorexia, nausea *Laboratory findings:* Serum magnesium below 0.65 mmol/L ECG showing prolonged QT intervals, widened QRS, flat T wave; ST depression	Monitor repiratory and cardiovascular status. Assess clients receiving digitalis for digitalis toxicity. Hypomagnesemia increases the risk of toxicity. Take protective measures when there is a possibility of seizures. • Assess the client's ability to swallow water before initiating oral feeding. • Initiate safety measures to prevent injury during seizure activity. • Carefully administer magnesium salts as ordered. Encourage clients to eat magnesium-rich foods, if permitted (e.g., whole grains, meat, seafood, and green leafy vegetables). Refer clients to alcohol treatment programs, as indicated.
Hypermagnesemia		
Abnormal retention of magnesium, as in: • Renal failure • Adrenal insufficiency Treatment with magnesium salts	Peripheral vasodilation, flushing Nausea, vomiting Muscle weakness, paralysis Hypotension, bradycardia Depressed deep-tendon reflexes Lethargy, drowsiness Respiratory depression, coma Respiratory and cardiac arrest, if hypermagnesemia is severe *Laboratory findings:* Serum magnesium above 1.05 mmol/L ECG showing prolonged PR and QT interval; an atrioventricular (AV) block may occur	Monitor respiratory and cardiovascular status. Monitor vital signs and level of consciousness when clients are at risk. If patellar reflexes are absent, notify the physician. Advise clients who have renal disease to contact their care provider before taking over-the-counter drugs.

muscles, depend on magnesium. Imbalances may go unrecognized in hospitalized clients. **Hypomagnesemia** occurs more frequently than hypermagnesemia. Chronic alcoholism is the most common cause of hypomagnesemia. Magnesium deficiency can aggravate the manifestations of alcohol withdrawal, such as delirium tremens (DTs). **Hypermagnesemia** often is iatrogenic, that is, a result of overzealous magnesium therapy.

CHLORIDE Because of the relationship between sodium ions and chloride ions (Cl^-), imbalances of chloride commonly occur in conjunction with sodium imbalances. **Hypochloremia** is a decreased serum chloride level, in adults a level below 95 mmol/L, and is usually related to excess losses of chloride ions through the GI tract, kidneys, or sweating. Hypochloremic clients are at risk for alkalosis and may experience muscle twitching, tremors, or tetany.

Conditions that cause sodium retention also can lead to a high serum chloride level or **hyperchloremia**, in adults a level above 105 mmol/L. Excess replacement of sodium chloride or potassium chloride are additional risk factors for high serum chloride levels. The manifestations of hyperchloremia include acidosis, weakness, and lethargy, with a risk of dysrhythmias and coma.

PHOSPHATE The phosphate anion (PO_4^-) is found in ICF and ECF. Most of the phosphorus (P^+) in the body exists as PO_4^-. Phosphate is critical for cellular metabolism because it is a major component of ATP.

Phosphate imbalances frequently are related to therapeutic interventions for other disorders. Glucose and

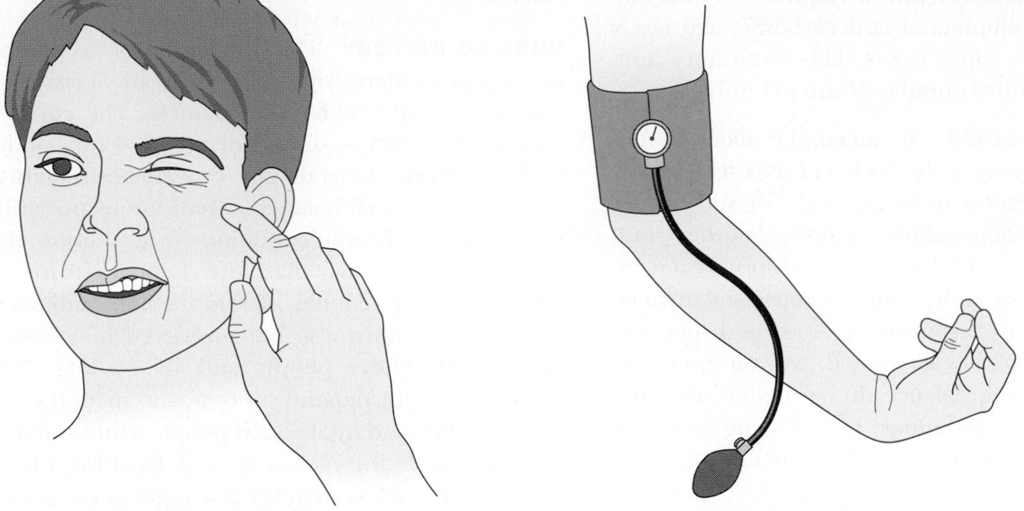

FIGURE 43.13 **A:** Positive Chvostek's sign; **B:** positive Trousseau's sign

(From **Medical Surgical Nursing: Critical Thinking in Client Care,** *3rd ed., by Priscilla LeMone and Karen M. Burke, © 2004. Reproduced with the permission of Pearson Education, Inc., Upper Saddle River, New Jersey.)*

insulin administration and total parenteral nutrition can cause phosphate to shift into the cells from extracellular fluid compartments, leading to **hypophosphatemia**. Alcohol withdrawal, acid-base imbalances, and the use of antacids, such as Gelusil, Maalox, or Mylanta, that bind with phosphate in the gastrointestinal tract, are other possible causes of low serum phosphate levels. Manifestations of hypophosphatemia include paresthesias, muscle weakness and pain, mental changes, and possible seizures.

Hyperphosphatemia occurs when phosphate shifts out of the cells into ECF, for example, because of tissue trauma, chemotherapy for malignant tumours, or renal failure, or when excess phosphate is administered or ingested. Infants who are fed cow's milk are at risk for hyperphosphatemia, as are people using phosphate-containing enemas or laxatives. Clients who have high serum phosphate levels may experience numbness and tingling around the mouth and in the fingertips, muscle spasms, and tetany.

Acid-Base Imbalances

Acid-base imbalances generally are classified as *respiratory* or *metabolic* according to the underlying cause of the disorder. Carbonic acid levels are normally regulated by the lungs through the retention or excretion of carbon dioxide, and problems of regulation lead to respiratory acidosis or alkalosis. Bicarbonate and hydrogen ion levels are regulated by the kidneys, and problems of regulation lead to metabolic acidosis or alkalosis. Healthy regulatory systems will attempt to correct acid-base imbalances, a process called **compensation.**

RESPIRATORY ACIDOSIS Hypoventilation and carbon dioxide retention cause carbonic acid levels to increase and the pH to fall below 7.35, a condition known as **respiratory acidosis**. Serious lung diseases, such as asthma and COPD, are common causes of respiratory acidosis. Central nervous system depression caused by anaesthesia or a narcotic overdose can sufficiently slow the respiratory rate so that carbon dioxide is retained. When respiratory acidosis occurs, the kidneys retain bicarbonate to restore the normal carbonic acid to bicarbonate ratio. Recall, however, that the kidneys are relatively slow to respond to changes in acid-base balance, so this compensatory response may require hours to days to restore the normal pH.

RESPIRATORY ALKALOSIS When a person hyperventilates, more carbon dioxide than normal is exhaled, carbonic acid levels fall, and the pH rises to greater than 7.45. This condition is termed **respiratory alkalosis** Psychogenic or anxiety-related hyperventilation is a common cause of respiratory alkalosis. Other causes include fever and respiratory infections. In respiratory alkalosis, the kidneys will excrete bicarbonate to return the pH to within the normal range. Often, however, if the cause of the hyperventilation is eliminated, the pH returns to normal before renal compensation occurs.

METABOLIC ACIDOSIS When bicarbonate levels are low in relation to the amount of carbonic acid in the body, the pH falls and **metabolic acidosis** develops. One cause of metabolic acidosis is renal failure and the inability of the kidneys to excrete hydrogen ions and produce bicarbonate. Metabolic acidosis can also occur when too much acid is produced in the body, for example, in diabetic ketoacidosis or starvation when fat tissue is broken down for energy. Metabolic acidosis stimulates the respiratory centre, and the rate and depth of respirations increase. Carbon dioxide is eliminated and carbonic acid levels fall, minimizing the change in pH. This respiratory compensation occurs within minutes of the pH imbalance.

METABOLIC ALKALOSIS In **metabolic alkalosis**, the amount of bicarbonate in the body exceeds the normal 20 to 1 ratio. Ingestion of bicarbonate of soda as an antacid is one cause of metabolic alkalosis. Another cause is prolonged vomiting with loss of hydrochloric acid from the stomach. The respiratory centre is depressed in metabolic alkalosis, and respirations slow and become shallower. Carbon dioxide is retained, and carbonic acid levels increase, helping balance the excess bicarbonate. The risk factors, manifestations, and nursing interventions for acid-base imbalances are listed in Table 43.8.

Assessing

Assessing clients for fluid, electrolyte, and acid-base balance and imbalances is an important nursing care function. Components of the assessment include (1) the nursing history, (2) physical assessment of the client, (3) clinical measurements, and (4) review of laboratory test results.

NURSING HISTORY The nursing history is particularly important for identifying clients who are at risk for fluid, electrolyte, and acid-base imbalances. The current and past medical history should be checked for conditions, such as chronic lung disease or diabetes mellitus, that can disrupt normal balances. Medications prescribed to treat acute or chronic conditions (e.g., diuretic therapy for hypertension) may place the client at risk for altered homeostasis. Functional, developmental, and socioeconomic factors must also be considered in assessing the client's risk. Older people and very young children, clients who must depend on others to meet their needs for food and fluid intake, and people who cannot afford or do not have the means to cook food for a balanced diet (e.g., homeless people) are at greater risk for fluid and electrolyte imbalances. Common risk factors are listed in Box 43.3.

When obtaining the nursing history, the nurse needs to not only recognize risk factors but also elicit data about the client's food and fluid intake, fluid output, and the presence of signs or symptoms suggestive of altered fluid and electrolyte balance. The Assessment:

TABLE 43.8 Acid-Base Imbalances

Risk Factors	Clinical Manifestations	Nursing Interventions
Respiratory Acidosis	**Acute:**	
Acute lung conditions that impair alveolar gas exchange (e.g., pneumonia, acute pulmonary edema, aspiration of foreign body, near-drowning) Chronic lung disease (e.g., asthma, cystic fibrosis, or emphysema) Overdose of narcotics or sedatives that depress respiratory rate and depth Brain injury that affects the respiratory centre	Increased pulse and respiratory rates, dysrythmias Headache, dizziness Confusion, decreased level of consciousness (LOC) Convulsions Warm, flushed skin **Chronic:** Weakness Headache *Laboratory findings:* Arterial blood pH less than 7.35 $PaCO_2$ above 45 mm Hg HCO_3^- normal or slightly elevated in acute; above 26 mmol/L in chronic	Frequently assess respiratory status and lung sounds. Monitor airway and ventilation; insert artificial airway and prepare for mechanical ventilation, as necessary. Administer pulmonary therapy measures, such as inhalation therapy, percussion and postural drainage, bronchodilators, and antibiotics as ordered. Monitor fluid intake and output, vital signs, and arterial blood gases (ABGs). Administer narcotic antagonists, as indicated. Maintain adequate hydration (2–3 L of fluid per day), unless contraindicated.
Respiratory Alkalosis		
Hyperventilation caused by: • Extreme anxiety • Elevated body temperature • Overventilation with a mechanical ventilator • Hypoxia • Salicylate overdose	Complaints of shortness of breath, chest tightness Light-headedness with circumoral paresthesias and numbness and tingling of the extremities Difficulty concentrating Tremulousness, blurred vision *Laboratory findings (in uncompensated respiratory alkalosis):* Arterial blood pH above 7.45 $PaCO_2$ less than 35 mm Hg	Monitor vital signs and ABGs. Assist client to breathe more slowly. Help client breathe into a paper bag or apply a rebreather mask (to inhale CO_2). Treat underlying problem as ordered.

(continued)

TABLE 43.8 Acid-Base Imbalances *(continued)*

Risk Factors	Clinical Manifestations	Nursing Interventions
Metabolic Acidosis		
Conditions that increase nonvolatile acids in the blood (e.g., renal impairment, diabetes mellitus, starvation) Conditions that decrease bicarbonate (e.g., prolonged diarrhea) Excessive infusion of chloride-containing IV fluids (e.g., NaCl)	Kussmaul's respirations (deep, rapid respirations) Lethargy, confusion Headache Weakness Nausea and vomiting *Laboratory findings:* Arterial blood pH below 7.35 Serum bicarbonate less than 22 mmol/L $PaCO_2$ less than 35 mm Hg with respiratory compensation	Monitor ABG values, intake and output, LOC, and respiratory status. Administer IV sodium bicarbonate carefully, if ordered. Treat underlying problem, as ordered. Assess cardiovascular status.
Metabolic Alkalosis		
Excessive acid losses caused by: • Vomiting • Gastric suction Excessive use of potassium-losing diuretics Excessive adrenal corticoid hormones caused by: • Cushing's syndrome • Hyperaldosteronism Excessive bicarbonate intake from: • Antacids • Parenteral $NaHCO_3^-$	Decreased respiratory rate and depth Dizziness Circumoral paresthesias, numbness and tingling of the extremities Hypertonic muscles, tetany *Laboratory findings:* Arterial blood pH above 7.45 Serum bicarbonate greater than 26 mmol/L $PaCO_2$ higher than 45 mm Hg with respiratory compensation	Monitor intake and output closely. Monitor vital signs, especially respirations, LOC, and intake and output. Administer ordered IV fluids carefully. Treat underlying problem as ordered. Assess cardiovascular status.

Interview box provides examples of questions to elicit information regarding fluid, electrolyte, and acid-base balance.

PHYSICAL ASSESSMENT Physical assessment to evaluate a client's fluid, electrolyte, and acid-base status focuses on the skin, the oral cavity and mucous membranes, the eyes, the cardiovascular and respiratory systems, urinary gastrointestinal systems, and neurological and muscular status. Data from this physical assessment are used to expand and verify information obtained in the nursing history. The focused physical assessment is summarized in Table 43.9; refer to Tables 43.4 through 43.8 for possible abnormal findings related to specific imbalances discussed in this chapter.

CLINICAL MEASUREMENTS Three simple clinical measurements that the nurse can initiate are daily weights, vital signs, and fluid intake and output.

DAILY WEIGHTS Daily weight measurements provide a relatively accurate assessment of a client's fluid status. Significant changes in weight over a short time (e.g., more than 2 kg in a week or less are indicative of *acute* fluid changes. Each kilogram of weight gained or lost is equivalent to 1 L of fluid gained or lost. Such fluid gains or losses indicate changes in total body fluid volume, rather than in any specific compartment, such as the intravascular compartment. Rapid losses or gains of 5% to 8% of total body weight indicate moderate to severe fluid volume deficits or excesses.

To obtain accurate weight measurements, the nurse should balance the scale before each use and weigh the client (1) at the same time each day (e.g., before breakfast and after the first void), (2) with the client wearing the same or similar clothing, and (3) on the same scale. The type of scale (i.e., standing, bed, chair) should be documented.

Regular assessment of weight is particularly important for clients in the community and extended-care facilities who are at risk for fluid imbalance. For these clients, measuring intake and output may be impractical because of lifestyle or problems with incontinence. Regular weight measurement, either daily, every other day, or weekly, provides valuable information about the client's fluid volume status.

VITAL SIGNS Changes in the vital signs can indicate, or in some cases precede, fluid, electrolyte, and acid-base imbalances. For example, elevated body temperature may be a result of dehydration or a cause of increased body fluid losses.

BOX 43.3 COMMON RISK FACTORS FOR FLUID, ELECTROLYTE, AND ACID-BASE IMBALANCES

The following are some of the common risk factors for changes in homeostasis:

CHRONIC DISEASES AND CONDITIONS

- Chronic lung disease (COPD, asthma, cystic fibrosis)
- Heart failure
- Kidney disease
- Diabetes mellitus
- Cushing's syndrome or Addison's disease
- Cancer
- Malnutrition, anorexia nervosa, bulimia
- Ileostomy
- Dysphagia

ACUTE CONDITIONS

- Acute gastroenteritis
- Bowel obstruction
- Head injury or decreased level of consciousness
- Trauma, such as burns or crushing injuries
- Surgery
- Fever, draining wounds, fistulas

MEDICATIONS

- Diuretics
- Corticosteroids
- Nonsteroidal anti-inflammatory drugs (NSAIDs)
- Antibiotics
- Magnesium salts
- Antacids
- Laxatives
- Potassium supplements

TREATMENTS

- Chemotherapy
- IV therapy and total parenteral nutrition (TPN)
- Nasogastric suction
- Enteral feedings
- Mechanical ventilation

OTHER FACTORS

- Age: very old or very young
- Inability to access food and fluids independently

ASSESSMENT: INTERVIEW

Fluid, Electrolyte, and Acid-Base Balance

These questions can help the nurse elicit data about the client during the nursing history:

CURRENT AND PAST MEDICAL HISTORY

- Are you currently seeing a health-care provider for treatment of any chronic diseases, such as kidney disease, heart disease, high blood pressure, diabetes insipidus, or thyroid or parathyroid disorders?
- Have you recently experienced any acute conditions, such as gastroenteritis, severe trauma, head injury, or surgery? If so, describe them.

MEDICATIONS AND TREATMENTS

- Are you currently taking any medications on a regular basis, such as diuretics, steroids, potassium supplements, salt substitutes, or antacids?
- Have you recently undergone any treatments, such as dialysis, parenteral nutrition, or tube feedings, or been on a ventilator? If so, when, and why?

FOOD AND FLUID INTAKE

- How much and what type of fluids do you drink each day?
- Describe your diet for a typical day. (Pay particular attention to the client's intake of foods high in sodium content, of protein, and of whole grains, fruits, and vegetables.)
- Have there been any recent changes in your food or fluid intake, for example, as a result of following a weight-loss program?
- Are you on any type of restricted diet?
- Has your food or fluid intake recently been affected by changes in appetite, nausea, or other factors, such as pain or difficulty breathing?

FLUID OUTPUT

- Have you noticed any recent changes in the frequency or amount of urine output?
- Have you recently experienced any problems with vomiting, diarrhea, or constipation? If so, when, and for how long?
- Have you noticed any other unusual fluid losses, such as excessive sweating?

FLUID, ELECTROLYTE, AND ACID-BASE IMBALANCES

- Have you gained or lost weight in recent weeks?
- Have you recently experienced any symptoms, such as excessive thirst, dry skin or mucous membranes, dark or concentrated urine, or low urine output?
- Do you have problems with swelling of your fingers, hands, feet, or ankles? Do you ever have difficulty breathing, especially when lying down or at night? How many pillows do you use to sleep?
- Have you recently experienced any of the following symptoms: difficulty concentrating or confusion; dizziness or feeling faint; muscle weakness, twitching, cramping, or spasm; excessive fatigue; abnormal sensations, such as numbness, tingling, burning, or prickling; abdominal cramping or distension; heart palpitations?

Tachycardia is an early sign of hypovolemia. Pulse volume will decrease in FVD and increase in FVE. Irregular pulse rates may occur with electrolyte imbalances. Changes in respiratory rate and depth may cause respiratory acid-base imbalances or act as a compensatory mechanism in metabolic acidosis or alkalosis.

Blood pressure, a sensitive measure to detect blood volume changes, may fall significantly with FVD and

TABLE 43.9 Focused Physical Assessment for Fluid, Electrolyte, or Acid-Base Imbalance

System	Assessment Focus	Technique	Possible Abnormal Findings
Skin	Colour, temperature, moisture	Inspection, palpation	Flushed, warm, very dry Moist or diaphoretic Cool and pale
	Turgor	Gently pinch up a fold of skin over sternum or inner aspect of thigh for adults, on the abdomen or medial thigh for children	Poor turgor: Skin remains tented for several seconds instead of immediately returning to normal position
	Edema	Inspect for visible swelling around eyes, in fingers, and in lower extremities	Skin around eyes is puffy, lids appear swollen; rings are tight; shoes leave impressions on feet
		Compress the skin over the dorsum of the foot, around the ankles, over the tibia, in the sacral area	Depression remains (pitting): see scale for describing edema in Figure 43.11
Mucous membranes	Colour, moisture	Inspection	Mucous membranes dry, dull, pale in appearance; tongue dry and cracked; edema
Eyes	Firmness	Gently palpate eyeball with lid closed	Eyeball feels soft to palpation
Fontanelles (infant)	Firmness, level	Inspect and gently palpate anterior fontanelle	Fontanelle bulging, firm Fontanelle sunken, soft
Cardiovascular system	Heart rate	Auscultation, cardiac monitor	Tachycardia, bradycardia; ECG changes; dysrhythmias
	Peripheral pulses	Palpation	Weak and thready; bounding; absent
	Blood pressure	Auscultation of Korotkoff's sounds BP assessment lying and standing	Hypotension; hypertension Postural hypotension
	Capillary refill	Palpation	Slowed capillary refill
	Venous filling	Inspection of jugular veins and hand veins	Jugular venous distention; flat jugular veins; poor venous refill
Respiratory system	Respiratory rate and pattern	Inspection	Increased or decreased rate and depth of respirations; use of accessory muscles
	Lung sounds	Auscultation	Crackles
Neurological	Level of consciousness (LOC)	Observation, stimulation Glasgow coma scale (GCS)	Decreased LOC, lethargy, stupor, or coma, change in GCS score
	Orientation, cognition	Questioning	Disoriented, confused; difficulty concentrating
	Motor function	Strength testing	Weakness, decreased motor strength
	Reflexes	Deep tendon reflex (DTR) testing	Hyperactive or depressed DTRs
	Abnormal reflexes	Chvostek's sign: Tap over facial nerve about 2 cm anterior to tragus of ear (see Figure 43.13A)	Facial muscle twitching including eyelids and lips on side of stimulus
		Trousseau's sign: Inflate a blood pressure cuff on the upper arm to 20 mm Hg greater than the systolic pressure, leave in place for 2 to 5 minutes (see Figure 43.13B)	Carpal spasm: contraction of hand and fingers on affected side

(continued)

TABLE 43.9 Focused Physical Assessment for Fluid, Electrolyte, or Acid-Base Imbalance *(continued)*

System	Assessment Focus	Technique	Possible Abnormal Findings
Urinary and gastrointestinal systems	Intake/output	Measurement of intake of oral or parenteral fluids	Fluid intake or urinary output less than normal
		Output: urine, liquid stool, vomit, drainage from a wound or operative site, drainage from a nasogastric tube	Excess losses from a surgical drain or vomiting
		Auscultate bowel sounds	High-pitched bowel sounds or absent bowel sounds
		Palpate bladder and abdomen	Firm bladder indicating possible distention

hypovolemia or increase with FVE and overhydration. *Postural,* or *orthostatic, hypotension* may also occur with FVD and hypovolemia.

To assess for orthostatic hypotension, measure the client's baseline blood pressure and pulse in a supine position. Allow the client to remain in that position for 3 to 5 minutes, leaving the blood pressure cuff on the arm. Stand the client up and immediately reassess the blood pressure and pulse. For a client who is too dizzy or weak to stand, assess supine and then sitting with legs dangling. A drop of 10 mm Hg to 15 mm Hg in the systolic blood pressure with a corresponding drop in diastolic pressure and an increased pulse rate (by 10 or more beats per minute) is indicative of orthostatic or postural hypotension.

FLUID INTAKE AND OUTPUT The measurement and recording of all fluid intake and output (I & O) during a 24-hour period provides important data about the client's fluid and electrolyte balance. Generally, intake and output are measured for hospitalized at-risk clients.

The unit used to measure intake and output is the millilitre (mL). To measure fluid intake, nurses convert household measures, such as a glass, cup, or soup bowl, to metric units. Most agencies provide conversion tables since the sizes of dishes vary from agency to agency. Such a table is often provided on or with the bedside I & O record. Examples of equivalents are given in Box 43.4.

Most agencies have a form for recording I & O, usually a bedside record on which the nurse lists all items measured and their quantities per shift. Recording the specifics of intravenous fluids, such as the type of solution, additives, time started, and amounts absorbed are often noted on the I & O record.

It is important to inform clients, family members, and all caregivers that accurate measurements of the client's fluid intake and output are required, explaining why and emphasizing the need to use a bedpan, urinal, commode, or in-toilet collection device (unless a urinary drainage system is in place). Instruct the client not to put toilet tissue into the container with urine. Clients who wish to be involved in recording fluid intake measurements need to be taught how to compute the values and what foods are considered fluids.

BOX 43.4 COMMONLY USED FLUID CONTAINERS AND SAMPLE VOLUMES

Water glass	200 mL
Juice glass	120 mL
Cup	180 mL
Soup bowl	
Adult	180 mL
Child	100 mL
Teapot	240 mL
Creamer	
Large	90 mL
Small	30 mL
Water pitcher	1000 mL
Jell-O, custard dish	100 mL
Ice cream dish	120 mL
Paper cup	
Large	200 mL
Small	120 mL

Note: Measurements vary with agencies.

To measure *fluid intake,* the nurse records each fluid item taken (if the client has not already done so) specifying the time and type of fluid. All the following fluids need to be recorded:

- *Oral fluids.* These include water, milk, juice, soft drinks, coffee, tea, cream, soup, and any other beverages. Include water taken with medications. To assess the amount of water taken from a water pitcher, measure what remains and subtract this amount from the volume of the full pitcher. Then, refill the pitcher.
- *Ice chips.* Record these as fluids at approximately one-half the volume of the ice chips. For example, if the ice chips fill a cup holding 200 mL and the client consumed all the ice chips, the volume consumed would be recorded as 100 mL.
- *Foods that are or tend to become liquid at room temperature.* These include ice cream, sherbet, custard, and gelatin (Jell-O). Do *not* measure foods that are pureed because purees are simply solid foods prepared in a different form.

- *Tube feedings.* Remember to include the water instilled as a rinse at the end of intermittent feedings or during continuous feedings.
- *Parenteral fluids.* The exact amount of intravenous fluid administered is to be recorded, since some fluid containers may be overfilled. Blood transfusions are included.
- *Intravenous medications.* Intravenous medications that are prepared with such solutions as normal saline (NS) and are administered as an intermittent or continuous infusion must also be included (e.g., ceftazidime 1 g in 50 mL of sterile NS). Most intravenous medications are mixed in 50 mL to 100 mL of solution.
- *Catheter or tube irrigants.* Fluid used to irrigate urinary catheters, nasogastric tubes, and intestinal tubes must be measured and recorded, if not immediately withdrawn.

To measure *fluid output,* measure the following fluids (remember to observe appropriate infection prevention and control precautions):

- *Urinary output.* Following each voiding, pour the urine into a measuring container, observe the amount, and record it and the time of voiding. For clients with retention catheters, empty the drainage bag into a measuring container at the end of the shift (or at prescribed times, if output is to be measured more often). Note and record the amount of urine output. In intensive care areas, often, urine output is measured hourly. If the client is incontinent of urine, estimate and record these outputs. For example, for an incontinent client, the nurse might record "Incontinent 3 times" or "Drawsheet soaked in 30 cm diameter." A more accurate estimate of the urine output of infants and incontinent clients may be obtained by first weighing diapers or incontinence pads that are dry, and then subtracting this weight from the weight of the soiled items. Each gram of weight left after subtracting is equal to 1 mL of urine. If urine is frequently soiled with feces, the number of voidings can be recorded, rather than the volume of urine.
- *Vomitus and liquid feces.* The amount and type of fluid and the time need to be specified.
- *Tube drainage,* such as gastric or intestinal drainage.
- *Wound drainage* and *draining fistulas.* Wound drainage can be recorded by documenting the type and number of dressings or linen saturated with drainage or by measuring the exact amount of drainage collected in a vacuum drainage (e.g., Hemovac) or gravity drainage system.

Fluid intake and output measurements are totalled at the end of the shift (every 8 to 12 hours), and the totals are recorded in the client's permanent record. In intensive care areas, the nurse may record intake and output more frequently. Usually, the nurses on night shift total the amounts of I & O recorded for each shift and record the 24-hour total.

To determine whether the fluid output is proportional to fluid intake or whether there are any changes in the client's fluid status, the nurse (1) compares the total 24-hour fluid output measurement with the total fluid intake measurement, and (2) compares both with previous measurements. Urinary output is normally equivalent to the amount of fluids ingested; the usual range is 1500 mL to 2000 mL in 24 hours, or 40 mL to 80 mL in 1 hour (0.5 mL/kg/h). Clients whose output substantially exceeds intake are at risk for deficient fluid volume. By contrast, clients whose intake substantially exceeds output are at risk for fluid volume excess. In assessing the client's fluid balance, it is important to consider additional factors that can affect intake and output. The client who is extremely diaphoretic or who has rapid, deep respirations has fluid losses that cannot be measured but must be considered in evaluating fluid status.

When a significant discrepancy exists between intake and output or when fluid intake or output is inadequate (for example, a urine output of less than 500 mL in 24 hours or less than 0.5 mL/kg per hour in an adult), this information should be reported to the appropriate member of the health-care team.

LABORATORY TESTS Many laboratory studies are conducted to determine the client's fluid, electrolyte, and acid-base status. Some of the more common tests are discussed here.

SERUM ELECTROLYTES Serum electrolyte levels are often routinely ordered for any client admitted to hospital as a screening test for electrolyte and acid-base imbalances. Serum electrolytes also are routinely assessed for clients at risk in the community, for example, clients who are being treated with a diuretic for hypertension or heart failure. The most commonly ordered serum tests are for sodium, potassium, chloride, magnesium, and bicarbonate ions. Normal values of commonly measured electrolytes are summarized in Box 43.5.

Some agencies use a diagram format for keeping track of the client's electrolytes when documenting in his or her progress notes. See Figure 43.14.

COMPLETE BLOOD COUNT (CBC) The complete blood count (CBC), another basic screening test, provides information about the hematocrit. The **hematocrit** is the

BOX 43.5 NORMAL ELECTROLYTE VALUES FOR ADULTS

Venous blood	
Sodium	135–145 mmol/L
Potassium	3.5–5.0 mmol/L
Chloride	95–105 mmol/L
Calcium (total)	2.2–2.58 mmol/L
Calcium (ionized)	1.0–1.15 mmol/L
Magnesium	0.65–1.05 mmol/L
Phosphate (phosphorus)	0.97–1.45 mmol/L
Serum osmolality	280–300 mmol/kg water

Note: Normal laboratory values vary from agency to agency.

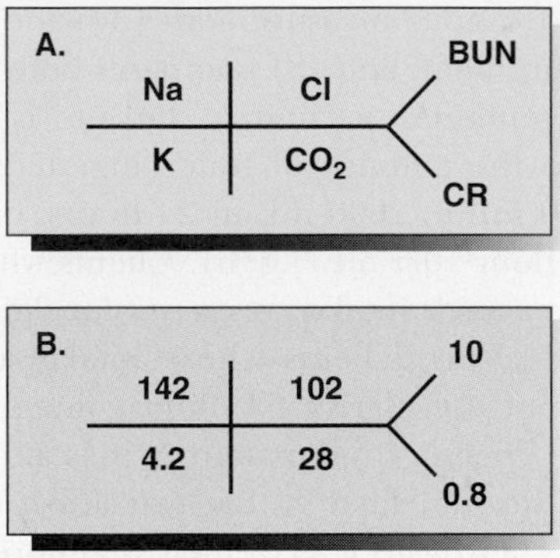

FIGURE 43.14 **A:** Format for a diagram of serum electrolyte results; **B:** example that may be seen in documentation notes

portion of blood plasma that is composed of erythrocytes (red blood cells [RBCs]). Because the hematocrit is measured in relation to plasma, it is affected by changes in plasma volume. Thus, the hematocrit increases with severe dehydration and decreases with severe overhydration. Normal hematocrit values are 0.37 to 0.49 (males) and 0.36 to 0.46 (females).

OSMOLALITY *Serum osmolality* is a measure of the solute concentration of the blood. The solutes included are sodium ions, chloride, bicarbonate, proteins, glucose, and urea. Serum osmolality can be estimated by doubling the serum sodium because sodium and its associated chloride ions are the major determinants of serum osmolality. Serum osmolality values are used primarily to evaluate fluid balance. Normal values are 280 mmol/kg to 300 mmol/kg. An increase in serum osmolality indicates a fluid volume deficit; a decrease reflects a fluid volume excess.

Urine osmolality is a measure of the solute concentration of urine. The particles included are nitrogenous wastes, such as creatinine, urea, and uric acid. Normal values are 500 mmol/kg to 800 mmol/kg. An increased urine osmolality indicates a fluid volume deficit; a decreased urine osmolality reflects a fluid volume excess.

URINE PH Measurement of urine pH can be obtained by laboratory analysis or by using a dipstick on a freshly voided specimen. Because the kidneys play a critical role in regulating acid-base balance, assessment of urine pH can be useful in determining whether the kidneys are responding appropriately to acid-base imbalances. Normally, the pH of the urine is relatively acidic, averaging about 6, but a range of 4.5 to 8 is considered normal. In metabolic acidosis, urine pH decreases as the kidneys excrete hydrogen ions; in metabolic alkalosis, the pH increases.

URINE SPECIFIC GRAVITY **Specific gravity** is an indicator of urine concentration that can be performed quickly and easily. Normal specific gravity ranges from 1.010 to 1.025. When the concentration of solutes in the urine is high, the specific gravity rises; in very dilute urine with few solutes, it is abnormally low.

Urine sodium and chloride excretion are indicators of renal perfusion and can provide useful information about a client's fluid status. With hypovolemia, aldosterone will be secreted. This will cause reabsorption of sodium and chloride, which will result in decreased levels of sodium and chloride, less than 20 mmol/L.

ARTERIAL BLOOD GASES **Arterial blood gases (ABGs)** are performed to evaluate the client's acid-base balance and oxygenation. Arterial blood is used because it provides a truer reflection of gas exchange in the pulmonary system than does venous blood. Because a high-pressure artery is used to obtain blood, it is important to apply pressure to the puncture site for at least 5 minutes after the procedure to reduce the risk of bleeding or bruising.

Six measurements are commonly used to interpret arterial blood gases (Simpson, 2004):

1. pH, a measure of the relative acidity or alkalinity of the blood. The greater the number of hydrogen ions, the more acidic the solution is. The normal range for pH is narrow, and death may ensue with pH values below 6.8 or above 7.8.
2. PaO_2, the partial pressure exerted by oxygen dissolved in the plasma of arterial blood; an indirect measure of blood oxygen content. This measure, representing one of the two forms in which oxygen is transported in the blood, accounts for only about 3% of oxygen content in the blood.
3. $PaCO_2$, the partial pressure of carbon dioxide in arterial plasma; the respiratory component of acid-base determination. Carbon dioxide is regulated by the lungs, and the $PaCO_2$ is used to determine whether an acid-base imbalance is respiratory in origin.
4. Bicarbonate (HCO_3^-) is a measure of the metabolic component of acid-base balance.
5. Base excess (BE), a calculated value of bicarbonate levels, also reflective of the metabolic component of acid-base balance. If the number is preceded by a plus sign, it is a base excess and indicates alkalosis; if preceded by a minus sign, it is a base deficit and indicates acidosis.
6. Oxygen saturation (SaO_2), the percentage of hemoglobin saturated (combined) with oxygen. This represents the other form in which oxygen is transported in the blood and accounts for about 97% of the oxygen in the blood. Pulse oximetry can also be used to measure oxygen saturation. This noninvasive procedure measures SpO_2. Measuring oxygen saturation by using pulse oximetry is detailed in Skill 28.7 (page 697).

Normal ABG values are listed in Box 43.6. Changes seen in common acid-base imbalances are summarized in Table 43.10. Note that although the PaO_2 and SaO_2 are important for assessing respiratory status, they generally do not provide useful information for assessing acid-base balance and so are not included in this table.

TABLE 43.10 Arterial Blood Gas Values in Acid-Base Disorders

Disorder		ABG Values
Respiratory acidosis	pH	< 7.35
	$PaCO_2$	> 45 mm Hg (excess CO_2 and carbonic acid)
	HCO_3^-	Normal; or > 26 mmol/L with renal compensation
Respiratory alkalosis	pH	> 7.45
	$PaCO_2$	< 35 mm Hg (inadequate CO_2 and carbonic acid)
	HCO_3^-	Normal; or < 22 mmol/L with renal compensation
Metabolic acidosis	pH	< 7.35
	$PaCO_2$	Normal; or < 35 mm Hg with respiratory compensation
	HCO_3^-	< 22 mmol/L (inadequate bicarbonate)
Metabolic alkalosis	pH	> 7.45
	$PaCO_2$	Normal; or > 45 mm Hg with respiratory compensation
	HCO_3^-	> 26 mmol/L (excess bicarbonate)

BOX 43.6 NORMAL VALUES OF ARTERIAL BLOOD GASES (ABGs)

pH	7.35–7.45
PaO_2	80–100 mm Hg
$PaCO_2$	35–45 mm Hg
HCO_3^-	22–26 mmol/L
Base excess	–2 to +2 mmol/L
O_2 saturation	95%–100%

Note: Normal laboratory values vary from agency to agency.

When evaluating ABG results to determine acid-base balance, it is important to use a systematic approach such as the one outlined in Box 43.7.

Diagnosing

NANDA International (2007) includes the following diagnostic labels that relate to fluid and acid-base imbalances:

- *Deficient Fluid Volume:* Decreased intravascular, interstitial, or intracellular fluid (this refers to dehydration, water loss alone without a change in sodium)
- *Excess Fluid Volume:* Increased isotonic fluid retention
- *Risk for Imbalanced Fluid Volume:* A state in which an individual is at risk of a decrease, increase, or rapid shift from one to the other of intravascular, interstitial, or intracellular fluid (this refers to body fluid loss, gain or both).
- *Risk for Deficient Fluid Volume:* At risk for experiencing vascular, cellular, or intracellular dehydration
- *Impaired Gas Exchange:* Excess or deficit in oxygenation or carbon dioxide elimination at the alveolar-capillary membrane

Fluid, electrolyte, and acid-base imbalances affect many other body areas, and, as a consequence, may be the etiology of many other nursing diagnoses, such as the following:

- *Impaired Oral Mucous Membrane* related to deficient fluid volume
- *Impaired Skin Integrity* related to dehydration or edema
- *Decreased Cardiac Output* related to hypovolemia or cardiac dysrhythmias secondary to electrolyte imbalance (K^+ or Mg^{2+})
- *Ineffective Tissue Perfusion* related to decreased cardiac output secondary to deficient fluid volume or edema
- *Activity Intolerance* related to hypervolemia
- *Risk for Injury* related to calcium shift out of bones into extracellular fluids
- *Acute Confusion* related to electrolyte imbalance

Planning

When planning care, the nurse identifies nursing interventions that will assist the client to achieve these broad goals:

- Maintain or restore normal fluid balance
- Maintain or restore normal balance of electrolytes in the intracellular and extracellular compartments
- Maintain or restore pulmonary ventilation and oxygenation
- Prevent associated risks (tissue breakdown, decreased cardiac output, confusion, other neurological signs)
- Maintain or repair renal function

Examples of NIC interventions related to fluid, electrolyte, and acid-base balance include the following (Bulechek, Butcher, Dochterman, 2008):

- Acid-base management
- Electrolyte management
- Fluid monitoring
- Hypovolemia management
- Intravenous (IV) therapy

Specific nursing activities associated with each of these interventions can be selected to meet the individual needs of the client.

BOX 43.7 INTERPRETING ABGs: A FOUR-STEP GUIDE

Nurses must use a systematic approach when evaluating ABG results:

1. Look at each number separately.
   - Label the pH:
     - If the pH is less than 7.35, the problem is acidosis.
     - If the pH is greater than 7.45, the problem is alkalosis.
   - Label the $PaCO_2$:
     - If the $PaCO_2$ is less than 35 mm Hg, more CO_2 is being exhaled than normal and indicates alkalosis.
     - If the $PaCO_2$ is greater than 45 mm Hg, less CO_2 is being exhaled than normal and indicates acidosis.
   - Label the bicarbonate:
     - If the HCO_3^- is less than 22 mmol/L, HCO_3^- levels are lower than normal, indicating acidosis.
     - If the HCO_3^- is greater than 26 mmol/L, HCO_3^- levels are higher than normal, indicating alkalosis.
2. Determine the cause of the acid-base imbalance.
   - Look at the pH: is it acidosis or alkalosis?
3. Determine whether the origin of the imbalance is respiratory or metabolic.
   - Check the $PaCO_2$ and HCO_3^-: which one *matches* the same acid-base status as the pH?

EXAMPLE

pH = 7.33 (acidosis)
$PaCO_2$ = 55 (acidosis)
HCO_3^- = 29 (alkalosis)
Cause of imbalance
(hint: look at pH) = acidosis
$PaCO_2$ (acidosis) *matches* the pH (acidosis) = respiratory problem
Client has respiratory acidosis.

4. Look for evidence of compensation.
   - Look at the value that does *not* match the pH.
   - If it (e.g., $PaCO_2$ or HCO_3^-) is within normal range, there is no compensation.
   - If it (e.g., $PaCO_2$ or HCO_3^-) is above or below normal range, the body is compensating.

EXAMPLES

a. In respiratory acidosis (pH < 7.35, $PaCO_2$ > 45 mm Hg), if the HCO_3^- is greater than 26 mmol/L, the kidneys are retaining HCO_3^- to minimize the acidosis: renal compensation.

b. In respiratory alkalosis (pH > 7.45, $PaCO_2$ < 35 mm Hg), if the HCO_3^- is less than 22 mmol/L, the kidneys are excreting HCO_3^- to minimize the alkalosis: again, renal compensation.

c. In metabolic acidosis (pH < 7.35, HCO_3^- < 22 mmol/L), if the $PaCO_2$ is less than 35 mm Hg, CO_2 is being blown off to minimize the acidosis: respiratory compensation.

d. In metabolic alkalosis (pH > 7.45, HCO_3^- > 26 mmol/L), if the $PaCO_2$ is greater than 45 mm Hg, CO_2 is being retained to compensate for excess base: again, respiratory compensation.

Note: If the value that doesn't match (e.g., $PaCO_2$ or HCO_3^-) is above or below normal and the pH is within normal range, the body has completely compensated. Complete compensation takes time to develop and is the result of a chronic condition (e.g., chronic respiratory acidosis with COPD).

Nursing activities to meet goals and outcomes related to fluid, electrolyte, and acid-base imbalances are discussed in the next section. These include (1) monitoring fluid intake and output, cardiovascular and respiratory status, and results of laboratory tests; (2) assessing the client's weight; the location and extent of edema, if present; skin turgor and skin status; specific gravity of urine; and level of consciousness and mental status; (3) fluid intake modifications; (4) dietary changes; (5) parenteral fluid, electrolyte, and blood replacement; and (6) other appropriate measures, such as administering prescribed medications and oxygen, providing skin care and oral hygiene, positioning the client appropriately, and scheduling rest periods.

PLANNING FOR HOME CARE To provide for continuity of care, the client's needs for assistance with care in the home need to be considered. Home care planning includes assessment of the client's and family's resources and abilities for care, and the need for referrals and home health services. The Assessment: Home Care box describes the specific assessment data required to establish a home care plan. On the basis of the data gathered in assessment of the home situation, the nurse individualizes the teaching plan for the client and family (see the Teaching: Home Care box on page 1398).

Implementing

PROMOTING WELLNESS Most people rarely think about their fluid, electrolyte, or acid-base balance. They know it is important to drink adequate fluids and consume a balanced diet, but they may not understand the potential effects when this is not done. Nurses can promote clients' health by providing wellness teaching that will help them maintain fluid and electrolyte balance. See the Teaching: Wellness box related to fluid and electrolyte balance on page 1399.

ENTERAL FLUID AND ELECTROLYTE REPLACEMENT Fluids and electrolytes can be provided orally in the home and hospital if the client's health permits, that is, if the client is not vomiting, has not experienced an excessive fluid loss, and has an intact gastrointestinal tract and gag and swallow reflexes. Clients who are unable to ingest solid foods may be able to ingest fluids.

FLUID INTAKE MODIFICATIONS *Increased* fluids (ordered as "push fluids") are often prescribed for clients with actual or potential fluid volume deficits arising, for example, from mild diarrhea or mild to moderate fevers. *Restricted* fluids may be necessary for clients who have fluid retention (fluid volume excess) as a result of renal failure, heart failure, syndrome of inappropriate antidiuretic hormone (SIADH), or other disease processes.

ASSESSMENT: HOME CARE

Fluid, Electrolyte, and Acid-Base Balance

Assess for the following:

CLIENT

- *Risk factors for imbalances:* The client's age, medications required, such as diuretic therapy or corticosteroids, and presence of chronic diseases, such as diabetes mellitus, heart disease, lung disease, or dementia (see Box 43.3)
- *Self-care abilities for maintaining food and fluid intake:* Mobility; ability to chew and swallow, to access fluids and respond to thirst, to purchase food and prepare a balanced diet
- *Current level of knowledge (as appropriate):* Prescribed diet, any fluid restrictions, activity restrictions, actions and side effects of prescribed medications, regular weight monitoring, gastric tube care and enteral feedings, central line or peripherally inserted central venous catheter care, and parenteral fluids and nutrition

FAMILY

- *Caregiver availability, skills, and responses:* Availability and willingness to assume responsibility for care, knowledge and ability to provide assistance with preparing food and maintaining adequate intake of food and fluids, knowledge of risk factors and early warning signs of problems
- *Family role changes and coping:* Effect on financial status, parenting and spousal roles, social roles
- *Alternative potential primary or respite caregivers:* For example, other family members, volunteers, church members, paid caregivers or housekeeping services; available community care (e.g., adult daycare), senior centres

COMMUNITY

- *Current knowledge of and experience with community resources:* Home care agencies, organizations that offer financial assistance or assistance with food preparation, Meals on Wheels or meal services (e.g., at senior centres, homeless shelters), pharmacies, home intravenous services, respiratory care services

Fluid restrictions vary from "nothing by mouth" to a precise amount ordered by a physician. The restriction of fluids can be difficult for some clients, particularly if they are experiencing thirst. Guidelines for helping clients to increase fluid intake are shown in Practice Guidelines 43.1 and to restrict fluid intake are shown in Practice Guidelines 43.2.

DIETARY CHANGES Specific fluid and electrolyte imbalances may require simple dietary changes. For example, clients receiving potassium-depleting diuretics need to be informed about foods with high potassium content (e.g., bananas, oranges, and leafy greens). Some clients with fluid retention need to avoid foods high in sodium. Most healthy clients can benefit from foods rich in calcium.

ORAL ELECTROLYTE SUPPLEMENTS Clients can benefit from oral supplements of electrolytes, particularly when a medication that affects electrolyte balance is prescribed. Supplements may also be used when dietary intake is inadequate for a specific electrolyte or when fluid and electrolyte losses are extreme as a result of excessive perspiration.

Corticosteroids and many diuretics can cause too much potassium to be eliminated through the kidneys. For clients taking these medications, potassium supplements may be prescribed. Instruct clients taking oral potassium supplements to take the medication with juice to mask the unpleasant taste and reduce the possibility of gastric distress. Emphasize the importance of taking the medication as prescribed and seeing their health-care provider on a regular basis. Because hyperkalemia can have serious cardiac effects, clients should never increase the amount of potassium being taken without a physician's order to do so. In addition, inform clients that most salt substitutes contain a salt of potassium, so it is important to consult with the health-care provider before using salt substitutes.

People who ingest insufficient milk and milk products benefit from calcium supplements. The recommended daily allowance for calcium is 1000 mg to 1500 mg. It is generally recommended that postmenopausal women take 1500 mg of calcium per day to reduce the risk of osteoporosis. Long-term use of corticosteroid drugs can also cause calcium loss from the bones, and calcium supplements may help reduce this loss. Clients who are predisposed to developing renal calculi and who take supplemental calcium need to maintain a fluid intake of at least 2500 mL per day (unless contraindicated) to reduce the risk of kidney stones, which are commonly composed of calcium salts.

Although routine supplements for other electrolytes generally are not recommended, clients who have poor dietary habits, who are malnourished, or who have difficulty accessing or eating fresh fruits and vegetables may benefit from electrolyte supplements. A daily multiple vitamin with minerals may achieve the desired goal. People who engage in strenuous activities in a warm environment need to be encouraged to replace the water and electrolytes that are lost through excessive perspiration by consuming a commercial sports drink, such as Gatorade, or another commercial fluid and electrolyte solution.

Liquid nutritional supplements are often given to clients who are malnourished or have poor eating habits. They are used with frequency in older adults to bolster nutritional status and caloric intake. It is very important to read the label on the product and to be aware of the contents of the supplement. Some of them are very high in protein and high in potassium, which may be contraindicated in an individual with impaired renal function.

TEACHING: HOME CARE

Fluid, Electrolyte, and Acid-Base Balance

After the assessment of the home situation, the nurse individualizes the teaching plan:

MONITORING FLUID INTAKE AND OUTPUT

- Teach and provide the rationale for monitoring fluid intake and output to the client and family, as appropriate, and how to monitor fluid intake and output. Include instructions for using a commode or collection device (*urine hat*) in the toilet, emptying and measuring urinary catheter drainage, or counting or weighing diapers.
- Instruct and provide rationale for regular weight monitoring to the client and family. Weigh at the same time of day, after voiding, using the same scale, and with the client wearing the same amount of clothing.
- Educate and provide rationale to the client and family regarding when to contact a health-care professional, such as in the cases of a significant change in urine output; any change of 2.5 kg or more in a 1- to 2-week period; prolonged episodes of vomiting, diarrhea, or inability to eat or drink; dry, sticky mucous membranes; extreme thirst; swollen fingers, feet, ankles, or legs; difficulty breathing, shortness of breath, rapid heartbeat; and changes in behaviour or mental status.

MAINTAINING FOOD AND FLUID INTAKE

- Instruct the client and family about any diet or fluid restrictions, such as a low-sodium diet. Contact a dietitian to provide appropriate teaching.
- Teach family members the rationale for offering fluids regularly to clients who are unable to meet their own needs because of age, impaired mobility or cognition, or other conditions, such as impaired swallowing because of a cerebrovascular accident.
- If the client is receiving enteral fluids or intravenous (parenteral) fluids at home, teach and provide the underlying rationale to caregivers about proper administration and care. Contact a home health or home intravenous service to provide services and teaching.

SAFETY

- Instruct and provide the rationale to the client regarding the need to change positions slowly, if appropriate, especially when moving from a supine to a sitting or standing position.
- Inform (with rationale) the client and family about the importance of good mouth and skin care.
- Teach the client to change positions frequently and to elevate the feet on a stool when sitting for a long period.
- Teach the client and family how to care for intravenous access sites or gastric tubes. Include instructions about what to do if tubes become dislodged.

MEDICATIONS

- Emphasize the importance of taking medications as prescribed.
- Instruct clients taking diuretics to take the medication in the morning. If a second daily dose is prescribed, they should take it in the late afternoon to avoid disrupting sleep in order to urinate.
- Inform clients about any expected side effects of prescribed medications and how to handle them (e.g., if a potassium-depleting diuretic is prescribed, increase intake of potassium-rich foods; if taking a potassium-sparing diuretic, avoid excess potassium intake, such as by using salt substitute).
- Teach clients when to contact their health-care provider, for example, if they are unable to take a prescribed medication or have signs of an allergic or a toxic reaction to a medication.

MEASURES SPECIFIC TO CLIENT'S PROBLEM

- Provide instructions and rationale specific to the client's fluid, electrolyte, or acid-base imbalance, such as the following:

  a. Deficient fluid volume

  b. Risk for deficient fluid volume

  c. Fluid volume excess

REFERRALS

- Make appropriate referrals to home care or community social services for assistance with resources, such as meal preparation and food, intravenous infusions and access, enteral feedings, and homemaker or home health aide services to help with the activities of daily living.

COMMUNITY AGENCIES AND OTHER SOURCES OF HELP

- Provide information about companies or agencies that can provide durable medical equipment, such as commodes, lift chairs, or hospital beds, for purchase, for rental, or free.
- Provide a list of sources for supplies, such as catheters and drainage bags, measuring devices, tube feeding formulas, and electrolyte replacement drinks.
- Suggest additional sources of information and help, such as the local hospital dietitian, wellness centre, or public health office.

PARENTERAL FLUID AND ELECTROLYTE REPLACEMENT Intravenous (IV) fluid therapy is essential when clients are unable to take food and fluids orally. It is an efficient and effective method of supplying fluids directly into the intravascular fluid compartment and replacing electrolyte losses. Intravenous fluid therapy is usually ordered by the physician or nurse practitioner. The nurse is responsible for administering and maintaining the therapy and for teaching the client and significant others how to continue the therapy at home if necessary.

INTRAVENOUS SOLUTIONS Intravenous solutions can be classified as isotonic, hypotonic, or hypertonic. As described earlier, most IV solutions are isotonic, having

TEACHING: WELLNESS

Promoting Healthy Fluid and Electrolyte Balance

Nurses should teach clients how to maintain homeostasis:

- Consume 2000 mL to 2500 mL water daily, unless contraindicated.
- Avoid excess amounts of foods or fluids high in salt, sugar, and caffeine.
- Eat a well-balanced diet. Include adequate amounts of milk or milk products to maintain bone calcium levels.
- Limit alcohol intake because it has a diuretic effect.
- Increase fluid intake before, during, and after strenuous exercise, particularly when the environmental temperature is high, and replace lost electrolytes from excessive perspiration as needed with commercial electrolyte solutions.
- Maintain a healthy body weight.
- Learn about and monitor side effects of medications that affect fluid and electrolyte balance (e.g., diuretics) and ways to handle side effects.
- Recognize possible risk factors for fluid and electrolyte imbalance, such as prolonged or repeated vomiting, frequent watery stools, or inability to consume fluids because of illness.
- Seek prompt professional health care for notable signs of fluid imbalance, such as sudden weight gain or loss, decreased urine volume, swollen ankles, shortness of breath, dizziness, or confusion.

the same concentration of solutes as blood plasma. Isotonic solutions are often used to restore vascular volume. Hypertonic solutions have a greater concentration of solutes than plasma; hypotonic solutions have a lesser concentration of solutes. Table 43.11 provides examples of IV solutions and nursing implications.

IV solutions can also be categorized according to their purpose. *Nutrient solutions* contain some form of carbohydrate, such as dextrose or glucose, and water. Water is supplied for fluid requirements and carbohydrate for calories and energy. For example, 1 L of 5% dextrose provides 170 calories. Nutrient solutions are

PRACTICE GUIDELINES 43.1

Facilitating Fluid Intake

Guidelines	Rationales
Explain to the client the reason for the required intake and the specific amount needed.	This explanation promotes understanding and may enhance compliance.
Establish a 24-hour plan for the client for ingesting the fluids. For the hospitalized or long-term-care client, half the total volume is given during the day shift, and the other half is divided between the evening and night shifts, with most of that ingested during the evening shift. For example, If 2500 mL is to be ingested in 24 hours, the plan may specify 7–3 (1500 mL); 3–11 (700 mL); and 11–7 (300 mL).	Distributing fluid intake throughout waking hours and in conjunction with usual meal times helps to ensure the required fluids are ingested.
Set short-term outcomes that the client can realistically meet. Examples include ingesting a glass of fluid every hour while awake or a pitcher of water by 12 noon.	The client can be positively reinforced for achieving the desired outcome; if the outcome is not achieved, then alternative strategies can be tested to ensure the 24-hour fluid intake goal is achieved.
Identify fluids the client likes, and make available a variety of those items, including fruit juices and milk (if allowed). Coffee and tea consumption should be limited.	Fluids that are palatable to the client will enhance motivation; caffeinated beverages can have a diuretic effect.
Help clients to select foods that tend to become liquid at room temperature (e.g., gelatin, ice cream, sherbet), if these are allowed.	These foods contribute significantly to daily fluid intake.
For clients who are confined to bed, supply appropriate cups, glasses, and straws.	Fluid intake for these clients requires additional functional and safety requirements.
Make sure fluids are served at the appropriate temperature: hot fluids hot and cold fluids cold.	This ensures the palatability of the fluids.
Encourage clients, when possible, to participate in maintaining the fluid intake record.	Maintaining the intake record assists the client in evaluating the achievement of desired health outcomes.
Be alert to any cultural implications of food and fluids.	Some cultures restrict certain foods and fluids and view others as having healing properties.

PRACTICE GUIDELINES 43.2

Restricting Fluid Intake

Guidelines	Rationales
Explain the reason for the restricted intake and how much and what types of fluids are permitted orally. Many clients need to be informed that ice chips, gelatin, and ice cream, for example, are considered fluid.	This explanation promotes understanding and may enhance compliance.
Help the client decide the amount of fluid to be taken with each meal, between meals, before bedtime, and with medications. For the hospitalized or long-term-care client, half the total volume is scheduled during the day shift when the client is most active, receives two meals, and takes most oral medications. A large part of the remainder is scheduled for the evening shift.	Dividing the intake throughout the day will permit fluids with meals and evening visitors and avoid periods of thirst.
Identify fluids or fluid-like substances the client likes, and make sure that these are provided, unless contraindicated. A client who is allowed only 200 mL of fluid for breakfast, for example, should receive the type of fluid the client favours.	Having something the client likes will help ensure quality of life despite fluid restrictions.
Set short-term goals, that is, schedule a specified amount of fluid at 1- or 2-hour intervals between meals. Some clients may prefer fluids between meals only if the food provided at mealtime helps relieve thirst.	Scheduling may help make the fluid restriction more tolerable.
Place allowed fluids in small containers, such as a 120 mL juice glass to allow the perception of a full container; offer the client ice chips as an alternative.	Doing so can help make the fluid restriction seem less restrictive (e.g., half a glass of ice chips, when melted, is approximately one-quarter of a glass).
Provide frequent mouth care and rinses.	These reduce the thirst sensation.
Instruct the client to avoid ingesting or chewing salty or sweet foods (e.g., hard candy or gum).	These foods tend to produce thirst. Sugarless gum may be an alternative for some clients.
Encourage the client, when possible, to participate in maintaining the fluid intake record.	Maintaining the record assists the client in evaluating the achievement of desired health outcomes.

TABLE 43.11 Selected Intravenous Solutions

Type/Examples	Comments/Nursing Implications
Isotonic Solutions	
0.9% NaCl (normal saline) Lactated Ringer's or Ringer's Solution (balanced electrolyte solutions)	Isotonic solutions, such as NS and lactated Ringer's, initially remain in the vascular compartment, expanding vascular volume. Assess clients carefully for signs of hypervolemia, such as bounding pulse and shortness of breath.
5% dextrose in water (D5W)	D5W is isotonic on initial administration but provides free water when dextrose is metabolized, expanding intracellular and extracellular fluid volumes. D5W is avoided in clients at risk for increased intracranial pressure (IICP) because it can increase cerebral edema.
Hypotonic Solutions	
0.45% NaCl (half normal saline) 0.33% NaCl (one-third normal saline)	Hypotonic solutions are used to provide free water and treat cellular dehydration. These solutions promote waste elimination by the kidneys. Do not administer to clients at risk for increased intracranial pressure or third-space fluid shift.
Hypertonic Solutions	
5% dextrose in normal saline (D5NS) 5% dextrose in 0.45% NaCl (D5 1/2NS) 5% dextrose in lactated Ringer's (D5LR)	Hypertonic solutions draw fluid out of the intracellular and interstitial compartments into the vascular compartment, expanding vascular volume. Do not administer to clients with kidney or heart disease or clients who are dehydrated. Watch for signs of hypervolemia.

useful in preventing dehydration and ketosis but do not provide sufficient calories to promote wound healing, weight gain, or normal growth in children. Common nutrient solutions are 5% dextrose in water (D5W) and 5% dextrose in 0.45% sodium chloride ($D_5$1/2NS).

Electrolyte solutions contain varying amounts of cations and anions. Commonly used solutions are normal saline (0.9% sodium chloride), Ringer's solution (contains sodium, chloride, potassium, and calcium), and lactated Ringer's (contains sodium, chloride, potassium, calcium, and lactate). Lactate is metabolized in the liver to form bicarbonate (HCO_3^-). Saline and balanced electrolyte solutions are used to restore vascular volume, particularly after trauma or surgery. They also may be used to replace fluid and electrolytes for clients with continuing losses, for example, because of gastric suction or wound drainage.

Lactated Ringer's solution is an *alkalinizing solution* that may be given to treat metabolic acidosis. *Acidifying solutions,* in contrast, are administered to counteract metabolic alkalosis. Examples of acidifying solutions are 5% dextrose in 0.45% sodium chloride and 0.9% sodium chloride solution.

Volume expanders are solutions used to increase the blood volume following severe loss of blood (e.g., from hemorrhage) or loss of plasma (e.g., from severe burns, which draw large amounts of plasma from the bloodstream to the burn site). Examples of volume expanders are dextran, plasma, and human serum albumin.

VENIPUNCTURE SITES The site chosen for venipuncture varies with the client's age, the length of time the infusion is to run, the type of solution used (e.g., vesicant or irritant), condition of veins, physical and functional assessment, and patient preference (Registered Nurses' Association of Ontario [RNAO], 2004). For adults, veins in the hand and arm are commonly used; for infants, veins in the scalp and dorsal foot are often used. Larger veins are preferred for infusions that need to be given rapidly and for solutions that could be irritating (e.g., certain medications).

The metacarpal, basilic, and cephalic veins are commonly used for intermittent or continuous infusions (Figure 43.15B). The ulna and radius act as natural splints at these sites, and the client has greater freedom of arm movements for activities, such as eating. Although the basilic and median cubital veins in the antecubital space are convenient sites for venipuncture, they are usually used for obtaining blood samples, giving bolus injections of medication, and inserting a peripherally inserted central catheter (PICC) line (see Figure 43.15A). See Practice Guidelines 43.3 for vein selection and general tips for easier IV starts.

When long-term IV therapy or parenteral nutrition is anticipated, or the client is receiving IV medications that are damaging to vessels (e.g., chemotherapy, fluids with an osmolarity greater than 500 mOsm/L, such as parenteral nutrition), a **central venous catheter** may be inserted. Central venous catheters usually are inserted into the subclavian or jugular vein, with the distal tip of the catheter resting in the superior vena cava just above the right atrium (Figure 43.16). They may be inserted at the client's bedside, or for longer-term access, surgically inserted. Subclavian central venous catheters permit freedom of movement for ambulation; however, there is greater risk of complications, including hemothorax or pneumothorax, cardiac perforation, thrombosis, and infection. Assess the client closely for manifestations, such as shortness of breath, chest pain, cough, hypotension, tachycardia, and anxiety, after the insertion procedure.

With a **peripherally inserted central catheter (PICC)**, the catheter is inserted in the basilic or cephalic vein just above or below the antecubital space of the right arm. The tip of the catheter rests in the lower portion of the superior vena cava. The risk of pneumothorax is eliminated with PICC. These catheters frequently are used for

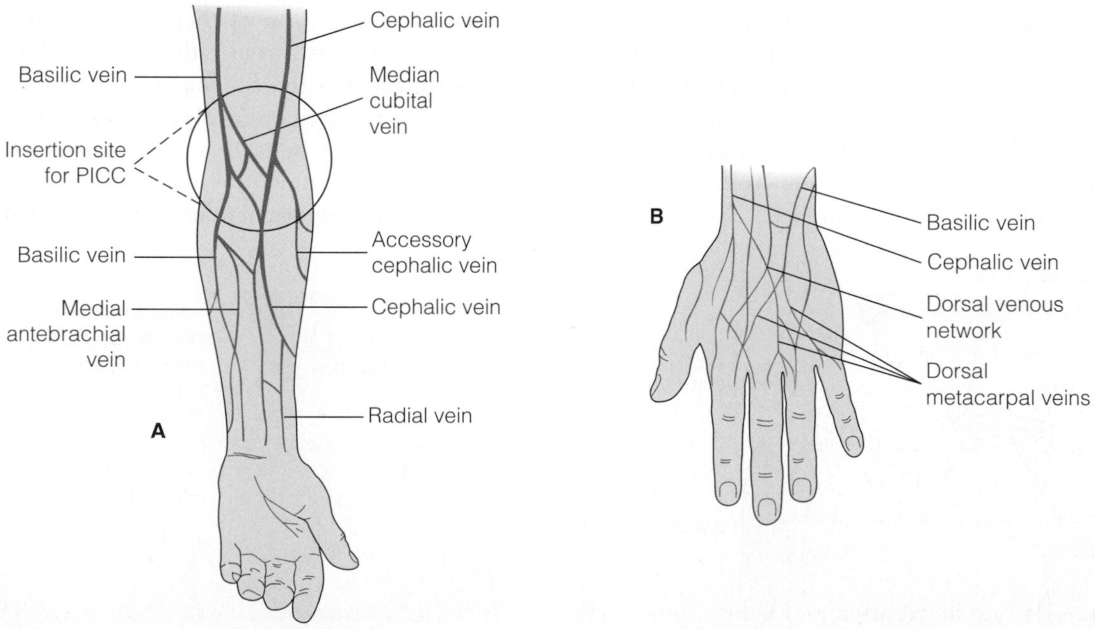

FIGURE 43.15 Commonly used venipuncture sites: **A:** arm; **B:** hand; **A** also shows the site used for a peripherally inserted central catheter (PICC)

PRACTICE GUIDELINES 43.3

Vein Selection

Guidelines	Rationales
Use distal veins of the arm first.	Distal vein selection provides for more proximal alternatives if subsequent venipuncture is required; if proximal veins are used first and they become sclerosed, all access to distal veins will be blocked.
Use the client's nondominant arm, whenever possible.	This helps to ensure that the client can continue to perform the activities of daily living.
Select a vein that is (1) easily palpated and feels soft and full; (2) naturally splinted by bone; and (3) large enough to allow adequate circulation around the catheter.	These factors ensure ease of insertion and patency once the catheter is in the vein.
Avoid using veins that are in areas of flexion (e.g., the antecubital fossa); are highly visible; are damaged by previous use, phlebitis, infiltration, or sclerosis; are continually distended with blood, knotted, or tortuous; or are in a surgically compromised or injured extremity (e.g., following a mastectomy).	These situations can involve impaired circulation and cause discomfort for the patient.
Consider client preference.	Having a choice helps to ensure client self-efficacy and nurse–patient partnership; the client can provide helpful input to ensure quality of life and care issues are addressed.

long-term intravenous access when the client will be managing IV therapy at home.

Implantable venous access devices or *ports* (Figures 43.17 and 43.18) are used for clients with chronic illness who require long-term IV therapy (e.g., intermittent medications, vesicants such as certain cancer chemotherapy, total parenteral nutrition, and frequent blood samples). The device is designed to provide repeated access to the central venous system, avoiding the trauma and complications of multiple venipunctures. Using local anaesthesia, implantable ports are surgically placed into a small subcutaneous pocket under the skin, usually on the upper anterior chest near the clavicle, and no part of the port is exposed. The distal end of the catheter is placed in the subclavian or jugular vein. Different kinds of implantable venous access devices are available and they may be tunnelled or nontunnelled.

Physical assessments that reveal lymphedema, tissue damage, or deformity can help determine site selection with efforts made to avoid any area that is already compromised. A client who requires crutches to function must, if at all possible, have a venipuncture site chosen that does not further impede mobility. Collaborating with the client and family in site selection not only enhances the client's self-efficacy but also ensures that any additional and relevant information is factored into the venipuncture site decision-making process (RNAO, 2004).

An alternative form of therapy, hypodermoclysis is sometimes used to treat adults with dehydration. **Hypodermoclysis** is the subcutaneous infusion of fluid, usually a solution containing electrolytes. This procedure does not require venous access and has been shown to be effective for the treatment of mild to moderate dehydration in adults, in particular those receiving home

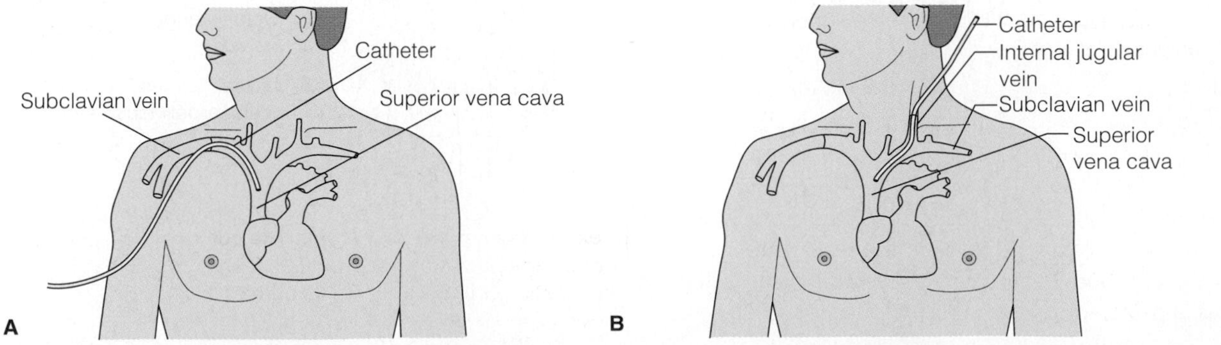

FIGURE 43.16 Central venous lines: **A:** subclavian vein insertion; **B:** left jugular insertion

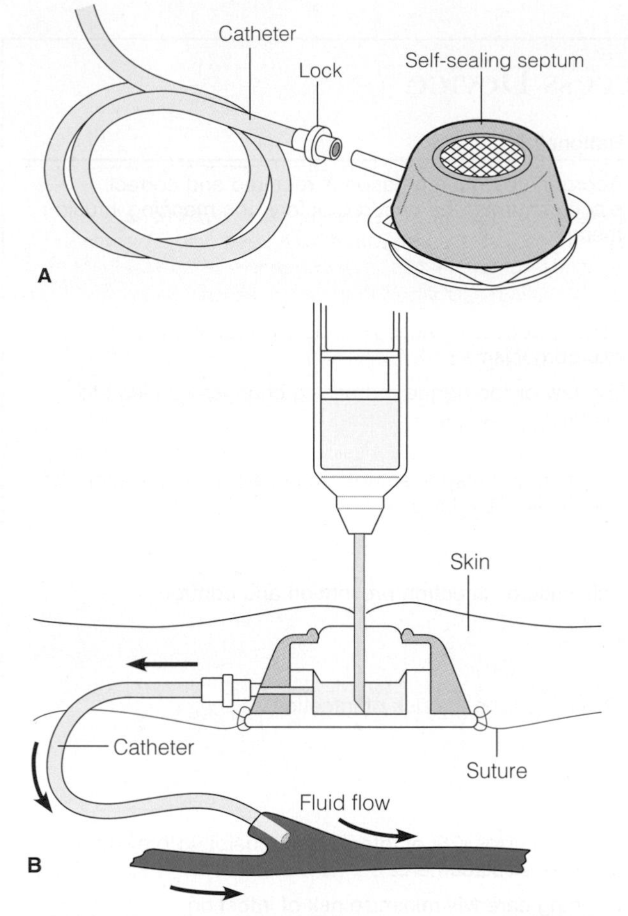

FIGURE 43.17 An implantable venous access device: A: components; B: the device in place

palliative care, and it can be performed at home by family members or a nurse. The fine-gauge device is inserted under the skin in such locations as the upper arm, chest wall, abdomen, or thigh. Site rotation is recommended every 3 to 7 days (Infusion Nurses Society, 2000).

Special precautions need to be taken with all central lines and venous access ports to ensure asepsis and catheter patency. Nursing care of clients with these devices is outlined in the Practice Guidelines 43.4.

INTRAVENOUS EQUIPMENT Because equipment varies according to the manufacturer, the nurse must become familiar with the equipment used in each particular agency.

Solution containers are available in various sizes (50 mL, 100 mL, 250 mL, 500 mL, or 1000 mL); the smaller containers are often used to administer medications. Most solutions are currently dispensed in plastic bags (Figure 43.19). However, glass bottles may need to be used if the medications to be administered are incompatible with plastic. Glass bottles require an air vent so that air can enter the bottle and replace the fluid that enters the client's vein. Some have a tube inside the bottle that serves as a vent; other containers without air vents require a vent on the administration set. Air vents usually have filters to prevent contamination from the air that

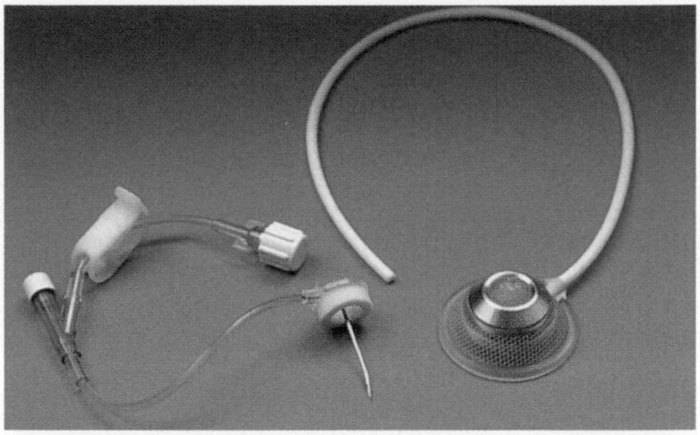

FIGURE 43.18 An implantable venous access device (right) and a Huber needle with extension tubing

enters the container. Air vents are not required for plastic solution bags because the bags collapse under atmospheric pressure when the solution enters the vein.

It is essential that the solution be sterile and clear. Cloudiness, evidence that the container has been opened previously, or leaks indicate possible contamination. Always check the expiration date on the label. Return any questionable or contaminated solutions to the pharmacy.

Infusion sets usually include an insertion spike, a drip chamber, a roller valve or screw clamp, tubing with secondary ports, and a protective cap over the needle adapter (Figure 43.20). The insertion spike is kept sterile and inserted into the solution container when the equipment is set up and ready to start. The drip chamber permits a predictable amount of fluid to be delivered. A commonly used drip chamber is the macrodrip, which delivers 10 to 20 drops per millilitre of solution. This information is found on the package. There are also

Evidence-Informed Practice

What Are Best Practice Guidelines for Maintaining Vascular Access Devices?

The Registered Nurses' Association of Ontario (2005) produced a document that outlines the best practices in caring for and maintaining vascular access devices. The guidelines are the result of a significant review of literature, critique of studies, and synthesis of a range of material on the topic. The final document gives detailed and concise recommendations for a range of venous access device issues, from cleaning solutions through taping procedures to frequency of tubing change.

NURSING IMPLICATIONS: This document provides an excellent resource for nurses. The concise and specific recommendations will ensure that knowledge transfer of research findings occurs in the clinical world.

Source: Based on *Care and Maintenance to Reduce Vascular Access Complications*, by the Registered Nurses' Association of Ontario, 2005, Toronto: Author.

PRACTICE GUIDELINES 43.4

Caring for Clients with a Venous Access Device

Guidelines	Rationales
On insertion, document the date; the site; the brand, gauge, and catheter length; the location of the catheter tip (verified by X-ray); the length of the external segment; and client teaching.	Appropriate documentation is required and correct placement must be ensured before commencing infusion therapy.
Site Care	
Use strict aseptic technique when caring for central lines and long-term venous access devices.	Venous access devices provide a portal of entry for microorganisms.
The frequency of dressing changes may vary from every 3 to 7 days, depending on the site. Dressings also should be changed when loose or soiled.	Too few or too frequent dressing changes can lead to infection.
Assess the site for any redness, swelling, tenderness, or drainage. Compare the length of the external portion of the catheter with its documented length. Obtain a chest X-ray to determine the catheter tip's position if in doubt.	Infection and displacement are possible complications of venous access devices.
Follow agency protocol for cleaning solutions and types of dressings; 2% chlorhexidine gluconate, 70% isopropyl alcohol or a combination of alcohol and acetone followed by povidone-iodine are commonly used to clean the port site.	This ensures infection prevention and control.
Before accessing the port, clean an area 5 cm in diameter around the site with an alcohol-acetone solution on a sterile cotton swab. Start at the centre of the port site, moving outward with a firm, circular motion. Follow with povidone-iodine solution. Allow the site to air dry.	This minimizes the risk of infection.
Secure the catheter, and cover the entry site and external portion of the catheter with an occlusive dressing.	This minimizes risk of infection and helps to prevent catheter displacement.
Provide routine care of the incision site for the implant device until it is healed. Once it heals, no care is necessary when the port is idle.	Ongoing care will minimize risk of infection.
Catheter Care and Flushing	
Change the catheter cap as indicated by protocol, usually every 3 to 7 days.	This minimizes risk of infection.
Flush the port with normal saline, a heparin flush solution (generally 10 units/mL), or as agency protocol recommends for the specific type of port being used. After infusing medications or solutions, flush the port with saline.	Flushing ensures patency and prevents contact between incompatible medications or fluids.
Using a 10 mL syringe, flush the catheter with a solution of 10 units of heparin after each use. The frequency of flushes between uses may vary from every 12 hours to once a week or less, depending on the type of catheter.	The syringe size ensures adequate pressure to deliver the flush without damaging the catheter. Note that the smaller the syringe, the greater the amount of pressure (Hadaway, 2006). The frequency of flushing varies with the size of the catheter gauge, the concentration of the flush fluid, and the nature of the catheter product.
Remember to flush all lumens for multiple-lumen catheters.	This helps maintain patency.
A needle with a 90-degree angle is generally used to access an implanted port for infusions. Stabilizing the port between the thumb and index finger of the nondominant hand, insert the needle through the centre of the port until the resistance of the platform is felt.	Specially designed needles are easier to stabilize and are more comfortable for the client.
To remove the needle after a treatment, again stabilize the port and use even pressure to withdraw the needle. Maintain positive pressure by withdrawing the needle as the last millilitre of flush solution is being instilled.	Stabilizing the port to promote client comfort. Positive pressure ensures catheter patency.
Flush idle implanted ports with heparinized saline in accordance with agency protocol or at least every 8 weeks.	Flushing ensures patency.

(continued)

PRACTICE GUIDELINES 43.4

Caring for Clients with a Venous Access Device *(continued)*

Guidelines	Rationales
Teaching Provide clients with the following instructions:	
• Do not allow anyone to take a blood pressure on the arm in which a PICC line is inserted. • Wear a MedicAlert tag or bracelet if the device is to be in place for a long period. • For a PICC, you do not need to restrict activities, except do not immerse the arm in water. Showering is allowed if the site and catheter are covered by an occlusive dressing. • For an implanted venous port, there are no activity restrictions, but remember that the port or catheter tip can become dislodged. Signs of a dislodged catheter tip include pain in the neck or ear on the affected side, swishing or gurgling sounds, or palpitations. Free movement of the port, swelling, or difficulty accessing the port may indicate port dislodgment. Notify the physician should any of these occur or if symptoms of infection develop.	Clients must learn many details related to the care of their catheter to ensure patency and minimize risk of displacement and infection.

Source: From "Getting a Line on Central Vascular Access Devices," by S. Masoorli & T. Angeles, 2002, *Nursing, 32*(4), pp. 36–43. Guidelines adapted with permission.

microdrip sets, which deliver 60 drops per millilitre of solution. The roller valve or screw clamp, which compresses the lumen of the tubing, controls the rate of the flow. The protective cap over the needle adapter maintains the sterility of the end of the tubing so that it can be attached to a sterile needle or catheter inserted in the client's vein.

Most infusion sets include one or more injection ports for administering IV medications or secondary infusions. Needleless systems reduce the risk of needlestick injury and contamination of the intravenous line. With a needleless system, a blunt cannula is inserted into a special injection port or adapter on the IV tubing to administer medications or secondary infusions (Figure 43.21). Many infusion sets include an inline filter to trap air, particulate matter, and microbes. A special infusion set may be required if the IV flow rate will be regulated by an infusion pump.

Catheters and *needles* are used for intravenous infusions. Over-the-needle catheters, also known as angiocaths, are commonly used for adult clients. The short catheter

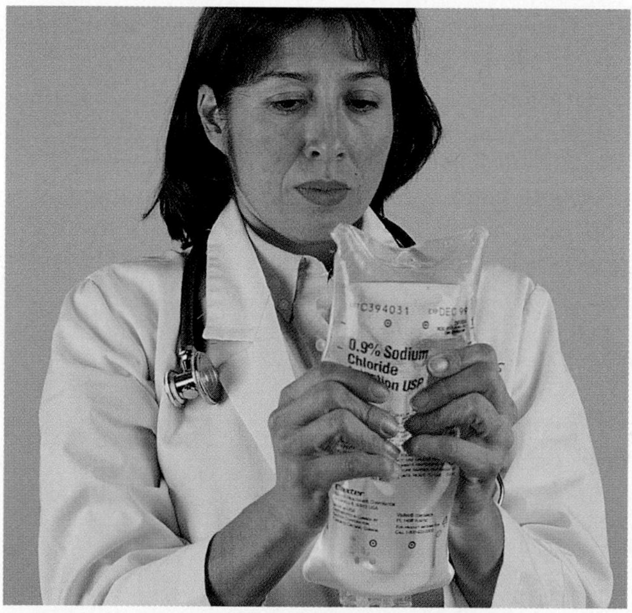

FIGURE 43.19 A plastic intravenous fluid container

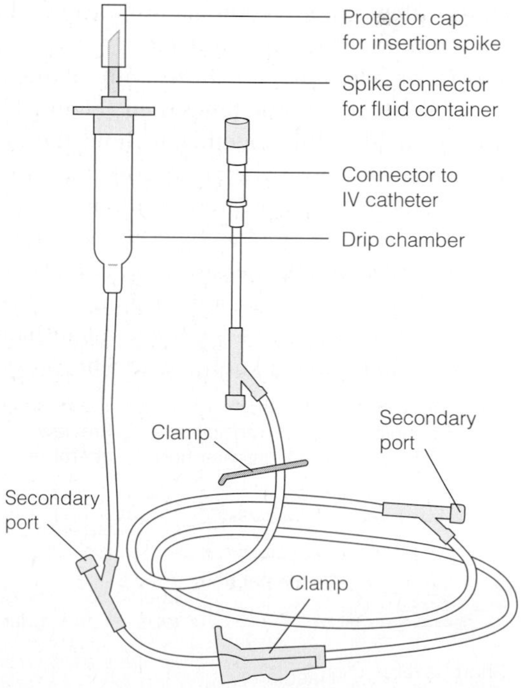

FIGURE 43.20 A standard IV administration set

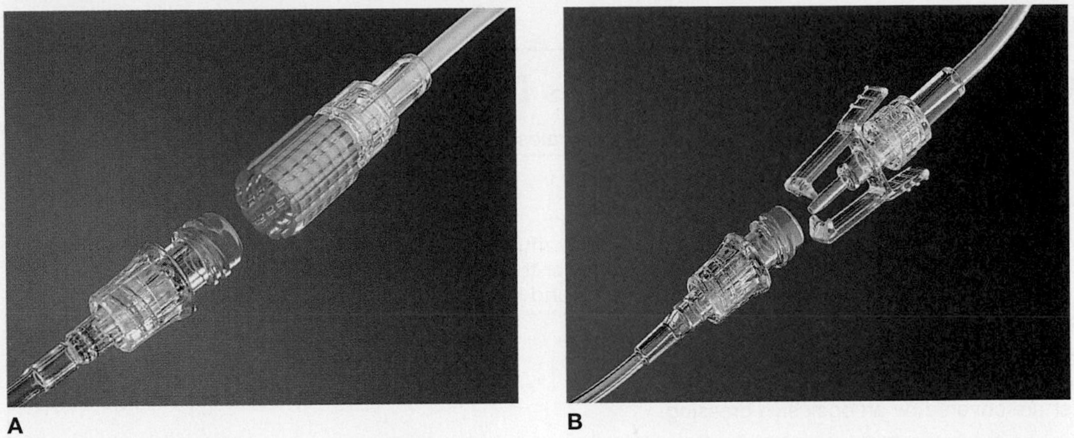

FIGURE 43.21 Cannulae used to connect the tubing of additive sets to primary infusions: **A:** threaded-lock cannula; **B:** lever-lock cannula

length is generally less than 7.5 cm. The plastic catheter fits over a needle used to pierce the skin and vein wall (Figure 43.22). Once inserted into the vein, the needle is withdrawn and discarded, leaving the catheter in place. Intravenous catheters allow the client more mobility and rarely *infiltrate,* that is, become dislodged from the vein and allow fluid to flow into interstitial spaces.

With the original over-the-needle catheters, the sharp stylet remained exposed until placed in a sharps container. This resulted in needle-stick injuries to nurses. A variety of safety devices on IV catheters are now available and their use is becoming a recommended standard of care (Canadian Vascular Access Association, n.d.). The safety devices can be either an active safety device that requires activation by the nurse or a passive safety device in which the safety feature is automatically activated after the stylet is removed from the catheter.

Butterfly, or wing-tipped, *needles* with plastic flaps attached to the shaft are sometimes used (Figure 43.23). The flaps are held tightly together to hold the needle securely during insertion; after insertion, they are flattened against the skin and secured with tape.

Intravenous poles are used to hang the solution container. Some poles are attached to hospital beds; others stand on the floor or hang from the ceiling. The height of most poles is adjustable. In the home, plant hangers, robe hooks, kitchen cabinet knobs, or an S-hook over the top of a door can be used to hang solution containers. The higher the solution container, the greater the force of the solution as it enters the client and the faster the rate of flow.

Starting an Intravenous Infusion Although the physician is generally responsible for prescribing IV therapy for clients, nurses initiate, monitor, and maintain the infusion. This is true not only in hospitals and long-term-care facilities but also increasingly in community-based settings, such as clinics and clients' homes. Nurses may be required to be certified for initiation of intravenous therapy by their employing agencies.

Before starting an infusion, the nurse determines the following:

- The type and amount of solution to be infused
- The exact amount (dose) of any medications to be added to a compatible solution
- The rate of flow or the time over which the infusion is to be completed

If solutions are prepared by the pharmacy or another department, the nurse must verify that the solution supplied exactly matches what the physician prescribed.

Understanding the purpose for the infusion is as important as assessing the client. For example, the nurse may question an order for 5% dextrose in water (D5W)

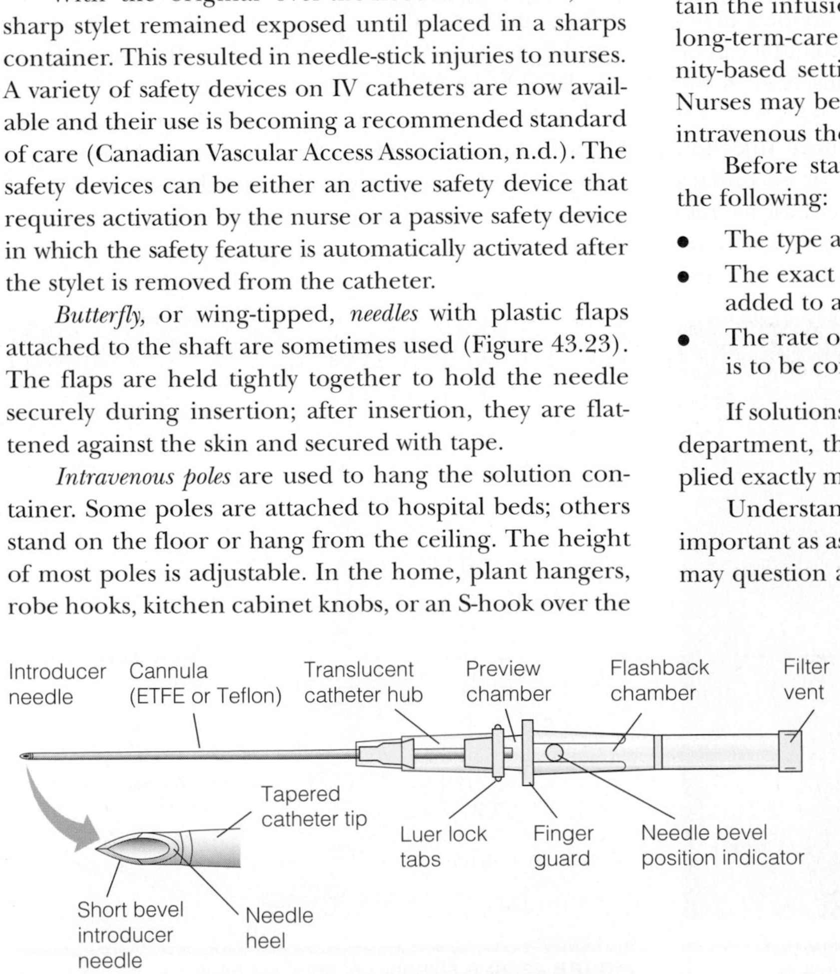

FIGURE 43.22 Schematic of an over-the-needle catheter

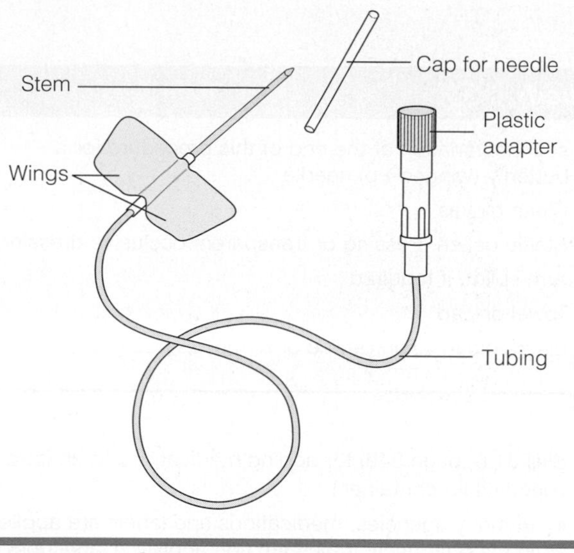

FIGURE 43.23 Schematic of a butterfly needle with adapter

at 150 mL/h if the client has peripheral edema and other signs of fluid overload.

To perform venipuncture and start an intravenous infusion, see Skill 43.1.

REGULATING AND MONITORING INTRAVENOUS INFUSIONS Orders for IV infusions can take several forms, such as "3000 mL over 24 hours"; "1000 mL every 8 hours × 3 bags"; "125 mL/h until oral intake is adequate." The nurse initiating the IV calculates the correct flow rate, regulates the infusion, and monitors the client's responses. Unless an infusion control device is used, the nurse manually regulates the drops per minute of flow by using the roller clamp to ensure that the prescribed amount of solution will be infused in the correct span. If the flow is incorrect, such problems as hypervolemia, hypovolemia, or inadequate medication administration can result. It is recommended that an infusion control device be used whenever possible, particularly with administration of medications.

The number of drops delivered per millilitre of solution varies with different brands and types of infusion sets. This rate, called the **drop factor** or **drip factor**, generally is printed on the package of the infusion set. Macrodrops commonly have drop factors of 10, 12, 15, or 20 drops/mL; the drop factor for microdrip is always 60 drops/mL (Figure 43.24, page 1412).

To calculate flow rates, the nurse must know the volume of fluid to be infused and the specific time for the infusion. Two commonly used methods of indicating flow rates are designating the number of millilitres to be administered in 1 hour (mL/h) and the number of drops to be given in 1 minute (gtt/min). Because 1 millilitre of fluid displaces 1 cubic centimetre of space, the volume to be infused in the first method can also be designated as cubic centimetres per hour (cc/h).

Millilitres per Hour Hourly rates of infusion can be calculated by dividing the total infusion volume by the total infusion time in hours. For example, if 1000 mL is to be infused in 8 hours, the number of millilitres per hour is

$$\frac{1000\text{ mL (total infusion volume)}}{8\text{ h (total infusion time)}} = 125\text{ mL/h}$$

Nurses need to check infusions at least every hour to ensure that the indicated millilitres per hour have infused. A strip of adhesive marking the exact time or amount to be infused can be taped to the solution con-

SKILL 43.1

STARTING AN INTRAVENOUS INFUSION

Before preparing the infusion, the nurse first verifies the prescription indicating the type of solution, the amount to be administered, the rate of flow of the infusion, and any client allergies (e.g., to tape, povidone-iodine, or latex). Agency policy should be checked.

PURPOSES

- To supply fluid when clients are unable to take an adequate volume of fluids by mouth
- To provide salts and other electrolytes needed to maintain electrolyte balance
- To provide glucose (dextrose), the main fuel for metabolism
- To provide water-soluble vitamins and medications
- To establish a lifeline for rapidly needed medications

ASSESSMENT

Assess the following:

- Vital signs (pulse, respiratory rate, and blood pressure) for baseline data
- Skin turgor
- Allergy to latex (e.g., tourniquet), tape, iodine
- Bleeding tendencies
- Disease or injury to extremities
- Status of veins to determine appropriate venipuncture site

Planning

- Before initiating the IV infusion, consider how long the client is likely to have the IV, what kinds of fluids will be infused, and what medications the client will be receiving or is likely to receive. These factors may affect the choice of vein and catheter size.

Equipment

- Infusion set
- Sterile parenteral solution

(continued)

SKILL 43.1

STARTING AN INTRAVENOUS INFUSion (*continued*)

- IV pole
- Moisture-permeable transparent dressing
- Tourniquet
- Antiseptic swabs (preferably 2% chlorhexidine gluconate)
- Intravenous catheter (for routine hydration or intermittent therapies, use 22- to 27-gauge catheters; for transfusion therapies, 20- to 24-gauge; for therapy for neonates or clients with very small, fragile veins, 24- to 27-gauge); see the Variation at the end of this procedure for a butterfly (winged-tip) needle
- Clean gloves
- Sterile gauze dressing or transparent occlusive dressing
- Arm splint, if required
- Towel or pad
- Electronic infusion device or pump, as necessary

IMPLEMENTATION

Preparation

Prepare the client.

- Before performing the procedure, introduce yourself and verify the client's identity by using agency protocol. Explain the procedure to the client. A venipuncture can cause discomfort for a few seconds, but there should be no discomfort while the solution is flowing. Use a doll to demonstrate for children, and explain the procedure to the parents. **Rationale: Pain and anxiety stimulate the sympathetic nervous system and trigger vasoconstriction and vasovagal reactions.**
- Unless initiating IV therapy is urgent, provide any scheduled care before establishing the infusion to minimize movement of the affected limb during the procedure. **Rationale: Moving the limb after the infusion has been established could dislodge the catheter.**
- Consider applying warm compresses to the site for 10 to 15 minutes before you attempt venipuncture. **Rationale: Warmth encourages vasodilation.**
- Make sure that the client's clothing or gown can be removed over the IV apparatus. Some agencies provide special gowns that open over the shoulder and down the sleeve for easy removal.

Performance

1. Perform hand hygiene and observe other appropriate infection prevention and control procedures.
2. Open and prepare the infusion set.
   - Remove the tubing from the container and straighten it out.
   - Slide the tubing clamp along the tubing until it is just below the drip chamber to facilitate its access.
   - Close the clamp.
   - Leave the ends of the tubing covered with the plastic caps until the infusion is started. **Rationale: This will maintain the sterility of the ends of the tubing.**
3. Spike the solution container.
   - Remove the protective cover from the entry site of the bag.
   - Remove the cap from the spike, and insert the spike into the insertion site of the bag or bottle (see ❶), following the manufacturer's instructions.
4. Apply a medication label to the solution container if a medication is added. Follow agency policy. (See Skill 31.8, page 849) for adding medications to an intravenous fluid container.)
   - In many agencies, medications and labels are applied in the pharmacy; if they are not, apply the label upside down on the container. **Rationale: The label is applied upside down so it can be read easily when the container is hanging up.**
5. Apply a timing label on the solution container.
   - The timing label may be applied at the time the infusion is started. Follow agency practice. See the discussion of regulating infusion flow rates and Figure 43.25 (page 1412).
6. Hang the solution container on the pole.
   - Adjust the pole so that the container is suspended about 1 m above the client's head. **Rationale: This height is needed to enable gravity to overcome venous pressure and facilitate flow of the solution into the vein.**
7. Partially fill the drip chamber with solution.
   - Squeeze the chamber gently until it is half full of solution (see ❷).
8. Prime the tubing.
   - Remove the protective cap and hold the tubing over a container. Maintain the sterility of the end of the tubing and the cap.
   - Release the clamp and let the fluid run through the tubing until all bubbles are removed. Tap the tubing if

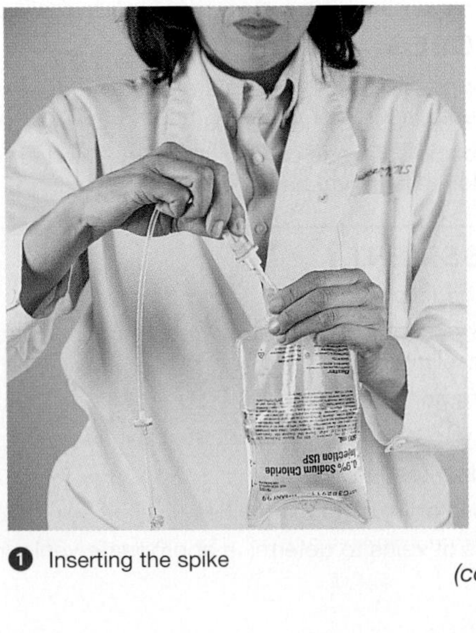

❶ Inserting the spike

(continued)

SKILL 43.1

STARTING AN INTRAVENOUS INFUSION *(continued)*

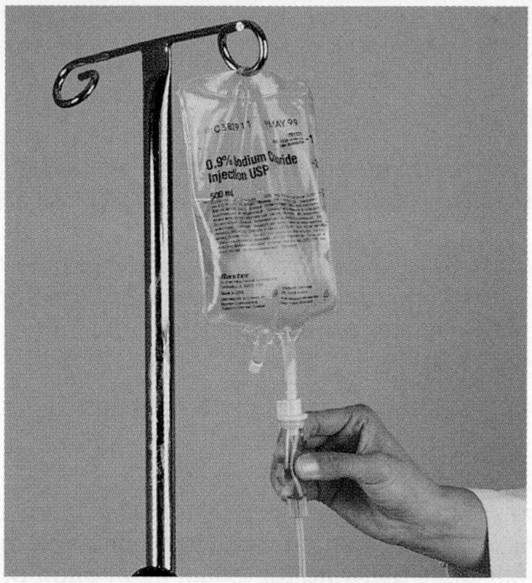

❷ Squeezing the drip chamber

necessary with your fingers to help the bubbles move. **Rationale: The tubing is primed to prevent the introduction of air into the client**.

- Air bubbles smaller than 0.5 mL usually do not cause problems in peripheral lines.
- Reclamp the tubing and replace the tubing cap, maintaining sterile technique.
- For caps with air vents, do not remove the cap when priming this tubing. The flow of solution through the tubing will cease when the cap is moist with one drop of solution.
- If an infusion control pump, electronic device, or controller is being used, follow the manufacturer's directions for inserting the tubing and setting the infusion rate.

9. Perform hand hygiene again just before client contact.

10. Select the venipuncture site.
    - Use the client's nondominant arm, unless contraindicated (e.g., mastectomy, fistula for dialysis, infection, injury). Identify possible venipuncture sites by looking for veins that are relatively straight, not sclerotic or tortuous, and avoiding venous valves. The vein should be palpable but may not be visible, especially in clients with dark skin. Consider the catheter length; look for a site sufficiently distal to the wrist or elbow that the tip of the catheter will not be at a point of flexion. **Rationale: Loss of lymph nodes with mastectomy may pose lymph drainage problems if the IV goes interstitial; sclerotic veins may make initiating and maintaining the IV difficult; joint flexion increases the risk of irritation of vein walls by the catheter**.
    - If the site is very hairy, remove hair by clipping with scissors. **Rationale: Shaving increases the risk of microabrasions, which can lead to infection**.
    - Place a towel or bed protector under the extremity to protect linens (or furniture if in the home).

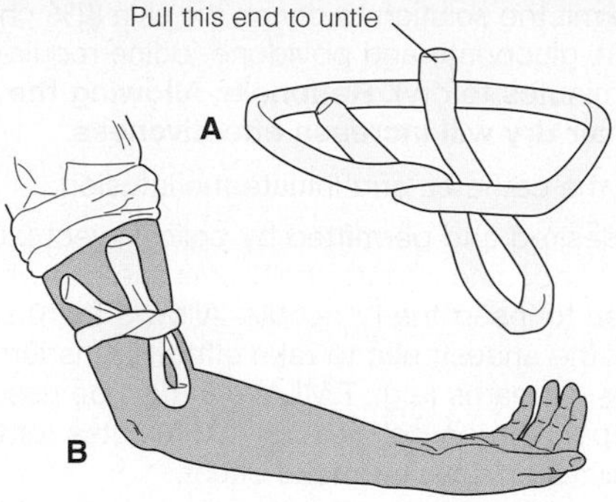

❸ Applying a tourniquet

11. Dilate the vein.
    - Place the extremity in a dependent position (lower than the client's heart). **Rationale: Gravity slows venous return and distends the veins. Distending the veins makes it easier to insert the needle properly**.
    - Apply a tourniquet firmly 15 to 20 cm above the venipuncture site (see ❸). Explain that the tourniquet will feel tight. **Rationale: The tourniquet must be tight enough to obstruct venous flow but not so tight that it occludes arterial flow. Obstructing arterial flow inhibits venous filling. If a radial pulse can be palpated, the arterial flow is not obstructed. Use the tourniquet on only one client. This avoids cross-contamination to other clients**.
    - If the vein is not sufficiently dilated:
      a. Massage or stroke the vein distal to the site and in the direction of venous flow toward the heart. **Rationale: This action helps fill the vein**.
      b. Encourage the client to clench and unclench the fist. **Rationale: Contracting the muscles compresses the distal veins, forcing blood along the veins and distending them**.
      c. Lightly tap the vein with your fingertips. **Rationale: Tapping may distend the vein**.
    - If the preceding steps fail to distend the vein so that it is palpable, remove the tourniquet and apply a warm towel to the entire extremity for 10 to 15 minutes. **Rationale: Warmth dilates superficial blood vessels, causing them to fill**. Then repeat step 11.

12. Put on clean gloves. **Rationale: Gloves protect the nurse from contamination by the client's blood**.
    - Clean the skin at the site of entry with a topical antiseptic swab (e.g., 2% chlorhexidine). Some institutions may use 70% isopropyl alcohol or 10% povidone-iodine swabs (check agency policy and see the Clinical Alert about swab preferences). Check for allergies to iodine or shellfish before cleansing skin with Betadine or iodine products.
    - Use a circular motion, moving from the centre outward for several centimetres. **Rationale: This motion carries microorganisms away from the site of entry**.

(continued)

SKILL 43.1

STARTING AN INTRAVENOUS INFUSION (*continued*)

- Permit the solution to dry on the skin (2% chlorhexidine gluconate and povidone-iodine require 2 minutes to dry). **Rationale: Allowing the solution to air dry will increase effectiveness.**

13. Insert the catheter, and initiate the infusion.
    - If desired and permitted by policy, inject 0.05 mL of 1% lidocaine intradermally over the site where you plan to insert the IV needle. Allow 5 to 10 seconds for the anaesthetic to take effect. Transdermal analgesic creams (e.g., EMLA) can also be used, depending on policy. Allow 30 minutes for the transdermal analgesic to take effect.
    - Use the nondominant hand to pull the skin taut below the entry site. **Rationale: This stabilizes the vein and makes the skin taut for needle entry. It can also make initial tissue penetration less painful.**
    - Holding the over-the-needle catheter at a 15- to 30-degree angle with bevel up, insert the catheter through the skin and into the vein in one movement. Sudden lack of resistance is felt as the needle enters the vein. Jabbing, stabbing, or quick thrusting should be avoided because it may cause rupture of delicate veins.
    - Once blood appears in the lumen of the needle or you feel the lack of resistance, lower the angle of the catheter until it is almost parallel with the skin, and advance the needle and catheter approximately 0.5 cm to 1 cm farther. Holding the needle portion steady, advance the catheter until the hub is at the venipuncture site. **Rationale: The catheter is advanced to ensure that it, and not just the metal needle, is in the vein.** The exact technique depends on the type of catheter used.
    - Release the tourniquet.
    - Put pressure on the vein proximal to the catheter to eliminate or reduce blood oozing out of the catheter. Stabilize the hub with thumb and index finger of the nondominant hand.
    - Remove the protective cap from the distal end of the tubing and hold it ready to attach to the catheter, maintaining sterility of the end.
    - Carefully remove the needle, engage the needle safety device, and attach the end of the infusion tubing to the catheter hub.
    - Initiate the infusion.

Note: If you miss the venipuncture, offer an honest explanation in a matter-of-fact and friendly manner. Think about what you can do to improve the next attempt, and explain what you'll do differently (if anything). It is generally recommended to limit your attempts to two; if unsuccessful after two tries, ask another member of the health-care team to try again a little later.

14. Dress and label the venipuncture site and tubing according to agency policy.
    - Secure the catheter using a sterile transparent dressing (see ❹) or according to agency policy. **Rationale: Transparent dressing secures the cannula while allowing for visual inspection of the insertion site (RNAO, 2005). This type of dressing can be left on for 48 to 72 hours, and then changed.**
    - Discard the tourniquet. Remove soiled gloves and discard appropriately.
    - Discard needle in sharps container.
    - Loop the tubing, and secure it with tape. **Rationale: Looping and securing the tubing prevent the weight of the tubing or any movement from pulling on the needle or catheter.**
    - Label the dressing with the date and time of insertion, type and gauge of needle or catheter used, and your initials (see ❺).
15. Ensure appropriate infusion flow.
    - Apply a padded arm board to splint the joint, as needed.
    - Adjust the infusion rate of flow according to the prescription.
16. Label the IV tubing.
    - Label the tubing with the date and time of attachment and your initials (see ❻). This labelling can also be done when the infusion is started. **Rationale: The tubing is labelled to ensure that it is changed at**

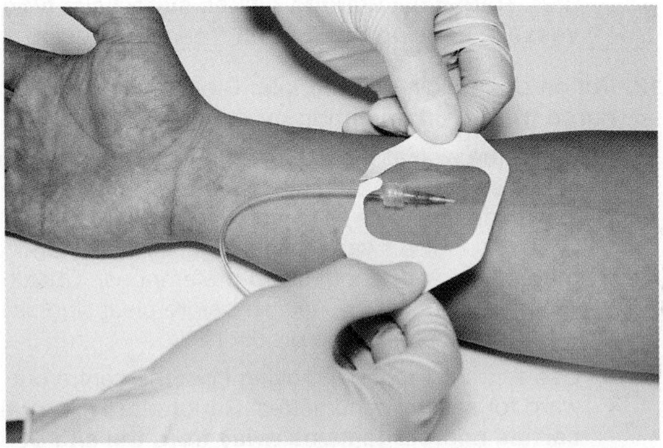

❹ Covering insertion site with transparent dressing

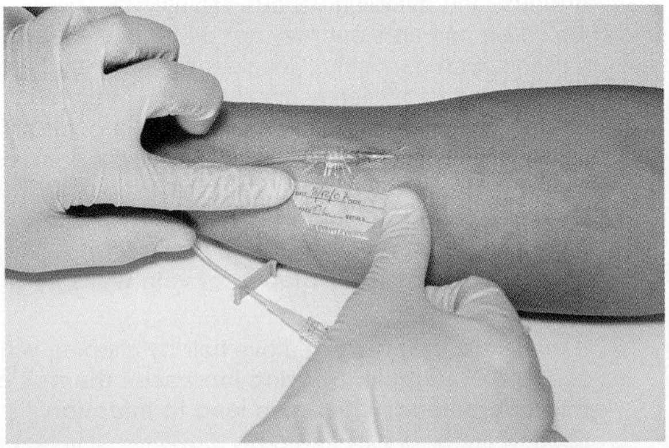

❺ Label IV site with date, time, size of catheter, and initials.

(continued)

SKILL 43.1

STARTING AN INTRAVENOUS INFUSION *(continued)*

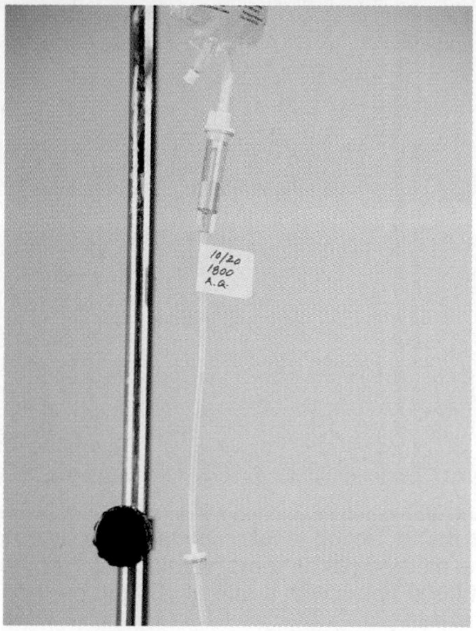

I.V. SET–*72* HRS.–ONLY
START DATE *9/11* HR. *0800*
DISCARD DATE *9/14* HR. *0800*
R.N. INITIAL *LA*

❻ Tubing labelled with date, time of attachment, and nurse's initials; also shown is a preprinted label

regular intervals (i.e., every 24 to 72 hours, according to agency policy).

17. Document relevant data, including assessments.
   - Record the start of the infusion on the client's chart. Some agencies provide a special form for this purpose. Include the date and time of the venipuncture; amount and type of solution used, including any additives (e.g., kind and amount of medications); container number; flow rate; type, length, and gauge of the needle or catheter; venipuncture site; how many attempts were made, and location of each attempt; the type of dressing applied; and the client's general response.

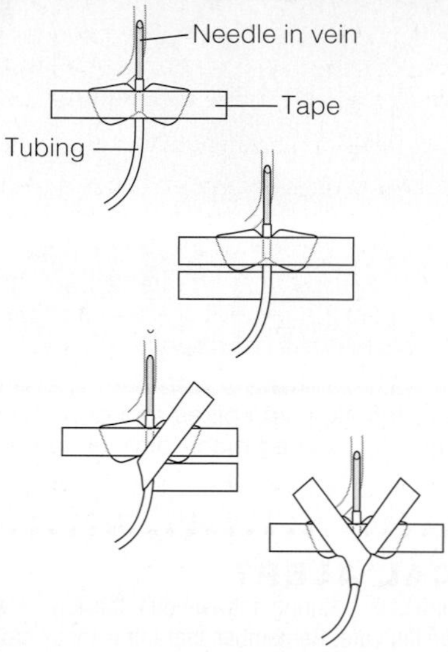

❼ Taping the butterfly needle by the chevron method

Variation: Inserting a Butterfly (Winged-Tip) Needle

- Hold the needle, pointed in the direction of the blood flow, at a 30-degree angle, with the bevel up, and pierce the skin beside the vein about 1 cm below the site planned for piercing the vein.
- Once the needle is through the skin, lower the needle so that it is almost parallel with the skin. **Rationale: Lowering the needle reduces the chances of puncturing both sides of the vein.**
- Follow the course of the vein, and pierce one side of the vein. Sudden lack of resistance can be felt as blood enters the needle.
- When blood flows back into the needle tubing, insert the needle to its hub.
- Release the tourniquet, attach the infusion, and initiate flow as quickly as possible. **Rationale: Attaching the tubing quickly prevents blood from clotting and obstructing the needle.**
- Secure the butterfly needle by taping it securely by the crisscross (chevron) method (see ❼). Place a small gauze square under the needle, if required. **Rationale: The gauze keeps the needle in position in the vein**

EVALUATION

Evaluate the following:

- Skin status at IV site (warm temperature and absence of pain, redness, and draining)
- Status of dressing
- IV flow rate consistent with that prescribed
- Ability to perform self-care activities and understanding of any mobility limitations
- Vital signs compared with baseline level

tainer. Some agencies make premarked labels available (Figure 43.25).

Drops per Minute The nurse initiating and monitoring an infusion must regulate the drops per minute to ensure that the prescribed amount of solution will infuse. Drops per minute are calculated by the following formula:

$$\text{Drops per minute} = \frac{\text{Total infusion volume} \times \text{Drop factor}}{\text{Total time of infusion in } \textit{minutes}}$$

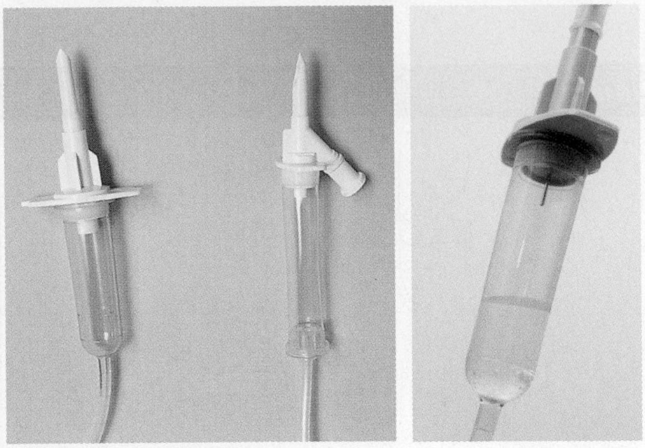

FIGURE 43.24 Infusion set spikes and drip chambers: unvented macrodrip, vented macrodrip, unvented microdrip

> **CLINICAL ALERT**
> Preventing infections during intravenous therapy is an important aspect of nursing care. Remember that intravenous catheter-related bloodstream infections are significantly lower when 2% chlorhexidine gluconate solution is used compared with the use of 10% povidone-iodine and 70% isopropyl alcohol swabs (LeBlanc & Cobbett, 2000; Rosenthal, 2006; Zitella, 2004). Chlorhexidine gluconate has antimicrobial features that last beyond the application time to provide additional protection. Antimicrobial ointments should *not* be applied to central or peripheral insertion sites as they promote fungal infections (RNAO, 2005).

In our previous example, if the requirements are 1000 mL in 8 hours and the drip factor is 20 drops/mL, the drops per minute should be

$$\frac{1000\text{ mL} \times 20\text{ gtt/mL}}{8\text{ h} \times 60\text{ min/h}} = 41.66\text{ gtt/min}$$

Approximating this rate as 42 drops/min, the nurse regulates the drops per minute by tightening or releasing the IV tubing clamp and counting the drops for 15 seconds, then multiplying that number by 4 (e.g., 10 to 11 drops/15 sec). A number of factors influence flow rate (see Box 43.8).

Devices to Control Infusions A number of devices are used to control the rate of an infusion. *Electronic infusion devices* (EIDs) regulate the infusion rate at preset limits. They also have an alarm that is triggered when the solution in the IV bag is low, when there is air in the tubing, or when the tubing is not high enough. The *Dial-A-Flo* inline device (Figure 43.26) is a regulator that controls the amount of fluid to be administered. Hospitals may stock the Dial-A-Flo for use in situations where a pump is not required but prevention of fluid overload is important. It is preset at the volume to be infused and can be attached at the time the infusion is set up or when the tubing is changed. Another variation is a *volume-control set,* or Volutrol, which is used if the volume of fluid administered is to be carefully controlled. The set, which

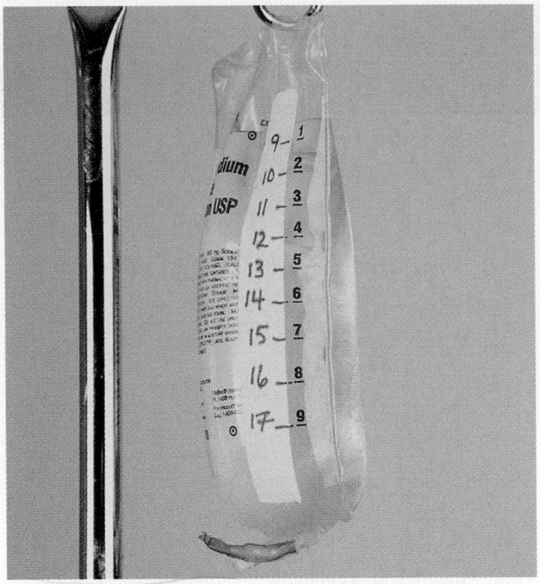

FIGURE 43.25 Timing label on an intravenous container. The first time marked (0900 hours) would be correct for a bag hung at 0800 hours with a rate of 100 mL per hour.

holds a maximum of 100 mL of solution, is attached below the solution container, and the drip chamber is placed below the set. Volume-control sets are frequently used in pediatric settings, where the volume administered is critical.

An *infusion pump* (Figures 43.27 and 43.28) delivers fluids intravenously by exerting positive pressure on the tubing or on the fluid. In situations where the fluid flow is unrestricted, the pump pressure is comparable to that of gravity flow. However, if restrictions develop (increased venous resistance), the pump can maintain the fluid flow by increasing the pressure applied to the fluid.

A *controller,* by contrast, operates solely by gravitational force. The delivery pressure depends on the height of the container in relation to the venipuncture site. The container must be at least 76 cm above the

BOX 43.8 FACTORS INFLUENCING FLOW RATES

Flow rates can be affected by a number of factors:

- *The position of the forearm.* Sometimes, a change in the position of the client's arm decreases flow. Slight pronation, supination, extension, or elevation of the forearm on a pillow can increase flow.
- *The position and patency of the tubing.* Tubing can be obstructed by the client's weight, a kink, or a clamp closed too tightly. The flow rate also diminishes when part of the tubing dangles below the puncture site.
- *The height of the infusion bottle.* Elevating the height of the infusion bottle a few centimetres can speed the flow by creating more pressure.
- *Possible infiltration or fluid leakage.* Swelling, a feeling of coldness, and tenderness at the venipuncture site may indicate infiltration.
- *Relationship of the size of the angiocath to the vein.* A catheter that is too large may impede the infusion flow.

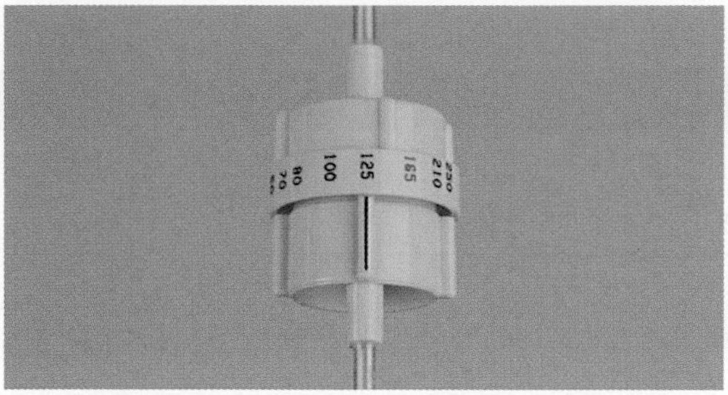

FIGURE 43.26 The Dial-A-Flo inline device

CLINICAL ALERT

A flow rate control device should be used when administering IV fluid to older adult or pediatric clients. Both of these age groups are especially at risk for complications of fluid overload, which can occur with rapid infusion of IV fluids.

venipuncture site for a controller to work. A controller does not have the ability to add pressure to the line and to overcome resistance to fluid flow.

Skill 43.2 outlines the steps involved in monitoring an intravenous infusion.

Changing Intravenous Containers, Tubing, and Dressings for Peripheral Intravenous Sites Intravenous solution containers are changed when a small amount of fluid remains in the neck of the container and fluid still remains in the drip chamber. However, all IV bags should be changed every 24 hours, regardless of how much solution remains, to minimize the risk of contamination. IV administration sets that do not contain lipids, blood, or blood products may be left in place for intervals of up to 96 hours without increasing the incidence of infection; tubing that contains lipids should be changed every 24 hours (Gillies et al., 2005). Agency policy and manufacturer's recommendations must also be considered in the decision-making process. Skill 43.3 provides guidelines for changing an IV solution container, tubing, and the IV site dressing.

When an IV infusion is no longer necessary to maintain the client's fluid intake or to provide a route for medication administration, the infusion is either discontinued and the catheter removed, or the catheter is left in place and converted to a saline or heparin lock. Guidelines for discontinuing an IV infusion are outlined in Skill 43.4, and guidelines for converting the catheter to a lock are outlined in Skill 43.5.

CHANGING PERIPHERAL INTRAVENOUS SITES The Public Health Agency of Canada (1997) guidelines established 3 days (72 hours) as the maximum time for a catheter to dwell in the same peripheral vein. When a vein is prone to phlebitis, the length of dwell should be even shorter (e.g., 48 to 72 hours) (Vanek, 2002). Clinical assessment of the site is ongoing and the intravenous site should be changed earlier than these guidelines in cases of infiltration, signs of infection, or severe discomfort.

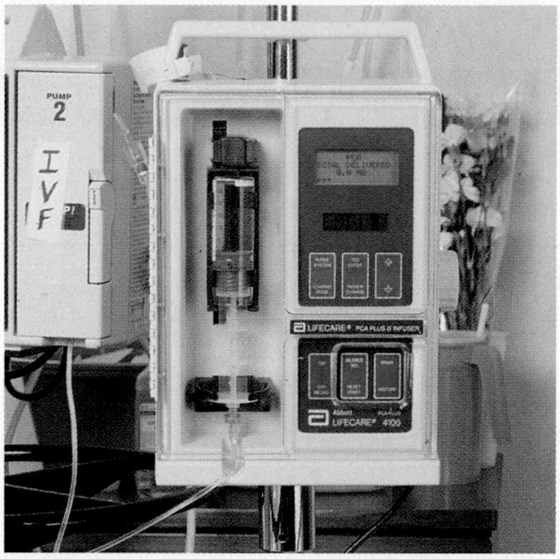

FIGURE 43.27 An intravenous infusion pump

BLOOD TRANSFUSIONS Intravenous fluids can be effective in restoring intravascular (blood) volume; however, they do not affect the oxygen-carrying capacity of the blood. When red and white blood cells, platelets, or blood proteins are lost because of hemorrhage or disease, it may be necessary to replace these components to restore the blood's ability to transport oxygen and carbon dioxide, to clot, to fight infection, and to keep ECF within the intravascular compartment. A blood transfusion is the introduction of whole blood or blood components into the venous circulation.

Blood Groups Human blood is commonly classified into four main groups (A, B, AB, and O). The surface of an individual's red blood cells (RBCs) contains a number of proteins known as **antigens** (substances capable of inducing the formation of antibodies) that are unique for each person. Many blood antigens have been identified, but the antigens A, B, and Rh are the most important in determining blood group or type. Because antigens

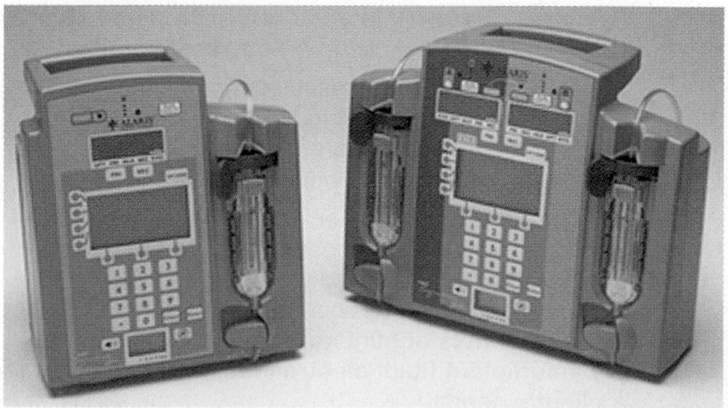

FIGURE 43.28 Programmable infusion pumps

SKILL 43.2

MONITORING AN INTRAVENOUS INFUSION

PURPOSES

- To maintain the prescribed flow rate
- To prevent complications associated with IV therapy

ASSESSMENT

Assess the following:

- Appearance of infusion site and the patency of system
- Type of fluid being infused and rate of flow
- Response of the client

IMPLEMENTATION

Preparation

1. Prepare the client.
   - Before performing the procedure, introduce yourself and verify the client's identity by using agency protocol. Explain the procedure to the client.
2. Gather the pertinent data.
   - From the physician's order, determine the type and sequence of solutions to be infused, and determine the rate of flow and infusion schedule.

Performance

1. Perform hand hygiene and observe other appropriate infection prevention and control procedures.
2. Ensure that the correct solution is being infused.
   - If the solution in incorrect, slow the rate of flow to a minimum to maintain the patency of the catheter. (If patient is at risk for developing an adverse reaction, infusion must be stopped.) **Rationale: Stopping the infusion may allow a thrombus to form in the IV catheter. If this occurs, the catheter must be removed and another venipuncture performed before the infusion can be resumed.**
   - Change the solution to the correct one. Document and report the error according to agency protocol.
3. Observe the rate of flow every hour.
   - Compare the rate of flow regularly, for example, at least every hour, against the infusion schedule. **Rationale: Infusions that are off schedule can be harmful to a client.**
   - If the rate is *too fast,* check agency policy. **Rationale: Solution administered too quickly may cause a significant increase in circulating blood volume (which is about 6 L in an adult). Hypervolemia may result in pulmonary edema and cardiac failure.**
   - Assess the client for manifestations of hypervolemia and its complications, including dyspnea; rapid, laboured breathing; cough; crackles in the lung bases; tachycardia; and bounding pulses.
   - If the rate is *too slow,* check agency practice. Some agencies permit nursing personnel to adjust a rate of flow by a specified amount. Adjustments above this rate may require a physician's order. **Rationale: Solution that is administered too slowly can supply insufficient fluid, electrolytes, or medication for a client's needs.**
   - If the rate of flow is 150 mL/h or more, check the rate of flow more frequently, for example, every 15 to 30 minutes.
4. Inspect the patency of the IV tubing and needle.
   - Observe the position of the solution container. If it is less than 1 m above the IV site, readjust it to the correct height. Recheck the rate of flow any time the height of the solution container is changed. **Rationale: If the container is too low, the solution may not flow into the vein because there is insufficient gravitational pressure to overcome the pressure of the blood within the vein.**
   - Observe the drip chamber. If it is less than half full, squeeze the chamber to allow the correct amount of fluid to flow in.
   - Open the drip regulator, and observe for a rapid flow of fluid from the solution container into the drip chamber. Then, partially close the drip regulator to re-establish the prescribed rate of flow. **Rationale: Rapid flow of fluid into the drip chamber indicates patency of the IV line. Closing the drip regulator to the prescribed rate of flow prevents fluid overload.**
   - Inspect the tubing for pinches or kinks or obstructions to flow. Arrange the tubing so that it is lightly coiled and under no pressure. Sometimes, the tubing becomes caught under the client's arm and the weight of the arm blocks the flow.
   - Observe the position of the tubing. If it is dangling below the venipuncture, coil it carefully on the surface of the bed. **Rationale: The solution cannot flow upward into the vein against the force of gravity.**
   - Lower the solution container below the level of the infusion site and observe for a return flow of blood from the vein. **Rationale: A return flow of blood indicates that the needle is patent and in the vein. Blood returns in this instance because venous pressure is greater than the fluid pressure in the IV tubing. Absence of blood return may indicate that the needle is no longer in the vein or that the tip of the catheter is partially obstructed by a thrombus, the vein wall, or a valve in the vein.**
   - Determine whether the bevel of the catheter is blocked against the wall of the vein. If it is blocked, pull back gently, turn it slightly, or carefully raise or lower the angle of insertion slightly by using a sterile gauze pad underneath to protect the skin and change the position of the catheter bevel.

(continued)

SKILL 43.2

MONITORING AN INTRAVENOUS INFUSION (*continued*)

- If leakage occurs, locate the source. If the leak is at the catheter connection, tighten the tubing into the catheter. If the leak cannot be stopped, slow the infusion as much as possible without stopping it, and replace the tubing with a new sterile set. Estimate the amount of solution lost.

5. Inspect the insertion site for fluid infiltration at least every hour.
   - When an IV needle becomes dislodged from the vein, fluid flows into interstitial tissues, causing swelling. This is known as *infiltration* and is manifested by localized swelling, coolness, pallor, and discomfort at the IV site.
   - If an infiltration is present, stop the infusion and remove the catheter. Restart the infusion at another site.
   - Apply a warm compress to the site of the infiltration. **Rationale: Warmth promotes comfort and vasodilation, facilitating absorption of the fluid from interstitial tissues.**
6. If the infiltration involves a vesicant drug (a drug that can cause tissue necrosis), it is called extravasation, and other measures may be indicated. Extravasated vesicant drugs can cause severe tissue injury or destruction. The extravasation of a vesicant drug should be considered an emergency (Hadaway, 2004).
   - Stop the infusion immediately. Disconnect the tubing as close to the catheter hub as possible and attempt to aspirate any drug remaining in the hub. If an injectable antidote is available, the catheter should remain in place.
   - The appropriate member of the health-care team should be notified and if ordered, the antidote administered.
   - The affected arm should be elevated and depending on the drug, heat or cold therapy should be implemented.
7. If infiltration is not evident but the infusion is not flowing, determine whether the needle is dislodged from the vein.
   - Gently pinch the IV tubing adjacent to the needle site. This will cause blood to flow (flash back) into the tubing if the needle is in the vein.
   - Use a sterile syringe of saline to withdraw fluid from the port near the venipuncture site. If blood does not return, discontinue the intravenous solution.
8. Inspect the insertion site for phlebitis (inflammation of a vein).
   - Inspect and palpate the site at least every 8 hours. Phlebitis can occur as a result of injury to a vein, for example, because of mechanical trauma or chemical irritation. Chemical injury to a vein can occur from intravenous electrolytes (especially potassium and magnesium) and some medications. The clinical signs of phlebitis are redness, warmth, and swelling at the intravenous site and burning pain along the course of a vein.
   - If phlebitis is detected, discontinue the infusion, and apply warm compresses to the venipuncture site as ordered and according to agency policy. Do not use this injured vein for further infusions.
9. Inspect the intravenous site for bleeding.
   - Oozing or bleeding into the surrounding tissues can occur while the infusion is freely flowing but is more likely to occur after the needle has been removed from the vein.
   - Observation of the venipuncture site is extremely important for clients who bleed readily, such as those receiving anticoagulants.
10. Teach the client ways to maintain the infusion system, for example:
    - Avoid sudden twisting or turning movements of the arm with the needle or catheter.
    - Avoid stretching or placing tension on the tubing.
    - Try to keep the tubing from dangling below the level of the needle.
    - Notify a nurse, if
      - **a.** The flow rate suddenly changes or the solution stops dripping
      - **b.** The solution container is nearly empty
      - **c.** There is blood in the IV tubing
      - **d.** Discomfort or swelling is experienced at the IV site
11. Document all relevant information.

EVALUATION

Evaluate the following:

- Amount of fluid infused according to the schedule
- Intactness of IV system
- Appearance of IV site (e.g., dry, tissue infiltration, discomfort)
- Urinary output compared with intake
- Tissue turgor; specific gravity of urine
- Vital signs and lung sounds compared with baseline data

promote *agglutination* or clumping of blood cells, they are also known as **agglutinogens**. The A antigen or agglutinogen is present on the RBCs of people with blood group A, the B antigen is present in people with blood group B, and both A and B antigens are found on the RBC surface in people with group AB blood. Neither antigen is present in people with group O blood.

SKILL 43.3

CHANGING AN INTRAVENOUS CONTAINER, TUBING, AND DRESSING

PURPOSES

- To maintain the flow of required fluids
- To maintain sterility of the IV system and decrease the incidence of phlebitis and infection
- To maintain patency of the IV tubing
- To prevent infection at the IV site and the introduction of microorganisms into the bloodstream

ASSESSMENT

Assess the following:

- Presence of fluid infiltration, bleeding, or phlebitis at IV site
- Allergy to tape, latex, or iodine
- Infusion rate and amount absorbed
- Blockages in IV system
- Appearance of the dressing for integrity, moisture, and need for change
- The date and time of the previous dressing change

Planning

Review the physician's orders for changes in fluid administration.

Equipment

- Container with the correct kind and amount of sterile solution, according to physician's orders
- Administration set, including sterile tubing and drip chamber
- Timing label
- Receptacle (e.g., a basin) for discarded fluid
- Sterile gauze square for positioning the needle

For the Dressing

- Clean gloves
- Sterile gauze or transparent dressing
- Adhesive remover
- Antiseptic swab (preferably 2% chlorhexidine gluconate)
- Cleansing solution as recommended by the agency (for example, normal saline)
- Moisture-permeable transparent dressing
- Towel

IMPLEMENTATION

Preparation

1. Prepare the client.
   - Before performing the procedure, introduce yourself and verify the client's identity by using agency protocol. Explain the procedure to the client.
2. Obtain the correct solution container.
   - Read the label of the new container.
   - Verify that you have the correct solution, correct client, correct additives (if any), and correct dose (number of bags or total volume ordered).
   - Check clarity of solution and expiry date.

Performance

1. Perform hand hygiene and observe other appropriate infection prevention and control procedures.
2. Set up the intravenous equipment with the new container, and label them.
   - See Skill 43.1, steps 2 to 9.
   - Apply a timing label to the container.
   - Prime the tubing.
   - Label the tubing as described in Skill 43.1.
3. Prepare the IV needle or catheter and the dressing equipment.
   - Prepare strips of tape as needed for the type of needle or catheter. For the butterfly needle, two or three strips of 7.5 cm tape are needed. For a catheter, transparent dressing can be used. **Rationale: These will be used later to secure the needle or catheter without covering the insertion site.**
   - Hang the pieces of tape, if using, from the edge of a clean table. **Rationale: This places the tape in readiness for use without disrupting the adhesive.**
   - Open all equipment: solution or swabs, dressing and adhesive bandage. **Rationale: This facilitates access to supplies.**
   - Place a towel under the extremity. **Rationale: This prevents soiling of bed linens.**
   - Apply clean gloves.
4. Remove the soiled dressing and all tape, except the tape holding the catheter or IV needle in place.
   - Remove old dressing one layer at a time. **Rationale: This prevents dislodgement of the catheter or needle in case tubing becomes entangled between layers of dressing.**
   - Remove adhesive dressings in the direction of the client's hair growth when possible. **Rationale: This minimizes discomfort when adhesive is removed from the skin.**
   - Discard the used dressing materials in the appropriate container.
5. Assess the IV site.
   - Inspect the IV site for the presence of infiltration or inflammation. **Rationale: Inflammation or infiltration necessitates removal of the IV needle or catheter to avoid further trauma to the tissues.**
   - Go to step 7, or discontinue and relocate the IV site, if indicated.
   - See Skills 43.1 and 43.4.

(continued)

SKILL 43.3

CHANGING AN INTRAVENOUS CONTAINER, TUBING, AND DRESSING (*continued*)

6. Disconnect the used tubing.
   - Place a sterile swab under the hub of the catheter. **Rationale: This absorbs any leakage that might occur when the tubing is disconnected.**
   - Clamp the tubing. With the fourth or fifth finger of the nondominant hand, apply pressure to the vein above the end of the catheter. **Rationale: This helps prevent blood from coming out of the needle during the change of tubing.**
   - Holding the hub of the catheter with the thumb and index finger of the nondominant hand, loosen the tubing with the dominant hand, using a twisting, pulling motion. **Rationale: Holding the catheter firmly but gently maintains its position in the vein.**
   - Remove the used IV tubing.
   - Place the end of the tubing in the basin or other receptacle.
7. Connect the new tubing, and re-establish the infusion.
   - Continue to hold the catheter, and grasp the new tubing with the dominant hand.
   - Remove the protective tubing cap, maintaining sterility, and insert the tubing end securely into the needle hub. Twist it to secure it.
   - Open the clamp to start the solution flowing.
8. Clean the IV site.
   - Start with adhesive remover to remove adhesive residue. **Rationale: Removal of adhesive residue facilitates adherence of the new dressing.**
   - Then, by using the solution recommended by agency policy, clean the site, beginning at the catheter or needle and cleaning outward in a 5 cm diameter. **Rationale: Cleaning in this manner prevents contamination of the IV site from bacteria on the peripheral skin areas. Antiseptics reduce the number of microorganisms present at the site, thus reducing the risk of infection.**
9. Retape the needle or catheter.
   - For a butterfly needle, apply strips of tape to the wings of the butterfly by using the crisscross (chevron) method (see ❼ in Skill 43.1).
   - Apply sterile gauze or transparent dressing over the site.
   - Remove gloves.
10. Label the dressing, and secure the IV tubing.
    - Place the date and time of the dressing change and your initials either on the label provided or directly over the top of the dressing.
    - Secure IV tubing with additional tape, as required.
11. Regulate the rate of flow of the solution according to the order on the chart.
12. Document all relevant information.
    - Record the change of the solution container, tubing, and dressing in the appropriate place on the client's chart. Also record the fluid intake, according to agency practice. Record the number of the container, if the containers are numbered at the agency. Also record your assessments.

EVALUATION

Evaluate the following:

- Status of IV site
- Patency of IV system
- Accuracy of flow

Preformed **antibodies** to RBC antigens are present in the plasma; these antibodies are often called **agglutinins**. People with blood group A have B antibodies (agglutinins); A antibodies are present in people with blood group B; and people with blood group O have antibodies to both A and B antigens. People with group AB blood do not have antibodies to either A or B antigens (Table 43.12). When blood is transfused, the blood group of the donor and recipient must match to avoid an antigen-antibody reaction and destruction (hemolysis) of RBCs.

RHESUS (RH) FACTOR The Rh factor antigen is present on the RBCs of approximately 85% of people. Blood that contains the Rh factor is known as Rh-positive (Rh^+) blood; when it is not present, the blood is said to be Rh-negative (Rh^-) blood. In contrast to the ABO blood groups, Rh^- blood does not naturally contain Rh antibodies. However, on exposure to blood containing Rh factor (e.g., an Rh^- mother carrying a fetus with Rh^+ blood, or transfusion of Rh^+ blood into a client who is Rh^-), Rh antibodies develop. Subsequent exposure to Rh^+ blood places the client at risk for an antigen-antibody reaction and hemolysis of RBCs.

TABLE 43.12 The Blood Groups with Their Constituent Agglutinogens and Agglutinins

Blood Type	RBC Antigens (Agglutinogens)	Plasma Antibodies (Agglutinins)
A	A	B
B	B	A
AB	A and B	—
O	—	A and B

SKILL 43.4

DISCONTINUING A PERIPHERAL INTRAVENOUS INFUSION

PURPOSE

- To discontinue an intravenous infusion when the therapy is complete or when the IV site needs to be changed

ASSESSMENT

Assess the following:

- Appearance of the venipuncture site
- Any bleeding from the infusion site
- Amount of fluid infused
- Appearance of IV catheter

Equipment

- Clean gloves
- Dry or antiseptic-soaked swabs, according to agency practice
- Small sterile dressing and tape

Planning

Review the physician's orders and check agency policy.

IMPLEMENTATION

Preparation

- Before performing the procedure, introduce yourself and verify the client's identity by using agency policy. Explain the procedure to the client.

Performance

1. Perform hand hygiene and observe other appropriate infection prevention and control procedures.
2. Prepare the equipment.
   - Clamp the infusion tubing. **Rationale: Clamping the tubing prevents the fluid from flowing out of the needle onto the client or bed.**
   - Loosen the tape or dressing at the venipuncture site while holding the needle firmly and applying countertraction to the skin. **Rationale: Movement of the needle can injure the vein and cause discomfort to the client. Countertraction prevents pulling the skin and causing discomfort.**
   - Put on clean gloves and hold a sterile gauze above the venipuncture site.
3. Withdraw the needle or catheter from the vein.
   - Withdraw the needle or catheter by pulling it out along the line of the vein. **Rationale: Pulling it out in line with the vein avoids injury to the vein.**
   - Immediately apply firm pressure to the site by using sterile gauze for 2 to 3 minutes. **Rationale: Pressure helps stop the bleeding and prevents hematoma formation.**
   - Hold the client's arm or leg above the body if any bleeding persists. **Rationale: Raising the limb decreases blood flow to the area.**
4. Examine the catheter removed from the client.
   - Check the catheter to make sure it is intact. **Rationale: If a piece of tubing remains in the client's vein it could move centrally (toward the heart or lungs) and cause serious problems.**
   - Report a broken catheter to the nurse in charge or physician immediately.
   - If the broken piece can be palpated, apply a tourniquet above the insertion site. Application of a tourniquet decreases the possibility of the piece moving until a physician is notified.
5. Cover the venipuncture site.
   - Apply the sterile dressing. **Rationale: The dressing continues the pressure and covers the open area in the skin, preventing infection.**
   - Note the amount of solution remaining in the IV solution container. Discard the IV solution container, and discard the used supplies appropriately.
6. Document all relevant information.
   - Record the amount of fluid infused on the intake and output record and on the chart, according to agency practice. Include the container number, type of solution used, time of discontinuing the infusion, and the client's response.

EVALUATION

Evaluate the appearance of the venipuncture site, pulse, respirations, skin colour, edema, sputum, cough, and urine output, and how the person feels physically and psychologically.

BLOOD TYPING AND CROSSMATCHING To avoid transfusing incompatible RBCs, both blood donor and recipient are typed, and their blood is crossmatched. *Blood typing* is done to determine the ABO blood group and Rh factor status. This test is also performed on pregnant women and neonates to assess for possible intrauterine exposure of the mother or baby to an incompatible blood type (particularly Rh factor incompatibilities).

Because blood typing determines only the presence of the major ABO and Rh antigens, *crossmatching* also is

SKILL 43.5

CHANGING A PERIPHERAL INTRAVENOUS CATHETER TO AN INTERMITTENT INFUSION LOCK

PURPOSE

- To permit IV administration of medications or fluids on an intermittent basis

ASSESSMENT

Assess the following:

- Patency of the IV catheter
- Appearance of the site (evidence of inflammation or infiltration)

Planning

Review the physician's order.

- A specific order may be written to convert an intravenous access to a heparin or saline lock. The order also may be implied, for example, IV fluids are to be discontinued but the client has orders for an IV antibiotic every 6 hours or is receiving analgesics intravenously.

Equipment

- Intermittent infusion cap or device
- Clean gloves
- Sterile gauze
- Sterile saline for injection (without preservative) or heparin flush solution (use caution in selecting correct concentration of heparin solution) using a 3 mL syringe with a 25-gauge needle, or a needleless infusion device
- Isopropyl alcohol wipe
- Tape
- Clean emesis basin

IMPLEMENTATION

Preparation

- Before performing the procedure, introduce yourself and verify the client's identity by using agency policy. Explain the procedure to the client and the reason for leaving the IV catheter in place. Changing an IV to a heparin or saline lock should cause no discomfort other than that associated with removing tape from the IV tubing.

Performance

1. Prepare the client and equipment.
    - Perform hand hygiene and observe other appropriate infection prevention and control procedures.
    - Assess the IV site (if visible) and determine the patency of the catheter (see Skill 43.2). If the catheter is not fully patent or there is evidence of phlebitis or infiltration, discontinue the catheter and establish a new IV site.
    - Expose the IV catheter hub, and loosen any tape that is holding the IV tubing in place or it will interfere with insertion of the intermittent infusion plug into the catheter.
    - Clamp the IV tubing to stop the flow of IV fluid.
    - Open the gauze pad, and place it under the IV catheter hub.
    - Open the alcohol wipe and intermittent infusion plug, leaving the plug in its sterile package.
2. Remove the IV tubing and insert the intermittent infusion plug into the IV catheter.
    - Put on clean gloves.
    - Stabilize the IV catheter with your nondominant hand, and use the little finger to place slight pressure on the vein *above* the end of the catheter. Twist the IV tubing adapter to loosen it from the IV catheter and remove it, placing the end of the tubing in a clean emesis basin.
    - Pick up the intermittent infusion plug from its package, and remove the protective sleeve from the male adapter, maintaining its sterility. Insert the plug into the IV catheter, twisting it to seat it firmly, or engage the Luer lock.
3. Instill saline or heparin solution per agency policy. **Rationale: Saline or heparin is used to maintain patency of the IV catheter when fluids are not infusing through the catheter.**
4. Tape the intermittent infusion plug in place using the chevron. **Rationale: Tape provides added security to prevent the infusion plug from coming out of the intravenous catheter. It also promotes comfort, preventing the plug from catching on clothing or bedding.**
5. Teach the client how to maintain the lock.
    - Avoid manipulating the catheter or infusion plug and protect it from catching on clothing or bedding. A gauze bandage, such as Kerlix or Kling, can be wrapped over the plug to protect it when it is not in use.
    - Cover the site with an occlusive dressing when showering; avoid immersing the site.
    - Notify the appropriate member of the health-care team if the plug or catheter comes out, if the site becomes red, inflamed, or painful, or if any drainage or bleeding occurs at the site.
6. Document all relevant information.

EVALUATION

Evaluate the patency of the catheter, the appearance of the site, and the ease of flushing.

TABLE 43.13 Blood Products for Transfusion

Product	Use
Whole blood	Not commonly used except for extreme cases of acute hemorrhage. Replaces blood volume and all blood products: RBCs, plasma, plasma proteins, fresh platelets, and other clotting factors.
Packed red blood cells (PRBCs)	Used to increase the oxygen-carrying capacity of blood in anemias, surgery, disorders with slow bleeding. One unit of PRBCs has the same amount of oxygen-carrying RBCs as a unit of whole blood.
Autologous red blood cells	Used for blood replacement following planned elective surgery. Clients donate their own blood 4 to 5 weeks before surgery for autologous transfusion.
Platelets	Replaces platelets in clients with bleeding disorders or platelet deficiency. Fresh platelets are most effective. Each unit increases the average adult's platelet count by about 5000 platelets/microlitre (Rosenthal, 2006).
Fresh frozen plasma	Expands blood volume and provides clotting factors. Does not need to be crossmatched (contains no RBCs). ABO compatibility must be confirmed. Each unit will increase the level of clotting factor by 2% to 3% in the average adult (Rosenthal, 2006).
Albumin and plasma protein fraction	Blood volume expander; provides plasma proteins.
Clotting factors and cryoprecipitate	Used for clients with clotting factor deficiencies. Each provides different factors involved in the clotting pathway; cryoprecipitate also contains fibrinogen.

TABLE 43.14 Transfusion Reactions

Reaction: Cause	Clinical Signs	Nursing Interventions*
Hemolytic reaction: incompatibility between client's blood and donor's blood	Chills, fever, headache, backache, dyspnea, cyanosis, chest pain, tachycardia, hypotension	1. Discontinue the transfusion immediately. 2. Maintain vascular access with normal saline, or according to agency protocol. 3. Notify the physician immediately. 4. Monitor vital signs. 5. Monitor fluid intake and output. 6. Send the remaining blood, a sample of the client's blood, and a urine sample to the laboratory. This should be done for all reactions, according to doctor's orders and agency policy.
Febrile reaction: sensitivity of the client's blood to white blood cells, platelets, or plasma proteins	Fever; chills; warm, flushed skin; headache; anxiety; muscle pain	1. Discontinue the transfusion immediately. 2. Give antipyretics, as ordered. 3. Notify the physician immediately. 4. Keep the vein open with normal saline solution.
Allergic reaction (mild): sensitivity to infused plasma proteins	Flushing, itching, urticaria, bronchial wheezing	1. Stop or slow the transfusion, depending on agency protocol. 2. Notify the physician. 3. Administer medication (antihistamines), as ordered.
Allergic reaction (severe): antibody-antigen reaction	Dyspnea, chest pain, circulatory collapse, cardiac arrest	1. Stop the transfusion. 2. Keep the vein open with normal saline. 3. Notify the physician immediately. 4. Monitor vital signs. Administer cardiopulmonary resuscitation (CPR), if needed. 5. Administer medications and oxygen, as ordered.
Circulatory overload: blood administered faster than the circulation can accommodate	Cough, dyspnea, crackles, distended neck veins, tachycardia, hypertension	1. Place the client upright with feet dependent. 2. Stop or slow the transfusion. 3. Notify the physician immediately. 4. Administer diuretics and oxygen, as ordered.
Sepsis: contaminated blood administered	High fever, chills, vomiting, diarrhea, hypotension	1. Stop the transfusion. 2. Keep the vein open with normal saline. 3. Notify the physician immediately. 4. Administer IV fluids, antibiotics, as ordered. 5. Obtain a blood specimen from the client for culture. 6. Send the remaining blood to the laboratory.

**Nurses should follow agency protocol regarding interventions. These may vary among agencies.*

necessary before transfusion to identify possible interactions of minor antigens with their corresponding antibodies. RBCs from the donor blood are mixed with serum from the recipient; a reagent (Coombs' serum) is added, and the mixture is examined for visible agglutination. If the recipient's serum does not contain antibodies to the donor's RBCs, agglutination does not occur, and the risk of a transfusion reaction is small.

Selection of Blood Donors Screening of blood donors is rigorous. Criteria have been established to protect the donor from possible ill effects of donation and to protect the recipient from exposure to diseases transmitted through the blood. Blood donors are unpaid volunteers. Potential donors may be declined if they have a history of hepatitis, convulsions, human immunodeficiency virus (HIV) infection (or risk factors for HIV infection), heart disease, most cancers, severe asthma, or bleeding disorders. Donation may be deferred for people with malaria or who have been exposed to malaria or hepatitis, or in situations of pregnancy, surgery, anemia, or high or low blood pressure, and if the donor is taking certain drugs.

Blood and Blood Products for Transfusion Not all clients require transfusion of whole blood; many times, transfusion of a particular blood component is more appropriate. Table 43.13 lists some of the common blood products that can be transfused.

Transfusion Reactions Transfusion of ABO or Rh incompatible blood can result in a **hemolytic transfusion reaction** with destruction of the transfused RBCs and subsequent risk of kidney damage or failure. Other forms of transfusion reaction can occur, including febrile reactions, allergic reactions, circulatory overload, and sepsis. Because the risk of an adverse reaction is high when blood is transfused, clients must be frequently and carefully assessed before and during transfusion. Many reactions become evident within 5 to 15 minutes of initiating the transfusion but they can develop any time during a transfusion; clients are closely monitored during the initial period of the transfusion. Stop the transfusion immediately if signs of a reaction develop. Possible transfusion reactions, their clinical signs, and nursing implications are listed in Table 43.14.

Administering Blood Special precautions are necessary when administering blood. When a transfusion is ordered, obtain the blood from the blood bank just before starting the transfusion. Do not store the blood in the refrigerator on the nursing unit; lack of temperature control can damage the blood. Once blood or a blood product is removed from the refrigerator, it has a limited amount of time in which to be administered (e.g., packed RBCs should not hang for more than 4 hours after being removed from the refrigerator). Follow agency policies for verifying that the unit of blood is correct for the client.

CLINICAL ALERT

Normal saline should always be used when giving a blood transfusion. If the client has an infusion of dextrose, stop that infusion and flush the line with saline before initiating the transfusion. Solutions other than saline can cause damage to the blood components.

Blood is usually administered through an 18-gauge or 19-gauge intravenous needle or catheter; using a smaller needle can slow the infusion and damage blood cells (although a smaller gauge needle may be necessary for small children or clients with small, fragile veins). A Y-type blood transfusion set with an inline or add-on filter is used when administering blood (Figure 43.29). One arm of the administration set connects to the blood, and normal saline (0.9% NaCl) is attached to the other arm of the Y-type set. Saline is used to prime the set and

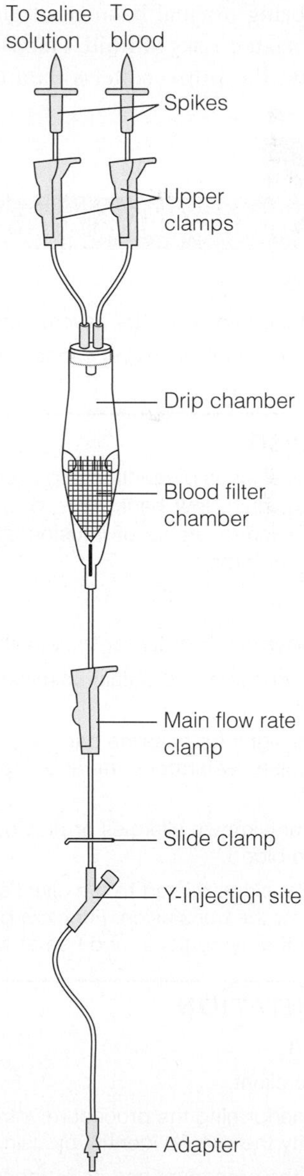

FIGURE 43.29 Schematic of a Y-set for blood administration

flush the needle before administering blood. It also provides a means to keep the vein open should a transfusion reaction occur. No other IV solutions should be administered with blood; they may cause the blood cells to clump or cause clotting. A transfusion should be completed within 4 hours of initiation, according to physician's orders and agency policy. The risk of sepsis increases if blood hangs for a longer period. Blood tubing is changed after every 4 to 6 units, per agency protocol; new intravenous tubing is used following a transfusion.

To initiate, maintain, and terminate a blood transfusion, see Skill 43.6.

Evaluating

By using the overall goals identified in the planning stage of maintaining or restoring fluid balance; maintaining or restoring pulmonary ventilation and oxygenation; maintaining or restoring normal balance of electrolytes; and preventing associated risks of fluid, electrolyte, and acid-base imbalances, the nurse collects data to evaluate the effectiveness of interventions. Examples of desired health outcomes for the identified goals are found in Table 43.15 (page 1425).

If desired outcomes are not achieved, the nurse, client, and support person, if appropriate, need to explore the reasons why before modifying the care plan. For example, if the outcome "Urine output is greater than 1300 mL per day and within 500 mL of intake" is not achieved, questions to be considered might include the following:

- Have other outcome measures for the goal of achieving fluid balance been met?
- Does the client understand and comply with planned fluid intake?
- Is all urinary output being measured?
- Are unusual or excessive amounts of fluid being lost by another route (e.g., gastric suction, excessive perspiration, fever, rapid respiratory rate, wound drainage)?
- Are prescribed medications being taken or administered as ordered?

SKILL 43.6

INITIATING, MAINTAINING, AND TERMINATING A BLOOD TRANSFUSION BY USING A Y-SET

PURPOSES

- To restore blood volume after severe hemorrhage
- To restore the oxygen-carrying capacity of the blood
- To provide plasma factors, such as antihemophilic factor (AHF) or factor VIII, or platelet concentrates to prevent or treat bleeding

ASSESSMENT

Assess for clinical signs of reaction (e.g., sudden chills, fever, nausea, itching, rash, low back pain, dyspnea); manifestations of hypervolemia; status of infusion site; vital signs; or any unusual symptoms.

Planning

- Verify the physician's order for transfusion.
- Verify client consent and obtain baseline data before the transfusion.
- Assess vital signs for baseline data, including blood pressure, pulse, respiratory rate and depth, and temperature.
- Determine any known allergies or previous adverse reactions to blood.
- Note specific signs related to the client's pathology and the reason for the transfusion. For example, for an anemic client, note the hemoglobin and hematocrit levels.

Equipment

- Blood product
- Blood administration set
- 250 mL normal saline for infusion
- IV pole
- Venipuncture set containing an 18-gauge or 19-gauge needle or catheter (if one is not already in place) or, if blood is to be administered quickly, a larger catheter (e.g., 14 gauge)
- Povidone-iodine solution or scrub pad (optional)
- Antiseptic swabs (preferably 2% chlorhexidine gluconate)
- Tape
- Clean gloves

IMPLEMENTATION

Preparation

1. Prepare the client.
   - Before performing the procedure, introduce yourself and verify the client's identity by using agency policy.
   - Explain the procedure and its purpose to the client. Instruct the client to report promptly any sudden chills, nausea, itching, rash, dyspnea, back pain, or other unusual symptoms.
   - If the client has an intravenous solution infusing, check whether the needle and solution are appropriate to administer blood. The preferred needle is an 18 gauge to 20 gauge, and the solution must be normal saline.

(continued)

SKILL 43.6

INITIATING, MAINTAINING, AND TERMINATING A BLOOD TRANSFUSION BY USING A Y-SET *(continued)*

Dextrose (which causes lysis of RBCs), Ringer's solution, medications and other additives, and hyperalimentation solutions are incompatible. See step 5 below if the infusing solution is not compatible.

- If the client does not have an IV solution infusing, check agency policies. In some agencies, an infusion must be running before the blood is obtained from the blood bank. In this case, you will need to perform a venipuncture on a suitable vein (see Skill 43.1) and start an IV infusion of normal saline.

Performance

1. Obtain the correct blood component for the client.
   - Check the physician's order with the requisition.
   - Check the requisition form and the blood bag label with a laboratory technician or according to agency policy. Specifically, check the client's name, identification number, blood type (A, B, AB, or O) and Rh group, the blood donor number, and the expiry date of the blood. Observe the blood for abnormal colour, RBC clumping, gas bubbles, and extraneous material. Return outdated or abnormal blood to the blood bank.
   - With another nurse (most agencies require an RN), compare the laboratory blood record (or according to agency policy) for the following:
     - **a.** The client's name and identification number
     - **b.** The number on the blood bag label
     - **c.** The ABO group and Rh type on the blood bag label
   - If any of the information does not match *exactly,* notify the charge nurse and the blood bank. Do not administer blood until discrepancies are corrected or clarified.
   - Sign the appropriate form and complete documentation with the other nurse, according to agency policy.
   - Make sure that the blood is left at room temperature for no more than 30 minutes before starting the transfusion (check agency policy). **Rationale: RBCs deteriorate and lose their effectiveness after 2 hours at room temperature. Lysis of RBCs releases potassium into the bloodstream, causing hyperkalemia**. Agencies may designate different times at which the blood must be returned to the blood bank if it has not been used. **Rationale: As blood components warm, the risk of bacterial growth also increases**. If the start of the transfusion is unexpectedly delayed, return the blood to the blood bank. Do not store blood in the unit refrigerator. **Rationale: The temperature of unit refrigerators is not precisely regulated, and the blood may be damaged**.
2. Verify the client's identity according to agency protocol (often, two nurses are required).
   - Ask the client's full name.
   - Check the client's arm band for name and ID number. Do not administer blood to a client who does not have an arm band.
3. Set up the infusion equipment.
   - Ensure that the blood filter inside the drip chamber is suitable for whole blood or the blood components to be transfused. Attach the blood tubing to the blood filter, if necessary. **Rationale: Blood filters have a surface area large enough to allow the blood components through easily but are designed to trap clots**.
   - Perform hand hygiene and observe other appropriate infection prevention and control precautions.
   - Put on gloves.
   - Close all the clamps on the Y-set: the main flow rate clamp and both Y-line clamps.
   - Hang the container on the IV pole about 1 m above the planned venipuncture site.
   - By using a twisting motion, insert the piercing pin (spike) into a container of 0.9% saline solution.
4. Prime the tubing.
   - Open the upper clamp on the normal saline tubing, and squeeze the drip chamber until it covers the filter and one-third of the drip chamber above the filter.
   - Tap the filter chamber to expel any residual air in the filter.
   - Remove the adapter cover at the tip of the blood administration set.
   - Open the main flow rate clamp, and prime the tubing with saline.
   - Close both clamps.
5. Start the saline solution.
   - If an IV solution incompatible with blood is infusing, stop the infusion, and discard the solution and tubing according to agency policy.
   - Attach the blood tubing primed with normal saline to the intravenous catheter.
   - Open the saline and main flow rate clamps, and adjust the flow rate. Use only the main flow rate clamp to adjust the rate.
   - Allow a small amount of solution to infuse to make sure there are no problems with the flow or with the venipuncture site. **Rationale: Infusing normal saline before initiating the transfusion also clears the IV catheter of incompatible solutions or medications**.
6. Prepare the blood bag.
   - Invert the blood bag gently several times to mix the cells with the plasma, according to agency policy. **Rationale: Rough handling can damage the cells**.
   - Expose the port on the blood bag by pulling back the tabs (see ❶).
   - Insert the remaining Y-set spike into the blood bag.
   - Suspend the blood bag.
   - Close the upper clamp below the IV saline solution on the Y-set.
   - Open the clamp on the blood arm of the Y-set and prime the tubing.
7. Establish the blood transfusion.
   - Close the upper clamp below the IV saline solution container. Open the upper clamp below the blood

(continued)

SKILL 43.6

INITIATING, MAINTAINING, AND TERMINATING A BLOOD TRANSFUSION BY USING A Y-SET (*continued*)

bag. The blood will run into the saline-filled drip chamber. If necessary, squeeze the drip chamber to re-establish the liquid level with drip chamber one-third full. (Tap the filter to expel any residual air within the filter.)

- Re-adjust the flow rate with the main clamp.

8. Observe the client closely for the first 5 to 10 minutes, remaining with the client. Assess frequently for the first 30 minutes after that.
   - Run the blood slowly for the first 15 minutes, at 20 drops per minute.
   - Note adverse reactions, such as chilling, nausea, vomiting, skin rash, tachycardia, or change in vital signs. **Rationale: The earlier a transfusion reaction occurs, the more severe it tends to be. Identifying such reactions promptly helps minimize the consequences.**
   - Remind the client to tell a nurse immediately if any unusual symptoms are felt during the transfusion.
   - If any of these reactions occur, report these to the nurse in charge, and take appropriate nursing action (see Table 43.14).
   - Change the IV administration set or flush IV administration line with normal saline thoroughly (according to agency policy) between units of blood products.
9. Document relevant data.
   - Record initiation of the blood transfusion, including vital signs, type of blood, blood unit number, sequence number (e.g., no. 1 of 3 ordered units), site of the venipuncture, size of the needle, and drip rate.
10. Monitor the patient.
    - Fifteen minutes after initiating the transfusion, check the client's vital signs. If there are no signs of a reaction, establish the required flow rate. Follow physician's orders and agency policy regarding length of time for transfusion. Most adults can tolerate receiving one unit of blood in 1.5 to 2 hours. Do not transfuse a unit of blood for longer than 4 hours.
    - Assess the client, including vital signs, every 30 minutes or more often, depending on the client's health status, until 1 hour after transfusion. If the client has a reaction and the blood is discontinued, send the blood bag and tubing to the laboratory for investigation of the blood.
11. Terminate the transfusion.
    - Perform hand hygiene and observe other appropriate infection prevention and control precautions.
    - Put on clean gloves.
    - If no infusion is to follow, clamp the blood tubing, and remove the needle. If another transfusion is to follow, clamp the blood tubing and open the saline infusion arm. Blood administration sets are changed within 24 hours or after 4 to 6 units of blood, per agency protocol.

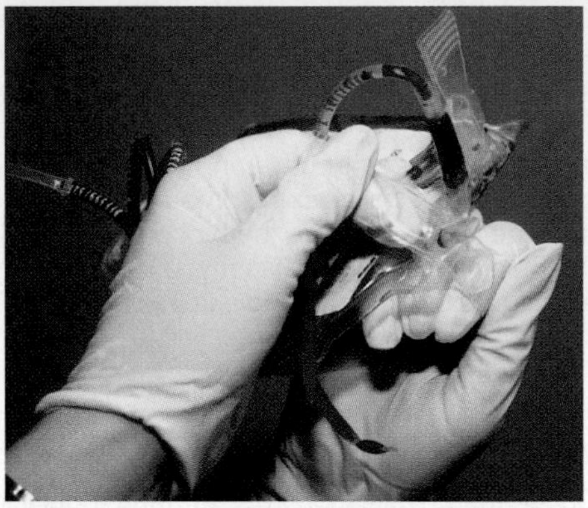

❶ Exposing the port on the blood bag by pulling back the tabs

    - If the primary IV is to be continued, flush the maintenance line with saline solution. Disconnect the blood tubing system, and re-establish the intravenous infusion by using new tubing. Adjust the drip to the desired rate. **Rationale: Often, a normal saline or other solution is kept running in case of delayed reaction to the blood.**
    - Discard the administration set according to agency practice. Needles should be placed in a labelled, puncture-resistant container designed for such disposal. Blood bags and administration sets should be bagged and labelled before being sent for decontamination and processing. See agency policy.
    - Remove gloves.
    - Again monitor vital signs.
12. Follow agency protocol for appropriate disposal of the blood bag.
    - On the requisition attached to the blood unit, fill in the time the transfusion was completed and the amount transfused.
    - Attach one copy of the requisition to the client's record and another to the empty blood bag.
    - Return the blood bag and requisition to the blood bank.
13. Document relevant data.
    - Record completion of the transfusion, the amount of blood absorbed, the blood unit number, and the vital signs and any signs and symptoms noted. If the primary intravenous infusion was continued, record connecting it. Also record the transfusion on the IV flowsheet and I & O record.

EVALUATION

Evaluate the following:

- Changes in vital signs or health status
- Presence of chills, nausea, vomiting, or skin rash

TABLE 43.15 Evaluation Goals and Outcomes: Fluid, Electrolyte, and Acid-Base Balances

Goal	Examples of Expected Health Outcomes
Maintain or restore normal fluid balance	Vital signs, including blood pressure, pulse, respirations, temperature, and central venous pressure, are within expected ranges Lung sounds are clear Urine output is greater than 1300 mL per day and within 500 mL of intake Skin turgor is elastic; tongue and mucous membranes are moist No edema is evident Thirst is absent Weight is within normal range for client Laboratory values within normal range (serum osmolality, serum sodium, hematocrit, urine specific gravity) Explains measures to prevent or treat fluid volume deficit or excess and symptoms that need to be reported to a health-care provider
Maintain or restore normal balance of electrolytes in the intracellular and extracellular compartments	Vital signs are stable and within expected ranges Alert; oriented to person, place, and time; speech clear Muscle strength is normal Absence of abnormal sensations, such as numbness, tingling around mouth or distal extremities Laboratory values within normal range (serum sodium, potassium, calcium, chloride, magnesium) Verbalizes measures to prevent future imbalances, including diet, medications
Maintain or restore pulmonary ventilation and oxygenation	Respiratory rate within normal range, no dyspnea or shortness of breath Demonstrates effective cough Lung sounds are clear Identifies specific factors leading to impaired airway clearance
Prevent associated risks (tissue breakdown, decreased cardiac output, confusion, other neurological signs)	Skin and mucous membranes are intact Skin is warm and pink Capillary refill is less than 3 seconds Lung sounds are clear Alert and oriented; no confusion evident

Case Study 43

Mr. Nelson, 74, was admitted to the hospital with a diagnosis of acute gastroenteritis following a three-day episode of fever and severe diarrhea. He is 178 cm tall and weighs 78 kg. His oral temperature is 38.7°C; pulse 98 and regular; respirations 32; and BP 106/86. His skin is flushed and diaphoretic. His lungs are clear to auscultation. His abdomen is tender throughout, and bowel sounds are hyperactive in all quadrants. His urine output is scanty and concentrated. He has an intravenous infusion of Ringer's solution infusing at 125 mL/h via an infusion pump.

Critical Thinking Questions

1. Predict the possible consequences of Mr. Nelson's fever, diarrhea, and diaphoresis on his fluid, electrolyte, and acid-base status.
2. Why do you think Ringer's solution was prescribed for Mr. Nelson rather than another type of fluid replacement, such as 5% dextrose in water?
3. Why is it important to monitor Mr. Nelson's intake and output?
4. Is it correct to assume that Mr. Nelson's intravenous infusion does not need to be monitored since it is being administered by an infusion pump? Why, or why not?
5. How would you know if Mr. Nelson was developing an acid-base imbalance related to his severe diarrhea?

After working through these questions, go to the MyNursingLab at **http://www.mynursinglab.com** to check your answers.

KEY TERMS

homeostasis
intracellular fluid (ICF)
extracellular fluid (ECF)
intravascular fluid
plasma
interstitial fluid
transcellular fluid
ions
electrolytes
cations
anions
mole
molarity
osmosis
solutes
crystalloids
colloids
solvent

osmolality
isotonic
hypertonic
hypotonic
osmotic pressure
colloid osmotic pressure (oncotic pressure)
diffusion
filtration
filtration pressure
hydrostatic pressure
active transport
insensible water loss
obligatory losses
renin-angiotensin-aldosterone system
acid
base
pH
buffer
acidosis
alkalosis
fluid volume deficit (FVD)
hypovolemia
third space syndrome
fluid volume excess (FVE)
hypervolemia
edema
dehydration
overhydration
hyponatremia
hypernatremia
hypokalemia
hyperkalemia
hypocalcemia
hypercalcemia
hypomagnesemia
hypermagnesemia
hypochloremia
hyperchloremia
hypophosphatemia
hyperphosphatemia
compensation
respiratory acidosis
respiratory alkalosis
metabolic acidosis
metabolic alkalosis
hematocrit
specific gravity
arterial blood gases (ABGs)
volume expanders
central venous catheter
peripherally inserted central catheter (PICC)
hypodermoclysis
drop factor (drip factor)
antigens
agglutinogens
antibodies
agglutinins
hemolytic transfusion reaction

CHAPTER HIGHLIGHTS

- A balance of fluids, electrolytes, acids, and bases in the body is necessary for health and life.
- The body fluid is divided into two major compartments: the intracellular fluid (ICF) inside the cells and extracellular fluid (ECF) outside the cells.
- Extracellular fluid is subdivided into three compartments: intravascular (plasma), interstitial, and transcellular. ECF constitutes about one-third of total body fluid.
- ECF is in constant motion throughout the body. It is the transport system that carries nutrients to, and waste products from, the cells.
- The percentage of total body fluids varies according to the individual's age, body fat, and gender. The younger the person, the higher the proportion of water in the body. The less body fat present, the greater the proportion of body fluid. Postadolescent females have a smaller percentage of fluid in relation to total body weight than do men.
- There are two types of electrolytes (ions): positively charged ions (cations) and negatively charged ions (anions).
- The principal ions of ECF are sodium and chloride; the principal ions of ICF are potassium and phosphate.
- Fluids and electrolytes move among the body compartments by osmosis, diffusion, filtration, and active transport.
- The major fluid pressures exerted as part of the movement of fluid and electrolytes from one compartment to another are osmotic pressure and hydrostatic pressure.
- The three sources of body fluid are fluids taken orally, food ingested, and the oxidation of food. Fluid intake is regulated by the thirst mechanism.
- Fluid output occurs chiefly through excretion of urine, although body fluid is also lost through sweat, feces, and insensible water loss.
- In healthy adults, measurable fluid intake and output should balance. The output of urine normally approximates the oral intake of fluids. Water from food and oxidation is balanced by fluid loss through the skin, respiratory process, and feces.
- A number of body systems and organs are involved in regulating the volume and composition of body fluids: the kidneys, the endocrine system, the cardiovascular system, the lungs, and the gastrointestinal system. The kidneys are the primary regulator of fluid and electrolyte balance.
- Hormones, such as antidiuretic hormone, the renin-angiotensin-aldosterone system, and the atrial natriuretic factor, are also involved in maintaining fluid balance.
- Fluid imbalances include (1) fluid volume deficit, also referred to as hypovolemia; (2) fluid volume excess, also referred to as hypervolemia; (3) dehydration, a deficit in water and increase in serum sodium level; and (4) overhydration, an excess of water and decrease in serum sodium level.
- The most common electrolyte imbalances are deficits or excesses in sodium, potassium, and calcium.
- The acid-base balance (pH) of body fluids is maintained within a precise range of 7.35 to 7.45.
- Acid-base balance is regulated by buffers that neutralize excess acids or bases; the lungs, which eliminate or retain carbon dioxide, a potential acid; and the kidneys, which excrete or conserve bicarbonate and hydrogen ions.
- Acid-base imbalance occurs when the normal 20-to-1 ratio of bicarbonate to carbonic acid is upset. Imbalances can be either respiratory or metabolic in origin; either can result in acidosis or alkalosis.
- Factors that influence an individual's fluid, electrolyte, and acid-base balance include age, gender, body size, environmental temperature, and lifestyle. Illness, trauma, surgery, and certain medications can place

individuals at risk for fluid, electrolyte, and acid-base imbalances.

- Fluid, electrolyte, and acid-base imbalance is most accurately determined through laboratory examination of blood plasma.
- Assessment relative to fluid, electrolyte, and acid-base balances includes (1) a nursing history; (2) physical examination; (3) measurement of body weight, vital signs, and fluid intake and output; and (4) various diagnostic studies of blood and urine.
- A nursing history includes data about the client's fluid and food intake; fluid output; signs of fluid, electrolyte, and acid-base imbalances; and medications, therapies, or disease processes that can disrupt these balances.
- NANDA International (2007) approved nursing diagnoses that relate specifically to fluid, electrolyte, and acid-base imbalances include *Deficient Fluid Volume, Excess Fluid Volume, Risk for Fluid Volume Imbalance,* and *Impaired Gas Exchange.*
- Other diagnoses that may be relevant are *Impaired Oral Mucous Membrane, Impaired Skin Integrity, Decreased Cardiac Output, Altered Tissue Perfusion, Activity Intolerance, Risk for Injury,* and *Acute Confusion.*
- In many instances, fluids and electrolytes are provided orally to clients who are experiencing or at risk of developing fluid deficits. The nurse needs to establish with the client a 24-hour plan for ingesting the necessary fluids and to respect the client's fluid preferences.
- For clients with fluid retention, fluids may need to be restricted; a schedule and short-term goals that make the fluid restriction more tolerable need to be developed.
- For clients experiencing excessive fluid losses, the administration of fluids and electrolytes intravenously is necessary. Meticulous aseptic technique is required when caring for clients with intravenous infusions.
- Preventing complications, such as infiltration, phlebitis, hypervolemia (circulatory overload), and infection, is an important aspect of intravenous therapy.
- The administration of blood transfusions involves accurately matching and identifying the blood for the individual, correctly identifying the recipient, and monitoring the client throughout the procedure for transfusion reactions.

ASSESS YOUR LEARNING

1. A nursing home resident has refused to eat or drink for several days and is admitted to the hospital. The nurse should expect which of the following findings?
   a. Increased blood pressure
   b. Weak, rapid pulse
   c. Moist mucous membranes
   d. Jugular vein distension
2. An older adult man brings his wife to the emergency department. He states that she has been vomiting and has had diarrhea for the past 2 days. She appears lethargic and is complaining of leg cramps. What should the nurse do first?
   a. Start an IV.
   b. Review the results of serum electrolytes.
   c. Offer the woman foods that are high in sodium and potassium content.
   d. Administer an antiemetic.
3. During a blood transfusion, the patient becomes anxious and complains of a headache and dyspnea. The nurse notes that the client is flushed. What should the nurse do first?
   a. Administer antihistamines as ordered.
   b. Discontinue the transfusion.
   c. Establish a second IV for emergency drugs.
   d. Start oxygen.
4. Which of the following ABG results indicates respiratory acidosis?
   a. pH 7.54; $PaCO_2$ 28 mm Hg; HCO_3^- 22 mmol/L
   b. pH 7.32; $PaCO_2$ 48 mm Hg; HCO_3^- 24 mmol/L
   c. pH 7.31; $PaCO_2$ 35 mm Hg; HCO_3^- 20 mmol/L
   d. pH 7.50; $PaCO_2$ 37 mm Hg; HCO_3^- 28 mmol/L
5. Mr. Blanchard, 42 years old, has been diagnosed with cancer and is being discharged with a peripherally inserted central catheter (PICC) for medication administration. What would the nurse teach Mr. Blanchard's family about working with a PICC?
   a. Inspect the area for redness and swelling on a daily basis.
   b. Flush the catheter daily.
   c. Use hydrogen peroxide to cleanse the site.
   d. Change the tubing every 24 hours.
6. Which of the following client statements indicates a need for further teaching regarding treatment for hypokalemia?
   a. "I will use avocado in my salads."
   b. "I will be sure to check my heart rate before I take my digoxin."
   c. "I will take my potassium in the morning after eating breakfast."
   d. "I will stop using my salt substitute."
7. An older adult man is admitted to the medical unit with a diagnosis of dehydration. Which of the following signs or symptoms are most representative of a sodium imbalance?
   a. Hyperreflexia
   b. Mental confusion
   c. Irregular pulse
   d. Muscle weakness
8. The client's arterial blood gas results are pH = 7.31; $PaCO_2$ = 35; HCO_3^- = 19. Which type of acid-base imbalance do these results indicate?
   a. Metabolic acidosis
   b. Respiratory acidosis
   c. Metabolic alkalosis
   d. Respiratory alkalosis
9. A client is admitted to the hospital for hypocalcemia. Nursing interventions relating to which system would have the highest priority?
   a. Renal
   b. Cardiac
   c. Gastrointestinal
   d. Neuromuscular

10. The nurse would assess for signs of hypomagnesemia in which of the following clients?

a. A client taking digoxin
b. A client with adrenal insufficiency
c. A client with bone cancer
d. A client with chronic alcoholism

*After working through these questions, go to the MyNursingLab at **http://www.mynursinglab.com** to check your answers and see explanations.*

SUGGESTED READINGS

Morris, C. G., & Low, J. (2008). Metabolic acidosis in the critically ill: Part 1. Classification and pathophysiology. *Anaesthesia, 63,* 294–301; and Morris, C. G., & Low, J. (2008). Metabolic acidosis in the critically ill: Part 2. Causes and treatment. *Anaesthesia, 63,* 396–411.

These two review articles provide detailed theory about acid-base balance and provide a comprehensive overview of metabolic acidosis.

Canadian Paediatric Society Nutrition and Gastroenterology Committee. (2006). Oral rehydration therapy and early refeeding in the management of childhood gastroenteritis. *Pediatrics Child Health, 11*(8), 527–531.

This position statement reviews the evidence supporting oral rehydration and gives important guidance for the assessment and management of dehydration in children.

Dillon, P. A., & Foglia, R. P. (2006). Complications associated with an implantable vascular access device. *Journal of Pediatric Surgery, 41,* 1582–1587.

This article is of relevance to pediatric nurses working with children who are receiving long-term therapy for such situations as infection or cancer care.

WEBLINKS

Canadian Association of Nephrology Nurses and Technologists

http://www.cannt.ca/about/overview

This is a group of health-care professionals with a commitment to specialized care of nephrology patients. The association promotes the dissemination of knowledge among those involved in the care of patients with renal disease.

The Kidney Foundation of Canada

http://www.kidney.ca

This foundation is a national volunteer organization dedicated to improving the health and quality of life of people living with kidney disease. The organization funds research and related clinical education, provides services for special needs of individuals, and actively promotes the awareness of organ donation.

Canadian Vascular Access Association (CVAA)

http://www.cvaa.info

This is a professional nursing organization dedicated to promoting standards for IV therapy and educational programs to enhance the care of patients requiring IV therapy. Note: this organization was previously named the Canadian Intravenous Nurses Association.

REFERENCES

Astle, S. M. (2005). Restoring electrolyte balance. *RN, 68*(5), 34–39.

Bulechek, G. M., Butcher, H. K., & Dochterman, J. C. (Eds.). (2008). *Nursing interventions classification (NIC).* St. Louis, MO: Mosby Elsevier.

Canadian Paediatric Society Nutrition and Gastroenterology Committee. (2006). Oral rehydration therapy and early refeeding in the management of childhood gastroenteritis. *Pediatrics Child Health, 11*(8), 527–531.

Canadian Vascular Access Association. (n.d.). *Mandatory use of safety devices for the prevention of sharps injury and exposure to body fluids.* Accessed July 7, 2008, from http://www.cvaa.info/Portals/0/documents/CINA%20POSITION%20PAPER%20ON%20SAFETY.doc

Chernecky, C. C., Macklin, K., & Murphy-Ende, D. (2006). *Fluid and electrolytes.* Philadelphia, PA: W.B. Saunders.

Gillies, D., O'Riordan, L., Wallen, M., Morrison, A., Rankin, K., & Nagy, S. (2005). Optimal timing for intravenous administration set replacement. *Cochrane Database of Systematic Reviews, 4,* Art. No.: CD003588.

Hadaway, L. C. (2004). Preventing and managing peripheral extravasation. *Nursing, 34*(5), 66–67.

Hadaway, L. (2006). Technology of flushing vascular access devices. *Journal of Infusion Nursing, 29*(3), 137–145.

Infusion Nurses Society. (2000). Infusion nursing: Standards of practice. *Journal of Intravenous Nursing, 23*(6S), S1–S88.

LeBlanc, A. & Cobbett, S. (2000). Traditional practice versus evidence-based practice for IV skin preparation. *Canadian Journal of Infection Control, 15*(1), 9–14.

NANDA International. (2007). *Nursing diagnoses: Definitions and classification, 2007–2008.* Philadelphia, PA: Author.

Public Health Agency of Canada. (1997). Preventing infections associated with indwelling intravascular access devices [Electronic version]. *Canada Communicable Disease Report, 23S8.* Retrieved June 17, 2008, from http://www.phac-aspc.gc.ca/publicat/ccdr-rmtc/97vol23/23s8/iiadb_e.html

Public Health Agency of Canada. (2007). *Osteoporosis—Info-sheet for seniors.* Retrieved July 7, 2008, from http://www.phac-aspc.gc.ca/seniors-aines/pubs/info_sheets/osteoporosis/pdf/osteo_e.pdf

Registered Nurses' Association of Ontario. (2004). *Assessment and device selection for vascular access.* Toronto: Author.

Registered Nurses' Association of Ontario. (2005). *Care and maintenance to reduce vascular access complications.* Toronto: Author.

Rosenthal, K. (2006). Intravenous fluids: The whys and wherefores. *Nursing, 36*(7), 26–27.

Schettler, A. E., & Gustafson, E. M. (2004). Osteoporosis prevention starts in adolescence. *Journal of the American Academy of Nurse Practitioners, 16,* 274–282.

Silverthorn, D. U. (2006). *Human physiology: An integrated approach* (4th ed.). Upper Saddle River, NJ: Prentice Hall.

Simpson, H. (2004). Interpretation of arterial blood gases: A clinical guide for nurses. *British Journal of Nursing, 13*(9), 522–528.

Vanek, V. W. (2002). The ins and outs of venous access: Part I. *Nutrition in Clinical Practice, 17*(2), 85–98.

Zitella, L. (2004). Central venous catheter site care for blood and marrow transplant recipients. *Clinical Journal of Oncology Nursing, 7*(3), 289–298.

UNIT 7

Promoting Psychosocial Health

CHAPTER 44
Self-Concept

CHAPTER 45
Sexuality and Sexual Health Practices

CHAPTER 46
Spirituality

CHAPTER 47
Stress and Coping

CHAPTER 48
Loss, Grieving, and Death

Chapter 44

Self-Concept

A primary focus of nursing is to provide care to the individual as a whole person. This care involves assessment and intervention with biopsychosocial, spiritual, and cultural needs in every context in which care is provided. Understanding psychosocial needs begins with assessment of the individual's self-concept.

Self-concept is a person's mental image of himself or herself. A positive self-concept is essential to a person's mental and physical health. How a person views himself or herself affects successful interaction with others. Individuals with a positive self-concept are better able to develop and maintain interpersonal relationships. Those who possess a strong self-concept are better able to accept or adapt to changes that occur over the lifespan. The ability to adapt to change increases resistance to psychological and physical illness.

The role of self-concept is significant in promoting and maintaining overall health. Nurses have a responsibility to assess clients for a negative self-concept and to identify possible causes in order to help them develop a more positive view of themselves. Individuals who have a poor self-concept may express feelings of worthlessness, self-dislike, or even self-hatred. They may feel sad or hopeless, and they may state they lack energy to perform even the simplest of tasks. These behaviours can result in deterioration of health status or interfere with healing when a person is physically ill.

OBJECTIVES

After studying this chapter, you should be able to

1. Identify and describe the four dimensions of self-concept
2. Describe the effects of Erikson's psychosocial tasks on self-concept and self-esteem
3. Identify six common factors affecting self-concept and some coping strategies
4. Describe how theory related to communication and the nurse–client relationship is used in the assessment of self-concept
5. Identify factors to consider in the assessment of each component of self-concept
6. Identify nursing diagnoses related to altered self-concept
7. Describe nursing interventions designed to achieve identified outcomes for clients with altered self-concept
8. Describe eight ways to enhance client self-esteem

Self-Concept

Self-concept involves all the self-perceptions—appearance, values, and beliefs—that influence behaviour and are referred to when using the words *I* or *me*. Self-concept is a complex idea that influences the following:

- How a person thinks, talks, and acts
- How a person sees and treats another person
- Choices a person makes
- A person's ability to give and receive love
- A person's ability to take action and to change things

A self-concept has four dimensions:

1. *Self-knowledge:* the knowledge that people have about themselves, including insights into abilities, nature, and limitations
2. *Self-expectation:* what people expect of themselves, which may be a realistic or an unrealistic expectation
3. *Social self:* how people are perceived by others and society
4. *Social evaluation:* the appraisal of the self in relationship to others, events, or situations

The nurse's awareness of his or her own self-concept is an important element in the accurate assessment and promotion of positive self-concept with clients. Nurses who understand the different dimensions of themselves are better able to understand the needs, desires, feelings, and conflicts of their clients. Nurses who feel positive about themselves are more likely to help clients meet their needs.

Self-awareness refers to the relationship between a person's perception of himself or herself and others' perceptions of that person. Thus, a nurse who is very self-aware has perceptions that are very congruent with how others see the nurse. Becoming more self-aware is a process that requires time and energy and is never complete. One important component of the process is **introspection**, which involves the nurse considering his or her own beliefs, attitudes, motivations, strengths, and limitations (Donnelly, 2004). In addition to using individual reflective exercises, the nurse gains insight into the self through working with other nurses who serve as mentors and by acting on constructive feedback obtained during regular performance reviews. The nurse can also respect others and avoid projecting his or her own beliefs onto others.

While in the caregiver role, the self-aware nurse must work to suspend judgment and focus on the needs of the client, even if those differ from those of the nurse. When conflicts arise, the nurse can analyze his or her reactions through introspection and by asking the following questions:

- "What is there in me that produces this kind of reaction in the client?"
- "Why do I react this way (fear, anger, anxiety, annoyance, worry)?"
- "Can I change the way I respond to this situation to be more helpful to the client?

The relationship between nurse and client is particularly important when assessing and intervening with self-concept needs and is *central* in the provision of effective nursing care. It is through the connection between nurse and client that the impact of psychosocial needs on health is *best* understood.

Hartrick (1997) emphasizes the importance of **relational practice** in which the nurse is focused on understanding the connection between nurse and client. She identifies five relational capacities that encourage the growth of a caring relationship:

1. *Initiative, authenticity, and responsiveness,* which involve active concern for others
2. *Mutuality and synchrony,* which refer to the experience and acknowledgment of similarities and differences
3. *Honouring complexity and ambiguity,* which is focused on the ability to acknowledge and respond to uncertainty that results from the complex human experience
4. *Intentionality,* which involves congruence between values that are held and the expression of values
5. *Re-imaging,* in which the nurse explores the structures and experiences that make up his or her life and the lives of clients

A relational practice approach is important in "helping people understand and clarify the meaning of their health and healing experience and in fostering the discovery of choice and power within those experiences" (Hartrick, 1997, p. 525).

Formation of Self-Concept

A person is not born with a self-concept; rather, it develops as a result of social interactions with others. Chapter 16 discusses the development of self-concept, including Erikson's stages of development, Piaget's cognitive developmental stages, and Havighurst's developmental tasks.

According to Erikson (1963), throughout life people face developmental tasks associated with eight psychosocial stages that provide a theoretical framework. The success with which a person copes with these developmental tasks largely determines the development of self-concept. Difficulty in coping results in self-concept problems at the time and, often, later in life. Table 44.1 lists examples of behaviours indicating successful and unsuccessful resolution of these developmental tasks.

The development of a self-concept has three broad steps:

1. The infant learns that the physical self is separate and different from the environment.
2. The child internalizes others' attitudes toward himself or herself.
3. The child and adult internalize the standards of society.

TABLE 44.1 Examples of Behaviours Associated with Erikson's Stages of Psychosocial Development

Stage: Developmental Tasks	Behaviours Indicating Positive Resolution	Behaviours Indicating Negative Resolution
Infancy: trust vs. mistrust	Requesting assistance and expecting to receive it	Being unable to accept assistance
	Expressing belief of another person	Refusing to provide a person with personal information
	Sharing time, opinions, and experiences	Restricting conversation to superficialities
Toddlerhood: autonomy vs. shame and doubt	Accepting the rules of a group but also expressing disagreement when it is felt	Failing to express needs
	Expressing own opinion	Not expressing own opinion when opposed
	Easily accepting deferment of a wish fulfillment	Overconcern about being clean
Early childhood: initiative vs. guilt	Starting projects eagerly	Verbalizing fear about starting a new project
	Expressing curiosity about many things	Apologizing and being very embarrassed over small mistakes
	Demonstrating original thought	Imitating others rather than developing independent ideas
Early school years: industry vs. inferiority	Completing a task once it has been started	Not completing tasks started
	Working well with others	Not assisting with the work of others
	Using time effectively	Not organizing work
Adolescence: identity vs. role confusion	Asserting independence	Failing to assume responsibility for directing own behaviour
	Planning realistically for future roles	Failing to set goals in life
	Establishing close interpersonal relationships	Accepting the values of others without question
Early adulthood: intimacy vs. isolation	Establishing a close, intimate relationship with another person	Remaining alone
	Making a commitment to that relationship, even in times of stress and sacrifice	Avoiding close interpersonal relationships
	Accepting sexual behaviour as desirable	
Middle-aged adults: generativity vs. stagnation	Being willing to share with another person	Talking about self instead of listening to others
	Guiding others	Showing concern for self in spite of the needs of others
	Establishing a priority of needs, recognizing both self and others	Being unable to accept interdependence
Older adults: integrity vs. despair	Using past experience to assist others	Demanding unnecessary assistance and attention from others
	Maintaining productivity in some areas	Not accepting changes
	Accepting limitations	Crying and being apathetic

The term **global self** refers to the collective beliefs and images a person holds about the self. It is the most complete description that individuals can give of themselves at any one time. It is also a person's frame of reference for experiencing and viewing the world. Some of these beliefs and images represent statements of fact, for example, "I am a woman"; "I am a father"; "I am short." Others refer to less tangible aspects of self, for instance, "I am competent"; "I am shy."

Each separate image and belief has a bearing on self-concept. However, self-concept is not simply the sum of its parts. The various images and beliefs people hold about themselves are not equal in weight and prominence. Each person's self-concept is like a piece of art. At the centre of the art are the beliefs and images that are most vital to the person's identity. They constitute **core self-concept**. For example, "I am very smart"; "I am female." Images and beliefs that are less important to the person are on the periphery. For example, "I am left-handed"; "I am not athletic."

People are thought to base their self-concept on how they perceive and evaluate themselves in these areas:

- Vocational performance
- Intellectual functioning
- Personal appearance and physical attractiveness
- Sexual attractiveness and performance
- How much they are liked by others
- Ability to cope with and resolve problems
- Independence
- Particular talents

Self-concept in these areas also extends to the choices people make and perceptions they have about their health. Persons with a strong positive self-concept about appearance are likely to value healthy behaviours and take action to maintain the health of their skin, hair, and body tone, for example. Persons with negative self-concepts may be less proactive about health-promotion and illness-prevention activities.

Maintaining and evaluating a self-concept is an ongoing process. Events or situations can change the level of self-concept over time. The basic self-concept includes how people see themselves and how they are seen by others. The accuracy of self-appraisal and the congruence between the evaluation of the self and others' evaluations are important factors that must be considered. Perceptions of the self are considered in relation to the **ideal self**, which is how a person should be or would prefer to be. The ideal self is the individual's perception of how he or she should behave based on certain personal standards, aspirations, goals, and values. Adults have some idea about their **perceived self**, that is, how they see themselves and how they are seen by others. Sometimes an individual's ideal self is realistic; sometimes it is not. When the perceived self is close to the ideal self, people are quite content with what they believe they already are. A discrepancy between the ideal self and the perceived self can be an incentive to self-improvement. However, when the discrepancy is great, low self-esteem can result.

Nurses, like most people, view themselves based on internal and external inputs acquired over many years. Their ability to appraise their own strengths, the desire to follow in the steps of role models, and the feedback received from colleagues and clients are some of the influences on the nurse's self-concept.

Components of Self-Concept

The self-concept has four components: personal identity, body image, role performance, and self-esteem.

Personal Identity

Personal identity is the conscious sense of individuality and uniqueness that is continually evolving throughout life. People often view their identity in terms of name, sex, age, race, ethnic origin or culture, occupation or roles, talents, and other situational characteristics (e.g., marital status and education).

Personal identity also includes beliefs and values, personality, and character. For instance, is the person outgoing, friendly, reserved, generous, or selfish? Personal identity thus encompasses both the tangible and factual, such as name and sex, and the intangible, such as values and beliefs. Identity is what distinguishes the self from others.

A person with a strong sense of personal identity has integrated body image, role performance, and self-esteem into a complete self-concept. This sense of identity provides a person with a feeling of continuity and a unity of personality. Furthermore, the individual sees himself or herself as a unique person.

Body Image

The image of physical self, or **body image**, is how a person perceives the size, appearance, and functioning of the body and its parts. Body image has both cognitive and affective aspects. The cognitive is the knowledge of the material body; the affective includes the sensations of the body, such as pain, pleasure, fatigue, and physical movement. Body image is the sum of these attitudes, conscious and subconscious, that a person has toward his or her body.

Body image includes clothing, makeup, hairstyle, jewellery, and other things intimately connected to the person (Figure 44.1). It also includes body prostheses, such as artificial limbs, dentures, and hairpieces, as well as devices required for functioning, such as wheelchairs, canes, and eyeglasses. Past and present perceptions and how the body has evolved over time are part of body image.

A person's body image develops partly from others' attitudes and responses to that person's body and partly from the individual's own exploration of the body. For example, body image develops in infancy as the parents or caregivers respond to the child with smiles, holding, and touching, and as the child explores its own body sensations during breastfeeding, thumb sucking, and the bath. Cultural and societal values also influence a person's body image.

The various information and entertainment media have played a part over the years in how individuals view themselves and others. The "ideal" person portrayed by the media is really an unrealistic goal for many. During adolescence, concerns related to body image are of paramount concern (see the Reflect on Primary Health Care box).

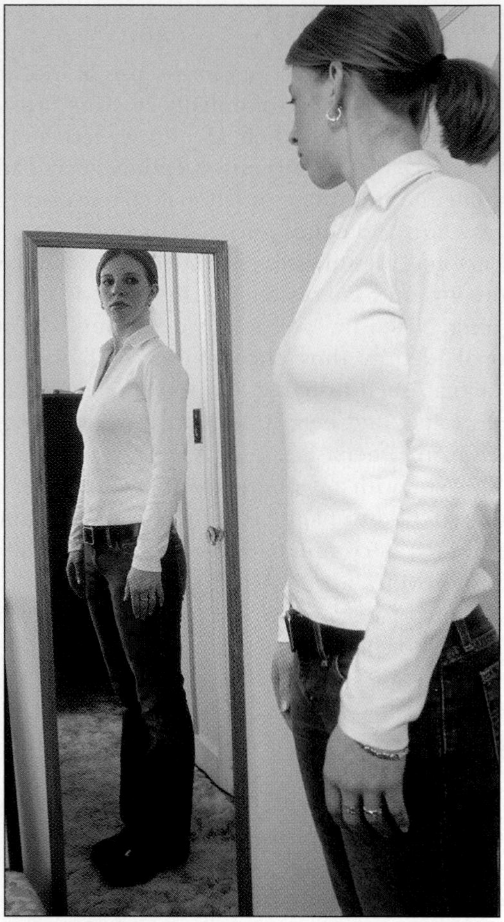

FIGURE 44.1 Body image is the sum of a person's conscious and unconscious attitudes about his or her body.

If a person's body image closely resembles that person's body ideal, the individual is more likely to think positively about the physical and nonphysical components of the self. The body ideal is greatly influenced by cultural standards. For example, in North America, the fit, well-toned body is admired.

Different parts of the body have different values for different people. For example, large breasts may be highly important to one woman and unimportant to another, or the occurrence of grey hair may be traumatic to one person and barely noticed by another.

A person with a healthy body image will normally show concern for both health and appearance. This person will be more likely to seek help if ill and will often include health-promoting practices in daily living. In contrast, a person with an unhealthy body image may neglect such activities as sleep and a healthy diet that are important to health.

The individual who has a body image disturbance may hide or not look at or touch a body part that is significantly changed in structure by illness or trauma. Some individuals also express feelings of helplessness, hopelessness, powerlessness, and vulnerability in relation to the body image changes that have occurred. These feelings can be so intense that self-destructive behaviour, such as overeating, undereating, or suicide attempts, may occur.

REFLECT ON PRIMARY HEALTH CARE

Public health nurses work collaboratively with teachers in school settings to develop sexual health education programs for preadolescent students. One of the activity components is to guide these students to develop a positive self-concept that will enable them to explore relationships and assertiveness, including ways to negotiate safe sex. This activity illustrates the principles of *health promotion* and *intersectoral collaboration*. Consider how nurses can implement the principle of *public participation* by engaging students to determine how best to deliver such sexual health education.

Role Performance

Throughout life, people undergo numerous role changes. A **role** is a set of expectations about how the person occupying one position behaves. **Role performance** relates what a person in a particular role does to the behaviours expected of that role. **Role mastery** means that the person's behaviours meet social expectations. Expectations, or standards of behaviour of a role, are set by society, a cultural group, or a smaller group to which a person belongs. Each person usually has several roles, such as husband, parent, brother, son, employee, friend, nurse, and church member. Some roles are assumed for only limited periods, such as client, student, and ill person. **Role development** involves socialization into a particular role. For example, nursing students are socialized into nursing through exposure to their instructors, practice experience, classes, laboratory simulations, and seminars.

To act appropriately, people need to know who they are in relation to others and what society expects for the positions they hold. **Role ambiguity** occurs when expectations are unclear, and people do not know what to do or how to do it and are unable to predict the reactions of others to their behaviour. Failure to master a role creates frustration and feelings of inadequacy, often with consequent lowered self-esteem.

Self-concept is also affected by role strain and role conflicts. People undergoing **role strain** are frustrated because they feel or are made to feel inadequate in or unsuited to a role. Role strain is often associated with sex-role stereotypes. For example, women in occupations traditionally held by men might be treated as having less knowledge and competence than men have in the same roles.

Role conflicts arise from opposing or incompatible expectations. In an interpersonal conflict, people have different expectations about a particular role. For example, a grandparent may have different expectations from the mother about how she should care for her children. In an **interrole conflict**, one person's or group's role expectations differ from the expectations of another person or group. For example, a woman who has little flexibility in her full-time job schedule has a role conflict if her husband expects her to handle all childcare problems. In a person-role conflict, role expectations violate the beliefs or values of the role occupant. For example, a nurse in a family planning clinic may be expected to advise couples about birth control methods that are inconsistent with the nurse's belief system regarding prevention or management of unwanted pregnancy. Role conflict can lead to tension, a decrease in self-esteem, and embarrassment if needs for achievement, independence, and recognition are unmet.

CLINICAL ALERT

According to Maslow, if an individual's love and belonging needs are met, they are more likely to achieve the need for self-esteem. Achieving this need is an important element in striving for self-actualization.

Self-Esteem

Self-esteem is a person's judgment of his or her own worth, that is, how that person's standards and performances compare with those of others and with his or her ideal self. If a person's self-esteem does not match the ideal self, then low self-concept results.

Self-esteem comes in two types: global and specific. **Global self-esteem** is how much a person likes himself or herself as a whole. **Specific self-esteem** is how much a person approves of a certain part of himself or herself. Global self-esteem is influenced by specific self-esteem. For example, if a man values his looks, then how he looks will strongly affect his global self-esteem. By contrast, if a man places little value on his cooking skills, then how well or badly he cooks will have little influence on his global self-esteem.

Self-esteem is derived from the self and others. In infancy, self-esteem is related to the caregiver's evaluations and acceptances. Later, the child's self-esteem is affected by competition with others. As an adult, a person who has high self-esteem has feelings of significance, feelings of competence, the ability to cope with life, and control over his or her destiny.

The foundation for self-esteem is established during early life experiences, usually within the family structure. However, an adult's level of overall self-esteem can change markedly from day to day and moment to moment. Severe stress—for example, stress related to prolonged illness or unemployment—can substantially lower a person's self-esteem. In health care, people who believe that their condition is viewed negatively by society may have lower self-esteem (Berge & Ranney, 2005). People frequently focus on their negative aspects and spend less time on their positive aspects. It is important that both strengths and weaknesses be identified.

Evidenced-Informed Practice

What Influences Adolescents' Self-Esteem?

Khanlou (2004) examined the global and current self-esteem levels of 550 secondary-school students in Canada. Eighteen percent of the respondents and 43.4% of respondents' parents were immigrants. Using a cross-sectional design, this survey examined the respondents' age, gender, cultural background, acculturating group, family circumstances, perception of support, and influences that promoted or challenged their current self-esteem. Results showed that a considerable portion of this study's participants had high self-esteem, with 27.6% of respondents having the highest global self-esteem level and 12.7% having the highest current self-esteem level. A significant gender difference occurred, with male adolescents having higher self-esteem than female adolescents. The findings suggested that self-esteem was generally promoted through lifestyle-oriented activities; however, its growth was largely influenced by the adolescents' relationships, school-related experiences, achievements, and attitudes toward themselves.

NURSING IMPLICATIONS: **The study findings can contribute to mental-health-promotion strategies in multicultural community settings. It is important for nurses, educators, and parents to recognize the individual, cultural, and environmental influences on adolescent mental health promotion and, in particular, on self-esteem development.**

Source: Based on "Influences on Adolescent Self-Esteem in Multicultural Canadian Secondary Schools," by N. Khanlou, 2004, *Public Health Nursing, 21*(5), pp. 404–411.

Factors That Affect Self-Concept

Many factors affect a person's self-concept. Major factors are stage of development, family and culture, stressors, resources, history of success and failure, and illness.

Stage of Development

As an individual develops, the conditions that affect the self-concept change. For example, an infant requires a supportive, caring environment, while a child requires freedom to explore and learn. An older adult's self-

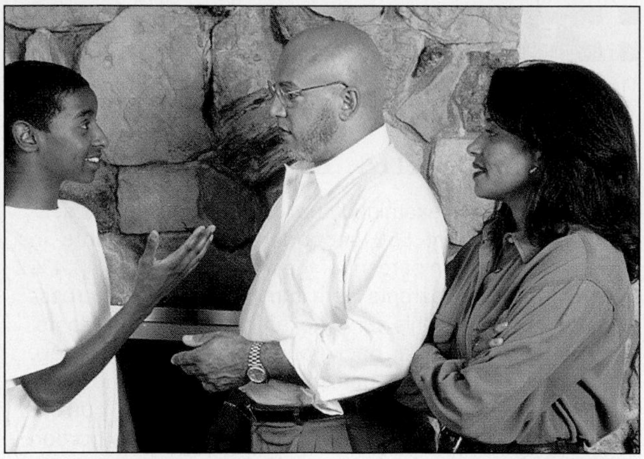

FIGURE 44.2 A child is often pulled in opposite directions by family and peer expectations.

concept is based on experiences and accomplishments in progressing through life's stages.

Family and Culture

A young child's values are largely influenced by the family and culture. Later on, peers influence the child and thereby affect the sense of self. When the child is confronted with differing expectations from family, culture, and peers, the child's sense of self is often confused (Figure 44.2). For example, a child may realize that his parents expect he will not drink alcohol and that he will attend religious services each Saturday evening. At the same time, his peers drink beer and encourage him to spend Saturday evenings with them.

Stressors

Stressors can strengthen the self-concept as an individual copes successfully with problems. Conversely, overwhelming stressors can cause maladaptive responses, including problematic substance use, withdrawal, and anxiety. A person's ability to handle stressors will largely depend on personal resources.

Resources

An individual's resources are internal and external. Examples of internal resources include confidence and values; external resources include a support network, sufficient finances, and organizations. Generally, the greater the number of resources a person has and uses, the more positive the effect on the self-concept.

History of Success and Failure

People who have a history of failure often come to see themselves as failures, whereas people who have a history of successes are more likely to have a positive self-concept. Individual judgment of success or failure is frequently determined by perceived **locus of control**. People with a strong internal locus of control believe that success is related to their own efforts in a situation and are more likely to adapt and change when the situation requires it. Individuals with an external locus of control feel they have less control over events in their lives and therefore are less likely to be motivated to change.

People with a positive self-concept tend to find contentment in their level of success, while having a negative self-concept can lead people to view their life situation as negative.

Illness

Illness and trauma can also affect the self-concept. A woman who has a mastectomy may see herself as less attractive, and the loss may affect how she acts and values herself. People respond to stressors, such as illness and alterations in function related to aging, in a variety of ways. Acceptance, denial, withdrawal, and depression are common reactions.

It is sometimes difficult to determine the direction of the relationship between self-concept and health. Some research has shown that persons with a positive self-concept may enhance their health because they are more likely to follow the health-care plan (Burkhart & Rayens, 2005). Other research shows that health conditions, including psychosocial situations, such as loss and grieving, have an impact on self-concept (Montpetit, Bisconti, & Bergeman, 2004). Thus, self-concept and health-related behaviour are intertwined.

Nursing Management

Assessing

A thorough assessment includes a psychosocial assessment of the client and the family or support person because this provides clues to actual or potential problems. The nurse assessing self-concept focuses on the four components: (1) personal identity, (2) body image, (3) role performance, and (4) self-esteem.

Before conducting a psychosocial assessment, the nurse must establish trust and a working relationship with the client. Guidelines for conducting a psychosocial assessment include the following:

- Create a quiet, private environment.
- Minimize interruptions if possible.

- Maintain appropriate eye contact.
- Sit at eye level with the client.
- Demonstrate an interest in the client's concerns.
- Indicate acceptance of the client by not criticizing, frowning, or demonstrating shock.
- Ask open-ended questions to encourage the client to talk rather than close-ended questions that tend to block free sharing.
- Avoid asking more personal questions than are actually needed.
- Minimize writing detailed notes during the interview because this can create client concern that confidential material is being "recorded" as well as interfere with your ability to focus on what the client is saying.
- Determine whether the family can provide additional information.
- Maintain confidentiality.
- Be aware of your own biases and discomforts that could influence the assessment.
- Consider how the client's behaviour is influenced by culture.

It is also important that the nurse identify any stressors that may affect aspects of the self-concept (see Box 44.1). Examples of stressors that can place a client at risk for problems with self-concept are shown in Box 44.2.

When stressors are identified, the nurse needs to determine how the client perceives the stressor. A positive, growth-oriented perception of stressful events reinforces self-worth; a negative, hopeless, defeatist perception leads to decreased self-esteem. The nurse should also explore the client's usual response to stress and determine whether this is effective by asking the client such questions as these:

- When you have a problem or face a stressful situation, how do you usually deal with it?
- Do these methods work?

BOX 44.1 CULTURALLY COMPETENT CARE: ASSESSING SELF-CONCEPT

It is the nurse's responsibility to use therapeutic communication and to remain sensitive to the effect that cultural influences will have on the client's behaviours and needs. Cultural background is not only assessed directly but also considered as a factor in the areas of self-perception, role relationships, major stressors, and coping strategies. In the area of behaviours that may suggest low self-esteem, nurses need to ask themselves the following question: Is this really a behaviour that would suggest a low self-esteem or is it part of the cultural behaviour of the client? In addition, consider whether the client might be experiencing cultural dissonance, a situation in which there are conflicting beliefs and attitudes between the client's culture and the one in which the client is living.

CLINICAL ALERT

The degree to which a stressor is perceived to affect self-concept varies from person to person. For example, whereas some people may respond to repeated failures by trying harder, others may give up.

PERSONAL IDENTITY When assessing self-concept, the information the nurse first needs is about the client's personal identity. This involves who the client believes he or she is. See the Assessment: Interview: Personal Identity box for examples of questions to ask.

BOX 44.2 STRESSORS AFFECTING SELF-CONCEPT

Many different stressors can interfere with a positive self-concept:

IDENTITY STRESSORS
- Change in physical appearance (e.g., facial wrinkles)
- Decline in physical, mental, or sensory abilities
- Inability to achieve goals
- Relationship concerns
- Sexuality concerns
- Unrealistic ideal self

BODY IMAGE STRESSORS
- Loss of body parts (e.g., amputation, mastectomy, hysterectomy)
- Loss of body functions (e.g., from stroke, spinal cord injury, neuromuscular disease, arthritis, declining mental or sensory abilities)
- Disfigurement (e.g., through pregnancy, severe burns, facial blemishes, colostomy, tracheotomy)
- Unrealistic body ideal (e.g., a muscular configuration that cannot be achieved)

SELF-ESTEEM STRESSORS
- Lack of positive feedback from significant others
- Repeated failures
- Unrealistic expectations
- Abusive relationship
- Loss of financial security

ROLE STRESSORS
- Loss of parent, spouse, child, or close friend
- Change in or loss of job or other significant role
- Divorce
- Illness
- Ambiguous or conflicting role expectations
- Inability to meet role expectations

ASSESSMENT: INTERVIEW

Personal Identity

The nurse can use the following questions to assess self-concept:

- How would you describe your personal characteristics? How do you see yourself as a person?
- How do others describe you as a person?
- What do you like about yourself?
- What do you do well?
- What are your personal strengths, talents, and abilities?
- What would you change about yourself if you could?
- Does it bother you a great deal if you think someone doesn't like you?

BODY IMAGE If a client has indications of a body image disturbance, the nurse should assess the client carefully for possible functional or physical problems. The disturbance may be a result of a present deformity or malfunction or an anticipated one. In addition to the stated responses about the problem, it is important to assess related behaviour. See the Assessment: Interview: Body Image box for examples of questions to ask about body image.

ROLE PERFORMANCE The nurse assesses the client's satisfactions and dissatisfactions associated with role responsibilities and relationships: family roles, work roles, student roles, and social roles. Family roles are especially important to people because family relationships are particularly close. Relationships can be supportive and growth producing or, at the opposite extreme, highly stressful if they contain violence or abuse. Assessment of family role relationships may begin with structural aspects, such as the number in the family group, ages, and residence locations. To obtain data related to the client's family relationships and satisfaction or dissatisfaction with work roles and social roles, the nurse might ask some of the questions shown in the Assessment: Interview: Role Performance box. Keep in mind, however, that questions need to be tailored to the individuals and their culture, age, and situation.

SELF-ESTEEM A nurse can ask the following questions to assess a client's self-esteem:

- Are you satisfied with your life?
- How do you feel about yourself?
- Are you accomplishing what you want?
- What goals in life are important to you?

It is important for the nurse to assess the client's cultural background first in order not to misinterpret specific behaviours. The following behaviours can indicate low self-esteem, but they can also be part of the client's cultural background:

- Avoids eye contact

ASSESSMENT: INTERVIEW

Body Image

Assessing body image is very important.

- Is there any part of your body you would like to change?
- Are you comfortable discussing your surgery?
- Do you feel different or inferior to others?
- How do you feel about your appearance?
- What changes in your body do you expect following your surgery?
- How have significant others in your life reacted to changes in your body?

ASSESSMENT: INTERVIEW

Role Performance

Use these questions as a base to construct questions to learn about the client's roles:

FAMILY RELATIONSHIPS

- Tell me about your family.
- What is your home like?
- How is your relationship with your spouse/partner/significant other [if appropriate]?
- What are your relationships like with your other relatives?
- How are important decisions made in your family?
- What are your responsibilities in the family?
- How well do you feel you accomplish what is expected of you?
- What about your role or responsibilities would you like changed?
- Are you proud of your family members?
- Do you feel as if your family members are proud of you?

WORK ROLES AND SOCIAL ROLES

- Do you like your work?
- How do you get along at work?
- What about your work would you like to change if you could?
- How do you spend your free time?
- Are you involved in any community groups?
- Are you most comfortable alone, with one other person, or in a group?
- Who is most important to you?
- Whom do you seek out for help?

- Stoops in posture and moves slowly
- Is poorly groomed and has an unkempt appearance
- Is hesitant or halting in speech
- Is overly critical of self (e.g., "I'm no good," "I'm ugly," or "People don't like me.")
- May be overly critical of others
- Is unable to accept positive remarks about self
- Apologizes frequently
- Verbalizes feelings of hopelessness, helplessness, and powerlessness, such as "I really don't care what happens," "I'll do whatever anyone wants," "Whatever is destined will happen"

Diagnosing

Three of the NANDA International (2007) nursing diagnostic labels relating specifically to the domain of self-perception and the classes of self-concept, self-esteem, and body image include the following (Carpenito-Moyet, 2008):

- *Disturbed Body Image*
- *Ineffective Role Performance*
- *Chronic Low Self-Esteem*

Examples of clinical applications of these diagnoses are shown in the Sample Care Plan.

Sample Care Plan for Chronic Low Self-Esteem

ASSESSMENT DATA

Nursing Assessment
George Kawazi, a first-year university student, is studying liberal arts and the sciences. George states that even though he attends all his classes and studies every day and on weekends, his grades do not please his father, who expects straight A's. "I've always had trouble measuring up to my father's expectations. He never thought I was as good as my older brother." George states, "I don't seem to do well at anything I try, I have no friends and no social life either." The nurse notes that George is poorly groomed and avoids eye contact in interactions.

Physical Examination

Height: 185 cm
Weight: 72.6 kg
Temperature: 37°C
Pulse: 84 bpm
Respirations: 20/min
Blood Pressure: 126/72 mm Hg

Diagnostic Data
Chest X-ray, CBC, and urinalysis all within normal ranges

Nursing Diagnosis
Chronic Low Self-Esteem related to unrealistic parental expectations (as evidenced by avoidance of eye contact, unkempt appearance, and statement: " I don't seem to do well at anything I try")

Client Goals
The client will demonstrate (1) an increased understanding of his negative evaluation of himself, and (2) increased feelings of self-worth.

Desired Health Outcomes

1. Demonstrate behaviour change to promote positive self-esteem
   a. Accept positive feedback from others
   b. Make eye contact in interactions with others
   c. Improve personal grooming
2. Verbalize understanding of negative evaluation of himself
   a. Identify personal strengths and limitations
3. Verbalize increased sense of self-worth

NURSING INTERVENTIONS AND SELECTED ACTIVITIES WITH RATIONALES* [*in italics*]

• Actively listen to and respect George.	*This promotes trust and acceptance.*
• Demonstrate and promote effective communication techniques.	*Effective communication increases the opportunity to receive positive validation from others.*
• Discuss George's perception of himself and encourage identification of misbeliefs and patterns of negative self-talk.	*Addressing these issues openly permits increased awareness of things that negatively affect self-esteem and provides opportunity for change.*
• Reinforce the personal strengths and positive self-perceptions that George identifies.	*Reinforcement promotes an increased sense of self-worth.*
• Assist George to challenge negative perceptions of self and performance.	*A reduction in negative thinking promotes an increase in self-esteem.*

EVALUATION
Goal met. George's grooming has improved and he is willing to make eye contact in verbal interactions with others. He has identified patterns of negative self-talk and is actively working to disrupt these patterns of thinking. George has developed a list of personal strengths and is able to identify realistic and achievable goals for himself based on these strengths.

*Interventions and activities selected are only a sample of those suggested in the *Nursing Interventions Classification (NIC),* by G. M. Bulechek, H. K. Butcher, and J. C. Dochterman (Eds.), 2008, St. Louis, MO: Mosby Elsevier, and should be individualized for each client.

Additional nursing diagnoses that may apply to clients with problems of self-concept include the following:

- *Disturbed Personal Identity*
- *Anxiety*
- *Impaired Adjustment* to changed physical functioning or appearance
- *Ineffective Coping* with role change related to death of spouse
- *Anticipatory Grieving* or *Complicated Grieving* related to change in physical appearance
- *Hopelessness*
- *Powerlessness*
- *Parental Role Conflict*
- *Readiness for Enhanced Self-Concept*
- *Disturbed Sleep Pattern*
- *Social Isolation*
- *Spiritual Distress*
- *Disturbed Thought Processes*

Planning

The nurse develops plans in collaboration with the client and his or her support system when possible, according to the client's state of health, level of anxiety, resources, coping mechanisms, and sociocultural and religious affiliation. The nurse who has little experience in intervening with clients with altered self-concept may want to consult with a more experienced nurse to develop effective plans. The nurse and client set goals to enhance the client's self-concept.

The goals established will vary according to the diagnoses and defining characteristics related to each individual. Examples of desired outcomes, interventions, and activities are shown in the Sample Care Plan box. Specific nursing orders associated with each of these activities can be selected to meet the individual needs of the client.

Implementing

Nursing interventions to promote a positive self-concept include helping a client to identify areas of strength. In addition, for clients who have an altered self-concept, nurses should establish a therapeutic relationship and help clients to evaluate themselves and make behavioural changes.

IDENTIFYING AREAS OF STRENGTH Healthy people often perceive their problems and weaknesses more easily than their assets and strengths. People with low self-esteem tend to focus even more on their limitations and to be aware of fewer strengths and many more problems. When a client has difficulty identifying personality strengths and assets, the nurse provides the client with a set of guidelines or a framework for identifying those personality strengths (Box 44.3).

Nurses can employ the following specific strategies to reinforce strengths:

- Stress positive thinking rather than self-negation.
- Notice and verbally reinforce client strengths.
- Encourage the setting of attainable goals.
- Acknowledge goals that have been attained.
- Provide honest, positive feedback.

ENHANCING SELF-ESTEEM Nurses assisting clients who have an altered self-concept must establish a therapeutic relationship. To do this the nurse must have self-awareness and effective communication skills. The following eight nursing strategies may help clients analyze the problem and enhance their self-concept:

- Encourage clients to appraise the situation and express their feelings.
- Encourage clients to ask questions.
- Provide accurate information.
- Become aware of distortions, inappropriate or unrealistic standards, and faulty labels in clients' speech.

BOX 44.3 FRAMEWORK FOR IDENTIFYING PERSONALITY STRENGTHS

Note past, present, and anticipated future participation in the following:

- Hobbies and crafts
- Expressive arts, such as writing, painting, sketching, or music appreciation
- Sports and outdoor activities, including spectator sports
- Education, training, and related areas (including self-education)
- Work, vocation, job, or position

In addition, determine the following:

- Sense of humour and the ability to laugh at self and take kidding
- Health status, including healthy aspects of body function and good health maintenance practices
- Special aptitudes, such as sales or mechanical ability; a green thumb; the ability to recognize and enjoy beauty; the ability to solve problems; a liking for adventure or pioneering; perseverance and the drive needed to get things done
- Relationship strengths, including the ability to make people feel comfortable, the capacity to enjoy being with people, the ability to be aware of people's needs and feelings, and the ability to listen
- Emotional strengths, including the capacity to give and receive warmth, affection, and love; the ability to control anger and to feel and express a wide range of emotions; and the capacity for empathy
- Spiritual strengths, such as faith (a belief in something for which there is no proof) and hope

- Explore clients' positive qualities and strengths.
- Encourage clients to express positive self-evaluation more than negative self-evaluation.
- Avoid criticism.
- Teach clients to substitute negative self-talk ("I can't walk to the store anymore") with positive self-talk ("I can walk half a block each morning"). Negative self-talk reinforces a negative self-concept.

Certain strategies vary depending on the age of the client (see the Lifespan Considerations box).

Lifespan Considerations

Enhancing Self-Esteem

CHILDREN

- Children build strong self-esteem if they develop five basic attitudes: (1) security and trust, (2) identity, (3) belonging, (4) purpose, and (5) personal competence.
- Security and trust are developed early in life; infants should not be left "to cry it out," for example, but should learn that they can rely on their parents to meet their needs promptly and consistently. With older children, trust and security are strengthened when adults spend time with them, listening, playing, reading, or just being there. Both emotional and physical contact, such as a hug, convey warmth and caring.
- Identity is developed when children are allowed to explore and experiment with the world around them and to express themselves as unique individuals in that world. They should be given opportunities to practise who they are. Preschoolers, for example, love to dress themselves and should be allowed to wear outlandish outfits (within limits of weather and safety) if they choose. Teenagers who try new hair colours and styles, some of which may upset their parents, are engaging in a crucial developmental step.
- Belonging is essential for all humans, and having a sense that others in your social network care about you, want you there, and benefit by your contribution is important to healthy self-esteem. Children gain this sense of belonging by being included in activities, by being praised for their efforts and achievements, and by being valued by parents, siblings, caregivers, and other adults. Parents should make an effort to catch their children doing well and praise them for it (e.g., "I like the way you share with your brother"). Children should also hear that they are valued just for being themselves (e.g., "I like doing things with you. Remember when we went to the park? Wasn't that fun?").
- Purpose and belonging are closely related. Children need opportunities to participate in the family and their community in order to discover what they can best contribute based on their strengths and skills. For example, a mother might say,. "Leo (age 4) is our actor. He is wonderful with costumes and can make any of us smile when he starts his routine." Leo may never become an actor, but he knows he makes a significant contribution to his family's well-being. He brings them joy.
- Personal competence grows as children identify and refine their skill sets. Children develop competence as they confront and solve problems, face challenges, expand their thinking, and are asked to do more than they think they can do. Adults must, however, provide children with support, guidance, appropriate assistance, and constructive feedback (including praise) in order to prevent the child from being overwhelmed. Too much frustration or uncertainty can lead to giving up, avoidance, lying, bullying, and other antisocial behaviours. If adults help children to accomplish goals that are important to them, children are more likely to develop a sense of personal competence and independence.
- Key ingredients for helping children develop high self-esteem are love, acceptance, firmness, consistency, and the establishment of expectations. Such qualities provide children with a safe, loving, supportive, and predictable world in which to live.

ADOLESCENTS

- Provide increasing levels of responsibility. Adolescents need to experience successes and failures and the consequences of their own behaviour.
- Encourage discussion about issues including problems and mistakes.
- Show appreciation for effort and contributions. Emphasize the process, not just the result.
- Ask for their opinions and suggestions.
- Encourage participation in decision making in areas that affect the adolescent. Show confidence in the teen's judgments.
- Avoid comparison with others, and avoid ridicule or punishment in front of others.
- Assist in the creation of realistic goals and standards.
- Adolescents often engage in volunteer activities in their schools or communities, helping them to identify their strengths and find meaning in their activities. Knowing that they have a purpose and make a difference gives them strong self-esteem.

ADULTS

- Explore the meaning of self-esteem and how the client's self-esteem has influenced past behaviours and actions (and can influence present and future plans and decisions).
- Assist the client in assessing the internal and external forces contributing to or weakening his or her self-esteem.
- Act in ways that demonstrate belief that the person can cope with the realities and demands of life and is worthy of experiencing joy and happiness.
- Avoid comparisons with other people.
- Discourage statements about the self that are negative.
- Encourage the use of affirmations to enhance self-esteem with such statements as "I like myself" or "I am a valuable person."
- Encourage associations with positive, supportive people.

(continued)

Lifespan Considerations (*continued*)

- Make positive statements about the person's past successes (major or minor).
- Help the person to make a list of his or her positive qualities and to review this list often.
- Suggest the person do things for others. Making a positive contribution enhances positive feelings of self-worth.

OLDER ADULTS

The older adult who becomes increasingly dependent can develop low self-esteem. Old age is frequently accompanied by changes, such as reduced income, decline in physical health, loss of friends and family, and retirement. In addition to those actions listed above for use with adults, nurses can use the following strategies to help older adults enhance their self-esteem:

- Encourage clients to participate in planning their own care.
- Listen carefully to their concerns.
- Help clients to identify and use their own strengths.
- Encourage them to participate in activities in which they can be successful.
- Communicate that the client is valued. Use the client's name and ask for advice.
- Encourage older adults to stay connected with their memories. Reminiscing by writing or recording an autobiography or by telling a story is an excellent way to do this.
- For older adults who are in hospitals or nursing homes, make sure that they are always shown respect and dignity and are provided privacy.
- Encourage creative activities to tap their resources. Examples are music, art, storytelling, quilting, and photography.
- Work with clients to establish goals in small steps that are achievable—this, in itself, can bolster self-esteem.

Evaluating

To determine whether client outcomes have been achieved, the nurse uses data collected during interactions with the client and significant others. If outcomes are not achieved, the nurse should explore the reasons why, considering such questions as the following:

- Have old situations recurred, triggering feelings or behaviours associated with low self-esteem?
- Have new stressful situations occurred with which the client feels unable to cope, resulting in continuing or recurrent low self-esteem?
- Are new or additional roles causing increased stress in adapting?
- Are significant others supporting the client adequately in attempts to improve self-esteem?
- Did the client follow through on referrals to appropriate agencies? Did the agencies provide the expected services?
- Were the client's expectations too high in relation to the time needed for successful resolution of self-esteem problems?

The nurse, client, and significant others need to understand that to change beliefs, feelings, and behaviours affecting self-esteem requires time and ongoing effort. Unlike many physical problems (e.g., wounds) where healing can be quickly observed, improving the self-concept can be a continuing concern and is not so easily evaluated. New crises can cause clients to doubt themselves and revert to former feelings of inadequacy. People can learn from each new situation and gain new strategies for feeling satisfied with themselves.

Case Study 44

Craig is a 20-year-old male university student who was involved in an automobile accident 3 days ago, suffering a traumatic amputation of his left lower leg. Craig's mother has remained with him since the accident and is very supportive. His father is grief stricken and having difficulty dealing with Craig's condition; Craig was captain of his university basketball team and had aspirations of becoming a professional athlete. Craig's condition is stable and he is being placed into a rehabilitation program immediately. Soon, he will be fitted for a leg prosthesis. Usually an outgoing individual, Craig is sombre and nontalkative. He does not look at his leg when dressings are being changed and he refuses to discuss his rehabilitation program.

Critical Thinking Questions

1. Given Craig's age, speculate about whether Craig's self-concept is at risk for being adversely affected by his disability.
2. What data suggest that Craig's self-esteem is being, or is at risk for being, negatively affected by his amputation?
3. What factors are likely to affect Craig's adaptation to his amputation and rehabilitation?
4. How would your interventions differ for a client with the same condition who was 70 years old?

5. How would your approach to this client change if he were from a different culture?
6. What other groups of clients, in addition to those with amputations, are at risk for the development of altered self-esteem or body image?

After working through these questions, go to the MyNursingLab at **http://www.mynursinglab.com** to check your answers.

KEY TERMS

self-concept
self-awareness
introspection
relational practice
global self
core self-concept
ideal self
perceived self
personal identity
body image
role
role performance
role mastery
role development
role ambiguity
role strain
role conflicts
interrole conflict
self-esteem
global self-esteem
specific self-esteem
locus of control

CHAPTER HIGHLIGHTS

- A positive self-concept is essential to a person's physical and psychological well-being.
- A person's self-perception can differ from the person's perception of how others see him or her and from the ideal self, that is, how the person would like to be.
- Interactions with significant others create the conditions that influence self-concept throughout life.
- When individuals are able to conceptualize the self, they begin a lifelong process of deciding whether and to what extent they are valuable and worthy.
- Individuals who grow up in families whose members value one another are likely to feel good about themselves.
- Factors affecting self-concept include development, family and culture, stressors, resources, history of success and failure, and illness.
- The nurse assesses four areas of self-concept: personal identity, body image, self-esteem, and role performance.
- Because a positive self-concept is basic to health, one of the nurse's major responsibilities is to help clients whose self-concept is disturbed to develop a more positive and realistic image of themselves.
- A trusting client–nurse relationship is essential for the effective assessment of a client's self-concept, for providing help and support, and for motivating client behaviour change.

ASSESS YOUR LEARNING

1. Julie, 10 years old, is newly diagnosed with diabetes mellitus type I. The nurse is assisting Julie and her family to understand this new diagnosis. Julie's parents are unsure if she should resume playing soccer. Julie cries and states, "I will never be normal again." What is the nurse's most appropriate response?
   a. "That's not true. Crying will only make you feel worse."
   b. "You are normal, Julie, even with diabetes."
   c. "Even with diabetes, you can still lead a normal life."
   d. "Other children have been diagnosed with diabetes."
2. Students who are juggling the responsibilities of work, school, and family are most likely to experience which of the following?
   a. Role ambiguity
   b. Role strain
   c. Role conflict
   d. Role enhancement
3. Which of the following is an appropriate desired health outcome for clients with situational low self-esteem?
   a. The client will demonstrate restored self-esteem.
   b. The client will consistently verbalize self-acceptance.

c. The client will teach adaptive skills.

d. The client will describe preoccupation with altered self.

4. An 89-year-old client states, "I'm a lost cause. I can't even stand long enough to cook my own meals anymore." Which of the following is the most appropriate response?

a. "That must be difficult. What things are you still able to do?"

b. "Well, that is to be expected at your age."

c. "Do you have someone else who can cook for you?"

d. "Are you a good cook?"

5. An adult who has failed to satisfactorily resolve the developmental task of adolescence—identity versus confusion—is most likely to show which of the following behaviours?

a. Asserts independence

b. Is unable to express personal desires

c. Has difficulty working as a member of a team

d. Goes along with the crowd in all activities

6. When asked to describe herself, a client newly diagnosed with a chronic illness describes only those roles involving others (e.g., wife, mother, medical assistant) and no personal hobbies or interests. Which of the following would be a priority nursing intervention for this client?

a. The nurse should encourage the client to identify how her treatment will affect her ability to perform those roles.

b. The nurse should encourage the client to explore the importance of and need for personal hobbies or interests.

c. The nurse should encourage the client to insist that her family be present while the treatment plan is being developed.

d. The nurse should encourage the client to go for psychological counselling for role performance in addition to her medical treatment.

7. You are caring for a client who has a nursing diagnosis of *Chronic Low Self-Esteem.* Which of the following behaviours is consistent with this diagnosis?

a. The client is assertive with authority figures.

b. The client consistently performs his family role of father.

c. The client works hard to achieve personal goals.

d. The client has difficulty making positive observations about himself.

8. Which of the following interventions are appropriate for a client with low or poor self-concept?

a. Encourage the client to compare herself with others.

b. Encourage the client to say positive things about herself.

c. Recommend the client avoid situations of having to care for others.

d. Communicate very low expectations of the client.

9. You are caring for a client with a diagnosis of *Low Self-Esteem* who is from a different cultural background. Which of the following nursing interventions best demonstrates awareness of the need to be sensitive to cultural differences?

a. Use therapeutic silence appropriately.

b. Avoid discussing issues of noncompliance.

c. Frequently use therapeutic touch to communicate with the client.

d. Have the client validate your perceptions of what the client is saying or doing.

10. You are caring for Mrs. J, a 65-year-old client with a history of demanding and aggressive behaviour. She reminds you of your grandmother. When you find yourself avoiding this client, you become concerned and seek out a colleague with whom to share your feelings about this situation. What does this behaviour best indicate?

a. An ineffective coping strategy

b. Insufficient knowledge about the client

c. Your lack of self-confidence in handling difficult clients

d. An appropriate response based on your awareness of your own behaviour

After working through these questions, go to the MyNursingLab at ***http://www.mynursinglab.com*** *to check your answers and see explanations.*

SUGGESTED READINGS

John, D., & MacArthur, C. T. (2004). *Self-esteem.* Research Network on Socioeconomic Status and Health. Retrieved October 15, 2007, from http://www.macses.ucsf.edu/Research/Psychosocial/notebook/selfesteem.html

This reading provides an overview of self-esteem in relation to health and socioeconomic status, measurements, and limitations.

Porr, C., Drummond, J., & Richter, S. (2006). Health literacy as an empowerment tool for low-income mothers. *Community Health, 29*(4), 328–335.

This article reinforces that health literacy is an important tool to equip low-income mothers with the necessary knowledge and skills to gain control over their lives and optimize the healthy development of their children.

WEBLINKS

Growing Healthy Canadians

http://www.growinghealthykids.com

This site contains a guide for positive child development developed around six perspectives, what is known about the factors that promote the healthy development of all children and youth, and the concept of developmental transitions; and four areas of focus: positive outcomes, important influences, multiple contributors, and effective strategies.

Public Health Agency of Canada

http://www.phac-aspc.gc.ca/new_e.html

This site provides access to a number of publications relevant to self-concept and self-esteem issues of Canadians across the lifespan. A search engine allows for easy access to articles and links.

REFERENCES

Berge, M., & Ranney, M. (2005). Self-esteem and stigma among persons with schizophrenia: Implications for mental health. *Journal of Long Term Home Health Care, 6,* 139–144.

Burkhart, P. V., & Rayens, M. K. (2005). Self-concept and health locus of control: Factors related to children's adherence to recommended asthma regimen. *Pediatric Nursing, 31,* 404–409.

Carpenito-Moyet, L. (2008). *Nursing diagnoses: Application to clinical practice* (12th ed.). Philadelphia, PA: Lippincott, Williams and Wilkins.

Donnelly, G. (2004). Thinking about feeling: The value of introspection. *Holistic Nursing Practice, 18,* 275.

Erikson, E. H. (1963). *Childhood and society* (2nd ed.). New York: Norton.

Hartrick, G. (1997). Relational capacity: The foundation for interpersonal nursing practice. *Journal of Advanced Nursing, 26*(3), 523–528.

Montpetit, M., Bisconti, T., & Bergeman, C. (2004). Self-concept in bereavement: Evidence for structural change. *Gerontologist, 44,* 572–573.

NANDA International. (2007). *Nursing diagnoses: Definitions and classification, 2007–2008.* Philadelphia, PA: Author.

Chapter 45

Sexuality and Sexual Health Practices

Any discussion on sexuality must begin with what sex is understood to be and how sexuality is assumed to be experienced and expressed. The word **sex** can be used to describe the anatomical differences between men and women. However, *sex* is often used to describe specific sexual behaviour, such as sexual intercourse. The words *sex* and *gender* are sometimes used interchangeably, and often incorrectly, to denote different aspects of sexual being.

Gender refers to the ways in which a person lives life that demonstrate or reflect masculinity and femininity. Gender is understood to define the notions of "woman" and "man" that are formed in response to a particular culture's expectation of the role, and it is a social construct. Although undoubtedly some interrelationship exists between biological sex and gender, gender is distinct from the categories of biological sex.

In Western society, people come to learn what it is to live a life as either male or female in a particular way. Shifting the understanding of gender beyond a biologically driven system allows for the recognition that people can live beyond the understanding of gender, such as those who are transgendered (Butler, 1990).

The *Canadian Guidelines for Sexual Health Education* defines **sexuality** as "a central aspect of being human throughout life and [encompassing] biological sex, gender identities and roles, sexual orientation, eroticism, pleasure, intimacy and reproduction. Sexuality is experienced and expressed

OBJECTIVES

After studying this chapter, you should be able to

1. Define sex, gender, sexuality, and sexual health
2. Understand how cultural, sociopolitical, and historical contexts influence sexual health
3. Appreciate the scope and diversity of human sexual experience, including sexual identity
4. Describe influences on and changes in sexual health throughout a person's life
5. Discuss conditions, circumstances, and treatments that can interfere with sexual desire, pleasure, and performance
6. Use the nursing process to devise a plan to promote sexual health practices
7. Understand the importance of client involvement in the generation of goals for desirable sexual practices

in thoughts, fantasies, desires, beliefs, attitudes, values, behaviours, practices, roles, and relationships. While sexuality can include all of these dimensions, not all of them are always experienced or expressed. Sexuality is influenced by the interaction of biological, psychological, social, economic, political, cultural, ethical, legal, historical, religious and spiritual factors" (Health Canada, 2003).

Sexual Orientation

Beliefs about the determinants of a person's sexual orientation are varied (see Figure 45.1). Some note that homosexual and heterosexual identities often begin in childhood. Discrepancy exists between the understanding of sexual orientation as having a genetic basis and the understanding of sexual orientation as being a result of social constructions, role training, and societal norms.

Although many attempts have been made to categorize lesbian women and gay men on the basis of their perceived commonalties, the differences between and among gay and lesbian persons are as pervasive as the differences between and among heterosexual persons. Health professionals should be aware of the stereotypes that are attributed to both heterosexual and homosexual appearances and behaviours. As advocates for sexual health, nurses have a responsibility to convey and to teach others to convey a nonjudgmental attitude regarding the expression of sexuality.

Gays and lesbians tend not to disclose their sexual orientation to health-care providers for fear of being judged or of not receiving the treatment they are entitled

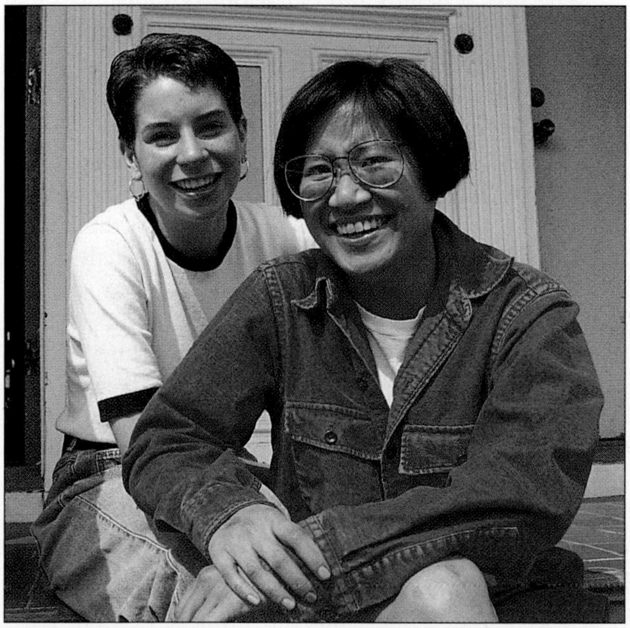

FIGURE 45.1 Many gay and lesbian relationships are based on long-term mutuality.

Evidence-Informed Practice

Lesbian Disclosure: Disrupting the Taken for Granted

In a qualitative inquiry, McDonald (2006) held conversations with 15 participants who self-identified as lesbian women. The participants talked about disclosure of their sexual orientation as an ongoing and repetitive experience in their lives. Participants revealed both the benefits and the limitations of disclosure. One of the tensions revealed in the study was between the societal pressure to disclose vulnerable truths and the sometimes deleterious effects of such disclosure, including social exclusion, isolation, discrimination, and stigmatization.

NURSING IMPLICATIONS: Nurses are challenged to consider the effects of societal beliefs and norms of heterosexuality, that is, the assumption that all people live in heterosexual arrangements, and to question the dominant categories of sexuality as adequate to speak to the realities of people's lives. Nurses need to consider the possibility that any given woman may be living a life outside heterosexuality and to engage with this reality as they encounter women as colleagues, clients, students, and research participants.

Source: Based on "Lesbian Disclosure: Disrupting the Taken for Granted," by C. McDonald, 2006, *Canadian Journal of Nursing Research, 38*(1), 42–57.

to (Stevens, 1995). *Homophobia*, a form of fear, and *heterosexism*, a form of prejudice, are two ways that health professionals' attitudes can interfere with the adequate delivery and assessment of health care. Lesbian and gay persons must also contend with the *heteronormative* (privileging heterosexuality as the norm) assumptions that underlie the health-care system (McDonald, 2006; Peterkin & Risdon, 2003).

The health experiences of lesbian, gay, and bisexual persons are like those of heterosexual persons, formed through the unique experiences of their individual lives. Experiences of sexual expression cannot be thought of as the same for individuals who name themselves lesbian, gay, bisexual, or heterosexual. Assumptions of particular sexual behaviour should not be drawn from the category of orientation that a client identifies with. Some persons who currently identify themselves as gay or lesbian have had previous sexual relationships with persons of the opposite sex. Persons who call themselves heterosexual may also engage in sexual behaviour with persons of the same sex. Some individuals who identify themselves as heterosexual or homosexual are celibate (McDonald, 2006).

Gender Identity

Western culture is deeply committed to the idea that there are only two genders. In some cases, gender is clear; in other cases, such as for transsexuals and cross-dressers, it is unclear.

Transsexuals

The medical profession considers **transsexuals** to have a condition called *gender dysphoria* (strong and persistent feelings of discomfort with the assigned gender) or *gender identity disorder*. For the transsexual person, sexual anatomy is not consistent with gender identity. Those who are born physically male but are emotionally and psychologically female are called male-to-female (MTF) transsexuals. Those who are born female but are emotionally and psychologically male are called female-to-male (FTM) transsexuals. Most transsexuals report that they have felt gender dysphoria since early childhood. They often suffer for many years and try to hide the situation from family and friends for fear of being considered mentally unstable. Being a transsexual puts women and men at extreme risk of the following:

- Being ridiculed and humiliated
- Being in constant jeopardy over getting and keeping a job
- Being asked to leave restaurants and stores without cause
- Being denied housing
- Being refused medical treatment, even to save their lives (Lips, 2005)

As self-understanding and acceptance increase, many transsexuals live part time or full time as members of the other sex. Cross-dressing (dressing in the clothing of the other sex) not only makes their outward appearance consistent with their inner identity and gender role but also increases their comfort with themselves. Their sexual orientation may be heterosexual, homosexual, or bisexual.

Cross-Dressers

Cross-dressers are typically males who cross-dress to express the feminine side of their personality. In most instances cross-dressers are not interested in permanently altering their bodies through surgical means. The majority of them are comfortable with their original birth gender identity and behaviour in their public and professional lives. Cross-dressing is a conscious choice and can occur at home or in public settings. Cross-dressing occurs more frequently in cultures in which males are expected to be strong, independent, and unemotional protectors. If the social climate is one with rigid gender roles, some men may need to express their gentleness and dependence by creating a separate world and female persona within that social climate (Barnett & Rivers, 2004).

Sexual Health

It is unlikely that any single definition of sexual health can capture the diversity of expressions of sexuality. **Sexual health** is "a state of physical, emotional, mental and social wellbeing in relation to sexuality: it is not merely the absence of disease, dysfunction or infirmity. Sexual health requires a positive and respectful approach to sexuality and sexual relationships, as well as the possibility of having pleasurable and safe sexual experiences, free of coercion, discrimination and violence. For sexual health to be attained and maintained, the sexual rights of all persons must be respected, protected and fulfilled" (Health Canada, 2003).

One limitation to our understanding of sexual health is that sexuality often comes to our attention as impairment, dysfunction, or illness. Although the focus on impairment of sexuality is an important part of a nurse's practice, it is inadequate to account for the range of experiences that are relevant to sexual health.

The sexual health and behaviour of individuals can also be compared with some perceived norm of health, without recognizing the influences of different social and cultural practices on the construction of these norms. For example, the media tends to approach sexual health with a normative attitude. In some cultures, sexual activity is presumed to imply only heterosexual intercourse, a conceptualization that narrows the understanding of what constitutes "normal" sexual activity.

Because sexuality and sexual functioning are aspects of health and well-being, they are a part of nursing care and may need to be assessed. Nurses should make their assessment nonjudgmentally, encouraging clients to discuss their concerns and offering suggestions to assist the return of sexual health. Questions that reduce heteronormative bias include the following:

- Are you in a relationship or a partnership? Who is that with, and what is your relationship with that person?
- Whom do you consider your immediate family?
- Over your lifetime, have your sexual partners been women, men, both, or neither?

- How would you like your partner or family to be involved in your care?

Clients prefer health-care professionals to initiate a discussion about sexual concerns, but many nurses expect clients to do this (Peterkin & Risdon, 2003). When no one introduces the topic of sexuality, the client is often left to resolve sexual concerns alone. Nurses require the following knowledge and skills to help clients in the area of sexuality:

- Self-knowledge and comfort with their own sexuality
- Acceptance of sexuality as an important area for nursing intervention and a willingness to work with clients who express their sexuality in a variety of ways
- Knowledge of basic sexuality, including how certain health problems and treatments can affect sexuality
- Ability to recognize the need of the client and family members to have the topic of sexuality introduced in verbal conversation, as well as through written or audiovisual materials
- Ability to create a safe and comfortable environment in which clients can discuss their sexual health

Each person's experience and expression of his or her sexuality is influenced by a unique combination of multiple factors. In planning an assessment of a person's sexual health, the nurse will consider the following:

- How does this person's race or ethnic origin influence the expression of sexuality?
- Do beliefs arising from ethnic, cultural, or religious ideologies create tension for this person in the experience with the health-care system?
- How does this person's location in a particular socioeconomic class influence experience or expression of sexual health?
- Does this person feel able to talk openly with me about particular sexual identity and health?

Sexuality throughout Life

Sexuality begins with conception and continues throughout life. Every society holds expectations about acceptable forms of sexual expression. Expectations of appropriate sexual behaviour are developed over time, they are not universal, and they may vary considerably with the cultural and ethnic background of individual clients.

It is important to be aware of ageist attitudes, which could lead to the assumption of *age-appropriate sexual expression.* Sexual expression is always grounded in the lived life of thc individual, regardless of chronological age. For example, the beginning and the ending of sexual desire is highly variable among cultures and among people within a culture.

Childhood

From birth, infants are assigned the biological sex of female or male and, by 3 years of age, begin to develop a gendered sense of themselves. Preschoolers become increasingly aware of their own and others' bodies. Body exploration and genital touching is normal and may begin in early childhood. Negative reaction to exploration of genitals and masturbation can lead to feelings of confusion about sexuality. Around age 9 or 10, the first physical changes of puberty begin: the development of breast buds in girls and the growth of pubic hair. As the adrenal glands mature, they produce more testosterone and estradiol, which contributes to the first experiences of sexual attraction to another person. Girls need to be taught about **menstruation** (monthly uterine bleeding) and related self-care.

Adolescence

During early adolescence (12 to 13 years), primary and secondary sex characteristics develop. In boys, the testes and scrotum increase in size, the skin over the scrotum becomes darker, pubic hair grows, and axillary sweating begins. Development of the genitals to adult size takes 5 to 6 years. In girls, the pelvis and hips broaden, breast tissues develop, pubic hair grows, axillary sweating begins, vaginal secretions become milky and change from alkaline to an acid pH, and vaginal flora change.

Young women should be taught about menstruation before adolescence. Although the mean age of menarche (the first menstrual period) is 12.5 years, the range of onset can vary between ages 9 to 16 years (Breslin & Lucas, 2003). Teenage women may have irregular menstruation initially. **Dysmenorrhea** (painful menstruation) is prevalent among adolescent females. They can be taught to be aware of subtle signs of impending menstruation, such as breast tenderness, water retention or bloating, or the appearance of skin eruptions or pimples. Young women should be counselled regarding the variety of feminine hygiene products available (e.g., tampons and sanitary pads) that are best for their lifestyles. Young women should be advised to wash their hands before inserting tampons, to change tampons frequently, and to use pads overnight to decrease the chances of infection.

Adolescence is the time when biological maturity occurs; it is also the time when many people become sexually active. Maticka-Tyndale (2001) points out that "sexual activity in the teenage years is not something new. It has been relatively common throughout history and continues to be common if we look across cultures" (p. 2). In most of the developed nations, the first experience of sexual intercourse is sometime during adolescence. Although the age of first intercourse for Canadians has gradually been decreasing, the mean age for first intercourse has been 17 years for both men and women since the 1960s. The average age at which both male and female Canadians have sex for the first time is 16.5 years (Roterman, 2005). In Canada, men under the age of 16 years are less likely than young men in other countries to have first intercourse. Canadian adolescents who are having intercourse at a younger age are likely to be Canadian-born youth who are from lower income households and who drop out of school. These groups tend to form a particular subset of youth, who are marginalized in a number of ways that may contribute to early sexual activity (Smylie, Medaglia, & Maticka-Tyndale, 2006).

Since half of Canadian youth are sexually active by the age of 17, it is imperative that adolescents have accurate and complete information regarding sexual health. This instruction should include education regarding the negotiation of sexual relationships, the use of contraception, and the prevention of sexually transmitted infections (STIs).

Gay, lesbian, and bisexual youth often remain *closeted* (not disclosing their sexual orientation) in their interactions with friends, family, and in school throughout adolescence. These young people continue to face rejection if they *come out* (disclose their orientation), with parental "rejection as extreme as being kicked out of the house and left to live on the streets" (Maticka-Tyndale, 2001, p. 13). During adolescence, many young people deal with issues of self-esteem, belonging, and identity; for lesbian, gay, and bisexual youth, these struggles are increased with the tensions of living in a heteronormative society and few visible role models for their development.

Human immunodeficiency virus (HIV) and acquired immune deficiency syndrome (AIDS) in Canada is spread mainly through intravenous drug use, and rates are rising among Aboriginals and women between the ages of 15 and 29. Although the highest number of new HIV and hepatitis C virus infections continues to be among gay men (45%), 27% of new infections are among women, who now make up more than 20% of the 58 000 Canadian people living with HIV or AIDS; many are unaware of their infections (Miller, Strathdee, Kerr, Li, & Wood, 2006).

Adulthood

During early adulthood, many people form emotional and sexual relationships and cohabitate with partners. Individuals establish their own value systems and develop lifestyles that reflect these personal values. Although some young adults partner in marriage and start to raise children, others cohabitate with sexual partners, live alone, or live with persons with whom they are not sexually involved.

Sexual activity is common throughout adulthood and includes not only sexual intercourse but also touching, masturbation, oral sex, sexual fantasies, and other sources of pleasure. Difficulties can arise in relationships because of differences in sexual desire and sexual response between individuals. Couples need to communicate their sexual needs to each other to support the growth and development of a successful intimate relationship.

Sexual desire and response are affected by social circumstances and biological changes throughout adulthood. During pregnancy, for example, some women and men express concerns about sexual intercourse. The Society of Obstetricians and Gynaecologists of Canada (2007) suggests that intercourse is generally safe in a healthy pregnancy up to the last month before delivery. The sexual lives of young adults are also affected by the demands of raising young children and the fatigue and stress of busy schedules.

During middle adulthood, both men and women experience decreased hormone production, causing the climacteric, usually called **menopause** in women. Most women experience menopause in the fifth decade of life. Women who report symptoms during perimenopause may experience hot flashes, vasomotor instability, sleep disturbances, vaginal dryness, mood changes, or skin, hair, and nail changes. The incidence of osteoporosis and cardiovascular lipid changes also increases following menopause.

Daniluk (1998) reported that "only a small percentage of women indicate that the cessation of menstruation and the secondary menopausal symptoms are particularly disruptive or debilitating. In fact, some women report a renewed sense of energy and creativity . . . like other transitions that occur throughout life, for most women, menopause is associated with both losses and gains. Each woman must incorporate these into her understanding of herself, as a woman, and as a sexual person" (p. 272). Similarly, Condon, (2004) talks of menopause as a time of renewed energy and focus, when midlife women "equipped with both the wisdom of their years and a new mix of hormones" (p. 507) take on new challenges. Menopause therefore should be viewed as a normal occurrence in the lives of women and not framed as a disorder that always requires medical intervention.

Troubling symptoms of menopause can, however, require intervention. Some changes in a woman's body can be effectively managed with nonprescription interventions, such as vaginal lubricants or moisturizers that increase lubrication and facilitate comfortable sexual contact. Vaginal lubrication and responsiveness to sex is also improved with continuing sexual activity. Administration of exogenous hormonal replacement therapy (HRT) is used to manage symptoms of menopause. Either oral or transdermal administration results in sustained estrogen blood levels. The decision to intervene with HRT should be made for each particular woman with consideration for the severity of her symptoms and should include a discussion of potential side effects of pharmacological intervention.

Andropause is the phase in men's lives in which they experience a gradual reduction in the production of

Lifespan Considerations

Sexuality

OLDER ADULTS

Sexuality in most older adults does not change as they get older, but their expression of it does. When they are comfortable with themselves, they can still relate to each other in a meaningful way. Sex-related changes of aging are outlined elsewhere in this chapter, as is a discussion of other contributing factors for problems related to sexual functioning. Nurses who are sensitive to these changes and challenges for older adults can be of great help in developing interventions to ease the problem and, at the same time, help older adults maintain their dignity and positive self-worth.

testosterone and sperm by the testes. Physical changes in men are less dramatic than in women. Men may, however, experience enlargement of the prostate leading to problems with voiding, a general loss of physical strength, and changes in the sexual response cycle. Although men may remain fertile into older adulthood, the ability to obtain and sustain an erection is affected by aging and the reduction in testosterone levels associated with aging.

Both women and men remain capable of and interested in sexual activity well into old age (see the Lifespan Considerations box). Older women remain capable of multiple orgasms, although as with men, the phases of the sexual response cycle may require longer to occur. As people age, the potential for obstacles to sexual intimacy increases, including chronic health conditions, such as diabetes or arthritis. These obstacles may require creative adaptation to facilitate a sexually satisfying relationship. Older adults are likely to experience social and relationship losses that affect their sexuality. These significant losses include the death of partners and the loss of privacy for those who eventually live with family or in long-term-care facilities.

Factors Influencing Sexuality

Many factors influence a person's sexuality. Discussed below are family, culture, religion, personal expectations and ethics, health and illness, and medications.

Family

For most people, the family is the earliest and most enduring social relationship. Families are the fabric of our day-to-day lives and shape the quality of our lives by influencing our outlooks on life, our motivations, our strategies for achievement, and our styles for coping with adversity. It is within our families that we develop our gender identity, body image, sexual self-concept, and capacity for intimacy. Through family interactions we learn about relationships and gender roles and our expectations of others and ourselves.

From earliest beginnings, children observe their parents and model themselves after these role models. If parents are able to share affection with each other and other family members, children will most likely become adults who are able to give and receive affection. If parents seldom hug, hold hands, or kiss each other, their children may become adults who are very uncomfortable with romantic touch. If family gender role behaviour is very rigid, arguments and hurt feelings will abound if a person from this system is partnered with a person who grew up in an androgynous family system. Family messages about sex range from "sex is so shameful it should not be talked about" to "sex is a joyful part of adult relationships."

Culture

Sexuality is structured and regulated by the individual's culture. For example, culture influences the sexual nature of dressing, rules about marriage, expectations of role behaviour and social responsibilities, and specific sex practices. Societal attitudes vary widely. Attitudes about childhood sexual play with the self or other children may be restrictive or permissive. Premarital and extramarital coitus may be unacceptable or tolerated. Polygamy (several partners) or monogamy (one partner) may be the norm.

Specific sex practices include puberty rites, body beautification, and female circumcision and genital mutilation. Puberty rites of adolescent males in native African and Australian cultures include circumcision (removal of the foreskin of the penis). Female body beautification carried out in some cultures (e.g., Democratic Republic of the Congo) to make the body more decorative involves the formation of keloids (scars) at 4 to 5 years of age from above the chest to the groin. Female circumcision or female genital mutilation, practised mostly in Africa even today, involves either excision of the clitoris, the labia minora, and the labia majora, or closure of the vagina (infibulation). The reasons for sexual mutilation vary. Infibulation may be done to guarantee the bride's virginity. Excision of the clitoris reduces sexual desire and vulnerability to temptation. In 1980, the World Health Organization and the United Nations Children's Fund (UNICEF) unanimously recommended that all forms of female circumcision be abolished.

Because clients (and colleagues) differ in their approaches to sexuality, nurses must be aware of and consider cultural factors when approaching sexual issues in health care. See Chapter 10 for additional information about culture. Some cultures have recognized gender roles beyond being a man and woman. These other gender roles can be referred to as third or fourth gender. In many Aboriginal groups, these persons are called *two-spirited.* Although the term is often used in reference to a gay, lesbian, or bisexual sexual orientation, the reference may also have a spiritual element to it. Historically called *berdache,* two-spirited people have held an important place in Aboriginal history. If a person discloses that she or he is two-spirited, the nurse would seek to understand the meaning that this holds for the client. The nurse might ask about the client's expression of her or his sexuality as a two-spirited person, how this experience is lived in daily life and relationships, or whether the person experiences difficulties in life in a predominantly heterosexual culture.

Religion

Religious beliefs influence sexual expression. They provide guidelines for sexual behaviour and acceptable circumstances for the behaviour, as well as prohibited sexual behaviour and the consequences of breaking the sexual rules. The guidelines or rules may be detailed and rigid or broad and flexible. For example, some religious ideologies dictate that forms of sexual expression other than male-female intercourse are unnatural and hold sexual activity before marriage to be unacceptable.

Some religious values conflict with the more liberal values of Canadian society. See Chapter 46 for additional information about religious values.

Personal Expectations and Ethics

Although ethics is integral to religion, ethical thought and ethical approaches to sexuality can be viewed separately from religion. Many individuals and groups have developed written or unwritten codes of conduct based on ethical principles. What one person views as bizarre, perverted, or wrong may be completely natural and right to another. Examples include masturbation, oral or anal intercourse, and cross-dressing. Many people accept sexual expression of various forms if it is performed by consenting adults, is practised in privacy, and is not harmful. Couples need to explore and communicate about various types of sexual expression to prevent domination of sexual decision making by one member of the couple.

Health and Illness

Healthy minds, bodies, and emotions are necessary for sexual wellness. Many health factors can interfere with a person's expression of sexuality.

HEART DISEASE Heart disease frequently influences sexual expression. Clients experiencing, or at risk for, myocardial infarction are often anxious about their sexuality and sexual activity. Concerns about the effect of sexual activity on the heart may cause people to restrict or avoid sexual activity. Education by health professionals can alleviate client fears following heart surgery or hospitalization for alterations in heart function. Suggestions about deciding when to resume activity based on reactions to exercise, avoiding sexual intercourse after eating large meals or consuming alcoholic beverages, choosing positions, and recognizing signs of distress can provide the couple with information that will help them make sexual activity decisions.

DIABETES MELLITUS Many men who have had diabetes mellitus for a long time develop erectile dysfunction related to neurologic and vascular changes associated with the disease process. Women who have diabetes may experience orgasmic dysfunction (loss of ability for orgasm), difficulty experiencing arousal, loss of vaginal lubrication, and painful intercourse related to a *Monilia* (yeast) infection of the vagina. The latter commonly occurs with diabetes.

SPINAL CORD INJURY Because the level of the injury to the spinal cord determines the effect on sexual functioning, individuals may be capable of erection and ejaculation and be fertile, may have psychogenic or reflexogenic genital arousal, or may have no physiological genital responses.

SURGICAL PROCEDURES Any surgical procedure has the potential to alter a person's body image, especially when the surgery involves mutilating, removing, or altering parts of the body. Examples include amputation of a leg, radical neck surgery, excision of large portions of the lower jaw, and ostomies. The impact is even greater when the surgery alters or removes body parts linked directly with sexual functioning (e.g., mastectomy, hysterectomy, and vaginal excision in women; orchiectomy [removal of the testicles] and penectomy [removal of penis] in men). Feelings of ugliness and loss of masculinity or femininity are common after these surgeries.

Many people have concerns about their reactions to their partners' surgical procedures. Having discussions with both individuals will provide facts in place of potentially erroneous beliefs about surgical procedures altering sexual behaviours. Many men fear that prostatectomy (removal of the prostate gland) can cause impotence, and they may delay seeking medical advice and treatment. Most surgical approaches for prostatectomy, however, do *not* result in impotence. Because of anatomical changes in the posterior urethra following a prostatectomy, retrograde ejaculation sometimes results; after ejaculation, the seminal fluid enters the bladder and is excreted in the urine, which affects fertility. In most instances, the man can resume sexual activity in 6 to 8 weeks. The client needs to know that the ejaculate will be decreased or absent and that the urine is often cloudy.

Some radical prostatectomies (e.g., radical perineal prostatectomy) performed for cancer of the prostate may cause impotence because of damage to the nerves responsible for producing erections. However, surgeons are now performing nerve-sparing radical prostatectomies that maintain sexual function in certain clients (Moore, Kubrik, Shea, & Kubrik, 1992).

JOINT DISEASE Joint disease can indirectly affect sexual function because of pain, stiffness, loss of joint motion, and fatigue. Such symptoms influence sexual motivation as well as sexual positioning and methods.

CHRONIC PAIN The chronic pain that accompanies many chronic illnesses often decreases sexual motivation. Altered positions for coitus may be necessary, and alternative ways to express sexual stimulation and warmth may need to be emphasized.

SEXUALLY TRANSMITTED INFECTIONS (STIs) Numerous sexually transmitted infections (STIs) exist. See Table 45.5 later in this chapter (page 1462). In some cases the presence of an STI in one partner induces fear of transmission in the other, resulting in abstinence of sexual contact. In some situations, the presence of an STI is unknown and transmission occurs without the knowledge of one or both persons involved.

MENTAL HEALTH AND ILLNESS A positive sexual self-concept (how a person values himself or herself as a sexual being) enables an individual to form intimate relationships throughout life. A negative sexual self-concept can prevent or impede the formation of relationships. A positive sexual self-concept enables an individual to be comfortable seeking pleasure and asking another to help satisfy sexual desires.

Body image, a central part of the sense of self, is constantly changing. Pregnancy, aging, trauma, disease, and therapies can alter an individual's appearance and functioning, which can affect body image. People who feel good about their bodies are likely to be comfortable with and enjoy sexual activity. People who have a poor body image may respond negatively to sexual arousal. A major influence on body image is the media's focus on a particular representation of physical attractiveness: slim, fit, and youthful bodies. Both women and men are vulnerable to the pressure to seek medical or surgical intervention to alter their attractiveness to align more closely to the images, such as large breasts, low body fat, and full heads of hair, represented in media.

Because the mind and thought processes are involved in sexual functioning, any impairment of the mind can affect sexual expression. For example, depression lowers libido and can affect both the depressed person and his or her partner. Some clients with mental disorders or brain injury behave in an inappropriate sexual manner, such as touching their genitals, removing their clothing, or seeking frequent sexual activity. Other clients, such as those with Alzheimer's disease, may not remember any previous sexual contact with their partners.

Medications

Many prescription medications have side effects that affect sexual functioning. See the section "Effects of Medications on Sexual Function" later in this chapter. Some people also take drugs to enhance sexual motivation. Amphetamines and cocaine enhance sexual motivation for some people for short periods. Lysergic acid diethylamide (LSD) and marijuana increase libido in some but inhibit it in others.

Sexual Desire and Pleasure

The sexual response is preceded by a period when sexual desire, more commonly known as **libido**, is dominant, perhaps as the result of environmental stimuli, and the individual becomes receptive to sexual activity. Sexually arousing stimuli, often called **erotic** stimuli, may be real or symbolic. In the right circumstances, imagination (sexual fantasy), sight, hearing, smell, and touch can all invoke sexual arousal. Libido fluctuates within each person and varies from person to person. The range of fluctuation in each individual is broad and is considered a problem only when the client (or someone interacting with the client) identifies it as interfering with the ability to have satisfying sexual interactions.

Sexual desire can be enhanced by various conditions and circumstances. Both males and females experience increased sexual motivation during puberty and adolescence as a result of hormonal and body changes. Certain drugs also increase libido. Several factors can also decrease sexual desire. Pregnancy can affect sexual desire if it is associated with physical discomfort, fear of injury to the fetus, or perceived loss of attractiveness. For about 4 weeks following delivery, libido is often reduced because of decreased vaginal lubrication, thinner vaginal walls, pain or fear of pain after an episiotomy, and a slower response to stimulation. Desire generally diminishes with general ill health, chronic diseases that cause disability or pain, and depression. Many prescription medications can also diminish sexual desire.

Sexual Arousal

Sexual arousal is enhanced by physical stimulation that involves touch or pressure to parts of the body and can be applied by the person himself or herself, by another's body contact, or by inanimate objects. Examples include kissing, stroking, hugging, squeezing, breast stimulation, manual stimulation of the genitals, oral-genital stimulation, and anal stimulation. Any of these may be engaged in for sexual pleasure on their own or as a prelude to genital intercourse. Physical stimulation us ed as a prelude to intercourse is called **foreplay** or **precoital stimulation**. Physical stimulation used for sexual pleasure is called **sex play**. Wide variations exist in the amount and types of physical stimulation used.

Manual self-stimulation is called **masturbation**. Reciprocal manual stimulation is called *mutual masturbation*. Stimulation of the penis generally produces a more erotic response than stimulation of the scrotum. The most common form of male masturbation is firm gripping and stroking of the shaft and glans of the penis. Light rubbing or tugging at the *frenulum* (the fold of tissue that connects the lower surface of the glans to the prepuce) can also produce sexual excitement. Whatever method is used, as sexual excitement increases, manipulation often becomes more rapid and intense, until **ejaculation** (expulsion of seminal fluid and sperm) occurs. After ejaculation, the glans penis is often hypersensitive to touch.

Stimulation of the *clitoris* is usually a major erotic focus for females. This highly sensitive area rarely requires direct stimulation. Rubbing pressure on the *mons pubis* (*mons veneris*), pulling or rubbing the clitoral hood (prepuce), or pulling on the labia stimulate the clitoral shaft and produce intensely erotic responses. Some women use external manipulation as well as insertion of fingers into the vagina to produce sexual excitement.

Manual stimulation of the genitals can be used to produce **orgasm** (climax of sexual excitement) or as a prelude to sexual intercourse.

Oral-genital stimulation has three forms: cunnilingus, fellatio, and soixante-neuf. **Cunnilingus** is oral stimulation (kissing, licking, or sucking) of the female genitals, including the mons pubis, vulva, clitoris, labia, and vagina. **Fellatio** is oral stimulation of the penis by licking and sucking. **Soixante-neuf** ("69") is simultaneous oral-genital stimulation by two persons. These practices, like other physical stimulation, can be engaged in for the pleasure they give, including orgasm, or as a prelude to genital intercourse. As with masturbation, no evidence shows that oral-genital contact is harmful.

Anal stimulation can be a source of sexual pleasure because the anus is richly innervated. Oral-anal stimulation is called **anilingus**. Stimulation can also be applied by hands or by sex aids, such as vibrators. Because the anus is associated with feces, many people do not include anal stimulation in their sexual repertoire.

Sexual Intercourse

The most common form of sexual activity for a heterosexual couple is genital intercourse, also known as **coitus** or **copulation**. Penile-vaginal intercourse can be both physically and emotionally satisfying. This kind of intercourse has a variety of positions; the most common is lying face to face (with female or male on top). Side-lying, standing, sitting, and rear-entry positions are also used. Side-lying, female-on-top, and rear-entry positions facilitate clitoral stimulation, either by penile or manual contact. The choice of intercourse positions and activities depends on physical comfort and beliefs, values, and attitudes about different practices.

During intercourse, the man moves the penis back and forth along the vaginal walls by rhythmic thrusting movements of his hips. At the same time the woman may move her own body to match the partner's hip movements. Movements continue until orgasm is achieved by one or both partners. Simultaneous orgasm is difficult to achieve. After coitus, caressing, hugging, and kissing can increase the shared intimacy. The other form of genital intercourse is **anal intercourse**, during which the penis is inserted into the anus and rectum of the partner. Anal intercourse is most commonly practised by gay men, but some heterosexual couples engage in it as well. Positions for anal intercourse are similar to those for penile-vaginal intercourse, with minor differences because of the position of the anus.

Current practice promotes the use of a condom in both forms of intercourse to prevent the transmission of disease. Because anorectal tissue is not self-lubricating, a lubricant must be used on the condom. Also, since normal bacterial flora from the bowel can produce infection in other parts of the body, the used condom should be removed and another applied before inserting the penis into other body orifices. Condoms are used for contraception as well as for preventing sexually transmitted infections. See the discussion of sexual health teaching later in this chapter.

Sexual Response Cycle

During sexual arousal, two primary physiological changes occur: **vasocongestion** (congestion of the blood vessels in the genital area) and **myotonia** (increased muscle tension). Table 45.1 summarizes the physiological changes associated with each of the phases of the sexual response cycle in both males and females. It is important to remember that many individual variations in this cycle fall within the norm.

Alternative Forms of Sexual Expression

Alternative forms of sexual expression include **voyeurism** (seeking sexual arousal by observing the body of another) and **sadomasochistic bondage** (sexual activities that involve inflicting pain or experiencing pain during sexual stimulation and can involve being tied up, hitting, whipping, pinching, scratching, and other activities). As long as these acts are performed with all parties consenting, these forms of sexual expression are not illegal. Safe

TABLE 45.1 Physiological Changes Associated with the Sexual Response Cycle

Phase of the Sexual Response Cycle	Signs Present in Both Sexes	Signs Present in Males Only	Signs Present in Females Only
Excitement or Plateau	Muscle tension increases as excitement increases Sex flush, usually on chest Nipple erection	Penile erection; glans size increases as excitement increases Appearance of a few drops of lubricant, which may contain sperm	Erection of the clitoris Vaginal lubrication Labia may increase 2 to 3 times in size Breasts enlarge Inner two-thirds of vagina widens and lengthens; outer third swells and narrows Uterus elevates
Orgasmic	Respirations may increase to 40 breaths per minute Involuntary spasms of muscle groups throughout the body Diminished sensory awareness Involuntary contractions of the anal sphincter Peak heart rate (110 to 180 bpm), respiratory rate (40/min or greater), and blood pressure (systolic 30 to 80 mm Hg and diastolic 20 to 50 mm Hg above normal)	Rhythmic, expulsive contractions of the penis at 0.8-sec intervals Emission of seminal fluid into the prostatic urethra from contraction of the vas deferens and accessory organs (stage 1 of the expulsive process) Closing of the internal bladder sphincter just before ejaculation to prevent retrograde ejaculation into bladder Orgasm can occur without ejaculation Ejaculation of semen through the penile urethra and expulsion from the urethral meatus The force of ejaculation varies from man to man and at different times but diminishes after the first two to three contractions (stage 2 of the expulsive process)	Approximately 5 to 12 contractions in the orgasmic platform at 0.8-sec intervals Contraction of the muscles of the pelvic floor and the uterine muscles Varied pattern of orgasms, including minor surges and contractions, multiple orgasms, or a simple intense orgasm similar to that of the male
Resolution	Reversal of vasocongestion in 10 to 30 min; disappearance of all signs of myotonia within 5 min Genitals and breasts return to their preexcitement states Sex flush disappears in reverse order of appearance Heart rate, respiratory rate, and blood pressure return to normal Other reactions include sleepiness, relaxation, and emotional outbursts such as crying or laughing	A refractory period during which the body will not respond to sexual stimulation; varies, depending on age and other factors, from a few moments to hours or days	

sex practices should still be included. **Pedophilia** (the sexual desire for or sexual acts involving children), however, is illegal in all cases.

Nurses may also care for clients who act out sexually or who are sexually aggressive toward or harass other clients or the nurse. Such behaviours infringe on the rights of others or are harmful to others. Nurses need to recognize this behaviour as unacceptable but also recognize it as a possible expression of a sexual concern or problem that the client may be experiencing.

Sexual Arousal Disorders

Sexual arousal refers to the physiological responses and subjective sense of excitement experienced during sexual activity. The ability to engage in genital intercourse is of great importance to most people. Many people experience transient problems with their ability to respond to sexual stimulation or to maintain the response. A smaller percentage of people experience long-standing problems.

Male Dysfunction

Three male dysfunctions are erectile dysfunction, premature ejaculation, and retarded ejaculation. **Erectile dysfunction**, more commonly referred to as **impotence**, is the inability of a man to achieve or maintain an erection sufficient for sexual satisfaction for himself or his partner. Erectile dysfunction can be caused by physiological or psychological factors. Physiological factors include (1) *neurological disorders* created by spinal cord injuries; injury to the genitals or perineal nerves; extensive surgery, such as abdominal-perineal bowel resections or radical perineal prostatectomy; diabetes mellitus; multiple sclerosis; and Parkinson's disease; and (2) *prolonged use of drugs,* such as alcohol, sedatives, heroin, antidepressants, antipsychotics (phenothiazines), and antihypertensives.

Psychological factors are often signalled by a sudden, rather than a gradual, onset. They may include (1) doubts about the ability to perform or about masculinity; (2) fatigue, anger, or stress; (3) traumatic early sexual experiences (e.g., rejection); and (4) boredom associated with the specific partner.

Premature ejaculation occurs when a man is unable to delay ejaculation long enough to satisfy his partner. "Long enough" usually means that ejaculation occurs after only very limited stimulation of the penis. Often, the ejaculation occurs either during penetration (of the vagina, mouth, or anus) or immediately thereafter. The condition can develop when the need for rapid orgasm or performance demands continue over time. To address the problem of premature ejaculation, many sex therapists advise couples to increase sexual communication and responsiveness and to decrease performance demands. The couple together practise *sensate exercises* (learning to enjoy the sensation of touch without attempting intercourse) and then work together to establish satisfying coitus.

Retarded ejaculation, or **ejaculatory incompetence**, is either the inability to ejaculate into the vagina or anus or a delayed ejaculation. Like erectile dysfunction, retarded ejaculation may have physical or psychological origins.

Female Dysfunction

Four female dysfunctions are orgasmic dysfunction, vaginismus, dyspareunia, and vulvodynia. **Orgasmic dysfunction** is the inability of a woman to reach orgasm. Orgasmic dysfunction can be caused by drugs, alcohol, aging, and anatomic abnormalities of the genitals. However, most cases have psychological causes, including hostility between partners, fear or guilt about enjoying the sexual act, and concern about performance. Therapy usually involves helping both partners to establish new attitudes about sex. Pelvic floor muscle exercises (Kegel exercises) can also increase the woman's capacity to achieve orgasm by increasing the strength of the pubococcygeus muscle. See Chapter 41 for an explanation of how to perform these exercises.

Vaginismus is the irregular and involuntary contraction of the muscles around the outer third of the vagina when coitus is attempted—that is, the vagina closes before penetration. Its causes can be severe sexual inhibition, often associated with early learning, or rape, incest, and painful intercourse. Treatment often involves sensate focus exercises and therapy to bring about psychological changes. In some instances, graduated vaginal dilators are used.

Dyspareunia describes pain experienced by a woman during intercourse as a result of inadequate lubrication, scarring, vaginal infection, or hormonal imbalance. Treatment—such as applying additional lubrication before intercourse—may correct the underlying cause.

Vulvodynia is a chronic vulvar discomfort or pain that is characterized by complaints of burning, stinging, irritation, or rawness of the female genitalia, affecting a woman's ability to engage in sexual activity. Neither the cause nor the cure is known.

Effects of Medications on Sexual Function

Many prescription medications and social drugs can affect sexual desire and response (see Table 45.2). These include central nervous system depressants, such as opiates; antianxiety agents, such as barbiturates and benzodiazepines; anticholinergic agents, such as atropine; cardiovascular agents, such as antiarrhythmics, antihypertensives, diuretics, and beta-blocking agents; antidepressants and antipsychotics; and social drugs, such as alcohol and marijuana.

Nursing Management

Assessing

Information about a client's sexual health status should always be an integral part of a nursing assessment. The amount and kind of data collected depend on the context of the assessment, that is, the client's reason for seeking health care and how the client's sexuality interacts with other problems. The nurse's professional

TABLE 45.2 Effects of Medications on Sexual Function

Medication	Possible Effects*
Alcohol	Moderate amounts: increased sexual functioning; chronic use: decreased sexual desire, orgasmic dysfunction, and erectile dysfunction
Alpha blockers	Inability to ejaculate
Amphetamines	Increased sex drive, delayed orgasm
Amyl nitrate	Reported enhanced orgasm; vasodilation, fainting
Anabolic steroids	Decreased sex drive, shrinking of testicles and infertility in men
Antianxiety agents	Decreased sexual desire; orgasmic dysfunction in women; delayed ejaculation
Anticonvulsants	Decreased sexual desire; reduced sexual response
Antidepressants	Decreased sexual desire; orgasmic delay or dysfunction in women; delayed or failed ejaculation; painful erection
Antihistamines	Decreased vaginal lubrication; decreased desire
Antihypertensives	Decreased sexual desire; erectile failure; ejaculation dysfunction
Antipsychotics	Decreased sexual desire; orgasmic dysfunction in women; delayed ejaculation; ejaculatory failure
Barbiturates	In low doses, increased sexual pleasure; in large doses, decreased sexual desire, orgasmic dysfunction, and erectile dysfunction
Beta blockers	Decreased sexual desire
Cardiotonics	Decreased sexual desire
Cocaine	Increased intensity of sexual experience; with chronic use, decreased sexual desire and sexual dysfunction
Diuretics	Decreased vaginal lubrication; decreased sexual desire; erectile dysfunction
Marijuana	As above for cocaine, but prolonged use reduces testosterone levels and reduces sperm production
Narcotics	Inhibited sexual desire and response; erectile and ejaculatory dysfunctions

*Nurses and clients must familiarize themselves with the specific medication prescribed or used, as effects vary in each category of drug.

preparation also influences the level of sexual health assessment.

Generally, the nurse conducts a sexual history as part of a complete assessment, or at these times:

- When a client is receiving care for pregnancy, infertility, contraception, or STI
- When the client's illness or therapy will affect sexual functioning (e.g., clients with diabetes, gynecological problems, heart disease)
- When the client is experiencing a sexual problem (e.g., erectile dysfunction)

NURSING HISTORY Many aspects of sexuality are integrated into the nursing history. For example, the need to collect data about erectile dysfunction in a male who has diabetes may be indicated in the review of the cardiovascular, neurological, and genitourinary systems (see the Nursing and Canadian Society box).

The screening process of the systems review allows the nurse and client to identify problem areas. For example, answers to the question "Do you have any concerns about the amount or regularity of your menstrual flow?" can give clues to the presence of problems not otherwise identified. A useful approach to psychosexual assessment is a review of sexual self-concept. Manner of dress, tone of voice, and comments about self and relationships with others can all give the nurse opportunities to explore issues of sexual self-concept more fully. Because illnesses and other health concerns can have a strong influence on sexual self-concept, assessment of these areas often provides the first clues to client concerns.

The Assessment: Interview box provides questions that the nurse can ask as part of the health history. Note that lead-in questions are asked before the questions about sexuality.

PHYSICAL EXAMINATION Physical examination of the female genitals and reproductive tract and the male genitals is part of a routine physical examination. See Chapter 27, sections on female genitals and inguinal lymph nodes and male genitals and inguinal area for details of the examination. If the client has not been examined within 1 year, or if data from the recent nursing history indicate a need, the nurse performs a physical examination. Nursing history data indicating the need for a physical examination include the following:

NURSING AND CANADIAN SOCIETY

Facts

A Canadian survey showed that staff activities and behaviours in addressing sexuality are influenced by explicit expectations (policies, job descriptions) and implicit expectations (accepted practices and the organizational culture) (Pyke, Rabin, Phillips, Moffs, & Balbirnie, 2002).

Chlamydia is the most frequently reported communicable disease in Canada. Although reported rates in Canada fell from 162 per 100 000 in 1992 to 123 per 100 000 in 1995, reported rates increased by 74% between 1997 and 2004 (Public Health Agency of Canada [PHAC], 2006).

The three nationally reportable STIs in Canada, chlamydia, gonorrhea, and infectious syphilis, are steadily increasing (Health Canada, 2003). Some of the potential social influences include the following:

- Sex is occurring at an early age, with a high rate of serially monogamous relationships.
- Sex is continuing later in life.
- Transmission of STIs associated with sexual activity (anal, oral, and vaginal) continue to be poorly understood by the public.
- Party drugs, such as ecstasy and crystal meth, are being increasingly linked to unsafe sexual behaviours.
- Anonymous partnering venues, such as the internet, are expanding.

Implications for Nursing Practice

Implicit and explicit expectations of particular workplaces will influence the degree to which clients' sexual health issues and educational needs are addressed by nursing staff.

Nurses need to remain vigilant to fluctuating changes in reported rates of sexually transmitted infections and to continue to educate clients about the use of safe sexual practices.

Nurses should be attentive to the shifting demographics of those contracting STIs and in particular to the emerging social behaviour that places people at risk for contracting STIs.

ASSESSMENT: INTERVIEW

Sexual Health History

Nurses must be comfortable taking a sexual health history from clients:

WOMEN

- When did your menstrual periods first begin, and when did you have your last menstrual period?
- What is the usual length of your period in days and usual amount of bleeding?
- Do you have any concerns about the amount or regularity of your menstrual flow?
- Are you having any burning with urination, any vaginal itching or discharge, midcycle spotting, pain with intercourse, or any other problems?
- Have you ever been pregnant? (Explore number and outcome of pregnancies, including miscarriages and induced abortions.)
- Do you regularly check your breasts for changes?
- Is there a history of breast or ovarian cancer in your family?
- Do you have a regular Pap test and mammogram?

MEN

- Are you having any difficulty with initiating urination, urinary frequency, or frequent urination at night?
- Are you having any itching or discharge from your penis?
- Do you know how to do testicular self-examination?
- How often do you do testicular self-examination?
- Is there a history of testicular cancer in your family?

MEN AND WOMEN

- Are you currently sexually active? With men, women, or both? With one or more than one partner?
- What do you do to protect yourself from infection when you are sexually active?
- Have you ever had a sexually transmitted disease?
- Have you noticed any discharge, lumps, or changes in colour, size, and shape of your genitals?
- Describe the positive and negative aspects of your sexual functioning.
- Do you have difficulty with sexual desire? arousal? orgasm? satisfaction?
- Do you experience any pain with sexual interaction?
- If there are problems, how have they influenced how you feel about yourself? How have they affected your partner? How have they affected the relationship?
- Do you expect your sexual functioning to be altered because of your illness?
- What are your partner's concerns about your future sexual functioning?
- Do you have any questions about your sexual health and functioning that I have not addressed?

- Suspicion of infertility, pregnancy, or an STI
- Reports of a discharge, a lump, or changes in the colour, shape, or size of a genital organ
- Changes in urinary function
- Need for Pap test
- Request for birth control

IDENTIFYING CLIENTS AT RISK Clients at risk for altered sexual patterns include those experiencing the following:

- Altered body structure or function caused by trauma, pregnancy, recent childbirth, anatomic abnormalities of the genitals, or disease
- Physical, psychosocial, or sexual abuse; sexual assault
- Disfiguring conditions, such as burns, skin conditions, birthmarks, scars (e.g., mastectomy), and ostomies
- Specific medication therapy that decreases sexual drive or causes erectile or ejaculatory dysfunction (see Table 45.2)
- Temporary or long-term impaired physical ability to perform grooming and maintain sexual attractiveness
- Value conflicts between personal beliefs and religious doctrine
- Loss of a partner
- Lack of knowledge or misinformation about sexual functioning and expression

Diagnosing

The NANDA International (2007) nursing diagnoses relating specifically to sexuality include the following (Carpenito-Moyet, 2008):

- *Ineffective Sexuality Patterns:* the state in which a person expresses concern regarding his or her sexuality
- *Sexual Dysfunction:* the state in which a person experiences a change in sexual function that is viewed as unsatisfying, unrewarding, or inadequate

Defining characteristics and contributing factors of these diagnoses were discussed earlier. Clinical applications of these diagnoses are shown in Table 45.3.

Nurses frequently diagnose a risk of one of the preceding two conditions because of risk factors in the client's database or because the client's illness, surgery, or therapies are associated with a high incidence of sexual concerns and problems.

Sexual problems can also be the etiology of other diagnoses, including the following:

- *Deficient Knowledge* (e.g., about conception, STIs, contraception, or normal sexual changes over the lifespan) related to misinformation and sexual myths
- *Pain* related to inadequate vaginal lubrication or effects of genital surgery
- *Anxiety* related to loss of sexual desire or functioning
- *Fear* related to history of sexual abuse or dyspareunia
- *Disturbed Body Image* (e.g., mastectomy) related to perceived sexual rejection by spouse

Planning

Goals to meet clients' sexual needs include the following:

- Maintain, restore, or improve sexual health.
- Increase knowledge of sexuality and sexual health.
- Prevent the occurrence of sexually transmitted infections.
- Prevent the spread of an existing STI.
- Increase satisfaction with the level of sexual functioning.
- Improve sexual self-concept.

TABLE 45.3 Clinical Application: Assessment Data Clusters and Related Nursing Diagnoses for Clients with Sexuality Problems

Data Cluster	Nursing Diagnosis
Marsha Ogilvy, 55 years old, reports vaginal burning and pain whenever she and her husband make love. Her last menses was 14 months ago. She says her husband is concerned about the lack of her usual response to lovemaking.	*Sexual Dysfunction* related to painful intercourse from inadequate vaginal lubrication
Georgina Honey, 49 years old, had a total mastectomy two weeks ago. She says, "I'm sure not going to be sexually appealing to my husband anymore. How on earth will he ever want to make love to me again? I feel like a lopsided oddity."	*Sexuality Pattern, Ineffective* related to body image disturbance secondary to mastectomy
Larry Stogryn, 52 years old, has a history of hypertension for which he has been taking an antihypertensive (reserpine [Serpasil]). He says he has lost interest in sex in the past few months, and when he does have sex, he has trouble keeping an erection.	*Sexuality Pattern, Ineffective* related to altered body function secondary to use of antihypertensive medication

Examples of specific desired outcomes related to some of these goals, although established in this phase, are provided in Table 45.6 in the "Evaluating" section of this chapter (page 1466). Nursing interventions to promote sexual health and function focus largely on the nurse's teaching role. For example, clients need to be taught about normal sexual function, the effects of medications on sexual function, the prevention of sexually transmitted diseases, and how to perform testicular self-examination and gain an awareness of what is normal for their breasts. In addition to teaching, nurses can do the following to help clients maintain a healthy sexual self-concept:

- Provide privacy during intimate body care.
- Involve the client's partner in physical care.
- Give attention to the client's appearance and dress.
- Give clients privacy to meet their sexual needs alone or with a partner within physically safe limits.

Implementing

The interventions the nurse selects are based on the data obtained from the client and the identified nursing diagnoses. Many interventions are directed at preventing problems the client is at risk for, providing information about sexual health, and counselling for altered sexual function.

Nurses require six basic skills to help clients in the area of sexuality:

- Self-knowledge of and comfort with their own sexuality
- Acceptance of sexuality as an important area for nursing intervention and a willingness to work with clients who express their sexuality in a variety of ways
- Knowledge of sexual growth and development throughout the life cycle
- Knowledge of basic sexuality, including how certain health problems and treatments can affect sexuality and sexual function and which interventions facilitate sexual expression and functioning
- Therapeutic communication skills
- Ability to recognize the need for all clients and family members to have the topic of sexuality introduced not only in written or audiovisual materials but also in a verbal discussion

CLINICAL ALERT

As a result of culture, age, gender, and personal characteristics, not every nurse will be comfortable discussing sex with every client. However, it is the nurse's responsibility to ensure that someone introduces the topic with the client.

PROVIDING SEXUAL HEALTH TEACHING Providing education for sexual health is an important component of nursing implementation (see the Reflect on Primary Health Care box). Many sexual problems exist as a result of sexual ignorance; many others can be prevented with effective sexual health teaching. Examples of important areas of teaching include (1) sex education, (2) responsible sexual behaviour, and (3) self-examination.

PROVIDING SEX EDUCATION Nurses can help clients to understand their anatomy and how their bodies function. For example, understanding the anatomy of the genitals may help women learn how their bodies respond to sexual stimulation. Both men and women need to learn the kind of stimulation that is pleasing and causes arousal. The importance of open communication between partners should also be encouraged. Women may also benefit from learning *Kegel exercises.* The benefits of Kegel exercises include increased pelvic floor muscle tone, increased vaginal lubrication during sexual arousal, increased sensation during intercourse, increased genital sensitivity, stronger gripping of the base of the penis, earlier postpartum recovery of the pelvic floor muscle, and increased flexibility of episiotomy scars (Berman & Berman, 2005). See the Teaching: Clinical box in Chapter 41 on Kegel muscle exercises (page 1287).

Physiological changes that occur during major developmental crises should be included as part of sexual health education. For example, the nurse needs to discuss the effects of puberty, pregnancy, menopause, and the male climacteric on sexual function. When clients experience illness or surgery that alters sexual function, the nurse needs to discuss effects of treatment (e.g., medications) and any changes that need to be undertaken to ensure safe sex (e.g., position changes or a safe time to resume sexual intercourse after a myocardial infarction).

Parents could also learn ways to answer questions and what information to provide for their children starting in the preschool years. Parents need to be the primary educators of children at an early age; however, peers, teachers, media, and toys also teach about sexual issues. See Box 45.1.

REFLECT ON PRIMARY HEALTH CARE

Sexual health education applies the principle of *health promotion* by aiming at prevention of STIs and unplanned pregnancies. Through *intersectoral cooperation*, sexual health information is integrated in the school curriculum, with public health nurses working closely with the teachers and the school board. Together, they design the best approaches, such as small groups, games, drama education, and use of the internet (appropriate technology) to meet the learning needs of the adolescents about sex, sexuality, and sexual health. Consider how the application of these primary health-care principles can transform the schools into caring communities for these young adults.

BOX 45.1 ADOLESCENT SEX EDUCATION

Teaching adolescents about sex education is an important task:

- School-based programs are an essential source of information on human sexuality and sexual health education for adolescents (Sex Information and Education Council of Canada, 2005).
- *Canadian Guidelines for Sexual Health Education* (Health Canada, 2003) notes that sexual health education should do the following:
  - Promote sexual health enhancement and positive interpersonal relationships in addition to the prevention of sexual health problems, such as unplanned pregnancies, transmission of STIs and HIV infection, and sexual exploitation and abuse.
  - Acknowledge and address the diverse needs of all students, including those who are transgendered, gay, lesbian, or bisexual.
  - Support informed decision making by providing individuals with the opportunity to develop the knowledge, personal insight, motivation, and behavioural skills that are consistent with each individual's personal values and choices.

Although awareness has increased about sexuality and sexual functioning, some people still hold certain myths and misbeliefs about sexuality. Many of these are handed down in families or are part of the beliefs in a particular culture. It is important that nurses learn about the beliefs clients hold and provide up-to-date information. See Table 45.4 for some common sexual myths and misbeliefs.

Responsible Sexual Behaviour Responsible sexual behaviour involves the prevention of sexually transmitted infections (STIs) and the prevention of unplanned pregnancy.

Prevention of STIs The prevention of STIs is an essential part of sexual health teaching, and it is the responsibility of health-care providers to maintain up-to-date knowledge of the prevention, symptoms, and treatment of STIs (see Box 45.2). Because the term *sexually transmitted infections* may elicit feelings of guilt, shame, and fear, some people are reluctant to seek health care. Clients need education about these diseases, preventive measures, and early treatment. Many STIs can be treated quickly and effectively. Others may have serious consequences.

Table 45.5 lists the common signs of STIs for which people should seek medical care. Methods for decreasing exposure to STIs are described in the Teaching: Wellness box on preventing STIs.

Prevention of Unplanned Pregnancies Prevention of unplanned pregnancies must be addressed not only with adolescents but also with couples who are timing their first birth and want to space children and limit family

TABLE 45.4 Common Sexual Misbeliefs

Misconception	Fact
Nearly all men over 70 years old are impotent.	Sexual desire and ability decrease very little after middle age.
Masturbation causes certain mental instabilities.	Masturbation is totally harmless.
Sexual activity weakens a person.	There is no evidence that sexual activity weakens a person.
Women who have experienced orgasm are more likely to become pregnant.	Conceiving is not related to experiencing orgasm.
A large penis provides greater sexual satisfaction to women than a small penis.	There is no evidence that a large penis provides greater satisfaction.
Alcohol is a sexual stimulant.	Alcohol is a relaxant and central nervous system depressant. Chronic alcoholism is associated with impotence.
Intercourse during menstruation is dangerous, i.e., it will cause vaginal tissue damage.	There is no physiological basis for abstinence during menses.
The face-to-face coital position is the moral or proper one.	The position that offers the most pleasure and is acceptable to both partners is the correct one.

BOX 45.2 SEXUALLY TRANSMITTED INFECTIONS AMONG CANADIANS

The following are some facts about STIs among Canadians:

- Human papillomavirus (HPV) is a virus that can manifest in different parts of the body that are vulnerable to infection; some forms of HPV are sexually transmitted. Particular strains of the virus have been linked to cervical cancer. It is estimated that 75% of Canadians will have a least one HPV infection in their lifetimes (Health Canada, 2007).
- HIV is the virus that causes AIDS. By the end of 2005, an estimated 58 000 Canadians were living with HIV infection and AIDS, 8000 more than at the end of 2002 (Health Canada, 2003).
- Hepatitis B is approximately 100 times more infective than HIV and carries with it a 15% to 25% risk of death from liver disease and damage. The prevalence in Canada is estimated at 0.7% to 0.9%; people who have unprotected sex with multiple partners are at high risk for contracting the infection (PHAC, 2004).

TABLE 45.5 Clinical Signs of Sexually Transmitted Infections

Disease	Male	Female
Gonorrhea	Painful urination; urethritis with watery white discharge, which may become purulent	May be asymptomatic or vaginal discharge, pain, and urinary frequency may be present
Syphilis	Chancre, usually on glans penis, which is painless and heals in 4 to 6 weeks; secondary symptoms: skin eruptions, low-grade fever, inflammation of lymph glands in 6 weeks to 6 months after chancre heals	Chancre on cervix or other genital areas, which heals in 4 to 6 weeks; symptoms same as for male
Genital warts (*Condyloma acuminatum*)	Single lesions or clusters of lesions growing beneath or on the foreskin, at the external meatus, or on the glans penis; on dry skin areas, lesions are hard and yellow-grey; on moist areas, lesions are pink or red and soft with a cauliflower-like appearance	Lesions appear at the bottom part of the vaginal opening, on the perineum, on the vaginal lips, on the inner walls of the vagina, and on the cervix
Herpes genitalis (herpes simplex of the genitals)	Primary herpes involves the presence of painful sores or large, discrete vesicles that last for weeks; vesicles rupture; recurrent herpes is itchy rather than painful; it lasts for a few hours to 10 days	Same as for males
Chlamydial urethritis	Urinary frequency; watery, mucoid urethral discharge	Commonly a carrier; vaginal discharge, dysuria (painful urination), urinary frequency
Trichomoniasis	Slight itching; moisture on top of penis; slight, early morning urethral discharge; many males are asymptomatic	Itching and redness of vulva and skin inside thighs; copious watery, frothy vaginal discharge
Candidiasis	Itching, irritation, discharge, plaque of cheesy material under foreskin	Red and excoriated vulva; intense itching of vaginal and vulvar tissues; thick, white, cheesy or curdlike discharge
Human immunodeficiency virus (HIV) and acquired immune deficiency syndrome (AIDS)	HIV attacks the person's immune system, diminishing the number of CD4 cells and lowering the person's resistance to opportunistic infections. A person is diagnosed with AIDS by the presence of 1 of the 21 opportunistic infections *or* a CD4 level of < 200. Symptoms can appear anytime from several months to several years after acquiring the virus. Symptoms include any of the following for which there is no other explanation: persistent heavy night sweats; extreme fatigue; severe weight loss; enlarged lymph glands in neck, axillae, or groin; persistent diarrhea; skin rashes; blurred vision or chronic headache; harsh, dry cough; thick grey-white coating on tongue or throat.	
Hepatitis B	Thirty percent of infected people show no symptoms. Where symptoms are present, they can include jaundice (yellowing of the skin and eyes), fatigue, loss of appetite, joint pain, abdominal pain, and general feelings of malaise.	
Human papillomavirus (HPV)	More than 100 types of HPV are known, some of which are sexually transmitted. Those viruses can cause anal-genital warts in men and women although infections are often asymptomatic. Another type of HPV, considered to be the high-risk type, is linked to cervical cancer in women and penile cancer in men. Although no tests are available for the detection of HPV, Pap testing can increase early detection of abnormalities or precancerous cells in the cervix.	

size (see Figure 45.2). Nurses need to be familiar with various contraceptive methods and their advantages, disadvantages, contraindications, effectiveness, safety, and cost. It is beyond the scope of this text to discuss contraceptives in detail. See Box 45.3 for the various methods of contraception.

SELF-EXAMINATION AND AWARENESS Early detection of cancer results in a greater chance of cure and less complex treatment. Clients need to be assured that most lumps discovered are not cancerous but that it is essential that all lumps or other detected abnormalities be checked by the client's health-care provider for accurate diagnosis. All nursing history assessments of clients need

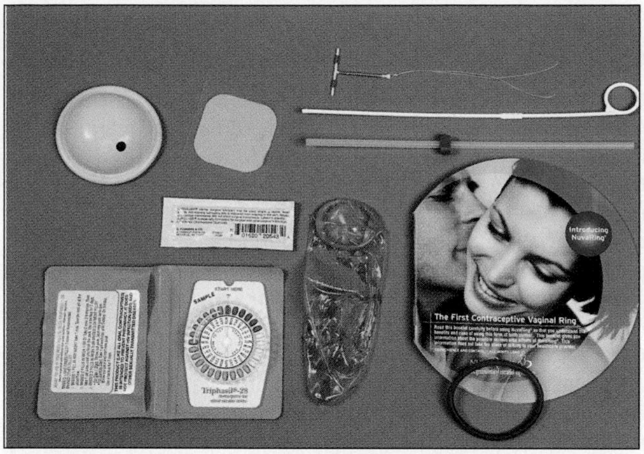

FIGURE 45.2 Methods of contraception

TEACHING: WELLNESS

Preventing Transmission of STIs

Clients need to know how to prevent STIs:

- Talk openly with partners about how to have safe sex and honestly discuss any history of an STI.
- Use condoms in all sexual relationships.
- Abstain from sexual activity with a partner *known* to have or *suspected* of having an STI.
- Report to a health-care facility for examination whenever in doubt about possible exposure or when signs of an STI are evident.
- When an STI is diagnosed, notify all partners and encourage them to seek treatment.
- Consider the use of vaccinations now available for hepatitis B and human papillomavirus (HPV).
- Women should have regular Pap tests for the early detection of STI-related cervical cell changes.

to include the client's understanding of breast awareness or testicular self-examination (TSE). Self-examination involves both inspection and palpation procedures and should be conducted regularly.

The Canadian Cancer Society (2008) and the Canadian Breast Cancer Foundation (2006) recommend that women be *familiar* with how their breasts *look and feel* normally and report any changes to their physicians (see the Teaching: Wellness box on breast awareness and mammography). Women need not follow a particular schedule or practice a standardized technique in examining their breasts. The Canadian Cancer Society recommends that women older than 40 have a clinical breast examination at least every 2 years and that women aged 50 to 69 have a mammogram every 2 years (see Skill 27.14: Assessing the Breasts and Axillae, page 618). Women younger than 40 and older than 70 can consult their health-care provider about any concerns.

BOX 45.3 METHODS OF CONTRACEPTION

Various methods are available to prevent unplanned pregnancies, some of which are more reliable than others:

- Abstinence
- Coitus interruptus (withdrawal of the penis before ejaculation)
- Fertility awareness (identification of the days of the month when conception could take place and abstaining during that time)
- Mechanical barriers: vaginal diaphragm, cervical cap, condom (male and female)
- Chemical barriers: insertion of spermicidal foams, creams, jellies, the sponge, or suppositories into the vagina before intercourse
- Intrauterine devices (IUDs)
- Hormonal: oral contraceptives (birth control pills), subdermal implants of synthetic progestin, morning after pills
- Surgical sterilization: tubal ligation and vasectomy
- Abortion

The best time for TSE is during or after a warm bath or shower, when the scrotal sac is relaxed (see the Teaching: Wellness box on TSE). Men should also be taught to inspect and palpate their chests because they have some glandular tissue beneath each nipple, a potential site for malignancy.

COUNSELLING FOR ALTERED SEXUAL FUNCTION

One technique nurses can use to help clients with altered sexual function is the PLISSIT model, developed by Annon (1974) for this purpose. The model involves four progressive levels represented by the acronym PLISSIT:

P Permission giving
LI Limited information
SS Specific suggestions
IT Intensive therapy

At each level, the nurse provides additional guidance and information to the client and, therefore, requires more specialized and specific knowledge and skill. All professional nurses should be able to function at the first three levels, described below.

PERMISSION GIVING Clients may feel that they need permission to be sexual beings, to ask questions, to show affection, and to express themselves sexually. Giving permission means that the nurse, by attitude or word, lets the client know that sexual thoughts, fantasies, and behaviours between informed consenting adults are allowed. Giving permission begins when the nurse acknowledges the client's spoken and unspoken sexual concerns and conveys the attitude that sexual concerns and needs are important to health and recovery.

TEACHING: WELLNESS

Breast Awareness and Mammography

BREAST AWARENESS

Women should become breast aware by following these five steps:

1. Know how your breasts normally look and feel.
2. Know what changes to look for.
3. Look and feel for changes.
4. Report any changes to a doctor or nurse.
5. Have regular mammograms if age appropriate or if recommended by a doctor.

Look and feel for the following changes by using the finger pads (tips) of the three middle fingers, moving in small circles, from the outside of the breast to the nipple, covering the surface (above and below) of each breast, including the armpit.

- Changes to the size or shape of one or both breasts
- Thickenings, dimples, or puckered skin of one or both breasts
- Unusual, persistent pain in the breast or armpit area
- Swelling under the armpit or below the collarbone
- Changes in the nipples, such as the shape or position of a nipple, a nipple turning inward, or crusting or scaling on a nipple

MAMMOGRAPHY

Mammography is a type of X-ray that can reveal changes inside your breasts that are too small to feel. Mammography also gives you and your doctor information about changes in your breasts that you find, or that a health professional finds during a physical examination of the breasts.

All women should discuss the risks and benefits of mammography with their doctor. Women between 50 and 69 years should have a mammogram every 2 years. If you are under age 50 or over 69 and are at a higher risk for breast cancer, you should discuss with your doctor when mammography may be appropriate for you.

Breast screening programs vary. All provinces and territories have breast cancer screening programs for women ages 50 to 69. They can make an appointment at a screening centre without a doctor's referral. Women outside that age range may need a referral.

Sources: Information adapted from *Be Breast Aware*, by the Canadian Breast Cancer Foundation, 2006, Toronto: Author. Retrieved May 19, 2008, from http://www.cbcf.org/breastcancer/bc_aware_fi.asp; and from *Signs and Symptoms of Breast Cancer*, by the Canadian Cancer Society, 2008, Toronto: Author. Retrieved May 19, 2008, from http://www.cancer.ca/ccs/internet/standard/0,3182,3172_10175_264799_langId-en,00.html

TEACHING: WELLNESS

Testicular Self-Examination

Testicular self-examination (TSE) can help detect testicular cancer early. All men should perform a TSE once each month from the time they are 15 years old. Ideally, you should examine your testicles during or after a hot bath or shower because the warmth will cause your testicles to descend and the skin of your scrotum to relax, making it easier to feel any lumps, growths, or tenderness.

- Choose one day of each month (e.g., the first or last day of each month) to examine yourself.
- Examine yourself when you are taking a warm shower or bath.
- Support the testicle underneath with one hand. Place the fingers of the other hand under the testicle and the thumb on top (this may be easier to do if the leg on that side is raised).
- Roll each testicle between the thumb and fingers of your hand, feeling for lumps, thickening, or any hardening (Figure 45.3). The testes should feel smooth.
- Palpate the epididymis, a cordlike structure on the top and back of the testicle. The epididymis should feel soft and not as smooth as a testicle.
- Locate the spermatic cord, or vas deferens, which extends upward from the scrotum toward the base of the penis. It should feel firm and smooth.
- By using a mirror, inspect your testicles for swelling, any enlargement, or lumps in the skin of the testicle.
- Report any lumps or other changes to your health-care provider promptly.

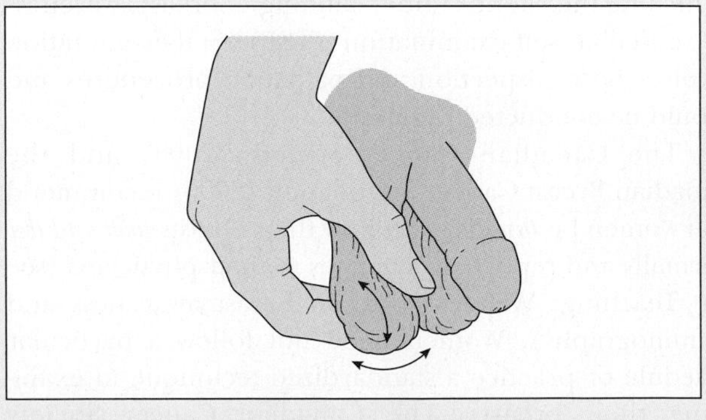

FIGURE 45.3 Rolling the testicle between the thumb and fingers

For example, the nurse might ask a client recuperating from a myocardial infarction the following questions:

- "Now that you're recuperating and you've had some time to sort out your feelings, have you thought about how your heart attack might alter your sex life?"
- "Have you and your partner discussed how you both feel about it?"

Limited Information Clients need accurate but concise information. The nurse might explain what is normal; how some medical conditions, treatments, injuries, or surgeries can affect sexuality and functioning; or how aging can affect sexuality and functioning.

Continuing with the preceding example, the nurse shares information and informs the client about how the myocardial infarction might affect the client's sex life, including the following:

- "Your heart attack will not alter your capacity for sexual response. Most people can resume intercourse in 4 to 6 weeks, but this should be confirmed by your doctor."
- "Many postcoronary clients fear sexual intercourse because of increased heart and respiratory rates associated with it. However, your prescribed program of progressive physical activity will also increase your tolerance for sexual activity."

Many clients recuperating from childbirth, for example, or a specific illness or disease (e.g., myocardial infarction) need instructions about safe sexual activities and the effects that therapy can have on sexual functioning. The following topics need to be considered:

- When sexual activity is safe
- Specific sexual activities that are unsafe and why
- Adaptations needed for resuming a satisfactory sexual life
- The side effects of prescribed medications on sexual functioning and the need to notify the physician for possible dose or medication adjustment should problems develop

Specific Suggestions At the level of specific suggestions, the nurse requires specialized knowledge and skill about how sexuality and functioning can be affected by a disease process or therapy and what interventions might be effective. The nurse offers suggestions to help the client adapt sexual activity to promote optimal functioning, such as what measures might be used to alleviate vaginal dryness, safe positions for intercourse following a total hip replacement, safe and unsafe sexual practices following a myocardial infarction, and ways to handle ostomy appliances, Foley catheters, casts, or other devices (e.g., prostheses) during sexual activity. Similarly, nurses on a cardiac unit need specialized knowledge about sexual readjustment during cardiac rehabilitation, and nurses working with clients with spinal cord injuries need information about the sexual consequences of spinal injuries at various levels.

Using the example of the client recuperating from a myocardial infarction, the nurse may offer the following suggestion:

- "Many people express concern about the stress of certain positions for intercourse, but you may use whatever position is comfortable for you and your partner, or try side-lying or partner-on-top positions."

DEALING WITH INAPPROPRIATE SEXUAL BEHAVIOUR

Nurses may encounter a variety of sexually inappropriate behaviours for a variety of reasons. The behaviour may be either aggressive or nonaggressive. Clients may act out sexually in the following ways:

- Exposing themselves
- Asking the nurse to provide intimate physical care, such as bathing genital areas, when they are capable of doing this themselves
- Touching or grabbing the nurse (e.g., on the breasts or buttocks); trying to pull the nurse into bed
- Making blatant sexual statements to the nurse
- Offering sex to the nurse
- Whistling; making comments about the nurse's attractiveness or desirability
- Making sexual comments to another client in the same room or to visitors about the "sexy" nurse or what they would like to do sexually with the nurse

Possible reasons for this inappropriate behaviour are as follows:

- Fear or anxiety over future ability to function sexually
- Unmet need for intimacy and sexual closeness because of hospitalization, injury, illness, treatment, lack of a partner, or lack of privacy
- Misinterpretation of the nurse's behaviour as sexual or provocative
- Need for reassurance that they are still sexual beings and still sexually attractive
- Need for attention
- Confusion: Neurologic impairment or trauma can lead clients to use profane sexual language, engage in masturbation, expose themselves, or inappropriately touch or grab at the nurse
- Need to control: Clients may be experiencing loss of control over their lives because of hospitalization, injury, or illness
- Need for power
- Belief that flirtatious behaviour is expected because of media portrayal of nurses as sexy, available, and experienced

Before implementing any nursing interventions, the nurse should first ensure that the behaviour *is* inappropriate and not an attempt to communicate a physical need. For example, clients may expose themselves if they are febrile, pull at the penis if a catheter is uncomfortable or irritating, or reach for the nurse if unable to communicate verbally. Nursing strategies to deal with inappropriate sexual behaviour are shown in Box 45.4.

BOX 45.4 NURSING STRATEGIES FOR INAPPROPRIATE SEXUAL BEHAVIOUR

Nurses sometimes have to deal with clients whose behaviour is sexually inappropriate:

- Communicate that the behaviour is not acceptable by saying, for example, "I really do not like the things you are saying," or "I see you are not dressed. I will be back in 10 minutes and will help you with breakfast when you get your clothes on."
- Tell the client how the behaviour makes you feel: "When you act like that toward me, I don't even want to come into your room. It makes it difficult for me to give you the kind of nursing care you need."
- Identify the behaviour you expect: "Please call me by my name, not 'Honey,'" or "I expect you to keep yourself covered when I am in the room. If you are feeling hot or something is uncomfortable, let me know, and I will try to make you more comfortable."
- Set firm limits: Take the client's hand and move it away, use direct eye contact, and say, "Don't do that!"
- Try to refocus clients from the inappropriate behaviour to their real concerns and fears; offer to discuss sexuality concerns: "All morning you have been making very personal sexual comments about yourself. Sometimes people talk like that when they are concerned about the sexual part of their life and how their illness will affect them. Are there things that you have questions about or would like to talk about?"
- Report the incident to your nursing instructor, charge nurse, or clinical nurse specialist. Discuss the incident, your feelings, and possible interventions.
- Ensure health-care team members relate to the client in a consistent manner, confronting the behaviour.
- Clarify the consequences of continued inappropriate behaviour (avoidance, withdrawal of services, no chance to help resolve underlying concerns of client).

Evaluating

The goals established during the planning phase are evaluated according to specific desired health outcomes also established during that phase. Examples of these are shown in Table 45.6. If any outcomes have *not* been achieved, the nurse should explore the reasons why with such questions as the following:

- Were risk factors correctly identified?
- Did the client convey all significant fears and concerns about sexuality?

TABLE 45.6 Evaluating Goals and Outcomes: Sexuality

Goal	Examples of Desired Outcomes
Increase knowledge of sexuality and sexual health	Describes male and female sexual anatomy and function accurately Identifies signs of STIs Identifies factors related to altered sexuality pattern or dysfunction due to disease condition Describes alternative modes of sexual expression required for disease condition or therapy
Prevent the occurrence of sexually transmitted infection	Identifies STI exposure risks Describes ways to avoid STIs Uses appropriate methods to control STI transmission Inquires about partner's STI status before sexual activity Is free of an STI
Prevent the spread of existing STIs	Recognizes the signs and symptoms of an STI Takes appropriate actions to control the STI Participates in screening for STI Uses available health services for STI treatment and complies with recommended treatment Notifies sexual partner(s) if STI infection exists
Increase satisfaction with level of sexual functioning	Verbalizes concerns about altered pattern of sexual functioning (e.g., body image, desirability as sexual partner, sexual stimulation pattern, sexual response) Reports satisfaction with sexual functioning Reports satisfaction with level of sexual relationship

- Was the client more comfortable following discussions about sexual matters?
- Did the client understand the nurse's teaching?
- Was the health teaching compatible with the client's culture and religious values?
- Was the client ready to deal with sexuality problems?

Case Study 45

Mr. Curry is a 50-year-old male who suffered a myocardial infarction 3 weeks ago. He is doing well and is in a cardiac rehabilitation program. His only medications consist of a daily Aspirin and an antihypertensive medication. During a routine checkup, you inquire how he is feeling and whether he is doing well on his medications. Reluctantly, he admits that he is having some sexual problems. You encourage further discussion of the matter by displaying interest and explaining that it is okay for him to share his concerns with you. Mr. Curry states that he is having some difficulty achieving erections but is more concerned that he will have another myocardial infarction if he engages in sexual activities.

Critical Thinking Questions

1. Speculate about Mr. Curry's reluctance to discuss his sexual concerns.
2. What factors influence nurses' abilities to discuss sexual concerns with their clients?
3. What is the relationship between health and sexual function?
4. How can you best intervene to help Mr. Curry?

After working through these questions, go to the MyNursingLab at **http://www.mynursinglab.com** to check your answers.

KEY TERMS

sex
gender
sexuality
transsexuals
cross-dressers
sexual health
menstruation
dysmenorrhea
menopause
andropause
libido
erotic
foreplay
precoital stimulation
sex play
masturbation
ejaculation
orgasm
cunnilingus
fellatio
soixante-neuf
anilingus
coitus
copulation
anal intercourse
vasocongestion
myotonia
voyeurism
sadomasochistic bondage
pedophilia
sexual arousal
erectile dysfunction
impotence
premature ejaculation
retarded ejaculation (ejaculatory incompetence)
orgasmic dysfunction
vaginismus
dyspareunia
vulvodynia

CHAPTER HIGHLIGHTS

- Sexuality is important in developing self-identity, interpersonal relationships, intimacy, and love.
- Sexuality involves physical, emotional, social, and ethical aspects of being and behaving.
- An understanding of the anatomy and physiology of the male and female genitals is essential for nurses.
- The components that contribute to the development of sexuality are numerous; both biological and psychological components exist at all ages.
- In adults, many secondary sexual problems are related to illnesses, injuries, and medical therapies.
- During the middle and later years, the genitals undergo physical changes. However, the desire and ability to maintain satisfying sexual relationships can remain.
- Assessing risk for, or actual, sexual problems is part of the initial nursing assessment. Assessment should also be carried out when clients or support people present cues that problems exist or when clients have an illness that could cause sexual problems.

- Nurses assess attitudes toward sexuality, including factors that affect attitudes and behaviours.
- An understanding of sexual stimuli and response patterns can help individuals have satisfying sexual relationships. This understanding is also vital for nurses to help clients with psychological problems, such as feelings of inadequacy, or medical problems, such as spinal cord injuries or myocardial infarctions.
- Common sexual problems of healthy adults are changes in libido, erectile dysfunction, premature ejaculation, retarded ejaculation, orgasmic dysfunction, vaginismus, dyspareunia, and vulvodynia.
- Illnesses that commonly affect sexuality include myocardial infarction and diabetes mellitus. Many surgical procedures, including mastectomy, hysterectomy, orchiectomy, and enterostomy, can also affect sexual abilities and sexual self-image.
- Nursing diagnoses for clients with sexual problems are related to many contributing factors, including altered body structure or function, lack of knowledge or misinformation about sexual matters, physical or psychological abuse, value conflicts, and loss or lack of a partner.
- Before assisting clients with sexual problems, nurses must acquire accurate information about sexuality, identify and accept their own sexual values and behaviours as well as those of others, and be comfortable acquiring and disseminating information about sexuality.
- Nursing interventions focus on teaching clients about sexual function and sexuality; responsible sexual behaviour that includes the prevention of STIs and unplanned pregnancies; self-examination of the testicles; and how to be breast aware.

ASSESS YOUR LEARNING

1. Breast cancer is one of the leading causes of death for Canadian women. Which of the following is the best method to routinely detect breast cancer for women 50 and older?
   - **a.** They should be aware of what their breasts look and feel like normally.
   - **b.** They should have a clinical breast examination monthly.
   - **c.** They should have a mammography every 2 years.
   - **d.** They should ask for blood tests for breast cancer genetic screening.
2. What is the best way for the nurse to promote safe sexual practices in a group of adolescents?
   - **a.** Provide condoms.
   - **b.** Encourage abstinence.
   - **c.** Teach ways to prevent pregnancy.
   - **d.** Teach safe sex practices.
3. Clients are unlikely to introduce the topic of sex with health-care providers for which of the following reasons?
   - **a.** They assume that health-care providers know little about sexual functioning.
   - **b.** Most clients have few, if any, questions or problems.
   - **c.** Female clients prefer to discuss problems with female health-care providers.
   - **d.** They are too embarrassed to introduce the topic of sex.
4. A client informs the nurse that he is a transsexual. Which of the following is most representative of this client?
   - **a.** Gonadal gender, internal organs, and external genitals are contradictory.
   - **b.** Sexual anatomy is not consistent with gender identity.
   - **c.** Sexual attraction is to individuals of both genders.
   - **d.** Gender identity is altered by acute psychosis.
5. In conducting client teaching, the nurse bases content on knowing that which of the following is true regarding masturbation?
   - **a.** People who masturbate are psychologically disturbed.
   - **b.** Masturbation by teenagers interferes with their academic achievement.
   - **c.** Most people do not masturbate after the teenage years.
   - **d.** Masturbation is a way people learn about their sexual response.
6. A male client is beginning an antidepressant medication. Which of the following should be included in the teaching?
   - **a.** "Your partner will be pleased because your sexual functioning is going to improve."
   - **b.** "You may find that your desire for sex will decrease while on this medication."
   - **c.** "Retrograde ejaculation is a common problem when taking antidepressants."
   - **d.** "Your skin will probably become supersensitive to touch, so you may need to change your activity during sex."
7. A 75-year-old male client reports decreased frequency of sexual intercourse although he does not express dissatisfaction or difficulty. He seems a little embarrassed by the discussion but is engaged and asks some questions. An appropriate nursing diagnosis would be which of the following?
   - **a.** *Sexual Dysfunction*
   - **b.** *Disturbed Body Image*

c. *Sedentary Lifestyle*

d. *Readiness for Enhanced Knowledge*

8. Which of the following outcomes may indicate the need for referral to a more highly skilled therapist?
   a. The client verbalizes methods of modifying sexual activity according to physical limitations.
   b. The client requests the phone number of a sex education support group.
   c. Suggestions given by the nurse are ineffective in reaching the desired goals.
   d. The client reports experimenting with new sexual activities.
9. A client reports having dyspareuna.Which of the following questions is the most appropriate for the nurse to ask?
   a. "Have you talked with your partner about this discomfort?"
   b. "Have you had these spasms since you became sexually active?"
   c. "Do you have pain before your period begins?"
   d. "Do your breasts swell large enough to need a larger bra?"
10. Including at least some sexual health history questions would be most relevant for clients taking which of the following?
    a. Anti-inflammatories (such as Aspirin or ibuprofen)
    b. Hypnotics (sleeping pills)
    c. Antihypertensives (blood pressure medications)
    d. Antihistamines (cold medications)

After working through these questions, go to the MyNursingLab at **http://www.mynursinglab.com** *to check your answers and see explanations.*

SUGGESTED READINGS

MacDonald, N., & Wong, T. (2007). Canadian guidelines on sexually transmitted infections, 2006. *Canadian Medical Association Journal, 176*(2), 175–176.

This edition includes a literature review and outlines practices for health-care professionals regarding STI prevention, counselling, screening, diagnosis, clinical management, reports to public health, and partner notification.

Neville, S., & Henrickson, M. (2006). Perceptions of lesbian, gay and bisexual people of primary healthcare services. *Journal of Advanced Nursing, 55*(4), 407–415.

This article reports on a national survey in New Zealand that explored people's perceptions of disclosure about lesbian, gay, and bisexual identity to their health-care providers. It concludes that nurses must provide appropriate and safe care for lesbian, gay, and bisexual people.

WEBLINKS

Public Health Agency of Canada

http://www.phac-aspc.gc.ca/std-mts/sti_2006/sti_intro2006_e.html

This site provides the publication Canadian Guidelines on Sexually Transmitted Infections, 2006 Edition*, for download.*

The Society of Obstetricians and Gynaecologists of Canada.

http://www.sexualityandu.ca

An initiative of Obstetricians and Gynaecologists of Canada, this website provides accurate and up-to-date information on sexual health and healthy sexuality.

Sex Information and Education Council of Canada

http://www.sieccan.org

This nonprofit association was established to promote education about human sexuality.

REFERENCES

Annon, J. (1974). *The behavioral treatment of sexual problems. Vol. 1. Brief therapy.* New York: Harper & Row.

Barnett, R., & Rivers, C. (2004). *Same difference.* New York: Basic Books.

Berman, L., & Berman, J. (2005). *Secrets of the sexually satisfied woman: Ten keys to unlocking ultimate pleasure.* New York: Hyperion Press.

Breslin, E., & Lucas, V. (2003). *Women's health nursing: Toward evidence-based practice.* St. Louis, MO: Saunders.

Butler, J. (1990). Perfomative acts and gender constitution: An essay in phenomenology and feminist theory. In S. Case (Ed.), *Performing feminisms, feminist critical theory and theatre* (pp. 270–282). Baltimore, MD: John Hopkins University Press.

Canadian Breast Cancer Foundation. (2006). *Be breast aware.* Retrieved May 20, 2008, from http://www.cbcf.org/breastcancer/bc_aware.asp

Canadian Cancer Society. (2008). *Early detection and screening for breast cancer.* Retrieved May 20, 2008, from http://www.cancer.ca/ccs/internet/standard/0,3182,3172_10175_74544430_langId-en,00.html

Carpenito-Moyet, L. (2008). *Nursing diagnoses: Application to clinical practice* (12th ed.). Philadelphia, PA: Lippincott, Williams and Wilkins.

Condon, M. (2004). *Women's health: An integrated approach to wellness and illness.* New Jersey: Pearson Education.

Daniluk, J. (1998). *Women's sexuality across the life span: Challenging myths, creating meanings.* New York: Guilford Press.

Health Canada. (2003). *Canadian guidelines for sexual health education.* Retrieved October 22, 2007, from http://www.phac-aspc.gc.ca/publicat/cgshe-ldnemss/pdf/guidelines_e.pdf

Health Canada. (2007). *It's your health: Human papillomavirus (HPV).* Retrieved June 21, 2007, from http://www.hc-sc.gc.ca/iyh-vsv/diseases-maladies/hpv-vph_e.html#ba

Lips, H. M. (2005). *Sex and gender* (5th ed.). Columbus, OH: McGraw-Hill.

Maticka-Tyndale, E. (2001). Sexual health and Canadian youth: How do we measure up? *The Canadian Journal of Human Sexuality, 10*(1–2), 1–17.

McDonald, C. (2006). Lesbian disclosure: Disrupting the taken for granted. *Canadian Journal of Nursing Research, 38*(1), 42–57.

Miller, C. L., Strathdee, M., Kerr, T., Li, K., & Wood, E. (2006). Factors associated with early adolescent initiation into injection drug use: Implication for intervention programs. *Journal of Adolescent Health, 38*(4), 462–464.

Moore, S., Kubrik, M., Shea, L., & Kubrik, N. (1992). Nerve-sparing prostatectomy. *American Journal of Nursing, 92,* 59–64.

NANDA International. (2007). *Nursing diagnoses: Definitions and classification, 2007–2008.* Philadelphia, PA: Author.

Peterkin, A., & Risdon, C. (2003). *Caring for lesbian and gay people: A clinical guide.* University of Toronto Press: Toronto.

Public Health Agency of Canada. (2004). *Hepatitis B fact sheet.* Retrieved June 21, 2007, from http://www.phac-aspc.gc.ca/hcai-iamss/bbp-pts/hepatitis/hep_b_e.html

Public Health Agency of Canada. (2006). *2004 Canadian sexually transmitted infections surveillance report: Pre-release.* Retrieved June 21, 2007, from http://www.phac-aspc.gc.ca/std-mts/stddata_pre06_04/tab1-2_e.htm

Pyke J., Rabin K., Phillips J., Moffs, J., & Balbirnie, M. (2002). Sexuality and the mental health client. *Canadian Nurse, 98,* 18–23.

Roterman, M. (2005). Sex, condoms, and sexually transmitted infections among young people. *Statistics Canada Report, 16*(3), 39–49.

Sex Information and Education Council of Canada. (2005). *Sexual health education in schools: Questions and answers.* Retrieved June 19, 2007, from http://www.sieccan.org/pdf/SHES_QA.pdf

Society of Obstetricians and Gynaecologists of Canada. (2007). *Pregnancy: Sex during pregnancy.* Retrieved June 28, 2008, from http://www.sexualityandu.ca/adults/sex-3.aspx

Smylie, L., Medaglia, S., & Maticka-Tyndale, E. (2006). The effect of social capital and socio-demographics on adolescent risk and sexual health behaviors. *Canadian Journal of Sexuality, 15*(2), 95–112.

Stevens, P. (1995). Structural and interpersonal impact of heterosexual assumptions of lesbian health care clients. *Nursing Research, 44*(1), 25–30.

Chapter 46

Spirituality

The nurse provides care not only for the physical body and mind but also for the client's spirit, soul, or inner essence. Assessing and responding to the client's spiritual needs can decrease suffering and aid in physical and mental healing (see the Nursing and Canadian Society box).

NURSING AND CANADIAN SOCIETY

Fact	Implications for Nursing Practice
About 75% of Canadians say they have spiritual needs: • 38% say spirituality is very important to them • 82% believe in God • 65% say they believe "God or a higher power cares for them personally" • 72% of Canadians pray (daily, 27%; rarely, 19%) • 84% of Canadians identify with a specific religion (Bibby, 2006)	Nurses should engage clients with basic assessment questions that include recognition of spirituality, and intervention should include interdisciplinary team-work with spiritual care professionals to address clients' spiritual and religious issues or needs.

OBJECTIVES

After studying this chapter, you should be able to

1. Compare and contrast the concepts of spirituality, religion, and faith as they relate to nursing and health care
2. Describe the spiritual development of the individual across the lifespan
3. Situate spiritual and religious care within the context of today's world views
4. List 10 characteristics of spiritual health
5. Recognize 11 factors associated with spiritual distress
6. Assess for spiritual resources and spiritual needs
7. Collaborate in interdisciplinary care planning and intervention
8. Identify desired outcomes for evaluating the client's spiritual health
9. Analyze the influence on health care of spiritual and religious beliefs about diet, dress, prayer and meditation, and birth and death

To implement spiritual care, nurses need to be skilled in multidimensional listening and in establishing trusting nurse–client relationships. Because involvement in spiritual care is personal for both the nurse and the client, nurses need to communicate with sensitivity and empathy, have a good understanding of their own spiritual and religious story, and understand how this can affect their ability to provide spiritual care. They also need to develop a broad concept of spirituality. Nurses cannot rely solely on their own spiritual practices; they need to be knowledgeable about various religious traditions and spiritual practices that express clients' spirituality.

A client's spirituality is complex and individual. Thus, clients need to be approached in light of their unique needs. Many clients have spiritual strengths that the nurse can nurture to help them attain or maintain a feeling of spiritual health, to recover from illness, and to face death peacefully. Likewise, many clients have had traumatic experiences that have wounded their spirits and will need interdisciplinary teamwork to facilitate spiritual health.

Spirituality, Religion, and Faith

Spirituality, religion, and faith are distinct entities, yet the words are often used interchangeably. The word *spiritual* derives from the Hebrew word *ruah* (wind) and the Latin *spiritus,* meaning "to blow" or "to breathe," and it has come to mean something that gives life or essence to the soul. Taylor (2002) summarized nursing definitions of spirituality since 1970. Burkhardt and Nagai-Jacobson (2002, p. 18) highlighted that "attempting to define spirituality is akin to trying to lasso the wind." According to Burkhardt (1993), spirituality is described as a belief in or relationship with some higher power, creative force, divine being, or infinite source of energy. For example, a person may believe in God, Allah, the Creator, or a Higher Power. Spirituality includes the following aspects (Burkhardt, 1993):

- Dealing with the unknown or uncertainties in life
- Finding meaning and purpose in life
- Being aware of and able to draw on inner resources and strength
- Having a feeling of connectedness with the self, others, and something beyond the self

"The spiritual dimension tries to be in harmony with the universe, strives for answers about the infinite, and especially comes into focus or sustaining power when the person faces emotional stress, physical illness, or death. It goes outside a person's own power" (Murray & Zentner, 1997, p. 107).

In this chapter, we draw on the work of Chui, Emblen, Van Hofwegen, Sawatzky, and Meyerhoff (2004) that describes **spirituality** as a universal human phenomenon revealing themes of existential reality, transcendence, connectedness, power, force, and energy. Characteristics of spirituality are listed in Box 46.1.

Although spirituality is a broad concept, **religion** is more practical and acts as a container or holding environment that offers ways to express spirituality. World religions serve as formal, socially recognized communities within which people share common values, beliefs, and practices (Clark & Olson, 2000). Diverse religious traditions provide guidance for believers in responding to life's questions and challenges. According to Vardey (1995), organized religions offer (1) a sense of community bound by common beliefs, (2) the collective study of sacred texts (the Torah, Bible, Koran, or others), (3) the performance of ritual, (4) the use of disciplines and practices, commandments, and sacraments, and (5) ways of taking care of the person's soul (such as fasting, prayer, and meditation). Many traditional religious practices and rituals are related to such life events as birth, transition from childhood to adulthood, marriage, illness, and death. Religious principles can also apply to matters of daily life, such as dress, food, social interac-

BOX 46.1 CHARACTERISTICS OF SPIRITUALITY

RELATIONSHIP WITH SELF

Inner strength and self-reliance

- Having self-knowledge (who you are, what you can do)
- Having positive attitudes (trust in self, trust in life and the future, peace of mind, harmony with self)

RELATIONSHIP WITH NATURE

Harmony

- Knowing about plants, trees, wildlife, weather
- Communing with nature (gardening, walking, being outside); preserving nature

RELATIONSHIP WITH OTHERS

- Sharing time, knowledge, and resources; reciprocating
- Caring for children, older adults, the sick
- Reaffirming the living and the dead (visiting, photos, cemetery meetings)

RELATIONSHIP WITH DEITY

Religious or nonreligious

- Using prayer-meditation
- Possessing religious articles
- Being in nature
- Participating in a faith community

Source: Adapted from "Characteristics of Spirituality in the Lives of Women in a Rural Appalachian Community," by M. Burkhardt, 1993, *Journal of Transcultural Nursing, 4,* pp. 12–18. Used with permission.

tion, menstruation, and sexual relationships. However, a person can follow certain religious practices and yet not internalize the symbolic meaning behind the practices.

Just as a rich language surrounds the concept of spirituality, a complex composition of terms is associated with religion. For example, an **agnostic** is a person who questions the existence of God or a supreme being, while an **atheist** does not acknowledge the existence of God. By contrast, some religions describe themselves as **theistic**, based on a belief in a higher power or God, with some believing in the existence of one God (**monotheism**) and others believing in more than one divine entity (**polytheism**).

Faith is a concept used to describe the relational essence of spirituality and religion as these are experienced in everyday life. Faith points to the need human beings have to connect with nature, family, various communities, and realities that transcend normal activities. Faith, then, can be described as "being in relationship with" the various others that make life meaningful, such as God, loved ones, and social contacts (Clark, 2000, p. 19). According to Fowler and Keen (1985), faith is universal—a feature of living, acting, and self-understanding. To have faith is to believe in or be committed to something or someone.

Fowler (1974) described faith as being present in both religious and nonreligious people. Faith gives life meaning, providing the individual with strength in times of difficulty. Westerhoff (1976) described faith as a way of being and behaving that evolves from a faith guided by parents and others during infancy and childhood to an owned faith that is internalized in adulthood and serves as a directive for action (see Table 46.1). For the client who is ill, faith—whether in a higher authority (e.g., God, Allah, Jehovah), in the self, in the health-care team, or in a combination of all—provides strength and trust.

Spiritual, Religious, and Faith Development

Like Westerhoff (1976), a number of other authors have contributed to the understanding of the concepts of spirituality, religion, and faith as **developmental** by highlighting stages through which people move over the course of their lifetime. Spiritual, religious, and faith development recognizes that growth across the lifespan not only includes but also needs to integrate spiritual experiences through reflection and articulation. Fowler and Keen (1985) used the image of "life maps" to describe faith as a journey. This image is helpful in assisting clients to see their lives in time (chronological dates) and space (geographical places) and to reflect on events that have occurred as they would reflect on various aspects of a journey.

Ford (1988) used the metaphor of "life spirals" by combining the faith development theory of James Fowler (1981) and the psychosocial theory of Erik Erikson (1963) to describe multidimensional holistic processes that occur as life transitions. The spiral is an ancient transcultural and multifaith image that is used all over the world to communicate connections that exist in chronological and situational spiritual experiences. In her spiral faith model (see Figure 46.1), Iris Ford (1988) depicted each spiral as a "cluster of opportunities" fashioned by "maturation, experience, and previous opportunities" (p. 15). One by one, and taken together, the 12 faith development spirals invite individuals and groups to face what life offers, both the positive and negative, with an attitude of hope.

TABLE 46.1 Westerhoff's Four Stages of Faith

Stage	Age	Behaviour
Experienced faith	Infancy and early adolescence	Experiences faith through interaction with others who are living a particular faith tradition
Affiliative faith	Late adolescence	Participates in activities that characterize a particular faith tradition; experiences awe and wonderment; feels a sense of belonging
Searching faith	Young adulthood	Through a process of questioning and doubting own faith, acquires a cognitive as well as an affective faith
Owned faith	Middle adulthood and old age	Puts faith into personal and social action and is willing to stand up for beliefs even against the nurturing community

Source: Adapted from *Will Our Children Have Faith?* (pp. 79–103), by J. Westerhoff, 1976, New York: Seabury Press.

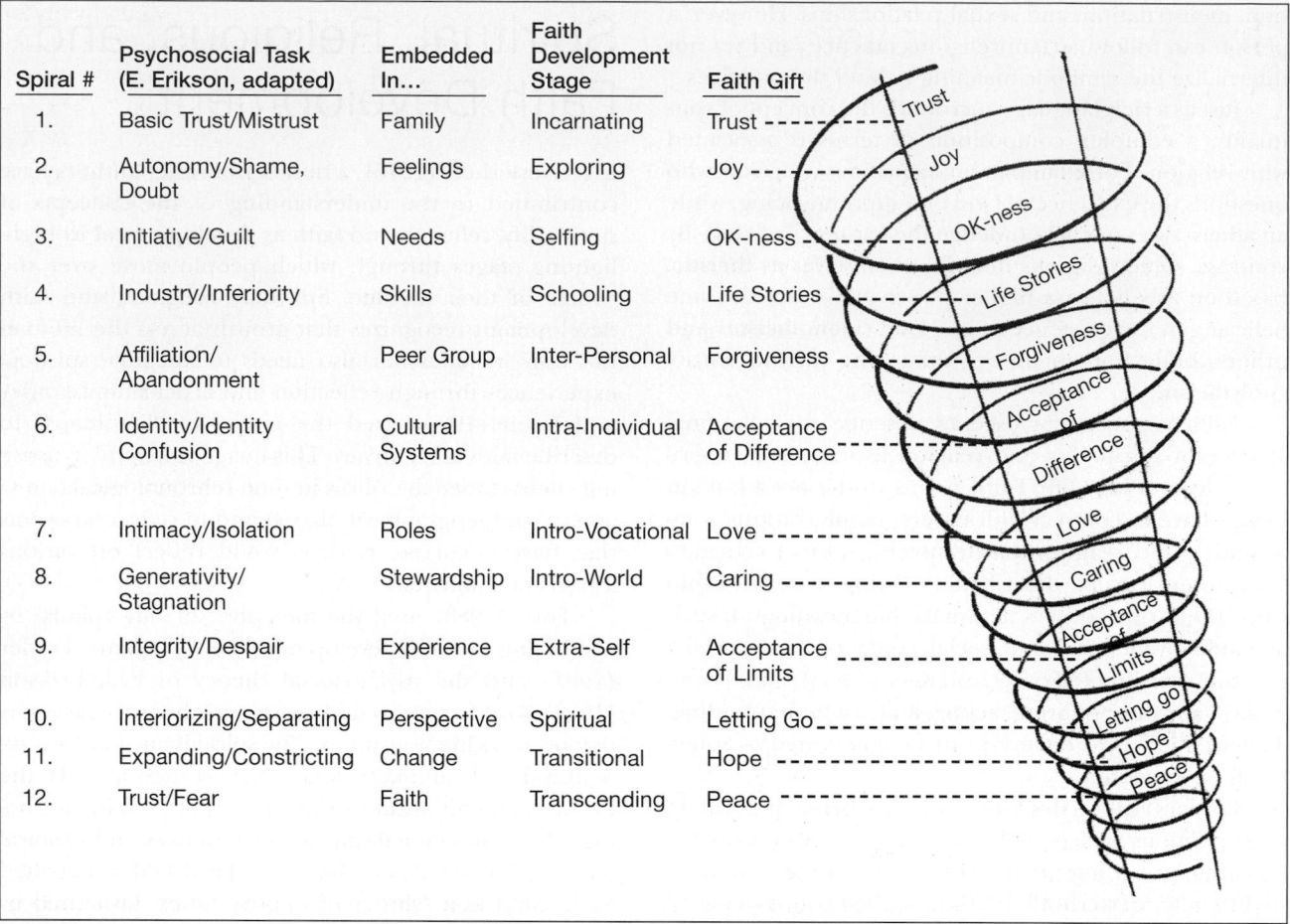

Spiral #	Psychosocial Task (E. Erikson, adapted)	Embedded In...	Faith Development Stage	Faith Gift
1.	Basic Trust/Mistrust	Family	Incarnating	Trust
2.	Autonomy/Shame, Doubt	Feelings	Exploring	Joy
3.	Initiative/Guilt	Needs	Selfing	OK-ness
4.	Industry/Inferiority	Skills	Schooling	Life Stories
5.	Affiliation/ Abandonment	Peer Group	Inter-Personal	Forgiveness
6.	Identity/Identity Confusion	Cultural Systems	Intra-Individual	Acceptance of Difference
7.	Intimacy/Isolation	Roles	Intro-Vocational	Love
8.	Generativity/ Stagnation	Stewardship	Intro-World	Caring
9.	Integrity/Despair	Experience	Extra-Self	Acceptance of Limits
10.	Interiorizing/Separating	Perspective	Spiritual	Letting Go
11.	Expanding/Constricting	Change	Transitional	Hope
12.	Trust/Fear	Faith	Transcending	Peace

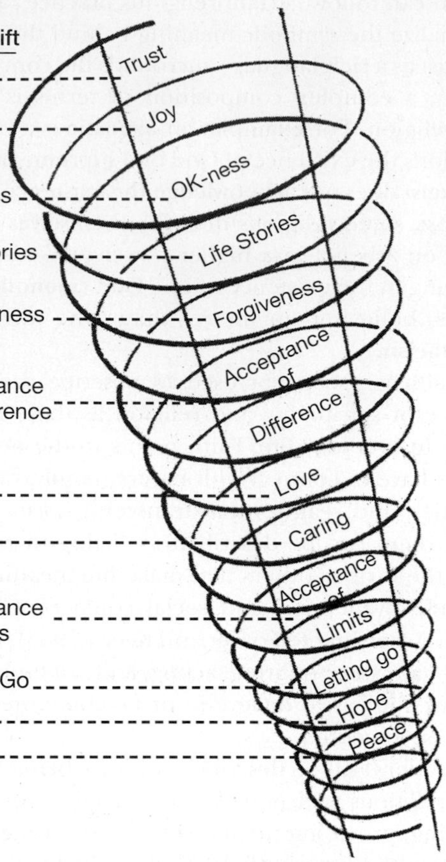

FIGURE 46.1 Spiral Faith Model

Source: From **Life spirals: The faith journey** *(pp. 19–20), I.M. Ford, 1988. Burlington, ON: Welch Publishing Company.*

A number of ancillary concepts are associated with the constructs of spiritual, religious, and faith development. Two worth mentioning are *hope* and *world view.* Hope, like faith, is a concept that also has a spiritual dimension. **Hope** was defined by Post-White and colleagues (1996) as a multidimensional concept that includes perceiving realistic expectations and goals, having motivation to achieve goals, anticipating outcomes, establishing trust and interpersonal relationships, relying on internal and external resources, having determination to endure, and being oriented to the future.

Hope is necessary for the individual to survive illness, loss, and other challenging life circumstances (Jevne, 1991). Grimm (1991, p. 511) stated that hope "is an interpersonal process that is created through trust and is nurtured by trusting relationships with others, including God." According to Stotland (1969, p. 1), "without hope, the individual is often dull, listless, and moribund." In the absence of hope, the client can give up, and illness—especially terminal illness—may progress more rapidly.

The other concept associated with the constructs of spiritual, religious, and faith development is **world view.** This concept derives from the German word *Weltanschauung* and aligns with various approaches to the term *environment* found in the nursing meta-paradigm. World view focuses attention on the context within which people move toward health. An individual's or a group's geographic location, psychosocial-spiritual circumstances and resources, and socioeconomic position contribute to their world view. These variables influence how people see and interpret the world insofar as they filter perceptions based on a person's or group's set of **beliefs, values,** and **assumptions** about life and the universe. Nurses need to notice and empathically engage the belief statements expressed by their clients in order to more fully understand the world view out of which they are operating.

Spiritual, religious, and faith development theories frequently draw on parallel theoretical considerations in the fields of philosophy, psychology, theology, and the social sciences. Early expressions of scholarly inquiry into spiritual, religious, and faith development used such terms such *philosophy of religion* and *religious psychology.* More recent literature includes recognition of the complexity of this topic area and acknowledges the need for interdisciplinary study (Andresen & Foreman, 2000).

Spiritual and Religious Care

Global events of the late twentieth and early twenty-first century changed health professionals' approaches to spiritual and religious care. With the decade of buildup to a new millennium came a great deal of reflection on historical, theological, and sociopolitical themes. Of particular note has been literature on millennialism, religious fundamentalism, and globalization, and the United Nations Millennium Declaration.

In a distinct series of computer and media events, Y2K gave evidence of how the functioning or nonfunctioning of electronic devices could influence every aspect of modern society, including health care. Y2K was the name given to computer software's inability to recognize dates after December 31, 1999. To save what was limited space when the programs were written, years were represented by only two-digit numbers.

Finally, the impact of terrorist attacks on the United States on September 11, 2001, combined with ongoing uncertainty and unpredictability related to terrorism, hotspots of military conflict, climate change, and pandemic threats, brought to the fore a renewed awareness of the interface among world religions, politics, and economics.

One health implication for spiritual and religious care today is the prominence of **generalized anxiety**—a state of mental uneasiness, apprehension, or dread that produces an increased level of arousal—and its potential to evoke spiritual distress in individuals as well as groups. The practical implications of these developments on spiritual and religious care by nurses include the need to think globally while acting locally, to realize that diverse subgroups or denominations exist within many world religions, to engage differing spiritual and religious perspectives with respectful inquiry, to recognize the health implications that flow out of clients' spiritual and religious views and practices, and to gain greater skill in assessing spiritual health and spiritual needs through interdisciplinary education and professional collaboration.

Spiritual Health and Spiritual Distress

Several concepts used in the literature speak about healthy spirituality. These include the ancient idea of *holiness,* as well as the more contemporary terms *wholeness, spiritual well-being, spiritual wellness,* and *spiritual health.* **Spiritual well-being** refers to harmonious interconnectedness, creative energy, and faith in a power greater than the self (Hood Morris, 1996). **Spiritual wellness** is "a way of living, a lifestyle that views and lives life as purposeful and pleasurable, that seeks out life-sustaining and life-enriching options to be chosen freely at every opportunity, and that sinks its roots deeply into spiritual values and/or specific religious beliefs" (Pilch, 1988, p. 31). **Spiritual health** is a feeling of being "generally alive, purposeful, and fulfilled" (Ellison, 1983, p. 332). Characteristics indicating spiritual well-being are shown in Box 46.2.

People enhance or nurture their spirituality in many ways. Some of these focus on development of the inner self or world; others focus on the expression of their inner essence to others or the outer world. Relating to the inner self or soul can be achieved through having an inner dialogue with a higher power or with the self; praying or meditating; analyzing dreams; communing with nature; listening quietly to music; or experiencing the inspiration of art, drama, or dance. The expression of a person's inner essence to others is manifested in loving relationships with and service to others; joy and laughter; and participation in spiritual or religious rituals.

Spiritual distress refers to a disturbance in or a challenge to a person's core value system that provides strength, hope, and meaning to life. Many factors are associated with spiritual distress: physiological problems, treatment-related concerns, or situational concerns. A fourth factor associated with spiritual distress is that of developmental transitions (Clark & Olson, 2000). Physiological problems include having a medical diagnosis of a terminal or debilitating disease or experiencing pain, the loss of a body part or function, or a miscarriage or stillbirth. Treatment-related factors include the recommendation for blood transfusions, surgery, dietary restrictions, amputation of a body part, or isolation. Situational factors can involve the death or illness of a significant other, barriers to or embarrassment at practising

BOX 46.2 CHARACTERISTICS INDICATIVE OF SPIRITUAL WELL-BEING

People with a sense of spiritual well-being usually display the following characteristics:

- Sense of inner peace
- Compassion for others
- Reverence for life
- Gratitude
- Appreciation of both unity and diversity
- Humour
- Wisdom
- Generosity
- Ability to transcend the self
- Capacity for unconditional love

Source: *Spiritual Dimensions of Nursing Practice,* by V. B. Carson, 1989, Philadelphia, PA: Saunders.

rituals (Carpenito-Moyet, 2008). NANDA International (2007) offered the following as defining characteristics of spiritual distress:

- Experiencing a disturbance in a personal belief system
- Questioning the meaning of life, death, or suffering
- Questioning the credibility of a personal belief system
- Demonstrating discouragement or despair
- Choosing not to practise usual religious rituals
- Having ambivalent feelings (doubts) about beliefs
- Not having a reason for living
- Feeling a sense of spiritual emptiness
- Showing emotional detachment for self and others
- Expressing concern (e.g., anger, resentment, fear) over the meaning of life, suffering, or death
- Requesting spiritual assistance for a disturbance in a belief system

Collaborating in Interdisciplinary Spiritual Care Planning and Intervention

With the benefits of increased awareness and interest in the topics of spirituality, religion, and faith, nurse practitioners—together with their interdisciplinary colleagues in chaplaincy, social work, psychology, rehabilitation sciences, and medicine—are in a position to examine the spiritual and religious values and assumptions that are embedded in health-care language and treatment paradigms. Helpful in this regard are the insights of Gottlieb and Ezer (1997) in their writing about the McGill model of nursing. They emphasized that understandings of health are learned within diverse family configurations, and these understandings can be engaged through professional activities that recognize clients' potential and resources for taking greater ownership of their health.

Foundational to the McGill model is the promotion of inquiry and an exploratory approach to data collection. This approach is conducive to interdisciplinary dialogue and can result in obtaining an overall profile of health. According to Olson (2000), health or wholeness can become "the goal toward which we strive during times of transition" including "health risks and health potentials as these exist in transitional times" (p. 224). A complete assessment of health risks and potentials requires the knowledge and skill of diverse health professionals. Each profession that includes spiritual care as central to its reason for being (i.e., chaplaincy) or associative to its optimal provision of care (i.e., nursing, social work, psychology, rehabilitation sciences, and medicine) needs to be included in assessing, planning, implementing, and evaluating processes. Learning skills of interdisciplinary assessment, dialogue, collaboration, and referral in the spiritual and religious care of clients is a developing topic in the literature.

According to Puchalski, Lunsford, Harris, and Miller (2006), for example, interdisciplinary spiritual care means that all health-care professionals on the team, including the chaplain, interact with one another to develop and implement the spiritual care plan for the patient in a fully collaborative model.

Analyzing Spiritual and Religious Practices Affecting Nursing Care

Spiritual holy days, sacred writings, spiritual symbols, prayer and meditation practices, rituals, and religious guidelines associated with diet, nutrition, dress, birth, and death are among the factors to consider when giving nursing care. Whenever these factors become obvious in their work with clients, nurses need to be aware that it is possible to impose personal spiritual beliefs on clients without intending to do so. Observing the following guidelines for ethical conduct in spiritual caregiving is essential. These guidelines for nurses were offered by Winslow and Winslow (2003):

- Seek a basic understanding of clients' spiritual needs, resources, and preferences (i.e., assess)
- Follow the client's expressed wishes regarding spiritual care
- Do not prescribe or urge clients to adopt certain spiritual beliefs or practices, and do not pressure them to relinquish such beliefs or practices
- Strive to understand personal spirituality and how it influences caregiving
- Provide spiritual care in a way that is in harmony with personal beliefs

HOLY DAYS A **holy day** is a day set aside for special religious observance. Most Christians observe Sunday as the Sabbath, while Jews and some Christians observe Saturday as the day of the week devoted to rest and worship. Muslims hold their congregational prayer on Fridays. These observances are in response to religious directives. Holy days can also be special days of celebration and feasting that occur once a year, such as Christmas and Easter (Christian), and Sukkoth or the Feast of Tabernacles (Jewish).

Solemn religious observances throughout the year may be referred to as high holy days and may include fasting, reflection, and prayer. Examples of such holy days are Rosh Hashanah and Yom Kippur (Jewish), Good Friday (Christian), and the month-long observance of Ramadan (Islam). Many religions require fasting, extended prayer, and reflection or ritual observances on sacred days; however, believers who are seriously ill are often exempt from such requirements. Many hospitals and health organizations facilitate ritual observances for clients and staff on holy days. For example, a hospital may provide fish or another nonmeat entree on Good Friday for Catholic clients. As many religions follow calendars that are different from the Gregorian calendar, a multifaith calendar can be used to identify the holy days of the various religious groups (Griffith, 1996).

SACRED WRITINGS Each religion has its sacred writings or scriptures, believed to be the thought or word of the Supreme Being and written by the appointed prophets or disciples. Usually, the rules or commandments for living are contained in the scriptures. For example, the Torah contains the body of wisdom and law for Jews, and the Bible contains the Gospels. Religious laws or commandments are often used as the basis for secular law, such as laws regarding committing murder or stealing. Religious law can affect a client's willingness to accept treatment suggestions. For example, blood transfusions are in conflict with the religious law of Jehovah's Witnesses. A religion's sacred writings also frequently tell the stories of the religion's leaders, kings, and heroes, such as the stories of Abraham and Solomon in both Jewish and Christian scriptures.

When people are ill or in crisis, they often gain strength and hope from reading religious writings. Examples of scriptural stories that can give comfort to clients are Job's suffering in both the Jewish and Christian scriptures and, in the Bible, Jesus healing people who were physically or mentally ill. See Box 46.3 for a list of sacred writings.

SPIRITUAL SYMBOLS Sacred symbols include jewellery, medals, amulets, icons, totems, or body ornamentation (e.g., tattoos) that carry religious or spiritual significance. They may be worn to pronounce a person's faith, to provide spiritual protection, or to be a source of comfort or strength. People may wear religious medals at all times, and they may want to wear them when they are undergoing diagnostic studies, medical treatment, or surgery. Catholics may carry a rosary for prayer, and Muslims may carry prayer beads.

People may have religious icons or statues in their homes, cars, or places of work as personal reminders of their faith or as part of personal places of worship or meditation. Hospitalized clients or long-term-care residents may want to have their spiritual icons or statues with them as a source of comfort.

PRAYER AND MEDITATION PRACTICES Prayer or meditation is a part of every religion. **Prayer** is a communication with God, Allah, Jehovah, or other Supreme Being in word or in thought. Prayers may be said in thankfulness (e.g., for health or healing), in supplication or request (e.g., for relief from pain and suffering, for a cure), or as communion or reflection. Dossey (1993) identified seven forms of prayer (see Box 46.4), all of which may be used when someone is experiencing illness or healing. Some religions have prescribed prayers that are printed in a prayer book, such as the Anglican or Episcopal Book of Common Prayer or the Catholic Missal. Some religious prayers are attributed to the source of faith; for example, the Lord's Prayer for Christians is attributed to Jesus, and the first sutra for Muslims is attributed to Mohammed.

Some religions require daily prayers or dictate specific times for prayer and worship, such as the five daily prayers, or Salat, of Muslims (performed facing east toward Mecca at dawn, noon, midafternoon, sunset, and evening); the daily Kaddish of Jews; or the seven canonical prayers of Catholics. People who are ill may want to continue or to increase their prayer practices (Moschella, Pressman, Pressman, & Weisseman, 1997). They may need uninterrupted quiet time and want to have their prayer books, rosaries, prayer beads, or other icons available to them.

Meditation is the act of focusing thoughts or engaging in self-reflection or contemplation. Some people believe that through deep meditation, they can influence or control physical and psychological functioning and the course of illness. See Chapter 15 for more discussion of meditation.

BELIEFS AFFECTING DIET AND NUTRITION Many religions have proscriptions regarding diet, including rules about which foods and beverages are allowed and which are prohibited. For example, Orthodox Jews may not eat shellfish or pork, and Muslims may not drink

BOX 46.3 SACRED WRITINGS

Christianity	Bible
Judaism	Torah
	Talmud
Islam: Muslim	Koran
Hindu	Ramayana
	Mahabharata
	Vedas
	Upanishads
Sikh	Granth
Buddhism	Vedas
Zoroastrianism	Avesta
	Gathas

BOX 46.4 FORMS OF PRAYER

Petition	Asking something for the self
Intercession	Asking something for others
Confession	Repenting wrongdoing and asking forgiveness
Lamentation	Crying in distress and asking for vindication
Adoration	Giving honour and praise
Invocation	Summoning the presence of the Almighty
Thanksgiving	Offering gratitude

Source: Adapted from *Healing Words: The Power of Prayer and the Practice of Medicine* (p. 5), by L. Dossey, 1993, New York: HarperSanFrancisco.

alcoholic beverages or eat pork. Mormons, or members of the Church of Jesus Christ of Latter-day Saints, may not drink caffeinated or alcoholic beverages. Older Catholics may choose not to eat meat on Fridays because of previous Catholic religious doctrine. Religious law may also dictate how food is prepared. For example, many Jewish people require **kosher** food, that is, food prepared according to Jewish law.

Some solemn religious observances are marked by fasting, which is the abstinence from food for a specified time. Some religions also restrict beverages; others allow drinking of water or other sustaining beverages on fast days. Examples of religions that observe fasting include Islam, Judaism, and Catholicism. During the month of Ramadan, devout Muslims eat no food and avoid beverages during daylight hours; the fast can be broken after sunset. Members of Jewish synagogues fast on Yom Kippur, the Day of Atonement; and devout Catholics may fast on Good Friday. Most religions lift the fasting requirements for seriously ill clients and believers for whom fasting may be a detriment to health, such as diabetic clients. Some religions may exempt nursing mothers or menstruating women from fasting requirements.

It is important for health-care providers to prescribe diet plans with an awareness of the client's dietary and fasting beliefs.

BELIEFS RELATED TO DRESS Many religions have laws or traditions that dictate dress. For example, Orthodox and Conservative Jewish men believe that it is important to have their head covered at all times and, therefore, wear a *yarmulke.* Orthodox Jewish women may wear a wig or scarf to cover their hair as a sign of respect. Muslim women may also cover their hair with a *hijab* (headscarf) in compliance with religious law.

Some religions require that women dress in a conservative manner, which may include not wearing sleeveless or low-cut tops and skirts that are above the knees. Some religions, for example, Islam, require that the body (torso, arms, and legs) be covered. Hospital gowns may make women who want to comply with religious dress codes uneasy and uncomfortable. Clients may be especially disconcerted when undergoing diagnostic tests or treatments, such as mammography, that require body parts to be bared.

BELIEFS RELATED TO BIRTH For all religions, the birth of a child is an important event giving cause for celebration. Many religions have specific ritual ceremonies that consecrate the new child to God.

When a Muslim child is born, "someone recites the call to prayer in the infant's ear" (Denny, 1993, p. 682). On the seventh day after birth, the child is named, and a tuft of hair is shaved from the head (Denny).

In the Christian faith, baptism and christening ceremonies may take place after the birth of a child to confirm that the "infant [was] born into a Christian family as part of the organism of the church" (Frankiel, 1993, p. 556). Christian parents of seriously ill infants may want baptism performed at birth by the chaplain.

In the Jewish religion, the ritual circumcision conducted on male children on the eighth day after birth is an expression of the religious bond between the prophet Abraham, his descendants, and their God. Following the circumcision by the ritually trained surgeon, called a *mohel,* the child is named. Girls are named in the synagogue on the Sabbath after the birth (Fishbane, 1993).

When nurses are aware of the religious needs of families and their infants, they can assist families in fulfilling their religious obligations. This help is especially important when the newborn is seriously ill or in danger of dying; some people believe that if religious obligations are not fulfilled, the infant will not be accepted into the community of the faithful after death.

BELIEFS RELATED TO DEATH Spiritual and religious beliefs play a significant role in the believer's approach to death, just as they do in other major life events. Many believe that the person who dies transcends this life for a better place or being.

Some religions have special rituals surrounding dying and death that must be observed by the faithful. Observance of these rituals provides comfort to the dying person and their loved ones. Some rituals are carried out while the person is still alive and can include special prayers, such as the Anointing of the Sick (previously referred to as the Last Rites), singing or chants, and reading of sacred scriptures. Many Muslims who are dying will want their body or head turned toward Mecca (Denny, 1993).

Some special religious observances must be followed after death. Griffith (1996, p. 18) suggested that "during a terminal illness, the client and family should be asked if any special procedures follow death." Some religions require that the body of the deceased be touched only by members of that faith. In both the Muslim (Denny, 1993) and the Jewish (Fishbane, 1993) religions, devout believers require that a ritual bath be given after death either by a family member or by a ritual burial society. Many religions require that a family member or other believer stay with the body at all times until it is buried or cremated. Religious symbols or objects should be treated with respect and kept with the body (Griffith, 1996). The nurse can support the family of the deceased by providing an environment conducive to the performance of death rituals.

Spiritual Health and the Nursing Process

Assessing

Data about a client's spiritual needs, spiritual and religious practices, and spiritual resources are obtained from

REFLECT ON PRIMARY HEALTH CARE

When examining the principles of primary health care, look at spiritual care as contributing to the principle of health promotion. Promoting health can be enhanced through the inclusion of spiritual elements in nursing care of the individual or family. This incorporation can be accomplished wherever the patient or client is encountered by the nurse and whatever the client's physical or mental health status.

the client's general history; through a nursing history; and by clinical observations of the client's behaviour, verbalizations, mood, and so on. Even when a particular religion is identified, nurses should never assume that a client follows all the practices of the stated religion. Individual assessment is required to determine the nature of spiritual needs, usual spiritual and religious practices, and available spiritual resources. Clients' spiritual needs can be as important to them as their health-care needs (see the Reflect on Primary Health Care box).

NURSING HISTORY The spiritual assessment is best taken once the nurse has developed a good relationship with the client or support person. The questions provided in the Assessment: Interview box can help begin the spiritual assessment process. In general, the nurse obtains data about the client's concept of a divine being, deity, or creative force; sources of hope and strength; religious and spiritual beliefs and practices; rituals; and any relationship perceived between spiritual beliefs and state of health.

A multitude of spiritual assessment tools have been developed from various disciplines and theoretical perspectives (Fitchett, 1993; O'Connor, Meakes, O'Neill, Prenner, VanStaalduinen, & Davis, 2005). These can be used as guides to assist practitioners in integrating spiritual assessment into overall health assessment. Spiritual assessment is also important when conducting family assessment and in planning family interventions. Specific guidelines have been developed for family spiritual development (Tanyi, 2006).

ASSESSMENT: INTERVIEW

Spirituality

Asking the following questions can help the nurse assess a client's spiritual needs:

- Are any particular religious or spiritual practices important to you? If so, could you please tell me about them?
- Will being in this health-care setting interfere with your religious or spiritual practices?
- In what ways is your faith important to you right now?
- In what ways can I help you carry out your faith? For example, would you like me to read your sacred writings to you or assist you with prayer or meditation?
- Would you like a visit from your faith group leader or a chaplain?
- What are your hopes and your sources of strength right now?

CLINICAL ASSESSMENT Cues to spiritual and religious preferences, strengths, concerns, or distress may be revealed by one or more of the following (Shelley & Fish, 1988; Sumner, 1998):

1. *Environment.* Does the client have a Bible, Torah, Koran, other prayer book, devotional literature, religious symbols (i.e., prayer beads, cross, Star of David), or religious get-well cards in the room? Does a faith community send flowers or worship service bulletins?
2. *Behaviour.* Does the client appear to pray before meals or at other times or read religious literature? Does the client have nightmares and sleep disturbances, or express anger at religious representatives or a deity?
3. *Verbalization.* Does the client mention a divine being, deity, or creative force, prayer, faith, the church, synagogue, mosque, temple, spiritual or religious leader, or religious topics? Does the client ask about a visit from the clergy? Does the client express fear of death, concern with the meaning of life, inner conflict about religious beliefs, concern about a relationship with the deity, questions about the meaning of existence, the meaning of suffering, or the moral or ethical implications of treatment options?
4. *Affect and attitude.* Does the client appear lonely, depressed, angry, anxious, agitated, apathetic, or preoccupied?
5. *Interpersonal relationships.* Who visits? How does the client respond to visitors? Do clergy visit? How does the client relate to other clients and nursing personnel?

Diagnosing

SPIRITUAL PROBLEMS AS THE DIAGNOSTIC LABEL NANDA International (2007) included the following diagnostic labels for clients with problems of spirituality:

- *Spiritual Distress* is "impaired ability to experience and integrate meaning and purpose in life through a person's connectedness with self, others, art, music, literature, nature or a power greater than oneself" (NANDA International, 2007, p. 186). Clinical examples of assessment data clusters and related nursing diagnoses are shown in Table 46.2.
- *Readiness for Enhanced Spiritual Well-Being* recognizes that spiritual well-being is the "ability to experience and integrate meaning and purpose in life through a person's connectedness with self, others, art, music, literature, nature or a power greater than oneself" (NANDA International, 2007, p. 189). Some people will respond to adversity with an

increased spiritual strength that provides hope and comfort.

- *Risk for Spiritual Distress* is defined by NANDA International (2007) as being "at risk for an impaired ability to experience and integrate meaning and purpose in life through a person's connectedness with self, other persons, art, music, literature, nature, and/or a power greater than oneself" (p. 188).

SPIRITUAL OR RELIGIOUS DISTRESS AS THE ETIOLOGY Spiritual distress can affect other areas of functioning and indicate other diagnoses. In these instances, spiritual distress becomes the etiology. Examples include the following:

- *Fear* related to apprehension about the soul's future after death and unpreparedness for death
- *Chronic or Situational Low Self-Esteem* related to failure to live within the precepts of faith
- *Disturbed Sleep Pattern* related to spiritual distress
- *Ineffective Coping* related to feelings of abandonment by God and loss of religious faith
- *Decisional Conflict* related to conflict between treatment plan and religious or spiritual beliefs

Planning

In the planning phase, the nurse identifies interventions to help the client achieve the overall goal of maintaining or restoring spiritual health so that spiritual strength, serenity, and satisfaction are realized. For example, goals may include the following:

- Maintains meaningful personal relationship with deity
- Maintains harmonious supportive relationships with others

Examples of desired outcomes to achieve each of these goals, although developed in the planning phase, are provided in Table 46.3 in the "Evaluating" section of this chapter (page 1484).

Planning in relation to spiritual needs should be designed to do one or more of the following:

- Help the client fulfill spiritual and religious obligations
- Help the client draw on and use inner resources more effectively to meet the present situation
- Help the client maintain or establish a dynamic, personal relationship with self, others, and a divine being in the face of unpleasant circumstances
- Help the client find meaning in existence and the present situation
- Promote a sense of hope
- Provide new spiritual resources

Implementing

Spiritual interventions promote health and healing (Tuck, 2004). Nursing actions to help clients meet their spiritual needs include (1) providing presence, (2) supporting spiritual and religious practices, (3) assisting clients with prayer and meditation, (4) referring clients to spiritual care professionals and faith group leaders, and (5) maintaining connections with others.

PROVIDING PRESENCE "Probably the greatest tool available to nurses for meeting spiritual needs is their own presence and an ability to touch another, both physically and spiritually" (Carson, 1989, p. 164). Being present means being willing to suffer with another, to offer and share oneself, and to gain insight into the client's meaning and purpose in life, sickness, and health. The nurse provides presence through the development of a personal relationship with the client, a relationship that enables the nurse to experience the client's uniqueness. The client, in turn, experiences the nurse's uniqueness. In providing presence, the nurse communicates a willingness to care, to listen, and to be available to the client. "Presence itself

TABLE 46.2 Clinical Application: Assessment Data Clusters and Related Nursing Diagnoses for Clients with Spiritual Distress

Data Cluster	Nursing Diagnosis
Marilyn Eckhardt, 72 years old, is crying, fingering her rosary, and voicing concern that she has not seen her priest for confession since being admitted to the hospital. She states that she is afraid to die without confessing her sins. She also states that she does not want to see the hospital chaplain, but rather her own priest, whose parish is about 18 kilometres away. The hospital record indicates that Ms. Eckhardt is Roman Catholic.	*Spiritual Distress* related to inability to practise spiritual ritual (confession with parish priest)
John Ames, 42 years old, is in a terminal state with an AIDS-related condition. He has become withdrawn but states to the nurse, "What have I done that God has punished me so?" The nurse observes religious literature on his bedside cabinet.	*Spiritual Distress* related to crisis of illness and impending death

touches the client's spirit, just as a cool hand might soothe a fevered brow" (Carson, 1989, p. 165).

The act of being present for clients involves qualities considered to be humanistic: compassion, kindness, honesty, love, gentleness, and patience. Being present to clients asks nurses to engage with others in times of uncertainty, not so much to fix or answer but to be in mystery with another. "Spiritual care-giving calls us to be with another in openness and love, creating a safe and sacred place in which to explore the questions, delve into the mystery, and seek meaning" (Burkhardt & Nagai-Jacobson, 2002, p. 50).

SUPPORTING SPIRITUAL AND RELIGIOUS PRACTICES
During the assessment of the client, the nurse obtains specific information about the client's spiritual and religious preference and practices. These will be considered when planning nursing care, especially when it is affected by client preferences and practices about birth, death, dress, diet, prayer, sacred symbols, sacred writings, and holy days. The Teaching: Wellness box outlines ways the nurse can help clients to continue their usual spiritual practices.

ASSISTING CLIENTS WITH PRAYER AND MEDITATION
Prayer involves a sense of love, connection, and a reaching out. It has many health benefits and healing properties (Dossey, 1996). It offers the following:

- Someone to talk to
- A sense of being loved unconditionally
- A sense of serenity and connection with something greater
- A way to develop compassionate behaviour

Clients may choose to participate in personal prayer or want community prayer with family, friends, or representatives of their faith. Likewise, meditation practices may be integral to a person's faith tradition. In such situations, the nurse's major responsibility is to ensure a quiet environment and privacy. Nursing care may need to be adjusted to accommodate periods for prayer and meditation.

Illness can interfere with some clients' ability to pray. Feelings of anxiety, fear, guilt, grief, despair, and isolation can produce barriers to relationships in general and in the relationship the person has with his or her deity. In these instances, clients may ask the nurse to pray with them. Prayers with clients should only be done when there is mutual agreement between the clients and those praying with them. Because prayer can take various forms, Carson (1989) offered the following guidelines:

- Ask the client to whom they pray and whether there is a special prayer that has personal significance. The client may be comforted by reciting such a prayer with the nurse.

TEACHING: WELLNESS

Supporting Religious Practices

IN HOSPITAL OR OTHER CARE CENTRE
Being able to continue their spiritual practices is important to many clients:

- Inform the client about religious services provided in the agency. Many agencies provide nondenominational religious services or several services for different denominations.
- Ensure opportunities for privacy for the client and family for prayer, meditation, or counsel. Many agencies have quiet areas for these purposes.
- Support the client's desire to have spiritual icons, statues, jewellery, or other religious items with him or her and protect them from damage or loss.
- With the client's permission, facilitate arrangements for the client's minister, priest, rabbi, or other spiritual adviser or healer to visit. Many hospitals also provide the services of an agency chaplain or a list of clergy to call when needed. Hospital chaplains can also be used as a resource for finding representatives for various religious groups.
- If sacraments or other rituals are to be performed by spiritual leaders or healers, prepare the client's room appropriately. For example, clear the bedside table, draw the bed curtains, and make sure there is a seat near the bedside for the religious counsellor.
- Make arrangements with the dietitian for dietary practices to be met. If the agency cannot accommodate the client's needs, ask the family to bring in their own food.
- Consult with the client, family, or spiritual adviser before removing special amulets, garments, or body hair for tests, treatments, or surgery. For example, Sikhism requires that men wear a turban 24 hours a day and have uncut hair. Some Sikhs, therefore, may refuse to have any body hair cut (e.g., for electrodes or an intravenous infusion).

IN THE HOME

- Explore resources available, such as audiotapes of weekly religious services, taped meditations or inspirational music, televised religious services, and clergy who routinely make home visits.
- Consult with family members to consider ways to help the client, such as reading scriptures on a regular basis, having prayer sessions, providing inspirational literature, and so on.

- Use a conversational type of prayer that reflects the client's concerns and needs. For example, "Please comfort Mrs. Wilson as she enters surgery. Lift her fear and in its place give her peace and strength. Let her know you are with her. . . ."
- Tell the client that you will say a private prayer if you are not comfortable praying out loud or if the client is uncomfortable with the spoken prayer.
- Offer to be with clients during private prayer or personal meditation.

Nurses who are unaccustomed to praying aloud or in public may find it helpful to have a formal prayer or a religious passage readily available. Because prayer can evoke deep feelings, the nurse needs to spend time with the client following a prayer to enable the client to express these feelings.

REFERRING CLIENTS TO SPIRITUAL CARE PROFESSIONALS AND FAITH GROUP LEADERS Sometimes, spiritual care is best referred to other members of the health-care team. Referrals can be made for hospitalized clients and their families through the hospital chaplain's office if one is available. Nurses in home and community health settings can identify spiritual resources by checking directories of community service agencies, telephone directories, or religious directories that describe available spiritual care professionals and the services provided through the religious community.

Many faith group leaders will provide assistance to members of their faith who are not members of their specific religious community. For example, a priest, a rabbi, an imam, or a minister may attend a client in the hospital or at home even though the person is not a member of the faith leader's local faith community.

Referrals may be necessary when the nurse makes a diagnosis of spiritual distress. In this situation, the nurse and spiritual care professional or faith group leader can work together to meet the client's needs. One situation the nurse may encounter is client refusal of necessary medical intervention because of religious tenets. In this case, the nurse encourages the client, physician, and spiritual adviser to discuss the conflict and consider alternative methods of treatment. The nurse's major role is to provide the information the client needs to make an informed decision and then to support the client's decision.

Referrals can also be made to parish nurses, registered nurses who function as members of a congregation's ministry team, combining nursing and health expertise in the context of a faith community's mission. They believe that spiritual health is the core of an individual's wellness and that it influences all aspects of well-being. Parish nurses build on the strengths of individuals, families, and the community, assisting and empowering them to become more active in their own health. They work in partnership with faith group leaders and congregational members to enable the faith community to become a place of health and healing (Clark & Olson, 2000; Solari-Twadell & McDermott, 1999).

MAINTAINING CONNECTIONS WITH OTHERS As human beings, our belonging needs are strong and our very survival depends on our connection with others (Burkhardt & Nagai-Jacobson, 2002). At times of stress and during illness these connections are even more important than when life flows along smoothly. The nurse can carry out important spiritual care interventions when facilitating clients' connections with loved ones in times of stress and illness. Being aware of the client's most significant relationships enables the nurse to seek ways to encourage these connections to promote health and healing. When actual connections with significant others are not possible, access to photos, phone calls, and electronic communication can be facilitated. It is also important to be aware of relationships that cause stress for the client. Nurses may need to offer support at times when these interactions are inevitable. Finally, assisting family members and friends with their questions and concerns about interacting with clients during times of illness and treatment can be an important nursing role.

See the Sample Care Plan for a care plan on spiritual distress.

Evidence-Informed Practice

What Does Spiritual Nursing Care Mean?

Carr (2008) examined the meaning of spiritual nursing care by interviewing 29 individuals. The participants included oncology nurses, patients, family members, and others. The analysis revealed that a core process within spiritual nursing care is developing a caring relationship. Although participants agreed that patients and families do seek spiritual care from nurses, they may not do so consciously or in a planned way; rather, the provision of spiritual care can develop out of the relationship. The results suggested that four qualities of nurses are very important for spiritual care: receptivity, humanity, competency, and positivity.

NURSING IMPLICATIONS: Spiritual care by nurses is a "whole and natural experience" arising out of the caring relationship, a "way of being" for the nurse (p. 697).

Source: Based on "Mapping the Processes and Qualities of Spiritual Nursing Care," by T. Carr, 2008, *Qualitative Health Research, 18*(5), pp. 686–700.

Evaluating

By using the measurable desired outcomes developed during the planning stage, the nurse collects data needed to judge whether client goals and health outcomes have been achieved. Examples of client goals and related health outcomes are shown in Table 46.3.

Sample Care Plan for Spiritual Distress

ASSESSMENT DATA

Nursing Assessment

Mrs. Sally Horton is a 60-year-old hospitalized homemaker who is recovering from a right radical mastectomy. Yesterday, she was told by her physician that because of metastases of the cancer, her prognosis is poor. This morning her primary nurse finds her tearful, stating she slept poorly and has no appetite. She asks the nurse, "Why is this happening to me? Perhaps it's because I have sinned in my life. I've not gone to church or spoken to a minister in several years. Is there a chapel in the hospital where I could go and pray? I'm terribly afraid of dying and what awaits me."

Physical Examination

Height: 165.1 cm

Weight: 54.0 kg

Temperature: 36.6°C

Pulse: 88 bpm

Respirations: 22/min

Blood Pressure: 146/86 mm Hg

Large surgical dressing right chest wall and axillary region, dry and intact. Slight edema right hand and arm.

Nursing Diagnosis

Spiritual Distress related to separation from religious rituals (as evidenced by questioning credibility of personal beliefs, depression, expressions of resentment and fear of death, requests for chapel visits).

Diagnostic Data	Normal	
RBC: 3.5×10^{12}/L	Female: 4.1–5.1 $\times 10^{12}$/L	Male: 4.5–5.3 $\times 10^{12}$/L
Hgb: 105 g/L	Female: 120–160 g/L	Male: 130–180 g/L
Hct: 0.35	Female: 0.36–0.46	Male 0.37–0.49

Client Goals

The client will regain a sense of spiritual satisfaction.

Desired Health Outcomes

1. Expresses desire to perform religious or spiritual practices
2. Visits with chaplain by day 2
3. Displays absence of feelings of anger and resentment by day 5
4. Verbalizes increase in psychological and spiritual comfort with illness, prognosis, and death

NURSING INTERVENTIONS AND SELECTED ACTIVITIES WITH RATIONALES *[IN ITALICS]**

Spiritual Support

• Be open to Mrs. Horton's feelings about illness and death.	*This honesty encourages expression of inner fears and concerns and teaches the client the value of confronting issues.*
• Assist her to properly express and relieve anger in appropriate ways.	*Anger can be a source of energy and its release a source of freedom when expressed in a constructive manner.*
• Use values clarification techniques to help Mrs. Horton clarify beliefs and values.	*Value conflicts often lead to confusion and indecision. Clarification of beliefs and values will help clients to base decisions on their most important values, including those that are spiritual in nature.*
• Listen carefully to her communication and develop a sense of timing for prayer or spiritual rituals.	*The nature of spiritual care may directly affect the speed and quality of recovery or redefinition of hope and finding of meaning in death.*
• Facilitate Mrs. Horton's use of meditation, prayer, and other religious traditions and rituals.	*Spiritual needs are sometimes overlooked or ignored. Recognizing and respecting the individual's spiritual needs is an important advocacy role for nurses.*
• Assure her that the nurse will be available to support her in times of suffering.	*Fidelity is essential in helping alleviate the client's fear of dying alone.*

Coping Enhancement

• Create an accepting, nonjudgmental atmosphere.	*This establishes rapport and the therapeutic relationship, which promotes communication and open expression.*
• Encourage verbalization of feelings, perceptions, and fears. Allow time for grieving.	*Being with the person who is suffering gives meaning to his or her experience.*
• Encourage her to list values that guide behaviour in various settings and types of situations.	*This exercise helps the client clarify values and beliefs by reflecting on past behaviours. Experience is a major source for value development.*

EVALUATION

Goal met. Mrs. Horton has been visited on several occasions by her minister. She reads scripture each day and has found consolation in reading the Book of Psalms. She states "God is merciful and will help me bear my suffering."

*Interventions and activities selected are only a sample of those suggested in the *Nursing Interventions Classification (NIC)*, by G. M. Bulechek, H. K. Butcher, and J. C. Dochterman (Eds.), 2008, St. Louis, MO: Mosby Elsevier, and should be individualized for each client.

TABLE 46.3 Evaluation Goals and Outcomes: Spiritual Well-Being

Goal	Examples of Desired Outcomes
Maintains meaningful personal relationships with deity	Verbalizes satisfaction with relationship with deity Carries out usual religious practices using resources available Expresses feelings of inner peace and spiritual fulfillment States faith provides strength to understand and endure suffering
Maintains harmonious, supportive relationships with others	Conveys warmth and compassion to family, friends, and others Shares thoughts, feelings, and faith with others

Case Study 46

Linh Van is a 32-year-old woman who received several units of blood following an automobile accident in the late 1980s. Five years ago she was diagnosed with AIDS (acquired immune deficiency syndrome) and is now in the hospital. She is very ill and you sense she is discouraged with the seriousness of her illness, but know from both your own experience and routine reports at change of staff that she does not speak about such matters. Ms. Van is a devout Buddhist, and you have noticed her daily practices of meditation and ritual. In light of her grave prognosis, including the probability of severe pain, you wonder about discussing the topic of spiritual care with her.

Critical Thinking Skills

1. On what basis are you sensing that Ms. Van is discouraged with the seriousness of her illness? Explain.
2. What does Ms. Van's silence in the face of her illness tell you about her spiritual beliefs?
3. How might Ms. Van's behaviour in the face of her illness and suffering be affected by her spiritual beliefs? by her religious beliefs?
4. How might a spiritual assessment be of benefit to both you and the client?
5. If you were to discuss the topic of spirituality and spiritual care with Ms. Van, what is the first question you might ask?

After working through these questions, go to the MyNursingLab at **http://www.mynursinglab.com** to check your answers.

KEY TERMS

spirituality
religion
agnostic
atheist
theistic
monotheism
polytheism
faith
developmental
hope
world view
beliefs
values
assumptions
generalized anxiety
spiritual well-being
spiritual wellness
spiritual health
spiritual distress
holy day
prayer
meditation
kosher

CHAPTER HIGHLIGHTS

- Clients have a right to receive care that respects their individual spiritual and religious beliefs, values, and practices.
- The spiritual needs of clients and support persons often come into focus at a time of illness. Spiritual beliefs and religious practices often help people accept illness and plan for the future.
- Spirituality and religion are distinct concepts. Spirituality is a broad concept that encompasses relationships with a divine being, deity, or creative force; with the self; with nature; and with others. Religion is more practical and acts as a container or holding environment that offers ways to express spirituality. Both spiritual and religious beliefs influ-

ence lifestyle, attitudes, and feelings about health, illness, and death.

- Spiritual health is described as a feeling of being generally alive, purposeful, and fulfilled. It is manifested by a person's communication that reveals meaning and purpose to existence, inner peace, trusting relationships, and inner strength that is directed toward ultimate values of love, meaning, hope, beauty, and truth.
- Spiritual distress refers to a disturbance in or a challenge to a person's core value system that provides strength, hope, and meaning to life. Possible factors in spiritual distress include physiological problems, treatment-related concerns, situational and developmental concerns. Spiritual distress can be reflected in a number of behaviours, including depression, anxiety, verbalizations of unworthiness, and fear of death.
- A spiritual assessment is best obtained after the nurse has developed a good relationship with the client. Information may be elicited about the client's concept of the deity or creative force, the client's source of hope and strength, the significance of spiritual or religious practices and rituals, and the relationship the client perceives between health and spiritual or religious beliefs.
- Home health nurses can observe cues in the home that may indicate client spiritual beliefs and practices. Nurses in community settings should be aware of spiritual and religious resources in the community and what services they provide.
- To implement spiritual care, nurses need to be skilled in establishing a trusting nurse–client relationship.
- Nurses can support clients' spiritual and religious practices if they understand needs related to holy days, sacred writings, spiritual symbols, prayer and meditation, diet practices, dress requirements or prohibitions, birth rituals, and death rituals.
- Nursing interventions that promote spiritual health include offering a supportive presence, supporting the client's spiritual and religious practices, assisting clients with prayer and meditation, referring clients to a spiritual care professional or faith group leader, and maintaining connection with others.
- Nurses need to be aware of their own spiritual beliefs in order to be comfortable assisting others.

ASSESS YOUR LEARNING

1. Mr. Marshall tells the nurse that his friend was killed in the all-terrain vehicle mishap. When the nurse is talking to Mr. Marshall about his feelings, he states, "I can't believe God can be so cruel. I am so angry and frustrated!" What should be the nurse's initial response?

a. Acknowledge Mr. Marshall's spiritual concerns.
b. Reassure Mr. Marshall that accidents are unavoidable.
c. Refer Mr. Marshall to a grief counsellor.
d. Ask whether Mr. Marshall would like to talk to a chaplain.

2. Mrs. Smith is an older adult residing in your skilled nursing facility. She is searching for a way to make life meaningful. When planning care for Mrs. Smith, which of the following nursing actions would be most beneficial?

a. Assess for depression.
b. Diagnose and document that the client has *Spiritual Distress.*
c. Keep the client busy with social activities.
d. Engage the client in a spiritual assessment.

3. Mr. Hussein, a Muslim patient, is given a grave prognosis. His wife asks the nurse for prayer support. Which of the following is the nurse's best initial response in determining further nursing interventions?

a. "May I call the chaplain?"
b. "I know your faith is important to you. My faith is important to me, too."
c. "How may I best help you in getting prayer support?"
d. "Isn't it wonderful that we have Jesus with whom we can share our concerns?"

4. A client reports, "Cancer is the best thing that has happened to me! It is making me appreciate life so much more." This statement fits best with which NANDA International diagnosis?

a. *Spiritual Distress*
b. *Risk for Spiritual Distress*
c. *Readiness for Enhanced Spiritual Well-Being*
d. *Cognitive Denial*

5. A dying client states, "Part of what makes dying hard is that I don't know for sure where I'm going. Nurse, what do you believe happens in the hereafter?" Which ethical guideline should guide your response?

a. Never share personal spiritual beliefs.
b. Share all spiritual beliefs, favouring none.
c. Share only your beliefs.
d. First, assess client beliefs.

6. A client in the emergency department needs red blood cells. She is a Jehovah's Witness, whose religious beliefs make it impossible for her to accept the prescribed blood transfusion. Which of the following statements would most likely lead to a resolution of this conflict?

a. "You must accept the transfusion or else leave the emergency department so others can receive care."

b. "Please accept the transfusion; you can ask for pardon after taking the blood."

c. "May I call a representative of your religion to facilitate discussion about alternative methods of treatment?"

d. "I understand your position. Without the transfusion you will die, but I'll be here to support you."

7. An 88-year-old Buddhist woman has just been admitted to a skilled nursing facility. She tells the nurse that she has been a spiritual practitioner for many years and hopes to continue her daily meditations. How should the nurse initially respond to this request?

a. "Tell me more about your daily meditation practice."

b. "I think there is a Buddhist temple listed in the phone book."

c. "I studied Buddhism in my world religions class in university."

d. "Unfortunately, you are our only Buddhist client."

8. Which of the following is an appropriate spiritual screening or assessment question?

a. "Tell me more about your religion."

b. "How can we support your spiritual and religious beliefs and practices?"

c. "How has your prayer experience been affected by your illness?"

d. "What do you see as the purpose or mission for your life?"

9. The mother of a pediatric client states, "I can't understand why God would allow this to happen to my innocent child!" Which NANDA International diagnosis is most accurate?

a. *Spiritual Distress* related to the search for meaning in a child's illness

b. *Impaired Religiosity* related to anger at God

c. *Ineffective Coping* related to anger

d. *Risk for Spiritual Distress* related to a threatened sense of hope

10. A client's spirituality is complex and individual. What is the main reason for assessing and responding to spiritual needs and resources in providing nursing care?

a. To uncover needs that could be referred to spiritual care professionals

b. To decrease suffering and aid in physical and mental healing

c. To fulfill nursing's obligation to do no harm

d. To be able to help clients observe their unique practices

After working through these questions, go to the MyNursingLab at ***http://www.mynursinglab.com*** *to check your answers and see explanations.*

SUGGESTED READINGS

Burkhardt, M., & Nagai-Jacobson, M. (2002). *Spirituality: Living our connectedness.* Albany, NY: Delmar.

This book focuses on helping health-care professionals nurture their own spirituality and recognize spiritual occurrences in everyday life in order to more effectively address the spiritual needs of their clients.

Callister, L. C., Semenic, S., & Foster, J. C. (1999). Cultural and spiritual meanings of childbirth: Orthodox Jewish and Mormon women. *Journal of Holistic Nursing, 17,* 280–295.

This study suggests that religious beliefs help women understand the meaning of childbirth and may offer coping strategies for them to deal with the experience and associated stresses.

Clark, M., & Olson, J. (2000). *Nursing within a faith community: Promoting health in times of transition.* Thousand Oaks, CA: Sage.

The authors provide a unique outlook on the theoretical underpinnings for faith community nursing from the perspective of theology and nursing.

Kirkham, S. R., Pesut, B., Meyerhoff, H., & Sawtzky, R. (2004). Spiritual caregiving at the juncture of religion, culture, and state. *Canadian Journal of Nursing Research, 36*(4), 148–169.

The findings of this study point to the need for health-care professionals to cultivate an internal space in which to provide spiritual care and to seek spiritual points of connection amid diverse faith and cultural traditions.

Olson, J. K., Paul, P., Douglass, L., Clark, M. B., Simington, J., & Goddard, N. (2003). Addressing the spiritual dimension in Canadian undergraduate nursing education. *Canadian Journal of Nursing Research, 35*(3), 94–107.

This study identified the extent to which the spiritual dimension is addressed in Canadian university undergraduate nursing curricula. Eighteen of the 29 eligible schools (62%) in Canada participated. The findings indicated that conceptions about spirituality were confusing and that the spiritual dimension is rarely defined or included in curricular objectives.

Ontario Multifaith Council on Spiritual and Religious Care. (2002). *Multifaith information manual: An authoritative guide to religious rights and accommodations.* Toronto: Author.

The *Multifaith Information Manual* is a creative response to the growing diversity of the Canadian population. Providers of care or service within institutional or community-based environments will find this manual an indispensable tool for managing religious diversity issues.

Taylor, E. J. (2002). *Spiritual care: Nursing theory, research, and practice.* Upper Saddle River, NJ: Pearson Education.

The innate and deeply personal nature of spirituality is emphasized in this text. It includes suggestions about spiritual caregiving, spiritual assessment, planning care, documentation, ethical concerns, and ways to nurture the spirit.

WEBLINKS

Canadian Association for Parish Nurse Ministry

http://www.capnm.ca

Parish nursing is recognized as an essential dimension in the integration of faith and health within diverse faith communities throughout Canada. The Canadian Association for Parish Nurse Ministry is committed to the development of parish nursing as a health and ministry resource within Canada.

Canadian Association for Pastoral Practice and Education

http://www.cappe.org

The Canadian Association for Pastoral Practice and Education (CAPPE) is a national multifaith organization that is committed to the professional education, certification, and support of people involved in pastoral care and pastoral counselling. CAPPE is concerned with a holistic approach to health care and personal development, with a special focus on spiritual and religious care.

Canadian Research Institute of Spirituality and Healing

http://www.crish.org

The Canadian Research Institute of Spirituality and Healing is a Canadian professional organization that promotes multidisciplinary research and education in spirituality, culture, healing, and health care. It was initiated in 2006 and is associated with regular international multidisciplinary conferences focusing on spirituality and health.

Multifaith Calendar

http://www.multifaithcalendar.com

The multifaith calendar stimulates dialogue and discussion for people of many cultures and faiths.

North American Interfaith Network

http://www.nain.org

The North American Interfaith Network (NAIN) is a nonprofit association of interfaith organizations and agencies in Canada, Mexico, and the United States. NAIN offers networking opportunities to persons of many religious traditions and numerous interfaith organizations.

Ontario Multifaith Council

http://www.omc.ca

The Ontario Multifaith Council on Spiritual and Religious Care is a nonprofit charitable organization representing a wide range of faith groups in Ontario. It is recognized as one of North America's largest organizations dedicated to advocacy of spiritual care and the protection of religious rights. This site includes a searchable multifaith library feature.

REFERENCES

Andresen J., & Foreman R. (2000). Methodological pluralism in the study of religion. *Journal of Consciousness Studies, 7*(11–12), 7–16.

Bibby, R. W. (2006). *The boomer factor: What Canada's most famous generation is leaving behind.* Toronto: Bastian Books.

Burkhardt, M. (1993). Characteristics of spirituality in the lives of women in a rural Appalachian community. *Journal of Transcultural Nursing, 4,* 12–18.

Burkhardt, M., & Nagai-Jacobson, M. (2002). *Spirituality: Living our connectedness.* Albany, NY: Delmar.

Carpenito-Moyet, L. J. (2008). *Nursing diagnosis: Application to clinical practice* (12th ed.). Philadelphia, PA: Lippincott.

Carson, V. B. (1989). *Spiritual dimensions of nursing practice.* Philadelphia, PA: Saunders.

Chiu, L., Emblen, J., Van Hofwegen, L., Sawatzky, R., & Meyerhoff, H. (2004). An integrative review of the concept of spirituality in the health sciences. *Western Journal of Nursing Research, 26*(4), 405–428.

Clark, M. (2000). Characteristics of faith communities. In M. Clark & J. Olson (Eds.), *Nursing within a faith community: Promoting health in times of transition* (pp. 17–29). Thousand Oaks, CA: Sage.

Clark, M., & Olson, J. (2000). *Nursing within a faith community: Promoting health in times of transition.* Thousand Oaks, CA: Sage.

Denny, F. M. (1993). Islam and the Muslim community. In H. Byron Earhart (Ed.), *Religious traditions of the world* (pp. 603–712). New York: HarperSanFrancisco.

Dossey, L. (1993). *Healing words: The power of prayer and the practice of medicine.* New York: HarperSanFranciso.

Dossey, L. (1996). *Prayer is good medicine. How to reap the benefits of prayer.* New York: Harper Collins.

Ellison, C. W. (1983). Spiritual well-being: Conceptualization and measurement. *Journal of Psychology and Theology, 11,* 330–340.

Erikson, E. (1963). *Childhood and society.* New York: Norton.

Fishbane, M. (1993). Judaism: Revelation and traditions. In H. Byron Earhart (Ed.), *Religious traditions of the world* (pp. 373–484). New York: HarperSanFrancisco.

Fitchett, G. (1993). *Assessing spiritual needs.* Minneapolis, MN: Augsburg.

Ford, I. M. (1988). *Life spirals: The faith journey.* Burlington, ON: Welch.

Fowler, J. W. (1974). Toward a developmental perspective on faith. *Religious Education, 69,* 207–219.

Fowler, J. W. (1981). *Stages in faith.* New York: Harper & Row.

Fowler, J., & Keen, S. (1985). *Life maps: Conversations in the journey of faith.* Waco, TX: Word Books.

Frankiel, S. S. (1993). Christianity: A way of salvation. In H. Byron Earhart (Ed.), *Religious traditions of the world* (pp. 484–601). New York: HarperSanFrancisco.

Gottlieb, L., & Ezer H. (Eds.). (1997). *A perspective on health, family, learning and collaborative nursing: A collection of writing on the McGill model of nursing.* Montreal: McGill University School of Nursing.

Griffith, J. K. (1996). *The religious aspects of nursing care.* Vancouver: Author.

Grimm, P. M. (1991). Hope. In J. L. Creasia & B. Parker (Eds.), *Conceptual foundations of professional nursing practice.* St. Louis, MO: Mosby-Year Book.

Hood Morris, L. E. (1996). A spiritual well-being model: Use with older women who experience depression. *Issues in Mental Health Nursing, 17,* 439–455.

Jevne, R. (1991). *It all begins with hope: Patients, caregivers and the bereaved speak out.* Philadelphia, PA: Innisfree Press.

Moschella, V. D., Pressman, K. R., Pressman, P., & Weissman, D. E. (1997). The problem of theodicy and religious response to cancer. *Journal of Religion & Health, 36*(1), 17–20.

Murray, R. B., & Zentner, J. B. (1997). *Nursing assessment and health promotion strategies through the life span* (6th ed.). Norwalk, CT: Appleton & Lange.

NANDA International. (2007). *Nursing diagnoses: Definitions and classification, 2007–2008.* Philadelphia, PA: Author.

O'Connor, T., Meakes, E., O'Neill, K., Prenner, C., VanStaalduinen, G., & Davis, K. (2005). Not well known, used little and needed: Canadian chaplains' experiences of published spiritual assessment tools. *Journal of Pastoral Care and Counselling, 59,* 97–107.

Olson, J. (2000). Health promotion during times of transition (pp. 223–232). In *Nursing within a faith community: Promoting health in times of transition.* Thousand Oaks, CA: Sage.

Pilch, J. J. (1988). Wellness spirituality. *Health Values, 12* (May/June), 28–31.

Post-White, J., Ceronsky, C., Kreitzer, M. J., Nickelson, K., Drew, D., Mackey, K. W., et al. (1996). Hope, spirituality, sense of coherence, and quality of life in patients with cancer. *Oncology Nursing Forum, 23,* 1571–1579.

Puchalski, C., Lunsford, B., Harris, M., & Miller, T. (2006). Interdisciplinary spiritual care for seriously ill and dying patients: A collaborative model. *Cancer Journal, 12*(5), 398–416.

Shelley, J. A., & Fish, S. (1988). *Spiritual care: The nurse's role* (3rd ed.). Downers Grove, IL: InterVarsity Press.

Solari-Twadell, P., & McDermott, M. A. (Eds.). (1999). *Parish nursing: Promoting whole person health within faith communities.* Thousand Oaks, CA: Sage.

Stotland, E. (1969). *The psychology of hope.* San Francisco, CA: Jossey-Bass.

Sumner, H. (1998). Recognizing and responding to spiritual distress. *American Journal of Nursing, 98,* 26–31.

Tanyi, R. A. (2006). Spirituality and family nursing: Spiritual assessment and intervention for families. *Journal of Advanced Nursing 53*(3), 287–294.

Taylor, E. (2002). *Spiritual care: Nursing theory, research, and practice.* Upper Saddle River, NJ: Pearson.

Tuck, I. I. (2004). Development of a spirituality intervention to promote healing. *Journal of Theory Construction and Testing, 8*(2), 67–71.

Vardey, L. (Ed.). (1995). *God in all worlds: An anthology of contemporary spiritual writings.* New York: Pantheon Books.

Westerhoff, J. (1976). *Will our children have faith?* New York: Seabury Press.

Winslow, G. R., & Winslow, B. W. (2003). Examining the ethics of praying with patients. *Holistic Nursing Practice, 17*(4), 170–177.

Chapter 47

Stress and Coping

Stress is a universal phenomenon. All people experience it. Parents refer to the stress of raising children; working people talk of the stress of their jobs; and students at all levels talk of the stress of school. Stress can result from both positive and negative experiences. For example, a bride preparing for her wedding or a graduate preparing to start a new job may have stress reactions to these positive experiences, and a husband concerned about caring for his wife and family following a diagnosis of cancer may experience similar stress reactions.

The concept of stress is important because it provides a way of understanding the person as a unified being who responds in totality (mind, body, and spirit) to a variety of changes that take place in daily life.

OBJECTIVES

After studying this chapter, you should be able to

1. Differentiate the concepts of stress as a stimulus, as a response, and as a transaction
2. Describe the three stages of Selye's general adaptation syndrome
3. Identify physiological, psychological, and cognitive indicators of stress
4. Differentiate four levels of anxiety
5. Outline behaviours related to specific ego defence mechanisms
6. Discuss types of coping and coping strategies
7. Identify essential aspects of assessing a client's stress and coping patterns
8. Explain nursing diagnoses related to stress
9. Describe interventions to help clients minimize and manage stress

Concept of Stress

Stress is a condition in which the person experiences changes in the normal balanced state. A **stressor** is any event or stimulus that causes an individual to experience stress. When a person faces stressors, responses are referred to as *coping strategies, coping responses,* or *coping mechanisms.*

Sources of Stress

Stress has many sources. They can be broadly classified as internal or external stressors, or developmental or situational stressors. *Internal stressors* originate within a person, for example, an infection or feelings of depression. *External stressors* originate outside the individual, for example, a move to another city, a death in the family, or pressure from peers. *Developmental stressors* occur at predictable times throughout an individual's life (Table 47.1). *Situational stressors* are unpredictable and can occur at any time during life. Examples of situational stressors include the death of a significant other, getting or losing a job, or an acute illness.

The degree to which any of these sources of stress has positive or negative effects can depend to some degree on an individual's developmental stage. For example, the death of a parent may be more stressful for a 12-year-old than for a 40-year-old. See the Lifespan Considerations box.

TABLE 47.1 Selected Stressors Associated with Developmental Stages

Developmental Stage	Stressors
Child	Resolving conflict between independence and dependence Beginning school Establishing peer relationships and adjustments Coping with peer competition
Adolescent	Accepting changing physique Developing relationships involving sexual attraction Achieving independence Choosing a career
Young adult	Getting married Leaving home Managing a home Getting started in an occupation Continuing education Rearing children
Middle adult	Accepting physical changes of aging Maintaining social status and standard of living Helping teenage children to become independent Helping aging parents
Older adult	Accepting decreasing physical abilities and health Accepting changes in residence Adjusting to retirement and reduced income Coping with death of spouse or partner and friends

Effects of Stress

Stress can have physical, emotional, intellectual, social, and spiritual consequences. Usually the effects are mixed, because stress affects the whole person. Physically, stress can threaten a person's physiological homeostasis. Emotionally, stress can produce negative or unconstructive feelings about the self. Intellectually, stress can influence a person's perceptual and problem-solving abilities. Socially, stress can alter a person's relationships with others. Spiritually, stress can challenge one's beliefs and values. Many conditions have been linked to stress (Figure 47.1).

Models of Stress

Models of stress help nurses to identify the stressor operating in a particular situation and to predict the individual's responses. Nurses can use the knowledge of these models to assist clients in strengthening healthy coping responses and in adjusting less healthy or unproductive responses. Three main models of stress are stimulus based, response based, and transaction based.

Stimulus-Based Models

In **stimulus-based stress models**, stress is defined as a stimulus, a life event, or a set of circumstances that arouses physiological or psychosocial reactions that may increase the individual's vulnerability to illness. In their classic work, Holmes and Rahe (1967) assigned a numerical value to 43 life changes or events. The most recent version of that scale includes 77 items (Miller & Rahe, 1997), and a shortened version (54 items, full stress and coping inventory completed in 15 minutes) was created more recently (Rahe & Tolles, 2002). The scale of stressful life events is used to document a person's relatively recent experiences, such as divorce, pregnancy, and retirement. In this view, both positive and negative events are considered stressful.

Lifespan Considerations

Stress and Coping

People experience stress at all stages of life:

INFANTS AND CHILDREN

- Children's perceptions of and responses to stress are dependent on their developmental stage. Infants sense stressors in their environment and respond in a diffuse way, often crying and clinging. Toddlers and preschool-age children may be frightened and react by withdrawing or losing control. School-age children and adolescents are more capable of thinking about incidents that cause stress (e.g., a catastrophic accident) and talking about them with adults.
- Temperament is a factor that influences how children respond to stress. An outgoing, low-sensitivity child, for example, is less likely than a timid, intense child to be upset by a family move to a different province.
- Anxiety disorders are the most common psychiatric disorders in children but are frequently unrecognized (Antai-Otong, 2003).
- As children grow, they are able to develop more coping skills to manage stressful situations. Nurses have an important role in teaching parents to recognize stress in their children and to help their children cope.

MIDDLE-AGED ADULTS

- Middle-aged adults are often called the *sandwich generation*. They find themselves caring for children or grandchildren and often caring for aging parents at the same time. When these activities become time and energy consuming, there is often not enough time left for attention to the self. Nurses need to be aware of this and assist in suggesting resources and effective planning to ease the strain.

OLDER ADULTS

- Older adults experience many losses and changes in their lives. The losses may be incremental and, over time, become stressful and possibly overwhelming. Changes in health, decreased functional ability and independence, need for relocation, loss of family and friends, and becoming a caregiver for a spouse or friend are a few of the stresses often experienced by older adults. Many of them have survived significant challenges in their earlier lives and have learned effective coping skills. Nurses can help them plan, evaluate their strategies, and learn new strategies, if needed. Informal and formal social supports are very important in learning to successfully live with these changes and stress.
- Some effective coping methods for older adults are exercise, learning different relaxation techniques, participating in activities, getting adequate nutrition and rest, and engaging in expressive creative activities, such as art, music, and journaling. Referral to community resources and supports should be done when appropriate. It is most important to see older adults as unique individuals, with unique past experiences and very specific needs as they age.

Other similar scales have been developed, but all such scales require caution because the degree of stress an event presents can be highly individual. For example, a divorce may be highly traumatic to one person and cause relatively little anxiety to another. In addition, many scales have not been tested for age, socioeconomic status, or cultural sensitivity.

Response-Based Models

Stress can also be considered as a response. This definition was developed and described by Selye (1956, 1976) as "the nonspecific response of the body to any kind of demand made upon it" (1976, p. 1). Schafer (1992, p. 9) defined stress as the "arousal of mind and body in response to demands made upon them."

Regardless of the cause, circumstances, or psychological interpretation of a demanding situation, Selye's stress response is characterized by the same chain or pattern of physiological events. This nonspecific response is called the **general adaptation syndrome (GAS)** or *stress syndrome.*

To differentiate the cause of stress from the response to stress, Selye created the term *stressor* (1976) to denote any factor that produces stress and disturbs the body's equilibrium. Because stress is a state of the body, it can be observed only by the changes it produces in the body. This response of the body, the stress syndrome or GAS, occurs with the release of certain adaptive hormones and subsequent changes in the structure and chemical composition of the body. Parts of the body particularly affected by stress are the gastrointestinal tract, the adrenal glands, and the lymphatic structures. With prolonged stress, the adrenal glands enlarge considerably; the lymphatic structures, such as the thymus, spleen, and lymph nodes, atrophy (shrink); and deep ulcers appear in the lining of the stomach.

In addition to adapting globally, the body can also react locally; that is, one organ or a part of the body reacts alone. This is referred to as the **local adaptation syndrome (LAS)**. One example of the LAS is inflammation. Selye (1976) proposed that both the GAS and the LAS have three stages: alarm reaction, resistance, and exhaustion (Figure 47.2).

ALARM REACTION The initial reaction of the body is the **alarm reaction (AR)**, which alerts the body's defences against the stressor, whether the stressor is heat, bacteria,

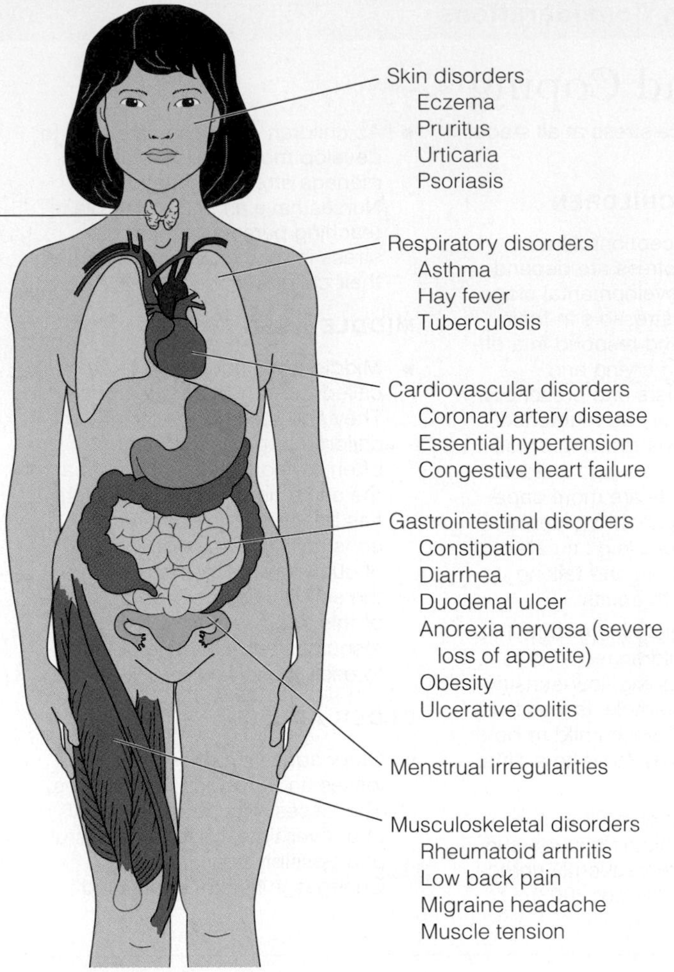

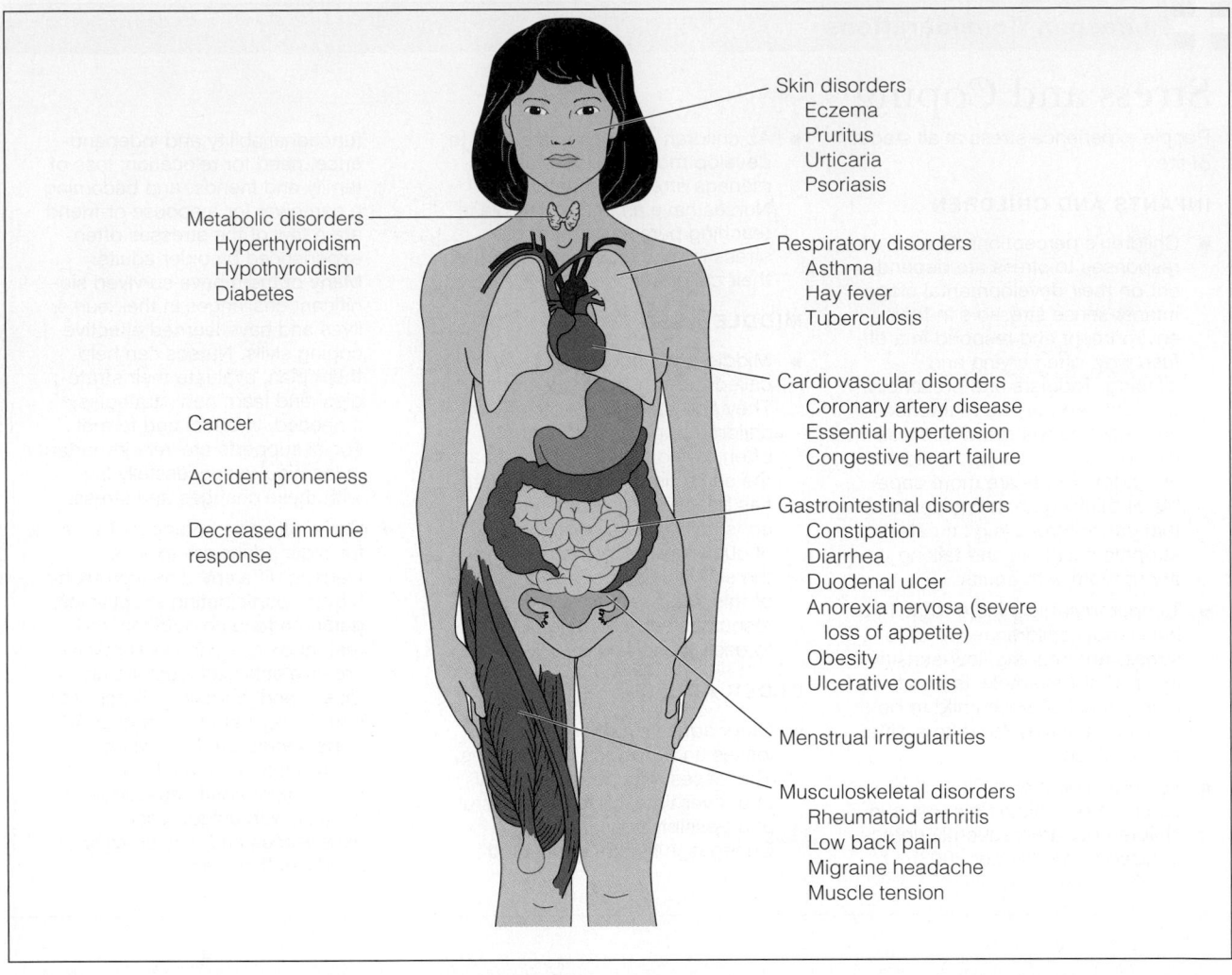

FIGURE 47.1 Some disorders can be caused or aggravated by stress.
(From **Health and Wellness: A Holistic Approach,** *9th ed. (p. 40), by G. Edin and E. Golanty, 2007, Boston, Jones & Bartlett. Adapted with permission.)*

or a verbal or physical attack from someone. Selye divided this stage into two parts: the shock phase and the countershock phase.

During the **shock phase** (Figure 47.2B), the stressor is perceived consciously or unconsciously by the person. Stressors stimulate the sympathetic nervous system, which in turn stimulates the hypothalamus. The hypothalamus releases corticotropin-releasing hormone (CRH), which stimulates the anterior pituitary gland to release adrenocorticotropic hormone (ACTH). During times of stress, the adrenal medulla secretes epinephrine and norepinephrine in response to sympathetic stimulation. Significant body responses to epinephrine include the following:

1. Increased myocardial contractility, which increases cardiac output and blood flow to active muscles
2. Bronchial dilation, which allows increased oxygen intake
3. Increased blood clotting
4. Increased cellular metabolism
5. Increased fat mobilization to make energy available and to synthesize other compounds needed by the body

The principal effect of norepinephrine is decreased blood to the kidneys and increased secretion of renin. Renin is an enzyme that hydrolyzes one of the blood proteins to produce angiotensin. Angiotensin tends to increase the blood pressure by constricting arterioles. The sum of all of these adrenal hormonal effects permits the person to perform far more strenuous physical activity than would otherwise be possible. The person is then ready for "fight or flight." This primary response is short-lived, lasting from 1 minute to 24 hours.

The second part of the AR is called the **countershock phase**. During this time, the changes produced in the body during the shock phase are reversed. Thus, a person is best mobilized to react during the shock phase of the AR.

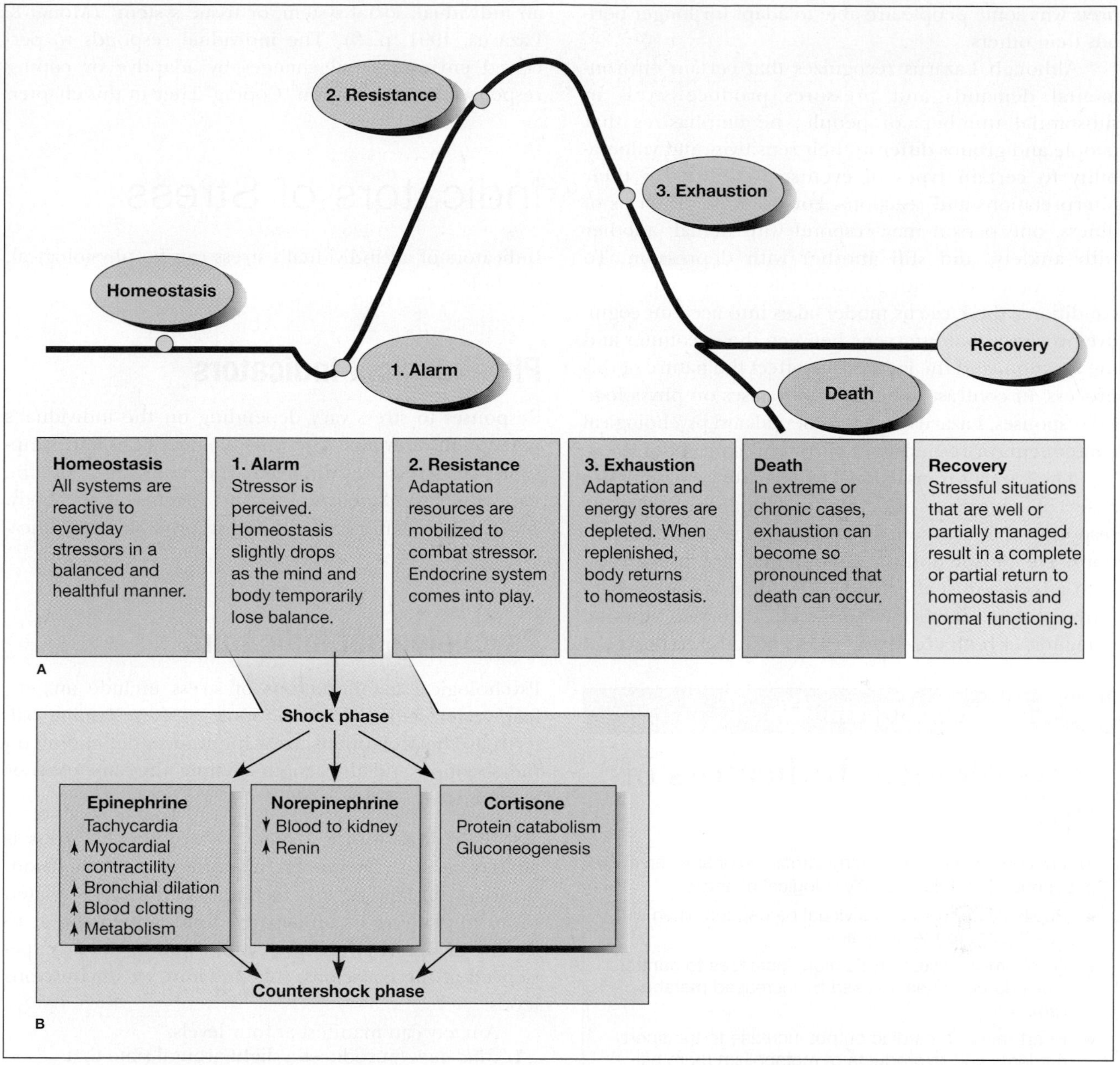

FIGURE 47.2 The three stages of adaptation to stress: The alarm reaction, the stage of resistance, and the stage of exhaustion

(A is from **Wellness: Concepts and Application,** *6th ed. (p. 298), by D. J. Anspaugh, M. Hamrick, and F. D. Rosato, 2005, New York: McGraw-Hill. Reprinted with permission.)*

STAGE OF RESISTANCE The second stage in the GAS and LAS syndromes, the **stage of resistance (SR)**, is when the body's adaptation takes place. In other words, the body attempts to cope with the stressor and to limit the stressor to the smallest area of the body that can deal with it.

STAGE OF EXHAUSTION During the third stage, the **stage of exhaustion**, the adaptation that the body made during the second stage cannot be maintained. This means that the ways used to cope with the stressor have been exhausted. If adaptation has not overcome the stressor, the stress effects may spread to the entire body. At the end of this stage, the body may either rest and return to normal, or death may be the ultimate consequence. The end of this stage depends largely on the adaptive energy resources of the individual, the severity of the stressor, and the external adaptive resources that are provided, such as oxygen.

Transaction-Based Models

Transactional theories of stress are based on the work of Lazarus (1966), who stated that the stimulus theory and the response theory do not consider individual differences. Neither theory explains which factors lead some people and not others to respond effectively, nor interprets why some people are able to adapt for longer periods than others.

Although Lazarus recognizes that certain environmental demands and pressures produce stress in substantial numbers of people, he emphasizes that people and groups differ in their sensitivity and vulnerability to certain types of events, as well as in their interpretations and reactions. For example, in terms of illness, one person may respond with denial, another with anxiety, and still another with depression. To explain variations among individuals under comparable conditions, the Lazarus model takes into account cognitive processes that intervene between the encounter and the reaction, and the factors that affect the nature of this process. In contrast to Selye, who focuses on physiological responses, Lazarus includes mental and psychological components or responses as part of his concept of stress.

The Lazarus **transactional stress theory** encompasses a set of cognitive, affective, and adaptive (coping) responses that arise out of person-environment transactions. The person and the environment are inseparable; each affects and is affected by the other. Stress refers to "any event in which environmental demands, internal demands, or both tax or exceed the adaptive resources of an individual, social system, or tissue system" (Monat & Lazarus, 1991, p. 3). The individual responds to perceived environmental changes by adaptive or coping responses. See the section "Coping" later in this chapter.

Clinical Manifestations

Physiological Indicators of Stress

When a person is experiencing stress, he or she can also experience the following physiological changes:

- Pupils dilate to increase visual perception when serious threats to the body arise.
- Diaphoresis (sweat production) increases to control elevated body heat caused by increased metabolism.
- Heart rate and cardiac output increase to transport nutrients and byproducts of metabolism more efficiently.
- Skin is pallid because of constriction of peripheral blood vessels, an effect of norepinephrine.
- Sodium and water retention increase because of the release of mineralcorticoids, which increases blood volume.
- Rate and depth of respirations increase because of dilation of the bronchioles, promoting hyperventilation.
- Urinary output decreases.
- Mouth may be dry.
- Peristalsis of the intestines decreases, resulting in possible constipation and flatus.
- For serious threats, mental alertness improves.
- Muscle tension increases to prepare for rapid motor activity or defence.
- Blood sugar increases because of release of glucocorticoids and gluconeogenesis.

Indicators of Stress

Indicators of an individual's stress can be physiological, psychological, and cognitive.

Physiological Indicators

Responses to stress vary depending on the individual's perception of events. The physiological signs and symptoms of stress result from the activation of the sympathetic and neuroendocrine systems of the body. The Clinical Manifestations box lists physiological indicators of stress.

Psychological Indicators

Psychological manifestations of stress include anxiety, fear, anger, and depression. Some of these coping patterns are helpful; others are a hindrance, depending on the situation and the length of time they are used or experienced.

ANXIETY AND FEAR A common reaction to stress is **anxiety**, a state of mental uneasiness, apprehension, dread, or foreboding or a feeling of helplessness related to an impending or anticipated unidentified threat to the self or significant relationships. Anxiety can be experienced at the conscious, subconscious, or unconscious levels.

Anxiety can manifest at four levels:

1. *Mild anxiety* produces a slight arousal state that enhances perception, learning, and productive abilities. Most healthy people experience mild anxiety, perhaps as a feeling of mild restlessness that prompts a person to seek information and ask questions.
2. *Moderate anxiety* increases the arousal state to a point where the person expresses feelings of tension, nervousness, or concern. Perceptual abilities are narrowed. Attention is focused more on a particular aspect of a situation than on peripheral activities.
3. *Severe anxiety* consumes most of the person's energies and requires intervention. Perception is further decreased. The person, unable to focus on what is really happening, focuses on only one specific detail of the situation generating the anxiety.
4. *Panic* is an overpowering, frightening level of anxiety causing the person to lose control. It is less frequently experienced than other levels of anxiety. The perception of a panicked person can be altered to the point where the person distorts events.

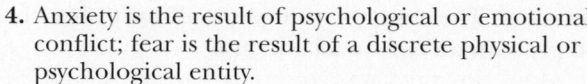

See Table 47.2 for indicators of these levels of anxiety.

Fear is an emotion or a feeling of apprehension aroused by impending or seeming danger, pain, or other perceived threat. The fear may be in response to something that has already occurred, in response to an immediate or current threat, or of something the person believes will happen. The object of fear may or may not be based in reality. For example, the beginning nursing student may be fearful in anticipation of the first experience in a client care setting. The student may fear that the client will not want to be cared for by the student or that the student might inadvertently harm the client.

Anxiety and fear differ in four ways:

1. The source of anxiety may not be identifiable; the source of fear is identifiable.
2. Anxiety is related to the future, that is, to an anticipated event. Fear is related to the present.
3. Anxiety is vague, whereas fear is definite.
4. Anxiety is the result of psychological or emotional conflict; fear is the result of a discrete physical or psychological entity.

CLINICAL ALERT

Mild or moderate anxiety motivates goal-directed behaviour. In this sense, anxiety can give rise to effective coping strategies. For example, mild anxiety generally motivates students to study. Excessive anxiety, however, often has destructive effects. For example, overwhelming anxiety can generate feelings of despair or depression.

ANGER **Anger** is an emotional state consisting of a subjective feeling of animosity or strong displeasure. People feel guilty when they feel anger because they have learned that to feel angry is wrong. However, anger can be expressed in a nonalienating verbal manner; it is then considered a positive emotion and a sign of emotional maturity because growth and beneficial interactions result from it.

A person's verbal expression of anger can be considered a signal to others of internal psychological discomfort and a call for assistance to deal with perceived stress. In contrast, *hostility* is usually marked by overt antagonism and harmful or destructive behaviour; *aggression* is an unprovoked attack or a hostile, injurious, or destructive action or outlook; and *violence* is the exertion of physical force to injure or abuse. Verbally expressed anger differs from hostility, aggression, and violence, but it can lead to destructiveness and violence if the anger persists unabated.

A clearly expressed verbal communication of anger, when the angry person tells the other person about the anger and carefully identifies the source, is constructive. This clarity of communication gets the anger out into the open so that the other person can deal with it and help

TABLE 47.2 Indicators of Levels of Anxiety

	Level of Anxiety			
Category	**Mild**	**Moderate**	**Severe**	**Panic**
Verbalization changes	Increased questioning	Voice tremors and pitch changes	Communication difficult to understand	Communication may not be understandable
Motor activity changes	Mild restlessness Sleeplessness	Tremors, facial twitches, and shakiness Increased muscle tension	Increased motor activity, inability to relax Fearful facial expression	Increased motor activity, agitation Unpredictable responses Trembling, poor motor coordination
Perception and attention changes	Feelings of increased arousal and alertness Uses learning to adapt	Narrowed focus of attention Able to focus but selectively inattentive Learning slightly impaired	Inability to focus or concentrate Easily distracted Learning severely impaired	Perception distorted or exaggerated Unable to learn or function
Respiratory and circulatory changes	None	Slightly increased respiratory and heart rates	Tachycardia, hyperventilation	Dyspnea, palpitations, choking, chest pain or pressure
Other changes	None	Mild gastric symptoms, e.g., "butterflies in the stomach"	Headache, dizziness, nausea	Feeling of impending doom Paresthesia, sweating

Sources: *Nursing Diagnosis: Application to Clinical Practice,* 11th ed. (pp. 97–109), by L. J. Carpenito-Moyet, 2006, Philadelphia, PA: Lippincott; and *Mental Health Nursing,* 5th ed. (p. 273), by K. L. Fontaine and J. S. Fletcher, 2003, Upper Saddle River, NJ: Prentice Hall.

alleviate it. The angry person gets it off his or her chest and prevents an emotional buildup.

DEPRESSION Depression is a common reaction to events that seem overwhelming or negative. **Depression**, an extreme feeling of sadness, despair, dejection, lack of worth, or emptiness, affects thousands of Canadians a year. The signs and symptoms of depression and the severity of the problem vary with the client and the significance of the precipitating event. Emotional symptoms can include feelings of tiredness, sadness, emptiness, or numbness. Behavioural signs of depression include irritability, inability to concentrate, difficulty making decisions, loss of sexual desire, crying, sleep disturbance, and social withdrawal. Physical signs of depression may include loss of appetite, weight loss, constipation, headache, and dizziness. Many people may experience short periods of depression in response to overwhelming stressful events, such as the death of a loved one or loss of a job; prolonged depression, however, is a cause for concern and may require treatment.

EGO DEFENCE MECHANISMS Ego **defence mechanisms** are unconscious psychological adaptive mechanisms or, according to Freud (1946), mental mechanisms that develop as the personality attempts to defend itself, establish compromises among conflicting impulses, and allay inner tensions. Defence mechanisms are the unconscious mind working to protect the person from anxiety. They can be considered precursors to conscious cognitive coping mechanisms that will ultimately solve the problem. Like some verbal and motor responses, defence mechanisms release tension. Table 47.3 describes these mechanisms and lists examples of their adaptive and maladaptive use.

Cognitive Indicators

Cognitive indicators of stress are thinking responses that include problem solving, structuring, self-control or self-discipline, suppression, and fantasy. *Problem solving* involves thinking through the threatening situation by using specific steps similar to those of the nursing process to arrive at a solution. The person assesses the situation or problem, analyzes or defines it, chooses alternatives, carries out the selected alternative, and evaluates whether the solution was successful.

Structuring is the arrangement or manipulation of a situation so that threatening events do not occur. For example, a nurse can structure or control an interview with a client by asking only direct, closed questions. This strategy avoids information or questions that may be threatening to the nurse's knowledge or values. Structuring, however, can be productive in certain situations. A person who schedules a dental examination semiannually to prevent severe dental disease is using productive structuring.

Self-control (discipline) is assuming a manner and facial expression that convey a sense of being in control or in charge, no matter what the situation is. When self-control prevents panic and harmful or unproductive actions in a threatening situation, it is a helpful response that conveys strength. Self-control carried to an extreme, however, can delay problem solving and prevent a person from receiving the support of others, who may perceive the person as handling the situation well, as cold, or as unconcerned.

Suppression is consciously and willfully putting a thought or feeling out of mind: "I won't deal with that today. I'll do it tomorrow." This response relieves stress temporarily but does not solve the problem. A person who keeps ignoring a toothache, pushing it out of mind fearing the pain of having a filling, will not relieve symptoms or find the solution.

Fantasy or *daydreaming* is likened to make-believe. Unfulfilled wishes and desires are imagined as fulfilled, or a threatening experience is reworked or replayed so that it ends differently from reality. Experiences can be relived, everyday problems solved, and plans for the future made. The outcome of current problems can also be fantasized. For example, a client who is awaiting the results of a breast biopsy may fantasize the surgeon saying, "You do not have cancer." Fantasy responses can be helpful if they lead to problem solving. For example, the client awaiting breast biopsy results might say to herself, "Even if the doctor says, 'You have cancer,' as long as the doctor also says it can be treated, I can accept that." Fantasies can be destructive and unproductive if a person uses them to excess and retreats from reality.

Coping

Coping can be described as dealing with change, successfully or unsuccessfully. A **coping strategy (coping mechanism)** is an innate or acquired way of responding to a changing environment or specific problem or situation. According to Folkman and Lazarus (1991), coping is "the cognitive and behavioural effort to manage specific external and/or internal demands that are appraised as taxing or exceeding the resources of the person" (p. 210).

Two types of coping strategies have been described: problem-focused and emotion-focused coping. *Problem-focused coping* refers to efforts to improve a situation by making changes or taking some action. *Emotion-focused coping* includes thoughts and actions that relieve emotional distress. Emotion-focused coping does not improve the situation, but the person often feels better. Both types of strategies usually occur together (Lazarus, 2000).

Coping strategies are also viewed as short term or long term. *Short-term coping strategies* can reduce stress to a tolerable limit temporarily but are ineffective ways to

TABLE 47.3 Defence Mechanisms

Defence Mechanism	Example(s)	Use/Purpose
Compensation Covering up weaknesses by emphasizing a more desirable trait or by overachievement in a more comfortable area.	A high school student too small to play football becomes the star long-distance runner for the track team.	Allows a person to overcome weakness and achieve success.
Denial An attempt to screen or ignore unacceptable realities by refusing to acknowledge them.	A woman, though told her father has metastatic cancer, continues to plan a family reunion 18 months in advance.	Temporarily isolates a person from the full impact of a traumatic situation.
Displacement The transferring or discharging of emotional reactions from one object or person to another object or person.	A husband and wife are fighting, and the husband becomes so angry he hits a door instead of his wife. A student gets a C on a paper and goes home and yells at the family.	Allows for feelings to be expressed through or to less dangerous objects or people.
Identification An attempt to manage anxiety by imitating the behaviour of someone feared or respected.	A student nurse imitates the nurturing behaviour she observes one of her instructors using with clients.	Helps a person avoid self-devaluation.
Intellectualization A mechanism by which an emotional response that normally would accompany an uncomfortable or painful incident is evaded by the use of rational explanations that remove from the incident any personal significance and feelings.	The pain over a parent's sudden death is reduced by saying, "He wouldn't have wanted to live disabled."	Protects a person from pain and traumatic events.
Introjection A form of identification that allows for the acceptance of others' norms and values into oneself, even when contrary to one's previous assumptions.	A 7-year-old tells his little sister, "Don't talk to strangers." He has introjected this value from the instructions of parents and teachers.	Helps a person avoid social retaliation and punishment; particularly important for the child's development of superego.
Minimization Not acknowledging the significance of one's behaviour.	A person says, "Don't believe everything my wife tells you. I wasn't so drunk I couldn't drive."	Allows a person to decrease responsibility for own behaviour.
Projection A process in which blame is attached to others or the environment for unacceptable desires, thoughts, shortcomings, and mistakes.	A mother is told her child must repeat a grade in school, and she blames this on the teacher's poor instruction. A husband forgets to pay a bill and blames his wife for not giving it to him earlier.	Allows a person to deny the existence of shortcomings and mistakes; protects self-image.
Rationalization Justification of certain behaviours by faulty logic and ascription of motives that are socially acceptable but did not, in fact, inspire the behaviour.	A mother spanks her toddler too hard and says it was all right because he could not feel it through the diapers anyway.	Helps a person cope with the inability to meet goals or certain standards.
Reaction Formation A mechanism that causes people to act exactly opposite to the way they feel.	An executive resents the bosses for calling in a consulting firm to make recommendations for change in the department but verbalizes complete support of the idea and is exceedingly polite and cooperative.	Aids in reinforcing repression by allowing feelings to be acted out in a more acceptable way.
Regression Resorting to an earlier, more comfortable level of functioning that is characteristically less demanding and responsible.	An adult throws a temper tantrum. A critically ill client allows the nurse to do the bathing and feeding.	Allows a person to return to a point in development when nurturing and dependency were needed and accepted with comfort.

(continued)

TABLE 47.3 Defence Mechanisms (*continued*)

Defence Mechanism	Example(s)	Use/Purpose
Repression An unconscious mechanism by which threatening thoughts, feelings, and desires are kept from becoming conscious; the repressed material is denied entry into consciousness.	A teenager seeing his best friend killed in a car accident becomes amnesic about the circumstances surrounding the accident.	Protects a person from a traumatic experience until he or she has the resources to cope.
Sublimation Displacement of energy associated with more primitive sexual or aggressive drives into socially acceptable activities.	A person with excessive, primitive sexual drives invests psychic energy into a well-defined religious value system.	Protects a person from behaving in irrational, impulsive ways.
Substitution The replacement of a highly valued, unacceptable, or unavailable object by a less valuable, acceptable, or available object.	A woman wants to marry a man exactly like her dead father and settles for someone who looks a little bit like him.	Helps a person achieve goals and minimizes frustration and disappointment.
Undoing An action or words designed to cancel some disapproved thoughts, impulses, or acts in which the person relieves guilt by making reparation.	A father spanks his child and the next evening brings home a present for him. A teacher writes an exam that is far too easy, then constructs a grading curve that makes it difficult to earn a high grade.	Allows a person to appease guilty feelings and atone for mistakes.

Source: *Mental Health Nursing,* 5th ed. (pp. 11–12), by K. L. Fontaine and J. S. Fletcher, 2003, Upper Saddle River, NJ: Prentice Hall. Reprinted with permission.

permanently deal with reality. They may even have a destructive or detrimental effect on the person. Examples of short-term strategies are using alcoholic beverages or drugs, daydreaming and fantasizing, relying on the belief that everything will work out, and giving in to others to avoid anger.

Long-term coping strategies can be constructive and realistic. For example, in certain situations, talking with others and trying to find out more about the situation are long-term strategies. Other long-term strategies include a change in lifestyle patterns, such as eating a healthy diet, exercising regularly, balancing leisure time with working, or using problem solving in decision making instead of anger or other unconstructive responses.

Coping strategies vary among individuals (see the Nursing and Canadian Society box) and are often

NURSING AND CANADIAN SOCIETY

Fact	Implications for Nursing Practice
According to a 2006 Ipsos Reid poll, half of Canadians feel that they have no control over their stress levels, especially when it comes to work and finances. Exercise and use of distraction, such as reading, were identified as helpful strategies.	Nurses can help people develop strategies for stress relief in areas over which they do have control. Something as prevalent as feeling out of control over stress levels indicates that nurses must assess this area when monitoring and intervening in client situations.
It is estimated that upward of 40% of Canada's peacekeepers returning from recent war efforts will experience some form of post-traumatic stress disorder (PTSD) or war-related stress (Veterans Affairs Canada, 2006).	Assessing for PTSD in returning servicepeople is relevant in determining the long-term effects of military service during wartime. Appropriate referral to Veterans Affairs Canada for a range of services will benefit those who suffer from PTSD.
The Canadian Mental Health Association (2005) offers tips on dealing with holiday stress. Although generally a time to celebrate, the holiday season can be particularly stressful for people who lack finances or social support. It can be a difficult time for people who are isolated or who have trouble coping with even minor changes in routine. The Canadian Mental Health Association notes an increased incidence of depression at Christmas.	Although many Canadians enjoy holiday festivities, nurses must be sensitive to the adverse effects of holiday seasons on people. Exacerbation of depression or suicidal ideation may be present in people who are overwhelmed with the demands and pressures of a holiday season.

related to the individual's perception of the stressful event. Three approaches to coping with stress are to alter the stressor, adapt to the stressor, or avoid the stressor. A person's coping strategies often change with a reappraisal of a situation. There is always more than one way to cope. Some people choose avoidance; others confront a situation as a means of coping. Still others seek information or rely on religious beliefs as a means of coping.

Coping can be adaptive or maladaptive. *Adaptive coping* helps the person to deal effectively with stressful events and minimizes the distress associated with them. *Maladaptive coping* can result in unnecessary distress for the person and others associated with the person or stressful event (Schafer, 1992). In nursing literature, effective and ineffective coping are often differentiated. *Effective coping* results in adaptation; *ineffective coping* results in maladaptation. Nurses may be able to teach clients coping skills.

Although coping behaviour may not always seem appropriate, the nurse needs to remember that coping is always purposeful. The effectiveness of an individual's coping is influenced by a number of factors, including the following:

- The number, duration, and intensity of the stressors
- Past experiences of the individual
- Support systems available to the individual
- Personal qualities of the person

If the duration of the stressors is extended beyond the coping powers of the individual, that person becomes exhausted and may develop increased susceptibility to health problems. Reaction to long-term stress is seen in family members who undertake the care of a person at home for a long period. This stress is called **caregiver burden** and produces such responses as chronic fatigue, sleeping difficulties, and high blood pressure. Prolonged stress can also result in mental illness. As coping strategies or defence mechanisms (see Table 47.3) become ineffective, the individual may have interpersonal problems, work difficulties, and a significant decrease in abilities to meet basic human needs. See Table 47.4 and the Reflect on Primary Health Care box.

TABLE 47.4 Examples of the Effects of Stress on Basic Human Needs

Need	Example
Physiological	Altered elimination pattern Change in appetite Altered sleep pattern
Safety and security	Expresses nervousness and feelings of being threatened Focuses on stressors and inattention to safety measures
Love and belonging	Isolated and withdrawn Becomes overly dependent Blames others for own problems
Self-esteem	Fails to socialize with others Becomes a workaholic Draws attention to self
Self-actualization	Preoccupied with own problems Shows lack of control Unable to accept reality

REFLECT ON PRIMARY HEALTH CARE

Reducing stressors in people's lives as well as helping them to cope with stress when it does occur is an excellent opportunity for *intersectoral coordination.* Individuals and families in crisis rely on the coordination of services across sectors so that their needs can be met in a timely and effective manner. An example of a coordinated approach in some communities occurs after police have been called to a home because of a domestic dispute. The police immediately file a report with the health and social services department of their community health centre so that follow-up can be made and underlying conflicts addressed.

Assessing

Nursing assessment of a client's stress and coping patterns includes (1) nursing history, and (2) physical examination of the client for indicators of stress (e.g., nail biting, nervousness, weight changes) or stress-related health problems (e.g., hypertension, dyspnea). When obtaining the nursing history of any client, the nurse poses questions about client-perceived stressors or stressful incidents, manifestations of stress, and past and present coping strategies. During the physical examination, the nurse observes for verbal, motor, cognitive, or other physical manifestations of stress. Remember, however, that clinical signs and symptoms may not occur when cognitive coping is effective.

In addition, the nurse should be aware of expected developmental transitions (predictable tasks that must be accomplished if the person is to grow psychologically as well as physically; see Chapters 17 to 19). This knowledge helps the nurse identify additional stressors that are present and the client's response to them. Table 47.1 provided an overview of developmental stressors. Questions to elicit data about the client's stress and coping patterns are shown in the Assessment: Interview box.

Evidence-Informed Practice

What Are the Links between Maternal Stress during Pregnancy and Behavioural Disturbances in Children?

Maternal stress during pregnancy has been linked to an increased incidence of spontaneous abortions and fetal malformations and lower infant birth weight. Attention span and neuromotor development are also thought to be affected by maternal stress. This Canadian study by Grizenko, Shayan, Polotskaia, Ter-Stepanian, and Joober (2008) looked at a large group of children, aged between 6 and 12 years, who were undergoing treatment for attention-deficit hyperactivity disorder (ADHD). The researchers measured the severity of ADHD symptoms in the children and then compared them with their mothers' reports of stress before, during, and after pregnancy. The results indicated that moderate to severe stressful experiences during pregnancy correlated with increased ADHD symptom severity in the children.

NURSING IMPLICATIONS: Nurses working with women during the perinatal period should assess their clients' experiences with stress. Nurses can help pregnant women anticipate stressful times and help them develop their resources and enhance their coping skills. Women who know that they had high levels of stress during their pregnancy and now have a child with behavioural problems may experience guilt and might need help to deal with this feeling.

Source: Based on "Relation of Maternal Stress during Pregnancy to Symptom Severity and Response to Treatment in Children with ADHD," by N. Grizenko, Y. R. Shayan, A. Polotskaia, M. Ter-Stepanian, and R. Joober, 2008, *Journal of Psychiatry & Neuroscience*, *33*(1), pp. 10–16.

ASSESSMENT: INTERVIEW

Stress and Coping Patterns

The nurse can use the following questions to learn about a client's stress and coping pattern:

- On a scale of 0 to 10, how would you rate the stress you are experiencing in the following areas?
  - a. Home
  - b. Work or school
  - c. Finance
  - d. Recent illness or loss of loved one
  - e. Your health
  - f. Family responsibilities
  - g. Relationships with friends
  - h. Relationship with parents or children
  - i. Relationship with partner
  - j. Recent hospitalization
  - k. Other (specify)
- How long have you been dealing with these stressors?
- How do you usually handle stressful situations? If the client does not adequately describe, prompt with the following:
  - a. Cry
  - b. Get angry
  - c. Talk to someone (Who?)
  - d. Withdraw from the situation
  - e. Control others or situation
  - f. Go for a walk or perform physical exercise
  - g. Try to arrive at a solution
  - h. Pray
  - i. Laugh, joke, or use some other expression of humour
  - j. Meditate or use some other relaxation technique, such as yoga or guided imagery
- How well does your usual coping strategy work?

Diagnosing

The NANDA International (2007) diagnostic labels related to stress, adaptation, and coping include the following:

- *Anxiety:* Vague, uneasy feeling of discomfort or dread accompanied by an autonomic response (the source often nonspecific or unknown to the individual); a feeling of apprehension caused by the anticipation of danger. It is an alerting signal that warns of impending danger and enables the individual to take measures to deal with a threat.
- *Caregiver Role Strain:* Difficulty in performing the caregiver role.
- *Compromised Family Coping:* Usually supportive primary person (family member or close friend) provides insufficient, ineffective, or compromised

support, comfort, assistance, or encouragement that may be needed by client to manage or master adaptive tasks related to his or her health challenge.

- *Decisional Conflict:* Uncertainty about course of action to be taken when the choice among competing actions involves risk, loss, or challenge to personal life values.
- *Defensive Coping:* Repeated projection of falsely positive self-evaluation based on a self-protective pattern that defends against underlying perceived threats to positive self-regard.
- *Disabled Family Coping:* Behaviour of significant person (family member or other primary person) that disables his/her capacities and the client's capacities to effectively address tasks essential to either person's adaptation to the health challenge.
- *Fear:* Response to perceived threat that is consciously recognized as dangerous.
- *Impaired Adjustment:* Inability to modify lifestyle/behaviour in a manner consistent with a change in health status.
- *Ineffective Coping:* Inability or risk of inability to manage internal and external stressors because of inadequate physical, psychological, behavioural, or cognitive resources.
- *Ineffective Denial:* Conscious or unconscious attempt to disavow the knowledge or meaning of an event to reduce anxiety/fear, but leading to the detriment of health.
- *Post-Trauma Syndrome:* A sustained maladaptive response to a traumatic, overwhelming event.
- *Relocation Stress Syndrome:* Physiological and/or psychosocial disturbance following transfer from one environment to another.

Defining characteristics and etiologies of these diagnostic labels were discussed earlier under clinical manifestations of stress. Clinical examples of assessment data clusters and related nursing diagnoses (*Anxiety* and *Decisional Conflict*) are shown in Table 47.5.

Planning

The nurse develops plans in collaboration with the client and significant support people, when possible, according to the client's state of health (e.g., ability to return to work), level of anxiety, support resources, coping mechanisms, and sociocultural and religious affiliation. The nurse who has little experience intervening with clients undergoing stress may want to consult with a clinical specialist or a more experienced nurse to develop effective plans. The nurse and client set goals to change the existing client responses to the stressor or stressors.

The overall client goals for persons experiencing stress-related responses are as follows:

- Decrease or resolve anxiety
- Increase ability to manage or cope with stressful events or circumstances
- Improve role performance

Examples of specific desired outcomes, although established in this phase, are provided in Table 47.6 in the "Evaluating" section of this chapter (page 1507).

Examples of interventions based on the Nursing Intervention Classification (NIC) system (Bulechek, Butcher, & Dochterman, 2008) include the following:

- Anxiety reduction
- Body image enhancement
- Caregiver support
- Coping enhancement
- Crisis intervention
- Decision-making support
- Role enhancement

Specific nursing activities related to each of these interventions can be selected to individualize client care. The Sample Care Plan uses NIC interventions and selected activities.

TABLE 47.5 Clinical Application: Assessment Data Clusters and Related Nursing Diagnoses: Stress and Coping Abilities

Data Cluster	Nursing Diagnosis
Darryl Johnson, a 47-year-old accountant, was admitted to the emergency department with a myocardial infarction. He says, "I'm scared about this. My dad died of a heart attack when he was 48 years old." He appears restless, questions everything that is going on, and is hyperventilating.	*Anxiety* related to change in health status and threat of dying
Sonia Park, a 33-year-old mother of three, returned to nursing after taking a refresher course. She says, "I'm so tired since I started work. I'm not keeping up with housekeeping the way I should, and I'm not spending as much time with the kids. I'm too tired to shop and go to my son's baseball game. Everyone is helping out and not complaining, but I just keep thinking they wish I still baked cookies and played more with them. I'm sure not sleeping well, and I'm having awful headaches."	*Decisional Conflict* related to work versus home responsibilities causing emotional and physical stress; possible uncertainty about course of action when the choice among competing actions involves risk, loss, or challenge to personal life values

Sample Care Plan for Ineffective Coping

ASSESSMENT DATA

Nursing Assessment
Amanda Crosby, a 55-year-old mother of four children, is hospitalized with breast cancer. She is scheduled for a modified radical mastectomy. Amanda was relatively healthy until she found a lump in her right breast 2 weeks ago. She and her husband are extremely anxious about the surgery. Amanda confides to the admitting nurse, "I can't stand the idea of having one of my breasts cut off; I don't know how I'm going to be able to even look at myself." Mr. Crosby informs the nurse that Amanda has been abusing alcohol since her diagnosis and neglecting her responsibilities as a mother. She is tearful and does not see how she will be able to continue her work as a dress designer.

Physical Examination
Height: 164 cm
Weight: 58 kg
Temperature: 37°C
Pulse: 88 bpm
Respirations: 16/minute
Blood Pressure: 142/88 mm Hg

Diagnostic Data
Chest X-ray negative, CBC and urinalysis within normal limits

Nursing Diagnosis
Ineffective Coping related to personal vulnerability secondary to mastectomy (as evidenced by verbalization of inability to cope, substance abuse, inability to meet role expectations)

Client Goal
The client will demonstrate effective coping strategies.

Desired Health Outcomes
Coping, as evidenced by often demonstrating ability to

1. Identify effective and ineffective coping patterns, including a reduction in the ineffective patterns
2. Report decrease in negative feelings
4. Verbalize a sense of control
5. Participate in activities of daily living postoperatively

Social support as evidenced by substantial reports of

1. Willingness to call on others for help
2. Emotional assistance provided by others

NURSING INTERVENTIONS AND SELECTED ACTIVITIES WITH RATIONALES* [*IN ITALICS*]

Coping Enhancement

- Provide an atmosphere of acceptance. *Establishing rapport is essential to a therapeutic relationship and supports the client in self-reflection. Recognizing problems and sharing feelings is best brought about in an atmosphere of warmth and trust.*
- Provide factual information concerning the diagnosis, treatment, and prognosis. *Factual information serves as a foundation for the individual in exploring feelings and alternative coping strategies. Clients who are experiencing stress often misunderstand facts and require frequent clarification so that appropriate conclusions can be drawn. Having valid information helps relieve stress.*
- Appraise Amanda's adjustment to changes in body image. *Alteration in body image may be a major issue for Amanda and should be explored to facilitate therapeutic intervention. Coping strategies often change with a reappraisal of the situation.*
- Arrange situations that encourage her autonomy. *Autonomy enhances a sense of control, personal achievement, and self-esteem.*
- Explore with her previous methods of dealing with life problems. *Present and past coping status assists both the client and the caregiver in capitalizing on successful methods, identifying ineffective strategies, and developing new skills more appropriate to the present situation. It also determines risk for inflicting self-harm.*
- Encourage verbalization of feelings, perceptions, and fears. *Open, nonthreatening discussions facilitate the identification of causative and contributing factors.*
- Encourage Amanda to identify her own strengths and abilities. *This identification assists the client to develop appropriate strategies for coping based on personal strengths and previous experiences. It improves self-concept and a sense of ability to manage stress.*
- Encourage Amanda to realistically describe changes in her role. *Individuals experiencing stress may have unrealistic perceptions or reality distortions. Helping Amanda clearly describe her role would be beneficial in developing realistic goals for role achievement.*
- Foster constructive outlets for anger and hostility. *The individual needs to channel potentially harmful emotions and physical energy into constructive behaviour.*

(continued)

Sample Care Plan for Ineffective Coping (*continued*)

Support System Enhancement

• Observe the degree of family support.	*Assessing family interactions serves as a basis for identifying Amanda's support systems or lack thereof.*
• Determine barriers to using support systems.	*Although adequate support systems may be available, Amanda may not be using them or may be using them ineffectively.*
• Involve significant others in the care and planning.	*Significant others can help Amanda in acknowledging the changes in her appearance and convey acceptance. They may also be able to help her identify her strengths and coping repertoire.*
• Discuss with concerned others how they can help.	*Supporting Amanda in acknowledging changes in her appearance conveys acceptance and provides a foundation for her to begin to adjust.*
• Discuss referral to a community-based breast cancer support group.	*Family and friends are often willing but unsure how to help. Identifying specific strategies, such as praise and encouragement, during rehabilitation and healing will promote acceptance of change.*

EVALUATION

The coping outcome was minimally met. Following surgery, Amanda was withdrawn. During bathing, she would not assist and turned her head away when the dressing was removed. She refused to learn how to manage the wound drain, discuss her feelings, or plan for the future. She did identify that alcohol was not an effective coping strategy. Because patients having a mastectomy are often only hospitalized for a few days, it may be that she requires more time to reach the desired outcome.

Social support outcome partly met. Amanda allows her husband to provide direct care and emotional support for her. She was discharged with her family, and a community nurse was consulted to care for and help her to cope with her ongoing issues. Amanda expressed an interest in receiving a call from the breast cancer support group member before deciding if she would attend an actual face-to-face meeting.

*Interventions and activities selected are only a sample of those suggested in the *Nursing Interventions Classification (NIC)*, by G. M. Bulechek, H. K. Butcher, and J. C. Dochterman (Eds.), 2008, St. Louis, MO: Mosby Elsevier, and should be individualized for each client.

Planning for Home Care

Clients who are experiencing stress may require ongoing nursing support or referral to community agencies that can provide support to meet client needs and enhance client coping. The determination of how much and what type of planning and home care follow-up is based in great part on the nurse's knowledge of how the client and family have coped with previous stressors and the nature of the present stressor. The Assessment: Home Care box describes data to be gathered for home care or follow-up assessment.

Implementing

Although stress is part of daily life, it is also highly individual; a situation that to one person is a major stressor may not affect another. Some methods to help reduce stress will be effective for one person; other methods will be appropriate for a different person. A nurse who is sensitive to clients' needs and reactions can choose those methods of intervention that will be most effective for each individual.

Encouraging Health-Promotion Strategies

Several health-promotion strategies are often appropriate as interventions for clients with stress-related nursing diagnoses. Among these are physical exercise, optimal nutrition, adequate rest and sleep, and time management.

EXERCISE Regular exercise promotes both physical and emotional health. Physiological benefits include improved muscle tone, increased cardiopulmonary function, and weight control. Psychological benefits include relief of tension, a feeling of well-being, and relaxation. Canadian health guidelines recommend adults accumulate 30 to 60 minutes of moderate physical activity most days. See Chapter 38 for more detailed information.

ASSESSMENT: HOME CARE

Stress and Coping

Nurses must assess clients and their families and whether they will need follow-up care after discharge:

CLIENT

- *Knowledge:* Client's understanding of the nature of the stressors
- *Current coping strategies:* Effectiveness of current coping strategies and willingness to learn new stress management techniques
- *Self-care abilities:* Physical, emotional, social, and financial ability to minimize associated stressors
- *Role expectations:* Client's perception of the need to return to prior roles and possible stressors associated with these roles

FAMILY

- *Knowledge:* Family members' and significant others' understanding of the nature of the client's stressors and their own relationship with client stressors
- *Family coping strategies:* Effectiveness of family members' and significant others' coping strategies and willingness to learn new stress management techniques
- *Role expectations:* Family members' and significant others' perception of the need for the client to return to family and work roles
- *Support people's availability and skills:* Family and significant others' sensitivity to the client's emotional and physical needs and ability to provide a supportive environment

COMMUNITY

- *Resources:* Availability of and familiarity with possible sources of assistance for stress management, such as massage therapists, religious or spiritual centres, physical care providers, support groups, and so on

NUTRITION Optimal nutrition is essential for health and for increasing the body's resistance to stress. To minimize the effects of a stress response (e.g., irritability, hyperactivity, anxiety), people need to avoid excesses of caffeine, salt, sugar, and fat, and deficiencies in vitamins and minerals. Guidelines for a well-balanced, healthy diet are detailed in Chapter 39.

REST AND SLEEP Rest and sleep restore the body's energy levels and are an essential aspect of stress management. To ensure adequate rest and sleep, clients may need help to attain comfort (such as pain management) and to learn techniques that promote peace of mind and relaxation. (See "Using Relaxation Techniques" later in this chapter.)

TIME MANAGEMENT People who manage their time effectively usually experience less stress because they feel more in control of their circumstances. Clients who feel overwhelmed often need help to prioritize tasks and to consider whether modifications can be made to decrease role demands. Some working mothers, for example, may need to consider delegating more tasks to family members or hiring part-time help. Controlling the demands of others is also an important aspect of effective time management because all requests made by others cannot always be met. Clients may need to learn to develop an awareness of which requests they can meet without undue stress, which ones can be negotiated, and which ones need to be declined. Feelings of control can also be enhanced when clients schedule a daily or weekly time to deal with specific tasks.

Time management must address both what is important to the client and what can realistically be achieved. For example, clients may need to consider whether a clean house and time spent with the children can both be accomplished satisfactorily and, if not, which is more important. Often, clients who are feeling overwhelmed need to re-examine the "should, ought, and must" approach to their actions and develop more realistic self-expectations.

Minimizing Anxiety

Nurses carry out measures to minimize clients' anxiety and stress. For example, nurses encourage clients to take deep breaths before an injection, explain procedures before they are implemented, including sensations likely to be experienced during the procedure, administer a back or neck rub to help the client relax, and offer support to clients and families during times of illness. General guidelines for helping clients who are stressed and feeling anxious are outlined in Box 47.1.

Mediating Anger

Often, nurses find clients' anger difficult to handle. Caring for the client who is angry is difficult for two reasons:

- Clients seldom state, "I feel angry or frustrated," or indicate the reason for their anger. Instead, they may refuse treatment, become verbally abusive or demanding, threaten violence, or become overly critical. Their complaints rarely reflect the cause of their anger.
- Anger from clients can elicit fear and anger in the nurse, who may respond in a manner that intensi-

BOX 47.1 MINIMIZING STRESS AND ANXIETY

The nurse can use these methods to help clients who are experiencing stress or anxiety:

- Listen attentively; try to understand the client's perspective of the situation.
- Provide an atmosphere of warmth and trust; convey a sense of caring and empathy.
- Provide factual information, as needed, to prepare clients for tests, treatments, and so on.
- Encourage clients to participate in the plan of care; give them choices about appropriate aspects of care.
- Stay with clients as needed to promote safety and feelings of security and to reduce fear.
- Control the environment to minimize additional stressors, such as by reducing noise, limiting the number of persons in the room, and providing care by the same nurse as much as possible.
- Help clients to do the following:
  - a. Determine situations that precipitate anxiety and identify signs of anxiety.
  - b. Verbalize feelings, perceptions, and fears as appropriate. Some cultures discourage the expression of feelings.
  - c. Identify personal strengths.
  - d. Recognize usual coping patterns and differentiate positive from negative coping mechanisms.
  - e. Identify new strategies for managing stress (e.g., exercise, massage, progressive relaxation).
  - f. Identify available support systems.
- Teach clients about the following:
  - a. The importance of adequate exercise, a balanced diet, and rest and sleep to energize the body and enhance coping abilities
  - b. The support groups that are available, such as Alcoholics Anonymous, Weight Watchers, or Overeaters Anonymous, and parenting and child abuse support groups
  - c. The educational programs that are available, such as time management, assertiveness training, and meditation groups

fies the client's anger, even to the point of violence. The majority of nurses respond in a way that reduces their own stress, rather than the client's stress.

Fontaine and Fletcher (2003) recommend the following strategies for dealing with clients' anger:

- Know and understand your own response to the feelings and expressions of anger.
- Accept the client's right to be angry; feelings are real and cannot be discounted or ignored.
- Try to understand the meaning of the client's anger.
- Ask the client what contributed to the anger.
- Help clients own the anger—do not assume responsibility for their feelings.
- Let clients talk about their anger.
- Listen to the client, and act as calmly as possible.
- After the interaction is completed, take time to process your feelings and your responses to the client with your colleagues.

Always ensure the safety of the client and others. Know the agency procedures to call for assistance from other staff or security personnel if you believe someone (including you) is in danger.

CLINICAL ALERT
A nurse who is concerned for his or her own safety while working with an angry client should withdraw from the situation or obtain support from another individual.

Using Relaxation Techniques

Several relaxation techniques can be used to quiet the mind, release tension, and counteract the fight-or-flight responses of GAS discussed earlier in this chapter. Nurses can teach these techniques to clients and then encourage clients to use them to control stress throughout life. Nurses can also encourage hospitalized clients to use these techniques when they encounter stressful situations in a hospital setting. Examples of these situations are (1) during childbirth, (2) postoperatively to cope with pain, and (3) before and during a painful procedure. Many agencies now have relaxation tapes available that the client can purchase, if desired. Some clients make their own recordings. Specific relaxation techniques are discussed in Chapter 15 and include the following:

- Breathing exercises
- Massage
- Progressive relaxation
- Imagery
- Biofeedback
- Yoga
- Meditation
- Therapeutic touch
- Music therapy
- Humour and laughter

Performing Crisis Intervention

A **crisis** is an acute, time-limited state of disequilibrium resulting from situational, developmental, or societal sources of stress. A person in crisis is temporarily unable to cope with or adapt to the stressor by using previous methods of problem solving. People in crisis generally have a distorted perception of the event, do not have adequate situational support, and do not have adequate coping mechanisms. Common characteristics of crises are shown in Box 47.2.

Crisis intervention is a short-term helping process of assisting clients to (1) work through a crisis to its resolution, and (2) restore their pre-crisis level of functioning. It is a process that includes not only the client in crisis but also various members of the client's support network. Crisis intervention is not the specialty of any one professional group. People who intervene in crises come from the fields of nursing, medicine, psychology, social work, and theology. Police officers, teachers, school guidance counsellors, and rescue workers, among others, are often on the spot in moments of crisis.

Because a state of disequilibrium is so uncomfortable, a crisis is self-limiting. However, a person experiencing a crisis alone is more vulnerable to unsuccessful negotiation than a person working through a crisis with help. Working with another person increases the likelihood that the person in crisis will resolve it in a positive way. Often, a state of crisis offers the individual or family great potential for growth and change.

The traditional steps of the nursing process correspond closely to the steps of crisis intervention. *Assessment* is the first phase of crisis intervention. The nurse or helper must focus on the person and the problem, collecting data about the client, the client's coping style, the precipitating event, the situational supports, the client's perception of the crisis, and the client's ability to handle the problem. Assessment is an essential and critical step of crisis intervention. This information is the basis for later decisions about how and when to intervene and whom to call. An individual's perception of the event and personal response will determine the nursing diagnoses. The most common nursing diagnoses for people in crisis are similar to those cited earlier in this chapter. In addition, such diagnoses as *Risk for Self-Directed Violence, Risk for Other Directed Violence, Rape Trauma Syndrome,* and *Hopelessness* may be appropriate. Effective *planning* for crisis intervention must be based on careful assessment and developed in active collaboration with the person in crisis and the significant people in that person's life.

Implementation involves crisis counselling and home crisis visits. **Crisis counselling** focuses on solving immediate problems and it involves individuals, groups, or families. Crisis intervention centres rely heavily on telephone counselling by volunteers who have professional consultation available to them. Also known as *hotlines* and often available around the clock, they allow callers to remain anonymous and test what it feels like to ask for assistance. The volunteers usually work within a protocol that indicates what information they need from the client to assess the crisis. Their goal is to plan steps to provide immediate relief and then long-term follow-up, if necessary.

Crisis home visits are made when telephone counselling does not suffice or when the crisis workers need to obtain additional information by direct observation or to reach a client who is unobtainable by telephone. Home visits are appropriate when crisis workers need to initiate contacts rather than waiting for clients to come to them, such as when a telephone caller is assessed to be highly suicidal or when a concerned neighbour, physician, or clergy member informs the agency of clients in potential crisis.

BOX 47.2 COMMON CHARACTERISTICS OF CRISES

Crises typically have the following characteristics:

- All crises are experienced as sudden. The person is usually not aware of a warning signal, even if others could "see it coming." The individual or family may feel that they have little or no preparation for the event or trauma.
- The crisis is often experienced as ultimately life threatening, whether this perception is realistic or not.
- Communication with significant others is often decreased or cut off.
- Perceived or real displacement from familiar surroundings or loved ones can occur.
- All crises have an aspect of loss, whether actual or perceived. The losses can include an object, a person, a hope, a dream, or any significant factor for that individual.

Managing Nurses' Stress

Nurses, like clients, are susceptible to experiencing anxiety and stress. Nursing practice involves many stressors related to both clients and the work environment: understaffing and increasing client care assignments, adjusting to various work shifts, being expected to assume responsibilities for which the nurse does not feel prepared, receiving inadequate support from supervisors and peers, visiting homes that are depressing, caring for dying clients, and so on.

Although most nurses cope effectively with the physical and emotional demands of nursing, in some situations, nurses become overwhelmed and develop

burnout, a complex syndrome of behaviours that can be likened to the exhaustion stage of GAS. The nurse with burnout manifests physical and emotional depletion, a negative attitude and self-concept, and feelings of helplessness and hopelessness.

Nurses can prevent burnout by using the techniques to manage stress discussed for clients. Nurses must first recognize their stress and become attuned to such responses as feelings of being overwhelmed, fatigue, angry outbursts, physical illness, and increases in coffee drinking, smoking, or other substance use. Once attuned to stress and personal reactions, it is necessary to identify which situations produce the most pronounced reactions so that steps can be taken to reduce the stress:

- Plan a daily relaxation program with meaningful quiet times to reduce tension (e.g., read a novel, listen to music, soak in a hot bath, or meditate).
- Establish a regular exercise program to direct energy outward (e.g., jog, play badminton, or join a dance class).
- Develop assertiveness techniques to overcome feelings of powerlessness in relationships with others. Learn to say no.
- Learn to accept failures—your own and others'—and make it a constructive learning experience. Recognize that most people do the best they can. Learn to ask for help, to show your feelings with colleagues, and to support your colleagues in times of need.
- Accept what cannot be changed. Every situation has certain limitations. Get involved in constructive change efforts if organizational policies and procedures cause stress.
- Develop collegial support groups to deal with feelings and anxieties generated in the work setting.
- Participate in professional organizations to address workplace issues.
- Seek counselling if indicated to help clarify concerns.

Evaluating

Using the desired outcomes developed during the planning stage as a guide, the nurse collects data needed to determine whether client goals and outcomes have been achieved. Examples of client goals and related outcomes are shown in Table 47.6.

If outcomes are not achieved, the nurse, client, and support people, if appropriate, need to explore the reasons why before modifying the care plan. Such questions as the following need to be considered:

- How does the client perceive the problem?
- Is there an underlying problem that has not been identified?
- Have new stressors occurred that interfere with successful coping?
- Were existing coping strategies sufficient to meet intended outcomes?
- How does the client perceive the effectiveness of the new coping strategies?
- Did the client implement the new coping strategies properly?
- Did the client access and use available resources?
- Have family members and significant others provided effective support?

TABLE 47.6 Evaluation Goals and Health Outcomes: Stress and Coping

Goal	Examples of Desired Outcomes
Decrease or resolve anxiety	Describes causes and level of anxiety Eliminates causes of anxiety, as appropriate Verbalizes feelings related to anxiety Decreases external stimuli when experiencing anxiety Verbalizes an increase in emotional and physical comfort
Improve ability to manage or cope with stressful events	Describes usual coping patterns Identifies personal strengths Develops new coping strategies for managing stress Plans coping strategies for stressful situations Uses effective coping strategies in managing anxiety Verbalizes a sense of control Reports decreased stress
Improve role performance	Describes realistic personal role expectations Reports strategies for role change, as appropriate Maintains role performance Performs family roles Performs effective work or school role Maintains social relationships

Case Study 47

Refer to the Sample Care Plan in this chapter and answer the following questions.

Critical Thinking Questions

1. If Amanda had been able to choose a lumpectomy rather than a mastectomy (less visible, smaller, potentially less "meaningful" tissue removal), would the nursing diagnosis and expected outcomes remain the same? Why or why not?
2. Does Amanda's situation reflect more of a stimulus-based or a response-based model of stress? Why?
3. While working with Amanda, she becomes very angry and says to you, "You don't understand. You've never had to go through this." How would you respond?
4. Based on the evaluation above, do you believe that Amanda is in crisis? What factors led to your decision? How does your view change the modifications indicated in her care plan?
5. Give one example of how Amanda might use the defence mechanisms described in Table 47.3. Explain whether this response is adaptive or maladaptive.

After working through these questions, go to the MyNursingLab at **http://www.mynursinglab.com** to check your answers.

KEY TERMS

stress
stressor
stimulus-based stress models
general adaptation syndrome (GAS)
local adaptation syndrome (LAS)
alarm reaction (AR)
shock phase
countershock phase
stage of resistance (SR)
stage of exhaustion
transactional stress theory
anxiety
fear
anger
depression
defence mechanisms
coping
coping strategy (coping mechanism)
caregiver burden
crisis
crisis intervention
crisis counselling
burnout

CHAPTER HIGHLIGHTS

- Stress is a state of physiological and psychological tension that affects the whole person, physically, emotionally, intellectually, socially, and spiritually.
- Models view stress as a stimulus, stress as a response, and stress as a transaction.
- Physiological responses to stress are described by the general adaptation syndrome (GAS) and the local adaptation syndrome (LAS).
- General adaptation syndrome (GAS) is a multisystem response to stress and involves three steps: alarm reaction, stage of resistance, and stage of exhaustion.
- Local adaptation syndrome (LAS) is a localized physiological response that also expresses the three stages of GAS. An example of LAS is the inflammatory response.
- Stress has physiological, psychological, and cognitive indicators. Physiological indicators are the result of increased activity of the sympathetic and neuroendocrine systems.
- Common psychological indicators are anxiety, fear, anger, and depression. Anxiety, the most common response, has four levels: mild, moderate, severe, and panic. Ego defence mechanisms, such as denial, rationalization, compensation, and sublimation, protect individuals from anxiety.
- Cognitive indicators or thinking responses to stress include problem solving, structuring, self-control (discipline), suppression, and fantasy.
- Coping strategies to deal with stress vary significantly among individuals. Strategies can be problem focused or emotion focused, long term or short term, and effective or ineffective.
- The effectiveness of individual coping depends on the number, duration, and intensity of the stressors; past experience; support systems available; and the personal qualities of the person.
- Prolonged stress and ineffective coping interfere with the meeting of basic needs and can affect physical and mental health.
- Nursing assessment of a client experiencing stress involves a nursing history to identify perceptions of and duration of stressors and coping strategies, and a physical examination for physical indicators of stress.

- Nursing interventions for clients who are stressed are aimed at encouraging health-promotion strategies (exercise, balanced diet, adequate rest and sleep, and time management), minimizing anxiety, mediating anger, teaching about specific relaxation techniques, and implementing crisis interventions, as needed.
- Because nursing practice involves many stressors related to both clients and the work environment, nurses are susceptible to anxiety and, in some cases, burnout. Like clients, they need to implement stress-reduction measures.

ASSESS YOUR LEARNING

1. After the death of several long-term clients, which of the following actions indicates that the nurse is demonstrating ineffective coping?
   - **a.** The nurse talks at length to her partner about the deaths.
   - **b.** The nurse keeps busy with other actions and doesn't think about the deaths for several days.
   - **c.** The nurse offers to work extra shifts for several weeks.
   - **d.** Several nurses schedule a group session with the agency clergy to discuss the deaths.

2. A 50-year-old client, newly diagnosed with diabetes mellitus, is to begin giving insulin injections. The nurse helps identify previously successful coping strategies that may be useful in the current situation. Which of the following stressors is closely related to the new stressor?
   - **a.** An interview for a new job
   - **b.** The death of a pet when the person was a teenager
   - **c.** The person's partner filing for a divorce
   - **d.** Starting to wear eyeglasses at age 30

3. Two people have been in a car accident and have similar injuries. According to the transaction-based model, their degree of stress from the accident would be which of the following?
   - **a.** Based on previous experience and personal characteristics
   - **b.** Very similar since they had the same stimulus
   - **c.** The identical physiological alarm reaction
   - **d.** Different depending on their external resources and support levels

4. A client who was informed of a cancer diagnosis assures the nurse he is fine. Which of the following is the most indicative physical evidence to the nurse of the client's stress?
   - **a.** Constricted pupils
   - **b.** Dilated peripheral blood vessels (flush)
   - **c.** Hyperventilation
   - **d.** Decreased heart rate

5. Immediately after the parents of a hospitalized child are informed that the child has leukemia, the father responds by continuing his usual work schedule, rarely visiting, and asking when the child can return to school. Of the following, which is the *least* likely to be an appropriate nursing diagnosis at this time?
   - **a.** *Ineffective Denial*
   - **b.** *Caregiver Role Strain*
   - **c.** *Fear*
   - **d.** *Compromised Family Coping*

6. A nurse has begun working with young adults. Which of the following would the nurse recognize as sources of stress common to that population? (Select all that apply.)
   - **a.** Getting married
   - **b.** Coping with aging parents
   - **c.** Starting a new job
   - **d.** Leaving the parental home
   - **e.** Accepting decreased physical abilities
   - **f.** Accepting a changing body structure

7. Which of the following would be the most important health-promotion strategy for a middle-aged male client who is experiencing stress because fear of a job layoff has led him to accept projects that require a great deal of international travel?
   - **a.** Exercise
   - **b.** Sleep
   - **c.** Nutrition
   - **d.** Time management

8. On entering the client's room for the first time, the nurse finds the client on the phone. Within the next few seconds, the client slams down the phone, sweeps everything off the overbed table, and demands that the nurse perform several duties "this very minute." Which of the following would be the most appropriate response for the nurse?
   - **a.** Tell the client, "I will return," and then leave the room.
   - **b.** Tell the client no care will be given until the screaming ends.
   - **c.** Begin providing needed care calmly and quietly.
   - **d.** Allow the client to complete venting and then respond calmly.

9. Mr. Jonas, 67 years old, will soon be discharged home from the cardiac unit. He indicates that he is concerned about his discharge because his home situation can be stressful. What strategy should the nurse employ to help him cope with stressful situations?

- **a.** Encourage him to plan his daily activities.
- **b.** Inform him that a nurse will visit him at home.
- **c.** Reassure him that stress is normal and that he should just rest.
- **d.** Have him practise a stress-reduction method that he has found effective.

10. Which of the following interventions best facilitates successful stress management with clients?

- **a.** Teaching relaxations techniques
- **b.** Suggesting talking with others
- **c.** Encouraging problem solving
- **d.** Promoting self awareness

After working through these questions, go to the MyNursingLab at ***http://www.mynursinglab.com*** *to check your answers and see explanations.*

SUGGESTED READINGS

Edgar, L., & Watt, S. (2004). Nucare, a coping skills training intervention for oncology patients and families: Participants' motivations and expectations. *Canadian Oncology Nursing Journal, 14*(2), 84–88.

This study looks at the effectiveness of an innovative nursing intervention program in a population dealing with a cancer diagnosis.

Sjöström-Strand, A. (2006). Women's descriptions of coping with stress at the time of and after a myocardial infarction: a phenomenographic analysis. *Canadian Journal of Cardiovascular Nursing, 16*(1), 5–12.

Women describe in their own words how they use different coping strategies to manage stress in their lives related to having had a myocardial infarction.

WEBLINKS

Canadian Mental Health Association

http://www.cmha.ca

This website contains educational information, links to multiple Canadian and international mental health sites, information regarding CMHA provincial and territorial locations (except Nunavut), and a discussion site.

Public Health Agency of Canada

http://www.publichealth.gc.ca

This website is funded by Health Canada and contains information on many health issues.

Centre for Addiction and Mental Health

http://www.camh.net

The Centre for Addiction and Mental Health site contains information on addictions, community health and education, mental health, and research at the centre.

REFERENCES

Antai-Otong, D. (2003). Anxiety disorders: Helping your patient conquer her fears. *Nursing, 33*(12), 36–41.

Bulechek, G. M., Butcher, H. K., & Dochterman, J. C. (Eds.). (2008). *Nursing interventions classification (NIC).* St. Louis, MO: Mosby Elsevier.

Canadian Mental Health Association. (2005). *Holiday angst hits everyone.* Retrieved June 1, 2008, from http://www.cmha.bc.ca/files/5-12-05.pdf

Folkman, S., & Lazarus, R. S. (1991). Coping and emotion. In A. Monat & R. S. Lazarus (Eds.), *Stress and coping* (pp. 207–227). New York: Columbia University Press.

Fontaine, K. L., & Fletcher, J. S. (2003). *Mental health nursing* (5th ed.). Upper Saddle River, NJ: Prentice Hall.

Freud, S. (1946). *The ego and the mechanisms of defense.* New York: International Universities Press.

Holmes, T. H., & Rahe, R. H. (1967). The social re-adjustment rating scale. *Journal of Psychomatic Research, 11*(August), 213–218.

IPSOS Reid. (2006). *Canada speaks: Half of Canadians (45%) feel they don't have enough control over their stress levels; finances (44%) and work (37%) are most common causes of stress.* Toronto: Author.

Lazarus, R. S. (1966). *Psychological stress and the coping process.* New York: McGraw-Hill.

Lazarus, R. S. (2000). Evolution of a model of stress, coping, and discrete emotions. In V. H. Rice (Ed.), *Handbook of stress, coping, and health: Implications for nursing research, theory, and practice* (pp. 195–222). Thousand Oaks, CA: Sage.

Miller, M. A., & Rahe, R. H. (1997). Life changes scaling for the 1990s. *Journal of Psychosomatic Research, 43*, 279–292.

Monat, A., & Lazarus, R. S. (Eds.) (1991). *Stress and coping* (3rd ed.). New York: Columbia University Press.

NANDA International. (2007). *Nursing diagnoses: Definitions and classification, 2007–2008*. Philadelphia, PA: Author.

Rahe, R. H., & Tolles, R. L. (2002). The brief stress and coping inventory: A useful stress management instrument. *International Journal of Stress Management, 9*, 61–70.

Schafer, W. (1992). *Stress management for wellness* (2nd ed.). Philadelphia, PA: Harcourt Brace Jovanovich.

Selye, H. (1956). *The stress of life*. New York: McGraw-Hill.

Selye, H. (1976). *The stress of life* (Rev. ed.). New York: McGraw-Hill.

Veterans Affairs Canada. (2006). *Post traumatic stress disorder (PTSD) and war-related stress*. Ottawa: Minister of Veterans Affairs.

Chapter 48

Loss, Grieving, and Death

Loss, grieving, and death are experienced by everyone at some time during their life. People may suffer the loss of valued relationships through life changes, such as moving from one city to another, separation, divorce, or the death of a parent, spouse, or friend. People may grieve changing life roles as they watch grown children leave home or when they retire from their lifelong work. The loss of valued material objects through theft or natural disaster can evoke feelings of grief and loss. When people's lives are affected by civil or national strife, they may grieve the loss of valued ideals, such as safety, freedom, and democracy.

In the clinical setting, the nurse encounters clients who are experiencing grief related to declining health, loss of a body part, terminal illness, or their impending death or that of a significant other. Nurses interact with dying clients and their families or caregivers in a variety of settings, from the demise of a fetus, to that of an adolescent victim of an accident, to that of an older adult client who finally succumbs to a chronic illness. Nurses must recognize the various influences on the dying process—legal, ethical, religious and spiritual, biological, and personal—and be prepared to provide sensitive, skilled, and supportive care to all those affected.

OBJECTIVES

After studying this chapter, you should be able to

1. Describe types and sources of losses
2. Describe the experience of grief as a response to loss that is individually experienced and expressed
3. Outline eight factors affecting grief responses
4. Identify measures that facilitate the journey of grief
5. List clinical signs of impending and of actual death
6. Describe the nurse's legal and moral responsibilities regarding end-of-life care and such issues as advance directives, artificial nutrition, and do not resuscitate orders
7. Describe six strategies for helping clients die with dignity
8. Identify nursing measures for care of the body after death
9. Describe the role of the nurse in working with families or caregivers of dying clients

Loss and Grief

Loss is an actual or a potential situation in which something that is valued is changed, no longer available, or gone. People can experience the loss of body image, a significant other, a sense of well-being, a job, personal possessions, beliefs, or a sense of self. Illness and hospitalization often produce losses.

Death is a fundamental loss, both for the dying person and for those who survive. Death is inevitable, and it is an experience that each person ultimately faces alone. Yet death, like loss, can stimulate people to grow in their understanding of themselves and others. Death can be viewed not simply as loss of life but also as the dying person's final opportunity to experience life in ways that bring meaning and fulfillment.

Types and Sources of Loss

The two general types of loss are actual loss and perceived loss. Both losses can be anticipatory. An **actual loss** can be identified by others and can arise either in response to or in anticipation of a situation. For example, a woman whose husband is dying may experience actual loss in anticipation of his death. A **perceived loss** is experienced by one person but cannot be verified by others. Psychological losses are often perceived losses in that they are not directly verifiable. For example, a woman who leaves her employment to care for her children at home may perceive a loss of independence and freedom. An **anticipatory loss** is experienced before the loss actually occurs.

Loss can be viewed as situational or developmental. The loss of a job, the death of a child, and the loss of functional ability as a result of acute illness or injury, for example, are unexpected situational losses. Losses that occur in the process of normal development—such as the departure of grown children from the home, retirement from a career, and the death of aged parents—are developmental losses that can, to some extent, be anticipated and prepared for. How individuals work through loss is closely related to their life stages and past experiences, personal and family resources, social support systems, and their beliefs about the loss itself.

Many sources of loss exist: (1) loss of an aspect of the self: a body part, a physiological function, or a psychological attribute, (2) loss of an object external to the self, (3) separation from an accustomed environment, and (4) loss of a loved or valued person.

ASPECT OF THE SELF The loss of an aspect of the self changes a person's body image, even though the loss may not be obvious to others. A face scarred from a burn is generally obvious to people; loss of part of the stomach or loss of ability to feel emotion may not be as obvious. The degree to which these losses affect a person largely depends on the integrity of the person's body image (part of self-concept). Any change that the person perceives as negative in the way he or she relates to the environment can be considered a loss of self. It should be noted that *self* is a culturally influenced concept; therefore, experiences of self-loss are particular to individuals and their particular cultural and personal influences.

Such losses as divorce can have a considerable impact. A divorce may mean loss of financial security, a home, daily routines, and a role as spouse. Therefore, even when the divorce was desired, the sense of loss can be substantial.

During old age, changes can occur in physical and mental capabilities. Again the self-image is vulnerable. Old age is the time when people usually experience many losses: of employment, of usual activities, of independence, of health, of friends, and of family.

EXTERNAL OBJECTS Loss of external objects includes (1) loss of inanimate objects that have importance to the person, such as the loss of money or the burning down of a family's house, and (2) loss of animate objects, such as pets that provide love and companionship.

FAMILIAR ENVIRONMENT Separation from an environment and people who provide security can result in a sense of loss. The 6-year-old is likely to feel loss when first leaving the usual environment to attend school. The university student who moves away from home for the first time also experiences a sense of loss.

LOVED ONES The loss of a loved one or valued person through illness, separation, or death can, among other experiences, create suffering. In some illnesses, a person may undergo personality changes that make friends and family feel they have lost that person.

Significant current research on grief indicates that the death of a loved one initiates a change in family relationships that constantly changes and evolves over time to bring new meanings to family members left behind (Moules, Simonson, Prins, Angus, & Bell, 2004). Making room for grief and death is not a popular concept (Moules et al., 2004). In past societies, death was considered a normal, natural event, and life was seldom long. In contemporary North American society, death is often denied. People may be uncomfortable talking about death and being around people who are dying. Sometimes, in an effort to escape the finality of death, people resort to extraordinary measures to prolong and preserve life.

The Experience of Grief

Grief has been explained in many of the early theorists' works as a process involving progression through a series of stages or phases requiring work or particular tasks that result in a final resolution of grief feelings. Out of this explanation, stage model theories, some of which are based on Kubler-Ross's (1969) work on death and dying, have provided one template for understanding the experience of grief. One criticism of stage model theories is that although they may provide some understanding, recognition, and language for the experience of grief, they may also serve to obscure unique and individual experiences of grief (Moules, 1998; Moules, Simonson, Fleiszer, Prins, & Glasgow, 2007; Moules et al., 2004). They can narrowly focus on psychological responses while overlooking social, spiritual, familial, and physical domains of the experience of grief. To understand grief as a staged experience can mistakenly invite the belief that grief occurs passively in expected sequences that disregard individual experiences and that fail to resonate with the experiences people actually undergo in grieving.

Martocchio (1985) discussed five clusters of grief, which exemplify common experiences in the grief response. These include shock and disbelief; yearning and protest; anguish, disorganization, and despair; identification in bereavement; and reorganization and restitution. Within these common experiences, however, there is no single correct way or timetable. Whether a person can successfully integrate the loss and how this is accomplished are related to that person's individual development and personal makeup. Individuals responding to the very same loss cannot be expected to follow the same pattern and schedule or reach the same outcome.

Another popularization of the experience of grief is that a normal grief reaction exists, as does an abnormal or unhealthy one. Grief that does not follow a predictable or an expected course is often described as abnormal, complicated, pathological, unresolved, chronic, morbid, prolonged, dysfunctional, exaggerated, or disenfranchised. This pathologizing view of any divergence of expected and typical responses to loss can serve to intensify the suffering of grief, and add, in addition to the experience of loss, a sense of personal failure and incompetence (Moules, 1998; Moules et al., 2004; Moules et al., 2007).

Furthermore, socially sanctioned notions about grief invite the idea that the work of grief resolution is to find a way to let go of the person who is lost and to say goodbye. Alternatively, White (1989) and Moules (1998; Moules et al., 2004; Moules et al., 2007) suggested that when people lose a loved one, they continue to feel in relationship to the person, and although the relationship is necessarily changed and altered through physical absence, it continues in their emotional and spiritual life. Grief then becomes the process of learning how to live with this new and changed relationship in such a way that it offers aspects of connection and comfort, rather than pain and suffering. Grief is an unwanted visitor that arrives within the context of the experience of loss. It sweeps into every domain of a person's life: biological, psychological, social, emotional, and spiritual. Grief endures in a way that shifts over time, eventually creating a mutable or changing and evolving but, most often, a lifetime relationship with the loss. Unwanted or not, this visitor, grief, takes up residence in lives.

In nursing work with the bereaved, the challenge then is to co-evolve a way to assist people in making room for grief in their lives in ways that open space for experiences other than suffering and in inviting people to remember their lost other and say hello to a new and changed relationship (Moules, 1998; Moules et al., 2004; Moules et al., 2007).

Experiences of grief can become complicated and can have potentially devastating effects on health. Among the symptoms that can accompany grief are anxiety, depression, weight loss, difficulties in swallowing, vomiting, fatigue, headaches, dizziness, fainting, blurred vision, skin rashes, excessive sweating, menstrual disturbances, palpitations, chest pain, dyspnea, and infection. The bereaved may also experience alterations in libido, concentration, and patterns of eating, sleeping, activity, and communication.

Although bereavement can threaten health, concurrent experiences within grief can enrich the individual with new insights, values, challenges, openness, and sensitivity. For some, the pain of loss, though diminished, recurs for the rest of their lives. For others, the pain shifts into a continuing experience of remembrance, connection, and even celebration of a life well lived and loved.

A complication that can result from the intense experience of grief is a continuing experience of only sadness, loss, or even depression that is not relieved over time and is not buffered with other experiences or a return to life and joy. Another source of conflict can stem from a held belief that all people experience grief in a similar way. This belief might lead family members to have expectations of one another that cannot be fulfilled and may invite a sense of alienation, isolation, or even conflict among those people who are expected to provide comfort and connection for one another.

Complicating an individual's experience of grief might be ambivalence, unresolved issues, or conflict with the lost person; a pervasive and unrelenting sense of guilt or responsibility; past experiences of loss; and the type, timing, and context of the loss (Herz Brown, 1989). Certain kinds of losses that are not synchronous with life-stage expectations, such as the loss of a child as opposed to an older parent, can (but do not necessarily) generate more intense experiences of grief (Cowles & Rodgers, 1991; Rolland, 2004) and have the potential for more complications in the experience.

Factors Influencing Loss and Grief

A number of factors affect a person's response to a loss or death. These factors include age, significance of the loss, culture, spiritual beliefs, gender, socioeconomic status, support systems, and the cause of the loss or death.

Nurses can learn general concepts about the influence of these factors on the grieving experience, but the constellation of these factors and their significance will vary from individual to individual.

AGE Age affects a person's understanding of and reaction to loss. With experience, people usually increase their understanding and acceptance of life, loss, and death.

People do not usually experience the loss of loved ones at regular intervals. As a result, preparation for these experiences is difficult. Coping with other losses in life, such as the loss of a pet, the loss of a friend, the loss of a job, and the loss of youth, can prepare people for the more severe loss of death.

CHILDHOOD Children differ from adults not only in their understanding of loss and death but also in how they are affected by the loss of others. The child's patterns progress rapidly; adult patterns of growth and development are generally stable. The loss of a parent or other significant person can threaten the child's ability to develop, and regression sometimes results. Assisting the child with the grief experience includes helping the child regain the normal continuity and pace of emotional development.

Some adults assume that children do not have the same need as an adult to grieve the loss of others. In situations of crisis and loss, children are sometimes pushed aside or protected from the pain. They can feel afraid, abandoned, and lonely. Careful work with bereaved children is especially necessary because experiencing a loss in childhood can have serious effects later in life.

EARLY AND MIDDLE ADULTHOOD As people grow, they come to experience loss as part of normal development. By middle age, for example, the loss of a parent through death seems a normal occurrence compared with the death of a younger person. Coping with the death of an aged parent has even been viewed as a necessary developmental task of the middle-aged adult.

The middle-aged adult can experience losses other than death. For example, losses resulting from impaired health or body function and losses of various role functions can be difficult for the middle-aged adult. How the middle-aged adult responds to such losses is influenced by previous experiences with loss, the person's sense of self-esteem, and the strength and availability of support.

LATE ADULTHOOD Losses experienced by older adults include loss of health, loss of mobility, loss of independence, and loss of work role. Limited income and the need to change living accommodations can also lead to feelings of loss and grieving.

For older adults, the loss through death of a longtime mate is profound. Although individuals differ in their ability to deal with such a loss, research suggests that health problems for widows and widowers increase during the first year following the death of the spouse (Richter, 1984). Because the majority of deaths occur among older adults and because the number of older people is increasing in North America, nurses will need to be especially alert to the potential problems of older adults who are grieving.

SIGNIFICANCE OF THE LOSS The significance of a loss depends on the perceptions of the individual experiencing the loss. One person may experience a great sense of loss over a divorce; another may find it only mildly disrupting. A number of factors affect the significance of the loss:

- The value placed on the lost person, object, or function
- The degree of change required because of the loss
- The person's beliefs and values

For older people who have already encountered many losses, an anticipated loss, such as their own death, may not be viewed as a highly negative loss, and they may be apathetic about it instead of reactive. More than fearing death, some may fear loss of control or becoming a burden.

CULTURE Culture influences an individual's reaction to loss. How grief is expressed is often determined by the customs of the culture. In the United States and Canada, unless an extended family structure exists, grief is handled by the nuclear family. The death of a family member in a typical nuclear North American family leaves a great void because the same few individuals fill most of the roles. In cultures in which several generations and extended family members either reside in the same household or are physically close, the impact of a family member's death may be softened because the roles of the deceased are quickly filled by other relatives.

Many North Americans appear to have adopted the belief that grief is a private matter to be endured internally. Therefore, feelings tend to be repressed and may remain unidentified. People who have been socialized to "be strong" and "make the best of the situation" may not express deep feelings or personal concerns when they experience a serious loss.

Some cultural groups value social support and the expression of loss. In some groups, the expression of grief through wailing, crying, physical prostration, and other outward demonstrations are acceptable and encouraged. Other groups may frown on demonstration as a loss of control, favouring a quieter and more stoic expression of grief. In cultural groups in which strong kinship ties are maintained, physical and emotional support and assistance are provided by family members.

SPIRITUAL BELIEFS Spiritual beliefs and practices greatly influence both a person's reaction to loss and a person's subsequent behaviour. Most religious groups have practices related to dying, and these are often important to the client and support people. For additional information, see Chapter 46. To provide support at a time of death, nurses need to understand the client's particular beliefs and practices. A part of a person's spirituality is represented in, and influences, the way that person makes meaning of the experience of loss. Asking questions of a spiritual nature is within the domain of nursing practice (Moules, 1999; Wright, 1997, 1999).

GENDER As mentioned earlier, the gender roles into which many people are socialized in North America affect their reactions at times of loss. Men are frequently expected to be strong and show very little emotion during grieving, whereas it is acceptable for women to show grief by crying. Gender roles also affect the significance of body image changes to clients. A man might consider his facial scar to be macho, but a woman might consider hers ugly. Thus, the woman, but not the man, would see it as a loss.

SOCIOECONOMIC STATUS The socioeconomic status of an individual often affects the support system available at the time of a loss. A pension plan or insurance, for example, can offer a widowed person or a person with disabilities a choice of ways to deal with a loss. A person who loses a hand and can no longer carry out work-related tasks may be able to pursue vocational re-education; a wealthy person whose spouse has died may decide to take a cruise or visit relatives in Europe. Conversely, a person who is confronted with both severe loss and economic hardship may not be able to cope with either.

SUPPORT SYSTEMS The people closest to the grieving individual are often the first to recognize and provide needed emotional, physical, and functional assistance. However, because many people are uncomfortable or inexperienced in dealing with losses, the usual support people may instead withdraw from the grieving individual. Also, support may be available when the loss is first recognized, but as the support people return to their usual activities, the need for ongoing support may be unmet. Sometimes, the grieving individual is unable or unready to accept support when it is offered.

CAUSE OF LOSS OR DEATH Individual and societal views on the cause of a loss or death can significantly influence the grief response. Some diseases are considered clean, such as cardiovascular disorders, and engender compassion; others may be viewed as repulsive and less unfortunate. A loss or death that is beyond the control of those involved may be more acceptable than one that is preventable, such as a drunk driving accident. Injuries or deaths occurring during respected activities, such as in the line of duty, are considered honourable, whereas those occurring during illicit activities may be considered the individual's just rewards.

Assessing

Nursing assessment of the client and family experiencing a loss includes three major components: (1) nursing history, (2) assessment of personal coping resources, and (3) physical assessment. During the routine health assessment of every client, the nurse poses questions regarding previous and current losses. The nature of the loss and the meaning of such losses to the client must be explored.

If the client has experienced a current or recent loss, greater detail is needed in the assessment. Because clients do not always associate physical ailments with emotional responses, such as grief, the nurse may need to probe to identify possible loss-related stresses. If the client reports significant losses, it is important to examine how the client usually copes with loss and what resources are available to assist the client in coping. Data regarding general health status; other personal stressors; cultural and spiritual traditions, rituals, and beliefs related to loss and grieving; and the person's support network will be needed in order to determine a plan of care (see the Assessment: Interview box).

In assessing the client's response to a current loss, the nurse may identify complications of grief that may be best treated by a health-care professional who is expert in assisting such clients. If the nursing assessment reveals severe physical or psychological signs and symptoms, the client should be referred to an appropriate care provider. Such complications include clinical depression, extensive social isolation and withdrawal, severe physiological symptoms, suicidal thoughts or urges, or unrelenting and oppressive sorrow that persists for prolonged periods and is not balanced by any relief or joy-filled experiences.

Implementing

The skills most relevant to situations of loss and grief are attentive listening, silence, open and closed questioning, paraphrasing, clarifying and reflecting feelings, and summarizing. Less helpful to clients are responses that give advice and evaluation, those that interpret and analyze, and those that give unwarranted reassurance. The offering of platitudes is often a temptation to those trying to comfort someone who is suffering a loss. Though well intended and often arising out of a loss for words, such platitudes as "It must have happened for a reason; you need to accept it," "Time heals all wounds," "Try not to think about it," "You'll get over it in time," or "Now you've got a little angel in heaven" serve only to contribute to messages that a visible grief is unhealthy and that grief is time limited (Moules & Amundson, 1997). These messages deny the right and need of the bereaved to fully experience, acknowledge, and express grief as a part of incorporating loss into their lives. What the nurse says or does is always best guided by the client and in response to the client's needs. Sometimes, a simple statement of "I am sorry for your loss," or a silent presence is what is most needed. To ensure effective communica-

ASSESSMENT: INTERVIEW

Loss and Grieving

The following questions can help the nurse determine a client's ability to cope with loss:

PREVIOUS LOSSES

- Have you ever lost someone or something very important to you?
- Have you or your family ever moved your home?
- What was it like for you when you first started school? moved away from home? got a job? retired?
- Are you physically able to do all the things you like to do? used to do?
- Has anyone important or close to you died?
- Do you think there will be any losses in your life in the near future?

PREVIOUS GRIEVING

- Tell me about (the loss). What was losing ________ like for you?
- Did you have trouble sleeping? eating? concentrating?
- What kinds of things did you do to make yourself feel better when something like that happened?
- Are there spiritual or cultural practices you observed when you had a loss like that?
- Whom did you turn to if you were very upset about (the loss)?
- How long did it take you to feel more like yourself again and go back to your usual activities?

CURRENT LOSS

- What have you been told about (the loss)? Is there anything else you would like to know or do not understand?
- What changes do you think this (illness, surgery, problem) will cause in your life? What do you think it will be like without (the lost object)?
- Have you ever experienced a loss like this before?
- Can you think of anything good that might come out of this?
- What kind of help do you think you will need? Who is going to be helping you with this loss?
- Are there any people or organizations in your community that might be able to help?

CURRENT GRIEVING

- Are you having trouble sleeping? eating? concentrating? breathing?
- Do you have any pain or other new physical problems?
- Are you taking any drugs or medications to help you cope with this loss?
- What are you doing to help you deal with this loss?

tion, the nurse must make an accurate assessment of what is appropriate for the client.

Communication with grieving clients needs to be relevant to meeting clients at the point of *their* needs, not the nurse's needs. To determine the point of a client's need, the nurse has to be willing to listen to the client's pain and suffering and not be tempted to try to take the pain away or heal it, even if such a thing were possible.

In addition to effective communication skills, a nurse can support and care in specific ways for a client experiencing loss. Of these, probably the most important is that the nurse "make room for grief" (Moules, 1998, p. 100). This means that the nurse accepts, facilitates, and normalizes the experience and expression of grief, which can be done through actions and attitudes:

- Be present, be comfortable with silence, and offer touch if the person indicates that would be comforting.
- Acknowledge pain and suffering.
- Encourage talk about the loss and the loved one, but accept it if clients cannot or do not want to do so.
- Explore and respect clients' racial, cultural, religious, personal, and family values in their expression of grief.
- Explore their support system and personal resources. Who is available to be with them? Who would be most helpful right now? Who can help them take care of practical arrangements and details?
- Assist clients and families in understanding that grief is expressed differently by different people and individuals cannot be expected to adhere to others' expectations of appropriate responses to grief.
- If children are involved, encourage family members to be truthful and to allow the children to participate in the grieving activities of others.
- Though maybe not at the time of the immediate loss, support clients in exploring the meaning they have made of their loss, how they have come to understand it or live with it, and how they have come to make room for a relationship with grief in their lives.
- Provide resource and support information, such as local grief support groups or counselling.

Dying and Death

The concept of death is developed over time, as the person grows, experiences various losses, and reflects on concrete and abstract concepts. In general, humans move from a childhood belief in death as a temporary state, to adulthood in which death is accepted as very real but also very frightening, and to older adulthood in which death may be viewed as more desirable than living with a poor quality of life. Table 48.1 describes some of the specific beliefs common to different age groups. The nurse's knowledge of these developmental stages helps in understanding some of the client's responses to a life-threatening situation.

TABLE 48.1 Development of the Concept of Death

Age	Beliefs and Attitudes
Infancy to 5 years	Does not understand concept of death
	Infant's sense of separation forms basis for later understanding of loss and death
	Believes death is reversible, a temporary departure, or sleep
	Emphasizes immobility and inactivity as attributes of death
5 to 9 years	Understands that death is final
	Believes own death can be avoided
	Associates death with aggression or violence
	Believes wishes or unrelated actions can be responsible for death
9 to 12 years	Understands death as the inevitable end of life
	Begins to understand own mortality, expressed as interest in afterlife or as fear of death
12 to 18 years	Fears a lingering death
	May fantasize that death can be defied, acting out defiance through reckless behaviours (e.g., dangerous driving, problematic substance use)
	Seldom thinks about death, but views it in religious and philosophic terms
	May seem to reach adult perception of death but be emotionally unable to accept it
	May still hold concepts from previous developmental stages
18 to 45 years	Has attitude toward death influenced by religious and cultural beliefs
45 to 65 years	Accepts own mortality
	Encounters death of parents and some peers
	Experiences peaks of death anxiety
	Death anxiety diminishes with emotional well-being
65+ years	Fears prolonged illness
	Encounters death of family members and peers
	Sees death as having multiple meanings (e.g., freedom from pain, reunion with already deceased family members)

End-of-Life Care for Older Adults

The aging of Canada's population has drawn attention to the necessity of an end-of-life care strategy that addresses the needs of the increasing proportion of older adults who die every year from causes other than cancer. Currently, cancer patients receive 90% of the available palliative care services, although they only represent 25% of those who die. Deaths caused by progressive chronic illnesses, such as congestive heart failure, chronic obstructive pulmonary disease, renal disease, and dementia, will increase. It is projected that by 2024, 20% of all Canadians will be 65 years of age and older (Martel & Malenfant, 2007). A paradox exists in Canada in that the numbers of older adults and people with chronic life-threatening illnesses are growing while downsizing in the health-care system continues and societal expectations of access to excellent care rise (MacDonald, 1998).

Older adults may have comorbid medical conditions that contribute an added symptom burden to the palliative care population. The presence of chronic medical conditions is associated with disability and increased health-care use, including institutionalization and hospitalization. Given the multisystemic nature of illness at the end of life, the pattern of symptoms is usually diverse and can include pain as well as dyspnea, dysphagia, edema, shortness of breath, and delirium. These will be discussed later in the chapter. Furthermore, the presence of existing comorbidities and disabilities renders older adults more susceptible to the complications of new illnesses and their treatments. The trajectory of death in older adults is also less predictable, encompassing many acute episodic illnesses that eventually result in a slow decline of functional and cognitive abilities.

Typically, family members meet care needs of older individuals and, more often than not, these individuals are women. Caregiver burden is well documented in the literature and includes a great number of depressive symptoms, anxiety, diminished physical health, financial problems, and disruption from work. Older adult patients requiring symptom care are more likely than younger patients to have an increased dependence on others for basic daily activity, such as bathing, meal preparation, eating, and ambulating. If the patient is confused or agitated, the burden is even greater, often requiring 24-hour care. For older adults with chronic illnesses, the duration of caregiving can be several years. When people have no family caregivers, or care needs become too great (as with Alzheimer's disease), patients are often placed in a long-term-care facility. Seventy-five percent of deaths today still take place in hospitals and long-term-care facilities (Canadian Hospice Palliative Care Association, 2004).

Responses to Dying and Death

"Understanding responses to death and dying begins with the recognition that dying individuals exist within a family system. The nurse considers the impact of the dying individual's illness on the whole family and the family's responses that affect the patient. Caring for the dying individual's family involves understanding family in the broadest sense. Family may include spouses and children, or those the dying individual defines as a 'significant other' who functions in supportive ways offering emotional, spiritual, and socioeconomic companionship and, possibly, intimate bonds" (Gilliss, Highly, Roberts, & Martinsen, 1989).

Both the client who is dying and the family members grieve as they recognize the loss. Literature is emerging on family factors thought to influence end-of-life decision making, including ways in which the acuity of onset or phase of the illness can intersect with family adaptation (Rolland, 2003, 2004). As well, families are thought to move in to and out of periods of relative closeness versus distance based on their characteristic style of adaptation and the phase of illness (Winchester Nadeau, 2001). Clinical literature (King, Shields, & Wynne, 2005; Qualls, 2000; Walsh & McGoldrick, 2004), and research (Kissane et al., 1996; Kissane, 2003; Weihs & Reiss, 1996) suggests that families have different levels of relational ability based on their history of shared experiences, as well as the strengths and vulnerabilities of individual family members.

Nurses and other health-care professionals must strive to understand the meaning of the grief experience to the dying individual and the family. Grieving can include feelings of fear, inability to focus, hopelessness without a sense of moving beyond the death, powerlessness, losing control over emotions, and despair and depression. People may also have many physical symptoms, including increased pulse and respirations, dry mouth, anorexia, difficulty sleeping, and nightmares. If meaningful care is to be provided to the dying individuals and their families, the nurse must understand their beliefs and values related to the experience, how the relationships fit together, and the many factors that affect the experience of dying and illness.

Caregivers, both professionals and support people, also are affected by the impending death. The ongoing responsibilities for providing physical, ethical, and emotional support to a dying person can create extreme stress for all providers in whatever setting care is provided (Seymour, 2001). Often, the length of time between a terminal diagnosis and when death will occur is unknown and the people supporting the dying person become fatigued and depressed and feel empty. They may feel anger because of lost time and resources for personal activities or attention for other people. The impending death can pose a challenge to family roles and day-to-day functioning. In this situation, the family may be unable to meet the physical, emotional, or spiritual needs of the members and may have difficulty communicating and problem solving.

Evidence-Informed Practice

What Guides Clinicians in Their Grief Work with Families?

In a second phase of a study on grief and grief interventions, Moules, Simonson, Fleiszer, Prins, and Glasgow (2007), examined the experiences of bereaved family members who had received care in a grief support program and explored the program clinicians' explanations of the work that they do with the bereaved. This research project was a two-phase hermeneutic interpretive study, based on the philosophy of Hans-Georg Gadamer (1989). Hermeneutics is the tradition, theory, and practice of interpretation and understanding in human contexts. In this phase of the study, three clinicians were selected from a grief support program on the basis of experience and willingness to be interviewed. The clinicians each volunteered one person with whom they had worked, who was also willing to be interviewed and who was likely able to offer useful data. No other selection criteria were employed. The six participants underwent individual interviews. The findings of this interpretive study suggest that it is not so much models of grief intervention but maps that most guide the clinicians—maps that are drawn out of experience and with awareness of their limitations. It is someone who is willing to step off the map that makes for the best travelling companion in the spiritual walk of grief.

NURSING IMPLICATIONS: Nurses need courage and willingness to walk alongside families in grief. Rather than seeing divergences from "normal" in grief reactions and experiences, nurses should accept a wide range of responses and acknowledge that grief is a complicated, complex, tangled experience. Nurses might consider the idea of grief as an experience of connection rather than of severance of a relationship.

Sources: Based on "The Soul of Sorrow Work: Grief and Therapeutic Interventions with Families," by N. Moules, K. Simonson, A. Fleiszer, M. Prins, and B. Glasgow, 2007, *Journal of Family Nursing, 13*(1), pp. 1–25; and *Truth and Method,* 2nd ed., by H. G. Gadamer, 1989 (J. Weinsheimer & D. G. Marshall, Trans.), New York: Continuum.

Nurses who have developed a close relationship with the dying individual and family may themselves experience a sense of loss and suffer with them as they care for them in the journey of dying (Raffin, 2002; Raffin Bouchal, 2007). Nurses who spend many hours, even days, with the dying individual and family "do not simply care for the dying individual's physical bodies, they also tend to their spirit, gently, respectfully, and knowingly" (Moules, 2000, p.4). The very nature of palliative care nursing is such that, every day, practitioners face some of the most fundamental and poignant issues confronting humanity (Perry, 1998). Nurses are invited to share in the intimate journey of living and dying where suffering is present. This sharing often entails a commitment of developing a meaningful relationship as a way to know and understand the dying experience. The relationship, although rewarding, often places the nurse in a vulnerable position. Nurses are affected by this position (Raffin, 2002; Raffin Bouchal, 2007).

Caring for the dying and the bereaved is one of the nurse's most complex and challenging responsibilities, bringing into play all the skills needed for care of the whole person—mind, body, and spirit. To care for the whole person, nurses must be aware of and comfortable with their own values and beliefs about death, dying, and suffering, as these will surely affect the care they are able to give others.

Legal and Moral Issues Related to End-of-Life Care

Many legal issues surround the event of death, including a legal definition as to when a person is considered clinically dead. Few jurisdictions in Canada provide a legislative definition of the moment of death. Physicians, until well into the twentieth century, concurred that a person was dead when all vital signs (pulse, respiration) had ceased. Since the last half of the twentieth century, medical technology has allowed physicians to sustain the lives of seriously ill individuals by means of artificial support that maintains blood circulation. As well, the advances of medical transplant technology have made possible transplantation of viable organs from deceased individuals to living recipients.

It has become apparent that the traditional medical criteria for determining the fact of death have become inadequate. In 1975, Manitoba became the first (and, so far, the only) province to enact a legal definition of death. The Manitoba Vital Statistics Act suggests that "the death of a person takes place at the time at which irreversible cessation of all that person's brain function occurs" (cited by Lazar, Shemie, Webster, & Dickens, 2001, p. 834). This definition conforms to the accepted medical practice. With this definition, the client still may be able to breathe but is irreversibly unconscious. People who support this definition of death believe that the cerebral cortex—which holds the capacity for thought, voluntary action, and movement—*is* the individual.

ADVANCE DIRECTIVES (LIVING WILLS) Individuals receiving health care sometimes worry that if they become incapacitated and unable to express their wishes, they will be hooked up to machines and receive treatment that they do not want. The Terry Schiavo case in the United States uncovered the complexity and possible issues people may face at the end of life. Advance directives have been suggested as one way to address this problem. The Canadian Nurses Association (CNA, 1998) and other sponsors produced a joint statement on advance directives for nurses' use in practice. **Advance directives** are "the means used to document and communicate a person's preferences regarding life-sustaining treatment in the event that they become incapable of expressing those wishes for themselves" (CNA, 1998, p. 1). Advance directives are commonly expressed in two ways: an instruction directive, or **living will**, which identifies what life-sustaining treatment a person wants in certain situations; or a **proxy directive**, which explains who is to make health-care decisions if the person becomes incompetent. A proxy directive is often referred to as a power of attorney for personal care (CNA, 1998). The CNA encourages nurses and other health-care professionals to communicate with clients regarding their health care and treatment to identify how clients want end-of-life issues to be addressed (CNA, 2000). A routine part of any admission to a hospital now includes inquiry about the client's advance directives; if they exist, they are included as part of the medical directives.

The legal right of each individual to decide future health care has been recognized by Canadian courts for some time and is also reflected in the Canadian Constitution. If the construction and the execution of the directive comply with the legal requirements set out by the province or territory in the individual's jurisdiction, then it will be legally binding (Tapp, 2006). It is necessary for nurses to be aware of the legal status of all types of advance directives in their province or territory. As outlined by the CNA (1998), some provinces and territories recognize only proxy directives as legally binding, while others recognize both proxy and instructional directives (Tapp, 2006). In addition, nurses need to become familiar with laws and documents regarding a person's competence to consent, issues regarding cardiopulmonary resuscitation (CPR), and issues at the end of life, as these are closely related to advance directives (Figure 48.1).

Health-care professionals, including nurses, are responsible for ensuring that advance directives are addressed, not only as an admission duty but also as a part of the ongoing communication among all members providing and receiving care. A significant part of this process is to discuss and obtain a statement of the indi-

Personal Directive

I, ______________________________, of __________________, Alberta, do hereby:
Appoint ______________________________, as my Agent; pursuant to the Personal Directives Act of Alberta. If (s)he predeceases me or is unavailable or unwilling to act, then I appoint ______________________________, to be my Alternate Agent. Any Agent appointed by me shall have full authority to interpret all personal and medical decisions, and the instructions below, even if they have no bearing upon the actual situation, should I be unable to make these decisions for myself.

Primary Agent	**Alternate Agent**
Agent's name: ____________________	Agent's name: ____________________
Agent's address: __________________	Agent's address: __________________
____________________________	
Home phone: ______________________	Home phone: ______________________
Work number: _____________________	Work number: _____________________

If at such a time the situation arises in which there is **no reasonable expectation of my recovery from severe physical or mental disability** to a state of meaningful interaction with loved ones, family and friends, I would like the following directions to be followed:

1. Measures of artificial life-support, in the above stated situation, that I refuse are:
   a. Cardiopulmonary resuscitation and admittance into an intensive care unit.
   b. Mechanical respiration when I cannot breathe by myself.
   c. Prolonged gastric tube or intravenous feeding when I am indefinitely unable to eat through my mouth.
   d. Antibiotic medication to treat or prevent infection.
   e. Other: ______________________________
2. I request to live my last days at home rather than a hospital, if my family agrees.
3. If any of my tissues or organs are healthy and useful for other people I give permission for all such donation, or as specified *during my life*:
4. I do wish to have medication mercifully administered to me in order to stop suffering even though this may shorten remaining life.

Dated at ____________________ in the Province of Alberta, this ________________
day of ________________, 20________.

______________________________ ______________________________

WITNESS'S SIGNATURE **MAKER'S SIGNATURE**

FIGURE 48.1 Sample advance directive appointing an agent and stating instructions
(From the Alberta Health Ethics Network)

vidual's personal values. This inquiry highlights the person's value system and beliefs about health, well-being, choice, and dignity. Identification of the person's values will enable the nurse to approach the client's hospital experience in a more holistic manner.

ARTIFICIAL NUTRITION AND HYDRATION Artificial nutrition and hydration (ANH) (non-oral means of administering nutrition to a patient) are common but controversial issues at the end of life. Although regularly used in certain populations, strong scientific evidence regarding the benefits of these therapies is lacking, making care decisions even more complex. Provision of food and fluids is a fundamental caregiving activity; issues arise when patients with progressive, life-limiting illness refuse or cannot take oral nourishment and fluids. Deciding whether or not to initiate ANH is an important conversation to have with patients and their families.

Artificial nutrition is an emotionally charged issue for many caregivers. Maintaining nutrition is a natural life-sustaining measure and a common part of the nursing role. Families often believe that their loved ones will suffer without nutrition. It is important for nurses and other health-care professionals to help family members understand that loss of appetite is an integral part of the dying process. Studies of terminally ill cognitively intact patients with anorexia have shown that they do not suffer hunger and that symptoms of thirst can be relieved with good oral hygiene, artificial saliva, and sips of water (Zerwekh, 1997).

Current literature suggests fluids should not be routinely administered to dying individuals or automatically withheld from them, but rather given based on the goals of care and a careful assessment of the client's comfort. A position statement by the CNA (2001) on futility stresses the importance of the health-care team working together to determine whether food and fluid are beneficial or harmful to a client. The following questions may help health-care professionals in thinking about the goals of care (Bennett Jacobs & Taylor, 2005; Ganzini, 2006): Will the client's well-being be enhanced by artificial nutrition? Are there symptoms that could be relieved or aggravated? Could hydration enhance the client's mental status or level of consciousness? Will it temporarily prolong the client's life? Is that what the client and family want? When food and hydration are administered for a prolonged period to a client who is not expected to improve, some nurses will view this care as extraordinary or heroic, whereas others will see it as humane. It is important to stress to families that dying individuals who are not receiving artificial nutrition or hydration will still be provided with adequate care.

EUTHANASIA The act of **euthanasia** can mean different things to different people. The word *euthanasia* comes from Greek words meaning "good death." The term is often used synonymously with the term **mercy killing**, a concept that has drawn much controversy over the years. Euthanasia has two forms: *active* and *passive*. These terms are meant to convey the difference between committing an act that causes death and omitting to take a life-sustaining act, allowing death to ensue.

The issue is an ethical one that remains unsettled. It revolves around two fundamental beliefs: the right of individuals to decide his or her own time and means of dying, and the equally strong argument that all measures must be tried before death is accepted. Often, it becomes a matter of to treat or not to treat.

A legal distinction, however, is made between acting and omitting to act. An action deliberately causing the death of another person is homicide; omitting treatment when it is futile or refused is not. The withholding or withdrawing of treatments and the provision of compassionate palliative care, even when life is shortened, is considered to be good and ethical medical practice (Lowy, Sawyer, & Williams, 1993). A discussion between the physician and family members to determine when treatment should be stopped or withdrawn is ethical and common practice. Patients and family members may request that a dying individual not be subjected to resuscitative measures in the event of death, in which case the physician should write "do not resuscitate (DNR) order" in the patient's chart.

Individuals who argue against euthanasia base their reasoning on the principle of the sanctity of life and on the traditional rules and laws prohibiting the taking of life except in situations of self-defence or war. Many are also concerned about the potential for abuse if euthanasia were to become legal. They see a law like this slipping (the slippery slope argument) to extend to such others as the chronically ill, the very old, and the demented.

Those individuals who support euthanasia believe that in some situations, life is not worth living. They believe that competent individuals should be given the right to end their life when it is burdened with physical, emotional, and psychological pain that it is no longer possible to eliminate. These individuals believe that sanctity of life is not an absolute principle and can be overridden out of respect for individual autonomy and for the dignity of human life.

Assisted suicide means helping someone to commit suicide. It differs from euthanasia in that the person choosing to die takes the action that directly causes death, rather than having a second person commit the act. The Criminal Code of Canada (CCC) prohibits intentional killing, regardless of the person's consent or desires, and this also applies to assisted suicide. Section 14 of the CCC states that "no person is entitled to consent to have death inflicted on him." And, according to section 241 of the CCC, "Every one who . . . aids or abets a person to commit suicide, whether suicide ensues or not, is guilty of an indictable offence."

DO NOT RESUSCITATE ORDERS Cardiopulmonary resuscitation (CPR) has become a standard intervention because of its potential benefits if implemented immediately. This standard, coupled with the lack of advance care planning, creates the routine use of CPR (Gilbert, Counsell, & Guin, 2001; Golin, Wegner, & Liu, 2000). The question of whether this intervention should be used for all patients at all times has been the topic of several research studies. The results indicate that CPR can do harm to certain patients (those with advanced age and the presence of comorbidities), bringing about a lesser quality of life (Brindley, Markland, Mayers, & Kutsogiannis, 2002; Robinson, 2002). Inappropriate use of CPR and inappropriate prolongation of life in general are among the most troubling issues for registered nurses (Storch, 2006). Nurses and others involved in resuscitative interventions with little perceived benefit may experience moral distress. Nurses and physicians in direct care roles often perform CPR on patients who might not have had the opportunity to articulate a preference for or against it. Alternatively, many times, the patient's age, history, and even personal directives are ignored to accommodate our "never give up attitude" (Lazaruk, 2006, p. 22).

When a client or surrogate has requested no CPR in the event of a respiratory or cardiac arrest, or if no medical benefit is apparent, a do not resuscitate (DNR) order can be written. Health-care institutions commonly have a policy for obtaining a DNR order. Approaching treatment decisions in palliative care, especially DNR orders, can be particularly troublesome for the team if advance directives are not available or are not followed. An ethical approach includes clarifying patient and family goals of care, balancing the potential burden and benefit of the proposed treatment, and, to some extent, considering the availability of resources for providing treatment. Health-care professionals need to consider the following question in their deliberations: Should resuscitation be presented as a treatment option when it almost certainly will not be successful? Advance care planning provides an opportunity for thoughtful consideration of CPR as an intervention.

The CNA (1995) issued a joint policy statement to provide guidance for developing policies on the appropriate use of CPR. The following principles are integral to the development of the CPR policy (pp. 2–3):

1. *Good health care requires open communication, discussion and sensitivity to cultural and religious differences among caregivers, potential recipients of care, their family members and significant others.*

2. *A person must be given sufficient information about the benefits, risks and likely outcomes of all treatment options to enable him or her to make informed decisions.*

3. *A competent person has the right to refuse, or withdraw consent to, any clinically indicated treatment, including life-saving or life-sustaining treatment. Competence can be difficult to assess because it is not always a constant state. A person may be competent to make decisions regarding some aspects of life but not others; as well, competence can be intermittent—a person may be lucid and oriented at certain times of the day and not at others. The legal definition and assessment of competence are governed by the provinces or territories. Facilities should be aware of the laws (e.g., capacity to consent and age of consent) regarding the assessment and documentation of incompetence.*

4. *When a person is incompetent, treatment decisions must be based on his or her wishes, if these are known. The person's decision may be found in an advance directive or may have been communicated to the physician, other members of the health care team or other relevant people. In some jurisdictions, legislation specifically addresses the issue of decision-making concerning medical treatment for incompetent people; the legislative requirements should be followed.*

5. *When an incompetent person's wishes are not known, treatment decisions must be based on the person's best interests, taking into account:*

   i. the person's known values and preferences;
   ii. information received from those who are significant in the person's life and who could help in determining his or her best interests;
   iii. aspects of the person's culture and religion that would influence a treatment decision; and,
   iv. the person's diagnosis and prognosis.

   In some jurisdictions legislation specifies who should be recognized as designated decision-makers (proxies) for incompetent people; this legislation should be followed. The term "proxy" is used broadly to identify those people who make a treatment decision based on the decision a person would have made for himself or herself (substitute decision-maker), people who help in determining what decision would be in the person's best interest and people whose appropriateness to make treatment decisions for the person is recognized under provincial legislation.

6. *There is no obligation to offer a person futile or nonbeneficial treatment. Futile and nonbeneficial treatments are controversial concepts when applied to CPR. Policymakers should determine how these concepts should be interpreted in the policy on resuscitation, in light of the facility's mission, the values of the community it serves, and ethical and legal developments. For the purposes of this document and in the context of resuscitation, "futile" and "nonbeneficial" are understood as follows. In some situations a physician can determine that a treatment is "medically" futile or nonbeneficial because it offers no reasonable hope of recovery or improvement or because the person is permanently unable to experience any benefit. In other cases the utility and benefit of a treatment can only be determined with reference to the person's subjective judgement about his or her overall well-being. As a general rule a*

person should be involved in determining futility in his or her case. In exceptional circumstances such discussions may not be in the person's best interests. If the person is incompetent the principles for decision making for incompetent people should be applied.

Families often need time to absorb information presented, seek additional information, discuss it among themselves, and observe that the client is not recovering before being able to accept a DNR decision. In ethical nursing practice, as in all areas of practice, respect for persons is a prime concern. Health-care professionals should frequently revisit their policies regarding interventions, such as CPR, especially in the context of a changing societal environment that recognizes the autonomy of the individual and encourages increased public discussion and participation in these issues. Decisions about CPR as an appropriate treatment option should be clearly identified on a client's record to make sure that all the involved health-care professionals are aware of these decisions (CNA, 1995).

Death-Related Religious and Cultural Practices

Various cultural and religious traditions and practices associated with death, dying, and the grieving process help people cope with these experiences. Nurses are often present through the dying process and at the moment of death. Knowledge of the client's religious and cultural heritage helps nurses provide individualized care to clients and their families, even though they may not participate in the rituals associated with death.

Dying in solitude is generally unacceptable in most cultures. In many cultures, people prefer a peaceful death at home rather than in the hospital. Members of some ethnic groups may request that health-care professionals not reveal the prognosis to dying clients. They believe the person's last days should be free of worry and pain. People in other cultures prefer that a family member (preferably a male in some cultures) be told the diagnosis so that the client can be tactfully informed by a family member in gradual stages or not be told at all. Nurses also need to determine whom to call and when, as the impending death draws near.

Beliefs and attitudes about death, its cause, and the soul also vary among cultures. Unnatural deaths, or bad deaths, are sometimes distinguished from good deaths. The death of a person who has behaved well in life may be considered less threatening based on the belief that the person will be reincarnated into a good life.

Beliefs about preparation of the body, autopsy, organ donation, cremation, and prolonging life are closely allied to the person's religion. *Autopsy,* for example, may be prohibited, opposed, or discouraged by Eastern Orthodox religions, Muslims, Jehovah's Witnesses, and Orthodox Jews. Some religions prohibit the removal of body parts and dictate that all body parts be given appropriate burial. The practice of *organ donation* varies among faiths. *Cremation* is discouraged, opposed, or prohibited by the Mormon, Eastern Orthodox, Islamic, and Jewish Orthodox faiths. Hindus, in contrast, prefer cremation and cast the ashes in a holy river. *Prolongation of life* is generally encouraged; however, some religions, such as Christian Science, are unlikely to use medical means to prolong life, and the Jewish faith generally opposes prolonging life after irreversible brain damage. In hopeless illness, Buddhists may permit euthanasia.

Nurses also need to be knowledgeable about the client's death-related rituals, such as last rites and administration of Holy Communion, chanting at the bedside, and special procedures for washing, dressing, positioning, and shrouding the dead. For example, in some cultures family members of the same sex wash and prepare the body for burial and cremation. Muslims customarily turn the body toward Mecca. Nurses need to ask family members about their preference and verify who will carry out these activities. Burial clothes and other cultural or religious items are often important symbols for the funeral. For example, faithful Mormons are often dressed in their temple clothes. Some Aboriginals may be dressed in elaborate apparel and jewellery and wrapped in new blankets with money. The nurse must ensure that any ritual items present in the health-care agency be given to the family or to the funeral home.

Assessment during the Transition of Active Dying

The nurse gets to know the dying individual's and family's beliefs, desires, and needs in the journey of dying. Through continued assessment the nurse also collects a complete patient and family history, which includes physical, emotional, social, and spiritual dimensions. In this relationship, the nurse becomes aware of the living and dying transitions that the dying individual and family experience. Knowing the dying individual and family allows the nurse to respond in a way that best supports their state of awareness, beliefs, and values about the dying journey. A classic research study by Glaser and Strauss (1965) uncovered themes related to the "awareness" and patterns of communication of impending death that nurses might observe in their practice: closed awareness, suspected awareness, mutual pretence, and open awareness.

In **closed awareness**, dying individuals, and perhaps families, are unaware of impending death. They may not completely understand why their loved one is ill and believe that he or she will recover. Sometimes health-care professionals are faced with situations in which families' cultural beliefs affect the decision of communicating a diagnosis or prognosis to the dying individual. Although the intention is to protect the dying individual, moral difficulties result for nurses and other health-care professionals whose values are different. As well, families and patients do not have the opportunity to communicate openly and to freely express their feelings, share the burden of grief, and plan realistically for the future. Nurses in this situation may feel an ethical burden as they are not able to communicate frankly and can feel that they are not upholding their own moral values of truthfulness or dignity.

In **suspected awareness**, dying individuals do not remain unaware for long. A deteriorating state of health, changes in physical appearance, and altered behaviours of family members and health-care professionals lead to suspected awareness. The dying individual senses that the information given is guarded, as families and health-care professionals do not want to abandon hope that remission is still possible. Feeling as if their trust has been undermined, dying individuals choose not to voice what they are sensing, and thus, communication becomes even more difficult.

With **mutual pretence**, dying individuals, families, and health-care professionals know that the prognosis is terminal but do not talk about it and make an effort not to raise the subject. Sometimes, dying individuals refrain from discussing death to protect their families from distress. Dying individuals may also sense discomfort on the part of health-care professionals and therefore do not bring up the subject. Mutual pretence permits dying individuals a degree of privacy and dignity, but it also places a heavy burden on them as they then have no one in whom to confide thoughts and fears.

With **open awareness**, dying individuals, families, friends, and health-care professionals know about the impending death and feel comfortable discussing it, even though it is difficult. This awareness provides dying individuals with opportunities to finalize affairs and have active involvement in preparing for their transition to death. Not all individuals can engage in open awareness.

Some believe that dying individuals acquire knowledge of their condition even if they are not directly informed. Another perspective is that many dying individuals remain unaware of their condition until the end. Regardless of the individual and family perspectives, nurses must acknowledge and remain open to all values and beliefs related to the awareness of dying.

Nursing care and support for the dying individual and family includes making an accurate assessment of the physiological signs of approaching death. In addition to signs related to the individual's specific disease, certain other physical signs are indicative of impending death. The four main characteristic changes are loss of muscle tone, slowing of the circulation, changes in respirations, and sensory impairment. See Box 48.1 for indications of impending clinical death.

BOX 48.1 SIGNS OF IMPENDING CLINICAL DEATH

Nurses must be able to recognize the signs of impending clinical death:

LOSS OF MUSCLE TONE

- Relaxation of the facial muscles (e.g., the jaw may sag)
- Difficulty speaking
- Difficulty swallowing and gradual loss of the gag reflex
- Decreased activity of the gastrointestinal tract, with subsequent nausea, accumulation of flatus, abdominal distension, and retention of feces, especially if opioids or tranquilizers are being administered
- Possible urinary and rectal incontinence because of decreased sphincter control
- Diminished body movement

SLOWING OF THE CIRCULATION

- Diminished sensation
- Mottling and cyanosis of the extremities
- Cold skin, first in the feet and later in the hands, ears, and nose (the client, however, may feel warm because of elevated body temperature)
- Decelerated and weaker pulse
- Decreased blood pressure

CHANGES IN RESPIRATIONS

- Rapid, shallow, irregular, or abnormally slow respirations; Cheyne-Stokes respirations (periodic breathing); noisy breathing, referred to as the *death rattle,* caused by the collection of mucus in the throat; mouth breathing, which leads to dry oral mucous membranes

SENSORY IMPAIRMENT

- Blurred vision
- Impaired sense of taste and smell

Various consciousness levels occur just before death. Some individuals are alert, whereas others are drowsy, stuporous, or comatose. Hearing is thought to be the last sense that is lost. As death approaches, the nurse assists the family and other significant people to prepare themselves. Depending, in part, on knowledge of the dying individual's state of awareness, the nurse asks questions that help identify ways to provide support before and after death. In particular, the nurse needs to know what the family expects to happen when the person dies so accurate information can be given. See the Assessment: Interview box for sample interview questions. When the family members know what to expect, they are better able to support the dying person and others who are grieving. In addition, they may be able to make certain decisions about events surrounding the death, such as whether they will want to view the body after death.

ASSESSMENT: INTERVIEW

The Dying Individual

Ask the spouse, partner, or significant others the following questions:

- Have you ever been close to someone who was dying?
- What have you been told about what may happen when death occurs?
- Do you have questions about what may happen at the time of death?
- Do you have questions about how we are caring for [the person] during these last days?
- How do you think you would like to say goodbye?
- How are you taking care of yourself during these times?
- Who can you turn to for help at this time?
- Is there anyone you would like us to contact now or when death occurs?

Planning a Peaceful Death

Major desires of dying individuals are (1) maintaining physiological and psychological comfort, and (2) achieving a dignified and peaceful death, which includes maintaining personal control and accepting declining health status. When planning care with these individuals, the dying person's bill of rights can be a useful guide (see Box 48.2).

Examples of specific desired outcomes, although established in the planning phase, are provided in Table 48.4 later in this chapter (page 1533).

Examples of nursing interventions for the dying individual include the following:

- Helping individuals die with dignity
- Meeting physiological needs
- Providing spiritual support
- Supporting the family
- Providing postmortem care

Planning for Home Care

Dying clients have been cared for in the home by nurses since early in the development of the profession. In Canada, the development of palliative care programs began in hospitals. This trend continued late into the 1990s, with up to 80% of deaths occurring at home (Wilson et al., 2001). Recently, a shift toward community care and more home deaths has occurred for various reasons, including increasing costs in hospital care, changing environments in hospitals that do not meet the needs of all patients, the growing expertise of health-care providers, and advancing technology that allows even complex care to be given at home. Growing numbers of patients and families are advocating for increased community care, and society has begun to value care for the dying and to embrace the expansion of a palliative care philosophy as paramount to quality end-of-life care.

A major factor in determining whether a person will die in a health-care facility or at home is the availability of willing and able caregivers. If the dying person wants to be at home, and the family or others can provide care to maintain symptom control and meet other basic needs of the dying individual, the nurse should facilitate a referral to home care services. Home care nurses and other inter-

BOX 48.2 THE DYING PERSON'S BILL OF RIGHTS

I have the right to be treated as a living human being until I die.

I have the right to maintain a sense of hopefulness, however changing its focus may be.

I have the right to be cared for by those who can maintain a sense of hopefulness, however changing this might be.

I have the right to express my feelings and emotions about my approaching death in my own way.

I have the right to participate in decisions concerning my care.

I have the right to expect continuing medical and nursing attention even though "cure" goals must be changed to "comfort" goals.

I have the right not to die alone.

I have the right to be free from pain.

I have the right to have my questions answered honestly.

I have the right not to be deceived.

I have the right to have help from and for my family in accepting my death.

I have the right to die in peace and dignity.

I have the right to retain my individuality and not be judged for my decisions which may be contrary to beliefs of others.

I have the right to discuss and enlarge my religious and/or spiritual experiences, whatever these may mean to others.

I have the right to expect that the sanctity of the human body will be respected after death.

I have the right to be cared for by caring, sensitive, knowledgeable people who will attempt to understand my needs and will be able to gain some satisfaction in helping me face my death.

Source: "The Dying Person's Bill of Rights," by A. J. Barbus, 1975, *American Journal of Nursing, 75*, p. 99. © 1975, American Journal of Nursing Company. Reprinted with permission from the *American Journal of Nursing*.

disciplinary team members will then conduct a full assessment of the home and the care provider's skills.

The issue of transfer of funds from hospital to homes, however, is not adequately addressed in all areas of Canada. Most home care programs do not fund 24-hour care over the long term, expecting that family members will do most of the care. Unless families are able to privately fund home care, including the cost of medications, home medical equipment and supplies, transportation, and respite services, the probability of staying at home until death is not always a reality.

Home care providers are typically characterized as formal or informal caregivers. As mentioned, family and friends (informal caregivers) provide the majority of the care, especially for older adults with multiple comorbidities requiring care for many years. Formal caregivers consist of all disciplines, the majority being registered nurses and personal care attendants or licensed practical nurses. Registered nurses are considered to be the coordinators of care, providing skilled assessments in pain and symptom management and providing direction for other nurses and paraprofessionals. Nurses provide the client and family with bereavement care. The goal and related nursing responsibilities for dying individuals is to assist them to a peaceful death. More specific responsibilities are the following:

- To provide relief from loneliness, fear, and depression
- To maintain the client's sense of security, self-confidence, dignity, and self-worth
- To maintain hope
- To help the client accept losses
- To provide physical comfort

Not all clients can manage or choose to remain at home. Individuals facing death need help accepting that they will have to depend on others. Some dying individuals require only minimal care and can be cared for at home; others need continuous care and attention and require the services of a hospital and palliative care interdisciplinary team. Families and dying individuals need support and guidance, well in advance of death, to plan for the transition to death. They need to consider what might happen and how and where they would like to die.

Helping Individuals Die with Dignity

Perhaps one of the most interesting and applicable ways for nurses to think about dignity when caring for dying individuals comes from the writings of Arthur Frank (2004). Frank's discussion of dignity is relational and places emphasis on the local nature of dignity, which conceptualizes it as "an event happening between persons, rather than a fixed quality" (p. 207). This postmodern understanding of dignity as *relational* places the value of dignity as a human experience in a different light. It serves to remind us that "caring is not a unidirectional administration of a standardized treatment. Care that takes dignity seriously is a dialogue" (p. 207).

Frank (2004) reminds us that caring requires the caregiver to reflect on his or her own values of care. Dignity is sustained in nurses' acts of caring; dignity can be enacted in silence. Dignity is inherent in the context of the nurse–client relationship. Nurses can facilitate care that allows for dying individuals to retain some control by making their own choices about the location of care (e.g., hospital, home, or hospice), times of appointments with health-care professionals, activity schedule, use of health-care resources, and times of visits from relatives and friends.

Many dying individuals want to be able to manage the events preceding death so they can die peacefully. Nurses can facilitate dialogue that opens possibilities for individuals to find meaning and completeness and to determine their own physical, psychological, and social priorities. Dying individuals often strive for self-fulfillment more than for self-preservation, and they need to find meaning in dying while continuing to live. Part of the nurses' challenge is to help facilitate day-to-day comfort and care so that the individual's transition to death is peaceful.

Sometimes nurses have difficulty discussing death with clients who are dying. Although it is natural for people to be uncomfortable discussing death, steps can be taken to make such discussions easier for both the nurse and the client. Callanan (1994) proposes the following strategies:

- Identify personal feelings about death and how they can influence interactions with clients. Acknowledge personal fears about death, and discuss them with a friend or colleague.
- Focus on the client's needs. The client's fears and beliefs may be different from the nurse's. It is important that the nurse avoid imposing personal fears and beliefs on the client or family.
- Understand the client and how the client copes. Talk to the client or the family about how the client usually copes with stress. Clients will use their usual coping strategies for dealing with impending death. For example, if they are usually quiet and reflective, they will become quieter and more withdrawn when facing terminal illness.
- Establish a communication relationship that shows concern for and commitment to the client. Communication strategies that let the client know you are available to talk about death include the following:

    a. Describe what you see, for example, "You seem sad. Would you like to talk about what's happening to you?"
    b. Clarify your concern, for example, "I'd like to know better how you feel and how I can help you."
    c. Acknowledge the client's struggle, for example, "It must be difficult to feel so uncomfortable. I

care about you and would like to help you be more comfortable."
  d. Provide a caring touch. Holding the client's hand or offering a comforting massage can encourage the client to verbalize feelings.
- Determine what the client knows about the illness and prognosis.
- Respond with honesty and directness to the client's questions about death.
- Make time to be available to the client to provide support, listen, and respond.

HOSPICE PALLIATIVE CARE Hospice or palliative care has emerged as a specialized field only within the past 30 years (Billings, 1998). The **hospice care** model was developed to address the specific needs of the dying and their families, so neglected by the medical system of care (see Figure 48.2). The modern hospice movement started in England in 1967 through the work of Dame Cicely Saunders and colleagues at St. Christopher's Hospice in London. The hospice movement came to North America in the mid 1970s, when Dr. Florence Wald, a nursing pioneer, led an interdisciplinary team to create the first American hospice (Wald, 1999). Typically, hospice care is for those individuals with a life expectancy of 6 months or less.

In the United Kingdom, a hospice is the building in which dying persons are cared for. In the United States, the term refers to a specific model for delivering palliative care. The **palliative care** model evolved from the traditional hospice perspective to address quality-of-life concerns for those patients living for prolonged periods with a progressive debilitating disease.

Historically, the terms *hospice* and *palliative care* in Canada were used in a variety of ways. The term *hospice* included a philosophy of care, often community-based, volunteer-driven programs providing care in the home, in a long-term-care facility, or in a freestanding hospice (Brenneis & Brown, 2006). New terminology in Canada was proposed in 2002. The words *hospice* and *palliative care* were combined to recognize the convergence of hospice and palliative care into one movement. The national organization for palliative care, which at that time was called the Canadian Palliative Care Association, adjusted its name to include the term **hospice palliative care**, becoming the Canadian Hospice Palliative Care Association (CHPCA) (Brenneis & Brown, 2006). See the Nursing and Canadian Society box.

Regardless of location or type of program, hospice palliative care is based on the principles of providing care to improve the dying individual's quality of life, rather than aiming for cure (Figure 48.3). The care is patient and family centred, focusing on needs and concerns that are most important to them. A hallmark of hospice palliative care since Cicely Saunders founded the modern hospice movement has been the combination of scientific rigour and personal concern. At St. Christopher's Hospice, Saunders developed an education program for palliative care that embraced three broad areas: (1) the science and techniques of pain management and symptom control; (2) the knowledge of psychosocial, social, and spiritual aspects of dying and grieving; and (3) self-knowledge on the part of caregivers, especially related to personal beliefs about death and loss (Barnard, Towers, Boston, & Lambrinidou, 2000). Hospice palliative care is always provided by a multidisciplinary team of primarily physicians, nurses, social workers, and chaplains.

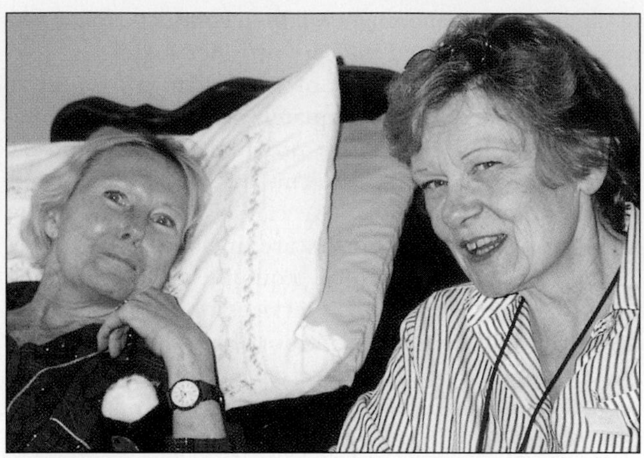

FIGURE 48.2 The patient and family are the "unit of care" in hospice palliative care.

MEETING THE PHYSIOLOGICAL NEEDS OF THE DYING INDIVIDUAL The physiological needs of people who are dying are related to a slowing of body processes and to homeostatic imbalances. Interventions include providing personal hygiene measures; controlling pain; relieving respiratory difficulties; assisting with movement, nutrition, hydration, and elimination; and providing measures related to sensory changes. See also Table 48.2.

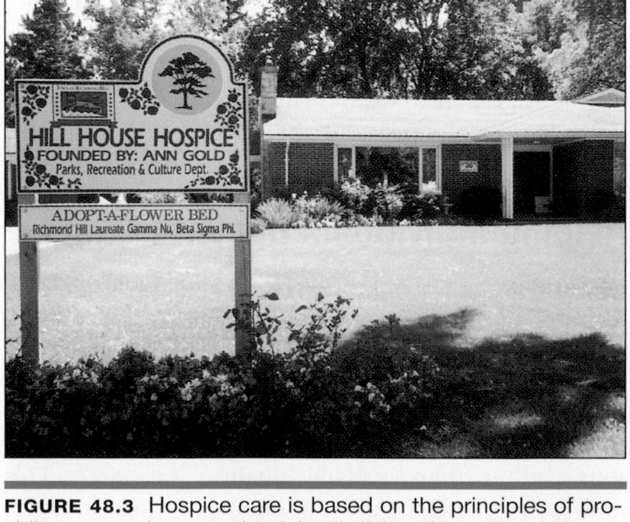

FIGURE 48.3 Hospice care is based on the principles of providing care to improve the dying individual's quality of life.

Nursing and Canadian Society

Fact	Implications for Nursing Practice
The Canadian Hospice Palliative Care Association (CHPCA) is the recognized national organization for leadership in palliative care. The mission of CHPCA is to promote palliative care awareness, education, and research, advocating at a national level for policy development, resource allocation, and support for caregivers.	Nurses need to be aware of the policy papers on nursing care of the dying that have been accepted by each professional association, in accordance with CHPCA standards.
Each province has a palliative care association that is linked to the CHPCA. The territories do not have their own associations yet.	Nurses interested in palliative care may want to consider membership in these associations.
The CNA board of directors has designated palliative care as a specialty, making it the twelfth discipline to gain that status. The first hospice palliative care nursing certification examination was offered in 2004.	In achieving hospice palliative care nursing certification in Canada, nurses share in the enhancement of hospice palliative care for all Canadians.

TABLE 48.2 Physiological Needs of Dying Persons

Problem	Nursing Interventions
Ineffective airway clearance	30° Fowler's position: conscious clients Lateral, throat suctioning: conscious clients Sims', 30° lateral, and lateral position: unconscious clients
Self-care deficit: bathing or hygiene	Frequent baths and linen changes, if diaphoretic Mouth care, as needed, for dry mouth
Impaired physical mobility	Assist client out of bed periodically, if client is able Regularly change bedridden client's position Support client's position with pillows, blanket rolls, or towels, as needed Elevate client's legs when sitting up to prevent pooling of blood
Imbalanced nutrition: less than body requirements	Antiemetics or small amount of alcoholic beverage to stimulate appetite Encourage liquid foods, as tolerated
Constipation	Dietary fibre, as tolerated Laxatives, as needed, to prevent constipation
Impaired urinary elimination	Skin care in response to incontinence of urine or feces Bedpan, urinal, or commode chair within easy reach Call light within reach for assistance onto bedpan or commode Absorbent pads placed under incontinent client; linen changed as often as needed Catheterization, if necessary Keep room as clean and odour free as possible
Disturbed sensory perception: visual, tactile	Clients prefer a well-lit room Hearing is not diminished; speak clearly and do not whisper Touch is diminished, but client will feel pressure of touch

SENSORY PERCEPTUAL NEEDS Changes in the level of consciousness may be the first symptom of dying, occurring over weeks or days. Changes may include **clouding of consciousness** or thought, drowsiness, **delirium**, **stupor** or unresponsiveness, **coma**, and, in some individuals, confusion or agitation. Consciousness is an integral aspect of being human; the ability to relate to others and the environment allows the individual an important sense of control. Even though individuals may have mentally accepted the fact that they are dying, the actual process of losing consciousness and the awareness of death may be a frightening experience. The fatigue and exhaustion of illness may prompt a wish of "falling asleep and not waking up." Others may struggle to continue to live and, thus, be very restless and unsettled until death. As the client's body slows down, the nurse must use the knowledge of normal physiological changes to prepare the client for death and lessen anxiety (see Table 48.3).

PAIN MANAGEMENT One of the greatest fears of dying individuals is that they will experience intense, unbearable pain. However, this fear is largely unfounded because the majority of patients with terminal illness can obtain pain relief. Nurses are critical members of the palliative care team, particularly when it comes to pain management (Paice & Fine, 2006). The prevalence of pain in the terminally ill varies by diagnosis and other factors. Approximately one-third of individuals actively receiving treatment for cancer and two-thirds of those with advanced malignant disease experience pain (Chang, Hwang, Feuerman, & Kasimis, 2000; Meuser et al., 2001; Morita, Ichiki, Tsunoda, Inoue, & Chihaa, 1998; Wells, 2000).

In studies of patients admitted to palliative care units, pain is often the dominant symptom, along with fatigue and dyspnea (Jenkins, Taube, Ken, Hanson, & Bruera, 1998; Ng & von Gunten, 1998). Pain control is essential because pain alters sleep, appetite, mobility, energy levels, and psychological functioning. Barriers to good pain relief are numerous and pervasive. Often,

TABLE 48.3 State of Consciousness in Dying Patients

A. Consciousness: To be fully conscious is to be aware of one's self and the surrounding environment. There are two aspects:

1. *Content.* The sum of mental processes, including the ability to discriminate among both the sensory inputs and the internal cognitive aspects.

2. *Arousal.* A state of wakefulness or alertness to external and internal processes.

B. Clouding of Consciousness: Defined as a reduced state of wakefulness or awareness.

1. *Mild Clouding.* For the terminal patient, fatigue and periods of drowsiness are not uncommon. After a period of rest, the patient remains fully conscious. Several other features may not be observed or appreciated by caregivers in the early part of this phase. These features include the following:

- Excitability and irritability, which alternate with drowsiness
- Startled by minor stimuli
- Easily distracted
- Misjudges sensory perception, especially visual
- Cannot think clearly or quickly

These features may be intermittent and mistaken for anxiety.

2. *Advanced or subacute confusional state.* In this phase, the intensity and persistence of the symptoms is increased. The patient is "confused."

- Stimuli are more consistently misinterpreted.
- Attention span is shortened.
- The patient is bewildered and has difficulty following commands.
- There is some disorientation to time and sometimes to place and person.
- Memory is faulty.
- Drowsiness is often prominent (may alternate with nighttime agitation).

3. *Delirium.* The next "lower" level of consciousness is delirium. Although defined and used here in the classical sense, the term is not consistently used in all practice settings where care of the dying is provided. The word has a connotation of being "crazy" and is inappropriate in working with dying patients. The next phases are referred to as lower levels of consciousness.

Symptoms at this level include the following:

- Intensified disorientation
- Misinterpretation of stimuli; often visual hallucinations
- Lucid periods that often alternate with delirium
- Delusions
- Loud, talkative, offensive, suspicious, or agitated behaviour

4. *Stupor.* Stupor is defined as a state in which the patient is unresponsive but briefly arousable, only during vigorous and repeated stimuli, and then immediately drifts back to unresponsiveness.

In this stage, the patient may moan or be briefly restless when being turned or when given skin care. Staff need to ascertain whether this "moaning" is due to insufficient pain control or simply being partially roused from a deeper level.

This is not a "withdrawn" state in which the patient, lying in a fetal position, is conscious but does not respond to people. In this type of case, the patient will initially appear to be in a stupor but is, in fact, conscious and just not responding to family or caregivers. Management (and prognosis) of this state is very different from that for the truly stuporous patient.

5. *Coma.* This is the true comatose state, defined as complete unarousable unresponsiveness or "the absence of any psychologically understandable response to external stimuli or inner need."

This is exemplified in a patient who is breathing on his own but is totally unarousable by any physical stimulus, such as pinching, heat or cold, and yelling or sudden noise. There is no intake by the patient.

Source: *Hospice Resource Manual. Volume 1: Medical Care of the Dying,* 3rd ed., by the Victoria Hospice Society, 1998, Victoria, BC: Author.

because of lack of education, misbeliefs, and attitudinal issues, these barriers prevent many individuals from receiving adequate pain relief (Parageon & Hailey, 1999).

Most nurses are educated in the observation and assessment of acute pain, which is very different from chronic pain. The dramatic signs and symptoms of acute pain warrant fast and immediate action. Outward signs of chronic pain are not as obvious and, therefore, may go untreated. Lack of expression does not mean lack of pain. Comprehensive assessment of pain is imperative. This must be conducted initially, regularly throughout treatment, and during any changes in the patient's experience of pain. Performing an individualized pain assessment is the first step to ensuring baseline data and continued treatment resulting in an improved quality of life for the dying individual.

Treatment of pain in older adults generally follows the same guidelines as in younger adults, with opioid therapy remaining the cornerstone of pain management. There is conflicting evidence on changes that occur in the nociceptive system with aging (Helme, Meliala, & Gibson, 2004). Even if nociceptive perception is decreased in older adults, diseases likely to cause chronic pain have a higher prevalence in older adults. These diseases include arthritis, polymyalgia rheumatica, atherosclerotic disease, zoster (shingles), and peripheral neuropathy. Pain assessment in older adults is often complicated by the existence of cognitive impairment. The cognitively impaired patient is often unable to express pain adequately or request analgesics; this increases the risk of undertreatment. The fear of precipitating or exacerbating a delirious episode by employing opioids in the management of pain may also lead to inadequate pain management.

Once the individual's pain has been assessed, an analgesic medication to control the pain is selected (opioid or non-opioid analgesic). The World Health Organization (1996) recommends the use of an analgesic ladder to assist with analgesic selection. With chronic pain, analgesics are generally most effective if administered regularly (or around the clock) rather than on an as-needed basis. Frequently, when patients receive a regular dose of medication, pain can break through and require additional doses to keep it under control. Opioid or controlled substances are used for managing moderate to severe pain. For primarily historical reasons, morphine is the strong opioid of choice. Non-opioid medications are commonly used to ease pain, lower fever, and manage mild to moderate pain.

Medications for pain management are not limited to analgesics; they can include corticosteroids, antidepressants, anticonvulsants, and anxiolytics, determined by the type of pain assessed. Other than medications for the control of pain, the nurse can offer therapeutic comfort measures, such as helping the patient relax, providing music, giving warm and soothing baths or a massage, and providing distraction. The presence of the nurse to ensure support, conversation, and genuine concern is most important and assists in the process of reducing pain and promoting comfort.

BREATHING NEEDS **Dyspnea** (shortness of breath) is an uncomfortable awareness of breathing. Like pain, dyspnea is a subjective sensation involving both the perception of breathlessness and the individual's reaction to it. The prevalence of dyspnea varies according to the disease. Approximately 50% of the general outpatient cancer population experiences some breathlessness, with this number rising to 55% to 70% in the terminal phase of the disease (Dudgeon, Kristjanson, Sloan, & Lertzman, 2001; Fainsinger, MacEachern, Hanson, Miller, & Bruera, 1991). In older adults, shortness of breath can be a symptom associated with chronic disease, such as emphysema and heart failure, or acute bronchopulmonary pneumonia.

Dyspnea, like pain, is multidimensional in nature, with physical symptoms and affective components, which are shaped by an individual's past experience with dyspnea (Dudgeon, 2006). Dyspnea, like pain, is not always evident to the observer. The nurse should inquire specifically about shortness of breath. Occasionally, dying individuals have physical signs of tachypnea and appear to be in distress; however, they may not feel dyspneic or distressed. The opposite can also occur, with individuals who are not tachypneic or in apparent respiratory distress describing feeling very short of breath. The extent of breathlessness experienced by a patient may or may not be related to the oxygen saturation level. Therefore, the patient's own assessment of the level of dyspnea may be a more reliable indicator than the oxygen saturation level. Dyspnea is, thus, a symptom that needs to be reported by the dying individual. A complete clinical assessment of dyspnea includes symptom history, including its temporal onset (acute or chronic), whether it is affected by positioning, its qualities, its associated symptoms, its precipitating and relieving events and activities, and its responses to medications. A past history of smoking, underlying lung or cardiac disease, concurrent medical condition, allergies, and details of previous medications or treatment should be elicited (Dudgeon, 2006).

The nurse provides many comfort measures to help relieve, decrease the perception of, and comfort the experience of dyspnea, including (1) administering medications, such as opioids, bronchodilators, and diuretics; (2) creating a therapeutic environment in which the individual engages in distraction therapy and relaxation exercises, is allowed to rest, or is allowed to be with family; (3) assisting the individual to a position that makes breathing easier (usually a high sitting position is best) and offering a fan to reduce the perception of breathlessness; (4) offering fluids and using a humidifier to loosen mucus so that coughing is easier; and (5) administering oxygen therapy by mask or nasal cannula. If the client is hypoxic, maintain oxygen saturation around 88% to 90%. The nurse has to be cautious in offering oxygen to a patient with chronic obstructive pulmonary disease (COPD); in these individuals, oxygen saturation should be kept around 90% or as ordered by the physician (Pereira & Bruera, 2001). Oxygen therapy relieves symptoms, improves exercise tolerance, and is the only therapy proven to prolong life in patients with COPD. It is important that the nurse offer these interventions early in the experience of dyspnea to reduce anxiety and improve quality of life.

The importance of teaching the dying individual and family cannot be overlooked. Strategies to relieve the acute experience of dyspnea include (1) using positioning and structured relaxation techniques, (2) knowing the signs and symptoms of an impending exacerbation, (3) using techniques to conserve energy and prioritize activities, and (4) understanding ways to maximize the effectiveness of medications, such as by using a spacer with inhaled drugs and taking an additional dose of the medications before activity, as ordered.

ACKNOWLEDGING AND STRENGTHENING SPIRITUALITY

Spirituality is an inherent, integrating, and, often, extremely valued dimension of the journey of dying for individuals and their families. Spirituality is immensely personal, abstract, and illusive in nature (Sinclair, Raffin, Pereria, & Guebert, 2006). Spiritual distress or *soul pain* is a common experience in those who are dying and, sometimes, an experience that is not addressed or understood. The experiences are complex, varied, and individual, and if left unaddressed, they may stifle the opportunity for growth, heighten the loss of a sense of meaning and purpose, and contribute to poorly controlled symptoms (Raffin, 2002).

The relationship between spirituality and religion is important for the nurse to understand, as each client and family will embrace a unique interconnection. A common understanding of the relationship presents spirituality as the overarching umbrella, with religion being only one of the many forms of spiritual expression. A review of the literature from many disciplines discusses religion as being correlated with an organized faith system, beliefs, worship, religious rituals, and relationship with a divine being (Sinclair, Pereira, & Raffin, 2006). Often, the experience of suffering prompts people, whether or not they see themselves as religious, to ask deeply spiritual questions and turn to God or a spiritual guide for solace. Even in the case of those who are avowedly religious, suffering can lead to questioning of fundamental beliefs (Anderson, 1989). To appreciate individual responses to suffering, it is imperative that the nurse attempt to understand the religious and spiritual views of the sufferer.

Spirituality delves into the nature of humanity and the deep mysteries of life (Sinclair, Raffin, et al., 2006). Nurses caring for dying individuals need to embrace values, meaning, and purpose; turn inward to the human traits of honesty, love, caring, wisdom, and compassion; help others to search for a higher authority, guiding spirit, or transcendence that is mystical; and help create healing of body, mind, and spirit that may or may not involve organized religion (Raffin, 2002). Nurses, in helping others find their expression of spirituality, need to allow for an open interpretation of what the individual considers to be divine or a transcendent Other.

Nurses have a responsibility not to impose their own religious or spiritual beliefs on a client but to respond to the client in relation to the client's own background and needs. Openness and honesty are most important in helping the client articulate needs and in developing a sense of caring and trust.

Specific interventions may include facilitating expressions of feeling, prayer, meditation, reading, and discussion with appropriate clergy or a spiritual adviser. It is important for nurses to establish an effective interdisciplinary relationship with other health-care professionals for quality patient and family care. Spirituality is inherently relational and shapes the care provided by palliative care professionals. Palliative care can also serve as a catalyst for interdisciplinary team members' own spiritual journeys (Sinclair, Raffin, et al., 2006). For a further discussion of spiritual issues, see Chapter 46. Death-related beliefs and practices of selected groups are discussed earlier in this chapter.

Evaluating the Process of Care

To evaluate the achievement of client goals, the nurse collects data in accordance with the desired outcomes established in the planning phase. Evaluation activities may include the following:

- Listening to the client's reports of feeling in control of the environment surrounding death, such as control over pain relief, visitation of family and support people, or treatment plans
- Observing the client's relationship with significant others
- Listening to the client's thoughts and feelings related to hopelessness or powerlessness

Finally, examples of goals and desired outcomes in fostering a peaceful death are shown in Table 48.4.

Caring for the Family

At no time is the family more important than during the times of death and dying. Nurses have an obligation not only to include the family in the care of the client but also to honour their wisdom, their beliefs, their wishes, and their needs. In this act of honouring, it is important to meet families at the point of their needs, rather than have set and unbending expectations of how family members will react to and involve themselves during the profound and difficult experience of watching a loved one die.

TABLE 48.4 Goals in Fostering a Peaceful Death

Goal	Examples of Desired Outcomes
Maintain personal control over present situation	Identifies areas of personal control
	Participates in self-care activities in accordance with health status
	Makes choices related to care and treatment
	Expresses sense of control over the present situation
Maintain comfort	Maintains physiological comfort
	Maintains psychological comfort
	Skin and oral tissues hydrated
	Absence of constipation or urinary retention
	Absence of restlessness
Accept declining health status	Shares values and personal meaning of life
	Verbalizes acceptance of situation
	Accepts limitations and seeks help, as needed

The most important thing a nurse can do to care for family members is to acknowledge them and include them. If the nurse shifts her or his thinking from considering the dying individual as the client to accepting the entire family as the client, then care becomes focused on the very significant event that is happening not just to the person but also to the entire family system.

Acknowledging family members includes consulting the family in terms of care of client and honouring their knowledge of the dying individual. It involves a collaborative evolution of ways in which the family needs to be involved and ways in which they prefer the nurse to assume care. For example, some family members want to be involved in physical care, whereas other family members are more comfortable with the nurse assuming these caring practices. It is important, in asking the family members' preferences, not to imply that the nurse has an expectation that they assume these acts, but rather that the nurse respects the family members' level of comfort. One way to approach this delicate establishment of roles and involvement would be to say to the family, "Sometimes family members like to be involved in the physical care of their ill members, and others prefer the nurse to assume these things. What would be most comfortable for you in this area?" Family members may want other kinds of involvement, rather than physical care, but be unsure of how to offer this. The nurse can help guide family members in knowing that it may be soothing to dying individuals to speak to them, read to them, hold their hands, or simply be present.

A part of what a nurse offers a family is a caring and compassionate presence. *Compassion* is defined as "suffering with." Though the nurse is not suffering as the family is, the nurse has in some ways entered the world of the family's suffering. "In entering the world of the one who is suffering, we do have to open space to where we listen to the pain, where we see, touch, and feel the pain" (Moules, 1999, p. 255). Nurses create a context in which family members feel as though they can be open about their pain, suffering, and grief. Nurses can offer information about the process of what is occurring and thereby walk alongside the family in understanding this experience (Raffin Bouchal, 2007).

When the individual dies, family members should be invited to spend time with the body (if they so desire) as this important ritual can serve as a significant event in making room for grief and grieving. Some people ask for mementos, such as locks of hair or other bodily reminders. Children should not be discouraged from being involved in this important ritual of viewing the body, and, at times, nurses can offer encouragement or even permission to families that it is appropriate to include children. Family members may have specific desires to participate in some care of the body, as in the case of a mother who asked to bathe her child one last time and dress him in special clothes. The nurse, in this instance, helped prepare clean towels and a basin for the mother, showing sensitivity in commenting that the water needed to be warmer, and then returning with warm water. The mother later reported that this simple act of kindness was of great comfort to her. In a health-care system that is often pushed for beds, the nurse may, at times, need to act as an advocate for families to ensure that they have all the time they need to spend with the body to begin saying goodbye to the physical presence of this person in their lives.

Postmortem Care

Rigor mortis is the stiffening of the body that occurs about 2 to 4 hours after death. It results from a lack of adenosine triphosphate (ATP), which is not synthesized because of a lack of glycogen in the body. ATP is necessary for muscle fibre relaxation. Its lack causes the muscles to contract, which, in turn, immobilizes the joints. Rigor mortis starts in the involuntary muscles (heart, bladder, and so on), then progresses to the head, neck, and trunk, and finally reaches the extremities.

Because the deceased person's family often wants to view the body and because it is important that the deceased appear natural and comfortable, nurses need to position the body, place dentures in the mouth, and close the eyes and mouth *before* rigor mortis sets in. Rigor mortis usually leaves the body about 96 hours after death.

Algor mortis is the gradual decrease of the body's temperature after death. When blood circulation terminates and the hypothalamus ceases to function, body temperature falls about 1°C per hour until it reaches room temperature. Simultaneously, the skin loses its elasticity and can easily be broken when removing dressings and adhesive tape.

After blood circulation has ceased, the red blood cells break down, releasing hemoglobin, which discolours the surrounding tissues. This discolouration, referred to as **livor mortis**, appears in the lowermost or dependent areas of the body.

Nursing personnel may be responsible for care of a body after death. Postmortem care should be carried out according to the policy of the hospital or agency. Because care of the body may be influenced by religious beliefs, the nurse should check the client's religion and make every attempt to comply. If the deceased's family or friends want to view the body, it is important to make the environment as clean and pleasant as possible and to make the body appear natural and comfortable. All equipment, soiled linen, and supplies should be removed from the bedside. Some agencies require that all tubes in the body remain in place; in other agencies, tubes may be cut to within 2.5 cm of the skin and taped in place; in others, all tubes are removed. Legal issues surrounding the death (e.g., coroner's case) may necessitate that all tubes remain in place.

Normally, the body is placed in a supine position with the arms either at the sides, palms down, or across the abdomen. One pillow is placed under the head and shoulders to prevent blood from discolouring the face by settling in it. The eyelids are closed and held in place for a few seconds so they remain closed. Dentures are usually inserted to help give the face a natural appearance. The mouth is then closed.

Soiled areas of the body are washed; however, a complete bath is not necessary because the body will be washed by the **mortician** (also referred to as an *undertaker*), a person trained in care of the dead. Absorbent pads are placed under the buttocks to take up any feces and urine released because of relaxation of the sphincter muscles. A clean gown is placed on the client, and the hair is brushed and combed. The top bed linens are adjusted neatly to cover the client to the shoulders. Soft lighting and chairs are provided for the family.

In the hospital, after the body has been viewed by the family, additional identification tags are applied. The body is wrapped in a **shroud**, a large piece of plastic or cotton material used to enclose a body after death. Identification is then applied to the outside of the shroud. The body is taken to the morgue if arrangements have not been made to have a mortician pick it up from the client's room.

Case Study 48

Jacob Frank, a 40-year-old father of two, lives in a small town in rural Alberta. Jacob, who has advanced prostrate cancer, has decided not to pursue further active chemotherapy. Jacob shares with the palliative home care nurse that his father died when he was only 8 years old. He recalls not being told that his father was very ill and that he was not permitted to attend the funeral service.

Critical Thinking Questions

1. How should the nurse respond to this information? In her conversation with Jacob, what should she explore further?
2. How can the nurse help Jacob clarify his beliefs and values about living and dying now that he is dealing with his own terminal illness?
3. What therapeutic interventions would be important for the nurse to explore with Jacob's family?

After working through these questions, go to the MyNursingLab at **http://www.mynursinglab.com** to check your answers.

KEY TERMS

loss
actual loss
perceived loss
anticipatory loss
grief
advance directives
living will
proxy directive
euthanasia
mercy killing
closed awareness
suspected awareness
mutual pretence
open awareness
hospice care
palliative care
hospice palliative care
clouding of consciousness
delirium
stupor
coma

dyspnea
rigor mortis
algor mortis
livor mortis
mortician
shroud

CHAPTER HIGHLIGHTS

- Nurses help clients deal with all kinds of losses, including loss of body image, loss of a loved one, loss of a sense of well-being, and loss of a job.
- Loss, especially loss of a loved one or a valued body part, can be viewed as either a situational or a developmental loss and as either an actual or a perceived loss (both of which can be anticipatory).
- Grieving is a normal, subjective emotional response to loss; it is essential for mental and physical and spiritual health. Grieving allows the bereaved person to cope with loss gradually and to accept it as part of reality.
- Knowledge of different stages or phases of grieving and factors that influence the loss reaction can help the nurse understand the responses and needs of clients, but recent research studies suggest that grief is an experience that is ongoing and changes over time, and involves a continuing relationship with the deceased.
- How an individual deals with loss is closely related to the individual's stage of development, personal resources, and social support system.
- Caring for the dying and the bereaved is one of the nurse's most complex and challenging responsibilities.
- Nurses' beliefs, values, and attitudes about death and dying directly affect their ability to provide care.
- Nurses must consider the entire family as requiring care in situations involving loss, especially death.
- Nurses must be knowledgeable about their responsibilities in regard to legal issues surrounding death: advance directives, euthanasia, and do not resuscitate orders.
- Dying clients require open communication, physical help, and emotional and spiritual support to ensure a peaceful and dignified death. They need to maintain a sense of control in managing the events preceding death.

ASSESS YOUR LEARNING

1. The hospice palliative care nurse educator is presenting a session to student nurses about the beliefs, attitudes, and practices essential to hospice palliative care. Which of the following best describes these practices?

a. Palliative care is best provided by an interdisciplinary team working collaboratively with the person and family to address physical, psychological, social, and spiritual concerns.

b. Palliative care is best provided by an interdisciplinary team working collaboratively with the person to address physical, emotional, and practical concerns.

c. Palliative care is best provided by the nurse and physician working with the person and family to address physical, psychosocial, and spiritual concerns related to dying.

d. Palliative care is best provided by an interdisciplinary team in a specialized setting working with the person and family to address identified social and emotional needs.

2. Which of the following is the best statement about DNR orders in advanced terminal illness?

a. Do not resuscitate orders are seldom appropriate. The principle of nursing is that all life is valuable and should be preserved at all costs.

b. When the disease progresses to the point that the heart stops beating or the person stops breathing, efforts to resuscitate will always fail and are an inappropriate use of resources.

c. Palliative care units do not have the capabilities to provide advanced life support. Therefore, people need to agree to a DNR on admission to the palliative care unit.

d. The goal of palliative care is to alleviate suffering and enhance quality of life. Resuscitation may prolong suffering and impede a peaceful death.

3. What is the best strategy the hospice nurse can use to support a person and family in making decisions and coping with advanced illness and the dying experience?

a. Assist the family to begin detaching from the dying person to help with the grieving process, allowing the team to provide appropriate care.

b. Facilitate the expression and understanding of the emotions of both the dying person and the family, allowing the person or family as much control as possible.

c. Facilitate discussions with the family about the dying person's roles within the family so that the family can make decisions about the dying experience.

d. Assess the person's or family's communication style and teach them the best communication strategies.

4. Which of the following is defined as the reaction to the loss of a loved person?
   a. Grief
   b. Mourning
   c. Bereavement
   d. Anticipatory grief

5. The hospice palliative care nurse has been following a client who is in bereavement. Which of the signs and symptoms might suggest grief that needs to be medically assessed?
   a. Crying at any time of the day without warning
   b. Continuing to experience sadness, loss, and depression not relieved over time or offset by periods of pleasure and joy
   c. Feeling pain and loss that reoccur with various memories and significant dates
   d. Experiencing grief that interrupts daily life activities and at certain times causes the bereaved person to withdraw

6. Which of the following is a characteristic of an advance directive?
   a. Writing one should occur only when the client is facing a life-threatening situation.
   b. Writing one involves exploring the client's goals and values if he or she should face a life-threatening event.
   c. Writing one typically does not involve family members.
   d. After one is written, it is signed by the client and not updated.

7. Which of the following is an experience of suffering at the end of life?
   a. It is often linked to an individual's search for meaning.
   b. It is alleviated with good symptom control.
   c. It is always understood when the sufferer searches for religious beliefs.
   d. It can always be alleviated by the nurse.

8. Dyspnea is defined as which of the following?
   a. A subjective sensation that appears only in certain diseases, such as COPD
   b. The medical term for hyperinflation of the chest
   c. A state that is always related to the patient's oxygen saturation level
   d. A subjective sensation involving both the individual's perception of breathlessness and his or her reaction to it

9. Which of the following is the most true statement about chronic pain at the end of life?
   a. It can be managed like acute pain, with opioid analgesics given as needed.
   b. Analgesics are most effective if administered regularly (around the clock), with breakthrough medication if needed.
   c. Once pain is stabilized, the routine of how analgesics are administered should not be altered.
   d. Chronic pain usually is treated with one type of medication that works best for the patient.

10. Mr. Hume, 64 years old, is a retired university professor. He has insulin-dependent diabetes and has required hemodialysis three times per week for the past year [for renal failure]. He has been admitted for an exacerbation of his condition. After working with his nephrologist and social worker, Mr. Hume decides he no longer wishes to continue with dialysis and is ready to die. What is the most appropriate action for the nurse to take?
    a. Tell Mr. Hume that this must have been a difficult decision and that she will continue to care for him.
    b. Notify Mr. Hume's son that his father has decided to discontinue dialysis.
    c. Try to convince Mr. Hume to continue with dialysis for another week.
    d. Share with Mr. Hume that her own father made the same choice a few years ago so she understands his decision.

After working through these questions, go to the MyNursingLab at ***http://www.mynursinglab.com*** *to check your answers and see explanations.*

SUGGESTED READINGS

Canadian Nurses Association, Canadian Medical Association, Canadian Health Care Association, Catholic Health Association of Canada, & Canadian Bar Association. (1995). *Joint statement on resuscitative interventions.* Ottawa: Authors; Canadian Nurses Association. (1998). *Advance directives: The nurse's role.* Ottawa: CNA; and Canadian Healthcare Association, Canadian Medical Association, Canadian Nurses Association, & Catholic Health Association of Canada. (2008). *Cardiopulmonary resuscitation.* Retrieved July 10, 2008, from http://www.cna-aiic.ca/CNA/practice/standards/cpr/default_e.aspx

The Canadian Nurses Association (CNA), as part of its mandate to address ethical issues affecting the practice of registered nurses, has prepared joint statements in collaboration with other national health-related organizations. In considering the range of issues related to end-of-life treatment, the CNA recommends that policy development be guided by this *Joint Statement on Resuscitative Interventions*

(1998) and by the *Joint Statement on Advance Directives* (1994). In 2008, the pamphlet on CPR was added to the CNA's standards and best practices' section of its website.

Johns, J. L. (1996). Advance directives and opportunities for nurses. *Image: Journal of Nursing Scholarship, 29,* 149–153.

The author reviewed the literature describing the role nurses have taken in the processes of advance directives. Both positive and negative outcomes of the process are described. Positive outcomes include increased discussions with clients regarding end-of-life decisions and greater ability to comply with clients' preferences. Negative outcomes involve the possible misinterpretation of advance directives as indicating that less care should be provided to the client who elects do not resuscitate status. Johns found few research studies on the effectiveness of advance directives and proposes a variety of potentially fruitful research questions.

Kuhl, D. (2002). *What dying people want: Practical wisdom for the end of life.* Toronto: Doubleday.

This book focuses on guidance, solace, and helpful strategies for people who are terminally ill and their families and caregivers. What dying people want includes ways to understand a doctor–patient relationship, guidance on how to hold a family meeting, an introduction to the process of life review, and direction in listening and in speaking your truth.

Northcott, H., & Wilson, D. (2008). *Dying and death in Canada* (2nd ed.). Aurora, ON: Garamond Press.

This book focuses on Canada and Canadian work in the area of dying and death. The book is written for students who want to learn about dying and death, for practitioners who work with the dying, and for the dying and bereaved themselves as well as the general public. The book explores the causes of deaths in Canada both historically and at present. It also examines the societal and cultural responses to death and dying. Most importantly, the book includes personal points of view of the dying and the bereaved.

WEBLINKS

Caregiver Network Inc.

http://www.caregiver.on.ca/content_main.html

Caregiver Network Inc. (CNI), the first of its kind in Canada, is a resource centre created to help caregivers of older adults and people who are ill. The goal of the network is to make caregivers' lives easier by providing information on the internet and in a newsletter (see CNI Services); education through the 13-part TV/video series "Caregiving with June Callwood"; the Canadian Aging and Caregiving Resource Guide; and personal assistance and support through seminar series, care management consulting service, the Caregiver Club, and Care Across the Border.

Canadian Hospice Palliative Care Association

http://www.chpca.net/about_us/mission_statement.htm

The Canadian Hospice Palliative Care Association (CHPCA) is the national association that provides leadership in hospice palliative care in Canada. The CHPCA uses collaboration and representation, increased awareness, knowledge and skills related to hospice palliative care of the public, health-care providers, and volunteers; development of national standards of practice for hospice palliative care in Canada; support of research on hospice palliative care; advocacy for improved hospice palliative care policy; resource allocation; and supports for caregivers to pursue excellence in care for persons approaching death so that the burdens of suffering, loneliness, and grief are lessened.

Hospice Association of Ontario End of Life Information Service

http://www.hospicelifeline.com

The Hospice Association of Ontario End of Life Information Service provides information about a wide range of hospice palliative care services and such resources as hospice palliative care programs, hospice palliative care units, community-based services, pain and symptom management, bereavement support services, and palliative care education.

Canadian Virtual Hospice

http://www.virtualhospice.ca

The virtual hospice is a network of information and support for people dealing with life-threatening illness and loss. The website does not offer direct medical advice or clinical care but does offer information and resources that may help people to better understand the physical, emotional, and spiritual aspects of their experiences. The Canadian Virtual Hospice is an interactive network designed to facilitate information exchange, communication, and mutual support among patients, their friends and family, health-care providers, and palliative care volunteers.

REFERENCES

Anderson, H. (1989). After the diagnosis: An operational theology for the terminally ill. *Journal of Pastoral Care, 43,* 141–150.

Barnard, D., Towers, A., Boston, P., & Lambrinidou, Y. (2000). *Crossing over: Narratives of palliative care.* New York: Oxford University Press.

Bennett Jacobs, B., & Taylor, C. (2005). Seeing artificial hydration and nutrition through an ethical lens. *Home Healthcare Nurse, 23*(11), 749–743.

Billings, J. (1998). What is palliative care? *Journal of Palliative Medicine, 1*(1), 73–81.

Brenneis, C., & Brown, P. (2006). International models of excellence: Palliative care in Canada. In B. Ferrell & N. Coyle (Eds.), *Textbook of palliative nursing* (2nd ed.) (pp. 1147–1159). New York: Oxford University Press.

Brindley, P., Markland, D., Mayers, I., & Kutsogiannis, D. (2002). Predictors of survival following in-hospital adult cardiopulmonary resuscitation. *Canadian Medical Association Journal, 167*(4), 343–348.

Callanan, M. (1994). Dealing with death: Breaking the silence. *American Journal of Nursing, 94,* 22–23.

Canadian Hospice Palliative Care Association. (2004). *Fact sheet: Hospice palliative care in Canada.* Ottawa: Author.

Canadian Nurses Association. (1995). *Policy Statement: Joint statement on resuscitative interventions.* Ottawa: Author.

Canadian Nurses Association. (1998). *Advance directives: The nurse's role.* Ottawa: Author.

Canadian Nurses Association. (2000). *End-of-life issues.* Ottawa: Author.

Canadian Nurses Association. (2001). Futility presents many challenges for nurses. *Ethics in Practice* series paper. Ottawa: Author.

Chang, V., Hwang, S., Feuerman, M., & Kasimis, B. (2000). Symptom and quality of life survey of medical oncology patients at a veterans' affairs medical center: A role for symptom assessment. *Cancer, 88,* 1175–1183.

Cowles, K. V., & Rodgers, B. L. (1991). The concept of grief: A foundation for nursing research and practice. *Research in Nursing & Health, 14*(2), 119–127.

Dudgeon, D. (2006). Dyspnea, death rattle and cough. In B. Ferrell & N. Coyle (Eds.), *Textbook of palliative nursing* (2nd ed.) (pp. 249–264). New York: Oxford University Press.

Dudgeon, D., Kristjanson, L., Sloan, J., & Lertzman, M. (2001). Dyspnea in cancer patients: Prevalence and associated factors. *Journal of Pain and Symptom Management, 21*(2), 95–102.

Fainsinger, R., MacEachern, T., Hanson, J., Miller, M., & Bruera, E. (1991). Symptom control during the last week of life on a palliative care unit. *Journal of Palliative Care, 7,* 5–11.

Frank, A. (2004). Dignity, dialogue and care. *Journal of Palliative Care, 20*(3), 207–211.

Ganzini, L. (2006). Artificial nutrition and hydration at the end of life: Ethics and evidence. *Palliative and Supportive Care, 4,* 135–143.

Gilliss, C. L., Highly, B. L., Roberts, B. M., & Martinsen, I. (Eds.). (1989). *Towards a science of family nursing.* Menlo Park, CA: Addison Wesley.

Gilbert, M., Counsell, C., & Guin, P. (2001). Determining the relationship between end-of-life decisions expressed in advance directives and resuscitation efforts during cardiopulmonary resuscitation. *Outcomes Management for Nursing Practice, 5*(2), 87–92.

Glaser, B., & Strauss, A. (1965). *Awareness of dying.* Chicago, IL: Aldine.

Golin, C., Wegner, N., & Liu, H. (2000). A prospective study of patient-physician communication about resuscitation. *Journal of American Geriatric Society, 48,* 52–60.

Helme, R., Meliala, A., & Gibson, S. (2004). Methodologic factors which contribute to variations in experimental pain threshold reported for older people. *Neuroscience Letters, 361*(1–3), 144–146.

Herz Brown, F. (1989). The impact of death and serious illness on the family life cycle. In B. Carter & M. McGoldrick (Eds.), *The changing family life cycle* (2nd ed.) (pp. 457–482). Needham Heights, MA: Allyn & Bacon.

Jenkins, C., Taube, A., Ken, T., Hanson, J., & Bruera, E. (1998). Initial demographic, symptom, and medication profiles in patients admitted to palliative care units. *Journal of Pain and Symptom Management, 16,* 163–170.

King, D. A., Shields, C. G., & Wynne, L. C. (2005). Family intervention and therapy with older adults. In B. J. Sadock & V. A. Sadock (Eds.), *Comprehensive textbook of psychiatry* (8th ed.) (pp. 3763–3769). Philadelphia, PA: Lippincott, Williams &Wilkins.

Kissane, D. W. (2003). Psychosocial morbidity associated with patterns of family functioning in palliative care: Baseline data from the family focused grief therapy controlled trial. *Palliative Medicine, 17,* 527–537.

Kissane, D. W., Bloch, S., Onghena, P., McKenzie, D., Synde, R., & Dowe, D. (1996). The Melbourne family grief study, II: Psychosocial morbidity and grief in bereaved families. *American Journal of Psychiatry, 13,* 659–666.

Kubler-Ross, E. (1969). *On death and dying.* New York: Macmillan.

Lazar, N., Shemie, S., Webster, G., & Dickens, B. (2001). Bioethics for clinicians: Brain death. *Canadian Medical Association Journal, 164*(6), 833–836.

Lazaruk, T. (2006). The CPR question. *Canadian Nurse, 102*(2), 22–24.

Lowy, F., Sawyer, D., & Williams, J. (1993). *Canadian physicians and euthanasia.* Ottawa: Canadian Medical Association.

MacDonald, N. (1998). Palliative care: An essential component of cancer control. *Canadian Medical Association Journal, 158,* 1709–1716.

Martel, L, & Malenfant, E. C. (2007). Portrait of the Canadian population in 2006, by age and sex: Findings. Retrieved October 31, 2008, from http://www12.statcan.ca/english/census06/analysis/agesex/index.cfm

Martocchio, B. C. (1985). Grief and bereavement: Healing through hurt. *Nursing Clinics of North America, 20,* 327–341.

Meuser, T., Pietruck, C., Radbruch, L., Stute, P., Lehmann, K., & Grond, S. (2001). Symptoms during cancer pain treatment following WHO guidelines: A longitudinal follow-up study of symptom prevalence, severity, and etiology. *Pain, 93,* 247–257.

Morita, T., Ichiki, T., Tsunoda, J., Inoue, S., & Chihaa, S. (1998). A prospective study on the dying process in terminally ill cancer patients. *American Journal of Hospice and Palliative Care, 15,* 217–222.

Moules, N. J. (1998). Legitimizing grief: Challenging beliefs that constrain. *Journal of Family Nursing, 4*(2), 142–166.

Moules, N. J. (1999). Suffering together: Whose words were they? *Journal of Family Nursing, 5*(3), 251–258.

Moules, N. J. (2000). Funerals, families and family nursing: Lessons of love and practice. *Journal of Family Nursing, 6*(1), 3–8.

Moules, N. J., & Amundson, J. K. (1997). Grief—An invitation to inertia: A narrative approach to working with grief. *Journal of Family Nursing, 3*(4), 378–393.

Moules, N., Simonson, K., Fleiszer, A., Prins, M., & Glasgow, B. (2007). The soul of sorrow work: Grief and therapeutic interventions with families. *Journal of Family Nursing, 13*(1), 1–25.

Moules, N., Simonson, K., Prins, M., Angus, P., & Bell, J. (2004). Making room for grief: Walking backwards and living forward. *Nursing Inquiry, 11*(2), 99–107.

Ng, K., & von Gunten, C. (1998). Symptoms and attitudes of 100 consecutive patients admitted to an acute hospice/palliative care unit. *Journal of Pain and Symptom Management, 16,* 307–316.

Paice, J., & Fine, P. (2006). Pain at the end of life. In B. Ferrell & N. Coyle (Eds.), *Textbook of palliative nursing* (2nd ed.) (pp. 131–153). New York: Oxford University Press.

Parageon, K., & Hailey, B. (1999). Barriers to effective cancer pain management: A review of the literature. *Journal of Pain and Symptom Management, 18,* 358–368.

Perry, B. (1998). *Moments in time: Images of exemplary nursing care.* Ottawa: Canadian Nurses Association.

Pereira, J., & Bruera, E. (2001). *Alberta palliative care resource book.* Edmonton: Alberta Cancer Board.

Qualls, S. (2000). Therapy with aging families: Rationale, opportunities and challenges. *Aging Mental Health, 4,* 191–199.

Raffin, S. (2002). *Accompanying the dying: Nurses create a moral space for suffering.* Unpublished doctoral dissertation, University of Alberta, Edmonton, Canada.

Raffin Bouchal, S. (2007). Moral meanings in caring for the dying. In N. E.

Johnston & A. Scholler-Jaquish (Eds.), *Meaning in suffering: Caring practices in the health professions. Vol. VI of interpretive studies in healthcare and the human sciences* (pp. 232–275). Chicago, IL: University of Wisconsin Press.

Richter, J. M. (1984). Crisis of mate loss in the elderly. *American Nursing Society, 6*(4), 45–54.

Robinson, E. M. (2002). An ethical analysis of cardiopulmonary resuscitation for elders in acute care. *AACN Clinical Issues, 13*(1), 132–144.

Rolland, J. S. (2003). Mastering family challenges in illness and disability. In F. Walsh (Ed.), *Normal family process* (3rd ed.) (pp. 460–489). New York: Guilford.

Rolland, J. S. (2004). Helping families with anticipatory loss and terminal illness. In F. Walsh & M. McGoldrick (Eds.), *Living beyond loss: Death in the family* (2nd ed.) (pp. 213–236). New York: WW Norton.

Seymour, J. (2001). *Critical moments—death and dying in intensive care.* Buckingham, UK: Open University Press.

Sinclair, S., Pereira, J., & Raffin, S. (2006). A thematic review of the spirituality literature within palliative care. *Journal of Palliative Medicine, 9*(2), 464–479.

Sinclair, S., Raffin, S., Pereira, J., & Guebert, N. (2006). Collective soul: The spirituality of an interdisciplinary palliative care team. *Palliative and Supportive Care, 4,* 13–24.

Storch, J. (2006). The CPR question: Commentary. *Canadian Nurse, 102*(2), 23–24.

Tapp, A. (2006). Advance directives. *Canadian Nurse, 102*(2), 26.

Wald, L. (1999). Hospice care in the United States: A conversation with Florence S. Wald. *Journal of the American Medical Association, 281,* 1683–1685.

Walsh, F., & McGoldrick, M. (Eds.). (2004). *Living beyond loss: Death in the family* (2nd ed.). New York: WW Norton.

Weihs, K., & Reiss, D. (1996). Family reorganization in response to cancer: A developmental perspective. In L. Baider & C. Cooper (Eds.), *Cancer and the family* (pp. 3–29). Oxford, UK: Wiley & Sons.

Wells, N. (2000). Pain intensity and pain interference in hospitalized patients with cancer. *Oncology Nursing Forum, 27,* 985–991.

White, M. (1989). Saying hello again: The incorporation of the lost relationship in the resolution of grief. In M. White (Ed.), *Selected papers* (pp. 29–36). Adelaide, AU: Dulwich Centre.

Wilson, D., Northcott, H., Truman, C., Smith, S., Anderson, M., Fainsinger, R., et al. (2001). Location of death in Canada: A comparison of 20th century hospital and non-hospital locations of death and corresponding population trends. *Evaluation and the Health Professions, 24*(4), 385–403.

Winchester Nadeau, J. (2001). Meaning making in family bereavement: A family systems approach. In M. Stroebe, R. Hansson, W. Stroebe, & H. Schut (Eds.), *Handbook of bereavement research: Consequences, coping and care* (pp. 329–348). Washington, DC: American Psychological Association.

World Health Organization. (1996). *Cancer pain relief and palliative care. Report of a WHO expert committee* (2nd ed.). Geneva, Switzerland: Author. WHO Technical Series #804.

Wright, L. M. (1997). Suffering and spirituality: The soul of clinical work with families. *Journal of Family Nursing, 39*(1), 3–14.

Wright, L. M. (1999). Spirituality, suffering, and beliefs: The soul of healing with families. In F. Walsh (Ed.), *Spiritual resources in families and family therapy* (pp. 61–75). New York: Guilford Press.

Zerwekh, J. (1997). Do dying patients really need IV fluids? *American Journal of Nursing, 97*(3), 26–30.

Appendix A

Laboratory Values

Abbreviations and symbols:

< = less than

> = greater than

fL = femtolitre (10^{-15} L)

IU = international unit

g = gram

mg = milligram (10^{-3} g)

μg = microgram (10^{-6} g)

ng = nanogram (10^{-9} g)

pg = picogram (10^{-12} g)

TABLE A.1 Hematology: Complete Blood Count with Clinical Implications

Component	Description	Normal Findings* (Adult)	Possible Causes of Abnormal Findings	
			Increased	**Decreased**
Erythrocyte (red blood cell [RBC] count)	The number of RBCs per litre of blood	M: 4.5×10^{12}/L to 5.3×10^{12}/L F: 4.1×10^{12}/L to 5.1×10^{12}/L	Primary polycythemia (e.g., polycythemia vera) Secondary polycythemia or erythrocytosis, usually caused by oxygen need (e.g., chronic lung disease, congenital heart defects)	Abnormal loss of erythrocytes Abnormal destruction of erythrocytes Lack of needed elements or hormones for erythrocyte production Bone marrow suppression
Hemoglobin (Hgb)	Composed of a pigment (heme), which contains iron, and a protein (globin)	M: 138 g/L to 180 g/L F: 120 g/L to 160 g/L	Polycythemia	Blood loss Hemolytic anemia Bone marrow suppression Sickle-cell disease
Hematocrit (Hct)	The hematocrit or packed cell volume (Hct, PCV, or crit) represents the proportion of RBCs to the plasma	M: 0.37 to 0.49 F: 0.36 to 0.46	Polycythemia Dehydration Burns	Blood loss Overhydration Dietary deficiency Anemia

(continued)

TABLE A.1 Hematology: Complete Blood Count with Clinical Implications *(continued)*

Component	Description	Normal Findings* (Adult)	Possible Causes of Abnormal Findings: Increased	Possible Causes of Abnormal Findings: Decreased
Red blood cell indices (RBC indices)				
Mean corpuscular volume (MCV)	The mean or average size of the individual RBC	M: 78 fL to 100 fL F: 78 fL to 102 fL	Liver disease Alcoholism Pernicious anemia	Iron deficiency anemia Lead poisoning
Mean corpuscular hemoglobin (MCH)	Amount of Hgb present in one cell	25 pg to 35 pg	Rarely seen	Iron deficiency anemia
Mean corpuscular hemoglobin concentration (MCHC)	The proportion of each cell occupied by Hgb	0.31 to 0.37	Rarely seen	Iron deficiency anemia
White blood cell count (WBC)	Count of the total number of WBCs in a litre of blood	4.5×10^9/L to 11×10^9/L	(Leukocytosis) Infection	(Leukopenia) Autoimmune disease
Differential count	The proportion of each of the five types of WBCs in a sample of 100 WBCs			
Neutrophils		55% to 70%	Stress Acute infection	Viral diseases Some drugs (e.g., chemotherapy, antibiotics such as nafcillin, penicillin, and cephalosporins) Radiation therapy
Lymphocytes		20% to 40%	Viral infection Mononucleosis Tuberculosis Chronic bacterial infections Lymphocytic leukemia	Adrenal corticosteroids and other immunosuppressive drugs Autoimmune diseases (e.g., lupus erythematosus) Severe malnutrition
Monocytes		2% to 8%	Chronic inflammatory disorders Tuberculosis Protozoan infections (e.g., malaria, Rocky Mountain spotted fever) Chronic ulcerative colitis	Drug therapy: Prednisone
Eosinophils		1% to 4%	Allergic reactions (e.g., asthma, hay fever, or hypersensitivity to a drug) Parasitic infestations (e.g., round worms)	Corticosteroid therapy
Basophils		0% to 2%	Leukemia	Acute allergic reaction Corticosteroids Acute infections

(continued)

TABLE A.1 Hematology: Complete Blood Count with Clinical Implications *(continued)*

Component	Description	Normal Findings* (Adult)	Possible Causes of Abnormal Findings	
			Increased	Decreased
Platelet count	Platelets are fragments of cytoplasm that function in blood coagulation	150×10^9/L to 350×10^9/L	Malignant tumours Polycythemia vera	Idiopathic (unknown cause) Thrombocytopenic purpura Viral infections AIDS Systemic lupus erythematosus Chemotherapy drugs Some types of anemia

*Normal laboratory values vary from agency to agency.

TABLE A.2 Hematology: Coagulation

Component	Normal Findings* (Adult)
Bleeding time	180 to 570 seconds
APTT (activated partial thromboplastin time)	24 to 36 seconds
PTT (partial thromboplastin time)	25 to 35 seconds
PT (prothrombin time)	11 to 13 seconds
INR (international normalized ratio)	0.81 to 1.2
Thrombin time	8 to 12 seconds
Fibrinogen	2 g/L to 4 g/L

*Normal laboratory values vary from agency to agency.

TABLE A.3 Normal Serum Electrolyte Values for Adults

Component	Normal Findings*
Sodium (Na^+)	135 mmol/L to 145 mmol/L
Potassium (K^+)	3.5 mmol/L to 5.0 mmol/L
Calcium (Ca^{2+}) (total)	2.2 mmol/L to 2.58 mmol/L
Calcium (ionized)	1.0 mmol/L to 1.15 mmol/L
Magnesium (Mg^{2+})	0.65 mmol/L to 1.05 mmol/L
Chloride (Cl^-)	95 mmol/L to 105 mmol/L
Phosphate (PO_4^-)	0.97 mmol/L to 1.45 mmol/L
Serum osmolality	280 mmol/kg water to 300 mmol/kg water

*Normal laboratory values vary from agency to agency.

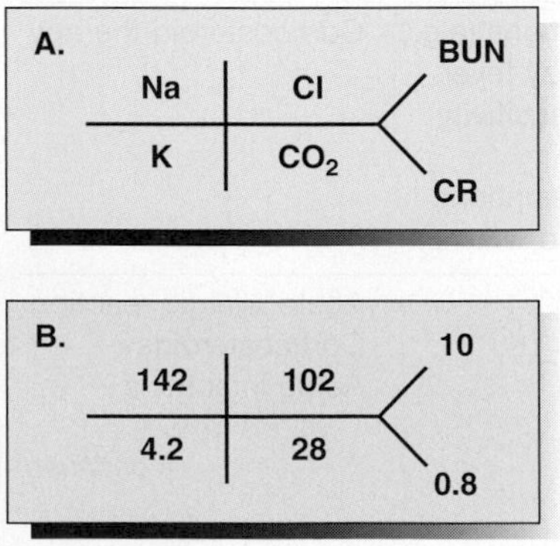

A: Format for a diagram of serum electrolyte results;
B: Example that may be seen in documentation notes

TABLE A.4 Blood Chemistry Tests with Clinical Implications

Test	Normal Findings* (Adult)	Significance	Possible Causes of Increased	Possible Causes of Decreased
Glucose Regulation**				
Random blood glucose (casual plasma glucose)	4 mmol/L to 6 mmol/L	Glucose provides body with energy; insulin produced by pancreas controls plasma glucose levels	Diabetes; stress response	Insulinoma; pancreatic disorders; liver disease; insulin overdose
FPG (fasting plasma glucose; no oral intake for 8 hours)	3.6 mmol/L to 5.7 mmol/L		6.1 mmol/L to 6.9 mmol/L: impaired fasting glucose (IFG); ≥ 7.0 mmol/L: diabetes mellitus	
OGT (oral glucose tolerance)	< 7.8 mmol/L	Blood glucose measured 2 hours after ingestion of 75 g glucose solution	7.8 mmol/L to 11.0 mmol/L: impaired glucose tolerance (IGT); ≥ 11.1 mmol/L: diabetes mellitus	Not applicable
Hemoglobin A_{1c} (HbA_{1c}) (also referred to as glycosylated hemoglobin)	4% to 6%	A measure of the blood glucose bound to hemoglobin; reflects the blood glucose levels during the prior 3 to 4 months	Diabetes mellitus	Hemoglobinopathy; invalid test in people with beta-thalassemia
Liver Function Tests				
ALT (alanine aminotransferase); formerly known as serum pyretic transaminase (SGPT)	M: 10 U/L to 55 U/L F: 7 U/L to 30 U/L	Marker of hepatic injury; more specific of liver damage than AST	Hepatitis; infectious mononucleosis; acute pancreatitis; acute myocardial infarction; heart failure	Not clinically significant
AST (aspartate aminotransferase); formerly known as serum gluctamic-oxaloacetic transaminase (SGOT)	M: 10 U/L to 40 U/L F: 9 U/L to 25 U/L	Found in heart, liver, and skeletal muscle; can also be used to indicate liver injury	Liver diseases (e.g., hepatitis, alcoholism, drug toxicity); acute myocardial infarction anemias, skeletal muscle diseases	Chronic renal dialysis; vitamin B6 deficiency
Albumin	35 g/L to 48 g/L; panic value: < 15 g/L	A protein produced by the liver	No pathology causes the liver to produce more albumin; an increased level reflects dehydration	Chronic liver dysfunction; AIDS; severe burns; malnutrition; renal disease; acute and chronic infections
Alkaline phosphatase	25 U/L to 100 U/L	Found in the tissues of the liver, bone, intestine, kidney, and placenta. Used as an index of liver and bone disease when correlated with other clinical findings	Liver disease; bone disease; hyperparathyroidism; myocardial infarction; chronic renal failure; heart failure	Malnutrition; pernicious anemia and severe anemias; hypothyroidism; magnesium and zinc deficiency (nutritional)

(continued)

TABLE A.4 Blood Chemistry Tests with Clinical Implications *(continued)*

Test	Normal Findings* (Adult)	Significance	Possible Causes of Increased	Possible Causes of Decreased
Ammonia	35 μmol/L to 65 μmol/L	The liver converts ammonia, a byproduct of protein metabolism, into urea, which is excreted by the kidneys	Liver disease, cirrhosis; Reye's syndrome; GI hemorrhage	Renal failure
Amylase	< 125 U/L		Hepatitis (acute and chronic)	Liver disease (cirrhosis, acute alcoholism)
Bilirubin	Total: 5.1 mmol/L to 17 mmol/L Direct: 0.0 to 3.4 mmol/L Indirect: 1.7 mmol/L to 17 mmol/L Panic value: > 20 mmol/L	Results from the breakdown of hemoglobin in the red blood cells; removed from the body by the liver, which excretes it into the bile	Total: Hepatitis; obstruction of the common bile or hepatic ducts; pernicious anemia; sickle-cell disease Direct: Cancer of the head of the pancreas; choledocholithiasis Indirect: Hemolytic anemias; drug toxicity; transfusion reaction	Not clinically significant
GGT (gamma-glutamyl transferase)	Men: 1 U/L to 94 U/L Women: 1 U/L to 70 U/L	Found primarily in the liver, kidney, prostate, and spleen; is more specific for the hepatobiliary system	Liver disease; alcohol abuse	Not clinically significant
Prothrombin	11 to 13 seconds Critical value: > 20 seconds for persons not on anticoagulants	A protein produced by the liver for clotting of blood	Liver disease, damage; vitamin K deficiency; obstruction of common bile duct; deficiency of factors II, V, VII, or X	Thrombophlebitis; malignant tumour
Cardiac Markers				
CK (creatine kinase)	Total: M: 38 U/L to 174 U/L F: 26 U/L to 140 U/L Isoenzymes: MM (CK_3): 96% to 100% MB (CK_2): 0% to 6% BB (CK_1): 0%	An enzyme found in the heart and skeletal muscles; has three isoenzymes: BB or CK_1, MB or CK_2, and MM or CK_3	Total: Acute myocardial infarction (MI); myocarditis; after open heart surgery; acute cerebrovascular disease, muscular dystrophy; chronic alcoholism CK Isoenzymes: MB (CK_2): Myocardial infarction; myocardial ischemia, angina pectoris	Not clinically significant

(continued)

TABLE A.4 Blood Chemistry Tests with Clinical Implications *(continued)*

Test	Normal Findings* (Adult)	Significance	Possible Causes of Increased	Possible Causes of Decreased
Myoglobin	5 ng/mL to 70 ng/mL	After an MI, serum levels of myoglobin rise in 2 to 4 hours, making it an early marker for muscle damage in MI	Myocardial infarction, angina, other muscle injury (e.g., trauma), renal failure, rhabdomyolysis	Rheumatoid arthritis; myasthenia gravis
Troponin I (cTnI) Troponin T (cTnT)	Troponin I: < 0.35 μg/L Critical value: > 1.5 μg/L Troponin T: < 0.2 μg/L	Cardiac troponin is highly concentrated in the heart muscle; this test is used in the early diagnosis of MI; after an MI, troponin I begins to increase in 4 to 6 hours and remains elevated for 5 to 7 days; troponin T begins to increase in 3 to 4 hours and remains elevated for 10 to 14 days	Troponin I: small infarct; myocardial injury Troponin T: Acute MI, unstable angina, myocarditis	Not clinically significant
Lipoprotein Profile				
Cholesterol	Desirable: < 5.19 mmol/L*** (5.2 mmol/L to 6.19 mmol/L = borderline high; > 6.20 mmol/L = high; > 7.21 mmol/L = extremely high)	This test is an important screening test for heart disease	Type II familial hypercholesterolemia; biliary cirrhosis; chronic renal failure; poorly controlled diabetes mellitus; alcoholism; diet high in cholesterol and fats	Severe hepatocellular disease; hyperthyroidism; malnutrition, chronic anemias, severe burns
HDL-C (high-density lipoprotein cholesterol)	Desirable: > 1.55 mmol/L (1.30 to 1.54: acceptable; 1.04 to 1.29 low is less desirable; < 1.04 very low and undesirable)	A class of lipoproteins produced by the liver and intestines; higher levels are beneficial.	HDL excess; chronic liver disease; long-term aerobic or vigorous exercise	Familial hypolipoproteinemia; hypertriglyceridemia (familial), poorly controlled diabetes mellitus, chronic renal failure
LDL (low-density lipoprotein)	< 2.5 mmol/L = target level for patients at high risk of coronary artery disease (CAD); < 3.5 = target level for patients at moderate risk of CAD; < 4.5 = target level for patients at low risk of CAD	Up to 70% of the total serum cholesterol is present in the LDL. Lower levels are beneficial.	Familial type 2 hyperlipidemia; Secondary causes can include a diet high in cholesterol and saturated fat, nephritic syndrome, multiple myeloma, diabetes mellitus, chronic renal failure	Hypolipoproteinemia; hyperthyroidism, chronic anemias, severe hepatocellular disease
Triglycerides	Desirable: 0.45 to 1.69 mmol/L	This test evaluates suspected atherosclerosis and measures the body's ability to metabolize fat	Hyperlipoproteinemia; liver disease; renal disease; hypothyroidism; pancreatitis; myocardial infarction	Malnutrition; hyperthyroidism, brain infarction, chronic obstructive lung disease

(continued)

TABLE A.4 Blood Chemistry Tests with Clinical Implications *(continued)*

Test	Normal Findings* (Adult)	Significance	Possible Causes of Increased	Possible Causes of Decreased
Renal Function				
Creatinine	44 µmol/L to 133 µmol/L	Produced as the result of protein metabolism (especially from muscles) and is excreted solely by the kidneys	Renal disease; rhabdomyolysis; heart failure; shock; severe dehydration	Low muscle mass (e.g., muscular dystrophy, debilitation); severe liver disease
Urea nitrogen (BUN = blood urea nitrogen)	3.6 mmol/L to 7.1 mmol/L	End product of protein metabolism	Renal disease; severe dehydration; heart failure; gastrointestinal bleed	Severe liver disease; celiac disease; severe malnutrition; overhydration

*Normal laboratory values vary from agency to agency.

**Source: "Definition, Classification and Diagnosis of Diabetes and Other Dysglycemic Categories," by the Canadian Diabetes Association Clinical Practice Guidelines Expert Committee, 2003, *Canadian Journal of Diabetes,* 27(Suppl 2), pp. S7–S9.

*** Source: "Recommendations for the Management of Dyslipidemia and the Prevention of Cardiovascular Disease: Summary of the 2003 Update," by J. Genest, J. Frohlich, G. Fodor, and R. McPherson, 2003, *Canadian Medical Association Journal, 169*(9), pp. 921–924.

TABLE A.5 Arterial Blood Gas

Component	Normal Findings (Adult)
pH (arterial)	7.35 to 7.45
Bicarbonate (HCO_3^-)	22 mmol/L to 26 mmol/L
$PaCO_2$	35 mm Hg to 45 mm Hg
PaO_2	80 mm Hg to 100 mm Hg
SaO_2 (oxygen saturation)	95% to 100%

TABLE A.6 Urine Analysis

Component	Normal Findings (Adult)
Colour, clarity	Straw, amber, transparent
Odour	Faint aromatic
Sterility	No microorganisms present
pH	4.5 to 8
Specific gravity	1.010 to 1.025
Glucose	None
Ketone bodies	None
Protein	None
Blood	None
Osmolality	500 mmol/kg to 800 mmol/kg

Appendix

Formulae

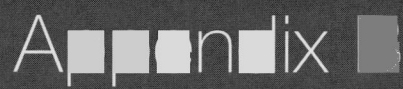

This appendix summarizes formulae that have been presented within the text.

Body Weight (see Chapter 39)

Body Mass Index (BMI)	BMI = weight (in kg/m^2) Normal: 18.5 to 24.5 (see Chapter 39)
Waist-to-hip ratio (WHR)	WHR = WC ÷ HC (WC = waist circumference; HC = Hip circumference) Normal: F: < 0.8 M: < 1.0

Circulatory Indices (see Chapter 42)

Cardiac output (CO)	CO = HR × SV (HR = heart rate; SV = stroke volume)
Mean arterial pressure (MAP)	MAP = CO × SVR (CO = cardiac output; SRV = systemic vascular resistance)
Ankle-brachial index (ABI)	ABI = posterior tibial *or* dorsalis pedis (whichever is highest) systolic pressure ÷ brachial artery systolic pressure

Fluid Requirements in Children (see Chapter 43)

Body weight 1 kg to 10 kg	100 mL/kg
Body weight 10 kg to 20 kg	1000 mL + 50 ml/kg for each kg above 10 kg
Body weight > 20 kg	1500 mL + 20 ml/kg for each kg above 20 kg

Intravenous infusion (see Chapter 43)

Millilitres per hour (mL/h)	mL/h = Total infusion volume ÷ Number of hours for infusion
Drops per minute (DPM; gtt/min)	DPM = (Total infusion volume × Drop factor) ÷ Total time of infusion in minutes

Medication dosage (see Chapter 31)

Desired quantity	(Dose on hand ÷ Quantity on hand) = (Desired dose ÷ Quantity desired *x*); *x* = (Quantity on hand × Desired dose) ÷ Dose on hand
Child dosages by using body surface area	Child's dose = (Surface area of child in m^2 ÷ 1.7 m^2) × Normal adult dose

Appendix C

Vital Signs

Temperature (see Chapter 28)

Hypothermia	< 36°C
Normal range	≥ 36°C to ≤ 38°C
Pyrexia	> 38°C to ≤ 41°C
Hyperpyrexia	> 41°C

Conversion formulae:

°C = (Fahrenheit temperature − 32) × 5/9

°F = (Celsius temperature × 9/5) + 32

Pulse and Respirations (see Chapter 28)

Age	Pulse (Average and Ranges)	Respirations (Average and Ranges)
Newborns (0–4 weeks)	130 (80–180)	35 (30–80)
< 1 year	120 (80–140)	30 (20–40)
1–4 years	110 (80–120)	25 (20–30)
5–8 years	100 (75–120)	20 (15–25)
9–10 years	70 (50–90)	19 (15–25)
11–19 years	75 (50–90)	18 (15–20)
20–64 years	80 (60–100)	16 (12–20)
≥ 65 years	70 (60–100)	16 (15–20)

Pulse Volume

3 Point Scale	Description of Pulse
0	Absent, not discernible
+1	Thready or weak, difficult to feel
+2	Normal, detected readily, obliterated by strong pressure
+3	Bounding, difficult to obliterate

4 Point Scale	Description of Pulse
0	Absent, not discernible
+1	Thready or weak, difficult to feel
+2	Normal, detected readily, obliterated by strong pressure
+3	Increased
+4	Bounding

Blood Pressure* (Adults) (see Chapter 28; Figure 28.17 for further detail)

Range	Interpretation
SBP ≤ 120 and/or DBP ≤ 80 mm Hg	Optimal
SBP < 130 and/or DBP < 85 mm Hg	Normal
SBP 130 to 139 mm Hg and/or DBP 85 to 89 mm Hg	High Normal
SBP ≥ 140 mm Hg and/or DBP ≥ 90 mm Hg	Hypertension
SBP 140 to 159 and/or DBP 90 to 99	Grade 1: Mild hypertension
SBP 160 to 179 and/or DBP 100 to 109	Grade 2: Moderate hypertension
SBP ≥ 180 and/or DBP ≥ 110	Grade 3: Severe hypertension

* Values based on *2008 CHEP Recommendations for the Management of Hypertension*, by the Canadian Hypertension Education Program, 2008, Ottawa: Author.

SBP = systolic blood pressure

DBP = diastolic blood pressure

Appendix D

2007–2008 NANDA International Approved Nursing Diagnoses

Activity Intolerance
Activity Intolerance, Risk for
Airway Clearance, Ineffective
Anxiety
Anxiety, Death
Aspiration, Risk for
Attachment, Parent/Infant/Child, Risk for Impaired
Autonomic Dysreflexia
Autonomic Dysreflexia, Risk for
Blood Glucose, Risk for Unstable
Body Image, Disturbed
Body Temperature: Imbalanced, Risk for
Bowel Incontinence
Breastfeeding, Effective
Breastfeeding, Ineffective
Breastfeeding, Interrupted
Breathing Pattern, Ineffective
Cardiac Output, Decreased
Caregiver Role Strain
Caregiver Role Strain, Risk for
Comfort, Readiness for Enhanced
Communication: Impaired, Verbal
Communication, Readiness for Enhanced
Confusion, Acute
Confusion, Acute, Risk for
Confusion, Chronic
Constipation
Constipation, Perceived
Constipation, Risk for
Contamination
Contamination, Risk for
Coping: Community, Ineffective
Coping: Community, Readiness for Enhanced Coping, Defensive
Coping: Family, Comprised
Coping: Family, Disabled
Coping: Family, Readiness for Enhanced
Coping (Individual), Readiness for Enhanced Coping, Ineffective
Decisional Conflict
Decision Making, Readiness for Enhanced
Denial, Ineffective
Dentition, Impaired
Development: Delayed, Risk for
Diarrhea
Disuse Syndrome, Risk for
Diversional Activity, Deficient
Energy Field, Disturbed
Environmental Interruption Syndrome, Impaired
Failure to Thrive, Adult
Falls, Risk for
Family Processes, Dysfunctional: Alcoholism
Family Processes, Interrupted
Family Processes, Readiness for Enhanced
Fatigue
Fear
Fluid Balance, Readiness for Enhanced
Fluid Volume, Deficient
Fluid Volume, Deficient, Risk for
Fluid Volume, Excess
Fluid Volume, Imbalanced, Risk for
Gas Exchange, Impaired
Grieving
Grieving, Complicated
Grieving, risk for Complicated
Growth, Disproportionate, Risk for
Growth and Development, Delayed
Health Behaviour, Risk-Prone
Health Maintenance, Ineffective
Health-Seeking Behaviours (Specify)
Home Maintenance, Impaired
Hope, Readiness for Enhanced
Hopelessness
Human Dignity, Risk for Compromised
Hyperthermia
Hypothermia
Immunization Status, Readiness for Enhanced
Infant Behaviour, Disorganized
Infant Behaviour: Disorganized, Risk for
Infant Behaviour: Organized, Readiness for Enhanced
Infant Feeding Pattern, Ineffective
Infection, Risk for
Injury, Risk for
Insomnia
Intracranial Adaptive Capacity, Decreased
Knowledge, Deficient (Specify)
Knowledge (Specify), Readiness for Enhanced
Latex Allergy Response
Latex Allergy Response, Risk for
Liver Function, Impaired, Risk for
Loneliness, Risk for
Memory, Impaired
Mobility: Bed, Impaired
Mobility: Physical, Impaired
Mobility: Wheelchair, Impaired
Moral Distress
Nausea

Neurovascular Dysfunction: Peripheral, Risk for
Noncompliance (Specify)
Nutrition, Imbalanced: Less than Body Requirements
Nutrition, Imbalanced: More than Body Requirements
Nutrition, Readiness for Enhanced
Oral Mucous Membrane, Impaired
Pain, Acute
Pain, Chronic
Parenting, Impaired
Parenting, Readiness for Enhanced
Parenting, Risk for Impaired
Perioperative Positioning Injury, Risk for
Personal Identity, Disturbed
Poisoning, Risk for
Post-Trauma Syndrome
Post-Trauma Syndrome, Risk for
Power, Readiness for Enhanced
Powerlessness
Powerlessness, Risk for
Protection, Ineffective
Rape-Trauma Syndrome
Rape-Trauma Syndrome: Compound Reaction
Rape-Trauma Syndrome: Silent Reaction
Religiosity, Impaired
Religiosity, Readiness for Enhanced
Religiosity, risk for Impaired
Relocation Stress Syndrome
Relocation Stress Syndrome, Risk for
Role Conflict, Parental
Role Performance, Ineffective
Sedentary Lifestyle
Self-Care, Readiness for Enhanced
Self-Care Deficit: Bathing/Hygiene
Self-Care Deficit: Dressing/Grooming
Self-Care Deficit: Feeding
Self-Care Deficit: Toileting
Self-Concept, Readiness for Enhanced
Self-Esteem, Chronic Low
Self-Esteem, Situational Low
Self-Esteem, Risk for Situational Low
Self-Mutilation
Self-Mutilation, Risk for
Sensory Perception, Disturbed (Specify: Auditory, Gustatory, Kinesthetic, Olfactory Tactile, Visual)
Sexual Dysfunction
Sexuality Pattern, Ineffective
Skin Integrity, Impaired
Skin Integrity, Risk for Impaired
Sleep Deprivation
Sleep, Readiness for Enhanced
Social Interaction, Impaired
Social Isolation
Sorrow, Chronic
Spiritual Distress
Spiritual Distress, Risk for
Spiritual Well-Being, Readiness for Enhanced
Spontaneous Ventilation, Impaired
Stress, Overload
Sudden Infant Death Syndrome, Risk for
Suffocation, Risk for
Suicide, Risk for
Surgical Recovery, Delayed
Swallowing, Impaired
Therapeutic Regimen Management: Community, Ineffective
Therapeutic Regimen Management, Effective
Therapeutic Regimen Management: Family, Ineffective
Therapeutic Regimen Management, Ineffective
Therapeutic Regimen Management, Readiness for Enhanced
Thermoregulation, Ineffective
Thought Processes, Disturbed
Tissue Integrity, Impaired
Tissue Perfusion, Ineffective (Specify: Cerebral, Cardiopulmonary, Gastrointestinal, Renal)
Tissue Perfusion, Ineffective, Peripheral
Transfer Ability, Impaired
Trauma, Risk for
Unilateral Neglect
Urinary Elimination, Impaired
Urinary Elimination, Readiness for Enhanced
Urinary Incontinence, Functional
Urinary Incontinence, Overflow
Urinary Incontinence, Reflex
Urinary Incontinence, Stress
Urinary Incontinence, Total
Urinary Incontinence, Urge
Urinary Incontinence, Risk for Urge
Urinary Retention
Ventilatory Weaning Response, Dysfunctional
Violence: Other-Directed, Risk for
Violence: Self-Directed, Risk for
Walking, Impaired
Wandering

Source: *Nursing Diagnoses: Definitions and Classification, 2007–2008*, by NANDA International, 2007, Philadelphia, PA: Author. Used with permission.

Index

A
abbreviations
accepted, 487
commonly used, 488*t*
dangerous abbreviations, 807*t*
in medication orders, 808*t*
abdomen
abdominal quadrants and underlying organs, 622*f*, 623*t*
abdominal regions, 623*f*, 623*t*
assessment, 624–629, 634
auscultation, 625
bowel sounds, 626
distension, 624
inspection, 625
landmarks, 624*f*
lifespan considerations, 630
palpation, 627–628
percussion, 626
peritoneal friction rubs, 626
vascular sounds, 626
abdominal breathing, 682, 1332, 1333
abdominal distension, 1234
abdominal thrust, 782
abnormal feces, 1229*t*
abnormal urine, 1273*t*
Aboriginal population, 254
berdache, 1452
colonialism, 261
common causes of death, 261
diabetes, 261
indigenous health-care system, 181
medicine wheel, 119
in nursing, 33
older adults, 348
restorative justice, 261–262
special health concerns, 261–262
suicide, 260
traditional Aboriginal medicine, 274
two-spirited, 1452
wellness, views of, 119
abrasion, 708*t*
absorption, 802
abuse
older adult abuse, 361–362
of women, 336
acceptance, 392
acceptance of pain, 998
accepted terminology and abbreviations, 487
access
electronic access to patient data, 501
to health care, 166–167
to hospitalized patient, 223–225
to information, 215
to literature, 506
accessibility, 11, **153,** 154*t*
accessory muscles of inspiration, 1311
accidental hypothermia, 666
accidents, 762
equipment-related accidents, 783
falls, 100
older adults, 359–360
procedure-related accidents, 783
toddlers, 317
accommodation, 299
accountability, 94–95, **541**
acculturation, 179
accuracy, 487–489
Achilles reflex, 639
acid, 1377
acid-base balance
see also fluid, electrolyte, and acid-base balances
acid-base imbalances, 1387–1388, 1388*t*, 1389*t*
disturbances, 1387–1388
factors affecting, 1376–1380
home care, 1396
regulation of, 1377–1378
acid-base imbalances, 1387–1388, 1388*t*, 1389*t*
acid-fast bacillus (AFB), 1324
acidifying solutions, 1401
acidosis, 1377
acknowledgment of pain, 998
acne, 708*t*
acquired immune deficiency syndrome (AIDS), 18, 1450
acquired immunity, 882–883, 882*t*
acrochordons, 569
action stage, 141
active-assistive ROM exercises, 1147
active immunity, 882
active involvement, 517–518
active living, 1104
active metabolite, 802
active ROM exercises, 1146
active transport, 1371
activity
see also exercise
and defecation, 1230
exercise and activity interventions. *See* exercise and activity interventions
external factors, 1115
factors affecting, 1114–1115
growth and development, 1114
home care, 1126
immobility, effects of, 1115–1121
and mental health, 1115
mobility problems. *See* mobility problems
normal movement, 1104–1110
nursing health history, 1121
and nutrition, 1114
personal values and attitudes, 1114–1115
physical activity, 1110, 1112
and physical health, 1115
prescribed limitations, 1115
tolerance, 1123–1124
and urinary elimination, 1268
activity-exercise pattern, 426, **1104**
Activity Intolerance (diagnostic label)
fluid, electrolyte, and acid-base balances, 1395
mobility problems, 1124–1125
nutritional status, 1196
respiratory and cardiovascular functions, 1328
sleep deprivation, 1091
activity-related affect, 140
activity theory, 355
activity tolerance, 1110
acts of commission, 765
acts of omission, 765
actual diagnosis, 431
actual loss, 1513
acupressure, 277–278, 1008
acupuncture, 277–278, 1009
acute confusion, 1071, **1072**
Acute Confusion (diagnostic label)
fluid, electrolyte, and acid-base balances, 1395
sensory perception problems, 1066
acute illness, 124
acute pain, 979, 980*t*, 982, 993, 994–996
Acute Pain (diagnostic label), 1040
acute sensory deficits, 1069–1071
acute wound, 928
adaptability, 388
adaptation, 299
adaptation model, 62–63
adaptation of thermal receptors, 969
adaptive coping, 1499
adaptive feeding aids, 1203
adaptive mechanisms, 292, 320
adaptive model, 119
addiction, 1000
additional precautions, 913–914
adequate intake, 1171
adherence, 516
adipose tissue, 1185
adjunctive therapies, 962
administering blood, 1421–1422
administration of medication. *See* medication administration
adolescence (12 to 18 years), 324
see also children
breasts and axillae, assessment of, 622
cognitive development, 326
defecation, 1229
developmental guidelines, 327
ejaculation, 324
gay and lesbian youth, 326
glandular changes, 324–325
health and physical activity, 122
health assessment and promotion, 327, 328
health problems, 326–327
leading causes of death, 326–327
menarche, 324
normal sleep patterns and requirements, 1084
nutrition, 1179
oral hygiene, 731
physical development, 324–325
physical growth, 324
psychosocial development, 325–326
puberty, 322, 324
safety measures, 770, 771–772
self-esteem, enhancement of, 1441
self-esteem, influences on, 1435
sex education, 1460–1463
sexual characteristics, 325
sexuality, 1449–1450
spiritual development, 326
suicide, 327
adolescent growth spurt, 324
adornments, 388–389
adults
apical pulse, 674*f*
computer use, 505
criteria for adulthood, 334
health and physical activity, 122
immunization schedules, 911*t*
middle-aged adults, 338–342
normal sleep patterns and requirements, 1084–1085
older adults. *See* older adults
oral hygiene, 731
self-esteem, enhancement of, 1441–1442
sexuality, 1450–1451
young adults, 334–338
advance directives, 1520–1522, 1521*f*
Advanced Nursing Practice: A National Framework (CNA), 94
adventitious breath sounds, 603*t*, **609, 1321**
adverse effects, 799
adverse event reporting, 103–104
adverse events, 763
advertising, and nutrition, 1175–1176
advocacy, 84–85, 240
aerobic exercise, 1111
aerosol spray, 858
aerosolization, 868
afebrile, 664
affective dimensions, 371
affective domain, 517
affective learning, 532
affective responses, 992

Affective subscale, 992
afterload, 1315
age
  and acid-base balance, 1378
  average daily urine output by age, 1269*t*
  and blood pressure, 687
  and body fluid, 1378
  and body temperature, 663
  and client education, 520
  and electrolytes, 1378
  and grief and loss, 1515
  pain, experience of, 987*t*
  and pulse rate, 672
  and safety, 764
  skin alterations, 707*t*
  surgical risk and, 1019
age-appropriate sexual expression, 1449
age of consent, 98
ageism, 349
agency fires, 773
agent, 120
agent-host-environment model, 120
agglutinins, 1417
agglutinogens, 1415
aggression, 1495
aging
  see also older adults
  attitudes toward, 349
  biological theories, 350*t*, 351
  and cognitive abilities, 357
  immune responses, 888
  medication administration and effectiveness, 818
  myths and realities of, 349*t*
  normal physical changes, 351*t*
  physiological aging, 351–355
  of population, 167
  and pressure ulcers, 931–932
  psychological aging, 355–357
agnostic, 1473
agonist, 802
agonist-antagonist analgesic, 999
agricultural injuries, 258
agriculture, 253, 256
air pollution, 1318
airborne precautions, 913, 914
airborne transmission, 886
alarm reaction (AR), 1491–1492
Alberta District Nursing Service, 5
Alberta Foundation for Nursing Research (AFNR), 40
Alberta nursing research, 40–41
albinism, 564
albumin, 942, 1193–1194
alcohol
  alcoholism, and middle-aged adults, 341
  and defecation, 1230
  and health-related problems, 260
  and nutrition, 1174–1175
  preoperative phase, 1022
  and sleep, 1086
alcohol-based hand rubs, 894, 1234
algor mortis, 1534
alignment, 1104–1105, 1114–1115
alkalinizing solution, 1401
alkalis, 1377
alkalosis, 1377
Allen, Moyra, 41, 66–67
allergies
  allergic responses, mild, 800*t*
  allergic wheal, 565*f*
  common food allergens, 1201
  drug allergy, 800
  food allergies, 1201
  intradermal injection for skin tests, 836–837
  preoperative phase, 1022
allodynia, 982
alopecia, 570
altered breathing patterns, 684, 1320–1321
altered nutrition, 1185–1186
Altered Oral Mucous Membrane (diagnostic label), 729, 730*t*
altered sexual function, 1463–1465
altered urinary elimination, 1269–1271
altered urine production, 1269
alternative care providers, 164, 164*t*
alternative health. *See* complementary and alternative health modalities
alternative medical systems
  Ayurveda, 273–274
  homeopathy, 274
  naturopathic medicine, 274
  traditional Aboriginal medicine, 274
  traditional Chinese medicine (TCM), 274
alternative medicine, 271
  see also complementary and alternative health modalities; complementary medicine
  balance, 272
  basic concepts, 272–273
  energy, 272
  healing environments, 272
  holism, 272
  humanism, 272
  spirituality, 272
altitude, 1318
alveolar gas exchange, 1311
alveolar hyperventilation, 1320–1321
Alzheimer's disease, 361
ambiguity, tolerance for, 378–379
amblyopia, 317
ambulation, 1041–1042, **1147**–**1152**
American Nurses Association, 415
amino acids, 1168
ammonia dermatitis, 708*t*
ampule, 829–**832**
anabolism, 1119, 1166
anaerobic exercise, 1111
anaesthesia, 650, 1032–1033, 1231
anal canal, 1227, 1228*f*
anal intercourse, 1454
anal phase, 316
anal sphincters, 1227, 1228, 1228*f*
analgesics, 999–1007
analysis, 433–434
anaphylactic reaction, 800
anaphylaxis, 1201
anatomical barriers, 880–881
Anderson frame, 750
andragogy, 516
andropause, 339, **1450**–1451
anemia, 1317
aneroid sphygmomanometer, 688, 690*f*
anger, 1495–1496
anger mediation, 1504–1506
angina pectoris, 1322
angiography, 1327–1328
angiotensin-converting enzyme (ACE) inhibitors, 1333
angle of Louis, 601
anilingus, 1454
animal-assisted therapy, 283
anions, 1369
anisocoria, 582
ankle flares, 934
ankle muscles, 632
ankle restraints, 788
anorexia, 1119, 1174
anorexia nervosa, 1179
anoscopy, 1236
antagonist, 802
anterior approach, 598
anterior axillary lines, 600
anterior ribs, 601*f*
anterior thorax, 607–608
anthropometric measurements, 1189–1193
antianxiety medications, 1097
antibiotic enemas, 1248
antibiotics, 1029
  IV antibiotics, 855–856
  and susceptibility to infection, 888
  systematic antibiotics, 939–940
antibodies, 882–883, **1417**
antibody-mediated defences, 882–883
anticholinergics, 1029
Anticipatory Grieving (diagnostic label)
  preoperative phase, 1022
  self-concept, 1440
anticipatory loss, 1513
anticoagulants, 1019
antidepressants, 1020
antidiarrheal medications, 1246, 1247
antidiuretic hormone (ADH), 1373–1374
antiembolism stockings, 1030–1032, 1358–1359
antiflatulent medications, 1246
antigens, 882, 1413
antigravity muscles, 1104
antihelix, 582–583
antihelmintic enemas, 1248
antihypertensive medications, 804, 1020
antimicrobial agents, 892
antiplatelet agents, 1020
antiseptic, 891, 891*t*, **892**
anuria, 1269
anus
  assessment of, 654–656, 658
  lifespan considerations, 656
anvil (ear), 583
anxiety, 1494
  antianxiety medications, 1097
  generalized anxiety, 1475
  levels of, 1494–1495, 1495*t*
  minimization of, 1504, 1505
  panic, 1494
  reducing, 998
  and sleep, 1085–1086
  and stress, 1494–1495
Anxiety (diagnostic label)
  fecal elimination, 1240
  pain, 993
  preoperative phase, 1021
  respiratory and cardiovascular functions, 1328
  self-concept, 1440
  sexual health status, 1459
  stress and coping patterns, 1500
  wounds, 946
aorta, 1315
aortic valve, 1313
apex, 611
apgar, 313, 314*t*
aphasia, 635
apical pulse, 672, 674*f*, 678–680
apical-radial pulse, 680–681
apnea, 683, 684, **1320**
apocrine glands, 324, 705
apothecaries' system, 811
appearance, 561–563
appendicitis, 881
appetite stimulation, 1202
applied research, 39
appropriateness of information, 489
aquamatic pad, 971
aquathermia pad, 971
aromatherapy, 275–276
arousal mechanisms, 1061, 1068
arrhythmia, 675
art therapy, 279
arterial adequacy test, 616
arterial blood gases (ABGs), 1327, **1394**–1395, 1396
arterial circulation, 1316
arterial disease, 936
arteries, 1315
arterioles, 1315
arthritis, 256
artificial airways, 1343–1349
artificial eyes (prosthesis), 745–746
artificial nutrition and hydration (ANH), 1522
artificial teeth, 731, 733–734
ascending colostomy, 1234–1235
ascultatory method, 691
asepsis, 871, **878**
aseptic technique, 898–899
Asepto syringe, 872
asphyxiation, 782
assault, 101
assertive communication, 407
assessing, 417
  see also assessment; assessment skills
  breastfeeding self-efficacy scale, 464
  cardiovascular functions, 1323–1328
  communication, 402–404
  data collection, 417–423
  described, 417
  documentation of data, 429
  educator, nurse as, 520–523

eye care, 743–744
fecal elimination, 1236–1238
fluid, electrolyte, and acid-base balances, 1388–1395
foot care, 721–722
general appearance and mental status, 561–563
immobility, 1124, 1124*t*
infection prevention and control, 917–918
intraoperative phase, 1033
loss, 1516
mobility problems, 1121–1124
nail hygiene, 726
nursing care plan, modification of, 461
nutritional status, 1186–1196
oral hygiene, 728–729
organization of data, 426–428
overview, 416*t*
pain, 988–993
patient safety, 766–768
postoperative phase, 1036–1039
preoperative phase, 1021
pressure sites, 941
pressure ulcers, 942
respiratory functions, 1323–1328
self-concept, 1436–1439
sensory perception problems, 1064–1066
sexual health status, 1456–1459
skin hygiene, 705–707
skin integrity, 928, 940
sleep, 1089–1091
spiritual health, 1478–1479
stress and coping patterns, 1499–1500
surgical wounds, 1046
tube feedings, 1216*t*
urinary elimination, 1271–1278
validation of data, 428–429, 428*t*
wounds, 940–945

assessment
see also assessing; examination; physical assessment
adolescence, 327, 328
complementary and alternative health modalities, use of, 283
cultural assessment, 191
emergency assessment, 417*t*
family assessment guide, 219
health of individuals, 143–144
home assessment parameters, 247
of individual health, 201–204
infants, 313–314
initial assessment, 417*t*
middle-aged adults, 341–342
neonates, 313–314
older adult abuse, 361–362
older adults, 358–359
preschoolers, 321
problem-focused assessment, 417*t*
reassessment, 457
risk assessment, 203–204
school-age children, 323–324
term, use of, 552
time-lapsed assessment, 417*t*
toddlers, 317, 318
transition of active dying, 1524–1525
types of, 417*t*
urine, 1271–1274
validation of assessment data, 144
vital signs. *See* vital signs
young adults, 337–338

assessment skills
abdomen, 624–629
anus, 654–656
apical pulse, 678–680
apical-radial pulse, 680–681
blood pressure, 692–695
body temperature, 669–671
breasts and axillae, 618–621
ears and hearing, 583–586
eye structures and visual acuity, 576–581
female genitals, 646–647
general appearance and mental status, 561–562
hair, 569–570
heart and central vessels, 612–615
inguinal lymph nodes, 646–647
male genitals, 651–653
mouth and oropharynx, 590–593
musculoskeletal system, 631–633
nails, 571–572
neck, 596–599
neurological system, 637–646
nose and sinuses, 588–589
oxygen saturation, 697–698
peripheral pulse, 675–678
peripheral vascular system, 615–617
rectum, 654–656
respiration, 684–685
skin, 566–568
skull and face, 573
thorax and lungs, 603–608

assimilation, 179, 299
assistance, need for, 457
assisted living centres, 162
assisting client to sit on side of bed, 1139–1140
assisting clients to ambulate, 1149–1152
assisting patients with meals, 1202–1204
Associated Professional Sleep Society, 1081
Association of College Honor Societies, 20
assumptions, 56, 374, 1474
Astanga yoga, 280
asthma, 1317
astigmatism, 574
asymptomatic infection, 884
at-risk aggregate, 143
atelectasis, 1037*t*, **1041,** 1119, **1311**
atheist, 1473
atherosclerosis, 1317
atomization, 868
atomizer, 868
atria, 1313
atrial natriuretic factor (ANF), 1374
atrioventricular (AV) node, 1314
atrioventricular values, 1313
atrophie blanche, 934
atrophy, 566*t*, **1116**
attention span and calculation, 637–646
attentive listening, 392–393
attitudes, 74
and body alignment and activity, 1114–1115
and communication, 392
and critical thinking, 377–379
that foster critical thinking, 371–374
toward aging, 349
attributes of professional caring, 67
audit, 463, 472
auditory aphasia, 635–636
auditory distraction, 1008
auditory stimuli, 1061
auricle, 582
auscultation, 561
auscultatory gap, 691
authoritarian leader, 538
authority, 541
autoantigen, 882
autocratic leaders, 538
autolytic debridement, 951
automated dispensing cabinet (ADC), 814
autonomic nervous system, 662
autonomous level, 300
autonomy, 16, **79, 124**
autonomy *versus* shame and doubt, 1432*t*
autopsy, 1524
awareness, 1061, 1062*t*
awareness of persons, 634
axillary crutch, 1154
axillary tail of Spence, 634
axillary temperature, 666*t*, 667, 671
Ayurveda, 273–274

B

Babinski reflex, 311, 639
baby boomers, 333, 542
baccalaureate nursing degrees, 16, **27,** 28–29, 32
bachelor of nursing (BN), 29
bachelor of science in nursing (BScN, BSN), 29
back injury, 1130
back massage, 1095–1096
bacteremia, 879, 884
bacteria, 880
bactericidal, 705
bactericidal preparation, 891
bacteriostatic preparation, 891
bag bath, 711
bagging, 914–915
balance, 272
ball-and-socket joint, 1106*t*, 1108*t*
bandages, 962, **963**–965, 967
Bandura, Albert, 300, 516
barbiturate sedative-hypnotics, 1097
barium enema, 1236
barium swallow, 1236
barrel chest, 602*f*, 1317
barriers to communication, 395, 396*t*
Bartholin's gland, 649*f*, 657
basal metabolic rate (BMR), 662, 1171
basal metabolism, 1119
base, 611, 1377
base of support, 1104
basic needs, 205–206
basic research, 39
basic three-part statements, 438
basic two-part statements, 438
bath grab bar, 718
bathing, 706, 710–717, 972
battery, 97, 101
Beale Code Approach, 253
beard care, 742
Beau's lines, 571
bed, moving clients in, 1134–1146
bed bath, 713–716
bed boards, 1130, 1131
bed cradles, 750
bed exit safety monitoring device, 777–779
bed-making, 750–757
bed rest, 1115
bedclothes, 1039
bedpan, 1243, 1244–1245, 1244*f*
bedside data entry, 496–497
bedtime rituals, 1094
behaviour
general behaviour, 561–563
health-seeking behaviours, 525
moral behaviour, 300
resistive behaviours, 398–399
behaviour change
enhancement of, 146, 147
harm reduction, 146–147
implementation, 145–147
stages, 141–143, 142*f*
behaviour modification, 531
behaviour-specific cognitions and affect, 139–141
behavioural effect questions, 223
behaviourism, 516
behaviourist theory, 300
behaviourists, 538
being present, 1480–1481
belching, 1234
beliefs, 74, 1474
about dress, 1478
about food, 1173
diet and nutrition, 1477–1478
related to birth, 1478
related to dying, 1478
spiritual beliefs, 1515–1516
belt restraints, 785, 786, 787
beneficence, 50, 80
Benner and Wrubel's primacy of caring, 384
Benner's stages of nursing expertise, 17
berdache, 1452
best practices, 94–95
bevel, 827
bibliographic systems and databases, 506
bicarbonate (HCO_3^-), 1376–1377
biceps, 631
biceps reflex, 638
bicultural, 179
bicuspid valve, 1313
Bier block, 1033
bilirubin, 1228
binders, 962–963, 965–967
biofeedback, 281
biohazard infectious materials, 915*f*
biolelectromagnetic therapies, 279
biological rhythms, 1081

biological system, 207
biological theories of aging, 350*t*, 351
biologically based treatments
  aromatherapy, 275–276
  dietary therapy, 276
  herbal medicine, 274–275
  herbal therapy, 274
  orthomolecular medicine, 276–277
biomedical health belief, 184
biophysical theory, 292
bioterrorism, 766, 767–768
biotransformation, 802
Biot's (cluster) respiration, 1321
birth, beliefs about, 1478
bisexuals
  closeted, 1450
  health experiences of, 1447–1448
black eye, 575
black wounds, 951
bladder, 629, 1265
bladder irrigation, 1298–1300
bladder training, 1285–1286
blanch test, 572
blended-mode learning, 264
blood, 1316–1317, 1421–1422
blood alterations, 1322–1323
blood area nitrogen (BUN), 1278
blood-borne pathogens, 921, 947
blood clots, 934–935
blood coagulation studies, 942
blood donors, 1421
blood flow, 910
blood glucose, measurement of, 1194–1195
blood groups, 1413–1417
blood pressure, 686, 1316
  ascultatory method, 691
  assessment of, 688–691, 692–695
  cardiac output, 686
  common errors in assessment, 692, 692*t*
  determinants of, 686
  diastolic pressure, 686
  direct (invasive monitoring) measurement, 691
  equipment, 688–690, 915
  factors affecting blood pressure, 687
  home care, 696
  hypertension, 688, 689*f*
  hypotension, 688
  Korotkoff's sounds, 691, 692
  lifespan considerations, 695–696
  maintaining a healthy blood pressure, 687
  mean arterial pressure (MAP), 1316
  measurement of, 686
  methods of measurement, 691
  noninvasive indirect methods, 691, 695
  palpatory method, 691, 694
  pulse pressure, 686
  sites, 690
  systemic vascular resistance (SVR), 686
  systolic pressure, 686
  thigh blood pressure, 690, 694–695
  white coat effect, 687
blood pressure cuff, 688, 689*f*, 690, 690*f*
blood products, 1421
blood tests, 1193–1196, 1325–1327
blood transfusions
  administering blood, 1421–1422
  blood donors, 1421
  blood groups, 1413–1417
  blood products, 1420*t*, 1421
  blood typing, 1418–1421
  crossmatching, 1418–1421
  described, 1413
  initiating, maintaining, and terminating a blood transfusion by using a Y-set, 1422–1424
  rhesus (Rh) factor, 1417
  transfusion reactions, 1420*t*, 1421
blood typing, 1418–1421
blood vessels, 1315–1316, 1316*f*, 1317, 1318
blood volume, 1322–1323
blue pigtail, 1204
body alignment, 1114–1115, 1122
body-based therapies. *See* manipulative and body-based therapies
body defences against infection
  imbalance between microorganisms and, 884
  impairment of, 886
  nonspecific defences, 880–882
  specific defences, 880, 882–883
  support defences of susceptible host, 909–911
body fluids
  see also fluid, electrolyte, and acid-base balances
  active transport, 1371
  balance, 1379
  components, 1368
  composition of, 1368–1370
  dehydration, 1381
  described, 1368
  diffusion, 1370–1371
  distribution of, 1368
  disturbances, 1380–1382
  edema, 1381
  enteral fluid and electrolyte replacement, 1396
  extracellular fluid (ICF), 1368
  factors affecting, 1376–1380
  filtration, 1371
  fluid imbalances, 1380–1382
  fluid intake, 1372
  fluid output, 1372–1373
  fluid volume deficit (FVD), 1380
  fluid volume excess (FVE), 1381
  fluid volume gains *vs.* losses, 1382*t*
  home care, 1396
  homeostasis, maintenance of, 1373–1374
  interstitial fluid, 1368
  intracellular fluid (ICF), 1368
  intravascular fluid, 1368
  lifespan considerations, 1379
  movement of, 1370–1371
  osmosis, 1370
  overhydration, 1382
  plasma, 1368
  regulation of, 1371–1374
  third space syndrome, 1380–1381
  total body fluid, 1368, 1368*f*
  transcellular fluid, 1368
body heat, and pressure ulcers, 931
body image, 1433–1434, 1438
body language, 388–390
body mass index (BMI), 563–564, **1185,** 1190–1191, 1192*t*
body mass index nomogram, 1191*t*
body mechanics, 1127–1129
body odour, 564, 710
body piercings, 118
body position. *See* positioning
body posture, 187
body preoccupation, 296–297
body substance, 912
body substance isolation (BSI), 912
body systems model, 427
body temperature, 662
  alterations in, 664–666, 664*f*
  assessment of, 666–671, 666*t*
  axillary temperature, 666*t*, 667, 671
  core temperature, 662
  estimated ranges, 662*f*
  factors affecting, 663–664
  home care, 669
  hypothermia, 665–666
  infrared thermometers, 667
  lifespan considerations, 671–672
  oral temperature, 666*t*, 670
  pyrexia, 664–665
  range of oral temperatures, 663*f*
  rectal temperature, 666–667, 666*t*, 670
  regulation of, 663
  skin temperature, testing, 559
  surface temperature, 662
  temperature scales, 669
  temperature sensation, 644
  temporal artery, 666*t*, 671
  tympanic membrane, 666*t*, 667, 671
  types of thermometers, 667–669
body transcendence, 296–297
body weight classification, 1192*t*
boiling water, 891
bolus dose, 1005
bone-conducted sound transmission, 583
bones, assessment of, 632
boomerang kids, 334
Borg scale of perceived exertion, 1111
bottle-mouth syndrome, 1177
bottle with drip chamber, 1213
boundary, 206
bowel diversion ostomies, 1234–1236
bowel incontinence, 1233–1234
Bowel Incontinence (diagnostic label), 1238
bowel movement. *See* defecation
bowel sounds, 626
bowel training programs, 1252
Bowman's capsule, 1264
brachial pulse, 673
bracing, 1008
Braden scale, 935*f*
bradycardia, 675, 684
bradypnea, 683, 1320
brand name, 796
breach of standard of care, 99
breast awareness, 1462, 1464
breast bud, 325
breast examination, 1462
breast milk, 1176
breast palpation, 620–621
breastfeeding self-efficacy scale, 464
breasts and axillae
  assessment of, 618–621, 633–634
  lifespan considerations, 621–622
breath sounds
  adventitious, 603*t*, 609
  altered breathing patterns and sounds, 684
  importance of, 683
  normal, 602*t*
breathing. *See* respiration
breathing needs, 1531–1532
brevity, 388
British North America Act, 153, 177
British Pharmacopoeia, 798
brokerage management model, 246
bromhidrosis, 564
bronchial tree, 1310
bronchial (tubular) breath sounds, 602*t*
bronchodilators, 1333
bronchoscopy, 1328
bronchovesicular breath sounds, 602*t*
Bronfenbrenner, Urie, 300
bruit, 622
brushing teeth, 731–734
bubbling sounds, 684
buccal, 804
buccal mucosa, 591
budget, 508
Buerger's test, 616
buffers, 1377
Building a Safer System (Leonard and NSCPS), 763
Building on Values (Romanow), 237, 499
bulbar conjunctiva, 576
bulimia nervosa, 1179
bulla, 565*f*
bullous pemphigoid, 565*f*
bundle branches, 1314
bundle of His, 1314
burden of proof, 103
bureaucratic leader, 539
burn, 773
burnout, 1507
butterfly needles, 1406

C

café-au-lait macules, 565*f*
caffeine
  and defecation, 1230
  and young adults, 337
calcium balance, 1119
calcium (CA^2), 1376, 1385
calcium channel blockers, 1333
callus, 721
caloric theory approach, 1171
caloric value, 1171
calorie, 1171
Campbell, Margaret, 65
Canada

cultural mosaic, 174–178
demographic profile, 174–175
families in, 215–218
health-care system. *See* health-care system
health in Canada, 125
health promotion, 135–136, 147–148
health-promotion initiatives in, 132–136
language, 175–176
life expectancy, 348
multicultural policy, 176–178
nursing history, 19
population density per square kilometre, 199
religion, 176
visible minorities, 176
Canada Act, 177
Canada Health Act
criteria, 153, 154*t*, 166
federal cost sharing, 153
passage of, 132
standards, 11
Canada Health Infoway, 499, 502
Canada's Food Guide. See Eating Well with Canada's Food Guide
Canadian Adverse Events Study, 765, 766, 813
Canadian Army Medical Corps (CAMC), 6
Canadian Association of Schools of Nursing (CASN), 13, 27, 31, 94
Canadian Association of Wound Care, 958
Canadian Association of Wound Care Quick Reference Guide, 930
Canadian Bill of Rights, 177
Canadian Cancer Society, 554
Canadian Charter of Rights and Freedoms, 177
Canadian Classification of Health Interventions (CCI), 500
Canadian Council on Health Services Accreditation (CCHSA), 166, 463, 766, 813
Canadian Diabetes Association, 1201
Canadian Federation of Nurses Unions (CFNU), 21
Canadian Food and Drugs Act, 797–798
Canadian Formulary, 798
Canadian Health Services Research Foundation (CHSRF), 40, 41
Canadian Hospice Palliative Care Association (CHPCA), 1529
Canadian Immunization Guide, 920
Canadian Institute for Health Information (CIHI), 500
Canadian Institutes of Health Research (CIHR), 40–41
Canadian Narcotic Control Act, 798
Canadian Nosocomial Infection Surveillance Program, 879
Canadian Nurse, 19, 46
Canadian Nurses Association (CNA)
certification, 30–31, 94
Code of Ethics for Registered Nurses. See CNA *Code of Ethics for Registered Nurses*
critical thinking, importance of, 377
described, 19
e-nursing strategy, 497
education, influence on, 30–31
electronic health record, benefits of, 500
entry-to-practice credential, 32
evidence-based decision-making, 503
framework, 11
funding for CNKN, 41
and health-care reform, 236
legal frameworks, 13
NurseONE, 46
nursing practice, description of, 9
nursing process, fundamental role of, 415
palliative care, 1529
and regulation of nurses, 94
safe practice, 34
Toward 2020: Visions for Nursing (CNA), 536
vision for change, 547
Canadian Nursing Knowledge Network (CNKN), 41
Canadian Nursing Students' Association (CNSA), 31
Canadian Patient Safety Dictionary, 763
Canadian Patient Safety Institute, 166, 813
Canadian Patient Safety Institute (CPSI), 763
Canadian Red Cross Society, 6
Canadian Registered Nurse Examination (CRNE), 27
Canadian Research Information Database, 46
Canadian Sleep Society, 1081
Canadian Triage and Acuity Scale, 158
cancer
early detection and screening guidelines, 554–555
leading causes of cancer morbidity, 336
middle-aged adults, 341
older adults, 362
pain, 982
in rural areas, 257
second-leading cause of death, 327
testicular cancer, 658
and young adults, 336–337
canes, 1152–1153
cannula, 827, 1338–1339
capacity, 97
capillary beds, 1315
capillary blood specimen to measure blood glucose, 1194–1195
capillary refill test, 616
capsules, 820
carative factors, 63
carbaminohemoglobin, 1312
carbohydrates, 1167–1168
carbon dioxide, 1311–1312
carbon monoxide, 782
carbon monoxide poisoning, 782
carbonic acid, 1312
cardiac arrest, 1360
cardiac conduction system, 1314–1315
cardiac cycle, 1315
cardiac disease, 360
cardiac monitoring, 1327–1328
cardiac nursing interventions, 1332
cardiac output, 672, 686, **1312,** 1314–1315, 1318, 1321–1322
cardiac veins, 1314
cardiopulmonary resuscitation (CPR), 1360
cardiovascular alterations, 1321–1323
cardiovascular changes, and aging, 354
cardiovascular complications, 122
cardiovascular disease (CD), 341, 1317
cardiovascular functions
assessing, 1323–1328
blood alterations, 1322–1323
cardiac monitoring, 1327–1328
cardiovascular alterations, 1321–1323
decreased cardiac output, 1321–1322
diagnosing, 1328
diagnostic studies, 1324–1327
environment, 1318
evaluating, 1360–1361, 1361*t*
factors affecting, 1317–1320
and gender, 1320
health status, 1319
impaired tissue perfusion, 1322
implementation. *See* oxygenation and circulation interventions
interview, 1323
lifespan considerations, 1317–1318
lifestyle, 1318–1319
nursing health history, 1323
pharmacological agents, 1319
physical assessment, 1324
planning, 1328–1330
specimens, 1324–1325
stress and coping, 1319
visualization procedures, 1327–1328
cardiovascular system
assessment of, 610–622
blood, 1316–1317
blood vessels, 1315–1316
cardiac conduction system, 1314–1315
central vessels, 612–615
coronary arteries, 1314
coronary circulation, 1314
exercise, benefits of, 1113
heart, 610–622, 1313–1314, 1313*f*, 1314*f*, 1316*f*
immobility, effects of, 1117–1118
physiology of the cardiovascular system, 1312–1317
care plans
nursing care plans. *See* nursing care plans
problem-oriented medical record (POMR), 475
sample care plans. *See* sample care plan
care settings
assisted living centres, 162
community health centres, 160
crisis centres, 163
daycare centres, 163
described, 158–159
extended-care (continuing-care) facilities, 162
general or specialist clinics, 161
home care, 160
hospice palliative care services, 163
hospitals, 161–162
lodges, 162
mutual support groups, 163
occupational health clinics, 161
for older adults, 350
patient safety, 765–766, 772–773
physicians' offices, 160–161
public health services, 159–160
rehabilitation centres, 162–163
retirement homes, 162
rural primary care, 163
self-help groups, 163
telehealth, 163
caregiver
perceptions of unsupportive interactions with others, 43
role of, 14, 240
caregiver burden, 1499
caregiver electronic record (CER), 502
Caregiver Role Strain (diagnostic label), 1500
caries, 317, **594**
see also dental caries
caring, 384
cultural care diversity and universality theory, 65, 384
for the dying, 10
and emotional closeness, 392
as essence of nursing, 9
human mode of being, 384
primacy of caring, 384
six Cs of caring in nursing, 385
theory of human care, 384
caring-healing health model, 64
caring moment, 64
caring theories, 79
caritas, 63
carminative enema, 1248
CARNA *Nursing Practice Standards,* 13
carotid arteries, 613–614, 622
carotid pulse, 673
carrier, 884
carrying out a physician's orders, 106–107
case law, 91
case management, 168
computer applications, use of, 505
models of, 246
case management model, 479–480
case managers, 168, 241
case method, 169
catabolism, 1119, 1166
cataracts, 353, 575
category-specific isolation precautions, 911
catharctics, 1245
catheter irrigations, 1298, 1393
catheters, 1289–1297, 1349, 1401–1402, 1405–1406
see also indwelling catheter
cations, 1368
causation, 99
ceiling dose, 999
ceiling effect, 999
cell-mediated defences, 883
cellular immunity, 883
cellular response, 881
cementum, 727
census rural area, 253
Centers for Disease Control and Prevention (CDC), 911

central apnea, 1088
central neuropathic pain, 980
central sensitization, 985
central venous catheter, 1401
central vessels
assessment of, 612–615, 622–630
lifespan considerations, 615
centre of gravity, 1104
centring, 272, 279
cephalocaudal growth, 291, **423**
cerebellum, 650
certification, 30–31, **94**
cerumen, 583
chain of infection
breaking the chain. *See* infection prevention and control
described, 884*f*
direct contact transmission, 886
etiological agent, 885
importance of framework, 884
portal of entry to the host, 886
portal of exit from reservoir, 885, 885*t*
reservoir, 885
reservoirs, 885*t*
route of transmission, 885–886
susceptibility of the host, 886–888
chains, 599
chair beds, 1131
chair exit safety monitoring device, 777–779
chairperson, 400
chairs
getting into, 1157–1158
getting out of, 1158
change, 544
change management models, 545–547
covert change, 545
developmental change, 545
driving forces, 546
Kotter's eight-step change process, 545–546
Lewin's theory of change, 545
overt change, 545
planned change, 545
Prochaska's transtheoretical model, 545
Quinn's theory of change, 545
resistance, dealing with, 546
restraining forces, 546
types of, 545
unplanned change, 545
vision for change, 547
change agent, 14, **544**–545
change management models, 545–547
change-of-shift report, 490
changing beds, 751–755
charismatic leadership, 539
chart, 470
charting, 470
charting by exception (CBE), 477–478
cheilosis, 729*t*
chemical agents, 881
chemical contaminants, 257
chemical debridement, 951
chemical dependency, problematic, 105
chemical disposable thermometers, 668, 668*f*
chemical name, 796
chemical restraints, 784
chemical thermogenesis, 662
chemoreceptors, 1312
chemotaxis, 881
Chess, Stella, 296, 297*t*
chest circumference, 309–310
chest deformities, 602*f*
chest landmarks, 599–601, 600*f*
chest movements, 684
chest shape and size, 601–609
chest tubes, 1356–1358
Cheyne-Stokes respiration, 684, **1321**
child abuse, 313
child safety restraint systems, 138
children
see also adolescence (12 to 18 years); infants (birth to 1 year); preschoolers (4 to 5 years); school-age children (6 to 12 years); toddlers (1 to 3 years)
abdomen, assessment of, 630
antiembolism stockings, 1032
anus, assessment of, 656
apical pulse, 674*f*
assisting clients to ambulate, 1152
bandages and binders, application of, 967
blood pressure, 695–696
body temperature, 672
catheterization, 1295
client education, 522
computer use, 505
dosages for, 812
ears and hearing, assessment of, 587
enema, administering, 1250
eyes and vision, assessment of, 582
female genitals, assessment of, 648
fluid and electrolyte balance, 1379
general survey, 562
and grief and loss, 1515
hair, assessment of, 570
health and physical activity, 122
health-care decisions, 376
health promotion, 148
heart and central vessels, assessment of, 615
home support following surgery, 502
illness prevention, 148
immunization schedules, 910*t*
infections, 887
inguinal lymph nodes, assessment of, 648
intradermal injections, 838
intramuscular injection, 848
male genitals and inguinal area, assessment of, 654
mask making, 279
medication administration, 816
metered-dose inhalers and nebulizers, 871
musculoskeletal system, assessment of, 633
nails, assessment of, 572
nasogastric tube, insertion of, 1208
neck, assessment of, 599
neurological system, assessment of, 645
normal sleep patterns and requirements, 1083–1084
ophthalmic instillations, 861
oral medications, administration of, 823
otic medications, 864
oxygen delivery equipment, 1341
oxygen saturation, 699
pain management, 1011
patient-controlled analgesia (PCA) pump, 1006
peripheral vascular system, assessment of, 617
positioning, moving, and turning clients, 1141
postoperative care, 1035–1036
preoperative teaching, 1027
pressure ulcers, 961
pulse, assessment of, 681
rectal medications, 868
rectum, assessment of, 656
respiration, 685
restraints, 789
safe play areas, in rural areas, 258–259
safety hazards, 764
seizure precautions, 780
self-esteem, enhancement of, 1441
and sexuality, 1449
skin, assessment of, 568
sputum and throat specimens, 1325
stress and coping, 1491
suctioning a tracheostomy or endotracheal tube, 1356
teaching tools for, 529
thorax and lungs, assessment of, 609
tube feeding, administering, 1216
urinary elimination, 1267
wound care, 961
chill phase, 664, 665
chiropractic therapy, 277
chlamydia, 1458
chloride (CL$^-$), 1376, 1386
CHNET-Works!, 505
choking, 782
cholesterol tests, 1194
CHPCN(C) (Certified in Hospice and Palliative Care Nursing (Canada)), 157
chronic cardiac pain, 1001
chronic confusion, 1072
Chronic Confusion (diagnostic label), 1066
chronic constipation, 1232
chronic diarrhea, 1251
chronic illness, 124
barriers to health care, 166
older adults, 360
and pressure ulcers, 932
Chronic Low Self-Esteem (diagnostic label), 1439
chronic obstructive pulmonary disease (COPD), 1317
chronic pain, 979–980, 980*t*, 982, 988, 993, 1453
chronic pustular psoriasis, 565*f*
chronic wound, 928
chronological age, 348
chyme, 1226
cicatrix, 882
circadian rhythms, 663, **1081**
circular turns, 964
circulating immunity, 882–883
circulating nurse, 1034
circulation, 1332
circulation status. *See* cardiovascular functions; oxygenation and circulation interventions
circulatory diseases, 256
circulatory problems, in postoperative phase, 1037*t*
Civil Code, 91
civil law, 91
clapping, 1334
clarity, 388
classical leadership theories, 538–539
classroom technology, 507
clean-catch urine specimens, 1274, 1275–1276
clean-contaminated wounds, 928
clean intermittent self-catheterization (CISC), 1297–1298
clean technique, 898
clean voided urine specimen, 1274
clean wounds, 928
cleaning, 889–891
cleansing baths, 711–712
cleansing enemas, 1246–1248
cleansing wounds, 945, 958–961
clear liquid diet, 1200, 1201
clear reasoning, 373
client, 9
see also patient
family unit as the client of care, 213
goals, 445–447
illness, impact of, 124
immunocompromised clients, 914
inpatient, 158
meaning of, 10
outpatient, 158
person in the context of the family, 213
preparation, for health assessment, 553–555
as primary source of data, 419
use of term, 198
client advocate, 14
Client-Centred Best Practice Guidelines Program (RNAO), 74
client-centred care, 198
see also individual care
client-centred model, 246
client contracting, 530
client data, 417–418
client education, 514
see also learning; teaching
age of client, 520
assessing, 520–523
children, 522
client support system, 521
client's understanding of health problems, 520
cultural practices, 520
diagnosing, 524–525
documenting, 532
economic factors, 520
evaluating, 531–532
health beliefs, 520
health literacy, 523
implementing interventions, 529–531
learning, 516–520
learning style, 520–521
lifespan considerations, 522

motivation, 522–523
nurse as educator, 520–532
nursing health history, 520–521
older adults, 522
physical examination, 521
planning, 525–528
readiness to learn, 521–522
reading level, 523
teaching, 515
client health outcomes, 429
client records, 470
see also documenting
accountability for, 472
auditing for quality assurance, 472
communication, 472
confidentiality of electronic health records, 471–472
as data source, 419
education and research, 472
ethical and legal considerations, 471–472
planning and continuity of client care, 472
purposes of, 472
recording guidelines, 486–489
clients' rights, 154
climacteric, 339
climate change, 167
clinical caritas processes, 63
clinical death, impending, 1525
clinical detective tool, 373*t*
clinical model, 119
clinical nurse specialist, 14
clinical record, 470
clinical spectrum of infection, 883–884
clitoris, 1454
clock system, 1203*f*
clogged feeding tubes, 1217–1218
closed awareness, 1524–1525
closed gravity drainage system, 1290
closed method, 907–909, 1298
closed questions, 421
closed surgery, 1018
closed system, 207
closed systems, 1211
closed-wound drainage system, 1050
closed wounds, 928, 1047–1049
clothing, 388–389
clouding of consciousness, 1529
clubbing, 571
cluster respiration, 1321
clustering cues, 436–437
CNA *Code of Ethics for Registered Nurses,* 49, 81, 84, 95, 106, 181, 240, 471
COACH, 500
coanalgesic, 1002
coarse crackles, 603*f*
cochlea, 583
Cochrane Library, 46
code of ethics, 16, **78,** 81
Code of Ethics for Registered Nurses (CNA), 49
cognitive, 516
cognitive abilities
and aging, 357
immobility and, 1121
cognitive awareness, and safety, 764
cognitive-behavioural interventions, 1009
cognitive development, 299
adolescence, 326
middle-aged adults, 340
neonates and infants, 312
preschoolers, 320
school-age children, 322–323
toddlers, 316
young adults, 335
cognitive domain, 517
cognitive impairments, 403
cognitive indicators of stress, 1496
cognitive-perceptual pattern, 426
cognitive skills, 456
cognitive theory, 299–300, **517**
cognitivism, 517
coitus, 1454
cold applications. *See* heat and cold applications
cold environment, 1318
colic, 313
collaboration, 244–246
collaborative care plans, 441–443
collaborative partnership, 244
collaborative problems, 432–433, 433*t*
collaborative relational stance, 222–223
collagen, 936
College and Association of Registered Nurses of Alberta (CARNA), 92
College of Nurses of Ontario (CNO), 74, 92, 93, 198, 377
College of Registered Nurses of British Columbia (CRNBC), 92, 93–94
colloid osmotic pressure, 1370
colloids, 1370
colloquial prayer, 282
colon, 1226
colonialism, 261
colonization, 179, 883–884, 939–940
colonoscopy, 1236
colostomy, 1234, 1235*f*
colostomy irrigation, 1257–1258
coloured food dye, 1214
coma, 1072, 1529
coma stimulation, 1073
comatose clients. *See* unconscious clients
come out, 1450
comfort, 385
intensity (type) of comfort, 385
measures, 385–386
needs, 385
in postoperative phase, 1036
promoting, for sleep, 1094–1097
comforting, 384
described, 384
process of, 384
commendations, 225–226
commitment, 385
committee members, 400
commode, 1243, 1244*f*
common food allergens, 1201
common law, 91
common-law relationships, 216–217
communicability, 880
communicable disease, 880
communication, 386
among health professionals, 407
assertive communication, 407
assessing, 402–404
barriers, 395, 396*t*
client communication, evaluation of, 405
client records and, 472
and collaboration, 246
congruent communication, 392
diagnosing, 404
education of client and support persons, 405
electronic communication, 390
evaluating, 405
group communication, 400–402
impaired communication, 404
Impaired Verbal Communication diagnosis, 1067
implementation of nursing interventions, 404–405
implementing interventions, 402–403
influencing factors, 390–392
intimate distance communication, 391
intrapersonal communication, 386
measures to enhance, 405
of a medication order, 808–809
message, 387
modes of communication, 387–390
nonverbal communication, 387, 388–390, 404
nurse communication, evaluation of, 405
nurse managers, 542
of nursing actions, 458
and nursing process, 402–406
with older adults, 403
planning, 404
process, 386–387
process recording, 405–406, 406*t*
receiver, 387
response, 387
and safety, 765
sender, 386
sensory deficits, 1070
style of communication, 403–404
therapeutic communication, 392–393, 394*t*
verbal communication, 387–388, 403–404
communication role, 14
communication style, 185–187
community agencies, 1040
Community and Hospital Infection Control Association - Canada (CHICA-Canada), 878
community assessor and evaluator, 241
community-based health care (CBHC), 238
approaches, 238–239
Canadian community health nursing practice model, 240*f*
collaboration, 244–246
community-based settings, 240–243
community health nursing, 239–240
continuity of care, 246–248
discharge planning, 246–248
features, 238
home assessment parameters, 247
referrals, 248
safety concerns, 243–244
workforce competencies, 244
community-based settings
community health centre nursing, 241
described, 240–243
forensic nursing, 242
home care nursing, 242–243
occupational health nursing, 242
parish nursing, 241
school health nursing, 241–242
community coalitions, 239
community health, and use of computer applications, 504–505
community health centre nursing, 241
community health centres, 160
community health nurses (CHNs), 239
community health nursing, 239–240
community health-promotion programs, 139
community initiatives, 238–239
community nutritional services, 1204
community outreach centres, 241
community safety, 765
community setting
nurse's role, 1198
skin hygiene assessment, 707
compassion, 385
compassionate stranger, 223
compensation, 1387
compensatory, 200
competence, 385
competencies
collaboration, 246
community and public health workforce competencies, 244
nurse managers, 541–543
nursing practice alterations in health competencies, 39
nursing practice health and wellness competencies, 39
professional practice competencies, 39
competent, 98
competent nursing practice, 34
competing demands, 141
competing preferences, 141
complaint process, 95
complementary and alternative health modalities
acupressure, 277–278
acupuncture, 277–278
alternative medical systems, 273–274
animal-assisted therapy, 283
aromatherapy, 275–276
assessment of use of, 283
biofeedback, 281
biolelectromagnetic therapies, 279
biologically based treatments, 274–277
chiropractic therapy, 277
dietary therapy, 276
energy therapies, 279
guided imagery, 280–281
herbal medicine, 274–275
herbal therapy, 274
horticultural therapy, 283
humour, 282–283
hypnosis, 280
manipulative and body-based therapies, 277–279

massage, 277
meditation, 280
mind-body interventions, 280–283
music therapy, 282
nursing role, 283–284
orthomolecular medicine, 276–277
pilates, 281–282
prayer, 282
progressive relaxation, 280
qigong, 278–279
reflexology, 277–278
Tai Chi, 278–279
yoga, 280
complementary medicine, 271
see also alternative medicine; complementary and alternative health modalities
complementary proteins, 1168
complete bed bath, 711
complete bed rest, 1115
complete blood count (CBC), 1325, 1393–1394
complete proteins, 1168
completeness of recording, 489
compliance, 516, 672
comportment, 385
comprehensiveness, 11, **153,** 154*t*
compress, 972
compromised, 431
Compromised Family Coping (diagnostic label), 1500–1501
compromised hosts, 886
computer-assisted instruction (CAI), 530–531
computer-assisted learning (CAL), 506–507
computer use, 505
computerized axial tomography (CAT) scans, 501
computerized billing, 508
computerized care plan, 441
computerized diagnostics, 501
computerized documentation, 478–479, 480
computers
see also nursing informatics
bedside data entry, 498–499
case management, 505
community and home health, 504–505
computerized diagnostics, 501
consumer informatics, 501–502
data collection and analysis, 509
documentation of patient status, 498–501
in education, 507
edutainment, 507
electronic access to patient data, 501
electronic health records, 499–501
evidence-based practice, 503
hospital information systems (HIS), 498
literature review, 508
management information systems (MIS), 498
in nursing practice, 498–505
in nursing research, 508–509
patient monitoring, 501
practice management, 503
problem identification, 508
research design, 508–509
research dissemination, 509
research grants, 509
simulations, 531
specific applications, 504–505
teaching and learning, 506–507
telehealth, 502–503
concept, 55
definitions of major concepts, 59
described, 59
concept maps, 370, 443, 444*f*, 447*f*, 1076*f*
conception, 308–309
conceptual framework, 55
purposes of, 60
vs. theory, 59–60
conceptual model, 55
conciseness of recording, 489
conclusions, 45
concrete operations phase, 322
concreteness, 399
concurrent audit, 463
condom catheter, 1287–1289
conduction hearing loss, 587, 662–663
condyloid joint, 1107*t*
conferring
nursing care conference, 491
nursing rounds, 492
confidence, 373, 385
confidential information, 104
confidentiality, 50, 104
electronic health records, 471–472
and email communication, 390
legal aspects of nursing, 104–105
conflict management, 543
confrontation, 399
confusion, 1071–1072
congestive heart failure (CHF), 1321
congruent communication, 392
conjunctivitis, 575
connections with others, 1482
conscience, 385
conscious sedation, 1033
consciousness, levels of. *See* level of consciousness
consciousness of caring or healing, 64
consent
age of consent, 98
components of consent, 97
disclosure of information, 97–98
informed consent, 98–99
obtaining consent, 97–98
preoperative consent, 1021
substitute decision makers, 99
types of consent, 97
consequence-based (teleological) theories, 78
consequentialist theory, 78
constant fever, 664
constipation, 1038*t*, 1120, 1168, 1230, **1231**–1232, 1243
Constipation (diagnostic label)
fecal elimination, 1238
nutritional status, 1196
Constitution Act, 1867, 91
consultative leaders, 538–539
consumer, 9
consumer demands, 17–18
consumer informatics, 501–502
Consumer Rights to Health Care, 155, 155*t*
contact lens care, 744–745, 745*f*
contact precautions, 913, **914**
contaminated wounds, 928
contamination, 939–940
contemplation stage, 141
contemplative prayer, 282
contemporary frameworks for care, 168–169
contemporary leadership theories, 539–540
contemporary nursing practice
consumer demands, 17–18
definitions of nursing, 8–9
demography, 18
economics, 17
family structures, 18
health promotion, 12–13
influencing factors, 17–18
nurse practice acts, 13
nursing practice standards, 13
nursing settings, 10–11
primary health care, 11–12
recipients of nursing, 9–10
role of the nurse, 12
science and technology, 18
scope of nursing, 10
women's movement, 18
context, 374
contextual awareness, 374
continence (bladder) training, 1285–1286
continent diversions, 1301–1302
contingency theorists, 539
continuing care facilities. *See* extended-care (continuing-care) facilities
continuing competence, 13
continuing nursing education, 34
to maintain competency, 34
in rural and remote areas, 33
continuity of care, 246–248, 1067
continuity theory, 355
continuous ambulatory drug delivery (CADD), 855
continuous-drip feeding, 1214
continuous feedings, 1211
continuous infusion by pump, 1005
continuous plus intermittent bolus, 1005
continuous positive airway pressure (CPAP), 1088, 1343, 1343*f*
continuous quality improvement (CQI), 463
continuous subcutaneous infusion, 1003
continuous sutures, 1051
continuum of care, 158
contraception methods, 1463
contract, 95
contractility, 1315
contractual arrangements in nursing
consent issues, 97–99
legal roles of nurses, 95–96
contractual obligations, 95
contractual relationships, 96
contracture, 1116
contralateral stimulation, 1008
controlled coughing, 1332, 1333
Controlled Drugs and Substances Act, 798
controller, 1412–1413
convection, 663
conventional level, 300, 323, 326, 340
cooling sponge bath, 972
coordinating, 541
coordinator, 241
coping, 1496
see also stress
adaptive coping, 1499
anger mediation, 1504–1506
anxiety, minimization of, 1504
assessing, 1499–1500
and cardiovascular functions, 1319
crisis intervention, 1506
diagnosing, 1500–1501
effective coping, 1499
emotion-focused coping, 1496
evaluating, 1507, 1507*t*
health-promotion strategies, 1503–1504
home care, 1503
implementing interventions, 1503–1507
ineffective coping, 1499
lifespan considerations, 1491
maladaptive coping, 1499
planning, 1501–1503
and preoperative phase, 1022
problem-focused coping, 1496
relaxation techniques, 1505
and respiratory functions, 1319
sample care plan for ineffective coping, 1502–1503
coping mechanisms, 1496
described, 201, 202–203, 1490
preschoolers, 320
coping responses. *See* coping mechanisms
coping strategies, 1496–1497
coping/stress-tolerance pattern, 426
copulation, 1454
cordotomy, 1010
core self-concept, 1432–1433
core temperature, 662
corn, 721
coronary angiography, 1327–1328
coronary arteries, 1314
coronary artery disease, 360
coronary circulation, 1314
correct spelling, 487
corticosteroids, 1020
costal (thoracic) breathing, 682
cotton applicators, 558*t*
coudé catheter, 1290
cough etiquette, 914
cough medications, 1334
cough reflex, 1310
cough suppressant, 1333
coughing, 684
coughing exercises, 1024–1027, 1041, 1332
counselling, 14
countershock phase, 1492
counting fingers (C/F), 581
course record management, 506
court testimony, 471
covert change, 545
cranial nerves
assessment of, 638, 646
functions and assessment methods, 636*t*

creams, 858
creatine kinase, 1327
creatinine, 1278
creatinine clearance, 1278
creativity, 369
  concept maps, 370
  described, 369–370
credentialing, 94
Credé's manoeuvre, 1289
credibility, 388
cremation, 1524
crepitation, 1123
crib net, 789
crises, 1506
crisis centres, 163
crisis counselling, 1506
crisis home visits, 1506
crisis intervention, 1506
critical analysis, 370
critical care settings, 214–215
critical incident, 104
Critical Incident Regulation (Saskatchewan), 103–104
critical pathways, 168, 443
critical thinking, 369, 542
  application to nursing practice, 374
  attitudes that foster critical thinking, 371–374
  clinical examples of, 375*t*
  concept maps, 370
  creating supportive environments, 379
  creativity. *See* creativity
  critical-thinking abilities, 370–371
  cultivating a questioning attitude, 379
  decision making, 376–377
  described, 369
  development of, 377–379
  and diagnostic process, 433
  expert critical thinker, 370
  importance of, 369
  mind map, 378*f*
  problem solving, 374–376
  self-assessments, 378
  standards of critical thinking, 374–377
  tolerance for dissonance and ambiguity, 378–379
critiquing, 46–49, 47*t*, 48*t*
cross-dressers, 1448
cross-training, 169
crossmatching, 1418–1421
crown, 727
crust, 566*t*
crutch gaits, 1156
crutch stance, 1156
crutches, 1154–1159
crying, 313
crystalloids, 1370
cues, 428, 434, 434*t*
cuffed tracheostomy tubes, 1345
cultural assessment, 191
cultural awareness, 179
cultural care
  see also culture
  barriers to cultural sensitivity and safety, 183
  Canada's cultural mosaic, 174–178
  communication style, 185–187
  conveying cultural sensitivity, 183–184
  cultural assessment, 191
  cultural care diversity and universality theory, 65
  cultural parameters for nursing, 184–190
  culturally competent care, 190–192
  culturally sensitive and safe care, 181–184
  death and dying practices, 189–190
  family patterns, 185
  health beliefs and practices, 184–185
  interpreters, 186
  Leininger's sunrise model, 182*f*
  negotiation, 192
  nonverbal communication, 187
  nutritional patterns, 188–189
  pain responses, 189
  space orientation, 188
  time orientation, 188
  verbal communication, 186–187
cultural care deprivation, 1063
cultural care diversity and universality theory, 65, 384
cultural competence, 180
cultural deprivation, 1063
cultural diversity, 216
Cultural Diversity (CNA), 165
cultural identity, 179
cultural mosaic
  demographic profile, 174–175
  history of migrations and immigration, 174
  language, 175–176
  multicultural policy, 176–178
  religion, 176
  visible minorities, 176
cultural safety, 180
cultural sensitivity, 179, 183–184
culturally competent care, 1437
culturally sensitive and safe care, 181–184
culture, 178–179
  see also cultural care
  characteristics of, 178
  and client education, 520
  components of, 178
  as concept, 178
  death-related practices, 1524
  eye contact, 390
  growth and development, 292
  health-care concerns, 180–181
  and learning, 519
  and loss and grief, 1515
  and medication action, 803
  naming systems, 185
  and nonverbal communication, 388
  and nutrition, 1173
  and pain, 986
  and preoperative phase, 1022
  related definitions and concepts, 178–181
  as risk factor, 203
  and self-concept, 1436
  and sensory perception problems, 1063
  and sexuality, 1451–1452
  subculture, 179
  transcultural teaching, 531
culture shock, 180
culture-specifics, 178
culture-universals, 178
cumulative effect, 800
Cumulative Index to Nursing and Allied Health Literature (CINAHL), 46
cunnilingus, 1454
curiosity, 373–374
curious listener, 222–223
current body weight (CBS), 1189
current data, 418
cutaneous stimulation, 1007
cyanosis, 564, 1320
cyclic feedings, 1211
cyst, 565*f*
cystic fibrosis, 1317
cystocele, 657
cystoscope, 1278
cystoscopy, 1278
cytokines, 881
cytology, 1324

D

dacryocystitis, 575
daily nursing assessment form, 478*f*
daily nursing care record, 481
daily pain diary, 993
daily weight measurements, 1389
dancing reflex, 311
dandruff, 737
data, 497
  analysis, 44–45, 434–437, 509
  bedside data entry, 496–497
  classifications, 500–501
  clustering, 436–437
  collection. *See* data collection
  comparison with outcomes, 459–460
  conflicting data, 437
  dietary data, 1187–1188
  documentation of data, 429
  electronic access to patient data, 501
  identification of gaps and inconsistencies, 437
  and nursing informatics applications, 497–498
  organization of, 426–428
  sources, 419–420
  standardization, 500–501
  vs. standards, 434
  validation of data, 428–429, 428*t*
data clusters, 523
data collection, 417
  and assessing, 417–423
  and computers, 509
  data sources, 419–420
  and evaluation process, 459
  hygiene practices, 707
  interview, 420–423
  methods, 420–424
  nursing health history, 418
  observation, 420
  physical examinations, 423, 424*f*
  in research process, 44
data warehousing, 506
database, 417, 474, 506
date of recording, 486
daycare centres, 163
daydreaming, 1496
daytime enuresis, 1270
deaf people, and sign language, 390
death and dying
  advance directives, 1520–1522, 1521*f*
  and aging, 357
  artificial nutrition and hydration (ANH), 1522
  assessment during transition of active dying, 1524–1525
  beliefs, 1478
  breathing needs, 1531–1532
  caring for the family, 1532–1533
  cause of, 1516
  cultural care, 189–190
  development of concept of death, 1518*t*
  do not resuscitate orders, 1523–1524
  dying person's bill of rights, 1526
  dying with dignity, 1527–1532
  end-of-life care for older adults, 1518–1519
  euthanasia, 1522
  evaluating process of care, 1532
  goals in fostering a peaceful death, 1533*t*
  home care, 1526–1527
  hospice palliative care, 1528
  infectious diseases, 878
  interview, 1526
  legal and moral issues, 1520–1524
  pain management, 1530–1531
  physiological needs of dying individual, 1528, 1529*t*
  planning a peaceful death, 1526
  postmortem care, 1533–1534
  religious and cultural practices, 1524
  responses to, 1519–1520
  sensory perceptual needs, 1529–1530
  signs of impending clinical death, 1525
  spirituality, 1532
  state of consciousness in dying patients, 1530*t*
debilitated clients, and oral hygiene, 734–736
debridement, 951
decision making, 376
  and collaboration, 246
  described, 376–377
  vs. problem solving, 374–375
decision-making framework, 377
decision tree, 437*f*
Decisional Conflict (diagnostic label), 1501
Declaration of Alma-Ata, 237
decode, 387
decontamination, 889–892
decreased, 431
decreased cardiac output, 1321–1322
Decreased Cardiac Output (diagnostic label)
  fluid, electrolyte, and acid-base balances, 1395
  respiratory and cardiovascular functions, 1328
decreased leukocyte count, 942
decubitus ulcers. *See* pressure ulcers
deductive reasoning, 371
deep breathing exercises, 1024–1027, 1041, 1332
deep palpation, 557, 559
deep sleep, 1082

deep tissue injury, 932, 934*f*
defaction reflex, 1120
defecation, 1227
see also fecal elimination
and activity, 1230
adolescents, 1229
anaesthesia, 1231
bowel diversion ostomies, 1234–1236
bowel incontinence, 1233–1234
common fecal elimination problems, 1231–1234
constipation, 1231–1232
described, 1227–1228
and development, 1228–1230
diagnostic procedures and, 1231
diarrhea, 1233, 1233*t*
diet and, 1230
encopresis, 1229
and exercise, 1243
factors affecting, 1228–1231
fecal impaction, 1232–1233, 1232*f*
flatulence, 1234
fluid intake, 1230
frequency of, 1227
habits, 1231
healthy defecation, 1242
medications, 1231
newborns and infants, 1228–1229
nutrition and fluids, 1243
older adults, 1230
and pain, 1231
paralytic ileus, 1231
pathological conditions, 1231
physiology of defecation, 1226–1228
and positioning, 1243
privacy, 1242
psychological factors, 1230–1231
regular defecation, promotion of, 1242–1243
school-age children, 1229
and surgery, 1231
timing, 1242–1243
toddlers, 1229
defence mechanisms, 292, 1496, 1497*t*
defences. *See* body defences against infection
defendents, 103
Defensive Coping (diagnostic label), 1501
defervescent stage, 664, 665
deficient, 431
Deficient Fluid Volume (diagnostic label), 1395
deficient knowledge, 525
Deficient Knowledge (diagnostic label)
accident prevention, 768
fecal elimination, 1239
foot hygiene, 722, 723*t*
oral hygiene, 729
pain, 994
patient safety, 768
preoperative phase, 1021
sexual health status, 1459
skin hygiene, 707
defining characteristics, 431–432
degenerative joint changes, 353
dehiscence, 937–939, 1046
dehydration, 1381
delayed primary intention healing, 934
delegating care, 95
delegation, 458, **543,** 544
delirium, 361, 1529
vs. dementia, 1073*t*
sensory perception, 1071
deltoid, 631
deltoid site, 844, 844*f*, 845*f*
demand feeding, 1176
dementia, 361, 1072
vs. delirium, 1073*t*
oral care, 736
Demerol, 999
democratic leaders, 538–539
demographic changes, 165–166
demographic profile, 174–175
demographic variables, 122
demography, 18, 255
denial, 1497*t*
dental caries, 728, 729*t*
see also caries
dental mirror, 558*t*
dentin, 727
dentists, 164, 164*t*
dentures, 731, 733–734
Denver Developmental Screening Test (DDST), 314
deontological theories, 78
dependent edema, 1118
dependent variable, 43
depression, 1496
antidepressants, 1020
postoperative depression, 1039*t*
sleep, 1085–1086
dermatological preparations, 806, 857–858
descending colostomy, 1235
descriptive statistics, 45
desired effect, 799
desired health outcome statements, 449
desired health outcomes, 445–450, 459, 460–461, 462
see also evaluation
determinants of health, 125, 126*t*, 135*t*, 705*t*
detoxification, 802
detrusor muscle, 1265
development, 290
see also growth and development
cognitive development. *See* cognitive development
and communication process, 391
of concept of death, 1518*t*
and defecation, 1228–1230
intrauterine development, 308–309
and medication action, 803
and medication administration, 816–818
moral development. *See* moral development
and nutrition, 1172–1173
and pain, 986–988
physical development. *See* physical development
prenatal development, 308–309
psychosocial development. *See* psychosocial development
and safety, 764
and self-concept, 1435–1436
and sensory perception, 1063
spiritual development. *See* spiritual development
stressors, 1490*t*
and urinary elimination, 1266–1267
developmental, 1473
developmental change, 545
developmental factors, 203
developmental guidelines
adolescence, 327
infants, 314
middle-aged adults, 342
older adults, 358–359
preschoolers, 321
school-age children, 323
toddlers, 318
young adults, 337
developmental milestones, 290
developmental screening tests, 314
developmental stage theories, 206
developmental task, 292, 294*t*
developmental theories, 428
developmental variations
feet, 720–721
hair, 737
teeth, 727–728
diabetes, 256, **261,** 910, 1322
diabetes mellitus, 1452
diagnosing. *See* nursing diagnosis
diagnosis, 156
see also nursing diagnosis
Diagnostic and Statistical Manual of Mental Disorders (DSM-IV-TR), 801
(diagnostic label)
fecal incontinence, 1231
transient incontinence, 1271
urinary incontinence (UI), 931, 1120, 1270–1271, 1285–1288
diagnostic labels, 431, **431,** 524–525
diagnostic procedures, 888, 1231, 1269
diagnostic process, 433–438
diagnostic statements, 438
diagnostic studies
cardiovascular functions, 1324–1327
fecal elimination, 1236–1238
respiratory functions, 1324–1327
sleep, 1091
Dial-A-Flo, 1412
diameter (of the shaft), 828
diapedesis, 881
diaper rash, 708*t*
diaphragmatic (abdominal) breathing, 682, 1332, 1333
diarrhea, 1233, 1233*t*, 1243, 1246, 1247, 1251
Diarrhea (diagnostic label), 1238
diastole, 610*f*, **615**–616, **1314,** 1315
diastolic pressure, 686
diet. *See* nutrition
diet as tolerated, 1201
diet history, 1188
dietary alterations, 1199
dietary data, 1187–1188
dietary fibre. *See* fibre
dietary reference intakes, 1170
dietary therapy, 276
dietitians, 164, 164*t*
difference questions, 223
diffusion, 1311, 1370–1371
digestion
carbohydrate, 1167
lipids, 1170
proteins, 1168
digital mucous cyst, 565*f*
digital removal of fecal impaction, 1251–1252, 1251*f*
digital sphygmomanometer, 688
digitalis glycosides, 1333
dignity, 49, 1527–1532
diminished cardiac reserve, 1117
diminished sensation, 931
diploma programs, 28
direct auscultation, 561
direct contact transmission, 886
direct (invasive monitoring) measurement, 691
direct percussion, 560
direct vasodilators, 1334
direct visualization techniques, 1236
directing, 541
directive interview, 420
directive leader, 538
dirty wounds, 928
Disabled Family Coping (diagnostic label), 1501
disaccharides, 1167
discharge note, 481–485
discharge planning, 246–248, **439,** 1040–1041
discipline, 94–95, 1496
disclosure, 97
disclosure of information, 97–98
discovery, 103
discovery techniques, 531
discrimination, 183
discussion, 470
disease, 123
arterial disease, 936
causation, 123
chronic diseases, 166
communicable disease, 880
infectious diseases, 878, 880
and medication action, 803
modification of diet for disease, 1201–1202
process, and blood pressure, 687
and susceptibility to infection, 888
venous disease, 936
disease prevention, 137, 137*t*
disease-specific isolation precautions, 911
disengagement theory, 355
dishes, 915
disinfectant, 891, 891*t*
disinfection, 891
displacement, 1497*t*
disposable bed bath, 711
disposable needles, syringes, and sharps, 915
disposable pads, 558*t*
disposal of soiled equipment and supplies, 914–915
dissonance, tolerance for, 378–379

distance education, 507
distant prayer, 282
distortion sores. *See* pressure ulcers
distraction, 1009
distribution, 802
Disturbed Body Image (diagnostic label)
  fecal elimination, 1239
  hair care, 738
  postoperative phase, 1040
  self-concept, 1439
  sexual health status, 1459
  urinary elimination problems, 1279
  wounds, 946
Disturbed Personal Identity (diagnostic label)
  self-concept, 1440
Disturbed Sensory Perception (diagnostic label)
  vs. Disturbed Thought Process, 1066
  sensory perception problems, 1066
Disturbed Sleep Pattern (diagnostic label)
  preoperative phase, 1022
  self-concept, 1440
Disturbed Thought Process (diagnostic label)
  chronic insomnia, 1091
  vs. Disturbed Sensory Perception, 1066
  self-concept, 1440
disuse atrophy, 1116
disuse osteoporosis, 1115
disuse syndrome, 1116*t*
diuresis, 1269
diuretics, 1020, 1230
diurnal (daytime) enuresis, 1270
diurnal variations, 663, 687
diversity, 179
divided colostomy, 1235, 1236*f*
divorce trends, 216–217
do not resuscitate orders, 1523–1524
doctoral programs, 29–30
documentation
  see also documenting
  of data, 429
  intraoperative phase, 1034
  of patient status, 498–501
documentation standards, 106
documentation systems
  case management model, 479–480
  charting by exception (CBE), 477–478
  computerized documentation, 478–479, 480
  focus charting, 477
  PIE, 476–477
  problem-oriented medical record (POMR), 474–476
  source-oriented record, 473–474, 473*t*
documenting, 470
  see also client records; documentation
  client education, 532
  discharge note, 481–485
  flowsheets, 481
  home care documentation, 486
  Kardex, 481
  long-term-care documentation, 486
  nursing activities, 480–486
  nursing care plans, 480–481
  progress notes, 481
domestic violence, 772
Doppler ultrasound stethoscope (DUS), 674, 674*f,* 677, 678–679, 690
dorsal position, 1132
dorsal recumbent position, 1131–1132, 1132*t*
dorsalis pedis, 674
dorsogluteal site, 843, 843*f*
dosage calculations, 811–812
dose designations, 807*t*
double-barreled colostomy, 1235, 1236*f*
Downey v. Rothwell, 100–101
downstream view, 125
drainable bowel diversion ostomy appliance, 1255–1257
drainage systems, 1356–1358
drains, 1039, 1050
drapes, 559*t*
draping, 556
dress, 1478
dressings
  damp gauze *vs.* advanced dressings, 962
  gauze dressings, 954*t*
  hydrocolloid dressings, 954–957
  moist transparent wound barrier dressing, 955–956
  peritoneal dressings, 966–967
  postoperative phase, 1039
  purposes, 951
  secured dressings, 957
  sterile dressing, 1047–1049
  surgical dressings, 1047
  transparent films, 952–954
  types of, 952–956, 952*t*
drip factor, 1407
driving forces for change, 546
drop factor, 1407
droplet nuclei, 886
droplet precautions, 913, 914
droplet transmission, 886
drops per minute, 1411–1412
drug allergy, 800
drug dependence, 801
drug interaction, 276, **800–801**
drug legislation
  application to nursing practice, 798–799
  Canadian Food and Drugs Act, 797–798
  Controlled Drugs and Substances Act, 798
  described, 796–798
  drug standards, 798
  Marihuana Medical Access Regulations (MMAR), 798
drug misuse, 801
drug-resistant bacteria, 1234
drug tolerance, 800, 1000
drug toxicity, 799–800
drug use. *See* problematic substance use
drugs
  see also medication; pharmacology
  actions of, in the body, 801–802
  adverse effects, 799
  classifications, 796
  drug allergy, 800
  drug interaction, 276, 800–801
  drug misuse, 801
  drug-nutrient interactions, 1175*t*
  drug preparations, 797*t*
  drug standards, 798
  drug tolerance, 800
  drug toxicity, 799–800
  drug use. *See* problematic substance use
  effects of, 799–802
  and erectile dysfunction, 1456
  factors affecting medication action, 802–804
  illicit drugs, 801
  pharmacodynamics, 802
  pharmacokinetics, 802
  primary effect, 799
  routes of administration, 804–806, 805*t*
  secondary effect, 799
  side effect, 799
  therapeutic actions of drugs, 800*t*
  therapeutic or desired effect, 799
dry heat, 969
ductus arteriosis, 1317
dullness, 560
Dunn's high-level wellness grid, 120
duration, 561
duty, 99
dyads, 400
dying. *See* death and dying
dying person's bill of rights, 1526
dying with dignity, 1527–1532
dynamic exercise, 1110–1111
dysesthesia, 982
dysmenorrhea, 1449
dyspareunia, 1456
dysphagia, 1174, 1202
dyspnea, 354, 684, **1321, 1531**–1532
dysrhythmia, 675, 1322
dysuria, 1270

E

e-nursing strategy. *See* nursing informatics
ear
  see also hearing
  assessment of, 582–589
  hygiene, 746–748
  inner ear, 583
  irrigation, 863
  lifespan considerations, 587
  middle ear, 583
  otic instillations, 861–864
  parts of, 582–583, 583*f*
ear infections, 317
eardrum, 582
earlobe, 582
early adulthood. *See* young adults (20 to 40 years)
early historians of nursing, 3
early training
  before establishment of training schools, 3
  first official training school, 4
  push for formal training, 4
ease, 385
Eating Well with Canada's Food Guide, 1173, 1177, 1179, 1179*f,* 1180, 1182, 1182*f,* 1184, 1188, 1200
eccrine glands, 324, 705
echocardiogram, 1328
ecologic theory, 300
ecomap, 220
economic change, and aging, 356
economic factors, and client education, 520
economics
  and contemporary nursing practice, 17
  and health-care system, 165
  and nutrition, 1174
  rural health framework, 255
ectoderm, 308
edema, 564, 930, 1118, 1193, **1381**
education. *See* client education; nursing education
educator role, 14, 240–241, 520–532
edutainment, 507
effective coping, 1499
effective leadership, 540
effectiveness, 543
effectors, 663
efficiency, 543
ego, 292
ego differentiation, 296
ego preoccupation, 297
ego transcendence, 297
eight-step change process, 545–546
ejaculation, 324, 1454
ejaculatory incompetence, 1456
elasticity of the arterial wall, 675
elbow restraints, 789
elder abuse, 361–362
elective health problem, 158
elective surgery, 1018
electric health technologies, 497
electric pads, 971
electrical hazards, 782–783
electrocardiogram (ECG), 1327
electrolyte imbalances, 1382–1387, 1383*t,* 1384*t,* 1385*t,* 1386*t*
electrolyte solutions, 1401
electrolytes, 1368
  see also fluid, electrolyte, and acid-base balances
  active transport, 1371
  balance, 1379
  composition, 1368–1369, 1369*f*
  diffusion, 1370–1371
  disturbances, 1382–1387
  electrolyte imbalances, 1382–1387, 1383*t,* 1384*t,* 1385*t,* 1386*t*
  enteral fluid and electrolyte replacement, 1396
  factors affecting, 1376–1380
  filtration, 1371
  functions, 1375*t*
  home care, 1396
  lifespan considerations, 1379
  movement of, 1370–1371
  normal electrolyte values for adults, 1393
  osmosis, 1370
  regulation of, 1374–1377, 1375*t*
  serum electrolytes, 1393
electronic access to patient data, 501
electronic communication, 390
electronic health records (EHRs), 471–472, **499**
electronic infusion devices (EIDs), 1412

electronic medical records (EMRs), 499
electronic patient records (EPRs), 499
electronic thermometer, 668, 668*f*
elimination. *See* fecal elimination; urinary elimination
elimination half-life, 801
elimination pattern, 426
email, 390
emboli, 1041
embolus, 1038*t,* **1118**
embryonic phase, 308
emergencies, and older adults, 362
emergency assessment, 417*t*
emergency surgery, 1018
emergent health problem, 158
emerging pathogens, 914
emigration, 881
emmetropic, 319
emotions
  emotional stress, and sleep, 1085–1086
  and learning, 518–519
  and safety, 765
empathetic listening, 399
empathy, 399
empiricist tradition, 57
employee performance, enhancement of, 542
employment contracts, 95–96
Employment Equity Act, 177
empowerment, 42, **137**
empty calories, 1167
enamel, 727
encoding, 386
encopresis, 1229
end colostomy, 1235, 1235*f*
end-of-life care, 157
  legal and moral issues, 1520–1524
  for older adults, 1518–1519
endocardium, 1313
endoderm, 308
endotracheal tubes, 1344, 1345, 1353–1356
enemas, 1246–1250, 1247*t*
energy, 272
energy balance
  caloric theory approach, 1171
  chronic energy imbalance, and obesity, 1178
  described, 1171
  Glycemic Index approach, 1172
energy therapies, 279
enteral, 804
enteral access devices, 1204–1209
enteral feedings, 1210–1216
enteral fluid and electrolyte replacement, 1396
enteral medications, 818–825
enteral nutrition (EN), 1204
  clogged feeding tubes, 1217–1218
  enteral access devices, 1204–1209
  enteral feedings, 1210–1216
  gastrostomy devices, 1208
  gastrostomy feeding, administering, 1214–1215
  home care, 1217
  jejunostomy devices, 1208
  jejunostomy feeding, administering, 1214–1215
  medication through a feeding tube, 1216–1217
  nasoenteric tube, 1208
  nasogastric tube, 1204–1208, 1209
  risks, 1217
  testing feeding tube placement, 1209–1210
  tube feeding, administering, 1211–1214
entoderm, 308
entry to practice, 32
entry-to-practice, 32
enuresis, 1266, 1270
environment
  and acid-base balance, 1378–1379
  agent-host-environment model, 120
  and body fluids, 1378–1379
  and body temperature, 663–664
  cardiovascular functions, 1318
  and communication process, 392
  and electrolytes, 1378–1379
  growth and development, 292
  hygienic environment, 749–757
  for learning, 518
  manipulation of, 404
  and medication action, 803
  and pain, 988
  preparation, for health assessment, 555–556
  respiratory functions, 1318
  restful environment, 1094
  and safety, 765–766
  sensory perception problems, 1065
  and sleep, 1086
  temperature, 1378–1379
  young adults and environmental exposure, 337
Environment Canada, 667
environmental comfort needs, 385
environmental control programs, 139
environmental management, 919
environmental restraints, 784
enzymatic debridement, 951
enzymes, 1167
epicardium, 1313
epidural, 806
epidural catheter, 1006*t*
epidural (peridural) anaesthesia, 1033
EpiPen, 1201
epistemology, 56
Epp, Jake, 132
Epp Report, 132–133, 136
equianalgesia, 1001
equilibrium, 200
equipment
  blood pressure, 688–690
  disposal of soiled equipment and supplies, 914–915
  intravenous equipment, 1403–1406
  parenteral medications, 825–828
equipment-related accidents, 783
equitable health care, 254
erectile dysfunction, 1456
Erikson, Erik, 294–295, 296*t,* 1473
Erikson's stages of psychosocial development, 1432*t*
erosion, 566*t*
eructation, 1234
erythema, 564, 708*t*
erythrocytes, 1312
eschar, 932
essential amino acids, 1168
essential fatty acids, 1169
essential nutrients
  macronutrients, 1167–1170
  micronutrients, 1170–1171
essential oils, 276, 276*t*
estimated average requirement, 1171
ethical decision making, 81–82
ethical decision making models, 82
ethical obligations, 77–78
ethical practice in nursing, 78
ethics, 56, 78
  autonomy (respect for persons), 79
  beneficence, 50, 80
  code of ethics, 49, 78, 81
  confidentiality, 50
  enhancement of ethical practice, 85
  ethical soundness of study, 43
  euthanasia, 83
  fidelity, 80
  full disclosure, 50
  inclusiveness, 50
  informed consent, 49–50
  justice, 50, 80
  medical futility, 83
  moral principles, variations in application, 83
  nonmaleficence, 50, 79–80
  nursing ethics, 80–81
  principle-based ethics, 79–80
  privacy, 50
  relational ethics theories, 80–81
  respect for human dignity, 49
  right of self-determination, 50
  rights of human subjects, 49–50
  selected issues in nursing, 82–84
  top health-care ethics challenges, 73
  Tri-Council Policy Statement, 49
  veracity, 80
  vulnerable persons, 50
ethics of care, 80–81
ethnic, 179
  see also ethnicity
  ethnopharmacology, 803, 804
  older adults, 348
ethnic identity, 179
ethnic values, and pain, 986
ethnicity
  see also ethnic
  and medication action, 803
  and nutrition, 1173
ethnocentrism, 183, 272
ethnographic research, 44
ethnopharmacology, 803, 804
ethnorelativity, 183
ethylene oxide gas, 891
etiological agent, 885
etiology, 123, 431
eudaimonistic model, 119
eupnea, 683, 1320
eustachian tube, 583
euthanasia, 83, **1522**
evaluation, 458
  see also assessment skills
  checklist, 462*t*
  client education, 531–532
  communication, 405
  comparison of data with outcomes, 459–460
  components, 459
  data collection, 459
  death and dying, 1532
  desired health outcomes, 459
  drawing conclusions, 461
  eye care, 746
  fecal elimination, 1258*t,* 1259
  fluid, electrolyte, and acid-base balances, 1422, 1425*t*
  foot care, 726
  hair care, 742
  infection prevention and control, 918–919
  intraoperative phase, 1034
  of learning, 531–532
  mobility problems, 1159, 1160*t*
  nail hygiene, 727
  nursing audit, 463
  nursing care plan, 461–463
  nutritional status, 1218, 1219*t*
  oral hygiene, 736, 737*t*
  outcome evaluation, 463
  overview, 416*t*
  oxygenation and circulation interventions, 1360–1361, 1361*t*
  pain management, 1010–1011
  patient safety, 790
  postoperative phase, 1053, 1054*t*
  preoperative phase, 1032
  process evaluation, 463
  process of evaluating client responses, 459–463
  quality assurance, 463
  quality improvement, 463
  quality of nursing care, 463
  relating nursing actions to goals or outcomes, 460–461
  relationship to other nursing process phases, 458–459
  self-concept, 1442
  sensory perception problems, 1074–1075, 1074*t*
  sexual health status, 1466–1467, 1466*t*
  skin hygiene, 720
  sleep, 1097–1098, 1098*t*
  spiritual health, 1482, 1484*t*
  stress and coping, 1507, 1507*t*
  structure evaluation, 463
  of teaching, 532
  urinary elimination, 1302–1303, 1303*t*
  wounds, 967–968, 968*t*
evaluation statement, 459–460
evidence-based practice, 39
  see also evidence-informed practice
evidence-informed practice, 39
  advancements in, and health-care system, 164–165

bath grab bar, location of, 718
being listened to, importance of, 65
breastfeeding self-efficacy scale, reliability of, 464
cancer among the Woodland Cree of northern Saskatchewan, 180
caregiver perceptions of unsupportive interactions, 43
child safety restraint systems, correct use of, 138
chronic diarrhea in HIV clients, 1251
chronic diseases, and heath care, 166
competencies related to use of evidence in practice, 39
and computers in nursing practice, 503
concept maps, and critical thinking, 370
electronic patient records, 479
empowerment for new graduate nurses, 42
ethical practice in nursing, 78
ethnicity, and perceptions of health, 349
family nursing, and mental illness care, 214
feeding following surgery, 1020
financial stress, impact of, 297
grief work, 1519
health-care workers and handwashing, 879
hearing impairment, effect of, 311
humour in palliative care unit, 203
immunization programs in nontraditional settings, 243
inflammatory bowel disease, and diet, 527
influences on adolescent self-esteem, 1435
informed consent issues, 98
lesbian disclosure, 1447
look-alike vials, 817
maternal stress during pregnancy, 1500
mental health problems, living with, 341
natural health product-drug interactions, 276
nutrition, and prevention of constipation, 1168
older adults and walking, 774
oral temperature readings, 667
patient treatment preferences, eliciting, 405
prevention of falls at home, 124
routine screening programs, 634
rural and remote areas, and continuing education, 33
rural nursing practice, 263
self-management program, and chronic cardiac pain, 1001
skin tears, 959
smoking cessation best practice guidelines, 1318
spiritual nursing care, meaning of, 1482
stretching before exercise, 1110
stroke impairments, 1072
urinary incontinence, and self-care strategies, 1285
violence against women, and sleep, 1086

evisceration, 937–939, 1046
exacerbation, 124
examination
see also physical assessment
auscultation, 561
eyes, 573–574
inspection, 556
methods of examination, 556–561
neurological system, 635
palpation, 556–560
percussion, 560
speculum examination, 657
use of term, 552
Excess Fluid Volume (diagnostic label), 1395
excessive dryness, 708*t*
excessive dryness of the buccal mucosa, 729*t*
excessive noise, 782
excoriated areas, 592
excoriated mucosa, 729*t*
excoriation, 566*t*
excretion, 802
exercise, 1110
benefits of, 1111–1114
and blood pressure, 687
and body temperature, 663
coughing exercises, 1024–1027, 1041
deep breathing exercises, 1024–1027, 1041
and defecation, 1243
exercise and activity interventions. *See* exercise and activity interventions
home care, 1126
intensity, 1111
Kegel exercises, 1286–1287
leg exercises, 1024–1027, 1041
nursing health history, 1121
pelvic floor muscle exercises (PFME), 1286–1287
and pulse rate, 672
relaxation response (RR), 1114
sensate exercises, 1456
stress and coping, 1503
stretching before exercise, 1110
types of, 1110–1111
exercise and activity interventions
ambulation, 1147–1152
assisting clients to ambulate, 1149–1152
back injury, prevention of, 1130
body mechanics, 1127–1129
lifting, 1127–1129
mechanical aids for walking, 1152–1159
moving and turning clients in bed, 1134
pivoting, 1129
positioning clients, 1130–1133
preambulatory exercises, 1149
pulling, 1129
pushing, 1129
ROM exercises, 1146–1147
transferring clients, 1134–1146
exhalation, 682, 682*f*
exocytosis, 883
exosystem, 300
expanded career roles, 15
expanded practice, 262
expansion of consciousness, 65
expected outcome, 445
expectorants, 1333
experimental design, 44
expert critical thinker, 370
expiration, 682
express consent, 97
expressive aphasia, 637
expressive communication problems, 404
extended-care (continuing-care) facilities, 162
external auditory meatus, 583
external (condom) catheter, 1287–1289
external eye structures, 576–579
external respiration, 682
external sphincter, 1227
external stimuli, 1061
external urinary drainage devices, 1287–1289
extinction, 645, 650
extracellular fluid (ICF), 1368
extraocular muscle tests, 580
exudate, 882, 937
exudate production, 882
eye
see also eye care; vision
anatomic structures, 574*f*
artificial eyes (prosthesis), 745–746
assessment of, 572–582
common refractive errors of the lens, 574
external structures, 574*f*
eye structures, assessment of, 576–581
hygiene, 743–746
inflammatory visual problems, 575
lacrimal apparatus, 574*f*
lifespan considerations, 582
protection against infection, 881
eye care
artificial eyes (prosthesis), 745–746
assessing, 743–744
comatose clients, 744
contact lens care, 744–745, 745*f*
diagnosing, 744
evaluating, 746
eye safety, 744
eyeglass care, 744
general eye care, 746
implementing interventions, 744–746
interview, 743
nursing health history, 743
ophthalmic instillations, 858–861
physical assessment, 744
planning, 744
eye charts, 574–575, 575*f*
eye contact, 390
eye movement, 187
eye safety, 744
eyeglass care, 744
eyeglasses, 574
eyesight loss, 259–260
eyewear, 896–898, 898

F

face, assessment of, 572, 573, 574
face masks, 895–898
face scales, 990, 991*f*
face tent, 1338–1339, 1341
facemask, 1338–1341
facial expression, 187, 389–390
facial sinuses, 587*f*
facilitation
of support, 145–146
and working phase, 399
facilitator, 241
facilities management, 508
facts, 371*t*
fad, 1173
failure, history of, 1436
failure to thrive, 312–313
fair-mindedness, 372
faith, 302, 1473
development of, 1473–1474
spiral faith model, 1474*f*
Westerhoff's four stages of faith, 303*t*, 1473*t*
faith group leaders, 1482
fall-risk prediction, 779
falls
broken bones as cause, 776
Get Up and Go (GUG) Test, 776
in health-care agencies, 776–777
prevention of, 774–779
preventive measures, 775*t*
risk factors, 775*t*
false imprisonment, 101
false-negative results, 1238
false-positive results, 1238
family, 212
see also family nursing
assessment guide, 219
Canadian families, 215–218
common-law relationships, 216–217
cultural diversity, 216
culturally competent care, 192
and death and dying, 1532–1533
divorce trends, 216–217
expectations for involvement in care, 215
families providing care, 217–218
family support, possibilities for, 218–220
and growth and development, 291
illness, impact of, 125, 220–221
illness, impact on, 221–222
income, 217
involvement in health care, 215
marriage trends, 216–217
mobility, 216
parenting trends, 216–217
patterns, and cultural care, 185
and self-concept, 1436
and sexuality, 1451
strengths, 225–226
stress, 213
types of, 212
understanding families, 218–222
family farms, 255
family nursing, 212
see also family
access to the hospitalized patient, 223–225
Canadian contributions to, 215
challenges, 212–213
collaborative relational stance, 222–223
commending family and individual stance, 225–226
critical care settings, 214–215
described, 212–213
development of, 213–215
evaluation, 228

family involvement in health care, 215
family support, creating and encouraging, 226–227
illness narratives, 225
individuals in hospital care, 214
maternal and child nursing, 214
mental health nursing, 214
nursing care of families, 222–228
offering information, 226
pediatric nursing, 214
public health, 214
reflective questions, 223
respite from caregiving, suggesting, 227–228
family structures, 18
family support, 226–227
family unit, 207
family unit as the client of care, 213
fantasy, 323, 1496
fasciculation, 635
fat-soluble vitamin, 1170
Fatigue (diagnostic label)
insomnia, 1091
respiratory and cardiovascular functions, 1328
fatty acids, 1169
fear, 1495
reducing, 998
and stress, 1494–1495
Fear (diagnostic label)
respiratory and cardiovascular functions, 1328
sexual health status, 1459
stress and coping patterns, 1501
feasibility, 42–43
febrile, 664
fecal elimination
see also defecation
assessing, 1236–1238
bowel incontinence, 1233–1234
bowel training programs, 1252
common fecal elimination problems, 1231–1234
constipation, 1231–1232
diagnosing, 1238–1240, 1239*t*
diagnostic studies, 1236–1238
diarrhea, 1233, 1233*t*
digital removal of fecal impaction, 1251–1252, 1251*f*
enemas, 1246–1250
evaluation, 1258*t*, 1259
factors affecting defecation, 1228–1231
fecal impaction, 1232–1233, 1232*f*
fecal incontinence pouch, 1252–1253
feces inspection, 1236
flatulence, 1234, 1252
home care, 1241–1242
implementing interventions, 1242–1258
interview, 1237
laboratory tests, 1237–1238
nursing history, 1236
ostomy management, 1253–1258
physical examination, 1236
physiology of defecation, 1226–1228
planning, 1240–1242
preoperative phase, 1028
promotion of regular defecation, 1242–1243
sample care plan, 1240–1241
stool specimens, 1237
teaching about medications, 1245–1246
testing feces for occult blood, 1238
visualization techniques, 1236
fecal impaction, 1232–1233, 1232*f*, 1251–1252, 1251*f*
fecal incontinence, 931, 1231, **1233**–1234
fecal incontinence pouch, 1252–1253
feces, 1226, 1228, 1229*t*, 1373
feces, liquid, 1393
feces inspection, 1236
feces testing, 1238, 1239
federal health departments, 159
feedback, 200, 387, 518
feeding bag, 1212
feeding patients, 1202–1204
feeding tube. *See* tube feeding
feet
assessment of, 722*t*
developmental variations, 720–721
hygiene. *See* foot hygiene
muscles, 632
fellatio, 1454
female circumcision, 1451
female dysfunction, 1456
female genital mutilation, 1451
female genitals
assessment of, 646–647, 656–658
lifespan considerations, 647–648
Tanner stages of development, 648*f*
femoral pulse, 673
fetal alcohol syndrome (FAS), 309
fetal phase, 308
fetal safety, 764
fever, 662, **664**–665, 672
fever spike, 664
fibre, 1167, 1230
fibrinogen, 882, 934
fibromyalgia, 981
fibrous (scar) tissue, 882
fidelity, 80
fifth vital sign, 988
figure-eight turns, 965
filtration, 1371
filtration pressure, 1371
finance, 508
financial stress, 297
fine crackles, 603*f*
fine motor tests, 640–643
fine muscle coordination, 316
finger muscles, 631
finger-to-nose tests, 640–641
fingers to fingers test, 641
fingers to thumb test, 642
firearms, 783
fires, 773–774
first intention healing, 934
first-level managers, 540
first marriages, 216
First National Nursing Research Conference, 39–40
first-pass effect, 802
fish, consumption of, 1184
fissure, 566*t*, **722**
fistulas, draining, 1393
fit checking, 898
fit testing, 898
fixation, 293
flaccid, 1115, 1289
flail chest, 684
flashlight, 558*t*
flatness, 560
flatulence, 1234, 1246, 1252
flatus, 1226–1227
flossing, 731–734
flowsheets, 481
fluid, body. *See* body fluids
fluid, electrolyte, and acid-base balances
assessing, 1388–1395
diagnosing, 1395
dietary changes, 1397
enteral fluid and electrolyte replacement, 1396
evaluating, 1422, 1425*t*
fluid intake modifications, 1396–1397
home care, 1396, 1398
implementing interventions, 1396–1422
oral electrolyte supplements, 1397
parenteral fluid and electrolyte replacement. *See* intravenous (IV) fluid therapy
planning, 1395–1396
wellness, promotion of, 1396
fluid balance, 1036–1039
fluid imbalances, 1380–1382
fluid intake
see also hydration
artificial nutrition and hydration (ANH), 1522
and body fluids, 1372
defecation, 1230, 1243
enteral fluid replacement, 1396
facilitation of (practice guidelines), 1399
fluid, electrolyte, and acid-base balances, 1392–1393
indwelling catheter, 1295
infection prevention and control, 910
measurement of, 1392–1393
modifications, 1396–1397
perioperative patients, 1028
restrictions, 1400
urinary elimination, 1267, 1281–1283
fluid output, 1372–1373, 1392–1393
fluid volume deficit (FVD), 1380, 1380*t*
fluid volume excess (FVE), 1381, 1381*t*
fluid volume gains *vs.* losses, 1382*t*
fluroscopic examination, 1236
flush phase, 664, 665
foam swabs, 734
focus charting, 477
Foley catheter, 1290
folic acid, 1180
fontanelles, 310
food
see also nutrition
allergies, 1201
beliefs about, 1173
for clear liquid, full liquid, and soft diets, 1201
common food allergens, 1201
labels, 1183
potassium-rich foods, 1376
safety, 1177
that becomes liquid at room temperature, 1392
Food and Drug Regulations, 797
food-borne illness, 1200
food diary, 1188
food-frequency record, 1188
foot boot, 750, 1131
foot hygiene
assessment, 721–722
diagnosing, 722, 723*t*
evaluating, 726
implementing interventions, 724
interview, 721
planning, 724
skill, 724–725
teaching, 725–726
foot reflex areas, 278*f*
footboard, 750, 1131
foramen ovale, 1317
forearm crutch, 1154
forensic nursing, 242
foreplay, 1454
formal care plan, 440
formal leader, 537
formal operations stage, 326, 335
four-point alternate gait, 1156–1157, 1156*f*
Fowler, James, 302, 302*t*, 1473
Fowler's position, 1131
frail elderly, 348
frail older adults, 348
frailty, 348
framework for population health, 134, 134*f*
Freedom of Information and Protection of Privacy Act, 471
frenulum, 1454
Freud, Sigmund, 292–294, 295*t*
friction, 929
friction rub, 603*f*
full agonists, 999
full disclosure, 50
full liquid diet, 1200–1201, 1201
functional age, 348
functional health patterns, 426, 427
functional method, 169
functional strength, 1110
Functional Urinary Incontinence (diagnostic label), 1279
functional vision tests, 581
funding
for nursing research, 40–41
research grants, 509
fungi, 880
funnel chest, 602, 602*f*
future-oriented questions, 223

G

gag reflex, 1325
gait, 389, **1122**

gaiter area, 934
gardening, 283
gas, 891
gastritis, 881
gastrocolic reflex, 1230
gastrointestinal changes, and aging, 354
gastrointestinal problems, in postoperative phase, 1038*t*
gastrointestinal suction, 1042–1046
gastrointestinal system
  and benefits of exercise, 1113
  immobility, effects of, 1120
gastrostomy, 1208, 1234
gastrostomy feeding, 1214–1215
gastrostomy tube, 824–825
gate control theory (GCT), 984–985
gauge, 828
gauze dressings, 954*t*
gay and lesbian
  berdache, 1452
  closeted, 1450
  disclosure of sexual orientation, 1447
  health experiences of, 1447–1448
  homophobia, 1447
  social relationships, and aging, 356
  two-spirited, 1452
  youth, 326
gender, 1446
  and acid-base balance, 1378
  and blood pressure, 687
  and body fluid, 1378
  and cardiovascular functions, 1320
  and communication process, 391
  and electrolytes, 1378
  and loss and grief, 1516
  and medication action, 803
  and nutrition, 1173
  and pulse rate, 672
  and respiratory functions, 1320
  as risk factor, 203
gender identity
  cross-dressers, 1448
  transsexuals, 1448
general adaptation syndrome (GAS), 1491
general anaesthesia, 1032
general appearance, 561–563
general clinics, 161
general survey
  appearance and behaviour, 561–563
  body mass index, 563–564
  height, 563–564
  lifespan considerations, 562
  vital signs, 563
  waist circumference, 563–564
  weight, 563–564
general systems theory, 206
generalists, 263
generalized anxiety, 1475
Generation X, 333, 542
Generation Y, 333, 542
generativity, 340
generativity *versus* stagnation, 340, 1432*t*
generic name, 796
genetic inheritance, 291
genetics
  and medication action, 803
  pharmacogenetics, 803
genital stages, 293
genitals
  and aging, 354
  female genitals, 646–647
  male genitals, 651–654
genogram, 218–219, 219*f*
genuineness, 399
geography, rural, 254–255
geragogy, 516
Gerontological Nursing, 350
gerontological nursing, 350
gerontology, 350
Gesell, Arnold, 292
gestures, 187, 390
Get Up and Go (GUG) Test, 776
Gilligan, Carol, 300–302
gingiva, 728
gingivitis, 594, 728, 729*t*
glandular changes, 324–325
Glasgow coma scale, 635*t*
glaucoma, 575
gliding joint, 1109*t*
global self, 1432
global self-esteem, 1435
global warming, 167
glomerulus, 1264
glossitis, 594, 729*t*
gloves, 559*t*, 895, 896–898
gloves, sterile, 905–907, 908–909
glucagon, 1168
glucose tests, 1196, 1278
glycemic control, 910
Glycemic Index (GI), 1172, 1172*t*, 1201
glycemic level, 1172
glycogen, 1167–1168
glycogenesis, 1168
goal statements, 449
goals, 445–450, 460–461
  see also evaluation
good food, bad food approach, 1173
good Samaritans, 106
goodness of fit, 296
Goodwill, Jean Cuthand, 5
Gordon's typology of functional health patterns, 426, 427
Gould, Roger, 297–298
gowns, 895, 896–898
graduate nursing education, 29
granulation tissue, 882, 936
grief, 1513
  and aging, 357
  experience of, 1513–1514
  factors influencing grief, 1514–1516
  interview, 1517
grip strength, 631
gross hearing acuity tests, 585–586
gross motor skills, 316
grounded theory, 44
grounding, 272
group, 400
  dyads, 400
  effective *vs.* ineffective groups, 401*t*
  group dynamics, 400
  growth groups, 402
  self-awareness groups, 402
  self-help groups, 401–402
  task groups, 400
  teaching and learning groups, 400
  therapy groups, 402
  types of health-care groups, 400–402
  work-related social support groups, 402
group communication, 400–402
group dynamics, 400
group teaching, 530
growth
  see also growth and development
  cephalocaudal growth, 291
  and health-care system, 165–166
  physical growth, 324
  proximodistal growth, 291
growth and development
  see also development; growth; lifespan development
  application of concepts to nursing practice, 302
  behaviourist theory, 300
  biophysical theory, 292
  and body alignment and activity, 1114
  cognitive theory, 299–300
  ecologic theory, 300
  hearing impairment, 311
  influencing factors, 291–292
  moral theories, 300–302
  principles of, 291
  psychosocial theories, 292–298, 298*f*
  social learning theory, 300
  spiritual theories, 302
  stages of, 292, 293*t*
growth groups, 402
guaiac test, 1238
guided imagery, 280–281
gums, 591–592
gustatory stimuli, 1061

H

habit training, 1285
hair
  assessment of, 564–570, 569–570, 737–738
  developmental variations, 737
  lifespan considerations, 570
  shaving, and preoperative phase, 1029
hair care
  assessing, 737–738
  beard and moustache care, 742
  diagnosing, 738
  evaluation, 742
  implementing interventions, 739–742
  planning, 738–739
  providing hair care for clients, 739–740
  safety razor, 743
  shampooing the hair, 740–742
hair loss, 737
half-life, 801
halitosis, 729*t*
hammer (ear), 583
hamstrings, 632
hand hygiene, 892–894, 895
hand movements (H/M), 581
hand restraints, 785, 786–787
The Handbook for Canada's Physical Activity Guide to Healthy Active Living, 1104, 1111
handwashing, 879, 892–894
harm, 99
harm reduction, 146–147
Hatha yoga, 280
haustra, 1226
haustral churning, 1227, 1227*f*
haustral shuffling, 1227
Havighurst, Robert, 292, 294*t*
hazard prevention
  carbon monoxide poisoning, 782
  choking or suffocation, 782
  electrical hazards, 782–783
  excessive noise, 782
  falls, 774–779
  firearms, 783
  fires, 773–774
  poisoning, 781
  radiation, 783
  scalds and burns, 773
  seizure, 779–781
hazardous material, 915
head
  assessment, 572
  bones of, 572*f*
  circumference, 309–310, 315
  ears and hearing, 582–589
  eyes and vision assessment, 572–582
  face, 572, 573
  lymph nodes, 595*t*
  mouth and oropharynx, 590–594
  nose and sinuses, 588–590
  skull, 572, 573
head injuries, 1231
head moulding, 310
head-to-toe assessment, 553
headache, 981
healing. *See* wound healing
healing environments, 272
healing garden, 283
healing through touch, 277
healing touch, 279
health, 117
  agent-host-environment model, 120
  and body alignment and activity, 1115
  and Canadians, 125
  determinants of health, 125, 126*t*, 135*t*, 705*t*
  downstream view, 125
  growth and development, 292
  individual health, 199–204
  models of health and wellness, 119–121
  and nutrition, 1174
  personal definition, 117
  and physical activity, 122
  population health initiatives, 135*t*
  prevention, levels of, 121
  in rural areas. *See* rural health care
  and sexuality, 1452–1453
  and sleep, 1085

Smith's models of health, 119
surgical risk and, 1019
upstream view, 125
WHO definition, 117
health appraisal, 202
health assessment. *See* assessment; physical assessment
health behaviour change. *See* behaviour change
health belief model, 122–123 (HBM)
health beliefs, 202, 520
health beliefs review, 144
Health Canada, 1177, 1184, 1214
health care
access to, 166–167
categories of, 156–158
categories of need for, 157–158, 157*t*
changes in health-care needs, 31–32
chronic diseases, 166
health-care ethics challenges, 73
levels of, 157
providers of, 163–164
and rights, 154–156
types of, 156–157
health-care-associated infections, 878–879, 879*t*
health-care delivery, in rural areas, 262–264
health-care organizations
see also care settings
assisted living centres, 162
community health centres, 160
crisis centres, 163
daycare centres, 163
extended-care (continuing-care) facilities, 162
general or specialist clinics, 161
hospice palliative care services, 163
hospitals, 161–162
lodges, 162
occupational health clinics, 161
physicians' offices, 160–161
public health services, 159–160
rehabilitation centres, 162–163
retirement homes, 162
specialization of, 166
types of, 158–163
health-care reform, 236–238
health-care settings. *See* care settings
health-care system, 152
access issues, 166–167
aging of population, 167
case management, 168
climate change, 167
contemporary frameworks for care, 168–169
and demographic changes, 165–166
economics and, 165
electronic health records and, 499–500
essential conditions, 11
evidence-based care, advancements in, 164–165
evolution of, 168
factors affecting, 164–167
federal cost sharing, 153
growth and, 165–166
health care, categories of, 156–158
health-care organizations and care settings, 158–163
homeless populations, 167
indigenous health-care system, 181
nursing delivery methods, 169
patient-focused care, 168–169
political and other leadership, 167
professional health-care system, 181
rights and health care, 154–156
technological advancements, 164–165
uneven distribution of services, 166
women's health, 167
Health Council of Canada, 499
health education, 137, 146
health educator, 241
health field concept, 117, **132,** 132*f*
health history
and health promotion, 143
nursing health history. *See* nursing health history
health information services, 504
health literacy, 523
Health on the Net (HON) Foundation, 502
Health Outcomes for Better Information and Care (HOBIC), 501
health-perception/health-management pattern, 426
health problems
adolescence, 326–327
client's understanding of, 520
elective health problem, 158
emergent health problem, 158
identification of, 437–438
infants, 312–313
mental health problems, 360
middle-aged adults, 340–341
neonates, 312–313
older adults, 359–362
preschoolers, 320
school-age children, 323
and surgical risk, 1020
toddlers, 317
urgent health problem, 158
young adults, 335–337
health professionals
communication among, 407
as data source, 419
handwashing and, 879
teaching, 515
Health Professions Act, 93
health promoter, 241
health promotion, 137, 156
adolescence, 328
assessment of individual health, 143–144
Canadians' health, 147–148
coping mechanisms, 203
defining health promotion, 137–138
development of initiatives in Canada, 132–136
vs. disease prevention, 137*t*
environmental control programs, 139
Epp Report, 132–133
evaluation of plan, 147
framework for population health, 134, 134*f*
health-promotion plans, 144–145, 145*f*
vs. health protection, 137*t*
health risk appraisal, 138
healthy communities movement, 133
implementation of behaviour change, 145–147
implementation strategies, 133
infants, 313–314, 315
information dissemination, 138
integrated model of population health and health promotion, 136*f*
Jakarta Declaration, 135–136
Lalonde Report, 132
lifespan considerations, 148
lifestyle and behaviour change programs, 138–139
mechanisms, 133
middle-aged adults, 341–342
neonates, 313–314, 315
nurses, role of, 12–13, 143–147
and nursing, 10
nursing process, 143–147
older adults, 358–359
Ottawa Charter for Health Promotion, 133, 135
partnerships in health, 133
Pender's health-promotion model, 139–141
population health-promotion model, 135
post-World War II, 132
preschoolers, 321
public participation, 133
school-age children, 323–324
sites for health-promotion activities, 139
stages of health behaviour change, 141–143, 142*f*
Strategies for Population Health, 134
toddlers, 315, 317
Toronto Charter for a Healthy Canada, 135–136
transtheoretical model, 141–143, 142*f*
types of programs, 138–139
wellness assessment programs, 138
wellness nursing diagnoses, 144
young adults, 337–338
health-promotion model (HPM) (Pender), 139–141, 140*f*
health-promotion models, 121–123
health-promotion strategies, 1503–1504
health protection, 137, 137*t*
health records. *See* client records
health restoration, 156–157
health risk appraisal, 138
health-risk appraisal (HRA), 143–144
health-seeking behaviours, 525
health status
cardiovascular functions, 1319
preoperative phase, 1022
respiratory functions, 1319
and safety, 764
healthier communities, 238
healthy breathing, 1331
healthy cities, 238
healthy communities movement, 133
healthy diet, 1180–1183
healthy heart, 1331
healthy sensory function, 1068
hearing
see also ear
assessment of, 582–589
changes, and aging, 353
conduction hearing loss, 587
hearing loss in rural areas, 259
impaired hearing, 1071
impairment, and growth and development, 311
lifespan considerations, 587
mixed hearing loss, 587
newborns and infants, 310
preschoolers, 319
school-age children, 322
sensorineural hearing loss, 587
sensory aids, 1070
sound transmission, 583
toddlers, 315
hearing aids, 746–748
heart
assessment of, 610–622
congenital heart defects, 1322
heart failure, 360
lifespan considerations, 615
location, 611
neck arteries and veins, 611*f*
physiology of, 1313–1314, 1313*f*, 1314*f*, 1316*f*
sounds, 610*f*, 611, 611*t*, 615–618
heart attack, 1321
heart disease, 1452
heart failure, 1321
heart rate, 1315
heat and cold applications
adaptation of thermal receptors, 969
application, 969–972
contraindications, 970
local effects of cold, 968
pain management, 1008
physiological responses, 968–969, 968*t*
rebound phenomenon, 969
selected indications, 970*t*
systemic effects of heat and cold, 968
temperatures for, 969*t*
thermal tolerance, 968–969
heat balance, 662
heat exhaustion, 664
heat stroke, 664
heave, 611
heel down opposite shin test, 642
heel-toe walking, 640
height
general survey, 563–564
preschoolers, 319
school-age children, 322
toddlers, 315
Heimlich manoeuvre, 782
Heimlich valve, 1357
helix, 582
helminths, 880
helper T cells, 883
helping relationship
characteristics of, 397
described, 397
development of, 397, 400
introductory phase, 397–399
phases of, 397–400, 398*t*

preinteraction phase, 397
termination phase, 399–400
working phase, 399
hematocrit, 386, 1312, 1393–1394
hematoma, 937
Hemoccult test, 1238
hemodynamics, 1328
hemoglobin, 1312, 1326
hemoglobin level, 942, 1193
hemolytic transfusion reaction, 1421
hemoptysis, 684, 1325
hemorrhage, 937, 1037*t*
hemorrhagic exudate, 937
hemorrhoids, 1227, 1227*f*
hemostasis, 934
hemothorax, 1357
Henderson, Virginia, 8–9, 62
herbal medicine, 274–275, 1020
herbal preparations, 275*t*
herbal therapy, 274
hereditary factors, 203
heredity, 888
hernia, 658
heteronormative, 1447
heterosexism, 1447
hierarchy of needs, 204–205, 427
high-density lipoproteins (HDLs), 1170
high enema, 1248
high-fidelity simulation, 33
high-Fowler's position, 1131, 1332
high-level wellness grid, 120
high spinals, 1033
hinge joint, 1107*t*, 1109*t*
hip abduction, 632
hip adduction, 632
hip circumference (HC), 1191–1192
hip muscles, 632
hirsutism, 570, 708*t*, **738**
histamine-receptor antagonists, 1029
historical data, 417–418
historical perspective
Canada's laws, 91–92
Canada's migrations and immigration, 174
historical nursing practice, 3–8
nursing research, 39–40
history of the health-care system, 152–153
HIV clients, and chronic diarrhea, 1251
holism, 199–200, **272**
Holism and Evolution (Smuts), 200
holistic, 199–200
holistic health, 272
holistic health belief, 184
holistic health care, 272
holy day, 1476–1477
home assessment parameters, 247
home care
ability and activity problems, 1126
activity and exercise, 1126
antiembolism stockings, 1032
bandages and binders, application of, 967
bed or chair exit safety monitoring device, 779
blood pressure, 696
body temperature, 669
catheterization, 1295
cleaning a closed wound, 1049
death and dying, 1526–1527
described, 160
drainable bowel diversion ostomy appliance, 1257
enema, administering, 1250
fecal elimination, 1241–1242
fluid, electrolyte, and acid-base balances, 1396, 1397
gastrointestinal suction, 1045
hearing aids, 747
hygiene, 708, 717
infection prevention and control, 918, 919
intradermal injections, 838
IV antibiotics, 855–856
medication administration, 823–824
metered-dose inhaler (MDI), 870
mobility problems, 1125
nutrition, 1199
nutritional status, 1198
oxygen equipment, 1342
oxygen saturation, 699
oxygenation, 1330–1332
pain, 996, 997
patient-controlled analgesia (PCA) pump, 1007
positioning, moving, and turning clients, 1141
postoperative instructions, 1028
postoperative phase, 1039, 1040–1041
during preoperative phase, 1022
pressure ulcers, 946
pulse, 681
removal of sutures or staples, 1053
respiration, 686
respiratory and cardiovascular functions, 1329
restraints, 790
safety, 765–766
seizure precautions, 781
sensory perception disturbances, 1067
skin hygiene, 707, 710
sterile field, 900
stress and coping, 1503, 1504
subcutaneous injection, 841
suctioning a tracheostomy or endotracheal tube, 1356
tube feeding, 1217
urinary elimination problems, 1280–1281, 1282–1283
urine specimens, 1276
wound care, 919, 961–962
wounds, 946–947
home care documentation, 486
home care nursing, 242–243
home fires, 773–774
home hazard appraisal, 766
home health nurse (HHN), 239
homeless populations, 167
homeopathy, 274
homeostasis, 200–201, **1367,** 1373–1374
homeostatic drive, 1081, 1082
homeostatic function, 1081
homeostatic regulators, 201*f*
homophobia, 1447
homosexual. *See* gay and lesbian
hope, 1474
Hopelessness (diagnostic label), 1440
hordeolum (sty), 575
hormones, and body temperature, 663
horticultural therapy, 283
hospice care, 1528
hospice palliative care, 157, 163, **1528**
hospices, 10
hospital beds
bed cradles, 750
described, 749
footboard or foot boot, 750
intravenous poles, 750
making beds, 750–757
mattresses, 749
occupied beds, 755–757
side rails, 749–750
unoccupied beds, 751–755
hospital care, 214
hospital diploma programs, 27–28
hospital gown, 711
hospital information system (HIS), 498
hospitals
as care setting, 161–162
environmental distractions, reducing, 1094
host, 120
hostility, 1495
hot and cold packs, 971
hot environment, 1318
hot water bag, 971
household measures, 809
hub, 827
huff coughing, 1332, 1333
The Human Act of Caring (Roach), 67
human caring theory, 63–64
human dignity, 49
human immunodeficiency virus (HIV), 1450
human mode of being, 384
human papilloma virus (HPV), 337
human resources
management of, 542
and nursing informatics, 507
human systems theories, 207
humanism, 517
humanist, 272
humidifiers, 1332–1333
humoral (circulating) immunity, 882–**883**
humour, 282
in communications, 388
mind-body interventions, 282–283
in palliative care unit, 203
hydration, 1042, 1332–1333
see also fluid intake
hydraulic lift, 1146
hydrocolloid dressings, 954–957
hydrostatic pressure, 1371
hygiene, 704
determinants of health and, 705*t*
ears, 746–748
eyes, 743–746
feet, 720–726
hair care, 737–742
hand hygiene, 892–894, 895
home care, 708, 717
and infection prevention, 910
mouth, 727–736
nails, 726–727
nose, 749
perineal-genital care, 718–720
preoperative phase, 1028–1029
skin, 705–720
hygienic environment
environment, 749
hospital beds, 749–757
noise, 749
room temperature, 749
supporting, 749–757
ventilation, 749
hyperalgesia, 982
hypercalcemia, 1385
hypercapnia, 1320
hypercarbia, 1320
hyperchloremia, 1386
hyperemia, 881
hyperesthesia, 650
hyperglycemia, 1172
hyperhidrosis, 564
hyperinflation, 1350
hyperinsulinemia, 1172
hyperkalemia, 1384
hypermagnesemia, 1386
hypernatremia, 1383
hyperopia, 574
hyperopic, 319
hyperoxygenation, 1350
hyperphosphatemia, 1387
hyperpyrexia, 664
hyperresonance, 560
hypersomnia, 1088
hypertension, 688, 689*f*, 1317, 1322
hyperthermia, 664–**665**
hypertonic solutions, 1218, 1247, **1370**
hypertrophy, 1111–1112
hyperventilation, 683, 684, **1320**–1321
hypervolemia, 1323, **1381**
hypnosis, 280
hypocalcemia, 1385
hypochloremia, 1386
hypodermic syringe, 826
hypodermoclysis, 1402–1403
hypoesthesia, 650
hypoglycemia, 1172
hypokalemia, 1383–1384
hypomagnesemia, 1386
hyponatremia, 1383
hypophosphatemia, 1387
hypoproteinemia, 930
hyposmolar imbalance, 1382
hypostatic pneumonia, 1119
hypotension, 688
hypothalamic integrator, 663
hypothermia, 359, 665–666
hypothesis, 43
hypothetical questions, 223
hypotonic solutions, 1247, **1370**
hypoventilation, 683, 684, **1321,** 1387

hypovolemia, 673, 1037*t*, **1380**
hypovolemic shock, 1037*t*
hypoxemia, 1320
hypoxia, 1312, 1320
hypoxic drive, 1312

I

"I" statements, 407
iatrogenic disease, 801
ice bags, 971
ice chips, 1392
ice collars, 971
ice gloves, 971
ICN Code of Ethics for Nurses, 81
ICU psychosis, 1071
ICU syndrome, 1071
id, 292
ideal body weight (IBW), 1186
ideal self, 1433
identification, 320, 1497*t*
identity, establishment of, 325
identity *versus* role confusion, 1432*t*
idiosyncratic effect, 800
ileal conduit, 1301
ileocecal valve, 1226
ileostomy, 1234
illicit drugs, 801
illness, 123
acute illness, 124
chronic illness, 124, 166
client, impact on, 124
effects of, 124–125
family, impact of, 221–222
family, impact on, 125, 220–221
the individual, impact on, 200
infectious diseases, 878
lifespan considerations, 148
and medication action, 803
remission, 124
and self-concept, 1436
sensory perception problems, 1064
and sexuality, 1452–1453
and sleep, 1085
illness narratives, 225
illness prevention, 10, **156**
illness-wellness continuum, 120–121
imagination, 320
Imbalanced Nutrition diagnosis, 1196
imitation, 516
immediate postanaesthetic phase, 1034–1035
Immigration Act, 177
immobility
assessing, 1124, 1124*t*
effects of, 1115–1121
and pressure ulcers, 930
problems related to, 1124
immobilization, 1008
immune status, 888
immune system
and aging, 355
and benefits of exercise, 1113
immunity, 882–883, 882*t*
immunization schedules, 910*t*, 911*t*
immunizations, 888
immunization programs, 243
infection prevention and control, 910–911
young adults, 337
immunocompromised clients, 914
immunoglobulins, 882–883
impaired, 431
Impaired Adjustment (diagnostic label)
self-concept, 1440
stress and coping patterns, 1501
Impaired Gas Exchanges (diagnostic label)
fluid, electrolyte, and acid-base balances, 1395
respiratory and cardiovascular functions, 1328
impaired hearing, 1071
Impaired Home Maintenance (diagnostic label), 1067
Impaired Memory (diagnostic label), 1066
impaired olfactory sense, 1071
Impaired Oral Mucous Membrane (diagnostic label), 1395
Impaired Physical Mobility (diagnostic label)
mobility problems, 1125
pain, 994
Impaired Skin Integrity (diagnostic label)
fluid, electrolyte, and acid-base balances, 1395
hair care, 738
intraoperative phase, 1033
wounds, 945, 946
impaired tactile sense, 1071
Impaired Tissue Integrity (diagnostic label), 946
impaired tissue perfusion, 1322
Impaired Urinary Elimination (diagnostic label), 1279
impaired verbal communication diagnosis, 404
Impaired Verbal Communication (diagnostic label), 1067
impaired vision, 1070–1071
impairments to communication, 402–403
impending clinical death, 1525
implantable venous access devices or ports, 1402
implementing (interventions)
see also assessment skills; nursing interventions
client education, 529–531
communication, 404–405
communication of nursing actions, 458
delegation, 458
described, 455–456
determination of nurse's need for assistance, 457
exercise and activity interventions. *See* exercise and activity interventions
eye care, 744–746
fecal elimination, 1242–1258
fluid, electrolyte, and acid-base balances, 1396–1422
foot care, 724
hair care, 739–742
infection prevention and control, 918
intraoperative phase, 1034
loss, 1516–1517
nail hygiene, 727
nursing care plan, modification of, 462
nursing interventions, 457–458
nutritional status, 1198–1218
oral hygiene, 730–736
overview, 416*t*
pain. *See* pain management
patient safety. *See* patient safety
postoperative phase, 1041–1054
precautions, 914–916
preoperative phase, 1023–1032
process of implementing, 456–458
reassessment of client, 457
relationship to other nursing process phases, 456
respiratory and cardiovascular functions. *See* oxygenation and circulation interventions
self-concept, 1440–1442
sensory perception problems, 1067–1073
sexual health status, 1460–1466
skills, 456
skin hygiene, 710–720
sleep, 1094–1097
spiritual health, 1480–1482
stress and coping patterns, 1503–1507
supervision, 458
urinary elimination, 1281–1302
wound care, 947–967
implications, 45
implied consent, 97
impotence, 1456
impulse conduction, 1061
in-service education, 34
in-service programs, 34
in-the-canal (ITC) aid, 747
in-the-ear aid (ITE, or intra-aural), 747
inactive metabolite, 802
inappropriate sexual behaviour, 1465–1466
incentive spirometers, 1334, 1335
inclusiveness, 50
income, 217, 356
incomplete proteins, 1168
inconsistencies, 437
incontinence
bowel incontinence, 1233–1234
fecal incontinence, 931, 1233–1234
and pressure ulcers, 931
urinary incontinence, 1285
incontinent diversions, 1301
independence
and aging, 356
need for, 325
of thought, 372
independent variable, 43
indigenous health-care system, 181
indirect auscultation, 561
indirect contact transmission, 886
indirect percussion, 560
indirect visualization techniques, 1236
individual care
assessment of individual health, 201–204
developmental stage theories, 206
holism, 199–200
homeostasis, 200–201
hospital care, 214
illness, impact of, 200
individual health, 199–204
individuality, 199
needs theories, 204–206
nursing process, 204
systems theories, 206–207
terminology, 198
theoretical frameworks, application of, 204–207
individual strengths, 225–226
individuality, 199
individualized care plans, 440
individuals
assessment of individual health, 143–144
characteristics and experiences, 139
health-promotion plans, 144–145, 145*f*
induced hypothermia, 666
inductive reasoning, 371
industry *versus* inferiority, 322, 1432*t*
indwelling catheter
catheter-associated urinary infections, prevention of, 1296
changing catheter and tubing, 1296
described, 1290
dietary measures, 1295
fluids, 1295
home care, 1295
nursing interventions, 1280–1297
ongoing assessment, 1296
perineal care, 1295
removal, 1296–1297
selection of appropriate catheter, 1291
urethral urinary catheterization, 1291–1294
indwelling catheter specimen, 1277
ineffective, 431
Ineffective Airway Clearance (diagnostic label)
mobility problems, 1125
pain, 993
postoperative phase, 1040
respiratory and cardiovascular functions, 1328
Ineffective Breathing Pattern (diagnostic label)
postoperative phase, 1040
respiratory and cardiovascular functions, 1328
ineffective coping, 1499
Ineffective Coping (diagnostic label), 1501
pain, 994
self-concept, 1440
Ineffective Denial (diagnostic label), 1501
Ineffective Health (diagnostic label), 994
Ineffective Health Maintenance (diagnostic label), 1040
Ineffective Individual Coping (diagnostic label), 1091
Ineffective Protection (diagnostic label), 1033
Ineffective Role Performance (diagnostic label), 1439
Ineffective Sexuality Patterns (diagnostic label), 1459
Ineffective Tissue Perfusion (diagnostic label)
fluid, electrolyte, and acid-base balances, 1395
intraoperative phase, 1033
respiratory and cardiovascular functions, 1328
infants (birth to 1 year)
abdomen, assessment of, 630
anus, assessment of, 656
bathing, 706, 713–717
blood pressure, 695
body temperature, 671–672
breasts and axillae, assessment of, 621–622

catheterization, 1295
cognitive development, 312
defecation, 1228–1229
developmental guidelines, 314
ears and hearing, assessment of, 587
enema, administering, 1250
eyes and vision, assessment of, 582
face, assessment of, 574
female genitals, assessment of, 647–648
fluid and electrolyte balance, 1379
food safety, 1177
general survey, 562
hair, assessment of, 570
health assessment and promotion, 313–314, 315
health problems, 312–313
heart and central vessels, assessment of, 615
immunization schedules, 910*t*
inguinal lymph nodes, assessment of, 647–648
intramuscular injection, 848
male genitals and inguinal area, assessment of, 653
medication administration, 816
moral development, 312
motor development, 312*t*
musculoskeletal system, assessment of, 633
nails, assessment of, 572
nasogastric tube, insertion of, 1208
neck, assessment of, 599
neurological system, assessment of, 645
normal sleep patterns and requirements, 1083–1084
nutrition, 1176–1177
ophthalmic instillations, 861
oral hygiene, 730
oral medications, administration of, 823
otic medications, 864
oxygen delivery equipment, 1341
oxygen saturation, 699
pain management, 1011
peripheral vascular system, assessment of, 617
physical development, 309–311
positioning, moving, and turning clients, 1141
pressure ulcers, 961
psychosocial development, 311–312
pulse, assessment of, 681
rectal medications, 868
rectum, assessment of, 656
respiration, 685
restraints, 789
safety measures, 768, 769
seizure precautions, 780
skin, assessment of, 568
skull, assessment of, 574
social development, 312*t*
sputum and throat specimens, 1325
stress and coping, 1491
suctioning a tracheostomy or endotracheal tube, 1356
thorax and lungs, assessment of, 608–609
tube feeding, administering, 1216
urinary elimination, 1266, 1267
wound care, 961

infected wounds, 928

infection, 878, 937
see also pathogen
additional precautions, 913–914
anatomical barriers, 880–881
antibody-mediated defences, 882–883
asymptomatic infection, 884
body defences against, 880–883
carrier, 884
cell-mediated defences, 883
chain of infection. *See* chain of infection
clinical spectrum of, 883–884
health-care-associated infections, 878–879, 879*t*
as imbalance, 884
inflammatory responses, 881–882
interview of clients at risk, 917
isolation precautions, 911–912
lifespan considerations, 887
local infection, 884
nonspecific defences, 880–882
nosocomial infections, 878
occupational health issues, 919–920
organisms causing infections, 880
pathophysiology of, 883
physiological barriers, 880–881
prevention, during intravenous (IV) fluid therapy, 1412
prevention and control. *See* infection prevention and control
risk for infection, 920*t*
routine practices, 912–913
septicemea, 884
specific defences, 880, 882–883
subclinical infection, 884
systemic infection, 884
transport of clients with, 915–916
urinary infection, 1120
and wound healing, 939–940
wound healing, complication of, 937

infection-control practitioners (ICPs), 920–921

infection prevention and control
see also infection
additional precautions, 913–914
antimicrobial agents, 892
aseptic technique, 898–899
assessing, 917–918
cleaning, 889–891
cough etiquette, 914
described, 888–889
diagnosing, 918
disinfection, 891
disposal of soiled equipment and supplies, 914–915
emerging pathogens, 914
evaluation, 918–919
hand hygiene, 892–894, 895
handwashing, 892–894
home care, 919
immunocompromised clients, 914
implementing interventions, 918
isolation precautions, 911–912, 916
microorganisms, elimination of, 889–892
multi-drug resistant organisms, 914
nursing interventions that break chain of infection, 889*t*, 890*t*
nursing responsibility for, 916–919
personal protective equipment (PPE), 894–898
planning, 918
practical issues for implementation of precautions, 914–916
radiation, 892
reduction of transmission, 892–909
reservoirs, elimination of, 889–892
routine practices, 912–913
as shared responsibility, 921–922
sterile field, 899*t*, 900–905
sterile technique, 899–909
sterilization, 891
support defences of susceptible host, 909–911
wound healing, 947

infectious agent, 878

infectious diseases
communicable disease, 880
death and illness, 878

inferences, 371*t*, **428**

inferiority, feelings of, 916

inflammation, 881

inflammatory bowel disease, 527

inflammatory phase, 934–936

inflammatory responses, 881–882

inflatable artificial sphincter, 1253*f*

influence, 540

informal care plan, 439–440

informal leader, 537–538

informatics. *See* nursing informatics

information, 497
see also nursing informatics
access to, 215
appropriateness, 489
confidential information, 104
disclosure, 97–98
information dissemination, 138
limited information, 1465
and nursing informatics applications, 497–498
offering information, 226

information dissemination, 138

information systems, 498

informed, 98

informed consent, 49–50, **97**, 98–99

infrared thermometers, 667, 668, 668*f*

infusion pump, 1412

infusion sets, 1403–1405

ingestion, 1226

ingrown nail, 572, **722**

inguinal area, 653–654

inguinal lymph nodes, 646–648, 656–658

inhalation, 682, 682*f*, 806

inhibiting effect, 800

initial assessment, 417*t*

initial planning, 439

initiative *versus* guilt, 319, 1432*t*

injections
see also parenteral medications
ampule, 829–832
intradermal injections, 835–838
intramuscular injections, 842–848, 842*f*
mixing medications in one syringe, 834–835
preparation of injectable medications, 829–833
subcutaneous injections, 838–841
vials, 829–833

injury, 256, 762
adverse events, 763
agricultural injuries, 258
deep tissue injury, 932, 934*f*
intentional injuries, 763
middle-aged adults, 341
needle-stick injuries, prevention of, 828–829
primary industry injuries, 258
unintentional injuries, 762–763
young adults, 335

inner ear, 583

inpatient, 158

input, 207

insensible heat loss, 663

insensible water loss, 663, 1372–1373

insight, 372

insoluble fibre, 1167

insomnia, 1087–1088

Insomnia (diagnostic label)
pain, 994
respiratory and cardiovascular functions, 1328
sleep problems, 1091

inspection, 556

inspiration, 682

instillations
described, 806
nasal instillations, 864–865
ophthalmic instillations, 858–861
otic instillations, 861–864
rectal instillations, 867–868
vaginal instillations, 865–867

Institute for Philosophical Nursing Research, 58

Institute for Safe Medication Practices Canada (ISMP Canada), 806

institution-based centres, 241

instrumental-relativist orientation, 323

instrumentation, for health assessment, 556, 558*t*

insufficient handwashing, 879

insulin, 1167
"clear before cloudy," 835
insulin syringes, 826, 838–839
mixing, 835
and surgical risk, 1020

insulin resistance, 1172

insulin syringes, 826, 838–839

intact skin, 928

integrated health-care system, 238

Integrated Pan-Canadian Healthy Living Strategy, 1104

integrated team model, 246

integrative medicine, 271
see also alternative medicine; complementary medicine

integrator, 241

integrity, 372

integrity *versus* despair, 355, 1432*t*

integument
described, 564
hair, 564–570

nails, 570–572
physiological aging, 351–353
skin, 564
integumentary system, and immobility, 1120
intellectual courage, 372
intellectual disabilities
older adults, 349
intellectual distraction, 1008
intellectual humility, 372
intellectual standards, 374*t*
intellectualization, 1497*t*
intensity, 561
intention tremor, 635
intentional injuries, 763
intentional torts, 101–103
intentional wounds, 928
interatrial pathways, 1314
intercessory prayer, 282
intercostal retraction, 684
intercourse, 1454
interdependence mode, 63
interdisciplinary approaches, 262
interdisciplinary spiritual care planning and intervention, 1476
intermittent feedings, 1210–1211
intermittent fever, 664
intermittent infusion devices, 856
intermittent intravenous infusions, 850–852
internal respiration, 682
internal sphincter, 1227
internal stimuli, 1061
International Council of Nurses (ICN), 9, 13, 19, 81
International Nursing Index, 46
International Nursing Review, 19
International Parish Nurse Resource Centre, 241
internationally educated nurses, 27
Internet
caregiver electronic record (CER), 502
consumer informatics, 501–502
criteria for evaluation of health information, 502*t*
patient portals, 502
research, 46
interpersonal attitudes. *See* attitudes
interpersonal concordance, 323
interpersonal influences, 140
interpersonal relations model, 62
interpersonal skills, 456
interphalangeal joints, 1107*t*, 1109*t*
interpreters, 186
interpretive tradition, 57
interprofessional approaches, 262
interprofessional collaboration, 169
interprofessional cooperation, 244–246, **245**
interprofessional education, 33
interrole conflict, 1435
interrupted sutures, 1051
interstitial fluid, 1368
intertarsal joints, 1109*t*
interventricular septum, 1313
interview, 420
activity and exercise, 1121
body image, 1438
cardiovascular functions, 1323
clients at risk for infections, 917
directive interview, 420
dying individual, 1526
eye care, 743
fecal elimination, 1237
fluid, electrolyte, and acid-base balances, 1390
foot care, 721
hair care, 737
history of current pain experience, 990
loss and grieving, 1517
nondirective interview, 420–421
oral hygiene, 728
personal identity, 1438
planning, 422
preoperative assessment data, 1022
questions, types of, 421–422
respiratory functions, 1323
role performance, 1438
sensory-perceptual functioning, 1065
setting, 422
sexual health history, 1458
skin care, 707
sleep disturbances, 1090
stages of, 422–423
stress and coping patterns, 1500
urinary elimination, 1272
intestinal distension, 1234
intestinal movements, 1227*f*
intimacy, 334
intimacy *versus* isolation, 1432*t*
intimate distance communication, 391
intonation, 387
intra-arterial, 806
intra-articular, 806
intracardiac, 806
intracellular fluid (ICF), 1368
intractable pain, 980, 982
intradermal, 806
intradermal injections, 835–838
intramuscular injections, 842–848, 842*f*, 1003
intraoperative phase, 1018
anaesthesia, types of, 1032–1033
assessing, 1033
diagnosing, 1033
documentation, 1034
evaluating, 1034
implementing interventions, 1034
planning, 1033–1034
positioning, 1034
surgical skin preparation, 1034
intraosseous, 806
intrapersonal communication, 386
intrapleural, 806
intrapleural pressure, 1311
intrapulmonary pressure, 1311
intrasmuscular, 806
intraspinal, 806
intraspinal delivery, 1004–1005, 1004*f*
intrathecal, 806
intrauterine development, 308–309
intravascular fluid, 1368
intravenous block, 1033
intravenous equipment, 1403–1406
intravenous hyperalimentation (IVH), 1218
intravenous infusion without a pump, 711, **806**
intravenous infusions. *See* intravenous (IV) fluid therapy
intravenous (IV) fluid therapy
blood transfusions, 1413–1422
catheters, 1401–1402
changing catheter to intermittent infusion lock, 1419
changing intravenous containers, tubing and dressings, 1413, 1416–1417
devices to control infusions, 1412–1413
discontinuing peripheral intravenous infusion, 1418
drops per minute, 1411–1412
factors influencing flow rates, 1412
importance of, 1398
infections, prevention of, 1412
intravenous equipment, 1403–1406
intravenous solutions, 1398–1401, 1400*t*
millilitres per hour, 1407–1411
monitoring intravenous infusions, 1407–1413, 1414–1415
peripheral intravenous sites, changing, 1413
regulating intravenous infusions, 1407–1413
starting an intravenous infusion, 1406–1407, 1407–1411
vein selection, 1402
venipuncture sites, 1401–1403
venous access device, 1404–1405
intravenous medications
adding medication to intravenous fluid containers, 849–850
described, 848–856
as fluid intake, 1393
home care, 855–856
intermittent infusion devices, 856
intermittent intravenous infusions, 850–852
intravenous push (IVP), 852–855
large volume infusions, 848
needleless systems, 851, 851*f*
opioids, 1003
secondary intravenous lines, 851*f*
volume-control infusion sets, 852
intravenous poles, 750, 1406
intravenous push (IVP), 852–855
intravenous pyelography (IVP), 1278
intravenous solutions, 1398–1401, 1400*t*
introductory phase, 397–399
introjection, 320, 1497*t*
introspection, 1431
intuition, 376
invasion of privacy, 102–103
invasive monitoring, 691
invasive (open) surgery, 1018
involuntary urination. *See* urinary incontinence (UI)
ions, 1368
iritis, 575
iron-deficiency anemia, 1176–1177
irrigation, 871
bladder irrigation, 1298–1300
catheter irrigations, 1298, 1393
closed method, 1298
colostomy irrigation, 1257–1258
described, 806
ear irrigations, 863
frequently used solutions, 958
gastrointestinal tube, 1045
open irrigation, 1298
syringes, 871–872, 871*f*
tube irrigants, 1393
urinary irrigations, 1298–1300
vaginal, 866–867
wound cleansing, 958, 960–961
ischemia, 929, 1322
isokinetic (resistive) exercises, 1111
isolation, 253
isolation precautions, 911–912, 916
isometric (static or setting) exercises, 1111
isotonic (dynamic) exercises, 1110–1111, **1370**
isotonic imbalances, 1380
isotonic solutions, 1247, **1370**

J

jacket restraints, 785, 787
Jakarta Declaration, 135–136
jaundice, 564
jejunostomy, 1208, 1234
jejunostomy feeding, 1214–1215
joint disease, 1453
joint movements, 1105, 1105*t*, 1106*t*
joints
appearance and movement of, 1122–1123
assessment of, 632
degenerative joint changes, 353
immobility, effects of, 1116
range of motion (ROM), 1105
Joseph Brant Memorial Hospital v. Koziol, 96
Journal of Nursing Scholarship, 20
judge-made law, 91
judgments, 371*t*
jugular veins, 614, 624
justice, 50, **80,** 261–262

K

Kardex, 481
[kcal], 1171
Kegel exercises, 1286–1287
keloid, 566*t*, **937**
ketones, 1278
keyhole surgery, 1018
kidneys, 1264, 1264*f*, 1373–1374
kilocalories, 1171
kilojoule, 1171
kinesthetic, 1061
kinesthetic sensation, 644
knowledge, 497
deficient knowledge, 525
and nursing informatics applications, 497–498
Kock pouch, 1301
Kohlberg, Lawrence, 300, 301*t*
koilonychia, 571
Korotkoff's sounds, 691, 692
kosher, 1478
Kotter's eight-step change process, 545–546
Kundalini yoga, 280

Kussmaul's respiration, 684, **1321**
kyphosis, 353, 602*f*

L

Laboratory Centre for Disease Control, 911
laboratory data, 917–918, 942
laboratory records, 419
laboratory specimens, 915
laboratory tests
 fecal elimination, 1237–1238
 fluid, electrolyte, and acid-base balances, 1393–1395
 for nutritional status, 1193–1196
laboured breathing, 683
lactated Ringer's, 1401
lactose intolerance, 1174
lactose maldigestion, 1174
laissez-faire leader, 539
Lalonde, Marc, 117
Lalonde Report, 132, 136
language
 assessment, 635–637, 637
 diversity of, in Canada, 175–176
language deficits, 402
lanugo, 308, 737
laparoscopic surgery, 1018
large-bore nasogastric tubes, 1204
large calorie (Calorie, kilocalorie, [kcal]), 1171
large intestine, 1226–1227, 1226*f*, 1227*f*
large volume enemas, 1247
laryngeal mirror, 558*t*
laryngoscopy, 1328
larynx, 1309–1310
late adulthood. *See* older adults
latency stages, 293, 322
lateral (side-lying) position, 1132–1133, 1133*t*
Latex Allergy Response (diagnostic label), 768
laughter, 282–283
lavage, 871
 see also irrigation
law, 91
 see also legal aspects of nursing
 battery, 97
 case law, 91
 civil law, 91
 common law, 91
 functions of the law in nursing, 91
 history of Canada's laws, 91–92
 judge-made law, 91
 negligence, 97
 precedents, 91
 source of Canada's laws, 91–92
 statutory law, 91–92
 tort law, 91
law and order orientation, 323, 340
law of similar, 274
lawsuit, 103
laxative abuse, 1245
laxatives, 1230, **1231,** 1245–1246, 1246*t*
lazy-eye, 317
leader, 537
 autocratic (authoritarian, directive) leaders, 538
 bureaucratic leader, 539
 democratic (participative, consultative) leader, 538–539
 laissez-faire (nondirective, permissive, ultra-liberal) leader, 539
leadership
 charismatic leadership, 539
 classical leadership theories, 538–539
 contemporary leadership theories, 539–540
 effective leadership, 540
 formal leader, 537
 informal leader, 537–538
 leader *vs.* manager roles, 537*t*
 leadership style, 538–539, 539*t*
 role, 14
 shared leadership, 540
 situational leadership, 539
 theories, 538–540
 transactional leadership, 539
 transformational leadership, 539–540
leadership style, 538–539, 539*t*
leading question, 422
LeaRN Canadian Registered Nurse Examination (CRNE) Readiness Test, 506
learning, 516
 see also client education
 active involvement, 517–518
 affective learning, 532
 barriers to, 519*t*
 and cultural barriers, 519
 and emotions, 518–519
 environment, 518
 evaluating learning, 531–532
 factors affecting learning, 517–520
 feedback, 518
 motivation, 517
 nonjudgmental support, 518
 physiological events, 519
 psychomotor ability, 519–520
 readiness to learn, 517
 relevance, 518
 repetition, 518
 from simple to complex, 518
 theories, 516–517
 timing, 518
learning need, 516, 524–525
learning outcomes, 525–526, 527
learning style, 520–521
learning theories
 behaviourism, 516
 cognitive theory, 517
 humanism, 517
least restraint, 784
Lebel v. Roe, 102
leg exercises, 1024–1027, 1041
legal aspects of nursing
 see also law
 advanced directives, 1521–1522
 artificial nutrition and hydration, 1522
 certification, 94
 confidentiality, 104–105
 consent issues, 97–99
 credentialing, 94
 do not resuscitate orders, 1523–1524
 end-of-life care, 1520–1524
 euthanasia, 1522
 expansion of role of registered nurses, 94
 legal protections in nursing practice, 106–108
 legal roles of nurses, 95–96
 licensure, 94
 nursing legislation in Canadian provinces and territories, 93*t*
 privacy, 104–105
 problematic substance use and chemical dependency, 105
 registration, 94
 regulatory bodies, 92–94
 regulatory considerations, 92–94
 reporting crimes, torts and unsafe practices, 108
 restraints, use of, 784–785
 selected aspects of professional regulation, 94
 selected categories of laws affecting nurses, 92*t*
 students, legal responsibilities of, 108–109
 tort liability in nursing, 99–104
 vicarious liability, 96
legal protections in nursing practice
 carrying out a physician's orders, 106–107
 legal precautions for nurses, 107
 professional liability insurance, 106
 provision of safe, competent nursing care, 107
 quality documentation, 106
legal prudence, 489
legal right to practice nursing, 27
legal roles of nurses, 95–96
legibility of recording, 486
legislation, 91, 177, 796–799
 see also legal aspects of nursing
Leininger, Madeleine, 65, 384
Leininger's sunrise model, 182*f*
length of newborn, 309
length of toddler, 315
lesbian. *See* gay and lesbian
lesions, 569
leukocytes, 881, 1326
leukocytosis, 881
leukotriene modifiers, 1333
level of consciousness, 635*t*, 638, 646, 1036, 1530*t*
levels of management, 540
leverage, 1129
Levin tube, 1204, 1205*f*
Lewin's theory of change, 545
liability
 professional liability insurance, 106
 vicarious liability, 96
libido, 292, 1453
lice, 738
licensed practical nurses (LPN)
 defined, 10
 licensed practical nursing programs, 30
 Practical Nurses Canada, 20
 recognition of, 27
 regulation of, 13
 role, 10
licensing examination, 27
licensure, 94
lichenification, 566*t*
life expectancy, 348
life spirals, 1473
life stress review, 144
lifespan considerations
 abdomen, assessment of, 630
 antiembolism stockings, 1032
 anus, assessment of, 656
 assisting clients to ambulate, 1152
 bandages and binders, application of, 967
 bathing, 706
 blood pressure, 695–696
 body temperature, 671–672
 breasts and axillae, assessment of, 621–622
 cardiovascular functions, 1317–1318
 catheterization, 1295
 client education, 522
 communication with older adults, 403
 complementary health modalities, 279
 computer use, 505
 ears and hearing, assessment of, 587
 enema, administering, 1250
 eyes and vision, assessment of, 582
 face, assessment of, 574
 female genitals, assessment of, 647–648
 fluid and electrolyte balance, 1379
 general survey, 562
 hair, assessment of, 570
 health-care decisions, 376
 health promotion, 148
 heart and central vessels, assessment of, 615
 infections, 887
 inguinal lymph nodes, assessment of, 647–648
 intradermal injections, 838
 intramuscular injection, 848
 male genitals and inguinal area, assessment of, 653–654
 metered-dose inhalers and nebulizers, 871
 musculoskeletal system, assessment of, 633
 nails, assessment of, 572
 nasogastric tube, insertion of, 1208
 neck, assessment of, 599
 neurological system, assessment of, 645–646
 nutritional variations throughout the lifespan, 1176–1180
 ophthalmic instillations, 861
 oral hygiene, 730–731
 oral medications, administration of, 823
 otic medications, 864
 oxygen delivery equipment, 1341
 oxygen saturation, 699
 pain management, 1011
 patient-controlled analgesia (PCA) pump, 1006
 peripheral vascular system, assessment of, 617
 positioning, moving, and turning clients, 1141
 postoperative care, 1035–1036
 preoperative teaching, 1027
 pressure ulcers, 961
 pulse, assessment of, 681
 rectal medications, 868
 respiration, 685
 respiratory functions, 1317–1318
 restraints, 789
 safety hazards, 764

safety measures, 768–772
safety problems, 772
seizure precautions, 780
self-esteem, enhancement of, 1441–1442
sexuality, 1449–1451
skin, assessment of, 568–569
skull, assessment of, 574
sputum and throat specimens, 1325
stress and coping, 1491
suctioning a tracheostomy or endotracheal tube, 1356
thorax and lungs, assessment of, 608–609
tube feeding, administering, 1216
urinary elimination, 1267, 1268*t*
wound care, 961
wound healing, 939
lifespan development
adolescence (12 to 18 years), 324–328
middle-aged adults (40 to 65 years), 338–342
neonates and infants (birth to 1 year), 309–315
older adults. *See* older adults
preschoolers (4 to 5 years), 319–321
school-age children (6 to 12 years), 322–324
toddlers (1 to 3 years), 315–318
young adults (20 to 40 years), 334–338
lifestyle
and acid-base balance, 1379
and body fluids, 1379
cardiovascular functions, 1318–1319
and electrolytes, 1379
and nutrition, 1173–1174
respiratory functions, 1318–1319
and safety, 764
sedentary lifestyle, 1178
sensory perception problems, 1064
and sleep, 1086
and wound healing, 939
lifestyle and behaviour change programs, 138–139
lifestyle assessment, 143
lifestyle factors, 204
lift, 611
lifting, 1127–1129
light palpation, 557
light perception test, 581
light-touch sensation, 642–643
likelihood of action, 123
limb restraints, 785, 787
limited information, 1465
line of gravity, 1104
linens, 915
lipids, 1169–1170
lipodermatosclerosis, 934
lipoprotein, 1170
lips, 591
liquid feces, 1393
liquid medication, 820–821
listening
attentive listening, 392–393
empathetic listening, 399
literature, 419–420, 506
literature review, 508
liver
palpation, 628–629
percussion, 627
living wills, 1520–1522
livor mortis, 1534
lobule, 582
local adaptation syndrome (LAS), 1491
local anaesthesia, 1032
local effects of cold, 968
local health agencies, 160
local infection, 884
local infiltration, 1033
locus of control, 1436
lodges, 162
Lofstrand crutch, 1154
logical positivism, 41
logrolling, 1134, 1138–1139
long-term-care documentation, 486
long-term coping strategies, 1498
long-term goals, 449
long-term memory, 357
look-alike health product names, 796
look-alike vials, 817
loop, colostomy, 1235*f*
lordosis, 1122
loss, 1513
actual loss, 1513
anticipatory loss, 1513
of aspect of the self, 1513
assessing, 1516
cause of, 1516
external objects, 1513
factors influencing loss, 1514–1516
of familiar environment, 1513
implementing interventions, 1516–1517
interview, 1517
of loved one, 1513
perceived loss, 1513
significance of, 1515
sources of, 1513
types of, 1513
love and belonging needs, 204
low-birth-weight babies, 308
low-density lipoproteins (LDLs), 1170
low enema, 1248
low-Fowler's, 1131
low literacy levels, 523
Low Self-Esteem (diagnostic label)
nutritional status, 1196
urinary elimination problems, 1279
low spinals, 1033
lower airway, 1309
lower extremity ulcers, 934
lubricant, 559*t*
lung compliance, 1311
lung recoil, 1311
lung scan, 1327
lungs. *See* thorax and lungs
lymph nodes
inguinal lymph nodes, 646–648, 656–658
neck, 595*f*, 595*t*, 596–597, 599
lymphocyte count, total, 1194
lysis, 883

M

maceration, 931
Mack, Theophilus, 4
Mack Training School, 28
macrominerals, 1170
macronutrients, 1167
carbohydrates, 1167–1168
lipids, 1169–1170
proteins, 1168–1169
macrophages, 881
macules, 565*f*
magnesium (MG^2), 1376, 1385–1386
magnetic resonance imaging (MRI), 501
magnetic therapy, 279
maintenance stage, 141
major surgery, 1019
making beds, 750–757
maladaptive coping, 1499
male dysfunction, 1456
male genitals
assessment of, 651–653, 658
lifespan considerations, 654
Tanner stages of development, 651*t*
Malette v. Shulman, 101
malignancies, 336–337
malleus, 583
malnutrition, 1185, 1186
mammography, 1464
Man-Living-Health: A Theory for Nursing (Parse), 64
management
see also manager
accountability, 541
authority, 541
coordinating, 541
directing, 541
functions, 541
levels of management, 540
organizing, 541
planning, 541
principles of management, 541
responsibility, 541
risk management, 541
management information system (MIS), 498
manager, 537
see also management
building and managing teams, 542–543
communication skills, 542
competencies, 541–543
conflict management, 543
critical thinking, 542
employee performance, enhancement of, 542
first-level managers, 540
levels of management, 540
middle-level managers, 540
networking, 542
resource management, 542
role of, 14, 537*t*
skills, 541–543
time management, 543
upper-level managers, 540
manipulative and body-based therapies
acupressure, 277–278
acupuncture, 277–278
chiropractic therapy, 277
massage, 277
qigong, 278–279
reflexology, 277–278
Tai Chi, 278–279
manubrium, 601
Margaret Scott Nursing Mission, 5
margination, 881
Marihuana Medical Access Regulations (MMAR), 798
marijuana, 798
marriage trends, 216–217
mask making, 279
masks. *See* face masks
Maslow, Abraham, 204, 427, 1435
mass peristalsis, 1227, 1227*f*
massage, 277, 1007–1008, 1095–1096
masses, characteristics of, 557
master's programs, 29
mastoid, 583
masturbation, 325, **1454**
maternal and child nursing, 214
maternal factors, 308
maternal stress during pregnancy, 1500
mattress interrupted sutures, 1052–1053
mattresses, 749, 1131
maturation phase, 936–937
maturity, 338
maximization of benefit, 50
McGill Model of nursing, 66–67
McGill pain questionnaire, 991, 992*t*
meal assistance, 1202–1204
mean, 45
mean arterial pressure (MAP), 1316
measurement systems, 809–812
measures of central tendency, 45
measures of variability, 45
meatus, 1265
mechanical aids for walking, 1152–1159
mechanical debridement, 951
mechanical loads, 929–930
meconium, 1228
median, 45
medical diagnosis, 432, 433*t*
see also diagnosis
medical futility, 83
medical narratives, 225
medical record keeping, 498–501
medical records, 419
medical records management, 507–508
Medical Service to Settlers in Quebec, 5
medical therapies, 888
medical treatment plan, 445
medication, 795
see also drugs; medication administration; pharmacology
abbreviations used in medication orders, 808*t*
antianxiety medications, 1097
antidiarrheal medications, 1246, 1247
antiflatulent medications, 1246
antihypertensive medications, 804
and blood pressure, 687
and cardiovascular functions, 1319
children, dosages for, 812
communication of a medication order, 808–809
cough medications, 1334

dangerous abbreviations, symbols and dose designations, 807*t*
and defecation, 1231
dosage calculations, 811–812
enteral medications, 818–825
essential parts of a drug order, 808
factors affecting medication action, 802–804
for fecal elimination, 1245–1246
forms of, 796
history of, and surgical risk, 1019–1020
intravenous medications, 848–856
measurement systems, 809–812
and nutrition, 1174
oral medications, 818–823
oxygenation and circulation interventions, 1333–1334
parenteral medications. *See* parenteral medications
parts of a prescription, 808, 809
preoperative phase, 1022, 1029
prescriptions, 806–809
psychotropic medications, 804
and pulse rate, 672
and respiratory functions, 1319
routes of administration, 804–806, 805*t*
sedative-hypnotic medications, 1097
sensory perception problems, 1064
sexual function, effects on, 1456, 1457*T*
and sexuality, 1453
and sleep, 1087
sleep medications, 1097
and susceptibility to infection, 888
through a feeding tube, 1216–1217
topical medications. *See* topical medications
types of drug preparations, 797*t*
types of medication prescriptions, 807–808
and urinary elimination, 1268
and wound healing, 939
medication administration
and aging, 818
developmental considerations, 816–818
enteral medications, 818–825
gastrostomy medications, 824–825
home care, 823–824
look-alike vials, 817
medication administration records, 809, 810*f*
medication dispensing systems, 813–814
medication history, 813
medication reconciliation, 813
nasogastric medications, 824–825
opioids, 1003–1005
oral medications, 818–823
parenteral medications. *See* parenteral medications
process, 814–816
safe administration, 812–818
ten "rights" of medication administration, 817
three checks, 816
topical medications. *See* topical medications
medication administration records, 809, 810*f*
medication cabinet, 814
medication cart, 813–814
medication dispensing systems, 813–814
medication error, 99–100
medication history, 813
Medication Reconciliation Project, 813
medication record, 481
medication room, 814
medicine wheel, 119
meditation, 280, 1477, 1481–1482
meditative prayer, 282
MEDLINE, 46
megavitamin therapy, 277
melanin, 564
melanotic freckles, 568
memory
and aging, 357
assessment of, 637
Impaired Memory diagnosis, 1066
long-term memory, 357
recent memory, 357
sensory memory, 357
short-term memory, 357
men
andropause, 339, 1450–1451
beard and moustache care, 742
climacteric, 339
genitals, assessment of, 651–653, 658
nocturnal emissions, 1084
perineal-genital care, 719–720
Tanner stages of development, 651*t*
urogenital tract, 650*f*
menarche, 324
menopause, 338, 1450
described, 338–339
and sleep, 1085
menstruation, 1449
mental health
and body alignment and activity, 1115
middle-aged adults, 341
older adults, 360
and pressure ulcers, 931
rural areas, issues in, 260
and sexuality, 1453
status. *See* mental status
mental health nursing, 214
mental illness, 214
mental status
assessment, 561–563, 635–646
attention span and calculation, 637–646
language, 635–637
memory, 637
orientation, 637
preoperative phase, 1022
sensory perception problems, 1064
and surgical risk, 1020–1021
mentor, 542
meperidine, 999
mercury in fish, 1184
mercury thermometer, 667
mercy killing, 1522
mesoderm, 308
mesosystem, 300
message, 387
metabolic acid-base imbalances, 1387
metabolic acidosis, 1387–1388
metabolic alkalosis, 1388
metabolic pool, 1169
metabolic substances in urine, 1278
metabolic syndrome, 1172
metabolic system
and benefits of exercise, 1113
immobility, effects of, 1119
metabolism, 802, 1119, 1166
carbohydrate, 1167
lipids, 1170
proteins, 1168–1169
metabolites, 802
metacarpophalangeal joints, 1107*t*
metaparadigm, 59
metatarsophalangeal joints, 1109*t*
metered-dose inhaler (MDI), 868, 869—870, 871
metric system, 809, 811
Metropolitan School of Nursing, 30
microbial load, 884
microminerals, 1170
micronutrients, 1167, 1170–1171
microorganisms, 881, 884, 889–892
see also infection
microsystem, 300
micturition, 1266
see also urinary elimination
micturition reflex, 1267
mid-arm circumference (MAC), 1192–1193, 1193*f*
mid-arm muscle circumference (MAMC), 1193
mid spinals, 1033
midaxillary line, 600
midclavicular lines, 599–600
middle-aged adults (40 to 65 years)
alcoholism, 341
cancer, 341
cardiovascular disease, 341
cognitive development, 340
developmental guidelines, 342
and grief and loss, 1515
health assessment and promotion, 341–342
health problems, 340–341
injuries, 341
mental health, 341
moral development, 340
nutrition, 1180
obesity, 341
physical development, 338–339, 339*t*
psychosocial development, 339–340
safety measures, 770, 772
spiritual development, 340
stress and coping, 1491
middle ear, 583
middle-ear infection. *See* otitis media
middle-level managers, 540
midsternal line, 599
midstream urine specimens, 1274
millennial generation, 542
millilitres per hour, 1407–1411
mind-body interventions
animal-assisted therapy, 283
biofeedback, 281
guided imagery, 280–281
horticultural therapy, 283
humour, 282–283
hypnosis, 280
meditation, 280
music therapy, 282
pilates, 281–282
prayer, 282
progressive relaxation, 280
yoga, 280
mind map, 378*f*
minerals, 1170
minimally invasive surgery, 1018
minimization, 1497*t*
minimization of harm, 50
minor surgery, 1019
miosis, 582
misbeliefs about pain, 998
mitral insufficiency, 1322
mitral valve, 1313
mitt restraints, 785, 786–787, 786*f,* 787–788
mixed apnea, 1088
mixed-colour wounds, 951
mixed hearing loss, 587
mobility, 216, 764, **1104,** 1124–1125
see also movement
mobility problems
see also activity
assessing, 1121–1124
evaluating, 1159, 1160*t*
exercise and activity interventions. *See* exercise and activity interventions
home care, 1125
physical examination, 1122–1124
planning, 1125
mode, 45
modelling, 516
models for delivery of nursing, 169
modes of care, 13
modes of communication, 387–390
modification of diet for disease, 1201–1202
modulation, 983
moist heat, 891
moist transparent wound barrier dressing, 955–956
moist wound healing, 947
molarity, 1369
mole, 1369
monosaccharides, 1167
monotheism, 1473
monounsaturated fatty acids, 1169
mons pubis, 1454
mons veneris, 1454
moral, 300
moral agents, 82
moral behaviour, 300
moral development, 300
adolescence, 326
Kohlberg's stages, 301*t*
middle-aged adults, 340
neonates and infants, 312
older adults, 357
preschoolers, 320
school-age children, 323
toddlers, 317
young adults, 335
moral issues, and end-of-life care, 1520–1524
moral principles, 83

moral theories, 78
consequence-based (teleological) theories, 78
described, 300–302
principle-based ethics, 79–80
principles-based (deontological) theories, 78
relationships-based (caring) theories, 79
utilitarianism, 78
morality, 300
Moro reflex, 311
mortality risks, in rural health care, 256
mortician, 1534
mother tincture, 274
motivation, 517
client education, 522–523
and sleep, 1087
motor aphasia, 637
motor development
neonates and infants, 311, 312*t*
preschoolers, 319
school-age children, 322
toddlers, 316
motor function, 639–640, 649–650
motor vehicle collisions, 259
moustache care, 742
mouth
anatomic structures of, 590*f*
assessment of, 590–594
common problems, 729*t*
developmental variations, 727–728
hygiene practices. *See* oral hygiene
movement
see also mobility
capabilities and limitations, 1123
normal. *See* normal movement
prescribed limitations, 1115
moving, 1024–1027, 1041–1042
moving clients in bed, 1134, 1135–1136
mucous membrane contact, 920
mucus blanket, 1310
multi-drug resistant organisms, 914
Multiculturalism Act, 176–178
multidose vial, 830, 833
multiparous, 657
mummy restraints, 789
muscles
activity, and heat production, 662
antigravity muscles, 1104
assessment of, 631–632
mass and strength, 1123
strength, 631–632
tone, and urinary elimination, 1268
muscular pump, 1316
musculoskeletal system
assessment of, 631–633, 634–635
exercise, benefits of, 1111–1113
immobility, effects of, 1115–1116
lifespan considerations, 633
music therapy, 282
mutual masturbation, 1454
mutual pretence, 1525
mutual respect, 246
mutual support groups, 163
mydriasis, 582
myocardial infarction (MI), 1321
myocardium, 1313
myopia, 574
myopic, 319
myotonia, 1454
mythic-literal stage, 323

N

nail hygiene, 726–727
nails
abnormality, 571
assessment of, 570–572, 571–572
ingrown nail, 572, 722
lifespan considerations, 572
normal nail, 571*f*
parts of, 570*f*
texture, 571
naming systems, 185
NANDA-I nursing diagnosis, 429–433, 430*f*, 455, 1196
NANDA International, 524–525
narcolepsy, 1088
narrative
described, 81
illness narratives, 225
medical narratives, 225
narrative charting, 473, **473**
narrative notes, 474*f*
nasal cannula, 1338–1339
nasal instillations, 864–865
nasal speculum, 558*t*
nasoenteric feeding tubes, 1205*f*
nasoenteric tube, 1208
nasogastric tube, 824–825, **1204**–1208, 1209
nasopharyngeal airways, 1344
nasopharyngeal suctioning, 1350, 1351–1353
nasotracheal suctioning, 1351–1353
National Formulary, 798
A National Framework for Continuing Competency Programs for Registered Nurses (CNA), 34
National Patient Safety Goals, 766–767
National Sleep Foundation, 1080–1081
Native Access Program to Nursing/Medicine (NAPN/M), 33
natural health products (NHPs), 271, 273, **275,** 276
natural resources, 253
naturalistic paradigm, 41
naturopathic medicine, 274
nausea, 1038*t*
nebulizers, 868, 871
neck
arteries and veins, 611*f*
assessment of, 596–599
lifespan considerations, 599
lymph nodes, 595*f*, 595*t*, 596–597, 599
major muscles of, 594*f*
muscles, 596
structures of, 595*f*
necrotic tissue, 1321
needle-stick injuries, 828–829
needleless systems, 851, 851*f*
needles, 827–828, 915, 1405–1406
needs
basic needs, 205–206, 1499*t*
comfort needs, 385
hierarchy of needs, 204–205
love and belonging needs, 204
physiological needs, 204
physiological needs of dying individual, 1528, 1529*t*
safety and security needs, 204
self-esteem needs, 204
sensory perceptual needs, 1529–1530
stress, and, 1499*t*
needs theories, 204–206
negative feedback, 200
negligence, 97, 99–101
negotiation, 192
neobladder, 1301–1302
neonates
cognitive development, 312
defecation, 1228–1229
health assessment and promotion, 313–314, 315
health problems, 312–313
lanugo, 737
moral development, 312
motor development, 312*t*
newborn screening, 313–314
normal sleep patterns and requirements, 1083
nutrition, 1176–1177
physical development, 309–311
psychosocial development, 311–312
safety measures, 768, 769
social development, 312*t*
nephrostomy, 1301
nerve block, 1009–1010, **1033**
nervous system plasticity, 985
networking, 542
neurectomy, 1010
neurogenic bladder, 1271
neuroleptanalgesic agents, 1029
neurological disorders, 1456
neurological system
appropriateness of questions and tests, 635
assessment of, 637–646
cranial nerves, 636*t*, 646
examination, described, 635
levels of consciousness, 646
lifespan considerations, 645–646
mental status, 635–646
motor function, 649–650
reflexes, 648–649
sensory function, 650
neuromusculoskeletal changes, and aging, 353
neuropathic pain, 980, 982
neutral question, 422
neutralization of virus, 883
newborn discharge summary, 482*f*
newborn screening, 313–314
newborns. *See* neonates
Newfoundland Outport Nursing and Industrial Association (NONIA), 5
Newman, Margaret, 65
NIC nursing intervention label, 453
NIC taxonomy, 454*t*
nicotine. *See* smoking
Nightingale, Florence, 4, 8, 27, 39, 60
Nightingale Training School for Nurses, 27
Nightingale's environmental theory, 60–62
nitrates, 1333
nitrogen balance, 1119, **1169**
nociception, 982
nociceptive pain, 982
nociceptors, 982
nocturia, 1269
nocturnal emissions, 1084
nocturnal enuresis, 1266
nocturnal frequency, 354, 1267
nodule, 565*f*
noise
excessive noise, 782
in hygienic environment, 749
nondirective interview, 420–421
nondirective leader, 539
nonessential amino acids, 1168
nonexperimental design, 44
nonjudgmental collaborator, 223
nonjudgmental support, 518
nonmaleficence, 50, 79–80
nonmetropolitan regions, 253
nonpharmacological invasive therapies, 1009–1010
nonpharmacological pain management, 1007–1009
nonproductive cough, 684
nonrebreather mask, 1340, 1340*f*
nonspecific defences, 880–882
nonsteroidal anti-inflammatory drugs (NSAIDs), 1001–1002
nonverbal communication, 187, **387,** 388–390, 404
norm, 434
normal breath sounds, 602*t*
normal feces, 1228, 1229*t*
normal flora, 877
normal movement
alignment and posture, 1104–1105
coordinated movement, 1110
joint mobility, 1105
normal saline, 1401
normal urine, 1273*t*
normocephalic, 572
normocephaly, 309
northern, 253
northern nursing practice, 262
nose
assessment of, 588–590
hygiene, 749
nosocomial infections, 878
notations on records, 487
nothing per ora (NPO), 1200
noxious, 982
noxious stimuli, 983*t*
NREM (non-rapid-eye-movement) sleep, 1082
nulliparous, 657
numerical rating scales (NRSs), 990, 991*f*
nurse
categories, 10
as delegator, 543, 544
as educator, 520–532

as employee or contractor for service, 95–96
expanded career roles, 15
and health promotion, 143–147
as leader, 537–540
legal roles of, 95–96
as manager, 540–543
as provider of service, 95
recognized categories of nurses, 27
role of the nurse, 12
roles and functions, 14–15
stress management, 1506–1507
telepractice, role in, 504
nurse administrator, 14
nurse educator, 14
nurse informaticist, 500
nurse-manager, 14
nurse managers. *See* manager
nurse midwife, 14
nurse practice acts, 13
nurse practitioner (NP)
core competencies, 15
described, 15
nurse practitioner programs, 29
recognition of, 27
nurse researcher, 14
NurseONE, 46, 504
Nurses (Registered) and Nurse Practitioner Regulation, 93
nursing
and advocacy, 84–85
definitions of, 8–9
and health promotion, 143–147
Henderson's definition of nursing, 62
nursing delivery methods, 169
philosophy in, 57
primary nursing, 12
recipients of, 9–10
scope of, 10
nursing administration
budget and finance, 508
facilities management, 508
human resources, 507
medical records management, 507–508
utilization review, 508
Nursing and Health Care, 65
nursing assessment, 426
nursing associations. *See* nursing organizations
nursing audit, 463
nursing care conference, 491
nursing care plans
collaborative care plans, 441–443
computerized care plan, 441
continuation, 461–463
development of, 439–443
documentation, 441*f*
documenting, 480–481
and evaluation, 461–463
modification, 461–463
sample, 452–453
see also sample care plan
standardized approaches to care planning, 440–443
standardized care plans, 442*f*, 480–481
student care plans, 441
termination, 461–463
traditional care plan, 480
writing, 451–452
nursing conceptual models, 426–428
nursing data base form, 426
nursing delivery methods, 169
nursing diagnosis, 431
actual diagnosis, 431
basic three-part statements, 438
basic two-part statements, 438
cardiovascular functions, 1328
client education, 524–525
clustering cues, 436–437
vs. collaborative problems, 432–433, 433*t*
communication, 404
data analysis, 434–437
defining characteristics, 431–432
described, 429
diagnostic labels, 431
diagnostic process, 433–438
diagnostic statements, 438
errors, avoidance of, 438
eye care, 744
fecal elimination, 1238–1240, 1239*t*
fluid, electrolyte, and acid-base balances, 1395
foot care, 722, 723*t*
formulation of, 435*t*
and goals or desired health outcomes, 449
hair care, 738
health problems, identification of, 437–438
infection prevention and control, 918
intraoperative phase, 1033
vs. medical diagnosis, 432, 433*t*
mobility problems, 1124–1125
nail hygiene, 726
NANDA-I nursing diagnosis, 429–433, 430*f*
nursing care plan, modification of, 461
nursing diagnosis, 429, 431
nutritional status, 1196
oral hygiene, 729
overview, 416*t*
pain, 993–994
patient safety, 768
possible nursing diagnosis, 431
postoperative phase, 1039–1040
preoperative phase, 1021–1022
related factors, 432
respiratory functions, 1328
risk nursing diagnosis, 431
risks, identification of, 437–438
self-concept, 1439–1440
sensory perception problems, 1066–1067
sexual health status, 1459, 1459*t*
skin hygiene, 707
skin problems, 709
sleep problems, 1091, 1092*t*
spiritual health, 1479–1480, 1480*t*
stress and coping patterns, 1500–1501, 1501*t*
syndrome diagnosis, 431
types of nursing diagnoses, 431
urinary elimination, 1279*t*
urinary elimination problems, 1279
wellness nursing diagnosis, 431
wounds, 945–946
nursing education
baccalaureate nursing degrees, 16, 27, 28–29, 32
certification, 30–31
changes in health-care needs, 31–32
changing demographics in nursing programs, 32–33
classroom technology, 507
and client records, 472
competent nursing practice, 34
computer-assisted learning (CAL), 506–507
continuing education in rural and remote areas, 33
continuing education to maintain competency, 34
described, 27
diploma programs, 28
distance education, 507
doctoral programs, 29–30
early training. *See* early training
educational programs, types of, 27–30
entry to practice, 32
evaluation and computers, 506
graduate nursing education, 29
hospital diploma programs, 27–28
in-service education, 34
interprofessional education, 33
issues facing nursing education, 31–34
licensed practical nursing programs, 30
literature access and retrieval, 506
master's programs, 29
nurse practitioner programs, 29
nursing associations, influence of, 30–31
nursing informatics in, 505–507
programs leading to or continuing basic RN education, 28–30
recognized categories of nurses, 27
registered practical nursing programs, 30
registered psychiatric nursing programs, 30
rural and remote practices, 264
shortage crisis, 32
student and course record management, 506
technological advancements, 33
nursing ethics, 80–81
nursing health history
activity and exercise history, 1121
cardiovascular functions, 1323
client education, 520–521
current pain experience, 989–992
data collection, 418
described, 426
eye care, 743
fecal elimination, 1236
fluid, electrolyte, and acid-base balances, 1388–1389
foot care, 721
hair care, 737
infection prevention and control, 917
nutritional status, 1188–1189
oral hygiene, 728
patient safety, 766
preoperative phase, 1021
respiratory functions, 1323
sensory perception problems, 1064
sexual health status, 1457
skin integrity, 928, 940
spiritual health, 1479
urinary elimination, 1271
nursing history. *See* nursing health history
nursing informatics, 497
see also computers
advanced practice in, 497
computers in nursing practice, 498–505
computers in nursing research, 508–509
consumer informatics, 501–502
goal of, 497
information systems, 498
interrelationships of data, information and knowledge, 497
nursing administration, 507–508
in nursing education, 505–507
nursing informatics in, 507–508
Nursing Intervention Classifications (NIC), 1196
nursing interventions
see also implementing (interventions)
breaking the chain of infection, 889*t*, 890*t*
criteria for selection, 451
endotracheal tubes, 1345
epidural catheter, 1006*t*
ethnopharmacology, implications of, 804
facilitation of communication, 404–405
fever, 665
hypothermia, 666
implementing interventions, 457–458
indwelling catheter, 1280–1297
interdisciplinary spiritual care planning and intervention, 1476
isotonic fluid volume deficit, 1380*t*
NIC nursing intervention label, 453
nursing care plan, modification of, 462
nutrition for older adults, 1181*t*
older adults, 362
patient safety, 768
selection of, 450–451
sensory perceptual alteration, 1074–1075
types of, 450–451
Nursing Interventions Classifications (NIC), 452–455
Nursing Labour Market in Canada: An Occupational Sector Study (CNA), 32
nursing organizations
see also specific nursing organizations
Canadian Nurses Association, 18–19
Canadian psychiatric nursing professional organizations, 21*t*
influence on education, 30–31
International Council of Nurses, 19
licensed (registered) practical nurses, 20
provincial and territorial practical nurse professional organizations, 20*t*
provincial and territorial registered nursing associations, 19*t*
registered psychiatric nurses, 20
Sigma Theta Tau International Honor Society of Nursing, 19–20
specialty organizations, 20
unions, 21

Nursing Outcomes Classification (NOC), 447–448, 448*t*
nursing philosophies. *See* philosophy
nursing practice
alterations in health competencies, 39
drug legislation, application of, 798–799
health and wellness competencies, 39
practice guidelines. *See* practice guidelines
nursing practice standards, 13
nursing process, 374, 412
see also assessment skills
in action, 413*f*
assessing, 417–429
characteristics, 415–417
and communication, 402–406
critical thinking, 375*t*
vs. decision-making process, 377*t*
diagnosing, 429–438
educator, nurse as, 520–532
evaluation, 458–463
health promotion, 143–147
implementing interventions, 455–458
individual care, 204
overview, 415–417, 416*f*, 416*t*
phases of, 375*t*, 415
planning, 439–455
spiritual health, 1478–1484
summary of, 464
vs. teaching process, 515*t*
use of, 415
nursing profession
autonomy, 16
code of ethics, 16
criteria of profession, 16
nursing as profession, 15
professional organization, 16
self-regulation, 15–16, 16
service orientation, 16
socialization to nursing, 16–17
specialized education, 16
well-defined body of knowledge, 16
nursing regulatory bodies, 13
nursing research, 39
applied research, 39
approaches, 41–42
basic research, 39
and client records, 472
computers in, 508–509
critiquing research, 46–49, 47*t*, 48*t*
data collection and analysis, 509
dependent variable, 43
dissemination of, 509
ethnographic research, 44
grounded theory, 44
history of nursing research, 39–40
hypothesis, 43
independent variable, 43
linking theory, practice and research, 40
literature review, 508
locating nursing research findings, 46
phenomenology, 44
pilot study, 44
population, 44
problem identification, 508
problem solving, 39
qualitative research, 41–42
quantitative research, 41
reliability, 44
research-based nursing practice, 39
research design, 44, 508–509
research grants, 509
research journals in nursing, 46
research process, 42–46
rights of human subjects, 49–50
sample, 44
support for nursing research, 40–41
validity, 44
Nursing Research, 46
nursing rounds, 492
nursing science, 39
nursing settings, 10–11
nursing sister, 6
nursing theories. *See* theory
nutrient solutions, 1399
nutrients, 1166
carbohydrates, 1167–1168
drug-nutrient interactions, 1175*t*
lipids, 1169–1170
macronutrients, 1167–1170
micronutrients, 1167, 1170–1171
proteins, 1168–1169
nutrition, 1166
see also food; nutritional status
adolescents, 1179
and advertising, 1175–1176
and alcohol consumption, 1174–1175
altered nutrition, 1185–1186
artificial nutrition and hydration (ANH), 1522
beliefs about food, 1173, 1477–1478
body alignment and activity, 1114
cardiovascular functions, 1319
constipation, prevention of, 1168
cultural care, 188–189
and culture, 1173
and defecation, 1230, 1243
drug-nutrient interactions, 1175*t*
Eating Well with Canada's Food Guide. See Eating Well with Canada's Food Guide
and economics, 1174
enteral nutrition (EN), 1204–1218
and ethnicity, 1173
factors affecting nutrition, 1172–1176
fetal development, 308
and fluid, electrolyte, and acid-base balances, 1397
food labels, 1183
and gender, 1173
growth and development, 292
and health, 1174
indwelling catheter, clients with, 1295
and infection prevention, 910
inflammatory bowel disease, 527
lifespan variations, 1176–1180
lifestyle, 1173–1174
malnutrition, 1185, 1186
and medication action, 803
and medications, 1174
middle-aged adults, 1180
neonates to 1 year, 1176–1177
and older adults, 1180
overnutrition, 1185
parenteral nutrition, 1204, 1218
personal preferences, 1173
portion grid, 1183*f*
in postoperative phase, 1042
preoperative phase, 1028
preschoolers, 1177
and pressure ulcers, 930, 948
and psychological factors, 1176
recommendations, 1184
and religion, 189
religious practices, 1173
respiratory functions, 1319
sample care plan, 1197–1198
school-age children, 1178–1179
serving sizes, 1182–1183
and sleep, 1086–1087
stage of development, 1172–1173
standards for a healthy diet, 1180–1183
stress and coping, 1504
surgical risk and, 1019
teaching healthy nutrition, 1199–1200
and therapy, 1174
toddlers, 1177
total enteral nutrition (TEN), 1204
undernutrition, 1185
and urinary elimination, 1267
vegetarian diets, 1184–1185
wound healing, 939, 947
and young adults, 1179–1180
nutritional assessment, 1186, 1187*t*
nutritional deficiencies, 1190*f*
nutritional-metabolic pattern, 426
nutritional screening, 1187
nutritional status
see also nutrition
anthropometric measurements, 1189–1193
assessing, 1186–1196
assisting patients with meals, 1202–1204
blood tests, 1193–1196
diagnosing, 1196
dietary data, 1187–1188
enteral nutrition (EN), 1204–1218
evaluating, 1218, 1219*t*
health history, 1188–1189
home care, 1198
implementing interventions, 1198–1218
laboratory tests, 1193–1196
nutritional assessment, 1186, 1187*t*
nutritional deficiencies, 1190*f*
nutritional screening, 1187
parenteral nutrition, 1204, 1218
physical examination, 1189
planning, 1196–1198
resistance to infection, 888
risk factors for nutritional problems, 1188
special community nutritional services, 1204
special diets, assisting with, 1200–1202
stimulation of appetite, 1202
thyroid function, 1196
urinary tests, 1196
weight gain or loss, percentage of, 1189–1193
nutritional supplements, 276
nutritionists, 164, 164*t*
nutritive enemas, 1248
nutritive value, 1166

O

obesity
and blood pressure, 687
in childbearing women, 336
chronic energy imbalance, 1178
middle-aged adults, 341
prevention, 1178
sedentary lifestyle, 1178
and susceptibility to infection, 888
treatment, 1178
objective, 445
objective data, 419
obligatory losses, 1373
observation, 420
obstructed airway, 1321
obstructive apnea, 1088
obstructive sleep apnea, 1321
occult (hidden) blood, 1238, 1239, **1278**
occupational exposure, 919–920, 921
occupational health clinics, 161
occupational health nursing, 242
occupational therapists, 164, 164*t*
occupations, and rural health framework, 256
occupied beds, 755–757
OECD predominantly rural regions, 253
OECD rural communities, 253
Official Languages Act, 177
official name, 796
oil-based lotions, 858
ointments, 858
older adults
see also aging
abdomen, assessment of, 630
Aboriginal older adults, 348
accidents, 359–360
advocates, 348
antiembolism stockings, 1032
anus, assessment of, 656
assisting clients to ambulate, 1152
attitudes toward aging, 349
bandages and binders, application of, 967
bath grab bar, 718
bathing, 706
blood pressure, 696
body temperature, 672
breasts and axillae, assessment of, 622
cancer, 362
cardiac disease, 360
care settings, 350
catheterization, 1295
characteristics, in Canada, 348–349
chronic disabling illness, 360
client education, 522
and cognitive abilities, 357
communication with, 403
computer use, 505
constipation, 1230

constipation, prevention of, 1168
defecation, 1230
delirium, 1071
dementia, 361
developmental guidelines, 358–359
developmental tasks, 355
ears and hearing, assessment of, 587
emergencies, 362
end-of-life care, 1518–1519
enema, administering, 1250
ethnic older adults, 348
eyes and vision, assessment of, 582
female genitals, assessment of, 648
fluid and electrolyte balance, 1379
frail older adults, 348
general survey, 562
gerontological nursing in Canada, 350
and grief and loss, 1515
hair, assessment of, 570
health and physical activity, 122
health assessment, 556
health assessment and promotion, 358–359
health-care decisions, 376
health problems, 359–362
health promotion, 148
heart and central vessels, assessment of, 615
illness prevention, 148
increasing number of, 167
infections, 887
inguinal lymph nodes, assessment of, 648
with intellectual disabilities, 349
intramuscular injection, 848
male genitals and inguinal area, assessment of, 654
medication administration, 816–818
mental health problems, 360
moral development, 357
musculoskeletal system, assessment of, 633
nails, assessment of, 572
neurological system, assessment of, 645–646
normal sleep patterns and requirements, 1084–1085
nursing interventions, 362
nutrition, 1180, 1181*t*
older adult abuse, 361–362
oral medications, administration of, 823
osteoarthritis (OA), 360
oxygen saturation, 699
pain management, 1011
patient-controlled analgesia (PCA) pump, 1006
peripheral vascular system, assessment of, 617
physiological aging, 351–355
positioning, moving, and turning clients, 1141
postoperative care, 1036
preoperative teaching, 1027
pressure ulcers, 961
problematic substance use, 360–361
psychological aging, 355–357
pulse, assessment of, 681
rectum, assessment of, 656
respiration, 685
safety hazards, 764
safety measures, 771, 772
self-esteem, enhancement of, 1442
skin, assessment of, 568–569
skin alterations due to aging, 707*t*
special groups of older Canadians, 348–349
spiritual development, 358
sputum and throat specimens, 1325
stress and coping, 1491
strokes, 360
suctioning a tracheostomy or endotracheal tube, 1356
Tai Chi, 279
thorax and lungs, assessment of, 609
tube feeding, administering, 1216
urinary elimination, 1266–1267
walking, 774
warmth in bed, 1097
wound care, 961
olfactory sense, impaired, 1071
olfactory stimuli, 1061
oliguria, 1269
omega-3 fatty acids, 1169
omega-6 fatty acids, 1169
oncotic pressure, 1370
one-point discrimination, 644, **650**
one-strip method, 1348–1349
ongoing planning, 439
onset of action, 801
ontology, 56
open awareness, 1525
open-handed questions, 421
open irrigation, 1298
open method, 906–907
open surgery, 1018
open system, 207
open systems, 1211
open wounds, 928
Operating Room Nurses Association of Canada, 1029
ophthalmic, 858
ophthalmic instillations, 858–861
ophthalmoscope, 558*t*
opinions, 371*t*
opioid adverse effects, 1000
opioid antagonists, 1000
opioid delivery, 1003–1005
opioids, 999–1001, 1029
opportunistic pathogen, 880
opsonization, 883
oral, 804
oral administration of opioids, 1003
oral electrolyte supplements, 1397
oral fluids, 1392
oral-genital stimulation, 1454
oral hygiene
assessing, 728–729
assisting clients with oral care, 731–735
diagnosing, 729
evaluating, 736, 737*t*
identification of at-risk clients, 729
implementing interventions, 730–736
lifespan considerations, 730–731
planning, 730
special oral hygiene, 734–736
teeth, care of, 731
oral medications, 818–823
oral opioids, 821
oral suctioning, 1350
oral temperature, 666*t*, 667, 670
organ donation, 1524
Organisation for Economic Co-operation and Development (OECD), 253
organizing, 541
orgasm, 1454
orgasmic dysfunction, 1456
oriental massage, 277
orientation, 637
orientation phase, 397–399
oropharyngeal airways, 1344
oropharyngeal suctioning, 1351–1353
oropharynx, 590–594
orthomolecular medicine, 276–277
orthopnea, 684, **1321**
orthopneic position, 1131
orthostatic hypotension, 354, 688, 1117, 1152, 1392
osmolality, 1370, 1394
osmolar imbalances, 1380
osmosis, 1370
osmotic pressure, 1370
ossicles, 583
osteoarthritis (OA), 360
osteoblasts, 1112
osteoclasts, 1112
osteoporosis, 353, 1114
ostomy, 1234
anatomic location, 1234–1235, 1235*f*
appliances or pouching systems, 1254*f*
changing an ostomy appliance, 1255–1257
colostomy irrigation, 1257–1258
construction of the stoma, 1235
drainable bowel diversion ostomy appliance, 1255–1257
management of, 1253–1258
odour control, 1254
permanence, 1234
pouch clamp, application of, 1254*f*
stoma and skin care, 1253–1257
types of, 1234
otic, 861
otic instillations, 861–864
otitis media, 259
otoscope, 558*t*, **582**
Ottawa Charter for Health Promotion, 133, 135, 136, 239
outcome evaluation, 463
outpatient, 158
outpatient surgical clients, 1024
output, 207
outreach programs, 239
overhydration, 1382
overnutrition, 1185
overt change, 545
overweight, 1185
overweight clients, 1199–1200
oximeter, 1091
oxygen
described, 1308
fetal demands for, 308
transport of, 1311–1312
oxygen delivery systems, 1337–1341
oxygen equipment, 1342
oxygen hood, 1341
oxygen saturation, 696–699
oxygen tent, 1341
oxygen therapy, 1336–1337
oxygenation, 1330–1332
oxygenation and circulation interventions
artificial airways, 1343–1349
cardiac nursing interventions, 1332
cardiopulmonary resuscitation (CPR), 1360
chest tubes and drainage systems, 1356–1358
circulation, promotion of, 1332
deep breathing and coughing, 1332
evaluating, 1360–1361, 1361*t*
home care, 1331
hydration, 1332–1333
incentive spirometers, 1334
medications, 1333–1334
oxygen delivery systems, 1337–1341
oxygen therapy, 1336–1337
oxygenation, promotion of, 1330–1332
percussion, vibration, and postural drainage (PVD), 1334–1336
suctioning, 1349–1356
vascular nursing interventions, 1332
venous stasis, prevention of, 1358–1359
oxygenation status. *See* oxygenation and circulation interventions; respiratory functions
oxyhemoglobin, 1312

P

pace, 387, **1122**
pain, 979
acute pain, 979, 980*t*, 982, 993, 994–996
affective responses, 992
age variations and, 987*t*
alleviating factors, 991
assessing, 988–993
associated symptoms, 991–992
behavioural responses, 992–993
cancer pain, 982
central mechanisms, 983–984
central neuropathic pain, 980
central sensitization, 985
chronic pain, 979–980, 980*t*, 982, 988, 993, 1453
clinical manifestations, 981
concepts, 982
daily living activities, effect of, 992
daily pain diary, 993
and defecation, 1231
developmental stage, 986–988
diagnosing, 993–994
environment, effect of, 988
ethnic and cultural values, 986
factors affecting experience of pain, 986–988
fifth vital sign, 988
gate control theory (GCT), 984–985
history of current pain experience, 989–992
home care, 996, 997

implementing interventions. *See* pain management
intensity, 981, 990–991
interview, 990
intractable pain, 980, 982
location, 989–990
management. *See* pain management
McGill pain questionnaire, 992*t*
meaning of, 988
mechanisms, 982–988
modulation, 983
nature of, 979–982
nervous system plasticity, 985
neuropathic pain, 980, 982
nociceptive pain, 982
past pain experiences, 988
pattern, 991
perception, 983–984
peripheral mechanisms, 982–983
peripheral neuropathic pain, 980
peripheral sensitization, 985
phantom pain, 982
physiological basis, 983*t*
physiological responses, 992–993
planning, 994–996
precipitating factors, 991
prevention, 998–999
proprioceptive reflex, 986, 986*f*
quality, 991
radiating pain, 980
referred pain, 980
reluctance to report pain, 989
research, 978–979
responses to, 985–986
self-report measures, 990–991
somatic pain, 980
support people, 988
sympathetically maintained pain, 980
transduction, 982–983
transmission, 983
types of, 979–981
visceral pain, 980
and wounds, 940
Pain (diagnostic label), 946, 1459
pain management, 996
acceptance of pain, 998
acknowledgment of pain, 998
acupressure, 1008
acupuncture, 1009
assisting support persons, 998
barriers, 997–998
coanalgesic, 1002
cognitive-behavioural interventions, 1009
concepts, 982
contralateral stimulation, 1008
coping resources, 992
cutaneous stimulation, 1007
death and dying, 1530–1531
distraction, 1009
equianalgesic dosing, 1001
evaluating, 1010–1011
heat and cold applications, 1008
immobilization, 1008
key strategies, 998–999
lifespan considerations, 1011
massage, 1007–1008
misbeliefs about non-opioids, 1002*t*
misbeliefs about pain, 998
nonpharmacological invasive therapies, 1009–1010
nonpharmacological pain management, 1007–1009
nonsteroidal anti-inflammatory drugs (NSAIDs), 1001–1002
opioid analgesics, 999–1001
patient-controlled analgesia (PCA), 1005–1007
pharmacological pain management, 999–1007
physical interventions, 1007–1008
placebo response, 1002–1003
postoperative phase, 1041
preemptive analgesia, 998–999
prevention of pain, 998–999
psychoeducation, 1009
reducing fear and anxiety, 998
relaxation response, 1009
routes for opioid delivery, 1003–1005
self-management program, and chronic cardiac pain, 1001
teaching, 997
transcutaneous electrical nerve stimulation (TENS), 1008
pain responses, and cultural care, 189
pain sensation, 643
pain threshold, 982
pain tolerance, 982
palates, 593
palliative care, 1528
palliative care unit, 203
pallor, 564
Palmar grasp reflex, 311
palpation, 556–560
palpatory method, 691, 694
Pan-Canadian Health Information Privacy and Confidentiality Framework, 500
panic, 1494
Pap (papanicolaou) test or smear, 337, 649*f*
papular drug eruption, 565*f*
papule, 565*f*
paradigms, 56–57
paradoxical breathing, 684
paralysis, and communication, 403
paralytic ileus, 1231
paramedical technologists, 164, 164*t*
parasites, 880
parasomnias, 1087, 1089
paraurethral glands. *See* Skene's glands
Parental Role Conflict (diagnostic label), 1440
parenteral, 806
parenteral fluid and electrolyte replacement. *See* intravenous (IV) fluid therapy
parenteral fluids, 1393
parenteral medications
ampule, 829–832
described, 825
equipment, 825–828
intradermal injections, 835–838
intramuscular injections, 842–848, 842*f*
intravenous medications, 848–856
mixing medications in one syringe, 834–835
needle-stick injuries, prevention of, 828–829
needles, 827–828
prefilled unit-dose systems, 827
preparation of injectable medications, 829–833
subcutaneous injections, 838–841
syringes, 825–827, 826*f*
vials, 829–833
parenteral nutrition, 1204, 1218
parenting trends, 216–217
paresis, 1115
paresthesia, 650
parish nursing, 241
paronychia, 572
parotid gland, 590
parotitis, 594, 729*t*
Parse, R.R., 64
Parsons, Tarcott, 117
partial agonists, 999
partial bath, 711
partial pressure, 1311
partial rebreather mask, 1340, 1340*f*
partially complete proteins, 1168
participative leaders, 538–539
passive immunity, 882
passive ROM exercises, 1147, 1148
past pain experiences, 988
pastes, 858
patch, 565*f*
paternalism, 80
pathogen, 877
see also infection
blood-borne pathogens, 921, 947
emerging pathogens, 914
opportunistic pathogen, 880
pathogenicity, 880
pathological conditions
and defecation, 1231
and urinary elimination, 1268–1269
pathological fractures, 353
pathology, and pulse rate, 673
pathophysiology of infection, 883
patient, 9
see also client
meaning of term, 9–10
use of term, 198
patient-controlled analgesia (PCA), 1005–1007
patient-controlled epidural analgesia (PCEA), 1005
patient-focused care, 168–169
patient-generated subjective global assessment (PG-SGA), 1187
patient monitoring, 501
patient portals, 502
patient safety
assessing, 766–768
awareness, 765
bioterrorism, 766, 767–768
care settings, 765–766
community safety, 765
diagnosing, 768
equipment-related accidents, 783
evaluating, 790
factors affecting, 764–766
in health-care setting, 772–773
in the home, 765
home care, 765–766
home hazard appraisal, 766
lifespan considerations, 764
National Patient Safety Goals, 766–767
nursing history, 766
oxygen therapy, 1336
physical examination, 766
planning, 768
preoperative phase, 1029–1030
prevention of specific hazards. *See* hazard prevention
procedure-related accidents, 783
report on, 103
restraints, 783–790
risk-assessment tools, 766
safety measures across the lifespan, 768–772
safety problems across the lifespan, 772
sensory perception problems, 1068, 1070–1071
stretchers, 1141, 1142
wheelchairs, 1141, 1142
workplace safety, 765
Patient Safety Law: From Silos to Systems, 103
patient safety movement, 198
Pavlov, Ivan, 516
peak plasma level, 801
Peck, Robert, 296
pectus carinatum, 602, 602*f*
pectus excavatum, 602, 602*f*
pedagogy, 516
pedal pulse, 674
pediatric nursing, 214
pediculosis, 738
pedophilia, 1455
peer groups, 326
peer review, 463
pelvic floor, 1265
pelvic floor muscle exercises (PFME), 1286–1287
Pender, Nola, 139
Pender's health-promotion model, 139–141
penis
assessment of, 652
development of, 651*t*
penlight, 558*t*
Penrose drain, 1050
Peplau, Hildegard, 62
Perceived Constipation (diagnostic label), 1238
perceived loss, 1513
perceived self, 1433
percentage of weight gain or loss, 1189–1193
perception, 357, 983, 1061
of pain, 983–984
sensory perception. *See* sensory perception
perceptions
benefits of action, 140
and communication process, 391
individual perceptions, 122
and individuality, 199
of unsupportive interactions with others, 43

perceptual changes, and aging, 353–354
percussion, 560, 1334–1335
percussion, vibration, and postural drainage (PVD), 1334–1336
percussion hammer, 558*t*
percussion sounds and tones, 560*t*
percutaneous, 856
percutaneous endoscopic gastrostomy (PEG), 1208
percutaneous endoscopic jejunostomy (PEJ), 1208
performance improvement (PI), 463
perfusion, 630
perfusion scan, 1327
peri-care, 718–720
pericardium, 1313
peridural anaesthesia, 1033
perineal-genital care, 718–720, 1295
periodic limb movements of sleep (PLMS), 1088–1089
periodontal disease, 728, 729*t*
perioperative care
  see also surgery
  intraoperative phase, 1032–1034
  postoperative phase, 1034–1054
  preoperative phase, 1021–1032
  surgery, types of, 1018–1021
perioperative period, 1017
peripheral blood vessels, 1318
peripheral intravenous infusion, 1418
peripheral intravenous sites, 1413
peripheral mechanisms, 982–983
peripheral neurofibromas, 565*f*
peripheral neuropathic pain, 980
peripheral perfusion, 616
peripheral pulse, 672, 675–678
peripheral sensitization, 985
peripheral vascular system
  assessment of, 615–617, 630–633
  lifespan considerations, 617
peripheral veins, 616
peripherally inserted central catheter (PICC), 1401–1402
peristalsis, 1227, 1227*f*
peritoneal dressings, 966–967
peritoneal friction rubs, 626
permanence of recording, 487
permanent colostomies, 1234
permanent teeth, 728*f*
permission giving, 1463–1465
permissive leader, 539
perseverance, 373
persistent quality improvement (PQI), 463
person in the context of the family, 213
personal appearance, 388–389
personal digital assistants (PdAs), 497
personal distance, 391
personal health counsellor, 241
Personal Health Information Protection Act, 471
personal hygiene, 704
  see also hygiene
personal identity, 1433, 1437
Personal Information Protection and Electronic Documents Act, 471
personal power, 540
personal preferences, 1173
personal protective equipment (PPE), 894–898
personal space, 391
personal values, 74, 1114–1115
personality, 292
  and sensory perception problems, 1064
  strengths, identification of, 1440
Pew Health Professions Commission, 244
pH, 1394
pH, 1377–1378
phagocytes, 881
phallic stage, 320
phantom pain, 981, 982
pharmacists, 164, 164*t*
pharmacodynamics, 802
pharmacogenetics, 803
pharmacokinetics, 802
pharmacological agents. *See* medication
pharmacological pain management
  coanalgesic, 1002
  equianalgesic dosing, 1001
  nonsteroidal anti-inflammatory drugs (NSAIDs), 1001–1002
  opioid analgesics, 999–1001
  patient-controlled analgesia (PCA), 1005–1007
  placebo response, 1002–1003
  routes for opioid delivery, 1003–1005
pharmacology, 795
  see also drugs; medication
  drug classifications, 796
  drug legislation, 796–799
  forms of medications, 796
  key concepts, 796
  look-alike health product names, 796
  sound-alike health product names, 796
pharmacopoeia, 798
pharynx, 1325*f*
phenomenology, 44
phenylketonuria (PKU), 314
philosophy
  empiricist tradition, 57
  epistemology, 56
  ethics, 56
  interpretive tradition, 57
  meaning of, 56
  in nursing, 57
  ontology, 56
  overview of selected nursing philosophies, 58–59
  paradigms or world views, 56–57
  primary areas of inquiry, 56
  selected nurse philosophers, 58*t*
phosphate (PO_4-), 1376, 1386–1387
phospholipids, 1170
physical activity, 1110, 1112
physical agents, 881
physical assessment
  see also assessing; assessment
  abdomen, 624–629, 634
  activity and exercise, 1122–1124
  anus, 654–656, 658
  auscultation, 561
  breasts and axillae, 618–621, 633–634
  cardiovascular functions, 1324
  central vessels, 612–615, 622–630
  draping, 556
  ears and hearing, 582–589
  examination methods, 556–561
  eye care, 744
  fecal elimination, 1236
  feet, 721–722, 722*t*
  female genitals, 646–647, 656–658
  fluid, electrolyte, and acid-base balances, 1389, 1391*t*
  general survey, 561–564
  hair, 564–570, 737–738
  head. *See* head
  head-to-toe assessment, 553
  heart, 610–622
  infection prevention and control, 917
  inguinal lymph nodes, 646–647
  inspection, 556
  instrumentation, 556, 558*t*
  integument, 564–572
  male genitals, 651–653, 658
  motor function, 649–650
  mouth and oropharynx, 590–594
  musculoskeletal system, 631–633, 634–635
  nails, 570–572
  neck, 596–599
  neurological system. *See* neurological system
  nose and sinuses, 588–590
  nutritional status, 1189
  older adult, 556
  oral hygiene, 728
  palpation, 556–560
  patient safety, 766
  percussion, 560
  peripheral vascular system, 615–617, 630–633
  positioning, 556, 557*t*
  preoperative phase, 1021
  preparing the client, 553–555
  preparing the environment, 555–556
  rectum, 654–656, 658
  reflexes, 648–649
  respiratory functions, 1324
  sensory function, 650
  sensory perception problems, 1064
  sequence of assessment, 553
  sexual health status, 1457
  skin, 564
  skin integrity, 928, 940
  sleep, 1091
  specific client situations, 554*t*
  thorax and lungs, 599–609
  urinary elimination, 1271
  vital signs. *See* vital signs
physical attending, 393
physical comfort needs, 385
physical dependence, 801, **1000**
physical development
  adolescence, 324–325
  middle-aged adults, 338–339, 339*t*
  neonates and infants, 309–311
  preschoolers, 319
  school-age children, 322
  toddlers, 315–316
  young adults, 334
physical examination
  see also physical assessment
  client education, 521
  and health promotion, 143
physical examinations, 423, 424*f*
physical growth, 324
physical health assessment. *See* physical assessment
physical interventions, 1007–1008
physical preparation for surgery, 1028–1029
physical restraints, 784
physicians, 164, 164*t*
physicians' offices, 160–161
physiological aging
  cardiovascular changes, 354
  gastrointestinal changes, 354
  genitals, changes in, 354
  immune system, 355
  integument, 351–353
  neuromusculoskeletal changes, 353
  normal physical changes, 351*t*
  perceptual changes, 353–354
  pulmonary changes, 354
  sensory changes, 353–354
  urinary changes, 354
  usual aging, 351
physiological barriers, 880–881
physiological events, and learning, 519
physiological mode, 63
physiological needs, 204
physiological needs of dying individual, 1528, 1529*t*
physiology
  of cardiovascular system, 1312–1317
  of defecation, 1226–1228
  of the respiratory system, 1309–1312
  of sleep, 1081–1083
  of urinary elimination, 1264–1266
physiotherapists, 164, 164*t*
Piaget, Jean, 299–300, 299*t*, 517
PIE, 476–477, 476*f*
pigeon chest, 602, 602*f*
piggyback, 850
pilates, 281–282
pillows, 1131
pilot study, 44
pinna, 582
piston syringes, 958
pitch, 561
pitting edema, 1381
pivot joint, 1106*t*
pivoting, 1129
place, 253–254
placebo response, 1002–1003
placenta, 308
plain interrupted sutures, 1052
plan of care. *See* nursing care plans
planned change, 545
planning, 541
  see also assessment skills
  an interview, 422
  cardiovascular functions, 1328–1330
  client education, 525–528

communication, 404
continuity of care, 1067
death and dying, and home care, 1526–1527
described, 439
desired health outcomes, 445–450
discharge planning, 439, 1040–1041
eye care, 744
fecal elimination, 1240–1242
fluid, electrolyte, and acid-base balances, 1395–1396
foot care, 724
goals, 445–450
hair care, 738–739
infection prevention and control, 918
initial planning, 439
intraoperative phase, 1033–1034
mobility problems, 1125
nail hygiene, 726–727
nursing care plan, modification of, 461
nursing care plans, 439–443
nursing interventions and activities, 450–451
Nursing Interventions Classifications (NIC), 452–455
Nursing Outcomes Classification (NOC), 447–448, 448*t*
nutritional status, 1196–1198
ongoing planning, 439
oral hygiene, 730
overview, 416*t*
pain, 994–996
patient safety, 768
peaceful death, 1526
postoperative phase, 1040–1041
preoperative phase, 1022
priority setting, 444–445, 446*t*
process, 444–452
respiratory functions, 1328–1330
self-concept, 1440
sensory perception problems, 1067
sexual health status, 1459–1460
skin hygiene, 709–710
sleep, 1091–1093
spiritual health, 1480
standardized approaches to care planning, 440–443
stress and coping patterns, 1501–1503
types of, 439
urinary elimination, 1279–1281
wounds, 946–947
writing plan of care, 451–452
plant proteins, 1185
plantar reflex, 311, 639
plantar warts, 722
plaque, 565*f*, 594, 728
plasma, 1368
plateau, 801
plateau phase, 664, 665
pleadings, 103
pleural space, 1310
pleximeter, 560
plexor, 560
PLISSIT model, 1463–1465
pneumatic pressure devices, 1359
pneumonia, 1037*t*
pneumothorax, 1356
point of maximal impulse (PMI), 611, 672
poisoning
carbon monoxide poisoning, 782
prevention, 781
policies, 440
policy, 253
political leadership, 167
polycythemia, 1326
polydipsia, 1269
polysaccharides, 1167
polysomnography, 1091
polytheism, 1473
polyunsaturated fatty acids, 1169
polyuria, 1269
popliteal pulse, 674
population, 44, 167
population health initiatives, 135*t*
population health-promotion model, 135, 136
portability, 11, 154*t*
portability, 153
portable electric suction units or pumps, 1046
portal of entry to the host, 886
portal of exit from reservoir, 885, 885*t*
position sensation, 644
positional power, 540
positioning
changes in, and pulse rate, 673
and defecation, 1243
exercise and activity interventions, 1130–1133
health assessment, 556, 557*t*
intraoperative phase, 1034
turning client to lateral or prone position in bed, 1136–1137
wound healing, 947–948
positive feedback, 200
positive reinforcement, 516
positron emission tomography (PET) scans, 501
possible nursing diagnosis, 431
post-mastectomy pain, 981
Post-Trauma Syndrome (diagnostic label), 1501
postanaesthesia care unit (PACU), 1018
postanaesthetic recovery room (PARR), 1018
postconventional level, 300, 326, 335, 340
posterior approach, 598
posterior axillary line, 600
posterior ribs, 601*f*
posterior thorax, 604–606
posterior tibial pulse, 674
postformal thought, 335
postherpetic neuralgia, 981
postmortem care, 1533–1534
postoperative depression, 1039*t*
postoperative ileus, 1038*t*
postoperative instructions, 1028
postoperative phase, 1018
assessing, 1036–1039
coughing exercises, 1041
deep-breathing exercises, 1041
diagnosing, 1039–1040
diet, 1042
evaluating, 1053, 1054*t*
home care, 1039, 1040–1041
hydration, 1042
immediate postanaesthetic phase, 1034–1035
implementing interventions, 1041–1054
leg exercises, 1041
moving and ambulation, 1041–1042
pain management, 1041
planning, 1040–1041
potential postoperative problems, 1037*t*
preparation for ongoing care, 1035
suction, 1042–1046
surgical dressings, 1047
suture, 1051–1053
urinary elimination, 1042
wound care, 1046–1053
wound drains and suction, 1050
postoperative regimen, 1024
postural drainage, 1335
postural hypotension, 1392
postural tonus, 1104
posture, 389, 1104–1105
posture of involvement, 393
potassium (K^+), 1375–1376, 1383–1384
potassium-rich foods, 1376
potentiating effect, 800
powder, 858
power, 540
Powerlessness (diagnostic label)
respiratory and cardiovascular functions, 1328
self-concept, 1440
Practical Nurses Canada, 20
practice guidelines
antidiarrheal medications, 1247
bandaging, 963
bedpan, giving and removing a, 1244–1245
bladder training, 1286
catheter-associated urinary infections, prevention of, 1296
common pressure sites, assessing, 941
facilitation of fluid intake, 1399
gastrostomy medications, 824–825
nasogastric medications, 824–825
normal voiding habits, maintenance of, 1284
passive ROM exercises, 1148
prevention of falls in health-care agencies, 776–777
restraints, application of, 785–786
restricting fluid intake, 1400
skin preparations, 858
smoking cessation best practice guidelines, implementation of, 1318
vein selection, 1402
venous access device, 1404–1405
wound cleansing, 959
practice management, 503
prayer, 282, 1477, 1481–1482
prealbumin, 1194
preambulatory exercises, 1149
precautions
additional precautions, 913–914
airborne precautions, 913, 914
contact precautions, 913, 914
droplet precautions, 913, 914
implementation of, 914–916
isolation precautions, 911–912, 916
routine practices, 912–913
precedents, 91
preceptor, 542
precoital stimulation, 1454
preconceptual phase, 316
precontemplation stage, 141
preconventional level, 300, 317, 323
precordium, 610*f*
precordium, 611
predicted outcome criterion, 445
preemptive analgesia, 998–999
prefilled unit-dose systems, 827
pregenital stages, 293
pregnancy
breasts and axillae, assessment of, 622
conception, 308–309
fish, consumption of, 1184
folic acid, 1180
maternal stress during pregnancy, 1500
prenatal development, 308–309
trimesters, 308
unplanned pregnancies, prevention of, 1461–1462
prehelping phase, 397–399
preinteraction phase, 397
prejudice, 183
preload, 1315
premature ejaculation, 1456
premature infant pain profile (PIPP), 993
premoral level, 300
prenatal development, 308–309
preoperative consent, 1021
preoperative phase, 1017
antiembolism stockings, 1030–1032
assessing, 1021
diagnosing, 1021–1022
evaluating, 1032
home care, 1022
implementing interventions, 1023–1032
interview, 1022
physical preparation, 1028–1029
planning, 1022
preoperative consent, 1021
preoperative teaching, 1023–1027
safety protocols, 1029–1030
screening tests, 1021, 1023*t*
sequential compression devices (SCD), 1032
vital signs, 1030
preoperative regimen, 1024
preoperative skin preparation, 1029
preoperative teaching, 1023–1027
preparation stage, 141
prepubertal changes, 322
presbycusis, 353, 1063
presbyopia, 353, 574
preschoolers (4 to 5 years)
see also children
cognitive development, 320
developmental guidelines, 321
health assessment and promotion, 321
health problems, 320
moral development, 320
normal sleep patterns and requirements, 1084

nutrition, 1177
oral hygiene, 730–731
physical development, 319
psychosocial development, 319–320
safety measures, 768–771
spiritual development, 320
urinary elimination, 1266
prescribed limitations to movement, 1115
prescription, 796, 806–809
prescription drugs. *See* medication
pressure sites, 941
pressure sores. *See* pressure ulcers
pressure ulcer scale for healing (PUSH) tool, 937, 938*f*
pressure ulcers, 929
see also wounds
advanced age, 931–932
assessing, 942
Braden scale, 935*f*
chronic medical conditions, 932
classification, 932
decreased mental status, 931
diminished sensation, 931
etiology of, 929
excessive body heat, 931
fecal and urinary incontinence, 931
home care, 946
immobility, 930
inadequate nutrition, 930
incidence and prevalence, 929
lifespan considerations, 961
mechanical loads, 929–930
pressure ulcer scale for healing (PUSH) tool, 937, 938*f*
prevention, 946, 948–950
reverse (down) staging, 932
risk-assessment tools, 932
risk factors, 929–932
RYB colour code, 950–951
staging system, 932, 933*f*
supportive devices, 948–950, 949*t*
treatment, 950–951
unstageable pressure ulcers, 932
prevention
back injury, 1130
catheter-associated urinary infections, 1296
constipation, 1168
disease prevention, 137, 137*t*
of falls, 774–779
food-borne illness, 1200
hazard prevention. *See* hazard prevention
illness prevention, 10, 148, 156
infection prevention and control. *See* infection prevention and control
levels of, 121
needle-stick injuries, 828–829
obesity, 1178
poisoning, 781
pressure ulcers, 946, 948–950
primary prevention, 121
secondary prevention, 121
sensory deprivation, 1069
sensory overload, 1068–1069
tertiary prevention, 121
tooth decay, 730
unplanned pregnancies, 1461–1462
urinary tract infection, 1283–1284
venous stasis, 1358–1359
previous surgery, and susceptibility to infection, 888
primacy of caring, 384
primary care
described, 12
vs. primary health care, 12, 237, 237*t*
primary health care, 236
vs. primary care, 12, 237, 237*t*
vs. primary nursing, 12
principles of, 11–12, 236
primary hypertension, 688
primary industry injuries, 258
primary intention healing, 934
primary nursing, 12, **169**
primary prevention, 121
primary sexual characteristics, 325
primary skin lesions, 564, 565*f*
primary sleep disorders, 1087
primary source of data, 419
primary union healing, 934
principle-based ethics, 79–80
principled level, 300, 326
principled reasoning, 335
principles-based (deontological) theories, 78
Principles of Biomedical Ethics (Beauchamp and Childress), 79
principles of management, 541
priority changes, 445
priority setting, 444–445, 446*t*
privacy, 104
during defecation, 1242
electronic health records and, 499–500
invasion of privacy, 102–103
and learning, 518
legal implications, 104–105
right to, 50
prn order, 807
problem-focused assessment, 417*t*
problem list, 474–475, 475*f*
problem-oriented medical record (POMR), 474–476
problem-oriented record (POR), 474–476
problem solving, 39, 374
described, 375
intuition, 376
and stress, 1496
teaching, 531
trial and error, 375
problem statement, 477
problematic substance use, 801
meaning of, 260
nursing and, 105
older adults, 360–361
in rural areas, 260
young adults, 336
procedure-related accidents, 783
procedures, 440
process evaluation, 463
process recording, 405–406, 406*t*
Prochaska's transtheoretical model, 545
proctoscopy, 1236
proctosigmoidoscopy, 1236
productive cough, 684
productivity, 543
profession, 15
see also nursing profession
professional health-care system, 181
professional liability insurance, 106
professional organization, 16
professional practice competencies, 39
professional regulation, 13
professional socialization, 16–17
professional values, 74
professionalization movements, 5
progress notes, 475–476, 476*f*, 481
progressive relaxation, 280
projection, 1497*t*
proliferative phase, 936
prolongation of life, 1524
prompted voiding, 1285–1286
prone position, 1132, 1133*t*
proprioception, 1110
proprioceptive reflex, 986, 986*f*
proprioceptors, 649
prostheses, care of, 1029
protein-calorie malnutrition, 1186
protein in urine, 1278
proteins, 1168–1169, 1169
protocols, 440
protozoa, 880
provider-driven model, 246
provincial and territorial practical nurse professional organizations, 20*t*
provincial and territorial regulatory bodies, 92–94
provincial and territory health departments, 160
proximodistal growth, 291
proxy directive, 1520
psoriasis vulgaris, 565*f*
psychiatric nursing professional organizations, 21*t*
psychoeducation, 1009
psychological aging
death and grieving, 357
described, 355
economic change, 356
independence, 356
relocation, 356
retirement, 355–356
self-esteem, 356
social relationships, 356
psychological factors
defecation, 1230–1231
erectile dysfunction, 1456
and medication action, 803
and nutrition, 1176
psychological homeostasis, 200–201
psychological indicators of stress, 1494–1496
psychological problems, in postoperative phase, 1039*t*
psychological system, 207
psychomotor, 456
psychomotor ability, and learning, 519–520
psychomotor domain, 517
psychomotor skills, 532
psychoneurological system
and benefits of exercise, 1113–1114
immobility, effects of, 1120–1121
psychosocial development, 1432*t*
adolescence, 325–326
middle-aged adults, 339–340
neonates and infants, 311–312
preschoolers, 319–320
school-age children, 322
toddlers, 316
trust *versus* mistrust, 311
young adults, 334–335
psychosocial factors, and urinary elimination, 1267
psychosocial needs, 916
psychosocial theories, 292–298, 298*f*
psychospiritual comfort needs, 385
psychotropic medications, 804
puberty, 322, 324
pubic hair
assessment of, 652
development of, 648, 648*f*, 651*t*
pubic lice, 738
public administration, 11, **153,** 154*t*
public distance, 391
public health
changing focus in, 132
family nursing traditions, 214
services, described, 159–160
workforce competencies, 244
Public Health Agency of Canada (PHAC), 878, 911, 1180
public health nurse (PHN), 239
PubMed, 46
pulling, 1129
pulmonary angiography, 1328
pulmonary changes, and aging, 354
pulmonary edema, 1321
pulmonary embolism, 1037*t*, 1322
pulmonary function tests, 1325
pulmonary veins, 1315
pulmonary ventilation, 1310–1311
pulmonary volumes and capacities, 1326*t*
pulmonic valve, 1313
pulp cavity, 727
pulse, 672
apical pulse, 672, 673, 674*f*, 678–680
apical-radial pulse, 680–681
assessment, 674–681
bounding pulse, 675
brachial pulse, 673
carotid pulse, 673
factors affecting pulse rate, 672–673
feeble pulse, 675
femoral pulse, 673
full pulse, 675
home care, 681
lifespan considerations, 681
palpation, 674
pedal pulse, 674
peripheral pulse, 672, 675–678
point of maximal impulse (PMI), 672
popliteal pulse, 674
posterior tibial pulse, 674

pulse sites, 673–674
radial pulse, 673
temporal pulse, 673
thready pulse, 675
variations, by age, 673*t*
weak pulse, 675
pulse deficit, 680
pulse oximeter, 696–697, 697*f*
pulse oximetry, 699
pulse pressure, 686
pulse rhythm, 675
pulse volume, 675
puncture injuries, 828–829
puncture wounds, 920
pureed diet, 1201
Purkinje fibres, 1314
purosanguineous discharge, 937
pursed-lip breathing, 1332, 1333
purulent, 882
purulent exudate, 937
push fluids, 1396
pushing, 1129
pustular psoriasis, chronic, 565*f*, **882**
pustule, 565*f*
pyogenic bacteria, 937
pyorrhea, 594, 728
pyrexia, 664–665
pyrogens, 881

Q

Q scan, 1327
qigong, 278–279
quadriceps, 632
qualifiers, 431
qualitative designs, 44
qualitative research, 41–42
critique of, 48*t*
designs, 44
quality, 561
quality assurance, 463, 472
quality assurance review, 508
quality improvement (QI), 463
quality of nursing care, 463
quality practice environments, 84–85
quantitative research, 41
critique of, 47*t*
designs, 44
quasi-experimental design, 44
questions
to elicit medical and illness narratives, 225*t*
reflective questions, 223, 224*t*
Quiet Revolution, 4
Quinn's theory of change, 545

R

RACE, 773
race, 179
and blood pressure, 687
as risk factor, 203
racism, 183
radial pulse, 673
radiating pain, 980
radiation, 662, 892
radiation injury, 783
radiographs, 1236
radiotherapy, 1174
rales, 603*f*
range, 45
range of motion (ROM), 1105, 1146–1147
rational beliefs, 372
rationale, 441
rationalization, 1497*t*
RBC indices, 1326
reaction formation, 1497*t*
reactive hyperemia, 929
Readiness for Enhanced Nutrition (diagnostic label), 1196
Readiness for Enhanced Self-Concept (diagnostic label), 1440
Readiness for Enhanced Spiritual Well-Being (diagnostic label), 1479–1480
readiness to learn, 517, 521–522
reading level, 523
reasoning process, 373
reassessment, 457
rebound phenomenon, 969
receiver, 387
recent memory, 357
receptive aphasia, 635
receptive communication problems, 404
receptive portal of entry, 885–886
receptor, 1061
recipients of nursing, 9–10
reciprocal, 227
recommended dietary allowance, 1170–1171
reconstitution, 830
record, 470
recording, 470
recording guidelines, 486–489
recording mistake, 487
records of therapies by other health professionals, 419
rectal instillations, 867–868
rectal route, 1004
rectal temperature, 666–667, 666*t*, 670
rectocele, 657
rectum, 654–656, 658, 1227, 1228*f*
rectus femoris site, 844–845, 845*f*
recurrent turns, 965
red wounds, 951
reddened mucosa, 729*t*
reduction of transmission, 892–909
referral source, 241
referral summary, 481–485
referrals, 248, 1040–1041, 1482
referred pain, 980
reflection, 378
reflective questions, 223, 224*t*
reflex, 648
assessment of, 638–639, 648–649
neonates and infants, 311
reflex hammer, 558*t*
Reflex Urinary Incontinence (diagnostic label), 1279
reflexology, 277–278
reflux, 1265
regeneration, 882, 934
regional anaesthesia, 1032–1033
regional health departments, 160
Regional Health Services Act (Saskatchewan), 103–104
Registered Nurses' Association of Ontario (RNAO), 10, 74, 94, 198, 503, 763
registered nurses (RN)
defined, 10
delegation, 543
expansion of role of, 94
programs leading to or continuing from basic RN education, 28–30
recognition of, 27
role, 10
registered practical nurse (RPN)
defined, 10
Practical Nurses Canada, 20
recognition of, 27
registered practical nursing programs, 30
regulation of, 13
role, 10
Registered Psychiatric Nurses of Canada, 20
registered psychiatric nurses (RPNs)
defined, 10
recognition of, 27
Registered Psychiatric Nurses of Canada, 20
registered psychiatric nursing programs, 30
regulation of, 13
role, 10
registration, 94
regression, 316, 1497*t*
regular diet, 1200
regularity, 1230
regulation, 13
regulation of professionals, 13
regulatory bodies, 92–94
regurgitation, 1176, 1322
rehabilitation, 156–157
rehabilitation centres, 162–163
Reiki, 279
relapsing fever, 664
related factors, 432
relational ethics theories, 80–81
relational practice, 1431
relational stance, 222–223
relationship orientation, 538
relationship power, 540
relationships
and communication process, 392
the helping relationship, 397–400
relationships-based (caring) theories, 79
relaxation, and sleep, 1094–1097
relaxation response, 1009
relaxation response (RR), 1114
relaxation techniques, 1505
relevance, 388, 518
reliability, 44
relief, 385
religion, 1472
in Canada, 176
death-related practices, 1524
and diet, 189
and nutrition, 1173
religious care, 1475–1478
religious development, 1473–1474
religious practices affecting nursing care, 1476–1478
sacred writings, 1477
and sexuality, 1452
religious care, 1475–1478
religious distress, 1480
religious practices affecting nursing care, 1476–1478
relocation, and aging, 356
Relocation Stress Syndrome (diagnostic label), 1501
REM (rapid-eye-movement) sleep, 1082
remission, 124
remittent fever, 664
remote, 253
see also rural health care
remote nursing practice, 262
removal of sutures, 1051–1053
renal calculi, 1119
renal regulation, 1378
renal ultrasonography, 1278
renin-angiotensin-aldosterone system, 1374
reparative phase, 882
repetition, 518
report, 470
change-of-shift report, 490
telephone orders, 491
telephone reports, 491
Report of 2005 Dialogue on Advanced Nursing Practice (CNA), 94
reporting
see also report
crimes, torts and unsafe practices, 108
guidelines, 108
repression, 320, 1498*t*
research, 42
see also nursing research
research-based nursing practice, 39, 48
research design, 44, 508–509
research ethics board (REB), 49
research grants, 509
research journals in nursing, 46
research problem, 42
research process
communication of the research, 45–46
data analysis, 44–45
data collection, 44
define study's purpose, 43
formulation of research question, 43–44
interpretation of findings, 45
pilot study, 44
review of literature, 43
selection of population, sample and setting, 44
selection of research design, 44
state a research problem, 42–43
research question, 43–44
researchability, 42
researcher/research consumer, 15
reservoirs, 885, 885*t*, 889–892
resident
meaning of, 10
use of term, 198
resident flora, 877, 883–884
resident organisms, 877, 878*t*

residual urine, 1274
resistance to change, 546
resistive behaviours, 398–399
resistive exercises, 1111
resonance, 560
resources
  allocation, 158
  management of, 542
  and self-concept, 1436
respect, 392, 399
respect for persons, 79
respiration, 682, 1308
  altered breathing patterns, 684, 1320–1321
  altered breathing sounds, 684
  assessment of, 683, 684–685
  breath sounds. *See* breath sounds
  control of, 683
  deep respiration, 683
  depth, 683
  exhalation, 682, 682*f*
  external respiration, 682
  factors affecting respirations, 683
  home care, 686
  inhalation, 682, 682*f*
  internal respiration, 682
  lifespan considerations, 685
  mechanics of breathing, 682–683
  normal respiration, 1320
  regulation of breathing, 682–683
  shallow respiration, 683
  variations, by age, 673*t*
respiration rate, 683
respirators, 895–898
respiratory acid-base imbalances, 1387
respiratory acidosis, 1387
respiratory alkalosis, 1387
respiratory alterations, 1320–1321
respiratory arrest, 1360
respiratory character, 683
respiratory diseases, 256
respiratory functions
  altered breathing patterns, 1320–1321
  assessing, 1323–1328
  cardiac monitoring, 1327–1328
  diagnosing, 1328
  diagnostic studies, 1324–1327
  environment, 1318
  evaluating, 1360–1361, 1361*t*
  factors affecting, 1317–1320
  and gender, 1320
  health status, 1319
  hypoxia, 1320
  implementation. *See* oxygenation and circulation interventions
  interview, 1323
  lifespan considerations, 1317–1318
  lifestyle, 1318–1319
  nursing health history, 1323
  obstructed airway, 1321
  pharmacological agents, 1319
  physical assessment, 1324
  planning, 1328–1330
  respiratory alterations, 1320–1321
  sample care plan, 1329–1330
  specimens, 1324–1325
  stress and coping, 1319
  visualization procedures, 1327–1328
respiratory inhalation, 868–871
respiratory movement, 1118
respiratory pattern, 683
respiratory problems
  postoperative phase, 1037*t*
  rural areas, 257
respiratory pump, 1316
respiratory quality, 683
respiratory regulation, 1312, 1377–1378
respiratory rhythm, 683
respiratory secretions, 1118
respiratory system
  alveolar gas exchange, 1311
  and benefits of exercise, 1113
  immobility, effects of, 1118–1119
  organs in respiratory tract, 1309*f*
  physiology of the respiratory system, 1309–1312
  pulmonary ventilation, 1310–1311
  respiratory regulation, 1312
  structure of respiratory system, 1309–1310, 1309*f*
  transport of oxygen and carbon dioxide, 1311–1312
respiratory therapists, 164, 164*t*
respiratory tract infections, 317
respite care, 227–228
response, 387, 516
response-based stress models, 1491–1493
responsibility, 541
responsibility for physician's orders, 106–107
responsible sexual behaviour, 1461–1462
rest, 1080
  bed rest, 1115
  history, 1089
  in preoperative phase, 1029
  promotion of, 1095
  restful environment, 1094
  sample care plan, 1092–1093
  stress and coping, 1504
resting energy expenditure (REE), 1171
resting tremor, 635
restless legs syndrome (RLS), 1089
restorative justice, 261–262
restoring health, 10
restraining forces for change, 546
restraints, 783
  alternatives, 784
  applying restraints, 785–786, 787–789
  chemical restraints, 784
  and death, 784
  environmental restraints, 784
  home care, 790
  kinds of, 785–787
  least restraint, 784
  legal implications, 784–785
  physical restraints, 784
  selection of, 785
restricted fluids, 1396
retarded ejaculation, 1456
retention, 1267
retention catheter. *See* indwelling catheter
retention enema, 1248
retention sutures, 1051
reticular activating system (RAS), 1061, 1081
retirement, 355–356
retirement homes, 162
retrograde pyelography, 1278
retrospective audit, 463
return-flow enema, 1248
reverse (down) staging, 932
review of systems, 423, 424*f*
review of the literature, 43
Rh factor, 1417
rhesus (Rh) factor, 1417
rheumatic fever, 1317
rhizotomy, 1010
rhonchi, 603*f*
right of self-determination, 50
rights
  clients' rights, 154
  Consumer Rights to Health Care, 155, 155*t*
  dying person's bill of rights, 1526
  and health care, 154–156
  of human subjects, 49–50
  of medication administration, 100
  right of self-determination, 50
  ten "rights" of medication administration, 817
rigor mortis, 1533
Ringer's solution, 1401
risk assessment, 203–204
risk-assessment tools, 766, 932
risk factors, 143, 431
  acid-base imbalances, 1388*t*, 1389*t*, 1390
  atherosclerosis, 1322
  body mass index, 1192*t*
  electrolyte imbalances, 1383*t*, 1390
  falls, 775*t*
  fluid imbalances, 1380*t*, 1381*t*, 1390
  fluid volume deficit, 1380*t*
  fluid volume excess (FVE), 1381*t*
  nutritional problems, 1188
  pressure ulcers, 929–932
  and related factors, 432
  various factors, described, 203–204
  waist circumference, 1192*t*
Risk for Activity Intolerance (diagnostic label), 1125
Risk for Aspiration (diagnostic label)
  intraoperative phase, 1033
  patient safety, 768
Risk for Caregiver Role Strain (diagnostic label), 1279
Risk for Constipation (diagnostic label), 1238
Risk for Deficient Fluid Volume (diagnostic label), 1239
  fluid, electrolyte, and acid-base balances, 1395
  intraoperative phase, 1033
  postoperative phase, 1040
  urinary elimination problems, 1279
Risk for Disuse Syndrome (diagnostic label), 1125
Risk for Excess Fluid Volume (diagnostic label), 1279
Risk for Imbalanced Body Temperature (diagnostic label), 1033
Risk for Imbalanced Fluid Volume (diagnostic label), 1395
Risk for Imbalanced Nutrition (diagnostic label), 1196
Risk for Impaired Gas Exchange (diagnostic label), 1091
Risk for Impaired Skin Integrity (diagnostic label)
  fecal elimination, 1239
  foot hygiene, 722, 723*t*
  sensory perception, 1067
  urinary elimination problems, 1279
  wounds, 945
Risk for Infection (diagnostic label)
  eye care, 744
  foot hygiene, 722
  hair care, 738
  infection prevention and control, 918
  mobility problems, 1125
  nail hygiene, 726
  nutritional status, 1196
  postoperative phase, 1040
  urinary elimination, 1279
  wounds, 946
Risk for Injury (diagnostic label)
  eye care, 744
  fluid, electrolyte, and acid-base balances, 1395
  mobility problems, 1125
  postoperative phase, 1040
  sensory perception problems, 1067
  somnambulism, 1091
Risk for Latex Allergy Response (diagnostic label), 768
Risk for Perioperative-Positioning Injury (diagnostic label), 1033
Risk for Poisoning (diagnostic label), 768
Risk for Spiritual Distress (diagnostic label), 1480
Risk for Suffocation (diagnostic label), 768
Risk for Transmission of Infection (diagnostic label), 918
Risk for Trauma (diagnostic label), 768
risk management, 541
risk nursing diagnosis, 431
risks
  of enteral nutrition (EN), 1217
  identification of, 437–438
  surgery, 1019–1021
ritual prayer, 282
Roach, Simone, 67, 384
roentgenography (X-ray), 1236
role ambiguity, 1434
role conflicts, 1434–1435
role confusion, 325
role development, 1434
role function mode, 63
role mastery, 1434
role of the nurse in health promotion, 143–147
role performance, 1434–1435, 1438
role-performance model, 119
role-relationship pattern, 426
role strain, 1434
roles, and communication process, 392
roller bandages, 963–965
ROM exercises, 1146–1147
Romanow Commission. *See Building on Values* (Romanow)

Romberg test, 639
room temperature, 749
rooting reflex, 311
Rosenstock's and Becker's health belief model, 122–123
roughage, 1167
route of transmission
  airborne transmission, 886
  droplet transmission, 886
  indirect contact transmission, 886
  reduction of transmission, 892–909
  vector-borne transmission, 886
  vehicle-borne transmission, 886
routes for opioid delivery, 1003–1005
routes of administration, 804–806, 805*t*, 808
routine order, 807
routine practices, 912–913
routine screening programs, 634
Roy, Callista, 62–63
Roy's adaptation model, 426
rubber bulb syringe, 872
rugae, 1265
rules of civil procedures, 103
rural, 253, **253**
rural and small town, 253
rural health care
  Aboriginal communities, special concerns in, 261–262
  agricultural injuries, 258
  cancer, 257
  chemical contaminants, 257
  continuing nursing education, 33
  demography, 255
  elements of rural health framework, 254–256
  expanded practice, 262
  eyesight, loss of, 259–260
  geography, 254–255
  health-care delivery issues, 262
  health issues, 256–261
  health of rural residents, 256–262
  hearing loss, 259
  mental health issues, 260
  mortality risks, 256
  motor vehicle collisions, 259
  nursing education, 264
  nursing practice issues, 262–264
  occupations, 256
  place, 253–254
  primary industry injuries, 258
  problematic substance use, 260
  respiratory problems, 257
  safe play areas for children, 258–259
  space, 253–254
  suicide, 260–261
  telehealth, 264
  time, 253–254
  water safety, 257–258
  zoonoses, 258
rural nursing practice, 262–264
rural postal codes, 253
rural primary care, 163
RYB colour code, 950–951

S

sacred symbols, 1477
sacred writings, 1477
saddle joint, 1108*t*
sadomasochistic bondage, 1454
Safe Kids Canada, 763, 773
safe play areas for children, 258–259
Safer Healthcare Now!, 763, 813, 1029
safety
  in community health nursing, 243–244
  patient safety. *See* patient safety
  safety and security needs, 204
safety belt, 787
safety razor, 743
safety strap body restraints, 786
Salem sump tube, 1204, 1205*f*
salivary glands, 592, 1324
sample, 44
sample care plan
  altered bowel elimination, 1240–1241
  chronic low self-esteem, 1439
  ineffective airway clearance, 1329–1330
  ineffective coping, 1502–1503
  nutrition, 1197–1198
  rest, 1092–1093
  sensory perception, 1074–1075
  sleep, 1092–1093
  spiritual distress, 1483
  urinary elimination, 1280–1281
sandwich program, 28
sanguineous (hemorrhagic) exudate, 937
sanguinous, 882
***Saskatchewan Critical Incident Reporting Guideline,* 104**
Saskatchewan Registered Nurses' Association (SRNA), 92, 198
saturated fatty acids, 1169
scabies, 738
scald, 773
scales, 566*t*
scapular lines, 600
scar, 566*t*, 882
scar tissue, 882, 937
school-age children (6 to 12 years)
  see also children
  breasts and axillae, assessment of, 622
  cognitive development, 322–323
  defecation, 1229
  developmental guidelines, 323
  health assessment and promotion, 323–324
  health problems, 323
  moral development, 323
  normal sleep patterns and requirements, 1084
  nutrition, 1178–1179
  oral hygiene, 730–731
  physical development, 322
  psychosocial development, 322
  safety measures, 770, 771
  spiritual development, 323
  urinary elimination, 1266
school health nursing, 241–242
school health-promotion programs, 139
science, 18, 56
scientific health belief, 184
scientific inquiry, 57
scientific method, 57
scoliosis, 602*f*
scope of nursing, 10
scope of practice, 13
screening examination, 423, 424*f*
screening tests, 1021, 1023*t*
scrotum
  assessment of, 652–653
  development of, 651*t*
scrub nurse, 1034
SDAT (Senile Dementia of the Alzheimer's Type), 361
seasonal affective disorders, 1082
sebaceous glands, 324–325
seborrheic keratosis, 568
sebum, 325, 705
secondary hypertension, 688
secondary intention healing, 934
secondary prevention, 121
secondary sexual characteristics, 325
secondary skin lesions, 564, 566*t*
secondary sleep disorders, 1087
secondary source of data, 419
secured dressings, 957
sedative-hypnotic medications, 1097
sedatives, 1029
sedentary lifestyle, 1178
Sedentary Lifestyle (diagnostic label), 1125
seizure, 779–781
seizure precautions, 779–781
self-actualization, 204
self-assessments, 378
self-awareness, 1431
self-awareness groups, 402
Self-Care Deficit (diagnostic label)
  eye care, 744
  foot hygiene, 722, 723*t*
  grooming, 738
  hair care, 738
  nail hygiene, 726
  oral hygiene, 729, 730*t*
  postoperative phase, 1040
  sensory perception problems, 1067
  skin hygiene, 707, 709
  urinary elimination problems, 1279
self-concept, 1431
  areas of strength, identification of, 1440
  assessing, 1436–1439
  body image, 1433–1434, 1438
  components of, 1433–1435
  core self-concept, 1432–1433
  culturally competent care, 1437
  and culture, 1436
  described, 1431
  developmental stage, 1435–1436
  diagnosing, 1439–1440
  evaluating, 1442
  factors affecting, 1435–1436
  and family, 1436
  formation of, 1431–1433
  history of success and failure, 1436
  ideal self, 1433
  and illness, 1436
  implementing interventions, 1440–1442
  loss of aspect of the self, 1513
  maintaining and evaluating, 1433
  nursing management, 1436–1442
  perceived self, 1433
  personal identity, 1433, 1437
  planning, 1440
  of preschooler, 319–320
  and resources, 1436
  role performance, 1434–1435, 1438
  sample care plan for chronic low self-esteem, 1439
  self-esteem, 1435, 1438–1439, 1440–1442
  stressors, 1436, 1437
self-concept mode, 63, 316
self-control, 1496
self-esteem, 356, 1120–1121, **1435,** 1438–1439, 1440–1442
Self-Esteem Disturbance (diagnostic label), 709
self-esteem needs, 204
self-examination and awareness, 1462–1463
self-help bed bath, 711
self-help groups, 163, 401–402
self-identity, 199
self-managed care model, 246
self-perception/self-concept pattern, 426
self-regulation, 15–16, 16, **200**
self-report pain measures, 990–991
self-talk, 386
semi-Fowler's position, 1131, 1332
semicircular canals, 583
semilunar valves, 1313
semiprone position, 1134*t*
sender, 386
senile lentigines, 568
sensate exercises, 1456
sense of autonomy, 316
sensorimotor phase, 316
sensorineural hearing loss, 587
sensoristasis, 1061
sensors, 663
sensory abilities, 315
sensory aids, 1069, 1070
sensory alterations, 1061–1063
sensory aphasia, 635
sensory changes, and aging, 353–354
sensory deficits, 402–403
sensory deficits, 1062–1063
sensory deprivation, 916, **1062,** 1065, 1066, 1069
sensory function, 650
sensory memory, 357
sensory overload, 1062, 1065, 1066, 1068–1069
sensory perception, 1061
  acute sensory deficits, management of, 1069–1071
  arousal mechanisms, 1061, 1068
  assessing, 1064–1066
  client safety, 1068, 1070–1071
  components of sensory-perceptual process, 1061
  concept map, 1076*f*
  the confused client, 1071–1072
  continuity of care, 1067

culture and, 1063
developmental stage, 1063
diagnosing, 1066–1067
environmental stimuli, 1068–1069
as etiology, 1066–1067
evaluating, 1074–1075, 1074*t*
factors affecting sensory function, 1063–1064
home care, 1067
illness, 1064
impaired hearing, 1071
impaired olfactory sense, 1071
impaired tactile sense, 1071
impaired vision, 1070–1071
implementing interventions, 1067–1073
lifestyle, 1064
medication, 1064
personality, 1064
planning, 1067
promotion of healthy sensory function, 1068
promotion of use of other senses, 1069–1070
sample care plan, 1074–1075
sensory aids, 1069
sensory alterations, 1061–1063
sensory deficits, 1062–1063
sensory deprivation, 1062, 1065, 1066, 1069
sensory overload, 1062, 1065, 1066, 1068–1069
stress, 1063
the unconscious client, 1072–1073
sensory-perceptual alterations, 764
sensory reception, 1061
sensory receptors, 663
separation anxiety, 316
septicemea, 884
sequence of events, 489
sequential compression devices (SCD), 1032, 1359–1360
serosanguineous exudate, 937
serous, 882
serous exudate, 937
serum electrolytes, 1393
serum osmolality, 1370, 1394
serum protein analysis, 942
serum proteins, 1193–1194
service management model, 246
service orientation, 16
serving sizes, 1182–1183
set point, 664
setting exercises, 1111
severe acute respiratory syndrome (SARS), 123
sex, 1446
sex education, 1460–1463
sex play, 1454
sex roles, 325
sexual activity, 325
sexual arousal, 1453–1454, **1456**
sexual arousal disorders
female dysfunction, 1456
male dysfunction, 1456
medication, effect of, 1456, 1457*T*
sexual behaviour, inappropriate, 1465–1466
sexual characteristics, 325
sexual desire and pleasure, 1453–1455
Sexual Dysfunction (diagnostic label), 1459
sexual expression, 1449
sexual expression, alternative forms of, 1454–1455
sexual function, altered, 1463–1465
sexual health, 1448–1449
sexual health status
assessing, 1456–1459
at-risk clients, identification of, 1459
diagnosing, 1459, 1459*t*
evaluation, 1466–1467, 1466*t*
implementing interventions, 1460–1466
interview, 1458
planning, 1459–1460
sex education, 1460–1463
sexual intercourse, 1454
sexual misbeliefs, 1461
sexual orientation, 1447–1448
sexual response cycle, 1454, 1455*t*
sexuality, 1446
adolescence, 1449–1450
adulthood, 1450–1451
children, 1449
and culture, 1451–1452
experience of, 1446–1447
factors influencing sexuality, 1451–1453
and family, 1451
health and illness, 1452–1453
and medications, 1453
nursing and, 1458
personal expectations and ethics, 1452
PLISSIT model, 1463–1465
and religion, 1452
sexual expression, alternative forms of, 1454–1455
throughout life, 1449–1451
sexuality-reproductive pattern, 426
sexually transmitted infections (STIs), 336, 1453, 1458, 1461, 1462*t*, 1463
shaft, 827
shaken baby syndrome (SBS), 313
shampooing the hair, 740–742
shared governance, 540
shared leadership, 540
sharp debridement, 951
sharps, 915
shearing, 929–930
shock phase, 1492
short-term coping strategies, 1496–1498
short-term goals, 449
short-term memory, 357
shortage crisis, 32
shower, 712, 716–717
shower seat, 706*f*
shroud, 1534
sibilant wheeze, 603*f*
side effect, 799
NSAIDs, 1001
opioids, 1000
side-lying position, 1132–1133, 1133*t*
side rails, 749–750
Sigma Theta Tau International Honor Society of Nursing (STTI), 19–20, 46
signature, 808
signature on recording, 487
significance of loss, 1515
signs, 419
silent generation, 542
simple facemask, 1340, 1340*f*
simplicity, 387–388
Sims' position, 1133, 1134*t*
single-dose vial, 830
single order, 807
single stoma, 1235
single use of a gown, 895
sinoatrial (SA or sinus) node, 1314
sinuses, 587*f*, 588–590
situational influences, 140–141
situational leadership, 539
sitz bath, 972
six Cs of caring in nursing, 385
Skene's glands, 549*f*, 657
skills
adding medication to intravenous fluid containers, 849–850
ampules, preparation of medications from, 831–832
antiembolism stockings, 1030–1031
assessment skills. *See* assessment skills
assisting client to sit on side of bed, 1139–1140
assisting clients to ambulate, 1149–1152
back massage, 1095–1096
bathing an adult or pediatric client, 713–717
bed or chair exit safety monitoring device, 777–778
brushing and flossing teeth, 731–734
cannula, facemask or face tent, oxygen administration using, 1338–1339
capillary blood specimen to measure blood glucose, 1194–1195
changing intravenous containers, tubing and dressings, 1416–1417
changing peripheral intravenous catheter to intermittent infusion lock, 1419
clean-catch urine specimen, collection of, 1275–1276
cleaning closed wound and applying sterile dressing, 1047–1049
continuous positive airway pressure (CPAP), 1343
discontinuing peripheral intravenous infusion, 1418
drainable bowel diversion ostomy appliance, changing, 1255–1257
enema, administering, 1248–1250
external (condom) catheter, application of, 1287–1289
foot care, 724–725
gastrointestinal suction, 1043–1045
gastrostomy feeding, administering, 1214–1215
hair care, 739–740
handwashing, 892–894
hearing aid, 747–748
hydrocolloid dressings, 956–957
initiating, maintaining, and terminating a blood transfusion by using a Y-set, 1422–1424
intradermal injection for skin tests, 836–837
intramuscular injection, 846–847
intravenous push (IVP), use of, 853–855
irrigating a wound, 960–961
jejunostomy feeding, administering, 1214–1215
logrolling, 1138–1139
mixing medications in one syringe, 834–835
moist transparent wound barrier dressing, 955–956
monitoring intravenous infusions, 1414–1415
moving client up in bed, 1135–1136
nasogastric tube, insertion of, 1205–1208
nasogastric tube, removal of, 1209
occupied beds, changing, 755–757
ophthalmic instillations, 858–861
oral care for unconscious client, 735–736
oral medications, administration of, 819–822
oropharyngeal, nasopharyngeal, and nasotracheal suctioning, 1351–1353
otic instillations, 861–863
perineal-genital care, 718–720
personal protective equipment, 896–898
restraints, application of, 787–789
seizure precautions, 779–780
sequential compression device, application of, 1359–1360
shampooing the hair of client confined to bed, 741–742
starting an intravenous infusion, 1407–1411
sterile field, establishing and maintaining, 901–905
sterile gloves, 906–907, 908–909
sterile gown, 907–909
subcutaneous injection, 839–841
suctioning a tracheostomy or endotracheal tube, 1353–1356
teaching moving, leg exercises, deep breathing, and coughing, 1024–1027
tracheostomy care, 1346–1349
transferring between bed and chair, 1142–1145
transferring between bed and stretcher, 1145–1146
tube feeding, administering, 1211–1214
turning client to lateral or prone position in bed, 1136–1137
unoccupied beds, changing, 751–755
urethral urinary catheterization, 1291–1294
vaginal instillations, 865–867
vials, preparation of medications from, 832–833
wound drainage specimen, 944–945
skin
assessment of, 564, 566–568
body odour, 564, 710
breakdown, 1120
colour and temperature, in postoperative phase, 1036
common problems, 708*t*
function, 928
intact skin, 928
integrity, 928, 940, 946–947, 1287

intradermal injection for skin tests, 836–837
lesions, describing, 569
lifespan considerations, 568–569
maceration, 931
prevention of breakdown, 927
reduced skin turgor, 1120
sensitivity, 710
tears, prevention and treatment, 959
trauma, avoiding, 948
wound/skin documentation sheet, 943*f*
skin applications, 857–858
skin contact, 920
skin-fold thicknesses, 1192
skin hygiene
agents commonly used on skin, 711
assessing, 705–707
assessment data clusters, 709
bathing, 710–717
bathing skills, 713–717
diagnosing, 707–708
evaluating, 720
general principles of skin care, 710
hygiene, 705–720
implementing interventions, 710–720
nursing diagnosis, 709
ostomy, 1253–1257
perineal-genital care, 718–720
planning, 709–710
and pressure ulcers, 948
skin preparation
practice guidelines, 858
preoperative skin preparation, 1029
surgical skin preparation, 1034
skin temperature, testing, 559
Skinner, B.F., 300, 516
skull, assessment of, 572, 573, 574
sleep, 1080
adolescents, 1084
adults, 1084–1085
and alcohol, 1086
assessing, 1089–1091
back massage, 1095–1096
bedtime rituals, 1094
circadian rhythms, 1081
comfort and relaxation, 1094–1097
deep sleep, 1082
diagnosing, 1091, 1092*t*
diagnostic studies, 1091
and diet, 1086–1087
and environment, 1086
evaluating, 1097–1098, 1098*t*
excessive sleep, 1088
factors affecting, 1085–1087
health and illness, 1085
history, 1089
homeostatic drive, 1082
homeostatic function of sleep, 1081
implementing interventions, 1094–1097
infants, 1083–1084
and lifestyle, 1086
and medications, 1087
and motivation, 1087
newborns, 1083
normal sleep patterns and requirements, 1083–1085
NREM (non-rapid-eye-movement) sleep, 1082
older adults, 1085
physical examination, 1091
physiology of sleep, 1081–1083
planning, 1091–1093
in preoperative phase, 1029
preschoolers, 1084
promotion of, 1095
REM (rapid-eye-movement) sleep, 1082
restful environment, 1094
sample care plan, 1092–1093
school-aged children, 1084
sleep cycles, 1082–1083
sleep diary, 1090–1091
sleep medications, 1097
slow-wave sleep (SWS), 1082
and smoking, 1087
Stage I, 1082
Stage II, 1082
Stage III, 1082
Stage IV, 1082
stages, 1082
states, 1082
and stimulants, 1086
stress and coping, 1504
teaching sleep habits, 1094
toddlers, 1084
violence against women, and sleep, 1086
sleep apnea, 1088, 1320
sleep architecture, 1082
sleep deprivation, 1089
sleep diary, 1090–1091
sleep disorders
hypersomnia, 1088
insomnia, 1087–1088
narcolepsy, 1088
parasomnias, 1087, 1089
periodic limb movements of sleep (PLMS), 1088–1089
primary sleep disorders, 1087
restless legs syndrome (RLS), 1089
secondary sleep disorders, 1087
sleep apnea, 1088
sleep medications, 1097
sleep-rest pattern, 426
slough, 932
slow-wave sleep (SWS), 1082
small-bore nasoenteric tubes, 1204
small calorie, 1171
small volume enemas, 1247
smell
neonates and infants, 311
toddlers, 315
Smith's models of health, 119
smoking
preoperative phase, 1022
and sleep, 1087
smoking cessation best practice guidelines, 1318
and susceptibility to infection, 888
sneeze reflex, 1310
Snellen chart, 575
soak, 972
SOAP, 476, 476*f*
SOAPIER, 475–476, 476*f*
soapsuds enemas, 1247
social arrangements, 56
social comfort needs, 385
social contract orientation, 340
social distance, 391
Social Isolation (diagnostic label)
respiratory and cardiovascular functions, 1328
self-concept, 1440
sensory perception problems, 1067
urinary elimination problems, 1279
social learning theory, 300
social relationships, and aging, 356
social resources, 1022
Social Sciences and Humanities Research Council (SSHRC), 40
social support, 143
see also support
and loss and grief, 1516
sensory perception problems, 1065–1066
support persons. *See* support people
social support systems, 143
social system, 207
social workers, 164, 164*t*
socialization, 16–17
socioeconomic status, and loss and grief, 1516
sociological factors, 203
sociopsychological variables, 122
Socratic questions, 370, 371
sodium intake, and blood pressure, 687
sodium (NA^+), 1375, 1382–1383
soft diet, 1201
soiled equipment and supplies, 914–915
soixante-neuf ("69"), 1454
soluble fibre, 1167
solutes, 1370
solution containers, 1403
solvent, 1370
somatic pain, 980
Somwar v. McDonald's Restaurants of Canada, 102
sonorous wheeze, 603*f*
sordes, 594, 729*t*
sound-alike health product names, 796
sound transmission, 583
source-oriented record, 473–474, 473*t*
space, 253–254
space orientation, 188
spastic, 1115
special diets, 1200–1202
special orders, in preoperative phase, 1029
specialist clinics, 161
specialist-generalists, 263
specialty organizations, 20
specific defences, 880, 882–883
specific gravity, 1278, 1394
specific self-esteem, 1435
specific suggestions, 1465
speculum examination, 657
speech
neonates and infants, 311
preschoolers, 320
spelling, 487
sphygmomanometer and cuff, 558*t,* 688
spinal anaesthesia, 1033
spinal analgesia, 1004–1005
spinal cord injuries, 1231, 1452
spinal cord stimulation (SCS), 1010
spiral faith model, 1474*f*
spiral reverse turns, 964–965
spiral turns, 964
spiritual beliefs, 1515–1516
spiritual care, 1475–1478
spiritual care professionals, 1482
spiritual development
adolescence, 326
described, 1473–1474
middle-aged adults, 340
older adults, 358
preschoolers, 320
school-age children, 323
toddlers, 317
young adults, 335
spiritual distress, 1475–1476, 1480, 1483
Spiritual Distress (diagnostic label)
self-concept, 1440
spiritual problems, 1479
spiritual facts, 323
spiritual health, 143, 1475, 1478–1484
spiritual practices affecting nursing care, 1476–1478
spiritual symbols, 1477
spiritual system, 207
spiritual theories, 302
spiritual well-being, 1475
spiritual wellness, 1475
spirituality, 272, 1472
characteristics of, 1472
and death and dying, 1532
preoperative phase, 1022
spiritual care, 1475–1478
spiritual development, 1473–1474
spiritual practices affecting nursing care, 1476–1478
spit, 1324
spitum specimen, 1324–1325
sponge bath, 972
sputum, 1324
stage of exhaustion, 1493
stage of resistance (SR), 1493
stairs
going down, 1159
going up, 1158
stance phase, 1122
standard, 434
standard deviation, 45
standard precautions, 912
standardized care plans, 440, 442*f,* 480–481
standards for a healthy diet, 1180–1183
standards of care, 95, 99, 440
standards of practice, 13, 94–95
standing order, 440, 807
stapes, 583
staples, 1053
starches, 1167
stat order, 807
Statement of Claim, 103

Statement of Defence, 103
static exercises, 1111
statutes, 91
statutory law, 91–92
stenotic, 1322
stepping reflex, 311
stereognosia, 322
stereognosis, 644, **650, 1061**
stereotyping, 183
sterile dressing, 1047–1049
sterile field, 899*t*, **900**–905
sterile gloves, 905–907, 908–909
sterile gowns, 895, 907–909
sterile technique, 899–909
sterilization, 891
sternocleidomastoid, 631
sternum, 601
sterols, 1170
stertor, 684
stethoscope, 558*t*, 674
stimulants, and sleep, 1086
stimulation of appetite, 1202
stimulus, 1061
stimulus-based stress models, 1490–1491
stirrups, 583
stoma, 1234, 1235, 1253–1257
stomatitis, 594, 729*t*
stool, 1226
stool specimens, 1237
storage
  carbohydrates, 1167–1168
  lipids, 1170
  protein, 1169
strabismus, 317
straight abdominal binder, 966
Strategies for Population Health, 134
street drugs, 801
strength-oriented diagnoses, 144
strengths, 437–438
stress, 1490
  see also coping
  anger mediation, 1504–1506
  anxiety, minimization of, 1504
  assessing, 1499–1500
  basic human needs, effects on, 1499*t*
  and blood pressure, 687
  and body temperature, 663
  burnout, 1507
  and cardiovascular functions, 1319
  caregiver burden, 1499
  cognitive indicators, 1496
  crisis intervention, 1506
  diagnosing, 1500–1501
  disorders caused or aggravated by, 1492*f*
  effects of, 1490
  emotional stress, and sleep, 1085–1086
  evaluating, 1507, 1507*t*
  financial stress, 297
  health-promotion strategies, 1503–1504
  home care, 1503
  implementing interventions, 1503–1507
  indicators, 1494–1496
  and infection prevention, 910
  lifespan considerations, 1491
  maternal stress during pregnancy, 1500
  minimization of, 1505
  models of stress, 1490–1494
  nurse's stress, 1506–1507
  physiological indicators, 1494
  planning, 1501–1503
  psychological indicators, 1494–1496
  and pulse rate, 673
  relaxation techniques, 1505
  and respiratory functions, 1319
  response-based stress models, 1491–1493
  sensory perception problems, 1063
  sources of, 1490
  stimulus-based stress models, 1490–1491
  three adaptation stages, 1493*f*
  transaction-based stress models, 1493–1494
stress electrocardiography, 1327
Stress Incontinence (diagnostic label), 1279
stress syndrome, 1491
stressors, 888, 1436, 1437, 1490, **1490,** 1490*t*
stretchers, 1141, 1142
stretching before exercise, 1110
stridor, 603*f*, 684, **1321**
stroke, 360, 1322
stroke impairments, 1072
stroke volume (SV), 1315
structural deficits, 403
structural variables, 122
structure evaluation, 463
structuring, 1496
student care plans, 441
student record management, 506
students
  educational programs. *See* nursing education
  legal responsibilities of, 108–109
study's purpose, 43
stupor, 1529
sty, 575
subarachnoid block (SAB), 1033
subclinical infection, 884
subculture, 179
subcutaneous, 806
subcutaneous administration of opioids, 1003
subcutaneous emphysema, 1358
subcutaneous injections, 838–841
subjective data, 418, 419
sublimation, 1498*t*
sublingual, 804
sublingual salivary gland, 590–594
submandibular gland, 590
substance use
  problematic. *See* problematic substance use
  start of, 260
substernal retraction, 684
substitute decision makers, 99
substitution, 1498*t*
subsystems, 206
success, history of, 1436
sucking reflex, 311
suction, 1042–1046, 1050
suction catheters, 1349
suctioning, 1349–1356
sudden infant death syndrome (SIDS), 313
sudoriferous (sweat) glands, 705
suffocation, 782
sugars, 1167
suicide, 256
  Aboriginal population, 260
  adolescence, 327
  in rural areas, 260–261
  young adults, 335–336
sulcular technique, 731
sundown syndrome, 1071, 1085
sunrise model, 182*f*
superego, 292
supervision, 458
supine position, 1132
supplements, 276
support
  see also social support
  client education, 521
  to facilitate communication, 404–405
  nonjudgmental support, 518
  spiritual and religious practices, 1481
support devices, 1131
support people
  assisting, 998
  as data source, 419
  pain, 988
support systems. *See* support
supportive devices, for pressure ulcer prevention, 948–950, 949*t*
suppository, 1246
suppression, 1496
suppressor T cells, 883
suppuration, 937
suprapubic catheter, 1300
suprasternal retraction, 684
suprasystems, 206
surface anaesthesia, 1033
surface temperature, 662
surface tension, 1311
surfactant, 1311
surgery
  see also perioperative care; surgical procedures
  and defecation, 1231
  degree of risk, 1019–1021
  degree of urgency, 1018
  elective surgery, 1018
  emergency surgery, 1018
  invasive (open) surgery, 1018
  level of invasiveness, 1018–1019
  major surgery, 1019
  minimally invasive surgery, 1018
  minor surgery, 1019
  outpatient surgical clients, 1024
  purpose, 1018
  surgical site marking method, 1030
  types of, 1018–1021
  urgent surgery, 1018
surgical dressings, 1047
surgical masks, 898
surgical procedures
  see also surgery
  advancements in, 164–165
  and sexuality, 1452*1453
  and urinary elimination, 1269
surgical skin preparation, 1034
surgical wounds, 1046–1053
Survey of Nursing Education in Canada (Weir), 28
susceptible host, 886–888, 909–911
suspected awareness, 1525
suspension-based lotion, 858
sustained maximal inspiration devices (SMIs), 1334
suture, 1051–1053
sutured wounds, 942
sutures, 310
sweat, 1373
sweat glands, 705
swing phase, 1122
swing-through gait, 1157
swing-to gait, 1157
symbols, 489*f*, 807*t*, 1477
sympathectomy, 1010
sympathetic stimulation, 662
sympathetically maintained pain, 980
symptom management, 419
syndrome diagnosis, 431
syndrome of inappropriate antidiuretic hormone (SIADH), 1382
synergistic effect, 800
syringes, 825–827, 826*f*, 871–872, 871*f*, 915, 958, 1212–1213
system hierarchy, 206*f*
systematic antibiotics, 939–940
systemic effects of heat and cold, 968
systemic infection, 884
systemic vascular resistance (SVR), 686, 1316
systems theories, 206, 206–207
systole, 610*f*, **615, 1314**
systolic pressure, 686

T

T-cell system, 883
tablets, 820
tachycardia, 675, 1390
tachypnea, 683, 684, **1320**
tactile discrimination, 644–645
tactile distraction, 1008
tactile sense, impaired, 1071
tactile stimuli, 1061
Tai Chi, 278–279
taking action, 399
talk test, 1111
tandem, 850
Tanner stages of development, 648*f*, 651*t*
target heart rate, 1111
tartar, 594, 728
task groups, 400
task orientation, 538
task power, 540
taste
  neonates and infants, 311
  preschoolers, 319
  toddlers, 315
tattoos, 118
teaching, 515
  see also client education
  abdominal breathing, 1333

about medications for fecal elimination, 1245–1246
assessment of stool for occult blood, 1239
behaviour modification, 531
breast awareness, 1464
canes, using, 1153
children, 529
choosing content, 526–527
client contracting, 530
clients with low literacy, 523
in the community, 515
computer-assisted instruction, 530–531
controlled and huff coughing, 1333
cough medications, use of, 1334
crutches, use of, 1155
discovery techniques, 531
electrical hazards, reducing, 783
evaluation of, 532
fecal elimination, 1242
foot care, 725–726
group teaching, 530
guidelines, 529–530
health personnel, 515
healthy breathing, 1331
healthy defecation, 1242
healthy fluid and electrolyte balance, promotion of, 1399
healthy heart, promotion of, 1331
healthy nutrition, 1199–1200
hygiene, 717
identification of clients requiring teaching, 524
incentive spirometers, use of, 1335
maintaining a healthy blood pressure, 687
mammography, 1464
metered-dose inhaler, use of, 869—870
vs. nursing, 515*t*
nutrition for older adults, 1181
nutrition recommendations for Canadians, 1184
organizing learning experiences, 527–528
orthostatic hypotension, control of, 1152
pain management, 997
patient-controlled analgesia (PCA) pump, 1007
patients and their families, 515
pelvic floor muscle exercises (Kegels), 1287
poisoning, prevention of, 781
postoperative instructions, 1028
preoperative instructions, 1024
preoperative teaching, 1023–1027
priorities, 525
problem solving techniques, 531
promotion of rest and sleep, 1095
pursed-lip breathing, 1333
safety measures throughout the lifespan, 769–771
sample teaching plan, 526
skin integrity, 946–947
sleep habits, 1094
special teaching strategies, 530–531
supporting religious practices, 1481
teaching strategies, 527, 528*t*, 530–531
testicular self-examination, 1464
tools, 527, 529
tooth decay, prevention of, 730
transcultural teaching, 531
urinary elimination, 1282–1283
walkers, using, 1154
written teaching aids, 523
teaching and learning groups, 400
teaching strategies, 527, 528*t*
team nursing, 169
teams, building and managing, 542–543
tears, 881
technical skills, 456
technological advancements
and health-care system, 164–165
high-fidelity simulation, 33
and nursing education, 33
web-based technology, 33
technology
and contemporary nursing practice, 18
and health promotion, 13
teeth
see also oral hygiene
assessment, 591
brushing and flossing, 731–734
care of, 731
dentures, 731, 733–734
developmental variations, 727–728
permanent teeth, 728*f*
temporary teeth, 727*f*
tooth decay, prevention of, 730
telangiectasias, 569
telehealth, 163, **264, 502**–503
telehealth projects, 241
telemedicine, 264
teleological theories, 78
telephone orders, 491
telephone reports, 491
telepractice, 504
temperament, 291, 297*t*
temperature. *See* body temperature
temperature scales, 669
temperature sensation, 644
temperature-sensitive tape, 668, 668*f*
temporal artery, 666*t*, 671
temporal artery (TA) thermometer, 668–669, 669*f*
temporal pulse, 673
temporary colostomies, 1234
temporary consistency modifications of diet, 1200
temporary teeth, 727*f*
ten "rights" of medication administration, 817
tender point, 981
TENS, 1008
tension pneumothorax, 1358
teratogen, 309
terminal colostomy, 1235
termination phase, 399–400
termination stage, 143
terminology, accepted, 487
territoriality, 391
tertiary intention, 934
tertiary prevention, 121
testes, 651*t*
testicular cancer, 658
testicular self-examination, 336, **658,** 1464
testicular self-examination (TSE), 1463
testing feeding tube placement, 1209–1210
theistic, 1473
theoretical frameworks
family nursing, 213
individual care, 204–207
theory, 56
Allen's McGill Model of nursing, 66–67
Campbell's UBC model of nursing, 65–66, 66*f*
vs. conceptual framework, 59–60
consequence-based (teleological) theories, 78
described, 59
Henderson's definition of nursing, 62
Leininger's cultural care diversity and universality theory, 65
moral theories, 78–81
Newman's expansion of consciousness, 65
Nightingale's environmental theory, 60–62
overview of selected nursing theories, 60–67, 61*t*
Parse's theory of human becoming, 64
Peplau's interpersonal relations model, 62
principles-based (deontological) theories, 78
purposes of nursing theories, 60
relationships-based (caring) theories, 79
Roach's attributes of professional caring, 67
Roy's adaptation model, 62–63
Watson's human caring theory, 63–64
theory of human care, 384
therapeutic actions of drugs, 800*t*
therapeutic baths, 712
therapeutic communication, 392–393, 394*t*
therapeutic effect, 799
therapeutic massage, 277
therapeutic touch (TT), 279
therapy, and nutrition, 1174
therapy groups, 402
thermal receptors, 969
thermal tolerance, 968–969
thermometer, 558*t*, 667–669, 915
third space syndrome, 1380–1381
Thomas, Alexander, 296, 297*t*
thoracic breathing, 682
thorax and lungs
adventitious breath sounds, 603*t*
assessment of, 599–609
breath sounds, 602*t*, 603*t*, 609
chest deformities, 602*f*
chest landmarks, 599–601
chest shape and size, 601–609
configurations of, 601*f*
lifespan considerations, 608–609
normal breath sounds, 602*t*
Thorndike, Edward, 516
three-point gait, 1157, 1157*f*
three-way Foley catheter, 1290
thrill, 622–623
throat culture, 1325
thrombophlebitis, 1037*t*, **1041, 1118**
thromboplastin, 882
thrombus, 1037*t*, **1041, 1118**
throughput, 207
thyroid function, 1196
thyroid gland, 597–598
thyroxine output, 662
ticks, 737–738
tidal volume, 683, 1311
time, 253–254
time management, 543, 1504
time of recording, 486
time orientation, 188
timed urine specimen, 1274–1277
timing
of administration of drug, 804
and communication, 388
defecation, 1242–1243
and learning, 518
of recording, 486
tinea pedis, 722
tissue oxygenation, 910
toddlers (1 to 3 years)
see also children
cognitive development, 316
defecation, 1229
developmental guidelines, 318
food safety, 1177
health assessment and promotion, 317, 318
health problems, 317
normal sleep patterns and requirements, 1084
nutrition, 1177
oral hygiene, 730
physical development, 315–316
psychosocial development, 316
safety measures, 768, 769
toe or heel walking, 640
toileting, assisting with, 1283
tolerable upper intake level, 1171
tolerance, 1000
tongue blades (depressors), 559*t*
tonic neck reflex, 311
tonicity, 1370
tonsils, 593
topical, 806
topical medications
irrigations, 871–872
nasal instillations, 864–865
ophthalmic instillations, 858–861
otic instillations, 861–864
percutaneous route of absorption, 856
rectal instillations, 867–868
respiratory inhalation, 868–871
skin applications, 857–858
vaginal instillations, 865–867
topical (surface) anaesthesia, 1033
Toronto Charter for a Healthy Canada, 135–136
tort, 99
tort law, 91
adverse event reporting, 103–104
battery, 97
described, 99
intentional torts, 101–103
lawsuit, 103
negligence, 99–101
patient safety, 103
reporting torts, 108

tortfeasor, 92
total character, 199
total enteral nutrition (TEN), 1204
total iron-binding capacity (TIBC) test, 1194
total lymphocyte count, 1194
total parenteral nutrition (TPN), 1218
total quality management (TQM), 463
Total Urinary Incontinence (diagnostic label), 1279
touch
  neonates and infants, 311
  school-age children, 322
  toddlers, 315
touching, 187
Toward 2020: Visions for Nursing (CNA), 536
toys, 915
trachea, 597
tracheal tugging, 684
tracheostomy, 1344–1349
tracheostomy care, 1346–1349
tracheotomy, 1344
trademark, 796
traditional Aboriginal medicine, 274
traditional care plan, 480
traditional Chinese medicine (TCM), 274
traditional medicine, 184–185, 273
tragus, 583
trait theorists, 538
tranquilizers, 1020, 1029
transaction-based stress models, 1493–1494
transactional leadership, 539
transactional stress theory, 1494
transcellular fluid, 1368
transcendence, 385
transcultural nursing, 179
  see also cultural care
transcultural teaching, 531
transcutaneous electrical nerve stimulation (TENS), 1008
transdermal patch, 857, 857*f*, 858, 1003–1004
transduction, 982–983
transfats, 1169
transfer belts, 1141
transferrin, 1194
transferring between bed and chair, 1142–1145
transferring between bed and stretcher, 1145–1146
transferring clients, 1134–1146
transformational leadership, 539–540
transfusion, blood. *See* blood transfusions
transfusion reactions, 1420*t*, 1421
transient incontinence, 1271
transient ischemic attack (TIA), 1322
transmission, 983
transmission-based precautions, 912
transmission route. *See* route of transmission
transnasal administration, 1003
transparent films, 952–954
transpersonal caring, 64
transport of clients with infection, 915–916
transsexuals, 1448
transtheoretical model, 141–143, 142*f*, 545
transverse colostomy, 1235
trapezius, 631
Travis' illness-wellness continuum, 120–121
treated wounds, 942
treatment, 156
tremor, 635
Tri-Council Policy Statement on Ethical Conduct for Research Involving Humans, 49
triadic questions, 223
trial and error, 375
triangle position, 1156
triangular arm sling, 966
triangular fossa, 583
triceps, 631
triceps skin fold (TSF), 1192, 1193*f*
trigeminal neuralgia, 981
triglycerides, 1170
trigone, 1265
trimesters, 308
tripod (triangle) position, 1156
troponin, 1327
true pathogen, 880
trust, 246, 399
trust *versus* mistrust, 311, 1432*t*
truth, 80
tub bath, 712, 716–717
tub seat, 706*f*
tube drainage, 1393
tube feeding
  administering, 1211–1214, 1216
  assessing patients, 1216*t*
  clogged feeding tubes, 1217–1218
  fluid intake, 1393
  home care, 1217
  medication, administering, 1216–1217
  placement, 1209–1210
tube irrigants, 1393
tuberculin syringe, 826
tubes, 1039
Tui Na, 277
tumour, 565*f*
tunica intima, 1315
tunica media, 1315
tunics, 1315
tuning fork, 558*t*
turgor, 1120
turning clients in bed, 1134, 1136–1137
24-hour fluid balance record, 481
24-hour food recall, 1188
twill tape, 1348–1349
two-point alternate gait, 1157, 1157*f*
two-point discrimination, 644, **650**
two-spirited, 1452
two-strip method, 1348
tympanic membrane, 582, 666*t*, 667, 671
tympanites, 1038*t*
tympany, 560

U

UBC model of nursing, 65–66, 66*f*
ulcer, 566*t*, 934
  see also pressure ulcers
ultra-liberal leader, 539
unconscious clients
  coma stimulation, 1073
  eye care, 744
  oral hygiene, 734–736
  sensory perception problems, 1072–1073
unconscious mind, 292
undermining, 942
undernutrition, 1185
undertaker, 1534
underweight clients, 1200
undoing, 1498*t*
unintentional injuries, 762–763
unintentional wounds, 928
unions, 21
United Nations Children's Fund (UNICEF), 1451
United States Pharmacopeia (USP), 798
universal precautions (UP), 912
universality, 11, **153,** 154*t*
unoccupied beds, 751–755
unplanned change, 545
unplanned pregnancies, prevention of, 1461–1462
unregulated care providers (UCP), 543, 544
unsafe practices, 108
unsaturated fatty acids, 1169
unstageable pressure ulcers, 932
unsupportive interactions with others, 43
untreated wounds, 940
upper airway, 1309
upper-level managers, 540
upstream view, 125
urea, 1196
ureterostomy, 1234, 1301
ureters, 1264–1265
urethra, 1265
Urge Urinary Incontinence (diagnostic label), 1279
urgent health problem, 158
urgent surgery, 1018
urinary catheterization, 1289–1290
urinary changes, and aging, 354
urinary creatinine, 1196
urinary diversions, 1301–1302
urinary drainage devices, 1287–1289
urinary elimination
  and activity, 1268
  altered urinary elimination, 1269–1271, 1270*t*
  altered urine production, 1269, 1270*t*
  anuria, 1269
  assessing, 1271–1278
  average daily urine output by age, 1269*t*
  clean intermittent self-catheterization (CISC), 1297–1298
  continence (bladder) training, 1285–1286
  developmental factors, 1266–1267
  diagnosing, 1279, 1279*t*
  and diagnostic procedures, 1269
  diuresis, 1269
  dysuria, 1270
  enuresis, 1270
  evaluating, 1302–1303, 1303*t*
  external urinary drainage devices, 1287–1289
  factors affecting voiding, 1266–1269
  fluid intake, 1267, 1281–1283
  food intake, 1267
  home care, 1280–1281, 1282–1283
  implementing interventions, 1281–1302
  indwelling catheter specimen, 1277
  indwelling catheters, nursing interventions for, 1280–1297
  infants, 1266
  interview, 1272
  irrigations, 1298–1300
  lifespan considerations, 1267, 1268*t*
  medications, 1268
  muscle tone, 1268
  neurogenic bladder, 1271
  nocturia, 1269
  normal and abnormal urine, characteristics of, 1273*t*
  normal urinary elimination, maintenance of, 1281–1283
  normal voiding habits, maintenance of, 1283, 1284
  nursing history, 1271
  older adults, 1266–1267
  oliguria, 1269
  pathological conditions, 1268–1269
  pelvic floor muscle exercises (PFME), 1286–1287
  physical assessment, 1271
  physiology of urinary elimination, 1264–1266
  planning, 1279–1281
  polydipsia, 1269
  polyuria, 1269
  postoperative patients, 1042
  preschoolers, 1266
  psychosocial factors, 1267
  residual urine, 1274
  sample care plan, 1280–1281
  school-age children, 1266
  skin integrity, maintenance of, 1287
  suprapubic catheter care, 1300
  surgical procedures, 1269
  teaching, 1282–1283
  toileting, assisting with, 1283
  urinary catheterization, 1289–1290
  urinary diversions, 1301–1302
  urinary frequency, 1269
  urinary hesitancy, 1270
  urinary incontinence, 1270–1271
  urinary incontinence management, 1285–1288
  urinary output, 1271–1273
  urinary retention, 1271, 1289–1290
  urinary tract infections, prevention of, 1283–1284
  urinary urgency, 1269–1270
  urine, assessment of, 1271–1274
  urine specimens, collection of, 1274–1277
  urine testing, 1277–1278
  visualization procedures, 1278
urinary frequency, 1269
urinary hesitancy, 1270
urinary incontinence (UI), 931, **1120, 1270**–1271, 1285–1288
urinary infection, 1120
urinary output, 1271–1273, 1393
urinary pH, 1278
urinary problems, in postoperative phase, 1038*t*
urinary reflux, 1120

urinary retention, 1038*t*, **1120,** 1268, **1271,** 1289–1290
Urinary Retention (diagnostic label), 1279
urinary stasis, 1119
urinary system
  and benefits of exercise, 1113
  immobility, effects of, 1119–1120
urinary tests, 1196
urinary tract
  anatomical structures of the urinary tract, 1264*f*
  bladder, 1265
  kidneys, 1264, 1264*f*
  pelvic floor, 1265
  ureters, 1264–1265
  urethra, 1265
urinary tract infection (UTI), 1038*t*, 1283–1284
urinary urea nitrogen, 1196
urinary urgency, 1269–1270
urination, 1266
  see also urinary elimination
urine
  assessment, 1271–1274
  output, 1372
  pH, 1394
  specific gravity, 1394
  testing. *See* urine testing
urine hat, 1272*f*
urine osmolality, 1394
urine specimens, 1274–1277
urine testing
  glucose tests, 1278
  ketones, 1278
  kits, 1277–1278
  metabolic substances in urine, 1278
  occult blood, 1278
  protein in urine, 1278
  specific gravity, 1278
  urinary pH, 1278
urogenital tract, male, 650*f*
urticaria, 565*f*
usefulness of a study, 42
usual aging, 351
usual body weight (UBW), 1189
utilitarianism, 78
utility, 78
utilization review, 508
uvula, 593

V

V scan, 1327
vaccination, 888
vacuum-assisted closure (VAC), 962
vagina
  defences against infection, 881
  perineal-genital care, 718–720
vaginal cream, 866
vaginal foam, 866
vaginal instillations, 865–867
vaginal jelly, 866
vaginal speculum, 558*t*
vaginal suppository, 866
vaginismus, 1456
validation, 428–429, 428*t*
validity, 44
Valsalva manoeuvre, 1117, 1120, 1232
valuables, care of, 1029
value-belief pattern pattern, 426
value set, 74
value system, 74
values, 73, 1474
  and communication process, 391
  personal values, 74
  professional values, 74
  transmission, 74
values clarification, 74
  care situations, clarification of values in, 77
  client values, clarification of, 75–77, 76*t*
  nurse's values, clarification of, 75
Vanier Institute of the Family, 212
vaporization, 663
variability, 45
variance, 45, 480*t*
variances, 479
vascular nursing interventions, 1332
vascular response, 881
vascular sounds, 626
vasocongestion, 1454
vastus lateralis site, 843–844, 843*f*, 844*f*
vector-borne transmission, 886
vegetarian diets, 1184–1185
vegetarians, 1185
vehicle-borne transmission, 886
vein selection, 1402
venipuncture sites, 1401–1403
venous access device, 1404–1405
venous disease, 936
venous return, 1316
venous stasis, 1358–1359
venous thrombosis, 1332
venous vasodilation and stasis, 1117–1118
ventilation, 682, 749, 1310–1311
ventilation scan, 1327
ventricles, 1313
ventrogluteal site, 842, 843*f*
Venturi mask, 1340–1341, 1340*f*
venules, 1315
veracity, 80
verbal communication, 186–187, **387**–388, 403–404
verbal rating scales (VRSs), 990
vernix caseosa, 308
vertebrae line, 600
vesicle, 565*f*
vesicostomy, 1301
vesicular breath sounds, 602*t*
vest restraints, 785–786
vestibule, 583
vials, 829–833
vibration, 1335
vicarious liability, 96
Victorian Order of Nurses, 5, 239
videoconferencing, 507
violence, 1495
violence against women, and sleep, 1086
Virginia Henderson International Nursing Library, 46
virions, 883
virtue, 80
virulence, 880
virulence factors, 880
viruses, 880
visceral, 1061
visceral pain, 980
viscosity, 686
visible minorities, 176
vision, 540
  see also eye
  amblyopia, 317
  assessment of, 572–582
  changes in, and aging, 353
  clock system, 1203*f*
  emmetropic, 319
  eyesight loss in rural areas, 259–260
  functional vision tests, 581
  hyperopic, 319
  impaired vision, 1070–1071
  lifespan considerations, 582
  myopic, 319
  newborns and infants, 310
  preschoolers, 319
  school-age children, 322
  sensory aids, 1070
  strabismus, 317
  toddlers, 315, 317
vision for change, 547
visual acuity, 573, 576–581
visual analogue scales (VASs), 990
visual aphasia, 637
visual distraction, 1008
visual fields, 573–574
visual stimuli, 1061
visualization procedures
  cardiovascular functions, 1327–1328
  fecal elimination, 1236
  respiratory functions, 1327–1328
  urinary elimination, 1278
vital capacity, 1118, 1317
vital signs, 661
  blood pressure, 686–696
  body temperature, 662–672
  fifth vital sign, 988
  fluid, electrolyte, and acid-base balances, 1389–1392
  general survey, 563
  oxygen saturation, 696–699
  postoperative phase, 1036
  preoperative phase, 1030
  pulse, 672–681
  respirations, 682–686
  times to assess vital signs, 662
vital signs graphic record, 477*f*
vitamin, 1170
vitiligo, 564, 569
voiding, 1266
  see also urinary elimination
volume-control infusion sets, 852
volume-control set, 1412
volume expanders, 1401
voluntariness, 97
vomiting, 1038*t*
vomitus, 1393
voyeurism, 1454
vulnerable persons, 50
vulvodynia, 1456
Vygotsky, Lev, 296

W

waist circumference (WC), 563–564, **1191**–1192, 1192*t*
waist-to-hip ratio (WHR), 1191–1192
walkers, 1153–1154
walking, 774, 1147–1152
walking aids, 1152–1159
walking gait, 639
walking reflex, 311
wall suction units, 1046
warmth, 392
warmth in bed, 1097
warty lesions, 568
water excess, 1382
water safety, 257–258
water-soluble vitamin, 1170
Watson, Jean, 63–64, 384
web-based technology, 33
weight
  at birth, 309
  gain, and sleep, 1086–1087
  general survey, 563–564
  infants, 309
  preschoolers, 319
  school-age children, 322
  toddlers, 315
weight-bearing exercise, 1112–1113
weight change, 1190
weight gain or loss, percentage of, 1189–1193
Weir, George, 28
Weir Report, 30
well-being, 117–118
wellness, 117
  Aboriginal views of, 119
  Dunn's high-level wellness grid, 120
  fluid, electrolyte, and acid-base balances, 1396
  maintaining a healthy blood pressure, 687
  models of health and wellness, 119–121
  and nursing, 10
  prevention, levels of, 121
  spiritual wellness, 1475
  tooth decay, prevention of, 730
  Travis' illness-wellness continuum, 120–121
wellness assessment programs, 138
wellness centres, 241
wellness nursing diagnoses, 144
wellness nursing diagnosis, 431
Westerhoff, John, 302, 303*t*
Westerhoff's four stages of faith, 303*t*, 1473*t*
wheal, 565*f*
wheelchair safety, 1141, 1142
wheeze, 684
whistle-blowers, 108
white blood cell count, 1326
WHMIS system of labelling, 784*f*, 915
women
  abuse of women, 336
  female genital mutilation, 1451

genitals, assessment of, 646–647, 656–658
issues, and health-care system, 167
menopause. *See* menopause
obesity in childbearing women, 336
perineal-genital care, 719
pregnancy. *See* pregnancy
pubic hair development, 648, 648*f*
and urinary tract infection (UTI), 1283–1284
violence against women, and sleep, 1086
women's movement, 18
work-related social support groups, 402
work-role preoccupation, 296
workforce competencies, 244
working phase, 399
Workplace Hazardous Materials Information System (WHMIS). *See* WHMIS system of labelling
workplace safety, 765
worksite health-promotion programs, 139
World Health Organization (WHO), 117, 132, 273, 878, 1451
world views, 56–57, **1474**
World War I, 5, 153
World War II, 6–7, 153
wound cultures, 942, 944–945
wound drainage, 937
wound drainage specimen, 944–945
wound healing
blood-borne pathogens, 947
colonization, 939–940
complications, 937–939
contamination, 939–940
dehiscence with possible evisceration, 937–939, 1046
delayed primary intention healing, 934
factors affecting wound healing, 939–940
factors to consider, 953
hemorrhage, 937
infection, 937, 939–940
infection prevention, 947
inflammatory phase, 934–936
lifespan considerations, 939
and lifestyle, 939
maturation phase, 936–937
and medication, 939
moist wound healing, 947
nutrition, 939, 947
phases of, 934–937
positioning, 947–948
primary intention healing, 934
proliferative phase, 936
regeneration of tissues, 934
secondary intention healing, 934
supporting wound healing, 947–948
tertiary intention, 934
types of, 934
types of wound care products, 952*t*
wound drainage, types of, 937
wounds
acute wound, 928
adjunctive therapies, 962
assessment of, 940–945
bandages, 962–965
binders, 962–963, 965–967
black wounds, 951
Canadian Association of Wound Care Quick Reference Guide, 930
chronic wound, 928
classification by depth, 928
clean-contaminated wounds, 928
clean wounds, 928
cleansing, 945, 958–961
closed wounds, 928, 1047–1049
contaminated wounds, 928
damp gauze *vs.* advanced dressings, 962
diagnosing, 945–946
dirty or infected wounds, 928
drainage, 937, 1050, 1393
dressings, 951–957
evaluating, 967–968, 968*t*
healing. *See* wound healing
heat and cold applications, 968–972
home care, 919, 946–947, 961–962
implementing interventions, 947–967
intentional wounds, 928
irrigation and packing, 958, 960–961
laboratory data, 942
lifespan considerations, 961
lower extremity ulcers, 934
mixed-colour wounds, 951
open wounds, 928
pain, 940
planning, 946–947
in postoperative phase, 1038*t*, 1046–1053
pressure sites, 941
pressure ulcers, 928–933
red, 951
suction, 1050
supporting and immobilizing, 962–967
surgical dressings, 1047
suture, 1051–1053
sutured wounds, 942
treated wounds, 942
types of, 928, 929*t*
unintentional wounds, 928
untreated wounds, 940
wound bed preparation paradigm, 958
wound cultures, 942, 944–945
wound drainage specimen, 944–945
wound/skin documentation sheet, 943*f*
yellow wounds, 951
wrist muscles, 631
wrist restraints, 788
Writ of Summons, 103
written teaching aids, 523

X

X-ray examination, 1327

Y

Y-set, 1422–1424
yarmulke, 1478
yellow wounds, 951
yoga, 280
young adults (20 to 40 years)
abuse of women, 336
caffeine intake, 337
cognitive development, 335
developmental guidelines, 337
environmental exposure, 337
and grief and loss, 1515
health assessment and promotion, 337–338
health problems, 335–337
immunizations, 337
injuries, 335
malignancies, 336–337
moral development, 335
nutrition, 1179–1180
obesity in childbearing women, 336
physical development, 334
problematic substance use, 336
psychosocial development, 334–335
safety measures, 770, 772
sexually transmitted infections (STIs), 336
spiritual development, 335
suicide, 335–336

Z

Z-track technique, 845, 846–847
zoomer, 333
zoonoses, 258

Photo Credits

Chapter 1 1.1 – Hôtel Dieu, Quebec. From Gibson, J., Mathewson, M. (1947). *Three Centuries of Canadian Nursing*. Toronto: McMillian; 1.2 – Library and Archives Canada C-022763. Reproduced with the permission of the Minister of Public Works and Government Services Canada, 2007; 1.3 – Library and Archives Canada e00241890. Reproduced with the permission of the Minister of Public Works and Government Services Canada, 2007; 1.4 – Library and Archives Canada, e002504605/ISN 576855. Reproduced with the permission of the Minister of Public Works and Government Services Canada, 2007; 1.5 – Victorian Order of Nurses; 1.6, 1.7 – From Gibson, J., Mathewson, M. (1947). *Three Centuries of Canadian Nursing*. Toronto: McMillian; 1.8 – Courtesy of the Wilberforce Heritage Guild; 1.9 – Courtesy Mrs. A. Elizabeth Pecknold, held by the AMS Nursing History Research Unit, University of Ottawa; 1.10 – Courtesy of Cynthia Toman, AMS Nursing History Research Unit, University of Ottawa; 1.11 – Courtesy of NS Eva R. Wannop, Toronto. Held by the AMS Nursing History Research Unit, University of Ottawa; 1.12 – © Elena Dorfman/Addison Wesley.

Chapter 5 5.1 – Faculty of Nursing, the University of Calgary.

Chapter 11 11.2 – (Top left) © Anne W. Krause/CORBIS/MAGMA; (Bottom left) Kevin Kornemann/Taxi; (Right) Digital Vision.

Chapter 13 13.2 – Kristen Knibbs; 13.3 – Tetra Images/Alamy.

Chapter 15 15.2 – Yoav Levy/Phototake, NYC.

Chapter 17 17.2 – © Elena Dorfman/Addison Wesley; 17.4 – Jane Wattenburg/Addison Wesley; 17.7 – © Elena Dorfman/Addison Wesley; 17.8 – © Elena Dorfman/Addison Wesley.

Chapter 18 18.1, 18.2 – © Elena Dorfman/Addison Wesley.

Chapter 19 19.1, 19.2 – © Elena Dorfman/Addison Wesley

Chapter 21 21.2 – © Alain McLaughlin/Addison Wesley; 21.4 – © Elena Dorfman/Addison Wesley; 21.5 – © Alain McLaughlin/Addison Wesley; 21.6 – Faculty of Nursing, The University of Calgary.

Chapter 23 23.6 – Mike English/MediChrome; 23.7 – Diane Clare.

Chapter 24 24.1 – Scott Camazine/Alamy; 24.2, 24.3, 24.4, 24.5 Courtesy of Sutter Health.

Chapter 25 25.1 – © Alain McLaughlin/Addison Wesley; 25.3 – © Elena Dorfman/Addison Wesley.

Chapter 26 26.1 – © Alain McLaughlin/Addison Wesley.

Chapter 27 27.1 – © Richard Tauber/Addison Wesley; Table 27.3 – © Elena Dorfman/Addison Wesley; 27.2, 27.3 – © Richard Tauber/Addison Wesley; 27.4 – © Elena Dorfman/AddisonWesley; 27.5 – © Richard Tauber/Addison Wesley; 27.8, ❶–❼ *Dermatology Secrets in Color*, 2nd ed., by J. E. Fitzpatrick and J. L. Aeling, 2001, Philadelphia, PA: Hanley & Belfus, Inc., ❽ reprinted with permission from the American Academy of Dermatology. All rights reserved; Skill 27.6 ❶–❺ © Richard Tauber/Addison Wesley, ❻ Patrick Watson, Pearson Education/PH, ❽–❿ Patrick Watson, Pearson Education/PH; Skill 27.7 ❸ Patrick Watson, Pearson Education/PH; ❺–❼ Patrick Watson, Pearson Education/PH; Skill 27.8 ❶ © Elena Dorfman/Addison Wesley; Skill 27.9 ❶–❹ © Elena Dorfman/Addison Wesley; Skill 27.10 ❶–❸ © Elena Dorfman/Addison Wesley; Skill 27.11 ❶, ❺ © Elena Dorfman/Addison Wesley; Skill 27.14 ❷–❸ Patrick Watson/Pearson Education/PH; Skill 27.15 ❶–❾ © Elena Dorfman/Addison Wesley; Skill 27.16 ❶ © Elena Dorfman/Addison Wesley; Skill 27.17 ❶–❻, ❽, ❿–⓰ © Elena Dorfman/Addison Wesley; ❼, ❾ Al Dodge, Pearson Education/PH; ⓱ Patrick Watson, Pearson Education/PH; 27.38 Patrick Watson.

Chapter 28 28.5 – © Elena Dorfman/Addison Wesley; 28.7, 28.8 – © Jenny Thomas Photography/Addison Wesley; 28.9 – Copyright © Exergen Corporation. All rights reserved; Skill 28.1 ❶–❸ Patrick Watson; ❹ © Jenny Thomas Photography/Addison Wesley; ❺ Copyright © Exergen Corporation. All rights reserved; 28.10, 28.11 – Patrick Watson; 28.14 – © Elena Dorfman/Addison Wesley; Skill 28.2 ❶C © Richard Tauber/Addison Wesley; Skill 28.3 ❶–❸ Patrick Watson; ❹–❺ © Elena Dorfman/Addison Wesley; 28.19 – © Elena Dorfman/Addison Wesley; 28.20 – Patrick Watson; 28.25 – © Elena Dorfman/Addison Wesley; 28.26, 28.27 – Courtesy of Nonin Medican, Inc.

Chapter 29 29.1, 29.2 – © Jenny Thomas Photography/Addison Wesley; 29.3, 29.4, 29.5 – Sara Daniels; Skill 29.1 ❶–❺, ❼, ❾ Al Dodge/Pearson Education/PH College; ❻ Patrick Watson; ❽ © Jenny Thomas Photography/Addison Wesley; Skill 29.4 ❶–❼ Al Dodge/Pearson Education/PH College; Skill 29.1 ❶ © Elena Dorfman/Addison Wesley; 29.11 – Sara Daniels; Skill 29.7 ❶ © Jenny Thomas Photography/Addison Wesley; 29.13 – David Parker/Science Photo Library/Photo Researchers, Inc.; 29.14 – Lester Lefkowitz/Corbis; 29.16 B, C – Jane Schemilt/Science Photo Library/Photo Researchers, Inc.; Skill 29.9 ❶–❷ Al Dodge/Pearson Education/PH College, ❸–❹, ❼ Patrick Watson; ❽ © Alain McLauglin/Addison Wesley; Skill 29.10 ❶–❺ Al Dodge/Pearson Education/PH College.

Chapter 30 30.1 – (top left) Courtesy of Tony Freeman/PhotoEdit, (top right) Jerry Marshall, (bottom left) Grantpix/Photo Researchers Inc., (bottom right) Michael Newman/PhotoEdit; 30.3 – © 2002 Hill-Rom Services, Inc. Reprinted with permission. All rights reserved; Skill 30.1 ❶ Courtesy of Alert Care, Mill Valley, CA, ❷ Courtesy of J.T. Posey, Co.; 30.4 – © Elena Dorfman/Addison Wesley; 30.7 – © Jenny Thomas Photography/Addison Wesley; 30.9 – © Jenny Thomas Photography/Addison Wesley; Skill 30.3 ❷ Al Dodge/Pearson Education/PH College, ❸ © Jenny Thomas Photography/Addison Wesley; 30.10 – Roy Ramsey/Pearson Education/PH College,

Chapter 31 31.10 A, B – Elena Dorfman; 31.13 A–C – Shirlee Snyder; Skill 31.1 ❸ Elena Dorfman, ❹ Patrick Watson; 31.16 – Patrick Watson; 31.18 – Patrick Watson; 31.19, 31.20 A–C, 31.22, 31.23 – Elena Dorfman; 31.27 A–B – © Richard Tauber/Addison Wesley; 31.28 A–C – Patrick Watson; Skill 31.2 ❶ Jenny Thomas, ❷ Patrick Watson; Skill 31.3 ❶–❸ Patrick Watson; Skill 31.4 ❶–❹ Patrick Watson; Skill 31.6 ❷ Elena Dorfman; 31.32 – Custom Medical Stock Photo, Inc.; 31.33 – Jenny Thomas; 31.34, 31.35, 31.36 – Custom Medical Stock Photo, Inc.; 31.41 – Custom Medical Stock Photo, Inc.; Skill 31.8 ❶–❸ Elena Dorfman; 31.44 – A: Photograph reprinted courtesy of (BD) Becton, Dickson and Company and courtesy of Baxter Healthcare Corporation. All rights reserved; Photo B: Photograph reprinted courtesy of (BD) Becton, Dickson and Company and courtesy of Baxter Healthcare Corporation. All rights reserved; Skill 31.9 ❶, ❸–❹ Jenny Thomas, ❷ Photograph reprinted courtesy of (BD) Becton, Dickson and Company; 31.47 – Courtesy of Baxter Healthcare Corporation. All rights reserved; 31.48 – From *Pharmacology for Nurses: A Pathophysiologic Approach* (p. 38), by Adams, Josephson, & Holland Jr., 2005, Upper Saddle River, NJ: Pearson Education; Skill 31.10 ❷–❸ Jenny Thomas; Skill 31.11 ❷ Jenny Thomas, ❸ Patrick Watson; 31.54 – Courtesy of Mabis Healthcare, Inc.; 31.56 – Courtesy of Trudell Medical International; 31.57, 31.58 – Jenny Thomas.

Chapter 32 32.2 – © A. Davidhazy/Custom Medical Stock Photo Custom Medical Stock Photo; Skill 32.1 ❶–❺ © Alain McLaughlin/Addison Wesley; Skill 32.2 ❶, ❸–❺ Al Dodge/Pearson Education/PH College, ❷ © Alain McLaughlin/Addison Wesley; Skill 32.3 ❶–❹, ⓮ Al Dodge/Pearson Education/PH College, ❺–❻ Elena Dorfman, ❼–❽, ❿–⓫ Patrick Watson, ⓬–⓭ Alexandra Truitt & Terry Marshall; Skill 32.4 ❶–❹ Al Dodge/Pearson Education/PH College; Skill 32.5 ❶–❺ © Alain McLaughlin/Addison Wesley; 32.3 – Health Canada, Workplace Hazardous Materials Information System, http://www.hc-sc.gc.ca/hecs-sesc/whmis/whmis_symbols.htm.

Chapter 33 33.1 – Line art from Clinical Practice Guideline, Pressure Ulcers in Adults: Prediction and Prevention (pp. 16–17), by U.S. Department of Health and Human Services, PPPPUA Pub. No. 92-0047, 1992, Rockville, MD: Public Health Service, photos from Cory Patrick Hartley, RN; 33.2 – © Educational Images/Custom Medical Stock Photo; 33.4 – Copyright © NPUAP, 2003. Reprinted with permission; 33.7 – Courtesy of Gaymar Industries, Inc.; 33.8 – Courtesy of Ease; 33.9 – KinAir MedSurg. Courtesy of KCI Licensing, Inc., San Antonio, TX; 33.10 – Courtesy of Hill-Rom Services, Inc. Reprinted with permission. All rights reserved; 33.12 – © Jenny Thomas/Addison Wesley; Skill 33.4 ❶ Shirlee Snyder; 33.16 – V.A.C. ATS Therapy System courtesy of KCI Licensing, Inc., San Antonio, TX; 33.17, 33.18 – Elena Dorfman/Addison Wesley; 33.24 – Patrick Watson; 33.25, 33.26 – © Richard Tauber/Addison Wesley.

Chapter 34 34.9 – Dr. Michael English/Custom Medical Stock Photo, Inc.; 34.13 – © Jenny Thomas Photography/Addison Wesley.

Chapter 35 Skill 35.1 ?–∏ Elena Dorfman; Skill 35.2 ❶–❷ © Elena Dorfman/Addison Wesley; 35.4 – Elena Dorfman/Addison Wesley; 35.9 – Jenny Thomas; 35.10 – Richard Tauber/Addison Wesley.

Chapter 36 36.2 – Richard Tauber/Addison Wesley.

Chapter 38 38.31 – Patrick Watson; 38.41 – EZ Way, Inc.; 38.42 – © Ronald Wittek/dpa/Corbis; 38.43 – Wright Products, Inc.; Skill 37.1 ❶ Richard Tauber/Addison Wesley; Skill 38.3 ❹–❺ Jenny Thomas Photography/Addison Wesley; Skill 38.5 ❷–❸ Elena Dorfman/Addison Wesley, ❹ Jenny Thomas Photography/Addison Wesley; Skill 38.7 ❶–❹ Elena Dorfman/Addison Wesley; 38.56 – Jenny Thomas Photography/Addison Wesley; 38.68, 38.69, 38.70 – Richard Tauber/Addison Wesley.

Chapter 39 39.6 – A, B Centers for Disease Control and Prevention (CDC), C Custom Medical Stock Photo, Inc., D Pearson Education/PH College; 39.8, 39.9 – © Elena Dorfman/Addison Wesley; 39.13 – © C. R. Bard, Inc. All rights reserved; 39.14 – Courtesy of Ross Products Division of Abbott Laboratories, Columbus, Ohio; Skill 39.2 ❶ © Elena Dorfman/Addison Wesley; 39.17 – © 2002 Kimberly-Clark Worldwide, Inc.; 39.18 – © Elena Dorfman/Addison Wesley; Skill 39.4 ? Ross Products Division, Abbott Laboratories. Used with permission.

Chapter 40 40.9 – Cory Patrick Hartley, San Ramon Regional Medical Center, San Ramon, CA; 40.12 – Elena Dorfman; 40.14 – © Jenny Thomas Photography/Addison Wesley; 40.15 – © Elena Dorfman/Addison Wesley; Skill 40.1 ❸ © Elena Dorfman/Addison Wesley; 40.18, 40.20, 40.21 – Permission to use these copyrighted images has been granted by the owner, Hollister Incorporated; Skill 40.2 ❶–❷, ❹ Cory Patrick Hartley, San Ramon Regional Medical Center, San Ramon, CA, ❸, ❺ Courtesy of Convatec, a Bristol-Meyers Squibb Company.

Chapter 41 41.7 – © Jenny Thomas Photography/Addison Wesley; Skill 41.2 ❶, ❸ Courtesy of Bard Medical Division; 41.11, 41.12, 41.13, 41.14 – Courtesy of Bard Medical Division; Skill 41.3 ❶ Courtesy of Bard Medical Division; Skill 41.4 ❷ Courtesy of Bard Medical Division.

Chapter 42 42.6 – © Elena Dorfman/Addison Wesley; 42.13, 42.14 – © Richard Tauber/Addison Wesley; 42.16, 42.17 – Shirlee Snyder; 42.19 – © Jenny Thomas Photography/Addison Wesley; 42.20, 42.21 – © Elena Dorfman/Addison Wesley; 42.22 – © Richard Tauber/

Addison Wesley; 42.23 – Jenny Thomas; 42.27 – © Don Gabara/PhototakeUSA.com; 42.33 – © Elena Dorfman/Addison Wesley; 42.34 – Courtesy of Portex Inc., Keene, NH; Skill 42.3 ❶ Elena Dorfman, ❷, ❺ Jenny Thomas; 42.38 Jenny Thomas; Skill 42.5 ❶–❷ Jenny Thomas; 42.40 – Pleur-evac® Chest Drainage System. Reprinted with permission from Genzyme Biosurgery, Cardiothoracic Division, Fall River, MA; Skill 42.6 ❶ Jenny Thomas.

Chapter 43 43.11A – Richard Tauber; 43.19 – Elena Dorfman; 43.21 – Reprinted courtesy of (BD) Becton, Dickson and Company and courtesy of Baxter Healthcare Corporation. All rights reserved; Skill 43.1 ❶–❷ Elena Dorfman, ❹–❺ Patrick Watson, ❻ Elena Dorfman; 43.25, 43.26 – Elena Dorfman; 43.27 – Jenny Thomas; 43.28 – Courtesy of Alaris Medical Systems, Inc., San Diego, CA.

Chapter 44 44.2 – Jonathan Nourak/PhotoEdit.

Chapter 45 45.1 – Elena Dorfman.

Chapter 48 48.1, 48.2 – Courtesy of Hill House Hospice, Richmond Hill, Ontario.

Skill Boxes

SKILL 27.1 Assessing General Appearance and Mental Status 561
SKILL 27.2 Assessing the Skin 566
SKILL 27.3 Assessing the Hair 569
SKILL 27.4 Assessing the Nails 571
SKILL 27.5 Assessing the Skull and Face 573
SKILL 27.6 Assessing the Eye Structures and Visual Acuity 576
SKILL 27.7 Assessing the Ears and Hearing 583
SKILL 27.8 Assessing the Nose and Sinuses 588
SKILL 27.9 Assessing the Mouth and Oropharynx 590
SKILL 27.10 Assessing the Neck 596
SKILL 27.11 Assessing the Thorax and Lungs 603
SKILL 27.12 Assessing the Heart and Central Vessels 612
SKILL 27.13 Assessing the Peripheral Vascular System 615
SKILL 27.14 Assessing the Breasts and Axillae 618
SKILL 27.15 Assessing the Abdomen 624
SKILL 27.16 Assessing the Musculoskeletal System 631
SKILL 27.17 Assessing the Neurological System 637
SKILL 27.18 Assessing the Female Genitals and Inguinal Lymph Nodes 646
SKILL 27.19 Assessing the Male Genitals and Inguinal Areas 651
SKILL 27.20 Assessing the Anus and Rectum 654
SKILL 28.1 Assessing Body Temperature 669
SKILL 28.2 Assessing a Peripheral Pulse 675
SKILL 28.3 Assessing an Apical Pulse 678
SKILL 28.4 Assessing an Apical-Radial Pulse 680
SKILL 28.5 Assessing Respirations 684
SKILL 28.6 Assessing Blood Pressure 692
SKILL 28.7 Measuring Oxygen Saturation 697
SKILL 29.1 Bathing an Adult or Pediatric Client 713
SKILL 29.2 Providing Perineal-Genital Care 718
SKILL 29.3 Providing Foot Care 724
SKILL 29.4 Brushing and Flossing the Teeth 731
SKILL 29.5 Providing Oral Care for an Unconscious Client 735
SKILL 29.6 Providing Hair Care for Clients 739
SKILL 29.7 Shampooing the Hair of a Client Confined to Bed 741
SKILL 29.8 Removing, Cleaning, and Inserting a Hearing Aid 747
SKILL 29.9 Changing an Unoccupied Bed 751
SKILL 29.10 Changing an Occupied Bed 755
SKILL 30.1 Using a Bed or Chair Exit Safety Monitoring Device 777
SKILL 30.2 Implementing Seizure Precautions 779
SKILL 30.3 Applying Restraints 787
SKILL 31.1 Administering Oral Medications 819
SKILL 31.2 Preparing Medications from Ampules 831
SKILL 31.3 Preparing Medications from Vials 832
SKILL 31.4 Mixing Medications by Using One Syringe 834
SKILL 31.5 Administering an Intradermal Injection for Skin Tests 836
SKILL 31.6 Administering a Subcutaneous Injection 839
SKILL 31.7 Administering an Intramuscular Injection 846
SKILL 31.8 Adding Medications to Intravenous Fluid Containers 849
SKILL 31.9 Administering Intravenous Medications Using IV Push 853
SKILL 31.10 Administering Ophthalmic Instillations 858
SKILL 31.11 Administering Otic Instillations 861
SKILL 31.12 Administering Vaginal Instillations 865
SKILL 32.1 Hand Washing 892
SKILL 32.2 Donning and Removing Personal Protective Equipment (Gloves, Gown, Mask, Eyewear) 896
SKILL 32.3 Establishing and Maintaining a Sterile Field 901
SKILL 32.4 Donning and Removing Sterile Gloves (Open Method) 905
SKILL 32.5 Donning and Removing Sterile Gloves (Closed Method) 907
SKILL 33.1 Obtaining a Wound Drainage Specimen for Culture 944
SKILL 33.2 Applying and Removing a Moist Transparent Wound Barrier Dressing 955
SKILL 33.3 Appling a Hydrocolloid Dressing 956
SKILL 33.4 Irrigating a Wound 960
SKILL 35.1 Teaching Moving, Leg Exercises, Deep Breathing, and Coughing 1024
SKILL 35.2 Applying Antiembolism Stockings 1030
SKILL 35.3 Managing Gastrointestinal Suction 1043